Oxford Medical Publications

Oxford Textbook of Public Health

Editors

Roger Detels
Professor and Chair, Department of Epidemiology, UCLA School of Public Health, University of California, Los Angeles, USA

James McEwen
Professor, Department of Public Health, University of Glasgow, UK

Robert Beaglehole
Professor of Community Health, Department of Community Health, Faculty of Medical and Health Sciences, University of Auckland, New Zealand

Heizo Tanaka
Director-General, National Institute of Health and Nutrition, Tokyo, Japan

Production team

Project Editor Roberta Nichols
Indexer Christine Boylan
Production Editor Lisa Blake
Design Manager Claire Walker
Text Designer Jonathan Coleclough
Illustrations by Technical Graphics Department, Oxford University Press
Publisher Helen Liepman

Oxford Textbook of

Public Health

Fourth Edition

Edited by

Roger Detels,
James McEwen,
Robert Beaglehole,
and Heizo Tanaka

OXFORD
UNIVERSITY PRESS

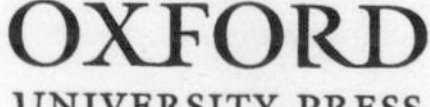

Great Clarendon Street, Oxford OX2 6DP

Oxford University Press is a department of the University of Oxford.
It furthers the University's objective of excellence in research, scholarship, and education by publishing worldwide in

Oxford New York

Auckland Bangkok Buenos Aires Cape Town Chennai
Dar es Salaam Delhi Hong Kong Istanbul Karachi Kolkata
Kuala Lumpur Madrid Melbourne Mexico City Mumbai Nairobi
São Paulo Shanghai Taipei Tokyo Toronto

and an associated company in Berlin

Oxford is a registered trade mark of Oxford University Press in the UK and in certain other countries

Published in the United States
by Oxford University Press Inc., New York

First Edition 1984
Second Edition 1991
Third Edition 1997
Fourth Edition 2002 (Reprinted in paperback 2004)

A catalogue record for this title is available from the British Library

Library of Congress Cataloguing in Publication Data
(Data available)

ISBN 0 19 263041 5 (Hardback; only available as a three-volume set)
ISBN 0 19 850959 6 (Paperback; only available in 1 volume)

Typeset by Mendip Communications Ltd., Frome
Printed in Italy by LegoPrint s.r.l.

Preface to the Fourth Edition

In the new millennium many old public health problems persist even as new problems present new challenges, despite the continuing development of new technologies and strategies. Poverty and deprivation continue to be the underlying causes of less than optimal health. Public health professionals are increasingly recognizing that public health cannot operate in a vacuum but must interact with the other organizations involved in promoting political and economic well-being. The situation at the beginning of the twenty-first century underscores the constantly changing nature of health threats to the public and the need for public health to remain a dynamic, scientifically grounded, and innovative field of endeavour.

The fourth edition of the *Oxford Textbook of Public Health* reflects the many changes that have occurred in the field of public health since the third edition. The scope of the textbook has been expanded to include issues relevant to developing as well as developed countries. The textbook also presents strategies to resolve current public health problems and anticipate new ones.

As in previous editions, our objective in the fourth edition has been to present the breadth and depth of the complex field of public health, to underscore persisting, resurging, and new public health problems, to update the methods of public health, and to identify the changing public health agenda for the resolution of these problems. The editors have encouraged the authors to give their own perspectives on the topic assigned to them. We feel that this policy stimulates debate, ensures an ongoing dynamic approach to public health problems, and ultimately advances the field.

Some public health professionals in the last few decades of the twentieth century thought that infectious diseases had been controlled. The indiscriminate use of antibiotics for both humans and animals, and in some regions the neglect of basic public health principles, has resulted in a resurgence of old previously controlled infectious diseases such as tuberculosis, diphtheria, and gonorrhoea. In addition, new diseases have been identified, such as hantavirus disease and bovine spongiform encephalitis, many of them resulting from human alteration of the environment and interference with the natural food chain. Controlling these emerging infectious diseases will be a difficult new challenge (see Chapter 2.6). On the optimistic side, however, poliomyelitis is close to being eradicated and measles has been put on the public health agenda as the next target for global eradication.

Recently, there have been numerous efforts to prioritize, focus, and target specific public health efforts to maximize their effectiveness. One strategy that has been proposed to prioritize the major diseases and conditions is to use disability-adjusted life years, which take into consideration quality of life as well as mortality (see Chapter 2.9). This strategy, which uses subjective as well as objective criteria to measure the burden of a specific disease, has caused some controversy. Public health still fails to make its case for the primacy of prevention over treatment of prevention failures, resulting in an imbalance in funding between public health and curative medicine. Given the chronic lack of funds for public health, more emphasis is being placed on the cost-effectiveness of public health interventions (see Chapter 7.6). Other public health leaders speak of the need for using a comprehensive rather than a disease/risk factor targeting approach for mounting public initiatives (see Chapter 12.9). In the latter half of the twentieth century there has also been an increasing awareness of the need to involve and mobilize the public itself in determining, prioritizing, and implementing public health initiatives in both developing and developed countries if these initiatives are to succeed (see Chapter 12.11). There is increasing concern over the issue of inequalities both between developed and developing countries and within these countries (Chapters 12.3 and 12.4).

A major change in the fourth edition of the *Oxford Textbook of Public Health* is the expanded scope to include public health issues confronting the developing as well as the developed world. As life expectancy increases in many developing countries, more people are developing those chronic diseases which have been a major burden in developed countries for many decades. Unlike the developed countries, however, these countries still carry the burden of infectious diseases which have been greatly reduced in developed countries. Compounding these problems are the extremely limited resources available to developing countries which, despite international assistance, still bear most of the cost of their public health initiatives. One cannot deal with the problems of developing countries, however, without recognizing the disastrous impact of HIV/AIDS on these countries, especially in sub-Saharan Africa (see Chapter 9.14). In many of these countries the average life expectancy has dropped by more than 20 years, reversing all the gains of the previous two decades and widening the gap between the rich and poor countries. Yet, because of the rapid advances in travel and communications, the developed world is threatened in new ways and thus cannot afford to ignore the problems of the developing world. To present the issues of the developing world we have invited public health leaders from developing countries to write these chapters to ensure that their perspective is heard (see Chapters 1.3, 1.4, 3.3, 3.4, 6.9, 7.9, 11.2, 11.9, and 12.11).

The fourth edition of the *Oxford Textbook of Public Health* concludes with a chapter by Frank Sorvillo, James R. Greenwood, and Roger Detels (Chapter 12.13) who discuss new public health threats associated with bioterrorism.

To the extent that we have succeeded in our objectives for the fourth edition of the *Oxford Textbook of Public Health* we are indebted to the many knowledgeable experts who have contributed their expertise and wisdom.

Finally, we wish to thank the technical editors, Ms Janet Whitehouse, and Mrs Roberta Nichols and our assistants, Ms Jean Savage and Mrs Adrienne Girvan, for the enormous task of chasing authors, keeping track of the progress of the various chapters, and ensuring that the tables, figures, and copyright permissions were all in order. Finally, we wish to thank Ms Helen Liepman of the Oxford University Press for her encouragement and enthusiasm during every step of the process.

March 2002

R.D.
J.McE.
R.B.
H.T.

Preface to the Third Edition

For the third edition of the *Oxford Textbook of Public Health*, we have undertaken a major revision of both the overall content and individual chapters. Our objective is to ensure the continuing relevance of the Textbook in the rapidly changing field of public health, and update the methods and the accomplishments in the field, its problems, and the changing agenda required to meet these and other emerging challenges. As in the previous editions, we describe the philosophy and underlying principles, the methods used for the investigation of public health problems, and solutions. In addition, the Textbook presents the moral basis for striving for better health for all in the face of increasing fiscal and political pressures to reduce governmental support for the measures needed to ensure the right of all to health.

The Textbook is intended to be a comprehensive reference source for postgraduate students in the field, but is also written to provide insights for those not primarily in public health who may need access to its expertise. The Textbook, a comprehensive review of this diverse field, should be included in the library of every major institution concerned with public health and community based, population based medicine.

Since the publication of the second edition of the *Oxford Textbook of Public Health*, considerable changes have occurred in the problems which public health must address. The editors have recruited leading authorities to present and discuss these new challenges to promoting the health of the public. There are also many examples of new challenges.

The epidemic caused by the human immunodeficiency virus has matured, spread, and established a new focus in Asia, destroying our complacency about having conquered infectious diseases. New and re-emerging organisms, such as drug-resistant strains of tuberculosis and Hanta and Ebola viruses, have potential epidemic consequences.

Efforts to improve the quality of the environment, and the need to sustain it for future generations, have gained momentum, but so also have efforts to reduce the laws and regulations essential to the preservation of a safe environment. Improvements have been realized in the quality of the environment in many developed countries. In most developing countries, however, the deterioration of the environment, especially in the major cities, has reached a point at which the quality of life for those forced to live in them has declined to an unacceptable level.

The World Health Organization's slogan, 'Health for all', developed from the Alma Ata Conference in 1978, emphasizes the need for equity in access to health services. The US 'Healthy People 2000: National Health Promotion and Disease Prevention Objectives' (DHHS 1990) and the British 'Health of the Nation' (Secretary of State for Health 1992) both include health goals for improved health among the poor, as well as for the general population. Other countries have developed similar targets but at the same time, the expenditure on medical care has risen in many countries, making the goal of equity even more difficult to achieve. The rapid increase in effective, but costly, medical technology has forced even the wealthiest of the developed countries of North America, Europe, and Asia to debate the issues of access to medical care and the limitations of the public purse to provide all clinical services demanded. One approach used in the United States to limit medical area costs has been 'managed care' which is, in reality, 'managed costs'. The United Kingdom and other countries have established a 'purchaser/provider' approach to introduce an element of competition to the provision of medical care in an effort to provide quality medical care to all the population within the constraints of a limited budget and burgeoning and expensive medical technology.

Ham, in the chapter on public policies and strategies in the United Kingdom, discusses some of the ways that 'rationing' has been introduced into the National Health System in that country. The state of Oregon, in the United States, has introduced the concept of 'priorities' in providing medical services in that state's medical programme for the poor. President Clinton tried unsuccessfully to introduce a national health care system which would include all Americans, but was defeated by political forces concerned primarily with budget issues. The dilemma of how to provide equitable services to an entire population of the highest quality with increasing expectations and demands has not been satisfactorily resolved in any country, but is still on the agenda and will remain there, as William Foege points out so eloquently in his chapter on 'Future Challenges to Public Health'.

Violence has emerged as a leading cause of death among young males in the United States and is thus a major contributor to years of healthy life lost. The epidemic of violence is an issue that will require new initiatives by society building on the research and practice of public health.

Many of the problems addressed in the previous two editions, which focused primarily on public health in developed countries, are also problems of the developing countries, especially those in transition to becoming developed countries. These countries must now grapple with the combined problems of both developing and developed countries. We have, therefore, considered the impact of these issues for developing as well as for developed countries.

We have retained the three volume organizational structure of the second edition of the *Oxford Textbook of Public Health*. The first volume deals with the scope of public health, including its development, philosophy, and the changes that have occurred. The second volume presents the methods and disciplines used to identify, quantify, and provide answers to health problems. The third volume presents applications of public health sciences to the resolution of the major public health problems occurring in the 1990s and public health functions critically required to achieve the objectives outlined in volume one.

We have presented the breadth and the depth of the field, as well as the contributions of the many disciplines which are an integral part of the armamentarium of public health scientists and practitioners. We realize that this is a formidable task. To the extent that we have succeeded, we are indebted to the knowledgeable experts who have contributed to the third edition.

Finally, we wish to thank the technical editors, Mrs Anna McNeil and Ms Laurel Kelly, our secretaries, Ms Jean Savage, Ms Jean Knight, and Ms A.M.A. Girvan, for the enormous task of compiling the chapters and obtaining computer disks in the appropriate computer language, or translating those that weren't into the computer language of the Textbook, and to Ms Julie Hoare, of the Oxford University Press, for her enthusiasm, support, and advice.

June 1996

R.D.
W.W.H.
J.McE.
G.S.O.

DEDICATION

The editors dedicate the fourth edition of the *Oxford Textbook of Public Health* to

Professor Walter W. Holland
CBE, MD, FRCP, FFPHM

Walter Holland was the founding editor of the *Oxford Textbook of Public Health.* He was also the founding chair of the Department of Clinical Epidemiology and Social Medicine, which subsequently became the Department of Public Health Medicine, at St Thomas' Medical School, London. For almost 40 years Walter Holland has been a leader in the field of public health, dedicating his professional career to improving health for all people while at the same time promoting high standards for public health professionals. He has made major contributions as a scholar, as a researcher, as a policy advisor, and as a mentor for public health leaders worldwide. He has received too many honours to enumerate here, but notably served as the President of the Faculty of Public Health Medicine and as President and Secretary of the International Epidemiological Association. He was also the founding editor of the *International Journal of Epidemiology*. As the current editors of the *Oxford Textbook of Public Health*, we are particularly grateful for his kind guidance and support in producing the fourth edition. In recognition of his significant and enthusiastic contributions to the advancement of the field of public health we dedicate this edition of the *Oxford Textbook of Public Health* to him.

Contents

The scope of public health

The methods of public health

5 Information systems and sources of intelligence

6 Epidemiological and biostatistical approaches

7 Social science techniques

8 Environmental and occupational health sciences

The practice of public health

9 Major health problems

10 Prevention and control of public health hazards

List of contributors

J.H. Abramson Emeritus Professor of Social Medicine, Hebrew University–Hadassah School of Public Health and Community Medicine, Hebrew University, Jerusalem, Israel

Michael Adler Professor of Genitourinary Medicine, Department of Sexually Transmitted Diseases, Royal Free and University College Medical School, University College London, UK

Lin An Associate Professor of Maternal and Child Health, Health Science Centre, Beijing University, Beijing, People's Republic of China

Roy Anderson Professor of Infectious Disease Epidemiology and Head of the Department of Infectious Disease Epidemiology, School of Medicine, Imperial College of Science, Technology, and Medicine, London, UK

Samara Asma Director, WHO Collaborating Center on Smoking and Health, Centers for Disease Control and Prevention, Atlanta, Georgia, USA

M. Christopher Auld Assistant Professor and Alberta Heritage Population Health Inspector, Department of Economics, University of Calgary, Canada

Dean Baker Professor and Director, Center for Occupational and Environmental Health, University of California, Irvine, California, USA

Joanne Barton Senior Lecturer in Child and Adolescent Psychiatry, University of Glasgow, UK

Robert Beaglehole Professor of Community Health, Department of Community Health, Faculty of Medical and Health Sciences, University of Auckland, New Zealand

Richard Beasley Professor and Director, Wellington Asthma Research Group, Wellington School of Medicine, Wellington, New Zealand

Carol Bellamy Executive Director, UNICEF, New York, USA

Ruth L. Berkelman Professor of Epidemiology, Rollins School of Public Health, Emory University, Atlanta, Georgia, USA

Douglas W. Bettcher Coordinator, Framework Convention on Tobacco Control, World Health Organization, Geneva, Switzerland

Paolo Boffetta Chief, Unit of Environmental Cancer Epidemiology, International Agency for Research on Cancer, Lyon, France

Ann Bostrom Associate Professor, School of Public Policy, Georgia Institute of Technology, Atlanta, Georgia, USA

James D. Bowen Assistant Professor, Neurology, University of Washington, Seattle, Washington, USA

Paul Brennan Scientist, Unit of Environmental Cancer Epidemiology, International Agency for Research on Cancer, Lyon, France

Lester Breslow Professor of Public Health, UCLA School of Public Health, University of California, Los Angeles, California, USA

Norman E. Breslow Professor of Biostatistics, University of Washington, Seattle, Washington, USA

Gro Harlem Brundtland Director General, World Health Organization, Geneva, Switzerland

James W. Buehler Associate Director for Science, National Center for HIV, STD, and TB Prevention, Centers for Disease Control and Prevention, Atlanta, Georgia, USA

Sir Kenneth Calman Vice-Chancellor and Warden, University of Durham, UK

Susan D. Cochran Professor of Epidemiology, UCLA School of Public Health, University of California, Los Angeles, California, USA

Frances Cowan Senior Lecturer in Genitourinary Medicine, Department of Sexually Transmitted Diseases, Royal Free and University College Medical School, University College London, UK

George Davey Smith Professor of Clinical Epidemiology, Department of Social Medicine, University of Bristol, UK

Peter Davis Professor of Public Health, Christchurch School of Medicine and Health Sciences, University of Otago, Christchurch, New Zealand

Bonnie Dean Associate Researcher, Southern California Injury Prevention Research Center, UCLA School of Public Health,University of California, Los Angeles, California, USA

Katherine DeLand Legal Officer, Tobacco Free Initiative, World Health Organization, Geneva, Switzerland

Don C. Des Jarlais Director of Research, Edmond de Rothschild Foundation, Chemical Dependency Institute, Beth Israel Medical Center, New York; Professor of Epidemiology and Social Medicine, Albert Einstein College of Medicine, New York, USA

Roger Detels Professor and Chair, Department of Epidemiology, UCLA School of Public Health, University of California, Los Angeles, USA

Ana V. Diez Roux Assistant Professor of Medicine and Epidemiology, College of Physicians and Surgeons, and Mailman School of Public Health, Columbia University, New York, USA

Cam Donaldson Svare Chair in Health Economics, Alberta Heritage Senior Scholar and Canadian Institutes of Health Senior Investigator, Departments of Community Health Sciences and Economics, University of Calgary, Canada

Jeroen Douwes Senior Research Fellow, Centre for Public Health Research, Massey University, Wellington, New Zealand

R.S. Downie Professor of Moral Philosophy, University of Glasgow, UK

Mohammed Dualeh Senior Public Health Officer, Health and Community Development Section, UNHCR, Geneva, Switzerland

Shah Ebrahim Professor of the Epidemiology of Ageing, University of Bristol, UK

Matthias Egger Senior Lecturer in Epidemiology and Public Health Medicine, Department of Social Medicine, University of Bristol, UK

M.J.G. Farthing Executive Dean and Professor of Medicine, University of Glasgow, UK

Elaine M. Faustman Professor and Associate Chair, Department of Environmental Health Director, Institute for Risk Analysis and Risk Communication, School of Public Health and Community Medicine, University of Washington, Seattle, Washington, USA

Manning Feinleib Research Professor, Department of Medicine, Georgetown University Medical Center, Washington, DC, USA

Josep Figueras Research Director, European Observatory on Health Care Systems/WHO, Copenhagen, Denmark

Baruch Fischhoff Professor, Department of Social and Decision Sciences, Department of Engineering and Public Policy, Carnegie–Mellon University, Pittsburgh, Pennsylvania, USA

Sev. S. Fluss Special Adviser, Council for International Organizations of Medical Sciences, Geneva, Switzerland

William H. Foege Department of International Health, School of Public Health, Emory University, Atlanta, Georgia, USA

Natalie Freeman Associate Professor of Environmental and Community Medicine, Robert Wood Johnson Medical School, Piscataway; Member, Environmental and Occupational Health Sciences Institute, Piscataway, New Jersey, USA

Julio Frenk Executive Director, Evidence and Information for Policy, World Health Organization, Geneva, Switzerland

Ralph R. Frerichs Professor of Epidemiology, UCLA School of Public Health, University of California, Los Angeles, California, USA

Lawrence M. Friedman Special Assistant to the Director, National Heart, Lung, and Blood Institute, Bethesda, Maryland, USA

Tom Fryers Visiting Professor of Public Mental Health, Department of Psychiatry, University of Leicester, UK; Visiting Lecturer, International and Public Health, New York Medical College, New York, USA

Stanley Gelbier Professor of Dental Public Health, Guy's, King's and St Thomas' Dental Institute, London, UK

Gary Giovino Senior Research Scientist, Department of Cancer Prevention, Epidemiology, and Biostatistics, Roswell Park Cancer Institute, Buffalo, New York, USA

Vivek Goel Professor, Departments of Public Health Sciences and Health Policy, Management and Evaluation, University of Toronto, Canada

Lynn Goldman Bloomberg School of Public Health, Johns Hopkins University, Baltimore, Maryland, USA

Bernard D. Goldstein Dean, Graduate School of Public Health, University of Pittsburgh, Pennsylvania, USA

Lawrence Green Director, Office of Extramural Prevention Research, Public Health Practice and Program Office, Centers for Disease Control and Prevention, US Department of Health and Human Services, Atlanta, Georgia, USA

Michael Greenberg Associate Dean, E.J. Bloustein School of Planning and Public Policy, Rutgers University, New Brunswick, New Jersey, USA

Sander Greenland Professor, Department of Epidemiology, UCLA School of Public Health, University of California, Los Angeles; Department of Statistics, College of Letters and Science, University of California, Los Angeles, California, USA

James W. Greenwood Director, Office of Environment, Health and Safety, and Adjunct Associate Professor of Epidemiology, UCLA School of Public Health, University of California, Los Angeles, USA

Emily Grundy Reader in Social Gerontology, London School of Hygiene and Tropical Medicine, London, UK

Sofia Gruskin Assistant Professor on Health and Human Rights, François-Xavier Bagnoud Center for Public Health and Human Rights, Harvard School of Public Health, Cambridge, Massachusetts, USA

Davidson R. Gwatkin Principal Health and Poverty Specialist, World Bank, Washington, DC, USA

Christopher Hamlin Professor of History, University of Notre Dame, Indiana, USA

Nicolette Hart Department of Sociology, University of California, Los Angeles, California, USA

A. J. Hedley Professor of Community Medicine, University of Hong Kong, Hong Kong

Basil S. Hetzel Chairman Emeritus, International Council for Control of Iodine Deficiency Disorders, Women's and Children's Hospital, North Adelaide, Australia

David Heymann Executive Director, Communicable Diseases, World Health Organization, Geneva, Switzerland

Charles Hillier Regional Epidemiologist, Communicable Disease Surveillance Centre (Wales), UK

M. Hobbs Associate Professor in Public Health, University of Western Australia, Perth, Australia

H. Hoffmeister Professor of Epidemiology and Former Director, Robert Koch Institute, Berlin, Germany

Walter W. Holland Emeritus Professor of Public Health Medicine, University of London; Visiting Professor, LSE Health and Social Care, London School of Economics, London, UK

Robert L. Hubbard Director, Institute for Community-Based Research, National Development and Research Institute Inc., Raleigh, North Carolina; Adjunct Professor, Department of Psychiatry, Duke University, Durham, North Carolina, USA

David J. Hunter Professor of Health Policy and Management, School for Health, University of Durham, UK

Hiroyasu Iso Associate Professor, Institute of Community Medicine, University of Tsukuba, Ibaraki, Japan

Dean T. Jamison Fellow, Fogarty International Center of the US National Institutes of Health; Professor of International Health Economics, University of California, Los Angeles, California, USA

K. Jamrozik Professor of Primary Care Epidemiology, Imperial College of Science, Technology and Medicine, London, UK; Visiting Professor in Public Health, University of Western Australia, Perth, Australia

Stephen Jan London School of Hygiene and Tropical Medicine, London, UK

Jerry Jeyaratnam Consultant Occupational Physician, Colombo, Sri Lanka

Jennifer L. Kelsey Professor, Department of Health Research and Policy, Stanford University, Stanford, California, USA

Don Kyoun Kim Professor of Preventive and Occupational Medicine, College of Medicine, Pusan National University, Pusan, Korea

Robert Kim-Farley World Health Organization Representative to India, World Health Organization, New Delhi, India

David Koh Professor and Head, Department of Community, Occupational and Family Medicine, Faculty of Medicine, National University of Singapore, Republic of Singapore

Yoshihiro Kokubo Post-Doctoral Researcher, Department of Preventive Cardiology, National Cardiovascular Center, Osaka, Japan

Jess F. Kraus Professor of Epidemiology. Southern California Injury Prevention Research Center, UCLA School of Public Health, University of California, Los Angeles, California, USA

Walter A. Kukull Professor and Director, National Alzheimer Coordinating Center, School of Public Health and Community Medicine, University of Washington, Seattle, Washington, USA

Prayura Kunasol Former Director-General, Department of Communicable Disease Control, Ministry of Public Health, Nonthaburi; Senior Advisor, Thai AIDS Vaccine Evaluation Group, Mahidol University, Bangkok, Thailand

T.H. Lam Professor of Community Medicine, University of Hong Kong, Hong Kong

Philip J. Landrigan Professor and Chair, Department of Community and Preventive Medicine, Mount Sinai Medical Center, New York, USA

M.J.S. Langman Honorary Professor of Medicine, University of Birmingham, UK

Khanchit Limpakarnjanarat Adjunct Director, HIV/AIDS Collaboration, Department of Medical Services, Ministry of Public Health, Tivanon Road, Nonthaburi, Thailand

Paul J. Lioy Professor of Environmental and Community Medicine, Robert Wood Johnson Medical School, Piscataway; Associate Director, Environmental and Occupational Health Sciences Institute, Piscataway, New Jersey, USA

R.F.A. Logan Professor of Clinical Epidemiology, School of Community Health Sciences, University of Nottingham, UK

A.D. Lopez Co-ordinator, Epidemiology and Burden of Disease, Global Programme on Science for Health Policy, World Health Organization, Geneva, Switzerland

Adetokunbo O. Lucas Adjunct Professor of International Health, Harvard University, Cambridge, Massachusetts, USA; Visiting Professor, London School of Hygiene and Tropical Medicine, University of London, UK

Jeff Luck Department of Health Services, UCLA School of Public Health, University of California, Los Angeles, California, USA

Russell V. Luepker Mayo Professor and Head, Division of Epidemiology, School of Public Health, University of Minnesota, USA

Martin McKee Professor of European Public Health, London School of Hygiene and Tropical Medicine, London, UK

A.J. McMichael Professor and Director, National Center for Epidemiology and Population Health, Australian National University, Canberra, Australia

J.P. Mackenbach Professor of Public Health, Faculty of Medicine and Health Sciences, Erasmus University, Rotterdam, The Netherlands

G. B.M. Mensink Senior Researcher, Risk Assessment Methods, General Epidemiology, Robert Koch Institute, Berlin, Germany

Anthony B. Miller Head, Division of Clinical Epidemiology, Deutsches Krebsforschungszentrum, Heidelberg, Germany; Professor Emeritus, Department of Public Health Sciences, University of Toronto, Canada

Craig Mitton Canadian Health Services Research Foundation Postdoctoral Research Fellow, Centre for Health and Policy Studies, University of Calgary, Canada

Gavin Mooney Division of Health Sciences, Curtin University, Perth, Australia

Myfanwy Morgan Reader in Sociology of Health, Guy's, King's and St Thomas' School of Medicine, King's College London, UK

Donald E. Morisky Professor and Vice Chair, Department of Community Health Sciences, UCLA School of Public Health, University of California, Los Angeles, California, USA

Arno G. Motulsky Emeritus Professor of Medical Genetics, Department of Medicine, Division of Medical Genetics, University of Washington, Seattle, Washington, USA

C.J.L. Murray Executive Director, Evidence and Information for Policy, World Health Organization, Geneva, Switzerland

Son N. Nguyen World Bank, Washington, DC, USA

Norman Noah Professor of Public Health and Epidemiology, London School of Hygiene and Tropical Medicine; Consultant Epidemiologist, PHLS Communicable Disease Surveillance Centre, London, UK

D. James Nokes Senior Lecturer, Department of Biological Sciences, University of Warwick, UK

Don Nutbeam Head of Public Health, Department of Health, London; Visiting Professor in Public Health, London School of Hygiene and Tropical Medicine, London, UK

Jørn Olsen Professor and Head, Danish Epidemiology Science Centre, University of Aarhus, Denmark

Gilbert S. Omenn Executive Vice President for Medical Affairs, Professor of Internal Medicine, Human Genetics, and Public Health, University of Michigan, Ann Arbor, Michigan, USA

Stephen Palmer Mansell Talbot Professor of Epidemiology and Public Health, University of Wales College of Medicine, Cardiff, UK

William Parry-Jones (deceased) Formerly Professor of Child and Adolescent Psychiatry, University of Glasgow, UK

Neil Pearce Professor and Director, Centre for Public Health Research, Massey University, Wellington, New Zealand

Corinne Peek-Asa Associate Professor of Occupational and Environmental Health and Epidemiology, University of Iowa Injury Prevention Research Center, College of Public Health, Iowa City, Iowa, USA

Wiput Phoolcharoen Director, Health Systems Research Institute, Nonthaburi, Thailand

Louise Potvin Associate Professor of Social and Preventive Medicine, University of Montreal, Canada

John Powles University Lecturer in Public Health Medicine, University of Cambridge, UK

Deborah Prothrow-Stith Professor of Public Health, Harvard School of Public Health, Boston, Massachusetts, USA

Denis J. Protti Professor of Health Informatics, School of Health Information Science, University of Victoria, British Columbia, Canada

Michael J. Puma Principal Research Associate, Education Policy Center, The Urban Institute, Washington, DC, USA

Laura Punnett Professor, Department of Work Environment, University of Massachusetts Lowell, Massachusetts, USA

Marilyn Jacobs Quadrel Manager, Environmental Technology Division, Pacific Northwest National Laboratory, Richland, Washington, USA

Uton Muchtar Rafei Regional Director, World Health Organization Regional Office for Southeast Asia, New Delhi, India

Margaret Reid Reader, Department of Public Health, University of Glasgow, UK

Peter G. Robinson Senior Clinical Lecturer, Dental Public Health and Oral Health Services Research, Guy's, King's and St Thomas' Dental Institute, London, UK

Milton I. Roemer (deceased) Formerly Professor of Public Health, UCLA School of Public Health, University of California, Los Angeles, USA

Ruth Roemer Adjunct Professor Emeritus, UCLA School of Public Health, University of California, Los Angeles, USA

Robin Room Professor and Director, Centre for Social Research on Alcohol and Drugs, Stockholm University, Stockholm, Sweden

Kenneth J. Rothman Professor of Epidemiology, Boston University School of Public Health, Boston University School of Medicine, Boston, Massachusetts, USA

Amit Roy Assistant Professor of Environmental and Community Medicine, Robert Wood Johnson Medical School, Piscataway; Member, Environmental and Occupational Health Sciences Institute, Piscataway, New Jersey, USA

Julia Royall Chief, International Programs, and Project Director, Multilateral Initiative on Malaria Telecommunications Network, National Library of Medicine, National Institutes of Health, Bethesda, Maryland, USA

Roland Salmon Consultant Neurologist, Poole Hospital NHS Trust, Poole, UK

Jonathan Samet Professor and Chairman, Epidemiology Director, Institute for Global Tobacco Control, Bloomberg School of Public Health, Johns Hopkins University, Baltimore, Maryland, USA

Rodolfo Saracci Director of Research in Epidemiology, National Research Council, Pisa, Italy; Consultant, Unit of Environmental Cancer Epidemiology, International Agency for Research on Cancer, Lyon, France

Eleanor B. Schron Nurse Scientist, Clinical Trials Scientific Research Group, National Heart, Lung, and Blood Institute, Bethesda, Maryland, USA

Sharon Schwartz Associate Professor of Epidemiology, Mailman School of Public Health, Columbia University, New York, USA

John C. Scott President, Center for Public Service Communications, Arlington, Virginia, USA

Ego Seeman Associate Professor of Medicine, Austin and Repatriation Medical Centre, University of Melbourne, Australia

Robert D. Sege Associate Professor of Pediatrics, Tufts University School of Medicine, Boston, Massachusetts, USA

Than Sein Director, Evidence and Information for Policy, World Health Organization Regional Office for Southeast Asia, New Delhi, India

Beatrice J. Selwyn Associate Professor of Epidemiology, School of Public Health, University of Texas Health Sciences Center at Houston, Texas, USA

Phil Shackley Lecturer in Health Economics, Sheffield Health Economics Group, University of Sheffield, UK

Paul Shears Senior Lecturer, Liverpool School of Tropical Medicine, Liverpool, UK

Prakash S. Shetty Professor of Human Nutrition, London School of Hygiene and Tropical Medicine, London, UK

Elliott C. Siegel Associate Director for Health Information Programs Development, National Library of Medicine, National Institutes of Health, Bethesda, Maryland, USA

Chitr Sitthi-Amorn Professor of Epidemiology, College of Public Health, Chulalongkorn University, Bangkok, Thailand

Frank Sorvillo Chief of Public Health Records and Research, County of Los Angeles Department of Health Services, Los Angeles, California, USA

MaryFran Sowers Professor, Department of Epidemiology, School of Public Health, University of Michigan, Ann Arbor, Michigan, USA

John Spicer Associate Professor, School of Psychology, Massey University, Palmerston North, New Zealand

Howard Spivak Professor of Pediatrics and Community Health, Tufts University School of Medicine, Boston, Massachusetts, USA

Jonathan A.C. Sterne Senior Lecturer in Medical Statistics, Department of Social Medicine, University of Bristol, UK

Donna F. Stroup Associate Director for Science, National Center for Chronic Disease Prevention & Health Promotion, Centers for Disease Control and Prevention, Atlanta, Georgia, USA

Ezra Susser Professor of Epidemiology and Psychiatry, Mailman School of Public Health and New York State Psychiatric Institute, Columbia University, New York, USA

Heizo Tanaka Director-General, National Institute of Health and Nutrition, Tokyo, Japan

Daniel Tarantola Senior Policy Adviser to the Director-General, World Health Organization, Geneva, Switzerland

Allyn L. Taylor Health Policy Adviser, World Health Organization, Geneva, Switzerland

Prasert Thongcharoen Emeritus Professor of Microbiology, Faculty of Medicine, Siriraj Hospital, Mahidol University, Bangkok, Thailand

Keith Tones Emeritus Professor of Health Education, Leeds Metropolitan University; Senior Associate Lecturer, Nuffield Institute for Health, University of Leeds, UK

Freya Tyrer Project Manager, MRC Clinical Trials Unit, London, UK

Peter Tyrer Professor of Community Psychiatry and Head of Department of Public Mental Health, Division of Neuroscience and Psychological Medicine, Imperial College of Science, Technology and Medicine, London, UK

Arthur C. Upton Clinical Professor of Environmental and Community Medicine, University of Medicine and Dentistry of New Jersey — Robert Wood Johnson Medical School, New Brunswick, New Jersey, USA

Friedrich Vogel Emeritus Professor of Human Genetics, University of Heidelberg, Germany

Shaoxian Wang Professor of Maternal and Child Health, Health Science Centre, Beijing University, Beijing, People's Republic of China

Anthony B. Ward Consultant/Senior Lecturer in Rehabilitation Medicine, North Staffordshire Hospital and University of Keele; Director, North Staffordshire Rehabilitation Centre, Stoke on Trent, UK

Noel S. Weiss Professor, University of Washington, and Member, Fred Hutchinson Cancer Research Center, Seattle, Washington, USA

Suwit Wibulpolprasert Deputy Permanent Secretary, Ministry of Public Health, Nonthaburi, Thailand

Marilyn Wise Director, Australian Centre for Health Promotion, Department of Public Health and Community Medicine, University of Sydney, Australia

Virginia Wiseman London School of Hygiene and Tropical Medicine, London, UK

Zunyou Wu Professor and Director of the Department of Behavioral Intervention, National Center for AIDS Prevention and Control, Chinese Academy of Preventive Medicine, Beijing, People's Republic of China

Derek Yach Executive Director, Noncommunicable Diseases and Mental Health, World Health Organization, Geneva, Switzerland

Gonghuan Yang Professor, Chinese Academy of Preventive Medicine, Institute of Epidemiology and Microbiology, Beijing, People's Republic of China

Tetsuji Yokoyama Research Associate, Department of Epidemiology, Medical Research Institute, Tokyo Medical and Dental University, Tokyo, Japan

Nobuo Yoshiike Chief, Research Planning and Evaluation, National Institute of Health and Nutrition, Tokyo, Japan

Shun-Zhang Yu Prevention Medicine Institution, Shanghai Medical University, Shanghai, People's Republic of China

Paul Zimmet Professor of Diabetes, Monash University, Melbourne, Australia

1

The development of the discipline of public health

1.1 Current scope and concerns in public health

Roger Detels and Lester Breslow

Introduction

Public health is the process of mobilizing and engaging local, state, national, and international resources to assure the conditions in which people can be healthy. In the nineteenth and early twentieth centuries health problems reflected primarily faecal contamination of water supplies and the widespread undernutrition, crowding, and exhaustion associated with early industrialization. These conditions resulted in a high prevalence of tuberculosis, enteric infections, infant mortality, and acute respiratory diseases. In response, communities, provinces, and nations developed successful ways of dealing with these important problems through public action to promote health. From the outset, public health embraced both social action and scientific knowledge. This partnership meant linking the antipoverty (reform) movement with the findings from epidemiological and bacteriological investigations, for example, to combat such diseases as tuberculosis and typhoid fever.

Now, at the beginning of the twenty-first century, these problems persist in many parts of the world, but another set of health problems, including new infectious diseases and major non-communicable diseases, confront the United Kingdom, Japan, the United States, and other highly industrialized nations, and they have also emerged as important problems in many of the developing countries. These non-communicable diseases stem from an overly rich diet, cigarette use, excessive alcohol consumption, too little physical activity, and other conditions that typify the way many people now live. In developing countries communicable diseases are still a major cause of death. Increasing numbers of people in these countries, however, are now encountering relative affluence for the first time and thus are beginning to suffer the same health consequences as people in developed countries. This chapter broadly presents the current scope and concerns of public health as well as issues that confront public health organizations in both industrialized and developing societies. Subsequent chapters will present specific topics in greater detail.

The first part of this chapter outlines the major health problems facing the world today, including infectious diseases, chronic diseases, trauma, and mental health. Determinants of health, such as nutritional problems, environmental hazards, and disorders resulting from lifestyle choices are discussed in the second part. The third part presents the scientific strategies that public health uses to cope with the problems, including strategies basic to public health, such as epidemiology, and those that are borrowed and modified from other disciplines, including the social, biological, and physical sciences. The four major public health strategies for influencing health—preventing disease and promoting health, improving medical care, promoting health-enhancing behaviour, and controlling the environment—are outlined in the fourth part. The fifth section presents the techniques for applying these scientific approaches to public health problems, and the final section discusses the interaction of the various governmental and voluntary actions aimed at improving the health of communities.

Public health is only one of the major influences on a community's health. The basic economic and social conditions of existence directly impact people's level and mode of living and thus constitute the foundation of health. These conditions limit and, to a considerable extent, determine the resources that can be devoted specifically to health promotion and disease intervention. Prevailing economic and social conditions also affect health in ways beyond the level of living and the concomitant ability of people to obtain the necessities of healthy life. Strong economic forces expressed in agriculture, manufacturing, commerce, and politics, for example, may sway people to use tobacco and thus injure their health.

The magnitude and success of public health efforts will vary both in time and place in different areas of the world. Nevertheless, the principles of public health remain the same. The actions that should be taken are determined by the nature and magnitude of the problems affecting the health of the community. What can be done will be determined by scientific knowledge and the resources available. What is done will be determined by the social and political situation existing at the particular time and place.

Health problems

Health problems vary considerably in the different parts of the world. Although communicable diseases once dominated the scene, the non-communicable diseases in recent years account for six out of seven deaths in the developed world and about half of all deaths in the developing world (Table 1).

Communicable disease

Infectious diseases account for 25 per cent of deaths worldwide (Fig. 1). Forty-eight per cent of deaths among people 0 to 44 years of age occur from an infectious disease (Fig. 2). Even in the developed countries of the world infectious diseases are the third most common cause of death. Sixty-three per cent of deaths in children worldwide are due to infectious diseases (Fig. 3). Clearly, infectious diseases remain a major public health challenge in the modern world.

Table 1 Distribution of deaths by broad cause group and region, 1990

	Deaths (thousands)				
	Total	**Group I**	**Group II**	**Group III**	**Group II/group I ratio**
World	50 467	17 241	28 141	5084	1.6
Developed	10 912	667	9411	834	14.1
Developing	39 554	16 573	18 730	4251	1.1

Group I: communicable, maternal, perinatal, and nutritional conditions.

Group II: non-communicable diseases.

Group III: injuries.

Source: WHO (1996).

In the past decade the leading infectious diseases worldwide in terms of both death and disability have been acute respiratory infections, AIDS, diarrhoeal diseases, tuberculosis, malaria, and measles (Fig. 4). These diseases can be treated effectively and can be largely prevented through relatively simple means. In fact, all have been substantially reduced in some parts of the world.

Factors which contribute to the persistence of infectious diseases include poverty and social inequalities, illiteracy, the low status of women, inadequate nutrition, poor sanitation, inadequate housing, rapid urbanization, failure to implement known preventive strategies, changing lifestyles which promote greater social and sexual mixing, limited access to health care, and inadequate surveillance systems.

The major infectious disease problems in developed countries (and increasingly in developing countries) are related to changing lifestyles, better survival of immunologically compromised individuals, and overuse/misuse of antimicrobial agents. Increased acceptance of multiple sexual partners and use of recreational drugs in both developed and developing countries have led to the current epidemic of sexually transmitted infections, including HIV/AIDS which have been exacerbated by the emergence of resistant strains of gonorrhoea and syphilis. People who have had their bone marrow or other organs replaced, or who are on chronic steroid treatment, are more susceptible to infectious disease agents.

Unstable political conditions in countries such as Rwanda and the former Yugoslavia have created increased numbers of refugees amongst whom infectious diseases spread rapidly. Another group of migrant people especially vulnerable to disease results from emphasis on manufacturing as a means for developing countries to increase income. The development of factories leads to increasing urbanization and migration of the rural poor to the industrial centres in search of jobs. The new migrants often must live in poor housing resulting in crowding and poor sanitation. Furthermore, many of the temporary migrants to urban areas leave their families in the villages, but engage the services of commercial sex workers and, thus, become at risk for sexually transmitted infections and HIV/AIDS.

Poverty remains one of the most important cofactors for infectious diseases in both developed and developing countries. Crowding, poor nutrition, limited access to health care, uncontrolled reproduction, and low educational levels, which are common amongst the poor, cause increased exposure and susceptibility to infectious disease agents and increased likelihood of death from them. Poor children are less likely to be immunized, to attend well-baby clinics, and to be introduced to medical attention early in the course of illness when intervention is most likely to be effective.

The advances that we have seen in the past decades have been due largely to the provision of safe drinking water, better handling of

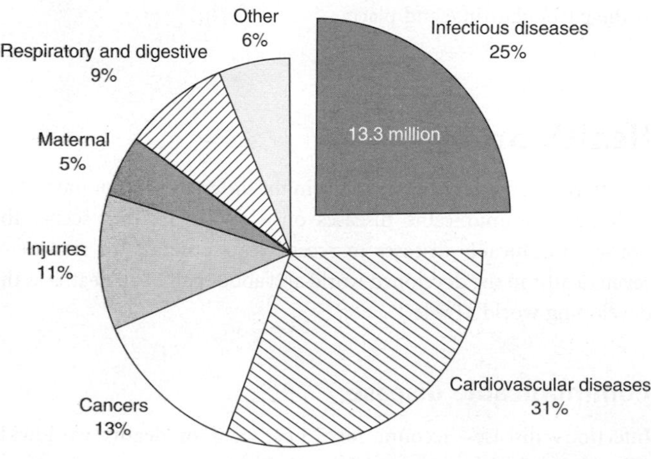

Fig. 1 Leading causes of death. (Source: WHO 1999.)

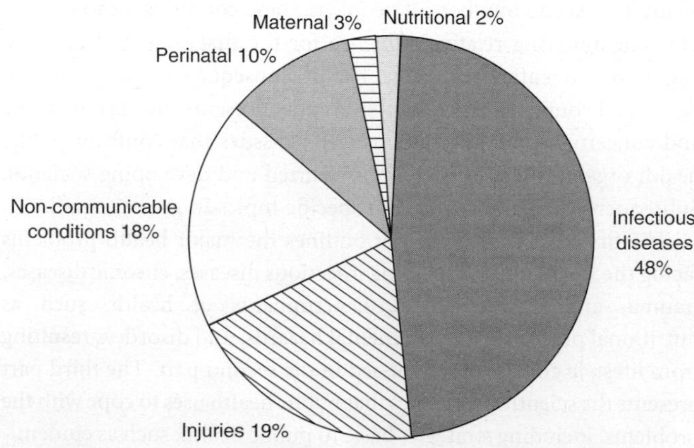

Fig. 2 Main causes of death among people 0 to 44 years of age. (Source: WHO 1999.)

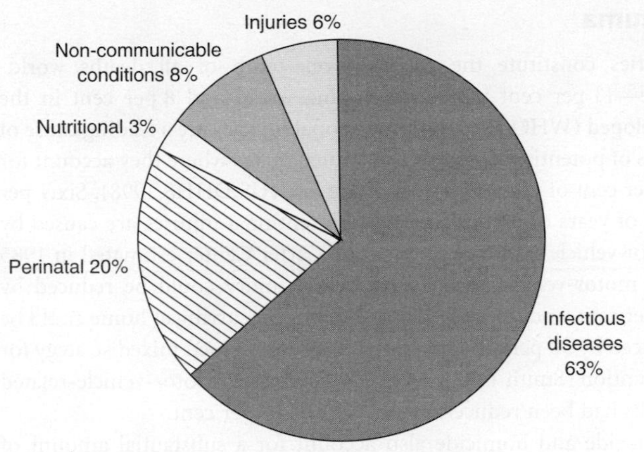

Fig. 3 Main causes of death amongst children. (Source: WHO 1999.)

sewage, development and effective use of vaccines, improved personal hygiene, health education, and improved nutrition. Nonetheless, all of these simple strategies to reduce and prevent infectious diseases have not yet reached many people of the world, especially the rural poor and the urban slum dwellers.

Control of existing or known infectious diseases, however, is inadequate to ensure the health of the public. New diseases are continually emerging. The most dramatic recent example was the discovery of AIDS in 1980 and the recognition 3 years later that it was due to an infectious agent. AIDS is now the second leading cause of death from infectious diseases worldwide and the third leading infectious cause of disability-adjusted life years. Other agents that have emerged in the last two decades include hantavirus and nipah virus. New variants of an existing agent causing human disease include the H5N1 influenza strain that erupted in Hong Kong in 1998 and required the slaughter of millions of poultry. The discovery of a new variant of bovine spongiform encephalitis in cattle in the United Kingdom required the slaughter of thousands of cows and caused the implementation of trade restrictions and political tensions between the United Kingdom and its trading partners. A variant of emerging diseases is the development of drug-resistant variants of common agents such as gonorrhoea and tuberculosis induced by overuse and misuse of antimicrobials. Because of rapidly increasing world travel, control of infectious diseases, including emerging diseases, is going to require multisectorial international co-operation. New technologies are being developed to recognize new agents. An example is the National Molecular Subtyping Network for Foodborne Disease Surveillance (PulseNet), which is a molecular subtyping network in the United States. These types of efforts will need to be implemented internationally as well.

While public health advances have resulted in dramatic reductions in the incidence of infectious diseases in most countries, for example the elimination of poliomyelitis from North and South America, public health professionals need to be continually alert to the emergence of new agents, new manifestations of previously known agents, and the presence of groups in the population that are particularly susceptible to disease through poverty or other factors. The control of infectious diseases in the future will require the continued use of often difficult but proven public health strategies including improvement in living conditions, more effective health education messages to induce behaviour changes, the continued development of new technologies for identification and control of infectious agents, the development of new drugs for treatment and prevention, and improved access to the means, such as condoms, to prevent transmission of infectious agents.

Dr Gro Harlem Brundtland, the Director-General of the World Health Organization (**WHO**), has said recently that 'Illness and death from infectious diseases can be, in most cases, avoided at an affordable cost' (WHO 1999). As in all of public health, what is needed is the commitment of the public to that goal and a willingness to commit the necessary resources.

Non-communicable disease

Beginning in the nineteenth and continuing throughout the twentieth century, industrialization and commercialization have vastly changed the way people live and, correspondingly, the nature of their health problems. This change becomes apparent in examining the leading causes of death in the United States in 1900, 1950, 1990, and 1997 (Table 2). Coronary heart disease, the major epidemic of the twentieth century in the heavily industrialized nations, reached a peak around 1960, and declined rapidly thereafter; and cancer mortality has been falling in the United States since 1990. Still, these two conditions remain the leading causes of death in most of the developed nations. Moreover, in the developing countries where infectious diseases have predominated, coronary heart disease and other chronic diseases are now coming to the fore (Table 3).

Moving beyond mortality and its trends, another system of evaluating the impact of disease and other factors affecting survival has recently been introduced: years of potential life lost. This term usually indicates the total number of years of life lost before a certain age due to various causes of death (Table 4). Thus, causes of death that tend to occur in early life (such as injuries) are weighted more heavily than

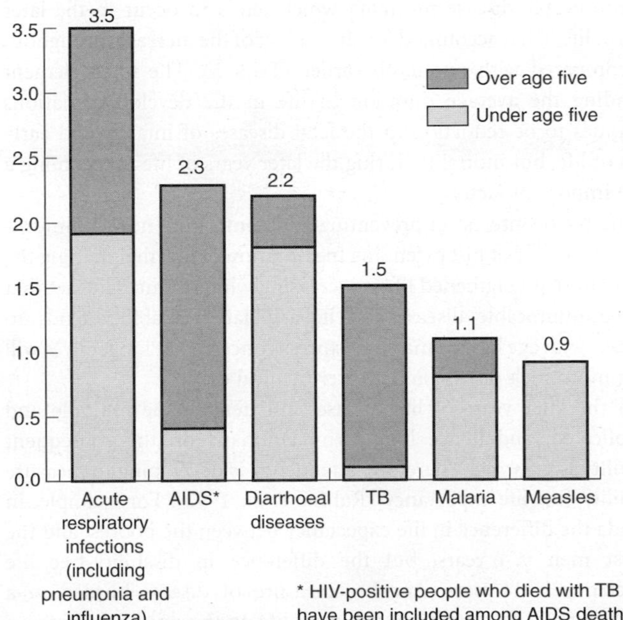

Fig. 4 Leading infectious killers. (Source: WHO 1999.)

Table 2 Leading causes of death in the United States (1900, 1950, 1990, 1997)

	Rate*			
	1900	**1950**	**1990**	**1997**
Diseases of heart	167	307	152	131
Malignant neoplasms	81	125	135	126
Cerebrovascular disease	134	89	28	26
Chronic obstructive lung disease	–	4	20	13
Motor vehicle injuries	–	23	19	16
Diabetes mellitus	13	14	12	13
Pneumonia and influenza	210	26	14	13
HIV infection	–	–	10	6
Suicide	11	11	12	11
Homicide and legal intervention	1	5	10	8

*Age-adjusted per 100 000.

Sources: McGinnis and Foege (1993); US DHHS (1999).

those that occur later in life. Furthermore, years of potential life lost is also dependent on the age distribution of the population; populations with higher proportions of young people have a greater years of potential life lost than populations with smaller proportions of young people, even if the age-specific rates by cause of death are the same for the two populations. Nonetheless, this is a useful measure for decision makers to estimate the public health impact of the various causes of death in order to plan prevention strategies.

The years of potential life lost measure, however, tends to obscure the fact that since 1950 the increase in life expectancy in the industrialized world beyond 65 years has accounted for a much greater proportion of the expanded longevity than during the first half of this century; in recent decades because of reductions in non-communicable disease mortality which tends to occur in the later years of life, it has accounted for almost half of the increase throughout life compared with one-tenth earlier (Table 5). The main element extending the average duration of life in the developing nations continues to be reduction in the fatal diseases of infancy and early years of life, but mortality during the later years of life is becoming a more important factor.

The major interest in preventing and controlling non-communicable disease is not just extending the duration of life; maintaining the quality of that lengthened life is increasingly important. The fact that non-communicable disease and its associated disability tends to increase with age has led many to express concern that longer lives will bring more such disease and greater medical costs.

In the later years of life diseases also tend to be multiple and complicated, and hence long term; emphasis on the consequent disability is growing. Therefore, a tendency is developing to measure disability-free life expectancy (Robine *et al.* 1992). For example, in Canada the difference in life expectancy between the poorest and the richest men is 6 years, but the difference in disability-free life expectancy is 14 years. Another measure of disease burden in a population is the disability-adjusted life year which combines a measure of premature mortality with a measure of life impairment due to disability (WHO 1996).

Trauma

Injuries constitute the cause of one-tenth of all deaths worldwide—11 per cent in the developing world and 8 per cent in the developed (WHO 1996). Unintentional injuries are a leading cause of years of potential life lost in the United States where they account for 15 per cent of years of potential life lost (US DHHS 1998). Sixty per cent of years of life lost due to unintentional injuries are caused by motor vehicle traffic accidents. The Carter Center estimated in 1985 that motor-vehicle-related deaths and injury could be reduced by 75 per cent, and injuries due to accidents occurring at home could be reduced by 50 per cent, by applying a broad-based mixed strategy for prevention (Smith 1985). As of 1996, however, motor-vehicle-related deaths had been reduced by only about 10 per cent.

Suicide and homicide also account for a substantial amount of years of potential life lost (Table 4). The rates of suicide and homicide, however, are not evenly distributed within a population, tending to occur more amongst young males and at different rates in the various racial groups (US DHHS 1998). In the United States, suicide amongst white males, for example, is responsible for 1.4 times as many years of potential life lost as amongst African-American males. Suicide is a major cause of premature death in most developed countries, especially in northern Europe and Scandinavia. Unfortunately, the causes for suicide are not well understood and satisfactory predictors of who will commit suicide have not been developed, making the development of preventive strategies particularly difficult. Often suicides amongst young people tend to occur in clusters.

Although declining, homicide remains a major public health problem in the United States where it is currently the leading cause of death amongst young African-American males aged 15 to 24 years; in 1996 it was nine times more common amongst them than amongst white males in that age group (US DHHS 1998).

Table 3 Proportions of mortality, selected causes, in high income, and low and middle income nations of the world, estimates for 1998

	High income[a] (% total)	**Low and middle[b] income (% total)**
Ischaemic heart disease	23.5	12.0
Cerebrovascular disease	11.1	9.2
Other cardiovascular disease	10.1	7.3
Malignant neoplasms	25.1	11.3
HIV/AIDS	0.4	4.9
Diarrhoeal diseases	0.1	4.8
Other infectious and parasitic diseases	1.0	11.4
Acute lower respiratory infections	3.8	6.9
Unintentional injuries	4.1	6.9
All other causes	20.8	25.3
Total	100	100

[a]Total high-income population, 907 828.

[b]Total low- and middle-income population, 4 976 748.

Source: WHO (1999).

Table 4 Potential years of life lost before age 75 for selected causes of mortality in the United States (1980 and 1997)

Causes of mortality	Years of potential life lost[a] 1980	1997
Malignant neoplasms	1815	1524
Disease of heart	1877	1190
Motor vehicle injuries	1011	661
HIV infection	–	209
Homicide and legal intervention	461	369
Suicide	403	378
Cerebrovascular disease	303	207
Chronic obstructive lung disease	141	159
Diabetes mellitus	115	150
Chronic liver disease and cirrhosis	259	142

[a]Years lost before age 75 per 100 000 population under 75 years of age, age-adjusted.
Source: US DHHS (1999).

As advances in public health over the last decades have caused declines in many major diseases, injuries have become a major public health problem that must be resolved; they are particularly important because they often affect the young disproportionately. The public health agenda for the twenty-first century must therefore address more intensively than before the issue of premature mortality due to trauma. Improvements in roads, seat belt laws, and improved car design have reduced injuries and death due to motor vehicle traffic accidents, and improvements in such everyday items as design of ladders have reduced accidents in the home. Better planning may not prevent disasters but it has, and can still further, reduce the damage from them. Forums for resolution of international differences and long-standing ethnic hatreds are gaining prominence but armed conflict over such matters has continued throughout the twentieth century, resulting in huge mortality tolls and other health tragedies.

More vigorous applications of intervention strategies should further reduce deaths and injuries from all types of trauma, but the nature of many factors causing death and injury from many types of trauma are still unknown. Further success in reducing injuries will therefore require multidisciplinary research to find the causes of these various types of injury. Such research should identify strategies that can be used for effective intervention programmes.

Table 5 Life expectancy at birth and at 65 years of age in the United States (1900, 1950, 1997)

	At birth	Gain	At 65 years	Gain
1900	47.3	20.9	11.9	2.0
1950	68.2	8.3	13.9	3.8
1997	76.5		17.7	

Source: US DHHS (1999).

Mental disorders

The concept of mental disorders has been expanding to include not only psychoses, neuroses, and mental retardation, but also alcoholism, dependency disorders, child abuse, and learning disabilities. Progress in understanding these disorders, especially the biological basis for many of them and what can be done about them, is accelerating. The discovery of syphilis as the cause of general paresis, and nutritional deficiency as the cause of pellagra, were early notable achievements. One can add the more recent identification of a specific genetic abnormality (trisomy 21) and lead intoxication as key factors in mental retardation, and the inappropriate use of drugs, especially in older people, as the cause of a vast amount of mental disorder. Also, pharmacotherapy in recent years has been proving remarkably effective in the treatment of increasingly recognized depression, thus relieving a tremendous burden from the lives of many people.

Despite considerable progress in elucidating the aetiology and therapy of mental disorders, however, the public health response has not kept pace with the huge problem they represent. The lag in implementing what can be done about mental disorders seems partly to reflect the lingering hostile attitude towards 'strange' people. Rather than simply placing them in custodial institutions and thereby excluding them from society, a more enlightened approach has developed in recent decades with more effective prevention and therapy. For example, treatment of syphilis prevents general paresis, Down's syndrome may be avoided through acting on amniocentesis results; and appropriate use of pharmaceuticals will minimize many cases of psychoses, particularly depression, which accounts for about one-sixth of the years lived with disability worldwide (WHO 1996).

The problem of mental disease is not diminishing. Increased longevity amongst people with congenital forms of mental retardation means more life years with that disorder, and lengthened life amongst older people is enlarging the problem of dementia, including Alzheimer's disease and arteriosclerosis of the brain.

Significant developments in the past few decades towards prevention and treatment of mental disorders include the following:

(1) increased numbers of mental health professionals and the increased range of services that they can provide;

(2) understanding that personal and community support systems can help individuals with mental health problems;

(3) awareness that early intervention may avoid chronicity;

(4) advances made in understanding the biological mechanisms of mental disorders;

(5) development of drugs for effective treatment of depression, one of the most common mental disorders.

The means to provide the mentally ill with the rights taken for granted by the vast majority of people in industrialized nations are now becoming available. Assuring these rights to those suffering from mental illness must become part of the public health agenda together with efforts to assure widespread application of the growing means of dealing with the problem.

Determinants of health

Nutrition

Diet has been scientifically and extensively linked to disease. The relationship between high-fat diets and coronary heart disease, and between undernutrition and infectious diseases, has been well established. Thus, the health of a community depends both on the adequate availability of safe food and the intelligent consumption of it.

Seventy-five years ago the major nutritional problems throughout the world were lack of adequate, safe, and affordable supplies of food, inadequate understanding of dietary needs, and widespread ignorance concerning the relationship of nutrition to health and disease. Most people, even in the developed countries, were not aware of the need for a balanced diet including components from several major food groups. Essential foods were often not available because of poverty, transportation, and distribution problems. For example, fresh fruits and other major sources of vitamin C were often unobtainable in northern climates for many months of the year. Finally, providing safe foods—uncontaminated by parasites, bacteria, and viruses—was difficult in the absence of refrigeration and pest control.

The high prevalence of infective and parasitic disease conditions led to undernutrition and, in turn, made individuals more susceptible to infectious disease agents because of their compromised nutritional status. For example, individuals with *Ascaris* infection could be undernourished in the face of what appeared to be an adequate diet, making them more susceptible to infection by other disease agents.

Most of the nutritional problems of 75 years ago have now been resolved in the developed nations through improved technology and education about nutrition. However, these problems persist in most developing countries and even amongst some groups of people in developed countries; for example, the poor and new migrants from developing countries who often lack both the fundamental knowledge of nutrition and the resources to purchase healthful food.

The major nutritional problem in developed countries now appears to be excessive consumption of fats, especially saturated and 'trans' fatty acids, refined carbohydrates, and salt, and inadequate consumption of fibre and cereals. This situation promotes diseases such as coronary heart disease, diabetes, hypertension, and dental caries. The United States National Health and Nutrition Survey documented a startling increase in obesity amongst American adults aged 20 to 70 years during the 1980s (Kuczmarski *et al.* 1994). The prevalence jumped from about 25 per cent, already high, during 1960 to 1980, to 33 per cent in 1990. The prevalence is even higher amongst the elderly and some other segments of the population and carries profound non-communicable disease and medical cost implications. Nutritional problems, moreover, are not confined to the developed countries; developing countries in transition also suffer from problems of overnutrition in the wealthier segments of their populations. Thus, developing countries suffer a double burden due to both overnutrition and undernutrition.

Another problem in developed countries is food faddists who advocate unhealthy diets especially to those wishing to lose weight. These diets lead to nutritional imbalances that can cause severe disease. Also, modern agricultural practices may not always lead to safer food. For example, the practice of adding hormones and antibiotics to animal feed may induce disease, including more rapid development of organisms resistant to current antibiotics. More research needs to be done to assure that modern technology to increase productivity does not lead to problems in consumers.

Appropriate nutrition can be assured through monitoring of populations using questionnaires, anthropometric measurements such as ponderal index, skinfold thickness, and height/weight indices; through education about the need for a properly balanced diet, particularly amongst expectant mothers, parents of small children, and amongst the elderly in whom nutritional problems are more likely to occur; and assurance of adequate, affordable food supplies. Finally, there are opportunities for intervention through nutritional fortification of common foods, such as the addition of vitamin D to milk and vitamins to bread. Adequate nutrition, however, requires sufficient income to buy healthy foods and, thus, alleviation of extreme poverty is essential for improved nutrition.

Environmental and occupational hazards

In the early part of the twentieth century public health professionals were concerned with ensuring the provision of biologically safe water and food to the public, and the safe removal of sewage and rubbish. The hazards of exposure to such substances as asbestos, lead, and radiation were unrecognized.

Systems are now in place in most developed countries to ensure biologically safe water and foods, and the proper removal of sewage and waste. However, the outbreak in 1993 of *Cryptosporidium* in the water supply in Milwaukee, Wisconsin, demonstrates the need for continued vigilance. Despite having the means to control pollution, many cities in the developed world and most of those in the developing world still suffer from levels of air pollution which are harmful, especially to children (Detels *et al.* 1991). Many lakes remain unfit for swimming and recreational use, and even the oceans adjacent to most major urban areas are still unsafe not only due to biological contamination, but also to chemical contamination. Even ground water in rural agricultural areas may be contaminated by concentrations of pesticides.

The environmental problems of importance in developed countries are now due largely to the explosion of technology over the last several decades. The production of chemicals in the United States has increased over 200-fold since 1940. This has been accompanied by a tremendous increase in the number of chemicals to which the public is exposed. As developing countries develop industries they too become polluted by chemicals.

> An example of the impact of these chemicals is the global warming due to the depletion of the ozone layer caused by the use of hydrofluorocarbons as aerosol propellants. Warming of only a few degrees will result in creating more ecosystems which are hospitable for deadly diseases such as malaria and dengue. (WHO 1999)

The impact of these chemicals is reviewed in Chapter 8.5.

The issue of environmental equity has been raised both within countries and between developing and developed countries. The poor, particularly minorities, are more likely to live in areas that are exposed to high levels of pollutants in the air, water, and soil (Rios *et al.* 1993). In their effort to produce cheaper goods for sale to wealthy nations developing countries have largely ignored the impact that rapid industrialization has had on their environments. Industrial areas in developing countries are now amongst the most polluted areas of the planet. Ironically, the cost of rescuing the environment will probably far exceed the cost that would have been incurred had environmental safeguards been incorporated during the process of industrialization.

Workers are subject to especially high concentrations of pollutants in the workplace. Unfortunately, health effects from pollutants may occur years after exposure and are therefore difficult to document. These health effects may be the result of cumulative burdens of chemicals in tissues or the disposition of chemicals in parts of the body that are not readily available for evaluation (e.g. the brain). A major threat to workers arises from exposure to substances not yet identified as hazardous and the reluctance of workers to wear cumbersome protective devices (Chapter 7.4). More research is needed to identify the potential health effects of acute and chronic exposure to a wide range of substances in the general environment, the food chain, and the workplace.

Safeguarding the health of the public requires regulation of pollutants. The establishment of acceptable levels of pollutants is complicated by two factors. The first is the difficulty of establishing dose–response relationships, particularly for effects with a long incubation period. The second is the economic burden that often results from regulatory actions. Whereas intervention in infectious diseases has met with enthusiastic support from the public, control of toxic substances in the environment has been supported by the public only recently. Inadequate understanding of the relationship between chemical pollutants and resultant disease, and the expense related to surveillance, regulation, and control of toxic substances has deterred action. Because stringent controls may increase costs, and even unemployment, regulation often rests more with the courts and legal procedures than on scientific expertise and judgement.

Resolution of important issues confronting society may themselves introduce health hazards. For example, the need to develop more energy efficient housing has increased the levels of pollutants such as radon and formaldehyde in homes, which, in turn, increases the potential for the occurrence of related diseases. In addition, certain personal habits may promote the action of specific toxic substances. For example, the likelihood of developing lung cancer from exposure to asbestos is increased about sevenfold in smokers, and is also increased in the non-smoker exposed to passive smoke.

Protecting the health of the public against environmental and occupational hazards in the future will depend on the following:

(1) continued research into the acute and long-term health effects of thousands of substances being released into the environment;

(2) surveillance of the occurrence of these hazards in the environment including the workplace;

(3) development and implementation of techniques for eliminating, reducing, or neutralizing these hazards;

(4) convincing the public of the need for implementing the necessary safeguards;

(5) laws to mandate the implementation of measures for controlling hazardous exposures.

Since such efforts will sometimes be both expensive and unpopular, careful consideration should be given to seeking to implement only those regulations that will have a high probability of yielding a positive recognizable effect on the health of the community.

Growing recognition of lifestyle

Although environmental measures and medical care have prevented much disease and improved health in recent decades, it is becoming increasingly apparent that individuals themselves play a substantial role in determining their own health. They do so through decisions about their diet, use of tobacco and alcohol, and other aspects of living. These decisions are largely influenced by the milieu in which people live. Spectacular achievements in microbiology and other biomedical sciences have evoked widespread and deserved admiration; unfortunately, these achievements have tended to obscure the important influence of lifestyle on health. The circumstances of life and how people respond to these circumstances are still the major determinants of health.

Evidence indicating that disability can be mitigated, rather than being an inevitable consequences of an ageing population, comes from studies in Alameda County, California (Breslow and Breslow 1993). The same health-related practices that predict longevity (not smoking, moderate or no alcohol, sleeping 7 to 8 h per day, exercising at least moderately, maintaining a moderate weight, eating breakfast and other regular meals) also predict freedom from disability and to the same extent (Fig. 5). Thus it appears that social conditions and ways of living influence disability as well as mortality patterns. The disabilities that now affect older people may subside in future generations along with mortality rates as social conditions and ways of living change.

In urban slums of developed countries as well as in developing countries, far too many people still live in extremely restricted circumstances that limit their scope of life. Most people in industrialized societies, however, have access to possibilities of consumption that, especially if followed to certain extremes, can generate serious health problems. The choices that people make when exposed to cigarettes, excessive amounts of alcohol and calories, reduced physical demand, and similar situations, exert a profound influence on whether they will suffer and die prematurely from lung cancer, coronary heart disease, diabetes, cirrhosis, chronic lung disease, trauma, or other current major causes of illness and death. Cigarette smoking alone is considered responsible for more than 400 000 (about one-fifth of all) deaths annually in the United States (McGinnis and Foege 1993). Obesity is another common and increasing factor (Kuczmarski *et al.* 1994).

Such health-related habits do not develop in a vacuum. The extent to which a person acquires them depends on circumstances such as the advertising and price of alcohol as well as cigarettes. Hence, social policy on these matters becomes an important public health issue. In this connection public health practitioners assure their credibility by advocating only those changes in lifestyle that are supported by scientifically sound studies.

A second aspect of lifestyle significantly associated with health embraces people's relationships to their social support systems. Considerable evidence links health to marital status, degree of closeness to friends and relatives, and social group involvement. Such social connections are highly associated with mortality and this association is largely independent of physical health status, health practices, use of health services, socioeconomic status, age, sex, and race (Berkman and Syme 1979).

Population

Success in public health initiatives, particularly in controlling infectious diseases, has reduced death rates worldwide with a resultant

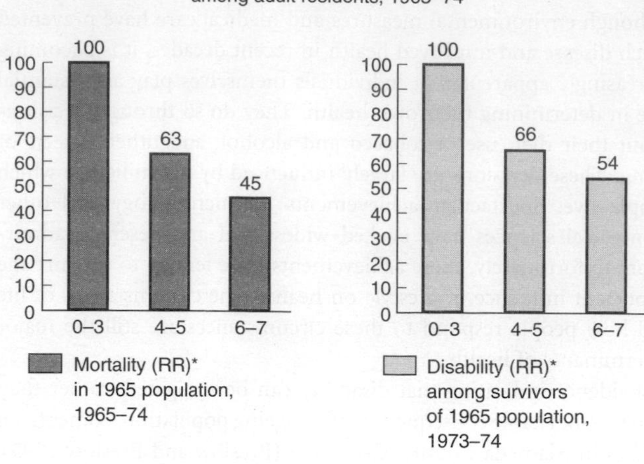

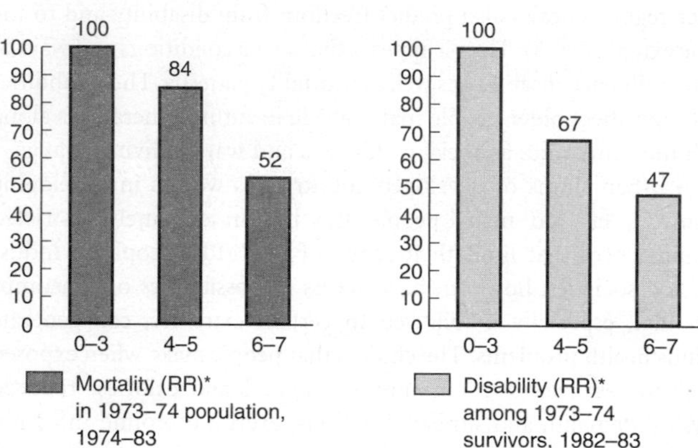

Fig. 5 Mortality, disability, and health practices amongst adult residents in Alameda County, California, 1965 to 1983. (Source: Breslow and Breslow 1993.)

increase in longevity, yielding significant population growth. In developed countries the decline in mortality took place gradually with a commensurate decline in birth rates as survival of infants increased. In developing countries the drop in mortality has occurred over a shorter time period and without a commensurate drop in birth rates. This has resulted in rapidly expanding populations, often in those countries where food and other vital resources are most limited. India, for example, has tripled its population since independence in 1947 and is expected to become the most populous country in the world within the first few years of this millennium. Overpopulation is a major cause of poverty and disease and is considered by many to be the most pressing public health problem.

Currently the less developed countries are expanding their populations four times as rapidly as the developed countries. These countries also have a much higher proportion of younger people, which means that the higher birth rates are likely to continue for at least the next several decades. However, the recent epidemic of AIDS, which affects primarily adults of child-bearing age, may have some impact in areas of high endemicity, such as southern and central Africa, where as much as 20 to 30 per cent of women of child-bearing age may be infected.

It is clear that unless efforts to control population growth are successful, the population of the earth will outstrip its ability to sustain itself despite the rapid advances in the agricultural sciences. Therefore, a major public health effort must be directed at controlling population growth. These efforts must include: the continued development and implementation of more effective and safe contraceptive methods, education efforts, both in the need for contraceptives and in their correct use, and the political commitment of the public and political leaders. The 1994 World Congress on Population brought together scientists and political and religious leaders to propose mutually agreeable policies for control of population growth (United Nations International Conference on Population and Development 1994). The goal is achievable as has been demonstrated by China with the development and enforcement of the one-child policy.

Conversely, in the more developed countries where population growth has declined to replacement levels or less, the proportion of elderly people has increased as the proportion of those in the productive years has decreased, introducing new problems. In the United States, for example, the social security system was designed on the assumption that the younger, and mostly working, population would be large enough relative to those over 65 years of age to provide support for the latter. This assumption may not hold in the future and is the subject of vigorous debate by the United States Congress and the President. Such shifts in age distribution in both developed and developing countries must be anticipated and their potential adverse effects recognized and prevented.

Income

The poor, in both developing and developed countries, are more prone to disease because their low income causes them to have poor nutrition and to be chronically exposed to unsanitary conditions. Furthermore, their low income limits their access to health care resulting in chronic disability from treatable diseases and conditions. In addition, the poor also often lack access to education and are more likely to be illiterate. Thus, it is difficult to reach them with health messages. Moreover, the poorly educated lack the social power to improve health conditions and access to health care.

Scientific approaches

Effective public health actions are based on scientifically derived information about factors influencing health and disease. The basic sciences of public health are epidemiology and biostatistics, but their effective use depends in turn on the knowledge and strategies derived from the biological, physical, social, and demographic sciences, including vital statistics.

Epidemiological strategies

Epidemiology is the core science of public health and preventive medicine. It is the scientific method used to describe the distribution, dynamics, and determinants of disease and health in human populations. Although there are many definitions, the Greek root of the word epidemiology delineates well the scope of the discipline: 'The study of that which is upon the people.' John Last in *A Dictionary of*

Epidemiology (1995) has defined epidemiology as 'the study of the distribution and determinants of health related states or events in specified populations and the application of this study to the control of health problems' (Last 1995). The epidemiologist seeks to identify those characteristics of people, the agents of disease, and the environment which determine the occurrence of disease and health. In order to accomplish that objective, the epidemiologist describes:

(1) disease occurrence (time characteristics);

(2) the population affected (person characteristics);

(3) the nature of the environment in which the disease is occurring (place characteristics), which contribute to knowledge about the natural history of the disease and ways to control it. For example, epidemiologists have observed that coronary heart disease occurs to a greater extent amongst middle-aged and older men who overeat, have high blood pressure, smoke cigarettes, do little exercise, have a family history of heart disease, and live in a developed country.

The science of epidemiology has many applications in public health as well as in medicine. These include:

(1) establishing the natural history of a disease in a population, for example, the impact of potent antiretroviral therapy on delaying the onset of AIDS and death amongst people infected with HIV;

(2) describing the natural history of infection and disease in the individual, for example the acute, asymptomatic, symptomatic, and clinical disease stages of HIV/AIDS;

(3) describing the clinical picture of disease, for example, who gets the disease, who dies from the disease, what is the outcome of the disease or infection, and what are the most effective treatments;

(4) identifying the risk factors for disease, for example the relationship of specific environmental conditions such as air pollution on the risk of developing respiratory conditions;

(5) identifying precursors of disease, for example the relationship of high blood pressure to stroke, cardiovascular disease, and kidney disease;

(6) identifying the major public health problems in a community, for example surveillance for the prevalence of specific diseases that are treatable or represent a threat to the health of the community;

(7) evaluating the effectiveness of intervention programmes, for example the impact of condom promotion on prevalence of HIV and sexually transmitted infections in a community or nation;

(8) investigating an outbreak of unknown aetiology, for example the cause of an epidemic of wasting disease in northern Luzon, Philippines.

For studying these matters, epidemiologists must have good information on the occurrence of disease, on the relevant characteristics of the population, and of the environment in which the disease is occurring. The need for this information has stimulated the development of health information systems for co-ordinating existing sources of data and guiding the development of essential new sources of information relevant to the health of the community.

Epidemiologists depend to a considerable extent upon comparing disease frequencies in different populations. Numbers of deaths are often the most readily available statistics for comparison. To make these comparisons it is necessary to estimate rates of disease occurrence or deaths due to specific causes. Information about populations is usually obtained from periodic censuses, or sometimes by a survey of a probability sample of the population. Rates that depend on census data are likely to be increasingly inaccurate with the number of years which have elapsed since the census data were collected. In addition, detailed information on populations derived from a periodic census is often not available for a year or more following the actual collection of the data. Information on population characteristics may be obtained at more frequent intervals by examining an appropriately selected probability sample of a population. This information can be particularly useful at times distant from the date of collection of census data.

The potential of epidemiology for documenting disease occurrence and developing and testing hypotheses has expanded rapidly over the last several decades. This advance is a result not only of the rapid development of computer technology but also because of the entry into the field of individuals whose major discipline is epidemiology. Although non-medical doctors, especially in the United Kingdom, made several significant contributions to epidemiological methodology (e.g. the great biostatistician, Bradford Hill) prior to the last decade, the majority of epidemiologists in the United States and United Kingdom were medical doctors who took an additional year or more of training in epidemiology to supplement their biomedical training. Now it is recognized that both medical and non-medical doctor epidemiologists are essential to the field: medical doctors for their clinical/biological expertise, and non-medical doctors because they are more likely to have expertise in methodological and statistical strategies.

Over the last several decades there has been a rapid increase in the number of techniques that distinguish factors that are truly related to disease from those factors that are related only indirectly to disease and, thus, may confound a true causal association. Greenland and Rothman discuss strategies to overcome these methodological problems in Chapters 6.10 and 6.11. Pearce and others have recently suggested that the concern for good methodology, however, has blurred the primary purpose of epidemiology to study the major public health diseases and issues in populations as opposed to individuals (Pearce 1996). The capacity of the epidemiologist for ascertaining the distribution, dynamics, and determinants of disease depends upon the availability of several other scientific disciplines. Laboratory procedures derived from chemistry, biochemistry, microbiology, and immunology, for example, can be used for obtaining information about the environment, the agents of diseases, and the changes that occur in humans. Conversely, epidemiology looks to statistics for mathematical methodologies that describe the strength of correlations amongst the multiple factors that may promote the occurrence of disease, and to the social sciences for techniques for obtaining accurate information from respondents as well as for assessing the influence of psychosocial factors on health and disease. Increasingly, epidemiologists and biostatisticians are working together to provide models of disease occurrence which can be used to predict trends of disease in the future—information which is extremely useful to public health planners.

In summary, rapid advances in the field of epidemiology have resulted from new epidemiological methods to reduce problems of bias and confounders as well as from the availability of new techniques in biostatistics, the laboratory sciences (microbiology, chemistry, and engineering), and the social sciences. Epidemiology will continue to draw upon these disciplines to help provide the basic information needed for the development and implementation of effective public health strategies for disease control and health promotion.

Biostatistics

Biostatistics is the science used to quantify relationships observed in public health and medicine. Through the correct application of biostatistical techniques, public health professionals can test and quantify the magnitude of the relationship of a factor or factors to the health of the community.

Advances in epidemiological methodology have been accompanied by rapid progress in biostatistics, particularly the development of computer technology. Through its application, biostatisticians have developed multivariate techniques to sort out the independent relationship of multiple factors to disease occurrence while simultaneously observing the relationship of these variables to each other. Sophisticated techniques for the analysis of events in relation to time are enhancing the value of the cohort study design. Because the computer can process massive amounts of information rapidly, it has been possible to develop and test mathematical models that describe hypothetical relationships and disease outcomes based on a variety of assumptions. The degree to which the actual occurrence of disease matches the model confirms or refutes these relationships. These models can be used to predict the future course of disease both in the individual and in the community. Both are useful for public health administrators responsible for allocation of scarce resources.

These new statistical techniques have been used to determine the strength of a relationship between a suspected risk factor and disease occurrence or causation, and to determine the efficacy of preventive strategies such as vaccines and health education, the level of efficacy of drugs through clinical trials, and the future course of epidemics. Through further development of biostatistical strategies and innovative computer methodology, the potential of statistics to contribute to public health will be even greater.

Biological and physical sciences

The laboratory sciences have long played an essential role in public health. Many of the new advances leading to the control of infectious diseases depend upon microbiology to provide new techniques to identify and isolate disease agents, to describe relevant variations within a group of agents (e.g. polio types 1, 2, and 3), to describe host variations in susceptibility to disease, and to identify markers of prior infection or exposure. The rapid expansion of vaccines to prevent viral diseases reflects new procedures for isolating viruses using cell cultivation techniques that were developed in the late 1930s. These cell culture techniques facilitated the manufacture of live vaccines using attenuated viruses, that is, viruses that have lost their virulence characteristics for humans but not their capacity for stimulating immunity. Recently, microbiologists have fragmented disease agents into specific components and selected those that are responsible for the protective immune response. Vaccines are now also being developed that utilize genetic recombination and synthetic peptide chains (NIAID 2000). It is likely that within the next few years vaccines based on DNA will become a reality. New techniques have been developed for identifying levels of viral DNA and RNA in cells and serum. These techniques can be used to provide new insights into the early stages in the infective process, to identify chronic diseases that have a viral aetiology, and to guide therapy.

Startling as these recent developments in microbiology and immunology have been, equally important contributions to public health continue to come from the laboratory sciences of chemistry, biochemistry, and engineering. These disciplines provide information about the levels of pollutants in the air, water, and soil which is used by epidemiologists to determine their health effects. The studies of the chemical interactions of primary pollutants in the atmosphere led to the discovery that the products of these interactions, such as photochemical oxidants, can cause permanent compromise of lung function. Physical scientists continue to develop monitors that can measure specific pollutant exposures even at the personal level. Knowledge of chemical interactions has also led to the development of catalytic converters which have played a major role in reducing pollutant levels due to vehicle exhaust emissions in urban areas. Further advances in the physical sciences can be expected to provide a more healthful environment in the future.

Advances in the laboratory sciences can be rapidly translated into new techniques for identifying infection and disease, as well as environmental and occupational hazards. For the epidemiologist they provide tools to identify and measure disease agents and knowledge which leads to the development of testable hypotheses. Thus, these new advances often lead to new techniques and strategies for intervention and control of threats to the public health.

Behavioural and social sciences

In addition to their influence on choice of exercise, levels of personal hygiene, eating patterns, and alcohol consumption in disease occurrence, behavioural factors also determine the response to illness, particularly to subtle manifestations of disease. Thus, they significantly affect the ability of the individual to live in a healthy way and to respond to disease. The role of the behavioural and social sciences (including psychology, sociology, and anthropology) in public health is therefore increasing as the nature of disease problems is changing. Experience with HIV/AIDS as well as cardiovascular disease and cancer over the past few years dramatically illustrates the need for changing types of behaviour that promote disease occurrence (Fauci 1996; Mann and Tarantoloa 1996).

Behavioural science techniques have proved valuable in understanding important influences on health. Social science, particularly its relationship to statistics in developing survey methodology and its increasing application to smaller population groups, for example, has greatly enhanced our capacity to discriminate the possible connections of behaviour and ecological factors to disease and thus to discern trends that are highly important to public health. Psychological investigations of people's knowledge and attitudes yield insight into the habitual and lifestyle practices that are related to health and often suggest ways of promoting health. Sociological investigation of group processes that determine a community's norms and values, and adherence to them, likewise leads to an understanding of how people behave and how they can be influenced to follow a healthy lifestyle. Anthropology elucidates the cultural traditions that affect what people do in everyday life and suggests approaches to health promotion specific to various cultural groups.

Within the field of public health, health education draws upon these disciplines to develop effective techniques for cultivating health-promoting behaviour (Green and Kreueter 1998). As emphasized above, the social milieu largely determines the choices that people make. Economic and other social conditions of life profoundly impact what people do about health-related actions. Lifestyle does not consist of behaviour elements selected by individuals in a void but depends upon their life circumstances. Hence public health must be concerned with the social conditions in which people live and direct substantial effort towards their improvement on behalf of health. The social sciences provide knowledge that guides analytic effort, in that regard, as well as for organizing and managing appropriate interventions; and they therefore contribute to formulating and implementing policy for public health.

Demography, vital statistics, and health information

Demography delineates the nature of populations, focusing on trends such as growth in their various segments, i.e. the excess of births over deaths, and immigration over emigration. Public health statistics are concerned with information about the health of populations. Both fields are devoted to satisfying social concerns about people. Mutual interest in factors such as those determining fertility illustrates the continuing interrelationships of public health and demography.

John Graunt is commonly considered the father of vital statistics because of his early studies of the Bills of Mortality in London and a parish town in Hampshire. He collected and examined the birth and death records maintained by parish clerks from 1603 to 1662 (Graunt 1662). From that work he drew important inferences about the population and its health. He analysed mortality, including infant mortality, seasonal variation of deaths, and longevity, as well as fertility and the excess of male births. His studies laid the groundwork for what has become vital statistics, which now include:

(1) births and the rates of their occurrence in various segments of the population;

(2) fertility, i.e. the ratio of births to women aged 15 to 49 years;

(3) mortality, including deaths amongst infants and in subsequent ages, as well as trends, specific causes, and determinants of deaths;

(4) migration patterns.

Information about health may be obtained through aggregated data from vital statistics, surveys, disease reporting, and disease registries as well as demographic statistics. Computer technology facilitates analysis of such data in relation to the characteristics of people affected. In addition, information from other sources can be linked to the occurrence of health events, thus providing additional information about factors in these events.

Data concerning non-lethal diseases are more difficult to obtain than the birth and death information that must be recorded by law. In the United States, the Centers for Disease Control and Prevention publishes a *Morbidity and Mortality Weekly Report*, which contains information on certain diseases, obtained through reporting from local health departments. Hospital discharge abstracts and summaries provide further information. Special surveys for specific diseases or factors affecting health may be carried out, in addition to ongoing national health surveys administered to a probability sample of the population. Cancer registries in several countries provide information about changing trends in cancer occurrence, mortality, treatment effectiveness, and duration of survival. Comparable data registries are also being developed for diabetes, coronary heart disease, congenital malformations, and other chronic diseases.

Programmatic scope of public health

Goal setting

Success in achieving the WHO's objective of eradicating smallpox throughout the world and, more recently, its initiative to eradicate poliomyelitis by 2005 (which has already been accomplished in the western hemisphere), have inspired other efforts to set and popularize explicit goals in public health (WHO 2000). For example, in 1980 the United States Department of Health and Human Services established specific objectives for 1990 in various health domains and a data collection and publication process to track progress in meeting the objectives (US DHHS 1980). It also delineated the measures necessary to reach those objectives. Based on experience with that venture, the agency set new goals in priority areas for the year 2000 (US DHHS 1991). For some specific objectives the trends have been on track, but for others, such as obesity, the trend was in the wrong direction. New goals for health priorities are now being formulated for the year 2010 (Table 6) (Institute of Medicine 1999).

Prevention of disease and promotion of health

The ultimate goal of public health has always been and remains the prevention of disease and the promotion of health in communities. Attention to quality of life is also growing, and represents a more positive goal than the traditional target of disease control in the health field (Breslow 1999). Although great strides have been made towards that goal, many conditions still cause considerable unnecessary deterioration in the quality of life as well as in disability and premature death. Furthermore, many people in both the developed and the developing world have not yet benefited from the public health achievements of the twentieth century. A major goal of public health in the developed countries in the future, therefore, will remain the prevention of diseases such as cancer, heart disease, trauma, and AIDS, which are currently responsible for most premature mortality and diminished quality of life. Achieving that goal requires assurance that public health advances reach those groups of people still suffering heavily from morbidity and mortality that can be avoided using current knowledge and technology. These include the poor and those not yet adequately integrated into the mainstream of society. In developing countries, reduction of infectious diseases and malnutrition often still must take priority, but increasingly, reduction of chronic diseases, accidents and trauma, and environmental threats to health are becoming goals there as well.

Prevention can be achieved through:

(1) emphasizing preventive aspects of medical care, such as immunizations and screening for selected conditions;

(2) health education and behavioural modification, including social influences on these aspects of health;

Table 6 Core list of candidate leading health indicators for Healthy People 2010

A	**Health and disease outcomes**
1	General physical well being
2	Infant mortality
3	Death rates from preventable causes
4	Disability-free survivorship
5	Self-reported health status
6	Sexually transmitted diseases
7	HIV
8	Cancer
9	Low birth weight
10	Cardiovascular disease
11	Asthma or chronic obstructive pulmonary disease
12	Hip fractures or osteoporosis
13	Injury
14	Diabetes
15	Disability days
B	**Preventive health behaviours**
1	Unintended pregnancies
2	Immunizations
3	Tobacco use
4	Physical activity
5	Alcohol use
6	Substance abuse
7	Appropriate body weight
8	Nutrition
C	**Mental health**
1	Psychological status
D	**Health system access**
1	Physical accessibility
2	Poverty
3	Health literacy
4	Education levels
E	**Ecological**
1	Air quality
2	Iatrogenesis
3	Firearm death and injury rates
4	Violence
5	Homelessness
6	Motor vehicle death and injury rates

Source: Institute of Medicine (1999).

(3) control of the environment for health;

(4) cultivating political will for public health initiatives.

Medical care

Beginning with Bismarck, the Western nations have generally provided medical care of varying kinds and degree as a social benefit to industrialized workers. In most countries care has also been extended to others, particularly to families of workers, the elderly, and the poor. The British National Health Service, for example, covers the whole population. Conversely, the United States relies mainly on private arrangements for employed people, and large-scale governmental assistance for health-care services goes only to the elderly and the poor, while one-sixth of the population has no coverage.

Medical care can be examined from several perspectives: medical and economic, for example, as well as from the standpoint of public health. The medical profession, reflecting both the centuries-old tradition of healing, as well as recent advances in medical science, looks upon medical care as the principal means to relieve suffering and restore health in individuals. Economists view medical care in terms of its cost and therefore are concerned about the increasingly large expenditures for it. Public health considers medical care to be one means of protecting and improving the health of people, but also is vigilant about its cost and financing, especially in so far as that constitutes a barrier to health care for some groups. Public health's focus on medical care emphasizes its potential for enhancing a community's health, with its cost a consideration in the same sense that environmental protection raises financial issues. Public health usually does not assume responsibility for the actual delivery of health care to the individual, but is concerned with the quality, access, and equity of the care that is provided.

Provision of medical services is usually determined in a specific country by cultural and traditional patterns, although these medical service patterns are constantly evolving. Thus, in the United Kingdom the individual general practitioner with a panel of patients comprises the predominant care module, with referral to the hospital consultant as necessary. However, a current trend is for general practitioners to work within group practice prepayment plans; for example, in the United States the former lifelong doctor–patient relationship is often replaced by health centres or clinics where the patient may be seen by a primary care doctor, by some specialists, such as paediatricians, general internists, or obstetricians, who see patients only during certain limited periods of their lives, and, to a growing extent, by free-standing emergency medical services. The number and type of various medical service arrangements and payment methods are rapidly expanding in the United States.

Public health relies upon doctors primarily to achieve preventive medical care. Thus, public health agencies have organized immunization activities and often maternal and child health services both through existing sources of medical care, and, where necessary, through direct provision of these services. In recent decades these efforts have contributed to spectacular achievements in control of communicable disease, for example the eradication of smallpox and the extensive control of poliomyelitis.

Curative services, however, generally receive funding priority over preventive services on the grounds of urgency. Most doctors and medical care agencies adhere to what may be termed the complaint–

response system of medicine; patients are encouraged to recognize and bring their health complaints to the doctor, whose response is to diagnose and treat any illness that may be present. Prevention, if advocated at all, is usually a minor consideration.

A new system of medical care that gives priority to promoting health and preventing disease has been slowly emerging. The health of individuals is monitored through periodic appraisal geared to age and other factors that determine both current and future prospects of health. Thus, infant care concentrates on growth, appearance of defects, immunization status, and any necessary corrective action to assure the healthiest possible development. When a person has reached 50 years of age, the focus shifts to blood pressure, weight-to-height ratio, blood sugar, blood cholesterol, cancer detection, cigarette and alcohol consumption, and other physical and behavioural characteristics. Many industrial leaders in the United States have started to provide health risk assessment and health counselling services for their employees. Arrangement for these services at or in connection with work is one of the fastest growing aspects of medical care in the United States (Fielding 1989).

While medical care services have absorbed a rapidly increasing proportion of total expenditures for all goods and services in some developed nations, the developing world has not had the resources to commit to such an effort. Vast numbers of people can thus receive only the most elementary medical services, if any. Furthermore, as medical education advances in the developing nations, a substantial number of doctors seek training in the high-tech training centres around the world. Those returning to their native countries then try to introduce the procedures they have learned, but these are pertinent and available mainly to the élite in their societies. That circumstance aggravates the tendency to spend the money largely on curative services rather than on the huge backlog of needed preventive services in the developing world. Use of community health workers, i.e. people recruited from the communities themselves and trained to promote health, as developed in several countries, may help to alleviate the problem.

In addition to the relative emphasis that should, worldwide, be accorded preventive *vis-à-vis* curative efforts, several other issues currently affect the public health approach to medical care. Previously many procedures and drugs have come into widespread use without sufficient consideration of their effectiveness. Initiatives are now underway, for example, by the Medical Research Council and the Departments of Health and Social Security in the United Kingdom, and the Congressional Office of Technology Assessment in the United States, to establish better systems for evaluating the effectiveness of medical technologies, including drug regimens, as well as to shorten the interval between the development of a drug and its licensing.

These initiatives reflect concern about the rapidly rising cost of medical care in the Western nations and about features with questionable, or even negative, relevance to health. Another rising issue is the efficiency of medical service, that is, how the best possible quality of medical care be provided within a given amount of resources. New facilities for 'ambulatory surgery', for example, make it possible to carry out many procedures without the extra expense entailed in admission to a hospital. Organizing medical personnel into groups, as well as providing incentives to personnel, offer possibilities for increasing the productivity of medical services. However, another cost-related issue is the extent to which medical resources should be used for highly expensive procedures and devices, such as heart replacement, that benefit only a few people at great expense. Recently, managed care organizations, which are private for-profit organizations, have become popular as a cost-effective strategy for providing care. Managed care organizations emphasize primary care, but the primary care doctor and a review board in them also act as the gatekeeper for seeing specialists and reducing costs. This latter role has raised questions about the quality of care delivered by managed care organizations which may limit referrals to specialists deemed necessary by primary care doctors as well as their patients.

Limited resources, together with the application of expanding technology for dubious gains, are forcing consideration of the ethical as well as the health and economic consequences of medical care. Resistance is growing to the technological prolongation of life when the quality of life has deteriorated beyond the point where it is worth saving. The state of Oregon, in the United States, has even introduced the concept of limiting funding for very expensive procedures to patients who fit certain criteria deemed to make the procedure cost-effective.

The principal aims of public health in the immediate future must be to find an appropriate balance between the provision of (a) sophisticated, technology-dependent health care at an affordable cost; (b) curative, complaint-driven medicine; and (c) preventive/health promotion services. The ideal balance will be partly determined by the resources that the country can devote to medical care. In developing countries greater emphasis should be placed on cost-effective preventive/health-promotion services than on expensive curative complaint-driven care.

Influencing behaviour

As noted above, the circumstances of life and the way people live largely determine their health. Thus a prime responsibility for public health is to develop effective strategies to promote healthful conditions and lifestyles. One approach is to assure that local, national, and even international milieux favour healthful behaviour, as in the various national and WHO campaigns against cigarette smoking and the worldwide struggle to promote breast feeding of infants. Such activities, however, often result in confrontation with powerful entrenched economic interests. Tactics in the struggle to turn public policies explicitly towards the side of health, therefore, must be high on the public health agenda.

Another approach is the so-called medical model: that is, using the doctor–patient relationship, or analogues of it, through a one-to-one or sometimes a small-group effort in a health-oriented environment to guide individuals towards healthful behaviour. It offers promise particularly when people have, or can be induced to have, concern about particular health problems such as cancer or heart disease, and then are willing to undertake the indicated habit changes. Doctors often have been reluctant to devote the effort needed, partly because of their discouragement with the results. Positive change, however, can be achieved with adequate protocols (Manley *et al.* 1991).

A third approach is to use the community intervention model for promoting more healthful behaviour. Particularly in developing countries people tend to consider themselves primarily as a member of a family and a community. Changing established community norms can, therefore, often influence people to adopt healthier behaviours. Community intervention can be initiated by identifying the leaders or trend setters in a community and enlisting their assistance in influencing the members of their community.

Environmental control

Attempts to control pollution of the environment, including the occupational setting, are complicated by the problem of identifying those pollutants that pose health hazards to humans. With the hundreds of new chemicals that are being introduced into the environment yearly this is a very difficult task. Many pollutants, such as radiation, have no apparent immediate effect on humans but can cause disease after many years of chronic and persistent exposure. Some pollutants may cause disease by accumulating in the body. However, the accumulation of these substances may occur in parts of the body, such as the bone, in which it is difficult to measure levels.

A highly desirable approach to control is to obtain the voluntary co-operation of industry as has been partially achieved in some developed countries in the control of air pollution. However, control mechanisms, which are often expensive, are seldom voluntarily adopted by industry, particularly in developing countries in which maintaining a competitive edge requires minimal production costs. Legislation is often used to achieve health-protecting environmental practices in developed countries. Controlling pollution in developing countries may be more difficult to achieve. McMichael addresses the issue of environmental policy in Chapter 2.7.

In the middle decades of the twentieth century the Western nations became increasingly aware of threats to health occurring through contamination of the environment. This concern led the United States, for example, to adopt the National Environmental Act in 1969, which directed the federal government to plan policies in the light of the effect that these policies would have on the environment. The National Environmental Act was followed in the next decade by a series of legislative actions creating regulatory agencies directed at protection of the environment and especially reduction of pollutants.

The economic downturn of the economy in the late 1990s, which first appeared in Asia, has precipitated serious challenges to maintaining and improving the quality of the environment, especially in developing countries and countries in transition. Even maintaining existing safeguards in the face of economic constraints has been difficult. Countries such as Myanmar and China have not limited massive logging for commercial use. The disastrous floods in eastern China in 1998 have been attributed to the loss of the forests in the watershed that form the origin of the Yangtze River.

In the future, innovative approaches, such as combining the control of wastes and the development of new energy sources and techniques for recycling waste products, will be needed. An example of this is the use of recharged waste water to augment existing limited water supplies. More cost-effective strategies for control of pollutants are needed. The public needs more education about the importance of preserving the environment and the need to monitor the environment constantly for new threats such as the destruction of forests and the introduction of new pollutants.

In summary, the programmatic scope of public health embraces preventive, medical, behavioural, and environmental measures designed to improve health at the community level. Although particular agencies and personnel address specific aspects of community health, public health embraces the whole range of these activities.

Public health strategies

Surveillance and monitoring

The backbone of public health strategy is the development, implementation, and maintenance of an accurate reliable health information or surveillance system. Donald A. Henderson, who led the successful campaign to eliminate smallpox, has said that 'surveillance serves as the brain and nervous system for programmes to prevent and control disease.' The elimination of smallpox from the world would not have been possible without effective surveillance. Surveillance can be used to establish the extent and distribution of a disease and the prevalence of risk factors or behaviours for disease in the population, to monitor the trends of disease or health factors in the community, to establish appropriate programme priorities and allocate resources, and to evaluate the impact of intervention strategies.

Surveillance systems can include information on the occurrence of infectious and chronic diseases, environmental information (including occupational exposures), behavioural characteristics of the population, and availability of medical facilities. It has become increasingly apparent that many infectious and chronic diseases and risk factors for them are determined by human behaviour. Thus, to implement effective intervention strategies it is necessary to know the behavioural characteristics of the population, including their sexual behaviour, and whether it is changing over time. To be most useful, information must be collected on a regular basis and reported rapidly while action in response to the information is still likely to be effective, particularly for infectious diseases and hazardous environmental/occupational exposures. Tardy information about disease outbreaks or sudden environmental exposures such as radiation hazards, for example, precludes the early implementation of effective intervention procedures when they are most likely to be effective. Surveillance systems are expensive to implement and maintain so it is important that they be evaluated periodically to assure that they remain cost-effective and are providing the information which is essential for the resolution of contemporary problems.

The most extensive experience in surveillance work has concerned the communicable diseases. There are fewer mechanisms for reporting chronic diseases, other than mortality. Currently, surveillance for environmental hazards and occupational exposures is even less satisfactory than surveillance for either infectious or chronic diseases. Most urban areas in developed countries have systems for monitoring quality of air and quality of water for human consumption, although provisions for monitoring new contaminants, such as cadmium and magnesium, have been inadequate. Considerable attention also needs to be directed to surveillance of recreational waters, toxic dump sites, and radiation sources. In addition, workers continue to be exposed to unsafe working conditions, particularly in small industries which are more difficult to monitor and regulate. Until permanent information systems which provide reliable, accurate, and rapid reporting of all principal factors affecting community health can be implemented, effective programmes cannot be fully realized. Implementation of effective surveillance is particularly difficult in developing countries that have limited resources or fewer health professionals with the necessary expertise. Yet, it is developing countries that have the greatest need for information on the prevalence of disease and risk factors for disease.

Intervention

Effective intervention forms the heart of public health efforts to protect communities from health hazards. These efforts include reducing the number of individuals vulnerable to infectious and chronic diseases, treating people early in the course of disease, modifying the environment, and promoting healthy behaviour of both communities and individuals.

Technological advances play a key role in developing effective intervention programmes, but often implementation of these programmes depends on the use of innovative epidemiological strategies, behavioural modification of individual lifestyles, and changing the political will of the community. For example, a satisfactory vaccine for smallpox existed for centuries before eradication was made possible by changing from an untargeted mass vaccination approach to an active surveillance and containment strategy supported by adequate resources. Legislation to control tobacco use by increasing the tax (and therefore the price) of tobacco products, restricting advertising for them and the places they can be used, denying access to youngsters, and requiring warning labels can change the whole social milieu regarding tobacco use and thus reduce it substantially, as has happened in California. Likewise, reduction of air pollution has been achieved by legislation requiring necessary corrective action after inspection of vehicles for pollutant levels and curtailing industrial pollution of the atmosphere.

Epidemiological research has identified many risk factors for cardiovascular disease, but implementation of intervention strategies to reduce these risk factors depends on convincing people to alter their basic habits such as diet and exercise. Methods for prevention of most sexually transmitted diseases, including AIDS, are well known, and treatment of many of them has been available for decades. Nonetheless, efforts to reduce the incidence of these diseases have been largely unsuccessful because of the difficulty of modifying this most intimate aspect of lifestyle. The source of many of the pollutants affecting the major cities of both the developed and the developing world are known, but techniques to reduce these pollutants involve major expenses by both the public and industry, and often cause inconvenience for the public.

Intervention through legislation typically invokes strong resistance, but that resistance can be overcome as has been demonstrated with the reduction of water and air pollution in Los Angeles through legislation that regulates industrial wastes and vehicle emissions. Changing the public's concept of what is socially acceptable can result in change, as has been demonstrated by the current attitude towards smoking in the United States and the current attitude towards vehicles that obviously pollute the environment in many cities of the developed world.

In summary, successful public health intervention is the result of technical advances coupled with the use of innovative epidemiological strategies, education of the public about the need for intervention, implementation of effective behavioural modification techniques, and induction of the political will.

Evaluation

An essential component of public health strategies is evaluation. The effectiveness of surveillance and intervention programmes changes over time due to changes in the incidence of disease, the development of new health hazards, and the development of new technologies for measurement and control. Thus, evaluation should be an ongoing, integral part of all public health surveillance and intervention programmes. For many years vaccination of all people in the United States against smallpox persisted even though the risk of an adverse outcome was greater from the vaccine than the risk of acquiring smallpox. Ultimately, the worldwide eradication of smallpox eliminated the need for vaccination against that disease. Since any immunization is associated with some adverse reactions, continued use must provide more benefit than risk. Because this ratio changes in relation to many factors, the relationship must continually be re-evaluated.

The effectiveness of different strategies of community intervention for promotion of healthy lifestyles can also be evaluated. Numerous studies have demonstrated, for example, that providing information about health hazards is seldom sufficient to motivate people to change their lifestyle.

Evaluation of environmental intervention has progressed less rapidly, partly because of the need for appropriate technology to identify and measure levels of pollutants in air, water, land, and the workplace, and partly because of the difficulty in identifying disease outcomes that may take years of chronic exposure. There is a need for earlier markers of disease processes resulting from exposure to pollutants which would permit faster evaluation. The cost of implementing environmental controls means that the public will be unlikely to pay for controls that have not been evaluated and demonstrated to result in improvement in health.

In summary, surveillance, intervention, and evaluation are the backbone of public health strategies to prevent disease, eliminate health hazards, and promote health in the community.

Organization of public health

Government structure

Organization of health services, both public and private, is largely conditioned by the cultural, political, and organizational patterns of the countries in which they are located. Thus in the United Kingdom and many European countries a national health service covers preventive, community, and clinical health services. Conversely, in the United States the tendency has been towards state and local governmental autonomy in environmental and health education services and medical care for the indigent population. Clinical services have been left principally in the private sector with federal governmental payments only for limited segments of the population.

United States

The United States constitution provides for the states to relinquish only those governmental powers that are essential to maintain the union. Accordingly, state and local governments historically have taken the main responsibility for public health, with most programmes being conducted at the local level under state regulation and only broad directions and incentives provided by the federal government. Thus the local jurisdictions (the county, city, or township), through authority delegated from the states, typically have undertaken communicable disease surveillance and control, maternal and child health services, environmental surveillance and control, and other traditional public health activities.

The role of the federal government in public health has evolved for the most part on a piecemeal basis. Usually it has assumed responsibility for meeting those needs not otherwise met by private, local, or state agencies. Generally, these initiatives have been categorical in nature, directed primarily at specific disease problems, such as cancer, or towards segments of the population, such as the poor. Exceptions to this approach have been the creation of the National Institutes of Health, the major research funding source in the United States, certain regulatory agencies such as the Environmental Protection Agency and the Food and Drug Administration, and the agencies and programmes stemming from the 1935 Social Security Act, the basic social security legislation for the nation.

Healthy People 2000, the National Promotion and Disease Prevention Objectives (US DHHS 1991), and other United States government documents do not have the force of legislation but serve as important guidelines and encouragement for local health agencies. The role of the federal government thus remains largely to suggest and encourage actions (sometimes with specific subsidies) that are either implemented (or ignored) at the local level.

Europe

In the European nations the philosophy of central control of public health has predominated, perhaps because of their smaller size and more homogeneous populations. The majority of the European nations have a national health scheme that is administered federally. Thus, to a larger degree than in the United States, public health activities are implemented centrally through an organized system.

The presence of a national health scheme, however, has not guaranteed more effective public health programming. Often the agencies within these federal governments do not command the respect and resources accorded the clinical components and therefore are not as effective as they could be. Also, many European countries lack schools of public health or their equivalents to prepare professionals for public health careers. Nonetheless, equity in access to medical care has generally been greater in the European systems than in the United States.

Whatever the government structure for public health, the need for good management is increasingly recognized. The responsibility for handling budgets that are often substantial, complex organizations involving many different categories of people, and maintaining effective relationships with a wide array of health agencies as well as other bodies, requires great managerial skill. The inadequate preparation in management skills of many health professionals who have previously occupied public health administrative posts has induced some governing authorities to call upon 'managers' rather than public health experts for the key positions in public health. This is increasingly true in the United States. Too often, public health administration has been reduced to budget control or complying with already adopted laws and regulations. As a result, little attention is given to analysing health problems or devising innovative solutions. The ideal is to combine the talent for leadership in public health with managerial skill.

Developing countries

In the developing countries the organization of public health is determined to a greater extent by economic and developmental considerations. Governments in developing countries tend to provide health services, although not at the level of sophistication available in the developed countries. In most of the developing countries responsibility for public health is usually assumed by the federal government through its Ministry of Health. Typically, a network of public health centres is established at the provincial and local levels, for example, the establishment of a network of anti-epidemic stations in China which are under the broad direction of the federal government. Often these provincial and local centres provide not only the usual public health services, but also provide care at local and provincial hospitals. The poorest of the developing countries also depend to a great extent upon support from non-governmental organizations and international agencies such as the WHO. These organizations do not always share the same vision of public health as the individual countries. Furthermore, they tend to provide assistance for specific diseases or subpopulations which often distort the priorities for health efforts. Health must compete with other governmental priorities for limited resources and often comes out second best. Because of the pressing need to address disease problems, particularly infectious disease problems, and the economic constraints under which they must operate, very few developing countries have developed plans for safeguarding the environment and assuring that it is healthy. Finally, there is often a shortage of health professionals trained in modern public health to design and implement effective public health programmes.

In summary, the organization of public health in various countries appears to be largely determined at every level—local, state, and national—by economic, cultural, and historical factors resulting in a wide array of often complex organizational arrangements.

Non-governmental public health agencies

Voluntary health agencies have flourished in the United States and to a somewhat lesser extent in Europe. They tend to be organized around specific entities: for example, the American Cancer Society, the American Heart Association, and the American Lung Association. Their success has encouraged the development of many more such groups, devoted to practically all the major diseases and several lesser ones.

Typically organized at the national level in the United States, with state divisions and local chapters, these voluntary health agencies bring together health professionals who are leaders in their particular fields and interested members of the public. They involve millions of people in fund raising for, and operation of, disease control activities. In this way they have contributed much to the level of enlightenment and activity concerning health, particularly in the United States. Their programmes usually include support of health research, professional education, public education, and demonstration services devoted to their own particular disease category.

These voluntary health agencies have become a considerable force in public health. They are able to operate with fewer constraints than governmental departments in the developed nations and thus have often broken new ground in the field. The American Heart Association and the American Cancer Society, for example, have been particularly active in bringing the concepts of risk factors and healthy lifestyles before the American public.

In the developing nations non-governmental organizations have played an even more important role in promoting health. Often governments in developing countries are constrained from specific activities by political and economic limitations. Non-governmental agencies, because they are not subject to these constraints, often play a key role in disease intervention and promotion of health. In the poorest countries, however, the health ministries must sometimes subjugate their health priorities to those of the non-governmental organizations because the latter have the funds and the freedom to implement activities that the governments cannot. In extreme cases the different non-governmental organizations may have conflicting health agendas making the setting of priorities by local public health professionals very difficult. Internationally, the increasing importance of non-governmental organizations in assisting the poorest countries to attack their major health problems is reflected in the number of non-governmental organizations recognized and affiliated with the WHO.

Another force in developing public health policy has been private foundations such as the Robert Wood Johnson Foundation, the Pew Memorial Fund, the Kellogg Foundation, the Rockefeller Foundation, and, most recently, the Gates Foundation and the California Wellness Foundation. These foundations support studies and trials of various approaches to health care, medical education, and public health. Thus they often point the way towards new ventures in public health. The Rockefeller Foundation, for example, has fostered an international network of doctors in clinical epidemiology by sponsoring selected training programmes in medical schools in developing countries. This has had a major impact both in promoting epidemiology and in increasing its profile within medical schools in the participating countries. By supporting programmes and studies with particular social and medical implications, these foundations will probably continue to play an important role in influencing public health policy.

Summary

The scope of public health in the last part of the twentieth century has expanded greatly (Fielding 1999). Not only have the number of recognized health hazards to the public increased, the strategies available to solve them have grown commensurately. Public health has borrowed and adapted knowledge from the physiological, biological, medical, physical, behavioural, and mathematical sciences, and has been quick to recognize the potential of new fields such as the computer sciences for improving, safeguarding, maintaining, and promoting the health of the community.

As the major communicable diseases have been brought under control through public health measures, more effort has been directed at chronic disease control, mental health, assuring a safe environment, reduction of accidents, violence, and homicide, and promotion of healthy lifestyles in developed countries. Although developing countries must continue to address persisting infectious diseases, they increasingly suffer from the ills of developed countries, particularly degradation of the environment. The biological sciences remain an important underpinning element of public health, but the contributions of the physical, mathematical, and behavioural sciences are increasingly recognized. As in the past, improvements in the health of the public in the future will be achieved by inducing public awareness and concern, which results in behaviour change, and the introduction and passage of effective legislation and regulations that are implemented by professionals committed to the principles of public health.

The previous effectiveness of such efforts, and the realization of the cost-effectiveness of preventive strategies for promoting and maintaining health, have brought renewed attention to public health and have set the stage for a new public health revolution.

References

Berkman, L.F. and Syme, S.L. (1979). Social networks, host resistance, and mortality: a nine-year follow-up study of Almeida County residents. *American Journal of Epidemiology*, **109**, 186–204.

Breslow, L. (1999) From disease prevention to health promotion. *Journal of the American Medical Association*, **281**, 1030–3.

Breslow, L. and Breslow, N. (1993). Health practices and disability: some evidence from Alameda County. *Preventive Medicine*, **22**, 86–95.

Detels, R., Tashkin, D.P., Sayre, J.W., ***et al.*** (1991). The UCLA Population Studies of Chronic Obstructive Respiratory Disease (CORD): X. A cohort study of changes in respiratory function associated with chronic exposure to SO_x, NO_x, and hydrocarbons. *American Journal of Public Health*, **81**, 350–9.

Fauci, A.S. (1996). AIDS in 1996; much accomplished, much to do. *Journal of the American Medical Association*, **276**, 155–6.

Fielding, J.E. (1989). Frequency of health risk assessment activities at US work-sites. *American Journal of Preventive Medicine*, **5**, 73–81.

Fielding, J.E. (1999) Public health in the twentieth century; advance and challenges. *Annual Review of Public Health*, **20**, xiii–xxx.

Graunt, J. (1662). *National and political observations mentioned in a following index, and made upon the bills of mortality.* Printed by Thomas Roycroft for John Martin, James Allestry, and Thomas Dicas, London. Reprinted (1939), Johns Hopkins Press, Baltimore, MD.

Green, L.W. and Kreueter, M.W. (1998). *Health promotion planning: an education and environmental approach*, (3rd edn). Mayfield Publishing, Mountain View, CA.

Institute of Medicine (1999). *Leading health indicators for healthy people 2010, Second Interim Report.* Committee on Leading Health Indicators for Healthy People 2010, Division of Health Promotion and Disease Prevention, Institute of Medicine. National Academy Press, Washington, DC.

Kuczmarski, R.J., Flegal, K.M., Campbell, S.M., and Johnson, C.L. (1994) Increasing prevalence of overweight amongst United States adults: the National Health and Nutrition Examination Surveys, 1960 to 1991. *Journal of the American Medical Association*, **272**, 205–11.

Last, J.M. (ed.) (1995). *A dictionary of epidemiology*, (4th edn). Oxford University Press.

McGinnis, J.M. and Foege, W.H. (1993). Actual causes of death in the United States. *Journal of the American Medical Association*, **270**, 2207–12.

Manley, M., Epps, R.P., Husten, C., Glynn, T., and Stropland, D. (1991). Clinical intervention in tobacco control. *Journal of the American Medical Association*, **286**, 3172–84.

Mann, J.M. and Tarantola, D. (ed.) (1996). *AIDS in the world.* Oxford University Press.

NIAID (National Institute of Allergy and Infectious Diseases) Division of AIDS (2000). *Vaccine concepts/designs.* Website: www.niaid.nih.gov/aids/vaccine/concepts.htm

Pearce, N. (1996). Traditional epidemiology, modern epidemiology and public health. *American Journal of Public Health*, **86**, 678–83.

Rios, R., Poje, G.V., and Detels, R. (1993). Susceptibility to environmental pollutants among minorities. *Toxicology and Industrial Health*, **9**, 797–820.

Robine, J.-M., Blanchet, M., and Dowd, J.E. (ed.) (1992). *Health expectancy: studies on medical and population subjects, No. 54.* Office of Population Census and Surveys, London.

Smith, G.S. (1985). Measuring the gap for unintentional injuries: the Carter Center health policy project. *Public Health Reports*, **100**, 565–8.

United Nations International Conference on Population and Development (1994). *Programme of action.* Cairo, Egypt.

US DHHS (United States Department of Health and Human Services) (1980). *Promoting health/preventing disease: objectives for the nation.* DHHS (PHS) publication No. 79-55071, US Government Printing Office, Washington, DC.

US DHHS (United States Department of Health and Human Services) (1991). *Healthy people, national health promotion and disease prevention objective.* US Government Printing Office, DHHS publication No. (PHS) 91-50212, Washington, DC.

US DHHS (United States Department of Health and Human Services), National Center for Health Statistics (1998). *Health, United States, 1998.* US Government Printing Office, Washington, DC.

US DHHS (United States Department of Health and Human Services), National Center for Health Statistics (1999). *Health, United States, 1999.* US Government Printing Office, Washington, DC.

WHO (World Health Organization) (1996). *The global burden of disease* (ed. C.J.L. Murray and A.D. Lopez). WHO, Geneva, Switzerland.

WHO (World Health Organization) (1999). *Report on infectious diseases. Removing obstacles to healthy development* (publication code: WHO/CDS/99.1). WHO, Geneva, Switzerland.

WHO (World Health Organization) (2000). *Global polio eradication initiative strategic plan 2001–2005* (publication code: WHO/Polio/00.05). WHO, Geneva, Switzerland.

1.2 The history and development of public health in developed countries

Christopher Hamlin

Introduction

Much more than is usually realized, public health is both a central and a problematic element of the history of the developed world—here conceived as Europe and the 'Neo Europes', i.e. the set of nations in broad latitude bands in the northern and southern hemispheres in which European institutions and biota have been particularly successful (Crosby 1986). It could be argued that a history of these regions in the last three centuries has broadly been a history of their health. It is in health terms that our lives are most profoundly different from those of our ancestors. We live longer; fewer parents experience the death of their young children and fewer adults experience the gradual 'consumption' of pulmonary tuberculosis; affluence and transportation mean most of us are no longer subject to periodic famines, and much less subject to epidemics of deadly infectious diseases, though we are less confident about that than we were two decades ago. Nor are most of us wracked with chronic pain, with abcesses, or induced deformities; most of us do not see life as a continuously painful experience and death as a merciful release, a view that is found fairly commonly in books of theology from three centuries ago (Browne 1964).Our health is adversely affected by aspects of the world we have built and the ways we choose to live individually and communally. A good deal is known about how to prevent those effects even if we do not always do so. Nonetheless, an expectation of health, and a preoccupation with it, are hallmarks of modernity. The freedom of action that ideally characterizes the lives of individuals in the developed world is predicated on health; so much of the agenda of development concerns health, that this transformation in health has some claim as one of the monumental changes in human history. It might be argued that economic and political progress are subordinate to securing health—they are means; health, which surely translates into life, liberty, and the pursuit of happiness, is the end.

If health is what we are all striving for, why is public health so invisible a part of our past? Until recently historians have been unconscionably negligent in investigating its history. Few general texts give it much attention (but see McNeill 1976); vast gaps in our empirical knowledge remain, and there is little good comparative work (but see Baldwin 1999; Porter 1999). Compared with the grand dramas of history, public health can seem a marginal function of modern society, representing little diversity, and nothing controversial. After all, we provide medicine, collect and evaluate demographic data, test water, and keep cities clean in roughly similar ways, according to the conventions of science, technology, and public administration that developed mainly in the nineteenth century. This view partly reflects a distortion of the history of public health by the modern professions and institutions of public health, which have often found it prudent to reduce the significance of the fact that they are necessarily political, even if their business is politics by medical means.

Public health is treated more broadly in this chapter, by examining actions taken in the name of a public to protect or improve the health of the public in general. Even that story is complicated by ambiguities—conceptual, causal, and definitional. Questions of what 'health' is, of what we mean by 'public', and of what we understand to be the proper domain of 'public health' are now, and have always been, contested matters. To define public health as that part of health that is the responsibility of the state does not help us to define these terms as what constitutes the state varies in time and place. However broadly or narrowly we define 'health', it will probably be admitted that many things that the public does will affect the public's health. Hence a central issue will be the enigmatic relationship between that universal goal, the health of the public, and public health—as profession, science, component of public administration, and vision (Rosen 1958; Fee 1993; Porter 1999). Within that framework there will be more diversity, contingency, complexity, and controversy in its history than is usually apparent. Ultimately, however, there can be no single historical narrative. A history of public health is necessarily part of an ongoing conversation about a systematic endeavour that is both rational and moral. Inevitably the story we tell will depend on what public health is conceived to be, yet our notions of public health will themselves be a product of the evolution of the professions and institutions we have inherited, and of the myths, memories, and sensibilities that sustain them.

Themes and problems in the history of public health

It will help at the outset to recognize several of the most troublesome issues that face any historian of public health. Amongst these are the following.

The units of public health: states and publics

1. *The public and the state.* 'State' and 'public' are not always interchangeable terms. The state, concerned with population, may arrive at different health-related policies from a public sphere of groups of citizens, carrying out a rational and critical dialogue amongst equals.

2. *The diversity of states.* Even when there arose widely accepted reasons of state and agendas of state responsibility, not every state was in the position to act on them. The focus of public health was quite often at the level of local states, whose responsibility and jurisdiction were often unclear or overlapping. However, the state itself became an artificial unit for addressing global problems, and those beyond the merely human.
3. *Goals of the state.* While health is now thought of in terms of the biological autonomy of individuals, that has rarely, and only recently, been the goal of programmes of public health. Health has meant a good supply of labour or of soldiers, control of excess population, protection of élites, enhancement of the genetic stock of a population, or environmental stability.

The condition that is truly health

1. *The definition of health.* The combating of epidemic infectious diseases has often seemed the core of public health. When we go beyond these diseases, questions arise of what level and kind of physical and mental well being the state should guarantee or require of its citizens, and of the status of health as a source of imperatives in competition with other imperatives such as the market, the environment, or individual liberty. What sort of normality will a society insist upon?
2. *The problem of causation of disease.* In a broad sense, diseases have many causes—personal, social, cultural, political, and economic, as well as biological. Amongst the multiple antecedents that converge in the production of epidemic or endemic disease, there are numerous opportunities to intervene. Notions of rights that must be respected, or of political or technical practicality, narrow that list. Discussion of cause has often included notions of responsibility or preventability—of where in a social system there is flexibility, of who or what must change to prevent disease.
3. *Equality and rights—race, class, gender.* The idea of 'health for all' disguises the fact that the interests of the public have not always been the interests of all of its members. Public health actions have often reflected, and sometimes exacerbated, a view of the world in which some groups were seen primarily as a threat to others. Often views of the standards of health that were matters of state differed for different groups: key divisions were by sex, by age (infants, working adults, and the aged all had a different status), by wealth, and by race, religion, or historical heritage (indigenous people had a different status from colonial rulers). Whether the public's response to disease was to advise, aid, or condemn, or to imprison, banish, or kill, reflected the allocation of rights and the distribution of power more than the status of the biological threat.

The health that is truly public

1. *Health and public health.* Most modern states have in principle distinguished aspects of health that are the business of the public from those that are for the individual to pursue in the medical marketplace, although the borders have been drawn in many different ways.
2. *Medical and non-medical public health.* Whilst public health has evolved into a subdivision of medicine with minimal and subordinate inclusion of the ancillary disciplines of engineering and the social sciences, the fact that health has been improved by many non-medical factors—economic prosperity, town planning, architecture, religious and humanitarian charity, the power of organized labour, and even broader political changes resulting in the greater availability of political or economic rights—suggests that any comprehensive account of improved health must include non-medical factors.
3. *Health as authority.* Given the amorphous nature of the concept of health and its status as the supreme good of human existence, it has been attractive as an imperative for political action. If other 'reasons of state' carry more immediacy, public health has better claim to the moral high ground because it is seen to be universal and apolitical, exactly the qualities that make it attractive to act politically in the name of health.

These questions are too many to address individually in this chapter, but they inform what follows. The history of public health in the developed world can be conceived in terms of three relatively distinct missions: public health as reaction to epidemics, as a form of police, and as a means of betterment. Public health was first reactive. Faced with the threat of an epidemic, European states closed borders and ports, instituted fumigation, shut down piggeries, and isolated victims. The second is public health as police. It is probably the case that wherever humans live in communities customs arise for the regulation of behaviour and the maintenance of the communal environment. Gradually much of the enforcement of these community standards became medical. The control of food adulteration or prostitution, of the indigent and the transient, or concern over dung or smoke overlapped with the control of epidemics, but went well beyond it, and occurred in normal as well as in epidemic times. Last to arise was public health as a proactive political vision for the improvement of the health of all. Even into the nineteenth century the view was widespread that remarkably high urban or infant death rates were inevitable. A proactive public health involved a determination that normal conditions of health, if they could be improved, were not acceptable conditions of health. That this sensibility changed was due partly to technical achievements, such as smallpox inoculation and later vaccination, and to better demographic information, due also to a more optimistic view of the possibility of human progress. Such visions sustained the building of comprehensive urban water and sewerage systems before there was wide acceptance that these needed to be universal features of cities; such visions have periodically led public health to venture beyond recognizably medical bounds, to recognize, for example, nuclear warfare or gun violence as public health problems.

The public health of epidemic crisis: reaction

Regardless of their virulence and pervasiveness, epidemic (and even more so, endemic diseases) do not necessarily warrant comment or action—they may simply be acknowledged as part of life. For a public to decide to fight an epidemic it must believe it can do something to mitigate it. A belief in the possibility of effective action is a prerequisite for public health; one of the most intriguing problems in its history is the emergence of that belief. It does not coincide with the replacement of supernatural by natural explanations of disease causation. 'Will-of-

God' explanations of disease have sometimes incited public action, but on other occasions implied abject resignation. Similarly, naturalistic explanations, attributing epidemics to a mysterious element in the atmosphere or, as in the case of classical conceptions of smallpox, to a normal process of fermentation in the growing body, have on some occasions been taken as proof that we can do nothing beyond giving supportive care and on other occasions sanctioned preventive public action. In each case assessments of technical and political practicality are mixed with assessments of propriety—is taking such action part of our cultural destiny?

These issues are already evident in the first European account of a widely fatal epidemic, the unidentified plague that struck Athens in 430 BC. Athenians both recognized contagion and acknowledged a duty to aid the afflicted, Thucydides informs us, but these recognitions did not translate into expectations of prevention, mitigation, or escape (Thucydides 1950; Longrigg 1992). Few fled; on the contrary, the epidemic was exacerbated by an influx from the countryside. While it was appreciated that those who survived the disease were unlikely to take it again, and some hoped it would bring permanent immunity from all afflictions, the main response was to accept one's fate. The disease was attributed to seasons, as well as to gods, and said to have been prophesied. Such resignation would be central in the moral philosophies of the Roman world, Stoicism and Epicureanism, both of which taught one to accept what was fated or necessary (Veyne 1987). Later writers in the Christian world attributed the failure of Islam to take active steps against plague to such an outlook. While classical Islamic doctors developed a science of hygiene to a remarkable degree, it did not follow that one should apply that knowledge in an epidemic: if plague came that was Allah's will. To fight it would be futile and impious; one's duty was to trust (Dols 1977; Conrad 1992).

In contrast, the response to epidemic disease in the medieval Christian Latin countries was activist. One could prevent disease from taking hold in a community, or extinguish it if it did, or at least avoid it personally. This activism had many targets, reflective of the syncretism of medieval Latin culture. In the Old and New Testaments alone, disease had a multiplicity of conflicting significations. It represented the dispensation of God to an individual, perhaps as punishment or a test. To act against disease by intervening to help others stricken by a dangerous epidemic was an act of devotion. If one died in such a situation that was a sign of grace; if one did not die, and helped to save others, that was equally a sign of grace. The laws of hygiene in the Pentateuch permitted a naturalistic interpretation of disease. Unclean acts or other transgressions, like failing to isolate lepers from society, generated the retribution of disease, perhaps through God's appointed secondary or natural causes. Disease might even be naturally communicative; in such a case, communal decisions to maintain the levitical laws were means not only of acting against potential epidemics but of maintaining the police of the community and perhaps of augmenting its welfare (Douglass 1966; Winslow 1980; Amundsen and Ferngren 1986; Dorff 1986). Such views would become widespread amongst nineteenth-century sanitarians.

The two diseases that did spur medieval Europeans to comment and react were leprosy and the plague. Whilst it is difficult to assess how much leprosy there was in medieval Europe, the common view is that there was a vast over-reaction, in terms of both investment in institutions to house victims of the disease—there were said to be several thousand leprosaria—and of detecting and isolating cases to prevent transmission of the disease. In keeping with the prominence of leprosy in the Bible, the professionals who diagnosed it were churchmen, not medical men. The diagnosis was a loose one; it might be based on skin blemishes alone. Often it involved an accusation. It led to the expulsion of the victim from ecclesiastical and civil society, symbolized in a ceremony resembling a funeral. Subsequently, no one was to touch or come near the leper or to touch what the leper touched. The theory of contagion provided the rationale for such action, but Skisnes has argued that the clinical characteristics of the disease itself—for example, its slow development, the visible disfigurement it produced—triggered such a reaction (Skisnes 1973; Brody 1974; Richards 1977; Carmichael 1997). Even if leprosy precautions did embody empirical knowledge of contagion, it, like most other diseases, belonged to the sphere of providence. While leprosy was sometimes seen as a punishment of sin, it might also reflect grace: God's singling out of an individual to bear a particular burden of suffering.

The prototypical institutional responses to epidemic disease, however, were those that arose in response to plague. The first wave of plague, the Black Death, spread across Europe from 1347 to 1351, and thereafter the disease returned to most areas about once every two decades for the next three centuries. This was a catastrophic disease, with case-fatality rates ranging from 30 to nearly 100 per cent depending on the strain of plague, the means of transmission, and the immunological state of the population. Plague and accompanying diseases reduced the European population by roughly a third in the fourteenth century and were responsible for only a very slow population growth during the following two centuries. As with leprosy, the aetiology of plague and the associated means of prevention and mitigation of the disease were conceived in terms of divine will and natural process, though even more clearly than with leprosy the distinction is misleading: Nature, whether in the courses of the stars, in meteorological phenomena, or in the process of contagion, was God's instrument (Nohl 1926; Ziegler 1969).

It is clear that in many communities the coming of plague was unacceptable. It could not be reconciled with the usual course of events, but indicated some fundamental violation of the cosmos, of an order which included human society. Boccaccio, whose *Decameron* is a document of the Black Death, testifies to one form of activism—a discarding of social convention and religious duty, a devil-may-care indulgence in the present founded in the recognition that life was short and the future uncertain. Those who could often fled plague-ridden places. Others, taking the view that the plague reflected God's just anger with hopelessly corrupt civil and ecclesiastical authority, saw a clear need to take charge of matters temporal and spiritual, to cleanse themselves, the state, and the church. Righteousness would end the plague. Thus the plague precipitated a social crisis, as would epidemics of other diseases in subsequent centuries. Beyond the massive disruption caused by high mortality and morbidity and an interruption of commerce and industry, the loss of faith in the conventions and institutions of society was a critical blow. Why respect property or family or communal obligations, pay taxes, invest money, or tolerate rivals and others? Latent tensions within society had an excuse to become active.

When people acted precipitately and independently, civil and ecclesiastical institutions were threatened, and it is in their responses that we clearly see the emergence of public health as a form of public authority. For a state, to act in a crisis was to keep the state going; one maintained authority by acting authoritatively. If some state actions were rational in terms of naturalistic aspects of theories of the plague, the viability of civic authority itself was probably more crucial than any lives they might save.

All these issues are evident in the manifold responses to plague from the mid-fourteenth to the early eighteenth century. Particularly in Germany, the response to the Black Death was to challenge civil and ecclesiastical authority. In 1349, lay flagellant groups paraded from town to town, giving public penitential performances to end the plague. While they were usually well received, and while their practices were not unorthodox, they did draw attention to what the Church had failed to do, and Pope Clement VI condemned the movement. But the state response to such actions was not uniform, for medieval and early states were not monoliths, but fragile alliances of multiple levels and kinds of authority, existing in continual tension with one another. In Basel, the majority Christian population blamed the plague on Jews—either it came by direct divine action because Jews had been allowed to live in the town, or through a natural agent with which the Jews had presumably poisoned the town's water. The town's Jews were rounded up, sequestered on an island, and burned. Here it was a local state, the town council, that took the action. Its credibility was at stake; it needed to be seen to act boldly to secure an end to the epidemic; its action built on pre-existing antisemitism. But to the central state, the Holy Roman Empire, such actions against one group of its subjects verged on anarchy. Emperor Charles IV condemned the persecution and asserted on the basis of medical and religious authority that the Jews were not responsible for the plague (Ziegler 1969).

In contrast, the approaches to plague prevention and control developed in the next two centuries in the Italian city states were humane, focused mainly on naturalistic intervention, and probably relatively successful. Plague control measures emerged out of a tradition of close municipal management, and in a cosmopolitan intellectual environment. Italy, after all, was the main European centre for receiving Galenic and Islamic medical knowledge. Included were concepts of hygiene, disease causation, and the purifying of enclosed spaces. The preventive measures taken in Italian city states were eclectic. They included the development of the 40-day hold on ships or other traffic coming from potentially infected places (the quarantine), the isolation of victims (and families of victims), and numerous means of purifying the air and/or destroying contamination: bonfires, burning sulphur, burning clothes and bedding, washing surfaces with lime or vinegar, killing or removing urban animals. Such actions were predicated on an understanding that the disease moved from place to place through some medium or media, possibly involving, though probably not limited to, person-to-person contact. But while the eclecticism of this response is certainly indicative of uncertainty about how plague spread, the actions do show a responsive civil authority (Cipolla 1979, 1992). Indeed, in some ways plague prevention initiatives were themselves a means of state growth. Plague control required officials to oversee quarantine or isolation procedures. It required a staff to disinfect, and a structure to gather information on health conditions in remote ends of the state. An embassy, which in the high Middle Ages signified an official visit by one state to another, became in the Italian city states the permanent presence of one state in the territory of another. Its initial purpose was to monitor the public health in the host country and to send word home if plague broke out (Cipolla 1981; Slack 1985).

The patterns and practices of the plague form the core of the catalogue of public responses to later epidemics of other diseases—flight, the exacerbation of social tensions leading to scapegoating, a heightening of religious seriousness (often combined with a collapse of normal customs and obligations), and a mix of pragmatic efforts to disinfect people, places, goods, or the environment, and to isolate victims or potentially contagious strangers (Briggs 1961). The particular mix of these actions reflected the current state of debate between proponents of atmospheric theories, including miasmatic theories, which located the origins of the epidemic in some unusual state of air, and of contagionist theories, which emphasized various forms of interpersonal transmission, and presumed that epidemics could spread only as far as infected humans (or human products) carried them (Ackerknecht 1948).

Thus, in the nineteenth century the series of cholera pandemics which arrived in Europe in the early 1830s brought forth accusations by the poor that the rich were poisoning them (particularly the doctors who wanted their bodies for teaching and research), and by the rich that the poor wantonly persisted in living in disease-nurturing squalor. It also engendered calls for public fasts, pure living, and declamations against sinful society, and a variety of attempts to disinfect, quarantine, and isolate (Briggs 1961; Rosenberg 1962; McGrew 1965; Durey 1979; Delaporte 1986; Richardson 1988; Evans 1990; Snowden 1995). In nineteenth-century America, the response to yellow fever and malaria was regular flight and the abandonment of cities during the summer by those who could afford to do so (Ellis 1992; Humphreys 1992). The summer home, in cooler, cleaner, and higher ground, became a mark of upper-middle-class life.

Significant new elements of that pattern entered in connection with efforts to control epidemics of three other diseases: venereal diseases, particularly syphilis, smallpox, and a mix of diseases including typhus, typhoid, and relapsing fever that was known as continued fever.

Whether syphilis came to Europe from America or Africa, or had been present in Europe in milder form (perhaps labelled as leprosy), is a question that has been much debated. What is clear is that a virulent epidemic known often as the French disease or pox began to spread quickly in the last years of the fifteenth century, and can be traced to the intercourse between Italian prostitutes and French and Spanish soldiers during the siege of Naples in 1494. The connection of the disease with sex was made quickly, partly because of the initial symptoms on the external genitalia—the more expressive German term *lustseuche* had been adopted by 1510. As had not been the case with plague or leprosy, syphilis represented a serious epidemic disease that constituted a state problem, particularly because it affected military strength, but which was not susceptible to large-scale public action. It was further complicated by having variable symptoms and effects, having a long course during parts of which it was not clearly manifest, and varying in contagiousness and virulence. If syphilis was to be controlled, states must prevail on individuals to avoid behaviours that spread the disease. One might expect that the moral opprobrium that went with contracting a disease that was usually acquired through illicit sexual contact to have had some role in discouraging such practices, but it did not. For an adventurous young man, a case of pox was a cost of doing business, even a badge of achievement. The disease was deemed curable, chiefly through mercurial treatments. While there are suggestions that by the eighteenth century syphilis had become something to hide (though not necessarily for moral reasons), such was not the case during the sixteenth century, when the disease was spreading rapidly (Arrizabalaga 1993; Arrizabalaga *et al.* 1997).

State attention shifted from cure to prevention only in the eighteenth century, partly because syphilis was becoming more clearly distinguished from other venereal conditions and as the varied phenomena of tertiary syphilis were becoming more evident. While the European states varied significantly in the priority they put on syphilis as a public problem, their approaches did not vary greatly: the disease was to be controlled by regulating prostitutes, who were regarded as the reservoir that maintained the contagion. Such approaches may well have had a significant effect in controlling the disease, but they exposed tensions between state and individual rights that have since become common in public health. Such conflicts developed first in the United Kingdom following the first Contagious Diseases Act of 1862, even though its programme against venereal disease was much smaller than that of France, where prostitution regulation was a central feature of public hygiene. The British Act allowed the police in designated garrison towns to arrest and inspect women presumed to be prostitutes and to confine infected women in hospital. It led to a sustained campaign for repeal that was ultimately successful in 1885. The repealers represented a broad coalition. Some objected that the legislation was morally indefensible because it acquiesced in the immoral industry of prostitution, others that it singled out women as responsible for a problem that was as much the responsibility of the men who used the services of prostitutes, while still others objected that the practice of arresting women was arbitrary (except with respect to class) and stigmatized working-class women who were not prostitutes (Walkowitz 1980; McHugh 1982).

The problem that the British parliament faced stemmed from liberal principles of human rights. Ironically, the Contagious Diseases Acts had been touted as respecting rights—the rights of men: the state would inspect women because male soldiers and sailors would not put up with genital inspection. Nor should they be expected to in a state in which the male franchise was broadening and the public was becoming increasingly uneasy with declarations that part of its population existed as cannon fodder. But recognizing the rights of men simply made it all the more clear that they were not accorded to women.

The issues that arose in combating venereal diseases arose in a more general way with regard to smallpox. While the ninth-century doctor Al-Razi had viewed smallpox as a normal childhood condition, a particularly dangerous part of growing up, it had become more virulent in fifteenth and sixteenth century Europe (Clendening 1942). By the eighteenth century it was accounting for 10 to 15 per cent of deaths. It was then widely recognized as a contagious disease of childhood, one sufficiently deadly that many parents exposed young children to it if it were present. Sooner or later one would be exposed—the older child who died from it was a time investment lost; the younger one who survived was subsequently immune. Accordingly, the practice arose in many parts of the world to induce smallpox. Whilst folk therapeutics owed nothing to medical statistics, it was recognized that some means of inducing the disease made it significantly less virulent. Mortality rates of 25 per cent or more might drop to a few per cent. Notwithstanding assertions that such practice defied providence, and its inherently counterintuitive character, such logic and experience had much to do with the relatively rapid acceptance of inoculation after 1721, when it was introduced into Western Europe by Lady Mary Wortley Montagu, a particularly well-connected aristocrat, who had observed the process in Turkey. It was taken up first in the British Isles; its subsequent spread elsewhere depended on the patronage of royalty and nobility, on increases in the safety of the procedure, especially when carried out by the most highly skilled practitioners, and the acquiescence of at least a segment of the medical profession (Miller 1957; Razell 1977; Hopkins 1983).

In 1798 the English practitioner Edward Jenner made immunization significantly safer by introducing the practice of vaccination with cowpox. Increasingly, smallpox prevention, which had hitherto been a personal matter, became a state concern. Presumably, the institutions that orchestrated quarantines could also ensure universal vaccination. But here too there was ambiguity: in whose interests were vaccination programmes to be undertaken? England began offering free vaccination in 1840, made it compulsory in 1853, and instituted fines for non-compliance in 1873. The initial assumption that all would take advantage of this free medical service proved unfounded; as the authorities sought to give the vaccination laws more teeth, they encountered growing opposition and decreasing rates of compliance. In 1898 antivaccinationists achieved permission for conscientious objectors to forego having their children vaccinated. The opposition was able to show that the dangerous procedure was not carried out everywhere with sufficient skill or care; and a real decline in smallpox meant decreasing risk to the unvaccinated. But mandatory vaccination also exposed underlying tension between the state and the public: in an atmosphere of distrust of the state, the more insistent the state became, the more convinced became the public that the state's actions were not in its interests (Porter and Porter 1988; Baldwin 1999; Brunton, in press).

It is important to emphasize that for most of the history of the West, efforts to combat epidemic disease had not reflected any sense of obligation to the health of individuals. At stake was the military, commercial, and cultural welfare of the state; the welfare of individual subjects (a better term than 'citizens' for much of the period) was incidental. While states devoted substantial resources to enforcing quarantines and other health regulations (and absorbed considerable costs in lost commerce), it would be misleading to think of them acting in some quasi-contractual way as agents of groups of individuals who had recognized that public actions were necessary to secure their own health. Whilst many places had town or parish doctors, and while there was often an expectation that the state take steps to protect the welfare of its subjects (such as making food affordable in times of dearth), early modern political theorists recognized no obligation of the state to protect the health of individuals. What was at risk in an epidemic was the state itself: the collection of taxes, the maintenance of defence, the continuance of commerce, and even the orderly transfer of property at a time of high mortality.

Perhaps nowhere was the tension between individual and state so great as in the combating of what was called continued fever. Typhus, typhoid, relapsing fever, and yellow fever were amongst the several epidemic diseases that appeared or became increasingly prominent in the aftermath of the Black Death. This 'continued fever' was endemic as well as epidemic, and amidst vast disagreement about classification and cause, there was general agreement about its frequent association with social catastrophe and squalor—with war, jails, pestilence, famine, and overcrowded slums (Wilson 1978; Smith 1981; Geary 1995; Hamlin 1998). But while it was often associated with class, it did not limit itself to the poor. It could spread from poor to rich, whether by person-to-person contact or by diffusion through some environmental medium from the hovels of the poor to the mansions of the wealthy. But, as would later be the case with tuberculous diseases, it was not clear that one could disentangle any single factor from the many conditions of poverty, nor did medical men necessarily think it made sense to try. The public action that might be taken was the comprehensive improvement of living conditions—the prevention of overcrowded dwellings; the insurance of sufficient food, fuel, and clothing; the provision of personal and environmental cleanliness, a safe work place, and a non-exhausting work day—in short, all the physical and social changes that would produce a sound human being (Hamlin 1992, 1998; Pickstone 1992). Yet such far-reaching actions to defend the state threatened also to transform it, and in essential ways—in its social distinctions, its institutions of property, even in the political rights it recognized. When the young Prussian radical doctors Rudolph Virchow and Sebastian Neumann investigated a typhus outbreak in Silesia in 1848, they argued that liberal political and economic reforms were the antidote to the squalor which caused the epidemic (Rosen 1947).

The public health of communal life: police

Beyond the response to epidemic outbreaks of specific diseases, Western societies had from early times taken steps to regulate their communities for the common good or the public peace. By the eighteenth century, the term generally used for such efforts was 'police', but the control of crime was only a small part of it. 'Police' referred to actions taken at all levels of government; indeed it referred generally to matters of internal order, i.e. to all aspects of government other than military and diplomatic affairs, the raising of funds, import and export duties, land tenure, and civil litigation. Police functions included:

- enforcing basic rules of sanitation, building construction, and public morality
- caring for the poor and for abandoned children and orphans
- regulating hours and modes of work
- the conduct of markets and the quality of the commodities sold in them
- marriage and midwifery
- the watering and treatment of cattle
- travellers and prostitutes
- times, places, and depths of burial
- taking steps to prevent fire and injury
- investigating accidental deaths and other forensic matters
- keeping population statistics
- regulating medical practice.

Sometimes town or public doctors were involved in these police measures, and some of them—like forensic diagnosis—were concerned with overtly medical matters, but at least as often doctors were part of the problem to be regulated.

The issues under the heading of police constituted problems at various levels: for individuals as property owners, towns as corporate entities, and regional or national states. Public health, in the sense of a recognized obligation to protect the health of the people through public regulation, was only rarely the rationale for police, though improvement in the public's health was probably the result. Some matters of police represented public means for the resolution of disputes between individuals as property owners, such as those that arose when the drainage, smoke, or dung of one person's premises encroached on anothers. At a municipal level, a widespread concern with the policing of the marketplace reflected the town's dependence on its markets. The privileges of trade and industry within a town were rarely free; a concern with the quality of foods and drugs reflected less a worry about the health of consumers than a concern with fair competition, consumer satisfaction, and the long-term profitability of the market. And it was in the interest of guilds, like the medical guilds, to keep out outsiders—the regulation of medical practice was in the self-interest of established practitioners, but was done under the auspices of maintaining the quality of public medical care. Finally, at the state level, concern with midwifery, nutrition, or demographic statistics did not necessarily reflect concern with individuals. Early modern statecraft equated state with population. In the crudest forms of that equation that population was understood as cannon fodder.

The character of institutions of police varied considerably, though most medieval European towns had some kind of institution(s) to carry out the tasks listed above. They reflected the nature of the state. In medieval Islamic towns, a muhtasib, an appointee of the caliph (or in early modern Spain a mutasaf) oversaw public morals and commerce, but also regulated medical and veterinary practice, refuse disposal, water supply, the cleansing of the public baths, and the licensing of prostitutes (Karmi 1981; López-Piñero 1981; Palmer 1981). In England, where the state was weak and towns strong, some of the police institutions reflected the bottom-up character of dispute resolution that would evolve into common law. Much of public police was built around the concept of nuisances, which included conditions offensive to health and sensibility, like concentrations of pig manure or butchers' waste, as well as antisocial forms of behaviour. Amongst medieval English institutions of local government were the leet juries (groups of citizens who biannually perambulated through the town and 'presented' the nuisances they found to the magistrates, who would order abatement), and the courts of sewers, which acted similarly in trying to resolve conflicts about drainage. Whenever a landowner altered drainage patterns, others were affected, often deleteriously. The sewers court was a means of minimizing those adverse effects and compensating for damage when they were unavoidable. In a similar way London's Assize of Nuisances managed disputes between neighbours about the location and cleansing of privies (Webb and Webb 1922; Redlich and Hirst 1970; Chew and Kellaway 1973; Leongard 1989; Novak 1996).

It is clear that the business of the public police did affect health in many ways and also that it covered much of what would later belong to the domain of public health. Mainly, however, the concern was with amenity, morality, and public order. But while the motives and contexts of police initiatives were broader than public health matters, health, understood in its broadest sense, was by no means absent from the police agenda. Within the frameworks of Hippocratic and Galenic medicine, amenity was not clearly distinct from health: to feel well was to be well; unpleasant sights or smells, noises or incidents, even if they led to nothing we would recognize as a serious disease, injured health. Concepts of specific diseases and environmental vectors were far in the future; notwithstanding the occasional speculation, like that of the Italian doctor Girolamo Fracastoro that each disease might be the product of an invisible living seed, most medical men were not thinking about individual diseases in a way that would encourage them to look for discrete distinguishing causes. Because amenity, order, and health were so closely linked, a medical rationale could provide a basis for social action on behalf of a community.

Too little is known about the operation of these institutions. What is known suggests that their performance varied enormously. It also suggests that the popular image of the premodern town as a filthy and ungoverned place is misleading. There may well have been filth in the streets, but clearly in some cases it was put there at prescribed hours of the day prior to the rounds of the municipal street sweepers who would collect it for manure or otherwise dispose of it. Many urban cottage industries—dyeing, soap making, the treating of leather or textiles—did use unpleasant animal products; complaints about them often reflect the struggle between classes over control of the urban environment, with wealthy merchants or professionals appealing to universal standards of sensibility and health to enhance their status over those who worked in what Guillerme calls the fermentation industries (Guillerme 1988; Kearns 1988).

Two examples of the ongoing legacy of such institutions of police can be seen in the regulation of the food supply and the central place of 'nuisances' in public health (at least Anglo-American public health). The fight for pure food and drugs that developed in the later nineteenth century is often seen as an early manifestation of consumerism and equally the product of advances in chemistry, microscopy, and bacteriology as applied to foods. Currently, the regulation of the food supply is one of the most common duties of public health departments—efficient inspection of meat- and milk-processing plants and institutional kitchens is regarded as an essential component of a civilized society. There were changes in the late nineteenth century in the recognition of a wider range of food contaminants, and due to the need to grapple with a more ingenious group of food adulterers, whose doings were better hidden by an increasingly complicated system of food production and distribution. But the concerns of consumers with food safety and their view that food inspection was a duty of government was old and widely shared. The concern of many medieval food inspection officers was with honest weights and measures, but quality was always implicit—the just measure did not satisfy if the ale was diluted. Whilst there might not always be objective ways of determining food quality, consumers knew: the records of civil discord are packed with the trashing of shops and the thrashing of vendors (Disraeli 1926).

Traditions of market regulation affected public health more broadly. Concern about water quality in metropolitan London, for example, reflected consumer outrage at high prices and poor quality and quantity well before there was any epidemiological evidence that such water was causing cholera. Equally, public willingness to accept that epidemiological evidence was tied to anger at paying too much for an irregular and visibly dirty water supply (Hamlin 1990). It is also likely, though difficult to show, that the ready acceptance of the new scientific forms of food inspection in the late nineteenth century reflected consumer expectations that the service was necessary and appropriate for government to undertake.

In the case of environmental nuisances too, institutions of public health took over from long-standing institutions for settling civil disputes. The term 'nuisance', drawn from the Anglo-French for annoyance, is peculiar to the English common law tradition, but analogous concepts operated in other cultures. 'Nuisance' referred to an accusation, and later to the legal determination, that actions on one person's property or in the public domain interfered with another's enjoyment of the rights of property, which included a right to enjoy health (Blackstone 1892; Novak 1996; Hamlin, in press). While in earlier centuries the concept had been very broad—including excessive noise, disturbances of the peace, the blocking of customary light—by the middle of the nineteenth century urban dung, human and animal, and action against nuisances acquired a basis in statute law that supplemented its status in civil law. Beginning with the first English Nuisances Removal Act of 1847, passed in expectation of the return of cholera, doctors, and later a new functionary called an inspector of nuisances (later a sanitary inspector) were charged with identifying nuisances and taking steps to have them removed (Wilson 1881; Hamlin, in press). The legislation reflects concern that a legal tradition built upon the power of property was unsuited to a situation in which most property was not occupied by its owners, and that one which depended upon an outrage to sensibility was unsuited in a situation in which peoples' sensibilities were insufficiently attuned to the particular states of environment presumed to be associated with cholera. But while this change was an emergency response to cholera, its effects were more far reaching; in effect, it represented the investing of community standards in a permanent institution with enforcement powers, rather than leaving them to be worked out, incident-by-incident, through the common law of nuisance and tort. The inspectors of nuisances did not restrict themselves to the causes of cholera; they and their successors responded to community complaints, which sometimes were primarily aesthetic. They became the defenders of the ever rising and increasingly universal standards of middle-class life, and however far their activities might stray from any direct relation to disease control, the inspectors carried the authority of public health (Hamlin 1988, 1994; Kearns 1991). Towards the end of the nineteenth century some epidemiologists, recognizing that the tracing of cases and contacts provided a more exact means of disease control, suggested that concern with these broad measures of environmental quality was an unjustified expense that deflected the attention of public health departments from what really mattered (Casseday 1962; Rosenkrantz 1974). In some cases they were effective in severing sanitation and public works from public health, but often they found that the public, which tended to support clean streets and pleasant neighbourhoods, continued (and continues) to appeal to public health as justification for their concern. Here too, medicine, however distantly it might be linked to the environmental condition under scrutiny, gave public action a legitimacy that would otherwise have been difficult to create.

The medicalization of public police that these examples suggest was clearly underway by the middle of the eighteenth century. The concept of medical police arose first in Germany and Austria, later in Scotland, Scandinavia, Italy, and Spain; in France the rough equivalent was *hygiene publique*. In America and in England the term and concept never really caught on. Medicine's rise to prominence reflected an alliance between medical practitioners who sought state patronage and the 'enlightened despots'—rulers who, like Austria's Joseph II, sought a science of good government that would significantly strengthen their states. Increasingly, rulers like Joseph felt obliged to test their policies against some tenets of rationality; health seemed to offer a well-defined arena of rational government, a set of means to improve the state and to measure the progress of that improvement (Rosen 1974*a*, *b*). How much the regulation of personal behaviour could improve the health of soldiers and sailors was becoming recognized; why not practice the same techniques on the rest of society? The effect of this medicalization was to move matters of police further from the realm of local social relations—for example, the determination and enforcement of community standards over cleanliness or food quality—and towards that of scientific rationality.

The classic text of eighteenth century medical police is Johann Peter Frank's six volume *System einer Vollständingen Medicinischen Polizey*, or *A System of Complete Medical Police*, which appeared between the 1779 and 1819 (Frank 1976). Frank (1745–1821) had a distinguished career as a medical professor and a public health and hospital administrator, mainly in Vienna. He began his giant work with a discussion of reproductive health (two volumes), including suggestions for the regulation (and encouragement) of marriage, prenatal care, obstetrical matters, and infant feeding and care. He turned then to diet, personal habits, public amusements, and healthy buildings. The fourth volume covered public safety, which involved everything from accident prevention to the injuries supposedly inflicted by witches, the fifth volume dealt with safe means of interment, and the sixth with the regulation of the medical profession. In Frank's cameralist view, anything that adversely affected health was a matter for public policy and an appropriate subject for regulation—rights, traditions, property, and freedoms, had no status if they interfered with the welfare of the population.

In its most far-reaching definitions, modern public health approaches the domain of a comprehensive police. It also recognizes that a wide range of factors are implicated in health conditions—current public health concerns include the effects of violent entertainment, the prevention of gun violence, and the conditions of the work place. But in modern liberal democracies, much of what Frank saw as the obvious business of the state is deeply problematic. For, in the nineteenth century, public health shifted radically in mission and constituency. It became less a means of maintaining the state, and more a means by which the state served its sovereign citizens with an (increasing) standard of health that they (increasingly) took as a right of citizenship.

The public health of human potential

The emergence of a public health that is not merely reactive or regulative, but that takes as its goal the reduction of rates of preventable mortality and morbidity, is a product of the eighteenth century. It is also one of the most remarkable changes of sensibility in human history. Its causes are complex but poorly understood. It clearly required the development both of knowledge of the problem and of the means to solve it. The concepts of preventable mortality and excess morbidity required being able to show that death and illness existed at much higher rates in some places than in others. Whilst there were a few attempts in seventeenth and eighteenth century Europe to determine local bills of mortality they were too few to provide a basis for comparison. In contrast, by the late nineteenth century annual mortality rates were an important focus of competition amongst English towns. The central government's public health officials, notably John Simon, chief medical officer of the Privy Council from 1857 to 1874, badgered towns with poor showings to analyse the reasons for their excess mortality and to take appropriate action (Brand 1965; Lambert 1965; Eyler 1979; Wohl 1983). By the end of the century, and during the twentieth century, reliable morbidity statistics were available to provide a better understanding of the remediable causes of disease. The gathering and analysis of such data has become a central part of modern public health.

The mission of prevention was also tied to a very real growth in knowledge of the means of prevention. The widespread adoption of inoculation and, after 1800, of vaccination for smallpox was the first clearly effective means to intervene decisively to prevent a deadly disease. Initially through the development of the numerical method and the cultivation of pathological anatomy in the Paris hospitals in the first decades of the nineteenth century, and subsequently through bacteriological and later serological methods, infectious diseases were distinguished and their discrete causes and vectors identified (Ackerknecht 1967; Bynum 1994). Such recognition led ultimately not only to the 'magic bullet' thinking of vaccine development; it also underwrote campaigns to improve water quality and provide other means of sanitation, and sometimes, as with tuberculosis and typhoid, programmes to identify, monitor, and regulate carriers.

Yet these factors alone cannot account for the widespread conviction that human health could, and must be, significantly improved. They are means, not ends. Whatever the symbolic significance of effective action against smallpox in boosting confidence, vaccination successes did not imply that all infectious diseases were amenable to a similar strategy. In most cases the new medical knowledge did not precede the determination to improve the health of all but was developed in the process of achieving that goal. A great deal of success was achieved despite quite erroneous conceptions of the nature of the diseases and their causes. The great sanitary campaign against urban filth (based on a vague and flexible concept of pathogenic miasms) is the best known example.

Recognition of differential mortality was not new in the early 1800s, but it did not necessarily convey a need for action. That there was a mortality penalty associated with poverty, infancy, and urban living was clear; but some regarded the town as a necessary corrective to the overfecundity of the countryside, and characterized the poor as occupying a fixed station in life whose biological characteristics included higher mortality than the virtuous middle classes (though not necessarily than the profligate aristocracy) amongst compensating benefits (like less anxiety and a simple, healthy, diet) (Sadler 1830; Weyland 1969). And even humane and optimistic writers saw infant mortality rates of 25 per cent or more as providential (Roberton 1827). To the influential eighteenth-century Lutheran clergyman Christoph Christian Sturm, God's providence was evident in the symmetry of the curve of mortality by age: mortality rates were high amongst the very young and very old, and low in between (Sturm 1832). This is in contrast with the modern sensibility which admits no justifiable reason (beyond, perhaps, the climatic factors that determine the range of some disease vectors) for differential mortality or morbidity.

The age of liberalism: health in the name of the people 1790 to 1880

The rise of liberalism changed all this. Whilst 'liberalism' covered a wide range of philosophical, political, economic, and religious ideas, at its heart were notions of individual freedom and responsibility, and usually, of equality in some form. In 1890, when John Simon, the pioneer of English state medicine, surveyed progress in public health during the past two centuries in his *English Sanitary Institutions*, he included a lengthy chapter on the 'New Humanity'. In it he covered the antislavery movement, the rise of Methodism, growing concern about cruelty to criminals and animals, legislation promoting religious freedom, the replacement of patronage by principle as the motor of parliamentary democracy, the introduction of free markets, the rationalization of criminal and civil law, and efforts towards international peace. Simon saw little need to explain how this concerned public health; he was sketching a fundamental change in 'feeling' that underlay changes in public health policy.

> Society had become readier than before to hear individual voices which told of pain or asked for redress of wrong; abler ... to admit that justice does not weight her balances in relation to the ranks, or creeds, or colours, or nationalities of men.

No longer were humans so much cannon fodder; the best policies were those which maximized 'human worth and welfare' (Simon 1890; compare with Pettenkofer 1941; Coleman 1974; Haskell 1985).

What Simon recognized was that with the granting of equal political and economic rights and responsibilities, it had become impossible to see health status as the birthmark of class, race, or sex. Nineteenth-century French and English liberals recognized that some—particularly women, children, or the poor—still suffered ill health disproportionately owing to the workings of the labour market, but they saw such consequences as incidental, accidental, and often, as temporary; in principle all had an equal claim to whatever version of human and health rights a society was prepared to recognize. As Simon also recognized, this change in feeling was both cause and product of the widening distribution of the political power it sanctioned.

And yet liberalism was no clear and compact doctrine, and its implications for public health were, and still are, by no means clear. Few of the pioneers of liberal political theory bothered to translate human rights into terms of health. They wrote mainly with middle-class men in mind, and saw the threats to life, liberty, and property as political rather than biosocial. The expansion (or translation) of political rights into rights to health was gradual, piecemeal (it has never been the rallying cry of revolution), complicated, and even fundamentally conflictual—it was and is not always the case that the choices free individuals make will be compatible with protecting the public's health, or even their own. Concern with public health arose accidentally, and quite differently and at different times in the developed nations. At the beginning of the twenty-first century an obligation to maintain and/or improve the health of all citizens exists only in varying degrees in the politics of developed nations.

Many early liberals found health rights hard to recognize because so much of public health had been closely associated with the medical police functions of an overbearing state. In revolutionary France the first instinct was to free the market in medical practice by abolishing medical licensing, a policy quickly recognized as disastrous for maintaining the armies of citizen-soldiers who were protecting the nation (Foucault 1975; Riley 1987; Weiner 1993; Brockliss and Jones 1997). Even after new, meritocratic and science-based medical institutions had been established, the cadre of public health researchers that it fostered—at the time the world's leaders in public health epidemiology—found it difficult to conceive how their findings of the preventable causes of disease could be translated into proposals for preventive legislation. Poverty, and to some degree working and living conditions, were dictated by the market; government mandates would induce dependence or simply shift the problem elsewhere. Thus France was the scientific leader in public health for the first half of the nineteenth century without finding a viable political formula for translating that knowledge into prevention (Coleman 1982; LaBerge 1992).

In early nineteenth-century Britain the ideas of T.R. Malthus led a broad range of learned public opinion, liberal and conservative, to similar conclusions. Disease was amongst the natural checks that kept population within the margins of survival. Successful prevention of disease would be temporary only; it would postpone an inevitable equilibration of the food–population balance that would occur through some other form of human catastrophe (Dean 1991; Hamlin 1998). Malthusian sentiment blocked attempts to establish foundling hospitals. Notwithstanding the fact that such institutions were notoriously deadly to their inmates, it was felt that their existence encouraged irresponsible procreation—faced with full economic responsibility for their actions, men (or women, depending on how one viewed the prevailing legal arrangements for child support) would stifle their urges (McClure 1981).

By 1850, in both France and England it was no longer possible to maintain what for many was a complacent and convenient faith in the welfare-maximizing actions of a completely free society. A number of factors shattered this faith. Firstly, no government ever adopted the programme of the early nineteenth-century liberals in full. In central, eastern, and southern Europe the old concerns of state security continued to govern their public health. In Sweden and later France, concern about a state weakened by depopulation fostered attention to the health and welfare of individuals. Secondly, working-class parties, while often generally sympathetic with political liberalism, saw no advantage in economic liberalism. Often they demanded adherence to the moral economy of the old order, which damped fluctuations in grain prices and backed up the working conditions that craft guilds had established. Most important is that many liberals themselves arrived at what is properly called a biosocial vision, a concept of society which recognized that it was impractical, inhumane, and injudicious to impose economic and political responsibilities on people who were biologically incapable of meeting those responsibilities: liberty had biological prerequisites.

These considerations were central to debates in France and Britain in the 1830s and 1840s. Governments in both countries were apprehensive about revolution and wary of an alienated underclass, urban and rural, of people who could not be trusted with political rights and seemed immune to the incentives of the market. Such people represented a reservoir of disease, both literal physical disease and metaphorical social disease, that could infect those clinging precariously to the lower rungs of the respectable working classes. Reformers proposed somehow to transform these dangerous classes, usually with Bibles, schools, or experimental colonies. Such was the political background against which Edwin Chadwick (1800–1884), secretary of the English bureau charged with overseeing the administration of local poor relief, developed 'the sanitary idea' in the late 1830s (Finer 1952; Lewis 1952; Chadwick 1965; Richards 1980; Hamlin 1998). Chadwick justified public investment in comprehensive systems of water and sewerage on the grounds that saving lives—particularly of male breadwinners—would be recompensed in lowered costs for the support of widows and orphans. But he also suggested that sanitation would remoralize the underclass, and for many supporters this was its most important feature. Politically, sanitation was a brilliant idea, since every other general reform was deeply controversial: proposals for religion and education were plagued by sectarianism; calls to improve welfare by allowing free trade in grain (leading to lower food prices) ran afoul of powerful agricultural interests; proposals for regulating working conditions were unacceptable to powerful industrial interests. Notwithstanding complaints that towns be permitted to undertake it in their own way and their own good time, sanitation achieved remarkable popularity in nineteenth-century Britain as the locus of hope not just for improved health, but in general, for a prettier, happier, and better world.

In treating insanitation as the universal cause of disease, Chadwick hoped to establish a public health that was truly liberal. He sought to deflect attention from other causes of disease, such as malnutrition and overwork, for these were areas of great potential conflict between public health and liberal policy. For many, the liberty of the free (and in the case of women unmarried) adult to bargain in the market for labour without state intervention to limit hours or kinds of work was axiomatic. And the need for food was to be the spur for work and self-improvement. Interventions by what has recently been called a 'nanny state' seemed to imply an obligation to the state and to affirm the desirability of dependence and subjugation. There were grounds for such concern: the relations of political status to health were fraught with ambiguity. Frank had written passionately of misery as a cause of disease amongst the serfs of Austrian Italy, but had not advocated the elimination of serfdom. Virchow argued in 1848 that liberal political rights were the answer to typhus in Silesia while in Scotland W.P. Alison argued on the contrary that too rigorous a liberal regime was the cause of poverty-induced typhus (Frank 1941; Rosen 1947; Weindling 1984; Hamlin 1998).

For about a generation, from 1850 to 1880, sanitation was unchallenged in Britain (and in much of its empire) as the keystone of improved health. Chadwick's campaigns led to a series of legislative acts, beginning with the Public Health Act of 1848 and culminating with a comprehensive act in 1875, that established state standards for urban sanitation and a bureau of state medicine, staffed by medical officers in central and local units of government and charged with detecting, responding to, and preventing outbreaks of disease (Wohl 1983). Outside Britain, sanitation did not have the same purchase. While continental towns and states took on sanitary projects for a variety of pragmatic reasons, adopting eventually the English paradigm of a water-centred sanitary system, the sanitary idea did not dominate public health (Simson 1978; Göckenjan 1985; Goubert 1989; Labisch 1992; Münch 1993; Ramsay 1994; Hennock 2000; Melosi 2000). They concerned themselves more with establishing networks of local medical officers and with controlling the transmission of contagious diseases through the regulation of travel and prostitution. Through the 1880s, the United States remained an exceptional case, coming closest to following a policy that an individual's health was a private matter alone. The national government maintained a system of marine hospitals along the coasts and navigable rivers, but less for controlling the spread of epidemics than for relieving ports of the burden of caring for sick seamen. In the early 1880s it established a National Board of Health to advance knowledge on public health issues of common import, but despite a superb research performance, it was scrapped within a few years on the grounds that public health was the business of the individual states (Duffy 1990). Often dominated by rural interests, many state legislatures had little enthusiasm for public health. Louisiana, which established a state board of health to combat yellow fever, was an exception (Ellis 1992). Towns and cities were more active, but often only sporadically, taking steps when faced with epidemics. States that did establish boards of health usually focused on specific problems rather than on public health generally: in Massachusetts the allotment of pure water resources was a key issue; elsewhere it was food quality, care for the insane, vital statistics, or the threat of immigrants (Rosenkrantz 1972; Shattuck 1972; Kraut 1994). In Michigan concern about kerosene quality (it was being adulterated with volatile and explosive petroleum fractions) and arsenical wallpaper dyes spurred the establishment of a state board of health in 1873 (Duffy 1990).

1880 to 1970: the golden age of public health?

By the 1880s the classic liberalism of the first half of the nineteenth century was giving way to a resurgent statism. The European nations, the United States, and later Japan competed for colonies and international influence. If the newly liberated or the newly enfranchised had some claim to a right to health, they also had a duty to the state to be healthy. In most of the industrialized nations there was renewed interest in monitoring social conditions. While the emerging techniques of empirical social research gave this inquiry the aura of quantitative precision, the surveys disclosed little that was distinctly new about the lives or health of the mysterious poor, the usual targets of public health and social reform. Much of it seemed new, however, because it now registered as problematic. For example, the enormous contribution of infant deaths to total mortality had long been clear, but only towards the end of the century did infant mortality, persistently high even in relatively well-sanitized Britain, become a problem in itself as distinct from an indicator of sanitary conditions in general. The health conditions of women too, and of workers, began to command attention in a way that they had not done previously.

While these newly recognized public health problems partly reflected the changing distribution of political power, they also reflected anxiety about the nation's vulnerability, and even the decadence of its population. Worried about the strengths of their armies, states like Britain discovered in the 1890s that too few of those they would call up were competent to be mobilized, and they attributed the problem to a vast range of causes: poor nutrition (coupled with lack of sunlight in smoky cities), bad sanitation, bad mothering, and bad heredity (Soloway 1982; Pick 1989; Porter 1991*a*, 1999). Epidemics of smallpox following the Franco-Prussian War of 1870 and again in the 1890s disclosed the gaps in vaccination programmes (Baldwin 1999; Brunton, in press). The usual response was to redouble the state's efforts to take responsibility for the immune status of its population. The persistence of syphilis registered at a new level of unacceptability (Brandt 1985; Baldwin 1999).

This led to an expanded public health, one highly successful in terms of reduced mortality and morbidity. It was undertaken jointly in the name of the state and the people, but it involved the regulation of an individual's life—home, work, family relations, recreation, sex—that went beyond the medical police of the previous century. From a contemporary standpoint such intimate regulation of the individual by the state may seem overbearing, but, with some notable exceptions, the populations of developed countries accepted it as an appropriate and even desirable role for the state.

New diseases, or old diseases that were (or seemed) more prevalent or virulent, new institutions for the practice of public health medicine, and advances in medical and social science contributed to this new relation between states and people. During the 1860s a long-standing analogy of disease with fermentation matured into the germ theory of disease as the research of Louis Pasteur and John Tyndall made clear the dependence of fermentation on some microscopic living ferment (Pelling 1978; Worboys 2000). During the 1880s, primarily through the work of emerging German and French schools of determinative bacteriologists, it became possible to distinguish many microbe species from one another, to ascertain the presence of particular species with some degree of confidence, and therefore to link individual species with particular diseases (Bulloch 1938). Through serological tests developed in the succeeding decades, the presence of a prior infection could be determined, regardless of whether anyone had noticed symptoms. Notwithstanding the increasing recognition of the many ways microbial agents of disease were transmitted from person to person, the effect of the rise of the germ theory was to focus attention on the body that housed and reproduced the germ—for example, the well-digger working through a mild case of typhoid—even when there were alternative strategies (water filtration or, by the second decade of the twentieth century, chlorination) that protected the public reasonably well most of the time (Hamlin 1990). The general interest in the human as germ bearer and culture medium brought with it an emphasis on the labour-intensive business of case-tracing, of keeping track not only of those who showed symptoms of the disease but also those with whom they had contact (Winslow 1980; Coleman 1987). In the key diseases of typhoid fever, syphilis, and tuberculosis concern with the inspection and regulation of people was exacerbated by the recognition that not all who were infected were symptomatic. The case of 'Typhoid Mary' Mallon, the asymptomatic typhoid carrier who lived for 26 years as an island-bound 'guest' of the City of New York, is notorious, but it was also important in the working out of both legal limits and cultural sensibilities with regard to the trade-off between civil rights and public health (Leavitt 1996). Newly virulent forms of diphtheria and scarlet fever, deadly childhood diseases transmitted person to person or by common domestic media, also gave immediacy to decisive public health intervention.

Such monitoring could not have occurred without a large rank and file of local public health officers. It was during the late nineteenth century that public health was identified as a distinct division of medicine and that most of the developed countries solidified a reasonably complete network of municipal and regional public health officers: in Germany, the *Kreisartz*; in France, the *Officier de Santé*; and in Britain, the Medical Officer of Health, assisted by the sanitary inspector. Increasingly these officers worked as part of hierarchical national health establishments to which they reported local health conditions and from which they received expert guidance. While preceding generations of public doctors had often been drawn from the ranks of undercapitalized young doctors, beginning in the mid-1870s many were specially trained and certified for public health work (Novak 1973; Watkin 1984; Acheson 1991; Porter 1991*b*). A commitment to public health was increasingly incompatible with ordinary medical practice, not so much because of its specialized knowledge, but because it was built upon a quite different ethic. There had long been economic tension between public and private medicine in areas of practice like vaccination, in which public authorities either took over entirely or inadequately compensated private practitioners for services that had traditionally been part of the ordinary medical marketplace (White 1991; Brunton, in press). But monitoring healthy carriers and those who might be susceptible to disease introduced a new regime of medicine—one which responded to an ethic of public good, even if there were no client-defined complaint. Effectively, bacteriology, epidemiology, and associated measures of immunological status redefined disease away from patient complaint. The healthy carrier might see no need to seek medical care, but to the public health doctor that person was a social problem. On occasion private doctors were appealed to for a diagnosis (bronchitis, pneumonia) that would protect one from the health officer's diagnosis of tuberculosis, which would bring loss of employment and social stigma (Smith 1988).

Rivaling the germ theory as the major motif of public health thinking from the 1890s to the 1930s was the application of the emerging science of heredity to the improvement of the human populations, the science and practice of eugenics (Paul 1995; Kevles 1995). Whether or not eugenic concerns were the source of the greatest anxiety about the public's health is debatable, but they were the locus of the greatest hope for health progress, the home of a residue of utopianism that had coloured the medical police and sanitary literature. Even more than other forms of public health, eugenics exposed a class, and sometimes a racial, division that had long been a part of public health: much of public health practice was predicated on a distinction between those, usually the poor, who were seen to represent the objects of public health efforts and those, often the well to do, who authorized intervention, whether to improve the lot of the poor, to protect 'society', or perhaps even to block the physical or moral contagia that might infect their own class (Kraut 1994; Anderson 1995). Eugenics appealed mainly to those with wealth and power: those others who were to improve their lot rarely identified heredity as the source of their unfortunate circumstances.

Such an attitude is reflected in the most infamous application of the eugenic viewpoint, the attempt by Nazi Germany to exterminate Jews and other 'races' regarded as inferior and unfit not only to intermarry with so-called 'true Aryans', but even to survive. While historians' views of the origins of the Holocaust differ, some of the immediate precedents for a state policy of negative eugenics—the prevention of the reproduction of those regarded as unfit—came from the sterilization laws that American states had begun to pass in the first decade of the century. The American laws focused on persistent immorality or criminality, and on what was called 'feeble-mindedness'. In Germany the acceptance of sterilization translated rather easily into the acceptance of euthanasia of the permanently institutionalized, and on to the extreme measures of the death camps, which were understood to be medical facilities. Even during the Holocaust the prevailing rationality remained that of public health: the trade-off between individual rights and the welfare of the state was a part of the working moral world of the public health officer. Just as an excision of corrupt or cancerous matter might be necessarily to maintain the body of the individual, so too it might be necessary to maintain the health of the body that was the nation (Lifton 1986).

The horrors of the extreme version of eugenics practiced in Nazi Germany have discredited eugenics to such a degree that it is difficult to recapture how central it seemed to reformers of the left as well as the far right. It appealed for a number of reasons. Firstly, it explained the failure of prior reforms, particularly sanitation, which was to have effected the thorough physical and moral renewal of the lower classes. Secondly, it seemed to be implied by Darwin's discoveries, which were themselves founded on deep familiarity with the successes of selective animal breeding of the agricultural revolution of the previous two centuries. Those discoveries seemed particularly applicable within the utilitarian framework of the new statism: the task of governments was to reverse the trend towards decadence and produce uniform, reliable humans. Such concerns became powerful especially for nations that perceived themselves to be in demographic crisis, like Sweden, which was experiencing depopulation and persistent tuberculosis, and the United States, where successive groups of immigrants found reasons to deplore the effects on the nation of the next immigrant group (Johannisson 1994; Kraut 1994; Broberg and Roll-Hansen 1996). Finally, it flattered those who held power and prominence by assuring them that this was no accident. It offered a simple explanation, one resistant to empirical falsification, of all that was wrong, and a simple remedy for improvement based on the formula of more sex for those who should breed (sometimes with new partners) and less for those regarded as inferior.

Eugenics sanctioned an enormous range of practices. Whilst eugenists focused attention on the human genotype and urged the inadequacy of public health programmes that ignored heredity, they were by no means uniformly dismissive of social and environmental reforms. These were needed to allow the better stock to fulfil its potential and because many believed that nurture *could* affect nature: heredity might be a limiting factor, but significant reforms were needed to fulfil hereditary potential. In almost every country in which eugenics was prominent—the United States, Britain, Japan, Germany, Russia, Brazil, and Argentina—eugenics fitted into a comprehensive concept of social hygiene, albeit one that translated rather easily into racial hygiene (Schneider 1990; Porter 1991; Stepan 1991; Gallagher 1999).

A third element of this phase of the development of public health was the rise of nutritional science. Whilst the effects of food on health had broadly been central to Western medicine throughout its history, and whilst it was no mystery that poor food led to poor health, a science of nutrition that discriminated the particular effects of particular foods only began to develop in the second half of the nineteenth century and chiefly in the new institutes of agricultural science where animal diets were being studied (Carpenter 1994). Most important was the link of several clinically distinct conditions with a deficit in trace substances in the diet. Particularly remarkable were Goldberger's association of pellagra in the American south with a too heavy reliance on maize, and the recognition of the roles of vitamin D and sunlight in the emergence of rickets. By the 1930s public health included attention to a varied diet which ensured adequate vitamins (Etheridge 1972; Kunitz 1988; Apple 1996). Diet, like genes, loomed in the public imagination as the cause of all troubles, and a universal source of hope.

Thus, during this golden age of public health, people in the developed world learned to fear three malign entities: the invisible germs of disease, which might come through the most casual contact; the mysterious genes in their gonads; and the peculiar set of trace nutrients that their food might not contain. Their health and survival depended on all these, yet governments could control them only partially; successful control depended on behaviour. Hence a significant role of public health was to educate, advise, and admonish. The citizen, particularly the female citizen, was now being asked to uphold a new standard of cleanliness and to clean things that were not visibly dirty with new kinds of disinfectants. It became important to exercise new prudence in choosing a mate and controlling sexuality. A doctor was required to see whether the baby was being properly fed (Apple 1987; Hoy 1995; Tomes 1998).

Ignorance heightened these hygienic demands. It was clear from tuberculin tests, for example, that exposure to tuberculosis was widespread, in some places nearly universal, but far from clear what was required for exposure to evolve into pulmonary consumption: whether it was a matter of concentrated exposure, the victim's own constitution, or the diet and environment. All seemed plausible; the advice of public health authorities (who were concerned with infected cases and with their potential for infecting others) involved every aspect of life. It was not simply a matter of not spitting, but of disinfecting eating utensils, clothes, and bedclothes; transforming relations with a spouse, family, and coworkers; and changing diet, leisure activities, and the climate of dwellings (Newsholme 1935; Dubos and Dubos 1987; Smith 1988; Barnes 1995).

It has seemed remarkable to some modern historians that these long lists of seemingly exhausting and impossible hygienic expectations, each with no guarantee of health, did not trigger widespread resentment, victim-blaming, and excessive violations of rights (Armstrong 1983). Four factors are important: firstly, this was an age stunned by scientific and technical achievement and lacking for the most part a critical vocabulary for mediating expert advice. Secondly, it was an age of mass aspiration to middle-class standards of living, which were manifested in health, behaviour, and cleanliness. Thirdly, all this was taking place against the backdrop of falling mortality and morbidity, and increasing domestic comfort. Fourthly, these efforts were redolent with the ethos of the progressive development of the community and the state (Lewis 1986).

The return of liberalism, 1970 to the present day: lifestyle, environment, and welfare

The decades following the Second World War brought a marked shift in the focus of public health and the expectations of the public. In the developed world, the infectious diseases that had so long been the chief focus of public health receded, with polio being the last of the shock epidemics to fall victim to immunizations, antibiotics, or epidemiological or environmental control (Rogers 1990). With the conquest of fascism and the subsequent decline of communism, liberalism re-emerged. This was symbolized in the mission statement of the World Health Organization (**WHO**) that health and welfare were the birthright of all (WHO 1968). It was the obligation of states to deliver that right to their populations, who now, at least in the developed world, were made up of those who saw themselves as individual free agents, perhaps diverse in culture but equal in rights. In such a situation the conflict between the imperatives of public health and civil rights re-emerged. It remains the most formidable issue that public health faces.

The retreat of infectious disease made clearer the failure of the developed nations to grapple with chronic diseases, some of which were the price of longer lifespans (Fox 1993). Some of these were clearly conditions that could be prevented by changes in behaviour: epidemiological studies in the 1950s and 1960s showed the deadly effects of good living—of smoking and a rich diet (Marks 1997; Porter 1999). A new set of personal disciplines emerged to control lifestyle diseases and prevent accidents—as well as not smoking, avoiding fats, recreational drugs, and alcohol, exercising one's heart and shedding weight, and using condoms (not to mention flossing and straightening one's teeth), one was to use seat belts and child harnesses, cope with child-proof caps on medicine bottles, and accept a fluoridated water supply. All these measures met with objections in terms of their intrusion into personal liberty or on culture, or because they were found to be irksome or unpleasant.

Another feature of postwar public health concern was the shift from individual hygiene back to the environment (Hays 1987; Gottlieb 1993). To many, these heart diseases and cancers, along with other diseases and pathological conditions that seemed even more serious—for example, other forms of cancer, birth defects, lowered sperm counts—had broader structural causes and could be prevented only by comprehensive changes in the physical and social environment (Epstein 1979). Thus part of the liberal resistance to public health imposition was the argument that a focus on disciplining lifestyles came at the cost of attention to grander and more serious political issues (Tesh 1987; Turshen 1987).

While this new environmentalism had links with the nineteenth-century view of public health as environmental improvement, there were greater differences. The fear of insidious invisible radiation or the toxic chemicals that might lurk in numerous consumer products reflects the terror of germs or invisible odourless miasmas which germs replaced; however, the blame was quite differently directed. The new problems of environmental public health were those in which individuals were victimized by corporate oligopolies and by the governments they influence. While Chadwick and his associates had warned of vested interests, such as those that perpetuated slum housing, nineteenth-century environmental health problems had a communal character that was missing from the twentieth. Everyone in a nineteenth-century town produced excrement, smoke, ash, and rubbish; the great problem was to find within the community the will and means to act collectively (Wohl 1977; Kearns 1988). Few in a twentieth-century community produced radiation or toxic chemical waste, and the reasons why nothing was done about these seemed all too clear. Public health had failed in its police function; an institution that had evolved to stop the selling of spoiled food by the individual grocer or restauranteur could not cope with the conglomerate that sold goods whose harmful effects were less obvious and slower to appear but which might be much more widely distributed.

The result was an increasingly adversarial relationship between the people and the public health institutions that were supposedly safeguarding their health. To the degree that governments were seen as colluding with the proliferation of these dangerous materials, institutions of public health, as departments of government, were implicated too (Brown and Mikkelsen 1990, Edelstein 1988; Steneck 1984). Even the establishment of new departments of environmental protection, though it might be a means to apply new kinds of expertise to problems of environmental health, did not fundamentally alter the climate of distrust. Public health again became a matter for grassroots political agitation with the emergence of neopopulist Green parties, whose platforms gave prominent attention to health as part of environmental good, and who put their marginality to established governments at the centre of their appeal to the electorate.

Such a focus on bad environmental policy even informed the response to AIDS and to other new infectious diseases, like Ebola fever, that appeared in the 1980s and 1990s. While it became clear that these diseases could be largely controlled through the traditional means of changes in personal behaviour and isolation or restriction of the activities of victims, these recognitions were not fully reassuring. They did little to deflect demand for a vaccine, or the investment of hope in curative medicine. They too could be seen as environmental diseases, caused by environmental changes that had allowed animal viruses to acquire secondary human hosts for whom they were highly virulent. Chief amongst these changes was the unwise exploitation of tropical forests by an international oligopoly that put profit ahead of prudence (Garrett 1995).

Even those diseases most closely linked to lifestyle choice could be attributed to the broader social environment. People smoked, drank, used drugs, ate too much or vastly too little, practised unsafe sex, spent hours immobilized before televisions absorbing images of violence, hit their spouses and children, or shot their coworkers or themselves because they could no longer cope. To expect disciplined personal behaviour from alienated people living in a stressful world was unrealistic, and the institutions of public health should recognize this. But the critics were ambivalent as to what such an analysis implied. For some, the obvious response was to remake a society whose support structures were more consistent with the health behaviours it wished to promote. How absurd, for example, for a state to subsidize the production of tobacco and the addiction to it of people in other nations, whilst blaming its own citizens for smoking. For others such a response sounded like an even more invidiously intrusive state, bent on removing not only the means by which we satisfied unhealthful temptations, but also the temptations themselves. In this 'critical public health' view the lifestyle agenda was suspicious as the public health agenda of the untrustworthy state, not of its people. It was not clear that the personal benefits of delayed or denied gratification were worth it: perhaps one should just enjoy life and rely on the miracles of modern medicine for redemption (Petersen and Lupton 1996).

This view, together with the emergence of widespread cancers and other chronic illnesses for which there was no clear preventive strategy, including the debilitating conditions of ageing, raised the question of why supportive and curative medical care did not form a part or priority of public health. It also raised the question of how far reaching the health obligations of the liberal state were to its citizens. This issue had vexed public health practitioners throughout the liberal era, though it had often been suppressed because it was seen as too politically volatile. In socialist or social democratic politics, or where the legacy of medical police remained strong (even when adopted, as in Sweden, by a democratic polity), there was often no clear boundary between public health and the public medical care most people demanded and received (Porter 1999). But elsewhere the recognition that public health was bound up in the larger issue of human welfare, which in turn included the rest of medical care, was problematic. Many of the newly prominent diseases were not infectious; they could be experienced privately without disturbing community or state, hence the reactive and police rationales for public health did not apply. But they did disrupt the fulfilment of human potential, and could justly take their place amongst the demands citizens could make of their governments.

In France, Germany, and Russia public health services had emerged from, and had remained closely linked to, medical services for the poor (Labisch 1992; Ramsey 1994; Solomon 1994). In mid-nineteenth century England, Edwin Chadwick, notwithstanding his own post as chief administrator of relief to the poor and the existence of a comprehensive national network of poor law medical officers, had deliberately severed public health (which he equated with sanitary engineering and saw as exclusively preventive) from the second-rate medical care that was offered to the poor, more on grounds of humanity than expectations of effectiveness. (It was hoped that they would thereby willingly pay for something better.) Chadwick's English successors, while moderating the focus on sanitary engineering, retained a distinction between public health medicine and social welfare, which seemed to them only marginally medical and to have more to do with the moral chastisement of the feckless or the warehousing of the incompetent or neglected (Hamlin 1998). In Ireland, by contrast, an integrated system of public health, welfare, and medical care did emerge during the late nineteenth century, but more by accident than design (Cassell 1997). At the end of the nineteenth century, the Fabian socialists presented British parliament with a clear choice. The Fabians (mainly Beatrice Webb) proposed a much expanded scheme of prevention, though one which made even greater demands on personal and social behaviour as the price the citizen must pay for greater guarantees from the state. The liberals, whose view prevailed, would not discipline personal hygiene, but offered instead an insurance plan to pay for the medical care needed by stricken working men (Fox 1986; Eyler 1997). It was a policy acceptable to the rank and file of the medical profession and that retained and reinforced the split between public health and medicine.

Subsequent efforts to expand state responsibility for health into matters of care and cure have generally worked when medical professions have seen them as advantageous, yet the relationship between even this expanded public medicine and the broader questions of social welfare remain problematic (Starr 1982; Fox 1986). The kinds of objections that were made to Webb's scheme still arise: however laudable prevention as a goal, ironically, as we have seen with the concerns about lifestyles and the environment, the strategies and priorities of the preventive public health of the last two centuries have not always been those most desired by the masses of people. To many, it has seemed that if the state was going to discipline behaviour for its own purposes, those who suffered that imposition deserved compensation for their trouble when things still went wrong. Such logic was clearest in compensating veterans of wars. It underwrote the postwar establishment of Britain's National Health Service, which would provide 'health for heroes' and sustains the Veterans Administration medical system in the United States. Thus what some have complained of as an unrealistic demand for risk-free living, in which people demand a political right to complete freedom of action without accepting responsibility for the consequences (as if one could somehow live free of one's biological self), may be better understood as a complaint about the fairness of the basic social contract of modern societies.

This problem of the relationship between the institutions of public health and the citizenry on whose behalf they claim to act is the greatest challenge currently facing public health in the developed world. That the problems that confront both public health and regular medical practice often stem from a wide range of social causes is plain. That it is so difficult to develop political will to respond to these problems is not chiefly a matter of epidemiological uncertainty. Such pathological phenomena are clearly the product of many causes on many levels and accordingly there are numerous points of access where defensible preventive measures might be taken. But almost all of them are likely to intrude on what are claimed as personal or cultural rights, and almost always attempts to act will be met with the response that it is fairer to act elsewhere. In such cases, epidemiology necessarily requires a large supplement, not from ethics so much as from a moral and political philosophy that must be acceptable to an increasingly diverse community. Without such a foundation, public health is forced to take refuge in science that is frequently challenged; but at the same time, it is not clear that the professional and educational institutions of public health, or the legal, political, and administrative structures that create and maintain it, will be able to initiate and implement a satisfactory enquiry about how these conflicting rights are to be adjudicated.

References

Acheson, R. (1991). The British diploma in public health: birth and adolescence. In *A history of education in public health: health that mocks the doctors rules* (ed. E. Fee and R. Acheson), pp. 44–82. Oxford University Press.

Ackerknecht, E.H. (1948). Anticontagionism between 1821 and 1867. *Bulletin of the History of Medicine*, **22**, 562–93.

Amundsen, D. and Ferngren, G. (1986). The early Christian tradition. In *Caring and curing: health and medicine in the Western religious traditions* (ed. R. Numbers and D. Amundusen), pp. 40–64. Macmillan, New York.

Anderson, W. (1995). Excremental colonialism: public health and the poetics of pollution. *Critical Inquiry*, **21**, 640–69.

Apple, R. (1987). *Mothers and medicine: a social history of infant feeding, 1890–1950.* University of Wisconsin Press, Madison, WI.

Apple, R.D. (1996). *Vitamania: vitamins in American culture.* Rutgers University Press, New Brunswick, NJ.

Armstrong, D. (1983). *The political economy of the body.* Cambridge University Press.

Arrizabalaga, J. (1993). Syphilis. In *The Cambridge world history of human disease* (ed. K. Kiple), pp. 1025–33. Cambridge University Press.

Arrizabalaga, J., Henderson, J., and French, R. (1997). *The great pox: the French disease in Renaissance Europe.* Yale University Press, New Haven, CT.

Baldwin, P. (1999). *Contagion and the state in Europe, 1830–1930.* Cambridge University Press, New York.

Barnes, D. (1995). *The making of a social disease: tuberculosis in nineteenth-century France.* University of California Press, Berkeley, CA.

Blackstone, W. (1892). *Commentaries on the laws of England.* Strouse, New York.

Brand, J.L. (1965). *Doctors and the state: the British medical profession and government action in public health, 1870–1912.* Johns Hopkins University Press, Baltimore, MD.

Brandt, A. (1985). *No magic bullet: a social history of venereal disease in the United States since 1880.* Oxford University Press, New York.

Briggs, A. (1961). Cholera and society in the nineteenth century. *Past and Present*, **19**, 76–96.

Broberg, G. and **Roll-Hansen, N.** (ed.) (1996). *Eugenics and the welfare state: sterilization policy in Denmark, Sweden, Norway and Finland.* Michigan State University Press, East Lansing, MI.

Brockliss, L. and Jones, C. (1997). *The medical world of early modern France.* Clarendon Press, Oxford.

Brody, S. (1974). *The disease of the soul; leprosy in medieval literature.* Cornell University Press, Ithaca, NY.

Brown, P. and Mikkelsen, E. (1990). *No safe place: toxic waste, leukemia, and community action.* University of California Press, Berkeley, CA.

Browne, Sir Thomas (1964). Religio medici. In *Religio Medici and other works.* Clarendon Press, Oxford.

Brunton, D. *Political medicine: the construction of vaccination policy across Britain, 1800–1871.* University of Rochester Press, in press.

Bulloch, W. (1938). *The history of bacteriology.* Oxford University Press, New York.

Bynum, W.F. (1994). *Science and the practice of medicine in the nineteenth century*. Cambridge University Press.

Carmichael, A. (1997). Leprosy: larger than life. In *Plague, pox, and pestilence* (ed. K. Kiple), pp. 50–7. Barnes and Noble, New York.

Carpenter, K. (1994). *Protein and energy: a study of changing ideas in nutrition*. Cambridge University Press.

Cassedy, J. (1962). *Charles V. Chapin and the public health movement*. Harvard University Press, Cambridge, MA.

Cassell, R.D. (1997). *Medical charities, medical politics: the irish dispensary system and the poor law, 1836–1872*. Royal Historical Society/Boydell Press, Woodbridge, Suffolk.

Chadwick, E. (1965). *Report on the sanitary condition of the labouring population of Great Britain*. Edinburgh University Press.

Chew, H. and Kellaway, W.E. (ed.) (1973). *London Assize of Nuisance, 1301–1431: a calendar*. London Record Society, London.

Cipolla, C. (1979). *Faith, reason, and the plague in seventeenth century Tuscany*. Norton, New York.

Cipolla, C. (1981). *Fighting the plague in seventeenth-century Italy*. University of Wisconsin Press, Madison, WI.

Cipolla, C. (1992). *Miasmas and disease: public health and the environment in the pre-industrial age* (trans. Elizabeth Potter). Yale University Press, New Haven, CT.

Clendening, L. (1942). *Source book of medical history*. Dover Publications, New York.

Coleman, W. (1974). Health and hygiene in the *Encyclopedie*: A medical doctrine for the bourgeoisie. *Journal of the History of Medicine*, **29**, 399–421.

Coleman, W. (1982). *Death is a social disease: public health and political economy in early industrial France*. University of Wisconsin Press, Madison, WI.

Coleman, W. (1987). *Yellow fever in the north: the methods of early epidemiology*. University of Wisconsin Press, Madison, WI.

Conrad, L. (1992). Epidemic disease in formal and popular thought in early Islamic society. In *Epidemics and ideas: essays on the historical perception of pestilence* (ed. T. Ranger and P. Slack), pp. 77–99. Cambridge University Press.

Crosby, A. (1986). *Ecological imperialism: the biological expansion of Europe, 900–1900*. Cambridge University Press.

Dean, M. (1991). *The constitution of poverty: toward a genealogy of liberal governance*. Routledge, London.

Delaporte, F. (1986). *Disease and civilisation, the cholera in Paris, 1832*. MIT Press, Cambridge, MA.

Disraeli, B. (1926). *Sybil, or the Two Nations* (introduction by Walter Sichel). Oxford University Press.

Dols, M. (1977). *The Black Death in the Middle East*. Princeton University Press.

Dorff, E. (1986). The Jewish tradition. In *Caring and curing: health and medicine in the Western religious traditions* (ed. R. Numbers and D. Amundusen), pp. 5–39. Macmillan, New York.

Douglas, M. (1966). *Purity and danger: an analysis of the concepts of pollution and taboo*. Routledge, London.

Dubos, R. and Dubos, J. (1987). *The white plague: tuberculosis, man and society*. Rutgers University Press, New Brunswick, NJ.

Duffy, J. (1990). *The sanitarians: a history of American public health*. University of Illinois Press, Urbana, IL.

Durey, M. (1979). *The return of the plague: British society and cholera, 1831–2*. Gill and MacMillan, Dublin.

Edelstein, M. (1988). *Contaminated communities: social and psychological impacts of residential toxic exposure*. Westview, Boulder, CO.

Ellis, J.H. (1992). *Yellow fever and public health in the New South*. University Press of Kentucky, Lexington, KY.

Epstein, S. (1979). *The politics of cancer* (revised edn). Anchor, New York.

Etheridge, E. (1972). *The butterfly caste: a social history of pellagra in the South*. Greenwood Press, Westport, CT.

Evans, R.J. (1990). *Death in Hamburg: society and politics in the cholera years, 1830–1910*. Penguin Books, London.

Eyler, J.M. (1979). *Victorian social medicine: the ideas and methods of William Farr*. Johns Hopkins University Press, Baltimore, MD.

Eyler, J. (1997). *Sir Arthur Newsholme and state medicine, 1885–1935*. Cambridge University Press.

Fee, E. (1993). Public health, past and present: a shared social vision. In *A history of public health* (ed. G. Rosen) (expanded edition), pp. ix–lxvii. Johns Hopkins University Press, Baltimore, MD.

Finer, S.E. (1952). *The life and times of Sir Edwin Chadwick*. Methuen, London.

Foucault, M. (1975). *The birth of the clinic*. Vintage, New York.

Fox, D. (1986). *Health policies, health politics: British and American experience, 1911–1965*. Princeton University Press.

Fox, D. (1993). *Power and illness: the failure and future of American health policy*. University of California Press, Berkeley, CA.

Frank, J.P. (1941). Academic address on the people's misery. *Bulletin of the History of Medicine*, **9**, 88–100.

Frank, J.P. (1976). *A system of complete medical police; selections from Johann Peter Frank*. Johns Hopkins University Press, Baltimore, MD.

Gallagher, N. (1999). *Breeding better Vermonters*. University Press of New England, Hanover, NH.

Garrett, L. (1995). *The coming plague: newly emerging diseases in a world our of balance*. Penguin, New York.

Geary, L. (1995). Famine, fever, and the bloody flux. In *The Great Irish Famine* (ed. C. Póirtéir), pp. 74–85. Mercier Press, Dublin.

Göckjan, G. (1985). *Kurieren und Staat Machen: Gesundheit und Medizin in der burgerlichen welt*, p. 19. Suhrkamp, Frankfurt am Main.

Gottlieb, R. (1993). *Forcing the spring: the transformation of the American environmental movement*. Island Press, Washington, DC.

Goubert, J.P. (1989). *The conquest of water* (trans. A. Wilson). Polity Press, London.

Guillerme, A. (1988). *The age of water: the urban environment in the north of France, AD 300–1800*. Texas A & M University Press, College Station, TX.

Hamlin, C. (1988). Muddling in Bumbledom: local governments and large sanitary improvements: the cases of four British towns, 1855–1885. *Victorian Studies*, **32**, 55–83.

Hamlin, C. (1990). *A science of impurity: water analysis in nineteenth century Britain*. Adam Hilger/ University of California Press, Bristol/Berkeley, CA.

Hamlin, C. (1992). Predisposing causes and public health in the early nineteenth century public health movement. *Social History of Medicine*, **5**, 43–70.

Hamlin, C. (1994). Environmental sensibility in Edinburgh, 1839–1840: the 'Fetid Irrigation' Controversy. *Journal of Urban History*, **20**, 311–39.

Hamlin, C. (1998). *Public health and social justice in the age of Chadwick: Britain 1800–1854*. Cambridge University Press.

Haskell, T. (1985). Capitalism and the origins of the humanitarian sensibility. *American Historical Review*, **90**, 339–61, 547–66.

Hays, S. (1987). *Beauty, health, and permanence: environmental politics in the United States, 1955–1985*. Cambridge University Press.

Hennock, E.P. (2000). The urban sanitary movement in England and Germany, 1838–1914: a comparison. *Continuity and Change*, **15**, 269–96.

Hopkins, D. (1983). *Princes and peasants: smallpox in history*. University of Chicago Press.

Hoy, S. (1995). *Chasing dirt: the American pursuit of cleanliness.* Oxford University Press, New York.

Humphreys, M. (1992). *Yellow fever and the South.* Rutgers University Press, New Brunswick, NJ.

Johannisson, K. (1994). The people's health: public health policies in Sweden. In *The history of public health and the modern state* (ed. D. Porter), pp. 165–82. Rudopi, Amsterdam.

Karmi, G. (1981). State control of the physician in the Middle Ages: an Islamic model. In *the town and state physician in Europe from the Middle Ages to the Enlightenment* (ed. A. Russell), pp. 63–84. Herzog August Bibliothek, Wolfenbüttel.

Kearns, G. (1988). Private property and public health reform in England, 1830–1870. *Social Science and Medicine*, **26**, 187–99.

Kearns, G. (1991). Cholera, nuisances, and environmental management in Islington, 1830–1855. In *Living and dying in London* (ed. W.F. Bynum and R. Porter), pp. 94–125. Wellcome Institute for the History of Medicine, London.

Kevles, D. (1995). *In the name of eugenics: genetics and the uses of human heredity.* Harvard, Cambridge, MA.

Kraut, A. (1994). *Silent travelers: germs, genes, and the 'immigrant menace'.* Basic Books, New York.

Kunitz, S. (1988). Hookworm and pellagra: exemplary diseases in the New South. *Journal of Health and Social Behavior*, **29**, 139–48.

LaBerge, A. (1992). *Mission and method: the early-nineteenth- century French public health movement.* Cambridge University Press.

Labisch, A. (1992). *Homo hygienicus: Gesundheit und Medizin in der Neuzeit.* Campus, New York.

Lambert, R. (1965). *Sir John Simon and English social administration.* McGibbon and Kee, London.

Leavitt, J. (1996). *Typhoid Mary: captive to the public's health.* Beacon Press, Boston, MA.

Leongard, J. (ed.) (1989). *London viewers and their certificates, 1508–1558: certificates of the sworn viewers of the City of London.* London Record Society, London.

Lewis, R.A. (1952). *Edwin Chadwick and the public health movement, 1832–1854.* Longmans Green, London.

Lewis, J. (1986). *What price community medicine? The philosophy, practice, and politics of public health since 1919.* Wheatsheaf Books, Brighton.

Lifton, R. (1986). *The Nazi doctors: medical killing and the psychology of genocide.* Basic Books, New York.

Longrigg, J. (1992). Epidemic, ideas and classical Athenian society. In *Epidemics and ideas: essays on the historical perception of pestilence* (ed. T. Ranger and P. Slack), pp. 21–44. Cambridge University Press.

López-Piñero, J.M. (1981). The medical profession in sixteenth-century Spain. In *The town and state physician in Europe from the Middle Ages to the Enlightenment* (ed. A. Russell), pp. 85–98. Herzog August Bibliothek, Wolfenbüttel.

McClure, R. (1981). *Coram's children: the London Foundling Hospital in the eighteenth century.* Yale University Press, New Haven, CT.

McGrew, R. (1965). *Russia and the cholera, 1823–1832.* University of Wisconsin Press, Madison, WI.

McHugh, P. (1982). *Prostitution and Victorian social reform.* Croom Helm, London.

McNeill, W. (1976). *Plagues and peoples.* Anchor Doubleday, New York.

Marks, H. (1997). *The progress of experiment: science and therapeutic reforming the United States, 1900–1990.* Cambridge University Press.

Melosi, M. (2000). *The sanitary city: urban infrastructure in America from colonial times to the present.* Johns Hopkins University Press, Baltimore, MD.

Miller, G. (1957). *The adoption of inoculation for smallpox in England and France.* University of Pennsylvania Press, Philadelphia, PA.

Münch, P. (1993). *Stadthygiene im 19 und 20 Jahrhundert.* Vandenhoeck und Ruprecht, Göttingen.

Newsholme, A. (1935). *Fifty years in public health: a personal narrative with comments.* Vol. 1, *The Years Preceding 1909.* George Allen and Unwin, London.

Nohl, J. (1926). *The Black Death.* Allen and Unwin, London.

Novak, S. J. (1973). Professionalism and bureaucracy: English doctors and the Victorian public health administration. *Journal of Social History*, **6**, 440–62.

Novak, W. J. (1996). The people's welfare: law and regulation in nineteenth-century America. University of North Carolina Press, Chapel Hill, NC.

Palmer, R. (1981). Physicians and the state in post-medieval Italy. In *The town and state physician in Europe from the Middle Ages to the Enlightenment* (ed. A. Russell), pp. 47–62. Herzog August Bibliothek, Wolfenbüttel.

Paul, D.B. (1995). *Controlling human heredity: 1865 to the present.* Humanities Press, New Jersey.

Pelling, M. (1978). *Cholera, fever, and English medicine, 1825–1865.* Oxford University Press.

Petersen, A. and Lupton, D. (1996). *The new public health: health and self in the age of risk.* Sage, London.

Pettenkofer, M. (1941). *The value of health to a city* (trans. with an introduction by H.E. Sigerist). Johns Hopkins University Press, Baltimore, MD.

Pick, D. (1989). *Faces of degeneration: a European disorder, c. 1848–1918.* Cambridge University Press.

Pickstone, J.V. (1992). Dearth, dirt, and fever epidemics: rewriting the history of British 'public health', 1780–1850. In *Epidemics and ideas: essays on the historical perception of pestilence* (ed. T. Ranger, and P. Slack), pp. 125–48. Cambridge University Press.

Porter, D. (1991*a*). 'Enemies of the race': biologism, environmentalism, and public health in Edwardian England. *Victorian Studies*, **34**, 159–78.

Porter, D. (1991*b*). Stratification and its discontents: professionalization and conflict in the British public health service, 1848–1914. In *A history of education in public health: health that mocks the doctor's rules* (ed. E. Fee and R. Acheson), pp. 83–113. Oxford University Press.

Porter, D. (1999). *Health, civilization and the state.* Routledge, London.

Porter, D. and Porter, R. (1988). The politics of prevention: anti-vaccinationism and public health in nineteenth century England. *Medical History*, **32**, 231–52.

Ramsey, M. (1994). Public health in France. In *The history of public health and the modern state* (ed. D. Porter), pp. 45–118. Rudopi, Amsterdam.

Razzell, P. (1977). *The conquest of smallpox: the impact of inoculation on smallpox mortality in eighteenth century England.* Caliban, Firle.

Redlich, J. and Hirst, F. (1970). *The history of local government in England, being a reissue of Book I of Local government in England, second edition, with an introduction and epilogue by Bryan Keith-Lucas.* Augustus Kelley, New York.

Richards, P. (1977). *The medieval leper and his northern heirs.* Rowman and Littlefield, Totowa, NJ.

Richards, P. (1980). State formation and class struggle. In *Capitalism, state formation, and Marxist theory* (ed. P. Corrigan), pp. 49–78. Quartet, London.

Richardson, R. (1988). *Death, dissection, and the destitute.* Penguin, London.

Riley, J.C. (1987). *The eighteenth century campaign to avoid disease.* Macmillan, London.

Roberton, J. (1827). *Observations on the mortality and physical mangement of children.* Longman, Rees, Orme, Brown, London.

Rogers, N. (1990). *Dirt and disease: polio before FDR.* Rutgers University Press, New Brunswick, NJ.

Rosen, G. (1947). What is social medicine: a genetic analysis of the concept. *Bulletin of the History of Medicine*, **21**, 674–733.

Rosen, G. (1958). *A history of public health.* MD Publications, New York.

Rosen, G. (1974*a*). Cameralism and the concept of medical police. In *From medical police to social medicine: essays on the history of health care* (ed. G. Rosen), pp. 120–41. Science History, New York.

Rosen, G. (1974*b*). The fate of the concept of mecical police, 1780–1890. In *From medical police to social medicine: essays on the history of health care* (ed. G. Rosen), pp. 142–58. Science History, New York.

Rosenberg, C. (1962). *The cholera years: the United States in 1832, 1849, and 1866.* University of Chicago Press.

Rosenkrantz, B. (1972). *Public health and the state: changing views in Massachusetts, 1842–1936.* Harvard University Press, Cambridge, MA.

Rosenkrantz, B.G. (1974). Cart before horse: theory, practice and professional image in American public health, 1870–1920. *Journal of the History of Medicine*, **29**, 55–73.

Sadler, M. (1830). *The law of population, being a treatise in six books, in disproof of the superfecundity of human beings, and developing the real principle of their increase.* John Murray, London.

Schneider, W.H. (1990). *Quality and quantity: the quest for biological regeneration in 20th century France.* Cambridge University Press.

Shattuck, L. (1972). *Report of a general plan for the promotion of public and personal health, devised, prepared, and recommended by the commissioners ... relating to a sanitary survey of the state.* Arno, New York.

Simon, J. (1890). *English sanitary institutions, reviewed in their course of development, and in some of their political and social relations.* Cassell, London.

Simson, J. v. (1978). Die Flussverungsreinigungsfrage im 19. Jahrhundert. *Vierteljahrschirft für sozial- und wirtschaftgeschichte*, **65**, 370–90.

Skisnes, O. (1973). Notes from the history of leprosy. *International Journal of Leprosy*, **41**, 220–37.

Slack, P. (1985). *The impact of the plague in Tudor and Stuart England.* Routledge and Kegan Paul, London.

Smith, D.C. (1981). Medical science, medical practice, and the emerging concept of typhus. In *Theories of fever from Antiquity to the Enlightenment* (ed. W.F. Bynum and V. Nutton), pp. 121–34. Wellcome Institute for the History of Medicine, London.

Smith, F.B. (1988). *The retreat of tuberculosis 1850–1950.* Croom Helm, London.

Snowden, F. (1995). *Naples in the time of cholera 1884–1911.* Cambridge University Press.

Solomon, S.G. (1994). The expert and the state in Russian public health: continuities and changes across the revolutionary divide. In *The history of public health and the modern state* (ed. D. Porter), pp. 183–223. Rudopi, Amsterdam.

Soloway, R.A. (1982). *Birth control and the population question in England, 1877–1930.* University of North Carolina Press, Chapel Hill, NC.

Starr, P. (1982). *The social transformation of American medicine.* Basic Books, New York.

Steneck, N. (1984). *The microwave debate.* MIT Press, Cambridge, MA.

Stepan, N. (1991). *The hour of eugenics: race, gender, and nation in Latin America.* Cornell University Press, Ithaca, NY.

Sturm, C.C. (1832). *Sturm's reflections on the works of god, and his providence throughout all nature.* Woodward, Philadelphia, PA.

Tesh, S.N. (1987). *Hidden arguments: political ideology and disease prevention.* Rutgers University Press, New Brunswick, NJ.

Thucydides (1950). *The history of the Peloponnesian War* (trans. R. Crawley). E.P. Dutton, New York.

Tomes, N. (1998). *The gospel of germs: men, women, and the microbe in American life.* Harvard University Press, Cambridge, MA.

Turshen, M. (1987). *The politics of public health.* Rutgers University Press, New Brunswick, NJ.

Veyne, P. (1987). The Roman Empire. In *A history of private life. I: From Pagan Rome to Byzantium* (ed. P. Veyne) (trans. A. Goldhammer), pp. 222–32. Belknap Press of Harvard University Press, Cambridge, MA.

Walkowitz, J. (1980). *Prostitution and Victorian society: women, class and the state.* Cambridge University Press.

Watkin, D. (1984). The English revolution in social medicine, 1889–1911. Unpublished PhD thesis, University of London.

Webb, S. and Webb, B. (1922). *English local government from the Revolution to the Municipal Corporations Act: statutory authorities for special purposes.* Longmans Green, London.

Weindling, P. (1984). Was social medicine revolutionary? Rudolph Virchow and the Revolution of 1848. *Bulletin of the Society for the Social History of Medicine*, **34**, 13–18.

Weiner, D. (1993). *The citizen-patient in Revolutionary and Imperial Paris.* Johns Hopkins University Press, Baltimore, MD.

Weyland, J. (1969). *The principles of population and production as they are affected by the progress of society with view to moral and political consequences* (orig. 1816). Augustus Kelley, New York.

WHO (World Health Organization) (1968). *Constitution of the World Health Organization in WHO Basic Documents*, (19th edn). WHO, Geneva.

White, K. (1991). *Healing the schism: epidemiology, medicine and the public's health.* Springer, New York.

Wilson, F.R. (1881). *A practical guide for inspectors of nuisances.* Knight, London.

Wilson, L. (1978). Fevers and science in early nineteenth century medicine. *Journal of the History of Medicine*, **33**, 386–407.

Winslow, C.A. (1980). *The conquest of epidemic disease: a chapter in the history of ideas* (orig. 1943). University of Wisconsin Press, Madison, WI.

Wohl, A. (1977). *The eternal slum: housing and social policy in Victorian London.* Edward Arnold, London.

Wohl, A.S. (1983). *Endangered lives: public health in Victorian Britain.* Harvard University Press, Cambridge, MA.

Worboys, M. (2000). *Spreading germs: disease theories and medical practice in Britain, 1865–1900.* Cambridge University Press.

Ziegler, P. (1969). *The Black Death.* Harper Torchbooks, New York.

1.3 The history and development of public health in developing countries

Than Sein and Uton Muchtar Rafei

Introduction

Historical reviews of the development of medicine and public health form the basis of our knowledge. Such reviews may provide valuable insights that can contribute to the solution of present and future health problems. Thus, it is useful to regard the evolution of public health from the earliest times as an essential element in modern public health education. Barton (1979) described the development of the health sciences over five major areas: empirical health, basic science, clinical science, public health science, and political science. Ko Ko U (1986) set the tone for integrated health in *Public Health Myths, Mysticism and Reality*, describing the progress of health development across each of these areas. A study by the Institute of Medicine in the United States (1988) indicated that there had been a growing demand for public health, as a profession, as a governmental activity, or as a commitment to society. The study also indicated that public health was not clearly defined, fully understood, or adequately supported. Public health, as it was expressed, was needed to focus on improving conditions that had a bearing on the health of the people. The goals of public health in broad terms should be to identify problems that affect entire communities or populations, to marshal support to address these problems, and to ensure that the solutions are implemented. Frenk (1993), Curtis and Taket (1996), Detels and Breslow (1997), and many others later defined both the national and international perspectives of the current and future scope and concerns in public health. A series of national, regional, and international conferences, seminars, and workshops have been organized by the World Health Organization (**WHO**), and recently many other international bodies have been organized on the role of public health in health development in the twenty-first century.

Detels and Breslow (1997) defined public health in simple terms as the process of mobilizing local, state, national, and international resources to ensure the conditions in which people can be healthy. Historically, public health efforts meant health development to be undertaken by the government as a public sector activity. Public health action was sometimes seen as health interventions addressing more than one individual, such as community hygiene, sanitation, and water supply, health education, maternal and child health care, immunization and nutrition promotion, or disease control activities. The people who carried out such measures were known as public health workers. Commonly, public health covered promotive, preventive, curative, and rehabilitative health measures. Most of the steps previously undertaken by governments included actions to promote and protect the health of the people through segregation, quarantine, prohibition, and other sanitary and hygienic practices that were considered to be public health measures. Disease and environmental control measures or food and drug control carried out by government agencies are considered to be public health activities. Similarly, necessary legislative acts and bylaws proclaimed to control various health problems have been regarded as public health measures. Later, the connotation of the term 'public' was widened to encompass the involvement of people together with the government in health development efforts. This concept of a wider public role in health development has become more prevalent today when both non-communicable and infectious diseases present the major public health problems. Without the full involvement of the population, the control of these diseases becomes ineffective.

Public health problems were historically known as the diseases or conditions that particularly affected large numbers of people leading to either death or disability. They were usually socially interpreted, but not all people saw the same reality. Diseases like malaria, tuberculosis, cholera, and HIV/AIDS, respiratory infections, injuries and trauma, cancer, and problems such as maternal and infant deaths have been identified as major public health issues in the 1990s, likely to continue into this new millennium. In the late 1990s, the concepts of the essential public health functions emerged within the context of health sector reforms undertaken in many developing countries (Bettcher *et al.* 1998). The functions of public health should be understood as comprehensive as they are linked to each other. The essence of public health is that it deals with the health of the population in its totality.

This chapter traces the historical development of comprehensive public health in the context of over 140 developing countries, of which about one-third are classified as the 'least developed'. The first part of the chapter deals with the development of public health before the twentieth century, especially how public health in the former colonial countries was developed and the impact on health of globalization of trade during the colonial era. It also documents the efforts of developing countries leading to the establishment of an international health organization. The second part presents the attempts made by the developing countries, as soon as they achieved independence from colonial rule. The chapter highlights how these countries tried to cope with the prevailing high morbidity and mortality conditions, including their major public health achievements and failures in preventing and controlling communicable and non-communicable diseases which are of global importance.

The third part of the chapter deals with the change in the concept of public health from narrow disease control interventions to multi-sectoral approaches. This coincides with the period when most countries joined the Health for All movement, which adopted the primary health care approach for reaching the universal goal of health for all by 2000. At the end of the twentieth century, developing countries were moving towards the new era of public health development, but suffering the double burden of diseases—both infectious and chronic problems—while their health systems tried to function with limited investments from both internal and external sources. The new phenomenon of globalization has made more complex challenges to the development of public health in this new millennium. The chapter also covers different phases of public health in different parts of the world. Examples are presented of how communities and countries have mobilized themselves to ensure the health and prosperity of their people. The success of public health measures depends on adhering to the basic principles of equity, social justice, and partnerships.

Early public health

Empirical public health

Since ancient times, human life has been threatened with diseases of all kinds. Historical records from the Egyptian, Roman, Greek, Indian, and Mayan civilizations reveal the dreadful nature of infectious diseases and how they were overcome. The teachings of Lord Buddha, as well as the Bible, the Koran, and Judaic literature, covered various aspects of personal hygiene and other public health practices, including civic duties. Sanitation measures were enforced through royal decrees (Sigerist 1951).

Diseases like syphilis, malaria, leprosy, tuberculosis, smallpox, measles, plague, and cholera were rampant in all parts of the world for many centuries. Most diseases occurred locally, killing thousands in certain years. The concept of 'disease' had been postulated within the limited 'scientific' knowledge available. Traditional medicine focused on management of illnesses at the individual rather than the public level. The spread of diseases due to contact amongst people or due to hereditary transmission was, however, recognized centuries ago. The treatise on economics and government by Kautilya (around 300 BC), during the early Maurya dynasty in India, showed how a king ensured the health and prosperity of his subjects through various measures and regulations. Heavy punishments were imposed on those guilty of adulteration of food, sexual violence, or of littering the streets. The royal proclamation also prescribed rules establishing brothels and entertainment centres (Rangarajan 1992). Quarantine and prohibition were major measures used historically to protect the transmission of diseases and remain as public health measures used by governments in many countries.

Sir Jeremy Bentham, Thomas Southwood Smith, Edwin Chadwick, Sir John Simon, John Snow, and William Farr stimulated public health conscience and principles in the early eighteenth century. Victorian sanitarians of the pre-Pasteur era mainly conformed to the theory that diseases related to decaying organic matter and its vaporous emanations or 'miasma' (Paneth *et al.* 1998). Max von Pettenkoffer, one of the pioneers of public hygiene, also developed modern public health principles in the same period. He believed that an agent in cholera evacuations became ineffective only after it had spent an extended period in the earth and entered the ground water. He experimented by attempting to drink by himself a glass of water containing rice-water evacuations of a cholera patient, and showed no major effect (Guthrie 1946). However, most historians of health development have related the development of modern public health to the advent of the basic medical sciences in the nineteenth century. The discovery of the microscope, animal cells and bacteria, chemicals and other substances, and other scientific knowledge and skills, including those related to the basic statistical and epidemiological methods, had provided the basis for scientific explanation of the causes of diseases and illnesses as well as their mode of transmission. The Industrial Revolution in the twentieth century encouraged social interest in the prevention and control of diseases. With increasing ability to identify the causal factors for disease, the interest in social, environmental, and political aspects of diseases and their prevention grew tremendously.

Owing to the scarcity of records, the health situation of the world in the early centuries is little known. However, a few records available from Asia, Europe, and the Middle East have made it possible to determine how diseases occurred and spread around the world, and what the early efforts were to control them. With the expansion of commerce, diseases spread from one area to other regions along the trade routes. For example, epidemics of smallpox and measles were reported in China between AD 37 and AD 653. These were due to importation from the northwest regions through migration. One Chinese record showed that around AD 640, bubonic plague was common in Kwangtung but rare in the inner provinces. The global pandemic of plague in the mid-fourteenth century, usually referred to as the 'Black Death', took the lives of 25 million people in Europe alone. Plague remained endemic in many countries and also spread both east and west causing millions of deaths (McNeill 1977).

Colonial public health

Trading around the world during the eighteenth and nineteenth centuries for the exploration and exploitation of natural resources led to the discovery of new territories in different parts of the world. Europeans and Americans were engaged in intense rivalry with each other for colonial possessions. In order to expand their control, these colonial powers made massive shifts of people from one continent to another, using both military and economic force. Thousands of Africans and Asians were brought to the Americas during the eighteenth and nineteenth centuries to work on the plantations in the southern part of the present-day United States or at the railway construction sites in the western or northern parts of the country. Later, they were brought to the islands of the West Indies and to South and Central Americas, and made to work in large plantations as well as in mining industries. Similarly, large numbers of people from the Indian subcontinent were shipped to Africa and other parts of Asia and the Pacific Islands. The colonials established their own administrative, legal, and medical care systems with varying degrees of autonomy and authority. The American government established a military medical corps in the nineteenth century to protect the American army, which had been expanding to new territories, as well as to protect the American commercial establishments in Mexico and other Latin American countries. Similarly, the Dutch, Portuguese, British, French, and Spanish colonial rulers first established a series of hospitals and dispensaries amongst the army establishments and later in other commercial places. The Indian Medical Service in British India and the Gold Coast Medical Department in Ghana are good examples of this (Harrison 1994; Mills 1998). Medical teams were brought in from the home countries or hired from other nations.

To protect the health of their own people and the workers, colonial rulers established laws similar to those in their home countries. Specific public health legislation varied with each colonial power, but definite imprints of them still exist. For instance, the Public Health Acts, Local Government Act, Civil Registration Act, Factory Acts, Food Adulteration Act, Vaccination Act, and Contagious Diseases Acts have remained in force for many decades. Some are in place today in many countries in Asia, the Pacific, the Americas, and Africa, where the British, Spanish, French, American, or Dutch colonies existed. European countries adopted Bismarck's model of national social health insurance scheme, which later spread to other countries, especially in the Americas and Asia. The public health measures enforced under those public laws and regulations made a greater impact in these countries. In most countries, expatriates managed administrative and commercial activities. Some colonial powers introduced their social and cultural identity, mainly through religious groups and their educational systems. Most of the educational systems were designed to meet the administrative and commercial interests of the colonial powers. These systems also created a supply of administrative and clerical staff for assisting in the management, administration, and commercial activities of the colonial rulers (Jaggi 1979*b*).

European and American religious missionaries also embarked on expeditions around the world along with the colonial powers. Many of them, having allopathic medical backgrounds, established 'Western' medical care institutions as well as general educational systems, including nursing and medical schools. These missionaries established medical clinics or dispensaries at first and, later, hospitals in the colonial countries. The introduction of allopathic and homoeopathic medicines by these missionaries resulted in the first exposure and increasing access by people in these countries to so-called 'Western' medical care. Clinical and practical training for the management of tropical diseases and the prevention and control of such diseases became major subjects for training medical professionals and public health workers who had to serve in tropical countries (Uragoda 1987; Harrison 1994). The late eighteenth century saw an increasing momentum in public health education with the establishment of undergraduate and postgraduate courses designed specifically for public health, first in the home countries and later in the colonies. Pioneer public health schools were established in the colonial countries in the late nineteenth and early twentieth centuries, in order to function as centres for the development of public health policies, and to train people who had to serve in the tropics. These schools not only provided academic teaching, but also conducted research in tropical diseases. Discoveries of causative organisms and ways of stopping transmission of malaria and sleeping sickness, through clinical and public health intervention research studies initiated by these schools, led to the application and adoption of preventive and curative measures. Through the support of the Rockefeller Foundation, the London School of Tropical Medicine was transformed into the London School of Hygiene and Tropical Medicine in 1920, expanding the scope of research and teaching on tropical medicine, medical statistics, and epidemiology (Wilkinson and Power 1998). Spain also established its National School of Public Health in 1924 and introduced a public health component into its comprehensive rural medical care network.

Similar public health educational and research institutions, such as the Calcutta School of Tropical Medicine and Hygiene and the All-India Institute of Hygiene and Public Health, also in Calcutta, were established in British India in the early 1920s in order to carry out public health training and research in the region. The Haffkine Institute in Mumbai (Bombay), the King Institute of Preventive Medicine in Chennai (Madras), the Central Vaccine Research Institute in Kasauli, the National Institute of Communicable Diseases in Delhi (previously known as the Malaria Institute of India), the Indian Research Fund Association (later redesignated as the Indian Council of Medical Research), and the National Institute of Nutrition in Hyderabad were the exemplary research and teaching institutions established at that time (Jaggi 1979*a*). Similar educational and research institutions were established in the colonial and other independent countries, such as Thailand, the Philippines, Malaysia, Singapore, Hong Kong, Indonesia, Sri Lanka, Ghana, Nigeria, South Africa, Mexico, Brazil, and so on. These institutions of public health education worked closely with their counterparts in Western nations in order to strengthen the knowledge on disease causation, mainly with the support of the Rockefeller Foundation and colonial governments. These institutions also helped their own countries to improve the capacity of local public health administrators.

However, the actual development of public health and medical care services for the general public remained rudimentary in these former colonial countries and territories. Moving millions of people to totally unfamiliar areas had led to a high incidence of death and disability. These displaced people frequently died due to smallpox, malaria, yellow fever, typhus, typhoid, and cholera, or were disabled due to yaws, leprosy, and syphilis. Infectious diseases posed formidable obstacles in the colonization of new areas. The development of science and technology in the early twentieth century, especially in the area of physics, microbiology, biochemistry, pharmacology, and other diagnostics led to an explosion of its application in public health practices. Radio and telephone also facilitated communication amongst people. Some newspapers and magazines had a global reach. The colonials launched a major international public health initiative in the prevention and control of smallpox through vaccination, first amongst the people working in the colonial administration and later amongst the workers employed. Another notable experience was the massive community health development projects for the prevention and control of communicable diseases, mainly initiated through the support of the Rockefeller Foundation in a few Asian and Latin American countries. The attempt was aimed at developing pilot disease control projects that could be replicated in other parts of the world (Foster and Anderson 1978).

Foundation of international public health

International public health efforts actually intensified in the early eighteenth century when European nations applied protective legislative measures to prevent importation of epidemic diseases by trading ships. It became obligatory for all incoming ships, prior to unloading passengers and cargo, to follow strict quarantine measures. Later, business interests in these countries clashed with concern by governments for the health of their own population. The First International Sanitary Conference, organized by 12 European nations in Paris in 1851, tried to work out solutions for the 'Defense of Europe'. This was the first attempt to reach a consensus on drafting international quarantine regulations (Howard-Jones 1974*a*).

For the next 50 years, a series of similar international sanitary conferences were held but failed to produce an international sanitary code. The reasons for delaying international consensus were partly due to the non-availability of a sound scientific basis for the prevention and control of epidemics, and partly to the vested political and commercial interests of each colonial power. The Eleventh International Sanitary Conference, held in Paris in 1903, was a major milestone in international health as it was the first international sanitary convention for the prevention and control of three epidemics: plague, cholera, and yellow fever. Based on this convention, the French Government hosted the first international health office, called *L' Office International d' Hygiene Publique* (**OIHP**) in 1907 in Paris. At its inception, the main objective of OIHP was to protect Europe against three notifiable diseases (Howard-Jones 1974*b*). Ultimately, in 1911, the tasks of OIHP were expanded as the first truly international health agency, to monitor and report the outbreaks of the three notifiable diseases, and to provide general public health information on measures taken to combat these diseases through a monthly bulletin (McNeill 1977).

Around the time of the establishment of the League of Nations, major epidemics, including the great influenza pandemic of 1918, were rampant in various parts of the world and some infectious diseases, such as cholera and plague, were threatening to become pandemics. The League had to cope with many other postwar rehabilitation problems and the Paris-based OIHP was unable to deal with such pandemics even with its originally assigned tasks. Based on the proposal of the Brazilian delegation, the League of Nations agreed, in 1920, to the establishment of an international health organization. Finally, after intensive negotiations between the League, the colonial rulers, and other countries, the League of Nations Health Organization was formed in 1923 (Howard-Jones 1977). The League of Nations Health Organization was originally assigned to handle international health matters relating to both technical assistance and clearing-house functions. The epidemiological information service of the League of Nations Health Organization was strengthened through regional bureaux in Washington, Alexandria, Singapore, and Sydney, in addition to the service provided by OIHP. A series of basic clinical and field research studies on medicine and public health were also undertaken. These were done by organizing various committees or commissions of leading public health experts in a wide range of subjects, such as malaria, tuberculosis, leprosy, maternal and child health, health systems, and medical education. In addition to its research promotion function, the League of Nations Health Organization provided technical advice as well as technical assistance to countries and promoted international medical education, including postgraduate education in public health. It also organized international health conferences, conventions, and study tours (WHO 1967).

As early as the 1930s, health administrators had expressed their concerns on the health status of mass populations, especially of those living in rural areas. The international health conferences organized by the League of Nations Health Organization in the early 1930s provided a forum for sharing experiences on public health development in the countries under colonial rule, especially those in Asia and Africa. The Intergovernmental Conference of Far-Eastern Countries on Rural Hygiene, held in 1937 at Bandoeng (Bandung), The Netherlands East Indies (Indonesia), was a cornerstone in public health and rural health development in Asia (League of Nations Health Organization 1937). The Conference, while noting the rampant conditions of communicable diseases and nutritional deficiency disorders in rural areas, studied the public health interventions of the participating countries. It also defined the central role of health in development, and emphasized the need for integrating health care and intersectoral action, which is now the current view. The countries recognized the heavy socio-economic costs of diseases. They also recognized that the adoption of possible approaches, such as bringing maternal and child health care, hospitals, and health centres nearer to the people could prevent death and disability. However, the onset of the devastating Second World War delayed effective follow-up of the Bandung Conference principles. Many developing countries became battlefields. These countries experienced destruction, destitution, and disease, as well as human misery and suffering, with a very heavy death toll. In addition, there were a series of epidemics of smallpox, cholera, typhus, and malaria. Large displacements of people and the existence of very little or no public health infrastructure or public utility distribution systems resulted in more epidemics. The situation was further accentuated by famines, which took many lives.

Implementation of the International Health Institution

The spirit of international solidarity, peace, security, and tranquillity, immediately after the Second World War, led to the creation of intergovernmental organizations like the United Nations and its specialized agencies. The original draft of the United Nations Charter did not include health. The Brazilian and Chinese delegations, however, submitted a joint declaration to the United Nations to include health in its Charter. They also called for an international conference whose purpose was to foster consensus to establish an international health organization, and to bring this organization under the aegis of the United Nations Economic and Social Council. With the unanimous approval at the first United Nations General Assembly, a landmark international health conference was held in New York in June and July 1946. At this conference, a total of 61 nations, many of which were still under colonial rule, approved the Constitution of the WHO on 22 July 1946. This initiated the establishment of the WHO as a specialized agency of the United Nations. After ratification by the member governments, the WHO Constitution came into force on 7 April 1948, and the WHO officially came into being. Attainment by all people of the highest possible level of health was its constitutional mandate. The WHO's main functional roles are directing and co-ordinating international health work and providing advice and advocacy on international health development. The WHO is also given authority to adopt international regulations, to set international standards for biological and pharmaceutical agents, as well as other diagnostic procedures and products, and to adopt international conventions and agreements (WHO 1992). Since then, the membership of the WHO has grown to over 190 countries and territories. The WHO has worked with great harmony for over 50 years, through its six regional organizations and its headquarters, as a single international health organization.

Science-oriented public health

Development of basic health services

Former colonial countries saw the end of the Second World War as the beginning of the end of colonial rule. They all hoped for national development and believed that the period would bring peace and relief from suffering and shortages, through liberation from colonialism. There were strong nationalist movements and political agitations in all countries, preventing the reimposition of colonial rule. Within a few years, many countries achieved independence. They all started reconstruction work for immediate economic growth and social development, to catch up with the technological advances in the colonial powers.

A few countries in Asia, the Pacific, and Africa entered the post-Second World War period in a relatively calm and favourable economic position for reconstruction and rehabilitation. A few others, however, were challenged by their own internal ethnic conflicts. Many developed countries demonstrated special consideration for the welfare and economic development of their former colonies. During the first few decades after independence, developed countries had assisted newly independent developing countries, especially those devastated by the war, through multilateral and bilateral aid programmes in order to support reconstruction and rehabilitation. The United Nations General Assembly launched a programme of international economic co-operation in 1961. This programme, known as 'the United Nations Development Decade', was aimed at promoting self-sustaining growth and social advancement. While the countries aimed for sustainable development, the tensions and turmoil of another war, the Cold War, gripped the world. The separation of the Communist blocs (East Europe) from the capitalist states (Western Europe and the United States) created an environment marked by political and social tensions as well as confrontations and conflicts.

These early days of the reconstruction period were termed as the age of contradiction and opportunity. It was a time of increasing affluence in the developed countries, in stark contrast to the relentless march of poverty amongst the less fortunate majority in the rest of the world. The period was also termed as the age of opportunity that saw remarkable scientific and technological advancements which opened up limitless vistas and unlimited possibilities for solving the age-old problems of poverty and disease (Gunaratne 1977). The various inventions and innovations during and following the Second World War provided tremendous impetus for the application of science and technology. These included the jet aircraft, microwave instruments, radar, and other telecommunication facilities, including satellites. The discovery and mass production of quinine, dichlorodiphenyltrichloroethane (**DDT**), penicillin, and sulphonamides, the development of newer and effective vaccines and other drugs to prevent and control communicable diseases, the introduction of birth-control pills and injectables, the introduction and use of computers, and the improvement in imaging technologies (X-ray and CT scanning) facilitated advanced applications in public health practices. Advances in microbiology and immunology contributed greatly to the development of vaccines and diagnostic technologies. An outstanding achievement in the field of food and nutrition was the virtual disappearance of large-scale famines from many developing countries. Timely intervention of Green Revolution initiatives in the 1960s, in order to produce high-yielding varieties of grains with higher standards of farming techniques and good seeds, enhanced agricultural output, promoted self-sufficiency, and increased exports.

After gaining independence, many countries adopted ambitious plans for socio-economic development, including health. Health-care facilities, however, were almost non-existent in the post-Second World War period. There were a few professionals for health care and most were expatriates. Many countries thus initiated reviews of their national health situations and formulated long-term development plans. In India, the Bhore Committee was established in 1945 to review the health situation and to recommend improvements in the Indian health system. In Myanmar, the Sorrenta Villa Plan in 1947 and the Pyidawtha Plan in 1950 were drawn up for achieving rapid socio-economic growth, including the expansion of health and education immediately after the war. Similar socio-economic plans were initiated by other developing countries.

Regional co-operation for socio-economic and cultural development was also sought in order to increase intercountry collaboration. For example, the Colombo Plan for Cooperative Economic and Social Development in Asia and the Pacific was conceived at the Commonwealth Conference, held in Sri Lanka, in January 1950. The Colombo Plan proved to be a valuable source of technical and financial assistance to the participating countries, in the area of economic and social development and national capacity building, including health. During the same period, different bodies for regional social and economic co-operation were established in quick succession, such as the Council for Mutual Economic Assistance, the Commonwealth Association, and the Common Markets for Central America and Caribbean. Similarly, in the 1980s, the Association of Southeast Asian Nations, the South Asian Association for Regional Co-operation, and other regional political, social, and economic co-operation organizations were established. These regional political and economic groupings were organized with the aim of having common markets and co-operation in socio-economic and cultural areas amongst neighbouring developing countries, sometimes in alliance with developed nations. In order to support economic development activities, regional development banks were also established. The developed countries got together and formed the Organization for Economic Co-operation and Development in 1961. Many developed countries also established their own development agencies, such as the Australian Agency for International Development, the Danish International Development Agency, the German Agency for Technical Co-operation, the Japan International Co-operation Agency, the Norwegian Agency for International Development, the Overseas Development Administration of the United Kingdom (later renamed as the Department for International Development), and the United States Agency for International Development.

Immediately after the Second World War—with advice and support from the WHO, the United Nations International Children's Emergency Fund (**UNICEF**), other United Nations agencies, and multilateral and other bilateral donors—developing countries started building up health systems infrastructures based on a network of hospitals and health centres. Minimally trained basic health workers ran these centres, especially in the rural areas. Expansion of basic health services was made through national public health projects on maternal and child health, school health, environmental sanitation, nutrition, and so on. During the early 1950s most countries adopted the Beveridge model of national health and social welfare policy and they initiated 'free' health services for all. Health-care facilities such as hospitals, health centres, or dispensaries, managed by medical doctors, were very few and were mainly concentrated in towns and cities. These facilities essentially were an expansion of the institutions already established during the colonial period.

Training of different categories of health auxiliaries, such as health assistants, medical assistants, health visitors, nurses, midwives, vaccinators, sanitary workers, community educators, laboratory technicians, pharmacists, and compounders, was initiated by the establishment of paramedical training institutes. These workers were deployed to serve at the various health institutions, especially those established in the rural areas. A number of rural health development and demonstration centres were also established in many countries. The Kalutara rural health project in Sri Lanka, the pilot project of the Aung San demonstration rural health unit in Myanmar, and the Singur rural health project in India were a few of them. The development of human resources for health, especially by creating medical, nursing, and other paramedical schools, was more intense between the 1950s and 1970s. Most countries did not have adequate personnel with appropriate professional training. Myanmar, Malaysia, and Sri Lanka even had to arrange for medical doctors from abroad to serve in their hospitals and educational institutions. Training institutions and related field training centres were established later to meet the local demand.

Exactly 20 years after the Bandung Conference in 1937, another international rural health conference was organized in New Delhi, India, in October 1957, this time under the auspices of the WHO. This conference reviewed and analysed a wide range of subjects: the concepts and functioning of rural health services, the training and use of multipurpose village workers, the enhancement of prevention and control of epidemic and endemic diseases, the utilization of local resources and promoting intersectoral action, and the participation of local people, including formation of village health committees. The conference recognized that the rural health centres were the basic health units where comprehensive health care could be provided to the rural population, and that they should be strengthened (WHO 1957).

Maternal and child health services in developing countries were very rudimentary during the early 1950s and the 1960s. Only a few countries had an administrative authority for maternal and child health matters at the central government level. Maternal and child health services were mainly provided through health clinics and centres employed with briefly trained midwives or auxiliary nurse–midwives. Maternal and infant mortality remained at higher levels in some countries, compared with others that had experienced high women's status in society and better access to health care and other essential services. With advice and support from the WHO and UNICEF, developing countries started establishing separate maternal and child welfare departments in the early 1950s and the 1960s. With financial and technical inputs by the United Nations and other partners, the numbers of maternal and child health centres expanded rapidly. However, experience within a few decades showed that the vertical approach of opening maternal and child health centres and deploying maternal and child health workers alone did not serve the purpose of improving accessibility. Countries recognized the importance of providing comprehensive basic health care while focusing on the problems of mothers and children. Excessive pregnancies, inappropriate timing and spacing of pregnancies, poor health and nutritional status of the mother, inadequate care during pregnancy and childbirth, and poor educational levels of mothers were identified as the main factors responsible for most maternal and infant mortality, as well as serious morbidity amongst women and children. The United Nations International Women's Decade (1976–1985) helped to increase awareness of these problems. The tragedy was that maternal health had received far less attention than child health (Rosenfield and Maine 1985).

Figure 1 shows the decline in trends in infant mortality rates in developing and developed countries in the last 20 years. The persisting relatively high levels of infant and maternal mortality and morbidity, and rapid population growth during the last three decades in developing countries, have added a heavy burden to improving the social and economic status of these countries. More food, more schools and health centres, and more funds from the government were needed to cope with the burden.

In the 1960s, most countries started adopting a comprehensive population policy in which family planning was the main strategy. Even though technology was available, only 9 per cent of women in the developing countries had access to contraceptive services in 1965. Concerted efforts of many governments with full support of international multilateral and bilateral agencies, including voluntary organizations, had resulted in the use of the contraceptive pill increasing to 50 per cent by 1990. Nonetheless, wide geographical variations still persisted. The proportion of couples using some form of contraception was approximately 75 per cent in China and East

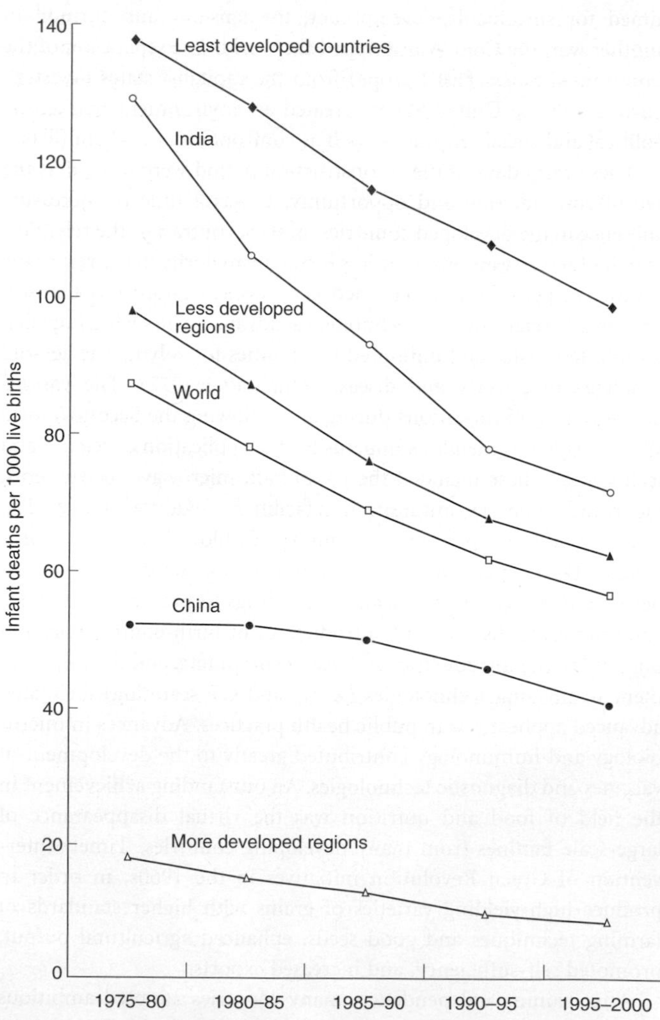

Fig. 1 Trends of infant mortality rates for selected countries and country groups, 1980 to 2000.

Asia, just over 50 per cent in Latin America, about 30 per cent in South Asia, and less than 15 per cent in Africa (UNICEF 1991). A majority of women in most developing countries were aware of the health risks posed by frequent pregnancies, and thus of the importance of birth spacing, but this awareness was not easily translated into action.

The Green Revolution, which began in the 1960s, impacted positively on the supply of food and nutrition. In contrast, it also created some distortion in the availability of food. Initially the Green Revolution focused less on pulses and vegetables, which were the main source of food energy in Asian and African diets, and completely neglected the development of horticulture. Thus, with seasonal shortage of vegetables, vitamin A deficiency was widespread in Asia (Gopalan 1992). Despite this drawback, the increase in food production globally resulted in substantial reductions in the number of people with inadequate access to food, from 35 per cent in the 1970s to 21 per cent in the 1990s. The average daily per capita dietary energy supplies increased from less than 9.7 kJ in 1960 to 11.4 kJ in 1990 (WHO 1998*a*). However, hunger and malnutrition continued to be the most devastating problems in the developing countries. Nearly 30 per cent of people in the world's poorest nations are currently suffering from one or more of the multiple forms of malnutrition (WHO 1999*b*). The nutritional status of an individual depends not only on food production and the availability of food but also on food consumption. Protein-energy malnutrition, the major nutritional deficiency disease of developing countries, is due to inadequate energy intake, leading to wasting and stunting. In the 1960s, the prevailing view on protein-energy malnutrition was that it was primarily a problem of protein deficiency and that the solution lay in the distribution of protein-rich foods and protein concentrates. Research in developing countries during this period showed that protein-energy malnutrition was mainly due to calorie deficiency. It took another 10 years for this concept to be accepted by Western institutions (WHO 1986). The prevalence of underweight amongst children under 5 years of age in developing countries had declined from 46 per cent in 1975 to 31 per cent in 1995, but progress was not uniform. Estimates in 1995 indicated that 206 million children were stunted and 49 million wasted in developing countries. The continuing burden of malnutrition is rooted within poverty, underdevelopment, and inequality. However, regional trends suggest that there may be additional reasons behind protein-energy malnutrition's persistence. The risk of being malnourished, as measured by weight, is 1.2 times higher in Asia than in Africa, and three times higher in Africa than in Latin America (WHO 1998*b*). Over two-thirds (72 per cent) of an estimated 206 million malnourished children, as measured in terms of height for age (stunted), live in Asia (especially southern Asia), while 25.6 per cent are found in Africa and only 2.3 per cent in Latin America (WHO 1999*b*).

The essential food factors, 'vitamins', identified by Frederick Hopkins in 1906, led the way towards nutrition research and promotion. Deficiency diseases in micronutrients, such as vitamins and minerals, had been well-known public health problems since those days and these diseases were more widespread than protein-energy malnutrition. Around 1999, an estimated 5 billion people had iron deficiency. The prevalence of anaemia was highest (over 50 per cent) in pregnant women and preschool children in developing countries. Iodine-deficiency disorders and iron-deficiency anaemia have profound effects on human health and development, including increased maternal and neonatal mortality, impaired health and development of infants and young children, limited learning capacity, impaired immune function, and reduced productive capacity. Apart from inadequate dietary intake of iron, poor bioavailability of iron from cereal-based diets and high worm infestations were mainly responsible for iron-deficiency anaemia.

Estimates in 1995 indicated that iodine-deficiency disorders were significant public health problems in 118 countries, with approximately 43 million people affected by some degree of brain damage. Fifty per cent of these handicapped people lived in South and Southeast Asia. Universal iodization of salt, advocated by the WHO and UNICEF as the main eradication strategy for the control of iodine-deficiency disorders, has been successful in most countries. For example, Bhutan, a land-locked Himalayan kingdom, witnessed a remarkable drop in the prevalence of iodine-deficiency disorders from 65 to 14 per cent within a decade, using a multisectoral approach which included adequate distribution of iodized salt, monitoring the iodine content at various points of distribution and at the consumers' homes, and promoting social mobilization (WHO 1999*a*).

Hundreds of thousands of children are going blind every year as a result of vitamin A deficiency. WHO estimates in 1999 showed that around 250 million children were affected by vitamin A deficiency globally. After extensive field clinical trials in developing countries, vitamin A supplementation programmes were introduced on top of the programmes for the promotion of breast feeding and dietary improvement, with the support of United Nations and bilateral agencies. Many countries adopted the vitamin A deficiency supplementation programme as part of their national immunization programmes, though questions were raised about its technical soundness. Although there was a 30 to 60 per cent reduction from the 1985 level by 1995, vitamin A deficiency remains a public health problem in many countries (WHO 1999*a*).

Simple nutrition education of mothers, protection and promotion of breast feeding, dietary improvement, supplementation, and fortification, good nutrition surveillance, making vegetables accessible at affordable prices, and early diagnosis and treatment of childhood illnesses, such as measles, acute respiratory infections, and diarrhoea, were the combination of interventions identified to reduce nutrition deficiency disorders. Improving food availability and providing adequate quantities of safe and nutritious food were the long-term goals. Recognizing the magnitude of the problem, the International Conference on Nutrition, organized jointly by the WHO and the Food and Agriculture Organization in Rome in 1992, pledged to reduce severe and moderate malnutrition amongst children under 5 years of age to half of the 1990 level by the year 2000. By mid-1999, a total of 152 countries and five territories (representing 91 per cent of the WHO's member states) had finalized or drafted their national plans of action for nutrition. Most of them continued the process of development, implementation, and monitoring of intensified strategies for the promotion of nutrition. There was a decline in the global prevalence of protein-energy malnutrition from 37.4 per cent in 1980 to 26.7 per cent in 1999 (WHO 1999*b*).

Promotion of environmental sanitation was also given the same priority as the development of basic health services in the early days of public health development in developing countries. Developed countries had shown from their experience in the eighteenth and nineteenth centuries that improvements in personal hygiene and environmental sanitation could prevent and control the spread of communicable diseases, especially water-borne and vector-borne diseases. Environmental sanitation work started with the deployment of public health officers, sanitary workers, inspectors, and engineers to promote the provision of safe water supply and adequate sanitation facilities, particularly in rural areas. Insufficient financial resources, inappropriate application of technology, and lack of community involvement, however, hindered progress. Municipal and local authorities could not provide adequate water supply as well as simple and proper sanitary facilities in urban or rural areas. A WHO survey, carried out in 1970 in 91 developing countries, showed that only 29 per cent of the total population had access to a safe drinking water and only 50 per cent of the urban population had access to a safe water supply. The access to adequate sanitation facilities was even worse, particularly in the rural areas (WHO 1998*b*).

Disease prevention and control campaigns

While attempts were made up until the 1970s to consolidate the patchy public health services and expand the basic health services facilities available, the application of scientific and technological advances in the prevention and control of communicable diseases and other public health problems began. This led to the introduction of special control campaigns in the areas of maternal and child health, nutrition, school health, environmental sanitation, occupational health, and infectious diseases. The launching of national projects for the control of major infectious diseases followed in parallel with the development and expansion of basic health services. Disease control campaigns were initiated with the new scientific and technological advancements, better understanding of disease aetiology, and the availability of appropriate tools for successful intervention. Developed nations also helped developing countries to contain infectious diseases at their source rather than through quarantine restrictions.

The WHO, UNICEF, and other United Nations agencies, together with international non-governmental organizations, such as the Rockefeller Foundation and the Save the Children Fund, promoted global disease control campaigns against major epidemic diseases. Demonstration projects were established in different corners of the world to identify appropriate disease prevention and control strategies. International experts were recruited and assigned to these projects. National experts were also trained through fellowships and on-the-job training. Many educational and research institutions were established to cope with emerging needs. The following sections highlight a few successes and failures in the prevention and control programmes against certain tropical diseases.

Yaws

The control of yaws (*Framboesia tropicana*) is amongst the great success stories of public health. The discovery that this painful disabling disease could be controlled by arsenic and bismuth compounds accelerated the control efforts of yaws before the Second World War. Mass campaigns were carried out in different parts of the world. Nevertheless, owing to the inaccessibility of such treatment and inadequate epidemiological knowledge, the prevalence of yaws remained high in most countries in Africa, Asia, the Pacific, and Latin America until the 1950s. The WHO and UNICEF initiated a global control project against yaws as early as 1948. Mass treatment campaigns using long-acting penicillin and the increasing accessibility of the local populace to Western medical facilities transformed the situation. In the early 1950s, there were an estimated 20 million cases of yaws worldwide, half of them in Asia. Using mass treatment with penicillin as a weapon for cure, the global programme had eliminated yaws as a major public health problem by the early 1970s. Only a few scattered foci of infection persisted in Latin America, the Pacific, and South and Southeast Asia.

Malaria

The spectacular success of the global yaws control programme provided a boost to other disease control campaigns. There were 110 to 115 million cases of malaria with about a million deaths in Southeast Asian countries alone during the 1950s. It was estimated that nearly 40 per cent of people in that region were at risk of contracting malaria annually, and that malaria accounted for more than 6 per cent of deaths from all causes. Economic losses due to malaria were also considerable. Most governments invested large amount of funds and human resources in its prevention and control. The discovery of quinine and aminoquinolines, as well as a better understanding of malaria transmission and vector biology at the local level, helped in improving prevention and control strategies. Prior to DDT (a long-lasting insecticide), a variety of preventive and curative measures had been tried. Bioenvironmental measures against vectors were not effective in many countries owing to the lack of adequate investment and supervision. At the same time, access to antimalaria drugs was also limited because of insufficient health-care facilities.

During the early 1950s, the WHO demonstrated in various pilot projects that residual spraying of human dwellings with DDT insecticide and the effective treatment of malaria cases with 4-aminoquinolines could interrupt the transmission of malaria effectively and efficiently. Encouraged by successful pilot projects, assured of massive support from international and bilateral agencies, and as recommended by the WHO, many governments launched large-scale national malaria control campaigns that expanded progressively in scope and coverage. National malaria institutes were also established in order to provide technical direction, research development, and training. Some countries adopted large-scale national malaria eradication campaigns using insecticide-based control strategy as the main approach.

Initially, national DDT-based malaria control or eradication programmes in most countries were a dramatic success. The reduction in the number of malaria cases was spectacular. Even from the experience of Southeast Asian countries, the malaria cases declined from over 100 million in 1950 to a low of 230 000 in 1965. The incidence of malaria in these countries also decreased from 40 000 per 100 000 population to less than 5. Some countries benefited from the transfer of technology in the domestic production of DDT. Later, the United Nations Expanded Programme of Technical Assistance (the precursor of the present-day United Nations Development Programme) joined the global effort for malaria eradication by creating a Malaria Special Account. Despite this effort, the erratic supply of DDT and inadequate planning and supervision of spraying operations led to increasing resistance amongst malaria vectors. The substantial amount of DDT and spraying equipment required for large-scale operations was beyond the means of developing countries, as were personnel and transport requirements. The technical problems of insecticide-resistant mosquitoes, and later drug resistance amongst malaria parasites, also increased. Despite this drawback, there was the beneficial effect of the use of DDT spraying on the control of a chronic systemic disease—visceral leishmaniasis (kala-azar)—which was highly endemic in Central and South Asia, Latin America, and Africa. By the early 1960s, kala-azar had completely disappeared in many areas (WHO 1992).

Leprosy

This oldest and widely prevalent disease was well recognized by the developing countries because of its chronic symptoms and signs. It affected individuals at their most productive period and imposed a significant social and economic burden on society. In the absence of effective control methods, people with leprosy were isolated from others. Discovery of the sulphone drug dapsone (diamino-diphenyl-sulphone or DDS) in 1943, and its availability for leprosy treatment, provided a welcome boost to leprosy control. With the active collaboration of highly endemic countries and with full support from international non-governmental organizations, the WHO and UNICEF jointly initiated the global leprosy control programme in the early 1950s. The main strategies adopted were early case detection through mass screening and treatment with dapsone, together with health education. Millions of leprosy cases were detected and given long-term dapsone therapy. Many leprosy cases were relieved of symptoms and discharged from the register after long years of treatment with dapsone. For many leprosy patients, the 1960s and subsequent decades brought hope and promise (WHO 1992).

Sexually transmitted diseases

In the early days, venereal diseases or sexually transmitted diseases, especially syphilis (lues), were regarded as the diseases of Europeans. Historic literature in Asia (India, China, and Japan) referred to syphilis as *Farangi Roga* (the Sanskrit for 'foreigners' disease'); fifteenth-century Indian literature refers to this disease as 'Portuguese disease'. Limited information showed that sexually transmitted diseases had been rampant amongst the populace in Asia since those early periods. Treatment in those days was with mercury compounds for a prolonged period, which led to the saying, 'Two hours with Venus and two years with Mercury'. The community intervention studies for venereal disease control with penicillin in Europe showed good results in the 1940s. The use of long-acting penicillin in 1948 as the main treatment strategy changed the outlook for the control of syphilis and other endemic treponematoses, including yaws (WHO 1992). A few pilot venereal disease control projects were initiated in developing countries in the 1950s to identify appropriate community intervention strategies. These included early case detection, effective contact tracing, early treatment, continuous surveillance, and health education. With the success of these demonstration projects, many developing countries started national venereal disease/sexually transmitted disease control projects. However, the effectiveness of these projects was short-lived. Availability of effective treatment conveyed a false sense of public health security, which ignored the increasing prevalence of prostitution, promiscuity, and homosexuality. Rapid urbanization, industrialization, and migration of labourers further contributed to promoting syphilis and other sexually transmitted diseases.

Cholera

This acute bacterial disease is one of the notifiable diseases under the International Health Regulations because of its severity and easy spread. Public health experience during the eighteenth and nineteenth centuries showed that provision of adequate sanitation and safe drinking water, having adequate personal and food hygiene, and appropriate quarantine measures could contain cholera effectively. The use of new therapeutic methods and newer antibiotics, supported by adequate rehydration therapy and early case detection, demonstrated that many deaths from cholera could be averted. The development of a cholera vaccine in the 1950s also helped to arrest further spread of cholera. A new cholera biotype, *eltor*, appeared in 1961 in Indonesia and invaded all of Asia, creating waves of epidemic. This *eltor* epidemic took thousands of lives and affected millions of people for more than two decades. By the 1990s, it had spread to other regions and caused major public health crises in Africa and the Americas. Although the development of a newer cholera vaccine is in progress, a newer bacterial strain, *Vibrio cholerae* 0139, has been identified in India and other parts of Asia and has spread slowly to other parts of the world (WHO 1978*a*).

Public health successes

The greatest success achieved by developing countries in the twentieth century was the prevention and control as well as the ultimate eradication of smallpox, a dreadful communicable disease that had existed since antiquity. As a public health preventive measure, inoculation of pus taken from smallpox cases into healthy people had been practised in Asia since ancient times. This method of variolation spread to Europe and other parts of the world in the seventeenth century. It was then simplified and widely used for the prevention and control of smallpox. In 1796 Edward Jenner introduced a modified technique of variolation by using cowpox material. The scientific community in Europe slowly accepted the results of this experimentation by Jenner. Later, mass inoculation using cowpox material (called vaccination) was introduced extensively, in Britain first and then in all of Europe and other parts of the colonial world. The vaccine material, dried on thread, glass, or ivory points, was despatched to all parts of the world. Wider acceptance of mass vaccination had resulted in smallpox ceasing to be a major threat in most countries of Europe and the Americas in the early twentieth century (Henderson 1997). Although the colonial rulers introduced vaccination against smallpox, the coverage of vaccination to the population in their colonies was inadequate. Control could not be achieved on account of the variable purity and potency of the vaccine as well as poor vaccination techniques. Non-availability of large quantities of safe smallpox vaccine and the absence of appropriate methods of preserving it in hot climates were major impediments (Kiat 1978). Thus, even a century after the discovery of smallpox vaccination, the disease continued to rage throughout the developing countries.

Early in the twentieth century, the French, later followed by the Dutch, produced large quantities of freeze-dried smallpox vaccine, and these were supplied annually to their own colonies in Africa and Asia. The Lister Institute in London further improved the technology of freeze-dried vaccine production in the early 1950s. Since then, large-scale commercial production of a stable freeze-dried smallpox vaccine has spread to other developed countries and later to the newly independent developing countries. Early in the 1950s, the WHO advocated a worldwide smallpox vaccination campaign, aimed at the eradication of the disease. However, many countries were sceptical about the global campaign, mainly because of inadequate supply of vaccines and inaccessibility of health services to a large proportion of the population. After reviewing the global situation, including technical and logistic feasibility, the WHO recommended launching the Eradication of Smallpox Programme at the World Health Assembly in 1958 through resolution WHA11.54 (WHO 1964). This time, all members pledged to fight against smallpox with the guidance and supervision of the WHO. Although the tension between the two superpowers—the United States and the then USSR—was at its height around 1960, they, together with other developed countries, agreed to work with the WHO to fight smallpox (Henderson 1998).

Some countries had already achieved smallpox eradication status before 1960 through routine and extensive vaccinations backed by legislation and mass campaigns. Initially, the strategy for control was to increase routine smallpox vaccination coverage through mass campaigns. Based on the recommendations of the WHO Expert Committee on Smallpox, many developing countries resolved to eradicate smallpox with intensified mass vaccination as the main strategy (WHO 1964). Beginning in 1960, mass smallpox vaccination campaigns were launched in all endemic countries. The WHO, with the support of developed countries, helped them by extending technical assistance and logistic support. In Myanmar, the 3-year rounds of primary vaccination strategy, alternating mass vaccination in one-third of the country in each round, had been used to cover the entire population without heavy investment. The introduction of the jet injector and bifurcated needles for mass vaccination had a great impact on expanding coverage. Indonesia succeeded in eradicating smallpox using the mass vaccination strategy. Its experience of having a special programme of village-to-village searches for cases, using the smallpox recognition cards and providing rewards for reporting and educating the people, made a significant impact on smallpox eradication efforts in Asia as well as globally. Other countries adopted similar approaches in order to intensify their efforts (WHO 1978*a*). The experience of the smallpox eradication campaigns in Western and Central Africa in the mid-1960s showed that smallpox epidemics could be successfully contained, through a surveillance–containment strategy (active case detection and mass vaccination around cases), even when the incidence was high and relatively few people were vaccinated (Foege *et al.* 1971; Fenner *et al.* 1988).

India launched a massive public health campaign called Operation Smallpox Zero in the early 1970s. The last case of smallpox occurred in India in May 1975 (Basu *et al.* 1979). Bangladesh, Bhutan, and Nepal also launched similar 'zero-transmission-targeted' eradication campaigns and, after 1975, reported no cases. The last case of smallpox in Asia was reported in Bangladesh in October 1975. The last cases of smallpox in Africa were reported in the late 1970s, mainly in the eastern parts. The last naturally acquired human case of smallpox in the world was reported in Somalia in October 1977. The global International Commission on Smallpox Eradication gave its final report to the 33rd World Health Assembly in May 1980. Based on the findings of the Commission, the World Health Assembly made a declaration that the world was free from natural transmission of smallpox. This was the most spectacular public health achievement in the twentieth century (WHO 1992).

Gaps between the 'haves' and the 'have-nots'

Great efforts made by governments and international organizations had helped in reducing the burden of many epidemic and endemic diseases, and strengthened the health-care delivery systems. Many diseases ceased to be major public health problems globally. However, the Joint WHO/UNICEF worldwide empirical study in 1975 (Djukanovic and Mach 1975) showed that approximately two-thirds of the population in the developing countries did not have reasonable access to any permanent form of health care. Health-care facilities were mostly concentrated in urban areas. Poor organization and management of the existing health facilities further compounded the situation. Since the educational institutions relevant for health workers were not properly developed, human resources for hospitals and health centres had to rely on poorly qualified people or foreign health workers. Professionals graduating from local educational institutes were not eager to work in rural areas. These professionals sometimes opposed new types of paramedical health workers on the grounds that providing medical care was too important and too complex to be left in the hands of less trained or differently trained personnel, and that it would be dangerous to do so. Inadequacy and maldistribution of resources for health services was another obstacle. Government investment in health care remained low for decades, compared with other sectors. Loans or grants from foreign sources had been used mainly for building specialized or large general hospitals, and procuring sophisticated equipment. In general, there was not much expansion of public health facilities like small rural hospitals, maternity homes, or rural health centres. Compounding these problems was the duplication of efforts by health workers functioning under many vertical programmes of disease control campaigns. There was weak development of the concept of a comprehensive health system. The central health administration had taken over the major authority and executive responsibilities, thus preventing effective and adequate delivery of services at the periphery. The integration of specialized disease control programmes into general health services moved slowly; most of them remained as autonomous bodies after more than three to four decades of operation. There was little co-ordination in planning and management between the health and health-related sectors, as well as between various sections of the health sector itself. Much of the health planning was done at the central level without closer involvement of the people responsible for implementation (WHO 1978*b*).

In most countries, a high proportion of people, especially those in rural areas, had no access to even minimum essential health care. Many were also prone to diseases due to a hostile environment, poverty, and the lack of knowledge of preventive measures. There were glaring contrasts in health status between developed and developing countries as well as within developing countries. According to the 1971 data, life expectancy at birth was 43 years in Africa and 50 years in Asia, while it was 71 in Europe and North America. Infant and maternal mortality rates were steadily declining in many developing countries, but remained high on account of a few countries showing a slow decline. Up to the mid-1980s, the situation remained unchanged. The average life expectancy at birth in the developing countries was around 55 years, and in Africa and some parts of Asia it was only 50 years.

Infant mortality in most developing countries was 10 to 15 times higher than in the developed world. Most deaths in the developing countries resulted from infectious and parasitic diseases. The high occurrence of such diseases was closely related to specific socio-economic and environmental health conditions, and impeded overall socio-economic development. The proportion of gross national product spent on health ranged from 1 to 6 per cent in many developing countries as compared to more than 10 per cent in the developed world. Another reason was the decision to continue the colonial systems of health care. Since many developing countries had acquired health-care institutions from their colonial rulers, their first attempt at health development after becoming independent was to continue running the existing facilities and building similar health infrastructures, mainly in towns and cities.

On a different note, the use and promotion of traditional medicine and medical practices was almost abandoned in most developing countries during and after the colonial days, even though these have been used as alternatives for health care for thousands of years. These alternative health care systems included the *Ayurveda*, *Siddha*, *Unani-Tibbi*, Chinese, Tibetan, and others. Herbalists, bonesetters, and spiritualists also practised non-formalized systems of traditional medicine. Most of the traditional medical practitioners had been trained through informal systems of education. In addition, home remedies, yoga, nature cure, and homoeopathy were also used in many countries, and there were millions of such practitioners all over the world. As soon as the developing countries achieved independence, they started promoting traditional medicine through new legislation. They established formal educational institutions and accorded recognition to the services of traditional medicine practitioners. A few countries set up national control bodies and central departments under their health ministries or under separate ministries to promote the development of traditional medicine. Some countries promoted research and development on traditional medicine.

During the late 1970s, at the time of intensification of primary health care, many countries recognized the importance of traditional medicine. They began to develop it in conjunction with 'modern' medicine. National programmes for the development of traditional medicine were initiated as a complementary strategy for promoting primary health care. Some countries even attempted integrated health care delivery so that the basic health staff could provide both traditional and allopathic systems at the same facility. People still saw traditional medicine as an alternative to modern health care for individuals rather than as a public health measure. Newer findings on the use of various types of traditional medicine and traditional practices led to the understanding that many of these could be used as public health interventions. These traditional medicines and practices were related to good personal hygiene, healthy behaviour, and proper nutrition for the protection and prolongation of life. Much more research needs to be undertaken for establishing the effectiveness of traditional medicine and practices. Furthermore, there is a need for continued research on the application of traditional medicine in the promotive and preventive aspects of health, especially in view of the expansion in public health interventions.

Political public health

Socialized public health

The 1970s and 1980s were regarded globally as economically and politically unstable decades. There were armed conflicts within and between countries and ethnic groups in various parts of the world. Of these, the war in the Middle East in 1973 had serious consequences on the world economy due to the oil crisis. Developing countries continued to face traditional health problems, such as high morbidity and mortality, as a result of maternal and childhood diseases, infectious diseases, and malnutrition and, at the same time, they were not able to cope with the rapidly increasing population. There was too much focus on technological advancements and the use of technical interventions. Dominance of the biomedical science approach, without adequate focus on the community, led to the failure of many mass disease control campaigns.

By 1970, developing countries and the international community at large had become increasingly aware that, despite 20 years of large foreign investments and top-down development efforts, the socio-economic status of the people, including their health status, had not risen to the desired level. Many countries, especially those that had achieved independence in the late 1960s and the 1970s, were still struggling for socio-economic growth. While the New World economic order was being formulated, a new philosophy of public health development with the principles of social justice and equity slowly evolved.

The initial ideas of social medicine or the social dimension of public health had emerged around the early twentieth century. Lord Dawson made a statement in 1919 that 'preventive and curative medicine cannot be separated in any sound principle and in any scheme of medical science. They must be together in close co-ordination' (Ko Ko U 1996). Professor Winslow defined public health as 'the science and art of preventing disease, prolonging life, and promoting physical health and efficiency through organized community efforts'. This definition was continuously debated as to whether it should fall in preventive medicine or public health. The social medicine concept emerged as a new discipline in the late 1940s and the early 1950s. Sir John Ryle described social medicine as deriving its inspiration more from the field of clinical experience, seeking always to assist the discovery of common purpose for remedial and preventive services (Ryle 1943). The leaders of both clinical medicine and public health questioned the polarization of curative and preventive medicine and specialization in each field as if they were mutually exclusive. Social medicine, as a new discipline taking inspirations from clinical experience, conceptualized by Iago Galdston (the United States), Sir John Ryle (the United Kingdom), and René Sand (Belgium) in the early and mid-1950s, failed for various reasons and the social medicine movement was overtaken by other developments. The concept of risk factors as determinants of disease returned strongly later (Ko Ko U 1996).

New knowledge about non-communicable diseases, such as cancer, diabetes, and tobacco-related diseases, became available in the late 1950s and the 1960s. The social and behavioural aspects of diseases were also recognized and many social interventions were proposed as part of health promotion. Without considering the basic concept of social medicine, many medical universities and faculties converted their departments or schools of public health into units for preventive and social medicine. Instead of teaching either social medicine or conventional public health, educational institutions considered public health to be the same as preventive and social medicine. Most of the associated changes were more of a change in designation than in the evolving concept of public health.

Many health planners came to believe that the task before them required fitting clinical medicine into a social context because of the political needs and demands of the community, the widening gaps between health needs and available resources, and the rising pressure of societal factors. Socialized health care had become the most reasonable, workable, and acceptable approach. Virchow had stated during the mid-1880s that medicine was a social science, and politics was medicine on a large scale (Ko Ko U 1996). Over the years, the definition of health and the means of attaining it were widely debated. The relationships between health and poverty were debated in an effort to find appropriate solutions. People became more aware of the social and economic determinants impacting health. Empirical evidence was collected from both the developed and the developing world. The value of health as a fundamental human right and its attainment as an essential social goal were firmly recognized. The need to rationalize the allocation of financial resources and deployment of staff was voiced. There was a consensus that vast numbers of the population remained vulnerable and a large proportion needed essential health care. A strong national commitment was required to expand and strengthen national health systems in order to ensure the greatest health benefit to the greatest number of people at the lowest cost. Mahler said, 'Without health, life has little quality, for even if health is not everything, without it the rest is nothing'. As a result of debates on the links between health and social, environmental, economic, and political factors, there were many comments on the need to give a political dimension to international public health (WHO 1992).

The Health for All movement

These debates yielded fruitful results when, in 1977, the World Health Assembly adopted the historic resolution on 'Health for All by the Year 2000'. It had been clarified at the very beginning that Health for All did not mean that everyone in the world would be healthy and receive treatment for all ailments. It also did not mean that nobody would be sick or disabled. Health for All by the year 2000 meant that, by 2000, people would use better approaches than they had before for preventing and controlling diseases and alleviating unavoidable illness and disability. They would find better ways of growing up, growing old, and dying gracefully. It was intended that there would be an even distribution of health resources. Essential health care would be accessible to all individuals and families, in an acceptable and affordable way, and with their full involvement. The adoption of the universal goal of Health for All helped many countries to recognize new ways of reaching higher health status and to place greater emphasis on adherence to health goals (WHO 1978*a*).

While almost all countries aimed at the universal goal of Health for All, they also realized that the gap was widening between the health 'haves' in the affluent countries and the health 'have-nots' in the developing world. The obstacles in closing such wide gaps in health status were clearly recognized by the world community at the international conference jointly organized by the WHO and UNICEF, at Alma-Ata in the then USSR, in September 1978. This conference was another landmark in public health development and heralded a new era. After detailed deliberations, the conference agreed on the ground-breaking Alma-Ata Declaration (WHO 1978*b*). This Declaration called for urgent action by all governments, health and development workers, and the world community, to protect and promote the health of all the people of the world, using the primary health care approach.

The underlying principles of health development such as equity, community involvement, appropriate technology, and a multisectoral approach were further expanded and broadened at this conference. Health as a fundamental human right was reaffirmed and every country was asked to aim at the attainment of the highest possible level of health as the most important universal social goal. Governments needed to incorporate and strengthen primary health care within their national development plans with special emphasis on rural and urban development programmes and the co-ordination of the health-related activities of different sectors. The principles of basic health services, such as accessibility, availability, acceptability, and appropriateness of health services, were retained. Primary health care was seen as a practical, scientifically sound, and socially acceptable approach. Keeping in view the need for providing essential health care to the unserved and underserved population, primary health care was expected to promote actions to reach out to these populations (WHO 1978*b*).

Developing countries saw the Alma-Ata primary health care conference as an opportunity for restructuring their health systems to reach the goal of Health for All by 2000. They formulated new health policies and strategies, as well as plans of action to launch and sustain primary health care. With the full support of United Nations agencies and bilateral and multilateral donors, the countries attempted to organize and manage comprehensive national health systems within the Health for All and primary health care framework. They tried to manage health resources better in order to expand their health systems. Many started emphasizing primary health care as a major public health approach in their national health development plans. Some countries concentrated on a few health-care interventions, while others tried to encompass as many elements as possible in their public health development. A few others made attempts to address the quality aspects of health-care services and programmes.

A series of innovative approaches aimed at intensifying primary health care were organized. UNICEF concurrently advocated a comprehensive child survival approach, which was later presented to the United Nations as child survival protection and development. The WHO had emphasized health systems development with the focus on strengthening district health systems based on primary health care. The Health for All movement in the 1970s and the 1980s resulted in many more public health interventions in developing countries. The accessibility of major elements of primary health care had risen to over 80 per cent of the people in most countries. Yet, progress with respect to coverage of mothers and children with appropriate health care or the promotion of safe water supply and adequate sanitation remained too slow in most countries, particularly the least developed ones. In these countries, trained health personnel had attended to less than 25 per cent of childbirths. The trend of expansion in curative care continued to be stronger than ever; more and more hospitals (including major specialty and subspecialty hospitals) were established at the expense of prevention and promotion.

There was considerable reorganization of comprehensive health systems based on the primary health care approach in most developing countries. During implementation, success in integrating health care was of varying degrees. Some difficulties still persist. For example, despite widespread acceptance by national health administrations of the idea of 'integration', there were many practical operational constraints in undertaking the transformation from semi-autonomous 'vertical' or 'selective' health development programmes, coexisting with the general health services, to an integrated health infrastructure. On many occasions, especially when reviewing or planning disease control programmes, alternatives were sought between an apparently selective approach to health development (vertical health system) and a systematic integrated approach (comprehensive health system). Many countries, using both approaches, had demonstrated positive and negative consequences, depending upon the socio-economic circumstances and the availability of basic health infrastructure. Resource constraints and external pressure forced governments to be more selective in health development. The issues for them were: (a) whether the selective health-care interventions gave priority attention to those types of health problems affecting the poor and the underprivileged populations; (b) whether their health systems addressed all essential health-care functions; (c) whether the country could emphasize comprehensive health care while, at the same time, protecting the technical quality and efficiency of specialized or selective health programmes.

Most nationwide health development programmes promoted increasing community awareness and the creation of active and effective mechanisms for community involvement. Many successful programmes showed that the conventional approach of merely extending basic health services had proved inadequate. It was also proving economically impossible to bear the cost of extension and expansion of public sector health services to the entire population in the face of resource constraints. Large-scale use of health volunteers, after receiving a minimal training programme, proved successful in many countries. These community health volunteers constituted a third force of human resources for health. With their involvement in community health action, many public health interventions—such as disease prevention and control, immunization, maternal and child health care including nutrition promotion, health education, treatment of minor ailments, and environmental health promotion—were undertaken.

Empowering the communities, including local leaders for health action and also through links with other development sectors, had proved successful. Such public health initiatives also received international attention and recognition. The WHO, with the support of partners, promoted the primary health care and Health for All movements by instituting the Sasakawa Health Prize, the Health for All medals, and other forms of recognition. Individuals, groups of experts, local and national institutions, and international associations were amongst the recipients of such coveted prizes and recognition.

The public health experience in the decades of the 1970s and 1980s gave rise to one notable programme—the expanded programme of immunization. This global expanded programme of immunization, initiated by the WHO and UNICEF, has been termed by many as the 'silent public health revolution' of the twentieth century. When the expanded programme of immunization was launched in 1974, fewer than 5 per cent of children under 5 years of age in developing countries were being immunized against major childhood diseases. Nearly 5 million young children were dying every year of measles, tetanus, whooping cough, diphtheria, tuberculosis, and poliomyelitis—childhood diseases that could be prevented by simple and effective immunizations. With the inspiration following successful smallpox eradication efforts, the WHO/UNICEF promoted the expanded programme of immunization to protect all children of the world from the six main vaccine-preventable diseases. The goal of universal childhood immunization was set for attempting to immunize globally 80 per cent of all children less than 2 years of age by the turn of the century. Until the early 1980s, this universal childhood immunization goal seemed impossible to many countries. Nevertheless, concerted efforts by many developing countries in the 1980s and the 1990s achieved remarkable results (Fig. 2).

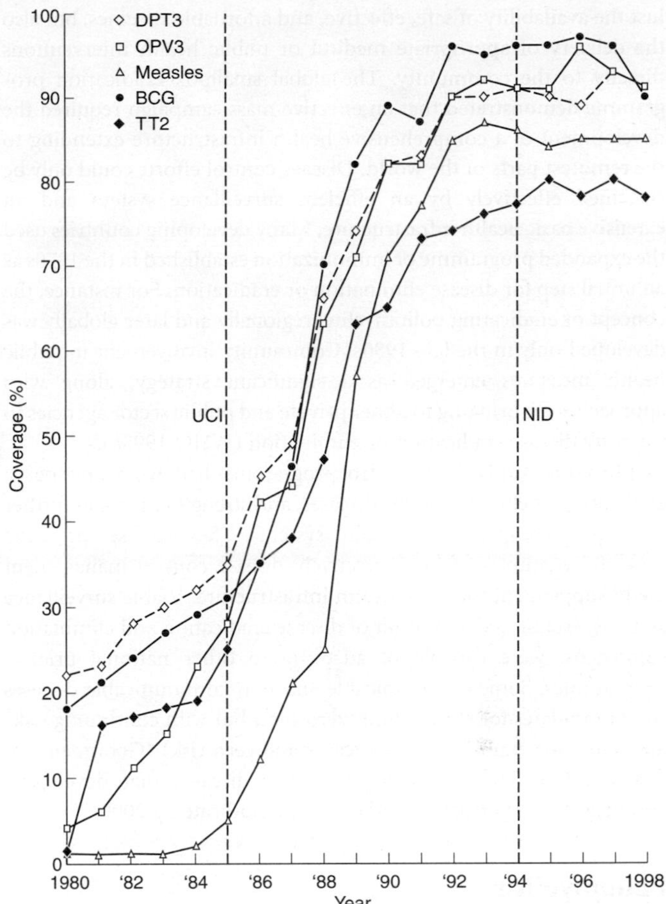

Fig. 2 Trends in immunization coverage in the WHO Southeast Asia region, 1980 to 1998.

This significant achievement was witnessed not only in the WHO Southeast Asia region but also throughout the world, and was made possible due to the full support of the WHO and the United Nations agencies, bilateral and multilateral donors, and international and national non-governmental organizations. In 1990, 80 per cent of all children in the world were successfully immunized against six major vaccine-preventable diseases before they reached the age of 2 years. Immunization coverage in developing countries alone was estimated at 85 per cent for a third dose of poliomyelitis vaccine, 83 per cent for combined diphtheria, pertussis, and tetanus (**DPT**), 90 per cent for tuberculosis (bacille Calmette–Guérin or **BCG**), and 79 per cent for measles vaccine. As a result, the lives of approximately 2 million children were saved. This outstanding coverage was possible because of improvements in the production, transport, and storage of vaccines. A major boost to increasing coverage was also provided by extended social mobilization efforts (UNICEF 1989; WHO 1993).

Eradication and elimination of disease

In the 1980s, the eradication of smallpox aroused the world's interest to adopt eradication and elimination of many diseases as plausible public health strategies. A number of candidate diseases have been examined for possible eradication or elimination. This required not just the availability of safe, effective, and affordable vaccines, but also the delivery of appropriate medical or public health interventions directly to the community. The global smallpox eradication programme demonstrated that an effective mass campaign required the development of a comprehensive health infrastructure extending to the remotest parts of the world. Disease control efforts could only be sustained effectively by an efficient surveillance system and an extensive basic health infrastructure. Many developing countries used the expanded programme of immunization established in the 1970s as an initial step for disease elimination or eradication. For instance, the concept of eradicating poliomyelitis regionally and later globally was developed only in the late 1980s. Community involvement in public health measures emerged as a significant strategy, along with approaches for bringing together private and public sector agencies to intensify disease eradication or elimination (WHO 1998*b*).

Most successful disease control programmes had two main aspects: eradicating or eliminating the diseases, and strengthening and further developing comprehensive health systems. The successes provided powerful examples of how effectively disease control management could supplement the basic health infrastructure. Viable surveillance systems, established as a result of disease eradication and elimination campaigns, were capable of adapting to other national priority programmes. Some communicable and non-communicable diseases were candidates for elimination (zero cases but with continuing risk) and some for eradication (zero cases and zero risk) (Goodman and Foster 1998). The following are a few diseases that developing countries had prioritized to eliminate or eradicate by 2000.

Poliomyelitis

The 41st World Health Assembly in 1988 resolved that the global eradication of poliomyelitis by 2000 represented not only a fitting challenge to undertake, but also an appropriate goal at the end of the twentieth century (WHO 1992). With the increasing coverage of the national expanded programme of immunization/universal childhood immunization programmes, poliomyelitis had been eradicated from the Americas and many other parts of the world by 1991. Yet, many countries in Asia and Africa reported large numbers of cases, infected by wild poliovirus. They also had continuing low coverage of immunization because of inadequate supply of vaccines, lack of appropriate basic health staff, and poorly managed programme implementation. Figure 3 shows the trends of polio immunization coverage amongst different sets of countries from 1980 to 1996.

In the wake of the poliomyelitis eradication programme, an additional significant strategy emerged with intensive advocacy by the WHO—national immunization days. The national immunization day strategy, adopted in polio-endemic countries, supplemented the routine coverage for all children under 5 years of age on certain fixed dates of the year. Usually, national immunization days were spread over 2 or 3 days, or even 4 or 5 days in highly endemic areas, about 4 to 6 weeks apart, during periods of good weather every year for 4 to 5 successive years. Polio cases reported in China dropped from 5000 in 1990 to zero in 1995, as a result of organizing national immunization days in 1993 and 1994. During 1996, in addition to the 500 million routine immunizations to children under 1 year old, a record of 450 million children (almost half of the world's children under 5 years of age) were immunized with polio vaccine during these national immunization day campaigns. In Sri Lanka, for example, a one-day

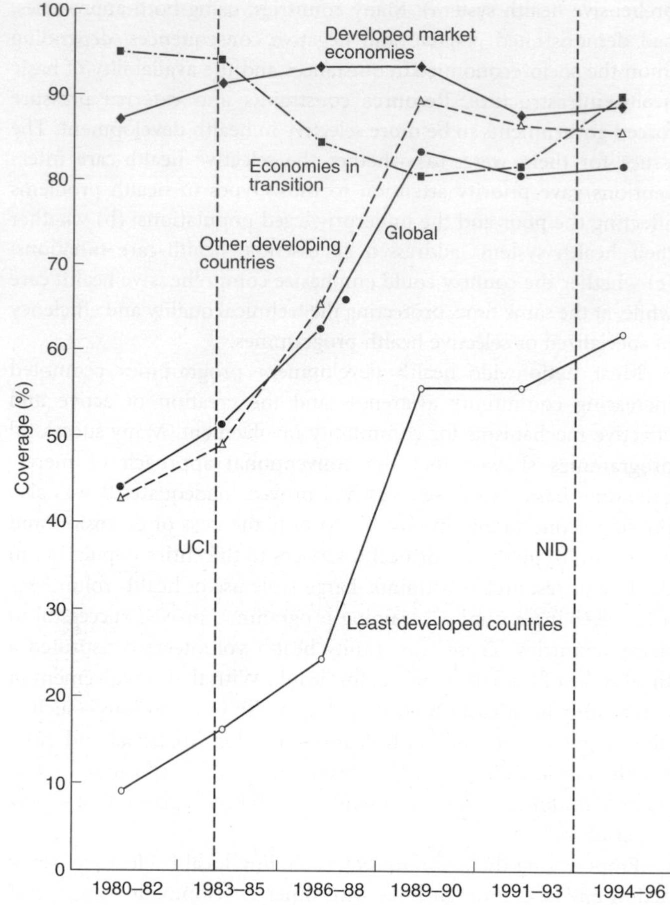

Fig. 3 Percentage of infants immunized against poliomyelitis in countries of different economic groups, 1980 to 1996.

truce—day of tranquillity—was agreed in the midst of civil strife in parts of the country, to enable thousands of children to be immunized. Since then, a number of strife-torn countries have followed similar approaches (Bland and Clements 1998).

Surveillance of acute flaccid paralysis in endemic countries has been intensified through good vigilance, proper case investigation, and prompt laboratory support. A majority of countries around the world are now free from polio infection. Poliomyelitis is on the verge of eradication in a few countries in Asia and the Pacific, but the major reservoir of wild poliovirus transmission remains in South Asia and sub-Saharan Africa. The WHO and UNICEF have urged the leaders of the countries where polio persists to intensify their campaign to eradicate it (WHO/UNICEF 2000). An extraordinary effort to intensify campaigns is required using stronger political will as well as national and international resources. Until the remaining area where transmission of wild poliovirus still occurs is made free from the virus, everybody in the world is at risk. Successful efforts to eradicate wild poliovirus from the world could represent the greatest achievement in public health in the first years of this new millennium (WHO 1998*b*).

While success may be achieved in the polio eradication efforts, there are reports of disturbing declining trends in routine immunization. The donor-driven national expanded programme of immunization, which has been organized solely for the purpose of improved immunization coverage, were short-lived following withdrawal of donor inputs. Each country needs to adopt a strategy for sustainable immunization programmes. Experience has shown that the coverage of pregnant mothers with tetanus toxoid vaccination never reached expected levels in most developing countries. Similarly, there has been a decline in measles vaccination coverage. Intensified efforts are needed to achieve the elimination of measles and tetanus. With the advocacy of the World Bank in 1993, many national programmes started adopting the 'expanded programme of immunization plus'. Vaccines against mumps, meningitis, rubella, hepatitis B, hepatitis C, *Haemophilus* influenza, and yellow fever were added to national immunization programmes. Yet, these additional vaccines were not readily available in many developing countries where they were needed most.

Leprosy

The new goal of eliminating this ancient chronic disease, by the end of the twentieth century, stems from the emergence and extensive adoption of an effective multidrug therapy in the 1990s. With multidrug therapy, many leprosy patients were cured and the total number of infectious cases reduced within a shorter period, thereby interrupting transmission. Early detection and prompt treatment with multidrug therapy has prevented disabilities, thus reducing the burden of disability. Around 1985, there were 10 to 12 million leprosy cases in 122 countries, half of them in South and Southeast Asia. Of these, India alone had an estimated 4 million patients. By 1990, the number had come down closer to 7 million leprosy patients globally. With increasing multidrug therapy coverage, there was a remarkable reduction of registered leprosy cases from 5.4 million in 1985 to 3.7 million in 1990, representing a decrease of 31.5 per cent (WHO 1993). Thus, in 1991, the world community resolved to eliminate leprosy as a public health problem by the year 2000 (Noordeen *et al.* 1996). Generous contributions were made by the International Federation of Anti-Leprosy Associations, the Nippon Foundation of Japan, the United Nations and its specialized agencies, multilateral and bilateral donors, and other philanthropic societies, through necessary financial, material, and human resources, to facilitate all endemic countries to achieve this ambitious goal. As a result, the geographical coverage of multidrug therapy had improved tremendously and the leprosy cases had decreased significantly. By mid-1999, about 1 million leprosy cases remained in the world, mainly concentrated in 24 countries, mostly in South Asia and sub-Saharan Africa. The majority of cases are still in a few states in India. If the current trend is sustained and intensified, the goal of leprosy elimination will be achieved.

Dracontiasis

Dracontiasis (guinea-worm disease, caused by *Drancunculus*) is a parasitic infestation aggravated by poor sanitation and hygiene. Before 1980, there were more than 10 million cases per year in Africa and South Asia. With accelerated efforts to provide safe drinking water and sanitation facilities during the International Drinking Water Supply and Sanitation Decade, the case load of 3.3 million in 1986 was reduced to 1 million by the early 1990s, despite the fact that there was no drug for this disease. In 1991, the World Health Assembly called for the eradication of dracontiasis by 2000. Since then, the endemic countries have adopted control strategies, such as clean water supply, community awareness, and involvement in surveillance and case containment, and larval control with the addition of cash incentives to identify cases. The number of endemic villages decreased tremendously in most endemic countries. Pakistan, for instance, claimed eradication status in 1997, while India was declared free of the disease in January 2000. It is expected that most endemic countries except Sudan will soon be certified dracontiasis-free. The achievement of global eradication is expected in the early twenty-first century.

Onchocerciasis

Onchocerciasis (river blindness) is a highly debilitating disease caused by the filarial worm transmitted by female blackflies in the tropical countries of Africa, Latin America, and the Arabian Peninsula. The WHO, the World Bank, the United Nations Development Programme (**UNDP**), the Food and Agriculture Organization, and a coalition of more than 20 donors and agencies sponsored the global Onchocerciasis Control Programme, initiated in endemic countries in 1974. An estimated 36 million people in West Africa have been protected from the disease. The main attempt at that time was to break the cycle of transmission by eliminating the vector. In 1990, some 86 million people were still at risk and about 18 million were infected. A million people were visually impaired and over 350 000 were blind as a consequence of infection. Almost 95 per cent of those infected were in Africa. The control programme was converted into an elimination campaign in the Americas in 1991 and in Africa in 1996. The new strategy adopted was to eliminate severe pathological manifestations of the disease and to reduce morbidity through wider use of case management with an effective microfilirial drug (ivermectin). The pharmaceutical industry pledged to provide adequate quantities of ivermectin at no cost for as long as the disease persisted as a public health problem. Still, many endemic developing countries could not implement their disease control programmes owing to lack of financial resources to maintain staff and logistic support. With sustained national commitments, completed case treatment, selective vector control, and mass health education campaigns as well as sustained international support, global elimination of onchocerciasis as a public health problem is envisaged in the next few years (WHO 1998*b*).

Emerging and re-emerging diseases

The last two to three decades have witnessed the re-emergence of a number of communicable and non-communicable diseases. Simultaneously, many new or previously unrecognized infections or disease conditions, such as HIV/AIDS and viral hepatitis C, are reported in both developed and developing countries. Complacency towards the prevention and control of many infectious diseases, such as tuberculosis, dengue and dengue haemorrhagic fever, malaria, and plague, in the last three decades resulted in disease control programmes being neglected in many countries. The main factors aggravating this situation were the change in human demographics and job opportunities (mass migration), human behaviour (e.g. sexual relations), improvement in technology and industry (air-conditioning, food processing and preservation, and so on), environmental degradation, microbial adaptation and resistance, the continued legacy of financial and resource constraints, and the breakdown of public health measures (especially surveillance). The latter factors were most common in developing countries, especially during periods of civil strife and natural disasters. Thousands of people were displaced, disabled, or died due to infectious diseases during natural disasters or ethnic conflicts. As a result, a number of diseases or conditions that had been controlled have re-emerged and many new ones have emerged, causing grave concern in developing countries.

HIV/AIDS

AIDS was unknown before 1981; the causal organism, HIV, was discovered in 1983. HIV infection emerged as an explosive pandemic by the mid-1980s, and is by far the most profound infectious disease of the latter half of the twentieth century. It will continue as the most devastating disease of the twenty-first century. Every year a million people are infected and most will die. As soon as the main modes of transmission of AIDS were identified, a global programme on AIDS was initiated in the mid-1980s by the WHO, with the full support of the World Bank, United Nations agencies, and other interested partners. After a decade, its work was consolidated into a new United Nations AIDS Control Programme, which was co-sponsored by United Nations agencies and their development partners.

In the absence of an effective vaccine, the main strategies of global and national HIV/AIDS control programmes were political advocacy, mass education including sex education, behavioural intervention and social mobilization, and integrated social development. Trends in AIDS incidence have differed in various parts of the world. The overwhelming majority of people with HIV and AIDS are in the developing countries of Asia and sub-Saharan Africa. In industrialized countries, the number of deaths due to AIDS has dropped rapidly due to increasing accessibility of proper care and expensive therapy. The progress in improving life expectancy over the past three decades in many developing countries has been reversed by HIV/AIDS, especially in the most severely affected countries (WHO 1999*c*). In Africa, HIV/AIDS has resulted in an increase in both infant and adult mortality. The impact on human development has gone beyond mortality, as the epidemic affects the sustainability of households and the socio-economic resources of communities (UNDP 1998). An effective vaccine is still a long way off and an effective drug therapy is also far too expensive to be widely applicable and accessible to developing countries, especially with the forthcoming implementation measures under multilateral trade agreements, such as TRIPS (the agreement on Trade-related Aspects of Intellectual Property Rights, one of the multilateral trade agreements). The problem of HIV/AIDS is likely to become even worse in the early part of the twenty-first century unless more effective public health interventions are identified and implemented.

Tuberculosis

Tuberculosis emerged as a globally dangerous infection in 1993. At the end of the twentieth century, it became one of the major leading causes of death globally, with 2 to 3 million deaths taking place each year. Annually, about 3 million cases occur in Southeast Asia and nearly 2 million in sub-Saharan Africa, with 340 000 cases in Europe. One-third of the incidence between 1994 and 1999 was attributed to HIV/AIDS. Effective tuberculosis case management, vaccination of infants with BCG, and preventive therapy were the main control strategies. The WHO promoted the use of the 'directly observed treatment, short-course' (**DOTS**) strategy for the effective management of infectious tuberculosis cases. More than 119 endemic countries had adopted this approach by 1998. When DOTS was introduced in 1993, no more than 2 per cent of active tuberculosis cases worldwide were being treated by this new method. By 1998, the DOTS population coverage had reached 43 per cent. The worldwide goal is to have universal DOTS coverage by the year 2005 and to achieve the target rapidly of treating 85 per cent of all active sputum-smear-positive tuberculosis cases successfully, and detecting 70 per cent of such cases. However, resource constraints and the lack of political commitment have hindered programme implementation, thus impeding coverage of all tuberculosis cases under DOTS (WHO 1998*b*, 2000*b*).

Plague

Improvement in sanitary measures, use of antibiotics and insecticides, and keeping good vigilance over dead rats (rat falls) resulted in a dramatic decline in the cases of human plague in many developing countries. Sporadic reporting of rat falls and bubonic plague cases has been noted in many parts of Asia, the Americas, and Africa in the last few decades. The outbreak of plague in India in 1994 created a wave of public panic around the world. Inadequate preventive and control measures caused India to lose a few billion dollars of export earnings. This and similar situations led to an increasing awareness of the relationship between international trade and health, especially the implications of health for multilateral trade agreements (Kinnon 1998).

Yellow fever

The largest epidemic outbreak of another internationally notifiable infectious disease, yellow fever, occurred in Ethiopia in the early 1960s, causing 30 000 deaths. Even though yellow fever can be prevented and controlled through effective immunization, the same number of deaths due to yellow fever persisted globally every year. The disease is still endemic in 34 African countries, including 14 of the world's poorest. Several countries in West Africa reported yellow fever outbreaks during 1994 to 1995. Some countries in South America are still at risk, and Peru reported an outbreak in 1995. At present, air travel is the easiest route of disease transmission. The presence of vectors and non-immune people could lead to a possible epidemic of yellow fever in various parts of the world. Thousands of lives could be lost unless a good surveillance system and higher immunization coverage are sustained.

Viral hepatitis B

Infection due to hepatitis B virus became a global health problem in the late 1980s. In 1990, more than 2000 million people, or two out of every five people on Earth, were affected with hepatitis B virus. About 350 million of them became chronically infected carriers, and of these, one-quarter were at high risk of serious illness and eventual death from cirrhosis of the liver and primary liver cancer (WHO 1998*b*). Although a safe and effective hepatitis B vaccine, the first and currently the only vaccine against a major human viral infection, has been available since 1982, the coverage of immunization with hepatitis B vaccine is still relatively low. The WHO and UNICEF recommended hepatitis B vaccination as an integral part of the national immunization programme. Over 90 countries, most of them in Asia, the Pacific

Islands, parts of South America, and sub-Saharan Africa, have had national programmes so far. Yet, some countries with a high prevalence of viral hepatitis due to hepatitis B virus, especially the developing countries in Asia, are not able to implement immunization of hepatitis B vaccine as a nationwide programme. The delay is due to lack of availability of appropriate and affordable hepatitis B vaccine. With sustained national and international commitments and the resource support of the international community, there is a possibility of achieving a high coverage of hepatitis B vaccine vaccination so that the disease can be eliminated by 2025 (WHO 1999*c*).

Malaria

Even after the integration of extensive eradication campaigns into national control programmes, malaria remains a major public health threat in about 100 countries, most of which are located in the tropics and subtropics. There are 300 to 500 million cases and 1.5 to 2.7 million deaths, 90 per cent of them reported in tropical Africa. Chloroquine-resistant *Plasmodium falciparum* infection, which appeared in Thailand and Colombia in the 1970s, spread to most countries of the tropical world. Recently, chloroquine-resistant *P. vivax* infection has also been reported in Sumatra and Oceania. Many countries had introduced multidrug therapy as the first- and second-line therapy for malaria. The malaria situation in Asia, especially in South and Southeast Asia, and also in some parts of the American and African regions, is alarming, with an increasing spread of multidrug-resistant *P. falciparum* infection. In addition, the vectors of malaria transmission are building resistance against a variety of insecticides. Inappropriate use of insecticides, the fluid movement of people in border areas and other malarial areas, and irrational use of drugs are the major factors for the continuing high prevalence.

Rapid deterioration in the malaria situation in many countries calls for greater efforts by governments of the endemic countries and the full support of the international agencies. In 1998, the WHO initiated a global programme called Roll Back Malaria, as a new health sector-wide partnership, to combat the disease at global, regional, country, and local levels. The programme anticipated a 50 per cent reduction in the number of deaths from malaria within a decade through better access by all people in malaria-affected areas to a range of effective interventions. Early detection and rapid treatment, multipronged interventions, well co-ordinated strategies, focused research, and the development of a dynamic social movement are the major strategies adopted in this global programme. Development partners would work together with the malaria-affected countries to achieve this new goal (WHO 1999*c*).

Diarrhoeal diseases and acute respiratory infections

Developing countries had adopted the prevention and control of diarrhoeal diseases and acute respiratory infections, mainly pneumonia, as part of major public health interventions, as these diseases have always been major causes of morbidity and mortality in infants and young children. Poor sanitation and housing conditions, including unclean and smoky kitchens, inadequate supply of safe water, and improper personal hygiene resulted in a high incidence of diarrhoeal diseases and acute respiratory infection. The total number of acute respiratory infection episodes in young children throughout the world has been estimated to be around 2000 million a year. A child in a developing country suffered from an average of two or three episodes of diarrhoea per year. This resulted in 1500 million episodes of illness, and more than 3 million deaths each year in children under 5 years of age. Acute respiratory infection added another 4.3 million deaths annually. Diarrhoea and acute respiratory infection cases accounted for two-thirds or more of outpatient and hospital admissions in most countries and they often required expensive medications (WHO 1998*b*).

The advent of inexpensive and effective oral rehydration therapy for diarrhoea and simplified case management for acute respiratory infection and other childhood illnesses in the early 1970s resulted in conceivable progress in implementing effective clinical interventions. Even so, progress has been very slow in promoting the integrated management of childhood illness. The action to impart the knowledge and skill to basic health workers on integrated management of childhood illness has required a lot of professional and financial resources. Though integrated management of childhood illness is low cost, simple, acceptable, and effective, only one-third of the developing world's families know about and have access to integrated management of childhood illness. Greater efforts are required to ensure that 80 per cent of the families in the developing countries have access to integrated management of childhood illness, in order to reduce the burden of diarrhoeal diseases and acute respiratory infection (WHO 1998*a*, *b*).

Non-communicable diseases

While infectious diseases continued to be a major public health problem, there were ominous signs that non-communicable diseases were increasingly prevalent in the developing world (Fig. 4).

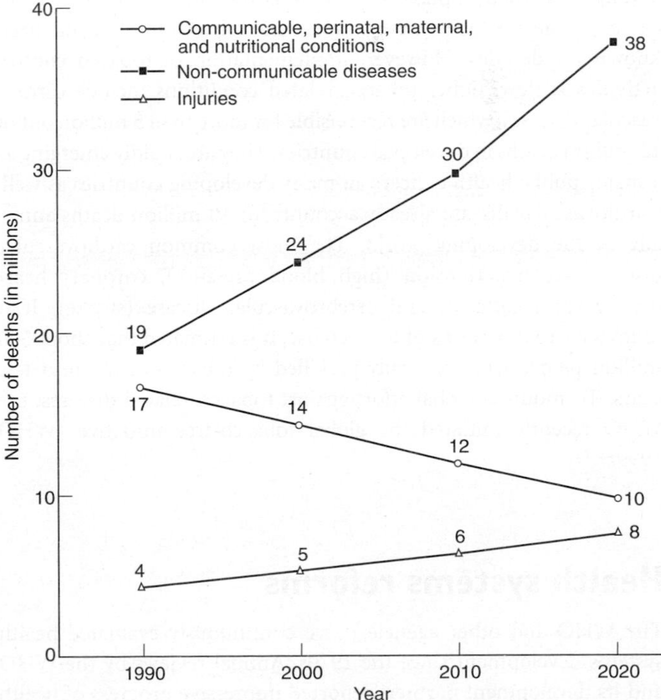

Fig. 4 Causes of death: distribution of deaths by main causes in developing regions for 1985, 1990, and 1997.

Improved longevity, together with changes in lifestyles and diets, and increased use of tobacco and alcohol, had contributed to a sharp rise in the incidence and prevalence of respiratory and cardiovascular disorders, malignancies, and mental illnesses. Many developing countries are not adequately prepared to tackle this double burden of diseases, as evidenced by relatively weak programmes for the prevention and control of non-communicable diseases. Recent estimates of global burden of disease and injury indicated that over 24 million people were expected to die due to non-communicable diseases in the developing world in the year 2000 (actual figures not yet published), and if uncontrolled, another 38 million will die by 2020 (Murray and Lopez 1996).

Although the discovery of insulin to treat diabetes was made in 1921, the disease was reported as an uncommon condition in the developing world. Current estimates indicate that 143 million people are affected with diabetic disease worldwide. The WHO estimates that by 2025 there will be about 300 million people with diabetes. The increase in the number of cases is mainly due to the demographic change and changing dietary patterns, lifestyles, and urbanization. With early diagnosis and effective management, diabetes can be controlled.

During the 1920s, George Papanicolaou introduced the Pap smear test for screening cervical and uterine cancer. This pioneering test is still used for identifying early cases of cervical and uterine cancer. Yet, this type of screening is rarely accessible to young and ageing women who are at greatest risk in rural areas of the developing world. An estimated 425 000 new cases of cervical cancer are diagnosed each year globally, most of them from urban areas. Regular periodic screening, early diagnosis, and prompt treatment can reduce mortality by 85 per cent (WHO 1998*b*).

Cancer of the lung was the highest-ranking cancer in 1997, both amongst the total population as well as the population aged 15 to 64 years. The link between lung cancer and tobacco smoking has been known for decades. However, implementation of tobacco control activities is slow. Other tobacco-related conditions include cardiovascular diseases, which are responsible for more than 5 million out of 12 million deaths in developed countries. They are rapidly emerging as a major public health concern in many developing countries as well. Cardiovascular disease already accounts for 10 million deaths annually in the developing world. The most common cardiovascular diseases are hypertension (high blood pressure), coronary heart disease (heart attack), and cerebrovascular disease (stroke). If it follows current patterns of tobacco use, it is estimated that about 500 million people will eventually be killed by tobacco in the next few years. To mount a global effort against tobacco-related diseases, the WHO recently initiated the global tobacco-free initiative (WHO 1999*c*).

Health systems reforms

The WHO and other agencies have continuously evaluated health systems development since the 1970s. Annual reviews by the WHO and its development partners reported impressive progress of health development in many countries. Concerns were expressed, however, on the widening gap in health status between and within countries. The following are the main factors that slowed down progress in implementing Health for All strategies using primary health care as the key approach:

(1) a lack of full understanding of the fundamental policies and principles of primary health care and Health for All applicable to national health systems development, which led to non-achievement of universal access to essential health care on a continuing basis;

(2) lack of co-ordination and collaboration between specific health intervention campaigns with the development of basic health infrastructure (district health systems development);

(3) difficulties in involving communities in health action;

(4) slow pace of integration of vertical disease control campaigns into the general health infrastructure;

(5) weak planning and management of health-care delivery, especially at the operational levels;

(6) imbalance and irrelevance of human resources for health.

Investments in health from government funds (from either internal or external resources) have declined in many developing countries. The same is also the case for investments by donor agencies in health. Donor support for the development of health systems is usually linked to specific objectives. Donors are generally keen on supporting selective public health intervention projects, especially for control of specific diseases. Thus, the gap between the principles of global solidarity at various international conferences and the implementation of those principles has remained very wide (WHO 1993, 1998*b*; Tarimo and Webster 1994; UNICEF 1996).

In the last decade, there has been widespread democratization in most developing countries. This has led to a certain amount of devolution of power and responsibility to the people, thereby increasing their involvement in the planning and management of development programmes, especially in social, environmental, and economic development. This change in overall government policy and organization, when undertaken, usually extended across all sectors. The World Bank, the International Monetary Fund, and many other multilateral and bilateral donors used these changes as a condition for extending their loans or grants. Many health sector reforms initiated by developing countries in the last few decades included decentralization or devolution as important strategy. However, the approach varied between countries depending on the extent of devolution and decentralization of authority, division of responsibility and resources, and the management capacity at each level of the health systems (Rafei 1993).

Evaluation reports showed that policy formulation and development, capacity building for planning and management at the local level, and the development of operational procedures are the main strategies being adopted to strengthen decentralization efforts. While training in management skills and knowledge are necessary, other facets, such as performance appraisals and quality assurance, including procedural reviews and revisions, delegation of authority and responsibility, assurance of accountability, and on-the-job training and problem solving, also usually need to be in place. Policy and organizational changes across all government sectors are also important for the success of decentralization.

Another trend in health systems development worldwide is the increasing role of the private—both for-profit and non-profit—sector. During the last few decades, the appropriate public and private mix in health systems has been extensively debated. This debate stemmed from the fact that the major proportion of health expenditure was from private sources and that governments could not increase their expenditure on health. The role of the private sector in health care was mainly concentrated in the area of provision of medical care, including health insurance. However, many private agencies are now involved in resource mobilization, health promotion, and also in preventing and controlling major health problems.

Various health systems reforms have been initiated during the last few years in both developing and developed countries in order to enhancing the optimal mix of private and public health provision. Some developing countries started with the introduction of user charges for both outpatient and inpatient care or the provision of private beds. Some had even attempted privatization of public health facilities, whereas others promoted the increasing involvement of private health-care providers in national health development. Some had introduced national health insurance schemes or expanded the existing social insurance coverage. The major changes introduced required the consumers to pay more for health care, especially in poorer countries (Creese 1994; Hanson and Berman 1998). The question of selecting an alternative option between the Beveridge and Bismarck models for health-care financing reform is still under debate. It is not a simple solution of choice, but how the most appropriate mix of the two models can fit within the existing socio-economic, political, and health situation in the country. Governments need to play a strong role in this decision.

Health research and development advance together with technological advancement. Previously, developing countries always relied on the results of research and development done by developed countries, especially in the area of science and technology. Nonetheless, many scientific breakthroughs actually came from experiences gained in developing countries, for example, malaria transmission, dengue vaccination, contraceptives, and multidrug therapy. Since its early years, the WHO has urged the promotion of research capability in developing countries. In the mid-1970s, after the establishment of regional and global advisory committees on medical research by the WHO, the scientific communities from the developing world have played significant roles in international research promotion and development. A series of research studies on the prevention and control of tropical diseases, the promotion of human reproduction including contraception and other fertility control measures, the strengthening of health systems, the protection of environmental health, the control of non-communicable diseases, and testing other essential health and medical care interventions have been initiated.

Partnerships in health research were established in the areas of cancer, human reproduction, and tropical diseases. The International Agency for Research on Cancer was established in 1965, under the aegis of the WHO, to conduct research on environmental biology and cancer. In 1972, the WHO launched a special programme of research, promotion, and development on human reproduction to meet the needs of the developing countries. Later, in 1988, the UNDP, the United Nations Population Fund, and the World Bank joined the WHO in this programme as co-sponsors. This Human Reproductive Research Programme made major contributions to the improvement of reproductive health, especially in the development of different methods of fertility regulation. Currently, a major network of over 110 institutions, mainly in developing countries, is involved in research on human reproduction. Over 1700 scientists from developing countries have been trained in various disciplines in human reproductive research and are participating in global research efforts.

The WHO, together with the UNDP and the World Bank, also established a special programme for research and training in tropical diseases in 1975. This programme concentrated initially on eight tropical diseases: leprosy, malaria, onchocerciasis, yellow fever, Chagas' disease, dengue/dengue haemorrhagic fever, and tuberculosis, all of which have been affecting millions of people in the tropics. Over the last 25 years, the Programme for Research and Training in Tropical Diseases has created more than 30 products related to drugs, diagnostics, and vector control tools, and has another 30 advances (including vaccines) in the pipeline. Research training grants have been provided to about 1000 scientists from developing countries to improve their scientific and research capabilities. After training and assuming influential positions in the ministries of health and national research institutions, many graduate scientists have introduced significant managerial, technical, and political changes (WHO 1999*c*).

In the innovation and intensification phases of primary health-care implementation during the post-Alma-Ata era, people working in public health realized that health systems research was an important tool for innovation. Many countries strengthened their health systems research units within the ministries of health. Some even established separate national institutes to provide appropriate scientific information to the decision-makers. Considerable progress was made in capacity building and capability strengthening in promoting health systems research. There was an enormous increase in the number of health systems research studies carried out. However, when compared with investments in basic science research, the budget allocations for health systems research remain relatively small.

The Ad Hoc Committee on Health Research, established by the WHO and interested development partners, in its report on Investing in Health Research and Development, concluded that the central problem in health research promotion and development was the '10/90' disequilibrium (WHO 1996). According to the WHO–World Bank study in 1990 on the burden of diseases (World Bank 1993), the top 20 diseases and their risk factors are affecting 90 per cent of the world population (Murray and Lopez 1996). An estimated US$ 56 billion was invested globally for health research, yet only 5 to 10 per cent was spent on health research on issues that affected the large majority of the world's population. The Ad Hoc Committee cautioned the global community of the enormous economic and social consequences to society as a whole of such misallocation of resources. This concern became even more important in the context of the public health challenges of the twenty-first century (GFHR 1999). The world community will need to increase efforts to complete the unfinished agenda for preventing unnecessary deaths, sickness, and disability. Essential public health interventions are needed to tackle new, emerging, and re-emerging health problems. A special effort is required to strengthen global capacity and capability to deal with the increasing burden of non-communicable diseases and conditions, and to promote healthy ageing. Both developed and developing countries need to work together to address the inequity and inefficiency of health systems. The successes of current and future efforts in health sector reforms demands international solidarity.

Technical co-operation amongst developing countries, as a mechanism for solidarity, emerged in the 1970s. The United Nations General Assembly in 1972 invited the UNDP Governing Council to identify the best ways of enabling developing countries to share their capabilities and experience, with a view to increasing and improving development assistance. The concept of technical co-operation amongst developing countries was soon recognized as an integral part of international co-operation for development. The United Nations and its agencies, including the WHO, took active steps to promote the concept and its application amongst developing countries. Within the intercountry and regional co-operation mechanisms, technical co-operation in health, through technical expertise, exchange of faculty members, training facilities, and other resources, was promoted. The meeting of health ministers of non-aligned and other developing countries, in 1984, further endorsed the technical co-operation amongst developing countries mechanism and even brought forth an initial plan of action on technical co-operation amongst developing countries for Health for All.

New public health

Public health transition

The final decades of the twentieth century witnessed rapidly changing political situations and severe economic upheavals, especially towards the end of the Cold War. Strong demands were made for pluralistic democracy, good governance, social justice, respect for human rights, and a clearly defined role of the state and for economic globalization. Social expectations and awareness increased in many developing countries. Primarily, progress and development depended on the inherent strength of a nation and its people, their ability to adopt new and appropriate patterns of behaviour, and to embrace social and other forms the freedom which they wished to pursue. The existing trends in developing countries are towards the adoption of more democratic forms of government, achieving peace and prosperity often after prolonged civil and military strife, dismantling of rigid central planning and economic systems, and adopting a more market-oriented economic approach. Many countries are actually preoccupied with domestic problems, but a few have been benefiting from a period of stability and sustainable growth. Such political and socio-economic changes are not achieved without painful choices. Costly repercussions in terms of civil disturbances and economic crises occurred in Eastern Europe, Africa, the Americas, and Asia.

Most developed nations and a few developing countries experienced demographic and epidemiological transitions. These countries had seen parallel reductions in birth and death rates. The age structure of their population had changed from the stage of numerous young and few elderly to nearly equal numbers in most age groups. While developed countries went through epidemiological and demographic transitions covering over two centuries, developing countries were experiencing the same transitions in decades (WHO 1999*c*). Enormous social, economic, and epidemiological changes rapidly followed the demographic transition. Added to this are the deteriorating environmental conditions that hinder sustainable development and human well being. People in developing countries are still not only exposed to traditional environmental health hazards, such as poor water supply and sanitation and inadequate food hygiene, but are also at high risk of the hazards of uncontrolled industrialization. Mismanagement of natural resources and poor living conditions in rural areas and urban slums have also led to higher risk of diseases from degraded environmental conditions (WHO 1997).

There is no doubt that people in developing countries are healthier than their counterparts a century ago. Life expectancy at birth in the least developed nations improved from 31 years in 1950 to 51 years in 1990. Compared with developed countries, which have a life expectancy at birth of more than 70 years, developing countries still have some way to go (WHO 1999*c*). The majority of developing countries in South Asia, the Pacific, Latin America, and sub-Saharan Africa still account for the major proportion of the global burden of communicable diseases. In addition to the higher prevalence of new, emerging, and re-emerging communicable diseases, the prevalence of non-communicable diseases like cancer, cardiovascular diseases, and other chronic degenerative diseases and conditions is also increasing. Inappropriate road conditions and inadequate control of traffic rules and vehicles in developing countries have resulted in high incidences of accidents and trauma. This double burden of disease has made it difficult for health policy-makers and administrators to decide on equitable allocation of scarce resources. Addressing this rapid epidemiological transition may be the biggest challenge for public health at the start of the new century. In addition, there were problems of implementing many international treaties and conventions in health-related areas. One notable example was the difficulty in implementing the biological and chemical weapons conventions. Eradication of smallpox in the human population is an outstanding achievement, but the final extinction of the smallpox virus remaining in a few laboratories has remained controversial from the scientific point of view. Able and dedicated scientists, the general public, and governments, together with the international community, have continued to play their part in meeting the challenge to address the problems associated with the combined burden of communicable and non-communicable diseases in developing countries (Kaplan 1999).

Globalization of public health

Globalization has been a phenomenon that is characterized by worldwide interdependence in all aspects—economic, political, social, and cultural. The transformation of local societies to a global society resulted in the blurring of territorial frontiers. An analysis of the impact of globalization in recent years is now available in the health and development literature (Frenk *et al.* 1997; Chen *et al.* 1999; Society for International Development 1999). It is accepted that globalization has enhanced opportunities for human advancement as well as economic and cultural growth of all peoples. It also offers great potential for achieving health for all. Global markets, finances, technology, knowledge, solidarity, and governance have the ability to improve the health of people everywhere. The UNDP and the World Bank have examined the opportunities and challenges for human and socio-economic development within the present context of globalization and localization, and suggested ways in which the global society should react to these issues, especially in the area of governance, markets, and sustainability (UNDP 1999; World Bank 1999). The threats and opportunities of public health have been analysed extensively within the context of globalization (Jamison *et al.* 1998; Walt 1998; Yach and Bettchner 1998; Berlinguer 1999; Navarro 1999). Similar policy and programme debates at various international arenas have dealt with the changing perception of decision-makers on national health development within the context of globalization, the possibility of exploiting technology advances, the need for national and global solidarity, and the need to sustain moral and social values.

Berlinguer used the term 'microbial unification of the world' for the phenomenon of the transmission of epidemics across countries and continents as part of globalization. Today, local control of the outbreak of a disease has become a global struggle. The rapidly increasing number of people travelling and migrating to neighbouring countries or across the world poses the threat of spread of communicable diseases. As disease agents know no physical boundaries, transmission can take place at any time anywhere in the world. With proliferation of information networks, the news of epidemic outbreaks spread globally almost instantaneously. Exaggerated and sensational news captured the audience rather than a true situation. The WHO, in consultation with its member states, is trying to address this problem by establishing a global disease surveillance system and also by revising the International Health Regulations. Debates continue on how this revision can be done within the framework of globalization.

Microbial and chemical hazards in food are of major concern worldwide. Certain infectious diseases, especially food-borne diseases like cholera, can be carried with food exports and tourism. If the preparation of food and food products is in accordance with good manufacturing practices, and no reported cases of infectious diseases are associated with the consignments, food imports should not be restricted. However, there are many trade-related cases from Asia, the Americas, and Africa where exports from the developing countries are restricted or sanctioned by developed nations because of the occurrence of infectious diseases. Peru lost over US$ 770 million during the 1991 cholera outbreak because of trade sanctions by several countries on imports of Peruvian fish and fishery products. Similarly, India lost around US$ 4000 million from export earnings because of the plague outbreak in a few states in 1994. Several African countries lost millions of dollars because of an embargo on certain fishery products during the cholera outbreaks in 1998 (Kinnon 1998; Miyagishima and Kaferstein 1998). In all these cases, the WHO provided appropriate information on disease outbreaks, and certified that there was no relationship between disease outbreaks and production of foodstuff. The WHO also suggested to the respective governments to apply protective measures based on scientific knowledge and evidence. These activities served to further the international harmonization of sanitary measures aimed at the protection of human life and health. The WHO could work closely with the World Trade Organization, with respect to the public health aspects of international trade disputes arising as a result of disease outbreaks. The WHO could also work with the World Trade Organization in revising the International Health Regulations, while the possibility of the International Health Regulations being formally recognized in future amendments of the multilateral trade agreements could also be explored. The international community needs to work together to ensure that reporting nations, mainly developing countries, are not unfairly penalized.

New facts of socialized public health

It is clear that health and economic development are mutually dependent. Policy-makers in both developed and developing countries are increasingly becoming concerned about finding equitable, realistic, and sustainable approaches for improving the health situation. Unfortunately, experience has shown that many governments in developing countries regard health expenditure by the public sector as purely a commodity of consumption and want to minimize it. The total spending on health proportionate to gross domestic product in these countries is still below 5 per cent. The main issue is not just the low percentage of expenditure, but also the lack of efficiency in the allocation of limited funds. International agencies have encouraged developing countries to set priorities and improve resource allocation.

The WHO has advocated a new paradigm for health that sees health as central to development and to the quality of life. Health development must be achieved through a dynamic yet harmonious balance between health in terms of consumption and health as an investment in the future of humankind (WHO 1992). The World Bank has initiated priority setting in health by introducing the notion of cost-effective public health intervention packages, tailored according to the public financial realities of each country (World Bank 1993). Many developing countries, especially those receiving substantial foreign investments in health, now design essential health-care packages as part of their national health-sector-wide programmes.

The two decades since the Alma-Ata Conference have shown that sustained progress of the Health for All movement using primary health care as the main approach towards achieving the universal goal of health for all is a complex and difficult task for many developing countries. A few developing countries in Asia, Latin America, and Africa showed that they could achieve major improvements in health outcomes while keeping the total public health spending at modest levels. Governments in these countries have consistent development policies and programmes for reaching the poor and the vulnerable populations with the most effective and appropriate preventive, promotional, and curative health interventions, in addition to other social services. The use of health volunteers in providing essential primary health care and also in expanding health knowledge was the success of the decade. Underprivileged people have access to health care (from providers of either public or private), where the right kind of health care is available for common ailments. This universal health-care coverage was one of the major strategies adopted at the Alma-Ata Conference.

In spite of the rapid expansion and improvement in health systems development over two decades, not all citizens in the developing countries have access to minimum essential health care. Many children in some isolated areas of the world are still missed for polio, measles, and tetanus immunizations. Many mothers deliver their babies unattended by trained personnel. A majority of tuberculosis or leprosy cases miss multidrug therapy. The challenge during this century is to ensure access of essential health care to all citizens of the world irrespective of their race, religion, citizenship, or residence. The WHO has advocated the 'new universalism in health': that health care must be compulsory for all, but it does not imply coverage for everything (WHO 1999*c*). Studies have indicated that out-of-pocket payment for any health care could penalize the poor and the underprivileged. Prepayment or any system of risk pooling allows a wide range of incentives for efficient purchase of services. Essential public health interventions can be efficient and effective in quality, and not dependent on who is providing. These essential interventions for each country may need to be defined based upon the health financing mechanisms, health systems infrastructures, social behaviour, and other aspects of socio-economic development.

Public health development in the last few centuries has explicitly shown the need for increasing interdependence between and amongst developed and developing countries, in order to promote the health of the people of the world. The health risks are shared by every citizen of the world and could also be seen as opportunities for improvement. Technological interventions for health care may not be the only solution; socio-economic and ethical dimensions are also relevant for successful implementation of such interventions. Debates have now been initiated on global governance of health. During the last 50 years, many international agencies (both within and outside the United Nations system) have emerged out of necessity to deal increasingly with international developmental issues, both in policy and programme terms, including health and other social development. Each of them has advantages.

Recently, the Director-General of the WHO defined a new role which the WHO could play as a step towards becoming a truly international as well as a global health organization (Robbins 1999; WHO 1999*c*). While the WHO's main mission remains the attainment for all people, of the highest possible level of health, it has further adopted a corporate strategic framework that will enable it to make the greatest possible contribution to world health through increasing its technical, intellectual, and political leadership (WHO 2000). The WHO would like to work with developing countries to focus global efforts to build healthy populations and communities. This will be achieved by addressing the excess burden of sickness and suffering resulting from both communicable and non-communicable diseases, especially in poor and marginalized populations. Partnerships will be established to sustain and support health system development so that equitable health outcomes are achieved and people's demands are met. The vision of the new universalism is realized through the development of an enabling policy and improved institutional environments, both nationally and globally.

The efforts of national and international communities should aim at promoting healthy living, reducing the double burden of disease, and making essential health care accessible to all. Since the Health for All movement, health, equity, and social justice remain the main theme of social policy priority. The social values and principles of solidarity, social justice, and ethics for primary health care and Health for All will be relevant now and in the future. All public health professionals and the international community need to sustain that vision. They need to commit and rededicate themselves to meeting the opportunities and challenges of health development in the twenty-first century.

References

Barton, W.L. (1979). Alma-Ata: signpost to the new health era. *World Health*, July, 10–4. WHO, Geneva.

Basu, Z., Jezek, Z., and Ward, N.A. (1979). *Eradication of small pox from India.* WHO Regional Publication Southeast Asia Series No. 5. WHO–SEARO, New Delhi.

Berlinguer, G. (1999). Globalization and global health. *International Journal of Health Services*, **29**, 579–95.

Bettcher, D.W., Sapirie, S., and Goon, E.H.T. (1998). Essential public health functions: results of international Delphi study. *World Health Statistics Quarterly*, **51**, 44–54.

Bland, J. and Clements, J. (1998). Protecting the world's children: the story of WHO's immunization programme. *World Health Forum*, **19**, 162–3.

Chen, L.C., Evans, T.G., and Cash, R.A. (1999). Health as a global public good. In *Global public goods* (ed. I. Kaul, I. Grunberg, and M.A. Stern). Oxford University Press, New York.

Creese, A. (1994). Global trends in health care reform. *World Health Forum*, **15**, 317–22.

Curtis, S. and Taket, A. (1996). *Health and societies: changing perspectives.* Arnold, London.

Detels, R. and Breslow, L. (1997). Current scope and concerns in public health. In *Oxford textbook of public health* (3rd edn) (ed. R. Detels, W.W. Holland, J. McEwen, and G.S. Omenn), Vol. 1, p. 3. Oxford University Press, New York.

Djukanovic, V. and Mach, E.P. (ed.) (1975). *Alternative approaches to meeting basic health needs in developing countries: a joint UNICEF/WHO study.* WHO, Geneva.

Fenner, F., Henderson, D.A., Arita, I., Jezek, Z., and Ladnyi, I.D. (1988). *Smallpox and its eradication*, pp. 473–516. WHO, Geneva.

Foege, W.H., Millar, J.D., and Lane, J.M. (1971). Selective epidemiologic control in small pox eradication. *American Journal of Epidemiology*, **94**, 311–15.

Foster, G.M. and Anderson, B.G. (1978). *Medical anthropology*, pp. 224–5. John Wiley, New York.

Frenk, J. (1993). The new public health. *Annual Review of Public Health*, **14**, 469–90.

Frenk, J., *et al.* (1997). The future of world health: the new world order and international health. *British Medical Journal*, **314**, 1404.

GFHR (Global Forum for Health Research) (1999). *The 10/90 Report on Health Research 1999.* GFHR, Geneva.

Goodman, R.A. and Foster, K.L. (ed.) (1998). Global disease elimination and eradication as public health strategies. Proceedings of a conference held in Atlanta, Georgia, United States, 23–25 February 1998. *Bulletin of the World Health Organization*, **76** (Supplement 2), 5–162.

Gopalan, C. (1992). *Nutrition in developmental transition in Southeast Asia.* Regional Health Paper, SEARO, No. 21, pp. 9–11. WHO–SEARO, New Delhi.

Gunaratne, V.T.H. (1977). *Challenges and response: health in Southeast Asia Region.* WHO–SEARO, New Delhi.

Guthrie, D. (1946). *History of medicine.* Lippincott, London.

Hanson, K. and Berman, P. (1998). Private health care provision in developing countries: a preliminary analysis of levels and composition. *Health Policy and Planning*, **13**, 195–211.

Harrison, M. (1994). *Public health in British India: Anglo-Indian preventive medicine 1859–1914.* Cambridge University Press.

Henderson, D.A. (1997). Edward Jenner's vaccine. *Public Health Reports*, **112**, 116–21.

Henderson, D.A. (1998). Smallpox eradication—a cold war victory. *World Health Forum*, **19**, 113–19.

Howard-Jones, N. (1974*a*). 1: The scientific background of the international sanitary conferences 1851–1938. *WHO Chronicle*, **28**, 159–71.

Howard-Jones, N. (1974*b*). 5: The scientific background of the international sanitary conferences 1851–1938. *WHO Chronicle*, **28**, 455–70.

Howard-Jones, N. (1977). 2: International public health: the organizational problems between the two World Wars. *WHO Chronicle*, **31**, 449–60.

Institute of Medicine, United States (1988). *The future of public health. Committee for the Study of the Future of Public Health. Division of Health Care Services, Institute of Medicine.* National Academy Press, Washington, DC.

Jaggi, O.P. (1979*a*) *History of science, technology and medicine in India.* Vol. 13: *Western medicine in India: medical education and research.* ATMA RAM, Delhi.

Jaggi, O.P. (1979*b*) *History of science, technology and medicine in India.* Vol. 14: *Western medicine in India: public health and its administration.* ATMA RAM, Delhi.

Jamison, D., *et al.* (1998). International collective action in health: objectives, functions, and rationale. *Lancet*, **351**, 514–17.

Kaplan, M.M. (1999). The efforts of WHO and Pugwash to eliminate chemical and biological weapons—a memoir. *Bulletin of the WHO*, **77**, 149–55.

Kiat, L.Y. (1978). *The medical history of early Singapore*, SEAMIC publication No. 14, pp. 221–35. SEAMIC, Tokyo.

Kinnon, C.M. (1998). World trade: bringing health into the picture. *World Health Forum*, **19**, 397–406.

Ko Ko U (1986). *Public health: myth, mysticism and reality*. WHO–SEARO, New Delhi.

Ko Ko U (1996). Closing the gaps in health care—a holistic approach to medical education. In *SEA regional conference on medical education*, 7–9 February 1996, pp. 152–67. Faculty of Medicine, Chulalongkorn University, Bangkok.

League of Nations Health Organization (1937). *Report of the intergovernmental conference of Far-Eastern countries on rural hygiene*, Bandoeng (Java), 3–13 August 1937. League of Nations Health Organization, Geneva.

McNeill, W.H. (1977). *Plagues and peoples*. Basil Blackwell, Oxford.

Mills, A. (1998). Health policy reforms and their impact on the practice of tropical medicine. *British Medical Bulletin*, **54**, 503–13.

Miyagishima, K. and Kaferstein, F.K. (1998). Food safety in international trade. *World Health Forum*, **19**, 407–11.

Murray, C.J.L. and Lopez, A.D. (ed.) (1996). *The global burden of disease: a comprehensive assessment of mortality and disability from diseases, injuries and risk factors in 1990 and projected to 2020*. Global Burden of Diseases and Injury Series, Vol. I. Harvard University Press, Cambridge, MA.

Navarro, V. (1999). Health and equity in the world in the era of 'globalization'. *International Journal of Health Services*, **29**, 215–26.

Noordeen, S.K., *et al.* (1996). Eliminating leprosy as a public health problem—is the optimism justified? *World Health Forum*, **17**, 109–44.

Paneth, N., *et al.* (1998). A rivalry of foulness: official and unofficial investigations of the London cholera epidemic of 1854, *American Journal of Public Health*, **88**, 1545–53.

Rafei, U.M. (1993). *Primary health care in changing world—Southeast Asia regional perspectives*. Paper presented at the 15th anniversary celebration of the Alma-Ata Conference on Primary Health Care, Almaty, 13–14 December 1993. WHO–SEARO, New Delhi.

Rangarajan, L.N. (ed.) (1992). *Kautilya: the arthashastra*. Penguin Books, New Delhi.

Robbins, A. (1999). Brundtland's World Health Organization: a test case for United Nations reform. *Public Health Reports*, **114**, 30–9.

Rosenfield, A. and Maine, D. (1985). Maternal mortality—a neglected tragedy. Where is the M in MCH? *Lancet*, **ii**, 83–5.

Ryle, J.A. (1943). Social medicine: Its meaning and scope. *British Medical Journal*, **ii**, 633–6.

Sigerist, H.E. (1951). *A history of medicine*. Vol. 1: *Primitive and Arabic medicine*. Oxford University Press, New York.

Society for International Development (1999). Responses to globalization: rethinking health and equity. *Development*, **42**, 1–158.

Tarimo, E. and Webster, E.G. (1994). *Primary health care concepts and challenges in a changing world: Alma-Ata revisited*. Current Concerns: SHS paper No. 7. Document WHO/SHS/CC/94.2. WHO, Geneva.

UNDP (United Nations Development Programme) (1998). *Human development report 1998*. UNDP, New York.

UNDP (United Nations Development Programme) (1999). *Human development report 1999*. UNDP, New York.

UNICEF (United Nations International Children's Emergency Fund) (1989). *States of the world's children, 1989*. Oxford University Press, New York.

UNICEF (United Nations International Children's Emergency Fund) (1991). *States of the world's children, 1991*. Oxford University Press, New York.

UNICEF (United Nations International Children's Emergency Fund) (1996). *States of the world's children, 1996*. Oxford University Press, New York.

Uragoda, C.G. (1987). *A history of medicine in Sri Lanka—from the earliest times to 1948*. Sri Lanka Medical Association, Colombo.

Walt, G. (1998). Globalization of international health. *Lancet*, **351**, 434–7.

Wilkinson, L. and Power, H. (1998). The London and Liverpool Schools of Tropical Medicine 1898–1998. *British Medical Bulletin*, **54**, 281–92.

WHO (World Health Organization) (1957). *Report on rural health conference, 14–26 October 1957*. Document SEA/RH/9. WHO–SEARO, New Delhi.

WHO (World Health Organization) (1964). *WHO Expert Committee on small pox: first report*. World Health Organization Technical Report Series, **283**, 9–11, 15, 24, 31.

WHO (World Health Organization) (1967). *Twenty years in Southeast Asia 1948–1967*. WHO–SEARO, New Delhi.

WHO (World Health Organization) (1978*a*). *A decade of health development in Southeast Asia 1968–1977*. WHO–SEARO, New Delhi.

WHO (World Health Organization) (1978*b*). *WHO, Alma-Ata 1978—Primary health care, Geneva, 1978*. HFA series No. 1. WHO, Geneva.

WHO (World Health Organization) (1986). *Regional Advisory Committee on Medical Research for Southeast Asia. Proceedings of the special session commemorating the tenth anniversary on 12 April 1985*. WHO Regional Publications, Southeast Asia Series No. 15. WHO, New Delhi.

WHO (World Health Organization) (1992). *WHO Collaboration in Health Development in Southeast Asia: 1948–1988*. WHO–SEARO, New Delhi.

WHO (World Health Organization) (1993). *Implementation of global strategy for Health for All by the year 2000: Eighth report on the world situation*, Vol. 1. WHO, Geneva.

WHO (World Health Organization) (1996). *Investing in health research and development: report of the Ad Hoc Committee on Health Research Relating to Future Intervention Options*. Document TDR/Gen/96.1. WHO, Geneva.

WHO (World Health Organization) (1997). *Health and environment in sustainable development: five years after the Earth Summit*. Document WHO/EHG/97.8. WHO, Geneva.

WHO (World Health Organization) (1998*a*). *Evaluation of the implementation of the global strategy for Health for All by the Year 2000, 1979–1996*. Document WHO/HST/98.2. WHO, Geneva.

WHO (World Health Organization) (1998*b*). *World Health Report 1998. Life in the twenty-first century: a vision for all*. WHO, Geneva.

WHO (World Health Organization) (1999*a*). *Health situation in the Southeast Asia Region 1994–1997*, p. 155. WHO–SEARO, New Delhi.

WHO (World Health Organization) (1999*b*). *Nutrition for health and development: progress and prospects on the eve of the twenty-first century*, Document WHO/NHD/99.9. WHO, Geneva.

WHO (World Health Organization) (1999*c*). *World health report 1999*. WHO, Geneva.

WHO (World Health Organization) (2000*a*). *A corporate strategy for the WHO Secretariat*. Report by the Director-General to the 105th Session of the Executive Board. Document EB105/3. WHO, Geneva.

WHO (World Health Organization) (2000*b*). *Global tuberculosis control*. WHO Report 2000. Document WHO/CDS/TB 2000.275. WHO, Geneva.

WHO/UNICEF (2000). *Final push in campaign to eradicate polio*. WHO Press Release WHO/1, 6 January 2000. WHO, Geneva.

World Bank (1993). *The world development report 1993: investing in health*. World Bank, Washington, DC.

World Bank (1999). *The World Development Report 1999/2000: entering the twenty-first century*. World Bank, Washington, DC.

Yach, D. and Bettcher, D. (1998). The globalization of public health. I: Threats and opportunities. *American Journal of Public Health*, **88**, 735–43.

1.4 Countries in economic transition: the history and development of public health in China and Korea

Don Kyoun Kim and Shun-Zhang Yu

Public health in China

'Prevention first—put the stress on prevention' is the motto of public health in China. This is not only the principal health strategy in China, but is also the basis of the ancient ideology of Confucianism. During the period 2838 to 2698 BC the origins of medicine in China were documented in a book called *Shen Nong Bencao*, which identified one hundred oriental herbs, thus establishing the art of Chinese medicine. Once the (unknown) author had tasted these herbs, and identified 70 different kinds of poisons in a single day, he drank tea to detoxify himself. Subsequently, Chinese people have claimed diuretic and rejuvenating properties for tea, and claim that it also reduces cholesterol levels. Since ancient times, Chinese people have used herbs and traditional medicine to cure diseases and have also established methods for prevention, especially the use of ideological proverbs of prevention. For example, the book of *Su Wen* (written around 900 BC during the Tang Dynasty), which is an important traditional Chinese medical text, noted that the wise man did not cure 'post-disease', but cured 'pre-disease'. This book used a dialogue format between the Emperor and Doctor Qihuang; they explained the principles of *yin* and *yang*, together with the aetiology, diagnosis, and treatment of diseases. In the books *Huai Nan Zi* and *Qian Jin Fang* it is argued that the best doctor solves the problem before disease strikes, the intermediate doctor cures the early disease symptoms, and the worst doctor deals with the full-blown condition. Therefore prevention is of utmost importance, and is ultimately better than cure.

There are many records of epidemics in ancient China. The book of *Su Wen* recorded that during the period 147 to 218 BC there were at least nine serious epidemics. Epidemics tended to continue for several years, with some lasting for more than 10 years, and they showed periodicity. During the Tang Dynasty (618–907 BC), leprosy patients were isolated. Later, during the Sung Dynasty (960–1127 BC), a type of human vaccine was commonly used to prevent smallpox, long before Edward Jenner (1749–1823) formally developed the variolar vaccine. People also perceived that they derived good health from drinking boiled water, using primitive pesticides, and disinfecting items of food and clothing by methods such as boiling, fumigating, and steaming. These were especially practised during the May festival. Sewers and lavatories were built in palaces and the homes of noble families before the Qin Dynasty (221–207 BC). The book of *Su Wen* records that, during the Northern Sung Dynasty (960–1127 BC), patients were stricken with mercury poisoning and suffered trembling; also, stone workers who cut into rock were found to suffered lung damage from the powder which was produced during their work. To help to promote health, Chinese people like to follow regular exercise regimes and to preserve their *yin–yang* balance by perfrming exercises such as *tai-chi* (Chinese boxing).

In the early days of the new China, infectious diseases were rife throughout the country. For example, 3400 cases of plague and 43 000 cases of smallpox were recorded in 1950, 100 000 cases of relapsing fever were documented in 1951, and 1.04 million cases of measles and 2.93 million cases of malaria were recorded in 1952. Schistosomiasis prevailed in 12 provinces and cities and 400 counties, with a total of 12 million patients. During that time the national mortality rate was 25 per thousand, infant mortality was 200 per thousand, and the average life expectancy was only 35 years. As a result the government issued a number of policy statements and called upon the people to put prevention first. Ideas included the need to control schistosomiasis and to eliminate four particular pests (mice, mosquitoes, flies, and cockroaches). To prevent infectious diseases, the people were called upon to live more cleanly, and to attain health and safety through individual measures.

By 1995, the national mortality rate had fallen to 7 per thousand, infant mortality was reduced to 33 per thousand, and average life expectancy had increased to 69 years. Most infectious diseases, such as smallpox, relapsing fever, typhus fever, and kalar-azar, were controlled or eliminated. The morbidity rate from notifiable infectious diseases was 185 per 100 000 in 1995. The acute wild-type poliomyelitis virus was under control in China by 1995, but the vaccination and monitoring programme is still continuing. Since the period 1993 to 1998 about 630 million children in China under 4 years of age have received the poliomyelitis vaccination. After 40 years of effort, schistosomiasis was eliminated in five provinces and cities, and was under control in 70.5 per cent of counties.

According to statistical data published in 1993, China has 22 per cent of the world's population but spends only 1 per cent of the global health budget. However, a large majority of the Chinese population now have access to basic health services at an affordable price. There are three main reasons for this.

1. By the late 1970s most of China's rural population had access to basic health services via a three-tiered health network consisting of regional health centres at the provincial, county, and town levels.
2. There are three medical insurance systems: medical care for workers, government welfare for governmental staff, and co-operative medical care, which is a community-based prepayment scheme for villagers.
3. 'Barefoot doctors' (now called rural doctors), who are trained as part-time health-care workers, work in 85 per cent of villages. The

barefoot doctors have led public health campaigns and provided basic curative care. They have also organized mass public health movements and initiated practical schemes like promoting the destruction of the snails which transmitted schistosomiasis.

Since the 1990s, China has been transforming itself into a 'socialist market economy'. This has involved evolving from collective to household agricultural production, phasing out price controls, reforming state-owned enterprises, creating a labour market, and developing new forms of enterprise ownership. Economic and gross national product has since increased rapidly and rural health services have been improving. The main changes have been a reduction in the reliance on state and collective funding, decentralization of public sector health services, and increased autonomy of health facilities.

During this period, rates of infectious disease have been falling, but chronic diseases have become more prevalent. According to the 1990s disability-adjusted life years analysis, the proportions of disability-adjusted life years for communicable, maternal, and perinatal disease were 6.3 per cent in Shanghai, 24.2 per cent in China, and 43.9 per cent globally. However, for non-communicable diseases these figures were 84.1 per cent, 58.9 per cent, and 40.9 per cent respectively. This means that non-communicable diseases have become a major health problem in China, especially in large cities. According to the standardized mortality rate in 1997, cancer ranked first among non-communicable diseases with a mortality of 72.3 per 100 000 (the three most prevalent cancers were of the lung, liver, and stomach), cerebrovascular disease ranked second (60.8 per 100 000), injury and toxication ranked third (27.4 per 100 000), and chronic obstructive pulmonary disease ranked fourth (26.15 per 100 000). After implementation of prevention measures leading to lifestyle changes, comparing rates in 1973–1975 with those in 1990–1992, oesophageal cancer decreased to 44.3 per cent and 14.2 per cent in urban and rural areas respectively, cervical cancer decreased to 78.2 per cent and 64.7 per cent, and nasopharyngeal cancer decreased to 39 per cent and 33 per cent. In urban areas, stomach and liver cancer also decreased to 20 to 30 per cent.

In the twenty-first century, the Ministry of Health intends to reorganize the three-tier health services, strengthen the programme of primary health care, and reform the medical care system (Bloom and Gu 1997). They want to focus on community health and promote more health measures concerned with ageing and younger people. Healthy cities will be used as examples for good chronic disease control, such as Qidong for liver cancer control, Ling Zhou for oesophageal cancer control, and Beijing for cerebrovascular disease control.

In 2001, the Chinese Ministry of Public Health decided to improve the medical care system. Firstly, all workers will establish a personal account for their own basic medical insurance, which is paid for by the employee and the employer. This personal account will pay for treatments such as outpatient visits and medicine for less serious illnesses. Secondly, 'low-level high-coverage' insurance means that the insurance system will provide cheap coverage for other common diseases. Most people will have this type of medical coverage, but other more expensive treatments will have to be covered by private medical insurance.

In 1997, China's immunization programme covered more than 95 per cent of children, including vaccines for bacille Calmette–Guérin (tuberculosis), poliomyelitis, diphtheria–tetanus–pertussis, and measles. Moreover, inoculation with the hepatitis B vaccine has been achieved in 96.6 per cent of infants in urban areas and 40 per cent in rural areas, with the carrier rate decreasing to 1 to 2 per cent in some cities. However, sexually transmitted diseases, hepatitis, diarrhoea, and HIV/AIDS have been increasing.

In the twenty-first century, the public health services in China will address and manage health issues, whilst the government addresses social and economic reform. Meanwhile, new problems are developing such as how to deal with the health problems associated with rural migration to the cities, how to collect surveillance data on health, and how to further enhance disease control systems.

Public health in Korea

Korea is a peninsula located on the eastern part of the Asian continent. It is bordered by the Aprok River, Mount Paektu, and the Tuman River of Manchuria, China proper, and the Martine Province of Siberia in the north. To the east it faces Japan and the Pacific Ocean beyond the Dong-Hae (the East Sea), and to the west it faces the Hwang-Hae (the Yellow Sea).

Korean culture has been greatly influenced by China, and medicine is no exception. Chinese medicine has been imported since ancient times, and so the Korean traditional medical literature is written in Chinese. However, continuous efforts have been made to develop traditional medicine based on Korean thought (Huh 1997).

In 1728, Western medicine began to be imported through the Chinese versions of Western medical almanacs published in China. The treatment of Koreans using Western-style medicine began in 1877, when the Japanese Navy set up Chaesaeng Hospital in Pusan, Korea, to treat Japanese residents. The medical missionaries who came to Korea in 1884 also contributed to the introduction of Western medicine.

In 1894 the administration system of health was reformed on the basis of Western medicine. The Korean government established the Bureau of Hygiene in the Ministry of Home Affairs, which was responsible for medicine, prevention of infectious diseases, and vaccination.

The teaching of Western medicine began with the establishment of government medical schools and municipal medical schools by the American Christian missions in 1899. However, in 1905 public health and medical education in Korea became dependent on Japanese medicine, which was based on German medicine.

Before the end of the Second World War (from 1910 to 1945) the Korean Public Health Service, particularly environmental hygiene and the prevention of infectious diseases, was operated by the hygiene section of the Japanese police. It was enforced as a military colonial policy, with the position of medical doctors being elevated in the field of health and quarantine. They made full use of their knowledge of modern medicine in the prevention of infectious diseases, the eradication of endemic diseases, and quarantine at sea ports (Cha 1984).

At the end of the Second World War, Korea was divided into North Korea and South Korea. In South Korea, the Department of Public Health and Welfare of the United States Military Government Office introduced a broader sense of public health. Since then, efforts have been made to introduce a modern public health system, but a lack of health experts as well as unfavourable economic and social conditions have resulted in serious problems in public health improvement.

Radical changes in the public health service were initiated in the Fourth Five-Year Economic Development Plan (1977–1981). For the past 30 years rapid industrial growth has brought continuous economic development and sociopolitical changes in all aspects of Korean society, including lifestyle. Such changes have affected the health of the Korean people, both directly and indirectly, and the prevalence and types of diseases experienced.

The increase in national income, improvement in hygiene and nutrition, and successful family planning have resulted in a reduction in the birth rate. The development of medical care and the enforcement of health insurance regulations have enabled more people to receive medical benefits. Conversely, industrialization, population growth, urbanization, the increase in vehicles, and serious environmental pollution have resulted in an increase in occupational diseases, industrial disasters, and traffic accidents. In addition, diet has changed to one high in fat and calories, and chronic diseases (e.g. heart disease, cancer, and diabetes), mental disorders, suicide, murder, and infectious diseases have all increased.

The next section describes the history and development of public health in Korea and its future.

Improved national health in Korea

Korean national health has been improved over the past 40 years with the increase in income, the improvement of living conditions, and the development of better public health (Cho *et al.* 1998).

The average life expectancy of Koreans increased from 52.5 years (51.1 years for men and 53.7 years for women) in the 1960s to 73.5 years (69.5 years for men and 77.4 years for women) in 1995, an increase of about 1 per cent per year (Cho *et al.* 1998).

The crude birth rate was about 40 per 1000 people before 1945, and then fell slowly until 1953. The baby boom after the Korean War increased the birth rate, which reached its highest level of 43 per 1000 in 1960. Family planning, which was enforced at the beginning of the 1960s, reduced the birth rate to 14.6 per 1000 by 1997, while the natural rate of increase was 9.3 per cent (National Statistical Office 1998*a*). The net reproductive rate was 2.3 in 1960, and declined to 1.6 in 1975. This success of national family planning attracted international attention.

The crude death rate was 20 to 25 per 1000 in the early 1940s. This rate fell temporarily after 1945, but increased to 30 per 1000 between 1950 and 1955 as a result of the Korean War. Social stability, economic rehabilitation, and the spread of a modern health service helped to reduce the death rate to 13 per 1000 in 1960, 8.8 per 1000 in 1965, 7.7 per 1000 in 1975, 7.3 per 1000 in 1990, and 5.3 per 1000 in 1997. The declining trend is predicted to continue for some time, but the crude death rate is expected to rise again because of the changing age structure of the population with increased numbers of elderly people.

The infant mortality rate was about 60 per 1000 babies between 1955 and 1960, 45 per 1000 in 1970, 10 per 1000 in 1991, and 9 per 1000 in 1995 (National Statistical Office 1998*a*). The rate is approaching that of developed countries, i.e. 5 to 10 per 1000 babies (WHO 1988). This decline was not achieved suddenly during any specific period, but gradually over a long period of socio-economic development.

Korea's proportional mortality indicator was between 25 and 26 per cent before 1945. This figure indicates high infant mortality and low life expectancy. The proportional mortality indicator continued to rise to 75.9 per cent in 1992 (National Statistical Office 1992*a*). This resulted in a change in the shape of mortality; the proportion of infant deaths declined while the proportion of elderly deaths rose.

The maternal mortality rate is closely related to nutrition and environmental hygiene, such as birthplace and parturition control, and the level of prepartum, delivery, and postpartum care. The maternal mortality rate in Korea was 30 per 100 000 people in 1990, and 20 per 100 000 in 1995 (National Statistical Office 1998*a*). This rate is lower than that of developing countries (100 per 100 000) but higher than that of developed countries (3–10 per 100 000) (World Health Statistics Annual 1988).

In the 1950s, the main cause of death was infectious diseases. This shifted to chronic degenerative diseases during the 1960s and 1970s. In the late 1970s, the main causes were chronic degenerative diseases such as malignant cancer, cerebrovascular diseases, hypertensive diseases, and chronic liver diseases due to the increased number of elderly people. The death rate due to traffic accidents increased markedly during the mid-1980s (Kim 1989). Causes of death are now distributed as follows: diseases of the circulatory system, 23.4 per cent; cancers, 22.2 per cent; accidents, 13.6 per cent; diseases of the digestive system, 6.6 per cent; diseases of the respiratory system and endocrine and metabolic disorders, 3.9 per cent (National Statistical Office 1997).

The proportion of chronic diseases rose from 20.5 per cent in 1992 to 29.5 per cent in 1995. Chronic diseases made up 55.4 per cent of all diseases in 1992, and 69.1 per cent in 1995 (Lee 1997). Peptic ulcer, gastritis, dental caries, arthritis, hypertension, and diabetes accounted for 43.5 per cent of all the chronic diseases suffered.

Korea's health expenditure was 2.28 per cent of the gross domestic product in 1975, 4.26 per cent in 1985, 5.15 per cent in 1990, and 5.89 per cent in 1996.

One Korean medical doctor was responsible for 2207 persons in 1975, 1690 persons in 1980, 1007 persons in 1990, and 735 persons in 1997. There was one hospital bed for 451 persons in 1988, and one bed for 423 persons in 1997. The number of persons per bed and per doctor is decreasing gradually (National Statistical Office 1998*b*).

The calorie intake per day was 9 kJ (2150 kcal) in 1970, 8.6 kJ (2052 kcal) in 1980, and 7.8 kJ (1868 kcal) in 1990 (Ministry of Health and Social Affairs 1994*a*). This decreasing trend was confirmed in several surveys of people of various ages (Kim *et al.* 1989, 1993; Yoon *et al.* 1990; Lee and Kim 1994).

Determinants of health in Korea

Socio-economic status

The population growth rate in Korea decreased from 3 per cent in 1960 to 1 per cent in 1995 as a result of the low birth rate which was achieved by the family planning programme as part of the economic development plan. This decreasing trend is expected to continue and the growth rate is predicted to be zero in 2028. After that, the population will decrease (Chang *et al.* 1996).

The gross national product per person was less than US$100 during the 1960s. Korea's recent remarkable economic growth increased annual personal income to US$802 in 1976, US$2242 in 1985, US$5883 in 1990, and US$10 037 in 1995. However, in 1997 it declined to US$9511.

The household distribution by monthly income in 1996 was as follows: the highest 21.8 per cent of households had a monthly income of US$1900 to 2500, the second highest 17.7 per cent had US$2500 to 3000, and the next 12.2 per cent had US$1500 to 1900 (National Statistical Office 1998*b*).

Working environment (Kim 1998)

The total number of workers in the 178 000 industrial plants employing five people or more was 6.6 million. Plants employing less than 50 workers accounted for 87.7 per cent of the total number of workplaces, and included 39.2 per cent of the total work force. Conversely, enterprises with more than 300 workers accounted for only 1.2 per cent of the total number of workplaces and 27.9 per cent of the total number of employees.

The increase in the number of workplaces and workers has resulted in an increase in industrial accidents and occupational diseases. According to the data from the Workers' Compensation Scheme, during the period 1970 to 1988 the number of plants and workers increased by factors of 7.5 and 4.7 respectively, and the total number of people injured, disabled, or killed as a result of industrial accidents increased by factors of 3, 5.2, and 3 respectively. Since then, accidents have gradually decreased due to preventive policies introduced by the government. In 1994, 82 352 (1.1 per cent) of a total of 7 273 132 people were injured in industrial accidents; of these, 29 907 (0.4 per cent) were disabled and 2678 (0.03 per cent) died. The average frequency rate and severity rate of industrial accidents were 4.7 and 2.9 respectively. This is attributable mainly to poor safety facilities in factories and insufficient training of workers. The frequency rates were higher in the mining and construction sectors and smaller industries. As for the causes of accidents, large industrial plants had higher accident rates due to power-driven machinery, while accidents in small plants were mostly related to work performance.

According to a nationwide annual medical examination reported in 1994, there were 8568 cases (1.3 per cent) of occupational diseases amongst 672 406 workers employed in hazardous working conditions and 129 842 cases (3.7 per cent) of non-occupational diseases in the 3 526 564 people examined. Major occupational diseases included pneumoconiosis, noise-induced hearing loss, occupational dermatitis, lead, chromium, mercury, carbon monoxide, and organic solvent intoxication, and diseases caused by heat, high barometric pressure, radiation, and vibration.

Educational attainment of the population aged 25 years or more is as follows (National Statistical Office 1998*b*): among males, 41.4 per cent are senior high school graduates, 26.6 per cent are university graduates, 17.8 per cent are primary school graduates or have not received any education, and 14.2 per cent are middle school graduates; among females, 35 per cent are primary school graduates or have not received any education, 34.8 per cent are senior high school graduates, 17.1 per cent are university graduates, and 13.1 per cent are middle school graduates.

The rate of housing supply in Korea increased annually from 71.2 per cent in 1980 to 72.4 per cent in 1990, 86 per cent in 1995, and 92 per cent in 1997 (National Statistical Office 1998*b*). Households by type of housing are as follows: detached dwellings decreased from 95 per cent in 1970 to 59.8 per cent in 1995; during the same period, apartments increased from 0.7 to 26.9 per cent, while town houses and apartment units in private houses increased from 3.6 to 8.8 per cent. During the past 15 years, the number of detached dwellings decreased while the number of apartments increased by a factor of 38.4 and town houses and apartment units in private houses increased by a factor of 2.4.

Nutrition

A national survey of nutrient intake has been completed annually since 1969. Furthermore, various health indices, the distribution of selected health parameters, and nutritional status have been estimated every 3 years since 1998.

In 1962, the Korean Food and Agriculture Organization, after consultaion with nutritionists, biochemists, and clinicians, published recommended dietary allowances for Koreans. The aim was to educate people to the fact that nutrition is very important for improving physical fitness. It has been revised every 5 years, and the sixth version was produced in 1995 (Moon 1995). The recommended dietary allowances are the level of nutrition that satisfies the basic nutritional requirements.

The daily energy intake was consistent at about 8.4 kJ (2000 kcal) between 1969 and 1998. The energy intake from grains decreased from 84 per cent in 1971 to 65.8 per cent in 1991.

The daily protein intake increased from 60 g in 1970 to 80 g in 1990. Half of this intake was from animal protein. The fat intake per day was 13 g in 1971 and 35.9 g in 1994. Intake of other nutrients, except for calcium and vitamins, is increasing. In a survey of nutrition in 1994, energy, calcium, vitamin A, and riboflavin were below the recommended levels (Ministry of Health and Social Affair 1994*a*). Fewer calories were obtained from carbohydrates, while more calories were obtained from protein and fat. This survey indicated that the average Korean consumed 85 per cent of the recommended energy allowance, 121.8 per cent of the recommended protein allowance, and 91 per cent of the recommended calcium allowance.

The problems of nutritional status in Korea are as follows: (a) a disproportionate nutrient intake among different income groups and among various districts; (b) poor care of expectant mothers, infants, and the aged who are too weak to take in nutrition; (3) lack of food-related policies based on the national nutrition conditions.

The patterns of the Korean diet are changing: dining out and consumption of meat and instant foods are increasing, while consumption of rice is decreasing. Differences by income, social strata, and geographical region lead to disparity between some sectors. In addition, various basic data for nutrition are not well understood. The government and the general public have little comprehension of nutrition. Early nutritional control for the improvement of national health has been weak (S.S. Choi 1999*a*).

Environmental conditions

Korea has always been dependent on agriculture. However, during Japanese rule of Korea (1910–1945), the munitions industry was given priority over resources. Most of the heavy industries, such as the metal-working and chemical industries, were in North Korea, while the light industries, such as textiles, food, and printing, were in South Korea (Cho 1979).

After the Second World War, political conflict, social insecurity, and the Korean War (1950–1953) destroyed almost all the industrial facilities in South Korea. However, development of heavy industries, such as the fertilizer, cement, and metal-working industries, began in the 1950s . In the early 1960s, industrial complexes were founded in Pohang, Ulsan, Sasang, and Kumi under the supervision of the national government, which promoted industrialization in Korea and rapidly developed the Korean economy. The use of large quantities of fossil fuel increased exhaust fumes from factories which had poor refining systems. The discharge of unpurified waste water into rivers emerged as a serious social problem by the end of the Second Economic Development Plan (1962–1966). In fact, it was when the United Nations adopted a human environment declaration at the International Conference of the Environment that the environmental problems in Korea first attracted international attention.

As humans we are a constituent of the ecosystem, yet we are the main cause of environmental destruction. It has been recognized that people themselves are responsible for the preservation of the environment and the control of resources. In order to discharge this responsibility, the following statement about environmental rights, 'All people have the right to live in a clean environment, and the government and the people should try to preserve the environment', was enacted as Article 35 in the Constitution of the Sixth Republic. At the same time, in 1963, the government enacted a law against environmental pollution and prepared to preserve the environment.

However, this law was ignored until 1976, because of the primacy of economic development that focused on quantitative growth. In 1977, laws regarding environmental preservation established systematic devices such as an establishment of environmental standards and the evaluation of environmental effects. In 1980, a governmental body, the Office of Environment, was established and subsequently became the Department of Environment. The laws regarding the preservation of the environment were changed completely to include laws regarding principles of environmental policy. These laws provided the foundation on which policies could be established regarding broad environmental control whilst taking into account both the ecology and the economy.

Since 1996, six pollutants (dust, sulphuric acid gas, carbon monoxide, carbon nitrogen, ozone, and lead) have been measured at 111 air pollution monitoring stations located in 47 cities all over Korea. Air pollution due to sulphuric acid gas and minute dust particles has decreased in the larger cities, but ozone levels have increased. Smog is a serious problem, and the solution has yet to be found. Owing to the increasing number of vehicles, increasing industrialization, and urbanization, noise has become a problem and the environmental standard for noise is exceeded in most geographical districts. In the future, noise pollution may become much more serious. Recently, noise pollution has increased due to the increase in air traffic.

In 1995, the Department of the Environment began enforcing an alarm system to reduce the damage by ozone gas. More important has been the effort to reduce the quantity of discharged ozone.

The distribution of sources of air pollution in 1994 was as follows: traffic, 47.5 per cent; industry, 29.5 per cent; electricity generation, 14.2 per cent; heating generation, 8.8 per cent. The main sources of water pollution are domestic sewage (12 638 000 m^3/day in 1994) and factory waste water (7259 000m^3/day in 1994). Any increase in sewage results in a further reduction in the water quality of rivers flowing through the larger cities (Ministry of Environment 1996). In addition, the increase in livestock industries and their waste accelerates the pollution of rivers in agricultural districts. Waste increases with economic development and improvements in the quality of life, but it has not been treated properly. Waste disposal is one of the most serious environmental problems requiring solution. Pollutants originating on land cause 80 per cent of the eutrophication of the sea. Wreckage of oil tankers and other large ships also damages fishing grounds.

The first water supply facilities in Korea, whose source was located at the Pummo Temple, were built by the Japanese in 1905 for the purpose of supplying water to ships. The first water supply facilities for the Korean population were built at Tuksom by American engineers in 1908. They used a slow-filtration method with a capacity of 12 000 t/day. As a result of the renovations in the 1950s after the Korean War and a population increase and rapid industrial development in the 1960s, water supply facilities have improved.

By the end of 1996, 83.6 per cent of the Korean population (about 38 820 000 people) were supplied with tapwater. The capacity of water supply facilities in Korea is 22 910 000 t/day. The distribution of water supply facilities by geographical districts is as follows: 98.1 per cent to the six large cities, and 1.9 per cent to small or medium-sized cities and to fishing and agrarian village districts. Most of the residents in the fishing and agrarian villages take drinking water from provisional water supply facilities and wells. The central or local government needs to exert more effort on expanding the water supply system.

In 1996 only 53 per cent of sewage in Korea was treated in disposal facilities. The government is planning to build 180 sewage disposal facilities in order to increase this figure to 70 per cent. Because of the high population density in Korea, the water from the upper reaches of rivers, with various types of sewage discharged into it, is collected as drinking water lower down. To improve this situation, 15 filtration plants on the four major rivers are changing their purification systems to an advanced disposal system using ozone or granular-activated carbon.

Lifestyle

Health behaviours may be divided into those that can threaten health and those that can promote health and prevent diseases. Behaviours that can threaten health include unhealthy eating, smoking, and drinking (S.S. Choi 1996; National Statistical Office 1998*b*).

Eating is the basic element of all health-promoting behaviours. In Korea, 60.7 per cent of the population have regular eating habits, but this proportion is decreasing amongst young people; 71.9 per cent regularly eat breakfast, but more and more young people generally skip breakfast. Eating between meals is known to be harmful to health, but 59.6 per cent of the Korean population enjoy between-meal snacks. This is much lower than in the West (70 per cent), but the proportion is increasing in the younger generation. While sweets are a serious problem for Westerners, spicy and salty food are a problem for Koreans; 52.7 per cent of the population enjoy spicy and salty food. Many Koreans consume supplementary nutrients such as high-calorie food or tonics: vitamins and minerals (22.6 per cent), oriental herbs (20.5 per cent), honey (18.6 per cent), black goat meat (7.2 per cent), Korean traditional mushrooms (5.7 per cent), and others (5.3 per cent). Males show a higher preference for supplementary nutrients than females. In addition, the elderly consume more supplements than young people.

National surveys show that the proportion of male smokers has remained steady at 73.2 per cent in 1992 and 73 per cent in 1995. In terms of smoking quantity, the proportion of male smokers who consume 10 to 20 cigarettes a day has decreased from 59 to 57.7 per cent, and the proportion of female smokers who consume less than 10 cigarettes or less a day has increased from 61.3 to 62 per cent.

Generally, smoking begins in the late teens or early twenties. Therefore antismoking education would be most effective during this period. Smokers who wish to quit smoking constitute 53.5 per cent of all smokers, and the number of non-smokers has been increasing in recent years. The number of male non-smokers is increasing rapidly.

Alcohol is known to be helpful in reducing the risk of myocardial infarction, improving the quality of life, and relieving stress. However, excessive alcohol use causes social, psychological, and physical problems. Social problems include low work productivity, divorce, and family conflicts. Psychological problems include insomnia, depression, suicide, amnesia, senile dementia, etc. Excessive drinking is also associated with hepatitis, gastrointestinal disorders, diabetes, obesity, hypertension, and other diseases (WHO 1990). Male adult drinkers decreased from 84.7 per cent in 1992 to 83 per cent in 1995, while female adult drinkers increased from 33 to 44.6 per cent during the same period. From the age of 20 onwards, the number of drinkers is similar to that of smokers, irrespective of age above the twenties. Non-drinkers who do not smoke make up 50.7 per cent of the population, while 75.6 per cent of drinkers also smoke. Furthermore, the more one drinks, the more one smokes.

The most effective health behaviours are regular physical exercise and regular eating habits. However, few Koreans take proper exercise. Koreans who exercise regularly made up 14.3 per cent of the population in 1992 and 18.1 per cent in 1995 (National Statistical Office 1998*b*). In urban areas, the proportion taking regular exercise was highest among young people. Most people who take physical exercise do so frequently and for long periods. The most common exercise activities are running, skipping, mountain climbing, walking, light gymnastics, swimming, and tennis.

Self-assessment of health is generally categorized as excellent, good, fair, poor, and very poor. In the national survey of the Korean population in 1992, 85.8 per cent of the respondents believed that they were healthy (excellent, 5.8 per cent; good, 40.7 per cent; fair, 35.3 per cent). In a subsequent survey in 1995, 80.6 per cent of the respondents believed they were healthy. The proportion of respondents who believed that they were unhealthy increased from 18.2 per cent in 1992 to 19.5 per cent in 1995.

Health care is an essential element in improving health. According to the 1995 survey, methods of improving health care included exercise (18.1 per cent), diet (17.4 per cent), moderation in smoking and drinking (5.3 per cent), and other activities (8.8 per cent); however, 42.7 per cent of the respondents did nothing. Compared with 1992, more people were interested in taking care of their health via exercise, diet, and bath or sauna treatments, which are seen as a form of exercise in Korea by promoting blood circulation and metabolism, and increasing the excretion of excess hormones and other waste materials.

Average weekly working hours

The average length of the working week in manufacturing industries was 49.8 h in 1990, 49.2 h in 1995, and 48.4 h in 1996. These figures shows that working hours have been decreasing in recent years, but are still longer than those in developed countries.

The population of Korea

The combined population of North and South Korea in 1925 was 19.5 million in 1925; in 1949, the population of South Korea alone was approximately 20 million (Hong 1979). Between 1944 and 1950 the population increased by about 4 million. This increase of over 40 per cent is based not only on simple natural increase, but also on social phenomena such as the return of Korean nationals from abroad (e.g. Japan and Manchuria) and defections from North Korea.

The Korean War resulted in a population decrease and displacement, and restricted the population growth rate to about 10 per 1000 between 1949 and 1955. Since 1953, the mortality rate has rapidly reduced, and Korea experienced an annual population growth rate as high as 28.8 per 1000 between 1955 and 1960.

During the last 50 years, rapid economic development and an increasing quality of life have resulted in a variety of population shifts. With a rapid decrease in death and birth rates, Korea experienced a demographic turnaround in 25 years similar to that undergone in a century in Western countries. Korea's population was 31 435 000 in 1970, 36 790 000 in 1975, 37 400 000 in 1980, 44 480 000 in 1985, and 44 609 000 in 1995. The respective mortality rate per 1000 during these periods was 9.8, 7.3, 6, and 5.4, the birth rate was 29.5, 24.6, 22.7, 16.2, and 15.8 respectively, and the natural increase was 19.7, 17.3, 15.4, 10.2, and 10.4 per cent respectively. Korea now has a similar population structure to that of developed countries.

The Korean government introduced a family planning programme as part of its Economic Development Plan in the early 1960s because of the high population density and Korea's limited territory and natural resources. In the early 1960s, Korea's fertility reached 6 per 1000 and the average life expectancy was 52.6 years. The structure of Korea's population was a typical pyramid shape, based on a high fertility rate and a high mortality rate. However, through social and economic development, together with the government's strong family planning programme, the fertility rate has been decreasing rapidly. The total fertility rate reached 2.1 in the mid-1980s, which is the substitution level for the population. Since then, Korea has maintained a low birth rate. Despite the fact that the government has made substantial cutbacks in the family planning programme, the total fertility rate in 1997 was 1.56 (Table 1) (National Statistical Office 1998*c*).

According to the National Statistical Office (National Statistical Office 1996), the fertility rate will remain below the substitution level of the population in the twenty-first century. The annual population growth rate is predicted to fall from 0.98 per cent, which was maintained between 1990 and 2000, to 0.68 per cent between 2000 and 2010, and to 0.34 per cent between 2010 and 2020. It will eventually reach zero by 2028. After that, the mortality rate will exceed the birth rate, resulting in a negative growth rate which will result in an absolute decrease in the population. The population will exceed 50 000 000 for the first time in 2008, and it will reach a maximum of 52 776 000 in 2028. The population shift was predicted to increase by 46.6 per cent between 1970 and 2000, and by 11.6 per cent between 2000 and 2030. It can be foreseen that the scale of the population shift will not be as large in the twenty-first century as before.

People aged 60 and over formed 3.9 per cent of the whole population in 1980, 5.0 per cent in 1990, and 6.6 per cent in 1998. This proportion can be expected to increase in the future to 9.9 per cent in

Table 1 Total annual national fertility in Korea (1960–1997)

Year	Total fertility rate	Year	Total fertility rate
1960	6.0	1990	1.6
1974	3.6	1993	1.8
1984	2.1	1996	1.7
1987	1.6	1997	1.56

Source: National Statistical Office (1998c).

2010, 13.2 per cent in 2020, and 19.3 per cent in 2030. The more older people there are in a society, the more money is required for social security provision such as pensions or medical care. The high cost of national medical services, and a critical demand for medical services for the aged, calls for the implementation of a new medical and welfare system for the elderly (E.Y. Choi *et al.* 1998).

Spectrum of diseases in Korea

Infectious diseases

The recent downward trend of acute infectious diseases showed that 3.7 people per 100 000 were affected in 1996. This trend has been continuing at this level during recent years. However, a particularly noteworthy phenomenon is that malaria has been increasing since 1994 (Ministry of Health and Welfare 1997).

Sixty-eight individuals were infected with cholera in 1995, and two were infected in 1996. The periods during which cholera was prevalent were short and there were no cholera-related deaths. Cholera in Korea typically occurs first along coastal areas and then spreads inland through the exchange of food, such as occurs in mourning houses, marriage ceremonies, etc. It is thought that cholera occurs in unclean coastal areas where sewage accumulates.

In the late 1960s there were over 4000 cases of typhoid fever, with a fatality rate of 1.48 per cent. However, the increase in Korea's gross national product and improvements in sanitation, together with the development of public health care, have resulted in a continuous reduction in the incidence and fatality rate of typhoid over the last 40 years. The annual incidence rate has decreased to 0.5 per 100 000 people since 1980. However, a report shows that there are still tens of thousands of patients annually, and thus the disease is still endemic.

In the 1950s, the average annual incidence of Japanese encephalitis was 2000, with a fatality rate of about 40 per cent. Since then, the incidence and fatality rate have continued to fall. Since 1985, only one of 25 patients has died from Japanese encephalitis.

In the 1990s, new infectious diseases have appeared or reappeared. Bacterial dysentery (in 1993), type A hepatitis (in 1994), and mumps (in the spring of 1998) are examples of reappearances. Since 1994, the number of cases of malaria has rapidly increased near the 38th Parallel (the border between North and South Korea). The reason for the reappearance of such infectious diseases is the continuous mutation of pathogenic micro-organisms, changes in population and social conditions, and the modification of the Earth's environment (B.Y. Choi 1999) (Table 2).

In 1996, there were five cases of cholera and 35 cases of tropical malaria in Koreans who had visited Southeast Asia or Africa; the first *Escherichia coli* 0157 patient appeared in 1988. Furthermore, increasing numbers of foreign infectious diseases are entering Korea.

Table 2 Number of cases of critically acute infectious diseases in Korea (1985–1996)

Disease	1985	1990	1994	1995	1996
Cholera	–	–	–	68	2
Typhoid fever	208	232	267	370	475
Bacterial dysentery	41	13	233	23	9
Measles	1283	3415	7883	71	65
Mumps	1237	2092	1874	430	254
Japanese encephalitis	–	1	3	–	–
Ep. haemorrhage	64	106	132	89	118
Leptospirosis	–	14	7	13	6
Malaria	–	–	20	107	356

Source: Ministry of Health and Welfare (1997).

Since the first HIV-positive patients were identified in Korea in 1985, the number has been growing annually, and reached 811 by June 1999, according to a report by the Ministry of Health and Welfare. Of the total cases reported, 133 resulted in death and 115 resulted in AIDS (Table 3). Seventy-six of the 811 cases were under epidemiological investigation or classified as of unknown cause. Of the remaining 735 cases, 696 were infected by sexual contact (95 per cent), 21 by blood transfusions (including transfusions received overseas), 17 by blood products, and one by vertical infection. Of the 696 patients infected by sexual contact, 230 had sexual relationships with foreigners, 292 had domestic heterosexual relationships, and 174 had homosexual relationships. HIV first appeared in Korea amongst foreigners, but the infection has now spread to domestic heterosexuals. It should be noted that a relatively high number of homosexual males are infected. No cases have been linked to blood transfusions or blood products in the last 2 years. This improvement is thought to have been achieved through the screening of blood donations, and an increase in the safety of blood transfusions and blood products. Fortunately, no cases of infection by intravenous injection have yet been reported. The best way to control infectious diseases is to establish a surveillance system and to improve the information network.

Chronic diseases

The mortality rate of infectious diseases has reduced significantly with improvements in housing conditions, nutrition, and medical care. However, the mortality rate of chronic degenerative diseases has been increasing rapidly. This trend will have a significant impact in the future, with the ageing of the population, changes in eating habits, an

Table 3 Cases of HIV infection and patients with AIDS in Korea

	1985–91	1992	1993	1994	1995	1996	1997	1998	Total
Total number infected with HIV	169	76	78	90	108	102	124	64	811
Number of women infected with HIV	23	4	7	12	19	12	17	10	104
Number of patients with AIDS	8	2	6	11	14	22	33	19	115

Source: National Health Institute (1998).

increase in the number of smokers, and a decrease in the amount of physical exercise.

Before 1970, infectious diseases were the greatest cause of death. However, the widespread use of antibiotics since the 1970s has resulted in a significant decrease in the number of deaths caused by infectious diseases.

In the early 1960s, the three major causes of death were diseases of the digestive system, such as diarrhoea and gastroenteritis, diseases of the respiratory system, such as pneumonia and influenza, and infectious and parasitic diseases. Malignant cancers were the fifth most significant cause of death. In 1970, the chief causes of death were diseases of the circulatory system. Malignant cancers were the fourth most significant cause of death while injury and poisoning were the fifth. In 1980, the most serious cause of death remained diseases of the circulatory system, cancer was the second, and injury and poisoning were the third. The order has remained unchanged until the present. However, recently, when the diseases of the circulatory system were divided into two categories (heart disease and cerebrovascular disease), the main cause of death became cancer. These three types of disease caused 61.9 per cent of all deaths in 1995 (Park 1998).

The number of Koreans who suffer from mental disorders is increasing due to rapid changes in living conditions and a more complicated social structure. At the end of 1996, the total number of people who suffered from mental disorders was estimated to be 993 000, or 2.16 per cent of the total population. Of all patients with mental illness, 115 000 (11.6 per cent) needed to be admitted to hospital. The prevalence rate of mental illness over a lifetime is 31.8 per cent in large cities, and 32 per cent in rural areas. The causes of mental illness in large cities and rural areas are alcohol misuse (21.7 per cent and 26.8 per cent), anxiety and somatoform disorders (7.4 per cent and 8 per cent), mood disorders (5.52 per cent and 3.07 per cent), and schizophrenia (0.12 per cent and 0.65 per cent) (Lee and Han 1986).

Trends in health policy in Korea

Between the end of the Second World War and the Korean War, the government was unable to increase investment in health care. Therefore most of the medical care was provided by non-governmental doctors who established the infrastructure of a health-care system through self-investment. The government had no policy for a desirable medical delivery system, but only developed policies for establishing a primary health care organization, disinfection, and medical aid.

The American Army Administration, which controlled the government of Korea after the Japanese occupation, judged that the prevention of illnesses was more effective than cure when supporting a country with limited resources for a public health system. Therefore the Administration declared the implementation of health care with a focus on the prevention of illnesses (American Army Administration Order No. 1, September 1945). A model health centre was established which began operation in October 1946. In 1958 the centre became the National Central Health Center but in 1959 it was dismantled. During its operation, this institution was a model for health-care programmes. It trained 330 health personnel, doctors, sanitary leadership members, and institution members, in addition to operating administrative training courses. After its dismantlement, the institution evolved into the National Health Research Institution (Kim 1984).

The National Health Care Law was enacted in 1951. More than 500 primary health care centres were built and operated. In 1953, 15 public health centres were established, and 471 primary health care centres were refurbished. As a result, health centres and primary health care offices were established in rural areas, but the government was unable to provide them with adequate support. After the enactment of the Health Centre Law in 1956, public health centres, governed by cities and provinces, were established and thus an infrastructure for country-wide preventive health care was put in place. However, because of political instability and financial limitations, the government allotted less than 1 per cent of the total government budget for health care, and this budget was only allocated to the control of acute infectious diseases, such as epidemic typhus, typhoid fever, smallpox, etc. (Yoo and Yang 1989).

The First Five-Year Economic Development Plan for the purpose of economic development began in 1962, but there was no investment in health-care development. However, although the governmental policies focused on economic development, a family planning policy was instituted.

The family planning programme as a health policy, which also helped to maximize economic development, formed the basis of governmental health programmes such as maternal and child health care and tuberculosis control. The Korean Family Planning Institute was established in 1961 as a non-governmental group. It organized the National Mothers' Meeting and allowed this organization to develop family planning. This was very successful, and became the basis on which non-governmental organizations participated in health-care programmes. Originally, the maternal and child health-care programme was only a part of the family planning policy whose primary purpose was population control. However, it was found that the family planning programme could be organized better as part of the maternal and child health-care programme, which steadily became more active from 1980 onwards as maternal and child health-care centres began to be established all over the country.

Control of tuberculosis was mainly in the form of tuberculosis prevention. In 1952 the government organized the BCG Vaccine Action Team, which toured cities and provinces in order to vaccinate elementary and preschool children. In 1965, in co-operation with the Tuberculosis Institute which was established in 1953, the team also began to survey the national tuberculosis situation.

At the time that the Health Center Law was revised in 1962, there was approximately one health centre per 100 000 people in cities, and one health centre per county (*kun*) in rural areas. From 1969, health subcentres were set up in towns (*eup*) and 'subcounties' (*myon*). However, the health centres and the health subcentres could not be fully activated because of a shortage of labour and facilities. In particular, the health centres followed the American model, focusing on preventive care and not providing clinical care. As a result, the health centres and the health subcentres were largely disregarded by patients. Also, because the main health programmes at the health centres were top-down programmes, these did not reflect regional characteristics. The American style of public health care relied on private sector investment, which was small, and the public perceived itself to have little input in administrative policies.

During the Second Five-Year Economic Development Plan (1969–1971), the government tried to increase production from industry, agriculture, and fisheries. The health-care policy during this period focused on eliminating or reducing factors disadvantageous for a rapidly growing economy. These factors included the prevention of acute infectious diseases, tuberculosis control, the enlargement of health-care services in rural areas, the qualitative improvement of food and medicine, training of health personnel, and family planning, including maternal and child health care.

The Third and Fourth Five-Year Economic Development Plans (1972–1976 and 1977–1981) focused on the social development of rural areas, and included social as well as economic development in an effort to reduce the income gap between urban and rural areas.

Under the banner of 'Self-Support, Diligence, and Co-operation', the nationwide *Saemael* (New Town) Movement, strongly supported by the government, was divided into four elements: production-based businesses (electrical, roads, irrigation, etc.), 'mental reformation' (morality and education), increasing income, and the improvement of environmental welfare. Rural residents were urged to participate in the movement actively and voluntarily, thus leading to improvements in their own society. Although the business priorities were different in each locality, the main objectives of this movement were to provide safe water and sanitary housing, including kitchens and bathrooms, and the management of child-care centres for agricultural regions (Yoo and Yang 1989).

Between 1962 and 1979 the annual income per household increased from US$147 to US$4840 in rural areas, and from US$190 to US$5460 in urban areas.

The primary developmental aims of the health system in the Fourth Five-Year Economic Development Plan were dissemination of medical services, reduction of infectious diseases, maintenance of maternal and child health care, improvement of national nutritional status, and the general improvement of living conditions.

From the late 1970s, health policies were implemented through medical insurance. In the mid-1970s, unequal sharing of medical benefits was a serious social problem related to the unequal distribution of the benefits of economic growth. From a political viewpoint, it was necessary to establish a policy to solve this problem. However, the execution of the policy was accompanied by problems of financial investment and a limitation of financial resources. Furthermore, the policy only applied to the employees of the conglomerates that could afford this expenditure. During this process, a set price for medical insurance was developed to secure affordable insurance.

As medical insurance gradually spread and came into effect nationwide in 1989, its cost became one of the most important issues in medical policy. The financial investment for public medical care, corresponding to the nation's economic power, grew continuously, and investment for creating facilities also steadily changed from the old privately controlled system to a government lending system. Governmental investment was also instituted as one of the most important policy measures.

Based on the new national medical insurance, a medical delivery system was also created. As a result, primary medical care began at clinics and health centres, as well as in secondary and tertiary general hospitals. This system was slowly put in place nationwide. From 1977, the government began to provide medical care for the poor.

From the end of the 1970s to the end of the 1980s, the government and some colleges tried to implement a model plan of primary health care. Family planning measures helped to realize this goal.

Rapid socio-economic development in the 1990s changed the trend of disease, and thus a new form of health policy was required. The recent trends in the causes of death differ from that of the past. Causes of death now resemble those in the West, i.e. a shift from respiratory and cerebrovascular disease to cancer and heart disease. To meet this changing trend in diseases, a health-care policy that was previously only focused on the treatment of diseases and which had a passive attitude to health care was forced to change by the late 1980s (Kim 1997).

To improve the recent patterns of harmful living, such as excessive drinking and smoking, the National Health Promotion Act was enacted in January 1995. This Act strengthened the health promotion programmes in such areas as health education, prevention service, and creating healthier living through improving individual health behaviours.

The Local Health Law was enacted in December 1996 to support the public health centres that were in charge of infectious disease control and family planning. The local public health centres became the central institutions for local people's health. In addition, the law added a national health promotion programme and a programme for chronic degenerative disease control, preparing the way for the introduction of autonomous local health programmes by clarifying national and local judicial responsibilities.

A law for elderly welfare was enacted in June 1981 for the prevention, early detection, and treatment of diseases, and for rehabilitation in the elderly. Korea is becoming an ageing society; 6.3 per cent of the total population were over 65 years old in 1997 (National Statistical Office 1998*b*). The law was reformed in August 1997 to address the issue of financial security for elderly people.

The government enacted and promulgated a pollution prevention law in 1963, but it did not become effective until 1976, when the Five-Year Economic Development Plan ended, because it centred on economic development. In 1977, the enactment and promulgation of the Environment Preservation Law established and controlled environmental standards and developed institutional equipment for the assessment of environmental effects. In 1990, the Environment Preservation Law was wholly revised as a basic environmental policy law, and it brought about a new phase of environmental control and laid the foundations for reasonable and comprehensive control measures of the environment.

Transition of non-governmental medical facilities

At the end of the Second World War, the Korean government was established through the American Army Administration. However, the Korean War destroyed Korea's economy and industry. As a result, health and medical care were neglected. Accordingly, health conditions were very poor, and even the existing facilities were not fully used because of the weak economy. Korean medical science, which had depended on Japan until the end of the Second World War, was introduced to American medical science, medical care system, and medical education after the Second World War. Thus the Korean medical establishment developed a health-care system which combined elements of both the Japanese and American approaches. Public medical institutions, which formed the core of the service during the Japanese colonial period, could not perform to their full capacity because of a shortage of doctors and obsolete facilities. Such limitations were caused by the government's lack of financial resources and management skills. Missionary hospitals were also in financial difficulties but, with the decline of public hospitals, they began to play a central role. The Pusan Gospel Hospital, the Seoul Sanitation Hospital, the Baptist Hospital, the Inchon Christian

Hospital, and the Wonju Christian Hospital were built in the 1950s. They also served a public function, and some of them became attached to universities. The Catholic Church established 15 small and large hospitals in a 20-year period beginning in the 1950s. The Red Cross developed smaller hospitals with less than 100 beds in eight areas including Seoul, and they took charge of medical care for the poor. Private medical institutions underwent large-scale growth and supported hospital care for the poor qualitatively and quantitatively until the end of the 1960s.

From the early 1960s, with the economy developing well, social insurance began to be introduced. The introduction of this insurance increased medical demand and led to an expansion of medical institutions. To solve the shortage of hospitals, the government provided financial aid and, in 1980, supported the building of private hospitals by establishing local private hospital programmes. Thus the structure of medical provision changed from public and missionary hospitals to private hospitals, and the scale and quantity of hospitals increased. Also, the purchase of expensive medical equipment increased rapidly.

However, many problems followed, such as an unbalanced distribution of health-care services in the regions, a rapid increase of health-care expenditure, and a shortage of doctors. Therefore, from 1984 onwards, the government tried to attract private hospitals to agricultural and fishing regions, which were experiencing the most severe shortage of hospitals, by restricting the number of hospitals that could be built in each region.

In the future, medical care services should be broadened to include poorer people and to ensure that a proper level of local health resources can be maintained.

Organization of public health in Korea

The Korean Public Health Administration system is composed of central and local health organizations. There is no direct link between them. Therefore all administrative systems that are composed of local autonomous groups constitute an artificial administrative system (S.S. Choi 1999*b*).

The Ministry of Health and Welfare is the central organization for the administration of health care at the national level, and it presides over such issues as the prevention of epidemics, regulation of medication, social welfare, medical security, pensions, domestic welfare, and others. It has no power over personnel or budgeting; as an administrative organization, it only provides technical support. Local health administration organizations are composed of the health departments of cities and provinces. In turn, each province is composed of bureaus under the health or social department and its health centres in administrative units: *si* (small city), *kun* (county), and *ku* (district, administrative unit of a large city). As units within the department, there are umbrella offices in each *eup* (town, administrative unit of a county with a large population), *myon* (subcounty, administrative unit of a county with a small population), and remote areas. The local health administrative organization has a dual system that is under the direct control of the Interior Ministry as part of the general administration. Under this system, the unique characteristics of health administration cannot be considered fully.

The national university hospitals that are directly or indirectly related to national health are administered by the Ministry of Education, police hospitals are administered by the Police Office, and medical centres of local corporations of cities or provinces are administered by the Interior Ministry. Because the central health administrative system is composed of various bodies, the functions and roles of the Ministry of Welfare and Health are restrained in the course of executing policies and therefore health and medical programmes have many problems with ineffectiveness and inefficiency.

The Central Health Administrative System

The Ministry of Health and Welfare is the central health administrative system of the government. The primary goal of the ministry is to improve the health of Korean citizens through the enactment of laws. The ministry is organized into two offices (planning and management, and social welfare policy), four departments (health policy, health promotion, health resource management, and pension insurance), three deliberation bureaus (social welfare deliberation, domestic welfare deliberation, and disability welfare deliberation), five centres (public information, inspection, technology co-operation, oriental medicine policy, and emergency planning), 27 divisions (including medical and medication policy, food policy, health promotion, prevention of epidemics, mental health, food and medication promotion, insurance policy, welfare of the elderly, child care, women's welfare, disability leadership), and nine bureaus with special responsibilities (including international co-operation, oriental medicine, and women's health).

The following institutions are attached to the Ministry of Health and Welfare: National Medical Center, National Health Center, National Health Safety Research Institute, National Social Welfare Training Center, five national psychiatric hospitals, National Sorok-Island Hospital, National Rehabilitation Center, two national tuberculosis centres, National Homesickness Management Office, 13 national quarantine offices, Food and Medicine Safety Agency, and six food and medicine agencies.

There are also 32 related groups, including the Korean Medical Association, the Korean Pharmacy Association, the Korea Red Cross, the Korea Association of the Elderly, the Korea Medical Insurance Union, the National Pension Management Corporation, the Korea Research Institute for Health and Society, and the Korea Health Management Association.

Local health organizations

Health administration organizations at the level of cities and provinces exist in Seoul, other metropolitan areas, and all provinces. The Ministry of Health and Welfare, as the central health administration organization, connects all public health centres for each city, county, and district.

Public health centres operating in cities, counties, and districts form the core national health organizations in Korea. The public health centres were established as local autonomous governments by an ordinance based on the public health centres. According to the ordinance, Seoul and all other metropolitan areas should have a centre in each district, and all other cities should have a centre in each town and county. In October 1997, there were a total of 245 centres—228 public health centres and 17 health medical centres. The business of public health centres is managed and controlled by the head of the local government, and the internal organizations and divisions are managed by the Direct Rules and Affairs Division of the public health centres. Decisions made at this level are based on local government policy, and the contents may differ amongst cities, counties, or districts.

Health and medical organizations in towns and subcounties are as follows. The town and subcounty should aim to establish one public health subcentre, based on a publicly decided law at each town and subcounty. As of October 1997, there were 1314 public health subcentres. The chief of the public health centre should be a qualified doctor. He or she is in charge of the area's business and directs its programmes, supervises personnel, and guides the health and medical business of the subcentre.

Villager's health centres are established in agricultural and fishing villages to care for the health of people living in those areas. These areas either do not have doctors, or they may have one for short periods of time. The public health centres in these areas are the lowest level of care and, as of 1997, there were a total of 2034 such centres. The public health practitioners in these centres are nurses and midwives whose qualifications are regulated by the Ministry of Health and Welfare based on the governor's ordinance. They have a 24-week period of on-the-job training, during which they can perform minor medical services.

Korea's medical policy

Korea's medical security system is composed of medical insurance, worker's compensation insurance, and medical aid.

Medical insurance

In 1963, Korea's medical insurance was enhanced by the enactment of a medical insurance law. However, its effects were generally insignificant, except for serving as a useful model for private businesses, because the national average annual income per household was only about US$100 at that time. A practical role was played by the second amendment, which was enacted at the end of December 1976.

Compulsory medical insurance began in 1977 for workers in companies with over 500 employees and in public corporation complexes. This was also the first year of the Fourth Five-Year Economic Development Plan, which centred on social development. Although it was mandatory, it was the beginning of social insurance.

The Insurance Law for Government Employees and Private School Teachers was promulgated in December 1977, and insurance businesses catering for government employees and private school teachers began to be established from January 1979. The coverage of insurance for employees in the private sector was extended from companies with more than 300 workers, to those more than 100 workers, and finally to those more than five workers.

While employees who had a regular cash income joined the medical insurance programme, self-employed workers or villagers living in agricultural or fishing areas could not join. This resulted in further social problems in the 1980s.

The government operated a pilot programme for regional medical insurance in 1981 and 1982, and, as a result, regional medical insurance for the self-employed in urban areas was etablished in 1988. In 1989, the programme was extended to city dwellers. By a series of such processes, national medical insurance was initiated.

When the national medical insurance law was passed in 1997, regional medical insurance and insurance for government employees and private school teachers were also established starting in October 1998.

The benefits of medical insurance are twofold:

- benefits in kind (medical care benefits, maternity benefits)
- cash benefits (medical care expenses, maternity expenses, funeral expenses).

The medical care benefit is given for the diagnosis, medication, provision of care materials, treatment, hospital admission, nursing care, transportation, and for sickness and injuries. Originally sickness benefits for diseases other than pulmonary tuberculosis were given for 330 days a year, but this was increased to 365 days a year in 2000. The benefit in kind for delivery is given for childbirth in medical institutions. The benefit in cash for delivery and care is paid only when the allowance in kind cannot be given because of unavoidable circumstances. The funeral benefit is paid in cash to the person who is responsible for the funeral service when an insured person or one of his supportees dies.

The medical insurance fee is between 3 and 3.2 per cent of the standard monthly income of government employees, private school teachers, and employees in the private sector. Employers and employees each pay 50 per cent of the fee. For private school teachers, the owner of the private school pays 30 per cent and the government pays 20 per cent of the medical insurance fee, while the teachers pay 50 per cent. The self-employed in rural and urban areas pay the fee by grade (from 1 to 50 classifications according to their income and assets).

Reimbursement of doctors' and hospital fees are largely based on a fee-for-services schedule, which is determined by the government.

An experimental project using diagnosis-related groups was tried in 1997. The system is being partly introduced into medical services in 2000. Under this system an insured individual will pay a part of the medical fee when an actual medical service is received (patient co-payment), in addition to a medical insurance fee.

Medical claims review and payment of medical care fees is a third-party payment system in which medical services for the medical practitioner or medical facilities are not owned by the insurer. The medical service providers are reimbursed by the insurer on the basis of a fee-for-services through the insurance medical care institution.

Medical aid

Before 1976, the Medical Aid Project in Korea provided free medical services on the basis of the National Assistance Act. However, the practical results were not satisfactory. In order to spread medical benefits to people of low income, the Medical Aid Act was promulgated in 1977 and medical aid was begun. The Medical Aid Law was promulgated in December 1977, and the enforcement ordinance of the law was established in May 1978. The previous regulations of medical aid were abrogated while the enforcement regulations of the medical insurance law were put into effect in September 1978.

The purposes of the Medical Aid Law are to provide medical services to those who cannot support themselves or who have a low income, and to improve national health and social welfare. This law mandates medical aid institutions to provide medical services to people who need livelihood assistance under the National Assistance Act. This includes those aged 60 years and above, the infirm, those below 18 years of age, expectant and nursing mothers, men disabled by incurable diseases, the mentally or physically handicapped, and others who cannot support themselves.

The people who need medical aid are divided into two classes.

- Class I: people in nursing or welfare facilities, victims of disasters, national heroes, human cultural assets, North Korean defectors, and patients with sexually transmitted diseases.
- Class II: self-support recipients with livelihood assistance.

The range of medical aid includes diagnosis, medical treatment, surgical treatment for all kinds of illnesses and injury, childbirth, other treatments, supply of medicine or medical material, hospital admission, nursing, transfer, and other medical measures.

The method of imposing medical charges depends on the class of medical aid. All class I medical charges, including both outpatient and hospital admission treatments, are paid by the government. In class II, all medical charges for outpatient treatments are paid by the government. Charges below 100 000 won (Korean currency) for treatment during hospital admission are paid for by the patient. If charges exceed 100 000 won, the government provides an interest-free loan which is repaid by instalments within 1 to 3 years.

City and provincial governments have established medical aid foundations, which are supported by government aid, surpluses, proceeds from the foundation, and other sources.

Occupational accident compensation insurance

The Korean Constitution guarantees workers three primary rights: the right to work, an equal right to share profits, and protection for the unemployed. However, the laws underpinning these rights have not been established. Occupational accident compensation is provided to the workers by a collective contract, not by the law.

The Labour Standard Law for the health and safety of workers was enacted in May 1953. This law prescribed a system of no-fault compensation for workers' occupational accidents. However, mismanagement by employers and a heavy burden of compensation for serious accidents drove the insurance companies into bankruptcy. The law could not achieve effective results and was unhelpful.

The Occupational Accident Compensation Insurance Law was enacted in 1963, when economic development through industrialization was a primary aim of Korea, and was enforced in 1964. This law was enacted to compensate occupational accidents fairly and quickly, and to reduce the burden on employers who could not provide accident compensation for large numbers of victims at the same time.

When the law was initially enforced, the insurance was managed by the government. Mine companies and manufacturing companies, which employ more than 500 workers, are legally required to buy the insurance policy.

An allowance for medical care was provided for hospital stays of longer than 11 days, and compensation for absence from work was 60 per cent of the average wage. Since then, the benefit has increased, and since 1982 the length of hospital stay qualifying for the medical care allowance has been reduced to 4 days. In 1989, compensation for absence from work was increased to 70 per cent of average wages. In 1992, workplaces employing more than four workers were required to buy the policy. Since 1995, the Korean Industrial Safety Complex has taken over management of the insurance.

The insurance premium depends on the total wage bill of the company which the policy holder manages and the type of company. Occupational accident compensation is provided for injuries and death, the causes and results of which are directly related to work. As of 1998 this insurance covers six kinds of allowance: medical care, absence from work, mental or physical handicap, survivor's pension, pension for injuries and diseases, and funeral expenses.

Medical care services in Korea

Health resources

Personnel expenses constitute 40 to 60 per cent of hospital budgets in Korea. The management of human resources is vital to the success of the promotion of health within Korea. Satisfactory health and medical services require a full supply and proper and effective management of well-trained health and medical human resources. This will help the national health and medical project to be executed satisfactorily with proper expenditure.

Health and medical human resources licensed by the Medical Service Act include medical doctors, dentists, oriental medical doctors, midwives, and nurses. Those who are licensed by the pharmacy laws include pharmacists and oriental medical pharmacists. The Medical Service Act prescribes 26 types of medical specialists and four types of special nurses, with additional nursing assistants, paramedics, massagers, and so on. Emergency service workers are licensed by the Emergency Service Law, nutritionists and cooks by the Food Sanitation Law, sanitarians and sanitary engineers by the Sanitarian Law, and veterinarians by the Veterinary Law.

As of 1997, on average there is one medical doctor for 735 people, one herbal doctor for 4951 people, one dentist for 2990 people, one pharmacist for 1004 people, and one nurse for 135 people.

All health and medical human resources, including medical doctors, have been increasing rapidly, but poor management of these resources will become a serious problem in the future. The increase in medical facilities is slower than that of human resources, so that there is unsatisfactory employment of medical personnel.

As of 1996, medical institutions employed 74.6 per cent of licensed medical doctors, 75 per cent of licensed dentists, 75.9 per cent of oriental medical doctors, 38.7 per cent of nurses, 13.6 per cent of midwives, 40.6 per cent of medical technicians, 26.8 per cent of medical records officers, and 31.5 per cent of nursing assistants.

The number of people served by one medical doctor or one dentist in Korea is larger than in developed countries. However, the present supply of medical human resources is considered to be sufficient to meet future demands. The supply of nurses, including nursing assistants, is close to the level in developed countries.

Specialists are defined as those who take a training course in internship and residency at a hospital or medical institution designated by the government after obtaining a medical licence according to the Medical Service Act, and who subsequently pass the qualifying examination of the Korean Medical Association.

The purpose of the medical specialty system is to encourage doctors to receive intensive and complete training in clinical specialities, and to continue to acquire new medical knowledge in order to upgrade the quality of medical care services and improve health care. There were 26 specialties and 34 726 specialists in 1996. This represents a 4.1-fold increase in the number of specialties compared with that of 1980. The number of specialists has increased, and the proportion of specialists amongst doctors has also increased since 1993. In 1996, 58.2 per cent of licensed doctors were specialists. The distribution of specialties is as follows: 14.2 per cent of specialties in internal medicine, 10.6 per cent of specialties in general surgery, 10.1 per cent of specialties in obstetrics and gynaecology, 8.4 per cent of specialties in paediatrics, and 8.3 per cent of specialties in family medicine.

Compared with medical doctors, pharmacists are outdated. According to the Medicinal Service Law, the specialization of dispensary and medical practice began to be implemented in 2000. Pharmacists will be in charge of dispensing medicine and will not be permitted to do so without a medical doctor's prescription. The number of pharmacies will decrease, and a considerable number of pharmacists will become unemployed.

Almost all kinds of medical technicians and assistants are becoming outdated. Medical assistant services will have to be specialized, and continuous training is needed for them to meet the needs of specialized assistant services.

Medical facilities are places where health and medical services are provided, and are a substructure of the national health and medical system. They include medical institutions under the Medical Service Law, rural health and medical centres, health centres, health sub-centres under the Health Service Center Law, and health clinics under the Temporary Law for Promotion of Agricultural and Fishing Villages.

Medical institutions are classified into general hospitals, other hospitals, and clinics. This classification is also applied to dental institutions and oriental medical institutions.

The third class of medical institutions has 262 general hospitals, which provide hospital admission, and diagnosis and treatment of more serious diseases. The second class of medical institutions has 456 hospitals, and the first class of medical institutions has 15 876 clinics. There are 49 sanitoriums, 9243 dental hospitals or clinics, 6446 oriental medical hospitals, 220 dispensaries or clinics, and 148 midwifery clinics in Korea (National Statistical Office 1998*b*).

The medical facilities have several problems. Firstly, the expansion in their number was achieved by non-governmental health insurance funds and therefore was dependent on private citizens. This interferes with the formulation and execution of a national health policy. A second problem is the regional difference in the increase of the number of institutions. A third problem is that unclear distinctions of services and functions between medical facilities creates wasteful expenditure. Fourthly, improvement in the quality and efficiency is slower than the expansion in the quantity of medical facilities.

Medical delivery system

The national health and medical system has always been considered as the core of primary policy in every establishment of long-term health projects. The establishment of a medical delivery system has been interrupted by disparate elements of public medical care, a lack of regional health planning, the unclear role of larger hospitals and clinics, and the lack of an economic transfer system.

The introduction of medical insurance resulted in a rapid increase in the demand for medical care, and in patient preference for large hospitals. The era of the national medical insurance system began with the medical insurance of the urban self-employed.

A patient-referral system was also introduced. Under this system, the country was divided into eight large and 142 middle-sized areas of medical care. Medical institutions were classified into the primary, secondary, and tertiary classes for the allocation of roles. The patients could choose primary or secondary medical institution care. The tertiary institution admitted patients with medical requests issued by the doctors of the primary or secondary institutions. If a patient chose any other primary or secondary institution outside his own geographical area without special permission from the insurer, he could not claim the allowance for the medical care. However, this restriction did not apply to emergency care and delivery. Any tertiary institution could provide primary medical services in six specialist fields, such as family medicine, ophthalmology, dermatology, rehabilitation medicine, and dentistry. The ultimate aim of this policy was to make the most of medical resources and to reduce medical costs.

The division of medical care areas was abolished in October 1998, and anyone can now receive medical services at any time in any area. Role allocation was not well established amongst the primary, secondary, and tertiary medical institutions, which led to excess competition and excessive preference of patients for larger hospitals. This problem is expected to be solved in the future. Medical-related systems should be improved to control human resources and facilities, and to meet the demands of health and medical care. The efficient use of human resources, health facilities, and medical care requires various plans, including the proper allocation of their functions and roles.

Public health services in Korea

Family planning

The Korean family planning project was started by Christian missionaries and medical doctors in Wonsan and Wonju in the 1920s, and in Inchon in the 1930s. They initiated a birth control and contraception campaign for peasant women, but it did not attract much interest. Meanwhile, the Korean Mothers Association, which was established in 1958, adopted and developed education about family planning as one of its own projects. This was the first systematic campaign of family planning in Korea.

The overpopulation of developing countries was one of the main causes of the vicious circle of poverty. Beginning in 1960, the government adopted a population policy as part of its economic development. The development of family planning achieved remarkable success in curbing population growth. Korea has become one of the countries with a very low birth rate. Its fertility rate has been below the population replacement level since the mid-1980s. The composition of the population is similar to that of developed countries which has made a great contribution to Korean's economic development.

In 1962, all the health centres throughout the country set up family planning consultation offices, and employed licensed nurses or midwives. At the same time, the Health Centre Law was revised to add consultation and education of family planning to the services of health centres. In 1963, the Law of Maternal and Child Health was established and provided the legal foundation of the Family Planning Project. This provided for legal abortion. In 1964, the section of family health was established under the city or provincial governments which took charge of the family planning project of the regional area. The association of family planning organized its branches with more than 30 members in city and county areas, and in individual workplaces.

The campaign for family planning spread rapidly all over the country, financed and supported by the government and other institutions.

When the Family Planning Project was adopted as a governmental policy, Korea had a rate of contraception of 4 to 9 per cent and was suffering an increasing crisis of population growth rates of 30 per cent. However, the contraception rate increased to 20 per cent in 1966,

25 per cent in 1971, 55 per cent in 1979, and 79 per cent in 1991. Contraception by intra-uterine device, condoms, vasectomy, and oral contraceptive pills increased in the early 1970s. Contraception by fallopian tube ligation increased to 4.1 per cent in 1976, 31.6 per cent in 1985, and 35.5 per cent in 1991. It is one of the most common forms of contraception (National Statistical Office 1992*b*). Vasectomies increased to 11 per cent in 1988, but were still less than a third of the fallopian tube ligations. At the same time, oral contraception decreased from the high point of 9 per cent in 1974 to 3 per cent in 1991 and 1.8 per cent in 1997. The change in contraceptive methods was brought about by the government's efforts to encourage permanent sterilization.

The high rate of contraception decreased the total birth rate rapidly to 6 per cent in 1960, 4.7 per cent in 1971, 2.7 per cent in 1982, and 1.7 per cent in 1997. The nationwide survey of birth rate and family health in 1988 shows that 91 per cent of all children who were born in 1987 were the first or second child (Cho *et al.* 1997). The age distribution of parturient mothers also changed. In 1960, 3.1 per cent of parturient mothers were below 19 years old and 24.2 per cent were over 35 years of age, whereas in 1987 these figures decreased to 0.9 per cent and 2.8 per cent respectively. However, parturient mothers aged between 20 and 34 years old increased from 72.7 per cent in 1960 to 96.35 per cent in 1987.

The interval between deliveries has shortened. A woman born in 1945 delivered her first baby on average 16.8 months after marriage, and the interval between the deliveries of her first and second child was 29.5 months on average.

Maternal and child health

The Maternal and Child Health Project of the Ministry of Health and Welfare covers a wide range of child-health-related issues at all stages of growth from birth, including pregnancy. The coverage of the project is dependent on medical resources and finances. The potentially dangerous areas of antenatal care, perinatal care, and neonatal care are the main work of the project.

The health of both mother and child is closely related to the environment of the household, such as living or financial conditions, familial relationships, and lifestyle. Especially important is the father's health, educational background, and job as regards his financial condition; also closely related to the family's living conditions are his diet and the degree of interest in health. Recently, the Maternal and Child Health Project has included all family members.

Financial support for the Maternal and Child Health Project was very small in Korea. The administrative support of the government was also very small; the Administration Office for Maternal and Child Health was established at the Ministry of Health and Social Affairs in 1972. It was composed of two sections: maternal and child health, and family planning. However, it was abolished in 1981 and replaced by the smaller division of family health. Subsequently, the section of maternal and child health was abolished, and was replaced by the division of life and health. At the time of restructuring of the government system in 1998, the Division of Health of Regional Areas was established under the Department of Health Resources Management, and it took charge of maternal and child health.

Maternal mortality rate and causes of death

According to the statistics of the Ministry of Health and Social Affairs, the maternal mortality rate was 4.2 per 10 000 people in 1980, 3.4 per 10 000 in 1985, and 3 per 10 000 between 1988 and 1992 (Ministry of Health and Social Affairs 1994*b*). The national survey in 1997 showed that it was 2 per 10 000 between 1995 and 1996 (Han *et al.* 1997). According to a national survey of the birth rate and the maternal mortality rate, the maternal mortality rate was 1.82 per 10 000 neonates at 219 general hospitals throughout the country (Park and Hwang 1993). This mortality rate is twice as high as that of developed countries, and one-fifteenth that of developing countries.

According to the 1993 death statistics, the causes of maternal death that were direct, as opposed to indirect, made up 85.7 per cent (National Statistical Office 1994). Analysis of maternal death between 1980 and 1988, using data collected at 22 university hospitals and seven general hospitals, revealed that direct causes of maternal death made up 79 per cent, while indirect causes were 15.4 per cent, and unknown causes 5.6 per cent. Hypertensive disorders made up 42.4 per cent, most of which were eclampsia and pre-eclampsia. Haemorrhagic disorders were 42.2 per cent, and infectious diseases 15.6 per cent (Han *et al.* 1997)

A national survey (Moon *et al.* 1985) has shown that 80.9 per cent of maternal deaths were direct, and 19.1 per cent were indirect. The direct causes were haemorrhagic disorders (25.7 per cent), hypertension (16.3 per cent), embolism (15.6 per cent), and infection 1.4 per cent. This reveals differences from past experience.

Most of the deaths caused by pregnancy-induced hypertension can easily be prevented with early detection and treatment of the disease through antenatal care. Most of the deaths caused by haemorrhagic and infectious diseases can be prevented with a well-established system of first aid. The maternal death rate could be reduced to that in developed countries because almost all deliveries are performed at medical institutions.

Antenatal care is a preventive service in which the health of a pregnant woman and her fetus is periodically checked. It promotes the safe delivery of a healthy baby by providing health-care education and risk assessment to the expectant mother.

In 1985, 56.2 per cent of pregnant women received antenatal care within the first trimester (Moon *et al.* 1985), and this increased rapidly to 65.6 per cent in 1988 (Moon *et al.* 1989) and 89.4 per cent in 1994 (Hong *et al.* 1994). The average frequency of antenatal care was four visits in 1983 and 10 visits in 1994 (Hong *et al.* 1994).

The rate and frequency of antenatal care, and the time to the first antenatal visit, have improved. However, 18.6 per cent of pregnant women did not receive antenatal care within the first trimester of the third pregnancy and 32.7 per cent had an educational background below elementary school (National Economic Planning Board 1983). This must to be improved.

The Maternal and Child Health Law prescribes that a city or county official must issue a document of maternal and child health to those who inform them of their pregnancy. Few inform officials of their pregnancy in accordance with the provision; instead, most of the medical institutions issue the document at the time of antenatal care. In the national sampling survey, 86.9 per cent of pregnant women were document holders and 74.7 per cent carried the documents at every antenatal treatment (Hong *et al.* 1994).

Parturition is a physiological phenomenon which causes danger to both the pregnant woman and the fetus. Well-trained specialists and a hygienic environment are required to care for and deliver babies safely. The recent rate of delivery at medical institutions with specialists and facilities increased dramatically from 35.8 per cent in

1975 to 75.2 per cent in 1985 and 99.7 per cent in 1997, reaching the level of developed countries (Cho *et al.* 1997).

The rate of antenatal care has reached almost 100 per cent, but that of postnatal care remains low. In the 1988 national sampling survey, the rate of postnatal care was 52.3 per cent, while that of antenatal care was 88.5 per cent. There was a large gap between those living in urban areas and those in rural districts; the rate of postdelivery diagnoses was 57.5 per cent in urban districts, but only 37.3 per cent in rural districts. In the 1997 survey, these rates improved to 81 per cent throughout the country, with 81.7 per cent in urban districts and 77.8 per cent in rural districts (Cho *et al.* 1997; Moon *et al.* 1989). The government should continue to issue the maternal and child health document, and do its best to encourage deliveries at medical institutions and the provision of antenatal and postnatal care.

Health of infants

The infant mortality rate and causes of death

The infant mortality rate in Korea was 61.8 per 1000 in 1965, 53 per 1000 in 1970, 41.4 per 1000 in 1975, 13.3 per 1000 in 1985, and 12.8 per 1000 in 1990 (Ministry of Health and Social Affairs 1994*b*). The mortality rate of infants who were born in 1993 and died within a year was 9.9 per 1000 (Han *et al.* 1996).

The infant mortality rate in developed countries is on average below 10 per 1000, while that of developing countries is 102 per 1000 (Han *et al.* 1996). The rate in Korea is higher than that in developed countries but lower than that of developing countries, which means that more effort must be made to reduce it.

The Maternal and Child Health Law requires that medical institutions report neonatal deaths and stillbirths. According to the report, premature birth and low birth weight babies were 23.4 per cent in 1990 and 41.8 per cent in 1992, and are on the increase. Congenital anomaly caused 20.1 per cent of the deaths in 1990 which declined to 19 per cent in 1992, but it is now increasing again (Park and Hwang 1993).

Congenital anomaly caused 36 per cent of infant deaths after the neonatal period, and perinatal problems, such as fetal growth retardation, prematurity, hypoxia, and delivery asphyxia, caused 14 per cent of the deaths in 1993 (UNICEF 1995). Another survey showed that intra-uterine fetal growth retardation occurred in 25.3 per cent of deaths, neonatal breathing difficulty in 16.4 per cent, and congenital anomaly in 15.9 per cent (Han *et al.* 1996).

In developed countries, about two-thirds of infant deaths occur during the neonatal period, and half of all infant deaths happen within a week of birth. The deaths were caused by premature birth, intra-uterine fetal growth retardation, and congenital anomaly.

Fetal body weight at the time of birth is an important factor upon which survival probability depends. It is closely related to the health of the mother before and during pregnancy. It is known that in developed countries, such as the United States and the United Kingdom, the infant mortality rate is 1 per cent for those of normal weight, 3 to 5 per cent for those weighing less than 2500 g, and 45 to 55 per cent for those weighing less than 1500 g (Park and Hwang 1993).

Reports from 64 general hospitals throughout the country in 1966 revealed that the birth rate of infants who weighed less than 2500 g was 9.8 per cent (Han *et al.* 1996) and a little higher than 6 to 6.5 per cent in another survey (Bae and Kim 1997). This difference suggests that most pregnant women in critical condition are treated at general hospitals.

The mortality rate of infants in 1993 was 8 per 1000 babies and that of children below 5 years old was 9 per 1000, while that of 1 to 4 year olds was 1 per 1000 (Han *et al.* 1996).

According to the statistics of formal death notices, 2023 children aged 1 to 4 years old are reported to have died in 1993, and their death rate was 77 per 100 000 in their age group (National Statistical Office 1994). This is equivalent to a rate of 3 per 1000, excluding neonatal deaths, but is higher than that reported by UNICEF (1995). Considering these statistics, the mortality rate of Korean children (10 per 1000) is lower than that of 30 developed countries.

The causes of 1966 of 2023 deaths reported in 1993 were clearly revealed. The causes of 1012 cases (51.5 per cent) were injuries and poisoning, of which 458 were traffic accidents, 246 (12.5 per cent) were due to congenital anomaly, 143 (7.3 per cent) were due to malignant cancer, and 134 (6.8 per cent) were due to non-inflammatory diseases of the central nervous system (National Statistical Office 1994).

Maternal feeding

The national sample survey shows that the rate of maternal breast feeding was 68.9 per cent in 1982, 59 per cent in 1985, and 48.1 per cent in 1988. It decreased sharply to 11.4 per cent in 1994, and increased slightly to 14.1 per cent in 1997. The rate of artificial feeding increased from 15.6 per cent in 1985 to 18 per cent in 1988, and from 27.9 per cent in 1994 to 33.4 per cent in 1997 (Cho *et al.* 1997).

Various factors caused the rate of maternal feeding to be low, including urban dwelling, high educational background, high income, young age, the first baby, employed mothers, delivery at medical institutions above the class of hospitals, delivery by Caesarean section, care of babies in a nursery room in which the mother and her baby are kept apart, and low birth weight (Kim and Park 1988; Park *et al.* 1990; Shin and Park 1992).

Mental health services

Psychiatric diseases are difficult to cure in the short term, and their complete cure rate is also low. They cause both economic and emotional problems for the patient and the family. More special clinics are needed for psychiatric diseases, to provide better medical services for patients, and to establish an effective system for early detection, treatment, and after-care of psychotic diseases.

The Mental Health Law, which was established in 1995 and implemented in December 1996, is intended to help patients with psychiatric diseases to access medical services and to return to society. It also aims to remove infringement of the patient's human rights during long-term hospital admission, and to lay the legal and institutional foundation of the mental health services (Ministry of Health and Welfare 1997).

The government has so far only aimed to provide mental health services by treating patients in psychiatric clinics which were to be expanded, not as a part of the regional mental health service. The expansion of mental health facilities was developed in three directions. Firstly, the zones of mental health service were established around psychiatric hospitals, and exisitng psychiatric hospitals were extended and new ones were built. Also, the number of beds in private psychiatric hospitals increased greatly. Secondly, general hospitals in 1989 were placed under an obligation to establish psychiatric departments, and the psychiatric departments of general hospitals were greatly expanded. Thirdly, unlicensed psychiatric asylums which were already in existence were upgraded to legal asylums, and new asylums were built.

In 1993, the Ministry of Health and Social Affairs began to focus on developing regional mental health services. Considering the universal trend and theoretical results of community psychiatry, the Korean policy of mental health should be provided on a regional basis. Without a strong policy, the mental health service cannot meet the social demands of confining psychotic patients to psychiatric hospitals.

The statistics from the data of medical insurance and medical aid allowances reveal that the annual prevalence rate of the treatment of psychiatric diseases was estimated to be 2.73 per 100 000 people in 1993. The prevalence rate of schizophrenia was 22.8 per 100 000, while that of mood disorder was 78.4 per 100 000. The rate of neurosis and other non-psychotic disorders was higher, but their symptoms and functional problems are not as serious and so they are not on the immediate agenda of the regional project of mental health.

The prevalence rate of psychiatric diseases of medical aid beneficiaries is twice as high as that of those with medical insurance. Specifically, the prevalence rate of psychoses such as schizophrenia, mood disorder, organic brain syndromes, alcoholism, or drug abuse among people receiving medical aid is much higher than that among those with medical insurance (S.S. Choi 1999*c*).

Facilities for the return of psychotic patients to society should be established to provide appropriate rehabilitation training programmes, such as occupational therapy and activities of daily living, and to help the patients adapt themselves to society and live independently. The activation of a mental health service project in a community needs specialists in mental health at regional health centres, who will be in charge of the prevention of psychiatric diseases and rehabilitation training for patients returning to society. With these efforts, a gradual deinstitutionalization of the patients could be accomplished.

Occupational health services

The Korean occupational health services were developed on the basis of the Labour Standard Law (1953) and the Occupational Accidents Compensation Insurance Law (1963). Later, the Occupational Safety and Health (1981) and the Prevention of Pneumoconiosis and Protection of Workers Diseased by Pneumoconiosis Law (1984) provided an institutional framework and made a great contribution to the stabilization of the occupational health project.

Health examination is divided into two types: general health examination and special health examination. Each has a primary (screening) and secondary (precise) function in the examination of health. In particular, in a special health examination, the list of topics covered was selected on the basis of hazardous factors in the workplace.

A regional allocation of special health examinations was adopted, with the medical institutions in the region taking responsibility for them. Health service providers, such as medical doctors, nurses, and industrial hygienists, were appointed according to the type and size of the work place. Mining and manufacturing companies with more than 1000 workers should appoint a doctor, a nurse, or an industrial hygienist. Other types of companies with more than 2000 workers should employ a full-time health manager. Small companies with between five and 49 workers comprised 85.8 per cent of all workplaces, and their workers made up 34.3 per cent of the total workforce.

The Occupational Safety and Health Law underwent major revision in 1989. It now requires that a proxy agent of occupational health services should be in charge of the occupational health service at workplaces with 50 to 300 workers, and that a medical doctor, two nurses, and two industrial hygienists are provided for every 1500 workers at 150 workplaces. The agent is responsible for all occupational health services, including environmental evaluation of workplaces, prevention planning against occupation-related diseases, and health education. Meanwhile, occupational health services at workplaces with between five and 50 workers are supported by government subsidy, as in 1993.

Special health examinations are carried out periodically every year according to the Occupational Safety and Health Law. The results show that the prevalence rate of observed occupational diseases is 1 to 2 per cent, and that the rate of pneumoconiosis is 43 to 76 per cent of all workers with observed occupational diseases. The rate of those afflicted by pneumoconiosis is 2.2 to 3.8 per cent of all workers at dusty workplaces, and pneumoconiosis and occupational hearing problems constitute 97 to 98 per cent of all occupational diseases.

The Korean occupational health service project should be converted gradually from prevention of occupational diseases to health promotion for all workers. The working conditions in smaller companies are much worse than those in larger companies, and it is difficult for their workers to be provided with health services by occupational health specialists. Health services for workers in smaller companies should be supported financially by a government subsidy and effective development of occupational health services should be accomplished nationwide.

Summary

Changes in the risk factors affecting human health, the epidemiology of disease, and the demands and use of health and medical care services have accompanied the changes in the population and the economic and social structure in Korea. Improvements have been occurring over the past 40 years in socio-economic conditions, nutrition, living conditions, and lifestyle, together with a beneficial reduction in population growth. As a result, Korea is now experiencing a variety of new problems related to health services.

In order to deal with the risk factors affecting health and the epidemiology of disease, health policies should aim to improve the management and control of unhealthy eating habits and lifestyles. They should also aim to address such diverse health problems as accidents, poisoning, psychiatric disorders, environmental pollution, and natural disasters, rather than concentrating on diseases of a single aetiology, such as the infectious diseases.

In the present system of health services, the structure of medical human resources, the functions of medical institutions, and the allowance systems of medical insurance are centred around the treatment of disease. However, resources should be allocated to the effective prevention of disease and to services for health promotion. Medical care systems should pursue these policies at low cost whilst maintaining high levels of effectiveness. Systems should be improved with regard to human resource and facilities management, and controlled to meet increasing demands. Policies to raise the efficiency of health services, which make clear the allocation of functions between the various institutions and people working in health facilities, should be outlined.

The system of information and statistics should be improved to establish a scientific and reasonable policy of health and medical care. Local governments lack the ability and the special knowledge required to deliver and control health services.

A system of information management should be established at every level of local government, and local governments should themselves have the ability to establish and implement reasonable plans concerning local health.

The success of the Korean family planning project contributed to changing the population pattern into a structure more like that of developed countries, and this project should continue. The maternal and child health project should be transferred to the family health project, which deals with the health of all family members. The system of issuing documents pertaining to maternal and child health will still be useful. In addition, a project to encourage hospital delivery and antenatal and postnatal care should be developed further. The project of mental health services should be changed to a regional basis. A powerful policy of mental health can change the social demand to isolate psychotic patients. Local government needs to support efforts to help their return to society and to active independent living in order to promote deinstitutionalization. The project of occupational health services should transfer its emphasis from prevention of occupational diseases to promotion of health for workers. The project of occupational health services for workers at smaller companies still needs a government subsidy.

Today, the whole world is interested in developing the quality of life. The national demand for improvement in quality of life is growing stronger together with a general rise in household incomes. The government has the responsibility of creating conditions under which people recognize that they are responsible for their own health, and that they can and should take care of themselves.

References

Bae, C.W. and Kim, M.H. (1997). Neonatal statistics of Korea in 1996: collective results of live-births, neonatal mortality, and incidence of discharge against medical advice at 64 hospitals. *Journal of the Korean Society of Neonatology*, **4**, 133–68.

Bloom, G. and Gu, X.Y. (1997). Introduction to health sector reform in China. *Institute of Development Studies Bulletin*, **28**, 1–11.

Cha, C.H. (ed.) (1984). Preventive medicine in 1950–1960. In *Korean medical history (1884–1983)*, pp. 472–5. Medical Press, Seoul.

Chang Y.S., Cho, N.H., and Moon, H.S. (1996). *The changes of population with size and structure by new population estimation and policy issues*, pp. 52–3. Korean Institute for Health and Social Affairs, Seoul.

Cho, K.S. (1979). *Industrial health*, p. 18. Soomoon Press, Seoul.

Cho, N.H., Kim, D.K., Cho, A.J., and Suh, M.K. (1997). *1997 national fertility and family health survey report*, pp. 174–87. Korean Institute for Health and Social Affairs, Seoul.

Cho, N.H., Moon, H.S., and Kim, S.K. (1998). *The recent trends and the countermeasures in population*, pp. 274–5. Korean Institute for Health and Social Affairs, Seoul.

Choi, B.Y. (1999). Bacterial dysentery. *The Korean Society of Preventive Medicine 1999 Symposium*, pp. 1–30. Korean Society of Preventive Medicine, Seoul.

Choi, E.Y., Kim, J.S., and Lee, W.B. (1998). *Health care system in Korea.* Korean Institute for Health and Social Affairs, Seoul.

Choi, S.S. (ed.) (1996). Life style and health behavior. In *Preventive medicine and public health* (2nd edn), pp. 624–7. Gyechuk Press, Seoul.

Choi, S.S. (1999*a*). The status of Korean nutritional health administrative system. In *Preventive medicine and public health* (3rd edn), pp. 768–71. Gyechuk Press, Seoul.

Choi, S.S. (1999*b*). The public health organization and health administrative system. In *Preventive medicine and public health* (3rd edn). Gyechuk Press, Seoul.

Choi, S.S. (1999*c*). The status and practice of public health in Korea. In *Preventive medicine and public health* (3rd edn), pp. 918–19. Gyechuk Press, Seoul.

Han, Y.J., To, S.L., Lee, S.W., Lee, H.B., and Lee, M.W. (1996). *A study on mortality level and causes of death in infant.* Korean Institute for Health and Social Affairs, Seoul.

Han, Y.J., Toh, S.L., Park, J.H., and Lee, S.W. (1997). *The estimation of maternal mortality ratio and analysis of causes of maternal death.* Korean Institute of Health and Social Affairs, Seoul.

Hong, S.W. (1979). *Population and population policy in Korea*, p. 157. Korean Institute of Development, Seoul.

Hong, M.S., Lee, S.Y., Chang Y.S., Oh, Y.H., and Kae, H.B. (1994). *1994 national fertility and family health survey report*, pp. 175–85. Korean Institute of Health and Social Affairs, Seoul.

Huh, J. (1997). *Search for Asian traditional medicine*, pp. 68–74. HanWool Books, Seoul.

Kim, D.J. (1984). A study on medical history. In *Centennial of modern medicine in Korea (1885–1994)*, pp. 4–9. Medical Press, Seoul, Korea.

Kim, J.S. (1989). Perspective and transition of death causes among Koreans. *Korean Journal of Epidemiology*, **11**, 175–82.

Kim, J.S. (1997). The background and future problems in regulation of health promotion in Korean. *Health and Welfare Policy Forum*, **12**, 67–9.

Kim, D.K. (1998). Today's occupational health in Korea. *Journal of Epidemiology*, **8** (Supplement 1), 41.

Kim, K.J. and Park, J.H. (1988). Comparison of feeding practice of mothers in urban and rural area. *Korean Journal of Public Health*, **14**, 63–74.

Kim, B.H., Youn, H.Y., and Choi, K.S. (1989). A study on nutritional status of elementary school children attending rural type school lunch programs in Yongin Gun, Gyunggi Province. *Korean Journal of Nutrition*, **22**, 70–83.

Kim, Y.K., You, M.Y., and Kim, Y.D. (1993). Nutrition knowledge and nutritional status of upper elementary school children attending rural type school lunch programs. *Korean Journal of Nutrition*, **26**, 982–7.

Korean Institute for Health and Social Affairs (1995). *The status of utility of medical care and health in Korea.* Korean Institute for Health and Social Affairs, Seoul.

Lee, S.Y. (1997). Korean health and political problem. *Health and Welfare Policy Forum*, **11**, 5–12.

Lee, C.K. and Han, J.H. (1986). The epidemiological study of mental disorders in Korea. *Seoul Journal of Psychiatry*, **11** (Supplement 1), 190–200.

Lee, H.Y. and Kim, S.H. (1994). Effects of nutritional status of Korean adults on lipid metabolism with age. *Korean Journal of Nutrition*, **27**, 23–45.

Ministry of Environment (1996). *Environmental statistics year book*, pp. 20–1. Ministry of Environment, Seoul.

Ministry of Health and Social Affairs (1994*a*). *National nutrition survey report.* Ministry of Health and Social Affairs, Seoul.

Ministry of Heath and Social Affairs (1994*b*). *Year book of health and social affairs.* Ministry of Heath and Social Affairs, Seoul.

Ministry of Health and Welfare (1972). Class I communicable diseases: number of cases and deaths, morbidity and case fatality by year. In

Yearbook of health and welfare, p. 4. Ministry of Health and Welfare, Seoul.

Ministry of Health and Welfare (1997). *Yearbook of health and welfare.* Ministry of Health and Welfare, Seoul.

Moon, S.J. (1995). *Recommended dietary allowances for Korea* (6th revision), p. 3. Korean Society for Nutrition, Seoul.

Moon, H.S., Lee, Y.J., Oh, Y.H., and Lee, S.Y. (1985). *1985 national fertility and family health survey report.* Korean Institute of Population and Health, Seoul.

Moon, H.S., Lee, Y.J., Oh, Y.H., and Lee, S.Y. (1989). *1988 national fertility and family health survey report.* Korean Institute of Population and Health, Seoul.

National Economic Planning Board (1983). *Social indicators in Korea*, p. 181. National Economic Planning Board, Seoul.

National Health Institute (1998). The information of infectious disease. *Communicable Diseases Monthly Report*, **8**.

National Statistical Office (1992*a*). *Annual report on population statistics.* National Statistical Office, Seoul.

National Statistical Office (1992*b*). Contraceptive practice rate. In *Social indicators Korea*, p. 104. National Statistical Office, Seoul.

National Statistical Office (1994). *Annual report on the cause of death statistics*, pp. 238–41. National Statistical Office, Seoul.

National Statistical Office (1996). *The future estimated population. Economic development after 1961: an overview.* National Statistical Office, Seoul.

National Statistical Office (1997). *Annual report on the cause of death statistics.* National Statistical Office, Seoul.

National Statistical Office (1998*a*). *Annual report on vital statistics (1970–1997)*, p. 61. National Statistical Office, Seoul.

National Statistical Office (1998*b*). *Social indicators in Korea.* National Statistical Office, Seoul.

National Statistical Office (1998*c*). Total fertility rate (1960–1997). *Population and housing census (including foreigners).* National Statistical Office, Seoul.

Park, C.H. (1998). To escape from diseases. *The Korean Society for Preventive Medicine Symposium Proceedings.* Korean Society for Preventive Medicine, Seoul.

Park, I.H. and Hwang, N.M. (1993). *Challenges and directions of development in the maternal health policies.* Korean Institute of Health and Social Affairs, Seoul.

Park, I.H. and Hwang, N.M. (1994). *The status of breast feeding practice and recommended policy.* Korean Institute of Health and Social Affairs, Seoul.

Park, J.H., Je, M.H., Chun, B.Y., and Cho, S.E. (1990). Cohort infant mortality rate of Gunwee and Hapchun counties and MCH center in Taegu. *Korean Journal of Preventive Medicine*, **23**, 87–97.

Shin, H.O. and Park, J.H. (1992). Breast feeding rates, advantage and disadvantages of rooming-in and nursery care perceived by mothers. *IL-Sin Christian Hospital Monograph*, **7**, 243–57.

UNICEF (1995). *The state of the world's children*, pp. 66–80. UNICEF, Geneva.

WHO (World Health Organization) (1988). *World health statistics annual.* WHO, Geneva.

WHO (World Health Organization) (1990). Management of drinking problems. In *WHO regional publications, Europeans, Series, No. 32.* WHO, Geneva.

Yoo, S.W. and Yang, J.M. (1989). *An outline of medical care*, pp. 104–6. Soomoon Press, Seoul.

Yoon, B.Z., Kang, H.W., Cho, K.S., and Son, K.H. (1990). A study on life style of elderly in rural area. *Journal of the Korean Academy of Family Medicine*, **28**, 66–86.

2

Determinants of health and disease

2.1 Overview and framework

Robert Beaglehole

Introduction

This chapter begins by providing an overview of the context for public health practice at the beginning of the twenty-first century with an emphasis on the current phase of economic globalization. The next section summarizes models of the determinants of health and disease relevant to public health research and practice, and provides a conceptual framework of these determinants incorporating both global and local perspectives. Finally, the major categories of the determinants of health status are briefly reviewed; the other chapters in this section explore these determinants in detail.

The public health context

A major transition in the health of human populations is occurring. Firstly, there have been broad gains in life expectancy over the past half-century and fertility rates are declining. Secondly, the profile of major causes of death and disease is being transformed; the pattern of infectious diseases has become more labile with new and old epidemic diseases emerging, and the burden of non-communicable disease is increasing. Finally, health inequalities between rich and poor are increasing both within and among countries.

The prospects for the future health of populations depend to an increasing extent on the processes of globalization and the emergence of global environmental changes in response to the burden of economic activity (McMichael and Beaglehole 2000). In addition to the immediate causes of disease, there are profound influences on population health status from social, economic, political, and environmental processes at multiple levels. The improvements in the health profile of developed countries over the past two centuries have resulted from both broad-based changes in the social, economic, and physical environment, in human ecology, and, to a lesser extent, from deliberate public health and medical interventions. In developing countries, health gains have begun more recently in the wake of increased literacy, family spacing, improved nutrition and vector control, assisted by the application of public health knowledge about sanitation, vaccination, and the management of infectious diseases (Powles 1992).

Public health is 'the art and science of preventing disease, promoting health, and prolonging life through the organised efforts of society' (Committee of Inquiry 1998). There are two major themes underlying the modern public health task. Firstly, as social and material inequalities within a society generate health inequalities, an important public health task is to identify through research the underlying determinants of these health inequalities. That knowledge must then be applied, in part through professional practice, to the development of health supporting social policies. Secondly, longer-term changes in the structure and conditions of the social, economic, and natural environments, at both the local and the global levels, affect the level and sustainability of good health within populations. The scope of contemporary public health practice includes the health consequences of rapid urbanization, demographic change, the globalization of economic, social, and cultural relations, and human-induced global environmental changes. To be most effective, modern public health research and practice should be based on an up to date understanding of the broad determinants of the health and disease status of human populations.

Models of the determinants of health

Over the last 50 years there have been important shifts in the manner in which the determinants of health are viewed. Four distinct, but overlapping, perspectives on the determinants of health can be identified:

- the biomedical view
- the lifestyle approach
- the broad socio-economic approach
- the population health view.

The biomedical paradigm emerged towards the end of the nineteenth century based on bacteriological discoveries. This paradigm is still dominant. It is based on the strength of the molecular and genetic sciences and is characterized by adherence to 'objective' sciences and the search for causes of specific disease in individuals and their constituent parts. The huge investment in the human genome project typifies this view of human health and its determinants.

The Lalonde Report to the Canadian government in 1974 began the modern era of health promotion by proposing a broader view of health (Lalonde 1974). The report asserted that positive health was not attainable for the majority of the population through a concentration of public health funds on personal services. The report described the health field in terms of four fields: human biology, environment, lifestyle, and health-care organization. Unfortunately, the emphasis rapidly shifted to the role of individual lifestyles in determining health status.

The 1986 Ottawa Charter emphasized the role of factors outside the health-care sector and, in particular, the social and economic determinants of population health status (Ottawa Charter 1986). This view did not gain widespread acceptance outside of the public health and health promotion communities.

Since the early 1990s and in response to the fiscal crisis affecting health-care systems worldwide, the 'population health model' has received increasing support (Evans *et al.* 1994). This model has replaced the earlier 'health promotion' model as a guiding framework for health policy and practice. The central message of the population health model is that health in human societies, as opposed to individual health status, is powerfully influenced by the wealth-generating capacity of a nation and the manner in which this wealth is distributed. The central assertions of this model are as follows:

- the major determinants of human health status are cultural, social, and economic factors at both the individual and population levels
- these factors are independent of medical care input at the population level
- societies that enjoy a high level and relatively equitable distribution of wealth enjoy a higher level of health status
- at the individual level, health status is determined by the social and economic environment and the way in which this environment interacts with individual psychological resources and coping skills.

Contemporary evidence in support of the population health model and of the prime importance of wealth and prosperity comes from Japan, which has the world's highest life expectancy at birth yet spends only a relatively small percentage of gross domestic product on the health system (Marmot and Davey Smith 1989). Another important strand of the model is the evidence from the Whitehall studies in the United Kingdom on the role of relative poverty in producing major health inequalities. The social determinants of these inequalities appear to be of more importance than the role of the major risk factors (smoking, elevated blood pressure and cholesterol levels, and physical inactivity) for non-communicable diseases (Marmot and Wilkinson 1999). The focus on social and economic determinants of health in the population health model is a welcome contrast to the mainstream biomedical model of health. However, the population health model has several limitations; in particular it downplays the importance of targeted public health interventions and the effects of improved living and working conditions in increasing life expectancy over the last 150 years (Szreter 1988). Clearly, wealth generation alone was insufficient to increase health status: public health and social reforms more generally were also involved. For example, the contemporary role of medical services in relieving suffering, enhancing quality of life generally, and improving life expectancy, particularly in poor countries, over the last 50 years is also underemphasized as described in Chapter 2.8. There is evidence that a medically based and high-risk approach to the primary prevention of non-communicable disease can be successful, even if it is not cost-effective (Hunick *et al.* 1997). Also, as far as the Japanese evidence is concerned, there appear to be large hidden costs in the private (home care) sector that is largely provided by women.

Another limitation of the population health model is that it underplays the importance of the current phase of economic globalization for public health practice (Hayes *et al.* 1994).

The links between wealth and health are obviously more complex than represented in the model. In fact, a high level of wealth at a national level is not a necessary prerequisite for high population health status. The final limitation is the lack of attention given to the importance of community involvement in health affairs.

Global and local determinants of health

The determinants of health are broad, extend from genetic influences to the social, cultural, and economic environment, and include manifold pathways by which these various factors operate to influence health and disease status at both the population and individual levels. The preferred model of the determinants of health is dynamic and interactive and adopts a life course approach to health status recognizing the complexity of the interplay between prenatal, early, and later life influences on the development and maintenance of health and disease states. This model is far removed from the more usual and more circumscribed 'medical model', which is based on a restricted biological view of disease aetiology and concentrates on the endstages of the disease production process.

The preferred model of the determinants of population health status places greater emphasis on both the role of the new global economy and its associated developments and on the role of people and communities. The new interconnected global economy has a major influence on and interacts with environmental, social, and cultural determinants of health (Fig. 1).

Economic 'globalization' has been a long-evolving feature of a world dominated by Western society. For example, the onset of the twentieth century was a time of vigorous free trade, subsequently curtailed in the aftermath of the First World War. Contemporary globalization differs in both the scale and comprehensiveness of change, and in the associated decline in the nation-state's capacity to set social policy. The West's post-Second World War international 'development project' anticipated national convergence towards the model of Western democratic capitalism. Since the early 1980s, that project has evolved towards a globally deregulated free-market economy. These globalizing processes, in turn, have become a major determinant of national social and economic policies (Gray 1998).

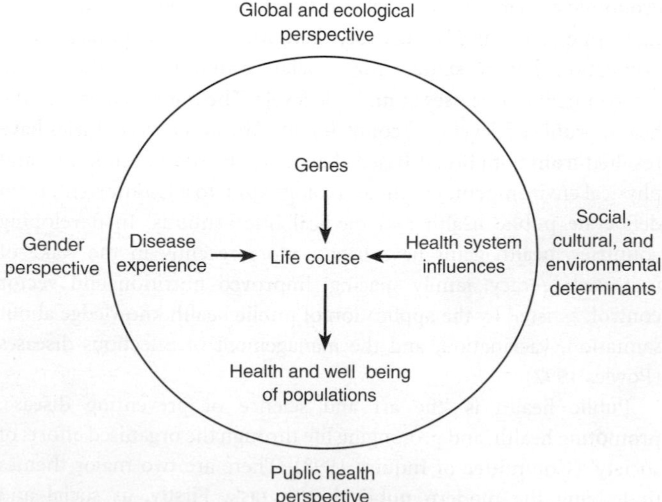

Fig. 1 The determinants of the health of populations.

Thus, although responsibility for health care and the public health system remains with national governments, the fundamental social, economic, and environmental determinants of population health are becoming increasingly supranational. It is evident that this current global configuration of liberal economic structures and constrained social policies promotes social dislocation, economic inequalities, and political instability, each adversely affecting public health. Unless the moderating role of the state or of international agencies is strengthened, increasing competition for the world's limited natural resources could become increasingly damaging to intercountry relations, local and global environments, and population health (UNEP 1999).

From a public health perspective, globalization is a mixed blessing (McMichael and Beaglehole 2000). On the one hand, accelerated economic growth and technological advances have undoubtedly enhanced health and life expectancy in most populations. At least in the short to medium term, material advances allied to social modernization and various health-care and public health programmes have yielded impressive gains in overall population health status.

On the other hand, aspects of globalization are jeopardizing population health through the erosion of social and environmental conditions, the global division of labour, the exacerbation of the rich–poor gap between and within countries, and the accelerating spread of consumerism. The primary health risks, reflecting the central impacts of globalization on social and natural environments, include the following.

- Perpetuation and exacerbation of income differentials, both within and among countries, thereby creating and maintaining the basic, poverty-associated conditions for poor health.
- The fragmentation and weakening of labour markets as internationally mobile capital acquires greater relative power. The resultant job insecurity, substandard wages, and lowest-common-denominator approach to occupational environmental conditions and safety can jeopardize the health of workers and their families.
- The consequences of global environmental changes (includes changing atmospheric composition, land degradation, biodiversity depletion, spread of 'invasive' species, and dispersal of persistent organic pollutants).

Other more specific risks to population health status include the following.

- The spread of smoking-caused diseases as the tobacco industry globalizes its markets.
- The diseases of dietary excesses as food production and food processing becomes intensified and as urban consumer preferences are increasingly shaped by globally promoted and marketed images.
- The diverse public health consequences of the proliferation of private car ownership, as car manufacturers extend their marketing.
- The continuing and widespread rise of urban obesity, exacerbated by the above two developments.
- Expansion of international drug trade, exploiting the inner-urban underclass and, more generally, the alienation of some young people in the context of ineffectual national control efforts and institutional weaknesses.
- The infectious diseases that now spread more easily because of the distant and rapid connections around the world, the disruption of natural habitats, and the emergence of drug resistance.
- The apparent increasing prevalence of depression and mental health disorders in ageing and socially fragmented urban populations.

A major manifestation of the increasing scale of the human enterprise is the advent of global environmental changes. While not directly caused by the globalization processes, global environmental change reflects the increasing numbers of humans and the intensity of modern consumer-driven economies (McMichael and Powles 1999). Humankind is now disrupting, at a global level, some of the biosphere's life-support systems which provide environmental stabilization, replenishment, organic production, the cleansing of water and air, and the recycling of nutrient elements (Chapter 2.7). Earlier generations could take these environmental 'services' for granted in a less populated lower-impact world. Changes are now occurring in the gaseous composition of the lower and middle atmospheres. There is a net loss of productive soils on all continents, and depletion of most ocean fisheries and many of the great aquifers upon which irrigated agriculture depends. There is an unprecedented loss of whole species and many local populations. An estimated one-third of the world's stocks of natural ecological resources has been lost since 1970. These changes to the earth's basic life-supporting processes pose long-term risks to human population health.

The complementary global and people-centred approaches to understanding the determinants of health are key components of strategies for health improvement in the twenty-first century. The people-centred approach to public health has at its core the concept of empowerment, which means that the people of a community are in control of the public health process and are strengthened by it. The key to this approach is the adoption of a community development strategy where needs assessment and clear goals are central aspects (Raeburn and Rootman 1997).

There is a need for a balanced emphasis in both research and public health practice on the proximal, intermediate, and distal causes of health, disease, and disability. This balanced approach is in contrast to the more usual epidemiological approach that focuses on the proximal determinants, especially intrinsic biological and behavioural factors (McKinlay 1992).

The determinants of health and disease

Health is a social and cultural concept in addition to its fundamental biological characteristics. There are three basic sources of differences in the health of populations: hereditary determinants, socio-economic circumstances, and lifestyles and other behavioural factors. Gender differences span all three domains and cultural and political factors also play important parts in determining the health of populations.

Hereditary determinants

The effects of genetic factors on the various components of health and the ageing process are not yet well known. It has been estimated that only 20 to 25 per cent of variability in the time of death is explained by genetic factors (Christensen and Vaupel 1996). About 50 per cent of variation in human lifespan is attributable to survival attributes that are fixed for individuals by the time they are aged 30, but only a third to a half of this effect is thought to be due to genetic factors. The influence of genetic factors on the development of chronic conditions, such as coronary heart disease and diabetes, varies considerably. However, from a practical point of view, the environmental determinants of these conditions still offer the greatest scope for prevention and control efforts.

Socio-economic determinants

Social and economic determinants of health refer to a wide range of factors that include occupational status, work conditions and security, educational attainment, housing environment and tenure, and family circumstances (Marmot and Wilkinson 1999) (see also Chapter 2.2). It is likely that each of these factors acts differently on health at each stage of life. Cumulatively these factors play a major part in determining the 'social capital' available to both individuals and communities.

An important question is the extent to which the roots of health inequalities lie in socio-economic circumstances earlier in life, compared with current circumstances. From life-history studies of childhood and adolescence it appears that social factors probably operate in a cumulative fashion (Kuh and Ben-Shlomo 1997). There are significant social class differences in height, growth, and other aspects of physical development, as well as in the incidence of infectious and other diseases and risk of injury. Vulnerability to physical ill health in childhood and later adult life is associated with poor parental socio-economic circumstances and low levels of parental education and concern (Wadsworth 1997). Cross-sectional studies also show differences in mortality and morbidity as a function of socio-economic status, across various disease categories throughout the life span. Educational attainment and marital status have also been shown in several longitudinal studies to be powerful predictors of mortality. In addition, age, gender, and socio-economic status influence disability-free life expectancy (Robine *et al.* 1992).

The economic consequences of unemployment and retirement place many citizens in positions of financial vulnerability. As populations age, in both the developing and the developed worlds, the issue becomes how to keep older persons economically active within their respective societies. No community is exempt from the financial hardships experienced by ageing and unemployed populations. As populations stop working, they lose not only the economic but also the social and psychological benefits of activity and purpose. Men seem to be particularly sensitive to loss of work and retirement.

Lifestyles and other behavioural determinants

Behaviours such as smoking, physical exercise, activity in everyday life, alcohol consumption, diet, self-care practices, social contacts, and work-style are important contributing factors to population health status and variations in ill health with age (Chapter 2.3). Changes in the population levels of several of these factors, for example smoking and inappropriate dietary habits, are probably responsible for an important fraction of the increase in life expectancy in middle-aged people that have occurred over the last three decades in many Western countries (Chapters 2.5 and 10.1). These gains are a result of the major declines in cardiovascular disease death rates that began in the mid-1960s in the United States and have since been experienced in many other industrialized countries, although not yet to the same extent in eastern European countries (Beaglehole 1999) (see also Chapter 9.3).

General health education messages have had only a modest impact on changing these health determinants in people from disadvantaged social circumstances. Attempts to change people's health-related behaviour have been based on a superficial understanding of their social conditioning. The concept of prevention, like the concept of health, is a cultural and social construct. Interventions, therefore, have to be adjusted to different cultures and social circumstances and to the life experiences of different individuals, and have to take into account cohort and period effects and the powerful economic determinants of health, which are increasingly located at the transnational level. It will be increasingly important to locate prevention policies in the broad context of social and economic policy if current knowledge on the role of these health determinants is to be applied for the benefit of entire populations.

Gender-related determinants

Gender differences in health status are apparent throughout the lifespan and one expression of this is the feminization of later age. Several reasons have been suggested for these gender differences (Chapter 11.2). Prominent among these are behavioural factors such as cigarette smoking, alcohol consumption, and exposure to occupational hazards. Conversely, women have a higher prevalence of chronic conditions and disabilities, particularly in old age. The influence of social structures on health for women goes beyond causes related to conventional socio-economic differentials. More attention needs to be given to the reasons for men's shorter life expectancy and women's greater burden of sickness and disability. The important role of 'masculinity' in shaping men's expectations, behaviour, and thus health, requires further exploration and is likely to be as important as 'feminine' roles are in shaping the health of girls and women. Development of gender-specific health policies and health research is needed in all countries.

Cultural determinants

Different cultures assign different values to the parts people play at different ages within their societies. In certain cultures, older persons, for example, are assigned the tasks of government or other important duties and are regarded with great respect as community leaders. The particular impact of ageing on the health of indigenous older men is an under-researched area. It is known that most indigenous people, for example the New Zealand Maori, are severely disadvantaged from a health perspective. In industrialized cultures, older persons are often removed from the patterns of regular life when families are unable to fulfil caregiver roles, and are resettled in residential or skilled nursing institutions. Such environments can lead to diminished states of physical and psychological well being and mark the beginning of serious declines in health.

Political determinants

Political decisions shape the social and economic environments and the health systems that have important effects on the health of populations. Policies involving the organization and delivery of health services, national social security, and insurance programmes, for example, are major determinants of the health status of populations, and especially the young and old (Chapter 2.8). The collaboration of health advocacy groups in lobbying policy-makers and creating general awareness is a key element in promoting the health needs of specific communities. Non-governmental organizations provide health advocacy at the local, developmental level. Functioning in both developed and developing countries, these groups are vital members of the health improvement network, having direct access to populations and often also to the policy-making process.

Conclusion

This introductory chapter has illustrated the need for modern public health teaching, research, and practice to be grounded in both local and global perspectives on the determinants of health and disease in human populations. The challenges facing public health are great, and a comprehensive approach to health determinants will be necessary to achieve the full potential of all citizens of the world.

References

Beaglehole, R. (1999). International trends in coronary heart disease mortality and incidence rates. *Journal of Cardiovascular Risk*, **6**, 63–8.

Christensen, K. and Vaupel, J.W. (1996). Determinants of longevity: genetic, environmental and medical factors. *Journal of Internal Medicine*, **240**, 333–41

Committee of Inquiry into the Future Development of the Public Health Function (1998). *Public health in England*. Cmd 289. HMSO, London.

Evans, R.G., Morris, L.B., and Marmor, T.R. (ed.) (1994). *Why are some people healthy and others not?* De Gruyter, Berlin.

Gray, J. (1998). *False dawn. The delusions of global capitalism*. Granta, London.

Hayes, M.V., Foster, L.T., and Foster, H.D. (ed.) (1994). *The determinants of population health: a critical assessment.* University of Victoria, Victoria.

Hunick, M.G.M., Goldman, L., Tosteson, A.N.A., *et al.* (1997). The recent decline in mortality from coronary heart disease, 1980–1990. *Journal of the American Medical Association*, **277**, 535–42.

Kuh, D. and Ben-Shlomo, Y. (1997). *A life course approach to chronic disease epidemiology*. Oxford University Press.

Lalonde, M. (1974). *A new perspective on the health of Canadians.* Information Canada, Ottawa.

McMichael, A.J. and Beaglehole R. (2000). The changing global context of public health. *Lancet*, **356**, 495–99.

McMichael, A.J. and Powles, J.W. (1999). Human numbers, environment, sustainability and health. *British Medical Journal*, **319**, 977–80.

McKinlay, J.B. (1992). Health promotion through healthy public policy: the contribution of complementary research methods. *Canadian Journal of Public Health*, **83**, 11–19.

Marmot, M.G. and Davey Smith, G. (1989). Why are the Japanese living longer? *British Medical Journal*, **299**, 1547–51.

Marmot, M. and Wilkinson, R.G. (ed.) (1999). *Social determinants of health.* Oxford University Press.

Ottawa Charter for Health Promotion (1986). *Health Promotion*, **1**, iii–v.

Powles, J.W. (1992). Changes in disease patterns and related social trends. *Social Science and Medicine*, **35**, 377–87.

Raeburn, J. and Rootman, I. (1997). *People-centred health promotion*. Wiley, Chichester.

Robine, J.M., Michel, J.P., and Branch, L.G. (1992). Measurement and utilization of healthy life expectancy: conceptual issues. *Bulletin of the World Health Organization*, **70**, 791–800.

Szreter, S. (1988). The importance of social intervention in Britain's mortality decline c.1850–1914: a reinterpretation of the role of the public health. *Society for the Social History of Medicine*, **1**, 1–37.

UNEP (1999). *Global environment outlook 2000.* UNEP, Nairobi.

Wadsworth, M.E.J. (1997). Health inequalities in the life course perspective. *Social Science and Medicine*, **44**, 859–70.

2.2 Social, economic, and cultural environment and human health

Nicolette Hart

Human existence and the social environment

Human beings are complex organisms. Aside from the material complexity of the body itself, they possess the capacity to think, communicate, reason, feel emotion, hold beliefs, care for others, and act upon their environment in purposeful, productive, and destructive ways. The term social being denotes this sentient intelligent dimension of the human animal with its investment of social experience and cultural understanding. This investment represents the presence of the social environment within every person. It includes moral sentiments defining good and bad thoughts, feelings and conduct, ideologies including religious and secular beliefs, and knowledge as well as the entire repertoire of cultural symbols and their meaning, including language. As Peter Berger (1964) nicely expressed it, 'the human being resides in the social environment and the social environment resides within the human being'.

Society has an objective as well as a subjective reality. As a structure external to individuals, the social environment has many facets. Among the most important for public health is the cumulative impact that our species has made upon the natural world. This includes the exploitation of the world's territory and resources leading to the extinction of many other species and the damaging effects of efforts to improve human livelihood on global ecology. Humankind has altered the 'natural' environment extensively enough to disturb significantly both global climate and intercontinental ecology (Crosby 1986). This is the broadest global sense in which the habitat of modern humanity can be described as a social environment. There is no doubt that the process whereby humankind increased its dominion of nature has been associated with a 'great leap forward' in the health of the species, although there is a downside to this.

The period of most rapid change in human health status is equivalent to what historians call the Modern Era. This is the period since 1500 in which industrial capitalist urban civilization was born and disseminated throughout the world. The latest stage is the development of a spectacular technology of global communication ushering in the Internet Age. The ascent of capitalist civilization produced a 'great transformation' of the material conditions of human existence (Polanyi 1946). It was also associated with a process of European conquest and colonization of most of the world's territory, with the extinction of many other species as well as entire aboriginal peoples in some areas, with ferocious world wars, genocidal ethnic cleansing, and the development of a technology of mass destruction. On the plus side, the industrial mode of livelihood was born out of a scientific and technological revolution, which created the conditions for every (surviving) descendant of the human species to develop their potentiality to the full. The realization of this promise is so far restricted to developed nations and even there significant inequalities remain. In the era of industrial capitalist civilization, the volume of global material resources produced to support human life has risen beyond all previous measure, although their distribution among those peoples who survived the transition to the new global order is highly unequal. This is the first and foremost principle of the relationship between the social environment and human health.

Urban industrialism is the mode of livelihood created by the forces of market capitalism over the last two to three centuries. It is far and away the healthiest form of social organization known in human history. Although it has been directly associated with the formation of densely populated anonymous urban and suburban industrial communities, the health status of the populations who dwell in these places has risen to new record levels of vitality.

Among indicators used to measure the distribution of health in a population, only one—mortality—can be used with any degree of precision to study trends over time between and within societies. Alternative indicators—morbidity or stature—are more useful for studying intranational variation and even then they can only be used with caution. Morbidity is the most methodologically problematic of all possible health status indicators because, as a complex medico-sociological variable itself, its meaning is influenced by the same economic and normative factors that help shape health outcomes. Thus, for example, the higher morbidity recorded by women is probably more a reflection of gender norms dictating economic roles than any difference in the risk of disease. Men of working age appear to suffer lower rates of morbidity but higher rates of mortality, suggesting that the direct risk of disease itself is not perfectly correlated with the same factors that predispose people to see themselves as unhealthy or in need of medical advice or treatment (Hart 1982). Morbidity, whether self-reported or medically reported, has an important motivational aspect that limits its utility as an objective (rather than subjective) health status indicator. Stature is another possible objective measure of health status. It is closely correlated with longevity and has the additional advantage of being a measure of the living not the dead (Marmot *et al.* 1984; Floud *et al.* 1990). It has yet to become a routine health status indicator in official statistics and, although in time its use is likely to increase, so far few societies produce systematic series of height differentials in the population. Average height is not exclusively dependent on socio-economic factors, nor is it correlated with international longevity differentials. Although average height in Japan increased rapidly in the second half of the twentieth century, it remains below that of many other industrial populations whose rates of infant mortality and age-specific death are much less favourable. The rationale for using mortality to measure the distribution of health in a population is first and foremost the availability of data, both historical and contemporary. Age-specific mortality is a measure of human durability, and within a population it reflects the distribution of human vitality, immune status, and nutritional welfare. More research is needed on the links between mortality and lifetime morbidity; therefore mortality will continue to be used, with good reason, as the principal indicator of population health status.

In Tokyo, which is the capital of Japan and one of the most densely populated cities in the world, male and female longevities in 1999 were 76 and 82 years respectively and are projected to rise even higher in the decade ahead. The gap of 6 years favouring female over male longevity is close to the average found in all industrial populations. It reverses the direction of vital fortunes found in earlier human communities where gender differences in the average age of death favoured males by about 5 years (Cohen and Armelagos 1984).

Urban industrialism as a health revolution

Rising life expectancy is the best gauge of the health-promoting quality of urban industrialism. The northwestern corner of Europe, where the world's first urban industrial communities appeared in the nineteenth century, blazed the trail of the modern health revolution. In Sweden, the Netherlands, and Britain, more than two decades had been added to mean longevity before the antibiotic age commenced in the late 1940s. These nations developed the means—the knowledge, the technology, the political will—to make the city as, if not more, salubrious than the countryside. The transition may be dated to the 1920s. Before this rural communities in new industrializing nations contained most of the 'healthy' districts.

Subsequently, rural/urban health differences disappeared just as surely as urban/rural lifestyles converged in the industrializing nations of Western Europe and in Neo-European New World settlements. The term Neo-European was used by Alfred Crosby (1986) in his book *Ecological Imperialism* to depict the descent of the populations who colonized the temperate territories of the North America, Australia, and New Zealand.

The term 'healthy' districts was coined by William Farr (1885); they were not exclusively rural, but also included middle-class suburbs such as nineteenth-century Hampstead. The higher rate of death in urban areas reflected specific hygienic risks and also the higher poverty of resident labouring populations. The recent epidemiological history of less-developed (i.e. Third World) societies does not conform to the pattern established in Europe in the nineteenth and early twentieth centuries. By 1950, chemotherapy and modern vaccination had created a much more rapid and individuated means for avoiding the risk of infective and parasitic disease. As access to modern preventive medicine is much greater in metropolitan areas, the urban populations of developing countries tend to record better health status than their rural counterparts. Cities are also the places where urban governmental and administrative elites reside and where they provide for themselves and their retainers all the accoutrements of the Western lifestyle, including high-tech hospitals.

The health-generating potential of the modern city depends on the extent to which urban growth is a true product of industrialization. There are today many large sprawling cities in less-developed nations where living standards, environmental hygiene, and life chances are extremely poor. This urban development is specifically associated with the administrative/political functions of the nation-state and not necessarily connected to or reflective of fundamental processes of socio-economic development, which impact on the material conditions of the population at large. In these places, the ruling elite may enjoy a Western standard of living using scarce national resources to erect the infrastructure of a Western way of life, including hospitals equipped with the latest mechanical gadgets. These urban communities are not founded on a process of economic development, which incorporates the entire population, and they are not appropriately subsumed under the term urban industrial civilization. The latter development is a population-wide phenomenon that encompasses the living conditions of all citizens wherever they live. Even in rural areas, industrial peoples participate in the 'urban' lifestyle of the nation.

Modern urban society is healthier by far than any habitat spontaneously encountered in nature. The imaginary existence of the 'noble savage' and even his actual depiction by some modern day anthropologists (Sahlins 1974)—free of exploitation by others, free of repressive social moralities, free from the stresses and strains of clocks and timetables—romanticizes the life of our earliest human ancestors. Clues from Palaeolithic demography reveal the body of and industrial human to be twice as durable as that of his Stone Age ancestor. The respective comparison with Stone Age woman is even more favourable to her present-day counterpart (Roosevelt 1984). Whatever the measure—stature or longevity—life in modern society far exceeds the level of welfare achieved before the dawn of civilization, or at any subsequent point during the last 5000 years of recorded history.

The critical feature in the improvement of health, which accompanied the ascent of urban industrial civilization, was the virtual elimination of infective and parasitic disease. This is known as the epidemiological transition and its proportional causes remain a matter of academic controversy. Several factors contributed, among them improvements in: nutritional status, public and personal hygiene, living standards generally, the care of infants and children, and the status and rights of women. Although there is some evidence that the early technology of vaccination may have contributed to the decline of smallpox, the contribution of individual medical therapy was very limited and in some respects may even have been negative. The great transformation in human health was primarily the product of socially engineered changes in the environment; it was a matter of reducing the risks of exposure either by erecting barriers to infection or by raising the immune status of people.

The elimination of the threat of infective disease improved the durability of the human body and made way for a proportionate increase in degenerative disease. Degenerative disease is connected with the ageing of the human body and its various parts. Indeed, it might be thought of as a medical classification of the various processes by which human organs progressively lose their effectiveness. Fries and Crapo (1981) coined the term 'universal disease' to highlight this fact and to press home the point that postponement not prevention should be the goal of public health policy. In the present day, the social stratification of health status and survival (by nation, class, race, and gender) is a reflection of social inequalities in the postponement of universal disease allied to differential exposure to the risk of accidents and violence.

Global capitalism and the social environment of nation-states

Urban industrialism must not be thought of as an optional mode of social organization encountered in certain prosperous European, Neo-European (North America, Australia), and Asian nations. It is not simply a design for social organization to be admired, aspired to, and freely adopted. It is a worldwide system of social stratification, dominated by a 'rich man's club', which sets the terms for participation in the global economy.

Social stratification refers to the division of a population into a hierarchy defined by wealth and/or status. Stratification according to economic resources is called class, while status refers to social division based on cultural scales of value. In practice the two forms of stratification go hand in hand because the best resourced people exert a powerful influence over the construction of social meanings. An individual's location within a stratification order may vary according to the population frame of reference. A working-class Briton would be located near the apex of a global stratification order but near the bottom of the hierarchy in a national population.

Another way of putting this is that urban industrialism is a product of capitalism, which is the international system of financing production and trade, whose principal stimulus is the profit motive. Although some nations make more systematic attempts to regulate the capitalist forces of production and distribution within their territories (see below), capitalism recognizes no national boundaries.

Its international character is not a recent development. From its earliest beginnings the profit motive has been the most significant force in globalization. It sponsored the Columbian exchanges, the Atlantic slave trade, and the Louisiana Purchase, in its infancy, it may even be credited with stimulating the Black Death. The long shadow effects of early capitalist enterprise between the sixteenth and nineteenth centuries continues to haunt race relations globally. In the United States, they remain the leading factor shaping the pattern of health inequalities (see Figs 1 and 8 below).

Contemporary intercontinental and international health inequalities reflect patterns of uneven social and economic development, which are themselves the product of the historical circumstances of the emergence and evolution of industrial capitalist civilization and its colonial outreach. Industrial capitalism is a societal phenomenon. It is the third great mode of social organization in human history—the Palaeolithic, the agrarian, and the industrial. Its proximate origins are conventionally dated to the eighteenth century and the location of its birth is northwestern Europe. In the two succeeding centuries, it became a global phenomenon, eclipsing substantial alternative experiments with industrial social organization, in particular Eastern European communism. As we enter the third millennium, and as the People's Republic of China continues to pursue economic and social reforms designed to create a market society, there appear to be no significant alternative agendas for designing a 'productive' and prosperous social environment, although the healthiest less-developed nations/regions are conspicuously not those where market forces have been permitted to 'let rip' the social fabric of communal life (Jeffrey 1978).

Society and nation designating boundaries for the impact of the social environment on health

Until recently sociologists have tended to equate society with the nation-state, thereby producing a series of individual social formations for comparative analysis. Given that much of the evidence of the relationship between health and social relationships has been assembled within this framework, the nation-state is the default unit of comparison. However, the boundaries of a society and the social forces operating on human health cannot be assumed unproblematically to be contiguous with the boundaries of the nation-state. At an empirical level this fact has been known for centuries, as epidemiological exchange was the first dramatic, indeed devastating, evidence of the social forces of globalization in the early modern era. A growing body of scholarship in historical epidemiology testifies to the part played by disease as a force of historical change (Zinserr 1965; McNeill 1977; Watts 1997).

It is only very recently, however, that analytic sociological and political science perspectives have become sensitive to the fact that forces shaping social life do not originate and cannot be contained within individual nation-states. Even within national populations, there may be very significant regional variations in living conditions and health. The geography of health inequality has been monitored in Britain for over a century (OPCS 1978) and it shows no declining tendency (Dorling 1997). In the United States (Fig. 1) regional inequalities are so significant that health and survival chances in some regions are no better than in the less-developed nations of the Third World.

In 1990 a life expectancy gap of more than 15 years separated the worst and the best counties in the United States. Ironically, one of the unhealthiest counties, where male survival chances are below the level of many Third World communities, turns out to be Washington, DC—the capital of the richest nation in the world. This extraordinary observation is testimony to the power of race as a factor of health inequality, for Washington is a black city and it is race that primarily underlies the distribution in Fig. 1. Figure 1 is a striking demonstration that the social dimension of the environment overwhelms the natural/physical dimension, for it is evidently the persisting social inequalities from the legacy of slavery in the United States which ranks Washington as the second most unhealthy territory in the nation.

Knowledge of territorial differentials within nation-states highlights the difficulties of drawing the boundary for analysing the impact of the social environment on health. Even so, nationality is an empirically significant division in health status. A comparison between, for example, Japan and the United Kingdom demonstrates that significant variation is found among highly developed industrial nations (Marmot and Davey Smith 1989). Even among the dozen or so nation-states located within the neighbourhood of northwestern Europe, there are notable differences in mortality risk that appear to be strongly connected with varying patterns of gender relations and with distinctive national patterns of disease and premature death (Hart 1989*a*) (Fig. 2).

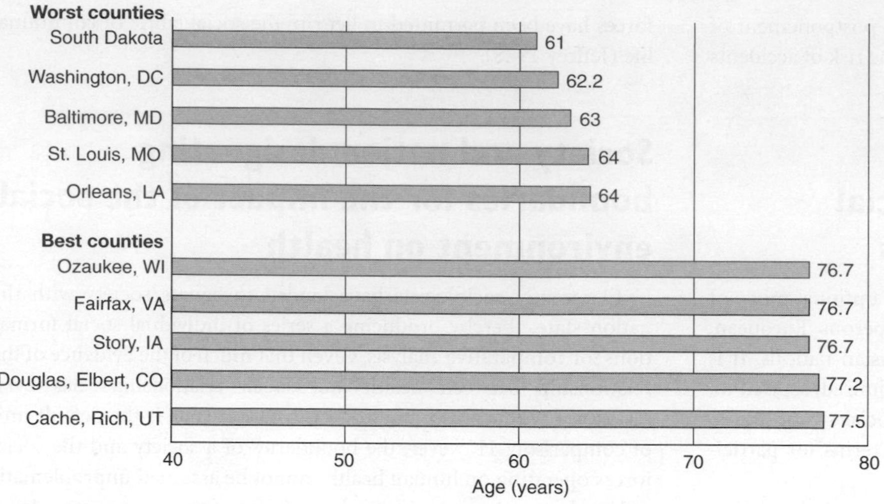

Fig. 1 Regional inequalities in health in the United States. (Data from Murray *et al.* 1998.)

The social environment and the expressive body

The range and scope of human qualities—psychic, emotional, somatic—virtually defies artificial scientific classification and anatomy, yet some sense must be made of the interactive sequences that make up the life process (James and Gabe 1996). The term 'expressive body' has been suggested as a means to capture the continuous and causally connected interchange between fundamentally different biochemical, psychological, and social processes entailed in human existence (Freund 1990). The question of how this interaction manifests itself in the processes of human development and daily interaction, and how it may be implicated in the processes of human vitality and disease are the most critical issues for the sociology of health and beyond that for the theory and practice of medicine (Evans *et al.* 1994).

The recognition that a socio-psychosomatic interchange plays a fundamental part in the health of human beings is a very old idea in medical thought, although it has taken a back seat to the biomechanical model in modern era.

Before the biomechanical paradigm began the ascent to its present contemporary pre-eminence, medical researchers and thinkers believed that this somatic dynamism must be powered by one or more vital spirits. For Plato, the heart was the source of the human spirit, although he also recognized the brain as the seat of reason (intellectual and sentient life) and the liver as the seat of appetite (the manufacturing base of the life process). A similar perspective frame of understanding was accepted from the times of Hippocrates (fifth century BC) to the eve of the modern mechanical era. William Harvey (1580–1656), a determined empiricist who first proved that the heart recycled the blood, remained committed to Platonic and Aristotelian ideas that vitality was a spirited phenomenon, that the body possessed a soul,

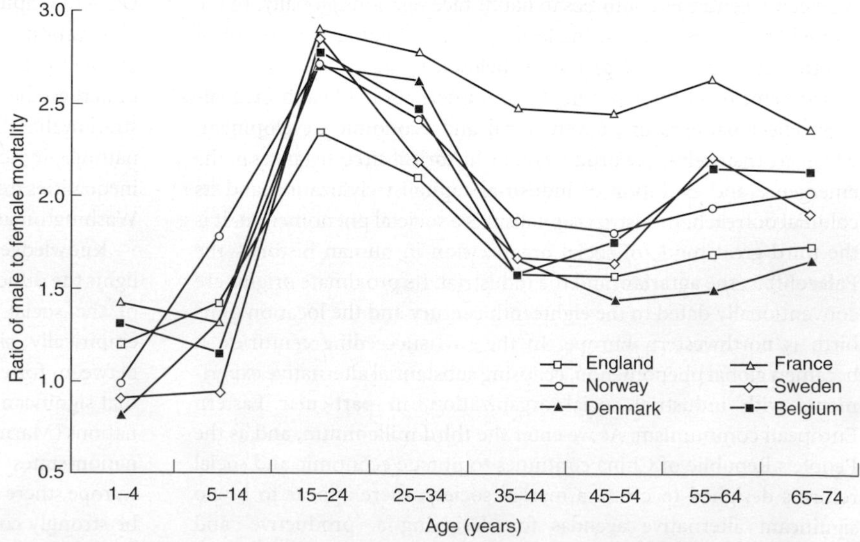

Fig. 2 Gender and survival in Western Europe.

and that physiological, emotional, and mental processes operated together in the management of somatic existence. These beliefs were the foundation of the Galenic paradigm, which captured and held the medical imagination in Europe from before the birth of Christ to the early modern era. They began to lose credibility in the sixteenth century as the machine age dawned. René Descartes is the figure most often associated with end of the Galenic paradigm in Western medical theory. His mechanical perspective left no room for the soul in bodily processes. In fact, Descartes rejected the idea that a human spirit directed bodily motion or function in any way at all. In the Cartesian paradigm, the soul did not even have a material existence. The human body was like a mechanical automaton powered by the heart and initially triggered by a divine switch. As Wear (1995, p. 340) puts it, '... Descartes' heart was like a mechanical engine which gave motion to the rest of the body. It was started by God, who put the initial heat into the heart, but God was acceptable to the mechanical philosophers'. Mind–body dualism was the legacy of Cartesian philosophy in medicine. It refers to the marked modern medical tendency to divide human experience into psychic and somatic arenas and to treat them autonomously. The depersonalized and socially anonymous body gradually became the most suitable object of observation and intervention.

The dominant contemporary paradigm of health is depicted as biological and mechanistic because of a virtually exclusive focus on the physiological and biochemical properties of human being and an associated tendency to objectify the body as a kind of machine which needs servicing, diagnosis and repair (McKeown 1976, p. xiv).

If the human body is a machine, it is far more sophisticated and versatile than any mechanism devised by humankind—an alimentary system transforms food fuel into energy and bodily repair materials, a sensory apparatus provides a continuous service of appraising and surveillance, an immune system works to repel noxious agents, a finely tuned muscular system permits motion and intricate movement, a brain and nervous system provides apparatus for learning, detection, judgement, speech, and communication, and a neuroendocrinal apparatus serves as an integrative mail service. All these extraordinary properties of the human being are interlinked by emotional mechanisms that articulate mental awareness and calculation with somatic and other vital processes.

This is medical materialism, and for much of the twentieth century it has nurtured an interventionist approach with a heavy reliance on machine technology and the biochemical manipulation of bodily processes. Although degenerative disease offers limited scope for curative intervention, the biomedical model has also spawned an energetic search for material risk factors, primarily elements of consumption or exposure deemed dangerous for survival. The next frontier for the biomedical paradigm is the decoding of the human genome, opening the door to the genetic manipulation of human tissue—ambitiously envisaged as the final solution for eliminating the material substance of disease. Although a knowledge of the massive influence of social organization and relationships on the distribution of health and disease within populations raises serious doubts about the future efficacy of genetic therapy for universal disease, there is no shortage of investors willing to fund the hugely expensive research effort required to anatomize human DNA. Fries and Crapo (1981) used the term 'universal disease' to highlight the normality of degenerate diseases.

The incentive is profit. The medico-industrial complex is the most profitable sector of contemporary global capitalism and private investment in genetic research is not the product of philanthropic impulse. Biogenetic companies are attractive to investors who hope to share in the profits expected from patenting the mysteries of the human genome and from the development of new techniques of biochemical intervention, which are expected to follow (Relman 1990).

The biomedical model embodies the materialist theory of disease and death. The human body is a material thing, disease has a real tangible appearance, and the most urgent and effective therapies are directed towards reversing or transforming pathogenic materiality. The aggregate impact of therapies developed through the biomedical paradigm on universal disease is surprisingly small. Faith is mostly sustained through a mystified understanding of medicine's past triumphs, an expectation that the future will yield rich rewards, and finally that this is the scientific, indeed the only sensible, approach to the management of human health in the modern era. In this perspective the body is abstracted from the other components of human experience—the emotional, the mental, and the social. Medical materialism shares a kindred spirit with sociological materialism, which also recognizes diet, living standards, working conditions, and housing (the material outcome of class, race, gender inequality) as the primary vectors of health and disease originating in the social environment.

The social theory of Karl Marx is known as materialism because he insisted that human beings are first and foremost material beings. This conclusion is based on the fact that the satisfaction of material needs in particular food is the primary requirement of daily existence. 'I eat, therefore I am'; my consciousness, my psychological state must therefore be secondary to my physical state. This classic blend of social and medical theory worked more effectively before and during the epidemiological transition; its explanatory limitations have been more exposed in the second half of the twentieth century as the mortal threat of acute and chronic infective and parasitic disease was substantially diluted in industrial societies. Even so, the direct impact of the material environment on the risk of disease and premature death remains a significant feature of the interaction between health and the social environment.

A 'holistic' conception of how the social environment impacts on human health calls for inclusion of all the life processes of human existence in the chain of causation. In other words, future progress in social medicine probably requires a substitution of the term social being for human body in order to decipher the epidemiological interaction of biochemical, emotional, psychological, and social life processes. Figure 3 charts the four principal components of human experience as a series of interacting spheres which show the potential array of categorically different forces implicated in the health of human beings.

Society is the surrounding sphere in Fig. 3. Its historically derived structure is the context for the biographical life of individuals. Soma is the corpus of the human being, the material substance that tends to be the exclusive focus of orthodox medical research and practice. Soma is a dynamic rather than a fixed thing. It literally emerges at conception through the bonding of sperm and ovum, and its dynamic potential is rapidly realized within a remarkable 20-week process of embryogenesis and organogenesis. Even before birth, fetal development appears to be powered by its own logic of physiological development

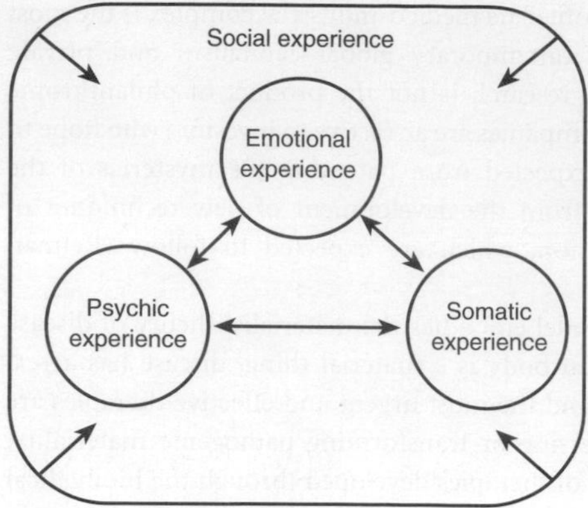

Fig. 3 The interactive processes of human health: society, psyche, emotion, and soma.

and is capable of adjusting to uterine constraints and opportunities (Barker 1994). The mature fetus is ready to attempt parturition at 40 weeks, although the dynamic of somatic growth (including weight gain and the achievement of stature) continues after birth until about the age of 16 years (Tanner 1978). When growth is complete, the human body 'works' to maintain life processes with minimal conscious management on the part of the sentient owner. The inherently dynamic character of the human body is evidenced in its apparently autonomous self-regulating and self-repairing properties. But the human body cannot survive without the sentient intervention of its owner or a caring parent or guardian.

Human existence entails a continuous process of mental calculation and communication, and much of it is based on the acquisition of cultural knowledge stored in the recesses of the mind. The ancients understood that the brain was the seat of reason and mental calculation. Modern researchers have gone much further in 'mapping' the various territories of the brain responsible for the government of human interaction and the inclusive formative activities of self, identity, intellect, personality, motivation, language, education, skill, knowledge, speech, and beliefs. Every minute of every day, the brain goes to work orchestrating decisions about appropriate action one after the other in rapid succession. Many of these decisions concern safety and have immediate vital relevance for ego and for other people. Modern urban society raises the stakes in this regard and at the same time reveals the enormous intellectual prowess of every human being, no matter what their measured IQ (Elias 1978). The safe operation of a modern freeway depends upon a vast interchange of skilful and sentient co-operation. Driving an automobile is a complex skill yet it is easily learned by an average human being, showing just how far many unskilled modern jobs underrate the potential capacities of the people who perform them (Blackburn and Mann 1979).

The intersection of mind and body is emotion. The fact that the body is emotionally reflexive is often witnessed in the course of social interaction even though human beings learn to manage and conceal the outward signs. The most visible manifestation is tears, a body fluid secreted in response to feelings of sadness, which reveals clearly how social events trigger biochemical bodily reactions (Katz 1999). The word expression meaning emission, release as well as verbal representation, captures the multifaceted character of communication, although the opportunity for catharsis is restricted by the etiquette of social interaction, which frequently dictates that emotional reactions be bottled up or otherwise transformed in polite society (Elias 1978). The body's emotional work might be consequently understood as the material equivalent of Freud's repressed unconscious. In this vein, we might conclude that rational man may be the primary victim if the requirement to withhold or disguise feelings is a cultural requirement more frequently imposed on the masculine than on the feminine social persona (Gilligan 1982).

A number of researchers have explored the possible contribution of managed emotions to the origins of modern disease (Totman 1979), and some have suggested that cultural variations in permissiveness of emotional response may explain distinctive national and ethnic epidemiological distributions (Arsenian and Arsenian 1948; Paulley 1975). These interactions open up a potentially vast field of socio-medical research, which some believe will prove particularly important in explaining persisting social inequalities in health (Sapolsky 1991). In Fig. 3, the tripartite structure of the human self is pictured by, located in, and encompassed by a social environment. Later in the chapter, considerable space is devoted to a delineation of the social environment as a series of macro- to microspheres enclosing and thereby shaping the unique biographical experience of individual human beings.

The Enlightenment planted two important ideas that shaped future research on the fate of individuals in society. The first draws an analogy with a *tabula rasa* to capture the plasticity of human formation and to illustrate the power of society's agents of socialization and child development—the family, the school, the church, the mass media, the medical system, and the state (Sagan 1996). Children will be what society wills them to be. The second recognizes that the composition of every human being represents a unique configuration of biographical contingencies; no one human being is ever the exact clone of another. The permutation of social, psychic, emotional, and somatic experience in a single person produces a unique configuration of human characteristics. At the same time, the macro- and microspheres of the social environment discharge a number of systematic forces, which either unify or divide the social group. Gender, race, and class are the pre-eminent axes of social stratification. They give rise to a series of overlapping hierarchies of social relationships that shape the context and outcome of everyday life. On a daily basis the expressive body experiences itself in and through these relationships, aiming for and sometimes, but not always, achieving material satisfaction, freedom from pain, emotional tranquillity, and self-reaffirmation (Collins 1990; Freund 1990; Williams 1998). In this ongoing way, society intersects with the psycho-emotional and biochemical processes that make up human existence. The multifaceted model of a human being captured in the concept of the expressive body offers a fruitful framework for surveying all the potential points of intersection between health and the social environment.

Macro- and micro-arenas of the social environment

The expressive body experiences the social environment as a series of enclosed spheres, which may possess insulating powers of varying magnitude. Figure 4 illustrates these relationships.

The outer and the inner rims of Fig. 4 represent a series of enveloping spheres around an inner core representing individual existence. Note that the human being is identified as a biographical

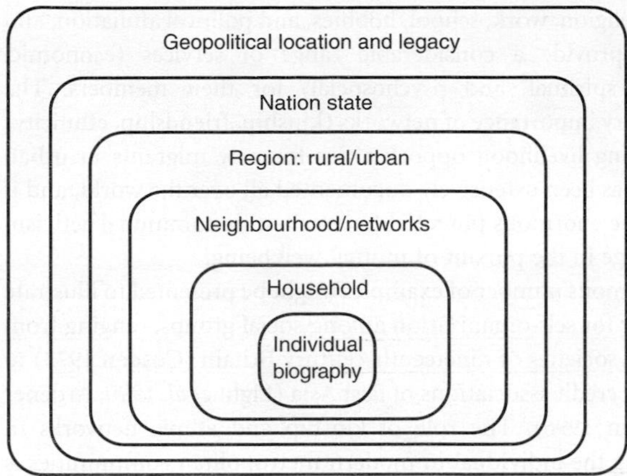

Fig. 4 Spheres of the social environment influencing individual biography.

phenomenon. The expressive body has its own unique physiological, psychic, and social histories, whose interaction determines the chances of survival. In the debate about the causes of systematic health inequalities within populations, the issue of biography has received considerable attention. Researchers have clashed over the relative importance of early 'formative' experience. There is a strong a priori case for assigning additional weight to the first two decades (including fetal life) in the formation of the expressive body. Apart from anything else, physical stature is determined by the age of about 16 to 17 years, and, as this is strongly correlated with survival rates within national populations, the quantity and quality of child rearing resources seems to be an unassailable ingredient of adult health experience (Tanner 1978). The work of David Barker and colleagues highlighting the very earliest fetal phases of human development has a growing influence on this debate (Barker 1994).

Another important point to note is that the outermost sphere extends the boundary of the social environment beyond the nation-state. The most significant and widest forms of health inequality originate in this outermost macrosphere, i.e. the global sphere. While a longevity gap of only a few years separates human durability between the industrial nation-states, the gap between more and less-developed societies is up to three decades. While these inequalities seem remote and disconnected to the experience of First World peoples, they are not. The process of industrialization was preceded by and depended on the expropriation and colonization of non-European territories, and living standards in First World nations still depend heavily on an unbalanced global trade in primary commodities and an unequal exploitation of the Earth's atmospheric, oceanic, and geological resources (Smith 1999).

Two of the enclosing spheres in Fig. 4 contribute disproportionately to the impact of the social environment on human health. These are the sphere of the nation-state and the sphere of the household, sociologically known as the public and private spheres of the social environment respectively. Societal development in the modern era may be equated with increasing enlargement of the scope of the public sphere. In pre-industrial societies (historic and contemporary), the public sphere is far less extensive in its outreach functions and the private sphere provides a far larger volume of individual material and emotional needs. The governance of social relationships within private life is subject to ecclesiastical and civil law but, in practice, a male authority figure in the private sphere enjoys a considerable 'natural right' to supervise and discipline his family and household. The historical facts of patriarchal domination in the private sphere explain why the private sphere is frequently singled out for analytical primacy in contemporary feminist analyses of gender inequality. The expansion of the public sphere is associated with a diminution of the idea of 'natural patriarchal rights' and an increase in legally defined individual rights. This is manifested in the increasingly interventionist role of the nation-state supervising relationships in the private sphere, in particular marriage and parenthood. Therefore the relative size and scope of the two spheres varies greatly between societies at different levels of social and economic development. The importance of the public sphere of the social environment will be discussed in greater detail shortly, with most attention given to industrial nation-states where it is highly developed.

Between the outer rim and the personal existence of the expressive body are a series of potentially insulating layers. The social institutions of the nation-state play an important part in either exposing or protecting life chances within their territories. This is the most important factor in the macrosocial environment. Nation-states are power structures. If they are democratically constituted, they ostensibly represent the interests and will of the people and their remit is to provide and manage a social infrastructure to safeguard the well being of the population. Public health legislation and institutions are a prime example of how the nation-state carries out this responsibility. Indeed the historical record of the first industrial societies indicates that pressures to inaugurate public health reforms played a crucial part in consolidating national governmental structures and public authorities in the late nineteenth century (Rosen 1958; Rosenberg 1975; de Swann 1988). This happened because private interests were neither disposed to inaugurate the integrated urban sanitation and communication projects that literally 'paved the way' for the healthy city nor possessed of sufficient territorial authority to do so. Modern governments interpret their responsibility for the public health in more or less expansive ways. Embracing a relatively narrow biomedical understanding of their responsibility for public health, they may see their remit as a duty to insure the population against the chances and consequences of disease by organizing access to comprehensive medical care. Among the mature industrial nation-states, the United States is the only exception to the rule that access to medical care should be set apart from the profit sector of the economy and organized by the national government. A broader sociomedical perspective on the public health reinforces a more integrated policy programme linking access to health care to income maintenance, full employment, and other social services (see below).

A regional sphere of the social environment is also distinguished in Fig. 4. This is more evident in nation-states with large territories and populations. In such cases, the national territory may represent past processes of geopolitical amalgamation involving distinct ethnic and linguistic communities. This legacy may be reflected in future patterns of race and ethnic stratification in the national population and in the distribution of health. This is true of many European nations, including Britain, Belgium, Spain, and France, and in each case regional health variations still bear the legacy of economic and cultural history. This refers to cultural legacies before the twentieth century (e.g. England, Wales, Scotland, Ireland).

The United States, which is the most populous industrial capitalist society, displays substantial regional inequalities in health and survival across its large territory. Strong hints of the way that this is articulated to the history of race relations in the United States are highlighted in Fig. 1, which also shows how, even within regions, other locality variables may be important in shaping survival chances. In the second half of the twentieth century, processes of migration, suburbanization, and deindustrialization combined to enhance the health risks of inner cities, rendering them once more (as in the late nineteenth century) the unhealthiest spaces in the national territory. Urban–rural inequalities in health today are far less a function of deficient sanitation and much more a direct reflection of real estate values and the impoverished economic status of the inner-city populations. These trends have enhanced the value of location variables as means of measuring the distribution of inequalities in health.

The sphere of networks and neighbourhood in Fig. 4 is the outer enclosure of the microsphere of the social environment. The term 'neighbourhood' suggests a propensity for fellowship among residentially contiguous households and individuals. In an earlier era this propensity may have found expression in the shared communal facilities, such as the local church, which could orchestrate supportive and charitable activity. Processes of secularization, allied to the increased mobility and growing diversity of local populations, has diminished the scope of the voluntary work performed by neighbours for one another through churches and other forms of local association. Even so, the neighbourhood still represents a potentially important agency of social support and social control, providing informal help and setting limits of tolerance for idiosyncratic, unruly, and, more importantly, aggressive behaviour in the local vicinity. This potential has generally been realized through informal mechanisms, and its effectiveness depends on the extent to which neighbours identify with and recognize a mutual responsibility to one another.

The extent of mutuality in a neighbourhood depends on a number of factors. Residential stability is one, shaping the opportunity for neighbours to get to know one another. The local age and sex structure determines how depopulated the neighbourhood becomes during the working day and physical/commercial neighbourhood features may either encourage or discourage pedestrian activity, which also shapes the chance of daily/weekly encounters and the formation of relationships between people who live near one another. In recent times, new formal mechanisms of mutual insurance have developed. The form they take depends on the prosperity of the community. More prosperous neighbourhoods have erected barriers and gates to regulate access to their property and private security firms to police it. In less prosperous communities, rising anxiety about the risk of crime and fear of strangers has encouraged neighbours to form watch committees to look out for and report suspicious persons and incidents. These developments may reflect the diminution of the informal power of local ties and increasing anonymity of modern life. In the latter sense, it is worth noting that the downside of 'old-style' close-knit ethnically homogeneous neighbourhood is that they may also operate as an instrument of intolerance, closing ranks to marginalize immigrants and to stigmatize unfamiliar and/or innovative lifestyles.

Even when the immediate residential environment is relatively anonymous, a significant layer of neighbourhood affiliation and support may still envelop the individual or household. Sociologists and anthropologists developed the concept of the social network to depict the ties that bind groups of people together in settings where individuals might otherwise appear socially isolated (Bott 1957). Networks may be organized around kinship, friendship, shared ethnicity, religion, work, school, hobbies, and political affiliation, and they may provide a considerable range of services (economic, emotional, spiritual, and psychosocial) for their members. The extraordinary importance of networks (kinship, friendship, ethnicity) in negotiating livelihood opportunities for new migrants in urban situations has been extensively documented all over the world, and it speaks to the enormous potential for small-scale communal activism and exchange in the pursuit of mutual well being.

An enormous number of examples might be presented to illustrate the capacity for self-organization among social groups, ranging from the friendly societies of nineteenth-century Britain (Gosden 1973) to the rotating credit associations of East Asia (Light *et al.* 1990; Ardener and Burman 1996). The role of kinship and ethnic networks in provisioning the individual in modern metropolitan communities is well documented by urban sociologists (Waldinger and Borzorgmehr 1996).

The contribution of supportive networks to personal health and survival is also very substantial. Social networks are enveloping sets of relationships through which individuals develop their identities, which in turn shape the motivation to act in accordance with a sense of self and lifestyle. Networks may thus act to reinforce both positive and negative patterns of 'health behaviour' (Cockerham *et al.* 1997). Bott (1957) made a simple yet striking sociological discovery about social networks in a study of the family in London in the 1950s. Using a 'knitting analogy', she showed that the tension of a family's social network was linked to the sexual division of labour in the household. Close-knit networks, where all participants know one another so that lines of affiliation cut across the entire network, were found in conjunction with a gender-segregated division of labour. Loose-knit networks, more anonymous with mutually exclusive lines of affiliation, were associated with a relatively gender-free division of family labour. Bott developed the terminology of segregated, complementary, and joint conjugal roles to depict variations in the marital relationship associated with close- and loose-knit networks. Joint conjugal roles are the centrepiece of companionate marriage in which gender division is significantly diluted. Husbands and wives participate together in work and leisure, and in the 1950s they were predominantly associated with middle-class family life. Companionate marriage is part of a trend of gender convergence in the twentieth century that carries major significance for health; the fact that its development is linked to social networks points to the wider epidemiological significance of these social groupings.

The 1950s was a fertile period for new theoretical insights about the scope for social affiliation in urban situations. Sociologists and historians had long imagined the industrial city to be a relatively anonymous environment—a social terrain created for the 'individuated social persona' of industrial capitalism free to devise his or her own lifestyle. The classic statement was Wirth's *Urbanism as a Way of Life* (1938). This view of the city as a site of social anonymity was always at some odds with ethnographic evidence gathered in studies of immigrant communities, especially in the United States (Lal 1990). Bott's (1957) research also pointed out that networks did not have to be close-knit and local to provide members with a sense of social connectedness and support in urban populations. As new means of communication emerged during the twentieth century, the scope for developing and maintaining far-flung networks has proportionately increased. If this trend has tended to diminish the significance of local close-knit networks in the management of everyday life, additional pressures may have been felt on the core relationship in the private sphere of life—marriage.

Research like Bott's exposed two problems with this conception. It emphasized the continued vibrancy of close-knit networks in urban industrial situations and the fact that the support they provided could act as a barrier to innovative behaviour. A loose-knit network offered more space for innovative development of lifestyle, such as gender-neutral conjugality, because the web of social affiliations was less dense and less able to sanction deviant, i.e. novel, behaviour. These insights hold important lessons for understanding the stimulus for and barriers to the development of innovative forms of 'healthy behaviour'.

A number of researchers have demonstrated the preservative effect of immersion in networks based on kinship, friendship, and local association, including church membership. One of the most quoted studies found a mortality differential of more than 2.5:1 between people who scored low and high on an index of social affiliation (Berkman and Syme 1979). This is profoundly important evidence of the interconnectedness of mind and body in society, revealing the severe limitations of the biomedical model approach to the explanation of systematic social variations in the postponement of universal disease (see above). However, social networks, particularly the close-knit variety, may also exert a negative effect on survival.

The gang is a close-knit social network, a setting within the microsocial environment in which young men seek to earn a 'respectable' identity by exposing themselves to an elevated risk of violent death (Courtwright 1996). This is one component of the pattern of excess male mortality in the second and third decades of a lifetime (see Fig. 2). The gang illustrates the sociology of death from accidental and violent causes, i.e. the way it is articulated to the social environment in a systematic and comprehensible fashion. The rate of violent death is not an aggregate of random events, however, it flows from class-based cultures of masculinity which construct the identities and motivations of adolescent and young adult men, propelling them into at-risk behaviours of varying severity. This is one example where social capital arising out of membership in social networks must be located on the deficit side of the health and survival equation (Buford 1993).

Thus membership of social networks may either enhance or diminish survival chances. Gang networks are an extreme example of the diminishing effect. A more routine instance of the negative health consequences of the social network is the barrier that membership may erect towards behavioural change. Once again it is easier to come up with examples of male social networks that have deleterious health consequences. The British television series *Men Behaving Badly* invariably involves the consumption of alcoholic beverages. The association has probably held from time immemorial and in diverse cultural settings everywhere. The reform of male drunkenness as a primary object of social and health improvement was associated with the Temperance Movement in Protestant nations in the nineteenth and early twentieth century. The extent of its success was partly a function of the rising consumption of cigarettes—tobacco was the best friend of temperance. Drinking and smoking are the two known primary contemporary medical risk factors that diminish survival chances, and shifting patterns of class consumption have made an important contribution to the worsening trend of class mortality gradients (Fig. 6). In the case of drinking, the decline of consumption involved separating men from customary patterns of male sociability, i.e. close-knit male social networks based on the pub. The consumption of alcohol among Protestant males fell steadily through the early twentieth century and one of the most important factors in the trend was the emergence of companionate marriage, which increasingly redirected male leisure away from the public house (the pub) and towards the private home (Hart 1989*b*).

The insulating properties of family relationships

The most significant layer of microsocial insulation between the individual and the outermost impersonal spheres of the social environment is the household or family. This is the private sphere of social life. Sociologists differ in their valuation of the private sphere as a font of emotional and psychic well being. Mid-twentieth-century structural functionalism associated with Talcott Parsons theorized it as an arena of intimacy and mutual interdependence set apart from the cash nexus, where services are provided free and relationships are not shaped by market principles.

Later feminist-influenced critiques were more likely to point to the scope for inequality in private-sphere relations and to highlight the family as a site of patriarchal privilege and female oppression (e.g. Barrett and McIntosh 1982). There is empirical support for both sides of this argument. The use of reasonable chastisement by male household heads to discipline wives and children was historically sanctioned by law in Western culture. Although resort to violence within the family has been progressively criminalized, reports of its incidence remain very high, and the private space of family life provides an ideal arena for its concealment. Observers disagree in their interpretation of contemporary statistics of domestic abuse. In the face of static or upward trends, more pessimistic accounts argue that, despite legal reform, nothing has changed. More optimistic accounts stress the difficulties of interpretation, seeing the same trends as evidence of rising intolerance of violent acts and the greater willingness of both victims and law-enforcement officers to report cases, apprehend perpetrators, and inflate statistics.

The original French version of structural functionalism developed by one of sociology's founders, Emile Durkheim, is rather less sentimental in its depiction of private-sphere relationships. The half-century separating Durkheim and Parsons saw substantial shifts in the conjugal relationship in the direction of what has been called companionate marriage. This social change coloured Parson's understanding of the essence of social relationships within the family, emphasizing sentimental over disciplinarian norms.

Whatever the relative merit of these opposed interpretations, there is a great deal of evidence pointing to the health-promoting potential of private-sphere relationships. Individuals of all ages living in contexts where they enjoy the unconditional commitment of parents, spouses, and siblings, or their non-kin equivalents, derive a substantial health dividend. Among these relationships, the clearest evidence exists for marriage. Married people of both sexes record death rates well below the rates of the unattached and the benefits rise with decreasing social class (OPCS 1978, p. 34).

Although there may be some selective (into and out of marriage) effect in the statistical record (Hu and Goldman 1990; Goldman and Hu 1993), the differential power of marital status promoting survival in different nations does not suggest that it may be simply explained as a statistical artefact. The most dramatic evidence of marriage's preservative effect has emerged recently in Eastern Europe. Here, in the midst of a health crisis linked to societal reconstruction and popularly associated with pollution, marital status has stood out as the most important means of insulating individual men and women from a sharply rising risk of death. This is further proof of the necessity of employing the expressive body as a model of human health as well as critical evidence that the microsocial environment offers a substantial means of insulation in contexts of societal stress, i.e. major upheaval in the outer public sphere of the social environment and even a deteriorating atmospheric environment (Hajdu *et al.* 1995; Watson 1995).

The anatomy of the social environment within the nation-state

How does the social environment vary between nations in ways that determine marginal differences in health status? To answer to this question, it is useful to build an anatomy of national society specifying the structural features of the environment for human development and survival. This is attempted in Fig. 5, which identifies three primary spheres of the social environment—economy, polity, and culture. In this chapter these three spheres encompassing economic, political, and cultural influences are subsumed under the heading of the social, which is taken as the comprehensive frame of analysis.

Economy in the social environment

Economy refers to social institutions concerned with the production and distribution of livelihood and the reproduction of the population.

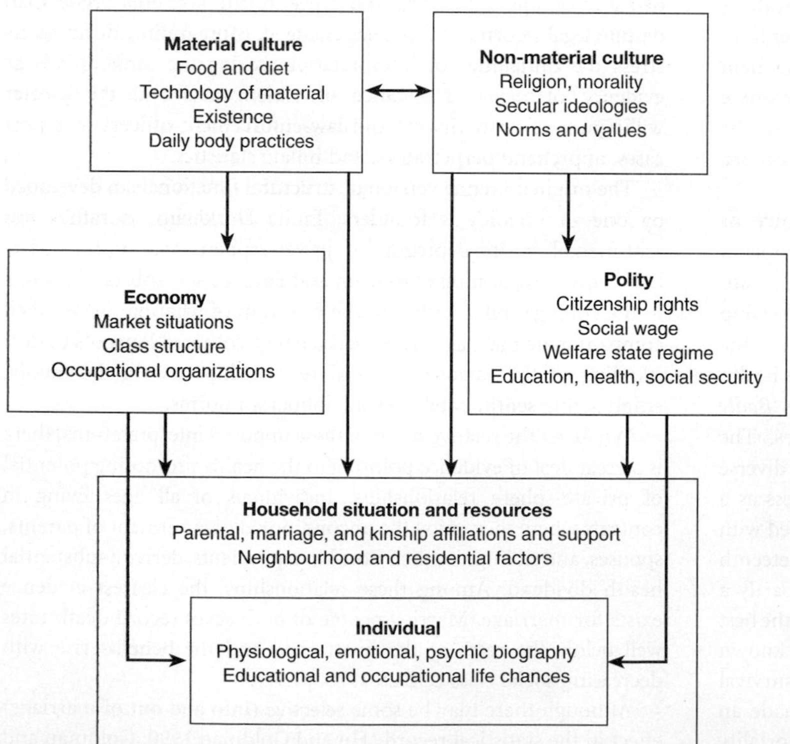

Fig. 5 Culture, economy, and polity as factors in human health.

The earliest economists (Smith, Malthus, Ricardo) were much more conscious of the fact that production and reproduction were two sides of the same coin. In the eighteenth century, demography (political arithmetic) was firmly established at the centre of economic analysis and nobody doubted that population was a primary factor of production and consumption (Rathbone 1924; Routh 1975). Their twentieth-century counterparts, focused on the international workings of the capitalist system, have long ago detached the material processes of making the next generation from their perspective of the logic of economic life. From the perspective of the public health, classical political economy is the more appropriate paradigm.

The economy includes the population organized into households and the work performed there (including procreation), the social institutions of the market and private property, the aggregate wealth of the population, including productive resources and plant in agriculture and manufacturing industries, occupational organizations, including trade unions and professions, and government legislation and regulatory agencies, including national treasuries, policy-making agencies, and occupational health and safety inspectorates. Economists use the term 'national income' to measure the aggregate earnings of a national economy, and sociologists use the term 'class' to refer to the hierarchy of wealth and income groups formed by its unequal ownership and distribution among the population. The term 'gross national product (**GNP**) per capita' refers to the value of national income divided by the number of people in the population. Measures of GNP always exaggerate average income because they assume that every one receives an equal share. In practice, the distribution of income is highly unequal in all industrial societies. Typically, a small but very rich group monopolizes a large share of national income, whereas a substantial proportion of the population receives income below the poverty standard. The last quarter of the twentieth century witnessed an accentuation of income inequality in Western capitalist societies. In the United States between 1965 and 1995, the share of total income going to the richest 5 per cent of the families in the national population increased from 15.5 to 20.1 per cent. Over the same period the upper quintile of the income distribution increased its share from 40 to 46 per cent. This redistribution to the very rich was accomplished mostly by tax-cutting measures at the expense of the lowest three quintiles. The income inequality trend in the United States is laid out in Table 1. It includes the Gini ratio, which indicates the proportion of income that would need to be redistributed to achieve parity between the five quintiles. In the four decades leading up to 1995, this increased from 0.356 to 0.426.

The growing research literature supporting the relative income hypothesis argues that the pattern of income inequalities laid out in Table 1 is the primary social vector of health inequality in industrial nation-states. Gravelle (1998) gives a succinct summary and critical evaluation of the relative income hypothesis.

Wilkinson (1992) regressed a combined estimate of male and female mortality on the distribution of family income for the nine OECD nations (Norway, Sweden. Switzerland, Netherlands, Austria, Canada, the United States, the United Kingdom, and Germany). He reported a correlation of 0.86 ($p < 0.001$) between life expectancy and the proportion of income received by the 70 per cent of the families with incomes below the third decile of the distribution. Inserting an additional control for GNP per capita increased the correlation to 0.91 per cent, enabling Wilkinson to suggest that three-quarters of the variation in longevity could be explained by differences in income inequality between the nine societies. Note the range of variations in the two correlated indices. Combined male and female life expectancy runs from about 73 to 76 years (a gap of 3 years), and the percentage of income going to the population below the upper three deciles of the income distribution varies from about 45 to 50 per cent (a range of 5 per cent). In regard to the latter, it must be noted that even in the most equal income distribution in the data set, only 50 per cent of the nation's income goes to 70 per cent of families.

Subsequent publications by the same author and by others stimulated by his example have now produced a considerable number of papers reporting mortality–income inequality relationships of varying size and strength between both nations and states within the United States (Kawachi *et al.* 1999). The accumulating body of evidence has also fed a round of theoretical speculation on the utility of income inequality as an index of social cohesion and/or social capital (Wilkinson 1996; Kawachi *et al.* 1999). The unhealthy society thesis is relatively easy to subject to empirical test, and hence the growing body of published findings support the early claim that income inequality measures the corrosive tendencies of the social environment, although few have managed to reproduce the scale of association claimed by Wilkinson (1992). However, there are some curious features to the reported findings that cast doubt on their robustness. Judge (1995) attempted to replicate Wilkinson's research using the same data and measures but added per capita income distribution in addition to the measure based on families. The use of per capita income greatly diminished the association between income inequality and life expectancy. For the population below the seventh decile of the income distribution, the correlation with life expectancy fell from 0.80 ($p > 0.001$) to 0.31 (not significant) when per capita measures were substituted for the family measure. Furthermore, still using the same data set, Judge also failed to find an association using alternative measures of income inequality such as the Gini coefficient. As Judge observes, the use of a measure of income distribution between families does not take account of differences in average family size between nations. Although Wilkinson (1995) has published a spirited response to this critique, he does not offer a persuasive explanation of why family income measures of inequality produce strongly significant associations while alternative measures do not. If the relative income hypothesis is valid and if the effect of income inequality is as strong as its proponents insist, one would expect to find robust results with all measures of income inequality on the same data set.

In this thesis, the issue is not about egalitarian versus inegalitarian societies—it is about marginal differences in extent of income inequality. The degree of income inequality varies between nation-states mainly in response to the relative autonomy of the market processes. The United States is probably the most unequal advanced industrial society, mainly because the market is a virtually sacred social institution and strong moral beliefs protect it from political intervention. Consequently, the social wage is very weakly developed. However, the general pattern of income inequalities depicted in Table 1 is a quite normal feature of all modern and postmodern industrial capitalist nations. An income distribution allocating about 5 to 6 per cent of total income to the poorest quintile and about 38 to 40 per cent to the richest is entirely orthodox.

Economic inequalities within nation-states are correlated with health and survival inequalities. The measurement of this effect over

Table 1 Trends in income inequality among families in the United States, 1965–95

Year	Lowest 20%	Second 20%	Third 20%	Fourth 20%	Highest 20%	Top 5%	Gini ratio
1965	5.2	12.2	17.8	23.9	40.9	15.5	0.356
1970	5.4	12.2	17.6	23.8	40.9	15.6	0.353
1975	5.4	11.8	17.6	24.1	41.1	15.5	0.357
1980	5.1	11.6	17.5	24.3	41.6	15.3	0.365
1985	4.6	10.9	16.9	24.2	43.5	16.7	0.389
1990	4.6	10.8	16.6	23.8	44.3	17.4	0.396
1995	4.2	10	15.7	23.3	46.9	20.1	0.426

Source: US Bureau of the Census International Database (http:\\www.census.gov).

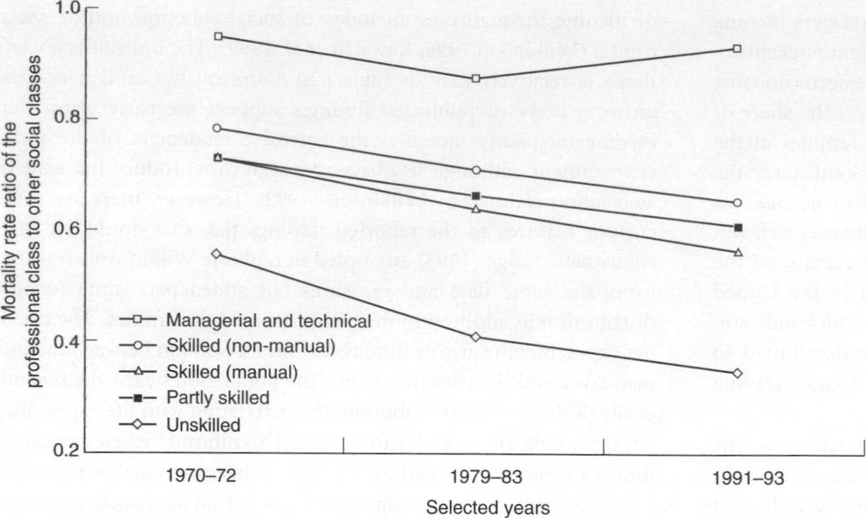

Fig. 6 Trends in health inequality by social class in England and Wales, 1970 to 1993.

the course of the twentieth century is best reviewed using British data because the National Statistical Office established a methodology for monitoring occupational and social class mortality differentials early in the twentieth century. In these data, occupation is a proxy for income. Figure 6 charts the trend of class inequality in health in England and Wales since 1921.

In 1970, there was a gap of about 7 years between the life expectancies of men classified in social class I and in social class V in Britain's occupational class structure (OPCS 1978). This scale of inequality was nothing new, although it appears disquieting to those who expected that the National Health Service would equalize the burden of disease and neutralize inequalities in the length of life. Note how this understanding is derived from an abstract biomedical model of health. Over the course of the twentieth century, the Registrar General's class divisions remained remarkably effective in identifying social inequalities in health, i.e. inequalities arising from the economic component of the social environment. The Registrar General's social class scale is a sixfold grouping of occupations according to their general standing in the community. This rather imprecise mode of classification is actually based on a status definition—the volume of social prestige associated with an occupation. However, the scale is also clearly economic, it depends on occupational skills and credentials that determine the price of labour and the security of livelihood in the market. Naturally, over the course of the century the occupational structure changed significantly in response to technological innovation and the growing global division of labour, which led to the export of manufacturing jobs and the substitution of imports for home-produced raw materials such as coal. These developments changed the nature of work to a substantial degree, but they do not appear to have exerted a proportional impact on health inequalities. A government working group, convened to review progress in the health of the population in 1980, concluded that the class gap in health in Britain had probably worsened during the last quarter of the twentieth century (DHSS 1980). Subsequent research has borne out this conclusion and shown that the effect is not restricted to the United Kingdom (Marmot and McDowell 1986; Valkonen *et al.* 1990; Pappas *et al.* 1993).

Social class measures inequalities in the distribution of a nation's wealth and annual income among the individuals and households who make up the population. It also includes inequalities in the relative cost of work to the individual worker, exposure to occupational hazards, occupational stressors, and hours of work. Class inequality has a number of forms, some more tangible than others. The most tangible is annual income and consumer power. This inequality is measured in material limitations on how people live and what kind of lifestyle choices they are empowered to make (Cockerham 1999). Related inequalities of occupational rights—protection and compensation for sickness, redundancy, and pensions—are equally important. The less intangible output of the class system is the distribution of status and prestige. The scale of differential earning and consumer power is simultaneously a scale of social worth. It denotes the value of the individual worker in the total scheme of things, sending crystal-clear messages that some are more worthy than others. Wilkinson (1996) identifies this psychosocial production of the economy as the more significant source of social inequality in health in post-epidemiological transition contexts. He suggests that hierarchical social relations arising from income inequality have emerged as the most potent source of biomedical risk in an otherwise prosperous social environment.

The economies of individual nation-states exhibit distinctive characteristics that reflect the peculiarities of their economic history, including, where appropriate, the particularities of the nation's transition to urban industrialism. Nations may exhibit economic specialisms that reflect geographical situation, geological resources, historical circumstances, or long-standing artisan or professional traditions. Sometimes, dramatic and destructive historical events can shift a national economy in new directions. This was the fate of Germany and Japan following their defeat in the Second World War. Both nations were brought to their knees by the combination of their own military ambitions and the subsequent Allied assault, leaving their industrial infrastructure severely damaged. As both were prevented from redeveloping their military capacity, their respective postwar programmes of technological research and development favoured the production of consumer goods in which they became global leaders. The victor nations (particularly the United States, France, and the United Kingdom), freed from the same restrictions, continued to put a premium on weapons research, ensuring that military production organized through highly developed capitalist industries remained a strong focus of the economy in these nations. The international arms trade is a highly profitable sphere of global capitalism with definite health and survival implications for national populations worldwide. The governments of less-developed nations are prolific consumers of Western armaments which are frequently used to police the nation-state and repress political opposition. The public health consequences of the international arms trade is a very important feature of global health inequalities. It enjoins the profits and material living standards of people engaged in armament production in prosperous nations with the death and disabilities endured by their deployment in less stable parts of the global social environment.

In a modern urban industrial nation, the economy is not autonomous; its operation is subject to forces emanating from the international capital market. Consequently, like a tsunami wave, economic events and trends on one side of the world can have knock-on effects on the other side where they are felt in the form of shifts (up and down) in the cost of living—in food, rents, interest, and wages. The international organization of economic life is a reminder that capitalism operates without consideration for the circumstances of individual nation-states. This may be one reason why reproductive issues have been removed from the economist's consciousness and relocated in a separate discipline—demography. The separation of society's two economic functions—production and reproduction—is a product of the individuating tendencies of industrial capitalism. It constitutes the critical flaw of capitalism as a model of effective organization of material existence within modern societies (Polanyi 1946).

The capitalist labour market is oriented to individuals rather than households. This feature has fuelled the enormous increase in personal autonomy experienced during the short but tumultuous history of capitalist civilization. Capitalist enterprises employ individuals, and the wages that they pay makes no allowance for the employee's household and family responsibilities. A single adult with no children earns the same as a married man or women with any number of dependents. The same effect is witnessed at the level of the nation-state; the capitalist market contains no institutional mechanism to articulate the nation's vital processes with its livelihood. Procreation is obviously a vital social function. The maintenance of a flow of people through the social fabric is a *sine qua non* of societal continuity. In precapitalist societies, production and reproduction were not distinguished. The household economy performed both social functions, and norms of kinship reciprocity made grandparents, parents, and children mutually interdependent.

Demographic historians have revealed how pre-industrial economies regulated the demographic process to protect the material conditions of existence. In England, this was achieved by severe sanctions against unmarried procreation and by varying the age at marriage. Late marriage age shortened the child-bearing career of the married female and operated as a preventive check on the rate of fertility (Wrigley and Schofield 1982).

The utilitarian logic of market capitalism is ultimately corrosive to the norms of family solidarity that underpinned the old procreative regime and wove it seamlessly with the livelihood system. The lack of any arrangement to orchestrate procreation with economic life goes unnoticed in capitalism's early development. In the short to medium term, the old cultural imperatives continue to propel men and women into marriage and procreative ventures. Over the long term, the old norms are eroded as the individual wage worker emerges as the free agent of his or her own destiny, and as public and private pension schemes replace the expectation that the elder generations can rely on material support from the younger generation in old age. This development fundamentally shifts the motivation for procreation replacing utilitarian logic with expressive sentiment, undoubtedly a less certain base for population replacement.

Child bearing and child rearing represent substantial opportunity costs in the adult female life career and, given the increased fragility of marriage (Fuchs 1988), women cannot count on the unfailing future support of the father to shoulder the labour requirements of parenthood and to fund the considerable additional expenses of bringing a child into the world. This is part of the explanation for the declining popularity of marriage and the falling rate of fertility that has accompanied women's incorporation in the labour force in recent decades. Ironically, the same process brings about a revaluation of children and childhood, which some observers include among the causes of the industrial era's health revolution (Shorter 1976; Zelizer 1985; Sagan 1996).

Analysis of the health consequences of the vital flaw in capitalist society is underdeveloped. Statisticians working within the social medicine tradition have relied on measures of social stratification based principally on male occupational life. In doing so, they accepted the reality of patriarchal power and the argument that the level of the breadwinner's wage was the primary determinant of household well being. The weakness here is the assumption of undifferentiated size. Material well being at home depends crucially on the ratio of people to space and resources. A manual worker's wage packet goes much further in a household of four than it does in one of eight. The size of the sibling group is a major factor of household living standard; it has never been properly represented in the measurement of class inequalities in health. The force of this criticism has strengthened in the second half of the twentieth century as rising rates of marital dissolution fuelled the contiguous rise of single parenthood. This demographic development spells economic hardship for a sizeable proportion of the female and child population; it underlies the trend towards the feminization of poverty in the recent decades. The health consequences are very substantial. A recent study carried out among lone parents in Sweden reported a 70 per cent excess mortality rate among women rearing children alone (Ringback Weitoft *et al.* 2000). That a differential of such scope was reported for Sweden, whose welfare provision is more generous and more people friendly than any other nation, testifies to some highly negative contemporary trends that have never received the attention they deserve in the health inequalities literature.

Polity in the social environment

The impact of the forces of market capitalism upon the livelihood and procreation of a national population is mediated by government policies represented as polity in Fig. 5. Polity includes the apparatus of government, including the legal system, the institutions of economic management, and the welfare state (education, child care, health care, social security). In democratic nations it also includes political parties and associated ideologies and policies of citizenship and social justice. The political consciousness/activism of a national population is a further resource of the social environment setting the probability for popular activism over citizenship and other vital issues of everyday life. Citizenship refers to the claims (legal, political, economic) that individuals make of the nation-state, and there is huge variation in its content across the global universe of nation-states. Among modern democratic nations, there is more variation in the content of economic, than of legal or political citizenship. While the latter respectively guarantees equality before the law and the right to vote (both are universal features of the world's mature capitalist nations), the former involves the guarantee of livelihood.

Economic citizenship refers to state recognition of the individual's right to income maintenance and other basic components of living standards such as health care. There is considerable national variation in the institutional mechanisms of economic citizenship. In the aftermath of the Second World War, most Western European nations developed a welfare state apparatus that involved establishing policies to protect individuals and households from impersonal market forces. It has often been observed that the vanquished nations in the First and Second World Wars got revolutions, while those connected with the winning side got welfare states (Mann 1993). Revolutions happen when ruling elites lose their credibility and/or when the population is mobilized, even armed, and motivated to capture the apparatus of the state. These conditions were met and played an important part in the Russian Revolution. The Russian example explains why warfare represents a vulnerable interlude for ruling elites and why the military is a formidable political force in politics in less-developed societies.

Revolutionary situations are very infrequent in developed societies. When they do occur, the opportunity may arise for a complete overhaul of the social environment. The opportunities for introducing even partial societal reform are also infrequent and connected to major national emergencies such as occurred during the First and Second World Wars. It is no accident that the impetus not to merely talk about but actually to create the institutions of the welfare state can be dated to the 1940s. In pacific times, the chances of achieving major reforms of the social environment are far less. The welfare state developments of Western Europe represent a constrained reform of the social environment, designed to protect the populace from the harsher economic effects of market capitalism without banning the system altogether. As a Marxist analysis would put it, they represent the ransom paid by the ruling class to allow the capitalist system to continue.

By the early twentieth century, the necessity for public intervention to regulate the effects of capitalism within national economies was keenly appreciated. It was associated with a growing critical literature on the limitations, indeed potential long-term non-viability, of capitalism. In this era, the sphere of economic policy was necessarily widening, partly through the roller-coaster tendencies of international capitalism and partly through the pressure of the newly enfranchised working class. This was the era of the Great Crash (another major disruption), which was for many a sure sign that capitalism was on its knees. It was also the social environment in which the English economist John Maynard Keynes forged his economic theory of capitalism and his plan to save it from self-destruction (Skidelsky 1994). His intervention was timely for, although the closing quarter of the nineteenth century saw an unprecedented increase in living standards, by the 1920s an expanding electorate was acutely aware that capitalism was an extremely risky mode of population livelihood (Garraty 1978). Many had first-hand experience of the fact that exclusive dependence on wage and salaried income and on the market for the purchase of basic subsistence, left nothing to fall back on during times of economic recession and unemployment. Before the welfare state, periodic capitalist recession produced significant subsistence crises for a large part of the working class. Keynes's solution to this inherent problem was to fashion the tools for government and multinational organizations to manage actively the capitalist economy both to save it from itself and to guarantee population livelihood. The management of the forces of capitalism within nation-states is a central purpose of government and the various institutions of the welfare state were designed to remove important areas of human well being, such as health from the pressures of market distribution.

The institutional structure of the welfare state is a fundamentally important part of the social environment in the mature urban industrial societies of Western Europe. It represents a halfway house to socialism—a series of mechanisms for guaranteeing individual livelihood and for safeguarding procreation within economies articulated to international capitalism. The guarantee of livelihood through the regulation of market forces within individual nations takes several forms. First, governments take responsibility for managing the business cycle to control the rate of economic growth, to balance the forces of supply and demand, and to protect national economic institutions from the winds of the global capitalist market. This is the preventive side of government policy. Ironically, nowadays it sometimes involves stimulating unemployment in order to cool an 'overheated economy', a solution unthinkable to earlier generations of politicians and populace with memories of the Great Depression. Other preventive policies orchestrated by the state are connected with maintaining the flow of and ensuring the subsistence needs and health of the population.

Most developed industrial nations have some sort of state-sponsored comprehensive health care system providing such services as family planning, prenatal care, obstetric assistance, and paediatric health care. These services developed in rudimentary form during the early twentieth century when the risk of infant death was as high as 1 in 10 even in the most prosperous nations. The development of infant welfare services was promoted by social reformers partly in response to eugenic speculation that the 'quality' of the race was being diminished by class-specific fertility decline and partly in response to sociomedical surveys charting the associations of infant mortality with poverty and low income (Dworkin 1987). The impulse for state intervention was the desire to improve the quality of the 'race' and in particular the nation's manhood. This was era when European governments were still quite prepared to sacrifice significant numbers of young men in military campaigns.

The nation-state's interest in promoting the developmental potential of the next generation is also manifested in publicly funded education. Compulsory education is a universal feature of urban industrial societies. In most places it came on to the statute books around the turn of the twentieth century partly in response to a felt need to educate recently enfranchised working-class voters. Reformers may also have been aware of the social control functions of schooling (keeping children off the streets and out of mischief), quite apart from its utility as a means for improving the literate and other skills of the work force, i.e. increasing the educational capital of the nation.

State intervention in the fields of both education and health care, whatever the ulterior motives, represent a significant investment in household living standards and a major opportunity for the state to play a part mitigating the impact of the market on the stratification order. Routh (1987) drew attention to early state initiatives in Sweden to eliminate unskilled occupations by actively promoting manufacturing firms that rely on skilled labour.

This 'active labour market policy', also known as the Rhen–Meidner model, was Sweden's own version of Keynesian economic management. It involved a permissive orientation to strong wage pressures designed to put low-wage firms out of business. Coupled with well-funded state-sponsored relocation and retraining packages and with state-subsidized credit for 'go-ahead' firms, it maintained full employment and worker flexibility in the postwar decades. The right to a job was recognized by the state, but not the right to remain in a current regressive occupational situation (Esping-Anderson 1990). The trade unions in concert with the government pledged to reshape the occupational hierarchy by eliminating the lowest rungs of unskilled work and upgrading the occupational status of the entire work force. This remarkable redesign of the occupational structure called for collaboration between the state, the employers, and the trade unions, which might only have been feasible in a Scandinavian social democracy or possibly in corporate Japan (Dore 1987).

The curative side of government's management of the economy involves distributing state benefits, pensions, and payments as substitutes for earned income and/or savings and insuring individuals and households against the threat of unemployment or other economic/health crisis. Social security is the general term and, except for the United States, it is also articulated within a state-sponsored system of comprehensive medical care. Social security and medical treatment have been interlinked in economic citizenship because ill health was always considered a primary cause of short-term unemployment and loss of earnings. Policy-makers reasoned that by providing free medical treatment and maintaining households through the economic crisis of illness, they could put an end to the relationship between disease and poverty. The classic statement of this relationship is found in the Beveridge Report which is the design document of the British welfare state. The National Health Service was the jewel in the crown of Britain's welfare state, although disillusion had set in by the last quarter of the twentieth century. Additionally, the health care system played a social control function certifying the legitimacy of sickness and eligibility for compensation. Existing welfare states were designed during the closing decade of the era of infections, when people still understood disease as an acute and reversible episode.

Nation-states vary significantly in the scope of their social security provision and in their willingness to allow spheres of the social environment to become commodified, i.e. defined as fair game for capitalist enterprise. This represents the variable content of economic citizenship, i.e. the social wage, between nation-states. The social wage is the value of goods and services distributed by the state, outside the market system. It is designed both to remove services which are vital to human development, such as health and education, from market processes of distribution and to insure households against the risk of unemployment and loss of earnings through sickness and retirement. International variation in the value of the social wage among industrial nations tends to reflect divisions of contemporary economic morality and political culture as these emerged from democratic struggles between social classes and other groups in the early industrial era. These struggles were a central factor of the historical development of the social environment in different nations, and as such there is a degree of stability in the way national governments are disposed to exercise their policy-making powers. It might be said that the contemporary politics of (especially economic) citizenship is the lasting legacy of the way class conflict was 'institutionalized' in different parts of Europe in the first half of the twentieth century.

Esping Anderson (1990) has identified three types of 'welfare state regime' among advanced industrial nations: liberal welfare state, corporate-statist welfare state, and social democracy.

The **liberal welfare state** is targeted on the poor and offers a minimum means-tested safety net with some modest universal benefits. The principal intention is to uphold the work ethic and protect the sanctity of the market mechanism. Consequently, the benefits distributed are associated with public charity and stigma rather than social rights. Liberal systems also typically extend tax benefits for private welfare provision to create market incentives for the development of profit-oriented welfare schemes such as personal equity plans. The aim is to reinforce the norms of personal initiative and self-sufficiency. The archetype is the United States, with Australia, Canada, and the United Kingdom not far behind.

The **corporate-statist welfare state** emerges from within pre-existing strong large states. The word 'corporate' refers to the distinctive groups or elites, such as the church, the military, and the bureaucracy, which are incorporated and wield power within the state apparatus. The welfare policies that follow preserve the interests of groups represented in the state and therefore preserve the status quo rather than serving as a force for equality or progressive change. Thus redistributive impact is minimal, and benefits are distributed in forms that protect existing institutions such as the church and the family. The principle of subsidiarity (i.e. state intervention only when the coping capacity of traditional institutions such as the family is exhausted) is a dominant feature of welfare policies of this type, but the association of benefits with charity is not so pronounced or stigmatizing as in the liberal regime. These regimes are found in the Catholic nations of Austria, France, Italy, Germany, and Spain.

The **social democracy** model of the welfare state is a peculiar fusion of liberalism and socialism, i.e. it promotes both freedom and equality (Esping Anderson 1990, p.2). The liberalism part is the goal of increasing individual choice and independence. These welfare states strive to offer women, in particular, the right to choose paid work over the household; consequently, they support a large social services sector—indeed, the very process of extending choice to women supports a huge job creation programme of new occupations to replace the labour lost in women's retreat from the private sphere. In effect, this development is a means of commodifying (paying for) domestic labour as women primarily take advantage of the new employment opportunities in child care and elderly care work. In their encouragement of employment, this type of state regime may also be described as a fusion of welfare and work.

Figure 7 compares the social class distribution of infant mortality in Sweden and in England and Wales to illustrate the potential health consequences of different welfare state regimes. In Sweden, a social democratic regime is associated with a virtual absence of class inequality; in England and Wales, a liberal regime preserves the familiar gradient along with the class inequalities which underpin it (Vagero and Lundberg 1989; Leon *et al.* 1992).

Social democratic regimes 'pre-emptively socialize the costs of family-hood' (Esping Anderson 1990). In other words, they may be

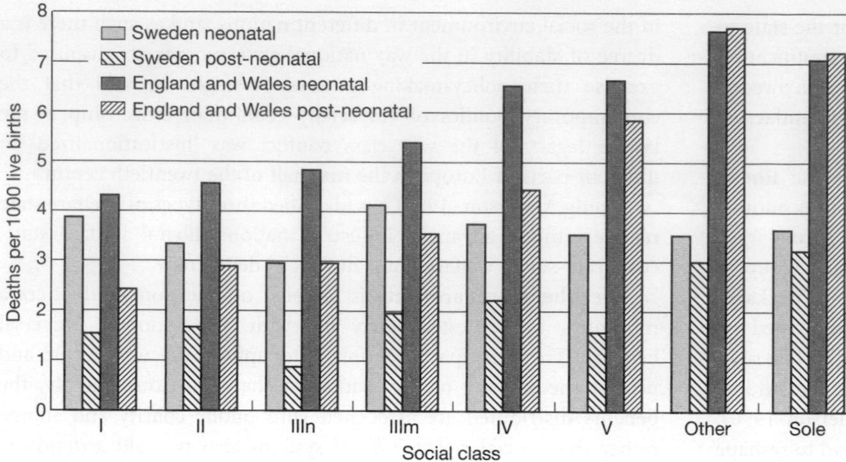

Fig. 7 Infant mortality in Sweden and England and Wales.

thought of as supplying the missing link between the logic of production and reproduction. In so doing they also sponsor female autonomy and redistribute resources from men to women and children as well as between the classes. There is no lingering association with public charity. Welfare benefits are set at middle-class standards of consumption. The aim is to level up and to unite the interests of all in the concept and practice of the social wage. A single social insurance system covers the entire population. This crowds out the market and reinforces a broad consensus in favour of state benefits which are widely perceived as universal social rights. The home of this type of regime is Scandinavia—it includes Sweden, Denmark, and Norway.

The three forms of welfare state regime represent different approaches to the need to compensate individuals, families, and households from the limitations of the labour market as a livelihood system. Their geographical distribution in Western Europe suggests that common cultural elements may have played a part in their foundation. Half a century or more after their establishment, the expectations that they have encouraged in the populace are now an important feature of the politicocultural landscape of Europe, acting to shape the level of political consciousness, the terms of political debate, and the mobilization of popular opinion behind government policies.

Culture in the social environment

Culture encompasses the way of life of a social group. It includes the symbols and tools of communication (linguistic, musical, artistic), the technology of communication and of livelihood, cuisine and culinary traditions, mode of dress, the method and style of construction, religious, moral and political beliefs and values, the ethics of interpersonal relationships, healing ideologies and practices, and marriage and kinship norms. The term 'ethnicity' is sometimes used interchangeably with the term 'culture' to refer to the defining characteristics of a social group or population, and there is a tendency to associate both terms with traditional folkways, although culture is now emerging as an important theoretical concept of modern sociology. Ideologies of gender and race are included under the heading of culture along with the norms of social relationships they prescribe. The latter may involve more or less overt forms of discrimination, which when accompanied by power differentials produce an axis of social stratification.

The measurement of gender inequalities in health in contemporary societies can be tricky. In a pre-industrial or industrializing social environment, the sex differential in mortality typically varies over the course of the lifetime. There is a substantial excess of male mortality in infancy and after middle age; female mortality is higher in childhood, adolescence, and during the childbearing years. This pattern is still typical of many less-developed societies where even the female infancy advantage is reversed. It disappears as a society modernizes. Excess male mortality becomes the statistical norm at all ages in a pattern that is found in all modern societies. With the evidence of historical hindsight, it may be deduced that the excess mortality of girls and young women in earlier eras and in contemporary pre-industrial populations is the product of social discrimination in favour of males. This judgement emerges from examining sex differences in survival among well-fed industrial populations where excess male mortality of at least 30 per cent is found in every age group. How other than through systematic differential female neglect could the apparent sex advantage be neutralized in former times? The usual answer to this question is childbirth. The 'natural' risk of maternal mortality is popularly and even professionally conceived as taking a huge toll of life before the emergence of obstetric medicine and procedures. In evoking a biological cause, this judgement equals sex not gender. It implies that the female body is a poorly developed instrument of procreation and that very large numbers of women lost their lives giving birth before the advance of modern obstetric medicine.

The contribution of maternal causes to female mortality before 1950 was much greater than it is today, but it was not large enough to explain the adverse ratio of female to male mortality in and before the nineteenth century (Schofield 1986; Loudon 1992). Nor could it explain the excess mortality of female infants and children. These unexplained features highlight the possibility that cultural norms of differential female neglect/deprivation might have underlain the typical pre-industrial pattern of sex mortality differentials. This is steadily eroded by the advance of industrialization, giving a strong impression that rising living standards impacting directly on the developmental growth processes of infants and children is the primary factor of change. If this is correct, the corollary is that pre-industrial norms of allocating nutritional resources within households may have systematically favoured male over the female offspring. The longer-term implication of these norms would be the impoverishment of the procreative prospects of the community, for the vitality of future generations depends on the growth chances of the female. In evaluating this cultural interpretation of sex mortality differentiation before the modern era, it is worth bearing in mind that we are not merely seeking to explain an absence of parity in childhood mortality risk, but a systematic reversal of what appears to be a 'natural' female advantage. A typical sex mortality differential among infants in an industrial population is 1.3:1 in favour of the female. The reversal of this advantage in conditions of nutritional scarcity strongly implies preferential male treatment. The probability that this was an important underlying cause is strengthened by our knowledge of sex-divided patterns of infant feeding and maternal care in pre-modern cultures of the twentieth century.

The foregoing interpretation is the leading example of gender as a factor of public health (Sen 1981; Shorter 1982). It is a routine sociodemographic feature of many less-developed societies. Differential female neglect, female infanticide, and even 'woman/widow slaughter' produce skewed sex ratios in a number of pre-industrial and industrializing communities today (Table 2). The effect of the unequal evaluation of the two sexes is not merely reflected in differential survival among the living but also makes its mark upon indices of reproduction—in particular, on fetal and infant mortality as the nutritional well being of the female child is an important factor of population health status. Gender discrimination in the allocation of food during the first decade of the lifetime results in a pattern of nutritional stratification within households, with serious implications for female childhood growth and later for fetal life chances (Barker 1994). Eliminating this situation does not necessarily require a feminist revolution, i.e. a rewriting of cultural norms to eliminate gender preferences. It can be accomplished through a systematic improvement in the conditions of nutritional status of the community as a whole. The cultural norms of male preference remain intact, but are they no longer manifested in nutritional status for as material scarcity gives way to sufficiency, if not affluence, male infants and children emerge as the more vulnerable sex with excess mortality rates of about 30 per cent. It is also possible for health status to improve even in the absence of material abundance if the ideological norms of gender inequality are reduced. This happened in Kerala, where a communist regime emerged from the collision of an indigenous matrilineal and a colonial patrilineal system. The British attempt to impose patrilineal legal rules on a matrilineal people in the early twentieth century acted to politicize the community and stimulated the establishment of a communist administration, which brought about a modern health revolution in a largely peasant society. Kerala is not among the most prosperous regions of India, but it is the healthiest and the female population is the most literate. In Table 2 the distribution of selected health status indicators in India during the 1990s shows just how powerful gender remains as a source of health stratification. Note how the sociodemographic profile of Kerala has more in common with a modern industrial society than with her territorial neighbours.

Race is another powerful cultural source of health inequality and, like gender, it is often thought of as a biological phenomenon (McBride 1991). The race differentiation of the human species in the twentieth century is the cultural product of late eighteenth- and nineteenth-century scholarship (Stepan 1982). The *Oxford English Dictionary* defines race as a social group descended from a common ancestor. Before the eighteenth century it was commonly used to

Table 2 Selected health status indicators for India

State	Sex ratio	Female literacy (%)	Male IMR	Female IMR	Male LE	Female LE
Andhra Pradesh	97.2	32.7	70	57	59.1	61.5
Assam	92.3		81	81	53.9	54.4
Bihar	91.1	22.9	68	72	58.4	56.4
Gujerat	93.4	48.6	58	58	58	60.5
Haryana	86.5	40.5	60	73	62.1	63.2
Karnataka	96	44.3	69	66	60.5	63.6
Kerala	*103.6*	*86.2*	*16*	*10*	*68.1*	*73.4*
Madhya Pradesh	93.1	28.9	106	107	53.8	53.2
Maharashtra	93.4	52.3	50	50	62	64.7
Orissa	97.1	34.7	118	101	55.8	55.1
Punjab	88.2	50.4	49	62	65.4	67.2
Rajasthan	91	20.4	82	81	56.2	56.7
Kamil Nadu	97.4	51.3	57	56	60.7	62.5
Uttar Pradesh	87.9	25.3	87	100	56.1	54.5
West Bengal	91.7	46.6	57	59	60.8	62.3

Sex ratio, number of females per 100 males.

IMR, infant mortality rate per 1000 live births; LE, life expectancy at birth.

Source: Velkoff and Adlakha (1998, p. 10).

designate class or status differences within a population. The inbred aristocracy of Europe perceived themselves as a branch of humanity set apart from the common people, whom they saw as a separate inferior race. Race became an anthropological classification during the nineteenth century as anthropologists in Darwinistic mode devised a definitive taxonomy of the human species (African, Asian, Caucasian) based on their continental origins and denoting their phenotypical characteristics. From within their European evolutionary perspective, the peoples of other continents were seen as weaker or inferior versions of humanity along a continuum of evolutionary progress. This was the ideological core of the great eugenic delusion; its legacy is racism, both pseudoscientific and popular. Today even the word race is blighted by association.

Race is perhaps the most powerful source of health inequality. This is true internationally and intranationally. If we operate with a continental racial division of humanity, the gap in life expectancy between different races is as much as 20 years. Within an industrial population containing significant representation of people with the same racial heritage, the survival gap is narrower but still the single most important source of health stratification. Table 3 lays out the key health status indicators for the six continents in 1996.

In a global perspective, the vital rates of Africa are the most disadvantaged. At the end of the twentieth century, life expectancy at birth is little more than five decades about the level achieved by northwestern Europe in 1900. African males were 11 years below the world average in 1996, and almost 20 years below the peoples of Europe and North America. The gap between Africa and the world's most prosperous regions is even wider for females. The mean global level of female life expectancy in 1996 was 64.7 years, African females were 12 years behind, compared with the European female average, they were 25 years below. These huge differentials are fundamentally associated with global inequalities in social and economic development, with political unrest, internecine ethnic struggles, civil war, and genocide. In the last quarter of the twentieth century Africa has also emerged as the epicentre of the global AIDS epidemic, an outcome which Hooper (1999) has linked to an anti-polio campaign, which dispensed a million experimental oral vaccines partly developed from chimpanzee kidney tissue.

The widespread administration of an experimental oral vaccine would not have been contemplated in a European population. In Hooper's (1999) gripping story of the possible connections between AIDS and European/North American public health efforts to develop an oral anti-polio vaccine in central Africa, researchers/practitioners clearly relaxed the standards they would have observed had the client population been European or North American. If Hooper's persuasive account proves correct, this would represent the most devastating case of medical negligence in human history.

By the end of the twentieth century, a rate of life expectancy of about five decades was highly atypical because by then most nations had traversed the epidemiological transition. That the peoples of Africa had not yet negotiated this watershed of health history must mean that the benefits (technological and material) of human progress had not been shared with this significant fraction of humanity. The observation does not hold for all social groups who live in Africa. The white farmers of East and South Africa descended from European settlers of the nineteenth and early twentieth centuries record life expectancy on a par with the contemporary European average. They inhabit the same ecological terrain as their African farmworkers but their life chances have kept pace with the European norm and are a century ahead of their black fellow citizens. The gap is a measure of the relative social and economic advantages of Africa's white former immigrant communities and it is testimony to the plasticity of human health and its responsiveness to relative economic and social well being.

By the end of the twentieth century, the population of the United States contained significant subpopulations of each of the global branches of humanity making it an appropriate context for measuring race inequalities in survival. Figure 8 charts race and sex differentials in survival in the American population in 1996 revealing the enormous gap in life chances between males and females of African-American descent and other races. Black males record the largest mortality excess but the chart also reveals a striking divergence in health between black females and white males. In every industrial population, male longevity lags behind female longevity by more than 6 years. In the United States race inequalities neutralize this socio-demographic universal, the life expectancy of a black female is approximately the same as a white male, an overall effect produced by disadvantaged mortality rates during the prime of life. The width of the gap in survival between black and white American citizens has changed relatively little during the course of the twentieth century. Black Americans lived for an average of 33 years in 1900, white Americans lived to a mean of 48 years. This was in the tubercular era, the early evening of the epidemiological transition. During the course of the twentieth century, the rate of mortality risk fell in both populations,

Table 3 Infant mortality and life expectancy in the global community in 1996

Global region	Male LE	Female LE	Male IMR	Female IMR
World	61.3	64.7	60.3	56.5
Africa	50.3	52.6	96.7	85.3
North America	69.8	75.7	23.6	18.9
South America	63.4	72.1	41.7	33.4
Asia	63.3	65.9	57.7	57
Europe	69.2	77.5	12.9	10.3
Oceania	69.8	75.1	28.1	23.8

IMR, infant mortality rate per 1000 live births; LE, life expectancy at birth.

Source: US Bureau of the Census International Database (http:\\www.census.gov).

principally through improvements in infant and child survival and through the continuing decline of infectious disease. Amidst all this progress, the gap between black and white persisted. The twentieth-century American longevity trend contains a simple but important empirical proof. It shows that race life expectancy differentials are not the product of eugenic potential, as they would have been conceived in the sociomedical racist ideology of 1910 (McBride 1991). Beginning from a lower level, African-Americans made relatively more progress in longevity during the last century. By 1996, they were approximately 15 to 16 years ahead of their ancestral populations in Africa but they remained 10 years behind their white compatriots. Once again we see the plasticity of human health and survival and the close correspondence between the social and economic standing of a racially defined population and its measured health status.

To a significant degree, the historical experience of African-Americans has been like a nightmare from which the group has only recently awakened and whose aftershocks are still felt in varying degree. During the twentieth century, African-Americans have made immense progress in the political struggle for social equality and in the process have dismantled institutional apartheid in American society. The Civil Rights Movement of the 1950s and 1960s is probably the most effectively organized and successful political struggle of American history and its long-term effect has been to diminish racist ideologies in the conduct of social life. However, the long shadow of race discrimination in the educational and occupational structures of American society has left an indelible mark on a large proportion of the African-American population, to which the continued gap in survival chances in Fig. 8 bears testimony.

Figure 8 also shows other significant race mortality differentials in the American population, which cannot be simply attributed to economic inequalities.

Other than in the black population, socio-economic race differentials in the United States census are not correlated with the pattern of mortality differentials in Fig. 8. The average income in the Asian and Hispanic populations is below the average white income.

Peoples of Asian descent in particular exhibit highly favourable health status. Compared with the continental averages displayed in Table 3, Asian-Americans are 12 to 15 years ahead of the population of Asia and they are as healthy as, if not healthier than, people who claim a 'white' racial heritage in the United States. This pattern suggests that health status is not a simple product of material living standards. Asian-Americans, principally Chinese and Japanese, are often depicted as the model minority of American society. During the twentieth century they have experienced upward mobility as an ethnic group overcoming institutional racism and discrimination, which was entrenched during the first half of the twentieth century, culminating in the internment of Japanese-Americans during the Second World War. During the closing decades of the twentieth century, the Asian-American population emerged at the top of the key indicators of achievement—life expectancy, education, occupation, and income. More recently, the population has become more diversified through the incorporation of immigrants from the Philippines, Laos, Vietnam, and Cambodia. This has tended to narrow the achievement gap between Asian-Americans and white Americans, although, even in its new diversity, the Asian-American community continues to stand out as the healthiest in the United States.

The social ascent of the Asian-American community as a whole suggests that economic factors on their own are not a sufficient determinant of above average health status. It is not a matter of explaining why selected talented people achieve above-average success; something is propelling the entire group towards greater prosperity, higher living standards, and longer life expectancy. This factor is clearly a property of the group norms falling under the heading of cultural or lifestyle factors. These include strong kinship solidarity, low divorce rates, stable family life, and a high value placed on education. These features of Asian-American values and lifestyle may be important preconditions for individuals to take advantage of opportunities in the American labour market, and they may exert equivalent influence over health and wealth.

The populations of modern industrial nations are seldom composed of a single ethnic group or characterized by a uniform homogeneous culture. Although the formation of the national state itself exerts a pressure towards national solidarity, shared identity, and therefore cultural uniformity, the survival and coexistence of a

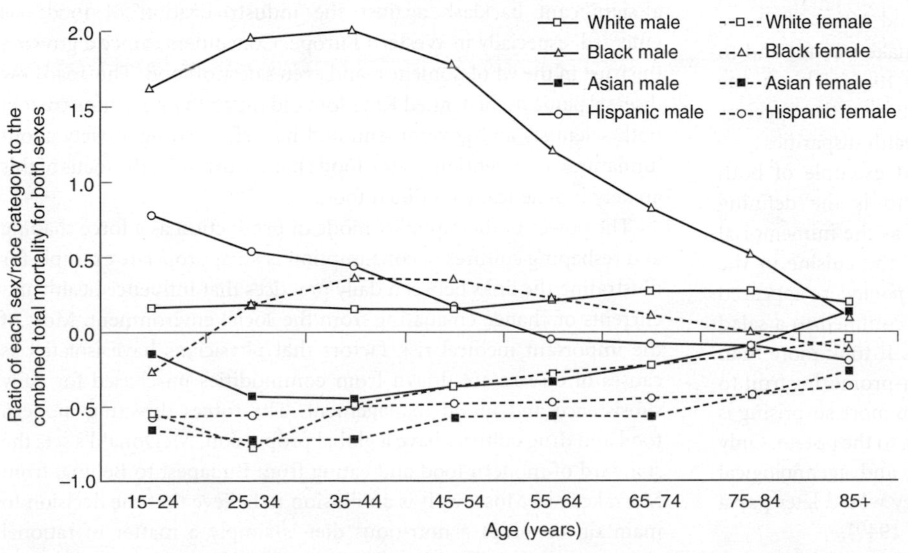

Fig. 8 Sex and race mortality differentials in the United States, 1995.

number of distinctive cultures is quite feasible. In recent decades, growing tolerance of cultural diversity has made it easier for ethnic subcultures to persist at least in some limited sense in mature nation-states. In newly emerging nation-states establishing their identity, the opposite conditions prevail and are manifested in ferocious struggles of ethnic cleansing with portentous public health consequences.

Cultural beliefs and practices, even within an ethnically homogeneous population, are the product of historical experience and frequently incorporate a diverse collection of other people's technology, food, language, and ideas. The English language is a blend of Germanic, Romance, and other languages. The Japanese use Chinese Kanji as their written script. These examples represent centuries of acculturation occurring through processes of migration, assimilation, trade, and conquest. Culture is clearly a blended historical phenomenon, and in the modern era the global pressure towards cultural uniformity is immense. It is felt most strongly within industrial nations fully articulated into the international capitalist economy, although virtually no corner of the globe is now immune to its influence. Culinary culture, the conception of what is good to eat (Harris 1985), reveals the enormous impact that global capitalism has exerted on the material culture of peoples worldwide. As diet is also a leading medical risk factor for universal disease, it provides an appropriate vehicle for illustrating what is involved in the relationship between health and culture.

The European diet, although regionally distinctive in many ways, has undergone a complete transformation in the modern era principally through the import and incorporation of New World foods. Although the voyages of the conquistadors were primarily stimulated by the quest for precious goods—gold and spices—the main material bounty brought to Europe, and thence to the rest of the world, was new crops, especially maize and the potato. New World staples, along with stimulants and narcotics, completely transformed the culinary and drug cultures of nineteenth-century Europe with important health and social implications in both the short and long term (Schivelbusch 1992). Today, tobacco is the single most important medical risk factor and it is worth reflecting that its consumption in Europe has a social history. The production of tobacco, along with sugar and cotton, bound the fate of the European industrial working class to that the indigenous peoples of America and Africa who were killed off and/or transported as slave labour to make way for and to work the plantations of the New World (Mintz 1985). This is one foundation of the urban industrial social environment that receives little attention in the contemporary debate on health disparities.

Diet and culinary traditions provide a good example of both cultural flexibility and inflexibility. The tomato is the defining ingredient of Italian cooking, which we think of as the immemorial ubiquitous ingredient, yet it only truly entered the cuisine in the nineteenth century (Toussaint-Samat 1994). The *pomodoro* appeared in Italy in the sixteenth century but its use was confined to a salad vegetable (as it remained in northern countries). It took more than two centuries for this highly nutritious and health-promoting fruit to be made the central ingredient of the cuisine. Even more surprising is the length of time it took for Europeans to latch on to the potato. Only the Irish quickly appreciated the nutritional and technological advantages of the New World crop, although they would later pay a heavy price for their cultural flexibility (Salaman 1949).

Irish agriculture became a virtual monoculture. The potato provided an economic rationale for subdividing land and maintaining rural communities at a very basic subsistence level. The consequence was a subsistence crisis of worse than medieval proportions when *Phytophthora infestans* destroyed the entire crop in 1845, with knock-on effects in the following years. There were as many as a million deaths in Ireland from the potato blight, which swept across Europe causing economic distress in all poor communities that had developed a dependence on the potato. The best source on the history of the potato is still Salaman's *History and Social Influence of the Potato* (Salaman 1949, pp. 188–345). The best historical image of the potato as a food of the poor is van Gogh's painting *The Potato Eaters*.

Elsewhere in Europe, the suspicion that potatoes were poisonous (it belongs to the same genus as the deadly nightshade) held fast for a number of centuries. Although it was grown as an ornamental plant and consumed as a delicacy by the rich, it did not become a field crop for human consumption until the late eighteenth century in most places. Slowly the potato caught on, first as animal or prison fodder, and then as a food of last resort in famines and among the poor. By the early twentieth century, the potato was a central feature of the urban industrial diet in northwestern Europe; its intensive cultivation saved the British population from food shortages during Hitler's blockade of transatlantic trade in the Second World War (Salaman 1949; Drummond and Wilbraham 1994).

The culinary cultures of industrial peoples have been further revolutionized in the last 50 years through international trade and investment. Fast-food and convenience food industries have transformed the content of meals and the manner of their preparation and consumption. In North America especially, the act of eating has been increasingly detached from its social context and broader purpose, and reduced to a functional activity that may be combined with other tasks in a tight time budget. In the process, not only food but the act of eating itself has been turned into a commodity, a thing to be bought and sold, stripped of its former commensal functions. The driving force in the dissolution of traditional culinary culture is the profit motive. Capitalism grows and prospers by invading and commodifying realms of social life previously outside its orbit. In the case of food and eating, its success is partly predicated on other processes detaching individuals from reliance on primary groups for the provision of daily subsistence. It is not all plain sailing. In recent years a significant backlash against the industrialization of food has emerged, especially in Western Europe. Consumers evince a growing mistrust in the wholesomeness and even safety of food. The 'mad cow disease' panic in the United Kingdom did much to undermine trust in both scientists and government, and has left a strong anxiety about 'unnatural' interventions in the food chain. Currently, the focus of this anxiety is genetically modified food.

The power of the capitalist mode of production as a force shaping and reshaping cultures of consumption is an appropriate example for illustrating the links between daily practices that influence health and currents of change emanating from the social environment. Most of the important medical risk factors that physicians have isolated as causes of disease are drawn from commodities purchased for daily subsistence and mood management. The forces directing modern food and drug cultures have a global propulsion. McDonald's sets the standard of modern food and eating from Budapest to Beijing, from Marrakech to Moscow. It is an illusion to believe that the decision to maintain or adopt a nutritious diet is simply a matter of rational choice on the part of the well-informed and appropriately educated consumer. As Harris (1985) puts it: 'Food must be good to think as well as good to eat and the global food industry makes no attempt to disguise its interests in shaping the perception of style in the matter of food and eating'.

Some nations appear to have been more successful than others at insulating traditional food cultures from the rationalizing forces of market capitalism. The Japanese diet is frequently held up as a food tradition especially suited to the needs of modern sedentary human (Marmot and Davey-Smith 1989), as is the Mediterranean diet (Spiller 1991). Both are claimed to diminish the pace of industrialism's leading universal disease—cardiovascular degeneration. Interestingly in both contexts, consumption of other seemingly dangerous commodities—cigarettes and alcohol—run directly opposite to modern health recommendations. The drinking culture of Japan has been held up as a stress-reducing strategy. Matsumoto (1970), searching the social environment for reasons for the low rates of coronary heart disease in Japan, settled on the consumption of sake in group settings:

> Drinking together remains for the Japanese an indispensable means of creating group intimacy accompanied by the greater release of emotions from everyday formalities. a man who will not partake of alcoholic drink with the group is one not to be trusted. (Matsumoto 1970, pp. 22–3)

This feature of Japanese culture is hardly unique. The same pattern of male sociability organized around the consumption of alcoholic beverages was widespread in Protestant Europe in the nineteenth and early twentieth centuries and remains intact in Eastern Europe, especially Russia, where it is currently seen as the principal proximate cause of the dramatic descent of life expectancy during the last quarter of the twentieth century. The drinking culture of northwestern, i.e. Protestant, Europe was reformed between 1850 and 1950 through an effective temperance campaign, which eventually forced legislation controlling the sale and consumption of alcohol. The Temperance Movement was an international phenomenon, principally located and successful in Protestant nations, and aimed at extending the new cultural values associated with the Protestant work ethic and sobriety to the male working class. Its ultimate success was connected to a number of other economic and cultural changes and also to a technological innovation—a machine for the mass production of cigarettes. Between 1870 and 1930, a substantial decline in the consumption of alcohol in Britain was matched by a concurrent increase in the consumption of cigarettes (Hart 1989*a*).

Cultural change with significant health consequences can occur in response to both external and internal pressures, and there may be both winners and losers from the process. In Britain, the declining consumption of alcohol by men may have resulted in less domestic violence and a strengthening of family finances with women and children as the principal beneficiaries. To the extent that it was also associated with the rise of smoking in men, the long-term effect may be measured in the rising trend of lung cancer and other smoking-related disease.

The reform of Protestant men's drinking culture was a multi-faceted process with a number of unintended consequences. If Matsumoto is right about Japan, one negative effect may have been to deprive the industrial male working class of a primary stress-reducing strategy. To an important degree this might be construed as the manifest intention—the imposition of a sober rational model of masculinity dedicated to his work. As Ehrenreich (1983) points out, the coronary-prone personality identified by American cardiologists in the mid-twentieth century bears more than a passing resemblance to the model of manhood associated with the Protestant ethic (Friedmann and Rosenhan 1968). This observation highlights the interwoven character of cultural forms, in this case gender relations, the organization of work, and patterns of narcotic consumption. It also reveals that cultural change occurs through initiatives in the political and economic realms and with the consent of the primary groups that orchestrate everyday life. In so doing, it changes the patterns of relationships within those groups.

Culture is an important feature of the social environment. It influences health in a number of ways. These include the following: religious beliefs and commitments shaping procreative ideologies and household formation; kinship sentiment, marriage, and the role of the family in processes of social support; industrial culture and the tenor of relationships in the workplace (Dore 1987); political culture and the differential insulating powers of welfare state regimes. Each of the examples listed here is the outcome of specific historical ingredients and contingencies, for culture is an inherently dynamic component of the social environment. The survival of a cultural form depends on public allegiance and its continued capacity to provide meaning and to shape motivation. Sustaining the loyalty of each new generation as it moves through the transition to adult life is the critical test; the emergence of oppositional youth cultures in the latter half of the twentieth century raised new challenges for sustaining distinctive national ways of seeing and acting upon the social environment.

Karl Marx reduced culture to an ideological superstructure resting upon and reflective of an economic base, which was the foundation of society. He predicted that the capitalist mode of production would destroy pre-existing cultural forms and install its own cultural superstructure. As the global market extends its reach over the territory of the globe, incorporating an expanding proportion of the world's population, the fate of traditional culture looks bleak from a Marxist perspective. International capitalism is a restless machine ever intent on substituting its own vision of the good life in opposition to lifestyles evolved from quite different origins. It is not just a matter of commercial interests marketing the Western way of life through Hollywood movies, popular music, Western consumer goods, blue jeans, and fast food. Equally important is the promise of economic autonomy and personal liberation from bonds of kinship. In this dual way, capitalism consciously and unconsciously maintains its mission to reshape humanity in its own image.

Against these formidable international economic and social forces for change, the resilience of authentic cultural forms depends crucially on the political infrastructure of nation-states, either singly or in combination (e.g. the European Union), and on the mobilization of political initiatives to maintain an independent power over the development of the social environment and the use of public policy to direct change in ways that protect the health of the population. The profession of public health operates within the social environment and is a potentially powerful factor of health promotion. It was among the founding features of polity, and the extent of its contemporary effectiveness depends on a savvy understanding of the source, range, and scope of influences emanating from the social environment and determining the people's health. This chapter has aimed to provide an overview of these influences and to encourage the profession to adopt an expansive framework of analysis incorporating economic, political, and cultural processes, which does not stop short at the boundary of the nation-state.

References

Ardener, S. and Burman, S. (1996). *Money-go-rounds: the importance of rotating savings and credit associations for women.* Berg, Washington, DC.

Arsenian, J. and Arsenian, J.M. (1948). Tough and easy cultures. *Psychiatry*, **11**, 377–85.

Barker, D. (1994). *Mothers, babies and diseases in later life.* BMA Publications, London.

Barrett, M. and McIntosh, M. (1982). *The anti-social family.* Verso, London.

Berger, P. (1964). *Invitation to sociology.* Penguin, Harmondsworth.

Berkman, L. and Syme, L. (1979). Social networks, host resistence and mortality: a nine year follow up study of Alameda county residents. *American Journal of Epidemiology*, **109**, 186.

Blackburn R. and Mann, M. (1979). *The working class in the labour market.* MacMillan, London.

Bott, E. (1957). *Family and social network.* Tavistock Press, London.

Buford, B. (1993). *Among the thugs.* Vintage Books, London.

Cockerham, W. (1999). *Health and social change in Russia and eastern Europe.* Routledge, London.

Cockerham, W., Rutten, A., and Abel, T. (1997). Conceptualizing contemporary health lifestyles: moving beyond Weber. *Sociological Quarterly*, **38**, 600–22.

Cohen, M.N. and Armelagos, G.J. (1984). *Paleopathology and the origins of agriculture.* Academic Press, New York.

Collins, R. (1990). Stratification, emotional energy and the transient emotions. In *Research agendas in the sociology of the emotions* (ed. T.G. Kemper). State University of New York Press, Albany, NY.

Courtwright, D.T. (1996). *Violent land: single men and social disorder from the frontier to the inner city.* Harvard University Press, Cambridge, MA.

Crosby, A.W. (1986). *Ecological imperialism: The biological expansion of Europe 900–1900.* Cambridge University Press.

de Swann, A. (1988). *In care of the state: Health care, education and welfare in Europe and the USA in the modern era.* Oxford University Press, New York.

DHSS (1980). *Inequalities in health: the report of a working group (the Black report).* Department of Health and Social Security, London.

Dore, R. (1987). *Taking Japan seriously: a confucian perspective on leading economic issues.* Stanford University Press.

Dorling, D. (1997). *Death in Britain: how local mortality rates have changed 1950s–1990s.* Joseph Rowntree Foundation, York.

Drummond, J.C. and Wilbraham, A. (1994). *The Englishman's food: five centuries of English diet.* Pimlico, London.

Dworkin, D. (1987). *War is good for babies and young children: a history of the infant and child welfare movement in England 1898–1918.* Tavistock Press, London.

Ehrenreich, B. (1983). *The hearts of men.* Anchor Books, New York.

Elias, N. (1978). *The civilizing process.* Blackwell, Oxford.

Esping-Anderson, G. (1990). *The three worlds of welfare capitalism* . Princeton University Press.

Evans, R.G., Barer, M.L., and Marmor, T.R. (1994). *Why are some people healthy and others not? The determinants of the health of populations.* Aldine de Gruyter, New York.

Farr, W. (1885). *Vital statistics* (reprinted 1975). Scarecrow Press, Metuchen, NJ.

Floud, R., Wachter, K., and Gregory, A. (1990). *Height, health and history: nutritional status in the United Kingdom 1750–1980.* Cambridge University Press.

Freund, P. (1990). The expressive body: a common ground for the sociology of the emotions and health and illness. *Sociology of Health and Illness* , **12**, 452–77.

Friedman, M. and Rosenman, R.H. (1968). The relationship of a behavior pattern to the state of the coronary vasculature. *American Journal of Medicine* , **44**, 525–37.

Fries, J.F. and Crapo, L.M. (1981). *Vitality and aging: implications of the rectangular curve.* Freeman, New York.

Fuchs, V. (1988). *Women's quest for economic equality.* Harvard University Press, Cambridge, MA.

Garraty, J. (1978). *Unemployment in history: economic thought and public policy.* Harper and Row, New York.

Gilligan, C. (1982). *In a different voice: Psychological theory and womens development.* Harvard University Press, Cambridge, MA.

Goldman, N. and Hu, Y. (1993). Excess mortality among the unmarried: a case study of Japan. *Social Science and Medicine*, **36**, 533–46.

Gosden, P.H.J.H. (1973). *Self help: voluntary associations in nineteenth century Britain.* Batsford, London.

Gravelle, H. (1998). How much of the relation between population mortality and the unequal distribution of income is a statistical artefact? *British Medical Journal*, **316**, 382–5.

Hajdu, P. McKee, M., and Bojan, F. (1995). Changes in premature mortality differentials by marital status in Hungary and England and Wales. *European Journal of Public Health*, **5**, 529–56.

Harris, M. (1985). *Good to eat: riddles of food and culture.* Simon and Schuster, New York.

Hart, N. (1982). Which is the weaker sex? *Radical Community Medicine* , **11**, 25.

Hart, N. (1989*a*). Sex, gender and survival: inequalities of life chances among european men and women. In *Health inequalities in Europe* (ed. A.J. Fox). Gower, London.

Hart, N. (1989*b*). Gender and the rise and fall of class politics. *New Left Review*, **175**, 19.

Hooper, E. (1999). *The river: a journey to the source of HIV and AIDS* . Little, Brown, Boston, MA.

Hu, Y. and Goldman, N. (1990). Mortality differentials by marital status: an international comparison. *Demography*, **27**, 233–50.

James, V. and Gabe, J. (1996). *Health and the sociology of the emotions* . Blackwell, Oxford.

Jeffrey, R. (1992). *Politics, women, and well-being: how Kerala became a model.* Macmillan, Basingstoke.

Judge, K. (1995). Income distribution and life expectancy: a critical appraisal. *British Medical Journal*, **311**, 1282–5.

Katz, J. (1999). *How emotions work.* Chicago University Press.

Kawachi, I., Kennedy, B., and Wilkinson, R. (1999). *The society and population health reader: income inequality and health.* New Press, New York.

Lal, B. (1990). *Romance of culture in an urban civilization.* Routledge, London.

Leon, D.A., Vagero, D., and Otterblad Olausson, P. (1992). Social class differences in infant Mortality in Sweden: a comparison with England and Wales. *British Medical Journal*, **305**, 687–91.

Light, I., Jung Kwuon, I., and Zhong, D. (1990). *Korean rotating credit associations in Los Angeles.* Center for Pacific Rim Studies, Los Angeles, CA.

Loudon, I. (1992). *Death in childbirth: an international study of maternal care and maternal mortality.* Clarendon Press, Oxford.

McBride, D. (1991). *From TB to AIDS: epidemics among urban Blacks since 1900.* State University of New York Press, Albany, NY

McKeown, T. (1976). *The role of medicine: dream, mirage or nemesis* ? Nuffield Provincial Hospitals Trust, London.

McNeill, W.H. (1977). *Plagues and peoples.* Doubleday, New York.

Mann, M. (1993). *The sources of social power: the rise of classes and nation-states, 1760–1914*, Vol. 2. Cambridge University Press.

Marmot, M.G. and Davey-Smith, G. (1989). Why are the Japanese living longer? *British Medical Journal*, **299**, 1547–51.

Marmot, M.G. and McDowell, M.E. (1986). Mortality decline and widening health inequalities. *Lancet*, **i**, 274.

Marmot, M.G., Shipley, M.J., and Rose, G.A. (1984). Inequalities in death—specific explanations of a general pattern. *Lancet*, **ii**, 1003.

Matsumoto, Y.S. (1970). Social stress and coronary heart disease in Japan. *Milbank Memorial Fund Quarterly*, **48**, 9–36.

Mintz, S. (1985). *Sweetness and power: the place of sugar in modern history*. Penguin, Harmondsworth.

Murray, C.J.L., Michaud, C.M., McKenna, M.T., and Marks, J.S. (1998). *US patterns of life expectancy by county and race 1965–94*. Harvard Center for Population and Development Studies, Cambridge, MA.

Office for National Statistics (1997). *Social focus on families*. HMSO, London.

OPCS (1978). *Occupational mortality 1970–72*. HMSO, London.

Pappas, G., Queen, S., Hadden, W., and Fisher, G. (1993). The increasing disparity in mortality between socio-economic groups in the United States 1960 and 1985. *New England Journal of Medicine*, **229**, 103–8.

Paulley, J.W. (1975). Cultural influences on the incidence and pattern of disease. *Psychotherapy and Psychosomatics*, **26**, 2–11.

Polanyi, K. (1946). *The great transformation*. Beacon Press, New York.

Rathbone, E. (1924). *The disinherited family* (reprinted 1949). Allen and Unwin, London.

Relman, A.S. (1990). The new medical-industrial complex. In *The sociology of health and illness: critical perspectives* (ed. P. Conrad and R. Kern). St Martins Press, New York.

Ringback Weitoft, G., Haglund, B., and Rosen, M. (2000). Mortality among lone mothers in Sweden: a population study. *Lancet*, **355**, 1215–19.

Roosevelt, A.C. (1984). Population, health and the evolution of subsistence. In *Paleopathology and the origins of agriculture* (ed. M.N. Cohen and G.J. Armelagos). Academic Press, New York.

Rosen, H. (1958). *A history of public health*. MD Publications, NewYork.

Rosenberg, C. (1975). *The cholera years:the United States in 1832, 1849, and 1866*. University of Chicago Press.

Routh, G. (1975). *The origin of economic ideas*. Sheridan House, New York.

Routh, G. (1987). *The occupations of the people of Great Britain 1801–1981* . Macmillan, Basingstoke.

Sagan, L. (1996). *The health of nations*. Basic Books, New York.

Sahlins, M. (1974). *Stone Age economics*. Tavistock Press, London.

Salaman, R. (1949). *The history and social influence of the potato* . Cambridge University Press.

Sapolsky, R. (1991). Poverty remains. *Science*, September–October, 8–10.

Schivelbusch, W. (1992). *The tastes of Paradise: a social history of spices, stimulants and intoxicants*. Pantheon, New York.

Schofield, R. (1986). Did the mothers really die? Three centuries of maternal mortality. In *The world we have gained* (ed. L. Bonfield, R.S. Smith, and K. Wrightson), pp. 231–60. Oxford University Press.

Sen, A. (1981). *Poverty and famines: an essay in entitlement and deprivation*. Clarendon Press, Oxford.

Shorter, E. (1975). *The making of the modern family*. Basic Books, New York.

Shorter, E. (1982). *A history of women's bodies*. Penguin, Harmondsworth.

Skidelsky, R. (1994). *The economist as saviour: John Maynard Keynes 1920–1937*. Macmillan, London.

Smith, D. (1999). *The state of the world atlas*. Penguin, Harmondsworth.

Spiller, G.A. (1991). *The Mediterranean diet in health and disease* . Van Nostrand–Reinhold, New York.

Stepan, N. (1982). *The idea of race in science:Great Britain 1800–1980*. Archo Books, Hamden, CT.

Tanner, J.M. (1978). *From foetus into man: physical growth from conception to maturity*. Open Books, London.

Totman, R. (1979). *The social causes of illness*. Pantheon, New York.

Toussaint-Samat, M. (1994). *History of food*. Blackwell, Oxford.

Vagero, D. and Lundberg, O. (1989). Health inequalities in Britain and Sweden. *Lancet*, **ii**, 35–6.

Valkonen, T., Martelin, T., and Rimpela, A. (1990). *Socio-economic mortality differences in Finland 1971–85*. Central Statistical Office, Helsinki.

Velkoff, V.A. and Adlakha, A. (1998). *Women's health in India* . US Bureau of the Census, Washington, DC.

Waldinger, R. and Borzorgmehr, M. (1996). *Ethnic Los Angeles*. Russell Sage Foundation, New York.

Watson, P. (1995). Explaining rising mortality among men in Eastern Europe. *Social Science and Medicine*, **41**, 923–34.

Watts, S. (1997). *Epidemics and history: disease, power and imperialism* . Yale University Press, New Haven, CT.

Wear, A. (1995). Medicine in early modern Europe 1500–1700. In *The Western medical tradition 800 BC to AD 1800* (ed. L. Conrad, M. Neve, V. Nutton, R. Porter, and A. Wear). Cambridge University Press.

Wilkinson, R. (1992). Income distribution and life expectancy. *British Medical Journal*, **304**, 165–8.

Wilkinson, R. (1995). A reply to Ken Judge: mistaken criticisms ignore overwhelming evidence. *British Medical Journal*, **311**, 1285–7.

Wilkinson, R. (1996). *Unhealthy societies: the afflictions of inequality* . Routledge, London.

Williams, S. (1998). Capitalizing on the emotions. *Sociology*, **32**, 121.

Wirth, L. (1938). Urbanism as a way of life. *American Journal of Sociology* , **44**, 1–24.

Wrigley, A.J. and Schofield, R. (1982). *Population history of England* . Cambridge University Press.

Zelizer, V. (1985). *Pricing the priceless child: the changing social value of children*. Basic Books, New York.

Zinsser, H. (1965). *Rats, lice and history*. Bantam Books, New York.

2.3 Education, health promotion, and social and lifestyle determinants of health and disease

Lawrence W. Green and Louise Potvin

Introduction

Interactions of behaviour and environment are pervasive as determinants of health. Technological, engineering, biomedical, legal, and regulatory approaches to public health have sought to control behaviour and to protect people from the environment and from each other. These strategies have declared their victories, only to find new environmental or behavioural problems breaking out somewhere else as causes of ill health. Educational approaches to health provide, at the very least, a palliative solution when technological solutions await development, and a developmental solution when legal or regulatory solutions await an informed and activated electorate. Education enables people to take personal and collective action to protect themselves from environmental threats and to support or resist the development and distribution of technology and the passage of legislation.

In this chapter we attempt to focus on those complex behaviour–environment interactions, called lifestyle, which influence health, and the ways in which education shapes or modifies lifestyle. We use the term lifestyle to refer to any combination of specific practices and environmental conditions reflecting patterns of living influenced by family and social history, culture, and socio-economic circumstances. We know that a discrete behaviour can be influenced directly by health education targeted at individuals and groups. Lifestyle changes more slowly and usually requires some combination of educational, organizational, economic, and environmental interventions in support of changes in both behaviour and conditions of living. This combination of strategies defines health promotion for individuals and communities (Green and Kreuter 1999).

AIDS presents the obvious contemporary example of a disease awaiting a technological solution, and a lifestyle responding slowly to educational, organizational, economic, and environmental interventions and changes. Virtually every public health breakthrough has had an educational process that served the public until the technology was at hand and that helped the diffusion and application of that new technology. Unless, and until, an HIV vaccine is developed, society must depend on behavioural preventive measures to curb the spread of AIDS. Much of the behaviour in question with AIDS is not amenable to legal regulation because of its private nature. Thus education is a primary choice to control the spread of AIDS. The success of health education in filling that gap has been modest but not insignificant depending on the targeted population. Although impossible to attribute to a single programme, the early dramatic changes in sexual practices (general use of condoms) among men in organized urban gay communities appear to have been in response to health education programmes (Petrow 1990; Higgins 1991). Reviews also show evidence of a possible increase in the use of clean needles and safe sexual practices among intravenous drug users (Higgins *et al.* 1991; Fisher and Fisher 1992). Evidence that health education leads to the regular use of condoms among sexually active adolescents, however, has not held up consistently (Fisher and Fisher 1992). Changing some of the more complex lifestyles associated with AIDS in lower-risk populations will require more population-tailored health promotion interventions that address information–motivation–behavioural needs in the specific environmental contexts of the behaviours.

We start with a reductionist view of specific behaviours as they relate to health and disease, and then progress to the more complex sociocultural aspects inherent in the term lifestyle. Finally, we examine the functions of education in reducing disease and promoting health in populations or communities.

Specific behaviours and health

For many diseases, some behaviours clearly increase the risk of developing disease and can be considered proximal causes of disease. Other behaviours correlate with and precede better health, increased longevity, and decreased disease risk, although the causal link is more tenuous, warranting their inclusion with other more distal determinants. Examining the relationships between specific behaviours and specific indicators of health and disease status provides the foundation for assessing behavioural and lifestyle factors as health determinants.

Behaviours and disease—the causal links

Evidence from observational epidemiological studies, human experimental trials, and animal models, together with potential mechanisms of biological action, lead one to conclude that many behaviours are, in fact, contributing causes (causal risk factors) of specific diseases. The causal link is relatively easy to establish for single-agent communicable diseases, but much more difficult to identify for multiple-cause chronic diseases and conditions (Krieger 1994). We present three examples of evidence supporting causal links between behaviours and coronary heart disease: smoking, diet, and physical activity. These three examples illustrate that even in the absence of direct experimental evidence in humans, strong evidence of other types can be assembled for the steps in a causal chain from behaviour through physiological effects to disease.

Studies of the relationship between smoking and coronary heart disease provide strong evidence of a behaviour as a cause of a chronic disease. A plausible biological model has been available for a long time (Dawber 1960). Observational epidemiological studies, using a variety of designs ranging from cross-populational to cross-sectional to case–control to prospective, have found strong and consistent measures of association, the correct temporal sequence, and a dose–response relationship (Stamler 1992). In addition, randomized trials that include smoking cessation programmes provide experimental evidence for smoking as a cause of coronary heart disease. In both the Multiple Risk Factor Intervention Trial (**MRFIT**) and a British trial on the effect of smoking reduction, the number of smokers decreased significantly after a smoking cessation programme, and many of them remained abstinent after several years (Ockene *et al.* 1990; Rose and Colwell 1992). Both studies have shown a decrease in coronary heart disease mortality: 13 per cent after 20 years in the British trial (Rose and Colwell 1992), and 12 per cent after 10.5 years in MRFIT (Ockene *et al.* 1990). In addition, when smokers at baseline from the experimental and control groups were pooled, quitters had a significant decrease in their risk of mortality from coronary heart disease compared with non-quitters (Ockene *et al.* 1990; Kuller *et al.* 1991).

Evidence that consumption of saturated fat and cholesterol are contributing causes of coronary heart disease has come from numerous ecological studies showing a correlation between dietary fat and coronary heart disease mortality and incidence rates (Keys 1970; McGill 1979). Other studies have shown that a high serum cholesterol level increases the risk of coronary heart disease development (Pooling Project Research Group 1978; Stamler *et al.* 1986; Andersen *et al.* 1987*a*), that changes in dietary saturated fat and cholesterol lead to changes in serum cholesterol (Mensink and Katan 1992), and that lowering the serum cholesterol level decreases the occurrence of coronary heart disease (Frick *et al.* 1987). A direct demonstration of the diet–heart hypothesis by a true experimental study may never occur because of the large sample size, the sustained differential changes needed between control and intervention groups, and the long-term follow-up required for such a trial. However, the strong evidence that exists for each step in a causal chain from diet to coronary heart disease has led to major national recommendations that diet be a first-line approach to reduce blood cholesterol to prevent disease (NHLBI 1990, 1993; US Department of Health and Human Services 1991).

The relationship between physical activity and coronary heart disease is the third example. Evidence that physical inactivity is a causal risk factor for coronary heart disease comes from biological effects of exercise on cardiovascular physiology, observational epidemiological studies, and randomized controlled trials of physical activity and physiological coronary heart disease risk factors. The biological effects of exercise training to enhance cardiovascular health are well established (McArdle *et al.* 1986). Epidemiological evidence shows consistent and relatively strong associations, the correct temporal sequence, and a dose–response relationship between physical activity level and coronary heart disease (Powell *et al.* 1987; Berlin and Colditz 1990; Blair *et al.* 1993). Observational epidemiological studies and randomized controlled trials have demonstrated the beneficial effects of physical activity on blood pressure (Arroll and Beaglehole 1992) and on blood lipids and lipoproteins (Haskell 1986; Lokey and Tran 1989), which have, in turn, been causally linked with subsequent coronary heart disease. Strong evidence exists for the steps in a causal chain.

Many causal risk factors are not themselves behaviours, but have determinants that are behaviours; in these cases the behavioural determinants can be considered as indirect risk factors that act earlier in the causal pathway. For example, a combination of high caloric intake and low energy output are the behavioural determinants of obesity (Heath *et al.* 1991; Helmrich *et al.* 1991; Stern 1991). Obesity, in turn, has been found in prospective studies to be a risk factor for type 2 (adult-onset) diabetes (Bergstom *et al.* 1990).

Behaviours contribute to the prognosis of those diseases for which the stage of diagnosis or the compliance with prescribed regimens of treatment or self-care affects outcomes. For example, the prognosis of breast cancer depends on the stage of disease at which the woman obtains medical care, and the prognosis for type 1 (insulin-dependent) diabetes depends on the patient's compliance with his or her insulin prescriptions. Because behaviour is so central to disease outcomes, a large literature on patient education and patient compliance with medical regimens has been catalogued and subjected to meta-analyses (Mullen *et al.* 1985; D.G. Simons-Morton *et al.* 1992; Silagy and Ketteridge 1998).

Behavioural risk factors and the public's health

Behavioural determinants of health and disease status can be found for almost every disease through behavioural risk factors, or through behavioural factors that influence physiological risk factors, or through behavioural factors that influence treatment and prognosis.

The leading causes of death in developed nations are primarily chronic diseases and injuries. Deaths from infectious diseases in the last two decades have refocused public health attention, particularly on the HIV/AIDS epidemic (National Center for Health Statistics 1993). The 10 leading causes of death in the United States in 1997, their generally accepted behavioural and physiological risk factors (McGinnis and Foege 1993), and some behavioural determinants of the physiological risk factors are listed in Table 1. The list for other developed countries would differ only slightly and for those causes that are further down the list. For example, the three leading causes of death in Canada in 1991 were the same as in the United States, accounting also for a little less than two-thirds of the total number of deaths (Canadian Center for Health Information 1994). World Health Organization (**WHO**) estimates of the percentage of deaths from the four leading causes for the developed countries in 1980 were as follows (WHO 1990): cardiovascular disease, 48 per cent; cancer, 19 per cent; respiratory diseases, 7.5 per cent; accidents, 7.0 per cent.

The causes of death in developing countries differ markedly. WHO estimates of the four leading causes of death for the developing countries are: respiratory diseases, 21 per cent; infectious and parasitic diseases, 18 per cent; cardiovascular diseases, 16 per cent; perinatal mortality, 7 per cent (WHO 1990). Among the most striking differences in health indicators between the developed and the developing countries are the perinatal–juvenile mortality rates. The infant mortality rates, for example, range from less than 10 per 1000 live births in western European, North American, and other Pacific Rim countries to more than 150 among some developing countries. The probabilities of dying before the age of 5 years range from less than 12 per 1000 live births to more than 280 for the same comparison countries (WHO 1994). UNICEF (1993) estimates that 12.9 million

Table 1 The 10 leading causes of death in the United States (1997), their generally accepted behavioural (in italics) and physiological risk factors, and the behavioural determinants of the physiological risk factors

Causes of death (percentage of totals number of deaths in United States)	Selected risk factors	Behavioural determinants of physiological risk factors
Diseases of the heart	*Smoking*	
(31.4)	*Physical inactivity*	
	High serum cholesterol	High-fat diet
	Obesity	High-calorie diet
	Hypertension	High-salt diet
	Diabetes mellitus	High-calorie diet (obesity)
Malignant neoplasms	*Smoking*	
(23.3)	*High-fat diet*	
	Low-fibre diet	
	Physical inactivity	
	Sexually transmitted diseases	*Sexual behaviours*
Cerebrovascular diseases	Hypertension	*High-salt diet*
(6.9)	Atherosclerosis	*High-fat diet*
	Smoking	
Chronic obstructive pulmonary disease	*Smoking*	
(4.7)		
Accidents (including fires)	*Alcohol abuse*	
(4.1)	*Unsafe driving*	
	Seat-belt non-use	
	Smoking	
	Drug use	
Pneumonia and influenza	*Drug use*	
(3.7)	Immunization status	*Failure to receive immunization*
	Malnutrition	Diet
Diabetes mellitus	*Physical inactivity*	
(2.7)	Obesity	*High-calorie diet*
Suicide	*Alcohol use*	
(1.3)	*Hand gun use*	
	Drug use	
Nephritis and other kidney disease	*Alcohol abuse*	
(1.1)	*High-fat diet*	
	Exposure to toxic agents	
Chronic liver disease and cirrhosis	*Alcohol abuse*	
(1.1)		

Source: Hoyert *et al.* (1999).

children die each year, almost a quarter of them from diarrhoeal diseases and another 16 per cent from diseases that are preventable by proper immunization.

By 2020, according to WHO estimates, the tobacco epidemic is expected to kill more people than any single disease. Because it is a known or probable determinant of at least 25 diseases, and the most important determinant of some of the leading causes of death, tobacco use will cause nearly 18 per cent of all deaths in developed countries and 11 per cent in developing countries (WHO 1998). The majority of addicted tobacco users began their use while in their teenage years or earlier.

Even when the immediate causes of deaths are specific infectious or toxic agents, behaviours are important contributing determinants of the transmission of those agents. In an analysis involving 66 countries, Hertz *et al.* (1994) have shown that the three most important predictors of infant mortality rates are percentage of households with sanitation, total literacy rate, and the percentage of households without safe water. Clearly, the major public health needs in developing nations relate to the provision of immunization, access to a sufficient supply of clean water, and the installation of proper sanitation facilities (WHO 1979, 1981, 1986). However, these environmental measures achieve the intended health goals only to the extent that an informed population uses them properly. A report by the World Bank (1993) suggests that the single most important public health policy for developing countries lies in the improvement of the education of young girls. Better-educated women have fewer children, who tend to be healthier and, in turn, are better educated.

Examination of the recent trends in the richest of the developing countries provides evidence that improvement of the socio-economic situation is accompanied by a shift in mortality towards the 'civilization diseases' reviewed earlier. For example, in Mexico in 1991 infectious and parasitic diseases were only the fourth leading cause of death, following diseases of the heart (15.8 per cent), malignant neoplasms (10.0 per cent), and accidents (9.5 per cent). Developing countries are now the primary target for market expansion for the multinational tobacco companies. As living standards improve in these countries, deaths from cardiovascular diseases and lung cancer will probably increase considerably. Such trends for lung cancer have been reported for China, India, and Malaysia (Simpson and Ball 1992; WHO 1998).

The role of behavioural risk factors in chronic diseases has been studied primarily in developed nations. Their patterns of mortality make behaviour a legitimate target for health policy (Canada 1974; Epp 1986; McGinnis and Foege 1993). However, it is clear from the shift in causes of death as countries develop and from historical trends in morbidity and mortality in developed nations that attention to behavioural risk factors is warranted early in a nation's development. Health education needs to accompany environmental and policy interventions as well as economic development and basic education.

When one examines the generally accepted behavioural risk factors for disease, it readily becomes apparent that in developed nations a few categories of behaviours are related to a large proportion of deaths. At least one of the three main behavioural risk factors—smoking, dietary practices, and alcohol use—is causally related to each of the 10 leading causes of death in the United States. Active smoking is a risk factor for coronary heart disease (Manson *et al.* 1992; Bartecchi *et al.* 1994), diabetes (Rimm *et al.* 1993), stroke (Robbins *et al.* 1994), and adverse pregnancy outcomes, such as low birth weight, premature rupture of membranes, and abruptio placentae (Fox *et al.* 1994; Mittendorf *et al.* 1994). Passive smoking (i.e. exposure to environmental tobacco smoke), has been related to lung cancer and other respiratory diseases (Office of Health and Environmental Assessment 1992) in adults, and is an independent risk factor for coronary heart disease (Hertz *et al.* 1994). Exposure to environmental tobacco smoke in the home has been associated with asthma and other respiratory conditions, and with ear infections in infants and children (Office of Environmental Health Hazard and Assessment 1997)

Dietary factors are related to the development of atherosclerosis and coronary heart disease through serum cholesterol level (Hunninghake *et al.* 1993) and obesity (Manson *et al.* 1992). Fat intake is also related to colon cancer and possibly to prostate and breast cancer; fibre intake is associated with colon cancer, and fruit and vegetable intake is related to cancers of the lung, cervix, bladder, oral cavity, oesophagus, stomach, and colon (Austoker 1994*a*). Through body weight, dietary factors are also associated with diabetes mellitus (Colditz *et al.* 1990; Helmrich *et al.* 1991). Alcohol use is related to cirrhosis of the liver and other liver diseases (Anderson *et al.* 1993), suicide, homicide, and unintentional injuries (Petrakis 1987), congenital anomalies (Ogston and Parry 1992), and cancer of the mouth, pharynx, larynx, oesophagus, and liver (Austoker 1994*b*). The population attributable risk (i.e. the proportion of the disease in the population that can be attributed to the behavioural factor) can be estimated for many diseases, to the extent that strong evidence of causality exists. For example, the US Centers for Disease Control and Prevention (**US CDC** 1993) has used estimates of the relative risk and risk factor prevalence, taken from numerous epidemiological studies, to calculate the proportion of disease-specific deaths attributable to smoking in the United States in 1990. The proportion of deaths estimated to be attributable to active smoking or to exposure to environmental tobacco smoke in the United States are shown for various diseases in Table 2. These estimates represented a total of 418 690 deaths (Bartechi *et al.* 1994). Based on information about the causal associations between behaviours and health, and on the prevalence of

Table 2 Percentage of deaths attributable to cigarette smoking (population attributable risk) for selected leading causes of death in the United States in 1990[a]

Cause of death	%
Lung cancer (active smoking) (160–165)[b,c]	81.9
Bronchitis and emphysema (490–491)[b,c]	77.0
Cancer of the lip, oral cavity, and pharynx (140–149)[b]	77.0
Ischaemic heart disease (35–64 years old) (410–414)[b]	43.5
Atherosclerosis (440)[b]	35.5
Pneumonia and influenza (480–487)[b]	24.1
Cerebrovascular disease (430–438)[b]	16.2
Ischaemic heart disease (65 and older) (410–414)[b]	15.8
Lung cancer (160–165)[d]	2.0

[a]Numbers in parentheses are the causes of death for the denominators (Ninth Revision of the International Classification of Diseases).

[b]Perfect correspondence between codes in numerator and denominator.

[c]Slight differences between codes in numerator and denominator.

[d]Exposure to environmental tobacco smoke.

Sources: National Center for Health Statistics (1993); US CDC (1993).

health problems, McGinnis and Foege (1993) estimated that, in the United States, 19 per cent of all deaths in 1990 were attributable to smoking and 14 per cent to diet and activity patterns.

Complexity and determinants of behaviours

Despite the implied simplicity in identifying a few major behaviours accounting for the majority of deaths in developed countries, those behaviours are highly complex. Most behavioural risk factors, and health-care behaviours also, are the product of a variety of component behaviours, tasks, or actions. For example, food consumption has been said to confront most people with a chain of behaviours that includes procuring and selecting food, planning menus or selecting from a menu, preparing or ordering foods, and eating with literally hundreds of food-related choices, including where to shop or eat, what to purchase or prepare, how to season food, and with whom to eat (B.G. Simons-Morton *et al.* 1986). One can identify similar chains of component behaviours and behaviour-related choices for other health behaviours identified in Table 1.

Not only are health behaviours complex, but each behaviour has numerous influences or determinants. Factors that influence behaviours can be grouped into three major categories (Green and Kreuter 1999): predisposing, reinforcing, and enabling. Predisposing factors reside in the individual and include attitudes, values, and beliefs, but these are shaped over time by cultural and social reinforcing factors—the positive or negative feedback on or consequences of behaviour—such as peer acceptance or social disapproval. Enabling factors are generally conditions of the environment that facilitate the behaviour or, alternatively, create barriers to it.

Most behaviours have influences from all three categories. Some of the known and likely influencing factors for the three most important preventive health behaviours plus the important interacting health behaviour, physical activity, are shown in Table 3.

The influences on smoking initiation and cessation are numerous (Warner 1986*a*,*b*; D.G. Simons-Morton *et al.* 1991). Predisposing factors include attitudes about smoking and beliefs about and knowledge of the health effects of smoking. Reinforcing social factors include social support, peer influences, and cigarette advertising (providing vicarious reinforcement). Enabling factors include availability and cost of cigarettes.

A variety of factors influence dietary practices (B.G. Simons-Morton *et al.* 1986; Samuels 1990; Contento *et al.* 1993). These include both personal and cultural food preferences, perceived social acceptance, social context, availability and convenience of foods, and skills in menu planning, food purchasing, food selection, and food preparation.

Numerous factors influence alcohol use and abuse (Petrakis 1987; Zarek *et al.* 1987; B.G. Simons-Morton *et al.* 1990; Villas *et al.* 1993). Predisposing factors may include expectations about the effects of alcohol, psychological stress and low self-esteem, perceptions of invulnerability to adverse consequences of drinking such as losing one's job, being a child of an alcoholic, and early drinking experiences. Reinforcing factors include parent and peer influences, and may include advertising and modelling in the visual media. Enabling factors and barriers include availability or non-availability of non-alcoholic drinks, cost of alcoholic beverages, access to alcohol, and supervision of adolescents.

In addition to the three major behavioural risk factors for causes of mortality, every behaviour related to morbidity and well-being also has a variety of influences. Physical inactivity is a good illustrative example. It is not only a risk factor for coronary heart disease (Blair *et al.* 1993), but is also related to hypertension (Duncan *et al.* 1985; Arroll and Beaglehole 1992), osteoporosis (Lee 1991), and mental health (Emery and Blumenthal 1991), all of which are prevalent health problems in developed countries. The numerous influences on physical activity include beliefs about the importance of physical activity, attitudes about physical activity, motivation and self-discipline, accessibility of an exercise facility, skills in relapse prevention and goal setting, discomfort or inconvenience of exercise, and family support (D.G. Simons-Morton *et al.* 1988*b*; Custer and Doty 1992; Field and Steinfardt 1992).

In addition to the complexity of risk behaviours and their numerous determinants, the performance of each behaviour is interwoven with other behaviours and with socio-economic and cultural factors.

Socio-economic and cultural factors and health

To understand better the lifestyle determinants of health, one must examine the context within which behaviour occurs. That context includes contemporary personal interaction with family and other people and with complex organizations. The cultural context includes

Table 3 Some known and suspected influences on four major behavioural risk factors

Cigarette smoking	Dietary practices	Alcohol use/abuse	Physical inactivity
Knowledge of adverse health effects of smoking	Personal food preferences	Expectations of alcohol effects	Beliefs of physical activity benefits
Attitudes about smoking	Cultural food preferences	Child of alcoholic	Attitudes toward physical activity
Skills in smoking cessation/prevention	Perceived social acceptance of foods	Alternatives to alcohol	Self-motivation
Cigarette cost	Social context of eating	Psychological stress	Self-discipline
Availability of cigarettes	Availability and convenience of foods	Low self-esteem	Accessibility of exercise facility
Cigarette advertising	Skills in menu planning	Early drinking experience	Skills in relapse prevention
Peer influences to smoke	Skills in food preparation	Heavy social drinking	Skills in goal setting
Social support for non-smoking	Skills in food selection	Parent and peer influences	Enjoyability of physical activity
	Food advertising	Alcohol advertising	Family support
		Cost of alcohol	
		Availability of alcohol	
		Supervision of drinking	

the cumulative weight of these interactions over generations, as reflected in values and traditions related to behaviour.

The substantial evidence that socio-economic conditions are associated with health status is reviewed elsewhere. Culture plays an intimate role in the determination of health status, most clearly through health behaviours, but also apparently through traditional patterns of social support (Berkman and Syme 1979). In this section we review representative studies and major reports for an overview of the relationships between socio-economic status and health, socio-economic status and use of health-care services, and culture and health, in order to provide a context for the behavioural factors. This will lead us to the more complex sociocultural–behavioural–environmental construct known as lifestyle.

Education may be the most basic aspect of socio-economic status as presented here. Duncan (1961) described the relationship between the basic components (income, education, and occupation of socio-economic status): 'Education qualifies the individual for participation in occupational life, and pursuit of an occupation yields him a return in the form of income'.

Socio-economic status and mortality

This relationship is hardly new. Antonovsky (1967) reviewed the literature from the seventeenth century through to the early 1960s on the relationship between socio-economic status and mortality, including over 30 studies primarily from the European countries and the United States. In these studies socio-economic status was measured in a variety of ways, including type of occupation, median rental costs in census tracts, taxpayer status, and indices comprising education, occupation, and median family income. Antonovsky concluded that:

> Despite the multiplicity of methods and indices used in the 30-odd studies cited, and despite the variegated populations surveyed, the inescapable conclusion is that [socio-economic] class influences one's chance of staying alive. Almost without exception, the evidence shows that [socio-economic] classes differ on mortality rates.

People with lower socio-economic status have higher mortality rates. He observed that the greatest difference in mortality rates occurred during the middle years of life (the thirties and forties) which, he conjectured, may be due to differences in preventable (postponable) deaths between those with different socio-economic status.

Table 4 summarizes results from several studies conducted in developed countries, showing a persisting relationship between socio-economic status and mortality. National data show a consistent association between various indicators of socio-economic status and various indicators of mortality and longevity. In the United States in 1960, socio-economic status as measured by educational level (years of schooling completed) and by family income was inversely associated with mortality ratios (Kitagawa and Hauser 1973). In 1982, in the United Kingdom, the Black Report (Black *et al.* 1982) cited higher 1970 to 1972 mortality rates in occupational groups of lower socio-economic status for both males and females in all age groups. Morris (1979) reported that, in the United Kingdom in 1975 to 1976, all-cause mortality in men continued to be higher for occupational groups of lower socio-economic status. Wilkins *et al.* (1989) showed that household wealth (as defined by the household income weighted by the number of individuals in the household, the average income of the census tract, and the Statistic Canada low-income cut-off) correlated with the life expectancy at birth for both males and females, and more so for the former. Using data from the 1986 National Mortality Followback Survey and the 1986 National Health Interview Survey, Pappas *et al.* (1993) showed that the level of income is strongly inversely related to the age-adjusted death rates for men and women,

Table 4 Results from recent studies of socio-economic status and mortality

Reference	Population	Mortality indicator	Socio-economic status measures	Results
Wilkins *et al.* 1989	Canadian urban 1986	Life expectancy at birth	1st income quintile[a]	78.5
			2nd income quintile	78.1
			3rd income quintile	77.5
			4th income quintile	76.9
			5th income quintile	74.8
Pappas *et al.* 1993	American white men	Age-adjusted death rate	Income in excess of $25 000	2.4
	aged 25–64	per 1000	Income $19 000–$24 999	4.6
	1986		Income $15 000–$18 999	5.7
			Income $9000–$14 999	10.2
			Income less than $9000	16.0
Pappas *et al.* 1993	American black men	Age-adjusted death rate	Income in excess of $25 000	3.6
	aged 25–64	per 1000	Income $19 000–$24 999	4.7
	1986		Income $14 999–$18 999	9.8
			Income $9000–$13 999	10.8
			Income less than $9000	19.5

[a]Highest socio-economic status.

both black and white. All these studies show a persistent gradient. In all these studies, the advantages associated with better socio-economic conditions increase across the whole spectrum of each socio-economic indicator.

Studies comparing data from multiple points in time show different pictures for different countries. The results of Wilkins *et al.* (1989) show that the gap between the 'haves' and the 'have nots', as indicated by the age-adjusted death rates, remained fairly stable in Canada between 1971 and 1986. Over a longer period between 1960 and 1986, however, Pappas *et al.* (1993) have demonstrated an increase in that gap, which is more pronounced for men than for women.

A socio-economic differential for infant and childhood mortality has been observed in many studies. Early childhood death rates (ages 0–5 years) in Southampton, England, from 1977 to 1982 were higher in districts with high unemployment, poor housing, and single-parent families (Robinson and Pinch 1987). In Kentucky, rates in 1982 to 1983, adjusted for a variety of variables, were significantly higher in poor than in non-poor infants during the postneonatal period (Spurlock *et al.* 1987). In Canada, Wilkins *et al.* (1989) found that, in 1986, the infant mortality rate in the lowest quintile of wealth was almost double the infant mortality rate in the highest quintile. Leon *et al.* (1992) found that in Sweden, in 1985 to 1986, the relative risk of neonatal mortality was significantly higher (1.20) for manual compared with non-manual occupational classes; the post-neonatal mortality was also significantly higher (1.38). Even in countries such as Canada and Sweden with equitable health-care systems and welfare policy, people of lower socio-economic classes experience higher mortality.

An inverse socio-economic differential for cause-specific mortality has also been observed for many diseases. The Whitehall Study of British civil servants revealed gradients of mortality rates for coronary heart disease with the lowest rates among high-status occupations and highest mortality rates for the lowest-grade employees. Ischaemic heart disease mortality in the United Kingdom is higher in manual than in non-manual workers (Marmot and McDowall 1986; Pocock *et al.* 1987), and in New York City cancer mortality rates are higher in lower-income groups (Shai 1986). Wilkins *et al.* (1989) have calculated the specific age-adjusted mortality rates in 1986 for several diseases for different groups of Canadians defined by their relative wealth. Comparing the rates for people in various quintiles on wealth, they found an excess mortality (1.5 times greater) among the poorest quintile for infectious diseases, lung cancer, uterine cancer, alcoholism for males, obstructive respiratory diseases, cirrhosis, perinatal mortality, pedestrian accidents, suicides, and other types of accidents. Davey Smith *et al.* (1996) retrieved the mortality data of the 300 000 men enrolled in the MRFIT study during the 1970s. They found a consistent gradient relationship between the median family income of the zip code of residence at the time of enrolment and age-adjusted mortality rates from all causes as well as from cardiovascular diseases, lung cancer, diabetes, respiratory diseases, and cirrhosis.

Thus, it seems that the relationship between socio-economic status and health is not attributable to a threshold effect. On the contrary, those at the top of the hierarchy are better off than those just below them who are themselves better off than the others, and so on down to those at the very bottom. The gradient adheres whether the socio-economic measure is education, income, occupational status, or place of residence.

It was long believed that all the above patterns of socio-economic status are also reflected in white versus non-white differences in mortality. In the United States the black death rate exceeds the white death rate by 50 per cent (Andersen *et al.* 1987*b*). However, Keil *et al.* (1992) have shown that in Charleston, North Carolina, where both groups experienced a similar socio-economic gradient when controlled for socio-economic status, the all-cause mortality rates between 1960 and 1988 were the same for black men and for white men.

Most within-country studies have been conducted in developed nations; however, comparisons between nations provide a global perspective. In general, less developed countries with lower per capita incomes exhibit lower life expectancy and higher infant mortality rates than more developed countries with higher per capita incomes.

A number of recent studies have examined the relationship between mortality rates and various indicators of social inequalities in geographical areas varying in size from metropolitan areas (Lynch *et al.* 1998) to whole countries (Wilkinson 1992*a*,*b*; Wilkinson and Marmot 1998). These studies consistently showed that those areas where inequalities between those at the top of the social hierarchy and those at the bottom were the largest were also those in which the mortality gradient was the strongest (Wilkinson 1996). Similar findings were found with other indicators of social inequities such as differences in educational status (Kunst and Mackenbach 1994) or differences in social capital (Kawachi *et al.* 1997). Disparity within a given society, or relative deprivation, seems to be more influential than the absolute level of poverty.

Socio-economic status and morbidity

Morbidity is difficult to estimate at the level of populations. Studies using diagnosed cases in the numerator of a prevalence rate are very rare, and those that exist are restricted to a limited number of diseases. For population studies, more general and accessible indicators such as self-reported health, the number of days of sickness, or disabilities are usually preferred as measures of morbidity. The same gradient has been observed between socio-economic status and mortality across a wide variety of socio-economic and morbidity indicators and in various industrialized countries, as shown in Table 5.

The results of the 1990 Canadian Health Promotion Survey (Adams 1993) showed that men and women with a higher level of education self-rated their health as excellent or good in a much higher proportion than individuals with a lower education. The same gradient has also been observed for a socio-economic indicator based on the relative wealth of the household. House *et al.* (1990) reported that individuals with lower socio-economic status, as defined by a combination of income and education values, declared more than twice as many chronic conditions as individuals with higher socio-economic status. In addition, they were able to show that the excess of preventable morbidity in the lower socio-economic strata for middle-aged people is not counterbalanced by an excess delayed morbidity for people past the age of 75 in the high socio-economic strata. The relative protection associated with higher socio-economic status exists for all age groups.

The same gradient between morbidity and socio-economic status has also been observed in Scandinavian countries where the social security and welfare is such that social inequalities are minimized. Among men aged 25 to 74, the age-standardized proportion of people with limiting long-standing illness is more than double in people with

Table 5 Results from recent studies of socio-economic status and morbidity

Reference	Population	Morbidity indicators	Socio-economic status measures	Results
Marmot *et al.* 1991	British civil servants (male) aged 35–55 1985–88	Self-rated health percentage rating themselves 'average' or worse	Grade occupation I[a]	15.3
			Grade occupation II	19.5
			Grade occupation III	21.5
			Grade occupation IV	22.8
			Grade occupation V	27.5
			Grade occupation VI	33.7
North *et al.* 1993	British civil servants (male) aged 35–55 1985–88	Adjusted odds ratio Long sickness absence from work	Grade occupation I[a]	1.00
			Grade occupation II	1.75
			Grade occupation III	2.12
			Grade occupation IV	2.89
			Grade occupation V	3.95
			Grade occupation VI	6.44
Bor *et al.* 1993.	Australian cohort of children aged 5 years 1980s	Adjusted odds ratio Child sick 3 times or more in the past 6 months	No disadvantage	1.00
			Mild disadvantage	1.19
			Moderate disadvantage	1.41
			Chronic disadvantage	2.03
Adams 1993	American men and women aged 15 years and older 1990	Self-rated health percentage reporting excellent or very good	University schooling	74.0
			College schooling	65.7
			Secondary schooling	65.6
			Elementary schooling	49.5
House *et al.* 1990	American men and women aged 55-64 1986	Number of reported chronic conditions	Upper SES	0.95
			Upper middle	1.45
			Lower middle	1.59
			Lower SES	2.14
Lahelma *et al.* 1994	Scandinavian men aged 25–74 1986	Age-standardized percentage with limiting long-standing illness	Finland	
			Higher education	17.0
			Secondary education	29.0
			Basic education	38.0
			Norway	
			Higher education	11.0
			Secondary education	25.0
			Basic education	30.0
			Sweden	
			Higher education	11.0
			Secondary education	23.0
			Basic education	26.0

[a]Highest socio-economic status (SES).

elementary education compared with people with higher education. This is true for Finland, Norway, and Sweden and, although to a lower extent, for women as well as men (Lahelma *et al.* 1994). Two different analyses of the data generated by the Whitehall II study of civil servants in England show a clear association between the grade of the occupation and the percentage of people self-rating their health as average or worse (Marmot *et al.* 1991) and between the occupation and the odds ratios of recorded long sickness absence from work adjusted for age, several health behaviours, work characteristics, social circumstances, and demographic factors. Bor *et al.* (1993) observed that, by the age of 5 years, Australian children born in households with lower socio-economic status had poorer general health, were sick more often, experienced a greater number of persistent health conditions, and had more dental problems.

Socio-economic status and health-related behaviours

Many surveys conducted in a wide variety of industrialized countries on numerous behaviours have consistently produced results showing associations between socio-economic status and health behaviours. The poorer and the less educated an individual in developing countries, the more likely he or she is to engage in patterns of behaviours that are not conducive to health. In the Canadian Health Promotion Survey (Health and Welfare Canada 1993), the number of smokers is double in people with elementary schooling compared with people with university degrees, and ranges from 36 per cent among the very poorest to 25 per cent among the richest. The rates were 40 per cent among blue collar workers and 27 per cent among people in managerial/professional positions (Pederson 1993). The Whitehall II study (Marmot *et al.* 1991) shows a wide gap between the proportions smoking in the highest and the lowest occupational grades. Although the difference is not as great for women, the relationship between smoking and education varies only slightly when adjusted for age, sex, and ethnicity (Winkleby *et al.* 1990; Shea *et al.* 1991). Analyses of data generated by the major community trials in cardiovascular disease prevention showed that the dramatic drop in prevalence of smoking over the 1980s was more pronounced for people with higher education compared with people with lower education (Winkleby *et al.* 1992*b*; Luepker *et al.* 1993). The same trend has also been observed in Canada for the period 1985 to 1991 (Millar and Stephens 1993).

Reasons for relationships between socio-economic status and health

There are four general hypotheses about possible mechanisms that can explain the consistent relationships observed between socio-economic indicators and health indicators such as mortality and morbidity (Macintyre 1997) . The first states that the relationship is spurious and arises from the association of both socio-economic and health indicators with underlying genetic predisposition. By showing that the relationship between job status and health persists after adjustment for height and body-mass index, the Whitehall I and Whitehall II studies (Marmot *et al.* 1984, 1991) have contributed to rendering that hypothesis highly improbable.

The second explanation, referred to as the 'drift hypothesis', states that socio-economic conditions deteriorate as a result of poor health rather than the reverse. Results from longitudinal studies, however, demonstrate that this hypothesis alone cannot explain all of the association between socio-economic status and mortality/morbidity. Living conditions, as defined by the relative poverty of the area of residence, are moderately associated with the relative risk of mortality over subsequent years, after controlling for baseline health, health practices, and socio-demographic characteristics (Fox *et al.* 1986; Haan *et al.* 1987). It has also been observed that the socio-economic conditions experienced during childhood are independently associated with mortality and with health-affecting factors such as social isolation, health-promoting lifestyles, and working conditions in adult life (Peck 1994).

The third explanation is related to the diminished access to health care associated with poverty. Adler *et al.* (1994) have made a strong case that, even though access to health care is probably contributing to the association between socio-economic status and health, the socio-economic status–health gradient still persists in countries with universal health insurance coverage, as shown earlier here for Canada and Sweden.

Finally, the fourth and most plausible explanation is that components of socio-economic status are intertwined with crucial features of life that affect health: physical environment, social and cultural environment, development and socialization process, and the health-related behaviours (Adler *et al.* 1994). Even if this hypothesis of the social determinants of health seems to be most plausible there is a vigorous debate among researchers as to the mechanisms by which social circumstances affect health. Notable are the stress hypothesis (Brunner and Marmot, 1999), the cumulative risk through life course approach (Kuh *et al.* 1997; Wadsworth 1999), the social cohesion explanation (Wilkinson 1996, 1999; Muntaner and Lynch 1999), the mediator role of health-related behaviours (Green 1970*b*; Marmot *et al.* 1978; Stronks *et al.* 1996; Cavelaars *et al.* 1997), and the perspective developed by Link and Phelan (1995) and echoed by Potvin and Frohlich (1998). This latter view holds that social categories such as socio-economic status, gender, or race are associated with access to resources, patterns of relationships, and distribution of power that shape health and disease patterns in a population.

Socio-economic status, gender, and health

One important aspect of life circumstances whose relationship with health has been increasingly studied is gender. Research has demonstrated that men's and women's experience with health differ markedly (Chapman Walsh *et al.* 1995) and that these differences cannot be solely attributable to biological determinants related to sexual differentiation (Bird and Fremont 1991; Krieger *et al.* 1993). The social construct of gender, as opposed to the biological categories of sex, was designed to refer to cultural and social conventions, roles and behaviours assigned to men and women (Krieger 1996). These in turn shape the social, political, cultural, and economical circumstances experienced by men and women. Gender thus attempts to capture this differential experience men and women have of their environment and the possibilities and constraints associated with these differences (Krieger *et al.* 1993; Potvin and Frohlich 1998). A growing body of research is showing that some of these constraints and possibilities are interacting with the living conditions associated with socio-economic status to shape the health of people. The relationship between gender and health is a complex one.

Until recently research on gender differences and health in the industrialized world has demonstrated a consistent portrait: although women were living longer than men, they had higher rates of morbidity throughout their lives (Verbrugge 1985, 1989; Macintyre 1993). The universality of this picture, however, is now being challenged. Until industrialization, life expectancy was higher for men and still is in some less developed countries. In the Western world the women's relative advantage in mortality rate over men was increasing for most of the twentieth century (Macintyre and Hunt 1997). Furthermore, it seems that the direction of the differential morbidity in men and women varies according to specific conditions and to phases in the life-cycle (Macintyre *et al.* 1996; Lahelma *et al.* 1999). Recent studies examining health inequalities resulting from the interaction between socio-economic status and gender provided insightful results.

The correlation between socio-economic status and health appears to be stronger for men than for women; the gradient of health that parallels the gradient of socio-economic strata is generally steeper when applied to men (Koskinen and Martelin 1994; Stronks *et al.* 1995; Arber 1997; Arber and Cooper 1999). This interaction was observed for various health indicators such as mortality, body size, activity limitations, overall morbidity, and self-assessed health, and across several socio-economic status measures such as occupation, education, and income (Macintyre and Hunt 1997). There are, however, variations in this interaction effect. Some combinations of disease and socio-economic status indicators, for example, show similar correlation in men and women (Arber 1997). It seems also that the gradient of socio-economic status and health is similar for men and women in their twenties and thirties (Matthews *et al.* 1999) whereas in people aged 60 and over socio-economic differences in self-assessed health are weaker among women compared with men (Arber and Cooper 1999).

Although making sense of this interaction effect of gender and socio-economic status on health still challenges health sociologists (Macintyre and Hunt 1997), some explanations have been explored. First, differentials in employment status between men and women have been examined. Stronks *et al.* (1995) concluded that several aspects of the job market might explain the differential gradient between men and women. One aspect is the lower proportion of women in paid employment. A complementary explanation is the differential distribution of working conditions with lower-status occupations being more likely to involve physical health risk for men than women. These differences in occupational opportunities have already been suggested to explain the health differentials between men and women (Ross and Bird 1994). Second, Koskinen and Martelin (1994) have found that the interaction effect between gender and socio-economic status arises totally from the married population. In other marital status groups the relationship between socio-economic status and health is similar for men and women. Observing that the proportion of married women is similar across socio-economic status categories, whereas the proportion of married men increased with socio-economic status, the authors suggest that various factors affecting one's life situation such as social support may be at play. Third, the same study also pointed to the fact that the causes of death that show the strongest relationship with socio-economic status, such as unintentional injury and violence and diseases of the circulatory system, are also more common among men.

Some common causes of death in women such as breast cancer even show a reverse gradient, affecting more women in higher socio-economic status categories (Koskinen and Martelin 1994). Fourth, Kawachi *et al.* (1999) have examined the patterns of relationships at the state-aggregated level between indicators of women's emancipation status and gender-specific health indicators. They found a strong relationship between various indicators of women's emancipation status and women's health. Surprisingly, they found an even stronger relationship between indicators of women's emancipation status and men's health. In addition to reinforcing the evidence that men's differences in health are more sensitive to life circumstances than are women's (Hunt and Annandale 1999), these intriguing results may indicate that men's health status is more closely related to general inequalities in life circumstances.

Culture and health

Culture appears to play an independent part in health status (Corin 1994). Culture is intimately related to accepted social practices, many of which are in turn related to health and disease.

Epidemiological evidence for the impact of culture on health comes from the ecological studies of diet and coronary heart disease, mentioned earlier, and immigrant studies of cardiovascular disease. The ecological studies show clear cultural differences in both dietary practices and cardiovascular disease consequences. Studies of Japanese men living in Japan and emigrating to California revealed coronary heart disease and stroke rates comparable with those of the country of residence only in subsequent generations, whereas those emigrating to Hawaii had intermediate rates (Keys *et al.* 1958; Kato *et al.* 1973). The implications are that, as the Japanese became acculturated, they assumed both the dietary and cardiovascular patterns of the new country. This is a clear argument against the hypothesis that genetic factors have the dominant influence on heart disease, and for the hypothesis that cultural factors play a prominent part. Dietary factors appear to be powerfully influenced by culture (Rozin 1984)..

The Roseto study provides another example of the effects of culture on health. Early observations have shown that this ethnically homogeneous Pennsylvania community experienced a significantly lower mortality from myocardial infarction than the nearby community of Bangor despite a higher prevalence of hypertension and obesity and a similar proportion of smokers (Stout *et al.* 1964; Bruhn 1965; Lynn *et al.* 1967). These results were attributed to the apparent protective effect of a unique social, ethnic, and family cohesion in the community (Bruhn and Wolf 1979; Bruhn *et al.* 1982). It was also hypothesized that the 'Americanization' of the lifestyle in this originally close-knit traditional Italian community (Bruhn and Wolf 1979) would lead to a loss of their relative protection from myocardial infarction (Lynn *et al.* 1967). Recent analyses show that, in fact, Rosetans have lost that relative protection over the last two decades (Egolf *et al.* 1992). This loss was accompanied by an increase in the number of intermarriages of Rosetans with people of non-Italian descent, a decrease in social participation in Roseto, and an increase in the general wealth of the community, as the original Italian-born generation was gradually replaced by their ageing American-born offspring (Lasker *et al.* 1994).

Socio-economic status and lifestyle: the merging of perspectives

Lifestyle has emerged as a concept in modern discourse to describe in shorthand what Madison Avenue advertising agencies call market segments—groups or types of people differentiated by a set of consumption and other living patterns related to their income, education, occupation, gender, residence, and geopolitical and ethnic identification. This commercialization of the term is not totally unrelated to the social science origins of the concept. In the health field, however, the term has been used more variously. At one extreme, it describes discrete narrowly defined behaviour related to chronic diseases or health enhancement. This usage is associated with elements of individualism (Coreil and Levin 1984–5). At the other extreme, 'lifestyle' is used to describe the total social milieu including the 'psycho-socio-economic environment' as well as personal health behaviours (Hancock 1986).

As a behavioural concept, lifestyle generally implies more complex, repetitive (if not habitual) patterns of behaviour conditioned by culture and living standards but still under the control of the individual or family within their economic means. The public health application of this behavioural notion of lifestyle has tended to associate it with 'health-related' (e.g. food consumption patterns) as distinct from 'health-directed' (e.g. diet) behaviour (Steuart 1965; Gottlieb and Green 1987). As a sociopolitical and ecological concept, lifestyle reflects how categories of people sharing similar life circumstances interact with their social context (Rutten 1995; Green *et al.* 1996; Frohlich and Potvin 1999*a*). The public health application of this notion of lifestyle has been to seek policies and environmental regulations that would redirect lifestyle or 'make healthy choices the easier choices' (Epp 1986; WHO 1986; Green and Kreuter 1999).

Relationships among lifestyle factors

The concept of lifestyle as the interplay between habitual behavioural patterns and sociocultural conditions leads one to put into a broader context the reductionist examinations, presented in the first half of this chapter, of specific behaviours and specific measures of socio-economic status as they relate to health and disease. The dynamic interplay between the specific measures creates a complex and intricate system of social, economic, cultural, and behavioural factors, interwoven with disease risk factors and health status, and influenced by the health-care and physical environments. A simplified scheme of such a system is shown in Fig. 1.

Although such a complex system is extremely difficult (if not impossible) to study directly, parts of it can be, and have been, studied. Evidence for its existence comes from the relationships presented earlier between specific health behaviours and health, socio-economic factors and health, and culture and health.

Studies of the relationships among health behaviours have not been consistent in showing strong interrelationships between types of health-related behaviours (Green 1970*b*; Steele and McBroom 1972). The highest correlations observed were generally below 0.20 and were between smoking and alcohol use, alcohol use and exercise (Calnan 1989), and smoking and diet (Blaxter 1990). Given these low correlations, there is very little evidence supporting a one-dimensional concept of health-related behaviours (Calnan 1994). In fact, patterns of health-related behaviours, when observed, tend to vary by socio-economic characteristics such as income and education (Green 1970*a*; Townsend *et al.* 1988; Prattala *et al.* 1994). According to Calnan (1994), recent developments in the area of health-related behaviours have led to a shift in emphasis away from an individualized model that explains behavioural choices solely as a product of knowledge and beliefs. Recent research emphasizes the role of social circumstances in influencing individuals' behaviours. This implies that income and education are highly influential determinants of the health risk factors.

Nevertheless, findings support the role of education as the most basic component of socio-economic status as a determinant of health risk behaviours. Winkleby *et al.* (1992*a*) have systematically compared

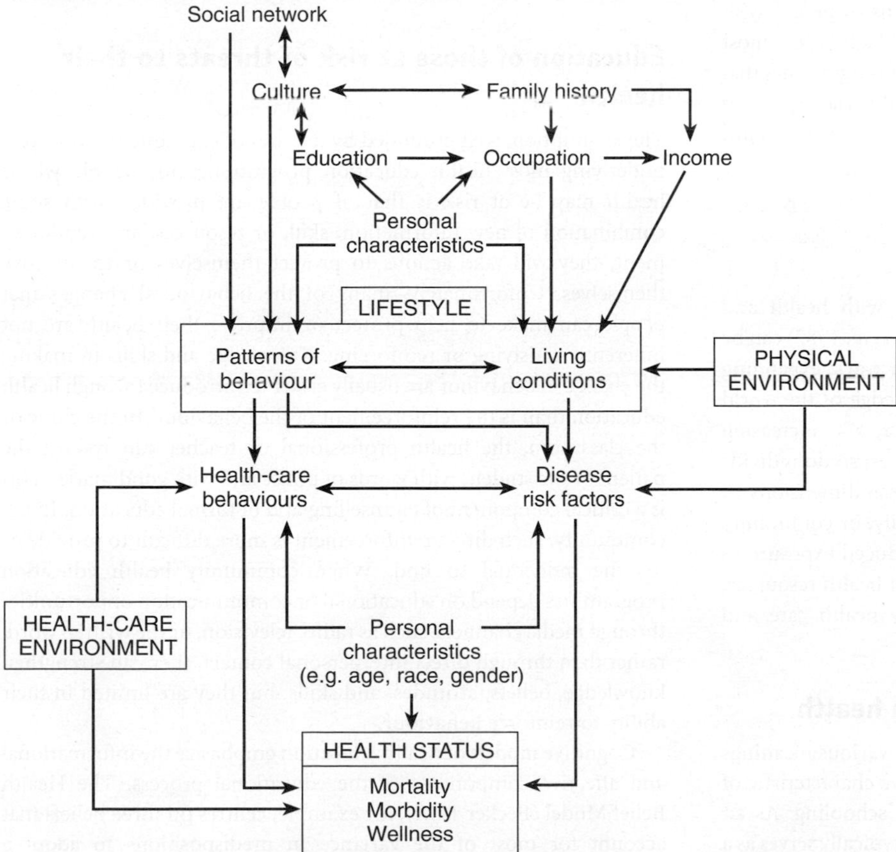

Fig. 1 Some interrelationship in the complex system of lifestyle, environment, and health status.

the relationships between different behaviours and three indicators of socio-economic status: education, income, and occupation. Education stands out as the indicator most consistently and highly correlated with health-related behaviours. Although education level is primarily a function of social, cultural, and economic circumstances, educational influence on lifestyles and health-related behaviours is clearly an important aspect of public health practice.

Education, socio-economic status, lifestyle, and the health agenda

Thus it seems quite clear that at least part of the relationship between socio-economic status and mortality and morbidity indicators is attributable to differences in behaviours and to differences in the environment. These differences in behaviours are strongly associated with the level of education and income. The body of knowledge presented above provides the basis for an ambitious health education agenda. The greatest gains in longevity will come from our efforts to reduce the number of premature preventable deaths among people from the lowest socio-economic classes. Wilkins *et al.* (1989) showed that, for 1986, 20 per cent of all potential years of life lost before the age of 75 was related to income differences for the urban population of Canada. This becomes as high as 44.5 per cent for injury deaths between the age of 25 and 44, and 39.8 per cent for deaths from circulatory diseases between 45 and 74.

The challenge for health professionals is to support behavioural modifications among the segments of the population with lower socio-economic status. The use of the mass media in educational campaigns is not sufficient to alter the risk patterns of people with lower socio-economic status for whom enabling factors are most problematic (Green and McAlister 1984). Ecological programmes that also address the environmental, organizational, and social aspects of health problems are more likely to succeed (Green *et al.* 1996; Richard *et al.* 1996; Green and Kreuter 1999)

Education and health

Education's powerful and pervasive correlations with health and health-related behaviour (Green 1970, 1972; Pincus *et al.* 1987) can be seen to operate through behaviour in at least four ways: expanding opportunities for the individual, increasing knowledge of the world and the options it offers, building self-confidence, and increasing specific skills and capabilities. As education advances, so do individuals, families, and the community on each of these dimensions of development. With education come personal, family, or community development, which result in improved health, reduced exposure to environmental threats to health, increased access to health resources, and increased purchasing power to buy primary health care and advanced medical care.

Channels of educational influence on health

The term education, like the term lifestyle, takes on various meanings depending on the context of its use. As a descriptive characteristic of individuals, it generally refers to years of formal schooling. As an epidemiological and demographic variable, it most typically serves as a surrogate measure of socio-economic status. As a family variable, education of the main earner often stands as an indicator of family's socio-economic status. Research generally shows, however, that the education of the female head of household is more influential in determining family health and the health behaviour of other family members (Green 1970, 1972; Mechanic 1979; Carmelli *et al.* 1986; Davis and Robinson 1988).

Education is also used as a term to describe organizations, social institutions, and the status of communities. Whole sectors of the community may be broadly identified as educational, as in 'the education establishment' or 'higher education'. Education is also a function of most social institutions and departments of government. It is in this latter context that the term 'health education' is used to describe the educational function of health agencies, but health education also has a place in a variety of different sites such as schools, churches, workplaces, and recreational facilities (Poland *et al.* 2000). The term health education applies to a wide range of approaches and topics relevant to health, including, for example, education in basic hygiene for children, safety education for children and youth, parent education for young adults, and chronic disease prevention and management in later adulthood. The various forms of health education occur through a variety of channels, some institutional and some interpersonal.

Health education can be defined as the combination of planned learning experiences to facilitate voluntary actions conducive to health (Green *et al.* 1986; Green and Kreuter 1999, p. 27). The actions may be of individuals to protect or promote their own health, of families to protect or promote the health of their members, or of organizational or community leaders and influential persons to change environmental conditions affecting health (see Chapter 7.3).

Education of those at risk of threats to their health

The assumption, well grounded by decades of experimental research, underlying most health education programmes for people whose health may be at risk is that, if people are provided with some combination of new information, skill, or resources, and reinforcement, they will take actions to protect themselves or to improve themselves. Unfortunately, many of the behavioural changes that people can make to help protect or improve their health are not inherently satisfying or reinforcing. Knowledge and skills in making the change in behaviour are usually easier to introduce through health education than is the reinforcement of the behaviour. In the clinic or the classroom, the health professional or teacher can reward the patient or the student with words of praise and with good marks. This is a critical component of counselling and of formal education. In the community, such direct reinforcement is more difficult to provide or for the individual to find. When community health education programmes depend on educational or communication opportunities through media channels, such as radio, television, or the written word, rather than through direct interpersonal contact, they can strengthen knowledge, beliefs, attitudes, and skills, but they are limited in their ability to reinforce behaviour.

Cognitive models of health education emphasize the informational and affective components of the educational process. The Health Belief Model (Becker 1974), for example, centres on three beliefs that account for most of the variance in predispositions to adopt a recommended health practice. These include a belief in susceptibility (or belief that you could have the disease and not know it in the case of undertaking screening or treatment for conditions such as hypertension), and a belief in the severity of the consequences of not taking action. The third belief influencing action is that the benefits of treatment or intervention will outweigh the costs (including social benefits and costs such as inconvenience, discomfort, or embarrassment). This model has been widely tested and found to have predictive validity (Becker 1974; Harrison *et al.* 1992).

Even the proponents of the Health Belief Model and other cognitive models that have proved useful in the development of health education interventions acknowledge that the task of behavioural change requires more than changing beliefs, attitudes, and perceptions (Harrison *et al.* 1992). These factors may produce strong desires to change, but without skills and resources the highly motivated individual will only be frustrated. Frustration leads to a need to deny the prior motivation, which leads to rationalization or other defence mechanisms that erect barriers to future attempts to convince the individual to change. Therefore, simplistic approaches to health education based entirely on information transfer can backfire in two ways. First, a result that is worse than being ineffective in changing behaviour for many people is aroused expectations and motivation that lead to frustration and disappointment when the target behaviour proves out of reach. Second, they may set up defence mechanisms in the disappointed individuals that make subsequent attempts to reach them with health messages more difficult.

A more promising alternative to information-only and fear-arousal approaches to health education is the combination approach referred to in the definition cited above. This approach recognizes that behaviour is complex and has multiple causes and sources of influence variously impinging on it. Motivation must be backed with skills and resources to enable the behavioural change, and with rewards or social support to reinforce it. These additional elements require upstream community organization, environmental changes, and training of professionals, family members, employers, or others to enable and provide social support for the behaviour (Green and Kreuter 1999; McKinley and Marceau 2000).

In addition to the rational model of education influencing cognitive predispositions, and enabling or reinforcing behaviour, an understanding of education influencing health through alternative routes that do not necessarily involve specific behaviour changes has been suggested (Lorig and Laurin 1985). Education may influence the process of social support, which can have a direct influence on health with changing health behaviour (Nuckolls *et al.* 1972; Berkman and Syme 1979). Education can also increase self-confidence, self-image, or self-efficacy, any of which might have an independent effect on health with or without behavioural change (Ewart *et al.* 1983; Kaplan *et al.* 1984).

Education for community development

Education can serve health at yet another level through the community development process or movements such as the Healthy Cities initiatives in Europe and Healthy Communities in North America. Here the function of education can be seen as more circuitous. Education arouses interest and increases the consciousness of the public about local issues or problems. The public then seeks more active participation in debating the priority that should be given to the problem and to optional solutions, and watches more vigilantly the process of governmental or institutional response. All these ways in which the public becomes more active in participating in community affairs have a ripple effect on the community's ability to solve other problems more effectively (Green 1986). With an active population, public agencies tend to be more responsive, elected and appointed officials tend to be more sensitive to public needs, and community organizations tend to be more co-operative in working with each other than in communities where the public waits for governmental and other organizations to provide all the leadership on health matters (Cottrell 1976; Goeppinger and Baglioni 1985). Community development leads to better schooling, which results in improved levels of education in the community, which comes full circle to the functions of education for health described above.

Education to influence environmental conditions

In addition to the education of people to influence their health behaviours and their socio-economic status, education also can be directed towards those people who have the power and authority to change the physical and health-care environments—environments that can influence health directly or that can enable health behaviours.

Organizations, communities, and governments establish more or less healthful environmental conditions through policies, practices, facilities, and resources. Those conditions are influenced by decision-makers such as managers, department heads, and administrators within organizations, legislators, regulators, enforcers, and agency administrators within local, state, and federal government, and community leaders. Education of the decision-makers is a crucial avenue for facilitating healthful environmental change (D.G. Simons-Morton *et al.* 1988*a*).

Approaches to influencing organizations, communities, and governments are often called something else, but always contain educational components. Such approaches include organizational change, consulting, social and political action, community organization, persuasive communication, and political process (e.g. lobbying) (D.G. Simons-Morton *et al.* 1988*a*; B.G. Simons-Morton *et al.* 1995; Green and Kreuter 1999; McKinlay and Marceau 2000).

Summary

Lifestyle is the combination of specific practices and environmental conditions reflecting patterns of living. These involve interactions between behaviours, environment, culture, and socio-economic status. Each of the factors that make up and influence lifestyle has been shown to affect health, illness, disability, and mortality. A pivotal variable in mediating these relationships is education. Environmental conditions are also important determinants of health status, and these conditions, in turn, influence and are influenced by behaviour and lifestyle.

Educational level is an integral part of the concept of socio-economic status and a crucial determinant of lifestyle. Education is also an important avenue for influencing specific behaviours, the environment, and the complex system of lifestyle, all of which influence health status. Education is crucial for achieving changes in personal behaviours, organizations, communities, and environments. Education can influence organizational, economic, and environmental supports that can contribute significantly to the protection and promotion of health.

References

Adams, O. (1993). Health status. In *Health and Welfare Canada. Canada's health promotion survey 1990: technical report* (ed. T. Stephens and D. Fowler Graham), p. 23. Ministry of Supply and Services, Ottawa.

Adler, N.E., Boyce, T, Chesney, M.A., *et al.* (1994). Socioeconomic status and health: the challenge of' the gradient. *American Psychologist*, **49**, 15.

Andersen, K.M., Castelli, W.P., and Levy, D. (1987*a*). Cholesterol and mortality: 30 years of follow-up from the Framingham Study. *Journal of the American Medical Association*, **257**, 2170–80.

Andersen, R.M., Mullner, R.M., and Cornelius, L.J. (1987*b*). Black–white differences in health status: method or substance. *Milbank Memorial Fund Quarterly*, **65** (Supplement 1), 71.

Anderson, P., Cremona, A., Paton, A., *et al.* (1993). The risk of alcohol. *Addiction*, **88**, 1493.

Antonovsky, A. (1967). Social class, life expectancy and overall mortality. *Milbank Memorial Fund Quarterly*, **45**, 31.

Arber, S. (1997). Comparing inequalities in women's and men's health: Britain in the 1990s. *Social Science and Medicine*, **44**, 773.

Arber, S. and Cooper, H. (1999). Gender differences in health in later life: the new paradox? *Social Science and Medicine*, **48**, 61.

Arroll, B. and Beaglehole, R. (1992). Does physical activity lower blood pressure: a critical review of the clinical trials. *Journal of Clinical Epidemiology*, **45**, 439–47.

Austoker, J. (1994*a*). Cancer prevention in primary care: diet and cancer. *British Medical Journal*, **308**, 1610–14.

Austoker, J. (1994*b*). Cancer prevention in primary care: reducing alcohol intake. *British Medical Journal*, **308**, 1549–52.

Bartecchi, C.E., MacKenzie, T.D., and Schrier, R.W. (1994). The human cost of tobacco use, Part 1. *New England Journal of Medicine*, **330**, 907.

Becker, M.H. (1974). The Health Belief Model and personal health behaviour. *Health Education Monographs*, **2**, 324.

Bergstrom, R.M., Newell-Morris, L.L., Leonetti, D.L., *et al.* (1990). Association of elevated fasting C-peptide level and increased intra-abdominal fat distribution with the development of NIDDM in Japanese-American men. *Diabetes*, **36**, 179.

Berkman, L.F and Syme, S.L. (1979). Social networks, host resistance, and mortality: a nine year follow-up of Alameda county residents. *American Journal of Epidemiology*, **109**, 186.

Berlin, J.A. and Colditz, G.A. (1990). A meta-analysis of physical activity in the prevention of coronary heart disease. *American Journal of Epidemiology*, **132**, 12–28.

Bird, C.E. and Fremont, A.M. (1991). Gender, time use, and health. *Journal of Health and Social Behavior*, **32**, 114.

Black, D., Morris, J.N., Smith C., and Townsend, P. (1982). *Inequalities in health: the Black Report* (ed. P. Townsend and N. Davidson). Penguin, Harmondsworth.

Blair, S, Powell, K., Bazzarre, T, *et al.* (1993). Physical activity. American Heart Association Prevention Conference III: Behaviour change and compliance, keys to improving cardiovascular health. *Circulation*, **88**, 1402.

Blaxter, M. (1990). *Health and lifestyles*. Routledge, London.

Bor, W., Naiman, J.M., Anderson, M., *et al.* (1993). Socioeconomic disadvantage and child morbidity: an Australian longitudinal study. *Social Science and Medicine*, **36**, 1053.

Bruhn, J.F. (1965). An epidemiological study of myocardial infarctions in an Italian-American community: a preliminary sociological study. *Journal of Chronic Disease*, **18**, 353.

Bruhn, J. and Wolf, S. (1979). *The Roseto story: an anatomy of health*. University of Oklahoma Press, Oklahoma City.

Bruhn, J.G., Philips, B.U., and Wolf, S. (1982). Lessons from Roseto 20 years later: a community study of heart disease. *Southern Medical Journal*, **75**, 575.

Brunner, E. and Marmot, M. (1999). Social organization, stress and health. In *Social determinants of health* (ed. M. Marmot and R.G. Wilkinson), p. 17. Oxford University Press.

Calnan, M. (1989). Control over health and patterns of health-related behavior. *Social Science and Medicine*, **26**, 435.

Calnan, M. (1994). Lifestyle and its social meaning. *Advances in Medical Sociology*, **4**, 69.

Canada (1974). *A new perspective on the health of Canadians (Lalonde Report)*. Department of National Health and Welfare, Ottawa.

Canadian Center for Health Information (1994). *Mortality summary list of causes, 1991*. Statistics Canada, Ottawa.

Carmelli, D., Swan, G.E., and Rosenman, R.H. (1986). The relationship between wives' social and psychologic status and their husband's coronary heart disease. *American Journal of Epidemiology*, **122**, 90.

Cavelaars, A.E.J.M., Kunst, A.E., and Mackenbach, J.P. (1997). Socio-economic differences in risk factors for morbidity and mortality in the European Community. *Journal of Health Psychology*, **2**, 353.

Chapman Walsh, D., Sorensen, G., and Leonard, L. (1995). Gender, health, and cigarette smoking. In *Society and health* (ed. B.C. Amick III, S. Levine, A.R. Tarlov, and D. Chapman Walsh), p. 131. Oxford University Press, New York.

Colditz, G.A., Willett, W.C., Stampfer, M.J., *et al.* (1990). Weight as a risk factor for clinical diabetes in women. *American Journal of Epidemiology*, **132**, 501.

Contento, I.R., Basch, C., and Shea, S. (1993). Relationship of mothers' food choice criteria to food intake of preschool children: identification of family subgroups. *Health Education Quarterly*, **20**, 227.

Coreil, J. and Levin, J. (1984–5). A critique of the life style concept in public health education. *International Quarterly of Community Health Education*, **5**, 103.

Corin, E. (1994). The social and cultural matrix of health and disease. In *Why are some people healthy and others not? The determinants of health populations* (ed. R.G. Evans, M.L. Barer, and T.R. Marmor), pp. 93–132. Aldine de Gruyter, New York.

Cottrell, L.S. (1976). *The competent community*. In *Further explorations in social psychiatry* (ed. B.H. Kaplan, R.N. Wilson, and A.H. Leighton), p. 195. Basic Books, New York.

Custer, S.J. and Doty, C.R. (1992). Assessment of self-motivation and selected physiological characteristics as predictors of adherence to exercise in a corporate setting. *Journal of Health Education*, **23**, 232.

Davey Smith, G., Neaton, J.D., Wentworth, D., *et al.* (1996). Socioeconomic differentials in mortality risk among men screened for the Multiple Risk Factor Intervention Trial: I. White men. *American Journal of Public Health*, **86**, 486.

Davis, N.J. and Robinson, R.V. (1988). Class identification of men and women in the 1970s and 1980s. *American Sociological Review*, **53**, 103.

Dawber, T.R. (1960). Summary of recent literature regarding cigarette smoking and coronary heart disease. *Circulation*, **22**, 164.

Duncan, J.J., Farr, J.E., Upton, J., *et al.* (1985). The effects of aerobic exercise on plasma catecholamines and blood pressure in patients with mild essential hypertension. *Journal of the American Medical Association*, **254**, 2609.

Duncan, O.D. (1961). Occupational components of educational differences in income. *Journal of the American Statistical Association*, 56, 783.

Egolf, B., Lasker, J., Wolf, S., and Potvin, L. (1992). The Roseto effect: a 50-year comparison of mortality rates. *American Journal of Public Health*, **82**, 1089.

Emery, C.F. and Blumenthal, J.A. (1991). Effects of physical exercise on psychological and cognitive functioning of older adults. *Annals of Behavioral Medicine*, **13**, 99.

Epp, J. (1986). Achieving health for all: a framework for health promotion. *Health Promotion International*, **1**, 419.

Ewart, C.K., Taylor, C.B., Reese, L.B., and DeBusk, R.F. (1983). The effects of early myocardial infarction exercise testing on self-perception and subsequent physical activity. *American Journal of Cardiology*, **51**, 1076.

Field, L.K. and Steinfardt, M.A. (1992). The relationship of internally directed behavior to self-reinforcement, self-esteem, and expectancy, values for exercise. *American Journal of Health Promotion*, **7**, 21.

Fisher, J.D. and Fisher, W.A. (1992). Changing AIDS-risk behavior. *Psychological Bulletin*, **111**, 455.

Fox, A.J., Goldblatt, P.O., and Jones, D.R. (1986). Social class mortality differentials: artefact, selection, or life circumstances. In *Class and health: research and longitudinal data* (ed. R.G. Wilkinson), p. 35. Tavistock Publications, London.

Fox, S.H., Koepsell, TD., and Daling, J.R. (1994). Birth weight and smoking during pregnancy—effect modification by maternal age. *American Journal of Epidemiology*, **139**, 1008.

Frohlich, K.L. and Potvin, L. (1999*a*). Collective lifestyles as the target for health promotion. *Canadian Journal of Public Health*, **90** (Supplement 1), S11.

Frohlich, K.L. and Potvin, L. (1999*b*). Health promotion through the lens of population health: toward a salutogenic setting. *Critical Public Health*, **9**, 211.

Frick, M.H., Elo, M.O., Haapa, K., *et al*. (1987). Helsinki Heart Study: primary-prevention trial with gemfibrozil in middle-aged men with dyslipidemia. Safety of treatment, changes in risk factors, and incidence of coronary heart disease. *New England Journal of Medicine*, **317**, 1237–45.

Goeppinger, J. and Baglioni, A.J., Jr (1985). Community competence: a positive approach to needs assessment. *American Journal of Community Psychology*, **13**, 507.

Gottlieb, N.H. and Green, L.W. (1987). Ethnicity and lifestyle health risk: some possible mechanisms. *American Journal of Health Promotion*, **2**, 37.

Green, L.W. (1970*a*). Manual for scoring socioeconomic status for research on health behavior. *Public Health Reports* **85**, 815.

Green, L.W. (1970*b*). *Status identity and preventive health behaviour*. Pacific Health Education Reports, No. 1. University of California School of Public Health, Berkeley, CA.

Green, L.W. (1986). The theory of participation: a qualitative analysis of its expression in national and international policies. In *Advances in health education and promotion* (ed. W.B. Ward, Z.T. Salisbury, S.B. Kar, and J.G. Zapka), Vol. 1, Part A, p. 211. JAI Press, Greenwich, CT.

Green, L.W. and Kreuter, M. (1999). *Health promotion planning: an educational and ecological approach* (3rd edn). Mayfield, Palo Alto, CA.

Green, L.W. and McAlister, A.L. (1984). Macro-intervention to support health behavior: Some theoretical perspectives and practical reflections. *Health Education Quarterly*, **11**, 322.

Green, L.W., Wilson, A., and Lovato, C.Y. (1986). What changes can health promotion produce and how long will they last? Trade-offs between expediency and durability. *Preventive Medicine*, **15**, 508.

Green, L.W., Richard, L., and Potvin, L. (1996). Ecological foundations of health promotion. *American Journal of Health Promotion*, **10**, 270.

Haan, I., Kaplan, G.A., and Camacho, T. (1987). Poverty and health. Prospective evidence from the Alameda County Study. *American Journal of Epidemiology*, **125**, 989–98.

Hancock, T. (1986). Lalonde and beyond: looking back at 'A new perspective on the health of Canadians'. *Health Promotion: An International Journal*, **1**, 93.

Harrison, J.A., Mullen, P.D., and Green, L.W. (1992). A meta-analysis of studies of the Health Belief Model. *Health Education Research*, **7**, 107.

Haskell, W.L. (1986). The influence of exercise training on plasma lipids and lipoproteins in health and disease. *Acta Medica Scandinavica Supplementum*, **711**, 25–37.

Health and Welfare Canada, Stephens, T., and Fowler Graham, D. (ed.) (1993). *Canada's health promotion survey 1990: technical report*. Minister of Supply and Services, Ottawa.

Heath, G.W., Wilson, R.H., Smith, J., and Leonard, B.E. (1991). Community-based exercise and weight control: diabetes risk reduction and glycemic control in Zuni Indians. *American Journal of Clinical Nutrition*, **53**, 1642S.

Helmrich, S.P., Ragland, D.R., Leung, R.W., and Paffenbarger, R.S. (1991). Physical activity and reduced occurrence of non-insulin-dependent diabetes mellitus. *New England Journal of Medicine*, **325**, 147.

Hertz, E., Hebert, J.R., and Landon, J. (1994). Social and environmental factors and life expectancy, infant mortality, and maternal mortality rates: results of a cross-national comparison. *Social Science and Medicine*, **39**, 105.

Higgins, D.L., Galavoiti, C., O'Reilly, K.R., *et al*. (1991). Evidence of the effect of HIV antibody counselling and testing on risk behaviors. *Journal of the American Medical Association*, **266**, 2419.

Higgins, M. (1991). Risk factors associated with chronic obstructive lung disease. *Annals of the New York Academy of Sciences*, **624**, 7.

House, J.S., Kessler, R.C., and Herzog, A.R. (1990). Age, socioeconomic status, and health. *Milbank Quarterly*, **68**, 383–411.

Hoyert, D.L., Kachanek, K.D., Murphy, S.L. (1999). Deaths: final data for 1997. In *National vital statistics report*; Vol. 47, No. 19. National Center for Health Statistics, Hyattsville, MD.

Hunninghake, D.B., Stein, E.A., Dujovne, C.A., *et al*. (1993). The efficacy of intensive therapy alone or combined with lovastatin in outpatients with hypercholesterolemia. *New England Journal of Medicine*, **328**, 1213.

Hunt, K. and Annandale, E. (1999). Relocating gender and morbidity: Examining men's and women's health in contemporary Western societies. Introduction to special issue on gender and health. *Social Science and Medicine*, **48**, 1.

Kaplan, R.M., Atkins, C.J., and Reinsch, S. (1984). Specific efficacy expectations mediate compliance in patients with COPD. *Health Psychology*, **3**, 223.

Kato, H., Tillotson, J., Nichaman, M.Z., *et al*. (1973). Epidemiological studies of coronary heart disease and stroke in Japanese men living in Japan, Hawaii, and California. Serum lipids and diet. *American Journal of Epidemiology*, **97**, 372.

Kawachi, I., Kennedy, B. P., Gupta, V., and Prothrow-Stith, D. (1999). Women's status and the health of women and men: A view from the States. *Social Science and Medicine*, **48**, 21.

Kawachi, I., Kennedy, B.P., Lochner, K., *et al*. (1997). Social capital, income inequality, and mortality. *American Journal of Public Health*, **87**, 1491.

Keil, J.E., Sutherland, S.E., Mapp, R.G., and Tyroler, H.A. (1992). Does equal socio-economic status in black and white men mean equal risk of mortality. *American Journal of Public Health*, **82**, 1133–6.

Keys, A. (1970). Coronary heart disease in seven countries. *Circulation*, **41** (Supplement 1), 1.

Keys, A., Kimura, N., Kusukawa, A., *et al*. (1958). Lessons from serum cholesterol studies in Japan, Hawaii, and Los Angeles. *Annals of Internal Medicine*, **48**, 83.

Kitagawa, E.M. and Hauser, P.M. (1973). *Differential mortality in the United States: a study in socioeconomic epidemiology*. Harvard University Press, Cambridge, MA.

Kuller, L.H., Ockene, J.K., Meilahn, E., *et al*. (1991). Cigarette smoking and mortality, MRFIT Research Group. *Preventive Medicine*, **29**, 638.

Koskinen, S. and Martelin, T. (1994). Why are socio-economic mortality differences smaller among women than among men? *Social Science and Medicine*, **38**, 1385.

Kuh, D., Power, C., Blane D., *et al*. (1997). Social pathways between childhood and adult health. In *A lifecourse approach to chronic disease* *epidemiology* (ed. D. Kuh and Y. Ben-Shlomo), p. 169. Oxford University Press.

Kunst, A.E. and Mackenbach, J.P. (1994). The size of mortality differences associated with educational level in nine industrialized countries. *American Journal of Public Health*, **84**, 932.

Krieger, N. (1994). Epidemilogy and the web of causation. Has anyone seen the spider? *Social Science and Medicine*, **39**, 887.

Krieger, N. (1996). Inequality, diversity, and health: thoughts on 'race/ ethnicity' and 'gender'. *Journal of American Medical Women's Association*, **51**, 133.

Krieger, N., Rowley, D.L., Herman, A.A., Avery, B., and Phillips, M.T. (1993). Racism, sexism, and social class: implications for study of health, disease, and well being. *American Journal of Preventive Medicine*, **9** (Supplement), 82.

Lahelma, E., Manderbacka, K., Rahkonen, O., and Karisto, A. (1994). Comparison of inequalities in health: evidence from national surveys in Finland, Norway, Sweden. *Social Science and Medicine*, **38**, 517.

Lahelma E., Martikainen, P., Rahkonen, O., and Silventoinen, K. (1999). Gender differences in health in Finland: patterns, magnitude and change. *Social Science and Medicine*, **48**, 7.

Lasker, J.N., Egolf, B.P., and Wolf, S. (1994). Community social change and mortality. *Social Science and Medicine*, **39**, 53.

Lee, C. (1991). Women and aerobic exercise: directions for research development. *Annals of Behavioral Medicine*, **13**, 125.

Leon, D.A., Vagero, D., and Otterblad, O.P. (1992). Social class differences in infant mortality in Sweden: comparisons with England and Wales. *British Medical Journal*, **305**, 687.

Lokey, E.A. and Tran, Z.V. (1989). Effects of exercise training on serum lipid and lipoprotein concentrations in women: a meta-analysis. *International Journal of Sports Medicine*, **10**, 424–9.

Lorig, K. and Laurin, J. (1985). Some notions about assumptions underlying health education. *Health Education Quarterly*, **12**, 231.

Link, B.G. and Phelan, J. (1995). Social conditions as fundamental causes of disease. *Journal of Health and Social Behavior*, (special issue) 80–94.

Luepker, R.V., Rosamond, W.D., Murphy, R., *et al.* (1993). Socioeconomic status and coronary heart disease risk factor trends: The Minnesota Heart Health Survey. *Circulation*, **88**, 2172.

Lynch, J.W., Kaplan, G.A., Pamuk, E.R., *et al.* (1998). Income inequality and mortality in metropolitan areas of the United States. *American Journal of Public Health*, **88**, 1074.

Lynn, T., Duncan, R., Naughton, J., *et al.* (1967). Prevalence of evidence of prior myocardial infarction, hypertension, diabetes, and obesity in three neighboring communities in Pennsylvania. *American Journal of Medical Services*, **254**, 385.

McArdle, W.D., Katch, F.L., and Katch, V.L. (1986). *Exercise physiology: energy, nutrition, and human performance* (2nd edn). Lea and Febiger, Philadelphia, PA.

McGill, H.C. (1979). The relationship of dietary cholesterol to serum cholesterol concentration and to atherosclerosis in man. *American Journal of Clinical Nutrition*, **32**, 2664.

McGinnis, J.M. and Foege, W.H. (1993). Actual causes of death in the United States. *Journal of the American Medical Association*, **270**, 2207.

Macintyre, S. (1993). Gender differences in longevity and health in Eastern and Western Europe. In *Locating health: sociological and historical explanations* (ed. S. Platt, T.H. Scott, and G. Williams), p. 57. Avebury UK, Aldershot.

Macintyre, S. (1997). The Black Report and beyond: What are the issues. *Social Science and Medicine*, **44**, 723.

Macintyre, S. and Hunt, K. (1997). Socio-economic position, gender and health. *Journal of Health Psychology*, **2**, 315.

Macintyre, S., Hunt, K., and Sweeting, H. (1996). Gender differences in health: are things really as simple as they seem? *Social Science and Medicine*, **42**, 617.

Manson, J.E., Tosteson, H., Ridker, P.M., *et al.* (1992). The primary prevention of myocardial infarction. *New England Journal of Medicine*, **326**, 1406.

Marmot, M.G. and McDowall, M.E. (1986). Mortality decline and widening social inequalities. *Lancet*, **ii**, 274.

Marmot, M.G., and Wilkinson, R.G. (ed.) (1999). *The social determinants of health*. Oxford University Press.

Marmot, M.G., Rose, G., Shipley, M.J., *et al.* (1978). Employment grade and coronary heart disease in British civil servants. *Journal of Epidemiology and Community Health*, **32**, 244.

Marmot, M.G., Shipley, M.J., and Rose, G.A. (1984). Inequalities in death. Specific explanations of a general pattern? *Lancet*, **i**, 1003.

Marmot, M.G., Smith, G.D., Stansfeld, S., *et al.* (1991). Health inequalities among British civil servants: the Whitehall II study. *Lancet*, **337**, 1387.

Matthews, S., Manor, O., and Power, C. (1999). Social inequalities in health: are there gender differences? *Social Science and Medicine*, **48**, 49.

Mechanic, D. (1979). The stability of health and illness behavior: results from a 16-year follow-up. *American Journal of Public Health*, **69**, 1142.

Mensink, R.P. and Katan, M.G. (1992). Effect of dietary fatty acids on serum lipids and lipoproteins: a meta-analysis of 27 trials. *Arteriosclerosis and Thrombosis*, **12**, 911–19.

McKinley, J.B. and Marceau, L.D. (2000). To boldly go... *American Journal of Public Health*, **90**, 25.

Millar, W.T. and Stephens, T. (1993). Social status and health risk in Canadian adults: 1985–1991. *Health Reports*, **5**, 143.

Mittendorf, R., Herschel, M., Williams, M.A., *et al.* (1994). Reducing the frequency of low birth weight in the United States. *Obstetrics and Gynecology*, **83**, 1056.

Morris, J.N. (1979). Social inequalities undiminished. *Lancet*, **i**, 87.

Mullen, P.D., Green, L.W., and Persinger, G.S. (1985). Clinical trials of patient education for chronic conditions: a comparative meta-analysis of intervention types. *Preventive Medicine*, **14**, 753.

Muntaner, C. and Lynch, J. (1999). Income inequality, social cohesion, and class relations: a critique of Wilkinson's neo-Durkheimian research program. *International Journal of Health Services*, **29**, 59.

National Center for Health Statistics (1993). Advance report of final mortality statistics, 1991. *Monthly Vital Statistics Report*, **42** (Supplement).

NHLBI (National Heart, Lung and Blood Institute) (1990). *Population strategies reduction*, NIH Publication 90, p. 3047. National Institutes of Health, Bethesda, MD.

NHLBI (National Heart, Lung, and Blood Institute) (1993). *Detection, evaluation and treatment of high blood cholesterol in adults*, NIH Publication 93, p. 3095. National Institutes of Health, Bethesda, MD.

North, F, Syme, S.L., Feeney, A., Head, J., Shipley M.A., and Marmot, M.G. (1993). Explaining socioeconomic differences in sickness absence: the Whitehall II Study. *British Medical Journal*, **306**, 361–6.

Nuckolls, K.B., Cassels, J., and Kaplan, B.H. (1972). Psychosocial assets, life crisis and the prognosis of pregnancy. *American Journal of Epidemiology*, **95**, 431.

Ockene, J.K., Kuller, L.H., Svendsen, K.H., and Meilahn, E. (1990). The relationship of smoking cessation to coronary heart disease and lung cancer in the Multiple Risk Factor Intervention Trial (MRFIT). *American Journal of Public Health*, **80**, 954.

Office of Environmental Health Hazard Assessment (OEHHA), California Environmental Protection Agency (1997). *Health effects of exposure to environmental tobacco smoke*. Final report. Sacramento, CA.

Office of Health and Environmental Assessment (1992). *Respiratory, health effects of passive smoking: lung cancer and other disorders*. EPA/600/(6–90/0006F), US Environmental Protection Agency, Cincinnati, OH.

Ogston, S.A. and Parry, G.J. (1992). EUROMAC. A European concerted action: maternal alcohol consumption and its relation to the outcome of pregnancy and child development at 18 months. Results-strategy of analysis and analysis of pregnancy outcome. *International Journal of Epidemiology*, **21** (Supplement 1), S45.

Pappas, G., Queen, S., Hadden, W., and Fisher, G. (1993). The increasing disparity in mortality between socioeconomic groups in the United States, 1960 and 1986. *New England Journal of Medicine*, **329**, 103.

Peck, M.N. (1994). The importance of childhood socio-economic group for adult health. *Social Science and Medicine*, **39**, 553–62.

Pederson, L. (1993). *Tobacco use. Canada's health promotion survey 1990: technical report.* (ed. Health and Welfare Canada, T. Stephens and D. Fowler Graham), pp. 97–108. Minister of Supply and Services Canada, Ottawa.

Petrow, S. (1990). *Ending the HIV epidemic.* Network Publications, Santa Cruz, CA.

Petrakis, P.L. (ed.) (1987). *Sixth Special Report to the US Congress on Alcohol and Health from the Secretary of Health and Human Services, January 1987*, DHHS Publication No. (ADM) 87–1519. NIAA, Rockville, MD.

Pincus, T, Callahan, L.F, and Burkhauser, R.V. (1987). Most chronic diseases are reported more frequently by individuals with fewer than 12 years of formal education in the age 18–64 United States population. *Journal of Chronic Disease*, **40**, 865.

Pocock, S.J., Shaper, A.G., Cook, D.G., *et al.* (1987). Social class differences in ischaemic heart disease in British men. *Lancet*, **ii**, 197.

Poland, B., Green, L.W., and Rootman, I.R. (2000). *Settings for health promotion: linking theory and practice.* Sage, Thousand Oaks, CA.

Pooling Project Research Group (1978). Relationship of blood pressure, serum cholesterol, smoking habit, relative weight and ECG abnormalities to incidence of major coronary events: final report of the Pooling Project. *Journal of Chronic Disease*, **31**, 201.

Potvin, L. and Frohlich, K.L. (1998). L'utilité de la notion de genre pour comprendre les inégalités de santé entre les hommes et les femmes. *Ruptures, Revue Transdisciplinaire en Santé*, **5**, 142.

Powell, K.E., Thompson, P.D., Caspersen, C.J., and Kendrick, T.S. (1987). Physical activity and the incidence of coronary heart disease. *Annual Review of Public Health*, **8**, 253.

Prattala, R., Kaaristo, A., and Berg, M.A. (1994). Consistency and variation in unhealthy behaviour among Finnish men 1982–1990. *Social Science and Medicine*, **39**, 115.

Richard, L., Potvin, L., Kishuck, N., Prlic, H., and Green, L.W. (1996). Assessment of the integration of the ecological approach in health promotion programs. *American Journal of Health Promotion*, **10**, 318.

Rimm, E.B., Manson, J.E., Stampfer, M.J., *et al.* (1993). Cigarette smoking and the risk of diabetes in women. *American Journal of Public Health*, **83**, 211.

Robbins, A.S., Manson, J.E., Lee, I.M., *et al.* (1994). Cigarette smoking and stroke in a cohort of US male physicians. *Annals of Internal Medicine*, **120**, 458.

Robinson, D. and Pinch, S. (1987). A geographical analysis of the relationship between early childhood and socio-economic environment in an English city. *Social Science and Medicine*, **25**, 9.

Rose, G. and Colwell, L. (1992). Randomized controlled trial of anti-smoking advice: final (20-year) results. *Journal of Epidemiology and Community Health*, **46**, 75.

Ross, C.E. and Bird, C.E. (1994). Sex stratification and health lifestyle: Consequences for men's and women's perceived health. *Journal of Health and Social Behavior*, **35**, 161.

Rozin, P. (1984). The acquisition of food habits and preferences. In *Behavioral health: a handbook of health enhancement and disease prevention* (ed. J.D. Matarazzo, S.M. Weiss, J.A. Herd, *et al.*), p. 590. Wiley, New York.

Rutten, A. (1995). The implementation of health promotion: a new structural perspective. *Social Science and Medicine*, **41**, 1627.

Samuels, S.E. (1990). Project LEAN: a national campaign to reduce dietary fat consumption. *American Journal of Health Promotion*, **4**, 435.

Shai, D. (1986). Cancer mortality, ethnicity and socioeconomic status: two New York City groups. *Public Health Reports*, **101**, 547.

Shea, S., Stein, A.D., Basch, C.E., *et al.* (1991). Independent associations of educational attainment and ethnicity with behavioral risk factors for cardiovascular disease. *American Journal of Epidemiology*, **134**, 567–82.

Silagy, C. and Ketteridge, S. (1998). *Physician advice for smoking cessation* (Cochrane Review). The Cochrane Library, issue 2. Update Software, Oxford.

Simons-Morton, B.G., O'Hara, N.M., and Simons-Morton, D.G. (1986). Promoting healthful diet and exercise behaviors in communities, schools, and families. *Family and Community Health*, **9**, 1.

Simons-Morton, B.G., Brink, S.G., Parcel, G.S., *et al.* (1990). *Preventing acute alcohol-related health problems in adolescents and young adults.* Centers for Disease Control, Atlanta, GA.

Simons-Morton, B.G., Greene, W.H. and Gottlieb, N.H. (1995). Social change. *In Introduction to health education and health promotion* (2nd edn), p. 193. Waveland Press, Prospect Heights, IL.

Simons-Morton, D.G., Simons-Morton, B.G., Parcel, G.S., and Bunker, J.E. (1988*a*). Influencing personal and environmental conditions for community health: a multilevel intervention model. *Family and Community Health*, **11**, 25.

Simons-Morton, D.G., Brink, S.G., Parcel, G.S., *et al.* (1988*b*). *Promoting physical activity amoing adults: a CDC community intervention handbook.* Centers for Disease Control, Atlanta, GA.

Simons-Morton, D.G., Brink, S.G., Parcel, G.S., *et al.* (1991). Smoking control among women: needs assessment and intervention strategies. In *Advances in health education and promotion*, pp. 199–240. Jessica Kingsley, London.

Simons-Morton, D.G., Mullen, P.D., Mains, D.A., *et al.* (1992). Characteristics of controlled studies of patient education and counseling for preventive behaviors. *Patient Education and Counselling*, **19**, 175.

Simpson, D. and Ball, K. (1992). From observation to policy: smoking. In *Coronary heart disease epidemiology: from aetiology to public health* (ed. M. Marmot and P. Elliot). Oxford University Press.

Spurlock, C.W., Hinds, M.W., Skaggs, J.W., and Hernandez, C.E. (1987). Infant death rates among the poor and non poor in Kentucky, 1982 to 1983. *Pediatrics*, **80**, 262.

Stamler, J. (1992). Established major coronary risk factors. In *Coronary heart disease epidemiology: from aetiology to public health* (ed. M. Marmot and P. Elliott), p. 35–66. Oxford University Press.

Stamler, J., Wentworth, D., and Neaton, J.D., for the MRFIT Research Group (1986). Is the relationship between serum cholesterol and risk of premature death from coronary heart disease continuous and graded. Findings in 356,222 primary screenees of the Multiple Risk Factor Intervention Trial (MRFIT). *Journal of the American Medical Association*, **256**, 2823–8.

Steele, J. and McBroom, W. (1972). Conceptual and empirical dimensions of health behavior. *Journal of Health and Social Behavior*, **13**, 382.

Stern, M.P. (1991). Primary prevention of type II diabetes mellitus. *Diabetes Care*, **14**, 399.

Steuart, G.W. (1965). Health, behavior, and planned change. *Health Education Monographs*, **20**, 3.

Stout, C., Morrow, J., Brandt, E.N., and Wolf. S. (1964). Unusually low incidence of death from myocardial infarction in an Italian-American community in Pennsylvania. *Journal of the American Medical Association*, **188**, 845.

Stronks, K., Van de Mheen, H., Van den Bos, J., and Mackenbach, J.P. (1995). Smaller socio-economic inequalities in health among women: The role of employment status. *International Journal of Epidemiology*, **24**, 559.

Stronks, K., Van de Mheen, D., Loomanm C.W.N., *et al.* (1996). Behavioural and structural factors in the explanation of socio-economic inequalities in health: an empirical analysis. *Sociology of Health and Illness*, **18**, 653.

Townsend, P., Davison, N., and Whitehead, M. (1988). *Inequalities in health*. Penguin, Harmondsworth.

Verbrugge, L.M. (1985). Gender and health: an update on hypotheses and evidence. *Journal of Health and Social Behavior*, **26**, 156.

Verbrugge, L.M. (1989). The twain meet: empirical explanations of sex differences in health and mortality. *Journal of Health and Social Behavior*, **30**, 282.

UNICEF (1993). *The state of the world's children 1993*. Oxford University Press.

US CDC (US Centers for Disease Control) (1993). Cigarette smoking attributable mortality and years of potential life lost United States, 1990. *Morbidity and Mortality Weekly Reports*, **42**, 645.

US Department of Health and Human Services (1991). *Healthy people 2000: national health promotion and disease prevention objectives*. US Government Printing Office, Washington, DC.

Villas, P., Cardenas, M., and Jameson, C. (1993). Instrument development using the PRECEDE model to distinguish users/triers from non-users of alcoholic beverages. *Wellness Perspectives: Research, Theory and Practice*, **10**, 46.

Wadsworth, M. (1999). Early life. In *Social determinants of health* (ed. M. Marmot and R.G. Wilkinson), p. 44. Oxford University Press.

Warner, K.E. (1986*a*). *Selling smoke: cigarette advertising and public health*. American Public Health Association, Washington, DC.

Warner, K.E. (1986*b*). Smoking and health implications of a change in federal cigarette excise tax. *Journal of the American Medical Association*, **255**, 1028.

WHO (World Health Organization) Executive Board (1979). *Formulating strategies for Health for All by the Year 2000*. WHO, Geneva.

WHO (World Health Organization) (1981). *Global strategy for Health for All by the Year 2000*. WHO, Geneva.

WHO (World Health Organization) European Regional Office (1986). *Health promotion concepts and principles in action. A policy framework*. WHO, Copenhagen.

WHO (World Health Organization) (1990). *Prevention in childhood and youth adult cardiovascular diseases: time for action. WHO Technical Report 792*. WHO, Geneva.

WHO (World Health Organization) (1994). *World health statistics annual 1993*. WHO, Geneva.

WHO (World Health Organization) (1998). *Tobacco epidemic: health dimensions*. Fact Sheet No. 154, revised. WHO, Geneva.

Wilkins, R., Adams, O., and Brancker, A. (1989). Changes in mortality by income in urban Canada from 1971 to 1986. *Health Reports*, **1**(2), 137.

Wilkinson, R.G. (1992*a*). Income distribution and life expectancy. *British Medical Journal*, **304**, 165–8.

Wilkinson, R.G. (1992*b*). National mortality rates: the impact of inequality. *American Journal of Public Health*, **82**, 1082–4.

Wilkinson, R.G. (1996). *Unhealthy society. The afflictions of inequality*. Routledge, London.

Wilkinson, R.G. (1999). Income inequality, social cohesion, and health: clarifying the theory—A reply to Muntaner and Lynch. *International Journal of Health Services*, **29**, 525.

Wilkinson, R.G. and Marmot, M. (1998). *The solid facts*. World Health Organization, Geneva.

Winkleby, M.A., Fortman, S.P., and Barrett, D.C. (1990). Social class disparities in risk factors for disease: eight years prevalence patterns by level of education. *Preventive Medicine*, **19**, 1–12.

Winkleby, M.A., Jatulis, D.E., Franck, E., and Fortman, S.P. (1992*a*). Socio-economic status and health: how education, income, and occupation contribute to risk factors for cardiovascular disease. *American Journal of Public Health*, **82**, 816–20.

Winkleby, M.A., Fortman, S.P., and Rockhill, B. (1992*b*). Trends in cardiovascular risk factors by educational level: the Stanford Five City Project. *Preventive Medicine*, **21**, 592–601.

World Bank (1991). *World development report. Special population issues*. World Bank, Washington, DC.

World Bank (1993). *World development report 1993. Investing in health*. Oxford University Press, New York.

Zarek, D., Hawkins, J.D., and Rogers, P.D. (1987). Risk factors for adolescent substance abuse. *Pediatric Clinics of North America*, **34**, 481.

2.4 Human and medical genetics

Friedrich Vogel and Arno G. Motulsky

Recent developments in human and medical genetics

During recent decades, human genetics has seen enormous progress. Up to the late 1950s, many traits with simple monogenic modes of inheritance were already known. Most of them were hereditary diseases, usually rare. However, twin and family studies indicated a genetic component for more common complex diseases. So-called 'empiric risk' figures to predict recurrence risks were useful for genetic counselling in such instances, but the nature of the underlying genetic variability was largely unknown. In the 1950s, methods for microscopic study of human chromosomes were developed, and the normal chromosome number was established to be 46 (Tijo and Levan 1956). Soon afterwards, some previously unexplained birth defects were found to be due to numerical or structural chromosomal aberrations; for example, Down syndrome as trisomy 21, the Klinefelter syndrome as 47,XXY, and the Turner syndrome as 45,X. Many different structural defects of chromosomes were discovered as deletions, or translocations (Vogel and Motulsky 1996). In the late 1960s, amniocentesis followed by analysis of fetal cells suspended in the amniotic fluid was shown to be useful for genetic, in most instances cytogenetic, diagnosis of various fetal anomalies. Together with improvements in the biochemical and molecular characterization of monogenic diseases, this development led to an increased demand for genetic diagnosis and counselling, mainly in industrialized countries such as North American and western Europe, but later in other parts of the world as well. To meet this demand, many genetic counselling centres were established.

In the early 1970s, a scientific revolution began. The concept of 'molecular disease' had been proposed in 1949 by Pauling and his coworkers when they discovered that sickle cell anaemia was caused by a genetically determined, electrophoretically detectable defect of the haemoglobin molecule (Pauling *et al.* 1949). In the 1970s, methods were developed for studying the genetic material (DNA) directly (Watson *et al.* 1987, 1992; Gelehrter and Collins 1990; Vogel and Motulsky 1996). This led to the discovery of many DNA genetic polymorphisms, that is, variants without phenotypic effects that were usually located outside coding DNA sequences. As such variants are inherited as Mendelian traits, they are useful markers for localizing genes by genetic linkage studies. The chromosomal localization or position of a disease-producing gene can often be demonstrated by showing linkage with such a DNA marker. A new methodology of defining genetic disease—positional cloning—now became possible. This approach allowed isolation of the gene followed by determination of the nature of the various mutations that interfered with gene function. This approach has become a highly successful strategy for identifying genes and for elucidating their mechanism of action. A total of about 7000 genes had been mapped by March 2001 as compared with fewer than 3000 in 1994 (World Wide Web URL http://www.ncbi.nlm.nih.gov/omim; see also McKusick (1986, 1987, 1988, 1994)). This success with localization of single genes has raised hopes that similar approaches could identify genes involved in complex diseases of multifactorial origin. In principle, linkage studies should permit identification of the major genes involved in the causation of such diseases, especially when combined with modern methods of genetic epidemiology such as segregation analysis (for a review of computerized analytical systems, see Fischer *et al.* (1996)). So far, the results of such studies in complex diseases (except for certain monogenic subtypes) have been disappointing. However, the approach remains sound and has been applied successfully to genetic counselling and prenatal diagnosis for monogenic diseases.

Human genetics and disease

Chromosomal diseases

Chromosomes consist of a continuous DNA structure and of certain histone and non-histone proteins. The microscopically visible chromosomes transport the genetic material and normally guarantee a regular distribution of DNA to daughter cells in cell division. As a rule, human chromosomes are studied in metaphase (that is, after replication of the DNA double helix), but immediately before the replicated chromosomes are distributed to the two daughter nuclei. Recently developed methods of 'chromosome painting' permit the study of chromosomes in interphase, that is, when the nucleus does not divide (Vogel and Motulsky 1996). However, most diagnostic chromosome studies are being performed on metaphase chromosomes of readily available blood lymphocytes. In short-term cultures, lymphocytes are first induced to divide and are then stained and photographed. Individual chromosomes can be identified by their length, shape, and banding pattern. The respective chromosomes of all nucleated cells in an individual (such as fibroblasts) are identical and can be studied in a similar manner to lymphocytes.

Trisomies

The most common numerical anomalies are the trisomies—a chromosomal complement is present in triplicate rather than in duplicate. In most instances, such trisomies are caused by an error during reduction division (meiosis). Normally, the number of chromosomes is reduced by half (in humans, from 46 to 23) to form germ cells; two chromosomes that should be distributed to daughter cells may stick together ('non-disjunction') and remain in one cell, making that egg (or sperm) became a trisomic fertilized egg. Most trisomies lead to a severely malformed embryo; as a rule, such an embryo is spontaneously miscarried during the first trimester of pregnancy. According to international statistics, about 15 per cent of recognized pregnancies end in spontaneous abortion and about 50 per cent of these are caused by various chromosomal aberrations. Many of them are trisomies. The high proportion of postnatal survival in trisomy 21 (Down syndrome) is an exception (about 25 per cent of affected fetuses), reflecting the small size of this chromosome, carrying relatively few genes.

The incidence of Down syndrome (trisomy 21) is about 1 in 700 live births; trisomy 21 is caused by non-disjunction of chromosomes within maternal germ cells in about 80 per cent of cases. Other autosomal trisomies include trisomy 13 and trisomy 18, which are much rarer and lead to much more severe malformations causing spontaneous abortions or early death postnatally. X-chromosomal trisomies include the XXY (Klinefelter syndrome) and XXX conditions and are often associated with mild mental retardation.

The risk of having a child with trisomy due to maternal non-disjunction increases with advancing age of the mother; a 45-year-old mother has a 10-to 20-fold risk of giving birth to a trisomic child as compared with a woman of 20. Therefore, the incidence of trisomies in various populations depends critically on the age distribution of the reproducing female population.

Public health policy considerations regarding amniocentesis

In most developed countries, prenatal diagnosis (amniocentesis or chorionic villus biopsy) is offered to pregnant women of 'advanced' maternal age to detect Down syndrome, thereby allowing the option of pregnancy termination. The selected 'cut-off' age for performing prenatal diagnosis varies in different countries. In the United States, an age of 35 years is generally chosen. In some European countries, a somewhat older age is selected, for example 36, 37, or 38 years. Since fewer women initiate pregnancies as they become older, the total number of antenatal procedures becomes smaller as the 'cut-off' age becomes higher. However, as older women have more affected fetuses, the proportion of detected cases rises. For instance, the incidence of trisomy 21 at amniocentesis is about 1 in 250 at 35 years, 1 in 150 at age 37 years, 1 in 100 at age 39 years, and 1 in 60 at 41 years. The selection of the cut-off age becomes a difficult issue of public health policy. Delaying the age for antenatal diagnosis becomes less expensive for publicly supported health services by reducing the number of antenatal procedures. However, as most cases of Down syndrome in a population are born to mothers younger than 35 years of age, fewer affected fetuses among the entire population of all pregnant women will be detected. In a pluralistic health service scheme such as that in the United States, many younger women select amniocentesis at an age younger than 35 years in order to reduce their chances of having a child with Down syndrome. In the European health system that has grown out of the belief that the state has some responsibility for the health of its citizens (Häfner 1999), stricter regulations exist—especially regarding payment for diagnostic efforts. The rate of uptake for amniocentesis usually does not reach 50 per cent of women above the recommended cut-off age. The highest rates have been observed in Denmark where about two-thirds of women above the age of 35 undergo the procedure (Galjaard 1994). These considerations point to the desirability of simple screening tests (such as low levels of α-fetoprotein and detection and (hopefully) analysis of embryonic cells in the maternal blood) to detect trisomies in women of all maternal ages (see below).

Other chromosomal anomalies

Structural chromosomal aberrations are much rarer than trisomies. In deletions, part of a chromosome is lacking. In reciprocal translocations, chromosome parts are exchanged between chromosomes. The resulting phenotypes depend on whether chromosomal material is lacking or is increased, and differ with the chromosomes involved. Different chromosome anomalies have some features in common (Table 1). A detailed description of such chromosomal syndromes has been given by Schinzel (1984).

A group of chromosomal anomalies known as contiguous gene syndromes were discovered when some unusual phenotypes suggesting simultaneous transmission of two or more genetic diseases were analysed at the DNA level. In these instances, no chromosomal defect could be seen by conventional techniques. However, the method of fluorescence *in situ* hybridization may permit a diagnosis. Such patients often suffer from signs of more than one hereditary disease (for example, X-linked Duchenne muscular dystrophy and chronic granulomatous disease). Molecular studies in such cases reveal a deletion spanning more than one gene but not extensive enough to be discovered by conventional microscopic studies.

Monogenic diseases

This category comprises conditions that are conventionally called 'hereditary diseases'. They follow Mendel's laws and are sometimes referred to as Mendelian diseases. If a heterozygote (that is, a person carrying one mutant gene) shows the anomalous phenotype, the mode of inheritance is dominant. Such a disease will be transmitted from one parent to 50 per cent of the offspring on average. This transmission occurs irrespective of gender. In autosomal recessive inheritance, the abnormal phenotype occurs in homozygotes only, that is, when both homologous chromosomes carry a mutation in the same gene. Hence both parents must be (at least) heterozygous for this gene. Within such families, both parents are unaffected; among their

Table 1 Common findings in autosomal chromosome abnormalities

Low birth weight (small for date)
Mental and physical retardation
Multiple malformations
Dysplasia of ears, hands
Facial dysmorphology
Dermatoglyphic anomalies

Adapted from Fuhrmann and Vogel (1983).

children, there is a ratio of one affected homozygote to three unaffected children (two of which will be heterozygous). As both parents have to carry a mutation in the same gene, it is not surprising that children from matings between relatives (such as first cousins who have inherited the abnormal gene from a common ancestor) run an increased risk of being affected, particularly if the gene is very rare.

These modes of inheritance are observed if the mutant gene is located on one of the 22 pairs of autosomes. If the mutant gene is located on the X chromosome, the mode of transmission is influenced by the mechanism of sex determination. Women have two X chromosomes, men carry only one X chromosome. Hence males carrying a single X-linked recessive gene will show the mutant phenotype; they are referred to as hemizygotes. In contrast, heterozygous females for recessive X-linked traits will usually be unaffected clinically but transmit the mutant gene to 50 per cent of their sons who will then be affected. Transmission from father to son cannot occur with X-linked inheritance.

The various Mendelian modes of inheritance suggest different biochemical mechanisms. Recessive diseases are often caused by enzyme defects. Heterozygotes produce about half the amount of enzyme protein compared with the normal homozygotes. In most instances, this reduced amount is sufficient for the maintenance of normal function (but see Vogel (1984)). Mendelian dominance (that is, manifestation of a clinical abnormality in heterozygotes) requires a more complex interaction between the gene products of the two alleles. Such interaction occurs, for example, if a protein is needed for building a structure. To give an example from daily experience, a wall that is built from 50 per cent normal and 50 per cent defective bricks will be defective. Examples are dominant diseases that are caused by the presence of an abnormal collagen, an important component of connective tissue. Patients with osteogenesis imperfecta suffer, among other clinical signs, from frequent bone fractures after trivial trauma. Other mechanisms of Mendelian dominance have been discussed elsewhere (Vogel and Motulsky 1996).

Non-Mendelian mechanisms

The phenomenon of anticipation has been observed by perceptive physicians for about a century. Certain diseases, such as myotonic dystrophy, tend to have an earlier onset and a more severe course in successive generations. For a long time human geneticists tried to explain this finding as reflecting bias, because it did not fit the theoretical model of Mendelian transmission. More recently, however, it has become possible to explain anticipation by a novel type of mutation. Certain genes contain sequences of many DNA base triplets. For unknown reasons, this system becomes unstable, and the number of triplets tends to increase from one generation to the next. This phenomenon leads to earlier onset and a more severe course of such diseases (Sutherland and Richards 1995). The number of diseases caused by such triplet amplifications is still increasing. In most of them, the function of the nervous and/or muscular system is impaired.

Another non-Mendelian phenomenon is genomic imprinting. The manifestations of certain mutations in offspring may vary with the sex of the parent who carries the mutant gene. In some instances, the mutant gene must be transmitted through the maternal germ line in order to lead to the mutant phenotype; in others, it has to pass the paternal line (Hall 1990; Sapienza and Hall 1995). Such observations show that the maternal and paternal genomes do not always contribute equally to the phenotype of the child. Further analysis of anticipation and genomic imprinting promises new insights into the genetic determination of embryonic development.

Mutations and hereditary diseases

About 1 per cent of all newborns suffer, or will suffer later in life, from an autosomal dominant or X-linked recessive disease (United Nations Scientific Committee on the Effects of Atomic Radiation (**UNSCEAR**) 1986, 1988, 1992). Within this group the dominantly inherited hypercholesterolaemias are among the most common; about 1 in 500 individuals carry a mutation for this condition, which strongly predisposes to an early onset of coronary heart disease. Matings between two such heterozygotes may occur, so that homozygous children are observed occasionally. They usually suffer from coronary heart disease in childhood or adolescence (Goldstein *et al.* 1995). Reproduction by heterozygotes for this type of hypercholesterolaemia is hardly impaired, as the first clinical signs among heterozygotes only occur at the age of about 40 or 50 years or even later. Thus most people have already had their children. For this reason, almost all persons carrying this gene have inherited it from one parent, and new mutations are extremely rare. This also holds true for Huntington disease for the same reason as the average age at onset is between about 40 and 50 years. However, many other dominant or X-linked diseases have severe clinical manifestations that prevent reproduction. Examples are acrocephalosyndactyly, a severe dominantly inherited malformation syndrome, and the X-linked recessive Duchenne type of muscular dystrophy, a progressive muscular disease with death at about age 20. If such a severe disease is dominantly inherited, the affected individuals are, as a rule, unable to transmit the mutant gene to the next generation. Thus the great majority of patients are 'sporadic' cases, and are the only affected persons in their families. The conclusion that a dominant mutation is responsible for the disease is based on three arguments.

1. Reproduction is observed occasionally, and in these rare instances a 1 : 1 ratio of affected and unaffected offspring is observed.
2. The probability of many (not all) dominant mutations increases with the age of the father. This increase is not as pronounced as that with the mother's age in trisomies, and its extent appears to differ somewhat between mutations. However, the risk for a man of 45 of fathering a child with such a mutant autosomal dominant phenotype may be four to five times as high as that for a man of 25. This paternal age effect has a strong influence on the population incidence of such diseases. If identical mutation rates are assumed, the risk of having a child with a disease caused by such a mutation in Pakistan has been estimated to be almost twice that in Bulgaria, simply because more men have children at a relatively advanced age in Pakistan (Modell and Kuliev 1990) (Table 2) (the United States is similar to Bulgaria).
3. The third and most direct argument is direct demonstration of a mutation in the responsible gene. Of course, this requires direct knowledge of this gene, but the evidence is now available for an increasing number of such genes (Vogel and Motulsky 1996). Many such mutations are point mutations in the strictest sense, that is, only one base pair of the approximately 6 to 7 × 10^9 base pairs in the diploid human genome (46 chromosomes) is mutated. Other mutations are deletions spanning a part of the

Table 2 Relative mutation rates in European countries in relation to father's age

Country and year	Fathers more than 35 years old (%)	Relative mutation rate*
Bulgaria 1980	7.3	1.22
GDR 1980	8.5	1.22
Czechoslovakia 1978	9.6	1.27
Hungary 1980	10.2	1.28
Belgium 1978	11.6	1.33
Scotland 1980	12.0	1.34
Poland 1980	12.1	1.35
Netherlands 1979	12.9	1.38
France 1980	14.9	1.43
England and Wales 1979	15.4	1.44
Finland 1980	16.0	1.45
Denmark 1980	17.6	1.47
Luxembourg 1980	17.8	1.47
Norway 1980	17.6	1.47
Iceland 1980	21.1	1.53
Northern Ireland 1978	19.0	1.53
Switzerland 1979	20.0	1.53
Sweden 1980	23.4	1.53
Malta 1980	19.8	1.54
FRG 1980	22.2	1.57
Spain 1980	23.6	1.64
Italy 1978	24.1	1.64
Greece 1979	24.3	1.69
Spain 1966	33.5	1.69
Pakistan 1968	46.1	2.67

*The rate is 1 when all fathers are less than 30 years old.

From Modell and Kuliev (1990).

affected gene (see Cooper and Krawczak (1993) for a detailed report on the molecular basis of human mutations). Newly discovered mutations are being documented in databases such as the Human Gene Mutation Database (Cardiff) (http://www.uwcm.ac.uk/uwcm/mg/hgdm0.html), which has links to many disease-specific registries.

In X-linked recessive diseases that prevent male patients from reproduction (such as Duchenne muscular dystrophy) only about a third of the affected patients are 'sporadic' cases; in the majority, the mutant gene is transmitted by the clinically unaffected heterozygous mothers. This is of practical importance because potential female carriers in such families often request genetic counselling and prenatal diagnosis. Here, risk determination must be supported by DNA studies regarding the presence or absence of the mutation or, if the mutation is unknown, by family studies using DNA markers that segregate together with the mutation.

The fraction of new mutants among patients having a disease that is caused by a dominant or X-linked recessive mutation is proportional to the degree to which this disease reduces reproduction of these patients, that is, to the severity of natural selection against this mutant. In diseases where early death prevents reproduction, most instances are cases who owe their disease to a fresh mutation (Table 3). When the mutation rates (that is, the probabilities of mutations in germ cells) can be estimated from epidemiological data in human populations, mutation rates per fertilizing germ cell and per generation have been estimated to range from somewhat less than 10^4 to about 10^6 (Vogel and Rathenberg 1975). However, there is good evidence that some mutations leading to hereditary diseases have a lower frequency (Stevenson and Kerr 1967).

The mutation rates for some dominant mutations are assumed to have decreased in recent generations, as fewer 'older' fathers, who produce more mutant sperm, have offspring in modern populations. However, a possible (small) increase may be anticipated because of more exposure to possibly mutagenic agents, such as ionizing radiation or mutagenic chemicals (see below). Selection is also changing for some diseases, mainly because of medical intervention. In the X-linked haemophilias, for example, patients are now being treated successfully with clotting factor preparations. This means higher reproduction rates and, with a constant mutation rate, a higher incidence. A counterbalancing factor could be genetic counselling and prenatal diagnosis followed by pregnancy termination, which could lead to fewer affected individuals in future generations.

Another example is retinoblastoma, the malignant eye cancer of children. About 40 per cent of sporadic cases are due to a new germ cell mutation transmitted to children. Until about 130 years ago, almost all affected children died. Today, however, at least 80 per cent survive due to surgical or radiation treatment and lead a normal life. If the mutation rate remains the same, successful therapy will lead to a substantial increase in the disease (Vogel 1979). Genetic counselling and prenatal diagnosis are likely to counteract this trend. In many dominant and X-linked conditions, a trend towards increase of a

Table 3 Approximate percentages of patients affected by new mutations in autosomal dominant disorders

Acrocephalosyndactyly	95
Achondroplasia	80
Tuberous sclerosis	80
Multiple endocrine neoplasia type 2B	50
Neurofibromatosis	40
Marfan syndrome	40
Myotonic dystrophy	25
Multiple endocrine neoplasia type 2A	6–9
Huntington disease	1
Adult polycystic kidneys	1
Familial hypercholesterolaemia	1

From Sankaranarayanan (1998).

disease is unlikely as no treatments are yet available. Examples are acrocephalosyndactyly, achondroplasia, and osteogenesis imperfecta.

Frequencies of hereditary diseases

Whereas autosomal dominant and X-linked diseases have similar rare frequencies in most populations, this is not the case in autosomal recessive conditions. These diseases only occur if the patient is homozygous for a mutant gene; the risk for homozygosity increases with increasing genetic similarity of his or her parents, and as a rule, with the degree of their biological relationship. The increased incidence of these diseases among children from matings between first cousins is the best-known example, but the principle also holds for more remote degrees of relationship. Therefore, frequencies for autosomal recessive diseases depend largely on the breeding structure of the population. In a relatively small (and, for a long time in the past, more or less isolated) population a mutant gene might become relatively common just by chance ('genetic drift'), but it might also have had a selective advantage at some time in the past. The more common a gene is among heterozygotes, the more the risk increases that two heterozygotes will mate and produce homozygous offspring. This risk is particularly high in populations originating from relatively small 'founder' groups that have lived in relative isolation for several generations. Examples from the North American continent are the French Canadians in Quebec (Scriver 1992) and the Amish of Pennsylvania. In such 'isolate' populations, a given mutation was introduced by a single founder and increased in frequency with subsequent expansion of the population.

In contrast, the high incidence of sickle cell anaemia among Africans and their descendants elsewhere in the world is an example of selection. Falciparum malaria was hyperendemic in Western and Central Africa, and heterozygotes for the sickle cell gene had a selective advantage by dying less frequently from the endemic infection. The high incidence of Tay–Sachs disease and several other recessive diseases among Ashkenazi Jews has not been explained conclusively. Recent evidence makes a founder effect most likely (Motulsky 1995). The proportion of consanguineous matings, particularly first-cousin matings, has decreased in the last 100 years from a few per cent to a few per thousand. This trend presumably has appreciably reduced the number of patients suffering from autosomal recessive diseases—even below the rate expected from genetic equilibrium between new mutations and selective disadvantage of affected homozygotes. Therefore, industrialized Western countries are currently enjoying a situation in which the incidence of autosomal recessive diseases is as low as it probably ever has been in human history. UNSCEAR has estimated this incidence at about 0.1 per cent of newborns. The actual frequency is likely to decrease further, as prenatal diagnosis with pregnancy termination has become possible in an increasing number of such diseases. However, consanguineous matings are still common in some populations of developing countries—especially in Arab countries and in parts of India. In such consanguineous matings, in addition to autosomal recessive diseases the rates of congenital malformations among children and, according to some reports, the rates of stillbirths, abortions, and neonatal deaths are increased due to homozygosity of mutant genes that are transmitted from common ancestors of the two mates (Vogel and Motulsky 1996). Considerations of public health alone would argue for discouraging consanguineous matings to prevent ill health. Yet, the custom of consanguineous marriages in societies where they are common is an important and integral part of their culture. The institution of public health policy to reduce such marriages, therefore, needs to be carefully considered.

Complex multifactorial anomalies and diseases

In many diseases, there are neither a microscopically visible chromosomal aberration nor a simple monogenic mode of inheritance. Familial aggregation and a higher concordance of monozygotic compared with dizygotic twins point to a contribution of genetic factors. Three broad disease groups can be distinguished: birth defects, common chronic diseases, and mental diseases.

Birth defects

Some malformation syndromes are caused by a numerical or structural chromosomal aberration (see above). In a few others, a monogenic mode of inheritance can be demonstrated. Most often, however, neither explanation holds true. Sometimes a slight familial aggregation is observed. The model of multifactorial inheritance in combination with a threshold effect is sometimes invoked. Exogenous agents such as exposure to a radiation, teratogenic drugs, or viral infections during early pregnancy can rarely be demonstrated. Sometimes a malformation could be the result of entirely random events without specific genetic or environmental causes. Statistics on the incidence of birth defects in various populations exist, but, owing to differences in definitions and ascertainment, the results are difficult to compare. More reliable data are available from Hungary, which has had a system of direct ascertainment, registration, and extensive study of birth defects since about 1970 (Czeizel and Sankaranarayanan 1984) (Table 4). Data from many other populations have been collected in the *World Atlas of Birth Defects*, the first edition of which was published in 1998 by the International Center for Birth Defects in co-operation with the European Registration of Congenital Anomalies and the World Health Organization. But for many countries, even some of the industrialized countries of the West, sufficiently reliable data are not available.

Common chronic diseases

Details of the common chronic diseases are given by King *et al.* (1992). Many people, unless killed by an injury or an acute infection, die from chronic diseases, including coronary heart disease, cancers, diabetes, high blood pressure, and others. Coronary heart disease and diabetes illustrate the principle of aetiological heterogeneity; such diseases are caused by different aetiologies, but manifest with similar phenotypes. Typically, a genetic predisposition combined with environmental influences causes the disease. We illustrate this with diabetes mellitus.

Diabetes

There are several types of diabetes: type 1 and type 2 diabetes are most common. Type 1 diabetes often manifests during childhood or adolescence. The onset often follows an acute viral infection that appears to precipitate the destruction of insulin-producing islet cells in the pancreas, often by an autoimmune mechanism. Therapy requires insulin substitution. There is a strong association with HLA

Table 4 Relative frequencies (per 10 000 births) of congenital anomalies in the United States, Hungary, and British Columbia, Canada

Congenital anomaly	Prevalence[a] per 10 000 births			
	USA among	Hungary among		British Columbia
	Total births	Total births	Live births	among live births
Anencephaly and spina bifida	17.4	16.6	10.3	9.2
Other anomalies of the nervous system	35.2	14.6	11.4	7.9
Anomalies of the eye	23.6	3.2	3.2	7.8
Anomalies of ear, face, and neck	14.9	4.7	4.6	6.0
Cardiovascular anomalies	86.5	80.8	79.2	42.6
Anomalies of the respiratory system	14.1	2.8	2.8	1.5
Cleft palate and cleft lip	27.3	14.8	14.5	17.5
Anomalies of the digestive system	61.7	27.8	27.8	17.6
Anomalies of the genital organs and urinary system	115.5	93.7	90.9	27.5
Musculoskeletal and skeletal anomalies	438.0	314.2	312.7	66.2
Anomalies of the integument	101.4	7.6	7.4	2.4
Chromosomal anomalies	16.1	12.6	12.6	14.1
Other and unspecified anomalies	12.8	21.5	20.0	1.9
Total	945.5	614.9	597.4	222.2

[a]The US prevalence figures refer to the number of congenital anomalies (and not the number of affected individuals); the figures for the other two are based on the numbers of affected individuals.

Adapted from Czeizel and Sankaranarayanan (1984).

types (DR3 and DR4). A major gene locus in the HLA region (chromosome 6p) has been identified by linkage studies. Another locus near the insulin gene (11p), as well as other less certain predisposing loci, has also been detected (see also Davies *et al.* 1994).

Type 2 diabetes usually manifests in middle or advanced age, often associated with obesity and overnutrition. The specific genes involved are not known but are under active investigation. Contrary to type 1 diabetes, concordance of monozygotic twins borders on 100 per cent. Relatives are frequently affected; however, except for rare autosomal dominant subtypes (such as mature onset diabetes of the young), monogenic inheritance cannot be demonstrated. Type 2 diabetes disappeared almost completely under conditions of undernutrition in central Europe near the end and after the Second World War. In contrast, the frequency of type 1 diabetes did not change during this period when severe food shortages were widespread. These observations demonstrate the importance of food intake in the pathogenesis of type 2 diabetes. Many individuals do not appear to be genetically equipped to cope with overnutrition. Insulin therapy is usually not required in type 2 diabetes; weight reduction, exercise, and occasionally drug therapy are sufficient. Type 2 diabetes is an excellent example of how a disease may appear to be largely genetically determined from a geneticist's point of view, whereas, for a nutritionist, this condition is a typical product of environmentally determined overnutrition in Western affluent societies. Both views are correct!

Some decades ago Neel (1962) proposed the hypothesis that type 2 diabetes might be caused by a 'thrifty genotype'. He suggested that the gene or genes underlying diabetes might be an adaptation to long-lasting conditions of food shortage and starvation. Genes that increased mobilization of carbohydrate may have enabled their carriers to survive and reproduce. There is circumstantial evidence in favour of this hypothesis. India is a country in which the majority of the population have suffered for a long time from food shortages. Indians who have emigrated and are living under affluent conditions have a higher frequency of type 2 diabetes. Among some Amerindian tribes, diabetes and obesity also have become very common under the conditions of the current Western American diet. Type 2 diabetes, despite its genetic determination, can often be prevented by avoiding overnutrition.

Many rare forms of diabetes also exist. Often, diabetes is only one part of a more complex syndrome. Rare mutations affecting the insulin molecule or insulin receptors have been identified. Such findings are typical for many 'complex' diseases. Upon detailed clinical and pathophysiological study, rare types can be distinguished from the more common variety. Monogenic modes of inheritance are often identified in the rarer subtypes and may aid in the elucidation of the more frequent forms. Familial hypercholesterolaemia is an example (Goldstein *et al.* 1995).

Table 5 (Czeizel *et al.* 1988) gives some data on lifetime prevalence of some common chronic diseases in Hungary.

Mental diseases and mental retardation

The third group of complex diseases comprises mental diseases and mental retardation (Propping 1989; Tsuang and Faraone 1990, 2000; Gottesman 1991; Vogel and Motulsky 1996). Their significance for public health is high.

Table 5 Some multifactorial diseases in Hungary (1977–81)

Disease	Lifetime prevalence per 10 000	Mean age of onset (years)	Mean age at death (years)
Acute myocardial infarction, other acute and subacute forms of ischaemic heart disease	359	50	68.0
Graves' disease	65	45	67.1
Diabetes mellitus	427	58	70.4
Gout	18	25	69.9
Glaucoma	160	55	76.0
Asthma	249	35	67.4
Peptic ulcer	460	45	68.2
Cholelithiasis	94	35	71.6
Kidney stones	90	45	70.6
Psoriasis	39	20	72.3
Rheumatoid arthritis	131	40	70.3
Ankylosing spondylitis	19	23	67.2
Allergic rhinitis	360	25	72.6
Atopic dermatitis	60	18	72.2

Adapted from Czeizel *et al.* (1988).

Major psychoses

The two main groups of mental diseases are schizophrenia and affective disorders, which appear to represent separate diagnostic entities with little overlap. The world-wide incidence of schizophrenia is about 0.5 to 1 per cent. The concordance rate is much higher in monozygotic than in dizygotic twins, but varies between studies and as a rule is higher when rates in twins of institutionalized index patients are compared with twin registry data of entire populations (mainly in Scandinavian countries). As an overall average, about 50 per cent of monozygotic pairs tend to be concordant for clinically verified schizophrenia. Other relatives are also more frequently affected than members of the general population, but such familial aggregation of schizophrenia could also be caused by pathogenic factors in the family environment. Evidence in favour of a genetic interpretation of the twin and family data was provided by various adoption studies. Children of schizophrenic parents who were adopted at a very young age by mentally healthy couples showed the same frequency of schizophrenia as children who had lived in a family with one affected parent. Studies of this type and comparisons of mothers and fathers of schizophrenic adoptees excluded intrauterine maternal influences. However, the operation of genetic factors does not mean that the environment is not important at all. After all, the concordance of monozygotic twins is only 50 per cent, allowing considerable opportunities for environmental or as yet unexplored endogenous and random factors. Life events such as loss of a parent or partner, loss of a job, a major somatic disease, and many other factors may trigger the outbreak of schizophrenia. The 'vulnerability' concept, which emphasizes complex interactions between genetic factors and negative life experiences, is popular among psychiatrists.

Within the affective disorders two groups can be distinguished: manic-depressive (or bipolar) disease and simple depression. In manic-depressive disease, episodes of mania are observed in addition to episodes of depression. Among relatives, persons with typical manic-depressive manifestations are observed side by side with others who only suffer from depressions. Concordance of monozygotic twins for affective disorders is of the order of about 70 per cent. The population incidence is slightly lower than that of schizophrenia. In families of probands with endogenous depression, mainly depressions are found; empirical risks are slightly lower than in relatives of manic-depressive patients. The incidence of endogenous depressions is difficult to determine. There is a continuum ranging from transient mood fluctuations to severe depressive episodes without readily recognizable external causes.

Epidemiological studies of entire populations have yielded a surprisingly high prevalence of rates of, mostly transient, psychiatric symptoms that, according to psychiatric criteria in the United States and Western Europe, would have required some form of therapy. However, only a small fraction of these individuals is seen by psychologically or psychiatrically trained caregivers. The severity of the symptoms, the socio-economic and educational status, and general economic conditions determine whether such therapy is obtained.

Alcoholism

From a public health point of view, alcoholism is particularly important. In industrialized Western countries, several per cent of the population can be regarded as alcoholics. Much alcoholism has an environmental explanation: if alcoholic drinks were not available at relatively low prices, alcoholism would be less widespread. Another reason is inducement to social drinking by group pressure. Family, twin, and adoption studies suggest the role of genetic susceptibility factors in alcoholism (Omenn and Motulsky 1972; Omenn 1988;

Propping 1992), but no specific genes have been identified. The reaction of the brain, as assessed by EEG (Propping 1977; Vogel 2000), appears to be one such factor. Persons exhibiting relatively regular α waves in their resting EEGs do not show a major change of EEG patterns after moderate alcohol intake. In contrast, individuals with a poorly developed α rhythm often develop a regular α pattern under such conditions. They 'feel much better' after alcohol intake and therefore may be more susceptible to the development of alcoholism.

A genetic variant of the enzyme aldehyde dehydrogenase, which determines the second step in the metabolic decomposition of alcohol, is particularly common in Oriental populations (about 50 per cent among Japanese). The variant enzyme acts more slowly than the 'normal' type, leading to the accumulation of acetaldehyde after alcohol intake. The resultant 'flushing' (red face, perspiration, increased heart rate, malaise) appears to deter gene carriers from drinking excessively as concluded from the very low frequency of this variant among Japanese alcoholics compared with controls (Harada *et al.* 1982; Shibuya 1988). Therefore, this common polymorphism appears to protect against alcoholism and alcoholic liver disease, and can be considered as an antialcoholism gene.

Mental retardation

Another group of conditions of great societal significance is mental retardation. It is useful to distinguish between mild (high grade, subcultural) and severe (low grade, mental deficient) individuals. If an IQ of less than 69 is taken as a criterion of mental retardation, the mild variety comprises about 2 to 3 per cent of the population. Only about 0.25 per cent are categorized as severely affected (IQ < 50). The mild group generally shows a high concordance of monozygotic twins and a high incidence of similar cases in the family; they can be interpreted as constituting the lower end of the bell-shaped IQ distribution in the population. The severely mentally deficient group is very heterogeneous. It comprises patients who have suffered intrauterine or postnatal brain damage, those with chromosomal aberrations such as Down syndrome (trisomy 21), and many others. Mental retardation is also one of the relatively constant common clinical signs of autosomal chromosomal aberrations. Some autosomal dominant diseases (for example, tuberous sclerosis) and many autosomal recessive conditions contribute to the pool of the many Mendelian disorders that cause mental retardation.

In recent years, X-linked mental retardation has attracted special attention (Sutherland and Richards 1995). It had been known for some time that severe mental retardation is much more common in males than in females, but this observation was explained by assuming ascertainment biases. We now know that a great number of X-linked types of mental retardation exist. One common type, often associated with a characteristic facial physiognomy, is characterized by a microscopically visible attenuation at the tip of the long arm of the X chromosome (fragile X). This common defect has an incidence of 1 in 4000 (Tariverdiau and Vogel 2000). It is the second most common single genetic condition causing mental retardation, after Down syndrome. The mutation causing this anomaly is an amplification of a base triplet, similar to the basic defect in myotonic dystrophy and in Huntington disease. This amplification only occurs in the female germ line (Vogel and Motulsky 1996). It is not entirely clear why the fragile X syndrome is so common. In addition to a high mutation rate, a selective advantage of female heterozygous carriers by increased reproduction in earlier times has been discussed.

Patients with any type of severe mental retardation pose a societal problem, as many of them need to be taken care of during their entire lifetime. Individuals and families with mild and borderline mental retardation are increasingly requiring attention and social aid. In rural societies of the past, it was easy to find adequate jobs for such individuals—simple farm and garden work. In modern industrialized societies, such work is increasingly done by machines and it is becoming more difficult to find suitable and adequately paid occupations. The medical geneticist can aid families by offering prenatal diagnosis. This is possible for Down syndrome, familial chromosomal aberrations such as various translocations and the fragile X syndrome, and the many autosomally recessive metabolic defects diagnosed with biochemical and/or DNA methods.

Novel methods to study complex diseases

So far, only traditional methods of genetic analysis—twin, family, and adoption studies—have been mentioned. Molecular genetics has provided new and efficient tools such as linkage studies using DNA markers with subsequent isolation of disease genes and their mutations. This strategy has proved successful for analysis of genes and mutations determining many hereditary diseases with simple Mendelian modes of inheritance. Under such modes of inheritance, each individual, based on phenotype, can be attributed to a specific genotype. The LOD score method for linkage study is used to localize the mutant gene to a chromosome; the likelihood of linkage (or cosegregation) of a marker gene and a disease gene compared with no linkage is estimated (Ott 1991). If the mode of inheritance is not definite, the 'affected sib pair' method or, more generally, the 'affected family member' method, as well as the examination of 'haplotype sharing' are preferred, but the sample sizes required are much larger than those needed for the classical LOD score method. The principle of these methods is based on the increased probability that two family members who are affected with the same hereditary or partially hereditary disease will also share part of the haplotypes of other genetic variants—especially DNA markers that are located on the same chromosomes—as the mutant genes responsible for this disease. The probability for such haplotype sharing is higher, the closer such markers are located to the disease gene in question (Van der Meulen and te Meerman; in Edwards *et al.* 1997). In addition to linkage studies, the principle of haplotype sharing can also be used for studying the origin and age of mutant genes in populations (te Meerman and Van der Meulen 1997). Geneticists are now applying this approach to pedigrees with many complex classic diseases and the major psychoses. Improvements of the basic strategy are being sought by studying extensive pedigrees suggesting autosomal dominance, or investigating families in relatively isolated populations.

Cancers

In Western societies, about 25 to 30 per cent of the population will die from malignant neoplasias such as various cancers and leukaemias. Many cancers appear to have an environmental cause, and an individual's lifestyle influences morbidity, as shown by the temporal trend of the age-specific mortality of certain cancers over recent decades. Cancer of the stomach has become much rarer, whereas lung cancer has seen a marked increase, first in males and later in females, definitively related to cigarette smoking. The decrease of stomach cancer is most probably due to improved food hygiene. Viral infection can also predispose to cancer. Many primary liver carcinomas are observed in countries where hepatitis B infection is common. The Epstein–Barr virus is associated with Burkitt's lymphoma in Western Africa.

What is the role of genetics? Concordance figures in monozygotic twins are not impressive and are not very much higher than in dizygotic twins. Modest familial aggregation is frequently observed but might be entirely environmental in origin. Nevertheless, impressive pedigrees suggesting autosomal dominant inheritance for certain 'cancer families' have been published.

The elucidation of the genetics of retinoblastoma—a malignant eye tumour—provided a clue to the genetic pathogenesis of cancer in general. About 40 per cent of all sporadic cases are caused by an autosomal dominant gene mutation that can be transmitted to the next generations. About 60 per cent of such patients suffer from bilateral retinoblastoma. The remaining 40 per cent are unilateral. All non-inherited cases are unilateral; they do not transmit the mutant gene to their offspring. Both the inherited and the non-inherited varieties are relatively rare (about 1 in 15 000 to 20 000) (Knudson 1971; Vogel 1979; Vogel and Motulsky 1996), suggesting an explanation that was confirmed later by direct molecular studies. The carriers of the inherited type are heterozygous for a germinal gene mutation in all their body cells, including the retina. The product of the normal allelic partner of this gene normally appear to prevent tumour formation. However, a somatic mutation in this allelic partner gene in a retinal cell abolishes its normal tumour suppressor function. When this happens in a person who already carries the germinal mutation, cell divisions proceed in an uncontrolled way and retinoblastoma develops. In the non-inherited form, these same tumour suppressor genes have to undergo a somatic mutation on both homologous chromosomes in the same cell in order to produce a tumour. The probability of two such rare events in one cell is much smaller than the probability of a single event. In familial adenomatous polyposis, which is rare, the large bowel is studded with epithelial polyps. Sooner or later, one or several will develop into a cancer. The various molecular events have been analysed carefully: a single mutation of a tumour suppressor gene is usually not sufficient; mutations of several such tumour promoter and suppressor genes are required for tumour development (Kinzler and Vogelstein 1995).

Cancers: somatic genetic diseases

Cancers can be considered as a special type of genetic disease. Sometimes, a single inherited mutation may segregate in a family and somatic mutations of the previously normal partner allele will set the stage for tumour formation. Early age at onset and bilateral tumours in paired organs (eyes, breast) are often observed. All cancers appear to have a mutational origin in a single cell. In contrast, for most cancers, somatic mutations occur in the affected individual only and are not inherited from parent to child.

Several breast cancer genes (Br-CA1 and Br-CA2) and colon cancer genes (mismatch repair genes) have recently been identified as being responsible for 5 to 10 per cent of all cases of breast and colon tumours, respectively. The cancers are not always specific for a given origin; additional malignancies are sometimes seen, such as ovarian cancer with the Br-CA1 gene mutation. Characteristically, not all persons who inherit the germinal cancer gene develop tumours, as the required additional somatic mutations do not always occur.

Cytogenetics of cancers

A specific chromosomal aberration in chromic myeloid leukaemia was found in the 1960s: a translocation between chromosomes 9 and 22 (the Philadelphia chromosome). This was the first example of a unique and specific chromosome aberration in neoplastic tissue. Irregular and non-specific abnormalities of cell division causing various chromosomal abnormalities are common in malignant cells and appear to be secondary effects. However, tumour-specific chromosomal aberrations are increasingly found—mainly in leukaemias, but in some solid tumours as well (Andrews *et al.* 1994). A translocation may lead to irregular growth and a malignancy if a gene necessary for an important step of oncogenesis comes under the control of an unrelated regulatory gene. For example, lymphomas are observed when genes coding for immunoglobulin components such as κ or λ chains are positioned close to such control genes.

Molecular applications to cancer therapy and prevention

So far, the results of ongoing molecular studies have had no direct influence on cancer therapy. However, experimental attempts at somatic gene therapy for cancer are being studied. Examples are the introduction of normal tumour suppressor genes or of genes that aim to stimulate immune destruction of the tumour. Leukaemias can now be treated by eliminating all cells within the haematopoietic system by massive irradiation or cytostatic treatment, and transplantation of stem cells from an individual with a compatible HLA phenotype—preferably a sibling. Molecular studies, preferably using the polymerase chain reaction method, are now able to find out whether all mutant cells were eliminated, or if a few of them have remained and might cause a relapse (van Dongen *et al.* 1998).

Molecular insights are also being applied to cancer prevention. Relatives of patients whose breast or colon cancers are caused by single mutant germinal genes detectable by molecular techniques are at high risk and warrant testing. Subjects found to carry the mutant genes need surveillance with more conventional methods, such as mammography and colonoscopy. Molecular tests need to be standardized before general introduction. Moreover, as several different genes and many different mutations at a given tumour gene may be responsible in different affected families, methods need to be developed to detect these mutations. Testing of family members (who may have risks as high as 50 per cent) has a much higher priority than testing in the general population, even for relatively high-frequency tumour genes (for example, about 1.5 per cent of the Ashkenazi Jewish population are heterozygotes for one of three breast cancer genes). Many problems abound. It will be difficult to convey to prospective testees that a negative test for a given breast cancer gene, for example, does not exclude the development of the more common non-familial type of breast cancer.

The recent developments in cancer genetics show how the concepts of cancer genes and their mutations explain the phenomenon of malignant growth. Genetics of families and populations are now being supplemented by the study of the genetics of cell populations.

Genetics as a basic science of medicine and public health

Medicine and public health are more than scientific fields. They are professions that deal with the causes and management of disease, but need science for optimal practice. In the early nineteenth century, pathology was the leading science of medicine. In the late nineteenth century, pathology was supplemented by bacteriology, which offered for the first time a rational aetiological concept of disease. A specific single cause explained microbial infections. This was great progress, as it opened the way for causal therapy, which finally arrived in the middle of the twentieth century with the development of chemotherapy and antibiotics.

During the last two decades human genetics has assumed the role of major paradigm in medicine. First, many monogenic diseases could be explained by mutations of enzymes or various proteins. This advance had immediate therapeutic consequences, allowing successful treatment by removing a noxious metabolite or by substituting a protein that was lacking. An example of the first strategy is the phenylalanine-restricted diet in phenylketonuria; the second strategy is epitomized by factor VIII substitution in haemophilia A. The development of cytogenetics identified the fundamental cause of many birth defects as chromosomal defects, but the mechanisms by which chromosomal aberrations determine complex phenotypes remain a challenge for research in developmental genetics. In recent years, the genetic material and the genes themselves became accessible to analysis, allowing direct elucidation of defects in genetic diseases, including cancers. These developments in molecular and cellular biology have brought genetic concepts and methods into biomedical research in general. The genetic paradigm has become the major conceptual framework within which biomedical research is currently being performed. The term 'molecular medicine' is increasingly applied to such work.

Genetic variability in the 'normal' range

Genetic polymorphisms and disease

A polymorphism is a monogenic trait that exists in the population in at least two phenotypes (and presumably at least two genotypes), neither of which is rare, that is, neither of which occurs with a frequency of less than 1 to 2 per cent. Often we find more than two alleles and more than two phenotypes for a single locus. The first human polymorphism was the ABO blood group discovered in 1900. ABO, Rh, and other blood groups are genetic differences of surface antigens of red blood cells. Polymorphisms of serum proteins and various enzymes are also known. A very important group of polymorphisms comprises the surface antigens of cells (such as lymphocytes) involved in the immune response (major histocompatibility complex); these highly polymorphic HLA types are particularly interesting because they are largely responsible for the rejection of organ and skin transplants if the HLA types of donor and recipient are not carefully matched (Tiwari *et al.* 1987). Organization of matching of immunologically compatible organs such as kidneys, hearts, or livers has become a major international endeavour; special organizations have been founded, for example Eurotransplant in Leiden (The Netherlands).

DNA polymorphisms

In addition to polymorphisms that are detected by phenotypic variation, there are many heritable differences in the base sequence of the DNA that do not influence the phenotype and can be detected only by direct studies of DNA. Most such DNA polymorphisms are found outside coding genes. They may consist simply of an exchange of single DNA base or involve variation in numbers of repeated dinucleotides or trinucleotides. Methods for identification include the use of one or other of many different restriction endonucleases that cut DNA sequences specifically recognized by each one of these enzymes. The most popular method at present is the use of the polymerase chain reaction to amplify the dinucleotide or trinucleotide variants.

DNA polymorphisms are utilized for many practical problems, such as identification of individuals for forensic purposes in criminal investigations or for identifying disputed paternity. In medical genetics, their main use is for linkage investigations in families. Association studies of polymorphic DNA markers with diseases are often carried out by comparing affected patients with controls. If a gene responsible for a disease cosegregates with the marker gene among patients, linkage may be present, but the interpretation of such findings is often difficult because of genetic heterogeneity of the disease and other complexities such as ethnic differences between patients and controls. Currently, major interest centres on the discovery of single nucleotide polymorphisms (**SNPs**) that occur with a frequency of 1 in 1000 nucleotide base pairs. Complete maps of the thousands of SNPs distributed over the genome should be helpful for both association and linkage studies.

Expressed polymorphisms

Polymorphisms at the phenotypic level may have a direct influence on susceptibility to 'complex' diseases; they may contribute to the multifactorial complex of genes involved in causation. The best-known examples are the ABO blood groups and the HLA system. Many diseases are slightly more common in carriers of certain ABO blood types than in others (Vogel and Motulsky 1996). Group A is found more frequently in cancers of the stomach, salivary glands, mouth and pharynx, and ovary, as well as in thrombotic diseases. Group O is more common in peptic ulcers. Moreover, there is evidence that some infectious diseases had ABO blood group associations at a time when treatments were unavailable. The total contribution of such genes to the disease aetiology is small. Associations with certain HLA types are observed mainly for diseases involving autoimmune processes. The strongest association has been found between ankylosing spondylitis and HLA B27. The risk for this disease among carriers of this HLA type is almost 90 times as high as that of other HLA types. Another disorder with a very strong, but unexplained, HLA association is narcolepsy (for a full tabulation of studies, see Tiwari and Terasaki (1985)). An increasing number of genetic polymorphisms—especially those of genes involved directly or indirectly in the various defence mechanisms against infective agents—have been shown to lead to differences in the response to infective agents, for example, course and outcome of infectious diseases (Hill 1996; Vogel and Motulsky 1996). This aspect of medical genetics appears to be relatively neglected—probably because, at present, infectious diseases are playing a minor part in morbidity and mortality in Western countries, where most medical geneticists are working. But in developing countries, infectious diseases are still very important. Therefore, a shifting of emphasis to this field among scientists of these countries would be worthwhile (Vogel 1998). Owing to increasing resistance of germs to antibiotics, infections are becoming increasingly dangerous in the Western world as well.

Genetic variability in reaction to drugs: pharmacogenetics

The pioneers of human genetics during the first decades of the twentieth century, such as Garrod and Haldane, hinted that inherited biochemical variation might explain unusual reactions to drugs and foods. In the 1950s, a few abnormal untoward reactions to drugs were shown to be caused by a genetically determined variation of enzymes (Motulsky 1957). Mutations of the enzyme glucose-6-phosphate dehydrogenase explained haemolytic reactions caused by ingestion of fava beans and by a variety of drugs, including the antimalarial agent primaquine. Variation in the enzyme pseudocholinesterase was found to cause prolonged apnoea on administration of suxamethonium, a drug widely used to relax muscles during surgery. Genetic differences in acetyltransferase activity explained marked individual differences in the blood level of isoniazid, a drug often used in tuberculosis therapy. Genetic variation in a component of the P-450 system of the liver (which is involved in the metabolism of foreign substances) causes defective oxidation of a wide variety of drugs, with certain adverse reactions. A variety of other monogenic pharmacogenetic traits have been described (Evans 1993; Vogel and Motulsky 1996).

In addition to these monogenic traits, a series of twin studies has shown that genetic factors are involved in the metabolism of many other drugs, as measured by plasma concentration, half-life, and other parameters. Among them are such frequently used drugs as antipyrine, dicumarol, aspirin, halothane, and others. Hence genetic variation in drug metabolism is a widespread and regularly observed phenomenon. If untoward drug reactions occur, genetic variation should be considered as one of the possible explanations.

Genetic variation in the reaction to food and other environmental factors: ecogenetics

Alcohol intake

One of the drugs for which genetic variation in metabolism has been demonstrated by repeated twin studies is ethanol. Ethanol is usually ingested for pleasure as an alcoholic drink. There are wide individual differences not only in alcohol metabolism, but also in its effects on the brain (see Chapters 10.2 and 10.3).

Lactose digestion polymorphism

Another ecogenetic polymorphism affects lactose digestion (Flatz 1992). The disaccharide lactose occurs widely in nature, but large amounts are found only in mammalian milk. To be absorbed, lactose must be hydrolysed to glucose and galactose. This is achieved by lactase, an enzyme located at the surface of intestinal cells. In all lactose-producing mammals, intestinal lactase activity is high during the suckling period, declines after weaning, and remains low in adolescent and adult animals. The human species was long considered an exception to this rule as high lactase activity appeared to be expressed throughout the lifetime. However, early studies had been performed among individuals of European origin who do maintain such intestinal lactase activity during adult life. With widespread population screening, it was found that most non-European adult humans had low lactase activity similar to other adult mammals.

Family studies have shown persistence of lactase production in adults to be genetically determined as a Mendelian dominant trait. This means that homozygotes or heterozygotes for the lactase persistence allele (LAC*P) digest lactose as adults. The genetic mechanism of persistence of lactose expression in the intestine is unknown. A regulatory gene is probably responsible. In most populations, both alleles (LAC*P and LAC*R for lactose restriction) are present. The frequency of poor lactose digesters (LAC*R/LAC*R) ranges between 1 and 96 per cent. Populations in subtropical Africa, Eastern Asia, Australia, and native Americans have frequencies of poor lactose digestion of between 90 and 100 per cent. A high rate of persistent lactose absorption is found only in populations who depend on milk from their animals—desert people in Arabia and northern Africa—as well as western and central Europeans. Most southern and eastern Europeans exhibit an intermediate distribution with frequencies of 'malabsorbers' ranging from about 30 to 90 per cent. The precise reasons for these enormous differences are largely unknown. Most observers agree that natural selection must have played a part. Arabian and African populations largely depend on milk for their protein supply, so that those who inherited a gene allowing absorption of lactose after weaning may have had a higher chance of survival. This explanation is less likely for Europe, as survival in northern Europe never appeared to depend critically on the milk supply. Protection of the gene for persistent lactose absorption (Lac*P) against vitamin D deficient rickets, which was common in central and northern Europe, has been suggested.

Lactose-containing foods lead to increased peristalsis, colonic irritation, and diarrhoea in subjects with lactose malabsorption. However, clinically significant signs are rare, as affected individuals usually reduce their milk consumption. Some well-intended support programmes for children, for example in Africa, have been disappointing because children fed too much milk developed diarrhoea. This polymorphism is a good example of how relative the concepts 'normal' and 'abnormal' are. Lactose absorption in adults, which was first regarded as normal, turned out to be the exception when the trait was studied globally. Lactose malabsorption appeared abnormal at first, but was later shown to be the rule among most populations of the world.

Mutagenic agents

Ionizing radiation

Further discussion can be found in various UNSCEAR reports, Sankaranarayanan (1988), Neel and Schull (1991), and Vogel (1992).

The fact that energy-rich radiation can influence mutations was first established in 1927 in *Drosophila*. 'Classical' radiation genetics developed from these results. When DNA was identified as the genetic material, it was soon demonstrated that the genetic material of all living beings is susceptible to radiation-induced damage. Extensive studies on the mouse have elucidated the principles of radiation mutagenesis for the mammalian genome. The mouse data, together with results from direct observations on spontaneous and induced mutations in humans, have been used by international committees to estimate the potential genetic effects of radiation in human populations and to predict genetic damage in relation to a radiation dose. Often, the so-called 'doubling dose' is estimated, that is, the radiation dose that doubles the spontaneous mutation rate, assuming that radiation has occurred more than about 8 to 12 weeks before fertilization. Tables 6 and 7 show recent estimates provided by two international committees (UNSCEAR and the Committee on the Biological Effects of Ionizing Radiation (**BEIR**)). The estimates agree fairly well regarding the induction of chromosomal aberrations and monogenic diseases. The estimates on malformations and complex diseases remain vague at best (for the available data and a detailed discussion, see Czeizel and Sankaranarayanan (1984), Czeizel *et al.* (1988, 1990), and Vogel (1992)).

Most estimates cited in Tables 6 and 7 are based on studies in mice. Directly observed information from humans is rare. A large body of data from human beings became available from follow-up studies of the survivors of the atomic bombings in Hiroshima and Nagasaki in August 1945. Joint American and Japanese research teams are continuing to study survivors, as well as their offspring born after the bombing. Direct teratogenic effects of microcephaly and mental retardation were observed in fetuses irradiated during the 18th to 25th weeks of fetal life. Search for mutations in survivors' germ cells initially utilized offspring parameters such as stillbirths, major malformations, and death during early life. Later, additional end-points were introduced, such as chromosomal studies and inherited protein variation (Neel and Schull 1991). The result can be summarized in one sentence. Despite the fact that about 70 000 children were examined and that all possible statistical biases were considered with painstaking precision, no definite genetic effects among the offspring could be proved.

Assuming that such effects must have occurred, as in all other species, a genetic doubling dose was estimated from the small but statistically insignificant differences in 'untoward pregnancy outcomes' and early mortality of children of irradiated survivors compared with controls. These doubling doses were higher (about 200 rem for acute radiation and about 400 rem for chronic radiation) than those estimated from earlier mouse studies. More recently, a reassessment of the mouse data suggests no difference between the species. No such estimates were possible for the most well-defined human data, chromosomal aberrations, and protein variants, as children of the irradiated group had even fewer untoward results than the non-irradiated control group. In any case, it can be reasonably concluded that ionizing radiation in doses that modern populations (including occupational groups exposed to low-level radiation) might receive have few untoward effects on the health of future generations. Similar conclusions were reached in less rigorous studies of offspring of populations in India and China who had lived for generations on ground containing radio-active isotopes (Vogel 1992). More recent studies seem to show that ionizing radiation causes mainly larger deletions outside of transcribed genes; therefore, its effects are mostly not visible in the phenotype of offspring (Sankaranarayanan 1999; Sankaranarayanan and Chakraborty 2000*a,b,c*). But studies on offspring of Japanese atomic bomb survivors largely failed to show any increase of mutations that change DNA markers (Neel 1995). Exposure to very high radiation doses will either kill the individual or lead to sterility by killing germinal stem cells and, therefore, does not damage future generations. These findings do not mean that radiation protection should be neglected, as there will always be an additional finite risk of mutations for offspring.

Most importantly, definitive risks to the irradiated atom bomb survivors themselves were detected. Clearly, increased risk for leukaemias was demonstrated a few years after atomic bombing and for solid malignant tumours 15 to many years later. The cancer risk was highest with radiation exposure at young ages. These and other data permit some recommendations to be made for radiation protection.

1. Radiation should be kept to a minimum.

2. If radiation therapy is necessary and protection of gonads is technically impossible, a time period of at least 8 weeks—even

Table 6 Radiation risk estimates for genetic diseases: estimated increase per 100 rem (1 Sv) low-dose rate radiation (UNSCEAR estimates)

Disease classification	Current incidence per million live births	Effect of 1 Sv per generation (additional cases)		
		First generation	Second generation	Equilibrium
Autosomal dominant and X-linked	c. 10 000	1500	1300	10 000
Autosomal recessive	c. 2500	5	5	1500
Chromosomal				
Due to structural anomalies	c. 400	240	96	400
Due to numerical anomalies	c. 3400	Probably very small		
Congenital anomalies	c. 60 000	Not estimated		
Other multifactorial diseases	c. 600 000	Not estimated		
Totals of estimated risk		1700	1400	1200

Adapted from Vogel (1992).

Table 7 Radiation risk estimates for genetic diseases: estimated increase per 1 rem (0.01 Sv) low-dose rate radiation (BEIR estimates)

Type of disorder	Current incidence per million live-born offspring	Additional cases/1 million live-born offspring/rem/generation	
		First generation	Equilibrium
Autosomal dominant			
Clinically severe	2500	5–20	25
Clinically mild	7500	1–15	75
X-linked	400	< 1	< 5
Recessive	2500	< 1	Very slow increase
Chromosomal			
Unbalanced translocations	600	< 5	Very little increase
Trisomies	3800	< 1	10–100
Congenital abnormalities	20 000–30 000	10	10–100

Adapted from Vogel (1992).

Note that the BEIR estimates are given per 0.01 Sv (= 1 rem) whereas the UNSCEAR estimates are given per 1 Sv (= 100 rem). The actual load per 30 years (= 1 Generation) is in the order of magnitude of 20.05–0.6 Sv.

better, 3 months—should elapse between the end of exposure to ionizing irradiation and fertilization. This avoids fertilization of germ cells that have been irradiated in a postmeiotic state of development, when they are particularly susceptible to genetically relevant radiation damage.

3. In women, the days immediately around fertilization are particularly dangerous, and so any radiation exposure should be avoided at that time.
4. Radiation in general should be avoided during pregnancy. If radiation exposure with low dosage (such as after diagnostic radiography or isotope diagnostic procedures) has occurred in early pregnancy, the fetal risks are extremely small.

Chemical mutagens

A second possible source of genetic damage to future generations are chemical mutagens. These are strongly reactive substances that are able to react with DNA to cause genetic alterations. Many agents are used in medical therapy as cytostatic agents. As their cytostatic action is based on interaction with DNA, potential mutagenic effects can hardly be avoided without compromising the desired therapeutic effects. However, such drugs are mostly used on patients who either have already reached their postreproductive age or will not have any more children because of poor health (Vogel and Jäger 1969). There is much concern about so-called environmental mutagens, that is, substances present in small doses due to many different chemical sources in environmental pollution. Numerous naturally occurring chemicals have been shown to be mutagenic in bacterial test systems used as surrogate models for chemical mutagenesis (Ames *et al.* 1990). Mutagenous assay results are important for risk assessment (see Chapters 8.8 and 8.9). Nature appears to have endowed our species with mechanisms that protect against mutagenic influences. We agree with Ames *et al.* (1990) that the potential of chemical mutagenesis has been exaggerated, but few direct data exist and unpleasant surprises remain possible.

Applications of genetic knowledge in medical practice

Further discussion can be found in Fuhrmann and Vogel (1983), Harper (1993), and Vogel and Motulsky (1996).

Assessment of genetic risks and genetic counselling

The potentially most important application of genetic knowledge for public health is genetic counselling. This activity consists of an accurate diagnosis, an assessment of genetic risks by appropriate information regarding these risks, and a discussion of the various reproductive options. Diagnosis may be technically complex and may require various procedures, particularly a variety of biochemical and molecular tests, including study of fetal cells following prenatal diagnosis. Making diagnosis may be difficult, but various reference books (McKusick 1994) and websites are now available (http://www3.ncbi.nlm.nih.gov/omim) (Fischer *et al.* 1996). Counselling has to start with the construction of a family chart or pedigree. Even clinically similar or identical diseases may have different modes of inheritance, with different consequences for the risk. Risk assessment may be simple, but sophisticated statistical techniques are sometimes required to integrate the various data. Genetic counselling usually requires expert knowledge. Apart from the scientific and technical aspects necessary for optimal genetic counselling, the genetic counsellor must be empathic and sensitive to the many psychological aspects raised by the genetic problems facing a family or a patient.

Genetic counselling is indicated for increased risks of occurrence of a disease or birth defect in a family. This may be evident if the counsellee or a close relative suffers from a disease for which a genetic cause is known or can be assumed, if the counsellee is at risk of being a healthy carrier of a disease gene, or if the two partners are close relatives such as first cousins. Often, a couple have already had a child with a birth defect or genetic disease and are concerned regarding the recurrence risk for the next child. An increased risk may also exist if the affected patient is the only diseased person in an otherwise healthy family (for example, in autosomal recessive diseases, dominant new mutation, trisomy 21, and various multifactorial diseases).

Chromosomal study is a common diagnostic test. The main indications are as follows.

1. Suspected Down syndrome: even if the clinical picture is definite, chromosome studies are indicated as recurrence risk is higher for translocation Down syndrome than for free trisomy 21.
2. Disturbances of sex development, for example, Klinefelter's (XXY) and Turner's (X0) syndromes.
3. Combinations of various anomalies, such as small size for date, retarded mental and motor development, multiple birth defects, and dysmorphic face and/or other body parts.
4. Suspected X-linked mental retardation.
5. Habitual abortions, to rule out translocations (after other causes have been excluded).

In order to make meaningful plans for appropriate cytogenetic study, the chromosome laboratory needs precise data on the clinical and genetic aspect of the case under study.

Prenatal diagnosis

Further details are given by Harper (1993) and Becker *et al.* (1995).

Non-invasive tests

Prenatal diagnosis may involve non-invasive as well as invasive methods. The most frequently used non-invasive technique is ultrasonic examination of the fetus. In some countries, particularly in Europe, ultrasonic examination has become a routine procedure that is performed in each pregnancy. Precise assessment of the gestational age and fetal position is possible in early pregnancy. Later studies permit the detection of abnormal fetal growth as well as of a growing number of birth defects. Interpretation of abnormal ultrasound patterns requires considerable experience. Ideally, a suspicious finding should lead to referral to specialist ultrasonographers with experience in fetal pathology in centres with high-quality ultrasound equipment.

A frequently used non-invasive prenatal test is α-fetoprotein screening in the blood of pregnant women. Based on the levels of α-fetoprotein, often supplemented with biochemical tests such as chorionic gonadotropin and unesterified oestriol (triple-marker screening), it is possible to recognize an increased risk for several malformations, including neural tube defects (increased α-fetoprotein level), Down syndrome (decreased α-fetoprotein level), and others. If such abnormal biochemical patterns are found, careful ultrasound study and amniocentesis to verify a diagnosis of neural tube defect by study of α-fetoprotein and other biochemical parameters in the amniotic fluid needs to be performed. Some authors are recommending maternal α-fetoprotein blood screening for all pregnant women as the method is harmless and can help in the recognition of several fetal abnormalities. The large number of false-positive as well as false-negative tests with this approach justifies some scepticism (Andrews *et al.* 1994), and there is no general agreement regarding the institution of such programmes in all countries. In the United States, over 2 million pregnant women (about half of all pregnancies) are said to undergo maternal α-fetoprotein testing every year.

Invasive tests

The most common invasive procedures are amniocentesis and chorionic villus sampling. Amniocentesis is carried out at 14 to 16 weeks of gestation and samples cells of fetal origin in the amniotic fluid. Chorionic villus biopsy is performed between 9 and 12 weeks of gestation. The risk of fetal loss following amniocentesis ranges between 0.5 and 1 per cent and is somewhat higher for chorionic villus biopsy, which has the marked advantage of being carried out early in pregnancy. The most common indications for amniocentesis or chorionic villus biopsy are maternal age above 35 (see above), Down syndrome or any other chromosomal aberration syndrome in a previous child, balanced translocation in one parent, neural tube defect in a previous child and/or in one of the parents, and monogenic hereditary disease where prenatal diagnosis (DNA or biochemical) is possible.

Organization of genetic counselling

The organization of genetic counselling and prenatal diagnosis differs in various countries of the world. In The Netherlands, for example, both activities are concentrated in a few centres in which all facilities are available. Health insurance does not pay for activities outside these centres. In Germany, genetic counselling and prenatal units exist in all university institutes of human genetics; there are about 30 such units for a population of more than 80 million. In addition, qualified doctors are permitted to perform genetic counselling and/or certain routine genetic diagnostics tests, which therefore tend to be shifted from university institutes to private practice.

In the United States, genetic counselling and prenatal centres exist in most medical schools as well as in many larger hospitals. Counselling prior to routine prenatal diagnosis (that is, as carried out for maternal age indications) is usually performed by obstetricians or their nurse assistants prior to the procedure. However, such personnel are only recently beginning to be well informed about medical genetics. Counselling for other than routine indications is usually performed by qualified medical geneticists (MD level) and increasingly by genetic counsellors, who have been trained in human and medical genetics and its practical applications for 2 years following a 4-year college education. These genetic counsellors often work in centres with a team that includes medical geneticists (MD level), biochemical and molecular geneticists (PhD level), and cytogeneticists (PhD level), but a growing proportion is attached to health maintenance organizations and to groups of obstetricians and/or paediatricians. These new professionals have filled an important gap in the provision of genetic services, particularly to population groups which, because of geographical location and other reasons, have not had access to expert genetic advice.

It has been recommended that one genetic and prenatal diagnosis unit should serve a population of a million. Location in or affiliation with a university hospital is a frequent and useful arrangement. A variety of personnel are required. Several medical geneticists, ideally with different special knowledge in various subareas of medical genetics and various clinical specialties, are desirable. Non-doctoral genetic counsellors or specially trained nurses are needed to deal with the many problems of patient communication and follow up. Expert PhD scientists, together with a certain number of technicians, are required to carry out the many different types of laboratory studies.

As in other fields of medicine, quality control is essential. This is relatively easy for laboratory work such as for chromosomal or DNA diagnosis. Here, it has become customary in many countries that licensing agencies or scientific or professional societies distribute anonymous specimens to the laboratories and compare results (Andrews *et al.* 1994).

Quality control for genetic counselling is more difficult but requires that personnel engaged in this practice must have undergone supervised training and, ideally, certification by examination. This is available in the United States where a specialty board of medical genetics exists for clinical genetics as well as for several aspects of laboratory genetics (cytogenetics, biochemical genetics, and molecular genetics). A different board for non-doctoral genetic counsellors has also been established. Primary care practitioners, obstetricians, paediatricians, internists, and oncologists will require more training in genetics and genetic counselling in medical schools and during postgraduate training in order to advise patients about the meaning and interpretation of the many new genetic tests that are becoming available.

Public health or community genetics

Aspects of human and medical genetics described so far are mainly the concern of the medical profession, including biologists, non-medical biochemists, and other helpers in research and medical practice. In recent years, however, emphasis has shifted toward studies on clinically healthy persons, individual differences in disease susceptibilities, and appropriate diagnostic and preventive measures in the 'normal' population (Modell and Kuliev 1989). Conferences are being held that centre around these problems, and a new journal *Community Genetics* has been founded. In an inaugural editorial of this journal L.P. ten Kate (1998) described these problems as follows:

> Community genetics ... encompasses all activities to enable the identification of people ... with increased genetic risk who want to acquire this knowledge in order to make informed decisions. [It] minimizes the number of people who would like to know that they are at increased risk, but do not know yet. However, we should not bargain on ethical principles of autonomy, doing good and not harm, justice, and providing equal access and solidarity.

Disease susceptibilities and individual risks have also been considered increasingly in other areas of medical genetics; it is the major difference that phenotypically healthy population groups are now being approached actively, and are offered genetic services. One major offer of this kind is genetic screening.

Genetic screening

Genetic screening involves the study of all individuals of a population or population group for the presence of a certain genetic variant, disease, or carrier state (Vogel and Motulsky 1996). Such screening is generally recommended if effective treatment or preventive measures are possible. Neonatal screening of newborns for phenylketonuria is the best-known example. This condition is one of the most common inborn errors of metabolism (about 1 in 12 000 births in populations of European origin) and is carried out in most European countries and in the United States. The enzyme defect leads to a build-up of phenylalanine in the body, including the brain, which results in profound mental retardation. Diagnosis involves measurement of phenylalanine level in a small drop of blood on filter paper. Restriction of phenylalanine from the diet in affected infants permits normal development. Another treatable condition that is screened neonatally is hypothyroidism, which is frequently not genetic in origin. Such programmes have been successful in that initial screening is followed by specific tests that are sensitive and specific. The required treatments are highly successful and prevent severe mental retardation. Even though these diseases are relatively rare, most European countries and the United States have introduced neonatal screening for these conditions.

Many other diseases have been suggested for testing newborn infants. These include conditions such as sickle cell anaemia, Duchenne muscular dystrophy, and cystic fibrosis. Sickle cell anaemia testing of newborns has been widely performed in the United States as early detection allows antibiotic therapy to prevent infant and childhood mortality. As racial identification of specimens is difficult, all newborns are tested for sickle cell anaemia.

No effective curative or preventive treatment is available for Duchenne muscular dystrophy, but newborn testing has been occasionally recommended to identify carrier mothers for genetic counselling. There is no general agreement regarding this recommendation. Some authoritative groups feel that identification of genetic disease in children for purposes of genetic counselling in the parent should never be carried out. More studies with emphasis on the psychosocial aspects are required.

Cystic fibrosis testing of newborns that might allow earlier treatment has not been definitely shown to affect the natural history of the disease and, therefore, is not generally recommended. Various other inborn errors in metabolism such as maple syrup urine disease, galactosaemia, and homocystinuria are being screened in some areas, but these conditions are very rare and the required metabolic treatment is not successful in all cases. Rigorous pilot studies that are clearly labelled as such should be required before newborn testing for a given condition is generally recommended as a service procedure. Even though such pilot studies need to involve a large number of newborns, a clear distinction must be maintained between such quasi-experimental programmes compared with generally recommended screening studies for all newborns.

Heterozygote screening

Another type of screening deals with heterozygote detection of relatively common recessive diseases to identify matings at risk of producing affected offspring. Among Ashkenazi Jews, 3 to 5 per cent of the population are heterozygotes for the autosomal recessive Tay–Sachs disease. Screening for the carrier state of the gene during pregnancy, or ideally even earlier, offers the possibility of avoidance of the disease, such as by prenatal diagnosis of couples where both partners are carriers. Tay–Sachs disease has become extremely rare among Jews in the United States and Israel by using this approach followed by pregnancy termination. Other recessive diseases common in this population such as Canavan's disease are now being added. The thalassaemias are very common in many populations of tropical and subtropical areas, for example, in the islands of Sardinia and Cyprus. A screening programme for heterozygous carriers of β-thalassaemia with subsequent prenatal diagnosis in couples at risk has led to a reduction of affected homozygotes by about 70 to 80 per cent. Attempts at screening for the sickle cell gene among the African-American population of the United States have been less successful. Insufficient information and failure to discriminate between the common sickle trait and the rare sickle cell anaemia have led to serious misunderstandings and even to discrimination of carriers on the job market. 'Population screening for haemoglobin disorders thalassaemias and sickle cell (thalassaemias and sickle cell disorders) has been practised on a large scale for over 20 years, and basic concepts and methods of community genetic have developed within this framework' (Modell and Kuliev 1998).

Screening for the cystic fibrosis gene, particularly in northern and central European populations, is sometimes recommended as cystic fibrosis is common in these populations (1 in 2000 births). The current life expectancy for a child with cystic fibrosis is about 30 or, with optimal medical care, about 40 years; the disease is not as devastating as phenylketonuria, Tay–Sachs disease, or β-thalassaemia. As a practically feasible genotyping programme does not detect all potential mutations among persons of central and northern European origin, an affected child may be born despite the fact that one (or even both) parents tested negative. Different sets of testing panels for cystic fibrosis mutations need to be used in other populations as the frequency of mutations differs in various ethnic groups. These reasons and the considerable expense of running a programme that needs to be carried out on the entire Caucasian population have led to restraint in instituting population screening for cystic fibrosis.

To arrive at a clearer picture of a complex situation, various approaches, together with their advantages and disadvantages, have been discussed (Decruyenaere *et al.* 1998; Schmidtke 1998). A 1997 National Institutes of Health consensus group recommended testing of pregnant women under certain, restrictive conditions, but did not recommend a general population screening for cystic fibrosis. In the opinion of Schmidtke (1998), there remain 'many unresolved, and perhaps unresolvable, psychological and ethical problems.' Therefore, in his opinion, 'a CF [cystic fibrosis] carrier screening program is premature at the best'.

Other screening

Much more extended genetic screening can be envisaged in some future scenarios. It appears likely that we shall have the power to predict a wide variety of specific risks and health hazards based on genetic testing. A committee of the Institute of Medicine of the National Academy of Sciences of the USA strongly recommended against combining many different tests at one time, such as at birth (Andrews *et al.* 1994). Tests for untreatable diseases should not be combined with tests for preventable or treatable conditions. Children should not be screened for any disorders unless treatment or prevention during childhood is available.

Gene therapy

Somatic gene therapy (treatment of certain genetic diseases and types of cancer by manipulation of certain genes in body cells outside the germ line) falls into the wide field of medical therapy; it has little impact on public health policy (except, of course, the large amount of money that would be necessary). Recently, however, some scientists (especially molecular biologists) have discussed gene therapy in germ cells not only for the treatment of diseases, but for improving certain abilities of 'normal' individuals. Most medical geneticists are much more conservative. For the prevention of diseases, such manipulations are not necessary; selection of appropriate zygotes after pre-implantation diagnosis would achieve the same goal. However, in some countries, manipulation of early zygotes by such a procedure is prohibited by law. Attempts at improvement of human individuals by manipulating normal germ cells meets with many technical and ethical problems that require much more extensive discussion. The purpose of public health genetics is not genetic improvement of human beings—it is not eugenics. Rather, human suffering from illness and disease should be diminished by intelligent and careful utilization of genetic knowledge.

References

Ames, B.N., Profet, M., and Gold, L.S. (1990). Dietary pesticides (99.99 per cent of all natural) and nature's chemicals and synthetic chemicals: comparative toxicology. *Proceedings of the National Academy of Sciences of the USA*, **87**, 7777–86.

Andrews, L.B., Fullarton, J.E., and Holtzman, N.A. (1994). *Assessing genetic risks*. National Academy of Sciences Press, Washington, DC.

Becker, R., Fuhrmann, W., Holzgreve, W., and Sperling, K. (1995). *Pranatale Diagnostik und Therapie*. Wiss Verlagsgesellschaft, Stuttgart.

BEIR (Committee on the Biological Effects of Ionizing Radiation). (1990). *Health effects of exposure to low levels of ionizing radiation (BEIR V)*. National Academy of Sciences Press, Washington, DC.

Cooper, D.N. and Krawczak, M. (1993). *Human gene mutation*. BIOS Scientific, Oxford.

Czeizel, A. and Sankaranarayanan, K. (1984). The load of genetic and partially genetic disorders in man. I. Congenital anomalies: estimates of detriment in terms of years of life lost and years of impaired life. *Mutation Research*, **128**, 73–103.

Czeizel, A., Sankaranarayanan, K., Losence, A., *et al.* (1988). The load of genetic and partially genetic diseases in man. II. Some selected common multifactorial diseases: estimates of population prevalence and of detriments in terms of lost and impaired life. *Mutation Research*, **196**, 254–92.

Czeizel, A., Sankaranarayanan, K., and Szondi, M. (1990). The load of genetic and partially genetic diseases in man. III. Mental retardation. *Mutation Research*, **232**, 291–303.

Davies, J.L., Kawaguchi, Y., Bennett, S.T., *et al.* (1994). A genome-wide search for human type 1 diabetes susceptibility genes. *Nature*, **371**, 130–6.

Decruyenaere, M., Evers-Kieboms, G., Denayer, L., and Welkenhuysen, M. (1998). Uptake and impact of carrier testing for cystic fibrosis. *Community Genetics*, **1**, 23–35.

Edwards, J.H., Pawlowitzki, I.H., and Thompson, E. (1997). *Genetic mapping of disease genes*. Academic Press, London.

Evans, D.A.P. (1993). *Genetic factors in drug therapy. Clinical and molecular pharmacogenetics*. Cambridge University Press.

Fischer, C., Schweigert, S., Spreckelsen, C., and Vogel, F. (1996). Programs, databases and expert systems for human geneticists—a survey. *Human Genetics*, **97**, 129–37.

Flatz, G. (1992). Lactase deficiency: biological and medical aspects of the adult human lactase polymorphism. In *The genetic basis of common disease* (ed. R.A. King, J.I. Rotter, and A.G. Motulsky), pp. 305–25. Oxford University Press.

Fuhrmann, W. and Vogel, F. (1983). *Genetic counseling*. Springer-Verlag, New York.

Galjaard, H. (1994). Genetic technology in health care: a global view. *International Journal of Technology Assessment in Health Care*, **10**, 527–45.

Gelehrter, T.D. and Collins, E.S. (1990). *Principles of medical genetics* . Williams and Wilkins, Philadelphia, PA.

Goldstein, J.L., Hobbs, H.H., and Brown, M.S. (1995). Familial hypercholesterolemia. In *The metabolic and molecular bases of inherited diseases* (ed. C.R. Scriver, A.L. Beaudet, W.S. Sly, and D. Valle), pp. 1981–2030. McGraw-Hill, New York.

Gottesman, II. (1991). *Schizophrenia genes. The origin of madness* . W.H. Freeman, New York.

Häfner, H. (1999). Ideengeschichte der Gesundheitspflege. In *Gesundheit, unser hochstes Gut?* (ed. H. Häfner), pp. 5–28. Springer-Verlag, Berlin.

Hall, J.G. (1990). Genomic imprinting: review and relevance to human diseases. *American Journal of Human Genetics*, **46**, 857–73.

Harada, S., Agarwal, D.P., Goedde, H.W., ***et al.*** (1982). Possible protective role against alcoholism for aldehyde dehydrogenase isozyme deficiency in Japan. *Lancet*, **ii**, 827.

Harper, P.S. (1993). *Practical genetic counselling*. Wright, Bristol.

Hill, A.V.S. (1996). Genetics in infectious disease resistance. *Current Opinions in Genetics and Development*, **6**, 348–53.

Institute of Medicine (1992). *Advances in understanding genetic charges in cancer: impact on diagnosis and treatment decisions in the 1990s*. National Academy of Sciences, Washington, DC.

King, R.A., Rotter, J.I., and Motulsky, A.G. (1992). *The genetic basis of common diseases*. Oxford University Press, New York.

Kinzler, K.W. and Vogelstein, B. (1995). Colorectal tumors. In *The metabolic and molecular bases of inherited diseases* (ed. C.R. Scriver, A.L. Beaudet, W.S. Sly, and D. Valle), pp. 643–63. McGraw-Hill, New York.

Knudson, A.G., Jr (1971). Mutation and cancer: statistical study of retinoblastoma. *Proceedings of the National Academy of Sciences*, **68**, 820–4.

Levy, H.L. (1973). Genetic screening. *Advances in Human Genetics*, **4**, 1–104.

McKusick, V.A. (1986). The morbid anatomy of the human genome: a review of gene mapping in clinical medicine, Part 1. *Medicine*, **65**, 1–33.

McKusick, V.A. (1987). The morbid anatomy of the human genome: a review of gene mapping in clinical medicine, Parts 2 and 3. *Medicine*, **66**, 1–63, 237–96.

McKusick, V.A. (1988). The morbid anatomy of the human genome: a review of gene mapping in clinical medicine, Part 4. *Medicine*, **67**, 1–19.

McKusick, V.A. (1994). *Mendelian inheritance in man*. Johns Hopkins University Press, Baltimore, MD.

Modell, B. and Kuliev, A. (1989). Impact of public health on human genetics. *Clinical Genetics*, **36**, 206–98.

Modell, B. and Kuliev, A. (1990). Changing paternal age distribution and the human mutation rate in Europe. *Human Genetics*, **86**, 198–202.

Modell, B. and Kuliev, A. (1998). The history of community genetics: the contribution of the haemoglobin disorders. *Community Genetics*, **1**, 3–11.

Motulsky, A.G. (1957). Drug reactions, enzymes and biochemical genetics. *Journal of the American Medical Association*, **165**, 835–7.

Motulsky, A.G. (1995). Jewish diseases and origins. *Nature Genetics* , **9**, 99–101.

Neel, J.V. (1962). Diabetes mellitus: a 'thrifty' genotype rendered detrimental by 'progress'? *American Journal of Human Genetics*, **14**, 353–62.

Neel, J.V. (1995). New approaches to evaluating the genetic effects of the atomic bombs. *American Journal of Human Genetics*, **57**, 1263–6.

Neel, J.V. and Schull, W.J. (1991). *The children of atomic bomb survivors* . National Academy Press, Washington, DC.

Omenn, G.S. (1988). Genetic investigations of alcohol metabolism and of alcoholism. *American Journal of Human Genetics*, **43**, 579–81.

Omenn, G.S. and Motulsky, A.G. (1972). A biochemical and genetic approach to alcoholism. *Annals of the New York Academy of Sciences*, **197**, 16–23.

Ott, J. (1991). *Analysis of human genetic linkage* (revised edn). Johns Hopkins University Press, Baltimore, MD.

Pauling, L., Itano, H.A., Singer, S.J., and Wells, I.C. (1949). Sickle cell anemia: a molecular disease. *Science*, **110**, 543–8.

Propping, P. (1977). Genetic control of ethanol action on the central nervous system. *Human Genetics*, **35**, 309–34.

Propping, P. (1989). *Psychiatrische Genetik*. Springer-Verlag, Berlin.

Propping, P. (1992). Alcoholism. In *The genetic basis of common disease* (ed. R.A. King, J.I. Rotter, and A.G. Motulsky), pp. 837–65. Oxford University Press.

Sankaranarayanan, K. (1988). Prevalence of genetic and partially genetic diseases in man and the estimation of genetic risks of exposure to ionizing radiation. *American Journal of Human Genetics*, **42**, 651–62.

Sankaranarayanan, K. (1998). Ionizing radiation and genetic risks. IX. Estimates of the frequencies of Mendelian diseases and spontaneous mutation rates in human populations: a 1998 perspective. *Mutation Research*, **411**, 129–78.

Sankaranarayanan, K. (1999). Ionizing radiation and genetic risks. X. The potential 'disease phenotypes' of radiation-induced genetic damage in humans: perspectives from human molecular biology and radiation genetics. *Mutation Research*, **429**, 45–83.

Sankaranarayanan, K. and Chakraborty, R. (2000*a*). Ionizing radiation and genetic risk. XI. The doubling dose estimates from the mid-1950s to the present and the conceptual change to the use of the human data on spontaneous mutation rates and mouse data on induced mutation rates for doubling dose calculations. *Mutation Research*, **453**, 107–27.

Sankaranarayanan, K. and Chakraborty, R. (2000*b*). Ionizing radiation and genetic risk. XII. The concept of 'potential recoverability correction factor' (PRCF) and its use for predicting the risk of radiation-inducible genetic disease in human live births. *Mutation Research*, **453**, 129–81.

Sankaranarayanan, K. and Chakraborty, R. (2000*c*). Ionizing radiation and genetic risk. XIII. Summary and synthesis of papers VI to XII and estimates of genetic risks in the year 2000. *Mutation Research*, **453**, 183–97.

Sapienza, C. and Hall, J.G. (1995). Genetic imprinting in human diseases. In *The metabolic and molecular bases of inherited diseases* (ed. C.R. Scriver, A.L. Beaudet, W.S. Sly, and D. Valle), pp. 437–58. McGraw-Hill, New York.

Schinzel, A. (1984). *Catalogue of unbalanced chromosome aberrations in man*. DeGruyter, Berlin.

Schmidtke, J. (1998). A commentary on the NIH consensus development statement 'Genetic testing for cystic fibrosis.' Appendix: conclusions and recommendations of the NIH consensus development statement on genetic testing for cystic fibrosis. April 14–16, 1997. *Community Genetics*, **1**, 53–6.

Scriver, C.R. (1992). What are genes like that doing in a place like this? Human history and molecular prosopography. In *Genetic diversity among Jews: diseases and markers at the DNA level* (ed. B. Bonné-Tamir and A. Adam), pp. 3219–29. Oxford University Press.

Shibuya, A. (1988). Genotypes of alcohol metabolizing enzymes in Japanese with alcoholic liver diseases: a strong association of the usual Caucasian type aldehyde dehydrogenase (ALDH) with the disease. *American Journal of Human Genetics*, **43**, 744–8.

Stevenson, A.C. and Kerr, C.B. (1967). On the distribution of frequencies of mutation in genes determining harmful traits in man. *Mutation Research* , **4**, 339–52.

Sutherland, G.R. and Richards, R.I. (1995). Single tandem repeats and human genetic disease. *Proceedings of the National Academy of Sciences of the USA*, **92**, 3636–41.

Tariverdiau, G. and Vogel, F. (2000). Some problems in the genetics of X-linked mental retardation. *Cytogenetics and Cell Genetics*, **91** , 278–84.

te Meerman, G.J. and Van der Meulen, M.A. (1997). Genomic sharing surrounding alleles identical by descent: effects of genetic drift and population growth. *Genetic Epidemiology*, **14**, 1125–30.

ten Kate, L.P. (1998). Editorial. *Community Genetics*, **1**, 1–2.

Tiwari, J. and Terasaki, P.I. (1985). *HLA and disease associations* . Springer-Verlag, New York.

Tiwari, J., Terasaki, P.I., and Mickey, M.R. (1987). Factors influencing kidney graft survival in the cyclosporine era: a multivariate analysis. *Transplantation Proceedings*, **19**, 1839–41.

Tjio, H.J. and Levan, A. (1956). The chromosome numbers of man. *Hereditas* , **42**, 1–6.

Tsuang, M.T. and Faraone, S.V. (1990). *The genetics of mood disorders* . Johns Hopkins University Press, Baltimore, MD.

Tsuang, M.T. and Faraone, S.V. (2000). Genetics of schizophrenia. Seminars in Medical Genetics. *American Journal of Medical Genetics*, **97**, 1–106.

UNSCEAR (United Nations Scientific Committee on the Effects of Atomic Radiation). (1986). United Nations, New York.

UNSCEAR (United Nations Scientific Committee on the Effects of Atomic Radiation). (1988). United Nations, New York.

UNSCEAR (United Nations Scientific Committee on the Effects of Atomic Radiation). (1992). United Nations, New York.

UNSCEAR (United Nations Scientific Committee on the Effects of Atomic Radiation). (1993). *Sources and effects of ionizing radiation*. United Nations, New York.

Van der Meulen, M.A. and te Meerman, G.J. (1997). Association and haplotype sharing due to identity by descent, with an application to genetic mapping. In *Genetic mapping of disease genes* (ed. J.A. Edwards, I.H. Pawlowitzki, and E. Thompson), pp. 115–35. Academic Press, London.

Van Dongen, J.J.M., Seriu, T., Panzer-Grunmayer, E.R., *et al.* (1998). Prognostic value of minimal residual disease in acute lymphoblastic leukaemia in childhood. *Lancet*, **352**, 1731–8.

Vogel, F. (1979). Genetics of retinoblastoma. *Human Genetics*, **52**, 1–54.

Vogel, F. (1984). Relevant deviations in heterozygotes of autosomal recessive diseases. *Clinical Genetics*, **25**, 381–415.

Vogel, F. (1992). Risk calculations for hereditary effects of ionizing radiation in humans. *Human Genetics*, **89**, 127–46.

Vogel, F. (1998). Gedanken über die Zukunft der Humangenetik. *Medizinische Genetik*, **10**, 33–9.

Vogel, F. (2000). *Genetics and the electroencephalogram*. Springer-Verlag, Berlin.

Vogel, F. and Jäger, P. (1969). The genetic load of a human populations due to cytostatic agents. *Human Genetics*, **7**, 287–304.

Vogel, F. and Motulsky, A.G. (1996). *Human genetics: problems and approaches*. Springer-Verlag, Berlin.

Vogel, F. and Rathenberg, R. (1975). Spontaneous mutation in man. *Advances in Human Genetics*, **5**, 223–318.

Watson, J.D., Hopkins, N.H., Roberts, J.W., *et al.* (1987). *Molecular biology of the gene*. Benjamin Cummings, Menlo Park, CA.

Watson, J.D., Gilman, M., Witkowski, J., and Zoller, M. (1992). *Recombinant DNA*. W.H. Freeman, New York.

WHO (World Health Organization) (1998). *World atlas of birth defects* . WHO, Geneva.

2.5 Food and nutrition

Prakash S. Shetty

Introduction

The general notion that the study of nutrition is merely aimed at providing a balanced diet for the populace is no longer adequate. Concepts of what constitutes a 'balanced diet' have changed markedly and it is not even an issue relating to the achievement of the 'recommended levels' of nutrients in the diet. Nutrition is a complex subject that biologically relates to nutrient–gene interactions and the induction of such diseases as diabetes mellitus, coronary heart disease (**CHD**), and cancers, and even to such conditions as asthma and impaired brain development. Nutrition also deals with the social, economic, and cultural issues related to making the right food choices and to purchasing and eating the 'correct' types of food in the 'appropriate' quantities, as well as the factors that determine this aspect of essential daily human activity and behaviour. Thus, just as our gradual acquisition of the knowledge of microbiology influenced our understanding of infectious diseases, which in turn led to preventive measures for the population at large, so the historical advances in the field of nutrition have led to a more coherent understanding of the patterns of and the prevention of food and nutrition related diseases of public health importance throughout the world.

Fluctuations in disease rates depend on environmental factors that include food and nutrition as one of the primary determinants. Nutrition is now recognized as a major determinant of a wide range of diseases of public health importance worldwide. In the developing world, numerous deficiency diseases persist, especially in the rural areas, which are the result of essential nutrient deficiencies in the daily diet. These now coexist with the increasing presence of diet-related chronic diseases in the adult typically seen only in industrialized, developed countries. Significant changes in the patterns of disease and the causes of premature death within a population have little to do with advances in curative medicine and therapeutics. The changes in health depend largely on the environmental changes, which include changes in social and economic conditions, the implementation of immunization programmes, improvements in women's social and educational status within the society and changes in agriculture and food systems and in the availability of food. These changes are, in turn, influenced by governmental regulations and global trade that affect agricultural practices and the industrial sector and thus affect individual lifestyles. Short-term national policies that seek to maximize economic activity and promote international trade and foreign exchange earnings, ignore the impact of these measures on health. Most of these environmental influences operate through changes in the provision and access to hygienic and nutritious food; the availability of uncontaminated water, clean housing, sanitary surroundings, and lack of exposure to environmental toxins. Economic development is thus normally accompanied by improvements in the quantity and quality of a nation's food supply. An increasingly recognized feature of these changes involves a nutritionally mediated improvement in the body's resistance to infections and the mutual interdependence of the immune and nutritional state of the population probably explains the remarkable gains in public health in Britain the twentieth century (McKeown 1976).

These quantitative and qualitative changes in our food patterns, which lead to such dramatic changes in life expectancy, often also result in the problems of diet-related non-communicable diseases, but these problems are not inevitable. The diet-related chronic diseases occur typically in middle and later adult life and can, as in central and eastern Europe, undermine the gains in life expectancy. These chronic diseases of the developed populations are traditionally regarded as manifestations of excess intake and self-indulgence in an 'affluent' society. In practice, some of these chronic diseases may be compounded by relatively deficient intakes of some nutrients. Thus, a 'balanced' diet has to be viewed in a more sophisticated way when considering the disease patterns of adult life.

Nutrition has re-emerged as being of fundamental importance in public health after having been in the doldrums for many decades. Nutritional issues were seen in industrialized and developed societies as relating to deficiency diseases that were conquered in the early part of this century while continuing to persist in the poor, developing countries. Now, however, food and nutrition are recognized as often the principal environmental component affecting a wide range of diseases of public health importance throughout the world. These diseases reflect the cumulative impact of subtle pathophysiological processes developing over a lifetime. These interactions within a society are often seen as reflecting individual genetic susceptibility, but the different disease patterns of groups living on different diets are manifestly a societal reflection of the impact of dietary factors. The display of nutrient–gene interactions is evident, for example, in obesity, alcoholism, cardiovascular disease, non-insulin-dependent diabetes mellitus (**NIDDM**), many gastrointestinal disorders, neural-tube defects, and the most prevalent cancers. As clinical studies and molecular epidemiology unravel the basis for genetic susceptibility to these disorders, physicians interested in metabolic medicine are eventually forced to look for the gene inducers or repressors, which then prove to be of dietary or environmental origin. Societal features that determine human behaviour and economic well being as well as climate, tradition, culture, and the role of women, all affect food patterns and dietary practices. These are the features that need to be recognized when considering public health rather than simply the epidemiological aspects of dietary disease. This chapter seeks to take a global view of diet in public health terms and so nutritional deficiency disorders as well as other diet-related diseases of public health importance will be considered. This is particularly important because deficiency diseases are rampant in several parts of the world and yet co-exist in the same country with chronic adult diseases usually found in affluent, developed societies. Vitamin deficiencies continue to manifest themselves in refugee camps, and the threat of starvation and dietary inadequacy resulting in malnutrition rapidly emerges in wartime and during conflict situations.

Intrauterine growth retardation and low birth weight

Intrauterine growth retardation (**IUGR**) resulting in low birth weights constitutes a major public health problem in developing countries. The recent WHO Technical Report (1995) recommended that the 10th percentile of a sex-specific, birth weight-for-gestational-age distribution be designated for the classification of small-for-gestational-age infants (**SGA**). It is difficult to establish with certainty in all cases whether the reduced weight at birth is the result of *in utero* growth restriction. However, in populations in developing countries with a high incidence of SGA the likelihood is that this is largely the result of IUGR. Hence in this context, the definition of IUGR should be infants born at term (i.e. > 37 weeks of gestation) with a low birth weight (i.e. < 2500 g). The causes of IUGR are multiple and involve many different factors. The most important determinant of infant weight at birth is the maternal environment of which nutrition is the single most important factor. Poor maternal nutritional status at conception and inadequate maternal nutrition during pregnancy can result in IUGR. Short maternal stature, low maternal body weight and body mass index (**BMI**) at conception, and inadequate weight gain during pregnancy are factors that are associated with IUGR. In developing countries IUGR is closely related to conditions of poverty and chronic undernutrition of economically disadvantaged mothers. According to current WHO estimates (de Onis *et al.* 1998) 16.4 per cent of infants born in developing countries have birth weights below 2500 g of which 11.0 per cent are low birth weight due to IUGR. South Asia (i.e. the countries of the Indian subcontinent) has the highest incidence of low birth weights (< 2500 g) at 28.3 per cent, of which 20.9 per cent is attributable to IUGR.

Low birth weights and IUGR are associated with increased morbidity and mortality in infancy. It is estimated that term infants weighing less than 2500 g at birth have a four times increased risk of neonatal death as compared with infants weighing between 2500 and 3000 g and 10 times higher than those weighing between 3000 and 3500. The risk of morbidity and mortality in later infancy is also considerably high in these low birth weight infants. In developing countries this is largely due to increased risk of diarrhoeal disease and respiratory infections. Barker's studies (1995) have consistently demonstrated a relationship between low birth weight and later adult disease and provide an important aetiological role for fetal undernutrition in amplifying the effect of risk factors in later life in the development of chronic diseases such as heart disease and diabetes mellitus in adult life.

Protein–energy malnutrition

The clinical conditions of childhood malnutrition are widely recognized as kwashiorkor, marasmus, and the mixed condition of marasmic kwashiorkor. These severe forms of malnutrition are, however, the tip of an iceberg of widespread mild and moderate childhood undernutrition within the community. The dominance of the three forms varies from country to country and this seems to reflect the weaning practices and staple foods of the area as well as the likelihood of recurrent infections. Kwashiorkor presents a variety of clinical features depending on the region of the world. Children are characteristically oedematous with a moon face, a scaling crazy-pavement pigmentation, and ulceration of the skin with sparse thin reddish hair. Clinically, they are morose and lethargic, and they have a large liver and often appreciable amounts of trunkal and limb fat, which obscures an atrophied muscle mass. The condition is associated with high mortality, is often accompanied by infections and was originally classified as the outcome of selective protein deficiency (Waterlow 1992). It can occur in epidemic form once a measles outbreak affects a society living on a low-protein staple diet (e.g. cassava, yam, plantain, or banana), but additional features may be the exposure to toxins such as aflatoxin. The impact of iron overload from the ready absorption of bacterial iron leading to marked free-radical damage in a liver, which is limited in free-radical scavengers derived from the diet (e.g. glutathione and vitamins E and C), also seems important (Briend and Golden 1993). The measles infection not only can induce diarrhoea with protein loss, but further protein can be lost through the skin as amino acids or transferred to boost lymphocyte and antibody production. Thus, a relative deficiency of amino acids for glutathione or protein production may still be important and the immune and inflammatory capacity of the malnourished child is impaired.

The marasmic form of protein–energy malnutrition is that of a wizened, shrivelled, growth-retarded, and skeletal child who is often alert and with normal-coloured but shrivelled skin. Mortality rates in marasmus are lower than in kwashiorkor but if overfed early with too high a sodium intake the marasmic child may become oedematous and simulate the mixed syndrome of marasmic kwashiorkor.

Diarrhoeal disease and malnutrition

Apart from these classic and extreme conditions there are millions of children with chronic diarrhoea who fail to respond completely to the usual treatment for acute gastroenteritis. The 5 million or more deaths per year from diarrhoeal diseases have been reduced by about half, but it is now becoming clear that the residual problem is essentially nutritional in origin. A vicious circle is established whereby an intestinal infection in a young child leads to anorexia, intestinal damage with malabsorption, and secretory diarrhoea, which then does not remit because the poor nutritional state of the child maintains the immunological deficit and this impairs the recovery of the intestine. These malnourished children with diarrhoea typically have more pronounced potassium depletion and are very sensitive to sodium retention.

Traditionally, children, particularly in Africa and Asia, fail to thrive once they have succumbed to an infectious disease, and they then languish, responding poorly to standard therapy and failing to grow even when presented with supposedly adequate amounts of food. New treatment schemes are now being developed based on the recognition that intestinal bacterial overgrowth is common and that for recovery to take place it is necessary to provide the full complement of minerals and vitamins (Golden *et al.* 1995). Once the child has re-equilibrated its fluid and electrolyte balance, the need is not only for the full supply of minerals and vitamins but also for adequate amounts of readily swallowed energy-dense feeds. This is often best met by adding oil, which is energy dense to the diet. The manufacture of oil-rich products for rehabilitating children in Third World countries is hampered by their tendency to oxidize, but locally produced food oils can make an extremely valuable contribution to increasing the energy density of the diet. New nutrient-to-energy ratios for the supplementary feeding of children and adults have been recently devised (Golden *et al.* 1995) and preliminary observations suggest that these new formulations can boost growth rates. Shifting strategies of rehabilitation by coping with malnourished children at home rather than in rehabilitation centres clearly show the cost–benefit advantages of home care to both mother and child (Khanum *et al.* 1994).

Assessment of undernutrition in children in the community

Undernutrition in childhood is characterized by growth failure, resulting in a body weight that is less than ideal for the child's age. Hence, in children, assessment of growth has been the single most important measurement that best defines their health and nutritional status. Measures of height and weight are, therefore, the commonly used indicators of the nutritional status of the child. Classification of childhood malnutrition based on height, weight, and age thus continues to be the backbone of nutritional assessment methods for both population and individual assessments. The set of guidelines for expressing children's nutritional status in a community has recently been revised by the World Health Organization (WHO 1995). There is increasing evidence that children throughout the world when well fed and free of infection tend to grow at similar rates whatever their ethnic or racial origin, and healthy children everywhere can, when fed appropriately, be expected to grow on average along the 50th percentile of a reference population's weight and height for age. Table 1 summarizes the methods for assessing a child's nutritional status using anthropometry by expressing both height and weight as standard deviations or *Z*-scores from the median reference value for the child's age. Thus a normal range corresponds to the third and 97th percentile (i.e. ±2 SD or ±2 *Z*-scores). By expressing data in this way, using relatively simple computer programs, it is possible to express the weight and height data for all children across a wide age range in similar *Z*-score units and thereby produce a readily understandable comparison of the extent of growth retardation at different ages and in different societies.

A deficit in height is referred to as 'stunting' whereas a deficit in weight-for-height as 'wasting'. These two measures are subsumed in the less helpful original designation of a child's failure to grow in terms of weight-for-age. Clearly this measure includes both the wasting and stunting features but fails to distinguish the important differences between the two. Wasting can occur on a short-term basis in response to illness with anorexia or malabsorption or because the child goes hungry for several weeks. Therefore changes in weight-for-height reflect the impact of short-term changes in nutritional state. Growth in height, however, is much more of a cumulative index of long-term health because growth in length or height stops immediately a child develops an infection and the subsequent growth may be slow during the recovery period. Increasing evidence suggests that a child normally grows in spurts for reasons that remain obscure. Energy intake is not a crucial determinant of height as popularly considered. The energy cost of growth and weight gain is only 2 to 5 per cent of total energy intake once the child is 1 year of age. Impairment or slowing of height growth classically occurs in many communities at the time of weaning and up to about 2 years of age and affects a large proportion of children in many developing countries. Once the children have failed to maintain their proper growth trajectory they tend to remain on the lower percentile and 'track' at this low level for many years.

Table 1 Diagnostic criteria for undernutrition in children and adults

Childhood undernutrition[a]	
Underweight	Low weight for age
Stunted	Low height for age
Wasted	Low weight for height
Adult undernutrition	
Grade I	BMI 17.0–18.49
Grade II	BMI 16.0–16.99
Grade III	BMI <16.0

[a]Low weight defined as more than 2 SD below the WHO–NCHS reference value.

Source: Shetty (1994).

Table 2 Prevalence and numbers of children with malnutrition in developing countries of Latin America, Asia, and Africa

	Latin America	Asia	Africa
Underweight			
Prevalence (%)	11.9	42.0	27.4
Number (×10[6])	6.5	154.1	31.6
Stunted			
Prevalence (%)	22.2	47.1	38.6
Number (×10[6])	12.1	172.8	44.6
Wasted			
Prevalence (%)	2.7	10.8	7.2
Number (×10[6])	1.5	39.6	8.3

Prevalence is expressed as the percentage more than 2 SD below the WHO–NCHS reference value. Data were obtained in the period 1990–1992 and are restricted to nationally representative surveys in developing countries from the three continents with more than 70 per cent of children covered in the sampling. Note the much higher prevalence rates of stunting than wasting. Thailand and North African data show less malnutrition than in the rest of their regions with rates closer to those seen in Latin America.

Source: de Onis *et al.* (1993).

Surveys throughout the world (Table 2) demonstrate the very high prevalence of stunting in Asian children who begin to fall behind the reference height percentiles by 6 months of age. Their continued stunting may reflect not only their lower nutrient intakes from local diets but also the constant impact of infection, mostly from infected water and food. The dramatic effect of ridding a child of a gastrointestinal infection is shown by the remarkable spurt in height when Jamaican children with a trichuris worm infection are dewormed (Callender *et al.* 1993). Within 2 weeks of treatment, sensitive measures of skeletal growth demonstrate a surge in long bone formation. Thus, the stunting of children may prove to be the result of a complex interaction between the quality plus quantity of the child's food intake and the burden of chronic low-grade intestinal, respiratory, and other infections. The persistence of infections is in part a reflection of the immune deficit in malnutrition, and deficiencies of many vitamins (e.g. vitamin A) and minerals (e.g. zinc) are clearly associated experimentally and clinically with an excess susceptibility to infection. The infection itself, however, places increased demands on nutrient requirements and often leads to anorexia (Stephenson *et al.* 1993); thus mechanistically nutrition and infection are intertwined as demonstrated several decades ago. Wasting and stunting are two types of nutritionally mediated growth deficits in childhood. Wasting indicated by a low weight for height can occur at any age. Stunting is seen when a child's height is low for their age and reflects poor nutrition during the early growth period, which is often the result of infectious episodes during this period. Physical stunting is associated with poor mental development and socio-economic deprivation. Stunting is more common in South Asia and seems to be related to the high incidence in low birth weight (i.e. < 2500 g) in this region.

Cognitive and mental development and malnutrition

A largely neglected issue of immense societal and public health importance is the issue of brain development and learning in undernourished children in developing societies. Grantham-McGregor (1995) has demonstrated that children who are stunted and living in deprived circumstances in Jamaica develop poorly and have major deficits in intellectual and cognitive development and social behaviour. In a series of controlled studies she has shown that children's scholastic ability in their teens can be strongly influenced by interventions in the second and third year of life. Children who are involved in simple parent-assisted play with the use of primitively constructed blocks, which can be assembled in a stack or sequence, learn early to improve their mental processing in non-verbal skills. By supplementing their diet with extra food rich in nutrients, the children's mental development is again improved but the combination of extra food and mental stimulation has an effect in boosting mental development, which is so remarkable that the combined 'therapy' allows children almost to catch up with the mental development of those reared in a very advantageous environment. Furthermore, imposing this combined 'therapy' on children for a mere 1 year when they are 6 months to 3 years of age leads to a long-term gain discernible in children's scholastic performance many years later.

The dependence of brain development on good nutrition has been recognized for decades with iodine deficiency in its extreme form leading to fetal retardation and the syndrome of cretinism. Even if cretinism is avoided, postnatal iodine deficiency can lead to such a slowing of mental processing that lethargy results with permanent impairment of mental development because of the need for adequate nutrition during the critical periods of brain development. Similarly, Pollitt (1991*a*, *b*) has now clearly demonstrated that anaemia induced by iron deficiency can permanently handicap children at a crucial time in their development even though iron deficiency *per se* is not enough to produce demonstrable deficiency. Experimentally, however, iron is required for the synthesis of many cerebral enzymes, so a biochemical basis for selective nutrition effects on mental processing is clear. Thus, selective nutrient deficiencies can lead to impaired brain function and this, therefore, raises the issue of whether food-deprived, stunted children in the Third World are capable of being rehabilitated with a complete diet or only need two to three nutrients. Grantham-McGregor's (1995) studies show that food that stimulates longitudinal bone growth also stimulates brain development, thus implying a more generic demand for a range of nutrients if mental function is to improve.

These studies of childhood nutrition and brain development have profound public health significance. Until now one has hesitated to infer that many groups in Third World societies are mentally less able as a result of nutritional insults. Yet 20 to 60 per cent of the children living in Third World countries are physically stunted. Anaemia in childhood is extremely common and iodine deficiency threatens 10 per cent of the world's children. In this context, therefore, we need to recognize that the human capital of Third World societies is limited by inadequate provision for the upbringing of children. This then becomes of huge economic and public health significance as adults who are slow and less able to adapt may become a societal burden rather than an asset. These examples illustrate the importance of food and nutrition in the development of human capital in developing societies of the Third World.

Iron deficiency

Iron deficiency is probably the most common nutritional deficiency disorder in the world. The highest prevalence figures for iron deficiency are found in infants, children, teenagers, and women of childbearing age. Hence it is a major public health problem with adverse consequences especially for women of reproductive age and for young children. The predominant cause of iron deficiency worldwide is nutritional, the diet failing to provide for the body's requirements of iron. In tropical countries, intestinal parasitosis exacerbates iron deficiency by increasing the loss of blood from the gastrointestinal tract. The increase in malaria in these countries further contributes to the anaemia. A low intake of iron and/or its poor absorption then fails to meet the enhanced demands for iron and anaemia results.

The consequences of iron deficiency are numerous as iron plays a central part in the transport of oxygen in the body and is also essential in many enzyme systems. Not only does iron deficiency affect neurotransmitter systems in the brain with changes in behaviour, such as attention, memory, and learning in infants and small children, but iron deficiency also negatively influences the normal defence systems against infection. T-lymphocyte function, phagocytosis, and the killing of bacteria by neutrophilic leucocytes are affected. In pregnant women iron deficiency contributes to maternal morbidity and mortality, and increases risk of fetal morbidity, mortality, and low birth weight (Viteri 1997). Long-standing iron deficiency in general terms also results in a reduction in physical working capacity and productivity of adults both in agricultural and industrial work situations. These functional impairments are economically important.

Iron deficiency disorders encompass a range of body iron depletion states. The least severe is diminished iron stores diagnosed by decreased serum ferritin levels and are not usually associated with adverse physiological consequences. Iron deficiency without anaemia is severe enough to affect the production of haemoglobin without haemoglobin levels falling below clinical criteria indicative of anaemia. This condition is characterized by decreased transferrin saturation levels and increased erythrocyte protoporphyrin. The major clinical manifestation of iron deficiency is iron deficiency anaemia (**IDA**). IDA seems to be a particular problem of Africa and South and Southeast Asia (Table 3), and the dominant cause is nutritional iron deficiency. Even in industrialized, developed countries the prevalence of iron deficiency anaemia varies between 2 and 8 per cent. In Africa, Asia, and South America, the trend in availability of iron in diet has been deteriorating so it is not surprising that iron deficiency anaemia continues to be a massive public health problem throughout the world. The availability of iron in the diet for absorption is affected by both the form of iron and the nature of foods concurrently ingested. Iron exists in the diet in two forms: 'haem iron' it is found only in animal sources and is readily available for absorption and is not influenced by other constituents of the diet, and 'inorganic iron' is not readily available and is strongly influenced by factors present in foods ingested at the same time. Both animal foods and ascorbic acid (vitamin C) promote the absorption of inorganic iron. Diets that are primarily cereal and legume-based may contain much iron but, in the absence of co-factors such as ascorbic acid, they may provide only a low level of available iron. Concern about iron deficiency is an important nutritional reason for recommending the consumption of at least some meat as well as foods with a substantial content of ascorbic acid for populations who eat predominantly a cereal-based diet.

WHO is active in developing strategies to combat iron deficiency. These strategies include iron supplementation, iron fortification of certain foods, dietary modification to improve the bioavailability of dietary iron by modifying the composition of meals, and parasitic disease control. Iron and folate supplementation programmes for pregnant women are currently widely implemented in several countries; 49 countries have a universal preventive supplementation policy during pregnancy. Iron supplementation aimed at pre-school or school-aged children are being carried out in 23 countries. Fortification of foods with iron is a preventive measure aimed at improving and sustaining adequate iron nutrition over a longer term. Many industrialized countries such as Canada, the United Kingdom, and the United States have fortified foods with iron and more recently five large studies in developing countries have demonstrated the effectiveness of iron fortification of foods provided these programmes are based on careful planning and follow well established guidelines (Viteri 1997). Improvement in the supply, consumption, and the bioavailability of iron in food is an important strategy to improve the iron status of populations. The bioavailability of iron in foods is influenced by the composition of the meal and food preparation methods. The consumption of ascorbate-rich foods enhances iron absorption while limiting the content of phytate, which inhibits iron absorption, will improve iron bioavailability from the diet. Malaria and intestinal parasites (especially hookworm) are important contributors to IDA in endemic areas. In populations where hookworm is prevalent, effective treatment of this helminth infection has reduced IDA in school age children (Stoltzfus *et al.* 1997).

Iodine deficiency

The term 'iodine deficiency disorder' (**IDD**) refers to a complex of effects arising from iodine deficiency. The mountainous areas of the

Table 3 Prevalence of anaemia and numbers affected (in millions) in different regions of the world

WHO regions[a]	Children				Women (15–49 years)				Men	
	0–4 years		5–14 years		Pregnant		All women		(15–59 years)	
Africa	33.1%	(35.5)	52%	(85.2)	46.9%	(9.6)	37.9%	(57.6)	28%	(41.9)
Non-industrialized Americas	22.9%	(13)	36.9%	(39.5)	39%	(3.8)	31%	(44.9)	11%	(15.8)
South-east Asia	52.7%	(93.8)	63.9%	(207.8)	79.6%	(22.2)	60%	(218.6)	42.4%	(184.8)
Eastern Mediterranean	38.3%	(28.1)	30.8%	(37.9)	63.9%	(8.8)	51.1%	(60.6)	32.7%	(41.5)
Non-industrialized West Pacific	14.7%	(19.7)	56.9%	(156)	38.5%	(9.4)	33.8%	(152.9)	36%	(172.5)
Total all regions	34%	(190)	53%	(526)	56%	(54)	43%	(535)	34%	(456.5)

Numbers in millions are given in parentheses.

[a]As defined in the *World Health Report* (WHO 1997).

Data from ACC–SCN (1997).

world are likely to be iodine deficient because the rain leaches the iodine from the rocks and soils. The most severely deficient areas are the Himalayas, the Andes, the European Alps, and the vast mountainous regions of China. Although iodine deficiency is likely to occur in all those elevated regions subject to glaciation and high rainfall that run off into rivers, it also occurs in flooded river valleys of eastern India, Bangladesh, and Burma. The Great Lakes basins of North America are also iodine deficient. Excessive intakes of goitrogens in food (due to the excessive consumption of cassava or the brassica group of vegetables) and in water (water-borne goitrogens in Latin America) as well as the deficiency of certain trace elements in the soil or food chain (such as selenium) may interfere with the uptake and metabolism of iodine in the body and can thus cause or amplify the effects of iodine deficiency.

The prevalence of IDD varies globally and at present is confined to developing countries, largely because public health initiatives such as iodization of salt have been introduced in the developed, industrialized Western world. Iodine deficiency and goitre are still prevalent, however, in central and eastern Europe. According to a recent WHO Report (1990), in developing countries alone about 1000 million (1 billion) are at risk of IDD, of which 200 million are suffering from goitre, 5 million have gross cretinism with mental retardation while another 15 million suffer from lesser degrees of mental defect. The estimated proportion of population at risk of IDD and their recent trends in the different regions of the world is summarized in Table 4.

IDD in humans is predominantly the result of a primary deficiency of iodine in the diet. Both water and foods are sources of iodine with marine fish being the richest source of iodine. Milk and meat are also rich sources of iodine. Fruits, legumes, and vegetables as well as fresh water fish are also important additional sources. Plant foods are likely to show a reduced content of iodine if the iodine content of the soils in which they are grown is low. Goitrogens in the diet are of secondary importance as aetiological factors in IDD. More recently it has been shown that staple foods consumed largely by rural populations of developing societies, such as cassava, maize, sweet potatoes, lima beans, etc., contain cyanogenic glucosides that release a goitrogen thiocyanate. Cassava is now implicated as an important contributor to iodine deficiency and results in endemic goitre and cretinism in non-mountainous Zaire and in Sarawak in Malaysia. There is also increasing evidence that selenium deficiency in the soil can result in manifestations of IDD in the presence of modest iodine deficiency as selenium is an important trace element, which is essential for thyroid metabolism. Selenium deficiency is now increasingly recognized as an aetiological factor in the IDD in several regions of China.

Table 4 Proportion of total population at risk of iodine deficiency disorders by region in the 1990s

WHO region	Population at risk of IDD (%)	
	1993	1997
Africa	32.8	23.4
Americas	23.1	6.6
Eastern Mediterranean	42.6	30.3
Europe	16.7	10.7
Southeast Asia	35.9	14.4
Western Pacific	27.2	9.8
Total	28.9	13.7

Data from WHO–UNICEF–ICCIDD (1993) and WHO (1997).
Source: ACC–SCN (1997).

Iodine is readily absorbed from the diet and forms a very important element in the synthesis of thyroid hormones in the body. Thyroid hormones are essential for normal growth and development. Just prior to birth, the levels of the biological active tri-iodothyronine (T_3) increase and prepare the organism for the transition from intrauterine to extrauterine life. Failure to synthesize sufficient T_3 as a result of iodine deficiency may be a factor in the stillbirths that occur as a part of the spectrum of IDD in humans. Thyroid hormone deficiency leads to severe retardation of growth and maturation of all organs. The brain is particularly susceptible to damage during the fetal and early postnatal periods. It is now confirmed that the thyroidal control of neonatal brain development is more important than fetal brain development as early and optimal thyroid hormone treatment after birth can lead to substantial improvement in thyroid function. The spectrum of IDDs in humans, from the fetus to the adult, have been outlined recently by Hetzel (1987).

The public health initiatives for correcting iodine deficiency require the provision of adequate iodine to the individual. This has been achieved by one of several methods:

Iodization of salt has been the most favoured method and has greatly reduced the prevalence of IDDs in Switzerland, the United States, Yugoslavia, and New Zealand. Since its first successful introduction in the 1920s in Switzerland (Burgi *et al.* 1990) successful programmes have been more recently reported in Central and South America, in Europe (Finland), and in Asia (China and Taiwan). However, several developing countries have encountered problems with their salt iodization programmes because it is difficult to produce and maintain enough high-quality iodized salt for large populations such as in India. The extra costs of iodized salt and problems with its availability and distribution to remote regions can also be a problem. These issues may be compounded by cultural prejudices about the use of iodized salt and the loss of iodine with cooking if salt is not added after cooking.

Iodized oil injections have been used to prevent goitre and cretinism in New Guinea (Pharoah and Connolly 1987). Iodized oil is suitable for mass programmes and can be carried out alongside mass immunization programmes. These methods have been successful in China, Indonesia, and Nepal. The major problems with iodized oil are the cost, the initial discomfort, and the likely potential disadvantage associated with the transmission of hepatitis B and human immunodeficiency virus with the use of needles. The need for a primary health care team to inject the iodized oil can be a further disadvantage.

Iodized oil by mouth may be an effective alternative and has been tried as a single oral dose for children in South America and Burma. Oral iodized oil has also been tried in women and primary health centres can readily administer this scheme. However, the effects of oral iodized oil seem to last for only half as long as a similar dose of injected iodized oil. They do not, however, suffer from the disadvantages of iodized oil injections so it is a preferred method for use in remote areas.

The IDDs are excellent examples of nutritional deficiency disorders of public health importance that can readily be abolished if mass community programmes are undertaken.

Vitamin A deficiency

Vitamin A deficiency leads to night blindness and xerosis (dryness) of the conjunctiva and cornea, disrupts the integrity of their surface and causes corneal clouding and ulceration, and may lead to blindness in children. Xerophthalmia continues to be a major cause of childhood blindness despite the intensive prevention programmes of the last two decades. It is a widespread problem and the parts of the world most seriously affected include South and East Asia, and many countries in Africa, Latin America, and the Near East (Fig. 1). The WHO (1991) estimated that between 6 and 7 million new cases of xerophthalmia occur every year, with about 1 in 10 of these children suffering corneal damage. Of these, 60 per cent are dead within a year and of the survivors 25 per cent are totally blind, whereas 50 to 60 per cent are partially blind. It is thus estimated that 3 million children under the age of 10 years are blind from deficiency of vitamin A at any one time. More recent estimates of the prevalence of clinical vitamin A deficiency indicates a considerable improvement with reduction of between 31 per cent and 57 per cent in prevalence in the various regions of the world (UNICEF 1997).

An additional 20 to 40 million people suffer from mild or subclinical deficiency of vitamin A, which we now recognize as having serious consequences for survival as vitamin A deficiency (**VAD**) is now known to decrease the child's resistance to infections and increase mortality. Even before eye signs of VAD are detectable, changes in the surface linings of the gastrointestinal and respiratory tracts occur along with changes in cell-mediated immunity and these can increase the risk of morbidity and even mortality associated with infections in children. More recent evidence suggests that VAD may be associated with increased maternal morbidity and even mortality. Vitamin A is also now known to be involved in fetal development, haematopoiesis, spermatogenesis, appetite, and physical growth.

Vitamin A is the parent of a class of compounds called retinoids. Provitamin A carotenoids, chiefly β-carotene, are also included in the vitamin A family. Preformed vitamin A is chiefly found in dairy products such as milk, butter, cheese, egg yolk, in some fatty fish, and in the livers of farm animals and fish. Carotenes are generally abundant in yellow fruits (papayas, mangoes, apricots, peaches) and vegetables (carrots). Absorption of vitamin A is about 80 per cent complete in the presence of an adequate fat intake, while the absorption of carotenoids is highly bile salt dependent. Vitamin A (retinol and retinoic acid) plays a very important part in the body in cellular development and differentiation. Retinol also plays a vital part in normal vision, particularly by the rods in the retina. Thus, one of the earliest manifestations of vitamin A deficiency is night blindness.

There is now increasing evidence that vitamin A supplements in deficient populations can reduce morbidity, mortality, and blindness. Xerophthalmia has become less prevalent in recent years in hyperendemic areas such as Indonesia and India. Intervention strategies that may have contributed to this include periodic megadose vitamin A supplementation either in the form of capsules, syrup, or as an injected dose. However, this method of intervention should only be intended as a short-term measure to save sight and lives on a large scale (West and Sommer 1985). The fortification of dietary items that are universally consumed (e.g. sugar) in Central America (Arroyave *et*

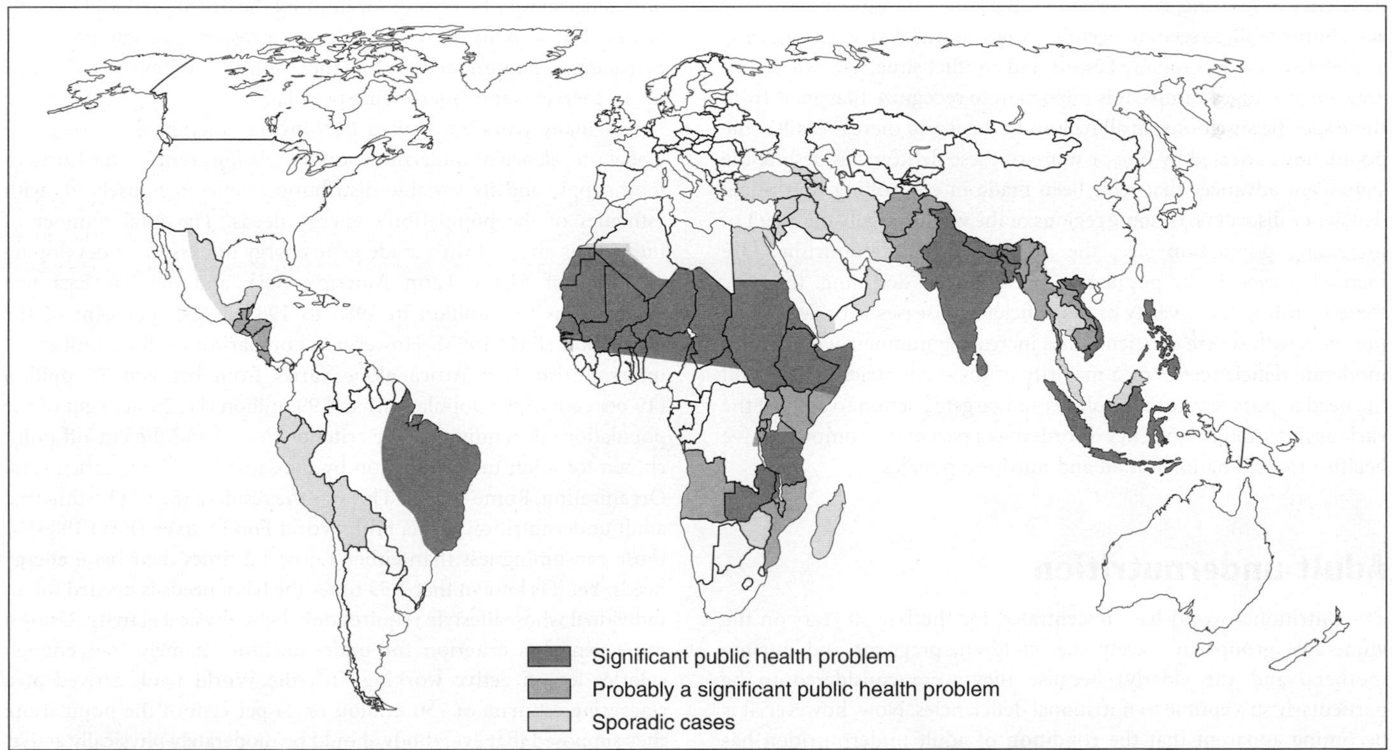

Fig. 1 The geographical distribution of xerophthalmia (vitamin A deficiency) in 1987. (Source: WHO Study Group 1990.)

al. 1981) and monosodium glutamate in Indonesia (Muhilal *et al.* 1988) have had a favourable impact on the vitamin A status of the whole population. The problems with food fortification are essentially logistical and technological. Food supplies from different regions of the world show limited vitamin A availability, but the problem is exacerbated by a tendency to withhold vegetables and fruits from children and from pregnant and lactating women for cultural and other reasons. In Asia, there is a particular problem because the average availability of vitamin A is less than that required by the population; the problem is also exacerbated by the maldistribution within the population of foods rich in vitamin A. Nutrition education is the only answer when vitamin A deficiency develops despite vegetable sources of the vitamin being in plentiful supply. These foods are not incorporated into the diets of young children and mothers because of either lack of knowledge or cultural biases. Nutrition education together with practical advice and help with growing cheap nutritious vegetables in home kitchen gardens may help eradicate vitamin A deficiency. Horticultural approaches are increasingly recognized for their effectiveness and potential sustainability in improving not only vitamin A status, but also micronutrient status generally. The importance of combining increased vitamin A levels in the food supply with nutrition education and appropriate social marketing that promotes consumption by vulnerable groups within populations cannot be underestimated. Economic development and poverty reduction programmes are likely to improve the socio-economic status and may indirectly contribute to reducing the problem of VAD.

So far this chapter has dealt with only some of the more important nutritionally determined deficiency disorders of public health importance. It is important to recognize that segments of populations in the world suffer from other nutritional disorders such as those due to the deficiency of fluoride, zinc, selenium, B group vitamins, and ascorbic acid. Some of these seem to occur during seasonal deficiencies in their availability and accompany famine and conflict situations when they are seen in refugee camps. It is important to recognize that apart from these specific situations, in all regions of the world there are still some populations affected by one or more of these deficiencies despite the significant advances that have been made in controlling nutritional deficiency disorders. In some regions of the world, largely the result of increasing population size, the numbers of undernourished are increasing even if the population prevalence is declining. In many there is shift in the severity of the deficiency diseases with decreasing numbers with severe deficiency and increasing numbers with mild to moderate deficiencies. For a majority of these countries there is still the need to pursue vigorous policies and targeted action to combat the various nutritional deficiency disorders as a part of the comprehensive health-oriented national food and nutrition policies.

Adult undernutrition

The nutritional world has concentrated for the last 50 years on the vulnerable groups in society (i.e. children, pregnant and nursing mothers, and the elderly) because they were considered to be particularly susceptible to nutritional deficiencies. Now, however, it is becoming apparent that the condition of adult undernutrition has been neglected and this may have profound significance for Third World development. One simple measure of undernutrition in adults is adult weight in relation to height. A United Nations Working Party recommended that BMI, defined as body weight (in kilograms) divided by the square of the height (in metres), may be the most suitable index (James *et al.* 1988). The choice of BMI as the likely objective index for the assessment of nutritional status of adults was based on the observation that BMI was consistently highly correlated with body weight (a proxy for the available energy stores within the body) and was relatively independent of the stature or height of the individual. Adults with a BMI <18.5 are considered to be chronically undernourished and the same BMI cut-offs apply to both males and females (Table 1). These criteria for different degrees of undernutrition, based on BMI, are not only a sensitive index of adult nutritional status but also allow variations in weight in relation to socio-economic status, dietary intakes and seasonal fluctuations in the availability of food in the community to be demonstrated (Shetty and James 1994). Below a BMI of 17.0 considerable impairment of physical well being and exercise capacity are evident with individuals becoming more lethargic and susceptible to illness. The ability to promote and sustain effective agricultural productivity, particularly in rural societies, may therefore be limited by the vigour and well being of the adults on whom the vulnerable in society depend. Thus, it is now important to consider adult undernutrition as well as the problems of childhood.

These anthropometric measures of adult undernutrition as well as childhood malnutrition now provide an opportunity for objective measures of the prevalence of undernutrition worldwide. In practice, children and adults may adapt to a shortage of food by reducing their physical activity without changing their body weight. Thus, measures of the prevalence of low weight-for-height provide only a minimum index of underfeeding; physical activity is fundamental to children's play and exploration and therefore to their mental development. Similarly, in adults physical activity is desirable not only for physiological well-being and for limiting the development of chronic disease but also to allow societies to prosper through physically demanding economic activity and those sound developments that rely on an energetic and enterprising population.

For many years the United Nations has attempted to assess the global prevalence of undernutrition by relating complex measures of food supply and its variable distribution between households with estimates of the population's energy needs. The total number of individuals afflicted with inadequate energy intakes in 87 developing countries of Africa, Latin America, Asia, and the Far East was estimated as 512 million in 1983 to 1985 or 21.5 per cent of the population (FAO 1995). However, a comparison of the numbers of undernourished in Africa alone varies from between 70 million (19 per cent of the population) and 99 million (i.e. 25 per cent of the population) depending on the criteria selected and the cut-off point chosen for adult undernutrition by the same Food and Agricultural Organization, Rome (**FAO**). This was the result of the FAO estimating adult undernutrition for its Fifth World Food Survey (FAO 1985) as those consuming less than either 1.4 or 1.2 times their basal energy needs. Yet it is known that 1.55 times the basal needs is needed for an individual whose lifestyle requires only light physical activity. Using a more generous criterion for undernutrition, namely 'not enough calories for an active working life', the World Bank arrived at a staggering estimate of 730 million or 34 per cent of the population: they supposed that everybody should be moderately physically active. Reliable global estimates of adult undernutrition are now based on objective anthropometric indicators. However, anthropometric sur-

Table 5 Percentage distribution of undernourished adult population

	Adult chronic undernutrition (%)		
	Grade I	Grade II	Grade III
Latin America			
Brazil	4.2	0.9	0.5
Peru	2.6	0.2	0.2
Asia			
China	7.4	3.9	1.0
India	25.7	12.7	10.2
Africa			
Ghana	13.3	3.9	2.8
Morocco	5.4	1.1	0.5
Tunisia	3.0	0.6	0.3

Adapted from Shetty and James (1994).

veys of the nutritional status of adults with objective assessments of the numbers of undernourished adults are rare because the issue of adult undernutrition in the developing regions of the world has also largely been ignored until recently. Table 5 provides some data compiled recently by the FAO for some countries in Asia, Africa, and South America based on the use of BMI (Shetty and James 1994).

Public health initiatives that deal with this malnutrition worldwide have to recognize that the basic causes of malnutrition are clearly political and socio-economic factors. Revolutions in the twentieth century in Russia and China resulted in great improvements in food supplies for the whole population. Agricultural revolutions such as the Green Revolution have also increased food availability and helped meet the food needs of the population. However, poverty is often the basis of a failure to obtain food even when it is available. A recent review by the World Bank (Reutlinger 1982) has emphasized that the most important determinants of hunger in developing countries are personal levels of income and the prices individuals must pay for food. Accelerated food production will alleviate hunger only to the extent that the scarce resources used in the process reduce poverty and lower food prices more than they would if used in other ways. Thus food entitlement decline is a more important force in sustaining poverty and undernutrition than a decline in the availability of food in poor developing societies.

Diet and chronic non-communicable diseases

The evidence relating diet to chronic non-communicable diseases such as cardiovascular disease, NIDDM, and cancers comes from population-based epidemiological investigations and from controlled trials. Animal experiments and *in vitro* tests on tissues have also contributed to our understanding of the relationship between diet and disease. Descriptive population-based epidemiological investigations yield valuable data that lead to important hypotheses, but they cannot be used alone to establish the causal links between diet and disease. The most consistent correlation between diet and chronic diseases have emerged from comparisons of populations or segments of population with substantially different dietary habits. Analytical epidemiological studies, such as cohort studies and case–control studies, that compare information from groups of individuals within a population usually provide more accurate estimates of such associations. It is important to recognize when examining population-based epidemiological data relating diet to disease that every population consists of individuals who vary in their susceptibility to each disease. Part of this difference in susceptibility is genetic. As the diet within a population changes in the direction that measures the risk of the specific disease, an increasing proportion of individuals, particularly those most susceptible to the risk, develop the disease. As a result of this interindividual variability in the interaction of diet with an individual's genetic make-up and therefore the individual's susceptibility to disease, some diet–disease relationships are difficult to identify within a single population. In experimental clinical studies and controlled trials, long exposures may be required for the effect of the diet as a risk factor to be manifest. Strict inclusion criteria for participants may have to be adopted in order to show the effect with small numbers in a reasonable length of time. These in turn may restrict the study to homogeneous samples and thus may limit the applicability of results to the population at large. Despite these limitations, when carefully designed studies show repeated and consistent findings of an association between specific dietary factors and a chronic disease, they generally indicate a cause-and-effect relationship.

Diet and cardiovascular diseases

The most common cardiovascular diseases that are diet-related are CHD and hypertension.

Coronary heart disease

CHD emerged as a burgeoning public health problem in Europe and North America after the Second World War and by the end of the 1950s had become the single major cause of adult death. Although the earliest observation relating diet, plasma cholesterol level, and CHD was made in 1916 it was the approximately fivefold difference in CHD rates among the various developed countries and the intrapopulation variations in rates, by socio-economic class, ethnicity, and geographical location that brought to our attention the dietary basis of CHD. The marked changes in CHD rates in migrant populations that moved across a geographical gradient in CHD risk provided further evidence of the environmental nature of the causative factor, i.e. a change in diet and lifestyle. As the evidence began to mount, the WHO Expert Committee on Prevention of CHD (1982) concluded, after reviewing the existing knowledge, that the data on the relationship between blood cholesterol and the risk of CHD and the relationship of lipids in the diet and blood met the criteria for an epidemiological association to be termed causal. These data were, of course, backed by a plethora of intervention trials in volunteers, clinical studies, and a wide range of animal experiments demonstrating the effects of diet on coronary artery atherosclerosis.

The relationship between dietary factors and CHD was supported by the results of the Seven Country Study (Keys 1980). The saturated fat intake varied between 3 per cent total energy in Japan and 22 per cent in Eastern Finland while the 15-year CHD incidence rates varied between 144 per 10 000 in Japan and 1202 per 10 000 in eastern

Finland. The annual incidence of CHD among 40 to 59-year-old men initially free of CHD was 15 per 100 000 in Japan and 198 per 100 000 in Finland (Keys 1980). Measurement of food consumption by the people in 16 well-defined cohorts in seven countries and its correlation with 10-year incidence rate of CHD deaths provided further support for this causal association. The strongest correlation was noted between CHD and the percentage of energy derived from saturated fat (Fig. 2), whereas total fat was not significantly correlated with CHD.

In the Seven Country Study, the serum total cholesterol values were 165 mg/dl in Japan and 270 mg/dl in eastern Finland, and suggested that the variation in serum total cholesterol levels between populations could be largely explained by differences in saturated fat intake and CHD incidence. On a population basis, the risk of CHD seems to rise progressively within the same population with increases in plasma total cholesterol (Fig. 3). Observational studies suggest that one population with an average total cholesterol level 10 per cent lower than another will have one-third less CHD and a 30 per cent difference in total cholesterol predicts a fourfold difference in CHD (WHO Study Group 1990). The Seven Country Study showed a strong positive relationship between saturated fat intake and total cholesterol level; populations with an average saturated fat intake between 3 per cent and 10 per cent of the energy intake were characterized by serum total cholesterol levels below 200 mg/dl and by low mortality rates from CHD. As saturated fat intakes increased to greater than 10 per cent of energy intake a marked and progressive increase in CHD mortality was noticed.

Several prospective studies have shown an inverse relation between high-density lipoprotein cholesterol (**HDL**) and CHD incidence. However, HDL cholesterol levels are influenced by several non-dietary factors and HDL levels do not contribute to explain differences in CHD mortality between populations; dietary influences on HDL levels are poorly recognized but include the terpenes, such as menthol, found in spices. Their influence on population differences in HDL levels seems, however, to be small. HDL levels are increased by alcohol, slimming, and by physical activity. The role of different unsaturated fatty acids (e.g. monounsaturated and n-3 and n-6 polyunsaturated fatty acids) and their role in the prevention of CHD are unclear.

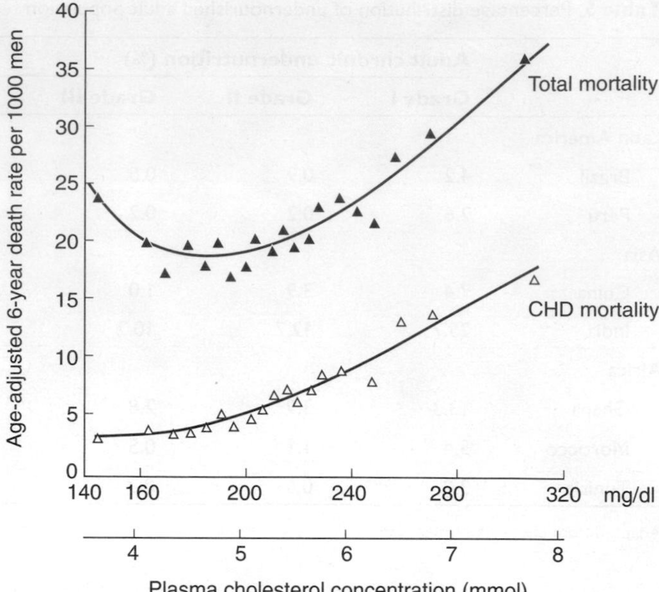

Fig. 3 Within-population relationship between plasma cholesterol and CHD mortality, and between plasma cholesterol and total mortality. (Source: Martin et al. 1986.)

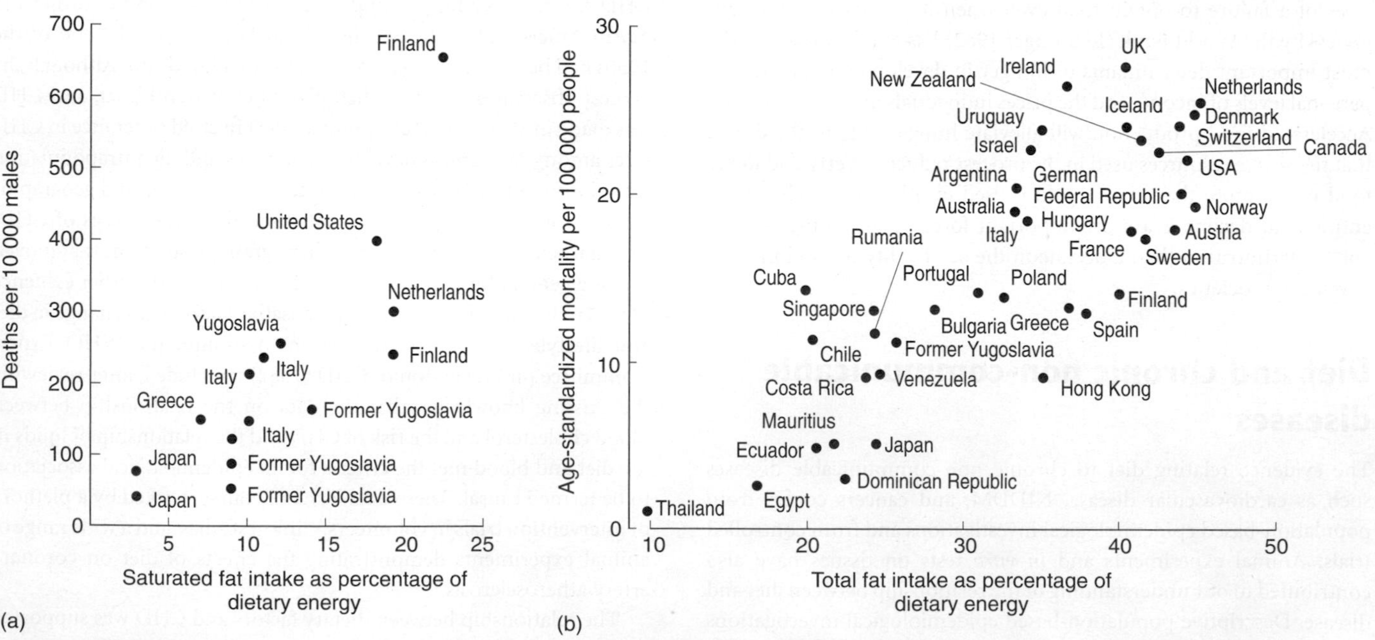

Fig. 2 (a) The association between the saturated fat content of food supply and CHD. More than one data point is shown for some countries because data from more than one year have been used to construct the diagram. (b) The association between total food supply fat content and breast cancer. (Source: WHO Study Group 1990.)

Populations who have high intakes of mono-unsaturated fatty acids (from olive oil) or have diets rich in n-3 polyunsaturates of marine origin (such as Eskimos) also have low CHD rates. There is emerging evidence that some isomers of fatty acids, such as *trans*-fatty acids may contribute to increasing the incidence of CHD by increasing low-density lipoprotein (**LDL**) cholesterol levels, by interfering with essential fatty acid metabolism, and by enhancing the concentrations of the lipoprotein Lp(a), which, in genetically susceptible people, seems to be an additional risk factor through mechanisms that include an antiplasminogen effect to limit fibrinolysis.

Other dietary components (e.g. dietary fibre or complex carbohydrates) seem to influence serum cholesterol levels and the incidence of CHD through complex mechanisms. Population subgroups consuming diets rich in plant foods with a high content of complex carbohydrates have lower rates of CHD; vegetarians have a 30 per cent lower rate of CHD mortality than non-vegetarians and their serum cholesterol levels are significantly lower than that of lacto-ovo-vegetarians and non-vegetarians. Alcohol consumption also reduces the incidence of CHD. A number of observational studies suggest that light-to-moderate drinkers have a slightly lower risk of CHD than abstainers. However, the relationship between alcohol intake and CHD is complicated by changes in blood pressure and also the nature of the alcoholic drink. The presence of phenolic compounds in red wine may contribute to the benefits of drinking red wine as compared with alcohol consumption *per se* in reducing the incidence of CHD.

Of the various risk factors shown in Fig. 4, the risk of CHD in individuals is dominated by three major factors: high serum total cholesterol, high blood pressure, and cigarette smoking (WHO 1982). There is also a synergism between risk factors, with the Japanese notable for their high smoking rates and hypertension but very low cholesterol levels; smoking and hypertension are particularly dangerous in societies and individuals with high cholesterol levels. Body-weight changes induced by dietary and lifestyle changes (e.g. in levels of physical activity) are strongly related to changes in serum total cholesterol, blood pressure, and obesity. Obesity in turn is strongly related to diabetes mellitus, both of which are risk factors for CHD.

There is now general agreement on the strategies that need to be adopted to reduce both the frequency and extent of the risk factors of CHD. The nutritional approach is aimed at reducing obesity, lowering blood pressure, lowering total and LDL cholesterol, and increasing HDL cholesterol. It is possible to adopt a population strategy recommending a range of dietary principles that are likely to facilitate attaining one or more of these objectives. Current recommendations take into consideration both the entire spectrum of cardiovascular risks, including effects on thrombosis as well as providing a holistic approach to recommending a healthy diet that will reduce all chronic, non-communicable diseases, including cancers. These recommendations include lowering total fat intake to between 30 and 35 per cent of total calories, restricting saturated fat intake to a maximum of 10 per cent of total calories, and to increase intakes of complex carbohydrates

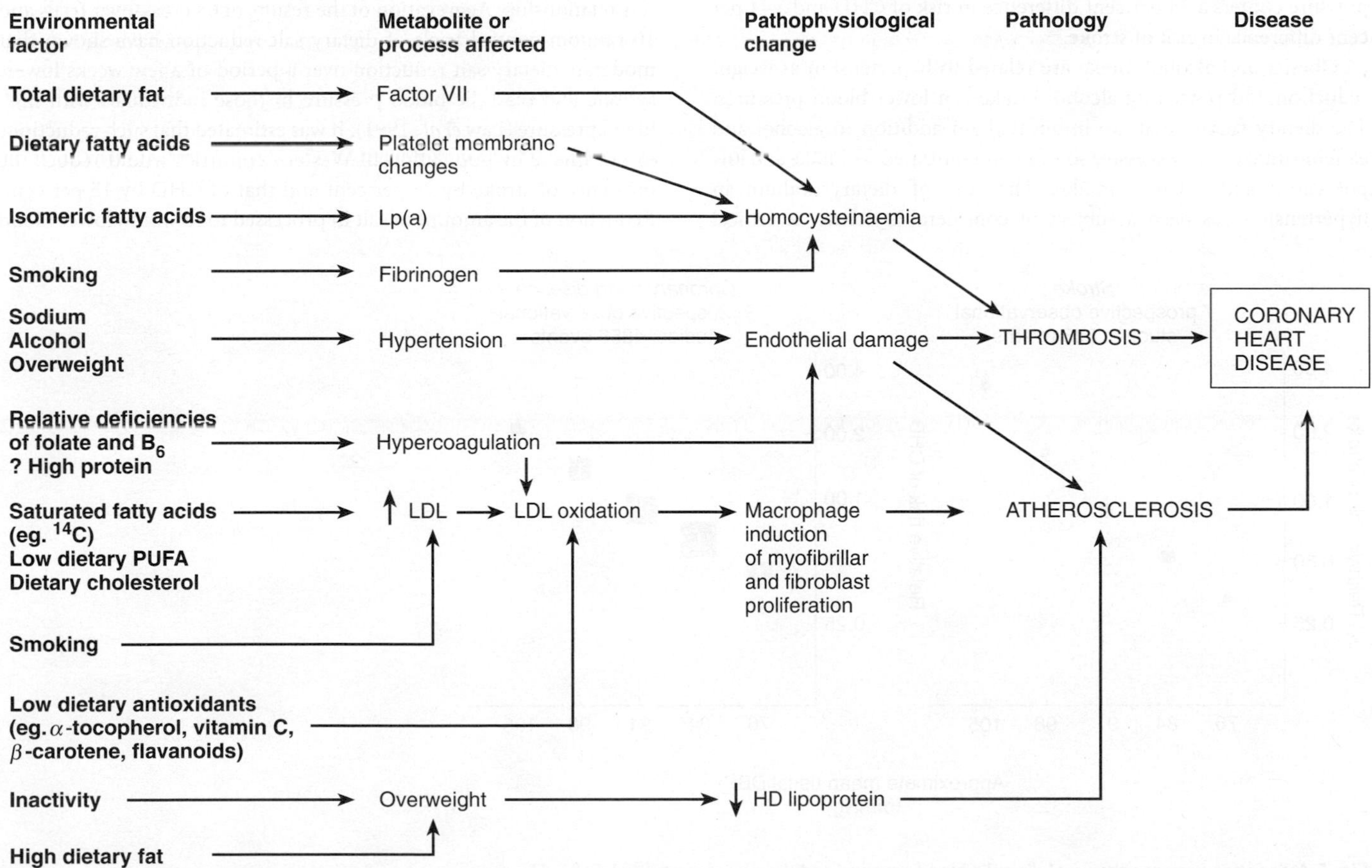

Fig. 4 The multiple dietary factors responsible for the pathophysiological changes leading to CHD. (Source: Scottish Office Home and Health Department 1993.)

or dietary fibre. Translated into food components this would mean reducing in particular animal fat intake and intake from hydrogenated and hardened vegetable oils and increasing the consumption of cereals, vegetables, and fruits.

Considerable controversy continues about the advisability of reducing cholesterol levels either in populations or in individuals, and much harm has been done by public health specialists and cardiologists who adopt a public stance questioning the benefits and highlighting the dangers of dietary change. Yet repeated expert government and WHO reports have consistently advocated a change in Western societies. Law *et al.* (1994) have recently undertaken a further set of meticulous analyses and suggested that dietary change is beneficial even for people in their seventh and eighth decades. Much of the confusion arises because drug trials of cholesterol lowering have been included and this confuses the picture because of increased rates of non-cardiovascular deaths linked to the drug used.

Hypertension and stroke

The risk of CHD and stroke increases progressively throughout the observed range of blood pressure (Fig. 5) based on nine major studies conducted in a number of different countries (MacMohan *et al.* 1990). From the combined data it appears that there is a fivefold difference in CHD and a 10-fold risk of stroke over a range of diastolic blood pressure of only 40 mmHg. Appropriate statistical analysis indicates that a sustained difference of only 7.5 mmHg in diastolic blood pressure confers a 28 per cent difference in risk of CHD and a 44 per cent difference in risk of stroke.

Obesity and alcohol intake are related to hypertension as weight reduction and restricting alcohol intake can lower blood pressures. The dietary factors that are implicated (in addition to alcohol and caffeine intakes) are excessive sodium and saturated fat intake and low potassium and calcium intake. The role of dietary sodium in hypertension has been a subject of considerable debate. A critical review of 27 published studies concluded that there was the relationship between intakes of salt and the prevalence of hypertension (Glieberman 1973). However, in the majority of studies the methods for assessing both dietary sodium and blood pressure were inadequate. The Intersalt study (Intersalt Cooperative Research Group 1988) compared standardized blood pressure measurements with 24-h urinary sodium excretion in 10 000 individuals aged 20 to 59 years in 32 countries and showed that populations with very low sodium excretion (implying low sodium intakes) had low median blood pressures, a low prevalence of hypertension and no increase in blood pressure with age. Although sodium intake was related to blood pressure levels and also influenced the extent to which blood pressures increased with age, the overall association between sodium, median blood pressure, and the prevalence of hypertension was less than significant.

A number of explanations have been put forward to explain why meticulous studies such as the Intersalt study (Intersalt Cooperative Research Group 1988) underestimate the relationship between dietary sodium and blood pressure. These include among others: unreliability of assessing dietary intake of sodium accurately; genetic variability; the contribution of other factors such as obesity and alcohol intake. Recent meta-analysis of published studies have correlated blood pressure recordings in individuals with measurements of their 24-h sodium intake (Law *et al.* 1991) and also seem to suggest that this association increases with age and with the initial blood pressure. The results of intervention trials of sodium restriction also tend to support this relationship. Aggregation of the results of 68 cross-over trials and 10 random control trials of dietary salt reduction have shown that moderate dietary salt reduction over a period of a few weeks lowers systolic and diastolic blood pressure in those individuals with high blood pressure (Law *et al*. 1991). It was estimated that such reductions in salt intake by population in Western countries would reduce the incidence of stroke by 26 per cent and that of CHD by 15 per cent. Reduction of the amount of salt in processed food would lower blood

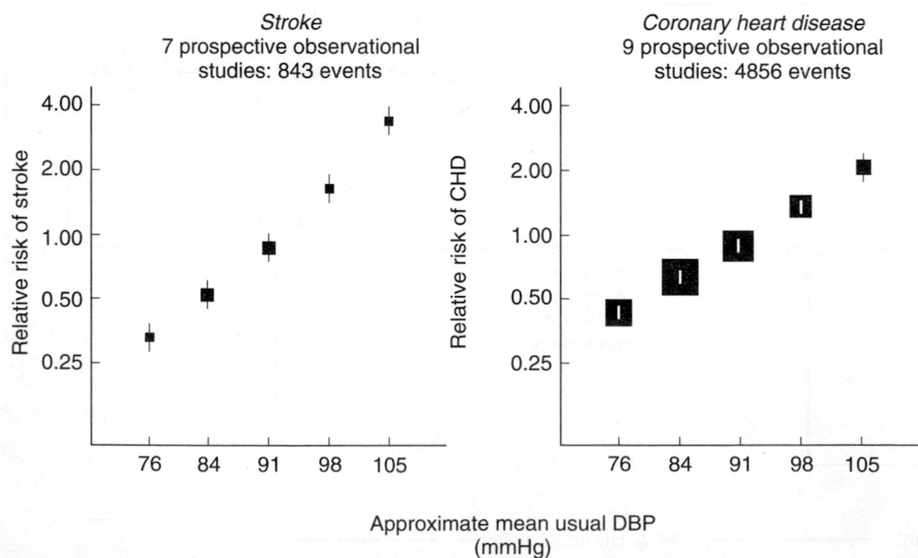

Fig. 5 Association between the usual diastolic blood pressure and the risk of stroke and CHD. The size of the boxes is proportional to the amount of information in each DBP category. The vertical bars denote 95 per cent confidence limits. Values of the mean usual DBP were estimated from later measurements in the Framingham Study. (Source: MacMahon *et al.* 1990.)

pressure even further and would prevent as many as 70 000 deaths per year in the United Kingdom. Results of therapeutic trials of drug therapy also support the fact that the incidence of stroke can be reduced if blood pressure is lowered, although the beneficial effect of lowering the incidence of CHD is lower than expected.

The other dietary component that has been investigated by the Intersalt Study (1988) has been potassium. Urinary potassium excretion, an assumed indicator of intake, was negatively related to blood pressure as was the urinary sodium-to-potassium concentration ratio. It has also been observed that potassium supplementation reduces blood pressure in both normotensive and hypertensive subjects (Cappucio and MacGregor 1991). Some, but not all, cross-sectional and intervention studies suggest a beneficial effect of calcium intake on blood pressure. Epidemiological studies also consistently suggest lower blood pressures among vegetarians than non-vegetarians independent of age and body weight. These studies may also support the role of other dietary components, i.e. vegetarian diets rich in complex carbohydrates are also rich in potassium and other minerals while some unknown components in animal products, possibly protein or fat, may influence blood pressure adversely in well-nourished populations.

Nutritional intervention is likely to reduce the occurrence of hypertension and the consequent complications of stroke and CHD in the community, as vividly demonstrated in Finland where the average blood pressure has fallen by nearly 10 mmHg and the prevalence of hypertension is only a quarter of what it was. In association with population falls in average cholesterol levels, CHD and stroke rates in Finland have fallen dramatically as the population's diet was transformed to change its fat content and to more than double the average vegetable and fruit intakes. The decline in CHD and stroke rates was predominantly dependent on the fall in cholesterol and blood pressure levels, respectively, and these changes occurred despite increasing obesity rates.

Diet and cancers

Although the relationships between specific dietary components and cancers are less well established than that between diet and cardiovascular disease, the overall impact of diet on cancer incidence appears to be significant. It is now widely accepted that one-third of human cancers could relate directly to some dietary component (Doll and Peto 1981) and it is probable that diet plays an important part in influencing the permissive role of carcinogens on the development of many cancers. Thus up to 80 per cent of all cancers may have a link with nutrition.

Evidence that diet is a determinant of cancer risk comes from several sources. These include correlation between national and regional food consumption data and the incidence of cancers in the population. Studies on the changing rates of cancer in populations as they migrate from a region or country of one dietary culture to another have contributed to many important hypotheses. Case–control studies of the dietary habits of individuals with and without a cancer and prospective studies as well as intervention studies have provided evidence for the effects of diet on cancer.

The section below summarizes only those cancers where the role of diet or a nutrient is reasonably well established. Many other cancers in which diet may have a possible role have not been discussed at length as the aim is not to make this section exhaustive and all inclusive.

Cancers of the gastrointestinal tract may be influenced by the diet. The intake of alcohol appears to be an independent risk factor for oral, pharyngeal, and oesophageal cancer. Consumption of salted fish, preserved, and fermented foods containing nitrosamines as weaning foods or from early childhood may introduce a substantial risk of nasopharyngeal cancer. Several studies have demonstrated a positive association between oesophageal cancer and several dietary factors, which include low intakes of vitamins A and C, riboflavin, nicotinic acid, calcium, and zinc. In dietary terms the associations are with low intakes of lentils, green vegetables, and fresh fruits. Like nasopharyngeal cancers, the risk of oesophageal cancers is also positively related to increased intakes of highly salted foods and fermented, mouldy foods containing N-nitroso compounds. Stomach cancer is also associated with diets comprising large amounts of smoked and salt-preserved foods, which may contain precursors of nitrosamines, and low levels of fresh fruit and vegetables, which may contain nutrients that possibly inhibit the formation of nitrosamines. Colon cancer is the third most common form of cancer and the incidence rates are high in western Europe and North America, whereas they are low in sub-Saharan Africa (Boyle *et al.* 1985). Almost all the specific risk factors of colon cancer are of dietary origin. International comparisons indicate that diets low in dietary fibre or complex carbohydrates and high in animal fat and animal protein increase the risk of colon cancer. The original hypothesis of the protective effect of dietary fibre was based on clinical observations. In Southern Africa, for instance, the consumption of large amounts of plant-based foods was associated with the large faecal weight and the virtual absence of large bowel cancer. A hypothesis was then proposed that suggested that increasing intakes of dietary fibre increased faecal bulk and reduced transit time. Later, it has been argued that this mechanism may not be relevant to colorectal carcinogenesis (Kritchevsky 1986). The epidemiological data relating dietary fibre intakes to colorectal cancer are largely equivocal despite the demonstration by several studies of the existence of an inverse relationship between the intake of foods that are rich in dietary fibre and colon cancer risk. The large majority of studies in humans have found no protective effect of fibre from cereals but have found a protective effect of fibre from vegetables and possibly fruits (Willett 1989). Diets rich in fibre are also rich sources of nutrients such as antioxidant vitamins and minerals with potential cancer inhibiting properties. Vegetarian diets seem to provide a protective effect from the risk of colon cancer and the effects may be mediated by intakes of vitamin A and its precursor β-carotene.

Epidemiological studies consistently show that fat intake is positively related to colorectal cancer risk. Energy intakes also seem to be consistently higher in cases with colorectal cancer than in comparison groups and many studies have hitherto failed to show an energy-independent effect of fat intake. More recently Willett *et al.* (1990) have shown, after adjusting for total energy intake, that the consumption of animal fat was found to be associated with increased colon cancer risk. They also demonstrated that the trend in risk was highly significant when the relative risk of different quintiles of fat intake was related to the risk of large bowel cancer. The risk was not, however, associated with vegetable fat but with the consumption of saturated animal fat. The study by Willett *et al.* (1990) thus provided good epidemiological evidence relating the consumption of saturated fat and meat intake as risk factors for colon cancer. Recent case–control studies of Chinese people in North America and China have confirmed that increasing total energy intake and specifically from saturated fat increases the risk of colon cancer (Whittemore *et al.* 1990).

In summary, dietary factors seem to be important determinants of colon cancer risk. An effect of saturated fat intake appears to exist independently of energy intake. Meat intake also increases risk; an effect that may not be independent of saturated fat intake, although it is likely that products of cooking meat may be mutagenic. Dietary fibre from vegetable sources may also be protective and reduce risk, whereas the possible protection from the consumption of cereal fibres seems to be uncertain.

Primary liver cancers have been correlated worldwide with mycotoxin (aflatoxin) contamination of foodstuffs. The primary causal factor for lung cancer, a leading cause of death among men, is cigarette smoking. However, several studies have shown an interactive effect between cigarette smoking and low frequency of intake of green and yellow vegetables rich in β-carotene. In prospective studies, the frequency of the consumption of foods rich in β-carotene has been inversely associated with lung cancer risk. Dietary fats and dietary cholesterol have also been positively associated with lung cancer risk.

Breast cancer is a common cause of death among women both in the United States and in the United Kingdom. Correlation studies have provided evidence of a direct association between breast cancer mortality and the intake of calories and dietary fat, and specific sources of dietary fat such as milk and meat. The evidence for the role of dietary factors in the causation of female breast cancer has been gleaned both from animal experiment studies and a range of epidemiological studies. Cross-cultural ecological studies have provided evidence of the association of fat intake with breast cancer risk (Fig. 2). Neither case–control studies nor prospective studies reported to date provide unequivocal support for the association between fat intake and risk of breast cancer in postmenopausal women. The most recent analysis has found no association between fat intake and intake of dietary fibre and breast cancer risk in either pre- or postmenopausal women (Willett *et al.* 1992). Other dietary factors that may be implicated are vegetable consumption, which may be protective, whereas a modest increase in risk has been consistently seen with increased alcohol intake in women.

International incidence and mortality data generally show a positive correlation of prostate cancer with the incidence of other diet-related cancers. Inter- and intracountry analyses show a positive correlation with total fat intake whereas vitamin A and β-carotene emerge as protective factors. The strength of association between selected foods, food processing, and nutrients in the diet and cancers is summarized in Table 6. The evidence suggests that a high intake of total fat in the diet, more specifically the intake of saturated fats of animal origin are associated with an increased risk of cancers of the colon and breast. Diets high in plant foods, especially green and yellow vegetables and fruits, are strongly associated with a lower incidence of a wide range of cancers, including lung, colon, oesophagus, and stomach. Such diets tend to be low in saturated fat, high in complex carbohydrate and fibre, and rich in several antioxidant vitamins, including vitamin A and β-carotene. Sustained and consistent intake of alcohol is also associated with cancers, in particular those of the upper alimentary tract. Dietary factors thus seem to be important in the causation of cancers at many sites and dietary modifications may reduce cancer risk. However, at present, it is difficult to quantify the contribution of diet to total cancer incidence and mortality.

Although the associations between diet and risk of cancers at various sites are not always conclusive, and the underlying mechanisms poorly understood, the available current evidence can be used to initiate public health strategies to prevent cancer. It seems quite clear that there is a link between fat, particularly saturated fat intake and colon cancer. This is a consistent finding and it can be concluded that if a population were to reduce its intake of fat (both total and saturated), then a reduction in colon cancer, and possibly breast cancer, can be expected. The recommendation is to lower total fat

Table 6 Associations of foods, food processing and nutrients on risk of cancer

	Vegetables, fruits	Cereals, starches, fibre	Meat	Animal fats (total and saturated)	Obesity	Physical Activity	Contaminants in food	Alcohol	Salt and salting	Cooking
Mouth and pharynx	– – –							+++		
Larynx	– –							+++		
Oesophagus	– – –							+++		
Lung	– – –			+		–		+		
Stomach	– – –	–							++	+
Colon and rectum	– – –	–	++	+	+	– – –[a]		++		+
Liver	–						++[b,c]	+++		
Breast	– –	–	+	+	++	–		++		
Bladder	– – –									

Adapted from World Cancer Research Fund (1997).

–, Possible decrease in risk; +, possible increase in risk; – –, probable decrease in risk; ++, probable increase in risk; – – –, convincing decrease in risk; +++, convincing increase in risk.

[a]Colon cancer only.

[b]Grilling and barbecuing.

[c]Aflatoxin contamination.

intake to between 30 and 35 per cent of total energy—a recommendation that is consistent with dietary goals to reduce cardiovascular risk. Another likely preventive measure is to increase the consumption of fruits and vegetables. Innumerable studies have helped conclude that the consumption of higher levels of vegetables and fruits is associated consistently with the reduced risk of cancer in most sites. Vegetables and fruits are exceptional sources of a large number of potentially anticarcinogenic agents including vitamin A and carotenoids, vitamins C and E, selenium, dietary fibre, and a whole range of chemical compounds such as flavonoids, phenols, and plant sterols. Much of their protective effect is unknown or poorly understood. The WHO and the more recent World Cancer Research Fund report (1997) recommends intakes of 400 g/day of fruit and vegetables (excluding potatoes) as a reasonable dietary goal to aim for.

Diet, lifestyles, and obesity

Obesity is one of the most important public health problems and the prevalence of obesity is increasing in the developed, industrialized world. Table 8 summarizes the prevalence rates of obesity among the adults of several countries in the world. Even in developing countries of the Third World, relatively affluent and urbanized communities are showing a rapidly increasing prevalence of obesity among adults.

Being overweight and obese is normally assumed to indicate an excess of body fat. Like adult undernutrition, BMI is used as an indicator of choice to diagnose obesity in adults and Table 7 outlines the diagnostic criteria for overweight and obese infants, children, adolescents, and adults (WHO 1995, 1998). Recent recommendations of the WHO consultation include the suggestion that a BMI of between 18.5 and 24.9 in adults be considered as the appropriate weight for height. A BMI between 25 and 29.9 is indicative of being overweight and possibly a pre-obese state, whereas obesity is diagnosed as BMI >30.0. The main health risk of obesity is premature death due to heart disease and hypertension and other chronic diseases. In the presence of other risk factors (both dietary and non-dietary), obesity increases the risk of CHD, hypertension, and stroke. In women, obesity seems to be one of the best predictors of cardiovascular disease. Longitudinal studies have demonstrated that weight gain, both in men and women, is significantly related to increases in cardiovascular risk factors. Weight gain was strongly associated with increased blood pressure, elevated plasma cholesterol and triglycerides, and hyperglycaemia (fasting and postprandial). The distribution of fat in the body in obesity may also contribute to increased risk. Swedish studies have shown that high waist-to-hip ratios (i.e. fat predominantly in the abdomen and not subcutaneous) increase the risk of heart disease and diabetes, although more recent follow-up over the longer term has not always supported this claim. The coexistence of diabetes among the obese is also an important contributor to morbidity and mortality in obese individuals. Obesity also carries an increased risk of gallbladder stones, breast and uterine cancer in females, and possibly prostate and renal cancer in males. Body-weight increase (with increased BMI) is also associated with increasing mortality in both smokers and non-smokers.

Table 7 Diagnostic criteria for overweight and obesity in infants, children, adolescents, and adults

Infants and children (all ages)	Weight-for-height +2 Z-scores
Adolescents	
Overweight	BMI-for-age 85th percentile
Obese	BMI-for-age 85th percentile of BMI plus Triceps-for-age 90th percentile of TSkf Subscapular-for-age 90th percentile of SSSkf
Adults:	
Normal weight range	BMI 18.5–24.9
Overweight or pre-obese	BMI 25.0–29.9
Obese	
Grade I	BMI 30.0–35.9
Grade II	BMI 35.0–39.9
Grade III	BMI 40.0

Tskf, triceps skinfold; SSSkf, subscapular skinfold.

Adapted from WHO (1995, 1998).

Table 8 Prevalence rates of obesity (BMI 30.0) among adults

Country	Age range (years)	Obesity prevalence (%)	
		Male	Female
USA (1991)	20–74	19.7	24.7
Canada (1991)	18–74	15.0	15.0
England (1995)	16–64	15.0	16.5
Netherlands (1995)	20–59	8.4	8.3
Finland (1991/93)	20–75	14.0	11.0
Sweden (1988/89)	16–84	5.3	9.1
Czechoslovakia (1988)	20–65	16.0	20.0
West Germany (1990)	25–69	17.0	19.0
Australia (1989)	25–64	11.5	13.2
Japan (1993)	20+	1.7	2.7
China (1992)	20–45	1.2	1.6
Brazil (1989)	25–64	6.0	13.0
Kuwait (1994)	18+	32.0	44.0
Saudi Arabia (1990/93)	15+	16.0	24.0
United Arab Emirates (1992)	17+	16.0	38.0

Adapted from WHO (1998).

Several environmental factors, both dietary and lifestyle related, contribute to increase obesity in communities. Social and environmental factors that either increase energy intake and/or reduce physical activity are of primary interest. Changes in the environment that affect the levels of physical activity among children and adults may contribute to the development of obesity. Changes both in the food consumed and the changes in the patterns of eating behaviour may contribute to increased intakes of energy well beyond one's requirements. Increased intake of dietary fat provides energy-dense food, which may not contribute to the efficient regulation of appetite and food intake. Excess fat is more readily stored while fibre-rich complex carbohydrates tend to bulk the meal and limit intakes. International and national comparisons reveal that obesity increases as the fat percentage of calories in the diet increases (Fig. 6). Patterns of eating, particularly snacking between meals and frequent snacks, may contribute to increased intakes. However, overwhelming evidence seems to support the view that much of the energy imbalance that is responsible for the epidemic of obesity in modern societies is largely the result of dramatic reductions in physical activity levels (both occupational and leisure time) when food availability is more than adequate.

Preventive measures to deal with the increasing prevalence of obesity worldwide has to start very early. Primary preventions may have to be aimed at primary school children. This includes nutrition education of children and parents and dealing with problems of school meals, snacking, levels of physical activity, and other issues. Public health initiatives should include attempts to tackle all social and environmental issues that may contribute to the increasing energy and fat intakes and the reducing physical activity levels. As the issues are too complex, attempts have to be made to address issues related to transportation policies, work site facilities for exercise, and several other factors that contribute to this complex problem.

Non-insulin-dependent diabetes mellitus

NIDDM is a chronic metabolic disorder that occurs in middle adulthood and is strongly associated with an increased risk of CHD. NIDDM has to be distinguished from insulin-dependent diabetes as well as from gestational diabetes of pregnancy. Obesity is a major risk factor for the occurrence of NIDDM; the risk being related both to the duration and the degree of obesity. The occurrence of NIDDM in a community appears to be triggered by a number of environmental factors such as sedentary lifestyle, dietary factors, stress, urbanization, and socio-economic factors. Certain ethnic or racial groups seem to have a higher incidence of NIDDM; these include Pima Indians, Nauruans, and South Asians (i.e. Indians, Pakistanis, and Bangladeshis). NIDDM also seems to occur when the food ecosystem rapidly changes, for example urbanization of Australian Aborigines or the adoption of Western dietary patterns by Pima Indians.

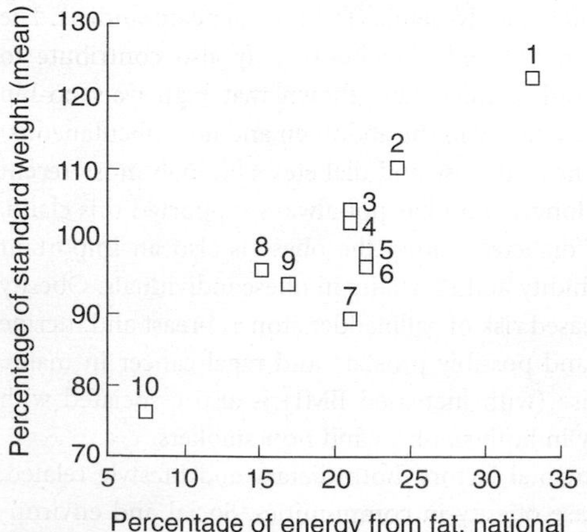

Fig. 6 Percentage of standard adult body weights in relation to national fat consumption figures in 10 countries: 1, Uruguay; 2, Venezuela; 3, Costa Rica; 4, Nicaragua; 5, Honduras; 6, Panama; 7, Malaya; 8, Guatemala; 9, El Salvador; 10, East Pakistan. (Source: Lissner and Heitmann 1995.)

The cause of NIDDM is unclear, but it seems to involve both an impaired pancreatic secretion of insulin and the development of tissue resistance to insulin. Excess weight and obesity, particularly the central or truncal distribution of fat accompanied by a high waist-to-hip ratio and a high waist circumference seems to be invariably present with NIDDM. Hence the most rational and promising approach to preventing NIDDM is to prevent obesity. Weight control is hence of fundamental importance in both a population strategy for the primary prevention of this disorder but is also essential to tackle high-risk individuals in this group. Physical activity also helps improve glucose tolerance by weight reduction and also by its beneficial effects on insulin resistance. Diets high in plant foods are associated with a lower incidence of diabetes mellitus. Vegetarians have a substantially lower risk than non-vegetarians of having NIDDM.

Expert groups have provided dietary recommendations for both the primary prevention of NIDDM, the management of diabetes and the reduction of secondary complications, which include CHD risk and renal, ocular, and neurological complications of diabetes. Prevention of weight gain and reduction of obesity is the key to minimizing the prevalence of NIDDM and its attendant complications and risks. Increasing levels of physical activity also help. The specific dietary recommendations include providing diets with carbohydrates providing 55 to 60 per cent of energy, maximizing content of complex carbohydrates and dietary fibre (maximize to 40 g of fibre) and reduction of simple sugar intakes. In addition, the general recommendations for fat (total fat more than 30 per cent calories, and saturated fat less than 10 per cent of calories) are also emphasized due to the associated high risk of CHD in individuals with NIDDM. The factor of prime importance is to achieve and maintain a desirable body weight and, if possible, to prevent weight gain in the first place.

Diet and osteoporosis

The increase in numbers of elderly in the populations of the developed world has seen an increase in health problems of the elderly, which affects their quality of life. Fracture of the hip is an important health problem, particularly among postmenopausal women. Fractures occur in the elderly following what appear as relatively trivial falls when there is osteoporosis and the density of the bone is reduced. Bone density increases in childhood and adolescence and reaches a peak at about 20 years of age. Bone density falls from menopause in women and from about the age of 55 years in men. The variation in bone density between individuals is large and of the order of ±20 per cent. As bone density declines with increasing age, those that attain high levels of peak bone mass at the end of adolescence and retain higher levels of bone density during adulthood become osteoporotic with advancing age much more slowly than those with lower bone densities to start with. Hence the range of factors that influence the attainment of peak bone density may play a crucial part in the development of osteoporosis and the occurrence of fractures as age advances.

Several factors determine the onset of osteoporosis; they include the lack of oestrogen in postmenopausal women, degree of mobility, smoking, and alcohol intake. Calcium intake is a likely dietary determinant that may contribute to the onset and degree of osteoporosis. Evidence from some countries, such as Yugoslavia, tends to indicate that the osteoporosis of bones that predisposes to fractures may be diet related as the fracture rate is halved among individuals in the higher calcium intake range as compared with those on low calcium diets. However, there are regions where the lower rates of fracture due to osteoporosis are associated with lower calcium intakes. For example, the rates are lower in Singapore as compared with the United States, although the calcium intakes are lower than the United States. The traditional emphasis on calcium intakes possibly reflects the recognition of its importance in contributing to the density of bone during growth and the need for attaining dense bones at the peak of adult life. High protein and high salt diets are known to increase bone loss, whereas calcium supplements, well above what may be considered physiological, in postmenopausal women, may help to reduce the rate of bone loss and slow down the development of osteoporosis.

It is generally believed that populations in developing countries are at less risk of developing osteoporosis. This is in spite of low calcium intakes, and it may be related to the fact that they do more physical work, smoke less, drink less alcohol, and have diets that are generally not high in protein or salt content. However, osteoporosis is seen in developing countries in regions where low intakes of dietary calcium are associated with high fluoride intakes. No osteoporosis occurs if high intakes of fluoride are accompanied by dietary intakes of calcium, which are also high.

Diet and dental caries

Dental caries is a common disease of the teeth that results in decay of the tooth surface, usually beginning in the enamel. An essential feature in the causation of dental caries is dental plaque, which is largely made up of microorganisms. Dietary sugars diffuse into the dental plaque where they are metabolized by the microorganisms to acids, which can dissolve the mineral phase of the enamel causing dental decay. The process is, however, much more complex and is related to the quantity and quality of saliva produced in the mouth among other factors.

The evidence relating diet to dental caries is vast and has been well reviewed (Rugg-Gunn 1993). The overwhelming evidence indicates that sugars are cariogenic. There is good correlation between the sugar supply (in grams per person per day) and the occurrence of dental caries in 12 year olds when data from 47 countries were compiled (Sreebny 1982). The consumption of refined sugar is a recent phenomenon in many parts of the world and seems to have been accompanied by an increase in dental caries in communities that were hitherto free of the problem. Fifty-five cross-sectional studies correlating an individual's sugar consumption with the incidence of dental caries has demonstrated significant correlations between the two, particularly among young children. It also appears that the consumption of sugars between meals is associated with a marked increase in caries while consumption of sugars with meals is associated only with a small increase. Sucrose seems to be the predominant dietary agent that is cariogenic, although the current emphasis is on the consumption of all free sugars, particularly between meals. Despite suggestions that starch is also cariogenic, careful analysis of epidemiological data from several countries suggests that a much closer relationship exists between dental caries and free sugars than between caries and starchy cereal foods. Fresh fruit, although it contains intrinsic sugars, has a lower cariogenic potential while fruit juices are cariogenic, which may be related to the added sugars in fruit juices or from the lack of adequate salivary stimulation. Food may also contain protective factors that may prevent the occurrence of dental caries. This includes a sufficient daily ingestion of fluoride. Inorganic phosphates in the diet also seem to protect against dental caries.

Prevention of dental caries can be achieved by health education aimed at the individual, beginning in infancy. Avoidance of the addition of free sugars to bottle feeds and milk and fruit drinks are a must. An adequate intake of fluoride is desirable quite early in life. During childhood and adolescence, the restriction of the three major sources that contribute to two-thirds of our intake of sugars (i.e. confectionery, table sugar, and soft drinks) will help reduce the increment of caries in childhood. At local and national level, the main public interventions should include fluoridation of water supply, labelling of foods, and possible changes in agricultural policies that promote the production of free sugars.

Diet and non-cancerous conditions of the large bowel

There are several chronic disorders of the large bowel that are frequently associated with a typical 'affluent' diet, which is low in dietary fibre content. This includes diverticular disease, haemorrhoids, and constipation. Constipation occurs when the daily faecal weight falls below 100 g and is associated with slower intestinal transit times. A linear relationship has been demonstrated between non-starch polysaccharide intake in the diet and mean daily stool weights. There is now evidence that the starch content of the diet, particularly if it is cooked and refrigerated after cooking, seems to influence faecal weights and transit times. Thus increasingly both the non-starch polysaccharide and starch intakes reduce the chances of constipation.

Emerging food and nutrition issues of public health concern

Over the last decade several issues of public health concern related to food and nutrition have emerged both in the developed, industrialized West and in developing societies of the world. These include the problems related to the microbiological safety of foods, the frightening prospect of an epidemic of spongiform encephalopathies, concerns related to genetically modified (GM) foods, issues related to labelling of processed foods, and the emerging epidemic of diet-related chronic diseases and obesity in developing societies. Some of these issues will be dealt with briefly in this section.

Food safety

Food safety refers to whether food is safe for human consumption and hence lacking in biological and chemical contaminants that have the potential to cause illness. The increasing concern over the safety of foods in the developed world is a paradox in that the epidemiological evidence on the safety of foods is quite contrary to the perceptions of the public and the media that the food available now is less safe than it used to be. The improvements in public health have virtually eradicated primarily food-borne infections that were until recently associated with considerable morbidity and mortality. The common food-borne diseases currently encountered are usually associated with mild self-limiting gastroenteritis. Studies of risk perception suggest that the public becomes alarmed by health threats that are disproportionate to the actual risk associated with the disease and this public concern is fuelled by the media, which make health issues into media health scares depending on the newsworthiness of the incidents.

There have been several food-borne epidemics in the developed world that have raised concerns about food safety in recent years. These include, for instance, the *Salmonella enteritidis pt4* (*Se4*) epidemic. This was attributed to the ability of *Se4* to invade the oviduct of poultry and get deposited in the albumin of the egg. At the consumer level the outbreak of the infection was linked to the use of raw egg in recipes or cross-contamination from raw to cooked foods. *Campylobacter* infection is the most common food-borne disease in the United Kingdom and the increase in its incidence may partly be explained by the better ascertainment and reporting of cases associated with this infection. The more recent food scare was the emergence of *Escherichia coli 0157* in Scotland. The emergence of this food-borne infection that caused several deaths include changes in husbandry and the movement of livestock as well as the rapid growth of the fast food industry and poor food hygiene in these environments. *Listeria* is another cause of food-borne disease, which is a good example of the role of international trade and globalization in the spread of food-borne diseases.

In the developing world the issues of food safety are related to microbiological agents that contaminate food and water and spread disease rapidly in the warm humid environments of these countries aided by the improper food hygiene practices, poor environmental sanitation, and inadequate regulation of food-related commerce. The safety of foods in the developing world is also compromised by the presence of toxins such as aflatoxins, which result from contamination with mycotoxins due to poor food storage practices or due to cyanogens in the diet due to inadequate preparation of staple foods such as cassava. In addition, the food chain in these poor countries is contaminated by pesticide and chemical residues thus compromising the safety of the food consumed by the populations in these countries.

Food, the bovine spongiform encephalopathy epidemic, and Creutzfeldt–Jakob disease

The most recent public health concern related to food in the United Kingdom and Europe has been the epidemic of bovine spongiform encephalopathy (**BSE**) with about 170 000 cases diagnosed among cattle by 1998 and the likelihood of over a million cattle having been infected with the causative agent, with most of them slaughtered and eaten before they showed clinical signs of the disease. The concern among consumers was the probability of the link between BSE and the new variant of Creutzfeldt–Jakob disease (**nvCJD**) due to the infection of humans with the agent responsible for the epidemic of BSE in cattle in the United Kingdom. The key risk factor identified in the case of BSE was the use of commercial concentrate feed and, in particular, the feeding of meat and bone meal as a protein-rich dietary supplement to calves. In the 1980s, largely the result of commercial pressures, changes were made in the rendering process of waste tissues of cattle and sheep. As a result, it is likely that a strain of scrapie (a transmissible spongiform encephalopathy endemic in British sheep) may have crossed from sheep to cattle in the meat and bone meal and adapted itself to infect cattle. An alternate explanation is that the infective agent of BSE was endemic at a low level and that the recycling of rendered waste from cattle allowed it to spread more widely and cause the epidemic in cattle. Whatever the probable cause the changes in the rendering process and the recycling of waste for feed created the right environment for an epidemic of disease to occur among cattle. The consumption of the meat of infected cattle is probably responsible for the increase in incidence of CJD which was diagnosed in young adults and teenagers as nvCJD. Epidemiological evidence strongly links the BSE epidemic with the increasing incidence of nvCJD, although it is not clear given the long incubation period of the disease what the extent of the epidemic is likely to be in the future. BSE and nvCJD are good examples of changes in the food chain influencing the infective process, which is likely to be food-borne, and resulting in considerable controversy and consumer pressure to regulate the food industry more tightly.

Genetically modified foods

Another issue that has emerged over recent years and has created a considerable degree of controversy is the use of biotechnology to produce GM foods. Genetic modification of food crops can be used to reduce food losses by increasing resistance to drought, frost, diseases, and pests, and help control weeds and reduce postharvest losses. Biotechnology can improve the nutritional value of foods, for example, by increasing protein or micronutrient content or by reducing saturated fat content. They could help slow down ripening so that foods retain their quality much longer. Biotechnology can increase both the yield and the quality of crops grown on existing farmland and thereby reduces pressure on wildlife habitats. In the developed world, particularly in the United Kingdom and Europe, the opposition to GM foods is based largely on ecological arguments that raise concerns regarding the ecological damage that may follow large-scale use of GM crops. In the poor, developing countries the concerns are more related to the use of the 'terminator gene' technology and the dependence on the large multinationals for seeds and chemicals that the small farmers will inherit. At the heart of this controversy and the raging debate is the gulf between plant breeders, seed, and agrochemical industries who promote biotechnology and the campaigners who argue that GM technology may have hazardous consequences on the environment. This is a debate replete with numerous paradoxes (Dixon 1999) and the climate of mistrust, some of it associated with the not too recent BSE and nvCJD scare, is obscuring the real issues and clouding objective decisions from being made with regard to the production and consumption of GM foods.

Food labelling

An important source of information for the consumer about the food on the supermarket shelf is the label on a food product. Food labels provide information that may be of interest to the consumer, especially with regard to the added chemicals (additives, pesticide residues, colouring and flavouring agents, and preservatives), fats, sugars, and energy content. Although, about two-thirds of shoppers claim to read the information on the labels of new or unfamiliar food products to check their contents, this interest in labels does not mean that consumers always understand the information on the labels. Consumers are even more confused by the nutrition information panel that appears on many food labels.

Food label information is usually designed by experts. A prototype label produced by the Codex Alimentarius Commission of the WHO–FAO which is the organization charged with advising on international food standards. This prototype is followed by Food Standards Committees around the world. According to this prototype the nutrients (energy, carbohydrate, protein, and fats) are listed according to their amounts per serving and per 100 g. Most consumers, however, have hardly any idea of what a 100-g serving is, or for that matter what a normal or average serving is. A further problem is that these labels designed by experts is also beset with problems of terminology. An example is the term 'carbohydrate' that covers a wide range of compounds, including sugars and starches, which have quite different health-related properties. Health benefits or nutritional claims are also not meant to be part of the food labels and they also do not provide information to cover ecological and ethical issues, which may be of concern for some consumers. More recently, the need to highlight the source or origin of foods and in particular the labelling of GM sources of the food product has been a serious concern of consumers. Food labelling is an important issue of public health concern and despite the considerable progress made so far there is much to be achieved.

Functional foods

New food products are being marketed as health-enhancing or illness-preventing foods. These are called functional foods, 'pharma-foods', 'nutriceuticals', or novel foods. Functional foods are generally defined as food products that deliver a health benefit beyond providing nutrients. The health benefits of functional foods may be conferred by a variety of production and processing techniques that include: fortification of certain food products with specific nutrients, using phytochemicals and active micro-organisms, and by genetic modification of foods. The topic of functional foods is complex and controversial. An assumption implicit in the functional foods and health benefit claims is that the food supply needs to be fixed or doctored (or medicalized) on public health grounds. The assumption, therefore, is that the current food supply is in some way deficient, that the habitual diets are inadequate, and that a technological fix will solve the problem. Thus the emerging debate viewed from the perspective of the proponents of functional foods is that these novel foods may reduce health care expenditure by promoting good health and that functional foods are a legitimate nutrition education tool, which will help inform consumers of the health benefits of certain food products. The opponents on the other hand rightly state that it is the total diet that is important for health. They believe that the functional foods are a 'magic bullet' approach, which enables manufacturers to indulge in marketing hyperbole, exploit consumer anxiety, and essentially blur the distinction between food and drugs.

Emerging epidemic of diet-related chronic diseases and obesity in developing societies

One of the important issues that is of considerable public health concern in developing countries is the emerging epidemic of diet-related chronic diseases and obesity in the midst of the persisting problem of malnutrition among children and adults. This burgeoning problem of obesity and adult-onset chronic diseases such as CHD, hypertension, and NIDDM and an increase in the incidence of certain cancers is determined by a range of factors that include changes in the diet and lifestyles. Most developing countries, particularly those in rapid developmental transition are in the midst of a demographic and epidemiological transition. Economic development and industrialization is accompanied by rapid urbanization. These developmental forces are bringing about both changes in the social capital of these societies as well as increasing availability of food and changing lifestyles. The changes in food and nutrition are both quantitative and qualitative; there is not only access to more than adequate food among some sections of the population, but also a qualitative change indicative of an increase in fat intake. Lifestyle changes are suggestive of a reduction in physical activity levels, which promote the onset of obesity. Urbanization by migration, economic growth, and the globalization of trade is increasing income disparities, which further contributes to the problem. The poor consumer resistance and inadequate regulation compromises food safety and increases contaminants in the food chain. All these factors contribute in a complex manner to fuel the epidemic of diet-related non-communicable diseases that are likely to emerge as a serious public health problem in the twenty-first century.

Food and nutrition in the prevention of diseases of public health importance

The public health approach to the prevention of nutrition and diet-related diseases requires the adoption of health-oriented nutrition and food policies for the whole population. In most developing countries, the first priority must be ensuring the production or procurement of adequate food supply and its equitable distribution and availability to the whole population along with the elimination of the various forms of nutritional deficiencies, which include protein–energy malnutrition, and vitamin, mineral, and trace-element deficiencies. Efforts must also be made to improve the quality of the food, which includes ensuring food safety while reducing spoilage and contamination of foods as well as diversifying the availability and use of foods. In agrarian societies, consideration must be given to the short- and long-term effects of agricultural policies that affect the income and buying power of the small producers. Particular attention needs to be paid to the impact the promotion of cash crops has on the availability and ability to procure the principal staples in the diet. Special attention needs to be paid to the feasibility of fortification of foods to deal with localized or widespread deficiencies of iodine and iron, as a mass intervention measure.

In developed countries, the burgeoning costs of tertiary health care related to the diagnosis and management of the increasing occurrence and the associated morbidity of chronic diet-related diseases has had an impact. There is an increasing recognition of the need for prevention-oriented health and nutrition policies and changes in behaviour and lifestyle to reduce the occurrence of these diseases. Some developed countries have been active in the field of public education using national dietary guidelines as a major stimulus. It is important to remember that nutrition education of the public operates in the area where advice is given on a balance of probabilities, rather than irrefutable evidence or any degree of certainty. There is bound to be information that does not fit in with the consensus view as the consensus is based on the balance of the available evidence. It is thus possible to apparently appear to refute the expert viewpoint, which often seems to be a popular thing to do. It is important to recognize that the causes of these chronic diseases are complex and dietary factors are only a part of the explanation. Individuals differ in their susceptibility to the adverse health effects of specific dietary factors or deficiencies of others. Within the context of public health the focus is the health of the whole population and interventions are aimed at lowering the average level of risk to the health of the whole population.

Changes in consumer preferences have emerged, initially among the upper socio-economic and educated masses. The media attention, along with the behavioural changes in food preferences and food choices are in turn influencing the industry in the modification of the systems for food production and processing. However, progress in changing consumer behaviour and preferences is by its nature intrinsically rather slow and has until recently largely occurred without support from public policies in any but the health sector. The process of changing unsatisfactory dietary practices and thus promoting health is not easy to achieve both socially and politically. Despite these limitations the occurrence of and mortality associated with some diet-related chronic diseases such as CHD have declined reflecting possible changes in lifestyles of the population.

The dynamic relationship between changes in a population's diet and changes in its health is reflected well in two critical situations. One is the changes in disease and mortality profiles of migrant populations moving from a low-risk to a high-risk environment. An example of this is the change in disease pattern of the Japanese migrants to the United States. The other more important and rapid change is seen within a country as rural to urban migration occurs or more frequently as a developing country undergoes rapid industrialization and economic development and in the process acquires a dietary change characteristic of the latter and also the disease, morbidity, and premature mortality profile of a developed country. Several other developing countries have urban pockets of affluent diet and lifestyles and similar disease burdens in the midst of problems typical of a poor developing country. Such countries in transition, such as India and Brazil, bear the dual burdens of diseases of affluence and the widespread health problems of a poor country. Developing countries can hence benefit by learning from the experience of dietary change and adverse health effects characteristic of the developed world. In the former countries the aim should be to avoid the diseases and premature deaths related to the affluent diet and lifestyle. By recognizing this problem, governments of developing countries can gain for their people the health benefits of avoiding nutritional deficiencies without encouraging at the same time the development of diet-related non-communicable diseases that invariably accompany economic and technological development.

It is thus possible for a country to achieve a reduction in infant and childhood mortality and an increase in life expectancy by means of the pursuance of health and nutrition policies that aim to provide adequate and equitable access to hygienic and nutritious food and to minimize at the same time the occurrence of diet-related chronic diseases. This in turn will help avoid the social and economic costs of morbidity and premature death in middle age—a period of highest economic activity and productivity to the nation and to society at large. If such a socially and economically desirable goal is to be achieved, then national governments in both developing and developed countries must aim towards achieving a population-based dietary change by providing suitable dietary guidelines (WHO Study Group 1990). In the pursuance of this objective, the FAO and WHO jointly convened a consultation in 1995, the overall purpose of which was to establish the scientific basis for developing and using food-based dietary guidelines (**FBDGs**) (FAO–WHO 1996).

The development of food-based dietary guidelines

FBDGs are developed and used in order to improve the food consumption patterns and nutritional well-being of individuals and populations. Guidelines would be needed by all countries given the important part that food and dietary practices play in nutrition-related disorders; both due to deficiencies or excesses. FBDGs can address specific health issues without the need to understand fully the biological mechanisms that may link constituents of food and diet with disease. However, FBDGs do take into account the considerable epidemiological data linking specific food consumption patterns with a low or high incidence of certain diet-related diseases.

Disseminating information and educating the public through the FBDGs is a 'user-friendly' approach as consumers think in terms of foods rather than nutrients. They provide a means for nutrition education mostly as foods for the public. They are intended for use by individual members of the general public, are written in ordinary language, and, as far as possible, avoid the use of technical terms in nutritional science. FBDGs will vary with the population group and has to take into account the local or regional dietary patterns, practices, and culture. It is important to recognize that more than one dietary pattern is consistent with good health. This will enable the development of food-based strategies that are appropriate for the local region and take the local dietary practices into consideration.

FBDGs can serve as an instrument of nutrition policies and programmes. As they are based directly on diet and health relationships of particular relevance to the individual country or region, they can help address those issues of public health concern, whether they relate to dietary insufficiency or dietary excess. Food and diet are not the only compone000nts of a healthy lifestyle and it is important that other relevant messages related to health promotion are integrated into dietary guidelines.

References

ACC–SCN (1997). *Third report on the world nutrition situation* . Sub-Committee on Nutrition, WHO, Geneva.

Arroyave, G., Mejia, L.A., and Aguilar, J.R. (1981). The effect of vitamin A fortification of sugar on serum vitamin A levels of pre-school Guatemalan children: a longitudinal evaluation. *American Journal of Clinical Nutrition* , **34**, 41–9.

Barker, D.J.P. (1995). Fetal origins of coronary heart disease. *British Medical Journal*, **311**, 171–4.

Boyle, P., Earidze, D.G., and Simans, M. (1985). Descriptive epidemiology of colo-rectal cancer. *International Journal of Cancer*, **36**, 9–18.

Briend, A. and Golden, M.H.N. (1993). Treatment of severe child malnutrition in refugee camps. *European Journal of Clinical Nutrition*, **47**, 9–18.

Burgi, H., Supersaxo, Z., and Selz, B. (1990). Iodine deficiency diseases in Switzerland one hundred years after Theodor Kocher's survey. A historical review with some new goitre prevalence data. *Acta Endocrinologia*, **123**, 577–90.

Callender, J., Grantham-Mcgregor, S., Walker, S., and Cooper, E. (1993). Developmental levels and nutritional status of children with trichuris dysentery syndrome. *Transactions of the Royal Society for Tropical Medicine and Hygiene* , **87**, 528–9.

Cappucio, F.P. and MacGregor, G.A. (1991). Does potassium supplementation lower blood pressure? A meta-analysis of published trials. *Journal of Hypertension* , **9**, 465–73.

de Onis, M., Monteiro, C., Akre, J., and Clugston, G. (1993). The worldwide magnitude of protein-energy malnutrion: an overview from the WHO Global database on child growth. *Bulletin of the World Health Organisation*, **71**, 703–12.

de Onis, M., Blossner, M., and Villar, J. (1998). Levels and patterns of intrauterine growth retardation in developing countries. *European Journal of Clinical Nutrition*, **52**, S5–15.

Dixon, B. (1999). The paradoxes of genetically modified foods. *British Medical Journal*, **318**, 547–8.

Doll, R. and Peto, R. (1981). *The causes of cancer.* Oxford University Press.

FAO (1985). *The fifth world food survey 1985.* Food and Agricultural Organization, Rome.

FAO (1995). *Dimensions of need: an atlas of food and agriculture.* Food and Agricultural Organization, Rome.

FAO–WHO (1996). *Preparation and use of food-based dietary guidelines* . World Health Organization, Geneva.

Glieberman, L. (1973). Blood pressure and dietary salt in human populations. *Ecology of Food and Nutrition*, **2**, 143–56.

Golden, M.H.N., Briend, A., and Grellety, Y. (1995). Report of a meeting on supplementary feeding programmes with particular reference to refugee populations. *European Journal of Clinical Nutrition*, **49**, 137–45.

Grantham-McGregor, S. (1995). A review of studies of the effect of severe malnutrition on mental development. *Journal of Nutrition*, **125**, 2232S–8S.

Hetzel, B.S. (1987). Progress in the prevalence and control of iodine deficiency disorders. *Lancet*, **ii**, 266–7.

Intersalt Cooperative Research Group (1988). Intersalt: an international study of electrolyte excretion and blood pressure. *British Medical Journal* , **298**, 920–4.

James, W.P.T., Ferro-Luzzi, A., and Waterlow, J.C. (1988). Definition of chronic energy deficiency in adults. Report of Working Party of IDECG. *European Journal of Clinical Nutrition*, **42**, 969–81.

Keys, A. (1980). *Seven countries: A multivariate analysis of death and coronary heart disease.* Howard University Press, Cambridge, MA.

Khanum, S., Ashworth, A.H., and Huttly, S.R.A. (1994). Controlled trial of three approaches to the treatment of severe malnutrition. *Lancet*, **344**, 1728–32.

Kritchevsky, D. (1986). Diet nutrition and cancer. The role of fibre. *Cancer*, **58** (Supplement 8), 1830–6.

Law, M.R., Frost, C.D., and Wald, N.J. (1991). By how much does dietary salt reduction lower blood pressure? *British Medical Journal*, **302** , 811–24.

Law, M.R., Wald, N.J., and Thompson, S.G. (1994). By how much and how quickly does reduction in serum cholesterol concentration lower rate of ischaemic heart disease ? *British Medical Journal*, **302**, 811–24.

Lissner, L. and Heitmann, B.L. (1995). Dietary fat and obesity: evidence from epidemiology. *European Journal of Clinical Nutrition*, **49**, 969–81.

McKeown, T. (1976). *The modern rise of population.* Edward Arnold, London.

MacMohan, S., Peto, R., Cutler, J., *et al.* (1990). Blood pressure, stroke and coronary heart disease. *Lancet*, **335**, 65–774.

Martin, M.J., Hulley, S.B., Browner, W.S., *et al.* (1986). Serum cholesterol, blood pressure and mortality: implications from a cohort of 361 662 men. *Lancet*, **ii**, 933–6.

Muhilal, P.D., Idjrodinata, Y.R., and Karyadi, D. (1988). Vitamin A fortified monosodium glutamate and health, growth and survival of children: a controlled field trial. *Americal Journal of Clinical Nutrition*, **48**, 1271–6.

Pharoah, P.O.D. and Connolly, D.C. (1987). A controlled trial of iodinated oil for the prevention of endemic cretinism: a long term follow-up. *International Journal of Epidemiology*, **16**, 68–73.

Pollit, E. (1991*a*). Effects of diet deficient in iron on the growth and development of preschool children. *Food and Nutrition Bulletin*, **13**, 110–18.

Pollitt, E. (1991*b*). Iron deficiency and cognitive function. *Annual Review of Nutrition*, **13**, 521–37.

Reutlinger, S. (1982). World Bank research on the hunger dimension of the food problem. *Research News, World Bank*, pp. 3–4.

Rugg-Gunn, A.J. (1993). *Nutrition and dental health.* Oxford University Press.

Scottish Office Home and Health Department (1993). *The Scottish diet: report of a working party to the Chief Medical Officer in Scotland.* The Scottish Office, Edinburgh.

Shetty, P.S. (1994). Assessing malnutrition in the community. *The Biochemist*, **16**, 21–4.

Shetty, P.S. and James, W.P.T. (1994). *Body mass index: an objective measure for the estimation of chronic energy deficiency in adults.* FAO Food and Nutrition Paper. Food and Agricultural Organization, Rome.

Sreebny, L.M. (1982). Sugar availability, sugar consumption and dental caries. *Community Dentistry: Oral Epidemiology*, **10**, 1–7.

Stephenson, L.S., Latham, M.C., Adams, E.J., Kinoti, S.N., and Pertet, A. (1993). Physical fitness, growth and appetite of school boys with hookworm, *Trichuris trichuria,* and *Ascaris lumbricoides* infections are improved four months after a single dose of albendazole. *Journal of Nutrition*, **123**, 1036–46.

Stoltzfus, R.J., Chwaya, H.M., Tielsch, J.M., Schulze, K.J., Albonico, M., and Savioli, L. (1997). Epidemiology of iron deficiency anaemia in Zanzibari schoolchildren: the importance of hookworms. *American Journal of Clinical Nutrition*, **65**, 153–9.

UNICEF (1997). *State of the world's children.* UNICEF, New York.

Viteri, F.E. (1997). Iron supplementation for control of iron deficiency in populations at risk. *Nutrition Reviews*, **55**, 195–209.

Waterlow, J.C. (1992). *Protein-energy malnutrition.* Edward Arnold, London.

West, K.P. and Sommer, A. (1985). Delivery of oral doses of vitamin A to prevent vitamin A deficiency and nutritional blindness. *Food Reviews International*, **1**, 355–418.

Whittemore, A.S., Wu-Williams, A.H., Lee, M., *et al.* (1990). Diet, physical activity and colorectal cancer among Chinese in North America and China. *Journal of the National Cancer Institute*, **82**, 915–26.

WHO (1991). *Prevention of childhood blindness.* World Health Organization, Geneva.

WHO (1995). *Physical status: the use and interpretation of anthropometry* . World Health Organization, Geneva.

WHO (1997). *World health report.* World Health Organization, Geneva.

WHO (1998). *Obesity: Preventing and managing the global epidemic.* Report of a WHO Consultation on obesity. World Health Organization, Geneva.

WHO Expert Committee (1982). *Prevention of coronary heart disease* . Technical Report Series. World Health Organization, Geneva.

WHO Study Group (1990). *Diet, nutrition and the prevention of chronic disease.* WHO Technical Report Series 797. World Health Organization, Geneva.

WHO–UNICEF–ICIDD (1993). *Micronutrient Deficiency Information System (MDIS). Global prevalence of iodine deficiency disorders.* MDIS Working paper. Joint WHO–UNICEF–ICIDD publication.

Willett, W.C. (1989). The search for causes of breast and colon cancer. *Nature*, **338**, 389–94.

Willett, W.C., Stampfer, M.J., Colditz, G.A., Rosner, B.A., and Speitzer, F.E. (1990). Relation of meat, fat and fibre intake to the risk of colon cancer in a prospective study among women. *New England Journal of Medicine*, **323**, 1664–72.

Willett, W.C., Hunter, D.J., Stampfer, M.J., ***et al.*** (1992). Dietary fat and fibre in relation to role of breast cancer. *Journal of American Medical Association*, **268**, 2037–44.

World Cancer Research Fund (1997). *Food, nutrition and the prevention of cancer: a global perspective.* World Cancer Research Fund and American Institute for Cancer Research, Washington, DC.

2.6 Infectious agents

David Heymann

> Illness and death from infectious diseases can in most cases be avoided at an affordable cost. It is in the interest of all that these obstacles to development be removed. Because of drug resistance, increased travel and the emergence of new diseases, there may only be a limited time in which to make rapid progress.
>
> Dr Gro Harlem Brundtland, Director-General (WHO 1999)

The infectious disease situation at the end of the twentieth century

Introduction

Throughout history, human populations have experienced major epidemics of infectious diseases, often resulting in large numbers of deaths, panic, disruption of trade, and political instability. At the same time, the majority of infectious disease mortality has been caused by endemic diseases such as malaria, tuberculosis, HIV, acute respiratory infections, acute diarrhoeal diseases, and measles—a phenomenon that continues today. While all infectious diseases have the potential to spread, it is the rapid nature of the spread of those with epidemic potential and their high mortality rate in newly affected populations that attracts the greatest attention.

Infectious diseases are termed endemic when they have a stable pattern of occurrence in a given population. Epidemics are defined as the occurrence of an infectious disease greatly in excess of expectation. Some endemic diseases cause epidemics if they spread to unprotected or previously unexposed populations, witnessed by a recent and highly fatal outbreak of cholera which caused well over 3000 deaths after its reintroduction into Latin America in 1991. Endemic diseases can also become epidemic when the mode of transmission changes, especially in the event of nosocomial outbreaks of initially endemic diseases such as hepatitis B. At the same time, many diseases now labelled endemic in certain populations have begun with severe exponential epidemics, becoming endemic only after the highly susceptible risk populations had become infected, thus leaving future risk populations to perpetuate transmission at a lower rate. The HIV epidemic is an example of an infectious disease that has become endemic in some countries and geographic areas while in others it still reaches and causes epidemics in previously unexposed populations.

International public health movements of the late nineteenth century identified the issues of poverty, overcrowding, and poor sanitation as providing fertile ground for infectious diseases, especially in urban areas. Despite these discoveries, the development of effective treatments and vaccines in the first two-thirds of the twentieth century led to erroneous hopes that most infectious disease mortality would be greatly decreased, if not eradicated. But the interrelationship between poverty, health, and development remains a major factor in the continuing threat of infectious diseases. Up to 45 per cent of deaths in low-income countries during 1998 are thought to have been due to an infectious disease, while worldwide 48 per cent of premature deaths (those under the age of 45 years) are thought to have an infectious aetiology (Fig. 1).

The fight against infectious diseases worldwide is therefore far from won. Since the early 1990s, the international public health community has been warning against a fatal complacency which is costing millions of lives every year (13.3 million out of a worldwide total of almost 54 million deaths in 1998), most among the poorest of the poor. Populations remain permanently at risk of the recurrence of epidemics which can to a certain extent be predicted, but also of new pathogens whose occurrence and impact on human health are not known. A good example is influenza, which is an ever-present threat. The last pandemic (defined as a disease which is epidemic worldwide) of highly virulent influenza is thought to have killed over 20 million people within a year, in 1918 to 1919. Another global pandemic of a highly virulent strain of influenza is foreseen, but its timing cannot be predicted. If it occurs, it will spread more rapidly than before owing to increasing and more rapid international travel, and it will have the potential to kill a larger number of people. A similar scenario cannot be excluded with yellow fever in central and western Africa, or malaria and dengue in areas where the diseases are not yet endemic. At the same time, the potential impact of newly identified infectious agents is a subject of continued epidemiological study.

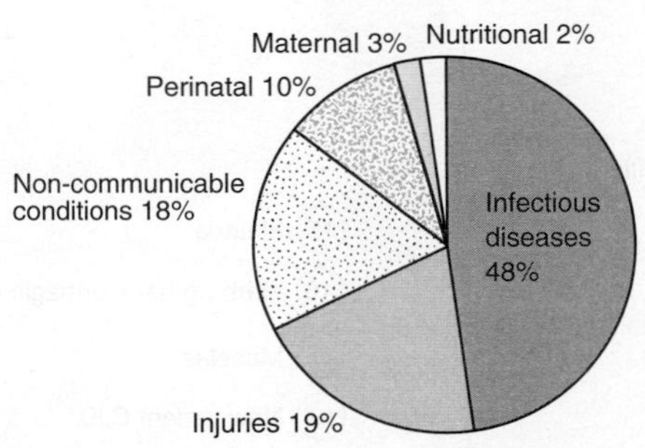

Fig. 1 Premature deaths in low-income countries.

Emerging and re-emerging infections

Over the past three decades, over 30 emerging infections have been newly identified in humans. They range from the Marburg, Ebola, and nipah viruses to the more common rotavirus, hepatitis C virus, and HIV. During this same time period, known infections such as tuberculosis, diphtheria, cholera, meningitis, dengue, yellow fever, and plague have re-emerged.

The term emerging infection, first widely used in the early 1990s, refers to newly identified and previously unknown infectious agents that cause public health problems either locally or internationally. The term re-emerging infection refers to infectious agents that have been known for some time, had fallen to such low levels that they were no longer considered public health problems, and are now showing upward trends in incidence or prevalence worldwide. The number of emerging and re-emerging infectious agents appears to have increased during the past 30 years, while infectious diseases known for centuries continue to cause a heavy burden of suffering, disability, and death.

Emergence and re-emergence of infectious agents have occurred throughout the world, and there have been dramatic reversals in formerly positive trends in infectious disease control, as well as many unexpected outbreaks (Fig. 2).

By 1995 the problem of infectious diseases had become so politically important that the World Health Assembly, health ministers representing the 191 member countries of the World Health Organization (**WHO**), urged all countries to strengthen surveillance of infectious diseases in order to detect re-emerging infectious diseases promptly, to identify emerging infections, and to respond more appropriately to both epidemic and endemic infectious diseases.

Re-emerging infections—reversals in trends

During a 3-year period in the early 1990s, a major epidemic of diphtheria occurred in the newly independent states of Eastern Europe. Whereas in 1980, Europe had accounted for less than 1 per cent of diphtheria cases reported worldwide, it reported almost 90 per cent of cases in 1994. The newly independent states have also reported a dramatic increase in sexually transmitted infections over the past decade, where there has been a 15 to 30 per cent increase in syphilis reported between 1989 and 1995, with rates in the Russian Federation increasing by 40 per cent.

The number of reported cholera cases increased nearly 100 per cent in 1998 as compared with 1997, on all continents. Africa was the most affected, with 72 per cent of the global total and 29 countries reporting cases out of a total of 74 worldwide (Fig. 3). In the Americas, the number of cases had declined up to 1997 after the disease had re-emerged along the Peruvian coastline in 1991, but another resurgence was recorded in 1998. Cholera caused by *Vibrio cholerae* 01 biotype *eltor*, a strain which first appeared in Indonesia in 1961, has now spread worldwide, causing major epidemics. In 1992, *V. cholerae* 0139 was first detected in the Bay of Bengal and has since been identified in 10 other Asian countries.

Epidemic meningococcal meningitis is highly transmissible and has a high case-fatality rate. The disease is characterized by severe

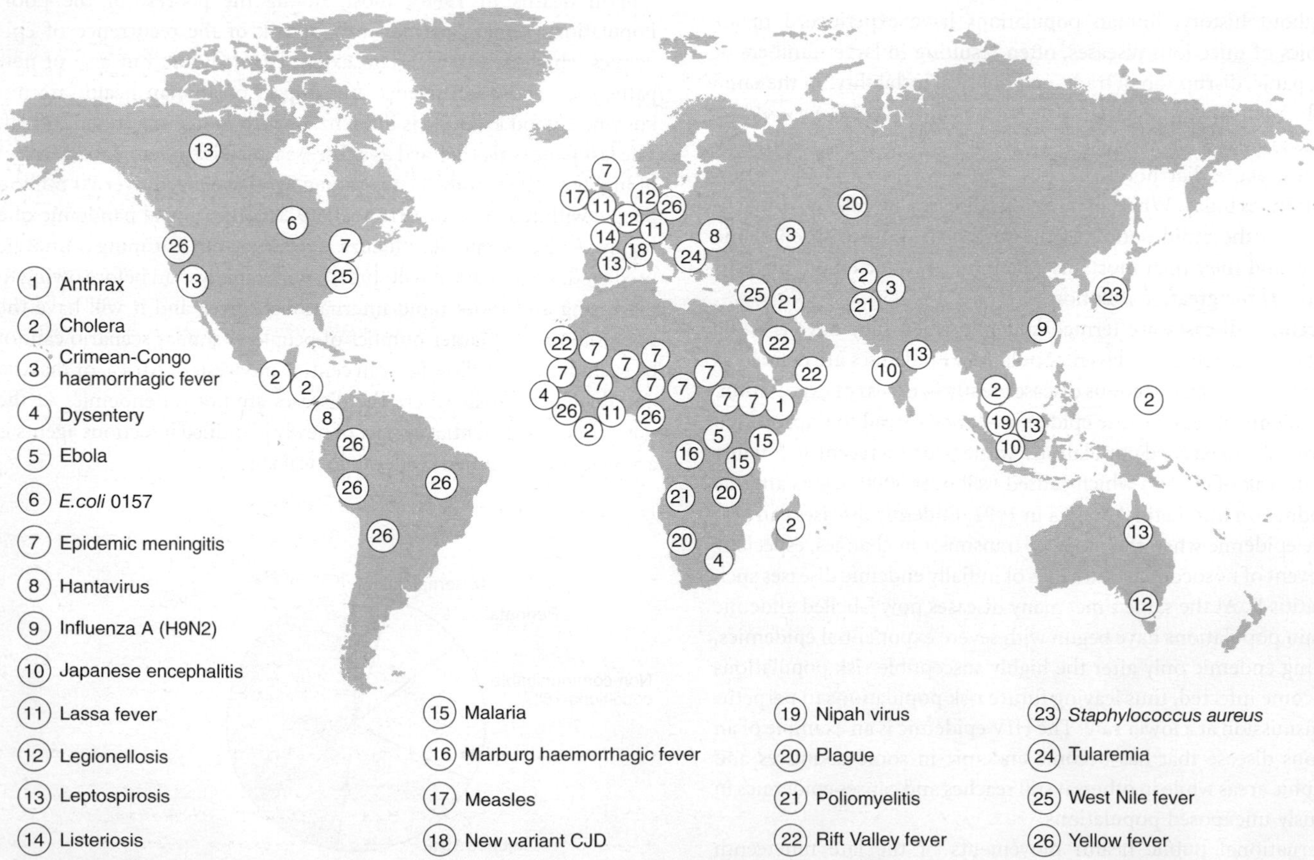

Fig. 2 Recent unexpected outbreaks of infectious diseases.

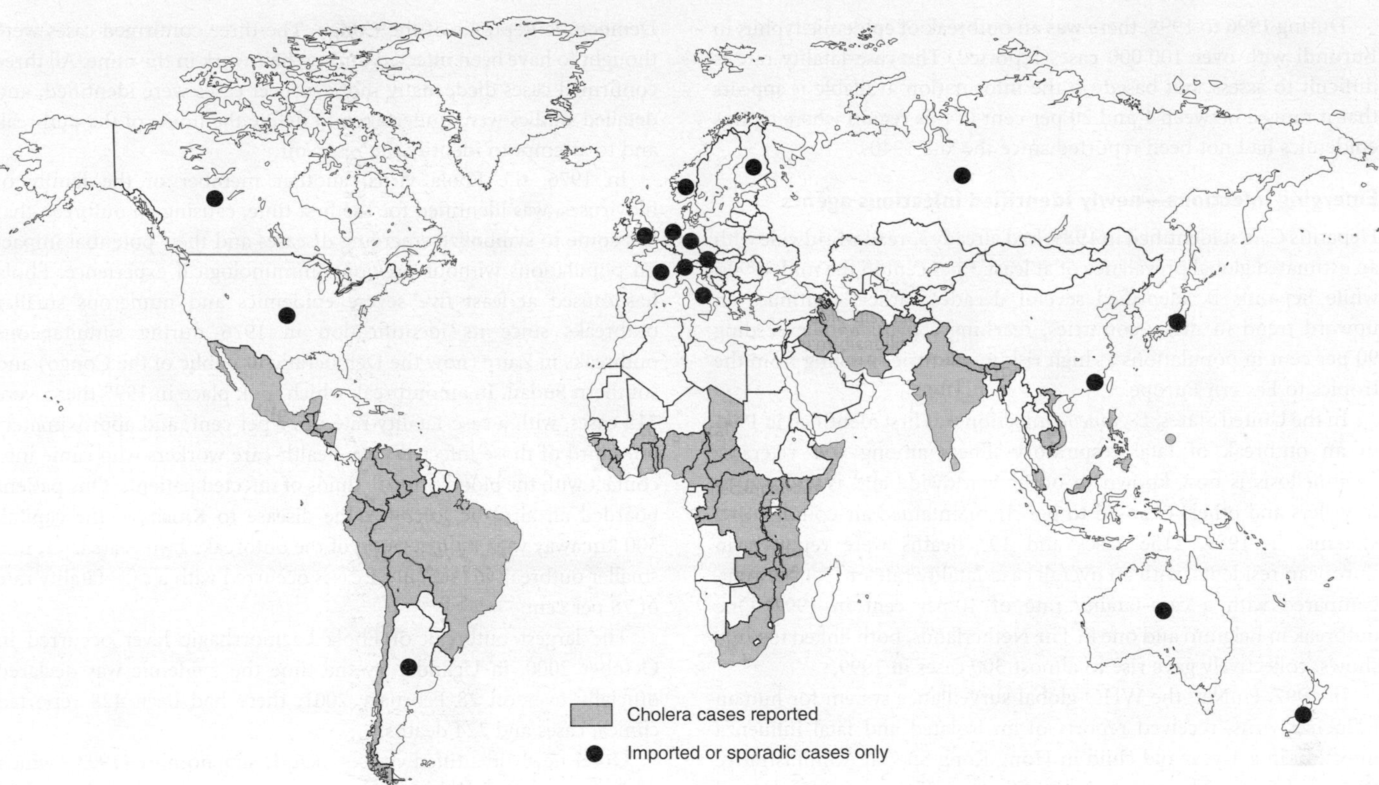

Fig. 3 Countries/areas reporting cholera in 1998.

recurring epidemics which devastate communities. While epidemic meningitis strikes people of all ages all over the world, the countries most at risk are in sub-Saharan Africa where the infection primarily affects young children. In 1997 to 1998, over 300 000 cases of meningococcal disease were reported to the WHO from the African meningitis belt, which stretches from Ethiopia to Senegal, and includes all or part of at least 15 countries, with an estimated population of 300 million.

Over the past 40 years, the number of reported cases of dengue/dengue haemorrhagic fever has increased 20-fold to nearly 515 000 in the period 1990 to 1998 when compared with the previous 9-year

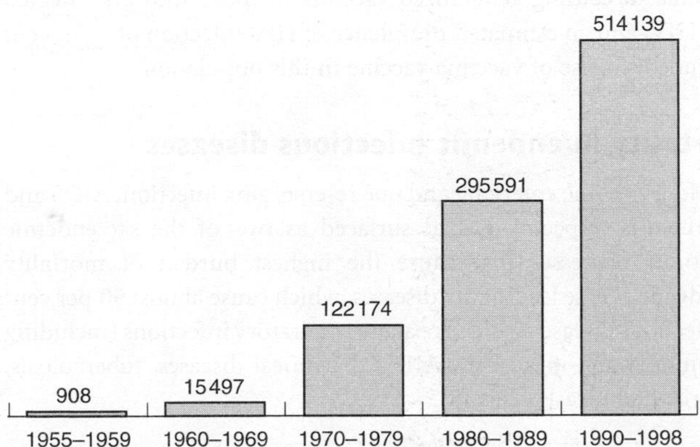

Fig. 4 Increase in average number of dengue cases reported annually, 1995 to 1998.

period (Fig. 4). Regions most affected were Latin America and south-eastern Asia.

Between 1990 and 1998, 11 countries in Africa (Benin, Burkina Faso, Cameroon, Côte d'Ivoire, Gabon, Ghana, Kenya, Liberia, Nigeria, Senegal, Sierra Leone) reported 9370 cases and 1707 deaths from yellow fever, while 1698 cases and 794 deaths were reported from six countries/areas in Latin America (Bolivia, Brazil, Colombia, Ecuador, French Guiana, and Peru).

Japanese encephalitis is the most important form of viral encephalitis in Asia, thought to cause at least 50 000 cases of clinical disease and 10 000 deaths each year, mostly among children. The high case-fatality rate and frequent neuropsychiatric sequelae in survivors make Japanese encephalitis a considerable public health problem in many Asian countries. Close to 3 billion people are now living in Japanese encephalitis endemic regions. In recent decades, outbreaks of Japanese encephalitis have occurred in several previously non-affected areas, and a small outbreak was recently reported from islands in the Torres Strait off the Australian mainland.

Epidemics of rodent or human plague have continued to occur during the past 30 years. In 1994, for example, human plague reappeared in Malawi, Mozambique, and India—after a 15- to 30-year absence. The total number of human plague cases reported to the WHO by 14 countries in 1997 was 5419, of which 274 were fatal. This represented an increase over 1996, when 3017 cases were notified from these same countries, and considerably exceeded the average annual of 1920 cases, 168 deaths for the previous 10 years. Over the last decade, 72 per cent of cases and 79 per cent of plague deaths were reported from Africa.

During 1996 to 1998, there was an outbreak of epidemic typhus in Burundi with over 100 000 cases reported. The case-fatality rate is difficult to assess, but based on the information available it appears that it ranged between 1 and 20 per cent in this region where typhus epidemics had not been reported since the late 1940s.

Emerging infections—newly identified infectious agents

Hepatitis C, first identified in 1989, had already spread worldwide with an estimated global prevalence of at least 3 per cent in the mid-1990s; while hepatitis B, identified several decades earlier, continues an upward trend in many countries, reaching a prevalence exceeding 90 per cent in populations at high risk in countries ranging from the tropics to Eastern Europe.

In the United States, *Legionella* infection was first identified in 1976 in an outbreak of fatal respiratory illness among war veterans. Legionellosis is now known to occur worldwide and is a threat to travellers and others exposed to poorly maintained air-conditioning systems. In 1999, 2136 cases and 193 deaths were reported in European residents, with an overall case-fatality rate of 13.1 per cent, compared with a case-fatality rate of 10 per cent in 1997. One outbreak in Belgium and one in The Netherlands, both linked to trade shows, collectively gave rise to almost 300 cases in 1999.

In 1997, FluNet, the WHO global surveillance system for human influenza virus, received reports of an isolated and fatal influenza infection in a 3-year-old child in Hong Kong Special Administrative Region of China. The virus was identified as influenza A (H5N1), and was associated with epidemics of avian influenza with high fatality rates in live poultry markets. By the end of 1997, a total of 18 human infections had been confirmed, 6 (33 per cent) of which were fatal. Twelve of the 18 developed complications of which seven were severe pneumonia. In 1999, FluNet received reports of another new influenza virus, A (H9N2), isolated from two human cases in Hong Kong, and no further spread was known to have occurred.

In 1996, the occurrence in the United Kingdom of 10 cases of an apparently new variant of Creutzfeldt–Jakob disease was linked to the epidemic of bovine spongiform encephalopathy among cattle. As of the end of September 2000, at least 84 people in the United Kingdom, one in Ireland, and three in France have contracted variant Creutzfeldt–Jakob disease. Accurate prediction of the future number of variant Creutzfeldt–Jakob disease cases is not possible, but the possibility of a significant and perhaps geographically diverse epidemic occurring over the next two decades cannot be excluded.

Since first being recognized as a human pathogen in 1982, enterohaemorrhagic *Escherichia coli* has gained increasing importance as a human pathogen. The best known serotype, *E. coli* 0157 H7, has been responsible for recent large food-borne outbreaks in Japan, Scotland, and the United States, placing heavy demands on medical and public health response systems while causing major political concern about food safety.

Unquestionably one of the most important emerging infections is HIV. First identified in the early 1980s, it has rapidly spread worldwide, affecting over 33 million people. The epidemic characteristics of HIV at the end of the twentieth century are described below.

The Marburg virus, a member of the filovirus family, was first recognized in 1967 when laboratory workers in Germany were infected by handling monkeys imported from Uganda. Since then, there have been reports of sporadic cases in 1975, 1980, and 1987. The most recent outbreak took place in 1999 amongst gold miners in the Democratic Republic of the Congo. The three confirmed cases were thought to have been infected during their work in the mine. All three confirmed cases died, many more suspect cases were identified, and detailed studies were undertaken to define the limits of the outbreak and to attempt to identify the reservoir.

In 1976, the Ebola virus, another member of the family of filoviruses, was identified for the first time, causing an outbreak that has come to symbolize emerging diseases and their potential impact on populations without previous immunological experience. Ebola has caused at least five severe epidemics and numerous smaller outbreaks since its identification in 1976 during simultaneous outbreaks in Zaire (now the Democratic Republic of the Congo) and southern Sudan. In an outbreak which took place in 1995 there were 315 cases, with a case-fatality rate of 77 per cent, and approximately one-third of those infected were health-care workers who came into contact with the blood or body fluids of infected patients. One patient boarded an airplane, carrying the disease to Kinshasa, the capital, 500 km away with no extension of the outbreak. Two years later, in a smaller outbreak in Gabon, 61 cases occurred with a case-fatality rate of 78 per cent.

The largest outbreak of Ebola haemorrhagic fever occurred in October 2000, in Uganda. By the time the epidemic was declared officially over on 28 February 2001, there had been 428 reported clinical cases and 224 deaths.

Other newly identified viruses include sine nombre (1993), which caused an outbreak of hantavirus pulmonary syndrome in the United States (50 cases, case-fatality rate over 75 per cent), Hendra virus, first identified in Australia in 1994, and nipah virus, first identified in 1999 and responsible for 155 confirmed cases in Malaysia.

Interaction of emerging and known infectious diseases

The interaction of infectious diseases is dynamic and at times synergistic, best exemplified in the interaction of endemic infectious diseases with HIV. The increase in active pulmonary tuberculosis and its role as an HIV-associated infection is a prime example. Another example is leishmaniasis, where dual infection with HIV causes increased visceral dissemination and severity. A further example is an extensive outbreak of human monkeypox in 1996 to 1997 in the Democratic Republic of the Congo. Prior to HIV, vaccination with vaccinia would have been the intervention of choice to prevent a continued epidemic. Vaccinia vaccine is now known to have the potential of causing generalized vaccinia in those who are infected with HIV, and an estimated prevalence of HIV infection of 7 per cent precluded the use of vaccinia vaccine in this population.

Mortality in endemic infectious diseases

By mid-1999, one emerging and one re-emerging infection, AIDS and tuberculosis respectively, had surfaced as two of the six endemic infectious processes that cause the highest burden of mortality worldwide. These leading six diseases, which cause almost 90 per cent of infectious disease deaths, are acute respiratory infections (including pneumonia and influenza), AIDS, diarrhoeal diseases, tuberculosis, malaria, and measles (Fig. 5).

Acute respiratory infections

Acute respiratory infections are estimated to have caused approximately 3.5 million deaths in 1998, 99 per cent of which occurred in

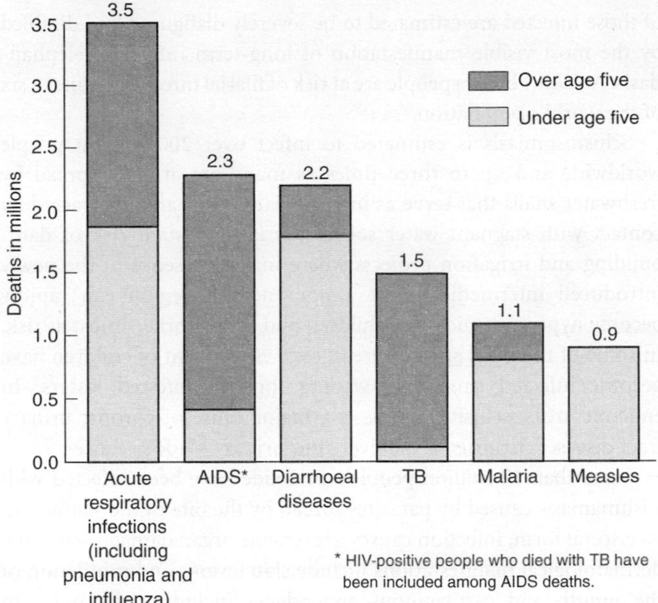

Fig. 5 Leading causes of death from infectious diseases in all ages worldwide, 1998.

developing countries, among children aged under 5 years. Pneumonia causes more childhood deaths than any other infectious disease process, mostly in children with low birth weight or those whose immune systems are weakened by other diseases or malnutrition. Exposure to smoke from indoor cooking fires likewise appears to be a major risk factor for pneumonia in children. Leading infectious agents causing childhood pneumonia are *Streptococcus pneumoniae* and *Haemophilus influenzae* type B.

There is very little information available on mortality from influenza in developing countries. However, in the United States alone, it is estimated that influenza kills 10 000 to 40 000 people in an average influenza season, mostly infants and adults aged over 60 years. During the 1968 influenza season, over 40 000 influenza deaths were recorded in another industrialized country, France, in the space of 2 months.

AIDS

By the end of 1999, 33.6 million people were living with HIV/AIDS worldwide; during 1999, 5.6 million people (including 570 000 children aged under 15 years) became infected.

By the end of 2000, it was estimated that a total of 21.8 million adults and children (including 3 million in 2000) had died because of HIV/AIDS since the beginning of the epidemic. During 2000, 5.3 million (including 600 000 children aged below 15 years) became infected. HIV infections are now almost equally distributed between men and women, with an estimated 18.2 million men aged 15 to 49 years living with HIV/AIDS. HIV/AIDS continues to spread in all regions of the world. The positive sign of a decrease in new infections in sub-Saharan Africa is offset by the increase in AIDS morbidity and mortality. Many African countries are experiencing the full impact of the epidemic, including its economic and demographic consequences. Epidemics of HIV infections continue to occur among injecting drug users in eastern Europe. An increasing number of HIV-positive people can, however, live longer and healthier lives due to antiretroviral therapies.

Asia continues to have relatively low prevalence rates. There are an estimated 6 million adults and children living with HIV/AIDS in Southeast Asia.

In 1999, Eastern Europe and Central Asia have seen the sharpest increase in HIV infections. Most of the 360 000 people living with HIV/AIDS in these countries have been infected through injecting drug use.

Diarrhoeal diseases

Diarrhoeal diseases are estimated to have caused approximately 2.2 million deaths during 1998, the majority of which took place among children under 5 years of age living in developing countries. The most common cause is infection with rotavirus, often occurring at the time of weaning. Death is a result of dehydration. Other causes of diarrhoeal disease include cholera, shigellosis, salmonellosis, *E. coli*, yersiniosis, giardiasis, campylobacteriosis, and enteroviruses other than rotavirus. In addition to its high mortality rates, diarrhoeal disease imposes heavy nutritional waste on children under 5 years of age who survive infection, especially in deprived areas where sanitation is poor, hygiene inadequate, and drinking water unsafe.

Tuberculosis

During 1999 there were an estimated 8.4 million new cases of tuberculosis—up from 8 million in 1997—adding to the estimated 2 billion people worldwide with latent tuberculosis infection. This rise is due largely to a 20% increase in incidence in African countries most affected by the HIV/AIDS epidemic (WHO 2001). Tuberculosis accounts for 2.3% of the global burden of disease (WHO 2000), and is among the most common causes of death in young women.

Co-infection with HIV significantly increases the risk of developing tuberculosis (Raviglione *et al.* 1997). Countries with a high prevalence of HIV, particularly those in sub-Saharan Africa, have witnessed a profound increase in tuberculosis, with reported incidence rates increasing two- or threefold in the 1990s (WHO 2001).

As for other infectious diseases, the poor and marginalized in developing countries are the worst affected: 95 per cent of all cases and 99 per cent of all tuberculosis deaths occur in developing countries, where 75% of cases are in the most economically productive age group (15 to 54 years old).

Malaria

Estimates of malaria mortality for 1998 suggest that approximately 3000 people died each day of the year from malaria, mostly due to *Plasmodium falciparum*. Three out of four of those who died from malaria were children, who are at great risk of cerebral manifestations. One of the sequels of repeated malaria infections is chronic anaemia, mostly affecting women and children. Of the estimated 1.1 million malaria deaths in 1998, most occurred in sub-Saharan Africa, where malaria accounts for almost one in five of all childhood deaths. Worldwide, over 275 million malaria infections are thought to have occurred in 1998. Women are especially vulnerable to malaria infection during pregnancy when infection is associated with an increase in spontaneous abortions, stillbirths, and low-birth-weight babies.

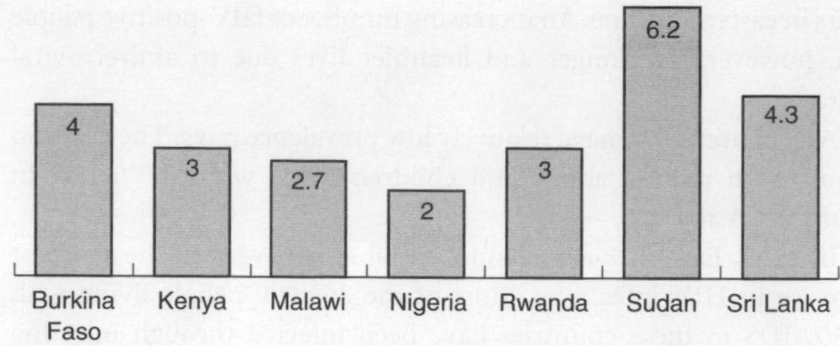

Fig. 6 Estimated average number of working days lost by adults for one episode of malaria (best available data).

Measles

The measles virus is among the most infectious pathogens known. Although great progress has been made in measles prevention because of a vaccine with an over 95 per cent efficacy, it remains a major cause of childhood mortality in developing countries, where it is thought to have caused approximately 900 000 deaths during 1998. Most at risk are young children who are protected during the first 9 to 12 months of life by placentally passed measles antibody, but who rapidly become susceptible to infection after its disappearance.

The high mortality from these six infectious diseases is an obstacle to economic development. Factors related to these diseases are also obstacles to development. The AIDS epidemic alone has left over 8 million orphans who must often depend on society for support. Families risk high debt through lost earnings and high health-care costs, trapping them in a vicious circle of poverty and ill health. One tuberculosis case alone has been shown to lead to a 30 per cent loss of household income, while recent studies in six African countries and one in Asia have shown that the average number of days of work lost because of an acute episode of malaria ranges from 2 to 6 days (Fig. 6).

Disability in endemic infectious diseases

In addition to mortality, the scale of individual pain, suffering, and disability from infectious diseases is immense, and chronic protein depletion and anaemia are common sequelae of many infectious diseases. At any one time, hundreds of millions of people—mainly in developing countries—are affected by infectious diseases either directly because of illness associated with acute infection, or indirectly because they are caregivers of those with illness or have severe postinfection disabilities.

For those suffering from infectious diseases associated with severe and long-term disability, there is often discrimination, stigmatization, shame, and anguish. At the same time those who are disabled are often unable to work, and thus are not only unable to provide resources for the family but become a burden to those who consequently become less productive themselves. The main infectious diseases which cause long-term disability are lymphatic filariasis, schistosomiasis, leishmaniasis, trachoma, onchocerciasis (river blindness), African trypanosomiasis (sleeping sickness), leprosy, dracontiasis (guinea-worm disease caused by *Dracunculus medinensis*), Chagas' disease, and intestinal parasites.

Lymphatic filariasis is estimated to be the second most important cause of long-term disability worldwide, after mental illness. The prevalence of chronic infection with lymphatic filariasis at the end of 1998 has been estimated at 120 million. Over 40 million (33 per cent) of those infected are estimated to be severely disfigured and disabled by the most visible manifestation of long-term infection, elephantiasis. At least 1 billion people are at risk of filarial infection—one in six of the world's population.

Schistosomiasis is estimated to infect over 200 million people worldwide and up to three times as many are at risk. Spread by freshwater snails that serve as intermediate hosts, and contracted by contact with stagnant water sources, it is a constant risk of dam-building and irrigation projects where in the presence of the newly introduced intermediate host a non-endemic region can rapidly become hyperendemic, with children and rural workers most at risk. In some of the most affected areas, over 90 per cent of children have become infected simply by wading through infested waters. In endemic areas, schistosomiasis is a major cause of chronic urinary tract disease, cirrhosis of the liver, and urinary bladder cancer.

More than 12 million people worldwide have been infected with leishmaniasis caused by parasites spread by the bite of the sandfly. In its visceral form, infection causes irreversible organ damage, while the dermatological manifestations include skin lesions and mutilation of the mouth and cartilaginous appendages including the nose. In countries such as India and Sudan there has been a sharp increase in visceral leishmaniasis as a result of coinfection with HIV. *Leishmania*–HIV coinfection also occurs in European countries, mainly among injecting drug users.

An estimated 5.6 million people today have been blinded or visually disabled by the sequelae of trachoma infection, and an additional 154 million are thought to have been chronically infected during 1998—mainly in Africa and Asia. The disease is transmitted by person-to-person contact, and amplified by poor hygiene.

Over 85 million people in Africa, Latin America, and the Arabian peninsula are at risk of infection with onchocerciasis. This parasitic disease is transmitted by the blackfly and causes visual impairment, blindness, and severe unrelenting pruritis due to the presence of microfilaria in the skin. Pruritis can be so intense that it results in open lesions from scratching, often followed by superinfection and suppuration.

In sub-Saharan Africa, 55 million people in 36 countries are at risk of infection with African trypanosomiasis, commonly referred to as sleeping sickness. The *Trypanosoma* are transmitted from the animal reservoir to humans by the tsetse fly, and chronic infection results in sleeping sickness manifested by debilitating illness and decrease in mental alertness. Without treatment, infection is fatal, and in some of the worst affected countries over half of the inhabitants in some villages are infected.

Infection with Hansen's bacillus (*M. leprae*), the cause of leprosy, results in significant disability in many countries in Africa, Latin America, and Southeast Asia. Approximately 800 000 cases of leprosy are detected each year, and current efforts are underway to decrease its prevalence to less than 1 per 10 000 during the coming 5 years.

Dracontiasis, or guinea-worm disease, is caused by a parasite transmitted by drinking infested water in regions where water is scarce and people with infection wade in that water which is also used for other household purposes including drinking. The mature worm, up to 1 m long, emerges through the skin, often in the lower leg, where it causes excruciating pain and disabling infections, and from where it deposits its eggs when in contact with water. The infection also causes severe arthralgia, fever, and vomiting. Over 78 000 cases were reported worldwide in 1998, mainly in Sudan, Nigeria, and Ghana. Efforts to eradicate dracontiasis are underway, with the major burden of disease remaining in southern Sudan.

Chagas' disease occurs only in Latin America, where it was estimated that up to 18 million people were infected in 1998. Some 120 million people live in areas at risk. Primarily transmitted by the blood-sucking *Triatoma* bug (family Reduviidae) that is infected with *Trypanosoma cruzi*, the parasite can also be transmitted by transfusion of contaminated blood and from mother to child at birth. It is estimated that the proportion of blood that is used for transfusion and is infected is over 50 per cent in some cities. Over one-third of those infected develop chronic disease, and about 30 per cent of them have incapacitating cardiac damage. Chagas' disease is the leading cause of cardiac death among young adults in some parts of South America. Others suffer intestinal and peripheral nerve damage.

Serious disability is also caused by sexually transmitted infections. In 1995, four sexually transmitted infections—gonorrhoea, *Chlamydia*, syphilis, and *Trichomonas*—accounted for an estimated 333 million new cases of curable sexually transmitted infections. In addition to acute suffering, syphilis and gonorrhoea result in serious sequelae worldwide. Acute gonorrhoeal infection has been shown to facilitate HIV transmission and infection, and untreated infections can thus prolong the period of increased transmissibility. Untreated gonorrhoeal infections also result in acute peritonitis, salpingitis, and infertility. Sequelae of untreated syphilis, known for centuries, include cardiac damage and aneurysm.

Infectious diseases and cancer

Epidemiological studies have shown that infection with viruses, bacteria, and parasites may be the initiating event in the later development of cancer, and that up to 85 per cent of some types of cancer can be attributed to an earlier infection. It is further estimated that at least 15 per cent of new cancers each year could be avoided if the associated preceding infectious process could be prevented.

According to estimates, mostly based on preliminary studies, approximately 550 000 cases of stomach cancer are attributable to *Helicobacter pylori* each year, representing approximately 55 per cent of stomach cancer worldwide. Sexually transmitted infection of the cervix with human papilloma virus is thought to be responsible for an estimated 83 per cent of cervical cancers, while approximately 82 per cent of liver cancers are attributable to infection with the hepatitis B and/or C virus. In countries where schistosomiasis is endemic, up to 4 per cent of new cases of bladder cancer have been linked to the presence of eggs of the adult parasite in the urinary bladder.

Causes and consequences of emergence, re-emergence, and spread of infectious diseases

The eradication of smallpox in the late 1970s boosted the already growing optimism that infectious diseases were no longer a threat, at least to developed countries. This optimism had prevailed since the 1950s, a period that saw unprecedented development of new vaccines and anti-infective drugs, and encouraged a transfer of resources and public health specialists away from infectious disease control. Optimism is now being replaced by an understanding that:

(1) climate and environmental changes result in the spread of infectious agents to new areas;

(2) transmission of infectious agents from animals to humans is occurring with increasing frequency, especially as humans exploit new ecological zones;

(3) poverty and the weakening of health infrastructures after political changes, or as a result of natural disasters or civil strife and war, are major causes of the resurgence of infectious diseases;

(4) uncontrolled urbanization and population displacement lead to concentrations of human populations in conditions that favour major epidemics (for example, urban slums or refugee camps);

(5) human behaviour can amplify the transmission of infectious agents;

(6) rapid development of anti-infective drug resistance is greatly facilitated by the misuse of antibiotics;

(7) globalization of travel and trade has markedly increased the potential for the spread of infectious diseases.

Climate and environmental changes

Alterations to the environment, whether natural or man-made, contribute to the emergence and re-emergence of infectious diseases. They range from localized warming with resultant extension of vector-borne diseases to deforestation that forces animals into closer human contact in search of food, increasing the possibility for infectious agents to breach the species barrier between animals and humans. Such changes have occurred on almost every continent. Most at risk are the over 500 million people who live in poverty and in ecologically fragile regions.

Health impact of El Niño

During the late 1990s, interest grew in the links between El Niño (and other extreme weather events) and human health. The longest single El Niño period on record occurred from 1990 to 1995. El Niño and similar weather disturbances affect human health mainly as a result of the natural disasters they trigger and the related outbreaks of infectious diseases.

The best-documented links exist between weather variations thought to be due to El Niño and the incidence of vector-borne diseases (for example, malaria or Rift Valley fever) and epidemic diarrhoeal diseases, particularly cholera. The resurgence in cholera cases in the Americas in 1998 was primarily attributable to the continuing effects of major disasters caused by the El Niño phenomenon and Hurricane Mitch. The increase in cholera cases on all continents in 1998 is similarly thought to be related to similar changes which have created conditions favourable for cholera outbreaks worldwide. The devastation of water and sanitation systems which has resulted from these naturally occurring phenomena is so severe that it is likely to take decades before the infrastructure and basic services in some of the affected regions regain their previous levels, thus continuing to favour outbreaks of diarrhoeal and other water-borne infectious diseases.

Recent outbreaks of Rift Valley fever, a vector-borne disease that principally infects livestock, have occurred in eastern Africa on almost every occasion that there has been excessive rainfall. Concurrent with the 1997 El Niño, areas of northeastern Kenya and southern Somalia experienced rainfall which was 60 to 100 times heavier than normal—the heaviest recorded rainfall since 1961. The rains are thought to have caused an increase in Rift Valley fever virus-infected eggs of *Aedes* mosquitos to hatch in the floodwaters. In the outbreak of Rift Valley fever that followed, which inflicted heavy livestock losses, there were an estimated 89 000 human cases with approximately 250 deaths, the largest recent outbreak of this disease.

Other weather patterns and disease outbreaks

The band of desert in sub-Saharan Africa, in which epidemic *Neisseria meningitidis* subgroup A infections traditionally occur, has enlarged as drought spreads south, so that countries such as Uganda and the United Republic of Tanzania now experience epidemic meningitis.

Current evidence suggests that in tropical and subtropical regions, influenza viruses circulate all year round, and that migrating aquatic birds transport viruses from these regions to the temperate zones during migration. More generally, outbreaks of diseases tend to follow temperature and precipitation patterns which affect the ability of influenza vectors such as birds to survive. New research into the links between specific weather patterns and outbreaks of Ebola haemorrhagic fever are examining the relationship between the clustering of reported outbreaks and climatic factors. Although the animal host of the Ebola virus remains elusive, it is hoped that by pinpointing specific regional and temporal 'trigger' weather events, it might be possible to establish the consequent animal behaviour which brings the host species into contact with humans under certain circumstances.

Global warming

Unprecedented changes taking place in the global climate because of greenhouse gas emissions could have even more wide-ranging effects on illness and death from infectious diseases. Global climate change is gradual and complex, and the environmental consequences are difficult to predict. A global mean temperature increase of 1 to 2°C would enable mosquitos to extend their range to new geographical areas, leading to increases in malaria and other mosquito-borne diseases, especially in populations living just outside areas endemic to these diseases. The proportion of the world's population at risk for malaria, currently estimated at 2.4 billion, could increase from 45 per cent in 1998 to 60 per cent by 2050 if global warming continues at the current estimated rate. The estimated annual number of deaths from malaria would inevitably rise as well, and control measures that might have been affordable and cost-effective at the end of the twentieth century could become impossible to implement. Some of the other vector-borne diseases potentially affected by global climate change include lymphatic filariasis, dengue, leishmaniasis, and Chagas' disease.

Transmission of infectious agents from animals to humans

Over two-thirds of emerging infections identified during the 1990s are known to have originated from animals—both wild and domestic species. Some are believed to have emerged from animals living in tropical rainforests or elsewhere in close proximity to humans, where micro-organisms have succeeded in crossing the species barrier to humans directly from an animal reservoir, or through an intermediary vector. The origins of some outbreaks of infectious agents, the Marburg and Ebola outbreaks for example, remain a mystery in spite of intensive research, but both are thought to have animal sources somewhere in the cycle of transmission to index cases. One was a single case of Ebola in a scientist working in Côte d'Ivoire who dissected a chimpanzee later known to be infected with the Ebola virus. A recent outbreak of Ebola in Gabon, associated in time and place with the butchering of a chimpanzee by the 19 index cases, adds credibility to this hypothesis.

Emerging influenza infections in humans have been associated with geese, chickens, and pigs. The influenza virus A (H5N1) that was isolated in 1997 from geese and chickens in Hong Kong Special Administrative Region of China was shown to be related to viruses isolated in the early 1990s in ducks in China and chickens in Italy. Likewise, the influenza A (H9N2) virus isolated in China in 1999 was similar to swine viruses isolated in Hong Kong Special Administrative Region of China in 1998. An influenza virus which had hitherto only been isolated in swine, A (H3N2), was detected for the first time in a human in 1999. In each of these instances the viruses were not able to transmit easily from human to human and did not become established in human populations as did others earlier in the century.

The majority (93 per cent) of people infected in the 1999 outbreak of viral encephalitis in Malaysia were people involved directly in the pig farming industry. The outbreak had a double aetiology: the re-emergence of the Japanese encephalitis virus and the emergence of a second, newly identified, neurotropic virus later named nipah.

An outbreak of West Nile like fever which caused five deaths in New York City in 1999 was thought to have been caused by transmission of the virus from birds to humans through mosquitos. Although West Nile virus is commonly found in humans and other vertebrates in Africa, western Asia, and eastern Europe, this was the first time it was detected in the western hemisphere. How the virus reached the area is the topic of great speculation, but its source had not been ascertained by the time of writing.

Animal displacement in search of new sources of food after deforestation or climate change can bring them into closer contact with human settlements and populations not previously in contact. One example is Lassa fever, first identified in West Africa in 1969, and now known to be transmitted to humans from food supplies contaminated with the urine of rats in search of food away from a natural habitat that can no longer support their needs. An outbreak of sine nombre virus in the United States in 1993 was linked to drought that likewise brought rodents into closer contact with humans, permitting transfer of this animal virus to humans.

Finally, humans themselves penetrate or modify formerly unpopulated regions, and come closer to animal reservoirs or vectors of infectious disease. Outbreaks of malaria, yellow fever, and leishmaniasis continue to be linked to the men who work in the rainforest cutting trees, and recent importation of yellow fever into Switzerland, the United States, and Germany have resulted from tourist excursions deep into the rainforests where yellow fever is enzootic.

Lapses in food production, handling, and processing also result in transmission of infectious agents from animals to humans. Outbreaks of food-borne infections such as salmonellosis and *E. coli* 0157 are regularly linked to faulty food processing practices, as has been new variant Creutzfeldt–Jakob disease associated with bovine spongiform encephalopathy in the United Kingdom. As lifestyles change, more people eat meals prepared outside the home, and insufficient training in food handling constitutes another major factor responsible for the rise in food-borne disease incidence.

Poverty, neglect, and the weakening of health infrastructure

More than one in four of the world's population are estimated to be living in poverty—over a billion of them with incomes of less than US$1 a day. Industrialized countries are not free of poverty, and 100 million people in industrialized countries live below the poverty line. These poor populations are a major reservoir of infectious diseases, and a source of continued transmission. In many developing countries poverty leads to malnutrition, a key factor that affects health, and malnutrition in turn increases the severity of infectious diseases such as pneumonia, malaria, measles, and diarrhoeal diseases—the major killers of young children. In 1997 it was estimated that over 160 million children were moderately or severely malnourished, and it is therefore not surprising that malnutrition is an associated factor in over half of all childhood deaths.

A child born in a developing country today has a 1000-fold greater chance of not being vaccinated and dying from measles than a child born in an industrialized country. This is clearly reflected by the fact that children born in Singapore during 1999 were likely to live 40 years longer than children born in Sierra Leone.

Effective public health policies save resources and can be effectively implemented even where poverty predominates. Over the years, cost-effective strategies have been developed for the prevention and control of the major infectious diseases. When implemented effectively, these strategies can decrease death and suffering caused by infectious diseases. Yet many governments fail to ensure that these strategies receive enough funding to succeed. In some cases, this is because health budgets are unrealistically small, and because the advocacy skills needed to increase them are lacking. In other cases, it is because health spending is poorly prioritized, often misplaced in curative rather than preventive infrastructure, and therefore not addressing the most urgent health threats. Finally, it is because some of the technologies available are out of the reach of governments and the majority of those willing to purchase health care with their own resources.

The strategy of integrated management of childhood illnesses, developed over the past 20 years, is a cost-effective means of preventing childhood mortality associated with acute diarrhoeal and respiratory infections and malaria, yet it has only been adopted by 57 of the 120 countries for which it is deemed appropriate. In none of those countries where it has been adopted is it being implemented nationwide. Expansion of integrated management of childhood illnesses and other cost-effective strategies in countries that have adopted them is slowed by weak public health infrastructure resulting in unequal distribution of supplies or difficulties in retaining qualified health workers.

Malaria is a particular risk for women during pregnancy. Pregnant women are more likely to die from malaria—either during pregnancy or the immediate postpartum period. Chronic anaemia resulting from repeated malaria infections is associated with low-birth-weight infants. To prevent this and other sequelae, it is recommended that pregnant women in high-risk malaria areas be treated presumptively for malaria at intervals to decrease parasite loads. Yet fewer than one in five are treated. Lack of funds are often cited as the reason, and failure to develop adequate health delivery systems is the result.

HIV prevention efforts targeted at youth, especially sex education in schools or other settings, has been demonstrated to be effective in preventing HIV infection. But in 171 countries worldwide, sex education of youth is not routinely provided, often because of unfounded fears that it will cause increased sexual activity among them. In countries where it is taught, girls are often not reached because they are excluded from secondary education.

On average, health expenditure in 1994 in low-income countries was US$16 per capita. Some of the poorest countries in the world provide no more than US$7 per capita for health care annually—making it difficult to ensure that even the most basic health needs are met. By comparison, average health expenditure in high-income countries during the same year was more than US$1800 per capita. Low-income countries spend 4 per cent of gross domestic product per capita on health, half the amount spent by wealthier countries. In many poor countries, spending is even lower. In Cameroon, Indonesia, Nigeria, and Sri Lanka, for example, it is less than 2 per cent of gross domestic product.

Some of the poorest countries fail to commit the resources necessary to purchase even the inexpensive vaccines available through the WHO and the United Nation International Children's Emergency Fund (**UNICEF**). Hepatitis B vaccine, for example, has now been introduced to childhood vaccination programmes in over 100 countries, but countries in areas where hepatitis B prevalence is highest—sub-Saharan Africa, Southeast Asia, and Eastern and Central Europe—have not yet included hepatitis B vaccine in childhood immunization programmes, even at the preferential price of US$0.50 to 1 per dose. Widespread use of hepatitis B vaccine could, in future generations, markedly decrease the prevalence of people chronically infected with hepatitis B, currently estimated at 350 million worldwide. The result would be decreased prevalence of hepatitis B, and decreased cirrhosis and hepatic carcinoma, two sequelae of chronic hepatitis B infection. At the end of the twentieth century two-thirds of the world's population still live in areas with high prevalence of hepatitis B, a fully vaccine-preventable infection.

Similarly, yellow fever vaccine has been available since 1937 but is currently not used in some of the countries most at risk. These countries, mainly in sub-Saharan Africa, are also among the world's poorest, and are those that have seen the steady increase in yellow fever reported since the late 1980s.

Weakening public health infrastructure for infectious disease surveillance and control, the result of under-resourced health ministries, is evidenced by such failures as mosquito control in Latin America and Asia with the re-emergence of dengue, failure of vaccination programmes in eastern Europe which contributed to the re-emergence of epidemic diphtheria and polio, and neglect of yellow fever vaccination which has facilitated the yellow fever outbreaks in Latin America and sub-Saharan Africa. It is also clearly demonstrated by high levels of hepatitis B and nosocomial transmission of other pathogens such as HIV in the former USSR and Romania, and by repeated nosocomial amplification of outbreaks of Ebola in the Democratic Republic of the Congo where needles, syringes, and failed barrier nursing methods drove transmission of Ebola and amplified outbreaks in 1976 and 1995 into major epidemics.

Increased funding for health care, however, does not necessarily decrease the prevalence of infectious diseases. In some developing countries, 60 per cent or more of government health expenditure is devoted to meeting the operating costs of urban hospitals and high-technology equipment that facilitates, but is not required for, patient management. For the cost of a few expensive procedures in such institutions, lives could be spared by preventive or curative interventions for infectious diseases among populations without access to the most basic health care. An outbreak of acute respiratory infection in a mountain area of Afghanistan in 1999, for example, continued for several months before it was reported, but was immediately controlled when adequate medical services were made available. Almost 800 million people worldwide lack access to basic health services.

The interrelationships between poverty, health, and development are so intertwined that it is impossible to address one without the others. Improvements in community health depend on sustainable development. At the same time, health is a minimum requirement for development. Infectious diseases remain a major obstacle to economic development in many countries because of the mortality and disability they cause. Premature deaths among the educated workforce, such as those that are occurring as a result of the AIDS epidemic, can take a generation to compensate. People with such disabilities as elephantiasis resulting from lymphatic filariasis, or trachoma- or onchocerciasis-associated blindness, cost the economy double in terms of both their lack of contribution to the workforce and their demands on the workforce for financial support. Intestinal parasites in women and children continue to cause severe debilitating anaemia in women, resulting in unsafe deliveries and postpartum illness, and decreased verbal fluency and cognitive skills in children.

In addition to the indirect costs associated with premature death and disability, or because of temporary absence from work, the cost of treatment for single or repeated bouts of an infectious disease such as malaria, for example, can be significant. In Nigeria, it has been estimated that subsistence farmers spend as much as 13 per cent of total household expenditure on malaria treatment each year. This economic output for malaria, heavy in itself, is compounded by absence from farming activities, which are most intense during the rainy season when malaria transmission is at its height, or the absence from work of another family member to take care of a child or adult sick with malaria.

The social and psychological impact of disabilities from infectious diseases often lead to marginalization, the destruction of marriages, family, and social relationships, and further obstructing economic development. Disabilities such as elephantiasis and blindness are involved, but in recent history no more important example of marginalization because of an infectious disease has occurred than AIDS. But AIDS has also been associated with other important obstacles to development. AIDS prevention strategies are much more difficult to implement where basic literacy skills are absent. At the same time, efforts to increase literacy have become a difficult struggle in many countries where schoolteachers have been among those at increased risk of HIV infection. In the United Republic of Tanzania, for example, the investments in education required to yield expected standards have been increased substantially because of high AIDS mortality among teachers. Additionally, 20 per cent fewer children attend school because parents are ill or dying with AIDS and therefore unable to pay school fees.

Uncontrolled urbanization and population displacement

The growth of densely populated cities with substandard housing, unsafe water, and poor sanitation place a great burden on public health services. Whereas in 1950 there were only two urban centres in the world with populations greater than 7 million, by 1990 this number had risen to 23, with increasing populations in and around all major cities challenging the capacity of existing sanitary systems and public housing. In Africa, Asia, and Latin America, at least 600 million urban dwellers live in substandard homes or neighbourhoods. People living in these neighbourhoods are at greater risk of infectious disease.

The link between environmental quality and health is critical. Over 10 per cent of all preventable ill health is estimated to be due to poor environmental quality—conditions such as substandard housing, overcrowding, indoor air pollution, poor sanitation, and unsafe water. The breakdown of sanitation systems in large coastal cities in Africa, Asia, and Latin America has facilitated the transmission of cholera, shigellosis, and intestinal parasites, and it is estimated that over a billion people worldwide lack access to safe drinking water—further increasing their vulnerability to diarrhoeal and intestinal parasitic diseases.

Traditional housing and substandard living conditions are likewise important factors leading to acute respiratory infections in children. Approximately 700 million people—mainly women and children in poor rural areas—inhale harmful smoke from burning wood and other fuels each day, and it is among this population that the risk of acute respiratory infections, especially pneumonia, is greatest.

Civil strife and political conflict are also major impediments to public health. In addition to destroying health infrastructures, they result in large numbers of homeless people living in refugee camps or less structured settings. If basic preventive services such as vaccination do not reach these populations, diseases which could easily be controlled become outbreaks. Negotiations with warring parties are sometimes necessary to ensure that national immunization days for polio eradication can be carried out.

The number of refugees and displaced people has increased ninefold over the past two decades. In 1996, it was estimated that as many as 50 million people worldwide had been uprooted from their homes. These refugees and displaced people are especially vulnerable to disease, forced to live in overcrowded insanitary conditions where the risk of outbreaks of water-borne diseases such as cholera and shigellosis are amplified. The movement of people as refugees and displaced people has also been shown to facilitate the spread of infectious diseases to new geographical areas, placing populations living in these regions at risk. In sub-Saharan Africa, for example, HIV is spread by migrant workers who congregate in urban areas where prevention is not promoted, and who then carry infection to their villages when they return home to families, and by lorry drivers who buy sex at or near truck stops on their way across the continent.

Human behaviour

A clear example of the impact of human behaviour in the emergence and re-emergence of infectious diseases is the increase in gonorrhoea and syphilis during the late 1970s, and the emergence and amplification of HIV worldwide—all directly linked to unsafe sexual practices. Other examples of the important relationship of human behaviour to infectious diseases are described throughout this chapter. They are related to lifestyle and include changes in agricultural and food production patterns which permit food-borne infectious agents to enter human populations, increased international travel for business or leisure which exposes humans to infectious diseases to which they ordinarily would not have exposure, and the outdoor activity and residential locations closer to forest and water that increase the risk of human exposure to animals or insect vectors.

Anti-infective drug resistance

Shortly after penicillin became widely available in 1942, Fleming warned of the potential importance of resistance and by 1946 a hospital in the United Kingdom had reported that 14 per cent of all *Staphylococcus aureus* infections were resistant to penicillin. By 1950 resistance in hospitals had increased to 59 per cent, and by 1990 penicillin-resistant *S. aureus* had attained a prevalence of greater than 80 per cent in hospitals and the community. At the same time resistance of *S. aureus* to other antimicrobials occurred with great rapidity, and by 1999 deaths were attributed to multiresistant staphylococcal infection in four children living in the United States. By 1999 it had become clear that bacteria, viruses, and parasites are all capable of rapidly developing or acquiring resistance to anti-infective agents, causing a decrease in the cost-effectiveness of treating most major infectious diseases.

In the early 1970s *N. gonorrhoeae* resistant to the usual doses of penicillin was introduced into Europe and the United States from Southeast Asia where it is thought to have first emerged. By 1999, *N. gonorrhoeae* resistance to penicillin had become global, and strains resistant to all major classes of antibiotics had been identified wherever these antibiotics had been widely used, with some countries in the Western Pacific region having registered quinolone resistance levels up to 69 per cent.

During the 1970s chloroquine-resistant *P. falciparum* malaria became highly prevalent in Southeast Asia, and by 1999 it had spread worldwide, as had high-level resistance to two second-line drugs, sulfadoxine-pyrimethamine and mefloquine.

The dramatic upsurge in the spread of drug resistant microbes over the past decade is undermining today's efforts to control infectious diseases. As diseases once thought to be under control become increasingly resistant to the arsenal of available drugs, the spectre of incurable infectious diseases looms large. In addition to requiring increased length of treatment, with more expensive, and in some instances more toxic, anti-infective drugs or drug combinations, a doubling of mortality has been observed in some resistant infections. At the same time fewer new anti-infective drugs reach the market, in part due to the high cost of new drug development, and the risk of developing a new anti-infective drug which may itself become ineffective before investment in its development is recovered. In fact, as the twentieth century came to a close, no new class of antibiotic had been marketed for human use since the 1960s (Fig. 7).

Although antimicrobial resistance affects industrialized and developing countries alike, its impact is far greater in developing countries. The switch from normally less expensive first-line drugs to second- or third-line drugs involves a dramatic escalation in the price of treatment. In some of the poorest countries, the cost of lengthy treatment and replacement drugs means that some diseases are too expensive to treat. Gonorrhoea, once easily treated in sub-Saharan Africa by penicillin or tetracycline, now requires more expensive drugs to which government health budgets do not commit. The resultant chronic gonorrhoeal infections lead to increased levels of infertility among young women, and chronic gonorrhoeal infections amplify the HIV epidemic by continuing to facilitate HIV transmission and infection throughout Africa.

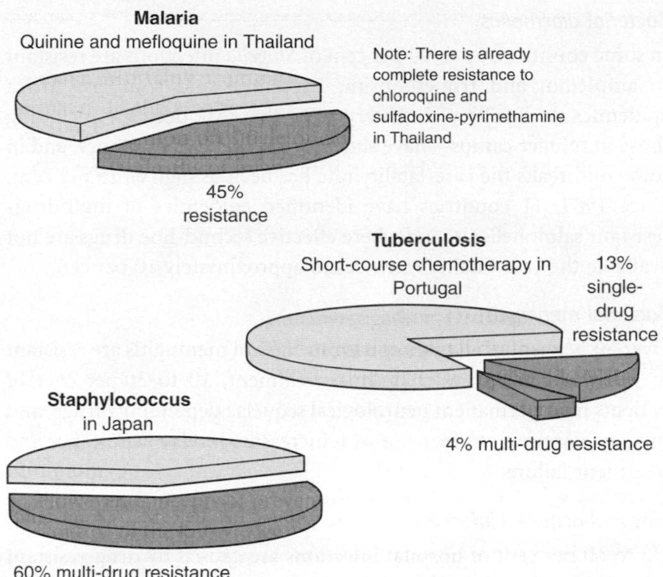

Fig. 7 Antimicrobial resistance, 1997.

In low-income countries, the cost of curing multidrug-resistant tuberculosis is as high as US$1500 to 4000, out of reach of health budgets. In Southeast Asia the cost of treating a child for meningococcal meningitis has been shown to increase from US$20 to 110 when second-line anti-infective drugs are required, while the cost of treating lower respiratory infections—the most frequent cause of childhood death—increases from US$5 to 40 for a course of antibiotics.

Major diseases affected

The effectiveness of anti-infective drugs against five of the six major infectious disease killers—tuberculosis, malaria, pneumonia, bacterial diarrhoeas, cholera, and HIV—is severely compromised by resistance, as is their effectiveness in most other common infections.

Tuberculosis

A 1997 report on antituberculosis drug resistance identified 'hot zones' of resistance around the world where over 5 per cent of tuberculosis infections are resistant to the most commonly prescribed drugs. In some countries in Eastern Europe more than 20 per cent of tuberculosis patients were found infected with multidrug-resistant organisms, and among prisoners in the Russia Federation up to 40 per cent of tuberculosis infections were found to be multiresistant.

Malaria

Chloroquine—once the first-line treatment for malaria—is no longer effective in curing malaria infections in over 80 of the 92 countries where malaria is a major public health problem. At the same time, mosquitos worldwide show resistance to the most commonly used insecticides including pyrethroids and dichlorodiphenyltrichloroethane (DDT).

Pneumonia

In some countries, up to half of all pneumococcal infections are resistant to penicillin. With increased treatment failures in children with pneumococcal pneumonia, mortality from this once easily treated infection is increasing.

Bacterial diarrhoeas

In some countries, up to 90 per cent of *Shigella* infections are resistant to ampicillin and trimethoprim. In central and southern Africa epidemics of bacillary dysentery over the past decade—including those in refugee camps—have shown resistance to quinolones, and in some outbreaks the case-fatality rate has been as high as 15 per cent. Since 1989, 11 countries have identified epidemics of multidrug-resistant salmonellosis, and where effective second-line drugs are not available the case-fatality rate rises to approximately 10 per cent.

Bacterial meningitis

Over 50 per cent of all cases of meningococcal meningitis are resistant to penicillin. Even under optimal treatment, 10 to 30 per cent of patients have permanent neurological sequelae depending on age, and this rate continues to increase with increasing levels of resistance and treatment failure.

Hospital-acquired infection

Up to 60 per cent of hospital infections are caused by drug-resistant microbes worldwide, and in the United States alone it is estimated that approximately 14 000 hospital patients die each year from nosocomially transmitted drug-resistant bacteria.

Causes of resistance

Numerous factors lead to anti-infective resistance by favouring selection of resistant strains of micro-organisms, while at the same time resistant genes can be transferred genetically from one bacterium to another through the spread of resistant plasmids.

Wrong prescribing practices

Widespread misuse of anti-infective drugs in human medicine is a major factor in selection of resistant micro-organisms. Misuse occurs in developing and industrialized countries alike. Overprescribing adds unnecessary anti-infective drugs to the environment, while prescribing anti-infective drugs in doses lower than required helps select out those organisms with resistance that are then passed on to others. In Canada and the United States, studies indicate that approximately half of all outpatient prescriptions for antibiotics are unnecessary, and in a recent study of patients in hospital in Thailand, 36 per cent of patients who received an anti-infective drug had no laboratory-confirmed infection. In a similar study in Vietnam, over 70 per cent of patients with a laboratory-confirmed infection were given antibiotics in doses lower than recommended by national infection treatment guidelines. The lack of simple diagnostic tests suitable for use at peripheral health facilities in most developing countries necessitates treatment of syndromes presumptively rather than based on diagnosis, further increasing anti-infective drug use.

Non-adherence by patients

Where anti-infective drugs are correctly prescribed, patient non-adherence to the correct dosage and/or number of days of treatment often occurs, especially once the symptoms disappear. In addition, antibiotics can be bought without a prescription in many developing countries resulting in self-medication that is often at incorrect dose and duration.

Counterfeit drugs

Counterfeit anti-infective drugs are commonplace in many developing countries; some are bogus and contain no active ingredient, while others contain non-standardized amounts of the active ingredient either due to intentional cost saving or lack of quality control during manufacture. As well as resulting in treatment failure and at times in death, counterfeit anti-infective drugs with reduced and non-standardized amounts of active ingredients contribute to the problem of drug resistance by selecting out resistant strains.

Use of anti-infective drugs in animals and plants

Anti-infective drugs are not only used in humans. They are used in animals for treatment as growth enhancers, non-specifically added to animal feed. They are also used in horticulture in temperate countries, sprayed on fruit trees to prevent blight, and in tropical countries to prevent blight on crops such as rice and orchids. Current estimates are that approximately 50 per cent of all anti-infective drugs are used in animal husbandry including fisheries. Although the full effect of anti-infective drug use in animals on human health is not yet fully known, there is growing evidence that anti-infective drug resistance developing in animals contributes to the problem of resistance in humans. Better understanding is required of the implications of antibiotic pressure and selection of resistant strains in animals, and of the genetic interaction between zoonotic and human pathogens. There is, however, scientific evidence that four multiresistant bacteria infecting humans (*Salmonella*, *Campylobacter*, enterococci and *E. coli*) are directly linked to resistant organisms in animals, and there is growing consensus worldwide that anti-infective drugs used in humans should not be used as growth-enhancement additives to animal feed.

Globalization of travel and trade

In the Middle Ages infectious agents were often the cause of high mortality rates among sailors and their passengers travelling in insanitary and crowded conditions. They were carried by animal vectors such as rats which transported plague from one continent to another on board ships. Today infectious agents travel worldwide by plane—carried by airline passengers in a matter of hours. A passenger can be infected on one continent and travel to another while still asymptomatic to the infectious agent, and then become sick and expose passengers and populations at the destination. As the number of international airline passengers has soared from 2 million a year in 1950 to over 1.4 billion today, the world has been slow to recognize the implications for public health (Fig. 8).

In 1988, a clone of multiresistant *Streptococcus pneumoniae* first isolated in Spain was shortly thereafter identified in Iceland. Another clone of multiresistant *S. pneumoniae*, also first identified in Spain, was subsequently found in seven different countries on three continents. A study conducted by the Ministry of Health of Thailand of 411 exiting tourists in 1996 showed that 11 per cent had an acute infectious disease, mostly diarrhoeal but also respiratory infections, malaria, hepatitis, and gonorrhoea. Failure to suspect and diagnose an infection such as malaria in a person with fever after returning home is not an uncommon death-provoking event among travellers.

Airborne infections such as pneumonic plague, influenza, and tuberculosis are easily spread in crowded airport lounges, on airplanes or by passengers after arrival at their destination. In the United States in 1977, over 70 per cent of the passengers on board an airliner were infected with influenza by a fellow passenger; in 1978 poliovirus was imported to Canada by Western Europeans who had refused polio vaccination, resulting in an outbreak of paralytic disease with 11 cases.

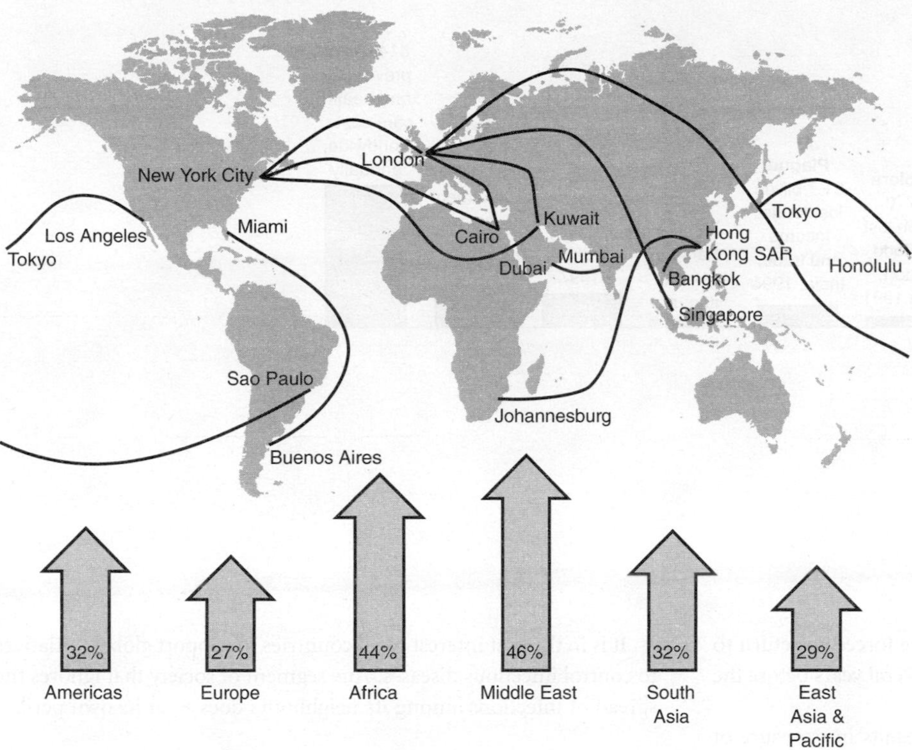

Fig. 8 Most popular air routes between continents (1997) and percentage increase in international arrivals between 1993 and 1997.

In the early 1990s, a flight attendant with active tuberculosis is thought to have infected up to 23 fellow crew members over the course of several flights, while in 1996, a health worker in South Africa was infected with Ebola by a patient who had entered the country to seek medical care during an outbreak in Gabon.

Malaria infections and deaths regularly occur in Europe and North America following unrecognized infection in blood transfusions and more commonly after a one-off bite from an imported mosquito near international airports. Brussels, Geneva, London, and Oslo have all reported recent cases of such airport malaria, as have the United States and Canada. In 1985, the tiger mosquito—normally found in Asia—slipped unnoticed into the United States inside a shipment of water-logged used tyres from Asia. Within 2 years tiger mosquitos—capable of transmitting yellow fever, dengue, and other diseases—were found in 17 states. In 1991, a ship thought to have carried contaminated water from Asia in its ballast tanks caused the cholera epidemic in Peru that spread rapidly throughout South and Central America resulting in reports of over 11 000 deaths.

Outbreaks and epidemics of infectious diseases have far-reaching economic and political consequences, at times out of reasonable proportion with their true threat to human health.

The response to infectious disease outbreaks requires an immediate investigation and containment activities, at times placing great financial demands on countries at the expense of routine endemic disease prevention and control measures. In recent epidemics of meningococcal meningitis in sub-Saharan Africa vaccine, antibiotic, and logistic support required massive inputs of funding from national governments and international donors. The countries most affected by the epidemic were those who had the greatest difficulty in responding appropriately, and routine health services and other important activities were disrupted as the health system attempted to cope.

Global media coverage of infectious disease outbreaks in remote and distant locations can trigger unjustified fear among populations for whom the threat is negligible. The collective imagination is fuelled by media stories such as those that have recently speculated on the origins of the Ebola virus, or on how West Nile like virus entered North America, and by fear of intentional use of infectious agents in terrorism or war. The resulting economic losses resulting from such reactions are significant indirect costs of infectious diseases, in addition to the direct costs to economies in lost earnings as a result of the disability and death they cause among those of working age.

The consequence of an outbreak with widespread and sensational reporting on trade and tourism is often immediate. In Peru in 1991, reports of a cholera epidemic resulted in a loss of US$770 million, almost one-fifth of normal export earnings in the trade and tourism sectors as countries banned seafood imports and tourism decreased.

Seven years later, when cholera outbreaks were reported from the Horn of Africa, embargoes were again placed on fishery products originating from these countries, with consequential loss of economic revenues estimated as high as US$36 million in one of the countries involved. Yet another infectious disease outbreak, an epidemic of plague in India, resulted in severe economic losses estimated unofficially at US$1.7 billion. Hotel bookings in India fell by 20 to 60 per cent immediately after media reports were published, and one airline reported losses of over US$1 million during the first week after reports. In countries throughout the world airports were closed to aeroplanes arriving from India, imports of foodstuffs were blocked,

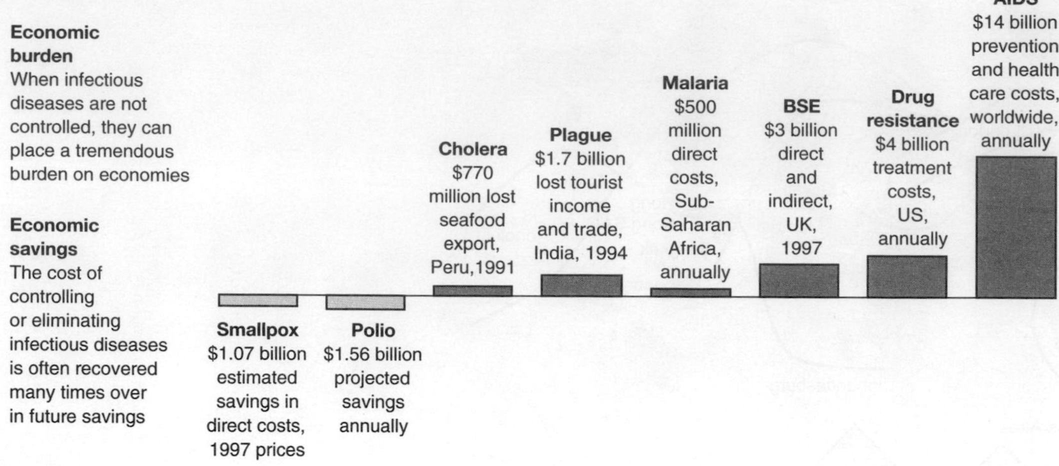

Fig. 9 Economic burden of infectious diseases, 1990s.

and in some countries Indian guest workers were forced to return to India even though they had not been there for several years before the plague epidemic occurred (Fig. 9).

Globalization of the food supply regularly results in exposure of humans, through foods purchased locally, to pathogens native to remote parts of the world. The risk of *V. cholerae* transmission associated with trade in certain food products is considered very small; to date there has been no documented outbreak of cholera resulting from commercially imported food from countries where cholera is endemic. But other infectious agents have clear potential to spread internationally in foodstuffs, creating major negative impact on economies. Recent examples include the epidemics of influenza in Hong Kong, nipah virus in Malaysia, and bovine spongiform encephalopathy in the United Kingdom, which resulted in the mass destruction of poultry, pigs, and cattle respectively. Concern occurs over the safety of a range of goods that are prepared from animals or animal products, ranging from cosmetics to biological agents.

Unjustified embargos, protectionism, and other political issues related to infectious diseases can lead to a severe strain on diplomatic relations between countries. A recent example occurred in 1999 when France refused to allow the importation of beef from the United Kingdom on the grounds that available scientific evidence was not sufficient to guarantee consumer safety from the threat of bovine spongiform encephalopathy. The perception of the potential use of the smallpox virus as a bioweapon has recently prevented the destruction of the remaining stocks of variola virus and continues to cause serious tensions between countries that wish destruction and those who do not. The unexplained appearance of a West Nile like virus in New York led to speculation in the media that it might have been released deliberately, again raising uncertainty and fear for national security and providing fertile ground for tensions between countries.

Infectious diseases occur in every country. Old scourges such as tuberculosis and diphtheria have occurred in explosive epidemics in industrialized countries of Eastern Europe during the 1990s. A 1996 outbreak of polio in Albania, Greece, and the Federal Republic of Yugoslavia showed how easily an infectious disease can be reintroduced to countries once free of the disease if immunization coverage is allowed to drop.

It is in the best interest of all countries to support global initiatives to control infectious diseases. Any segment of society that ignores the spread of infections among its neighbours does so at its own peril.

Solutions to infectious disease problems

At the beginning of the twenty-first century it is clear that new infectious agents will continue to emerge. Known infectious agents will continue to be transmitted—in some instances to re-emerge at greater incidence than previously while in others to decrease to lower incidence. Moreover, the effectiveness of existing anti-infective drugs will continue to decrease. At the same time new anti-infective drugs under development offer hope, new vaccines are adding to those that have successfully controlled many childhood infections, and the potential of the genomic research agenda is becoming a reality as information about the genome begins to be applied to further drug and vaccine development.

However, most of the 13 million deaths and untold disabilities estimated to have occurred from infectious diseases in 1998 could have been prevented using the tools we have available today. Vaccines offer solid immunity to infectious agents, and anti-infective drugs can still be effectively applied to most infections. The use of these existing tools has been largely responsible for the advances in the control of infectious diseases made to date (Table 1). But the window of opportunity for their cost-effective use is closing, and they must be applied now to reduce infectious diseases and ensure healthy economic development.

Based on decades of operational study of existing technologies, it is generally agreed that infectious-disease-related mortality and disability could be greatly decreased if political support were strengthened to exploit fully the following proven strategies for infectious disease control:

(1) eradication, elimination, and intensified control through global public–private sector partnerships;

Table 1 Affordable health services for developing countries, 1990s

Disease	Intervention	Prevention or treatment costs (US dollars)	Annual cost per capita (1990) (US dollars)
AIDS	Treatment of sexually transmitted diseases	$14 for a year's supply of condoms	$0.20
	Prevention programmes		$1.70
Tuberculosis	DOTS strategy	$20 for 6 months of medicines	$0.60
Malaria	Prevention	$10 for a bednet treated with insecticide	Being determined
Measles	Immunization	$0.26 to administer one dose of measles vaccine	$0.50
Diarrhoeal diseases	Integrated management of childhood illness	$0.33 for oral rehydration salts	Being determined
Acute respiratory infections	Treatment of pneumonia	$0.27 for 5 days of antibiotics	

Source for per capita spending World Development Report (1993). Source for prevention or treatment costs: WHO (1999).

DOTS, directly observed treatment, short course.

(2) promotion of a core set of interventions that use proven cost-effective strategies and are selected based on national infectious disease priorities;

(3) working across government sectors to ensure sustainability and synergy in public health activities;

(4) expansion of surveillance and response systems to alert the world and respond to unexpected outbreaks and emergences of new infectious diseases;

(5) strengthening international agreements and regulations to ensure maximum international public health security with minimal interference in travel and trade;

(6) investment in research and development of diagnostic tools, drugs and vaccines to improve prevention and control.

Eradication, elimination, and intensified control

Eradication is the interruption of transmission of an infectious agent and its disappearance from nature. Only one infectious disease—smallpox—has been eradicated. Efforts to eradicate smallpox began in 1966 when ministers of health from around the world resolved in the World Health Assembly to utilize maximally vaccination with the vaccinia vaccine to eradicate smallpox within the coming 10 years. The initial strategy of smallpox eradication was mass vaccination of the entire population. This gradually shifted to a search and containment strategy, with active surveillance to search for and identify cases of smallpox that were then isolated in their homes, which became the central focus for mass vaccination of populations living in households in the near vicinity. In 1966 at the start of the eradication programme, smallpox was endemic in 30 countries, the other countries having eliminated smallpox by routine vaccination. During 1966 alone, smallpox virus was estimated to cause disease in 10 to 15 million worldwide, among whom 1.5 to 2 million were thought to have died, while survivors were left with severe facial scarring, and in some instances corneal scarring with blindness.

However, the eradication of smallpox has raised serious political and scientific issues. In spite of a recommendation made by the World Health Assembly in 1990 that remaining stocks of variola virus be destroyed, the debate continues and the decision as to when destruction will actually occur is still pending consensus within the scientific and political communities.

To eradicate an infectious disease a combination of factors is required. There must be no known animal reservoir, and disease must result in solid life-long immunity with no long-term carrier state. At the same time there can be no subclinical manifestation of infection that could result in continued transmission, and case detection must be relatively simple. Above all a highly effective, stable, and easily administered vaccine or curative drug must be available, which, in the case of the vaccine, must confer long-term protection. Smallpox eradication was certified by the WHO in 1980, and in addition to the morbidity and mortality that have been prevented, savings have been substantial because smallpox vaccination is no longer required. A study in the United States during the immediate posteradication period demonstrated that because the United States no longer needed to vaccinate its population against smallpox, and support those who suffered the rare but severe neurological side-effects associated with the vaccine, an amount equal to its investment in the global smallpox eradication programmes was being saved every 29 days.

At the end of the twentieth century, two more diseases—poliomyelitis and guinea-worm disease—are on the verge of eradication (Fig. 10). In 1988, the World Health Assembly resolved to eradicate polio globally by the year 2000 by calling for maximum use of the trivalent oral polio vaccine which was developed during the 1950s. Substantial progress in implementing the recommended polio eradication strategies was reported from all endemic countries in the subsequent decade, achieving and maintaining high routine coverage with oral poliovirus vaccine, conducting national immunization days to decrease poliovirus circulation rapidly, establishing sensitive surveillance systems for the detection of polio cases and identifying the poliovirus, and carrying out mopping-up vaccination activities to eliminate the last remaining reservoirs of poliovirus transmission.

While progress has been dramatic in many countries, significant obstacles remain in the early twenty-first century, particularly in 14 priority countries that represented global poliovirus reservoirs

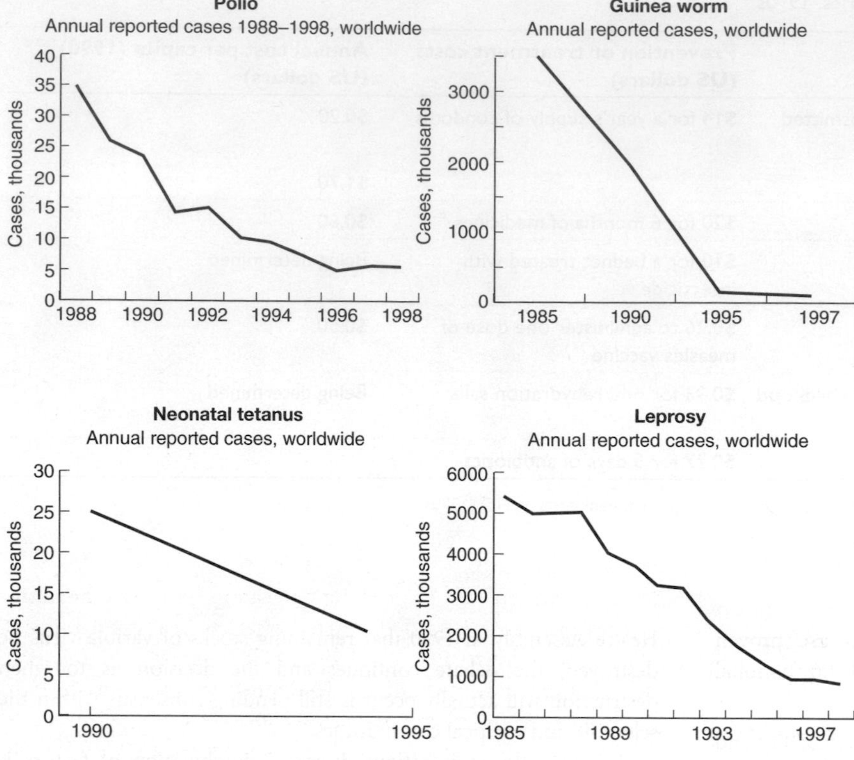

Fig. 10 Diseases close to eradication/elimination, 1999.

because of insufficient national commitment or political conflict (Fig. 11). At the same time, three geographical regions had eliminated poliovirus or were close to doing so: the Americas had interrupted polio transmission during 1991 and has been polio-free since then, the Western Pacific region has not detected poliovirus since 1997, and poliovirus transmission in Europe was confined to southeastern Turkey.

Reaching the global polio eradication goal required the planned acceleration of eradication activities during the year 2000 in the remaining major foci of poliovirus transmission in the densely populated global reservoir countries of southern Asia and Africa—Bangladesh, Democratic Republic of the Congo, Ethiopia, India, Nigeria, and Pakistan.

The World Health Assembly resolved to eradicate dracontiasis (guinea-worm disease) in 1991. Between 1989 and 1998, the number of cases were reduced from almost 900 000 to just under 80 000. Strategies for eradication include filtering of drinking water and education about the infection and its means of transmission, and by 1999 only 15 countries reported cases. By the end of 1999 it appeared that guinea-worm transmission had been interrupted in Asia, and the remaining endemic areas in Africa remained a formidable challenge either because of decreasing government commitment or unstable political situations making operations difficult.

Although there were just two eradication programmes being implemented at the end of 1999, several more infectious diseases were gradually being brought under control worldwide by elimination programmes, or by programmes of intensified control. Elimination is defined as the reduction in incidence or prevalence of an infectious disease to a level which is more manageable within the existing health systems (Fig. 10). Unlike diseases targeted for eradication, once a disease elimination target is reached continued control measures are required. For some of the diseases targeted for elimination the question remains as to whether, once these diseases are brought to low levels, interruption of transmission will occur spontaneously as occurred for several infectious diseases in industrialized countries. Intensified control is similar to elimination, with a resolution of health ministers for increased commitment, but with no elimination target.

The neonatal tetanus elimination strategy was adopted by the World Health Assembly in 1989, with a target for 1993 of less than 1 case per 1000 live births. The estimated global number of neonatal tetanus cases decreased from 510 000 in 1990 to 355 000 in 1997, with a corresponding decrease in mortality, using vaccination of pregnant women with tetanus toxoid and provision of safe delivery services to all pregnant women as the primary strategies. The goal at the end of 1999 was to achieve this targeted incidence in each health district of all countries by 2000.

In 1991, the World Health Assembly resolved to eliminate leprosy as a public health problem by 2000, elimination being defined as prevalence less than 1 case per 10 000 population. By the end of 1999, of the 122 countries which were highly endemic for leprosy in 1985 prior to the WHO resolution, 98 had reached the elimination target at the national level and were working to achieve this target in all health districts by the end of 2000. Leprosy prevalence worldwide has thus been reduced by 85 per cent using an active search strategy to identify people with leprosy who are then provided free treatment with multidrug therapy.

At the end of 1999 the majority of the global leprosy burden was concentrated in 24 countries where the leprosy elimination target had

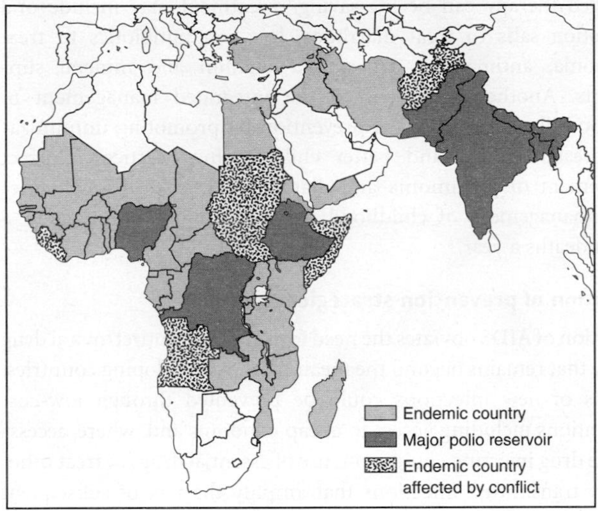

Fig. 11 Global polio situation, April 1999.

not been reached, within limited and difficult to access geographical areas in these countries as well as in some of those countries that had reached the global target.

In 1997 the World Health Assembly adopted a resolution calling for the global elimination of lymphatic filariasis as a public health problem. The elimination target resolved is 2015, and the elimination strategy uses simple safe inexpensive periodic delivery of albendazole and ivermectin or diethycarbamazole to kill the parasite in populations at risk of infection. By the end of 1999, 10 countries had begun elimination programmes with momentum expected to increase in the early twenty first century.

In 1991, six countries in Latin America have made a political commitment to interrupt transmission of Chagas' disease. The strategy for elimination is screening of blood donations and vector control. Transmission was interrupted in Uruguay in 1997 and in Chile in 1999.

In 1989 the World Health Assembly resolved an intensification of prevention activities to reduce measles morbidity and mortality by 90 and 95 per cent, respectively, by 1995 using measles vaccine. During 1997 it was estimated that approximately 31 million measles cases and 1 million associated deaths had occurred worldwide, and by the end of 1997 measles morbidity and mortality worldwide had been reduced by 74 and 85 per cent, respectively, when compared with prevaccine rates (Fig. 12). By 1998 measles mortality was estimated to have decreased from 1 million in 1997 to 800 000, and by the end of 1999 all countries in the Americas and in the western Pacific had reached the morbidity and mortality reduction goals, and Europe had reached the mortality reduction goal. At the end of 1999, 99 per cent of the remaining measles mortality continued to occur in the least developed countries.

The onchocerciasis control programme, which began in 11 countries in West Africa in 1974, has protected an estimated 36 million people from infection and sequelae such as severe pruritis and blindness. The programme, which uses strategies for control of the insect vector and mass distribution of the antiparasitic drug ivermectin to populations at risk of infection, was extended in 1996 to an additional 19 African countries where the disease is endemic. In 1991, an onchocerciasis control programme for the Americas was launched in six Latin American countries, with the aim of decreasing severe pathological manifestations and reducing morbidity through the distribution of ivermectin. It is expected that the onchocerciasis control programmes will have maximum public health impact early in the twenty-first century.

In 1998 the World Health Assembly resolved to give high priority to intensifying tuberculosis control, and in 1999 it resolved to intensify malaria control. From these two resolutions, two worldwide partnerships in public health have developed: the Stop Tuberculosis Initiative and Roll Back Malaria. These two global partnerships promote proven prevention and control strategies at the country level, and have the following global functions:

(1) removing obstacles to expansion of prevention and control strategies;

(2) composite work planning with partners;

(3) global level advocacy and social mobilization;

(4) resource mobilization.

The partnerships for eradication, elimination, and intensified control programmes provide both technical and financial resources to countries. Their strength lies in forging alliances with donor governments, ministries of health in developing countries, international development banks, foundations, the private sector, civil society, United Nations agencies, and non-governmental organizations. Rotary International, a private sector service organization, has raised US$500 million to purchase vaccine for the polio eradication programme and to help to equip a refrigerated cold chain for vaccine transport, and has used its global network of over 28 000 clubs in 155 countries to enlist volunteers to carry out immunization campaigns. Merck provides ivermectin for onchocerciasis elimination, Glaxo SmithKline provides albendazole for the elimination of leprosy, Novartis provides multidrug treatment for leprosy, and Pfizer provides azithramycin for the treatment of trachoma. Loans from the World Bank are strategically aimed at eradication, elimination, and intensified control, while the recent launch of the New Medicines for Malaria Venture—a joint initiative by the public and private sectors to develop new antimalarial drugs—is a visionary example of efforts to harness greater public and private sector collaboration in developing new products for use in developing countries. In this venture, industry provides its technical expertise for research and development while risk-taking is provided through public sector funding, with a goal of developing one new drug for malaria treatment every 5 years.

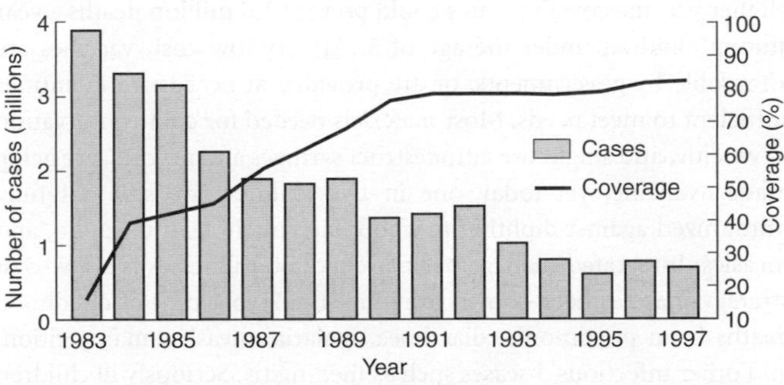

Fig. 12 Measles cases and vaccination coverage worldwide, 1986 to 1997.

Effective use of a core set of interventions

Operational study of existing health technologies during the past several decades has identified cost-effective interventions for the prevention and control of infectious diseases. Government commitment to their use, even in areas of extreme poverty, will prevent infectious disease mortality and disability. A core set of these cost-effective interventions, from which a selection must be made to respond to evidence-based national or subnational disease priorities, includes interventions such as those that follow.

Insecticide-impregnated bednets

One in four childhood deaths from malaria could be prevented if children at risk slept under bednets at night to avoid mosquito bites. Bednets dipped in an insecticide cost about US$10 each, and a supply of insecticide to re-treat the net costs between 50 cents and $1 per year. 'Dip-it-yourself' kits are now available for re-treating the nets at home, and the pyrethroid insecticides used have been shown to be safe. Social marketing and community participation in bednet programmes serve to create demand for this affordable intervention and ensure its sustainability.

Directly observed treatment, short course

Expansion of directly observed treatment, short course (**DOTS**) to greater number of people could avert millions of tuberculosis deaths. This highly effective health-care strategy involves detection of tuberculosis cases through low-cost sputum smear tests, followed by 6 to 8 months of treatment with a combination of inexpensive drugs. A key component is regular ongoing support to the patient that includes observation to ensure that treatment is correctly followed and follow-up sputum tests to determine whether treatment has been successful. DOTS can detect and cure disease in up to 95 per cent of infectious patients, even in the poorest countries.

DOTS not only drastically reduces deaths by increasing the cure rate of tuberculosis treatment, it also cuts the transmission of infection and prevents the development of multidrug-resistant forms of the disease. DOTS has been evaluated by the World Bank to be one of the most cost-effective of all health interventions, as an investment of only about US$3 is required per year of healthy life saved, making it one of the best buys available to health and finance ministries. Since the introduction of the DOTS strategy in the early 1990s, the world has witnessed remarkable progress in global tuberculosis control.

Childhood immunization

Higher vaccine coverage rates could prevent 1.6 million deaths a year among children under the age of 5. At very low cost, vaccines are affordable by governments, or are provided at no cost in quantities sufficient to meet needs. Most materials needed for cold conservation of vaccine, and single-use autodestruct syringes and needles, are being made available, yet today one in five children are still not fully immunized against diphtheria, whooping cough, tetanus, polio, and measles. Integrated management of childhood illnesses is a low-cost strategy that has been shown to reduce the 70 per cent of childhood deaths from pneumonia, diarrhoea, malaria, measles, malnutrition, and other infectious diseases such as meningitis. Seriously ill children often suffer from more than one condition at the same time or in rapid sequence, making exact diagnosis difficult. For these children, combined therapy can be life-saving. Treatment may include oral rehydration salts to treat diarrhoea, low-cost antibiotics to treat pneumonia, antimalarial drugs, and vitamin and mineral supplements. Another key focus of the integrated management of childhood illnesses strategy is prevention by promoting immunization, breast feeding, and better child-feeding practices. Correct management of pneumonia and diarrhoeal diseases through integrated management of childhood illnesses could prevent up to 3 million deaths a year.

Promotion of prevention strategies against AIDS

Prevention of AIDS obviates the need for expensive antiretroviral drug therapy that remains beyond the means of most developing countries. Millions of new infections could be prevented through low-cost interventions including access to cheap condoms and, where necessary, safe drug injecting equipment, use of essential drugs to treat other sexually transmitted infections that amplify the risk of subsequent infection with HIV, HIV testing and counselling which can lead to safer sex, counselling and support for HIV-positive pregnant women and mothers along with antiretroviral drugs, counselling on safe alternatives to breast feeding, and sex education at school and beyond. For those who are infected with HIV, well-targeted low-cost care strategies can have a major impact on the suffering and must be better provided.

Increasing availability of essential drugs and vaccines

Increasing drug and vaccine access requires health infrastructure strengthening to the very periphery of the health-care system in order to decrease the current estimate of one-third of the world's population that lacks regular access to essential life-saving drugs. Drugs may be too expensive for those on the lowest incomes, or they may not be available in countries or health systems. In Africa it is estimated that in the poorest countries less than half the population has access to the basic drugs they need (Fig. 13).

Ways of increasing access to essential drugs and vaccines require strengthening of national health infrastructure, and inadequacy or breakdown of health-care services is one of the main obstacles to ensuring the availability of essential drugs. Resources being spent on health services must not be wasted. Logistics infrastructures which had been built up by the smallpox eradication programme, for example, disappeared with the disease and debate continues about the long-term effect of those resources in strengthening health infrastructure. The logistics and momentum created by global programmes must be used to strengthen routine health systems.

Clear priorities must be set for prevention and control based on epidemiological analysis and feasibility with existing resources and opportunities, and with careful assessment of the cost-effectiveness and potential for sustainability of the proposed interventions.

But increased access to essential drugs and vaccines does not only require strengthening of infrastructure. It also requires more rational use of those drugs that are available so that their maximum effectiveness is achieved. User-friendly packaging of drugs, for example, is a low-cost way of increasing patient adherence to antimalarial drug therapy. Studies in Ghana show that over 80 per cent of patients given a course of antimalarial drugs packaged in a numbered blister pack finished the course of treatment. Of those receiving loose unpackaged drugs—the way they are usually dispensed in developing countries—only 65 per cent completed the treatment. A

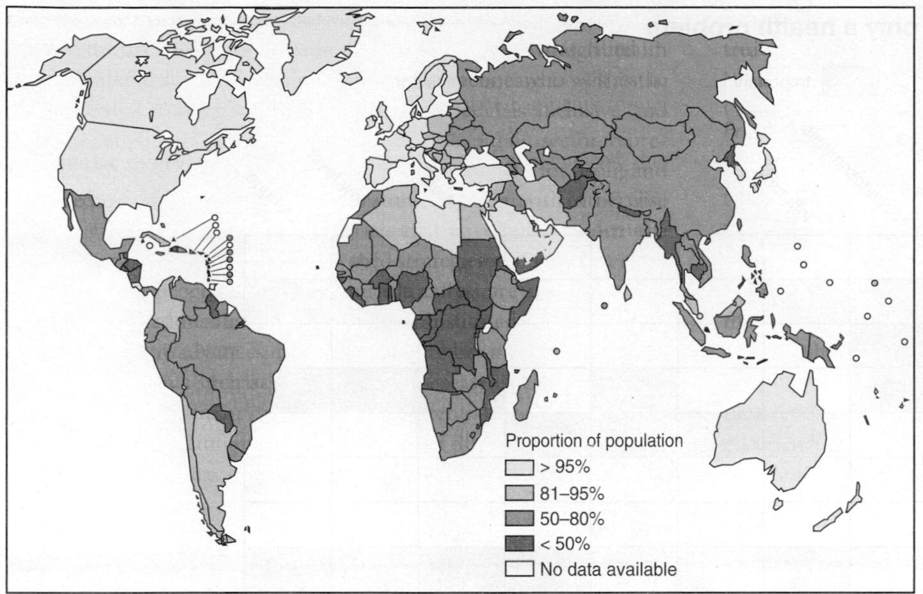

Fig. 13 Population with regular access to essential drugs in 1996 (1997 estimates).

simple packet of fast-acting drugs made widely available to parents—together with training to recognize malaria symptoms—could save the lives of many children with severe malaria.

Inexpensive vitamin and mineral supplements can also save lives, and by giving children vitamin A supplements along with other preventive services, deaths from measles and diarrhoea can be reduced. Malaria deaths among children can likewise be reduced through the use of iron supplements to treat anaemia. These inexpensive supplements, and life-saving anti-infective drugs, must be made available where they are needed.

Working across government sectors

Many key determinants of health, and the causes of emergence and re-emergence of infectious diseases that result in the increasing incidence and prevalence of endemic infectious diseases—as well as the solutions—lie outside the direct control of the health sector. Other government sectors involved are those dealing with sanitation and water supply, environmental and climate change, education, agriculture, trade, tourism, transport, industrial development, and housing (Fig. 14). Yet many developing, and some industrialized, countries lack the capacity to ensure co-ordinated action among the health sector and key sectors other than health. Failure to take account of the health impact of other sectors adds to the lack of funds and inadequate application of existing cost-effective tools to fight infectious diseases, and unless a broad multisectoral approach to health is ensured, prevention and control remain tenuous.

The critical need for collaboration between health and other sectors has been highlighted most recently by efforts to prevent AIDS. A few governments have attempted to reduce individual vulnerability to AIDS through a cross-sectoral approach that influences infrastructure development plans, laws, education, labour policies, and the exercise of human rights, for example, in an effort to create an environment that makes it easier for people to avoid AIDS. In some countries the approach has involved providing incentives to enable girls to finish secondary educatión, boosting job and educational opportunities for women to break the cycle of economic and sexual dependency, and ending the criminalization of marginalized groups such as sex workers and injecting drug users. It has also involved the conduct of impact assessments for development projects to foresee ways in which schemes could fuel the epidemic—through accelerating the pace of urbanization, for example, or splitting up families through creating the need for a migrant labour force.

Expansion of surveillance and response systems

Many networks throughout the world provide information about infectious disease occurrences. These networks include non-governmental organizations such Médecins sans Frontières, electronic discussion groups such as Promed, and search engines for infectious disease information from the World Wide Web such as those maintained by the Global Public Health Information Network. They also include laboratory and epidemiologist networks such as the WHO collaborating centres, the Training in Epidemiology and Intervention Public Health Network, and the Association of South-East Asian Nations. Together these networks are a powerful means of obtaining the information that leads to a co-ordinated international response and enhanced international public health security.

Epidemic intelligence is the constant receipt and validation of information about suspected or confirmed infectious disease outbreaks that is received from these networks worldwide. Once the information has been validated, key public health professionals must be informed of those confirmed and unconfirmed outbreaks that are of potential international public health importance. At the same time active and appropriate response must occur, ranging from local containment measures to an investigation and containment by a highly specialized international team. Recent outbreaks such as the human monkeypox outbreak in the Democratic Republic of the

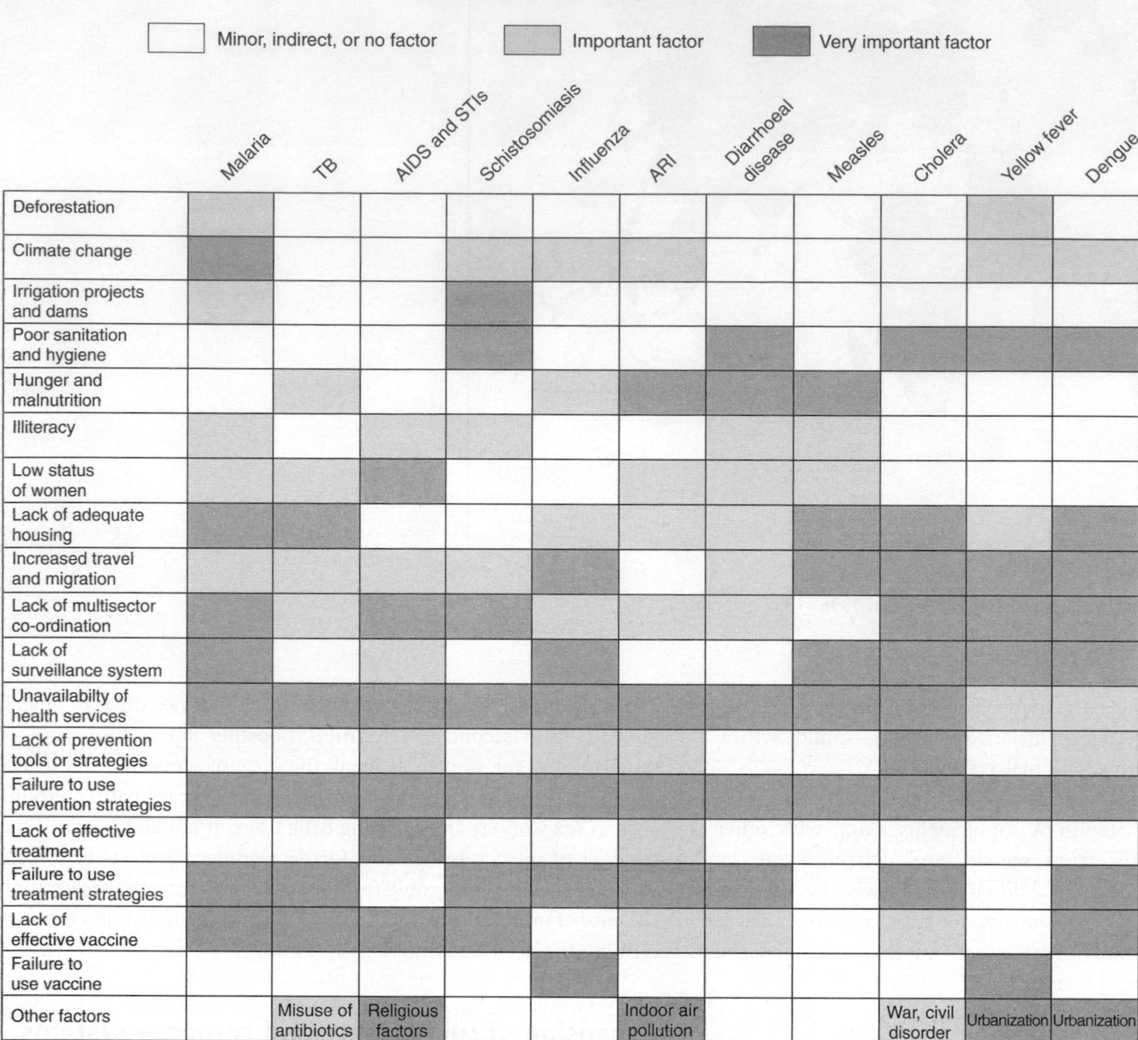

Fig. 14 Determinants of health: TB, tuberculosis; STIs, sexually transmitted infections; ARI, acute respiratory infections.

Congo reported by the Médecins sans Frontières network, the outbreak of influenza A (H5N1) in Hong Kong Special Administrative Region reported by the WHO Flunet, and the outbreak of highly fatal respiratory disease in Afghanistan reported by Global Public Health Information Network all led to partnerships of national and international public health experts for co-ordinated investigation and containment. In all three of these outbreaks, and in many more during the past 3 years, detection and response have forged partnerships between scientists in developing and industrialized countries that continue to strengthen and ensure greater public health security (Fig. 15).

Since infectious disease outbreaks will continue to occur, often in countries without the capacity to respond fully, the challenge is to build national epidemic preparedness before outbreaks occur. Investment must be made now if adequate systems are to be put in place. The metaphor of the fire service is a good illustration—it is impossible to build a fire service while trying to respond to the fire.

Essential tools to ensure epidemic preparedness include surveillance standards and stronger multidisease surveillance systems, preidentified partners for outbreak response, strengthened laboratory capacity, and training in field epidemiology.

Surveillance networks that have been built for one infectious disease must be expanded to include others. Those systems built with eradication or elimination programmes are examples, and are usually well funded so that the vital search for final cases and certification activities are possible. The acute flaccid paralysis surveillance system established for polio eradication in Myanmar, for example, was expanded in 1999 to include surveillance for measles and neonatal tetanus; and the laboratory networks for polio surveillance in sub-Saharan Africa have routinely been expanded to other viral diseases such as yellow fever. In sub-Saharan Africa acute flaccid paralysis surveillance systems are likewise being strengthened by the provision of field epidemiology and public health laboratory training.

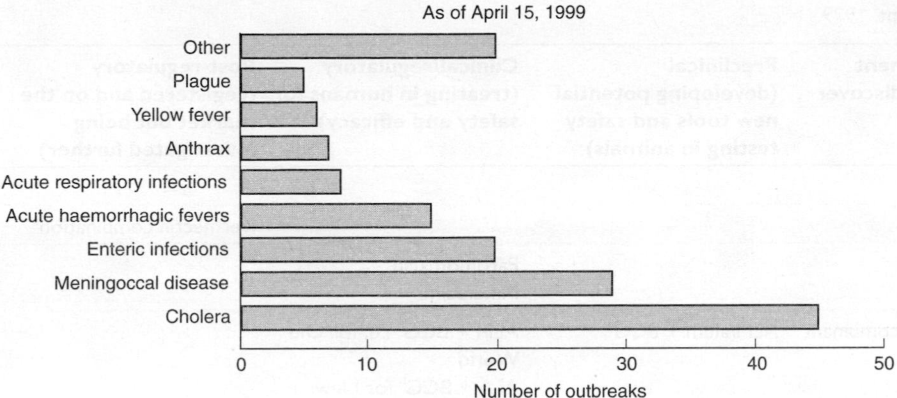

Fig. 15 Reported outbreaks of known infectious diseases, 1998 to 1999.

Strengthening international agreements and regulations

Attempts at agreement and regulation to prevent the spread of infectious diseases were first recorded in 1377 in quarantine legislation to protect the city of Venice from plague-carrying rats on ships from foreign ports. Similar legislation in Europe, and later in the Americas and other regions, led to the first international sanitary conference in 1851 which laid down a principle for protection against the international spread of infectious diseases: maximum protection with minimum restriction. Uniform quarantine measures were determined at that time, but a full century elapsed, with multiple regional and inter-regional initiatives, before the International Sanitary Rules were adopted, in 1951. These were amended in 1969 to become the International Health Regulations which are implemented by the WHO.

The International Health Regulations provide a universal code of practice which ranges from strong national disease detection systems and measures of prevention and control including vaccination, to disinfection, disinsection, and deratting of public conveyances, and sanitary norms at ports of entry. Currently the International Health Regulations require reporting of three infectious diseases—cholera, plague, and yellow fever. But when these diseases are reported, the Regulations are often wrongly applied, resulting in disruption of international travel and trade, and huge economic losses.

Many infectious diseases, including those which are new or re-emerging, are not covered by the International Health Regulations even though they have great potential for international spread. Because of the problematic application and disease coverage of the International Health Regulations, the World Health Assembly has requested a revision and updating of the Regulations so that they are better adapted to the control of infectious diseases in the twenty-first century. The revised Regulations are expected to replace reporting of specific diseases (for example cholera) by reporting of disease syndromes with high mortality, such as epidemic haemorrhagic fever. They will have a broader scope to include all infectious diseases of international importance, and will clearly indicate what measures are appropriate internationally, as well as those which are inappropriate. It is envisaged that the revised International Health Regulations will strengthen global alert and response to ensure maximum protection against infectious diseases with minimum restriction on world traffic and trade.

Investment in research

Despite their importance, infectious diseases come low on the global health research and development agenda. In 1992, global spending on health research was US$56 billion—less than 4 per cent of total global expenditure on health. Of that, no more than 10 per cent was allocated to research relating to the health needs of developing countries—mainly infectious diseases.

The combined investment in research and development into acute respiratory infections, diarrhoeal diseases, and tuberculosis—which kill over 7 million people a year—was US$133 million (about 0.2 per cent of global spending on health research and development). Yet these three diseases together account for almost one-fifth of the global disease burden. Malaria, which accounts for 3 per cent of the disease burden globally and almost 10 per cent in sub-Saharan Africa, fared as poorly—attracting about 0.1 per cent of research funds.

In contrast to the limited funds available, the research needs for infectious diseases are vast. Some of the research needed involves cutting-edge science—sequencing the genome of the major disease-causing microbes, for example, or discovering ways of slowing the spread of anti-infective-drug resistance. Other critical research needs include the discovery of new affordable drugs, vaccines, and diagnostic tests. In some cases, these are needed to lower costs, improve compliance, and replace drugs that have been compromised by resistance.

Equally important is the need for research to find ways of making more widespread and better use of existing cost-effective tools such as vaccines, multidrug therapy, bednets, and an integrated approach to childhood illness. Meanwhile, research is also needed to understand better the causes of the disease burden in individual countries, so that health systems can respond effectively to needs in the most cost-effective way. An urgent need is to develop new low-cost anti-infective drugs to replace those that have become ineffective due to resistance (Table 2).

Table 2 New drugs and vaccines under development, 1999

	Pre-development (research to discover new tools)	Preclinical (developing potential new tools and safety testing in animals)	Clinical/regulatory (treating in humans for safety and efficacy)	Post-regulatory (registered and on the market but being investigated further)
Chagas' disease	SCH 56592[a]			
Onchocerciasis/lymphatic filariasis	Moxidectin[a]			Ivermectin combination[a]
Leishmaniasis	PX 6518[a]		Paromomycin[a] Miltefosine[a]	
	ALA + IL-12 recombinant cocktail[b]	ALM/alum + BCG[b]	ALM + BCG[b] i.d. for Old World ALA + BCG[b] for New World MLA [b] i.m. for New World	
Schistosomiasis	Paramyosin + ????[b] GST (SJ26) GST (SJ28)[b]		GST + alum (Sh28)[b]	
Malaria	Synthetic endoperoxides[a] Choline uptake inhibitors[a]		Arteether[a] i.m. Artesunate [a] i.r. Pyronaridine[a] CPGN/DAP[a]	
	EBA-175 SERA[b] RAP-1, [b] RAP-2[b] MSP-1,[b] 19 kDa MSP-1,[b] 42 kDa Pfs-25 + alum, 6.8[b]		SPf66 + alum[b] SPf66 + OS21[b] AMA-1 + SEPPIO[b] RTS-S[b]	
Sleeping sickness	CGP 40 215[a] SIP10-1029 analogues[a]			Eflornithine[a]

Note: These are examples of just a few of the many drugs and vaccines under development for infectious diseases.

[a]Drug.

[b]Vaccine.

Source: WHO (1999).

Making better use of existing tools

In the short term, a great deal can be achieved through research into ways of improving the use of existing tools—one of the most neglected areas of research. This includes the need to improve the home management of malaria and other childhood diseases, and to provide clear information about prompt referral for severely ill children. Research is also needed to find ways of ensuring that newer more expensive vaccines such as those against *H. influenzae* type b and hepatitis B—which have proved successful in the industrialized countries—can now be introduced into developing countries.

Diagnostic tests

Research is needed to develop low-cost rapid diagnostic tests to improve the accuracy of diagnosis and accelerate the start of appropriate treatment. Although rapid diagnostic dipstick tests for malaria are in the final stages of development, they are currently too expensive for widespread use in developing countries. Tests are also needed for tuberculosis, gonorrhoea, and sleeping sickness for use in developing countries.

New diagnostic tests for sexually transmitted infections could help prevent their spread, ensure prompt and more effective treatment, and provide a valuable weapon in the fight against HIV/AIDS. The currently available tests are too expensive for use in developing countries and laboratory analysis is not always available. Simple diagnostic tests are also required for other diseases, including tuberculosis and malaria.

New drugs

It is now urgent to develop new drugs to treat diseases like malaria, tuberculosis, and pneumonia which are rapidly becoming resistant to first-line drugs. Without a new generation of low-cost drugs, some diseases could become serious treatment problems in countries which have not been able to purchase more expensive second-line drugs. Also needed are new combination therapies to treat diseases such as lymphatic filariasis, river blindness, and malaria—using more than one drug to increase effectiveness and lower the risk of developing drug resistance. Other priorities include a new oral drug which could help reduce deaths from visceral leishmaniasis and a new non-injectable quick-acting drug to treat severe cases of malaria. One promising new product (a combination of chlorproguanil and dapsone) is an oral treatment for cases of uncomplicated malaria in Africa. Another is a suppository (artesunate) for malaria sufferers who are too sick to take oral medication. It is fast-acting, easy to administer, and can 'buy time' for people with severe malaria living in remote areas who might not survive the journey to hospital.

New low-cost drugs that could improve compliance with drug therapy by shortening the course or simplifying the treatment are also needed. The drop-out rates for DOTS therapy for tuberculosis, for example, could be greatly improved if the multidrug therapy could be combined in a single tablet and the length of treatment reduced from the minimum 24 weeks now required. For leprosy, efforts are being made to develop new drugs which could both increase the effectiveness and shorten the duration of multidrug therapy.

New vaccines

Top of the global priority wish-list in vaccine development are vaccines against acute respiratory infections, diarrhoeal diseases, HIV/AIDS, malaria, tuberculosis, and dengue. Of these, a vaccine against HIV/AIDS is arguably the most important since no cure exists and mortality is high.

Advances in genetic engineering have produced vaccine contenders that should simplify immunization, boost the performance of existing vaccines, and protect children against diseases which are not yet vaccine-preventable. New vaccines against tuberculosis, malaria and acute respiratory infections could provide the first line of defence against drug-resistant microbes. The successful sequencing of the genome of the tuberculosis-causing microbe in 1998 was a major breakthrough that is expected to shed more light on which genes cause tuberculosis and to speed up the development of a more effective vaccine. Meanwhile progress in microbial genetics is also driving the development of new, improved vaccines against meningococcal meningitis, dengue fever, and Japanese encephalitis.

Efforts must also be made to reach the one in five children who are still not immunized each year through national immunization programmes. This includes efforts to lower vaccine delivery costs, simplify the administration of vaccines, and reduce the number of immunization contacts needed. In addition to the need to develop new or improved vaccines, research is under way to simplify the administration of existing vaccines, reduce delivery costs, and boost immunization coverage. This includes research into ways of reducing the number of immunization contacts that are needed through combining several vaccines in a single dose and combining several booster doses in a single slow-release dose. Another priority is the development of new safer ways of delivering vaccines—orally or nasally—that minimize the risk of injection hazards.

Summary

The rapid economic and scientific advances of the twentieth century for controlling infectious diseases can be built upon, and the impact of infectious diseases can be cut dramatically. With the emergence of new infectious agents, the re-emergence of those we know, and the rapid development of anti-infective drug resistance, the windows of opportunity to use these advances cost effectively are closing. Increased commitment is required for their use, and for the research necessary in the future.

Further reading

Anonymous (1999). *Research on Legionella epidemic—preliminary report of 21 June 1999.* Dutch Royal Institute for Public Health and Environment.

Anonymous (2000). HIV/AIDS. *Weekly Epidemiological Record*, **75**, 379–83.

Anonymous (2000). *Legionella* infection. *Weekly Epidemiological Record*, **75**, 347–52.

Ashford, W.A., *et al.* (1976). Penicillinase-producing *Neisseria gonorrhoea. Lancet*, **ii**, 657–8.

Aswapokee, N., *et al.* (1990). Pattern of antibiotic use in medical wards of a university hospital, Bangkok, Thailand. *Review of Infectious Diseases*, **12**, 136–41.

Baron, R.C., *et al.* (1983). Ebola virus disease in southern Sudan: hospital dissemination and intrafamilial spread. *Bulletin of the WHO*, **61**, 997–1003.

Bax, R.P. (1997). Antibiotic resistance: a view from the pharmaceutical industry. *Clinical Infectious Diseases*, **24** (Supplement 1), S151–3.

Breman, J.G., *et al.* (1978). The epidemiology of ebola haemorrhagic fever in Zaire, 1976. In *Ebola haemorrhagic fever* (ed. S.R. Pattyn). Elsevier, Amsterdam.

CDC (Centers for Disease Control and Prevention) (1993). Update—hantavirus pulmonary syndrome, United States, 1993. *Morbidity and Mortality Weekly Report*, **42**, 816–20.

CDC (Centers for Disease Control and Prevention) (1999). *Fact sheets on West Nile encephalitis.* CDC, Atlanta, GA.

Fraser D.W., *et al.* (1977). Legionnaire's disease: description of an epidemic of pneumonia. *New England Journal of Medicine*, **297**, 1189–97.

Goma Epidemiology Group (1995). Public health impact of Rwandan refugee crisis. What happened in Goma, Zaire, in July 1994? *Lancet*, **345**, 339–44.

HABITAT (United Nations Centre for Human Settlements) (1996). *An urbanizing world: global report on human settlements.* UNCHS, Geneva.

Holmberg, S.D., *et al.* (1987). Health and economic impact of antimicrobial resistance. *Review of Infectious Diseases*, **9**, 1065–78.

Infectious Disease Society of America (1999). Ebola: the virus and the disease. *Journal of Infectious Diseases*, **179** (Supplement 1).

Lederberg, J., Shope, R.E., and Oaks, S.C. (ed.) (1992). *Emerging infections—microbial threats to health in the United States.* Institute of Medicine, Washington, DC.

Lester, S.C., *et al.* (1990). The carriage of *Escherichia coli* resistant to antimicrobial agents by healthy children in Boston, in Caracas, Venezuela and Qin Pu, Chinal. *New England Journal of Medicine*, **323**, 285–9.

Levy, S.B. (1992). *The antibiotic paradox—how miracle drugs are destroying the miracle.* Plenum Press, New York.

Medeiros, A.A. (1977). Evolution and dissemination of β-lactamases accelerated by generations of β-lactam antibiotics. *Clinical Infectious Diseases*, **24** (Supplement 1), S19–45.

Monath, T.P. (1975). Lassa fever: review of epidemiology and epizootiology. *Bulletin of the WHO*, **52**, 577–92.

Munoz, R., *et al.* (1991). Intercontinental spread of a multiresistant clone of serotype 23F *Streptococcus pneumoniae. Journal of Infectious Diseases*, **164**, 302–6.

Payne, D. (1989). The history and development of the WHO standard *in vivo* and *in vitro* systems for the sensitivity of *Plasmodium falciparum* and other human plasmodia to antimalarial drugs. PhD Thesis, University of London.

Phillips, I. (1976). β-lactamase producing penicillin-resistant gonococcus. *Lancet*, **ii**, 656–7.

Pisani, P, Parkin, D.M., Munoz, N., and Ferlay, J. (1997). Cancer and infection: estimates of the attributable fraction in 1990. *Cancer Epidemiology, Biomarkers and Prevention*, **6**, 387–400.

Preston, R. (1999). West Nile mystery. *New Yorker*, 18 and 25 October.

Raviglione, M.C., Harries, A.D., Msiska, R., Wilkinson, D., and Nunn, P. (1997). Tuberculosis and HIV: current status in Africa. *AIDS*, **11** (Supplement), S115–23.

Robertson, S.E., *et al.* (1996). Yellow fever—a decade of emergence. *Journal of the American Medical Association*, **276**, 1157–62.

Sato, P.A. (1989). Review of AIDS and HIV infection: global epidemiology and statistics. *AIDS*, 3 (Supplement 1), S301–7.

Soares, S., *et al.* (1993). Evidence for the introduction of multiresistant clone of 6B *Streptococcus pneumoniae* from Spain to Iceland in the late 1980s. *Journal of Infectious Diseases*, **168**, 158–63.

Walsh, J.F., *et al.* (1993). Deforestation: effects on vector-borne diseases. *Parasitology*, **196** (Supplement), S55–75.

Wasserheit, J.N. (1994). Effect of changes in human ecology and behaviour patterns of sexually transmitted diseases, including human immunodeficiency virus infection. *Proceedings of the National Academy of Sciences of the USA*, **91**, 2430–5.

Webster, R.G. and Bean, W.J. (1998). Evolution and ecology of influenza viruses: interspecies transmission. In *Textbook of influenza* (ed. K.G. Nicholson, R.G. Webster, and A.J. Hay). Blackwell Science, Oxford.

WHO (World Health Organization) (1978*a*). Ebola haemorrhagic fever in Sudan, 1976. Report of a WHO/international team study team. *Bulletin of the WHO*, **56**, 247–70.

WHO (World Health Organization) (1978*b*). Ebola haemorrhagic fever in Zaire. Report of an international commission. *Bulletin of the WHO*, **56**, 270–93.

WHO (World Health Organization) (1995). *World health report. Bridging the gap.* WHO, Geneva.

WHO (World Health Organization) (1996). *World health report. Fighting disease, fostering development.* WHO, Geneva.

WHO (World Health Organization) (1998). *World health report. Life in the twenty-first century: a vision for all.* WHO, Geneva.

WHO (World Health Organization) (1999). *Removing obstacles to healthy development.* WHO, Geneva.

WHO (World Health Organization) (2000). *World health report 2000. Health systems: improving performance.* WHO, Geneva.

WHO (World Health Organization) (2001). *Global tuberculosis control.* WHO report, WHO, Geneva.

Will, R.G. (1996). A new variant of Creutzfeldt–Jakob disease in the UK. *Lancet*, **347**, 921–5.

2.7 The environment

A. J. McMichael

Introduction

The meaning of the word 'environment', applied to human health, is elastic. Conventionally it refers to the various external factors that impinge on human health, via exposures that are usually shared between members of communities or whole populations and that are predominantly involuntary (that is, not under the control of individuals). The scope of 'environmental exposures' is usually confined to physical, chemical, and microbiological agents that are able to induce pathological effects. Occupational exposures, especially in the wage-paid workplace, are an important subset of 'environmental exposures'—although the specialized topic of the occupational environment is usually treated separately (see Chapter 8.6).

The roles of housing quality, material circumstances, and socio-economic status in the determination of disease patterns have claimed increasing attention from epidemiologists. These considerations invite a more inclusive definition of 'environment', one that embraces the built environment, social and economic relations, and the patterns of living that flow from those circumstances. This comprehensive view of the environment is illustrated in Fig. 1, which also shows examples of types of health problems that arise in relation to the various facets and interactive combinations of environmental influences. While recognizing the fundamental importance of the social environment as a determinant of human health, and as a dimension of humankind's complex ecology, this chapter will not develop that aspect further.

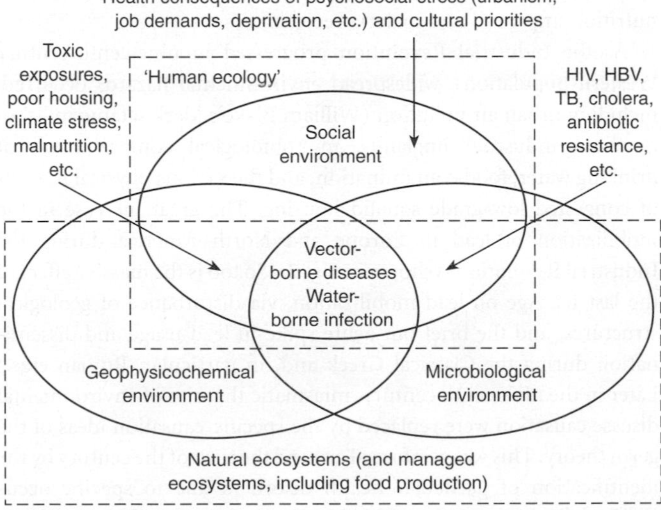

Fig. 1 The major components of 'the environment'. Examples of environmental diseases and disorders are shown, emphasizing that most arise from the interplay of several aspects of the environment.

History of environmental health in Western society

Concern over environmental conditions has been a driving force in the historical evolution of public health. Indeed, the origins of the modern discipline of epidemiology are substantially grounded in studies of environmental health problems before the twentieth century, in particular: toxic contaminants in locally brewed alcoholic drinks, the patterns of cholera occurrence in London, mortality gradients between different residential areas and socio-economic groups, and some specific occupational exposures. The history of 'environmental health' in Western countries was, throughout those centuries, dominated by infectious diseases. That remains true in low-income countries today, where around two-fifths of all deaths are due to infectious disease.

Over the broad sweep of history, radical changes in human ecology and the pattern of contacts between civilizations have largely determined the turbulent tides of infectious diseases and the changing nutritional profiles of populations. The microbiological environment has been transformed over the past 10 000 years as, first, human societies opted for settled farming and herding, and, later, as emerging civilizations with their own distinctive disease pools made commercial and military contact with one another (McNeill 1976). The gradual 'domestication' of epidemic infections, via coevolutionary adaptations of microbe and human host, and the attainment of famine-free food supplies in Europe over the past seven to eight centuries laid the foundations for a healthier living environment.

Historians discern several distinct stages in Western society's relationships to nature. During much of the seventeenth and eighteenth centuries, long-standing ideas persisted about disease arising from nature as God's judgement on the human condition. The weight of religious authority and the inertia of folklore fostered a generally passive and fatalistic approach to environmental adversity. The wages of sin were disease. However, during those centuries new philosophical perspectives were emerging as the foundations of modern empirical science was being laid in Western Europe. Francis Bacon argued for scientific enquiry based upon empirical observation and comparison. Descartes, having differentiated the human mind from the body, propounded a reductionist framework for studying the external world—a world which, as a machine-like entity, was amenable to disassembly. Newton elucidated the laws of physical motion, light, and gravity. Other scientists revealed various other basic laws of the natural world. With the rapid growth of this Enlightenment thinking and knowledge, the rise of inductive logic, and the application of utilitarianism to the fruits of scientific enquiry, a more 'activist' approach to managing and changing the environment emerged.

One consequence of this more interventionist philosophy was the rise of the 'social hygiene' movement in Europe, originating in France in the late seventeenth century (Riley 1987). This movement 'sought to cleanse the environment, to reduce its pathogenic properties and its capacity to promote epidemics' (Riley 1987). Major social expenditures were required to undertake these ambitious infrastructural development and clean-up projects, ranging from the draining of marshes, the removal of urban refuse, and the improvement of roadways. Governments were persuaded, sometimes grudgingly, that such investments would lead to gains in the health of workforces and to increases in the amount of arable land—and therefore to higher productivity, more taxes, and fuller treasury coffers (Shahi *et al.* 1997).

Environmental health issues in the nineteenth century

Following the convulsion of the French Revolution at the end of the eighteenth century, more humane and egalitarian social ideologies emerged early in the nineteenth century. It was increasingly recognized that the well being and health of populations were affected by their social and physical environment—and that often there were resultant infectious disease risks throughout the social ranks. There was much talk of 'miasmas' (foul emanations arising from decay and putrefaction), especially within urban environments. Following the crisis of urban industrial blight and increased mortality in the 1830s in Britain, the Sanitary Idea emerged and became, temporarily, linked with ideas of urban sustainability—including ideas of recycling sewage, maintaining fertile adjoining soils, attaining local self-sufficiency in food production, and achieving full employment. The proposal for 'garden cities' became popular in England, partly inspired by the prospect of minimizing miasmas that were presumed to arise from crowded polluted dark urban environments. This new belief in the possibilities for enlightened collective action, for the general technocratic management of nature, challenged the inherent selfishness of the *laissez-faire* ideology of the age.

From around the mid-nineteenth century, however, 'environmental health' increasingly became a topic of formalized research, pursued by biomedical scientists. Statistics were collected on exposures, disease, and deaths. Public authorities were urged to ameliorate particular offending places to reduce the risks to health. The spectacular rise of bacteriology in the 1880s caused further divergence from the earlier ecological perspective. Microbes were deemed to be the primary cause of disease. This powerful new germ theory, along with new theories of cell biology and heredity, new concern over micronutrient deficiencies, and the medicalization of child-bearing and child-rearing all refocused the health sciences on the individual. Ideas of shared environmental exposures and their risks to health receded.

There has been protracted debate over how best to explain the declining mortality rates in Britain over the past two centuries, a mortality that was dominated by infectious diseases until the second quarter of this century. McKeown (1976) gives most of the credit to improvements in social and environmental factors, arguing in particular that gains in nutrition strengthened human biological defences against the ever-present infectious diseases of early industrial city life. The improvements in food and nutrition flowed from the modern agricultural revolution, with mechanization, diversification of food species, cross-breeding of plant and animal species to increase yields, and more efficient transport networks. Improved housing quality, safe water supplies, increasing literacy, and better domestic hygiene gave further important protection to infants and children against infectious agents. While many commentators have broadly concurred with McKeown, others have championed the role of deliberate public health interventions (Szreter 1988). In France, for example, substantial gains in life expectancy emerged first in Lyon (in the 1850s), then Paris (1860s and 1970s, albeit more protractedly), and then Marseille (around 1890) in direct association with improved public water supply and sanitation in each of those cities.

These improvements in population nutrition, in attributes of the urban environment, and general social progress fostered, beginning in Europe in the nineteenth century, the first broad-based public health revolution. Various health gains arose incidentally, as consequences of changes in human social organization and economic practices. For example, the increased supplies of cattle fodder (alfalfa and turnips) that followed the mechanization of European agriculture from the mid-eighteenth century stimulated an increase in cattle herds. Not only did this lead to a dietary increase in animal protein but it also caused a reduction in human malaria, since the anopheline mosquitoes prefer their blood-meals from bovids rather than from hominids. This unplanned health benefit was further boosted by the fact that the malaria parasite (*Plasmodium*) cannot complete its lifecycle in cattle as it does in humans (McNeill 1976). Thus, without the deliberate intent of public health practitioners, the population's nutrition improved and malaria receded.

As the Industrial Revolution progressed in nineteenth-century Western populations, widespread environmental hazards occurred, including urban air pollution (William Blake's 'dark satanic mills' of northern industrial England), microbiological contamination of drinking water, food contamination, and the various physical hazards of congested low-grade squalid housing. The great increase in the mobilization of lead in Europe and North America during the Industrial Revolution is shown in Fig. 2. (So too is the massive effect of the last Ice Age on lead mobilization, via disturbance of geological structures, and the brief but acute spike in lead usage and dissemination during the Classical Greek and, in particular, Roman eras.) Later in the nineteenth century, miasmatic theories of environmental disease causation were replaced by the specific-causation ideas of the germ theory. This was reinforced around the turn of the century by the identification of particular health disorders due to specific occupational exposures such as pitchblende (uranium oxide ore) mining and working in the dyestuffs industry, and by recognition of specific micronutrient deficiencies. Hence the notion of specific causation of specific diseases became dominant.

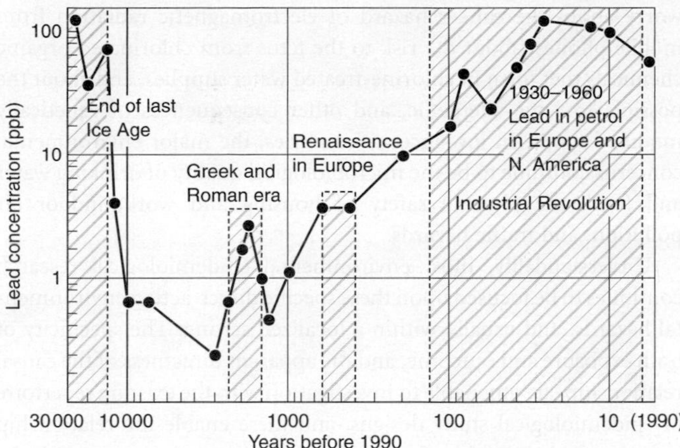

Fig. 2 Variations in the amounts of lead mobilized into the environment, as reflected in Greenland ice-core concentrations over the past 20 000 years. Note the effects of glaciation, the extensive use of lead during the classical Roman era, and the rise of environmental lead levels in association with the industrial revolution over the past two centuries. (Data from Delmas and Legrand 1998.)

Environmental health issues in the twentieth century

The germ theory, which was later qualified by an increasing appreciation of the modulating influences of environmental conditions and endogenous host characteristics, held sway during the early decades of the twentieth century. New knowledge about the vector-based transmission of major diseases such as malaria, schistosomiasis, dengue fever, yellow fever, trypanosomiasis (African sleeping sickness), leishmaniasis (kala-azar), and onchocerciasis (river blindness) led to new environmental management strategies, predominantly in the tropical and subtropical regions. This included the spraying of mosquito breeding sites with dichlorodiphenyltrichloroethane (**DDT**), the control of surface water, the curtailment of certain types of vegetation, and the control of alternative mammalian host species.

The spread of industry and motorized transport systems in the early part of the twentieth century hugely increased the inventory of human-made environmental chemical exposures. As noted in Fig. 2, it also contributed to the marked rise in environmental lead exposures. Various notorious urban air pollution episodes occurred during the middle decades of the century. These were an important stimulus to the new generation of environmental legislation in Western countries during the 1960s and 1970s. In the latter half of the twentieth century, led particularly by environmental regulatory agencies in the United States and drawing on the predominant model of specific causation, a reductionist and quantitative mode of research and risk management has prevailed. The approach has been essentially of an itemizing kind, with emphasis on identifying specific diseases attributable to specific environmental exposures. In the light of that research and the ensuing quantitative risk assessments, official exposure standards have been set for a long succession of specific environmental agents. The task has proved endless.

Meanwhile, in the latter third of the twentieth century we became aware of an additional dimension of hazard resulting from human-made environmental contaminants. In her influential book *Silent Spring*, Carson (1962) argued that pervasive forms of environmental contamination by non-biodegradable bioaccumulating pesticides were ecologically damaging. Non-human species and whole ecosystems were being adversely affected; humans, argued Carson, were therefore on notice that such chemicals could have ripple effects throughout nature, eventually impinging on human biology and well being.

In the 1970s we became increasingly aware of acid rain. Environmental health hazards were thus transcending landscapes, crossing boundaries, and growing in scale. In the 1980s, suspicions arose about the health consequences of cumulative exposures to various families of environmental contaminants, especially the long-lived ('residual') chlorinated hydrocarbons and several of the heavy metals. Evidence from animal species, if not from humans, indicated that such exposures could disrupt the workings of the immune system, reproductive system, and neurological system. This increasing emphasis on thinking about ecological and biological systems, within the framework of 'environmental health', were harbingers of today's systems-oriented concerns about larger-scale environmental change, ecological disruption, and their impacts on human population health.

Categories of environmental exposure

External environmental exposures can be conveniently classified in a two-by-two table, differentiating exposures according to whether they are natural or human-made phenomena, or whether they are of local or global scale. Our modern preoccupation is with human-made environmental hazards. Historically, however, preindustrial concerns focused more on aspects of the natural environment. This was memorably encapsulated by Hippocrates, writing nearly two and a half millennia ago in *Airs, Waters, Places*.

> [C]onsider the seasons of the year, and what effects each of them produces . . . then the winds, the hot and the cold, especially such as are common to all countries, and then such as are peculiar to each locality . . . concerning the waters which people use, whether they be marshy and soft, or hard and running from elevated and rocky situations, and then if saltish and unfit for cooking . . .

Natural versus human-made environmental hazards

Natural environmental influences remain relevant today. They include extremes of weather, locally circulating infectious agents, physical disasters, and local micronutrient deficiencies that reflect soil composition. For example, almost one-fifth of the world population lives on ancient, leached, and often mountainous soils which are deficient in iodine. This puts many such populations at risk of dietary iodine deficiency disorders, including goitre, reproductive impairment, and congenital disorders including cretinism, deafness, and neuromuscular disorders (Hetzel and Pandav 1994). Likewise, there are pockets of exposure to selenium deficiency in China and elsewhere, causing Keshan disease of the heart muscle in young adults and Kashin–Beck disease of bones and joints in older people (Appleton *et al.* 1996). In recent years it has become apparent that there is widespread exposure to arsenic from both soil and water, causing skin lesions, cardiovascular disorders, and various cancers in south-west Taiwan, the Obuasi region of Ghana, and parts of South

America. The problem of arsenic-containing groundwater has reached extreme proportions in Bangladesh and West Bengal where there is increasing reliance on deep tubewells—as an alternative to faecally contaminated surface waters (Mazumder *et al.* 1998).

While most of these natural environmental health hazards can be defined and studied on a local scale, some have a larger dimension. For example, the quasi-periodic El Niño events, occurring every 5 to 7 years, entail a worldwide perturbation of climatic patterns that originate in natural oceanic-atmospheric fluctuations in the eastern Pacific region. These events often lead to environmental disasters and disturbances which, conditional on the vulnerability profile of local populations, pose various physical, microbiological, and other types of hazards to human health (Epstein 1999; Kovats *et al.* 1999).

The distinction between natural and human-made environmental hazards is not always clear. Several experiences in India in recent decades are illustrative, where natural environmental/nutritional health hazards have unexpectedly improved or become worse following human interventions in the wider environment (Gopalan 1999). Such interventions can disturb geochemical processes in soil and water, causing altered human ingestion of certain metals and trace elements. Pellagra (tryptophan deficiency) was alleviated in the 1980s by basic, economically driven changes in India's production and market price of alternative cereal grains. Wheat and, to a lesser extent, rice substantially displaced pulses and jowar. Meanwhile, goitre and intellectual stunting due to dietary iodine deficiency increased their geographic range because the spread of irrigation and the expansion of sugar-cane production both depleted soil iodine levels.

Local versus global environmental hazards

Today, the topic of 'environmental health' must accommodate a further larger-scale dimension of external environmental influence. This type of health hazard arises from the disruption of the Earth's ecological and geophysical systems and processes. This disruption jeopardizes the flow of nature's 'goods and services': climatic stability, food yields, the supply of clean and fresh water, and the healthy functioning of biotically diverse natural ecosystems that recyle nutrients, cleanse air and water, and produce useful materials (Daily 1997). The disruption of these systems can affect population health in more diverse, and often less direct and less immediate, ways than those of specific conventional environmental hazards that pose direct local hazards via injury, toxicity, nutritional deficiency, or infection (Last 1992).

The distinction between these two categories of environmental influences upon health is perhaps best characterized as a difference in the scale of environmental change and in the immediacy and directness of action. The conventional 'environmental health' focus of epidemiologists and public has been on hazards that arise from local human-made environmental indiscretions. In the popular view, prototypical environmental health events include the disasters of Chernobyl, Bhopal, Seveso, Love Canal, Minamata Bay, and the London smog of 1952. In contrast, global environmental changes entail disruptions of complex ecological and geophysical systems.

In industrialized countries attention over the past 50 years has been directed predominantly to the plethora of chemical contaminants entering air, water, soil, and food, along with various physical hazards such as ionizing radiation, non-ionizing radiation, urban noise, and road trauma. As technologies evolve and as levels of consumption rise, the list of candidate hazards seems endless. In the 1990s we began to worry about the cancer hazard of electromagnetic radiation from mobile phones, about the risk to the fetus from chlorinated organic chemicals that form in chlorine-treated water supplies, and about the possible toxicity, allergenic, and other consequences of genetically modified foods. In low-income countries, the major environmental concerns continue to be the microbiological quality of drinking water and food, the physical safety of housing and work, indoor air pollution, and traffic hazards.

Understandably, most environmental epidemiological research continues to be focused upon these specific direct-acting environmental hazards, and usually within a localized setting. The specificity of both exposure and outcome, and the apparent directness of the causal relationship, are amenable to investigation with the existing repertoire of epidemiological study designs, and these enable the relationship between varied levels of individual or group exposure and the probability of some specified health outcome to be determined. Dose–response relationships are described, usually via statistical modelling. Then, if the causal interpretation is convincing, the estimated dose–response relationship can be used to guide directly the setting of standards and regulations. There is now a need to extend the repertoire of epidemiological research and risk assessment methods to accommodate the study of the health impacts of larger-scale environmental change and ecological disruption.

Contribution of environmental exposures to global burden of disease

The relative importance of 'environmental' exposures as a cause of human disease and premature death remains contentious. In industrialized countries the main concern in recent decades has been with the succession of chemical contaminants entering the air, water, soil, and food, and with various physical hazards such as ionizing radiation, non-ionizing radiation (electricity transmission), urban noise, and road trauma. Typical examples of quantifiable environmental health relationships include those between benzene exposure and leukaemia, blood lead concentration and IQ, and tropospheric ozone and asthma attacks. In less developed countries, the persisting environmental concerns are with the microbiological quality of drinking water and food, the physical safety of housing and work, indoor air pollution, exposure to the elements (especially during extreme weather events), and the hazards on chaotic local roads.

Assessing the contribution of environmental exposures to the global burden of disease is difficult for several reasons. Firstly, our knowledge about disease aetiology is incomplete. Secondly, the environmental exposure being assessed is often a moving target: many of today's diseases are primarily the result of yesterday's exposures. Consider, for example, how the mixture of urban air pollution, ever changing over time as technologies and transport systems evolve, is likely to affect the incidence of chronic respiratory disease over the course of several decades. Thirdly, environmental exposures affect not just the occurrence of disease, but may also affect the subsequent clinical management and eventual health outcome.

Depending on the definitions and assumptions used, estimates of the environmental contribution to the global burden of disease vary. An assessment conducted for the fifth anniversary of the Rio de Janeiro Earth Summit estimated that about 25 per cent of the global burden of disease and premature death, as measured in disability-adjusted life years, was caused by environmental hazards, including the workplace environment (WHO 1997). Smith *et al.* (1999), in a recent comprehensive analysis that encompassed disease initiation, progression, and case outcome, estimate that 25 to 33 per cent of the global burden of disease and premature death is attributable to direct environmental risk factors. Using published dose–response data for major exposure–disease relationships, Murray and Lopez (1999) have estimated (Table 1) that around one-quarter of the global burden of disease is due to 'environmental exposures' (at all ages), including around one-sixth of the total burden in young people (birth to 14 years).

Some caution is needed in the choice of the health risk coefficients that are incorporated in this type of calculation. In particular, there are some environmental exposures that vary on both a short-term and long-term basis. Ambient temperature is one such exposure: it varies on a daily basis, a seasonal basis, and (with incipient climate change) on a decadal scale. Likewise the concentrations of various air pollutants vary over short periods. This day-to-day variation in exposure levels presents a challenge to environmental epidemiologists: How do the biological impacts of acute fluctuations in exposure relate to the induction of chronic disease by prolonged exposure to above-average levels?

The answer is that we do not yet really know. In general, it is easier to estimate the health risks associated with acute fluctuations in the exposure than to study the long-term health consequences of sustained exposure. Hence, daily time-series studies within single populations, particularly studies of mortality, have become prominent within air pollution epidemiology. The regression-based risk coefficients from these studies have then been widely used to estimate the excess annual mortality within a population with a specified average level of air pollution. Yet such calculations are inappropriate (McMichael *et al.* 1998), since daily time-series data provide no direct information about the extent of life-shortening associated with the excess daily deaths (many of which result from exacerbation of well-advanced disease, especially cardiovascular disease). Therefore, such data cannot contribute to the estimation of the effects of prolonged exposure to air pollution upon chronic disease incidence and death rates—even though that latter category of effect is of much greater public health importance. (Indeed, a comparative risk assessment carried out for The Netherlands (de Hollander *et al.* 1999) estimates that the health-impairing effect of chronic exposure to air-borne particulates is at least an order of magnitude greater than the effect of short-term exposures.) The long-term effects are best estimated via cohort studies. Time-series studies can identify the acute toxic effects, and can assist in identifying the most noxious pollutants, but they cannot quantify the long-term health impacts of air pollution.

Before reviewing the scope of local, and then global, environmental health hazards, the major research strategies, and some of the distinctive needs of this topic area, will be summarized.

Environmental health research: some specific issues

Scope, strategies, and policy interface

The prime task of environmental epidemiological research is to elucidate causal relations between environmental exposures and

Table 1 Estimated proportion of global burden of illness, injury, and premature mortality attributable to environmental exposures, measured with a common unit (disability-adjusted life year (DALY))

Disease/injury	Global DALYs (thousands)	Environmental fraction[a] (%)	Percentage of all DALYs	
			All ages	0–14 years
Acute respiratory infections	116 696	60	5.0	4.50
Diarrhoeal diseases	99 633	90	6.5	6.10
Vaccine-preventable infections	71 173	10	0.5	0.49
Tuberculosis	38 426	10	0.3	0.04
Malaria	31 706	90	2.1	1.80
Injuries				
Unintentional	152 188	30	3.3	1.60
Intentional	56 459	Not estimated		
Mental health	144 950	10	1.1	0.08
Cardiovascular diseases	133 236	10	1.0	0.12
Cancer	70 513	25	1.3	0.11
Chronic respiratory diseases	60 370	50	2.2	0.57
Total of these diseases	973 350	33	23.3	15.4
Total other diseases	403 888		76.7	84.6
Total all diseases	1379 238		100.0	100.0

[a]For example, in the first row the estimated proportion of all DALYs incurred by acute respiratory infections that is attributable to environmental exposures is 60%. In contrast, for tuberculosis (fourth row), only 10% of DALYs are deemed to be due to environmental exposures.

Data from Murray and Lopez (1996).

impaired states of health. It also seeks to quantify risks to populations, to develop appropriate interventions to reduce environmental risks to health, and to evaluate the effectiveness of such intervention. Epidemiology is the basic quantitative science of environmental health research. The concepts and methods of epidemiology are addressed in detail in Part 6. In essence, epidemiological research describes and explains variations and temporal changes in the pattern of illness and disease between and within populations. Most environmental epidemiology is observational (non-experimental), and this imparts certain well-known challenges to research design and data interpretation. Where health benefit is anticipated from interventions that reduce environmental exposures, experimental studies can be carried out.

Historically, epidemiology has played a crucial and largely self-sufficient role in identifying the environmental health hazards posed by relatively high levels of exposure, such as heavy air pollution (e.g. the London smog of 1952), heavy metals (especially in the occupational setting) in air, water, and food, solar ultraviolet irradiation, and environmental tobacco smoke. Those early studies were mostly done in industrializing countries, where research expertise existed and where there were technical and information resources available. Increasingly, the spotlight of attention is shifting to environmental exposures in low-income countries and in former communist countries undergoing rapid social and economic transition (often with a background of extensive environmental pollution and degradation). In low-income countries there is commonly a compounded range of environmental exposures. There are environmental health hazards arising from traditional practices (such as the use of solid fuels and biomass for domestic heating and cooking, and the consumption of fungal toxins in stored foods in tropical regions); those that continue to arise from microbiological contamination of water, food, and soil; and those that are now emerging via industrialization, the extension of mining and oil extraction, forest clearance and irrigation, urbanization, and the rapid increase in private car ownership.

Many environmental exposures occur at dose rates and total doses that are low compared to occupational exposures and personal habits such as cigarette smoking. This situation presents the epidemiologist with the difficult task of detecting modest increments in risk. Yet the importance of these external environmental exposures is threefold.

1. The exposures often impinge on a large proportion of people within the population, thereby resulting in a large aggregate health impact (this is a socio-economic criterion), i.e. while the individual 'risk' is small, the population 'effect' may not be.
2. The exposures are encountered on an essentially involuntary, and often unequal, basis (an ethical criterion).
3. The exposures are amenable to control at source (a practical criterion).

There are several other characteristic features of environmental epidemiological research. Firstly, many types of environmental exposures (such as drinking-water fluoride levels or urban air pollution levels) impinge fairly evenly over whole communities, which makes the individual-level comparison of health impacts difficult. Secondly, any one particular environmental exposure is likely to be accompanied by other environmental exposures. This results, at least, in the need to take account of confounding effects—and the combined exposures may mean that there are significant biological interactions. Thirdly, modern understanding of the subtle and complex processes of development and functioning of various organ systems—especially the central nervous system, immune system, and reproductive system—have led to an awareness of how environmental exposures may induce 'subclinical' impairment of those systems.

In the light of these complexities environmental health research increasingly is undertaken in an interdisciplinary fashion. For example, research into the effect of low-level environmental lead exposure on the cognitive development of young children has required the integrated consideration of the results of epidemiological studies, animal experimental research, and neuropathological and molecular toxicological studies. The development of molecular biology over the past several decades has yielded many new techniques for measuring 'internal' exposure, especially in relation to carcinogenesis. Molecular biological markers are also useful for measuring putative biological mechanistic phenomena (which strengthens the basis for causal inference) and, in some situations, as early preclinical biological outcomes.

Other key issues in environmental epidemiology

Units of 'exposure': collective versus individual exposure

Environmental exposures, as discussed above, often impinge approximately equally on most or all members of a community. Hence, many epidemiological studies have depended on comparing groups of people defined by area of residence, city, or occupation. Even where it is likely that there is moderate exposure difference between individuals, because of interindividual behavioural variation, it is often difficult in practice to estimate those exposure differences. Notwithstanding the implications of many textbooks, the reflex discounting of population-level ('ecological') studies is inappropriate. There is impressive historical precedent for the informativeness of such an approach, such as Snow's comparison of cholera death rates in adjoining suburbs in mid-nineteenth century London (Snow 1855). Furthermore, various environmental epidemiological questions are essentially of a 'population' kind. For example: How does the mortality impact of heatwaves differ between coastal and midcontinental urban populations? Are migrant populations at increased risk of childhood leukaemia because of their encounter with unfamiliar local viruses?

Time lags between exposure and outcome

A recurring difficulty in environmental epidemiology, especially in relation to chronic disease outcomes, is that many exposures change over time. In effect, today's health events may be primarily the result of exposure in earlier decades. It is well documented, for example, that the composition and level of air pollution has changed in most cities over recent decades. Therefore cross-sectional correlations of levels of community exposure to air pollution and disease rates may be misleading. The phenomenon of temporal trends in exposure variables is not limited to the environmental realm; the same applies to dietary habits, oral contraceptive formulation, and so on. However, there is a particular temptation in environmental epidemiology to examine readily available cross-sectional data.

The time-lag question also arises in relation to the study of acute effects. Is the mortality toll of a heatwave greatest on the day of maximum temperature, or one or two days later? To answer this sort of question it is necessary to test a succession of different short-term lag periods.

Total exposure assessment

To estimate the health risk associated with an environmental exposure agent it is necessary to consider all the ways it might reach people. Some pollutants can readily reach people through several different routes. Therefore, if exposure assessment is based on environmental sampling it may be necessary to sample several media. For example, airborne lead pollution, arising mainly from leaded fuel in motor vehicles, can spread through the environment via air, water, soil, and food. Even though the original emissions of lead may have only been to air, exclusive attention to that route would greatly underestimate the actual total exposure—and it is the latter that determines the risk to health.

This problem can either be tackled by multimedia measurements or by the use of some integrating biological measure. Examples of the latter include blood lead concentration, adipose tissue dioxin concentration, and breast-milk concentrations of polychlorinated biphenyls.

Spatial analysis

Many of the relationships being investigated in environmental epidemiology depend on the analysis of spatial relations. Simple techniques entail, for example, the use of concentric circles around point sources of environmental pollutants or of residential distance from main highways. As the amount and quality of information on the spatial distribution of the exposure hazard, and of its sources, increases, along with the equivalent information on the distribution of health outcome measures, so the possibilities increase for formal spatial analysis (Lawson *et al.* 1999). Geographic information systems afford an analytic technique for identifying spatial relationships via the integration of 'layers' of spatial data about one or more exposures, other confounding or modifying factors, and health outcomes. In situations that entail a mix of input variables of quantitative, ordered, and nominal types, multivariate ordination techniques such as non-metric multidimensional scaling ordination are becoming increasingly widely used. A range of research strategies has evolved over the past decade for the study of 'small-area' environmental epidemiological statistical analysis (Elliott *et al.* 1992). Improved techniques for smoothing data and for dealing with autocorrelation and outlier observations are now available. The use of these various techniques has been facilitated by the rapid increases in computing power.

There is a largely untapped wealth of historical and current spatial environmental data, much of it from satellite remote-sensing. There is the opportunity, indeed need, for the public health sciences to become more integrated with the relevant scientific networks, and to learn about and access these resources. Global 'observing systems' were created during the 1990s, with detailed data on the world's land surfaces (terrestrial systems), oceans, and atmosphere. These are auspiced within the United Nations family of organizations. Other regional or national environmental data sets are also available, particularly from the well-resourced American agencies such as the National Aeronautical and Space Administration and the National Oceanic and Atmospheric Administration.

Specific toxicity versus generic organ system effects

Most toxicological studies and most environmental epidemiological studies aim to characterize effects and risks associated with specific exposure agents. When such exposures yield specific avoidable clinical outcomes (e.g. bladder cancer, renal failure, encephalopathy), then this approach makes good sense. However, there has been increasing recognition that certain organ systems can be cumulatively, adversely, affected by multiple exposures over time. Such exposures can result in immune system suppression, endocrine disruption, and cognitive impairment.

Both the immune system and the endocrine system entail complex interactive networks of organs, cells, and chemical messengers. It is not surprising that many exogenous organic chemicals can cause metabolic perturbation of these systems. Those are not so much 'toxic' as 'pharmacological' effects. There is accruing evidence that implicates organochlorine pesticides and other organic chemicals such as butyltin in suppression of the human immune system (WRI 1998; Whalen *et al.* 1999). There is suggestive, but inconclusive, evidence of a decline in sperm count over the past 50 years (Sharpe and Skakkebaek 1993), although the interpretation of the evidence is hampered by the constituent datasets being neither representative nor standardized. Plausibility comes from various observations of impaired fertility and reproduction in other mammals, birds, and fish.

There has been specific concern about the possible involvement of endocrine-disrupting xeno-oestrogens in breast cancer in women. Some organochlorine compounds such as DDT (especially its metabolite dichlorodiphenyldichloroethylene) may have weak oestrogenic effects and are therefore suspected of increasing the risk of hormone-dependent cancers, particularly breast cancer in women (Davis *et al.* 1998). Breast cancer is the most common cancer among women in many Western countries and most of the major risk factors for breast cancer, such as early menarche, late menopause, nulliparity, late conception of the firstborn, and hormone replacement treatment, suggest that oestrogen is important in the pathogenesis of breast cancer. However, the results from studies of breast cancer in relation to environmental exposures to organochlorine compounds have been inconsistent.

Risk assessment: the research–policy interface

The increasing awareness within educated communities about the potential health risks posed by ambient environmental exposures has brought an increased expectation that governments will assess risks, prescribe standards, and ensure environmental risk management. Epidemiologists have therefore become increasingly engaged at this research–policy interface, seeking to summarize the range of published research findings, to derive dose–response relationships, and to identify critical levels of exposure.

Methods of quantitative risk assessment have evolved over the past two decades, particularly within the United States—and particularly in relation to exposure agents deemed to be causes of cancer (Samet *et al.* 1998; Corvalan *et al.* 1999; Nurminen *et al.* 1999). Proponents proclaim the merits of quantitative risk assessment as a successful social application of otherwise disparate results of a myriad of epidemiological and toxicological studies. Critics indicate the problems in averaging across epidemiological studies, the uncertainty of the form of dose–response functions, the difficulties of extrapolating between dose ranges and species, and the questionable assumption that single factors act independently of one another. The lack, or imprecision, of epidemiological data within parts of the exposure range of interest often necessitates supplementation with, or reliance on, animal toxicological data (McMichael and Woodward 1999).

Quantitative risk assessment, in its fullest form, enables the current or future burden of disease attributable to a particular profile of exposure, within an entire population, to be estimated. Thus, for a specified urban population, we may estimate how many episodes of asthma are attributable to an annual pattern of daily fluctuations in specified air pollutants. Or we may estimate the total sick days resulting from that asthma, or the total loss of productive working days. It is then possible to extend the analysis to estimate the economic costs to the population. Indeed, if the preventability of asthma is sufficiently well understood, cost–benefit analysis can titrate the 'savings' from averted asthma episodes against the costs of reducing the pollutant levels. This extension of quantitative risk assessment into the realm of cost–benefit analysis has highlighted the need for a common metric, applicable to disparate health outcomes. The disability-adjusted life year has recently been promoted and widely used as one such common metric that enables 'comparative risk assessment' (Murray and Lopez 1999). A recent example of how such an approach can facilitate the comparison of environmental risks and guide the choice of environmental interventions has been published by de Hollander *et al.* (1999), showing, for example, that the long-term effects of particulate air pollution account for almost 60 per cent of the total environment-attributable health loss in The Netherlands.

There is an important extension to this item. As we recognize the prospect of large-scale environmental declines that are likely to jeopardize the well being and health of future generations, so we encounter an ethical problem. How do we weigh the health needs of future generations against the manifest needs of the present generation? Unavoidably, there must be a trade-off since generalized and globally equitable economic development today, based on current technologies and patterns of consumption, will greatly increase the pressures on the biosphere. Indeed, some would argue that unless it is shown that obligations to future generations differ qualitatively from those to the present generation, our undoubted first priority must be to deal with existing problems—buoyed by the hope that solutions to future sustainability will emerge. The argument is morally and philosophically complex, but it is one that will be eased by improved assessments of the range and magnitude of likely future impacts on human population health. As ever, social policy-making will be assisted and enhanced by fuller information and more extensive risk assessments.

Profiles of hazardous ambient environmental exposures

Overview

The advent of the new environmentalism in Western societies, during the latter third of the twentieth century, has been associated with widespread reductions in various forms of environmental pollution. Sulphate and particulate air pollution has declined, largely in response to legislative and regulatory initiatives; likewise acid rain has been curbed, the use and release of heavy metals has decreased, pesticide use has been constrained (and DDT banned), and the nuclear power industry has become more tightly controlled. These were the sorts of environmental issues that were prominent at the agenda-setting United Nations Conference on the Human Environment in Stockholm in 1972.

Meanwhile, car usage and urban transport systems in general, and hence exhaust emissions, have proliferated. The rise of photochemical-oxidant air pollutants (especially ozone), and the increase in fine particulates (especially from diesel engines) have posed particular risks to cardiovascular and respiratory health. Food production methods have tended to become intensified and the long-distance transport of fresh and processed foods has increased. Both developments have been associated with an apparent rise in the occurrence of episodes of microbiological and chemical contamination of food (McMichael 1999*a*). The occurrence of bovine spongiform encephalopathy ('mad cow disease') in the United Kingdom, and its subsequent transmission to humans as new variant Creutzfeldt–Jakob disease, illustrates well the sort of unexpected public health consequence that can arise from aberrant methods of intensified livestock production.

In low-income countries the profile of environmental exposures is more mixed, reflecting the 'old' and the 'new'. Microbiological hazards, especially in drinking water, remain widespread in rural populations, shanty towns, and urban slums: approximately 40 per cent of the world's population still lack safe drinking water and 60 per cent lack sanitation. Domestic air pollution levels are often high, especially where biomass fuels or coal are used for heating and cooking. In consequence, high rates of infant and child mortality from diarrhoeal diseases and acute respiratory infections persist (Wang and Smith 1999). Meanwhile, as industries proliferate, as chemical-intensive agriculture spreads, and as cities fill with cars, trucks, and buses, so the ambient environment acquires a range of additional physical, air-borne, water-borne, and food-borne hazardous exposures. The combination of population pressures and economic intensification is placing increasing stresses on local environments and these result in both immediate environmental hazards and in the longer-term depletion of natural resource stocks, alteration of physicogeochemical cycles (e.g. the public health problem of arsenic-contaminated groundwater from deep tubewells sunk throughout Bangladesh and West Bengal), and disruption of ecological systems.

As we enter the twenty-first century, more than half of all people are living in urban environments. This statistic will continue to rise during the coming several decades as *Homo sapiens* becomes an urbanized species. It is important to think about the urban environment as a 'habitat', as a system of interacting conditions, exposures, and processes—physical, chemical, and microbiological; demographic, social, and cultural. It will suffice, in this chapter, to mention just a few of the distinguishing features of the ever-evolving urban environment.

The urban environment

Contemporary sources of hazards

The modern urban configuration—which is both variable and evolving in countries around the world—comprises industrial activities, concentrated transport systems, intensive waste generation, and fluid and often novel patterns of social relations and interactions. This configuration poses various environmental risks to health. Some of the risks may be overt, as with road trauma or the increase in asthma hospital admissions during air pollution crises. Others, however, are non-acute and more insidious. Environmental lead exposure, which blunts young children's intelligence, is a good example of the latter type of urban exposure. The best estimate, based on cohort studies in Western populations, is that children whose blood lead concentrations during early childhood differ by around 10 μg/dl have a resultant difference of 2 to 3 IQ points, relative to an expected population mean of 100 (Tong and McMichael 1999). Such exposure differentials typically occur between the top and bottom quintiles of children within the urban environment.

The material quality of housing is another important dimension of the urban environment. It appears to be an important determinant of seasonal patterns of morbidity and mortality. For example, the older housing stock in the United Kingdom is a likely contributor to the well-documented above-average excess of winter mortality in that country relative to most other European countries. Housing quality, including dampness, may contribute to early-life exposure to fungal spores and to house dust mites, both of which are likely initiators of asthmatic predisposition in children.

The three contrasting examples of urban environmental hazards discussed below all reflect basic aspects of our urban living style and environment. They are urban air pollution, the various physical and social hazards of transport systems, and the vulnerability of inner-urban populations to heatwaves.

Urban air pollution

Urban air pollution has, in recent decades, become a worldwide public health problem. The earlier industrial/domestic air pollution from coal burning has been replaced by pollutants from motorized transport which form photochemical smog in summer and episodes of heavy haze of particulates and nitrogen oxides in winter.

Studies relating ambient air pollution levels to health risks were, until the 1970s, largely confined to examining particular extreme episodes of very high outdoors air pollution levels (e.g. the famous London smog of 1952). These episodes were associated with a marked increase in total mortality, especially cardiovascular and respiratory deaths, and with various respiratory disorders. More recently, long-term follow-up studies of populations exposed at different levels of air pollution, especially particulates, indicate that the higher the background levels of exposure the greater the mortality risk (Dockery *et al.* 1993; Pope *et al.* 1995).

In China, urban air pollution with particulates and sulphur dioxide is increasing sharply. The main source of pollution is the industrial use of coal, with its relatively high sulphur content. However, emissions from domestic cooking and heating fuels are also increasing. Indeed, nationally, the much greater health hazard is from indoor air pollution (Smith *et al.* 1999). The World Bank has recently assessed that morbidity and mortality in Chinese cities will increase steeply over the coming two decades. On current industrialization trends, it has been estimated that premature deaths will increase from around 200 000 to over half a million per year by 2020, while chronic bronchitis cases and annual bouts of respiratory symptoms are expected to triple (World Bank 1997).

An interesting contemporary policy application of these risk estimates is in assessing the avoidable health impacts attendant upon reduction of fossil fuel combustion undertaken to mitigate greenhouse gas emissions. Worldwide, it has been estimated that 7 million premature deaths could be avoided by 2020 if there were worldwide compliance with the level of carbon dioxide emission reduction recommended in the Kyoto Protocol (WGPHFFC 1997). Related estimations for China indicate that, if that country were to comply with the carbon dioxide emission cutbacks of the Kyoto Protocol, then by 2020 the annual avoidance of premature deaths from ambient (external) air pollution in China would be in the range of 2000 to 16 000 (Wang and Smith 2000). Furthermore, the equivalent number of avoidable deaths for the simultaneous reductions in indoor exposure (where coal is currently the main domestic fuel and exposures are often extreme) would be a vast 50 000 to 500 000. The width of those ranges reflects both the existence of alternative technological approaches to emission reductions and the uncertainties of the dose-specific risks to health.

Epidemiologists have developed a diverse and increasingly sophisticated set of methods for assessing the health impacts of air pollution. Nevertheless, the issue remains constrained by difficulties in exposure assessment, by the uncertain differentiation between acute and chronic effects, by the need to elucidate interactive effects between coexistent air pollutants that are often highly correlated, and by the fact that the profile of air pollution keeps evolving as human activity patterns change.

Transport systems

As modern cities grow in size, transport systems become a prominent feature of the environment. In various of Europe's main cities, public transport systems were established many decades ago before the rising counterpressure of privately-owned cars. Hence there are undergound train systems in many cities, and extensive tram-car networks in a few (such as Amsterdam). Car ownership and travel has increased spectacularly over the past 50 years, in much of the world. Indeed, in the second quarter of the twentieth century, the oil, tyre, and automobile industries in the United States took deliberate collective action to buy up and dismantle most of the nation's urban light-rail systems, thus making the future safe for the private car (Newman and Kenworthy 2000). In many of the cities of eastern and southeastern Asia, rapid unplanned growth in private car ownership has created serious environmental health problems (including the escalation of lead pollution). Road networks and highways have become dominant influences on urban topography, and they often subdivide and fracture communities. There are two sides to this ledger: privately owned cars create new opportunities and freedoms, while also creating new social and public health problems (McMichael 1996).

In addition to the well-known environmental problems of exhaust gas emissions—comprising various noxious gases that cause local air pollution, gases that contribute to acid rain, and the release of the greenhouse gas carbon dioxide—the other major public health detriments of car-based transport systems are as follows.

1. Fatal and non-fatal injuries of car occupants, pedestrians, and cyclists. The global annual total of deaths caused by traffic now approaches 1 million, and the death rates are growing most rapidly in many of the world's poorer countries as urban traffic proliferates.

2. Physical disruption of neighbourhoods. This contributes to social fragmentation and isolation. In conjunction with (1) above, this physical dominance of roads and traffic diminishes levels of physical activity, particularly in young schoolchildren who are constrained from walking to school and from exploring and playing in their local residential environments. This is an important contributor to the emerging problem of obesity in urban populations everywhere.

3. Chronic increases in noise levels, with disturbance of sleep patterns and exacerbations of social tensions.

Thermal stress: urban vulnerability and mortality

Severe heatwaves adversely affect health. This is particularly so in the centre of large cities, where temperatures may be higher than in the suburbs and the surrounding countryside, and where the relief of night-time cooling may be reduced. These manifestations of the 'heat island' effect are due to the heat-retaining concrete, asphalt, and masonry structures of most inner cities, the physical obstruction of cooling breezes, and the lack of parks and trees. Note that much of the problem is a micro-ecological one, reflecting the form and materials of urban design.

The 1990s was the warmest decade on record (that is, since the mid-nineteenth century), and, from proxy measures of temperature, for at least the last eight centuries. In July 1995, more than 460 extra deaths were certified as due to the effects of the extreme heatwave in Chicago in July, when temperatures reached 40°C (Semenza *et al.* 1996). Studies of such episodes elsewhere in North America and Europe have shown that those most vulnerable to heat-related illness and death are the elderly, the sick, and the urban poor. In the Chicago heatwave, the rate of heat-related death was much greater in those living in poorly ventilated apartment-block housing (Semenza *et al.* 1996). That same high pressure system subsequently affected the United Kingdom. An estimated 768 extra deaths (an approximately 10 per cent excess) occurred during the ensuing 5-day heatwave in England and Wales, relative to the equivalent period in 1993–1994 (Rooney *et al.* 1998). In Greater London, where daytime temperatures were higher (and where there was lesser cooling at night), mortality increased by around 15 per cent during the heatwave.

These studies have underscored the mix of determinants of mortality excess during heatwaves: the urban environment itself as part of modern human ecology, the cultural and technological adaptation to coping with heat (cities in northern Europe and northern United States cope less well than do southern cities), and the circumstances or characteristics of certain individuals that render them particularly vulnerable.

Urban populations: ecological footprints and sustainability

There is another qualitatively different dimension to the topic of urban populations and environmental health. Urban populations play the dominant role in the mounting pressures that currently jeopardize the sustainability of current human ecology. Cities have increasingly large 'ecological footprints' (Rees 1996). There are undoubted ecological benefits of urbanism, including economies of scale, shared use of resources, and opportunities for reuse and recycling. Equally, though, there are great 'externalities'. Urban populations depend on food grown elsewhere, on raw materials (timber, metals, fibre, and so on) and energy sources (especially fossil fuels) extracted from elsewhere, and on disposing their voluminous wastes elsewhere.

Urban populations thus depend on the natural resources of ecosystems that, in aggregate, are vastly larger in area than the city itself. The highly urbanized Netherlands consumes resources from a total surface area 15 times larger than itself. Folke *et al.* (1996) have studied the renewable resource appropriations by the cities of the Baltic Sea region. The estimated consumption of resources (wood, paper, fibres, and food (including seafood)) by 29 cities depends upon a total area many hundred times greater than their combined area. Similarly, Rees (1996) has estimated that the almost half-million residents of Vancouver, Canada, occupying just 11 400 hectares, actually use the ecological output and services of 2.3 million hectares (Table 2)—a ratio of 207:1.

Viewed prospectively, the sustainability of the world's urban populations and their health thus depends on the continued productivity of, and other 'services' provided by, those distant ecosystems. Yet, even so, the magnitude of the environmental externalities of urbanism is growing. The externalities include massive urban contributions to the global accumulation of greenhouse gas, stratospheric ozone depletion, land degradation, local aquifer depletion, and coastal zone destruction. The urbanized developed world, with approximately one-fifth of the world population, currently contributes around three-quarters of all greenhouse gas emissions (IPCC 1996).

Simple arithmetic reveals that the Earth is not large enough to support, sustainably, a future population of 8 to 10 billion living at the level of energy and material consumption of today's Western middle-class populations. A radical 'greening' of social structures, urban design, and technology, with an emphasis on energy efficiency and on reuse and recycling, is required (McMichael and Powles 1999). Shifts in literate consumer preferences and behaviours, via a market place that is socially regulated to ensure that pricing internalizes the full environmental costs, will be a necessary and important input to this process.

'New and resurgent' infectious diseases: a global phenomenon

Infectious diseases receded in Western countries throughout the latter nineteenth and most of the twentieth century. Initially, this was largely the result of urban sanitation, improved housing design, personal hygiene, antisepsis in clinical medicine, and the advent of vaccination. The antibiotic era consolidated this increasing suppression of infectious disease as a source of serious morbidity and mortality. However, the receding tide apparently turned during the last quarter of the twentieth century. As the turn of the century approached there was much talk of 'new and resurgent' infectious diseases (de Cock and Greenwood 1998).

In 1996, the annual WHO Health Report stated that: 'Until relatively recently, the long struggle for control over infectious diseases seemed almost over. . . Far from being over, the struggle to control infectious diseases has become increasingly difficult. . . The result

Table 2 Ecological footprints of Vancouver and the Lower Fraser Basin

Geographic unit	Population	Land area (ha)	Ecological footprint (ha)	Overshoot factor
Vancouver City	472 000	11 400	2360 600	207
Lower Fraser Basin	2000 000	830 000	10 000 000	12

Source: Rees (1996).

amounts to a global crisis'. This hyperbolic language aside, something unexpected has recently happened to patterns of infectious disease. An unusually large number of new or newly discovered infectious diseases have been recorded in the past 25 years, including rotavirus, cryptosporidiosis, legionellosis, the Ebola virus, Lyme disease, hepatitis C, HIV/AIDS, hantavirus pulmonary syndrome, *Escherichia coli* 0157, cholera 0139, toxic shock syndrome (staphyloccal), and others (Morse 1995; Heymann and Rodier 1997).

There are unusually large-scale influences on infectious disease patterns (Wilson 1995). Populations are becoming interconnected economically, culturally, and physically, enhancing the mixing of people, animals, and microbes from all geographical areas. Human mobility has escalated dramatically, in volume and speed, between and within countries. Long-distance trade facilitates the geographical redistribution of pests and pathogens. This has been well illustrated in recent years by the HIV pandemic, the worldwide dispersal of rodent-borne hantaviruses, and the rapid dissemination of a new epidemic strain of bacterial meningitis along routes of travel and trade (Morse 1995).

Rapid urbanization is expanding the traditional role of cities as gateways for infectious diseases. Population movement from rural areas into cities, and the amplified urban–rural, interurban, and intraurban contacts, is opening new vistas of opportunity to otherwise marginal microbes. This probably assisted the launch of the otherwise poorly-transmissible HIV/AIDS virus in the 1980s (Morse 1995). Likewise, the modern global spread of dengue and dengue haemorrhagic fever (the latter reflecting the increasing geographic overlap of the four viral serotypes) has been aided by the urban expansion of breeding sites for the *Aedes* mosquito vector. In addition to the ongoing microbial genetic evolution in response to antibiotic use, changes in contemporary human ecology have intensified much of the 'microbial traffic' and thus increased the probability that potential human pathogens will find an ecologically supportive pathway or niche (Morse 1993).

Urbanism and the relaxation of traditional cultural norms is yielding newer and freer patterns of human behaviour, including sexual activities and illicit drug use. Modern medical manoeuvres create new ecological opportunities for viruses and prions; hospital admission practices have done similarly for various bacteria (e.g. the *Proteus* and *Pseudomonas* genera). Over the past 50 years antibiotics have been used widely and often unwisely (including for livestock and agricultural purposes), thus helping to nurture a new generation of drug-resistant organisms. Likewise, we have inadvertently bred pesticide-resistant mosquitoes, thereby facilitating the dissemination of malaria, yellow fever, dengue fever, and many other vector-borne diseases (Chapin and Wasserstrom 1981).

Infectious disease patterns are also affected by the intensification of food production and processing methods. The notorious bovine spongiform encephalopathy/Creutzfeldt–Jakob disease ('mad cow disease') episode in the United Kingdom is a particular example of this problem. On a more familiar front, the reported rates of food poisoning have increased in Western countries during the past two decades, and have almost doubled in the United Kingdom between the mid-1980s and mid-1990s (WHO 1997). The spread of the potentially fatal toxin-producing *E. coli* 0157 in North America and Europe in the mid-1990s appears to have accompanied beef imported from infected cattle in Argentina (where the rates of human infection with *E. coli* 0157 are reportedly higher than in Western countries).

The environmentally disruptive impact of technological innovation—whether industrial, agricultural, or medical—in the course of several decades of linear Western-style national economic development in the developing countries made clear that large-scale human interventions in the natural environment often adversely affect infectious disease patterns (Heyneman 1984). Large dams, irrigation schemes, land reclamation, road construction, and population resettlement programmes (as currently occurring in Indonesia) have often potentiated the spread of malaria, dengue fever, schistosomiasis, and trypanosomiasis (Kloos and Thompson 1979; Inhorn and Brown 1990).

Patterns of infectious diseases are widely influenced by land clearance activities in populous regions of the developing world and by the extension of irrigation. In the Sudan, for example, schistosomiasis appeared within several years of the start of the Gezira scheme, a large irrigated cotton project (Fenwick *et al.* 1981). Various viral haemorrhagic fevers have emerged over the past several decades as intensified land clearance and habitat disruption, especially in South America, have exposed human populations to new viruses that previously circulated exclusively within wilderness ecosystems. For example, the Junin virus, causing Argentine haemorrhagic fever, naturally infects wild rodents (the mouse *Callomys callosus*). However, the extensive conversion of grassland to maize cultivation in recent decades, stimulating a proliferation of the virus-bearing mice, has exposed farm-workers to this 'new' virus.

Meanwhile, casting a longer shadow over the future prospects for human health is the possibility that changes in the world's climate, the continued loss of biodiversity, and the persistence of large pockets of urban and rural poverty in a market-driven global economy will sustain, even increase, the occurrence of infectious diseases. By the late twentieth century, the ecological complexion of life on *Earth* had begun rapidly changing. This globalization of our economic activities and culture, worldwide urbanization, increasingly rapid and long-distance mobility, growth in refugee movements, and the intensification of food-producing systems, are creating a world of increasing opportunity for established and potential human pathogens.

Environmental health research: the wider dimensions

Humankind's unprecedented disruption of various of the Earth's natural systems at the global level (Vitousek *et al.* 1997; Lubchenco 1998) reflects the combined pressure of rapidly increasing population size and a high-consumption, energy-intensive, and waste-generating economy. During the last quarter of the twentieth century we have begun to see evidence of a general weakening of the world's life-supporting systems and processes (Loh *et al.* 1998; Watson *et al.* 1998). The resultant risks to population health pose a special research challenge.

These environmental changes, including depletion of stratospheric ozone and long-term changes in global climatic patterns, entail unusually large spatial scales. They also entail temporal scales that extend decades, or further, into the future. Some entail irreversible changes. While some direct impacts on health would result, such as the health consequences of increased floods and heatwaves due to global climate change, or increases in skin cancer due to ozone depletion, many of the impacts would result from the disruption of the ecological processes that are central to food-producing ecosystems or to the ecology of infectious-disease pathogens. Therefore a central research task is to develop mathematical models for carrying out scenario-based health risk assessments that refer to future anticipated scenarios of environmental change.

Over the past three decades, a growing appreciation of ecological relationships and the new insights into the complex interdependencies intrinsic to the biosphere have begun to reshape our understanding of the environmental and ecological influences on the well being, indeed the sustainability, of human societies. The modern agendas for environmental health research and policy now extend beyond the identification, study, and management of specific localized physicochemical and microbiological hazards. We must include the systems-based study, and the sustainable management, of the environment as a life-supporting habitat.

Intertwined relationships: environment, population, poverty, and health

The relationships between ambient environmental conditions, socioeconomic circumstances, demographic change and human health are complex and multidirectional. Some of the relationships are immediate: for example, poverty today causes malnutrition tomorrow. Other relationships involve long time lags; for example, current poverty contributes to the need to clear local forests for fuel and to farm marginal lands, and these actions often lead to ecological attrition and hunger in the future. Time lags aside, there is no simple linear causal chain connecting these variables. Population pressure and poverty among rural populations often lead to land degradation and deforestation, with consequences for supplies of food and materials, and within the urban environment they predispose to many other adverse environmental exposures (physical hazards, high exposures to polluted air, and unsafe drinking water), especially in urban slum-dwellers. Poverty influences fertility rates, and vice versa. Environmental degradation often causes further impoverishment—for example, by reducing food yields, depleting fuel-wood, or potentiating destructive floods—and it can also impair health via increased exposure to vector-borne infectious disease (especially following habitat disruption), nutritional deficiencies, and toxic environmental pollutants.

In many African, Asian, and Latin American countries, the average life expectancy is 20 to 30 years less than for rich Western countries (WHO 1999). Infectious diseases remain the main killer, particularly in children below the age of 5 years. Much of this health deficit in poor developing countries reflects the widespread poverty, adverse social consequences of export-oriented economic development, and environmental adversity caused by exploitation of natural resources. The plight of sub-Saharan Africa, with its entrenched poverty and marginalization from the global economy, illustrates well these complex relationships. With two-thirds of the world's poorest countries, trends in the region's health, education, and material living standards have reversed in the past two decades and are continuing to fall (Logie and Benatar 1997). Meanwhile, environmental pressures have increased widely, with deforestation, desertification, and the erosion of Africa's relatively vulnerable soils. More than half the population still lacks safe water and 70 per cent of people lack proper sanitation. Infant mortality rates are over 50 per cent higher than in the world's other low-income, developing countries. Malaria and tuberculosis are widespread and increasing, while in parts of central, southern, and eastern Africa one in three pregnant women are HIV positive. Logie and Benatar (1997) assess that the two-way relationship between poverty and ill health erodes African economic productivity by at least one-sixth.

These statistics aside, it remains intrinsically difficult to confirm or refute the widely-assumed 'vicious spiral' link between poverty, environment, and health. It is certain that both poverty and environmental degradation, via independent pathways, increase the risks to health. It is also clear that there is a strong, albeit complex, relationship of income level to environmental quality. For many important environmental pollutants, as populations undergo an increase in average income there is an inverted U-shaped curve. This is known as the 'environmental Kuznets curve' (Grossman 1995). Initially, the pollutant loads increase. Then as wealth, literacy, and political liberalism increase, negative feedback processes ensue and societies take action to reduce the release of those environmental pollutants. However, the indices of several of the larger-scale forms of environmental degradation (such as carbon dioxide emissions) display a clear tendency to a continuing increase. These are the 'global common' problems, such as greenhouse gas emissions, for which there is no immediate negative feedback in terms of adverse social impact, health consequences, or market signals. The difference is illustrated in Fig. 3.

In most low-income countries, a 'dual profile' of health and disease is now emerging. Rapid and poorly regulated increases in extractive and manufacturing industries typically result in environmental degradation, including air and water pollution, while also increasing the rates of occupational injury and disease (Shahi *et al.* 1997; Pearce 1996). Meanwhile, the persistence of widespread poverty, lack of safe water and sanitation, and urban crowding ensures the continuation of infectious diseases, especially as a source of childhood mortality. Indeed, recent analyses that have sought to compare the world's poorest people (as opposed to the conventional aggregation of the world's poorest countries) with the richest reveal the continued predominance of infectious disease as a cause of disease burden and premature death (Farmer 1999; Gwatkin *et al.* 1999). Meanwhile, in the urbanizing portions of developing countries, changes in demography (increased life expectancy, decreased fertility) and environmental conditions are transforming the profile of health and disease—illustrated by the increasing prevalence of obesity, hypertension, cigarette smoking, sedentary lifestyle, exposure to ambient air pollution, and the hazards of urban traffic. Chronic non-infectious diseases are increasing alongside the persistence of infectious diseases.

At the beginning of the twenty-first century, various sub-Saharan African countries and parts of South Asia continue to face recurring or worsening 'subsistence crises'. This situation reflects the excessive weight of ever-increasing population numbers and environmental pressures on the nation's local resource base, unbuffered by the accrued wealth, trading connections, and political power that high-income countries have (King *et al.* 1995). In the likely absence of greatly accelerated economic and social development some of these disadvantaged countries face a prospect of further environmental deterioration, resource depletion, uncontrolled urbanization, persistent poverty, and continuing great public health deficits. This, in effect, is a classic Malthusian problem wherein local population needs exceed local environmental carrying capacity (King and Elliott 1996). Such a population can survive, in the short term, by 'ecological deficit

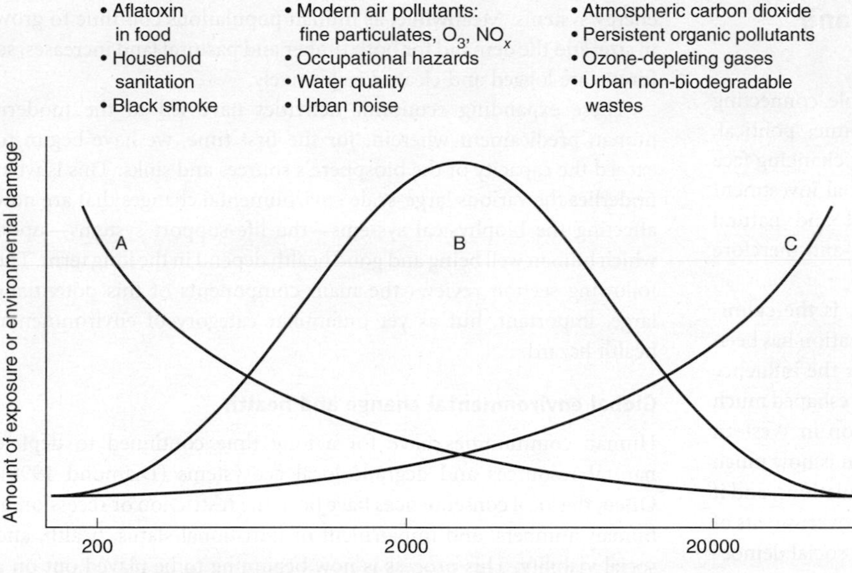

Fig. 3 The rise and fall of levels of local environmental pollutants in association with increasing population wealth (the Kuznets curve). As societies become richer and acquire higher expectations, so negative feedback via evolving policies and regulatory action leads to reductions in pollutant levels. However, this type of feedback operates less immediately and less strongly in relation to regional and global environmental changes, the resolution of which requires collective action across diverse populations and jurisdictions.

budgeting'—that is, by depleting 'stocks' of material, energy, and biotic resources to subsidize deficient existing 'flows'. Furthermore, in today's increasingly connected world, these local pressures can be partly offset with international aid and refugee flows, albeit often too late and too little. This has happened recently with Rwanda, Somalia, and parts of West Africa—and may yet occur in India, Bangladesh, and Pakistan where populations are still increasing, land pressures are mounting and environmental conditions are declining (Cassen and Visario 1999).

Meanwhile, more remarkably, the process of ecological deficit budgetting has recently assumed a global dimension (Rees 2000). On any reasonably comprehensive accounting basis it appears that meeting the needs of the current total world population, with its high levels of consumption and waste generation, depends to a substantial extent on the depletion of global stocks of resources and on the overloading of environmental 'sinks' (e.g. greenhouse gas accumulation in the lower atmosphere) (Loh *et al.* 1998; UNEP 1999). This is an extraordinarily important and unprecedented crossroads for humankind to have reached, and it has great implications for the future levels and sustainability of human population health (McMichael and Powles 1999).

We are only slowly perceiving the extent of this deficit-budget dilemma. Its resolution will require more than just a few clever technical fixes (such as the rehabilitation of nuclear power generation and the worldwide diffusion of genetically modified higher-yielding crops). While such technological advances may relieve pressures and extend the biosphere's effective carrying capacity, a generalized and more radical 'greening' of technologies is needed such as, for example, methods of reducing global carbon dioxide emissions by around two-thirds (McMichael and Powles 1999). The degree of required change will not easily be achieved by the accretion of marginal technical advances. Furthermore, reliance on technical fixes is a risky approach that can lead to mishaps—or to unexpected outcomes. (For example, the chlorofluorocarbons, discovered in the 1920s as inert gases useful for refrigeration, undergo a surprising character change in the extreme cold of the stratosphere where they react with ozone molecules.) Therefore, in addition to the undoubted environmental 'lightening' gains that technical improvements can make, the wholesale solution of our global environmental problems level will require great collective, and equitable, action.

Social scientists regard that type of co-operation as intrinsically very difficult for human societies to achieve (Caldwell 1990). In particular, human societies generally find it difficult to achieve co-operation whenever substantive changes in social priorities, cultural values, and technological modes are required. This difficulty has been well illustrated by the complex forging and the aftermath of the Kyoto Protocol, adopted under the United Nations Framework Convention on Climate Control in 1997, and which committed developed countries to making small cuts (5 per cent on average) in their national emissions of carbon dioxide. In responding to the threat of global environmental changes, supranational collective action must overcome the self-interested rigidities of national sovereignty, strong vested corporate interests, cultural diversity, the grievances of the very poor against the minority of the very rich in an increasingly unequal world, and today's dominant philosophies of neoliberalism, individual rights, and the superiority of the marketplace as rational arbiter of social choices. Caldwell, a historian, has observed of this particular contemporary challenge: 'The co-operative task would require behavior that humans find most difficult: collective self-discipline in a common effort' (Caldwell 1990).

Globalization, environmental impacts, and health

The world is undergoing a rapid and seemingly inexorable 'connecting up'. This connectedness is occurring in the economic, political, cultural, physical, and electronic realms. The resultant changing face of economic structures, production, trade, and financial investment has various important consequences for the social and natural environments within which human populations live—and therefore for health (McMichael and Beaglehole 2000).

This contemporary process, now massive in scale, is the culmination of a longer historical process. Economic globalization has been underway for the past 500 years, predominantly under the influence of European civilization, as trade and colonialism have reshaped much of the world, and created the basis for industrialization in Western countries—and now elsewhere. Economic globalization is now much more comprehensive in its embrace of the world's populations, and it is distinctively a creature of liberalized market forces. Governments of high-income countries, custodians of mixed-economy social democracies a short few decades ago, are now wedded via increasingly powerful international agreements and regulations to the primacy of deregulated markets, to the importance of 'free trade', and to the need to compete in an open global economy.

One important consequence is that new pressures are being put upon various aspects of the world's environment as the scale and reach of economic activity increases. The spread of large-scale agribusiness and monoculture crop production is exacerbating soil erosion and land degradation. Freer access to the world's forests by logging companies is creating problems of erosion, flooding, and silting of reservoirs. The continued building of large dams not only displaces many millions of people, but creates breeding sites for various infectious disease vectors, and carries the risk of occasional massive dam-break disasters. The expansion of long-distance trade creates new opportunities for the spread of pests and pathogens, as evidenced by the introduction of the mosquito species *Aedes aegypti*, via cargoes of used tyres from Asia to South America, the United States, and parts of Africa (Morse 1995). More generally, the dissemination of invasive species of plants and animals around the world is disrupting ecosystems and, in many cases, affecting the prospects for local health via effects on infectious disease transmission and local food production. The spread of the water hyacinth (introduced from Brazil) over much of Lake Victoria, in eastern Africa, has amplified the breeding sites for schistosomiasis-spreading water snails and diarrhoeal bacteria (Epstein 1998).

Economic globalization, and the segmentation of the world manufacturing workforce, has created a number of local environments with high levels of hazardous occupational and residential exposures. The creation, via taxation incentives to large corporations, of special 'export industrial zones' in China, Brazil, and various other low-income countries has spawned chemically and physically hazardous living environments for many poorly paid urban-fringe workers and their families (La Dou 1992).

An associated consequence of this increasingly intensive globalization of economic activity is the escalation in energy use for industrial production, car-based urban transport, long-distance trade, and increased long-distance human mobility. The resultant growth in combustion of fossil fuels is occurring in a world in which the prevailing harsh competitive economic realities do not allow longer-sighted investment in the development of alternative low-carbon energy systems. Meanwhile, as human populations continue to grow in size, and the demand for both timber and pastoral land increases, so forests are logged and cleared respectively.

These expanding economic activities have led to the modern human predicament wherein, for the first time, we have begun to exceed the capacity of the biosphere's sources and sinks. This is what underlies the various large-scale environmental changes that are now affecting the biophysical systems—the life-support systems—upon which human well being and good health depend in the long term. The following section reviews the main components of this potentially large, important, but as yet unfamiliar category of environmental health hazard.

Global environmental change and health

Human communities have for a long time continued to deplete natural resources and degrade local ecosystems (Diamond 1998). Often, the local consequences have been the restriction or recession in human numbers, and impairment of nutritional status, health, and social viability. This process is now beginning to be played out on a much larger scale. Some of the longer-term consequences for the health of human populations could be commensurately more serious. The scale of human impact on the environment has increased rapidly over the past two centuries, as human numbers have expanded and as the material intensity and energy intensity of economic activity has increased. Global economic activity increased 20-fold in the twentieth century. Meanwhile, in absolute terms, the human population has been growing faster than ever in the last 25 years, capping a remarkable fourfold increase from 1.6 to 6 billion during the twentieth century (Raleigh 1999). The last 3 billion have been added in 14, 13 and, most recently, 12 years respectively. While we remain uncertain of the Earth's human 'carrying capacity' (Cohen 1995), it is expected that the world population will approximate to 9 billion by around 2050, and will probably stabilize at around 10 to 11 billion by the end of the twenty-first century.

Over the past century or so, the typical localized symptoms of human environmental impact have been urban industrial air pollution, chemical pollution of waterways, and the various manifestations of urban squalor in rich and poor countries. These local health hazards are now being supplemented with the health risks posed by changes to some of the planet's great biophysical systems. Humankind is beginning, unintentionally and at a global level, to alter the conditions of life on Earth—even though we remain largely uncertain, even ignorant, of the long-term consequences (McMichael 1993; Vitousek *et al.* 1997; Watson *et al.* 1998). Several ambitious global assessments have estimated that we are now in significant and increasing 'ecological deficit', with a manifest decline in natural environmental and ecological resource stocks (Wackernagel and Rees 1996; Loh *et al.* 1998).

The central issue here is that the underpinnings of human health are being perturbed or depleted. The sustained good health of any population, over time, requires a stable and productive natural environment that yields assured supplies of food and fresh water, that has a relatively constant climate in which climate-sensitive physical and biological systems do not change for the worse, that retains its richness of biodiversity (a source of both present and future value), and that promotes secure livelihoods in agriculture, pastoralism, and fishing along with those in urban professions, trades, and crafts. For the human species, as a 'social animal' *in extremis*, the richness, texture, and stability of the social environment is also important to population health.

Some of these environmental stresses are likely to cause tensions between human communities, leading to conflict and hence to damage to the population's health (Homer-Dixon 1994). For example, Ethiopia and the Sudan, upstream of Nile-dependent Egypt, increasingly need the Nile's water for their own crop irrigation. Around the world, many other river systems are shared uneasily between neighbours in unstable regions; these include the Ganges, the Mekong, the Jordan, and the Tigris and Euphrates (Gleick 1998). Approximately 40 per cent of the world's population, living in 80 countries, now face some level of water shortage. Thus, as we leave the most war-scarred and arms-profiteering century on record, the prospect of international conflict because of the tensions caused by environmental decline, dwindling resources, and ecological disruption continues to cast a long shadow over the prospects for human health.

Challenges to science

The assessment of the risks to population health from global environmental change require several complementary research strategies. Recent research experience in relation to both stratospheric ozone depletion and tropospheric climate change, as sources of risks to human health, is illustrative. Research into the health impacts of these environmental changes can be conducted within three domains.

1. By reference to analogue situations which, as manifestations of existing natural climatic variability, are deemed likely to foreshadow future aspects of climate change.
2. By seeking early evidence of changes in health risk indicators or health status occurring in response to actual climate change. Special attention should be paid to climate-sensitive early-responding phenomena.
3. By using existing empirical knowledge and theory to conduct integrated mathematical modelling (or other forms of integrated assessment) of likely future health outcomes. This is referred to as scenario-based health risk assessment.

Most of the formal assessment of the health impacts of global environmental changes has, to date, focused on the issue of climate change. These have predominantly been assessments of potential health impacts, referring to processes anticipated to occur over future decades. However, for some types of health impact it may soon be possible to observe early changes. For example, if the trend of increasing world temperature since the 1970s continues, then statistically detectable trends in annual heatwave-attributable deaths may soon emerge. There is, thus, an important role for empirical research.

Conversely, scenario-based health risk assessment requires us to apply, via mathematical modelling, our current knowledge and theory to future environmental scenarios. Therein lies a central problem for scientists, policy-makers, and the general public. Science classically operates empirically, via observation, interpretation, replication, prediction, and, as necessary, hypothesis modification. However, having initiated an unintentional global experiment entailing large-scale environmental and ecological changes we cannot sensibly plan to wait decades for sufficient empirical evidence to enable us to describe the health consequences. That would be too great a gamble with an uncertain future. Therefore, to guide society's transition to the future, we must carry out scenario-based health risk assessment. This must be tempered by the realization that we cannot expect to anticipate all the resultant feedbacks, threshold-based phenomena, and surprise outcomes (Levins 1995)—including under conditions in which climate change interacts with other complex biophysical and ecological systems. In these circumstances, as mentioned earlier, it is essential that policy-making comply with the Precautionary Principle, as enunciated at the 1992 United Nations Conference on Environment and Development in Rio de Janeiro. That policy states that, where the consequences of environmental change are uncertain but potentially serious, perhaps irreversible, then that scientific uncertainty does not justify delaying precautionary preventive action.

The Precautionary Principle moves our thinking towards the realm of uncertainty-based decision-making. In this realm, action is prudently taken in light of what we do not know, and often cannot expect to know, before it may be too late to take corrective action. This mode of decision-making sits in contradistinction to the hard-won edifice of evidence-based quantitative risk assessment as the familiar scientific driver of social policy. The particular and important need to understand and apply uncertainty-based decision-making arises from the increasingly large, but uncertain, risks posed by human-induced changes in large, complex, dynamic environmental systems.

Main forms of global environmental change

The two best-defined 'global environmental changes'—the depletion of stratospheric ozone by the emission of ozone-destroying gaseous emissions (especially chlorofluorocarbons) and the accumulation of heat-trapping greenhouse gases in the lower atmosphere—each entail changes in 'global commons'. That is, although the gaseous emissions arise from diverse localized sources, in all continents, their environmental impact is of a diffuse globalized kind. Thus these local emissions result in integrated global changes. These changes entail a range of hazards to human population health, some of which are beyond direct assessment from existing scientific knowledge (McMichael 1993); this necessarily extends the environmental health research agenda.

Global climate change

The Second Assessment Report of the United Nations Intergovernmental Panel on Climate Change (IPCC 1996) concluded that: 'The balance of evidence suggests a discernible human influence on global climate.' The Third Assessment Report (IPCC 2001) concluded more firmly that most of the warming (approximately 0.4 °C) since 1975 has been due to humankind's emissions of greenhouse gases, and that this incipient climate change has begun to alter many physical systems (glaciers, sea ice, permafrost, and rainfall patterns) and many simple biotic processes (flowering time, bird nesting, insect hatching, polewards movement of animal and plant species, and crop-growing seasons). Trends in greenhouse gas emissions will, in the Intergovernmental Panel on Climate Change's assessment, cause an increase in average world temperature of approximately 2 to 3 °C over this century.

The anticipated health risks from climate change are of different complexion from the more familiar localized environmental health risks due to toxic chemical pollutants. The health effects of climate change would encompass direct and indirect, immediate and delayed effects (McMichael and Haines 1997). While some health outcomes in some populations would be beneficial—for example, some tropical regions may become too hot for mosquitoes or other disease vector organisms, or winter cold-snaps may become milder in temperate zones—most health effects would be adverse. This conclusion follows from the fact that long-term changes in background climatic conditions would alter the functioning of various biophysical and ecological systems that underpin human population health. Thus, the main health consequences would arise from systemic disturbances to the infrastructure of the biosphere.

The anticipated direct health effects include changes in mortality and morbidity from thermal extremes, the respiratory health consequences of altered exposures to photochemical pollutants and aeroallergens (spores, moulds, and so on), and the physical hazards of any resultant increases in storms, floods, and droughts.

Indirect health effects would include alterations in the range and activity of vector-borne infectious diseases (e.g. malaria, dengue fever, and leishmaniasis—the last of these is already present in southern Europe). Predictive mathematical modelling has suggested (Fig. 4) that the geographic zone and seasonality of potential transmission of malaria, and of dengue fever, might increase in many parts of the world (IPCC 1996; McMichael and Haines 1997). In temperate Europe, climate-sensitive vector-borne infections include tick-borne encephalitis and Lyme disease.

Other indirect effects would include altered transmission of person-to-person infections (especially summer season food-poisoning and water-borne pathogens), the nutritional health consequences of regional changes in agricultural productivity in poorly-resourced populations, and the various physical and psychological health consequences of rising sea levels and population displacement. Diffuse public health consequences would be likely to result from migration and the loss of employment caused by the disruptive effects of climate change upon various economic sectors and vulnerable populations.

Stratospheric ozone depletion

Higher in the atmosphere, depletion of stratospheric ozone by human-made gases such as chlorofluorocarbons is already occurring. Ambient levels on the ground of ultraviolet irradiation are estimated to have increased consequently by up to 10 per cent at mid-to-high latitudes over the past two decades (Basher *et al.* 1994). Via the Montreal Protocol of 1987, updated in the 1990s, the release of many of these gases has been curtailed. However, a problem remains with illegitimate sales and with the escalating production of halons by China and other low-income countries temporarily exempted from the production ban.

Scenario-based modelling, integrating the processes of emissions accrual in the stratosphere, consequent ozone destruction, increased ultraviolet ray flux, and cancer induction, indicates that European and American populations will experience a 5 to 10 per cent excess in skin cancer incidence during the middle decades of this century (Slaper *et al.* 1996). Similar modelled projections have been made for other fair-skinned populations living in Australia and New Zealand (Martens 1998).

Biodiversity loss and invasive species

As human demand for space, materials, and food increases, so populations and species of plants and animals are being extinguished increasingly rapidly. An important consequence for humans is the disruption of ecosystems such that 'natural goods and services' decline (Daily 1997). Biodiversity loss also means that we are losing, prior to their discovery, many of nature's chemicals and genes—of the kind that have already conferred enormous medical and health improvement benefits. Myers (1997) estimates that five-sixths of nature's medicinal tropical vegetative goods have yet to be recruited for human benefit.

Meanwhile, 'invasive' species are spreading into new non-natural environments via intensified human food production, commerce, and mobility. These changes in regional species composition have many consequences for human health. For example, as mentioned above, the choking spread of water hyacinth in eastern Africa's Lake Victoria, introduced from Brazil as a decorative plant, has provided a microenvironment for the proliferation of diarrhoeal disease bacteria and water snails that transmit schistosomiasis (Epstein 1998).

Impairment of food-producing ecosystems

The increasing pressures from intensified agricultural and livestock production are stressing the world's arable lands and pastures. At the beginning of the twenty-first century an estimated one-third of the world's previously productive land has been seriously damaged by erosion, compaction, salination, waterlogging, and chemical pollution that destroys organic content (WRI 1998). Similar pressures on the world's ocean fisheries have left most of them severely depleted or stressed. Unless an environmentally benign and socially acceptable way of using genetic engineering to increase food yields is found, we face a future struggle to produce sufficient food for humankind.

Modelling studies that allow for future trends in trade and economic development have been used to estimate the impacts of climate change upon cereal grain yields (representing two-thirds of world food energy). Globally, a slight downturn of around 2 to 4 per cent appears likely, but this would be substantially greater in food-insecure regions in South Asia, the Middle East, North Africa, and Central America (Parry *et al.* 1999). Such downturns would increase the number of malnourished people in the world, which already approximates to 800 million people.

Other global environmental changes

Freshwater aquifers in all continents are being depleted of their ancient 'fossil water' supplies. Agricultural and industrial demand, amplified by population growth, often greatly exceeds the rate of natural recharge. Water-related political and public health crises loom in several regions within decades, including the Middle East, northern Africa, and parts of south Asia. India, which had a supply of 5500 m^3 per person per year in 1950 currently has around 1800 m^3 per person (close to the recognized minimum requirement), and this will fall by a further quarter over the coming 25 years (Cassen and Visario 1999). Climate change may reduce supplies further in much of India.

Various semi-volatile organic chemicals (such as polychlorinated biphenyls) are now known to be disseminated worldwide via a sequential 'distillation' process in the cells of the lower atmosphere, thereby transferring chemicals from their usual origins in low to mid latitudes to high, indeed, polar latitudes (Watson *et al.* 1998). In

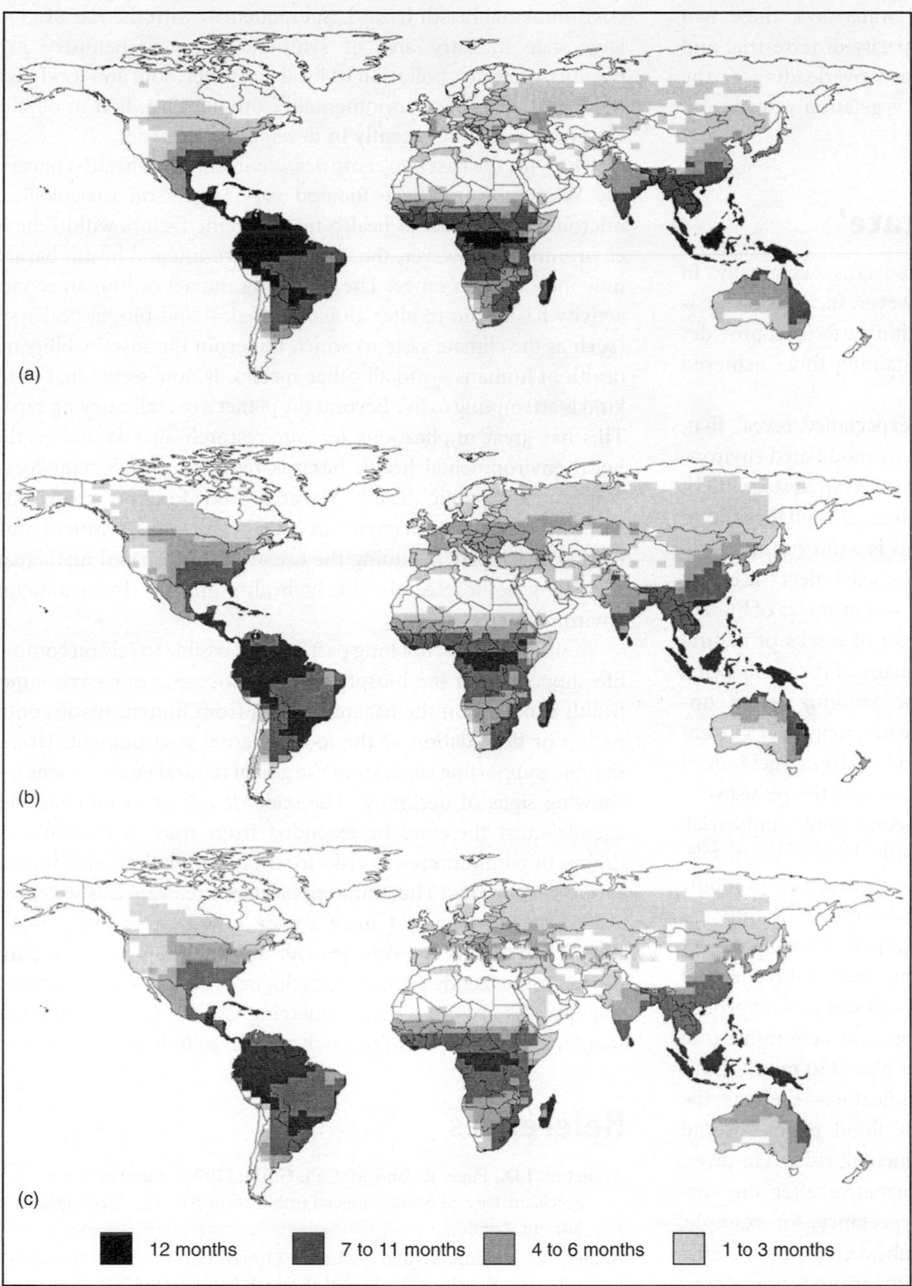

Fig. 4 Changes, relative to the present (a), in the annual transmissibility (number of months) of falciparum malaria under two scenarios of climate change: unmitigated emissions (b) and constrained emissions leading to carbon dioxide stabilization at 550 ppm. (c). These maps have been produced by integrated mathematical modelling, which links modelled future climate scenarios to a model of how the malaria system (mosquito and *Plasmodium*) responds to changes in temperature and rainfall (based on McMichael *et al.* (1999*b*)). The next step in this linked modelling (not shown here) is to estimate the additional numbers of people at risk of malaria under these future climate scenarios. In future, more complex modelling will take account of estimated trends in population vulnerability as a function of social, economic, demographic, and technological changes.

consequence, increasing levels of these chemicals are present in polar mammals and fish, and in traditional human groups who depend upon those food sources. Environment-polluting chemicals are no longer just an issue of local toxicity.

Finally, humankind is rapidly changing the cycling of major elements through the biosphere. Since the 1940s there has been a sixfold increase in the global annual human 'fixation' of nitrogen (that is, nitrogen that has been converted from inert form to biologically active nitrate and ammonium ions). This amount now exceeds the annual natural yield of 'fixed' nitrogen. Most of this increase derives from the use of nitrogenous fertilizers. Likewise, we have markedly altered the geochemical cycling of sulphur. By affecting the acidity and nutrient balances of the world's soils and waterways, these two chemical changes are likely to impair the capacity of terrestrial and aquatic food-producing systems. The nitrogen overloading of the biosphere is beginning to affect patterns of vegetation growth and various crop-plant pests and diseases.

Health as a 'sustainable state'

Population health is conventionally measured cross-sectionally, in tally-card fashion, as an 'achieved' entity. However, such a measure is an integration of past activities and consumption patterns; it provides no information about the possibility of sustaining those achieved levels in the future.

These generalized gains in human life expectancy reveal that, recently, the life-supporting capacity of the man-modulated environment has been increasing. But at what future cost? At what stage might depletion of the world's ecological and biophysical capital rebound against the health of human populations? This is a difficult question for scientists to answer. In principle, the answer will reflect the extent to which the ongoing health gains reflect increases in stocks of human and social capital, as opposed to the depletion of stocks of natural capital (McMichael and Powles 1999). Since many of the Earth's vital life-supporting systems appear now to be coming under unprecedented stress, the question assumes greater weight. If current trends continue, will long-term risks to human health emerge? Indeed these risks will tend to increase so long as human societies persist with an economy that entails a linear, waste-generating, 'industrial' metabolism. Such a metabolism is at odds with the circular metabolism of the rest of nature (wherein every output becomes an input.

The development of indicators of sustainability will be difficult. The uncertainties surrounding the prognostic criteria of sustainability and which are inherent in estimations of the potential health effects of ecological disruption are such that a pluralist, and sceptical, approach is desirable. As we acquire fuller understanding of the determinants of ecological sustainability we will become better placed to monitor our changing circumstances. Some types of indicators—such as the proportion of settled populations living in flood plains—would provide information about future environmental risks. However, many 'indicators' would only become informative after the sustainabilty threshold had been passed. Life expectancy, for example, may continue to increase if we persist in subsidizing our material needs by depleting natural capital (soil fertility, groundwater stores, biodiversity, atmospheric constancy, and so on). The challenge to public health scientists, social scientists, and environmental scientists in assisting society to foresee population health risks, and to make the transition to sustainable living successfully, is great.

Conclusion

In the Western world, in the eighteenth century, the dominant and age-old environmental health hazard facing the mass of people was malnutrition and famine, along with endemic childhood infectious diseases and recurrent epidemics. After the 1740s, in Europe, malnutrition and famines receded as the modern agricultural revolution began. The extreme urban crowding, insanitary conditions, and working-class poverty due to early industrialization in the nineteenth century resulted in infectious diseases becoming the pre-eminent environmental health hazard. Subsequently, with the rise of modern large-scale industry and of synthetic organic chemistry in the twentieth century, pollution of local air, water, soil, and food became the major focus of environmental health concern, first in developed countries and more recently in developing countries.

Thus, for the past two centuries, environmental health concerns in the Western world have focused very largely on toxicological or microbiological risks to health from specific factors within the local environment. However, the scale of environmental health hazards is now increasing in range. The escalating impact of human economic activity has begun to alter global ecological and biophysical systems (such as the climate system) which underpin the sustainability of the health of humans—and all other species. It now seems that humankind is attempting to live beyond the planet's overall carrying capacity. This has great implications for our research agenda and methods. Local environmental health hazards remain an important focus of concern for public health research and for risk management. Meanwhile, the tools of environmental health risk assessment must be further developed, including the use of scenario-based mathematical modelling to foresee the likely health impacts from anticipated environmental changes.

In simpler times, not long past, it was possible to rely on continuing life support from the biosphere, while focusing our environmental health concerns on the hazards arising from human-made contamination or degradation of the local external environment. However, that life-supporting capacity of the global natural environment is now showing signs of declining. The scale of our environmental health agenda must therefore be extended from risks to particular local groups or communities, to risks to whole populations and, indeed, to future generations. This thinking has extra relevance as we enter the age of the genome and must decide how best to apply this new molecular genetic knowledge. As Rudolf Virchow, the famous German nineteenth-century pathologist and public health advocate, might well have said of these emerging issues—this type of environmental health will be politics writ very large indeed.

References

Appleton, J.D., Fuge, R., and McCall, G.J.H. (1996). *Environmental geochemistry and health.* Special publication No. 113. Geological Society, London.

Basher, R.E., Zheng, X., and Nichol, S. (1994). Ozone-related trends in solar UV-B series. *Geophysical Research Letters*, **21**, 2713–16.

Caldwell, L.K. (1990). *Between two worlds: science, the environmental movement and policy choice.* Cambridge University Press.

Carson, R. (1962). *Silent spring.* Houghton Mifflin, New York.

Cassen, R. and Visario, P. (1999). India: looking ahead to one a half billion people. *British Medical Journal*, **319**, 995–7.

Chapin, G. and Wasserstrom, R. (1981). Agricultural production and malaria resurgence in Central America and India. *Nature*, **293**, 181–9.

Cohen, J. (1995). *How many people can the Earth support?* Norton, New York.

Corvalan, C.F., Kjellstrom, T., and Smith, K.R. (1999). Health, environment and sustainable development: identifying links and indicators to promote action. *Epidemiology*, **10**, 656–60.

Daily, G.C. (ed.) (1997). *Nature's services. Societal dependence on natural ecosystems.* Island Press, Washington, DC.

Davis, D.L., Axelrod, D., Bailey, L., Gaynor, M., and Sasco, A. (1998). Rethinking breast cancer risk and the environment: the case for the Precautionary Principle. *Environmental Health Perspective*, **6**, 523–9.

De Cock, K. and Greenwood, B. (ed.) (1998). *New and resurgent infections. Detection and management of tomorrow's epidemics.* Wiley, Chichester.

De Hollander, A.E.M., Melse, J.M., Lebret, E., and Kramers, P.G.N. (1999). An aggregate public health indicator to represent the impact of multiple environmental exposures. *Epidemiology*, **10**, 606–17.

Delmas, R.J. and Legrand, M. (1998). Trends recorded in Greenland in relation with Northern Hemispheric anthropogenic pollution. *IGBP Global Change Newsletter*, **36**, 14–17.

Diamond, J. (1998). *Guns, germs and steel. The fate of human civilizations.* Jonathan Cape, London.

Dockery, D.W., Pope, C.A., and Xu, X. (1993). An association between air pollution and mortality in six US cities. *New England Journal of Medicine*, **329**, 1753–9.

Elliott, P., Cuzick, J., English, D., and Stern, R. (ed.) (1992). *Geographical and environmental epidemiology: methods for small area studies.* Oxford University Press.

Epstein, P.R. (1998). Weeds bring disease to the east African waterways. *Lancet*, **351**, 577.

Epstein, P.R. (1999). Climate and health. *Science*, **285**, 347–8.

Farmer, P. (1999). *Infections and inequalities. The modern plagues.* University of California Press, Berkeley, CA.

Fenwick, A., Cheesmond, A.K., and Amin, M.A. (1981). The role of field irrigation canals in the transmission of *Schistosoma mansoni* in the Gezira Scheme, Sudan. *Bulletin of the World Health Organization*, **59**, 777–86.

Folke, C., Larsson, J., and Sweitzer J. (1996). Renewable resource appropriation. In *Getting down to Earth* (ed. R. Costanza and O. Segura). Island Press, Washington, DC.

Gleick, P.H. (1998). *The world's water. The biennial report on freshwater resources 1998–1999.* Island Press, Washington, DC.

Gopalan, C. (1999). The changing epidemiology of malnutrition in a developing society: the effect of unforeseen factors. *Bulletin of the Nutrition Foundation of India*, **20**, 1–5.

Grossman, G. (1995). Pollution and growth: what do we know? In *The economics of sustainable development* (ed. I. Goldin and L.A. Winters). Cambridge University Press.

Gwatkin, D.R., Guillot, M., and Henneline, P. (1999). The burden of disease among the poor. *Lancet*, **354**, 586–9.

Hetzel, B.S. and Pandav, C.S. (1994). *SOS for a billion. The conquest of iodine deficiency disorders.* Oxford University Press, Bombay.

Heymann, D.L. and Rodier, G. (1997). Reemerging pathogens and diseases out of control. *Lancet*, **349**, 8–9.

Heyneman, D. (1984). Development and disease: a dual dilemma. *Journal of Parasitology*, **70**, 3–17.

Homer-Dixon, T.F. (1994) Environmental scarcities and violent conflict: evidence from cases. *International Security*, **19**, 5–40.

Inhorn, M.C. and Brown, P.J. (1990). The anthropology of infectious disease. *Annual Reviews of Anthropology*, **19**, 89–117.

IPCC (Intergovernmental Panel on Climate Change) (1996). *Climate change. Report of Working Group I, 1995* (ed. J.T. Houghton, L.G. Meira Filho, B.A. Callander, *et al.*). Cambridge University Press.

IPCC (Intergovernmental Panel on Climate Change) (2001). *Climate change 2001: the scientific basis. Climate change 2001: impacts, adaptations and vulnerability.* Cambridge University Press.

King, M. and Elliott, C. (1996). Averting a world food shortage: tighten your belts for CAIRO II. *British Medical Journal*, **313**, 995–7.

King, M., Elliott, C., and Hellberg, H. (1995). Does demographic entrapment challenge the two-child paradigm? *Health Policy and Planning*, **10**, 376–83.

Kloos, H. and Thompson, K. (1979). Schistosomiasis in Africa: an ecological perspective. *Journal of Tropical Geography*, **48**, 31–46.

Kovats, R.S., Bouma, M., and Haines, A. (1999). *El Niño and health.* WHO/SDE/PHE/99.4, WHO, Geneva.

La Dou, J. (1992) The export of industrial hazards to developing countries. In *Occupational health in developing countries* (ed. J. Jeyaratnam). Oxford University Press.

Last, J.M. (1992). Global environment, health and health services. In *Maxcy Rosenau Last. Public health and preventive medicine* (ed. J.M. Last and R.B. Wallace), pp. 677–86. Appleton Lange, Norwalk, CT.

Lawson, A., Biggeri, A., Boehning, D., Lesaffre, E., Viel, J-F., and Bertollini, R. (1999). *Disease mapping and risk assessment for public health.* Wiley, Chichester.

Levins, R. (1995). Preparing for uncertainty. *Ecosystem Health*, **1**, 47–57.

Logie, D.E. and Benatar, S.R. (1997). Africa in the 21st century: can despair be turned to hope? *British Medical Journal*, **315**, 1444–6.

Loh, J., Randers, J., MacGillivray, A., *et al.* (1998). *Living planet report, 1998.* WWF International, Switzerland.

Lubchenco, J. (1998). Entering the century of the environment: a new social contract for science. *Science*, **279**, 491–7.

McKeown, T. (1976). *The modern rise of population.* Academic Press, New York.

McMichael, A.J. (1993). *Planetary overload: global environmental change and the health of the human species.* Cambridge University Press.

McMichael, A.J. (1996). Transport and health: assessing the risks. In *Health at the crossroads: transport policy and urban health* (ed. T. Fletcher and A.J. McMichael), pp. 9–26. Wiley, Chichester.

McMichael, A.J. (1999*a*). Dioxins in the Belgian food chain: chickens and eggs. *Journal of Epidemiology and Community Health*, in press.

McMichael, A.J. (1999*b*). Urbanisation and urbanism in industrialised nations, 1850–present: implications for human health. In *Urbanism, health and human biology in industrialised countries* (ed. L. Schell and S. Ulijasek), pp. 21–45. Cambridge University Press.

McMichael, A.J. and Beaglehole, R. (2000). The changing global context of public health. *Lancet*, **356**, 495–9.

McMichael, A.J. and Haines, A. (1997). Global climate change: the potential effects on health. *British Medical Journal*, **315**, 805–9.

McMichael, A.J. and Powles, J.W. (1999). Human numbers, environment, sustainability and health. *British Medical Journal*, **319**, 977–80.

McMichael, A.J. and Woodward, A.J. (1999). Quantitative estimation and prediction of human cancer risk: its history and role in cancer prevention. In *Quantitative estimation and prediction of human cancer risks* (ed. S. Moolgavkar, D. Krewski, and L. Zeise), pp. 1–10. IARC Scientific Publications No. 131, Oxford University Press.

McMichael, A.J., Anderson, H.R., Brunekreef, B., and Cohen, A. (1998). Inappropriate use of daily mortality analyses for estimating the longer-term mortality effects of air pollution. *International Journal of Epidemiology*, **27**, 450–3.

McMichael, A.J., Bolin, B., Costanza, R., *et al.* (1999*a*). Globalization and the sustainability of health: an ecological perspective. *BioScience*, **49**, 205–10.

McMichael, A.J., Kovats, R.S., Martens, W.J.M., Nijhof, S., de Vries, P., and Livermore, M. (1999*b*). Comparative scenarios of climate change and health: modelling future patterns of malaria and thermal stress. In *Global climate change and its impacts* (ed. G. Jenkins), pp. 24–7. Department of the Environment, London.

McNeill, W. (1976). *Plagues and people.* Doubleday, New York.

Martens, W.J.M. (1998). *Health and climate change: modelling the impacts of global warming and ozone depletion.* Earthscan, London.

Martens, W.J.M., Kovats, R.S., Nijhof, S., *et al.* (1999). Climate change and future populations at risk of malaria. *Global Environmental Change*, **9** (Supplement), S89–107.

Mazumder, D.N.G., Haque, R., Ghosh, N., *et al.* (1998). Arsenic levels in drinking water and the prevalence of skin lesions in West Bengal, India. *International Journal of Epidemiology*, **27**, 871–7.

Morse, S.S. (1993). Examining the origins of emerging viruses. In *Emerging viruses* (ed. S. Morse). Oxford University Press, New York.

Morse, S.S. (1995). Factors in the emergence of infectious diseases. *Emerging Infectious Diseases*, **1**, 7–15.

Murray, C.J. and Lopez, A. (1996). *Global burden of disease.* Harvard School of Public Health, Cambridge, MA.

Murray, C.J. and Lopez, A. (1999). On the comparable quantification of health risks: lessons from the Global Burden of Disease Study. *Epidemiology*, **10**, 594–605.

Myers, N. (1997). Biodiversity's genetic library. In *Nature's services. Societal dependence on natural ecosystems* (ed. G. Daily), pp. 255–73. Island Press, Washington, DC.

Newman, P. and Kenworthy, G. (1999). *Cities and sustainability: overcoming automobile dependence.* Island Press, Washington, DC.

Nurminen, M., Nurminen, T., and Corvalan, C.F. (1999). Methodologic issues in epidemiologic risk assessment. *Epidemiology*, **10**, 585–93.

Parry, M., Rosenzweig C., Iglesias, A., Fischer, G., and Livermore, M.T.J. (1999). Climate change and global food security: a new assessment. *Global Environmental Change*, **9** (Supplement), S51–68.

Pearce, N. (1996). Traditional epidemiology, modern epidemiology, and public health. *American Journal of Public Health*, **86**, 678–83.

Pope, C.A., Thun, M.J., Mohan, M., *et al.* (1995). Particulate air pollution as a predictor of mortality in a prospective study of US adults. *American Journal of Respiratory and Critical Care Medicine*, **151**, 669–74.

Raleigh, V.S. (1999). World population and health in transition. *British Medical Journal*, **319**, 981–4.

Rees, W. (1996). Revisiting carrying capacity: area-based indicators of sustainability. *Population and Environment*, **17**, 195–215.

Rees, W. (2000). Patch disturbance, ecofootprints, and biological integrity: revisiting the limits to growth (or why industrial society is inherently unsustainable). In *Ecological integrity in the world's environment and health* (ed. D. Pimentel, L. Westra, and R. Noss), pp. 139–56. Island Press, Washington, DC.

Riley, J.C. (1987). *The eighteenth-century campaign to avoid disease.* St Martin's Press, New York.

Rooney, C., McMichael, A.J., Kovats, R.S., and Coleman, M. (1998). Excess mortality in England and Wales during the 1995 heatwave. *Journal of Epidemiology and Community Health*, **52**, 482–6.

Samet, J.M., Schnatter, R., and Gibb, H. (1998). Invited commentary: epidemiology and risk assessment. *American Journal of Epidemiology*, **148**, 929–36.

Semenza, J.C., Rubin, C.H., Falter, K.H., *et al.* (1996). Heat-related deaths during the July 1995 heatwave in Chicago. *New England Journal of Medicine*, **335**, 84–90.

Shahi, G.S., Chen, L., Levy, B.S., Binger, A., Kjellstrom, T., and Lawrence, R.S. (1997). A historical perspective. In *International perspectives on environment, development, and health. toward a sustainable world* (ed. G.S. Shahi, B.S. Levy, A. Binger, T. Kjellstrom, and R.S. Lawrence), pp. 21–47. Springer, Basel.

Sharpe, R.M. and Skakkebaek, N. (1993). Are oestrogens involved in falling sperm counts and disorders of the male reproductive tract? *Lancet*, **341**, 1392–5.

Slaper, H., Velders, G.J.M., Daniel, J.S., de Gruijl, F.R., and van der Leun, J.C. (1996). Estimates of ozone depletion and skin cancer incidence to examine the Vienna Convention achievements. *Nature*, **384**, 256–8.

Smith, K., Corvalan, C., and Kjellstrom, T. (1999). How much global ill health is attributable to environmental factors? *Epidemiology*, **10**, 573–84.

Snow, J. (1855). *On the mode of communication of cholera.* Churchill, London.

Szreter, S. (1988). The importance of social intervention in Britain's mortality decline *c.* 1850–1914: a re-interpretation of the role of public health. *Social History of Medicine*, **1**, 1–37.

Tong, S. and McMichael, A.J. (1999). The magnitude, persistence and public health significance of cognitive effects of environmental lead exposure in childhood. *Journal of Environmental Medicine*, **1**, 103–10.

UNEP (United Nations Environment Programme) (1999). *Global environment outlook 2000.* Earthscan, London.

Vitousek, P.M., Mooney, H.A., Lubchenco, J., and Melillo, J.M. (1997). Human domination of Earth's ecosystems. *Science*, **277**, 494–9.

Wackernagel, M. and Rees, W. (1996). *Our ecological footprint. Reducing human impact on the Earth.* New Society Publishers, Canada.

Wang, X. and Smith, K.R. (2000). Secondary benefits of greenhouse gas control: health impact in China. *Environmental Science and Technology*, **33**, 3056–61.

Watson, R.T., Dixon, J.A., Hamburg, S.P., Janetos, A.C., and Moss, R.H. (1998). *Protecting our planet. Securing our future. Linkages among global environmental issues and human needs.* UNEP, USNASA, World Bank, Washington, DC.

WGPHFFC (Working Group on Public Health and Fossil-Fuel Combustion) (1997). Short term improvements in public health and global-climate policies on fossil-fuel combustion: an interim report. *Lancet*, **350**, 1341–9.

Whalen, M.M., Loganahtan, B.G., and Kannan, K. (1999). Immunotoxicity of environmentally relevant concentrations of butyltin on human natural killer cells *in vitro*. *Environmental Research*, **81**, 108–16.

WHO (World Health Organization) (1997). *Health and environment in sustainable development. Five years after the Earth Summit.* WHO, Geneva.

WHO (World Health Organization) (1999). *World health report 1999. Making a difference.* WHO, Geneva.

Wilson, M.E. (1995). Infectious diseases: an ecological perspective. *British Medical Journal*, **311**, 1681–4.

World Bank (1997). *Clear water, blue skies: China's environment in the new century.* World Bank, Washington, DC.

WRI (World Resources Institute) (1998). *1998–99 world resources. A guide to the global environment. environmental change and human health.* Oxford University Press.

2.8 Medical care and public health

K. Jamrozik and M. Hobbs

> To assist us to come safely into this world and comfortably out of it, and during life to protect the well and care for the sick and disabled. (McKeown 1979)

Introduction

This chapter examines the role of medical care services as a determinant of the level of health experienced in a particular community. The discussion is deliberately limited to personal medical services that are delivered in a one-to-one setting. As well as emergency medical or surgical care, rehabilitation, and palliative measures, such personal medical services can include a range of preventive activities such as health education, immunization, and family planning. In considering the entire range of activities designed to maintain or improve the health of a given population, a distinction is drawn between personal medical care services of the type described and, on one hand, measures for protecting health such as provision of clean water, waste disposal, quarantine, and food standards, and, on the other hand, community-wide health promotion activities such as advertising campaigns or creation of public facilities for exercise. Clearly, proper control of certain health problems, such as infectious diseases, requires a co-ordinated approach containing elements of health protection, health promotion, and personal medical care services. In practice, however, these three different activities are overseen by separate parts of the health service or even by separate governmental departments. It is therefore meaningful to examine the effect on the health of the population of personal medical services, even if this fragmented approach is somewhat remote from the ideal one.

The approach of this chapter is based on assessment of the impact of personal medical care services on health in three stages corresponding to the past, the present, and the future. These provide different challenges because the data that are available or potentially available to examine the impact of personal medical services at each stage are qualitatively very dissimilar. To consider the historical dimension—to answer the question 'What have personal medical services contributed to the state of health that we enjoy at present?'—is not only to reflect on what has been achieved, but also to identify those areas where humankind is reaching 'the flat of the curve' and further gains, in terms of further reductions at least in mortality, are likely to be small or expensive or both. With regard to the present and the future, to those charged with the planning and delivery of health services, identification of which of a number of possible initiatives might be truly useful in terms of improving health or reducing disease is at least as important as being able to demonstrate that programmes already in place are effective. Some appear to pay an obvious and direct dividend in terms of benefit to health, but it is less easy to be certain whether others justify the corresponding investments.

How best to measure health is a matter of central importance to this chapter but this is not a simple task. Instead, the second part of this chapter is built around five key questions that should inform the planning and delivery of health services to whole communities—'Who lives there?', 'What health problems do they have?', 'What health services already exist?', 'How are the existing health services performing?', and 'Are there any special features of the population or situation that need to be taken into account?' Consideration of the overall gains in health already made provides an opportunity to review the basic tools and a number of approaches to the measurement at least of ill health. The evaluation of the effects of single, readily identifiable components within complex systems of medical care is also discussed as this is a key practical issue. This section therefore includes a series of case studies of the evaluation of medical care using the various approaches and types of data previously identified. Several of the examples are drawn from Western Australia, but the principles they illustrate have wide application.

The third part of the chapter is devoted to the assessment of proposals for new services. This task is slowly becoming easier as it is accepted that new health services and strategies should be introduced only after rigorous assessment via randomized trials, first under tightly controlled conditions, and later under conditions that resemble everyday practice more closely. Debate continues, however, as to the applicability of the randomized trial to situations where the outcome of interest is rare and the validity of using observational data to chart the diffusion and impact of new methods in health care. The final section of the chapter is a brief discussion of what the future for the evaluation of medical care might hold, including areas that require further developmental work before a comprehensive overview can be obtained of the effect of medical care on health.

Historical overview

Western industrialized nations invested heavily in health protection long before medical care services began to develop into the highly organized and elaborate systems that we see today. While it is true that hospitals and various kinds of individual practitioners have been providing personal medical care services in these countries for many years, quarantine regulations date back at least to the fifteenth century (Burnet and White 1972) and the state became embroiled in the campaign to provide basic water supplies and sanitation at the beginning of the nineteenth century. In the United Kingdom, governments had provided hospitals for the poor but state involvement in the provision of universal personal medical care services is usually dated to the inception of systematic antenatal care in the early 1900s.

There have been many achievements since that time. Immunization has led to the eradication of smallpox worldwide (Fenner 1980) and, in the developed countries, the virtual control of poliomyelitis, diphtheria, tetanus, and measles. Substantial progress has been made towards reduction in morbidity from rubella and the congenital abnormalities it causes. Through the exigencies of two World Wars and several other major conflicts, substantial improvements have been made in the management of injury, and in restorative surgery and rehabilitation. In the field of reproduction, large advances have occurred in the control of fertility and in obstetric and neonatal care; it is now possible to contemplate radical programmes for population control as part of public health. Modern anaesthesia and parenteral therapy have greatly increased the safety of emergency surgery and have extended the scope of restorative surgery. New drugs have led to the successful treatment of many bacterial conditions, although multiple-drug resistance is now a growing problem. Developments in pharmacology have also contributed significantly to improved prognosis in surgery for injuries and emergencies. Certain malignant tumours of childhood and testicular cancer are now curable and substantial relief, if not cure, can be provided for many of the more common cancers of adults and for psychoses, epilepsy, diabetes, ischaemic heart disease, and some forms of arthritis. New prosthetic devices have opened the door to surgery for conditions previously associated with major disability and handicap. Advances in methods for diagnosis have supported many of these developments in treatment, and the theory and practice of screening asymptomatic individuals for risk factors or early evidence of disease have steadily become more sophisticated.

In parallel with technical advances there have been major changes in the philosophy of the provision of health care and in the structure of health systems. In most developed countries the concept of universal access to essential medical care, regardless of means, has been accepted. Even though systems of payment differ, most health care is heavily subsidized by governments and the principle of charity no longer applies (Kohn and White 1976; Maxwell 1981; Roemer and Roemer 1981). To be effective, medical care must be efficacious and access to it must be unimpeded.

Hospital and professional structures have changed to reflect increases in specialized knowledge in medicine. This has led to improvement in technical care but at the expense of holistic care. Conversely, previous shortcomings in relation to the care of the chronically sick are now becoming recognized and are slowly being redressed. For example, geriatric medicine, pioneered in the United Kingdom, has greatly increased insights into the care of the disabled aged (Brocklehurst 1975), which is timely, given the rapid expansion of the elderly population. New concepts for multidisciplinary services have been developed and put into practice in both hospital and community settings, although some remain to be properly evaluated. The hospice movement has drawn attention to the relief of pain and discomfort as a legitimate primary objective in health care, and palliative medicine has emerged as a clearly defined area of specialized care (Hillier 1988). Not only has the scope of medical care been broadened, but access to medical services has been greatly increased.

The relationship between declining mortality in the nineteenth and early twentieth centuries and medical care measures has been extensively reviewed by McKeown (1965, 1979). He provides convincing evidence that improvements in health as measured by falling mortality rates during that time had little to do with personal medical care. This chapter is therefore restricted to the examination of the effects of medical care on health during the last 80 years, the era of 'scientific medicine'.

That the advances in medical care described above have made an important contribution to health in the second half of the twentieth century would appear to be self-evident to many people. Despite this common view, some writers have seriously questioned the benefits of medicine. The most radical views have been expressed by Illich (1975), who suggested that apart from the direct iatrogenic consequences of some medical treatments, the overall approach of the medical and allied professions to health issues—defined as health 'problems'—and the ways they are thought about and discussed have broader negative repercussions for both individual patients and society at large. These views are probably shared by only a small minority, but other observers, including McKeown (1979) and Cochrane (1971), have also drawn attention to the fallacies inherent in some beliefs about the contribution of medical care to health. McKeown argued that much of the fall in mortality during the nineteenth century was due to social changes and, therefore, that any further improvements in health seen now should not automatically be attributed to modern medical care. Rose (1985, 1992) made the point that the health of individuals significantly reflects the norms of lifestyle and behaviour of the population in which they live.

Concerned because of escalating cost of health care, and in particular because of the unrestrained introduction of new medical technologies, many other writers have since used McKeown's arguments in relation to mortality to question the value of modern medicine, even though McKeown (1979) took a much broader view of how the benefits of medical care should be assessed. Since the 1970s, the focus of debate has shifted considerably, so that the concern is now about the marginal cost-effectiveness and cost-benefit of different aspects of medical care. Moreover, 30 years on, the assertion that there is little or no relationship between levels of mortality and the introduction of various medical interventions must be seriously questioned.

Cochrane was more concerned to show that the benefit of much medical care activity is unproven and should be carefully reappraised, partly to ensure that unsafe procedures are discontinued and partly to ensure that resources for medical care are employed in the most effective and efficient ways. In a widely quoted aphorism he asserted: 'It is surely a great criticism of our profession that we have not organised a critical summary, by specialty or subspecialty, updated periodically, of all randomised controlled trials' (Cochrane 1979). This challenge has now been accepted and a worldwide network, the Cochrane Collaboration (Chalmers and Haynes 1994), has been established to undertake systematic reviews of the evidence relating to the benefits of all aspects of medical care.

Writers such as Illich, McKeown, Cochrane, and Rose have broadened the focus from the direct benefits of health care to the indirect effects, adverse effects as well as beneficial effects, and social effects in groups as well as biological effects in individual patients.

Health services that are at all effective can have profound effects at the population level. For example, slowing population growth by successful control of fertility may lead to major improvements in the social environment in favour of health. In contrast, declining mortality without an associated reduction in fertility can lead to rapid growth in a population, which, by overtaxing the social and physical environments, is eventually counterproductive as far as health is concerned. Concomitant falls in fertility and mortality, while stabilizing population growth, will also produce the type of demographic transition observed in industrial countries and this, in turn, will produce entirely new patterns of morbidity with relative increases in the dependent aged and reductions in the dependent young.

As far as direct adverse effects are concerned, the rapid development of new methods of treatment has produced many dramatic and salutatory lessons that must caution us against unqualified enthusiasm for the presumed benefits of modern medicine. While thalidomide is perhaps the landmark example, there are unresolved questions pertaining to many other drugs including oral contraceptives, hormone replacement therapy, and calcium-channel blockers, drugs to which many people worldwide are or have been exposed, and to procedures such as electroconvulsive therapy and laparoscopic surgery. Questions about the balance of risks and benefits apply equally to established programmes and to new interventions.

Assessment of the current contribution of medical care to the health of populations

Evaluation of existing systems of medical care is one of five key questions that should inform the planning and delivery of health services to populations, be they a settled and affluent community, refugees inhabiting a makeshift border camp, the population of a school, a gaol or a cruise ship, or a military formation on active duty. The full set of questions is: 'Who will use the services?', 'What health problems do they have?', 'What health services already exist?', 'How are the existing health services performing?', and 'Are there any special features of the population or situation that need to be taken into account?' These questions are considered here in this order because it is impossible to judge whether health services are performing well and appropriately without knowing the size and nature of the population they serve, the level and pattern of need, and the resources that are available. At a very broad level, such as a developing versus an industrialized country, a given set of general principles for the provision and evaluation of medical care is likely to have wide application, but the wise practitioner will always take care to gather and use intelligence on special features of the local population that should also be taken into account.

Features of the population served

While it seems obvious that the age, sex, and ethnic structure of a population, along with its geographical and occupational distribution, are likely to be fundamental determinants of its level and pattern of need for, and use of, health services, these basic data are too often ignored or surprisingly difficult to find. National census data are frequently available at least to the level of local government area or county, but health services, be they general practices, infant welfare clinics, or hospitals, are not necessarily confined by these administrative boundaries. The principal risk here is not that ill-defined denominators complicate accurate measurement of activity and need in the health system, but that unmet need in subgroups of the population defined by one of the demographic characteristics already mentioned is overlooked. Aggregating data to larger geographic units for which the populations are well described can overcome the former, but is no substitute for careful collection and analysis of more local information (Rissel *et al.* 1996). An example here is the problem of osteomalacia (rickets) in the relatively small South Asian population of Glasgow, Scotland, recognition of which prompted a successful campaign of vitamin D supplementation (Goel *et al.* 1981). At the same time, needs assessment based upon measurement of the gap between current experience of (ill) health in a community and some predetermined target level may be a simplistic basis on which to set priorities for the allocation of health resources (Mooney 1998).

What health problems currently exist?

Any rational approach to the assessment of the impact of medical care on health requires that we have basic knowledge about the incidence, prevalence, and natural history of the problems that collectively comprise ill health. Unfortunately, our understanding of these aspects of ill health is often rudimentary. Another of the difficulties of measuring the benefits of medical care lies in the fact that most readily available data relating to health or medical services were collected for other purposes. The types of data generally available for monitoring health and the performance of health services are reviewed elsewhere in this book. Here the main classes of data in relation to their possible use in assessing the contribution of medical care to health are reviewed briefly.

Mortality data

Mortality data have the great advantage that they are collected in a relatively uniform way in different countries and are available for the whole period in which effective medical care has evolved. Such data are therefore of central importance in making broad comparisons of health status between countries and between different periods since 1900. Mortality data can be used to derive other useful indices such as life expectancy and potential years of life lost, but they do have some shortcomings as indicators of the state of health of populations. To begin with, they are subject to variations caused through changes in diagnostic practice and in coding and classification procedures so that, at the level of individual diseases, it is often not possible to provide valid trends over time or to make comparisons between countries. Mortality data also do not directly reflect the need for medical care associated with conditions, such as mental illness, which cause significant morbidity but are infrequent causes of death. Nevertheless, trends in mortality may be a useful surrogate for changes in morbidity as well as demonstrating actual gains in years of life.

The use of mortality data to plan and assess the impact of changes in medical care is subject to special difficulties in the area of confounding. As the general economic situation of a country improves allowing progressively more money per head of population to be invested in health services, so it is likely that the average standard of living, including housing and nutrition, also improves. It then becomes impossible, *post factum*, to ascribe any improvement in overall mortality rates to increases in total expenditure on medical care because changes in the other likely determinants of general health usually have not been monitored and because their actual effects on health and mortality are indirect and very difficult to measure.

The potential importance of confounding is exemplified by comparisons of trends in perinatal mortality and in mortality rates from ischaemic heart disease in developed countries over the period since the Second World War, for which there is strong evidence for contributions from both social change and medical intervention. The impact of medical care on perinatal mortality and ischaemic heart disease is further discussed below.

Disease registers

Compilation of registers of certain diseases tends to be reviewed as a research function by those with responsibility for delivery of services and as a service activity by agencies that fund biomedical research. Thus funding of registers is a perennial problem facing those who can see their potential, but only one of several challenges that registers present. Other recurring issues include achieving and maintaining complete ascertainment, in order that selection bias does not affect cases that are registered; the trade-off between the volume of data to be collected for each registered case and the completeness of the data; and the need for consistent and accurate application of definitions for each item of information that is recorded. Collection of information about patients for purposes not immediately related to the medical care that they require is subject to increasing and increasingly bureaucratic scrutiny. The involvement of multiple institutions and hence of their ethics committees poses a real threat to the continued use of name-identified population-based registers for the study of particular health problems, and identification of inefficiencies in the health system and of hazards in occupational and general environments as well as in health-care institutions (Jamrozik and Kolybaba 1999).

Once established, registers have many uses, several of which are of direct relevance to the planning and evaluation of medical care. For example, the incidence, severity, and outcome of a particular condition may reflect all of preventive, curative, and rehabilitative programmes. In any case, these parameters are needed for informed planning of health services. Registers may also serve as a source of cases for controlled trials or for detailed studies of the management of a condition or of its causes. It would be wasteful to develop a register corresponding to every aspect of medical care, but priorities for monitoring health problems by this method can be defined. Thus registers are especially useful for monitoring problems that are preventable, to help to ensure that knowledge already available is applied appropriately, problems that are extremely cost-intensive, since marginal increases in the efficiency of care for such conditions should result in savings that are relatively large in absolute terms, and problems that are important causes of disability if not mortality, since they contribute to a significant and ongoing need for care.

Cancer registries exemplify many of these issues, with a legal duty on medical practitioners to notify newly diagnosed cases of malignancies other than non-melanocytic skin cancer now established in many jurisdictions. In a well-developed health system, ascertainment and objective confirmation of relevant cases are usually easy to achieve. In contrast, many registers do not routinely collect or validate information on the stage of the cancer at presentation, despite this being a key datum in clinical decision-making about the management of patients. Because they are very difficult to collect, even fewer registries are able to provide data on the outcome of individual cases, thus complicating routine population-wide evaluation of oncological care.

Community surveys

Intensive community studies such as those in Framingham (Dawber *et al.* 1951; Dawber 1980), Busselton (Curnow *et al.* 1969) and North Karelia (Puska *et al.* 1985), which measure the incidence and prevalence of specific health problems, provide a basis for detailed epidemiological studies of various forms of health-care intervention. However, most studies of this type are necessarily restricted to a narrow range of causes of ill health in small communities and are therefore of limited use in assessing the impact of medical care on a wider front. In addition, as exemplified by the Nurses' Health Studies (Colditz *et al.* 1997), the populations and settings in which they are conducted may not be typical of national populations and conditions, adding to the difficulty of extrapolating results concerning medical care, even if it is valid to extrapolate results regarding risk factors and aetiological relationships.

General health surveys

More general sample surveys of illness and disability in the community such as the health component of the General Household Survey in the United Kingdom, the National Health Interview Survey and associated National Health and Nutrition Examination Survey in the United States, and the National Health Surveys in Australia, have provided insight into levels of treated and untreated sickness and disability in the community as well as into illness behaviour. However, the types of questions that can be asked in surveys using non-medical interviewers are limited, with the result that the information obtained may be too general for the purpose of relating the effects of medical care to the health of the community. Changes in the survey instruments over time and variations in response according to characteristics such as age, ethnic group, and economic and educational status, may make interpretation of trends and geographical differences difficult. The problems of using various measures of health status in the United States for this purpose have been extensively reviewed by Wilson and Drury (1984).

Health service utilization data

The universality, historical continuity, and comparability across populations of morbidity data are all limited. Compared with mortality data, the quality of morbidity data is suspect as it is dependent firstly on the quality of medical records, and, secondly, the records themselves tend to be coded and processed at several locations, whereas in most countries the coding of mortality data is relatively centralized and subject to greater quality control. In addition, although hospital morbidity data lend themselves reasonably well to coding using the International Classification of Diseases, which was originally intended for use in classifying deaths, other systems have had to be developed for data collected in general practice, for example, or to distinguish between impairment, disability, and handicap. Translation from one of these systems to another is not always straightforward. Even so, morbidity data have the potential to fill in some of the gaps in mortality data.

The most commonly used measures of morbidity such as hospital statistical collections or data generated from general practice are in fact measures of service utilization rather than measures of the level of illness in the community. Data of this kind may obviously be affected by factors that are quite independent of true need, such as changes in clinical practice, availability of resources, and general factors that affect access to medical care of all types. While measures of utilization are important if they can indicate the extent of diffusion of interventions shown to be efficacious (or not efficacious) in randomized controlled trials, most hospital morbidity data systems record only that contact with the hospital occurred and the nature of the problem, a smaller number record which operative procedures, if any, were performed, and only a minority record information on other aspects of investigation or management of the patient's condition. Nevertheless, an appropriately designed and maintained hospital morbidity data system may be invaluable for monitoring the incidence of common and important problems such as major injuries and infections, and non-fatal acute myocardial infarction, as well as the extent of uptake of cost-intensive procedures such as organ transplants.

Morbidity data frequently measure episodes of care or occasions of consultation rather than people treated. Record linkage offers one means of overcoming this, providing person-based statistics relating to hospital use, while cross-linkage with mortality data allows for the study of survival following admission to hospital for a selected condition or surgical procedure (Acheson 1967; Gelding *et al.* 1987; Goldacre 1987). Opportunities for this type of analysis are extremely limited, with record linkage being extensively developed only in Canada, Scotland, and Oxford, and some capability available in Sweden, Denmark, Finland, and Western Australia. Even so, the use of morbidity data as one source of information for disease registers, and as a starting point for *ad hoc* studies for planning and assessing the effect of medical care, should be kept in mind. In Perth, Australia, for example, linked morbidity and mortality data have been used retrospectively to study trends in incidence and survival in acute coronary disease, parameters which reveal much about the medical care received both by people at risk of developing ischaemic heart disease and by those who have developed symptoms (Hobbs *et al.* 1984; Martin *et al.* 1984, 1987*a*, *b*).

Data from general practice

The technical problems relating to consistent capture and coding of data from general practice are even greater than those relating to hospital morbidity statistics. It is difficult to recruit general practitioners to continuing studies, and compliance with collection of data is likely to be low. Most studies of illness or treatment using general practice records have therefore been based on selected practices that may not be fully representative. It follows that data from general practice of most value derive from special broad-based but time-limited investigations which have specific goals such as the study of adverse effects of oral contraceptives undertaken by the Royal College of General Practitioners (1974).

Nevertheless data from general practice have other important potential uses in planning, assessing, and improving medical care. Given appropriate records and, in particular, the possibility of defining clearly the population served by a given practice (as is the case in the British system of capitation where, theoretically, all people are registered and only with one practice), it is at least possible to measure the proportion of the target group which has received a particular service. This is an important step on the way to determining the impact on health of that medical care activity. For example, Mak and Straton (1993) have described the establishment and operation of a cervical cytology register based in the single general practice in Fitzroy Crossing in the remote North-West of Australia. The setting is unusual because of the large distances involved—two-thirds of women screened in the first year of operation lived more than 20 km from the township—and because 80 per cent of the population served are Aboriginal Australians, many of whom do not read English. Initial contact and recall for screening of many of the women on the register is therefore verbal and opportunistic. Despite this, 54 per cent of women aged 15 to 69 years in the population were screened in the first year of operation of the register, indicating that the programme was likely to meet its target of screening all eligible women biennially. More importantly, one-quarter of women screened in the first year had never had a Pap smear taken previously. In addition to monitoring coverage of the target group, the quality of smears collected is reviewed regularly. As Mak and Straton (1993) note, the incidence and mortality from cervical cancer is significantly higher in Aboriginal women than in the remainder of the Australian population. Their study shows how responses to such problems can be designed, implemented, and evaluated using simple data collected in general practice.

What health services already exist?

Existing health services can be classified according to target group and function. Thus, there are community-wide services intended to protect and promote health, and personal medical services concerned with prevention, cure, restoration, and palliation. Personal medical services can be further classified according to level, that is, into primary, secondary, and tertiary services. To fulfil its function each component of the health system requires appropriate numbers and types of personnel plus the buildings, equipment, transport, and information and communication systems that together constitute the infrastructure. What constitutes an 'appropriate' level of provision of human and other resources presupposes a clear and shared view of an optimal state of health and of the kinds of services needed to achieve and maintain that state. Universal provision of adequate food, water, and sanitation is an agreed goal but one that is yet to be realized in much of the world. In contrast, in the industrialized countries, health protection systems concerned with the food and water supply and with sanitation are frequently taken for granted and their importance only rediscovered when human error, war, natural disaster, or union action leads to interruption of services. Nevertheless, there is more agreement about minimum goals for environmental health than about the optimal numbers of doctors or hospital beds per head of population. The sources of disagreement include the fact that demand for health services is probably boundless and the tensions between philosophical arguments about access, equity, and basic human rights, on the one hand, and vested bureaucratic and professional interests in rationing services or numbers of practitioners, on the other. Given finite resources in the health system, it is legitimate that advocates of new or expanded services are challenged to demonstrate the efficacy and cost-utility or marginal cost-effectiveness of the changes they are proposing. This principle is already well-established in several countries in relation to subsidized provision of pharmaceuticals and is likely to be applied more widely in the health system in the future.

How are the existing health services performing?

Introduction

Evaluation of the contribution to health of medical services already in place is one of the key issues facing those charged with meeting the role of medicine defined by McKeown. Traditionally, most aspects of medical care have been evaluated and funded on the basis of measures of activity rather than beginning with an assessment of need, making an initial investment, and then determining whether the health of the community in which the service was delivered has improved to the extent expected. The assumption that medical institutions that are busy must be doing good is now being questioned. Several developments have contributed to this change in outlook. Firstly, it has been realized that successful completion of a course of treatment does not necessarily mean a return to the premorbid state and that it is necessary to check that the latter has in fact occurred. This has led to greater emphasis on quantifiable outcomes of health care, and it may be that the increasing attention attracted by controlled clinical trials, with their need to define endpoints unambiguously, has also influenced this trend. A second development, also related to the increasing influence of clinical trials as well as to the writings of Cochrane (1971, 1979) and others, is greater scrutiny of the actual diagnostic and therapeutic strategies employed in medical care and of the extent to which they are supported by good scientific evidence rather than empirical observations or deductions from 'first principles'. When coupled with questions about value for money, such scrutiny becomes searching indeed. A third factor is probably the rise of epidemiology and, in parallel with this enlarging body of theory and practice, a burgeoning capability to store, process, and analyse data. Previously, the simple measures of what health services actually did were all that it was possible to collect and it was not easy to assess, for example, the impact on the health of the local community of particular units within a large hospital. Finally, a prolonged period during which the governments of many countries were committed to 'economic rationalism' meant that public services of all kinds came under intense scrutiny in attempts to improve their efficiency.

It is inevitable that the performance of health services will be subject to ever-closer examination because they constitute such a large part of social expenditure and their cost rises faster than the cost of living. The disciplines of epidemiology and health economics have now developed sophisticated tools for evaluating medical care, but the comprehensive sets of data on health and outcomes of health services that are required for an exhaustive examination are not routinely collected in any community. Many questions might be answered if registers of certain diseases were available but special studies may still have to be undertaken to evaluate other particular aspects of medical care.

Even so, in order to evaluate medical services presently operating, an appropriate conceptual framework which embraces all of the activities of health care and which describes the desired outcomes in relation to each of these must first be established. Secondly, the technical problems involved in measuring the extent to which these benefits are achieved must be considered. This leads to a review of the data that are required and that are currently used to assess the performance of health services because, where the most appropriate resources are not available, evaluation of need for and performance of medical care is often attempted by pressing into service data that are collected routinely but intended for other purposes. This section then concludes with a series of case studies of the evaluation of medical care. The examples are drawn from across the full range of activities in medical care and have been deliberately selected to illustrate the use of the different types of data discussed above. The common thread that links them is the need to evaluate for a whole population the impact of medical care for a health problem which is either common or is associated with serious consequences.

A conceptual framework for the evaluation of medical care

This chapter has followed McKeown's (1979) classification of the functions of personal health-care services into those that contribute to the prevention, cure, or mitigation of disease and subdivided the latter into measures that aim to restore function and those that are solely palliative in intent. Clearly each of these main categories can be further subdivided down to the level of separate and distinct clinical activities. An illustrative schema is depicted in Table 1. This is by no means exhaustive but it serves to illustrate the complexity of the medical task on the one hand, and the equally complex task of determining suitable measures of outcome for the various components of medical care, on the other. When discussing the contribution of medical care to health it is important to specify both which of the above functions is in question and the nature of the expected benefit. The latter may be a reduction in the incidence or prevalence of specific health problems, reduction in overall mortality or premature loss of life, reduced suffering, or improved quality of life. Quite different measures are required to assess the impact of a preventive programme (measured by the absence of disease), of acute care, as in the management of injuries (not only reduction of mortality but also absence of residual disability), or the management of chronic illness (prolongation of life in some instances and also minimization of pain and restriction of function). To define all of the activities that form part of medical care and their potential contribution to the health of populations is beyond the scope and purpose of this discussion. Nevertheless it should be noted that under models for funding health services such as those which separate owners, funders, purchasers, and providers, this exhaustive approach will be required if there is to be a meaningful attempt to relate funding to specified outcomes. For the present, we will draw upon the framework illustrated in Table 1 for examples that illustrate the range of benefits expected from health-care systems in industrialized countries.

Problems in assessing the performance of medical care services

Apart from the establishment of an appropriate conceptual framework for considering the benefits of health services, the most fundamental problems are difficulties in defining and measuring need for medical care and in devising suitable measures of its effects.

Firstly, it is obvious that benefits of health care can be determined only if the size and nature of the health problem in question can be clearly defined. In other words, a baseline must be established against which changes in frequency or severity of disease can be measured. Much has been written about the need for more satisfactory and comprehensive measures of health status that could be used to define specific needs for medical care and to determine the impact of various types of care at the population level (Fingerhut *et al.* 1980; Murnaghan 1981; Hunt *et al.* 1986; Bergner and Rothman 1987). The volume of this literature is in itself testimony to the difficulties involved and to the fact that answers to the problem remain elusive.

Secondly, while it is possible to examine outcomes of disease in biological terms, it is difficult to measure its personal and social impact. Biological states that can be measured and classified as disease do not necessarily correspond to a subjective experience of illness or to a socially acknowledged sick role (Hunt *et al.* 1986). As discussed by Butler and Vaile (1984), there are several aspects to social outcomes. For example, are benefits considered in terms of the productive capacity of the individual, the impact of disability on families, or the

Table 1 A framework for the evaluation of medical care

Function	Intervention	Broad effect (examples)	Outcome measures
Preventive medicine	Control of fertility	Reduction in family size; increased birth spacing	Fertility; infant and maternal mortality
	Dietary supplementation	Prevention of specific deficiency disorders	Incidence and prevalence of deficiency
		Increased resistance to infectious disease (e.g. measles)	Mortality from communicable disease
		Prevention of birth defects	Birth prevalence of neural tube abnormalities and associated long-term disability
	Immunization	Reduced incidence of communicable diseases and associated mortality and long-term disability	Infant and childhood mortality Prevalences of flaccid paralysis (postpolio), disability with congenital rubella syndrome, and ?epilepsy
	Screening	Reduction in congenital malformations	Birth prevalence of Down's syndrome and neural tube defects
		Earlier detection of precancerous states and selected cancers	Incidence of cervical cancer; earlier detection of and improved survival from cervical and breast cancer
		Earlier detection and improved management of hypertension and other vascular disorders	Prevalence of people with controlled hypertension; incidence of stroke and the prevalence of associated disability
Curative medicine	Obstetric management and neonatal intensive care	Reduction in maternal and perinatal mortality and morbidity; reduced prematurity and low birth weight	Maternal and perinatal mortality; prematurity and low birth weight; other perinatal complications in mothers and babies
	Acute medical care	Treatment of acute infections	Mortality and long-term sequelae from acute infections
	Acute surgical care	Treatment of acute surgical emergencies	Incidence of complications
	Management of injury	Reduced case-fatality and longer-term disability due to injury	Case-fatality in common surgical emergencies; prevalence of injury-related disability
Restorative care	Medical treatment	Improvement in functional status as the result of medical treatment for various chronic medical conditions; such as anaemia, various deficiency states, cardiac failure, renal failure, psychiatric disorders, etc.	Proportions of affected individuals with symptoms controlled or ameliorated; measures of physical and mental function; levels of independence
	Rehabilitation	Restoration of function following conditions such as stroke and various forms of injury	Prevalence of potentially disabling conditions and measures of disability and/or dependence in affected people
	Corrective surgery	Reduction in pain and discomfort and in impairments and disabilities associated with congenital, acquired, and degenerative disorders; e.g. corrections of skeletal deformities, joint prostheses, lens replacement, vascular surgery, cardiac pacemakers	Prevalence of potentially correctable and of individuals who have received putative of corrective surgery; levels of function in people with and without corrective procedures
Palliative care	Relief of symptoms in non-life-threatening chronic conditions	Reduction in discomfort, improved productivity (including social role) in people with conditions such as emotional and psychiatric disorders, atopic conditions, migraine, arthritis	Prevalence of non-life-threatening chronic conditions and the proportion of those affected receiving relief from medications and other forms of therapy; the proportion of affected individuals able to fulfil desired social roles
	Terminal care	Reduction in pain and other suffering associated with terminal illnesses such as cancer, AIDS, muscular dystrophy; counselling for affected individuals and their families	The proportion of individuals with terminal illness who receive adequate relief of symptoms counselling; other measures of performance relating to the palliative care function in hospitals, nursing homes, and palliative care services

Source: Australian Bureau of Statistics (1998b)

opportunity costs of expending resources on this type of care rather than on some other service which might yield greater benefit overall to the community? Although the case for particular programmes of preventive and acute care of proven effectiveness might be regarded as beyond doubt, they may not be assets if the opportunity costs are high.

An important issue in assessing health outcomes is the assessment of personal benefit—the extent to which the change produced by medical care is valued by the subject. Here it is essential to recognize the difference between extension of life and its quality. The latter is necessarily a matter of subjective judgement, but whose judgement?

The need for measures to help us ensure that medical care results in better quality of life, if not necessarily a longer life, has been championed by Katz (1987), himself a pioneer of measures of physical function (or activities of daily living) that may be used in assessing outcomes of rehabilitation. The importance of describing function, as opposed to describing disease, was also stressed by a Scientific Group of the World Health Organization (WHO 1984) who advocated that 'loss of autonomy should be used broadly as an endpoint in epidemiological studies of the relationships among specific diseases, impairments and handicaps'.

In a review of progress in the assessment of quality of life, Spitzer (1987) underlined the difference between generally accepted measures of health status, which may distinguish between the healthy and ostensibly healthy, and measures of quality of life, which are used in situations of established illness and disability. He conceded that some overlap in these approaches may be necessary in the transition zone between the ostensibly healthy and the definitely ill, and also noted the need for a hierarchy of measures extending from the conceptual level, to the operational level, and finally to targets for specific clinical interventions. At the higher level, he suggested that, to be of value, any generic instrument must cover the domains of physical and mental function, emotional and mental state, the burden of symptoms and perception of health, and sense of well being. At the clinical level, there is the additional need for 'hypothesis-determined functional measures for clinical evaluation', specific for particular diseases and perhaps applicable to treatments or to different areas of activity, whether these be preventive, therapeutic, or restorative in nature. For example, Fletcher *et al.* (1987) stressed the need to include appropriate measures of quality of life in randomized controlled trials of drugs used in the treatment of cardiovascular diseases.

Trying to measure the effects on quality of life of many different medical problems and interventions is another challenge. Use of a single method for all situations stands to provide comparability at the cost of insensitivity to subtle effects on quality of life of particular diseases or treatments, while the converse applies to the numerous problem-specific scales. Some widely used generic instruments such as the SF-36 (Short Form Health Survey with 36 items) address several different dimensions of function and well being but do not yield a single measure of utility, thereby complicating the weighting of years of life gained by their quality or the level of ongoing disability.

Another difficulty is that medical care is usually provided by generic services. The objectives of such services are not explicitly defined in terms of prevention, cure, or care and it is therefore difficult to identify, let alone quantify, the components of medical care that are devoted to each of these functions, or, as health economists would wish, to apportion costs to them. Problems are also encountered in moving from a consideration of the benefits of specific treatments for specific diseases to the aggregate benefit of medical services applied to the whole population. Thus it is beyond debate that many diseases have been reduced or eliminated through immunization, that obstetric care has minimized the likelihood of maternal and perinatal mortality or morbidity, that surgery for injuries and particular abdominal emergencies may be life-saving, and that drugs developed in the past 80 years offer the prospect of a cure or substantial relief of symptoms in many illnesses. Yet, the lack of valid measures of outcome and difficulty in controlling for confounding make a formal and overall evaluation of established medical care services impossible. Proxy measures of outcome are therefore frequently used. Arising from the classic paper of Donabedian (1966), measures of 'structure', such as numbers of beds per head of population, and of 'process', such as numbers of admissions to hospital, have become widely accepted as alternatives to measures of outcome in assessment of the performance of health services.

How measures of structure and process relate to unmet need or to the true contribution of medical care to health is not immediately clear. Ultimately, using such variables to assess medical care is likely to yield misleading conclusions if some nexus between them and the effectiveness of care is not established. But this has rarely been done, and many of the current norms and standards for health services have been determined mainly by historical precedent rather than through explicit rational processes. Uncritical acceptance of measures of structure and process for the assessment of health services carries dangers because of the complacency that it may engender in removing the apparent need for true measures of outcome. Yet, as the preceding discussion indicates, 'outcome' itself is a complex notion extending beyond the simple died–survived dichotomy to encompass concepts such as disability and quality of life. How to combine multiple measures of outcome for a single condition, what weight to give to each, and whether the weights are, or should be, different for different populations are all very active areas of research and publication.

Assessing the present performance of medical care services

In evaluating the performance of health services already in place, there is clearly a need to go beyond measures of structure and process to examine direct indicators of health and ill health. However, in so far as they reflect levels of health, many of the statistical systems mentioned above always have some element of lag, making an up-to-the-minute assessment impossible, and it is a truism that data collected today on survival and quality of life in the long term must reflect not current patterns of investigation and treatment but those that were in vogue at the time that the patients first became ill. While cross-sectional surveys of the population and registers of specific diseases have the potential to provide data that are more up to date and can be very useful in exploring fully the levels, patterns, and short-term impact of medical activity, including the extent of application of new treatments, it may be years before the outcome of medical care for particular problems is seen clearly. Evaluation of screening for colorectal cancer is a case in point (Mandel *et al.* 1993).

Mooney *et al.* (1986) suggested that, rather than assess the performance and impact of the health system as a whole, or at the other extreme, the benefit from treatment of individual diseases, it is possible to identify and examine specific functions or 'programmes' performed by particular sectors of the health-care system as illustrated in Table 1. These may be further divided into subprogrammes each with its own explicit goals relating to particular problems of certain client groups. For example, immunization services might constitute a 'programme' with various subprogrammes concerned with delivery of vaccines for particular infectious agents to defined subgroups of the population. The assumption is made that all of the individual medical care activities undertaken by a given programme contribute, either directly or indirectly, to the achievement of its goals—in this case, minimizing morbidity and mortality from vaccine-preventable diseases, and this assumption obviates the requirement to identify the contribution of each individual activity to reaching the goals.

In contrast, Kessner *et al.* (1973) advocated detailed study of the performance of health services for selected sentinel or tracer conditions and Rutstein *et al.* (1976) developed an equivalent approach concerning certain avoidable causes of death. Thus, one way to evaluate a specific programme may be to assess carefully the extent to which the goals of one of its constituent subprogrammes are being achieved. The inference here is that if, for example, the incidence of measles in a population is consistently very low and the sporadic cases seen are almost entirely attributable to infections imported from outside, one might conclude not only that the effort to prevent measles is working well, but also that the whole programme to control vaccine-preventable diseases is effective, at least in childhood. It may also be concluded that a wider range of preventive services for infants and children are probably reaching their targets. Clearly the extent to which it is possible to extrapolate in such a fashion will be a matter of judgement informed by local knowledge, but the converse situation is illustrative. If, despite investment of significant financial and human resources, the incidence of measles failed to fall or to stay low in a particular community, one would legitimately have concerns not only about measles and other vaccine-preventable diseases, but also about whether all kinds of preventive services were reaching infants and young children.

In keeping with this approach of starting with a specific service and making judicious inferences about wider programmes, examples are given below of ways in which mortality data and data on morbidity from hospitals, general practices, special registers of diseases and cross-sectional surveys can be used to evaluate particular aspects of medical care.

Data currently used to assess the benefits of medical care

Mortality data

Global approaches based on mortality from all causes combined The work of McKeown (1965, 1979) has demonstrated that the major proportion of the decrease in mortality rates in the United Kingdom since the early nineteenth century was probably due to improvements in nutrition, water supply, and housing, with relatively minor contributions from specific medical interventions, including immunization. On the basis of earlier trends, McKeown suggested that at least some part of the continuing decline in mortality following the development of effective medical care would still have occurred without the advent of scientific medicine. The fact that mortality rates in middle-aged and elderly men demonstrated little improvement during most of the twentieth century, even after effective medical measures became available, has also been cited as evidence that medical care has contributed little to the decline in mortality.

However, as suggested by Levine *et al.* (1983), further sharp declines in mortality rates in males and females of all ages that have occurred recently in some countries indicate a need to review this interpretation. Firstly, it must be noted that mortality in females in several countries has continued to improve throughout most of the twentieth century. For example, since 1900, expectation of life in Australian females has increased at all ages but the trend has accelerated in the past 40 years. Expectation of life at birth also increased in Australian males, albeit at a slower rate than in females. Between 1932–1934 and 1974, as in other developed countries, there was no improvement in male life expectancy from the age of 60 years. Since then, expectancy of life at all ages in males has increased at a rate comparable with that in females (Australian Bureau of Statistics 1998*a*,*b*). Figures 1 and 2 summarize the percentage decline in the risk of dying between selected ages in Australia since the 1930s, that is, since a period generally recognized to predate the introduction of effective medical care.

Evidence from consideration of major causes of death separately Analysis of subgroups of causes of death also provides evidence of the impact of medical care. Morris (1967) has shown that mortality in men in England and Wales would have declined continuously if there had not been increases in deaths from lung cancer and ischaemic heart disease of such proportions as to swamp an underlying downward trend in mortality from other causes. While certain writers have suggested that the apparent increases in lung cancer and ischaemic heart disease were due to statistical artefact (Stehbens 1987), the subsequent marked decline in mortality from ischaemic heart disease in some countries (Epstein and Pisa 1979; Thom *et al.* 1985; Uemura and Pisa 1985; Dobson 1987), and downturn of mortality from lung

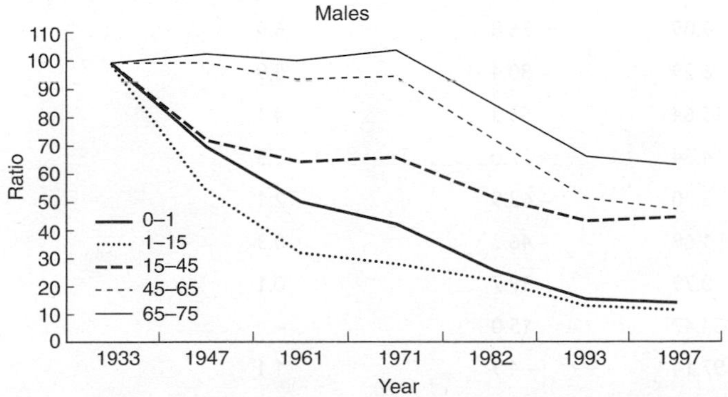

Fig. 1 Change in mortality in Australia since the 1930s (males). (Data from Australian Bureau of Statistics 1998*b*).

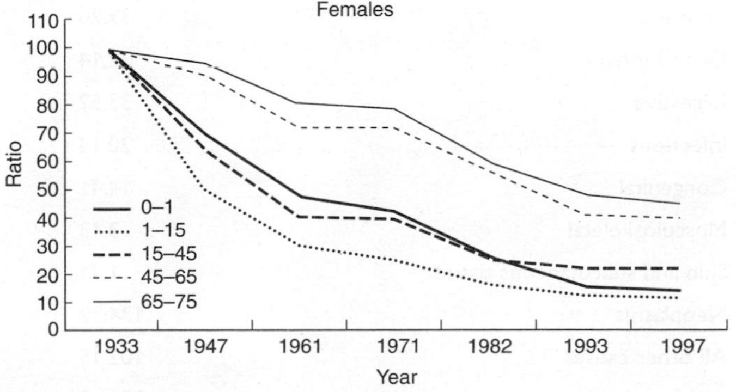

Fig. 2 Change in mortality in Australia since the 1930s (females). (Data from Australian Bureau of Statistics 1998*b*).

cancer in others (Doll and Peto 1981), attest to the epidemic nature of these diseases. Although the fall in mortality from ischaemic heart disease in countries such as Australia, Finland, New Zealand, and the United States, and the more recent appearance of the same phenomenon in most countries in Western Europe (Epstein and Pisa 1979; Uemura and Pisa 1985), are not necessarily related to medical care, by the same argument, the earlier intractability in male mortality rates cannot be used as evidence against benefits from medical care.

Data from Western Australia in Tables 2 and 3 and Fig. 3(a), show that, apart from recent improvements in mortality from ischaemic heart disease, impressive reductions in mortality rates have occurred in the past 50 years across most broad categories of disease as well as across all age and sex groups. With the exception of deaths due to malignant neoplasms, the mortality rate fell in virtually all major categories of disease subsumed in the chapters of the International Classification of Diseases. In both males and females, the greatest proportion of this improvement by far was attributable to falls in mortality from circulatory diseases (Tables 2 and 3). However, reductions in mortality rates from injuries, perinatal disorders, genitourinary diseases, disorders of the digestive system, and infectious diseases each made substantial contributions to the decline in males, while in females, perinatal disorders, injuries, respiratory diseases, disorders of the digestive system, and genitourinary diseases contributed much of the remaining improvement. Less frequent causes of death which showed marked relative improvements include diseases of the skin and subcutaneous tissues in both sexes, congenital and musculoskeletal disorders in males, and infectious diseases, disorders of pregnancy, labour and puerperium, endocrine disorders, and diseases of the blood and blood-forming tissues in females.

Substantial though these changes may be, trends in overall age-standardized mortality rates obscure the complexity of different rates of change in specific age groups or specific diseases. More detailed examination of the latter is helpful in understanding some of the multiple factors that may be contributing to general improvements in mortality. For example, modest changes in age-standardized total mortality rates for respiratory diseases conceal larger improvements in people under the age of 45 years and rising rates or mixed trends at older ages (Fig. 3(b)). One explanation for these findings is that mortality from acute respiratory infections has declined at younger ages, due at least partly to the use of antibiotics, while mortality due to chronic, smoking-related, and industrial respiratory diseases in older age groups has proved less tractable.

Similarly, with regard to mortality from disorders of the digestive system, the contributions of marked improvements in people aged under 25 have been accompanied by smaller decreases at later ages due to rising mortality from cirrhosis of the liver. Discounting the latter, it is clear that mortality from digestive disorders has fallen at all ages (Fig. 3 (c)). As several authors, including McKeown (1979) and Beeson (1980), have suggested, it is likely that this is due principally to advances in medical and surgical care. Further improvements are possible with the recognition by Marshall and Warren (1984) that peptic ulcer is largely an infectious disease which can be treated simply with antibiotic therapy, thereby probably reducing the need for elective surgery and the risks of perforation or life-threatening haemorrhage. Mortality from genitourinary diseases also decreased at all ages (Fig. 3(d)), but presumably for different reasons: under 15 years of age because of a decline in acute nephritis, in adults from 15 to 64 years of age due to improvements in the management of chronic renal failure, and in males aged 65 years and over because of lower mortality associated with obstructive uropathy.

Trends in mortality from injuries (Fig. 3(e)) are more difficult to interpret. Because of the disproportionately heavy impact of vehicular crashes and suicide in younger adults, and to a lesser extent, the middle-aged, improvement in mortality from injuries was greater in children under the age of 15 years and in people over 64 years of age. Reduced mortality from injuries in children may be due to a number of improvements in prevention. Conversely, lower rates in the elderly could reflect improvements in medical care for conditions such as fractures of the proximal femur due to falls, which constitute the largest single cause of admission to hospital for injury in this age

Table 2 Change in mortality in Western Australia 1953–1957 to 1993–1997 (males)

Condition/system	1953–1957 rate[a]	1993–1997 rate[a]	Relative change (%)	Proportion of decline (%)
Circulatory	467.64	187.77	– 59.8	63.7
Injury	110.37	56.40	– 48.9	12.3
Perinatal	39.20	9.09	– 76.8	6.9
Genitourinary	32.14	6.29	– 80.4	5.9
Digestive	33.52	15.64	– 53.3	4.1
Infections	20.14	4.64	– 77.0	3.5
Congenital	14.41	5.20	– 63.9	2.1
Musculoskeletal	3.13	1.68	– 46.3	0.3
Skin and subcutaneous tissue	1.31	0.79	– 39.7	0.1
Neoplasms	134.32	154.47	15.0	–
All other causes	102.15	97.14	– 4.9	1.1
All causes	958.33	539.11	– 43.7	–

[a]Age-standardized rates per 100 000.

Source: Australian Bureau of Statistics (1998*b*)

Table 3 Change in mortality in Western Australia 1953–1957 to 1993–1997 (females)

Condition/system	1953–1957 rate[a]	1993–1997 rate[a]	Relative change (%)	Proportion of decline (%)
Circulatory	321.8	110.8	– 65.6	71.9
Perinatal	29.3	7.8	– 73.3	7.3
Injury	33.8	19.8	– 41.3	4.8
Respiratory	34.8	23.0	– 33.9	4.0
Digestive	21.5	10.2	– 52.7	3.9
Genitourinary	13.2	4.5	– 66.3	3.0
Infections	8.0	2.9	– 63.9	1.7
Endocrine	15.2	11.6	– 23.6	1.2
Pregnancy	3.4	0.1	– 96.8	1.1
Haematological	2.5	1.1	– 55.0	0.5
Skin and subcutaneous tissue	1.6	0.7	– 55.5	0.3
Neoplasms	101.3	100.4	– 0.9	0.3
All other causes	27.2	32.4	19.1	–
All causes	613.6	325.3	– 47.0	–

[a]Age-standardized rates per 100 000.

Source: Australian Bureau of Statistics (1998*b*).

group. Since 1971, the age-standardized rates of admission for these fractures in Western Australia have remained unchanged, but in people over the age of 55 years, case fatality at 1 month has fallen from 7.1 to 3.6 per cent in females and from 16.6 to 6.6 per cent in males (Hockey and Hobbs 1990).

In virtually all of the examples discussed above, a range of non medical as well as medical factors could have contributed to lower mortality rates. Clearly there is no way of quantifying these various effects. Nor is it necessarily true that the changes are replicated elsewhere. Nevertheless, as Kleinman (1982) suggested, there may still be lessons to learn from closer scrutiny of mortality rates for the past 50 years.

Contribution of medical care to reductions in specific causes of death

An alternative to relating trends in total mortality or in mortality from major causes of death to medical care is to examine the possible benefits of specific treatments for specific diseases on a case-by-case basis and then to sum the total effects. For example, Reid and Evans (1970) assessed the possible effects of changes in drug therapy on mortality rates of selected non-communicable diseases in the United Kingdom, while Mackenbach and Looman (1988) documented the relationship between changes in the rate of decline in mortality from infectious diseases from 1911 to 1978 and the introduction of antibiotics in the years following the Second World War.

While this approach has not so far been applied over a wide range of diseases, Beeson (1980) used subjective judgement to compare the efficacy of medical treatments for a large range of diseases in 1975 with the impact of measures in use in 1927. Emphasizing also the increased scope and safety of surgery and improved care of severe injuries, including burns, that result from antibacterial drugs and other technical improvements, he concluded that 'substantial advances have been made along the whole frontier of medical treatment' and that 'a patient today is likely to be treated more effectively, to be returned to normal activity and to have a better chance of survival than fifty years ago'. This qualitative assessment falls far short of what we require to know about the effects of medical care on health, but it is an approach that might be furthered by the combination of meta-analysis of the effects of specific medical interventions with good epidemiological data on the incidence, prevalence, and the natural history of the corresponding diseases and on the treatment received by representative samples of relevant patients.

A further example of assessment of specific areas of medical care is that provided by the Reports of Confidential Inquiries into Maternal and Perinatal Deaths in the United Kingdom, which have attempted to distinguish between inevitable deaths and those associated with possibly preventable factors (Department of Health 1998*a*,*b*). Rutstein *et al.* (1976) adopted a similar approach for broader causes of death, on the basis that the frequency of selected, potentially preventable causes of death could be used as a measure of the performance of medical services. With the advice of an expert panel, these authors constructed a list of conditions where, in general, death should not occur if appropriate medical care is given. The original intention was to use the list for the purposes of medical audit. It was recognized, however, that death rates based on aggregated causes of death potentially preventable by medical intervention could be used to monitor the overall performance of the health-care system. Clearly not all causes of deaths will be preventable, and while some authors continue to refer to those that are as 'preventable' deaths, others have preferred the term 'amenable' deaths. Charlton *et al.* (1983) in the United Kingdom developed this concept further and examined variations among Area Health Authorities in mortality from 14 conditions selected from Rutstein's original list and representing 6.5 per cent of all deaths. The list included some conditions such as appendicitis and cholecystitis, where prevention of death confers an all-of-life benefit, and others, such as hypertensive disease and stroke, where intervention may lead only to death being deferred.

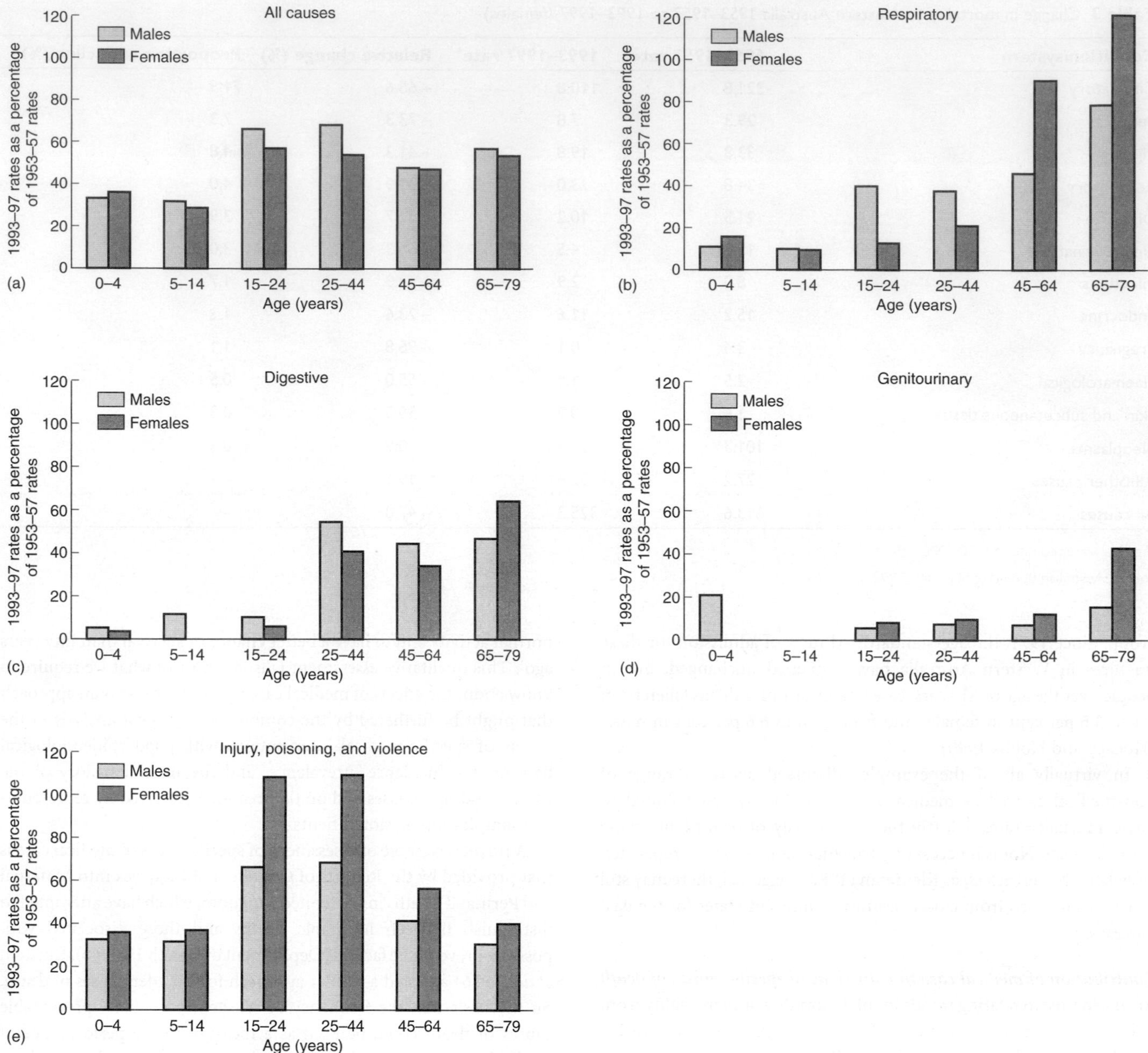

Fig. 3 (a) Change in mortality in Western Australia 1953–1957 to 1993–1997 (all causes). (b) Change in mortality in Western Australia 1953–1957 to 1993–1997 (respiratory causes). (c) Change in mortality in Western Australia 1953–1957 to 1993–1997 (digestive disorders). (d) Change in mortality in Western Australia 1953–1957 to 1993–1997 (genitourinary diseases). (e) Change in mortality in Western Australia 1953–1957 to 1993–1997 (injuries, poisoning, and violence).

This work provided the stimulus for a number of further studies of mortality amenable to medical care, culminating with the publication of atlases of preventable mortality for countries of the European Community (Holland 1988, 1993). These studies have been of two general kinds: those that have attempted to relate changes in amenable mortality over time to the introduction and diffusion of medical interventions; and those that have sought to find a relationship between regional variation in amenable mortality and the provision of health services. Studies in the former category are summarized in Table 4.

The first major exploration of long-term trends in amenable mortality was undertaken by Charlton and Velez (1986) who undertook a comparative study of contemporaneous trends in the United States, the United Kingdom, France, Italy, Japan, and Sweden. Similar studies were undertaken by Pokilanen and Eskola (1986) in Finland, Mackenbach *et al.* (1988, 1990) in The Netherlands, and Gil and Rathwell (1989) in Spain. More recently the same method has been applied to the European Community as a whole (Carstairs 1993), separately to Ireland (Barry 1992) and Scotland (Carstairs 1993), and independently in New Zealand (Malcolm and Salmond 1993), Quebec

Table 4 Average annual decline in amenable and non-amenable mortality in selected countries

	Country	Years	Population	Number of years	Age[a]	Number of conditions	Average annual decline (%) Amenable	Non-amenable	Amenable fraction at start (%)
Charlton and Velez (1986)	England and Wales	1956–80	M + F	24	0–64	10	2.93	0.17	17.3
	USA	1956–80	M + F	24	0–64	10	3.27	0.30	15.8
	France	1956–80	M + F	24	0–64	10	4.17	0.87	15.3
	Japan	1956–80	M + F	24	0–64	10	5.17	2.31	33.3
	Italy	1956–80	M + F	24	0–64	10	3.46	0.77	19.7
	Sweden	1956–80	M + F	24	0–64	10	3.85	0.13	15.9
Mackenbach et al. (1988, 1990)	Netherlands	1950–84	F	34	0–74	35	6.00	2.00	42.0
			M	34	0–74	35	6.00	0.00	42.0
Pokolainen and Eskola (1986)	Finland	1969–81	M + F	12	0–64	22	7.95	2.26	42.9
Malcolm and Salmond (1993)	New Zealand (non-Maori)	1968–87	F	19	0–64	19	3.19	1.04	14.2
			M	19	0–64	19	4.97	1.30	8.0
Gil and Rathwell (1989)	Spain	1960–84	M + F	24	0–64	13	4.40	0.93	NA
Carstairs (1993)	Scotland	1974–85	M + F	6	0–64	13	6.23	1.65	30.8
	European Community	1974–86	M + F	6	0–64	13	6.23	1.29	20.2

F, female; M, male.

[a]Age range for specific conditions variable within the inclusive age range.

(Pampalon 1993), Sweden (Westerling and Smedby 1992), and Greenland (Bjerregaard and Juel 1990). As shown in Table 4, in all of the studies with comparable presentation of data, substantially greater declines have been observed in amenable causes of death compared with remaining causes of death. This was taken by most of the authors to indicate that medical care had contributed to declining mortality, even though the absolute benefits could not be separated from those due to other non-medical factors.

While the relative changes have been considerable, absolute effects on mortality are also an important consideration. In the studies included in Table 4, amenable causes of death initially accounted for about 15 to 20 per cent of total deaths but subsequently fell to about 11 per cent in European countries, a useful but only a modest improvement in terms of mortality from all causes. Moreover, most studies have been restricted to people under the age of 65 years.

Conversely, studies of trends in amenable mortality by Mackenbach *et al.* (1988, 1990) extended the selection of causes of death (to 35, compared with 14 on Rutstein's original list) and included deaths in people up to the age of 75 years. Amenable deaths, including deaths in infants, accounted for 42 per cent of all deaths, or 35 per cent if deaths in infants were excluded. More importantly, Mackenbach and coworkers sought to relate variation in the rate of change in particular groups of deaths to the period in which specific and relevant medical interventions were introduced. In general, the findings consistently support a relationship between medical care and lower mortality. The results strengthen considerably the case for an appreciable effect of medical care on declining mortality in developed countries in recent decades.

In contrast to these studies of national trends, those that have attempted to relate regional variation in amenable deaths to intranational variations in health services have been inconclusive. Charlton *et al.* (1983) in the United Kingdom found wide variation between health areas in causes of amenable mortality that persisted after adjustment for social factors. They suggested that this should be examined further in relation to levels of provision of health services, an approach disputed by Carr-Hill *et al.* (1987). Mackenbach *et al.* (1989) also found marked regional variation in amenable mortality in The Netherlands, but the relationship between this and variation in the supply of health services was weak and inconsistent. Similarly, the *European Atlas of Preventable Mortality* reveals differences between countries that persist after taking into account a number of social indicators associated with variation in deaths from all causes and in non-preventable mortality. These persisting differences are too large in absolute terms to be credibly attributed to differences in standards of medical care.

A number of further caveats are necessary in relation to the interpretation of declining amenable mortality. The first is that, as already intimated, the extent of change is likely to be influenced by the selection of both the particular causes of death and the age range considered. For example, hypertensive diseases and stroke tend to dominate trends in amenable deaths, even though these two conditions have not necessarily shown the greatest relative declines. From data in the first and second editions of the *European Community Atlas of 'Avoidable Death'* (Holland 1988, 1993), total mortality declined by 7.8 per cent, mortality from hypertension and cerebrovascular disease declined by 20.9 per cent, while mortality from all other amenable causes of death declined by over 30 per cent. However, hypertensive diseases and stroke accounted for over 80 per cent of amenable deaths in both periods and contributed nearly three-quarters of the decline in mortality from amenable causes. All non-amenable causes declined by 4 per cent.

The second consideration is that mortality from at least some of the amenable causes of death was falling and may have continued to decline without the benefits of medical care. Conversely, some deaths that were previously not preventable may now have become amenable to medical intervention. Thus the list of causes of amenable mortality will need to be modified over time as effective interventions become available for conditions not previously amenable to medical care. For example, the second edition of the *European Community Atlas of 'Avoidable Death'* (Holland 1993) recognized that medical intervention may have some effect on mortality from both ischaemic heart disease and cancer of the breast. While only a part of mortality from these conditions is likely to be prevented by currently available interventions, in absolute terms these effects could overshadow the gains relating to other, less common, amenable causes of death. The possible savings in deaths from these two conditions are discussed below.

A third question relates to the need to distinguish between deaths that indicate the standard of medical care and those, such as deaths caused by smoking, that reflect broader national health policies concerned with prevention. The example of smoking also highlights the issue of lag time. Even if a totally effective method of helping people to stop smoking were to become universally available today, deaths caused by smoking would continue to occur in former smokers for at least another 20 years (Doll and Peto 1981; Peto *et al.* 1992).

Finally, one should distinguish between reduced mortality from acute conditions that provide benefits for the whole of life, compared with deferment of death from chronic illnesses which may be associated with changes in the prevalence of people with disability. For example, aggressive resuscitation may save the life of a premature baby but the patient may never function normally. It is thus not only the reduction in mortality that is important; the quality of the years of life gained must also be taken into account.

Trends in mortality from ischaemic heart disease In the studies described above, stroke was regarded as a cause of amenable mortality but ischaemic heart disease was not considered as such until the second edition of the *European Community Atlas of 'Avoidable Death'* (Holland 1993). With hindsight, it can now be appreciated that mortality from ischaemic heart disease is not only potentially amenable to various forms of medical treatment, but also that the magnitude of this benefit is potentially so large as to overshadow the improvements in mortality from other causes. For example, we have shown in Tables 2 and 3 that, between 1953 and 1993, mortality from circulatory diseases in Western Australia declined by over 50 per cent in both males and females, and accounted for nearly two-thirds of the total improvement in mortality in that period. It is now well documented that mortality from ischaemic heart disease began to fall in the United States, Canada, Australia, and New Zealand from the late 1960s and has since more than halved. A similar decline was not observed in Western Europe until at least a decade later, while mortality from ischaemic heart disease is still rising in some Eastern European countries (Epstein and Pisa 1979; Thom *et al.* 1985; Uemura and Pisa 1985; Dobson 1987; Tunstall-Pedoe *et al.* 1999).

The reasons for this fall in mortality from ischaemic heart disease are unclear, but there is evidence to suggest that it has been associated with both a decline in the incidence of acute ischaemic events (Goldberg *et al.* 1987; Elveback *et al.* 1981; Martin *et al.* 1984; Stewart *et al.* 1984; Tunstall-Pedoe *et al.* 1999), and improved short- and long-term survival following acute myocardial infarction (Gomez-Marin *et al.* 1987; Thompson *et al.* 1988; Hopper *et al.* 1989; Hammar *et al.* 1992). The first of these associations suggests that there has been an improvement in the risk factors for ischaemic heart disease. The second observation is consistent with an effect from medical treatment. However, these explanations are not independent, as medical treatment in people with hypertension or subacute ischaemic heart disease could pre-empt or defer the development of acute ischaemic events, while improved survival following myocardial infarction could be due to a change in the natural history of the disease associated with an improvement in risk factors in the general population.

Thus, some authors such as Dwyer and Hetzel (1980), Marmot (1985), and Dobson (1987) have linked the decline in mortality from ischaemic heart disease to changes in lifestyle factors such as diet and smoking or to changes in treatment of hypertension, while others have attributed at least part of the decline to direct treatment of ischaemic heart disease. Goldman and Cook (1984), for instance, suggested that 60 per cent of the decline was due to changes in lifestyle and the remainder to medical care. Beaglehole (1986), using similar methods, estimated that 42 per cent of the decline in ischaemic heart disease in New Zealand could be attributed to medical care.

It is clear from randomized controlled trials that medical and surgical treatment can reduce mortality from ischaemic heart disease. What is uncertain is the impact that such innovations in treatment have had on mortality at the level of whole populations, or the extent to which the recent improvements in mortality from ischaemic heart disease can be attributed to medical care.

Studies based on disease registers

Obstetric and neonatal care The major objectives of modern obstetric and neonatal practice include the reduction of perinatal loss and of the prevalence at birth of major, disabling defects. Whereas 40 years ago both of these problems appeared to be intractable, perinatal mortality has improved dramatically and there are now credible prospects for substantial reductions in the prevalence of birth defects or their consequences. In both instances, a range of interventions, including primary prevention, screening, and medical and surgical treatment are involved. The study of these problems requires the maintenance of registers for the systematic recording of birth defects and to integrate information relating to maternal and infant health during pregnancy, labour, and at least the perinatal period.

Although antenatal care is usually thought of as serving a purely preventive function, in practice it operates as a screening system to identify pregnancies at high risk of poor fetal or maternal outcome in order that the 'full force' of the obstetric services can be brought to bear early, before irreversible problems develop. Most obstetric activity is therefore fundamentally curative in intent, in that it seeks to recognize and terminate established disease processes rather than to prevent them from ever starting.

Historically, standards of obstetric and neonatal care, together with levels of reproductive fitness, have been assessed by monitoring maternal and perinatal mortality. Maternal mortality is now so low in most developed countries that it makes a negligible contribution to total mortality in females and is of doubtful value as a measure of outcome in obstetric care (Department of Health 1998*b*). Through the *Confidential Inquiries into Maternal Mortality* (Department of Health 1998*a*, *b*) it is apparent that most of the deaths that still occur under the general rubric of 'complications of childbirth, pregnancy, and the puerperium' are related more to social and maternal factors or to abortion, than to obstetric care *per se*. There is much evidence to suggest that the virtual elimination of maternal mortality has been due to factors such as improved maternal fitness, stature, and nutrition in early life, together with better education, control of fertility, and, in many countries, more liberal attitudes to termination of pregnancy with a subsequent reduction in illegal abortions. But there is equally strong evidence, again from the *Confidential Inquiries into Maternal Mortality* , that certain avoidable causes of maternal death have been eliminated through the disciplined application of modern obstetric and anaesthetic techniques.

With the marked decline in maternal mortality, attention has turned to the assessment of preventable factors in perinatal deaths. The relatively high frequency of these compared with maternal deaths dictates the need to focus attention on deaths which are likely, *a priori*, to be associated with potentially avoidable factors. For example, the Perinatal Mortality Committee in Western Australia has excluded perinatal deaths associated with lethal malformations and concentrated its attention on singleton stillbirths weighing 2000 g or more and neonatal deaths of infants weighing at least 1500 g at birth, and, for multiple births, stillbirths weighing 1500 g or more and neonatal deaths of infants weighing 1000 g or more (Health Department of Western Australia 1987).

In 1986 approximately 20 per cent of perinatal and infant deaths met the above criteria for full investigation. Of these cases 14.8 per cent, representing 3.4 per cent of total perinatal deaths, were associated with potentially avoidable factors. Thus it appears likely that in most developed countries, perinatal mortality, like maternal mortality previously, has declined to something approaching an irremediable minimum.

However, concepts of preventability must clearly be considered in the context of the knowledge and medical practices of the day. Thus it is now evident that a sizeable proportion of cases of anencephaly could be prevented by women taking supplements of folic acid during the periconceptual period (Bower *et al.* 1998). Furthermore, the birthweight limits for preventability now used are considerably lower than those used by Baird *et al.* (1954) in their studies of perinatal mortality in Aberdeen in the 1950s and may need to be reduced still further in the future. This change is emphasized particularly by the accelerated decline in neonatal mortality that has occurred in developed countries in the past two decades in association with the development of neonatal intensive care and, more recently, intrauterine and intrapartum fetal monitoring.

In Western Australia, perinatal mortality fell from 28 per 1000 births in 1970–1975 to 9 per 1000 in 1987–1991 (Stanley and Waddell 1985; Gee 1988, 1992). The improvement occurred in all components of perinatal mortality. The effect was most marked initially in the case of intrapartum stillbirths and neonatal deaths, with subsequent marked improvement in antepartum stillbirths (Table 5). Approximately 20 per cent of the fall in neonatal mortality after 1970 can be attributed to improvement in the distribution of birth weights but, as shown in Table 6, the greatest part is due to improved survival in lower-birth-weight babies, during a period in which there have been marked changes in neonatal intensive care. Similarly, the decline in both antepartum and intrapartum stillbirths has occurred in association with new methods for monitoring intrauterine growth in late pregnancy and fetal distress during labour.

A concern relating to the development of neonatal intensive care and consequent survival of babies with very low birth weight who

Table 5 Changes in stillbirths, neonatal, and postneonatal infant mortality rates in Western Australia (1970–1991)

	Stillbirth rate (per 100 total births)		**Infant mortality rate (per 1000 live births)**	
	Antepartum	**Intrapartum**	**Neonatal**	**Postneonatal**
1970–75	10.3	2.2	12.8	5.5
1976–81	7.8	1.3	8.0	3.8
1982–86	5.6	0.8	5.1	3.4
1987–91	3.8	1.4	3.8	3.2
Decline (%)	63.1	36.3	70.3	41.8

Sources: Stanley and Hartfield (1979); F. J. Stanley (1986, unpublished data); Gee (1988, 1992).

Table 6 Changes in birth weight specific neonatal mortality rates per 1000 live births in Western Australia (excluding lethal malformations) from between 1971 and 1974 to 1987 and 1991

Birth weight (g)	1971–74	1975–78	1980–84	1987–91
1000–1499	526	252	137	31
1500–1999	141	79	37	7
2000–2499	35	18	17	3
2500–2999	7.5	6.0	2.3	1.2
3000–3499	3.3	3.7	2.3	0.6
3500+	2.4	1.8	1.0	0.5

Data not available for 1979.

Sources: Stanley and Hartfield (1979); F. J. Stanley (1986, unpublished data); Gee (1988, 1992).

would previously have died, is the potential for increases in long-term morbidity and disability, resulting particularly from cerebral damage. Stanley and Watson (1992) reviewed the incidence of cerebral palsy in Western Australia over the period of falling neonatal mortality described above. They found no increase in the birth-weight-specific incidence of cerebral palsy, but observed an overall increase in cases of approximately 5 per cent due to the combined effects of the relatively high frequency of cerebral palsy in low-birth-weight babies and their improved survival.

In summary, maternal mortality has become obsolete as a measure of obstetric outcome in developed countries, probably due to a combination of general improvements in maternal health and better medical care. Furthermore, perinatal mortality is now also approaching a level where only very large studies will have any chance of detecting additional improvements, and the contribution of improved obstetric and paediatric care to this trend would appear to be beyond question. However, there is some evidence that this reduction in mortality has been associated with an overall increase in the prevalence of long-term disability in children of low birth weight, underlining the necessity for taking into account a number of different measures of outcome, including those relating to adverse as well as beneficial effects.

Birth defects The prospects for the prevention of birth defects have been reviewed by Czeizel *et al.* (1993). In a comprehensive analysis based on the prevalence of individual birth defects (as recorded in the Hungarian Congenital Abnormality Registry) and the effectiveness of a range of interventions relevant to each, they estimated that 70 per cent of birth defects could be prevented or successfully treated. The figure fell to 60 per cent if congenital dislocation of the hip, which has an unusually high prevalence in Hungary, was excluded. The authors state that their estimates are probably conservative as they do not allow for the potential benefit of improved ultrasonography applied routinely during pregnancy. Conversely, frequent ultrasound examinations during pregnancy do not lead to improved obstetric outcomes (Newnham *et al.* 1993). Nevertheless, the interventions considered by Czeizel *et al.* (1993) included avoidance of pregnancy as the result of genetic counselling, avoidance of teratogens (particularly rubella), termination of pregnancy in association with estimation of serum α-fetoprotein, human chorionic gonadotrophin, and oestriol, amniocentesis, and ultrasonography, and medical treatment and early neonatal surgery for remediable conditions detected by neonatal screening. They did not include periconceptional supplementation of the maternal diet with folate.

The convergence of several of the above measures is seen in the prevention of neural tube defects. Clinical trials have now clearly established a substantial protective effect of dietary supplementation with folate in preventing both recurrent and first occurrences of neural tube defect, if folate is given before conception and early in pregnancy (Medical Research Council 1991; Czeizel and Dudas 1992; Lumley *et al.* 1999); the benefits of routine screening of maternal serum α-fetoprotein during pregnancy have been well established in some communities; and there is evidence of increasing termination of affected fetuses as the result of wider use of ultrasonography in pregnancy and growing community acceptance of this type of intervention. In the United Kingdom, there were dramatic declines in the birth prevalence of both anencephaly and spina bifida between 1970 and 1987 (Fig. 4), during the period in which screening programmes became generally available, although it was not possible from available data to determine the precise proportion of the decline that could be attributed to screening and termination of pregnancy (Wald and Cuckle 1992). The prevalence has stabilized at 8 per 10 000

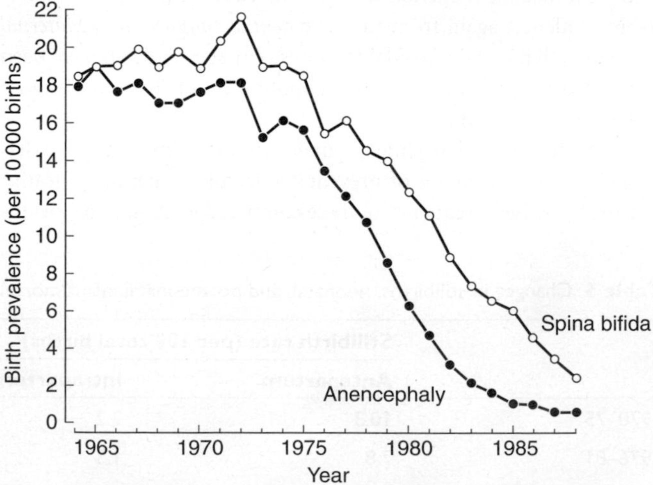

Fig. 4 Birth prevalence of anencephaly and spina bifida in England and Wales from 1964 to 1968 (data from the Office of Population Censuses and Surveys adjusted for estimated under-reporting). (Source: Wald and Cuckle 1992.)

live and stillbirths during the 1990s, down from 34 per 10 000 two decades previously (Murphy *et al.* 1996). Similar improvements occurred in South Australia (Chan *et al.* 1993), where a population-based screening programme has been in operation since 1982. The proportion of women screened increased from 52 per cent in 1983 to 81 per cent in 1986–1991, while the proportion of affected pregnancies detected increased progressively to 90 per cent in 1990–1991. Termination of affected pregnancies also rose from low levels in 1978–1979 to 80 per cent in 1990–1991. In contrast, in the States of Western Australia, Victoria, and Tasmania, where there was no such programme (Bower *et al.* 1993*a*, *b*), there was a slow increase in the termination of affected pregnancies from less than 10 per cent in 1980–1982 to 40 per cent in 1989. Throughout this period, the overall frequency of neural tube defects (including terminations as well as completed pregnancies) in all States remained unchanged at approximately 20 per 10 000, but it has since fallen by about one-third in Western Australia (Bower *et al.* 1997, 1998).

Control of infectious disease by immunization Modern developments in immunization have seen the global eradication of smallpox and the virtual elimination of poliomyelitis in some populations. Promising results have been achieved with both measles and rubella immunization, although both present problems in relation to vaccine failure and hence optimal vaccination routines. An essential component of global programmes for the control and eradication of communicable disease is the maintenance of information systems which record both levels of immunization in the target populations and the frequency of major disease endpoints, such as death in the case of measles and tetanus, flaccid paralysis in the case of poliomyelitis, birth defects in the case of rubella, and primary hepatoma in the case of hepatitis B.

In reviewing the WHO Expanded Program on Immunization, Kim-Farley (1992) asserted that at current levels of immunization, with the proportion children receiving three doses of diphtheria–pertussis–tetanus (**DPT**) and polio vaccine estimated as 80 per cent in 1990, 3.2 million deaths from measles and 450 000 cases of paralytic poliomyelitis are prevented annually. Nevertheless, there are an estimated 1.2 million deaths from measles and 120 000 cases of paralytic poliomyelitis that might be saved if full immunization is achieved. Among the targets of the programme were the reduction, by 1995, of 90 per cent of deaths from measles compared with levels prior to the immunization programme, and the global eradication of poliomyelitis by 2000. In contrast to the favourable estimates of coverage by polio and DPT vaccines, only 38 per cent of newborn infants are protected against neonatal tetanus by maternal immunization in countries where this disease is a public health problem. The programme nevertheless had a target for the elimination of neonatal tetanus by 1995. To support achievement of these goals, the programme promoted further improvement in structures for primary care, improved immunization schedules, the introduction of more effective vaccines, and further improvements in surveillance systems.

While worldwide eradication of measles and rubella is not yet a realistic goal, the efficacy of immunization in terms of the major sequelae of infection can be judged. For example, Stanley *et al.* (1986) demonstrated that the inception of a universal immunization programme for young teenage girls is the most likely explanation for an observed decline in the frequency of congenital rubella syndrome in Western Australia. Vaccination of schoolgirls aged 12 or 13 years began in 1971 (when the proportion immunized was 75 per cent), and acceptance had increased to 88 per cent by 1983. The observed 'background' frequency of congenital rubella in Western Australia was approximately 20 per 100 000 live births from 1968 onwards, but rose sharply in association with epidemics of rubella in 1970 and 1974 (Fig. 5). At the latter time, the first girls to have participated in the programme would have been 15 years old. Over the subsequent years, the frequency of congenital rubella syndrome in Western Australia fell to approximately 5 per 100 000 live births (Condon and Bower 1993; Bower *et al.* 1993*a*, *b*) and only a single case was observed in the 3 years from 1995 to 1997 (Bower *et al.* 1998). In 1990–1991, 95 per cent of women attending the major obstetric hospital in Western Australia demonstrated serological immunity to rubella, with over 97 per cent of Australian-born women seropositive. There is therefore strong presumptive evidence that a specific medical care activity has virtually eliminated one source of lifelong and at times life-threatening disability in the target community. However, the examples provided by the rubella vaccination programme in Western Australia and the measles eradication campaign in the United States (Mitchell and Balfour 1985) are relatively straightforward compared with the problems encountered in assessing the impact of more complex medical care activities where the relationship between the intervention and the outcome is less specific.

Screening mammography Records of breast cancer from a population-based cancer registry can be used to predict the likely impact of screening mammography and therefore can be used to determine whether mammography is having a potentially useful impact on the pattern of breast cancer at diagnosis in that population. Table 7 presents data on breast cancer in Western Australia (total population 1.9 million). In 1989, when 9 per cent of the 584 invasive breast cancers were first detected by mammography (Jamrozik *et al.* 2000), 36.1 per cent of tumours were stage I at diagnosis, that is, the tumour itself was confined to the breast tissue and did not involve the overlying skin or underlying muscle, there was apparently no involvement of lymph nodes and no distant metastases. Such tumours are potentially curable and are almost always treatable by breast-conserving surgery rather than mastectomy. The average size of all invasive tumours diagnosed in 1989 was 22.7 mm.

Universal mammographic screening has been progressively introduced in Australia since 1989 but, under current policies, it is offered only to women aged 50 to 69 years, with some self-referral of other women and selective screening of women of other ages who are at high

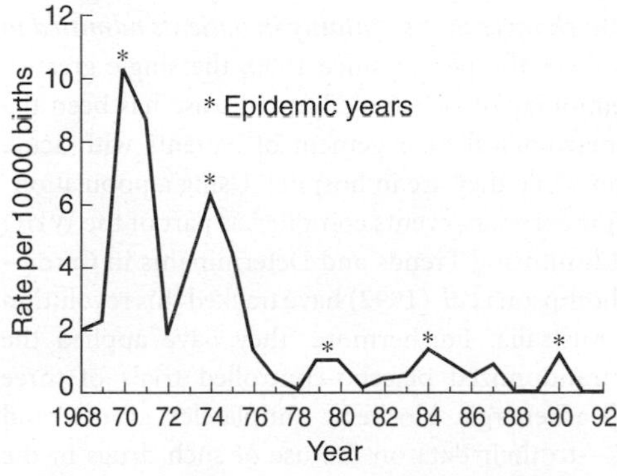

Fig. 5 Birth prevalence of congenital rubella syndrome in Western Australia 1968 to 1992. (Sources: Stanley *et al.* 1986; Bower *et al.* 1993*a*.)

Table 7 Potential impact of screening mammography in Western Australia

Scenario	Proportion of all cases detected by mammography (%)	Proportion of all tumours at stage I (%)	Average size of all tumours (mm)
Actual 1989	9.2	36.1	22.7
Actual 1994	34.5	55.1	20.0
100% mammography coverage[a]	66.0	64.7	18.3
70% mammography coverage[a]	50.9	52.2	19.9

[a]Refers to coverage in the target age group of 50–69 years.

Source: Bennett and Magnus (1994).

risk of developing breast cancer. The third line of the table shows that if all women in the target age group were screened and all breast cancers detected by mammography or presenting clinically in that age group were stage I cases, the overall proportion of these tumours in 1994 would have increased to 64.7 per cent and the average size of all tumours would have fallen to 18.3 mm. A more realistic scenario is that mammography might have the same effect on size and stage but that only 70 per cent of eligible women undergo screening. In this case, 52.2 per cent of tumours diagnosed in 1994 would be stage I and the average size of all tumours would be 19.9 mm. In fact, in 1994 55.1 per cent of all cases were stage I at detection, and the average size of tumours had fallen to 20.0 mm (Jamrozik *et al.* 2000).

Thus, increasing access to and participation in mammographic screening is reflected in an increasing proportion of all malignant breast tumours detected by this method and in a reduction in the average size and clinical stage of the tumours at presentation. In addition the proportion of tumours that are malignant but not yet invasive (*in situ* ductal carcinomas) should also increase. Progress in reaching such intermediate endpoints has been monitored in Western Australia from data collected by a population-based cancer register covering the community in which mammography is being introduced. Confirmation of the appearance of such trends provides important evidence that the benefits on mortality from breast cancer of mammographic screening demonstrated previously in randomized controlled trials are likely to be shared by the target community. Conversely, failure to see such changes in the data from the register would raise important questions about the implementation of the screening programme.

Uptake of β-blockers, fibrinolytic therapy, and antiplatelet agents in myocardial infarction; changes in case-fatality in patients admitted to coronary care units Over the period since 1980, the single greatest change in the epidemiology of ischaemic heart disease has been the change in the pharmacological management of patients with acute myocardial infarction while they are in hospital. Using a population-based register of major coronary events compiled as part of the WHO MONICA Project (Monitoring Trends and Determinants in Cardiovascular Disease), Thompson *et al.* (1992) have tracked this revolution in Perth, Western Australia. Furthermore, they have applied the results of previous randomized placebo-controlled trials of three classes of drugs—β-adrenergic blockers, antiplatelet agents, and thrombolytic agents—to their data on the use of such drugs in the population under study to estimate the impact on coronary mortality expected from the earlier experiments.

As may be seen from Fig. 6, the period from 1984 to 1990, inclusive, witnessed major increases in the use of each of the three classes of agent, while the use of calcium-channel blockers, which have not been tested as extensively as the other drugs in relatively unselected cases of suspected acute myocardial infarction, first increased slightly but then fell significantly.

Thompson *et al.* (1992) estimate that changes in the use of thrombolytic agents, aspirin, and β-blockers should have reduced early case-fatality after acute myocardial infarction in their population by 7.6 per cent, 17.4 per cent, and 5.2 per cent respectively. Since these agents exert their influences via different and independent mechanisms, one potentially can add these figures and suggest that case-fatality should have improved by 30 per cent. However, this figure will only apply to the proportion of patients who survive long enough after the onset of acute coronary symptoms to receive one or more of the treatments. With approximately two-thirds of coronary fatalities occurring before the patient reaches hospital, and further deaths occurring very soon after arrival at hospital, the impact of the major changes in pharmacological management of acute myocardial infarction will be 'diluted' considerably. Even so, this conclusion itself has implications for improving health services further since it throws into perspective the importance of early recognition and early presentation for treatment of patients with acute coronary symptoms.

Studies based on community surveys

Population prevalence of impairments, disabilities, and handicaps Periodic population surveys of disability and handicap are undertaken

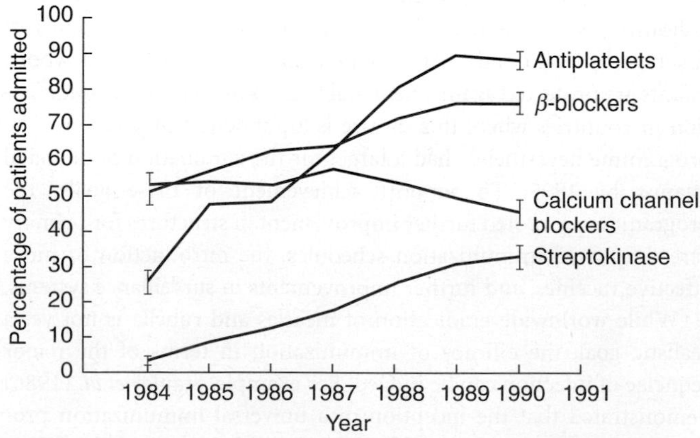

Fig. 6 Trends in the use of β-blockers, calcium-channel antagonists, antiplatelet agents (predominantly aspirin), and streptokinase in the hospital treatment of acute myocardial infarction. Vertical bars represent 95 per cent confidence intervals. (Source: Thompson *et al.* 1992.)

by the Australian Bureau of Statistics (1982, 1990) using the conceptual framework embodied in the International Classification of Impairments, Disabilities and Handicaps (WHO 1980). Under this classification, a disability is defined as 'a restriction or lack of ability to perform an activity normally, for example, less than full use of arms and fingers', while a handicap is defined as 'the cultural, economic and social consequences of disability, for example, needing assistance getting dressed'. Changes in the prevalence of disability and handicap revealed in the surveys of 1981 and 1988 (which used identical questions) have been reviewed by McCallum (1990). The overall level of reported disability and handicap rose by 31 and 49 per cent, respectively. These changes were more marked in the age group 65 to 84 years, with disabilities increasing by 52 per cent and handicaps by 72 per cent. The principal causes of disability in both surveys were circulatory disease, musculoskeletal diseases, loss of hearing, loss of vision, and mental disorders. The age- and sex-specific changes in prevalence of these disorders are reproduced in Fig. 7. Increases in prevalence of disability related to circulatory disease, loss of hearing, and musculoskeletal diseases occurred in both sexes and in most age groups. The prevalence of loss of vision increased in people over 75 years, but was generally less in people under 75 years. Changes in the prevalence of mental disorders were variable. As McCallum states, it is uncertain whether the overall increases in the prevalence of disability are due to increases in relevant risk factors, or whether they are due to deferment of death.

The increase in disability related to circulatory disease is in marked contrast to the dramatic decline in mortality from these diseases in Australia since the late 1960s. It is possible that increased diagnosis of various forms of circulatory disease, and hence greater awareness of such diseases in the respondents, could have contributed to the increase in reported prevalence of disability. However, the observation is also consistent with improved long term survival in people with cardiovascular disease as noted previously. The extent to which these changes are actually associated with handicap or impaired quality of life is uncertain, but Czarn *et al.* (1992) have reported that only a minority of survivors of working age have paid employment following acute myocardial infarction. These findings illustrate the need for careful studies to determine the extent to which gains in years of life from medical care are offset by a reduction in the quality of life.

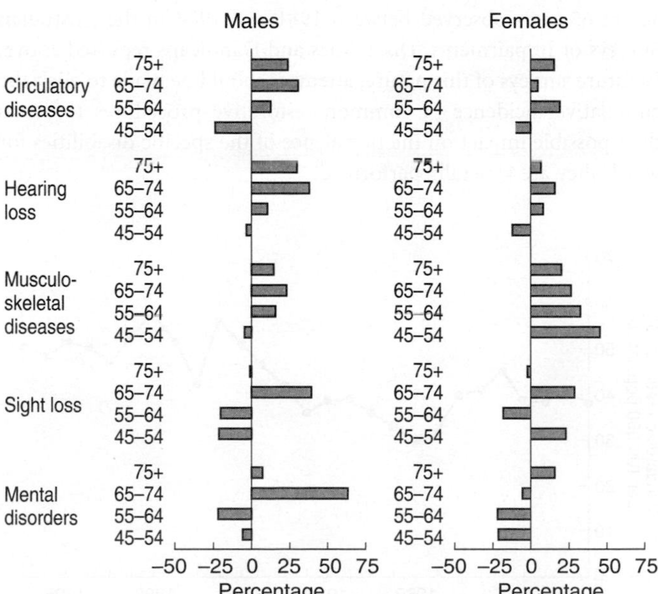

Fig. 7 Changes in prevalence ratios of disabling conditions in Australia, 1981 to 1988, in people 45 years and over. (Source: McCallum 1990.)

Detection and treatment of hypertension In common with New Zealand, Canada, and the United States, mortality from ischaemic heart disease has been falling in Australia since the late 1960s (National Heart Foundation of Australia 1998). Since a change in the incidence of acute myocardial infarction due to a change in the prevalence or severity of risk factors could be contributing to the downwards trend in mortality, whether detection and management of individuals with avoidable risk factors has improved is of considerable interest. In the Australian setting, the best set of data in which to examine trends in risk factors has been compiled by a private charity, the National Heart Foundation. The Foundation has conducted major surveys of risk factors in residents of the capital city of each of the six states in 1980, 1983 and 1989. These reveal significant decreases in mean blood pressure in both sexes as well as a significant fall in the prevalence of hypertension (Bennett and Magnus 1994). The latter has been accompanied by significant decreases in the prevalence of both previously undocumented hypertension, indicating improved detection, and inadequately treated hypertension, along with potentially important increases in the prevalence of hypertension that is treated and controlled (Table 8). Thus, these surveys not only reveal trends in mean blood pressure and the prevalence of hypertension that would contribute to a continuation of the fall in mortality from ischaemic heart disease but they also provide important data indicating the impact of previous programmes of professional and public education.

Studies based on hospital utilization data

Orthopaedic and ophthalmic surgery in the aged Since 1970 greatly improved anaesthesia and the development of prosthetic devices have led to a wide range of surgical procedures for the prevention or correction of disability and handicap. These include improved methods for internal fixation of fractures, arthroplasty, ophthalmic procedures, valvular surgery, arterial grafting, cardiac pacing, and organ transplantation.

Two of the principal objectives in care of the aged that can be readily related to quality of life are the maintenance of mobility and of independence in activities of daily living. Particular conditions that threaten these and are amenable to surgery include fractures of the proximal femur, osteoarthrosis in the hip, and impairment of vision.

Total hip replacement is undertaken in osteoarthrosis, for both relief of pain and restoration of mobility, and following some fractures of the proximal femur. From both clinical and economic points of view the procedure has been judged to be highly effective (Attenborough 1977; Harries and Sledge 1990). As a consequence, demand for total hip replacement continues to increase and far exceeds previous predictions based on earlier studies of the prevalence of osteoarthrosis (Williams *et al.* 1994). For example in the North West Thames Region of the United Kingdom, rates for hip arthroplasty in people over the age of 65 years increased by approximately 50 per cent between 1978 and 1984 (Rajaratnam *et al.* 1990), while in Western Australia, rates increased slowly from 1972 to 1986 and then rose steeply by approximately 40 per cent by 1992. They have since stabilized but, with a growing population in late middle-age and old age, this still represents an increase in the absolute numbers of

Table 8 Trends in the prevalence of hypertension in Australia in people aged 25–64 years (1980–1989)

Category of hypertension	Men			Odds ratio[a] (95% CI)	Women			Odds ratio[a] (95% CI)
Undetected	11.1	7.0	6.6	0.57 (0.47, 0.68)	4.4	2.8	2.1	0.48 (0.35, 0.65)
Treated but not controlled	11.5	10.7	7.3	0.60 (0.50, 0.72)	10.6	7.8	4.8	0.43 (0.35, 0.53)
Treated and controlled[b]	4.1	4.6	4.9	1.26 (0.97, 1.63)	6.4	6.7	7.1	1.20 (0.97, 1.49)
Total	26.7	22.4	18.8	0.62 (0.54, 0.71)	21.4	17.3	13.9	0.60 (0.52, 0.69)

[a]Prevalence odds ratio adjusted for age and survey design factors (95% confidence limits).

[b]Systolic blood pressure <160 mmHg and diastolic blood pressure <95 mmHg.

operations being performed (Fig. 8). Some measure of the proportion of elderly people who may ultimately benefit from this procedure can be judged from studies conducted in the United States in 1986 (Sharkness *et al.* 1993) and in the United Kingdom in 1991 (Williams *et al.* 1994) of the prevalence of people who have received the operation, as summarized in Table 9. In the former study the prevalence of people having undergone the procedure was 1.1 per cent in those aged 65 to 74 years and 2.4 per cent in those aged 75 years and over. In the study in the United Kingdom the equivalent proportions were 3.5 and 7.5 per cent. Comparative studies of rates for surgical procedures (Holman and Brooks 1987; Rutkow and Starfield 1984; Schacht and Pemberton 1985) generally show that the rates for any given operation in the United States at least equal if not exceed those in the United Kingdom. As rates for hip replacement are still rising, it would appear that a significant proportion of people over the age of 75 years, possibly of the order of 10 per cent, might eventually benefit from this procedure. On this basis, arthroplasty of the hip may be judged to play an important role in maintaining mobility and independence in old age.

Surgical treatment of cataract provides a further example of an elective procedure in which continuing improvements in techniques and in prostheses have been accompanied by continuing rises in the rate of replacement procedures. Previously, the frequency of cataract operations was tempered by concerns for intraocular complications and problems in some patients with visual adjustment following operation (Jaffe 1978). Such difficulties have been greatly reduced by refinements in surgical technique and by the development, in the early 1980s, of flexible prosthetic lenses that are inserted directly into the lens envelope. Improved postoperative function and the ability to perform the operation under local anaesthesia as a day case have led to a more liberal attitude to cataract surgery, with the majority of procedures in many centres now being performed under local anaesthesia in day hospitals. Thus, having been relatively stable from 1974 to 1980, rates for lens surgery in Western Australia have increased by a factor of almost 4 between 1980 and 1998 with no sign that they will stabilize (Fig. 9). To some extent this increase may have been brought about by earlier intervention, as it is no longer considered necessary to wait for cataracts to 'mature' or for vision to deteriorate in both eyes as was frequently the case before the era of lens replacement. At the anecdotal level, impairment of vision sufficient to result in the loss of a driving licence is commonly the motivation for lens surgery.

Restoration of mobility and vision in the elderly are clearly matters of considerable importance. While the data shown here fall mainly into the category of process measures, it is of interest to note the general reduction in disability due to loss of vision in people under the age of 65 years observed between 1981 and 1988 in the Australian Surveys of Impairments, Disabilities and Handicaps reported above. In future surveys of this nature, attempts should be made to elicit the cumulative incidence of common restorative procedures to assess their possible impact on the prevalence of the specific disabilities for which they are generally performed.

Table 9 Prevalence (%) of hip replacement (unilateral or bilateral) in the United States and the United Kingdom

	65–74 years	75+ years
United States 1988[a] (M+F)	1.1	2.4
United Kingdom 1991[b]		
M	4.1	8.8
F	2.7	5.2
M + F	3.5	7.5

Sources: [a]Sharkness *et al.* (1993); [b]Williams *et al.* (1993).

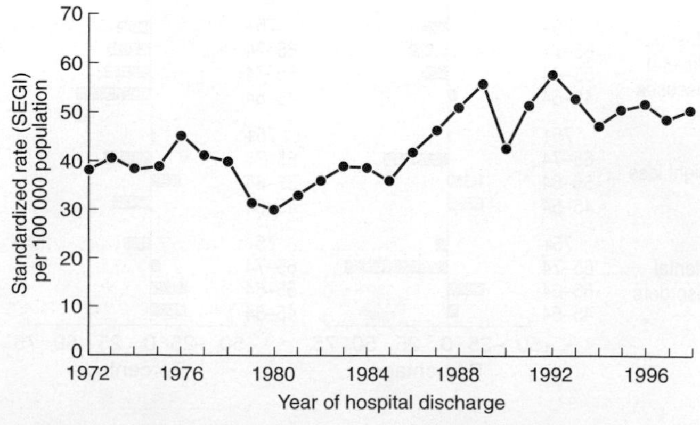

Fig. 8 Trends in hip replacement surgery in Western Australia 1972–1998.

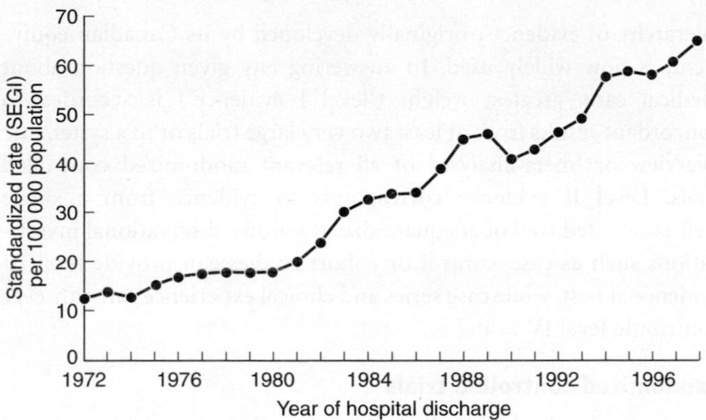

Fig. 9 Trends in surgery for cataract in Western Australia 1972–1998.

Palliative care Palliative care may be defined broadly as the alleviation of symptoms of disease without curing the disease, which is undoubtedly the longest standing function of medicine. Indeed much of medical care is still concerned with relief of symptoms of common, incurable diseases or disabilities, whether or not these are associated with life-threatening illness. Thus the term 'palliation' may relate to the medical response to conditions that range from highly prevalent 'nuisance' disorders, such as headache or allergic rhinitis, to pain or loss of function with less common but more disabling conditions such as rheumatoid arthritis, or pain, loss of function, depression, and anxiety associated with terminal illness such as cancer, and to the distress and disruption to the family associated with these problems. Through detailed studies, medical care can be shown to provide very significant relief from many disorders individually, but it is difficult to find an appropriate index of benefit that can be applied to the whole range of such problems as they affect entire communities.

It is ironic, therefore, that palliative care, as one of the newest specialties in medicine (Hillier 1988), has had to be redefined. This stems from the increase in the prevalence of chronic or intractable illness on the one hand, and, on the other, the inability of generic services, which have an essentially curative focus and philosophy, to deal adequately with the dying. As Higginson (1993) has noted in a review of past changes and future trends in palliative care, modern hospices emerged in response to poor treatment given by conventional providers of care. Thus there is now general acceptance of Doyle's (1987) definition of palliative care as 'the total (physical, emotional and spiritual) care of patients with life-threatening disease and their families. The focus is both the quality of the remaining life of the patient and the support of families and friends'.

Higginson (1993) also suggests that while palliative care was concerned formerly with the care of patients with terminal illness, this has now broadened to include the care of those who have life-threatening illnesses but are not imminently dying. This change in emphasis has important implications for the selection of patients for palliative care services. When the concern previously was for patients with terminal illness, the majority of patients were those dying from cancer. If services are to be concerned with patients from the point of diagnosis, as proposed by the WHO Expert Committee (1990), the spectrum of conditions accepted for palliative care services will be much broadened and the volume of patients supported by such services at any point in time, dramatically increased. The Expert Committee recognized that this would require significant redeployment of resources. The potential scale of such a development inevitably raises one of the long-standing issues surrounding palliative care—whether this extended role should be accepted by palliative care services as they now exist, or whether the palliative care function should be 'reintegrated' into generic services through, for example, the establishment of palliative care support teams (Higginson 1993) and appropriate modifications of the curricula of schools of medicine and nursing.

Studies of the cost of medical care at the end of life, principally in the United States, have been reviewed by Scitovsky and Capron (1986). These authors concluded that medical care in the last year of life accounts for 20 to 30 per cent of total expenditure on health care. The question then arises as to whether this expenditure represents unjustified use of technology and other costly measures. One argument for the further development of hospice and palliative care services is that they provide cost-effective alternatives to conventional care. However, in reviewing hospice care in the United States, Torrens (1985) noted that such services are frequently costly because of the intensive support that they provide. He concluded that evidence that hospice care is cost-effective compared with conventional care was equivocal. Conversely, Higginson (1993), when reviewing experience in the United Kingdom, concluded that 'hospice and specialist home care services are at least as effective as and probably more acceptable and efficient than conventional care'. It is noted, however, that this conclusion is based on relatively small studies, which do not allow us to determine the true extent of community benefit provided by palliative care services.

These contrary conclusions point, perhaps, as much to the difficulty of assessing the benefits of palliative care, and lack of evidence based on controlled trials, as to its true value as an activity of medical care. There are clearly major conceptual, technical, and ethical difficulties in measuring both the physical and social dimensions of the effects of chronic and terminal diseases and the changes that might occur as the result of medical intervention. The importance of dealing with this problem is now well recognized and much progress has been made, as discussed for example, in the proceedings of the Portugal Conference on Measuring Quality of Life in Clinical and Epidemiological Research (Katz 1987; Spitzer 1987).

Special problems in particular populations

Insightful provision and planning of health services (or any other services) for a whole community requires a thorough knowledge of that community. A straightforward area of difficulty concerns languages and literacy. Access to medical care and to information about health will be greatly impeded if a sizeable proportion of the community speaks a different language from the dominant one or is unable to read signs and printed information. Addressing differences in spoken and written language requires professional interpreters and that staff understand and appreciate that use of interpreters of convenience, such as members of a patient's family or of the hospital's support staff, may actually compound problems of communication through such individuals being perceived as inappropriate by the patient.

Challenges relating to differences in culture can be both more subtle and more far-reaching than those related to language. Apart from dietary rules, the most obvious examples of differences in cultural norms influencing medical care are those relating to the roles of the two sexes and rules regarding the sex of the practitioner whom each may consult during illness or for preventive care. However, all of the major events of life—birth, marriage, reproduction, retirement, death, and bereavement—are likely to have attached cultural prescriptions which, if ignored, may add to distress or even lead to services not being used. Refugees may experience the sharpest differences of language and culture, and they tend to make heavy demands on health services because of the combination of a lack of material and social resources, the psychological consequences of an often sudden and unplanned exodus from their homes, and the physical and mental trauma associated with the events that precipitated their flight.

Human characteristics aside, certain populations are dominated by extremes of distance or weather that inevitably shape both provision of and access to health services. The continental United States and Australia are not dissimilar in size, for example, but the one has cities scattered throughout its interior while virtually all sophisticated medical services are located on the coast of the other. Thus, provision of free mammographic screening for breast cancer in Australia has necessitated the development of mobile services that go to the women at risk rather than expect women to come to them.

In addition to patterns of place and person, time is a factor that should be borne in mind when planning health services. Worldwide, the absolute and proportionate numbers of elderly people are growing very rapidly, with enormous potential consequences in terms of need for curative and restorative health services for chronic non-communicable diseases. The impact of HIV disease is yet to be fully felt, tuberculosis is once again a growing problem, and the morbidity and premature mortality associated with smoking will continue to increase for at least another generation (Peto *et al.* 1992). These trends have timescales longer than the lifetimes of most governments, but the inevitability of their impact on health and health services obliges planners and administrators to obtain the best available information on both the current position of a given community with regard to these problems and the likely future developments.

Assessment of proposed new services

Introduction

A systematic approach to the evaluation of new services, both during their development and following their general introduction, holds the promise of avoiding many of the difficulties now faced by those trying to establish whether aspects of routine medical care that are already in place truly are effective. Here Cochrane (1971) was a leading advocate of the need for randomized trials of new medical strategies, while Sackett *et al.* (1991) have emphasized the difference between efficacy—whether a strategy works under ideal conditions—and effectiveness—whether it works under the conditions of everyday practice.

Assessment of efficacy

Many decisions that need to be made in running health services relate not to the overall impact of the 'health endeavour' but to the adoption or discontinuation of single, narrowly-defined strategies for preventing or dealing with particular problems. In this situation, evidence from good clinical experiments is more helpful than any other, not least because it is usually the most valid. This has been recognized by the United States Preventive Services Task Force (1996) whose 'hierarchy of evidence', originally developed by its Canadian equivalent, is now widely used. In answering any given question about medical care, greatest weight ('level I evidence') is accorded to concordant results from at least two very large trials or to a systematic overview or 'meta-analysis' of all relevant randomized controlled trials. Level II evidence corresponds to evidence from a single well-conducted trial of adequate size. Rigorous observational investigations such as case–control or cohort studies can provide level III evidence at best, while case series and clinical experience can only ever contribute level IV evidence.

Randomized controlled trials

Despite randomized controlled trials having become so common and influential, certain of the fundamental precepts on which they are based are still not widely understood. It is therefore worth reiterating some of the key principles relating to such studies here even though there are now many textbooks dedicated entirely to the design, execution, and analysis of these experiments. Randomization itself is the most basic of these principles as, subject to the play of chance, the process of allocating participants to treatments at random should balance known and unanticipated confounding variables across the study groups, leaving exposure to different interventions as the only systematic difference between them. Thus, systematic differences in outcome may logically be ascribed to differences in the way that the participants were managed rather than to some other factor. Less widely understood is that most randomized controlled trials are testing policies, that is, they are designed to answer questions of the kind: 'All other things being equal, should my policy in a particular situation be to employ strategy A or B?' The method of the controlled trial can therefore be applied to diagnostic and screening activities as well as to therapeutic strategies, to interventions other than drugs, and to whole communities as well as to individuals. A third key principle is analysing the results of trials on the basis of 'intention to treat'. In practice, trial protocols almost always make allowance for the clinical imperative, meaning that some participants never receive the treatment to which they were allocated and others begin on the allocated treatment but subsequently cross over to the other treatment or withdraw from the study altogether because the clinical circumstances of the particular individual change. Nevertheless, the least biased assessment of the question of policy that the trial was designed to answer comes from including all recruited patients in the analysis, regardless of their later withdrawal or cross-over, and including them in the study group to which they were originally allocated. This intention-to-treat approach avoids introducing selection bias (since participants who withdraw or cross over are not random subsamples of all participants allocated to particular treatments) and is conservative in that it helps to avoid reaching an incorrect conclusion that one strategy under test is superior to the other.

From this discussion it can easily be seen that properly conducted trials account for all patients who are ever recruited to them. As Sackett *et al.* (1991) point out, they should also report adverse as well as positive effects of each strategy under test, and distinguish between clinical and statistical significance (since a sufficiently large study will render the smallest of differences in outcome significant at the 5 per cent level). To be useful, reports of trials need also to describe the participants carefully in order that the reader can judge whether the population that took part in the experiment is sufficiently similar to his or her own to be reasonably confident that the local population would experience the same outcome from the same intervention. Finally, the treatment or intervention itself must be described in adequate detail for it to be replicated by someone who wishes to introduce that strategy in his or her own practice.

Systematic overviews

The medical and public health literature is laden with otherwise well-designed and well-conducted trials that have failed to demonstrate clear differences between the strategies under test. Not infrequently this occurs because 'miracle cures' are unlikely to be found in populations that already enjoy sophisticated health services, and therefore any advances in care are likely to be small. However, for common problems such as cardiovascular disease, such small increments in prevention or treatment are potentially very important because they 'translate' into many episodes of illness avoided or lives saved. A good trial may detect such a clinically important effect but fail to declare it as statistically significant because the trial is too small and thus lacks statistical power. Common reasons for such situations include overestimation, in the design phase of the study, of both the likely benefits of a given strategy and the rates of recruitment, and greater than anticipated cross-over during the conduct of the trial itself.

The technique of systematic overview, sometimes called meta-analysis, was developed to bring together all randomized controlled trials addressing a given question. It provides a summary figure of what they reveal, in aggregate, regarding two strategies for dealing with the same clinical problem. The statistical validity of the technique has been the subject of some debate, but there is general agreement that it rests on reasonable assumptions when the true clinical effects are small. Like all statistical techniques, meta-analysis needs to be used with care. Overviews based on analyses of data for individual patients participating in relevant trials are generally held to be preferable to those that combine summary data for groups of participants but, ideally, either type of review is followed by one or two major controlled trials that are sufficiently large to provide unambiguous confirmation or refutation of its findings. Failing that, well-conducted overviews are becoming increasingly influential as guides to which strategies for improving health are efficacious, and the number of such overviews appearing in the literature is climbing sharply as the Cochrane Collaboration gathers momentum.

The second International Study of Infarct Survival (**ISIS-2**) trial of fibrinolytic therapy and aspirin in the management of suspected acute myocardial infarction (ISIS-2 Collaborative Group 1988) is an early example of the sequence of numerous small trials followed by a systematic overview and then a definitive large study. The trial employed a two-by-two factorial design to test the effects of streptokinase and aspirin, separately and in combination, on short-term (35-day) case-fatality after acute myocardial infarction. Systematic overviews of data from the previous smaller studies had indicated that each treatment was effective (Yusuf *et al.* 1985; Antiplatelet Trialists Collaboration 1988) but, with some 17 000 patients enrolled, ISIS-2 was several times larger than any of the earlier trials and its results were convincingly unambiguous. In turn, ISIS-2 has been followed by a further meta-analysis of the effects of thrombolytic therapy in suspected myocardial infarction (Fibrinolytic Therapy Trialists' Collaborative Group 1994). The new overview has been very helpful in clarifying answers to important clinical questions about the efficacy of thrombolytic therapy when a patient presents relatively late after the onset of symptoms with consequent delay in the inception of treatment. The appropriate use of aspirin and related agents also continues to be explored via meta-analyses (Anti-Platelet Trialists' Collaboration 1994).

The technique of systematic overview has now been applied in a wide variety of fields. For example, the Early Breast Cancer Trialists' Collaborative Group (1992) has published an overview of the results of randomized controlled trials of adjuvant treatment for potentially curable breast cancer that began recruiting patients before mid-1985. Four principal modalities of treatment were examined—hormonal therapy with tamoxifen, ovarian ablation, chemotherapy, and immunotherapy—with the smallest analysis, that for ovarian ablation with or without chemotherapy, still including 1817 women. In total the overview covered 75 000 women, 42 per cent of whom had died or experienced a recurrence of breast cancer by the time that the data were analysed. This total was estimated to account for 90 per cent of women ever recruited to a randomized controlled trial in early breast cancer, but it can also be put in perspective by considering that a general medical oncologist working on a mixed service might see a maximum of 100 new patients with breast cancer each year, or 3000 in a working lifetime. Thus, the overview can be equated with the clinical experience that might be accrued in 25 professional working lifetimes. While the treatment of individual patients should always be influenced by the particular clinical circumstances, as a guide to general policy in the management of patients with early breast cancer, the evidence provided by such overviews must be regarded as compelling. As more data and longer follow-up accrue and further cycles of analysis are completed, clear answers to other questions of central importance in the management of breast cancer are being obtained (EBCTCG 1998).

Major overviews of obstetric and neonatal practice have also been completed and published (Chalmers *et al.* 1985; Enkin *et al.* 1989).

Increasingly, these efforts to bring together and review all available evidence are being translated into preparation and publication of 'guidelines' for clinical practitioners, sometimes accompanied by lay equivalents. For example, in 1995, the National Health and Medical Research Council in Australia released a pair of publications relating to the management of early breast cancer (NHMRC 1995*a*,*b*). It is perhaps insufficiently understood, however, that being based on randomized controlled trials, level I and II evidence is derived from patients for whom there was clinical equipoise. Thus, 'guidelines' founded on such evidence should not necessarily inform the decisions about cases where there are compelling clinical reasons to adopt or avoid one of the possible strategies available for management of the patient's problem.

Evaluation of the effectiveness of new strategies

It is one thing to demonstrate, via one or more large randomized controlled trials or via a systematic overview, that a particular strategy for the prevention, investigation, or management of a certain condition is efficacious, and another to show that it is effective under the conditions of everyday practice. There are many reasons why a strategy that works well in a 'clinical laboratory' can be a failure in the field. Failure to maintain 'the cold chain' leading to worse than expected results from early immunization programmes in tropical developing countries is an example familiar to many. Good practice in clinical trials, therefore, is that a study that successfully demonstrates efficacy is followed by another that is designed to confirm effectiveness. Even then, assuming that the second study is also successful, there remains the challenge of ensuring that the findings become widely known and adopted, and that the anticipated benefits do flow through to the relevant population. On occasion and particularly when a specific therapeutic agent is shown to be harmful, the problem can be solved easily, in this case, by prompt withdrawal of the product from sale. Tracking the adoption of beneficial advances and the extent to which their potential benefits are realized is no less important but frequently is more difficult.

Diffusion of the innovation

There is a large sociological literature on the ways that new ideas and techniques spread through a population, and a smaller but growing number of papers on the diffusion of innovation in medical practice. For some operations and drugs, uptake of the new approach can be monitored via routinely collected statistics such as hospital morbidity data or records of subsidized prescriptions. However, pitfalls also abound in using such systems for this purpose. Official coding systems for surgical procedures are updated infrequently, leading to old rubrics being adapted to accommodate new operations, making trends difficult to follow, and to different parts of the health system solving the same 'problem' in different ways, making data from different institutions or regions difficult to compare. For example, because the procedure did not have a unique rubric in the manuals used to code surgical procedures, Mattes *et al.* (1997) had to search the casebooks of radiology departments in several different hospitals in Western Australia to track trends in the use of thrombolysis in acute peripheral arterial obstruction. While a particular operation may be specific to a certain medical condition, there are frequently multiple indications to prescribe the same pharmaceutical, leading to confusion as to the exact reason or reasons underlying changes in sales figures. A case in point here is the extension of the permitted indications for prescription of H_2-receptor blocking agents, known as H_2-antagonists, from peptic ulcer only to include gastric reflux. Coupled with the wide indications for the use of antibiotics, this change prevents Australian data on the sales of histamine antagonists being used to monitor the replacement of antisecretory therapy for peptic ulcer by treatment intended to eradicate *Helicobacter pylori*. Similarly, the multiple indications for use of each of β-adrenergic blockers and calcium-channel antagonists mean that aggregate data on sales of these agents cannot be used to monitor changes in the management of hypertension. In the absence of routinely compiled data of information concerning the indications for using a particular strategy, one is obliged to study trends in the uptake of new, efficacious treatments via serial cross-sectional surveys or special registers.

Impact of the innovation

Data showing increased use of a particular strategy only provide circumstantial evidence that the population is experiencing the benefits of the new approach; the definitive proof comes with evidence that the pattern of the relevant health outcome has changed as far and as fast as one would expect given the extent and speed of diffusion of the innovation and its efficacy or effectiveness as indicated by previous controlled trials. Ideally, this evidence is gathered in the form of data on exposure to the strategy and the eventual outcome in the same individual. Failing this, ecological comparisons of condition-specific use of the approach and an appropriate, and preferably unique, outcome may provide indirect evidence. An example of the latter method is the link between trends in Western Australia in use of thrombolytic therapy and angioplasty for peripheral arterial disease, on the one hand, and falling rates of amputation of the lower limb, on the other (Mattes *et al.* 1997). Here, the two new treatments have unique codes when they are used for peripheral vascular disease and amputations for vascular insufficiency are readily distinguished in routine hospital morbidity data from those following trauma via inspection of a field denoting the presence or absence of an external cause for the patient's problem.

Compared with the sophistication of systematic overviews and large multicentre double-blind placebo-controlled trials, using ecological studies to assess the spread and impact of new strategies in medical care is a very imperfect science, although it does have an important role in generating new questions and hypotheses for further controlled studies (Rigg *et al.* 1999). Demonstrating that medical care is effective as well as efficacious is an essential activity at the very core of accounting for the massive public investment that the health system represents. As initiatives such as the Cochrane Collaboration develop and their influence expands, energy and resources will have to be found to maintain and extend collections of data in which evidence can be sought that new developments in care are being followed by improvements in health.

Conclusion

The impact of personal medical services on the health and survival of individuals seems readily apparent. With modern investigations and treatments, patients are now regularly saved and make very good recoveries from infections, injuries, and a variety of other conditions that were almost uniformly fatal even a few years ago. Surprisingly, it is more difficult to demonstrate conclusively the impact of these medical advances on the health of whole communities. Health is more than the avoidance of death, yet mortality statistics are our principal tool for the assessment of historical trends in disease and its management. Not only are mortality statistics subject to artefacts arising from changes in classification and in coding practice, but trends in them are confounded by general improvements in the overall standard of living. Nevertheless, mortality rates for most developed countries show increasing life expectancy with decreases (and certain increases) in particular causes of death that are so large as to seem unlikely to be due to artefacts.

Whatever the impact on overall health of past developments in medical care, the pressing matters are to evaluate existing health services, to identify and withdraw those that are not effective, and to redeploy the resources that they were consuming to implement new programmes of proven worth. This must be built upon a foundation of detailed knowledge and understanding of the population for which services are being provided, the health problems that that population faces and the resources that one has available for mounting a response to those problems. As many medical strategies have never been subjected to controlled trials, evaluating those presently in use frequently requires judicious inferences to be drawn from routinely collected data on morbidity and mortality, careful analysis of information from special registers, and sometimes special surveys of health problems, disability, and quality of life. This approach is undeniably piecemeal but it is also true that health services tend to evolve via adjustments at the margins rather than by full-scale revolutions.

Looking to the future, there is the promise that the imperfect pragmatism of today will be replaced by much more rigorous science tomorrow. The randomized controlled trial has become widely accepted as the method for establishing the efficacy of particular medical strategies, whether they be the choice between investment in prevention now or treatment later, between expectant observation or immediate and active investigation of some clinical problem, or between surgical or pharmaceutical management of the patient's complaint or some combination of these and other modalities of treatment. Demonstrated efficacy is not the end of the matter, however, as what may work well under the selected and tightly controlled conditions of a research centre may be a failure in everyday practice. Controlled trials establishing efficacy therefore must be complemented by others confirming effectiveness and, in turn, these must be followed by further studies to check that the new strategies have been taken up and applied appropriately and that the expected benefits, in terms of mortality, morbidity, or quality of life, are being seen. All elements of this sequence need to be put in place if we are to be confident that medical services are indeed improving health.

References

Acheson, E.D. (1967). *Medical record linkage.* Nuffield Provincial Hospsitals Trust and Oxford University Press, London.

Antiplatelet Trialists Collaboration (1988). Secondary prevention of vascular disease by prolonged antiplatelet treatment. *British Medical Journal*, **296**, 320–31.

Antiplatelet Trialists' Collaboration (1994). Collaborative overview of randomised trials of antiplatelet therapy–I: Prevention of death, myocardial infarction, and stroke by prolonged antiplatelet therapy in various categories of patients. *British Medical Journal*, **308**, 81–106.

Attenborough, C.G. (1977). Arthritis in the elderly. In *Geriatric orthopaedics* (ed. M.B. Devas), p. 77. Academic Press, London.

Australian Bureau of Census and Statistics (1982). Handicapped Australia 1981. Catalogue no. 4343. Australian Bureau of Statistics. Australian Government Publishing Services, Canberra.

Australian Bureau of Census and Statistics (1990). *Disability and handicap in Australia 1988.* Catalogue no. 4120. Australian Bureau of Statistics. Australian Government Publishing Services, Canberra.

Australian Bureau of Statistics (1998*a*). *The Australian year book.* Catalogue number 1301. Australian Bureau of Statistics, Canberra.

Australian Bureau of Statistics (1998*b*). *Life tables. Deaths in Australia. Annual reports from 1978.* Catalogue number 3302. Australian Bureau of Statistics, Canberra.

Baird, D., Walker, J., and Thomsen, A.M. (1954). The causes and prevention of still births and first week deaths. *Journal of Obstetrics and Gynaecology of the British Empire*, **61**, 433.

Barry, J. (1992). Avoidable mortality as an index of health care outcome: results from the *European Community Atlas of 'Avoidable Death'. Irish Journal of Medicine*, **161**, 490–2.

Beaglehole, R. (1986). Medical management and the decline in mortality from coronary heart disease. *British Medical Journal*, **292**, 33.

Beeson, P.B. (1980). Changes in medical therapy during the past half century. *Medicine*, **49**, 79.

Bennett, S.A. and Magnus, P.M. (1994). Trends in cardiovascular risk factors in Australia. *Medical Journal of Australia*, **161**, 519–27.

Bergner, M. and Rothman, R.L. (1987). Health status measures: an overview and guide for selection. *Annual Review of Public Health*, 8, 191.

Bjerregaard, P. and Juel, K. (1990). Avoidable deaths in Greenland 1968–1985: variations by region and period. *Arctic Medical Research*, **49**, 119–27.

Bower, C., Forbes, R., Rudy, E., Evan, A., and Stanley, E. (1993*a*). *Report of the birth defects register of Western Australia, 1980–92.* Health Department of Western Australia, Perth.

Bower, C., Raymond, M., Lumley, J., and Bury, G. (1993*b*). Trends in neural tube defects, 1980–89. *Medical Journal of Australia*, **158**, 152–4.

Bower, C., Rudy, E., Ryan, A., and Grace, L. (1997). *Report of the Birth Defects Registry of Western Australia 1980–1996.* King Edward Memorial Hospital, Perth.

Bower, C., Ryan, A., Rudy, E., and Grace, L. (1998). *Report of the Birth Defects Registry of Western Australia 1980–1997.* King Edward Memorial Hospital, Perth.

Brocklehurst, J.C. (ed.) (1975). *Geriatric care in advanced societies.* MTP Press, Lancaster.

Burnet, M. and White, D.O. (1972). *Natural history of infectious disease.* Cambridge University Press.

Butler, J.R. and Vaile, S.B. (1984). *Health and health services.* Routledge and Kegan Paul, London.

Carr-Hill, R.A., Hardman, G.E., and Russell, I.T. (1987). Variations in avoidable mortality and variations in health care resources. *Lancet*, **i**, 789–92.

Carstairs, V. (1993). Avoidable deaths in countries of the European Community and in Scotland. *Health Bulletin*, **51**, 151–7.

Chalmers, I. and Haynes, B. (1994). The Cochrane Collaboration (editorial). *British Medical Journal*, **309**, 969–70.

Chalmers, I., Enkin, M., and Keirse, M.J.N.C. (1985). *Effective care in pregnany and childbirth.* Oxford University Press.

Chan, A., Robertson, E.F., Haan, E., Keane, R.J., and Ranieri, E. (1993). Prevalence of neural tube defects in South Australia, 1966–91: effectiveness and impact of prenatal diagnosis. *British Medical Journal*, **307**, 703–6.

Charlton, J.R.H. and Velez, R. (1986). Some international comparisons of mortality amenable to medical intervention. *British Medical Journal*, **292**, 295–301.

Charlton, J.R.H., Hartley, R.M., Silver, R., and Holland, W.W. (1983). Geographical variations in mortality from conditions amenable to medical intervention in England and Wales. *Lancet*, **i**, 691–6.

Cochrane, A.L. (1971). *Efficiency and efficiency: random reflections on health services.* Nuffield Provincial Hospitals Trust, London.

Cochrane, A.L. (1979). 1973–1971: a critical review, with particular reference to the medical profession. In *Medicines for the year 2000.* Office of Health Economics, London.

Colditz, G.A., Manson, J.E., and Hankinson, S.F. (1997). The Nurses' Health Study: 20-year contribution to the understanding of health among women. *Journal of Women's Health*, **6**, 49–62.

Condon, R.J. and Bower, C. (1993). Rubella vaccination and congenital rubella syndrome in Western Australia. *Medical Journal of Australia*, **158**, 379–82.

Curnow, D.H., Cullen, K.J., McCall, M.G., Stenhouse, N.S., and Welborn, T.A. (1969). Health and disease in a rural community. *Australian Journal of Science*, **31**, 281.

Czarn, A.O.S., Jamrozik, K., Hobbs, M.S.T., and Thompson, P.L. (1992). Follow-up care after acute myocardial infarction. *Medical Journal of Australia*, **157**, 302–5.

Czeizel, A.E. and Dudas, I. (1992). Prevention of the first occurrence of neural-tube defects by periconceptional vitamin supplementation. *New England Journal of Medicine*, **327**, 1832–5.

Czeizel, A.E., Intody, Z., and Modell, B. (1993). What proportion of congenital abnormalities can be prevented? *British Medical Journal*, **306**, 499–503.

Dawber, T.R. (1980). *The Framingham study: the epidemiology of atherosclerotic disease*. Harvard University Press, Cambridge.

Dawber, T.R., Gilcin, M.E., and Moore, E.E. (1951). Epidemiological approaches to heart disease: the Framingham study. *American Journal of Public Health*, **41**, 279.

Department of Health (1998*a*). *Why some babies die: report on confidential enquiries into maternal deaths in the United Kingdom, 1994–1996*. HMSO, London.

Department of Health (1998*b*). *Confidential enquiries into maternal deaths 1994–1996*. HMSO, London.

Dobson, A.J. (1987). Trends in cardiovascular risk factors in Australia, 1986–1983: evidence from prevalence surveys. *Community Health Studies*, **11**, 2.

Doll, R. and Peto, R. (1981). *The causes of cancer: quantitative risk of cancer in the United States today*. Oxford University Press.

Donabedian, A. (1966). Evaluating the quality of medical care. *Millbank Memorial Fund Quarterly*, **44**, 169.

Doyle, D. (1987). Education and training in palliative care. *Journal of Palliative Care*, **2**, 5–7.

Dwyer, T. and Hetzel, B.S. (1980). A comparison of trends in coronary heart disease in Australia, USA, England and Wales with reference to three major risk factors—hypertension, cigarette smoking and diet. *International Journal of Epidemiology*, **9**, 65.

EBCTCG (Early Breast Cancer Trialists' Collaborative Group) (1992). Systemic treatment of early breast cancer by hormonal, cytotoxic, or immune therapy. *Lancet*, **339**, 1–15, 71–85.

EBCTCG (Early Breast Cancer Trialists' Collaborative Group) (1998). Tamoxifen for early breast cancer: an overview of the randomised trials. *Lancet*, **351**, 1451–67.

Elveback, L.R., Connolly, D.C., and Kurland, L. (1981). Coronary heart disease in residents of Rochester, Minnesota. II. Mortality, incidence and survivorship, 1950–1975. *Mayo Clinic Proceedings*, **56**, 665.

Enkin, M., Keirse, M.J.N.C., and Chalmers, I. (1989). *A guide to effective care in pregnancy and childbirth*. Oxford University Press.

Epstein, E. and Pisa, Z. (1979). International comparisons in ischaemic heart disease mortality. In *Proceedings of the conference on the decline in coronary disease mortality* (ed. R.J. Havlik and M. Feinleib), NIH Publication No. 79-1610, p. 58. United States Department of Health Education and Welfare, Bethesda, MD.

Fenner, R. (1980). Smallpox and its eradication. In *Changing disease patterns and human behaviour* (ed. N.E. Stanley and R.A. Joske), p. 215. Academic Press, London.

Fibrinolytic Therapy Trialists' (FTT) Collaborative Group (1994). Indications for fibrinolytic therapy in suspected acute myocardial infarction: collaborative overview of early mortality and major morbidity results from all randomised trials of more than 1000 patients. *Lancet*, **343**, 311–22.

Fingerhut, L.A., Wilson, R.W., and Feldman, J.J. (1980). Health and disease in the United States. *Annual Review of Public Health*, **1**, 1.

Fletcher, A.E., Hunt, B.M., and Bulpitt, C.J. (1987). Evaluation of quality of life in clinical trials of cardiovascular disease. *Journal of Chronic Diseases*, **40**, 557–66.

Gee, V. (1988). *Perinatal statistics in Western Australia. Annual report of the Western Australian Midwives Notification System*. Health Department of Western Australia, Perth.

Gee, V. (1992). *Perinatal statistics in Western Australia. Annual report of the Western Australian Midwives Notification System*. Health Department of Western Australia, Perth.

Gelding, J., Vivian, S.P., Baines, C.J., and Baldwin, J.A. (1987). Analytical methods of time-sequenced linked records. In *Textbook of medical record linkage* (ed. J.A. Baldwin, E.D. Acheson, and W.J. Graham), p. 55. Oxford University Press.

Gil, L.M. and Rathwell, T. (1989). The effect of health services on mortality: amenable and non-amenable causes in Spain. *International Journal of Epidemiology*, **18**, 652–7.

Goel, K.M., Sweet, E.M., Campbell, S., Attenburrow, A., Logan, R.W., and Arneil, G.C. (1981). Reduced prevalence of rickets in Asian children in Glasgow. *Lancet*, **ii**, 405–7.

Goldacre, M.J. (1987). Implications of record linkage for health services management. In *Textbook of medical record linkage* (ed. J.A. Baldwin, E.D. Acheson, and W.J. Graham), p. 305. Oxford University Press.

Goldberg, R.J., Gore, J.M., Alpert, J.S., and Dalen, J.E. (1986). Recent changes in attack and survival rates of acute myocardial infarction (1975–1981): the Worcester Heart Attack study. *Journal of the American Medical Association*, **255**, 2774.

Goldman, L. and Cook, E.E. (1984). The decline in ischaemic heart disease mortality rates: an analysis of the comparative effects of medical interventions and changes in lifestyle. *Annals of Internal Medicine*, **101**, 825.

Gomez-Marin, O., Folsom, A.R., Kottke, T.E., *et al.* (1987). Improvement in long-term survival among patients hospitalized with acute myocardial infarction, 1970 to 1980. The Minnesota Heart Survey. *New England Journal of Medicine*, **316**, 1353–9.

Hammar, N., Larsen, F.F., Sandberg, E., Alfredsson, L., and Theorell, T. (1992). Time trends in survival from myocardial infarction in Stockholm County 1976–1984. *International Journal of Epidemiology*, **21**, 1090–6.

Harries, W.H. and Sledge, C.B. (1990). Total hip and total knee replacements (first of two parts). *New England Journal of Medicine*, **323**, 725–8.

Health Department of Western Australia (1987). The seventh annual report of the Perinatal and Infant Mortality Committee of Western Australia and the annual report of the Maternal Mortality Committee for 1986, Statistical Series No. 7. Health Department of Western Australia, Perth.

Higginson, I. (1993). Palliative care: a review of past changes and future trends. *Journal of Public Health Medicine*, **15**, 3–8.

Hillier, R. (1988). Palliative medicine. A new specialty (editorial). *British Medical Journal*, **297**, 874–5.

Hobbs, M.S.T., Hockey, R.L., Martin, C.A., Armstrong, B.K., and Thompson, P.L. (1984). Trends in ischaemic heart disease mortality and morbidity in Perth Statistical Division. *Australian and New Zealand Journal of Medicine*, **14**, 381.

Hockey, R.I. and Hobbs, M.S.T. (1990). *Report on femoral neck fractures in Western Australia, 1971–1988*. University of Western Australia, Department of Public Health, Perth.

Holland, W.W. (ed.) (1988). *European Community atlas of 'avoidable death'*. Commission of the European Communities Health Services Research Series 3. Oxford University Press.

Holland, W.W. (ed.) (1993). *European Community atlas of 'avoidable death'* (2nd edn) Commission of the European Communities Health Services Research Series 6. Oxford University Press.

Holman, C.D.J. and Brooks, B.H. (1987). *Surgical procedures in Western Australia. An analysis of surgery type in 1985 and trends in surgical procedure rates 1972–1985*. Occasional paper No. 15. Health Department of Western Australia, Perth.

Hopper, J.L., Bhupendra, P., Hunt, D., and Chan, W.W.C. (1989). Improved prognosis since 1969 of myocardial infarction treated in a coronary care unit. *British Medical Journal*, **299**, 892–6.

Hunt, S.J., McEwen, J., and McKenna, S.P. (1986). *Measuring health status*. Croom Helm, London.

Illich, I. (1975). *Medical nemesis: the expropriation of health*. Marion Boyars, London.

ISIS-2 Collaborative Study Group (1988). Randomized trial of intravenous streptokinase, oral aspirin, both, or neither among 17 187 cases of suspected acute myocardial infarction. *Lancet*, **ii**, 320–31.

Jaffe, N.S. (1978). Cataract surgery—a modern attitude toward a technological explosion. *New England Journal of Medicine*, **299**, 235.

Jamrozik, K. and Kolybaba, M. (1999). Are ethics committees retarding the improvement of healthcare services in Australia? *Medical Journal of Australia*, **170**, 26–8.

Jamrozik, K., Byrne, M.J., Fitzgerald, C., *et al.* (1993). Breast cancer in Western Australia in 1989: 1. Presentation. *Australian and New Zealand Journal of Surgery*, **63**, 617–23.

Jamrozik, K., Byrne, M.J., Dewar, J.M., *et al.* (2000). The impact of mammographic screening on breast cancer in Western Australia. *Medical Journal of Australia*, **172**, 203–6.

Katz, S. (1987). The science of quality of life (editorial). *Journal of Chronic Diseases*, **40**, 459–63.

Kessner, D.M., Kalk, C.E., and Singer, J. (1973). Assessing healing quality: the case for tracers. *New England Journal of Medicine*, **288**, 189.

Kim-Farley, R. and the WHO Expanded Programme on Immunization Team (1992). Global immunization. *Annual Review of Public Health*, **13**, 223–38.

Kleinman, J.C. (1982). The continued vitality of vital statistics. *American Journal of Public Health*, **72**, 125.

Kohn, R. and White, K.L. (ed.) (1976). *Health care. An international study. Report of the World Health Organization/International Collaborative Study of Medical Care Utilization*, p. 125. Oxford University Press.

Levine, S., Feldman, J.J., and Elinson, J. (1983). Does medical care do any good? In *Handbook of health care and the health professions* (ed. D. Mechanic), p. 394. Free Press, New York.

Lumley, J., Watson, L., Watson, M., and Bower, C. (1999). Periconceptional supplementation with folate and/or multivitamins to prevent neural tube defects (Cochrane Review). In *The Cochrane Library*, Issue 1. Update Software, Oxford.

McCallum, J. (1990). Health and the quality of survival in older age. In *Australia's health, 1990. The second biennial report of the Australian Institute of Health.* Australian Government Publishing Service, Canberra.

Mackenbach, J.P. and Looman, W.N. (1988). Secular trends of infectious disease mortality in the Netherlands, 1911–1978: quantitative estimates of changes coinciding with the introduction of antibiotics. *International Journal of Epidemiology*, **17**, 618–24.

Mackenbach, J.P., Looman, C.W.N., Kunst, A.E., Habema, J., Dik, E., and van der Maas, P.J. (1988). Post-1950 mortality trends and medical care: gains in life expectancy due to declines in mortality from conditions amenable to medical interventions in the Netherlands. *Social Science in Medicine*, **27**, 889–94.

Mackenbach, J.P, Kunst, A.E., Looman, C.W.N., Habema, J., Dik, E., and van der Maas, R.J. (1989). Regional differences in mortality amenable to medical intervention in The Netherlands: a comparison of four time periods. *Journal of Epidemiology and Community Health*, **42**, 325–32.

Mackenbach, J.R., Bouvier Colle, M.I., and Jougla, E. (1990). Avoidable mortality and health services: a review of aggregate data studies. *Journal of Epidemiology and Community Health*, **44**, 106–11.

McKeown, T. (1965). *Medicine in modern society.* Allen & Unwin, London.

McKeown, T. (1979). *The role of medicine: mirage or nemesis?* Nuffield Provincial Hospitals Trust, London.

Mak, D.B. and Straton, J.A.Y. (1993). The Fitzroy Valley Pap Smear Register: cervical screening in a population of Australian Aboriginal women. *Medical Journal of Australia*, **158**, 163–6.

Malcolm, M.S. and Salmond, E. (1993). Trends in amenable mortality in New Zealand 1968 1987. *International Journal of Epidemiology*, **22**, 469–74.

Mandel, J.S., Bond, J.H., Church, T.R., *et al.* (1993). Reducing mortality from colorectal cancer by screening for fecal occult blood. Minnesota Colon Cancer Control Study. *New England Journal of Medicine*, **328**, 1365–71.

Marmot, M.G. (1985). Interpretation of trends in coronary heart disease mortality. *Acta Medica Scandinavica*, **701** (Supplement), 58.

Marshall, B.J. and Warren, J.R. (1984). Unidentified curved bacilli in the stomach of patients with gastritis and peptic ulceration. *Lancet*, **i**, 1311–15.

Martin, C.A., Hobbs, M.S.T, and Armstrong, B.K. (1984). The fall in mortality from ischaemic heart disease in Australia: has survival after mvocardial infarction improved. *Australian and New Zealand Journal of Medicine*, **14** (Supplement), 435.

Martin, C.A., Hobbs, M.S.T, and Armstrong, B.K. (1987*a*). Estimation of myocardial infarction mortality from routinely collected data in Western Australia. *Journal of Chronic Diseases*, **40**, 661.

Martin, C.A., Hobbs, M.S.T, and Armstrong, B.K. (1987*b*). Identification of non-fatal myocardial infarction from hospital discharge data in Western Australia. *Journal of Chronic Diseases*, **40**, 1111.

Mattes, E., Norman, P.E., and Jamrozik, K. (1997). Falling incidence of amputations for peripheral occlusive arterial disease in Western Australia between 1980 and 1992. *European Journal of Vascular and Endovascular Surgery*, **13**, 14–22.

Maxwell, R.J. (1981). *Health and wealth. An international study of health care spending.* Lexington Books, Toronto.

Medical Research Council (1991). Vitamin Study Research Group. Prevention of neural tube defects: results of the Medical Research Council Vitamin Study. *Lancet*, **338**, 131–7.

Mitchell, C.D. and Balfour, H.H. (1985). Measles control: so near and yet so far. *Progress in Medical Virology*, **31**, 1.

Mooney, G. (1998). 'Communitarian claims' as an ethical basis for allocating health resources. *Social Science and Medicine*, **47**, 1171–80.

Mooney, G.H., Russell, E.M., and Weir, R.D. (1986). *Choices for health care.* Macmillan, London.

Morris, J.N. (1967). *Uses of epidemiology.* Churchill Livingstone, Edinburgh.

Murnaghan, J.H. (1981). Health indicators and information systems for the year 2000. *Annual Review of Public Health*, **2**, 299.

Murphy, M., Seagroatt, V., Hey, K., *et al.* (1996). Neural tube defects 1974–1994. Down but not out. *Archives of Disease in Children, Fetal and Neonatal Edition*, **75**, F133–4.

National Heart Foundation of Australia (1998). *Heart facts report—1996.* National Heart Foundation, Canberra.

Newnham, J.P., Evans, S.F., Michael, C.A., Stanley, F.J., and Landau, L.I. (1993). Effects of frequent ultrasound during pregnancy: a randomised controlled trial. *Lancet*, **342**, 887–91.

NHMRC (National Health and Medical Research Council) (1995*a*). *Clinical practice guidelines for the management of early breast cancer.* Australian Government Publishing Service, Canberra.

NHMRC (National Health and Medical Research Council) (1995*b*). *Early breast cancer: a consumer's guide.* Australian Government Publishing Service, Canberra.

Pampalon, R.T. (1993). Avoidable mortality in Quebec and its regions. *Social Science in Medicine*, **37**, 823–31.

Peto, R., Lopez, A.D., Boreham, J., Thun, M., and Heath, C. Jr (1992). Mortality from tobacco in developed countries: indirect estimation from national vital statistics. *Lancet*, **339**, 1268–78.

Pokolainen, K. and Eskola, J. (1986). The effect of health services on mortality: declines from amenable and non-amenable causes in Finland, 1969–81. *Lancet*, **i**, 199–202.

Puska, P., Tuomilehto, J., and Salonen, J.T. (1985). Ten years of the North Karelia project. *Acta Medica Scandinavica*, **701** (Supplement), 66.

Rajaratnam, G., Black, N.A., and Dalziel, M. (1990). Total hip replacements in the National Health Service: is need being met? *Journal of Public Health Medicine*, **12**, 56–9.

Reid, D.D. and Evans, J.G. (1970). New drugs and changing mortality from non infectious disease in England and Wales. *British Medical Bulletin*, **3**, 191.

Rigg, J.R.A., Jamrozik, K., and Myles, P.S. (1999). Evidence-based methods to improve anaesthesia and intensive care. *Current Opinion in Anaesthesiology*, **12**, 221–7.

Rissel, C., Ward, J., and Sainsbury, P. (1996). An outcomes approach to population health at the local level in NSW: practical problems and potential solutions. *Australian Health Review*, **19**, 23–39.

Roemer, M.T. and Roemer, R.J. (1981). *Health care systems and comparative manpower policies.* Marcel Dekker, New York.

Rose, G. (1985). Sick individuals and sick populations. *International Journal of Epidemiology*, **14**, 32–8.

Rose, G. (1992). *Strategy of preventive medicine.* Oxford University Press.

Royal College of General Practitioners (1974). *Oral contraceptives and health.* Pitman Medical, London.

Rutkow, I.M. and Starfield, B.H. (1984). Surgical decision making and operative rates. *Archives of Surgery*, **119**, 899.

Rutstein, D.D., Berenberg, W., Chalmers, T.C., Child, C.G., Fishman, A.P., and Perrin, E.B. (1976). Measuring the quality of medical care. A clinical method. *New England Journal of Medicine*, **294**, 582.

Sackett, D.I., Haynes, R.B., Guyatt, G.H., and Tugwell, P. (1991). *Clinical epidemiology: a basic science for clinical medicine* (2nd edn). Little, Brown, Boston, MA.

Schacht, P.J. and Pemberton, A. (1985). What is unnecessary surgery? Who shall decide issues of consumer sovereignty, conflict and self regulation. *Social Science and Medicine*, **20**, 199.

Scitovsky, A.A. and Capron, A.M. (1986). Medical care at the end of life: the interaction of economics and ethics. *Annual Review of Public Health*, **7**, 59.

Sharkness, M., Hamburger, S., Moore, R.M., and Kaczmarek, R.G. (1993). Prevalence of artificial hip implants and use of health services by recipients. *Public Health Reports*, **108**, 70–5.

Spitzer, W.O. (1987). State of science 1986: quality of life and functional status as target variables for research. *Journal of Chronic Diseases*, **40**, 465–71.

Stanley, F.J. and Hartfield, M.J. (1979). *Livebirths and perinatal mortility in Western Australia 1976–78.* Report of NH and MRC Research Unit in Epidemiology and Preventive Medicine and Department of Health and Medical Services, Western Australia.

Stanley, F.J. and Waddell, V. (1985). Changing patterns of perinatal and infant mortality in Western Australia: implications for prevention. *Medical Journal of Australia*, **143**, 379.

Stanley, F.J. and Watson, L. (1992). Trends in perinatal mortality and cerebral palsy in Western Australia, 1967 to 1985. *British Medical Journal*, **304**, 1658–63.

Stanley, F.J., Sim, M., Wilson, G., and Worthington, S. (1986). The decline in congenital rubella syndrome in Western Australia: an impact of the school girl vaccination programme? *American Journal of Public Health*, **76**, 35.

Stehbens, W.E. (1987). An appraisal of the epidemic rise of coronary heart disease and its decline. *Lancet*, **i**, 606.

Stewart, A.W., Beaglehole, R., Fraser, G.E., and Sharpe, D.N. (1984). Trends in survival after myocardial infarction in New Zealand, 1974–81. *Lancet*, **ii**, 444.

Thom, T.J., Epstein, F.H., Feldman, J.J., and Leaverton, P.E. (1985). Trends in total morbidity and mortality from heart disease in 26 countries from 1950 to 1978. *International Journal of Epidemiology*, **14**, 510.

Thompson, P.L., Hobbs, M.S.T., and Martin, C.A. (1988). The rise and fall of ischaemic heart disease in Australia. *Australian and New Zealand Journal of Medicine*, **18**, 327.

Thompson, P.L., Parsons, R.W, Jamrozik, K., Hockey, R.L., Hobbs, M.S.T., and Broadhurst, R.J. (1992). Changing patterns of medical treatment in acute myocardial infarction: observations from the Perth MONICA study 1984–1990. *Medical Journal of Australia*, **157**, 87–92.

Torrens, P. (1985). Hospice care: what have we learned? *Annual Review of Public Health*, **6**, 65.

Tunstall-Pedoe, H., Kuulasmaa, K., Mahonen, M., Tolonen, H., Ruokokoski, E., and Amouyel, P. (1999). Contribution of trends in survival and coronary-event rates to changes in coronary heart disease mortality: 10-year results from 37 WHO MONICA project populations. Monitoring trends and determinants in cardiovascular disease. *Lancet*, **8**, 1547–57.

Uemura, K. and Pisa, Z. (1985). Recent trends in cardiovascular disease mortality in 27 industrialized countries. *World Health Statistics Quarterly*, **38**, 142.

US Preventive Services Task Force (1996). *Guide to clinical preventive services* (2nd edn). Williams and Wilkins, Baltimore, MD.

Wald, N. and Cuckle, H. (1992). Antenatal screening and diagnosis. In *Epidemiology and control of neural tube defects* (ed. J.M. Elwood, J. Little, and J.H. Elwood), pp. 711–26. Oxford University Press.

Westerling, R. and Smedby, B. (1992). Trends in 'avoidable' mortality in Sweden, 1974–1985. *Journal of Epidemiology and Community Health*, **46**, 489–93.

Wilson, R.W. and Drury, T.E. (1984). Interpreting trends in illness and disability: health statistics and health status. *Annual Review of Public Health*, **5**, 83.

WHO (World Health Organization) (1980). *International classification of impairments, disabilities, and handicaps.* WHO, Geneva.

WHO (World Health Organization) (1984). *Uses of epidemiology in aging. Report of a scientific group.* Technical report series 706. WHO, Geneva.

WHO (World Health Organization) (1990). *Cancer pain relief and palliative care. Report of an expert committee on pain relief.* Technical report series 804. WHO, Geneva.

Williams, M.H., Newton, J.N., Frankel, S.J., Braddon, E, Barclay, E., and Gray, J.A.M. (1994). Prevalence of total hip replacement: how much demand has been met? *Journal of Epidemiology and Community Health*, **48**, 188–91.

Yusuf, S., Collins, R., Peto, R., *et al.* (1985). Intravenous and intracoronary fibrinolytic therapy in acute myocardial infarction: an overview of results on mortality, re-infarction and side effects from 33 randomized controlled trials. *European Heart Journal*, **6**, 556–83.

2.9 Assessing health needs: the Global Burden of Disease Study*

C. J. L. Murray and A. D. Lopez

Introduction

The epidemiological transition and rapid changes in disease patterns have posed serious challenges to health-care systems and forced difficult decisions about the allocation of scarce resources. Epidemiological information is often required at all levels of health systems, and compilations of mortality and morbidity statistics at the national and subnational levels have been published by many countries for several decades. However, prior to the Global Burden of Disease Study which began in 1992, there had been no comprehensive efforts to provide comparable regional and global estimates and projections of disease and injury burden based on a common methodology and denominated in a common metric.

One of the major goals of the Global Burden of Disease Study was to facilitate the inclusion of non-fatal health outcomes into debates on international health policy, which had largely drawn on the mortality data available in countries, much of it referring to children. Secondly, there was a need to decouple epidemiological assessment from advocacy so that estimates of the mortality or disability from a condition are developed as objectively as possible. In addition, there was a need to quantify the burden of disease using a measure that could then be used for cost-effectiveness analysis. The Global Burden of Disease Study method quantifies not merely the number of deaths but also the impact of premature death and disability on a population, combining these measures into a single unit of measurement of the overall burden of disease in the population. The Study also presented the first global and regional estimates of disease and injury burden attributable to certain risk factors for disease, such as tobacco, alcohol, poor water and sanitation, and unsafe sex. Quantifiable estimates and projections of disease and injury burden from various exposures to specific disease and injuries, measured in a comparable fashion, are required if information on comparable assessments is to guide health policy debate.

Measuring disease burden

The incorporation of the burden of premature mortality and disability into one summary measure requires a common metric. Since the late 1940s, researchers have generally agreed that time is an appropriate currency: time (in years) lost through premature death, and time (in years) lived with a disability. A range of such time-based measures has been used in different countries, many of them variants of the so-called quality-adjusted life year. For the Global Burden of Disease Study, an internationally standardized form of the quality-adjusted life year was developed, called the disability-adjusted life year. The disability-adjusted life year expresses years of life lost to premature death and years lived with a disability of specified severity and duration. One disability-adjusted life year is the equivalent of one lost year of healthy life. Here, a premature death is defined as one that occurs before the age to which a person could have expected to survive if he or she were a member of a model population with a life expectancy at birth approximately equal to that of the world's longest-surviving population—Japan.

To calculate total disability-adjusted life years for a given condition in a population, years of life lost and years lived with disability for that condition must each be estimated, and then summed. For example, to calculate disability-adjusted life years incurred through road traffic accidents in India in 1990, the total years of life lost in fatal road accidents must be added to the total years of life lived with disabilities by survivors of such accidents, weighted by the severity of the disability. For the Global Burden of Disease Study, 1990 was chosen as the base year for estimating disease burden.

Summary measures of population health

Over the past 30 or so years, several indicators have been developed to adjust mortality to reflect the impact of morbidity or disability. These summary measures of population health fall into two basic categories, health expectancy and health gap (Murray *et al.* 1999) (Fig. 1). Within the former category, Sullivan (1971) first suggested weighting life expectancy to measure the health of a population using a single indicator, disability-free life expectancy. Disability-free life expectancy incorporates a dichotomous weighting scheme, that is, it does not account for varying levels of severity. Wilkins and Adams (1983) suggested a more sensitive weighting scheme based on functional limitations, leading to the disability-adjusted life expectancy approach.

As a summary measure of the burden of disability from all causes in a population, disability-adjusted life expectancy has two advantages (Murray and Lopez 1996*a*) over other summary measures. The first is that it is relatively easy to explain the concept of a lifespan without disability to a non-technical audience. The increasing popularity of health expectancy indicators among policy-makers has been documented (van de Water *et al.* 1996; Barendregt *et al.* 1998). The second is that it is easy to calculate disability-adjusted life expectancy using the Sullivan method which relies on prevalence data.

* The authors are extremely grateful to Brodie Ferguson for his assistance in preparing this chapter.

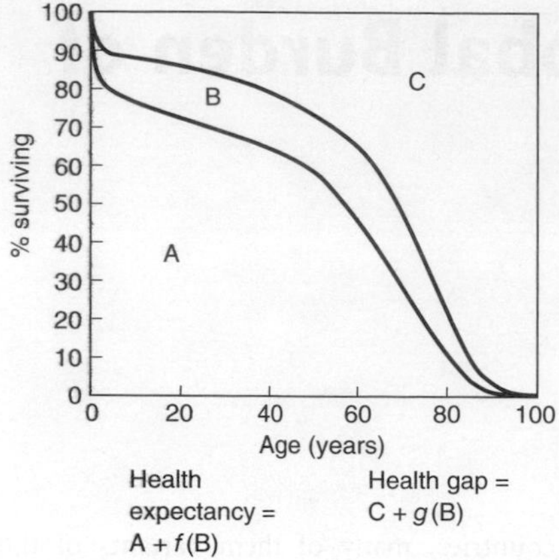

Fig. 1 A typology of summary measures.

The disability-adjusted life year is an example of a particular type of health gap summary measure which allows the disaggregation of overall disease burden into the burden attributed to specific diseases, injuries, or exposures. In the Global Burden of Disease Study, the aim was to develop a measure based on explicit and transparent value choices that may be readily debated and modified. Overall, the disability-adjusted life year used in the Global Burden of Disease Study is an egalitarian measure in that it is built on the principle that only two characteristics of individuals that are not directly related to their health, their age and their sex, should be taken into consideration when calculating the burden of a given health outcome in that individual. Other characteristics, such as socio-economic status, race, or level of education are not considered.

Constructing disability-adjusted life years: social value choices

To assess premature mortality, the Study utilized a standard life table for all populations, with life expectancies at birth fixed at 82.5 years for women and 80 years for men. A standard life expectancy allows deaths at the same age to contribute equally to the burden of disease irrespective of where the death occurs. Alternatives, such as using different life expectancies for different populations that more closely match their actual life expectancies, violate this egalitarian principle. As life expectancy is rarely equal for men and women, the Global Burden of Disease Study assigned men a lower reference life expectancy than women. However, since much of the difference between men and women is determined by men's higher exposure to various risks such as alcohol, tobacco, and occupational injury, rather than purely biological differences, this choice could be modified in future revisions of the Study.

If individuals are forced to choose between saving a year of life for a 2-year-old and saving it for a 22-year-old, most prefer to save the 22-year-old. A range of studies confirms this broad social preference to weight the value of a year lived by a young adult more heavily than one lived by a very young child or an older adult. Adults are widely perceived to play a critical role in the family, community, and society. It was for these reasons that the Global Burden of Disease Study incorporated age weighting into the disability-adjusted life year. It was assumed that the relative value of a year of life rises rapidly from birth to a peak in the early twenties, after which it steadily declines.

Individuals commonly discount future benefits against current benefits similarly to the way that they may discount future dollars against current dollars. Whether a year of healthy life, like a dollar, is also deemed to be preferable now rather than later, is a matter of debate among economists, medical ethicists, and public health planners, since discounting future health affects both measurements of disease burden and estimates of the cost-effectiveness of an intervention. There are arguments for and against discounting. In the Global Burden of Disease Study, future life years were discounted by 3 per cent per year. This means that a year of healthy life bought for 10 years hence is worth around 24 per cent less than one bought for now, as discounting is represented as an exponential decay function. Since the impact of discounting is significant, the findings of the Global Burden of Disease Study were published based on disability-adjusted life years with and without discounting. Discounting future health reduces the relative impact of a child death compared with an adult death. Another effect is that it reduces the value of interventions that provide benefits largely in the future, such as vaccinating against hepatitis B, which may prevent thousands of cases of liver cancer, but some decades later.

In order to quantify time lived with a non-fatal health outcome and assess disabilities in a way that will help to inform health policy, disability must be defined, measured, and valued in a clear framework that inevitably involves simplifying reality. There is surprisingly wide agreement between cultures on what constitutes a severe or a mild disability. For example, a year lived with blindness appears to most people to be a more severe disability than a year lived with watery diarrhoea, while quadriplegia is regarded as more severe than blindness. These judgements must be made formal and explicit if they are to be incorporated into measurements of disease burden.

Two methods are commonly used to formalize social preferences for different states of health. Both involve asking people to make judgements about the trade-off between quantity and quality of life. This can be expressed as a trade-off in time (how many years lived with a given disability a person would trade for a fixed period of perfect health) or a trade-off between persons (whether the person would prefer to save 1 life year for 1000 perfectly healthy individuals or 1 life year for perhaps 2000 individuals in a worse health state).

The Global Burden of Disease Study developed a protocol based on the person trade-off method. In a formal exercise involving health workers from all regions of the world, the severity of a set of 22 indicator disabling conditions—such as blindness, depression, and conditions that cause pain—was weighted between 0 (perfect health) and 1 (equivalent to death). These weights were then grouped into seven classes where class 1 has a weight between 0 and 0.02 and class VII a weight between 0.7 and 1. Subsequent valuation exercises carried out in various cultures have closely matched the results of the original Global Burden of Disease exercise (Table 1).

In essence, the weight is set by the number of people with a given condition whose claim on a fixed health-care budget is equal, in the judgement of a participant, to that of 1000 healthy people. For example, if the participant judges that 1000 entirely healthy people would have an equal claim on the resources as 8000 people with some severe disability, the weight assigned to that particular disability is equal to 1 – (1000/8000), or 0.875. If 1000 entirely healthy people were judged to have an equal claim on the resources as 2000 people with a

Table 1 Pearson's correlation coefficients for median disability weights for 10 exercises, based on 14 conditions common to all exercises

	Int. I	Nether.	Maghreb	Japan	GBD	Int. II	CDC	Brazil	Mexico	Int. III
International I	1.00									
Netherlands	0.98	1.00								
Maghreb	0.96	0.96	1.00							
Japan	0.94	0.88	0.91	1.00						
GBD	0.97	0.96	0.98	0.92	1.00					
International II	1.00	0.98	0.96	0.93	0.97	1.00				
CDC	0.99	0.99	0.95	0.90	0.95	0.98	1.00			
Brazil	0.95	0.91	0.90	0.93	0.91	0.94	0.94	1.00		
Mexico	0.96	0.92	0.92	0.96	0.92	0.96	0.93	0.97	1.00	
International III	0.98	0.95	0.92	0.93	0.93	0.97	0.98	0.97	0.96	1.00

CDC, Centers for Disease Control (United States); GBD, Global Burden of Disease (Study); Int., international.

particular, less severe, disability, the weight assigned would be equal to 1 – (1000/2000), or 0.5.

For the Global Burden of Disease protocol, each participant is asked two versions of the person trade-off question: one about extending life for people in a given health state versus extending life for healthy people, and the second about giving health back to people in a given health state versus extending life for healthy people. Two questions are asked because people's answers to each one are invariably inconsistent with the other, and the process of making them consistent forces the participant to think through the implications of their decision in greater depth.

The implications of choosing between the claims of different groups in a society are profound, so the process of setting weights cannot be undertaken lightly. The Global Burden of Disease Study protocol is a deliberative process in which a comparatively small group of participants (between eight and twelve) are confronted with the implications of their decision, encouraged to discuss their choices with their peers, and allowed to revise their initial choices. Once the 22 indicator conditions have been weighted, the participants assigned the remaining conditions across the seven classes.

Sensitivity analyses

To gauge the impact of changing these social choices on the final measures of disease burden, the Global Burden of Disease Study assessments were recalculated with alternative age weighting and discount rates, and with alternative methods for weighting the severity of disabilities. Overall, the rankings of diseases and the distribution of burden by broad cause group are largely unaffected by age weighting and only slightly affected by changing the method for weighting disability. Changes to the discount rate, by contrast, may have a more significant effect on the overall results. A higher discount rate results in an increased burden in older age groups, while a lower discount rate results in an increased burden in younger age groups. Changes in the age distribution of burden, in turn, affect the distribution by cause, as communicable and perinatal conditions are most common in children while non-communicable diseases are most common in adults. The most significant effect of changing the discount and age weights is a reduction in the importance of several psychiatric conditions.

Ultimately, however, the accuracy of the underlying basic epidemiological data from which disease burden is calculated will influence the final results much more than the discount rate, the age weight, or the disability weighting method. If, for example, estimates of the incidence of blindness are off by a factor of 2, then the results, whatever the social value choices used in the metric, will be substantially incorrect. We conclude that much more effort needs to be invested in improving the basic epidemiological data than in analysing the effects of what are eventually minor adjustments to the particular summary measure of population health employed.

Estimating mortality and disability

Classification

As most developing countries still have only limited information about the distribution of causes of death in their populations, a primary objective of the Global Burden of Disease Study has been to develop comprehensive internally consistent mortality estimates worldwide for each major cause in 1990. Deaths were classified using a tree structure, in which the first level of disaggregation comprises three broad cause groups as follows.

Group I comprised communicable, maternal, perinatal, and nutritional conditions (*International Classification of Diseases (10th revision)* (**ICD-10**) codes A00–B99, G00, N70–N73, J00–J06, J10–J18, J20–J22, H65–H66, O00–O99, P00–P96, E00–E02, E40–E46, E50, D50). (For an explanation of these codes in terms of disease and injury entities, see WHO (1992).)

Group II comprised non-communicable diseases (ICD-10 codes C00–C97, D00–D48, D51–D89, E03–E07, E10–E16, E20–E34, E51–E89, F00–F99, G03–G99, H00–H61, H68–H95, I00–I99, J30–J99, K00–K92, N00–N64, N75–N99, L00–L99, M00–M99, Q00–Q99).

Group III comprised injuries (ICD-10 codes V01–Y89).

Each group was then subdivided into categories: for example, cardiovascular diseases and malignant neoplasms are two subcategories of group II. Beyond this level, there are two further disaggregation levels such that 107 individual causes from the ninth revision of the ICD (ICD-9) can be listed separately.

Consistent with the goal of providing disaggregated estimates of disease burden to assist priority setting in the health sector, estimates were prepared by age and sex and for eight broad geographic regions of the world: Established Market Economies, Formerly Socialist Economies of Europe, China, India, Latin America and the Caribbean, Middle-Eastern Crescent, Other Asia and Islands, and sub-Saharan Africa.

Estimating regional mortality patterns

The Study arrived at mortality estimates by cause by drawing on the following four broad sources of data.

Vital registration systems

Cause of death data certified by a doctor have been assembled through vital registration systems for over 100 years in some European countries. Data were available for 1990 or thereabouts for about 70 countries.

Sample death registration systems

In China, a set of 145 Disease Surveillance Points, representative of both urban and rural areas, and covering about 10 000 000 people, provides useful mortality data. In India, Maharashtra State provides full medical certification for at least 80 per cent of urban deaths, while a rural surveillance system including more than 1300 primary health-care centres nationwide was used to assess broad rural patterns of mortality.

Epidemiological assessments

Epidemiological estimates exist for specific causes in different regions. These estimates combine information from surveys on the incidence or prevalence of the disease with data on case-fatality rates for both treated and untreated cases.

Cause of death models

These are based on the fact that the broad cause structure of mortality is closely related to the level of mortality in a population. Such models estimate the distribution of deaths by cause in a population from historical studies of mortality patterns in countries with vital registration. The models developed for the initial Global Burden of Disease Study drew on a data set of 103 observations from 67 countries between 1950 and 1991, and were used primarily to provide plausibility bounds on estimates derived from epidemiological assessments.

Vital registration data, corrected where necessary for under-registration, were used to construct regional model life tables for those regions where registration was complete or virtually complete. For other regions, sex/age-specific mortality rates were estimated from survey and census data using conventional demographic techniques.

Assessing disability

A disease or injury may have multiple disabling effects, or sequelae. For example, diabetes may result in diabetic vascular disease, retinopathy, or amputation. To estimate the total burden of disability, the Study measured the amount of time lived with each of the various disabling sequelae of diseases and injuries, in both treated and untreated states, and weighted for their severity, in each population. In all, 483 disabling sequelae of disease and injuries were analysed for the Study, for all regions and age groups, and for both sexes.

Calculating the number of years lived with a disabling condition requires information about its incidence, the average age of onset, the average duration of the disability, and the severity weight for the condition. Epidemiological experts were requested to estimate each of these variables for each condition based on an in-depth review of published and unpublished studies. For each sequela, prevalence, case-fatality, remission, and mortality were estimated. This information allowed correction of the preliminary estimates for internal consistency, that is, ensuring that the estimated prevalence was consistent with estimated incidence and vice versa. Consistency was validated using DISMOD software which was specifically developed for the Study (Fig. 2). (DISMOD is a computer model (DISease MODel) which allows for simultaneous estimation of age patterns of basic epidemiological parameters, such as incidence, prevalence, case-fatality, and duration, based on knowledge of a limited set of these variables.) When inconsistencies were detected, epidemiological experts were asked to revise their initial estimates. The final disability estimates were the result of several rounds of revision in a process lasting nearly 5 years.

The number of years lived with a given disability for each individual were calculated from the incidence of the disability, with the 'stream' of disability arising from it measured from the age of onset, for the estimated duration of the disability, multiplied by the condition's severity weight. To calculate the years lived with disability due to a condition in any given population, the number of years lived with disability lost per incident case must be multiplied by the number of incident cases. A case of asthma, for example, carries a disability weight of 0.1 if untreated and 0.06 if treated. If the annual incidence of asthma in males aged 15 to 44 years is 1 million cases, the untreated proportion is 35 per cent, and the average duration is 7 years, then this sequela alone is estimated to cause 664 000 years lived with disability for that demographic group. Unlike the estimates of years of life lost, not all sequelae of all conditions could be explicitly assessed for years lived with disability. Estimates for conditions not explicitly considered were made on the basis of information about the ratio of total premature mortality to disability for each broad cause group.

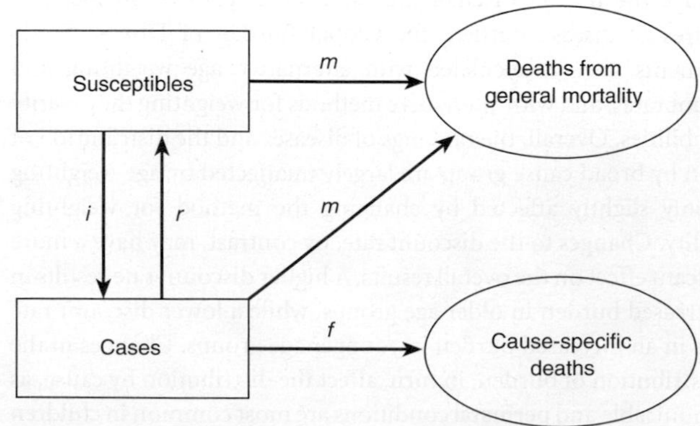

Fig. 2 Basic relationships between susceptibles, cases, and deaths used in developing DISMOD.

The global burden of disease in 1990: main findings

The results of the Study demonstrate clearly that disability plays a central role in determining the overall health status of a population. Yet that role has until now been almost invisible to public health. The leading causes of disability are shown to be substantially different from the leading causes of death, which has considerable implications for the practice of judging a population's health from its mortality statistics alone.

A key aim of the Global Burden of Disease Study was to quantify the burden of fatal and non-fatal health outcomes in a single measure, the disability-adjusted life year. This section presents the main results of the assessments of overall burden for each region. (More detail on the age–sex–cause and sequelae patterns can be found in Murray and Lopez (1996*b*).) To calculate disability-adjusted life years due to each disease or injury in a given year and population, the years of life lost through all deaths in that year were added to the years of life expected to be lived with a disability for all new cases of disease or injury occurring in that year, weighted for the severity of the condition.

Regional imbalances in the burden of disease

Sub-Saharan Africa and India together accounted for more than 40 per cent of the total global burden of disease in 1990, although they make up only 26 per cent of the world's population. In contrast, the Established Market Economies and the Formerly Socialist Economies of Europe, with about a fifth of the world's population between them, together bore less than 12 per cent of the total disease burden. China emerged as substantially the most 'healthy' of the developing regions, with 15 per cent of the global disease burden and a fifth of the world's population. This means that about 579 years of healthy life were lost for every 1000 people living in sub-Saharan Africa, compared with just 124 for every 1000 people in the Established Market Economies (Fig. 3).

In terms of the risk of dying, the Study found a sevenfold higher risk of child death (that is, a newborn dying before the age of 15 years) in sub-Saharan Africa compared with a newborn in the Established Market Economies (Fig. 4). This extraordinary excess mortality in many developing regions must remain a priority for global health programmes. Somewhat surprisingly, the risk of adult death in the Formerly Socialist Economies of Europe region, at least for males, was higher than in any other region of the world, except Africa (Fig. 5). This largely reflects the rapid increase in adult male death rates in Russia since 1987. In 1990, mortality at these ages (15 to 59 years) was still rising rapidly in Russia, reaching a peak in 1994. Since then, the probability of death between the ages of 15 and 60 has declined as rapidly as it rose. The trends for females are qualitatively similar, though less extreme.

In addition, the Global Burden of Disease Study has provided support for the theory that people in high-income low-mortality populations not only live longer, but remain healthier for longer as well. In recent years, researchers have been divided between those who argue that ill health is compressed into the last few years of life in these populations, and those who argue that longer life merely exposes people to a longer period of poor health. The results suggest that older people in the developed world are healthier than their counterparts in developing countries. It was also found that babies born in sub-Saharan Africa could expect to spend about 15 per cent of their lifespan disabled, compared with just 8 per cent for babies born in the Established Market Economies. A 60-year-old person in sub-Saharan Africa can expect to spend about half of his or her remaining years with a disability, whereas the same person in the Established Market Economies is likely to spend just one-fifth of those years disabled. The results suggest that the proportion of the lifespan lived with a disability falls as life expectancy rises.

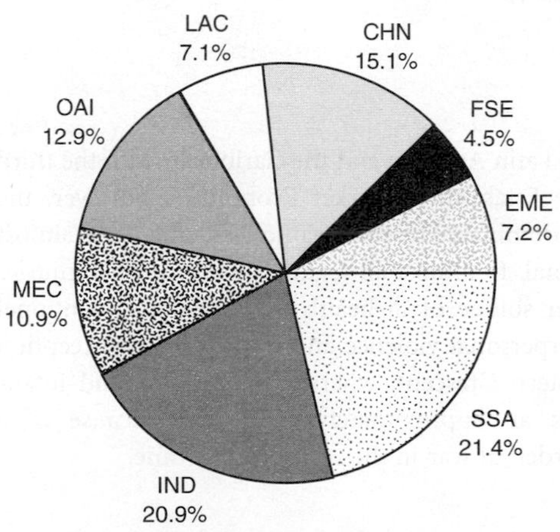

Fig. 3 Distribution of disability-adjusted life years by region, 1990.

Major causes of disease burden

While the leading causes of disease burden in 1990, namely lower respiratory infections, diarrhoeal diseases, and perinatal causes, may come as no surprise, the fact that depression was the fourth leading cause was perhaps unexpected (Table 2). Indeed, the Study showed that the burden of psychiatric conditions had been heavily underestimated. Of the 10 leading causes of disability worldwide (in years lived with disability) in 1990, five were psychiatric conditions: unipolar depression, alcohol use, bipolar affective disorder, schizophrenia, and obsessive–compulsive disorder. Unipolar depression alone was responsible for more than 1 in every 10 years of life lived with a disability worldwide. Altogether, psychiatric and neurological conditions accounted for 28 per cent of all years lived with disability, compared with 1.4 per cent of all deaths and 1.1 per cent of years of life lost. The predominance of these conditions is by no means restricted to the rich countries, although their burden is highest there. They were the most important contributors to years lived with disability in all regions except sub-Saharan Africa, where they still accounted for 16 per cent of the total.

Alcohol use was the leading cause of male disability, and the tenth largest in women, in developed regions. More surprisingly, perhaps, it was also the fourth largest cause in men in developing regions. The remaining important causes of years lived with disability were

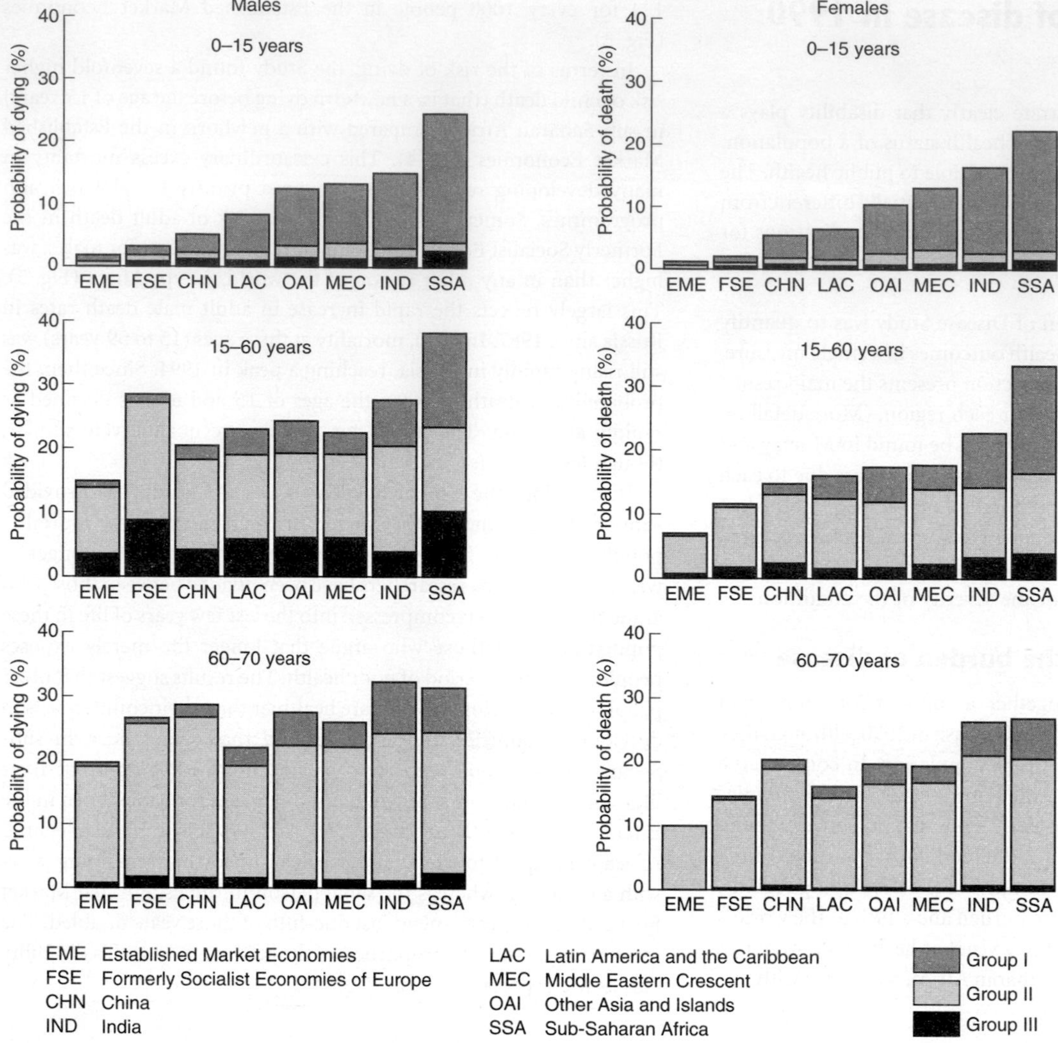

Fig. 4 regional probabilities of death for males and females by age and group, 1990.

anaemia, falls, road traffic accidents, chronic obstructive pulmonary disease, and osteoarthritis.

The traditional causes of disease burden in developing societies—communicable diseases, maternal and perinatal conditions, and nutritional deficiencies—remain of major concern in the 1990s. Even though these group I conditions accounted for only 7 per cent of the burden in the Established Market Economies and less than 9 per cent in the Former Socialist Economies, they nevertheless made up more than 40 per cent of the total global burden of disease in 1990, and almost half the burden (49 per cent) in developing regions. In sub-Saharan Africa, 2 out of every 3 years of healthy life lost were due to group I conditions. Even in China, where the epidemiological transition is far advanced, a quarter of years of healthy life lost were due to this group. Worldwide, five out of 10 leading causes of disease burden (as measured by disability-adjusted life years) are group I conditions: lower respiratory infections (pneumonia), diarrhoeal disease, perinatal conditions, tuberculosis, and measles.

The burden of injury in 1990 was highest in the Formerly Socialist Economies of Europe, where almost 19 per cent of all burden was attributed to this group of causes. China had the second largest injury burden, followed by Latin America and the Caribbean with the third largest. Even in the Established Market Economies, however, the burden of injuries—dominated by road traffic accidents—was almost 12 per cent of the total. In almost all regions, unintentional injuries were a much greater source of ill health in 1990 than intentional injuries such as interpersonal violence and war. The only exception was the Middle-Eastern Crescent, where unintentional and intentional injuries took an approximately equal toll because of a particularly high burden of war in the region at the time.

Sex differences in disease burden

Although girls and boys suffer from broadly similar health problems in infancy and early childhood, striking sex differences emerge in adults. Firstly, and most obviously, women suffer disproportionately from their reproductive role. Although the burden of reproductive ill health is almost entirely confined to the developing regions, it is so great that, even worldwide, maternal conditions make up three out of the ten leading causes of disease burden in women aged 15 to 44. In developing regions, five out of the ten leading causes of disability-

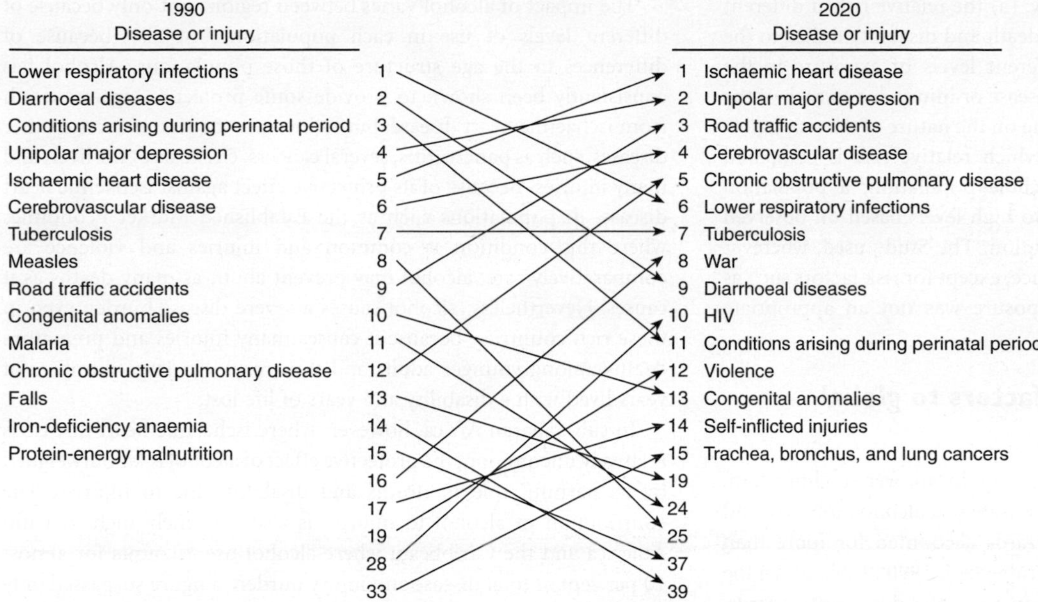

Fig. 5 Change in the rank order of disease burden for 15 leading causes worldwide, 1990 to 2000.

adjusted life years are related to reproductive ill health, including the consequences of unsafe abortion and *Chlamydia* infection. However, the Study revealed that poor reproductive health is not the only concern for women. In both developing and developed regions, depression is women's leading cause of disease burden. In developing regions, suicide is the fourth. Thus, while programmes to reduce the burden of poor reproductive health among women must remain a high priority in the future, their psychological health deserves greater attention as well. For men aged 15 to 44, road traffic accidents are the greatest cause of ill health and premature deaths worldwide, and the second greatest in developing regions, surpassed only by depression. Alcohol use, violence, tuberculosis, war, bipolar affective disorder, suicide, schizophrenia, and iron-deficiency anaemia make up the remainder of the list in developing countries. Until only recently, road traffic accidents in developing regions have received relatively little attention from public health specialists.

Table 2 Ten leading causes of disability-adjusted life years (DALY) worldwide for both sexes, 1990

	Disease or injury	DALYs (millions)	Cumulative (%)
1	LRI	112.9	8.2
2	Diarrhoeal diseases	99.6	15.4
3	Perinatal conditions	92.3	22.1
4	Depression	50.8	25.8
5	IHD	46.7	29.2
6	Stroke	38.5	32.0
7	Tuberculosis	38.4	34.8
8	Measles	36.5	37.4
9	Road traffic accidents	34.3	39.9
10	Congenital anomalies	32.9	42.3
	All causes	1379.2	

IHD, ischaemic heart disease; LRI, lower respiratory infections.

The global burden of disease in 1990: assessment of risk factors

Exposure to particular hazards, such as tobacco, alcohol, unsafe sex, or poor sanitation, can significantly increase individual risk of developing disease. These hazards, or risk factors, are significant contributors to the total global disease burden and health policy-makers need accurate information on their impact in order to devise effective prevention strategies. Until recently, however, there have been few attempts to measure the burdens of these risk factors, or to express them in a currency that can be compared directly with the burdens of individual diseases. The Global Burden of Disease Study assessed, for the first time, the mortality and loss of healthy life that can be attributed to each of 10 major risk factors in each region. These risk factors are malnutrition, poor water supply, sanitation, and personal/domestic hygiene, unsafe sex, tobacco use, alcohol use, occupation, hypertension, physical inactivity, illicit drug use, and air pollution.

Assessing risk factor burden

The burden of disease or injury in a population that can be attributed to past exposure to a given risk factor is, essentially, an estimate of the burden that could have been averted in the population if that particular risk factor had been eliminated. More precisely, this is defined as the difference between the currently observed burden and the burden that would be observed if past levels of exposure had been equal to a specified reference distribution of exposure. In general, to calculate this, it is necessary to know: (a) the relative risk at different levels of exposure for each cause of death and disability linked to the factor; (b) the distribution of different levels of exposure in the population; and (c) the burden of disease or injury due to each of the causes linked to the factor. Depending on the nature of the risk factor, the reference distribution against which relative risk is compared could be zero exposure for the whole population, a population distribution of exposure from low to high levels based on observed populations, or an arbitrary distribution. The Study used, wherever possible, zero exposure as the reference, except for risk factors such as hypertension, where clearly no exposure was not an appropriate reference standard.

The contributions of risk factors to global burden

Of the 10 risk factors studied, the most significant were malnutrition, poor water, sanitation, and hygiene, unsafe sex, alcohol, tobacco, and occupation. Together, these six hazards accounted for more than one-third of total disease burden worldwide in 1990 (Table 3). Of the six, malnutrition and poor sanitation were the dominant hazards, responsible for almost a quarter of the global burden between them. Unsafe sex and alcohol each contributed approximately 3.5 per cent of the total disease burden, closely followed by tobacco and occupation hazards with just under 3 per cent each. These are comparable to the disease burden due to tuberculosis or measles. As might be expected, major inequalities exist between regions and between men and women in the burdens of most risk factors. For example, the ill health consequences of unsafe sex—which include both infections and the complications of unwanted pregnancy—are borne disproportionately by women in all regions. In young adult women in sub-Saharan Africa, unsafe sex accounts for almost one-third of the total disease burden. Tobacco and alcohol, owing to longer exposures, caused their heaviest burdens in men in the developed regions, where the two together accounted for more than one-fifth of the total burden in 1990. In Asia and other developing regions, the rapid increase in tobacco use over the past few decades is expected to kill many more people in the coming decades than have so far died in the developed regions.

The impact of alcohol varies between regions not only because of different levels of use in each population, but also because of differences in the age structure of those populations. Alcohol has consistently been shown to provide some protection against death from ischaemic heart disease, but to increase the risk of several other diseases, such as pancreatitis, several cancers, cirrhosis of the liver, and many injuries. Because of its protective effect against ischaemic heart disease, in populations such as the Established Market Economies where this condition is common and injuries and violence are comparatively rare, alcohol may prevent about as many deaths as it causes. Nevertheless, alcohol causes a severe disease burden even in these rich countries, because it causes many injuries and premature deaths among younger adults and thus results in large numbers of years lived with a disability and years of life lost.

In sub-Saharan Africa, however, where ischaemic heart disease is relatively uncommon, the protective effect of alcohol is far outweighed by its harmful role in deaths and disability due to injuries. The contribution of alcohol to injuries is also extremely high in Latin America and the Caribbean, where alcohol use accounts for almost 10 per cent of total disease and injury burden, a figure surpassed only in the developed regions. Ultimately, alcohol is estimated to have caused about three-quarters of a million more deaths in 1990 than it averted, with more than four-fifths of the excess deaths in the developing regions.

Diseases as risk factors for other diseases

In addition to estimating disease and injury burden from risk factors such as tobacco and alcohol, it is important to recognize that several diseases may be factors for other diseases. The full impact of these conditions needs to be evaluated if public health priorities are to be appropriately guided. For example, diabetes mellitus strongly increases an individual's risk of developing ischaemic heart disease and stroke, while infection with hepatitis B virus increases the risk of developing liver cancer and cirrhosis of the liver. Traditional methods of assessing deaths by the single underlying cause fail to capture these relationships. In the Global Burden of Disease Study, a short list of well-studied conditions were evaluated as risk factors. We estimated

Table 3 Contribution of 10 risk factors to the global burden of disease and injury in 1990

Risk factor	Deaths (thousands)	As % of total deaths	DALYs (thousands)	As % of total DALYs
Malnutrition	5881	11.7	219 575	15.9
Poor water supply, sanitation, and personal and domestic hygiene	2668	5.3	93 392	6.8
Unsafe sex	1095	2.2	48 702	3.5
Tobacco	3038	6.0	36 182	2.6
Alcohol	774	1.5	47 687	3.5
Occupation	1129	2.2	37 887	2.7
Hypertension	2918	5.8	19 076	1.4
Physical inactivity	1991	3.9	13 653	1.0
Illicit drugs	100	0.2	8467	0.6
Air pollution	568	1.1	7254	0.5

DALY, disability-adjusted life year.

Table 4 Estimated impact of selected conditions viewed as risk factors, 1990

Disease	Deaths			DALYs		
	Direct attributable burden (both sexes)	Total attributable burden (both sexes)	Direct/ total	Direct attributable burden (both sexes)	Total attributable burden (both sexes)	Direct/total
Chagas' disease	19.2	49.2	0.39	0.6	1.6	0.40
Hepatitis B, C	106.4	818.7	0.13	2.1	13.3	0.16
Tuberculosis	1959.6	1959.6	1.00	38.2	39.8	0.96
Diabetes	579.4	2758.9	0.21	11.0	26.3	0.42
Cataracts	11.0	1104.4	0.01	7.5	17.9	0.42
Glaucoma	6.6	330.5	0.02	2.6	5.8	0.44
Onchocerciasis	0.0	18.6	0.00	0.9	1.2	0.76
Trachoma	0.0	103.1	0.00	1.0	2.0	0.51
Unipolar major depression	0.0	786.5	0.00	51.0	69.8	0.73
Sexually transmitted diseases	231.4	413.3	0.56	18.7	25.3	0.74

DALY, disability-adjusted life year.

how much of the total disease burden would be averted in each region's population if the condition were eliminated. The most dramatic differences between directly coded and total burden are for diabetes, hepatitis B, and hepatitis C (Table 4).

The global burden of disease projections from 1990

To plan health services effectively, policy-makers need to know how health needs might change in the future. To meet this need, the authors have developed projections of mortality and disability for each 5-year period from 1990 to 2020, by cause, for all regions and both sexes. The findings have considerable implications for public policy.

Projection methods

Rather than attempt to model the effects of the many separate direct, or proximal, determinants of disease from the limited data that are available, it was decided to model mortality change as a function of a limited number of socio-economic variables: (a) income per capita, (b) the average number of years of schooling in adults, termed 'human capital', and (c) time, a proxy measure for the secular improvement in health in the twentieth century that partly resulted from accumulating knowledge and technological development. These socio-economic variables show clear historical relationships with mortality rates; for example, income growth is closely related to the improvement in life expectancy that many countries achieved in the twentieth century. Because of their relationships with death rates, these socio-economic variables may be regarded as indirect, or distal, determinants of health. In addition, a fourth variable, tobacco use, was included because of its overwhelming impact on health, using information from more than four decades of research on the time lag between persistent tobacco use—measured in terms of 'smoking intensity'—and its effects on health (Peto *et al.* 1992).

Death rates for all major causes based on historical data for 47 countries covering the period 1950 to 1991 were related to these four variables to generate the projections. A separate model was used for HIV and modifications for the interaction between HIV and tuberculosis. Three projection scenarios were developed using different projections of the independent variables.

Mortality projections

In all regions, life expectancy at birth is expected to increase for women. By 2020, infant girls born in the Established Market Economies may expect to survive to almost 88 years. For men, life expectancy will grow much more slowly, mainly because of the impact of the tobacco epidemic. Nevertheless by 2020, males born in sub-Saharan Africa, whose life expectancy at birth was below 50 in 1990, may expect to reach 58 years. (This projection, made before the massive effects of the HIV/AIDS epidemic were known, has since been revised downwards.) Males born in Latin America and the Caribbean, who in 1990 could have expected to live to 65, may expect to reach 71 years. However, for men in the Formerly Socialist Economies of Europe, life expectancy is not expected to increase at all between 1990 and 2020. This is partly due to the fact that life expectancy was falling in 1990, so that any positive change is likely to be merely recovering to the 1990 position.

In young children and adolescents under the age of 15 years, the risk of death is projected to decline dramatically in all regions, falling by about two-thirds in sub-Saharan Africa and India. In adult women, too, the risk of death is expected to fall in all regions. Men in the Formerly Socialist Economies of Europe and China, because of the tobacco epidemic, may expect a higher risk of dying between the ages of 15 and 60 than they do today. In other regions, the risk of death for men in this age group is expected to fall, but more modestly than in women. Remarkably, by 2020, men of this age group in the Formerly Socialist Economies of Europe could face a higher risk of death even than men in sub-Saharan Africa.

Deaths from communicable, maternal, and perinatal conditions and nutritional deficiencies (group I) are expected to fall from 17.3 million in 1990 to 10.3 million in 2020. As a percentage of the total burden, group I conditions are expected to drop by more than half, from 34 to 15 per cent. This projected reduction overall, despite increased burdens due to HIV and tuberculosis, runs counter to the now widely accepted belief that infectious diseases are making a comeback worldwide. It partly reflects the relative contraction of the world's 'young' population; the age group under the age of 15 years is expected to grow by only 22 per cent between 1990 and 2020, whereas the cohort of adults aged between 15 and 60 is expected to grow by more than 55 per cent. In addition, the projection reflects the observed overall decline in group I conditions over the past four decades owing to increased income, education, and technological progress in the development of antimicrobials and vaccines. Even under the pessimistic scenario, in which both income growth and technological progress are expected to be minimal, deaths from these conditions are still expected to fall slightly to 16.9 million.

Clearly, it should not be taken for granted that the progress of the past four decades against infectious diseases will be maintained. It is possible, for example, that antibiotic development and other control technologies will not keep pace with the emergence of drug-resistant strains of important microbes such as *Mycobacterium tuberculosis*. If such a scenario were to prove correct, and if, in addition, case-fatality rates were to rise because of such drug-resistant strains, the gains of the present century could be halted or even reversed. The evidence to date nonetheless suggests that, as long as current efforts are maintained, group I causes are likely to continue to decline.

While group I conditions are expected to decline overall, deaths from non-communicable diseases are expected to climb from 28.1 million deaths in 1990 to 49.7 million in 2020, an increase of 77 per cent in absolute numbers. In proportionate terms, group II deaths are expected to increase their share of the total from 55 per cent in 1990 to 73 per cent in 2020. These global figures do not reveal the extreme nature of the change that is projected in some developing regions because they incorporate the projections for the rich nations, which show little change. In India, deaths from non-communicable diseases are projected to almost double, from about 4 million to about 8 million a year, while group I deaths are expected to fall from almost 5 million to below 3 million a year. In the developing world as a whole, deaths from non-communicable diseases are expected to rise from 47 per cent of the burden to almost 70 per cent.

The steep projected increase in the burden of non-communicable diseases worldwide is largely driven by population ageing, augmented by the large numbers of people in developing regions who are now exposed to tobacco. It is important to note that ageing will result in a rise in the absolute numbers of cases of non-communicable diseases and in their increased share of the total disease burden for the population as a whole, but not in any change to the rates of those diseases in any given age group. As studies in the Established Market Economies show, the age-specific rates of some important non-communicable diseases, such as ischaemic heart disease and stroke, have been falling steadily for at least two decades. Whether these rates are also falling in other regions is much less clear. However, any age-specific decrease in the rates of these diseases that may also emerge in low-income countries is likely to be outweighed by the large and demographically driven increase in the absolute numbers of adults at risk for these diseases, augmented by the tobacco epidemic. As with non-communicable diseases, deaths from injury are also expected to rise for mainly demographic reasons. Young adults are generally exposed to greater risks of injury.

Leading causes of disease burden in 2020: projections

When disability is taken into account as well as death, a different view of the future emerges—and one that emphasizes adult health problems still further. By 2020, the disease burden due to communicable diseases, maternal and perinatal conditions, and nutritional deficiencies is expected to fall to a fifth of the total. The burden attributable to non-communicable diseases, accordingly, is expected to rise sharply, and the burden from injuries is also expected to rise to equal that of group I conditions.

In 1990, the three leading causes of disease burden were, in descending order, pneumonia, diarrhoeal diseases, and perinatal conditions. The three conditions projected to take their place by 2020 are ischaemic heart disease, depression, and road traffic accidents. Pneumonia is expected to fall to sixth place, diarrhoeal diseases to ninth, and perinatal conditions to eleventh. Notably, measles, currently in eighth place, is expected to drop to twenty-fifth. However, not all infectious diseases are expected to decline, despite the projected overall decline of group I conditions. Tuberculosis is expected to remain at its current level of seventh place, a substantial source of disease burden for the foreseeable future. Of equally great concern is the finding that HIV, currently twenty-eighth in the ranking, will be in the top 10 by 2020 (Fig. 6).

As with the 1990 assessments, neuropsychiatric conditions emerge as a highly significant component of global disease burden when disability, as well as death, is taken into account. The projections show that psychiatric and neurological conditions could increase their share of the total global burden by almost half, from 10.5 per cent of the total burden to almost 15 per cent in 2020. This is a larger proportionate increase than that for cardiovascular diseases.

By 2020, the burden of disease attributable to tobacco is expected to outweigh that caused by any single disease. From its 1990 level of 2.6 per cent of all disease burden worldwide, tobacco is expected to increase its share to just under 9 per cent of the total burden in 2020, compared with just under 6 per cent for ischaemic heart disease (part of which is due to tobacco), the leading projected disease. This is a global health emergency that many governments have yet to confront.

The burdens of several important types of injury are also likely to increase because of the growth of the adult fraction of the population. For example, young men are the group most frequently involved in road traffic accidents, so if the proportion of young adults in the population increases sharply, road traffic accidents are likely to increase too. Indeed, according to the baseline projection, road traffic accidents could rise to third place from ninth worldwide. Violence, currently nineteenth, could rise as high as twelfth place and suicide could climb from seventeenth to fourteenth place.

Not surprisingly, these changes are not expected to be evenly dispersed worldwide. The total number of lost years of healthy life in the Established Market Economies is likely to fall slightly, while it will increase slightly in the Formerly Socialist Economies of Europe. Strikingly, however, sub-Saharan Africa's future looks disturbingly poor despite the decline in the burden of group I conditions that currently dominate its health needs. Overall, the region faces an increase in the number of lost years of healthy life between 1990 and 2020, due mainly to a steep projected rise in the burden of injuries from road accidents, war, and violence.

Recent health trends in the 1990s: implications for the Global Burden of Disease Study projections

The original Global Burden of Disease Study projections were based on data and information about health conditions worldwide in the late 1980s/early 1990s. At that time, two major epidemics were affecting the health of large population groups: the HIV epidemic, particularly in Africa, which killed an estimated 300 000 people worldwide in 1990 but had, by that time, infected millions more, and the explosive increase in adult mortality rates in Russia and neighbouring countries, particularly from cardiovascular diseases and injuries, and particularly among men. Making projections in the context of such dramatic epidemiological trends is extremely hazardous, as recent trends have confirmed.

The 1990 Global Burden of Disease Study's HIV/AIDS projections have severely underestimated the spread of the epidemic in sub-Saharan Africa, particularly southern Africa. By 1999, HIV/AIDS was estimated to have killed 2.2 million Africans, several times more than projected on the basis of what was known in 1990. Whether the disease burden will continue to rise, and how far, is uncertain and new projection methods are being developed to forecast the epidemic better, particularly in Africa.

The other large uncertainty in the projections, namely adult mortality in the Formerly Socialist Economies of Europe, has confounded epidemiologists with the dramatic change in mortality risks during the 1990s. Death rates are now falling markedly in most large countries in this region, and, if they continue to do so, the 1990 forecasts will prove to be unduly pessimistic. It is too early to decide whether or not the recent declines in mortality are the beginning of a long-term secular trend in mortality.

Progress in refining the Global Burden of Disease Study approach

Measuring and valuing health

One of the major innovations of the Global Burden of Disease Study was the attempt to measure and value states of health worse than perfect health in a comparable fashion across various societies. This presupposes a common conceptual framework and measurement strategy. In particular, the key domains of health that need to be assessed and the minimum number of items and response categories needed to measure them need to be decided. Self-report instruments currently in use lack cross-cultural comparability, with the result that the measurement of health in various populations is largely not comparable. The development and operation of a conceptual framework to measure and describe health in a way that improves comparability across populations is a key challenge for burden of disease research (Murray and Lopez 2000).

The issue of comorbidity is another measurement problem to emerge from the original Global Burden of Disease Study where further methodological work is required. In the Study, comorbid conditions were valued separately and time spent with these combined states was valued as the sum of the individual state valuations. This additive model is clearly problematic. More data are required on the prevalence of major comorbidities in order to avoid multiple attribution in health state valuations.

The process of valuing health states worse than perfect health entails a number of methodological choices ranging from which measurement methods to use to the choice of respondents. In particular, the empirical assessment of health state valuations from large population surveys in different countries would greatly increase the representativeness of disability weights applied in the assessment of the global burden of disease. Research on measuring health state valuations in more than a dozen countries in all regions has begun at the World Health Organization (**WHO**) and such population-based valuations are being collected for use in future iterations of the Global Burden of Disease Study.

Comparative risk assessment

The Global Burden of Disease assessment of the magnitude of risk factors illustrated the power of comparing risk factor burden with the burden of specific diseases and injuries. Such comparisons are an effective means of drawing the attention of decision-makers to the magnitude of health problems caused by various distal socio-economic, proximal, or physiological variables. In future efforts at comparative risk factor assessment, the number of variables examined will be expanded to include distal determinants. One clear method of improving future revisions of the Global Burden of Disease Study is to standardize the methods for risk factor assessment.

In order to standardize terminology and permit comparable assessments of disease burden due to various exposures, Murray and Lopez (1999) have proposed a series of criteria for future risk factor assessments. A key distinction is made between attributable burden (from past exposures) and avoidable burden (due to future exposures).

In addition, given the very different traditions in risk factor epidemiology, depending on the specific risk factor under study, recent efforts have focused on standardizing the approach to defining and measuring population distributions of exposure. In future, estimates of disease and injury burden will be assessed by comparing current exposure (and hazards) to a 'counterfactual' distribution of exposure strictly defined in the same fashion for all exposures being assessed. One obvious counterfactual is the population distribution of exposure which results in the theoretical minimum risk for the entire population. For most risk factors (for example, tobacco use, illicit drugs) this minimum risk counterfactual will be 100 per cent of the population having zero exposure, but for others (for example, cholesterol, hypertension), the theoretical minimum is not so obvious and may be derived from different perspectives (for example, lowest empirical observation, animal studies).

Other counterfactuals, defined in exactly the same way for all risk factors, could also be developed, such as reducing the population distribution of exposure to a level which is 'feasible' or even 'plausible' given current knowledge. Whatever distribution is chosen to assess risk factor burden, it is critical that the same definition is applied across all risk factors to improve comparability.

Most standardized approaches are also developed to ensure that relative risk estimates control, as far as possible, for obvious confounding, and where this has not been rigorously applied in the epidemiological literature, adjustment methods have been proposed similar to those used by Peto *et al.* (1992) for tobacco. The standardization framework being applied for risk factor burden also includes common guidelines for judging causality and for extrapolating relative risks from one population to another, and from younger to older ages.

Efforts to compile age–sex regional distributions of exposure and age–sex-specific relative risk are being led by the Burden of Disease Team and WHO. First results of this revised global Comparative Risk Factor Assessment project are expected in 2001.

Conclusion

The Global Burden of Disease Study has provided a new and much needed strategy to estimate current and projected health needs. In particular, it has shown that non-communicable diseases are rapidly becoming the dominant causes of ill health in all developing regions except sub-Saharan Africa, it has revealed the extent to which mental health problems have been underestimated worldwide, and it has shown the significance of injuries as a problem for the health sector in all regions. The findings pose new and immediate challenges to policy-makers and are certain to provoke debate. Ultimately, the Study's impact will be judged in two ways: firstly, by the degree to which it stimulates other researchers to apply the same rigorous methods of measuring disease burden in all regions; secondly, to the extent that it changes priorities for public health in the decades ahead.

References

Barendregt, J.J., Bonneux, L., and van der Maas, P.J. (1998). Health expectancy: from a population health indicator to a tool for policy making. *Journal of Aging and Health*, **10**, 242–58.

Murray, C.J.L. and Lopez, A.D. (ed.) (1996*a*). *The Global Burden of Disease: a comprehensive assessment of mortality and disability from diseases, injuries, and risk factors in 1990 and projected to 2030.* Global Burden of Disease and Injury Series, Vol. 1. Harvard University Press, Cambridge, MA.

Murray, C.J.L. and Lopez, A.D. (1996*b*). *Global health statistics: a compendium of incidence, prevalence and mortality estimates for over 200 conditions.* Global Burden of Disease and Injury Series, Vol. 2. Harvard University Press, Cambridge, MA.

Murray, C.J. and Lopez, A.D. (1999). On the comparable quantification of health risks: lessons from the Global Burden of Disease Study. *Epidemiology*, **10**, 594–605.

Murray, C.J. and Lopez, A.D. (2000). Progress and directions in refining the global burden of disease approach: a response to Williams. *Health Economics*, **9**, 69–82.

Murray, C.J.L., Salomon, J.A., and Mathers, C. (1999). *A critical examination of summary measures of population health.* GPE Working Paper Series. WHO, Geneva.

Peto, R., Lopez, A.D., Boreham, J., Thun, M., and Heath, C., Jr (1992). Mortality from tobacco in developed countries: indirect estimation from national vital statistics. *Lancet*, **339**, 1268–78.

Sullivan, D.F. (1971). A single index of mortality and morbidity. *HSMHA, Health Reports*, **86**, 347–54.

Van de Water, H.P., Perenboom, R.J., and Boshuizen, H.C. (1996). Policy relevance of the health expectancy indicator: an inventory of European Union countries. *Health Policy*, **36**, 117–29.

WHO (World Health Organization) (1992). *International statistical classification of diseases and related health problems (10th revision)*, Vol. 1. WHO, Geneva.

Wilkins, R. and Adams, O. (1983). Health expectancy in Canada, late 1970s: demographic, regional and social dimensions. *American Journal of Public Health*, **73**, 1073–80.

3

Public health policies

3.1 Overview of policies and strategies

Walter W. Holland

The prime aim of health policies worldwide has been the maintenance and improvement of the health status of populations. This implies an understanding of human health and disease in order to determine the major biological, political, social, environmental, and lifestyle factors influencing health status and the burden of disease. The risk factors which influence health differ between countries, and the examples in this book illustrate their investigation, influence on health, and methods of control. Thus policies for health will be influenced by different factors in each country and region. Although it may appear that the problems addressed in this chapter are mainly concerned with developed countries, it is important to emphasize that the issues are the same in all countries at all stages of development. Public health problems in the developing world may appear different and greater, but the principles and methods for solution are the same.

Health status

The health of most of the populations of the developed world has never been better. Powles (1992) has dealt comprehensively with the changes in disease pattern and related social trends. He has shown changes in disease patterns that have occurred and are occurring in different parts of the world and has attempted to relate these to changes in social and other environmental factors. Both this study and others have shown a great increase in non-communicable diseases in the developing world together with the abatement of the mortality from infectious diseases. At the same time, in the developed world, we have seen a diminution in the frequency of infectious diseases and a great extension of the length of life with consequent increase in the diseases that are associated with old age, cancer, stroke, heart disease, arthritis, and others. These have serious implications in terms of the measures employed for the prevention of disease and improvement in the quality of life.

There is a major argument as to whether the extension of life is merely associated with an extension of time of disability or whether it is an extension of good quality of life. That argument still rages (Fries 1980; Davies 1985) and a definitive answer is not available although it is suggested that major disability, at least, has not increased with increasing longevity (Fries 1998).

Of more worrying concern have been the changes in disease pattern and recurrence of conditions, virtually unknown in recent times in the developed world, in Eastern Europe. An example is the enormous increase in the incidence of diphtheria in Russia (Public Health Laboratory Service 1994).

With the reduction of common infectious diseases in the developed world new hazards have arisen, for example HIV and AIDS.

In all countries there has been an extension of life, but this has been particularly evident in developed areas. This has important implications for health policies; the problems are mainly concerned with the elderly, rather than children. In the elderly quality of life is more important than extension of life; thus policies will be concerned with such matters as mobility, social contacts, and relief of pain, rather than with acute treatments.

Health services

As the health of most of the populations of the developed world has improved, complaints and concerns with the health services have risen. All health systems face the challenges of demographic change (ageing of the population), increasing population mobility, growing social exclusion, costly new therapeutic techniques, and rising public demands and expectations. While all these place mounting pressure on service provision at a time that public spending is under tight constraints, there are new opportunities for prevention and treatment, there is growing interest in prevention and health promotion, and the quality, as well as quantity, of life is generally improving.

The public has widely different views on the quality of health services, ranging from 95 per cent considering that health services are good in France to only 25 per cent in Greece (Ferrara 1993). All countries face similar problems as follows:

(1) inequalities in both health status and health service provision between different geographic areas and social groups;

(2) variations in the utilization of services for similar conditions (for example hysterectomy);

(3) difficulties in the apportionment of limited resources to different strategies (for example prevention versus cure, or cure versus care) or between services (for example cardiac services versus renal services);

(4) many of the problems are related to lifestyle behaviour and political/economic issues (for example cigarette smoking).

These issues have recently been described in detail for the countries of the European Union (Abel-Smith *et al.* 1995; Holland and Mossialos 1999).

The following chapters all illustrate the approaches adopted in individual countries to cope with these dilemmas. Most people accept that difficult choices need to be made. Most concentrate on the provision of health services, but health services in themselves do relatively little to bring about an improvement in the health status of populations. Environmental factors, such as housing, traffic, and employment, and behavioural factors, such as smoking, diet, and alcohol consumption, probably make greater contributions. Nonetheless, health services have an essential role in improving quality of life and can produce specific valuable improvements in other aspects of health status.

Organization and financing

The promotion of services to improve health by those working in public health and the influence that can be brought to bear on the management and administration of all services are important contributions to health service planning. Most health systems in developed countries have well-developed mechanisms for funding and provision. The problems in developing and developed countries may differ widely. In the former, health services are usually well organized in the urban areas, with deficits in the rural areas. But there are also problems in the former. In many developing countries most doctors are paid by the state, and are not well paid. However, opportunities usually exist for doctors in urban areas to supplement their income by private practice, which leads to great difficulties and disparities both between different groups of practitioners as well as between different areas in a country. There are also problems relating to the distribution of health workers caused by migration to developed countries. This may have grave implications for the supply and quality of health services. Different solutions are being developed; one suggestion is that all doctors who provide clinical services should be in private practice, and only those in public health and/or health planning should be employed by the state at a reasonable salary.

Although this problem also exists in developed countries, it does not have such an impact on the delivery of basic health services. Countries differ, however, in their ability to use these structures to initiate broad policies to maximize the population's health. All health systems operate within a framework of national law. In some countries, such as the United Kingdom, the state is clearly visible as a regulator and provider of services. In others, legislation creates an environment in which doctors, hospitals, and insurance agencies operate with less visible state intervention. The ability of health services to co-operate with other agencies varies but it is less where there is little formal control beyond legislation of the health system itself. Most countries have endorsed the World Health Organization (**WHO**) *Health for All* charter but there is great variation in implementation in national and local policies. The state is involved in all health systems in varying degrees:

(1) as legal regulator of the arrangements for patients to receive medical care and doctors to receive remuneration;

(2) as a contributor to health-care financing, either through formal taxes or through quasi-taxes such as compulsory social insurance;

(3) as a guardian to ensure that the correct balance of resources is used to achieve optimum population health.

Health care may be conceived in an economic framework as an exchange of goods. Patients seeking medical care are making demands while doctors are supplying services. However, there are ways other than medical treatment of using resources to improve population health and the priorities of medical practice emphasizing technical over social models of care do not always provide optimal health benefits. There is a role in all health-care systems for an overview of resource allocation, health policy, and population health outcomes; this is the task of health commissioning.

Health commissioning (administration)

Health commissioning needs to take into account the following factors:

(1) improvement in health status (for example targeting smokers to reduce smoking should result in fewer cases of ischaemic heart disease);

(2) risk reduction (for example, as above, reducing the number of smokers in a population);

(3) services and protection needed to achieve improvements in health and reduction of risks (for example product labelling);

(4) data needs for monitoring the achievement of the tasks identified (discussed in detail by Holland (1995)).

The prerequisites for achieving these goals need to be clear. The best model for this is that developed in The Netherlands (Ministry of Health, Welfare and Cultural Affairs 1993) which considers that health is seen as 'the possibility for every member of society to function normally and to participate in social life'. Thus the need for health care is 'to enable an individual to share, maintain and if possible improve his or her life together with other members of the community.' This implies that necessary health care is that which allows the individual to be a full participant in society. This societal perspective is a little different from the individual perspective, where health is seen as the balance between what the individual wants to do and what the individual can do, or the professional approach, where health is the absence of disease. The Dutch model is the best one to follow in the arena of public health choices. Within that framework it is necessary to consider the place of public health. For that the current British definition is helpful as discussed below.

Role of public health

> Public Health is the science and art of preventing disease, prolonging life, promoting health through the organised efforts of society. Public Health Medicine is that branch of medicine which specialises in public health. Its chief responsibilities are the surveillance of the health of the population, the identification of its health needs, the fostering of policies which promote health and the evaluation of health services. (Acheson 1988)

For the proper application of these principles it is essential to appreciate the methods to be used. Epidemiology, which is the science fundamental to the study and practice of public health, increases the understanding of the determinants of health and disease and the knowledge of their occurrence in populations and groups. Such information indicates the action that can be taken to prevent disease and promote health by health education or social policies which aim to modify behaviour, prophylactic procedures like immunization, screening for identification of those at special risk or in need of special care, and protection against specific environmental hazards. Preventive programmes also need to be monitored to determine whether they are achieving their objectives, at what cost, and how they may need to be modified.

A further function is the study of the nature and extent of disease and disability in the population and how this varies with age, sex, economic and social circumstances, occupation, and environment. Information on the patterns of disease is essential in defining health needs and tasks for health services and in setting priorities. It also allows the review of the services as they now are and the identification of those who do and do not use them so that the need for new services or the modification of the present ones can be judged. In addition, it is necessary to evaluate how effective the services are in helping the community in cure and care, in the relief of suffering, the maintenance of working capacity, rehabilitation of the disabled, and lowering of death rates. It also needs to assess how efficient the services are in using the community's resources. Both aspects are critical in assuring value for money and are an integral part of health service management and resource planning—the more so since technology is always offering expensive new options.

Thus the problems for which public health action is required include:

(1) outbreaks of disease caused by infectious or toxic agents, for example smallpox, typhoid, food poisoning, bovine spongiform encephalopathy, radiation, and so on;

(2) problems arising from social and environmental issues such as inadequate housing, unemployment, poverty, abortion, fluoridation of water, and global environmental and population issues (McMichael and Powles 1999; Raleigh 1999);

(3) behavioural concerns such as smoking, excessive consumption of alcohol, drug abuse, and insufficient exercise;

(4) health service issues including assessment of health-care needs and outcomes, and the effectiveness and efficiency of particular services.

Public health, as a discipline, should not become involved in the direct management of clinical services in the community or within institutions—it lacks the expertise essential for these tasks. Its prime responsibilities are to promote health and to prevent and control disease. It thus has responsibility for surveillance and for the planning and co-ordination of measures that promote and maintain health. It must be involved in the planning and distribution of clinical services in accordance with measures of need and demands and the assessment of effectiveness.

Assurance of appropriateness

Few countries, at present, appear to have developed an organizational framework whereby these principles and methods are systematically applied.

In considering the provision of services for health it is important to be clear about what is to be achieved. In most countries it is now accepted that everyone who needs health care must be able to obtain it. However, that is not always the rule, as is shown in the following chapters.

The form and content of the right to health care are the result of a series of political and social compromises. As the Dutch *Report on Choices in Health Care* emphasizes, responsibility for others, the ideal of equality, and the social benefits of good public health have encouraged the belief that people are responsible for their own health, and are free to choose how to use health care and which risks they are willing to take (Ministry of Welfare, Welfare and Cultural Affairs 1993). The fusion of such different starting points has always brought strain to the design of health-care systems. That these strains are limited in the determination of rights is partly due to a pragmatic coupling between equality and freedom of choice so that, in principle, everyone has equal rights to virtually all of the facilities of health care. People do not need everything they want and not all needs for health care are equally important. There is a need for health-care services to maintain or restore health, for care and nursing of impaired health, or to relieve suffering. The concept of health is therefore the most appropriate standard to determine as to when there is a need for health care.

A definition of 'health' is the ability to function normally. In this definition there will be a need for health care when people are restricted in their normal functioning or when there is a threat of such restriction. Such a need is more essential when the restriction is greater or threatens to be greater. From a community-oriented view of health this is an incomplete statement. Health has a value in itself because it allows a people to participate in social life and to develop themselves. The more health problems restrict a person's possibilities in society the more the need for health care and the more necessary the health care.

As stated above there are a variety of approaches to health. From the perspective of the individual, health is linked to self-determination or autonomy. To be healthy is to be able, as an individual, to achieve in society what one has chosen to aim for. Whether that is possible depends on one's physical, material, and psychological resources but also on what one wishes to achieve. Health can be described as a balance between what people want and what they can achieve. Thus there will be differences in how individuals express a desire for health care.

From the medical professional perspective, health is the absence of disease and is seen as a deviation from normal biological function. In this definition there is a clear distinction between health care for the sick and social services for people who are not sick, where health care must be seen as professionally given care provided on the basis of indications defined objectively by the provider.

The effectiveness of care is also defined objectively with the most important criteria being danger to life and the extent of normal biological function. Biological functions seem ultimately to be directed at survival and reproduction. From that perspective demands can be sorted according to gravity and it is possible to distinguish necessary from less necessary care.

From the community-oriented approach health is seen as the possibility of every member of the society to function normally. The choices are made at the level of society because individual health is linked to the possibility of participation in social life. Care is thus necessary when it enables an individual to share, maintain, and if possible improve his or her life together with other members of the community. Individual preferences in needs are not given priority here. The central question is which care is necessary from the point of view of the community. Of course this question is not answered in the same way by all communities. There are three points of departure: the fundamental equality of people, the fundamental need for the protection of human life, and the principle of solidarity. Thus the major aim of any such system is the improvement of health and the ability to participate within society. If one accepts this Dutch model, then it is possible to define the different types of care that need to be provided in a variety of ways.

The WHO (Europe) has recently (WHO 1999) discussed the key areas specifically for public health. These can be summarized as understanding health and disease, measuring health status, appropriate disease surveillance and control, promoting health and well being, evaluating and improving health outcomes, intersectoral and collaborative working, and advocacy and communications. These define the role of public health within a health system which includes health care and ensures that appropriate decisions are made.

Criteria, access, and utilization

The first criterion that needs to be established is whether care is necessary or not. The second criterion is the effectiveness of the services provided, the efficiency with which they are provided, and whether the individual could take responsibility for providing them.

These principles are established in some way or another in most health systems. They are thus concerned with improvement of health status, risk factor reduction, and improvement of services and protection.

In most developed countries there is now a split between provision and purchasing for health care. The relative role of those who purchase health care varies between countries. In most private insurance systems, what is insured constitutes what is bought; however, in those that have managed care, or purchasing authorities, these institutes decide what care should be purchased and where it should be obtained. It is thus feasible to introduce health-care systems that consider the improvement of health on a societal basis. The characteristic that prevents medical care becoming an ordinary market, from an economic viewpoint, is that the receivers of services are often unable to make informed choices about care. Patients make many of the key choices over health care, whether their feelings and symptoms indicate that they are ill, and whether to consult a doctor.

There are wide variations between the different methods of organization and responses of individuals to health care. Similarly, doctors do not perform uniformly. Individual doctors vary in their action when faced with similar patients and make different decisions for patients with similar conditions. In both the National Health Service and social insurance systems, doctors are gate-keepers to resources. They legitimize a patient's claim for services. Health systems seek to influence doctors' decisions broadly, for example in the level of remuneration given to a particular service.

As indicated, in all systems it is crucial that there is interaction between the different sectors of society. Health can only be improved through changes in the environment, through occupation, including agriculture as well as health services and education, and unless there is some degree of co-ordination between these activities the optimal distribution of resource will be lacking. This also has an important impact on the improvement of health which is the aim of most national health systems. Most systems have now come to terms with the fact that they cannot only treat established disease but also have to be concerned with the improvement of health and the prevention of disease.

International trends in health care

Abel-Smith *et al.* (1995) have reviewed trends in health care. They note that there is a worldwide trend towards giving every citizen in a country the same rights to health care. If President Clinton had followed through recent health proposals made in the United States, this would also have been the case in America. There has not been much of a decline in public financing of health care quantitatively, whether by compulsory insurance contribution or taxation. There is some trend towards consumers making a contribution in the forms of copayments, for example prescription charges. Some countries are following the trend set by the United Kingdom in 1978 (Department of Health and Social Security 1976) of distributing resources on a geographical per head of population basis.

Some countries are encouraging people to take out private insurance or even to contract out of the public system.

Most countries are attempting to improve efficiency and effectiveness by introducing charters for waiting times. These indicate the right to be treated within a given time and reduce travel times by locating services in individual practices or locations rather than concentrated in a few large centres; however, some specialist services (for example, cancer) are only provided in a limited number of institutions. All countries and political regions have become concerned with quality and effectiveness and a few, for example the European Union, have developed indices of outcome (Holland 1997).

Provider–purchaser model for both public health and personal health services

The separation of commissioning and providing services discussed above theoretically enables better decisions to be made over which services to provide within a limited budget. Theoretically, it should also be possible to balance preventive, curative, and rehabilitative services. For this to be effective an adequate knowledge of the epidemiology, including the natural history, of conditions is necessary. However, this is not possible for more than a small number of conditions, although a few, such as coronary heart disease, chronic obstructive lung disease, and lung cancer, may represent a large proportion of the disease burden in a particular population.

Coronary heart disease may be used as an example. The prevalence of the various stages of the disease can be ascertained in a defined population by appropriate epidemiological studies or estimated by extrapolation from studies in equivalent populations. Incidence figures for each stage of the condition are obtained in the same way. Many of the factors responsible for the development of coronary heart disease, for example smoking cigarettes, blood pressure, and poor diet, are known. Evidence of the effectiveness of various approaches to prevention, for example advice to school children not to start smoking, counselling adults who smoke to stop when they attend the doctor, banning cigarette advertising, and so on, is known (or required). Evidence of the effectiveness and procedures to be used for the treatment of the early stages of diseases such as angina is available.

It is thus possible to devise an appropriate model of the requirement for different treatment strategies like the use of aspirin, thrombolytics, and anticoagulants, and the need for efficient ambulance services, coronary care beds, and so on. Finally, knowledge is available of the appropriate rehabilitative services that are effective after a myocardial infarction.

From this complex model it is thus possible to consider the balance of resources to be devoted to, or invested in, the development of effective methods to both reduce the burden of coronary heart disease as well as to improve the outcome of those who develop the condition.

Obviously this scheme is idealistic so far, but it remains the underlying rationale for the separation of purchasing and providing health services. Managed care, now so popular in the United States, is an example of this type of separation. All these models rely on the development of knowledge of the effective methods of treatment or prevention of a condition.

The problem in all countries is that, although the effectiveness of many procedures or treatments is known, understanding of many common ailments, for example arthritis, is still poor. Thus all countries are involved in a variety of schemes to identify cost-effective methods of investigation, prevention, treatment, and rehabilitation (Holland and Mossialos 1999).

The role of public health in the determination of priorities

The role of public health is in the determination of priorities among these possibilities for improving health. Theoretically, the role of public health is clear in almost all the systems described here. It has the necessary tools to describe the problems and to devise appropriate mechanisms for their solution. In all the systems, however, the ability for public health to influence health policy is limited. Few of the countries described have effective mechanisms to influence individual health behaviours (for example the smoking of cigarettes) or to consider investment in non-health activities (for example education or employment) which are known to have more profound effects on health status than the use of medical care services (Black 1980; Acheson 1998). Nonetheless, the framework and structures currently being devised, coupled with concerns about the environment and demography, as well as increasing fiscal constraints in all systems, is forcing all countries to begin to confront these issues.

Previously, decisions on expenditure and treatment were largely controlled by those who were providing services. The treatment or service delivered to an individual or community was rarely questioned. With improvements in educational attainments and rising costs of medical procedures all societies have begun to question health expenditure. Thus decisions on priorities have become more explicit and democratic. Most countries have begun to debate how and what should be done; for example, should preventive services be provided to all the population or should heart transplants be available on demand (dependent on a sufficient supply). As a result, most countries have also begun to spend resources more effectively and to examine ethical issues involved in the setting of priorities and supply of services. All these issues are raised in the following chapters, and common threads are beginning to emerge.

Conclusion

The chapters describing the policies and strategies of various countries demonstrate the progress that has been made not only in the control of disease but also in the delivery of services. Most countries demonstrate a willingness to consider a wider perspective in the provision of health services than purely concern with treatment activities. Most have developed mechanisms for beginning to address the problem of inequalities and deprivation, with one notable exception (the United States). Most are facing the problem of increasing costs of medical care by rational deliberations and are beginning to consider alternative approaches, including an increased investment in public health research, in order to be able to introduce appropriate and effective preventive strategies.

References

Abel-Smith, B., Figueras, J., Holland, W., Mckee, M., and Mossialos, E. (1995). *Choices in health policy; an agenda for the European Union.* Dartmouth, Aldershot.

Acheson, E.D. (Chairman) (1988). *Public health in England. Report of the Committee of Inquiry into the Future Development of the Public Health Function.* HMSO, London.

Acheson, E.D. (1998). *Independent inquiry into inequalities in health.* HMSO, London.

Black, D. (1980). *Inequalities in health.* Department of Health and Social Security, London.

Davies, A.M. (1985). Epidemiology and the challenge of aging. *International Journal of Epidemiology*, **14**, 9–19.

Department of Health and Social Security (1976). *Sharing resources for health in England. Report of the Resource Allocation Working Party.* HMSO, London.

Ferrera, M. (1993). *EC citizens and social protection: main results from a Eurobarometer survey.* Commission of the European Communities, Brussels.

Fries, J.F. (1980). Aging, natural death, and the compression of morbidity. *New England Journal of Medicine*, **303**, 130–5.

Fries, J.F. (1998). Reducing cumulative lifetime disability: the compression of morbidity. *British Journal of Sports Medicine*, **32**, 193.

Holland, W.W. (1995). Achieving an ethical health service: the need for information. *Journal of the Royal College of Physicians, London*, **29**, 325–34.

Holland, W.W. (Project Director) (1997). *EC atlas of 'avoidable death'* (3rd edn), pp. 1–2, Oxford Medical Publications.

Holland, W. and Mossialos, E. (ed.) (1999). *Public health policies in the European Union.* Ashgate, Aldershot.

McMichael, A.J. and Powles, J.W. (1999). Human numbers, environment, sustainability and health. *British Medical Journal*, **ii**, 977–80.

Ministry of Health Welfare and Cultural Affairs (1993). *Report on choices in health care.* Ministry of Health Welfare and Cultural Affairs, The Hague.

Powles, J. (1992). Changes in disease patterns and related social trends. *Social Science and Medicine*, **35**, 337–87.

Public Health Laboratory Service (1994). Diphtheria in Russia and Eastern Europe. *Communicable Disease Report Weekly*, **4**, 47.

Raleigh, V.S. (1999). World population and health in transition. *British Medical Journal*, **2**, 981–4.

WHO (World Health Organization) (1999). *The changing role of public health in the European region.* EUR/RC 49/10 and EUR/RC 49/Conf. Doc./6 Appendix 1. WHO, Geneva.

3.2 Public health policy in developed countries*

John Powles

Politics is a strong and slow boring of hard boards. It takes both passion and perspective. (Weber 1921)

Introduction

The scope and purpose of public health policy is implicit in widely used definitions of public health. The Acheson Report in England defined it (following Winslow) as:

> The science and art of preventing disease, prolonging life and promoting health through organised efforts of society. (Secretary of State for Social Services 1988)

Public health policies are thus the policies that guide these 'organised efforts' to protect and improve health—and the real interest in policy is the prospect that it might make a difference to the public's health. Although policy is mainly the province of governments (national, regional, and local), civic organizations such as professional bodies and major health charities along with supranational bodies, such as the World Health Organization (**WHO**) and the World Bank, are also involved. This chapter is limited to 'developed countries', excluding countries in transition from socialism. These can be regarded as equivalent to the 'high-income' category used by the World Bank: the countries of Western Europe, Canada, the United States, Australia, New Zealand, Israel, Singapore, and Japan (excluding Taiwan and various small states for which data are less readily available).

Assessing the effects of policy

It is paradoxical that the greatest interest in public health policy now exists in developed countries where the benefits of public health activity may seem least apparent. In other times and places, the value of this endeavour could seem clear. Thus in 1890 John Simon could look back on half a century of sanitary reform in England and confidently attribute declining mortality from infectious causes to the organized efforts to clean up the cities and towns (Simon 1890). Or, if one were to take 'lower-middle' income countries in today's world, three- to fourfold differences in child mortality rates are associated with substantial differences in the coverage achieved by public health programmes. Countries that are 'good performers' in reducing child mortality (such as El Salvador, Jordan, and Sri Lanka) have higher immunization coverage and larger proportions with safe water supplies—suggesting that public health programmes are making important contributions to declines in child mortality (McMichael and Powles 1999).

Analogous attempts to demonstrate the value of public health endeavour in lowering mortality levels in developed countries soon run into difficulties. In examining changes in life expectancy over the last two decades, there is some, unsurprising, evidence of 'catch-up' with countries starting at lower levels tending to show greater gains (Fig. 1). Outliers, relative to the trend, are as 'good performers' Japan, France, Singapore, Canada, and Australia, and as 'poor performers' Denmark, Norway, the United States, The Netherlands, and Portugal. It is not at all plausible that these 'poor performers' have lagged behind and lost rank just because they underinvested in public health endeavours. (Life expectancy at birth in these countries is not significantly related to income per person.)

There are three major impediments to relating overall mortality levels in rich countries to their public health endeavours. Firstly, there are no readily available measures of the 'independent variable'—the amount of 'organised effort' to prevent disease and injury that has actually been taking place. Secondly, variation in adult mortality levels is strongly influenced by the timing and magnitude of two major overlapping epidemics: (a) diseases caused by tobacco smoking, and (b) vascular diseases. Both of these have proved relatively insensitive, in the short term, to the effects of identifiable public health endeavours. Thirdly, variations in mortality levels in middle to late life represent the lagged effects of changes in disease determinants over preceding decades and these temporal relationships are not easy to specify or quantify. Illumination is thus unlikely to come from analyses employing short time frames and highly aggregated disease groupings. A sharper focus is needed on different types of policy responses to different types of public health problems, if useful lessons are to be drawn. A fourfold classification for this heuristic purpose is set out in Table 1. Note that this is a classification for operational programmes directed towards major components of the avoidable burden of disease. It does not adequately cover important maintenance functions, nor the 'infrastructure' needed to support operational programmes. Nor does it address social inequalities in health. (This last topic will be touched on later.) Furthermore, the examples will not be discussed comprehensively but rather used to illustrate points that may be of wider significance in understanding the relation of public health policies to health levels in developed countries.

* The author is grateful to Nick Day for the examples relating to HIV transmission and the decline in sudden infant death syndrome, and to Daniela de Angelis for the model data on HIV in England.

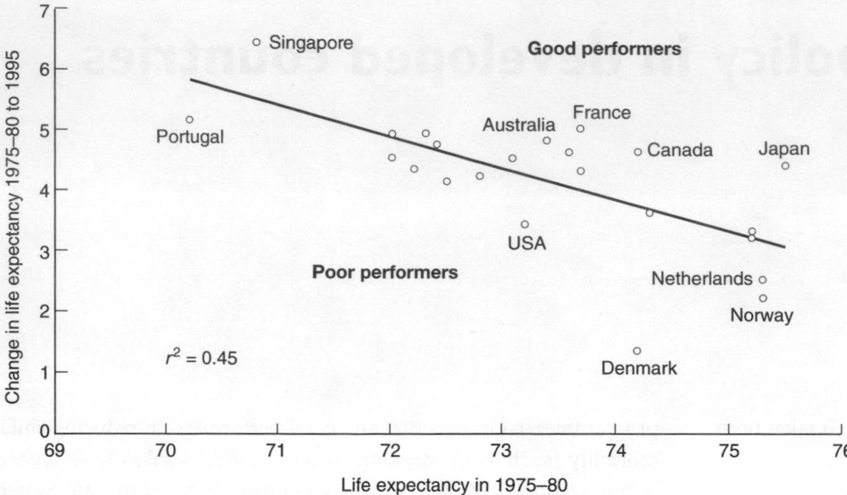

Fig. 1 Change in life expectancy at birth for both sexes combined between 1975/1980 and 1995 by starting level, high-income countries. (Data from World Resources Institute 1998.)

Table 1 Classification of public health problems by the predominant type of response needed

	Administrative measures applied to whole populations	Technical procedures applied to individuals	Large-scale change in behaviour	Unsolved
Nature	Problems amenable to specific measures administered by public agencies and requiring little public involvement for their effect	Problems where 'organised efforts' are used to enhance population coverage by clinical procedures of defined efficacy and feasibility	Problems whose solution requires large-scale behavioural change, typically requiring supporting institutional changes	Problems without clearly defined solutions within current social and economic arrangements
Examples[a]	*Fluoridation of water supplies*	Immunization	*HIV infection*	*Disease attributable to declining physical activity and obesity*
	Regulation of the sale and use of hazardous chemicals	*Programmes to enhance the detection and control of high blood pressure*	*Road traffic injuries*	Asthma and allergic diseases
	Regulation of occupational hazards; making roads safer	Cancer screening	*Disease attributable to smoking*	*Effects (still uncertain) of large-scale ecological disruption*
			Disease attributable to dietary composition	

[a]Examples in *italics* are discussed further in the text.

Examples of policies to improve health

Administrative means: fluoridation

Fluoridation of water supplies provides a classic illustration of public health improvement by administrative means; its limited implementation may yield lessons in public health politics and economics.

In 1929, a dentist in Colorado, in the United States, observed that mottled tooth enamel (which he suspected was associated with the water supply) was associated with fewer dental caries. The factor in the water supply was soon identified as fluoride. During the 1930s, inverse associations between fluoride concentrations in the water supplies of 21 cities and a newly developed quantitative index of dental caries (decayed, missing, and filled teeth) were reported. Caries prevalence declined as concentrations of natural fluoride in the water supply approached 1 ppm, with little additional benefit at higher concentrations. In 1945 community intervention trials of the effects of adjusting fluoride levels to 1 to 1.2 ppm began in four pairs of cities, with one pair in Canada. After 13 to 15 years caries was reduced by 50 to 70 per cent in the experimental cities compared with the controls. Official recommendations for the fluoridation of community water supplies were formalized in the United States in 1962 and the proportion of the population receiving fluoridated water from community supplies rose from 40 per cent in the mid-1960s to around 56 per cent in 1992. Over this same period, the mean decayed, missing, and filled teeth among all 12-year-olds fell dramatically from around 4 to just over 1. With time, the observed effects of water fluoridation have lessened as those without such supplies get fluoride from other sources, including toothpaste and drinks and foods manufactured in fluoridated areas (Division of Oral Health 1999).

It has been estimated that for large cities in the United States, the (undiscounted) costs of fluoridated water per individual over a lifetime are of the order of $10 (American dollars used throughout this chapter). By contrast, the lifetime costs of restoring a carious tooth could exceed $1000. Fluoridation is thus one of the most cost-effective preventive measures available (US Department of Health and Human Services and Batelle 1995).

Despite this attractiveness, the expansion of fluoridation slowed in the United States in the 1980s and 38 per cent of the American population served by community water supplies was still not benefiting from fluoridation in 1992 (Division of Oral Health 1999). In the United Kingdom, only 10 per cent of the population receives fluoridated water and no fluoridation schemes have been implemented since 1985 (British Dental Association 1999). Failure to fluoridate needs explanation.

In both the United States and the United Kingdom fluoridation enjoys the support of around 70 to 75 per cent of respondents to national opinion surveys (American Dental Association 1999; British Dental Association 1996). However, implementation requires local decisions and these have frequently been blocked by opponents. In the United States, local referenda have been lost because opponents have been more committed and better organized than proponents. Legal challenges in the lower courts have also obstructed progress, though the highest courts have upheld none. In the United Kingdom, privatization of the water companies created an additional obstacle with several water companies refusing to implement fluoridation when requested by the local health authorities (British Dental Association 1996).

The vocal minority opposed to fluoridation rest their claims on health risks that have repeatedly failed to be substantiated (National Research Council 1993). Their continued currency attests to the widespread, and perhaps increasing, distrust of technical manipulation of the human environment, also evident in the United Kingdom in the opposition to genetically modified foods. Popular sentiments tend to generalize, and well-founded observations on the progressive degradation of the living environment by industrial expansion may easily join together with ill-founded suspicions of particular technologies.

Fluoridation was not mentioned in the most important public health policy document produced by the British Conservative governments between 1979 and 1997 (Secretary of State for Health 1992) and was 'overlooked' in the incoming Labour government's discussion paper which claimed to be 'setting out a third way' in public health policy 'between the old extremes of individual victim blaming on the one hand and nanny state social engineering on the other' (Secretary of State for Health 1998). It appeared that the political aversion to 'engineering', as a means of health improvement, also encompassed civil engineering. The omission of explicit support for fluoridation was widely criticized and the final policy document promised 'to introduce a legal obligation on [privatized] water companies to fluoridate where there is strong local support for doing so'—assuming a satisfactory outcome from a newly commissioned review of the scientific evidence (Secretary of State for Health 1998).

Inaction on fluoridation in the United Kingdom between the mid-1980s and the late 1990s appears to have been partly a consequence of the ascendancy of neoliberal political ideas. Even the notionally social-democratic Blair Labour government (elected with an overwhelming majority in 1997) appeared, during its initial period of office, to be more afraid of accusations from its opponents that it favoured a 'nanny state' than of criticism from its own supporters that it was not using state powers to beneficial effect.

Fluoridation thus introduces several themes pertinent to the consideration of public health policy in rich countries. One is the power of research using quantitative methods, including experiments on whole communities, to expand the repertoire of effective means for controlling disease and injury. Another is the possibility of massive disjunctions between the cost-effectiveness of a preventive measure and the political feasibility of its implementation. Perceptions of risks and benefits held by vocal minorities may depart substantially from those of experts, and governments may be more sensitive to their reputations in the eyes of the press and other powerful bodies than they are to public opinion. Some observers see controversy and conflicts about risks as being typical of 'late modernity' (Giddens 1998).

Enhanced coverage with clinical procedures: control of high blood pressure

Raised blood pressure is a major contributor to risk of ischaemic heart disease and stroke, ranked respectively first and third as leading causes of disability-adjusted life years lost in rich countries (Murray and Lopez 1996). Meta-analyses of prospective studies have shown that a prolonged difference of about 5 mmHg in usual diastolic blood pressure is associated with a 21 per cent difference in risk of ischaemic heart disease and a 34 per cent difference in risk of stroke (MacMahon *et al.* 1990). All of the excess stroke risk appears to be reversible if blood pressure is lowered to target levels by medication and about half of the excess risk of heart attack may be reversible (Collins *et al.* 1990).

It is typically doctors who are expected to find cases of high blood pressure, to advise on drug and other therapies, and to help maintain control. Thus although all these processes also depend on the active co-operation of the public, high blood pressure provides the most important example of a persisting major public health problem that is being mainly addressed by professionally controlled measures applied to individuals.

The National High Blood Pressure Education Program adopted in the United States in 1972 is perhaps the best-known public health policy addressing high blood pressure (Joint National Committee 1997). Such policies have aimed to make case-finding more complete and control more effective. Progress has, rather confusingly, been monitored by using as a denominator individuals with blood pressures above 140/90 on a single occasion plus those reporting antihypertensive medication, and then calculating the percentages 'aware' that they have high (usual) blood pressure (which some of them will not have), are on treatment, or are controlled (Table 2). Despite their problems, these data show a substantial improvement in case-finding and control between the late 1970s and the late 1980s with little subsequent gain.

The Framingham Study cohorts have provided the opportunity to track changes over a longer time span, though in a population that is likely to be more health conscious than average. The proportion of those aged 45 to 74 who reported antihypertensive medication increased from 2 per cent in the 1950s to 25 per cent in the 1980s in males and from 6 to 28 per cent in females. Those with blood pressures above 160/100 measured on a single occasion (and irrespective of treatment status) fell from 19 to 9 per cent in the case of males and from 28 to 8 per cent in females. Greater proportionate declines occurred in progressively higher blood pressure strata and the prevalence of left ventricular hypertrophy fell markedly. These findings are consistent with other data indicating substantial secular declines, especially in severe hypertension (Mosterd *et al.* 1999).

In assessing the National High Blood Pressure Education Program as a public health programme, two questions need to be addressed. To what extent has the improvement in case-finding and management for high blood pressure been attributable to the 'organised effort' of the National High Blood Pressure Education Program? How much health benefit is attributable to the more effective clinical management of blood pressures?

Studies designed to answer the first question appear to have been very limited. In rural Kentucky a community high blood pressure control programme was run in two counties between 1979 and 1984 with a third county serving as control. In the intervention counties the percentage of 'hypertensives' whose blood pressure was controlled to below 140/90 rose from 37 to 53 per cent, with no change in the control county. Cardiovascular mortality fell in the intervention counties, while remaining constant in the control (Kotchen *et al.* 1986).

Some American observers believed, in the early 1980s, that 'the documented improvements in hypertension control since the beginning of the National High Blood Pressure Education Program must be considered a major contribution ... to the decline in cardiovascular mortality rates' (Lenfant and Roccella 1984). Between 1972 and 1994 in the United States, age-adjusted death certification rates for stroke fell by nearly 59 per cent and for ischaemic heart disease by 53 per cent. The fall in stroke was steepest in the early period and appears to have ceased in the early 1990s (Joint National Committee 1997).

Risk of stroke provides the more sensitive test of the benefits of enhanced control of high blood pressures because risk of stroke rises more steeply (and exponentially) with increasing blood pressure; furthermore, it is more completely reversed by treatment. For people aged 60 to 74, data from the American national health surveys show a substantial shift downwards in blood pressure distributions from the early 1960s to the most recent survey period around 1990. Because nearly all treated people stay above the median, reductions in the median provide a useful measure of shifts in the central tendency due to causes other than treatment; reductions in the mean, by contrast, will be due to both reductions in the central tendency and inward shrinkage of the top tail of the distribution. Median systolic pressures at ages 60 to 74 fell over this period by about 16 mmHg, from 148 to 132 mmHg. The shift in the upper tail of the distribution was more marked, with 90th centiles falling by about 30 mmHg—from around 191 to 160 mmHg. Some of this proportionally greater shift in the top tail could be attributable to the shrinkage of the distribution as the central tendency falls; for example, at ages 18 to 29, where the effects of medication are likely to be small, the 90th centile fell by 14 mmHg when the median fell by 8 mmHg (all estimates from smoothed distributions in Fig. 1 of Burt *et al.* (1995)). Nevertheless much of the fall in the prevalence of people at risk because of their high blood pressures can be assumed to have been due to enhanced clinical control of blood pressure.

Rose coined the term 'prevention paradox' to describe how, when risk is related monotonically to a quantitative attribute such as blood pressure, the interventions which offer most to the individuals at high risk contribute less to reducing the population burden of the disease

Table 2 Trends in awareness, treatment, and control of high blood pressure in people aged 18 to 74 years in the United States, 1976 to 1994

	Per cent of those either above 140/90 at time of survey or reporting antihypertensive medication		
	1976–1980	1988–1991[a]	1991–1994[a]
Aware that they have high blood pressure	51	73	68
Report taking antihyptertensive medication	31	55	53
Controlled (below 140/90 on survey day)	10	29	27

[a]These estimates are based on National Health and Nutrition Examination Survey III in which blood pressure was measured on two occasions.

Source: Joint National Committee (1997).

than do small downward shifts in the whole distribution (Rose 1985). Strachan and Rose (1991) reworked these analyses taking account of the misclassification of risk status when blood pressure is only measured on a single occasion. Because distributions of true (usual) blood pressures are not readily available they modelled them using data from the Whitehall Study with three alternative levels of intraindividual variation. Their models suggested that, assuming a reliability coefficient of 0.5, over 50 per cent of the population risk of fatal stroke attributable to true (usual) blood pressures higher than those in the lowest decile, was to be found in those whose true pressures were in the top decile. Yet, even in these apparently promising circumstances, a 'high-risk' case-finding strategy that correctly identified all in the true top decile, and that achieved an average reduction of 7.5 mmHg diastolic in all those offered treatment, would reduce stroke mortality only by about the same amount as would result from a 3-mmHg reduction in diastolic blood pressures across the whole distribution (Strachan and Rose 1991). Thus, although classification on the basis of usual blood pressures enhances the relative effectiveness of the 'high-risk' strategy in relation to stroke, it still remains modest when compared with downward shifts in the whole distribution of blood pressures.

No analyses of this kind appear to have been reported using data for the United States. However, earlier analyses of the contribution of hypertension treatment to the decline in stroke mortality between 1970 and 1980 placed it in the range of 6 to 25 per cent (Bonita and Beaglehole 1989).

In conclusion, the 'organised efforts' of the National High Blood Pressure Education Program will account for part of the improved case-finding and management for people with usual blood pressures above treatment thresholds. This improved management will account for part of the decline in the prevalence of people above treatment thresholds. The decline in the prevalence of people above treatment thresholds will account for part of the decline in stroke mortality attributable to raised blood pressures. Furthermore, given that MONICA (Monitoring of Trends and Determinants of Cardiovascular Diseases) results show that there are major determinants of stroke other than blood pressure (Stegmayr *et al.* 1997), it is also likely that all the causes of downward movements in blood pressure combined will have been only one part of the environmental changes contributing to declining stroke mortality.

Despite this cumulative diminution of the contribution of the National High Blood Pressure Education Program (in accordance with Rose's 'prevention paradox'), that contribution is still likely to have been very worthwhile because even small reductions in the heavy burdens imposed by heart attack and stroke will add up to a large benefit in absolute terms. Furthermore, the gains attributable to the National High Blood Pressure Education Program are notable for having been achieved within a pluralistic and organizationally diverse system of medical care.

This example also illustrates the main appeal of preventive strategies involving clinical procedures—their mode of action can be readily appreciated by practising doctors and their effectiveness at an individual level can be determined by randomized controlled trials—as well as the quantitative limitations of these strategies where risk is a continuously graded function of the determinant to be modified.

Behaviour change: HIV and sudden infant death

The epidemic of HIV infection in Europe followed that of the United States. The time course of the epidemic through the population of homosexual and bisexual males in England and Wales has been reconstructed by statistical modelling (de Angelis *et al.* 1998). The incidence of HIV infection appears to have peaked in 1983 and then to have fallen sharply (Fig. 2). These estimates are broadly consistent with the time trends shown by laboratory reports of hepatitis B infection in homosexual males, which peaked in 1984 but then showed a somewhat slower decline. Against the time course of the new infection rate can be set the timing of the formal control measures. Intensive 'social marketing' campaigns to promote changes to safer sexual practices were not launched by the British government until 1986 (Acheson 1993). It is thus likely that most of the change in sexual practices responsible for the sudden decline in HIV incidence after 1983 had occurred before the formal programme began. How is this to be explained? Almost certainly new knowledge about the dire consequences of HIV and how it was spread passed through both the general news media and through communication channels used especially by homosexual and bisexual communities. Because the epidemic in England substantially lagged behind that in the United States (perhaps by 3 years) there was an opportunity to learn from the United States where suspected modes of transmission had been identified as early as 1982, well before the identification of the virus in 1984 (US Department of Health and Human Services and Batelle 1995). From a societal point of view, this example shows the possibility of 'public health success without programmes'. In circumstances such as those surrounding the early HIV epidemic, the ability of formal public health programmes to contribute to health improvement may be limited by the need to await the building of a supporting political consensus. In the United States, a national household drop of an eight-page brochure, *Understanding Aids*, from the Surgeon General was not conducted until 1988.

The decline in sudden infant death syndrome in England illustrates the same point. The relationship between sleeping position and risk of sudden infant death syndrome was discussed in the letters pages of the *Lancet* during 1988 (Beal 1988), and this and other theories were widely discussed in magazines commonly read by mothers with young infants. Death rates from sudden infant death syndrome fell by more than a third in the 3 years before the British government's formal

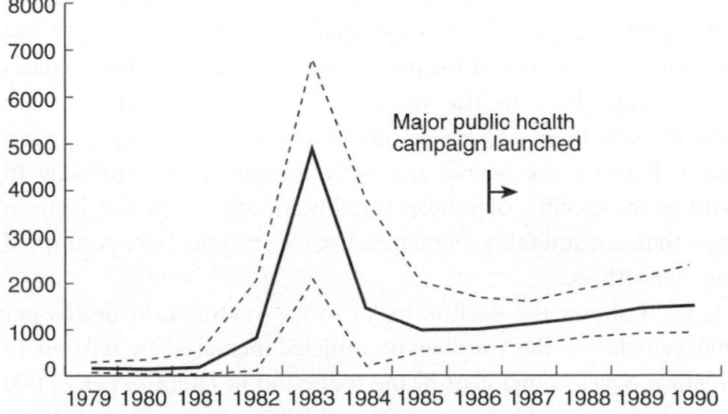

Fig. 2 HIV incidence in homosexual and bisexual males, England and Wales. Estimates by back-projection for 1979–1990 (with 95 per cent confidence interval) and timing of main public health campaign. (Source: D. De Angelis, personal communication.)

public health programme ('Back to sleep') began in December 1991 (OPCS 1988, 1995; Hiley and Morley 1994), again suggesting that mass behaviour change had occurred in response to new information flowing through the general mass media and, in an uncoordinated way, via health professionals. It is important to note in this case, however, that the rate of decline did accelerate sharply after the formal programme, with the rate halving in the following 12 months.

Thus, in highly literate and health-conscious populations, much, if not most, of the health benefit from new knowledge may flow more or less automatically from its dissemination through channels other than formal public health programmes; in these circumstances, it is the advance of public health science, perhaps even more than the strength of public health programmes, that sets the pace for health improvement (Dwyer and Ponsonby 1996). This is not to say that the incremental gain from formal programmes is typically negligible; it may still be very worthwhile relative to their typically modest resource requirements. But the main point to emerge from these examples is that the 'organised efforts' that have contributed most to reducing the burden of these diseases have been the research efforts. Thus, in developed countries, investment in the development of public health science is the most fundamental component of public health policy. In the cases of HIV and sudden infant death syndrome, the benefits flowing from scientific advance were realized largely without the aid of practising professionals. Therefore medicine and public health should not be understood just as domains of professional practice; they are, more fundamentally, cultural resources appropriated by all members of society—lay as well as professional. The mistake of confusing 'medicine' and 'public health' with the professional practice of these disciplines is commonly made, as in the title of a recent review of the benefits deriving from new knowledge: 'Medicine [used here to mean professional medicine] matters after all' (Bunker 1995).

Behaviour change: road traffic injuries

Traffic injuries rank fifth in their contribution to the burden of disease and injury in developed countries (Murray and Lopez 1996). Because of the short time lags between control measures and their expected effects, traffic injuries also provide a sensitive field in which to explore the relationship between policies, programmes, and effects.

Death rates from traffic crashes per unit registered vehicles follow a very general, and pronounced, downward trend as the number of motor vehicles increases in relation to population (Smeed's law: deaths/vehicle = 0.0003 (vehicles/population)$^{-0.66}$) (Smeed 1972). In the mid-1960s, two-thirds of 70 populations analysed by Smeed had rates within 40 per cent of his prediction. This implies that societies generally learn how to use motor vehicles more safely as both familiarity with them and the resources available for safety measures increase. Because the overall tendency is general, it is unlikely to depend on the specifics of policies variably adopted. However, it is also the case that, around this general trend, some societies have performed better than others.

Figure 3 shows the decline in Victoria, Australia, in deaths per 10 000 vehicles as the number of vehicles increased in relation to population. Over 80 per cent of the reduction in fatalities per 10 000 vehicles that occurred between 1920 and 1995 happened before 1970. During these five decades, Victoria generally had rates in excess of Smeed's prediction. Then, in a little more than two decades from 1970, it changed from being a relatively poor performer in this domain to being one of the best (Fig. 4).

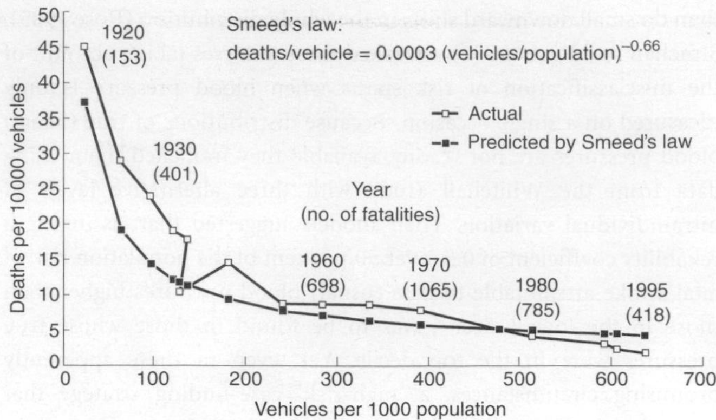

Fig. 3 The decline in traffic fatalities per 10 000 vehicles with increasing motorization, State of Victoria, Australia, 1920 to 1995. (Data from Smeed 1972; Hawthorne 1991.)

During the 1960s there had been a growing political consensus in Victoria that the loss of so many lives on the roads was unacceptable. In December 1970 it became the first jurisdiction in the world to make the wearing of seatbelts compulsory. A string of legislative measures followed, including random testing of the breath alcohol concentrations of drivers in 1977. After the decline in fatality rates faltered in the late 1980s, a very strong 'social marketing' campaign was launched in combination with intensive policing (Powles and Gifford 1993). The number of speed camera checks per year rose to eight per licensed driver and the proportion of vehicles recorded as speeding fell from 20 to 3 per cent. In 1994 1.6 million random breath tests were performed, a number equal to about half of the driving age population (Hendrie and Ryan 1995). Fatality rates fell sharply and have stayed down. During the early 1990s the Traffic Accident Commission, which carries all compulsory traffic injury insurance and makes 'no-fault' compensation payments to victims, spent several dollars per person on traffic accident prevention programmes, mainly of a 'social marketing' character, with intensive use of paid television advertising. Ten per cent of the spend was allocated to evaluation, from which the Traffic Accident Commission concluded that its benefits-to-costs ratio, from reduced injury claims, was at least 3 (Cameron and Newstead 1996). The ratio was larger still when estimates of the social costs of traffic injuries were used rather than average compensation payments. Thus effects that seem small relative to background trends may still be very worthwhile relative to the costs incurred.

Four points can be made as follows. Most of the very large secular declines in traffic injury deaths per unit vehicle (or distance travelled) observed around the world are likely to have occurred with a substantial degree of independence from the specific policies and programmes adopted in different political jurisdictions. Against this broad background trend, a second-order, but nevertheless important, degree of variation seems attributable to the intensity and nature of the control measures taken. In the relatively compact political environment of an Australian state, it was possible to build support for the escalation of control measures as less forceful measures proved inadequate to achieve widely desired goals—notwithstanding a political culture that valued personal independence. The comparative trend line for Britain (in Fig. 4), ending with rates among the lowest in Europe, shows that Victoria does not differ so much in the level it has attained as in its rate of improvement during two and a half decades of intensive political attention.

As an addendum, one may also note the powerful social benefits of having single substantial 'pots of gold' for dealing with leading sources of disease or injury. By linking the size of the 'pot' to the size of the problem—in this case by the level of compensation payments for traffic injuries—a resource is created that bears some commensurability with the public health challenge faced. The custodians of this fund can then gain social approbation both by reducing a recognized 'evil' and by reducing the financial levy needed to compensate for it. (Antismoking programmes funded by hypothecated tobacco taxes, as also exist in Victoria and in California, exploit an analogous link.)

Behaviour change: smoking

It is ironic that medicine provided the 'cultural bridge' that enabled tobacco use to be rapidly transferred from the exotic rituals of the Amerindian cultures to the everyday life of seventeenth century Europe. By explaining tobacco's properties within the contemporary humoral theories of well being, doctors such as the Sevillian Nicolas Monades provided what was to be the main (medical) justification for tobacco use until into the nineteenth century, when 'recreational' justifications came to the fore (Goodman 1993). With the advent of manufactured cigarettes in the late nineteenth century, tobacco use was made more convenient and more deadly. In the twentieth century, increased purchasing power resulting from economic development has been almost universally accompanied by widespread adoption of what is now known to be essentially an addiction to nicotine (Tobacco Advisory Group 2000). These epidemics of nicotine addiction can, on the experience of 'early adopters' such as England, be expected to last at least a century (Lopez *et al.* 1994). As a public health problem, cigarette smoking is thus distinguished not only by the great quantity of disease attributable to it—recently accounting, in the United Kingdom, for about a third of male and a quarter of female deaths between 35 and 69 years of age (Peto *et al.* 1994)—but also by the protracted time-scale over which it evolves. For example, it will be over half a century before the full health effects of onsets of nicotine addiction in today's adolescents will be manifest. Tobacco smoking is, in addition, a form of addiction that is both licit and extremely profitable.

The nature and magnitude of the health effects of cigarette smoking were mostly revealed by epidemiological studies conducted between the late 1940s and the mid-1960s. A question of interest is how this new knowledge (since much strengthened) has influenced the course of the smoking 'epidemic' and the epidemics of disease that have followed in its wake.

From around 1950 to the mid-1960s, new knowledge of the health effects of smoking flowed from scientists to the public mainly through the general news media. The Royal College of Physicians report in the United Kingdom in 1962 (Royal College of Physicians 1962) and the Surgeon General's report in the United States in 1964 (US Public Health Service 1964) were 'organised efforts' that nevertheless depended for their effects on such news coverage. A study of this process in the United States showed that the intensity of print media discussion of the risks of smoking was closely mirrored by adult smoking cessation rates through the 1950s and 1960s (J. Pierce, personal communication, 1999). The same group have also shown a close match between the intensity and targeting of commercial efforts and smoking uptake rates in adolescents (Pierce *et al.* 1994, 1998).

The intensification of 'organised efforts' to discourage tobacco smoking dates mainly from the 1970s. The main measures have included price increases (by specific taxes), requirements for warning labels on tobacco products and on advertisements, restrictions on smoking in public places, health education in schools, mass education and persuasion, enhanced advice (and assistance with cessation) from health professionals, and bans on advertising and other forms of promotion.

Attempts to assess the contribution of these measures to national trends in smoking prevalence (and, with appropriate lags, to national trends in attributable mortality) must take account of the fact that the onset of the epidemics of cigarette smoking, before its health effects were understood, took place at different times in different countries. In Europe, British males and females and Finnish males (but not females) were 'early adopters' of cigarette smoking (Lopez 1996). A general pattern of 'first in, first out' of the smoking epidemic might

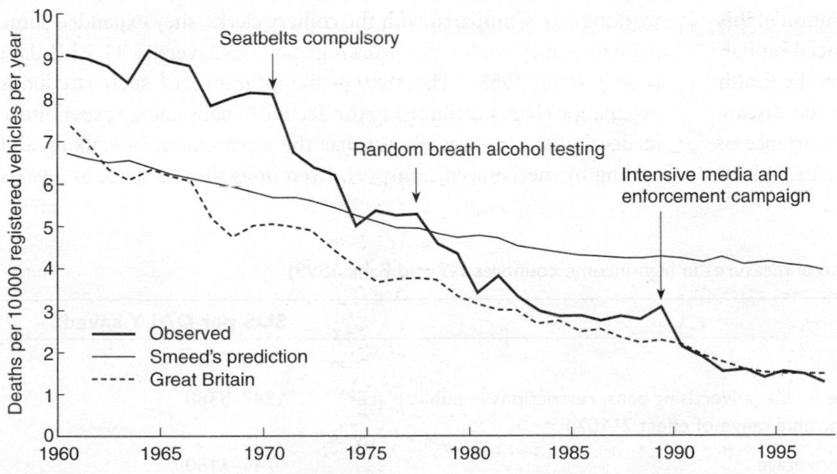

Fig. 4 Decline in traffic fatalities per 10 000 vehicles, 1960 to 1995, State of Victoria, Australia. (Data from VicRoads (1993); Smeed 1972; Department of the Environment, Transport and the Regions 1998.)

have been expected, to some extent independently of the relative strength of national counter-measures. Lung cancer mortality in early middle-age (ages 35–54 years) peaked in 1955 to 1959 in British males and in 1960 to 1964 in Finnish males. Falls since these peaks have exceeded 50 per cent and have recently been somewhat more rapid in Finland. It also happens that Finland (which banned tobacco advertising in 1978) (Harkin *et al.* 1997) and the United Kingdom have been among the leaders in efforts to reduce smoking. Finnish females, whose delayed smoking epidemic came to maturity during a period of tobacco control activity, have experienced a lung cancer mortality peak (at about 7 per 100 000 for those between 45 to 54 years old in 1990) less than one-third as great as that experienced by British females (about 27 per 100 000 for those between 45 to 54 years old in 1975) (Peto *et al.* 1994). The size of the smoking epidemic in British females was largely determined in the precontrol period (Lopez 1996). This pattern—of smoking epidemics having lower amplitudes when maturing in an environment of tobacco control activity—suggests that control measures are effective.

Based on systematic assessments of the effects of a number of tobacco control measures, a 1999 World Bank report concludes that tobacco control measures are highly cost-effective, with price increases by specific taxes giving the greatest yield (Table 3). The Bank is now a strong advocate of comprehensive tobacco control policies (Jha and Chaloupka 1999).

Against the generally favourable trends in adult smoking prevalences in high-income countries stand adverse trends since the late 1980s in smoking uptake by adolescents in a number of countries—the United States, Canada, Australia, the United Kingdom, and Austria (Hill *et al.* 1995; Gilpin and Pearce 1997; Harkin *et al.* 1997; Jarvis 1997; Spurgeon 1999). Responding appropriately to these reversals poses a number of challenges: the limited effectiveness of school-based programmes, especially those that are knowledge-based (US Department of Health and Human Services 1994), and the long time lag before substantial benefits will be experienced (as noted above). In the light of these, the World Bank document stresses the need to maintain an emphasis on smoking cessation in adults if benefits are to be seen in the next half century. Conclusions such as these may be supported by calculations of the discounted present value of future health states, which show that gains in the mid to distant future count for little today. An alternative appreciation of this situation is considered further below in the section on social capital.

In summary, cigarette smoking remains the leading public health problem in developed countries. It is without rival in the disease burden it generates. It also illustrates well the central importance of calendar time in the assessment of public health problems. Whilst peak smoking prevalences appear to have been lower in the higher educated strata in 'late-uptake' countries—where knowledge of health effects has had more opportunity to influence behaviour—high smoking prevalences among professional groups, such as Spanish doctors (Harkin *et al.* 1997), shows the limited effects of knowledge outside the context of comprehensive control policies and normative change. Reductions in attributable mortality within the next half century will need to come from encouraging and supporting cessation in current smokers. But if the course of the epidemic of nicotine addiction is to be curtailed, intergenerational transmission must also be minimized. The World Bank analyses show that resources allocated to tobacco control are nowhere commensurate with the magnitude of potential gains to health still to be won.

The history of efforts to reduce the damage to health caused by tobacco also illustrates how the development of quantitative methods has supported appropriate policy responses. It is striking that high-level policy debates in the United Kingdom during the 1950s and 1960s revolved around a largely illusory search for 'proof of causation' rather than estimation of how much was at stake (Pollock 1999). With the subsequent consolidation of epidemiological findings and their transmission to political and wider publics (Peto *et al.* 1994), quantitative assessments have become much more central to policy deliberations—reflecting again the preoccupation with 'risk' characteristic of 'late modern' societies.

Unsolved problems: physical inactivity and obesity

> Unless Prudence be a constant attendant on Opulence ... 'tis better living on a slender fortune. Richard Mead (1673–1754)

The material basis of modernization lies in the replacement of muscle, wind, and water power by energy mobilized through steam, electricity, and liquid hydrocarbons. Of the main adverse consequences for health, two—air pollution and transport injuries—have been largely brought under control. The third—the physiological consequences of declining energy expenditure—remains unsolved.

As recently as the mid-1950s many occupations still required substantial muscular exertion. Coal miners studied in Fife, Scotland, in 1952 had to walk over a mile to the underground coalface where they would hew and load 6 to 9 tons of coal onto a moving belt each working day. Compared with the colliery clerks, they expended some 3.6 more megajoules per working day (15.3 versus 11.7 MJ/day) (Garry *et al.* 1955). The virtual disappearance of such strenuous occupations has contributed to the decline in daily energy expenditure in developed countries. So too has the replacement of walking and cycling by mechanized transport. Even in as short a space as 7 years

Table 3 Estimates of the cost-effectiveness of tobacco control measures in high-income countries (World Bank 1999)

	$US per DALY saved[a]
Price increases of 10%	16–645
Non-price measures assumed to reduce smoking prevalence by 5% (advertising bans, restrictions in public places, information and counter-advertising, warning labels, etc.; plausible range of effect 2–10%)	1347–5388
Public provision of nicotine replacement therapy with 25% coverage	746–1160

DALY, disability-adjusted life year.

[a]Discounting at 3 per cent and summing over 30 years.

Source: Jha and Chaloupka (1999).

(1985 to 1992), there were substantial measurable declines in the distances walked and cycled by English children and corresponding increases in distances travelled by car (DiGuiseppi *et al.* 1997). The other side of the coin is the increase in time spent in 'activities' requiring little more than basal energy expenditure. School-aged children in the United States spent a mean of over 20 h/week watching television in the late 1980s (AC Nielson Company 1990, cited in Robinson *et al.* 1993).

Data, of known validity, on time trends in energy expenditure is generally unavailable for developed populations. Because of the technical difficulties involved, the measurement of total energy turnover in representative free-living individuals is a major challenge for contemporary public health surveillance. The 'doubly-labelled water' technique provides a gold standard but is too expensive for large-scale use. Individually calibrated heart rate monitoring is the next best but so far only one study has reported findings from a broadly representative study population (Wareham *et al.* 1997).

In the absence of data on trends in energy expenditure over time, data on recorded energy consumption may be used as a proxy, bearing in mind that such records tend to underestimate true intake and that an assumption of a roughly constant under-reporting bias over time is required. Data for English adults show substantial declines since the first 7-day weighed dietary intakes of the 1930s (Widdowson 1936; Widdowson and McCance 1936; Bingham *et al.* 1981; Prentice and Jebb 1995). Data abstracted from a large series of dietary studies in the United States show falls of around 17 per cent in recorded energy consumption of American adults (without adjustment for increasing body weight) between the 1940s and the early 1980s (Stephen and Wald 1990).

The Physical Activity Level is the ratio of total energy expenditure to basal metabolic rate (James and Schofield 1990). It is an important determinant of public health via two types of effect. Firstly, activity is directly protective of health (independently of its effects on body composition and of its contribution to aerobic fitness) (US Department of Health and Human Services 1996; Wareham *et al.* 2000). Secondly, as activity levels decline, the prevalence of obesity increases (Prentice and Jebb 1995).

The most dramatic evidence of the scale of public health problems associated with declining energy expenditure is the rise in obesity in most rich countries. The prevalence of obesity, defined as body mass index (weight in kilograms over height in meters squared) of 30 or more, doubled—from 10 to 20 per cent—in American men between 1960 and the early 1990s, with a particularly rapid increase over the latter part of this interval. In American females the absolute increase was similar but the proportional increase less, with a recent prevalence of around 25 per cent. In English men prevalence jumped from 6 to 15 per cent and in English women from 8 to 16.5 per cent between 1980 and 1995. Elsewhere trends have been less marked: in Dutch men prevalence has risen only modestly to 8.5 per cent since the mid-1980s and there has been no clear increase in Dutch women (WHO 1998). Whilst a high proportion of fat in the diet may also be contributing to obesity in rich countries (Jebb 1997), the recent secular rise in obesity in the United States has occurred concurrently with a decline in the proportion of dietary energy coming from fat (Stephen and Wald 1990).

The adverse effects of obesity are reasonably well quantified because body mass index is easily and reliably measured. In rich populations where adult deaths from infection are uncommon and a high proportion of deaths are from vascular causes, death rates among the obese are roughly double those for people of desirable weight for height (body mass index 20 to 25). A recent American review of physical activity and health concluded that 'health benefits appear to be proportional to the amount of activity' and noted that a quarter of American adults are 'not active at all' (US Department of Health and Human Services 1996).

In summary, recent declines in adult mortality in rich countries have, in most cases, been occurring in spite of adverse trends in one important health determinant. Declining physical activity merits recognition as a major unsolved public health problem.

The difficulty faced in solving this problem may be compared with that of changing the composition of the diet in order to favour health. Although there are hedonistic attractions in unhealthy dietary elements such as chocolate and ice cream, attractive alternatives that favour health are also available (for example, Mediterranean diets). However, exertion is not as attractive as indolence. During our evolutionary past, there was unlikely to have been a survival advantage in exertion in the absence of hunger or other immediate need. In this light, the origins of our problems with obesity and inactivity are profoundly social: they are a consequence not so much of individual misbehaviour as of our collective transformation of the way we provision society and the resulting marked reduction in the need for muscular exertion. However, it is still true that, within the material culture of late industrialism, some become obese while others do not and this leaves plenty of room for fatness to be attributed to moral failure. The individuals who find it hardest to avoid obesity are those who are genetically susceptible (Stunkard *et al.* 1986). Although no one can exercise moral responsibility in choosing their genes, those who become obese are heavily stigmatized. Some indication of the extensive efforts that citizens of rich countries are obliged to make to avoid becoming obese is that 64 per cent of American men and 78 per cent of American women reported in 1996 that they were making conscious efforts to lose or control weight (Serdula *et al.* 1999). (The desire to be thinner will have arisen from a mixture of concerns with both personal appearance and with health.) Given the apparent difficulties in achieving these objectives, it is not surprising that those who are most socially disadvantaged have the least success. The problems created by low energy turnover are thus also intimately connected with social inequalities in disease burdens.

Possible solutions to physical inactivity and obesity

Investment in new knowledge is a clear priority. Strategic importance, and the indications that solutions will not be easy, both indicate the need to establish physical activity and energy balance as high priorities in public health research. Given the rapid advances in identifying genetic susceptibility, preventive strategies will be needed at all levels—universal (for the whole population), selective (for the susceptible), and targeted (for those already affected) (WHO 1998). Assuming further research confirms the fundamental importance of low physical activity levels, the most feasible and attractive ways of increasing such activity will need to be found (Blair *et al.* 1996). The implications for institutional change are discussed further below.

Unsolved problems: sustainability

Averting harm to health from the disruption of the ecological systems on which human well being depends is unlike other public health challenges. The need for action cannot be inferred from empirical observations of previous harm from this source, but rather is to be inferred from highly uncertain models of what may happen in the future. Those who prefer to base decisions on 'science' rather than 'speculation' might be inclined to defer judgement until there has been time for the relevant models to be more thoroughly challenged, and the contributory evidence better marshalled. The argument against delay is that the interacting momenta of population increase and economic development are likely to result in 'overshoot and collapse' unless corrective action begins now. To a projected approximate doubling of the current world population one might add, for illustrative purposes, the fivefold increase in global income that would result from levelling world incomes (currently averaging about \$5000/person/year) up to current rich country levels (around \$25 000/person/year). Without any reduction in energy and resource use per unit of economic product this would translate to a $2 \times 5 = 10$-fold increase in the global 'material economy'. Even allowing for the likelihood of more efficient use of materials and energy, the point remains that it is not the ecological sustainability of the current global 'material economy' that is in question, but that of a several-fold multiple of it.

If attempts to extend the current pattern of energy and resource-intensive industrialism to the whole of an increasing human population are likely to come seriously unstuck, then the sooner the transition to more sustainable material culture is begun the better. A case for scaling down the quantum of ecological disruption per unit of economic product can be based more specifically on:

(1) evidence that productive activities are already adversely effecting major global meteorological systems, for example 'global warming' and stratospheric ozone depletion;

(2) evidence that the absolute scale of rich country material usage is unlikely to be generalizable;

(3) time trends in measurable effects on ecosystems.

Global warming

In order to limit the carbon dioxide build-up to a doubling of its preindustrial concentration (that is, from 275 to 550 ppm.)—a level which climatologists think would be tolerable—with a population of 10 to 11 billion by 2100, carbon dioxide emissions per person would need to be reduced to the levels of the 1920s (Wigley *et al.* 1996), a reduction of approximately two-thirds from today's level. The 1997 Kyoto Protocol was for an average 7 per cent cut, and restricted to developed countries.

Use of materials and absorption of wastes

Citizens of Germany, Japan, The Netherlands, and the United States use between 45 and 85 metric tons of materials per year. A majority of this is 'hidden' from commerce, for example mine tailings and soil erosion, and much of it occurs off shore: 'More than 70 per cent of the materials that flow through the Dutch economy….never touch Dutch soil' (World Resources Institute 1998). The kind of resource-intensive production that is commonplace in developed countries probably cannot be replicated in a large number of other countries without causing serious environmental harm. A target of halving the rate of global materials used in the coming decades while leaving room for economic development in low- and middle-income countries has been estimated to require a 90 per cent reduction, in rich countries, in the materials used per unit of economic product. Although this 'factor 10' reduction has been adopted as an objective by the Organization for Economic Co-operation and Development (Adriaanse *et al.* 1997), the magnitude of the transformations in productive technologies and consumption habits entailed do not appear to have penetrated far into either public or business opinion.

A related guide to the sustainability has been calculated as the amount of 'average' Earth's surface needed to 'produce the resources consumed and to assimilate the wastes generated by that population on a continuous basis'. Rees and others have estimated that most high-income countries have an ecological footprint several times larger than their national territories and that the total world population exceeds global carrying capacity by up to one-third (Rees 1999).

Effects on ecosystems

The 'living planet index' is one of the first systematic attempts to quantify the effects of human activity on natural ecosystems. It gives equal weight to three contributing indices: forest ecosystems (area of natural forest cover), freshwater ecosystems, and marine ecosystems (trends in the populations of 70 and 87 indicator species respectively). Set to 100 in 1970, it was estimated to have fallen to 68 by 1995—a clearly unsustainable rate of decline (Loh *et al.* 1998).

Ecological sustainability is an important issue for public health professionals: firstly, because it concerns the biological basis of human well being, whether or not the specific adverse health effects can be predicted with any confidence at this time; secondly, because 'organised efforts' will be needed to optimize health outcomes within 'ecologically-constrained' material economies; and thirdly, because the rethinking about economic life that is flowing from a concern with sustainability provides important leads to new ways of thinking about the connections between economic life and health. These are discussed further below.

Some issues emerging from examples considered

At the opening of this chapter seven public health topics were selected for further discussion. They were chosen to represent a variety of challenges to public health policy development, in the hope that a consideration of them would highlight important issues in this field. No claim to comprehensiveness is advanced. Four interim conclusions will be recapitulated before taking up a broader theme.

1. Governments may be more concerned to protect their reputations in the eyes of the press (and other powerful institutions) than to implement measures with high public support and dramatically favourable cost–benefit ratios (for example, fluoridation as an administrative measure to protect health).
2. Enhanced coverage with preventive measures applied to individuals appeals to doctors but may, in many circumstances, offer only modest gains in health (for example, the control of hypertension, illustrating the 'prevention paradox').
3. Formal programmes to promote change to healthier ways of life may have small (but still worthwhile) effects compared with the informal processes promoting such changes but both formal and informal processes depend critically on new knowledge (US Department of Health and Human Services and Batelle 1995). Investment in new knowledge is therefore the most fundamental component of public health policy (for example, changes from

sexual behaviours associated with HIV transmission, changes from infant care practices associated with sudden infant death, changes from high-risk driving practices, and cessation of cigarette smoking).

4. Combinations of regulatory measures (including taxation) and persuasion are likely to be more effective in changing behaviour than the latter alone, but these are only likely to be politically feasible where there is widespread public appreciation that stronger measures are needed if valued health gains are to be secured (for example, traffic injury reduction and smoking reduction).

The broader theme, to be taken up now, concerns the institutional underpinning of health protection within a given social order. Its importance was suggested in the above discussion of cigarette smoking and in the discussion of physical activity and ecological sustainability. Current discussion of the role of 'social capital' in the processes of economic and social development is taken as a starting point (Dasgupta and Serageldin 2000).

'Social capital'

The inability of quantitative predictors to account for the dramatic successes of the East Asian economies, or for the equally dramatic failures of economic transition in Russia, has focused attention on the institutional sources of these phenomena. In bodies such as the World Bank, attention is switching from a critique of the state as a displacer of markets to a desire to better understand why large-scale organizations function well in some circumstances but not in others, and how the development and effectiveness of state organizations can influence patterns of economic and social development (World Bank 1997, 1999; Dasgupta and Serageldin 2000). This interest has been sharpened by the generally poor performance of state institutions in sub-Saharan Africa and by the dire consequences of the collapse of state institutions in several 'global trouble spots'.

Economic collapse in Russia has been associated with perhaps the most severe deterioration in public health yet experienced in the industrialized world. Its institutional origins are therefore of interest to our theme, even if they remain poorly understood. Richard Rose has characterized contemporary Russia as an 'antimodern' society 'characterised by organisational failure and the corruption of formal organisations' (Rose 2000). Modern societies, by contrast, are to be distinguished by 'the predominance, in both the market and the state sectors, of social capital in the form of large, impersonal bureaucratic organisations operating according to the rule of law [citing Weber], such as IBM, commercial airlines, social security agencies, and universities. Even though informal networks can supplement or at times substitute for formal bureaucratic organisations, in modern society they are of much less importance than in a traditional or premodern society'. Soviet Russia was simultaneously 'overorganised' and 'underbureaucratised...in that the rule of law did not apply and the system encouraged people to create informal networks as protection against the state and to circumvent or subvert its commands'. This interpretation follows Max Weber in seeing bureaucratic rationalization as essential to the effective functioning of modern societies and is in strong contrast to the sociologically naive view that 'bureaucracy' is an unattractive characteristic of state organizations that can be dispensed with by privatization. (The attractiveness of bureaucracy is really a side issue. Weber himself was pessimistic: 'Not summer's bloom lies ahead of us, but rather a polar night of icy darkness and hardness, no matter which group may triumph externally now' (Weber 1991).)

The conclusions drawn by Putnam *et al.* (1993) from their detailed and prolonged investigation of the establishment of a regional tier of government in Italy have been particularly influential in the social capital literature. They found that the regional governments established in the early 1970s worked well in the north and badly in the south, despite their identical structures and equivalent legal and financial resources. The regional characteristics most closely associated with effective government were not those indicative of economic development but rather those indicative of a strong 'civic community': the empirical measures used were voting behaviour (including turnout, not preferences), newspaper readership, and density of sports and cultural associations. In the 'civic' regions, 'the community values solidarity, civic engagement, cooperation, and honesty. Government works'. The authors traced the origins of these different institutional inheritances back to the emergence of republican city governments in the late Middle Ages. In this interpretation, inherited stocks of social capital are important determinants of the good government and economic well being of today's citizens.

Against the background of these recent debates, there is clearly no need to be defensive or apologetic about the need to move beyond the quantitative evidence to discuss the institutional requirements for health protection (Breslow 1996). However, it should be acknowledged that public health strategies now need to be framed within a more strongly liberal (European sense) political culture in which respect for government is currently much less than it was in the early years after the Second World War. (Giddens (1998) cites a drop in the United States from 76 per cent in 1964 to 25 per cent in 1994 in the proportion of opinion poll respondents answering 'all' or 'most of the time' when asked 'How much of the time do you trust the government in Washington to do the right thing?'.) A related development is the shift in power away from national governments to supranational bodies above and regional governments below (World Bank 1999).

The three examples used to justify this detour to the social capital literature were tobacco smoking, inactivity, and ecological sustainability.

Smoking

It was noted above that quantitative analyses of the discounted present value of future health gains from increasing smoking cessation versus reducing smoking uptake would push policy emphases strongly towards the former. However, this matter can be approached differently by thinking of a society's institutional defences against tobacco smoking as part of its stock of 'health capital' and as a valuable asset to be accumulated and transmitted to future generations. To minimize the cumulative toll of tobacco smoking (the area under the epidemic curve) each generation will need to transmit strengthened institutional defences against cigarette smoking to the next, based in a sound popular understanding of its health risks, and including a strong disapproval of tobacco smoking. Such a process might be less likely in a society relying heavily on smoking cessation because most smokers who quit do so in middle-age. The intergenerational transmission of nicotine addiction is sensitive to smoking prevalences in young parents, and this will reflect both the general strength of tobacco control activities and, more specifically, the strength of measures directed to adolescents and young adults (Distefan *et al.*

1998; Farkas *et al.* 1999). Nor is it necessary to be too pessimistic about the responsiveness of adolescents to tobacco control measures: smoking initiation rates among American males aged 15 to 20 years halved between the 1950s and the 1980s and fell substantially in females after the mid-1970s (Gilpin *et al.* 1994). (Among American black adolescents, smoking had almost gone out of fashion by the late 1980s (McIntosh 1995). In respect of school-based programmes, those concentrating on teaching relevant social skills, rather than knowledge and norms, have generally been effective (US Department of Health and Human Services 1994).)

Inactivity

The problem of declining physical activity levels is embedded in the everyday realities of late industrialism. 'Labour-saving' investments have increased productivity and profits; they are unlikely to be abandoned. Scope will still need to be sought for inserting more activity back into the working day. Patterns of commuting to work reflect the patterns of investment in residential settlements and in transport infrastructure. Sprawling cities in North America and Australasia have dependence on the car 'built in'. Such massive investments cannot suddenly be undone. Moves towards walking and cycling will require a widespread public recognition that increasing daily activity is an inescapable requirement if optimum health levels are to be attained in rich countries. Without such recognition, the radical changes required will not be politically feasible. The health problems generated by declining physical activity levels in the late twentieth century thus bear this similarity to the increased transmissibility of infection recognized as a consequence of rapid urbanization in the second quarter of the nineteenth century. Effective solutions are likely to require an adaptive reconfiguration of urban life and government. Walking and cycling will need to be made more attractive and this is unlikely to happen without substantial investments in infrastructure (McCarthy 1999). The trend towards driving children to school is unlikely to be reversed unless parents can be more confident that their children are safe on the streets. Waking time spent at very low levels of physical activity, for example watching television, appears to be especially predictive of weight gain, at least in adolescents (Kimm *et al.* 1999). If children are to be diverted to outdoor play they will need attractive and secure environments.

Just as new competencies, born of new policies, were needed by local governments in order to protect nineteenth century urban dwellers from infection transmitted by water, food, and urban crowding (Szreter 1988), so is it likely that another renewal of local government will be required to foster activity patterns that are optimal for health. Via their connections with energy and resource use, there is a natural bridge between public health issues related to physical activity levels and those related to sustainability.

Sustainability

> [Society is a partnership] not only between those who are living, but between those who are living, those who are dead and those who are to be born.
>
> Edmund Burke, *Reflections on the revolution in France*, 1790 (cited in Giddens 1998)

To operate the idea of sustainability within economic analyses, attention needs to be diverted from measures of 'flow' (income) to measures of 'stock' (capital), including natural capital and human resources. Conventional national income ('flow') accounts are biased for this purpose in that they treat depletions of natural capital as income (as when a forest is cut down to make furniture), and are insensitive since they provide little indication of future legacies. The Environment Department of the World Bank has noted that if 'sustainable development is about leaving future generations more capital per capita than we have had, then the rate of genuine saving becomes a good measure of whether our aggregate activities are on a sustainable path' (Serageldin 1996). Genuine saving is evidenced by increases in a proposed broad measure of wealth combining the estimated values of natural and human resources along with those of produced assets (capital as traditionally considered). Human resources include the 'human capital' embodied in individuals (for example, health and education levels) and 'social capital' embodied in institutions, customs, and knowledge (Environment Department World Bank 1998).

Such a shift of emphasis from economic flows to stocks, especially of human and natural resources, helps to clarify the scope for enhancing health at any given level of income—an important objective if we are to maximize well being while minimizing flows of materials and energy. It is also in tune with the consistent empirical finding that human and social resources play a more important role in determining mortality levels than income. For rich countries, health evidently depends less on the consumption opportunities provided by income than on personal and social capacities to protect and enhance health.

Social institutions and health: psychosocial versus material emphases

> In direct contrast to German philosophy, which descends from heaven to earth, here we ascend from earth to heaven.
>
> Marx and Engels, *The German ideology*, 1846 (1959)

Much of the literature on 'social determinants of health' has an emphasis on 'psychosocial' phenomena—stress, the psychosocial environment at work, relative income, and social networks and support (see for example many of the contributions in Marmot and Wilkinson 1999)—and the role of such phenomena in generating inequalities in health. A shortcoming of this work is its inadequate recognition of the importance of major health determinants that are simultaneously social and material, that is, of phenomena that might alternatively be described as components of material culture. Mediterranean food cultures and the Russian drinking culture can be cited as examples of phenomena which are clearly anchored to the institutional inheritances of certain cultural regions (and therefore qualify as social rather than natural phenomena) and which are exerting powerful effects on recent mortality trends.

Being born into a Mediterranean culture might plausibly have a greater influence on one's risk of premature death from coronary disease than differential access to modern medical care or discretionary individual behaviours such as exercising or even smoking (Willett *et al.* 1995). It is striking that Albania, by far the poorest country in Europe but bordering the Mediterranean, has adult mortality levels substantially below those of richer ex-socialist states further east and north (Gjonca and Bobak 1997).

The catastrophic increase in adult mortality that befell Russia between the mid-1980s and around 1994—in contrast, for example, to Georgia or Armenia, which have suffered even greater falls in income (World Resources Institute 1998)—appears to be partly the result of a dramatic increase in binge drinking (Leon *et al.* 1997). This has clearly had important short-term determinants, including the political unsustainability of Gorbachev's anti-alcohol campaign and the deregulation of sales during economic liberalization, but the outcome is only explicable if local drinking customs are taken into account (White 1996).

This dependence of an individual's health prospects on their cultural inheritances is akin to the findings of Putnam *et al.* (1993), in the political domain, that the chances of being well governed and prosperous may depend substantially on place of birth. The effect of these inheritances is not static, but is continually projected forward by evolving material possibilities arising from economic development and by dynamic social processes. The rapid evolution of eating and drinking habits, for example, powerfully influences health trends. Mediterranean countries such as France, Italy, and Spain have enhanced their advantage in mortality levels from vascular causes as they have become more affluent, despite their rising fat consumption (Powles and Sanz 1999).

Public health institutions are inevitably concerned with changing consumption norms. The institutions that normatively regulate consumption are fundamental to the regulation of social and political life itself—'a society's notion of political order is a result of its evaluation of desire and identification of need (that which is socially necessary)' (Berry 1994). Since the eighteenth century, the dominant liberal idea has been that desires should be respected as the 'authentic voice of individual preference'. But not all: most jurisdictions make it illegal to use heroin and most place heavy ('luxury') taxes on tobacco. Contention about the acceptability of certain desires and the legitimacy of public action to suppress their fulfilment is close to the surface in many debates on public health policy.

Public health problems and public health investments

The opening discussion—questioning whether one can see in health trends, the effects of public health programmes—presumes that the programmes are always the cause and the health trends the effects. This is, of course, much too simple. Causes could, and probably often have, worked in the opposite direction, where it is the nature and magnitude of health problems experienced that has determined the strength of the public health response. Finland and Australia provide cases in point.

In the late 1960s mortality from vascular disease in middle-aged males in the Finnish province of North Karelia was far above levels in other developed countries and the risk of dying before the age of 65 approached 50 per cent. These risks were perceived, by the local people, as unacceptable and so they petitioned the national government to mount a preventive programme. From this the North Karelia Project was born and it, in turn, stimulated investment in public health institutions (Vartiainen *et al.* 1994). Despite its modest population, Finland now has over 700 staff in its National Institute of Public Health and it ranks at the top in its rate of publication in leading international epidemiological journals (Fig. 5). The fact that this substantial investment has not been sufficient to push Finland to the fore of 'good performers' in Fig. 1 (it lies just below the trend line) may mainly be due to the intrinsic difficulties Finns face in lowering their vascular mortality. Without such investment, Finland may have done substantially worse. Evaluative studies of the North Karelia Project itself suggest it was effective. Lung cancer mortality fell sooner there and has fallen further than elsewhere in Finland consistent with early results for changes in smoking prevalence (Puska *et al.* 1993). Conversely, the very poor performance of Denmark (Fig. 1) contrasts with its apparently heavy investment in public health science (Fig. 5), suggesting that science does not always find effective application.

Australia, like Finland, faced adverse mortality trends in the first two postwar decades with male life expectancy at birth falling during the 1960s. Death rates rose from coronary heart disease, car crashes, and suicide. A country which had been notable for its favourable mortality levels at the beginning of the century, which had experienced a long postwar economic boom, and which thought of its way of life as being especially favourable to health had to come to terms with a serious loss of rank in international health comparisons. Strong institutional responses evolved in relation to traffic injuries (discussed above), heart disease, and tobacco control (Powles and Gifford 1993). Through the 1980s there was a rapid expansion of masters level programmes in public health disciplines, with enrolment levels exceeding those in most (if not all other) high-income countries. These institutional developments have plausibly contributed to Australia's recent ranking as a relatively good performer in reducing overall mortality (Fig. 1).

The strong development of public health institutions oriented towards chronic disease control in countries such as Finland and Australia may be contrasted with experience in countries such as France, Italy, and Spain where the evolving nature of public health challenges has been different. Vascular mortality in these countries did not persist at high levels, but tended to fall, often rapidly; this brought down all-cause mortality rates and made the case for reinvigorating public health institutions to prevent less pressing chronic disease. In these countries traffic injuries, HIV, tobacco control, and the reduction of harm from alcohol use are among the most salient challenges.

The search for equality

Recent favourable trends in overall adult mortality have been accompanied by growing inequalities in states such as the United Kingdom, because mortality declines have been much greater in more favoured strata. In England and Wales, between 1977–1981 and 1987–1991, male life expectancy at 15 years of age increased from 58.8 to 60.5 years for people in professional and managerial occupations but only from 55.1 to 55.8 years for people in semiskilled and unskilled jobs; for females the respective trends were from 64.1 to 65.8 years and from 62 to 62.4 years (cited in Shaw *et al.* 1999). The causes of, and appropriate remedies for, these inequalities in health have been a major preoccupation in public health policy discussions in the United Kingdom (Black *et al.* 1980; Acheson 1998).

Comparisons of mortality differentials between males in manual and non-manual occupations across 11 European countries found them to be broadly similar (though somewhat greater in France and Finland) with 'no evidence that mortality differences are smaller in

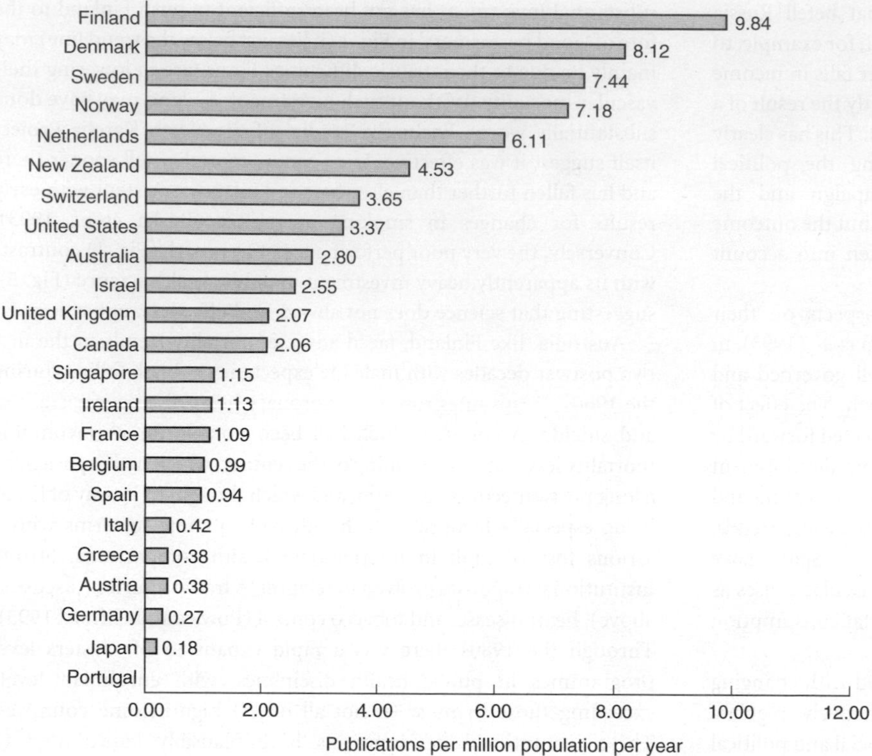

Fig. 5 Publications in the *American Journal of Epidemiology* plus the *International Journal of Epidemiology* classified by country of author's address, per million population, average for 1995 to 1998. (Author's calculations using Medline records.)

countries with more egalitarian socio-economic and other policies' (Kunst *et al.* 1998*a*). The causes of death contributing most to these differences did, however, vary markedly between countries: 'mortality from ischaemic heart disease was strongly related to occupational class in England and Wales, Ireland, Finland, Sweden, Norway, and Denmark, but not in France, Switzerland, and Mediterranean countries. In the latter countries, cancers other than lung cancer and gastrointestinal diseases made a large contribution to class differences in total mortality. Inequalities in lung cancer, cerebrovascular disease, and external causes of death also varied greatly between countries' (Kunst *et al.* 1998*b*).

Black *et al.* (1999) have articulated a 'materialist' interpretation of the cause of inequalities in the United Kingdom. This gives primacy to 'material deprivation' (both absolute and relative) and draws attention to the marked increase in income inequalities there between 1979 and 1995–1996; for example, over this period the number of people living in households with less than half the national average income increased from 4.5 to 12.2 million. However, the finding of Kunst *et al.* (1988*a*) that relative mortality inequalities are not less in countries with more equal income distributions does not support this interpretation. Furthermore, constrained consumption opportunities are not everywhere associated with high mortality levels: impoverished Cuba has lower adult male mortality than the United States, and Sri Lanka has adult male mortality levels comparable to some European countries (WHO 1999). Within Europe, Cretan villagers observed in the 1960s and 1970s in the Seven Countries Study had favourable mortality levels, despite their extremely frugal circumstances (Keys 1980). Thus, within some material cultures (all of which seem to have warm climates) it has become possible to attain low mortality on low incomes. The health effects of limited consumption opportunities therefore appear to depend strongly on the context in which consumption choices are made. Materialist explanations, if they are to be persuasive, need either to acknowledge their limited sphere of applicability ('northern commodity-intensive cultures'?) or, more informatively, to incorporate explicit reference to the kinds of differences between life in a Cretan village in the 1960s and life on housing estates in a British industrial city in the 1990s that are likely to be most important for health: for example, dietary traditions (related also to local food-producing possibilities), norms governing alcohol and tobacco use (and purchasing power for cigarettes), and obligatory daily energy expenditure. (The greater absolute poverty of the Cretans probably protected them from tobacco-attributable disease by limiting their tobacco consumption, especially prior to the Second World War.)

Given that the relative importance of causes contributing to mortality inequalities varies by country, responses should also differ. In France, where inequalities in males appear to be the greatest within Western Europe, chronic diseases related to the volume of alcohol consumed make a major contribution; policies to reduce consumption will therefore be important. In Finland, injuries related to drunkenness are more salient, indicating the need both for 'harm-reduction' policies (such as control of drunk driving), and for programmes to encourage a change away from the 'peak drinking' pattern. Measures to counter smoking are of primary importance in countries where a mature smoking epidemic is combined with a high background risk of vascular disease (roughly the 'northern' countries). (In countries at earlier stages in their smoking epidemics, programmes to encourage quitting may have the effect of increasing mortality inequalities. This does not mean that they should not be implemented.)

Jarvis and colleagues have shown for the United Kingdom that the current social gradient in smoking prevalence has been mainly created by greater rates of smoking cessation in the upper social strata: 'What we need to explain above all is not so much why poor people start smoking, but why they do not give it up' (Jarvis and Wardle 1999). Plasma cotinine levels among smokers show that nicotine dependence increases systematically with deprivation and that poor smokers obtain more nicotine per cigarette smoked. Using the indirect method of Peto *et al.* (1992) (in which lung cancer mortality is used as a measure of tobacco exposure to estimate the proportion of other deaths attributable to smoking), it is estimated that, in the United Kingdom, smoking-attributable deaths contribute about two-thirds of the excess mortality in the less favoured groups. The most obvious short-term policy response is to provide even greater assistance for quitting—including free or subsidized supplies of nicotine replacement therapy. In the long term, all measures that contribute to making tobacco use uncommon will have helped to reduce a major actual or potential cause of health inequality.

Making progress safe

Material progress both favours and harms health. It has been one of the main responsibilities of public health institutions to help resolve this ambivalence by countering the manifest and potential harms to health arising from material progress. This has enabled the net effect of affluence on health to approximate more closely towards its beneficial effect. In nineteenth-century Britain, industrialism did not impress as 'progress' until ways had been found to control the increase of fatal infection in the new industrial towns (Szreter 1997). In the twentieth century, the increased consumption opportunities generated by economic development has permitted a global epidemic of nicotine addiction which, especially when combined, in susceptible food cultures, with 'early dietary affluence', resulted in epidemic waves of tobacco-caused cancer and tobacco-amplified vascular disease. These epidemics were sometimes large enough, at least in males, to nullify substantially the beneficial effects of economic development on traditional infective killers of adults such as tuberculosis and pneumonia. Today, in many developed countries, these two related epidemics are in retreat. However, challenges and unsolved problems are ever renewed. As noted above, the uptake of tobacco smoking by young people has ceased declining in many developed countries and no plausible solution to the rising prevalence of obesity is in sight. The sustainability of industrialism in its current form, once it is generalized to the whole human population, is improbable. Although we cannot predict the exact ways in which the cumulative disruption of major ecological processes will rebound on our health, the likelihood of serious harm from this source is now substantial. Public health endeavour will continue to be an important determinant of what we are able to mean by 'progress' and of whether we shall be able to make it safe.

References

AC Nielson Company (1990). *Nielson report on television.* Nielson Media Research, New York.

Acheson, E.D. (1993). Behold a pale horse: a view from Whitehall. *PHLS Microbiology Digest*, **10**, 133–40.

Acheson, E.D. (1998). *Independent inquiry into inequalities in health.* HMSO, London.

Adriaanse, A., Bringezu, S., Hammond, A., *et al.* (1997). *Resource flows: the material basis of industrial economies.* World Resources Institute, Washington, DC; Wuppertal Institute; Netherlands Ministry of Housing, Spatial Planning, and Environment; National Institute for Environmental Studies, Japan.

American Dental Association (1999). *Fluoridation facts (revised).* American Dental Association, Chicago, IL.

Beal, S. (1988). Sleeping position and SIDS. *Lancet*, **ii**, 512.

Berry, C.J. (1994). *The idea of luxury: a conceptual and historical investigation.* Cambridge University Press.

Bingham, S.A., McNeil, N.I., and Cummings, J.H. (1981). The diet of individuals: a study of a randomly chosen cross section of British adults. *British Journal of Nutrition*, **45**, 23–35.

Black, D., Morris, J.N., Smith, C., and Townsend, P. (1980). *Inequalities in health: report of a research working group.* Department of Health and Social Security, London.

Black, D., Morris, J.N., Smith, C., and Townsend, P. (1999). Better benefits for health: plan to implement the central recommendation of the Acheson Report. *British Medical Journal*, **318**, 724–7.

Blair, S.N., Booth, M., Gyarfas, I., *et al.* (1996). Development of public policy and physical activity initiatives internationally. *Sports Medicine*, **21**, 157–63.

Bonita, R. and Beaglehole, R. (1989). Increased treatment of hypertension does not explain the decline in stroke mortality in the United States, 1970–1980. *Hypertension*, **13**, 169–73.

Breslow, L. (1996). Social ecological strategies for promoting healthy lifestyles. *American Journal of Health Promotion*, **10**, 253–7.

British Dental Association (1996). *Oral health, tooth decay and the need for water fluoridation (Parliamentary Briefing).* British Dental Association, London.

Bunker, J.P. (1995). Medicine matters after all. *Journal of the Royal College of Physicians of London*, **29**, 105–12.

Burt, V.L., Culter, J.A., Higgins, M., *et al.* (1995). Trends in the prevalence, awareness, treatment, and control of hypertension in the adult United States population. Data from the health examination surveys, 1960 to 1991 *Hypertension*, **26**, 60–9. (Erratum, *Hypertension*, **27**, 1192 (1996).)

Cameron, M. and Newstead, S. (1996). *Mass media publicity supporting police enforcement and its economic value.* Monash University Accident Research Centre, Melbourne.

Centers for Disease Control (1999). Fluoridation of drinking water to prevent dental caries. *Morbidity and Mortality Weekly Report*, **48**, 933–40.

Collins, R., Peto, R., MacMahon, S., Hebert, P., *et al.* (1990). Blood pressure, stroke, and coronary heart disease. Part 2: Short-term reductions in blood pressure: overview of randomised drug trials in their epidemiological context. *Lancet*, **335**, 827–38.

Dasgupta, P. and Serageldin, I. (2000). *Social capital: a multifaceted perspective.* World Bank, Washington, DC.

De Angelis, D., Gilks, W.R., and Day, N.E. (1998). Bayesian projection of the acquired immune deficiency syndrome epidemic. *Applied Statistics*, **47**, 449–98.

Department of the Environment, Transport and the Regions (1998). *Road accidents Great Britain 1997: the casualty report.* HMSO, London.

DiGuiseppi, C., Roberts, I., and Li, L. (1997). Influence of changing travel patterns on child death rates from injury: trend analysis. *British Medical Journal*, **314**, 710–13.(Erratum. *British Medical Journal*, **314**, 1385.)

Distefan, J.M., Gilpin, E.A., Choi, W.S., and Pierce, J.P. (1998). Parental influences predict adolescent smoking in the United States, 1989–1993. *Journal of Adolescent Health*, **22**, 466–74.

Dwyer, T. and Ponsonby, A.L. (1996). The decline of SIDS—a success story for epidemiology. *Epidemiology*, **7**, 323–5.

Environment Department, World Bank (1998). *Expanding the measure of wealth: indicators of environmentally sustainable development*. World Bank, Washington, DC.

Farkas, A.J., Distefan, J.M., Choi, W.S., Gilpin, E.A., and Pierce, J.P. (1999). Does parental smoking cessation discourage adolescent smoking? *Preventive Medicine*, **28**, 213–18.

Garry, R.C., Passmore, R., Warnock, G.M., and Durnin, J.V.G.A. (1955). *Studies on expenditure of energy and consumption of food by miners and clerks, Fife, Scotland, 1952*, pp. 1–69. HMSO, London.

Giddens, A. (1998). *The third way. The renewal of social democracy*. Polity Press, Cambridge.

Gilpin, E.A. and Pierce, J.P. (1997). Trends in adolescent smoking initiation in the United States: is tobacco marketing an influence? *Tobacco Control*, **6**, 122–7.

Gilpin, E.A., Lee, L., Evans, N., and Pierce, J.P. (1994). Smoking initiation rates in adults and minors: United States, 1944–1988. *American Journal of Epidemiology*, **140**, 535–43.

Gjonca, A. and Bobak, M. (1997). Albanian paradox, another example of protective effect of Mediterranean lifestyle? *Lancet*, **350**, 1815–17.

Goodman, J. (1993). *Tobacco in history: the cultures of dependence*. Routledge, London.

Harkin, A.M., Anderson, P., and Goos, C. (1997). *Smoking, drinking and drug taking in the European Region*. WHO Regional Office for Europe, Copenhagen.

Hawthorne, G. (1991). Pre-driver education. An evaluation of a traffic safety education program for senior students in Victorian post-primary schools. PhD Thesis, Monash University, Australia.

Hendrie, D. and Ryan, G.A. (1995). *Review of road safety practices in Australia and recommendations for Western Australia*. Road Accident Prevention Research Unit, Department of Public Health, University of Western Australia, Perth.

Hiley, C.M.H. and Morley, C.J. (1994). Evaluation of government's campaign to reduce risk of cot death. *British Medical Journal*, **309**, 703–4.

Hill, D., White, V., and Segan, C. (1995). Prevalence of cigarette smoking among Australian secondary school students in 1993. *Australian Journal of Public Health*, **19**, 445–9.

James, W.P.T. and Schofield, C. (1990). *Human energy requirements*. Oxford University Press.

Jarvis, L. (1997). *Smoking among secondary school children in 1996: England*. HMSO, London.

Jarvis, M.J. and Wardle, J. (1999). Social patterning of individual health behaviours: the case of cigarette smoking. In *Social determinants of health* (ed. M.G. Marmot and R.G. Wilkinson), pp. 240–55. Oxford University Press.

Jebb, S.A. (1997). Aetiology of obesity. *British Medical Bulletin*, **53**, 264–85.

Jha, P. and Chaloupka, F.J. (1999). *Curbing the epidemic: governments and the economics of tobacco control*. World Bank, Washington, DC.

Joint National Committee (1997). The sixth report of the Joint National Committee on prevention, detection, evaluation, and treatment of high blood pressure. *Archives of Internal Medicine*, **157**, 2413–46. (Erratum. *Archives of Internal Medicine*, **158**, 573 (1998).)

Keys, A. (1980). *Seven countries: a multivariate analysis of death and coronary heart disease*. Harvard University Press, Cambridge, MA.

Kimm, S.Y.S., Glynn, N.W., and Obarzanek, E. (1999). Obesity and its relationship to physical activity and inactivity during adolescence. *Abstracts of the 39th Annual Conference on Cardiovascular Disease Epidemiology and Prevention*, p. 10.

Kotchen, J.M., McKean, H.E., Jackson-Thayer, S., Moore, R.W., Straus, R., and Kotchen, T.A. (1986). Impact of a rural high blood pressure control program on hypertension control and cardiovascular disease mortality. *Journal of the American Medical Association*, **255**, 2177–82.

Kunst, A.E., Groenhof, F., and Mackenbach, J.P. (1998*a*). Mortality by occupational class among men 30–64 years in 11 European countries. EU Working Group on Socioeconomic Inequalities in Health. *Social Science and Medicine*, **46**, 1459–76.

Kunst, A.E., Groenhof, F., Mackenbach, J.P., and EU Working Group on Socioeconomic Inequalities in Health (1998*b*). Occupational class and cause specific mortality in middle aged men in 11 European countries: comparison of population based studies. *British Medical Journal*, **316**, 1636–42.

Lenfant, C. and Roccella, E.J. (1984). Trends in hypertension control in the United States. *Chest*, **86**, 459–62.

Leon, D.A., Chenet, L., Shkolnikov, V.M., *et al.* (1997). Huge variation in Russian mortality rates 1984–94: artefact, alcohol or what? *Lancet*, **350**, 383–8.

Loh, J., Randers, J., MacGillivray, A., Kapos, V., Jenkins, M., Groombridge, B., and Cox, N. (1998). *Living planet report, 1998*. WWF International, Gland, Switzerland; New Economics Foundation, London; World Conservation Monitoring Centre, Cambridge.

Lopez, A. (1996). The lung cancer epidemic in developed countries. In *Adult mortality in developed countries* (ed. A. Lopez), pp. 111–34. Oxford University Press.

Lopez, A.D., Collishaw, N.E., and Piha, T. (1994). A descriptive model of the cigarette epidemic in developed countries. *Tobacco Control*, **3**, 242–7.

McCarthy, M. (1999). Transport and health. In *Social determinants of health* (ed. M. Marmot and R.G. Wilkinson), pp. 132–54. Oxford University Press.

McIntosh, H. (1995). Black teens not smoking in great numbers. *Journal of the National Cancer Institute*, **87**, 564–5.

MacMahon, S., Peto, R., Cutler, J., *et al.* (1990). Blood pressure, stroke, and coronary heart disease. Part 1: Prolonged differences in blood pressure: prospective observational studies corrected for the regression dilution bias . *Lancet*, **335**, 765–74.

McMichael, A.J. and Powles, J.W. (1999). Human numbers, environment, sustainability and health. *British Medical Journal*, **319**, 977–80.

Marmot, M. and Wilkinson, R.G. (ed.) (1999). *Social determinants of health*. Oxford University Press.

Marx, K. and Engels, F. (1959). The German ideology (excerpts) (written 1846, trans. 1939). In *Marx and Engels: basic writings on politics and philosophy* (ed. L.S. Feuer), pp. 246–61. Doubleday, New York.

Mead, R. (1775). *The medical works of Richard Mead, M.D.* Alexander Donaldson and Charles Elliot, Edinburgh. (Reprinted by AMS Press, New York, 1978.)

Mosterd, A., D'Agostino, R.B., Silbershatz, H., *et al.* (1999). Trends in the prevalence of hypertension, antihypertensive therapy, and left ventricular hypertrophy from 1950 to 1989. *New England Journal of Medicine*, **340**, 1221–7.

Murray, C.J.L. and Lopez, A.D. (1996). *The global burden of disease: a comprehensive assessment of mortality and disability from diseases, injuries and risk factors in 1990 and projected to 2020*. Harvard School of Public Health on behalf of WHO and the World Bank. Harvard University Press, Cambridge, MA.

National Research Council (1993). National Academy of Sciences Committee on Toxicology. *Health effects of ingested flouride*. National Academy Press, Washington, DC.

OPCS (Office of Population, Censuses and Statistics) (1988, 1995). *OPCS Monitor*, Series DH3 Sudden Infant Deaths. OPCS, London.

Peto, R., Lopez, A.D., Boreham, J., Thun, M., and Heath, C.J. (1992). Mortality from tobacco in developed countries: indirect estimation from national vital statistics. *Lancet*, **339**, 1268–78.

Peto, R., Lopez, A.D., Boreham, J., Thun, M.J., and Heath, C., Jr (1994). *Mortality from smoking in developed countries, 1950–2000: indirect estimates from national vital statistics.* Oxford University Press.

Pierce, J.P., Lee, L., and Gilpin, E.A. (1994). Smoking initiation by adolescent girls, 1944 through 1988. An association with targeted advertising. *Journal of the American Medical Association*, **271**, 608–11.

Pierce, J.P., Choi, W.S., Gilpin, E.A., Farkas, A.J., and Berry, C.C. (1998). Tobacco industry promotion of cigarettes and adolescent smoking. *Journal of the American Medical Association*, **279**, 511–15. (Erratum. *Journal of the American Medical Association*, **280**, 422 (1998).)

Pollock, D. (1999). *Denial and delay: the political history of smoking and health, 1951–1964.* Action on Smoking and Health, London.

Powles, J.W. and Gifford, S. (1993). Health of nations: Lessons from Victoria, Australia. *British Medical Journal*, **306**, 125–7.

Powles, J.W. and Sanz, M.A. (1999). 'Arcadian bias' in discussions of the Mediterranean advantage. *Proceedings of the 15th International Scientific Meeting of the International Epidemiological Association*, p. 37. IEA, Florence.

Prentice, A.M. and Jebb, S.A. (1995). Obesity in Britain: gluttony or sloth? *British Medical Journal*, **311**, 437–39, 1568–9.

Puska, P., Korhonen, H.J., Torppa, J., *et al.* (1993). Does community-wide prevention of cardiovascular diseases influence cancer mortality? *European Journal of Cancer Prevention*, **2**, 457–60.

Putnam, R.D., Leonardi, R., and Nanetti, R.Y. (1993). *Making democracy work: civic traditions in modern Italy.* Princeton University Press.

Rees, W.E. (1999). Consuming the earth: the biophysics of sustainability. *Ecological Economics*, **29**, 23–7.

Robinson, T.N., Hammer, L.D., Killen, J.D., *et al.* (1993). Does television viewing increase obesity and reduce physical activity? Cross-sectional and longitudinal analyses among adolescent girls. *Paediatrics*, **91**, 272–80.

Rose, G. (1985). Sick individuals and sick populations. *International Journal of Epidemiology*, **14**, 32–8.

Rose, R. (2000). Getting things done in an anti-modern society: social capital networks in Russia. In *Social capital: a multifaceted perspective* (ed. P. Dasgupta and I. Serageldin), pp. 147–71. World Bank, Washington, DC.

Royal College of Physicians (1962). *Smoking and health.* Pitman Medical, London.

Secretary of State for Health (1992). *The health of the nation.* HMSO, London.

Secretary of State for Health (1998). *Our healthier nation: a contract for health. A consultation paper.* HMSO, London.

Secretary of State for Health (1999). *Saving lives: our healthier nation.* HMSO, London.

Secretary of State for Social Services (1988). *Public health in England: the report of the Committee of Inquiry into the future development of the Public Health Function* (D. Acheson, Chairman). HMSO, London.

Serageldin, I. (1996). *Sustainability and the wealth of nations. First steps in an ongoing journey.* Environmentally Sustainable Development Studies and Monographs Series No. 5. World Bank, Washington, DC.

Serdula, M.K., Mokdad, A.H., Williamson, D.F., Galuska, D.A., Mendlein, J.M., and Heath, G.W. (1999). Prevalence of attempting weight loss and strategies for controlling weight. *Journal of the American Medical Association*, **282**, 1353–8.

Shaw, M., Dorling, D., and Davey Smith, G. (1999). Poverty, social exclusion and minorities. In *Social determinants of health* (ed. M.G. Marmot and R.G. Wilkinson), pp. 211–39. Oxford University Press.

Simon, J. (1890). *English sanitary institutions, reviewed in their course of development, and in some of their political and social relations.* Cassell, London.

Smeed, R.J. (1972). The usefulness of formulae in traffic engineering and road safety. *Accident Analysis and Prevention*, **4**, 303–12.

Spurgeon, D. (1999). Studies reveal increased smoking among students in Canada. *British Medical Journal*, **319**, 1391A.

Stegmayr, B., Asplund, K., Kuulasmaa, K., Rajakangas, A.M., Thorvaldsen, P., and Tuomilehto, J. (1997). Stroke incidence and mortality correlated to stroke risk factors in the WHO MONICA Project. An ecological study of 18 populations. *Stroke*, **28**, 1367–74.

Stephen, A.M. and Wald, N.J. (1990). Trends in individual consumption of dietary fat in the United States, 1920–1984. *American Journal of Clinical Nutrition*, **52**, 457–69.

Strachan, D. and Rose, G. (1991). Strategies of prevention revisited: effects of imprecise measurement of risk factors on the evaluation of 'high-risk' and 'population-based' approaches to prevention of cardiovascular disease. *Journal of Clinical Epidemiology*, **44**, 1187–96.

Stunkard, A.J., Sorensen, T.I., Hanis, C., *et al.* (1986). An adoption study of human obesity. *New England Journal of Medicine*, **314**, 193–8.

Szreter, S. (1988). The importance of social intervention in Britain's mortality decline *c.* 1850–1914: a re-interpretation of the role of public health. *Journal of the Society for the Social History of Medicine*, **1**, 1–37.

Szreter, S. (1997). Economic growth, disruption, deprivation, disease, and death: on the importance of the politics of public health for development. *Population and Development Review*, **23**, 693–728.

Tobacco Advisory Group (2000). Royal College of Physicians. *Nicotine addiction in Britain.* Royal College of Physicians, London.

US Department of Health and Human Services (1994). *Preventing tobacco use among young people: A report of the Surgeon General.* Serial No. 017-001-00491-0. US Department of Health and Human Services, Public Health Service, Centers for Disease Control and Prevention, Atlanta, GA.

US Department of Health and Human Services (1996). *Physical activity and health: a report of the Surgeon General.* US Department of Health and Human Services, Centers for Disease Control and Prevention, Atlanta, GA.

US Department of Health and Human Services and Batelle (1995). *For a healthy nation: returns on investment in public health.* US Government Printing Office, Washington, DC.

US Public Health Service (1964). *Smoking and health: report of the advisory committee to the Surgeon General of the Public Health Service.* US Department of Health, Education and Welfare, Washington, DC.

Vartiainen, E., Puska, P., Jousilahti, P., Korhonen, H.J., Tuomilehto, J., and Nissinen, A. (1994). Twenty-year trends in coronary risk factors in North Karelia and in other areas of Finland. *International Journal of Epidemiology*, **23**, 495–504.

VicRoads (1993). *Road Traffic Accidents Involving Serious Casualties.* VicRoads, Melbourne.

Wareham, N.J., Hennings, S.J., Prentice, A.M., and Day, N.E. (1997). Feasibility of heart-rate monitoring to estimate total level and pattern of energy expenditure in a population-based epidemiological study: the Ely Young Cohort Feasibility Study 1994–5. *British Journal of Nutrition*, **78**, 889–900.

Wareham, N.J., Wong, M.-Y., and Day, N.E. (2000). Glucose intolerance and physical inactivity: the relative importance of low habitual energy expenditure and cardio-respiratory fitness. *American Journal of Epidemiology*, **152**, 132–9.

Weber, M. (1991). *Politics as a vocation* (originally published as *Politik als Beruf*, 1921, trans. by the editors). In *From Max Weber: essays in sociology* (ed. H.H. Gerth and M. Wright). Routledge, London.

White, S. (1996). *Russia goes dry: alcohol, state and society.* Cambridge University Press.

Widdowson, E.M. (1936). A study of English diets by the individual method, part I. Men. *Journal of Hygiene*, **36**, 269–79.

Widdowson, E.M. and McCance, R.A. (1936). A study of English diets by the individual method, part II. Women. *Journal of Hygiene*, **36**, 293–99.

Wigley, T.M.L., Richels, R., and Edmonds, J.A. (1996). Economic and environmental choices in the stabilization of atmospheric CO_2 concentrations. *Nature*, **379**, 240–3.

Willett, W.C., Sacks, F., Trichopoulou, A., *et al.* (1995). Mediterranean diet pyramid: a cultural model for healthy eating. *American Journal of Clinical Nutrition*, **61**, 1402S–6S.

WHO (World Health Organization) (1998). *Obesity: preventing and managing the global epidemic. Report of a WHO Consultation on obesity, Geneva 2–5 June 1997.* WHO, Geneva.

WHO (World Health Organization) (1999). *World Health Report 1999: Making a difference*. WHO, Geneva.

World Bank (1997). *The state in a changing world: world development report 1997*. Oxford University Press for the World Bank, New York.

World Bank (1999). *Entering the 21st century: World Development Report 1999/2000*. Oxford University Press for the World Bank, New York.

World Resources Institute (1998). United Nations Environment Programme, United Nations Development Programme, and World Bank. *World resources 1998–99*. Oxford University Press, New York.

3.3 Health policies in developing countries

Adetokunbo O. Lucas

At the close of the twentieth century, health policy-makers and practitioners in developing countries were approaching the future with cautious optimism. The enormous health gains in past decades have generated the expectation of continuing progress in the coming years. Lessons learnt from the application of existing knowledge and the promise of new health technologies raise hopes of further improvements in health as shown by declining mortality, increased expectation of life, and control of major endemic diseases (Table 1 and Fig. 1). This optimism is tempered by the threats posed by the emergence of new diseases and the continuing pressures on the health sector to meet the rapidly escalating costs of health services (WHO 1999). Although much progress has been made in the past few decades, many people in developing countries still do not have access to essential health care (Fig. 2).

Although developing countries have some features in common, there is considerable variation within the group with regard to the health situation and each country's capacity to deal with them. Economic growth in the more advanced developing countries have secured relatively large resources as compared with the least developed countries such that there is a 20-fold difference in national income as measured by gross domestic product between the most affluent developing countries and the poorest nations. Institutional capacity and human resources show the same diversity among developing countries. Although the health systems of these nations share some features, it is difficult to make generalizations that apply equally to all of these countries. One common feature is the large gap between the health needs and demands of the population, and the available resources. Whilst the least developed countries are still struggling to provide basic health services, the more advanced countries are endeavouring to meet the rising expectations and demands of their population for the most up-to-date high technology diagnostic tools and treatments. Much of the debate on health policy in developing countries revolves around this central issue of making the best use of limited resources in environments in which there is a wide gap between needs and resources, expectations and performance.

The process of policy-making for the health sector has become increasingly intricate. Health practitioners, policy-makers, and planners have to contend with three main issues: diversity, complexity, and change.

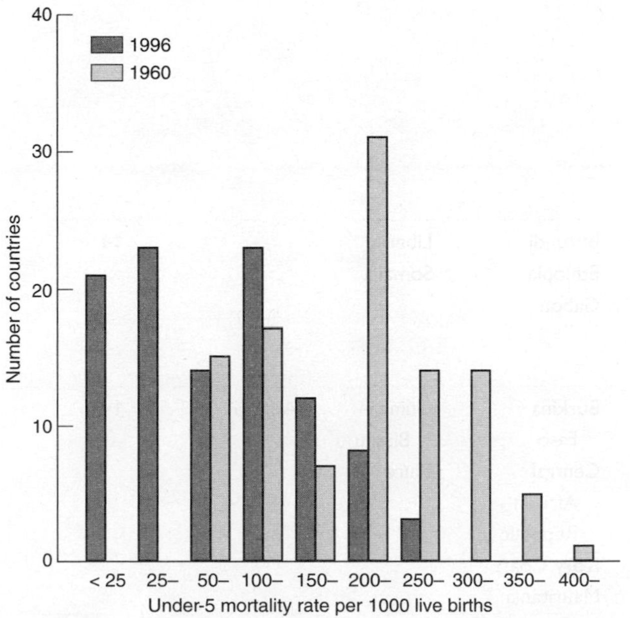

Fig. 1 The distribution of under-5 mortality rates in 1996 in 104 countries with under-5 mortality rates of 50 per 1000 live births and above in 1960.

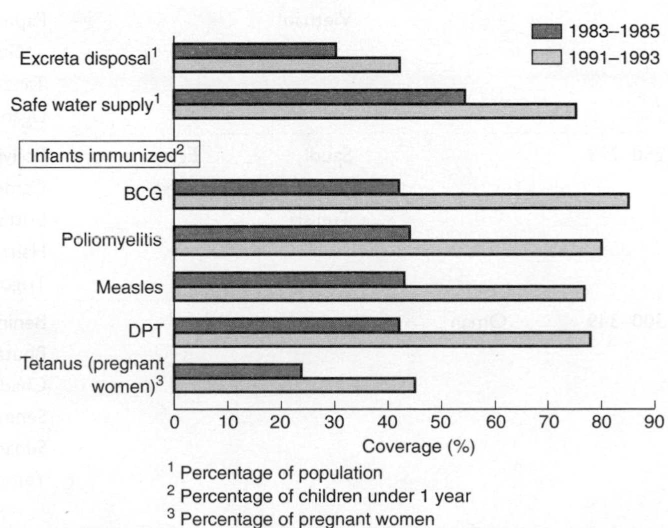

Fig. 2 Access to selected elements of primary health care, developing countries 1983 to 1985 and 1991 to 1993.

Table 1 Under-5 mortality rates (U5MR) in 1996 in 104 countries with under-5 mortality rates of 50 and above in 1960

U5MR in 1960	<25 (in 1996)	25–49 (in 1996)	50–99 (in 1996)	100–149 (in 1996)	150–199 (in 1996)	200–249 (in 1996)	250+ (in 1996)	Total in 1960
50–99	Bulgaria Cuba Greece Hong Kong Hungary Italy Jamaica Mauritius Poland Spain Trinidad and Tobago	Argentina Paraguay Romania Venezuela						15
100–149	Chile Costa Rica Kuwait Malaysia Panama Portugal S. Korea Sri Lanka	Colombia Jordan Lebanon Mexico N. Korea Philippines Thailand	Dominican Republic South Africa					17
150–199		Albania Ecuador	Brazil Botswana Mongolia Zimbabwe	Iraq				7
200–249	United Arab Emirates	Algeria China El Salvador Honduras Iran Syria Turkey Vietnam	Guatemala Indonesia Kenya Namibia Nicaragua Peru	Bangladesh Congo Ghana India Laos Lesotho Nepal Pakistan Papua New Guinea Tanzania Uganda	Cambodia Myanmar Nigeria Rwanda	Zambia		31
250–299		Saudi Arabia Tunisia	Egypt Libya	Bolivia Cameroon Eritrea Haiti Togo	Burundi Ethiopia Gabon	Liberia Somalia		14
300–349	Oman			Benin Bhutan Chad Senegal Sudan Yemen	Burkina Faso Central African Republic Ivory Coast Mauritania	Guinea–Bissau Zaïre	Angola	14
350–399					Madagascar	Guinea Malawi	Afghanistan Sierra Leone	5
400+						Mali		1
Total in 1996	21	23	14	23	12	8	3	104

Diversity

There is often great diversity within countries, as well as between and within different geographical areas. Ecological and geographical factors account for some of the variation in the pattern of distribution of health and disease but economic, social, and cultural determinants also contribute to the diversity. The association of poverty with poor health status is a consistent finding in both developed and developing countries.

Complexity

The explosion of new knowledge and innovative health technologies have markedly increased the complexity of health care. The expanding scope of prophylactic, diagnostic, and therapeutic options demands an increasing range of specific programmes with the associated need for specialist personnel, new categories of support staff, high-technology equipment, and infrastructure. Figure 3 illustrates the complex interaction of medical and non-medical factors that are involved in perpetuating the high maternal mortality rates occurring in the developing world. It also offers clues as to the package of interventions that are required to reduce maternal mortality (Box 1) (McCarthy and Maine 1992). The complex interaction of medical and non-medical factors in the dynamics of health and disease calls for a critical analysis of needs and opportunities as the basis of designing and managing health programmes. Rather than blindly attempting to deliver standardized prepackaged stereotyped interventions, health authorities should try to match the services to suit local needs. To complement medical inputs from the health sector it is necessary to mobilize intersectoral action because of the important influence of non-medical factors on health, such as:

- agriculture (food security and nutrition)
- education (especially women's education)
- waterworks and sanitation
- labour and industry (health of workers, pollution).

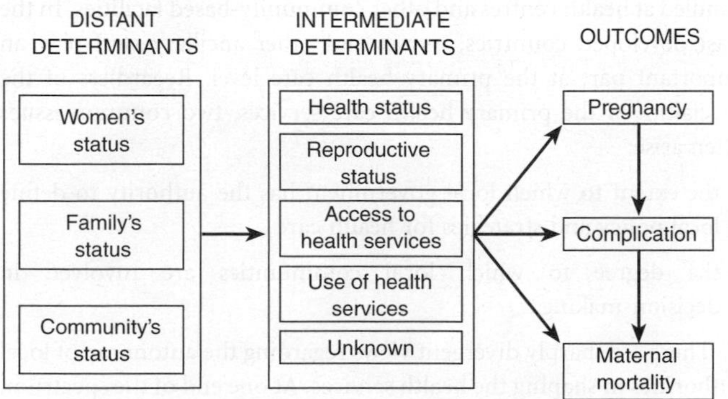

Fig. 3 The complex interaction of factors involved in the epidemiology of maternal mortality. (Source: McCarthy and Maine 1992.)

Box 1 Prevention of maternal mortality

- Half a million or more women die each year from complications of pregnancy and childbirth
- Most of these deaths occur in developing countries
- The clinical causes of the deaths are well known and are amenable to treatment
- These deaths occur against the background of intermediate and remote causes as illustrated in Fig. 3
- The prevention of maternal mortality must ultimately address all these issues but the interventions must be ranked in an appropriate order of priority and designed to suit the local circumstances
- In countries with very high maternal mortality rates, the highest priority should be assigned to improving emergency obstetric care; other interventions will include reduction of exposure to high-risk and unwanted pregnancies by the provision of family planning services, safe abortion, training and supervision of traditional birth attendants, and improvement of other aspects of maternal health services

Source: McCarthy and Maine (1992); McCarthy (1997).

Change

Policy-making in developing countries has to be fluid and dynamic to adapt strategies and programmes to the many changes that are occurring in the environment.

Epidemiological transition

As in developed countries, developing countries are undergoing epidemiological transition. The traditional health problems, such as childhood diseases and communicable diseases, are declining, whilst chronic diseases, such as cancers, cardiovascular diseases, diabetes, etc., are becoming increasingly prominent causes of morbidity and mortality. Many developing countries present a mixed picture with the persistence of infectious diseases compounded by malnutrition and the emergence of chronic diseases especially among the urban élite (Frenk *et al.* 1989). However, there is the constant threat of the emergence of new infections and the re-emergence of old diseases that were previously controlled, as shown respectively by the recent examples of HIV/AIDS and tuberculosis (Institute of Medicine 1992).

Epidemics and other emergencies

In addition to this slowly evolving epidemiological transition, more rapid changes occur in the form of epidemics and other acute problems, for example natural disasters (floods, drought, etc.).

Socio-economic variables

Changes in the economic and social situation in the country may have a profound effect on the health sector. Health policies have had to be modified in the light of rapid development in some countries and economic recession in others. In the immediate post-Second World

War era, macroeconomic policies emphasizing central planning and welfare programmes gained popularity. This trend has been reversed in recent decades, with national policies increasingly favouring free-market economy in place of welfare programmes and central control. These changes have important implications with regard to policies in health and other social sectors.

Major challenges and issues

Policy-making in the health sector of developing countries involves many complex problems. This chapter highlights seven critical issues:

(1) health reform with special emphasis on structural reform and decentralization;

(2) tools for policy-making—assessment of burden of disease, cost-effectiveness, and health accounts;

(3) financing health care—cost recovery schemes, user fees, and private insurance;

(4) public–private partnerships in the delivery and financing of health care and in drug policy;

(5) health research;

(6) international agencies such as the World Health Organization (**WHO**), the World Bank, the United Nations International Children's Emergency Fund (**UNICEF**), and bilateral donor agencies;

(7) equity in health.

Health reform: special emphasis on structural reform/decentralization

The rapid advances in health technologies, the increasing demands and expectations of populations, and the escalating costs of health care are challenging governments in both developed and developing countries. Governments are responding to these dramatic changes and the associated challenges by undertaking reforms of the health sector. In order to meet the needs and demands of their populations, they are redesigning mechanisms for delivering care and paying for the services (World Bank 1993).

Health reform has been defined as 'sustained purposeful change to improve efficiency, equity and effectiveness of the health sector' (Berman 1995). The decentralization of the planning and management of health services is a common feature of these reforms. Governments cannot efficiently manage the delivery of health care in large countries with dispersed populations. In a decentralized system, the central Ministry of Health can set national goals and targets, whilst devolving the responsibility for detailed management of the services to peripheral authorities—provincial, state, municipal, and local governments.

Models of decentralization

The exact details of decentralization vary from country to country. Although the idea of decentralization of health services has gained favour in recent years, there is no consensus on the ideal pattern for allocating functions, and sharing and dividing power, between the various levels of government. Some of the variations relate to the type of government (federal or unitary), but other factors, such as the size of country, political systems, and other variables, influence decisions about decentralization. A simple model considers the management of health services at three levels:

- primary health care through community level services and local referral hospitals
- provincial or state level co-ordinating services in defined geographical parts of the country
- setting up a ministry of health at central government level.

Decentralization involves allocating functions to provincial and local governments as well as defining their relationships with each other and with the central government.

Primary health care

The responsibility for community health care is usually devolved to local or municipal governments. In developed countries, primary health care is largely doctor based with the support of nurses and other paramedical staff; the aim is to provide comprehensive health care and associated social services through community-based facilities and referral hospitals.

In developing countries, the package of services that are delivered at this level were formerly labelled as 'basic health services' but were further refined into the eight elements of primary health care as defined at the Alma-Ata Conference (WHO 1978) including at least the following items:

- immunization against major infectious diseases
- education concerning prevailing health conditions
- promotion of food supply and proper nutrition
- adequate supply of safe water and basic sanitation
- maternal and child health care including family planning
- appropriate treatment of common diseases and injuries
- prevention and control of locally endemic diseases
- provision of essential drugs.

This list has been further elaborated to make more explicit items that were not clearly expressed such as family planning and reproductive health with maternal and child health, and the promotion of mental health.

The usual pattern of primary health care is a network of community-based services with appropriate back-up from referral hospitals which deal with difficult problems that cannot be effectively handled at health centres and other community-based facilities. In the least developed countries, nurses and other ancillary staff play an important part at the primary health care level. Regardless of the specialties of the primary health care services, two common issues often arise:

- the extent to which local government has the authority to define local policy and strategies for health care
- the degree to which local communities are involved in decision-making.

There are sharply divergent views regarding the autonomy of local authorities in shaping the health services. At one end of the spectrum, the WHO proposes integrated health care at the district level involving all health-care providers, both public and private, and all health systems, whether they are modern, traditional, orthodox, or non-orthodox. This model defines the district as the smallest planning unit for health care, involving community-based services through health centres and other institutions providing ambulatory care as well as the referral hospital (WHO 1987). The WHO model is inclusive and involves collaboration of all stakeholders: the public sector represented by the local government, the private sector (both for profit and non-profit), traditional healers, and other representatives of civil society. The hope is that the consensus that emerges from the interaction of these stakeholders would lead to the development of realistic health programmes that are culturally sensitive, financially sustainable, and capable of growth and expansion as the community develops (Tarimo 1991).

Some critics, who regard the WHO's approach as being too broad and therefore unrealistic, proposed an alternative strategy that aims at delivering a limited number of interventions of proven efficacy and cost-effectiveness, for example immunization and mass chemotherapy for some endemic infections (Walsh and Warren 1979; Warren 1988). UNICEF's GOBI-FFF plan and the World Bank's clinical and public health packages are examples of proposed cost-effective interventions (Box 2), which include measures on growth monitoring, oral dehydration, breast feeding, immunization (**GOBI**), family planning, female education, and supplementary feeding of pregnant women (**FFF**).

Box 2 Cost-effective public health and clinical packages recommended by the World Bank (World Bank Report 1993)

Public health package

- The expanded programme on immunization, including micronutrients (iron, vitamin A, and iodine) supplementation
- School health programmes to treat worm infections and micronutrient deficiencies and to promote health education
- Programmes to increase public knowledge about family planning and nutrition, about self-care or indications for seeking care, and about vector control and disease surveillance activities
- Programmes to reduce consumption of tobacco, alcohol, and other drugs; and AIDS prevention programmes with a strong sexually transmitted disease component

Clinical package

- Prenatal and delivery care
- Family planning services
- Treatment of tuberculosis
- Case management of sexually transmitted diseases

Rather than grant local authorities the right to define local priorities and strategies, this selective primary health care programme would require each community to conform to a centrally determined national programme, which is made up of a limited list of well-defined specific interventions. There is some danger that selective primary health care would merely recreate vertical programmes in which practitioners in the field would be required to implement prepackaged interventions blindly. An acceptable compromise would be to develop primary health care systematically using elements of UNICEF's GOBI-FFF plan, the World Bank's clinical and public health packages, and similar cost-effective interventions as building blocks of primary health care whilst retaining local flexibility and decision-making.

Provincial or state level provision

In federal states, health services are usually devolved to provincial authorities, which serve an intermediate role between the central government and the local health authorities; they develop regional policies and programmes in the context of the overall national policy and plans. They support, supervise, and co-ordinate the local health services and they provide services such as specialist hospitals that cannot be replicated in individual local government areas. Again, the question arises over the extent to which provincial health departments have the authority to undertake independent action in designing the services, and how they relate to the private sector and the civil society in drawing up their strategies and plans.

Central government provision

In a decentralized health service, the central government retains certain key functions, which may include the following:

- setting national goals and targets
- establishment of standards
- accreditation of training programmes
- registration of drugs
- national disease surveillance
- provision of highly specialized services including research
- emergency response to natural disasters and major epidemics
- international relations.

Formal protocols define the official relationships of the various health authorities but, ideally, the interactions should represent mutual support towards the achievement of the common goal.

Making decentralization work

Decentralization of health services is a common feature of the reform process that many countries are currently undertaking. Other elements in the reform package may include a variety of structural changes, new mechanisms for financing health care, redefined relationships with the private sector, and other policy changes. There is also much variation in the structure of decentralized services but regardless of the specific details, certain important issues need to be addressed as follows:

- autonomy
- financial resources
- professional and technical capacity
- information system
- other health-related sectors
- relationship with other health-care providers.

Autonomy

In federal states, constitutional authority may provide provincial governments with higher degrees of autonomy than is given to regional health authorities in unitary states. Provincial and local health authorities in unitary states may have the responsibility of implementing services under the direction of the central government with little authority to make changes in the programmes.

Financial resources

Decentralization of health services is generally accompanied by resource flows from the central government to peripheral authorities. The subvention from the central government may represent the bulk of the resources available to the local health authority but some authorities supplement central funds with revenue derived from local taxes and user fees. In general, local authorities that can raise funds through taxation and/or can retain revenue derived from user fees tend to have more autonomy in making decisions and fine tuning health policies to suit local needs.

Information system

Up-to-date information is an essential tool for the management of health services for identifying needs, designing services, and for monitoring performance as well as changes in health status (Rosen 1999). Ideally, the data should be disaggregated by the standard demographic indicators—age, sex, and marital status—but also by variables that may be relevant locally, for example ethnic group, race, religion, etc.

Professional and technical capacity

Local professional and technical capacity is an important issue in decentralized health systems. In order for the devolved services to function efficiently, the peripheral health authorities must have appropriate capacity for planning, implementing, and monitoring services. In particular, they must be able to gather and analyse relevant data as the basis for decision-making and monitoring. Many developing countries are in the process of building such capacity that is available in long established local authorities of developed countries. In any event, even in the most advanced countries, the resources of regional authorities and central government are sometimes required to fill the gaps in local capacity.

Other health-care providers

In addition to the public sector, private providers, both for profit as well as non-profit agencies, are involved in health care. In developing countries, traditional healers still play a prominent role and as in developed countries, practitioners of alternative medicine are also increasingly popular. Local health services relate vertically to regional and central authorities, which provide support for supplementing local capacity both for dealing with emergencies as well as for long-term interventions. They must interact horizontally with other local health authorities especially those that serve neighbouring areas. By sharing information, they can reinforce their programmes by learning from each other and they can also achieve economies of scale by sharing resources.

Other health-related sectors

The well-known effects of socio-economic and environmental factors on health dictate the need for intersectoral action. National policies in such sectors as education, agriculture, welfare, and environment are translated into action through provincial and local authorities. Decentralization of these health-related sectors would facilitate interaction with their colleagues in the health sector.

Tools for policy-making

Previously, policy-making in developing countries was largely determined by the dictates of influential experts rather than by objective analysis. In the immediate postindependence period, some developing countries copy models of health services in developed countries with particular emphasis on the construction of large tertiary hospitals. The high cost of maintaining such establishments often distort the national health budget leaving very little resources for supporting less expensive but highly effective community-based services. Because of severe resource constraints, developing countries should set clear priorities, and adopt policies that would help to achieve maximum improvement in health in return for minimum expenditure.

It was relatively easy to establish priority lists in the traditional epidemiological situation where a few major conditions, mainly acute infectious diseases, accounted for a high proportion of deaths. In such situations, it was possible to rank priorities by considering the mortality rates from specific acute infectious diseases or the prevalence of chronic disabling diseases like onchocerciasis (river blindness). As major epidemic and endemic conditions come under control, the process of priority setting has become more complex. The increasing pressure on policy-makers to base their decisions on sound evidence has led them to use three new types of tools:

- measurement of 'burden of disease'
- assessment of the cost-effectiveness of interventions
- analysis of national health accounts.

Burden of disease

Objective decisions in setting priorities require measurements of the impact of individual conditions and risk factors, and their amenability to control. What is required is an index that would summarize the impact of specific health problems in terms of disease, disability, and premature death. Early attempts to develop a summary index were based on the calculation of the number of useful days of life lost from premature death (mortality) and from disability (morbidity) (Ghana Health Assessment Project Team 1981). This approach was further refined to a new measure, the disability-adjusted life year (**DALY**) which combines losses from death and disability but also makes allowance for:

- a discount rate, so that future years of healthy life are valued at progressively lower level)
- age weights, so that years lost at different ages are given different values (Murray 1994*a*,*c*).

The WHO and the World Bank collaborated in a venture to measure the global burden of disease (Murray and Lopez 1996). Individual countries are being encouraged to measure their national burden of disease. Measurement of burden of disease using DALYs is proving a valuable tool but is rather a complex operation, particularly difficult in developing countries that lack reliable data about the frequency and distribution of various health problems. In such situations, estimates of DALYs are based on extrapolations from limited studies and rough approximations. However, attempts to calculate the national burden of disease draw attention to gaps in information that can be filled by improvements in the national health information systems. The DALY is proving a useful tool but more

Table 2 Global pattern of burden of disease in countries by income

Cause of loss of DALYs	DALYs lost (%)	
	High-income countries	**Low-income countries**
Group I: communicable diseases, maternal and perinatal conditions, and nutritional deficiencies	7834 (7.2)	557 694 (43.8)
Group II: non-communicable conditions	87 732 (81.4)	5007 631 (39.8)
Group III: injuries	12 739 (1.8)	208 934 (16.4)
All causes	108 305 (100)	1274 859 (100)
Population (thousands)	907 828	4976 748

work is required to refine and simplify it (Morrow and Bryant 1995; Hyder *et al.* 1998) (Table 2).

The DALY is used to:

- rank diseases and conditions by the burden of disease;
- estimate the cost-effectiveness of interventions by comparing the cost of averting a DALY.

Cost-effectiveness analysis enable policy-makers to compare different interventions for the same condition and select the interventions that give the largest gain in DALYs per unit cost (Murray 1994*a*). It also allows comparison of diseases and conditions by the availability of cost-effective interventions. It may provide clues on how modifications of interventions could make them more cost-effective.

National health accounts

Previously, policy-makers concentrated mainly on spending within the public sector, ignoring private spending through insurance, corporate arrangements, employees' schemes, and out-of-pocket expenditure. Health economists now obtain a more comprehensive view of health expenditures by compiling national health accounts. These analyses attempt to obtain an overview of health spending from all sources—public and private, corporate and personal—into comprehensive health accounts. The results affect the choices made within the public sector but also influence the public role in providing guidelines to the private sector and communities on the most cost-effective uses of their personal expenditure. The basic analysis consists of a matrix of elements as follows:

(1) the columns of the matrix list all sources of health spending—both public sources (taxation and national social insurance) and private sources including employment-based schemes, privately financed insurance, and out-of-pocket expenditure;

(2) the rows of the matrix show the distribution of expenditure for personal health care, public health and environmental sanitation services, and administration.

Disaggregating the items in the columns and rows generates more elaborate analyses, providing more detailed information about sources and spending. Thus, the analyses could show variations over time, by geography, by population subgroups, or any other variable that is relevant to policy-making (Berman 1997).

Financing health care

The wide margin between the public resources for health and the demands and expectations of the population is a common challenge to health authorities in developing countries. Governments should ensure that there is an adequate level of financing from public and private sources to develop and sustain the essential components of the health services. In some of the more advanced developing countries which have enjoyed economic boom in recent years, the health services have grown and are meeting many of the public demands. In the poorer nations, especially those that have experienced marked economic decline, there is increasing pressure on public spending for health and other social sectors. Macroeconomic policies advocated by the International Monetary Fund and other funding agencies have forced many governments to trim public spending on health and to reassess the allocation of their limited resources.

Under these circumstances, policy-makers are exploring approaches to increase the resources available for health, allocate the limited resources to target priority conditions and groups, and promote equity. Specifically, governments are endeavouring to:

- develop income-generating schemes
- promote supplementary sources of finance, for example privately financed insurance schemes.

Income generation

In the least developed countries, it is critically important to increase the financial resources if the health sector is to provide basic essential services. In the more advanced middle-income countries, the main issue is how to organize and manage a prepay system that is efficient and fair. In the high-income developing countries, the absolute quantity of funds is not the critical factor, rather it is often a question of using resources in the most cost-effective manner and promoting equity.

Many countries that previously offered health services at no cost or at highly subsidized rates are now imposing fees on users at the point of delivery. The aim is to generate additional income for use by the public sector, to enable the public sector to redistribute resources in favour of the poor, and to achieve increasing self-reliance for sustainable community health programmes.

Mobilizing additional resources for health

The main objective of user fees is to generate resources that can be used to expand the quantity and improve the quality of health services. These schemes are designed not only to recover some of the costs involved in providing the services but also to focus public resources on top priorities. In favour of user fees is the observation that free health services selectively subsidize the more affluent members of society.

This is particularly true for curative services in hospitals. The share of hospitals in total public recurrent expenditure in many developing countries ranges from 40 to 80 per cent, but only a small unrepresentative section of the population, the urban élite, benefits directly from these hospital services (Barnum and Kutzin 1993) (Fig. 4).

Redistribution of resources

User charges enable the public sector to reallocate the resources by withdrawing subsidies from those who can afford to pay and redirecting the savings to expand cost-effective public health services to the poor. The imposition of charges is based on the evidence from studies on health accounts that people already spend a considerable amount of private resources in paying for health care (Shaw and Griffin 1995).

Community financing

User fees have also been designed to promote self-reliance and make community health programmes sustainable. At the primary health care level, this manifests as charges for medications with a small profit margin that can be used to support local health services (Gbedonou *et al.* 1994; Diallo *et al.* 1996; Anderson 1998).

The imposition of user fees remains a contentious issue. The advocates of this policy claim that it is a progressive measure that promotes equity. Their analyses suggest that the public sector can derive additional revenue from clients who are willing and able to pay. The additional income can be used to improve the quality of services and to subsidize poor people who are exempted from payment (World Bank 1994; Shaw and Griffin 1995). Noting the sharp decline in the utilization of services when user fees are introduced, other workers regard such schemes as a regressive policy that further widens the gap between the rich and the poor (Ekwempu *et al.* 1990). Some of the concerns about equity can be met by carefully designed exemptions for certain people and for specific services.

Many lessons are being learnt in the development of these schemes. People seem more willing to pay if they perceive an improvement in the quality of services. Local institutions can deliver these improved services if they are able to retain some of the income generated from user fees. A major challenge is the administration of cost recovery schemes and the management of services to reflect the increased income.

Risk sharing through privately financed health insurance

The promotion of self-financed insurance schemes is a complementary policy; it is designed to make it easier for those who can afford to pay to share the risk, thereby protecting individuals and families against the effects of catastrophic illness or accident. The availability of

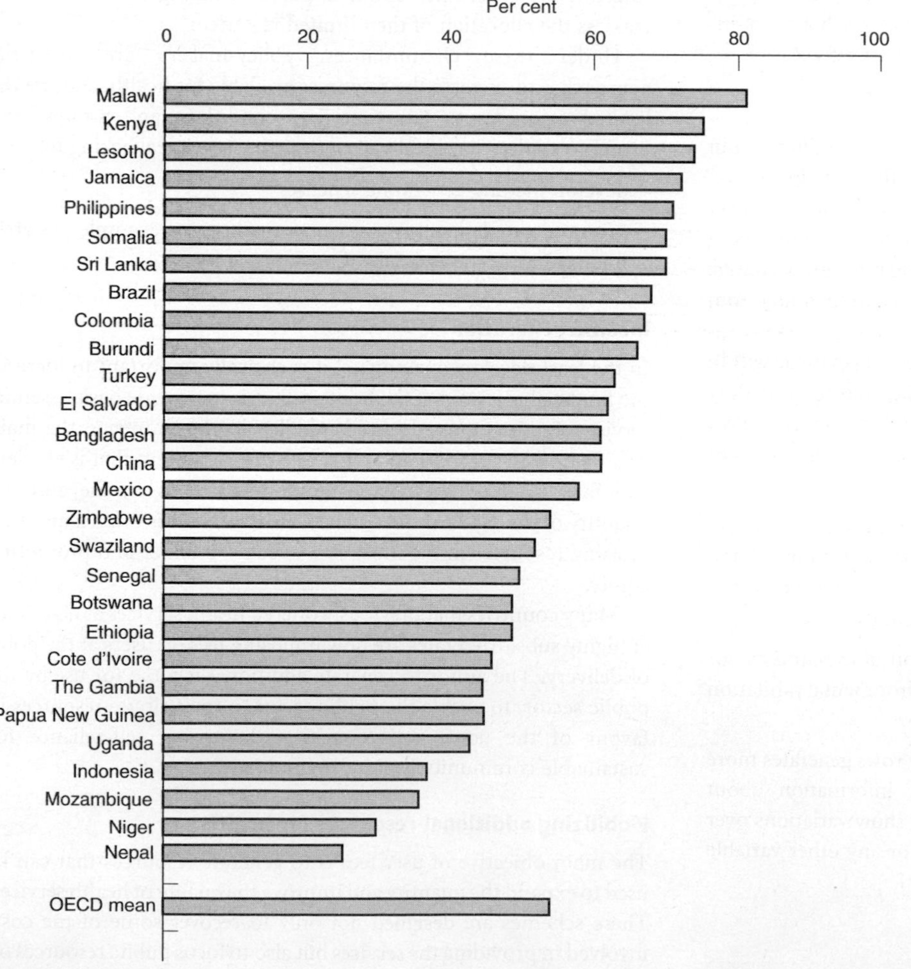

Fig. 4 The share of hospitals in total public recurrent expenditure.

personal insurance schemes facilitates the operation of cost recovery schemes in hospitals. Private insurance schemes would also promote the development of the private providers of hospital and other health services thereby reducing the pressure on public institutions.

In summary, the policy direction for financing health care in many developing countries is to ensure that those who can afford to pay cover health costs from their own resources. This enables the public sector to focus resources on top priority health issues and to target selectively the needs of the poor.

Public–private partnerships

The crisis in the health sector has induced governments in many developing countries to review the relationship of the public sector to the private sector. Specifically, policy-makers are exploring mechanisms to promote complementary involvement of the private sector in particular with regard to the delivery of health care and the provision of medical supplies. The WHO now strongly supports the promotion of public–private partnerships with the caveat that such partnerships should be mutually beneficial and must always benefit health (WHO 1998*a*,*b*).

Public–private partnerships in health-care delivery

The non-profit private sector—non-governmental organizations and religious-based medical missions—provides a variety of health services; often they target populations that are poorly served by the public sector and people with special needs such as leprosy and HIV/AIDS. Such services usually have the reputation of being very efficient; they are highly appreciated by the public who would use the fee based services from non-governmental organizations in preference to the free services offered by the public sector.

Another important source of health care are employment-related health schemes which provide health care for workers and their families. The employer may finance the cost of care by reimbursing their workers' medical expenses, or they may provide health care through company-based services or by contracting such services from private providers.

Relationships of the public sector with the for-profit private services have been more tentative but are now being encouraged. Now that many governments have abandoned the goal of providing comprehensive health care to the entire population, new policy directions favour the promotion of the private sector as providers of curative services to affluent sections of the population. For those who receive care from the private sector, the role of the government is to protect public interest by regulating the services and setting minimal standards for care. The fostering of private health insurance schemes facilitates the growth of the private sector by enhancing the ability to pay private providers.

Drugs and supplies

Drugs, vaccines, and other supplies take up a high proportion of public resources in the health services of developing countries. The WHO and other international agencies are assisting governments to improve their drug policies, and the procurement and management of pharmaceuticals through essential drug programmes. The goal is to ensure reliable availability of consistent supplies of basic remedies so that health institutions can consistently deliver cost-effective treatments. In collaboration with industry, governments are encouraged to select a list of the most cost-effective medicaments using inexpensive generic products as far as possible (WHO 1998*b*).

The high cost of some new drugs and vaccines limits the access of developing countries. For example, poor developing countries cannot afford to provide the expensive triple therapy for the management of HIV/AIDS nor can they introduce the *Haemophilus influenzae* and hepatitis B vaccines into their routine immunization programmes. New international initiatives, such as the Global Alliance for Vaccines and Immunization, aim to assist poor countries to have access to vaccines.

Health research

Previously, policy-making was based largely on intuitive opinions of experts but were not always backed by sound knowledge and objective analysis. There is now increasing pressure to make decisions on the basis of sound scientific knowledge. Evidence-based decision-making requires that relevant information be collected and analysed, and that essential research be conducted to elucidate issues.

Developing countries are paying increasing attention to the role of research in policy-making. Following the report of an independent Commission for Health Research for Development (1990), developing countries are being encouraged to improve the management of health research in support of their health services. The Commission recommended that each country should adopt the principles of Essential National Health Research as a strategy for planning, prioritizing, and managing national health research. The goal of Essential National Health Research is health development on the basis of social justice and equity; its content is the full range of biomedical and clinical research, as well as epidemiological, social, and economic studies (Table 3). Its mode of operation is inclusiveness, involving all stakeholders—research scientists, policy-makers and programme managers, and other representatives of civil society (Task Force on Health Research for Development 1991).

At the global level, there is concern that market-driven research and development effort largely ignores the needs of the poor. Only 10 per cent of 50 to 60 billion American dollars that is spent every year for health research is used for research on the health problems of 90 per cent of the world's people. A new entity, the Global Forum for Health Research (1999) has drawn attention to the '10/90' disequilibrium, and in collaboration with the WHO, the World Bank, private foundations, the pharmaceutical industry, non-governmental organizations, and other stakeholders, is seeking solutions to the problem. The central objective of the Global Forum is to help correct the 10/90 gap and focus research efforts on diseases representing the heaviest burden on the world's health, by improving the allocation of research funds and by facilitating the collaboration among partners both in the public and private sectors. One of the initiatives of the Forum is the Alliance for Health Policy and Systems Research. Following on studies initiated by the Ad Hoc Committee on Health Research Relating to Future Intervention Options (1996), the Global Forum is developing analytical tools for defining priorities for global health research. The Ad Hoc Committee introduced a five-step process in priority setting for health research as follows (Table 4).

Table 3 A simple classification of health research

Broad classification	Types of research	Goals	Disciplines involved
Country specific	1. Situation analysis	To define the distribution of health and disease	Epidemiology, statistics, sociology
		To identify determinants and risk factors	
	2. Health policy and systems research	To enhance the efficiency, effectiveness, and cost-effectiveness of health interventions	Management, economics, political science, communications science, other social sciences, etc.
		To provide the basis for developing and testing health policies including equity issues	
Global	3. Developmental	To develop new and improved technologies for diagnosis, prevention, and therapy	Biomedical sciences, clinical sciences, pathology, pharmacology, etc.
	4. Basic research	To advance knowledge of basic biology with particular reference to aspects that have a potential application in tackling human disease	Biomedical sciences
		To expand understanding of human behaviour, poverty, dynamics of social organization, and aspects of individual as well as group behaviour	Behavioural and social sciences
			Comparative health policy and health systems research

1. What is the burden of the disease/risk factor?
2. Why does the burden of disease persist? What are the determinants?
3. What is the present level of knowledge?
4. How cost-effective could future interventions be?
5. What are the resource flows for that disease/risk factor?

The research priorities are also derived from an analysis of the relative share of the burden that can or cannot be averted with existing technologies (Fig. 5):

- averted with current mix of interventions and population coverage
- avertable with improved efficiency
- avertable with existing but not cost-effective interventions
- cannot be averted with existing interventions.

International organizations and foreign donors

The WHO is recognized as the leading agency for health within the United Nations system. In recent years, other international agencies have increased their involvement in the health sector. UNICEF, through its child survival programme, provides massive input into the health sector often in collaboration with the WHO. Other United Nations agencies like the United Nations Fund for Population Action, the International Labour Organization, and the Food and Agricultural Organization have relevant programmes involving specific aspects of the health sector. Through its lending programme, the World Bank has now become the largest source of external finance for the health sector and has stimulated countries to develop more efficient and cost-effective health programmes.

Generally, these external agencies operate independently of each other but there have been some attempts at co-ordination and

Table 4 A practical framework for setting priorities in health research

Five steps in priority setting	Data and analytic requirements
What is the burden of the disease/risk factor?	Health status Assessment of the burden of disease (DALYs, QALYs, etc.)
Why does the burden of disease persist? What are the determinants?	Acquisition of knowledge about disease determinants
What is the present level of knowledge?	What is known today about existing and new potential interventions? How cost-effective are they?
How cost-effective could future interventions be?	Is research likely to produce more cost-effective interventions than the present ones?
What are the resource flows for that disease/risk factor?	Assessment of the public and private resource flows

QALY, quality-adjusted life year.

Source: Global Forum for Health Research (1999).

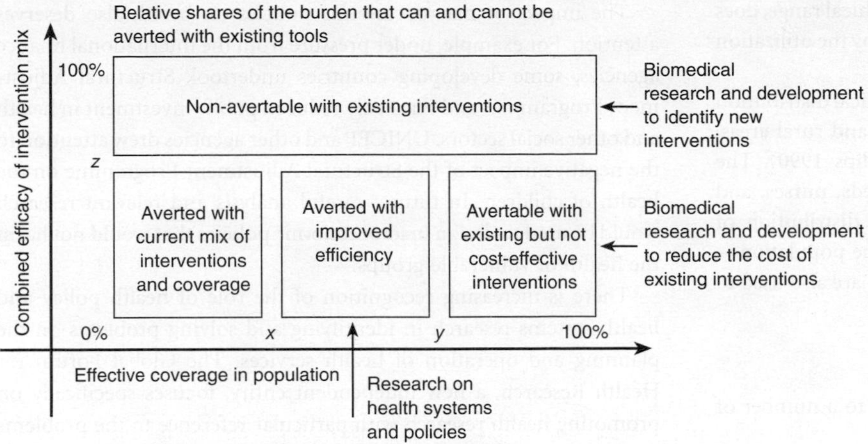

Fig. 5 Analysing the burden of a health problem to identify research needs. (Sources: Barnum and Kutzin 1993; Ad Hoc Committee on Health Research Relating to Future Intervention Options 1996.)

collaboration. UNICEF and the WHO have established mechanisms of collaboration including such formal mechanisms as the Task Force for Child Survival. The WHO also sometimes executes health programmes on behalf of other external agencies. A more ambitious attempt at interagency collaboration is the United Nations AIDS programme; six United Nations agencies jointly manage this programme for the global control of the HIV/AIDS epidemic.

A number of bilateral donor agencies have also expanded their involvement in the health sector. Some of these aid agencies now fund and support health programmes as part of their development assistance programme. The bilateral programmes vary considerably in their content, duration, and interaction with other external agencies. Some of them narrowly focus on the specific interest of the donor countries, for example family planning. There is, however, a new move to achieve more effective co-ordination of external aid through the mechanism of sectorwide expenditure planning. The idea is to develop a national programme, based on national priorities and funded from national resources supplemented by donor aid. All participating donors subscribe to the national plan and contribute their donation to a common basket.

Equity

> The existing gross inequality in the health status of the people particularly between developed and developing countries as well as within countries is politically, socially and economically unacceptable and is, therefore, of common concern to all countries.
>
> *Declaration of Alma-Ata* (WHO 1978)

Although equity in health is intuitively understood to reflect a sense of fairness and justice, the term is used to refer to related but non-identical concepts covering three main issues:

- health status of families, communities, and population groups
- allocation of resources
- access to and utilization of services.

Health status

Inequalities in health status occur commonly and are regarded as prima-facie evidence of inequities in the health-care system. Significant inequalities in health status are found even in the most affluent developed countries, with long traditions of national health services that are designed to provide universal coverage. (Black *et al.* 1998; Pollock 1999). A consistent finding is the strong association between poverty and poor health status as defined by such indicators as the expectation of life, the incidence of acute diseases and injuries, and the prevalence of chronic diseases and disabilities (Gwatkin 2000). This consistent association of poverty with poor health strengthens the case in favour of programmes for the alleviation of poverty as important strategies for health promotion.

Allocation of resources

Equity is also examined in terms of the allocation of resources to different sections of the population. On moral and ethical grounds, the objective of allocative equity is for public resources to be shared out in a fair manner (Taipale 1999). The simplest formula would be a uniform per capita allocation. However, if large differences in health status already exist, an equal allocation would tend to perpetuate the inequalities. It can be argued that it is the responsibility of governments to perform a redistributive function by allocating resources from the more affluent sector of society to meet the needs of lower-income individuals and families, so-called 'vertical equity'.

Access and utilization

Another view of equity is that everyone should have an equal opportunity of receiving care. This so-called 'horizontal equity' proposes that individuals in like situations should be treated in like manner. Access is often defined in terms of the availability of services and its geographical coverage but experience has shown that the potential access, that is the services are within geographical range, does not necessarily correspond to real access as measured by the utilization of services.

Marked disparities are often found in the geographical distribution of health facilities: between regions, between urban and rural areas, between rural areas, and within urban areas (Phillips 1990). The differential ratios of people per facility—hospital beds, nurses, and doctors—are used to measure the disparities. The distribution of health centres and other institutions in relation to the population—how far people have to travel to reach such facilities—are also used to indicate the uneven distribution of resources.

Optimization of equity

Optimization of equity requires conscious attention to a number of important issues:

- political commitment
- policy formulation
- allocation of resources
- intersectoral action
- community involvement
- information system
- monitoring of equity.

Political commitment

The political commitment of the government is the essential basis for promoting equity in health (Feachem 2000). The objective of equity in health fits well with the political philosophy in welfare states that have the clear goal of providing universal coverage of comprehensive health care for the entire population from birth to death. In such countries, the question is not whether the state should embrace equity in health but how to achieve this goal in practice. The situation is more difficult where the political outlook is dominated by free-market ideas, individual entrepreneurship, and market forces.

Political commitment is also required to correct the inequities that result from discrimination on the basis of gender, race, ethnic group, and religion. Often, inequalities in health status reflect the marginalization of disadvantaged groups (Brockerhoff and Hewett 2000).

The plight of indigenous populations in the Americas and Australasia is a special case. There is much variation in the commitment of the national governments to promoting equal socio-economic and political status to the indigenous populations. In extreme cases, erosion of their human rights borders on genocide.

Policy formulation

In weighing policy options, a good guideline would be to examine critically the expected impact of the selected option on equity. The formulation of health policies has to contend with a variety of pressures including the increasing demands of populations for more services, the desire to achieve maximal improvement in health of the populations served, and the need to contain costs. Reforms of the health sector aim at improving efficiency, effectiveness, cost-effectiveness, and equity. It is not always easy to reconcile these goals. For example, the delivery of care to the populations in remote areas is relatively expensive and less cost-effective than services to dense urban areas. However, in the interest of equity, health services should reach the underserved populations even in remote settings.

The impact of macroeconomic policies on health also deserves attention. For example, under pressure from the international finance agencies, some developing countries undertook Structural Adjustment Programmes and markedly reduced public investment in health and other social sectors. UNICEF and other agencies drew attention to the negative impact of the Structural Adjustment Programme on the health of children. In future, careful analysis and relevant research would be used to design macroeconomic policies that would not harm the health of vulnerable groups.

There is increasing recognition of the role of health policy and health systems research in identifying and solving problems on the planning and operation of health services. The Global Forum for Health Research, a new independent entity, focuses specifically on promoting health research with particular reference to the problems that affect the poor.

Allocation of resources

One aspect of equity is that the government should allocate financial resources fairly to the entire population. A simple demographic formula that allocates funds simply on population size may need to be adjusted to take note of the special needs of particular regions; otherwise, the uniform allocation may tend to perpetuate inequalities. Another source of inequity is the degree to which local authorities can raise additional funds through taxation and by retaining user fees. Again, the fact that the more affluent areas are able to raise much larger funds than the poorer areas may tend to widen the gap in the quantity and quality of health care.

Within the health budget, there is the difficult task of allocating resources to the needs of the various groups within the community (Castro-Leal *et al.* 2000; Makinen *et al.* 2000). With finite resources, even the most affluent nations have to accept limits to the services that the public sector can provide. Hence rationing is an inevitable feature of health planning. In the interests of equity and social justice, if economies have to be made, the burden should be fairly shared among various sectors of the community. Quantitative estimates of burden of disease and of the cost-effectiveness of various interventions help to rationalize the selection of priorities (Murray 1994*a,b,c*; Hyder *et al.* 1998). But a point is reached at which difficult choices cannot be made solely on the basis of objective measurements. At this stage, the debate must include philosophical and ethical considerations about the value of human life (Morrow and Bryant 1995).

Intersectoral action

The profound effects of socio-economic circumstances on health have been widely recognized. Social stratification as variously defined is also a prominent risk factor for ill health, reflecting the combined effects of income, education, and culture. The association between poverty and poor health is a consistent finding. The poor die young (Table 5) and their disease profile is largely dominated by communicable diseases, maternal and perinatal conditions, and nutritional deficiencies (Table 6). In developed countries, not only are they are at higher risk from the diseases of the poor but they also suffer more from the lifestyle health problems that are prominent in affluent communities—cancer, coronary heart disease, etc. Furthermore, with the increasing emphasis on free-market economy, the gap between rich and poor is widening. Improved quantity and quality of health care is

Table 5 Comparing some health indicators of the poor versus the better off in selected countries

Country	Percentage of population in absolute poverty[a]	Probability of dying per 1000				Prevalence of tuberculosis	
		Between birth and age 5 (females)		Between 15 and 59 (females)			
		Non-poor	Poor: non-poor ratio	Non-poor	Poor: non-poor ratio	Non-poor	Poor: non-poor ratio
Chile	15	7	8.3	34	12.3	7	8.0
China	22	28	6.6	35	11.0	13	3.8
Ecuador	8	45	4.9	107	4.4	25	1.8
India	53	40	4.3	84	3.7	28	2.5
Kenya	50	41	3.8	131	3.8	20	2.6
Malaysia	6	10	15.0	99	5.1	13	3.2

[a]Poverty is defined as income per capita less than or equal to $US1 per day adjusted for purchasing power.
Source: WHO (1999).

necessary but not sufficient to correct and prevent inequities in health status associated with poverty and social deprivation.

Discrimination against females is a global phenomenon but it varies in its intensity in different parts of the world. It extends through the entire lifecycle, ranging from selective abortion of females, discrimination in quality of health care for infants and children, access to education, and salary differentials based on gender. Discriminatory practices have direct and indirect effects on the health of women. It is often an underlying or aggravating factor in the frequency, severity, and outcome of some specific health problems. For example, poverty is a common cause of malnutrition in women in some parts of the world; not only does it predispose them to anaemia and other health problems but it also limits their access to health care. A common finding is the association between female education and various health indicators for themselves and their children (Cleland and Van Ginneken 1989; Harrison 1997).

The health sector must provide the leadership for mobilizing intersectoral action to achieve these three objectives:

- policies and programmes to alleviate poverty and social deprivation
- ensuring that people have the basic requirements for maintaining good health—food, safe and adequate water supply, sanitation, and housing
- guaranteeing access to affordable health care.

Community involvement

Decentralized health services need to devise mechanisms for obtaining informed opinions from the whole community through credible representatives of civil society. The involvement of communities in decisions that affect their health care is widely recommended: it does not often work effectively in practice. Even in developed countries, the communities are often unable to participate effectively in decision-making because:

- authorities may not consult them
- they lack relevant information
- the society may not be well organized.

Lack of consultation Health officials often make key decisions about health care with minimal consultation with the public. Decisions about priorities for allocation of resources are often handed down without informed participation of the client communities.

Lack of information The public often lack information that would enable them to make informed judgements about health-care issues. Often this is because the technical information and their significance are not presented in language that would inform the lay public. Occasionally, there is deliberate suppression of information by government officials, for example there is a tendency to cover up

Table 6 Distribution of deaths by cause in different population groups (1990)

Cause of death	Percentage of deaths		
	Entire global population	Poorest 20% of the global population	Richest 20% of the global population
Group I: communicable diseases, maternal and perinatal conditions, and nutritional deficiencies	34.2	58.6	7.7
Group II: non-communicable conditions	55.7	32.0	85.2
Group III: injuries	10.1	9.4	7.1

Source: Global Forum for Health Research (1999).

information about outbreaks of infectious diseases like cholera, HIV/AIDS, etc. Some governments invoke Official Secrets Acts and claims about sovereign rights and national security to justify their suppression of health information. Access to health information should be recognized as a human right (Lucas 1992).

Lack of effective organization of society Even in developed countries where the lay public is relatively sophisticated, the civil society is poorly organized with regard to health issues. Public opinion about health is often stage managed by vociferous single-issue lobbyists and by sensational reports in the tabloid press. In modern societies, a variety of special groups maintain watching briefs on specific issues of interest to them—cruelty to animals or to children, protection of the environment, of wildlife, of birds, etc. Such groups collect and disseminate information, lobby governments, and engage in advocacy. Health care does not usually attract such strong lobbies from the lay public. The public response tends to be ad hoc and episodic rather than being well considered and systematic. Furthermore, there is usually no effective leadership and representation of the civil society to provide credible representation of the public. When consultations take place, the powerful elite, the politically influential, and other privileged groups tend to dominate the debate drowning the quieter voices of the poor, the disadvantaged, and marginalized groups.

Information systems

In order to design services that are equitable and to monitor performance of health services, each health authority needs an appropriate management information system which must include measuring inequalities in health status and inequities in access to health care. The data-collecting instruments must be designed to take note of groups and subgroups especially vulnerable groups whose access to services is restricted by geographical, economic, social, and cultural factors. It should include the usual demographic indicators of age, sex, and marital status, as well as socio-economic indicators like race, ethnic origin, occupation, residence, and other social variables (Rosen 1999).

Special studies aimed at probing aspects of the operation of the health services with particular reference to the issue of equity, can usefully supplement routinely collected data. The studies should be designed not only to inform the debate on specific issues but also to provide clues about feasible solutions to the identified problems (Gakidou *et al.* 2000; Wagstaff 2000).

Monitoring and evaluation

The health system should include mechanisms for monitoring equity objectively. Interest in measuring equity has generated some useful tools and some valuable experience is accumulating. In the first instance, monitoring equity is the responsibility of health authorities at each level of care. They must build into their service sensitive indicators that would inform them of their performance with regard to equity and access to care.

In addition to such internal processes, it would be valuable to commission independent reviews of equity within the health system by groups outside the health departments. Another option would be to assign responsibility for a national equity watch to a local non-governmental organization.

With its strong commitment to this goal of equity and its accumulated knowledge and experience, the WHO may provide useful guidance to the national programme. Because some of the issues involved are politically sensitive, many governments would not welcome the direct involvement of external agencies in the review process.

Conclusion

The design and management of efficient health systems is one of the main challenges for developing countries in this century. The vast amount of information accumulated in recent decades provides valuable guidance to policy-makers. Not only must policy-making be knowledge based it must also be result oriented. Careful planning and skilled management can achieve good results even where financial resources are limited. The countries that have achieved good health at low cost challenge other countries to adapt and adopt relevant aspects of their policies. It is a painful irony that millions of children in developing countries are dying of diseases that can be controlled with simple, affordable interventions. Policy-makers must give high priority to strategies that will eliminate the major items of the unfinished agenda that still plague many developing countries. Many lives can be saved and much disability prevented by simple measures like boosting immunization programmes, ensuring access to adequate supplies of safe water and good sanitation, providing effective treatment for common childhood ailments, and ensuring skilled care during childbirth including emergency obstetric care. More daunting tasks include the pandemic of HIV/AIDS that is ravaging parts of the developing world but experience has shown that some progress can be made through the application of social and behavioural interventions without necessarily relying on expensive drugs or waiting for the promise of vaccines.

References

Ad Hoc Committee on Health Research Relating to Future Intervention Options (1996). *Investing in health research and development.* WHO, Geneva.

Andersen, E. (1998). Establishment of drug chests in commune health stations in Vietnam, Bamako Initiative. *South-east Asian Journal of Tropical Medicine and Public Health*, **29**, 628–35.

Barnum, H. and Kutzin, J. (1993). *Public hospitals in developing countries: resource use, cost, and financing.* Johns Hopkins University Press, Baltimore, MD.

Berman, P.A. (ed.) (1995). *Health sector reform in developing countries: making health development sustainable.* Harvard University Press, Cambridge, MA.

Berman, P.A. (1997). National health accounts in developing countries: appropriate methods and recent applications. *Health Economics*, **6**, 11–30.

Black, D., Morris, J.N., Smith, C., and Townsend, P. (1998). Better benefits for health: plan to implement the central recommendation of the Acheson Report. *British Medical Journal*, **318**, 724–7.

Brockerhoff, M. and Hewett, P. (2000). Inequality of child mortality among ethnic groups in sub-Saharan Africa. *Bulletin of the World Health Organization*, **78**, 30–41.

Castro-Leal, F., Dayton, J., Demery, L., and Mehra, K. (2000). Public spending on health care in Africa: do the poor benefit? *Bulletin of the World Health Organization*, **78**, 66–74.

Cleland, J. and Van Ginneken, J. (1989). Maternal schooling and childhood mortality. *Journal of Biosocial Science*, Supplement 10, 13–34.

Commission For Health Research For Development (1990). *Health research: essential link to equity in development.* Oxford University Press, New York.

Diallo, I., McKeown, S., and Wone, I. (1996). Bamako boost for primary care. *World Health Forum*, **17**, 382–5.

Ekwempu, C.C., Maine, D., Olorukoba, M.B., Essien, E.S., and Kisseka, M.N. (1990). Structural adjustment and health in Africa. *Lancet*, **336**, 56–7.

Feachem, R.G.A. (2000). Poverty and inequity: a proper focus for the new century. *Bulletin of the World Health Organization*, **78**, 1.

Frenk, J., Bobadilla, J.-I., Sepulveda, J., and Lopez-Cervantes, M. (1989). Health transition in middle-income countries: new challenges for health care. *Health Policy and Planning*, **4**, 29–39.

Gakidou, E.E., Murray, C.J.L., and Frenk, J. (2000). Defining and measuring health inequality: an approach based on the distribution of health expectancy. *Bulletin of the World Health Organization*, **78**, 42–54.

Gbedonou, P., Moussa, Y., Floury, B., Josse, R., Ndiaye, J.M., and Diallo, S. (1994). The Bamako initiative: hope or illusion? Observations on the Benin experience. *Sante*, **4**, 281–8.

Ghana Health Assessment Project Team (1981). A quantitative method of assessing the health impact of different diseases in less developed countries. *International Journal of Epidemiology*, **10**, 73–80.

Global Forum for Health Research (1999). *The 10/90 report on health research.* Global Forum for Health Research, Geneva.

Gwatkin, D.R. (2000). Critical reflection: health inequalities and the health of the poor: what do we know? What can we do? *Bulletin of the World Health Organization*, **78**, 3–18.

Harrison, K. (1997). The importance of the educated healthy woman in Africa. *Lancet*, **349**, 588.

Hyder, A.A., Rotllant, G., and Morrow, R.H. (1998) Measuring the burden of disease: healthy life-years. *American Journal of Public Health*, **88**, 196–202.

Institute of Medicine (1992). *Emerging infections: microbial threats to health in the United States.* National Academy Press, Washington, DC.

Lucas, A.O. (1992). Public access to health information as a human right. Proceedings of the International Symposium on Public Health Surveillance. *Morbidity and Mortality Weekly Report*, **41**, 77–8.

McCarthy, J. (1997). The conceptual framework of the PMM network. *International Journal of Gynecology and Obstetrics*, **59** (Supplement 2), S15–22.

McCarthy, J. and Maine, D. (1992). A framework for analyzing the determinants of maternal mortality. *Studies in Family Planning*, **23**, 23–33.

Makinen, M., Waters, H., Rauch, M., *et al.* (2000). Inequalities in health care use and expenditures: empirical data from eight developing countries and countries in transition. *Bulletin of the World Health Organization*, **78**, 55–65.

Morrow, R.H. and Bryant, J. (1995). Health policy approaches to measuring and valuing human life: conceptual and ethical issues. *American Journal of Public Health*, **85**, 1356–60.

Murray, C.J. (1994*a*). Cost-effectiveness analysis and policy choices: investing in health systems. *Bulletin of the World Health Organization*, **72**, 663–74.

Murray, C.J. (1994*b*). National health expenditures: a global analysis. *Bulletin of the World Health Organization*, **72**, 623–37.

Murray, C.J. (1994*c*). Quantifying the burden of disease: the technical basis for disability-adjusted life years. *Bulletin of the World Health Organization*, **72**, 429–45.

Murray, C.J.L. and Lopez, A.D. (ed.) (1996). *The global burden of disease. A comprehensive assessment of mortality and disability from diseases, injuries, and risk factors in 1990 and projected to 2020.* Global Burden of Disease and Injury Series, Vol. I. Harvard School of Public Health on behalf of the World Health Organization and the World Bank, Cambridge, MA.

Phillips, D.R. (1990). *Health and health care in the third world.* Longmans, Harlow.

Pollock, A.M. (1999). Devolution and health: challenges to Scotland and Wales. *British Medical Journal*, **319**, 94–8.

Rosen, M. (1999). Data needs in studies on equity in health and access to care—ethical considerations. *Acta Oncologica*, **38**, 71–5.

Shaw, R.P. and Griffin, C.P. (1995). *Financing health care in sub-Saharan Africa through user fees and insurance.* World Bank, Washington, DC.

Taipale, V. (1999). Ethics and allocation of health resources—the influence of poverty on health. *Acta Oncologica*, **38**, 51–5.

Tarimo, E. (1991). *Organizing and manging district health systems based on primary health care.* WHO, Geneva.

Task Force on Health Research for Development (1991). *Essential national health research. A strategy for action in health and human development.* United Nations Development Programme, Geneva.

UNICEF (1999). *The state of the world's children 1998.* UNICEF/Oxford University Press.

Wagstaff, A. (2000). Socioeconomic inequalities in child mortality: comparisons across nine developing countries. *Bulletin of the World Health Organization*, **78**, 19–29.

Walsh, J.A. and Warren, K.S. (1979). Selective primary health care; an interim strategy for disease control in developing countries. *New England Journal of Medicine*, **301**, 967–74.

Warren, K.S. (1988). Selectivity within primary health care. *Social Science and Medicine*, **26**, 899–902.

WHO (World Health Organization) (1978). *Declaration of Alma-Ata.* Report of the International Conference on Primary Health Care. Alma-Ata, 6–12 September 1978. WHO, Geneva.

WHO (World Health Organization) (1987). *Hospitals and health for all.* Report of a WHO Expert Committee on the Role of Hospitals at the First Referral Level. Technical report series No. 744. WHO, Geneva.

WHO (World Health Organization) (1998*a*). *Health for all in the twenty-first century.* WHO, Geneva.

WHO (World Health Organization) (1998*b*). *The use of essential drugs.* Eighth report of the WHO Expert Committee. Tenth model list of essential drugs. Technical report series, No. 882. WHO, Geneva.

WHO (World Health Organization) (1999). *The world health report 1999. Making a difference.* WHO, Geneva.

World Bank (1993). *World development report 1993: investing in health.* Oxford University Press, New York.

World Bank (1994). *Better health in Africa: experience and lessons learnt.* World Bank, Washington, DC.

3.4 Health policies in transition economies

Son N. Nguyen and Julio Frenk

Introduction

After defining the relevant terms, this chapter describes the profound socio-economic changes that have been happening in transition economies. Secondly, it reviews the recent health trends in these countries and their possible explanations. Thirdly, it provides an overview of the current state of health systems in transition economies and examines their health strategies. Emphasis is placed on the discussion of policies undertaken to reform health service and health finance in transition economies. Lastly, it raises issues to be considered in the formulation and implementation of future policies.

In this chapter, it would be impossible to examine in detail the situation in each of the 30 transition economies, so a more general approach is taken with a discussion on the common trends in health and health policies in transition economies. For country-specific discussion, the cases of China and Russia—the world's two largest transition economies—are focused upon. The chapter covers other transition economies, although in less detail. Much of what is analysed will no doubt continue to change in the near future.

Definition of transition economies

Generally, the term transition economy is used to refer to a country which is transforming from a predominantly state-owned centrally planned economy into a system with a free-market orientation and significant private ownership. Such transformation, which has been taking place in many countries around the world, is one of the most important historical events of the last 15 years and has dramatically changed the lives of hundreds of millions of people.

There is as yet no consensus on the official list of transition economies. Although a few other countries in Africa and Latin America may fall under this category, international agencies such as the International Monetary Fund and the World Bank tend to use the term exclusively for formerly communist economies (World Bank 1996; IMF 1998). However, unlike the World Bank, the International Monetary Fund excludes China and Vietnam from its list of transition economies, where economic change has not been accompanied by fundamental political reform. Since the changes in the health systems of China and Vietnam bear much resemblance to those in other former communist countries after the initiation of economic reform, these two countries should be included in the discussion on health policies in transition economies. Thus this chapter employs the World Bank's list of 30 transition economies, which encompasses the following:

- the newly independent states of the former Soviet Union (Armenia, Azerbaijan, Belarus, Estonia, Georgia, Kazakhstan, the Kyrgyz Republic, Latvia, Lithuania, Moldova, Russia, Tajikstan, Turkmenistan, Ukraine, and Uzbekistan)
- its former communist allies in Central and Eastern Europe (Albania, Bosnia, Bulgaria, Croatia, the Czech Republic, Herzegovina, Hungary, the former Yugoslav Republic of Macedonia, Poland, Romania, the Slovak Republic, Slovenia, and the Federal Republic of Yugoslavia)
- China
- Vietnam
- Mongolia.

There should be a clarification of two concepts: health in transition economies and health transition. The first term refers to the health situation during the transition process of former centrally planned economies, which in many cases means an acute crisis with a worsening of many health indicators. This will be discussed further below. Conversely, the second term (also known as epidemiological transition) describes complex long-term changes in the health and disease patterns of specific populations. These changes are usually closely related to major economic, social, and demographic transformations of societies. In its original formulation by Omran (1971), the epidemiological transition referred to a linear undirectional process of change from a pattern dominated by infectious diseases to one where chronic and degenerative ailments dominate. There have been modifications to the original theory, such as the possible overlapping of stages, the reversibility of the patterns of diseases, and the coexistence of pre- and post-transitional pathologies (Frenk *et al.* 1989).

It is notable that for the former Soviet Union and Central and Eastern Europe, the recent acute health crisis during the socio-economic transition has taken place against the backdrop of an on-going health transition during the last three decades. This health transition appears to have a new pattern of mortality which deviates from the collective experience of other developed countries and other middle-income countries in Latin America and Asia (Murray *et al.* 1992; Kingkade and Arriaga 1997).

Why do health policies in transition economies deserve a separate discussion?

The situation in transition economies is unique for two reasons. Firstly, the transition has opened up both enormous opportunities and challenges. In the long run, a free-market economy is expected to result in improvements in living standards and, ultimately, the health of the people through higher income growth and the provision of more resources for human welfare. Historically, income growth has been one of the most important factors, which explains the rise in life expectancy of a nation (World Bank 1993). However, in the short term, transformations often led to profound social, economic, and, in many countries, political upheavals that affected the welfare and health of many of its citizens. In this context, health strategies can help to ease or exacerbate the health problems of the transitional period. Secondly, sharing similar legacies of the previous health systems, transition economies are embarking on a health-care reform process by adopting policies that bear much resemblance in nature. During this reform process, these countries are also facing many common obstacles.

Social and economic contexts

One-third of the world's population live in transition economies. The two largest transition economies, China and Russia, rank numbers 1 and 6 in population terms, with 1230 million and 145 million inhabitants respectively. Variations exist among countries in transition in terms of levels of economic and human development (Fig. 1). For example, gross national product per capita ranges from US$310 in Vietnam to US$9840 dollars in Slovenia in 1997. Of all 30 transition economies, only one country (Slovenia) is in the high-income group. For the remaining transition economies, there are six upper-middle, 13 lower-middle, and 10 low-income countries (World Bank 1999). The Human Development Index, which is published by the United Nations Human Development Programme, quantifies a country's development level based on such factors as life expectancy, education, access to clean water, and adjusted gross domestic product. According to the 1995 Human Development Index, Slovenia and the Czech Republic are the only two transition economies ranked in the high human development group. All the remaining transition economies are in the medium category, with rankings ranging from 67 to 122 (out of 174 countries) (UNDP 1998).

Socio-economic transition in the former Soviet Union and Central and Eastern Europe

The countries of the former Soviet Union and Central and Eastern Europe started the rapid transformation into market economies in the early 1990s, and since then there has been a decade of tremendous change and challenge. Most of them had to undergo major social, political, and economic upheaval. For some, social change came in the form of a break-up into smaller states, or even wars.

Regarding the economic reform, the transformation in the former Soviet Union and Central and Eastern Europe was dramatic with the freeing up of prices, decentralization, and privatization. However, countries of the former Soviet Union and Central and Eastern Europe suffered from a profound fiscal crisis. While deep economic recession led to declining national incomes, effective mechanisms required to collect tax in a market economy were not yet in place. These two factors brought about falling government revenues in most countries of the former Soviet Union and Central and Eastern Europe (Ensor and Thompson 1998). As a result, there was a steep reduction in public expenditures, which in turn translated into a general deterioration of public services and erosion of social protection mechanisms. Severe economic recession has also led to high unemployment rates and widening income gap.

The situation is especially difficult for the former Soviet Union, where government revenue fell by more than 60 per cent between 1991 and 1995 (Ensor and Thompson 1998). Russia and the former republics of the Soviet Union in Central Asia have been particularly hard hit by the economic recession. Severe recession in the absence of

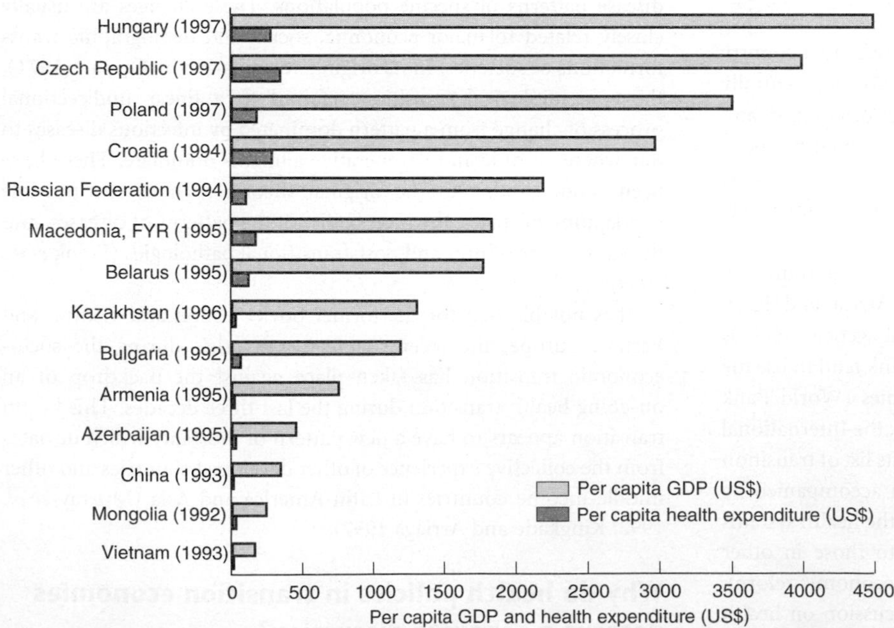

Fig. 1 Gross domestic product (GDP) and health expenditure per capita for selected transition economies, latest available year. (Source: World Bank 1999.)

reliable social safety nets make the poor extremely vulnerable. For example, Russia entered transition with 10 per cent of the population living below the then minimum consumption basket. Since that time, there has been a sharp increase in poverty, and by 1993 about 32 per cent of the population was living below the revised official poverty line (World Bank 1995*a*). In Kazakhstan, 73 per cent of the population lived below the minimum subsistence level in 1997, compared with 16 per cent in 1989. During the past 7 years, the number of people registered as officially unemployed has increased more than 60-fold in Kazakhstan, and the difference between the richest and the poorest in its population is now almost 20-fold (Almagambetova 1999).

Socio-economic transition in China and Vietnam

Compared with the situation in the former Soviet Union and Central and Eastern Europe, the transition process in China and Vietnam has been mostly economic and incremental in nature. In these two countries, economic change has not been accompanied by fundamental political reform and the transition has not led to acute social and political turmoil.

Although China introduced economic reform in the late 1970s, 10 years earlier than transition economies in Europe and central Asia, the pace of reform has been gradual. The formation of the free market began in the agricultural production and 5 years later spread to urban sectors. Chinese economic reform has succeeded in achieving continuous economic growth. The annual growth rate of the Chinese economy has been about 8 to 10 per cent for the last 10 years. Per capita gross domestic product (adjusted for inflation) increased by 7 per cent between 1980 and 1997 (World Bank 1999). The proportion of Chinese people living below the property line was only 6 per cent in 1997. Economic success has enabled China to maintain a better and more effective social safety net than Russia and other countries of the former Soviet Union (Liu *et al.* 1998).

In a move that closely mirrors the Chinese process, Vietnam cautiously implemented market-oriented reform in 1986 and it has been able to increase the real income of its people. Although for the last couple of years, Vietnam's growth, at a rate around 5 per cent, has not been as impressive as it was during the first 10 years of reform (when it was 8 per cent), the overall record of its reform policies has been fairly good.

Recent trends in health status of transition economies

Although variations in health exist among transition economies, in general they have all faced important health challenges during the transition period to free-market economies. The dramatic socio-economic disruptions have been reflected in recent changes of the health status of many transition economies.

Recent health trends in the former Soviet Union and Central and Eastern Europe

The health status of the former Soviet Union and Central and Eastern Europe started to lag behind that of Western Europe in the early 1970s. However, it was only during the early phase of transition in the early 1990s that a health crisis occurred in Eastern Europe with a level unprecedented in the peacetime history of industrialized countries in this century. For example, in the early 1970s, life expectancy of countries in the former Soviet Union and Central and Eastern Europe was 2 to 3 years shorter than that of the European Union. The difference in the early 1990s was more than 6 years (WHO 1994). Except in Albania (where data are not available), the Czech Republic, and Slovakia, increases in the number of avoidable deaths among adults males between 20 and 59 years of age were reported in all transition economies in Eastern Europe and these were chiefly responsible for the drop in life expectancy in such countries. Russia, Ukraine, Hungary, and Bulgaria experienced the most marked declines in male life expectancy (WHO 1999). In contrast to adults, there has been little change in childhood mortality during transition, though the former Soviet Union and Central and Eastern Europe are still lagging behind Western Europe in this health indicator (Koupilova and Leon 1998).

The Russian mortality crisis, with the greatest decline in life expectancy in the countries of the former Soviet Union and Central and Eastern Europe since 1990, is worth discussing in further detail. In only 4 years, from 1990 to 1994, life expectancy declined by 5 years and age-adjusted mortality rose by almost 33 per cent in Russia. The most dramatic change was in male mortality. During this period, male life expectancy dropped by 6 years (from 64 to 58), whereas female life expectancy fell by 3 years (from 74 to 71) (World Bank 1999). More than 75 per cent of the decline in life expectancy was attributed to increased mortality rates among adults from 25 to 64 years of age (Walberg *et al.* 1998). Overall, cardiovascular diseases (heart disease and stroke) and injuries accounted for 65 per cent of the decline in life expectancy. Increases in cardiovascular mortality accounted for 41.6 per cent of the decline in life expectancy for women and 33.4 per cent for men, while increases in mortality from injuries accounted for 32.8 per cent of the decline in life expectancy for men and 21.8 per cent for women (Notzon *et al.* 1998).

In the mid-1990s, health began to improve in some former Soviet Union and Central and Eastern Europe countries. Infant mortality and life expectancy improved in the Czech Republic, Hungary, Poland, and Slovenia. Health indicators also began to improve in Russia and some former Soviet Union countries (WHO 1999). However, experience in the past clearly demonstrated that major declines in health and life expectancy can take place rapidly (Notzon *et al.* 1998) and thus the recovery from the health crisis might be reversed in the event of a new economic recession.

Compared with the European Union, at the end of the 1990s, mortality in the former Soviet Union and Central and Eastern Europe is still significantly higher in many categories such as:

- most important causes of death
- preventable causes of death
- communicable diseases (especially in the poorer countries)
- chronic diseases
- injuries and suicides.

Age-standardized mortality rates for chronic diseases are extremely high when compared with European Union countries. The divide in mortality between Eastern Europe and the European Union is caused mainly by chronic diseases in adulthood. This fact is explained by lifestyle patterns in the former Soviet Union and Central and Eastern Europe which have the highest smoking prevalence rate for both sexes and the highest per capita cigarette consumption rate in the world

(WHO 1997; World Bank 1999). Recent significant increases in prevalence and level of consumption will worsen the smoking-attributable burden of diseases in the future.

With regard to communicable diseases, there was a resurgence of certain epidemics, notably the diphtheria outbreaks during the period 1991 to 1995, and the cholera epidemic in 1994 in Russia (Barr and Field 1996).

Recent health trends in China and Vietnam

Since the beginning of economic reform in the late 1970s, China's major health indicators have continued to improve. During this 20-year period, life expectancy increased from 67 to 70 years whereas infant mortality rate declined by almost 25 per cent. However, health gain in China has not always been maintained throughout the transition. In the early 1980s, for instance, infant mortality failed to keep up with the reduction rate achieved in the 1960s and 1970s (WHO 1999). Moreover, recent studies have shown that mortality in China is no longer improving in the manner of the previous decades, especially among working age males (Banister 1997). Thus, maintaining the improving trends in health status of its people in the years to come remains a great challenge for China.

Similarly, the overall health gain achieved in the previous decades has continued to improve in Vietnam since the introduction of market-oriented reform in 1986. However, many health indicators such as infant mortality rate and life expectancy are significantly greater than predicted for Vietnam's income level. As in the case of China, certain untoward health outcomes were also experienced in Vietnam during the transition period. For example, there was a significant increase in malaria deaths between 1980 and 1990 (Gudner 1995).

Emerging health problems in transition economies

Many transition economies have in common emerging health challenges brought about by an ageing population and an increasing burden of non-communicable diseases, which is mostly attributable to tobacco and alcohol use, injuries, and traffic accidents. All of these are taking place in the face of a continued burden of communicable diseases. In the discussion of new health problems for transition economies, comparison of Russia and China might be useful. Although China has been spared the mortality crisis which Russia is going through, both countries have experienced significant increases in injuries, suicides, substance abuse, and mental health problems during the transition period. The situation is more serious in Russia (Liu *et al.* 1998).

Possible explanations for the health crisis in transition economies of the former Soviet Union and Central and Eastern Europe

There has been a debate on the key determinants of recent changes in the health status of the former Soviet Union and Central and Eastern Europe countries. Many possible explanations have been examined such as:

- poor economic performance and widespread impoverishment
- break-up of the health system and deterioration of health-care services
- poor nutrition
- pollution
- increasing income disparities within transition economies
- psychological stress arising from economic and social instability and stress-related behaviour such as tobacco and alcohol abuse.

Researchers suggest that impoverishment is not a sufficient explanation. Obviously, it is not sufficient to depend solely on economic performance to bring about a health outcome. They also argue that contributions from the breakdown in health services, nutrition, and pollution are likely to be modest. Rather, much of the deterioration can be attributed to the impact of social and economic transition, exacerbated by a lack of social cohesion. For example, a study by Walberg *et al.* (1998) shows that in Russia there is a high correlation between the fall in life expectancy and three socio-economic indicators: labour force turnover (a measure of 'transition'), high crime rates (a proxy measure of social cohesion), and income inequality (Walberg *et al.* 1998). However, health behaviour, diet, and tobacco and alcohol consumption are also very important factors. While alcohol consumption is an important cause of premature death in Russia, as shown by the fact that Russia's life expectancy dramatically improved during Gorbachev's anti-alcohol campaign in 1985 to 1998 and then dropped after its relaxation (World Bank 1996), smoking seems to have the largest impact in the former Soviet Union as a whole (Bobak and Marmot 1996; Walberg *et al.* 1998).

There is still controversy about which is the chief contributor to the health crisis observed in most former Soviet Union and Central and Eastern Europe countries. Nevertheless, each of the above-mentioned factors is likely to play a role. Furthermore, the deterioration in health became manifest to some extent before the transition in the former Soviet Union and Central and Eastern Europe. Therefore, past health policies and the inherited health systems also seem to contribute to the health crisis in these transitional economies.

The former health-care systems in transition economies

Discussion of current health policies in transition economies is not complete without an examination of what they have inherited from the pre-existing health systems. Such a historical examination can provide explanations for the strengths and weaknesses of the current systems as well as a rationale for new health policies adopted by the governments.

An overview of the key components of a health-care system is useful for this discussion and can be found in Table 1. The former health systems in transition economies had a number of common features, which were the consequences of past health policies. Their advantages and disadvantages are summarized in Table 2. Although reform has been under way and new financing and management mechanisms have been introduced, numerous imprints of the former systems are still visible in many transition economies.

The former health systems were characterized by a strong commitment of the state to the health of the people. There were three major manifestations of this commitment in the way that the health systems

Table 1 Key components of a health-care system

Institutions	Health departments Health-care providers (public and private) Medical education institutions
Resources	Financing mechanisms Supporting human resources Information systems
Organizations that link institutions and resources	Associations of public health and health professionals, health-care providers, health profession schools
Management structures	

Source: Anderson (1989); Frenk (1994); Lassey *et al.* (1997).

were financed and organized. Firstly, before the transition, most countries had the model of free medical services for all, and this principle of universal access and equity was successful to some extent. Secondly, the states developed comparatively well-organized health-care systems with a strong emphasis on prevention. Thirdly, there was a build-up of a more extensive health-care infrastructure per capita in transition economies than in other countries at the same level of development. Thus, there exist comprehensive networks of health-care institutions and adequate numbers of staff in most transition economies as the legacy of past policies. Most transition economies now have higher ratios of doctors and hospital beds per population than the averages for their corresponding income group (Figs 2 and 3).

Besides the advantages mentioned above, the former health systems in transition economies suffered from a number of shortcomings. They were poorly maintained, with outdated management mechanisms. Years of rigid central planning and bureaucracy had led to limited efficiency and quality of the services and therefore the health systems were not operating to their full potential. Central planning, which placed great emphasis on meeting numerical targets and input indicators at the expense of quality and outputs, resulted in low-quality imbalanced physical infrastructure and staff in health care. For example, while many hospitals were constructed, investment in hospital equipment or other types of health facilities was neglected. Health professionals might have been abundant in numbers, yet many of them had low skills. Though some former Soviet Union countries had the highest ratios of doctors and beds to population in the world, supporting this massive infrastructure, especially in the event of a fiscal crisis, would not be feasible (Ensor and Thompson 1998).

In the former systems, the structure of primary care was specialist led, with patients either having direct access to specialists or being referred to the latter without receiving much care from general

Table 2 Strengths and weaknesses of the former health-care systems in transition economies

		Advantages	Disadvantages
Institutions		Extensive infrastructure	Hospital dominated Too many hospital beds Lack of equipment No competition No choice
Resources	Financing mechanisms	State-funded based on number of beds	Inadequate budget Long hospital stay Emphasis on curative care
		Universal access, free of charge	No financial autonomy Inefficiency Certain equity issues
	Human resources	Adequate numbers	Overstaffed Specialist-led Low efficiency and skills
Linking organizations		None (banned)	Weak links between resources and institutions No quality monitoring entity
Management		Centralized	Outdated management style No managerial autonomy or ownership

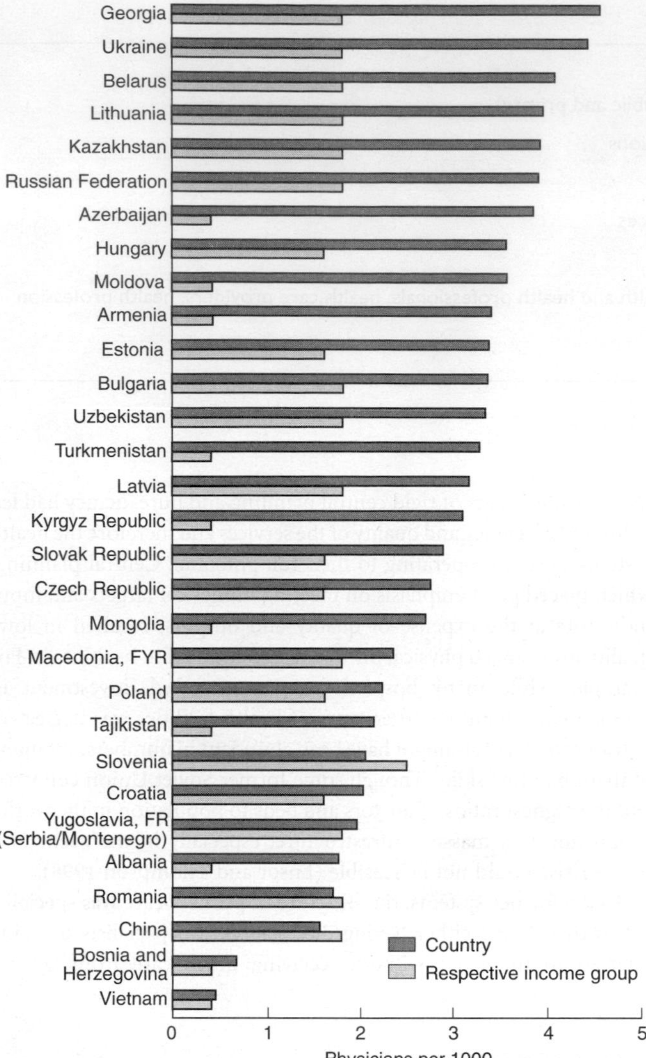

Fig. 2 Number of doctors per 1000 in transition economies compared with the respective income groups, 1994. (Source: World Bank 1999.)

practitioners. Thus, general practice was bypassed and eclipsed. As a result, currently in Russia, half of the district doctors (who are responsible for primary care of a district) are specialists (Toon 1998). Similarly, in Poland there is a shortage of family doctors, who are only able to cover 2 per cent of the population (Thompson 1998). Moreover, doctors were underpaid and became a socially and economically underprivileged group. As state employees, health professionals were paid irrespective of their efficiency and quality. Meanwhile, doctors, often without formal training in health management and administration, were running the system with an authoritarian management style. Many qualified health personnel became disillusioned with the system and started leaving the profession.

There were also equity issues with the former health systems. Despite the principle of universal access, the systems were not delivering equality as people in rural areas had lower access to health care than urban dwellers. In Vietnam, public subsidies for the richest quintile of the population were twice as much the amount spent on the poorest quintile (World Bank 1995*b*).

With regard to financing mechanisms, the old system relied on an inadequate state budget and a tightly centralized financial management structure in which the allocation of funds did not reflect local needs. Since providers were prepaid an amount based on the number of hospital beds and staff, there was no incentive for them to deploy resources efficiently. This resulted in large numbers of beds, long hospital stays, overuse of secondary-care facilities, and an emphasis on curative rather than preventive care. In Kazakhstan, for example, hospitals received 75 to 85 per cent of the health-care funds while the primary health-care system received only about 10 per cent of the overall budget (Almagambetova 1999).

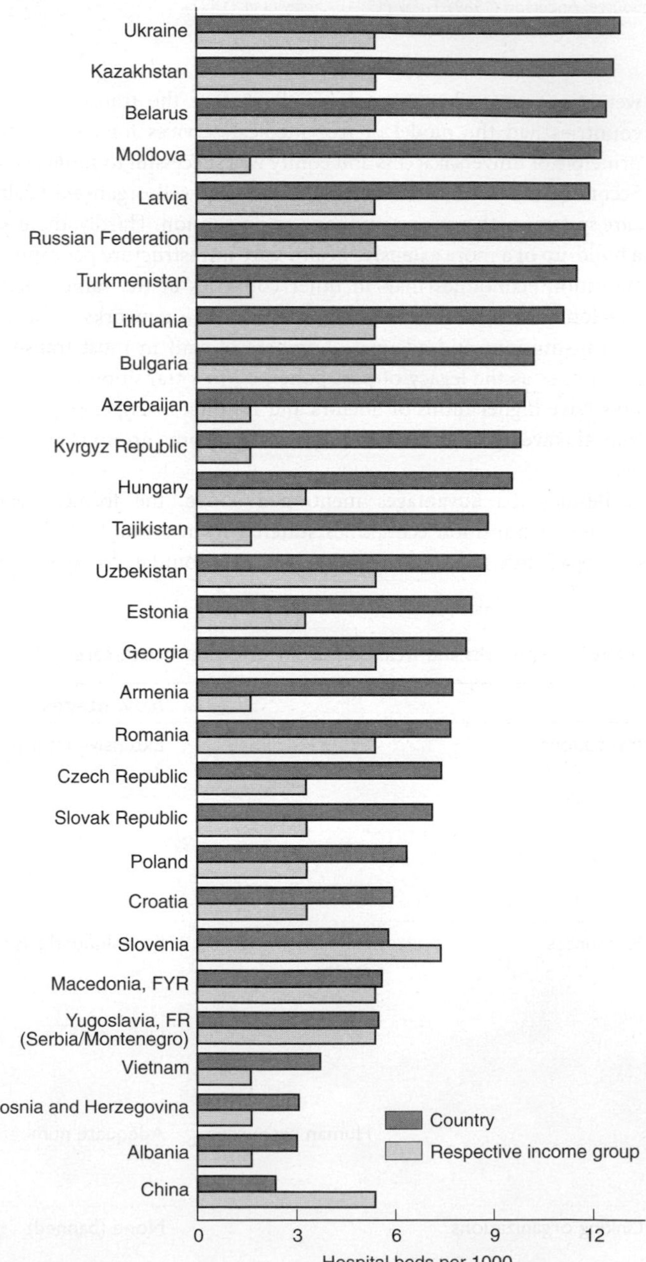

Fig. 3 Number of hospital beds per 1000 in transition economies compared with the respective income groups, 1994. (Source: World Bank 1999.)

For the above reasons, the old health systems failed to use resources to maximize gains in health outcomes and left negative impacts on the current systems. Coupled with the fiscal crisis, health systems in transition economies are struggling to cope with the current demand, especially with the extra burden exerted by the deterioration of health during the transition.

Policies to reform health-care systems in transition economies

As part of a major social restructuring, many transition economies have had to overhaul their health systems amid a health crisis associated with the transition as well as the pre-existing problems of the inherited health-care legacy. Just like the move towards democracy, the process of health reform, which has great social and economic implications, has not come without pain. The implementation of new health policies has resulted in a mixed record of both improvements and setbacks. One of the most difficult tasks is to reorganize health care and make it more cost-effective while ensuring its accessibility to those who need it most. Whether this can be done within the tight fiscal constraints in place during the transition to a market economy remains a great challenge. There appears to be conflict between long-term reform agendas and the short-term consequences that they brought about.

This section focuses on the key components of the health system in which transition economies are facing great challenges and important policies that have recently been implemented in response. They include policies to reform financing mechanisms, introduce privatization into health care, and overhaul the management structures.

Policies to reform the financing mechanisms of public health

Generally, to ease the fiscal crisis in the health sector, governments in transition economies are pursuing policies to create additional funding, reduce the range of services, scale down the massive infrastructure of the health sector, and change the way in which care is provided.

While the new finance mechanisms are not yet in place, governments in transition economies are now only able to contribute a small proportion of the health-care budget. With the health sector facing a fiscal crisis, most transition economies have departed—or plan to depart—from heath systems exclusively financed by governments. Efforts to reform health finance include the introduction of varying degrees of private funding instruments, such as medical insurance and direct user charges, and decentralization of health finance.

Introduction of private funding instruments

Medical insurance

Efforts to reform health finance in transition economies are usually led by the social health insurance initiative, which is viewed as an important source of funding for the cash-poor health sector. This reflects the government's efforts to depart from the traditional system of universal free health care that it no longer can afford. Many transition economy governments are pursuing this policy and, with the adoption of insurance laws, they have now switched from tax-funded health care to social health insurance. The most vulnerable populations, which include the elderly, the young, and the indigent, are usually covered by such social health insurance schemes.

Nevertheless, it has been argued that there may be other reasons to introduce health insurance besides the provision of additional revenue. Social insurance can catalyse organizational change and induce fundamental restructuring of provision. Revenue generated from health insurance will result in greater autonomy for the ministry of health and local health departments over expenditure allocation (Ensor and Thompson 1998).

Direct user charges

User charges have been legalized in many transition economies as another method to recover cost. However, there have been concerns that in the absence of appropriate regulatory structures, such charges can exacerbate inequity and inefficiency since a provider could abuse the system and oversubscribe medications and procedures in order to claim more revenues. For example, a survey in Kazakhstan, where such charges were instituted in 1995, suggested that inpatients bear up to 45 per cent of expenditure per patient in city hospitals (Ensor and Savelayeva 1998).

Decentralization of health finance

Historically, the ministry of finance had vertical control over the ministry of health for funding. The ministry of finance would provide finance to local medical facilities through local administrations and health departments, often bypassing the ministry of health. Usually based on the number of staff and the number of bed days in the previous year, funding flows from the ministry of health do not necessarily reflect the true local needs and expenditure though they are meant as a way of strictly controlling local spending.

The implementation of social insurance promotes fiscal decentralization. It gives the national ministry of health a degree of independence from the ministry of finance. With access to direct funding, the ministry of health is empowered and can develop a more influential role in directing health policy. Local health departments also have greater control over the allocation of local expenditures and thus take up more responsibilities (Ensor and Thompson 1998).

Implementation, results, and challenges

Despite recent reforms, health systems in many transitional economies remain predominantly publicly funded. In 1995, around 70 per cent of health expenditure in the former Soviet Union and Central and Eastern Europe are still covered by general tax revenues. Health expenditure as a percentage of gross domestic product in transition economies was higher than in developing countries at similar income levels (Goldstein *et al.* 1996). As shown in Fig. 4, health care consumes between 3 and 10 per cent of national income (gross domestic product) in transition economies where data are available.

There are three major challenges in the implementation of social insurance in transition economies. Firstly, collecting contributions, which is vital to the sustainability of a health insurance scheme, is a hurdle to many governments in the context of a falling tax base and ineffective tax collecting mechanisms. Evidence suggests that in many countries, revenue obtained from insurance has been lower and less stable than expected. In 1997, a year after the implementation of social health insurance in Turkmenistan, the collection rate was 66 per cent (Ensor and Thompson 1998). Secondly, a mechanism to pay health-care providers is another issue to tackle. In the absence of

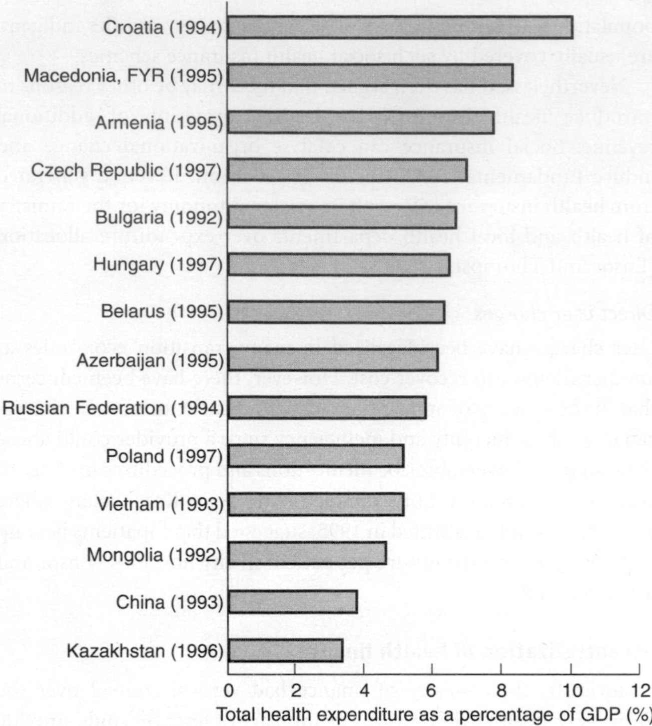

Fig. 4 Total health expenditure as a percentage of gross domestic product for selected transition economies, latest available year. (Source: World Bank 1999.)

appropriate regulatory structures, the fee-for-service method creates an incentive for providers to oversupply and leads to overspending of the social insurance scheme. The situation in the Czech Republic in 1992 after the introduction of fee-for-service in 1992 provides an example for this (Fig. 5) (World Bank 1996). Thirdly, there is a need to determine the right benefit package offered by the insurance scheme in terms of the items included and excluded from that package. In the case of Turkmenistan, the excess of the package resulted in escalating costs and a 100 per cent difference between reimbursement and contributions a year after the introduction of the voluntary health insurance system in 1996 (Ensor and Thompson 1998).

Adoption of payroll-based health insurance during the transition has been followed by a marked increase in health expenditure as a percentage of gross domestic product. This necessitates increased efficiency in public sector resource mobilization, explicit shift in cost burden to the active population, and complete introduction of financial incentives in the implementation of social insurance. It is critical that health insurance schemes should be made as effective as possible and based on sound economic and actuarial principles. The design of new health finance mechanisms should provide effective protection to vulnerable groups while, at the same time, encouraging the development of competition among providers. This requires a number of measures to increase revenue and make health expenditures more cost-effective.

Countries differ in their suitability for introducing health insurance. Using Shaw and Ainsworth's methodology, Ensor and Thompson ranked the feasibility of implementing health insurance in low- and middle-income countries according to four criteria: proportion of urban population, proportion of industrial workforce, population density, and per capita income (Ensor and Thompson 1998). Table 3 shows the results for transition economies. Consistent with these results, evidence shows that more industrialized countries like the Czech Republic, Estonia, and Hungary (which have high scores in the ranking) have implemented health insurance with relative success. Countries at the bottom of the ranking, like Vietnam and Turkmenistan, achieved very low coverage, especially in rural areas. As a result, sustainability of the health insurance scheme is a great challenge for transition economies with low suitability. For example, mandatory health insurance was introduced in Kazakhstan in 1996; however, the scheme was not sustainable, and it was cancelled 2 years later (Almagambetova 1999).

With a new emphasis on cost recovery, health services now tend to be available to those with the ability to pay. There have been concerns and evidence that private payment for health care, especially at the point of delivery, may be a barrier to access for the poor and reduce the utilization of health services. Analysis of a household survey in Kyrgyzstan shows that, in 1996, a quarter of those who were either sick or injured did not seek medical care because they could not afford it (Falkingham 1998). In Vietnam, outpatient consultation has declined by 50 per cent since the late 1980s, from 2.1 visits per capita in 1987 to 0.9 in 1993 (World Bank 1995*b*). For this reason, necessary government interventions are needed to provide health care for the indigent and public health services.

China offers interesting lessons for reform in health-care financing. It introduced social insurance reforms in the mid-1980s. With the new policies, health-care utilization rates for both urban and rural populations was significantly increased from the mid-1980s to the early 1990s (Chinese Ministry of Health 1994). The challenge is to finance and provide both public health and health-care services to the poor in the countryside, where 70 per cent of the population resides.

Hungary is experimenting with private health insurance, which was introduced in early 1999 as an alternative to the state health-care insurance. However, it has not been very successful because most people cannot afford it (Kovac 1999). Some analysts have warned of the threat of losing previous health gains if unrestrained market mechanisms are used to dominate the health-care sector in transition economies. Better results in terms of efficiency and equity are obtained

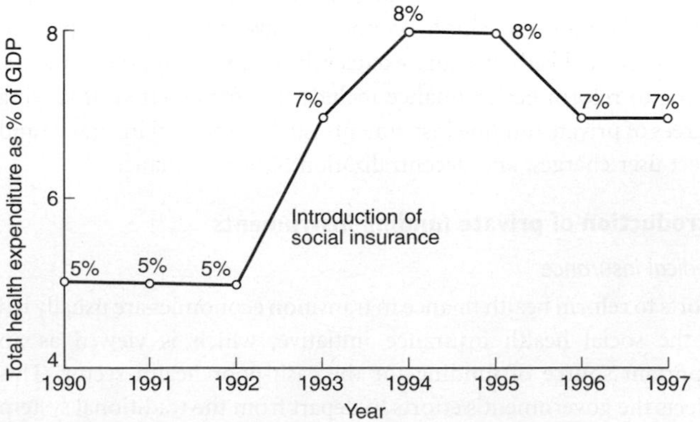

Fig. 5 Health expenditure rises after the introduction of social insurance: total health expenditure as a percentage of gross domestic product in the Czech Republic 1990 to 1997. (Source: World Bank 1996.)

Table 3 Feasibility of introducing insurance in transition economies

Score	Countries
3, 4	Belarus, Estonia
2	Czech Republic, Hungary, Latvia, Lithuania, Bulgaria, Ukraine
1	Slovenia, Poland, Russian Federation, Romania, Moldova
0	Armenia, Georgia, Kazakhstan, Uzbekistan
–1	Albania, Azerbaijan, Kyrgyzstan, China, Tajikistan
–2	Turkmenistan, Mongolia, Nigeria, Vietnam

Source: Adapted from Ensor and Thompson (1998).

through public insurance or tightly regulated non-commercial insurance (Evans *et al.* 1994; Burger *et al.* 1998).

To help governments prioritize essential services in the face of funding shortages, the World Bank recommends the adoption of a basic package of publicly funded services (World Bank 1993). Georgia has adopted this approach and, furthermore, has made it radical by making the publicly funded package of basic services available to the socially protected only; thus everyone else has to pay for their own health care.

Policies to reform health services

There is an urgent need to improve the quantity, quality, and mix of health services in transition economies while making them more efficient and equitable. Most transition economies are adopting similar policies enabling their health-care systems to depart from the model in which the state is the sole provider of health services, as well as making them more efficient, competitive, and decentralized.

Privatization of the health sector

Most transition economies have adopted legislation to legalize the involvement of the private sector in the production, trade, and distribution of drugs, medical equipment, and supplies as well as in the provision of health services. By doing this, transition economies have introduced market-oriented mechanisms into the health system, namely consumer choice and competition between different health-care providers.

Reform of management structures

This includes decentralization of health management, in which local health institutions are granted larger managerial autonomy and clearer ownership.

Reform of human resources

Financial incentives for health workers to improve quality and productivity are created by policies to introduce performance-based financial rewards. Reform efforts in medical education have been taken to introduce the concept of family practice and to train general practitioners.

Promoting cost-effectiveness of the delivery system

This is being accomplished by restructuring in favour of primary care, promoting general and family practice of medicine, and eliminating unnecessary hospital capacity and staff.

Establishment of linked organizations

One of the main features of the health system in a democratic society is the presence of organizations that serve as links between institutions and resources. These include associations of public health professionals, doctors, and other health-care workers, hospitals, health professional schools, and so on. Such organizations, once absent in the former health system, are now emerging in transition economies. One example is Romania where, after than 50 years of restrictions, professional associations, non-governmental organizations, and health advocacy groups have been allowed and are now actively contributing to the reform process (Ionescu *et al.* 1998).

Implementation, results, and challenges

The extent of success in implementing policies to reform health services varies among transition countries.

1. Data mostly available for the public sector indicate little significant restructuring of the public sectors health networks in most transitional economies.
2. Currently, there are not enough data to assess the impact of new policies on the improvement of quality and efficiency of care except in a few cases.
3. Privatization development has been rapid in the pharmaceutical and dentistry areas, slow in ambulatory care, and negligible for hospital care.
4. There have been many discussions on scaling down the massive infrastructure of the health-care system with such measures as reducing staff and closing hospitals. However, political constraints often prevent the successful implementation of such policies, except in Central and Eastern Europe where some success have been reported with decreases in number of hospital beds and average hospital stay (Berlin and Hunter 1998).
5. In some countries, there has been a gradual shift towards the model of general practice and primary care based on gatekeeping and integrated care. In Russia, a move towards general practice started in 1992.

The major challenges facing most transition economies include the following:

(1) disparity in access to health services between the rich and the poor, the rural and the urban;

(2) temporary market failure in the supply of heath care and drugs through weaknesses in regulations;

(3) resistance to the shift towards general practice from both the public, who are used to bypassing general practitioners, and the specialists, who feel that their jobs are threatened by the changes;

(4) regulation and quality control of both public and private services.

Public health and policies in transition economies

The inherited public health system

Historically, transition economies have a long history of well-developed public health programmes. However, the public health model is many former communist countries is the outdated vertical 'hygiene' model with a strong emphasis on sanitation, food, and water safety. With regard to health promotion and disease prevention, this old public health system does not encourage active participation of the population. People are simply expected to carry out the instructions of health professionals. Modern public health has demonstrated that this practice is not effective in bringing about behaviour change. Instead, it leads to a passive attitude, as people do not take personal responsibility for their own health. As a result, they do not actively participate in health promotion, disease prevention, or the healing process. Thus a departure from the old model of public health is needed for transition economies to cope with the increasing burden of behaviour-related chronic diseases.

Impact of transition on public health

Comprehensive health reform must include the public health component. Unfortunately, the public health function was neglected during the early phase of transition. Insurance and privatization-led health-care reform was higher on the political agenda and received more media and public attention in most transition economies. The transformation to the market-oriented finance mechanism has weakened the financing of public health function for two reasons. Firstly, as elsewhere in the world, there is competition between public health needs and individual health-care needs for funding, which became even more limited during the fiscal crisis. Secondly, in most transition economies, the general direction of health reform is towards decentralization of public sector services, privatization, recognition of patient choice, and introduction or increase of out-of-pocket expenses. Such application of market values to health care has created opportunities for improving the demand-focused health services.

Consequences of a weakened public health function

Thus, during transition, public health activities face major challenges which include the lack of funding and the ability to adapt public health systems to cope with the changing patterns of health risks and diseases. Even the good legacy of primary care has been eroded during transition. For example, in China, public financing of the Epidemic Prevention Service, the backbone of public health programmes, has fallen from 0.11 per cent of gross domestic product in 1978 to 0.04 per cent in 1993. This, together with fiscal decentralization, has reduced the capacity of public health programmes in China's poorer counties. Introduction of user fees has reduced demand for public health services such as preventive services and tuberculosis control (Liu *et al.* 1998). As a result, certain public health indicators, such as immunization coverage, deteriorated in many poorer areas in the early 1990s. Certain epidemic outbreaks were also traced back to breakdown in public health programmes (Liu *et al.* 1996).

Recent changes in public health policies

The need for public health reform is now being felt in many transition economies. The realization that public health cannot be left to unrestrained market forces in China was reflected in a landmark national health conference in December 1996 which adopted major policies to address public health problems (Chinese Ministry of Health 1997). In the former Soviet Union and Central and Eastern Europe, many countries, such as Lithuania, the Russian Federation, and Moldova, are seriously discussing comprehensive health policies and reviewing their public health services. Estonia now allots a proportion of heath insurance premiums for public health activities (Vienonen and Springet 1998).

Transition economies are facing two public health challenges. Firstly, since public health services are 'public goods', they should be state financed. Thus governments need to draw up mechanisms to fund public health activities from their tight health budget. Secondly, the single largest contributor to the health gap between Western Europe and transition economies in Eastern Europe is cardiovascular and cerebrovascular disease, for which the main risk factors are alcohol consumption, smoking, obesity, unhealthy diet, and lack of exercise. All these factors are more prevalent in the former Soviet Union and Central and Eastern Europe than in Western Europe, and one single factor, smoking, is far more prevalent. In fact, the former Soviet Union and Central and Eastern Europe have the highest smoking prevalence for males and females (41 per cent and 26 per cent respectively) among all World Bank regions. Smoking prevalence rates are also very high among males in the other transition economies in East Asia, China, and Vietnam, where about two-thirds of adult males are regular smokers (Jha and Chaloupka 1999). In this context, transition economies need to adopt and implement effective public health measures for the control of the large burden of behaviour-related mortality and disability.

Implications for health policy

1. Parallel to policies to privatize and decentralize the economy, there have been similar efforts in the health sector. However, health policies tended to follow or to be subservient to economic policies (Liu *et al.* 1998). Certain policies to reform health finance and health services have been adopted just to serve the economic–fiscal–political reform agenda without the consideration of improving health as the ultimate goal of health reform. The negligence of public health function in many transition economies is an illustration of this.
2. Better evidence is required to orient the formulation of sound health policies. Yet good policies are only the first step to successful health reform. Effective implementation of policies requires legislative and regulatory infrastructure as well as administrative capacity. In fact, health-care reforms in transition economies are facing similar challenges as other sector reforms. In this regard, there is an argument that institution building should received more attention as reform without the right regulatory framework is bound to fail (*Economist* 1999).
3. Reform should aim to enhance the performance of health systems by promoting equitable access to health services that are affordable, effective, well managed, of good quality, and responsive to the population.
4. Reform should also aim to secure sustainable health-care financing by mobilizing adequate levels of resources, establish broad-based risk-pooling mechanisms, and maintain effective control over public and private expenditure.
5. The establishment of schools of public health for training in health policy, economics, and management in countries where

they did not exist before is an important step towards a good health system in the long run.

6. In a democratic society, there is extensive involvement of the public in the formulation, implementation, and validation of health policies. Hence the development of the civil society in a transition economy is helpful for health reform. Representative democracy can be a major facilitator of civic trust and social capital and should be applied to the health sector as well (Szreter 1999).
7. The concept of self-responsibility in health should be introduced and reinforced in transition economies. This will also lead to greater participation of citizens in health promotion and disease prevention.
8. During the transition period, state intervention is a complex issue. On the one hand, the argument is that the role of the state (with its strategic planning and directing capacity) is more important than ever during the transition. On the other hand, there is a need for the state to embrace the concept of 'civil society' in health through communication and civic participation (Szreter 1999).
9. No health reform is comprehensive when the public health component is neglected.
10. A functioning health-care system must be maintained throughout the process of reform. Thus there is a need for policy-makers to adapt rapidly, and to design and implement strategies to minimize disruption in essential health services.
11. It is necessary to monitor carefully the health status of the population during the transition, especially among the marginal groups.
12. Many of the challenges faced by transition economies are shared by other countries. Learning from the successes and failures of others can make reform efforts more effective. International co-operation can help in the production and dissemination of sound evidence on health policies.

Conclusion

Historical evidence indicates that economic transformation, even with success and growth, can translate into social insecurities and health problems. Thus countries in Western Europe, Japan, the United States, and Australia had to endure severely compromised health when they first experienced industrialization in the nineteenth century (Szreter 1999). Similar disruptions can be observed a century later in many transition economies, especially Russia and other countries of the former Soviet Union, despite the improvement in medical technology and the new wealth of public health knowledge that has been achieved in the interim. The issue here is not whether transition economies should continue their reform process or not, since this has been historically proven necessary for the development of a country. Rather, it is about what the government can do to alleviate health problems through the adoption and implementation of sound policies. Since the health of a nation is strongly dependent on social, macroeconomic, and political stability, sound health policies have to go hand in hand with adequate economic policies and a set of measures to ensure a social safety net to protect the relatively deprived. Better health for the population should be the ultimate goal of health policies. Reforming health services and finance is just a means towards that end.

References

Almagambetova, N. (1999). Overhauling the health-care system in Kazakhstan. *Lancet*, **354**, 313.

Anderson, O.W. (1989). *The health service continuum in democratic states: an inquiry into solvable problem.* Health Administration Press, Ann Arbor, MI.

Banister, J. (1997). China: updated information on China's mortality trends. *Proceedings of IUSSP International Population Conference*, Beijing, pp. 1335–51. IUSSP, Liege.

Barr, D.A. and Field, M.G. (1996). The current state of health care in the former Soviet Union: implications for health care policy and reform. *American Journal of Public Health*, **86**, 307–12.

Berlin, A. and Hunter, W. (1998). EU enlargement—the health agenda. Public health challenges and opportunities. *EuroHealth*, **4**, 5–7.

Bobak, M. and Marmot, M. (1996). East–West mortality divide and its potential explanations: proposed research agenda. *British Medical Journal*, **17**, 421–5.

Burger, E.J., Jr, Field, M.G., and Twigg, J.L. (1998). From assurance to insurance in Russian health care: the problematic transition. *American Journal of Public Health*, **88**, 755–8.

Chinese Ministry of Health (1994). *Research on National Health service—an analysis report of the national health services survey in 1993.* Ministry of Health, Beijing.

Chinese Ministry of Health (1997). *Proceedings of the national health conference.* The People's Health Publishing House, Beijing.

Economist (1999). Sick patients, warring doctors. *Economist*, 18 September, p. 81.

Ensor, T. and Savelyeva, L. (1998). Informal payments for health care in the Former Soviet Union: some evidence from Kazakhstan. *Health Policy Plan*, **13**, 41–9.

Ensor, T. and Thompson, R. (1998). Health insurance as a catalyst to change in former communist countries? *Health Policy*, **43**, 203–18.

Evans, R., Maynard, A., Preker, A., and Reinhardt, U. (1994). Health care reform. *Health Economics*, **3**, 359.

Falkingham, J. (1998). Barriers to access? The growth of private payments for health care in Kyrgyzstan. *EuroHealth Winter*, **4**, 68–71.

Frenk, J. (1994). Dimensions of health system reform. *Health Policy*, **27**, 19–34.

Frenk, J., Bobadilla, J.L., Sepulveda, J., and Lopez, M. (1989). Health transition in middle-income countries: new challenges for health care. *Health Policy and Planning*, **4**, 29–39.

Goldstein, E., Preker, S.A., Adeyi, O., and Chellaraj, G. (1996). *Trends in health status, services, and finance. The transition in Central and Eastern Europe.* Technical paper No. 341. World Bank, Washington, DC.

Gudner, M. (1995). Health care in transition in Vietnam: equity and sustainability. *Health Policy Planning*, **10** (Supplement), 49–62.

IMF (International Monetary Fund) (1998). *World economic outlook: financial turbulence and the world economy.* IMF, Washington, DC.

Ionescu, A., Ionescu, A.A., Vinereanu, D., and Bruckner, I. (1998). Facing the challenge: reform and hardship in Romania's health care system. *EuroHealth*, **4**, 17–20.

Jha, P. and Chaloupka, F. (1999). *Curbing the epidemic: Governments and the economics of tobacco control.* World Bank, Washington, DC.

Kingkade, W.W. and Arriaga, E.E. (1997). Mortality in the new independent states: patterns and impacts. In *Premature death in the new independent states* (ed. J.L. Bobadilla, C.A. Costello, and F. Mitchell). National Academy Press, Washington, DC.

Koupilova, I. and Leon, D. (1998). Health of children and youth during the transition in Eastern Europe. *EuroHealth*, **4**, 10–12.

Kovac, C. (1999). Hungarians spurn private health insurance. *British Medical Journal*, **318**, 1370A.

Lassey, M.L., Lassey, W.R., and Jinks, M.J. (1997). *Health care systems around the world. Characteristics, issues, reforms.* Prentice Hall, Englewood Cliffs, NJ.

Liu, Y., Hu, S., Fu, W., and Hisao, W.C. (1996). Is community financing necessary and feasible for rural China? *Health Policy*, **38**, 155–71.

Liu, Y., Rao, K., and Fei, J. (1998). Economic transition and health transition: comparing China and Russia. *Health Policy*, **44**, 103–22.

Murray, C.J.L., Yang, G., and Quiao, C. (1992). Adult mortality: levels, patterns and causes. In *Adult health in developing countries* (ed. R.G. Feachem, T. Kjellstrom, C.J.L. Murray, M. Over, and M. Phillips). Oxford University Press, New York.

Notzon, F.C., Komarov, Y.M., Ermakov, S.P., Sempos, C.T., Marks, J.S., and Sempos, E.V. (1998). Causes of declining life expectancy in Russia. *Journal of the American Medical Association*, **279**, 793–800.

Omran, A.R. (1971). The epidemiological transition. A theory of the epidemiology of population change. *Milbank Memorial Fund Quarterly*, **49**, 509–38.

Szreter, S. (1999). Rapid economic growth and 'the four Ds' of disruption, deprivation, disease and death: public health lessons from nineteenth-century Britain for the twenty-first century China? *Tropical Medicine and International Health*, **4**, 146–52.

Thompson, S. (1998). Poland reforms its health system. *British Medical Journal*, **317**, 769.

Toon, P.D. (1998). Reforming the Russian health service. *British Medical Journal*, **317**, 741–2.

UNDP (United Nations Development Programme) (1998). *Human development report.* Oxford University Press, New York.

Vienonen, M.A. and Springet, J. (1998). Public health, primary health care and health insurance: how to bring the quest for health into the health sector reform in Central and Eastern Europe. *EuroHealth*, **4**, 17–20.

Walberg, P., McKee, M., Shkolnikov, V., Chenet, L., and Leon, D.A. (1998). Economic change, crime, and mortality crisis in Russia: regional analysis. *British Medical Journal*, **317**, 312–18.

World Bank (1993). *World development report 1993: investing in health.* Oxford University Press.

World Bank (1995*a*). *Poverty in Russia: an assessment.* Report 14110-RU. World Bank, Washington, DC.

World Bank (1995*b*). *Vietnam: poverty assessment and strategy.* Report 13442-VN. World Bank, Washington, DC.

World Bank (1996). *World development report 1996: from plan to market.* World Bank, Washington, DC.

World Bank (1999). *World development indicators.* World Bank, Washington, DC.

WHO (World Health Organization) (1994). *Health in Europe: the 1993/1994 Health for All Monitoring Project.* WHO Regional Publications, European Series, No. 56. WHO, Copenhagen.

WHO (World Health Organization) (1997). *Tobacco or health: a global status report.* WHO, Geneva.

WHO (World Health Organization) (1999). *WHOSYS: WHO statistical information system.* WHO, Geneva.

4

Law, ethics, and challenges

4.1 Health and human rights

Sofia Gruskin and Daniel Tarantola

Introduction

Since the creation of the United Nations over 50 years ago, international responsibility for health and for human rights has been increasingly acknowledged. Yet the actual links between health and human rights had not been recognized even a decade ago. Generally thought to be fundamentally antagonistic, these two worlds had evolved along parallel but distinctly separate tracks until a number of recent events helped to bring them together.

Conceptually one can point to the HIV/AIDS pandemic, to women's health issues, including violence, and to the blatant violations of human rights which occurred in such places as the Balkans and the Great Lakes region in Africa as having brought attention to the intrinsic connections that exist between health and human rights. Each of these issues helped to illustrate distinct, but linked, pieces of the health and human rights paradigm. While the relationship between health and human rights with respect to these and similar issues may always have made sense intuitively, the development of a 'health and human rights' language in the last few years has allowed for the connections between health and human rights to be explicitly named, and therefore for conceptual, analytical, policy, and programmatic work to begin to bridge these disparate disciplines and to move forward. In the last few years human rights have increasingly been at the centre of analysis and action in regard to health and development issues. The level of institutional and state political commitment to health and human rights has, in fact, never been higher. This is true within the work of the United Nations system but, even more importantly, can also be seen in the work of governments and non-governmental organizations at both the national and international level.

From HIV/AIDS and human rights to health and human rights

The importance of the HIV/AIDS pandemic as a catalyst for beginning to define some of the structural connections between health and human rights cannot be overemphasized. The first time that human rights were explicitly named in a public health strategy was only in the late 1980s, when the call for human rights and for compassion and solidarity with people living with HIV/AIDS was embodied in the first World Health Organization (**WHO**) global response to AIDS (WHO 1987). This approach was motivated by moral outrage but also, even more importantly, by the recognition that protecting the human rights of people living with HIV/AIDS was a necessary element of the worldwide public health response to the emerging epidemics. The implications of this call were far reaching. Framing this public health strategy in human rights terms—although initially focused on the rights of people living with HIV/AIDS rather than on the broad array of human rights influencing people's vulnerability to the epidemic—allowed it to become anchored in international law, thereby making governments and intergovernmental organizations publicly accountable for their actions towards people living with HIV/AIDS (Mann and Tarantola 1998). The ground-breaking contribution of this era lies in the recognition of the applicability of international law to HIV/AIDS issues and in the attention this approach then generated to the links between other health issues and human rights—and therefore to the ultimate responsibility and accountability of the state under international law for issues relating to health and well being (Mann *et al.* 1994).

International conferences and the United Nations system

The series of international conferences held in the past decade under the auspices of the United Nations system have also been of critical importance in helping to clarify the links between health and human rights. While all of these conferences, ranging from the World Summit for Children held in 1990 to the World Conference on Racism held in 2001, are relevant to health and human rights concerns, the two most crucial in articulating the health and human rights link were the 1994 International Conference on Population and Development and the 1995 Fourth World Conference on Women. These conferences brought together policy-makers, activists, and representatives from local, national, and international agencies, as well as government representatives. The negotiated documents resulted in the first concrete links between health and human rights in international consensus documents and helped to focus attention to the dual obligations of governments regarding both health and human rights (see in particular Chapters IV to VII of the *Report of the International Conference on Population and Development*, and Chapter IV (C) 'Women and health' and Chapter IV (I) 'Human rights of women' of the Fourth World Conference on Women (ICPD 1994; FWCW 1995)). These documents were of use to governments and others in shaping policy and programmatic work which explicitly dealt with these links, as well as to activists and non-governmental organizations in framing their advocacy for government responsibility for health in the human rights language of responsibility and accountability.

In recent years there has been a substantial increase in attention and resources devoted to implementation of health and human rights within virtually all United Nations development agencies and programmes, due in large part to these international conference processes. All of the organizations and agencies of the United Nations have, albeit to varying degrees, begun to consider the relevance of human rights to their work in the health field (Alston 1997). The 1997 Programme for Reform put out by United Nations Secretary-General Kofi Annan, however, has been most crucial in moving the United Nations system's conceptual attention to human rights towards implementation and action within their own work. The Programme for Reform designates human rights as among the core activities of the United Nations system (UN 1997*a*; UNGA 1997). The document states that human rights are to be understood to cut across the four substantive fields of the United Nations' work: peace and security, economic and social affairs, development co-operation, and humanitarian affairs. Each of the agencies with responsibility for health currently has policy documents at various stages of elaboration which concern health and human rights, and technical staff responsible for the integration or implementation of human rights into at least some aspects of their work, a situation that would have been unimaginable even a few years ago.

1. The United Nations International Children's Emergency Fund (**UNICEF**) has restructured its policy and programmatic framework around the Convention on the Rights of the Child (UNICEF 2000).

2. The Joint United Nations Programme on HIV/AIDS (**UNAIDS**) recognizes human rights as a theme relevant to all aspects of its policy and programme work; see *UNAIDS Strategic Plan 1996 to 2000* (revised December 1995), pp. 5, 6, and 13 where the importance of contextual factors that increase vulnerability to HIV/AIDS is recognized, including existing discrimination against certain groups, and where human rights are cited as core values and guiding principles for the mission of UNAIDS.

3. A Memorandum of Understanding now exists between the United Nations Development Programme and the Office of the High Commissioner for Human Rights (UNDP 1999).

4. The United Nations Development Programme Human Development Report for the year 2000 has an explicit focus on human rights, and the WHO is currently preparing its first strategy on health and human rights (WHO 1999*b*).

Likewise, the bodies of the United Nations system with responsibility for human rights are also paying increasing attention to health-related concerns. This is most easily seen in the recent attention to HIV/AIDS and reproductive health by the human rights treaty monitoring bodies (UNHCHR 1996, 1997, 1998*a*, *b*). However, this commitment extends to the recent appointment of two health-related focal points in the Office of the High Commissioner for Human Rights: one responsible for integrating HIV/AIDS issues into the work of the human rights bodies and structures, and the other serving as a general liaison for all health and human rights issues.

State and non-state actors entering the arena of health and human rights

Governments are also increasingly recognizing the relevance of human rights to their health and development work, and calling for technical assistance in the field of human rights. This is true in developing and industrialized countries alike. In Nepal, a comprehensive workshop was recently held on tuberculosis and human rights (WHO 1999*b*). An open debate in South Africa recently focused on the human rights implications of a proposed new regulation concerning AIDS reporting and AIDS-status disclosure to third persons (South Africa Government Gazette 1999). In Colombia, the Convention on the Elimination of All Forms of Discrimination Against Women is being used as a framework for mobilization around much of the work in family planning (Plata and Yanuzova 1993; Corporación Casa de la Mujer 1998). Within the United States, President Clinton issued an Executive Order in commemoration of Human Rights Day in 1998 that obliges the United States to respect and implement fully its obligations under the international human rights treaties to which it is a party and to 'promote respect for international human rights in our relationships with all other countries' (Clinton 1998). As a result, all United States federal agencies, including those with health-related responsibilities, have been directed to re-examine their policies and strategies from the perspective of international human rights standards.

Non-governmental organizations, such as Amnesty International and Human Rights Watch, are also increasingly considering the implications of the health and human rights connection for their own work. Non-governmental organizations that focus on health or development issues, many of which previously saw human rights as having little relevance to their work, are increasingly using not only the rhetoric of human rights but also its method of analysis to help shape their interventions. One prime example is the recent decision of the International Council of AIDS Service Organizations (**ICASO**) to name the promotion of human rights in the context of HIV/AIDS as one of its fundamental organizing principles (ICASO 1998). In addition, human rights non-governmental organizations are expanding their formerly tight focus on civil and political rights to pay increasing attention to economic, social, and cultural rights, including the right to health. These developments are helping to shape new forms of advocacy and to put increased pressure on governments to take responsibility for the health of their populations. The current challenge is to ensure that the increased rhetorical attention to rights translates into policies, national legislation, and actions that will effectively impact on the underlying conditions necessary for health, as well as the ways in which health policies, programmes, and services are conceptualized and delivered.

Academics and researchers are also increasingly finding the links between health and human rights to be of critical importance in expanding their domains of work (Alfredsson and Tomaševski 1998; Toebes 1999). Academic centres with an explicit focus on the links between health and human rights are beginning to appear in a number of places, some with a focus on specific substantive issues, and others concerned with health and human rights more broadly (for example, the François-Xavier Bagnoud Center for Health and Human Rights at the Harvard School of Public Health, as well as the Macfarlane Burnett Centre for Medical Research in Australia, the Programme on Gender, Sexuality, Health and Human Rights at the Mailman School of Public Health at Columbia University, The Netherlands Institute of Human Rights, and the Department of Community Health at the University of Cape Town, South Africa). In the last several years, institutions around the globe have begun to offer courses in health and human rights, international conferences on health and human rights have been held in a number of locations, and professional health journals such as *The Lancet*, the *Journal of the American Medical Association*, and the *American Journal of Public Health* have devoted space to exploring health and human rights issues (Brenner 1996; Sonis *et al.* 1996; Leaning 1997; Fluss 1999). The first course on health and human rights was offered at the Harvard School of Public Health in 1992. Since then, courses on health and human rights have been increasingly offered in countries such as the United States, France, Sweden, Brazil, South Africa, and Zimbabwe. Efforts are currently under way to document existing courses on health and human rights.

Understanding the implications of linking health and human rights is of increasing importance to policy-makers, government officials, and activists—indeed, to anyone concerned with health issues, human rights issues, or the links between the two (Marks 1997). This chapter demonstrates the relationship between health and human rights, and provides a glimpse of some of the conceptual, analytical, and practical approaches to bringing health and human rights together that are currently being explored. It begins by explaining the basic concepts and procedures of human rights, with specific emphasis on their relation to health. It goes on to explore the framework of health as it relates to human rights promotion and protection. The next section considers the reciprocal relationships between health and human rights, with an emphasis on the human rights impact of public health policies and programmes and the impact of neglect or violation of human rights on health. Attention is then given to suggested methods for increasing the synergy between health and human rights, both as a method of analysis and as an approach to the design, implementation, and evaluation of health policies and programmes. This last section offers a useful method for considering the practical application of health and human rights concepts to policy and programmatic work.

What are human rights?

While human rights thinking and practice has a long history, the importance of human rights for governmental action and accountability was first widely recognized only after the Second World War. Agreement between nation-states that all people are 'born free and equal in dignity and rights' was reached in 1945 when the promotion of human rights was identified as a principal purpose of the newly created United Nations (UN 1945). The United Nations Charter established general obligations that apply to all its member states, including respect for human rights and dignity. Then, in 1948, the Universal Declaration of Human Rights was adopted as a common standard of achievement for all peoples and all nations (UN 1948). The basic characteristics of human rights are that they are the rights of individuals, which inhere in individuals because they are human, that they apply to people everywhere in the world, and that they are principally concerned with the relationship between the individual and the state. In practical terms, international human rights law is about defining what governments can do to us, cannot do to us, and should do for us. For example, governments obviously should not do things like torture people, imprison them arbitrarily, or invade their privacy. Governments should ensure that all people in a society have shelter, food, medical care, and basic education.

The Universal Declaration of Human Rights can well be understood to be the cornerstone of the modern human rights movement. The preamble to the Universal Declaration of Human Rights proposes that human rights and dignity are self-evident, the 'highest aspiration of the common people', and the 'foundation of freedom, justice and peace'. 'Social progress and better standards of life' including the 'prevention of barbarous acts which have outraged the conscience of mankind', and, broadly speaking, individual and collective well being, are understood to depend upon the 'promotion of universal respect for and observance of human rights' (UN 1948). Although the Universal Declaration of Human Rights is not a legally binding document, nations have endowed it with a tremendous legitimacy through their actions, including invoking it legally and politically at the national and international levels. Portions of the Universal Declaration of Human Rights are cited in the majority of national constitutions drafted since it came into being, and governments often cite the Universal Declaration of Human Rights in their negotiations with other governments, as well as in their accusations against each other of violating human rights. A useful compilation can be found in Hannum (1998).

Under the auspices of the United Nations, more that 20 multilateral human rights treaties have been formulated since the adoption of the Universal Declaration of Human Rights. These treaties create legally binding obligations on the nations that have ratified them, thereby giving them the status and power of international law. Countries that become party to international human rights treaties accept certain procedures and responsibilities, including periodic submission of reports on their compliance with the substantive provisions of the texts to international monitoring bodies. The key international human rights treaties, the International Covenant on Economic, Social and Cultural Rights (UNICESCR 1966) and the International Covenant on Civil and Political Rights (UNICCPR 1966), further elaborate the content of the rights set out in the Universal Declaration of Human Rights and contain legally binding obligations for the governments that ratify them. As of January 2000, 142 countries had ratified the ICESCR and 144 had ratified the ICCPR. Together with the Universal Declaration of Human Rights and the United Nations Charter, these documents are often called the 'International Bill of Human Rights' (Humphrey 1976). Building upon these core documents, other international human rights treaties have focused on either specific populations (for example, the international Convention on the Elimination of All Forms of Racial Discrimination (UN 1965), the Convention on the Elimination of All Forms of Discrimination Against Women (UN 1979), and the Convention on the Rights of the Child (UNCRC 1989)), or on specific issues (for example, the Convention against Torture and other Cruel, Inhuman or Degrading Treatment or Punishment (UN 1984*a*)).

There are also regional human rights treaties, which essentially concern the same sets of rights but are only open for signature by states in the relevant region, such as the African Charter on Human and Peoples' Rights (1982), the American Convention on Human Rights (1969), and the European Convention on the Protection of Human Rights (1950). Only the Asian region does not contain such a treaty. Additionally, there are numerous international declarations, resolutions, and recommendations which, although not strictly binding in a legal sense, express the political commitment of governments to promote and protect human rights and provide broadly recognized norms and standards relevant to the topic at hand (for example, the Declaration on the Elimination of All Forms of Intolerance and of Discrimination Based on Religion or Belief (UN 1981, 1993*a*)).

In the past decade, the series of international conferences held under the auspices of the United Nations have, to a great degree, helped give recognizable content to many of the rights contained in the various human rights treaties. Out of each of these conference processes has come a declaration and programme of action reflecting the consensus of the nations of the world. Though technically 'non-binding' commitments, these documents demonstrate that there is a consensus of the world community that international human rights treaty norms encompass the relationship between health and human rights, including reproductive rights, and that there are steps that ought to be taken at the local, national, and international levels to advance these concerns.

While these conference declarations and programmes of action represent nothing more than the political commitments of the governments present at their inception, the fact that they are then adopted at the next session of the United Nations General Assembly gives them a degree of formal standing. Although the declarations and programmes of action from the 1994 International Conference on Population and Development (ICPD 1994) and the 1995 Fourth World Conference on Women (FWCW 1995) have been of particular relevance, the 1993 World Conference on Human Rights (UN 1993*c*, 1998*a*) and the 1995 World Summit for Social Development (UN 1995*b*) have also helped explicate the relevance of the health and human rights framework to government action. Individually and collectively, these documents have been of critical importance in helping to elaborate provisions relevant to vulnerable groups, women's human rights, and broader concepts of health and human rights. Those commitments have helped to create new approaches for considering the extent of government accountability for health issues, as well as for determining the content of health issues using a rights framework. In so doing, these conference documents are helping to clarify the evolving meaning of the relationship between health and human rights and the steps needed for implementation (Gruskin 1998).

A human rights perspective on health

The specific rights that form the corpus of human rights law are found in the international human rights documents. While it is possible to identify different categories of rights, it is also critical to rights discourse and action to recognize that all rights are interdependent and interrelated, and that individuals rarely suffer neglect or violation of a particular right in isolation. For historical reasons, the rights described in the human rights documents have been divided into civil and political rights on the one hand and economic, social, and cultural rights on the other. Civil and political rights include the rights to liberty, to security of person, to freedom of movement, to vote, and not to be subjected to cruel, inhuman, or degrading treatment or punishment or to arbitrary arrest or detention. Economic, social, and cultural rights include the rights to the highest attainable standard of health, work, social security, adequate food, clothing and housing, and education, and the right to enjoy the benefits of scientific progress and its applications. Although the Universal Declaration of Human Rights contains both categories of rights, these rights were artificially split into two treaties due to Cold War politics, with the United States championing civil and political rights, and the former Soviet Union those rights considered to be more economic, social, and cultural in nature (Steiner and Alston 1996). Since the end of the Cold War, acknowledgement of the indivisibility and interdependence of rights has, once again, become commonplace (UN 1993*c*). The Convention on the Rights of the Child, the first human rights treaty to be opened for signature after the end of the Cold War, is the only one so far to include civil, political, and economic and social rights considerations not only within the same treaty but within the same right. (See, in particular Article 6, which in guaranteeing the right to life includes both the more civil and political provision which states that 'every child has the inherent right to life' and the more economic and social provision in which 'State Parties shall ensure to the maximum extent possible the survival and development of the child' (UNCRC 1989).)

Health and government responsibility for health is codified in these documents in several ways. The right to the highest attainable standard of health appears in one form or another in most of them. More importantly, nearly every article of every document can be understood to have clear implications for health (Mann *et al.* 1994). While the rights to information, education, housing and safe working conditions, and social security, for example, are particularly relevant to the health and human rights relationship, specific reference must be made to three rights: the right to non-discrimination, the right to the benefits of scientific progress, and the right to health.

Non-discrimination

The principle of non-discrimination is key to human rights thinking and practice. Under international human rights law, all people should be treated equally and given equal opportunity. Within the international human rights framework, discrimination is a breach of a government's human rights obligations (Bilder 1992). Adverse discrimination occurs when a distinction is made against a person which results in their being treated unfairly or unjustly. In general, groups that are discriminated against tend to be those that do not share the characteristics of the dominant groups within a society. Thus, discrimination frequently reinforces social inequalities and denies equal opportunities. Common forms of discrimination include racism, gender-based discrimination, and homophobia. Each of the major human rights treaties specifically details the principle of non-discrimination with respect to race, colour, sex, language, religion, political or other opinion, national or social origin, property, birth, and, as it is called, 'other status'.

Governmental responsibility for this right includes ensuring equal protection under the law, as well as in relation to such issues as housing, employment, and medical care. The prohibition of discrimination does not mean that differences should not be acknowledged, only that different treatment must be based on objective and reasonable criteria. Although the international human rights documents do not explicitly prohibit discrimination on the basis of health status, the United Nations Commission on Human Rights has stated that 'all are equal before the law and entitled to equal protection of the law from all discrimination and from all incitement to discrimination relating to their state of health' (UN 1992*a*, 1993*b*; UNCHR 1994).

Right to enjoy the benefits of scientific progress

Closely allied to many of the issues relevant to health is the right to 'enjoy the benefits of scientific progress and its applications', recognized explicitly in the ICESCR, Article 15. This right includes governmental obligations for the steps necessary to conserve, develop, and diffuse science and scientific research, as well as freedom of scientific inquiry. The implications of this right for health issues have been explored recently with respect to access to drugs for the developing world, to name one important example (Lallemant *et al.* 1994; Reich 2000). In fact, this right is increasingly being cited by activist groups, non-governmental organizations, and others concerned by the large and growing disparities and inequities between wealthier and poorer populations regarding access to antiretroviral therapies and other forms of HIV/AIDS care. In addition, the relevance of this right to concerns about the development of vaccines that adequately respond to the specific needs of all populations, both in the North and the South, has recently been cited (Beloqui *et al.* 1998; Fluss and Little 1999). (See, for example, Statement from the Community AIDS Movement in Africa, presented at the Meeting on the International Partnership against HIV/AIDS in Africa, New York, United Nations Headquarters, 6–7 December 1999.) Unfortunately, while this right has long been recognized as relevant to governmental obligations under the ICESCR, its implications for health and health-related issues are only just beginning to be recognized.

The right to health

The human right to health should be understood, in the first instance, with reference to the description of health set forth in the preamble of the WHO Constitution and repeated in many subsequent documents (WHO 1946). Health is a 'state of complete physical, mental, and social well-being, and not merely the absence of disease or infirmity' (WHO 1946). This definition has important conceptual and practical implications, and it illustrates the indivisibility and interdependence of rights as they relate to health (Leary 1994; Tomaševski 1995*a*; Kirby 1999; Toebes 1999). Rights relating to discrimination, autonomy, information, education, and participation are an integral and indivisible part of the achievement of the highest attainable standard of health, just as the enjoyment of health is inseparable from that of other rights, whether categorized as civil and political, economic, social, or cultural. While the right to health has been set out in a number of international legal instruments, government obligations under this right are quite narrowly defined. As first elaborated in the ICESCR, the right is set forth only as 'the right to the highest attainable standard of physical and mental health', with obligations understood to encompass both the underlying preconditions necessary for health and the provision of medical care.

It is worth noting that the apparent tension between the broad definition of health proposed by the WHO, which includes the notion of social well being, and the more restrictive definition set out in the ICESCR reflects the very different purposes of these two documents. The WHO definition projects a vision of the ideal state of health as an eternal and universal goal to strive constantly towards, and has as its main purpose defining directions for the work of the Organization and its member states. The ICESCR definition differentiates the two attributes of health—physical and mental well being—and is specifically concerned with assigning particular responsibilities to the governmental health sector; it assigns obligations relevant to social well being to the same governments under other articles of the treaty. The right to health as stated in the ICESCR (Box 1) is the principal framework for understanding governmental obligations under the right to health.

Box 1 Article 12 of the United Nations International Covenant on Economic, Social and Cultural Rights (UNICESCR)

1. The States Parties to the present Covenant recognize the right of everyone to the enjoyment of the highest attainable standard of physical and mental health.

2. The steps to be take by the States Parties to the present Covenant to achieve the full realization of this right shall include those necessary for:
   (a) the provision for the reduction of the stillbirth rate and of infant mortality and for the healthy development of the child
   (b) the improvement of all aspects of environmental and industrial hygiene
   (c) the prevention, treatment, and control of epidemic, endemic, occupational, and other diseases
   (d) the creation of conditions which would assure to all medical service and medical attention in the event of sickness

Governmental obligations for health under international human rights law

Governments are responsible not only for not directly violating rights, but also for ensuring the conditions which enable individuals to realize their rights as fully as possible. This is understood as an obligation to respect, protect, and fulfil rights, and governments are legally responsible for complying with this range of obligations for every right in every human rights document they have ratified (Eide 1995*a*,*b*; Maastricht Guidelines on Violations of Economic, Social and Cultural Rights 1997).

Respecting, protecting, and fulfilling human rights

Governmental obligations towards ensuring that every individual enjoys the right to health are summarized below as an illustration of the range of issues relevant to respecting, protecting, and fulfilling all human rights.

1. Respecting the right means that a state cannot violate the right directly. A government violates its responsibility to respect the right to health when it is immediately responsible for providing medical care to certain populations, such as prisoners or the military, and it arbitrarily decides to withhold that care.

2. Protecting the right means that a state has to prevent violations of rights by non-state actors and offer some sort of redress that people know about and can access if a violation occurs. This means that the state would be responsible for making it illegal to deny insurance or health care automatically to people on the basis

of a health condition, and that they would be responsible for ensuring some system of redress that people know about and can access if a violation does occur.

3. Fulfilling the right means that a state has to take all appropriate measures—including but not limited to legislative, administrative, budgetary, and judicial—towards fulfilment of the right, including the obligation to promote the right in question. A state could be found to be in violation of the right to health if it failed to allocate sufficient resources incrementally to meet the public health needs of the communities within its borders.

In all countries, resource and other constraints can make it impossible for a government to fulfil all rights immediately and completely. The human rights machinery recognizes this and acknowledges that, in practical terms, a commitment to the right to health requires more than just passing a law. It will require financial resources, trained personnel, facilities, and, more than anything else, a sustainable infrastructure. Therefore, realization of rights is generally understood to be a matter of progressive realization of making steady progress towards a goal (ICESCR Article 2.1; Alston and Quinn 1987). The principle of 'progressive realization' is fundamental to the achievement of human rights. This is critical for resource-poor countries that are responsible for striving towards human rights goals to the maximum extent possible. It is also of relevance to wealthier countries in that they are responsible for respecting, protecting, and fulfilling human rights not only within their own borders, but through their engagement in international assistance and co-operation (UN 1984*b*).

Valid limitations on human rights

In spite of the importance attached to human rights, there are situations where it is considered legitimate to restrict rights in order to achieve a broader public good. As described in the International Covenant on Civil and Political Rights, the public good can take precedence to 'secure due recognition and respect for the rights and freedoms of others; meet the just requirements of morality, public order, and the general welfare; and in times of emergency, when there are threats to the vital interests of the nation' (ICCPR Article 4). Public health is one such recognized public good. (The specific power of the state to restrict right in the state of public health can be understood to be derived from Article 12 (c) of the ICESCR, which gives governments the right to take the steps they deem necessary for the 'prevention, treatment and control of epidemic, endemic, occupational and other diseases'.) Traditional public health measures have generally focused on curbing the spread of disease by imposing restrictions on the rights of those already infected or thought to be most vulnerable to becoming infected. In fact, coercion, compulsion, and restriction have historically been significant components of public health measures (Smith 1911; Schmidt 1995; Cohen 1998). Although the restrictions on rights that have occurred in the context of public health have generally had as their first concern protection of the public's health, it is also true that the measures taken have often been excessive. Interference with freedom of movement when instituting quarantine or isolation for a serious communicable disease—for example, Ebola fever, syphilis, typhoid, or untreated tuberculosis—is an example of a restriction on rights that may be necessary for the public good and therefore could be considered legitimate under international human rights law. Conversely, arbitrary measures taken by public health authorities that fail to consider other valid alternatives may be found to be abusive of both human rights principles and public health 'best practice'. In recent times, measures taken around the world in response to HIV/AIDS provides examples of this type of abuse (Cohen and Wiseberg 1990; UN 1992*a*, 1994; HRI 1998).

Certain rights are absolute, which means that restrictions may never be placed on them, even if justified as necessary for the public good. These include such rights as the right to be free from torture, slavery, or servitude, the right to a fair trial, and the right to freedom of thought. (See, for example, Article 4 of the ICCPR, which states that '[n]o derogation from articles 6, 7, 8 (paragraphs 1 and 2), 11, 15, 16, 18 may be made under this provision'.) Paradoxically, the right to life, which might at first glance appear to be inalienable, is not absolute; what is forbidden is the arbitrary deprivation of life. Interference with most rights can be legitimately justified as necessary under narrowly defined circumstances in many situations relevant to public health. (See, for example, Article 4 of the ICCPR, which states that '[i]n time of public emergency which threatens the life of the nation and the existence of which is officially proclaimed, the States Parties to the present Covenant may take measures derogating from their obligations under the present Covenant to the extent strictly required by the exigencies of the situation, provided that such measures are not inconsistent with their other obligations under international law and do not involve discrimination solely on the ground of race, colour, sex, language, religion or social origin'.)

Limitations on rights, however, are considered a serious issue under international human rights law, regardless of the apparent importance of the public good involved. When a government limits the exercise or enjoyment of a right, this action must be taken only as a last resort and will only be considered legitimate if the following criteria are met (UNECOSOC 1985).

1. The restriction is provided for and carried out in accordance with the law.
2. The restriction is in the interest of a legitimate objective of general interest.
3. The restriction is strictly necessary in a democratic society to achieve the objective.
4. There are no less intrusive and restrictive means available to reach the same goal.
5. The restriction is not imposed arbitrarily, i.e. in an unreasonable or otherwise discriminatory manner.

Whereas this approach, often called the Siracusa Principles because they were conceptualized at a meeting in Siracusa, Italy, has long been recognized by those concerned with human rights monitoring and implementation as relevant to analysing a government's actions, it has also recently begun to be considered a useful tool in a number of places by those responsible within government for health-related policies and programmes (WHO/UNAIDS 1999). This framework, although still rudimentary, may be helpful in identifying public health actions that are abusive, whether intentionally or unintentionally.

Human rights monitoring mechanisms relevant to health

The degree of governmental compliance with the obligations to respect, protect, and fulfil human rights are of direct relevance to the people affected, but they are also of interest to the international community. The accountability of governments for their legal commitments is monitored at the international level through the reporting process and, in many places, at the national level by governments themselves through the creation of commissions and ombudspersons, as well as by non-governmental organizations.

Reporting under the human rights treaties

As mentioned above, once a government has ratified a human rights treaty, it is obliged to report every several years to the specific body responsible for monitoring government action under that treaty. Governments are responsible for showing the ways that they are and are not in compliance with the treaty provisions, and must show constant improvement in their efforts to respect, protect, and fulfil the rights in question (UN 1996). Each of the treaty bodies meets several times a year to review a number of the government reports submitted. The process is very formal, with the government under review submitting a copy of its report approximately 2 months before the meeting. The report is officially presented at the meeting by a high-ranking government official, and the treaty body engages in formal dialogue with the country in question. Health-oriented United Nations institutions, such as the WHO, UNAIDS, or UNICEF, are invited to provide the treaty bodies with information on the state of health and the performance of health systems in the country under review. Non-governmental organizations can also submit informal reports (often termed shadow reports) providing additional information, as well as stating their views on the situations and issues at stake. At the conclusion of the session, the treaty body prepares concluding comments and observations, which are made part of the substantive record. These comments address the extent to which the government in question is in compliance with its treaty provisions and provide concrete suggestions for actions to be taken by the country in order for it to be found in compliance at its next review. While this process can be extremely useful, there is, unfortunately, a tremendous backlog, largely because governments are often late with their reports, and none of the treaty bodies meets for a sufficient amount of time each year to cover all of the countries that are responsible for reporting to it.

All of the human rights treaty bodies have expressed a commitment to exploring the implications of health broadly defined, as well as the specific issues raised by both HIV/AIDS and reproductive health concerns, for governmental obligations under the treaties (UNDAW 1996; UNHCHR 1996; Boerefon and Toebes 1998; UNFPA 1998). While several of the treaties contain specific health-related provisions, the added impetus to pay attention to health in the context of monitoring work can largely be attributed to the interest generated from international conferences and the political commitments made there about governmental responsibility for ensuring the human rights of individuals in relation to health.

For each of the human rights treaties, general guidelines for reporting provide guidance to governments as to how to present the information about their compliance with their obligations to the treaty bodies (UN 1996). The information requested by the treaty bodies concerning health-related issues explains what governments are doing with respect to both the underlying preconditions for health and the ways in which health policies, programmes, and services are designed and implemented. From a health perspective, however, the actual information requested under current requirements is largely insufficient to get at this range of issues. The general guidelines provided to governments for reporting on the right to health under the ICESCR are included in Box 2. They provide a concrete example of what the treaty body with primary responsibility for implementation of the right to health considers in determining if, and the degree to which, a government is in compliance with its obligations for the right to health.

The increasing links among the work of the treaty bodies, the United Nations specialized agencies, and non-governmental organizations are useful to the treaty monitoring process, but they are also beginning to contribute directly to the enhancement of the implementation of human rights at the country level by governments as well as other actors. The role of the technical and specialized agencies, funds, and programmes of the United Nations in the treaty monitoring process is growing, with respect to both provision of information and interactions with the treaty bodies and governments in question. This includes primarily UNICEF, UNAIDS, and the WHO but also, increasingly, the International Labour Organization, the United Nations Development Programme, and the United Nations Population Fund. These agencies and programmes have increasingly been providing the treaty bodies with statistical information and other data collected as part of their routine work concerning the country in question to assist the treaty bodies in their review of government compliance. They have also been providing treaty bodies with guidelines and other examples of 'best practice' they have produced, which can assist the treaty bodies in their analysis of the information provided by the government and in the drafting of their concluding comments and observations. To date, however, the input of these agencies has been somewhat uncoordinated, even within the same institution, often resulting in heavy servicing of some treaty bodies in some specific ways while virtually ignoring others. As a result, a country may be heavily questioned by one treaty body as to some specific aspect of their compliance with their health-related obligations under one treaty, but not questioned at all by another treaty body responsible for monitoring similar health-related obligations. In addition, owing to lack of resources and the relative newness of their engagement with this process, the United Nations agencies, funds, and programmes do not provide even the treaty bodies they do work with equivalent information on all countries reporting at a particular time. Thus, while one country may be heavily questioned by a treaty body as a result of information provided by a particular agency, the next country immediately under review may not even be questioned superficially on comparable issues. UNICEF has been involved in the treaty monitoring process in other ways as well. For example, it has expended considerable resources on helping governments to prepare their reports as well as increasingly framing technical assistance to countries according to the provisions of the Convention on the Rights of the Child (UNICEF 1998). This approach to the work of United Nations agencies and programmes at the country level has increasingly been considered of interest by the other technical agencies of the United Nations, especially UNAIDS and the WHO, and may help to frame some of their future work.

Non-governmental organizations have a critical role to play in monitoring government compliance with treaty provisions. Within countries, non-governmental organizations are increasingly using government obligations under the human rights treaties, as well as the concluding comments and observations of the treaty bodies, in their advocacy efforts. The input of non-governmental organizations is also

Box 2 Guidelines for reporting on Article 12 of the United Nations International Covenant on Economic, Social and Cultural Rights (UNICESCR) (UNECOSOC 1991; Alston 1991)

1. Please supply information on the physical and mental health of your population, both in the aggregate and with respect to different groups within your society. How has the health situation changed over time with regard to these groups? In case your government has recently submitted reports on the health situation in your country to the WHO you may wish to refer to the relevant parts of these reports rather than repeat the information here.

2. Please indicate whether your country has a national health policy. Please indicate whether a commitment to the WHO primary health care approach has been adopted as part of the health policy of your country. If so, what measures have been taken to implement primary health care?

3. Please indicate what percentage of your gross national product as well as of your national and/or regional budget(s) is spent on health. What percentage of those resources is allocated to primary health care? How does this compare with 5 years ago and 10 years ago?

4. Please provide, where available, indicators as defined by the WHO, relating to the following issues:
   (a) infant mortality rate (in addition to the national value, please provide the rate by sex, urban/rural division, and also, if possible, by socio-economic or ethnic group and geographical area. Please include national definitions of urban/rural and other subdivisions)
   (b) population access to safe water (please disaggregate urban/rural)
   (c) population access to adequate excrete disposal facilities (please disaggregate urban/rural)
   (d) infants immunized against diphtheria, pertussis, tetanus, measles, poliomyelitis, and tuberculosis (please disaggregate urban/rural and by sex)
   (e) life expectancy (please disaggregate urban/rural, by socio-economic group, and by sex)
   (f) proportion of the population having access to trained personnel for the treatment of common diseases and injuries, with regular supply of 20 essential drugs, within 1 hour's walk or travel
   (g) proportion of pregnant women having access to trained personnel during pregnancy and proportion attended by such personnel for delivery. Please provide figures on the maternity mortality rate, both before and after childbirth
   (h) proportion of infants having access to trained personnel for care.

(Please provide breakdowns by urban/rural and socio-economic groups for indicators (f) to (h).)

5. Can it be discerned from the breakdown of the indicators employed in paragraph 4, or by other means, that there are any groups in your country whose health situation is significantly worse than that of the majority of the population? Please define these groups as precisely as possible and give specifics. Which geographical areas in your country, if any, are worse off with regard to the health of their population?
   (a) During the reporting period, have there been any changes in national policies, laws, and practices negatively affecting the health situation of these groups or areas? If so, please describe these changes and their impact.
   (b) Please indicate what measures are considered necessary by your government to improve the physical and mental health situation of such vulnerable and disadvantaged groups in such worse off areas.
   (c) Please explain the policy measures your government has taken, to the maximum of available resources, to realize such improvement. Indicate time-related goals and benchmarks for measuring your achievement in this regard.
   (d) Please describe the effect of these measures on the health of the vulnerable and disadvantaged groups or worse-off areas under consideration, and report on the successes, problems, and shortcomings of these measures.
   (e) Please describe the measures taken by your government in order to reduce the stillbirth rate and infant mortality and to provide for the healthy development of the child.
   (f) Please list the measures taken by your government to improve all aspects of environmental and industrial hygiene.
   (g) Please describe the measures taken by your government to prevent, treat, and control epidemic, endemic, and occupational and other diseases.
   (h) Please describe the measures taken by your government to assure to all medical service and medical attention in the event of sickness.
   (i) Please describe the effect of the measures listed in subparagraphs (e) to (h) on the situation of the vulnerable and disadvantaged groups in your society and in any worse-off areas. Report on difficulties and failures as well as on positive results.

6. Please indicate the measures taken by your government to ensure that the rising costs of health care for the elderly do not lead to infringements on these persons' right to health.

7. Please indicate what measures have been taken in your country to maximize community participation in the planning, organization, operation, and control of primary health care.

8. Please indicate what measures have been taken in your country to provide education concerning prevailing health problems and the measures of preventing and controlling them.

9. Please indicate the role of international assistance in the full realization of the right enshrined in Article 12.

crucial at the international level in that they are able to provide treaty monitoring bodies with the necessary additional outside information on the action (or inaction) of the government in question, which can then be used by the treaty body in its dialogue with that government. Although non-governmental organizations are sometimes present during the formal dialogue, this information is most often presented in shadow reports. There is no formal mechanism, however, for ensuring that non-governmental organization information reaches the treaty bodies, and, unfortunately, non-governmental organizations generally do not co-ordinate with each other on the information they provide. At times, the same information about a particular situation has been presented to a treaty body from numerous sources, while other potentially critical information of a more general nature is never provided. In addition, many local non-governmental organizations are unaware of or lack access to the treaty monitoring process, resulting in a number of problems. Firstly, only the most publicized cases come to the attention of the monitoring body. Secondly, the lack of functioning non-governmental organizations in a majority of countries results in both a dearth of information from countries with some of the worst human rights records and a privileging of the information provided by well-established international human rights non-governmental organizations such as Amnesty International and Human Rights Watch, which have more contacts and closer relationships with the treaty body members than other organizations do. This last point is of particular concern in relation to health-related human rights issues, as these issues often fall outside the purview of mainstream human rights organizations, and therefore little alternative information on health-related issues reaches the relevant bodies (UNAIDS 1997). As a result, while the utility of the involvement of non-governmental organizations to this process is at this point undisputed, mechanisms for ensuring their involvement in a comprehensive way, particularly with respect to health-related information, still remain to be worked out.

General recommendations and general comments concerning health

In the past 5 years, there have been increasing efforts to draft authoritative interpretations of the right to health in order to ensure state responsibility and accountability with respect to health in a structured way. These authoritative interpretations have taken the form of general comments or general recommendations, which are drafted and endorsed by the treaty monitoring body in question and which form the basis of the treaty body's formal understanding of the content of a particular right or issue. These general comments or general recommendations then help to serve as a guide for governments concerning the issues that they must consider in making their periodic reports under the guidelines, for non-governmental organizations in their monitoring of governmental action and for the treaty bodies themselves in their dialogue and interaction with governments in the context of the monitoring process (UN 1996). While these comments and recommendations are meant only to provide interpretation, their formulation does have real implications for whether or not a government is judged to be in compliance with its treaty obligations. For example, the right to health as formulated in international treaties contains no mention of primary health care. This is mainly because the concept of primary health care had not yet been internationally recognized at the time that the ICESCR was drafted. While the guidelines for reporting contain substantive mention of primary health care, the relationship between a primary health care approach and government obligations under the treaty are not detailed. Thus, in the absence of a general comment or recommendation emphasizing a primary health care approach, it is difficult to judge a country that pays little or no attention to primary health care not to be in compliance with its health-related obligations.

Until very recently, no general comments or recommendations had been issued by any of the treaty bodies specifically related to health. In 1999, the United Nations Committee on the Elimination of Discrimination Against Women (**UNCEDAW**), which monitors governmental compliance under the Women's Convention, issued a General Recommendation on Health (UNCEDAW 1999), and in 2000 the Committee on Economic, Social and Cultural Rights, the body responsible for monitoring the ICESCR, issued a General Comment on the Right to Health (UNICESCR 2000). Nonetheless, a number of the general comments and recommendations previously issued by the treaty bodies have had clear health-related implications. These include the General Comments on disability (UN 1994), housing (UN 1997*b*), and food (UN 1995*a*) issued by the UNCESCR, and the General Recommendations concerning HIV/AIDS (UNCEDAW 1990*b*), female circumcision (UNCEDAW 1990*a*), and violence against women (UNCEDAW 1989) issued by the UNCEDAW.

At the outset of the twenty-first century, the translation of the right to health into guidelines and other tools useful to national and international monitoring of governmental and intergovernmental obligations is still in its infancy. The ICESCR General Comment on the Right to the Highest Attainable Standard of Health, which was adopted in 2000 (UNICESCR 2000), may help to provide some useful guidelines. In parallel, as described below, the WHO is developing a new set of tools and recommendations aimed at redirecting the attention given to monitoring global health indicators from disease-specific morbidity and mortality trends towards others that are more reflective of the degree to which health and human rights principles are respected, protected, and fulfilled (WHO 2000*c*). How and to what extent these instruments will be put to use and how effective they will be in advancing the health and human rights agenda has yet to be seen, but there are several factors that, even at this early stage, allow for guarded optimism. Firstly, the treaty bodies and international organizations concerned with health are doing this work based on open dialogue and a degree of collaboration that greatly exceeds the level and quality of interagency collaboration traditionally observed within the United Nations machinery. This is exemplified by the sharing of goals and the collective technical co-operation that has prevailed in the current processes of defining obligations and monitoring methods and standards relevant to health and human rights in the process of operationalizing both the international treaties and the recommendations promulgated at the international conferences (UNDAW 1996; UNDP 1998*b*; WHO 2000*b*). Potentially, this work will help not only to monitor what governments are doing, but also to build their capacity to incorporate health and human rights principles into their policies and programmes. In several countries, including Brazil, Thailand, and South Africa, human rights principles relevant to health have recently found their way into national legislation and new constitutions, thereby ensuring citizens the right to seek fulfilment of their right to care, for example, through national juridical means (Hannum 1998). As the methods and tools for monitoring and accountability of health-related issues mature, it is likely that cases of human rights violations related to health will increasingly be heard both within countries and at the regional and international level. (See, for example, *Open Door Counselling Ltd and Dublin Well Women's Centre Ltd* v. *Ireland*, 1992, 15 EUR. H.R. Report 244.) A focus on monitoring and redress of violations of the right to health is but one means of ensuring action using the human rights documents. Equally important are the steps being taken to build national and international capacity to develop and reform public policy and laws in line with international human rights norms and standards as they apply to health (UNFPA 1998). This work requires institutional changes, as well as capacity building within both governmental systems and international organizations. The Director-General of the WHO has cited the need to integrate efforts towards this goal, noting: 'Even when governments are well-intentioned, they may have difficulty fulfilling their health and human rights obligations. Governments, the WHO and other intergovernmental agencies should strive to create the conditions favorable to health, even in situations where the base of public finance threatens to collapse' (Brundtland 1998).

The process of 'mainstreaming human rights', currently well underway in the United Nations system, is specifically aimed toward this goal (UN 1997*a*). Mainstreaming human rights is 'the process of assessing the human rights implications of any planned action, including legislation, policies or programmes, in all areas and at all levels. It is a strategy for making human rights an integral dimension of the design, implementation, monitoring and evaluation of policies and programmes in political, economic and social spheres' (UN 1997*a*). Two examples illustrate how this is done. In the 1990s, UNICEF adopted the Convention on the Rights of the Child (**CRC**), thereby ensuring that their policy and programmatic work would be guided by the principles and standards established by the CRC, as well as the Convention on the Elimination of All Forms of Discrimination Against Women. The 1996 Mission Statement says explicitly that pursuit of the rights of children and women is a fundamental purpose of the organization. These efforts have led to a restructuring of UNICEF and a rights-based approach to all programming efforts at all levels of its work (UNICEF 1998). In the WHO, a similar process began in 1999 with the aim of defining the goals of human rights mainstreaming for their national and international health work (WHO 1999*c*). The process was begun following the 1998 World Health Assembly Resolution that set out the need to 'promote and support the rights and principles, actions and responsibilities enunciated in the [World Health Declaration] through concerted action, full participation and partnership, calling on all peoples and institutions to share the vision of health for all in the twenty-first century, and to endeavor in common to realize it' (WHO 1998*d*). In 2000, work began towards a strategy document which would incorporate health and human rights into the policy and programme work of the WHO. Towards this aim, health and human rights are considered relevant to each of the WHO's four strategic directions (WHO 1999*c*):

- reducing excess mortality, morbidity, and disability, especially in poor and marginalized populations
- promoting healthy lifestyles and reducing risk factors to human health that arise from environmental, economic, social, and behavioural causes
- developing health systems that equitably improve health outcomes, respond to people's legitimate demands, and are financially fair
- developing an enabling policy and institutional environment in the health sector and promoting an effective health dimension to social, economic, environmental, and development policy.

These strategic directions are discussed more extensively below with specific reference to their health and human rights implications. To pursue these directions, the WHO is proposing to contribute to the building of skills and knowledge within the WHO and within countries; to perform an internal review of its policies and programmes to verify their conformity with health and human rights principles; to further its co-operation with the Office of the High Commissioner for Human Rights and the treaty monitoring bodies; to disseminate information; and to develop and refine human rights-sensitive monitoring and evaluation processes applicable nationally and internationally.

A health perspective on human rights

As stated above, over 50 years ago, the Constitution of the WHO projected a vision of health as a state of complete physical, mental, and social well being—a definition of health that is more relevant today than ever (WHO 1946). It recognized that the enjoyment of the highest attainable standard of health was one of the fundamental rights of every human being and that governments have a responsibility for the health of their peoples, which can be fulfilled only through the provision of adequate health and social measures. The 1978 Alma-Ata Declaration (WHO/UNICEF 1979) called on nations to ensure the availability of the essentials of primary health care, including:

- education concerning health problems and the methods for preventing and controlling them
- promotion of food supply and proper nutrition
- an adequate supply of safe water and basic sanitation
- maternal and child health care, including family planning
- immunization against major infectious diseases
- prevention and control of locally endemic diseases
- appropriate treatment of common disease and injuries
- provision of essential drugs.

In 1998, the World Health Assembly reaffirmed the commitment of nations to strive towards these goals in a World Health Declaration that stressed the 'will to promote health by addressing the basic determinants and prerequisites for health' and the urgent priority 'to pay the greatest attention to those most in need, burdened by ill health, receiving inadequate services for health or affected by poverty' (WHO 1998*d*). These ambitious objectives of health development must be examined from the perspective of the role of governments in ensuring equal and equitable access to medical care and health promotion while striving to create the underlying conditions necessary for health.

This section begins with a discussion of the traditional dichotomy between the roles and functions of medicine and those of public health, which will help begin to frame the content of governmental obligations towards individuals and populations for health under international human rights law. Health will then be placed in the broader context of human development in order to underscore the relevance of a broad array of governmental obligations, well beyond the health sector, that may impact on health. The four strategic directions to health development mentioned above will then be presented as an approach relevant to the development of both a health and human rights analysis and monitoring and accountability. Finally, a new grouping of these issues will be proposed as an entry point into their analysis from a human rights perspective, leading to a pathway for action.

Medicine, public health, and human rights

Health as it connects to human rights analysis and implementation concerns two related but different disciplines: medicine and public health. Historically the territorial boundaries of medicine and public health reflected not only professional interest and skill, but also the environments within which these skills were practised: homes, clinics, hospitals, and clinical laboratories on the one hand; institutes, public health laboratories, offices, and field projects on the other (Detels *et al.* 1997). Recently, the apparent differences between the two professions—the first primarily understood to focus on the health of individuals, the second on the health of populations—have profoundly impacted the ways in which the relationship between health and human rights has been understood by different actors. From a rights perspective, this ancient division resulted in the assumption that, of the two, medicine was more concerned with the health and rights of the individual (for example, in creating conditions enabling a particular individual to access care), while the primary focus of public health was the protection of collective interests, even at the cost of arbitrarily restricting individual rights (Mann 1997*b*). For example, coercion and restrictions of rights had been critical to traditional smallpox eradication efforts (Fenner *et al.* 1988). Yet as the human rights approach has made increasingly clear, this stark differentiation between medicine and public health is no longer fully relevant either to human rights or to health. Although they apply different methods of work, both medicine and public health seek to ensure every person's right to achieve the highest attainable standard of health, and both have a strong focus on the individual. Medicine is more concerned with analysing, diagnosing, and treating disease, as well as preventing ill health in individuals through such methods as immunization, appropriate diet, or prophylactic therapies. Public health seeks to address health and ill health by focusing on individual and collective determinants, be they behavioural, social, economic, or other contextual factors.

Three sets of factors have contributed to blurring traditional boundaries between medicine and public health. Firstly, the transitions in health status through which many populations have been recently evolving have called for a closer understanding of the links between individual health, public health, and the environment (Shrader-Frechetter 1991; Gubler 1998). Current thinking about optimal strategies for disease control have evolved, as efforts to confront the most serious global health threats (including cancer, mental disorders, cardiovascular and other chronic diseases, reproductive and sexual health, infectious diseases, and violence) have increasingly emphasized the role of personal behaviour within a broad social context (Murray and Lopez 1996; WHO 1999*a*). The transition of the global disease burden from communicable to non-communicable diseases (which are heavily dependent on lifestyle), has evoked a medical need to care for patients in their own social contexts. There has been increasing understanding that behaviours and their social, economic, and cultural contexts are inextricably linked with the biology of health and disease, and are therefore relevant to individual care (Krieger and Sidney 1996).

Secondly, the tools and technologies of each field have been found to be of increasing utility to the other. For example, new technologies developed through biomedical research in such fields as immunology, molecular biology, and genetics are of increasing relevance to public health (Barry and Molyneux 1992; Andrews 1995; Aluwihare 1998). Scientific discoveries in molecular virology have provided tools that are as useful to individual diagnosis and care as they are to epidemiology, vaccine development, and public health programmes (Hunter 1999). Likewise, traditional public health tools, drawn from epidemiology, ecology, and social and behavioural sciences, have demonstrated their usefulness in deciphering powerful determinants of health and of disease outcomes, thus creating stronger bridges between biomedical care and public health interventions (Terragni 1993; Krieger and Zierler 1997).

Thirdly, the human rights framework has shown that the state's human rights responsibilities to respect, protect, and fulfil rights relating to health include obligations concerning both medicine and public health. In the context of a health and human rights analysis, a challenge to the now artificial dichotomy between medicine and public health is not merely rhetorical or of analytical interest; it also brings into play the range of obligations of the state towards every individual. The health and human rights paradigm is relevant to clinical practice, community health, large-scale health programme development, implementation, and policy. The synergistic health and human rights perspective aims to guarantee that every individual can achieve the highest attainable standard of physical, mental, and social well being. Human rights are progressively being understood to offer an approach for considering the broader societal dimensions and contexts of the well being of individuals and populations, and therefore to be of utility to all those concerned with health.

Globalization and health development

The definition of health enshrined in the WHO Constitution was an important step in helping to move health thinking beyond a limited biomedical- and pathology-based perspective towards the more positive domain of well being, understood to include recognition of individuals and their need to realize aspirations, to satisfy needs, and to change or cope with their environments. The societal dimensions of this effort were emphasized in both the Alma-Ata Declaration (WHO 1979) and the Ottawa Charter for Health Promotion (1986). The Alma-Ata Declaration describes health as a social goal whose realization requires the action of many social and economic sectors in addition to the health sector. The Ottawa Charter proposes that the fundamental conditions and resources for health are peace, shelter, education, food, income, a stable ecosystem, sustainable resources, social justice, and equity.

When the WHO was created to improve health 50 years ago, there were hopes that antibiotics and the progress achieved in vaccines and biomedical technology would provide the tools sufficient to enable individuals worldwide to reach the highest attainable standard of physical, mental, and social well being (Tomaševski 1995*b*). However, decades later, as reflected in both the Alma-Ata Declaration and the Ottawa Charter, it is clear that, regardless of the effectiveness of technologies, the underlying civil, cultural, economic, political, and social conditions at both a global and local level have to be addressed as well. The major determinants of better health are increasingly understood to lie outside the health system and to include better education and information, as well as fulfilment of an array of rights which are relevant to, but not intrinsically connected with, the right to health (Carrin and Politi 1996). Thus health requires attention to the increasingly complex relationship of people to their environment and an understanding of respecting, protecting, and fulfilling human rights as a necessary prerequisite for the health of individuals and populations.

Globalization and the direct and indirect impacts of intensifying global flows of money, trade, information, culture, and people on health and related aspects of human development, have brought out a new set of human rights issues (Brundtland 2000). These issues need particular attention, as they have largely been ignored. The process of globalization has proceeded at a much faster pace than the development of policies aimed at maximizing its benefits to human development and preventing or mitigating its harmful effects.

Globalization, and the privatization of the means of production and services that inherently accompanies it, can contribute to the advancement of health through the sharing of information, technologies, and resources, as well as through the competition it generates to provide more effective, more widely available, and higher-quality services. Globalization can create new employment opportunities in some populations or sectors of the economy, but at times may do so to the detriment of others. It can also stimulate the spread of health hazards and disease as a result of intensified population mobility, or through the worldwide marketing of harmful substances, such as tobacco and alcohol. If poorly conceived and monitored, globalization can contribute to the widening of inequalities by increasing the autonomy and well being of some sectors of the population while producing negative consequences for others without access to safety nets to support the fulfilment of essential needs (Cooper Weil *et al.* 1990; UN 1995*c*; WHO 1995; Al-Mazrou *et al.* 1997; Hallack 1999; Heggenhougen 1999; Brundtland 2000). In the wake of globalization and privatization, increasing attention must be paid to the role of non-state actors because they are now influencing the health and well being of people to an unprecedented extent, comparable even to the influence of governments (UNHCHR 2000). The role of the state is to ensure that all human beings are guaranteed their basic human rights, including the right to the highest attainable standard of health, whether this obligation is fulfilled directly through government-run services or through private intermediaries. Governmental roles and responsibilities are increasingly being delegated to non-state actors (for example, biomedical research institutions, health insurance companies, care providers, health management organizations, and the pharmaceutical industry) whose accountability for what they do, do not do, or should do about people's health is poorly defined and inadequately monitored. There is a universal need to reinforce the commitment and capacity of governments to ensure that actions taken by the private sector and other actors in civil society relevant to health and other aspects of human development, both within and outside the boundaries of nation-states, are informed by and comply with human rights principles. Current structures are generally insufficient for non-governmental organizations or governments to monitor effectively and hold corporations operating on a national scale accountable. This problem is compounded when these companies are multinational (Hossain 1999; Orford 1999; UNHCHR 2000).

Attention to health reveals that multinationals are more than agents of economic change whose decisions are increasingly affecting the distribution of wealth, the fabric of society, and the creation of conditions favourable to advancing health; they are also increasingly the institutions called upon by political and social forces to create and operate alternative mechanisms to extend health and social services and to make available new and affordable vaccines and drugs (Kolodner 1994). Yet because they are multinational, they largely escape the realm of legal accountability within states, and, while they may choose to adopt ethical guidelines and codes of conduct, there is no international human rights law that directly applies to them or to their actions. The fora where world issues are debated have expanded from assemblies of governments—for example, under the United Nations umbrella—to gatherings and congresses such as the Davos forum that give a prominent role to these non-state actors, demonstrating that the state and non-state actors leading the world economy have become inseparable partners. From a health and human rights perspective, the desirable forms and extent of responsibility for multinational actors within the international legal system have yet to be defined in ways that help to shape international trade agreements effectively and to ensure their accountability. This is the next and most important challenge in the world of human rights, and it will have far-reaching health consequences.

Strategic directions to better health

Human rights can help to provide an approach for redefining the ways in which governments and the international community as a whole are accountable for what is done and not done about the health of people (Mann *et al.* 1994). This requires an understanding of the content of the health issues most relevant to the health and well being of individuals and populations, as well as of those actions which ought to be taken at the national level to move towards health development.

As the approaches set out by the WHO are relevant to all its member states, this discussion will be framed around the strategic framework laid out by the WHO in its 1999 corporate strategy (WHO 1999*b*). From a strategic perspective, the issues relevant to health development can be understood to lie along four converging axes: (a) reducing excess mortality, morbidity, and disability; (b) promoting healthy lifestyles and reducing risk factors to human health that arise from environmental, economic, social, and behavioural causes; (c) developing health systems that equitably improve health outcomes, respond to people's legitimate demands, and are financially fair; (d) developing an enabling policy and institutional environment in the health sector while promoting an effective health dimension to social, economic, environmental, and development policy. Each of these approaches is briefly discussed below.

Reducing excess mortality, morbidity, and disability

Recent WHO information reveals that six preventable or curable diseases cause 90 per cent of infectious disease deaths worldwide, as well as half of all premature deaths, most of which occur in children and young adults living in developing countries (Murray and Lopez 1996; WHO 1999*a*). Reduction of excess mortality, morbidity, and disability calls for a combination of sound health interventions—some of a clinical nature, such as diagnosis and treatment of communicable and non-communicable diseases, and others building on large-scale programmes to inform, immunize, or apply population-based prophylactic therapies. From a health and human rights perspective, it is worth recognizing that the growing health disparity between the North and the South creates compelling needs both for every country to develop effective disease prevention and control programmes targeted to their specific needs, and for global sharing of technology and resources in order to enable poorer countries to accelerate progress in health development. Therefore, priority must be given both locally and globally to poor and marginalized communities.

Promoting healthy lifestyles and reducing risk factors to human health that arise from environmental, economic, social, and behavioural causes

Modern public health recognizes the influence of external factors on the ability of individuals to adopt healthy behaviours or to access care when ill health has set in. As stated above, health promotion is the process of enabling people to increase control over and improve their health. To do so, individuals or groups must be informed and able to identify and realize aspirations, satisfy needs, and change or cope with their environment. The concept of interventions aimed at reducing risk is familiar to those working on such health issues as HIV/AIDS and other sexually transmitted diseases, tobacco, and other types of substance use or occupational hazards (Mann *et al.* 1992; Mann and Tarantola 1996*b*,*c*; WHO 1998*b*). Risk reduction interventions can also bring attention to the inadequacy of public services to address such issues as reproductive health, access to safe blood transfusion, or access to clean water. Some authors have distinguished the notion of risk, defined as a statistical probability of suffering from ill health, from that of 'vulnerability', which impacts on risk via societal, programme-related, or individual factors (Mann and Tarantola 1996*b*, *c*; Tarantola 1998). Others have further extended this analysis by defining 'susceptibility' as the influence of external or individual factors on risk and 'vulnerability' as the degree to which individual, communities, or nations are able to cope effectively with the impacts of ill health (Barnett and Whiteside 1999). Still others have grouped these factors among the 'underlying preconditions for health', including policy, legal, and institutional environments, which have traditionally been dealt with as separate issues (Mann *et al.* 1994; Mann and Tarantola 1996*a*). All of these paradigms recognize the importance of integrating morbidity, mortality, and disability reduction programmes with interventions to mitigate or address the factors underlying the occurrence of these events. Reducing susceptibility or vulnerability requires understanding of who is affected and how and to what extent these people are exposed to and able to cope with the factors that impact on their health, and then designing interventions that can enable them to cope effectively. From a health and human rights perspective, this process is linked to the need to create conditions conducive to health through information, education, and the development or strengthening of health systems and social support programmes that promote healthy behaviours, impact on risk-taking behaviours, and increase individual and collective commitment and capacity to engage in these processes.

Developing health systems that equitably improve health outcomes, respond to people's legitimate demands, and are financially fair

In this context, 'health systems' can be understood as the set of public or private structures, services, actions, and people whose main aim is to promote health and prevent and treat disease. In order to progress towards these aims, health systems must be sufficiently accessible, efficient, and affordable, and of good quality (WHO 2000*d*). The WHO *World Health Report 2000* has proposed measures that reflect responsibility and create the grounds for accountability within health systems with regard to three dimensions of health: health outcome, fairness, and responsiveness (WHO 2000*d*). The responsibilities of health systems in relation to health outcomes largely determines the type of services, interventions, and technologies they offer. If analysed on the basis of health outcomes, the accountability demanded of health systems must take into consideration the capacity of these systems to recognize and respond to health issues, as well as such factors as personal behaviours or unforeseen social, economic, or environmental situations or events. From an accountability perspective, it is worth recognizing that some of these latter factors may impact on health outcomes but are beyond the responsibilities assigned to health systems. They must be taken into account in other ways—for example, in relation to governmental accountability for education, employment, freedom of movement or association, or in relation to other rights that impact on health.

Underlying this attention to the responsibility and accountability of health systems is the concept of equality, which implies that health systems are capable of defining and recognizing the characteristics and specific needs of populations within a nation who experience a disproportionate level of mortality, morbidity, and disability. This, in turn, requires that health data be collected and analysed with a degree of sensitivity and specificity sufficient to determine who is likely to require additional attention; what behaviours and practices have to be supported, induced, or changed; what service provisions have to be enhanced and in what ways; and what financial mechanisms are necessary to provide the safety nets necessary to ensure that those who need more actually receive more. Therefore, it follows that the information used to develop, monitor, and evaluate policies and programmes must accurately reflect characteristics that may be associated with discrimination and inequality, including sex, age, rural/urban location, and other relevant behavioural, social, or economic factors (Barton Smith 1998).

The WHO *World Health Report 2000* proposes that 'the way health care is financed is perfectly fair when the burden that health spending represents on the household, or its relative health financial contribution is identical for all households, independent of their income, their health status or their use of the health system' (WHO 2000*d*). Although the principle of fairness is not articulated as such in human rights treaties, it builds on an array of rights, such as non-discrimination, equality, and participation, that, together with obligations directly related to health, can be used to consider the responsibilities of governments for health systems. The financing of health systems must be considered from the perspective of competing human development priorities within a nation, as well as that of the intrinsic priorities within health systems themselves. No global benchmark can therefore be proposed to establish the minimum national spending for health systems, whether from public or private sources, and the debate must remain open as to the extent to which and the ways in which governments will invest in the health of their populations. Within health systems, the decisions concerning allocation of public funds for specific health initiatives can draw from epidemiological, economic, or political considerations and can use a variety of methods and processes, including cost-effectiveness analysis, as well as human rights considerations. The concept of financial fairness implies that these systems should enable all individuals to seek and receive services that are commensurate to their needs and economically affordable.

Finally, the concept of responsiveness imposes on health systems a requirement that they be sensitive to people's aspirations, needs, and demands with full respect for human rights, and that they offer support and services. The principles of non-discrimination, protection of confidentiality (privacy), and respect for people's dignity are central to both the design of health systems and to the attitude and practices of health providers. From a health and human rights perspective, each of the components considered necessary for health systems to improve health outcomes equitably raises additional issues to be considered from the perspective of governmental responsibility and accountability.

Developing an enabling policy and institutional environment in the health sector while promoting an effective health dimension to social, economic, environmental, and development policy

If it is clear that policies and practices within health systems may impact positively or negatively on health, it is also clear that policies and practices concerned with the broad spectrum of human development may also impact significantly on health status and health-seeking behaviours (Cooper Weil *et al.* 1990). A large-scale industrial project may, for example, create selective migratory movements that may result in accentuated health hazards, whether these are linked to inadequate working conditions, housing, or social or cultural uprooting (Shenker 1992; ILO 1996). The association between enhanced vulnerability to HIV/AIDS among migrant labourers and economically motivated mobility in Africa and Asia provides one example (UNAIDS/IOM 1998). Similarly, factors such as the amount of pollution that industries have generated, or the impact that the use of pesticides in agriculture has had on the health of some populations, imply that health impacts must be considered at all stages of human development programmes (McMichael 1993). From a health and human rights perspective, this requires attention to health impacts in the design of human development programmes; this would include preventing or counterbalancing their potential negative health effects, as well as ensuring that health indicators are built into the monitoring of human development initiatives (WHO 1992; Watson *et al.* 1998).

The four strategic elements of health as briefly described above provide a useful framework for analysing the interface between health and rights. Indeed, each of these elements involves governmental obligations that are relevant to policies and programmes directly impacting on health, as well as those more broadly concerned with human development.

Health development and human rights

While the above categorization of strategic directions for health is useful because it reflects the approach being taken by the WHO and is guiding the current global health agenda, a perspective of governmental human rights obligations towards health development emerges more clearly if these strategies are divided into the following three domains.

1. The highest attainable standard of health. This is measured by morbidity, mortality, and disability, by positive health measures of growth and development in children, and by demographic variables, reproductive health, healthy lifestyles, behaviours, and practices in adults. The focus here is on health outcomes affecting individuals and populations.
2. Access to health systems which provide affordable and good-quality preventive, curative, and palliative care services and related social support. The focus here is on health systems.
3. A societal and physical environment conducive to health promotion and protection, including access to education, information, and other positive expressions of rights necessary for health as well as protection from violence, environmental and occupational hazards, harmful traditional practices, and other factors that may impact directly and negatively on health. The focus here is on the societal and environmental preconditions for health.

The development and application of governmental policies transcends all three of these domains of health development and is equally relevant to governmental responsibilities both to promote and protect health and to respect, protect, and fulfil human rights (Roemer and Roemer 1990; UNDP 1998*a*). A systematic analysis of the responsibilities of governments for health, considered with respect to their obligations under international human rights law, begins to lead us towards the practice of health and human rights.

Recognizing the reciprocal impact of health and human rights

There are two approaches to analysing the relationship between health and human rights that help not only to illustrate their connection, but also to provide a framework for considering the implications of the health and human rights relationship for government responsibility and accountability (Mann *et al.* 1994). The first focuses consideration on the ways in which health policies, programmes, and practices can promote or violate rights in the ways they are designed or implemented. Health policies, programmes, and practices in and of themselves can promote and protect or, conversely, restrict and violate human rights, whether by design, neglect, or ignorance. The second approach examines how violations or lack of attention to human rights can have serious health consequences. The promotion, protection, restriction, or violation of human rights all can be seen to have direct and indirect impacts on health and well being. Looking at health through a human rights lens means recognizing not only the technical and operational aspects of health interventions but also the civil, political, economic, social, and cultural factors that surround them. These factors may include, for example, gender relations, religious beliefs, homophobia, or racism, which individually and in synergy influence the extent to which individuals are able to access services or to make and effect free and informed decisions about their lives—and, therefore, the extent of their vulnerability to ill health. Thus, health and human rights interact in numerous ways, both direct and indirect (Mann *et al.* 1994). Public health and human rights each recognize the ultimate responsibility of governments to create the enabling conditions necessary for people to make choices, cope with changing patterns of vulnerability, and keep themselves and their families healthy. Using human rights concepts, one can look at the extent to which governments are respecting, protecting, and fulfilling their obligations for all rights—civil political, economic, social, and cultural—and how these government actions influence both the patterns of mortality, morbidity, and disability within a population and what is done about them.

The impact of health policies, programmes, and practices on human rights

A human rights framework can help to identify potential burdens on the lives of individuals and populations that are created by health policies, programmes, and practices. An obvious example, as was recognized in the International Conference on Population Development Programme of Action, is demographic goal-driven family planning programmes, which may by their very nature violate basic human rights (ICPD 1994). More subtle human rights issues may arise from health programmes that fail to provide services to certain populations or are not appropriately tailored to meet the needs of marginalized groups (Altman 1998; Beyrer 1998; Jackson 1998; Stevens 1998; Wodak 1998).

Responsibilities for public health are largely carried out through policies and programmes promulgated, implemented, and, at the very least, supported by the state. Therefore, a human rights approach to public health requires analysis of every stage of the design, implementation, and evaluation of health policies and programmes. This section teases out some of the issues that a human rights analysis can raise at various stages of policy and programme design and implementation. HIV/AIDS, sexual health, and reproductive health will serve as primary examples in this section because, in recent years, these issues have been especially important in illuminating the impact that health policies and programmes can have on human rights.

Human rights considerations arise at the initial formulation of health policies and programmes. Relevant issues would be raised, for example, if a state decides to approach a health issue in a particular way but refuses to disclose the scientific basis of its decisions or permit any debate on its merits, or if a government wilfully or neglectfully fails to consult with members of affected communities in reaching its decisions, or in any number of ways refuses to inform or involve the public in policy or programme development. Human rights issues may also interact with the development of health policies and programmes when prioritization of certain health issues is based less on actual need than on existing discrimination against certain population groups (Gilmore 1996). This can occur when, for example, minor health issues that predominantly impact the dominant group are systematically given higher priority in research, resource allocation, and policy and programme development than other more major health problems. Restrictive laws and policies that deliberately focus on certain population groups without sufficient data, epidemiological and otherwise, to support their approach may raise an additional host of human rights concerns. Two examples might be policies concerning the involuntary sterilization of women from certain population groups that are justified as necessary for their health and well being (Lombardo 1996; Comite Latinoamericano para la Defensa de los Derechos de la Mujer 1999), and sodomy statutes criminalizing same-sex sexual behaviour that are justified as necessary to prevent the spread of HIV/AIDS (UNHRC 1994).

Human rights also need to be considered when choosing which data are collected to determine the type and extent of health problems affecting a population, as this choice has a direct impact on the policies and programmes that are designed and implemented (Zierler *et al.* 2000).The choice of issues to be assessed and the way in which a population is defined in these assessments are of primary relevance (Braveman 1998). A state's failure to recognize or acknowledge health problems that particularly impact on a marginalized group, or to consider the impacts of particular health issues on all members of a population, may not only violate the right to non-discrimination, but may also lead to neglect of necessary services, which in turn may adversely affect the realization of other human rights (Cook 1994; Hendriks 1995; Miller *et al.* 1995). Examples of this would include the almost complete lack of attention and resources devoted to the early detection of cervical cancer by a number of governments, or state-controlled reproductive health programmes that exist for some population groups but exclude certain marginalized communities from their consideration and outreach (WHO 1994*b*). Likewise, the scarcity or absence of HIV-related services in a number of places can well be understood to have resulted in a disproportionate burden of health consequences that could have been prevented or alleviated through simple and affordable prevention messages and methods of early diagnosis and treatment.

Once a decision is made that a particular health problem will be dealt with, human rights issues can come into play in both the articulation and the implementation of the health policy or programme. An example is programmes that provide contraception to young boys but deny access to young girls, with the stated rationale that access might prompt girls to be sexually active (Radhakrishna *et al.* 1997; Youth Research 1997). From a human rights perspective, this distinction can be understood to be treating young girls unfairly and unjustly on the basis of their sex. The prohibition of discrimination in the human rights documents does not mean that differences should not be acknowledged, but rather that different treatment must be based on reasonable and objective criteria (Cook 1992; Coliver 1995). Therefore, applying different approaches to girls and boys in policy and programme development must be based on a valid recognition of gender-related differentials in risk and vulnerability with respect to the particular health issue and with an attempt to minimize the influence of prescribed gender roles and cultural norms in making this determination (Moody 1989; Holder 1992).

The severity of the devastating tuberculosis epidemic in developing countries, and in marginalized communities in affluent nations, draws attention to the relevance of a human rights analysis for the implementation of a health policy and programme (Raviglione *et al.* 1995; WHO 1999*c*). While the directly observed therapy strategy (**DOTS**) is widely recognized for its efficacy in controlling tuberculosis, the issues raised by the very different ways this strategy is administered in different countries, and to different population groups, demonstrates how discrimination may be relevant to the ways in which health programmes are implemented (WHO 2000*a*). Many health practitioners argue that the speed with which tuberculosis is spreading and the potential impact of individual non-compliance to treatment are likely to aggravate both the spread of the disease and the currently observed prevalence of multiple-drug resistance (WHO 1998*c*). The DOTS strategy aims to combat this by enrolling patients diagnosed with active tuberculosis in a programme where drugs are administered under the direct observation of a care provider, rather than self-administered by the patient (WHO 1994*a*). The strategy requires frequent visits by patients to the site where drugs are administered, which can potentially involve work absenteeism and in some cases out-of-pocket travel expenses. In small communities, the strategy may also lead to breaches of the right to privacy, as frequent visits to a treatment point may be associated with the stigma commonly attached to the disease. In cases of non-compliance to regular treatment administered in this way, measures up to and including mandatory hospital admission may be taken to motivate defaulting patients to comply. There is ample evidence to suggest, however, that in a number of places the level of coercion exercised by health practitioners in the decision to apply DOTS, as well as in the application of mandatory institutionalization, is directly associated with the levels of discrimination against particular population groups within the society in question (Farmer *et al.* 1991; Bayer *et al.* 1993; Schmidt 1995; Efferen 1997; Heymann and Sell 1999).

Attention must also be given to whether health and social services take into account logistic, financial, and sociocultural barriers to access and enjoyment, as a failure to do so can result in discrimination in practice, if not in law (Focht-New 1996). This includes attention to the factors that may impact on service utilization, such as hours of service and accessibility via public transportation. Issues are also raised by decisions concerning the location of prevention and treatment services for certain health issues. An extreme example relates to the location of sexually transmitted disease diagnosis, prevention, and care services, which may be integrated into the reproductive health services generally available to women or offered only in centres dedicated to sexually transmitted disease prevention and treatment. Evidence suggests that individuals, and women in particular, are less likely to take advantage of sexually transmitted disease services that operate under this latter designation for fear of stigma and discrimination within the community if they are seen at the facility (Weiss and Gupta 1993; d'Cruz-Grote 1996).

Laws and policies that may seem neutral but neglect to detail sufficiently the steps necessary for their implementation may raise additional human rights issues. Illustrative of such a situation are laws and policies that mandate the reporting of HIV infection but fail to spell out the actors responsible for doing so, or fail to take into account a lack of infrastructure to ensure that privacy can be respected and that mechanisms for redress exist if breaches of confidentiality occur (Gruskin and Tarantola 2000). Indeed, collecting personal information from individuals about their health status (for example, HIV infection, cancer, or genetic disorders), or behaviours (for example, sexual orientation or the use of alcohol or other substances) has the potential for misuse by the state, whether directly or because this information is intentionally or inadvertently made available to others. In recent times the most explicit examples of the impact of misuse or neglect of privacy protections are found in the context of HIV/AIDS. Misuse of personal information related to HIV status has led to restrictions on the right to marry and found a family, and the right to work and education, as well as, in extreme cases, limitations on freedom of movement, arbitrary detention, or exile, and even cruel, inhuman, and degrading treatment. The release of information concerning a person's HIV status to others has, in many places, led to loss of employment and housing, as well as harassment and verbal and physical attacks (Cohen and Wiseberg 1990; Gruskin *et al.* 1996; UNDP 1998*b*).

Decisions on how data are collected have a direct influence on the policies and programmes that are put into place. For example, differentials determined by sex or gender roles in relation to HIV/sexually transmitted disease infection are generally not systematically considered in the collection and analysis of HIV/sexually transmitted disease epidemiological data, nor are they sufficiently studied or built into the design of prevention and care programmes. In countries where the HIV/AIDS pandemic has matured, some 15- to 16-year-old girls attending antenatal clinics for their first pregnancy are already infected with HIV, and no information is available as to the cause of this infection (that is, whether it involved sex or another mode of transmission) (Tarantola and Gruskin 1998). The degree to which gender factors influence the relative risk of becoming infected through various routes of transmission during childhood, and how they may influence patterns of access to care and the quality of care provided to boys and girls once HIV infection has set in, remains unknown. There has been very little attention to the general failure to differentiate by sex in the collection and analysis of epidemiological information on 'children' younger than 15. This raises a host of human rights concerns and may result in neglect of the very real differences between female and male adolescents in the prevention and care programmes that do exist.

Violations of the right to information in the context of health policies and programmes must be mentioned specifically, as these can have substantial health impacts (Freedman 1999). Examples include decisions by governments to withhold or block access to valid scientific information that would enable people to participate in the improvement of their health, avoid disease, or claim and seek better care. Such is the case for young women who become unwillingly pregnant or acquire sexually transmitted diseases because they are denied information considered too sexually explicit for them—even though they became pregnant or infected because they were sexually active (Alan Guttmacher Institute 1998; Dowsett and Aggelton 1999).

The health and human rights approach determines whether health policies, programmes, and practices are valid from both a public health and a human rights perspective (IFRCRC/FXBC 1999). The first step in this analysis will always be to determine the stated justification for the measure—and then to consider the framework set forth in the Siracusa Principles mentioned above (UNECOSOC 1985). In analysing health policies and programmes, as Jonathan Mann was fond of saying: 'Assume all health policies and programmes are discriminatory or restrictive of rights until proven otherwise' (Mann 1997*a*).

The impact of neglect of violations of human rights on health

When health is understood to include physical, mental, and social well being, it seems reasonable to conclude that the violation or neglect of any human right will impact adversely on health. While this is certainly true with respect to specific rights, such as non-discrimination or education, the impact of neglect or violation of rights is also compounded by the number of rights brought into question by any particular situation. The health impacts of certain severe human rights violations, such as torture, imprisonment under inhumane conditions, summary executions, and disappearances have long been understood. Much work has been done in this field, and efforts in this regard continue to expand. Such efforts include exhumations of mass graves to ascertain how people have died, the coding and matching of genetic information to reunite families separated during war and massive political repression, examination of torture victims to bring perpetrators to justice and to assist with asylum claims, and entry into prisons and other state-run institutions, such as detention centres, to assess health conditions and the health status of confined populations. The impacts on health of these human rights violations can be both obvious and subtle. For example, torture is a violation that causes immediate and direct harm to health. Yet only recently has the full impact of torture begun to be recognized, including the lifelong injury to the victim, the effects on the health of families and of entire communities, and the transgenerational damage (AI 1983; Goldfeld 1988). There is increasing recognition of the need to assess the duration and extent of the health impacts of such human rights violations, including the direct and immediate impact of being subjected to torture oneself, but also its severe and lifelong effects on survivors and the trauma associated with being forced to witness summary executions, rape, and other forms of torture and trauma perpetrated on others (Dawes 1990).

Health practitioners can—and in most cases do—have a strong positive influence on the promotion and protection of human rights within the populations they serve. Yet violations of human rights perpetrated by health professionals regularly occur. These include not only such egregious examples as doctor participation in torture and other severe violations of human rights, but also actions in the provision of treatment and care, for example when care providers make decisions concerning patient access to available prevention services, or when children with a chronic fatal disease or disability are denied immunization against measles and other preventable childhood infections (Savage 1998; UN 1998*b*; Ward and Myers 1999). In many countries, rich and poor, patients with diabetes, carcinoma, chronic renal syndrome, mental disability, haemophilia, or other severe health conditions may receive a lower standard of care than others not only with respect to the health issue in question but in general because their possibility of cure is regarded as limited (UN 1992*b*; Crofts *et al.* 1997).

A less obvious impact of neglect of human rights on health concerns the many children from poor or marginalized communities, where poor nutrition and ill health prevail, that have a below-average school enrolment and attendance rate and, as a result, below-average educational attainment (Swartz and Levett 1989; Brundtland 1999). The deprivation of these children from access to basic health services, coupled with the imposition of school fees, leads to a limitation of their ability to exercise their right to education, producing lifelong effects on their health and well being.

In addition to the impact of egregious violations of rights on health, the more subtle effects of neglect or violations of rights on health can also be considered. These would include exposures to ill health resulting from violations of such rights as work, free movement, association, and participation (Daniels *et al.* 1990; Berlinguer *et al.* 1996). The impact of neglect or violation of factors considered to form the underlying preconditions for health must also be considered. In addition to medical services, these have been understood to include such factors as adequate housing, education, food, safe drinking water, sanitation, access to information, and protection against discrimination. Understood in human rights terms, neglect of these rights, particularly in combination, can have serious negative consequences on health (Mann *et al.* 1994). No community is fully protected from neglect or violation of rights and its detrimental consequences to individual and public health (CESR 1999; UN 1999*a*, *b*). In particular, gender-based discrimination poses a pervasive threat to health. Girls and women who are denied access to education, information, and various forms of economic, social, and political participation are particularly vulnerable to the impact of discrimination on their health. This is true when discrimination is recognized, tolerated, acknowledged, or even condoned by governments, but also when it remains insidiously hidden or deliberately ignored behind an accepted status quo (Dixon-Mueller 1990; Sullivan 1995).

One example, drawn from the world of reproductive health, dramatically illustrates this point. There is now general acknowledgement that violations of human rights, including systematic gender discrimination, create an environment of increased risk in relation to women's health (Cook 1995; Berer 1999). In this context, it is necessary to consider those factors that are understood to influence directly the reproductive health of women. Access to information, education, and quality services is critical, as are services adequately targeted to respond to the needs of women of different ages and from different communities. Underlying all this is the impact that gender roles and gender discrimination have on both health status and service delivery (Doyal 1995; WHO 1998*a*). The relevance of human rights to this analysis becomes clear when considering the gaps and inequalities in services and structures in relation to the social roles that construct male and female identity. Equally important is how these factors play out at the policy and programme level in terms of reproductive health research, policy, financing, and service delivery. Traditional public health focused on the need for information, education, contraception, counselling, and access to quality services. These elements of health practice were, and still are, central to improving women's reproductive health. However, even if these services are available, an individual woman has to be able to decide when and how she is going to access these services. This implies that she has to have the ability to control and make decisions about her life.

In this example, considering the impact that violation or neglect of human rights has on health highlights the societal context that would hinder or empower an individual woman's ability to make and act on the free and informed choices necessary for her reproductive health. From a broader policy and programme perspective, this insight reveals that linking the human rights framework to health implies recognizing that individual health is largely influenced by one's environment. This means that the integration of human rights in the design, implementation, and evaluation of health policies and programmes is necessary not only because of a government's human rights obligations, but also in purely pragmatic public health terms. Thus, attention to the civil, political, economic, social, and cultural factors that are relevant to a person's life, such as gender relations, racism, or homophobia, and the ways this combination of factors projects itself into who becomes ill and what is done about it, is central to sound health and human rights practice.

The process of documenting evidence on the health impacts resulting from violations or neglect of human rights must be thorough and thoughtful because of the multifarious effects on health of human rights neglect or violations. The involvement of communities that are disproportionately affected by human rights violations in the development, implementation, and monitoring of decisions affecting them is crucial to mitigating these impacts. Affected individuals working together in defence or advocacy groups—be they concerned with breast cancer, diabetes, renal syndromes, haemophilia, chronic disabilities, or other health issues—have been effective in bringing to light some of the more subtle mechanisms that come into play in linking health status with the human rights violations to which people are subjected (Steingraber 1997; UNAIDS 1999).

Optimizing health and human rights in practice

A crucial step in optimizing the relationship between health and human rights is to conduct a systematic review of how and to what extent governmental policies and programmes are respectful of human rights and of benefit to public health. Such a review, presented in Box 3, is proposed as a critical first step in improving new and existing policies and programmes through assessment of their validity, applicability, and soundness, while addressing their practical implications from both human rights and public health perspectives. The suggested questions can be used by policy-makers and public health and other government officials to help in the development, implementation, and evaluation of more effective policies and programmes, and by non-governmental organizations and other concerned actors as an advocacy tool to hold governments accountable for the ways they are and are not in compliance with their international legal obligations to promote and protect both public health and human rights.

Box 3 Issues to be addressed in assessing policies and programmes. The following questions may serve as starting points to help guide this analysis (Gruskin and Tarantola 2000)

- What is the specific intended purpose of the policy or programme?
- What are the ways and the extent to which the policy or programme may impact positively and negatively on health?
- Using the relevant international human rights documents, what and whose rights are impacted positively and negatively by the policy or the programme?
- Does the policy or programme necessitate the restriction of human rights?
- If so, have the criteria/preconditions to restrict rights been met?
- Are the health and other relevant structures and services capable of effectively implementing the policy or programme?
- What system of monitoring, evaluation, accountability, and redress exist to ensure that the policy or programme is progressing towards the intended effect and that adverse effects can be acted upon?

The importance of the human rights framework to policies and programmes is that it can provide a method of analysis and a framework for action, which can then be used to help shape specific interventions aimed at reducing the impact of health conditions on the lives of individuals and populations. This approach requires work with the international human rights documents to determine the specific rights applicable to a given situation, and then considering how and to what extent morbidity, mortality, disability, risk behaviours, and vulnerability to ill health are caused or exacerbated by insufficient realization of human rights. This analysis will be most effective if done in partnership with people with substantive knowledge of human rights.

A second level of analysis can be created by recognizing the convergence of the three health domains described above (health outcome, health systems, and underlying conditions for health) with the three levels of governmental obligations that exist for each right—respect, protect, and fulfil (Table 1). Health practitioners will find this table most relevant to their work if they use the suggested health domains (first column of Table 1) as their entry point and then move to the right, seeking to identify how each level of governmental obligation can influence health policies and action within each of the three domains. Ultimately, such an analysis could be extended to examine how those approaches recognized as best health practice in each domain could contribute to the advancement of human rights with respect to each level of governmental obligation. The issues raised in Table 1 are not meant to be highly detailed, but simply to serve as examples of the issues this approach brings to light.

The questions proposed in Box 3 may be used to create an agenda for action to help guide the analysis of governmental obligations for health outcomes, health systems, and the societal preconditions for health proposed in Table 1. Human resource development in support of health requires that health training include the skills necessary to document and measure the health effects of neglect or violations of rights. Education and training of people working in human rights should likewise provide them with the skills necessary to analyse the complex relations between neglect or violation of rights and their health impact, in such a way that the information provided can be used to monitor and ensure government accountability. This joint approach is necessary if the health and human rights framework is to be practical and useful. Only when the many dimensions necessary for health are described, measured, and named in human rights terms can the full extent of the relationship between health and human rights be realized. Such a review offers a critical approach to assessing the validity, applicability, and soundness of new and existing policies and programmes, and to addressing their practical implications from both human rights and public health perspectives. Through this approach, the disciplines of health and of human rights come together most visibly, and national capacity building to ensure reasoned and sound analysis becomes a necessity.

Another dimension of developing the health and human rights relationship is the application of mechanisms, methods, and tools to monitor progress and shortcomings in implementation of health and human rights at the national and international level. An earlier section described the role of treaty bodies in engaging in dialogue with governments on their degree of compliance with their international legal obligations. The WHO, for its part, is developing monitoring methods and indicators that, although technically not binding on governments (with the exceptions of reporting under the International Health Regulations), set out international norms by which member states commit to abide in principle after passage at the World Health Assembly. Previously, the WHO's attempts to measure health on the national or international level selectively used morbidity, mortality, and disability indicators (WHO 1999*a*). This exercise was severely constrained by incomplete national data, differences in measurement methods across countries, and, even more importantly, an inability to relate health outcomes to the performance of health systems. Furthermore, most of these indicators were applied at a national aggregate level with insufficient attempts to disaggregate the data collected to reveal the disparities that exist within nations. It has been understood that measurement indicators and benchmarks that focus on the aggregate (national) level may not reveal important differentials that may be associated with a variety of human rights violations—in particular, discrimination.

Table 1 A pathway to health and human rights

Domains of health	Governmental obligations with respect to human rights		
	Respect	**Protect**	**Fulfil**
Health outcome	Government not to violate rights of people on the basis of their health status including in information collection and analysis, as well as in the design and provision of health and other services	Government to prevent non-state actors (including private health-care structures and insurance providers) from violating the rights of people on the basis of their health status including in the provision of health and other services	Government to take administrative, legislative, judicial, and other measures to promote and protect the rights of people regardless of their health status, including the generation of data concerning health outcomes for use in guiding health policies and the provision of health and other services, as well as providing legal means of redress that people know about and can access
Health systems	Government not to violate rights directly in the design, implementation, and evaluation of national health systems, including ensuring that they are sufficiently accessible, efficient, affordable, and of good quality for all members of the population	Government to prevent non-state actors (including private health-care structures and insurance providers) from violating rights in the design, implementation, and evaluation of health systems and structures, including ensuring that they are sufficiently accessible, efficient, affordable, and of good quality	Government to take administrative, legislative, judicial, and other measures including sufficient resource allocation and the building of safety nets, to ensure that health systems are sufficiently accessible, efficient, affordable, and of good quality, as well as providing legal means of redress that people know about and can access
Societal and environmental preconditions	Government not to violate the civil, political, economic, social, and cultural rights of people directly, recognizing that neglect or violations of rights impact directly on health	Government to prevent rights violations by non-state actors, recognizing that neglect or violations of rights impact directly on health	Government to take all possible administrative, legislative, judicial, and other measures, including the promotion of human development mechanisms, towards the promotion and protection of human rights, as well as providing legal means of redress that people know about and can access

Adapted from Tarantola and Gruskin (1998).

In order to improve the knowledge and understanding of health status and trends, and to relate these trends to health system performance, the WHO has developed the following five global indicators (WHO 2000*c*).

1. Healthy life expectancy: a composite indicator incorporating mortality, morbidity, and disability in a disability-adjusted life years measure. This indicator will reflect time spent in a state of less than full health.
2. Health inequalities: the degree of disparity in healthy life expectancy within the population.
3. Responsiveness of health systems: a composite indicator reflecting the protection of dignity and confidentiality in and by health systems, and people's autonomy (that is, their individual capacity to effect informed choice in health matters).
4. Responsiveness inequality: the disparity in responsiveness within health systems, bringing out issues of low efficiency, neglect, and discrimination.
5. Fairness in financing: measured by the level of health financing contribution of households.

The WHO has stated that it will collect this data through built-in health information systems, demographic and health surveys conducted periodically within countries, and other survey instruments. Data will thus be analysable by sex, age, race/birth (if warranted under national law), population groups (for example, indigenous populations), educational achievement, and other variables.

The WHO has also expressed its commitment to working with countries towards increasing their capacity to collect this information and also to determine additional data and targets that may be specifically suited to country-specific situations and needs. The WHO and other institutions concerned with health have stated their desire to use these data to assess trends in the performance of national health systems, inform national and international policies and programmes, make comparisons across countries, and monitor global health. This process is also intended to support the development of national benchmarks whereby targets will be set by individual governments with a view towards being able to compare their own health system performance with others, and to compare among regions and over time. These benchmarks will be chosen according to each country's set of health priorities and information needs (WHO 2000*c*).

The global indicators now being tested by the WHO, as well as its current efforts to enhance the capacity of member states to monitor their health performances, appear to be in line with human rights principles. These developments, coupled with the increasing attention to health by the bodies responsible for monitoring governmental compliance with their human rights obligations, are promising steps for the future development and application of the health and human rights framework.

Conclusion

This chapter has outlined the health and human rights framework as a pathway towards enhancing the value and impact of health work by health policy-makers, programme developers, practitioners, and students. It is hoped that increased attention to this fundamental relationship can open new avenues to human development, and by so doing, marshall new resources towards improving individual and population health. Keeping in mind the tools proposed in the previous section, there are three levels on which this new synergy can be recognized, applied, and monitored. The first concerns the development of adequate monitoring tools reflecting both health and human rights concerns; the second, the application of the health and human rights framework to health practice; and the third, the creation of a significant research agenda to advance our collective understanding of the health and human rights relationship.

Firstly, on the level of health best practice and international human rights law, evidence-based health policy and programme development can be guided by a systematic human rights analysis. This process involves significant efforts to ensure that the information that is sought, collected, and analysed brings attention to both trends and disparities, and that this information is used to address these gaps. This would include attention to the relative successes and failures of progress achieved towards global goals, such as those to which countries have subscribed in such forums as the World Health Assembly or through the international conference processes.

It is of critical importance that the WHO and the human rights treaty bodies are currently and simultaneously engaged both in the process of setting out global indicators and in defining approaches towards the development of country-specific benchmarks consistent with international knowledge, practice, and experience. The prevailing state of health and resource availability within individual countries must, nonetheless, be taken into account to allow trends and disparities to be measured in relation to individual benchmarks. While the existence of this work is encouraging, there is a need to further develop, test, and apply indicators that capture the disparities that may prevail within a population, as well as those that can begin to suggest the differences between government unwillingness and incapacity. Relevant indicators have been developed in the economics field, where the Gini coefficient, for example, is used as a measure of economic heterogeneity within a population (Kennedy *et al.* 1998). Disaggregation of data would allow the attributes on which discrimination is often based, including sex, age, prior health status, disability, birth, or social status, to be taken into account. Policies and programmes could then aim to advance the health of populations by setting out higher goals for the population as a whole, while bringing increased attention to reducing the gaps between those who enjoy better health and better services and those who, for political, civil, economic, social, or cultural reasons, are more vulnerable to ill health and to inadequate services and structures.

The second level on which health and human rights are beginning to converge is in ensuring that health systems and practice are sufficiently informed by human rights norms and standards. Sound formulation and implementation of health policies and programmes must seek to achieve the optimal balance between the promotion and protection of public health and the promotion and protection of human rights and dignity. Processes to arrive at this optimal balance can be built within national systems on the basis of the approach proposed in the previous sections, incorporating evidence collected in the ways suggested above and through participatory dialogues between decision-makers with expertise in public health, those with expertise in human rights, and concerned populations. The realization of such an approach requires additional efforts to create consultative mechanisms, as well as education and training in health and human rights.

Finally, the third level of convergence between health and human rights lies in the broad need for further research. Given that human rights are established, internationally agreed upon norms to which states have subscribed, the reciprocal impacts between human rights and health must be further researched and documented. There is a national and international obligation to increase research and documentation, as well as to conceptualize and implement policies and programmes that fully take these connections into account. The utility of this research will largely be predicated on the extent to which those with expertise in health collaborate with people knowledgeable about human rights in the conceptualization of their research agendas and in the steps necessary for carrying this work forward.

The challenges posed in linking health with human rights are immense. There is, however, increasing evidence that public health efforts that respect, protect, and fulfil human rights are more likely to succeed in public health terms than those that neglect or violate rights. National and international policy and decision-makers, health professionals, and the public at large all, to varying degrees, understand the fundamental links between health and human rights, and the way in which those links can provide new ways to analyse and conceive responses to health issues. To move the work of health and human rights forward will require building and strengthening the information and education available about human rights concepts and procedures. It will also require information exchange and stronger co-operation between those working on health and those working on human rights. When people are sufficiently knowledgeable about human rights, they will be able to identify the issues for which the synergy of human rights and health is critical, and to act accordingly. Human rights and health are progressing, in parallel, towards a common goal that will never be fully realized. Yet, together, they project a vision and an approach that may fundamentally and positively improve the lives of people everywhere in the world.

References

African [Banjul] Charter on Human and Peoples Rights (1982). OAU Document CAB/LEG/67/3 rev. 5, 21 ILM 58.

AI (Amnesty International) (1983). *Chile: evidence of torture.* AI Publications, London.

Alan Guttmacher Institute (1998). *Into a new world: young women's sexual and reproductive lives.* Alan Guttmacher Institute, New York.

Alfredsson, G. and Tomaševski, K. (1998). *A thematic guide to documents on health and human rights.* Martinus Nijhoff, Dordrecht.

Al-Mazrou, Y., Berkley, S., Bloom, B., *et al.* (1997). A vital opportunity for global health. *Lancet*, **350**, 750–1.

Alston, P. (1991). The international covenant on social, economic, social and cultural rights. In *Manual on human rights reporting*, pp. 63–5. United Nations Centre for Human Rights, UN Document HR/PUB/91/1.

Alston, P. (1997). What's in a name: does it really matter if development policies refer to goals, ideals or human rights? *SIM Special Issue*, **22**, 95–106.

Alston, P. and Quinn, G. (1987). The nature and scope of state parties' obligations under the international covenant and economic, social and cultural rights. *Human Rights Quarterly*, **9**, 165–6.

Altman, D. (1998). HIV, homophobia, and human rights. *Health and Human Rights*, **2**, 15–22.

Aluwihare, A.P.R. (1998). Xenotransplantation. Ethics and rights: an interaction. *Annals of Transplantation*, **3**, 59–61.

American Convention on Human Rights (1969). *OAS treaty.* Series No. 36, 1144 UNTS 123 entered into force 18 July 1978. In *Basic documents pertaining to human rights in the inter-American system*, OEA/Series LV/II.82 document 6 rev. 1 at 25.

Andrews, L.B. (1995). Genetic privacy: from the laboratory to the legislature. *Genome Research*, **5**, 209–13.

Barnett, T. and Whiteside, A. (1999). HIV/AIDS and development: case studies and conceptual framework. *European Journal of Development Research*, **11**, 200–34.

Barry, M. and Molyneux, M. (1992). Ethical dilemmas in malaria drug and vaccine trials: a bioethical persepective. *Journal of Medical Ethics*, **18**, 189–92.

Barton Smith, D. (1998). Addressing racial inequities in health care: civil rights monitoring and report cards. *Journal of Health Politics, Policy and Law*, **23**, 75–105.

Bayer, R., Dubler, N., and Landesman, S. (1993). The dual epidemics of tuberculosis and AIDS: ethical and policy issues in screening and treatment. *American Journal of Public Health*, **83**, 649–54.

Beloqui, J., Chokevivat V., and Collins, C. (1998). HIV vaccine research and human rights: examples from three countries planning efficacy trials. *Health and Human Rights*, **3**, 39–58.

Berer, M. (1999). Access to reproductive health: a question of distributive justice. *Reproductive Health Matters*, **7**, 8–14.

Berlinguer, G., Falzi, G., and Figà-Talamanca, I. (1996). Ethical problems in the relationship between health and work. *International Journal of Health Services*, **26**, 147–71.

Beyrer, C. (1998). Burma and Cambodia: human rights, social disruption, and the spread of HIV/AIDS. *Health and Human Rights*, **2**, 85–97.

Bilder, R.B. (1992). An overview of international human rights law. In *Guide to international human rights practice* (ed. H. Hannum) (2nd edn), pp. 3–18. University of Pennsylvania Press, Philadelphia, PA.

Boerefon, I. and Toebes, B. (1998). Health issues discussed by the UN treaty monitoring bodies. Netherland Institute of Human Rights. *SIM Special Issue*, **21**, 25–53.

Braveman, P. (1998). *Monitoring equity in health: a policy-oriented approach in low and middle class income countries.* Working Paper No. 3. WHO, Geneva.

Brenner, J. (1996). Human rights education in public health graduate schools. *Health and Human Rights*, **2**, 129–39.

Brundtland, G.H. (1998). The UDHR: fifty years of synergy between health and human rights. *Health and Human Rights*, **3**, 21–5.

Brundtland, G.H. (1999). Nutrition, health and human rights. *ACE/SCN Symposium on The Substance and Politics of a Human Right Approach to Food and Nutrition Policies and Programmes.* United Nations, Geneva.

Brundtland, G.H. (2000). Health in times of globalization. In *Health, the key to human development*, pp. 49–73. Campus-Verlag, Frankfurt.

Carrin, G. and Politi, C. (1996). *Exploring the health impact of economic growth, poverty reduction and public health expenditure.* Technical Paper No. 18. WHO, Geneva.

CESR (Center for Economic and Social Rights) (1999). Rights violations in the Ecuadorian Amazon. The human consequences of oil development. In *Health and human rights: a reader* (ed. J. Mann, S. Gruskin, M. Grodin, and G. Annas). Routledge, New York.

Clinton, W.J. (1998). United States Executive Order on Implementation of Human Rights Treaties. US Government Printing Office, Washington, DC.

Cohen, M.L. (1998). Resurgent and emergent disease in a changing world. *British Medical Bulletin*, **54**, 523–32.

Cohen, R. and Wiseberg, L. (1990). *Double jeopardy—threat to life and human rights: discrimination against persons with AIDS.* Human Rights Internet, Cambridge, MA.

Coliver, S. (ed.) (1995). The right to information necessary for reproductive health and choice under international law. In *The right to know: human rights and access to reproductive health information*, pp. 38–82. Article 19. University of Pennsylvania Press, Philadelphia, PA.

Comite Latinoamericano para la Defensa de los Derechos de la Mujer (1999). *Nada personal: reporte de derechos humanos sobre la aplicacion de la anticoncepcion quirurgica en el Peru, 1996–1998.* Comite de America Latina y el Caribe para la Defensa de los Derechos del la Mujer, Lima.

Cook, R.J. (1992). International protection of women's reproductive rights. *New York University Journal of International Law Politics*, **24**, 645–727.

Cook, R.J. (1994). *Women's health and human rights*, pp. 5–12. WHO, Geneva.

Cook, R.J. (1995). Gender, health and human rights. *Health and Human Rights*, **1**, 350–66.

Cooper Weil, D.E., Alibusan, A.P., Wilson, I.F., Reich, M.R., and Bradley, D.I. (1990). *The impact of the development policies on health.* WHO, Geneva.

Corporación Casa de la Mujer (1998). *Women's reproductive rights in Colombia: a shadow report.* Center for Reproductive Law and Policy (CRLP), New York.

Council of Europe (1950). *European Convention for the Protection of Human Rights and Fundamental Freedoms and its Nine Protocol.* ETS. No. 5.

Crofts, N., Louie, R., and Loff, B. (1997). The next plague: stigmatization and discrimination related to hepatitis C virus infection in Australia. *Health and Human Rights*, **2**, 86–97.

Daniels, C., Paul, M., and Rosofsky, R. (1990). Health, equity, and reproductive risks in the workplace. *Journal of Public Health Policy*, **11**, 449–62.

Dawes, A. (1990). The effect of political violence on children. A consideration of South African and related studies. *International Journal of Psychology*, **25**, 13–31.

d'Cruz-Grote, D. (1996). Prevention of HIV infection in developing countries. *Lancet*, **348**, 1071–4.

Detels, R., Holland, W., McEwen, J., and Omenn, G.S. (ed.) (1997). *Oxford textbook of public health* (3rd edn). Oxford University Press.

Dixon-Mueller, R. (1990). Abortion policy and women's health in developing countries. *International Journal of Health Services*, **20**, 297–314.

Dowsett, G. and Aggelton, P. (1999). Young people and risk-taking in sexual relations. In *Sex and youth: contextual factors affecting risk for HIV/AIDS*, pp. 10–56. UNAIDS Best Practice Collection, Geneva.

Doyal, L. (1995). *What makes women sick: gender and the political economy of health.* Rutgers University Press, New Brunswick, NJ.

Efferen, L.S. (1997). In pursuit of tuberculosis control: civil liberty vs. public health. *Chest*, **112**, 5–6.

Eide, A. (1995*a*). Economic, social and cultural rights as human rights. In *Economic, social and cultural rights: a textbook* (ed. A. Eide, C. Krause, and A. Rosas), pp. 1–40. Martinus Nijhoff, Dordrecht.

Eide, A. (1995*b*). The right to an adequate standard of living, including the right to food. In *Economic, social and cultural rights: a textbook* (ed. A. Eide, C. Krause, and A. Rosas), pp. 89–105. Martinus Nijhoff, Dordrecht.

Farmer, P., Robin, S., Ramilus, S.L., and Kim, Y.K. (1991). Tuberculosis, poverty, and 'compliance': lessons from rural Haiti. *Seminars in Respiratory Infection*, **6**, 254–60.

Fenner, F., Henderson, D.A., Arita, I., Jezek, Z., and Ladugi, T.D. (1988). *Smallpox and its eradication.* WHO, Geneva.

Fluss, S.S. (1999). A select bibliography of health aspects of human rights: 1984–1999. *Health and Human Rights*, **4**, 265–76.

Fluss, S.S. and Little, J. (1999). Vaccination and human rights. *Archives of Clinical Bioethics*, **2**, 79–85.

Focht-New, V. (1996). Beyond abuse: health care for people with disabilities. *Issues in Mental Health Nursing*, **17**, 427–38.

Freedman, L. (1999). Censorship and manipulation of family planning information: an issue of human rights and women's health. In *Health and human rights: a reader* (ed. J.M. Mann, S. Gruskin, M.A. Grodin, and G.J. Annas), pp. 145–78. Routledge, New York.

FWCW (Fourth World Conference on Women) (1995). *Action for equality, development and peace.* UN Document A/CONF.177/20/Rev. 1 (96.IV.13). UN, Geneva.

Gilmore, N. (1996). Drug use and human rights: privacy, vulnerability, disability, and human rights infringements. *Journal of Contemporary Health Law and Policy*, **12**, 355–447.

Goldfeld, A., Mollica, R.F., Pesavento, B., and Faraone, S. (1988). The physical and psychosocial sequelae of torture. *Journal of the American Medical Association*, **259**, 2725–9.

Gruskin, S. (1998). The highest priority: making use of UN conference documents to remind governments of their commitments to HIV/AIDS. *Health and Human Rights*, **3**, 107–42.

Gruskin, S. and Tarantola, D. (2000). HIV/AIDS, health and human rights. *Handbook for the design and management of HIV/AIDS prevention and care programs in resource-constrained settings.* Family Health International, Arlington, VA.

Gruskin, S., Tomaševski, T., and Hendriks, A. (1996). Human rights and responses to HIV/AIDS. In *AIDS in the world, II* (ed. J.M. Mann and D.J.M. Tarantola), pp. 326–40. Oxford University Press.

Gubler, D. (1998). Resurgent vector-borne diseases as a global health problem. *Emerging Infectious Diseases*, **4**, 442–50.

Hallack, J. (1999). *Globalization, human rights, and education.* IEP Contributions No. 33. UNESCO, Paris.

Hannum, H. (1998). The UDHR in national and international law. *Health and Human Rights*, **3**, 145–58.

Heggenhougen, K. (1999). Are the marginalized the slag-heap of globalization? Disparity, health and human rights. *Health and Human Rights*, **4**, 205–13.

Hendricks, A. (1995). A selected bibliography of human rights and disability. *Health and Human Rights*, **1**, 212–25.

Heymann, S.J. and Sell, R.L. (1999). Mandatory public health programs: to what standards should they be held? *Health and Human Rights*, **4**, 193–203.

Holder, A.R. (1992). Legal issues in adolescent sexual health. *Adolescent Medicine*, **3**, 257–68.

Hossain, K. (1999). Globalization and human rights: clash of universal aspirations and special interests. In *The future of international human rights* (ed. B.H. Weston and S.P. Marks), pp. 187–99. Transnational Publishers, New York.

HRI (Human Rights Internet) (1998). *Human rights and HIV/AIDS: effective community responses.* International Human Rights Documentation Network, Ottawa.

Humphrey, J. (1976) The international bill of rights: scope and implementation. *William and Mary Law Review*, **17**, 526.

Hunter, D.J. (1999). The future of molecular epidemiology. *International Journal of Epidemiology*, **28**, S1012–14.

ICASO (International Council of AIDS Organizations) (1998). *The ICASO plan on human rights, social equity and HIV/AIDS.* ICASO, Toronto.

ICPD (International Conference on Population and Development) (1994). *Programme of Action of the International Conference on Population and Development.* UN Document A/CONF.171/13. UN, Geneva.

IFRCRC/FXBC (International Federal of Red Cross and Red Crescent Societies and the François-Xavier Bagnoud Center for Health and Human Rights) (1999). The public health–human rights dialogue. In *AIDS, health and human rights: an explanatory manual*, pp. 39–47. IFRCRC/FXBC, Geneva.

ILO (International Labor Organization) (1996). Occupational safety and health. In *Globalization of the footwear, textiles and clothing industries: effects on employment and working conditions*, pp. 101–2. ILO, Geneva.

Jackson, H. (1998). Societal determinants of women's vulnerability to HIV infection in southern Africa. *Health and Human Rights*, **2**, 9–14.

Kennedy, B.P, Kawachi, I., Glass, R., and Prothrow-Stith, D. (1998). Income distribution, socioeconomic status, and self rated health in the United States: multilevel analysis. *British Medical Journal*, **317**, 917–21.

Kirby, M. (1999). The right to health fifty years on: still skeptical? *Health and Human Rights*, **4**, 7–24.

Kolodner, E. (1994). *Transnational corporations: impediments or catalysts of social development?* Social Summit Occasional Paper No. 5. United Nations Research Institute for Social Development, Geneva.

Krieger, N. and Sidney, S. (1996). Racial discrimination and blood pressure: the CARDIA study of young black and white women and men. *American Journal of Public Health*, **86**, 1370–8.

Krieger, N. and Zierler, S. (1997). The need for epidemiologic theory. *Epidemiology*, **8**, 212–14.

Lallemant, M., LeCoeur, S., Tarantola, D., Mann, J.M., and Essex, M. (1994). Anti-retroviral prevention of HIV perinatal transmission. *Lancet*, **343**, 429–30.

Leaning, J. (1997). Human rights and medical education. *British Medical Journal*, **313**, 1390–1.

Leary, V. (1994). The right to health in international human rights law. *Health and Human Rights*, **1**, 24–56.

Lombardo, P.A. (1996). Medicine, eugenics, and the Supreme Court: from coercive sterilization to reproductive freedom. *Journal of Contemporary Health Law and Policy*, **13**, 1–25.

McMichael, A.J. (1993). *Planetary overload: global environmental change and the health of the human species.* Cambridge University Press.

Maastricht Guidelines on Violations of Economic, Social and Cultural Rights (1997). *Human Rights Quarterly*, **20**, 691–705.

Mann, J. (1997*a*). *Human rights and health: a program designed specifically for health professionals.* Centers for Disease Control, Atlanta, GA.

Mann, J.M. (1997*b*). Medicine and public health, ethics and human rights. *Hastings Center Report*, **27**, 6–13.

Mann, J.M. and Tarantola, D.J.M. (1996*a*). From vulnerability to human rights. In *AIDS in the world II*, pp. 463–76. Oxford University Press, New York.

Mann, J.M. and Tarantola, D.J.M. (ed.) (1996*b*). Societal vulnerability: contextual analysis. In *AIDS in the world II*, pp. 444–62. Oxford University Press, New York.

Mann, J.M. and Tarantola, D.J.M. (ed.) (1996*c*). Vulnerability: personal and programmatic. In *AIDS in the world II*, pp. 441–3. Oxford University Press, New York.

Mann, J.M. and Tarantola, D.J.M. (1998). Responding to HIV/AIDS: a historical perspective. *Health and Human Rights*, **2**, 5–8.

Mann, J.M., Tarantola, D.J.M., and Netter, T.W. (ed.) (1992). Assessing vulnerability to HIV infection and AIDS. In *AIDS in the world*, pp. 577–602. Harvard University Press, Cambridge, MA.

Mann, J.M., Gostin, L., Gruskin, S., Brennan, T., Lazzarini, Z., and Fineberg, H. (1994). Health and human rights. *Health and Human Rights*, **1**, 6–23.

Marks, S.P. (1997). Common strategies for health and human rights: from theory to practice. *Health and Human Rights*, **2**, 95–104.

Miller, A.M., Rosga, A., and Satterthwaite, M. (1995). Health, human rights and lesbian existence. *Health and Human Rights*, **1**, 428–48.

Moody, H.R. (1989). Age-based entitlements to health care: what are the limits? *Mount Sinai Journal of Medicine*, **56**, 168–75.

Murray, C.J.L. and Lopez, A.D. (1996). The global burden of disease: a comprehensive assessment of mortality and disability from diseases, injury and risk factors in 1990 and projected to 2020. In *Global burden of diseases injury series*, Vol. I. Harvard School of Public Health on behalf of the WHO, Cambridge, MA.

Orford, A. (1999). Contesting globalization: a feminist perspective on the future of human rights. In *The future of international human rights* (ed. B.H Weston and S.P Marks), pp. 157–85. Transnational Publishers, New York.

Ottawa Charter for Health Promotion (1986). Presented at the First International Conference on Health Promotion, Ottawa.

Plata, M.I. and Yanuzova, M. (1993). *Los derechos humanos y la convencion sobre la eliminacion de todas las formas de discriminacion contra la mujer, 1979.* Profamilia, Bogotá.

Radhakrishna, A., Gringle, R., and Greenslade, F. (1997). Adolescent women face triple jeopardy: unwanted pregnancy, HIV/AIDS and unsafe abortion. *Women's Health Journal*, **2**, 53–62.

Raviglione, M.C., Snider, D.E., and Kochi, A. (1995). Global epidemiology of tuberculosis: morbidity and mortality of a worldwide epidemic. *Journal of the American Medical Association*, **273**, 220–6.

Reich, M.R. (2000). The global drug gap. *Science*, **287**, 1979–81.

Roemer, M. I. and Roemer, R. (1990). Global health, national development and the role of government. *American Journal of Public Health*, **80**, 1188–92.

Savage, T.A. (1998). Children with severe and profound disabilities and the issue of social justice. *Advanced Practical Nursing Quarterly*, **4**, 53–8.

Schmidt, T.A. (1995). When public health competes with individual needs. *Academy of Emergency Medicine*, **2**, 217–22.

Shenker, M. (1992). Occupational lung diseases in the industrializing and industrialized world due to modern pollutants. *Tubercle and Lung Disease*, **73**, 27–32.

Shrader-Frechette, K. (1991). Ethics and the environment. *World Health Forum*, **12**, 311–21.

Smith, S. (1911). The powers and duties of the board of health. *Social Diseases*, **2**, 9.

Sonis, J., Gorenflo, D.W., Jha, P., *et al.* (1996). Teaching of human rights in US medical schools. *Journal of the American Medical Association*, **276**, 1676–8.

South Africa Government Gazette (1999). R. 485. Draft law. *South Africa Government Gazette.*

Steiner, H. and Altston, P. (1996). *International human rights in context: law, politics and morals.* Oxford University Press.

Steingraber, S. (1997). Mechanisms, proof, and unmet needs: the perspective of a cancer activist. *Environmental Health Perspectives*, **105** (Supplement 3), 685–7.

Stevens, H. (1998). AIDS, not hearing AIDS: exploring the link between the deaf community and HIV/AIDS. *Health and Human Rights*, **2**, 99–113.

Sullivan, D. (1995). The nature and scope of human rights obligations concerning women's right to health. *Health and Human Rights*, **1**, 368–98.

Swartz, L. and Levett, A. (1989). Political repression and children in South Africa: the social construction of damaging effects. *Social Science and Medicine*, **28**, 741–50.

Tarantola, D. (1998). *Expanding the global response to HIV/AIDS through focused action.* UNAIDS Best Practice Collection, Geneva.

Tarantola, D. and Gruskin, S. (1998). Children confronting HIV/AIDS: charting the confluence of rights and health. *Health and Human Rights*, **3**, 60–86.

Terrangi, F. (1993). Biotechnology patents and ethical aspects. *Cancer Detection and Prevention*, **17**, 317–21.

Toebes, B. (1999). *The right to health as a human right in international law.* Intersentia-Hart, Antwerp.

Tomaševski, K. (1995*a*). Health rights. In *Economic, social and cultural rights: a textbook* (ed. A. Eide, C. Krause and A. Rosas), pp. 125–42. Martinus Nijhoff, Dordrecht.

Tomaševski, K. (1995*b*). Health. In *United Nations Legal Order*, Vol. 2 (ed. O. Schachter and C. Joyner), pp. 859–906. American Society of International Law and Cambridge University Press.

UN (United Nations) (1945). *UN charter*, adopted 26 June 1945, entered into force 24 October 1945, as amended by GA Res. 1991 (XVIII) 17 December 1963, entered into force 31 August 1966 (557 UNTS 143); 2101 of 20 December 1965, entered into force 12 June 1968 (638 UNTS 308); and 2847 (XXVI) of 20 December 1971, entered into force 24 September 1973 (892 UNTS 119). UN, New York.

UN (United Nations) (1948). *Universal declaration of human rights.* GA Resolution 217A (III), UN GAOR, Resolution 71, UN Document A/810. UN, New York.

UN (United Nations) (1965). *Convention on the elimination of all forms of racial discrimination.* UN GA Resolution 2106A(XX) UN, New York.

UN (United Nations) (1979). *Convention on the elimination of all forms of discrimination against women.* GA Resolution 34/180, UN GAOR, 34th Session, Supplement No. 46, at 193, UN Document A/34/46. UN, New York.

UN (United Nations) (1981). *Declaration on the elimination of all forms of intolerance and of discrimination based on religion or belief.* GA Resolution 36/55, UN GAOR 36th Session, UN Document A/RES/36/55 (1981). UN, New York.

UN (United Nations) (1984*a*). *Convention against torture and other cruel, inhuman or degrading treatment or punishment.* GA Resolution 39/45, UN GAOR, 39th Session, Supplement No. 51, at 197, UN Document A/39/51. UN, New York.

UN (United Nations) (1984*b*). *Progressive development of the principles and norms of international law relating to the new international economic order.* Report of the Secretary General, GA, Session 39, UN Document A/39/504/Add. 1. UN, New York.

UN (United Nations) (1992*a*). Commission on Human Rights, SubCommission on Prevention and Discrimination and Protection of Minorities. *Discrimination against HIV-infected people or people with AIDS.* UN Document E/CN.4/Sub.2/1992/10 (28 July 1992). UN, Geneva.

UN (United Nations) (1992*b*). United Nations General Assembly. *The protection of persons with mental illness and the improvement of mental health care.* Resolution Adopted by the General Assembly, UN Document A/RES/46/119. UN, New York.

UN (United Nations) (1993*a*). *Standard rules on the equalization of opportunities for persons with disabilities.* 85th plenary meeting 20 December 1993, UN Document A/RES/48/96. UN, Geneva.

UN (United Nations) (1993*b*). *Sub-commission on prevention and discrimination and protection of minorities discrimination against HIV-infected people or people with AIDS.* UN Document E/CN.4/Sub.2/1993/9 (23 August 1993). UN, Geneva.

UN (United Nations) (1993*c*). United Nations General Assembly. *Vienna declaration and programme of action. World Conference on Human Rights*, Vienna 14–25 June 1993, UN Document A/CONF.157/23. UN, New York.

UN (United Nations) (1994). Committee on Economic, Social and Cultural Rights (UNCESCR). *General Comment No. 5 (Eleventh Session). Persons with disabilities.* UN Document E/C.12/1194/13. UN, Geneva.

UN (United Nations) (1995*a*). Committee on Economic, Social and Cultural Rights (UNCESCR). *General comment No. 12 (Twentieth*

Session). The right to adequate food. UN Document E/C.12/1995/5. UN, Geneva.

UN (United Nations) (1995*b*). *Programme of action for the world summit for social development*, Copenhagen 6–12 March, UN Document A/CONF.166/9 (96.IV.8). UN, New York.

UN (United Nations) (1995*c*). *World economic and social survey 1995: current trends and policies in the world economy.* UN, New York.

UN (United Nations) (1996). *Manual on human rights reporting*, UN Document HR/PUB/96/1. United Nations Centre for Human Rights, Geneva.

UN (United Nations) (1997*a*). *Report by the Secretary General on programme for reform.* UN Document A/51/950. UN, New York.

UN (United Nations) (1997*b*). Committee on Economic, Social and Cultural Rights (UNCESCR). *General Comment No. 7 (Sixteenth Session). The right to adequate housing.* UN Document E/C.12/1991/4. UN, Geneva.

UN (United Nations) (1998*a*). *Coordination of the policies and activities of the specialized agencies and other branches of the United Nations system related to the coordinated follow-up to and the implementation of the Vienna Declaration Programme of Action.* Report of the Secretary-General, UN Document E/1990/60, June 1998. UN, New York.

UN (United Nations) (1998*b*). *Report of the United Nations Consultative Expert Group Meeting on International Norms and Standards Relating to Disability.* UN, New York.

UN (United Nations) (1999*a*). *Committee on Economic, Social and Cultural Rights (UNCESCR). Concluding observations. Cameroon.* E/C.12/1/Add.40. UN, Geneva.

UN (United Nations) (1999*b*). *Committee on Economic, Social and Cultural Rights (UNCESCR). Concluding observations. Mexico.* E/C.12/1/Add.41. UN, Geneva.

UNAIDS (Joint United Nations Programme on HIV/AIDS) (1997). *The UNAIDS guide to the United Nations human rights machinery.* UNAIDS, Geneva.

UNAIDS (Joint United Nations Programme on HIV/AIDS) (1999). *From principle to practice: greater involvement of people living with or affected by HIV/AIDS (GIPA).* UNAIDS Best Practice Collection, Geneva.

UNAIDS/IOM (Joint United Nations Programme on HIV/AIDS and the International Organization for Migration) (1998). Migration and AIDS. *International Migration*, **36**, 445–68.

UNCEDAW (United Nations Committee on the Elimination of Discrimination Against Women) (1989). *General Recommendation No. 12 (Eighth Session). Violence against women.* UN Document A/43/38. UN, New York.

UNCEDAW (United Nations Committee on the Elimination of Discrimination Against Women) (1990*a*). *General Recommendation No. 14 (Ninth Session). Female circumcision.* UN Document A/45/38. UN, New York.

UNCEDAW (United Nations Committee on the Elimination of Discrimination Against Women) (1990*b*). *General Recommendation No. 15 (Ninth Session). Avoidance of discrimination against women in national strategies for the prevention and control of acquired immunodeficiency syndrome (AIDS).* UN Document A/45/38. UN, New York.

UNCEDAW (United Nations Committee on the Elimination of Discrimination Against Women) (1999). *General Recommendation 24 on Women and Health*, EDAW/C/1999/I/WGII/WP2/Rev. 1. UN, Geneva.

UNCHR (United Nations Commission on Human Rights) (1989). *Non-discrimination in the field of health*, preamble, Resolution 1989/11 (2 March 1989). UN, Geneva.

UNCHR (United Nations Commission on Human Rights) (1994). *Protection of human rights in the context of HIV and AIDS.* UN Document E/CN.4/1994/L.60 (1 March 1994). UN, Geneva.

UNCRC (United Nations Convention on the Rights of the Child) (1989). *GA Resolution 44/25*, UN GAOR, 44th Session, Supplement No. 49, at 166, UN Document A/44/25. UN, Geneva.

UNDAW (United Nations Division for the Advancement of Women) with the United Nations Population Fund (UNFPA) and United Nations High Commissioner for Human Rights (UNHCHR) (1996). *Roundtable of Human Rights Treaty Bodies, with a Focus on Sexual and Reproductive Health and Rights.* UN, New York.

UNDP (United Nations Development Programme) (1998*a*). *Integrating human rights with sustainable development: a UNDP policy document.* UNDP, New York.

UNDP (United Nations Development Programme) (1998*b*). *Symposium on human development and human rights.* UN, New York.

UNDP (United Nations Development Programme) (1999). *Memorandum of understanding between the United Nations Development Programme and Office of the High Commissioner for Human Rights.* Survey of UNDP Activities in Human Rights, New York.

UNECOSOC (United Nations Economic and Social Council) (1985). *The Siracusa Principles on the limitations and derogation provisions in the international covenant on civil and political rights.* UN Document E/CN.4/1985/4, Annex. UN, Geneva.

UNECOSOC (United Nations Economic and Social Council (1991). *Revised general guidelines regarding the form and contents of reports to be submitted by states parties under articles 16 and 17 of the International Covenant on Economic, Social and Cultural Rights*, 17 June 1991. UN Document E/C.12/1991. UN, Geneva.

UNFPA (United Nations Population Fund) (1998). *Ensuring reproductive rights and implementing sexual and reproductive health programmes including women's empowerment, male involvement and human rights.* UNFPA, New York.

UNGA (United Nations General Assembly) (1997). *Renewing the United Nations: a programme for reform*, 14 July 1997, UN Document A/RE/52/12. UN, New York.

UNHCHR (United Nations High Commissioner for Human Rights) (1996). *Report of the Seventh Meeting of the Treaty Bodies.* UN Document A/51/482. UN, Geneva.

UNHCHR (United Nations High Commissioner for Human Rights) (1997). *Report of the Eighth Meeting of the Treaty Bodies.* UN Document A/52/507. UN, Geneva.

UNHCHR (United Nations High Commissioner for Human Rights) (1998*a*). *Report of the Ninth Meeting of Persons Chairing the Human Rights Treaty Bodies.* UN Document A/53/125. UN, Geneva.

UNHCHR (United Nations High Commissioner for Human Rights) (1998*b*). *Report of the Tenth Meeting of Persons Chairing the Human Rights Treaty Bodies.* UN Document A/53/432. UN, Geneva.

UNHCHR (United Nations Office of High Commissioner for Human Rights) (2000). *Business and human rights: a progress report.* UN, Geneva.

UNHRC (United Nations Human Rights Committee) (1994). *Fiftieth Session Communication*, No. 488/1992, CCPR/C/50/D/488/1992, 4 April 1994. UN, Geneva.

UNICCPR (United Nations International Covenant on Civil and Political Rights) (1966). *GA Resolution 2200 (XXI)*, UN GAOR, 21st Session, Supplement No. 16, at 49, UN Document A/6316. UN, New York.

UNICEF (United Nations International Children's Emergency Fund) (1998). *A human rights approach to UNICEF programming in children and women: what it is, and some changes it will bring.* UNICEF, New York.

UNICEF (United Nations International Children's Emergency Fund) (2000). *Mission statement*, March 2000. UN, New York.

UNICESCR (United Nations International Covenant on Economic, Social and Cultural Rights) (1966). *GA Resolution 2200 (XXI)*, UN GAOR, 21st Session, Supplement No. 16, at 49, UN Document A/6316 UN, Geneva.

Ward, C. and Myers, N.A. (1999). Babies born with major disabilities: the medical-legal interface. *Pediatric Surgery International*, **15**, 310–19.

Watson, R.T., Dixon, J.A., Hamburg, S.P., Janetos, A.C., and Moss, R.H. (1998). *Protecting our planet, securing our future.* United Nations Environment Programme and United States National Aeronautics and Space Administration.

Weiss, E. and Gupta, G.R. (1993). Women facing the challenges of AIDS: prevention and policy concerns. In *Women at the center: development issues and practices for the 1990s*, pp. 168–81. Kumarian Press, West Hartford, CT.

WHO (World Health Organization) (1946). *Constitution of the World Health Organization*, adopted by the International Health Conference, New York, 19 June–22 July 1946, and signed on 22 July 1946. WHO, Geneva.

WHO (World Health Organization, with UNICEF) (1979). *International conference on primary health care.* WHA 32.30. WHO, Geneva.

WHO (World Health Organization) (1987). *World Health Assembly, Resolution WHA 40.26, Global Strategy for the Prevention and Control of AIDS*, 5 May 1987. WHO, Geneva.

WHO (World Health Organization) (1992). *Our planet, our health.* Report of the WHO Commission on Health and Environment. WHO, Geneva.

WHO (World Health Organization) (1994*a*). *Framework for effective tuberculosis control.* Tuberculosis Programme, WHO/TB/94.179. WHO, Geneva.

WHO (World Health Organization) (1994*b*). *Women's health, towards a better world.* Report of the first meeting of the global commission on women's health. WHO/DGH/94.4, pp. 21–3. WHO, Geneva.

WHO (World Health Organization) (1995). *WTO: What's in it for WHO?* WHO Task Force on Health Economics Document WHO/TFHE/95.5. WHO, Geneva.

WHO (World Health Organization) (1998*a*). *Gender and health.* Technical Paper WHO/FRH/WHD/98.16. WHO, Geneva.

WHO (World Health Organization) (1998*b*). *Tobacco free initiative.* Executive Board, Provisional Agenda Item 3, 103rd Session, EB103/5. WHO, Geneva.

WHO (World Health Organization) (1998*c*). *WHO fact sheet*, No. 104. WHO, Geneva.

WHO (World Health Organization) (1998*d*). *World Health Assembly Resolution on the World Health Declaration*, WHA51/5 adopted by the fifty-first World Health Assembly, 1998. WHO, Geneva.

WHO (World Health Organization) (1999*a*). *Removing obstacles to healthy development.* WHO Report on Infectious Diseases, WHO/CDS/99.1. WHO, Geneva.

WHO (World Health Organization) (1999*b*). *WHO corporate strategy for the WHO Secretariat.* Executive Board Provisional Agenda Item 2, 105th Session, EB105/3. WHO, Geneva.

WHO (World Health Organization) (1999*c*). *World health report 1999—making a difference.* WHO, Geneva.

WHO (World Health Organization) (2000*a*). *The economic impacts of tuberculosis.* Ministerial Conference, the Stop TB Initiative 2000 Series WHO/CDS/STB/2000–5. WHO, Geneva.

WHO (World Health Organization) (2000*b*). *Informal consultation on mainstreaming human rights in WHO, 3–4 April 2000.* WHO, Geneva.

WHO (World Health Organization) (2000*c*). *World health report—2000.* WHO, Geneva.

WHO/UNAIDS (World Health Organization and the Joint United Nations Programme on AIDS) (1999). *Consultation on HIV/AIDS reporting and disclosure, 20–22 October 1999.* WHO, Geneva.

Wodak, A. (1998). Health, HIV infection, human rights, and injecting drug use. *Health and Human Rights*, **2**, 25–41.

Youth Research (1997). Naked wire and naked truths: a study of reproductive health risks faced by teenage girls in Honiara, Solomon Islands. *Pacific Aids Alert Bulletin*, **16**, 11–12.

Zierler, S., Cunningham, W.E., Andersen, R., *et al.* (2000). Violence victimization after HIV infection in a US probability sample of adult patients in primary care. *American Journal of Public Health*, **90**, 208–15.

4.2 Comparative national public health legislation*

Ruth Roemer and Milton I. Roemer

Public health law, like public health, concerns the health of populations as contrasted with the health of individuals. Thus, public health law concerns the legal aspects of providing preventive, curative, and rehabilitative services to populations, although public health law has an important impact on health protection and health care for individuals as well.

As the role of public health has expanded from its early function of preventing the spread of communicable diseases to encompass the development of resources, the organization and financing of the delivery of care, surveillance of the health-care system, health promotion, and overall protection of community health, so public health law and legislation have expanded to provide authorization, direction, and regulation of many fields of environmental and personal health services. As Grad has written, 'The reach of public health law is as broad as the reach of public health itself. Public health and public health law expand to meet the needs of our society' (Grad 1986).

This chapter begins by describing the functions of law and legislation in protecting the public health. Then several fields of public health law are examined, with comment on the general scope of law and legislation, methods of implementing law and policy, selected examples of legislation, and current legal issues.

In each field the review of the law is necessarily brief, and not all fields of public health law are covered. For further information, the reader is directed to the primary texts of the health laws of the world, published by the World Health Organization (**WHO**) in its quarterly journal, the *International Digest of Health Legislation* (now on the Internet), and to the many legal treatises, texts, journals, and reports of court decisions available in law libraries.

Perhaps a caveat or two are in order. Firstly, it should be noted that law and legislation can play a negative or a positive role with respect to public health. Some laws may be adverse to public health by imposing restrictions on health services based on the knowledge, social conditions, or fiscal constraints obtaining at the time that legislation was adopted. Such negative laws are illustrated by the criminal laws outlawing abortion that are being replaced by legalized abortion in most countries of the world (Cook 1989; Cook *et al.* 1999). Fortunately, laws also play a constructive role supportive of public health by authorizing measures to protect health, to increase access to health services, and to assure the quantity and quality of health care that a society needs. This chapter is replete with such examples.

Secondly, one should bear in mind that while law performs a technical function of expressing health policy and setting forth procedures for implementing it, the content of the law is determined by the nature and orientation of the political power in the country at any time and place. The element of political will is crucial to the enactment of health legislation. Legislation can serve as an instrument of change to improve health services and health protection but only if policy makers have the necessary political will.

Functions of health laws

Health laws perform various essential functions in protecting the health of populations.

1. Laws and legislation prohibit conduct that is injurious to the health of individuals and communities. Examples of this function are environmental health laws that prohibit the dumping of toxic chemicals in the environment, traditional public health legislation to prevent the spread of disease, laws to control drug abuse, laws regulating smoking in public places, and laws to regulate the quality of health care.
2. Health legislation authorizes programmes and services that promote the health of individuals and communities. Many diverse, categorical programmes authorized by law provide health services for specific people (mothers and children, the military, veterans, the mentally ill, the handicapped, the elderly), for specific diseases and conditions (heart disease, cancer, stroke, sexually transmitted diseases, mental illness and retardation, alcoholism and drug abuse, HIV/AIDS), and for specific services in various fields (environmental and occupational health, nutrition, mental health, dental health and ambulatory, hospital, and long-term care).
3. Legislation regulates the production of resources for health care. Laws authorize or provide financing for the construction of hospitals, health centres, and other health facilities. Legislation provides support for education of the health professions and occupations. Regulation of the production and importation and export of drugs, medical devices, and medical equipment and supplies is carried out under the authority of law. Financial support of research—the production of knowledge—may require legal action.

* The authors are deeply indebted to Mr S.S. Fluss, former Chief of Health Legislation at the WHO, Geneva, and Editor of the *International Digest of Health Legislation*, for information and insights generously provided over the years on health legislation of countries throughout the world.

4. Legislation provides for the social financing of health care. This function is carried out by laws establishing systems of national health insurance or a national health service. It is also expressed in government grants for specific health programmes, in the imposition of special taxes for health purposes, and in tax exemption for non-profit health facilities.
5. Legislation authorizes surveillance over the quality of health care. Examples of this function are licensure laws establishing minimum standards for health personnel and facilities, legislation providing for peer review of the quality of care, and financing programmes that regulate the quantity and quality of care. The judicial system, in handling malpractice suits, also carries out this function.

In the process of performing these various functions, health law faces the challenge inherent in all law—that of balancing the interests of the individual and the interests of society. This over-riding issue faced by legislators, administrators, and judges is both legal and ethical. To what extent may individual rights be curtailed in order to promote the general welfare? The answer to this question is 'It depends'. It depends on the importance of the governmental purpose, the degree of risk to the community, and the degree of intrusion on individual rights. It depends on the scientific and epidemiological evidence pertaining to the issue being legislated or litigated. It depends on the nature of the legal system and its protection of individual rights.

Environmental health and the law

Environmental sanitation was one of the earliest concerns of public health because of the basic need for a safe water supply and waste disposal in all societies. With the growth of industrialization, modern law to assure a healthful living and working environment has expanded to include control of air and water quality, regulation of domestic waste and industrial and agricultural effluents, management of solid waste disposal, control of marine pollution, regulation of radiation emissions, control of toxic substances in industry and the community, regulation of the use of pesticides in agriculture, and noise abatement. Each of these branches of environmental law is based on the need to protect the public health. In addition, other branches of environmental law, while not directed solely to protecting health, have an important impact on health and the quality of life. These include conservation of natural and environmental resources, land use control and regulations governing housing, and measures to meet population growth and power needs (Grad 1994).

Public health personnel are involved to varying degrees in each of these problems in environmental health. They may be called on to set standards for air and water quality, to treat water to make it potable, to add fluorides to a public water supply to prevent dental caries, to inspect factories for toxic chemicals, to enforce sanitation regulations in markets and restaurants, to develop solid waste disposal systems, and for other tasks. The size and complexity of environmental engineering, management, and control activities have caused principal responsibility for environmental regulation to be placed in non-health agencies with specialized scientific, engineering, and economic expertise in many countries, but public health personnel retain responsibility for managing the health component of environmental control. As they undertake their varied functions, public health environmentalists encounter legislation and regulations designed to control contaminants and prevent harm to the health of the community.

A number of mechanisms are used for environmental control. The most important of these is not a legal mechanism but rather economic measures that promote compliance with environmental standards. For example, an industry may find it cheaper to clean up its wastes than to pay the penalties for pollution. Or a government may find it advantageous to subsidize practices that will improve environmental quality.

Among the legal remedies used to implement environmental legislation are inspections and citations for violations of established standards of environmental quality, civil penalties for pollution, effluent charges, licensing of businesses and withdrawal of the license in the event of violation of standards, criminal prosecutions to punish violators, injunctions to prevent future harm, and seizure and forfeiture of property in cases of egregious pollution (Grad *et al.* 1971).

Examples of environmental legislation

Environmental health legislation may be either categorical or comprehensive. Categorical legislation deals with one type of problem, such as air or water quality or solid waste disposal. Comprehensive legislation is designed to provide integrated control of the many and often interrelated insults to the environment having an impact on health.

Choosing examples of categorical environmental legislation at random, one may cite as laws designed to protect health and safety in a specific field the 1996 legislation of Algeria and Djibouti promulgating water codes and specifying principles of water policy, including preservation of common resources, protecting the aquatic environment, and assuring the compatibility of water management and land use (Algeria 1996; Djibouti 1997). Virtually all countries have categorical legislation dealing with various specific aspects of environmental control to promote health.

Both industrialized and developing countries have also enacted comprehensive environmental legislation addressed to multiple aspects of the environment. In the United States, the National Environmental Policy Act of 1969 was designed to create a means for integrating and co-ordinating the many programmes affecting environmental protection (US 1969). An important provision of the legislation requires the filing of environmental impact statements before major federal projects with significant impact on the environment can be undertaken.

Impelled by the increasingly recognized threats to health from environmental pollution, many other countries have enacted comprehensive environmental legislation (for example, Sri Lanka 1981). An important provision of these laws is the requirement for an environmental assessment in advance of construction of a project to determine its effect on health and on physical and living conditions. The Canadian law establishing an environmental assessment process is designed to ensure that the environmental effects of projects receive careful consideration before responsible authorities take actions in connection with them, to encourage these authorities to take actions that promote sustainable development and thereby achieve or maintain a healthy environment and a healthy economy, and to ensure an opportunity for public participation in the environmental assessment process (Canada 1992). A statute of the Province of Ontario, Canada, allows any two people residing in Ontario who believe that an existing policy or regulation should be amended or repealed or that a new policy should be adopted to protect the environment apply to the Environmental Commissioner for review of that policy (Canada 1998).

As East European countries are making the transition from communism to capitalism, they have recognized that industrialization has been associated with serious degradation of the environment, and have consequently enacted broad environmental protection legislation. For example, Bulgaria's 1991 law provides for monitoring the state of the environment, assessment of environmental impacts, and development of environmental policy based on the reduction of hazards to human health and the environment and its relation to damages suffered and benefits lost (Bulgaria 1993). The Hungarian legislation on environmental impact assessments requires a forecast and evaluation of the changes in environmental conditions resulting from the activity; an estimate of the probable environmental, health, economic, and social consequences of the changes in the environmental conditions; a definition of measures to prevent, reduce, or avert possible pollution and damage; the methods for measuring and analysing environmental impacts in the course of the activity and the method for subsequent monitoring of these impacts after the activity ceases; and a map of the impact areas (Hungary 1993).

Many developing countries have adopted statutes or regulations under their environmental protection acts specifying functions to be performed to protect the environment (for example, planning, standard setting, studies of industry and trade, pollution control) (Burkino Faso 1994; Belize 1996; Indonesia 1998; Morocco 1998), requirements for environmental impact statements (Malawi 1998), and the organization and operation of a secretariat responsible for the environment or an advisory body on environmental policy (Cameroon 1997; Madagascar 1998).

Issues in environmental legislation

Many issues face policy-makers and public health administrators in the field of environmental control. Each of these issues merits lengthy analysis, which is not possible here. However, a brief mention of the issues shows the magnitude and complexity of the problems in this field.

A priority for all countries, both industrialized and developing, is to balance the interest in a healthful environment and the need for employment and industrial development. This conflict is exemplified by Algeria in its law on environmental protection which provides: 'National development implies the necessary equilibrium between the imperatives of economic growth and those on environmental protection and the preservation of the living conditions of the population' (Algeria 1984).

The tension between the need for economic growth and the need to protect the quality of the living environment underlies all regulation of environmental pollution.

Management of environmental problems requires a high degree of scientific knowledge and technical sophistication in various specialized fields. At the same time, the interrelations among the various ambient elements (for example, the impact of water pollution on land use) requires an intersectoral approach involving both health and non-health agencies. These environmental health interfaces and interactions have implications for the geographical jurisdiction of environmental agencies, for the responsibilities of various levels of government, for the functions of environmental health personnel, and for the role of public health personnel in large environmental management agencies (Goldsmith 1970; Roemer *et al.* 1971).

In the operation of any environmental management system, agencies responsible for regulating substances harmful to health face the difficult question of what limits exist on the agency's regulatory power in the light of scientific uncertainty. What are the powers of the agency if there are conflicting scientific opinions or if the evidence is based solely on epidemiological data (Grad 1994)? A case study of the court decision upholding the regulation by the United States Environmental Protection Agency restricting the amount of lead additives in gasoline provides important insights on the scope of judicial review and the role of the courts in cases of great technological complexity (Silver 1980).

The issue of how widely accepted a scientific process or theory must be to be admitted in evidence in a lawsuit arose in a case before the United States Supreme Court in 1993. The case involved not environmental issues but whether a drug prescribed for nausea during pregnancy caused birth defects. The decision has wide applicability to various kinds of cases involving scientific evidence (*Daubert* v. *Merrell Dow Pharmaceuticals Inc.* 1993).

The United States Supreme Court, by a vote of 7 to 2, rejected the test of 'general acceptance' of scientific evidence that has previously been applied and ruled that under modern rules of evidence adopted in the 1970s, particularly Rule 702 of the Federal Rules of Evidence, 'general acceptance' is not an absolute prerequisite to admissibility of scientific evidence. The Court's opinion stated that trial judges serve as gatekeepers to ensure that all scientific evidence admitted is not only relevant but reliable. Pertinent evidence based on scientifically valid principles will satisfy these requirements. While publication in a peer-reviewed journal is not essential for admissibility of evidence, such publication is a relevant, but not a dispositive, factor for a judge to consider in determining whether a method or technique is valid. Also, the known or potential rate of error may be considered. Justice Blackmun justified the gatekeeper role by pointing out that there are 'important differences between the quest for truth in the courtroom and the quest for truth in the laboratory. Scientific conclusions are subject to perpetual revision. Law, on the other hand, must resolve disputes finally and quickly.'

An innovative strategy used for obtaining scientific advice on complex and disputed questions in lawsuits is to establish a panel of scientists to study the question and advise judges and juries. Such a panel in federal class action lawsuits against silicone breast implant makers resulted in a finding that the breast implants did not cause the women's illnesses (National Science Panel 1998).

Finally, an issue that is assuming increasing importance in the field of occupational and environmental health is worker and community involvement in assuring a healthful working and living environment. In the United States, worker and the community right-to-know laws impose on employers and manufacturers the duty to disclose hazards in the workplace or activities involving toxic exposures (Ashford and Caldart 1985). These laws are not a substitute for enforcement of environmental protection laws, but they are an important aid to better regulation of the environment. The principle is embodied in an international convention, the Convention Concerning Occupational Safety and Health and the Working Environment, adopted by the International Labour Organization in 1981. The International Labour Organization Convention requires employers and workers and their representatives to co-operate in protecting occupational safety and health. Measures taken by the employer to protect occupational safety and health must be disclosed to workers' representatives, and the workers have a right to know all aspects of occupational safety and health associated with their work. The Convention also requires training of workers and their representatives in occupational safety and health (International Labour Organization 1981).

Regulation of food and drugs

Laws to prevent the adulteration of food and medicines originated centuries ago (Christoffel 1982). Today in industrialized countries, and to an increasing extent in developing countries, people are dependent on commercially produced food and manufactured drugs that they are unable to evaluate themselves. They must rely on governmental regulation of these goods.

Legislation related to nutritional quality and food safety regulates the hygienic standards for production and marketing of foods; control of equipment, utensils, and containers; hygiene and health of food handlers, storage, and vending places; methods of testing and inspection; requirements for labelling of contents and shelf-life; and advertising of foods. More specialized legislation deals with such matters as safety of food additives, including what additives are allowed, maximum permissible levels, and requirements for package labelling. These regulations include the requirement for iodization of salt to prevent goitre and in some countries labelling of foods for salt content to promote uniformity in definitions of low salt content.

Comprehensive drug control legislation, which exists generally in all industrialized countries and in many developing countries, provides authority to control the importation and production of drugs; the licensing of manufacturers, wholesalers, and distributors; drug registration; and the distribution, sale, labelling, advertising, and promotion of drugs. A national drug control programme regulates the quality, safety, and efficacy of prescription drugs and over-the-counter drugs and also shares in responsibility for control of narcotic drugs (Chapman 1976).

Enforcement of food and drug laws is carried out through inspections of the manufacturing process, recall or seizure of defective products, civil and criminal penalties for violations of established standards, and injunctions to prevent marketing of food and drugs found unsafe or unsanitary. Enforcement relies heavily on rule-making by the food and drug agency and on administrative hearings on violations of standards. Use of administrative law in this field so critical to health hastens the disposition of cases, provides expertise on the technical issues involved, and introduces flexibility in the process of adjudicating cases and designing sanctions.

Examples of food and drug legislation

In 1976, Norway became the first country in Western Europe to establish a national nutrition and food policy (Norway 1981–1982). Its objectives are to encourage healthful dietary habits, develop nutrition and food policy in accord with the recommendations of the World Food Conference, increase production and consumption of Norwegian food products, and improve self-sufficiency in food products. Numerous laws are implemented by various governmental agencies to these ends. The Food Control Coordinating Act of 1978 established a Food Control Board with representation from the various ministries and interests. The Inter-Ministerial Coordinating Committee on Nutrition (composed of leading civil servants in the Ministries of Fisheries, Consumer Affairs, and Government Administration; Trade, Industry, Church, and Education; Agriculture, the Environment, Health, and Social Affairs; and Foreign Affairs) is charged with defining tasks, preparing long-term plans, and implementing policies. The National Nutrition Council is composed of members who represent research and teaching in the fields of nutrition, diet, dietetics, food hygiene and technology, food production, and the food industry. The mandate of the Council is to advise the authorities, industrial organizations, large households, and food producers on nutrition and to disseminate information on diet. Implementation of the national nutrition policy thus depends on permanent interministerial bodies with well-staffed secretariats.

In addition, the national nutrition policy of Norway is elaborated through a health policy on nutrition which includes preventive work and training of personnel; agricultural, fisheries, and price policies that affect production and subsidies of foods; and a consumer and school policy to present an appropriate range of foods and develop sound attitudes towards diet and nutrition. The aim is to help the population consume more cereals, skimmed milk, fish, fruits, and vegetables, and less fat, sugar, and meat, and to substitute fish for some meat, starch for some sugar, and skimmed milk for most whole milk. The goals of the Norwegian nutrition policy are to motivate individuals to adopt a healthful diet, to improve food distribution in outlying districts, and to strengthen the rural economy by making farming more profitable and attractive (Klepp and Forster 1985).

Illustrative of comprehensive drug control programmes is the legislation of Australia, which regulates the manufacture, importation, sale, and distribution of drugs and also establishes a Pharmaceutical Benefits Scheme providing publicly financed prescribed drugs to the entire population (Roemer and Roemer 1976). About 90 per cent of all drugs prescribed in Australia are available on the approved list, and the patient generally pays only a flat $1 copayment, regardless of the cost of the prescription.

The Foods, Drugs and Devices, and Cosmetics Act of The Philippines provides for a comprehensive food and drug regulatory system governing various aspects of food and drug production and distribution, including standards and quality measures for these products, approval of new drugs, control of adulteration, labelling requirements, and licensing of manufacture, sale, and import and export of drugs (Philippines 1990). The 1995 decree of Bulgaria sets forth requirements relating to registration, clinical trials, manufacture, trade, import, and export of pharmaceuticals (Bulgaria 1996).

In contrast to comprehensive food and drug regulatory schemes are the numerous statutes dealing with specific issues in the field. For example, Indonesia requires all government hospitals and health centres to prescribe and use generic drugs for all patients and requires pharmacies to stock essential drugs, including generic drugs (Indonesia 1990). Increasing numbers of countries are enacting laws making the iodization of salt compulsory (Madagascar 1995; Côte d'Ivoire 1996; Morocco 1996; Tunisia 1996; Zaire 1996; Djibouti 1997; Philippines 1997). In the United States, voluntary labelling of the contents of foods, long unsatisfactory because of lack of uniformity and difficulty for consumers in interpreting the information, has been replaced by mandatory labelling (US 1991). Regulations of the Food and Drug Administration require nutrition labelling on most foods and specify the contents and format for nutrition information (US 1993*c*).

Issues in food and drug control

Control of such essential consumer products as food and drugs requires constant vigilance to monitor the safety and nutritional values of foods and the safety, efficacy, and quality of prescription and over-the-counter drugs. Public health agencies are concerned with surveillance of the production and marketing of both food and drugs, with labelling and advertising, and with provision of information to the consumers. Mandatory labelling of the sodium content of foods is a form of consumer education. Warning labels and package inserts in pharmaceuticals are an important part of patient education.

Drug regulation begins with establishing and implementing protocols for research on and testing of new drugs and proceeds to evaluate drugs for safety and efficacy. The process of evaluating animal and clinical data, and determining health risks from drug trials, may be quite protracted, so that regulatory agencies may be accused of unreasonable delays in approval of new drugs ('drug lag'). In 1992, perhaps partially impelled by the needs of patients with AIDS, the American Food and Drug Administration adopted new regulations to accelerate approval of certain new drugs and biological products for serious or life-threatening conditions, with provisions for any necessary continued study of the drugs' clinical benefits or with restrictions on use, if necessary (US 1993*d*).

Associated with the drug approval process is the determination of national policy governing the import and export of therapeutic drugs. The multiple national standards on acceptability of different drugs affects the availability of drugs in international trade—an increasingly critical problem in a shrinking world (Cook 1987). Fortunately, in 1975 the WHO established the Certification Scheme on the Quality of Pharmaceutical Products Moving in International Commerce. It regularly disseminates information on drugs and drug quality as certified by the competent authority of the exporting country that the product is safe for distribution or sale in the exporting country; furthermore, the plant at which the product is manufactured is subject to inspection showing that the manufacturer conforms to requirements for good practice in manufacture and quality control as recommended by the WHO (World Health Assembly 1989). Use of international standards is designed to alleviate problems related to variance in standards among countries.

Another issue addressed in national legislation is advertising of pharmaceuticals. Some countries restrict advertising of pharmaceuticals to professional journals and publications, allowing advertising in the mass media of only over-the-counter drugs (Bulgaria 1996; Iceland 1998; Niger 1998). Colombia, seeking to limit advertising of pharmaceuticals to established facts and to avoid exaggeration of benefits, partial truths, and fraud, provides that all advertising of pharmaceuticals is subject to prior authorization by the National Institute for Food and Drug Surveillance (Colombia 1998*b*).

A major problem on which there is great variation in the laws of different jurisdictions is that relating to product liability and compensation for adverse effects of drugs. The tension existing between the interest of the pharmaceutical industry in marketing new drugs, the interests of the consumer in compensation for damages suffered, and the interest of society in promoting development of pharmaceutical products and assuring their availability has led to varying solutions. These have included, to take the example of the United States, decisions holding the manufacturers strictly liable, with damages assessed according to their share of the market where the supplier of the drug could not be identified (*Sindell* v. *Abbott Laboratories* 1980), decisions holding a manufacturer liable only for failure to follow state-of-the-art manufacturing practices (*Brown* v. *Superior Court* 1988), and, in the case of vaccines, development of a no-fault federally funded compensation system for untoward outcomes of childhood immunizations (US 1986).

Finally, an increasingly important issue relates to regulation of drug prices. The high cost of drugs has led to the use of generic drugs and repeal of laws banning substitution of generic equivalents for brand name drugs prescribed by the doctor (DeMarco 1975). Another strategy for controlling drug costs in health-care programmes is development of a drug formulary or a list of essential drugs for which reimbursement is provided.

Licensure of health personnel

Licensing or registration laws for doctors were designed originally to protect the public against quacks, charlatans, and incompetent practitioners. Over the years the function of licensing laws for a wide variety of health professionals has expanded to specify minimum qualifications for practice, to regulate educational programmes, to define the scope of practice for each profession, and to set forth requirements for continued competence. Some licensing laws are mandatory, such as medical and dental practice acts, requiring all who practice the profession to be licensed and making it illegal to practice without a license. Voluntary or permissive licensing laws protect only the title and prohibit unlicenced personnel from holding themselves out as licensed personnel but do not require licensure in order to practice the profession. As professions grow in strength, voluntary licensure tends to be replaced by mandatory licensure.

While licensing or registration laws have been criticized as protecting the professions rather than the public and as creating monopolies of the licensed professions, all countries have a governmental system for regulating the qualifications of medical, dental, and a varying number of other health personnel. In some countries licensure may be granted without further examination on completion of an approved educational programme. In others a separate examination may be required after completion of the approved educational programme. In recent years, recognition of the capacity of licensing laws to do more than specify minimum qualifications for practice—to influence the geographic location of doctors, dentists, and others, to affect the proportions of generalists and specialists, to influence the pattern of practice, and to promote the continued competence of practitioners—has given them a new importance for the health professions.

Implementation of licensing laws is carried out by licensing boards composed originally largely of members of the profession to be licensed. In response to the demand for greater public accountability, members of other professions, consumers, and representatives of governmental agencies have been added to the boards in many countries.

The example of nursing licensing laws

To present some insight on the role of licensing laws in regulating the qualifications and functions of health personnel the example of nursing licensure is useful. Nursing practice acts generally provide for personal and educational qualifications of nurses, prescribe the content of nursing curricula, including practical experience, define the scope of nursing practice, specify grounds and procedures for disciplinary action, and provide for renewal of licenses.

As nursing education has been expanded and technology in health care improved, it became clear in the United States and in other countries that nurses were being underutilized. Although they were equipped by enriched training for new nursing roles, the licensing laws generally barred nurses from undertaking 'diagnosis and treatment', which were defined as medical functions. Beginning in 1971 the American states adopted various legislative strategies to authorize an expanded role for nurses (Bullough 1975). These included the following.

- Authorization by the medical and nursing licensing boards of expanded functions for nurses.
- Authorization by the medical and nursing licensing boards of amended definitions of professional nursing to include autonomous functions for nurses (New York 1972). (In 1972 the State of New York revised its definition of professional nursing as follows: 'The practice of the profession of nursing as a registered professional nurse is defined as diagnosing and treating human responses to actual or potential health problems through such services as case-finding, health teaching, health counseling, and provision of care supportive to or restorative of life and well-being and executing medical regimens prescribed by a licensed or otherwise legally authorized physician or dentist. A nursing regimen shall be consistent with and shall not vary any existing medical regimen.' Furthermore, in *Sermchief* v. *Gonzales* (Missouri Supreme Court 1983), the Missouri Supreme Court upheld the authority of nurses to perform diagnostic and treatment functions in family planning services under a modernized nursing practice act prescribing a broad spectrum of nursing functions qualified by the phrase 'including but not limited to'.)
- Authorization by the medical and nursing licensing boards of standardized procedures and protocols to authorize expanded nursing functions.
- Authorization by the medical and nursing licensing boards to allow individual doctors to delegate to nurses the right to diagnose and treat.

These legislative changes made in nursing practice acts in state after state expanded the contribution of nurses to patient care and made the profession of nursing more interesting and rewarding.

Legal barriers to extension of the nurse's role in developing countries are particularly grave because the nurse is often the only health professional available in rural areas to provide primary health care. Yet often the medical and pharmacy acts bar the nurse from diagnosing and treating and from prescribing medications. The nursing practice acts restrict not only the scope of nursing practice but also the training that nurses receive (WHO Study Group 1986). In order to alter this negative impact of the law, countries have enacted new statutes to reorient nursing education and to authorize functions for nurses that were formerly the exclusive province of the doctor. For example, in 1977 Senegal issued a decree adapting its nursing education to the needs of the country so that nurses will be prepared to serve the rural population (Senegal 1978). Also in 1977 the Ministry of Health of Israel authorized nurses to carry out certain kinds of medical activity, such as drawing blood for tests, immunizations, and suturing wounds (WHO Study Group 1986). In 1982 Dominica authorized its family nurse practitioners to prescribe drugs from the Dominica Nurse Practitioner Formulary (Dominica 1983). In 1998 Luxembourg issued regulations defining the preventive, curative, and palliative functions of the nurse (Luxembourg 1998).

Legal issues in regulation of personnel

The issue of scope of practice of health personnel recurs periodically as new types of health workers are introduced in a country, such as pharmacy technicians or acupuncturists, and as strengthened preparation of existing categories of personnel warrants expanded functions. A newly recognized need is the requirement for management personnel specialized in health-care administration (Morocco 1998*a*). In fact, an overriding issue in this field is how allied and auxiliary personnel should be credentialed, whether by a governmental mechanism, such as licensure or some form of officially required registration, or by a voluntary mechanism, such as certification by a professional association.

Another concern is to assure equitable and rational geographic and specialty distribution of health professionals. Some countries, such as Norway and Mexico, require doctors to contribute a period of service in an underserved area as a condition of licensure. Other countries, such as the United States, use governmental funding for medical education as leverage for specialty distribution and as an economic incentive for settlement in rural areas.

The development of distance learning and telemedicine for the training of personnel and the provision of medical care in remote areas have led to new programmes and legislation (Tunisia 1998).

The problem of assuring continuing competence has challenged many countries. Various strategies have been adopted, including voluntary and mandatory educational programmes, periodic re-examinations, and further clinical training. But no consensus has been reached on the best way to achieve the objective of updated knowledge and skills.

With the introduction of private medical practice in East European countries and Vietnam, new legislation specifies the conditions and rules governing private practice. Bulgaria, for example, requires medical specialists wishing to practice privately in their consulting rooms to register with the municipal council. Their scope of practice is limited: private practitioners are not authorized to perform abortions, to administer required immunizations, or to treat communicable diseases, which must be treated in a public health establishment (Bulgaria 1992). Vietnam requires that applicants seeking to open a private medical or dental practice, test laboratory, anaesthetic surgery establishment, convalescent or rehabilitation facility, maternity home, or birth control centre have at least 5 years of continuous practice at relevant consulting and treatment establishments (Vietnam 1996). Similar experience is prescribed for applicants seeking to open traditional medical clinics and traditional pharmacies. Traditional medical practices are required to keep medical records, observe public health sterilization and bacteria-killing regulations of the Ministry of Public Health, and refer patients with complications or who do not improve after long treatment to state-run medical establishments (Vietnam 1996).

Not only licensing laws but various other regulatory mechanisms affect the qualifications and functions of health personnel. These include the educational system, the policies of professional associations, the regulation of work settings, the requirements of payment programmes, and judicial decisions in malpractice suits and other legal cases. While licensing laws impinge directly on the qualifications and functions of health personnel, indirect influences through the methods of providing and paying for care can also shape the 'health' human resources component of a national health system.

Regulation of health-care facilities

Various mechanisms regulate the quality of the care provided by hospitals, health centres, and long-term care facilities—hospital licensing laws, requirements of the financing system, court decisions, actions of voluntary accrediting bodies, standards of professional associations for specialty training, and rules of the facilities themselves. Legislation sets minimum standards that facilities must meet in order to operate. Legislation also governs the planning, construction, and distribution of facilities.

The cornerstone of this multifaceted regulatory system is hospital licensure. Hospital licensing laws are important because such a large proportion of care—and care for serious illness—is provided in hospitals and because the costs of hospital and long-term care represent such a large proportion of health-care expenditures. As Somers has written, 'it is difficult to exaggerate the importance of the hospital in contemporary society' (Somers 1969).

Originally, hospital licensing laws were concerned solely with the physical conditions in the hospital—safety, sanitation, and space. But over the years health facility legislation has expanded to cover many types of health facility and to prescribe requirements to assure not only the safety of patients but also the quality of their care (Lander 1980). Government sets standards for both public and private institutions. The public purpose of health facilities and the public interest in their use are the basis for public regulation of private institutions. For non-governmental agencies and the private market, legislation may regulate performance to protect public health, may provide support, and may define inter-relationships of private institutions with government.

Implementation of hospital licensing laws is carried out through rule-making by governmental agencies, inspections of facilities, consultations to remedy deficiencies, administrative hearings, injunctions, denial of reimbursement, license suspension, and, if all else fails, through closure of the facility.

Examples of health-care facility regulation

In the United States hospital licensing laws are fairly recent, having been enacted in 1946 following the Second World War in response to the Hill–Burton Hospital Survey and Construction Act, which required states to specify minimum standards for facilities receiving federal subsidies.

Beginning in 1968 a number of states amended their hospital licensing laws to enact what were termed comprehensive laws encompassing both physical and patient care standards. For example, the modernized facility licensing law of New York State, enacted in 1969 (New York 1985), contains detailed provisions governing construction, financial reporting, and patient care. The law specifies, among other matters, requirements for ambulatory care, calls for a comprehensive evaluation of patients on a periodic basis, requires continuity of care when patients are referred outside the hospital, mandates full-time medical staffing in emergency rooms, specifies rules for surgical consultation, and requires general hospitals to admit patients in need of immediate hospital admission without advance enquiry as to their ability to pay. Thus, the provisions of modernized facility licensing laws have moved far beyond bricks and mortar.

In Bolivia, regulations issued in 1982 specify that establishments that provide health services (hospitals, clinics, laboratories, medical posts, and consulting rooms) must be licensed by the Ministry of Social Welfare and Public Health and conform to the requirements of the National Health Plan (Bolivia 1983). The services that various types of hospitals are required to provide are set forth. A Commission on Health Establishments is created, with power to review applications for planning and construction of health establishments in urban and rural areas. Such applications must include a study of the population to be served, classification of the population by age, sex, and occupation, foreseeable population changes in the next 20 years, health conditions in the area, numbers and kinds of health personnel available in the area, co-ordination with other health establishments, and conditions of funding (Bolivia 1983).

In Senegal, the law on hospital reform classifies public health hospitals as first, second, and third levels, assures patients free choice of practitioner and hospital, specifies that all shall have equitable access to care, and requires hospitals to take part in public health activities (Senegal 1998).

Issues in health-care facility regulation

A critical issue in health facility regulation is the authorized supply of beds, whether in public or private facilities and whether subsidized by public funds or not. Since the supply of beds is a major determinant of hospital utilization rates, under conditions of widespread insurance, the control of this supply is extremely important in the overall issue of health care cost containment (Roemer and Shain 1959).

Implementation of requirements for facility licensure is a prominent issue facing governmental agencies responsible for standards in health-care facilities. Frequent inspections and time-consuming consultations require trained staff, often in short supply. Although licensing statutes provide legal mechanisms for enforcement, less onerous strategies are generally preferred. Particularly in the field of long-term care, where often the need is to upgrade the quality of care, attaching standards of the facility to the financing mechanism is increasingly preferred as an effective sanction.

Even when implemented, the standards specified in a licensing law may be minimal standards rather than the most up-to-date requirements for patient care. To take account of the need to encourage higher standards than those required by the hospital licensing law, a voluntary accreditation system has long been established in the United States. The Joint Commission on Accreditation of Health Care Organizations periodically surveys hospitals and other health-care establishments and accredits those that meet its exigent standards.

Social financing of health care

Health services to individuals and communities may be financed in several different ways. Aside from expenditures by individuals and families for their personal benefit, there are several mechanisms for collective economic support. These are through charitable donations, general tax revenues, voluntary (non-governmental) insurance, mandatory or social insurance, and foreign aid.

Social insurance—also called social security—has been adopted by an increasing number of countries throughout the world (Social Security Administration 1997). Starting in Germany in 1883, in order to finance personal health services for low-wage industrial workers, this mechanism has spread to coverage of other types of person for a variety of benefits over the years.

The types of person covered have increased to those with higher earnings and having different types of occupation, such as in agriculture, transport, commerce, and other fields. The types of monetary benefit have also been increased from personal health services to maternity, old age, disability and death, work injury, unemployment, and family allowances.

As of 1997, the number of countries with designated types of social insurance programme were as follows (Social Security Administration 1997).

Old-age, disability, death	166 countries
Sickness and maternity	111 countries
Work injury	164 countries
Unemployment	68 countries
Family allowances	86 countries

Benefits for these risks consist of money for periods of time that vary among countries. Furthermore, among the 111 countries that provide for sickness and maternity, 93 also pay for the costs of medical care and/or hospital admission (Social Security Administration 1997, Table 1, p. xlv).

The patterns by which health services are delivered to beneficiaries differ among countries. In the industrialized countries, such as Germany and France, where these programmes have operated for the longest time, health services are usually delivered by private medical practitioners and allied personnel who are paid on a fee-for-service basis. In developing countries, where these programmes are younger, health services are usually delivered through more structured patterns, under which health personnel work on salaries in hospitals and health centres. This pattern prevails in Colombia, Peru, and most Latin American countries (Roemer 1991).

In some countries both of these patterns may operate in parallel. A beneficiary may seek service in an organized facility or seek care from a private practitioner who is paid by the insurance, usually along with a copayment by the patient. Such dual-choice policies exist in the health systems of most Latin American countries, as well as in the systems of Middle Eastern and Asian countries, such as Egypt, Iraq, and Malaysia (Roemer 1991).

The worldwide trend has been towards extension of social security protection for health services to larger proportions of national populations. In several countries, the extension has been to cover total national populations. This has occurred by evolution, as in the United Kingdom (Roemer 1991) or by revolution as in the former Soviet Union (Roemer 1991). By either route, when coverage has become universal, the financial support usually changes from social security to general tax revenues. With the latter arrangement, health expenditures are subject to greater planning and supervision.

Recent legislation in developing countries has extended coverage for health care by various means. In a country with an entrepreneurial health system as in The Philippines, the national health insurance programme seeks to provide all citizens of The Philippines with financial access to health services and to assure beneficiaries free choice of health provider, who is paid according to a fixed fee schedule (Philippines 1998). In Colombia, the Primary Health Care Plan of the General Health and Social Security System provides personal preventive services and community health promotion measures free of charge (Colombia 1998*a*). For treatment, beneficiaries may choose between public and private health care (Social Security Administration 1997).

The use of collectivized financing has gradually contributed to greater national expenditures for personal health services. The changing demographic composition of the population, with larger proportions of elderly people, is linked to effective reductions of mortality in the younger years. Also influential have been advanced technology, higher rates of health-care utilization at all ages, and prevention, which have enabled people to live longer even with disabilities. The rising proportion of national wealth, measured by gross national product per capita, being devoted to national health systems has also been associated with greater proportions of health expenditures being derived from public compared with private sectors of national economies (Roemer 1991).

Control of communicable diseases

Prevention of the spread of communicable diseases was one of the earliest functions of public health. In this effort, two types of law have been employed: laws to assure a sanitary environment (discussed above) and laws to regulate human conduct to control the spread of disease.

Turning off the Broad Street pump through which cholera was spread was an ideal public health measure because it cut off the source of the disease and benefited the whole population served by that water supply. In 1854, John Snow demonstrated that the distribution of deaths from cholera in London was from water in the River Thames that flowed to consumers through the Broad Street pump (Rosen 1958). Such a solution, however, is not always available. Therefore, other measures to prevent epidemics have been adopted. Such laws authorize public health officials to ascertain the incidence of communicable disease, to regulate the conduct of those who are infected, and to require measures to prevent its spread. Because these actions involve some restriction of the rights of individuals, the law in this field seeks to balance the need of society for protection against disease and the rights of the individual to privacy and liberty.

Traditional methods of preventing and controlling communicable disease have evoked statutory responses. To assist epidemiological investigation of the incidence of communicable diseases, laws mandating reporting to public health officials of specified communicable diseases by doctors, school authorities, and laboratories have been passed. To prevent and control communicable disease, the law provides for compulsory examination of individuals who are in a position to spread disease (for example, food handlers), and of individuals in whom communicable disease presents special hazards (for example, schoolchildren, applicants for a marriage license, pregnant women). A health officer also generally has power—although it is rarely exercised—to order a person suspected of being infected with a contagious disease to submit to a physical examination (Grad 1990). Similarly, rarely used today is the health officer's power to isolate and quarantine an infected individual, although the power continues on the statute books. The most important legal measure for control of communicable diseases is certainly compulsory immunization.

Statutes authorizing these measures for controlling communicable diseases generally provide a civil or criminal penalty for violators, but much preferred are other strategies for implementation of the laws, such as exclusion from school or work. Compliance with a specified immunization schedule may be required for school attendance, as in Ontario, Canada (Canada 1984*a*,*b*). Compulsory examinations may be required for a marriage license or to obtain a certain job, as in the United States (Grad 1990).

Examples of legislation to control communicable disease

In 1986 Finland enacted a comprehensive ordinance concerned with the prevention of communicable diseases through vaccination, distribution of antibody preparations and medicines, the provision of measures related to individuals and their environment that are intended to prevent the development or spread of communicable disease, early diagnosis, screening, and treatment, and medical rehabilitation. The duties of the National Board of Health, county councils, communes, hospitals, pathology laboratories, and Institute of Public Health are set forth in this comprehensive regulatory system to control communicable diseases (Finland 1987).

In 1988, Malaysia amended and consolidated into a single, comprehensive statute its various laws on the prevention and control of infectious diseases (Malaysia 1990). The statute provides for the declaration of an infected area, examination of vehicles arriving in Malaysia, required notification of infectious diseases to the health authorities, power of health officers to require treatment, immunization, isolation, observation, or surveillance, or any other measure necessary to control the disease, obligation of infected people not to spread the disease, and other matters (Malaysia 1990).

Trends in communicable disease control

Immunization and other measures to control communicable diseases are so well accepted that the principal problems in this field are spin-offs from effective immunization: the high cost of vaccines, the question of how to compensate those patients who suffer an untoward outcome of immunization, and providing treatment for tuberculosis in developing countries, now that leprosy is being eradicated (Lamb 1994), and in all countries in a time of AIDS (Bayer *et al.* 1992). These problems are handled in different fashions by the health and legal systems of each country.

Tension between protection of the public health and protection of the civil liberties of individuals is a feature of all communicable disease control. This tension was heightened as measures were developed to control the AIDS epidemic (discussed below). Prompted by this tension, a legal scholar in the United States re-examined the balance between collective and individual rights and found current public health laws in the United States inadequate for dealing with the issues (Gostin 1986). In order to provide health-care officials and agencies with the tools to balance individual rights against public health necessities, Gostin recommended revising American public health legislation to provide clearly stated criteria for defining 'public health necessity' to guide public health officials in the exercise of their powers, to assure strong protections of confidentiality in the collection and storage of public health information, and to authorize a graded series of less restrictive measures than currently exist, such as a community health order that can be adjusted to the particular risk to the public health presented by each case.

Legislation on HIV/AIDS

As with other communicable diseases, the epidemic of HIV/AIDS presents the classical public health problem of a conflict between the welfare of the community and the rights of the individual, but with significant differences. Like other sexually transmitted and communicable diseases, HIV/AIDS calls for measures to prevent its spread and also for protection of the privacy and other civil rights of people with the disease. But HIV/AIDS presents grave and different problems because as yet there is no cure and no vaccine for prevention. Also, the incidence of HIV/AIDS is concentrated in some countries in people who engage in certain high-risk activities (homosexual activity and intravenous drug use)—groups that are particularly vulnerable to discrimination.

Legislation has been a significant component of the response to the HIV/AIDS epidemic (Gostin and Curran 1987; WHO 1997). An early response to the epidemic was to require testing of all blood and blood products provided by blood donors and confidential reporting of results. A most effective measure to protect the blood supply was the public health strategy, often adopted without the necessity of legislation, of establishing alternate testing sites (that is, other than blood collection centres) enabling people seeking information on their antibody status to have confidential or entirely anonymous testing without endangering the blood supply.

Most jurisdictions having legislation on HIV/AIDS require reporting of cases of AIDS to a health agency. Some statutes classify AIDS as a sexually transmitted disease, as in the State of Idaho (United States), Chile, Guatemala, Iceland, and Sweden. Such an approach permits the testing of prostitutes and tracing of contacts to advise testing and provide counselling. In order to improve tracking of the epidemic, increasing numbers of jurisdictions require reporting of HIV positivity either by confidential names-based reporting or by a unique identifier (usually a number). Despite concern that names-based reporting will deter testing and treatment, experience with confidential names-based reporting of HIV shows that it has not deterred testing (Nakashima *et al.* 1998). Much of the HIV/AIDS legislation contains specific requirements to safeguard the confidentiality of information, and stringent systems have been put in place to prevent any breach of confidentiality.

Protection of the confidentiality of test results has conflicted with the need to protect other members of society. In order to cope with this problem, some laws provide for very limited disclosure of identifying information, for example, to a health-care professional engaged in the care of a patient with HIV/AIDS and to a medical facility that will receive blood, organs, semen, or breast milk from an HIV-positive individual. Some jurisdictions authorize a doctor to disclose positive HIV antibody status to an individual's spouse or sexual partner when the doctor has reason to believe that the individual will not inform the spouse or sexual partner.

A controversial legal issue concerns the recalcitrant patient or seropositive person who does not respond to education, counselling, medical direction, and community pressures to stop infecting others but knowingly exposes others to HIV infection. Legal remedies may exist in the general civil and criminal law. Regulations in the United Kingdom authorize an order by a justice of the peace to detain the patient if the justice is satisfied that the patient will not take proper precautions to prevent the spread of the disease (UK 1989).

Vast numbers of diverse laws relating to HIV/AIDS have been enacted worldwide. Fortunately, this legislation is readily available in a directory compiled and periodically updated by the WHO's Health Legislation Unit with the support of the Joint United Nations Programme on HIV/AIDS (WHO 1997). Organized by country, these laws cover a wide range of issues, including, among others, establishment of national committees to control HIV/AIDS or sexually transmitted diseases generally; screening of blood donors and maintenance of the safety of the blood supply; preventive measures and health education; testing for HIV and confidentiality of test results; required notification to public health authorities of cases of HIV and AIDS; provision of pharmaceuticals and medical care to patients with HIV/AIDS; and prohibition of discrimination against people with HIV/AIDS with respect to work, housing, education, and other matters.

As an example of recent legislation, the law of the Dominican Republic requires screening of blood donations, bans testing for HIV for work-related purposes, mandates sex education throughout schools and colleges, provides for public information messages, and requires hotels and motels to provide condoms in a conspicuous place without the customer having to ask for them (Dominican Republic 1998). Vietnam's legislation calls for measures for the prevention and control of drug abuse and prostitution as part of the campaign for HIV/AIDS prevention and control (Vietnam 1998). The law of Latvia specifies the functions of the National Centre for AIDS comprised of a service for epidemiological surveillance and a service for the diagnosis, treatment, and medical observation of AIDS (Latvia 1996).

An important support for national efforts to combat the AIDS epidemic is legislation of the European Community to implement a programme to assist the developing countries in their efforts to minimize the spread of HIV/AIDS and to help them cope with its impact on health and social and economic development (European Community 1997). The programme, for which specific aims and guiding principles are set forth, is to be directed primarily at the poorest and least developed countries and the most disadvantaged sections of developing countries. The measures to be taken include information and education for target groups; improved protection of the blood supply; increasing women's power of decision-making with respect to sexuality and reproductive health; strengthening health services, particularly primary health care; improving training for health personnel; combating discrimination against, and the social and economic exclusion of, people with HIV/AIDS; and combating the stigma attached to those living with the virus through public health information campaigns and the setting up of an appropriate legislative framework.

Issues in the control of the AIDS epidemic

The most controversial issue in the law governing AIDS is the extent to which screening for AIDS—the systematic application of the ELISA test and confirmatory supplemental tests to specific populations—should be undertaken. While some countries have mandated tests for particular groups, such as prisoners, prostitutes, or immigrants, or even, in some jurisdictions, intravenous drug users or applicants for a marriage license, the weight of authority favours voluntary testing accompanied by counselling for several reasons.

1. It encourages behaviour changes and notification of sexual contacts and people with whom needles have been shared.
2. It facilitates protection of privacy and therefore does not drive those who believe they may be infected to go 'underground'.
3. In a low-prevalence population a test with a high degree of sensitivity and specificity, as the serological tests for HIV antibodies are, will produce a large proportion of false-positive responses, causing great anxiety, providing misleading information, and requiring confirmatory tests.
4. In any testing system a certain number of false negatives will occur in the window of time before infection is manifested, which give a false sense of security and inhibit behaviour changes.

Therefore, the United Nations Global AIDS Program strongly favours voluntary testing, counselling, and protection of confidentiality. Mandatory testing without informed consent has no place in an AIDS prevention and control programme, the WHO states, because it violates the rights and dignity of individuals and is counterproductive to control of the epidemic (WHO 1992).

Advances in therapy may, however, increase the urgency of expanding testing. For example, the finding that zidovudine reduces the chance that an infected woman will pass the HIV virus to her fetus from 25 to 8 per cent led the United States Centers for Disease Control and Prevention (**CDC**) to recommend that all pregnant women be tested voluntarily early in pregnancy, with infected women offered zidovudine therapy (CDC 1998).

Another issue concerns precautions to prevent the transmission of HIV to health-care workers. The increasing prevalence of HIV increases the risk that health-care workers will be exposed to blood from patients infected with HIV. The CDC has issued an authoritative document emphasizing the need for health-care workers to consider all patients as potentially infected and to adhere rigorously to infection-control precautions. The response to the risk to health-care workers must be universal precautions (CDC 1987). In late 1991, the United States Occupational Safety and Health Administration adopted standards mandating universal precautions to protect workers from blood-borne diseases, including the requirement that the employer make available the hepatitis B vaccine and vaccination series to all employees who have occupational exposure, and postexposure prophylaxis and follow-up to all employees who have had an exposure incident. These detailed standards provide legal force in the United States to the recommendations of the CDC (US Department of Labor 1991). In a landmark decision in 1998, the United States Supreme Court held that a dentist may not discriminate against a person with asymptomatic HIV infection. The Americans with Disabilities Act prohibits discrimination against a person who suffers a disability that impairs a major life function. The Court held that the patient in this case suffered a disability that impairs the major life function of the ability to bear children (*Bragdon* v. *Abbott* 1998). The Court also rejected the dentist's claim that courts should defer to his assessment of the risk posed by HIV-positive patients. Instead, the Court ruled, deference should be given to the opinion of public health authorities, which the dentist could seek to rebut, because they are the ones best trained to assess risk. Subsequent lower court proceedings found the dentist unable to rebut public health's conclusion that HIV-positive patients could be safely treated in dentists' offices.

From the beginning of the AIDS epidemic the issues of privacy, confidentiality, and protection against discrimination have been prominent concerns. But, as Dr Stephen Joseph, Commissioner of Health of New York City 1986 to 1990, points out, AIDS constitutes a public health emergency which carries within it extraordinary civil liberties issues; it is not a civil liberties emergency which carries within it extraordinary public health issues (Joseph 1992). For this reason, the AIDS epidemic raises a double ethicolegal imperative: to prohibit and punish discrimination in employment, housing, health insurance, public accommodations, governmental services, and schooling solely because the person has AIDS or is believed to be seropositive and, at the same time, to expand and intensify the response to the public health emergency created by the epidemic.

Legislation on mental illness

If one were to select a single sector of health services to see the field of health law in microcosm, one should examine health services for the mentally ill. This sector illustrates with particular sharpness the conflict between health needs and legal rights, between protection of the patient and protection of society, and ways to resolve these conflicts.

The scope of legislation affecting the mentally ill is very broad. It includes laws governing admissions to mental hospitals, standards for mental health facilities and care of patients, organization of community mental health programmes, legal protection of the person and property of the mentally ill, the doctrines of the right to treatment and right to treatment in the least restrictive alternative setting, legal aspects of deinstitutionalization, and mental illness and the criminal defendant (Curran and Harding 1978). The discussion here is restricted to mental hospital admission laws.

With the advent of tranquillizers, the development of the concept of the open hospital and the therapeutic community, and increased awareness of the civil rights of patients, many jurisdictions have amended their centuries-old statutes governing criteria for hospital admission of the mentally ill. Definitions of who is mentally ill have moved away from vague standards, such as 'in need of care and treatment', to more precise standards, such as 'dangerous to others', 'dangerous to self', and 'gravely disabled'. In addition to changes in the grounds for admission, the procedures for admission have been modified to assure prompt and non-traumatic admission to mental hospitals when needed, to require periodic review of the need for continued hospital treatment, and to assure prompt discharge as soon as the patient is ready.

Many of the old commitment laws, as they were called, resemble criminal proceedings. They require a petition to the court, notice of hearing, representation by counsel, a hearing before a judge, often with a jury trial, testimony by witnesses, and even sometimes a written opinion by the judge as to the necessity for hospital admission. These laws, it was found, provided only the illusion of due process and actually were adverse to the health needs of patients in many cases for prompt and non-traumatic hospital admission (Association of the Bar of the City of New York 1962). Modern statutes have replaced this legalistic procedure with new administrative mechanisms for protecting both the health needs and the legal rights of mental patients. At the same time, since an individual's liberty is at stake in an involuntary admission to a mental hospital, the role of the courts in overseeing the propriety of retaining an individual in a hospital has been strengthened.

Examples of mental hospital admission laws

The first country to enact a modernized mental health law was the United Kingdom, which adopted legislation along lines recommended by the Royal Commission on the Law Relating to Mental Illness and Mental Deficiency in 1957. Previously in England and Wales, involuntary patients were admitted to mental hospitals on an order from a justice of the peace based on one medical certificate from a medical practitioner. This procedure was viewed as providing inadequate safeguards because the magistrate could not form any sound independent opinion on the patient's mental condition and because the judicial order associated mental hospital admission with the courts and with punishment of crime (Maclay 1960).

The Mental Health Act of 1959, applicable to England and Wales, abolished the judicial order and made compulsory admission, when necessary, a medical matter requiring two medical opinions, including one from a doctor with special experience (UK 1959). The doctors recommending compulsory detention must specify the grounds for their opinions and state whether alternative methods of dealing with the patient are available and, if so, why they are not appropriate and hospital admission is necessary. The hospital must confirm the need for hospital admission, and on the basis of these three certifications the hospital is authorized to retain the patient for specified time limits. Most importantly, an administrative agency to which patients and their families have access—the Mental Health Review Tribunal—is established in each hospital region, with power to review the appropriateness of hospital admission and to discharge the patient.

In 1983, 24 years after passage of the Mental Health Act, amendments to the law were adopted to strengthen protection of the civil rights of mental patients (UK 1983). These amendments require consent to treatment, assurance of patient rights (such as the right to visitors, to pocket money, and so on), and establishment of a Board of Visitors to provide surveillance of the quality of care in mental hospitals.

In the climate of opinion created by new methods of treatment of the mentally ill and new public attitudes towards mental illness, New York State revised its mental hospital admission law after an extensive study which found great variations, inequities, and injustices in the involuntary admission of patients to mental hospitals. The measures intended to protect the rights of patients had become a rubber stamp by the judges of the decisions of doctors (Association of the Bar of the City of New York 1962).

Accordingly, in 1964 the New York State Legislature unanimously passed a new Mental Hygiene Law (New York 1978). It abolished civil judicial certification of an involuntary patient to a mental hospital and provided that the initial admission of an involuntary patient to a mental hospital is a medical matter, on the application of a near relative or other interested person and on the recommendations of two doctors, with the concurrence of the admitting hospital. Immediate and periodic legal reviews of the propriety of hospital admission are required. The rights of the patient are protected by an arm of the court, the Mental Health Information Service, which faces towards the patient and his family to inform them of the patient's rights and alternatives, and towards the court to inform it of the patient's condition and alternative treatment resources.

A key feature of both the British and the New York laws is the functioning of a protective structure to provide representation of the patient's interests and needs. Both the British Mental Health Review Tribunal and the New York Mental Health Information Service, however, apply only to institutionalized people.

As deinstitutionalization has increased, so have the numbers of the mentally disabled in the community and many of them have become homeless. Recognition has grown of the need for similar protection of non-institutionalized mentally disabled people (Association of the Bar of the City of New York 1988). Simon Rosenzweig, who was one of the architects of the New York Mental Hygiene Law of 1964, proposed establishing an ongoing continuing legal service for the mentally disabled in the community. Such a service would differ from the service for institutionalized patients in that it would be concerned principally with entitlements to welfare, housing, treatment (including complaints as to treatment modes), access to ambulatory mental health centres, and so on. Rosenzweig envisaged a form of 'outpatient commitment', now quite common, to assure mental health care in the community and comport with constitutional rights to due process (McCafferty and Dooley 1990; Rosenzweig 1990).

Israel has enacted a law providing for an order for compulsory ambulatory treatment as an alternative to hospital admission or as a follow-up to hospital admission for patients meeting the requirements for involuntary hospital admission. The statute provides a right of appeal from an order for ambulatory treatment just as a right of appeal exists from an order for hospital admission (Israel 1992).

Issues in mental hospital admission laws

Modernized mental hospital admission laws reflect the revolution that has occurred in the care of the mentally ill. But not all problems have been resolved. What standard of proof should be required for involuntary hospital admission? Does the patient have a right to treatment or a right to refuse a particular kind of treatment? What safeguards are afforded for minors deemed in need of mental hospital admission (*Parham* v. *J.R. et al.*1979)? Probably in no field of health law is the conflict between the rights of the individual to liberty and confidential treatment and the right of society to protection from harm so sharp as in the field of mental illness.

To some extent, legislation can provide a solution for this dilemma. For example, the statute of Qatar contains a detailed patient's bill of rights protecting the patient's right to know about his or her illness, to give informed consent before any treatment, to refuse treatment, to have information about his or her case treated as confidential, to inspect his or her chart in the presence of the doctor, and to receive a reasonable continuity of care (Qatar 1989). The law of Albania provides restrictions on the use of physical restraints on mental patients (Albania 1997). But in the long run, resolution of this conflict in various contexts will depend on further advances in psychiatric diagnosis and treatment, and on imaginative legal strategies to protect the individual and society.

Legal problems in human reproduction

A priority for public health concerns the protection of the health of mothers and children. In all countries emphasis has been placed on prenatal and maternity care and on breast feeding, immunization, and well-baby care. A new dimension was added to maternal and child health efforts with the recognition of the importance of birth control and abortion to prevent unwanted pregnancy and assure proper child spacing. Deaths from illegal abortion were the largest single cause of maternal mortality in many countries and still are in some. According to the WHO, 20 million unsafe abortions each year result in 78 000 maternal deaths and hundreds of thousands of disabilities in women, with the majority occurring in developing countries (Cook *et al.* 1999).

To tackle the enormous toll in preventable maternal deaths from dangerous illegal abortion, a number of countries turned in the mid-twentieth century to legislation to shift abortion from the illegal to the legal sector of medical practice (Cook and Dickens 1988). To promote family planning programmes, laws were enacted removing barriers to access to birth control and providing educational and financial support for contraceptive services (for example, France, Germany, Italy, Morocco, and Spain) (Paxman 1980; Isaacs 1981; Mason *et al.* 1987). Laws also authorized voluntary sterilization, as in Japan, Panama, the Scandinavian countries, and Singapore (Isaacs 1981; Stepan *et al.* 1981). Statutes mandating sex education in schools were adopted (Roemer and Paxman 1985). Also, as another aspect of the woman's choice in reproductive matters, the law has been called on to authorize means to reduce infertility and has addressed alternative or assisted means of reproduction (Annas and Elias 1983; Andrews 1984; Annas 1984; Warnock Committee 1984; Swiss Institute of Comparative Law 1986).

These legal changes were not achieved without opposition. A minority of the population in a number of countries opposed legalized abortion and even attempted to restrict contraceptive and sex education programmes. Despite their efforts, advances in the technology of contraception, and changed social attitudes concerning sexual behaviour and the rights of women, have impelled modernization of the laws governing human reproduction.

Legislation on abortion

Abortion at the request of the woman or on a wide range of indications has been legalized in the most countries of the world, including China, India, Japan, the United States, and the former Soviet Union. It is allowed in the first 3 months of pregnancy in Austria, France, Germany, Denmark, and Italy. Abortion is authorized on social or sociomedical grounds in Barbados, Belize, the Scandinavian countries, and the United Kingdom, and it was legal in most of the countries of Eastern Europe before the end of the communist regimes. Many countries allow abortion on medical grounds, as in Algeria, Israel, and Switzerland. South Africa allows abortion on request of the woman during the first 12 weeks of pregnancy; from the 13th to the 20th week abortion is allowed if a doctor believes that the pregnancy poses a risk to the physical or mental health of the woman, there is a risk of a defective fetus, the pregnancy is the result of a sex crime, or the continued pregnancy would significantly affect the social or economic circumstances of the woman; after the 20th week abortion is allowed if two doctors or a doctor and a registered midwife determine that continued pregnancy would endanger the life of the woman, result in severe malformation of the fetus, or risk injury to the fetus (South Africa 1997).

In Colombia, Guatemala, Honduras, Nicaragua, Turkey, and Venezuela abortion is allowed only to save the life of the woman.

Abortion is prohibited in Chile, the Dominican Republic, Haiti, Panama, Paraguay, The Philippines, and Suriname. The reality in many countries where abortion is illegal or restricted is that it is nevertheless widely practised, often by doctors, and with acceptance by the public (David 1984; Mason *et al.* 1985; Cook and Dickens 1988; David and Pick de Weiss 1992; Cook *et al.* 1999).

Henshaw has analysed recent trends in abortion laws, from 1988 to 1993, in non-communist industrialized countries, the formerly communist countries of Eastern Europe, and developing countries (Henshaw 1994). Little change occurred in almost all the non-communist industrialized countries, which had fairly liberal laws. Three of these countries—Canada, France, and the United Kingdom—made minor changes liberalizing their laws. Belgium replaced its extremely restrictive law with one allowing women in a state of 'distress' to end their pregnancies during the first trimester. In Ireland, a decision of the Supreme Court held that, although the law prohibits abortion without exception, the procedure is permissible when the pregnant woman's life is endangered by physical health conditions or threat of suicide.

Before 1988 most of the formerly communist countries of Eastern Europe allowed abortion on request or for social indications. With the end of the communist regimes, three countries that had severe restrictions on abortion—Albania, Mongolia, and Romania—immediately authorized abortion on request. Bulgaria and Hungary liberalized their laws further. However, in Poland, the liberal 1956 law was repealed in 1993 by a law allowing abortions only in public hospitals on grounds of threat to life or health of the pregnant woman, serious and irremediable malformation of the fetus, and pregnancy resulting from rape or incest (David 1993). The Polish law was amended in 1996 and 1997 to allow abortion within the first 12 weeks of pregnancy only on the grounds of risk to the woman's physical or mental health or in pregnancy resulting from sex crimes (Cook *et al.* 1999). It is a crime punishable by imprisonment for up to 3 years to carry out a pregnancy termination in violation of the law or to encourage a woman to terminate her pregnancy in violation of the law (Poland 1997). Two other ex-communist countries—the Czech Republic and Serbia—restrict abortions by imposing fairly substantial fees (Henshaw 1994).

Among developing countries, Malaysia replaced a restrictive law with one modelled on the British statute allowing abortion if continuing a pregnancy involves more risk to the woman's physical or mental health than terminating it. Other developing countries that made minor changes liberalizing their laws are Botswana, Pakistan, Peru, and the Sudan (Henshaw 1994). In Indonesia, a family health law of 1992 provides that, in emergency cases, to save the life of a pregnant woman 'certain medical procedures' may be performed—a provision, according to the Indonesian Family Planning Association, designed to assure safe services and act as a compromise with those opposed to abortion (David 1993). Developing countries that increased their restrictions on abortion are Argentina, Chile, and Singapore (Henshaw 1994).

Issues in laws affecting human reproduction

The worldwide turnabout in the law governing birth control and abortion that has occurred in the last two decades has brought significant public health benefits to women and their families. Deaths from illegal abortion of desperate women faced with unwanted pregnancies have been prevented. Infant mortality and morbidity have been combated by improved spacing of pregnancies (Maine and McNamara 1985). Many adolescents have been able to defer child-bearing to a time more appropriate for parenting (Roemer 1985; Paxman and Zuckerman 1987). The development of medical abortion, with approval of mifepristone (RU-486) in several countries, provides a new option for pregnancy termination (Cook *et al.* 1999). A most significant advance in women's health—and in human rights—occurred with the enactment in Egypt and Ghana of statutes making it a crime to perform female circumcision (Ghana 1996; Egypt 1997).

Still, many problems remain. In many countries where abortion is still illegal or restricted, desperate women faced with unwanted pregnancies are driven to unsafe illegal abortions. Geographic access to family planning and abortion services is uneven. Financial access is a serious problem where universal financing of health services is not available. The shortage of abortion providers is a barrier to access to service. Required authorization by a spouse or a parent blocks or delays services. Further work is needed to prevent teenage pregnancy by improved sex education in the schools and improved access to contraceptive services and abortion. Constant vigilance is necessary to prevent restrictions in law or practice on the right of women to choose to terminate unwanted pregnancies. Finally, an unknown element in this field is the impact of the epidemic of AIDS on the use of condoms and on the option of abortion for seropositive women.

Legislative approaches to health promotion

The historical role of public health of preventing disease and disability received a new impetus in 1974 with the publication in Canada of the Lalonde Report, *A New Perspective on the Health of Canadians* (Lalonde 1974). This report launched a worldwide effort for health promotion, examining and improving the judgements that must be made by individuals in respect of their own living habits, by society in respect of the values it holds, and by governments in respect of both the funds they allocate to the preservation of health and the restrictions they impose on the population for whose well being they are responsible (Lalonde 1974).

How does health promotion differ from the time-honoured function of public health, the function of health education? Horowitz (1981) defines health education as consisting of any combination of learning experiences designed to facilitate voluntary adaptations of behaviour conducive to health. In contrast, health promotion is the process of advocating health to enhance the probability that personal, private, and public support of positive health practices will become a societal norm.

In this effort to establish societal norms that contribute to healthful lifestyles, legislation has proved to be an essential component. This does not denigrate the role of education, which is important to engender the motivation to change behaviour. That motivation, however, can be encouraged by societal norms and expectations which, in turn, are promoted by governmental policy expressed in legislation.

Prevention of motor vehicle accidents

The fields in which legislation can be directed to promoting health are many and varied. A high priority has been given to laws to prevent the enormous toll in death and disability from motor vehicle accidents.

These include laws setting standards for fitness to drive, mandating the use of child passenger restraint systems, seat belts, and motor cycle crash helmets, and requiring manufacturers of vehicles to instal air bags. With the technological innovation of blood alcohol measurement, stringent laws make the presence of a given level of alcohol in the blood a conclusive presumption of drunk driving entailing mandatory fines, jail sentences, license restriction, and rehabilitation programmes (California Vehicle Code 1985).

Control of alcohol abuse

Drunk driving laws are just one kind of law to control alcohol abuse. There are two major types of legislation: control of the availability of alcoholic beverages, and influencing drinking practices.

In the category of controlling the availability of alcohol are laws to control places of sale, hours of sale, and sales to minors, and to provide controls through taxation and prices (Moser 1980; Addiction Research Foundation 1981; Institute of Medicine 1982). While the evidence on the effectiveness of some of these measures is equivocal, it is generally agreed that decreasing the availability of alcohol is important. The experience of the Province of Ontario, Canada, showed that lowering the drinking age increased alcohol-related traffic accidents and admissions of teenagers to alcoholism and rehabilitation facilities (Addiction Research Foundation 1981; Single 1984). Increase in price of alcohol relative to income has been associated with a decline in consumption (Moser 1980).

In the category of regulating drinking practices are control of advertising, punishing public drunkenness, control of drinking and driving, education and information about alcohol, taxation policy, and counselling, treatment, and rehabilitation (Porter *et al.* 1986). Again, although evidence on the effectiveness of these measures is conflicting, there are indications that drinking practices can be affected by legislation, combined with education, provided the laws are enforced.

A notable advance in alcohol control policy is the 1985 law in the United States providing for mandatory label information on alcoholic beverages stating that women should not drink alcoholic beverages during pregnancy because of the risk of birth defects and that consumption of alcoholic beverages impairs the ability to drive a car or operate machinery, and may cause health problems (US 1993*b*). Most importantly, the pioneering 1991 French law bans all advertising of alcoholic beverages (France 1991).

Control of the tobacco epidemic

Tobacco use is the largest single avoidable cause of ill health and premature mortality in the world, accounting for an estimated 3 million deaths a year from smoking-related diseases. In response to the worldwide smoking epidemic, governments have intensified their efforts to control smoking by legislation, combined with education and smoking cessation programmes.

Two broad categories of laws have been enacted: laws to bring about changes in the production, manufacture, promotion, and sale of tobacco—laws to control the supply (or 'production') side—and laws to achieve changes in practices among smokers—laws to control the 'demand' (or 'consumption') side (Roemer 1993).

In the category of bringing about changes in the production, manufacture, promotion, and sale of tobacco are:

- control of advertising, sales promotion, and sponsorship of tobacco products
- requirements for health warnings and statement of tar and nicotine contents on cigarette packages and other tobacco products
- control of harmful substances in tobacco, such as tar, nicotine, and additives
- restrictions on sales to adults
- economic strategies relating to subsidies, crop substitution, and trade policies.

While all these measures contribute to a decline in tobacco consumption, the most important is control of advertising and sponsorship. The tobacco industry spends more than US$2 billion a year globally to lure consumers to its products, not counting the cost of indirect advertising through sponsorship of sports and cultural events by tobacco companies. Through advertising, the industry conveys the message, especially to young people, that smoking is associated with success, pleasure, relaxation, sports, freedom, beauty in nature, sophistication, virility, and sexuality. Moreover, the substantial revenues received by newspapers and magazines from advertising of tobacco products have a chilling effect on their editorial policies and deter publication of articles on smoking and health.

By 1991, 27 countries in the world had banned all advertising of cigarettes and 77 had enacted partial bans, some limiting the contents of advertisements to facts, barring the depiction of adolescents or children associated with sports, or restricting the amount of space devoted to advertising, and some imposing moderate partial bans prohibiting use of the electronic media for advertising of tobacco products or restricting the hours during which cigarettes may be advertised on television. Experience in the Scandinavian countries, particularly Finland and Norway, showed that total bans on advertising combined with strong antismoking policies lowered smoking rates markedly, particularly among young people (WHO 1987). A study of tobacco-promotion policies and consumption trends in 33 countries, commissioned by the New Zealand Toxic Substances Board, found that, when countries were grouped according to the degree of governmental restriction on tobacco promotion, the greater the degree of restriction, the greater the average annual fall in tobacco consumption (New Zealand Toxic Substances Board 1989). The alarming uptake in smoking by children and adolescents led Canada, Australia, New Zealand, and France to ban all advertising and promotion of tobacco products (Canada 1988; New Zealand 1990; Australia 1991; France 1991; Roemer 1993).

In the category of legislation to change smoking behaviour are:

- tax and price policies
- restricting smoking in public places
- restricting smoking in the workplace
- preventing young people from smoking (by prohibiting sales to minors and restricting sales of cigarettes from vending machines)
- mandating health education.

Experience in Canada, Hong Kong, the State of California (United States), and the United Kingdom has shown that raising taxes on tobacco decreases sales (Roemer 1993). An important report from

Finland confirms the need for substantial and repeated increases in taxes and prices of tobacco products if consumption is to be significantly reduced (National Board of Health of Finland 1985).

Compelling scientific evidence on the dangers of environmental tobacco smoke led the United States Environmental Protection Agency to classify environmental tobacco smoke as a group A human carcinogen, a classification used only when there is sufficient evidence from epidemiological studies to support a causal association between exposure to the agents and cancer (US Environmental Protection Agency 1993). Because of the Environmental Protection Agency's findings on the respiratory health effects of passive smoking, restrictions on smoking in public places and the workplace are of prime importance. Such legislation has been enacted at the national level of government, and it has also been successfully implemented when enacted by states and cities (Roemer 1988, 1993). These laws contribute to the creation of a non-smoking environment and the view that smoking is socially unacceptable. It is generally agreed that social acceptability is the ground on which the battle against the smoking epidemic will be decided.

In the United States, new impetus was given to tobacco control efforts by the following revelations in the mid-1990s (Hilts 1994*a–g*; Glantz *et al.* 1995, 1996):

- that the Philip Morris Company knew that tobacco was addictive 5 years before the United States Surgeon General declared tobacco an addictive substance
- that the tobacco industry abruptly terminated research to develop a 'safe' cigarette and concealed its findings on the addictiveness of tobacco
- that the Brown and Williamson Tobacco Company grew a genetically engineered tobacco in Brazil that more than doubles the amount of nicotine delivered, used it in five brands of cigarettes, including three brands labelled 'light', and has 3 million tons of it in warehouses in the United States.

In 1996, after a 2-year investigation, the United States Food and Drug Administration issued a determination that nicotine in cigarettes and smokeless tobacco is a drug and that these products are nicotine delivery devices subject to regulation by the Food and Drug Administration (US 1996). On 23 August 1996 President Clinton approved the Food and Drug Administration's regulations designed to reduce teenage consumption of tobacco by reducing easy access to and appeal of tobacco products (Federal Register 1996). In March 2000, the United States Supreme Court, by a vote of 5 to 4, held invalid these regulations on the ground that the Food and Drug Administration lacks jurisdiction to regulate tobacco. The dissent by Justice Stephen G. Breyer states: 'The upshot is that the court today holds that a regulatory statute aimed at unsafe drugs and devices does not authorize regulation of a drug (nicotine) and a device (a cigarette) that the court itself finds unsafe' (*Food and Drug Administration* v. *Brown and Williamson Tobacco Corp.* 2000).

The powerful evidence on the addictiveness of tobacco and the revelation of the industry's deception about the risk of smoking and the addictiveness of tobacco over the years have fuelled the wave of litigation that has been launched against the industry in the United States. Suits by state attorneys general to recover the costs of caring for patients with tobacco-induced diseases were settled in a series of stunning agreements. In 1997, Mississippi settled its suit for $3.3 billion to be paid over 25 years, Florida settled next for $11.3 billion, then Texas in 1998 for $15.3 billion, and Minnesota for $6.1 billion (Bloch *et al.* 1998). In November 1998, a multistate national settlement for $206 billion to be paid over 25 years was entered into with 46 states. It bars outdoor tobacco advertising nationally but also bars future claims against the industry that might be brought by state and local officials and gives the industry credit on its payments to the states if Congress enacts a tobacco tax in the next 4 years and turns the money over to the states (Torry 1998). Litigation continues, strengthened by industry documents showing that the tobacco companies lied to the public about the addictiveness and risks of smoking. On 7 July 1999 a jury in a class-action suit in Florida (the Engle case) returned a unanimous verdict holding all the defendant tobacco companies liable for the negligence and fraud of the industry. Although appeals will undoubtedly be taken, this decision makes the industry potentially liable for billions of dollars in damages (Weinstein and Levin 1999).

Most important for the control of the tobacco epidemic worldwide is the action of the WHO to develop an international regulatory authority to promote tobacco control. In 1996 the World Health Assembly adopted a resolution to initiate a Framework Convention on Tobacco Control to encourage the countries of the world to move towards comprehensive tobacco control policies (WHO 1996). (For further discussion of the Framework Convention on Tobacco Control see Chapters 4.3 and 10.1.)

In 1999 the World Health Assembly put in place the structures and process to move towards adoption of the Framework Convention, with May 2003 as the target date for adoption (WHO 1999). The WHO's leadership is designed to promote international co-operation and to energize national governments, regional associations, and non-governmental organizations to combat the largest single cause of preventable mortality and morbidity in the world.

Other health promotion legislation

To promote healthful nutrition, legislation may regulate the quantitative declaration of calories, fats, cholesterol, sodium, sugars, and other nutrients to promote safe and wholesome food, as discussed earlier. Legislation may also establish supplemental feeding programmes, such as school lunches and nutritional supplements for low-income pregnant women and infants, require use of unsaturated fats in commercially produced foods, subsidize the production of foods rich in unsaturated fats in order to lower the price, assist farmers to change cattle feed in order to produce beef low in saturated fats, and provide scientific, technical, and other assistance to agriculture and the food industry to enable them to shift as painlessly as possible to production of foods compatible with the 'prudent diet' (Terris 1983). These are ideal public health measures because they benefit whole populations and do not require individual behavioural change.

Another ideal measure is fluoridation of public water supplies to prevent dental decay. Community water fluoridation improves the oral health of an entire population regardless of socio-economic level, education, individual motivation, or the availability of dental personnel (Murray 1986).

Many of the problems discussed in connection with health promotion are manifestations of stress. Certainly, smoking and alcoholism are largely responses to stress. Stress is also produced by adverse environmental and life situations, such as poor working conditions, poor housing, and unemployment. Stress has so many causes that one needs to address specific problems to ascertain what legislation can do to alleviate them.

The list of health problems associated with stress is long and daunting. It includes drug abuse, depression, suicide, mental illness generally, child abuse, and family violence. Societal responses to these difficult problems lie in social institutions and programmes that can be assisted by legislation.

Examples of health promotion legislation

One could select many examples of legislation to promote health, such as legislation to assure product safety to prevent accidents in the home, laws to prevent road accidents, or laws to reduce alcohol consumption. The Norwegian national nutrition and food policy, discussed above, expresses an important policy to promote health. Two examples of laws to control the smoking epidemic are useful here.

In 1992, Thailand enacted two laws—the Tobacco Products Control Act and the Non-Smokers' Health Protection Act—to provide a comprehensive or multifaceted tobacco control policy. On the 'supply' side, the Thai Tobacco Products Control Act bans all advertising of tobacco products, requires health warnings on cigarette packages, bans the sale of tobacco products to people under 18, bans sales from vending machines, distribution of free samples, exchanges, and gifts of tobacco products, and bans manufacture and advertising of non-tobacco goods in imitation of tobacco products. Manufacturers and importers are required to report the contents of tobacco products to the Ministry of Public Health, which has authority to prohibit their sale or import if they fail to comply with prescribed standards. On the 'demand' side, the Thai Non-Smokers' Health Protection Act is designed to protect the health of non-smokers. It bans smoking in public places, authorizing designation of smoking areas in some public places (Health Systems Research Institute of Thailand 1995; Chitanondh 2000).

A single-purpose statute with a far-reaching impact is the 1987 Belgian Crown Decree banning smoking in all indoor places to which the public is admitted, including post offices, hospitals, schools, universities, homes for the elderly, theatres, concert halls, and sports arenas (Belgium 1987). In premises where the service to the public consists of furnishing food or drink, smoking may be allowed in a clearly defined part of the premises, but such permission may be denied if the premises are in buildings where students are taught, lodged, or cared for.

Issues in health promotion legislation

A number of general issues or recurring questions plague the field of legislation for health promotion.

1. How should the interest in social control and individual liberty be reconciled?
2. What types of legislative control are acceptable and effective?
3. How do various legislative approaches affect different socio-economic groups, and are they consistent with our notions of equity?
4. What legislative measures are effective in motivating individuals to change their behaviour? How do we evaluate them?
5. Who should bear the costs of risk-taking behaviour?
6. Are environmental measures available that lessen or eliminate the need for behavioural change?
7. What strategies for implementation of legislation are useful?
8. What is the responsibility of government for the people's health *vis-à-vis* powerful commercial interests?
9. How should one legislate in the face of scientific uncertainty?

Ethical issues in public health law

Ethics is a set of philosophical beliefs and practices concerned with questions of justice, fairness, equity, rights, allocation of resources, and costs. Law is a system of principles and rules devised by organized society for the purpose of controlling human conduct. Law may be described as a vital process or group of processes by which people living together in a society meet their common problems and solve them to promote the common good (Christoffel 1982; Wing 1985). Law and ethics converge because both are concerned with rights and duties.

Public health is concerned with ethics because, as Beauchamp (1985) points out, public health is concerned not only with explaining the occurrence of disease but also with ameliorating it, and public health is concerned with integrative goals expressing the commitment of the whole people to face the threat of death and diseases.

A well-known ethicist in the field of health in the United States, Daniel Callahan, has stated that the most significant development in the field of bioethics in the decade from 1970 to 1980 was the development of a closer interface between ethics and regulation (Callahan 1980). Formerly, ethics was discussed in terms of individual choice and personal morality. But we have come to examine ethical issues in terms of their legislative, regulatory, and judicial implications.

For example, Hutt, an eminent American expert in the field of food and drug regulation, has stated that all regulation of food and drugs and of the environment as a whole has emerged from our collective sense of societal ethic. He specifies the following five moral imperatives of government for its regulatory process (Hutt 1980):

- to protect the public from harm
- to preserve maximum individual choice
- to guarantee meaningful public participation in the decision-making process
- to promote consistent and dependable rules applicable to everyone
- to provide prompt decisions on all issues that arise in a regulatory context.

While ethical issues pervade much of governmental regulation of health services, in a few fields ethical issues predominate. These may be described as:

- clinical decision-making on life and death issues involving providing medical treatment to severely disabled neonates and continuing life-support measures for terminally ill and comatose patients
- regulation of clinical experimentation
- equitable allocation of all resources for health care, including scarce resources, such as equipment for kidney dialysis and organ transplants

- control of non-coital methods of human reproduction, such as *in vitro* fertilization and surrogate motherhood
- policies concerning genetic testing and use of genetic information.

A voluminous literature is available on each of these topics and on many others involving ethical issues (Ladimer and Newman 1963; Walters 1975; Reich 1978; Annas and Elias 1983; Capron 1983, 1984; Andrews 1984; Annas 1984; Warnock Committee 1984; Bankowski and Bryant 1985; Bankowski *et al.* 1989). It is not possible here to do justice to the complexities involved in any one of these issues. Sensitive and difficult questions are involved, such as the best interests of the child and the family, the length of life and the quality of life, assuring individual integrity and autonomy, protecting confidentiality, equitable distribution of resources, competition for scarce resources, and societal values in individual choice and collective conduct.

The development of law governing ethical issues has provided guidelines to doctors and has narrowed their sphere for making ethical judgements (Grad 1978). In fact, one of the most significant contributions of the law to this field is its capacity to create procedures and processes to resolve ethical questions in medicine and public health. Ethics committees of hospitals, ombudspeople to resolve disputes, patient advocates, review tribunals to monitor involuntary admissions to mental hospitals, protocols to govern care of the terminally ill, and manuals of procedures developed by the medical and nursing professions are all feasible mechanisms promoted and assisted by the law for resolving ethical issues in health care.

For the principal public health problem in the world—the threat of nuclear war—international law is crucial. No better illustration of the role of law in solving ethical problems can be found than efforts to achieve international agreements to stop the production and deployment of nuclear armaments and eventually to reduce conventional weapons of war. If peace in the world can be secured through international law, then other ethical problems in public health can surely follow.

Conclusion

Laws can generally be inspired by a sense of justice and right. Law provides the rules that all in society must abide by. Health law provides the regulatory system for patients, providers, and governments in the sphere of health protection and health services.

While the law may, in some instances, stand as a barrier to innovations in health service, in the main it has proved responsive to new scientific discoveries and to changed social and economic conditions. Where existing policies are inequitable or outmoded, the law has the capacity to serve as an instrument for change. If the outlines for change are uncertain, the law can facilitate the development of mechanisms for defining and achieving solutions.

Working in co-operation with public health experts, the health lawyer can assist and clarify the definition of sound health policy and can promote its implementation for the benefit of individuals and society.

References

Addiction Research Foundation (1981). *Alcohol, society and the state, a comparative study of alcohol control*, Vols 1 and 2. Addiction Research Foundation, Toronto.

Albania (1997). Law No. 8092 of 21 March 1996 on mental health. *International Digest of Health Legislation*, **48**, 332.

Algeria (1984). Law No. 83–03 of 5 February 1983 on environmental protection. *International Digest of Health Legislation*, **35**, 176.

Algeria (1997). Ordinance No. 96–13 of 15 June 1996 amending and supplementing Law No. 83–17 of 16 July 1983 promulgating the Water Code. *International Digest of Health Legislation*, **48**, 64.

Andrews, L.B. (1984). *New conceptions.* St Martin's Press, New York.

Annas, G.J. (1984). Making babies without sex: the law and the profits. *American Journal of Public Health*, **74**, 1415.

Annas, G.J. and Elias, S. (1983). Medico-legal aspects of a new technique to create a family. *Family Law Quarterly*, **17**, 199.

Ashford, N.A. and Caldart, C.C. (1985). The 'right to know': toxics information transfer in the workplace. *Annual Review of Public Health*, **6**, 383.

Association of the Bar of the City of New York in co-operation with the Cornell Law School (1962). *Mental illness and due process.* Report and Recommendations on Admission to Mental Hospitals under New York Law, Bertram F. Willcox, Director of Study. Cornell University Press, Ithaca, NY.

Association of the Bar of the City of New York (1988). Committee on Legal Problems of the Homeless, Report. *The Record*, **44**, 33.

Australia (1991). The Smoking and Tobacco Products Advertisements (Prohibition) Act. *International Digest of Health Legislation*, **42**, 48.

Bankowski, Z. and Byrant J.H. (ed.) (1985). *Health policy, ethics and human values. An international dialogue.* Council for International Organizations of Medical Sciences, Geneva.

Bankowski, Z., Barzelatto, J., and Capron, A.M. (ed.) (1989). *Ethics and human values in family planning.* Council for International Organizations of Medical Sciences, Geneva.

Bayer, R., Dubler, N.N., Greifinger, R.B., *et al.* (1992). *The tuberculosis revival; individual rights and societal obligations in a time of AIDS.* United Hospital Fund of New York.

Beauchamp, D.E. (1985). Community: the neglected tradition of public health. *The Hastings Center Report*, **15**, 28–36.

Belgium (1987). Crown Decree on the banning of smoking in certain public places, 31 March 1987. *International Digest of Health Legislation*, **38**, 542.

Belize (1998). The pollution regulations of 10 April 1996. *International Digest of Health Legislation*, **49**, 375.

Bloch, M., Daynard, R., and Roemer, R. (1998). A year of living dangerously—the tobacco control community meets the global settlement. *Public Health Reports*, **113**, 488.

Bolivia (1983). Regulations on public and private health establishments. *International Digest of Health Legislation*, **34**, 499.

Bragdon v. *Abbott* (1998). 524 US 624.

Brown v. *Superior Court of the City and County of San Francisco* (1988). Daily Appellate Report 4211. *Daily Journal*, 31 March.

Bulgaria (1992). Order No. 5 of 22 April 1991 on the conditions and rules governing the private practice of medicine. *International Digest of Health Legislation*, **43**, 719.

Bulgaria (1993). Decree No. 326 of 11 October 1991 promulgating the law on environmental protection. *International Digest of Health Legislation*, **44**, 701.

Bulgaria (1996). Decree No. 109 of 17 April 1995 promulgating the law on medicaments and pharmacies with regard to human medicine. *International Digest of Health Legislation*, **47**, 56.

Bullough, B. (1975). The third phase in nursing licensure: the current nurse practice acts. In *The law and the expanding nursing role*, pp. 153–70. Appleton-Century-Crofts, New York.

Burkino Faso (1998). Law No. 002/94/ADP of 19 January 1994. *International Digest of Health Legislation*, **49**, 376.

California Vehicle Code (1985). Sections 23152–3.

Callahan, D. (1980). Ethics and regulation. *The Hastings Center Report.* February, 25.

Cameroon (1997). Decree No. 96/224 of 1 October 1996. *International Digest of Health Legislation*, **48**, 382.

Canada (1984*a*). An Act (Chapter 41) to promote the health of pupils in schools. Dated 7 July 1982 (the Immunization of School Pupils Act, 1982), *International Digest of Health Legislation*, **35**, 57–9

Canada (1984*b*). Regulation made under the Immunization of School Pupils Act, 1982. Ontario Regulation 23/83. Dated 13 January 1983. *International Digest of Health Legislation*, **35**, 59–60.

Canada (1988). The tobacco products control act. An act (C-51) to prohibit the advertising and promotion and respecting the labeling and manufacturing of tobacco products. *International Digest of Health Legislation*, **39**, 858.

Canada (1993). An Act (Chapter 37) to establish a federal environmental process. *International Digest of Health Legislation*, **44**, 94.

Canada (Ontario) (1998). The Environmental Assessment Act. *International Digest of Health Legislation*, **49**, 690.

Capron, A.M. (1983). *Report of the President's Commission for the Study of Ethical Problems in Medicine and Biomedical and Behavioral Research.* US Government Printing Office, Washington, DC.

Capron, A.M. (1984). The new reproductive possibilities. Seeking a moral basis for concerted action in a pluralistic society. *Law, Medicine and Health Care*, **12**, 192.

CDC (Centers for Disease Control) (1987). Recommendations for prevention of HIV transmission in health-care settings. *Morbidity and Mortality Weekly Report*, **36** (Supplement), 2S.

CDC (Centers for Disease Control) (1998). Guidelines for treatment of sexually transmitted diseases. *Morbidity and Mortality Weekly Report*, **47**, 16.

Chapman, R.A. (1976). *Development of a national drug control agency. Need, legislative authority, responsibilities, organization, and operation.* WHO/PDT 76.1. World Health Organization, Geneva.

Chitanondh, H. (2000). *The passage of tobacco control laws: Thai Davids versus transnational tobacco Goliaths.* Thailand Health Promotion Institute, the National Health Foundation, Bangkok.

Christoffel, T. (1982). *Health and the law, a handbook for health professionals.* Free Press, New York.

Colombia (1998*a*). Resolution No. 4288 of 20 November 1996 defining the Primary Health Care Plan of the General Health and Social Security System. *International Digest of Health Legislation*, **49**, 453.

Colombia (1998*b*). Resolution No. 4536 of 9 December 1996, regulating advertising of medicaments. *International Digest of Health Legislation*, **49**, 521.

Cook, R.J. (1987). The United States export of 'pipeline' therapeutic drugs. *Colombia Journal of Environmental Law*, **12**, 39.

Cook, R.J. and Dickens, B.M. (1988). International developments in abortion laws. *American Journal of Public Health*, **78**, 1305.

Cook, R.J. (1989). Abortion laws and policies: challenges and opportunities. *International Journal of Gynecology and Obstetrics*, Supplement 3, 61–87.

Cook, R.J., Dickens, B.M., and Bliss, L.E. (1999). International developments in abortion law from 1988 to 1998. *American Journal of Public Health*, **89**, 579.

Côte d'Ivoire (1996). Making compulsory the iodization of salt intended for human and animal consumption in Côte d'Ivoire. Interministerial Order No. 18 H5/HC of 3 April 1996. *International Digest of Health Legislation*, **47**, 456.

Curran, W.J. and Harding, T.W. (1978). *The law and mental health: harmonizing objectives.* WHO, Geneva.

Daubert v. *Merrell Dow Pharmaceuticals, Inc.* (1993). 509 US 579, 113 S. Ct. 3786, 125 L. Ed. 2d 469.

David, H.P. (ed.) (1984). *Abortion research notes*, Vol. 13, Nos 1–2, pp. 1–2. Transnational Family Research Institute, Bethesda, MD.

David, H.P. (ed.) (1993). *Abortion research notes*, Vol. 22, Nos 1–2, pp. 2, 6. Transnational Family Research Institute, Bethesda, MD.

David, H. and Pick de Weiss, S. (1992). Abortion in the Americas. In *Reproductive health in the Americas* (ed. A.H. Omran, J. Yunes, J.A. Solis, and G. Lopez). Pan American Health Organization, Washington, DC.

DeMarco, C.T. (1975). *Pharmacy and the law*, p. 65. Aspen Systems Corporation, Maryland.

Djibouti (1997). Law No. 93/AN/95/3eL of 4 April 1996 promulgating the Water Code. *International Digest of Health Legislation*, **48**, 65.

Dominica (1983). An Act (No. 34 of 1982) further to amend the Medical Ordinance, Cap. 149. Dated 21 October 1982 (the Medical Amendment) Act 1982. *International Digest of Health Legislation*, **34**, 241.

Dominican Republic (1998). Law No. 55–93 of 19 May 1993. *International Digest of Health Legislation*, **49**, 619.

Egypt (1997). Order No. 261 of 8 July 1996. *International Digest of Health Legislation*, **48**, 318.

European Community (1997). Council Regulation (EC) No. 550/97 of 24 March 1997 on HIV/AIDS-related operations in developing countries. *International Digest of Health Legislation*, **48**, 161.

Finland (1987). Ordinance No. 786 of 31 October 1986 on communicable diseases. *International Digest of Health Legislation*, **38**, 244.

Food and Drug Administration v. *Brown and Williamson Tobacco Corp.* (2000). 529 US 120, 146 L. Ed. 2d 121, Sup. Ct. Reporter 1291.

France (1991). Law No. 91–32 of 10 January 1991 on measures to combat tobacco use and alcoholism. *International Digest of Health Legislation*, **42**, 44.

Ghana (1996). An Act to amend the Criminal Code to include the offence of female circumcision. *International Digest of Health Legislation*, **47**, 30.

Glantz, S.A. (1996). *The cigarette papers.* University of California Press, Berkeley, CA.

Glantz, S.A. *et al.* (1995). The Brown and Williamson documents. *Journal of the American Medical Association*, **274**, 219–55.

Goldsmith, J.R. (1970). Changing concepts of environmental health. *The education and training of engineers for environmental health.* WHO, Geneva.

Gostin, L.O. (1986). The future of public health law. *American Journal of Law and Medicine*, **12**, 461.

Gostin, L. and Curran, W.J. (ed.) (1987). AIDS law and policy. *Law, Medicine and Health Care*, **15**, 3–89.

Grad, F.P. (1978). Medical ethics and the law. *Annals of the American Academy of Political and Social Science*, **437**, 19.

Grad, F.P. (1986). Public health law. In *Maxcy-Rosenau Preventive Medicine and Public Health* (12th edn) (ed. J.M. Last). Appleton-Century-Crofts, New York.

Grad, F.P. (1990). Restrictions of the person. In *Public health law manual* (2nd edn). American Public Health Association, Washington, DC.

Grad, F.P. (1994). *Treatise on environmental law*, Vol. 1. Matthew Bender, New York.

Grad, F.P., Rathjens, G.W., and Rosenthal, A.J. (1971). *Environmental control: priorities, policies, and the law*, pp. 29–38. Columbia University Press, New York.

Health Systems Research Institute of Thailand (1995). *Thailand's tobacco control laws.* Bangkok.

Henshaw, S.K. (1994). Recent trends in the legal status of induced abortion. *Journal of Public Health Policy*, **15**, 165.

Hilts, P.J. (1994*a*). Philip Morris blocked paper showing addiction, panel finds. *New York Times*, April 1.

Hilts, P.J. (1994*b*). Scientists say Philip Morris withheld nicotine findings. *New York Times*, April 20.

Hilts, P.J. (1994*c*). Tobacco company was silent on hazards. *New York Times*, May 7.

Hilts, P.J. (1994*d*). Cigarette makers debated risks they denied. *New York Times*, 16 June.

Hilts, P.J. (1994*e*). Tobacco maker studied risk but did little about results. *New York Times*, 17 June.

Hilts, P.J. (1994*f*). Grim findings scuttled hope for 'safer' cigarette. *New York Times*, 18 June.

Hilts, P.J. (1994*g*). Cigarette company developed a potent gene-altered tobacco. *New York Times*, 22 June.

Horowitz, H.S. (1981). Promotion of oral health and prevention of dental caries. *Journal of the American Dental Association*, **103**, 141.

Hungary (1993). Government Decree No. 86–93 of 4 June 1993 on the provisional regulation of environmental impact assessment of certain activities. *International Digest of Health Legislation*, **44**, 716.

Hutt, P.B. (1980). Five moral imperatives of government regulation. *Hastings Center Report*, February, 29–31.

Iceland (1984). Law No. 74 of 28 May 1984 on the prevention of the use of tobacco. *International Digest of Health Legislation*, **35**, 772.

Iceland (1998). The Pharmaceutical Law (No. 93/1994) of 20 May 1994. *International Digest of Health Legislation*, **49**, 358.

Indonesia (1990). Regulation No. 085/Men. Kes./Per/I/1989 of the Ministry of Health for the Republic of Indonesia on the compulsory prescribing and/or use of generic drugs in Government health services. *International Digest of Health Legislation*, **31**, 469.

Indonesia (1998). Decree of the Minister of Industry and Trade No. 245/MPP/KEP/8/1996. *International Digest of Health Legislation*, **49**, 383.

Institute of Medicine (1982). *Legislative approaches to prevention of alcohol-related problems*. National Academy Press, Washington, DC.

International Labour Organization (1981). Convention concerning occupational safety and health and the working environment. Convention No. 155 adopted by the International Labour Conference on 22 June 1981. *International Digest of Health Legislation*, **32**, 549.

Isaacs, S.L. (1981). *Population law and policy, source materials and issues*. Human Sciences Press, New York.

Israel (1992). The treatment of mentally ill persons. Law, 5751–1991. *International Digest of Health Legislation*, **43**, 746.

Joseph, S.C. (1992). *Dragon within the gates: the once and future epidemic*. Carroll and Graf, New York.

Klepp, K.-I. and Forster, J. (1985). The Norwegian nutrition and food policy: an integrated policy approach to a public health problem. *Journal of Public Health Policy*, **6**, 447–63.

Ladimer, I. and Newman, R.W. (ed.) (1963). *Clinical investigation in medicine. Legal, ethical, and moral aspects, an anthology and bibliography*. Law-Medicine Research Institute, Boston University, Boston, MA.

Lalonde, M. (1974). *A new perspective on the health of Canadians, a working document*. Government of Canada, Ottawa.

Lamb, D. (1994). Leprosy nearly eradicated: African clinic to turn to TB. *Los Angeles Times*, July 16, A4.

Lander, L. (1980). Licensing of health care facilities. In *Legal aspects of health policy: issues and trends*, pp. 129–72 (ed. R. Roemer and G. McKray). Greenwood Press, Westport, CT.

Latvia (1996). Regulation No. 207 of 18 July 1995 laying down provisions concerning the National Centre for AIDS. *International Digest of Health Legislation*, **47**, 161.

Luxembourg (1998). Regulations of the Grand Duchy of Luxembourg of 21 January 1998 on the practice of the profession of nurse. *International Digest of Health Legislation*, **49**, 615.

McCafferty, G. and Dooley, J. (1990). Involuntary outpatient commitment: an update. *Mental and Physical Disability Law Reporter*, May/June, 277–87.

Maclay, W.S. (1960). The new Mental Health Act in England and Wales. *American Journal of Psychiatry*, **116**, 777.

Madagascar (1995). Interministerial Order No. 2413/94-MPCA/MIN SAN MRAD of 2 June 1994 specifying the Malagasy standard for edible salt and iodized salt. *International Digest of Health and Legislation*, **46**, 177.

Madagascar (1998). Decree No. 97–822 of 12 June 1997. *International Digest of Health Legislation*, **49**, 694.

Maine, D. and McNamara, R. (1985). *Birth spacing and child survival*. Center for Population and Family Health, Columbia University, New York.

Malawi (1998). Act No. 23 of 5 August 1996. *International Digest of Health Legislation*, **49**, 383.

Malaysia (1990). An Act (No. 342) to amend and consolidate the law relating to the prevention and control of infectious diseases and to provide for other matters connected therewith (the Prevention and Control of Infectious Diseases Act 1988). *International Digest of Health Legislation*, **44**, 49.

Mason, P.E., Yackle, J.F., and Stephan, J. (1985). *Annual review of population law, 1983*, Vol. 10, p. 74. United Nations Fund for Population Activities and Harvard Law School Library, Cambridge, MA.

Mason, P.E., Boland, R., and Stepan, J. (1987). *Annual review of population law, 1984*, Vol. 11. United Nations Fund for Population Activities and Harvard Law School Library, Cambridge, MA.

Missouri Supreme Court (1983). *Sermchief* v. *Gonzales*, 660 S.W. 2d 683 (Mo. banc 1983).

Morocco (1996). Decree No. 2-95-709 of 12 December 1995 on the iodization of salt intended for human consumption. *International Digest of Health Legislation*, **47**, 459.

Morocco (1998*a*). Decree No. 2-93-752 of 10 March 1994. Establishing the National Health Administration Institute to train senior managerial staff specialized in health administration to serve in public and private bodies. *International Digest of Health Legislation*, **49**, 612.

Morocco (1998*b*). Decree No. 2-93-809 of 24 May 1994. *International Digest of Health Legislation*, **49**, 695.

Moser, J. (1980). *Prevention of alcohol-related problems, an international review of preventive measures, policies, and programmes*. WHO and Addiction Research Foundation, Ontario.

Murray, J.J. (1986). *Appropriate use of fluorides for human health*, pp. 38–73. WHO, Geneva.

Nakashima, *et al.* (1998). Effect of HIV reporting on use of HIV testing in publicly funded counselling and testing programs. *Journal of the American Obstetrical Association*, **280**, 1421–6.

National Board of Health of Finland (1985). Advisory Committee on Health Education *An evaluation of the effects of an increase in the price of tobacco and a proposal for the tobacco price policy in Finland in 1985–87*. National Board of Health of Finland, Helsinki.

National Science Panel (1998). Summary Report: silicone breast implants in relation to connective tissue diseases and immunologic dysfunction.

New York (1972). New York Education Law title 8, article 139, sec. 6902.

New York (1978). NY Mental Hygiene L., sec. 9.01.

New York (1985). NY Public Health L., sec. 2805.

New Zealand (1990). The smoke-free environments act. *International Digest of Health Legislation*, **41**, 636.

New Zealand Toxic Substances Board (1989). *Health or tobacco: an end to tobacco advertising and promotion*, pp. 64–6. New Zealand Department of Health, Wellington.

News and Views (1990). European Community bodies adopt resolution on AIDS (1990). *International Digest of Health Legislation*, **41**, 348.

Niger (1998). Order No. 54/MSP/DPHL of 23 February 1998 determining the conditions governing the advertising of pharmaceutical products directed to the general public. *International Digest of Health Legislation*, **49**, 686.

Norway (1981–1982). Report No. 11 to the Storting (1981–2) of the Follow-Up on Norwegian Nutrition Policy. Recommendation of 10 July 1981. Ministry of Health and Social Affairs, Oslo.

Parham v. *J.R. et al.* (1979). 442 US 584 (1979); *Secretary of Public Welfare* v. *Institutionalized Juveniles*, 442 US 640.

Paxman, J.M. (1980). *Law and planned parenthood.* International Planned Parenthood Federation, London.

Paxman, J.M. and Zuckerman, R.J. (1987). *Laws and policies affecting adolescent health.* WHO, Geneva.

Philippines (1990). Executive Order No. 175 of 22 May 1987 further amending Republic Act No. 3720, entitled 'An Act to ensure the safety and purity of foods, drugs, and cosmetics being made available to the public by creating the food and drug administration which shall administer and enforce the laws pertaining thereto,' as amended, and for other purses. *International Digest of Health Legislation*, **41**, 470.

Philippines (1997). An Act (Republic Act No. 8172) promoting salt iodization nationwide. *International Digest of Health Legislation*, **48**, 166.

Philippines (1998). An Act (Republic Act No. 7875) of 14 February 1995 instituting a National Health Insurance Program for all Filipinos and establishing the Philippine Health Insurance Corporation for the purpose. *International Digest of Health Legislation*, **49**, 298.

Poland (1988). Law of 6 June 1997 promulgating the Penal Code. *International Digest of Health Legislation*, **49**, 607.

Poland (1997). Law of 30 August 1996 amending the law on family planning, protection of human fetuses, and the conditions under which pregnancy termination is permissible. *International Digest of Health Legislation*, **48**, 176.

Porter, L., Arif, A.E., and Curran, W.J. (1986). *The law and treatment of drug and alcohol-dependent persons, a comparative study of existing legislation.* World Health Organization, Geneva.

Qatar (1989). The mental health law 1989. *International Digest of Health Legislation*, **49**, 330.

Reich, W.T. (1978). *Encyclopedia of bioethics.* Free Press, New York.

Roemer, M.I. (1991). *National Health Systems of the World.* Vol. 1. *The Countries.* Oxford University Press, New York.

Roemer, R. (1985). Legislation on contraception and abortion for adolescents. *Studies in Family Planning*, **16**, 241.

Roemer, R. (1988). *Legislative strategies for a smoke-free Europe*, pp. 26–30. WHO Regional Office for Europe, Copenhagen.

Roemer, R. (1993). *Legislative strategies to combat the world tobacco epidemic* (2nd edn). WHO, Geneva.

Roemer, R. and Paxman, J.M. (1985). Sex education laws and policies. *Studies in Family Planning*, **16**, 219.

Roemer, R. and Roemer, M.I. (1976). *Health manpower in the changing Australian health services scene.* DHEW Publication (HRA) 76–58, pp. 7–8. US Department of Health, Education, and Welfare, Washington, DC.

Roemer, M.I. and Shain, M. (1959) *Hospital utilization under insurance.* Hospital Monograph Series No. 6, American Hospital Association, Chicago.

Roemer, R., Frink, J.E., and Kramer, C. (1971). Environmental health services: multiplicity of jurisdictions and comprehensive environmental management. *Milbank Memorial Fund Quarterly*, **49**, 419.

Rosen, G. (1958). *A history of public health.* MD Publications, New York (reissued 1993, Johns Hopkins University Press, Baltimore, MD).

Rosenzweig, S. (1990). The predicament of the mentally disabled in the community—the need for a protective structure. *New York State Bar Journal*, **1**, 26.

Senegal (1978). Decree No. 77–017 of 7 January 1977.

Senegal (1998). Law No. 98–08 of 2 March 1998 on hospital reform. *International Digest of Health Legislation*, **49**, 464.

Sermchief v. *Gonzales* (1983). 660 SW 2d 683.

Silver, L. (1980). An agency dilemma: regulating to protect the public health in light of scientific uncertainty. In *Legal aspects of health policy: issues and trends*, pp. 61–93 (ed. R. Roemer and G. McKray). Greenwood Press, Westport, CT.

Sindell v. *Abbott Laboratories* (1980). 26 Cal. 3d 588.

Single, E. (1984). International perspectives on alcohol as public health issue. *Journal of Public Health Policy*, **5**, 238.

Social Security Administration, Office of Research, Evaluation and Statistics (1997). *Social security programs throughout the world.* Research Report No. 65. SSA Publication No. 13-11805.

Somers, A.R. (1969). *Hospital regulation: the dilemma of public policy*, p. ix. Industrial Relations Section, Department of Economics, Princeton University.

South Africa (1997). An Act to determine the circumstances under which pregnancy may be terminated. *International Digest of Health Legislation*, **48**, 178.

Sri Lanka (1981). An Act (No. 47 of 1980) to establish a 'Central Environmental Authority (and) to make provision with respect to the powers, functions, and duties of that Authority; and to make provision for the protection and management of the environment and for matters connected therewith or incidental thereto. Dated 29 October 1980'. *International Digest of Health Legislation*, **32**, 565.

Stepan, J., Kellogg, E.H., and Piotrow, P.T. (1981). Legal trends and issues in voluntary sterilization. *Population Reports*, **9**, E75–102.

Swiss Institute of Comparative Law (1986). *Artificial procreation, genetics and the law.* Schulthess Polygraphischer Verlag, Zürich.

Terris, M. (1983). The complex tasks of the second epidemiologic revolution. *Journal of Public Health Policy*, **4**, 8.

Torry, S. (1998). Proposed tobacco settlement labeled too soft on industry. *Washington Post*, November 19.

Tunisia (1996). Decree No. 95-1633 of September 1995 on the requirement that throughout the territory of the Republic only salt that has been iodized may be marketed for human consumption. *International Digest of Health Legislation*, 47, 460.

Tunisia (1998). Order of the Minister of Public Health of 15 May 1996 on establishment and organization of the Technical Committee on Telemedicine. *International Digest of Health Legislation*, **49**, 302.

UK (1959). Mental Health Act (England and Wales), 7 and 8 Eliz. 2, Chapter 72, Section 5. *International Digest of Health Legislation* (1961), **12**, 207.

UK (1983). An Act (Chapter 51) to amend the Mental Health Act 1959 and for connected purposes, 28 October 1982. *International Digest of Health Legislation*, **34**, 524. Superseded by the Mental Health Act 1983. *International Digest of Health Legislation*, **34**, 536.

UK (1989). The Public Health (Infectious Diseases) Regulations 1988. *International Digest of Health Legislation*, **40**, 586.

US (1969). The National Environmental Policy Act 1969, PL No. 91–190, 83 Stat. 852, 42 USCA section 4321.

US (1986). National Childhood Vaccine Injury Act 1986, 42 USC 300aa-10 et seq., 100 Stat. 3755–3784 (PL 99–660), 14 November 1986.

US (1991). An Act (Public Law 101–535) to amend the Federal Food, Drug, and Cosmetic Act to prescribe nutrition labeling for foods, and for other purposes (the Nutrition Labeling and Education Act of 1990). *International Digest of Health Legislation*, **42**, 502.

US (1993*b*). Code of Federal Regulations Subpart C—*Health warning statement requirements for alcoholic beverages*, 27 CFR 16.20, 16.21.

US (1993*c*). Food labeling; mandatory status of nutrition labeling and nutrient content revision, format for nutrition label. Parts 1 and 101 of Title 21 (Food and Drugs) of the United States Code of Federal Regulations. *International Digest of Health Legislation*, **44**, 464.

US (1993*d*). New drug, antibiotic, and biological drug product regulations; accelerated approval. Parts 314 and 601 of Title 21 (Food and Drugs) of the United States Code of Federal Regulations. *International Digest of Health Legislation*, **44**, 325.

US (1996). US Food and Drug Administration, Department of Health and Human Services. Nicotine in cigarettes and smokeless tobacco is a drug and these products are drug delivery devices under the Federal Food, Drug and Cosmetic Act: Jurisdictional Determination. *Federal Register*, **61**.

US Department of Labor, Occupational Safety and Health Administration (1991). Code of Federal Regulations. *Bloodborne pathogens*, 29 CFR 1910.1030, Final Rule, Federal Register 64, 009 (6 December 1991).

US Environmental Protection Agency (1993). *Respiratory health effects of passive smoking: lung cancer and other disorders.* The report of the US Environmental Protection Agency, NIH Publication No. 93–3605. US Department of Health and Human Services, Bethesda, MD.

Vietnam (1996). Circular No. 7-BYT/TT of 30 April 1994 of the Ministry of Public Health guiding the implementation of the ordinance on private medical and pharmaceutical practice and Decree No. 6-CP of 29 January 1994 of the Government concretizing a number of articles of this ordinance in the area of private medical practice. *International Digest of Health Legislation*, **47**, 308.

Vietnam (1998). Government Decree No. 34-CP of 1 June 1996 guiding the implementation of the ordinance on the prevention and control of HIV/AIDS infection. *International Digest of Health Legislation*, **49**, 308.

Walters, L. (1975). *Bibliography of bioethics.* Center for Bioethics, Kennedy Institute, Georgetown University, Gale Research Company, Detroit, MI.

Warnock Committee (1984). *Report of the Committee of Inquiry into Human Fertilisation and Embryology* (Dame Mary Warnock, Chairperson). HMSO, London.

Weinstein, H. and Levin, M. (1999). Cigarette makers liable in Florida class-action case. *Los Angeles Times*, 8 July.

Wing, K.R. (1985). *The law and the public's health*, pp. 1–5. Health Administration Press, Ann Arbor, MI.

WHO (World Health Organization) Study Group (1986). *Regulatory mechanisms for nursing training and practice: Meeting primary health care needs.* World Health Organization Technical Report Series 738, p. 32. World Health Organization, Geneva.

WHO (World Health Organization) (1987). *Success against smoking, the story of four countries.* Tobacco or Health Programme, World Health Organization, Geneva.

WHO (World Health Organization) (1992). *Consultation on testing and counselling for HIV infection.* Global Programme on AIDS. World Health Organization, Geneva.

WHO (World Health Organization) (1996). *International framework convention on tobacco control.* WHA Res. 49.17. World Health Organization, Geneva.

WHO (World Health Organization) (1997). *Directory of legal instruments dealing with HIV infection and AIDS.* World Health Organization, Geneva.

WHO (World Health Organization) (1999). *Towards a WHO framework convention on tobacco control.* World Health Organization, Geneva.

World Health Assembly (1989). World Health Assembly adopts revised certification scheme for pharmaceutical products in international commerce. *International Digest of Health Legislation*, **40**, 261.

Zaire (1996). Interministerial Order No. 001 of 28 October 1993 regulating the promotion, quality control and marketing in Zaire of salt iodized in order to prevent disorders caused by iodine deficiency. *International Digest of Health Legislation*, **47**, 460.

4.3 International health instruments: an overview*

Allyn L. Taylor, Douglas W. Bettcher, Sev S. Fluss, Katherine DeLand, and Derek Yach

Introduction

No definition of international health law is accepted worldwide. As the eminent scholar Frank Grad has observed:

> Public health law does not come in a single, neat legislative package marked 'public health law'. It consists of many different types of legislation which have little in common except for the benign purpose of advancing public health. (Grad 1998)

This statement was undoubtedly written in the context of national health-care systems, but it is especially applicable to international public health law.

As Grad has observed, the field of international public health law encompasses increasingly complex concerns, including aspects of human reproduction, biomedical science and human reproduction/cloning, organ transplantation and xenotransplantation, infectious and non-communicable diseases, international trade and the control of safety of health services, food, and pharmaceuticals, and the control of addictive substances such as tobacco and narcotics. International public health law is linked with other areas of international concern. International labour law and occupational health and safety, environmental law and the control of toxic pollutants, arms control and the banning of weapons of mass destruction, nuclear safety and radiation protection, disabilities and human rights, and fertility and population growth are all related to public health (Grad 1998).

The breadth and depth of international health law at the beginning of the twenty-first century and its nexus with other realms of international concern is largely a result of globalization. Globalization is the process of increasing economic, political and social interdependence, and global integration that occurs as capital, traded goods, people, concepts, images, ideas, and values diffuse across state boundaries (Ruggie 1995). The roots of globalization can be traced back to the industrial revolution and the *laissez-faire* economic policies of the late nineteenth century. However, globalization at the beginning of the twenty-first century has assumed a magnitude and taken on patterns that are unprecedented in world history.

The global context of development has profound implications for public health and, concomitantly, the expansion of international health law as the lives of individuals are increasingly affected by transnational economic, social, scientific, and technological changes. As a result of the new globality, the domestic and international spheres of health policy are becoming more intertwined and inseparable. The domain of globalization includes many interconnected phenomena, risks, and opportunities that affect the sustained ability of health systems and the well being of populations of countries at all stages of development (Yach and Bettcher 1998*a*).

The development of binding global public health norms and commitments is becoming increasingly important as global interdependence accelerates and nations increasingly feel the need to co-operate to solve essential problems (Taylor 1992). Although international health law is still in a rudimentary stage of development relative to other fields of international concern, the health impact of globalization, both positive and negative, have become key global policy issues. Consequently, health development in the twenty-first century is likely to make wider use of international legal instruments to take advantage of the opportunities afforded by global change and to minimize the risks and threats associated with globalization.

At the same time, international health law remains very much concerned with the protection of human rights relating to physical and mental integrity (Abbing 1998). The domain of human rights in relation to health has expanded dramatically in the last 50 years, and tailored international instruments now address the rights of special populations, such as people with HIV/AIDS and disabilities, women, children, migrant workers, and refugees. International human rights law is also increasingly concerned with the human rights implications of advances in health technology, including human experimentation and biomedicine. It is well recognized, however, that human rights relating to health proclaimed in numerous instruments must be crystallized and operationalized if they are to affect national and international practice and that the human rights agenda of this century must move from the elaboration to the implementation of international norms.

This chapter focuses on international instruments ranging from binding treaties and conventions adopted under the auspices of international and regional organizations to non-binding instruments adopted under the auspices of such public international organizations as well as international non-governmental organizations and professional associations. It is concerned primarily with two complementary areas: the organizations under whose auspices international public health law and standards are developed, and international public health law and standards as they affect certain areas of health.

* The views expressed herein are those of the authors and do not necessarily reflect the views of the World Health Organization.

This chapter is not intended to be historical or comprehensive in perspective, rather it provides information on the current configuration of international public health law. Furthermore, space limitations prohibit systematic analysis of the effectiveness or efficacy of the instruments described. The reader is referred to the reference list at the end of this chapter for further information on international health law instruments. In addition, most of the organizations discussed in this chapter maintain websites where timely information on the instruments negotiated and adopted under their respective auspices can be obtained.

While it is not possible to discuss and clarify thoroughly the nature of the rules and process of international law within the confines of this chapter, it should be recognized that the rules of international law are very different in kind from those of municipal law as a consequence of the international legal system. Given the international political system of nation-states and the concept of state sovereignty, the sources of international law cannot be equivalent to those of municipal laws. Municipal rules generally derive from national constitutions, municipal statutes, executive regulations, and the decisions of municipal courts. Of course, some international organizations, such as the European Union, have established law-making structures that approach municipal-like sources, but, overall, formal international legislative and executive organs are fairly rare in the international system. Brownlie (1998), Higgens (1994), and Hiller (1994) provide thorough analyses of international law rules and processes.

It would have been impossible to write or conceive of this chapter without the pioneering work of four people. The late Norman Howard-Jones (1950, 1975), whose work on the early development of international public health law has almost biblical status for scholars in the field. Valentin Mikhailov (1984), whose legal treatise on the development of international health law has no real parallel in the English language. Michel Bélanger (1983, 1989) has made significant contributions to the field of international health law. Finally, Sev Fluss has made major and extensive contributions to the field of international health law are essential resources for all scholars in this field. This chapter draws upon Fluss's contribution to the third edition of the *Oxford Textbook of Public Health* (1997*b*).

Sources of international public health law: the contribution of international, regional, and non-governmental organizations

United Nations

Although the United Nations is not normally perceived as having a major role in health law, in fact, as shown in various sections of this chapter, numerous international conventions and non-binding instruments relevant to global public health have been adopted by or under the auspices of the United Nations. These include provisions dealing with discrimination in the field of health, rules governing the health and medical services to be provided to prisoners, mental health, medical ethics in certain contexts, measures to combat malnutrition, the rights of disabled people, the right to development (including the right to health), human rights and health, human rights in the population and reproductive health context, and various aspects of the protection of the human environment.

The legal foundation of the United Nations' activities in international health is based on its Charter and, in particular, those sections that describe the objectives of the United Nations. Article 55 of the Charter describes the goals that the United Nations has pledged to promote among its members:

- higher standards of living, full employment, and conditions of economic and social progress and development
- solutions of international economic, social, health, and related problems, and international cultural and educational co-operation.

Acting within the framework of the United Nations Charter, the General Assembly, for example, has the legal capacity to discuss and study international health concerns. Article 13 of the United Nations Charter commands the General Assembly to 'initiate studies and make recommendations ... promoting international cooperation in the ... health [field]'. The General Assembly also has the authority to make formal recommendations to the specialized agencies that those agencies are required to take into account. In addition, the General Assembly has the legal capacity to provide a forum for the negotiation of multilateral treaties. Article 13.1(a) empowers the General Assembly to 'initiate studies and make recommendations ... encouraging the progressive development of international law and its codification'. Although the General Assembly lacks express legislative powers, it has discharged its obligation to encourage the progressive development of international law and its codification by acting as a facilitator for the creation of international legislative rules through the traditional treaty-making process. The role of the General Assembly in international health law making is described by Taylor (1996).

As described in this chapter, a number of the specialized agencies, organs, and other bodies of the United Nations make a significant contribution to the development of international health law. The World Health Organization (**WHO**) is the United Nations specialized agency with the primary mandate to implement the aims of the Charter with respect to health.

Other United Nations bodies and organizations

Economic Commission for Europe

Established in 1947 as a United Nations organ, the Economic Commission for Europe was given the mandate of helping rebuild postwar Europe, develop economic activity, and strengthen economic relations between European countries and between them and other parts of the world. The Economic Commission for Europe has served as the forum for numerous conventions and other instruments relevant to the protection and promotion of human health including the following:

- 1979 Convention on Long-Range Transboundary Air Pollution and its protocols
- 1991 Convention on Environmental Impact Assessment in a Transboundary Context
- 1992 Convention on the Protection and Use of Transboundary Watercourses and International Lakes and its protocol
- 1992 Convention on Transboundary Effects of Industrial Accidents.

Food and Agricultural Organization

The Food and Agricultural Organization (**FAO**), the largest specialized agency within the United Nations system, was established in 1945 with the mandate to raise levels of nutrition and standards of living, to improve agricultural productivity, and to better the conditions of rural people. The Organization has developed a number of instruments directly and indirectly relevant to human health. The Food and Agricultural Organization collaborates with the WHO as a partner in the administration of the Codex Alimentarius Programme, which was initiated to promulgate food standards aimed at protecting consumer health and ensuring fair practices in the food trade. In collaboration with the United Nations Environment Programme, the Food and Agricultural Organization served as a forum for the adoption of the 1998 Convention on the Prior Informed Consent for Certain Hazardous Chemicals and Pesticides in International Trade, the most recent international instrument designed to promote health and environmental protection in international trade in chemicals and pesticides.

International Atomic Energy Agency

The International Atomic Energy Agency (IAEA) serves as the central intergovernmental forum for scientific and technical co-operation on nuclear issues and is the international inspectorate for the application of nuclear safeguards and verification measures covering non-military nuclear programmes. A related agency within the United Nations system, the International Atomic Energy Agency, currently has 128 member states. The International Atomic Energy Agency Statute was approved on 23 October 1956 by the Conference on the Statute of the International Atomic Energy Agency and entered into force on 29 July 1957.

The International Atomic Energy Agency has developed a number of conventions and codes dealing with nuclear safety. Those that have potential relevance to the protection of public health include the Convention on Early Notification of a Nuclear Accident (1986), the Convention on Assistance in the Case of a Nuclear Accident (1986), the Convention on Nuclear Safety (1994), and the Joint Convention on the Safety of Spent Fuel Management and on the Safety of Radioactive Waste Management (1997). Adede (1987) has written a definitive book on the 1986 Early Notification and Assistance Conventions.

The International Atomic Energy Agency, along with the Food and Agriculture Organization, the International Labour Organization, the Nuclear Energy Agency of the Organization for Economic Co-operation and Development, the Pan American Health Organization, and the WHO, jointly sponsored the recently updated International Basic Safety Standards for Protection Against Ionizing Radiation and for the Safety of Radiation Sources. Other relevant conventions and recommendations are discussed below in the sections dealing with nuclear safety and radiation protection in international public health law as it affects certain sectors of health.

International Labour Organization

The Geneva-based International Labour Organization (**ILO**) was founded in 1919 and is the only surviving entity created by the Treaty of Versailles. It became the first specialized agency of the United Nations in 1946. Articles 14 to 21 of the Constitution of the International Labour Organization (1919) enable that Organization to adopt conventions and recommendations. A substantial number of the 182 conventions and 190 recommendations developed under the auspices of the International Labour Organization as of 1999 have dealt with issues that are directly or indirectly related to human health. In fact, as early as October 1919, what was then known as the General Conference of the International Labour Organization adopted the Maternity Protection Convention, 1919 (this has since been superseded by the Maternity Protection Convention 1952). Other relevant conventions and recommendations are discussed below in the section dealing with occupational health in international public health law as it affects certain sectors of health.

International Maritime Organization

The London-based International Maritime Organization, originally established as the Intergovernmental Maritime Consultative Organization, is the United Nations specialized agency responsible for improving maritime safety and preventing pollution from ships. The International Maritime Organization has served as the platform for the development of numerous international instruments relevant to international public health, including:

- 1969 Convention on Civil Liability for Oil Pollution Damage
- 1972 Convention on the Prevention of Marine Pollution by Dumping of Wastes and Other Matter (London Ocean Dumping Convention)
- 1973 International Convention for the Prevention of Pollution from Ships, as modified by the Protocol of 1978
- 1990 International Convention on Oil Pollution, Preparedness, Response and Cooperation
- 1996 International Convention on Liability and Compensation for Damage in Connection with the Carriage of Hazardous and Noxious Substances by Sea.

United Nations Educational, Scientific and Cultural Organization

The Paris-based United Nation's Educational, Scientific and Cultural Organization (**UNESCO**), established in 1945, has the primary constitutional directive of promoting collaboration among member states in education, science, and culture. With six regional offices, UNESCO is one of the largest specialized agencies of the United Nations.

The first article of UNESCO's Constitution specifies that the purpose of the organization is to 'contribute to peace and security by promoting collaboration among nations through education science and culture in order to further universal respect for justice, for the rule of law, and for the human rights and fundamental freedoms which are affirmed for the peoples of the world'.

Biomedical science has been a particular emphasis of UNESCO for more than 25 years. The Organization held its first of many symposiums on social and cultural changes brought about by scientific progress in the early 1970s and has monitored the human rights implications of advances in genetic science for over a decade. In 1997 UNESCO served as the forum for the adoption of the Universal Declaration on the Human Genome and Human Rights.

United Nations Environment Programme

The United Nations Environment Programme (**UNEP**), established by General Assembly Resolution 2997 of 15 December 1972 and with headquarters in Nairobi, is the outcome of the 1972 United Nations Conference on the Human Environment, the Stockholm Conference. UNEP, which operates as a quasi-autonomous subsidiary organ of the

United Nations, has served as the forum of numerous multilateral environmental law instruments that have important implications for global public health. Some of the most significant are:

- the 1987 Cairo Guidelines for the Environmentally Sound Management of Hazardous Wastes
- the 1989 Code of Ethics on the International Trade in Chemicals
- the 1989 Basel Convention on the Control of Transboundary Movements of Hazardous Wastes and their Disposal
- the 1985 Vienna Convention for the Protection of the Ozone Layer and the 1987 Montreal Protocol thereto
- in collaboration with the Food and Agricultural Organization, the 1998 Prior Informed Consent Convention.

UNEP also provided substantive support and technical expertise to the 1992 United Nations Framework Convention on Climate Change and the United Nations Convention to Combat Desertification in those Countries Experiencing Serious Drought and/or Desertification, particularly in Africa. In addition, it served as the framework for the negotiation of a number of regional seas agreements designed to protect the marine environment.

UNEP is in the process of organizing intergovernmental negotiations for the development of new treaties relevant to international public health, including a legally binding instrument for certain persistent organic pollutants. In addition, UNEP is currently developing new instruments within the framework of conventions formerly negotiated or developed under its auspices. The most significant of these are a Protocol on Biosafety to the 1992 Convention on Biological Diversity, and a Protocol on Liability and Compensation for Damage Resulting from Transboundary Movements of Hazardous Wastes and their Disposal to the 1989 Basel Convention on the Control of Transboundary Movements of Hazardous Wastes and their Disposal.

World Health Organization

The WHO is the primary multilateral organization charged with protecting and promoting global public health. With headquarters in Geneva, six regional offices and 191 member states, the WHO is the largest international health organization and one of the largest specialized agencies of the United Nations.

Although the WHO is not the only international agency involved in health matters, it has a unique mandate to address global public health based on responsibilities assigned by relevant international instruments. Article 1 of the WHO's Constitution proclaims the fundamental objective of the 'attainment by all peoples of the highest possible level of health'.

The foundation of the WHO's unique obligation to promote global health is its affiliation with the United Nations system as a specialized agency. The structure of the relationships between the United Nations and the WHO is grounded in the United Nations Charter and, in particular, those sections that describe the objectives of the United Nations. Article 55 of the Charter describes the goals that the United Nations has pledged to promote among its members, including '(b) solutions of international, economic, social, health and related problems; and international cultural and educational co-operation'. As the specialized agency with the primary constitutional directive to act as the 'directing and co-ordinating authority on international health work', the WHO has the cardinal responsibility to implement the aims of the Charter with respect to health.

The first steps towards the creation of the WHO were taken at the United Nations Conference on International Organization, held in San Francisco from 25 April to 26 June 1945. During that conference, two delegations proposed convening an international health conference, with the objective of creating such an organization. Thereafter, the Economic and Social Council of the United Nations agreed to convene an international conference of members of the United Nations, with a view to establishing a single international health organization to replace pre-existing international health organizations, in particular the Health Organization of the League of Nations, the Paris-based International Office of Public Hygiene, and the United Nations Relief and Rehabilitation Administration. The ensuing conference was held in New York from 19 June to 22 July 1946, and the WHO's Constitution was signed on the final day, entering into force on 7 April 1948. Further details of the origins of WHO have been described by Fluss and Gutteridge (1993).

The WHO's Constitution confers authority upon the Organization to develop conventions under Article 19, regulations under Article 21, and recommendations under Article 23. The WHO has the legal authority under Article 19 to seek member state adoption of conventions or agreements with respect to any matter within the competence of the Organization. Historically, the WHO has not utilized its constitutional authority to develop binding international conventions (Taylor 1992). However, as described in the section on tobacco control below, the World Health Assembly (the supreme governing body of WHO) has recently activated Article 19 to authorize the negotiation of the WHO's first international convention, a proposed WHO framework convention on tobacco control.

The WHO also has the authority to adopt international regulations under Article 21 of its Constitution, which lays down that such regulations may concern:

- sanitary and quarantine requirements and other procedures designed to prevent the international spread of disease
- nomenclatures with respect to diseases, causes of death, and public health practices
- standards with respect to diagnostic procedures for international use
- standards with respect to the safety, purity, and potency of biological, pharmaceutical, and similar products moving in international commerce
- advertising and labelling of biological, pharmaceutical, and similar products moving in international commerce.

Article 23 confers further authority on the Assembly to make recommendations with respect to any matter within the Organization's competence. The WHO regularly formulates and adopts technical recommendations and guidelines that command attention because of the Organization's established reputation for technical expertise. Article 62 requires member states to report annually on action taken with respect to such recommendations, as well as with respect to conventions, agreements, and regulations, although this constitutional provision has never strictly been applied.

World Trade Organization

The Geneva-based World Trade Organization (**WTO**), formed at the conclusion of the Uruguay Round of the General Agreement on Tariffs and Trade (**GATT**) in 1994, is the primary international institution governing international trade: approximately 90 per cent of world trade is conducted pursuant to its rules. The initial Round of GATT (1947) called for the formation of the International Trade Organization to administer the multilateral agreement, but that organization was never formally established. The organizational features of GATT (1947) were therefore rudimentary, and it functioned primarily as a forum for negotiation. With the conclusion of the Uruguay Round in 1994, the GATT contracting parties took a major step towards strengthening the international trade regime by establishing and formalizing the institutional status of the World Trade Organization, strengthening the trade dispute mechanisms, and broadening the World Trade Organization's jurisdiction.

The Uruguay Round brought about an overhaul of the international trade regime through the conclusion of a number of agreements addressing contemporary trade issues. The World Trade Organization Agreement has four annexes that contain the agreements reached in the Uruguay Round. The agreement was amended and incorporated into the new World Trade Organization agreement, including the case law and interpretive decisions. Now known as GATT (1994), the amended agreement, other agreements addressing non-tariff barriers to trade, trade in services, and a long list of understandings, declarations, decisions, and other texts are contained in the first Annex. Other World Trade Organization agreements covering trade in intellectual property as well as dispute settlement rules are contained in the second and third Annexes. These three sets of multilateral agreements were accepted by member states as a 'single package' during the Uruguay Round and therefore impose binding obligations on all member states. The fourth Annex, which contains the plurilateral agreements, are binding only on the World Trade Organization members who have accepted them.

The principal aim of the World Trade Organization is the reduction of barriers to trade. The general principles of the World Trade Organization include a commitment to achieving free trade and fair competition; limits on and eventual elimination of tariff and non-tariff barriers to trade; non-discriminatory treatment of all trading partners; the non-discriminatory treatment of domestically produced and foreign products; predictability by ensuring that trade barriers are not erected arbitrarily; negotiated elimination of trade barriers; the settlement of trade disputes; and opposition to retaliatory trade sanctions.

As described below, a number of the new World Trade Organization agreements have important implications for the protection and promotion of global public health. The most significant of these agreements are GATT (1994), the General Agreement on Trade in Services, the Agreement on the Application of Sanitary and Phytosanitary Measures, the Agreement on Technical Barriers to Trade, and the Trade-Related Aspects of Intellectual Property Rights Agreement.

Other international intergovernmental organizations

Organization for Economic Co-operation and Development

The forerunner of the Paris-based Organization for Economic Co-operation and Development (**OECD**) was the Organization for European Economic Co-operation, which was formed to administer American and Canadian aid under the Marshall Plan for reconstruction of Europe after the Second World War. Since it took over from the Organization for European Economic Co-operation in 1961, the OECD's mission has been to build strong economies in its member countries, improve efficiency, expand free trade, and contribute to development in industrialized as well as developing countries.

Article 5 of the December 1960 Convention on the OECD empowers it to make recommendations to its members. A substantial number of texts dealing with the environment and pharmaceutical and chemical safety have been developed under OECD auspices. Other areas of OECD concern which have relevance to global public health are biotechnology, food, agriculture, and fisheries, biodiversity, nuclear energy, and ageing.

Regional intergovernmental organizations

Benelux Economic Union and Nordic Council

The health-related texts adopted by the Committee of Ministers of the Benelux Economic Union relate to food safety, while those formulated by the five-member Nordic Council (Nordic Committee on Medicines) relate to the registration of pharmaceuticals.

Council of Europe

Article 1, Statute of 5 May 1949, of the 41-member Council of Europe states that the Council's aim is to 'achieve a greater unity between members for the purpose of safeguarding and realising the ideals and principles which are their common heritage and facilitating their economic and social progress'. This aim is to be pursued 'through the organs of the Council by discussion of questions of common concern and by agreements and common action in economic, social, cultural, scientific, legal and administrative matters and in the maintenance and further realisation of human rights and fundamental freedoms'. There is no explicit reference to health matters in this statute, but the Committee of Ministers has given a remit to various committees to deal with health issues.

In addition, 18 states of the Council of Europe are also members of the Partial Agreement in the Social and Public Health Field, concluded in 1959 and revised in 1996. The aim of the Partial Agreement public health activities is to protect consumers from contemporary health risks. Committees of experts provide the scientific basis for national and international regulations concerning products that have a direct or indirect impact on the human food chain (control of foodstuffs, nutrition, food safety, consumer health, food contact materials, flavouring substances), pesticides, pharmaceuticals, and cosmetics.

The Committee of Ministers has adopted many resolutions and recommendations dealing with matters related directly or indirectly to human health which are used by member states as the basis for corresponding national laws and regulations. They have addressed issues such as organ transplantation, protection of health and medical data, blood, and blood products, certain aspects of health care, genetic screening and testing, ethical, legal, and policy aspects of AIDS, food safety, pesticides, health professionals, mental health, and pharmaceuticals. Other instruments likely to have an impact on public health, at least in the member states of the Council of Europe, have been or are being developed under the auspices of the Steering Committee on Public Health.

Reference should also be made to the Convention on the Protection of Human Rights and Dignity with Regard to the Application of Biology and Medicine: the Convention on Human Rights and Biomedicine, opened for signature on 4 April 1997. A protocol to the Convention on the Prohibition of Cloning Human

Beings was opened for signature on 12 January 1998 and came into force in December 1999. In addition, the Council of Europe is in the process of preparing further protocols to the Convention on Human Rights and Biomedicine which will address organ transplantation, biomedical research, the protection of the human embryo and fetus, and problems relating to human genetics.

European Union

The Brussels-based European Union has a mandate under various articles of the Treaty of Rome, the Single European Act, the Maastricht Treaty, and the Treaty of Amsterdam. Bélanger (1985) has analysed the enabling provisions of the Treaty of Rome, the Single European Act, and the Maastricht Treaty from the standpoint of their relevance to the protection of public health in the European Community.

Of particular relevance to contemporary public health protection in the European Union is the Treaty of Amsterdam, signed by the European Union's political leaders on 2 October 1997 and entered into force 1 May 1999. The Treaty introduced major reforms for promoting high standards of public health. The Treaty of Amsterdam amended the Treaty Establishing the European Union by authorizing the organization to adopt measures directly aimed at ensuring a high level of human health protection. Pursuant to the new Article 152 of the Treaty Establishing the European Union, areas of co-operation between member states include not only diseases and major health scourges, but also all causes of danger to human health, as well as the general objective of improving health. The single Article 152 contained in Title XIII of the Treaty establishing the European Union comprises the following provisions.

1. A high level of human health protection shall be ensured in the definition and implementation of all Community policies and activities.
   (a) Community action, which shall complement national policies, shall be directed towards improving public health, preventing human illness and diseases, and obviating sources of danger to human health. Such action shall cover the fight against the major health scourges, by promoting research into their causes, their transmission, and their prevention, as well as health information and education.
   (b) The Community shall complement the Member States' action in reducing drugs-related health damage, including information and prevention.
2. The Community shall encourage cooperation between the Member States in the areas referred to in this Article and, if necessary, lend support to their action.
   (a) Member States shall, in liaison with the Commission, coordinate among themselves their policies and programmes in the areas referred to in paragraph 1. The Commission may, in close contact with the Member States, take any useful initiative to promote such coordination.
3. The Community and the Member States shall foster cooperation with third countries and the competent international organisations in the sphere of public health.
4. The Council, acting in accordance with the procedure referred to in Article 251 and after consulting the Economic and Social Committee and the Committee of the Regions, shall contribute to the achievement of the objectives referred to in this Article through adopting:
   (a) measures setting high standards of quality and safety of organs and substances of human origin, blood and blood derivatives; these measures shall not prevent any Member State from maintaining or introducing more stringent protective measures;
   (b) by way of derogation from Article 37, measures in the veterinary and phytosanitary fields which have as their direct objective the protection of public health;
   (c) incentive measures designed to protect and improve human health, excluding any harmonisation of the laws and regulations of the Member States.

The Council, acting by a qualified majority on a proposal from the Commission, may also adopt recommendations for the purposes set out in this Article.

5. Community action in the field of public health shall fully respect the responsibilities of the Member States for the organisation and delivery of health services and medical care. In particular, measures referred to in paragraph 4(a) shall not affect national provisions on the donation or medical use of organs and blood.

Other provisions of the Treaty of Amsterdam also have important implications for public health. For example, Title VI of the Treaty Establishing the European Union, as amended by the Treaty of Amsterdam, contains new measures to combat drug trafficking in the region. The Treaty of Amsterdam also includes formal recognition of human rights, including a new Article 13 to the Treaty on the European Union which provides for measures to combat disability discrimination. Furthermore, the Treaty of Amsterdam promotes the consolidation of environmental policy, emphasizing sustainable development, the consideration of environmental aspects in all sectoral policies, and the simplification of Community decision making.

A series of resolutions and other instruments relating to public health have been adopted by the Council of the European Union or other Community institutions. Of particular interest is Resolution 94/C 165/01 on the Framework for Community Action in the Field of Public Health, adopted by the Council of the European Union (2 June 1994). This Resolution recommended the establishment of a Community framework to enhance co-operation and co-ordination between member states for the protection of public health. It further emphasized that priority should be given to the establishment of Community programmes in cancer, drug dependence, AIDS, and other communicable diseases, and health promotion, education, and training, as well as disease surveillance and the collection of reliable and comparable health data. Following on this Resolution, a number of new programmes have been established within the identified priority areas as well as others. Included are programmes on health monitoring (1997 to 2001), pursuant to Decision No. 1400/97/EC of the European Parliament and of the Council of the European Union (30 June 1997); health promotion, information, education, and training (1996 to 2000), pursuant to Decision No. 654/96/EC of the European Parliament and of the Council of the European Union (29 March 1996); and the prevention of drug dependence (1996– 2000), pursuant to Decision No. 102/97/EC of the European Parliament and of the Council of the European Union (16 December 1996).

In June 1999, the Council of the European Union adopted Resolution 1999/C 200/01 on the future of organizational action in the field of public health. Following on the entry into force of the Treaty of Amsterdam on 1 May 1999, this Resolution recommended review of the internal organization and working methods of the European Union to achieve better co-ordination of its public health policies. It also recommended key challenges that should be addressed within a programme of action in the field of public health, including emerging and re-emerging threats to health; major health scourges; genetic, behavioural, and environmental determinants of health; growing health inequalities; quality assurance; demographic changes and the impact of ageing; social, economic, and political factors; and advances in research and the proliferation of new technologies, in particular biotechnology.

European Free Trade Association

The European Free Trade Association, which now has four members (Iceland, Liechtenstein, Norway, and Switzerland), has been active in the field of pharmaceuticals, having been responsible for the Convention on the Mutual Recognition of Inspections in respect to the Manufacture of Pharmaceutical Products (better known as the Pharmaceutical Inspection Convention) and for the Scheme for the Mutual Recognition of Evaluation Reports on Pharmaceutical Products (better known as the PER Scheme). Many countries that are not members of the European Free Trade Association have adhered to this Convention, originally signed in October 1970.

Organization of African Unity

The Organization of African Unity, with headquarters in Addis Ababa, Ethiopia, was established on 25 May 1963, and the Charter of the Organization was signed on that occasion by 32 independent African states. The purposes of the Organization include promoting the unity and solidarity of the African States; defending the sovereignty of members; eradicating all forms of colonialism; promoting international co-operation having due regard for the Charter of the United Nations and the Universal Declaration of Human Rights; and co-ordinating and harmonizing member states' economic, diplomatic, educational, health, welfare, scientific, and defence policies.

The treaty establishing the African Economic Union (Abuja, Nigeria, 3 June 1991) under the auspices of the Organization of African Unity includes Article 73 (Health), under which member states 'agree to promote and increase cooperation among themselves in the field of health'. To this end, they are to 'cooperate in developing primary health care, promoting medical research, particularly in the field of African traditional medicine and pharmacopoeia'. The Organization of African Unity adopted a Resolution on Bioethics (AHG/Res. 254 (XXXII)) in July 1996 and also served as the forum for the adoption of the Bamako Convention on the Ban of the Import into Africa and the Control of Transboundary Movement of Hazardous Wastes within Africa (30 January 1991).

Organization of American States

The Organization of American States, comprising 35 states from the region of the Americas and located in Washington, DC, is not typically thought of as having a strong mandate in international health law. Although the Organization of American States Charter does not specifically mention health as one of the purposes of the Organization, instruments developed under the auspices of the Organization of American States address regional public health concerns. Article 10(1) of the Additional Protocol to the Inter-American Convention on Human Rights in the Area of Economic, Social and Cultural Rights provides that '[e]veryone shall have the right to health, understood to mean the enjoyment of the highest level of physical, mental and social well-being'. Recent Organization of American States instruments with an important health component include the 1994 Inter-American Convention to Prevent and Punish Torture, the 1996 Inter-American Convention on the Prevention, Punishment and Eradication of Violence Against Women, and the 1998 Draft Inter-American Convention on the Elimination of All Forms of Discrimination Against People with Disabilities. The role of the Organization of American States in regional standard-setting is analysed by Gorove *et al.* (1999).

Pan American Health Organization

The Pan American Health Organization (**PAHO**), which serves as the WHO Regional Office for the Americas, administers the Pan American Sanitary Code, signed at Havana on 14 November 1924. Based in Washington, DC, in 1950 PAHO was recognized as a specialized Inter-American organization pursuant to the Charter of the Organization of American States.

The Constitution of PAHO specifies that the fundamental purposes of the Organization 'shall be to promote and coordinate efforts of the countries of the Western Hemisphere' to 'combat disease, lengthen life, and promote the physical and mental health of the people'. The 'objects' in the current version of the Pan American Sanitary Code include the prevention of the international spread of communicable infections of human beings, the promotion of co-operative measures for the prevention of the introduction and spread of disease into and from the territories of the signatory governments, the standardization of the collection of morbidity and mortality statistics by the signatory governments, and the stimulation of the mutual interchange of information that may be of value in improving the public health and combatting the diseases of humans (PAHO 1991).

Reference should be made to Resolution CSP25.R15 adopted by the Pan American Sanitary Conference in 1998, instructing PAHO to 'begin a study of the feasibility of preparing a regional convention against tobacco use' and to 'submit a progress report in 1999'. The legal authority of PAHO to adopt and promote conventions and the relationship of a regional convention on tobacco control to the proposed WHO Framework Convention on Tobacco Control is examined in the feasibility study commissioned by PAHO pursuant to Resolution CSP25.R15 (Gorove *et al.* 1999).

Non-governmental organizations

The principal non-governmental organizations whose statements and declarations have exerted an impact on national health law include the Council for International Organizations of Medical Sciences based in Geneva, the World Medical Association based in Ferney-Voltaire, France, the Commonwealth Medical Association based in London, the World Psychiatric Association, and various other organizations focusing on particular issues in the field of health care and/or bioethics. Recent products of these organizations include the Commonwealth Medical Association's Guiding Principles on Medical Ethics in Human Rights (1995) and the Declaration on the Role of Medical Ethics and Woman's Right to Health, including Sexual and Reproductive Health (1997). The following resolutions and statements were recently adopted by the General Assembly of the World Medical Association:

- Statement on Family Planning and the Right of a Woman to Contraception (1996)
- Statement on Professional Responsibility for Standards of Medical Care (1996)
- Resolution on Cloning (1997)
- Statement on Health Hazards of Tobacco Products (1997)
- Proposal for a United Nations Rapporteur on the Independence and Integrity of Health Professionals (1997)
- Resolution on Economic Embargoes and Health (1997)
- Declaration of Ottawa on the Right of the Child for Health Care (1998)
- Resolution on Medical Care for Refugees (1998)
- Declaration on Nuclear Weapons (1998).

International health instruments as they affect certain sectors of health

Ageing

The United Nations General Assembly has been active in the field of ageing and has adopted numerous programmes and resolutions in this field. Resolutions adopted during the last decade include:

- 1999 Resolution on the International Year of Older Persons
- 1998 Resolution on the International Year of Older Persons: Towards a Society for All Ages
- 1992 Proclamation on Ageing
- 1991 Resolution on the Implementation of the International Plan of Action on Ageing and Related Activities.

HIV/AIDS

In 1996, the United Nations undertook a major reform of the intergovernmental organizational framework for addressing AIDS. A new Joint United Nations Programme on HIV/AIDS (**UNAIDS**) based in Geneva, commenced in January 1996. UNAIDS supersedes the WHO Global Program on AIDS, which itself replaced the WHO Special Programme on AIDS.

The new organization, UNAIDS, is a partnership effort of six institutional cosponsors: the United Nations International Children's Emergency Fund (**UNICEF**), the United Nations Development Program, the United Nations Population Fund, UNESCO, the WHO, and the International Bank for Reconstruction and Development (World Bank).

The United Nations and its organs have adopted a series of international instruments on HIV/AIDS and HIV/AIDS-related discrimination, including Resolution 1999/49 on the Protection of Human Rights in the Context of HIV and AIDS, adopted by the Commission on Human Rights on 27 April 1999 and the Resolution on Discrimination in the Context of HIV or AIDS, adopted on 24 August 1995 by the United Nations Sub-Commission on Prevention of Discrimination and Protection of Minorities. In addition, the International Guidelines on HIV/AIDS and Human Rights were jointly issued by the Office of the United Nations High Commissioner for Human Rights and UNAIDS (UN 1998*c*). The guidelines are designed to provide an international framework for discussion of human rights and public health considerations in the context of HIV/AIDS at the national, regional, and international level. See Gostin and Lazzarini (1997) for a discussion of international human rights in the context of HIV/AIDS.

At the regional level, a substantial number of instruments relating to HIV/AIDS and HIV/AIDS-related discrimination have been adopted in Europe, starting with the Parliamentary Assembly of the Council of Europe Resolution 812 (1983) which, among other things, drew attention to various human rights issues raised by HIV/AIDS, including the dangers of discrimination against homosexuals and the need for respect for privacy of AIDS-related information.

The European Community has developed numerous texts establishing a regional strategy to address HIV/AIDS, including the European Parliament and Council Decision No. 1729/95 on the extension on the Europe against AIDS programme (19 June 1995) and Decision No. 647/96 (29 March 1996) on a programme of Community action on the prevention of AIDS and certain other communicable diseases within the framework for action in the field of public health (1996 to 2000). To facilitate global co-ordination, the Council of the European Union adopted Regulation No. 550/97 (24 March 1997) on HIV/AIDS-related operations in developing countries. The Organization of African Unity Declaration on the AIDS Epidemic of 19 June 1995 also established a regional approach to address the issue.

Since 1987 the WHO has developed a series of statements, recommendations, and the like, which have influenced the current configuration of HIV/AIDS legislation. Resolution WHA 41.24, adopted by the 41st World Health Assembly in May 1988, is an early instrument in the field. This Resolution specifically addressed the need to 'protect the human rights and dignity of HIV-infected people and people with AIDS...and to avoid discriminatory action against and stigmatization of them in the provision of services, employment and travel'.

Significant international and regional documents in this field appear in a listing generated by UNAIDS (1999). UNAIDS has also recently produced a guide to United Nations human rights machinery (1997). See the section on blood and blood products below for a discussion of blood safety in the context of AIDS.

Biomedical science

Dramatic advances in biomedical science during the past decade have triggered numerous initiatives at the international, regional, and non-governmental level, particularly in relation to human rights and human experimentation. Instruments that address bioethics and human experimentation are described below in the section on human experimentation.

Despite the extensive international activity in this area, there is still no legally binding global instrument that addresses the global implications of advances in genetic science. In November 1997, the UNESCO General Conference adopted the Universal Declaration on the Human Genome and Human Rights, the first global instrument to address a broad range of human rights and public health implications of advances in genetic science. The seven chapters of the Declaration cover such topics as human rights, research on the human genome, and co-operation between industrialized and developing countries. The Universal Declaration on the Human Genome and Human Rights was endorsed by the General Assembly in Resolution 53/152 of 9 December 1998.

At the regional level, the Council of Europe has developed the first legally binding regional instrument designed to preserve human rights through a series of principles and prohibitions against the misuses of biological and medical advances. The Council of Europe's Convention for the Protection of Human Rights and Dignity of the Human Being with Regard to the Application of Biology and Medicine: Convention on Human Rights and Biomedicine was opened for signature on 4 April 1997 and entered into force on 1 December 1999. Article 2 of the Convention proclaims that 'The interests and welfare of the human being shall prevail over the sole interest of society or science'. Substantive articles of the Convention address human rights in relation to genetic science, including free and informed consent, non-discrimination, scientific research, genetic counselling, and medical privacy. Notably, Article 13 of the Convention prescribes that interventions seeking to modify the human genome may only be undertaken for preventive, diagnostic, and therapeutic purposes and not to introduce modifications in the genome of any descendants. On 1 December 1999 a protocol to the Convention on the Prohibition of Cloning Human Beings entered into force. The Council of Europe has also developed a Draft Additional Protocol on the Transplantation of Organs and Human Tissues of Human Origin to the 1997 Convention on Human Rights and Biomedicine. The Draft Protocol was examined by the Steering Committee on Bioethics during its 15th meeting (7–10 December 1998) and authorized for publication for consultation purposes by the Committee of Ministers at its 658th meeting (2–3 February 1999). The Council of Europe is preparing additional protocols to the Convention on Human Rights and Biomedicine relating to organ transplantation, biomedical research, the protection of the human embryo and fetus, and problems relating to human genetics. The Council of Europe has recently issued a report on the Convention on Human Rights and Biomedicine (1998*b*).

On 8 July 1996, the Organization of African Unity adopted a Resolution on Bioethics (AHG/Res. 254 XXX.II). Finally, a Resolution on Bioethics and its Implications Worldwide for Human Rights Protection was adopted by consensus by the 93rd Inter-Parliamentary Conference of Inter-Parliamentary Union on 1 April 1995.

The WHO plays an important role in the ethical and public health discourse relating to biomedicine and has published guidelines on ethical issues in medical genetics and genetic services (WHO 1998*d*).

Fluss (1995, 1997*a*,*b*, 1998*a*) has recently examined the contributions of international law and international organizations to the field of bioethics and human rights. International human rights and bioethics is also examined by Le Bris *et al.* (1998) and Schwartz (1997). In addition, Taylor (1999) has analysed international standard setting in this field and UNESCO's Universal Declaration on the Human Genome and Human Rights.

Recent advances in genetics have also led to the development of resolutions and declarations at the non-governmental level. Reference should be made to the 1994 Declaration of Ixtapa adopted by the Council for International Organizations of Medical Sciences; the 1996 Statement on the Principled Conduct of Genetics Research adopted by the Human Genome Organisation; the 1996 Draft International Convention on the Human Genome prepared by the International Bar Association; and the 1992 Declaration on the Human Genome Project adopted by the World Medical Association.

Following the successful cloning of a sheep, numerous initiatives related to research on cloning and human health have been put forth. These include the Council of Europe's Additional Protocol on the Prohibition of Cloning Human Beings to the Convention on Human Rights and Biomedicine (1997), the World Medical Association Resolution on Cloning (1997), and the World Health Assembly Resolution 50.37 on Cloning in Human Reproduction (1997) and Resolution 51.10 on Ethical, Scientific and Social Implications of Cloning in Human Health (1998). The WHO has recently examined the implications of cloning for human health (WHO 1998*e*) and has developed draft guiding principles in this field (WHO 1999*a*).

Blood safety

Many international instruments exist in the area of blood safety. As early as May 1975, the 28th World Health Assembly adopted Resolution WHA 28.72 (Utilization and Supply of Human Blood and Blood Products), under which member states were urged, among other things, 'to enact effective legislation governing the operation of blood services and to take other actions necessary to protect and promote the health of blood donors and of recipients of blood and blood products' WHO (1994*b*). The WHO published Requirements for the Collection, Processing and Quality Control of Blood, Blood Components and Plasma Derivatives and the Consensus Statement on Screening of Blood Donations for Infectious Agents Transmissible through Blood Transfusion was developed by what was known as the Global Blood Safety Initiative and issued by the WHO in 1991.

Numerous instruments addressing blood safety have been adopted in Europe. In 1998 the Council of the European Union adopted Recommendation 98/463 on the suitability of blood and plasma donors and the screening of donated blood in the European Community. This Recommendation established standards for screening of blood donors, the screening of donations, and the recording of appropriate data to ensure the safety of blood and plasma donations and the transfusion process. Resolution 96/C 164/01 and Resolution 96/C 374/01, adopted by the Council of the European Union on 2 June 1995 and 12 November 1996 respectively, affirm the need to develop a strategy to promote self-sufficiency and safety of blood supplies in the European Community.

The Council of Europe has also developed and adopted a number of instruments dealing with the safety of blood and blood supplies. The Council of Europe *Guide to the preparation, use and quality assurance of blood components* (1999*b*) was adopted in 1995 as a technical appendix to Council of Europe Recommendation R (95) 15 on the preparation, use, and quality assurance of blood components and forms the basis for many national guidelines. Recommendation R (95) 14 addresses the protection of health of blood donors and recipients in blood transfusions. A recent Council of Europe publication reviews the history of blood transfusion in Europe and the legal framework in which it has developed (1998*a*).

Chemical safety

The 1998 Convention on the Prior Informed Consent for Certain Hazardous Chemicals and Pesticides in International Trade, adopted under the auspices of UNEP and the Food and Agricultural Organization, is the most recent international instrument designed to promote health and environmental protection in international trade in chemicals and pesticides. The Prior Informed Consent Convention codifies a voluntary programme on chemicals operated by Food and Agricultural Organization and UNEP since 1989, based on the amended London Guidelines for the Exchange of Chemical Information in International Trade and the International Code of Conduct on the Distribution and Use of Pesticides (Prabhu 1993).

The Convention on the Prior Informed Consent for Certain Hazardous Chemicals and Pesticides in International Trade covers pesticides and industrial chemicals that have been banned or severely restricted for health and environmental reasons by participating parties. Currently, 29 chemicals are included in the Prior Informed Consent Convention procedure. This Convention allows governments that import banned or severely restricted chemicals to make informed regulatory decisions about future imports and allows the global community to monitor and control trade in toxic substances. It also mandates that export of a chemical can only take place with the prior informed consent of the importing party. It specifically excludes certain groups of chemicals, such as narcotic drugs, radio-active materials, wastes, chemical weapons, pharmaceuticals, foods, and food additives.

There have also been recent developments in the international regime governing the transboundary movement of hazardous wastes pursuant to the 1989 Basel Convention on the Transboundary Movements of Hazardous Wastes and their Disposal. The Basel Convention establishes a notice and consent system for the transboundary movement of hazardous wastes. Subject to certain agreements, States Parties are generally prohibited from trading in wastes covered by the Convention with non-Parties. In September 1995, the Third Conference of the Parties adopted an amendment to the Convention that, when ratified by three-quarters of the Parties, will greatly restrict hazardous wastes exports from developed to developing countries. In addition, the Basel Protocol on Liability and Compensation was adopted on 10 December 1999. Reference should also be made to the Bamako Convention, developed under the auspices of the Organization of African Unity.

Other instruments in this field currently under development include a Biosafety Protocol to the 1992 Convention on Biological Diversity, which entered into force on 29 December 1993. The Convention on Biological Diversity is the first international instrument to address conservation of biological diversity and the equitable sharing of its benefits. Responding to the mandate of Article 19.3 of the treaty, in November 1995 the Second Conference of the Parties to the Convention initiated negotiation of a protocol to address any threat to the conservation and sustainable use of biodiversity posed by living, genetically modified organisms. The core function of the proposed protocol will be to enable importing nations to learn in advance of the possible entry of genetically modified organisms and thereby have the opportunity to prohibit importation.

Intergovernmental negotiations concluded in December 2000 on the development of a Draft Protocol to the Convention on Long-range Transboundary Air Pollution on Persistent Organic Pollutants. UNEP defines persistent organic pollutants as 'chemical substances that persist in the environment, bioaccumulate through the food web, and pose a risk of causing adverse effects on human health and the environment'.

Other existing instruments that exert an impact on national legislation in this area are the 1985 Vienna Convention for the Protection of the Ozone Layer and the 1987 Montreal Protocol on Substances that Deplete the Ozone Layer, both developed under the auspices of UNEP. The Montreal Protocol mandates that ratifying nations gradually reduce their consumption and production of certain ozone-depleting chemicals. The international ozone regime established by the Vienna Convention, widely considered a success story in international law making, is described at length by Benedick (1998).

Another highly significant instrument is the 1992 United Nations Framework Convention on Climate Change. The Climate Change Convention obligates all States Parties to develop inventories of their emissions (carbon dioxide, methane, nitrous oxide, and others) and includes a pledge by industrialized countries to aim to reduce their emissions to 1991 levels by the year 2000. The Climate Change Convention, however, did not impose a legally binding cap on greenhouse gas emissions. In December 1997, States Parties adopted the Kyoto Protocol to the Climate Change Convention, which establishes caps on the emissions of greenhouse gases from industrialized nations. The Kyoto Protocol also establishes market-based approaches for implementing these caps.

Child health

Concern for the health of children is expressed in numerous international instruments. The 1966 Covenant on Economic, Social and Cultural Rights provides for measures to be undertaken by States Parties to achieve full realization of the right to health, including in Article 12.2(a) 'the provision for the reduction of the stillbirth-rate and of infant mortality and for the healthy development of the child'.

Certain conventions developed under the auspices of the International Labour Organization relate to the protection of children from harmful work, the establishment of minimum ages to begin employment, and required conditions of employment. In 1999 the International Labour Organization General Conference adopted the Convention Concerning the Prohibition and Immediate Action for the Elimination of the Worst Forms of Child Labour. This convention seeks to eliminate and prohibit the worst forms of child labour, including slavery and all practices similar to slavery such as the compulsory recruitment of children into armed forces.

The most significant international instrument addressing children's health rights is the Convention on the Rights of the Child adopted by the United Nations General Assembly in Resolution 44/25 of 20 November 1989 and entered into force on 2 September 1990. Article 24 of the Convention, which addresses the children's health rights, is examined by Pais (1997), UNICEF (1998), and van Buren (1995).

Another important instrument is the World Declaration and Plan of Action, adopted at the 1990 World Summit for Children, which includes targeted reductions in infant and child mortality as well as targeted increases in access to basic services for health to be achieved in children's health by the year 2000.

At the regional level, the Additional Protocol to the American Convention on Human Rights in the Area of Economic Social and Cultural Rights (Protocol of San Salvador) contains several provisions relevant to children's health rights. Article 15(3)(c) provides that States Parties undertake to 'adopt special measures for the protection of adolescents in order to ensure the full development of their physical, intellectual, and moral capacities'. Garcia-Mendez (1998) has recently examined children's rights in Latin America, and the Council of Europe (1996*a*,*b*) has published reports on children's rights, including health rights, in Europe.

At the non-governmental level, the 1998 World Medical Association Declaration of Ottawa on the Rights of the Child to Health Care addresses a broad range of child health-care issues, including quality of care, informed consent and self-determination, confidentiality of medical data, child abuse, and health education.

Communicable disease control

Upon its establishment in 1948, the WHO inherited from its predecessor health organizations the responsibility for management of the international legal regime for the control of the international spread of disease. This regime was based on a series of international agreements and conventions dating from 1892. The revision and consolidation of these international sanitary conventions and agreements was undertaken by the WHO, starting in 1948. Regulations were first adopted by the Fourth World Health Assembly in 1951 as WHO Regulations No. 2, the International Sanitary Regulations (1951 Regulations).

The 1951 Regulations have been subject to a number of revisions, resulting generally from global improvements in knowledge and control of epidemic diseases. The 1951 Regulations were renamed the International Health Regulations in 1969. Last revised in 1981, the International Health Regulations are binding international law for all member states of the WHO (except Australia), subject to limited reservations by certain counties.

Fluss (1997*b*), retired chief of health legislation at the WHO, citing the WHO's former Legal Counsel, Frank Gutteridge, has observed that:

> The inconsistency of the earlier regime under the succession of conventions and agreements was apparent: none of these entirely replaced each other, they did not take account of new methods available for the control of the diseases they covered, and they were not framed to deal adequately with the greatly increased volume and speed of international traffic. For years, it has been pointed out that the need for the health control of international traffic could be obviated if the transmission of disease was stopped or reduced in the places where it principally occurred. However, this is a solution which cannot be obtained by an international instrument but only by improvement of the health conditions of the peoples of WHO's member states. Any attempt to control diseases by the imposition of barriers at frontiers is by definition fortuitous, since frontiers are political and do not necessarily constitute a natural barrier to the spread of infection. To obtain effective control of the international spread of diseases required sound epidemiological services with reliable disease surveillance and the frank and rapid exchange of information among national epidemiological services.

Although a considerable improvement over earlier conventions and agreements, the International Health Regulations have come under detailed scrutiny by scholars and practitioners. Recent critical commentary on the efficacy of the current version of the International Health Regulations has included recommendations to enhance co-ordination with the World Trade Organization on trade-related aspects of infectious diseases (Plotkin and Kimball 1997) and to develop an effective monitoring institution for the International Health Regulations (Taylor 1997). Following the WHO's adoption of a framework convention-protocol approach for global tobacco control, another commentator recommended applying a parallel international regulatory strategy for infectious disease control (Fidler 1999).

The WHO is revising the International Health Regulations into a working global alert system to adapt to changes in disease epidemiology and control and to substantial increases in the volume of international traffic (Gostin 1998). The WHO Secretariat expects that the revised International Health Regulations will be submitted for consideration for adoption at the May 2002 World Health Assembly. The WHO is consulting with the Members of the Committee on Sanitary and Phytosanitary Measures of the World Trade Organization to explore mechanisms that can minimize any conflict in the application of measures under the International Health Regulations and the Committee on Sanitary and Phytosanitary Measures Agreement (WHO 1999*b*). Both the Committee on Sanitary and Phytosanitary Measures Agreement and the International Health Regulations are concerned with minimizing interference with international trade and traffic because of unwarranted health measures.

In the administration of the regulations, the WHO has produced a number of publications for the use of its member states and others. The regulations are available in an 'annotated' edition which includes, in addition to the text of the articles, the format of international certificates of vaccination and other health documents required in international travel, as well as information and interpretations of the provisions. Information on the incidence of disease, including communicable diseases under surveillance, is published in the *Weekly Epidemiological Record*.

Disabled people

A number of provisions to protect the rights of disabled people are established in various United Nations and regional instruments. At the global level, the United Nations General Assembly Declaration on the Rights of Disabled Persons (1975) is an important early instrument in the field. In 1993, the General Assembly adopted the Standard Rules on the Equalization of Opportunities for Persons with Disabilities. Although they are non-binding, the Standard Rules reflect a political commitment on behalf of states to take action for the equalization of opportunities for people with disabilities and provide a basis for technical co-operation among states, the United Nations, and other international organizations.

The past decade has seen a rapid expansion in international standard setting in the field of disability by regional organizations. One of the most significant advances in international disability law is the Draft Inter-American Convention on the Elimination of All Forms of Discrimination Against Persons with Disabilities (1998), developed under the auspices of the Organization of American States. Although subject to a number of significant exceptions or exclusions, Article 3 of the Draft Convention mandates that States Parties adopt broad-based measures to eliminate discrimination against people with disabilities by both public and private entities. See also Article 18 of the Additional Protocol to the American Convention on Human Rights in the Area of Economic, Social and Cultural Rights (Protocol of San Salvador).

The Treaty of Amsterdam (1998) establishes significant measures to address the human rights of people with disabilities. It amends the Treaty on European Union to create a new Article 13 that prohibits discrimination on the basis of disability. The Intergovernmental Conference that negotiated the Treaty of Amsterdam sought an even stronger guarantee of the protection of the fundamental human rights of people with disabilities by including a declaration in the Final Act that states that the Community's institutions must take account of the needs of people with disabilities when adopting measures to approximate member states' legislation.

Important secondary sources on international disability law and policy include Leo *et al.* (1996), Cabrit (1996), and Despouy (1991).

Environmental protection

The vast field of international environmental law is not typically thought of as part of international public health law. But, as Kiss (1998) has noted:

> Admittedly, the convergence between human health and the environment was not obvious to everyone, at least not at the beginning. It should not be forgotten that the prime objective of the protection of the environment was the safeguard of nature, understood essentially as wild nature. The discovery of the problems of pollution affecting the oceans, continental waters and the atmosphere, now considered as natural resources—thus as elements perceived as being in a relationship with man—has broadened the horizons and fields of action for environmental protection.

Modern environmental hazards, including pollution of the seas, watercourses, lakes, and continental waters, air pollution, solid and hazardous waste accumulation and transfer, chemical and radiation hazards, climate change, transboundary air pollution, stratospheric ozone depletion, deforestation, and land degradation, to name a few, are widely recognized as having critical implications for global public health. In recent decades, the United Nations and its agencies, including the International Maritime Organization and UNEP, have taken the lead in bringing international environmental concerns to the attention of the world community and fostering global and regional co-operation through numerous binding and non-binding international instruments.

The conceptual link between the human health and environmental protection has been strengthened by the gradual recognition and integration of 'sustainable development' within the global environmental agenda. In 1987, the World Commission on Environment and Development defined 'sustainable development' as development that meets the needs of the present without compromising the ability of future generations to meet their own needs. UNEP, in Governing Council Decision 15/2 of May 1989, added that sustainable development requires 'the maintenance, rational use and enhancement of the natural resource base that underpins ecological resilience and economic growth and 'implies progress towards international equity'. The significance of sustainable development to international health law is aptly stated by Kiss (1998).

> A decisive step was taken at the end of the 1980s with the fusion between environment and development, given that health problems have long been considered as constituting an aspect of development. Principle One of the Declaration adopted at the United Nations Conference on Environment and Development (Rio de Janeiro, 3–14 June 1992), in affirming that human beings are at the centre of concerns for sustainable development—a concept that expresses the integration of environment and development—thus seals the alliance between preoccupations and measures concerning, on the one hand, human health and, on the other, the environment.

Although some aspects of international environmental law are addressed in other parts of this chapter, this formidable field and its relation to public health cannot be fully covered here. For recognized scholarship in international and regional environmental law see Birnie and Boyle (2001), Weiss (1989, 1993), Weiss *et al.* (1992), Kiss and Shelton (1991), and Sands (1991).

Food safety

The WHO collaborates with Food and Agricultural Organization in the administration of the Codex Alimentarius Programme, which was initiated to promulgate food standards to protect consumers' health and ensure fair practices in the food trade. The standards prescribe requirements pertaining to food hygiene, food additives, food contaminants, food labelling, and so forth. The Codex Alimentarius consists of standards, recommended codes of practice, and guidelines. A Codex standard sets out the required qualities of food commodities, as sold, in objective terms. The Codex Alimentarius Commission recommends the standards to the governments of the member states of the Food and Agricultural Organization and the WHO. Codex Codes of Practice and Codex Guidelines are advisory instruments, covering such matters as good manufacturing practices and nutrition labelling. These are sent to governments as recommendations. The legal basis for the Codex Alimentarius operations and the procedures it is required to follow are published in the procedural manual, which is currently in its 10th edition (FAO/WHO 1999).

The Codex Alimentarius standards have recently been incorporated as binding standards in the international legal regime for food trade. Expanding international trade in food has markedly increased the risk for cross-border transmission of infectious diseases and has led to rapid expansion in international food safety standard setting (Kaferstein and Abdussalam 1998). The Uruguay Round of Multilateral Trade Negotiations (1994) led to a number of multilateral agreements that entered into force in 1995 and incorporated agriculture, for the first time, under the operational rules of the multilateral trading system. Of particular importance for the trade in food are the Agreement on the Application of Sanitary and Phytosanitary Measures (SPS Agreement) and the Agreement on Technical Barriers to Trade (TBT Agreement) (Miyagishima and Kaferstein 1998).

The World Trade Organization agreements provide detailed rules and standards for determining what phytosanitary and sanitary measures are permitted, based upon risk assessment and scientific support, including the Codex Alimentarius. The TBT Agreement, which deals with aspects of food labelling and claims relating to health and nutrition, is designed to encourage the development of international standards, technical regulations, and conformity assessment systems to facilitate trade. Standards established by the Codex

Alimentarius are specifically recognized in Technical Regulations and Standards provisions contained in Article 2 of the TBT Agreement.

The Sanitary and Phytosanitary Measures Agreement is designed to promote free trade by ensuring that measures taken by countries to protect human, animal, or plant life or health are based on scientific evidence and are not used as pretexts to protect domestic markets from international competition. Central to the Sanitary and Phytosanitary Measures Agreement is the required use of established international standards, guidelines, or recommendations rather than domestic standards to promote international harmonization of measures. Regarding food safety, the Sanitary and Phytosanitary Measures Agreement specifically incorporates the standards, guidelines, and recommendations established by the Codex Alimentarius Commission.

The adoption of the Codex Alimentarius standards as norms for the purposes of the Sanitary and Phytosanitary Measures and TBT Agreements is of considerable significance: the Codex Alimentarius standards have become a central component of the legal framework within which world food trade is facilitated (FAO/WHO 1999). The implications of the World Trade Organization regime for food safety have recently been examined by Charnovitz (1997, 1998).

The Rome Declaration on World Food Security, adopted at the 1996 World Food Summit organized by the Food and Agricultural Organization reaffirms the 'right of everyone to safe and nutritious food, consistent with the right to adequate food and the fundamental right of everyone to be free from hunger'. Article 21 of the World Food Summit Plan of Action sets forth strategies and goals, amongst others, to improve the safety of the food supply.

Eide has extensively examined the relationship between nutrition and human rights (Eide *et al.* 1984, 1996).

It is not possible within the confines of this chapter to describe fully the food safety instruments developed by the European Community, primarily in the form of directives. However, Council Directive EC/222 (23 April 1990), as amended, on the deliberate release into the environment of genetically modified organisms is particularly noteworthy. Part C of the Directive establishes a Community procedure enabling the competent authority of a member state to give consent to placing products consisting of genetically modified organisms on the market.

Health services

There have been major developments in international standards for trade in health services in the past 5 years. With the conclusion of the Uruguay Round of Trade Negotiations and the establishment of the World Trade Organization, the World Trade Organization Member States adopted the General Agreement on Trade in Services (**GATS**), which has significant implications for health services. GATS is the first multilateral agreement to provide legally enforceable rights to trade in all services, subject to certain exceptions, including services provided in the exercise of governmental authority.

Although still relatively modest, trade in health-care services is growing rapidly and has considerable potential as a foreign-exchange earner for developing countries (Kinnon 1998; UNCTAD/WHO 1998). GATS also has potentially wide-ranging ramifications for international health services, as it addresses every possible means of supplying a service, including the right to set up a commercial presence. Health services sectors addressed by GATS include foreign direct investment in the health sector; health-care services for those who travel abroad for treatment: telemedicine; services provided abroad by expatriate health personnel; and medical training of foreign students. The World Trade Organization has recently published a document analysing the health services implications of GATS (WTO 1998*b*). Bettcher *et al.* (2000) have also recently examined the implications of the World Trade Organization regime for trade in health services.

Human experimentation

Of all the topics covered in this chapter, human experimentation may well be the area that has attracted the largest number of international efforts to address the ethical and legal dimensions. Perhaps the best-known formulation is that of the International Covenant on Civil and Political Rights (1966), Article 7 of which proscribes that 'no one shall be subjected without his free consent to medical or scientific experimentation'.

The 1947 Nuremberg Code, which was enumerated as part of a judgment at the trial of Nazi doctors in post-Second World War Germany, was the first international code to establish ethical standards for human experimentation. The principles of the Nuremberg Code have been embodied in many subsequent codes governing medical ethics and biomedical research. Numerous intergovernmental and non-governmental organizations have addressed issues surrounding medical and scientific experimentation, notably the World Medical Association in the Declaration of Helsinki (1989), the Council for International Organizations of Medical Sciences and the WHO in the International Guidelines for Ethical Review of Epidemiological Studies, and the WHO in the Guidelines for Good Clinical Practice for Trials on Pharmaceutical Products. The Declaration of Helsinki has recently been examined by Fluss (1999*a*).

Reflecting developments in biomedical research and bioethics over the past decade or so, recent international, regional, and non-governmental instruments have focused on human experimentation in the context of genetics research. Such instruments include UNESCO's 1997 Declaration on Human Rights and the Human Genome, the Council for International Organizations of Medical Sciences' 1993 International Ethical Guidelines for Biomedical Research Involving Human Subjects, and the Council of Europe's draft Protocol on Biomedical Research to the Convention on Human Rights and Biomedicine. The WHO has also addressed human experimentation in the *Proposed International Guidelines on Ethical Issues in Medical Genetics and Genetic Services* (WHO 1997*b*).

Human experimentation is also addressed in the field of humanitarian law and prohibited by numerous provisions of the 1949 Geneva Convention and the 1977 Protocols:

- Convention (I) for the Amelioration of the Condition of the Wounded and Sick in Armed Forces in the Field
- Convention (II) for the Amelioration of the Condition of the Wounded, Sick and Shipwrecked Members of Armed Forces at Sea
- Convention (III) Relative to the Treatment of Prisoners of War
- Convention (IV) Relative to the Protection of Civilian Persons in Time of War
- Protocol Additional to the Geneva Conventions of 12 August 1949, and relating to the Protection of Victims of International Armed Conflicts (Protocol I)

- Protocol Additional to the Geneva Conventions of 12 August 1948, and relating to the Protection of Victims of Non-International Armed Conflicts (Protocol II).

Many concepts and ideas that have arisen in the framework of human experimentation have been widely accepted in other areas of human health. Specifically, reference should be made to the 1978 Belmont Report, prepared by the United States National Commission for the Protection of Human Subjects of Biomedical and Behavioural Research, which consists of a set of ethical principles and guidelines for the protection of human subjects of research. These principles, well described by Gillon (1994), have been formulated and applied in different contexts. For example, Last (1992) has formulated them as follows in the context of public health, rather than biomedical research:

- respect for autonomy means concern about human dignity and freedom, the fundamental rights of the individual
- non-maleficence is the principle of not harming, derived from the ancient *maxim primum non nocere* (first do no harm); this may have had greater force in former times when medical care was often hazardous, but it remains relevant today
- beneficence is the principle of doing good, which members of the professions related to public health practice often believe to be the main function of health care
- justice in the ethical sense means natural justice, distributive justice—fairness, equality, and impartiality.

The Nuremberg Code and its significance for the contemporary framework for international standards on medical ethics and human experimentation has been examined in a collection of essays edited by Annas and Grodin (1992). In addition, reference should be made to a symposium edited by Dickens *et al.* (1991) and to Fluss (1998*b*) for national and international ethical guidelines for research on human populations.

Infant feeding and nutrition

In 1981 the World Health Assembly adopted the International Code of Marketing of Breast-milk Substitutes in the form of a recommendation under Article 23 of the WHO Constitution. The aim of the code is to contribute to the provision of safe and adequate nutrition for infants by protecting and promoting breast feeding and by ensuring the proper use of breast-milk substitutes when these are necessary, on the basis of adequate information and through appropriate marketing and distribution.

The Convention on the Rights of the Child (1989) recognizes the role of breast feeding in infant nutrition. Article 24(e) of the Convention specifies that State Parties shall take appropriate measures to 'ensure that all segments of society, in particular parents and children, are informed, have access to education and are supported in the use of basic knowledge of child health and nutrition, the advantages of breast feeding, hygiene and environmental sanitation and the prevention of accidents'. UNICEF has sought to operationalize the International Code of Marketing Breast-milk Substitutes by promoting it as a practical mechanism to fulfil State obligations under Article 24(e) with respect to State Parties that have ratified the Convention on the Rights of the Child (UNICEF 1997). In 1991, WHO and UNICEF launched the Baby-Friendly Hospital Initiative, a global advocacy campaign to encourage hospitals to adhere to measures to promote breast feeding.

The 1992 World Declaration on Nutrition and Plan of Action for Nutrition, products of the International Conference on Nutrition, reaffirmed the role of breast feeding in infant nutrition. Article 30 of the Plan of Action, adopted by 159 states, sets forth a detailed list of measures to promote breast feeding.

Difficulties in implementing the International Code of Marketing Breast-milk Substitutes and in promoting breast feeding are widely recognized (IGBM 1997). According to the WHO's Global Data Bank on Breast-Feeding, which covers 94 countries and 65 per cent of the world's infant population, only 35 per cent of infants worldwide are exclusively breast-fed at some point between birth and 4 months (WHO 1997*a*).

Shubber has recently published a comprehensive book on the International Code of Marketing Breast-milk Substitutes (1998).

Mental health

Perhaps the most important recent text at the global level is the Principles for the Protection of People with Mental Illness and the Improvement of Mental Health Care, adopted by United Nation General Assembly Resolution 46/119 of 17 December 1991. One of the Principles (23) provides that 'States should implement these Principles through appropriate legislative, judicial, administrative, educational and other measures'. At the European level, an important instrument in the field is Recommendation R (83) 2 of the Committee of Ministers of the Council of Europe (adopted on 22 February 1983) 'concerning the legal protection of persons suffering from mental disorder placed as involuntary patients'. On 12 April 1994, the Parliamentary Assembly of the Council of Europe adopted Resolution 1235 (1994) on psychiatry and human rights which affirms, 'the time has come for the member states of the Council of Europe to adopt legal measures guaranteeing respect for human rights of psychiatric patients'.

The WHO has developed guidelines intended to assist countries in the development of mental health legislation and other measures to protect the human rights of people with mental disabilities. These documents include *Guidelines for the Promotion of the Rights of Persons with Mental Disorders* (WHO 1995*a*) and *Mental Health Care Law: Ten Basic Principles* (WHO 1996*a*).

At the non-governmental level, provisions that may be useful in the development of mental health legislation are also contained in the Declaration of Madrid, approved by the General Assembly of the World Psychiatric Association on 25 August 1996.

Narcotics and psychotropic substances

There is a complex international regime governing narcotic and psychotropic substances. The three major global treaties in the field are the 1961 United Nations Single Convention on Narcotic Drugs and the 1972 Protocol amending that Convention; the 1971 United Nations Convention on Psychotropic Substances; and the 1988 United Nations Convention Against Illicit Traffic in Narcotic Drugs and Psychotropic Substances. The International Narcotics Control Board, an independent and quasi-judicial control organ established by the 1961 Single Convention on Narcotic Drugs, is the primary implementing agency of the United Nations narcotics conventions.

The three major United Nations drug control treaties are complementary. The 1961 Single Convention on Narcotic Drugs and the 1971 Convention on Psychotropic Substances are intended to ensure the availability of narcotic drugs and psychotropic substances for medicinal and scientific purposes and to prevent their distribution through illicit channels. These two treaties also include general provisions on illicit trafficking and drug abuse. The 1988 Convention Against the Illicit Traffic in Narcotic and Psychotropic Substances provides for comprehensive measures against drug trafficking, including the establishment of internationally recognized criminal offenses relating to drug trafficking and money laundering that are to be criminalized under the domestic laws of the parties to the Convention. It also provides a framework for international co-operation through, amongst other measures, extradition of drug traffickers, controlled deliveries, and transfer of proceedings. The Convention further requires that States Parties enact broad-based domestic laws providing for the confiscation of drug proceeds or instrumentalities used, intended to be used, or derived from the drug trafficking activities. In 1998 the United Nations published an official commentary on the 1988 Convention to assist states in interpreting and implementing the Convention (UN 1998*a*). The 1988 Convention and its implementation by States Parties is reviewed by Gurule (1998).

To assist States in giving effect to the United Nations drug control conventions, the United Nations International Drug Control Programme in Vienna has developed relevant model legislation on matters ranging from the classification of narcotic drugs to drug trafficking and international co-operation for civil and common law systems (UNDCP 1999).

In Resolution 51/64 of 12 December 1996, the General Assembly called for a special session to consider the fight against illicit narcotic drugs and psychotropic substances and related activities, and to propose new strategies, methods, practical activities, and specific measures to strengthen international co-operation in addressing the problem. At the General Assembly's 20th special session on countering the world drug problem, held on 8 to 10 June 1998, states adopted, without a vote, a Political Declaration, a Declaration on the Guiding Principles of Drug Demand Reduction, and a Resolution on Measures to Enhance International Cooperation to counter the world drug problem.

The WHO plays an important role in the implementation of United Nations psychotropic and drugs conventions by providing expertise in updating the list of drugs of abuse under the 1961 and Single Convention on Narcotic Drugs and the 1971 Convention on Psychotropic Substances.

Recent initiatives in Europe in this field include Decision 102/97/EC of the European Parliament and of the Council of the European Union (16 December 1996) adopting a programme of Community action on the prevention of drug dependence within the framework for action for public health (1996 to 2000); and Regulation 2046/97 of the Council of the European Union on North–South co-operation in the campaign against drugs and drug addiction.

Nuclear safety and radiation protection

Modern nuclear technology creates public health risks for all states: every state is potentially affected by the risk of radio-active contamination and the long-term health hazards resulting from radiation exposure. It is not possible within the confines of this chapter to discuss in full the numerous international and regional conventions and texts addressing nuclear energy and safeguards.

Both the United Nations and the International Atomic Energy Agency are primary actors in nuclear safety and radiation protection. The 1968 Treaty on the Non-Proliferation of Nuclear Weapons is intended to prevent the spread of nuclear weapons and weapons technology, to foster the peaceful uses of nuclear energy, and to further the goal of achieving general and complete disarmament. The treaty establishes a safeguards system under the responsibility of the International Atomic Energy Agency, which also plays a central role under the instrument in areas of technology and transfer for peaceful purposes. The Non-Proliferation of Nuclear Weapons Treaty, which was originally given a 25-year lifespan, was extended indefinitely in 1995 by the International Atomic Energy Agency Non-Proliferation of Nuclear Weapons Treaty Review and Extension Conference.

The central provision of the Non-Proliferation of Nuclear Weapons Treaty is Article III, which requires bilateral 'full scope safeguards' agreements with the International Atomic Energy Agency by all nuclear facilities of non-nuclear weapons states that are Non-Proliferation of Nuclear Weapons Treaty parties, and International Atomic Energy Agency safeguards in nuclear exports by any of its Parties. As of December 1998, 222 International Atomic Energy Agency safeguard agreements were in force with 138 states. In May 1997, the Board of Governors of the International Atomic Energy Agency approved an agreement to strengthen safeguards on peaceful nuclear activities. The new measures are designed to help the International Atomic Energy Agency detect undeclared nuclear activities, as well as to assist it in determining whether declared ones are being used for nuclear explosive purposes. The agreement, referred to as the Model Protocol, is in the form of a protocol to existing safeguards agreements between the International Atomic Energy Agency and individual states.

Article VII of the Non-Proliferation of Nuclear Weapons Treaty preserves the 'right of any group of States to conclude regional treaties in order to assure the total absence of nuclear weapons in their respective territories'. Recent regional initiatives to develop nuclear-free zones include the 1996 Treaty on the Nuclear-Weapon Free Zone in Africa (Pelindaba Treaty) adopted 11 April 1996, and the Treaty on the Southeast Asia Nuclear-Weapon-Free Zone (Bangkok Treaty) adopted 14 December 1995 and entered into force on 27 March 1997. The Treaty of Tiateloloco, or the Treaty of the Prohibition of Nuclear Weapons in Latin America, was concluded in 1967 and therefore predates the Non-Proliferation of Nuclear Weapons Treaty. However, it is an example of a regional agreement envisioned by Article VII.

The most recent United Nations instrument in this field is the Comprehensive Test Ban Treaty of 1996. This Treaty, which has not yet entered into force, requires States Parties to prohibit and prevent nuclear weapon test explosions or any other nuclear explosions. To facilitate compliance, the Comprehensive Test Ban Treaty established an international organization, the Comprehensive Nuclear Test-Ban Treaty Organization, and a multifaceted verification regime.

A series of treaties designed to moderate the ultrahazarous risks of nuclear energy through international regulation, transboundary co-operation, and liability for damage have been developed and adopted under the auspices of the International Atomic Energy Agency, including the following:

- 1963 Vienna Convention on Civil Liability for Nuclear Damage

- 1980 Convention on Physical Protection of Nuclear Material
- 1986 Convention on Early Notification of a Nuclear Accident
- 1986 Convention on Assistance in the Case of a Nuclear Accident
- 1994 Convention on Physical Protection of Nuclear Material
- 1994 Convention on Nuclear Safety
- 1997 Joint Convention on the Safety of Spent Fuel Management and on the Safety of Radioactive Waste Management.

In addition, in September 1997, governments took a significant step in improving the liability regime for nuclear damage by adopting a protocol to the 1962 Vienna Convention on Civil Liability for Nuclear Damage and a Convention on Supplementary Compensation for Nuclear Damage.

Under Article III.A.6 of its Statute, the International Atomic Energy Agency is authorized to establish or adopt standards of safety in collaboration with the competent organs of the United Nations and the specialized agencies concerned. The Board of Governors of the International Atomic Energy Agency first approved basic radiation standards in 1962 and issued revised versions of those standards in 1967 and 1982. In a jointly sponsored 1994 project with the WHO, PAHO, the Food and Agricultural Organization, the International Labour Organization, and the OECD–Nuclear Energy Agency, the International Atomic Energy Agency approved the International Basic Safety Standards for Protection Against Ionizing Radiation and for Safety of Radiation Sources (IAEA 1995). The Standards are supplemented by many International Atomic Energy Agency guides and supporting documents.

The development of new international standards for radiation safety has been described by González (1994) as 'the product of unprecedented co-operation'. It provides an almost paradigmatic example of how authoritative non-governmental bodies (and specifically the International Commission on Radiological Protection and the International Commission on Radiation Units and Measurements) influence United Nations entities in a process whose international endpoint is safety standards and whose general national endpoint is national legislation. The development of international safety standards for the management of radio-active wastes has been described by Warnecke and Saire (1994). In addition, the eminent scholar Paul Szasz (1970, 1991, 1992, 1994) has examined the role of the International Atomic Energy Agency and international instruments on nuclear safety and liability.

The numerous nuclear safety instruments adopted in the European region include European Council Directive 97/43/Euratom of 30 June 1997 on health protection of individuals against the dangers of ionizing radiation in relation to medical exposures and repealing Directive 84/466/Euratom; European Council Directive 89/618/Euratom of 27 November 1989 on informing the general public about health protection measures to be applied and steps to be taken in the event of a radiological emergency; and European Council Resolution of 8 June 1999 on the limitation of exposure of the general public to electromagnetic fields.

Occupational health

The key role in the development of international law in the field of occupational health has been played by the International Labour Organization. Conventions that have exerted a substantial influence on national legislation in this field as well as new conventions with relevance to occupational health include the following:

- Radiation Protection Convention 1960 (No. 115)
- Benzene Convention 1971 (No. 136)
- Occupational Cancer Convention 1974 (No. 139)
- Working Environment (Air Pollution, Noise and Vibration) Convention 1977 (No. 148)
- Occupational Safety and Health Convention 1981 (No. 155)
- Occupational Health Services Convention 1985 (No. 161)
- Asbestos Convention 1986 (No. 162)
- Chemicals Convention 1990 (No. 170)
- Night Work Convention 1990 (No. 171)
- Prevention of Major Industrial Accidents Convention 1993 (No. 174)
- Part-Time Work Convention 1994 (No. 175)
- Safety and Health in Mines Convention 1995 (No. 176)
- Home Work Convention 1996 (No. 177)
- Worst Forms of Child Labour Convention 1999 (No. 182).

In addition, there are many European Community directives on various aspects of occupational health.

Organ transplantation

A series of international instruments deal with various aspects of organ transplantation, with particular reference to measures to combat commerce in human organs. The first such measure dates from 1970, when the Committee on Morals and Ethics of the (international) Transplantation Society adopted a statement on the subject. In September 1985 the Council of the Transplantation Society proposed a series of guidelines for the distribution and use of organs from cadavers and living unrelated donors. In May 1978 the Committee of Ministers of the Council of Europe adopted Resolution R (78) 29 on 'harmonisation of legislations of member states relating to removal, grafting and transplantation of human substances' (*sic*). Numerous key issues in organ transplantation were addressed in the Final Text adopted by a Conference of European Health Ministers held in Paris on 16 to 17 November 1987, under the auspices of the then French Minister of Health and Family Affairs. Other important instruments are the Committee of Ministers 1997 Recommendation R (97) 16 on liver transplantation from living related donors and 1998 Recommendation R (98) 2 on the provision of haematopoietic progenitor cells.

The Council of Europe has prepared a Draft Additional Protocol on the Transplantation of Organs and Human Tissues of Human Origin to the 1997 Convention on Human Rights and Biomedicine. The Draft Protocol was examined by the Steering Committee on Bioethics during its 15th meeting (7 to 10 December 1998) and authorized for publication for consultation purposes by the Committee of Ministers at its 658th meeting (2 to 3 February 1999). This instrument is designed to define and safeguard the rights of organ and tissue donors, both living and deceased, and the rights of people receiving implants of organs and tissues of human origin. Article 2 limits the scope of the proposed treaty by specifically excluding organs and tissues removed from animals, blood and derivatives, reproductive organs and tissue, and embryonic and fetal organs and tissues (including embryonic stem cells). The transplantation of embryonic and fetal organs and tissues will be addressed in another draft protocol to the Convention being prepared on the protection of the human embryo and fetus.

Another regional initiative was the adoption of a Unified Arab Draft Law on Human Organ Transplants by the 12th session of the Council of Arab Ministers of Health (Khartoum, 14 to 16 March 1987).

The WHO has also been active in this field. The Guiding Principles of Human Organ Transplantation, which were adopted by the 44th World Health Assembly in May 1991 and other related activities, as well as relevant national legislation, have been published by the WHO (1991). In 1996, the WHO established a Task Force on Organ Transplantation to identify the medical, social, economic, ethical, and related issues involved in human organ transplantation. The work of the WHO Task Force is reviewed by Dickens (1998).

International efforts are also being made to address the ethical, legal, and public health dimensions of the rapidly moving field of xenotransplantation. Xenotransplantation involves the grafting of cell tissues or organs from non-human species into humans. The emphasis of the discussion on xenotransplantation has shifted from the rights and welfare of non-human source animals to deepening concern about the public health risk of transmission of disease (Daar 1999). In September 1997, for example, the Committee of Ministers of the Council of Europe adopted Recommendation R (97) 15 calling upon governments of member states to establish mechanisms for the registration and regulation of certain aspects of xenotransplantation to minimize the risk of transmission of diseases and infections. In 1999, the Parliamentary Assembly of the Council of Europe, in Recommendation 1399, called for the Committee of Ministers to work toward the development in all member states of a legally binding moratorium on clinical xenotransplantation and to consider the feasibility of elaborating a new protocol to the Convention on Human Rights and Biomedicine on xenotransplantation.

In 1997, a WHO meeting of global experts established a uniform set of recommendations on xenotransplantation consisting of technical and ethical guidelines to minimize the risk of infection, safeguard human dignity and human rights, and ensure animal welfare (WHO 1998*f*).

Patients' rights

There have been major developments in the formulation of international standards in patients' rights over the past decade, particularly in Europe. Emerging threats to the confidentiality of personal medical data resulting from the development of sophisticated biotechnology and medical information systems have hastened the elaboration of instruments designed to protect personal privacy and confidential medical information. For example, the Committee of Ministers Recommendation R (97) 5 to Member States on the protection of medical data, 13 February 1997, sets forth detailed standards for the collection, processing and confidentiality of medical data.

Other significant developments include the adoption of a Declaration on the Promotion of Patients' Rights in Europe, endorsed by a WHO European Consultation on the Rights of Patients (Amsterdam, 28 to 30 March 1994), which has been published by the WHO (1994*a*, 1995*b*). The Amsterdam Declaration on the Promotion of Patients' Rights recognizes the right of every citizen to respect, dignity, integrity, privacy, informed consent, confidentiality, care, and treatment. The Statement on the Promotion of Patients' Rights was adopted by the European Forum of Medical Associations and the WHO in Stockholm 1 to 2 February 1996, and the 1996 Statement on Professional Responsibility for Standards of Medical Care was adopted by the World Medical Association.

In addition, in an April 1999 meeting organized by the WHO, the Nordic Council of Minsters, and the Nordic School of Public Health, a new European network on patients' rights was launched by patients' organizations, health professionals, and ministries of health in the 38 countries of the WHO European Region.

Fluss (1994*a*), Chapman (1997), and Zielinski (1994) have examined international patients' rights issues.

Pharmaceuticals, medical devices, and cosmetics

A very large number of international texts deal with pharmaceuticals, medical devices, and cosmetics. The WHO has been active in the development of guidance to be used at the country level in the formulation of national laws and regulations dealing with medicinal drugs. The WHO Department of Essential Drugs and Medicines Policy develops and promotes international standards for safety, quality, and efficacy of biological and pharmaceutical products, and it disseminates drug regulatory information. In addition, the WHO Drug Action Programme supports countries in implementing policies and programmes to achieve the objectives of the revised drug strategy.

The Ethical Criteria for Medicinal Drug Promotion were endorsed by the World Health Assembly in a resolution adopted in May 1988, and in 1995 the WHO prepared Guidelines for Good Clinical Practice for trials on pharmaceutical products. In addition, the ninth WHO Model List of Essential Drugs was published in 1997 and work is in progress on the development of a WHO Model Formulary for Essential Drugs. In addition, the WHO Certification Scheme on the Quality of Pharmaceutical Products Moving in International Commerce is subscribed to by some 140 member States.

The WHO has also been actively involved in the so-called **ICH** process (i.e. the convening of a series of International Conferences on Harmonisation of Technical Requirements for Registration of Pharmaceuticals for Human Use), which provides a forum for regulatory authorities and experts from the pharmaceutical industry of the European Union, Japan, and the United States to address scientific and technical aspects of the marketing authorization of pharmaceutical products (Idänpään-Heikkilä 1994).

WHO publications, the quarterly *WHO Drug Information*, and the monthly *WHO Pharmaceuticals Newsletter*, provide current information on drug development, drug regulation, and drug regulatory decisions. A recent WHO report set forth international guidelines and other recommendations to assist national drug regulatory authorities in the quality control of pharmaceutical products (WHO 1996*b*). The WHO has recently published a study on the impact of the World Trade Organization Trade-Related Aspects of Intellectual Property Rights Agreement on global access to drugs (WHO 1998*a*). Bettcher *et al.* have examined the implications of Trade-Related Aspects of Intellectual Property Rights Agreement on access to medical technologies and pharmaceuticals in developing countries (Bettcher *et al.* 2000).

Tarabusi and Vickery (1998) have analysed globalization in the pharmaceutical industry.

Many directives dealing with pharmaceuticals have been developed under the auspices of the European Union, while the Council of Europe has developed a significant number of essentially non-binding recommendations dealing with pharmaceuticals. As mentioned previously, the European Free Trade Association is the intergovernmental organization responsible for the Pharmaceutical Inspection Convention, as well as subsidiary texts (including a scheme for the mutual recognition of evaluation reports on pharmaceutical products). A set of guidelines on good clinical trial practice is among the texts developed under the auspices of the Nordic Council (Nordic Committee on Medicines).

Significant European Union instruments include the Council Directive concerning medical devices (14 June 1993), the Council Resolution on the mutual recognition of the validity of medical prescriptions in member states (20 December 1995), the Council Resolution on medical plant preparations (20 December 1995), and the Council Resolution on generic medicinal products (20 December 1995). Recently, the European Commission has proposed the codification of a new European Parliament and Council Regulation on orphan medicinal products, drugs used for the diagnosis or treatment of diseases that occur in less than 5 per 10 000. The impact of new European authorization procedures has been analysed by Matthews and Wilson (1998).

Council of Europe resolutions in this field include Resolution AP (99) 1 on the classification of medicines which are obtainable only on medical prescription (superseding AP (95) 1); Resolution AP (96) 1 on the declaration of excipients present in pharmaceutical products (superseding Resolution AP (91) 1); Resolution AP (99) 2 on warning phrases for certain categories of medicines (superseding Resolution AP (92) 1); and Resolution AP (99) 1 on the classification of medicines which are obtainable only on medical prescription. In the field of cosmetics, the Council of Europe has published books addressing good manufacturing practices in cosmetics products (Council of Europe 1995, 1999*a*).

Refugees, detainees, and internally displaced people

A number of provisions designed to safeguard the health of people in detention or imprisonment are contained in various United Nations instruments, including the Standard Minimum Rules for the Treatment of Prisoners (1957, 1977); the Basic Principles for the Treatment of Prisoners (1990) (this text, adopted by the General Assembly, states that 'prisoners shall have access to the health services available in the country [of detention] without discrimination on the grounds of their legal situation'); the Body of Principles for the Protection of All Persons under Any Form of Detention or Imprisonment (1988); the United Nations Rules for the Protection of Juveniles Deprived of their Liberty (1990); and the Principles of Medical Ethics relevant to the Role of Health Personnel, Particularly Physicians, in the Protection of Prisoners and Detainees against Torture, and Other Cruel, Inhuman or Degrading Treatment or Punishment (1982). The United Nations Center for Social Development and Humanitarian Affairs has compiled international standards and norms in criminal justice (1992).

At the European level, in 1998 the Council of Europe Committee of Ministers adopted Recommendation R (98) 7 to member states concerning the ethical and organizational aspects of health care in prison. In addition, Tomasevski (1992) has described various other European standards.

The core international instruments addressing refugees and access to health care are the 1951 United Nations Convention Relating to the Status of Refugees and its 1967 Protocol, which expanded the geographic and temporal coverage of the Convention. These instruments are described by Helton (1994). Langren (1999) has examined the protections of the United Nations Convention in relation to regional and bilateral treaties in the field. Amnesty International produced a manual on United Nations human rights mechanisms and refugees (Amnesty International 1997). At the non-governmental level, the Resolution on Medical Care for Refugees, adopted by the World Medical Association in 1998. The rights of refugees and international law are examined in a recent compilation of essays edited by Nicholson and Twomey (1999).

The protection of internally displaced people has recently risen to the fore of the global human rights agenda. Internally displaced people are described by the United Nations High Commissioner for Refugees as people who have been forced to flee their homes suddenly in large numbers, as a result of conflict, internal strife, systematic violations of human rights, or natural or manmade disasters; and who are in the territory of their own country. The estimated 25 million internally displaced people worldwide, also called 'internal' refugees, have traditionally fallen outside the legal foundation for humanitarian assistance and the mandates of refugee and relief organizations because they have not crossed a border (Cohen 1994).

Resolutions of the United Nations General Assembly and the Security Council have increasingly moved towards establishing an entitlement of humanitarian assistance for internally displaced people whose governments are unable or unwilling to provide assistance. In Resolution 45/100 of 1990, the General Assembly affirmed the importance of humanitarian assistance and access and endorsed the establishment of relief corridors to provide assistance to people in need. The role of the Security Council in implementing humanitarian assistance for internally displaced people is described by Henkin (1994).

Although United Nations resolutions have moved in the direction of recognizing the rights of the internally displaced, no specific treaties currently exist in this field. To clarify the international structure for the protection of internally displaced people, the Commission on Human Rights, in Resolution 50/195 of 22 December 1995, and the United Nations General Assembly in Resolution 1996/52 of 19 April 1996, requested the preparation of an appropriate framework for the protection and assistance of the internally displaced. In 1998, the Representative of the Secretary-General of the United Nations completed the Guiding Principles on Internal Displacement, a non-binding document designed to provide information and guidance on international human rights law and international humanitarian law relevant to internally displaced people (United Nations 1998*b*). Principle 7(2) proclaims that authorities undertaking displacements 'shall ensure, to the greatest practicable extent ... that such displacements are effected in satisfactory conditions of safety, nutrition, health and hygiene'. Principle 19 addresses the rights of wounded, sick, and disabled internally displaced people to medical care, the special health needs of women, and the prevention of contagious and infectious diseases, including HIV/AIDS.

Reproductive health

The Programme of Action of the International Conference on Population and Development, adopted in Cairo on 13 September 1994, contains a formulation of reproductive rights and reproductive health. Principle 8 of that formulation states:

> Everyone has the right to the enjoyment of the highest attainable standard of physical and mental health. States should take all appropriate measures to ensure, on a basis of equality of men and women, universal access to health-care services, including those related to reproductive health care, which includes family planning and sexual health. Reproductive health-care programmes should provide the widest range of services without any form of coercion. All couples and individuals have the basic right to decide freely and responsibly the number and spacing of their children and to have the information, education and means to do so. (UN 1994*b*)

The Beijing Declaration, produced by the Fourth World Conference on Women in September 1995, also addresses reproductive rights. Article 17 of the Declaration provides 'The explicit recognition and reaffirmation of the right of all women to control all aspects of their health, in particular, their own fertility, is basic to their empowerment'. In addition, Article 12(1) of the Convention on the Elimination of all Forms of Discrimination Against Women guarantees women equal access to health care services, including family planning services and advice. Article 12(2) further provides that States Parties must ensure appropriate health services in connection with pregnancy, confinement, and the postnatal period.

The United Nations (1996) and the United Nations Population Fund (1997) have examined global reproductive rights and reproductive health (1996). In addition, Tomasevski (1994), and Issacs and Freedman (1992) provide an examination of international law and policy on reproductive rights.

The Council of Europe Convention on Human Rights and Biomedicine is the first treaty to address some of the implications of genetic advances for reproductive rights. Article 14 of the Convention prohibits the use of techniques of medically assisted procreation for the purpose of choosing a future child's sex, except where serious hereditary sex-related disease is to be avoided. In addition, the Council of Europe is developing an additional protocol to the Convention Human Rights and Biomedicine on the human embryo and fetus.

At the non-governmental level, instruments relating to reproductive rights are contained in the 1997 Declaration on the Role of Medical Ethics and a Woman's Right to Health, Including Sexual and Reproductive Health, produced by the Commonwealth Medical Association; the 1997 Recommendations on Ethical Aspects of Sexual and Reproductive Rights adopted by the International Federation of Gynecology and Obstetrics; the 1995 Statement on Ethical Aspects of Embryonic Reduction adopted by the 47th World Medical Assembly; the 1994 Recommendation on Donation of Genetic Material for Human Reproduction adopted by the International Federation of Gynecology and Obstetrics (**FIGO**) Committee for the Study of Ethical Aspects of Human Reproduction; and the 1996 International Planned Parenthood Federation Charter on Sexual and Reproductive Rights.

Fluss (1994*b*, 1997*b*) has reviewed some of the international instruments and texts that have addressed legal and ethical issues of reproductive rights. The WHO, in collaboration with the United Nations Development Programme, the United Nations Population Fund, and the World Bank Special Programme on Research, Development and Research Training in Human Reproduction, has also addressed the ethical aspects of fertility regulation methods.

Right to health

There are numerous provisions for health and health-related matters in international human rights instruments (Mann *et al.* 1994; Fluss 1999*b*). The principal international legal basis for the right to heath is found in the core instruments of international human rights law, the International Bill of Rights. The International Bill of Rights consists of the Universal Declaration of Human Rights (1948), the International Covenant on Economic, Social and Cultural Rights (1966), and the International Covenant on Civil and Political Rights (1966).

Article 25 of the Universal Declaration of Human Rights (1948) proclaims that:

> Everyone has the right to a standard of living adequate for the health and well-being of himself and of his family, including food, clothing, housing and medical care and necessary social services, and the right to security in the event of unemployment, sickness, disability, widowhood, old age or other lack of livelihood in circumstances beyond his control.

The Universal Declaration does not guarantee a right to health *per se*, but a right to health incident to an adequate standard of living. To evidence the legal obligation necessary to advance the rights proclaimed in the Universal Declaration, the United Nations promulgated two treaties, the International Covenant on Civil and Political Rights (1966) (**ICCPR**) and the International Covenant on Economic Social and Cultural Rights (1966) (**ICESCR**). As Henkin has observed, these two treaties 'legislate essentially what the Universal Declaration had declared' (Henkin 1990).

The Universal Declaration of Human Rights provides the normative basis for the most significant United Nations instrument guaranteeing a right to health, the ICESCR. Article 12.1 of the Covenant provides for 'the right of everyone to the enjoyment of the highest attainable standard of physical and mental health'. The ICESCR also provides, among other things, that each nation to the maximum extent of its resources, 'undertakes to take steps' to achieve the 'highest attainable standards of physical and mental health' for all individuals, without discrimination.

Article 12(2) of the Covenant identifies measures to be undertaken by member states to 'achieve the full realization of this right', including those necessary for:

- the provision for the reduction of the still-birth rate and infant mortality and for the health development of the child
- the improvement of all aspects of environmental and industrial hygiene
- the prevention, treatment, and control of epidemic, endemic, occupational, and other diseases
- the creation of conditions which would assure to all medical service and medical attention in the event of sickness.

Following the International Bill of Rights, the General Assembly and other organs of the United Nations have produced numerous declarations and treaties addressing the international right to health of particularly vulnerable populations, including women, children, and disabled and mentally impaired people. These instruments are discussed in elsewhere in this chapter.

The Vienna Declaration and Programme of Action, adopted by the World Conference on Human Rights (14 to 25 June 1993), includes passages that address health and health-related issues. The following passage is particularly noteworthy (UN 1993).

> Everyone has the right to enjoy the benefits of scientific progress and its applications. The World Conference on Human Rights notes that certain advances, notably in the biomedical and life sciences as well as information technology, may have potentially adverse consequences for the integrity, dignity and human rights of the individual, and calls for international cooperation to ensure that human rights and dignity are fully respected in this area of universal concern.

The United Nations regularly publishes compilations of all international (universal and regional) instruments in the field of human rights. Many of the relevant texts are also reproduced in Brownlie (1992). Amnesty International (1999) and Fluss (1999*b*) have recently published extensive bibliographies on select aspects of health and human rights.

With respect to regional instruments, Brownlie (1992) points out that the European Convention on Human Rights (1950) is essentially concerned with political and civil rights, and it was in 1961 that the European Social Charter was adopted to 'develop and protect social and economic rights'. The European Social Charter (Revised) entered into force on 7 January 1999. Item 11 of Part I of the new Charter states that 'everyone has the right to benefit from any measures enabling him to enjoy the highest possible standard of health attainable' and, in item 13, that 'anyone without adequate resources has the right to social and medical assistance'. Of particular importance is Article 11 (the right to protection of health).

> With a view to ensuring the effective exercise of the right to protection of health, the Contracting Parties undertake, either directly or in co-operation with public or private organizations, to take appropriate measures designed amongst others:
> (1) to remove as far as possible the causes of ill-health;
> (2) to provide advisory and educational facilities for the promotion of health and the encouragement of individual responsibility in matters of health;
> (3) to prevent as far as possible epidemic, endemic and other diseases.

The Charter includes provisions on the right to safe and healthy working conditions (Article 3), the right of children and young people to protection (Article 7), the right to social and medical assistance (Article 13), the right of employed women to protection of maternity (Article 8), and the right of physically or mentally disabled people to independence, social integration, and participation in the life of the community (Article 15).

In the Western Hemisphere, the principal human rights instrument is the American Declaration of the Rights and Duties of Man (1948), Article XI of which reads: 'Every person has the right to the preservation of his health through sanitary and social measures relating to food, clothing, housing and medical care, to the extent permitted by public and community resources'.

There are no specific health provisions in the American Convention on Human Rights (1969), although its Additional Protocol in the Area of Economic, Social, and Cultural Rights (1988) includes a section on the right to health (Article 10).

> 1. Everyone shall have the right to health, understood to mean the enjoyment of the highest level of physical, mental and social well-being;
> 2. In order to ensure the exercise of the right to health, the States Parties agree to recognize health as a public good and, particularly, to adopt the following measures to ensure that right;
> (a) primary health care, i.e. essential health care made available to all individuals and families in the community;
> (b) extension of the benefits of health services to all individuals subject to the State's jurisdiction;
> (c) universal immunization against the principal infectious diseases;
> (d) prevention and treatment of endemic, occupational and other diseases;
> (e) education of the population on the prevention and treatment of health problems; and
> (f) satisfaction of the health needs of the highest risk groups and of those whose poverty makes them the most vulnerable.

Other articles deal with the right to a healthy environment (Article 11), the right to food (Article 12), and the protection of the handicapped (Article 18).

The African Charter on Human and Peoples' Rights (1981) includes the following Article 16.

> 1. Every individual shall have the right to enjoy the best attainable state of physical and mental health.
> 2. States Parties to the present Charter shall take the necessary measures to protect the health of their people and the ensure that they receive medical attention when they are sick.

The preamble to the WHO's Constitution, the first international expression of a right to health, defines health as a 'state of complete, physical, mental and social well-being and not merely the absence of disease or infirmity'. The preamble further declares that '[t]he enjoyment of the highest attainable standard of health is one of the fundamental rights of every human being without distinction of race, religion, political belief, economic or social condition'.

Although there has been a proliferation of international and regional instruments proclaiming the right to health, none of these instruments has elaborated with legal specificity the scope of obligations and individual entitlements with respect to the right to health (Taylor 1992; Molinari 1998). Alston (1994) has put forward proposals on how the economic, social, and cultural rights set forth in the international covenant that addresses these rights could potentially become more effective.

The right to health is commonly viewed as implying a right to health services. Marmor (1991) suggests that 'almost all of the twentieth century debate over the right to health in fact has addressed issues concerning not health *per se* but the distribution of access to medical care'. Others suggest that a requirement to provide healthy living conditions is extremely vague and impossible to satisfy fully and that the rights relating to health set out in the international instruments are expressed in terms too general for them to be invoked as international rules before a domestic judge (von Wartburg 1979; Auby 1981; Hersch 1986). Giesen (1994) analyses the implications of the right to health care (see also Leary 1994; Mann *et. al.* 1994).

The WHO definition has not gone without other criticism. Daniels (1983) has suggested that the inclusion of the reference to social well being amounts to the 'over-medicalization' of the domain of social philosophy.

To restore to the WHO definition the integrity of its purpose, the member states of WHO defined the concept and vision of Health for All, when the 30th World Health Assembly declared that the main social target of governments and the WHO in the coming decades should be 'the attainment by all citizens of the world by year 2000 of a level of health that would permit them to lead a socially and economically productive life'. In the interpretation of this goal by governments and the WHO, the intention is that there is a health baseline below which no individuals in any country should find themselves, and that all peoples in all countries should have a level of health that would enable them to work productively and participate actively in the social life of the community in which they live.

Health for All was conceived as a process leading to progressive improvement in the health of people, not as a single finite target. It combines a set of strategies, plans of action, and managerial processes, with evaluation and monitoring, using indicators developed for this purpose (WHO 1981). The Global Strategy for Health for All by the Year 2000 relied on the concept of country-wide health systems based on primary health care as described in the report of the International Conference on Primary Health Care (WHO 1978). It proposed concerted action in the health and related socio-economic sectors following the principles of the Declaration of Alma-Ata, adopted in 1978 by the International Conference on Primary Health Care, which was jointly sponsored and organized by the WHO and UNICEF. The Declaration of Alma-Ata stated that primary health care was the key to attaining Health for All as part of overall development, and that the approach to attaining health development could be interpreted differently according to the social, economic, and health characteristics of each country.

In May 1995 the World Health Assembly, in Resolution WHA 48.16, requested the Director-General of the WHO to take the necessary steps to develop a new holistic global health policy.

Emerging from a 3-year consultative process, the 51st World Health Assembly, in May 1998, adopted a World Health Declaration stating that 'changes in the world health situation require that we give effect to the Health for All Policy for the 21st century'. The Health for All Policy for the 21st century notes that although the twenty-first century brings with it new threats and new opportunities, new approaches to overcome them are also becoming available. The globalization of trade, travel, technology, and communication could yield substantial benefits, provided serious adverse effects are addressed. In particular, global environmental hazards, and the globalization and mass marketing of harmful commodities, such as tobacco, require urgent attention.

The foundational role of certain values is emphasized in the updated Health for All policy. These core values are recognition that the enjoyment of the highest attainable standard of health is a fundamental human right ('the right to health'), continued and strengthened application of ethics to health policy, research, and service provision, implementation of equity-oriented policies and strategies that emphasize solidarity, and incorporation of a gender perspective into health policies and strategies. This policy approach emphasizes that these values are interlinked and should be incorporated into all aspects of health policy and strategy. The new policy for Health For All in the 21st Century succeeds the Health for All strategy launched in 1977, and will come into action fully within WHO member states and regions in 2002 to 2003. Health for All in the 21st Century is described by Antezana *et al.* (1998) and Yach (1996, 1997*a*, *b*).

Tobacco control

In 1999 the WHO set in motion a process to begin multilateral negotiations on a new treaty to circumscribe the global rise and spread of the tobacco pandemic. If adopted and brought into force, the WHO Framework Convention on Tobacco Control will be the first legally binding convention developed under the auspices of the WHO.

In response to the globalization of the tobacco pandemic, in 1995 the 48th World Health Assembly adopted Resolution WHA 48.11 which, among other things, requested the Director-General to report to the 49th World Health Assembly on the feasibility of developing an international instrument for tobacco control. Reference should be made to the feasibility study commissioned by the WHO calling for the development of a framework convention protocol approach to tobacco control (Taylor and Roemer 1996). On 30 November 1995, the Director-General submitted his report calling for the development of a framework convention-protocol approach to global tobacco control. In 1996, the 49th World Health Assembly, in Resolution WHA 49.17, requested the Director-General to initiate the development of a WHO Framework Convention on Tobacco Control.

In Resolution WHA 52.18 of May 1999, the 52nd World Health Assembly authorized a process leading to formal negotiations of the Convention and called upon member states to adopt the Framework Convention on Tobacco Control no later than May 2003. This Resolution established a Framework Convention on Tobacco Control Working Group to develop proposed draft elements of the Convention and complete its work by May 2000. It further established an intergovernmental negotiating body, which met for the first time in October 2000, to draft and negotiate the framework convention and possible related protocols.

The globalization of the tobacco pandemic and global control strategies is extensively described in Chapter 10.1. Reference should also be made to a number of recent articles that analyse the transnationalization of the tobacco pandemic and the potential role of the WHO Framework Convention on Tobacco Control and related protocols (Taylor 1996; Yach and Bettcher 1998*b*, 2000; Bodansky 1999; Joosens 1999; World Bank 1999; Taylor and Bettcher 2000).

In addition to the WHO framework convention process, a whole series of resolutions have been adopted by successive World Health Assemblies aimed at combatting smoking and other forms of tobacco consumption. These have been described in detail by Roemer (1993). Furthermore, a resolution adopted in October 1992 by the International Civil Aviation Organization addresses smoking restrictions on international passenger aircraft.

There have been various regional initiatives in tobacco control, including certain recommendations adopted under the auspices of the Council of Europe and a series of European Community directives as well as other instruments. Of particular importance is the 1998 Directive 98/43 of the European Parliament and the Council of the European Union on the approximation of the laws, regulations, and administrative provisions of the member states relating to the advertising and sponsorship of tobacco products. This Directive establishes measures gradually to phase out all direct tobacco advertising and promotion in the European Community. Mention should also be made of a series of resolutions on smoking and health issues adopted by the health ministers of the Arab States of the Gulf Area.

Trade and health

The conclusion of the Uruguay Round, marked by the Final Act (GATT 1994), transformed the General Agreement on Tariffs and Trade to a permanent organization, the World Trade Organization. The Multilateral Agreements establishing the World Trade Organization have been compared to a tricycle: 'a driver (World Trade Organization), two large wheels (the thirteen multilateral agreements on trade in goods and the General Agreement on Trade in Services), and a smaller one, the Agreement on Trade-Related Aspects of Intellectual Property' (Berrod and Gippini 1995). These agreements constitute a single undertaking (i.e. a single binding treaty), which must be accepted by members of the World Trade Organization. The World Trade Organization agreements represent a motor of trade liberalization in the global trading system, and a major force behind the globalization of trade in goods and services, information, and investment. Moreover, the global transformation of the world's trading order intersects with global public health in several areas (Kinnon 1995).

With respect to public health, Article XX(b) under the General Exceptions of the General Agreement on Tariffs and Trade (1947), allows 'each contracting party to set its human animal or plant life or health standards' if these restrictions do not represent an 'unjustifiable discrimination or a disguised restriction on international trade'. Under the single package of Multilateral Trade Agreements, Article XX (b) is part of GATT 1994, and in other multilateral agreements, for instance the Technical Barriers to Trade Agreement and the Agreement on Trade-Related Aspects of Intellectual Property similar provisions for the protection of human health and safety are included.

In several disputes on trade issues, Article XX(b) has been enlisted as a justification for restricting or barring trade. In 1990, Thailand referred to Article XX(b) in order to defend its import restrictions on cigarettes. The GATT dispute settlement Panel Report entitled 'Thailand—Restrictions on Importation of and Internal Taxes on Cigarettes' decided that 'GATT consistent measures could be taken to control both the supply of and demand for cigarettes, as long as they were applied to both domestic and imported cigarettes' without discrimination. In other words, comprehensive tobacco control measures, including excise tax increases and advertising bans, were permissible as long as they do not discriminate unduly between foreign and domestic products. The relationship between international trade law and tobacco control is described by Taylor *et al.* (2000).

Article XX(b) has also been referred to in other dispute settlement cases. For instance in 1991, under the old GATT dispute settlement procedure, Mexico complained that the United States could not embargo imports of tuna products from Mexico just because Mexican regulations on the method by which tuna was produced did not satisfy United States regulations. The United States Marine Mammal Protection Act sets standards within its jurisdiction for dolphin protection for fishing fleets catching yellowfin tuna. The GATT dispute settlement panel report found that trade action could not be taken by one country to enforce its own domestic regulations in another country, even if such measures were take to protect animal health. In the end, Mexico did not choose to pursue the case and the panel report was not adopted. Similarly, the United States prohibited imports of shrimp into the United States that were caught in a way which endangered sea turtles. The report released by the Appellate Body of World Trade Organization in October, 1998, stated that one World Trade Organization member could not 'impose its domestic environmental regulations on another member as long as certain safeguards are met'. This report has also not been formally adopted. Such restrictions on the imposition of extraterritorial public health measures/standards, as exemplified by these two cases, would, presumably, also apply to the protection of human public health.

The protection of human health has also been the subject of the World Trade Organization Dispute Settlement Body case on 'European Community Measures Concerning Meat and Meat Products (Hormones)'. In May 1996 the Dispute Settlement Body of the World Trade Organization established a panel on the request of the United States to investigate European Community measures regarding the hormone ban on United States bovine meat and meat products (WTO 1999*d*). Both the panel and the Appellate Body found that the hormones measures taken by the European Community violated the Agreement on Sanitary and Phytosanitary Measures (SPS Agreement) (WTO 1999*e*). Although this decision has not been readily accepted by the European Community, it clearly demonstrates the interface between global trade agreements and the protection of public health.

The globalization of food production and distribution, in conjunction with liberalization of world markets, has led to a ballooning of global food trade to US$266 billion in 1994, which represents an increase of 300 per cent over 20 years. With the growth of world food trade, the risks of infectious disease dissemination have increased accordingly. Therefore, the protection of human health is intimately linked to global trade in food and feedstuffs. International standards on food trade are discussed in the section on food safety in this chapter.

Another multilateral trade agreement with significant implications for public health is the Agreement on Trade-Related Aspects of Intellectual Property. This Agreement establishes minimum standards for governing the scope, availability, and use of intellectual property, including medical technologies and pharmaceuticals. The Trade-Related Aspects of Intellectual Property Agreement extends patent protection, including both product and process patenting, to a minimum of 20 years from the filing date. Under the Trade-Related Aspects of Intellectual Property Agreement, all members of World Trade Organization are given 1 year to fulfil their obligations under the agreement, developing countries are provided an additional 4-year grace period, plus an additional 5 years for countries that had not previously provided for patent protection. Least developed countries are provided a transitional period of 10 years. Discord has already erupted between some developed and developing countries over patent protection of pharmaceuticals, particularly in the context of

HIV/AIDS, and other aspects of the Trade-Related Aspects of Intellectual Property Agreement. In a recent World Trade Organization Dispute Settlement Panel, India-Patent Protection for Pharmaceutical and Agricultural Chemical Products, the United States complained that India was in breach of its obligations under the Trade-Related Aspects of Intellectual Property Agreement. The panel concurred with the United States, concluding that India had failed to ensure adequate mechanisms for ensuring product patents for pharmaceutical and agricultural chemical interventions (WTO 1997*b*).

Weapons systems

It is not possible within the confines of this chapter to cover the vast fields of arms control, peace, and security. Discussion is limited to contemporary international efforts to control the proliferation of particular types of weapons systems recognized as uniquely catastrophic for human health. In particular, global efforts to control nuclear weapons, biological weapons, chemical weapons, landmines, and excessively injurious conventional weapons is reviewed.

By eroding the traditional distinction between combatants and civilians, weapons of mass destruction, including biological, chemical, and nuclear weapons, have emerged as a significant public heath concern. International instruments relevant to nuclear non-proliferation are discussed in the section on nuclear safety and radiation protection above.

The most significant contemporary instrument relating to biological weapons is the 1972 Convention on the Prohibition of the Development, Prevention, and Stockpiling of Bacteriological (Biological) and Toxin Weapons and on their Destruction. The so-called Biological Weapons Convention prohibits the development or acquisition of biological agents or toxins, as well as weapons carrying them and means of their production, stockpiling, transfer, or delivery, except for prophylactic, protective, or other peaceful purposes. Biological weapons, which are agents designed to cause disease and death in humans, animals, and plants, span a wide range of potential infection causing organisms, promoted through various vectors and modes of dispersal. In 1994 an Ad Hoc Group was created to consider possible ways of strengthening the Convention. In 1996 the Ad Hoc Group was called upon to develop a verification protocol to the Biological Weapons Convention within 5 years in order to strengthen implementation of the Convention. The public health implications of biological weapons and efforts to regulate them are examined by Gould and Connell (1997).

Another class of weapons of mass destruction of significant public health concern are chemical weapons. Chemical weapons are poisonous or toxic compounds that are designed to kill or disable by direct effect on body organs and systems. Recognizing that existing treaties did not provide adequate safeguards to prevent the proliferation of chemical weapons, in January 1993 130 nations signed Chemical Weapons Convention. As of March 2000, 131 had ratified or acceded to the treaty. The Chemical Weapons Convention bans production, possession, or transfer of chemical weapons and requires destruction of existing weapons within 10 years after the treaty enters into force. An inspection/verification regime is included in the Convention's provisions.

International initiatives have recently focused on the control of antipersonnel landmines. Landmines are a unique weapons system in that they are victim-activated and may continue to cause death and injury decades after being sown. In December 1997 122 States signed the Convention on the Prohibition of the Use, Stockpiling, Production and Transfer of Anti-Personnel Mines and their Destruction (the Ottawa Treaty). This instrument, which is significant for being the first treaty to ban an entire class of weapons already in widespread use, is examined by Thakur and Maley (1999).

A key instrument in the field of conventional weapons is the 1980 Convention on Prohibitions or Restrictions on the Use of Certain Conventional Weapons which May Have Been Deemed to be Excessively Injurious or to have Indiscriminate Effects (**CCW**), which entered into force on 2 December 1983. The CCW does not contain any prohibitions on the use of specific weapons. Rather, provisions on the prohibition or restrictions on the use of certain weapons are elaborated in protocols to the Convention. Article 4(3) of the CCW proscribes that only states that have expressed their consent to be bound by at least two of these Protocols at the time of deposition of its instrument of ratification, acceptance or approval, or of accession may be bound by the Convention. The Conventional Weapons Convention and the first three protocols were adopted by States Parties, by consensus, on 10 October 1980. Protocols to the Convention include: the 1980 Protocol on Non-Detectable Fragments (Protocol I) (entered into force 2 December 1983); the 1980 Protocol on Prohibitions or Restrictions on the Use of Mines, Booby-Traps and Other Devices as amended on 3 May 1996 (Protocol II) (entered into force, as amended, 3 December 1998); the 1980 Protocol on the Prohibitions or Restrictions on the use of Incendiary Weapons (Protocol III) (entered into force 2 December 1983); and the 1995 Protocol on Blinding Laser Weapons (Protocol IV) (entered into force 30 July 1998).

Women's health

While the core instruments of international human rights law (the Universal Declaration, and the International Covenants on Civil and Political Rights and on Economic Social and Cultural Rights) declare that all people are entitled to human rights and fundamental freedoms without discrimination, international organizations have not, until recently, paid significant attention to issues of human rights affecting women, including health rights. The United Nations Commission on the Status of Women, a body established under the United Nations Charter in 1947, was until 1982 the only public international body devoted entirely to the pursuit of women's human rights.

A major accomplishment of the Commission on the Status of Women is the development of the Convention on the Elimination of All Forms of Discrimination Against Women (**CEDAW**), adopted by the General Assembly in 1979 and ratified by 130 states in December 1993. Article 12(1) of CEDAW provides that 'States Parties shall take all appropriate measures to eliminate discrimination against women in the field of health care in order to ensure, on a basis of equality of men and women, access to health care services, including those related to family planning'. The Committee on the Elimination of Discrimination Against Women, the body charged with monitoring the implementation CEDAW, has recently produced an extensive interpretation of Article 12 along with recommendations to governments (CEDAW 1999). On 6 October 1999 the General Assembly adopted an Optional Protocol to the Convention which creates a communications procedure to allow individuals and groups to submit complaints to the Committee against State Parties to the Protocol for grave or systematic violation of rights established by the Convention. The Optional Protocol has not yet entered into force.

Reference should also be made to the Beijing Declaration and Platform for Action adopted by the Fourth World Conference on Women, held in Beijing in September 1995 for an elaboration of women's health rights. In 1996 the General Assembly, in Resolution 50/203, specifically endorsed the Beijing Declaration and the Platform for Action, and called upon bodies of the United Nations system to implement the Platform for Action.

Violence against women in both the public and private spheres has recently attracted a number of international initiatives. Both CEDAW and the World Conference on Women Platform for Action recognize the right of women to be free from violence. The Committee on the Elimination of Discrimination Against Women in its General Recommendation 19 defines gender-based violence as 'violence directed against a women because she is a woman or that affects women disproportionately, as discrimination'. Such violence includes acts that inflict physical, mental and sexual harm or suffering, threats of such acts, coercion, and other deprivations of liberty (Llic and Corti 1997). Reference should also be made to the 1996 Inter-American Convention on the Prevention, Punishment and Eradication of Violence Against Women (Convention of Belem do Para), developed under the auspices of the Organization of American States.

Scholarly contributions in the field include Alfredsson and Tomasevski (1995), Cook (1994), and Schuler (1995).

Conclusion

To mark the 40th anniversary of the establishment of the WHO, the editors of the *International Digest of Health Legislation* organized a Round Table on the Future of International Health Law, which was published by the WHO in 1989. This consisted of lead contributions from Bélanger and Mikhailov as well as comments from five experts in the field.

In his contribution, Mikhailov was singularly forward-looking, expressing the view that international health law is a rapidly evolving branch of international law and commenting that:

> Although this may be unrealistic at the present time, and indeed even ridiculous, I for my part am convinced that the day will come when international health law will contain rules aimed at eliminating ... tobacco use ... which cause(s) enormous damage to health. Efforts to combat these scourges are being carried out in certain countries with varying degrees of success. One could in fact envisage that these efforts be made global in character and that an international law framework be developed. This would be difficult to achieve at the present time but could become a reality one day. Certain actions could indeed be carried out forthwith, examples being the development of conventions prohibiting advertising for tobacco products.

This was written 10 years before the 191 member states of 52nd World Health Assembly adopted, by consensus and without objection, a resolution to set in motion a process leading to the adoption of a WHO framework convention on tobacco control.

Grad (1998) has observed:

> The reach of public health law is as broad as the reach of the public health itself. Public health and public health law expand to meet the needs of our society. The scope and the reach of public health law have expanded enormously during the past fifty years and continue to expand today.

This chapter illustrates that the scope and depth of international health law has evolved dramatically in the last several decades and now encompasses increasingly complex concerns such as biotechnology, organ transplantation, and global trade in food, medicine, and health services. In addition, international health law now incorporates various other legal subjects, including environmental protection, arms control, and population control. The rapid development of binding international law and non-binding standards and guidelines endorsed and adopted by the world community provide a framework for global co-operation and co-ordination in an increasingly interdependent world.

Health development in the twenty-first century is likely to include expanded use of international norms, standards, and instruments. As the world becomes more interdependent, innovative global health development strategies are needed to address the increasingly complex and interrelated health problems. Globalization makes multilateral collective action, through the further development and refinement of international norms and standards, imperative to protect and promote world health.

Health development in the twenty-first century must take advantage of the opportunities afforded by global change and, at the same time, minimize the risks and threats associated with globalization so that the dramatic improvements in the health of the world's population achieved in the twentieth century can be maintained and advanced in the twenty-first.

References

Abbing, H.D.C. (1998). Health, human rights, and health law: the move towards internationalization, with special emphasis on Europe. *International Digest of Health Legislation*, **49**, 101–112.

Adede, A.O. (1987). *The International Atomic Energy Agency notification and assistance conventions in the case of a nuclear accident: landmarks in the multilateral treaty-making process.* Graham and Trotman, Boston, MA.

Alfredsson, G. and Tomasevski, K. (ed.) (1995). *A thematic guide to documents on the human rights of women: global and regional standards adopted by intergovernmental organizations, international non-governmental organizations and professional associations.* Martinus Nijhoff, Dordrecht.

Alston, P. (1994). The UN's human rights record: from San Francisco to Vienna and beyond. *Human Rights Quarterly*, **16**, 375–90.

Amnesty International (1997). *The UN and refugees' human rights: a manual on how UN human rights mechanisms can protect the rights of refugees.* Amnesty International, London.

Amnesty International (1999). Publications on health and human rights themes: 1982–1998. *Health and Human Rights*, **4**, 215–64.

Annas, G.J. and Grodin, M.A. (1992). *The Nazi doctors and the Nuremberg Code: human rights in human experimentation.* Oxford University Press, New York.

Antezana, F.S., Chollat-Traquet, C.M., and Yach, D. (1998). Health for all in the 21st century. *World Health Statistics Quarterly*, **51**, 3–6.

Auby, J.M. (1981). *Le droit de la santé*, p. 19. Presses Universitaires de France, Paris.

Bélanger, M. (1983). *Droit international de la santé.* Economica, Paris.

Bélanger, M. (1985). *Les Communautes Europennes et la Santé.* Presses Universitaires, Bordeaux.

Bélanger, M. (1989). *Droit international de la santé par les textes.* Berger-Levrault, Paris.

Benedick, R.E. (1998). *Ozone diplomacy: new directions in safeguarding the planet.* Harvard University Press, Cambridge, MA.

Berrod, F. and Gippini, F.E. (1995). The common institutional framework of the new world trade system. In *The Uruguay Round results: a European lawyer's perspective.* European Interuniversity Press, Brussels.

Bettcher, D.W. (1997). *Think and act globally and intersectorally to protect national health.* Document WHO/PPE/PAC/97.2. WHO, Geneva.

Bettcher, D.W. and Yach, D. (1998). The globalization of public health ethics? *Millennium Journal of International Studies*, **27**.

Bettcher, D.W., Sapirie, S., and Goon, E.H.T. (1998). Essential public health functions: results of the international Delphi study. *World Health Statistics Quarterly*, **51**, 44–54.

Bettcher, D.W., Yach, D., and Guindon, G.E. (2000). Global trade and health: key linkages and future challenges. *Bulletin of the World Health Organization*, **78**, 521–34.

Birnie, P.W. and Boyle, A.E. (2001). *International law and the environment* (2nd edn). Clarendon Press, Oxford.

Bodansky, D. (1999). *The framework convention-protocol approach. FCTC Technical Briefing Series.* Document WHO/NCD/TFI/99.1. WHO, Geneva.

Brownlie, I. (ed.) (1992). *Basic documents on human rights* (3rd edn). Oxford University Press.

Brownlie, I. (1998). *Principles of public international law.* Oxford University Press.

Cabrit, A. (1996). *Handicapés, tous vos droits (The full rights of the disabled)* (2nd edn). Héricy, Paris.

CEDAW (Committee on the Elimination of Discrimination Against Women) (1999). *Implementation of Article 21 of the Convention on the Elimination of All Forms of Discrimination Against Women: General Recommendation on Article 12: Women and Health.* Document CEDAW/C/1999/I/WG.II/WO.2/Rev.1. United Nations, New York.

Centre for Social Development and Humanitarian Affairs, United Nations Office at Vienna (1992). *Compendium of United Nations standards and norms in crime prevention and criminal justice.* United Nations No. E.92.IV.1. United Nations, New York.

Chapman, A.R. (ed.) (1997). *Health care and information ethics: protecting fundamental human rights.* Sheed and Ward, Kansas City, MO.

Charnovitz, S., (1997). The WTO, meat hormones, and food safety. *International Trade Reporter*, **14**, 1779–81.

Charnovitz, S. (1998). Environment and health under the WTO dispute settlement. *International Law*, **32**, 901–21.

Cohen, R. (1994). International protection for internally displaced persons. In *Human rights: an agenda for the next century* (ed. L. Henkin and J.L. Hargrove), pp. 17–48. American Society of International Law. Washington, DC.

Cook, R.J. (1994). *Women's health and human rights: the promotion and protection of women's health through international human rights law.* WHO, Geneva.

Council of Europe (1995). *Guidelines for good manufacturing practice of cosmetic products.* Council of Europe Publishing, Strasbourg.

Council of Europe (1996*a*). *Children's rights and child policies in Europe: new approaches, Leipzig 30 May to 1 June 1996.* Council of Europe Publishing, Strasbourg.

Council of Europe (1996*b*). *The rights of the child—a European perspective.* Council of Europe Publishing, Strasbourg.

Council of Europe (1998*a*). *Blood transfusion: half a century of contribution by the council of europe.* Council of Europe Publishing, Strasbourg.

Council of Europe (1998*b*). *Convention on Human Rights and Biomedicine.* Council of Europe Publishing, Strasbourg.

Council of Europe (1999*a*). *Comparative study of borderline products in the field of cosmetics.* Council of Europe Publishing, Strasbourg.

Council of Europe (1999*b*). *Guide to the preparation, use and quality assurance of blood components* (5th edn). Council of Europe Publishing, Strasbourg.

Daar, A.S. (1999). Animal to human organ transplants—a solution or a new problem? *Bulletin of the World Health Organization*, **77**, 54–61.

Daniels, N. (1983). Health care needs and distributive justice. In *In search of equity: health needs and the health care system* (ed. R. Bayer, A.L. Caplan, and N. Daniels), p. 13. Hastings Center, New York.

Despouy, L. (1991). *Human rights and disability: final report prepared by Leandro Despouy.* United Nations, Economic and Social Council, Commission on Human Rights, Geneva.

Dickens, B.M. (1998). World Health Organization guidelines on transplantation and the WHO task force. In *Organ allocation* (ed. J.L. Touraine *et al.*), pp. 83–94. Kluwer Academic, Boston, MA.

Dickens, B.M., Gostin, L., and Levine, R.J. (ed.) (1991). Research on human populations: national and international ethical guidelines. *Journal of Law, Medicine and Health Care*, **19**, 147–295.

Eide, A., *et al.* (ed.) (1984). *Food as a human right.* United Nations University, Tokyo.

Eide, A., Kracht, U., and Robertson R.E. (ed.) (1996). Nutrition and human rights. *Food Policy*, **21**.

Englert, Y. (1995). *Organ and tissue transplantation in the european union: management of difficulties and health risks linked to donors.* Kluwer Academic, Boston, MA.

FAO/WHO (Food and Agricultural Organization /World Health Organization) (1999). *Understanding the Codex Alimentarius.* FAO, Rome.

Fidler, D. (1999). *International law and infectious diseases.* Oxford University Press.

Fielding, L.E. (1996). Taking a closer look at threats to peace: the power of the Security Council to address humanitarian crises. *University of Detroit Mercy Law Review*, **73**, 551.

Fluss, S.S. (1994*a*). Comparative overview of international and national developments in regard to patients' rights legislation. In *Patients' rights: informed consent, access and equality* (ed. L. Westerhall and C. Phillips), pp. 439–71. Nerenius and Santerus, Stockholm.

Fluss, S.S. (1994*b*). Some international responses to legal/ethical issues in the field of fertility and the human embryo. In *Essays in honour of Jan Stepan on the occasion of his 80th Birthday* (ed. J. Bednarikova and F. Chapman), pp. 151–60. Swiss Institute of Comparative Law, Zurich.

Fluss, S.S. (1995). From bioethics to biolaw: an international overview 1984–1994 (Part II). In *Poverty, vulnerability and the value of human life: a global agenda for bioethics* (ed. Z. Bankowski and J.H. Bryant). Council for International Organizations of Medical Sciences, Geneva.

Fluss, S.S. (1997*a*). Contributions of international organizations. In *Bioethics: from ethics to law, from law to ethics*, pp. 189–204. Schulthess Ploygraphischer Verlag, Zurich.

Fluss, S.S. (1997*b*). International health law. In *Oxford textbook of public health* (3rd edn), Vol. 1, pp. 371–90. Oxford University Press.

Fluss, S.S. (1998*a*). An international overview of developments in certain areas. In *A legal framework for bioethics* (ed. C.M. Mazzoni), pp. 11–37. Kluwer Law International, Deventer.

Fluss, S.S. (1998*b*). The regulation of human experimentation: historical and contemporary perspectives. In *Research on human subjects: ethics, law and social policy* (ed. D.N. Weisstub), pp. 222–42. Elsevier Science, Oxford.

Fluss, S.S. (1999*a*) How the Declaration of Helsinki developed. *Good Clinical Practice Journal*, **6**, 18–22.

Fluss, S.S. (1999*b*). A select bibliography of health aspects of human rights. *Health and Human Rights*, **4**, 215–64.

Fluss, S.S. and Gutteridge, F. (1993). World Health Organization. In *International encyclopedia of medical law* (ed. R. Blanpain). Kluwer Law and Taxation, Deventer.

Garcia-Mendez, E. (1998). *Child rights in Latin America: from 'irregular situation' to 'full protection'.* UNICEF, Geneva.

Gervais, D. (1995). *The TRIPS Agreement: drafting history and analysis.* Sweet and Maxwell, London.

Giesen, D. (1994). Health care as a right: some practical implications. *International Journal of Medicine and Law*, **13**, 285–96.

Gillon, R. (ed.) (1994). *Principles of health care ethics*. Wiley, Chichester. [Contains chapters describing the perspectives of various religions and beliefs on the four principles.]

González, A.J. (1994). Radiation safety: new international standards. *IAEA Bulletin*, **36**, 2–11.

Gostin, L. (1998). Health legislation and communicable diseases: the role of law in an era of microbial threats. *International Digest of Health Legislation*, **49**, 221–39.

Gostin, L.P. and Lazzarini, Z. (1997). *Human rights and public health in the AIDS pandemic*. Oxford University Press.

Gould, R. and Connell, N.D. (1997). The public health effects of biological weapons. In *War and public health* (ed. B.S. Levy and V.W. Sidel), pp. 98–116. Oxford University Press/the American Public Health Association, Oxford.

Grad, F. (1990). *The public health law manual*. American Public Health Association, Washington, DC.

Grad, F. (1998). Public health law: Its forms, function, future and ethical parameters. *International Digest of Health Legislation*, **49**, 19–40.

Gurule, J. (1998). The 1998 UN convention against illicit traffic in narcotic drugs and psychotropic substances—a ten year perspective: is international cooperation merely illusory? *Fordham International Law Journal*, **22**, 74–120.

Helton, A.C. (1994). Refugees: an agenda for reform. In *Human rights: an agenda for the next century* (ed. L. Henkin and J.L. Hargrove), pp. 49–72. American Society of International Law, Washington, DC.

Henkin, L. (1990). *The age of rights*. Columbia University Press, New York.

Henkin, L. (1994). Humanitarian intervention. In *Human rights: an agenda for the next century* (ed. L. Henkin and J.L. Hargrove), pp. 49–72. American Society of International Law, Washington, DC.

Hersch, J. (1986). Human rights in Western thought: conflicting dimensions. *Philosophical Foundations of Human Rights*, p. 144. UNESCO, Paris.

Higgins, R. (1994). *Problems and process: international law and how to use it*. Oxford University Press, New York.

Hiller, T. (1994). *Principles of public international law*. Cavendish Publishing, London.

Howard-Jones, N. (1950). Origins of international health work. *British Medical Journal*, **i**, 1032–7.

Howard-Jones, N. (1975). *The scientific background of the international sanitary conferences, 1851–1983*. WHO, Geneva.

IAEA (International Atomic Energy Agency) (1995). *International Basic Safety Standards for Protection Against Ionizing Radiation and for the Safety of Radiation Sources*. IAEA Safety Series No. 115 IAEA, Vienna.

Idänpään-Heikkilä, J. (1993). Second International Conference on Harmonisation of Technical Requirements for Registration of Pharmaceuticals for Human Use, Orlando, Florida, 27–29 October 1993. *International Digest of Health Legislation*, **45**, 554–7.

IGBM (Interagency Group on Breast-feeding Monitoring) (1997). *Cracking the code: monitoring the international code of marketing of breast-milk substitutes*. IGBM.

Isaacs, S. and Freedman, L. (1992). *Reproductive health/reproductive rights: legal, policy, and ethical issues*. Ford Foundation, Oaxaca.

Joosens, L. (1999). *Improving public health through an international framework convention for tobacco control*. FCTC Technical Briefing Series. Document WHO/NCD/TFI/99.2. WHO, Geneva.

Kaferstein, F.K. and Abdussalam, M. (1998). *Food safety in the twenty-first century*. Proceedings of the 4th World Congress on Foodborne Infections and Intoxications, Berlin, Germany, June 1998.

Kaferstein, F.K., Motarjemi, Y., and Bettcher, D.W. (1997). Foodborne disease control: a transnational challenge. *Emerging Infectious Diseases*, **3**, 503–10.

Kinnon, C.M. (1995). *WTO: What's in it for WHO?* Document WHO/TFHE/99.5. WHO, Geneva.

Kinnon, C. (1998). World Trade: bringing health into the picture. *World Health Forum*, **19**, 397–406.

Kiss, A. (1998). Health legislation and the environment. *International Digest of Health Legislation*, **49**, 207–20.

Kiss, A. and Shelton, D. (1991). *International environmental law*. Ardsley, New York.

Langren, K. (1999). *Deflecting International Protection by Treaty: bilateral and multilateral accords on extradition, readmission and the inadmissibility of asylum requests*. United Nations High Commissioner for Refugees Working Paper No. 10.

Last, J.M. (1992). Ethics and public health policy. In *Maxcy–Rosenau–Last public health and preventive medicine* (13th edn) (ed. J.M. Last and R.B. Wallace), pp. 1187–96. Appleton and Lange, Norwalk, CT.

Le Bris, S., Knoppers, B.M., and Luther, L. (1997). International bioethics, human genetics, and normativity, *Houston Law Review*, **33**, 363–95.

Leary, V. (1994). The right to health in international human rights law. *Health and Human Rights*, **1**, 24–57.

Leo, J.M., Aarts, R., Burkhauser, V., and de Jong, P.R. (ed.) (1996). *An international perspective on disability reform*. Ashgate Publishing, Aldershot.

Llic, Z. and Corti, I. (1997). The convention on the elimination of all forms of discrimination against women. In *Manual on human rights reporting*. United Nations, Geneva.

Mann, J., Gostin, L., *et al.* (1994). Health and human rights. *Health and Human Rights*, **1**, 6–23.

Marmor, T. (1991). The right to health care. In *Rights to health care* (ed. T.J. Bole III and W.B. Bondeson). Kluwer, Dordrecht.

Matthews, D. and Wilson, C. (1998). Pharmaceutical regulation in the single European market. *Medical Law*, **17**, 401–27.

Mikhailov, V.S. (1984). *History of international health law* (in Russian). Far Eastern University Publishing House, Vladivostok. [The Russian term used for health more properly denotes *health protection* and corresponds, in fact, to the word used for *health* in the Russian name of the WHO.]

Miyagishima, K. and Kaferstein, F. (1998). Food safety in international trade. *World Health Forum*, **19**, 407–11.

Molinari, P.A. (1998). The right to health: from solemnity of declarations to the challenges of practice. *International Digest of Health Legislation*, **49**, 41–60.

Nicholson, F. and Twomey, P. (1999). *Refugee rights and realities: evolving international concepts and regimes*. Cambridge University Press.

Office of the UN High Commissioner for Human Rights (1998). UNAIDS, *HIV/AIDS and human rights: international guidelines*. United Nations, New York.

PAHO (Pan American Health Organization) (1991). *Basic documents of the Pan American Health Organization* (15th edn), pp. 1–5. Pan American Health Organization, Washington, DC.

Pais, M.S. (1997). The Convention on the Rights of the Child. In *Manual on human rights reporting*, pp. 393–504. United Nations, Geneva.

Plotkin, B.J. and Kimball, A.M. (1997). Designing the international policy and legal framework for emerging infectious diseases: first steps. *Emerging Infectious Diseases*, **3**, 1–9.

Prabhu, M. (1993). *Overview of international efforts to control toxic chemicals and industrial wastes*. Prepared for the Regional Workshop on Law and Legislation for the Management of Industrial Chemicals and Wastes in the CARICOM. Barbados, 21–23 October 1993. CARICOM.

Roemer, R. (1993). *Legislative action to combat the world tobacco epidemic* (2nd edn). WHO, Geneva.

Ruggie, R. (1995). At home abroad—abroad at home—international liberalization and domestic stability in the new world economy. *Millennium Journal of International Studies*, **24**, 447–70.

Sands, P. (1991). European Community environmental law: the evolution of a regional regime of international environmental protection. *Yale Law Review*, **100**, 2511.

Sands, P. (1995). *Principles of international environmental law*. Manchester University Press.

Schuler, M. (ed.) (1995). *From basic needs to basic rights: women's claim to human rights*. Women, Law and Development International, Washington, DC.

Schwartz, R. (1997). Bioethics policy looking beyond the power of sovereign governments. *Houston Law Review*, **33**, 1283–91.

Shubber, S. (1998). *The International Code of Marketing Breast-Milk Substitutes: an international measure to protect and promote breast-feeding*. Kluwer Law International, Boston, MA.

Szasz, P. (1970). Health and safety. In *The law and practices of the International Atomic Energy Agency*. IAEA, Vienna.

Szasz, P. (1991). Measuring liability for damage due to radioactivity. In *International law and pollution* (ed. D.B. Magraw), pp. 175–95. University of Pennsylvania Press.

Szasz, P. (1992). The IAEA and nuclear safety. *Review of European Community and International Environmental Law*, **1**, 165–72.

Szasz, P. (1994). International Atomic Energy Agency: Convention on Nuclear Safety. *International Legal Materials*, **33**, 1514–16.

Szasz, P. and Rainer, R. (1993). Health and safety. In *The law and practices of the International Atomic Energy Agency 1970–1980*, pp. 409–41. IAEA, Vienna.

Tarabusi, C.C. and Vickery, G. (1998). Globalization in the pharmaceutical industry, part. II. *International Journal of Health Services*, **28**, 281–303.

Taylor, A.L. (1992). Making the World Health Organization work: a legal framework for universal access to the conditions for health. *American Journal of Law and Medicine*, **18**, 301–46.

Taylor, A.L. (1996). An international regulatory strategy for global tobacco control. *Yale Journal of International Law*, **21**, 257–304.

Taylor, A.L. (1997). Controlling the global spread of infectious diseases: toward a reinforced role for the international health regulations. *Houston Law Review*, **33**, 1327–62.

Taylor, A.L. (1999). Globalization and bioethics: UNESCO and an international agenda to protect human rights and public health. *American Journal of Law and Medicine*, **25**, 479–541.

Taylor, A.L. and Bettcher, D.W. (2000). WHO Framework Convention on Tobacco Control: a global 'good' for public health. *Bulletin of the World Health Organization*, **78**, 920–9.

Taylor, A.L. and Roemer, R. (1996). *An international strategy for tobacco control*. Document WHO/PSA/96.6. WHO, Geneva.

Taylor, A.L., Chaleupka, F.J., *et al.* (2000). The impact of trade liberalization on tobacco consumption. In *Tobacco control in developing countries* (ed. P. Jha and F. Chaleupka). Oxford University Press, New York.

Thakur, R. and Maley, W. (1999). The Ottawa Convention on Landmines: a landmark humanitarian treaty in arms control? *Global Governance*, **5**, July–September.

Tomasevski, K. (1992). *Prison health: international standards and national practices in Europe*. Institute for Crime Prevention and Control, Helsinki.

Tomasevski, K. (1994). *Human rights in population policies: a study for SIDA*. Swedish International Development Authority, Stockholm.

UN (United Nations) (1993). Dated 12 July 1993, p. 6 (para. 11). Document A7/CONF/157/23. UN, Geneva.

UN (United Nations) (1994*a*). *Human rights: a compilation of international instruments*. Vol. 1 *Universal instruments*. Vol. 11. *Regional instruments*. UN, Geneva.

UN (United Nations) (1994*b*). *Programme of action adopted at the International Conference on Population and Development*. United Nations, New York.

UN (United Nations) (1996). *Reproductive rights and reproductive health: a concise report*. United Nations, New York.

UN (United Nations) (1998*a*). *Commentary on the United Nations Convention Against Illicit Traffic in Narcotic Drugs and Psychotropic Substances*. United Nations, New York.

UN (United Nations) (1998*b*). *Further promotion and encouragement of human rights and fundamental freedoms, including the question of the programme and methods of work of the commission: human rights, mass exoduses and displaced persons*. Report of the Representative of the Secretary General, Mr Francis M. Dneg, Guiding Principles on Internal Displacement, 11 February 1998. Fifty-fourth Session of the Commission on Human Rights., Item 9(d) of the Provisional Agenda. Document E/CN.4/1998/53/Add.2. UN, Geneva.

UN (United Nations) (1998*c*). *HIV/AIDS and human rights international guidelines: second consultation on HIV/AIDS and human rights, Geneva, 21–25 September 1996*. Document HR/PUB/98.1. United Nations, New York.

UNAIDS (Joint United Nations Programme on HIV/AIDS) (1997). *The UNAIDS guide to the United Nations human rights machinery*. UNAIDS, Geneva.

UNAIDS (Joint United Nations Programme on HIV/AIDS) (1999). Published on the UNAIDS website.

UNCTAD/WHO (United Nations Centre for Trade and Development/ World Health Organization) (1998). *International trade in health services: a development perspective*. Document UNCLAD/IT'D/TS.B/5. UNCTAD/WHO.

UNDCP (United Nations Drug Control Programme) (1999). *Working with governments and countries: model legislation*. UNDCP.

UNFPA (United Nations Population Fund) (1997). *The state of world population, 1997. The right to choose: reproductive rights and reproductive health*. UNFPA, New York.

UNICEF (United Nations Children's Fund) (1997). The international code of marketing of breastmilk substitutes as a practical aid to states parties in implementing the convention on the rights of the child. UNICEF Document prepared for the Working Group on Breast-feeding and Complementary Feeding, March 1997, Kathmandu, Nepal.

UNICEF (United Nations Children's Fund) (1998). *Implementation handbook for the convention on the rights of the child*. UNICEF, New York.

van Bueren, G. (1995). *The international law on the rights of the child programme international rights of the child, University of London*. Martinus Nijhoff, Dordrecht.

von Wartburg, W.P. (1979). A right to health? Aspects of constitutional law and administrative practice. In *The right to health as a human right* (ed. R.-J. Dupuy), pp. 112–21. Sijtoff and Noordhoff, The Hague.

Warnecke, E. and Saire, D.E. (1994).Safety standards for radioactive waste management: documenting international consensus. *IAEA Bulletin*, **36**, 2–11.

Weiss, E.B. (1989). *In fairness to future generations*. United Nations University Press, New York.

Weiss, E.B. (ed.) (1993). *Environmental change and international law*. United Nations University, New York.

Weiss, E.B., Szasz, P., and Magraw, D. (1992). *International environmental law: basic instruments and references*, Volume II. Transnational Publishers.

World Bank (1999). *Curbing the epidemic: governments and the economics of tobacco control*. World Bank, Washington, DC.

WHO (World Health Organization) (1978). *Declaration of Alma-Ata*. Report of the International Conference on Primary Health Care, Alma-Ata, USSR, 6–12 September 1978. 2. WHO, Geneva.

WHO (World Health Organization) (1981). *Global Strategy for Health for All by the Year 2000*. 34. WHO, Geneva.

WHO (World Health Organization) (1989). The future of international health law: a round table. *International Digest of Health Legislation*, **40**, 1–29.

WHO (World Health Organization) (1991). *Human Organ Transplantation: A Report on Developments Under the Auspices of WHO (1987–1991)*. WHO, Geneva.

WHO (World Health Organization) (1993). *Collaboration with the United Nations System-General Matters: Provisional Agenda Item 31.1. 20 April 1993.* Document WHA 46/25. WHO, Geneva.

WHO (World Health Organization) (1994*a*). European consultation on the rights of patients (Amsterdam, 28–30 March 1994) adopts declaration on the promotion of patients' rights in Europe. *International Digest of Health Legislation*, **45**, 410–19.

WHO (World Health Organization) (1994*b*). *WHO Technical Report Series, No. 840.* 34–99. WHO, Geneva.

WHO (World Health Organization) (1995*a*). *Guidelines for the Promotion of Human Rights of Persons with Mental Disabilities.* Document WHO/MNH/MND/95.4. WHO, Geneva.

WHO (World Health Organization) (1995*b*). *Promotion of the rights of patients in Europe.* WHO, Geneva.

WHO (World Health Organization) (1996*a*). *Mental health care law: ten basic principles.* Document WHO/MNH/MND/96.9. WHO, Geneva.

WHO (World Health Organization) (1996*b*). *WHO Expert Committee on Specifications of Pharmaceutical Preparations.* Document technical report series No. 863, 34th Report. WHO, Geneva.

WHO (World Health Organization) (1997*a*). *Implementation of Resolutions and Decisions: Report by the Director General (29 October 1997).* Document WHO/EB/101/10. WHO, Geneva.

WHO (World Health Organization) (1997*b*). *Proposed international guidelines on ethical issues in medical genetics and genetic services.* Report of a WHO meeting on ethical issues in medical genetics. Document WHO/HGN/GL/ETH/98. WHO, Geneva.

WHO (World Health Organization) (1998*a*). Globalization and access to drugs: implications of the WTO/TRIPS Agreement. Document WHO/DAP/98.9. WHO, Geneva.

WHO (World Health Organization) (1998*b*). *Health-for-All in the twenty-first century.* Document WHA 51.5. WHO, Geneva.

WHO (World Health Organization) (1998*c*). *The International Code of Marketing of Breast-Milk Substitutes: summary of action taken by member states and other interested parties 1992–1998.* Document WHO/NUT/98.11. WHO, Geneva.

WHO (World Health Organization) (1998*d*). *Proposed international guidelines on ethical issues in medical genetics and genetic services.* Report of a WHO meeting on ethical issues in medical genetics, Geneva 15–16 December 1997. Document WHO/HGN/GL/ETH/98.1. WHO, Geneva.

WHO (World Health Organization) (1998*e*). *Report by the Director-General: ethical, scientific and social implications of cloning in human health, 51st World Health Assembly, Provisional Agenda Item 20 (8 April 1998).* Document WHA/A51/6 Add. 1. WHO, Geneva.

WHO (World Health Organization) (1998*f*). *Report of WHO Consultation on Xenotransplantation.* Document WHO/EMC/ZOO/98.2. WHO, Geneva.

WHO (World Health Organization) (1999*a*). *Cloning in human health*: Report by the Secretariat. Document WHO/A52/12, 52nd World Health Assembly, 1 April 1999. WHO, Geneva.

WHO (World Health Organization) (1999*b*). Revision of the international health regulations public health and trade: comparing the roles of three organizations. *Weekly Epidemiological Record*, **25**, 123–201.

World Medical Association (1995). *Handbook of Declarations.* WMA, Ferney-Voltaire, France.

WTO (World Trade Organization) (1995*a*). *Selected World Health Organization activities relevant to the implementation of the WTO Agreement on the Application of Sanitary and Phytosanitary Measures. 15 November 1995.* Document G/SPS/W/37. WTO, Geneva.

WTO (World Trade Organization) (1995*b*). Thailand—restrictions on importation of and internal taxes on cigarettes. In *Analytical index: guide to GATT law and practice*, Volume I. WTO, Geneva.

WTO (World Trade Organization) (1997*a*). *European Communities—Measures Concerning Meat and Meat Products (Hormones): Notification of and Appeal by the European Communities under paragraph 4 of Article 16 of the Understanding on Rules and Procedures Governing the Settlement of Disputes (DSU).* 25 September 1997. Document WT/DS26/9. WTO, Geneva.

WTO (World Trade Organization) (1997*b*). *India-Patent Protection for Pharmaceutical and Agricultural Chemical Products: Report of the Appellate Body.* Document WT/DS50/AB/R. WTO, Geneva.

WTO (World Trade Organization) (1998*a*). *European Communities—Measures Concerning Meat and Meat Products (Hormones): Arbitration under Article 21.3c of the Understanding on Rules and Procedures Governing the Settlement of Disputes (Award of the Arbitrator Julio Lacarte-Muro).* 29 May 1998. WTO Document WT/DS26/15 and WT/DS48/13. WTO, Geneva.

WTO (World Trade Organization) (1998*b*). *Health and social services: background note by the Secretariat.* Council for Trade in Services S/C/W/50 (98-3558). WTO, Geneva.

WTO (World Trade Organization) (1999*a*). *Beyond the Agreements: 'The Tuna–Dolphin Dispute'.* WTO Website document.

WTO (World Trade Organization) (1999*b*). *European Communities—Measures Concerning Meat and Meat Products (Hormones).* 14 January 1999. WTO Documents WT/DS26/17 and WT/DS48/15. WTO, Geneva.

WTO (World Trade Organization) (1999*c*). *European Communities—Measures Concerning Meat and Meat Products (Hormones): Communication from the European Communities.* 12 May 1999. WTO Documents, WT/DS26/18, WT/DS48/16. WTO, Geneva.

WTO (World Trade Organization) (1999*d*). *European Communities—Measures Concerning Meat and Meat Products (Hormones): Original Complaint by the United States/ Recourse to Arbitration by the European Communities under Article 22.6 of the DSU decision of the arbitrators.* 12 July 1999. WTO Document WT/DS26/ARB. WTO, Geneva.

WTO (World Trade Organization) (1999*e*). *European Communities—Measures Concerning Meat and Meat Products (Hormones): Recourse by the United States to Article 22.2 of the DSU.* 18 May 1999. WTO Document WT/DS26/19.WTO, Geneva.

WTO (World Trade Organization) (1999*f*). *European Communities—Measures Concerning Meat and Meat Products (Hormones): Status Report by the European Communities.* WTO Documents: WT/DS26/17/Add. 1 and WT/DS48/15/Add. 1 (5 February, 1999; WT/DS26/17/Add. 2 and WT/DS48/15/Add. 2 (9 March 1999); WT/DS26/17/Add. 3 and WT/DS48/15/Add. 3 (16 April 1999), and WT/DS26/17/Add. 4 and WT/DS48/15/Add. 4. WTO, Geneva.

Yach, D. (1996). Renewal of the Health for All Strategy. *World Health Forum*, **17**, 321–49.

Yach, D. (1997*a*). Health for All in the Twenty-first Century. A global perspective. *National Medical Journal of India*, **10**, 82–9.

Yach, D. (1997*b*). The emerging role of public health law in the new policy for the 21st century. In *Souvenir 1997, International Conference on Global Health Law*, 5–7 December 1997. pp. 27–32. Indian Law Institute, New Delhi.

Yach, D. and Bettcher, D. (1998*a*). The globalization of public health. I: Threats and opportunities. *American Journal of Public Health*, **88**, 735–8.

Yach, D. and Bettcher, D. (1998*b*). The globalization of public health. II: The convergence of self-interest and altruism. *American Journal of Public Health*. **88**, 738–41.

Yach, D. and Bettcher, D. (2000). Globalization of tobacco marketing, research and industry influence: perspectives, trends and impacts on human welfare. *Tobacco Control*, **9**, 206–16.

Zielinski, H.L. (1994). *Health and humanitarian concerns: principles and ethics.* Martinus Nijhoff, Dordrecht.

4.4 Ethical principles and ethical issues in public health

K. C. Calman and R. S. Downie

Introduction

Let us begin by accepting the World Health Organization (WHO 1952) definition of the term 'public health' as modified by the Acheson Report (HMSO 1988): 'Public health is the science and art of preventing disease, prolonging life and promoting health through organised efforts of society'. This definition suggests that ethical problems can arise in public health over preventing disease and promoting health. 'Prolonging life', if it is not achieved by preventing disease or promoting health, is a matter for clinical medicine and will not be discussed separately in this chapter. Ethical issues may also arise over the 'organised efforts of society' and over what it means to say that public health is both a science and an art. This discussion is conducted under these headings and encompasses a wide range of ethical issues, including some with international implications.

Medical care ethics and public health ethics

From the time of Hippocrates until the 1960s, medical ethics (or health-care ethics or bioethics) was seen in terms of doctors' duties to patients. These duties have traditionally been thought of as those of not harming the patient (non-maleficence) and of helping the patient (beneficence). Although these principles of non-maleficence and beneficence were interpreted differently in different cultural contexts over the centuries, their exclusiveness was not seriously challenged until the appearance in the 1960s of the patients' rights movement. There were many influences on this movement but an important one was the general democratization of society in the post-Second World War period. The public generally wish to be involved in decisions which are going to affect them. This move to more openness and more consultation has influenced medicine as much as other branches of society. More specifically within medicine the rise of patients' rights movements was influenced by the exposure of abuses in medical research, when it emerged in the 1960s that in some cases informed consent was not being obtained for potentially dangerous research procedures. The result was that, first in the United States and then in the United Kingdom and elsewhere, research ethics committees or human subjects committees were established, which in turn influenced the medical approach to the doctor–patient relationship.

The concept which was adopted to encapsulate the idea of the rights of patients is 'autonomy'. Codes of medical ethics and philosophical discussion from the 1970s increasingly added 'respect for the patient's autonomous decisions' to the duties of non-maleficence and beneficence. To be autonomous is to be self-governing and self-determining. To respect people's autonomous decisions may seem highly desirable. However, the autonomy of the lion can give problems to the lamb! Consider, for example, women's issues. In some countries of the world women have few rights and are treated as second-class citizens. Gender-based violence is common. Genital mutilation is still practised in some places. Clearly in such cultures there is little respect for the autonomy of women. Racial and cultural differences must also be respected, but not to the extent that the rights of women are ignored.

Education is important here. The level of education of the population is closely related to health status. Female literacy, for example, is closely related to significantly reducing mortality in children under 5 years of age, and this is consistent with this relationship worldwide (Caldwell 1986; Sen 1999). Women make decisions about food, health, and lifestyle and are therefore the most important agents for change. Violence against women and the restriction of their roles are particular problems. These are problems of respecting autonomy in diverse cultural contexts.

In the 1960s the concept of justice entered the discussion of health-care ethics. This sometimes seemed to mean treating individual patients justly, say by observing their rights, and sometimes that autonomous patients were all equally entitled to equal shares in the distribution of health care. The latter emphasis is particularly important for public health. Indeed, it is arguable that justice (or equity) raises the most important of the ethical issues for public health. The information given in the first section shows just how variable the levels of health are between countries and within countries there are marked differences in health which can he correlated with differences in the distribution of resources (Whitehead 1987; HMSO 1998). In this context it is worth noting that the first two targets for the European Region of the WHO in the Health for All strategy for the twenty-first century are 'solidarity' and 'equity' with a reduction of inequalities, such is their importance.

In discussions of justice it is important to distinguish 'equity' and 'equality'. The two words have different meanings in relation to health and health care, yet they are often used interchangeably. Equity is about fairness and justice. It has an ethical dimension in that judgements need to be made in relation to society as a whole. It is concerned, therefore, with avoiding unfairness in opportunity and choice. Conversely, equality is about comparisons between the level of health or the ability of individuals and communities to access health care. There are some inequalities which are predictable, but could not be considered inequitable. For example, women live longer than men due to biological differences. This is an inequality but is not inequitable. Equality (and inequality) does not necessarily have an ethical base, though ethics might be relevant in health contexts in which there are neglected risk factors.

The distinction between equity and equality can best be described by looking at those factors which can influence health and health care. It is possible to divide inequalities into those which are unavoidable and, hence, where questions of equity do not arise, and those which might be avoided and thus raise issues of equity. It is useful to look at some examples (Whitehead 1990). In discussing these examples it is important to remember that what is 'unavoidable' at one point in history may become 'avoidable' at another.

Firstly, natural or biological variations such as age, sex, race, and genetic background could be considered as factors which cannot be changed and thus any inequalities related to them unavoidable. For example, older men have a higher incidence of heart disease than younger men, a clear example of an inequality. But no one would consider this related to inequity, except to the extent that risk factor reduction in the elderly has been neglected (Hermanson *et al.* 1988; Omenn 1990).

Secondly, lifestyle and behaviour, if freely chosen, can result in inequalities in health. As an example, cigarette smokers have a higher incidence of lung cancer than non-smokers. This is an inequality, but to the extent that it is created by choice, it might be considered not inequitable. Indeed selective uptake of health promotional initiatives, for example by middle-class groups, could even increase inequalities in health, but could not be considered as unfair, unless it could be established that health promotion is selectively targeted at these groups.

Thirdly, lifestyle and behaviour if not freely chosen and which results in poorer health, is likely to be considered as avoidable by society and thus unfair. Behaviours chosen through a lack of resources, housing conditions, overcrowding, dangerous working conditions, exposure to environmental hazards, or lack of adequate public health response, would be examples. Disabled people often suffer unfairness (inequity) which compounds their already unequal health.

Fourthly, inadequate access to health care or other public services might he inequitable if the cause were avoidable. For example, financial considerations which resulted in a failure to use transport might be one such factor. Another might be lack of access to information about services due to learning or language problems or the information not being available. This lack, or inequity, could lead to inequalities of access because of the restriction of choice and opportunity.

A further practical example of the problem of equity and equality is that of poverty. Why should it be so important? The simple answer to the question is that poverty, worldwide, is associated with poor health and has a profound effect on well being. The term poverty is often confounded by other related concepts such as deprivation, alienation, social exclusion, and maginalization. It explains many of the variations in health which occur across communities and countries. Yet from an ethical point of view why should some countries, groups, or individuals be disadvantaged in this way? This is one of the most important questions in public health today.

One key problem is to arrive at a definition of poverty. One way of doing so is to consider a number of statements which bring together many of the writings on this subject (Calman 1997).

Poverty is a term which describes the state of an individual or a community where there is a lack of resources which significantly affect health and well being. The lack of resources may include money, material possessions, emotional and psychological support, environmental protection, education, opportunities, shelter, housing, information and so on.

Poverty can be absolute or relative. Absolute poverty exists where the lack of resources may result in an inability to provide adequate food or shelter and the essentials of life which may result in a life threatening state. Relative poverty is measured by comparing individuals or groups and relating them to some norm, defined locally, nationally or internationally. However it is defined, it identifies a gap between what is and what might be, and thus the potential for improvement.

Poverty in any individual is not necessarily a static state and can change with age, employment, disability and other factors. Poverty is a reversible condition.

The key fact therefore is that poverty is not inevitable. There are no biological reasons why an individual or a group should suffer poverty. It is a consequence of social and economic factors and thus the major determining factor is a moral one. Why communities should be poor is not in the genes but in the way in which resources are distributed. This is why it is of such importance to public health. Something can, and could, be done to alleviate it. Tackling poverty is a complex issue and a wide range of different methods need to be employed. However, fundamental to it are the values of society and the will to see that something is done to provide equity of opportunity and a removal of the disadvantages which can result in so much ill health.

These examples illustrate that equity is about fairness and justice and implies that everyone should have an opportunity to attain his or her full potential for health. Inequalities exist in health and health care. Some of these are unavoidable and thus would not be classified as unfair or inequitable. Others are avoidable. It is this latter group, in which the inequalities are inequitable, to which further attention might be addressed.

So much is currently known about health and how to improve it, that the potential to change the health of people can and should be realized (Calman 1998; Townsend *et al.* 1992). There is a moral issue which needs to address the question of why we cannot implement existing knowledge to improve health. The public have an increased understanding of health issues, and a realization as to the determinants of health. The Internet, for example, provides rapid access to information, not all of it necessarily accurate, which allows them to see the choices and the potential for them and their families.

Another area of concern which raises questions of justice, is that of war. The ethical dimensions of war have been discussed throughout the centuries, often under the heading of the 'just' war. It may or may not be possible to establish that some wars are 'just', but the impact of war on health is clear and that impact creates injustice as much as removing it. In addition, the casualties in wars occur very disproportionately among the less advantaged.

Conversely, Nobel Laureate Amartya Sen points out that at times of national scarcity, such as wartime, nutrition and life expectancy at birth can actually improve even though the total supply of food per head declines. For example, in Britain during the wartime decades of 1911 to 1921 and 1941 to 1951 life expectancy increased by nearly 7 years as compared with 1 to 4 years in other decades. The incidence of undernutrition declined because of more effective food distribution and more equal sharing through rationing (Sen 1999).

For almost two decades discussions of medical ethics have been conducted in the United States and the United Kingdom very largely in terms of the four principles of non-maleficence, beneficence, respect for autonomy, and justice. Many influential textbooks have been and are being written, using these principles as the necessary and sufficient principles of humane discussion in medical ethics. In discussions of public health, the principle of utility, of maximizing the total benefits for the populations involved, must also be stressed. Some writers argue that the principle of utility underlies the others, that they are specific expressions of the single principle of utility. But this at once gives too little and too much emphasis to utility. It gives too little in that utility is not some submerged underlying principle, but is itself a first-order principle which can and must be used to guide decision procedures in ethics, particularly public health ethics. At the same time it gives too much emphasis, since utility is not the single ultimate principle but is one among others and indeed is often in conflict with the others. This is especially true of one important issue for public health medicine, namely rationing.

Some people may argue that rationing, while it raises important policy issues, does not raise ethical issues. The assumption of this position is that ethics only concerns the face-to-face situation. This view is inadequate. Questions of the supply and fair distribution of resources are matters of ethics and the general ethical principles which are relevant as those of utility and justice. Utility is the principle concerned with the maximizing of outcomes or preferences. In the old formulation it tells us, 'to seek the greatest happiness of the greatest number'. As such, the principle of utility says nothing about how the greatest happiness should be distributed. An aggregate of utility A might be greater than an aggregate of B, but we might still give our moral approval to the situation which produces B rather than A, on the grounds that in B the benefits are more fairly distributed.

The ethical problems which derive from the tension between justice (or equity) and utility arise in different areas of health care. One such is the area of health service provision. The level of provision of health services is of considerable importance particularly in relation to the balance between hospital and primary care, the use of resources to develop effective interventions, and the ability to deliver public health measures. The more recent development of high-cost procedures and treatments, such as new diagnostic techniques or drug therapies, show how rapidly the system of health care can be tested. A good example of the questions raised relating to access is the new drug Viagra, a treatment for impotence. Should such a drug be readily available when there are more 'serious' conditions which cannot be dealt with because of lack of funds? And is impotence a 'disease' which should be using public funds, or should the individual pay for it himself? These are issues which all governments are grappling with and the need to have an infrastructure, organization, and management to deal with such issues is all important.

How such decisions are taken is the subject of distributive justice. How do you decide what is fair or just? How can such decisions be put into practice? Decisions on such matters are difficult partly because such matters are complex and there may be no right answer. Choices do have to be made within fixed resources, and it is clear that the knowledge base is only one part of the decision-making process. For thousands of years such problems have been debated and there is general agreement that:

- each person should have an equal right to basic liberties such as freedom of speech, assembly, and thought
- each person has a right to equal opportunities, such as education.

If the resources are fixed then they could be distributed:

- to each person an equal share
- to each person according to individual needs
- to each person according to individual efforts
- to each person according to societal contributions
- to each person according to merit.

Very different choices would be made depending on the option selected. Such principles are generally mutually incompatible. Putting equity into practice is very difficult and depends on a consensus view as to the principles to be adopted from the list above. Health need is an obvious starting point followed by a consideration of the evidence available for intervention. Eventually a judgement will have to be made and, no matter how much care is taken to select the appropriate procedure, some are likely to be dissatisfied.

For most health-care systems primary care is the most important feature. It was enshrined as a basic principle by the WHO in the Declaration of Alma-Ata in 1978. The conflict in the use of resources in developing countries between primary care and the acute hospital sector may be of a different magnitude, but the issues are the same. How is it possible to ensure the most effective use of limited resources to benefit the greatest number of the population? The draining away of resources to specialist facilities instead of being directed towards primary care is particularly relevant.

For developing countries numerous interventions are known to be both effective and affordable. These include immunization, information on family planning and infant and maternal health, reductions in the use of alcohol and tobacco, improving air and water quality, treatment of tuberculosis with short courses of chemotherapy, the underpinning of an appropriate diet with vitamins, iodine, and iron, and use of the WHO essential drug list. All of this can be delivered within the primary care setting.

It can be argued that hospital services are needed, even in the poorest countries. However, it is necessary to ensure that the treatments are effective and the outcomes give value for money. The professional challenge in developing countries, as in developed countries, is to measure and evaluate outcomes of care. For this reason good management of the resources available is essential, and so one of the requirements in developing countries is to ensure that such management skills are available. Management skills are at their most effective when there is a balance between justice and utility in the distribution of resources.

In many countries there is a reassessment occurring of the structure and organization of health services to make them more effective and achieve value for money. Many different models are being tried; it is necessary to ensure that the lessons learned in one country are able to be used in others. International health organizations can be used to facilitate the sharing of such information to ensure the most efficient use of resources compatible with equity.

Sharing information can also guide the way in which money can be invested in health. Donor agencies and humanitarian organizations put large resources of money and skills into developing countries. In doing so it is essential that priorities are set to achieve the maximum health benefit. Some of the issues raised above about effective interventions are relevant. The balance between the allocation of limited resources to primary health care and hospital care would be an example. But who is to make these choices? The country itself or the donor agencies? There is no right answer to these questions; tact and diplomacy are as important as medical and economic knowledge. The autonomous decisions of the recipient countries must be respected, but the donor agencies must also have regard for utility and equity.

An example of this kind of problem is the ethical promotion of pharmaceuticals. In countries with limited resources, a source of effective drugs is essential. Such drugs need to be supplied as cheaply as possible and the use of expensive alternatives avoided. Heavy promotional campaigns can divert resources—hence the importance of the WHO Essential Drug Project to supply effective drugs as cheaply as possible to countries. This project is another example of the attempts by the WHO to give concrete expression to the principle of utility tempered by equity.

There is another area in which there can be tensions between utility and equity and that is in the measurement of quality in health care. Utility commits us to evaluating outcomes, setting targets, and auditing everything that can be audited. Evaluation programmes, under the umbrella of 'utility', require the introduction of scales and units of measurement.

What is not in measurable units tends to be regarded as unimportant. To put it differently and controversially, quality is interpreted in quantitative terms; consequently in some areas of health care where quality is not easily quantifiable, quality may be marginalized. For example, how is quality to be measured in the palliative area of health care? As a result of the desire to quantify (which is an implication of utility) there can be injustice in the evaluation of some services. Again, there are ethical problems here for public health medicine.

Hence, health-care ethics is best discussed in terms of five principles—non-maleficence, beneficence, respect for autonomy, justice, and utility. As we have seen, these principles can and frequently do conflict. In addition to the conflicts which can be found in any area of health-care ethics, there is a special problem in the area of public health. This special problem can be introduced by contrasting the clinician with the public health specialist.

The clinician is typically in a one-to-one relationship with a patient who has requested an interview because of a health-related problem. The clinical imperative is therefore that something must be done including the giving of advice. Conversely, the public health specialist does not have a specific patient with whom he or she is in a special relationship and has received no request from a patient. Therefore the public health specialist is making a judgement about what is in people's interests, whether they have requested it or not, and is dealing with populations, groups, or societies rather than individuals. The ethical consequences of these features are that public health generates problems concerned with issues such as paternalism and individual rights, and generates problems which are broadly (that is, non-party) political in their implications.

This issue becomes particularly clear in the communication of risk. While the patient and the doctor have an opportunity to discuss and explore choices and options, the public health professional has less opportunity to do so. The patient–doctor relationship allows an agreed plan to be drawn up based on the wishes of the patient and the knowledge and expertise of the doctor. For the public health professional such a process (unless you have a referendum on all public health issues) is not possible. Thus issues of trust and the methods of communicating risk are of particular relevance in public health, and especially where an outcome is uncertain.

Conversely, the distinction between the problems of the clinician and those of the public health doctor must not be exaggerated. Some potential clinical developments raise public health issues. Consider for example the ethical issues raised by the possibility of xenotransplantation. From the clinical point of view if xenotransplantation were to become a realistic treatment then there would be an immense benefit to the many thousands of patients worldwide in need of kidney and other organ transplants. But there is a real risk that new viruses might enter the human population via the source animals. This is especially likely in view of the immunosuppressed state of the recipients. Thus public health concerns are legitimate even if this is classed as a clinical development (HMSO 1997).

After this general introduction to ethical principles, the four areas of public health identified in the WHO definition above will be discussed, beginning with the claim that it is a 'science and an art'.

The science and art of public health

Practitioners in the field of public health include a variety of personnel such as doctors, environmentalists, educators, and managers. The core science which assists these practitioners is epidemiology. Some authors argue that epidemiology does not raise ethical problems because it is simply an attempt to gather information on health and disease, and information is ethically neutral. Unfortunately the matter is not so simple; ethical issues surely can enter epidemiology via the methods which are used to gather health statistics and the choice of subjects and populations for study. To illustrate, let us examine a controversy between a distinguished epidemiologist, Sir Richard Doll, and a distinguished writer on medical ethics, Dr Raanan Gillon (Gillon 1987).

Doll wished to carry out anonymous screening for the prevalence of HIV in blood sample taken in hospitals for other purposes. Apparently ethics committees have been reluctant to sanction such testing. In a letter to the *British Medical Journal* he wrote: 'How it can be unethical is incomprehensible, as it can do no possible harm to anyone and could do much good' (Doll 1987).

The method which Doll proposed was to wait until the blood samples had been tested for whatever reason they had originally been taken and then to make them anonymous, except that the donor's age, sex, and residential area would be noted. The samples would then be tested for an antibody to HIV. Samples would be obtained, for example, from antenatal clinics or casualty departments. The epidemiological justification was that it would provide some information on the prevalence and spread patterns of HIV. It could therefore be argued in favour of this proposal that it represents an 'organised effort of society' which might make some contribution to combating disease.

Gillon was not convinced. He pointed out that the proposal violated the Declaration of Helsinki, as endorsed in 1989, which sets out the principles which should govern medical research on human subjects. The code makes it explicit that subjects of research should be volunteers and should be adequately informed about the research. Indeed, the code explicitly contradicts the expressed view given by Doll quoted above by stating that 'in research on man the interests of science and society should never take precedence over considerations related to the well being of the subject'. In other words, the code is making absolute the principle of respect for autonomy.

An obvious answer to this particular dispute might seem to be to show respect for the autonomy of the research subject by obtaining consent for using the blood sample for epidemiological research. Various difficulties can be raised about the attempt to obtain consent in all such instances: that it is too cumbersome, that the results will be inaccurate if permission is refused, that testing without consent is common, that consent is implied by allowing the blood to be taken in the first place, and that ethical problems arise if the result is positive. Gillon (1987) made replies to all these arguments.

It is not our purpose to adjudicate on the issue, but to use this controversy as an example of the claim that even the scientific basis of public health—epidemiology—can raise ethical issues and these issues relate to basic principles and conflicts of health-care ethics.

The WHO definition speaks of the 'science and art' of public health. What is the 'art' and does it also raise ethical issues? The 'art' is understood as the art of persuading the public and the government to adopt policies which are derived from the scientific basis. This is discussed below when we consider the 'organised efforts of society', which is the final clause in the WHO definition. In the meantime we turn to the concept of prevention.

Prevention

To prevent is to intervene or to take steps in advance to stop something happening. It is easy to think that prevention must be an ancient concept of medicine. This is not the case. In earlier periods in history some diseases were thought to be inevitable, perhaps as a consequence of human sin and, while they might be avoided in individual cases, they could not be prevented. Indeed there is still confusion between prevention, which is the abolition or reduction of the incidence of the disease, avoidance, which is keeping clear of risk factors, and protection which may limit the spread of disease, for example by vaccination or immunization. Public health policy may encourage the prevention of malaria by swamp-clearing programmes, for example, and thus aim at the elimination of the source of the disease, or travellers may be prevented from catching the disease by avoiding certain geographical areas, or they may be protected against it by being given tablets. All these practices are loosely called 'prevention'. Of course, the categories will sometimes overlap. For instance, immunization or vaccination programmes, which are really protection programmes, may lead to a reduction in the incidence of a disease or even to its elimination, as in the case of smallpox. But this overlap does not always occur. The compulsory wearing of seatbelts is often regarded as a preventive measure. However, it does not prevent accidents; only good driving and safer roads and vehicles do that. It gives a measure of protection against the adverse effects of accidents (Blaney 1987).

The terminology is further confused because of the distinctions customarily drawn between prevention, where the intent is to reduce the sources and incidence of disease, secondary prevention, where the intent is to ameliorate the disease condition when it exists, and tertiary prevention, where the intent is to reduce complications in a disease state. These categories have often been criticized, but they remain in use. They are not used here, but look at some ethical problems which arise in the general area of prevention.

It might seem that there is no need to provide any ethical justification for prevention: it is self-evidently a good thing. While this may be true, the general public and governments do not always act as if it were so. From the point of view of government it seems that much more money goes in the direction of health care than of prevention, and from the point of view of the public there is often an attitude of scepticism towards many preventive measures and even more towards what is now called 'health promotion'. Prevention as a general policy therefore requires some justification.

There is an economic justification that prevention is usually cheaper than care, a medical justification that some diseases are probably not completely curable so their occurrence should be prevented, and an ethical justification that prevention avoids the pain, misery, and grief of disease. It is also possible to include the economic and the medical justifications in a wide sense of 'ethical justification'. As will be argued, however, this general ethical justification of prevention does not always apply to specific areas of prevention and even when it does there are those who argue that the benefits of prevention can be outweighed in some cases by the ethical costs.

From the example of the fluoridation of local water supplies, it was noted from the 1930s that there was a correlation between levels of fluoride in the drinking water and levels of dental caries. This suggested a preventive policy of introducing fluoride where the level was low. There were objections, on the grounds of undesirable side-effects, such as Down's syndrome and, more recently, cancer. However, in Britain the Report of the Working Party on Fluoridation of Water and Cancer (HMSO 1985) found no evidence for such claims and other scientific groups have reached the same conclusion. The ethical objection remains, however, that adding fluoride to the water supply can count as compulsory medication and, as such, it is a violation of individual rights as laid down in the United Nations Declaration of Human Rights. Rights, of course, are not inalienable and can be over-ridden when the survival of the public requires it. However, the question is whether the prevention of dental caries can count as a justification for ignoring rights. Note that there is really no solution to this dispute. One position or the other must be over-ruled (Knox 1987).

The issue of vaccination for rubella raises rather different issues. The vaccine for rubella works by providing a benefit to the children of those to whom it is given (preventing congenital defects due to infection during pregnancy). The vaccine can be given to girls only or to both girls and boys. If it is given to girls only there is little effect on the transmission or eradication of the disease. A 'girls only' policy is therefore a 'protection' rather than a 'prevention' measure. Conversely, if the vaccine is given to both girls and boys and if the uptake is over 90 per cent, it will constitute a preventive measure which will eventually lead to the eradication of the disease. However, if the second policy is followed and the uptake is low, say approximately 60 per cent, then a situation develops which is harmful to the children of the unvaccinated young female population, for they will be much less likely to develop natural immunity. The ethical issues are these. If the public wants the benefits of prevention, then it must also agree to a degree of compulsion to ensure a high uptake. If compulsion is ethically or politically unacceptable, then the best policy, to avoid harm, is to offer protection to those at risk. Again, there is no ethically correct answer; a choice must be made (Knox 1987).

Under the general heading of 'prevention' the ethical issue of contraception can be discussed. One of the major problems in the world at present is overpopulation. Methods of contraception are readily and cheaply available with very few adverse effects. Yet abortion continues to be used for contraceptive purposes in some countries, with serious health consequences for some women. In some countries religious views oppose the use of contraception in any form. This policy therefore moves the arguments for and against contraception from an individual to a national perspective. This is a good example of how the value system and beliefs of a nation or culture can affect the health of the population and complicate discussions of ethics. Unplanned parenthood and multiple pregnancies can have many negative health and social consequences and are closely related to the role of women in society.

Another public health activity which falls generally into the category of prevention is that of screening. Screening can be defined in various ways, but a simple definition is provided by Stone and Stewart (1994): 'Screening is a preventive activity which seeks to identify an unsuspected disease or pre-disease condition for which an effective intervention is available'. Screening is currently a fashionable medical activity. The demand for it is being encouraged by governments and by certain patients' organizations.

Politically it seems desirable because there is a belief that prevention saves money and successive governments have therefore set up various screening programmes. A national screening programme for cervical cancer was set up in the United Kingdom in 1964 and a programme for breast cancer was established in 1988 for women aged 50 to 64 years. The establishment of such programmes has been enthusiastically supported by various women's groups. Indeed, such is the current demand for screening that Shickle and Chadwick (1994), in a discussion of the ethics of screening, ask whether 'screeningitis' is an incurable disease.

It is possible to screen for many conditions, but screening programmes must satisfy ethical criteria. Firstly, they must satisfy the informed consent criteria for any sort of medical intervention. Secondly, since screening initiatives tend to be profession driven rather than individual driven, there is an additional responsibility for the professional to justify the intervention which may not have been requested. Thirdly, some screening procedures carry health risks and all of them are likely to be accompanied by discomfort, anxiety, and inconvenience for symptomless individuals. Fourthly, any screening programme carries with it the risks of the false-positive or false-negative result. Thus, screening requires as much ethical justification as other medical interventions. Moreover, since screening programmes can be expensive in the aggregate, they require evaluation.

It is interesting to note that, although the main growth of writing in the area of medical ethics began in the 1970s, the criteria for screening were drawn up by Wilson and Jungner (1968) and adopted by the WHO in 1968. These criteria are a sensible mixture of the medical, the ethical, the economic, and the democratic. They are listed below as Principles 1 to 10. The Ad Hoc Group on Screening Research (1992) added four principles which had already been proposed by Professor Haggard of the Medical Research Council Hearing Research Unit at Nottingham (Principles 11 to 14, below).

1. The condition sought should be an important health problem.
2. There should be an accepted treatment for patients with recognized disease.
3. Facilities for diagnosis and treatment should be available.
4. There should be a recognizable latent or early symptomatic stage.
5. There should be a suitable test or examination.
6. The test should be acceptable to the population.
7. The natural history of the condition, including development from latent to declared disease, should be adequately understood.
8. There should be an agreed policy on whom to treat as patients.
9. The cost of case finding (including diagnosis and treatment of patients diagnosed) should be economically balanced in relation to possible expenditure on medical care as a whole.
10. Case finding should be a continuing process and not a 'once and for all' project.
11. The incidental harm done by screening, and by the information (correct or otherwise) that it gives, should be small in relation to the total benefits from the screening–assessment–treatment system.
12. There should be agreed guidelines on whom to divulge the provisional and final results to, and on when and how this is best done; there should be transitional counselling support where necessary.
13. All screening arrangements should be periodically reviewed in the light of changes in demography, culture, health services, technologies, and the epidemiology of the target conditions.
14. Since 'cases' are not homogeneous, the balance of costs, benefits, and risks from screening, assessments, and treatments has to be worked out on a stratified (demographic or case types) basis.

Do the 'new genetics' raise special ethical problems for public health not covered by the general framework for screening outlined here? There seem to be several special ethical problems raised by the new genetics. Some of these are not particular problems for public health (BMA 1998). For example, there is a fear that the knowledge about human beings discovered by the new genetics is threatening to personal identity. The perception is that if we were to know the genetic code of an individual we would know all about them. This is, of course, an illusion. There is much more to personal identity than a genetic code. But we need not pursue the issue here since the problem it raises is not especially a problem for public health. Four ethical problems arising from genetic screening and testing which are related at least partly to public policy issues will be discussed. Generally the ethical problem raised by the new genetics is that genetic knowledge affects more than the individual tested. The problems affecting the family, employment, insurance, and eugenics will be highlighted.

Firstly, ethical problems which affect the family may vary in detail but they typically involve a conflict between the right of an individual that his or her privacy should be respected and sensitive information kept confidential, and the right of other members of the family to available information which might affect important decisions. This type of dilemma can be made more acute if some family members wish to be given information and others do not. The main ethical burden in this type of situation will fall on the health professional concerned. If the health professional takes the view that the information really is of importance to a family member then it is his or her duty to try to persuade the individual to allow the disclosure. Suppose, however, that the individual refuses consent for disclosure to other family members. May the duty of confidentiality be breached? Two factors might influence the argument in this situation. The first concerns the implications of the genetic information for other family members. If this is substantially damaging to other family members, then there may be a case for breaching confidentiality. No ethical rule is absolute and ethics is often a matter of weighing burdens and benefits. The second concerns the reasons someone might have for refusing consent to disclosure. If this reason is malicious, then this strengthens the case for over-riding the duty of confidentiality, but if it is a fear that the information might have compromising implications for paternity, then the ethical problems change. In their report *Genetic Screening: Ethical Issues* the Nuffield Council on Bioethics (1996) give the following example of this kind of dilemma.

> If information about non-paternity were not disclosed, a man who correctly believed himself to be the father of the child with a particular genetic status might make the wrong decision about having children. On the other hand, for the health professional to reveal such information might lead to harm to the woman concerned, not only because of the breach of confidentiality itself, but also because of its impact on the woman's relationship with the man involved. For this dilemma there are no easy answers.

Fortunately it is a dilemma which is not only the responsibility of the public health professional, but the implications if genetic information for other family members do raise matters of public policy and so are relevant to the concerns of public health. DNA testing of individuals or populations would raise the same issues.

A second area in which genetic screening has implications for public policy is employment. The implications can be both positive and negative. The positive aspect is that employees might be able to assess their ability to contract occupational diseases. This kind of information could enable employees to avoid occupations which are more likely to give rise to life-threatening or disabling disorders. Moreover, the information might assist employers to develop appropriate safeguards in the workplace. There is also the negative side in that some people might feel themselves debarred from occupations they wish to follow, and argue that they are personally willing to run the risk of occupational disorders. Indeed, it might be argued that this kind of genetic information could give rise to discrimination and stigmatization. But there is also the public interest side of the argument. Genetic screening might make it possible to identify individuals who are at risk of developing late-onset disorders which might make them a danger to the public. It is already accepted that certain conditions, such as epilepsy, render individuals ineligible for certain sorts of occupation, such as public service vehicle driving, and genetic screening might be regarded as an extension of this kind of public policy. But the ethical risks are clear.

A third area in which genetics has implications for public policy is health and life insurance. These issues are of a technical nature so they will only be mentioned here, and there is already a large literature on the topic. It is widely accepted that those seeking health or life insurance should be willing to submit to a medical examination. The question is: Why is a genetic test different? The main difference is that genetic tests may indicate a predisposition to a late-onset disorder and this may adversely affect a decision on whether a policy will be offered or the amount of the premium if it is offered. It might be said that it is unfair to expect insurance companies to carry avoidable risks in the current situation of commercial competitiveness. But the problem is that a genetic predisposition to a disease, such as breast cancer, is by no means a sure indicator of future ill health. All sorts of environmental and personal factors will also play a part. There is therefore a fear that insurance companies will misinterpret the information. The problem is partly actuarial, partly one of obtaining clear advice from genetic scientists, and partly one of justice in the sense of ensuring equality for both clients and insurers.

Finally, there is an ethical concern that the new genetics will provide the scientific basis for eugenics. The British Medical Association defines eugenics as: 'The study and practice of methods designed to improve the quality of the race, especially by selective breeding. This usually involves the coercion of individuals in terms of their reproductive choices in order to obtain a societal goal' (BMA 1998). A danger here is that eugenics can appear in a disguise. For example, in the United States compulsory sterilization of the inmates of state institutions was compared to programmes of compulsory vaccination which benefited the community (McLean 1994). The policy of the British Medical Association is that the focus of genetic services should be to enable individuals to make decisions in terms of their own values (BMA 1998). But perhaps this slightly simplifies the ethical situation in matters of reproduction. It may be ethically desirable that a pregnant woman should be made aware of the genetic nature of her future child (although even this is controversial) and it is understandable that some women may wish to terminate their pregnancy in the light of some genetic information. But granted the social pressures to produce a perfect child, and granted the pressure of the state to keep health-care expenditure to a minimum, there is at least a risk that mothers will feel obliged to terminate a pregnancy which is likely to result in a less than perfect child. No doubt it can be argued that this is an individual decision and is not eugenics, but social pressure can be a subtle matter, and even well-meaning health professionals can easily become agents of social control. The line between the ethics of clinical practice and the ethics of public policy eugenics is not clear. Not all public policies are publicly articulated and passed by state legislation. It is therefore possible that eugenics can be encouraged because it is seen as advice in the best interests of the mother and child. These issues will be debated more fully as national screening programmes for such genetic disorders as Down's syndrome become available.

Negative and positive health

The next task of public health medicine as defined by the WHO is that of prolonging life and promoting health. As stated above, if prolonging life is not an aspect of preventing disease or promoting health, then it is a matter for clinical medicine so will not be discussed here. Therefore this section concentrates on promoting health and begins by examining the conception of health held by the health promotion movement (Swedish Council for Planning and Co-ordination of Research 1994).

The literature of the new public health, and in particular health promotion, tends to have a complex view of the concept of health and to distinguish various elements within it.

The first concept of health is often defined negatively as the absence of ill health. However, 'ill health' is a complex notion comprising disease, illness, handicap, injury, and other related ideas. These overlapping concepts can be linked if they are seen on the model of abnormal, unwanted, or incapacitating states of a biological system.

The second idea of 'positive health' has appeared more recently in published reports. The origins of this idea are in the definition of health to be found in the preamble to the constitution of the WHO: 'Health is a state of complete physical, mental and social well being, and not merely the absence of disease or infirmity' (WHO 1946). It follows from this definition that 'well being' is an important ingredient in positive health.

A third idea in the concept of health is that of 'fitness'. Fitness in its most obvious sense refers to the state of someone's heart and lungs. To be fit in this sense is to have a place on a scale ranging from being able to climb stairs or run for a bus without getting out of breath to being able to run a marathon or climb Mount Everest. Fitness can also be used in a related but broader sense, which might be called the 'sociological' as opposed to the 'heart and lungs' sense. In the sociological sense of fitness a person is fit for some occupation or job. This means that people have the necessary health to enable them to perform the job or task adequately without, for example, too many days off work.

It is tempting to think of fitness as standing alongside well being as a component in positive health. But this is a mistake; fitness can be seen as part of either the negative or the positive dimensions of health. One is healthy if one is not ill or diseased; analogously one can be fit if one can perform the tasks of daily life, such as stair climbing, walking to and fro, luggage lifting, and so on, without undue physical stress. The analogue to positive well being is the fitness which enables a person to swim, ride a bicycle, climb a hill, and so on. Fitness, then, is best seen as a component of both negative and positive health rather than as a separate dimension to health.

The WHO definition refers to the 'mental and social' as well as to the physical. Nevertheless, the mental and social components of health are the poor relations of the health services and do not receive adequate attention. It is certainly true that mental health is most often taken to be the absence of mental ill health. The idea of positive mental health or mental well being is an obscure one and perhaps a dangerous one if it implies that eccentricity and single-mindedness are to be discouraged and the balanced and conformist personality encouraged.

The idea of 'social well being' is in fact just as obscure as that of mental well being, although at first sight it does not seem to be a difficult notion. What does it mean? In one sense 'social well being' refers to the skills and other abilities which enable people to form friendships and relate to other people in conversation and through the many different sorts of contacts which are part of ordinary social life. Sometimes these are called 'life skills' and the possession of them helps to create a sense of 'self-esteem' which is currently a fashionable concept in the literature of health education. Clearly, like fitness, social well being in this sense can be graded on a scale from negative to positive. It is a property of individuals and refers to their ability to cope in a social context; hence 'social well being' is an appropriate term.

Is it possible to link the absence of ill health and the presence of well being in a single concept of health in the manner of the WHO definition? This is not a rarified question because it affects the legitimate scope of health education. If well being is a component in the concept of health, then clearly health education has a much wider remit than it would otherwise have.

One important factor influencing this question is that ill health and well being cannot be related to each other as opposite poles on a linear scale. This approach has been tried by some theorists but it is not satisfactory, for it is logically possible (and not uncommon) for someone to have poor physical health but a high state of well being—as in the case of a terminal patient in a hospice who is supported by a caring staff and loving friends—or a good state of physical health but poor well being—as in the case of someone who has no diseases or illnesses but lacks friends, a job, and interests.

The fact that health (the absence of ill health) and well being cannot be related on a linear scale must raise the question of whether they are in fact two components of a single concept. It can be argued that they are aspects of a single concept (Downie *et al.* 1996). However, it may be preferable and less confusing conceptually to think of them as two overlapping concepts rather than as a single concept with two dimensions. Thus, the feeling of well being that a person has after an invigorating swim can fairly be described as a 'glow of health', but the well being or satisfaction that a person has after writing a chapter in a book, listening to a piece of music, or just playing an enjoyable game is less obviously related to concepts of health and more obviously related to the concepts such as 'enjoyment' and 'happiness'. Again, the well being that is created by moving someone to better housing is more obviously related to concepts of 'welfare' than to that of health. Our conclusion is that, while the concepts of health and well being overlap, they are distinct and cannot be combined into one concept. This point will be discussed again (see below).

It does not follow from the fact that well being is a different concept from health that health education has no bearing on it. To take analogous cases, a health educator, indeed a doctor, might reasonably be concerned with the process of ageing or with contraception. But neither getting older nor pregnancy constitutes ill health. In other words, just as the legitimate activities of a doctor may be wider than coping with ill health, so the legitimate activities of a health educator may be wider than anything reasonably called 'health'. The multi-faceted nature of health means that health promotional activities can be controversial (Antonovsky 1987).

Two types of intervention: an ethical contrast

The rise of the health promotion/education side of public health practice has led to a comparison with clinical medicine and to implications of the ethical superiority of health promotion, which can take place in a variety of settings other than the clinical. This matter requires investigation and it is useful to contrast the interventions typical of clinical medicine with those of health promotion.

What is called the 'biomedical' model of health presents health in negative terms as the absence of disease, injury, or disability and sees health interventions primarily in terms of 'treatments' for existing conditions. As Mencken (1923) wrote: 'The aim of medicine is surely not to make men virtuous; it is to safeguard and rescue them from their vices'. Conversely, it is sometimes suggested that the aim of health promotion is to make us virtuous. In terms of this contrast it is possible to compare medical interventions and health promotion as follows (Downie 1990).

Medicine characteristically bypasses our rational minds and treats us as causal mechanisms. In other words, characteristic medical treatments are biochemical or surgical, whereas health promotion characteristically attempts to enable people to understand their bodies and their environments. Medicine typically (but again by no means exclusively) stresses the curative or palliative, while health education stresses the preventive. Medicine stresses the doctor–patient or one-to-one relationship, whereas health promotion tends to have a broader societal perspective. Perhaps most fundamentally, medicine tends to be reductionistic in its assumptions—from the scientific study of disease processes on which it is based—whereas health promotion tends to be holistic in its assumptions.

But does it follow from these distinctions, if they contain at least some truth, that health promotion is in some way ethically superior to medicine? This by no means follows. There is a place for both approaches; they are or should be complementary. What does follow is that health promotion gives rise to an acute set of ethical problems because it is interfering with lifestyle. It therefore requires considerable ethical justification.

For any specific intervention (for example, legislation for clean water, a programme of immunization, restrictions on smoking in public places), the necessary precondition of implementation is that it will improve the health of the public and this improvement must be objectively demonstrable. In this context, as distinct from the clinical context, no patient is requesting intervention; experts are deciding that intervention is necessary and the onus is therefore on them to establish the need for intervention (Charlton 1993). According to this approach, effectiveness must be established by scientific means, such that all rational and competent judges can agree on the facts (Kelly and Charlton 1992). The most common technique for establishing effectiveness of this kind is, as described above, through the discipline of epidemiology, in which clear and certain conclusions may not always be obtainable.

This approach to health promotion in general applies in particular to prevention and to health protection. For example, it must be demonstrable that exercise or a low-fat diet are health determinants and that preventive measures such as screening are effective. In these areas some precision is possible but health promotion can reasonably be criticized ethically for 'gratuitous intervention' if it extends beyond its expertise in those areas (Skrabanek 1990). The importance of having measurable objectives for programme management and evaluation has been recognized in some official documents, for example, the United States Surgeon General's Report *Healthy People 2000* (1991), and in the United Kingdom the report of the Department of Health *Our Healthier Nation: Saving Lives* (HMSO 1999) or Tones and Tilfors (1994).

Health fascism, health imperialism, and self-absorption

A nastier variant of the 'gratuitous intervention' objection to health promotion is the 'health fascism' objection. It is that health promotion is attempting to impose a certain lifestyle on us whether we want it or not (Kelly and Charlton 1992).

While this way of putting the objection is exaggerated and over-dramatic, it has some elements of truth. The health promotion movement is value driven in a way in which medicine ordinarily is not. It is committed to the view that there are better and worse ways of living one's life, and that there are better and worse ways of organizing society and distributing its goods and services. In other words, health promotion has moral and political commitments. It is committed to encouraging the kinds of lifestyle which will bring about true well being. But this is not to say that there is only one correct way of leading one's life. The health promotion position is the modest one that some sorts of lifestyle and some social and political arrangements are much more likely than others to bring about true well being. A modest position of this sort is hardly health fascism.

Another version of the same objection claims that health promotion turns every good state into a matter of health. Health promotion is imperialistic. Those making the charge of health imperialism might argue that what in health promotion terms is 'positive health' is really just a name for a range of states which are as easily or better seen in other ways. For example, 'well being' is just another name for happiness and there are no professional skills which can reliably assist us in attaining happiness. Again, the idea of 'fitness' might he said to be a technical one, relative to specific ends, such as playing in the Premier League, but not one with an important bearing on health. The charge of health imperialism can also be directed at mental health. Mental illness may satisfy some of the criteria for illness (although even that has been disputed), but positive mental health might be said by critics to be a concept which attempts to annex the territory of the well adjusted to that of the healthy. For example, mental illnesses, such as depressions or obsessions, are incapacitating in a manner similar to that of physical illness, but to stress positive mental health might be seen as simply making a value judgement in favour of the conventional or the well balanced as opposed to the eccentric, as noted above.

The reply to the charge of health imperialism can be expressed in terms which are partly logical or philosophical and partly practical. There is a philosophical view argued by Plato which can be conveyed by the slogan 'Everything is what it is and not another thing'. According to this view it must either be true or false that well being and fitness are components of the concept of health. But concepts can be much more flexible. Indeed, it may only be concepts in exact sciences which are rigid and mutually exclusive. Many concepts overlap or are 'open-textured'. For example, the concept of an opera will overlap with that of a musical. Again, one and the same phenomenon can be seen in different ways for different purposes. For example, a morning assembly at school can be seen as an occasion for making announcements or as an expression of corporate identity. In like manner, for certain purposes or in certain contexts it is helpful to include well being and fitness in the concept of health, whereas in other contexts it might seem inappropriate to do so. For example, two people who have acknowledged their love for each other may experience states of well being, but it would be a comic distortion to construe this possibly fleeting feeling in terms of health. Thus there is no correct answer to the question 'Is well being really part of the concept of health?'

Turning to the activities which critics might claim represent the imperialism of health promotion, the same kind of conceptual flexibility is helpful. For example, suppose that a local authority builds a leisure centre with a swimming pool, gymnasium, squash courts, and so on. Is this a health promotional enterprise or not? Again, there is no one answer to this question. From one point of view it could be seen as contributing to prevention or health protection, fitness, or well being, but from another it might seem too solemn to see it in these terms; rather it is a centre where people can have fun. In the United States there is considerable debate about public funding for 'midnight basketball' for disadvantaged youth—with crime prevention, socialization, and health promotion aims intermingled.

It is helpful here to introduce the concept of health alliances. There are certain activities which are indisputably health promotion, but there are many others with which health promotion can form alliances. If health and health promotion can be seen in this logically and practically flexible way, then the charge of imperialism can be avoided.

An undue concern with physical health is a characteristic to be found in some present-day societies. But to see health as a positive good is not necessarily to commit oneself to self-absorption. It is certainly the view of the WHO that positive health is 'seen as a resource for everyday life, not the objective of living' (WHO 1984). The point is that positive health is a value, not the supreme value. It makes perfectly good sense to weigh health against other values; sometimes it will be reasonable to give precedence to health and sometimes not. For example, someone with a stressful lifestyle might give up a job—perhaps at some personal economic cost or even to the detriment of service to others—on the grounds that his or her health was suffering. Equally, someone might reasonably sacrifice health for another value, such as dedication to a life of scholarship or service to others. To say that health is a value and makes a claim is by no means to say it is the supreme value or requires self-absorption. The question which is posed here is that of the purpose of health. Is it a means, or an end? Is the purpose of health to be one component of quality of life and well being, or is it more than that, and something which must be attained at all costs? The answer to such a question is directly relevant to questions of autonomy, utility, and the distribution of resources to individuals or populations, and to health care, transport, the environment or defence, and other publicly funded programmes. It brings up questions of equity and the variations in health which exist in all societies.

Health commercialism and health indoctrination

It is often said in objection to health promotion that it attempts to bypass autonomy and to sell health like a commodity. In this it might be said to resemble the advertisements for the unhealthy products which it is opposing (Williams 1984).

In reply to this argument it is possible to question the premise that autonomy is something which everyone in fact possesses. People can be victims of all sorts of social processes and be lacking in power. For example, as the advertising of tobacco and alcohol becomes progressively more difficult in some countries, so the manufacturers have turned their attention to the developing world and the huge markets which are opening up. As the countries become more affluent, so the consumption of such products increases with consequential long-term adverse health effects. Another example concerns breast milk substitutes. All health authorities are clear about the value of breast feeding for the mother and the baby. However, considerable pressure was brought to bear on mothers in developing countries to use breast milk substitutes. Not only was this more expensive, but the health benefits of breast feeding were lost. International action was required. The WHO resolved that states ensure that there be no free or subsidized substitute which would affect breast feeding practice. This may seem to be merely a political compromise, but it may nevertheless be an effective way of implementing an ethically defensible position.

In view of the political and commercial power of the antihealth forces in society, health must be presented in as attractive a way as possible or health education will fail totally. If health educators confine themselves strictly to the rational, critical approach to education, then it is preferable to depict health education as an element within a larger health promotion movement concerned with health advocacy, legislative change, fiscal reform, and the mobilization of community interests, as well as education narrowly conceived.

The tension between the ethical requirement to be person respecting, and the practical necessity to be effective, is addressed from an interesting point of view in the literature of self-help groups. The growth of self-care groups concerned with every conceivable malady and involving both the sufferers and their relatives has been a notable development during the last decade. These movements avoid the charge of paternalism commonly still made against every branch of health care, including health education. Apart from ethical considerations, self-care organizations seem to be effective within their limits. They may benefit, however, from a professional health educator to advise and facilitate. Advising and facilitating are indeed important roles for health education.

The 'organised efforts of society'

The final clause in the WHO definition is that public health medicine is to obtain its results 'through the organised efforts of society'. How is this to be interpreted and what ethical issues arise from this interpretation? Is it just a metaphor to speak of 'society' bringing about health? One obvious answer to this question is that to speak of 'society' bringing about health is a roundabout way of referring to our elected political representatives. This section therefore begins by looking at the role of the state in health care concentrating on health legislation.

Firstly, a person's right to exercise autonomy may be legitimately curtailed by health legislation when he or she is suffering from certain sorts of infectious disease or mental illness such that the interests or health of others are liable to be harmed. There is no difficulty about the acceptance of this restriction in general terms. The problems arise over the more detailed application. For example, a topical question concerns the nature and extent of the restrictions which should he placed on sufferers from AIDS or the extent of justifiable investigation or reporting of those who may be HIV positive (Walters 1988). Again, it is controversial how far those who are mentally ill should be detained against their will or what sort of treatment they should have if they are detained.

Pressure for legislation is generated as more becomes known about how diseases are transmitted. For example, the dangers of 'passive smoking' are now appreciated and other sorts of environmental pollution are now known to cause or exacerbate diseases such as asthma. There is therefore a case for curbing the freedom of both individuals and corporate bodies, such as industries, in the name of the autonomy of other individuals. This issue is a source of much political debate. Some countries have banned smoking in many public places and various 'watchdogs' keep a close eye on the consequences of the operation of the nuclear power industry. Although there can be political debate about applications of the 'preventing harm to others' idea, the general principle is clear and acceptable.

These problems become more acute when considering the international dimension of health. In a developed country like the United Kingdom international aspects have several implications. The first relates to communicable disease and with the case of transport now that the possibility of transmission to different populations is becoming increasingly easier. Movement for business, leisure, or migration of populations is occurring on a scale as never before. The great plague, cholera, and influenza epidemics of the past, and AIDS, tuberculosis, and malaria in the present, show just how vulnerable the world is to such infections. The introduction of quarantine in Italy and France in the fourteenth century were the earliest attempts to control such infections and there is still ethical justification for certain sorts of boundary control for health reasons.

The need for international legislation is also apparent in environmental issues, the most recent and serious of which was the radio-active release in Chernobyl. But environmental problems regularly cross international boundaries as the effects of acid rain and global warming make clear. The need to ensure that there is an environmental impact assessment of economic growth has been set out in a series of programmes of 'sustainable development'.

Has the state any justification for using fiscal policy or for passing legislation to promote positive health or well being? A strong argument for maintaining that a government does have a duty to promote positive health can be found in the preamble to the Constitution of the WHO (1946), which asserts that there is a right to positive health. In ambitious terms it states 'The enjoyment of the highest attainable standard of health is one of the fundamental rights of every human being without distinction of race, religion, political belief, economic or social condition' (WHO 1946). If this is a fundamental right, then presumably there is a correlative duty laid upon governments to implement it. In other words, acceptance of the WHO Constitution commits states to health and welfare policies. How far such policies can be implemented no doubt turns on the wealth of the country, but there can be no doubt that wealthy Western nations are committed to implementing fiscal and legislative policies to enhance positive health.

A health alliance which has been shown to be helpful in developing community awareness is that between health promotion services and community arts. Several projects have taken place in the United Kingdom and have been favourably evaluated. For example, the Bristol Area Specialist Health Promotion Service reports on projects in photography, the visual arts, and drama (Hecht 1996). Also, Bromley by Bow has ongoing community arts and health projects (Bromley by Bow 1995–1996). The central message from these and similar projects is that disease and ill health cannot be eradicated by narrowly medical means; they must be tackled in a community context with the approval of the community. In other words, the development of public health needs alliances, and the arts are a vital and ethically acceptable ally. The ancient Greeks recognized this when they made Apollo god of both medicine and the arts.

To argue that there is a duty on governments to promote health for its own sake still leaves some questions unanswered. Supposing there is such a duty, can it be implemented other than at the expense of individual autonomy?

It is easy to slip into the error of regarding all legislation on the model of the criminal law—as restrictive prohibition backed by sanction. But this is an oversimplified way of looking at some health legislation. For example, legislation may require public bodies to make provision for the disabled. This is more aptly seen as a positive creation of new opportunities than as negative prohibition. There are legal requirements on factory owners to restrict unpleasant pollutants and on car manufacturers to ensure certain safety standards. Indeed, there is an enormous range of health legislation with a positive slant. Whereas this may diminish the freedom of some groups in society, it certainly extends the freedom of the majority and improves their quality of life (Pinet 1987).

If autonomy is considered in this way, then health legislation is not removing individual autonomy but rather enhancing it. In improving the general quality of life, legislation can add to our autonomy. This is obviously the case when considering the example of provision for the disabled, but it is true also of antipollution legislation and many other types of health legislation.

So far this section has concerned the role of the state and health legislation. But there is much more to the 'organised efforts of society' than legislation. The five principles which the WHO (1984) sees as the basis of health promotion are as follows.

1. Health promotion involves the population as a whole in the context of their everyday life, rather than focusing on people at risk for specific diseases.
2. Health promotion is directed towards action on the causes or determinants of health.
3. Health promotion combines diverse but complementary methods or approaches, including communication, education, legislation, fiscal measures, organizational change, community development, and spontaneous local activities against health hazards.
4. Health promotion aims particularly at effective and concrete public participation.
5. While health promotion is basically an activity in the health and social fields, and not a medical service, health professionals—particularly in primary health care—have an important role in nurturing and enabling health promotion.

How is 'concrete public participation' to be interpreted? What is the ethical importance of this approach?

One way to understand this idea is to think of society not in terms of the individuals who make it up, but in terms of the institutions, practices, customs, political arrangements, and social class relationships which give it structure. From this point of view, people are related to each other by the structures of their society, and indeed part of their identity is created by these social structures. It would then be possible to evaluate society in terms of the ways in which its social structures tend to produce health in the people who belong to that society. Just as the 'atmosphere' in a school or hospital can be praised as one of well being, so the social structures of an entire society might be said to make for or detract from health or well being.

Some theorists with firm attachments to individualism might prefer to understand the health of society as referring to health determinants rather than health itself. For example, they might agree that a society with marked social class gradients and corresponding gradients in the distribution of ill health is one with a tendency to create ill health in individuals. Thus, in terms of this approach, if we speak of an 'unhealthy society' we are simply speaking metaphorically about the determinants, such as poor housing and diet, that have helped to produce poor health states in individuals. Other thinkers might be prepared to extend language and to maintain that it is not a metaphor to characterize social relationships and structures as being themselves unhealthy. It is perhaps self-indulgent to pursue this theoretical question here, but it is one way of making sense of the phrase 'the organised efforts of society' in the WHO (1952) definition or 'effective and concrete public participation' as the WHO (1984*b*) described it later.

To the extent that there is exclusive emphasis on the state delivery of health care to individuals, there is the invitation to see health as a commodity to be supplied by the state. The same is true if health is thought of as a commodity bought by private health insurance. But health is not in any sense a commodity. Health and well being are a set of relationships among citizens. As Beauchamp (1987) wrote:

> Collective goods are ultimately a set of relationships among the citizens of a community, relationships in which the community as a whole participates to obtain desired benefits. These collective goods include aggregate states of welfare or well being, including declining rates of disease and premature deaths; efforts to limit the resources society devotes to personal health services; shared and common access to a good like medical care to foster the sense of community and membership in the group itself. And finally, there are those highly important collective goods, shared or common beliefs and values.

It is possible to add a legal system to Beauchamp's list and in particular one designed to stimulate social responsibility. Indeed, it is plausible to suggest that the increasing government intervention on drink-driving issues has encouraged a greater social awareness about the dangers of alcohol more generally and, thus, a greater sense of community and individual responsibility. In a similar way, legislation designed to assist disabled or handicapped people can also increase a sense of community responsibility for those groups. In other words, in so far as health legislation and other governmental health policies are directed at increasing community awareness, as distinct from being directed at the good of specific individuals, it is not paternalistic.

Environment, risk, and health

There is a very considerable amount of interest at present in the relationship between the environment and health, and this brings with it its own ethical problems. Pollution, air quality, urban issues, rural development programmes, housing, and genetically modified crops are only a few of the problems. Chemical and radio-active waste disposal is a major problem for all countries.

The ethical issues raised relate to many of the topics discussed above such as autonomy, utility, paternalism, and inequity. Two important questions involve who decides on such issues and how the public becomes involved.

The more specific topic which relates to the environment is that of risk, its assessment, its management, and its communication to the public. The ethical dimension relates particularly to the use of the Precautionary Principle and when and how it should be invoked. Essentially the Precautionary Principle is invoked when a product or process is considered potentially harmful and is therefore banned or eliminated. Several implications follow. The first is that the scientific data may be incomplete and thus the decision is based on uncertainty and a judgement is required. In most instances, therefore, the evidence cannot be used alone to make a decision—other factors are involved. The questions this raises concern who is to make the decision, and how it is to be done. A further consequence of invoking the Precautionary Principle is that legislation introduced will inevitably reduce choice, and those who break the rules will be punished. Two simple examples of this would be the introduction of compulsory seatbelts and safety helmets for motor cycles. Both reduce freedom and the individual is punished if he or she does not comply. There is therefore an issue of human rights and of justice. It is not difficult to extrapolate this to major health and safety problems, pollution incidents, and food legislation. On the one hand, it is easy to perhaps 'invoke the Precautionary Principle', and on the other to consider the consequences of doing this every time a potential problem arises. This is where the ethical dimension becomes important and where the value base needs to be clear.

The public are naturally concerned about such risks and their perceptions need to be taken into account in the judgements made (Bennett and Calman 1999). Science can only partially answer the questions; it is a particularly difficult role to make a judgement. The public health professional is often in this role without the benefit either of evidence or of having the time to consult the public fully. In the words of Hippocrates 'Life is short, and the art long; the occasion fleeting and judgement difficult. The physician must not only be prepared to do what is right himself, but also to make the patient, the attendants and externals co-operate.' The role of the public health professional can be difficult, especially around the ethical issues described here and elsewhere in this textbook.

Conclusion

The issues described in this chapter highlight a number of general ethical principles which are of relevance in improving the health of a population. They are illustrated by being applied to the basic issues which need to be addressed in any country which wishes to see the health of its citizens improved. The issues include social and economic problems, the intersectoral nature of action, the role of women, the level of education of the population, the organization of health services, the way resources are allocated, and the national and international importance of health legislation. It has been shown that these issues can be discussed in terms of the ethical principles of non-maleficence, beneficence, respect for autonomy, and justice. But these traditional bioethical principles must be supplemented by the ethical principle of utility to take into account the severe resource problems of the contemporary world.

References

Ad Hoc Group on Screening Research (1992). *Report to the health services and public health research board.* MRC, London.

Antonovsky, A. (1987). *Unravelling the mystery of health.* Jossey-Bass, San Francisco, CA.

Beauchamp, D. (1987). Life-style, public health and paternalism. In *Ethical dilemmas in health promotion* (ed. S. Doxiadis), pp. 69–81. Wiley, Chichester.

Bennett, P. and Calman, K.C. (ed.) (1999). *Risk, communication and the public health.* Oxford University Press.

Blaney, R. (1987). Why prevent disease? In *Ethical dilemmas in health promotion* (ed. S. Doxiadis), pp. 47–56. Wiley, Chichester.

BMA (British Medical Association) (1998). *Human genetics: choice and responsibility.* Oxford University Press.

Bromley by Bow (1995–1996). *Bromley by Bow Centre annual report.* Bromley by Bow Centre, London.

Caldwell, J.C. (1986) Routes to low mortality in poor countries. *Population and Development Review,* **12.**

Calman, K.C. (1997). Equity, poverty and Health for All. *British Medical Journal,* **314**, 1187–8.

Calman, K.C. (1998) *The potential for health.* Oxford University Press.

Charlton, B. (1993) Public health medicine—a different kind of ethics. *Journal of the Royal Society of Medicine*, **86**, 194–5.

Doll, R. (1987). A proposal for doing prevalence studies of AIDS. *British Medical Journal*, **294**, 244.

Downie, R.S. (1990). Ethics in health education: an introduction. In *Ethics in health education* (ed. S. Doxiadis), pp. 3–18. Wiley, Chichester.

Downie, R.S., Tannahill, C., and Tannahill, A. (1996). *Health promotion: models and values.* Oxford University Press.

Gillon, R. (1987). Testing for HIV without permission. *British Medical Journal*, **294**, 821–3.

Hecht, R. (ed.) (1996). *Talk now.* Bristol Specialist Health Promotion Service, Central Health Clinic, Bristol.

Hermanson, B., Omenn, G.S., Kronmal, R.A., and Gersh, B.J. (1988). Beneficial six-year outcome of smoking cessation in older men and women with coronary artery disease. *New England Journal of Medicine*, **319**, 1365–9.

HMSO (Her Majesty's Stationery Office) (1985). *Report of the Working Party on Fluoridation of Water and Cancer: a review of the epidemiological evidence.* HMSO, London.

HMSO (Her Majesty's Stationery Office) (1988). *Acheson Report. Public health in England.* Report of the Committee of Inquiry into the future development of the public health function. HMSO, London.

HMSO (Her Majesty's Stationery Office) (1997). *Report by the Advisory Group on the Ethics of Xenotransplantation of Animal Tissue into Humans.* Department of Health, Norwich, HMSO, London.

HMSO (Her Majesty's Stationery Office) (1998). *Independent inquiry into inequalities and health.* Report of the Independent Inquiry into Inequalities and Health. Chairman: Sir Donald Acheson. HMSO, London.

HMSO (Her Majesty's Stationery Office) (1999). *Our healthier nation: saving lives.* Department of Health, HMSO, London.

Kelly, M.P. and Charlton, B.G. (1992). Health promotion: time for a new philosophy? *British Journal of General Practice*, **42**, 223–4.

Knox, E.G. (1987). Personal and public health care: conflict, congruence or accommodation? In *Ethical dilemmas in health promotion* (ed. S. Doxiadis), pp. 59–68. Wiley, Chichester.

McLean, S.A.M. (1994). *Law, ethics and the human genome project.* SSC Biennial Lecture. Society of Solicitors in the Supreme Court of Scotland, Edinburgh.

Mencken, H.L. (1923). *Prejudices: third series.* Jonathan Cape, London.

Nuffield Council on Bioethics (1996). *Genetic screening: ethical issues.* Nuffield Council on Bioethics, London.

Omenn, G.S. (1990). Prevention and the elderly: what are appropriate policies. *Health Affairs*, **9**, 80–93.

Pinet, G. (1987). Health legislation, prevention and ethics. In *Ethical dilemmas in health promotion* (ed. S. Doxiadis), pp. 83–97. Wiley, Chichester.

Sen, A. (1999) *Development as freedom.* Oxford University Press.

Shickle, D. and Chadwick, R. (1994). The ethics of screening: is 'screeningitis' an incurable disease? *Journal of Medical Ethics*, **20**, 12–18.

Skrabanek, P. (1990). Why is preventive medicine exempted from ethical restraints? *Journal of Medical Ethics*, **16**, 187–90.

Stone, D. and Stewart, S. (1994). *Towards a screening strategy for Scotland.* Scottish Forum for Public Health Medicine, Glasgow.

Swedish Council for Planning and Co-ordination of Research (1994). In *Health promotion and prevention* (ed. P.-E. Liss and N. Nikka). FRN, Stockholm.

Tones, B.K. and Tilfors, S. (1994) *Health education: effectiveness and efficiency.* Chapman & Hall, London.

Townsend, P., Davidson, N., and Whitehead, M. (1992). *Inequalities in health.* Penguin Books, Harmondsworth.

United States Surgeon General's Report (1991). *Healthy people 2000. National health promotion and disease prevention objectives.* Department of Health and Human Services, Public Health Service. US Government Printing Office, Washington, DC.

Walters, L. (1988). Ethical issues in the prevention and treatment of HIV infection and AIDS. *Science*, **239**, 597–603.

Whitehead, M. (1987). *The health divide: inequalities in health in the 1980s.* Health Education Council, London.

Whitehead, M. (1990). *The concepts and principles of equity and health.* WHO European Regional Office, Copenhagen.

WHO (World Health Organization) (1946). *Constitution.* WHO, New York.

WHO (World Health Organization) (1952). *Expert Committee on Public Health Administration.* Technical Report Series No. 55. WHO, Geneva.

WHO (World Health Organization) (1984). *Health promotion. A discussion document on the concepts and principles.* WHO, Copenhagen.

WHO (World Health Organization) Regional Office (1994). *Health in Europe. The 1993/1994 Health for All monitoring report.* WHO Regional Office, Copenhagen.

Williams, G. (1984). Health promotion—caring concern or slick salesmanship? *Journal of Medical Ethics*, **10**, 191–5.

Wilson, J.M.G. and Junger, G. (1968). *Principles and practice of screening for disease.* WHO, Geneva.

4.5 Challenges to public health leadership

William H. Foege

Introduction

> We can't know all of those cut down needlessly for lack of public health action in the past. But they continue to bear witness through our work to improve the future.

The new millennium begins with high expectations for public health. The spectacular health improvements of the past 50 years have given the profession confidence to try new approaches and to solve other problems. No one can be sure that the public health structures that exist will continue. But, as we proceed into the third century of public health activities, beginning in 1798 with Jenner's introduction of the vaccine, the responsibility to take action to improve the health of people, the belief in the primacy of preventive measures, and the idea of 'going to scale' with actions that benefit all individuals, are part of our understanding of quality health practice.

It is possible to predict, based on recent experience, what some of the challenges will be for public health leaders of the future. They continue to expand, but are not all of equal importance. The following account indicates the author's view of the most important. While the basic challenges of public health, such as equity and prevention, will remain constant, changes in science, changes in the problems themselves, and changes in social norms will add topics to the list. Furthermore, if the future is as exciting as the recent past, it is impossible to visualize many of the challenges to be faced by future health officers or the relative importance of those challenges. For example, those receiving their public health training up to the 1960s found that few of their mentors predicted an increase in serious infectious disease problems, much less the specific cases of Lassa fever, toxic shock syndrome, legionnaires' disease, HIV/AIDS, Ebola virus, or nipah virus (Gibbs 1999). The epidemic of drugs and violence which now causes such anguish was not part of the public health lexicon in earlier decades. The role of tobacco was not yet understood in the 1950s when a National Cancer Institute employee was quoted as saying, 'If excessive smoking actually plays a role in the production of lung cancer, it seems to be a minor one' (*New York Times*, 14 April 1954). It was still possible to be lulled in 1963, when a surgeon reported, 'For the majority of people, smoking has a beneficial effect' (I. Macdonald, *Newsweek*, 18 November 1963). The public health implications of nosocomial infections were only slowly being revealed and a healthy breakfast could be viewed, without even a second thought, in terms of whole milk, eggs, and bacon. The widening gap between the rich and the poor, both internationally and nationally, with its profound public health implications, was not part of the world thought to have been ushered in after the Second World War. One certainty is that the future will be no more static than the past.

Over-riding challenges

'Do no harm'

This first rule of medicine applies to all public health professionals. Despite a host of difficulties in interpreting incomplete information, the challenge is to make sufficient decisions with insufficient data. The public health practitioner shoulders the burden of potential harm for large numbers of people if incorrect decisions are made and, in addition, faces a problem not encountered in clinical medicine. In medical practice new findings are replicated or confirmed before they become accepted as standards. In public health, the duty to share findings may cause changes that make it impossible to replicate them. For example, a study in the 1970s (Shands *et al.* 1980), which found an increased risk of toxic shock syndrome associated with the use of a particular brand of tampons caused the withdrawal of that tampon from the market. Therefore it became impossible to repeat the study. The public health officer will be faced, at times, with the need to make definitive decisions based on a single study, even before all questions are answered, and with the knowledge that there will not be a second chance to revisit the issue.

Even medical journals, which often refuse to accept articles containing information already made public, have come to accept that public health information that has been released in the *Weekly Epidemiological Record* of the World Health Organization (**WHO**), or the *Morbidity and Mortality Weekly Report* of the American Centers for Disease Control and Prevention (**CDC**), must be held to a different standard. The public health officer therefore must strive to do no harm, work in a transparent environment that encourages public scrutiny, and at the same time accept the fact that it may be impossible to repeat a study for additional clarification.

The search for equity

The philosophical basis for science is to discover truth and to combat ignorance. The philosophy driving the medical practitioner is to bring that truth to bear on every patient seen. However, the underlying philosophy behind public health is to apply the best knowledge available for the improvement of the health of everyone; therefore social justice is the basis for all public health activities. While a clinician can have a success with every patient seen, public health successes are always relative. Available knowledge is never actually applied in every country and every sector of the population within a country. The differences in morbidity and mortality rates between black and white people in the United States, as well as the disease differences between market economies and developing areas of the world, become measures of our failure to achieve equity.

The exception, to date, has been the elimination of smallpox. The entire population worldwide, and all who will be born in the future, have and will benefit from the knowledge and practice of smallpox vaccination. While the free-market system has been demonstrated to provide great social benefits, a challenge for public health officers is to determine when the market system is not conducive to good health and where deliberate decisions are required to improve public health. The market system failed to provide the public with protection against smallpox. After 170 years of vaccine availability, it required a global resolution for public health workers to achieve the goal of equity. For a dozen years, from 1966 to 1977, the combined efforts of public health workers around the world resulted in elimination of the virus from human populations. This required a systematic search for all outbreaks and eventually every individual case of smallpox, followed by the protection of every person at risk of contact with those harbouring the smallpox virus. Now, despite the cessation of smallpox vaccination, the world has not seen a case for around 25 years. This is not only a refreshing example of the power of public health but also a reminder of the need to keep equity at the centre of all public health activities (Ogden 1987; Fenner *et al.* 1988). The equity issue for smallpox has now entered a new arena. Is it possible to safeguard people for all time by destroying all samples of the virus still in storage? If not, can we guard against accidental escape or intentional use of the virus in biological warfare? It is not certain that collective social and political wisdom can keep pace with public health accomplishments.

Soon guinea-worm disease (dracontiasis) and poliomyelitis will be added to the list of diseases eliminated. Again, deliberate decisions were required to determine the size of the problem and to organize systematic interventions which will eliminate each problem for all time. Nonetheless, although these efforts are satisfying, public health success remains largely relative—an indictment of our control of this challenge.

The Task Force for Disease Eradication has reviewed a list of infectious and non-infectious diseases to determine other areas which could benefit all current and future populations (MMWR 1993). Previous efforts have concentrated on determining which diseases could be eliminated given current scientific knowledge. This recent attempt used a radically different approach, which was to determine what the barriers to elimination would be for each condition. This provided a new perspective, raised other possibilities for action, and provided a research agenda designed to overcome the barriers for each condition. An example is found with measles. Participants agreed that the single greatest barrier to worldwide eradication of measles is the narrow window of opportunity for immunization between the waning of maternal antibodies in the child and exposure to wild measles viruses. Therefore a high-priority research approach is to create a vaccine that is not inactivated by maternal antibody and yet can stimulate a newborn's immune system to produce protective antibodies. Such a disciplined approach should make it possible to eliminate dozens of diseases systematically. The provision of equity in public health will then become more than an exception.

The daughter of the brilliant naval officer Admiral Ernest J. King once described her father as: 'the most even-tempered man in the Navy. He is always in a rage' (Cutler 1994). Public health leaders must be seen as the most predictable people in health, always insisting on equity.

Effective use of the information

Effective use of information requires collecting the information, analysing the significance of the information, and responding appropriately. The difficulty in living up to an effectiveness standard is seen in the worldwide delivery of public health programmes. Measles-related deaths continue to occur 35 years after an effective vaccine has become widely available. Disability due to the poliovirus is still a fact of life for many people in Africa and India, even 45 years after the introduction of an effective vaccine. Partial success in reducing the toll of morbidity and mortality from a condition often hides the inefficiency of efforts and the fact that with the resources available greater reductions in suffering should have been possible. Within the challenge of effective information use is the challenge of using the tools made available by the digital revolution. It is now possible to collect and link information that has importance for the understanding and prediction of morbidity and mortality from a wide variety of sources. These include electronic sensors that report on air, water, and sewage. Information can be gathered from hospitals, clinics, and laboratories, as well as from devices on people, vehicles, toilets, and satellites which can be variously used to predict outbreaks of disease, characterize new clinical syndromes, detect antibiotic resistance patterns, or determine disease spread. Risk factor surveillance data can be gathered on smoking, seatbelt use, unhealthy eating patterns, or substance abuse, and can be used to predict health patterns months, years, and even decades in the future.

Daily summaries of analysis, computer-mediated weekly rounds for all ministries of health, electronic consultation, distance diagnostic assistance, and interactive computer training will provide a public health service without walls that will effectively serve the entire globe. Local practitioners will have all the benefits of the best expertise available in the world. Interventions that are inadequate at the local level will trigger assistance with minimum delay. 'Inaccessible' will cease to be a term used in public health.

These new techniques will only increase the challenges for public health officers as they provide guidance for the public. Information on diet, fibre, fat, caffeine, micronutrients, and so on will become greater and more confusing to interpret. Information on prenatal care or risks to the fetus, mushrooming information on the relationship of specific genes to specific diseases, and developmental findings will provide public health officers with new power but also new responsibilities: 'There is a tendency to mistake data for wisdom, just as there has always been a tendency to confuse logic with values, intelligence with insight' (N. Cousins, unpublished speech, August 1995). The challenge to the public health officer is to provide wisdom, values, and insight.

The primacy of prevention

Few ideas attract such support in the abstract and neglect in fact. On the day that a person receives a diagnosis of lung cancer he or she would give their entire financial portfolio to erase that diagnosis. But a week earlier they are still willing to accept the risks of smoking. Prevention is a primary obligation of public health, not because it saves money, although it will in some cases, but because it prevents suffering, improves the quality of life, and improves the efficiency of systems. From Hippocrates, who said that the function of protecting and developing health must rank even above that of restoring it when it is impaired, to Gandhi who said, 'I am hard-hearted enough to let the sick die...if you can tell me how to prevent others from falling sick' (V. Ramalingaswami, personal communication, 1990), society has been given advice on the importance of prevention. Even so, health budgets (global, national, local, and personal) provide the evidence of human immunity to such wise words.

In November 1984, the Carter Center sponsored a conference entitled 'Closing the Gap' (Amler and Dull 1987). Each of 15 areas, such as cardiovascular disease, injury, diabetes, and so on, was examined to see what levels of morbidity and mortality could be expected in the United States if the skills and knowledge of the condition, already available, could be applied. The findings of the conference indicated that if current knowledge in primary, secondary, and tertiary prevention were used, immediate and significant changes would be seen in both morbidity and mortality rates. As an example, it was concluded that, despite continuing improvements in mortality rates and an ever-increasing life expectancy, two of every three deaths in the United States are premature, given what is known about delaying such deaths. Of the 12 million years of life lost each year in the United States due to deaths before the age of 65, more than 8 million are lost needlessly, even with the current state of knowledge. While expensive endstage care in intensive care units is continuing to be provided, low-cost preventive procedures that could add quality years to life are failing to be provided.

A revisit of the above approach in 1990 showed little change in the United States and demonstrated that almost 40 per cent of deaths are caused by three factors, all potentially within the control of individuals who wish to change their risk of premature death (McGinnis and Foege 1993). Almost 20 per cent of all deaths (about 400 000) were due to tobacco. An additional 300 000 deaths (14 per cent of the total) were the result of diet, and 100 000 deaths, 5 per cent of the total, were associated with alcohol. Such opportunities to improve the quality of life through the practice of prevention make the lack of effective action in this area a continuing frustration and challenge for public health leaders.

The primacy of prevention requires an attitude that it is never too late and at the same time knowing that the best return is realized when actions are taken early. Richard Feynman once said that it takes very little energy to scramble an egg, but science is powerless to reverse that simple process. It takes very little to scramble a brain or to destroy nerve cells with poliovirus. Science is powerless to reverse those processes because the arrow of time moves only in one direction, but we are capable of preventing the event.

Taking a global approach

A frequently used African quotation says: 'It takes an entire village to raise a child'. It may have been possible in the past for that statement to be both true and sufficient. Now, the truth is that it takes the whole world to raise a child. It is not possible to get through a day without making use of the products of a hundred countries. Medicine is dependent on the findings of scientists from around the world and interdependent in the application of those findings. At the memorial service for Dr Jonas Salk in 1995, Dr Charles Merieux reminded those in attendance that the interdependence crosses both geography and time. He talked of the eighteenth century work of Edward Jenner on vaccinia in England, continued by Louis Pasteur in the nineteenth century on vaccinations, and expanded by Jonas Salk in the twentieth century in the United States with his work on vaccinology.

The concept is not new. Polybius reminded us more than 2000 years ago that the world is an organic whole where everything affects everything else. Public health leaders ignore this concept at their peril. Infectious disease examples abound and are most easily appreciated. The United States saves its entire investment in global smallpox eradication every 3 months. Despite this demonstration, it is exceedingly difficult to get investments in global health. The country saves more each year because of smallpox eradication than our entire annual contribution to the WHO. This does not prevent the American government from withholding payment of dues in some years for political purposes. It is anticipated that similar savings will follow the eradication of poliomyelitis (Bart and Foulds 1992).

Measles importations constantly challenge attempts to interrupt measles transmission in the United States. Indeed, it appears that measles transmission has actually been interrupted in the United States and genotypic characteristics of current outbreaks now show that all current strains are the result of importations. This indicates that even without a vaccine that can be used in the presence of maternal antibody, elimination of the disease is possible if the degree of effort expended within the United States is applied in other areas. The Pan-American Health Organization is now demonstrating that measles elimination in the entire hemisphere is possible. However, global eradication would be required to protect this investment, making it obvious why the public health officer must take a global approach to even local problems. Importations of dengue fever, cholera, typhoid, and other infectious diseases are a constant threat, and when they occur they always involve a local health jurisdiction.

Global concern is required for travellers to other areas of the world. They are subjected to diarrhoeal agents and sexually transmitted diseases, as well as to malaria and other parasitic diseases. Both the popular and scientific press are now paying considerable attention to emerging infections and their implications globally (Preston 1994).

However, the interactions extend beyond the risk of infectious diseases being imported to the United States or travellers becoming ill. The improved health of populations in developing countries makes that country a better market for American products and at the same time decreases the ultimate price of goods going from that country to American markets. Therefore health in developing countries has an impact on market conditions that affect the American economy. Inequities that are easily seen as ultimately untenable within a family or a community have counterpart implications within a nation or between nations. Sometimes such market impacts require an understanding of long incubation periods. As Maclean once wrote: 'Coming to recognize you are wrong is like coming to recognize you are sick. You feel bad long before you admit you have any of the symptoms and certainly long before you are willing to take your medicine' (Maclean 1992). Coming to recognize we are wrong when we tolerate disparities of health does not come easily.

Local health officers make the best decisions for their area of responsibility if they consider the disease problem in its global context and if they are contributing to and utilizing a surveillance system that reflects the entire ramifications of the problem. The need is so great that we must, at every opportunity, support the involvement of the United States in global health endeavours, whether through United

Nations agencies, voluntary groups, or bilateral government programmes.

Establishing objectives and standards

Objectives and standards are so much a part of the commercial world as well as a staple part of management literature that it is difficult to believe that the United States had no health objectives for itself until 1978. At that time, the United States Public Health Service initiated a process to develop objectives for the nation for the year 1990. An initial meeting in Atlanta, Georgia, was attended by national, state, and local health workers. They attempted to reach consensus on more than 220 specific health objectives (Public Health Service 1980). These objectives became a guideline for budget planning as well as the basis for monthly reviews by the Public Health Service in an attempt to improve health and also to improve on the objectives and the tracking of progress. By 1990, about half of the objectives had been reached. Of far more importance was the fact that a process had been developed that allowed for collective decision-making on the determination of objectives that could guide public health actions.

Similar health objectives have been developed by countries under the auspices of the WHO as the result of the Summit for Children held at the United Nations on 30 September 1990. The Summit provided an agreed blueprint by country leaders that has been used for immunization, nutrition, and other aspects of child health. The world is now in need of a new agreement on what will be collectively sought in terms of health objectives for all children.

In the United States the importance of establishing such a process was made very clear by the release of objectives for the year 2000 (Public Health Service 1990). The new objectives were better, more realistic, and more easily tracked because of the previous experience with the 1990 objectives. The 2010 objectives are even more comprehensive and increasingly measurable.

The selection of objectives and priorities is a major step forward. In addition, health departments need standards to know whether their organizations are likely to achieve those objectives. It has been said that the improvement of civilization has finally required codification of the lessons learned into laws that guide future health professionals. Likewise, the improvement of the health of the public is dependent on determining what works and then developing standards that guide future actions. The development of standards is not without its difficulties. In 1994, 14 October was celebrated in the United States as World Standard Day. However, celebrations were held on 13 October in Finland and 18 October in Italy (*Economist*, 15 October 1994)!

The American Public Health Service, together with the United States Conference of City Health Officers, the National Association of County Health Officers, the Association of State and Territorial Health Officials, and the American Public Health Association published the first edition of *Community Preventive Health Services Model Standards* in 1979 (Secretary of Health, Education and Welfare 1979). As with maintenance, this is an area that requires eternal vigilance. It is an embarrassment to the public health community to acknowledge the degree to which standards have been developed for many other endeavours. Even baseball has better standards than public health. It is possible for a coach to know, with precision, the standards for a ballpark, bats, balls, and the rules of play. It is also possible to know whether a player is measuring up to the compensation level agreed on. It is possible for the public to know in great detail how well dozens of teams have done in meeting these standards, and thousands of workers spend their lives tracking and polishing both standards and activities. It is therefore difficult to understand why it is so hard to give similar attention to the standards of public health workers and programmes where the results could lead to improved health, extended life, and increased quality of life.

High-priority challenges

Defining the boundaries of public health

Until recently, public health was almost synonymous with infectious disease control. While this is undoubtedly an overstatement, little attention was given to injuries, violence, chronic diseases, environmental concerns, obesity, or other conditions. Failure to identify these fields as being within the legitimate concern of public health prevented the full development of intervention strategies. In 1977, the CDC assembled a committee to look at patterns of morbidity and mortality in the United States, and then to advise the Center on the top 12 or so priorities to be addressed. Major changes date from this review. Not only did the CDC begin using the concept of both mortality and premature mortality to analyse deaths, but it also became obvious that some major problems were being ignored by the public health community, primarily because there was no 'tradition' of including such conditions within the definition of public health. For example, while heart disease, cancer, and stroke were the three leading causes of death in the United States, changing the question from 'How many years are lost?' to 'How many years are lost prematurely?' provided a new perspective. (While there was a desire to use the median life expectancy age for this determination, the need to change each year was a drawback. Age 75 might have provided a useful cut-off for the United States, but age 65 was finally selected with the idea that, despite all its drawbacks, it would facilitate comparisons with other countries.) This approach disclosed that three of the five leading causes of premature death involved intentional or unintentional injuries. After considerable review by programme managers, the CDC used the recommendations of this committee to reorganize around health problems such as infectious diseases, chronic diseases, environmental health problems, and occupational health problems. Eventually, a Center for Injury Control and Prevention was formed, even though the Department of Health and Human Services was not convinced that injury was a public health problem. Demonstrating that public health is the concern of everyone, the initial funding for the Center came from an appropriation given to the Department of Transportation, on the condition that it be transferred to the CDC to use for an injury centre. Congressman William Lehman was the architect of this approach, which was used for 3 years until the Department of Health and Human Services included funding in its own budget.

The tradition is changing. If tradition is the genetics of our beliefs, it becomes important to mould the new public health traditions with care. In the past two decades, health officers have become surprisingly comfortable dealing with a vast array of both old and new problems. This includes instituting surveillance on both health problems and risk factors, examining the health problems associated with guns and alcohol, promoting changes in diet, evaluating toxic spills, or using molecular biology to investigate hospital infections. On the one hand, there is a concern over where this progression will stop. On the other hand, it is equally clear that: 'We are involved in a field that most fully exemplifies the integration of mind, body and spirit. No human activity lies outside our interest' (Ademola 1965).

For example, experiences in the past 50 years are strongly supportive of the idea that the health of the public improves when political leaders are responsive to their constituents. Accountability is an important component of improved public services. While dictators may achieve short-term health advantages, long-term improvements are favoured by people having the ability to articulate health objectives and secure a leadership interested in such goals. The open society that characterizes democracies, and holds leaders accountable, provides for a healthy society. Democracy becomes an asset to public health leaders, and the encouragement of democratic structures and procedures becomes one of the obligations of public health.

Redefining the boundaries, with the inclusion of a range of new problems, places new challenges on the use of public health approaches. For example, while traditional public health practice has been based on working with health workers, hospitals, clinics, and so on, the challenge of violence requires new partnerships. Public health workers must collaborate with, and seek information from, police, traffic safety personnel, the justice system, schools, and even weapons manufacturers. Intervention techniques must involve all segments of society, including the news media, faith groups, and politicians. The price of this larger vision is more responsibility to make networks meaningful and productive.

What other health problems should be benefiting from the full range of public health talents? One example, raised by Richmond and Eisenberg (1991), concerns the possibility that mental health could be improved by more intimate involvement with public health. As more mental health conditions are found to have a biological basis and are yielding to treatment modalities, there has been a movement from the labour-intensive concentration on a relatively small number of people with the most serious illnesses, to concern with population-based approaches which include people suffering from depression, addiction, and other common conditions. This involves sampling or surveillance systems. At the same time, public health has become increasingly involved in the behavioural sciences as it seeks greater insight into AIDS, other infectious diseases, smoking, addiction, and violence. Therefore public health workers are becoming more comfortable in dealing with the problems of mental health. It appears an attractive time to combine the changes in both disciplines and to approach mental health as a public health problem, with national surveillance, prevention programmes, interventions, and evaluations to see whether it is possible to make significant gains in the level of mental health experienced by an entire nation.

Improving the definition of public health problems

The approaches of surveillance and epidemiological analysis, followed by appropriate interventions and evaluation, have led to dramatic improvements in some conditions, such as the vaccine-preventable diseases. Yet comprehensive surveillance systems are lacking, and there are major gaps in the ability to access the information base available through hospitals, clinics, and doctors. Society's health burdens are not quantified in ways that are understandable and allow for meaningful comparisons, and systematic methods of comparing the costs and effectiveness of various intervention strategies are lacking. All this could be changed if modest resource increases were available from local, state, and national governments, thus improving the ability to diagnose national health problems, to quantify the burden of disease imposed by various conditions, and to detect threats from other geographical areas.

In 1993, the World Bank published the *World Development Report* (World Bank 1993), part of an annual series produced by the Bank, but the first devoted to health. As part of the report they attempted to quantify disease by combining morbidity and mortality into a single number which they called disability-adjusted life-years (**DALYs**). An incidence approach was used, combining the premature loss of years for people dying in 1990 with the loss of healthy years that resulted from illness in 1990. Various morbid conditions were given values equivalent to some percentage of death, thereby providing a universal unit of measurement (see Chapter 2.9).

While not perfect, the approach is a major step forward in rationalizing the approach to health financing and interventions. For example, the report calculated the total burden of disease for the world in 1990 to be a loss of 1.4 billion DALYs. It was then possible to measure the impact of any given condition on that total. Tuberculosis was found to be responsible for the loss of 46 million DALYs or about 3.4 per cent of the total. AIDS accounted for about 1.5 per cent of the total and neuropsychiatric conditions for 7 per cent of the total. The first step in public health improvement has always been the ability to identify and measure the conditions to be targeted and never has the ability of measurement been as great as now. The problem is that few public health departments have risen to the challenge of using such quantifiable approaches.

In 1990, 24 conditions each accounted for more than 1 per cent of the total global burden of disease. That information already provides help in deciding which conditions should receive the greatest attention. For example, falls, vehicle injuries, homicide, suicide, and war each accounted for more than 1 per cent of the 1990 burden. When combined, these five conditions of intentional and unintentional injury were second only to respiratory diseases as a cause of distress or ill health. The size of the problem provides a compelling argument for public health engagement in the field of intentional and unintentional injury.

The predictable and salutary result of the World Bank approach is the identification of what needs to be improved to make the DALY concept more useful. Anand and Hanson (1997, 1998) have pointed out the equity consequences of the approach. With new attention to equity, quality, age, and consensus on weighting, a useable and fair method is possible both to measure the burden of disease and to help make decisions on resource allocation.

Defining public health problems goes far beyond placing quantities on disease outcomes. Defining risk factors or generic conditions responsible for ill health is also necessary and is often the key for planning logical interventions. At times the risk factors will be discrete and suggest a specific intervention, such as vitamin A, iodine, or folic acid. At other times the risk factor may be important for a variety of illnesses and yet defy easy intervention strategies. For example, studies from various countries now implicate poverty as a risk factor for many disease conditions. It is not just a problem of extreme poverty but rather a continuum, with poverty being 'dose related'. This appears to hold true for various cultures, with death rates increasing for most conditions as income decreases. It is at this point that one is tempted to call for a limit on the dimensions of public health, yet it is realized that few risk factors are as powerful. Therefore the public health workers of today have no alternative but to become involved in poverty reduction activities, education, attempts at empowerment, and safety nets of various kinds.

Many have provided reasons why society should not tolerate poverty. Aristotle called poverty the parent of revolution. Martin Luther King said that poverty is 'socially as cruel and blind as the practice of cannibalism at the dawn of civilization'. In 1424, the Chinese Emperor Hongxi stated: 'Relieving people's poverty ought to be handled as though one were rescuing them from fire or saving them from drowning. One cannot hesitate' (*Seeds Magazine*, July 1994). But only in recent years has the public health cost been appreciated. Public health leaders now have two excellent arguments for engaging the battle on poverty. Firstly, the resulting ill health has been a cost to society in terms of health care, lost work, and decreased productivity. Secondly, the poor actually subsidize the lifestyle of middle- and upper-income people by providing goods and services at a minimum wage. This is an issue of equity.

In the face of a historic understanding of the evils of poverty and a more recent appreciation of the ill health which results from it, the unhappy finding is that it is now apparent that the poverty problem is becoming worse. *The State of the World's Children 1995* (Grant 1995) provides two clear but seemingly conflicting pictures. On the one hand, health has never been better. Life expectancy has continued to improve to the highest levels ever seen, infant mortality rates are declining around the world, birth rates are going down, and disease-specific rates are improving for a variety of conditions. On the other hand, the gap between rich and poor has never been greater. Not only is the difference in the disease rate between the two increasing but the number of people in the poverty category is increasing, both in the United States and globally.

How can the two conditions coexist? Average figures continue to improve for the middle and especially the upper classes, which improves the average for the entire population, while averages move much less for the lowest socio-economic groups, and not at all for those at the bottom. In fact, the worst health conditions in the world are as bad as any seen this century. For example, the death rate during the first month of existence of the Rwandan refugee camps was estimated to have been about 9 per cent (M. O'Toole, personal communication, 1993), two to three times as high as in January 1942 during the worst month of the siege of Leningrad in the former USSR.

Bluestone (unpublished talk, 10 May 1995) has discussed the wage compression seen in the United States following the Second World War when the greatest improvement in wages was seen in the lowest quintile. The situation has now gone from wage compression to wage dispersal and he states, 'If anything is fundamental to the modern era, this is it'. In the United States, the percentage of wealth owned by the top 1 per cent of the population is actually increasing, having reached almost 40 per cent of the total wealth. The unrestrained market system is not the answer to many public health problems. This being the case, it appears that a challenge for public health workers will be to determine where interventions are required to overcome the disease-inducing tendencies of the market-place—a problem which will be greater in the future than before. The implications involve health and equity, both public health concerns.

Selecting priorities

Health will always be relative, as will resources. Therefore one of the challenges of the public health officer is to obtain the best return on invested resources. This remains a combination of weighing factual information, including prevalence, incidence, severity, death rates, age of cases, and type and cost of interventions, with the less tangible impressions of the population, judgements of public health workers, and influences of the political processes. While decisions will always involve both art and science, the desire is to increase the factual content of decisions.

Again, the *World Development Report 1993* (World Bank 1993) contains some of the most helpful information available on providing quantifiable techniques for measuring the burden of disease, whether examining a particular disease, a collection of diseases, a geographic area, or an age group. Using the DALY as the common outcome measure for various disease conditions, it is possible to calculate the resources needed to gain one unit of benefit through investments in various interventions. The report indicates that health gains are achieved at relatively low cost, for instance, in programmes providing vitamin A supplementation, immunization, and chemotherapy for tuberculosis. It is now possible to compare immunization, AIDS prevention, and water chlorination with cancer therapy or highway safety programmes. It is also possible to provide increased sophistication in presenting programmes to decision-makers in rough priority order.

But challenges for health professionals remain. The words 'disability-adjusted life-year' themselves seem to provide a barrier to effective use. 'Disability' is seen as too negative and 'adjusted' leads to suspicion among people outside the discipline of public health who may be concerned about what is hidden if something is adjusted. As mentioned above, both problems are being addressed by the increasing use of 'healthy life-years' saved or lost. Remaining problems involve reaching consensus on the weighting of values for morbid conditions and ages as well as the challenge of incorporating certain aspects of quality. While the approach is useful in comparing the presence or absence of disease, it is more difficult to quantify, for example, the feeling of well being which may attend high levels of physical activity, or satisfaction with contributions to society or the accomplishment of a quality job. Nevertheless, the World Bank has catapulted public health into a new era of quantifying the burden of disease and encouraging rational decision-making in selecting intervention strategies. Such an approach has already shown that 75 per cent of the disease burden affecting children of developing countries can be prevented by effective and inexpensive interventions. Quantification helps to provide a powerful moral argument for implementation.

What is not yet possible is to cost all parts of the infrastructure, such as surveillance, health education, research, or evaluation. But even in these areas, measuring the disease burden can be helpful. To illustrate, the selection of research priorities can be improved by comparing the burdens imposed. Vaccine-preventable diseases continue to extract a major toll despite proven methods for preventing the infections. Applied research aimed at better delivery of the tools available, as well as behavioural science research to seek better utilization of services, is indicated. Conversely, certain cancers or infectious and parasitic diseases, as well as violence, still require the attention of basic researchers. Despite all the limitations, however, the ability to make a case for priorities in public health is much improved, if still underutilized.

The incorporation of behavioural sciences into public health

From the first inoculation of cowpox material, on 14 May 1796, to protect James Phipps from smallpox, the delivery and utilization of public health knowledge has required information exchange and behavioural modifications. Recent decades have accelerated the process with a new understanding that we require knowledge of behaviour to understand the transmission of infectious diseases, the process of addiction to tobacco, alcohol, and other substances, the significance of eating patterns, and the dynamics of violence. Furthermore, the interventions for the major public health problems of the day have been hampered by a paucity of knowledge on how people act, why they make decisions, and the types of reward systems required to influence behaviour.

Of all the benefits of the medical science revolution which characterize the twentieth century—new drugs, organ transplantation, intensive care units, surgical techniques, vaccines, imaging devices—surely none is as extraordinary as the power given to individuals to influence their own health. Information on tobacco, diet, exercise, sun screens, micronutrients, and dozens of other conditions now inundate people through health newsletters, magazines, newspapers, and television. The ability to modify and improve one's health exceeds the entire ability of the health-care system to repair that health when lost. In theory, unlike wealth, which tends to pool in the hands of a small percentage of the population, information on health should be a great equalizer. As with time, it should be available in equal amounts for the benefit of all. In practice this simply does not happen; as with wealth, those who already have the use of information acquire more. Public health practitioners have the challenge of designing research which makes knowledge both useful and useable for a much broader segment of the population.

Previously, public health practitioners have often failed to acknowledge the need for assistance from the behavioural scientists. The field of public health will increasingly see anthropologists, psychologists, psychiatrists, sociologists, ethicists, and theologians with joint degrees in epidemiology, statistics, or health-care management.

Resource generation

Despite the significant return on investments in public health programmes, it has never been easy to appropriate adequate resources. Intensive care units continue to attract budgets. Prevention requires a conceptual understanding that is not required of funders when they agree to provide money for the setting of bones or the treatment of heart attacks. In addition to the conceptual differences, personal freedom intrudes on issues surrounding lifestyle, and this in turn leads to controversy which is not seen when funding hospital care. Water fluoridation, and at times even chlorination, also encourage controversy. Even the foundation programme of modern public health, immunization, is not free of controversy. In the United States a strong anti-immunization movement has developed, encouraged by parents who have difficulty weighing risks because they no longer remember or have not seen the disease tragedies inflicted by poliomyelitis, measles, *Haemophilus* influenza, meningitis, and pertussis, and groups who believe that such programmes conflict with personal freedom. To compound this problem, public health writers often hold public health programmes to different standards than health-care delivery by evaluating their benefit–cost ratios. Some programmes actually save more money than the programme costs; however, most public health programmes are undertaken because they delay death, improve quality of life, or spare people the suffering of disease. Conversely, health-care delivery programmes are held to cost-effectiveness standards after a decision is made that a health benefit is useful. The same standard should be used to evaluate public health programmes.

Five approaches could be pursued to improve public health resources. Firstly, as already indicated, a conscious effort by public health leaders to quantify the burden of disease, followed by attempts to evaluate the cost-effectiveness of interventions, would greatly improve the transparency and the credibility of public health programmes. Such an approach could make public health competitive with health-care delivery which would then be required to make similar calculations.

Secondly, in the cases where financial returns exceed the investments, as is the case with immunization programmes, the programmes should become entitlements and not compete with other health budget items. To do otherwise is to agree to spend more money and simultaneously to have more suffering. While the number of such programmes would be small, it would greatly simplify public health financing to have such programmes dealt with separately.

Thirdly, public health resources should be indexed to total health expenditures. Only in this way can public health be assured of competing. The great debate would then concern the percentage of the total health expenditure which would go to public health. Since the percentage of total health expenditure which is going to public health programmes is reducing, public health leaders would be advised to accept, with alacrity, the current percentage level. This would help public health in the future.

Fourthly, the experiments with tobacco taxes in California, Canada, and elsewhere have been very encouraging. Such funds should not be seen as core or dependable funds since the great hope would be to decrease smoking rates and thereby decrease such revenues in the future. However, they do provide an approach to public health problems where the problem itself helps to fund its own solution.

Fifthly, public health officers should take full responsibility for educating policy-makers as well as the public about the costs and benefits of public health actions (see the discussion below on utilizing the political structure).

The challenge of better management

Whether or not a group of people benefit from a given body of public health knowledge is the responsibility of management. Can that knowledge be managed for the health benefit of recipients? The public health field needs to increase the amount of managerial expertise transmitted to public health specialists, but also needs to attract more management experts into the field. The training of public health managers (public health advisors) at the CDC has been an exemplary programme. To use the example of smallpox eradication again, the scientific techniques were developed in the eighteenth century. While there were modifications in the vaccine and in the method of administration, the reason that smallpox disappeared from the world in the 1970s was because of the introduction of management approaches to the problem. Surveillance systems were put in place, target areas were determined, logistics systems were instituted, intervention teams were trained, personnel policies were developed, operations were decentralized in dozens of countries, hundreds of states or provinces, and thousands of counties, and evaluations were conducted to make continuing corrections in the strategy and tactics. Public health advisors deserve much of the credit for these innovations. Smallpox eradication was a managerial success.

Likewise, as the late executive director of the United Nations International Children's Emergency Fund (**UNICEF**), James Grant, used to point out, the immunization of 80 per cent of the world's children by 1990 was the largest peacetime project in history (UNICEF Board Meeting, April 1993). It is an example of co-ordinated global management which requires billions of contacts between children and a health-care system every year. The ability to deliver these health benefits on such a large scale has encouraged UNICEF, the WHO, and others to continue the development and expansion of services for diarrhoeal disease control, acute respiratory infection control, micronutrient provision, guinea-worm eradication, onchocerciasis control, and other services. The major global health programmes have been, and will continue to be, dependent on skilled managers as well as on the biological and social sciences.

Skilled management requires an intact and adequate infrastructure. For much of the world this is a continuing barrier to better public health. Even in developed countries the attraction of health-care delivery often blinds resource decision-makers to the importance of public health infrastructures. Michael Osterholm once pointed out that fire departments at airports have no difficulty with funding even if they go for decades before they are needed. Their importance is obvious. Public health leaders have the challenge to make daily public health protection so obvious that infrastructure resource support becomes as compelling as fire-department support.

Evaluation

As noted above, continuing improvement of the health of people in the aggregate requires accurate measurement of the burden of disease in order to determine priorities. Often avoided is the careful measurement of changes in this burden as the result of interventions. Rational investment in health programmes is dependent on comparing the healthy years of life saved by the various possible interventions. Therefore evaluation is not just an important management tool for increasing the efficiency of a given programme, but also an effective method of comparing programmes and deciding on future interventions.

A challenge to public health leaders is to make this case for evaluation. Resource shortages often result in shifting resources from evaluation to other operations, and it requires tenacity to demand a measure of the impact of interventions. In smallpox eradication in India, the decisive change in disease burden from smallpox came when it was possible to evaluate every outbreak for such characteristics as days between the onset of the first case and the reporting of the outbreak, time from report to the arrival of control teams, time from the onset of control activities to the onset of the last case, number of secondary outbreaks, and so on. With such information available, it was possible to change tactics rapidly, to train additional people, and to measure the effectiveness of each action.

This same value of evaluation is now being seen in the global poliomyelitis eradication programme where standards have been developed for national immunization days, surveillance for acute flaccid paralysis, the collection of stool specimens for laboratory analysis, the speed of reporting, and so on. Programme standards encourage evaluation and the immediate detection of problem areas.

Other challenges

Changing public perceptions of public health

The science revolution is often pictured in terms of intensive care units, molecular biology, and organ transplantation. All are dramatic and part of the truth. However, if the most significant implication of the great increase in scientific knowledge is the power it gives each individual to control risks and influence their own health destiny, then it follows that public health must learn how to make individuals active participants in public health rather than targets of public health programmes. The leading causes of death in the United States, mentioned above, are tobacco, diet, and alcohol. Increasingly, these are also becoming the most significant factors in global health. To be able to influence the three most significant causes of death through personal actions is an incredible gift that was not available 40 years ago. When we add information on injury prevention, cancer prevention, micronutrients, exercise, sun injury to the skin, vaccinations, oral rehydration, and a host of other actions which can be exercised by the individual, it is clear that the age of science has given power to people. This concept has not been conveyed adequately, and fatalism is still the norm for large parts of the population both in the United States and throughout the world.

Indeed, fatalism may be one of the major detractors from life quality throughout history. However, because of this new power, never has the gap been greater between what people could do to improve health and what they actually do. Therefore one challenge is to find ways to enrol everyone as a participant in using this vast knowledge bank person by person, day by day. It is an interesting concept to see everyone as members of this knowledge bank, with free access to the information and with unlimited withdrawals not only allowed but rewarded.

Privacy issues and public health

Many public health activities require acquiring personal identifiers. For example, to provide booster doses of vaccine requires a record showing that a child has received the primary series. The movement of families to different geographical areas or to different clinics within a geographical area requires the ability to share such basic health information. The challenge is to provide adequate protection to individual children by making such information available only to those who need to know, and at the same time to provide adequate protection to other children by identifying those who need follow-up immunizations. Procedures are developing but are not yet adequate even for this relatively simple public health task. All Kids Count, a programme funded by the Robert Wood Johnson Foundation, encourages innovation in developing tracking systems and is having success in developing approaches that use computer networks and co-operation between public health systems and private providers. One by one, the programme has solved hardware and software problems, the enrolment of all children at birth, the provision of records in real time to new providers if the child moves or simply changes the location of care, and the problems of simplicity in record-keeping and providing security.

The situation becomes more complex when tracking infectious diseases where it is necessary to identify potential contacts. This now involves one or more additional people, often in most sensitive ways. Sexually transmitted diseases have required contact tracing, as in the case of syphilis, and since the disease can be effectively treated with penicillin, the custom has been to secure identifying information on contacts and to then locate, counsel, test, and treat as indicated. The agreement has been much more difficult in the case of AIDS where effective treatment was late in developing.

Even situations that seem straightforward to public health workers often involve privacy concerns. In the 1970s, the CDC investigated several dozen deaths associated with the use of the Liquid Protein Diet (Sours *et al.* 1981). The families of the deceased had been interviewed with the belief that the information would be held confidential. When a United States Senate Committee requested the names of the women, the CDC was informed by lawyers for the Committee that Congress was not subject to the privacy laws it had passed for the remainder of the country! Although the Senate Committee eventually dropped their request, such issues have not been settled in a satisfactory way. Some of the best efforts of public health professionals must be invested in finding an acceptable balance between the needs of individuals and the needs of society, as efficient ways of using the available science are developed for the benefit of everyone.

Utilizing the political structure

Public health improvements ultimately depend on a political decision. Public health leaders require more experience with the political system, need to develop better programmes to educate political leaders, and need to encourage public health professionals to go into politics.

Learning the political process was simpler in the past. Fewer interventions were possible, concerns for privacy and personal rights were much lower, and much less suspicion of government existed. In addition, health officers were often in their jobs for long periods of time, maintaining their positions even with changes of administration. Now the average state health officer often has a tenure of 2 or 3 years, must quickly learn the guidelines for operating with a congressional and executive system, and must provide a compelling argument for appropriation of funds at a time when medical care costs are continuing to increase and general revenue has stagnated.

The need to educate political leaders cannot be overstated. On the assumption that they wish to make correct decisions and that they want to improve life for their constituents, the absence of good decisions may be due to lack of information, incorrect information, or the inability of the political leader to interpret the information. Any of those scenarios involves a failure of the public health community. In 1987, Congress voted to lift the national 55 miles/hour speed limit. Much of the momentum for this change was provided by political leaders from states with lower population densities and long distances to travel between towns. At the same time Baker *et al.* (1987) had demonstrated that mortality as a result of automobile crashes is inversely related to population density. The differences in mortality are major. Counties with a low population density may have an increase in death rate not of 100 per cent but of 100-fold! Congress over-rode the scientific evidence. Despite all the improvements in the design of roads, the design of cars, and the safety equipment that is becoming standard, the number of deaths on the highway increased in 1994 and again in 1995. An easy response is to point out that the denominator, miles driven, has increased significantly and that the rate of death has continued to decrease. While this is true, the potential decrease in mortality was not being realized. The lesson of 1987, 'It is not only a failure of Congress to obtain and use the appropriate facts but also a failure of the health professions to convey their knowledge to policy makers. The total system, science and policy, has once again failed to provide a protection level that could pass any reasonable peer review' (Foege 1987), continues to be applicable.

One of the most impressive displays of incorporating the power structure was seen with the Children's Summit held on 30 September 1990 at the United Nations headquarters in New York. UNICEF provided the encouragement for this meeting of 71 heads of state to plan a programme for children's health in the final decade of the twentieth century. The foundation was set at a meeting in Bangkok in March 1990, when United Nations agencies, bilateral agencies, non-governmental organizations, and ministers of health determined the health objectives that they thought would be achievable if political commitments were made (Task Force for Child Survival 1990). Six months later, heads of state met and, in an awesome display of positive peer pressure, they were each given a few minutes to summarize what they had done for the health of children in their country and what they planned to do over the next decade. Agreements were then reached on global goals (UN 1990), including the eradication of poliomyelitis and guinea worm as well as specific goals on reducing measles mortality, improving nutritional status, and improving education levels. The decade goals were in turn refined by deciding what achievements would be needed by 1995 if the objectives were to be met by the year 2000. A review was undertaken in January 1994 (Task Force for Child Survival and Development 1994) which revealed remarkable progress in the areas selected. Child health has clearly improved because of the summit meeting and the commitments made by country leaders. Many countries have periodic reviews, some even under the direction of the head of state. The impact of the summit was a remarkable improvement in child health programmes and child health indices. However, sustainability is difficult to institutionalize. As the decade ends some of the most hopeful results are being reversed. Immunization rates have declined in many African countries and vaccine-preventable outbreaks have occurred in the former Soviet countries. Iodine deficiency in children has returned in some countries, and general nutritional deficiency rates are unacceptably high in both Africa and Asia.

Despite the problems, the early success of the Children's Summit has led to attempts at other summits to engage political leaders in a variety of problems. The Environmental Summit in Rio de Janeiro, the Population Summit in Cairo, and the Social Summit in Copenhagen are examples of such efforts. The advantages of the world concentrating on a single topic for a period of time are obvious. The disadvantages include the logistics involved, the fatigue of government agencies in involvement in almost a summit per year, and the inability of the media to concentrate on more than a handful of heads of state at one time. An alternative should be explored to combine the benefits of attention to a single subject with the involvement of many political leaders. For example, would there be benefits to following up the Population Summit in Cairo, or any of the other summits, by providing each interested head of state with a few minutes to address the world on how his or her country is doing in providing maternal health programmes, family planning programmes, and education for girls, as well as on the innovations they plan for empowering women? Twice a week, a global television programme could feature such a leadership forum and political leaders would discover an acceptable way to secure global attention. Within 18 months, 150 world leaders would have had the opportunity to state their views, provide positive peer pressure, raise the stakes, and undoubtedly provide new ideas and impetus for stabilizing population in the world. Could this provide a format for widespread agreement to tackle other shared global problems?

Application of new tools

A host of new tools and approaches require evaluation. The power of the computer in public health is only just beginning to be appreciated. Computer networks which automatically report on microbial isolations and resistance patterns throughout the world could improve knowledge on how and why antibiotic and antiparasitic resistance develops and provide suggestions on control strategies. Global surveillance systems could provide clues to improve knowledge of disease patterns, speed up the development of eradication strategies, and at the same time provide protection to the people.

The combination of techniques for sorting cells and various techniques for recognizing differences between organisms, together with the ability to store computer profiles for every organism, raises the possibility of being able to recognize micro-organisms instantaneously and thereby diagnose infectious diseases. While of considerable importance in routine public health work, such potential is of crucial importance in treating meningitis or other infectious diseases where the outcome is dependent on the speed of appropriate therapy.

The small and predictable rate of mutations of viruses is already proving useful in dating specimens. For example, polioviruses mutate at a known rate, and one country, in working up an outbreak of poliomyelitis, was able to prove that the specimens were not collected in 1994 but, rather, 5 years earlier. This led to the discovery of laboratory contamination of current specimens with viruses which had been isolated in the laboratory during the earlier outbreak in 1989. Such precision, with its considerable importance during poliomyelitis eradication efforts, would not have been possible even a decade ago. Likewise, the ability to track an outbreak through sophisticated characterization of the virus not only provides information on the spread of disease but also provides the ability to notify the country of origin that they have a disease problem. It is the ability to provide such detailed characterizations of viruses that has made it clear that measles transmission was interrupted in the United States and current measles problems are the results of importations of the disease from other countries.

One challenge in public health today, given the increasing gaps between rich and poor, is to find innovative ways to present standard deviations with the clarity now characterizing presentations of means or averages. If public health, in its attack on poverty, is to concentrate on 'trickle-up' effects which will result from attention to the most disadvantaged, it must find persuasive ways to highlight the gaps and show the rates of increase or decrease of such gaps.

Other challenges involve providing generic solutions which do not require daily decisions by every individual, such as the advantages of water chlorination, iodized salt, and food fortification. One example is the value of quality protein maize (corn) (Anonymous 1988) with increased levels of lysine and tryptophan. The introduction of this strain in Ghana is beginning to impact the incidence of kwashiorkor. The recent development of rice strains with vitamin A and iron is a forerunner of quality foods of all types. Similar advances in low-fat foods, other micronutrients, and antioxidants would provide advantages that no amount of education could match. Even well-motivated people 'know more than they live'.

Another challenge is to link pleasurable activities to the daily decisions that must be made for better health. For example, many people find certain types of exercise enjoyable but not always sufficiently convenient to be habit-forming. If attention could be given to making such activities possible, emphasis could be on positive rather than negative messages. To become addicted to racquetball, swimming, tennis, or some similar activity changes self-image, reduces weight, reduces blood pressure, provides motivation to stop smoking, and adds other positive changes as the quality of daily life is improved. The organization of programmes by public health departments to combine the provision of facilities by employers, faith groups, and communities with flexible hours at work could be an important aspect of public health programmes of the future.

A final challenge to be mentioned under the use of new tools is to identify ways of extending public health activities without major additional resources. Faith groups have a strong history of providing health services through hospitals and clinics. Many cities in the United States have a St Joseph's Hospital or a Baptist Hospital as a reminder of that heritage. As faith groups increasingly sell their health facilities to for-profit agencies, they are not necessarily undertaking other health work to substitute for that loss. The findings of recent decades, that individuals can do much to change their health destinies, provides an ideal low-technology activity for faith groups to continue health work without the requirement of high-technology equipment and capital expenditures. The incorporation of the interest and resources of faith groups into public health activities provides them with a new avenue to fulfil their genuine concern with health, and indeed in most cases their obligation to be involved with health. It also provides them with an opportunity to demonstrate a concern for the community that goes far beyond a desire to proselytize. In addition, it provides to public health programmes the involvement of multiple organizations already in the community, trusted by their members, and well suited to education of how best to live. Programmes that incorporate smoke-enders programmes, Alcoholics Anonymous, aerobics, diet management, health education, mental health options, organized athletics for children and adults, the use of facilities, and so on provide opportunities for public health that increased resources alone would not match. Such coalitions could provide a major impact on public health.

Improving public health research

In 1985, international child health advocates met in Cartagena, Colombia, to discuss progress in global childhood immunization. Included in the meeting was a discussion of what should be desired in immunization programmes based on a survey of immunization workers who were asked for their conclusions on the major barriers to immunization coverage. The focus on barriers made clear that there were difficulties with the vaccines themselves, such as the requirement for booster doses, the need for refrigeration, the varying windows during which each vaccine could be given, and the need to separate vaccines in different syringes. There were also equipment difficulties such as the problem of sterilizing needles and syringes, problems with refrigeration, and the quantities of sterile diluent required. Finally, there were major barriers in the behavioural area, both in insuring appropriate behaviour of immunization teams when it came to sterilizing equipment, using the correct dosage, discarding impotent vaccine, and so on, and also with the behaviour of parents who had difficulties responding to such a demanding schedule which involved bringing children to immunization sites on many different occasions.

The examination led to a listing of what would be desirable for immunization if there were no restraints. Answers included immunization by the oral route to eliminate needles and syringes, vaccines that required no refrigeration, vaccines that required no booster doses and were capable of providing life-long protection with a single dose, vaccines that could be physically combined or at least all given at a single visit, and vaccines that could be given any time after birth, free of adverse side-effects (Task Force for Child Survival 1986). With such a vaccine there could be high coverage, since repeat visits are not required, and it would be possible to contemplate such possibilities as measles eradication.

Eventually, the Children's Vaccine Initiative was developed with the collaboration of the WHO, UNICEF, the World Bank, the United Nations Development Programme, the Rockefeller Foundation, research institutions, universities, and vaccine producers. The objective was to provide a systematic approach capable of bringing together the abilities and talents of research and global organizations all focused on achieving the vision of 'perfect' vaccines. At the end of the century there was a great effort to find an ideal method of organizing the project: while the objectives are clear, organization is more difficult. The agencies that created the Children's Vaccine Initiative are trying to form a new global consortium that will include global agencies, vaccine manufacturers, other parts of the business community, foundations, developing countries, and others who have a genuine concern for the task of bringing science into the service of children, by developing a better global immunization programme.

A second example concerns the deaths of children due to firearms. A conference sponsored by the Carnegie Corporation began with the objective of determining how to reduce such deaths through concerted public health and community action. Discussions finally focused on the fact that any reduction of deaths still left a percentage of deaths that could not be justified. Finally the group reached a consensus that the objective must be to avoid the loss of even one child and that research must start from the assumption that every death is avoidable. The resulting report, *Not Even One* (Carter Center 1994), includes a plan for the approach to such an objective, including the investigation of every childhood firearm death to determine which things went wrong and how such problems could be eliminated in the future. The journey may be extended, but the objective is clear and the research needs evolve from that clarity.

Utilizing the health-care delivery system for prevention

The health-care delivery system is not able to organize national approaches to surveillance, analysis, intervention of community programmes, and many of the duties of public health departments. Likewise, public health departments are not ideally suited to the provision of comprehensive medical care. However, both systems could be strengthened by better co-ordination. Specifically for the public health community, great opportunities are available to improve disease prevention through health-care delivery programmes. Increasingly, health delivery programmes are being monitored by employers who are eager to go beyond price comparisons to compare health outcomes. This has led to the development of an evaluation tool known as the Health Plan Employer Data and Information Set (**HEDIS**). In the absence of many health outcome measures, the system relies heavily on process measurements, many of them prevention methods such as immunization coverage rates, mammography rates by age, percentage of women receiving Pap smears, and so on. The list continues to improve as health-care delivery programmes implement HEDIS programmes. The opportunity is available for public health leaders to assist in improving this and other 'report cards', thereby incorporating the powerful and massive health-care delivery system in a focus on prevention.

Firstly, keeping the focus on outcomes may be one of the most influential roles for public health leaders. Health-care reform in the United States was debated around the wrong issues. From the beginning the discussion placed highest priority on access, cost, and quality. Access is only a process measure that provides no assurance of better health in itself. For years, all children in the United Kingdom had access to immunizations and yet the immunization coverage rates lagged behind those in the United States. When the United Kingdom changed the focus from access to outcome and rewarded practitioners who immunized 90 per cent of the children in their practice, immunization rates suddenly increased. If health outcome was made an important requirement in a health-care system, access would be found to be required but insufficient. Secondly, for reasons given above, prevention provides the best quality of life and should be the second measure of a health-care system. Thirdly, quality should be sought after. Fourthly, the most cost-effective approach should be the goal. Public health professionals could still influence the ultimate debate on health-care reform by moving the agenda from access, quality, and cost to health outcome, prevention, quality, and cost. At the same time it is worth providing our best effort to define the positive health outcomes that are most useful for tracking health-care delivery.

The challenge of optimism

New risks become evident with changes in technology, emerging infections capture the headlines, war and violence are daily events, social capital dissolves, and the poor see no hope. Pessimism and cynicism seem to be not only acceptable but required as both an explanation of the past and a premature condemnation of the future. As the actor Lily Tomlin has said, 'No matter how cynical you become, it is never enough to keep up'.

In the midst of this, public health leaders must provide a balance. There are things beyond the control of public health professionals but they will be judged on how they respond to what can be altered. Two imperatives drive the promotion of optimism. Firstly, the past record of public health success is impressive. Whether overall indices such as infant mortality and life expectancy, specific risks such as the incidence of poliomyelitis, measles, or strokes, or the information available to individuals for improving their own health are examined, optimism is justified.

Secondly, the ability to see and predict the future is not given alone to epidemiology but is a wonderful attribute of epidemiology. This ability to predict hazards and intervene before they occur—to improve the future—is one of the great burdens of public health, and a reason for optimism.

A man was told by a fortune teller that he would be very poor and very unhappy until he was 45 years of age. Grasping at that straw he asked what would happen when he was 45. He was told, 'You will get used to it'. The job of public health professionals is to convince the world that it does not have to get used to preventable illness, premature mortality, environmental pollution, and poverty.

Predicting the predictable future

It is not realistic to believe that public health professionals should predict what could not be expected. Only in general can it be known that new organisms will appear; it cannot be known specifically which organisms they will be. However, it is very easy to predict that resistant organisms will appear whenever a new antibiotic or antiparasitic agent is introduced. Likewise, it seems unreasonable to have foreseen the full implications of DDT when it was first introduced, the intelligence-reducing impact of lead, or even the toll which would be extracted by the invention of the automobile.

However, the fact that the most lethal agent in the world is tobacco is an indictment of our current ability and desire to predict. People have lacked the will to make the inevitable public health consequences of smoking sufficiently vivid. The toll of tobacco is astounding, is ever increasing, and is the leading generic cause of death in the United States and in the rest of the world. Three million lives end prematurely every year because of tobacco use, and it is expected that the global figure will reach 10 million a year before a plateau is observed.

How could we have been so ineffective in making use of the information available? The basic risk information has been available for around 50 years and widely available since the first Surgeon General's report on smoking 35 years ago. The major problems resulting from tobacco, their approximate frequency, the difficulty in stopping smoking, the power of advertising, and the rate of increase in use of tobacco products have been known for many years. Yet the public health community was passive in allowing morally corrupt systems and individuals to promote the use of such products for their own financial gain. It will be one of the most perplexing mysteries for future historians to understand how societies with high levels of scientific expertise, analytical inclinations, communication abilities, demonstrated interest in health for people in the aggregate, and repeated claims to be concerned about the health and well being of children could have allowed money and power to blind the entire society to the importance of health.

It is important to understand how to make the use of tobacco a true choice rather than a daily millstone around the neck of smokers. If false advertising of tobacco could be eliminated, sales to minors adequately controlled, and a share of tobacco revenues used to protect children, then a decision to smoke could be delayed until adulthood and a true choice would be possible.

Civilization is finally measured by how people treat each other. It is not measured by the splendour of corporate offices or the texture of a politician's suit. We simply failed, as public health professionals, to predict the future in an appropriate way, and in so doing have allowed a small consortium of tobacco executives and politicians to wreak a vengeance on the world that equates each year to the annual death toll under the Nazis.

Epidemiology is one of the most powerful predictors of risk that the world possesses. The analysis of a handful of cases of poliomyelitis in 1955 was able to show that one vaccine was contaminated but that others could be used without fear. Even the second wave of cases due to those who contracted poliomyelitis from the contaminated vaccine was predicted with accuracy. Public health leaders are challenged to use such tools to provide a vision, a decade or two into the future, regarding what can be expected based on various policies. This should estimate the impact of decisions regarding tobacco, diet, alcohol use, violence, immunization policies, micronutrient use, investments in the education of young people, economic policies, family planning policies, environmental approaches, job programmes, and many other activities that impinge on the health and quality of life of people in the aggregate.

Protecting the future

Maclean reports that his father used to say: 'One of the chief privileges of man is to speak up for the universe' (Maclean 1992). It is not enough to predict the future. Public health has the opportunity, expertise, challenge, and privilege to speak up for the protection of the future. The other side of possessing a predictor of risk is the requirement to respond appropriately. The over-riding concept to bring to such a responsibility is the conviction that the vast majority of the public which we serve, has not yet been born. While public health plans may extend for 10 or 20 years, the audience is a future generation. It is imperative, in the words of the Carter Center Interfaith Health Program, to 'balance the world's future needs with the world's current deeds' (Interfaith Health Program 1994).

The study of Greek History leaves several indelible conclusions. The levels of writing, architecture, art, and government were awesome—but they were lost. It does not matter how advanced our public health practices become if provisions are not made about how to improve and maintain them. They can be lost.

The usual roles are easy to visualize. Together with other groups, it is important to be conscious of the impact of current actions on future populations, their numbers as well as their attributes, on the physical environment, including the ozone layer, rainforest preservation, acid rain, biodiversity, and sustainability, and on the social environment that they inherit. Furthermore, deliberate policies that protect the future must be aimed at, even if that requires current investment and sacrifice.

But there may be a role for public health that goes beyond the obvious. A concerted effort to understand and reduce violence could have a decisive role in improving the quality of life on a community level. Historically, the two major reasons for premature death have been infectious diseases and violence. Only recently has there been hope that violence can be reduced, and that hope has come through public health. It is only a few decades since Kemp *et al.* (1962) published the first article on the battered child, revealing the dark side of society that had been part of our heritage but long ignored or denied. Once faced, it has led to policies that alert medical personnel, teachers, and others to signs of violence against children and has resulted in the protection of many children. This, in turn, has provided a look at violence through the age spectrum involving children, spouses, parents, other family members, and friends. Now public health accepts its role in looking at violence in general. The resulting involvement with the entire spectrum of violence will inevitably lead to a better understanding of the dynamics, and a reduced impact on society. While the long-term impact of abuse and violence seems apparent, some scientific evidence is now available that links adverse health effects in adults with abuse in childhood (Felitti *et al.* 1998). Post-traumatic stress disorder may be a product of such abuse and 'the battered child syndrome' may be followed by a 'battered adult syndrome' (Foege 1998).

Could public health have an impact on the larger stage of violence, i.e. the violence practised between ethnic groups, religious groups, or nations? We may already be in the early stages of such an impact. Durant, reflecting on the unity of spirit that characterized Americans during the Second World War, asked how that spirit could be captured globally. He reached the conclusion that the world would not be willing to work in unity unless they feared an alien invasion, a common enemy.

This theory appears to have had an impact in the 50-year struggle to deal constructively with nuclear weapons. A scant decade ago nuclear weapons were arguably the single greatest risk that the world faced. That risk has not disappeared, but the superpowers have begun to discuss how to safeguard arsenals and how to decrease the number of weapons held by each side. The reason for this attempt to change the risk is a result of many things, including the work of such groups as the International Physicians for the Prevention of Nuclear War. But a major reason was that nuclear weapons became a surrogate for an alien invasion. Everyone felt vulnerable, and the weapons that had defined enemies became a common enemy.

In smaller ways, smallpox was a common enemy and eradication became possible, not just because it was scientifically possible but because it became a surrogate for an alien invasion. Guinea worm and poliomyelitis now have roles to play in organizing the world for common action. Certainly the environment and population pressures are beginning to be seen as common problems.

In 1995, a ceasefire was arranged in Sudan by former President Carter. The basis for the agreement was an attempt to improve health services to populations on both sides of the fighting, specifically against disease problems of both local and international significance such as poliomyelitis, guinea worm, and onchocerciasis, and problems involving children. During the ceasefire, work concentrated on those problems but also included the administration of measles vaccine, oral rehydration salts, and vitamin A. The result was not only the protection of thousands of children from a variety of diseases, but also the education of village workers to improve water supplies, to protect against blindness due to onchocerciasis, and to treat children for diarrhoea. Of even more long-term importance was the development of mechanisms for public health work that could exist even if fighting resumed. On a national scale disease was used as the surrogate for an alien invasion; it became a common enemy.

On the basis of these local and national examples, public health professionals, with the leadership of the WHO, UNICEF, and the United Nations agencies, should embark on a deliberate programme to define the common disease enemies. Then, with programmes on disease control, population, environment, education, poverty, and so on, global programmes could inspire co-operation, trust, a sense of accomplishment, and a 'high-pressure system' that displaces the usual vectors for discord. It is not an impossible legacy to leave for the future, fulfilling the hope of Jonas Salk that we would learn to be good ancestors.

References

Ademola, G. (1965). *Harvard School of Public Health yearbook.* Harvard University Press, Cambridge, MA.

Amler, R. and Dull, H. (1987). *Closing the gap.* Oxford University Press.

Anand, S. and Hanson K. (1997). Disability-adjusted life years: a critical review. *Journal of Health Economics*, **16**, 685–702.

Anand, S. and Hanson K. (1998). DALYs: efficiency versus equity. *World Development*, **26**, 307–30.

Anonymous (1988). *Quality protein maize.* National Academy Press, Washington, DC.

Baker, S.P., Whitefield, R.A., and O'Neill, B. (1987). *Geographic variations in motor vehicle occupant mortality.* Johns Hopkins School of Hygiene and Public Health, Baltimore, MD.

Bart, K. and Foulds, J. (1992). The cost and cost–benefits of poliomyelitis eradication. In *Proceedings of theWorld Conference on Poliomyelitis and Measles, New Delhi* (ed. E. Kurstak). International Comparative Virology Organization, Montreal.

Carter Center (1994). *Not even one: a report on the crisis of children and firearms.* Carter Center, Atlanta, GA.

Cutler, T.J. (1994). *The Battle of Leyte Gulf, 23–26 October.* Harper, New York.

Felitti, V.J., Anda, R.F., Nordenberg, D., *et al.* (1998). The relationship of childhood abuse and household dysfunction to many of the leading causes of death in adults: the Adverse Childhood Experiences (ACE) Study. *American Journal of Preventive Medicine*, **14**, 245–58.

Fenner, F., Henderson, D., Arita, I., Jezek, Z., and Ladnyi, I. (1988). *Smallpox and its eradication.* WHO, Geneva.

Foege, W.H. (1987). Highway violence and public policy. *New England Journal of Medicine*, **316**, 1407–8.

Foege, W.H. (1998). Adverse childhood experiences: a public health perspective. *American Journal of Preventive Medicine*, **14**, 354–5.

Gibbs, W.W. (1999). Trailing a virus. *Scientific American*, August, 80–7.

Grant, J. (1995). *The state of the world's children 1995.* UNICEF/Oxford University Press.

Interfaith Health Program (1994). *Program objectives.* Carter Center, Atlanta, GA.

Kempe, C.H., Silverman, F.N., Steele, B.F., Droegemueller, W., and Silver, H.K. (1962). The battered child syndrome. *Journal of the American Medical Association*, **181**, 17–24.

McGinnis, J.M. and Foege, W.H. (1993). Actual causes of death in the United States. *Journal of the American Medical Association*, **270**, 2207–11.

Maclean, N. (1992). *Young men and fire.* University of Chicago Press.

MMWR (1993). Recommendations of the International Task Force for Disease Eradication, December 31. *Morbidity and Mortality Weekly Report*, **42**.

Ogden, H. (1987). *CDC and the smallpox crusade.* US Department of Health and Human Services, Washington, DC.

Preston, R. (1994). *The hot zone.* Random House, New York.

Public Health Service (1980). *Promoting health/preventing disease: objectives for the nation.* US Department of Health and Human Services, Washington, DC.

Public Health Service (1990). *Healthy people 2000: national health promotion and disease prevention objectives.* US Department of Health and Human Services, Washington, DC.

Richmond, J. and Eisenberg, L. (1991). Putting the public back in public health and mental back in mental health. *Journal of Biological Psychiatry*, 1 September.

Secretary of Health, Education and Welfare (1979). *Model standards for community preventive health services. Report to the United States Congress.* US Government Printing Office, Washington, DC.

Shands, K., Schmid, G., Dan, B., ***et al.*** (1980). Toxic-shock syndrome in menstruating women: association with tampon use and *Staphylococcus aureus* and clinical features in 52 cases. *New England Journal of Medicine*, **303**, 1436–42.

Sours H., Frattali V., Feldman R., ***et al.*** (1981). Sudden death associated with very low calorie weight reduction regimens. *American Journal of Clinical Nutrition*, **34**, 453–61.

Task Force for Child Survival (1986). *Protecting the world's children. Report from October 1985 Meeting, Cartagena, Colombia*, pp. 165–76. Task Force for Child Survival, Atlanta, GA.

Task Force for Child Survival (1990). *Protecting the world's children: a call for action. proceedings of the 4th International Child Survival Conference, Bangkok, March 1–3 1990.* Task Force for Child Survival, Atlanta, GA.

Task Force for Child Survival and Development (1994). *Achieving health: new perspectives on integrated services and their contributions to mid-decade goals. Proceedings of the Task Force for Child Survival and Development, New Delhi, February 2–4 1994.* Task Force for Child Survival, Atlanta, GA.

UN (United Nations) (1990). *World declaration on the survival, protection and development of children and plan of action for implementing the world declaration on the survival, protection and development of children in the 1990s.* United Nations, Geneva.

World Bank (1993). *World development report.* Oxford University Press.

5

Information systems and sources of intelligence

5.1 The application of information science, technology, and management to public health

Denis J. Protti

Introduction

The field of public health has greatly benefited in the past and will benefit even more in the future from the effective application of the principles of information science and information management, and the effective implementation of information technology. Public health practitioners have at times been required to avail themselves of technology and systems designed to meet the requirements of the private sector or the acute care medical sector. As Friede *et al.* (1994) point out, public health information requirements are different and their needs unique. In the traditional clinical setting, the focus is on the single patient; in the public health setting, the focus is on the population.

Numerical information systems developed for patient care or the clinical laboratory are typically oriented towards facilitating the entry and review of a single record or of several hundred records of subjects in a study. In contrast, public health practitioners often need to examine thousands of records, although they may not need detailed information for each individual but only summary information about the population. In addition, holders of data are often eager to share selections of their data with others, and to engage in collaborative studies.

Textual information systems that describe the experimental medical literature are easily accessed through MEDLARS (Medical Literature Analysis and Retrieval System) and software packages such as Grateful Med. In contrast, searching the corresponding public health literature is difficult because government publications at all levels are not listed in Index Medicus, are not centrally stored, and have extremely variable formats and lengths. A further complicating factor is the paucity of public health oriented keywords in the Medical Subject Headings (MeSH) system; hence making the public health literature available in full text searchable form is an important way to provide access to it (Friede *et al.* 1994).

The data analysis needs of the clinically based epidemiologist often differ from those of public health professionals in health departments. The clinically based epidemiologist collects and analyses data from chart reviews and clinical trials, and needs software that supports non-parametric statistics and time-series analysis. However, the public health worker collects data from surveillance systems, population-based surveys, and outbreak reports and needs software that can be used to perform standardization, fit mathematical models to disease patterns, analyse data from complex surveys, and draw maps.

The most significant difference is perhaps in the area of communications. The clinician needs to communicate with patients, the clinical laboratory, and colleagues who are typically close by. The amount of information to share is often small (a status, a recommendation) and urgency is often high; telephones and beepers fit these needs. Conversely, the public health practitioner needs to communicate with colleagues in the state or district laboratory, federal agencies, and research collaborators at many geographically separated sites; large groups may be called upon to make decisions. The amount of information to share is often large but urgency is rarely high. E-mail and video teleconferencing are often more appropriate technologies that fit these needs.

Information science

Before exploring the application of information management principles and the impact of information technology in the field of public health, it is important first to understand the foundations on which information science is built.

Information

The most universal definition of information comes from philosophy—information is knowledge for the purposes of taking effective action (Meadow 1979). In his original treatise on cybernetics, Wiener (1948) compared the acquisition and processing of information in human beings and animals with the similar activity in the control of machines and other activities. Many have attempted to define information. A few examples follow:

- an increment of knowledge
- an interpretation of external stimuli
- increasing the state of knowledge of a recipient
- a reduction in uncertainty, following communication
- any physical form of representation, or surrogate of knowledge, or of a particular thought, used for communication
- a measure of one's freedom of choice when one selects a message
- recorded experience that is, or can be, used in decision-making.

The last definition is that of Churchman (1971) who postulated that recorded experience becomes information only when it is or can be applied to a decision process. Hence it is possible to have access to large amounts of descriptive raw data but yet have little or no information. In an engineering or information theory sense, information is the capacity of a communications channel, a measurable quantity that is independent of the physical medium by which it is conveyed. Applying this theory to Churchman's definition enables the measurement of the amount of information than can be obtained from a particular piece of raw data or descriptive material. In an 'information system' sense, information is generally considered to be data (raw material) that has been processed into a form that is meaningful to the recipient and is of real or perceived value in current or prospective decisions. Wiener regarded communication between the component parts of a community as vital to its activities. He saw an information system as the means by which the necessary communication can be established and maintained.

There appears to be no consensual definition of information. Information is a complex concept, and simplistic views of it lead to simplistic decisions. In a world of uncertainty, information reduces uncertainty. It changes the probabilities attached to expected outcomes in a decision situation and therefore has value in the decision process. It is so closely related to the concepts of thought, values, knowledge, and environment, that it is often difficult to isolate and adequately define 'information'. Cybernetics, which is concerned with the use of information to effect certain control actions, is but one of many fields which claims to study information.

Information theory

Wiener (1948) first suggested information theory. His contention that any organism is held together by the possession of means for acquisition, use, retention, and transmission of information denotes a biological sense of information. In their paper, 'A mathematical theory of communication', Shannon and Weaver (1960) provided the foundation for measuring information (in a non-semantic sense). Their concern was not with meaning, or the semantic aspects of information, but with the engineering problems of transmitting it. Information theory, as ascribed to by Shannon and Weaver, is only concerned with the factors that determine whether or not a message has been exactly or approximately transferred between a source and the destination. The principal elements of Shannon and Weaver's communications system can be delineated as follows.

1. Information source: the originator of the messages, which are to be transferred to the destination. There are an almost unlimited variety of permissible message types. Typewriter-like systems use sequences of letters. Bank cheques are messages, which are composed of letters and numbers.
2. Transmitter: operates on the message to transform it into a signal form, which can be transmitted over the communication channel (path).
3. Channel: the communication path over which the signal is transmitted to the receiver.
4. Receiver: usually performs the inverse function of the transmitter to yield a reconstruction of the message.
5. Destination: the intended termination of the message transfer.

A noise source is included in the model as unwanted signals in one form or another perturbs all systems. There is a distinction between noise and distortion. Distortion is caused by a known (even intentional) operation and can be corrected by an inverse operation. Noise is random or unpredictable interference. Shannon and Weaver identified three levels of problems in a communication system:

1. Technical accuracy: just how accurately are the message symbols transferred from the message source to the destination?
2. Semantic accuracy: how accurately is the semantic meaning of the messages transferred from the message source to the destination? These semantic problems are concerned with how closely the destination interprets the knowledge conveyed by the message to the knowledge intended by the sender.
3. Effectiveness: how effectively does the received message control the system in the intended fashion?

The primary motivation for communication within a system is to instruct selected subsystems to take some course of action. Effectiveness is closely related to semantic accuracy, and the two problems cannot always be completely dissociated. In fact, it is not uncommon to discover situations in which it is either entirely impossible or meaningless to separate the three problem levels. No real communication can take place unless the transmitter and the receiver are making use of compatible codes or schemes for symbolic representation of information, for example a bridge player failing to 'catch' and respond in an appropriate manner to his partner's bidding signal.

Information science

Although information science is not a direct descendant of information theory, many of its practitioners do attempt to retain the spirit of information theory by making information the central concept and by providing precise definitions of what it is. In information theory, the concept of information was never meant to express the meaning of a message; Shannon and Weaver, in fact, clearly stated that semantic concepts were quite irrelevant to the problem. Yet to many, information science is interested in the meaningfulness of information and in the usefulness of information to the user. It is a field of study which investigates how systems, humans, and/or machines retrieve information rather than just receive information. Humans are active rather than passive; they search for information for a specific purpose and do not just wait to process it, should it happen to pass by (Radford 1978).

Webster's Dictionary defines 'information science' as the collection, classification, storage, retrieval, and dissemination of recorded knowledge, treated both as a pure and an applied science. Although Webster's considers 'informatics' to be synonymous with information science, the literal translation of the French term *informatique* and the German term *informatik* is 'the rational scientific treatment, notably by computer, needed to support knowledge and communications in technical, economic, and social domains'. The significant difference between the English and European definitions is the latter's inclusion of the computer. It should also be noted that the European definitions of informatics make no explicit claim to its being a science.

The field of information science is perhaps best exemplified by Meadow (1979) who views it as a study concerned with:

- the nature of information and information processes
- the measurement of information (including its value) and information processes
- the communication of information between humans and information machines
- the organization of information and its effect on the design of machines, algorithms, and human perception of information

- human behaviour in respect to the generation, communication, and use of information
- the principles of design and measurement of the performance of algorithms for information processing
- the artificial intelligence applied to information processing.

Before discussing the broader concept of information science in public health, a historical review of the term medical informatics is in order.

Medical informatics

Over the past 25 years, many have published their impressions and opinions as to what constitutes the field of medical informatics. One of the first to use the term was Reichertz (1973), a doctor, who defined medical informatics as the science of analysis, documentation, steering, control, and synthesis of information processes within the health-care delivery system, especially in the classical environment of hospitals and medical practice.

Over 25 years ago, Shires and Ball (1975) confidently wrote that '[t]he year 1975 will be noted as the year in which medical informatics became accepted as a legitimate term used to describe activities involved in assembling, correlating and making effective use of information and decision making in health care delivery'. Moehr *et al.* (1979) also observed that informatics as a science does not fit into the conventional classification of sciences: it neither belongs to the natural sciences—its objects are not phenomena of nature—nor is it a part of mathematics. It is not a human science nor is it one of the classical engineering sciences. In their opinion, informatics deals with investigating the fundamental procedures of information processing and the general methods of the application of such procedures in various application areas.

Another doctor, Levy (1977) defined medical informatics as the acquisition, analysis, and dissemination of information in health-care delivery processes. He concluded that on the grounds of relevance and direct appropriateness to modern medicine, informatics is a proper basic medical science. Van Bemmel (1984), who wrote that medical informatics comprises the theoretical and practical aspects of information processing and communication, based on knowledge and experience derived from processes in medicine and health care, expressed a similar view. This definition is tempered somewhat by Hannah (1985) who reported that nurses continue to consider the term 'medical' to be synonymous with the word doctor. A relatively new but highly related term is that of nursing informatics. In using the term, Hannah refers to the use of information technologies in relation to any of the functions which are within the purview of nursing and which are carried out by nurses. As evidenced by the above definitions, the term medical informatics on the one hand appears to be confined to the clinical practice of medicine while on the other it encompasses the broader notion of health and health-care delivery. The term public health informatics is now surfacing as evidenced by the National Forum 'Accessing Useful Information: Challenges in Health Policy and Public Health' held at the New York Academy of Medicine in March 1998.

Health information science

After an extensive review of the literature and a critical analysis of the aims and objectives of the University of Victoria's new baccalaureate degree programme in health information science, Protti (1982) defined health information science as the study of the nature of information and its processing, application, and impact within a health-care system. This definition was not intended to be unique and mutually exclusive of the work of others. Rather it was an attempt to broaden the Reichertz domain of hospitals and medical practice to encompass all of health care. Health information science is to information science as health economics is to economics. An economist is one who specializes in the social science concerned chiefly with the description and analysis of the production, distribution, and consumption of goods and services. A health economist, upon familiarizing himself with the institutions, participants, and concepts of health, illness, and disease, analyses economic phenomena in health-care delivery and resource management settings. Similarly, a computer scientist is concerned with the science of properties, representation, construction, and realization of algorithms. A medical computer scientist is concerned with the application of these concepts to medical science and medical practice. To be effective, he or she must have more than a passing acquaintance with concepts of diagnosis and treatment of disease.

An engineer is concerned with the application of science and mathematics by which the properties of matter and the sources of energy in nature are made useful to many in structures, machines, products, systems, and processes. A biomedical engineer is concerned with the capacity of human beings to survive and function in abnormally stressing environments and with the protective modification of such environments.

In keeping with Meadow's views, a health information scientist or health informatician should therefore be concerned with:

- the nature of information and information processes in all aspects of health promotion, detection, and delivery of care
- the measurement of information and information processes
- the organization of information and its effect on the performance of health practitioners, researchers, planners, and managers
- the communication of information between patients, health-care providers, administrators, evaluators, planners, and legislators
- the behaviour of patients, health-care providers, administrators, planners, and legislators, in respect to the generation and use of information.

Many of health information science's conceptual foundations are borrowed from other fields such as mathematics, economics, psychology, engineering, sociology, and biology. It is a discipline which is not distinctively different from those in subject content, but is different in outlook. Information science in health is concerned with the individual and group behaviour of health-care personnel in their interaction with information and with the technology, which processes information.

Information technology

What are the major issues surrounding this complex and rapidly changing subject? To what extent will information technology affect the public health profession over the next 20 years? Rather than presume to have definite answers, this section will raise questions which readers will have to answer for themselves.

The section is structured so as to develop the following premises:

- information technology is part of the larger domain of 'technology'
- the impact that informatics will have on public health can be seen by observing the impact technology is having on society.

Although technologies such as hydroponics, genetic engineering, and nuclear fission are important in the overall scheme of things, they will not be discussed in this section.

One must resist the temptation to predict unrealistically. A little more than a hundred years ago, the American Press Association organized a group of 74 leading authors, journalists, industrialists, business leaders, engineers, social critics, lawyers, politicians, religious leaders, and other luminaries of the day to give their forecasts of the world 100 years later. Among the most striking features of the 1893 forecasts is the remarkable paucity of predictions that actually came true. Some of them seem outlandish and completely disconnected from reality—but fervently believed by their authors (Denning 1999). Predictions of what the world will be like 30 to 40 years from now are easy—the predictors need not worry about being around to defend their views. The nearer to the present, the more difficult the task for the political, social, economic, and emotional issues which influence change are much more apparent. This section will attempt to identify the issues which will probably affect public health over the next 5 to 10 years. The extent to which one agrees with someone else's views of the future is very much influenced by one's own view of the past and present, and by how well one understands the issues and is challenged or threatened by their implications. One consolation is that all health professionals have to wrestle with the same questions.

The evolution of information technology

Information technology is not a new phenomenon. It has been around since the beginning of time. It entails people communicating with each other, and recording their thoughts, ideas, and actions for others to read or hear. The broad definition of information technology includes:

- computers (mainframes to workstations, desktop personal computers, and multimedia)
- telecommunications (switching systems to faxes)
- networks (local area and wide area)
- document reproduction
- artificial intelligence and speed recognition expert systems.

In understanding information technology in a modern context, it is important to realize that the electronic computer is only one component in an elaborate and highly differentiated infrastructure. This infrastructure has grown through a succession of generations of computers, each of which represent a major change in technology. During the 8-year span of each computing generation (the first generation started in the late 1940s and the fifth in the early 1980s), revolutionary changes have taken place that correspond to those taking place over some 70 years or more in the aircraft industry. If we were to draw parallels to the rapid and massive advancements, aircraft would be able to go 100 times faster, a $200 000 home would cost $20 000, and colour televisions would cost $20.

The definition of generations in terms of electronic device technology captures important aspects of computing technology such as cost decreases, size decreases, power increases, and so on. However, it fails to account for the qualitative changes that have given computing its distinct character in each generation. The change from mechanical to electronic devices made it possible to store programs as data and enabled the use of computers as a general-purpose tool and then the development of programming language compilers. The transistor made reliable operation possible and enables routine electronic data processing and then interactive time-sharing. Integrated circuits reduced costs to the level where computers became commonplace and made possible the personal computer dedicated to the single user.

Each generation represents a revolution in technology with a qualitatively different impact. Each generation subsumes the capabilities of that preceding it, providing very much better facilities at very much lower cost, and adding new capabilities not possessed by the previous generations. One of the innovative new capabilities has been in the area of knowledge-based systems. The products stemming from breakthroughs in this area are expert systems, which simulate some of the processes of the human mind, knowledge representation, and inference, allowing expertise to be encoded for a computer and made widely available. This has generated a new industry based on creating expert systems to make the practical working knowledge of a human expert in a specific subject area such as medicine widely available to those without direct access to the original expert.

Technology and society

Society is experiencing its second major revolution in less than 200 years. The first was the Industrial Revolution of the nineteenth century, which saw the substitution of mechanical processes for human muscles. It changed the nature of work, though not the size of the workforce, and with it society's view of human values. The spinning-jenny may have done the work of 1000 women, but hundreds of thousands were eventually needed in the mills. The automobile may have put the horse out of business, but Henry Ford saw to it that many more mechanics were needed than blacksmiths, many more oil industry personnel than haymakers. Although it had a significant impact on the nature of work, the Industrial Revolution did provide untold opportunities for the individual to hold a job at some level. Even if the job was classified as unskilled labour, the person still had an identity as a breadwinner, and could feel a sense of worth from that. If that industrial job was classified as skilled labour, the person had not only the benefits of the unskilled labourer, but in addition a higher job status. As a rule, every major technological advance destroys the civilization that existed at the time of its introduction into everyday life. The steam engine pushed us out of the field, in huge crowds in darkened halls; television returned us to our own darkened living rooms. The compass and chronometer made intercontinental travel possible, the airplane makes it trivial, and advances in communications technology may make it unnecessary.

The second major revolution is the so-called electronic or information revolution in which electronic circuits are being substituted for human mental skills. The electronic revolution is not only replacing the mental processes of the unskilled labourer, but is creating a genuine human value dilemma for technologists, managers, and professionals. Technology is changing everyone's job. What is both exciting and frightening is that the rate of change does not appear to be diminishing. As put by Kaiser:

> We are at the cusp of a new century, but the alteration we are about to undergo is much more than a change in digits. It is far greater than the incremental steps—in science, art or engineering—that each century has so far brought us. It will be a quantum leap in consciousness, a dramatic step forward. The Internet, the electronic global brain, is behind this revolution. It will bring us to a new consciousness because it will allow us to share all the information we are able to gather from cultures past and present. And this sharing of information, this global conversation, will change the consciousness of the planet. (Kaiser 1999)

The fundamental economic activities of our society—agriculture and the multitude of extractive, manufacturing, and service industries—continue, but a new decision-making process increasingly influences them. Vastly more information (on markets, costs, techniques, other options) is being made available to decision-makers because of the information technology now available. This information is being eagerly sought because more informed decisions, be they in politics, operating factories, hospitals, public health agencies, or any organization, are likely to produce better results. The electronic revolution has made robotics a reality. The development and use of intelligent robots, which perform delicate tasks that once could have been done by thinking human beings, is increasingly commonplace in manufacturing sectors of society. Robotics is beginning to be introduced into health care. How long before they become commonplace?

While the industrial age found its symbol in the factory, the symbol of the information age is the computer, which can hold all the information in the Library of Congress in a machine the size of a small refrigerator. Alternatively, its proper symbol may be a robot, a machine capable of supplementing age-old manual labour and liberating human beings from the most arduous and repetitive tasks. Perhaps its symbol is the direct broadcast satellite, which can send television programmes directly into homes around the globe. Telephone companies the world over are joining forces under the banner of the Integrated Services Digital Network (**ISDN**), which is described as the key to linking all the elements of the information age. ISDN is several things at the same time, but it will allow every home and organization to receive simultaneously voice, computing, and video signals on a telephone line.

A popular way of looking at information technology is in terms of its utility. The most frequently used reasoning to justify purchases of information technology goes as follows: labour expenses are high and getting higher, computer expenses are low and getting lower; it then logically follows that one should always trade an expensive commodity, such as labour, for an inexpensive commodity, such as computers. One of the resulting dilemmas is that value has become less personal and more social or group-oriented. In a technological society, the individual has the potential of becoming insulated against ethical and moral decisions as these responsibilities are projected onto society itself. For people whose identities have been embedded in their jobs, traditional culture provides no guidelines to help them value themselves after they have been more or less excluded from the productive parts of society.

The evolution of the health-care industry

The future of the health-care industry is not the same in all parts of the world. In many parts of the world, the health-care industry is struggling to satisfy the most basic and fundamental of needs. In other parts of the world, the rapid advances in medical science are putting strains on governments to provide the best possible care, given the limited resources available. In the United States and the United Kingdom, the future of the health-care industry is quite clear—the future is competition. Competition is not new, nor is it unique to the Americans and the British; competition has always existed in terms of institutional pride, quality of care, staff prestige, and reputation. In the United States and the United Kingdom, competition is being redefined to include price and marketing as important factors and the key to being competitive is how well information is provided and used.

The increasing emphasis on competition has spurred the movement towards 'alternate-site' medicine, that is the delivery of health care outside the traditional, and costly, hospital setting. Of particular interest is the role technology plays in this new movement. Diagnoses that were once run in the hospital or in the large clinical laboratories are now being performed in doctors' offices in minutes and at a fraction of the cost charged by the large automated laboratories. Increasing numbers of surgical procedures are now performed routinely in outpatient day surgery units and in private surgical centres. Technological advances such as the lithotriptor replace complex and costly major surgery, along with its 10- to 12-day hospital stay, with a 1-day procedure, which 'shatters' rather than removes kidney stones. Medical costs are also being reduced by treatments that can be performed by many patients at home.

The market—which includes not only the drugs used in the treatment but also auxiliary equipment, such as small programmable pumps—now consists primarily of special nutritional products and services (aimed at patients with abnormal digestive systems), kidney dialysis, and continuous intravenous drug administration. Home therapies will almost certainly embrace such intractable disorders as Alzheimer's disease and many forms of physical rehabilitation. One company markets a home chemotherapy system for cancer patients, many of whom would normally have to receive anticancer drugs in a hospital or doctor's office. Patients who are healthy enough to live at home can often use a continuously administered prepackaged drug or combination of drugs. The drugs are contained in a small plastic pouch that is attached to a catheter. A portable programmable pump delivers the drugs at a slow constant rate. One of the advantages to this approach is that the steady infusion of such drugs often eliminates the side-effects, such as nausea, that usually accompany large doses.

The benefits of such procedures, moreover, extend well beyond lower costs. Recovery or remission rates for many patients are dramatically reduced in the familiar and comfortable home environment. A lens implant in the eyes of a 75-year-old woman allows her to continue to live independently in the home and community, which is meaningful to her. The quality of life is infinitely 'better' than moving to a home for the blind in a nearby town or city. Neonatal intensive care units are allowing life to be continued in hundreds of cases in which death would have been a certainty 25 years ago. Microcomputing technology is providing artificial voices for those who cannot speak, workstations for the sightless, and communication for those paralysed by stroke. The elderly, handicapped people, and others with high-risk medical conditions can find a new level of security when their hospitals use a computer and the telephone system to guarantee them almost instant response in an emergency. The list grows with each passing year. What are the implications of these trends on the public health practitioner?

Communications technology

Perhaps the form of modern information technology which will most affect the public health practitioner in the future, is communications technology. The advances in telecommunications are matching the speed of those of computing technology. More importantly the cost of this form of technology is now dropping—after years of overpricing. This drop in cost is no more evident than in the explosion of the Internet.

The Internet

What is it?

> What railroads were to America in the 19th century and superhighway systems were in the 20th, high bandwidth networks are in the 21st century. (Mitchell Kertzmay, CEO Powersoft Corporation)

Ask for a definition of the Internet and, depending on whom you ask, you will get either a simplistic answer or one that is long, detailed, and mainly incomprehensible. The simplest way to describe the Internet is with one word—communication. The Internet is often called a network of networks (Plucauskas 1994). It provides a vehicle for networks of all kinds and individual stand-alone computers to intertwine to form a global network, which connects people the world over. Exactly how many people is not easy to determine. In 1994, it was reported that the number of users with access to the Internet was growing at 10 per cent per month; forecasts were that by the turn of the century there may be 1 million networks, 100 million computers, and 1 billion users on the Internet (Smith and Gibbs 1994). In 1998, it was reported that the number of Internet users outside the United States was growing at an average annual rate of 70 per cent, and would surpass users in the United States by 2002. At that time, there were currently 60 million Internet users worldwide, of whom 68 per cent were in the United States and Canada. Worldwide, the total number of Internet users will reach 228 million by 2002 (Ohlson 1998).

As of July 1999, 205 countries or territories had at least one connection to the Internet. Thus only four new countries joined the Internet in the first 6 months of 1999. This is a diminished Internet spread rate, because there are not many new countries to join. Estimates of the number of people on the Internet seem to range between 50 and 80 million people worldwide, with 3 to 5 million users in Europe. But all that is available are estimates (just as there are only estimates of how many people watched a particular television show). There is no precise way to count the number of people on the Internet.

The users are connected to small local area networks in their offices where they share files and e-mail. Increasingly, these local area networks are being connected to form groups of thousands of computers that are linked across large areas, sometimes referred to as wide area networks. The speed at which one can do things on the Internet is remarkable, not because it is particularly speedy, but because it enables one to travel around the world in seconds. The lure of the Internet is communication and access. People who want to exchange ideas and develop knowledge are increasingly doing it on the Internet (for example, librarians whose job it is to find documents, books, and other materials now share their catalogues through the Internet).

The system that has grown into the Internet was originally designed by the United States military in 1969 under the name Advanced Research Projects Agency. The first Advanced Research Projects Agency configuration involved four computers and was designed to demonstrate the feasibility of building networks using computers dispersed over a wide area. Each computer communication point or node on the Internet is able to pass information on to the next node. Information on the Internet is controlled using a set of data communications standards known as the transmission control protocol/Internet protocol. Protocols are agreed upon methods of communication used by computers similar to the way people have protocols for communicating. The specifics of transmission control protocol are complex (and highly technical) and beyond the scope of this chapter. Suffice it to say that the transmission control protocol/Internet protocol is designed to ensure that every piece of information finds the most direct route to its destination. The hundreds of thousands of nodes around the Internet form a web in which information can travel, thus eliminating the need for central communication switches and means that as long as at least two nodes are in contact, the network will remain operational.

There is no single owner, or even a formal coalition that actually 'owns' the Internet. The various subnetworks have owners who recognize that having connections to other networks either enhances their mission or makes their services more desirable. The only group that 'runs' the Internet is the Internet Society. The Internet Society is a professional membership society with more than 150 organizational and 6000 individual members in over 100 countries. It provides leadership in addressing issues that confront the future of the Internet, and is the organization home for the groups responsible for Internet infrastructure standards, including the Internet Engineering Task Force and the Internet Architecture Board. A common stake in maintaining the viability and global scaling of the Internet binds the Society's individual and organizational members. They comprise the companies, government agencies, and foundations that have created the Internet and its technologies as well as innovative new entrepreneurial organizations contributing to maintain that dynamic. Its Board of Trustees elected by its membership around the world governs the Society.

Internet tools

There are many different ways to send and receive information across the Internet. There are also many recent publications that provide in-depth descriptions. Many are available for free around the Internet or can be purchased in the ever-growing number of computer sections in bookstores. The ability to access different tools depends on the type of Internet account and the sophistication of the interfaces users employ to log on (connect) to the Internet.

E-mail is and probably always will be the most common use of the Internet. It allows Internet users to send and receive messages from around the world. Requests for database searches and the result posted to an account can also be done by e-mail. E-mail is also used to join electronic mailing lists (called listservers) on specific topics of interest. E-mail is used to transfer text, program files, spreadsheets, and even photographic images. Messages can be sent and received in hours at most and often within minutes; it is no wonder that most e-mail users refer to the regular postal service as 'snail mail'.

E-mail is based on the fundamental concept of store-and-forward technology. The store part refers to a message being added to a storage system by the message's originator. When the recipient is ready the message is forwarded for retrieval. The beauty of this technique is that the recipient does not have to be available when the originator sends the message. This enables the e-mail system to select how the message will move from the place where it is first stored to the place where it is retrieved (forwarded to the user).

It is becoming increasingly easy to find anyone on the Internet—even if one does not know his or her e-mail address. Internet addresses are in two parts, a 'domain' name and a user name separated by an '@' sign. The domain name (more correctly called a hierarchical name) consists of the name of the machine on which the user has an account, along with the network groups and subgroups leading to that computer, thereby giving that machine a unique identification which enables the Internet software to determine where to deliver the message. Delivering the message to the addressee is then up to the named computer. The computer's name is chosen locally and is often colourful or thematic. User names can be cryptic. They are often composed of first initial and last name but can be shortened to a nickname or identifying numbers. All Internet alphanumeric addresses are actually aliases for numeric addresses, such as 134.6.4.187. The alphanumeric addresses are used because, even though they can be hard to interpret, they are easier than the numeric names. Machines on the Internet called name servers handle the translation of alphanumeric names into numeric addresses. To bypass the cumbersome Internet address of a person or persons, many mail programs enable users to create aliases. Aliases are particularly helpful when e-mail is sent to a group of people.

E-mail is such an inexpensive form of communication, and it is so easy to send copies of messages to long distribution lists, that recipients may get much mail which is of little or no value to them. As a result, new filtering software is being developed to help sort the wanted from the unwanted mail. Users can develop their own filtering rules (such as, if from 'boss', display immediately) and can modify them at any time. Techniques such as assigning points to messages to indicate their importance is another variation of the same theme to make e-mail communications among groups more effective—to get relevant information to the recipients with less waste of time on the part of both senders and recipients.

Usenet newsgroups are Internet bulletin boards that are similar to listservers but require the use of software known as a newsreader. There are thousands of Usenet groups and listservers for discussion of medical and health-related topics. A number of groups have already put up information relating to community and public health issues. The Institute of Maternal and Child Health policy at the University of Florida has provided information through the Maternal and Child Health Network. The topics include items such as vaccination requirements, injury prevention summaries, school health information, and child health policy documents. Internet resources for the hearing impaired, including newsletters, software, and demographic data, are available through a number of sites. As well as providing services for the hearing impaired, the Internet can be used as an enabling technology, especially for individuals who are homebound or live in an institution. Other types of community health information available include breast cancer support and poison control information.

The potential of the Internet for public health cannot be overstated. The World Health Organization (**WHO**) says it receives as many as five unconfirmed rumours a week of new infectious disease outbreaks, by telephone, newspaper, or e-mail. Each rumour is then investigated and a rumour/outbreak list is sent out electronically on a need-to-know basis to relevant personnel at the WHO, its collaborating centres, and other public health authorities. These reports, however, are not intended for public consumption. The WHO will only post news of an outbreak on the public web page of the Emerging and Communicable Diseases (**EMC**) after confirmation. Because confirmation often requires sending specimens to a laboratory that may be outside the country of origin, the WHO system is notoriously slow at alerting the world at large to outbreaks.

Public health experts who want their news immediately have learned to rely on a web site known as ProMED-Mail (the name represents Program for Monitoring Emerging Diseases). Founded by New York State Health Department epidemiologist Jack Woodall, ProMED-Mail is an Internet e-mail based system connected by satellite to ground stations and Internet nodes throughout the world. Anyone can subscribe. In the 4 years since it went online, ProMED-Mail has grown from 40 subscribers in seven countries to 15 000 in 150 countries and is now considered by experts to be an indispensable, although not wholly reliable, medium for transmitting news of outbreaks and connecting health experts to the far corners of the globe (ProMED-Mail http://www.healthnet.org) (Taubes 1998).

However, it is not devoid of controversy. The fact that ProMED provides such rapid access is a great strength, yet that same rapidity of access can breed problems with quality control—these are the two sides of a coin in the electronic age. ProMED staff are overworked and underfunded, and they cannot fact-check every entry that is made. This unavoidable situation led to criticism that ProMED-Mail disseminates rumours. David Heymann, who directs the WHO's Division of EMC, calls ProMED a 'very valuable service', but adds that the WHO does not participate in their discussions, because the organization is 'not in a position to discuss rumors with the general public'. The WHO goal, he says, is to get the rumours and check them out (Anonymous 1998).

On the increasingly common applications of the Internet for public health is Public Health Focus Team (http://pelican.gmpo.gov/pubhealt.html) whose purpose is to facilitate actions to minimize adverse health effects resulting from consumption of seafood harvested from the Gulf of Mexico or from contact with its waters. The Health Canada web site (http://www.hc-sc.gc.ca/english/promo.htm) is but one of many similar ones around the world designed to assist the public at large to readily access information on healthy living and health promotion.

Another Internet tool is Telnet with which users can log in to other computers around the Internet. Through Telnet a person can access other computer sites using his or her own computer as a terminal. This is particularly useful for accessing medical libraries and other health-care database systems that are linked to the Internet.

File transfer protocol is the method by which specific computers transfer data or files around the Internet. Files can be simple text, usually known as ASCII files, or more complex data such as graphics or computer programs, known as binary files. The ability to pull down a file, to get data, or to run a program (if the file is executable) is vital for people doing research and development work. The Internet transfers files at a rate of millions of bytes per second, and with the coming of the National Research and Education Network, that will soon be upgraded to gigabytes (thousands of millions of bytes) per second. File transfer protocol can do more than just retrieve files. It can be used to transfer files to remote machines from a given computer. To make it a practical tool, file transfer protocol includes commands of listing directories, listing files in directories, changing directories, and getting information about what is being done and setting parameters for how the operations will be done. Many pieces of free software can be obtained from around the Internet via anonymous file transfer protocols, which allow users to log in to file transfer protocol sites where they do not have accounts. These anonymous file transfer protocol sites together contain millions of files that add up to terabytes of information.

The World Wide Web is the newest and perhaps the most powerful Internet service. It provides links to information via hypertext and, for those who have the proper type of Internet access, it can bring multimedia Internet to the desktop. Hypertext provides links to other information sources through selected, or highlighted words within a text. A person simply chooses the highlighted word to receive further facts on the topic of interest. The links could be of data located on the same machine or anywhere else on the Internet. According to one study, the World Wide Web is estimated to contain approximately 800 million pages of publicly accessible information. As if the Web's immense size was not enough, it continues to grow at an exponential rate, tripling in size every 2 years.

The two basic approaches to searching the Web are search engines and subject directories. Search engines allow the user to enter key words that are run against a database (most often created automatically, by 'spiders' or 'robots'). Based on a combination of criteria (established by the user and/or the search engine), the search engine retrieves World Wide Web documents from its database that match the key words entered by the searcher. It is important to note that the search engine is not searching the Internet 'live', as it exists at this very moment. Rather, it is searching a fixed database that has been compiled some time previous to your search. While all search engines are intended to perform the same task, each goes about this task in a different way, which leads to sometimes amazingly different results. Factors that influence results include the size of the database, the frequency of updating, and the search capabilities. Search engines also differ in their search speed, the design of the search interface, the way in which they display results, and the amount of help they offer.

In most cases, search engines are best used to locate a specific piece of information, such as a known document, an image, or a computer program, rather than a general subject. Examples of search engines include:

- AltaVista (http://www.altavista.com)
- Excite (http://www.excite.com)
- FAST (http://www.alltheweb.com)
- Google (http://www.google.com)
- HotBot (http://www.hotbot.com)
- Infoseek (http://infoseek.go.com)
- Northern Light (http://www.northernlight.com).

The growth in the number of search engines has led to the creation of 'meta' search tools, often referred to as multithreaded search engines. These search engines allow the user to search multiple databases simultaneously, via a single interface. While they do not offer the same level of control over the search interface and search logic as do individual search engines, most of the multithreaded engines are very fast. Recently, the capabilities of meta tools have been improved to include such useful features as the ability to sort results by site, type of resource, or domain, the ability to select which search engines to include, and the ability to modify results. These modifications have greatly increased the effectiveness and utility of the meta tools. Popular multithreaded search engines include:

- Dogpile (http://www.dogpile.com)
- Metacrawler (http://www.go2net.com/search.html)
- ProFusion (http://www.profusion.com)
- SavvySearch (http://www.savvysearch.com).

Subject-specific search engines do not attempt to index the entire Web. Instead, they focus on searching for websites or pages within a defined subject area, geographical area, or type of resource. Because these specialized search engines aim for depth of coverage within a single area, rather than breadth of coverage across subjects, they are often able to index documents that are not included even in the largest search engine databases. For this reason, they offer a useful starting point for certain searches.

Subject directories are hierarchically organized indexes of subject categories that allow the web searcher to browse through lists of websites by subject in search of relevant information. They are compiled and maintained by humans and many include a search engine for searching their own database. Subject directory databases tend to be smaller than those of the search engines, which means that result lists tend to be smaller as well. However, there are other differences between search engines and subject directories that can lead to the latter producing more relevant results. For example, while a search engine typically indexes every page of a given website, a subject directory is more likely to provide a link only to the site's home page. Furthermore, because their maintenance includes human intervention, subject directories greatly reduce the probability of retrieving results out of context.

Because subject directories are arranged by category and because they usually return links to the top level of a website rather than to individual pages, they lend themselves best to searching for information about a general subject, rather than for a specific piece of information. Examples of subject directories include:

- LookSmart (http://www.looksmart.com)
- Lycos (http://www.lycos.com)
- Magellan (http://magellan.excite.com)
- Open Directory (http://dmoz.org)
- Yahoo (http://www.yahoo.com).

Owing to the Web's immense size and constant transformation, keeping up with important sites in all subject areas is humanly impossible. Therefore a guide compiled by a subject specialist to important resources in his or her area of expertise is more likely than a general subject directory to produce relevant information and is usually more comprehensive than a general guide. Such guides exist for virtually every topic. For example, Voice of the Shuttle (http://vos.ucsb.edu) provides an excellent starting point for humanities research. Just as multithreaded search engines attempt to provide simultaneous access to a number of different search engines, some websites act as collections or clearing houses of specialized subject directories. Many of these sites offer reviews and annotations of the subject directories included and most work on the principle of allowing subject experts to maintain the individual subject directories. Some clearing houses maintain the specialized guides on their own website while others link to guides located at various remote sites. Examples of clearing houses include:

- Argus Clearinghouse (http://www.clearinghouse.net)
- About.com (http://about.com)
- Virtual Library (http://www.vlib.org).

Hooking up to the Internet

Not all Internet connections are the same; some allow users only to access certain types of Internet tools and are available in host-based dial-up interfaces. Other, usually commercial, Internet connections can enable users to employ Windows- or Macintosh-based software to access the Internet. Although these commercial connections can be more expensive than other options, the ease of use that these interfaces offer make them an attractive option, especially for first-time users. The three most common methods of accessing the Internet are through a university affiliation, via a community access bulletin board known as Freenet, or through a commercial service provider.

Universities

Universities were the first large-scale users of the Internet; thus virtually all schools within a typical university have some form of Internet connectivity. Students, faculties, and groups with university affiliations may be eligible for some level of Internet connectivity through their institution. Most universities will give those who are eligible an account on a computer, which has a connection to the Internet. Dialling in to another machine at the university generally accesses university Internet accounts over a modem on a personal computer either at home or on campus. University accounts can be a good place to start to navigate the Internet, especially if they are available for free as part of a university affiliation—most universities do not expect their users to pay for the Internet access. However, difficulties mastering unfriendly interfaces and lack of user support have been known to cause problems for university-based users.

Freenets

Freenets are community-based electronic bulletin boards that allow users Internet access. Freenets are relatively new tools, but more are coming on-line every month. The Freenet system is menu driven and is set up with the novice user in mind. They are, as the name implies, free to use; however, donations are strongly encouraged to help offset operating costs. As well as being able to attain local information, including health-care resources, registered users can access e-mail and other Internet tools. Freenets are not intended for business or commercial ventures and users are limited in the scope of tools they can use. For example, the use of file transfer protocol and Telnet are limited on most Freenets.

Commercial Internet accounts

Commercial service prices can vary greatly depending on the provider and the type of services used. The four most common types of Internet access that commercial providers supply are as follows:

1. Dial-up host access—similar to a university account with access through a text-based computing environment. However, interfaces and user support may be better.
2. Dial-up serial line Internet protocol and point-to-point protocol access—serial line Internet protocol and point-to-point protocol allow full Internet access over a modem and telephone line; thus users can employ interfaces that reside directly on their own computer. This is especially useful for neophytes because it means they can make use of Windows and Macintosh graphical interfaces, many of which are free to access Internet tools. Serial line Internet protocol and point-to-point protocol can also be used with multimedia Internet through the World Wide Web and browsers such as Mosaic.
3. Dedicated serial line Internet protocol and point-to-point protocol access—in this case a dedicated serial line Internet protocol and point-to-point protocol account is open for use 24 hours a day.
4. Dedicated link—used to connect an entire local area network to the Internet and/or be connected to computer(s), which will act as Internet information servers. These links can be quite expensive and are usually only feasible at an organizational level.

Conclusion

The Internet was originally developed so that science and research could share resources. To a great extent, communications in the form of e-mail and discussion groups have overshadowed the Internet use for resource sharing. Although the traditional methods of scholarly communication—presentations at conferences, publishing of papers in journals, and so on—have not been eliminated, they are being recognized as inadequate for current research needs. The Internet distributes information in a way that is infinitely more flexible and more timely. Findings, papers, and information can be instantly shared and discussed.

The Internet can provide an innovative solution for meeting a variety of communication needs within the public health communications. As services and tools expand and improve, more ways of applying the technology will continue to be found; the Internet will probably soon become a service from the telephone company. It is, however, important to remember that the Internet is not about technology, it is about people. The tools and applications are only as valuable as the people they enable and empower to communicate.

Computer-based group support systems

There are a varied and growing number of computer-based group support systems including computer conferencing, video and audio teleconferencing, document interchange services, meeting support tools, and group decision support. Perhaps the most common group support system aimed at increasing the effectiveness of communication amongst individuals is computer conferencing.

Computer conferencing

Computer conferencing is a teleconference that uses computers, software, and communications networks to allow groups of people to exchange ideas, opinions, and information (McNurlin and Sprague 1989). The people in a teleconference may all be located in the same building, or they can be scattered worldwide. Each user signs on to the teleconference (via a terminal or personal computer) at his or her own convenience; there is no need for members of the group to be using it simultaneously, although they may do so if they choose.

Although similar in some ways, computer conferencing systems are different from other types of computerized communication, such as e-mail, bulletin boards, and information retrieval services. E-mail is essentially a one-to-one (or one-to-many) form of communication. Moreover, after a message has been read, it is generally deleted; there tends to be little or no storage of messages. Bulletin boards provide storage but are designed mainly for posting notices for other people to read a one-to-many type of communication. Information retrieval services provide a stored database that users can retrieve from but cannot change.

Computer conferencing systems typically include not only e-mail and bulletin boards but also many-to-many communications, by allowing all participants to join topics and enter comments on the subject being discussed. They provide storage; comments are not deleted after being read. In joining one or more conferences, each time the person logs on, the system tells them how many messages have been entered in those particular conferences since the last time, and will deliver those messages one at a time. If one gets tired of a conference, one can leave it and not receive any more messages from it. Computer conferencing allows the setting up of subconferences for discussing some aspect of the general subject in more detail. Some systems also allow voting, to indicate consensus of opinion.

The benefits of computer conferencing include:

- fast exchange of information
- less formality
- encourages more stimulating ideas
- provides a written record of discussions
- convenient, use it at any time
- non-interruptive
- avoids telephone tag and slowness of mail
- handles a dispersed group as easily as a local one
- branching allows for special interest discussions and limits junk mail
- late joiners can catch up easily
- users can settle matters without face-to-face meetings
- users like its collaborative nature
- supports group interaction, valuable for project management
- encourages chance meetings of people with shared interests
- fosters cross-fertilization of ideas
- managers can participate and be more proactive
- allows large numbers of people to interact as equals.

Video conferencing

Video conferencing technology is becoming an affordable reality that can substantially increase communications productivity. The products being developed to support 'personal conferencing' exploit the power and availability of the workstation and the capabilities of interfaces such as Microsoft Windows, Presentation Manager, X Windows, and Motif. They allow users on either end to share moving video images, voice communications, documents, and even applications across the 'new' digital ISDN phone service or over common high-speed local area networks and wide area networks such as Ethernet or Token Ring. They now even work over public data networks such as the Internet (Linthicum 1994). In New Zealand 5 years ago it was estimated that there were around 30 to 40 users of video conferencing. Now it is estimated that around 300 New Zealand organizations dial into video conferencing with systems that range from around US$17 500 to US$70 000. Payback time has become more attractive as managers identify savings in travelling time, which over time can be put into other business areas (Tapsell 1998).

The multimedia revolution is making the presence of speakers and microphones on workstations commonplace. The new mini video cameras are less intimidating than camcorders. The picture that these cameras produce and the sound quality from the audio equipment are surprisingly good. The price of these systems ranges from US$500 to US$20 000, depending on the features and the platform supported.

Video conferencing still has network problems and, until 1993, when desktop units came along, conference rooms systems cost upwards of US$60 000; portable units started at US$25 000 (Strauss 1994). A research report estimated that there were just 14 000 desktop units installed worldwide at the end of 1993, but it expected that the number would soar to 1.96 million by the end of 1998. Even in view of AT & T's arrangement with Intel to create a personal conferencing gateway, universal video calling does not seem likely for a few years. However, innovative use of the technology is giving early users a competitive edge. As an example, most banks have television cameras at their automated teller machines for security purposes. Some are turning that camera into a two-way videoconference application and staffing the bank remotely. They let customers interact with bank personnel and do all of their banking around the clock at considerably less expense than keeping branch offices open. MEDITrust pharmacy (http://www.meditrust.com), a Canadian mail-order pharmaceutical firm, has created a virtual pharmacy. It puts a video/phone/data kiosk in a convenience store, connects it to a pharmacist at a remote site over ISDN lines, and sends medicines by mail. The kiosk scans the prescription so that the pharmacist can give advice, stamps the prescription filled, and processes the credit card order. Medicine is sent to a customer's home by 2-day special mail service. The convenience store may be in a rural village too small to support a full pharmacy. Employers are considering offering their staff a similar service from the company offices.

Group decision support systems

Until recently most of the work in decision support systems has been to help individuals make decisions. However, increasingly in all sectors, and particularly so in public health, decisions are not made by individuals—instead groups of people are involved. Rather than support only communication between members of group, group decision support systems have features and functions that help these groups form a consensus or come to a decision (McNurlin and Sprague 1989).

The desired design of a group decision support system typically includes several features or characteristics. Each participant is able to work independently of the others, and then publicly release or demonstrate his or her personal work. When personal work is released, all group members are able to retrieve and view it. Similarly, each member is able to retrieve and view the work performed by the group as a whole.

Elements of a group decision support system include a database, a group decision support systems model base, specialized application packages, a good user interface, plus the 'people' component. The people include not only the participants but also a group facilitator who is responsible for the smooth operation of the group and who may also serve as the operator of the computerized system. Additional features typically include numerical and graphical summarization of ideas and votes, programs for specialized group procedures (such as calculating weights of different alternatives), anonymous recording of ideas, formal selection of a leader, handling progressive rounds of voting, and eliminating redundant input.

Undoubtedly the supporting of communications and decision-making will merge as researchers and developers from both areas begin supporting both. For example, rooms for video conferencing focus on communication support and seldom have workstations to support consensus building. Likewise, group decision rooms with workstations for each participant seldom have video conferencing capability to support dispersed groups. As the tools and technology improve, it is expected that group support will move beyond problems or decisions that are familiar to the participants to sensitive decisions, crisis decisions, confrontation decisions, and even 'regular' day-to-day decisions.

Data capturing technology

When the first portable computers (now called notebooks or laptops) arrived on the scene 10 years ago, these 15-kg units were considered saviours for users who needed to take their computers with them. As size began to decrease and the portable computer's power began to increase, more and more people began to enjoy the benefits of computing 'on the go'. The notebook is now full featured enough to function as the main computer for many users—all in a package that can weigh approximately 2 kg. Future notebook users can expect to see more features added with no gain in size or weight.

Firstly, lighter materials will be developed that will keep the weight down and more functionality will be integrated into the motherboards, so that additional add-ons are not required. The monochrome screen has disappeared as production yields increase and prices decrease on active-matrix colour LCD displays. Secondly, while nickel–metal hydride batteries are replacing traditional nickel–cadmium cells, lithium batteries are just emerging and are offering longer life and less weight. One of the most important developments in notebooks is the advent of the PCMCIA (Personal Computer Memory Card International Association) card. PCMCIA presents a new paradigm of computing that extends the portability of notebook computers.

These credit-card-sized devices offer 'plug-and-play' convenience. They can also be inserted and removed without turning off the computer. PCMCIA cards are available for a variety of functions, including network cards, memory expansion, storage fax/modems, sound cards, and so on. PCMCIA cards have become a regular feature on desktop machines as well. One future scenario has users simply moving their data and applications back and forth between machines on a PCMCIA. Another popular option is the notebook docking station combination. The docking station will become more of a common accessory as users take the components out of their notebooks and plug them into the station at the office or home to obtain the benefits of a larger monitor, external keyboard, alternate pointing devices, better sound, or link onto a network. One aspect of notebook computing is the palmtop computer, which is an even smaller device capable of data connection in the field. Nurses are already using this form of technology, as are physiotherapists, chiropodists, and health visitors in the North West Anglia Health Care Trust in Peterborough in the United Kingdom. Once users have adjusted their work patterns and behaviours, they report that the palmtop leads to a more professional and business-like approach to the job, enabling them to rationalize the workload and manage their time more efficiently, thereby offering a higher standard of patient care than was previously possible (Bradford 1994).

Finally, voice recognition is not far away. This technology has been used for sometime in the field of radiology and is now beginning to appear in other aspects of medicine. Computer systems are now being delivered with speech boards. For dictation systems to run effectively requires a multitasking system that lets several programs run at the same time. One of the programs just sits and listens to what one is saying, looking for either command phrases or phrases to dictate. Doctors testing these new systems find the system accurate and capable of supporting dictation at 60 to 70 words per minute (Mullin 1994). They are finding that it saves time and provides more control over clinical notes, bypassing the normal transcription process.

Data storage and retrieval technology

The power of information technology rests in its ability to process instructions very quickly. One aspect of this increased speed relates to a computer's ability to store and retrieve data quickly. Primary storage is part of the computer's central processing unit and is generally referred to as memory. Conversely, secondary storage is physically separated from the central processing unit. A type of secondary storage that is becoming increasingly common and affordable is the optical disk (Hicks 1993).

One type of optical disk shares the same technology as the digital compact disk players used with stereo systems and is referred to as a CD-ROM (compact disk read-only memory). Originally, data could be written on them only once; however, there are now erasable versions. The primary advantage of optical disks is large storage capacity at low costs; some of them cost less than $10 and hold 200 to 2000 megabytes (1 gigabyte) of data. Five hundred megabytes is the equivalent of 300 000 double-spaced typewritten pages, or the entire *Encyclopaedia Britannica* several times over.

Optical disks are used for storing large volumes of data, including photographs that are not changed often. The Medline CD-ROM, available in most medical libraries, is a well-known medical example. A number of medical specialties receive their journal references on CD-ROMs and access the material at home on their personal computers. SAM-CD is the CD-ROM version of *Scientific American*'s reference book on internal medicine. *Scientific American* sends out a CD-ROM every 3 months with the new data (including photographs) in place and ready to use. The *Compendium of Pharmaceuticals and Specialties* is available on CD-ROM, which offers users the power of the computer in conducting complex searches in a matter of seconds. New and more flexible software is being developed, as CD-ROM technology will soon become a standard component of all personal computers, much as hard disks became standard in the late 1980s. In the world of high-speed technology, CD-ROM drives are considered slow; the average access time is 1 s and the average transfer rate is only 300 000 bits of data per second. The newer WORM (write-only read-many) technology is being packaged in multifunction drives or 'jukeboxes' and has access times as fast as 45 ms. Still, this is also 'too slow', and not far away is holography, a technique for recording and then reproducing a complete image of a three-dimensional object and the next great technology in data storage. In August 1994, researchers at Stanford University reported the first digital holographic storage system. The team believes that 120 billion bytes can be stored per cubic centimetre using digital holographic storage and access rates will be significantly faster than today's technology.

Information management

Given the 'information revolution' our society is experiencing, it is not uncommon to assume that 'information' infers only the involvement of computers and communication technology. In organizational settings, one often further assumes that the major issue involved is the introduction of information technology within the organization. What is often overlooked is that the introduction of information technology in an organization is much more of a social than a technical process. If the people involved in information management are to co-ordinate the acquisition and provision of information effectively, they must understand how people process information, both as individuals and as members of organized groups or units. The real challenges in implementing successful information systems are those of managing people and their perceptions.

Information systems

An information system connects, classifies, processes, and stores data, and retrieves, distributes, and communicates data to decision-makers. This processed data may or may not then be transformed into information by the human decision-maker. In an organizational setting such systems are often called management information systems. This view was promulgated by Davis (1983) when he defined a management information system as an integrated man–machine system for providing information to support the operations, management, and decision-making functions in any organization. The system uses computer hardware and software, manual procedures, management and decision models, and a database. In many ways, information systems are an extension of the study of organizations, organizational systems, organizational behaviour, organizational functions, and management. An organization is an administrative and functional structure of human resources, material, and natural and information resources co-ordinated in some manner to achieve a purpose.

Since the 1990s, the once traditional organization has quickly been replaced by the 'virtual corporation' (Davidow and Malone 1992). Whether real or virtual, any organization is held together by the methodologies of acquiring, processing, retaining, transmitting, and utilizing information. The purpose of an information system is to support managerial activities of all types at all levels of an organization. An organizationally based information system acquires, processes, stores, and transmits raw material which is usually a mixture of (a) factual data, (b) material that has been subjected to interpretation in its passage through the system, and (c) other content that is openly acknowledged to be the opinions, judgements, and observations of individuals both within the organization and outside it. The value of this material, that is information, depends upon the use to which it can be put. Measuring information, decision-making, and productivity in information processing is an unresolved problem. Information is an essential commodity and a unique resource. It is often not depreciable and a 'purchaser' may not be able to determine the value of an information item without examining it. Information is not a 'free good'. It is a resource no less essential to the survival of an organization than are personnel, material, and natural resources. Information is a resource that must be conserved, recycled, and protected. As with any other resource, it must be managed.

Increasingly, organizations are coming to accept this premise and hence look for people who view information management from in 'information science' versus a 'computer science' perspective. The two perspectives are related but by no means the same. People with computer science backgrounds tend to be more concerned with computer hardware and software. Their formal education had a strong theoretical and mathematical basis, with particular emphasis in algorithm development. They probably have a thorough grounding in the study of the implementation of algorithms in programming languages which operate on data structures in the environment of hardware. They usually have had little exposure to information requirement analysis and organizational considerations. They have greater expertise in programming, system software, and hardware. People with such a technical background tend to be more machine and technology focused.

People with an information science background or orientation tend to be more concerned with people and the nature of information and information processes in the organization. They are more likely to assess the value of information and its effect on the performance of the decision-makers within the organization. In a health-care setting, they are more likely to be aware of how and why information is communicated between patients, clients, health-care providers, epidemiologists, administrators, evaluators, and planners. The use to which these people put information is the most critical criteria of success of information systems, whether computer based or not.

Managing information

If information is to be managed, someone has to be the information manager. The future will place new demands for information systems in public health environs. Information exchange between health-care facilities, governments, and other constituencies is becoming more prevalent, and the need for individuals within an organization to share and use the same information is becoming much more common. In this new climate, new professions are emerging—those of health information managers. These individuals will become active in planning, designing, implementing, managing, developing, and deploying information systems to meet the needs of rapidly changing health-care systems. These information systems will vary in complexity from simple central registers, to hospital and/or community data abstracting, and on to complex interinstitutional networked decision support systems. In health-care settings information is needed to support decisions that relate to:

- promoting wellness, preventing illness, and curing or ameliorating disease
- monitoring, evaluating, controlling, and planning health-care resources
- formulating health and social services policy
- advancing knowledge through research and disseminating knowledge through education.

An information manager is any individual within an organization who has been given the responsibility to manage the organization's information. Given the information revolution that today's society is experiencing, it is not uncommon to assume that information infers the involvement of computers and communication technology. In organizational settings, one often further assumes that the major issue involved is the introduction of information technology within the organization. As noted above, what is sometimes overlooked is that the introduction of information technology is much more a social than a technical process. If information managers are to co-ordinate the acquisition and provision of information effectively, they must understand how people process information both as individuals and as members of organized groups or units. They will need to have excellent interpersonal skills in order to teach, motivate, convince, and influence a variety of people. The real challenges in implementing successful information systems are those of managing people and their perceptions. Information managers will be agents of change—a bridge between older systems and models, and newer technologies and techniques. No matter where they are positioned in the organization, they are usually expected to develop planning processes for aligning all information systems to the strategic direction, objectives, and structure of the organization. This entails co-ordinating all information systems within the organization including computing services, minicomputers and microcomputers, records rooms, office automation, management engineering, voice communication, and other related areas. Determining the investment to be made in information systems and providing a rigorous and disciplined framework for evaluating information benefits versus information costs is also a part of the job. Specific standards and guidelines need to be established for the definition, measurement, use, and disposition of information so that all segments within the organization are operating within the same framework. It is often left to the information manager to explain information technology and the need for new systems to staff at all levels of the organization. This critical educational role is often carried out in conjunction with the development of policies and procedures that ensure the co-ordination and justification of request for personal computers, terminals, office automation devices, and various software packages.

These responsibilities can often be onerous, and those who succeed possess excellent interpersonal, written, and verbal communication skills (that is, an ability to function effectively at the board, senior and middle management, and operational levels of the health-care facility). Effective information managers understand the organization's mission and the business that it is in. They also understand the complexity and dynamics of health-care delivery, are able to function in multidisciplinary teams and environments, appreciate 'small p' and 'capital P' politics, and are able to assess political situations. To be effective information managers, they have to be 'doers'. They have to be able to demonstrate short-term success while making progress on the long-range information systems requirements. To do so they must understand the present and future capabilities of information technology, be technologically credible to their peers and staff, and be able to plan the effective use of information technology in the organization.

Information systems are people and information systems that create change. Information managers must be able to manage change, which includes a sincere appreciation of the effects of change on people. They must be willing and able to teach and educate a wide variety of individuals at all levels of the organization, none of which can be done without having a positive attitude towards users. Effective information managers demonstrate leadership through effective listening, team building, and consensus building. They are creative, innovative, and have a vision of the future. Most of all, they have an honest concern for the organization's most critical resource—its people.

The health of a nation depends to a certain extent on how well organizations use the resources available to them to promote wellness, prevent illness, and cure disease. The health of an organization depends to a large extent on the effectiveness of the decisions made by its staff; effective decisions require effective managers and information systems, which produce reliable and useful information. The health of an information system is a function of how well it has been defined, designed, implemented, operated, and maintained. Keeping the organization's information systems healthy is the role of the information manager regardless of his or her title.

Organizational transformation

In 1992, Scott Morton and his colleagues at the Massachusetts Institute of Technology's Sloan School of Management Research published a textbook entitled *The Corporation of the '90s* (Scott Morton 1992). The work was a 5-year multimillion-dollar research programme on how organizations can make better use of information technology.

A consortium of Massachusetts Institute of Technology faculty and 12 corporate and public sector sponsors contributed financial resources, advice, and their workplaces as experimental sites. The group's focus was about how new technologies are changing the way people work and the way organizations will collaborate and compete. The major findings have had a significant impact on a multitude of organizations in both the private and public sectors around the world, including the United Kingdom's National Health Service (**NHS**). The Massachusetts Institute of Technology findings are summarized under the following headings.

Fundamental changes due to changes in information technology

Information technology is enabling fundamental changes in the way work is done. The degree to which a person is affected is determined by how much their work is based on information; that is, information on what product to make or service to deliver and how to do it (production task), as well as when to do it and in conjunction with whom (co-ordination task). The impact on production work is apparent in:

- physical production—affected by robotic, process control, intelligent sensors
- information production—affected by data processing computers for clerical tasks such as invoicing
- knowledge production—affected by computer-assisted design/computer-assisted manufacturing.

What is less well known is that the new information technology is permitting a change in the economics and functionality of the co-ordinating process as distance can be shrunk towards zero as far as information flow is concerned. Time can shrink to zero or shift to a more convenient point. Organizational memory, as exemplified by the common database, can be updated by anyone and made available to all authorized users. New 'group work' and team concepts combine all three aspects of co-ordination: distance, time, and memory. The increasing availability of information technology can fundamentally change management work as relevant and timely information on changes in the external environment and the organization's view of the environment affects the direction dimension. Relevant and timely information on measuring the organization's performance against critical success factors affects the control dimensions. The second aspect of control is interpreting such measures against the corporate plan and determining what actions to take.

Integration of business functions

Information technology is enabling the integration of business functions within and between organizations. Public and private telecommunication networks are making the principle of 'any information, at any time, anywhere, and at any way you want to look at it' economically feasible. The boundaries of organizations are becoming more permeable; where works gets done, when, and with whom is changing. Electronic integration is surfacing in the following forms:

- within the value chain—land area networks permit 'teams' to work together on a common product
- end-to-end links of value chains between organizations—electronic data interchange and 'just-in-time' systems are shifting the boundaries of an organization to include elements of other organizations thereby creating a 'virtual' organization
- value chain substitution via subcontract or alliance—permit an organization to take advantage of (mutual) economies of scale and unique skills of its partner organization.

Electronic integration is removing unproductive buffers and leveraging expertise.

Shifts in the competitive climate

Information technology is causing shifts in the competitive climate of many industries. Information technology is introducing unprecedented degrees of simultaneous competition and collaboration between firms. It is becoming increasingly important to know when to support standards and when to try to pre-empt competitors by establishing a proprietary *de facto* standard. The benefits do not flow from the mere use of information technology but arise from the human, organizational, and system innovations that are added on to the original business benefit. Information technology is merely an enabler that offers an organization the opportunity to invest vigorously in added innovations if it wishes to stay ahead of its competitors.

New strategic opportunities

Information technology presents new strategic opportunities for organizations that reassess their mission and objectives. Organizations are going to go through three distinctive stages as they attempt to respond to their changing environments.

1. Automate—reduce the cost of production, usually by reducing the number of workers. As an example, scanners, bar code, and universal product codes are being introduced for more than identifying goods.
2. Informate—what happens when automated processes yield information as a byproduct. This necessitates that knowledge workers develop new skills to work with new information tools; it often entails new ways of thinking.
3. Transform—a stage characterized by leadership, vision, and a sustained process of organization empowerment. It includes the broad view of quality but goes beyond this to address the unique opportunities presented by the environment and enabled by information technology.

Production workers will become analysers, a role offering a different level of conceptual skill from what was needed before as a 'doer' or machine minder; it will require an ability to see patterns and understand the overall process rather than just looking at controlling information on a screen.

Successful application of information technology will require changes in management and organizational structure Information technology is enabling a break-up or disintegration of traditional organizational forms, multiple skills can be brought together at an arbitrary point in time and location. The ability of information technology to effect co-ordination by shrinking time and distance permits an organization to respond more quickly and accurately to the marketplace. This not only reduces assets that the organization has tied up but improves quality as seen by the customer. The 'metabolic' rate of the organization, that is, the rate at which information flows and decisions are made, is speeding up and will become faster in the next millennium. The measurements, rewards, incentives, and required skills all require rethinking in the new information technology-impacted world.

Management of public health organizations: global competition

A major challenge for management in this millennium will be to lead their organizations through the transformation necessary to prosper in the globally competitive environment. Management must ensure that the forces influencing change move through time to accomplish the organization's objectives. Evidence to date is that, at the aggregate level, information technology has not improved profitability or productivity. Some of the reasons are:

- benefits are there but simply not visible
- improvement is in lower prices or better quality
- investment in information technology is necessary to stay in business
- the external world is demanding more
- use of information technology in low pay-off areas
- information technology is laid on top of existing services
- no cost reduction, just cost replacement.

To go through the transformation process successfully, organizations must have a clear business purpose and a vision of what the organization is to become; a large amount of time and effort must be invested to enable the organization to understand where it is going and why. The organization must have a robust information technology infrastructure in place, including electronic networks and understood standards; the organization must invest heavily and early enough in human resources—all employees must have a sense of empowerment. Last, but by no means least, understanding one's organizational culture and knowing what it means to have an innovative culture is the first key step in a move towards an adaptive organization.

Case study: the United Kingdom's NHS information management and technology strategy

One public service organization which has adopted the Massachusetts Institute of Technology findings as a cornerstone to its corporate strategy, is the United Kingdom's NHS. The goal of the NHS Management Executive is to create a better health service for the nation in three ways:

- ensuring services are of the highest quality and responsive to the needs and wishes of patients
- ensuring that health services are effectively targeted so as to improve the health of local populations
- improving the efficiency of the services so that as great a volume of well-targeted effective services as possible is provided from the available resources.

The July 1992 White Paper, *The Health of the Nation* (Department of Health 1992), identified five priority areas and established key targets such as:

- reducing deaths from coronary heart disease in the under-65 age group by at least 40 per cent by the year 2000
- reducing cervical cancer by at least 20 per cent by the year 2000
- reducing suicides by at least 15 per cent by the year 2000
- reducing gonorrhoea by at least 20 per cent by 1995
- reducing deaths from accidents among children under 15 by at least 33 per cent by 2005.

A strengthened information and research capability at central and regional levels was an essential component of the business plan. Expanded or new health surveys and epidemiological overviews to improve baseline statistics on the health of the population would be undertaken. A Central Health Outcomes Unit would lead on developing and co-ordinating work on assessment of health outcomes. Information systems, which enable adequate monitoring and review, would be developed including a public health information strategy (Ranade 1994). Such was the case in 1992 under a Conservative government. In May 1997, a new Labour government was elected and the policies changed. One of their first efforts was the White Paper *Saving Lives: Our Healthier Nation* (http://www.doh.gov.uk/ohn/execsum.htm). In it they rejected the previous government's scatter-gun targets. Instead they set tougher (their term) but attainable targets in priority areas by the year 2010:

- cancer: to reduce the death rate in people under 75 by at least a fifth
- coronary heart disease and stroke: to reduce the death rate in people under 75 by at least two-fifths
- accidents: to reduce the death rate by at least a fifth and serious injury by at least a tenth
- mental illness: to reduce the death rates from suicide and undetermined injury by at least a fifth.

The NHS Information Management and Technology Strategy

In 1992, any public health information strategy was to be a part of the NHS Information Management and Technology Strategy, which was to respond to the business needs of the NHS to see best benefit and value for money from information management and technology investment. It was to set the direction for computerization and information sharing across the NHS into the next century. The Strategy was intended to ensure that the implementation of information systems in the NHS was co-ordinated and managed to achieve maximum potential benefits for patients, clinical staff, management, and administrative staff.

The Strategy was intended to support better care and communication through the appropriate use of information management and technology. It was to provide a framework for the connection and exchange of data (Keen 1994). Whether or not it achieved these goals is outside the purview of this chapter. In the opinion of some it failed, while others hold the view that critical infrastructure elements were indeed put into place.

In September 1998, the Labour government released its own information strategy entitled *Information for Health: an Information Strategy for the Modern NHS, 1998–2005* (http: www.NHSIA.NHS.UK/). The purpose of this information strategy is to ensure that information is used to help patients receive the best possible care. The Strategy will enable NHS professionals to have the information they need both to provide that care and to play their part in improving the public's health. The Strategy also aims to ensure that patients, carers, and the public have the information necessary to make decisions about their own treatment and care, and to influence the shape of health services generally.

The government has set out the following specific objectives to be delivered through the implementation of this strategy over the period 1998 to 2005:

- to ensure that patients can be confident that the NHS professionals caring for them have reliable and rapid access, 24 hours a day, to the relevant personal information necessary to support their care
- to eliminate unnecessary travel and delay for patients by providing remote on-line access to services, specialists, and care, wherever practicable
- to provide access for NHS patients to accredited independent multimedia background information and advice about their condition
- to provide every NHS professional with on-line access to the latest local guidance and national evidence on treatment, and the information they need to evaluate the effectiveness of their work and to support their professional development
- to ensure the availability of accurate information for managers and planners to support local Health Improvement Programmes and the National Framework for Assessing Performance
- to provide fast convenient access for the public to accredited multimedia advice on lifestyle and health, and information to support public involvement in, and understanding of, local and NHS policy development.

NHS Information Management and Technology Principles

The five key principles of the 1998 Strategy are exactly the same as those of 1992.

1. Information will be person based. Priority will be given to person-based systems where data is connected as part of the process of care. Such systems will hold a health-care record for each individual, which can be uniquely referenced to that person's new English NHS number and thereby shared with other systems that use the same identifying key.
2. Systems are to be integrated. Wherever possible information should be entered into a computer only once; seamless care needs seamless information. After that it should be available to authorized NHS employees, with steps taken to protect confidential information from unauthorized access.
3. Information will be derived from operational systems. Whenever possible, information is to be captured at the point of delivery of care, from systems used by health-care professionals in their day-to-day work. There should be little need for different systems to record management information. Information for management purposes (administrative, financial, research, and so on) should be derived from operational point-of-care systems. Data not connected in a way that helps clinical professionals do their jobs better will not be clinically acceptable and will not be usable for other purposes.
4. Information must be secure and confidential. While recognizing the need for sharing and accessibility of information across organizations, all systems must recognize and respect the principles of privacy, security, and confidentiality. Great care is being taken to ensure that all the data held in a computer will be available only to those who need to know it and are authorized to know it.
5. Information will be shared across the NHS. Common standards and NHS-wide networking will allow computers to communicate so that information can be shared between health-care professionals and organizations, again subject to security and the safeguard of confidentiality.

The specific targets of the new 1998 Strategy are:

- reaching agreement with the professions on the security of electronic systems and networks carrying patient-identifiable clinical information
- developing and implementing a first generation of person-based electronic health records, providing the basis of life-long core clinical information with electronic transfer of patient records between general practitioners
- implementing comprehensive integrated clinical systems to support the joint needs of general practitioners and the extended primary care team, either in general practitioner practices or in wider consortia (for example, primary care groups/primary care trusts)
- ensuring that all acute hospitals have the ability to undertake patient administration, including booking for planned admissions, with an integrated patient index linked to departmental systems, and capable of supporting clinical orders, results reporting, prescribing, and multiprofessional care pathways
- connecting all computerized general practitioner practices to NHSnet
- providing 24-hour emergency care access to relevant information from patient records
- using NHSnet for appointment booking, referrals, discharge information, radiology and laboratory requests, and results in all parts of the country
- the development and implementation of a clear policy on standards in areas such as information management, data structures and contents, and telecommunications, with the backing and participation of all key stakeholders
- community prescribing with electronic links to general practitioners and the Prescription Pricing Authority
- routinely considering telemedicine and telecare options in all Health Improvement Programmes
- offering NHS Direct services to the whole population
- establishing local Health Informatics Services and producing costed local implementation strategies
- completing essential national infrastructure projects including the networking infrastructure, national applications, and so on
- opening a National Electronic Library for Health with accredited clinical reference material on NHSnet accessible by all NHS organizations
- planning and delivering education and training in informatics for clinicians and managers.

As a result of yet another round of reforms in the United Kingdom, there is a fundamental change in emphasis of Health Authority information responsibilities (from contracting to public health and service effectiveness) and a need to establish a two-way flow of information between the NHS and the communities it serves. This suggests that the development of Health Authorities' information capability may need specific attention in the implementation programme for the new NHS, the public health White Paper (in due course), and the implementation of this strategy. The effective use of the informatics skills of current public health practitioners will be particularly important.

Health Authorities and their directors of public health already have access to a variety of nationally produced public health, epidemiological, and mortality data. The data presented in the Public Health Common Data Set is of particular value. The new National Framework will supplement this for assessing performance, which is currently being road-tested. However, the range of the data available needs to be extended if the vision of *Our Healthier Nation* and the consequent increased responsibilities are to be met. The information that may be needed to assess resistance to antibiotics is an example of the need to keep information requirements under review.

Conclusion—questions to be answered

Every individual has their own view, their own perception of the world around them. This view is a result of their individual backgrounds, cultures, education, and values. Everyone does not perceive that technology will affect them in the same way. As recently as 1994, a survey of nursing students found that over 95 per cent of them felt that they would never speak to a computer or use an expert system. Yet even at that time, voice recognition technology had moved out of the research laboratory and expert systems were routinely being used in a growing number of sectors including health care.

We are witnessing not only the automation of clerical activities, but also the automation of thoughtful technical and clinical work. What are the consequences? Will the responsibility for the production of reliable information rest more with rules incorporated in equipment and on established procedures than on a health professional's judgement? The acute care sector of health care is undergoing dramatic and radical changes in delivery and management, many of which are the result of new technologies and the realities of modern-day fiscal constraints. The acute care sector is under increasing pressure to account for its actions and to justify its decision-making and its use of resources. Health-care organizations worldwide are in the process of re-engineering and changing the way people do their work.

Is the same degree of change and accountability occurring in the public health sector? Will the public health information systems, which currently support financial accounting and programme delivery, be expected to allow costs to be matched to services provided and monitor productivity? Will the public health practitioner of the future be a multiskilled individual whose method of working is dramatically different than today? If not, why not?

References

Anonymous (1998). Epidemiology at the Web café. *Technology Review*, **101**, 54.

Bradford, A. (1994). Palmtop practitioners. *British Journal of Healthcare Computing*, **10**, 12–13.

Churchman, C. (1971). *The design of inquiring systems*. Basic Books, New York.

Davidow, W.H. and Malone M.S. (1992). *The virtual corporation: lessons from the world's most advanced companies*. Harper, New York.

Davis, G. (1983). Evolution of information systems as an academic discipline. *Administrative Sciences Association of Canada Conference Proceedings*, pp. 185–9. WBC Press, Vancouver.

Denning, P. (1999) *Talking back to the machine*. Copernicus Books, New York.

Department of Health (1992.) *The health of the nation*. Cmnd 1986, HMSO, London.

Friede, A., *et al.* (1994). CDC WONDER: a co-operative processing architecture for public health. *Journal of American Medical Informatics Association*, **1**, 303–12.

Hannah, K. (1985). *Current trends in health informatics: implications for curriculum planning*. Computers in Nursing, North Holland, Amsterdam.

Hicks, J. (1993). *Management information systems: a user perspective*. West Publishing, New York.

Kaiser, L. (1999). Quantum leaps in healing. *Health Forum Journal*, **42**, 50.

Keen, J. (ed.) (1994). *Information management in health services*. Open University Press, Buckingham.

Levy, A.H. (1977). Is informatics a basic medical science? In *Medinfo 1977 Proceedings* (ed. D. Shires and H. Wolfe), pp. 979–81. North Holland, Amsterdam.

Linthicum, D. (1994). Tommy, can you see me? *Open Computing*, September, 67–8.

McNurlin, B.C. and Sprague, R.H. (1989). *Information systems in management practice*. Prentice Hall, Englewood Cliffs, NJ.

Meadow, C.T. (1979). Information science and scientists in 2001. *Journal of Information Science*, **1**, 217–21.

Moehr, J.R., *et al.* (1979). Four specialized curriculums for medical informatics—review after 6 years of experience. *Proceedings of the International Conference in Medical Computing*, Springer-Verlag, Berlin.

Mullin, S. (1994). Start talking to your computer—three physicians rate IBM's speech recognition system. *Canadian Medical Informatics*, **1**, 16–17.

Ohlson, K. (1998) Non-United States Net users to dominate by 2002. *Computer World*, July 16.

Plucauskas, M. (1994). Internet and medicine part 11: hooking up and using the Internet. *Canadian Medical Informatics*, **1**, 28–30.

Protti, D.J. (ed.) (1982). A new under-graduate program in health informatics. *AMIA Congress 1982 Proceedings*, pp. 241–5. Masson, San Francisco, CA.

Radford, K.J. (1978). *Information for strategic decisions*. Reston, New York.

Ranade, W. (1994). *A future for the NHS: health care in the 1990s*. Longmans, Harlow.

Reichertz, P. (1973). Protokoll der Klausurtangung Ausbildungsziele. *Methoden in der Medizinischen Informatik*, **2**, 18–21.

Scott Morton, W. (ed.) (1992). *The corporation of the '90s*. Harvard University Press, Cambridge, MA.

Shannon, C.E. and Weaver, W. (1960). *The mathematical theory of communication*. University of Illinois Press, Urbana, IL.

Shires, D. and Ball, M. (1975). Update on educational activities in medical informatics. *Proceedings of the 5th Annual Conference of the Society for Computer Medicine*, pp. 52–4. Washington.

Smith, R. and Gibbs, M. (1994). *Navigating the Internet*. SAMS Publishing, Indiana.

Strauss, P. (1994). Beyond talking heads: videoconferencing makes money. *Datamation*, 1 October, 38–41.

Tapsell, S. (1998). Telling it like it is with teleconferencing. *Management*, **45**, 65.

Taubes, G. (1998). Virus hunting on the web. *Technology Review*, **101**, 50.

van Bemmel, J.H. (1984). The structure of medical informatics. *Medical Informatics*, **9**, 175–80.

Wiener, N. (1948). *Cybernetics*. Prentice Hall, Englewood Cliffs, NJ.

5.2 Information systems and community diagnosis in developing countries*

Chitr Sitthi-Amorn

Outline

This chapter outlines the importance of information in the planning, monitoring, and evaluation of health problems, their determinants, intervention options, and evaluation of health intervention in a community. It argues for at least five objectives of the health actions, which determine what types of information are needed. A general framework for information and community diagnosis is given which includes defining the community, agreeing on the indicators, determining the sources and methods of obtaining the information, and using the information to predict the current situation as well as future trends. Each of the sources or methods used for information gathering (routine reports, surveillance, survey and special studies, rapid survey, contact tracing, and vital registration and census) has inherent strengths and weaknesses. Therefore a combination of approaches for collecting information for community diagnosis is necessary. Despite the availability of several approaches to developing an information system, some technological limitations for a community diagnosis exist and are also discussed. Finally, a comparison is made between information systems in developed and developing countries, which partly reflect the different emphasis in the operation of health-care systems as well as differences in available resources for community diagnosis.

Introduction

Information is the basis for planning for a rational allocation of resources to cope with public health problems. Information should shed light on health situations, help to set priorities, appraise options, develop and implement programmes, and monitor and evaluate actions to determine whether they adequately address the situations. Information is the essence of the planning process. Decision-makers balance evidence from information with their values and the imperatives to arrive at the best choices. Information includes what is measured, what is not measured, and what is inherently unmeasurable. Most information systems, which rely on information technology, collect measurable quantifiable information possibly at the expense of less explicit soft and qualitative information. Therefore, an appropriate mix of measurable and intangible information will be needed. Although the information is rarely perfectly accurate, its accuracy can be enhanced through the development of a clear operational definition, training and motivating the enumerators, and interaction with stakeholders to standardize interpretations.

The definition of a community can have many interpretations such as a neighbourhood or a collection of people in similar geographical circumstances. A community also refers to a group of people who share the same stakes and common interests such as trade unions, those who are mobilized around a given activity, or the users of health services. Some have even expanded the definition of a community to include those employed in a workplace, the population of a nation, or a civil society. In this chapter, a community can encompass several interpretations such as a village, subdistrict, district, province, or nation. A fundamental requirement of an information system is to enhance the ability of decision-makers to employ evidence-based actions and enhance their roles in solving problems of a community however defined. A community is not a static entity; therefore any meaningful information system for the diagnosis of community problems requires a dynamic interaction between the members of the community and the managers of information systems. It is important to make the best use of updated information and interpret information into meaningful strategic options that reflect the reality of health and health-care systems in a given community or society. Any information produced should then be fed back to the community to enhance their future involvement. This feedback can then be the driving force in linking information to actions because the community will press for the kind of information they can use.

Public health policy-makers and health-care managers need timely, useful, and balanced information (quantifiable and intangible) for the diagnosis of health needs, their determinants, and trends to achieve effective planning and monitoring of health-care interventions. New challenges to public health have highlighted the importance of community involvement in defining problems and in coping with them. These challenges include globalization and its impacts on environment, the relationship between trade and health, emerging diseases, the market orientation of health-care system, and changes in behaviour and lifestyles. There are several ways to obtain health information for the diagnosis of communities including routine health facility reporting, screening, surveillance, special large-scale surveys, rapid surveys, contact tracing, and census. These methods vary depending on the objectives, investment, and utilities available.

The objectives of public health actions

An overall objective of community diagnosis is to estimate the magnitude of the health problems and their determinants as well as to

* The author wishes to acknowledge partial support by the Thailand Research Fund. The continuous support and encouragement of Professor Roger Detels is deeply appreciated.

analyse trends and changing paradigms of these problems and determinants. Because the community consists of heterogeneous groups, the overall objective needs to be expanded to include many value-laden issues such as health needs and determinants, equity, responsiveness to expectation, efficiency, protection of individuals, and fairness. The results of community diagnosis can then be used as evidence for discussion among the stakeholders in the community, balancing the values of the various stakeholders in setting priorities and making decisions for resource allocation acceptable to the community. The priorities and decisions for control should take into account not only the current status of health but also the impact that controls may have on health of the future generation.

The priorities and decisions for control depend not only on the indicators used for the diagnosis but also on the expressed or unexpressed values of a health system. Recently, the World Health Organization (**WHO**) suggested some possible value-laden objectives of a health system. Indicators for these value-laden objectives are being developed for better measurements of how well a health system has achieved its objectives. The possible value-laden objectives of a health system include (a) improving average health status and reducing the burden of illnesses, (b) reducing health inequities, (c) responding to the legitimate expectations of individuals, (d) improving the efficiency of health system, and (e) protecting individuals and enhancing fairness (WHO 2000*a*).

Improving average health status and reducing the burden of illnesses

Improving average health status and reducing the burden of illnesses as measured by life expectancy, death rates by age groups, disease or morbidity rates, and the measurement of the burden of illness combining mortality and morbidity are important functions of public health professionals. Indicators for the measurement of risk factors to explain mortality and morbidity have also been developed.

There are changes occurring in the burden of illnesses resulting from population growth both in developing and developed countries. In addition, demographic and epidemiological transitions can influence trends of ill health in a nation or community. Lifestyle changes are associated with illnesses such as cardiovascular diseases and the epidemics of HIV infection and tobacco use. Owing to globalization, there are many things in the future that will change health and the burden of illnesses in a community. The current decline in communicable disease mortality in many areas of the world may reverse due to drug resistance and new pathogens. Therefore, the mortality and morbidity rates from various diseases will be the backbone of information needed for health planning.

Reducing health inequities

Equity is particularly important if planning involves allocation of resources for health from the government budget that comes mainly from taxation. The agencies implementing the plans can be the government or non-governmental organizations supported by the government. In contrast, the private health system does have more responsibility to satisfy individuals who pay for their services, rather than the responsibility for reducing inequities. Therefore, the reduction of health inequities as an indicator does not apply to the private as much as to the government system.

Health inequality is linked to the agenda of poverty and material deprivation. The WHO has developed a set of measures for health inequalities including social, household, and individual differences in health. For example, male life expectancy differs greatly among various regions of the United States. Health inequalities differ between various regions of the world with different stages of human development as exemplified by the health status in Mexico compared with that of the United States and Japan. The distribution of life expectancy at birth estimated from large numbers of small area studies showed that life expectancy is most equally distributed in Japan. In both Mexico and the United States, the distribution of life expectancy between areas was wider, indicating more inequity between population groups. The inequity is particularly significant for men (WHO 2000*a*) Measuring inequalities gives health a central theme in the development agenda.

In terms of investment in research, there is also a 10/90 disequilibrium between global health expenditures for research and the burden of illness (Commission on Health Research for Development 1990). This report found that less than 10 per cent of global health research funds were spent on 90 per cent of health problems in developing countries. Thus, information on these parameters will be needed to plan a more balanced allocation of resources according to need.

Responding to the legitimate expectations of individuals

The legitimate expectations of individuals reflect an attempt to fulfil their right to health services because they are citizens of a country and community. Legitimate expectations do not include expectations based on self-interest at the expense of the public. Examples of legitimate expectations include the provision of emergency services and services with high public health values such as immunization, preventive and promotive services, and the treatment of infectious diseases.

One measure of the response to the legitimate expectations of individuals is satisfaction with services. Satisfaction has multiple dimensions including access, cost, and quality of care. There is a significant difference in the satisfaction with health systems between countries. Satisfaction with health services in the community can also be compared within regions in countries and between the public and private sectors.

Improving the efficiency of health system

The efficiency of a health system depends on the allocation of resources to services with high public health values (allocative efficiency) and the provision of technically efficient services (technical efficiency) including clinical services. Technical efficiency involves the use of cost-effective services and some form of competition and market mechanism, and therefore can apply readily to the private sector. Measures to improve the efficiency of a health system may be in conflict with measures to reduce inequities. Nevertheless, measures to reduce inequities using public resources must also be efficient. This gives rise to the notions of hierarchy of objectives in community diagnosis. It is difficult to prescribe the optimal mix between equity, efficiency, and satisfaction with services. The challenges are to use the available resources to best achieve health system goals agreed upon by the society.

There are variations in health-care expenditures with respect to the gross domestic product of countries. Thailand spends more on health as a percentage of gross domestic product than Malaysia but has a lower life expectancy and higher infant mortality than Malaysia. Theoretically, the private sector can enhance the efficiency of health care through the provision of good services at a competitive price. However, it is not known whether the changing proportion of the private sector correlates with efficiency (Newbrander 1997) because the public sectors of countries have monitored the pricing and quality of private services with differing levels of rigour. Some information for planning health care has to involve centralized efforts to monitor service standards and to protect the public. Information is needed to monitor financing, provide services at public and private facilities, and to enable the public to make appropriate choices.

Protecting individuals and enhancing fairness

Protecting individuals and enhancing fairness are two important goals of health. Citizens of a country have a right to a certain level of health regardless of whether they are rich or poor. Rights to health promotion services, disease prevention such as immunization, treatment of emergencies, and acute infections are some examples. Governments can involve the stakeholders to determine the level of health all citizens will have within the constraints of limited resources.

Each of the objectives can serve to indicate directions for the development of variables to measure the current health situation as well as to assess changes with time. A good variable has to be reliable, valid, sensitive to change, and credible to the stakeholders.

Although fulfilment of many of these objectives would lead to similar decisions, this may not be true for all cases. For example, coping with inequity by focusing on the health of the underprivileged groups to enhance social justice will require different decisions than improving the average health status of both the élites and the underprivileged groups of the society.

Without clear objectives of the health system, the demand for good information missing in the information system can be used as an excuse not to plan a programme. One important argument for not using information for planning is that information is not accurate and basing a decision on incomplete information can do more harm than good. Therefore, a clear objective will identify the minimum information needed to make decisions. A clear objective will help focus on the improvement of an information system to enhance its utility to meet the objective. A balance can then be struck to see whether a minimum level of useful information exists for the decision. In the case of inadequate information, efforts to collect additional information through a rapid survey or focus group discussions can fill an information gap in planning.

Components of information systems for planning health care

The major components of health care which will need systematic information for planning include information about (a) health situations and needs, (b) the availability of resources to deal with those needs including the various approaches to organizing and financing of the resources, (c) the organization and capacity to take those resources and convert them into services (that is, the performance of the system: efficacy, effectiveness, efficiency, quality, and decision analysis), (d) variation of use, and practice with their implication on equity to access and coverage, (e) the impact on health outcome, and (f) the consequences of health-care financing on politics, the economy, and society as well as on the welfare of the entire population.

The users and contributors of information for health planning can be policy analysts, health-care providers, epidemiologists, social scientists, and economists, among others. The gatherers and users of health information are often different people at different levels of the health-care system. For policy decisions, policy analysts will need information to facilitate policy recommendations. Those who provide health services and have the task of being accountable for the services they provide should also be involved in the development of an information system. The general areas outlined above differ among developed and developing countries, not with respect to the problems themselves but rather to the emphasis given to each of them.

The measurement of needs

With respect to the measurement of needs, it is important to understand current needs, trends, and types of services needed (promotive, preventive, curative, and rehabilitative), including both objective and subjective needs. The differentiation between need, demand, and utilization is also crucial (Box 1).

Box 1 Health care need

- Current needs:
  - real need versus want
  - effective demand
  - use
  - prioritization
- Trends, for example in AIDS and related conditions, ageing trade
- Types: promotive, preventive, treatment, rehabilitation
- Validity and objectives of data sources

Real needs are those that require appropriate fulfilment and they may be both felt or unfelt. Demand is generated by felt need, and needs and demands require effective provisions. Effective provisions represent the capacity of the health systems to satisfy the real needs within the technological and other resources of the society. Use is not the same as effective provision although it is easier to measure. This is fundamental to the author's approach to the problem. Utilization reflects the perception of health need, individual reaction to symptoms of ill health, resources that the individual must invest to acquire the service, ability of the facilities to provide the service, and benefits that the providers of service expect to generate. It does not tell us what volume of service is optimal. It is important to know what volume of health services should be consumed, not just how they are actually consumed, to decide upon the likely benefit of a particular investment. Without appropriate data, decision-makers might focus on ineffective provisions without meeting needs. A needs-based system is difficult to establish but is essential to allow people to be more responsible for what they do in terms of their own health.

Current needs only represent part of the picture in planning of health services. The health system has to be more aggressively involved in the trends of diseases such as HIV infection and AIDS, with the emphasis on finding more effective means of delivering educational and other preventive programmes which highlight high-risk activities. With the new industrialized trends of developing countries, occupational diseases will be increasingly important. The current trend of population demographics may require a greater emphasis on the needs of the elderly who may claim a greater share of the funds provided by the various health-care schemes.

In the analysis of the types of effective provision, it is necessary to understand the need to establish a balance between preventive and promotive strategies versus treatment and rehabilitation.

It is important to develop an information system in both developed and developing countries to measure incidence and prevalence of objective and subjective needs as well as the use of specific types of health services to fulfil those needs.

Fulfilment of non-health needs can also lead to health improvement. For example, the role of women in determining the health and life prospects of their children is crucial. It is therefore important to find ways to assure women's health through nutrition, education, gender equality, and health practices. How can social and other non-health interventions interrupt the vicious circle of poverty, health, and the lack of social development? This area will remain important for future research.

Information about the organization and financing of a health service

The organizational arrangements for health-care financing and delivery are also important components of an information system to ensure universal coverage and equity of access.

The organization

Ideally, the structure that should be involved in a health service system are the public health facilities, the private sector, other communities, the workplace, and families and individuals. Major activity is currently occurring in the public sector, particularly the ministries of public health. Information about other components of a health system must also be sought. So-called 'unqualified' personnel or 'minimally trained community-based health-care workers' for workplace communities, family support, and self-care, can be trained to become resources for health-care currently provided by higher level professionals (Box 2).

Appropriate personnel requirement is also an important issue. It is important to identify the appropriate proportion, type, qualifications, and distribution of personnel required to support the health-care financing schemes. How much should currently 'unqualified' personnel be trained to support the system? What is the role of informal care and self-care?

Privatization will not facilitate universal access to health care. It will, however, affect the financing and payment system. More active work and more cross-cultural comparisons are needed in this respect, particularly where more privatization is developing in many countries, including those in Eastern Europe. Information will be needed to monitor the extent to which these trends can alter the basic relationship between patients and health-care professionals resulting in an impact on health and the quality of services as well as on the livelihood of people.

Box 2 The structure and the organization of a health system

- Structures
    - public: ministries of public health, local government offices
    - private sector
    - workplace
    - home
- Personnel requirement
    - specialist/generalists
    - nurses
    - currently 'unqualified'
    - informal care
    - self-care
- Population being served
    - based on workplace
    - based on residence
    - other
- Co-ordination

Finally, although some resources are needed for mounting and co-ordinating an information system, it is important that the proportion of resources allocated to co-ordination not be so substantial as to jeopardize other activities. However, the information base to do such analyses may not exist and therefore may need to be constructed.

Information on financing

The framework for analysis of the financing of health services is depicted in Box 3.

The factors affecting the various sources of health-care financing mechanisms vary between countries. In this complex situation, it is important to resolve questions over who pays, who receives payment,

Box 3 Financing of health systems

- Who pays?
    - insurance scheme
    - employers
    - government (welfare)
- Pay for how much?
    - total
    - percentage of gross national product
    - trends
- Pay for what?
    - types of services
    - levels of services
    - specific activities
- Pay to whom?
- Basis of payment
    - fees for services
    - capitation
    - co-payment

what is being paid for, who eventually benefits, and how to ensure sharing and pooling of the risk of ill health to attain a certain degree of equity.

In order to monitor and determine the appropriate emphasis of the programme, the total amount of payment under the various health-care financing schemes, its trends, the relative proportions of the various schemes, and the percentage of gross national product used for each scheme need to be assessed.

The relative contribution of the various health-care financing schemes for preventive, promotive, curative, and rehabilitative care is also important to guide the setting and monitoring of the appropriate proportion of these various services. Related to these issues is the relative contribution of health-care financing schemes to the various levels of services: primary health care, primary medical care, secondary medical care, and tertiary medical care.

The basis for payment under the health-care financing schemes will be important for determining the rate and the appropriateness of utilization of services.

The alternative models

Each of the alternative models has their strengths and weaknesses. Each of them may be considered appropriate for meeting the needs of health services, depending on the situation. However, there are some common targets of all models of financing. These are equity, efficiency, stability, sustainability, administrative feasibility, health impact, as well as impacts on the socio-economic and political systems of a society. As there are numerous ways of organizing resources, alternative models have to be developed, tested, and compared.

Resource allocation and utilization of services

In allocating resources, it is important to define practice variations and use variations (including issues of acquisition, diffusion, use, and control of access to health technology). Practice variations result from the decisions of providers while use variations are the consequences of consumer behaviour (Box 4).

Variations of service provision can depend on which scheme is used to pay health-care providers (for example, fee-for-service scheme or capitation). The rate of certain procedures might be inappropriately increased if the fee-for-service scheme is adapted to the point that the financing system cannot be sustained because of a greater emphasis on treatment than prevention. In Australia, for example, the rates of obstetric intervention in private patients have been higher than for non-private patients (Roberts *et al.* 2000). The views of specialists differ on whether or not to perform cancer genetic testing and carry out prophylactic hysterectomies when patients prove positive (Matloff *et al.* 2000). If coverage refers to the degree to which effective provision is given to those who have real need, it is not always true that more services lead to more coverage. Conversely, hospitals may avoid providing standard services if they are costly, or may not join the health-care financing schemes programme if a capitation scheme is in place. If the hospitals fail to provide high-cost but already proven efficacious and standard care because the services are too expensive, certain ethical issues may arise. A good information system should be able to identify these issues.

On the one hand, people who are covered by private health-care financing schemes might overutilize health resources because they perceive that it is their right to obtain services. On the other hand, people might underutilize services under certain health-care financing schemes because they may perceive that they are receiving inferior care.

Services that are overutilized might lead to inequitable access to services of other low-income groups. If coverage refers to the degree to which effective provisions are given to those who have real needs for services, it is not always true that more services lead to more coverage.

An information system has to associate appropriate population denominators with the numerators, particularly where the people in a catchment area can use many different financing schemes for the same health condition. In this general area, the topics of national relevance are those of access, equity, and coverage as they relate to factors including income, age, sex, and occupation.

Health system performance

Measures of health system performance are becoming increasingly important as the financial demands of health care have put increasing pressures on national economies (Box 5). Although some of the most exciting work is taking place in developed countries, much is happening in developing countries as well. The field of epidemiology has made a great contribution to public health and health-care research. Epidemiology, political mapping, decision analysis, health system economics, and evidence-based practice have helped revolutionize the practices of medicine and public health. Epidemiology, however, supplements but does not replace basic sciences. The major problem for measuring health system performance is the availability of data. Information systems therefore need to be strengthened to be able to track the performance of public health interventions.

Box 4 Resource allocation and use

- Practice variations among providers
  - special 'track'
  - over or under prescription of technologies
  - provider satisfaction
- Variations among users
  - underuse
  - overuse
  - user satisfaction
- Access, equity, coverage
  - among social insurance clients
  - among clients of other insurance schemes
- Allocative efficiency

Box 5 Health system performance

- Efficacy
- Effectiveness
- Operative efficiency
- Clinical decision analysis
- Outcome and epidemiology of medical care

It is not only the expensive technology of public health and clinical medicine that is subjected to the analysis of health system performance, but the very inexpensive and moderately priced everyday practices also need to be evaluated. Information systems are needed to track preventive activity such as immunization programmes, screening for chronic diseases, availability of early treatments, and risk factor counselling.

Decision-makers and health providers must have the skill to evaluate their own decisions and practices, and to be more accountable in their decisions. The design of a good information system should empower these practitioners to ask questions about public health interventions. Such an empowerment should lead not only to heightened expectation and demand for quality and accessibility at reasonable cost, but also create an environment in which the information system for public health decisions has reason to grow. A more systematic approach to information systems is needed. Information and technology gaps between developed and developing countries in this area need to be narrowed. Only then can the strategies to define an optimal health care for all be achieved.

It is important to make providers accountable for their services. This requires information support. Information should not be an exercise that can only be performed in university faculties. The task of the specialists in information systems is to make the methods as accessible as possible. The emphasis in much of information system research in the decade ahead will shift from a traditional study of inputs (for example, personnel, facilities, procedures, appliances, drugs, and so on) to the evaluation of health-care output and performances.

Information on health outcomes

Outcomes of care are usually measured using mortality and morbidity rates. While these are important indicators, they do not take into account the impact of illnesses and death on the individuals and their families as well as on the economic and social well being of the society. The death of a child in a family might have very different consequences from the death of the mother; in many societies, such as those in Africa, the death of a mother might lead to the death of other children and disintegration of the whole family. Deaths of young adults have more impact on the production of the society than deaths of the incapacitated elderly. Therefore the definition of outcome of care needs to take into consideration the lifetime consequences of illnesses, impact of illnesses and death on other family members, the well being of society, and productivity (Box 6).

Defining outcomes of care

An exciting feature of health-care analysis is the ability to access information to measure outcome, for example measures of functional health status and well being. This field has previously not received enough attention. More people are doing research on what it means to have certain physical limitations. Functional health status is complex and the study of it can provide important information. More research on quantitative measures of well being, including the quality-adjusted life year, is needed. It is hoped that methods will be developed to measure these not only in individuals but also in communities.

Box 6 Health outcomes

- Definition
  functional status
  well being
- Health status measures
  single index from aggregates
  utilities
  preferences

Health status measurement

Far more attention needs to be spent than previously on health status measurements including (a) the aggregation of various health indicators into single indices, (b) deriving the utilities and preferences for various health states, (c) the measure of possible health states across the various health conditions, (d) the measure of health status in children and the elderly (most of the current measures of health status apply to adults), and (e) evaluation of clinical treatments and changes in health-care delivery.

Information of development policies affecting health

A public health system is very different from a health-care system. The public health system needs to provide information on development policies that can affect health. These include policies on the macroeconomy, agriculture, energy, and housing (Box 7).

Box 7 Development policies affecting health

- Macroeconomic
- Agriculture
- Industrial
- Energy
- Housing

Planning a public health system requires information on the ecology and environment, schools, workforce, social care, housing, and alternative energy sources in addition to information about the performance and integration of various levels of health care as described above. Public expenditures and subsidies to stimulate macroeconomic growth may be done at the expense of support for essential drugs, employment programmes for the poor, and so on. Agricultural development can exploit land use, which can change biodiversity and thereby promote emerging diseases and resistant strains of micro-organisms. Agricultural development can also affect the short- and long-term health of migrants and local people through the use of pesticides and acute poisoning. Improvement in irrigation systems can change the lifecycle of vectors and complicate water-borne diseases. An information system to monitor work safety and pollution should go along with the development of industrial policy. To promote safe energy, information is needed on the sources of energy (for example, the effect of hydropower on deforestation and health), consumption of energy for cooking, household use, transport, and pollution standards by industries, and pricing policy related to the use of safe energy. Information on housing policy can cover issues such as health problems in slums and government housing, safety of high rise buildings, availability of public services, cost of rent compared to cost of food, and hygiene standards.

The general framework for community diagnosis

Defining the community

The first task to define health and disease burden in a given community is to define the target community. This can be a country, province, district, or state, but might be a more defined geographical region, such as an urban inner city, or a socially defined group, such as poor communities, women in the reproductive age range, pregnant mothers, infants, young adults, or the elderly. The target population should be broad enough to cover all subgroups relevant for the assessment of health situations outlined by the objectives such as equity of access to care. If the target population is not well defined at the outset, there could be a tendency for the subgroups from whom data are easily obtained to be over-represented. For example, disease patterns from hospital data under-represent those who have limited access to hospitals.

Health indicators

The definition of indicators is a pre-requisite for the development of an effective information system in community diagnosis. Indicators have to reflect the kind of decisions which will be needed to estimate the burden of illness and the strategies for control.

Positive and negative health

Ideally, health indicators should reflect both the positive and negative aspects of health status. The new definition of health by the WHO includes the physical, mental, social, and spiritual aspects of health. Many attempts have been made to develop measures of quality of life as a proxy of positive health (e.g. the WHO quality of life instrument (Anonymous 1995)). Positive health measures have not been widely used in developing countries partly due to cultural influence on the expectations of people. Poor people in developing countries are more likely to accept the limitation and be satisfied with poorer health than their counterparts in wealthier countries.

Good health tends to be unnoticed until obvious symptoms from diseases have occurred. The concept of the 'burden of risk' can be brought to the attention of public health officers if there is a method to modify the course of presymptomatic illness. Thus screening for hypertension is an essential public health tool because of the possibility of modifying the course of hypertension and preventing stroke. Screening for diseases can be a part of community diagnosis if a cost-effective intervention is available for modifying the course of the disease once identified at screening.

In most developing countries, health information systems are principally oriented towards negative aspects of health because of the relative ease of their measurement. People will seek help from the health-care system when they become ill. The main health indicators are expressed in terms of crude age-adjusted or age-specific mortality rates (such as infant mortality rates, mortality for children under 5, or maternal mortality rates), disease-specific morbidity rates, and life expectancy at birth. Mainly because diseases have different natural histories and impacts, other indicators have been developed. Examples include potential years of life lost, quality-adjusted life years gained, disability-adjusted life years, healthy life years lost, and disabilities and quality of life index (Murray and Lopez 1996; Hyder and Morrow 1998). Debate has continued over the assumptions that these measures make, such as the relative values of time lived at different ages and the application of discounting rates over time. Many maintain that the implications of age weighting and discounting are unacceptable. Those who disagree with allotting relative values to time find it difficult to trade healthy years by giving less weight to future generations in favour of the present generation. Those who agree with age weighting and discounting feel that such methods of weighting and discounting are consistent with the necessary allocation of resources, for reasons of cost-effectiveness, and with avoidance of giving less value to childhood death. In view of this debate, it is important for developing countries to focus on the development of information that can measure mortality and morbidity rates with some degree of certainty. These standard indicators can later be transformed to calculate other newer indicators after agreement has been reached over the various methods.

Sources of information and the methods that can be used for community diagnosis

Information for community diagnosis can come from many sources (Box 8). Examples include routine reporting from health facilities, surveillance, screening, special surveys, contact tracing, vital registration, and a combination of several methods including using qualitative information to define variables and continued surveys of the nature and extent of the problems once the variables are defined.

The details of these approaches are addressed in the next section.

Box 8 Sources of information and methods for community diagnosis

- Routine reporting from health facilities
- Surveillance including active, passive, and sentinel surveillance
- Screening
- Special surveys
- Rapid surveys
- Contact tracing
- Vital registration
- A combination of several methods

Trend analysis

Information can be gathered and analysed for changes over time. Trends in the health status of a nation and a community involve demographic transition, urbanization, education expansion, changing status of women, economic transformation, politics, technological innovation, and global integration including the international transfer of risk (for example, pollution and global epidemics), trade liberalization, and shared learning leading to accelerated development and interdependencies. Assessing trends can be done in terms of health situations, burden of illnesses, and risk behaviours (Ungchusak *et al.* 1996; Kitsiripornchai *et al.* 1998; Mills *et al.* 1998), and can be used to assess the effectiveness of an intervention (Muller *et al.* 1995).

Characteristics of community diagnosis

The basis of community diagnosis is to learn whether the community has achieved the objectives proposed by the policy and programmes in use. There are several desirable characteristics for community diagnosis:

- ability to address important problems amenable to practical control
- ability to identify most of the target health events
- adequacy in reflecting changes in distribution of events over time, place, and person
- having a clearly defined population, data collection, data flow, analysis, interpretation, and feedback
- orientation towards appropriate action
- being participatory, uncomplicated, sensitive, timely, and inexpensive.

Sources of information and methods for community diagnosis

Routine reporting system

In developing countries, death registrations are incomplete and disease notification is unreliable. The information most readily available is from health facilities such as clinics and hospitals. The number or proportions of patients who seek care are commonly presented to indicate the burden of illness. This method has particular appeal because of its simplicity and low cost. Routine reporting from hospitals and health facilities can give useful information on the health status and burden of illness of a target catchment area to plan and monitor health services if survey information is not available or gives incomplete information. For example, the burden of illnesses and priority ranking of disease in Ghana has been based mainly on the routine information obtained from hospital facilities (Ghana Health Assessment Project Team 1981).

Information from routine reporting of the HIV seroprevalence among heroin users derived from different regions of a country can shed light on the rate of HIV infection at an early stage of infection (Table 1).

Information from the routine report of a key facility for the treatment of drug-dependent patients of Thanyarak Hospital (Thailand) indicated that the spread of HIV seroprevalence among drug users occurred first in the central region of Thailand including Bangkok, followed by the north, the south, and the northeast.

Routine reporting from health facilities has frequently been used to identify disease trends for health problems associated with stigmatization such as drug dependence and HIV/AIDS as shown in Fig. 1.

When the information obtained from male addicts in one facility (that is, among new cases, revisited cases, and non-heroin addicts) was analysed, the seroprevalence among the new cases showed a declining trend (Fig. 2). Conversely, the seroprevalence rates among the old cases and the non-heroin addicts (not injecting) were stable. These trends suggested a possible change in the behaviour of the new cases of heroin injectors, which may have been due to a successful campaign by the authorities.

Similarly, the routine reporting of the hill tribes people seeking treatment for drug dependence at the key Northern Drug Dependence Treatment Center (Thailand) showed a constant increase in the proportion of heroin users among this traditional people who used to smoke opium over the years as shown in Fig. 3. There was a rising trend of the percentage of injecting drug users among the hill tribespeople, indicating a shift in drug use pattern from opium smoking to heroin use first by smoking and later via injection. The higher percentage of injecting drug users compared with the percentage of heroin users since 1992 suggested that the hill tribespeople also injected other drugs.

The increase in the percentage of heroin users seeking treatment has corresponded with an increase in HIV-positive prevalence among the hill tribe population up to 1994 as shown in Table 2. Despite the limitations discussed below, routine reporting can generate useful information for planning if analysed and interpreted with care.

Limitation of routine reporting: measuring utilization of services versus health needs

In developing countries, events reported depend on the use of facilities. This gives rise to a distorted picture of health problems in the community since many who need services do not have access to health facilities due to geographical, financial, cultural, and other barriers, or when the coverage of the population by such services is incomplete. It has been demonstrated that between one-third and two-thirds of diabetic and hypertensive people in a community either did not know that they had the diseases or did not seek hospital care (Wadsworth *et*

Table 1 Provinces with HIV seropositive drug users classified by region (Thanyarak Hospital: December 1987 to December 1988)

	Number of provinces with HIV+ addicts and total number of HIV+ addicts per region			
	Central region	Northern region	Northeastern region	Southern region
Oct–Dec 1987	8	1	–	–
Jan–Mar 1988	15	8	–	1
Apr–Jun 1988	21	10	4	2
Jul–Sep 1988	23	11	7	6
Oct–Dec 1988	25	13	8	8
HIV+ cases (*n*)	603	103	11	32

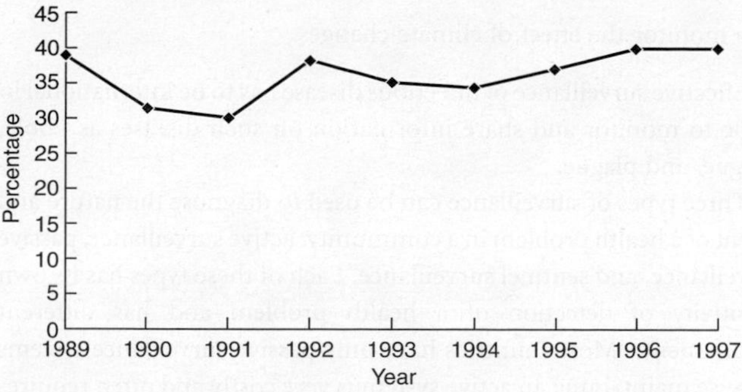

Fig. 1 Percentage of HIV-positive people among injecting drug users collected from routine reporting data from drug dependence treatment facilities at the Thanyarak Hospital, July 1989 to December 1997. (Data from V. Poshyachinda 1997, personal communication.)

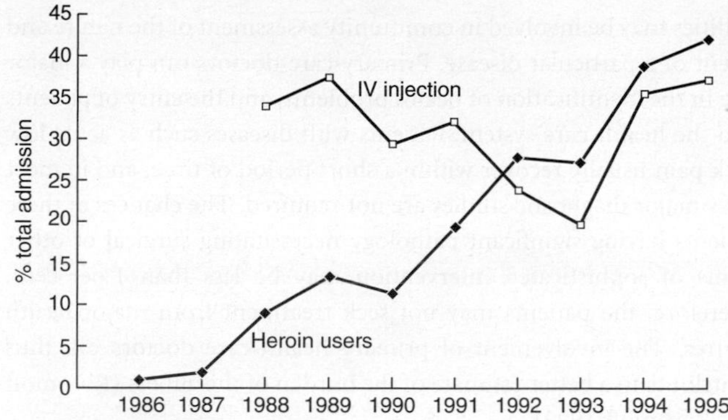

Fig. 3 The percentage of heroin users and the percentage of injecting drug users among the hill tribespeople seeking care at the Northern Drug Dependence Treatment Centre (Thailand): 1986 to 1995. (Data from V. Poshyachinda 1997, personal communication.)

al. 1971; Sitthi-Amorn *et al.* 1989). In addition, because the services provided by the various levels of health care are uncoordinated due to poor referral systems, one patient could seek care from several places and therefore be counted many times, leading to an overestimate of the burden of illnesses. Many factors can affect why patients use or do not use services including the reputation of health facilities, difficulty of access to facilities, and client perception of the seriousness of their illness. Thus, in using routine reporting, it must be remembered that the information available is not perfect and that the information needed may not be obtainable. A review of the information system must be done periodically to ensure that the information system provides the information desired for planners to meet the defined objectives of the health system.

Routine reporting is most useful in capturing most cases if a condition produces severe symptoms, and if the natural history of the condition is long enough to permit seeking treatment. Thus, a collation of routine hospital records can be used to produce cancer registries capturing most cancer cases in a community because most patients with cancer will have severe enough symptoms before death to seek treatment from health facilities. Conversely, a large proportion of myocardial infarction patients will die outside health facilities and therefore the records from health facilities alone will underestimate the true magnitude of the burden of illness from this condition. Likewise, reports from health facilities will underestimate cases of diarrhoea since many people only have mild symptoms and will not seek care.

The methods for detection of specific diseases between health facilities can create biased estimates in a routine reporting system. For example, differences in the incidence, prevalence, and mortality from coronary heart disease are observed between and within countries. In addition to the differing levels of risk factors between communities, these differences are also believed to be related to the different application of technology in health-care facilities. Medical care for acute myocardial infarction has changed significantly in the past decades, with the development of new methods for diagnosis and treatment. Although widely known, these technologies are not consistently applied for reasons of availability and cost, as well as local medical cultures and traditions (Luepker and Herlitz 1999).

To cope with the difference between utilization of major health facilities and the actual health need, an extended network of health

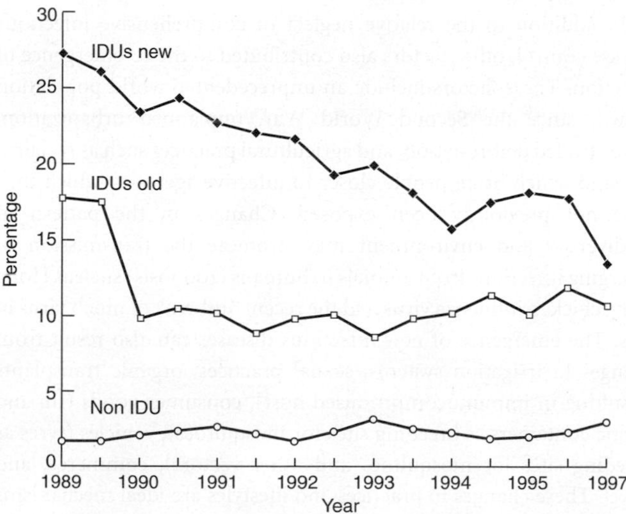

Fig. 2 Percentage of HIV-positive people among new injecting drug users, readmission cases of injecting drug users, and non-injecting drug users, at the Thanyarak Hospital, July 1989 to December 1997. (Data from V. Poshyachinda 1997, personal communication.)

Table 2 HIV seropositive prevalence among hill tribe heroin and opium users (Northern Drug Dependence Treatment Centre, 1992 to 1995)

	HIV seroprevalence[a] (%)			
	1992	**1993**	**1994**	**1995**
Heroin				
Smoking	4.6 (388)	4.4 (387)	14.1 (199)	8.1 (346)
Injecting	20.6 (92)	24.3 (74)	55.3 (99)	37.3 (204)
Opium users				
Smoking	2.3 (1274)	3.2 (951)	7.1 (451)	2.5 (710)
Injecting	–	–	–	5.9 (51)

[a]Number in sample given in parentheses.

facilities may be involved in community assessment of the nature and extent of a particular disease. Primary care doctors can play a major role in the identification of health problems, and the entry of patients into the health-care system. Patients with diseases such as acute low back pain usually recover within a short period of time, and in most cases major diagnostic studies are not required. The chances of these patients having significant pathology necessitating surgical or other forms of sophisticated intervention may be less than 1 per cent. Therefore, the patients may not seek treatment from major health centres. The involvement of primary health-care doctors can thus contribute to a better estimate of the burden of this illness (Rosomoff and Rosomoff 1999).

Outreach based on the samples defined in a health facility can also be used to determine the possible source of community infections. For example, in determining whether secondary cases of tuberculosis resulted from those dying in health facilities, a retrospective review of all cases of tuberculosis reported within a specified period was combined with a prospective evaluation of the molecular characteristics of new tuberculosis cases. The study revealed that cases of tuberculosis diagnosed after death did not appear to be significant sources of tuberculosis in the community (DeRiemer *et al.* 1999).

Efforts should be made to improve the quality of routine systems and to make use of innovative analyses of routine information because of the simplicity and potential usefulness of routine reporting systems (Kitayaporn *et al.* 1994, 1996*a*,*b*; Mastro and Kitayaporn 1998). Unfortunately, in many countries, significant progress in this direction is not expected. Therefore it is important to supplement routine reporting systems with other methods of estimating the burden of illnesses including screening, surveillance, special surveys, rapid surveys, and contact tracing.

Surveillance

Surveillance is considered a tool for community diagnosis of diseases which have the potential to become an epidemic, thus affecting many people in the community or internationally. Surveillance has been traditionally applied to the control of infectious diseases. The new paradigms of public health require that surveillance include the detection of toxins, hazardous chemicals, and genetically modified products. Of particular importance are the diseases transmitted from animals to humans, such as the outbreak of chicken influenza virus in Hong Kong and nipah virus in Malaysia. The influenza strains transmitted from birds to humans can cause widespread infection. Thus, surveillance has to be supplemented with strategies to detect the transmission of species-specific infections, which occur between humans and animals.

Depending on the nature of the diseases, surveillance can be active, passive, or targeted periodically towards special groups seeking treatment from sentinel sites. To be effective, a surveillance system must be integrated with other measures to take control of the spread of diseases under surveillance. The role of surveillance is:

- to monitor secular and long-term trends of diseases and public health issues
- to provide early warning for disease outbreaks
- to evaluate prevention and control programmes
- to monitor the effect of climate changes.

Effective surveillance of infectious disease has to be international in scope to monitor and share information on such diseases as Ebola, dengue, and plague.

Three types of surveillance can be used to diagnose the nature and extent of a health problem in a community: active surveillance, passive surveillance, and sentinel surveillance. Each of these types has its own sensitivity of detection of a health problem and has different requirements. Most countries have only passive surveillance systems because maintaining an active system is very costly and often requires some sophisticated laboratory support. Considerable infrastructure and human resources are required to maintain a sentinel surveillance system.

Traditionally, the main use of surveillance systems has been to monitor epidemics of infectious diseases. Recently, surveillance has been increasingly used to detect toxins, such as pesticides in human milk and lead in the blood of children, as well as deficiencies of trace elements such as vitamin A, zinc, folic acid, and iodine in adults.

The world has recently seen increases in diseases and epidemics in others that were once controlled. Since the middle of the twentieth century, antibiotics combined with improved sanitation, housing, nutrition, and vaccines have led to a dramatic drop in many infectious diseases that once killed millions (WHO 2000*b*). By the early 1960s, infectious diseases began to be controlled and these campaigns were so successful that many predicted their potential eradication. This created complacency among public health officials, policy-makers, and the public, which led to many policy and technical problems such as a decline in political and economic support for infectious disease programmes. This has led to the development of drug-resistant microbes, resistant vector strains, and the re-emergence of diseases once under control. There has been a decay of infrastructures and a shortage of trained personnel to deal with major infection control. One of the most important problems has resulted from the neglect of prevention in favour of using the 'magic bullet' or the 'high-technology/quick-fix' solution.

In addition to the relative neglect of comprehensive infectious disease control, other factors also contributed to the re-emergence of infection. These factors include an unprecedented world population growth since the Second World War, unplanned urbanization, uncontrolled deforestation, and agricultural practices such as reclaiming land which bring people closer to infective agents to which they have not previously been exposed. Changes in the pattern of biodiversity and environment may promote the transmission of emerging infections from animals to humans (zoonosis) such as Hong Kong chicken influenza virus and the recent outbreak of nipah virus in pigs. The emergence of new infectious diseases can also result from changes in irrigation systems, sexual practices, organic transplants (resulting in immunocompromised host), consumer goods (tin and plastic containers as breeding sites for mosquitoes), vehicles (tyres as breeding sites for mosquitoes and other vectors), commerce, and travel. These changes in practices and lifestyles are ideal mechanisms of constantly redistributing pathogens around the world.

Other factors include genetic changes in aetiological agents such as influenza (change in strains), development of antibiotic-resistant microbes and insecticide-resistant vectors, and an increase in vector-borne disease in general (through various hosts). These possible scenarios will need more research before scientists can fully understand the influence of genetic factors of micro-organisms on transmission potential.

Climate changes are imputed to help spread infectious disease but strong evidence to support this notion has yet to be found. The El Niño phenomenon has been imputed to have caused the spread of dengue in Indonesia and Thailand. Since dengue epidemics can be caused by many factors, the relative contribution of climate to the spread of diseases still needs to be clarified. Thus research is needed to see whether the degree of efforts to strengthen surveillance systems is needed in areas where more severe climate changes occur.

Surveillance can give information for policy-makers to act on which will help to reverse the trend of infectious diseases. Regulations and controls should be targeted at population growth, urbanization, and deforestation. Stronger emphasis must be placed on strengthening public health policy and public health rules that have been deregulated to give more rights to individuals but consequently, might harm the public at large. A better balance between individual rights and the good of the community must be established.

The public health infrastructure (including surveillance systems) in many countries, particularly in the developing world, must be improved, including personnel and laboratory facilities to deal with the major infectious diseases.

A key strategy is to rethink disease prevention from the public health standpoint, emphasizing disease prevention that includes such strategies as general hygiene, vaccines, vector control, public outreach, and education.

Surveillance systems for effective infectious disease prevention must provide information to promote:

- effective emergency responses to outbreaks of disease
- public and professional outreach to communicate important information effectively to key stakeholders such as the public, doctors, and government officials
- effective community-based preventive strategies.

Active surveillance: a case study from India

Plague in India is a useful example to highlight the need for international co-operation and surveillance. In the first 25 years of the twentieth century, India lost about 12 million people to plague. The government launched an effective control programme, and in the 1950s plague was mostly brought under control. In 1959, plague had been eliminated from India, and in 1966, India was declared plague free. Subsequently, very little effort related to the control of plague was carried out. There was no laboratory doing diagnostic work for plague. In August 1994, an outbreak of pneumonic plague began in Maharashtra and moved into the city of Surat by September. The surveillance system did not pick it up. No one knew about it, not even the WHO. People started dying of pneumonic types of haemorrhagic diseases in Surat, an industrialized city of several million people. Some doctors consulted their old books and realized that it could be pneumonic plague. They sent samples to the laboratory for diagnosis, but the laboratory could not diagnose it. This created confusion, uncertainties, and a lack of confidence among medical communities. People panicked and 500 000 people fled the city of Surat. The WHO contacted the United States Centers for Disease Control (**CDC**) for assistance in identifying the microbes because it had the only functional plague diagnostic laboratory in the world. The CDC sent references and diagnostic kits to 15 countries in Southeast Asia and Europe. The WHO and the CDC were working blind and had to assume the worst. People from Surat fled to Madras, Bombay, and other cities worldwide, spreading the problem. There were reports about the spread in New Delhi and Pakistan, and the CDC worked with the WHO to intensify surveillance. Fortunately, rumours about the spread to other countries worldwide proved to be a false alarm and there were no cases identified from countries outside India. In retrospect, it was discovered that there was an outbreak of plague in Maharashtra and a few cases in Surat. There was no transmission to Bombay, New Delhi, Madras, and Calcutta. The lack of laboratory diagnosis capability had caused an epidemic of panic. There was a loss of 2 billion American dollars from the Indian economy and probably several billion dollars from the global economy. What should have been a focal public health event turned into a worldwide emergency. The WHO is not a policing organization and its actions are limited if countries do not want to co-operate.

The goals of active surveillance include:

- to detect without delay the introduction of change in incidence of a specific disease agent: active surveillance has to be disease specific although there are some exceptions
- to alert pubic health officials early about the epidemic—an early warning system (the emphasis is on the pre-epidemic period as opposed to the epidemic period)
- to assess the extent of the risk of transmission of a particular disease
- to estimate and monitor the effectiveness of control activities.

Active surveillance usually has to be laboratory based. The case definitions of an active system can vary. Case definitions can be non-specific in the pre-epidemic period but become more specific during the epidemic as the incidence increases. There must be standardized sample collection and reporting. The surveillance tool must be convenient and easily transportable (Frerichs *et al.* 1994; Cassol *et al.* 1996*a*,*b*).

When a clear disease definition is not available, syndromes can be used to cover multiple diseases. For example, although the basic diagnosis of dengue has to be laboratory based, a syndromic approach may also be used to increase case detection. The syndromic approach for dengue consists of three surveillance systems: clinic doctors, fever alert, and sentinel hospitals. When a syndromic approach is used, the case definition is very non-specific but should later be supplemented with more definite diagnostic techniques. In the case of dengue, the clinics and the hospital will be asked to submit to the laboratory information on a quarter of their viral syndromes every week. Fever alert allows blood to be taken for laboratory confirmation within 24 hours. Hospital deaths of all viral syndromes should similarly be laboratory confirmed and ideally autopsied (difficult in many countries). Individually, none of the three approaches is sensitive but collectively they become so. Clearly, the laboratory is critical to this type of effort.

The laboratory must be able to (a) conduct routine surveillance for priority diseases important in the area, (b) focus on epidemic transmissions of priority diseases, and (c) recognize new diseases, natural disasters, imported diseases, and bioterrorism.

At a minimum the laboratory should be able to conduct surveillance on priority diseases. If it is not capable of detecting the broad spectrum of new and other infections there must be some reference laboratory in the region such as a WHO reference laboratory where samples can be sent for identification and confirmation. Ideally, every country should have a national laboratory with satellite laboratories at the district and local levels. However, this can be beyond the means of poor countries. A more efficient way of sharing existing resources is to map out existing laboratory facilities in a region, co-ordinate sharing and standardization among them, and develop new facilities, which might be needed in the region. WHO reference laboratories should be capable of a wide array of diagnostic procedures. The WHO can also link up with other sophisticated laboratories such as the CDC in the United States.

Every national laboratory should have some well-trained personnel, enough facilities, equipment, and basic microbiology capacity. State-of-the-art technology such as the polymerase chain reaction assay is important but not as important as basic microbiology, which has frequently been ignored. The capacity to perform polymerase chain reactions at the expense of basic microbiology is a mistake because sophisticated equipment inappropriately used can create data that are misleading.

A mechanism should be in place to ensure quality assurance so that people have confidence in laboratory results.

Once an infection has been identified, the standard public health measures must be actively applied such as the identification of individuals, implementation of quarantine, implementation of sanitary regulations, the sacrifice of infectious sources such as animals, and measures to heighten precautions by individuals at risk. With acute emerging virus infections, there might not be time to develop vaccines and to find a treatment. In such cases, public health precautions will be the key coping measures. With bacterial infections, available antibiotics can be resorted to, some of which may be helpful.

Another example to highlight the importance of the laboratory is the concern for yellow fever. Yellow fever is a time bomb. An increase of yellow fever has occurred in Europe and the United States. This means that it can also be taken to Asia, and might remain there undetected because of insufficient laboratory capability. In the 1930s, there were major epidemics of yellow fever in Latin America. In 1947, the Pan American Health Organization implemented an *Aëdes aegypti* eradication programme to control the epidemics of yellow fever and dengue. By 1970, they had eradicated cases in much of Central and South America but they then abandoned the programme. *Aëdes aegypti* began to reinvade tropical America. There is the highest risk in 50 years for the occurrence of yellow fever in urban areas. If urban yellow fever begins to occur in Latin America with 300 million people, it will spread to other urban areas, particularly those with populations of over 1 million. This may also happen in Asia owing to ease of transport and travel. When this happens, the medical and public health communities might impute the illness to dengue, malaria, or leptospirosis. Therefore, the laboratory must be able to distinguish yellow fever from other diseases so health professional can react quickly and appropriately.

Passive surveillance

Passive surveillance is most useful for monitoring long-term secular trends but is relatively insensitive to tracking epidemics. Most countries have a passive surveillance system. The key components of a passive surveillance system include the use of standardized case definitions and a standardized reporting system.

Passive surveillance relies on doctors and health officials to report diseases and therefore is very insensitive for predicting epidemics. Constant communications, reference, and referral, together with political and economic support, are all crucial components of both active and passive surveillance systems.

Effective emergency response: a necessary complementary measure for surveillance An effective emergency response is an important element necessary for the effective prevention of the spread of infectious diseases. Good co-ordination between epidemiologist, laboratory personnel, and professionals in the field is critical. Effective control has to be disease specific. Knowledge about the dynamics of transmission is essential. Furthermore, there must be strong community involvement for sustainability and a real-time response and timely policy decisions. Even when a surveillance system has predictive capability, many policy-makers do not believe the surveillance data and, as a result, do not respond to the data quickly enough. Therefore, laboratory capability must be credible and understandable so that rapid decisions are made in real time rather than after the epidemic spreads or peaks.

Outreach: empowering the community to be integrated in surveillance diagnosis and control Outreach is an area where public health has failed. Despite the availability of health education materials by public health specialists for all kinds of diseases and health problems, people usually ignore them. Social scientists and medical anthropologists who know how to communicate with the community should be encouraged to play a greater role in developing health education messages. The use of the 'scatter-gun' approach, having one message for all recipients with diverse ethnosocial background, is unlikely to succeed. Education messages should be targeted at different groups, particularly the medical community (epidemiologists and doctors who must be well versed in diagnosis, treatment, and disease prevention), who use them to reach the public. The public must accept their own responsibility and not rely on the government to do everything. Government officials must make an honest assessment of what the epidemiologists have to say and must not have 'selective hearing', for example questioning epidemiological data to protect local tourism.

An integrated community-based approach must have common ownership and an emphasis on disease prevention. The approach must take advantage of all the updated technology and instruments available to cope with the epidemic and prevent disease. People must have a role in the programme and in setting the priorities of the programme. Government officials must not simply tell people how to do things. Without community ownership there is no sustainability. Policy decisions have to support a community-based approach.

Sentinel surveillance

A sentinel surveillance system can help to identify rapidly changing health problems in a country or community (Box 9).

Box 9 Selecting sentinel sites

- Not necessarily representative sites
- Likely to identify problems
- High enough case load
- Staff capacity and willingness
- Data reliable
- High-quality diagnostic capabilities

A good example is surveillance for HIV/AIDS to monitor the effectiveness of intervention programmes in Thailand.

In sentinel surveillance, the main objective is not to achieve representativeness of a health problem or an epidemic of the entire population. Rather, the objective is to track an approximate pattern or trend of the situation on which to base interventions. Sentinel surveillance allows monitoring of trends in specific groups within the community. Thus in Thailand, monitoring the year of first use of heroin can provide an estimate of when the next heroin epidemic may occur. Sentinel surveillance has been able to monitor the pattern of HIV infection among the people engaging in high-risk activity such as drug addicts, commercial sex workers, those infected with sexually transmitted diseases, expectant mothers, and military conscripts (Nopkesorn *et al.* 1998).

The results of sentinel surveillance must be interpreted with care. The critical factor is the issue of population change among different samples to estimate the magnitude of health problems. A prevalence of 40 per cent of HIV-positive people among drug addicts may give the impression that the situation of HIV spread has been stabilized. New cases of HIV-positive people among military recruits can give a better estimate of the trend in HIV-related problems in a country or community. However, the interpretation may be invalid if the rate of new infection equals the rate among the addicts who disappeared from the detection of the sentinel surveillance system either through migration or death.

Screening

The objective of a screening programme is to detect health problems at an early stage and link the problems with services which are effective in modifying the natural history of the diseases or to prevent cases with specific diseases such as HIV infection from spreading infection to non-infected contacts.

The target for screening can be the general public as well as those engaged in high-risk activity. Genital chlamydial infection is a common sexually transmitted infection that is often asymptomatic, but is associated with long-term morbidity in many women. Early infection can be diagnosed reliably using non-invasive methods and treated effectively with antibiotics. Screening for genital chlamydial infection in high-risk settings, such as genitourinary medicine and abortion clinics, has already been documented (Stephenson 1998). Screening in the wider community also needs to be evaluated since chlamydial infection is widely distributed among young sexually active people who may have little contact with health services. Studies are in progress to assess the acceptability of different screening approaches for both women and men in the community, and to compare the performance of newer diagnostic techniques. The cost-effectiveness of community-based screening for reducing morbidity needs to be evaluated empirically in randomized trials to encourage a coherent, evidence-based screening policy (Stephenson 1998).

Investments in national screening programmes should be based on benefits to the people who are found to be positive who can then be given intervention treatment or monitoring. Ideally, the evidence of such benefits should be strong such as evidence from a randomized control trial. In the United Kingdom, a national programme to screen newborn infants for phenylketonuria was introduced in 1969, followed in 1981 by a similar programme for congenital hypothyroidism. Decisions to start these national programmes were informed by evidence from observational studies. Subsequent national registers of diseases were used to measure the impact of the screening programmes. Differences and changes in infrastructure and standard instruments for screening within and between screening facilities over time can result in inconsistent policies and inequitable access to effective screening services, as well as to problems in the comparability of information. More recent developments in tandem mass spectrometry have made it technically possible to screen for several inborn errors of metabolism in a single analytical step. However, the availability of the instrument should not prompt decisions for screening. In fact, for each of these conditions, evidence is required that the benefits of screening outweigh the harm, ideally informed by evidence from randomized controlled trials. Setting a priority on what conditions should be formally evaluated can be an important challenge to the public health, clinical, and scientific communities (Dezateux 1998). Screening programmes have the potential to reduce the burden from mortality, morbidity, and disability, and to improve quality of life and livelihood, but they also have the potential to cause harm. A set of criteria will be needed to identify worthwhile screening programmes, develop strategies, and mount effective implementation that is agreed upon by stakeholders. A much more critical approach to screening is now being adopted. Efforts are being made to ensure that new programmes of proven benefits that are acceptable to the public, are effectively and equitably implemented in the community particularly if the resources from such a screening programme come from taxation. This issue will stimulate further discussion and debate among important stakeholders (Peckham and Dezateux 1998).

In developing an expensive screening programme, one criterion is to redefine the unacceptable by the stakeholders particularly the community. For example, the community might decide that it is unacceptable to have children infected with HIV. If so, couples will be encouraged to be screened and counselled for HIV infection if they decide to have a child. It is imperative to strengthen the community-based programme. Unless healthy populations and healthy communities decide to be involved, screening programmes will not be very effective. The communities must be encouraged to help providers and decision-makers help themselves.

Survey and special studies

The objective of a special survey is to gain insight into the nature and extent of a problem in a defined community. The problems to be surveyed may be suggested by information from routine reporting and the surveillance system. Surveys and special studies can answer a particular question relevant to a community when routine systems cannot yield adequate information for action. Members of the community can be involved in such a survey not only as collectors of data or joint explorers of local conditions but also as partners in interpreting the data and in determining systematically how to manage a problem. The community can also shed light on the cultural meaning attached to a disease or a condition (MacQueen *et al.* 1996; Van Landingham *et al.* 1997). An understanding of the survey results as seen from the standpoint of the people will enhance an understanding of the problem and improve the dissemination of the results of surveys to the community and thus empower the community groups. Primary health care workers can be the most important group to engage in the dissemination of information to the individuals. In the Philippines, health-care workers learn to identify the mosquitoes responsible for the spread of malaria and help conduct and read blood smears.

One example of a survey is to assess whether universal condom use to reduce the spread of HIV infection was effective as suggested by routine surveillance (Mastro and Limpakarnjanarat 1995). A survey was conducted and showed that a low rate of condom use occurred in lower social class commercial sex workers, construction workers, and poor truck drivers. The seroconversion rates of HIV among these sex workers was shown to be on the rise (Sawanpanyalert *et al.* 1994; Mastro and Limpakarnjanarat 1995; Kilmarx *et al.* 1998). Many commercial sex workers did not use condoms if they were entertaining 'regular customers', if they drank, or if they believed that healthy people had no risk of HIV transmission (Vanichseni *et al.* 1993). The special survey was an important supplement to the information gathered from routine surveillance for designing effective control strategies.

A special survey was also conducted among housewives in Thailand to clarify the reasons for a rise in HIV infection in pregnant women. The survey showed that there was a significant difference in attitude between the Thai housewives who were HIV positive and those who were HIV negative. Those who were HIV positive were not confident at discussing HIV disease with their partners. They were also less likely to tell their partners first if they were infected (Suwanagool *et al.* 1995). Special surveys also helped to clarify the risk of perinatal transmission (Shaffer *et al.* 1999), and the rate of discordance of HIV status between pregnant women and their partners (Siriwasin *et al.* 1998). This special study helped to design a public health campaign aimed at addressing the increase in HIV prevalence among pregnant women discovered from the sentinel surveillance system.

Training of interviewers and enumerators for valid data collection is required for epidemiology studies. Qualitative data to identify variables meaningful to a community, reflecting their voices, and bringing in the human dimension of a problem can be a powerful complement to epidemiological surveys which highlight differences between groups. Therefore, public health surveys and special studies have embraced methods from the social sciences in the identification of variables for surveys as well as the interpretation, dissemination, and use of results.

Large-scale health surveys conducted by government agencies, which record information on a large number of health-related variables, are available for analysis. The information can be applied to estimate demographic profiles associated with possible lifestyles and biochemical determinants of diseases. It can also estimate the probability of receiving some clinical services and screening according to the type of health insurance, the probability of receiving a digital rectal examination, and the effectiveness of community intervention to encourage positive lifestyles such as smoking cessation (Graubard and Korn 1999). Special studies which follow cohorts can detect changes in epidemics and behavioural factors (Limpakarnjanarat *et al.* 1999).

Rapid surveys

The objective of a rapid survey is to collect information required to make decisions to cope with urgent health problems when the true nature and extent of the problem is unknown. Large surveys are usually expensive and cannot be done frequently or timely enough to assess or evaluate health problems in a specific area. Furthermore, it is unwise to infer the results of a large general population survey for local planning (Smith 1989). A rapid survey can be used to collect population-specific information on health situations, on possible determinants of disease, and on knowledge, perceptions, and cultural aspects of illnesses. A typical rapid survey can be carried out by sampling 30 clusters of seven to ten respondents (or households), each covering 200 to 300 household interviews (Henderson and Sunaresan 1982; Frerichs and Tar Tar 1989). These methods have been used to assess the status of immunization, family planning, and use of antenatal services.

Contact tracing

Contact tracing is particularly useful when information from routine systems and surveillance suggests the need for a clarification of the pattern of the spread of diseases (Box 10). It is also useful to estimate acute illness episodes and disease problems among illegal migrants and mobile ill-defined populations such as tourists and migrant workers. The purposes of contract tracing (community visiting team) are to confirm the diagnosis, determine the extent of secondary transmissions, and estimate the pattern of risk behaviours.

Box 10 Purpose of contact tracing

- Confirm diagnosis and find causes
- Behaviour risk estimates
- Estimate magnitude of problems
- Identify possible control measures
- Identify where/to whom to apply control measures
- Recommend control measures

Contact tracing can lead to more cases contacting the patients who failed to come to receive service from the health-care system and thus increases the validity of the estimates of the magnitude of problems. In addition, better targeting of control measures can be a desirable outcome, leading to increased efficiency of the health system.

Contact tracing was carried out for heroin users seeking treatment from Samutprakarn Hospital in Thailand (Table 3) to identify the magnitude of needle-sharing behaviours among the confirmed addicts.

Through contact tracing, drug use and needle sharing were identified as a mode of spread of HIV infection from the urban to rural

Table 3 Drug use and travel pattern of 731 injecting heroin users treated at Samutprakarn Hospital

Ever travel and stay over night in other province	38.9%
Reasons for travelling	
Holiday/sociocultural ceremonies	45.6%
Occupational/personal business	39.5%
Visiting friends/relatives	16.8%
Drug injection while travelling	59.5%
Needle sharing	24.7%
Borrowed from someone	6.3%
Lent to someone	10.6%
Borrowed from and lent to someone	7.8%

areas. The result gave rise to the design of a prevention programme aimed at reducing needle sharing among addicts during travel. Contact tracing could also document the spread of HIV infection among convicts through needle sharing in prisons.

International travel can be one of the major modes of transmission of HIV. Estimates of contacts of tourists with sex workers, beach boys, and massage parlour attendants through surveys and contact tracing can help clarify the magnitude and pattern of disease transmission (Mulhall *et al.* 1993). Migration also occurs across borders for jobs in construction, factories, logging, and commercial sex work (Asian Research Center for Migration 1999).

Vital registration and census

Vital registration relies on the requirement by law to report health events including birth and death. These figures can be obtained from the national statistical offices and relevant departments such as health, welfare, education, and the ministry of interior. Many countries also have periodic censuses every 10 years.

There are examples in developing countries where events are under-reported due to the lack of quality assurance of the reporting system, even to document all deaths. For example, the accuracy of perinatal and infant mortality rates in most developing countries is questionable. The perinatal and infant mortality rates in a rural district of Thailand as measured from surveys were compared with the official statistics to assess accuracy. All stillbirths and 45 per cent of infant deaths were unregistered (Lumbiganon *et al.* 1990).

In addition, the inaccurate enumeration of deaths and inadequate medical certification of deaths in developing countries limits the ability to infer the cause of death, particularly in those occurring outside hospital or clinical settings. In Thailand, the causes of mortality were defined only in about 40 per cent of all deaths. Verbal autopsy and lay reporting have been used as methods for estimating the causes of death (Snow and Marsh 1992; Kleinman 1978) through data gathered from relatives and friends. Verbal autopsy has been widely used for the diagnosis of causes of child mortality. Standard criteria have been developed for the diagnosis of common causes of childhood mortality to allow a comparison of the results of different studies (Bang and Bang 1992). Such standard criteria will be needed to acquire data on cause-specific mortality for evaluating disease prevalence and for targeting, monitoring, and measuring the impact of interventions.

A combination of several methods: an example

All academic disciplines for community diagnosis have both strengths and weaknesses. To solve a public health problem adequately requires inputs from several disciplines and approaches either through composing multidisciplinary teams or training public health researchers to move beyond disciplinary boundaries.

A combination of several methods has been used to understand the epidemics of HIV infection in Thailand. An epidemic among drug users was predicted by routine reporting from various drug dependency treatment centres (Ministry of Public Health 1997). In addition, routine information from drug dependency treatment facilities also suggested the spread of the epidemic from Bangkok to the provinces and from the urban to rural areas. Different incidence rates occurred in various geographical areas at any point in time. The HIV epidemic in specific regional areas, such as the hill tribes drug user population discussed above, most likely occurred at different times from 1987 to at least 1995 if not after (Beyrer *et al.* 1997). HIV infection in non-injecting drug users consistently persisted due to sexual behaviour. Contact tracing showed that travelling, needle sharing, and imprisonment interfere with intervention efforts to stop the spread of HIV infection. Periodic special surveys showed that a reduction of risk behaviours such as needle sharing could be achieved in a relatively short time with timely implementation of appropriate interventions. They also documented the epidemiological evolution of HIV-1 subtypes B and E among heterosexuals and injecting drug users in Thailand (Limpakarnjanarat *et al.* 1998; Poshyachinda 1993*a*,*b*). Moreover, routine reporting and sentinel surveillance supported the notion that the prevalence among injecting drug users in the rural population and minority groups was still low when preventive interventions were introduced. Nonetheless, the prevalence in these populations increased to the level of Bangkok and the central region.

Sentinel surveillance has demonstrated the development of infective pools of HIV infection among intravenous drug users and commercial sex workers in Thailand. Special surveys and contact tracing among the clients of sexually transmitted disease clinics and among the migrant workers helped clarify the transmission among the high-risk and socially deprived groups. Also, through the sentinel surveillance of pregnant women visiting antenatal clinics, military conscripts, blood donors, and outpatient clinics, the epidemic was shown to have spread from the infective pool and high-risk populations to the general population, and subsequently demonstrated the reduction of the rate of the epidemic through effective control (Fig. 4). The story of an information system and various methods for community diagnosis of HIV infection has emphasized the need for a combination of approaches to understand the evolution of a public health problems as well as the effectiveness of control measures. It also showed the value of various types of information system in explaining aspects of epidemics leading to effective control.

Finally, the information system and attempt at community diagnosis will only be possible if done in concert with political commitment and effective administration and planning which balances the evidence and values collected from different stakeholders within the society (Phoolcharoen *et al.* 1998*a*,*b*).

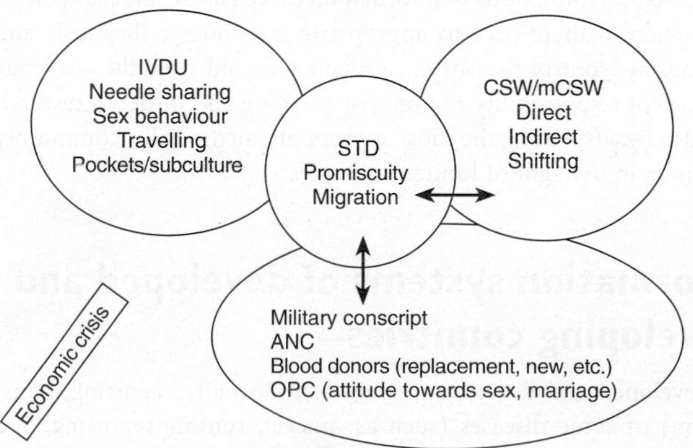

Fig. 4 Model of transmission of HIV infection in Thailand derived from various methods of community diagnosis. IVDU, intravenous drug user; STD sexually transmitted disease; CSW, commercial sex worker; ANC, antenatal clinics; OPC, outpatient clinics.

Technological limitations of information systems and community diagnosis

Even if the data for community diagnosis are valid, methodological advances are still needed to help set priorities for health needs.

Estimates of lifetime effects on individuals with particular health problems

Many health measures such as person years of life lost, healthy days of life lost, disability-adjusted life years, and quality-adjusted life years attempt to introduce time dimensions to the evaluation of health and diseases. These measures are not likely to correspond to social preferences and social investment in the individuals before death occurs. The social preferences probably vary between cultures and therefore an attempt to make global estimates using common measures might not be valid to compare burden of illness. Particular care must be used if these measures affect the allocation of resources across countries.

Effects of health problems of individuals on their relatives

The loss of the main source of income through death is not equivalent to the death of a dependent in a family. Therefore, deaths will not be equal among members of a household depending on many factors. These include the changes in social status caused by widowhood or orphanhood, changes in the dependency ratios of the household, and the reallocation of work responsibilities between household members. Other significant factors are the reallocation of domestic responsibilities, changes in major sources and the levels of income of the household in which deaths occur, changes in ownership and indebtedness, and expenditure due to medical bills or funeral costs.

Therefore, the community needs to be consulted to see whether the community diagnoses accurately reflect their perceptions of the values given to deaths and illnesses, particularly when decisions on the allocation of limited resources will be based on such a diagnosis.

Universities have a definite role in helping to overcome the technological limitations of information as well as to guide and direct the society with respect to appropriate community diagnosis and appropriate control measures. Academics should meet the challenge and accept responsibility not only by teaching and in-depth research but also by advocating the most appropriate methods for community diagnosis in the light of limited resources.

Information systems of developed and developing countries

In developed and developing countries, mortality reporting, registrations of some diseases (such as cancer), routine reporting, and census data have been the main sources of information used to estimate the burden of health problems. These generally have been supplemented by household surveys and periodic population-based survey such as the National Health Examination Survey, the National Health and Nutrition Examination Survey, the Health and Welfare Survey, contact tracing, and several population surveillance systems of notifiable diseases.

However, the most significant difference between the information systems of developed and developing countries is the accuracy of routine statistics, particularly with respect to the cause of mortality. Thus, in Thailand, data collected for cause of death suffered from under-reporting. In addition, nearly half of the reported deaths were classified under ill-defined causes (Samutharaks *et al.* 1997). Even when deaths occur in hospitals, only a small percentage undergo autopsy (less than 10 per cent for large hospitals in Thailand). In some developed countries, linking records of repeat events occurring in individuals has been used to reduce the errors in recording the cause of deaths, dramatically reducing validity problems (Archeson 1966). As to the validity of morbidity data, even Western countries have variable notification of infection, with poorer notification for milder infection (Benjamin 1968). For diseases like cancer with a much longer natural history, most patients are likely to be registered.

The chief challenge of information systems in developed countries is how to ensure that the pressure of new but untested technology does not dictate the acquisition of high-technology equipment to track the operation of managed care. Recently, large budgets have been allotted to information systems in large health-care networks such as the Kaiser-Permanente's Northern California Region ($1 billion over 7 years), Health Care Sacramento ($27.5 million over 5 years), and Sutler Health ($150 million over the next 7 years) (Morrissey 1995). How much the gain in health will mirror the extent of the increase in the efficiency of service delivery remains to be investigated. Moreover, there is a tendency for further investment in telemedicine and the expansion of fibre-optic capacity. This trend will complicate how information systems are used to track the allocation of resources and appropriate reimbursement for patient care. Whether the incremental increase in the investment in information systems will produce a proportional gain in health of the community is a valid and as yet unanswered question.

Developing countries must not be trapped into investing in high technology for sophisticated information systems beyond their needs. Some guidelines might be useful for decisions on the effective information system projects. Firstly, the involvement of the system users from the beginning is desirable for establishing a clear and realistic goal. Secondly, a complete review for existing solutions must be in place before deciding on investing in high technology. Thirdly, some assurance of adequate support and continuity from the vendor must be obtained since developing countries will be very dependent on the support system. Finally, the reality of the organizational constraints on the systems must be taken into account, for example, the adequacy of human resources to operate the system. Therefore, it is important to 'think big' (holistic manner), 'start small' (adopt an evolutionary not a 'big bang' approach), and 'act rationally' according to the need to advance the objectives of the health-care system (Wyatt 1994).

However, developing countries must invest in resources to capture essential information on health problems and trends (the resources used, utilization, costs, and outcomes of public health problems) to decide whether an investment in health care will yield the outcome described in the objectives of the health-care system. An information system is not for gathering information via sophisticated technology. It is for giving evidence to stakeholders to solve health problems with an accepted method of conflict resolution.

References

Anonymous (1995). The World Health Organization quality of life assessment (WHOQOL): position paper from the World Health Organization. *Social Science and Medicine*, **41**, 1403–9.

Archeson, R. (1966). *Medical record linkage.* Oxford University Press.

Asian Research Center for Migration (1999). *Recent trends in international migration in Asia.* Chulalongkorn University Printing House, Bangkok.

Bang, A.T. and Bang, R.A. (1992). Diagnosis of causes of childhood deaths in developing countries by verbal autopsy: suggested criteria. *Bulletin of the WHO*, **70**, 499–507.

Benjamin, B. (1968). *Health and vital statistics.* Allen and Unwin, London.

Beyrer, C., Celentano, D.D., Suprasert, S., *et al.* (1997). Widely varying HIV prevalence and risk behaviours among the ethnic minority peoples of northern Thailand. *AIDS Care*, **9**, 427–39.

Cassol, S., Weniger, B.G., Babu, P.G., *et al.* (1996*a*). Detection of HIV type 1 env subtypes A, B, C, and E in Asia using dried blood spots: a new surveillance tool for molecular epidemiology. *AIDS Research in Human Retroviruses*, **12**, 1435–41.

Cassol, S.A., Read, S., Weniger, B.G., *et al.* (1996*b*). Dried blood spots collected on filter paper: an international resource for the diagnosis and genetic characterization of human immunodeficiency virus type-1. *Memorias do Instituto Oswaldo Cruz*, **91**, 351–8.

Commission on Health Research for Development (1990). *Health research: essential link to equity in development.* Oxford University Press.

DeRiemer, K., Rudoy, I., Schecter, G.F., Hopewell, P.C., and Daley, C.L. (1999). The epidemiology of tuberculosis diagnosed after death in San Francisco, 1986–1995. *International Journal of Tuberculosis and Lung Disease*, **3**, 488–93.

Dezateux, C. (1998). Evaluating newborn screening programmes based on dried blood spots: future challenges. *British Medical Bulletin*, **54**, 877–90.

Frerichs, R.R. and Tar Tar, K. (1989). Computer-assisted rapid surveys in developing countries. *Public Health Reports*, **104**, 14–23.

Frerichs, R.R., Silarug, N., Eskes, N., *et al.* (1994). Saliva-based HIV-antibody testing in Thailand. *AIDS*, **8**, 885–94.

Ghana Health Assessment Project Team (1981). A quantitative method of assessing the health impact of different diseases in less developed countries. *International Journal of Epidemiology*, **10**, 73–80.

Graubard, B.I. and Korn, E.L. (1999). Analyzing health surveys for cancer-related objectives. *Journal of the National Cancer Institute*, **91**, 1005–16.

Henderson, R.H. and Sunaresan, T. (1982). Cluster sampling to assess immunization coverage: a review of experience with a simplified method. *Bulletin of the WHO*, **60**, 253–60.

Hyder, A.A. and Morrow, R.H. (1998). Steady state assumptions in DALYs: effect on estimates of HIV impact. *Journal of Epidemiology and Community Health*, **53**, 43–5.

Kilmarx, P.H., Limpakarnjanarat, K., Mastro, T.D., *et al.* (1998). HIV-1 seroconversion in a prospective study of female sex workers in northern Thailand: continued high incidence among brothel-based women. *AIDS*, **12**, 1889–98.

Kitayaporn, D., Uneklabh, C., Weniger, B.G., *et al.* (1994). HIV-1 incidence determined retrospectively among drug users in Bangkok, Thailand. *AIDS*, **8**, 1443–50.

Kitayaporn, D., Kaewkungwal, J., Bejrachandra, S., Rungroung, E., Chandanayingyong, D., and Mastro, T.D. (1996*a*). Estimated rate of HIV-1-infectious but seronegative blood donations in Bangkok, Thailand. *AIDS*, **10**, 1157–62.

Kitayaporn, D., Tansuphaswadikul, S., Lohsomboon, P., *et al.* (1996*b*). Survival of AIDS patients in the emerging epidemic in Bangkok, Thailand. *Journal of AIDS and Human Retrovirology*, **11**, 77–82.

Kitsiripornchai, S., Markowitz, L.E., Ungchusak, K., *et al.* (1998). Sexual behavior of young men in Thailand: regional differences and evidence of behavior change. *Journal of AIDS and Human Retrovirology*, **18**, 282–8.

Kleinman, A. (1978). Culture, illness and care: clinical lessons from anthropology and cross cultural research. *Annals of Internal Medicine*, **88**, 251–8.

Limpakarnjanarat, K., Ungchusak, K., Mastro, T.D., *et al.* (1998). The epidemiological evolution of HIV-1 subtypes B and E among heterosexuals and injecting drug users in Thailand, 1992–1997. *AIDS*, **12**, 1108–9.

Limpakarnjanarat, K., Mastro, T.D., Saisorn, S., *et al.* (1999). HIV-1 and other sexually transmitted infections in a cohort of female sex workers in Chiang Rai, Thailand. *Sexually Transmitted Infection*, **75**, 30–5.

Luepker, R.V. and Herlitz, J. (1999). Differences in the treatment of acute myocardial infarction between regions of countries and the impact on prognosis. *Journal of Cardiovascular Risk*, **6**, 77–87.

Lumbiganon, P., Panamonta, M., Laopaiboon, M., Pothinam, S., and Patithat, N. (1990). Why are Thai official perinatal and infant mortality rates so low? *International Journal of Epidemiology*, **19**, 997–1000.

MacQueen, K.M., Nopkesorn, T., Sweat, M.D., Sawaengdee, Y., Mastro, T.D., and Weniger, B.G. (1996). Alcohol consumption, brothel attendance, and condom use: normative expectations among Thai military conscripts. *Medical Anthropology Quarterly*, **10**, 402–23.

Mastro, T.D. and Kitayaporn, D. (1998). HIV type 1 transmission probabilities: estimates from epidemiological studies. *AIDS Research in Human Retroviruses*, **14** (Supplement 3) S223–7.

Mastro, T.D. and Limpakarnjanarat, K. (1995). Condom use in Thailand: how much is it slowing the HIV/AIDS epidemic? *AIDS*, **9**, 523–5.

Matloff, E.T., Shappell, H., Brierley, K., Bernhardt, B.A., McKinnon, W., and Peshkin, B.N. (2000). What would you do? Specialists' perspectives on cancer genetic testing, prophylactic surgery and insurance discrimination. *Journal of Clinical Oncology*, **18**, 2484–92.

Mills, S., Ungchusak, K., Srinivasan, V., Utomo, B., and Bennett, A. (1998). Assessing trends in HIV risk behaviors in Asia. *AIDS*, **12** (Supplement B), S79–86.

Ministry of Public Health (1997). *Health in Thailand 1995–1996.* Bureau of Health Policy and Planning. Ministry of Public Health, Nonthaburi.

Morrissey, J. (1995). Building networks to stay competitive. *Modern Healthcare*, August 21, 150–4.

Mulhall, B.P., Hu, M., Thompson, M., *et al.* (1993). Planned sexual behaviour of young Australian visitors to Thailand. *Medical Journal of Australia*, **158**, 530–5.

Muller, O., Sarangbin, S., Ruxrungtham, K., Sittitrai, W., and Phanuphak, P. (1995). Sexual risk behaviour reduction associated with voluntary HIV counselling and testing in HIV infected patients in Thailand. *AIDS Care*, **7**, 567–72.

Murray, C.J. and Lopez, A.D. (1996). The incremental effect of age-weighting on YLLs, YLDs, and DALYs: a response. *Bulletin of the WHO*, **74**, 445–6.

Newbrander, W. (1997). *Private health sector growth in Asia: issues and implications.* Wiley, Chichester.

Nopkesorn, T., Mock, P.A., Mastro, T.D., *et al.* (1998). HIV-1 subtype E incidence and sexually transmitted diseases in a cohort of military conscripts in northern Thailand. *Journal of AIDS and Human Retrovirology*, **18**, 372–9.

Peckham, C.S. and Dezateux, C. (1998). Issues underlying the evaluation of screening programmes. *British Medical Bulletin*, **54**, 767–78.

Phoolcharoen, W. (1998). HIV/AIDS prevention in Thailand: success and challenges. *Science*, **280**, 1873–4.

Phoolcharoen, W., Ungchusak, K., Sittitrai, W., and Brown, T. (1998). Thailand: lessons from a strong national response to HIV/AIDS. *AIDS*, **12** (Supplement B), S123–35.

Poshyachinda, V. (1993*a*). Drugs and AIDS in Southeast Asia. *Forensic Science International*, **62**, 15–28.

Poshyachinda, V. (1993*b*). Drug injecting and HIV infection among the population of drug abusers in Asia. *Bulletin of Narcotics*, **45**, 77–90.

Roberts, C.L., Tracy, S., and Peat, B. (2000). Rates for obstetric intervention amongst private and public patients in Australia: population-based descriptive study. *British Medical Journal*, **321**, 137–41.

Rosomoff, H.L. and Rosomoff, R.S. (1999). Low back pain. Evaluation and management in the primary care setting. *Medical Clinics of North America*, **83**, 643–62.

Samutharaks, B., Wecharak, P., Kongkamned, R., and Sitthi-amorn, C. (1997). *Quantitative assessments of disease impact on society: a conceptual approach to prioritization and agenda setting of health problems for policy determination in Thailand.* College of Public Health, Chulalongkorn University, Bangkok.

Sawanpanyalert, P., Ungchusak, K., Thanprasertsuk, S., and Akarasewi, P. (1994). HIV-1 seroconversion rates among female commercial sex workers, Chiang Mai, Thailand: a multi cross-sectional study. *AIDS*, **8**, 825–9.

Shaffer, N., Roongpisuthipong, A., Siriwasin, W., *et al.* (1999). Maternal virus load and perinatal human immunodeficiency virus type 1 subtype E transmission, Thailand. Bangkok Collaborative Perinatal HIV Transmission Study Group. *Journal of Infectious Disease*, **179**, 590–9.

Siriwasin, W., Shaffer, N., Roongpisuthipong, A., *et al.* (1998). HIV prevalence, risk, and partner serodiscordance among pregnant women in Bangkok. Bangkok Collaborative Perinatal HIV Transmission Study Group. *Journal of the American Medical Association*, **280**, 49–54.

Sitthi-amorn, C., Chandraprasert, S., Bunnag, S.C., and Plengvidhya, C.S. (1989). The prevalence and risk factors of hypertension in Klong Toey slum and Klong Toey government apartment houses. *International Journal of Epidemiology*, **18**, 89–94.

Smith, G.S. (1989). Development of rapid epidemiological assessment methods to evaluate health status and delivery of health services. *International Journal of Epidemiology*, **19** (Supplement 4).

Snow, B. and Marsh, K. (1992). How useful are verbal autopsies to estimate childhood causes of death? *Health Policy and Planning*, **7**, 22–9.

Stephenson, J.M. (1998). Screening for genital chlamydial infection. *British Medical Bulletin*, **54**, 891–902.

Suwanagool, S., Chaiyakul, P., Ratanasuwan, W., Pechthanom, L., and Chaisilwattana, P. (1995). HIV-1 infection among low income women attending a Siriraj sexually transmitted disease clinic: sociodemographic differentials. *Journal of the Medical Association of Thailand*, **78**, 355–61.

Ungchusak, K., Rehle, T., Thammapornpilap, P., Spiegelman, D., Brinkmann, U., and Siraprapasiri, T. (1996). Determinants of HIV infection among female commercial sex workers in northeastern Thailand: results from a longitudinal study. *Journal of AIDS and Human Retrovirology*, **12**, 500–7. (Erratum *Journal of AIDS and Human Retrovirology*, **18**, 192 (1998)).

Van Griensven, G.J., Limanonda, B., Ngaokeow, S., Ayuthaya, S.I., and Poshyachinda, V. (1998). Evaluation of a targeted HIV prevention programme among female commercial sex workers in the south of Thailand. *Sexually Transmitted Infection*, **74**, 54–8.

Vanichseni, S., Des Jarlais, D.C., Choopanya, K., *et al.* (1993). Condom use with primary partners among injecting drug users in Bangkok, Thailand and New York City, United States. *AIDS*, **7**, 887–91.

Van Landingham, M., Grandjean, N., Suprasert, S., and Sittitrai, W. (1997). Dimensions of AIDS knowledge and risky sexual practices: a study of northern Thai males. *Archives of Sexual Behaviour*, **26**, 269–93.

Wadsworth, M.I., Butterfield, B.J.H., and Blaney, R. (1971). *Health and sickness: the choice of treatment.* Tavistock Publications, London.

WHO (World Health Organization) (2000*a*). *The world health report 2000: health systems—improving performance.* WHO, Geneva.

WHO (World Health Organization) (2000*b*). *The world health report on infectious diseases.* WHO, Geneva.

Wyatt, J.C. (1994). Clinical data systems. 3. Developing and evaluating clinical data systems. *Lancet*, **344**, 1682–8.

5.3 The revolution in electronic communication and public health

Elliot R. Siegel, Julia Royall, and John C. Scott

Introduction

Advances in computing, information, and communications are dramatically transforming the health sciences, and they underpin the very means for generating new knowledge and aid in its rapid utilization by scientists and health workers in the field. Investigators in basic research need access to databases and repositories. Developers of new vaccines, drugs, and diagnostics need access to discussion groups for product development work and co-ordination of clinical trials. Published literatures are readily identifiable and accessible through computer databases. Electronic versions of printed journal articles are sought especially where library resources are poor. Epidemiologists engaged in vector control and surveillance programmes use geographic information systems and satellite-based remote sensing technologies. It is highly desirable that collaborating units, within countries and around the globe, maintain contact through e-mail and other electronically mediated means of communication that are becoming increasingly possible over the Internet. New modes of communication and publication, particularly electronically linked World Wide Web sites, provide a central means for identifying and networking with fellow researchers and public health workers, and accessing related scientific resources.

Scientists and public health workers in developing regions face particular challenges in accessing the products of this revolution in electronic communication. Traditional dial-up telephone connections can be slow, unreliable, and costly. More dependable solutions can include microwave, a point-to-point option that uses radio waves, and very small aperture terminals which communicate via geostationary satellites. Commercial development of low Earth orbiting satellite systems may be another promising option in the years ahead. Obtaining regulatory approval in some countries can be a significant impediment for very small aperture terminal and other wireless solutions. However, progress has been realized in recent years wherein full Internet connectivity has become a reality in most major cities in the developing world. This has been partly fuelled by special communications initiatives undertaken by donor agencies, and the growth of in-country public and private sector providers of commercial Internet services. Yet access in remote regions is still problematic. A case study based of the Multilateral Initiative on Malaria illustrates the promise and challenges of connecting malaria research and control sites in sub-Saharan Africa to the Internet, thus providing support for a viable and sustainable human and technical infrastructure.

The Internet

The Internet is a global network of interconnecting computer networks first developed over 25 years ago. This 'network of networks' allows any computer attached to it to communicate with any other computer using the same Internet protocol. From its start as a research network supported largely by American government agencies, the Internet has evolved to become a ubiquitous and largely unregulated carrier of data, images, voice, and full motion video available at the click of a button to users worldwide. The proliferation of low-cost personal computers with rapidly expanding memory capacity, coupled with increasingly affordable high-bandwidth telecommunications technology available at locations both accessible and inaccessible by wires, have together combined to produce a remarkable revolution in electronic communication.

In 1973, the United States Defense Advanced Research Projects Agency initiated a research project at several universities to develop communication protocols which would allow networked computers to communicate transparently across multiple linked packet networks. This was called the Internetting Project and the system of networks, which emerged from the research, was called the 'Internet' (National Research Council 1999). The system of protocols became known as transmission control protocol/Internet protocol. The Internet was designed partly to provide a communications network that would work even if some of the sites were destroyed by nuclear attack. If the most direct route was not available, 'routers' would direct traffic around the network via alternate routes.

In 1986, the United States National Science Foundation developed NSFNET, a major backbone capable of switching information 'packets' at speeds of 45 million bits per second (Mbps). The National Aeronautics and Space Administration (**NASA**) and the United States Department of Energy contributed additional backbone facilities. In Europe major international backbones such as NORDUNET were established. Commercial network providers worldwide soon entered the market and offered Internet backbone and access support on a competitive basis to any interested party. By the end of the decade, the Internet grew to include some 5000 networks in over three dozen countries, serving 700 000 host computers used by 4 million people. These numbers can only be grossly approximated today as virtually every country participates in the Internet revolution. The interested reader is referred to the Internet Society website where an excellent history of these developments may be found online, often in the words of the people who made the history, including Vint Cerf, Robert Kahn, Jonathan Postel, and Stephen Wolff (http://www.isoc.org).

The World Wide Web

When computer experts, engineers, and scientists first used the early Internet, there was nothing user-friendly about it. The need existed for a tool which would unify Internet access for the general computer user population, a group which had become accustomed to graphical user interfaces, pointing-and-clicking, and simple commands masking complex software functions. This need prompted the creation of the World Wide Web in 1991 at the European Center for Nuclear Research in Switzerland (**CERN**).

The concept implemented by Tim Berners-Lee along with Robert Cailliau at CERN sought to develop a system of links between different sources of information (Berners-Lee *et al.* 1994). Parts of a file would be made up into nodes which, when called up, would link the user to other related files. They devised a document format called Hypertext Markup Language, a variant of one used in the publishing industry since the 1950s, and released it as a new Internet protocol, the hypertext transfer protocol. Like e-mail 20 years earlier, the World Wide Web quickly diffused from the physics community at CERN to become the new 'killer application' for the Internet (National Research Council 1999). In 1993, Marc Andreessen and his team at the United States National Center for Supercomputing Applications provided a major impetus to the protocol's utility. The graphical browser Mosaic was developed and later commercialized by Andreessen when he founded Netscape. Microsoft's full-scale entry into the browser, server, and Internet service provider market has accelerated the shift to a commercially based Internet, especially timely with the diminution of funding by the United States government agencies in 1995.

On-ramps to the information superhighway

In the meantime, high-speed connections to the Internet—permitting faster web browsing and downloading of ever-larger datasets—is proceeding apace. Dial-up modems operating at speeds of 56 thousand bits per second (kbps) are widely supported by commercial Internet service providers serving homes and offices, but these are generally not fast enough to carry multimedia, such as sound and video, except in low quality. New technologies, such as cable modems and digital telephone lines that are continuously connected to the Internet are becoming increasingly available and offer relatively low-cost access to bandwidth in excess of 1 Mbps. Satellite broadcasting, discussed in some detail below, provides services at lesser speed (typically 128 kbps) but has the capacity to reach underserved regions of the world where wired communications lines are economically unfeasible or physically impractical due to distance, terrain, and climate. In contrast, large institutional users in the industrialized countries (that is, businesses, universities) routinely subscribe to broadband services offering shared Internet connections to literally hundreds of individual users wired together via local area networks, at speeds ranging from 1.5 (t_1) to 45 (t_3) Mbps.

In parallel to what is sometimes now referred to as the 'commodity Internet', we are seeing the development of a complementary 'next generation Internet' intended to serve the needs for higher levels of bandwidth by scientific and research communities. These on-ramps to the next generation Internet are capable of operating at speeds of 155 Mbps, and offer connection to the very high performance Backbone Network Service. Launched in 1995, the very high performance Backbone Network Service is a National Science Foundation-funded nationwide network supporting supercomputing centres and research institutions, a model having its roots in the original Internet a decade earlier. Some segments of the American very high performance Backbone Network Service are now operating at 622 Mbps (known as OC-12), with one link at 2.5 billion bits per second (Gbps) (OC-48) between San Francisco and Los Angeles. International consortia are working towards extending very high performance backbone network services worldwide.

Factors limiting use of the Internet

The American National Research Council underscores the increasing popularity of the Internet in health and health care, and the ability of the Internet to revolutionize the health sector by connecting people, information, and services from anywhere across the country, and around the globe (National Research Council 2000). At the same time, its report identifies a number of fundamental factors concerning security that can limit the use of the Internet in health applications, as well as technical limitations in the capability of the Internet itself.

Health information can be extremely personal and sensitive. Systems designed to transmit patient medical records across the Internet or to allow remote access to a patient's medical record, for example, must have strong built-in security protections to ensure that the information remains confidential and is not intentionally or unintentionally altered. The limiting factor, from a health perspective, is the difficulty in verifying the identity of people communicating across the network and accessing sensitive information. Large organizations can overcome this problem by using digital credentials, or certificates, that can be verified by most web browsers. But mechanisms are not in place for distributing such credentials to everyone who might use the Internet for health purposes. This problem is referred to as an 'authentication' problem, and one proposed solution is the establishment of a ubiquitous public key infrastructure.

Another element of security is network availability. If the Internet is to be routinely used for critical health functions such as retrieving medical records, users must be sure the network is available 24 hours a day, 7 days a week. However, situations can arise in which denial-of-service can take place by so-called 'hacker' attacks. A combination of research and development, and the adoption of best practices, can achieve improvement of overall reliability by network operators and system administrators.

Quality of service can be variable. Enormous variations in download times can exist due to variations in congestion—across the Internet, at the source website, and at the user's location. This can be a critical barrier for health applications that require downloading of large image files or videos. A recent evaluation study of end-to-end Internet performance revealed that local bottlenecks at the user's site, rather than inadequate bandwidth on the backbone links, was the source of most of the congestion problems at the United States and international sites studied (Wood *et al.* 1998).

High-speed user access may be problematic in many locations where the health need is greatest. Broadband access via cable modems, digital subscriber lines, and wireless communications is not available in many areas that need them most. Rural areas that could benefit from telemedicine services tend to be the last to acquire broadband services, and many inner city locations are often unable to afford local connections. These issues, and others cast under the general rubric of the 'digital-divide' are addressed elsewhere in this chapter.

Public health information content on the Web

Despite these limitations, the Internet and the World Wide Web have become a major resource for health-related information for health professionals and, increasingly, for members of the general public. In 1999 an estimated 30 million Americans used the Internet to search for health-related information, many of them accessing consumer-oriented health websites created especially for the non-health professional user. Proponents of these sites make the case that the Internet can dramatically improve the public's health by making information available to consumers in a more tailored and targeted fashion than is possible with other media. They also see the Internet as offering a means of changing personal behaviours, such as diet and exercise habits, in a way that will improve health. (One-third of these individuals also purchased prescription drugs and other health products as part of yet another revolution in electronic commerce, a discussion of which is beyond the scope of this chapter.) The appetite for authoritative and reliable health information on the Internet is large and growing. Approximately 600 000 searches each day from more than 120 000 different users are carried out on just one popular health information website (National Research Council 2000).

Thousands of health-related websites are presently available. Many provide convenient and often free access to bibliographic reference databases previously available in printed and/or limited electronic form. Others offer newly created digital versions of full-text journal articles directly from their publishers or by document delivery services. Still others provide information on specific health topics by leading medical specialty and lay organizational groups. Non-commercial websites geared to the public, patients, and their caregivers include MedlinePlus (http://www.MedlinePlus.gov) and a newly developed comprehensive listing of clinical trials supported by the American National Institutes of Health (http://www.ClinicalTrials.gov). An entirely new category of communication, spawned by the Internet itself, provides a venue (sometimes called a 'chat room') for the anonymous discussion of health problems by patients and their families.

Such ease of access does come with a price, however. The contents of these Internet-accessible resources may be of uneven quality and questionable validity (Silberg *et al.* 1997). An international initiative, the Health on the Net Foundation (http://www.hon.ch), offers a voluntary certification programme whereby information providers on the Web may elect to adhere to a code of conduct attesting to the reliability and credibility of the medical and health information available on their sites. A 'seal of approval' is awarded and may be prominently displayed for the assurance of users.

Examples of databases broadly relevant for the public health community include the American National Library of Medicine's Medline (http://nlm.nih.gov), which contains more than 9 million references to biomedical journal articles published in 3900 journals since 1965. The PubMed system offers a simple search interface that can also provide direct links to publishers' websites for the full-text articles referenced in Medline. The Biosis Biological Abstracts (http://www.biosis.org) offers a comprehensive and complementary reference source to the life science journal literature.

Specialized information resources abound as well. Those pertinent to the concerns of environmental health workers, for example, include the TOXNET (http://sis.nlm.nih.gov) cluster of databases for toxicology data (for example, Hazardous Substances Data Bank), toxicology literature (for example, TOXLINE), and toxic release information collected by the Environmental Protection Agency. Other resources are initially released on CD-ROM but are created to be accessible on the Web when connectivity becomes more widely available in regions not now well served. An example is the Virtual Disaster Library, which is produced by the Pan American Health Organization's Latin American and Caribbean Center on Health Sciences Information. The Virtual Disaster Library contains more than 250 publications in English and Spanish on disaster preparedness, mitigation, and response.

Use of electronic information resources by the AIDS community is particularly noteworthy. It has been especially quick to realize the benefits of Web technology and the Internet as a means to access and provide a cost-effective and rapid means for AIDS service organizations to disseminate new and authoritative information, and to communicate with difficult to reach clients. Patients living with AIDS and health workers serving the HIV/AIDS community have numerous Internet resources available to them, including literature references (for example, AIDSLINE), drug information (for example, AIDS-DRUGS), clinical trials (for example, AIDSTRIALS), and electronic gateway services and treatment guidelines (http://hivinsite.ucsf.edu). Many health institutions and community-based organizations offer their own information services on the Web, many of which are geared to particular ethnic, cultural, or the sexual preferences of their intended users (Kuromilya and Bauer 1998). The University of Washington, in collaboration with the National Library of Medicine, is connecting 16 American Indian and Alaskan native communities to the Internet. The aim is to improve access to social and health resources, emphasizing HIV/AIDS (http://www.tribalconnections.org).

In 1999, a major experiment in scientific communications was initiated by the National Institutes of Health in collaboration with authors and members of the international publishing community (Marshall 1999). PubMed Central (http://www.pubmedcentral.nih.gov) contains two separate collections of life science research and related materials. One consists of the contents of peer-reviewed journals, deposited as soon after publication as the journals are willing to make publicly available without charge. The other will contain articles that have been submitted directly by authors and that have undergone screening. Not without controversy, PubMed Central may be the cornerstone of a new era of publishing in the sciences, or evolve into a somewhat different approach to electronic publishing not yet defined. In any case, such an experiment reflects the frustration of authors with the present system, and the opportunities offered by the new technologies that will transform the landscape of scientific communications (Caelleigh 2000).

In short, the Internet and the World Wide Web offer unprecedented opportunities for the exchange of all manner of public health information around the globe. Accessible and affordable telecommunications technology is the means by which connectivity to the Internet is achieved and all forms of communication may occur.

Telecommunications technology for developing regions

The almost daily improvement in telecommunications and information technology is fuelled partly by the realization that low-cost, easy to access, and easy to use systems are available. No better example of these rapidly developing technologies exists than the Internet. Though not yet universally available, the Internet is moving in that direction. The increasing utility of mobile portable communications, linked with various terrestrial distribution systems and peripheral technologies, will help to ensure growth of Internet use in the public health sector (Scott *et al.* 1997).

Epidemiologists and a host of other professional disciplines have long appreciated the benefits of interactive real-time telecommunications links. Realizing these benefits has been a challenge in many areas of the world, however. In urban centres of countries with highly developed economies (locations that provide the economic stimulus frequently needed to motivate the development of new technologies) some of these systems can be found operating. But in remote areas of these same countries, and in developing countries in general, if such networks are available at all, they are not yet likely to be widely spread.

Telecommunications systems mediated by international satellite links will in the near future provide an attractive technical solution in many instances. Geostationary satellite systems are readily available now; low Earth orbiting systems deploying multiple satellites capable of supporting interactive communication are literally on the horizon. Other communication modalities are available and should be utilized in the meantime (Acosta and Scott 1999). A brief description of these follows, with a contextual view of their relative utility for the disaster and emergency relief community given as examples.

Terrestrial telecommunication

'Plain old telephone service'

Traditional terrestrial telecommunications services, the most characteristic of which is telephone service provided via 'telephone wires', have been costly to install, difficult to repair, and vulnerable to disasters, particularly in remote areas of developing countries. Telephone systems in difficult terrain or climates or in undeveloped areas are notoriously unreliable. If even one 'telephone pole' is incapacitated in a terrestrial network, all communications past that point are affected until that pole and its connection to the system can be repaired. Thus, although they may play a role in the early phases of disaster planning and warning, terrestrial communications cannot be relied upon for continuous use during a disaster event.

Even if the telephone system is not damaged by the disaster event, it is likely to be made unreliable or unusable because of heavy demand by the affected population. Outages (service interruptions) due to overloaded circuits can last anywhere from several hours to several weeks. Dial tones can also be affected by power outages and overloads, and this can be a further obstacle to disaster management.

The Disaster Relief Communications Foundation (http://www.reliefweb.int) recommends that health sector disaster managers should develop and maintain good working relationships with local and national telecommunication service providers and work with them to develop disaster services and emergency protocols based on infrastructure at hand. National governments should be strongly encouraged to strengthen their terrestrial telecommunications infrastructure and make it resilient to the type of disasters to which their area is vulnerable. Until that time, disaster managers should not rely solely on these systems for onset and acute phases of response.

Radio communications

Radio systems offer many advantages in the developing world. However, while operational costs are low, the costs of installing and maintaining an efficient system can be high. In most countries medical and other community lifeline sectors maintain some type of radio link, although each service tends to operate its own system independent of the others. There is a wide range of available technology and possible uses. A brief summary of some the systems is given below.

High-frequency single-sideband units

Communication in the field is most frequently conducted over long distance using high-frequency radio. This communication is point to point and permits voice and low-speed data communications between and among fixed installations at field headquarters and regional offices. Mobile high-frequency single-sideband units can also be used in a similar manner (although by definition 'mobile' units are considered to be permanent installations in vehicles), as can transportable units which are integrated communications packages designed to be deployed at single locations at short notice.

A significant advantage of high-frequency single-sideband networks is that hardware costs are minimal and use is free. A disadvantage is that, because of its wide use, it is difficult to get allocation of the dedicated high frequencies required to operate. High-frequency transmissions are also subject to propagation effects that occur both daily and seasonally.

Effective distance of high-frequency voice communications is from 2000 to 10 000 km, typically sufficient for communications between field operations and national headquarters. The use of advanced technology, namely the Pactor Level 2, Clover, and other data modes, along with the use of enhanced modems, permit effective data communications worldwide.

VHF hand-held radio communication

For short-distance communication (within cities and within geographic regions of approximately 100 km) use of VHF hand-held radios is ubiquitous among national authorities, United Nations agencies, and non-governmental organizations for communication between and among staff. Like high-frequency radios for longer distance, VHF radios are relatively inexpensive to purchase and free to operate. However, the use of VHF equipment is subject to the delivery of a license with a limited number of assigned frequencies, a process that requires a significant amount of negotiation with local telecommunications authorities. In the absence of regular telephone communications these VHF radios provide a basic and vital administrative function. Another important function is security and maintaining contact with staff travelling from one part of a city to another.

Amateur radio operators

Amateur radio operators have historically been the first group to establish and operate communications networks locally for governmental and emergency officials during and immediately following a disaster. Amateur radio facilities can generally be characterized as having a high survival capability. Although amateur radio operators are most likely to be active after disasters that damage regular lines of communication such as power outages and destruction of telephone lines, they frequently support the delivery and relay of predisaster and warning information. Amateur radio operators are generally well motivated, willing, and prepared to work under extreme conditions encountered during acute emergencies, where both solid technical knowledge and the ability to improvise are required. Although most 'ham' radio operators belong to organized groups and show a great sense of discipline and responsibility, the accuracy of their reports may vary widely. Direct close co-ordination of these groups by emergency telecommunications managers is critical to avoid the danger of transmitting inaccurate, unconfirmed, or unreliable information.

Governments license amateur or ham radio operators in most countries. Some governments severely restrict the use of amateur radio operators. The International Amateur Radio Union co-ordinates the activities of amateur services and actively supports their introduction in those countries where the value has not yet been fully recognized.

Radio paging service

Radio paging is increasingly common in most countries. Its coverage, which can range from local to international, is of unquestionable value to disaster managers. Access and reliability of these systems during periods of disaster depends on a variety of factors. These range from the availability of telephone, cellular, and/or satellite lines to interconnect and operate the system, through independent sources of electrical power, and the quality (that is, robustness) of the actual paging transmitter.

While the majority of paging systems are one-way and do not guarantee delivery to the recipient, 'one-and-a-half way' systems (message receipt acknowledgement) and two-way systems are emerging, often with e-mail links.

In countries where there are sizeable global systems for mobile communications (that is, mobile telephone) penetration, traditional paging systems have been supplanted by the short message service built-in to the global system for mobile communication protocols.

Limited resources may not make possible the routine use of pagers. If a paging service is available the possibility of leasing the service for essential personnel in disaster situations should be considered. It must be kept in mind that most radio paging services rely on terrestrial infrastructure that is vulnerable during disasters. This is the case to a lesser extent with satellite-based paging systems.

Satellite communications

Fixed satellite service

Early satellite communications service and infrastructure were developed first within urban areas with large populations. Then, largely through rapid advancements in space technology, population centres were connected. Early communication satellites developed in response to the demand for their services. They were designed to provide the most powerful coverage and greatest service to the most populated areas.

Furthermore, the phenomenon of television resulted in an increased requirement for greater satellite capacity that was, again, dedicated largely to population centres. Because the technology of these early fixed satellite services did not provide for powerful transmitters, large, complex, and expensive Earth stations had to be used to receive signals from the satellites and send signals to them. Their use, therefore, was as regional or national gateways for major telecommunications trunking services and for television distribution. They are still mostly limited to communications within and between capital cities and large urban areas.

Space segment providers and satellite designers soon recognized the increasing need to reduce the size and expense of the ground hardware and launched a new generation of services that relied on more versatile and powerful satellites. Because these new satellites transmitted more powerful signals, the new ground hardware size and power requirements were significantly reduced.

The capital cost for hardware and the recurrent cost of satellite time were also reduced. In practical terms this meant a move from stationary to transportable Earth stations (*not* portable). These changes in service made possible the advent of very small aperture terminals. The applicability for very small aperture terminal services could include linking, in a permanent or semipermanent network, national health sector disaster managers. This is still relatively costly and it still must be remembered that, as with terrestrial telecommunications links, fixed satellite service infrastructure is susceptible to damage or destruction at the onset of the disaster. Unlike its terrestrial counterparts, however, if one link goes down all others are not affected.

Global mobile personal communications by satellite

Within 3 to 5 years there will probably be several low Earth orbit satellite systems covering the whole world in addition to the existing geosynchronous satellite networks. They will consist of betwen one and as many as 325 satellites per system, and will be part of a new category of service, global system personal communication by satellite. These systems offer the health sector the promise of easy-to-use, reliable, and affordable communications that was not possible 5 years ago.

These emerging systems will have a wide range of capabilities ranging from narrowband (data only) to broadband (making possible video, voice, and data) communications. Global system personal communication by satellite technologies will probably be of such low cost as to be affordable to all sectors and thus should be of great interest to health sector managers.

Despite their promise, in the near future health professionals should be cautious when deciding what new and emerging technologies to use and invest in. A safe bet is to explore a mix of technologies, including but not limited to new global system personal communication by satellite services, until such time as their strengths and weaknesses have been proven.

Mobile satellite service

Mobile satellite services were first developed for maritime applications and now are broadly used for aeronautical and land-based purposes as well.

Mobile satellite services are less expensive than traditional fixed satellite services. They are easily transportable and are not technologically dependent on terrestrial telecommunications infrastructure. They are far less vulnerable to natural disasters and, because they can be used reliably to send data or call anywhere in the world, their use in the field has grown rapidly.

Although lower in cost than fixed systems, they are not inexpensive, and are still used almost exclusively by United Nations agencies and the larger non-governmental organizations. Although some national/domestic systems are available, the most widely used—and the only system available worldwide at this time—is the international consortium INMARSAT.

Additional systems at either end of the technology and cost spectrum are rapidly becoming available. These range from Iridium, featuring hand-held telephones that allow for voice calling from anywhere in the world, to Orbcomm, which offers low data messaging and data collection from fixed sites or hand-held units on a worldwide basis.

E-mail services

Communication by e-mail has undergone explosive growth. Initially, it was possible to communicate within closed networks, but with the opening of the Internet to the civilian world, millions of individuals and institutions can exchange information from almost any point on the planet. E-mail requires a computer with a modem, access to telephone or other telecommunications service, an account with an Internet service provider, and some training.

The Internet has become very useful in the health sector to support medical care as well as many aspects of public health including disease prevention and health promotion. It is inexpensive to use compared with traditional communication systems. The service makes it possible to contribute and use information on websites about disasters, form discussion groups and 'virtual' conferences among institutions worldwide, and send documents and graphics. It allows free exchange of information among interested parties, with a minimum of bureaucratic restrictions.

It should be understood, however, that most Internet service providers in the developing world rely on terrestrial telecommunications infrastructure and therefore Internet service is vulnerable during disasters. This is an issue not only in so far as the Internet may be relied upon to be a communications tool, but also because Internet users have become accustomed to 'storing' valuable data on the servers located at their institution or at their Internet service provider. The safety of these data may be in jeopardy during disasters or other emergencies.

Public health applications of telecommunications technology

Significant targets of opportunity exist for the application of new electronic communications tools to support the detection of public health threats, prepare for their management, and act to ameliorate their consequences. The Internet may be used beneficially to support new applications addressing public health surveillance, data integration, and the detection of bioterriorist attacks (National Research Council 2000).

The American public health system is hierarchically organized around community, state, and federal efforts. Each of these jurisdictions collects different data and shares them in different ways. Where the systems interact with one another, such as doctors and laboratories reporting the occurrence of communicable diseases (for example, tuberculosis), the Internet could vastly improve upon present paper-based methods that are fraught with errors and delays.

The Internet could also help public health officials to better integrate available data to improve data analysis and health monitoring. Vertically integrated disease-specific systems that serve traditional public health functions may result in extensive duplication, with a patient's clinical information residing in several different systems that do not interconnect. The Internet could be a powerful technical tool to realign these programmes and allow better integration of data for monitoring public health.

The use of biological weapons by terrorists could inflict life-threatening illnesses on a large scale and, unlike explosions or chemical releases, could easily escape immediate notice. Days or weeks may go by before symptoms are produced, delaying recognition of a widespread problem. Initial clinical reports, for example, would need to be aggregated at a high enough level for a geographical pattern to emerge and a problem to be detected. The American Centers for Disease Control (**CDC**) is developing an Internet-based network to facilitate information collection from testing laboratories, and to support interactive collaboration among public health officials and multimedia distance training (CDC 1998).

Already in general use are remote sensing and early warning systems. Telemedicine applications continue to make important progress in overcoming technical and organizational barriers relating to reimbursement, licensure, and demonstrable cost–benefit effects. These limitations are less critical for use in developing regions and for disaster mitigation, the contexts in which they are discussed below.

Remote sensing and early warning

Early warning or early detection systems consist of telemetry between remote sensing or detection devices, and scientists involved with the specific phenomenon, for example, seismologists. The telecommunication component of these applications provides data, usually via dedicated telecommunications systems, making scientists and public health workers aware of the occurrence of a disaster and its parameters, or its potential characteristics. Many communities and countries are putting in place disaster preparedness plans that are supported by remote sensing technologies that go beyond disaster response, to disease prevention and control following disaster.

Remote sensing technologies can help to assess and communicate the areas of damage and the extent of damage. An accurate description of the location, and estimated number of people and types of facilities affected, enable a coherent response and plan for the institution of public health measures. They can also help better distribute resources throughout an area, and help to inform health and medical facilities of the likelihood of epidemics and other adverse public health consequences of a disaster.

Among the growing number of examples is health monitoring and disease forecasting and control by health sector disaster managers. Baseline surveillance data on endemic disease distribution in an area provided by geographic information systems can be used to assess the nature of disease threats to displaced people and enable public health action, such as immunization, to be taken to protect groups at risk. These types of data may also be used to evaluate the evolution of eventual outbreaks or epidemics, and to adapt disease control strategies.

The 1990 Baguio City earthquake in the Philippines provides an example. In the wake of the earthquake, the Philippines Department of Health issued a warning of the potential spread of typhoid fever, diarrhoea, amoebiasis, and cholera that had developed in refugee encampments in the area. By employing public warning systems, health authorities appealed to the public to co-operate with measures designed to check the incidence of these deadly diseases (Scott 1998).

Epidemiologists engaged in vector control and surveillance programmes also use geographic information systems and satellite-based remote sensing technologies. An example that illustrates the complimentarity of space-based communications, global positioning, and remote sensing technologies and other developing technologies, such as geographic information systems, is a project conducted in Chiapas, Mexico, in the early to mid-1990s. A co-operative effort of the Centro de Investigation de Paludismo and several teaching institutions in the United States, this was a model programme that addressed a potential health disaster caused by malaria-carrying mosquitoes (Beck *et al.* 1997).

With support from NASA, this project developed a landscape approach to using remote sensing and geographic information systems technologies to discriminate between villages at high and low risk for malaria transmission, as defined by the abundance of *Anopheles albimanus* mosquitoes.

Satellite data for an area in southern Chiapas were digitally processed to generate a map of landscape elements. Geographic information system processes were used to determine the proportion of mapped landscape elements surrounding 40 villages where data had been collected identifying an abundance of *Anopheles albimanus* mosquitoes. Analysis of the data indicated that rainfall and growth of vegetation could be correlated with malaria vector production, and that changes in these parameters can be monitored and quantified by remote sensors. Thus, changes in mosquito populations could be predicted and malaria controlled by the use of remote sensing images to monitor changes in these key environmental parameters. With data from 1985 and 1987, the programme team successfully demonstrated that remotely sensed spectral data can be used to predict, with an accuracy of 90 per cent, which rice fields would become heavy producers of malaria-carrying mosquitoes 2 months before peak production. Beck *et al.* (1997) predicted that, if employed on a large scale, this discovery can lead to economical and precisely targeted malaria control programmes. Such a programme is now under way in sub-Saharan Africa where the MARA project is mapping malaria risk by integrating spatial malaria and environmental datasets, and producing maps of the type and severity of malaria transmission (Snow *et al.* 1996).

Many countries of the world, including many developing countries, currently have a relatively high level of health disaster preparedness. What is frequently missing is information technology infrastructure and specific technical assistance required to implement appropriate applications that will strengthen local and regional services. Access to telecommunications and information technologies that can serve to connect key regional health sector agencies in a preparedness network (Scott 1998) could permit:

- support for maintaining effective co-ordination and co-operation between and among national and regional organizations (public as well as private) in the implementation of national disaster management plans
- maintenance of current inventories of human, material, and institutional resources in the medical care area
- preparation and presentation of national and international workshops and courses on topics ranging from refugee health care and emergency sanitation to administration of health relief and hospital disaster preparedness
- preparation and dissemination of technical manuals, audiovisual training material, simulation exercises, and access to epidemiology and other health science articles and databases
- 'on-line' access to short-term services of experts in disasters as they relate to primary health care, health services management, disease surveillance and control, water supply and sanitation, mental health, and nutrition.

Telemedicine

Telemedicine can be defined as the use of telecommunications technologies that provide and support health care when distance separates the participants. At the simplest level of technology, the most commonplace telemedicine application is the 911 emergency call number in the United States. Other applications, such as telesurgery, involve exotic technologies and procedures that are still in the experimental stage. In between are applications that employ telemetry (for example, between ambulance and emergency department personnel), patient monitoring in the home, teleradiology, and consultations involving all manner of voice, image, and video configurations (Institute of Medicine 1996).

Telemedicine consultation frequently brings to mind an image of two-way high-resolution video interaction for clinical consultation. This is perhaps too limiting; a broader conception extends this definition to include applications of telecommunications and information technology for health. For it is health—not just curative relief, but preparedness and population-based public health as well—that will benefit from telemedicine. Furthermore, it is a broad spectrum of applications that ultimately will justify the capital investment and recurrent cost of the infrastructure.

In disaster situations, for example, a variety of applications can be valuable. In the acute phase, there seems to be little use thus far for telemedicine consultations between first responders and colleagues outside the disaster site, where triage is the priority. Once the most acute phase is over, consultation with specialists becomes important when there is time to deal with more complex cases and diagnostic problems. However, implementation of that advice by a local health provider or first responder may require technical support beyond what is available in the field. Conversely, there are numerous positive applications of telemedicine in disaster scenarios (Scott 1997, 1998).

In December 1988, a major earthquake struck the Republic of Armenia, causing widespread destruction and devastation, leaving much of Armenia's health-care delivery in ruins. NASA, under the auspices of the United States/USSR Joint Working Group on Space Biology and Medicine, developed a link using space-based communications technology to provide medical consultations. The project was named Telemedicine Spacebridge to Armenia. Later that summer, the same communications network was extend to provide assistance to burn victims of a gas explosion in Ufa, in the former USSR.

Remaining in operation for nearly 3 months, the Spacebridge provided an opportunity for 209 patients to be presented to clinicians at several United States medical centres via the satellite-based communications network. During the 12 weeks of the Spacebridge operations, 247 Armenian and Russian and 175 American medical professionals participated in 34 clinical sessions on a variety of clinical disciplines, including rehabilitation medicine, reconstructive surgery, burn management, sanitation and epidemiology, preventive medicine, and post-traumatic stress, among others.

The use of the Spacebridge for medical consultations resulted in 54 altered diagnoses, nearly 26 per cent of the total patient consultations. The participants judged that the format and quality of transmission of video was successful and beneficial. These results suggest that interactive consultation by remote specialists can provide valuable assistance to on-site doctors and favourably influence clinical decisions in the aftermath of major disasters (Nicogossian *et al.* 1989).

In recent years the American Department of Defense has been engaged in humanitarian initiatives in Somalia, Haiti, Macedonia, Bosnia, and Kosovo. They have deployed INMARSAT and fixed satellite terminals to support emergency telemedicine applications in each case. Interactive telemedicine consultations have been instrumental in saving the lives of soldiers and injured civilians. These *ad hoc* efforts have helped diagnose infectious disease parasites, and have helped doctors deployed in advance to treat injured military personnel locally, avoiding costly evacuations for treatment of non-life-threatening injury or illness.

In the United States permanent telemedicine systems have been established on a statewide and regional basis. The East Carolina University telemedicine programme, for example, has improved access to care for hundreds of patients in rural areas. Rural doctors can reach medical specialists using secure Web-based links transmitting voice and video, enabling them to make more accurate assessments for patient management. Patient travel time, effort, and expense are also significantly reduced. Emergency care has benefited as well. Swift consultation by emergency doctors can determine the need for trauma team mobilization or air evacuation. By reducing the need for helicopter transport, telemedicine can greatly reduce the cost of emergency care (Harr *et al.* 1997).

This existing telemedicine infrastructure was put to the test in September 1999 when hurricane Floyd struck North Carolina with torrential rain and flooding. Food, water, and medical supply lines were cut off. The emergency situation was greatly exacerbated by medical and environmental concerns stemming from extensive livestock deaths and damage to sewage treatment plants. The Telemedicine Center at East Carolina University School of Medicine set up four emergency telemedicine systems in area shelters isolated by flood waters and hurricane damage. Airlifting telemedicine equipment into these areas and using military vehicles to move between sites, they were able to set up videophones at each of these makeshift clinics. Upon arrival of the telemedicine teams, three of the four shelters were without phones in their makeshift clinical rooms. Amateur radios were used to work with the emergency operations centre and temporary telephone lines were pulled to establish the telemedicine links.

Within the first day at the clinics, the telemedicine team was able to establish functional telemedicine links and provide crash course training sessions for the already fatigued volunteer clinic staff. The telemedicine links were used immediately. The primary uses were communication between medical staff and triage of chronically ill patients. Over time, the systems were able to help relieve the load on doctors, who are only needed at the sites intermittently, and the links also lightened medical personnel traffic on the helicopters so that they could be used to transport food and supplies (D.C. Balch, personal communication, 1999).

The case for Internet connectivity in Africa

Nowhere has the challenge to effective communications been greater than in Africa. At the beginning of the 1990s, SatelLife's HealthNET system succeeded in establishing a low Earth orbiting satellite service that enabled health professionals in developing countries, including seven in Africa, to send and receive e-mail. It used a 'store-and-forward' sequence that corresponded to the timing and footprint of the satellite's periodic overflight (Royall 1998). But full Internet connectivity, permitting real-time interactive information exchange was essentially non-existent on the continent, outside of South Africa. Mike Jensen, a chronicler of Internet connectivity in Africa, documents the rapid growth of the Internet in recent years (http://www3.sn.apc.org). At the end of 1996, only 11 countries had local access, but by 1999 only Congo, Eritrea, and Somalia were still without local services. Estimates place the number of African users at 1.5 million, with two-thirds in South Africa alone, and the remaining one-third allocated among the continent's nearly 750 million people. On a relative basis, this represents one Internet user for every 1500 people, compared with a world average of one for every 38 people, and a North American and European average of one in every four people.

Internet access in Africa is still confined largely to the capital cities. More widespread access has been constrained by a number of factors: low density of telephone lines and the poor quality of an ageing copper infrastructure, expensive international connections for Internet service providers, and a tight control over the telecommunications and Internet market which frequently remains under monopolistic state control. Rural areas, where the majority of the population lives and research stations are frequently located, have poor access to telephones. Lack of a stable power supply and a lack of personnel able to maintain sophisticated computer and telecommunications equipment compound this (Jensen and Bennett 1999). These factors all combine to create an enormous barrier to the use of modern communication technology for the support of new research and public health control measures that have recently been directed at malaria, a newly re-emergent infectious disease having disastrous consequences for the peoples of sub-Saharan Africa.

The Multilateral Initiative on Malaria in Africa

The malaria crisis

Three million deaths per year (mostly children), one death every 20 s, had a punishing impact on the health and economy of Africa. This is the cost of malaria as a re-emergent infectious disease in Africa.

Traditional means of malaria prevention and treatment are failing due to drug resistance, insecticide resistance, and new and dramatically different patterns of disease transmission.

The fundamental goals of the Multilateral Initiative on Malaria

In a landmark conference held in Dakar, Senegal, in January 1997, 125 malaria experts from 35 countries, 50 from 22 African countries, came together to seek means to strengthen and sustain, through collaborative research and training, the capability of malaria-endemic countries in Africa to carry out research to develop or improve tools for malaria control. An essential goal of Multilateral Initiative on Malaria is to enhance the capacity of African scientists to do research in Africa. The Dakar participants identified access to communications and information resources as an essential means to that end. At a minimum these should enable African scientists to communicate electronically with colleagues in Africa and the North, and to access scientific information from libraries, remote databases, and on the Internet (http://niaid.nih.gov).

Communications as an enabling resource

Investigators in basic research need access to databases and repositories. Access to genetic sequence databases such as GenBank and BLAST (http://ncbi.nlm.nih.gov) are essential for the complete genome sequencing of malaria parasites that will provide the basis for rational approaches to the design and development of vaccines and new drugs. Similarly, the new Malaria Research and Reference Reagent Resource Center (MR4) will provide access to parasite, vector, and human host reagents and standardized assays using well-characterized renewable reagents (http://www.malaria.mr4.org).

Developers of new vaccines, drugs, and diagnostics need access to e-mail and discussion groups for product development work, and co-ordination of clinical trials with research colleagues within countries and abroad, and with testing sites in the field (http://www.mimcom.net and http://www.malaria.org).

Published literature is readily identifiable and accessible through computer databases, such as Medline and Biological Abstracts. Electronic versions of printed journal articles are sought, especially where library resources are poor. The newly announced PubMed Central system promises to greatly expand easy and affordable access to full-text journal articles available on the Internet in the future.

Epidemiologists engaged in vector control and surveillance programmes use geographic information systems and satellite-based remote sensing technologies. The multicentred collaborative MARA project is mapping malaria risk in Africa by integrating spatial malaria and environmental datasets, and producing maps of the type and severity of malaria transmission (Snow *et al.* 1996).

It is highly desirable that collaborating research and control units maintain contact through e-mail and other electronically mediated means of communication that are easily supported over the Internet.

New modes of communication and publication, particularly electronically linked World Wide Web sites, provide a central means for identifying and networking with fellow researchers, and accessing related scientific resources. The Medical Research Council of South Africa's National Health Knowledge Network (http://www.healthnet.org.za), and the European Commission-supported SHARED system for knowledge management are two noteworthy examples (http://www.shared.de).

The Communications Working Group

In the months following the Dakar conference, a Communications Working Group was organized under the leadership of the American National Library of Medicine, a component of the National Institutes of Health, and formally launched in Bethesda, Maryland, in January 1998. The Communications Working Group is a collaborative undertaking seeking to promote cost sharing and partnership. Sustainability of its work is of paramount concern and is predicated on the principle that the cost of communications should be borne as a necessary part of the research enterprise.

The Communications Working Group seeks to enhance communications between African scientists and with colleagues worldwide by creating telecommunications links to the Internet that permit African scientists to participate fully in the work of the international research community. This includes access to the contents of the electronic databases and networks described above. The support of informatics training and knowledge management skills is also essential to develop a library infrastructure for collection development and document delivery. Improved communications will also promote interaction between scientists and communities involved in research and control (Royall *et al.*, in press).

Building new partnerships

Like the Multilateral Initiative on Malaria itself, the Communications Working Group is diverse in membership and collective experience. It brings together African malaria research scientists and control workers; African governmental agencies and academic institutions; and representatives of the major Multilateral Initiative on Malaria research and donor agencies. These include the National Institutes of Health, the Institut Pasteur, the Wellcome Trust, the CDC, the Walter Reed Army Institute of Research, the National Naval Medical Research Institute, the World Health Organization Special Programme for Research and Training in Tropical Diseases and Regional Office with Responsibility for Africa Region, the World Bank, and the United States Agency for International Development. The inclusion of African health information professionals and telecommunications experts in the Communications Working Group helps to inform the malaria research community of the considerable number of technical considerations that must be addressed, while giving the technical community an appreciation for the scientific research needs that will benefit from improved communications. These experts also share prior experiences and lessons learned, as they comprise individuals and organizations that have contributed significantly to earlier communications infrastructure development efforts in Africa.

Methods of operation

Under American National Library of Medicine leadership, the Communications Working Group undertakes on-site assessments and technical consultations at selected malaria research laboratories in Sub-Saharan Africa. Candidate sites are prioritized on the basis of funding availability, and the presence of local leadership and on-site expertise capable of assuming responsibility for supporting initial and sustained infrastructure development efforts. Current and planned malaria research and/or control activities at the site are characterized for the purpose of identifying needed or enhanced communications capabilities. The team assesses the status of local information and communications technology and their Internet service providers, along with specific geographical or other local conditions that could impact on recommended technical solutions for achieving the desired level of Internet connectivity. Detailed technical specifications, budgets, and work plans are developed that address recommended technical solutions which may take the form of wireless links or very small aperture terminal satellite ground stations. The need for local area networks, file servers, and upgraded computer workstations may become part of the site assessment.

More than wires and dishes

The American National Library of Medicine has been fortunate to assemble an expert technical team, and new Multilateral Initiative on Malaria partners, from the international telecommunications community, medical informatics, and library community. Achieving full Internet connectivity at geographically remote malaria research sites is a difficult undertaking in its own right. It also calls for the need to train users in equipment operation and the skills needed to utilize newly accessible electronic information resources, including local and regional library services.

Preliminary plans are underway to put in place and support journal article lending arrangements that are centred in southern, central/eastern, and western Africa, with back-up access to major DOCLINE libraries in the United States and Europe. DOCLINE is an interlibrary loan request routing and order referral system long maintained in the United States by the National Library of Medicine, and recently extended internationally to promote more efficient sharing of medical information worldwide. DOCLINE libraries are committed to serving the medical library resource needs in their country or region, with back-up services provided by other DOCLINE libraries and, ultimately, the National Library of Medicine.

Accomplishments

Malaria Research and Training Center, Bamako, Mali. Direct microwave connection (56 kbps) to the local Internet service provider installed in 1998. Collections of the University of Mali library are undergoing enhancement to support its function as a DOCLINE library for the West Africa region. Partnering institutions include the National Institutes of Health and its National Institute of Allergy and Infectious Diseases, the American National Library of Medicine, the University of Mali, the Mali Ministry of Health, USAID, and the World Bank.

CDC/Kenya Medical Research Institute, Kisian, Kenya. Installed very small aperture terminal groundstation in 1999 linking the research site to a London hub and Internet backbone (64 kbps downlink and 32 kbps uplink) via the Intelsat801 satellite. Registered the Internet domain name (mimcom.net) for Kenya and other Multilateral Initiative on Malaria locations for e-mail addresses. Developed a World Wide Web site. Partner institutions: the National Institutes of Health, the American National Library of Medicine, and the CDC.

Wellcome Trust/Kenya Medical Research Institute, Kilifi, Kenya. Very small aperture terminal installation follows the Kisian arrangement, with shared services provided by the same vendor (Redwing Satellite Solutions). Partner institutions: the National Institutes of Health, the American National Library of Medicine, the Wellcome Trust, and Oxford University.

Walter Reed Army Institute of Research, Nairobi, Kenya. Very small aperture terminal installation in 2000 supports several collaborating and independent research efforts in the region. Partner institutions: the American National Library of Medicine, the Walter Reed Army Institute of Research, the CDC, the Kenya Medical Research Institute, the United States Library of Congress, and the Wellcome Trust.

Navrongo Health Research Center and Noguchi Memorial Institute, Accra, Ghana. Very small aperture terminal installations at both locations completed at the end of 1999. Infrastructure follows the Kenya arrangement, with shared very small aperture terminal services supporting malaria vaccine trials. With these additional locations in place, incoming bandwidth increased to 128 kbps for all sites on the 'Multilateral Initiative on Malaria.Network'. Partner institutions: the American National Institute of Allergy and Infectious Diseases, the American National Library of Medicine, the American Naval Medical Research Institute (**NAMRI**), and USAID.

National Institute for Medical Research, Dar-es-Salaam, Ifakara, and Amani, Tanzania. Site assessment plans completed in early 2000. Technical solution calls for a wireless connection (64 kbps) from the Dar headquarters to the local Internet service provider, with very small aperture terminal groundstations at the two remote sites. Model expands on the Kenya arrangement, with shared resources and greater bandwidth allocation consistent with local needs. Installation scheduled in 2000. Partner institutions: the National Institutes of Health and the American National Library of Medicine.

University of Yaounde, Cameroon. Site assessment plans competed for a wireless connection (64 kbps) from the remote malaria research station to the university's campus-wide fibre-optic network. Partner institutions: the National Institutes of Health and the American National Library of Medicine.

University of Zimbabwe, Harare, Zimbabwe. Facilitated wireless connection (64 kbps) to a very small aperture terminal link at the newly established WHO/AFRO headquarters. Literature holdings of medical library enhanced to support functions of a DOCLINE library for the East Africa region. Partner institutions: the National Institutes of Health, the American National Library of Medicine, and the British Medical Association.

South Africa Medical Research Council, Cape Town, South Africa. Existing DOCLINE services expanded to southern Africa region. Partner institutions: the American National Library of Medicine and medical libraries of South Africa.

Institut Pasteur, Dakar, Senegal. A dedicated leased line (64 kbps) to the Universite Cheikh Anta Diop. Partner institution: the Pasteur Institute, Paris.

Conclusion

As we enter the new millennium, we can be assured that the pace of change in information and communications technology will continue unabated. Changes that formerly took 3 to 5 years are now accomplished in less than half that time. Yet, the evidence of a widening gap between the information 'haves' and 'have-nots' is clear. Some of this is generational and will be overcome with the natural progression of time and training. A far greater threat lies in income and educational disparities, particularly along the North–South divide.

The communications connectivity work being carried out in the context of the Multilateral Initiative on Malaria is addressing this gap, albeit in a focused mode that limits these efforts to malaria research sites located in a limited number of countries in sub-Saharan Africa. But it is this focus that makes the task possible to finish, and hopefully sustainable. It is also the concept of partnership and a shared vision that shapes the ultimate formula for success. In Kenya, for example, the National Institutes of Health, the National Library of Medicine, the CDC, and the Wellcome Trust have come together in partnership. Each of these organizations separately, and together, has determined that access to the Internet and the World Wide Web is essential to their mission of malaria control and eradication. Moreover, the pooling of financial resources has made it possible to purchase broadband satellite capacity that would not be affordable by any one institution acting alone. The two Kenya Medical Research Institute sites, in Kisian and Kilifi, are sharing bandwidth and responsibility for the underlying communications infrastructure where, formerly, there was very little professional interaction at all. Communication has brought these scientists and health professionals together and very much in keeping with the spirit of that first Multilateral Initiative on Malaria meeting in Dakar.

Partnership and collaboration can make a difference in closing the information access gap, not just in the remote outreaches of Africa but in other locations separated by great distances and the uneven distribution of wealth. Research agencies, donor organizations, and non-government organizations acting in concert can achieve results far greater than each acting independently. This is a lesson that, no doubt, can benefit many other endeavours of importance to the public health community.

Lastly, this chapter has dealt with the specific communication tools that are supporting new directions and applications in the field of public health. The fascination of how it all happens will dim as people preoccupy themselves more with the application itself, and require more from the technology to serve that application. Health care, disaster relief, and the nature of research itself will gradually transform and be transformed by these tools in unimaginable ways. That is the way of all revolutions.

Box 1 Useful Internet websites

http://www.isoc.org
http://www.medlineplus.gov
http://www.clinicaltrials.gov
http://www.hon.ch
http://www.nlm.nih.gov
http://www.biosis.org
http://www.sis.nlm.nih.gov
http://www.hivinsite.ucsf.edu
http://tribalconnections.org
http://www.pubmedcentral.nih.gov
http://www.reliefweb.int
http://www3.sn.apc.org
http://www.niaid.nih.gov
http://www.malaria.mr4.org
http://www.mimcom.net
http://www.malaria.org
http://healthnet.org.za
http://www.shared.de

References

Acosta, E. and Scott, J. (1999). Communications and transport. In *Health management of natural disasters*, Publication No. 407. Pan American Health Organization, Washington, DC.

Beck, L.R., Rodriguez, M.H., Dister, S.W., *et al.* (1997). Assessment of a remote sensing-based model for predicting malaria transmission risk in villages of Chiapas, Mexico. *American Journal of Tropical Medicine and Hygiene*, **56**, 99–106.

Berners-Lee, T., Cailliau, R., and Luotonen, A. (1994). The World Wide Web. *Communications of the ACM*, **37**, 76.

Caelleigh, A.S. (2000). PubMed Central and the new publishing landscape: shifts and tradeoffs. *Academic Medicine*, **75**, 4–10.

CDC (Centers for Disease Control and Prevention) (1998). *Strengthening community health protection through technology and training: The Health Alert Network.* CDC, Atlanta, Georgia.

Harr, D.S., Balch, D.C., and McConnell, M.E. (1997). Next generation telemedicine; the future is now. *North Carolina Medical Journal*, **58**, 398–401.

Institute of Medicine (1999). *Telemedicine: a guide to assessing telecommunications in health care.* National Academy Press, Washington, DC.

Jensen, M. and Bennett, M. (1999). Connectivity in Africa, the challenges and lessons learned. In *MIM African Malaria Conference* (ed. C. Davies and B. Sharp). B-46. Editions Durban, South Africa.

Kuromilya, K. and Bauer, R. (1998). Building a community-based infrastructure for AIDS dissemination on the net: two years later. *International Conference on AIDS*, **12**, 747.

Marshall, E. (1999). National Institutes of Health's online publishing venture ready for launch. *Science*, **285**, 1466.

National Research Council (1999). *Funding a revolution: government support for computing research.* National Academy Press, Washington, DC.

National Research Council (2000). *Networking health: prescriptions for the Internet.* National Academy Press, Washington, DC.

Nicogossian, A., Rayman, R., Sarkissian, A., and Nikogossian, H. (1989). *United States/USSR Telemedicine Spacebridge to Armenia and Ufa.* National Aeronautics and Space Administration, Washington, DC.

Royall, J. (1998). SatelLife—linking information and people: the last ten centimetres. *Development in Practice*, **8**, 85–90.

Royall, J., Siegel, E.R., and Bennett, M. Wires, webs, and MIMcom.Net. *African Journal of Medicine and Medical Sciences*, in press.

Scott, J. (1997). Telemedicine in disaster applications. *Stop Disasters*, **32**, 19–21.

Scott, J. (1998). Applications of telecommunications and information technology for humanitarian health initiatives. In *Proceedings of Pacific Medical Technology Symposium-PACMEDTek.* (ed. R. Nelson, A. Gelish, and S. Mun). IEEE Computer Society, Los Alamitos, CA.

Scott, J., *et al.* (1997). *Report on earth observation, hazard analysis and communications technology for early warning.* United Nations International Decade for Natural Disaster Reduction Early Warning Programme, IDNDR Secretariat, Geneva.

Silberg, W.M., Lundberg, G.D., and Musacchio, R.A. (1997). Assessing, controlling, and assuring the quality of medical information on the Internet 2. *Journal of the American Medical Association*, **277**, 1244–5.

Snow, R.W., Marsh, K., and le Sueur, D. (1996). The need for maps of transmission intensity to guide malaria control in Africa. *Parasitology Today*, **12**, 455–7.

Wood, F.W., Cid, V.H., and Siegel, E.R. (1998) Evaluating Internet end-to-end performance: overview of test methodology and results. *Journal of the American Medical Informatics Association*, **5**, 528–45.

5.4 Applications of information systems to public health

Jeff Luck

Introduction

A **health information system** in the broadest sense is comprised of data as well as procedures to collect, store, analyse, transfer, and retrieve that data. The data may be stored in paper and/or electronic form, and the collection, analysis, transfer, and retrieval may be performed by human beings or electronic information technology, but usually by some combination of both. Information technology consists of computers, the networks and telecommunications systems that connect them, and the software that operates the computers and networks. Dramatic advances in all aspects of information technology are driving profound changes in organizations and societies.

The ultimate purpose of a public health information system is to convert raw data into information that can be used for decision-making. One major challenge in developing information systems for public health is the great diversity of data that must be captured (demographical, clinical, geographical, administrative, financial) and the diversity of sources from which it originates (patients, health providers, laboratories, hospitals, restaurants, and so on). A second challenge is the number and diversity of users of public health information, including policy-makers, public health professionals, managers, community-based organizations, and the population at large. The emerging discipline of **public health informatics** addresses these challenges by the 'systematic application of information and computer science and technology to public health practice, research, and learning' (O'Carroll *et al.* 2000; Yasnoff *et al.* 2000) (http://www.nlm.nih.gov/pubs/cbim/phi2001.html).

Information systems are at the core of all public health activities. This chapter reviews how information systems, especially those that employ electronic information technology, are applied in public health, and how those applications are changing as information technology evolves. In addition, it describes some of the important types of **information resources**, such as population survey data files, that are produced by public health information systems.

Advances in information technology and information systems

Computer hardware

Computer hardware is becoming continuously more powerful. Moore's law is an observation that the number of transistors that can be packed onto a semiconductor chip doubles every 18 months, with corresponding increases in computer power. Since manufacturing costs do not rise nearly as fast, the price per unit of computing power continues to plummet. The capacity of disk storage devices has risen by more than 50 per cent per year for several years, yielding even more dramatic reductions in the price per unit of electronic data storage. These trends have resulted in affordable shared server computers, powerful desktop computers costing less than US$500, portable computers of equivalent power but higher cost, and a growing range of small handheld computers.

Networks and telecommunications

Computers are increasingly being connected to each other via networks: local area networks within buildings, wide-area networks within organizations with multiple locations, and the Internet worldwide. Wide-area networks and the Internet use the publicly available telecommunications infrastructure. The benefits of this increasing interconnection are summarized by Metcalfe's law, which states that the value of a computer network grows exponentially by the number of computers connected to it, since every new computer can access, and be accessed by, every other computer on the network.

The transmission capacity of a computer network, measured in amount of data transferred per unit of time, is referred to as the network's bandwidth. Owing to rapid construction and the development of more powerful computerized network switching devices and technologies such as fibre optics, the available bandwidth of networks is growing at a dramatic rate, with concomitant drops in price. The result is that people connected to the robust computer networks found in universities and large corporations take for granted practically instant access to information from computers around the world. Technologies such as cable modems and digital subscriber line telephone service are now making this high bandwidth and low cost available to homes.

Within a decade, most of the population of many industrialized countries will have routine low-cost access to bandwidth sufficient for real-time video and audio communication. Portable and handheld computers will be able to access networks via wireless connections, albeit at lower bandwidth. Bandwidth availability in developing countries will vary widely, both across countries and between urban and rural areas. However, the dropping price of wired, fixed wireless, and satellite telecommunications will provide more and more developing country locations with bandwidth sufficient to support important information systems applications.

Software

Computers require elaborate specialized instructions to store, process, display, and share data. These instructions or programs are known as software. Since software is only a type of information, the marginal cost of duplicating it is nearly zero. However, the writing and testing of software is a very labour-intensive process conducted by skilled programmers. Therefore advances in individual software programs are less dramatic than the increases in hardware and network capabilities, but a new program can be distributed to millions of users in weeks at minimal cost. For example, easy-to-use browser software distributed free enabled the explosion of network and Internet use in the last half of the 1990s.

Software now exists for thousands of applications, including database creation and maintenance, quantitative analyses (e.g. scientific, statistical, epidemiological, financial), communications, management, and entertainment. New software is being written and disseminated continuously worldwide to take advantage of advances in computer hardware and telecommunications.

Public health activities supported by information systems

In order to describe applications of information systems to public health, it is necessary to choose a framework for discussing each of the diverse activities of public health. Such frameworks have been developed from several different perspectives.

The Institute of Medicine (1988) identified three major categories of activities carried out by local health departments: assessment, policy development, and assurance. More specifically, this means that a local health department monitors and assesses health problems and resources of populations within its geographical jurisdiction, promotes healthy behaviours, ensures and promotes a healthy environment, and assures preventive and curative health services. To accomplish these tasks effectively, the health department must be able to manage its own and its contractors' activities efficiently, evaluate its numerous public health programmes, and involve the community at all stages.

Local health departments accomplish these general goals by carrying out a number of different programmes, each requiring its own organizational unit and specialized expertise. Many of these programmes are mandated by national and/or state law. For example, Title 17 of the California Code of Regulations mandates that county or city health departments offer at least the following services: vital statistics registration, health education, communicable disease control, maternal and child health promotion, environmental health and sanitation, a public health laboratory, nutrition, chronic disease prevention and mitigation, social factors (including community planning), occupational health, family planning, and public health nursing. Health departments often conduct programmes that reduce other risks to the public's health, including tobacco control, substance abuse prevention and treatment, injury and violence prevention, and oral health promotion. Finally, health departments often also manage facilities that provide personal health services, although these may not fall under the definition of public health activities in the strictest sense.

State and national government health agencies establish broad health policies, set mandates for local health departments, aggregate and disseminate health data collected from local jurisdictions, fund some public health programmes, and carry out national population surveys. In some countries, state and national health departments operate some programmes directly.

Internationally, the World Health Organization (**WHO**) identifies global health priorities, carries out programmes within countries and across borders (such as malaria prevention or health systems strengthening), and collects and disseminates a wide range of country-specific health information.

Applying information systems in public health activities

Public health is a data-intensive field. Paper-based information systems can be found in public health programmes in any country. In industrialized countries, information technology has been applied in public health programmes for decades. Initially, centralized computers were used to aggregate and analyse data collected in the field. Desktop computers made it possible for increasingly sophisticated analyses to be performed on a distributed basis, and telecommunications links allowed the electronic transmission of data. Management and some clinical functions in laboratories, clinics, and hospitals were also computerized. Nevertheless, the actual collection of data in the field and in most facilities is still accomplished with paper records. Recently, many public health organizations and some health departments have begun using the Internet for information dissemination.

Other industries, including banking, transportation, and health insurers, followed a similar path, beginning with centralized automation and moving incrementally to distributed processing and networks. However, the mutually reinforcing advances in all aspects of information technology are creating huge new opportunities to collect, analyse, and share information more rapidly, cheaply, and effectively. Therefore private-sector firms have now moved on to the phase of completely re-engineering their processes to take advantage of these information technology capabilities (Hammer 1990).

While these same benefits could accrue to public health agencies in industrialized countries, they have not yet taken advantage of information technology to transform fundamentally how they accomplish their missions. The reasons include their organizational inertia as government agencies, the above-mentioned challenges of diverse data and users, and limited funds for investment in information systems upgrading. Building upon successful applications in other industries, public health agencies could use information technology to improve operations in several ways. Firstly, core public health activities, ranging from data collection in the field to transmission, analysis, and dissemination, can be fully computerized. Personal health services providers are moving in this direction, with a fully electronic medical record as the ultimate goal (Dick *et al.* 1997). Such automation ensures that data are shared more quickly, analysed more easily, and are also available to multiple users simultaneously. Secondly, information systems can be implemented to manage more efficiently administrative activities such as procurement, contracting, human resources, and financial management. These systems can be modelled closely on successful similar systems in other industries. Thirdly, data from information systems in different public health programmes can be aggregated and linked together in centralized databases to facilitate population-level analyses, policy development, and dissemination to a wide range of users.

In other industries, re-engineering processes to take advantage of information technology capabilities has resulted in dramatic efficiency and performance improvements, better customer service, and more effective analyses of company-wide data to formulate management strategy. In public health, the fundamental goals will not be changed by information technology, nor will the basic activities such as disease surveillance, treatment, education, facility inspection, and epidemiological analysis. However, innovative agencies will probably transform how those activities are performed. For example, geographical analyses of disease patterns have been essential to public health since John Snow's work (http|://www.ph.ucla.edu/epi/snow.html). Geographical information systems (**GIS**) software that make it possible to combine and display geographically coded data very easily are just beginning to be widely available to public health professionals.

Outline of this chapter

The outline for this chapter's discussion of information systems applications to public health is a synthesis of the frameworks for public health activities presented above. It describes how information systems support a wide range of public health activities, emphasizing current, emerging, and potential uses of information technology. In some cases, the actual data (such as surveys) are described in some detail. Most examples are from industrialized countries due to the greater penetration of information technology there, but several developing country applications are noted. The topic areas are as follows.

- Data collection: vital statistics, population surveys, disease surveillance, facility-based data collection, data from providers and payers.
- Clinical and management information systems: hospitals and clinics, public health programmes, telemedicine, quality-of-care measurement.
- Data analysis and policy development: computerized statistical and epidemiological analyses, health indicators, GIS, linked databases, data warehousing
- Data access and dissemination: public health and medical literature, downloadable datasets, on-line query systems, information sharing among public health professionals, providing health data to community members
- Health training and education: distance learning, educational campaigns, curriculum development, specialized health information providers
- Challenges to applying information systems in public health: information technology and communications infrastructure, funding availability, privacy and confidentiality protections, information technology development challenges.

Data collection

All public health activities rely on accurate population health data, including data on events such as mortality, population health status and behaviour, communicable disease case and treatment reports, and utilization of health-care services. Each of these major types of data is usually collected by a specialized public health programme, using its own customized information systems. The types of data, the programmes that collect them, and the information systems used, are described in this section.

Vital statistics

Natality and mortality are the main categories of vital statistics information. Each birth and death event is recorded, so that vital statistics registries are an ongoing census of these events in the population. Additional data items about each event, such as race/ethnicity of a newborn's parents or causes of deaths, are also recorded in a standardized fashion. For example, the California death record has over 100 data items.

The collection of vital statistics data is highly computerized in industrialized countries. For example, the Automated Vital Statistics System (**AVSS**) is used to input birth and death data in all 58 counties in California. These records are aggregated at the state level. The National Center for Health Statistics (**NCHS**) compiles national-level natality and mortality data files in its National Vital Statistics System (**NVSS**). Summary and detail files from NVSS allow analyses of deaths by factors such as location, age group, race, gender, year, and cause of death (http://www.cdc.gov/nchs/about/major/dvs/mortdata.htm).

The American Census Bureau, as well as many state and county governments, use vital statistics data to make intercensal population projections because the Census Bureau only conducts a complete census every 10 years. Vital statistics can also be used for planning public health services. For example, the number, location, and characteristics of births can help project the need for children's health services. Mortality data are essential for planning disease prevention programmes.

Vital statistics activities lend themselves to computerization. In California, birth records are input to AVSS directly where births occur. In developing countries, accurate and complete recording of vital events, even with paper records, is the highest priority. However, regional registries can be computerized at modest cost, allowing data to be aggregated easily on a national basis; analyses and report generation can then be computerized as well.

Population surveys

Although vital statistics are collected as a census, many other important types of information necessary for public and health services research analyses are collected from surveys of representative samples of the population of a nation or region. This includes information on the determinants of health, the health status and needs of communities, health services access and insurance coverage, and health behaviours.

Given the diverse types of information to be gathered, industrialized countries conduct a broad spectrum of health surveys, each designed to collect specific data from a defined population. Some of the major national health surveys in the United States are briefly described below as examples of the data collection methods employed and the resulting information resources available for public health analyses.

1. The National Health Interview Survey (**NHIS**) is conducted by the NCHS. This in-person survey, conducted annually, targets a nationally representative cluster sample of 40 000 households. In addition to underlying demographic data on each household, the NHIS collects data on health status and health services utilization, including acute and chronic conditions, activity limitations due to health problems, insurance coverage, and utilization of outpatient and inpatient health services. Specialized modules, covering topics such as cancer prevention and control, are added periodically (http://www.cdc.gov/nchs/nhis.htm).
2. The National Health and Nutrition Examination Survey (**NHANES**), also conducted by the NCHS, is a much more intensive survey of 5000 randomly sampled people annually.

Respondents complete interviews and in-depth physical examinations and testing. The data collected include diet, nutrition, health behaviours, and risk factors. This combination of behavioural and biomedical data from a nationally representative population allows prevalence estimates of diseases and risk factors, as well as analyses of the links between health behaviours and health status (http://www.cdc.gov/nchs/nhanes.htm).

3. The National Health Care Survey (**NHCS**) is composed of several surveys drawing data on patient characteristics and services utilization at a wide range of health provider organizations: hospitals, ambulatory surgery facilities, ambulatory care clinics, nursing homes, and hospices. These surveys are also conducted by the NCHS and draw their data from medical records at nationally representative samples of facilities; tens of thousands of records are reviewed in each survey. Some of the surveys are annual, others periodic (http://www.cdc.gov/nchs/nhcs.htm).

4. The Medical Expenditure Panel Survey (**MEPS**) is conducted by the Agency for Healthcare Research and Quality (**AHRQ**). This in-person survey follows panels of households over a 2.5-year period; households are selected as a subsample of households from the NHIS. Households provide detailed data on their insurance coverage and utilization of and payment for health services, as well as personal health information, allowing these data to be linked longitudinally. The household survey is supplemented by data collection at health providers and employers to provide a more complete picture of health insurance and health expenditures (http://www.meps.ahrq.gov/).

5. The Behavioral Risk Factor Surveillance System (**BRFSS**) is a telephone survey conducted by the Centers for Disease Control (**CDC**). The BRFSS is a concatenation of surveys conducted in each state, comprising over 150 000 interviews annually. Data are collected on a variety of health risk and behaviours, including tobacco and alcohol use, exercise and diet, chronic disease prevention and screening, and injury prevention. Individual states can add questions tailored to their public health needs (http://www.cdc.gov/nccdphp/brfss/index.htm).

6. Private foundations often conduct surveys that provide data useful for public health analyses. For example, the National Survey of America's Families (**NSAF**). Designed to assess the effect of policy changes such as welfare reform, the NSAF oversampled low-income households and collected a range of data on family demographics and welfare, including health. Primarily a telephone survey, the NSAF collects data from a nationally representative sample of over 44 000 households (http://newfederalism.urban.org/nsaf/).

Although comprehensive health surveys are also very useful in developing countries, resource constraints severely limit their scope and frequency. An ongoing series of Demographic and Health Surveys (**DHS**) has been funded primarily by the United States Agency for International Development (**USAID**). Dozens of surveys have been conducted in countries throughout the world. Each survey covers a nationally representative sample of about 5000 households, with data collected in person. Comparable instruments are used to gather data on health and nutrition, family planning, maternal and child health, child survival, HIV/AIDS, and reproductive health (http://www.measuredhs.com/).

For local health assessment and planning, rapid surveys with sample sizes of a few hundred can be conducted rapidly and inexpensively (Husein *et al.* 1993; Kipp *et al.* 1994; Satia *et al.* 1994). These advantages make rapid surveys especially attractive in developing countries, since a small trained staff and a simple microcomputer are essentially the only infrastructure needed. Rapid survey methods are described in more detail in Chapter 6.15.

Information systems are used to support all phases of survey design and execution in industrialized countries. In-person survey interviewers use portable computers, and computer-assisted self-interview software may be used to collect data on particularly sensitive topics. Telephone survey interviewers use automated questionnaires on computer-assisted telephone interview software (Aday 1996). These computerized data collection systems feed data directly into a computerized database of results. Other specialized software is used for other aspects of survey design, analysis, and management, including sample design, random digit dialling, call centre management, data cleaning and imputation, and calculation of weights (e.g. for non-response and adjustment to population proportions). Information systems for disseminating survey results via query systems and downloadable public use datasets are described later in this chapter. Copies of survey instruments and documentation can also be made available on the Internet, enabling users to analyse and interpret survey results correctly.

Telephone surveys, portable computers for field interviewers, and Internet dissemination of data may not be practical in developing countries. However, inexpensive computers can still significantly enhance efficiency when used to design the survey and manage data collection. Data from paper survey instruments can be key-punched at modest cost, allowing computerized data cleaning, analysis, and report preparation.

In future years, some surveys in industrialized countries will become even more computerized, collecting data over the Internet. Already, interactive data collection forms are straightforward to implement. However, Internet data collection will probably not supplant in-person or telephone methods, as the response rate to Internet surveys is expected to mirror the relatively low response rates of mail surveys.

Disease surveillance

Surveillance of communicable diseases is a fundamental public health activity (Drotman and Strassburg 2001). Surveillance techniques and information systems are discussed only briefly here, since they are the subject of Chapter 6.16.

In industrialized countries, laws require that several dozen communicable diseases be reported to local health departments by doctors, clinics, hospitals, and laboratories. These data are in turn reported to state/provincial health departments, and thence to national government health agencies. In developing countries with less robust health infrastructures, sentinel sites may be the focus of communicable disease reporting. These are facilities that provide services to a large enough population to capture significant numbers of patients with the target diseases and have the resources for ongoing data collection (Woodall 1988). Sampling from a network of carefully chosen locations can provide reporting representative of the population, as is done in China (Chunning 1992).

Even in industrialized countries, much of the communicable disease reporting is still accomplished by paper forms submitted to the local health department. There the data from the form are input into computerized databases, and reporting to state and national levels is often electronic. However, the initial paper form step is unreliable and can be too slow for rapid response to disease reports. For example, slow reporting hinders the identification of outbreaks of emerging infectious diseases, such as West Nile virus, thereby making responses less prompt and effective.

Large facilities with more comprehensive computerized information systems, such as laboratories and hospitals, are beginning to use electronic reporting in some jurisdictions. As more and more doctors' offices are connected to the Internet, and capabilities for secure Internet transmission of confidential information expand, more communicable disease reporting will move to that medium.

The CDC is developing a comprehensive electronic communicable disease reporting system, the National Electronic Disease Surveillance System (**NEDSS**), to address the shortcomings of the current communicable disease reporting systems in the United States (http://www.cdc.gov/od/hissb/docs.htmnedss). Its components will include the following:

- data standards for uniform generation, transmission, and aggregation of communicable disease reports
- record matching software to eliminate duplicate reports of the same case of a communicable disease
- a common user interface for all computerized CDC reporting systems
- standardized Internet-based secure transmission links from health departments to the CDC
- standardized data definitions to facilitate data sharing and analysis.

Facility-based data collection

Large facilities, particularly those operated or funded by government health agencies, can be required to report data on patients seen there. These data can be very useful in describing patterns of disease and treatment, as well as the underlying demographic data on patients. However, a major shortcoming of such data is that patients using the reporting facilities may not be representative of the population overall. This is a particular problem in developing countries, where access to health care is very limited and many people with diseases do not present to facilities for treatment. Nevertheless, in many countries these data are the best available (Cibulskis and Izard 1996).

The most appropriate use of facility-based data collection is the standardized reporting of procedures that are almost always performed at large facilities, or diseases almost always diagnosed or treated there. For example, in the United States, hospitals in 35 states are required to report data on inpatient discharges (Love 2000). Required data on each discharge includes length of stay, diagnosis, mortality, patient demographics, and payer. A state government department aggregates the data and removes personally identifiable data so that complete files can be made public. These data are then used for a range of management, health services research, and policy analyses.

However, inpatient discharge reporting does not capture all data on procedures because ambulatory surgeries are becoming more common, and are performed in free-standing centres as well as in hospitals. Therefore some states have now begun to require that ambulatory surgeries be reported as well, whether performed at hospital or at a centre certified by Medicare (Love 2000).

Cancer registries are another facility-based system that provides data of great value for cancer epidemiology, health services research, and environmental health analyses. For example, California requires that all diagnosed neoplasms be reported, along with treatment data and underlying patient demographics (http://www.ccrcal.org/). All hospital and facilities that treat cancer are required to file reports, as are doctors who treat cancer themselves. Reported data are aggregated at the state level, personally identifiable data are removed, and complete files made available for public use.

Facility-based data collection can be very information-technology intensive. Reported data is often compiled from clinical or management information systems at facilities, data is reported via tapes or electronic transmission of data files, central databases are large and complex, and data files are made publicly available in CD-ROM form or over the Internet.

Data collection from payers and providers

Data on disease patterns and health services utilization can be collected from payers, such as health insurers, or directly from providers when they are reimbursed by government health agencies. Payers who reimburse doctors and hospitals on a fee-for-service basis receive claims data for each outpatient encounter or inpatient stay. These data are limited in clinical and demographic detail because they are collected for billing purposes, but they can cover very large segments of the population. Data collection from providers can also be effective when a government payer requires encounter or discharge data to be submitted as a condition of receiving capitation or global budget allocations. However, since a claim for each encounter need not be submitted under a capitated payment system, ensuring that providers submit complete and timely data is a major challenge, and so the resulting datasets may not be fully complete. No matter how encounter data are collected, privacy concerns must be addressed by removing personally identifiable fields from data files.

Medicare is a near-universal health insurance programme for all American residents who are 65 years of age and older and/or disabled. It reimburses fee-for-service for over 80 per cent of its beneficiaries, and so the resulting claims data are quite comprehensive. The remaining beneficiaries are in enrolled health maintenance organizations (**HMOs**) which receive capitated payments; encounter data are not available for these people. The Health Care Financing Administration (**HCFA**) provides a 5 per cent sample of fee-for-service claims to approved users. These data are used for health services research and policy analyses (http://www.hcfa.gov/stats/pufiles.htmpufcat).

Medicaid is the American health insurance programme covering people in poverty. It is operated and financed jointly by state governments and the HCFA. Many states are attempting to reduce the programme's cost by moving Medicaid beneficiaries to HMOs.

Therefore the HCFA is now working with states, HMOs, and providers to obtain encounter data (http://www.hcfa.gov/medicaid/m2082.htm).

In the long term, electronic medical records will facilitate the capture and sharing of data by health providers. Ideally, data captured at the bedside or in a clinic can be electronically transmitted to central payer or government data repositories, and there aggregated across the entire population. However, for reasons discussed below, this vision is many years from practical realization.

Clinical and management information systems

Health providers—clinics, general practitioners, and hospitals—have historically used paper-based medical records to record clinical information. Hospitals in industrialized countries have computerized many administrative functions, as well as some clinical functions. Clinics have also automated some activities, such as appointment scheduling. These information systems are discussed in this chapter because they can contribute to public health in several ways: enhancing the efficiency and effectiveness of health facilities operated by government agencies, serving as rich sources of data on disease patterns and health services utilization, and providing data for health services quality measurement. This section also describes information systems which support the activities of public health programmes, and telemedicine systems to help deliver appropriate health-care services to isolated populations.

Hospitals and clinics

Hospitals have the most comprehensive information systems of any health services provider organizations, because they command resources and can clearly benefit from automation (Austin and Boxerman 1998). Most hospitals in the United States find it cost-effective to purchase complete information systems from commercial vendors, such as Siemens Medical Solutions Inc. or McKesson-HBOC, rather than develop them in house. These comprehensive hospital information systems automate admission, billing, purchasing, and other tasks, as well as some aspects of hospital-based clinical services, such as radiology, laboratory, and pharmacy.

Hospitals in wealthier developing countries are increasingly purchasing information systems as well. Nevertheless, purchasing and installing any such large information system is expensive and risky. The Pan-American Health Organization (**PAHO**) has recently published a very useful book that lays out in detail how to navigate through the process of defining requirements, selecting vendors, and implementing the information system (PAHO 1999).

Most clinics also purchase the information systems that automate functions like scheduling and claims submission. Medical records systems suitable for outpatient practice are being developed, but are only at the early stages of implementation (http://www.health-infosys-dir.com/yp_hc.htm).

The fully electronic medical record has been an elusive goal for over 20 years (Dick *et al.* 1997). Despite technological advances, the volume and diversity of health data have frustrated attempts to develop such systems. Incremental progress has been made, such as automating some hospital functions, providing computerized doctor order entry, and digitizing dictated reports such as hospital discharge summaries. However, doctors still resist taking the time to type, and variations in medical vocabulary make automated recognition of clinical concepts the most difficult technical challenge. However, installation of computers and networks throughout hospitals has made it possible for some institutions, such as the United States Veterans Administration, to assemble very comprehensive computerized medical records.

Use of the Internet to streamline transactions between provider organizations is increasing, and could significantly improve the efficiency and timeliness of health provider operations. Electronic data interchange is currently used to transmit routine transaction data such as claims data for payment, eligibility files from plans to providers, and electronic payments (Austin and Boxerman 1998). Broader business-to-business applications are the fastest growing application of the Internet in other industries, and health-care providers will probably follow the trend. The largest entity currently providing electronic data interchange and business-to-business services to health-care firms in the United States is Healtheon-WebMD (http://www.webmd.com/).

Public health programmes

As described above, local health departments in industrialized countries establish programmes to carry out their legally mandated functions, such as communicable disease control, environmental health, substance abuse prevention/treatment, and the public health laboratory. Each of these programmes may have its own information system, built upon a database containing information about people, facilities, and service providers with whom the programme interacts. These information systems are essential to the effective functioning of the programmes, and also provide essential data on the health of the underlying population, as the following examples show.

1. Information systems to support communicable disease investigation and treatment were discussed above under the topic of surveillance. These information systems are person-oriented, i.e. their major data elements are demographics of infected people and contacts, disease characteristics, provider IDs, and treatment status. Other person-oriented information systems support nutrition and maternal and child health promotion programmes.
2. Environmental health programmes carry out inspections of facilities that prepare food as well as other facilities that serve the population, such as public swimming pools. These information systems are facility-oriented rather than person-oriented. For example, Los Angeles County, California, has an Environmental Health Management Information System database of records of inspections carried out at facilities, including facility characteristics, violations found, sanctions applied, and dates of correction.
3. Substance abuse prevention and treatment programmes in the United States often accomplish their mission by funding contractors that provide services to people with substance abuse problems. For such programmes, an information system must be provider-oriented as well as person-oriented. That is, its database must contain contractor characteristics, number of clients served, funding, and contract status, as well as data describing the people under treatment.
4. The public health laboratory processes a very large number of specimens (hundreds of thousand per year) for a very wide range of diseases, providing results throughout the community as well

as to other public health programmes. Independent and hospital laboratories use transaction-oriented information systems to capture data electronically from instruments and store the results in a database. Public health laboratories can purchase and install these commercially developed systems with minimal customization.

These public health programme information systems currently rely on paper-based data collection in the field, although data collection in some public health facilities may be computerized. Each public health programme inputs the paper reports and maintains its own database. If paper reports are received and input by public health programmes in a timely manner, these systems can respond to public health hazards, such as communicable disease outbreaks, with adequate speed.

However, since timely input of paper forms is usually problematic, more data collection is likely to become electronic. For example, reporting of adverse health events by the public, such as foodborne illnesses contracted at restaurants, can easily be accomplished over the Internet (http://www.lapublichealth.org/phcommon/complaints/phcomp.cfm). As mentioned above, other disease surveillance activities can also be transitioned to the Internet. Public health field staff who collect large amounts of data, such as public health nurses administering directly observed therapy to tuberculosis patients, or food preparation facility inspectors, can input data to portable or handheld computers in the field, with wireless or network uploading to the central database. However, these systems are only in the early stages of development. They face many of the challenges that must be overcome by the electronic medical record, including diverse data arising from field encounters and variations in vocabulary, as well as the expense of equipping large field staffs with portable computers.

Health departments also perform many tasks generic to any large organization, including accounting and finance, human resource management, procurement, contracting, and equipment inventories. Information systems to perform these functions can be purchased from commercial vendors to other industries or government agencies, or developed by suppliers to those industries. In small health departments or in developing countries, desktop computer spreadsheets and database programs can be adequate to accomplish these functions.

Telemedicine

Information technology allows expert clinicians to treat patients at a distance, via telecommunications links. These telemedicine services range from voice telephone communication to videoconferencing and image transmission requiring very high-bandwidth connections (Field 1996; Reid 1996). Telemedicine may significantly improve public health by allowing facilities in poor or rural areas to access clinical expertise.

Telemedicine can be adopted to the available computing power and telecommunications bandwidth (D. Krasnow, 2000, unpublished work). The simplest use of telemedicine is the telephone service using voice and/or fax. For example, a nurse in a rural clinic can call an urban-based doctor for advice on how to treat a particular type of injury. After one or two consultations about such injuries, she will be able to treat them on her own. Similarly, a doctor in a remote clinic can fax a patient's history, physical examination, and test results to a medical school specialist, receiving the consultation results back the next day.

More sophisticated uses of telemedicine involve capturing images with a digital camera or scanned photograph, and transmitting them to an expert for consultation. For example, photographs of unusual dermatological lesions can be transmitted, with the dermatologist e-mailing back treatment instructions or further questions. The telephone service is adequate for transmitting still images. Inexpensive video cameras can also transmit images during real-time consultation, allowing the remote doctor to zoom in to examine the patient in greater detail. With a bandwidth of 384 kb/s or higher, real-time discussion between the patient and the remote doctor is possible.

Highly sophisticated applications of telemedicine are being developed in industrialized countries. Teleradiology is the most common, where images are transmitted for interpretation. Another ideal use of telemedicine is the treatment of rare diseases, where a remote expert doctor can prescribe treatment based on images. For example, neuroblastomas are rare ocular tumours in infants and are fatal if untreated. With a special handheld camera, images can be taken and transmitted to academic medical centres worldwide for evaluation and treatment recommendations.

Applications of telemedicine can combine simple and sophisticated technology (D. Krasnow, 2000, unpublished work). For example, retinal scans of diabetics can indicate the need for treatment to prevent blindness. However, existing retinal cameras are very large and expensive, and so the patient must go to the specialist. Affordable ophthalmoscopes that incorporate digital cameras are being developed, so that images can be taken in rural clinics or mobile units and then transmitted via the telephone service to specialists for evaluation. In rural populations with high diabetes prevalence, such as Native Americans, this capability could significantly improve secondary prevention of diabetes-related complications.

Cheaper computers and digital cameras, as well as more widespread high-bandwidth telecommunications, will foster the growth of telemedicine. Even developing countries are installing networks of sufficient bandwidth to support highly effective telemedicine, such as the ISDN links from Lima to regional hospitals in Peru.

In any country, technology is often the easiest part of telemedicine implementation. To achieve success, the people who use the systems must also be adequately trained and provided with appropriate incentives to use it. In addition, processes must be in place to integrate the use of the technology routinely into the provision of care (Krasnow and Rodrigues 1998).

Quality-of-care measurement

Improved quality in the delivery of health services contributes to public health by conserving resources and by improving the health of patients. Information systems are essential for efficiently measuring the quality of health services. In industrialized countries, quality measurements focus on all potential types of problems: underuse of efficacious procedures, overuse of procedures whose risks exceed their benefits, and misuse that leads to avoidable complications (Chassin 1998). In developing countries, underuse because of poor access to services is the overwhelmingly most severe problem, followed by misuse (Peabody *et al.* 1999). In addition, information systems will play an increasing role in improving the process of care.

Measurement of the quality of health care can be broken down into the measurement of three different aspects (Donabedian 1980; Blumenthal 1996; Brook *et al.* 1996).

- Structure: institutional capabilities and qualifications.
- Process: technical and interpersonal aspects of the care provided to patients.
- Outcome: patients' morbidity, mortality, functional status, and quality of life.

Structural aspects are the easiest to measure, but have only an indirect effect on outcomes. Information systems are used in constructing structural quality measures, for example monitoring doctor credentialling at hospitals.

Data to construct process measures can be derived from hospital or clinic information systems, and specialized analysis software used to analyse the resulting data. When process criteria are clearly linked to outcome improvements, such as prescribing β-blockers to patients following myocardial infarction, process measurements that fall short of goals directly indicate where quality improvement interventions should be targeted. Information systems can also be used for ongoing monitoring after interventions are implemented (Mclaughlin and Kaluzny 1999). Clinical information systems, especially computerized order entry systems or electronic medical records, can incorporate clinical practice guidelines. When properly designed and integrated into the organizational context of a clinic or hospital, such information systems can significantly improve the quality of care, for example by reducing the incidence of medication errors (Evans *et al.* 1998).

Health outcomes are what patients and providers ultimately want to improve, but measurement of outcomes must adjust for confounding risk factors, such as the severity of patients' underlying illnesses and the presence of comorbidities. Nevertheless, successful outcome measurements provide important policy and clinical data. For example, small-area variation studies have shown that rates of common surgical procedures vary greatly over small geographical distances, without correlation to the disease patterns of the underlying populations (Wennberg 1999). In New York State, clinical data have been collected and sophisticated statistical risk adjustment models applied to compare mortality after coronary artery bypass graft surgery at all hospitals in the state. Hospitals performing low volumes of the surgery were found to have higher risk-adjusted mortality. This measurement programme has been credited with improving outcomes by reducing the fraction of coronary artery bypass graft surgeries performed at lower-volume hospitals (http://www.health.state.ny.us/nysdoh/research/heart/heart.htm). Compiling data from facilities in sufficient clinical detail to construct risk-adjusted outcome measures requires sophisticated information systems.

Data analysis and policy development

The information systems described so far provide data that can be analysed to provide information for planning and policy development, including epidemiological studies, resource allocation decisions, program design and evaluation, and quality assessment. Specialized software has been developed to perform these analyses and make information available in formats usable by decision-makers and communities.

Computerized statistical and epidemiological analyses

Almost all statistical and epidemiological analyses in industrialized countries are now performed using computerized analysis software. The increase in memory storage capacity and processing power of desktop and portable computers enables even very large datasets to be analysed on inexpensive computers. The use of microcomputers in epidemiology is discussed in Chapter 6.15.

Powerful statistical programs such as SAS (http://www.sas.com/) can now be run on microcomputers. Other programs such as Stata (http://www.stata.com/) or SPSS (http://www.spss.com/spss10/index.htm) also offer very robust statistical analysis capabilities. Analysis of survey data requires special statistical procedures to account properly for the sample design, but survey data analysis programs like SUDAAN also run on microcomputers (http://www.rti.org/patents/sudaan/sudaan.html). Stata also offers some survey data analysis capabilities.

Epidemiology software is also available. The widely used EpiInfo program can be downloaded free from the Internet (http://www.cdc.gov/epiinfo/). This software performs a full range of epidemiological functions, and a basic mapping program (EpiMap) is also available at the same website. In conjunction with inexpensive microcomputers, such free software makes it feasible for analysts in almost any developing country to perform computerized data analyses.

Geographical information systems

A GIS is a database of different types of information, all linked to a common geographical co-ordinate system (http://wwwdb.csu.edu.au/division/dit/span/spatial_technology/gis/what_gis.html). For example, a GIS might include population characteristics and census area boundaries, or health facility locations and street maps. A GIS primarily displays data as maps, a very effective way to display large amounts of information in easily understandable form. Locations of events or facilities can be presented, or areas of the map colour coded, to indicate differing levels of a population characteristic. GISs are applicable to numerous aspects of public health (Yasnoff and Sondik 1999).

Inexpensive computers with the ability to generate complex graphics rapidly have made GIS technology widely available. Specialized software is used to compile the database and generate the maps. The two most common commercial GIS systems are distributed by the Environmental Systems Research Institute (**ESRI**) and MapInfo. While very powerful, these systems are relatively costly and require substantial user training to be used most effectively. EpiMap GIS software is freely available from the CDC (http://www.cdc.gov/epiinfo/index.htm), and is designed to link with EpiInfo. GIS capabilities are also built into many Internet sites. The American Census Bureau's Topological Integrated Geographic Encoding and Referencing (**TIGER**) mapping system allows users to generate maps of population characteristics derived from census data (http://www.census.gov/geo/www/tiger/index.html).

A GIS analysis consists of several steps. The first is to obtain basic geographical data layers, such as street grids, political or census boundaries, or pollution source locations. The next step is to geocode the health events of interest, such as deaths or reported communicable disease cases. In geocoding, each event is assigned a latitude/longitude co-ordinate, by which it will be related to other data layers. Geocoding is not a perfect process, however, since address data collected in surveys may be incorrect or garbled. After geocoding, maps displaying the desired data layers can be produced and refined. Individual events may be displayed as points on the map. Average values for defined areas, such as census tracts within a county or states within a nation, can also be used to colour code map regions. Maps can be modified interactively by the user to address particular health questions, by adding or subtracting layers, zooming in and out, or changing colour-coding schemes. GIS databases can perform other analyses in addition to producing descriptive statistical maps, such as comparing rates over time, calculating optimal locations for new facilities, or correlating disease patterns to pollution sources. Figure 1 is an example of pollution source locations in California's 'Silicon Valley', which could be correlated with geographical distributions of diseases potentially attributable to pollution.

Statistical and epidemiological methods must be properly incorporated into GIS analyses for public health. For example, disease rates in small geographical areas may be based on small numbers of cases, and therefore may be highly variable from year to year. Spatial statistical techniques have been developed to interpolate rates from observed data to locations between observations.

Health indicators

Indicator sets describe the health of a population in a summary fashion, including features such as the socio-economic environment, disease patterns, access to health services, and mortality. Indicators are useful for comparisons across populations, analyses of health trends over time, and development of policies to address a community's most important health problems. One example set is the core health indicators developed by PAHO, which it publishes for its member countries. Some of these indicators are listed in Table 1.

Developing an indicator report for a community is a multistep process (Durch *et al.* 1997) (see also Chapter 5.2). The first step is collaboration among stakeholders to choose the indicators to be measured, given the state of development and most pressing problems faced by the community. Secondly, data to calculate the indicators must be compiled from many different sources. For example, each of the data collection information systems described in this chapter might be a data source for one or more indicators. Thirdly, indicators must be calculated and published. Computers and networks are very useful in compiling and analysing the data and formatting it for presentation. Fourthly, policy-makers and community-based organizations can use the results as a basis for discussion, policy decisions, and resource allocation. However, once the process for collecting and analysing data is in place, future cycles are less labour intensive, and the data can be compared with the baseline period to evaluate the policies that are implemented.

Many indicator sets are available, which can be used to choose individual indicators and as templates for a community's own efforts. Examples include the following.

- The PAHO Core Health Data indicators are appropriate for comparisons both in and across developing countries.
- The United States government's Healthy People 2010 objectives establish goals for a broad range of public health objectives (http://www.health.gov/healthypeople/publications/default.htm).
- The Institute of Medicine book *Improving Health in the Community: A Role for Performance Monitoring* (Durch *et al.* 1997) describes the process by which communities develop indicator sets and contains extensive lists of potential indicators.
- The Health Plan Employer Data and Information Set (**HEDIS**) was developed to assess the quality of HMOs. While it has substantial shortcomings, it is the most widely used indicator set for comparing the quality of these organizations that are responsible for main-

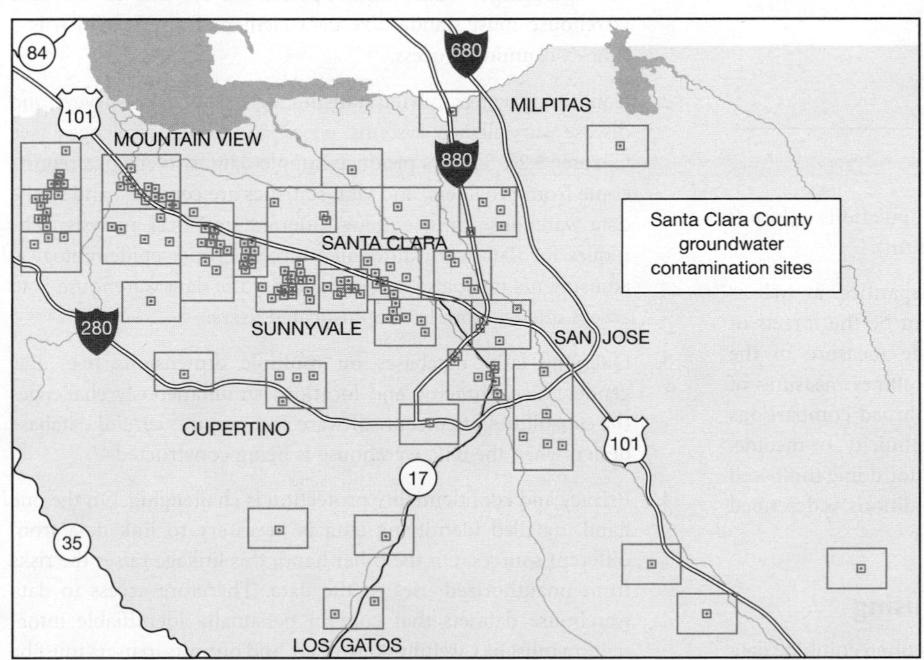

Fig. 1 Groundwater contamination sites in Santa Clara County, California ('Silicon Valley').

Table 1 Selected PAHO Core Health Indicators (http://www.paho.org/English/SHA/bsindcvr.htm)

Total population
Population growth rate
Percentage population urban
Birth rate
Death rate
Infant mortality rate
Life expectancy
Literacy rate
Percentage with access to safe water
Percentage with access to sewerage
National health expenditures as percentage of gross domestic product
Death rates
All causes
Communicable diseases
Malignant neoplasms
Circulatory system
External causes
Percentage under-5 deaths diarrhoeal
Percentage under-5 deaths acute respiratory
Communicable disease incidence
Measles
Cholera
Tuberculosis
Malaria
AIDS
Doctors, nurses, dentists per 10 000
Hospital beds per 1000
Immunization coverage in infants

taining the health of their covered populations (http://www.ncqa.org/Pages/Programs/HEDIS/index.htm).

Sets of health indicators highlight health disparities, as well as health system strengths and weaknesses, that can be the targets of policy initiatives, but do not provide a single measure of the population's health status. An indicator that combines measures of both morbidity and mortality is very useful for broad comparisons across communities defined by geography, race/ethnicity, or income. Disability-adjusted life-years (**DALYs**), a method for doing this based on disability weighting for diseases and health conditions, is described in detail in Chapter 2.9.

Linked databases and data warehousing

In-depth health policy and public health analyses often combine data on many different aspects of a population's health, such as those summarized by health indicator sets. However, compiling the raw data for these analyses is the most labour-intensive part of the effort, since it resides in information systems developed and maintained by separate public health programmes, other government agencies, hospitals, and clinics. Nevertheless, the benefits of comprehensive analyses can be worth the effort, for example, to investigate patterns of infant mortality by combining vital statistics and hospital discharge data.

Private firms face similar challenges, with information systems in different departments containing different aspects of information about the same customers. As a result, firms have created data warehouses that summarize data from operational information systems in different departments (Marietti 1997). Inexpensive server computers with large amounts of hard disk storage lower the hardware costs of building a data warehouse, and firms can use existing local area networks and wide-area networks to upload data to the data warehouse. Specialized software is necessary to query these very large databases efficiently, and to provide a user interface that supports users ranging from managers to professional analysts.

Public health organizations could use data warehouses to aggregate data from different programmes, as well as from providers and payers, to assemble an overall picture of population health. Such a data warehouse would be of use to researchers, community-based organizations, and providers, in addition to analysts and managers in health departments. For example, data warehouses could provide currently unavailable comprehensive data for public health priority setting and resource allocation (UCLA 1997).

Despite this great promise, several technological and organizational challenges must be overcome before public health data warehouses can become widespread.

1. Different information systems have different formats for data such as personal identifiers, geographical locations, and medical terminology. (Data can be aggregated more easily in a health-care payer than in public health organizations, since the payer has a unique identifying number for each enrolled member.) Therefore the uploading of data from operational systems to the data warehouse must standardize data element formats, which is a time-consuming process.

2. Combining data from vital statistics registries, health surveys, and disease surveillance systems poses additional challenges (see Chapter 5.2). Surveys produce sample data, surveillance reports come from providers, and vital statistics are censuses, and so the data warehouse must employ different statistical analysis techniques for data from different sources. Proper epidemiological adjustments must also be automated if the data warehouse is to accept queries from less sophisticated users.

3. Querying large databases on multiple dimensions (e.g. age, gender, race/ethnicity, and location) simultaneously challenges the capabilities of current software and requires careful database design when the data warehouse is being constructed.

4. Privacy and confidentiality protection is challenging. On the one hand, detailed identifying data is necessary to link data from different sources. On the other hand, this linkage raises the risks from unauthorized uses of the data. Therefore access to data warehouse datasets that contain personally identifiable information must be carefully controlled, and outputs to users must be screened for confidentiality protection (e.g. by suppressing data for small cell sizes).

5. Gaining community stakeholder co-operation in sharing data from sources outside the public health organization, such as hospitals or health plans, can be difficult (Multnomah County Health Department 1999).

Some important steps are being taken towards the development of public health data warehouses. The Population Health Information System (**POPULIS**) in Manitoba aggregates data from many different sources to provide comprehensive population health data (Roos *et al.* 1996); Canada's single-payer health insurance system helps nurture the necessary co-operation among stakeholders. In the United States, some states, such as Wisconsin, have developed datasets on many aspects of population health that could be linked together (http://badger.state.wi.us/agencies/oci/ohci/). Finally, the on-line query systems discussed below can be incremental steps to full data warehouses.

Data access and dissemination

The Internet has made a vast array of public health information available worldwide at the click of a mouse. Once information has been collected or created, dissemination via the Internet is much faster and simpler than by print or physical digital media such as CD-ROMs. Types of public health information available on line include documents (e.g. books, papers, reports, brochures), downloadable datasets, and query systems. Each of these types of information is described in more detail below. Internet data access tools vary in sophistication from those intended for analysts with advanced training to ones targeted at the general public.

A special type of information resource, the centralized index or bibliography, has been developed to make all these information sources easily accessible to users. The broadest indexes are the Internet 'search engines'. These are databases of web page content, compiled by software that automatically accesses and catalogues all types of web pages. Users can perform simple or complex keyword searches of all these web pages simply by accessing the search engine's main web page. For example, Google (www.google.com) indexes over 1 billion web pages and has a sophisticated algorithm to rank search results by likely relevance to the user's query. Portals are indexes targeted at users in specific disciplines. MDConsult (www.mdconsult.com) provides a wide range of medical information to doctors, including news summaries and searchable databases of journals and clinical practice guidelines. Some portals (including MDConsult) charge a membership fee for full access to their content. Bibliographies of Internet resources in particular disciplines are often maintained by libraries or non-profit organizations, and can offer users very efficient access to relevant websites. Useful bibliographies of public health Internet resources are provided by the University of California at Berkeley (www.lib.berkeley.edu/PUBL/Internet.html), Johns Hopkins University (http://support.jhsph.edu/sph/intresources/), and the University of Iowa (http://www.lib.uiowa.edu/hardin/md/).

Internet data access requires relatively little information technology infrastructure: a microcomputer, either direct connection to a local area network connected to the Internet or a telephone line and modem to connect to an Internet service provider, and several pieces of inexpensive software, including a browser program (such as Netscape or Microsoft's Internet Explorer), the free Adobe Acrobat Reader (http://www.adobe.com/products/acrobat/readermain.html) to read documents in .pdf format, e-mail software, word-processing and spreadsheet software to open downloaded files, and virus detection/removal software to protect against harmful computer viruses attached to downloaded files.

Increased availability of these tools and of high-bandwidth telecommunications will make Internet public health resources available to more users, and will allow access to larger and more interactive databases. Conceptually, and soon practically, any product that can be put in digital format can be shared via the Internet.

Public health and medical literature

More and more of the published academic and policy literature relevant to public health is becoming available on-line. The largest resource for accessing the biomedical, public health, and health services research literature on-line is the United States National Library of Medicine (**NLM**). NLM's bibliographic database, Medline, is now accessible via the Internet (http://www.ncbi.nlm.nih.gov/entrez/query.fcgi). Full citations and abstracts can be downloaded.

The full text of journals and books is also increasingly available on-line. The *Morbidity and Mortality Weekly Report* published by the CDC, an essential tool for dissemination of public health data, is now fully available via the Internet (http://www.cdc.gov/mmwr/). Some prominent medical journals, such as the *British Medical Journal*, are freely accessible in full text. Others, such as the *New England Journal of Medicine*, make abstracts and some articles available free, but require a subscription fee for complete access. Ovid (http://www.ovid.com) is a service that provides the full text of a large number of journals in return for a licensing fee. Universities and other organizations also make medical textbooks available on line to staff and students. Electronic versions of these reference materials can be better than print versions, offering more frequent updates and fully searchable text. Finally, government agencies can make their reports, which are in fact public goods, available on line. The American Institute of Medicine (http://www.nap.edu/) has begun making many of its books accessible this way.

Downloadable datasets

Public-use versions of many datasets from vital statistics registries or surveys are being made available for downloading via the Internet. Others are available in magnetic tape or CD-ROM format for a fee and/or under confidentiality restriction agreements. This section will focus on datasets available via the Internet.

Demographic data for many geographical regions can be downloaded, and are fundamental inputs to public health analyses. For example, data on the age and gender of residents within specified geographical boundaries are necessary to calculate mortality or disease prevalence rates. The Data Extraction System at the United States Census Bureau Internet site (http://www.census.gov/) provides access to a public-use versions of data from the decennial census as well as from other ongoing surveys of income and other population characteristics. Users define the parameters of the data that they require, i.e. variables and geographical boundaries, and receive the dataset by e-mail. Other demographic data, such as vital statistics on births and deaths, can also be accessed on line. One example is the United States NCHS National Death Index (part of the NVSS) described above.

Data obtained from many of the health surveys and disease surveillance systems described above are also available via the Internet.

For example, public-use datasets from several United States NCHS surveys and other national surveillance systems are available via the dedicated Internet data portal CDC WONDER (http://wonder.cdc.gov/). After choosing a survey or type of surveillance data, users receive a dataset that meets the parameters they define, through a process similar to that described above for the American census data. DHS surveys provide comparable high-quality data for many developing countries, and these datasets are also available for download (http://www.measuredhs.com/). For users wishing to learn about downloadable data sources available on particular topics, the University of Michigan maintains a list of numerous such resources (http://www.lib.umich.edu/libhome/Documents.center/sthealth.html).

On-line query systems

Analysts with the necessary training and software can manipulate downloaded datasets to answer their particular questions. However, users without such training, including managers, policy-makers' staffs, and other public health practitioners, often need quantitative information about population health as inputs to their decision-making. For example, information about rates of different diseases is essential for the rational allocation of limited resources across programs designed to prevent those diseases. On-line query systems can provide answers directly to users logged on via local area network, wide-area network, or the Internet. These information systems are much more flexible than printed reports, which show only a few of the many potential ways to present large datasets. They accept structured queries, usually via a system of dialogue boxes that prompt users to define the parameters of their query.

A wide range of types of data are being made available in this fashion, including demographics, health indicators, and health services utilization. For example, several American states offer population and demographics query capabilities. Figure 2 is an example of such a dialogue box from a population data query system offered by the Utah Department of Health (http://hlunix.hl.state.ut.us/hda/population/). The PAHO core health indicators described above can be queried via the Internet (http://www.paho.org/English/SHA/ihomeibs.htm). An example output is shown in Fig. 3. The AHRQ offers an Internet query system called HCUPnet (http://www.ahrq.gov/data/hcup/hcupnet.htm) for hospital utilization data collected as part of its Healthcare Quality and Utilization Project (**HCUP**). This system is an example of a sophisticated but user-friendly query system. It offers outputs in time trends as well as in tabular form. In some cases, databases that can be downloaded can also be queried directly. An example of this is the database of results from DHS surveys from many developing countries (http://www.ahrq.gov/data/hcup/hcupnet.htm).

Underlying any interactive query system is a database of information categorized along the dimensions that can be queried. This may be a dataset composed of individual observations (such as vital statistics registries), or even multiple linked datasets as described above. Statistical analyses are performed by calling preprogrammed routines, which must also contain the necessary confidentiality and privacy protection conditions. Therefore, to provide faster response to users and to ensure confidentiality, many query systems draw their responses from large, preformatted summary tables.

To serve users who are not trained analysts effectively, the user interface of an interactive query systems should be as simple as possible to learn. To be as useful as possible, they should provide not only cross-sectional output tables, but also time trends and bar charts for comparisons over time and across groups. Maps can also be used, both to select geographical regions as part of a query and to display results by colour-coding map regions.

Information sharing among public health professionals

The Internet greatly improves the efficiency with which public health professionals can share information on best practices. Such sharing is especially important in public health, because while development of new procedures and programmes is costly and time-consuming, public health professionals in different cities, states, and countries usually perform very similar functions and can borrow ideas from each other easily.

The simplest way for individual professionals to share information via the Internet is a USENET e-mail newsgroup. In this method, people who share an interest in a specific topic subscribe to an e-mail list. All members of the list receive the questions, answers, and notices

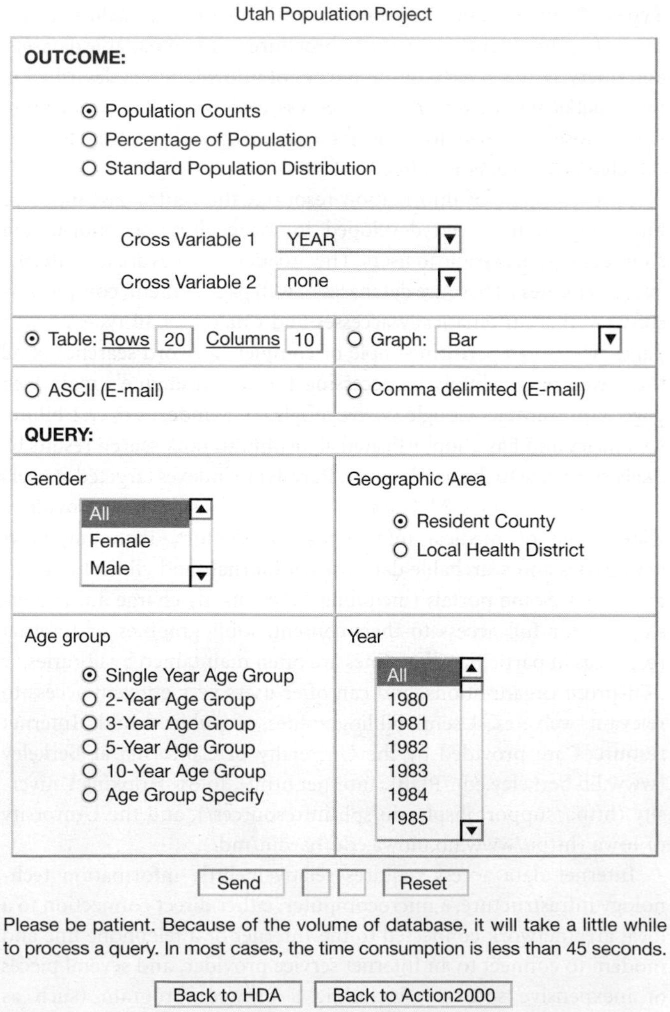

Fig. 2 Utah population projection. (Source: Utah Department of Health.)

Core Data for the Americas
(updated: Sep/1998)

Indicator	Argentina	Brazil	Chile	Colombia	Venezuela
C.18–Estimated death rates due to ischemic heart disease	71.8	71.2	59.0	67.5	64.8
male	88.7	84.0	63.3	70.1	75.2
female	55.4	58.6	54.9	66.4	54.1
45–64 years	95.9	167.4	69.6	150.9	168.3
65 years and over	576.7	898.1	747.0	1057.2	1110.6
male 45–64 years	158.8	234.8	100.0	183.9	238.5
male 65 years and over	744.0	1026.8	872.6	1165.5	1297.7
female 45–64 years	37.7	104.0	40.9	118.8	99.8
female 65 years and over	456.8	793.0	658.1	963.8	954.8

Click one of these buttons to select other:

Indicators | Ind Groupings | Countries

or click the following button to export table:

Export data | Include notes

Fig. 3 Core data for the Americas (September 1998).

posted to the list by its members. For example, the author subscribes to such a list server of people sharing an interest in the design of state health surveys. Many common methodological issues and survey questions are posted and discussed by members. Some lists are moderated by their founders to make the list as useful as possible by weeding out inappropriate postings.

Community-based organizations in the same region or with shared goals can also easily share information and best practice ideas with each other. E-mail contacts are the simplest to set up. With more co-ordination, groups of community-based organizations can create, share, and update electronic inventories of health facilities, programmes, and other resources in their region, to facilitate referrals and collaboration.

More structured information sharing can be sponsored by government agencies or non-profit organizations. For example, several United States government and non-profit organizations have formed the 'Partners in Information Access for Public Health Professionals' programme (http://www.nnlm.nlm.nih.gov/partners/) to facilitate access to a variety of public health data sources. Sharing is also possible on an international level. The International Clearinghouse on Health Systems Reform Initiatives (**ICHSRI**) compiles information on health systems reform initiatives in developing countries (http://www.insp.mx/ichsri/). Users can access the site to learn about reform initiatives, compare them, and discuss related issues and challenges. In the coming years, improvements in automated language translation software may further widen the international sharing of best practices among governmental and non-governmental organizations.

Providing health data to community members

Individual members of the population are increasingly turning to the Internet as a source of health information. Tens of millions of Ameican residents are now doing so, and that number grows as Internet access expands (Wellner 2000). To the extent that consumers are thus better informed about disease prevention, health promotion, and the appropriate utilization of health services, the Internet will have a beneficial impact on public health. However, sites that contain inaccurate information or information biased due to commercial sponsorship pose a risk to the health of on-line consumers.

Government and non-profit organizations offer health information over the Internet as a public service. One of the best examples is the Cancer Information Service at the National Cancer Institute (http://cis.nci.nih.gov/). This site, and its associated toll-free telephone number, are extremely useful resources for consumers faced with the need to learn about cancer diagnosis and treatment. Local public health departments can also post information, such as advisories of health hazards, on their websites for easier access. The Internet is an ideal medium for publishing reference materials, and community resource guides are a reference that can assist those seeking health services. For example, the *People's Guide*, a comprehensive reference on how to obtain health and other social services in California, is available on line (http://www.peoplesguide.org/) as well as in print.

Numerous for-profit websites have been founded to provide health information to consumers. The business-to-consumer sites, such as DrKoop.com (http://www.drkoop.com/) and WebMD (http://shn.webmd.com/), offer a wide range of information on health promotion, specific conditions, and treatments. The best of these sites are easy to use, often contain well-researched and well-written information, and draw millions of viewers. However, they have struggled to find commercial sponsors to support their ongoing operations, and the long-term viability of many of these business-to-consumer sites is currently in doubt. Other for-profit health services providers, including health plans, doctor groups, and hospitals, also maintain websites. While these sites may contain useful health information, their primary purpose is marketing to new patients and providing services more efficiently to current patients.

Search engines and well-designed general health websites make it relatively easy for consumers to find information on the Internet about the health topics of interest to them. However, the quality of that information is not guaranteed, and most consumers are not trained to evaluate the validity of the information they access. For example, large numbers of ineffective or dangerous treatments are promoted via the Internet (http://www.familyInternet.com/quackwatch/). No uniform enforceable standards for health information quality have yet been developed, although some outlines for such standards are emerging (Winker *et al.* 2000). At the present time, consumers must still carefully evaluate the sponsorship and the source of health information they access via the Internet (Cooke 1999).

Health training and education

Information systems can enhance both training for public health professionals and health education programmes targeted at consumers. Information systems have been incorporated into consumer health education for many years, especially since inexpensive microcomputers began to offer powerful graphics capabilities. High-bandwidth network access will allow computerized educational content, including content that supports user interactivity, to be distributed even more widely. Overall, the basic health education and training methods are not likely to be replaced, but some of them may be transformed or expanded by the use of information technology and telecommunications (Chamberlain 1996).

This section will first discuss the application of information systems to distance learning, for training of public health professionals. It will then describe the effects of information technology and telecommunications on several modes of consumer health education, including campaigns, curriculum materials, and the exchange of information among groups with specialized health interests. (Internet dissemination of health information to consumers is discussed at the end of the previous section of this chapter. General principles of health education are presented in Chapter 7.3.

Distance learning

Distance learning is a relatively inexpensive way to teach many students in dispersed locations from a central locus of expertise, such as a school of public health or medicine. Given the shortage of adequately trained public health personnel, especially in rural areas and developing countries, it can be an important way to leverage limited public health resources. For example, the CDC and several partner organizations established the Public Health Training Network (**PHTN**) in 1993 to provide distance learning services for the state and local public health workforce. Over 1 million people have received training and information via PHTN to date (http://www.cdc.gov/phtn/).

Distance learning can be conducted in several different modes, with increasing degrees of interactivity (and cost): videotape or CD-ROM, Internet or print course materials, audio or video broadcast, and audio or video conferencing. Audio or video can be delivered via telephone lines, radio and television, satellite, local area networks or wide-area networks, or the Internet. Students can interact with the instructor using e-mail or on-line chat sessions. Several of these delivery modes and technologies can be combined in one program, such as Internet distribution of course materials, video delivery of lectures, and e-mail feedback to instructors.

Availability of cheaper and higher-bandwidth telecommunications should accelerate the application of the more interactive modes of distance learning in public health. For example, acceptable quality interactive video conferencing is possible using inexpensive computer-mounted video cameras and a transmission bandwidth of 384 kb/s, achievable using ISDN or digital subscriber line telephone lines (V.G. Winting, personal communication, 2000).

In industrialized countries, distance learning is increasingly focusing on video delivery or interactive video conferencing. For example, the four schools of public health in California installed video-conferencing equipment and dedicated ISDN lines to provide training to rural health departments in the state; webcasting capability is currently being added (V.G. Winting, unpublished data, 1999; J.M. Nunez, personal communication, 2000).

Less expensive delivery modes can still be effective, and are much more practical in developing countries. For example, downloadable curriculum materials for self study or for local trainers/teachers can be easily disseminated via the Internet. The Global Health Network Supercourse (Anonymous 1999) is a series of lecture materials on topics such as epidemiology, developed by participating public health faculty in many countries, that are made available worldwide via the Internet.

As mentioned above with regard to telemedicine, the technology component of distance learning is often not the most challenging. A useful framework for evaluating the practicality of a distance learning application is that the application must be simultaneously:

- available (i.e. technologically feasible in the context of a particular country)
- accessible to the target users (e.g. convenient to their workplaces)
- affordable.

If any one of these criteria is absent, the application is unlikely to succeed as planned (V.G. Winting, personal communication, 2000).

Educational campaigns

Health education campaigns are designed to convey a specific message, such as safe sex practices or smoking cessation, to a specific audience. These campaigns, one of the techniques broadly known as social marketing, are widespread in both industrialized and developing countries (Glanz *et al.* 1997). Their messages have traditionally been delivered using broadcast and print media, as well as community worker outreach. However, as Internet use expands, it makes possible the targeting of messages to narrower and narrower niche audiences. Commercial advertisers are increasingly using Internet advertising for this purpose, and health education campaigns can be expected to adopt this practice as well (D. Glik, personal communication, 2000).

Health journalism is another means of educating consumers. It is growing in prominence, with coverage of biomedical discoveries and public health themes. As more journalistic content is distributed via the Internet, health journalism is also likely to migrate there (D. Glik, personal communication, 2000). Similarly, entertainment media can be used to communicate health education messages, and expanded use of computerized entertainment should offer opportunities to deliver health education (D. Glik, personal communication, 2000).

Curriculum development

Computerized multimedia presentations, incorporating graphics and audio as well as text, are effective vehicles to present large amounts of information to target audiences. The viewer can proceed through the material at his or her own pace and replay sections as necessary. Interactive multimedia allow the viewer to make queries or answer questions posed by the software. Multimedia tools have been developed for several public health education topics, such as maternal and child health promotion (D. Glik, personal communication, 2000). Such tools can also be particularly helpful for patients with serious chronic health conditions. For example, they can teach preventive health behaviours to children with diabetes or asthma (Robitaille 2000).

Multimedia tools have mostly been distributed on CD-ROMs. These are cheap to manufacture and distribute, and can be played back on inexpensive microcomputers. They are usually used in institutional settings, such as clinics or hospitals, where the viewer can have access to a computer (D. Glik, personal communication, 2000). However, high-bandwidth networks and telecommunications make it possible to deliver large files easily, offering opportunities to distribute multimedia educational materials to much wider audiences via the Internet.

Nevertheless, creating the content itself will remain the bottleneck in developing effective multimedia health education materials (Chamberlain 1996). Crafting and testing messages and tailoring the interactive presentation requires experts in health education, graphics design, and video production. These skills are costly, and the development process is time-consuming. Although Internet dissemination makes the marginal cost of distribution negligible, substantial funding will still be required to design, produce, and test effective content.

Specialized health information providers

While the Internet can provide health information to the general population cheaply, it can be even more useful to people suffering from particular health conditions. These people, especially if they have physical disabilities or live in rural areas or small cities, previously had very limited opportunities to share knowledge and experiences with other people suffering from the condition. However, the Internet makes it possible to aggregate these small populations on a national or international basis. These on-line grassroots groups can provide education and mutual support, as well as be vehicles for political activism. Non-profit health organizations can also use their websites to disseminate educational information about the conditions or health issues they address.

Both websites and e-mail groups can be used for communication among these condition-specific on-line communities. Their numbers and membership can be expected to grow as Internet access expands throughout the world. At the time of writing, the Yahoo Internet directory lists over 8450 websites devoted to specific diseases and health conditions (http://dir.yahoo.com/Health/Diseases_and_Conditions/). Commercial enterprises can also arise to serve the needs of these communities, such as eBiocare.com, a pharmacy specializing in genetically engineered medications for people with six different health conditions (http://www.ebiocare.com/index.asp).

Challenges to applying information systems in public health

The previous sections have outlined many ways in which information systems can contribute to improving public health. Continued technological advancement and innovative applications of those technologies in organizations will certainly foster even more ideas in the years to come. However, several challenges must be overcome before this full potential can be realized. This final section summarizes some of those obstacles to more widespread application of information systems to public health.

Information technology and telecommunications infrastructure

Many of the potential advances described above will require improved and expanded information technology and telecommunications infrastructure, in both industrialized and developing countries. Applications in industrialized countries, such as multimedia health education or fully electronic disease surveillance systems, depend on the widespread availability of inexpensive high-bandwidth telecommunications, such as digital subscriber line telephone lines or cable television modems. In the United States, businesses and government agencies are installing these capabilities rapidly, but only a very small minority of households (less than 5 per cent) have them at present. In other industrialized countries, deployment of these telecommunications systems is much less advanced. Even within the United States, telecommunications infrastructure in rural areas and poor urban areas lags far behind that in wealthy urban areas.

In developing countries, even the availability of computers and reliable telephone service cannot be taken for granted in public health agencies or health-care provider organizations, let alone among the general population. However, even inexpensive computers and voice telephone connections can support appropriately tailored information systems applications with large benefits, such as Internet delivery of educational materials or voice-based telemedicine. Investments in computer hardware can be focused on leveraging the skills of trained analysts at regional and national levels. Information can be transferred among regions or to the national level using physical storage media. As described in Chapter 5.3, advances in wireless communications will allow important public health applications of information systems to proceed long before hardwired telecommunications services are universal.

Funding availability

In most industrialized countries, funding for the core public health activities of disease prevention and health promotion, as well as primary health care, have historically been underfunded in comparison to the provision of curative health services. In developing countries, the poverty of the population and limited government budgets for health make this funding misallocation even more severe.

Unfortunately, information systems development and implementation require significant initial investments in computer hardware, software development, network infrastructure, and training before benefits can begin to accrue. This will remain a major hurdle to the broader application of information systems in public health. Therefore public health leaders must become more knowledgeable about information systems (Yasnoff *et al.* 2000) and argue vigorously to policy-makers when the benefits of such investments clearly exceed the costs.

Privacy and confidentiality protection

Health data are among the most sensitive of personal information, and organizations that collect such data from individuals are obligated to protect it from unauthorized use or disclosure. However, wider applications of information systems in health care mean that more and more personal health data are available in electronic form, and are therefore subject to new and worrying disclosure risks. Public concerns over protecting the privacy of personal health data are especially strong in countries like the United States, where the majority of the population is not covered by universal health insurance.

Organizations that collect personal health data, including public health agencies, health services providers, and health financing organizations, must protect against three different types of confidentiality breaches.

1. Access to stored health information by unauthorized people. This is accomplished by controlling access to information systems with tools like passwords and restricted access to the most sensitive types of data.
2. Interception of information while it is being transmitted from the source to the collecting organization, or between organizations. This is accomplished using encryption technology.
3. Sharing of information among organizations without the originating person's full consent. The solution to this problem is not a technological one, but rather requires health organizations to adopt and enforce strict procedures with regard to sharing the information they have collected.

In the United States, federal legislation carrying significant penalties will soon establish the framework for the protection of consumer health information. The 'administrative simplification' provisions of the Health Insurance Portability and Accountability Act (**HIPAA**) of 1996 require that health organizations comply with national standards for the protection of health data and electronic sharing ('transactions') of that data. Regulations implementing this requirement were published in October 2000, and organizations have 2 years to comply. Almost any information system containing personal health data may be affected by HIPAA requirements (http://www.jhita.org/).

Data collected through vital statistics systems, disease surveillance, and health surveys is often highly sensitive and personally identifiable. However, there are important public health reasons for making these data as widely available as possible. Agencies that collect such data must therefore strike a balance between easy access and necessary privacy protection. Several techniques are employed to accomplish this. Access to complete data files should be restricted to authorized users working under clear confidentiality procedures. Public-use data files are stripped of all personal identifying information, such as name or address. Because combinations of individual characteristics (e.g. age, race, income, and education) can allow salient individuals to be identified in small population divisions, geographical identifiers in public-use datasets may be very general (e.g. state only). Users who wish to see lower-level detail, or to link different datasets, may be required to do so at special data centres, whose staff supervise analyses to prevent confidentiality breaches. In the future, it is possible that public access to some datasets will be allowed only via query systems, with even professional analysts being required to work through data centres to access complete datasets.

Information technology development challenges

Development and implementation of large information systems are risky in any industry. The technical sophistication, limited funding, and confidentiality requirements of public health information systems all increase the risk of failure if the development process is not well managed. Some risks can be mitigated by borrowing technologies, such as GIS, that have been refined in other industries. In addition, proven information systems development methods can be applied as successfully in public health as in any other industry. On the technical side, effective health services software development methodologies are well documented (Austin and Boxerman 1998; PAHO 1999). Organizational leadership skills are also necessary to prevent development problems in large information systems (Lorenzi and Riley 1995). While these methods are documented and proven, applying them correctly is a key responsibility of public health managers.

Conclusion

Despite the formidable challenges to overcome, broader application of information systems can improve our ability to achieve the goals of public health. Rapid technological evolution makes it impossible to predict future trends precisely, but what we can already realistically envision is remarkably exciting.

References

Aday, L.A. (1996). *Designing and conducting health surveys: a comprehensive guide.* Jossey-Bass, San Francisco, CA.

Anonymous (1999). The Global Health Network Supercourse: epidemiology, the Internet, and global health. *Telemedicine Journal*, **5**, 303–7.

Austin, C.J. and S.B. Boxerman (1998). *Information systems for health services administration.* Health Administration Press, Chicago, IL.

Blumenthal, D. (1996). Quality of health care. Part 1: What is it? *New England Journal of Medicine*, **335**, 891–4.

Brook, R.H., McGlynn, E.A., *et al.* (1996). Quality of health care. Part 2: Measuring quality of care. *New England Journal of Medicine*, **335**, 966–70.

Chamberlain, M.A. (1996). Health communication: making the most of new media technologies—an international overview. *Journal of Health Community*, **1**, 43–50.

Chassin, M.R. (1998). Is health care ready for Six Sigma quality? *Milbank Quarterly*, **76**, 565–91, 510.

Chunning, C. (1992). Disease surveillance in China. *Morbidity and Mortality Weekly Report*, **41**(Supplement), 111–22.

Cibulskis, R. and Izard, J. (1996). Monitoring systems. In *Health policy and systems deveopment: an agenda for research* (ed. J. Kanovsky). WHO, Geneva.

Cooke, A. (1999). Quality of health and medical information on the Internet. *Clinical Performance and Quality Health Care*, **7**, 178–85.

Dick, R.S., Steen, E.B., *et al.* (ed.) (1997). *The computer-based patient record: an essential technology for health care.* National Academy Press, Washington, DC.

Donabedian, A. (1980). *The definition of quality and approaches to its assessment.* Health Administration Press, Ann Arbor, MI.

Drotman, D.P. and Strassburg, M.A. (2001). Sources of data. In *Epidemiologic methods for the study of infectious diseases* (ed. J.C. Thomas and D.J. Weber). Oxford University Press.

Durch, J.S., Bailey, L.A., *et al.* (ed.) (1997). *Improving health in the community: a role for performance monitoring.* National Academy Press, Washington, DC.

Evans, R.S., Pestotnik, S.L., *et al.* (1998). A computer-assisted management program for antibiotics and other antiinfective agents. *New England Journal of Medicine,* **338,** 232–8.

Field, M.J. (ed.) (1996). *Telemedicine: a guide to assessing telecommunications in health care.* National Academy Press, Washington, DC.

Glanz, K., Lewis, F.M., *et al.* (ed.) (1997). *Health behavior and health education: theory, research, and practice.* Jossey-Bass, San Francisco, CA.

Hammer, M. (1990). Reengineering work: don't automate, obliterate. *Harvard Business Review,* **68,** 104–12.

Husein, K., Adeyi, O., *et al.* (1993). Developing a primary care information system that supports the pursuit of equity. *Social Science and Medicine,* **36,** 585–96.

Institute of Medicine (1988). *The future of public health.* National Academy Press, Washington, DC.

Kipp, W., Kielman, A., *et al.* (1994). Monitoring of primary health care services: an example from Western Uganda. *Health Policy and Planning,* **9,** 155–60.

Krasnow, D. and Rodrigues, R.J. (1998). International perspectives. *Telemedicine: practicing in the information age* (ed. S.F. Viegas and K. Dunn). Lippincott–Raven, Philadelphia, PA.

Lorenzi, N.M. and Riley, R.T. (1995). *Organizational aspects of health informatics: managing technological change.* Springer-Verlag, New York,

Love, D. (2000). State data sources. Presented at Association for Health Services Research Annual Meeting, Los Angeles, CA.

Mclaughlin, C.P. and Kaluzny, A.D. (1999). *Continuous quality improvement in health care: theory, implementatiion, and applications.* Aspen Publishers, Baltimore, MD.

Marietti, C. (1997). The data warehouse. New uses for old data. *Healthcare Informatics,* **14,** 93–6, 98, 100.

Multnomah County Health Department (1999). *Designing a public-private integrated health information system for use in local public health planning and policy development.* Multnomah County Health Department, Portland, Oregon.

O'Carroll, P., Yasnoff, W., *et al.* (ed.) (2000). *Public health informatics and information systems.* Aspen Publishers, Baltimore, MD.

PAHO (Pan American Health Organization) (1999). *Setting up healthcare services information systems: a guide for requirements, analysis, application specification, and procurement.* PAHO, Washington, DC.

Peabody, J.W., Rahman, M.O., *et al.* (1999). *Policy and health: implications for development in Asia.* Cambridge University Press.

Reid, J. (1996). *A telemedicine primer: understanding the issues.* Innovative Medical Communications, Billings, Montana.

Robitaille, S. (2000). Orphan technologies look for a home. *California Healthline.* http://www.chcf.org/features/index.cfm?itemID=1326

Roos, N.P., Black, C., *et al.* (1996). Population health and health care use: an information system for policy makers. *Milbank Quarterly,* **74,** 3–31.

Satia, J.K., Mavalankar, D.V., *et al.* (1994). Micro-level planning using rapid assessment for primary care health services. *Health Policy and Planning,* **9,** 318–30.

UCLA (1997). *Report of review of public health programs and services, Los Angeles County, Department of Health Services.* UCLA School of Public Health Technical Assistance Group, Los Angeles, CA.

Wellner, A.S. (2000). Casting the health.net. *American Demographics,* **22,** 46–9.

Wennberg, J.E. (1999). Understanding geographic variations in health care delivery. *New England Journal of Medicine,* **340,** 52–3.

Winker, M.A., Flanagin, A., *et al.* (2000). Guidelines for medical and health information sites on the Internet: principles governing AMA websites. *Journal of the American Medical Association,* **283,** 1600–6.

Woodall, J.P. (1988). Epidemiological approaches to health planning, management, and evaluation. *World Health Statistics Quarterly,* **41,** 2–10.

Yasnoff, W.A. and Sondik, E.J. (1999). Geographic information systems (GIS) in public health practice in the new millennium. *Journal of Public Health Management and Practice,* **5,** ix–xii.

Yasnoff, W.A., O'Carroll, P.W., *et al.* (2000). Public health informatics: improving and transformng public health in the information age. *Journal of Public Health Management and Practice,* **6,** 65–75.

Web page citations

http://badger.state.wi.us/agencies/oci/ohci/. 'Wisconsin Office of Health Care Information.' Wisconsin State Government. Accessed 6 October 2000. Updated 31 August 2000.

http://cis.nci.nih.gov/. 'Cancer Information Service.' National Cancer Institute. Accessed 7 October 2000. Updated 5 October 2000.

http://dir.yahoo.com/Health/Diseases-and-Conditions/. 'Diseases and Conditions.' Yahoo. Accessed 7 October 2000.

http://familyInternet.com/quackwatch/. 'Quackwatch.' Quackwatch. Accessed 7 October 2000. Updated 29 January 2000.

http://hlunix.hl.state.ut.us/hda/population/. 'Utah Population Projection.' Utah Department of Health. Accessed 7 October 2000.

http://newfederalism.urban.org/nsaf/. 'National Survey of America's Families.' Urban Institute. Accessed 6 October 2000.

http://shn.webmd.com/. 'WebMD.' WebMD. Accessed 7 October 2000.

http://support.jhsph.edu/sph/intresources/. 'Internet Public Health Resources.' Johns Hopkins University. Accessed 7 October 2000.

http://wonder.cdc.gov. 'CDC WONDER.' CDC WONDER. Accessed 7 October 2000.

http://www.ahrq.gov/data/hcup/hcupnet.htm. 'Healthcare Cost and Utilization Project.' Agency for Healthcare Research and Quality. Accessed 7 October 2000. Updated August 2000.

http://www.ccrcal.org/abouttheccr.html. 'California Cancer Registry.' California Cancer Registry. Accessed 6 October 2000.

http://www.cdc.gov/. 'Public Health Training Network.' Centers for Disease Control and Prevention. Accessed 7 October 2000.

http://www.cdc.gov/epiinfo/. 'Epi Info.Epi Map.' Centers for Disease Control and Prevention. Accessed 6 October 2000. Updated 5 June 2000.

http://www.cdc.gov/epiinfo/index.htm. 'Epi Info and Epi Map.' Centers for Disease Control and Prevention. Accessed 6 October 2000. Updated 5 June 2000.

http://www.cdc.gov/mmwr/. 'Morbidity and Mortality Weekly Report.' Centers for Disease Control and Prevention. Accessed 7 October 2000. Updated 6 October 2000.

http://www.cdc.gov/nccdphp/brfss/index.htm. 'Behavioral Risk Factor Surveillance System.' Centers for Disease Control and Prevention. Accessed 6 October 2000. Updated 28 September 2000.

http://www.cdc.gov/nchs/about/major/dvs/mortdata.htm. 'Mortality Data from the National Vital Statistics System.' Centers for Disease Control and Prevention. Accessed 6 October 2000. Updated 12 September 2000.

http://www.cdc.gov/nchs/nhanes.htm. 'National Health and Nutrition Examination Survey.' Centers for Disease Control and Prevention. Accessed 6 October 2000. Updated 25 July 2000.

http://www.cdc.gov/nchs/nhcs.htm. 'National Health Care Survey.' Centers for Disease Control and Prevention. Accessed and updated 24 July 2000.

http://www.cdc.gov/nchs/nhis.htm. 'National Health Interview Survey (NHIS).' Centers for Disease Control and Prevention. Accessed 6 October 2000. Updated 12 September 2000.

http://www.cdc.gov/od/hissb/docs.htmnedss. 'National Electronic Disease Surveillance System.' Centers for Disease Control and Prevention. Accessed 6 October 2000. Updated 9 August 2000.

http://www.census.gov/. 'U.S. Census Bureau.' US Census Bureau. Accessed 7 October 2000.

http://www.census.gov/geo/www/tiger/index.html. 'Topologically Integrated Geographic Encoding and Referencing system.' US Census Bureau. Accessed 6 October 2000. Updated 3 October 2000.

http://www.db.csu.edu.au/division/dit/span/spatial technology/gis/what gis.html. 'Geographic Information System.' Chicago State University. Accessed 6 October 2000.

http://www.drkoop.com/. 'Drkoop.' Accessed 7 October 2000.

http://www.ebiocare.com/index.asp. 'eBioCare.com.' eBioCare.com. Accessed 7 October 2000. Updated 5 October 2000.

http://www.google.com/. 'Google.' Google. Accessed 6 October 2000.

http://www.hcfa.gov/medicaid/m2082.htm. 'Medicaid Statistical Information System.' Health Care Financing Administration. Accessed 6 October 2000. Updated 17 May 2000.

http://www.hcfa.gov/stats/pufiles.htmpufcat. 'Public Use Files.' Health Care Financing Administration. Accessed 6 October 2000. Updated 29 September 2000.

http://www.health.gov/healthypeople/publications/default.htm. 'Healthy People 2010.' US Department of Health and Human Services. Accessed 6 October 2000.

http://www.health.state.ny.us/nysdoh/research/heart/heart.htm. 'Information for Researchers: Heart Disease.' New York State Department of Health. Accessed 6 October 2000. Updated October 2000.

http://www.insp.mx/ichsri/. 'International Clearinghouse of Health System Reform Initiatives.' Accessed 7 October 2000.

http://www.jhita.org/. 'Health Insurance Portability and Accountability (HIPAA).' Joint Healthcare Information Technology Alliance. Accessed 7 October 2000. Updated 20 July 2000.

http://www.lapublichealth.org/phcommon/complaints/phcomp.cfm. 'REPORT-A-PROBLEM PAGE.' LA PUBLICHEALTH.ORG Public Health Programs. Accessed 6 October 2000.

http://www.lib.berkeley.edu/PUBL/Internet.html. 'Public Health Resources the Internet.' UC Berkeley. Accessed 7 October 2000. Updated 25 September 2000.

http://www.lib.uiowa.edu/hardin/md/. 'Hardin Meta Directory of Internet Health Sources.' University of Iowa. Accessed 7 October 2000. Updated 5 October 2000.

http://www.lib.umich.edu/libhome/Documents.center/sthealth.html. 'Statistical Resources on the Web.' University of Michigan. Accessed 7 October 2000.

http://www.mdconsult.com/. 'MD Consult.' MD Consult. Accessed 6 October 2000.

http://www.measuredhs.com/. 'Demographic and Health Survey.' Accessed 6 October 2000.

http://www.meps.ahrq.gov/. 'Medical Expenditure Panel Survey.' Agency for Healthcare Research and Quality. Accessed 6 October 2000. Updated 24 February 2000.

http://www.nap.edu/. 'National Academy Press.' National Academy Press. Accessed 7 October 2000.

http://www.ncbi.nlm.nih.gov/entrez/query.fcgi. 'National Library of Medicine: PubMed.' National Center for Biotechnology Information. Accessed 7 October 2000.

http://www.ncqa.org/Pages/Programs/HEDIS/index.htm. 'Health Plan Employer Data and Information Set (HEDIS).' NCQA. Accessed 6 October 2000.

http://www.nlm.nih.gov/pubs/cbm/phi2001.html. 'Current Bibliographies in Medicine: Public Health Informatics.' National Library of Medicine. Accessed 23 July 2001. Updated April 2001.

http://www.nnlm.nlm.nih.gov/partners/. 'Partners in Information Access for Public Health Professionals.' Accessed 7 October 2000. Updated 23 March 2000.

http://www.ovid.com/. 'Ovid Technologies.' Ovid Technologies. Accessed 7 October 2000.

http://www.paho.org/English/SHA/bsindcvr.htm. 'HEALTH SITUATION IN THE AMERICAS: BASIC INDICATORS 1995–1998.' Pan American Health Organization. Accessed 6 October 2000.

http://www.paho.org/English/SHA/ihomeibs.htm. 'Pan American Health Organization.' Accessed 7 October 2000.

http://www.peoplesguide.org/. 'L.A. Coalition to End Hunger and Homelessness.' LA Coalition to End Hunger and Homelessness. Accessed 7 October 2000.

http://www.ph.ucla.edu/epi/snow.html. 'John Snow.' Department of Epidemiology, UCLA School of Public Health. Accessed 23 July 2001.

http://www.rti.org/patents/sudaan/sudaan.html. 'SUDAAN.' SUDAAN. Accessed 6 October 2000. Updated 31 March 2000.

http://www.sas.com/. 'SAS.' SAS Institute. Accessed 6 October 2000.

http://www.spss.com/spss10/index.htm. 'SPSS.' SPSS. Accessed 6 October 2000.

http://www.stata.com/. 'STATA.' STATA. Accessed 6 October 2000.

http://www.uiowa.edu/~geog/health/. 'Geographical Information Systems and Public Health.' The University of Iowa. Accessed 23 July 2001.

http://www.webmd.com/. 'WebMD.' WebMD. Accessed 6 October 2000.

6

Epidemiological and biostatistical approaches

6.1 Epidemiology: the foundation of public health

Roger Detels

The subsequent chapters in this section present detailed discussions of the principles and methods of epidemiology. This introductory chapter will attempt to define epidemiology, present ways in which epidemiology is used in the advancement of public health, and discuss the range of applications of epidemiological methodologies.

What is epidemiology?

There are probably as many definitions of epidemiology as there are epidemiologists, although every epidemiologist will know exactly what it is that he or she does! Defining epidemiology is difficult primarily because it does not represent a body of knowledge, as does, for example, anatomy, nor does it target a specific organ system, as does cardiology. Epidemiology represents a philosophical method of studying a health problem and can be applied to a wide range of problems, from transmission of an infectious disease agent to the design of a new strategy of health-care delivery. Furthermore, that methodology is continually changing as it is adapted to a greater range of health problems and more techniques are borrowed and adapted from other disciplines such as mathematics and statistics.

Maxcy, one of the pioneer epidemiologists of the twentieth century, offered the following definition: 'Epidemiology is that field of medical science which is concerned with the relationship of various factors and conditions which determine the frequencies and distributions of an infectious process, a disease, or a physiologic state in a human community' (Lilienfeld 1978). The word itself comes from the Greek *epi*, *demos*, and *logos*; literally translated it means the study (*logos*) of what is among (*epi*) the people (*demos*). Last, in the *Dictionary of Epidemiology*, has defined epidemiology as 'The study of the distribution and determinants of health-related states or events in specified populations, and the application of this study to the control of health problems'. Last's definition emphasizes that epidemiologists are not only concerned with disease but also with 'health-related events', and that ultimately epidemiology is committed to the control of disease. All epidemiologists, however, will agree that epidemiology concerns itself with populations rather than individuals, thereby separating itself from the rest of medicine and constituting the basic science of public health. Following from this, therefore, is the need to describe health and disease in terms of frequencies and distributions in the population. The epidemiologist relates these frequencies and distributions of specific health parameters to the frequencies of other factors to which populations are exposed in order to identify those that may be causes of a disease or promoters of good health. Inherent in the philosophy of epidemiology is the idea that ill health is not randomly distributed in populations, and that elucidating the reasons for this non-random distribution will provide clues regarding the risk factors for disease and the biological mechanisms that result in loss of health. Because epidemiology usually focuses on health in specifically human populations it is rarely able to provide experimental proof in the sense of Koch's postulates, as can often be done in the laboratory sciences. Epidemiology more often provides an accumulation of increasingly convincing indirect evidence of a relationship between health or disease and other factors. This process, referred to as causal inference (Chapter 6.11), includes considering an observed relationship in term of its strength, consistency, specificity, temporality, biological gradient, plausibility, coherence, and experimental evidence (Hill 1965).

Although they will differ on the exact definitions of epidemiology, most epidemiologists will agree that they try to characterize the relationship between the agent, the environment, and the host (usually human). The epidemiologist considers health to represent a balance among these three forces, as shown in Fig. 1.

Changes in any one of these three factors may result in loss of health. For example, the host may be compromised as a result of treatment with steroids, making him or her more susceptible to agents that do not ordinarily cause disease. Conversely, a breakdown in the water supply system may result in an increased exposure of people to hepatitis B, as happened some years ago when the main water supply of New Delhi, the River Jumna, was drastically reduced by drought. Finally, some agents may become more or less virulent over time—often because of the promiscuous use of antibiotics—thereby disturbing the dynamic balance among agent, host, and environment. Two examples are the cases of acute necrotizing fasciitis caused by *Streptococcus* A (Communicable Disease Surveillance Centre 1994) and the development of multidrug-resistant tuberculosis (Chapman and Henderson 1994).

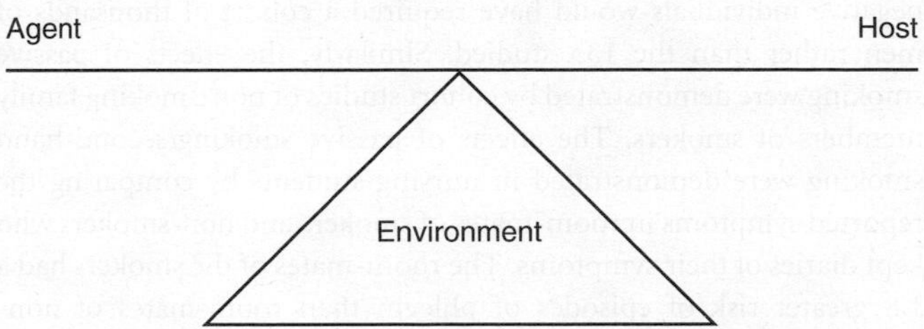

Fig. 1 The relationship between agent, host, and environment in epidemiology.

The epidemiologist uses another triad to study the relationship of agent, host, and environment: time–place–person. Using various epidemiological techniques described in subsequent chapters, the epidemiologist describes disease or disease factors occurring in the population in terms of characteristics of time (for example, trends, outbreaks, and so on), place (the geographic area in which the disease is occurring), and person (the characteristics of the affected individuals, for example age, gender, and so on) to elucidate the causative agent, the natural history of the disease, and the environmental factors that increase the likelihood of the host acquiring the disease. With this information the epidemiologist is able to suggest ways to intervene in the disease process to prevent disease or death.

Epidemiology has been described as the 'art of the possible'. Because epidemiologists work with human populations, they are rarely able to manipulate events or the environment as can the laboratory scientist. They must, therefore, exploit situations as they exist naturally to advance knowledge. They must be both pragmatic and realistic. They must realize both what is possible and what are the limitations of the discipline. Morris has said that the 'epidemiologic method is the only way to ask some questions..., one way of asking others and no way at all to ask many' (Morris 1975). The art of epidemiology is to know both when epidemiology is the method of choice and how to use it to answer the question.

Applying the epidemiological method to resolve a health question successfully can be compared to constructing a memorable Chinese banquet. It is not enough to have the best ingredients and to know the various Chinese cooking methods. The truly great Chinese chefs must be able to select the appropriate ingredients and cooking methods for each individual dish and, furthermore, must know how to construct the correct sequence of dishes to excite the palate without overwhelming it. These chefs create a memorable banquet by adding their creative genius to the raw ingredients and the established cooking methods. Similarly, it is not enough for the epidemiologist to know the various strategies and methods of epidemiology; she or he must be able to apply them creatively to obtain the information needed to understand the natural history of the disease. It is not enough to know what a cohort study is; the epidemiologist must know when the cohort design is the appropriate design for the question at hand, and then must apply that design appropriately and creatively. These skills make epidemiology more than a methodology. It is this opportunity for creativity and innovation that provides excitement for the practitioner and makes the successful practice of epidemiology an art.

For example, Imagawa *et al.* (1989) identified probable transient HIV-1 infection in men, implying clearance of the virus by the immune system of the men by focusing their viral isolation studies on relatively few HIV-1 antibody-negative homosexual men who had many different sexual partners. A simple cohort study of antibody-negative individuals would have required a cohort of thousands of men rather than the 133 studied. Similarly, the effects of passive smoking were demonstrated by cohort studies of non-smoking family members of smokers. The effects of passive smoking/second-hand smoking were demonstrated in nursing students by comparing the reported symptoms in room-mates of smokers and non-smokers who kept diaries of their symptoms. The room-mates of the smokers had a 1.8 greater risk of episodes of phlegm than room-mates of non-smokers (Schwartz and Zeger 1990). Colley *et al.* (1974), Tager *et al.* (1979), and Tashkin *et al.* (1984) demonstrated that children of smokers had lower levels of lung function than children of non-smokers. All of these investigators used traditional study designs, but demonstrated their creativity by applying that design to specific populations which were most likely to reveal a relationship if it existed.

Epidemiological studies rarely provide 'proof' of a causal relationship. Thus, there is continuing debate among epidemiologists about what constitutes adequate criteria for inferring a causal relationship from epidemiological studies (Rothman 1988). Hill (1965) suggested the following criteria for establishing a causal relationship: strength of association (statistical probability and risk ratio), consistency of finding across multiple studies, specificity of the relationship, temporality (outcome follows causation), biological gradient (a dose–response relationship), plausibility, coherence (consistency with prior knowledge), experimental evidence, and analogy (relationship hypothesized similar to that in known relationships). Susser has added to these criteria the ability of the observed relationship to predict other relationships correctly (Rothman 1988). The debate goes on, but the principle is the same: epidemiologic studies seldom provide 'proof' of a causal relationship in the sense of Koch's postulates, but may be used to reveal a possible relationship and build a convincing case that this relationship is causal.

Uses of epidemiology in support of public health

Epidemiology is the basic science of public health because it is the health science that describes health and disease in populations rather than in individuals, information essential for the formulation of effective public health initiatives to prevent disease and promote health in the community. Epidemiology can (a) describe the spectrum of the disease, (b) describe the natural history of the disease, (c) identify factors that increase or decrease the risk of acquiring disease, (d) predict disease trends, (e) elucidate mechanisms of disease transmission, (f) test the efficacy of intervention strategies, (g) evaluate intervention programmes, (h) identify the health needs of a community, and (i) evaluate public health programmes.

Describing the spectrum of the disease

Disease represents the endpoint of a process of alteration of the host's biological systems. Although many disease agents are limited in the range of alterations they can initiate, others, such as measles, can cause a variety of disease endpoints. For example, the majority of infections with measles virus result in the classical febrile disease with a blotchy rash, but the measles virus can also cause generalized haemorrhagic rash and acute encephalitis. Years after initial infection, measles can also cause subacute sclerosing panencephalitis, a fatal disease of the central nervous system.

Various types of epidemiological studies have been used to elucidate the spectrum of disease resulting from many agents and conditions. Cohort studies have been used to document the role of high blood pressure as a major cause of stroke, myocardial infarction, and chronic kidney disease. For rare diseases such as subacute sclerosing panencephalitis and multiple sclerosis, case–control studies have been useful to identify the role of the measles virus (Detels *et al.* 1973; Sullivan *et al.* 1984). Knowing the spectrum of disease that can result from specific infections and conditions allows the public health professional to design more effective intervention strategies; for example, education, screening, and treatment programmes to reduce the prevalence of high blood pressure will also reduce the incidence of myocardial infarction, stroke, and chronic kidney disease (Hypertension Detection and Follow-up Program Cooperative Group 1979).

Describing the natural history of disease

Epidemiological studies can be used to describe the natural history of disease, to elucidate the specific alterations in the biological system in the host, and to improve diagnostic accuracy. For example, cohort studies of individuals who were infected with HIV revealed that a drop in the level of T lymphocytes having the CD4 marker was associated with being infected with HIV, and that a further decline in CD4 cells was associated with developing clinical symptoms and AIDS (Detels *et al.* 1987; Polk *et al.* 1987). This observation stimulated immunologists to focus their research on the interaction of the immune system and HIV. From a clinical perspective, clinicians can target HIV-positive individuals who have declining CD4 cells for prophylactic treatment when it is most likely to be effective. Epidemiology can also be used to describe the impact of treatment on the natural history of disease. For example, a cohort study design was used to demonstrate the public health efficacy of combined highly active retroviral therapy on reducing both the incidence of AIDS and extending survival of those who already had the disease (Detels *et al.* 1998). Thus, describing the natural history of AIDS has assisted researchers to focus their studies and clinicians to use the limited treatment modalities available more effectively (Phair *et al.* 1992). The field of 'clinical epidemiology' applies research on the natural history of disease to improving the diagnostic accuracy of doctors in their clinical practice (Sackett *et al.* 1991).

Identifying factors that increase or decrease the risk of acquiring disease

Having specific characteristics increases the probability that individuals will develop disease. These 'risk factors' may be social (smoking, drinking), genetic (ethnicity), dietary (saturated fats, vitamin deficiencies), and so on. Knowing these risk factors can often provide public health professionals with the necessary tools to design effective programmes to intervene before disease occurs. For example, descriptive, cross-sectional, case–control, cohort, and intervention studies have all shown that smoking is the biggest single risk factor for ill health, because it is a major risk factor for cardiovascular disease, chronic respiratory disease, and many cancers (for example, of the lung, nasopharynx, and bladder). Thus, smoking is the leading cause of disability and death in developed countries, if not the world. Health education campaigns and other strategies to stop or reduce smoking, based on these epidemiological studies, are now a major public health activity in most countries.

Predicting disease trends

The ability to predict future epidemics provides the public health professional with the opportunity to muster the most effective forces to combat the disease. Descriptive studies of many infectious diseases, such as measles, polio, and influenza, have revealed a periodicity of pandemics and epidemics caused by them. Knowledge of these disease patterns has been useful to public health officials to prevent these epidemics.

Studies of the trends of HIV infection in those engaging in high-risk activities, and of changing frequency of high-risk activities, have permitted epidemiologists and statisticians to develop models that predict the number of cases of AIDS likely to occur in 5 to 10 years (Brookmeyer and Damiano 1989; Taylor 1989; Chin *et al.* 1990). This information is particularly useful for public health professionals who must anticipate future health-care needs.

Elucidating mechanisms of disease transmission

Understanding the mechanisms of disease transmission can suggest ways in which public health professionals can protect the public by stopping transmission of the disease agent. Epidemiological studies of the various arboviral encephalitides have incriminated certain species of mosquitoes as the vectors of disease and specific animals as the reservoirs for the viruses. For example, public health efforts in California to prevent western equine encephalitis have concentrated on control of the mosquito vector and vaccination of horses, which are a reservoir of the virus. Although an effective vaccine for smallpox had been available for almost two hundred years, eradication of the disease was not achieved until the recognition that the low infectivity of varicella virus and the relatively long incubation for development of smallpox could be used to develop a strategy of surveillance for cases, with identification and immediate vaccination of all susceptible contacts (containment). Using this containment strategy based on epidemiological principles, smallpox was eradicated through a world-wide effort in less than 10 years (Fenner *et al.* 1988).

Testing the efficacy of intervention strategies

A primary objective of public health is to prevent disease through intervention in the disease process. But a vaccine or other intervention programme must be proven to be effective before it is used in the community. Epidemiological studies (double-blind placebo-controlled trials) are a necessary step in developing an intervention programme, whether that programme is administration of a new vaccine, a behavioural intervention strategy to stop smoking, or a community intervention study to lower heart disease. Although it may be argued that injection of a saline placebo is no longer considered ethical, a proven vaccine, such as polio, can often be used as a placebo for a trial of a new vaccine for a different disease, as was used for trials of rubella vaccines in Taiwan (Detels *et al.* 1969). Widespread use of an intervention not subjected to epidemiological studies of efficacy may result in implementation of an ineffective intervention programme at great public expense and may actually result in greater morbidity and mortality because of an increased reliance on the favoured but unproved intervention and a reduced use of other strategies which are thought to be less effective but which are actually more effective.

Evaluating intervention programmes

Although an intervention such as a vaccine may have been demonstrated to have efficacy in double-blind trials, it may fail to provide protection when used in the community. Double-blind trials may demonstrate the 'biological efficacy' of the vaccine; but if the vaccine is not acceptable to the majority of the public, they will refuse to be vaccinated, and the 'public health efficacy' of the vaccine will be very low. For example, the typhoid vaccine provided some protection against small infecting inocula, but the frequency of unpleasant side-effects with the whole-cell vaccines and the need for multiple injections in the past influenced many people against being vaccinated (Chin 2000).

Another problem of inferring public health efficacy from small vaccine trials is that volunteers for vaccine trials may not be representative of the general public which needs to be protected against a specific disease. Thus broad-based intervention trials also need to be carried out, to demonstrate the acceptability and public health efficacy of a vaccine or other intervention to the population in need of protection.

Since there are adverse side-effects associated with any vaccine, ongoing evaluations of the cost–benefit relationship of specific vaccines are important. By comparing the incidence of smallpox with the incidence of adverse side-effects from the smallpox vaccine, Lane *et al.* (1969) demonstrated that more disease resulted from routine use of the vaccine in the United States than by transmission from imported cases.

There are several epidemiological strategies that can be used for ongoing evaluation of intervention programmes. Serial cross-sectional studies can be used to determine if there has been a change in the prevalence of disease or of indicators of health status over time. The cohort design can be used to compare incidence of disease in comparable populations receiving and not receiving the prevention programme. The case–control design can be used to determine if there are differences in the proportion of cases and non-cases who had the intervention programme.

Identifying the health needs of a community

To be effective in promoting the health of a community or country, health agencies must know what the major health problems of that community are and which subgroups in it are most affected. Cross-sectional studies will reveal the prevalence of disease in the community as well as in specific subgroups of the population, while surveillance programmes can identify trends in disease, infection, and/or health status over time. For example, the prevalence of HIV/AIDS is low in most developed countries, including the United States, but is disproportionately high in some subgroups such as African Americans and poorer communities. With this information, many health departments are now focusing their education, testing, and support programmes for HIV/AIDS on African-Americans and poorer communities.

Evaluating public health programmes

Departments of health are engaged in a variety of activities to promote the health of the community, ranging from vaccination programmes to clinics for the treatment of specific diseases in the poor. Ongoing evaluation of such programmes is necessary to assure that they continue to be cost-effective. Periodic review of routinely collected health statistics can provide information about the effectiveness of many programmes. For those programmes for which relevant statistics are not routinely available, cohort studies and serial cross-sectional studies of the incidence and changing prevalence of the targeted disease in the populations which are the intended recipients of these programmes can measure whether the programmes have had an impact and are cost-effective.

Applications of epidemiology

Specific epidemiological study designs are used to achieve specific public health goals. These goals range from identifying a suspected exposure–disease relationship to establishing that relationship, to designing an intervention to prevent it, and, finally, to assessing the effectiveness of that intervention. The usual sequence of study designs in the identification and resolution of a disease problem are:

- ecological studies
- cross-sectional (prevalence) surveys
- case–control studies
- cohort studies
- experimental studies.

There are, however, many exceptions to the application of this sequence of study designs, depending on such things as the prevalence and virulence of the agent and the nature of the human response to the agent.

The earliest suspicion that a relationship exists between a disease and a possible causative factor is frequently obtained from observing correlations between exposure and disease from existing data such as mortality statistics and surveys of personal or national characteristics. These can be correlations observed across geographical areas (ecological studies) or over time, or a combination of both. Many of the initial epidemiological investigations into chronic bronchitis used vital statistics data, particularly data on mortality. Case–control studies identified smoking as a possible causal factor for chronic bronchitis. Subsequent prevalence studies confirmed the relationship, as have cohort studies. Finally, a decline in respiratory symptoms of chronic bronchitis and a concurrent, but slower decline in lung function, has been observed in individuals who cease smoking (Colley 1991).

Although this is the usual sequence in which the various epidemiological study designs are applied, there are exceptions to this sequence. Furthermore, all study designs are not appropriate to answer all health questions. The usual applications of each of the different epidemiological study designs and the limitations of each are therefore presented briefly below and in greater depth in subsequent chapters.

Ecological studies (Chapter 6.2)

The use of existing statistics to correlate the prevalence or incidence of disease in groups or populations to the frequency or trends over time of suspected causal factors in specific localities has often provided the first clues that a particular factor may cause a specific disease. These epidemiological strategies, however, document only the co-occurrence of disease and other factors in a population; the risk factors and the disease may not be occurring in the same people within the population. These types of descriptive studies are inexpensive and relatively easy to do, but the co-occurrence observed may be due merely to chance. For example, the incidence of both heart disease and lung cancer has increased concurrently with the prevalence of automatic dishwashers in the United States. Few people, however, would attribute the increase in these two diseases to the use of automatic dishwashers. Thus, ecological studies must be interpreted with caution. Nonetheless, they often reveal important relationships and provide a strong rationale for undertaking more expensive analytical studies.

Cross-sectional/prevalence surveys (Chapters 6.3, 6.4, and 6.16)

Cross-sectional/prevalence surveys establish the frequency of disease and other factors in a community. Since they require the collection of data, however, they can be expensive. They are useful to estimate the number of people in a population who have disease and can also identify the difference in frequency of disease in different subpopulations. This descriptive information is particularly useful to health administrators who are responsible for developing appropriate and effective public health programmes. Cross-sectional studies can also be used to document the co-occurrence of disease and suspected risk factors not only in the population but also in specific individuals within the population. The cross-sectional study design is useful to study chronic diseases such as multiple sclerosis and chronic bronchitis, which have a high prevalence, but an incidence that is too low to make a cohort study feasible (Detels *et al.* 1978). Conversely, they are not useful for studying diseases that have a very low prevalence, such as subacute sclerosing panencephalitis. Cross-sectional studies are subject to problems of respondent bias, recall bias, and undocumented confounders. Also, unless historical information is obtained from all the individuals surveyed, the time relationship between the factor and the disease is not known. Furthermore, prevalence surveys identify people who have survived to that time point with disease and, thus, under-represent people with a short course of disease.

The cross-sectional study design is used in two special types of studies: field studies and surveillance. Field studies are usually investigations of acute outbreaks which require immediate identification of the causative factors if effective public health interventions are to be implemented in a timely fashion. Surveillance is the monitoring of disease- or health-related factors over time and uses serial cross-sectional surveys to observe trends. Surveillance is important to identify diseases that are becoming an increasing public health problem, to assure that diseases already brought under control remain under control, and to evaluate the impact of public health intervention strategies.

Case–control studies (Chapter 6.5)

The case–control study compares the prevalence of suspected causal factors between cases and controls. If the prevalence of the factor is significantly different in cases than it is in controls, it suggests that this factor is associated with the disease. Although case–control studies can identify associations, they do not measure risk. An estimate of relative risk, however, can be derived by calculating the odds ratio. Case–control studies are often the analytical study design used initially to investigate a suspected association. Compared to cohort and experimental studies, they are usually relatively cheap and easy to do. Cases can often be selected from hospital patients and controls either from hospital-admitted patients with other diseases or by using algorithms or formulas for selecting community (neighbourhood) or other types of controls, although selection bias is often a problem, especially when using either hospital-admitted cases or controls. The participants are seen only once, and no follow-up is necessary. Although time sequences can often be established for factors elicited by interview, they usually cannot be for laboratory test results. Thus, an elevation in factor 'B' may either be causally related, or it may be a result of the disease process and not a cause. Furthermore, factors elicited from interview are subject to recall bias; for example, patients are often better motivated for recall of events than controls because they are concerned about their disease. The case–control study is particularly useful for exploring relationships noted in observational studies. A hypothesis, however, is necessary for case–control studies. Relationships will be observed only for those factors studied. Case–control studies are not useful for determining the spectrum of health outcomes resulting from specific exposures, since a definition of a case is required in order to do a case–control study. Conversely, case–control studies are the method of choice for studying rare diseases. Case–control studies are often indicated when a specific health question needs to be answered quickly.

Cohort studies (Chapter 6.6)

Cohort studies follow defined groups of people without disease to identify risk factors associated with disease occurrence. Cohort studies have the advantage of establishing the temporal relationship between an exposure and a health outcome, and, thus, they measure risk directly. Because the population studied is defined on the basis of its exposure to the suspected factor, cohort studies are particularly suitable for investigating health hazards associated with environmental or occupational exposures. Furthermore, cohort studies will measure more than one outcome of a given exposure and, therefore, are useful for defining the spectrum of disease resulting from exposure to a given factor. Occasionally a cohort study is done to elucidate the natural history of a disease when a group can be identified that has a high incidence of disease but in which specific risk factors are not known. Although this cohort is not defined on the basis of a known exposure, questions are asked and biological specimens are collected from which exposure variables can be identified concurrently or in the future. Unfortunately, cohort studies are both expensive and time-consuming. Unless the investigator can define a cohort in which risk factors were measured at some time in the past and has assurance that the cohort has been completely followed up for disease outcome in the interim, the cohort design can take years to decades to yield information about the risks of disease resulting from exposure to specific factors. Assuring that participants remain in a cohort study for such long periods of time is both difficult and expensive. Furthermore, the impact of those who drop out of follow-up must be taken into account in the analysis and interpretation of cohort studies. Finally, exposures may vary over time, complicating the analysis of their impact. Because of the cost and complexity of cohort studies, they are usually done only after descriptive, cross-sectional, and/or case–control studies have suggested a causal relationship. The size of the cohort to be studied is partly dependent on the anticipated incidence of the disease resulting from the exposure. For diseases with a very low incidence, cohort studies usually are not feasible, either in terms of the logistics or of the expense of following very large numbers of people, or both. Cohort studies establish the risk of disease associated with exposure to a factor, but do not 'prove' that the factor is causal. The observed factor merely may be very closely correlated with the real causative factor or may even be related to the participants' choice to be exposed.

A variant of the cohort study which has become popular is the 'nested case–control' study (Gange *et al.* 1997). Cases which arise from a cohort study are compared to individuals followed in the cohort who have not developed disease using the usual case–control analytical strategies. The advantage of this type of study is that the exposure variables are collected before knowledge of the outcome and therefore are unlikely to be tainted by recall bias.

Experimental studies (Chapters 6.7 to 6.9)

Experimental studies differ from cohort studies because it is the investigator who makes the decision about who will be exposed to the factor based on the specific design factors to be employed (for example, randomization, matching, and so on). Therefore, confounding factors that may have led to the subjects being exposed in the cohort studies are not a problem in experimental studies. Because epidemiologists usually study human populations, there are few opportunities for an investigator to deliberately expose participants to a suspected factor. Conversely, intervention studies of individuals randomly assigned to receive or not receive an intervention programme that demonstrates a subsequent reduction in a specific health outcome in the intervention group do provide strong evidence, if not proof, of a causal relationship. Because of the serious implications of applying an intervention that may alter the biological status of an individual, intervention studies are not undertaken until the probability of a causal relationship has been well established using the other types of study designs.

Meta-analysis (Chapter 6.12)

A recent trend has been to combine similar studies to increase the power of the analysis because individual epidemiological studies rarely provide proof of causation and results of different studies can vary for a number of reasons, including small sample size. This strategy for data synthesis is known as 'meta-analysis'. It has been especially helpful in studying diseases with a low incidence or where different studies have given conflicting results.

Methodological issues (Chapters 6.10 and 6.11)

Epidemiological studies, because they deal with humans, are subject to problems such as bias (deviation of results from truth) due to the strategies of recruiting participants, or to differential recall among persons with and without disease and confounding due to factors which are associated with both the exposure variables and outcome variable under study. In the last several decades many new techniques have been developed to reduce the effect of these factors which can influence the outcome of a study and, in some instances, can cause apparent relationships to be observed which are false.

Summary

Epidemiology is the basic science of public health because it is the science that describes the relationship of health or disease with other factors in human populations. Furthermore, epidemiology is used to generate much of the information required by public health professionals to develop, implement, and evaluate effective intervention programmes for the prevention of disease and the promotion of health, such as the eradication of smallpox, the anticipated eradication of polio and guinea worm disease, and the recent decline in heart disease in most of the developed countries. Finally, it is the best strategy to evaluate the effectiveness of public health programmes.

Unlike pathology, which constitutes a basic area of knowledge, and cardiology, which is the study of a specific organ, epidemiology is a medical philosophy or methodology that can be applied to learning about and resolving a very broad range of health problems. The art of epidemiology is knowing when and how to apply epidemiological methods creatively to answer specific health questions; it is not enough to know what the various study designs and statistical methodologies are. The uses and limitations of the various epidemiological study designs have been presented to illustrate and underscore the fact that the successful application of epidemiology requires more than a knowledge of study designs and epidemiological methods. These designs and methods must be applied both appropriately and innovatively if they are to yield the desired information. The field of epidemiology has been expanding dramatically over the last two decades, as more epidemiologists have demonstrated new uses and variations of traditional study designs and methods. The uses of epidemiology will expand even more in the future as increasing numbers of creative epidemiologists develop new strategies and techniques of epidemiology.

References

Brookmeyer, R. and Damiano, A. (1989). Statistical methods for short-term projections of AIDS incidence. *Statistics in Medicine*, **8**, 23–34.

Chapman, S.W. and Henderson, H.M. (1994). New and emerging pathogens multiply resistant *Mycobacterium tuberculosis. Current Opinion in Infectious Diseases*, **7**, 231–7.

Chin, J. (2000). *Control of communicable diseases manual.* American Public Health Association, Washington, DC.

Chin, J., Sato P., and Mann, J. (1990). Projections of HIV infections and AIDS cases to the year 2000. *Bulletin of the World Health Organization*, **68**, 1–11.

Colley, J.R.T. (1991). Major public health problems; respiratory system. In *Oxford textbook of public health* (2nd edn) (ed. W.W. Holland, R. Detels, and G. Knox), (Volume 3), pp. 227–48. Oxford University Press.

Colley, J.R.T., Holland W.W., and Corkhill R.T. (1974). Influence of passive smoking and parental phlegm on pneumonia and bronchitis in early childhood. *Lancet*, **ii**, 1031–4.

Communicable Disease Surveillance Centre (1994). Invasive group A streptococcal infections in Gloucestershire. *Communicable Disease Report (England/Wales)*, **4**, 97–100.

Detels, R., Grayston, J.T., Kim, K.S.W., *et al.* (1969). Prevention of clinical and subclinical rubella infection: efficacy of three HPV-77 derivative vaccines. *American Journal of Diseases of Children*, **118**, 295–300.

Detels, R., McNew, J., Brody, J.A., and Edgar, A.H. (1973). Further epidemiological studies of subacute sclerosing panencephalitis. *Lancet*, **819**, 11–14.

Detels, R., Visscher, B.R., Haile, R.W., Malmgren, R.M., Dudley, J.P., and Coulson, A.H. (1978). Multiple sclerosis and age at migration. *American Journal of Epidemiology*, **108**, 386–93.

Detels, R., Visscher, B.R., Fahey, J.L., *et al.* (1987). Predictors of clinical AIDS in young homosexual men in a high-risk area. *International Journal of Epidemiology*, **16**, 271–6.

Detels, R., Munoz, A., McFarlane, G., *et al.* (1998). Effectiveness of potent antiretroviral therapy on time to AIDS and death in men with known HIV infection duration. *Journal of the American Medical Association*, **280**, 1497–1503.

Fenner, F., Henderson, D.A., Arita, I., Jezek, Z., and Ladnyi, I.D. (1988). *Smallpox and its eradication*. World Health Organization, Geneva.

Gange, S., Munoz, A., Schrager, L.K., *et al.* (1997). Design of nested studies to identify factors related to late progression of HIV infection. *Journal of Acquired Immune Deficiency Syndromes and Human Retroviruses*, **15** (Supplement), S5–9.

Hill, A.B. (1965). The environment and disease: association or causation? *Proceedings of the Royal Society of Medicine*, **58**, 295–300.

Hypertension Detection and Follow-up Program Co-operative Group (1979). Five-year findings of the hypertension detection and follow-up program. I. Reduction in mortality of persons with high blood pressure, including mild hypertension. *Journal of the American Medical Association*, **242**, 2562–71.

Imagawa, D.T., Lee, M.H., Wolinsky, S.M., *et al.* (1989). Human immunodeficiency virus type 1 infection in homosexual men who remain seronegative for prolonged periods. *New England Journal of Medicine*, **320**, 1458–62.

Lane, J.M., Ruben, F.L., Neff, J.M., and Millar, J.D. (1969). Complications of smallpox vaccination, 1968: national surveillance in the United States. *New England Journal of Medicine*, **281**, 1201–8.

Lilienfeld, D.E. (1978). Definitions of epidemiology. *American Journal of Epidemiology*, **107**, 87–90.

Morris, J.N. (1975). *Uses of epidemiology* (3rd edn). Churchill Livingstone, London.

Phair, J., Jacobson, L., Detels, R., *et al.* (1992). Acquired immune deficiency syndrome occurring within 5 years of infection with human immunodeficiency virus type-1: the Multicenter AIDS Cohort Study. *Journal of Acquired Immune Deficiency Syndromes*, **5**, 490–6.

Polk, B.F., Fox, R., Brookmeyer, R., *et al.* (1987). Predictors of the acquired immunodeficiency syndrome developing in a cohort of seropositive homosexual men. *New England Journal of Medicine*, **316**, 61–6.

Rothman, K.J. (ed.) (1988). *Causal inference*. Epidemiology Resources, Chestnut Hill, MA.

Sackett, D.L., Haynes, R.B., Buyatt, G.H., and Tugwell, P. (1991). *Clinical epidemiology, a basic science for clinical medicine*. Little, Brown, London.

Schwartz, J. and Zeger, S. (1990). Passive smoking, air pollution, and acute respiratory symptoms in a diary study of student nurses. *American Review of Respiratory Disease*, **141**, 62–7.

Sullivan, C.B., Visscher, B.R., and Detels, R. (1984). Multiple sclerosis and age at exposure to childhood diseases and animals: cases and their friends. *Neurology*, **34**, 1144–8.

Tager, I.B., Weiss, S.T., Rosner, B., and Speizer, F.E. (1979). Effect of parental cigarette smoking on the pulmonary function of children. *American Journal of Epidemiology*, **110**, 15–26.

Tashkin, D.P., Clark, V.A., Simmons, M., *et al.* (1984). The UCLA Population Studies of Chronic Obstructive Respiratory Disease: VII. relationship between parental smoking and children's lung function. *American Review of Respiratory Disease*, **129**, 891–7.

Taylor, J.M.G. (1989). Models for the HIV infection and AIDS epidemic in the United States. *Statistics in Medicine*, **8**, 45–58.

6.2 Ecological variables, ecological studies, and multilevel studies in public health research

Ana V. Diez Roux, Sharon Schwartz, and Ezra Susser

There has been much discussion in epidemiology about the utility of ecological studies in investigating the causes of disease. Epidemiology textbooks commonly appraise this study design as a crude attempt to ascertain individual-level relationships. It is argued that ecological studies should be limited to 'hypothesis generation', leaving the more esteemed process of 'hypothesis testing' to individual-level data. The limitations of ecological studies are generally attributed to the ecological fallacy, that is the well-established logical fallacy inherent in making inferences regarding individual-level associations based on group-level data (Morgenstern 1982, 1995; Piantadosi *et al.* 1988; Greenland 1992). However, in recent years, interest in potential ecological or group-level determinants of health has led epidemiologists to reconsider the utility and limitations of ecological studies (Susser 1994*a*,*b*). In this context, there has been renewed interest in the notion that group-level (or ecological) variables may provide information which is not always captured by individual level data (Schwartz 1994; Susser 1994*a*,*b*; Koopman and Lynch 1999), and in rethinking the ways in which these group-level constructs can be examined in epidemiological analyses. More broadly, there has been growing recognition of the need to consider multiple levels of organization (for example, from molecules to society) in studying the determinants of health and disease.

Many of the conceptual and analytical issues that arise when considering the uses of ecological studies and ecological variables derive from the presence of multiple levels of organization and nested data structures more generally. For example, many problems that arise when dealing with individuals nested within groups (for example, people nested within geographical areas), are also present when dealing with groups nested within larger groups (for example, states nested within countries), people nested within families, or multiple measurements on individuals over time (in this case the 'group' is the individual, and the 'individuals' are the measurement occasions). In fact the need to deal with multiple levels of organization is the norm rather than the exception in epidemiology.

The presence of multiple levels has several implications. Firstly, the units of analysis (or observations for which independent and dependent variables are measured) can be defined at different levels. The unit of analysis determines the level at which variability is examined. For example, a study with individuals as the units of analysis (that is, where each observation is an individual) can investigate the causes of interindividual variation in the outcome. A study with groups as the units of analysis (where observations are groups), can investigate the causes of intergroup variation in the outcome. A study involving repeated measures on individuals over time in which measures at different points in time are the units of analysis can investigate the causes of variability across measures. As will be shown, the use of units of analysis at one level to make inferences about the causes of variability at a different level leads to a series of methodological problems.

The second implication of the presence of multiple levels is that both independent and dependent variables can be conceptualized (and measured) at different levels. Constructs pertaining to a higher level may be important in understanding variability at a lower level, and, conversely, constructs defined at a lower level may be important in understanding variability at a higher level. For example, characteristics of the groups to which individuals belong may be important in explaining interindividual variability, and characteristics of individuals comprising the groups may be important in explaining intergroup variability. Analogously, when looking at multiple measures on individuals over time, individual characteristics may be important in understanding variability across measures, and factors specific to measurement occasions may be important in understanding interindividual variability.

This chapter discusses the use of ecological variables, ecological studies, and individual-level and multilevel studies in epidemiology within the broader context of the implications of multiple levels of organization for understanding disease aetiology. As discussed in the sections to follow, the particular research question investigated should guide decisions regarding the most appropriate unit of analysis (and level at which variability in the outcome is examined) as well as the relevant constructs to be investigated as predictors (and the levels at which they are defined and measured). Although the discussion will focus on the simple case of individuals nested within groups, it is generalizable to many other situations involving nested data structures, as noted above.

We begin by reviewing the classical distinction between ecological and individual-level studies made in epidemiology. Next, we review the sources of the 'ecological fallacy', placing this fallacy within the context of other fallacies which may arise when the presence of multiple levels is ignored. Finally, we review the full range of study designs available to investigators based on (a) the units of analysis (and the level at which variability is examined) and (b) the levels at which relevant constructs are defined and measured.

Ecological studies and studies of individuals

Epidemiology has traditionally distinguished two types of studies based on the units of analysis: ecological studies and studies of individuals. Ecological studies are studies in which groups are the units of analysis: both the dependent and the independent variables are measured for groups, and intergroup variability (and associations between independent and dependent variables across groups), are examined. For example, common ecological studies in public health involve measuring rates of disease for different geographic areas, and relating these rates to area social or physical characteristics (for example, measures of area median income, levels of air pollution, water hardness, radiation). Ecological studies are often cross-sectional with independent and dependent variables measured at the same point in time. However, ecological studies can also involve repeated measures on a group, or on several groups, over time, as in time-trend studies (Susser 1994*b*; Morgenstern 1995). For example, an ecological study could examine yearly incidence rates of disease for different regions over a 10-year period and investigate the relation of these incidence rates to area characteristics that do and do not change over time. Although not common in the epidemiological literature, ecological studies could also use a case–control approach, in which a sample of ecological cases (groups with a certain outcome, for example a disease rate above a certain level) are compared with a sample of ecological controls. Ecological studies could also involve the analysis of groups randomized to receive or not receive an intervention, as in randomized trials. In many ecological studies the predominant analytic approach involves the estimation of correlation coefficients between the group-level exposure and the group-level outcome. However, many other analytic approaches are also possible, including the estimation of other measures of association (such as rate differences or rate ratios) using linear or log-linear models (Morgenstern 1995).

In contrast, in individual-level studies (the studies commonly referred to under headings of 'study design' in epidemiological textbooks) the units of analysis are individuals: both independent and dependent variables are measured for individuals and interindividual variation (and associations between independent and dependent variables across individuals) are investigated. Based on their design, individual-level studies can be cross-sectional (when both independent and dependent variables are measured at the same point in time), cohort (when individuals free of the outcome at baseline are followed over time to compare risk of the outcome in exposed and unexposed), or case–control (when a sample of people with the outcome is compared with a sample of controls with regard to the presence of certain exposures).

The information these two study designs provide (and the information they lack) differs because the units of analysis are not the same. Ecological studies include information on group characteristics (which may sometimes summarize the characteristics of individuals in the group), but lack information on the cross-classification of individual-level characteristics within groups. For example, an ecological study may relate the percentage of smokers in different groups to mortality rates, but have no information on whether, within groups, smokers were actually the ones more likely to die. Conversely, individual-level studies focus on interindividual variation, and have information on individual-level characteristics but often lack information on characteristics of the groups to which individuals belong.

Uses of ecological studies in public health

Descriptive ecological studies in which rates of disease or death are compared over time or across geographic areas have been a staple of epidemiology for centuries (Susser 1973). Chadwick used an ecological approach in his famous *Report on the sanitary condition of the labouring population of Great Britain* in 1842 (Chadwick 1965). Table 1 shows a portion of Chadwick's Report, in which a drained area is compared with an undrained area at three parallel points in time. By comparing mortality rates over time in both communities (one drained and the other undrained), he was able to draw inferences regarding the relationship between drainage and ill health. Drainage was the 'exposure', mortality the outcome, and communities the units of analysis. With these findings Chadwick had grounds to institute a system of sanitation nationwide. Although the miasmatic theory of disease causation which Chadwick espoused (and which he believed was supported by his data) was later shown to be mistaken, the method of sanitation that Chadwick introduced was probably as important as any other single measure in modern times (Susser 1973).

Early in his studies, Snow also used an ecological approach in comparing cholera rates for London districts, and examining whether differences in these rates were related to differences in the sources of water (Susser 1973) (Table 2). The units of analyses were districts, and both the independent variable (source of water) and the dependent variable (cholera rates) were conceptualized and measured at the district level. At the beginning of this century, Goldberger *et al.* (1920) also used an ecological approach to demonstrate that pellagra was not 'an intestinal infection transmitted in much the same way as typhoid fever', as was argued by many at the time. These findings laid the groundwork for much of Goldberger and Sydenstricker's later work relating diet and economic conditions to pellagra in the southern United States (Terris 1964).

More recently, in the chronic disease era, ecological studies relating rates of cardiovascular disease across countries to risk factor prevalences (Keys' Seven Country Study) laid the foundation for future work on the epidemiology and causes of cardiovascular disease (Keys 1980). For example, data from the Seven Country Study showed a

Table 1 Death rates compared in three successive decades in a drained and an undrained town

The following was the proportion of deaths to the population in the two towns	Beccles	Bungay
Between 1811 and 1821	1 in 67	1 in 69
Between 1821 and 1831	1 in 72	1 in 67
Between 1831 and 1841	1 in 71	1 in 59

Chadwick says in conclusion 'You will therefore see that the rate of mortality has gradually diminished in Beccles since it has been drained, whilst Bungay, notwithstanding its larger proportion of rural population, has considerably increased'

Source: Chadwick (1965) (originally published in 1842).

Table 2 Showing the mortality from cholera, and the water supply, in the districts of London in 1849; the districts are arranged in the order of their mortality from cholera

District	Population	Deaths from cholera	Deaths by cholera to 10 000 inhabitants	Annual value of house and shop room to each person (£)	Water supply
Rotherhithe	17 208	352	205	4.238	Southwark and Vauxhall Water Works, Kent Water Works, and Tidal Ditches
St Olave, Southwark	19 278	349	181	4.559	Southwark and Vauxhall
St George, Southwark	50 900	836	164	3.518	Southwark and Vauxhall, Lambeth
Bermondsey	45 500	734	161	3.077	Southwark and Vauxhall
St Saviour, Southwark	35 227	539	153	5.291	Southwark and Vauxhall
Newington	63 074	907	144	3.788	Southwark and Vauxhall, Lambeth
Lambeth	134 768	1618	120	4.389	Southwark and Vauxhall, Lambeth
Wandsworth	48 446	484	100	4.839	Pump-wells, Southwark and Vauxhall, River Wandle
Camberwell	51 714	504	97	4.508	Southwark and Vauxhall, Lambeth
West London	28 829	429	96	7.454	New River
Bethnal Green	87 263	789	90	1.480	East London
Shoreditch	104 122	789	76	3.103	New River, East London
Greenwich	95 954	718	75	3.379	Kent
Poplar	44 103	313	71	7.360	East London
Westminster	64 109	437	68	4.189	Chelsea
Whitechapel	78 590	506	64	3.388	East London
St Giles	54 062	285	53	5.635	New River
Stepney	106 988	501	47	3.319	East London
Chelsea	53 379	247	46	4.210	Chelsea
East London	43 495	182	45	4.823	New River
St George's, East	47 334	199	42	4.753	East London
London City	55 816	207	38	17.676	New River
St Martin	24 557	91	37	11.844	New River
Strand	44 254	156	35	7.374	New River
Holborn	46 134	161	35	5.883	New River
St Luke, Kensington (except Paddington)	110 491	260	33	5.070	West Middlesex, Chelsea, Grand Junction
Lewisham	32 299	96	30	4.824	Kent
Belgrave	37 918	105	28	8.875	Chelsea
Hackney	55 152	139	25	4.397	New River, East London
Islington	87 761	187	22	5.494	New River
St Pancras	160 122	360	22	4.871	New River, Hampstead, West Middlesex
Clerkenwell	63 499	121	19	4.138	New River
Marylebone	153 960	261	17	7.586	West Middlesex
St. James, Westminster	36 426	57	16	12.669	Grand Junction, New River
Paddington	41 267	35	8	9.349	Grand Junction
Hampstead	11 572	9	8	5.804	Hampstead, West Middlesex
Hanover Square and May Fair	33 196	26	8	16.754	Grand Junction
London	2280 282	14 137	62	–	

Source: Snow (1936) (originally published in 1855).

clear relationship between the average proportion of calories derived from saturated fat and coronary heart disease mortality. Another recent example is provided by psychiatric epidemiology. Ecological studies have demonstrated that the incidence of acute transient psychoses varies dramatically across sociocultural settings. In the World Health Organization (**WHO**) Ten Country Study, for instance, the incidence of non-affective acute remitting psychosis was 10-fold higher in developing than in developed country settings (Susser and Wanderling 1994). These studies have led to testing of specific hypotheses about causation, including antecedent fever and culturally normative life events.

Much useful public health information has been obtained from ecological studies. However, as illustrated throughout this chapter, both studies of individuals and studies with groups as the units of analysis have their limitations. The degree to which a given study design is appropriate depends on the particular research problem. Snow's research provides an illustrative example. Four years after Snow's initial investigation (illustrated in Table 2), one of the companies, the Lambeth Company, had moved its waterworks to a point higher up on the Thames, thus obtaining a supply of water free from the sewage of London. This meant that within a single district, some houses were receiving water drawn from one place on the Thames and others were receiving water drawn from a different point. Thus, the district as the unit of analysis was no longer appropriate. In Snow's words 'To turn this grand experiment into account, all that was required was to learn the supply of water to each individual house where a fatal attack of cholera might occur' (cited in Susser 1973). Snow subsequently confirmed his original findings by examining the relation between source of water and cholera risk with households, rather than districts, as the units of analysis (Table 3).

The following two sections, which focus on 'fallacies' related to the existence of multiple levels of organization, discuss some of the limitations and potentialities of both ecological studies and studies of individuals. A discussion of the ecological fallacy begins these sections because it is the fallacy most commonly mentioned in epidemiology. How traditional studies of individuals may also be subject to other types of fallacies, which are less often discussed in the epidemiological literature, is then discussed.

The ecological fallacy

The post-Second World War emphasis in epidemiology in investigating interindividual variability, and the implicit assumption that all relevant predictors can be conceptualized as individual-level constructs, has led to a critique of ecological studies. This critique is based on the well-established ecological fallacy. The ecological fallacy is the fallacy of drawing inferences at the individual level (that is, regarding variability across individuals) based on group-level data. The most common example of the ecological fallacy involves situations in which group-level variables are used as proxies for unavailable individual-level exposures. For example, in order to study the relation between exposure to substance X and cancer in the absence of individual-level data, the prevalence of exposure to X in different areas is related to cancer rates in those areas. In this case, information is unavailable on exactly who is exposed to X and who is not, and so the area prevalence of X is used as a rough approximation for the exposure of each area resident. Since information is lacking on the joint distribution of exposure and outcome at the individual level (that is, it is unknown whether people who developed cancer were actually exposed to X) it is impossible to conclude that individuals exposed to X have a higher risk of lung cancer even if it is found that areas with higher per cent exposed to X have higher cancer rates. In addition, information is unavailable on other individual-level characteristics related to cancer which may also vary between areas and may confound the ecological relationship. Another example is provided by the relation between mean income and obesity when mean income is used as a proxy for individual-level income. Suppose that a researcher finds that, at the country level, higher mean income is associated with higher prevalence of obesity (or increased body mass index). If it is inferred that within countries higher income is associated with higher body mass index, the researcher may be committing the ecological fallacy, because within countries body mass index may always be higher in low-income than in high-income people. In addition, people living in countries with high mean income may differ from those living in countries with low mean income in terms of other individual characteristics related to body mass index.

Sources of the ecological fallacy

The ecological fallacy arises when associations between two variables at the group level (or ecological level) differ from associations between analogous variables measured at the individual level. An analysis of the reasons that lead to this difference is helpful in understanding what each type of study can or cannot reveal. These differences between individual-level and group-level associations were first described for correlation coefficients (Robinson 1950) but may also be present for other measures of associations such as linear regression coefficients (Morgenstern 1982). Because the use of correlation coefficients raises additional complexities (and because of its limitations as a measure of association), the following discussion will focus on linear regression coefficients as the main measure of association estimated at both the group and the individual level.

The example on income and obesity used above is schematically illustrated in Fig. 1. At the group or country level, mean body mass index increases with increasing mean income. At the same time, for individuals within countries, body mass index decreases with increasing individual-level income. This situation arises because

Table 3 Cholera death rates by company supplying household water

Company	Number of houses	Deaths from cholera	Deaths in each 10 000 houses
Southwark and Vauxhall Company	40 046	1263	315
Lambeth Company	26 107	98	37
Rest of London	256 423	1422	59

Source: Snow (1936) (originally published in 1855).

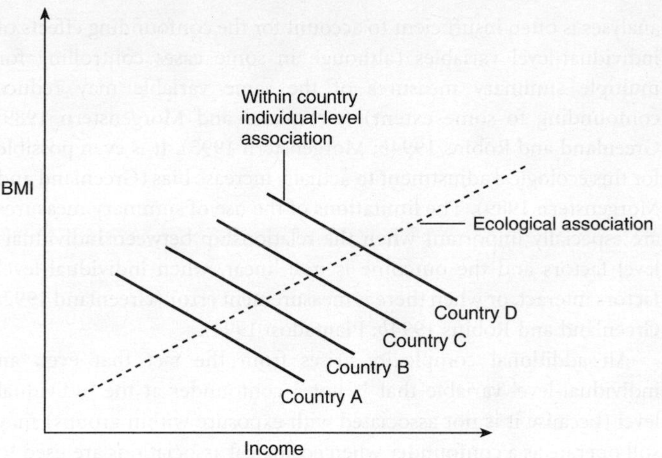

Fig. 1 Hypothetical associations of income with body mass index within and between countries. No interaction between mean country income and individual-level income.

group-level mean income is related to body mass index independently of individual-level income (or in other words because there is a group effect). People living in countries with higher mean income have generally higher body mass indexes than those living in countries with lower mean income, regardless of their individual-level income.

Another situation is depicted in Fig. 2, where the relation between individual-level income and body mass index differs by mean country income: in countries with higher mean income, individual-level income is strongly and inversely related to body mass index, whereas this relation is non-existent, or perhaps exists in the opposite direction, in countries with lower mean income. Here the group-level variable (average income of the country in which a person lives) modifies the effect of individual-level income on the outcome. In this case, group-level associations (the relation between mean country income and mean country body mass index) will also differ from individual-level associations (the relationship between individual-level income and individual-level body mass index). In addition, individual-level associations will differ from country to country, according to levels of mean country income. Thus, when a group-level variable is related to the outcome independently of the analogous variable measured at the individual level, or when the group-level variable modifies the effects of its individual-level analogue on the outcome, ecological associations (which express the relationship between group-level variables and group-level outcomes) will differ from the corresponding individual-level associations (which express the relationship between individual-level variables and individual-level outcomes) (Hammond 1973; Firebaugh 1978; Greenland and Morgenstern 1989; Levin 1995).

The concepts summarized above can also be expressed mathematically. Suppose that the 'true' relationship between country mean income, individual-level income, and individual-level body mass index is reflected in the following equation:

$$Y_{ij} = B_0 + B_1 X_{ij} + B_2 \bar{X}_j \quad (1)$$

where Y_{ij} is the body mass index for the ith individual in the jth country, X_{ij} is the income for the ith individual in the jth country, $\bar{X}_j$ is the mean X_{ij} in country j, B_1 is the mean difference in individual-level body mass index per unit difference in individual-level income, and B_2 is the mean difference in individual-level body mass index per unit difference in mean country income. Thus, body mass index for each individual is related not only to his or her own income, but also to the mean income for the country in which he or she lives. In the equation above, B_1 reflects the individual-level relation between X_{ij} and Y_{ij}. Since it is 'adjusted' for the group effect (to the extent that between-group differences are entirely captured by B_2) it is equivalent to the within-group effect of individual-level income (or the average within-group effect if this varies across groups). B_1 is what we would like to estimate in order to quantify the individual-level effect of X_{ij} on Y_{ij}. B_2 reflects the relation between mean country income ($\bar{X}_j$) and Y_{ij}, after controlling for X_{ij} (that is, the effect of mean country income on individual-level body mass index after controlling for individual-level income). (Equation (1) can also be modified to allow interactions between X_{ij} and $\bar{X}_j$ as shown in Fig. 2. For simplicity this situation will not be illustrated, but the discussion that follows applies as well.)

Suppose that instead of this full equation showing the relationship between body mass index and individual-level income and mean country income, we fit the ecological equation

$$\bar{Y}_j = B_{e0} + B_{e1} \bar{X}_j \quad (2)$$

where $\bar{Y}_j$ is the mean body mass index in country j, $\bar{X}_j$ is the mean income in country j, and B_{e1} is the mean difference in mean country body mass index per unit change in mean country income. (The subscript 'e' is used in this case because regression coefficients refer to ecological or group-level associations.) In this case B_{e1} reflects the ecological relation between mean country income ($\bar{X}_j$) and mean country body mass index ($\bar{Y}_j$). It is sometimes referred to as the between-group effect. Clearly, B_{e1}(the between-group effect) is not equivalent to B_1 (the within-group effect of $\bar{X}_{ij}$) or B_2 (the effect of $\bar{X}_j$) in eqn (1). In fact both the individual level within group effect (B_1) and the effect of mean $\bar{X}_j$ (B_2) are confounded in the ecological regression coefficient (B_{e1}).

Yet a third alternative is to fit a purely individual-level equation ignoring group membership:

$$Y_{ij} = B_{p0} + B_{p1} X_{ij} \quad (3)$$

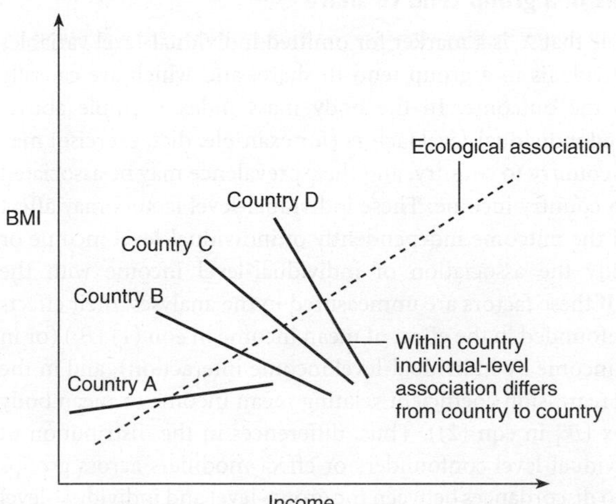

Fig. 2 Hypothetical associations of income with body mass index within and between countries. Mean country income interacts with individual-level income.

(The subscript 'p' is used in this case because regression coefficients refer to associations between individual-level variables pooled across groups.) B_{p1} reflects the effect of X_{ij} on Y_{ij} pooling across groups and ignoring group membership (it is unadjusted for any potential group effects). When group effects are present, B_{p1} will differ from B_1 (the within-group effect) in eqn (1), and will also differ from B_{e1} (the ecological effect of $\overline{X}_j$) in eqn (2). Both the within-group effects of X_{ij} and the effect of $\overline{X}_j$ on Y_{ij} are confounded in B_{p1}.

In the absence of group effects (for example, when B_2 in eqn (1) is zero) and when there is no interaction between $\overline{X}_j$ and X_{ij} (the group and individual-level variables), B_1 (within-group effect), B_{e1} (ecological effect), and B_{p1} (pooled individual effect) are all equivalent. However, in the presence of group effects B_e does not equal B_1 or B_{p1} (source of the ecological fallacy). In addition, B_{p1} does not equal B_{e1} or B_2. When group effects are present, B_{p1} will be a weighted average of B_1 and B_{e1}, and will lie between them, although the order of magnitude of B_1 and B_{e1} cannot be predicted (Piantadosi *et al.* 1988). Here it is important to note that, although results for correlation coefficients generally follow those for regression coefficients outlined above, individual-level (within-group) and ecological (between-group) correlation coefficients may differ even in the absence of group effects (that is, even when $B_1 = B_{e1} = B_{p1}$) (Hammond 1973; Piantadosi *et al.* 1988). This is because correlations also depend on the relative dispersion of X and Y (Piantadosi *et al.* 1988; Morgenstern 1982).

As illustrated above, ecological associations will differ from individual-level associations in the presence of group effects, that is when B_2 in eqn (1) does not equal zero (or when the interaction between X_{ij} and $\overline{X}_j$ in eqn (1) does not equal zero). The key to understanding the sources of the ecological fallacy therefore lies in specifying the conditions under which B_2 (the independent effect of $\overline{X}_j$) or the interaction between $\overline{X}_j$ and X_{ij} will differ from zero. Several different situations may result in non-zero values for B_2 or for the interaction term between X_{ij} and $\overline{X}_j$. These include situations where the group mean X_{ij} ($\overline{X}_j$) is a marker for omitted individual-level variables which individuals in a group tend to share, and situations where mean X_{ij} at the group level measures a different construct than $\overline{X}_{ij}$ at the individual level. Both situations will be discussed in more detail below.

$\overline{X}_j$ is a marker for omitted individual-level variables which individuals in a group tend to share

It is possible that $\overline{X}_j$ is a marker for omitted individual-level variables which individuals in a group tend to share, and which are causally related to the outcome. In the body mass index example above, unmeasured individual-level factors (for example, diet, exercise) may vary from country to country, and their prevalence may be associated with mean country income. These individual-level factors may affect the risk of the outcome independently of individual-level income or may modify the association of individual-level income with the outcome. If these factors are unmeasured in the analyses, their effects will be confounded in the effect of mean income in eqn (1) (B_2) (or in the mean income by individual-level income interaction), and in the ecological regression coefficient relating mean income to mean body mass index (B_{e1} in eqn (2)). Thus, differences in the distribution of these individual-level confounders or effect modifiers across groups may lead to discordances between the group-level and individual-level associations of income and body mass index. Summary ecological measures of these individual-level factors for each group are sometimes available (for example, per cent sedentary, or mean dietary fat). However, controlling for these summary measures in ecological analyses is often insufficient to account for the confounding effects of individual-level variables (although in some cases controlling for multiple summary measures of the same variable may reduce confounding to some extent) (Greenland and Morgenstern 1989; Greenland and Robins 1994*b*; Morgenstern 1995). It is even possible for this ecological adjustment to actually increase bias (Greenland and Morgenstern 1989). The limitations of the use of summary measures are especially important when the relationship between individual-level factors and the outcome is non-linear, when individual-level factors interact, or when there is measurement error (Greenland 1992; Greenland and Robins 1994*b*; Piantadosi 1994).

An additional complexity arises from the fact that even an individual-level variable that is not a confounder at the individual level (because it is not associated with exposure within groups) may still operate as a confounder when ecological associations are used to draw individual-level inferences, if it is ecologically associated with the exposure prevalence across groups (Greenland and Morgenstern 1989; Greenland 1992). Similarly, even weak effect modifiers at the individual level may lead to important differences between ecological and individual-level associations, if their prevalence differs across groups (Greenland and Morgenstern 1989). Conversely, a variable that is a confounder at the individual level (because it is associated with the exposure and the outcome within groups) may not confound the analogous ecological association if it is ecologically unassociated with the exposure across groups (Morgenstern 1995; Greenland and Robins 1994*b*) (that is, the grouping process itself may control for some confounding variables) (Morgenstern 1982). Brenner *et al.* (1992) have also shown that although non-differential misclassification of a binary variable seriously hinders the ability to control for that variable in individual-level studies, it does not always reduce the ability to control for that variable in ecological studies.

Although classical discussions of the ecological fallacy focus on omitted individual-level variables correlated with group membership as potential confounders, it is important to remember that when individual level variables are distributed differently across groups, group membership may hold clues as to the causes of the distribution of these variables. When individuals in a group tend to share individual-level characteristics (such as behavioural risk factors, for example) it may be that group membership (or certain group properties) plays a causal role in the appearance and distribution of these individual-level characteristics. Ultimately, the decision to conceptualize these individual-level variables as confounders or mediators depends on the specific research question being asked.

The absence of information on individual-level confounders (which may differ from group to group) and the limitations inherent in using ecological summaries (and interactions between ecological summaries) to control for individual-level confounders or non-linearities in the individual-level effects are the most common critiques of ecological studies in epidemiology. A key underlying assumption of these critiques (which often goes unstated) is that the ecological measures (for example, mean country income) and the individual-level measures (individual-level income) are indicators of the same construct; that is, if it were somehow possible to control for the unavailable individual-level information on other confounders and to fully capture non-linearities, it would be perfectly legitimate to infer things about how individual-level income is related to the outcome based on how mean country income is associated with it. But this assumption is not always true. Even if all possible individual-level confounders are controlled, ecological associations may differ from individual-level associations because the ecological measure of exposure and its individual-level namesake may be tapping into different constructs. This brings us to another important source of the ecological fallacy, discussed below.

$\bar{X}_j$ and X_{ij} measure different constructs

An alternative interpretation of Fig. 1 (or Fig. 2) is that country mean income and individual-level income are measuring different constructs, and country mean income is related to body mass index independently of its individual level analogue. Firebaugh (1978) has noted that 'The demystification of cross-level bias begins with the recognition that an aggregate variable often measures a different construct than its name-sake at the individual-level'. In this case, country mean income is a measure of a truly group-level attribute and not a proxy for individual-level data. Living in countries with high mean income places individuals at greater risk of having high body mass index regardless of their individual-level income (or modifies the relation between individual-level income and body mass index, as in Fig. 2). Thus mean country income is said to exert a contextual effect on body mass index. Both country-level and individual-level income provide distinct information, and both are needed to understand completely the distribution of body mass index. In this case, the origin of the ecological fallacy lies in assuming that the group-level measure is tapping into the same construct as the individual-level measure, when in fact it is not. Mean country income is associated with increased body mass index, after controlling for individual-level income, but within countries individual-level income is negatively associated with body mass index. In this situation the ecological fallacy can be thought of as a problem of construct validity; it arises because the aggregate measure is assumed to be measuring an individual-level construct when in fact it is measuring a group-level construct (Schwartz 1994).

The contextual effect of mean income may be mediated through a variety of different mechanisms. For example, countries with higher levels of mean income may rely to a greater extent on mass food production, and this may in turn be associated with higher fat contents, and higher fat in the diets of individuals. In addition the higher standard of living may be related to more sedentary occupations, higher frequency of food consumption outside the home, exposure to food advertisements, dieting behaviours, and so on. Since disease is defined in terms of dysfunctions of the body, in order to affect health, contextual effects must ultimately be mediated through individual-level processes (that is, through processes defined at a lower level of organization), just as the effects of individual-level behaviours, for example, are mediated through biological mechanisms. Mediators of a contextual effect do not necessarily involve the individual-level namesake of the group-level variable. In our body mass index income example, for instance, the contextual effect of mean income may work through individual level variables other than income. As in any epidemiological analysis, the extent to which contextual effects should be estimated before or after adjustment for individual-level factors depends on whether the latter are conceptualized as confounders or mediators.

A variant of the example above is when the ecological variable investigated is actually associated with another group-level attribute which exerts a contextual effect on the outcome. Thus, the ecological effect is actually the result of confounding by another group-level or ecological variable. For example, mean income may be a proxy for level of industrialization. It may be that level of industrialization, rather than mean income, that exerts an effect on body mass index. In this case, the observed contextual effect of mean income is the result of confounding by level of industrialization. The discordance between the group and individual effects of income arises because mean income is a proxy for level of industrialization, which is related to body mass index independently of individual-level income. This is an example of confounding, and is not only specific to ecological variables. It is directly analogous to the situation that arises when an individual-level association between a factor and a disease is due to confounding by a third factor.

The previous discussion (like typical discussions of the ecological fallacy) focuses on the situation where the independent variable at the group level is an aggregate of characteristics of individuals in the group. Thus the group-level variable (mean income) has an individual-level namesake (individual-level income). However, other ecological variables do not involve aggregates of individual-level data (for example, the existence of a certain law) and the problem of separating out contextual effects from individual-level effects of the variable (for example, the effects of mean country income from that of individual-level income) is not an issue. Ecological studies relating these types of predictors to outcomes may still be limited in their ability to draw individual-level inferences because of the absence of information on individual-level confounders or effect modifiers which may differ from group to group (similar to what we have discussed earlier).

In addition to the conceptual issues discussed above, there are statistical considerations which may lead to a discrepancy between estimates from ecological and individual-level studies. The example used throughout this section (country mean income, individual-level income, and body mass index) is based on a continuous individual-level dependent variable, and on the limitations inherent in using a linear ecological model as a proxy for a linear individual-level model. Additional complexities arise when the individual-level outcome is binary. The use of a linear regression ecological model as a proxy for a non-linear individual-level regression model may not always be appropriate. Fitting the aggregate or ecological regression model that directly corresponds to a non-linear individual-level regression model is not always simple or possible with available ecological data (see Greenland (1992) for details). Failure to specify correctly the ecological model to be used as a proxy for the individual-level model may be yet another source of differences between individual-level and aggregate-level regression coefficients. However, all the sources of the ecological fallacy described above may still be present even if the form of the ecological model is appropriate for the individual-level model it is attempting to proxy.

It is important to emphasize that the degree to which ecological and individual-level coefficients differ may vary from situation to situation. The logical possibility of the ecological fallacy should not be taken as evidence that the fallacy necessarily occurs in all cases (Greenland and Robins 1994*a*) or that when it occurs it has a critical impact. Some researchers have proposed strategies which may sometimes help reduce the ecological fallacy when drawing individual-level inferences from aggregate data, including selecting regions so as to minimize within-region variability and maximize between-region variability in individual-level exposure, comparing groups with similar covariate distributions, conducting sensitivity analyses, and comparing results based on different specifications of the ecological model (Greenland 1992), as well as other recently proposed statistical approaches (King 1997). Nonetheless the use of ecological associations as proxies for individual-level relationships is often problematic.

Other fallacies related to the existence of multiple levels

The ecological fallacy is only one of a set of possible 'fallacies' that derive from the existence of multiple levels of organization (Diez Roux 1998). Because, at least recently, epidemiologists have been mostly concerned with drawing inferences regarding the causes of interindividual variability, the ecological fallacy has received much more attention than its counterpart, the atomistic fallacy. The atomistic fallacy is the fallacy of drawing inferences regarding variability across groups based on individual-level data. The effect of an individual-level predictor on an outcome in a study of individuals is not necessarily the same as the effect of its group-level namesake on group-level outcomes. Thus the use of individual-level associations to draw inferences regarding group-level associations may also lead to incorrect inferences. In the body mass index example above, B_{p1} (the relation between individual-level income and body mass index pooling individuals across groups) does not equal B_{e1} (the ecological relation between country mean income and country mean body mass index). In addition, B_1 (the within-group effect of individual-level income) does not equal B_{e1} either. Moreover, the body mass index example includes multiple groups (countries) and individuals within them, but many individual-level studies only include individuals from a single group. Factors that explain variability across individuals within groups are not necessarily the same as those that explain variability across groups. For example, if stress levels are relatively invariant within groups (for example, communities or countries), stress may not be important in explaining variability in coronary heart disease within groups, but may be strongly associated with differences in coronary heart disease rates across groups. This is another reason why the use of individual-level data to infer group-level associations may lead to incorrect inferences.

Both the ecological and atomistic fallacies can be thought of as methodological problems inherent in drawing inferences at one level when the data are collected at another level. These fallacies arise when the conceptual model being tested corresponds to one level, but the data are collected at another level, or in Riley's words when 'the methods fail to fit the model' (Riley 1963). We have seen that the sources of these problems lie in (a) the lack of information on constructs pertaining to another level of organization and (b) the failure to realize that a variable defined and measured at one level of organization may tap into a different construct than its namesake at another level, and that constructs at both levels may be relevant to the outcome studied. Both of these issues indicate a more general problem which is that even when making inferences about a given level, other levels of organization may need to be taken into account. For example, the failure to consider group characteristics in drawing inferences regarding individuals, and the failure to consider individuals in drawing inferences regarding groups gives rise to another set of fallacies, which are closely related to the ecological and atomistic fallacies described above. In these fallacies (which have been termed the psychologistical or individualistic and sociologistical fallacies), although the level at which data are collected may fit the conceptual model being investigated, important facts pertaining to other levels have been ignored, in Riley's words 'the methods may fail to fit the facts' (Riley 1963).

Ignoring relevant group-level variables in a study of individual-level associations may lead to what Riley has termed the 'psychologistical fallacy', that is assuming that individual-level outcomes can be explained exclusively in terms of individual-level characteristics. For example, a study based on individuals might find that immigrants are more likely to develop depression than natives. But suppose this is only true for immigrants living in communities where they are a small minority. A researcher ignoring the contextual effect of community composition might attribute the higher overall rate in immigrants to the psychological effects of immigration *per se* or even to genetic factors, ignoring the importance of community-level factors and thus committing the psychologistic fallacy (Riley 1963; Valkonen 1969). (The term 'psychologistical fallacy' is not the most appropriate because the individual-level factors used to explain the outcome are not always exclusively psychological. Other authors have used the term 'individualistic fallacy', (Valkonen 1969) but because the term has also been used as a synonym of the 'atomistic fallacy' (Alker 1969; Scheuch 1969) it will be avoided here.)

Analogously, ignoring the role of individual-level factors in a study of groups may lead to what has been termed the sociologistical fallacy (Riley 1963). Suppose that a researcher finds that communities with higher rates of transient population have higher rates of schizophrenia, and he or she concludes that higher rates of transient population lead to social disorganization, breakdown of social networks, and increased risk of schizophrenia among all community inhabitants. But suppose that schizophrenia rates are only elevated for transient residents (because transient residents tend to have fewer social ties, and individuals with few social ties are at greater risk of developing schizophrenia). That is, rates of schizophrenia are high for transient residents and low for non-transient residents, regardless of whether they live in communities with a high or a low proportion of transient residents. If this is the case, the researcher would be committing the sociologistical fallacy in attributing the higher schizophrenia rates to social disorganization affecting all community members rather than to differences across communities in the percentage of transient residents, who are at higher risk because of individual characteristics.

Both the psychologistical and the sociologistical fallacies arise because relevant variables pertaining to other levels have been excluded from the model which led to an inappropriate explanation for the association. Although it is didactically useful to distinguish both sets of fallacies (ecological and atomistic versus psychologistical and sociologistical), they are closely interrelated and are essentially different manifestations of the same phenomenon: the failure to recognize that constructs defined at different levels may be important in understanding variability within a given level, and the failure to adequately distinguish constructs defined at different levels.

The types of fallacies are summarized in Table 4.

Table 4 Types of fallacies

Unit of analysis	Level of inference	Type of fallacy
Group	Individuals	Ecological
Individual	Groups	Atomistic[a]
Individual (relevant group-level variables excluded)	Individuals	Psychologistical[a]
Group (relevant individual-level variables excluded)	Groups	Sociologistical

[a]Also called individualistic by some authors.

Source: Diez-Roux (1998).

The full range of epidemiological studies

In considering the most appropriate study design to answer a given research question, investigators need to consider two issues. The first issue is the level of organization about which inferences are to be made. For example, is the interest in drawing inferences regarding causes of variation in the outcome among groups or among individuals? The answer to this question will determine the most appropriate unit of analysis. The second issue is the level of organization at which the constructs of interest in explaining the outcome are conceptualized and measured. The answer to this second question will determine the predictors to be investigated and the level at which they are conceptualized. Constructs relevant to health may be conceptualized, and measured, at different levels of organization (for example countries, states, neighbourhoods, peer groups, families, couples, people, measurement occasions). Factors defined at a higher level may be important in understanding variability at a lower level, and vice versa factors defined at a lower level may be important in understanding variability at a higher level. Decoupling the unit of analysis from the level of organization of the constructs investigated may be helpful in discussing the full range of studies available to epidemiologists and the advantages and disadvantages of each for a particular research question.

Clearly specifying the constructs of interest (as well as how they will be measured) is an important requirement of any study. Lack of clarity on exactly what constructs group-level or ecological variables are actually measuring underlies an important part of the confusion generated by the use of ecological studies in epidemiology, and the interpretation of group-level or ecological effects. The next section reviews the use of group-level variables in epidemiology based on the constructs which they are intended to be measuring. The study designs with different units of analysis are then considered in terms of the types of inferences that can be drawn from them and the types of constructs they are best suited to investigating.

Group-level variables in epidemiology

In this discussion of group-level variables the focus is on the generic example of 'individuals' nested within 'groups'. However, as previously noted, the issues discussed may pertain to many other situations (for example, neighbourhoods nested within states, countries nested within regions, siblings nested within families, repeated measures nested within individuals) where the 'higher' level can be thought of as the group (and higher-level variables as 'group' variables) and the lower level can be thought of as the 'individual' (and lower-level variables as 'individual-level' variables).

Group-level (higher-level) variables as proxies for individual-level (lower-level) variables

One of the most common uses of ecological variables in epidemiological studies is as proxies for individual-level variables, either because individual-level data are unavailable or because individual-level measurements are prone to measurement error. For example, in the absence of detailed information on smoking for individuals, median smoking levels in the area in which an individual lives may be used as a proxy. Of course, the use of these group-level proxies implies loss of information. It is not known whether a given person smokes or not; mean smoking levels in the area are used as an approximation. In this case the group-level measure is a second class alternative to the ideal individual-level measurement. The relevant construct (smoking) is defined at the individual level, but a group-level measurement is used as a proxy for it because direct individual-level measurements are unavailable. If a valid and reliable measure of individual-level exposure were available, it would be used instead.

Group-level variables are also used as proxies for individual-level data in cases in which individual-level measures are subject to a lot of measurement error, or when intraindividual variability makes a single measure a poor marker for the person's true exposure. For example, the mean yearly hours of sunlight in an area may be used as a proxy for individual-level exposure to sunlight and average per capita fat consumption in a group may be used as a proxy for the fat consumption of each member (due to limitations in characterizing an individual's fat intake based on a single one-day measurement). In these situations, the ecological measure is believed to be a better indicator of the 'true' individual-level exposure than the individual-level measure itself, because the ecological measure reduces the 'noise' associated with measurement error or intraindividual variation.

Group-level proxies for individual-level variables can be used in studies with individuals or groups as the units of analysis. Regardless of the study design in which they are used, the key assumption in the use of these variables is that the group-level measure is an adequate proxy for the individual-level construct; that is, even if there is measurement error, the construct that is being tapped into by the measure is an individual-level property rather than a group-level property. But this may not always be true; it is possible that the group-level measure is capturing information about a group-level attribute rather than (or in addition to) information about the individual-level characteristics of people comprising the group. For example, it is theoretically possible that areas with a higher percentage of smokers have higher cancer rates not only because smokers develop cancer, but also because there is something about areas with a high percentage of smokers (for example, the percentage of smokers may exert a contextual effect on cancer risk mediated, for example, through exposure to passive/second-hand smoke) which places everyone in the area at higher risk regardless of whether they smoke or not. Unless individual-level data are available, it may not be possible to differentiate the effects of individual-level smoking from the contextual effect of the percentage of smoking in the area (or other group-level properties associated with it). Thus, in considering the use of group-level variables as proxies of individual-level data, researchers may need to consider two issues: (a) the degree of measurement error in the individual-level construct inherent in using the group-level variable (for example, misclassification of smokers as non-smokers), and (b) the degree to which the group-level measure is tapping into a group-level construct rather than the individual-level construct it purports to proxy.

Group-level (higher-level) variables as measures of group-level (higher-level) constructs

Another application of ecological variables, much less common in epidemiology, is to measure group-level constructs. Variables that reflect the characteristics of groups have been classified into two basic types (Valkonen 1969; Lazarsfeld and Menzel 1971; Blalock 1984; Von Korff *et al.* 1992; Morgenstern 1995): derived variables and integral variables. Derived variables (also termed analytical or aggregate variables) summarize the characteristics of individuals in the group (means, proportions, and so on) (for example, percentage of people with incomplete high school, median household income). Although created through the aggregation of information from the individual members of a group, derived variables are group characteristics and may provide information distinct from their individual-level analogue. As discussed above, mean neighbourhood income and individual-level income are indicators of two distinct constructs, each of which may be important to health. Mean neighbourhood income may be a marker for neighbourhood-level factors potentially related to health (such as recreational facilities, school quality, road conditions, environmental conditions, types of foods available and their cost), and these factors may affect everyone in the community regardless of their individual-level income. Similarly, community unemployment levels may affect everyone in the community regardless of whether they are unemployed or not.

A special subset within derived variables is the average of the dependent variable within the group (Susser 1994*a*). As noted by Ross (1911) in his theory of happenings, for some types of events, the frequency of occurrence may depend on the number of individuals already affected. The prevalence of a given infection in the group to which a person belongs will affect his or her risk of infection, or may modify the relation between individual-level risk factors and the risk of disease (Halloran and Struchiner 1991; Koopman *et al.* 1991*b*; Koopman and Longini 1994). The classic concept of herd immunity is a variant of this notion: the prevalence of immunity in a community will determine whether an epidemic of disease does or does not occur, and will therefore influence a non-immune individual's risk of acquiring disease (Susser 1973). The contextual effect of the dependent variable's prevalence within a group may also be important in understanding other health outcomes. For example, the prevalence of obesity in a community may influence the likelihood that an individual is obese. This effect may operate through several different mechanisms. The prevalence of obesity may itself generate societal norms regarding acceptability and desirability of obesity, which may influence an individual's risk of being obese. In addition, the probability of adopting behaviours conducive to obesity (for example, certain types of diet or physical activity patterns) may be higher in situations where the behaviour is highly prevalent in the community. Although infrequently considered, these types of contextual effects may be of crucial importance in understanding the distribution (and causes) of health-related behaviours (smoking and alcoholism are two common examples).

Integral variables (also termed primary or global variables) describe group characteristics that are not derived from characteristics of its members (for example, the existence of certain types of laws, availability of health care, political system, or population density). Integral variables do not have analogues at the individual level. They may be discrete and dichotomous (for example, an intervention or a disaster, presence of a certain law), scaled and polychotomous (for example, social disorganization, intensity of newborn care), or continuous (for example, doctors per capita). A special type of integral variable refers to patterns and networks of contacts or interactions between individuals within groups. These patterns are derived from how individuals are connected to each other, and yet they are more than aggregates of individual characteristics. Lazarsfeld and Menzel (1971) have referred to these variables as structural variables, although the term structural effects has also been used to refer to the effects of group-level properties more generally (Blau 1960). Patterns of interconnections among individuals may be important determinants of individual risk, particularly for infectious diseases, but possibly for many other health outcomes as well (Koopman *et al.* 1991*a*; Koopman and Longini 1994; Koopman and Lynch 1999). In addition, these patterns of interconnections may modify the relation between certain individual-level attributes and risk of disease (Koopman *et al.* 1991*a*). These patterns of interactions can be summarized in the form of group-level attributes such as network size or structure (Lazarsfeld and Menzel 1971; van den Eeden and Huttner 1982). Just as other 'group-level' variables can refer to groups of various sizes, these patterns of interactions may characterize a whole continuum of groups depending on the particular research problem: large groups, smaller groups within larger groups, or even pairs of individuals.

When group-level variables are used to characterize group-level properties there is no ambiguity in defining whether individuals are or are not exposed (as there is when group variables are used as proxies for individual-level exposure data). The group-level variable (whether derived or integral) applies equally to all individuals within the group; for example, all are 'exposed' to living in a neighbourhood with high unemployment regardless of whether they themselves are employed, and all are 'exposed' to existing laws regarding seatbelt use. Thus the measurement error problem which may be present when group measures are used as proxies for measures of individual-level constructs is not present (although there may be measurement error in the measure of the group-level construct itself, as there may be for any measure). As discussed below, such group-level constructs can be investigated in studies with either individuals or groups as the units of analysis.

Study designs based on the units of analysis

Studies with groups as units of analysis

Studies with groups as the units of analysis (traditional ecological studies) are most appropriate when investigators are interested in explaining variation between groups and the constructs of interest can be conceptualized as group-level properties. As discussed above, these group-level properties may be derived or integral variables. Over the past few years numerous studies have examined the relationship between area measures of deprivation (a derived variable) and area mortality rates with geographic regions as the units of analysis (Townsend *et al.* 1988; Carstairs and Morris 1991). This analytical approach is most appropriate if the research question is formulated at the area (group) level and the main construct investigated (deprivation) is conceptualized as an area- or group-level attribute. Similar studies have examined the relation between area socio-environmental characteristics and the decline of coronary heart disease mortality rates in the United States (Wing *et al.* 1988): area socio-environmental characteristics are conceptualized as group attributes that affect all individuals living within the community and the interest lies in drawing inferences regarding differences between areas.

An example involving integral group-level variables is provided by studies relating national legislation restricting tobacco advertising in different countries to country smoking rates: a country-level construct is examined and the interest lies in drawing country-level inferences. Ecological designs may also be appropriate for the evaluation of the effects of group-level interventions on group-level outcomes (Morgenstern 1982). For example, a study may want to investigate the relationship between the introduction of a mass media campaign to prevent teenage smoking (an integral variable) and the prevalence of teenage smoking in the area. Because the mass media campaign may affect all community inhabitants (regardless of whether they actually saw the advertisements or not) through mechanisms involving diffusion, peer pressure, and so on, the intervention can be conceptualized as a group-level attribute.

As discussed above in the section on the ecological fallacy, these studies are limited in their examination of the role of individual-level constructs—as confounders, mediators, or effect modifiers of the group-level associations. In the example above, differences in the effects of the mass media campaign by individual-level characteristics (effect modification) could not be investigated. Neither could the impact of differences in individual exposures to the mass media campaign. In addition, in the case of ecological variables with individual-level analogues (for example, area unemployment and individual-level unemployment) studies with groups as the units of analysis cannot differentiate the contextual effect of the variable from its individual-level effect. For example, an ecological study relating area unemployment to rates of mental health outcomes could not differentiate whether the increased rate of mental illness is seen only in the unemployed or is present in all area inhabitants regardless of whether they are unemployed or not. However, from a public health perspective, the group-level association may itself be of great interest. Decreasing the unemployment rate would decrease the rate of mental illness whether the effect resulted from a group-level or individual-level construct or both. Similarly, the country-level relationship between income inequality and health may have important policy implications regardless of whether it is due to a contextual effect of income inequality, or to the fact that more unequal countries tend to have more people in the lower-income categories.

It is often argued that there is one situation in which ecological studies may be particularly useful, even when the intention is to draw individual-level inference (despite the potential for the ecological fallacy). This situation involves individual-level attributes with little within-group variation but large between-group variation. For example, if dietary fat is homogeneous within countries but varies greatly from country to country, an individual-level study restricted to individuals from a single country may find no association between dietary fat and cardiovascular disease, but an ecological study comparing country rates with country average fat intake may find a strong relationship. From this perspective, the advantage of the ecological study results purely from the fact that it is able to include more variability in the exposure of interest. (The same research question could be addressed in a study of individuals that included individuals from different countries and thus ensured sufficient variation in the exposure. But often this option is not feasible, whereas country-level measures may be available from standard sources.) Of course, the presence of significant between-country differences in diet raises the important question of why countries differ in diet to begin with, and suggests that the diet of individuals has important country-level determinants. Diet may be simply a mediator in the causal pathway relating country characteristics to cardiovascular disease. A study which concluded that differences between countries in cardiovascular disease are reducible to differences in the diets of individuals could be missing important disease antecedents.

Although they will not be discussed here in detail, studies with groups as the units of analysis are subject to many of the same analytical issues as individual-level studies with respect to bias, confounding, and establishment of temporality. In addition, these types of analyses raise additional methodological issues, such as the need to have adequate numbers of groups as well as enough individuals per group, the need to account for differences in the variability of outcomes (for example, rates) for the different groups due to the fact that they may be based on different numbers of observations, and the possibility of multicolinearity between the predictors examined (which is often more of a problem in ecological studies than in individual-level studies) (Morgenstern 1982). In addition, studies in which the units of analysis are geographic areas may need to use statistical methods to account for the fact that areas geographically closer to each other may tend to be more similar (in outcomes) than those more distant from each other (due to unmeasured factors that cluster in space), which leads to violation of the assumption of independence of observations (for example, see Clayton *et al.* 1993). This is identical to situations involving individuals nested within groups or repeat measures on individuals over time, in which residual correlation between outcomes may be present. Time-trend studies also raise additional methodological issues related to time-series analyses generally (Morgenstern 1995).

Studies with individuals as units of analysis

Traditional individual-level studies are most appropriate when investigators are interested in drawing inferences regarding variability across individuals, and all potential constructs of interest can be conceptualized as individual-level properties. The most common 'classic' epidemiological studies (for example, case–control studies of lung cancer and cohort studies of cardiovascular disease) are of this type. The assumption is that all constructs relevant to the outcome being studied are individual-level constructs.

Studies with individuals as the units of analysis and with information limited to individual-level constructs cannot examine the role of group-level constructs as antecedents of individual-level variables, as independent predictors of outcomes, or as confounders of individual-level associations. They cannot determine whether the effect of a given individual-level variable is only present in certain group contexts, or varies from group to group, as a function of group characteristics. In summary, they are unable to investigate the role of group-level factors in explaining variability in the outcome across individuals. In order to answer these questions, other types of analyses are needed.

Studies limited to individuals from a single group are clearly unable to examine the role of group-level constructs in causing the outcome (or in interacting with individual-level variables), because group-level properties are invariant within groups (Schwartz and Carpenter 1999). If group-level factors are important in causing the outcome, studies focused on a single group may fail to detect important disease determinants. In the dietary fat example mentioned above, it was noted that a study based on individuals from a single country would not detect dietary fat as a risk factor if it were invariant within countries. More fundamentally, the country-level factors that influence the range of fat intake is the salient variable that the individual-level study could not capture.

If the study involves individuals from many different groups, relevant group-level properties may be included in individual-level analyses. For example, group-level variables can be included in regression equations with individuals as the units of analysis. These types of analyses have been called contextual analyses (Blalock 1984; Iversen 1991). Susser (1994*a*) has referred to studies which investigate the effects of group-level variables on individual-level outcomes as mixed studies. This approach is still relatively uncommon in epidemiology perhaps partly because it is sometimes difficult to measure the group-level construct adequately, and cover the variation in this construct, in studies designed with individuals as the units of analysis.

A simple example of the type of regression model fitted in contextual analysis (for the linear case) is

$$Y_{ij} = b_0 + b_1 C_j + b_2 X_{ij} + e_{ij} \tag{4}$$

where Y_{ij} is the outcome for the *i*th individual in the *j*th group, C_j is the group-level variable, X_{ij} is the individual-level variable, and e_{ij} is the error term for the *i*th individual in the *j*th group. Contextual models can include multiple group-level and individual-level variables as well as their interactions. In the model shown above, b_1 estimates the effect of the group-level characteristic on the individual-level outcome (after adjustment for X_{ij}) and b_2 estimates the effect of the individual-level variable on the outcome (after adjustment for C_j). Contextual models can be used, for example, to investigate the effects of neighbourhood context on fertility outcomes by including characteristics of the neighbourhoods where individuals live (derived or integral variables) together with individual-level characteristics in individual-level regression models. Special methods may be required to account for non-independence of the outcomes within groups. Although contextual analysis can be used for simultaneous investigation of the effects of group-level and individual-level constructs in shaping individual-level outcomes, it does not allow examination of group-to-group variability *per se*, or of the factors associated with it. The unit of analysis remains the individual and only interindividual variation is examined.

Studies with both groups and individuals as the units of analysis (multilevel studies)

Recently, multilevel studies and multilevel analysis have emerged as new analytic strategies in several fields including education, sociology, demography, and public health (Mason *et al.* 1983; Bryk and Raudenbush 1992; Von Korff *et al.* 1992; DiPrete and Forristal 1994; Paterson and Goldstein 1995; Wu 1995; Duncan *et al.* 1998; Kreft and de Leeuw 1998). Multilevel studies simultaneously examine groups (or samples of groups) and individuals within them (or samples of individuals within them). Variability at both the group level and the individual level can be simultaneously examined and the role of group-level and individual-level constructs in explaining variation between individuals and between groups can be investigated. For example, a study may have information on a series of country-level characteristics (for example, gross national product, inequality in the distribution of income) and on the individual-level characteristics of a sample of individuals within each country (including health outcomes). Researchers may be interested in investigating how country-level and individual-level factors are related to health outcomes, as well as the extent to which between-country and between-individual variability in the outcomes are explained by variables defined at both levels. Thus, multilevel analysis allows researchers to deal with the microlevel of individuals and the macrolevel of groups or contexts simultaneously (Duncan *et al.* 1998). Multilevel models can be used to draw inferences regarding the causes of interindividual variation and the extent to which it is explained by individual-level or group-level variables, but inferences can also be made regarding intergroup variation, whether it exists in the data, and to what extent it is accounted for by group- and individual-level characteristics.

In the case of multilevel analysis involving two levels (for example, individuals nested within groups), the model can be conceptualized as a two-stage system of equations. The case for a normally distributed dependent variable is illustrated below. For reasons of simplicity the illustration will focus on the case of only one independent variable at the individual and one independent variable at the group level (although models can of course be extended to include as many independent variables as needed).

In the first stage, a separate individual-level regression is defined for each group:

$$Y_{ij} = b_{0j} + b_{1j} I_{ij} + \varepsilon_{ij} \qquad \varepsilon_{ij} \sim n(0, \sigma^2) \tag{5}$$

where Y_{ij} is the outcome variable for the *i*th individual in the *j*th group (or context), I_{ij} is the individual-level variable for the *i*th individual in the *j*th group (or context), b_{0j} is the group-specific intercept, and b_{1j} is the group-specific effect of the individual-level variable. Individual-level errors (ε_{ij}) within each group are assumed to be independent and identically distributed with a mean of zero and a variance of σ^2. The same regressors are generally used in all groups, but regression coefficients (b_{0j} and b_{1j}) are allowed to vary from one group to another.

In a second stage, each of the group- or context-specific regression coefficients defined in eqn (5) (b_{0j} and b_{1j} in this example) are modelled as a function of group-level variables:

$$b_{0j} = \gamma_{00} + \gamma_{01} C_j + U_{0j} \qquad U_{0j} \sim n(0, \tau_{00}) \tag{6}$$

$$b_{1j} = \gamma_{10} + \gamma_{11} C_j + U_{1j} \qquad U_{1j} \sim n(0, \tau_{11}) \tag{7}$$

$$\text{cov}(U_{0j}, U_{1j}) = \tau_{10}$$

where C_j is the group-level or contextual variable, γ_{00} is the common intercept across groups, γ_{01} is the effect of the group-level predictor on the group-specific intercepts, γ_{10} is the common slope associated with the individual-level variable across groups, and γ_{11} is the effect of the group-level predictor on the group-specific slopes.

The errors in the group-level equations (U_{0j} and U_{1j}), sometimes called 'macro errors', are assumed to be normally distributed with mean zero and variances τ_{00} and τ_{11} respectively. τ_{01} represents the covariance between intercepts and slopes; for example, if τ_{01} is positive, as the intercept increases the slope increases. Thus, multilevel analysis summarizes the distribution of the group-specific coefficients in terms of two parts—a 'fixed' part which is unchanging across groups (γ_{00} and γ_{01} for the intercept, and γ_{10} and γ_{11} for the slope) and a 'random' part (U_{0j} for the intercept and U_{1j} for the slope) which is allowed to vary from group to group.

By including an error term in the group-level equations (eqns (6) and (7)), these models allow for sampling variability in the group-specific coefficients (b_{0j} and b_{1j}) and also for the fact that the group-level equations are not deterministic (that is, the possibility that not all relevant macrolevel variables have been included in the model) (Wong and Mason 1985). The underlying assumption is that group-specific intercepts and slopes are random samples from a normally distributed population of group-specific intercepts and slopes (or equivalently, that the groups or macro errors are 'exchangeable') (Diprete and Forrister 1994).

An alternative way to present the model fitted in multilevel analysis is to substitute eqns (6) and (7) in (5) to obtain

$$Y_{ij} = \gamma_{00} + \gamma_{01}C_j + \gamma_{10}I_{ij} + \gamma_{11}C_jI_{ij} + U_{0j} + U_{1j}I_{ij} + \varepsilon_{ij}. \quad (8)$$

This final model is a random effects model (Hox and Kreft 1994). The model includes the effects of group level variables (γ_{01}), individual-level variables (γ_{10}), and their interaction (γ_{11}) on the individual-level outcome Y_{ij} (often called the 'fixed effects'). It also includes a random intercept component (U_{0j}), and a random slope component (U_{1j}), which, together with the individual-level errors ε_{ij}, comprise a complex error structure. Because of the presence of this complex error structure, special estimation methods must be used. Although multilevel or random effects models were first developed for continuous dependent variables, analogous methods have been developed or are under development other types of outcomes (Wong and Mason 1985; Goldstein 1995).

Multilevel models allow investigation of a variety of interrelated research questions. They allow separation of the effects of context (that is, group characteristics) and of composition (characteristics of the individuals in groups) (Duncan *et al.* 1998). Do groups differ in average outcomes after controlling for the characteristics of individuals within them? Are group-level variables related to outcomes after controlling for individual-level variables? Multilevel models can also be used to examine the effects of individual-level variables. Are individual-level variables related to the outcome after controlling for group-level variables? Do individual-level associations vary from group to group, and is this partly a function of group-level variables? Multilevel models also allow quantification of variation at different levels (for example, within group and between group) and the degrees to which variation is 'statistically explained' by individual-level and group-level variables. For example, is there significant variation in group-specific intercepts or slopes (do τ_{00} and τ_{11} differ significantly from 0)? How does this variability change as individual-level or group-level variables are added? What percentage of the variability in individual-level outcomes is between and within groups?

Although the terms contextual analysis and multilevel analysis have often been used synonymously (Van den Eeden and Huttner 1982; Mason *et al.* 1983), today's multilevel models are more general than early contextual models. Contextual effects models do not allow examination of group-to-group variability in outcomes as multilevel models do. In multilevel analysis, inferences can be drawn regarding differences among groups as well as differences among individuals, and the role of both group-level and individual-level constructs can be examined. In a sense, both groups and individuals are units of analysis, and both group-to-group and individual-to-individual variation are examined. Thus, multilevel studies provide a link between traditional ecological and individual-level studies. The advantages and limitations of multilevel models have been reviewed in several publications (DiPrete and Forristal 1994; Duncan *et al.* 1998; Diez Roux 2000).

The types of studies, the levels at which variability is examined, and the types of constructs which they are more suited to investigate are summarized in Table 5.

Conclusion

In public health research, both predictors and outcomes may be conceptualized at different levels of organization, and understanding outcomes at a given level may require taking into account information pertaining to levels above or below it. Each system can be thought of as nested within another level and dynamically interrelated with the levels above and below it. In addition, each level may acquire 'emergent' properties, unique characteristics confined to that level,

Table 5 Types of study designs used in public health based on unit of analysis, level at which variability is examined, and constructs most appropriately investigated

Type of study	Unit of analysis	Level at which variability is examined	Constructs investigated as potential 'causes' of variability	
			Group-level	Individual-level
Ecological	Groups	Groups (utility for interindividual variability limited)	Yes	Only group-level proxies
Individual level	Individuals	Individuals (utility for intergroup variability limited)	No (Yes in contextual)	Yes
Multilevel	Groups and individuals	Groups and individuals	Yes	Yes

which are different from the properties of its components. The selection of the appropriate study design should be based on the specific research question investigated, including the level of organization about which inferences are to be made, as well as the levels of organizations of the constructs of interest (including the main independent variables as well as potential confounders or effect modifiers of the association).

As noted above, many of the issues discussed in relation to generic 'individuals' and 'groups' are generalizable to other situations in public health involving 'lower levels' nested within 'higher levels'. Generic issues which are present across the continuum of 'levels' include limitations of using measures at a higher level as proxies for lower-level measures, the problems in making inferences regarding causes of variability at one level based on data collected at another level, and the need to consider multiple levels in drawing inferences at a given level. For example, in a study involving multiple measures on individuals over time the use of 'average' outcome and exposure measurements for individuals could lead to problems analogous to those described for the ecological fallacy. Similarly, both individual characteristics and occasion-specific (or time-specific) constructs may be important in understanding the outcome being studied. Indeed, the multilevel analysis methods described above as an alternative analytical approach which allows simultaneous examination of intergroup and interindividual variation, are suited to situations involving nested data structures generally (for example, multiple measures on individuals over time, patients nested within providers, neighbourhoods nested within regions). It is interesting to point out that analogous issues related to the existence of multiple levels of organization may also exist within individuals, for example, when looking at cells within tissues.

Problems related to the use of ecological studies and ecological variables in epidemiology often result from confusion regarding the level of organization to which the research question pertains, the level of organization at which the constructs of interest are defined and measured, and the sometimes inappropriate use of variables defined and measured at one level to proxy constructs defined at another level. Researchers must necessarily focus on certain aspects of the continuum of levels of organization and not all studies need (or can) span all levels. Rather than defending or criticizing one study design in favour of another, it is more useful to evaluate whether the level of analysis investigated and the constructs examined are appropriate for the specific question being asked. Because 'ideal' study designs are often not possible, the key lies in determining whether the particular design employed is 'good enough' for the question being asked. The issues reviewed in this chapter may be helpful in making this judgement.

References

Alker, H.R. (1969). A typology of ecological fallacies. In *Social ecology* (ed. M. Dogan and M.S. Rokkam), pp. 69-86. MIT Press, Cambridge, MA.

Blalock, H.M. (1984). Contextual-effects models: theoretical and methodological issues. *Annual Review of Sociology*, **10**, 353–72.

Blau, P.M. (1960). Structural effects. *American Sociology Review*, **25**, 178–93.

Brenner, H., Greenland, S., and Savitz, D. (1992). The effects of nondifferential confounder misclassification in ecologic studies. *Epidemiology*, **3**, 456–9.

Bryk, A.S. and Raudenbush, S.W. (1992). *Hierarchichal linear models: applications and data analysis methods.* Sage, Newbury Park, CA.

Carstairs, V. and Morris, R. (1991). *Deprivation and health in Scotland.* Aberdeen University.

Chadwick, E. (1965). *Report on the sanitary conditions of the labouring population of Great Britain.* Edinburgh University Press (originally published 1842).

Clayton, D.G., Bernardinelli, L., and Montomoli, C. (1993). Spatial correlation in ecological analysis. *International Journal of Epidemiology*, **22**, 1193–202.

Diez Roux, A.V. (1998). Bringing context back into epidemiology: variables and fallacies in multilevel analysis. *American Journal of Public Health*, **88**, 216–22.

Diez Roux, A.V. (2000). Multilevel analysis in public health research. *Annual Review of Public Health*, **21**, 171–92.

DiPrete, T.A. and Forristal, J.D. (1994). Multilevel models: methods and substance. *Annual Review of Sociology*, **20**, 331–57.

Duncan, C., Jones, K., and Moon, G. (1998). Context, composition, and heterogeneity: using multilevel models in health research. *Social Science and Medicine*, **46**, 97–117.

Firebaugh, G. (1978). A rule for inferring individual-level relationships from aggregate data. *American Sociology Review*, **43**, 557–72.

Goldberger, J., Wheeler, G.A., Sydenstricker, E., and Tarbett, R.E. (1920). A study of the relation of factors of a sanitary character to pellagra incidence in seven cotton-mill villages of South Carolina in 1916. *Public Health Report*, **35**, 1701–24.

Goldstein, H. (1995). *Multilevel statistical models.* Halsted Press, New York.

Greenland, S. (1992). Divergent biases in ecologic and individual-level studies. *Statistics in Medicine*, **11**, 1209–23.

Greenland, S. and Morgenstern, H. (1989). Ecological bias, confounding, and effect modification. *International Journal of Epidemiology*, **18**, 269–74.

Greenland, S. and Robins, J. (1994*a*). Accepting the limits of ecologic studies: Drs Greenland and Robins reply to Drs Piantadosi and Cohen. *American Journal of Epidemiology*, **139**, 769–71.

Greenland, S. and Robins, J. (1994*b*) Ecologic studies—biases, misconceptions, and counter-examples. *American Journal of Epidemiology*, **139**, 747–60.

Halloran, M.E. and Struchiner, C.J. (1991). Study design for dependent happenings. *Epidemiology*, **2**, 331–8.

Hammond, J.L. (1973). Two sources of error in ecological correlations. *American Sociology Review*, **38**, 764–77.

Hox, J.J. and Kreft, I.G. (1994). Multilevel analysis methods. *Sociological Methods and Research*, **22**, 283–99.

Iversen, G. (1991). *Contextual analysis.* Sage, Newbury Park, CA.

Keys, A. (1980). *Seven countries: a multivariate analysis of death and coronary heart disease.* Harvard University Press, Cambridge, MA.

King, G. (1997). *A solution to the ecological inference problem. Reconstructing individual behavior from aggregate data.* Princeton University Press.

Koopman, J.S. and Longini, I.M. (1994). The ecological effects of individual exposures and nonlinear disease dynamics in populations. *American Journal of Public Health*, **84**, 836–42.

Koopman, J.S. and Lynch, J. (1999). Individual causal models and population system models in epidemiology. *American Journal of Public Health*, **89**, 1170–4.

Koopman, J.S., Longini, I.M., Jacquez, J.A., *et al.* (1991*a*). Assessing risk factors for transmisson of infection. *American Journal of Epidemiology*, **133**, 1199–209.

Koopman, J.S., Prevots, D.R., Vaca Marin, M.A., *et al.* (1991*b*). Determinants and predictors of dengue infection in Mexico. *American Journal of Epidemiology*, **133**, 1168–78.

Kreft, I. and deLeeuw, J. (1998). *Introducing multilevel modeling.* Sage, London.

Lazarsfeld, P.F. and Menzel, H. (1971). On the relation between individual and collective properties. In *A sociological reader on complex organizations* (ed. A. Etzioni), pp. 499–516. Holt, Rinehart, and Winston, New York.

Levin, B. (1995). Annotation: accounting for the effects of both group- and individual-level variables in community-level studies. *American Journal of Public Health*, **85**, 163–4.

Mason, W., Wong, G., and Entwisle, B. (1983). Contextual analysis through the multilevel linear model. In *Sociological methodology 1983–1984* (ed. S. Leinhardt), pp. 72–103. Jossey Bass, San Francisco, CA.

Morgenstern, H. (1982). Uses of ecologic analysis in epidemiologic research. *American Journal of Public Health*, **72**, 1336–44.

Morgenstern, H. (1995). Ecologic studies in epidemiology: concepts, principles, and methods. *Annual Review of Public Health*, **16**, 61–81.

Paterson, L. and Goldstein, H. (1991). New statistical methods for analysing social structures: an introduction to multilevel models. *British Educational Research Journal*, **17**, 387–93.

Piantadosi, S. (1994). Invited commentary: ecologic biases. *American Journal of Epidemiology*, **139**, 761–71.

Piantadosi, S., Byar, D.P., and Green, S.B. (1988). The ecological fallacy. *American Journal of Epidemiology*, **127**, 893–903.

Rice, N. and Leyland, A. (1996). Multilevel models: applications to health data. *Journal of Health Service Research Policy*, **1**, 154–64.

Riley, M.W. (1963). Special problems of sociological analysis. In *Sociological research I: a case approach*, pp. 700–25. Harcourt, Brace, and World, New York.

Robinson, W.S. (1950). Ecological correlations and the behavior of individuals. *American Sociology Review*, **15**, 351–7.

Ross, R. (1911). *The prevention of malaria* (2nd edn). John Murray, London.

Scheuch, E.K. (1969). Social context and individual behavior. In *Social ecology* (ed. M. Dogan and S. Rokkam), pp. 133–55. MIT Press, Cambridge, MA.

Schwartz, S. (1994). The fallacy of the ecological fallacy: the potential misuse of a concept and its consequences. *American Journal of Public Health*, **84**, 819–24.

Schwartz, S. and Carpenter, K. (1999). The right answer for the wrong question: consequences of type III error for public health research. *American Journal of Public Health*, **89**, 1175–80.

Snow, J. (1936). On the mode of communication of cholera. In *Snow on cholera* (2nd edn). Commonwealth Fund, New York (originally published 1855).

Susser, M. (1973). *Causal thinking in the health sciences.* Oxford University Press, New York.

Susser, M. (1994*a*). The logic in ecological. I: The logic of analysis. *American Journal of Public Health*, **84**, 825–9.

Susser, M. (1994*b*). The logic in ecological. II: The logic of design. *American Journal of Public Health*, **84**, 830–5.

Susser, E. and Wanderling, J. (1994). Epidemiology of nonaffective acute remitting psychosis versus schizophrenia: sex and sociocultural setting. *Archives of General Psychiatry*, **51**, 294–301.

Terris, M. (1964). *Goldberger on pellagra.* Louisiana State University Press, Baton Rouge, LA.

Townsend, P., Phillimore, P., and Beattie, A. (1988). *Health and deprivation. Inequality and the North.* Routledge, London.

Valkonen, T. (1969). Individual and structural effects in ecological research. In *Social ecology* (ed. M. Dogan and S. Rokkam), pp. 53–68. MIT Press, Cambridge, MA.

van den Eeden, P. and Huttner, H.J. (1982). Multi-level research. *Current Sociology*, **30**, 1–178.

Von Korff, M., Koepsell, T., Curry, S., and Diehr, P. (1992). Multi-level research in epidemiologic research on health behaviors and outcomes. *American Journal of Epidemiology*, **135**, 1077–82.

Wing, S., Casper, M., Riggan, W., *et al.* (1988). Socioenvironmental characteristics associated with the onset of decline of ischemic heart disease mortality in the United States. *American Journal of Public Health*, **78**, 923–6.

Wong, G. and Mason, W. (1985). The hierarchical logistic regression model for multilevel analysis. *Journal of the American Statistics Association*, **80**, 513–24.

Wu, Y.-W. (1995). Hierarchical linear models: a multilevel data analysis technique. *Nursing Research*, **44**, 123–6.

6.3 Cross-sectional studies

J. H. Abramson

Introduction

This chapter deals with prevalence and other cross-sectional studies, that is, with surveys of the situation existing at a given time (or during a given period) in a group or population or a set of groups or populations. These surveys may be concerned with:

- the presence of disorders, such as diseases, disabilities, and symptoms of ill health
- dimensions of positive health, such as physical fitness
- other attributes relevant to health, such as blood pressure and body measurements
- factors associated with health and disease, such as exposure to specific environmental factors, defined social and behavioural attributes (including health practices and attitudes to health and health services), and demographic characteristics; the correlates may be determinants, predictors, or effects of health and disease states.

Such a study may be descriptive, analytical, or both. At a descriptive level it yields information about a single variable (AIDS, haemoglobin concentration, capacity to work, cigarette smoking, and so on) or about each of a number of separate variables, in a total study population, or in specific population groups. At an analytical level, it provides information about the presence and strength of associations between variables, permitting the testing of hypotheses about such associations.

Most cross-sectional studies are individual based, that is, they seek information about the individuals in the group or sample studied. There are also group-based ('ecological') surveys, which seek information about groups or populations (Chapter 6.2), and analytical surveys that operate at more than one level; in a Mexican study, for example, an association between dengue infection (the presence of antibodies) and exposure to *Aedes aegyptii* mosquitoes was not found at an individual level, but it was found when villages were compared (Koopman and Longini 1994).

Cross-sectional studies may be contrasted with incidence and other 'time-span' studies that require information relating to two or more points of time. The latter studies, which are discussed in later chapters, measure changes in status (for example, disease onset, growth, changes in blood pressure) or examine associations between variables with a defined temporal relationship, for example, between childhood experiences and health in adulthood, or between treatment and subsequent survival. The difference between cross-sectional surveys and these studies is often likened to the difference between snapshots and motion pictures.

This distinction is not, however, a rigid one. Although the essential feature of cross-sectional surveys is that they collect information relating to a single specified time, they are often extended to include historical information that can be easily collected at the same time. This may lead to the demonstration of statistical associations with past experience, for example, relationships between herpes simplex type 2 infection and the number of previous sexual partners and receptive anal intercourse (van der Laar *et al.* 1998), and a negative association (in Barbados residents aged under 70) between lens opacities and the regular use of nutritional supplements for at least a year (Leske *et al.* 1997). Field investigations of epidemics (Chapter 6.4) typically combine a cross-sectional approach (case-finding and the investigation of environmental and other hazards) with the collection of historical information (about possible exposures to infection). Cross-sectional studies in which cases are compared with controls are considered elsewhere (Chapter 6.5).

Current status, and not only historical information, may be indicative of past experiences, permitting consideration of possible aetiological processes. In a study of behavioural problems in school, for example, the lead content of the schoolchildren's milk teeth was used as an indicator of lead poisoning in early childhood (Needleman *et al.* 1979). Similarly, assays of iron, arsenic, zinc, and other trace elements in toenail clippings may be used as measures of the prior intake of these elements (Garland *et al.* 1996). But the temporal relationships of the variables studied in a cross-sectional study (which came first?) is usually uncertain, making causal inferences uncertain.

If cross-sectional studies are repeated, they may be used for the purpose of health surveillance to observe changes in the population's health status and its determinants. If there are enough surveys extending over a long enough period, they may be used to reconstruct the lifetime experience of birth cohorts. An analysis of successive surveys of smoking habits in Norway, for example, demonstrated the differences between the smoking habits of people born in different periods and the changes that occurred in specific birth cohorts (Ronneberg *et al.* 1994). Such appraisals are generally based on a comparison of graphs based on a rearrangement of the age-specific findings of successive studies. Ages at the time of the study are converted to birth dates, and birth-cohort graphs are then constructed by bringing together the data for each birth cohort and plotting them against age; also, the data for each age group can be plotted against year of birth or year of death (MacMahon and Pugh 1970). Birth-cohort effects can also be investigated by the median polish procedure (Selvin 1996)—a very simple exploratory data analysis technique that shows whether age and time trends alone can explain the findings—as well as by more elaborate statistical procedures.

The uses of cross-sectional studies can be categorized as follows.

1. The findings may be used to promote the health of the specific group or population studied; that is, the study can be used as a tool in community health care.
2. The study may contribute to clinical care.
3. The study may provide 'new knowledge'—generalizable inferences that can be applied beyond the specific group or population studied. This knowledge may relate, for example, to the aetiology of a disease or the value of a type of health care.

These uses are not mutually exclusive; a single study may fulfil more than one purpose.

This chapter briefly considers the terms **prevalence** and **incidence**, and then reviews the methods used in cross-sectional studies, paying special attention to rapid epidemiological appraisal (cluster surveys and rapid methods of data collection) and to statistical measures, including prevalence measures of various kinds. The next three sections give consideration to the uses listed above. The first of these sections, on uses in community health care, considers community diagnosis, surveillance, community education and community involvement, and the evaluation of a community's health care. The subsection on community diagnosis deals with studies of health status, determinants of health and disease, associations between variables (including the measurement of impact, risk markers, and community syndromes), and the identification of groups requiring special care. The section on uses in clinical practice briefly describes applications in individual and family care and in community-oriented primary care. The section on studies yielding new knowledge reviews studies of growth and development, studies of aetiology, and programme trials.

Prevalence and incidence

Prevalence refers to the number of individuals who have a given disease or other defined attribute at a specific time, as opposed to incidence, which is based on a count of events. The event may be the onset of a new disease, death, and so on.

The prevalence of a disease in a population at any point in time depends on the prior incidence of new cases and on the average duration of the disease from onset to recovery or death. This relationship is shown diagrammatically in Fig. 1, in which the contents of the container represent prevalence, and the time spent in the container is the duration of the disease.

If incidence and the average duration have remained constant over a long period (a condition seldom encountered in real life), point prevalence (defined below) is the product of the incidence rate of new cases per time unit *t* and the average duration of the disease (mean *t* per case).

For a disease that runs an episodic course, the point prevalence of active disease is (under certain assumptions) the product of the incidence rate, the average duration of an episode, and the average number of episodes per case (Von Korff and Parker 1980). For formulae expressing the change in point prevalence during a specified period, see Rothman and Greenland (1998, pp. 43–5).

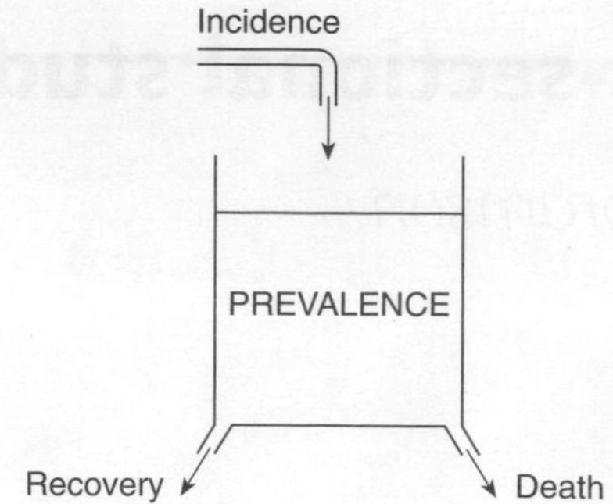

Fig. 1 Relationship between prevalence and incidence.

Methods

Like any other kind of study, a cross-sectional study can yield useful findings only if sound methods are used. At all stages—in the planning phase, during the collection of data, and when the data are processed and interpreted—there is a need for detailed attention to methods (Abramson and Abramson 1999) so as to minimize bias and ensure that the results will be as accurate as practical constraints permit. Simple rapid methods may be called for if resources are limited or speedy results are needed (see section on rapid epidemiologic assessment below).

Findings are obviously determined by the methods used, and different methods may yield very different findings. The prevalence of dementia in a large sample of elderly people in Canada, for example, varied from 3 to 29 per cent, depending on which commonly used set of diagnostic criteria was employed; only 1 per cent had dementia according to all six sets of criteria (Erkinjuntti *et al.* 1997). Similarly, the prevalence of benign prostatic hyperplasia in a community sample of men ranged, according to different definitions, from 4 to 19 per cent (Bosch *et al.* 1995). Guidelines for the critical appraisal of a prevalence study have been proposed by Loney *et al.* (1998); they suggest the following eight questions.

1. Are the study design and sampling method appropriate for the research question?
2. Is the sampling frame (from which subjects are selected) appropriate?
3. Is the sample size adequate?
4. Are objective, suitable and standard criteria used for measurement of the health outcome?
5. Is the health outcome measured in an unbiased fashion?
6. Is the response rate adequate? Are the refusers described?
7. Are the estimates of prevalence given with confidence intervals and in detail by subgroup, if appropriate?
8. Are the study subjects and the setting described in detail and similar to those of interest to you?

Cross-sectional studies may be performed in total target groups or populations, or in representative samples. Simple random sampling or systematic, stratified, or cluster sampling may be used.

Methods of collecting information can be broadly classified as follows.

1. Clinical examinations, special tests, and other observations.
2. Interviews and questionnaires. The subjects themselves may be questioned, or proxy respondents, for example, household informants may be used.
3. Clinical records and other documentary sources. Sources of information on the prevalence of diseases include hospital and other medical records, disease registers, records of routine examinations (in schools, prenatal clinics, army induction centres, health insurance schemes, and so on), and published statistics based on these or other records.

Disease prevalence may be studied in two stages, by using a screening test to identify people who are likely to have a given disease, and then subjecting them to more elaborate and specific tests.

Each method of data collection has its own advantages and limitations and carries its own possible biases. If information on the prevalence of a disease is obtained from hospitals, for example, people with mild disease are likely to be under-represented. The degree of bias may vary for different subgroups of the population as a result of variation in the accessibility or use of health services, or of differences between clinical services in their diagnostic and recording procedures. In a rural region in the United States, Anderson *et al.* (1988) found that 42 per cent of the cases of Parkinson's disease found in a survey based on screening questions and subsequent neurological examinations had not been diagnosed previously, and would have been missed by a survey based on medical records. Had people in institutions been omitted from the survey, a quarter of the cases would have been overlooked. The associations observed in a study of hospital or clinic patients may differ from those in the general population, if admission rates to the study group are connected with the variables whose associations are studied (Berksonian bias).

Since any method of case-finding may miss cases, it is often recommended that prevalence surveys should use more than one method, and combine the findings. The cases can be cumulated, or the total (including cases not found by any method) can be estimated by the 'capture–recapture' and related techniques (McCarty *et al.* 1993). These are methods originally used in estimating animal populations, where they are based on marking and releasing a batch of captured animals, and then seeing how many are recaptured in the next batch of animals caught.

Applied to two independent case-finding procedures that identify A and B cases respectively, with C cases common to both procedures, one formula for the estimated 'ascertainment-corrected' total number of cases is as follows:

$$[(A + 1)(B + 1)/(C + 1)] - 1.$$

In a study of childhood diabetes in Madrid, 451 cases were identified—432 by one procedure and 138 by another, with 119 common to both. The estimated total by the above formula was 501, with a 95 per cent confidence interval of 451 to 552. In a town in Japan, where the prevalence of type 2 diabetes mellitus among people aged 50 to 69 was 8.8 per cent according to a cross-sectional survey and 7.1 per cent according to a diabetes registry, the prevalence using the capture–recapture technique was 13.1 per cent (Sekikawa *et al.* 1999).

The capture–recapture approach is based on assumptions that are not always met. Its limitations are listed by Papoz *et al.* (1996). In particular, case-finding procedures are usually not independent. If cases ascertained by one method are especially likely to be identified by another method also, the calculated total will be an underestimate; and if cases ascertained by one method are likely to be missed by another, the total will be an overestimate.

This bias can be largely controlled by log-linear modelling (the multiple recapture census). This is a more elaborate technique that takes account of the observed dependencies between procedures (Fienberg 1972; Bishop *et al.* 1975), and can be used if there are three or more case-finding methods. Frischer *et al.* (1991) used this technique to estimate the number of injecting drug users in Glasgow, where 2006 cases were ascertained from three sources. The computed 'ascertainment-corrected' total was 13 050, a number that the authors reduced to 9424 to compensate for possible false-positive reports (95 per cent confidence interval, 6964–11 884). No method of estimation provides a fully satisfactory answer to the problem of incomplete ascertainment (Fienberg 1972; Armstrong and Hayes 1992; Kiemeney *et al.* 1994). If, for example, a certain type of case is 'uncatchable'—that is systematically missed by all procedures—no manipulation can estimate their number. If all cases have in fact been found, the computed total will be an overestimate.

In cross-sectional studies the common sources of selection bias (where the individuals for whom data are available are not representative of the target population) are failure to choose a representative sample and incomplete coverage of the sample or study group. Information bias (due to shortcomings in the gathering or handling of information) is often attributable to the lack of clear diagnostic criteria or other operational definitions, and to inconsistency in their application. In studies that set out to examine causal associations, bias is commonly caused by the respondents' or investigators' knowledge that there has been exposure to the putative cause, or that the putative effect is present. In a study of the association between coffee drinking and digestive symptoms, for example, a respondent who drinks much coffee and believes that this beverage causes digestive upsets may be more likely to recall and report symptoms, or an interviewer may tend to be more persistent when asking such a respondent about symptoms. Also, subjects who have symptoms and believe that these are caused by coffee may tend to provide a fuller (or exaggerated) account of their consumption of the beverage, and interviewers may tend to be especially persistent when questioning subjects whom they know to have symptoms. The subjects' awareness of their symptoms may also have led them to avoid coffee. These and other kinds of bias can be minimized by suitable survey procedures.

Some biases can be avoided, measured, or corrected during the analysis. Others cannot, but must still be taken into account when inferences are drawn from the findings.

As in other epidemiological studies, causal effects can be inferred from the findings of cross-sectional studies only after careful consideration has been given to the possibility of fortuitous and artefactual associations and confounding effects (Susser 1973; Rothman 1988; Rothman and Greenland 1998; Abramson and Abramson 2001). For example, associations between moderate or vigorous sports activities and low levels of blood pressure and other cardiovascular risk factors, observed in three cross-sectional surveys in Germany, could be taken as evidence for the preventive role of physical activity only after the effects of age, social class, body mass index, overall health, treatment for hypertension, activity at work, and other variables had been taken into account in the analysis (Helmert *et al.* 1994).

Rapid epidemiological assessment

Simple, undemanding, and inexpensive methods can often supply information that will adequately meet a study's purpose. Such methods are particularly useful if financial, human, and other resources are limited, as in developing countries and in many studies (in both developed and developing countries) carried out by practitioners in the context of community health services. They have special relevance in situations where it is important to obtain real-time results as a basis for programme decisions, and may be essential in mass emergencies, where health needs should be appraised within a day or two (Guha-Sapir 1991). Extensive surveys have been performed in 10 days, including the publication of lengthy reports (Frerichs and Tar 1989; Materia *et al.* 1995).

The evolution and use of rapid assessment methods are reviewed by Smith (1989), who points out that the introduction of these methods was a major factor responsible for the worldwide eradication of smallpox.

Simple methods will generally provide information that is less detailed and less accurate than would be provided by more elaborate methods. This need not matter, provided that the information meets the study's purposes, particularly if the alternative is no information at all. Care should be taken to avoid unnecessary inaccuracy, for example by giving due attention to the training of data collectors and by checking completed questionnaires and the coding of data.

Aspects of rapid survey methodology that are relevant to cross-sectional studies—cluster surveys and simplified methods of data collection—are discussed below. In addition, the appropriate use of computers can greatly speed up the performance and analysis of surveys, both in developed countries, where random-digit dialling and computer-assisted telephone interviewing may be useful techniques, and in developing countries, where changes in the cost and portability of computers have made them increasingly useful.

Uses of microcomputers are described in Chapter 6.15.

Cluster surveys

Two-stage cluster sampling has been advocated by the World Health Organization (**WHO**) Expanded Programme on Immunization since 1978 as a rapid, cheap, and accurate basis for surveys of immunization coverage (Lemeshow and Robinson 1985). It is based on the selection of a simple random sample not of individual subjects, but of groups or clusters of individuals. The method has been used for studies of specific diseases, service coverage, health service needs, and other topics. It can provide reasonably representative data, and has the advantages that it does not require a detailed sampling frame, it uses clusters of subjects who live close to one another, and it is so simple that subjects can be easily selected in the field with minimal technical support. Since clusters may contain people with similar characteristics, a representative sample requires a reasonably large number of clusters.

Cluster surveys following the Expanded Programme on Immunization pattern are based on the random selection of 30 or more villages, towns, sectors of cities, and so on, with the probability of inclusion being proportional to the cluster's size (it is possible for a large cluster to be selected more than once). The selection is easily done (Bennett *et al.* 1991; Abramson and Abramson 1999) if reasonably accurate population estimates are available. Strictly speaking, the subjects in each cluster should be chosen randomly, using a census. But, for simplicity, Expanded Programme on Immunization surveys use a modified method. One household in each cluster is randomly selected, preferably using a list or map; alternatively, the investigator can start at a central point, count the number of households (H) in a randomly-chosen direction (a spinning top or pencil can be used) from the central point to the border of the area, and then randomly choose a number from 1 to H to identify a household for selection. A preset number of subjects (for example, children of a defined age) is then studied in each cluster, starting with the selected household and moving on to the next one (the residence whose front door is closest) or perhaps the fifth-nearest household, until the quota is filled.

The number required in each cluster is decided by applying the usual method of estimating sample size for simple random sampling and then multiplying the result by the 'design effect' and dividing it by the chosen number of clusters. The design effect, which expresses the difference in precision between a cluster sample and a simple random sample of the same size, may be estimated from previous surveys (Bennett *et al.* 1991). A typical Expanded Programme on Immunization cluster survey that aims to provide an immunization coverage rate that is within 10 percentage points of the true rate, with 95 per cent confidence, might use seven non-randomly chosen subjects in each of 30 clusters. Computer simulation has shown that although this method yields overall results that are more biased and variable than those based on simple random sampling, it meets the above requirement in over 95 per cent of replications (Henderson and Sundaresan 1982; Lemeshow and Robinson 1985; Lemeshow *et al.* 1985). The results in specific clusters or in subsets of clusters cannot be relied on; analyses of a particular cluster are warranted only if the sample is large and not based on non-random selection. Comparisons of subsets of clusters may be feasible, as in an Indian survey that showed a higher level of immunization coverage in urban than in periurban areas and an especially low level in rural areas (Balraj *et al.* 1993). In a study of disease prevalence, the extent to which the disease is clustered may be of interest; a survey in Tanzania, for example, revealed clustering of trachoma within neighbourhoods in villages, not explicable by known risk factors (West *et al.* 1991). Simple methods of analysis are described by Bennett *et al.* (1991) and Frerichs (1989).

Computer simulations suggest that, in view of its ease and cheapness, cluster sampling with non-random selection in the second stage may be a reasonable choice even in analytical studies that use the ratio of two prevalence rates (for example, in people exposed and unexposed to a risk factor) to measure the strength of an association. But if the rates are large and their ratio is high, simple random sampling is much more successful in yielding a ratio within 0.1 of the true value and a confidence interval that includes the true value (Harris and Lemeshow 1991).

Approximate incidence rates can sometimes be derived from the prevalence findings. For example, lame children can be identified in a cluster survey, and the prevalence of lameness attributable to poliomyelitis can then be calculated, using criteria such as the presence of flaccid paralysis and intact sensation, with a history of an acute onset. Correction factors can then be applied to allow for the omission of upper limb paralysis, lethal cases, and complete recovery, and approximate poliomyelitis incidence rates can be computed (LaForce *et al.* 1980). Such a survey in Nigeria led to the estimate of at least 33 300 paralytic poliomyelitis cases annually in the period before an immunization programme was introduced (Babaniyi and Parakoyi 1991). In Burkina Faso, a cluster survey of this sort indicated a significant decrease in incidence, possibly because of immunization (Schwoebel *et al.* 1992). Incidence rates may also be estimated by obtaining a history of diseases or fatal conditions (for example, neonatal tetanus) that occurred in the households included in the clusters (Rothenberg 1985).

The main deficiency of the Expanded Programme on Immunization design arises from its non-use of random methods when selecting subjects, and its use of quota sampling for this purpose; results may be misleading if subjects with similar characteristics tend to live close to one another. Ways of mitigating the deficiencies include the use of the fifth-nearest instead of the nearest household, and splitting the community into quadrants and selecting a quarter of each cluster from each quadrant, starting at the centre point of the quadrant. A suggested 'not quite as quick but much cleaner alternative' to the Expanded Programme on Immunization design, aimed at retaining the advantages of ease and cheapness but making the procedure more rigorous and appropriate even for surveys that make multiple measurements, is based on the preselection of a 'target segment size'—the number of households to be surveyed for each cluster—instead of fixing the number of subjects needed in each cluster (Turner *et al.* 1996). Communities are selected randomly (as in the basic Expanded Programme on Immunization method) and then divided into equal segments, each containing approximately the required number of households; this requires a rough sketch map showing the households in the community. A segment of the community is then chosen at random, and all eligible individuals in all the households in the chosen segment are included in the sample. This method ensures that all households in the study population have approximately the same probability of being selected.

Simplified methods of data collection

Data collection may be simplified in various ways. The most obvious is to restrict the variables to those that are essential to meet the study's purposes (resulting in very short questionnaires or examinations) and to choose sources that are easily accessible—available records may, despite their deficiencies, contain enough information to obviate the need for a more demanding survey. Purposive sampling will often satisfy a study's needs. Patients attending a health facility, for example, may be deemed sufficiently representative of the total community to warrant their use (with reservations) as a study sample, and tests and interviews of antenatal clinic attenders and men attending outpatient clinics can provide useful information on the prevalence of sexually transmitted diseases in a refugee camp (Mayaud *et al.* 1992).

If available, simpler procedures can be chosen rather than more accurate but elaborate ones: for example, a rapid urine test for use in surveys of iodine deficiency (Rendl *et al.* 1998) or a simple test card for identifying people with low vision (Keeffe *et al.* 1996). Household food inventories (Patterson *et al.* 1997) or brief dietary questionnaires may supply enough information on dietary practices, rendering detailed dietary interviews unnecessary.

It may be decided to use simple proxy measures: for example, arm circumference or weight-for-height as easy and cheap indices of malnutrition in children (Velzeboer *et al.* 1983*a*, *b*), night blindness as a relatively easily measured surrogate for vitamin A deficiency (Sommer *et al.* 1980), or a characteristic depigmentation pattern ('leopard skin') as an index of the endemicity of onchocerciasis (Edungbola *et al.* 1987); or to appraise the burden of lymphatic filariasis by measuring the rate of infection of insect vectors (Pani *et al.* 1997) or by examining a small sample of men for hydroceles (Gyapong *et al.* 1996).

If the measures are simple, it is easy to train health workers or others in their use. Schoolteachers can measure weight and height with adequate precision, assistants can be taught simple cataract recognition (Venkataswamy *et al.* 1989), and traditional midwives have been taught to identify low birth weight babies by using a hand-held scale that shows a coloured signal if the weight is below 2.5 kg (Ritenbaugh *et al.* 1989). In Tanzania, a simple questionnaire on diseases and symptoms was administered by teachers to children in 245 schools; a comparison with urine tests showed that reports of haematuria or schistosomiasis had a high validity (Lengeler *et al.* 1991).

Cross-sectional methods—for example, for appraising child growth in a community—are obviously faster than longitudinal ones. Simple data on current infant feeding practices can, if appropriately analysed, rapidly provide a picture of the average duration of breast feeding and the age at introduction of supplements (Ferreira *et al.* 1996).

Where appropriate, rapid qualitative methods may be used. Qualitative (as opposed to quantitative) methods provide findings that are described in words rather than numbers. They are especially useful in the investigation of knowledge, attitudes, and practices—'beliefs and perceptions regarding health, the prevention and treatment of illness, and the utilization of traditional and biomedical health resources' (Scrimshaw and Hurtado 1987). Qualitative methods can provide 'culture specific maps [that] can help to improve the "fit" of programmes to people'. These maps show the presence of beliefs and behaviours, but not their numerical prevalence in the population (Scrimshaw and Hurtado 1987). A survey of patients who had a heart attack, for example, pinpointed the misconceptions (about heart attack symptoms) that contributed to delay in calling for medical help (Ruston *et al.* 1998), and a study of mothers in a population with a low breast feeding rate highlighted the role of seeing successful breast feeding by a relative or friend, rather than advice, as a determinant of the decision to breast feed (Hoddinott and Pill 1999). These methods have been termed 'rapid ethnographic assessment' (Smith 1989), 'rapid assessment procedures' (Scrimshaw and Hurtado 1987), and 'social research methods' (Smith and Morrow 1991).

Qualitative studies may be based on interviews and conversations with key informants and other members of the community, in which people can express their attitudes, perceptions, motivations, feelings, and behaviour; on observations in health-care facilities and the community at large; and on other methods (some of which require special training), such as focus group discussions, in which a small group of informants talk freely and spontaneously about themes considered important to the investigator (Khan *et al.* 1991), and the nominal group technique. Rapid methods of evaluating health care include surveys of people attending for care (clinic exit interviews) and checks on clinic facilities and supplies (Anker *et al.* 1993; WHO 1993). Guidelists for the collection of data on topics related to health and health care are provided by Scrimshaw and Hurtado (1987).

The nominal group technique, which was developed by Van de Ven and Delbecq (1972), is a useful method of obtaining a semi-quantitative picture of the views of a group of people: for example, professionals or laypeople who are invited to provide information on the problems of a specific community, or to suggest possible solutions (Abramson and Abramson 1999). The technique is so called because although the participants sit together, direct interaction is permitted only during specified phases of the process; hence during most phases this is a group 'in name only'. The Delphi procedure (Linstone and Turoff 1975) is a much more elaborate method.

Methods of validating the results of qualitative studies include 'triangulation', that is, the use of more than one qualitative method, to ascertain their common conclusions. Three suggested questions for use in appraising a qualitative study of beliefs and practices (Mays and Pope 1996) are as follows.

1. How well do the conclusions explain why people behave in the way they do?
2. How comprehensible would this explanation be to a thoughtful participant in the setting?
3. How well does it cohere with what we already know?

Qualitative and quantitative approaches may be regarded as complementary (Kroeger 1983). In a study of the reasons for incomplete childhood immunization in Haiti, for example, ethnographic methods were used to identify barriers to the use of preventive services, and these were then measured in a quantitative survey (Coreil *et al.* 1989). Qualitative methods can also be used as a follow-up to a quantitative study, to explain and expand the findings.

Statistical measures

The statistical measures used to summarize the findings of descriptive cross-sectional studies include means and standard deviations, medians, percentiles and other quantiles, measures of prevalence (see below), and other proportions. Ratios other than proportions are occasionally used: for example, the sex ratio (usually the male to female ratio) of people with a specific disease. Separate statistical measures may be provided for specific sex and age categories, ethnic groups, social classes, regions, and so on. Measures of association commonly used in analytical cross-sectional studies are described below.

If the study is based on a random sample, confidence intervals should be calculated in order to obtain an interval that has a high probability of containing the true value of the measure in the total target population. Confidence intervals are also often calculated even in the absence of a 'chance' process such as random sampling, to permit generalization to a broad 'reference' population, for example 'the nation's children', but in this instance the procedure is open to criticism.

Measures of prevalence

A measure of prevalence expresses the relative frequency of a disease or other qualitative attribute in a group or population; it is a proportion. The convenient and commonly used term 'prevalence rate' is disparaged by many experts who prefer to confine the term 'rate' to measures of the rapidity of change, and therefore use 'prevalence' or 'prevalence proportion' rather than 'prevalence rate', claiming that the latter is an impossible concept (Elandt-Johnson 1975).

There are a number of prevalence measures. Used without qualification, prevalence usually refers to a point prevalence, that is, the prevalence at a specified point of time. The point prevalence of a disease per 1000 population, for example, is calculated by the formula

$$\frac{\text{number of individuals with the disease at a specified point of time}}{\text{population at that time}} \times 1000.$$

The numerator is the total number of people who have the disease at the stated time, irrespective of when the disease commenced. The denominator is the total population (actual or estimated) at that time, including affected and unaffected people. A multiplier of 1000 or any other convenient or conventional multiple of 10 is used in order to eliminate awkward decimals—6.5 per 100 000 is easier to comprehend than the equivalent 0.000065.

The point of time to which prevalence refers need not be a fixed calendar time. The reference may be to a fixed point in the experience of each individual, for example, birth, entry to a job or army service, immigration, death, date of diagnosis, or (in a prevalence survey where interviews or examinations are staggered over a period) the date of examination. In such instances the formula is

$$\frac{\text{number of individuals with the disease at the time the individual is studied}}{\text{number of individuals studied}} \times 1000.$$

A measure expressing the frequency of a finding in an autopsy study is a point prevalence that refers to the time of death. This may be an indication of prevalence in the living, if the disorder does not affect the risk of dying or the probability of an autopsy, as in autopsy studies that showed that 45 per cent of young American soldiers killed in battle had coronary atherosclerotic lesions (MacNamara *et al.* 1971).

Like other measures, point prevalence may express the findings in a specific subgroup of the population; when so used, the numerator and denominator must both refer to the same population category. As an example, the sex- and age-specific point prevalence of a disease per 1000 men aged 45 to 64 years is calculated by the formula

$$\frac{\text{number of men aged 45–54 years with the disease at a specified point in time}}{\text{total number of men aged 45–54 years in the population at that time}} \times 1000.$$

Paradoxically, there are some point prevalences that can be accurately measured only by a longitudinal study. An example is the prevalence of congenital anomalies per 100 live births, which may be regarded as a point prevalence referring to the moment of birth. Many anomalies become manifest only weeks, months, or years after birth, so that reasonably full case-finding requires long-term follow-up.

Period prevalence refers to prevalence not at a single point in time but during a defined period (usually a specific year). Period prevalence (persons) represents the proportion of the population manifesting the disease at any time during the period. The formula is

$$\frac{\text{number of individuals manifesting the disease in the stated time period}}{\text{population at risk}} \times 1000.$$

The numerator is the number of people with the illness during the specified period, including those whose illness started earlier. The denominator is the average size of the total population during the specified period. It is often estimated by using the population at the middle of the period, or by averaging the size of the population at the beginning and end of the period. Other methods may be needed if the change in population size during the period was large and did not occur at an approximately even pace. It is usually more helpful to know the point prevalence at the beginning of the period and the incidence rate of new cases during the period, rather than the period prevalence.

There is also a type of period prevalence that refers not to a defined calendar period but to a defined period of the individual's life, for example, pregnancy or childhood. A study of a sample of healthy pregnant women in an American city, for example, revealed that the prevalence of reported physical battering during the current pregnancy was 8 per cent (Helton *et al.* 1987) and a cross-sectional study of men in England indicated that 5.3 per cent had experienced sexual abuse during childhood (Coxell *et al.* 1999).

The numerator of the little-used period prevalence (spells) is the number of spells (episodes) of an illness observed during the specified period (including episodes that commenced before the start of the period); the same person may be ill more than once. The denominator is the population at risk. For a short-term disease, this measure is usually similar to the incidence rate (spells).

Lifetime prevalence is a period prevalence referring to the whole of the subject's prior life. It differs from point prevalence only if the disorder is one that does not always persist. It refers to the presence of the disorder or of a scar, antibodies, historical or other evidence that the disorder was present in the past. The formula is

$$\frac{\text{number of individuals with evidence of the disorder (past or present)}}{\text{number of individuals studied}} \times 1000.$$

This measure is usually useful only if it refers to a specific age, and if valid information on prior occurrence is available. As an example, a cross-sectional study in Jerusalem revealed that the point prevalence of inguinal hernia among men aged 65 to 74 years was 30 per cent, whereas the lifetime prevalence (including men with scars of hernia repair operations) was 40 per cent (Abramson *et al.* 1978). It could be inferred that in this cohort the risk of developing a hernia, among men surviving to the age of 65 to 74 years, was 40 per cent. Such information would be of little value if the disorder were one with an important impact on mortality, such as cancer.

The lifetime prevalence of a disorder among the blood relatives of an index case may be used as a measure of familial risk, especially in genetic studies.

Measures of association

In analytical cross-sectional studies, the most commonly used measures of the association between two variables are odds ratios, rate ratios (for example, ratios of disease prevalences or of prevalences of exposure to a supposed causal factor) and rate differences (for example, differences between disease prevalences or prevalences of exposure). These measures are defined in Table 1, illustrated by fictional data on the association between exposure to fumes and headaches, based on a cross-sectional study in Denmark that found that reported exposure to fumes or chemicals at work was associated with the prevalence of reported headaches during a 1-year period. Table 1 also includes measures of the impact of exposure on the prevalence of headaches (assuming a causal association). Associations may also be measured by correlation and regression coefficients, differences between means, and other statistics.

A prevalence ratio of 1.8 means that the prevalence of the disease in exposed people is 1.8 times as high as in unexposed people. An exposure ratio of 1.74 means that exposure is 1.74 times as prevalent among people with the disease as it is among those free of it.

An odds ratio is the ratio of one odds to another. An odds is the ratio of the probability that something is so or will occur, to the probability that it is not so or will not occur; in Table 1, *a*/*b* is an odds in favour of the presence of headaches. The odds ratio (*ad*/*bc*) of 1.89 in Table 1 can be regarded as the disease odds ratio—the odds in favour of headaches are 1.89 times as high among people exposed to fumes (odds = *a*/*b*) as among those not exposed (odds = *c*/*d*). It can also be regarded as the exposure odds ratio—the odds in favour of exposure are 1.89 times as high among people with headaches (*a*/*c*) as among people free of headaches (*b*/*d*).

Odds ratios may be difficult to understand, and are easy to misinterpret. A survey of treatment decisions made by doctors presented with feigned patients with identical clinical pictures revealed that the odds ratio for referral for cardiac catheterization was 0.6 for black people, in comparison with white people (Schulman *et al.* 1999), and this was widely reported in the media in such terms as 'Doctors are only 60 per cent as likely to order cardiac catheterization for blacks as for whites'. The referral rates were 84.7 per cent and 90.6 per cent respectively, and the rate ratio corresponding to the odds ratio of 0.6 was 0.93 (Schwartz *et al.* 1999).

Opinions of the utility of odds ratios vary widely (Greenland 1987; Kahn and Sempos 1989; Lee 1994; Osborn and Carraruzza 1995; Selvin 1996; Zocchetti *et al.* 1997). Their useful features (using the numbers in Table 1 where possible) include the following.

1. Use of odds ratios facilitates comparisons of results from different kinds of study. Identical odds ratios can be expected in a study of a total population (or representative sample), a comparison of representative samples of people exposed and not exposed to fumes (yielding the disease odds ratio), and a comparison of representative samples of people with and without headaches (yielding the exposure odds ratio). The sampling fractions do not affect the value of the odds ratio; for example, the ratio remains 1.89 if the numbers in the 'factor absent' group are reduced to one-tenth ($c = 5$, $d = 85$). Under certain conditions, odds ratios from cross-sectional studies can be compared with odds ratios from time-span studies, and odds ratios derived from studies based on analyses of 2 × 2 tables can be compared with those derived from logistical regression analysis, whose regression coefficients are the natural logs of odds ratios.

2. The odds ratio for freedom from the disease is the reciprocal of the disease odds ratio. The disease odds ratio in Table 1 is 1.89, and the ratio of the odds in favour of freedom from headaches in exposed people (90/10) to the corresponding odds in unexposed people (850/50) is 0.53, which is 1/1.89. This does not hold true for the prevalence ratio; again comparing exposed and unexposed people, the disease prevalence ratio is 1.8, but the ratio of the freedom-from-headaches prevalences, that is the ratio of 90/100 to 850/900, is 0.95—which gives the impression of very little difference between exposed and unexposed people.

3. Observations in different population groups or strata are often combined by the Mantel–Haenszel procedure, multiple logistic regression analysis, or other techniques, on the assumption that the association has the same strength in each group. There is no problem with this concept if odds ratios are used to measure the association. But the concept of a common value for the prevalence

Table 1 Measures of association and impact (study of a population) using fictional data on headaches and exposure to fumes

Exposure to fumes	Disease present (headaches)	Disease absent (no headaches)	Total
Factor present	$a = 10$	$b = 90$	$a + b = 100$
Factor absent	$c = 50$	$d = 850$	$c + d = 900$
Total $a + c = 60$	$b + d = 940$	$n = 1000$	

Odds ratio = ad/bc = 1.89; this is the formula for both the disease odds ratio and the exposure odds ratio, which have the same value. It can also be calculated as bc/ad = 0.53 (the reciprocal of 1.89).

Disease odds ratio = the ratio of a/b (one disease odds) to c/d (another), or the ratio of c/d to a/b.

Exposure odds ratio = the ratio of a/c (one exposure odds) to b/d (another), or the ratio of b/d to a/c.

Rate ratios

Prevalence ratio = $[a/(a + b)]/[c/(c + d)]$ = 1.8 or $[c/(c + d)]/[a/(a + b)]$ = 0.56 (the reciprocal of 1.8).

Exposure ratio = $[a/(a + c)]/[b/(b + d)]$ = 1.74 or $[b/(b + d)]/[a/(a + c)]$ = 0.57 (the reciprocal of 1.74).

Rate differences

Prevalence difference = $a/(a + b) - c/(c + d)$ = 0.0444.

Exposure difference = $a/(a + c) - b/(b + d)$ = 0.07.

Number needed in unexposed group to avoid one case: 1/prevalence difference = 1/0.444 = 22.5.

Measures of impact

- If the factor is a risk factor:
  - excess risk among exposed = $a/(a + b) - c/(c + d)$ = 0.04
  - population excess risk = $(a + c)/n - c\ (c + d)$ 0.004
  - attributable fraction (exposed) = $[a/(a + b) - c/(c + d)]/[a/(a + b)] \times 100$ = 44.4 per cent
  - or (prevalence ratio − 1)/prevalence ratio × 100 = 44.4 per cent
  - attributable fraction (population) = $[(a + c)/n - c/(c + d)]/[(a + c)/n\ ] \times 100$ = 7.4 per cent
  - or [(prevalence ratio − 1) × E]/{1 + [(prevalence ratio − 1) × E]} × 100 = 7.4 per cent (where E = exposure rate in population).
- If the factor is a protective factor:
  - excess risk among unexposed = $c/(c + d) - a/(a + b)$
  - population excess risk = $(a + c)/n - a/(a + b)$
  - prevented fraction (exposed) = $[c/(c + d) - a/(a + b)]/[c/(c + d)] \times 100$
  - (this is also the preventable fraction % among the unexposed)
  - prevented fraction (population) = $[c/(c + d) - (a + c)/n]/[c/(c + d)] \times 100$
  - preventable fraction (population) = $[(a + c)/n - a/(a + b)]/[(a + c)/n] \times 100$.

ratio may be untenable if rates are high (Kahn and Sempos 1989). The prevalence ratio in Table 1, for example, is 1.8, but in a different stratum where the prevalence in the unexposed was 70 per cent, a prevalence ratio of 1.8 would be impossible—the highest possible ratio would be 100 per cent/70 per cent, or 1.4.

4. In aetiological studies of disease, the measure of interest is the ratio of the incidence in persons exposed and unexposed to a putative causal factor, and the odds ratio can sometimes serve as a proxy for this. The prevalence ratio can serve as an indicator of the risk ratio (cumulative incidence-rate ratio) in cross-sectional studies if the risk factor is no longer active: for example, a study of non-lethal birth defects in relation to some prenatal factor, or other studies of diseases with short and well-defined periods of risk, for example, of an epidemic of diarrhoeal illness after a social gathering (Kleinbaum *et al.* 1982; Rothman 1986).

If the prevalence ratio is not available—for example, if the study compares samples of people with and without the disease—an odds ratio is a good estimator of the prevalence ratio, provided that prevalence is low, and can therefore be used as an estimator of the risk ratio. Selvin (1996) suggests that 'low' here means a rate of under 10 per cent in each of the groups that are compared. The odds ratio and the prevalence ratio in Table 1 are fairly close (1.89 and 1.8); they would be closer (the odds ratio would also be 1.8) if the prevalence of headaches was only 1.8 per cent in exposed and 1 per cent in unexposed people.

The odds ratio can sometimes be interpreted as an incidence ratio even if the disease is not rare (Breslow 1982; Miettinen 1985; Rothman 1986; Pearce 1993). This applies to studies in which cases of a disease with a long risk period (like most chronic diseases) are compared with disease-free controls who are representative of the population from which the cases developed, and who at the time that they are studied can be regarded as possible future cases. In such a cross-sectional study the odds ratio is equivalent to the ratio of person-time incidence rates, provided that exposure can be assumed to precede the onset of the disease and not to affect the duration of the disease, and that the disease does not affect exposure status; this equivalence does not apply within narrow age categories, or if aetiological factors have changed in the course of time. The odds ratio can also be interpreted as the ratio of person-time incidence rates in a study comparing cases that develop during a given time with controls selected at the same times as the cases, and as a risk ratio if controls are sampled from the whole population at the beginning of follow-up.

Odds ratios and prevalence ratios based on samples tend to overestimate the true odds and prevalence ratios in the population sampled. This bias may be marked if the sample is small, and the use of estimators that offset the bias has been suggested. Jewell's (1986) low-bias estimator of the odds ratio is

$$ad/[(b + 1)(c + 1)]$$

or (conversely)

$$bc/[(a + 1)(d + 1)].$$

For the fairly large numbers in Table 1 the disease odds ratio becomes 1.83, instead of 1.89 by the usual formula. A disadvantage of this method is that the odds ratio for freedom from the disease is no longer the reciprocal of the disease odds ratio (Walter and Cook 1991); it becomes 0.48, which is 1/2.11. Jewell's low-bias point estimate of the prevalence ratio is

$$[a/(a + b)]/[(c + 1)/(c + d + 1)]$$

or (conversely)

$$[a/(a + c)]/[(b + 1)/(b + d + 1)]$$

(1.77 or 0.51 in this instance).

Studies of causal relationships generally use odds or other ratios, but differences, especially between prevalences, may be preferred to ratios when interest lies in the magnitude of a public health problem; for example, if we wish to estimate how many people in a population have headaches because of exposure to fumes, or to use this information in estimating treatment costs or impact on productivity. A useful measure based on the prevalence difference is the number needed to prevent one case, on the assumption that exposure is causal and can be avoided; this is the reciprocal of the prevalence difference. According to Table 1, 22.5 people are needed in the unexposed group to avoid one case.

In analytical cross-sectional studies that aim to explain as well as to describe associations, a variety of measures and techniques may be used to control confounding factors and determine whether other variables modify the association. The procedures range in complexity from stratification and standardization to sophisticated multivariate techniques that permit the simultaneous consideration of a large number of variables and their relationships. The findings in separate strata (for example, sex and age groups) are frequently combined by the Mantel–Haenszel or similar procedures to obtain odds ratios, rate ratios, or rate differences that control for the effects of the stratifying variable or variables; the summary measures should be used only after appraising the homogeneity of the findings in the strata in order to see whether they can be validly combined (Fleiss 1981; Selvin 1996; Abramson and Gahlinger 2001).

Uses in community health care

Cross-sectional studies can fulfil important functions in the health care of a community. They can contribute to the planning of services, to the effective implementation of care, and to decision-making on the continuation and modification of services. In this discussion, 'community' may be taken to refer to any aggregation of people for whose care a doctor, health-care team, agency, or authority is responsible; it may be a nation or region, a local neighbourhood, a list of registered patients, a defined group of schoolchildren or workers, inmates of an institution, and so on.

Separate consideration will be given to the use of cross-sectional studies in community diagnosis, in ongoing surveillance, in community health education and the promotion of community involvement, and in evaluation of the community's health care.

Community diagnosis

Cross-sectional studies can provide a major part of the epidemiological foundation for community diagnosis, that is, for determining the health status of a community and the factors that influence it. They can supply information on the nature, extent, and impact of health problems, as a basis for the identification of priorities and the planning of intervention. Such studies may relate to a broad spectrum of health states and their correlates, or may be limited in their scope.

Health status

Cross-sectional studies may yield useful information on a variety of dimensions of health and disease, including self-appraised health, mental health status, growth and development, physical fitness, the distribution of blood pressures, and so on. The following remarks refer only to the prevalence of disorders; the cross-sectional method for the study of growth and development is discussed below.

It must be remembered that prevalence, especially point prevalence, may provide an incomplete picture because of the under-representation of conditions with a short duration. These include not only the acute non-fatal diseases that constitute a considerable load for the health services, and acute episodes of long-term or recurrent diseases, but also severe and rapidly fatal conditions, such as fatal strokes and sudden deaths from coronary heart disease. This bias was strikingly illustrated during a famine in Chad in 1985, when a rapid assessment displayed no severe malnutrition in children and it was concluded that serious malnutrition did not exist; in fact many children were affected, but they died too soon to be included in the survey (Guha-Sapir 1991).

The most direct evidence of a need for improved secondary and tertiary prevention, at least for long-term diseases that are not rapidly fatal, is an unduly high prevalence of remediable disease that has not been diagnosed or that is untreated or inadequately treated. Prevalence surveys providing such information may be based on examinations, interviews, clinical files, or other documentary sources, or a combination of these. In Australia, a two-stage prevalence study found that almost a million adults had moderate or severe hearing impairment that would probably be helped by a hearing aid, which well over half were not using (Wilson *et al.* 1999). In Italy, a survey based on the Registry of the Blind showed that the rate of blindness was much higher in the south of the country than in the north; possible causes for the difference in blindness due to treatable conditions such as cataract and glaucoma included a regional difference in the quality or accessibility of care (Nicolosi *et al.* 1994).

Needs for primary prevention can be inferred from the presence of preventable disorders, that is, those whose incidence can be reduced by known preventive measures. For this purpose too, the prevalence data should be supplemented by data on incidence and mortality, both because diseases with a high fatality rate will otherwise be under-represented and because prevalent cases may be long-standing ones that do not reflect present preventive needs. A high prevalence of crippling due to poliomyelitis does not necessarily mean that current preventive procedures are ineffective. Information on the recent incidence of new cases is to be preferred for this purpose. If prevalence data are to be used, information should be sought on the duration of the disorder, so that the prevalence of disease of recent onset can be measured. In institutional settings where people who develop a disorder are especially likely to remain in the institution, prevalence data may overestimate the need for primary prevention. In a hospital, for example, patients who develop nosocomial infections are for this reason likely to have a longer hospital stay. A prevalence survey of such infections in a hospital may thus give an exaggerated idea of the need for primary prevention.

The use of highly valid measures of the presence of a disease often presents practical difficulties, and reliance may be placed on a proxy measure that is simple, cheap, and acceptable; a screening test may be used for this purpose.

The confidence interval of the prevalence of the disease can be estimated from the prevalence of the proxy attribute (Rogan and Gladen 1978).

Determinants of health and disease

Information on the prevalence of modifiable factors that are known to affect health is of obvious relevance to the planning of health care. These may be factors with broad effects on health, for example, dietary, infant rearing, smoking, and family planning practices and (presumably) the use of health services, and they may be factors that affect the risk of developing specific disorders. They may be factors relevant to the community at large, such as poverty, unemployment, or air pollution, or they may be relevant to specific subgroups, as in studies of bullying behaviour in schools (Forero *et al.* 1999). They may be risk factors, which increase the risk of ill health, or protective factors, for example, physical activity or specific immunity (natural or acquired) to a pathogenic agent.

Associations between variables

When associations are investigated in a cross-sectional study in the context of community health care, the focus may be placed on specific diseases, disabilities, or other health characteristics, in order to throw light on their determinants or predictors, or on specific risk factors or protective factors, in order to examine their associations with health and disease. In this context, the aim is usually to determine what causal factors or correlates (of those known to be potentially important) are active in the specific community, and to measure their impact. The primary aim is to obtain information that will be useful in practice, not to generate new knowledge about aetiology, although this may be a secondary gain. A cross-sectional survey of respiratory symptoms and exposure to tobacco smoke in schoolchildren in Hong Kong, for example, was undertaken not to reconfirm known aetiological relationships, but to examine the impact of active and passive smoking in this population, as a basis for policy decisions on tobacco control (Lam *et al.* 1998).

Attention may also be centred on the determinants of supposed risk or protective factors, as in studies of the determinants of cigarette smoking, the use of a health service, or compliance with medical advice, and on associations among diseases or other dimensions of health, or among determinants of health.

Measurement of impact

In a situation where it is believed that an association of a risk factor with the prevalence (or incidence) of a disease expresses a causal relationship, the factor's impact may be measured by the attributable (or aetiological) fraction in the population. This is the proportion of the disease in the population that can be attributed to exposure to the factor (Table 1). Among workers aged 20 to 64 years in a community in Jerusalem, for example, the fraction of the prevalence of varicose veins that could be attributed to work involving much standing was 16 per cent in each sex, after controlling for effects connected with age, region of birth, weight, and height (Abramson *et al.* 1981). Such values must be interpreted with caution, as part or all of the apparent causal effect may be due to other (uncontrolled) factors associated with the apparent causal factor. The attributable fraction among the exposed may also be of interest: 31 per cent of the prevalence of varicose veins in men whose work involved much standing could be attributed to their work posture; for women, this fraction was 32 per cent.

For a protective factor, the corresponding measures (Table 1) are the prevented fraction, which is the proportion of the hypothetical total prevalence that has been prevented by exposure to the factor, and the preventable fraction, which is the proportion of the observed prevalence that would be prevented if everyone was exposed to the factor. These fractions are sometimes termed the 'efficacy' of the protective factor, particularly with respect to vaccines.

Attributable, prevented, and preventable fractions are specific to a particular population, since they are influenced by the prevalence of the factor, and the factor's causal effect may be dependent on the prevalence of other factors. The fractions attributable to different causes can sum up to more than 100 per cent, since causes operate in conjunction, and their attributable fractions overlap (Rothman and Greenland 1998).

Measures of impact are generally more helpful as a basis for intervention and policy decisions than odds and prevalence ratios or other measures of association. It is more useful to know that according to a cross-sectional study, 26 to 43 per cent of various asthma-like symptoms in young women in towns in East Anglia were attributable to the use of gas for cooking, than to know that the odds ratios were about 2 (Brauer and Kennedy 1996; Jarvis *et al.* 1996). If the proportion exposed to a factor is high, the attributable risk may be much higher than might be guessed from the odds or prevalence ratio; for drinking alcohol (ever) and breast cancer, for example, the population attributable fraction according to a study in New York was 25 per cent and the odds ratio 1.4 (Bowlin *et al.* 1997).

Risk markers

Interest may not be confined to cause–effect relationships. Any attribute or exposure that is strongly associated with a disease or other disorder, even non-causally, has potential value as a predictor, provided that there is reason to believe that it precedes the appearance of the disorder. Such predictors may be used as risk markers to identify vulnerable individuals or groups. The risk marker may be a factor that itself influences the risk, or a precursor or early manifestation of the disorder, or it may be secondarily associated with the disorder because it is associated with a cause or precursor of the disorder.

Risk markers are best identified by longitudinal studies, but can also be detected by cross-sectional ones. A cross-sectional study in Singapore, for example, showed that over 80 per cent of people with corneal arcus (a grey circle around the cornea) at the age of 30 to 49 years had high serum low-density lipoprotein cholesterol levels (Hughes *et al.* 1992). In The Netherlands, a cross-sectional study showed that divorced people were less healthy than single, married, or widowed people, controlling for age, sex, whether living alone, and other variables (Joung *et al.* 1994). In Israel, a national cross-sectional study showed a high prevalence of morbidity among 17-year-olds who were extremely underweight or extremely overweight, suggesting the use of low or excessive weight as markers to trigger intervention at an earlier age (Lusky *et al.* 1996). The reasons for the associations with corneal arcus, divorcee status, and body weight are of interest and may be of practical importance, but are irrelevant to the decision whether to use these characteristics as risk markers.

The value of a risk marker or combination of risk markers depends on the following considerations.

1. Is its use practical? Questions of simplicity, acceptability, safety, convenience, cost, and resources must be considered.
2. Is detection of high risk likely to be beneficial? Are resources and techniques available for reducing the risk? Does the benefit outweigh any harm that intervention may cause? What is the predictive value of the risk marker, that is, what proportion of people with the marker are likely to have or develop the disease?
3. How prevalent is the risk marker? If more than half of the children in a community fall into a high-risk group, might it not be more efficient and possibly more effective to modify the routine care programme so as to give extra attention to all children?
4. What is the marker's sensitivity as a predictor? That is, what proportion of the individuals with the disorder will it identify? If this proportion is small, its value is limited.

The answers to these questions may vary in different contexts, as may the associations between specific factors and diseases. A given risk marker may be useful in one setting but not in another.

Community syndromes

The term 'community health syndrome' may be used to refer to diseases or other health characteristics found to occur together in a community. Examples described by Kark (1974, 1981), who introduced the community syndrome concept and emphasized its potential importance for the development of community health programmes, are a syndrome of malnutrition, communicable diseases, and mental ill health in a poor rural community undergoing rapid change, and the syndrome of hypertension, coronary heart disease, and diabetes frequently found in affluent communities characterized by nutritional imbalance and excesses, limited physical activity, and a drive for achievement.

The components of a syndrome may occur together because they possess shared or related causes, or because they are themselves causally inter-related. The syndrome points to a nexus of causal processes in the community. Even if this nexus is not completely understood, a health programme directed at the syndrome as a whole may be more effective and efficient than an endeavour to deal separately with the individual components.

Associations between diseases or other health states may be detected at a population level or (more convincingly) at an individual level, that is, by finding a tendency to affect the same persons. As an example of the latter approach, a study of coprevalence in Jerusalem revealed clustering of migraine and other common disorders characterized by complaints (rather than objective signs) (Abramson *et al.* 1982). These disorders were frequently associated with emotional symptoms and with family disharmony or other stressful situations, and people with one or more components of the syndrome made heavy use of medical services. This syndrome represented a considerable burden of discomfort for many individuals and their families, and there was no organized programme to deal with it.

Identification of groups requiring special care

Community diagnosis may focus not only on the community as a whole but on its component groups. Comparisons may identify groups for whom special care may be needed. This identification may be based on the presence of disorders, on screening tests that point to a high probability of having a disorder, on the presence of modifiable risk factors, and/or on the presence of known risk markers indicative of vulnerability and a need for preventive care.

A differential approach in community diagnosis is of basic importance for the identification of priorities and the allocation of resources. Sometimes simple descriptive findings suffice for these purposes, and in other circumstances the planning of effective care requires an understanding of the reasons for the differences found, requiring the use of analytical epidemiological techniques.

The detection of a high-risk or high-morbidity group does not necessarily mean that special care is indicated; this depends on the likely benefits, on what proportion of the community's cases or prospective cases is concentrated in the group, and on practical and other considerations.

Surveillance

Ongoing surveillance permits the identification of changes in health status and its determinants in the community, and updating of the community diagnosis. Repeated cross-sectional studies, as well as incidence studies, have a clear role, and are the only practicable method for some purposes, for example to detect changes in a community's health habits or blood pressure distributions. Surveys of different representative samples may be advisable for this purpose, rather than repeated investigations of the same sample, to avoid the possibility that participation in a survey may affect the subjects' behaviour, including their participation in health programmes and their responses in a later survey (Kroeger 1985; Puska 1991). In North Karelia, during 3 years of operation of a cardiovascular risk factor programme, men who were followed up longitudinally decreased their smoking by 11 per cent, whereas a comparison of the baseline data with a new representative sample showed a drop of only 7 per cent (Puska 1991). Repeated cross-sectional studies, like those of the WHO MONICA (Multinational Monitoring of Trends and Determinants in Cardiac Disease) project, yielded much information about changes in cardiovascular diseases and their risk factors in various countries (Tunstall-Pedoe *et al.* 1999).

Surveillance of the prevalence of chronic disorders may be based on repeated prevalence surveys, or on the use of a case register that is updated as new cases are found or old ones recover, die, or leave. Changes in the prevalence of chronic disorders may be important as an indication of changing needs for curative and rehabilitative care facilities.

Changes in the prevalence of a chronic disease cannot, however, be glibly taken to indicate changes in the risk of developing the disorder; for this purpose, incidence data should be used. There are a number of possible reasons for changes in prevalence. As illustrated in Fig. 1, the changes reflect the interplay of incidence, recovery, and fatality rates. They may be caused by changes in the demographic characteristics of the population as a result of ageing or inward or outward migration. Especially in studies of small local communities, prevalence may be influenced by a tendency of affected persons to leave or enter the neighbourhood.

Often, apparent changes in prevalence are artefacts caused by changes in methods of case identification (for example, the introduction of a case-finding programme), in the use of medical services, in diagnostic procedures or definitions, or in recording, notification, or registration practices. They may also be caused by incomplete updating of a case register.

Community education and community involvement

Community surveys can be used as tools for community health education. This may be done not only by communicating the findings and their implications to the community and its leaders, but also by using the educational potential of the survey situation itself, for example, by explaining to participants why the collection of specific information is important. If accurate results are required, such explanations should preferably be given after the information has been collected, to minimize bias in the responses.

An example is provided by the 'Know Your Body' programme, which aimed to motivate schoolchildren to adopt a healthier lifestyle (Williams *et al.* 1977). After the measurement of chronic disease risk factors, each child received a feedback of results in a 'health passport', together with explanations of desirable ranges for each test, in order to enhance the effect of the curriculum. Trials indicate that this programme effectively modified health knowledge, and had mixed effects on cardiovascular risk factors (Marcus *et al.* 1987; Walter *et al.* 1987; Tamir *et al.* 1990; Resnicow *et al.* 1993).

Involvement of key community members in the planning and conduct of a health survey may be a useful way to motivate them to a more active participation in the promotion of their community's health. A community's interest and involvement in its own health care may find expression in the performance of community self-surveys, even without the participation of professional health workers. Such surveys are usually simple descriptive ones, and may not collect very accurate or sophisticated information.

Evaluation of a community's health care

In the context of community health care, the purpose of an evaluative study is to yield a factual basis for decisions about the provision of care to a specific community. This kind of evaluative study, the programme review, can be contrasted with programme trials, which aim to provide generalizable inferences about the value of a given type of health programme. In programme reviews, considerable attention is given to evaluation of the process of care (the performance of activities by providers and recipients of care), as well as to measurements of desirable and undesirable effects, especially more immediate outcomes.

Certain findings that are used in the process of community diagnosis as indicators of needs for health care, such as a high prevalence of preventable or remediable disorders, may by the same token be seen as indicators of the value of past health care. In some instances a prevalence survey may reveal more direct evidence of the quality of previous care; for example, the quality of the dental work in subjects' mouths may be appraised, or the presence of inguinal hernia recurrences may be recorded (in one study, one in five operated hernias showed evidence of recurrence (Abramson *et al.* 1978)).

Evaluative judgements that relate to the subjects' prior health care as a whole, however, may be less helpful than those relating to recent or current health care, and especially to care in the context of a specific health programme or service. Studies might deal, for example, with compliance with medical advice (what proportion of hypertensives are taking the medicines prescribed for them?), with satisfaction with medical care, or with immunization status.

In these as in other studies, separate attention is usually paid to population subgroups. The impact of a health programme often varies with age, sex, social class, and other characteristics.

Evidence of change in health status or practices may be provided by repeated cross-sectional studies as well as by incidence and other longitudinal studies. It is usually assumed that such changes (or their absence) are, at least to some extent, reflections of programme effectiveness and not attributable only to outside influences. At the very least, the findings may indicate whether there is a need for more detailed evaluative study.

More rigorous proof that the change is attributable to the programme requires a comparison with controls. For example, the effectiveness of a breast-feeding promotion programme was confirmed by the finding that the prevalence of breast feeding rose much more than in a neighbouring community with no such programme (Palti *et al.* 1988).

Uses in clinical practice

Epidemiological studies serve important functions in clinical care. The role of cross-sectional studies are considered in individual and family care and in community-oriented primary care.

Individual and family care

Textbooks of clinical epidemiology emphasize that epidemiology is a basic science for clinicians, and demonstrate its use (Sackett *et al.* 1991). 'A great many routine clinical decisions about individual patient care . . . can only be based upon information from properly designed and executed studies in groups or populations' (Roberts 1977). The systematic use of properly appraised information is the central feature of what is increasingly becoming known as evidence-based medicine—'an approach that integrates the best external evidence with individual clinical expertise and patient choice' (Sackett *et al.* 1997).

Cross-sectional studies play a role here, if a modest one, since they can provide information on the prevalence of diseases and their symptoms and causes, the frequency distributions of biochemical and other measurements in the population and in patients with specific disorders, patterns of child growth, health practices, and so on. This information may be derived from any studies whose results can validly be generalized to the population in which the clinician works. A population study in Edinburgh, for example, that demonstrated the high prevalence, in people without varicose veins, of lower limb symptoms commonly attributed to varicose veins, cannot be ignored by a doctor anywhere who is considering the extirpation of varices in order to ameliorate symptoms (Bradbury *et al.* 1999).

Epidemiological information of this sort is seldom the fruit of the clinician's own labours, except in a context of community-oriented primary care (see below). Sometimes, however, even a doctor concerned only with individual patients may conduct what in effect are small-scale (usually cross-sectional) epidemiological surveys—for example, of a patient's contacts for evidence of a communicable disease, to reduce the patient's risk of reinfection. A family doctor, responsible for the care of whole families, may need to perform such investigations more often; the discovery that a patient has a condition with a known tendency to 'run in families' (for example, rheumatic heart disease, diabetes, amoebiasis, AIDS, or *Helicobacter pylori* infection) may be seen as a signal that the whole family should be surveyed.

Family diagnosis, the process of appraising a family's health status and the factors that affect it, is an exercise in small-group epidemiology, conducted by a family practitioner. Its aim is to determine a family's health needs as a basis for the planning of a family health programme. This involves elucidation of the family members' health status and appraisal of relevant features of the family life situation: for example, the family's structure and composition, the role performance and health-relevant behaviour of its members, relationships, material resources and their use, and the family's social and physical environment. At an analytical level, it involves appraisal of the ways in which family members' health may be affected by other members and by the family life situation.

Community-oriented primary care

Community-oriented primary care refers to the combination of the care of individuals and the care of the community as a whole, in a single integrated practice (Kark 1981; Abramson 1988; Kark *et al.* 1994; Kark and Kark 1999). The practitioner or team providing clinical care initiates or participates in specific community programmes that deal in a systematic way with the main health needs of the community and its subgroups. There is growing awareness of the potential of this form of integrated practice for improving health in both developing and developed countries (Connor and Mullan 1983; Nutting 1987; Gillam *et al.* 1994; Tollman and Friedman 1994; Rhyne *et al.* 1998).

Epidemiology is an indispensable basis for the planning, development, and evaluation of the community health programmes that characterize community-oriented primary care, and the uses (listed above) of cross-sectional studies both in community health care and in individual and family care are relevant to this form of practice.

Obviously, the information required for the practice of community-oriented primary care is not limited to the community served—evidence concerning the effectiveness of various methods of treatment and various community interventions may come from studies elsewhere, and a decision that a specific program is needed (for example, for the control of hypertension) may be based on findings in other or broader populations. But information about the specific community is always required, and the community-oriented primary care practitioner or team must ensure that this is collected, or a community orientation is likely to remain a well-meaning aspiration rather than a means of effecting demonstrable improvements in health.

Information about the community may have three foci, as follows.

1. A general picture ('getting to know the community'), whose purposes include identification of health problems that merit detailed study and possible action (a 'needs assessment') (Trompeter 1992), and appraisal of their possible causes and the resources and circumstances that may be relevant to their solution. Use is generally made of 'rapid' methods, based on easily available sources and qualitative research procedures.
2. A more detailed community diagnosis with respect to selected health problems and their determinants, in order to decide whether a programme is warranted (is there a sufficient 'case for action'?) and, if so, to aid in its planning and implementation, and provide baseline data for the measurement of the changes it is expected to produce.
3. Monitoring of programme activities and surveillance of change, leading to an evaluation of effectiveness.

Much of this information (but obviously, not all) is derived from cross-sectional studies. These do not necessarily refer to a fixed calendar time; the prevalence of a disease, for example, is usually determined by interviews or examinations that are staggered over a period. An important feature is that much of the information needed for community diagnosis, surveillance, and evaluation is generally obtained in the course of routine clinical care. The collection of data thus serves a double function. When a child is weighed or a question is asked about smoking or a diagnosis is made, the results may be used both in the management of the patient and as data for subsequent analysis at a group level. The data may be derived either from routine clinical procedures or from questions or tests specially added for epidemiological purposes. In a practice where periodic health examinations are conducted, these provide an especially useful opportunity for the collection of data for analysis.

This use of clinical data demands careful attention to methods of obtaining, recording, and retrieving data, to make the information as accurate and complete as possible.

Standardized procedures are required, and definitions and diagnostic criteria should be standardized as rigorously as possible. The collection of data by care providers in a care setting carries advantages and disadvantages. On the one hand, it may be relatively easy to obtain answers to awkward questions, and to achieve a high response rate. On the other hand, there are several sources of possible bias.

Except in groups with very high attendance rates (for instance infants and their mothers, pregnant women, and the elderly), there may be a need for supplementary survey procedures to obtain information about members of the community who have not attended for clinical care, and these people may be invited to attend, visited at home, or asked for information by mail or telephone.

If resources are available, information may also be obtained by special surveys. In a community-oriented primary care setting, these generally aim to provide information that will benefit individual participants as well as providing a basis for decisions at a community level. The WHO has published a practical guide to the conduct of simple epidemiological surveys at a district level (Vaughan and Morrow 1989).

Sampling is seldom appropriate, since one aim is usually to identify individuals who need care.

For chronic diseases, a common technique is the maintenance of a case register. This permits the calculation of prevalence rates or other epidemiological indices and may assist in monitoring the performance of tests and other activities, besides its use as a tool to ensure that patients receive the care they need.

The process of information collection can serve to promote community development and the community's involvement in its own care, which are usually defined as aims of community-oriented primary care.

Meetings with community leaders, designed to learn their opinions about health problems and their solutions, can stimulate interest and promote community action, as can surveys and feedbacks of survey findings. In some community-oriented primary care practices, focus groups have proved to be a valuable means not only of collecting data, but also of enabling the community to recognize its needs, so that it can mobilize to meet them (Plaut *et al.* 1993).

Studies yielding 'new knowledge'

Many cross-sectional studies are performed to expand the horizons of knowledge, rather than solely to promote the health of the specific groups or populations studied. They are 'research' studies that aim to yield generalizable inferences that are of broad applicability, not relevant only to a specific local context.

Studies of growth and development, and of aetiology and programme trials, are briefly considered. Other research topics include the natural history of health and disease (usually better investigated by time-span studies) and methodological issues. Cross-sectional studies are also commonly used in comparisons of diagnostic criteria and other operational definitions and of study methods, and to appraise the validity of screening tests and proxy measures.

Studies of growth and development

Growth and development, and age trends in the prevalence of disorders, can be studied cross-sectionally as well as longitudinally. The cross-sectional method compares different age groups observed at one point of time, whereas the longitudinal method makes repeated observations of a single cohort as its age changes. The cross-sectional method is simpler, but has limitations. It can provide information about average changes, but not about intraindividual changes or interindividual differences.

The main limitation of the cross-sectional method is that the age groups that are compared may differ in respects other than age, so that the effects of age and other influences may be confounded. There is always potential confounding of age changes with differences between birth cohorts, as the age groups that are compared must belong to different cohorts. Cohort differences in growth may be negligible, but they may be significant if cohorts were exposed to very different circumstances: for example, different infant-feeding or child-rearing practices, changes in economic prosperity, or war. As a result the cross-sectional method may yield a misleading picture. If there has been a secular increase in height, a cross-sectional study may show a decrease in average height throughout adult life, but young adults will be taller because they belong to a more recently born generation, not because they are younger. If a series of cross-sectional studies has been done, suitable rearrangement of the data may permit examination and comparison of the longitudinal changes in different cohorts.

In studies that include the middle-aged and elderly, selective survival may be important. The mean blood pressure may be lower in the very old, not because blood pressure tends to drop with age, but because hypertensive people are more likely to have died and thus left the study sample. Also, the validity of measures may vary with age. The results of a memory test in the elderly may reflect hearing ability, attentiveness, or depression, rather than memory capacity.

Studies of aetiology

Cross-sectional studies often provide useful guides to aetiological processes, especially with respect to influences on long-term disorders and relatively stable measurements and health habits. They have two features, however, that often restrict their value for the testing of causal hypotheses.

Firstly, any associations they reveal are with the presence, not the appearance, of the disorder or other variable studied. Transient or rapidly fatal cases are inevitably under-represented. The causes that determine the appearance of the disorder are confounded with those that influence its duration, and it may be difficult to draw clear inferences about either set of causes. As an example, a high frequency of the A2 human lymphocyte antigen was found in children with acute lymphocytic leukaemia, suggesting that this was a risk factor, but later studies showed that the antigen lengthened the children's lifespan, which was why prevalent cases included a high proportion who had the antigen (Rogentine *et al.* 1972, 1973; cited by Newman *et al.* 1988). Such confounding is relatively unimportant if the disorder studied is seldom fatal and has high chronicity, or data on lifetime prevalence are used. In such instances the main difficulty in a cross-sectional study is that the causal factors may no longer be apparent because of the time-lag since the initiation of the disease.

Secondly, in a strictly cross-sectional study the absence of information on time relationships may render it difficult to separate effects on a dependent variable from effects of the dependent variable. The influence of blood pressure, serum cholesterol, and cigarette smoking on the occurrence of myocardial infarction, for example, may be confounded with changes ensuing from the disease episode.

The demonstration in a cross-sectional study that fat abdomens (based on a comparison of waist with hip size) are associated with hypertension, hypertensive heart disease, and diabetes (controlling for sex, age, and ponderal index) is difficult to interpret without knowing which came first, the fat abdomen or the disease (Gillum 1987). The discovery of an inverse association in San Francisco's bus drivers between hypertension and reported job-related problems—a relationship that was not explained by confounding factors and was specific to hypertension (gastrointestinal, respiratory, and musculoskeletal problems were positively associated with the self-reported stressors)—was given two competing explanations. On the one hand, 'emotional states or coping mechanisms ... may play a role in the pathogenesis of hypertension through the repression of anger and hostility'. On the other, 'the hemodynamic consequences of elevated blood pressure may lead to a physiologic alteration of perception ... elevation in blood pressure reduces reactivity to noxious stimuli' (Winkleby *et al.* 1988).

There is no 'chicken-or-egg' (time-sequence) problem if the postulated cause is blood type or some other genetically determined characteristic or a long-past exposure or long-lived acquired attribute that can be assumed to precede the onset of the latent period of the disease being studied, or if a causal process in the opposite direction does not make sense. A study of postmenopausal women aged 45 to 61 in England, for example, showed that (controlling for numerous possible confounders) fast walking and climbing stairs were positively associated with bone mineral density measured in the femoral trochanter and in the whole body, and walking frequency was associated with a high bone density in the trochanter and the femoral neck, but only in women who walked fast (Coupland *et al.* 1999). The findings strongly support the hypothesis that these activities affect bone density, since a reverse causal association is untenable, and numerous possible confounders were controlled in the analysis. But even here, the possibility of confounding by some uncontrolled factor (for example, muscularity) that preceded and affected both bone density and activity patterns cannot be excluded.

The value of a cross-sectional study in the search for causes and precursors is limited whenever there is a possibility that the disease may change the subject's lifestyle, bodily functions and characteristics, or circumstances. To throw light on time sequences, cross-sectional studies are often extended to include historical information on times of disease onset or of other occurrences. Repeated cross-sectional studies of the same population can sometimes establish the order of events.

Cross-sectional studies may be fruitful sources of causal hypotheses for testing in time-span studies, even if, for one or other of the above reasons or because of possible bias or confounding, they do not themselves convincingly support a causal explanation. Here are three examples. The observation by Gregg (1941) that most of the mothers of a series of infants with congenital cataract had had rubella in pregnancy led to a series of studies that proved the causal relationship between rubella in early pregnancy and congenital anomalies. Secondly, a strong association between dietary diversity and anthropometric measures of nutritional status in Kenyan toddlers (Onyango *et al.* 1998) might be attributed either to the effect of diet on growth or to the effect of health status on the acceptance of new foods; the former explanation, which seems more likely, is open to testing in a cohort or intervention study. Thirdly, a cross-sectional study of American army veterans of the Persian Gulf War revealed a number of specific associations between symptoms and reported exposures (for example, to pesticides, anti-nerve-gas pills, and chemical and biological warfare agents), which the authors proposed to address by analysing the longitudinal data available for the subjects (Proctor *et al.* 1998).

Cross-sectional studies frequently demonstrate unexplained associations whose investigation in subsequent epidemiological or other studies might lead to important new knowledge. As an example, the most striking finding in a study of the prevalence of human T-lymphotropic virus type I infection in seven villages in Gabon (where this infection is endemic) was that prevalence was very much higher in the Kota-Obamba ethnic group (Le Hasran *et al.* 1994). No behavioural or other differences were found that could explain this high prevalence. Similarly, a study of young adults in the Antwerp region revealed large unexplained differences between small areas in the prevalence of respiratory symptoms (Wieringa *et al.* 1998). Associations of this kind pose aetiological riddles—findings awaiting an explanation.

A cross-sectional study may form the first stage of a time-span study, for which it provides baseline measurements of dependent and independent variables, and sometimes a sampling base. If the study is concerned with the incidence of a long-term disease, the baseline prevalence study identifies affected people, who may be followed up in order to study the natural history of the disease, but must be excluded from the population at risk of subsequently developing the disease. A cluster survey in a region of Tanzania, for example, provided information on the prevalence of HIV-1 infection in adults aged 15 to 34 years (the prevalence was 10 per cent, reaching 24 per cent in an urban zone), and seronegative individuals were re-examined 2 years later in order to determine the rate and correlates of seroconversion (Killewo *et al.* 1993).

Programme trials

Cross-sectional studies can have a role in studies that aim to provide generalizable conclusions and inferences about the value of a given type of health programme.

A simple way of testing the effectiveness of a programme is to compare the status of people who have and have not been exposed to it. In eight clinics in Lesotho, for example, a children's growth monitoring and nutrition education programme was evaluated by means of a cross-sectional study in which maternal knowledge about infant feeding was measured, and mothers were classified according to whether or not they had previously attended the clinic. Women who had attended were found to be more knowledgeable about the introduction of animal protein foods, the use of oral rehydration salts, and the method of weaning (Ruel *et al.* 1992). But an evaluative study based on simple comparison of the findings or changes seen in people who voluntarily participate or do not participate in a programme is generally unconvincing, as the comparison may be confounded by differences between the groups. It is difficult to be sure that the difference in the findings can be attributed to the difference in exposure to the programme. Perhaps women who were more knowledgeable, or more educable, were also more likely to attend the clinics. The possible confounding effects are not easy to control. In this study, the difference in knowledge remained apparent when a few easily measured possible confounders—maternal education, working status, parity, and the child's age—were controlled in the analysis. The authors correctly limited their conclusion to the statement that previous clinic attendance 'appeared to be' beneficial.

A similar approach is used in studies that aim to evaluate preventive and therapeutic procedures or programmes by comparing people who have experienced an unfavourable outcome with controls, to see whether they differ in their prior exposure to the procedure or programme. Such studies offer a relatively simple and rapid approach to evaluation (Smith 1989). But they present problems, particularly the possibility that the cases and controls may have differed in their initial characteristics (including prognostic factors) or eligibility for the procedure or programme, and care is required to control for confounding and other biases (Horwitz and Feinstein 1981).

To obtain convincing evidence of the effectiveness of a health programme that aims to modify the distribution of a characteristic in a population or to reduce the prevalence of a disease, it is necessary to measure the change in the population and to demonstrate that this can be attributed to the programme rather than to other causes. A trend shown by repeated cross-sectional studies adds to the force of the evidence—for example, in a population where the prevalence of anaemia in pregnant women was originally 12 per cent, and the introduction of an intervention programme was followed by a progressive drop to 8.8, then 3.3, then 1.6 per cent (Kark 1981). But the cause-and-effect relationship between a programme and its apparent outcome is always difficult to substantiate without observations of a comparison or reference population not exposed to the programme.

In trials of programmes directed at populations, it is unfortunately seldom possible to randomize. There is often little or no choice as to which population will be exposed to the programme under trial, and a restricted choice concerning a control population. Most programme trials are therefore quasi-experiments, in which the control group or groups are selected so as to be as similar as possible to the intervention group, and it remains necessary to control for possible confounders in the analysis. In a 5-year evaluation of the CHAD programme (Community Syndrome of Hypertension, Atherosclerosis and Diabetes) for the control of cardiovascular risk factors in a Jerusalem neighbourhood, for example, where cross-sectional studies revealed a significantly greater improvement in the exposed population than in a neighbouring control population, the confounders that were controlled included age, sex, education, and region of birth. The prevalence of some risk factors declined to some extent in the control population as well, apparently as a result of changes in awareness and health care—underlining the need for comparison groups in such studies. Over the next 18 years the essential features of the programme were adopted in the clinic serving the control population, and differences in risk factors became less obvious (Abramson *et al.* 1994). Difficulties in the evaluation of community programmes are discussed by Blackburn (1991), who stresses the need for studies involving more communities (possibly smaller), and preferably randomized.

The use of population samples in surveys designed to evaluate health programmes is discussed by Salonen *et al.* (1986), who compare the advantages and disadvantages of surveying separate samples on each occasion, compared with repeated surveys of the same samples.

Summary

This chapter has reviewed uses, methods, strengths, and weaknesses of cross-sectional studies. The essential feature of such surveys is that they collect information relating to a single specified time, but a time dimension is often introduced by the inclusion of easily collected historical information or by comparing successive studies so as to appraise changes in health status and its determinants, and their sequence.

Like other epidemiological studies, cross-sectional studies (descriptive and analytical) can both contribute to the health care of a specific group or community and serve as a research method for the attainment of generalizable new knowledge. These purposes, especially the first, can sometimes be met by the use of simple, undemanding, and inexpensive methods, such as cluster sampling; 'rapid epidemiological assessment' is especially relevant in situations (in both developed and developing countries) where resources are limited or results are required as a basis for programme decisions.

Cross-sectional surveys may be used in community diagnosis, ongoing surveillance, community health education and the promotion of community involvement, and evaluation of the community's health care, and they can contribute to the planning of services, the effective implementation of care, and decision-making on the continuation and modification of services.

In clinical practice, information derived from prevalence studies of the population in which a clinician works is of special pertinence. The performance of cross-sectional studies is often integrated with clinical care in the provision of community-oriented primary care, where (with other sources of information) they play an essential role in the planning, development, and evaluation of community health programmes.

Cross-sectional studies can contribute new knowledge on growth and development, birth-cohort effects, aetiology, the effectiveness of health programmes, the validity of screening tests, and other topics. Uncertainties concerning time relationships limit the value of cross-sectional studies in aetiological research, unless the causal factors are genetically determined ones, long-past exposures, or long-lived acquired attributes that can be assumed to precede the onset of the latent period of the disease under study.

Cross-sectional studies are a fruitful source of causal hypotheses for subsequent testing in other studies. A cross-sectional study may form the first stage of a longitudinal study, for which it provides baseline measurements of dependent and independent variables, and sometimes a sampling base.

References

Abramson, J.H. (1988). Community-oriented primary care: strategy, approaches and practice. *Public Health Reviews*, **16**, 35.

Abramson, J.H. and Abramson, Z.H. (1998). *Survey methods in community medicine: epidemiological research, programme evaluation, clinical trials* (5th edn). Churchill Livingstone, Edinburgh.

Abramson, J.H. and Abramson, Z.H. (2001). *Making sense of data: a self-instruction manual on the interpretation of epidemiologic data* (3rd edn). Oxford University Press, New York.

Abramson, J.H. and Gahlinger, P.M. (2001). *Computer programs for epidemiologists: PEPI 4.0.* Sagebrush Press, Salt Lake City, UT.

Abramson, J.H., Gofin, J., Hopp, C., Makler, A., and Epstein, L.M. (1978). The epidemiology of inguinal hernia. *Journal of Epidemiology and Community Health*, **32**, 59.

Abramson, J.H., Hopp, C., and Epstein, L.M. (1981). The epidemiology of varicose veins: a survey in western Jerusalem. *Journal of Epidemiology and Community Health*, **35**, 213.

Abramson, J.H., Gofin, J., Peritz, E., Hopp, C. and Epstein, L.M. (1982). Clustering of chronic disorders—a community study of co-prevalence in Jerusalem. *Journal of Chronic Diseases*, **35**, 221.

Abramson, J.H., Gofin, J., Hopp, C., Schein, M.H., and Naveh, P. (1994). The CHAD program for the control of cardiovascular risk factors in a Jerusalem community: a 24-year retrospect. *Israel Journal of Medical Sciences*, **30**, 108.

Anderson, D.W., Schoenberg, B.S., and Haerer, A.F. (1988). Prevalence surveys of neurologic disorders: methodological implications of the Copiah County study. *Journal of Clinical Epidemiology*, **41**, 339.

Anker, M., Guidotti, R.J., Orzeszyna, S., Sapirie, S.A., and Thuriaux, M.C. (1993). Rapid evaluation methods (REM) of health services performance: methodological observations. *Bulletin of the World Health Organization*, **711**, 15.

Armstrong, J.R.M. and Hayes, R. (1992) Estimating prevalence of injecting drug use in an urban population: limitations of the three-sample estimation procedure. *International Journal of Epidemiology*, **21**, 613.

Babaniyi, O. and Parakoyi, B. (1991). Cluster survey for poliomyelitis and neonatal tetanus in Ilorin, Nigeria. *International Journal of Epidemiology*, **20**, 515.

Balraj, V., Mukundan, S., Samuel, R., and John, T.J. (1993). Factors affecting immunization coverage levels in a district of India. *International Journal of Epidemiology*, **22**, 1146.

Bennett, S., Woods, T., Liyanage, W.M., and Smith, D.L. (1991). A simplified general method for cluster-sample surveys of health in developing countries. *World Health Statistics Quarterly*, **44**, 98.

Bishop, Y., Fienberg, S., and Holland, P. (1975) *Discrete multivariate analysis: theory and practice.* MIT Press, Cambridge, Massachusetts.

Blackburn, H. (1991). Community programmes in coronary heart disease prevention and health promotion: changing community behaviour. In *Coronary heart disease epidemiology: from aetiology to public health* (ed. M. Marmot and P. Elliott), p. 495. Oxford University Press.

Bosch, J.L., Hop, W.C., Kirkels, W.J., and Schroder, F.H. (1995). Natural history of benign prostatic hyperplasia: appropriate case definition and estimation of its prevalence in the community. *Urology*, **46** (3 Supplement A), 34.

Bowlin, S.J., Leske, M.C., Varma, A., Nasca, P., Weinstein, A., and Caplan, L. (1997) Breast cancer risk and alcohol consumption: results from a large case-control study. *International Journal of Epidemiology*, **26**, 915.

Bradbury, A., Evans, C., Allan, P., Lee, A., Ruckley, C.V., and Fowkes, F.G.R. (1999). What are the symptoms of varicose veins? Edinburgh vein study cross-sectional population survey. *British Medical Journal*, **318**, 353.

Brauer, M. and Kennedy, S.M. (1996). Gas stoves and respiratory health. *Lancet*, **347**, 412.

Breslow, N. (1982). Design and analysis of case–control studies. *Annual Reviews of Public Health*, **3**, 29.

Connor, E. and Mullan, F. (ed.) (1983). *Community oriented primary care: new directions for health service delivery*. National Academy Press, Washington, DC.

Coreil, J., Augustin, A., Holt, E., and Halsey, N.A. (1989). Use of ethnographic research for instrument development in a case-control study of immunization use in Haiti. *International Journal of Epidemiology*, **18**, S33.

Coupland, C.A.C., Cliffe, S.J., Bassey, E.J., Grainge, M.J., Hosking, D.J., and Chilvers, C.E.D. (1999). Habitual physical activity and bone mineral density in postmenopausal women in England. *International Journal of Epidemiology*, **28**, 241.

Coxell, A., Kink, M., Mezey, G., and Gordon, D. (1999). Lifetime prevalence. characteristics, and associated problems of non-consensual sex in men: cross-sectional survey. *British Medical Journal*, **318**, 846.

Edungbola, L.D., Alabi, T.O., Oni, G.A., Asaolu, S.O., Ogunbanjo, B.O., and Parakoyi, B.D. (1987). 'Leopard skin' as a rapid diagnostic index for estimating the endemicity of African onchocerciasis. *International Journal of Epidemiology*, **16**, 590.

Elandt-Johnson, R.C. (1975). Definitions of rates: some remarks on their use and misuse. *American Journal of Epidemiology*, **102**, 261.

Erkinjuntti, T., Ostbye, T., Steenhuis, R., and Hachinski, V. (1997). The effect of different diagnostic criteria on the prevalence of dementia. *New England Journal of Medicine*, **337**, 1667.

Ferreira, M.U., Cardoso, M.A., Santos, A.L., Ferreira, C.S., and Szarfarc, S.C. (1996). Rapid epidemiologic assessment of breastfeeding practices: probit analysis of current status data. *Journal of Tropical Pediatrics*, **42**, 50.

Fienberg, S.E. (1972). The multiple recapture census for closed populations and incomplete 2^k contingency tables. *Biometrics*, 59, 591.

Fleiss, J.L. (1981). *Statistical methods for rates and proportions* (2nd edn). Wiley, New York.

Forero, R., McLellan, L., Rissel, C., and Bauman, A. (1999). Bullying behaviour and psychosocial health among school students in New South Wales, Australia: cross-sectional survey. *British Medical Journal*, **319**, 344.

Frerichs, R.R. (1989). Simple analytic procedures for rapid microcomputer-assisted cluster surveys in developing countries. *Public Health Reports*, **104**, 24.

Frerichs, R.R. and Tar, K.T. (1989). Computer-assisted rapid surveys in developing countries. *Public Health Reports*, **104**, 14.

Frischer, M., Bloor, M., Finlay, A., *et al.* (1991). A new method of estimating prevalence of injecting drug use in an urban population: results from a Scottish city. *International Journal of Epidemiology*, **20**, 997.

Garland, M., Morris, J.S., Colditz, G.A., *et al.* (1996). Toenail trace element levels and breast cancer: a prospective study. *American Journal of Epidemiology*, **144**, 653.

Gillam, S., Plamping, D., McClenaham, J., Harries, J., and Epstein, L. (1994). *Community-oriented primary care.* King's Fund, London.

Gillum, R.F. (1987). The association of body fat distribution with hypertension, hypertensive heart disease, diabetes and cardiovascular risk factors in men and women aged 18–79 years. *Journal of Chronic Diseases*, **40**, 421.

Greenland, S. (1987). Interpretation and choice of effect measures in epidemiologic analysis. *American Journal of Epidemiology*, **125**, 761.

Gregg, N.M. (1941). Congenital cataract following German measles in the mother. *Transactions of the Australian College of Ophthalmology*, **3**, 35.

Guha-Sapir, D. (1991) Rapid assessment of health needs in mass emergencies: review of current concepts and methods. *World Health Statistics Quarterly*, **44**, 171.

Gyapong, J.O., Adjei, S., Gyapong, M., and Asamoah, G. (1996). Rapid community diagnosis of lymphatic filariasis. *Acta Tropica*, **61**, 65.

Harris, D.R. and Lemeshow, S. (1991). Evaluation of the Expanded Programme on Immunization survey methodology for estimating relative risk. *World Health Statistics Quarterly*, **44**, 107.

Helmert, U., Herman, B., and Shea, S. (1994). Moderate and vigorous leisure-time physical activity and cardiovascular disease risk factors in West Germany, 1984–1991. *International Journal of Epidemiology*, **23**, 285.

Helton, A.S., McFarlane, J., and Anderson, E.T. (1987). Battered and pregnant: a prevalence study. *American Journal of Public Health*, **77**, 1337.

Henderson, R.H. and Sundaresan, T. (1982). Cluster sampling to assess immunization coverage: review of experience with a simplified sampling method. *Bulletin of the World Health Organization*, **60**, 253.

Hoddinott, P. and Pill, R. (1999). Qualitative study of decisions about infant feeding among women in east end of London. *British Medical Journal*, **318**, 30.

Horwitz, R.I. and Feinstein, A.R. (1981). The application of therapeutic-trial principles to improve the design of epidemiologic research: a case-control study suggesting that anticoagulants reduce mortality in patients with myocardial infarction. *Journal of Chronic Diseases*, **34**, 575.

Hughes, K., Lun, K.C., Sothy, S.P, Thai, A.C., Leong, W.P., and Yeo, P.B. (1992). Corneal arcus and cardiovascular risk factors in Asians in Singapore. *International Journal of Epidemiology*, **21**, 473.

Jarvis, D., Chinn, S., Luczynska, C., and Burney, P. (1996). Association of respiratory symptoms and lung function in young adults with use of domestic gas appliances. *Lancet*, **347**, 426.

Jewell, N.P. (1986). On the bias of commonly used measures of association for 2 × 2 tables. *Biometrics*, **42**, 351.

Joung, I.M.A., van de Mheen, H., Stronks, K., van Poppel, F.W.A., and Mackenbach, J.P. (1994). Differences in self-reported morbidity by marital status and by living arrangement. *International Journal of Epidemiology*, **23**, 91.

Kahn, H.A. and Sempos, C.T. (1989). *Statistical methods in epidemiology* (2nd edn). Oxford University Press, New York.

Kark, S.L. (1974). *Epidemiology and community medicine.* Appleton-Century-Crofts, New York.

Kark, S.L. (1981). *The practice of community-oriented primary health care.* Appleton-Century-Crofts, New York.

Kark, S. and Kark, E. (1999). *Promoting community health: from Pholela to Jerusalem.* Witwatersrand University Press, Johannesburg.

Kark, S.L., Kark, E., Abramson, J.H., and Gofin, J. (ed.) (1994). *Atencion Primaria Orientada a la Comunidad.* Ediciones Doyma, Barcelona.

Keeffe, J.E., Lovie-Kitchin, J.E., Maclean, H., and Taylor, H.R. (1996). A simplified screening test for identifying people with low vision in developing countries. *Bulletin of the World Health Organization*, **74**, 525.

Khan, M.E., Anker, M., Patel, B.C., Barge, S., Sadhwani, H., and Kohle, R, (1991). The use of focus groups in social and behavioural research: some methodological issues. *World Health Statistics Quarterly*, **44**, 145.

Kiemeny, L.A.L.M., Schouten, L.J., and Straatman, H. (1994). Ascertainment corrected rates. *International Journal of Epidemiology*, **23**, 203.

Killewo, J.Z.J., Sandstrom, A., Raden, U.B., Mhalu, F.S., Biberfeld, G., and Wall, S. (1993). *International Journal of Epidemiology*, **22**, 528.

Kleinbaum, D.G., Kupper, L.L., and Morgenstern, H. (1982). *Epidemiologic research: principles and quantitative methods.* LifeTime Learning Publications, Belmont, CA.

Koopman, J.S. and Longini, I.M. Jr (1994). The ecological effects of individual exposures and nonlinear disease dynamics in populations. *American Journal of Public Health*, **84**, 836.

Kroeger, A. (1983). Health interview surveys in developing countries: a review of the methods and results. *International Journal of Epidemiology*, **12**, 465.

Kroeger, A. (1985). Response errors and other problems of health interview surveys in developing countries. *World Health Statistics Quarterly*, **38**, 15.

LaForce, F.M., Lichnevski, M.S., Keja, J., and Henderson, R.H. (1980). Clinical survey techniques to estimate prevalence and annual incidence of poliomyelitis in developing countries. *Bulletin of the World Health Organization*, **58**, 609.

Lam, T.H., Chung, S.F., Betson, C.I., Wong, C.M., and Hedley, A.J. (1998). Respiratory symptoms due to active and passive smoking in junior secondary school students in Hong Kong. *International Journal of Epidemiology*, **27**, 41.

Lee, J. (1994). Odds ratio or relative risk for cross-sectional data? *International Journal of Epidemiology*, **23**, 201.

Le Hasran, J.Y., Delaporte, E., Gaudebout, C., *et al.* (1994). Demographic factors associated with HTLV-I infection in a Gabonese community. *International Journal of Epidemiology*, **23**, 812.

Lemeshow, S. and Robinson, D. (1985). Surveys to measure programme coverage and impact: a review of the methodology used by the Expanded Programme on Immunization. *World Health Statistics Quarterly*, **38**, 65.

Lemeshow, S., Tserkovnyi, A.G., Tulloch, J.L., Dowd, J.E., Lwanga, S.K., and Keja, J. (1985). A computer simulation of the EPI survey strategy. *International Journal of Epidemiology*, **14**, 473.

Lengeler, C., Mshinda, H., de Savigny, D., Kilima, P., Morona, D., and Tanner, M. (1991). The value of questionnaires aimed at key informants, and distributed through an existing administrative system, for rapid and cost-effective health assessment. *World Health Statistics Quarterly*, **44**, 150.

Leske, M.C., Wu, S.-Y., Connell, A.M.S., Human, L., Schachat, A.P., and the Barbados Eye Study Grpup (1987). Lens opacities, demographic factors and nutritional supplements in the Barbados Eye Study. *International Journal of Epidemiology*, **26**, 1314.

Linstone, H.A. and Turoff, M. (ed.) (1975). *The Delphi method: techniques and applications.* Addison-Wesley, Reading, MA.

Loney, P.L., Chambers, L.W., Bennett, K.J., Roberts, J.G., and Stratford, P.W. (1998). Critical appraisal of the health research literature: prevalence or incidence of a health problem. *Chronic Diseases in Canada*, **19**, 170.

Lusky, A., Barell, V., Lubin, F., *et al.* (1996). Relationship between morbidity and extreme values of body mass index in adolescents. *International Journal of Epidemiology*, **25**, 829.

McCarty, D.J., Tull, E.S., Moy, C.S., Twoh, C.K., and LaPorte, R.E. (1993). Ascertainment corrected rates: applications of capture-recapture methods. *International Journal of Epidemiology*, **22**, 559.

MacMahon, B. and Pugh, T.F. (1970). *Epidemiology: principles and methods.* Little, Brown, Boston, MA.

MacNamara, J.J., Molot, M.A., Stremple, J.F., and Cutting, R.T. (1971). Coronary artery disease in combat casualties in Vietnam. *Journal of the American Medical Association*, **216**, 1185.

Marcus, A.C., Wheeler, R.C., Cullen, J.W., and Crane, L.A. (1987). Quasi-experimental evaluation of the Los Angeles Know Your Body program: knowledge, beliefs, and self-reported behaviours. *Preventive Medicine*, **16**, 803.

Materia, E., Imoko, J., Berhe, G., Dawuda, C., Omar, M.A., Pinto, A., and Guerra, R. (1995). Rapid surveys in support of district health information systems: an experience from Uganda. *East African Medical Journal*, **72**, 15.

Mayaud, P., Msuya, W., Todd, J., *et al.* (1992). STD rapid assessment in Rwandan refugee camps in Tanzania. *Genitourinary Medicine*, **73**, 33.

Mays, N. and Pope, C. (1996). *Qualitative research in health care.* BMJ Publishing, London.

Miettinen, O.S. (1985), *Theoretical epidemiology: principles of occurrence research in medicine.* Wiley, New York.

Needleman, H.L., Gunnoe, C., Levison, A., Reed, R., Pereshie, H., Maher, C., and Barrett, N. (1979). Deficits in psychologic and classroom performance of children with elevated dentine lead levels. *New England Journal of Medicine*, **300**, 689.

Newman, T.B., Browner, W.S., Cummings, S.R., and Hulley, S.B. (1988). Designing a new study: II. Cross-sectional and case-control studies. In *Designing clinical research* (ed. S.B. Hulley and S.R. Cummings). Williams and Wilkins, Baltimore, MD.

Nicolosi, A., Marighi, P.E., Rizzardi, P., Osella, A., and Miglior, S. (1994). Prevalence and causes of visual impairment in Italy. *International Journal of Epidemiology*, **23**, 359.

Nutting, P.A. (ed.) (1987). *Community oriented primary care: from principle to practice.* Health Resources and Services Administration, Public Health Services, Washington, DC.

Onyango, A., Koski, K., and Tucker, K.I. (1998). Food diversity versus breastfeeding choice in determining anthropometric status in rural Kenyan toddlers. *International Journal of Epidemiology*, **27**, 484.

Osborn, J. and Carraruzza, M.S. (1995). Odds ratio and relative risk for cross-sectional data. *International Journal of Epidemiology*, **24**, 464.

Palti, H., Adler, B., Flug, D., Shamir, Z., and Kark, S.L. (1977). Community diagnosis of psychomotor development in infancy. *Israel Annals of Psychiatry*, **15**, 223.

Palti, H., Valderama, C., Pugrund, R., Jarkoni, J., and Kurtzman, C. (1988). Evaluation of the effectiveness of a structured breastfeeding promotion programme integrated into a maternal child health service in Jerusalem. *Israel Journal of Medical Sciences*, **24**, 432.

Pani, S.P., Srividya, A., Krisknamoorthy, K., Das, P.K., and Dhanda, V. (1997). Rapid assessment procedures (RAP) for lymphatic filariasis. *National Medical Journal of India*, **10**, 19.

Papoz, L., Balkau, B., and Lellouch, J. (1996). Case counting in epidemiology: limitations of methods based on multiple data sources. *International Journal of Epidemiology*, **25**, 474.

Patterson, R.E., Kristl, A.R., Shannon, J., Hunt, J.R., and White, E. (1997). Using a brief household food inventory as an environmental indicator of individual dietary practices. *American Journal of Public Health*, **87**, 272.

Pearce, N. (1993). What does the odds ratio estimate in a case-control study? *International Journal of Epidemiology*, **22**, 1189.

Plaut, T., Landis, S., and Trevor, J. (1993). In *Successful focus groups* (ed. D.L. Morgan). Sage, Beverly Hills, CA.

Proctor, S.P., Heeren, T., White, R.F., *et al.* (1998). Health status of Persian Gulf War veterans; self-reported symptoms, environmental exposures and the effect of stress. *International Journal of Epidemiology*, **27**, 1000.

Puska, P. (1991). Intervention and experimental studies. In *Oxford textbook of public health* (2nd edn) (ed. W.W. Holland, R. Detels, and G. Knox), p. 177. Oxford University Press.

Rendl, J., Bier, D., Groh, T., and Reiners, C. (1998). Rapid urinary iodide test. *Journal of Clinical Endocrinology and Metabolism*, **83**, 1007.

Resnicow, K., Cross, D., and Wynder, E. (1993). The Know Your Body program: a review of evaluation studies. *Bulletin of the New York Academy of Medicine*, **70**, 188.

Rhyne, R., Bogue, R., Kukulka, G., and Fulmer, H. (1998). *Community-oriented primary care: health care for the 21st century.* American Public Health Association, Washington, DC.

Ritenbaugh, C.K., Said, A.K., Gaslal, O.M., and Harrison, G.G. (1989). Development and evaluation of a colour-coded scale for birthweight surveillance in rural Egypt. *International Journal of Epidemiology*, **18**, S54.

Roberts, C.J. (1977). *Epidemiology for clinicians*. Pitman Medical, Tunbridge Wells.

Rogan, W.J. and Gladen, B. (1978). Estimating prevalence from the results of a screening test. *American Journal of Epidemiology*, **107**, 71.

Rogentine, G.N., Yankee, R.A, Gart, J.J., Nam, J., and Trapani, R.J. (1972). HL-A antigens and disease: acute lymphatic leukemia. *Journal of Clinical Investigation*, **51**, 2410.

Rogentine, G.N., Trapani, R.J., and Henderson, E.S. (1973). HL-A antigens and acute lymphocytic leukemia: the nature of the HLA2 association. *Tissue Antigens*, **3**, 470.

Ronneberg, A., Lund, K.E., and Hafstad, A. (1994) Lifetime smoking habits among Norwegian men and women born between 1890 and 1974. *International Journal of Epidemiology*, **23**, 267.

Rothenberg, R.B. (1985) Observations on the application of EPI cluster methods for estimating disease incidence. *Bulletin of the World Health Organization*, **63**, 93.

Rothman, K.J. (1986). *Modern epidemiology*. Little, Brown, Boston, MA.

Rothman, K.J. (ed.) (1988). *Causal inference*. Epidemiology Resources, Chestnut Hill, MA.

Rothman, K.J. and Greenland, S. (1998). *Modern epidemiology* (2nd edn). Lippincott–Raven, Philadelphia, PA.

Ruel, M.T., Habicht, J.-P., and Olson, C. (1992). Impact of a clinic-based growth monitoring programme on maternal nutrition knowledge in Lesotho. *International Journal of Epidemiology*, **21**, 59.

Ruston, A., Clayton, J., and Calnan, M. (1998). Patients' action during their cardiac event: qualitative study exploring differences and modifiable factors. *British Medical Journal*, **316**, 1060.

Sackett, D.L., Haynes, K.B., and Tugwell, P. (1991). *Clinical epidemiology: a basic science for clinical medicine*, (2nd edn). Williams and Wilkins, Baltimore, MD.

Sackett, D.L., Richardson. W.S., Rosenberg, W., and Haynes, R.B. (1997). *Evidence-based medicine: how to practice and teach EBM*. Churchill Livingstone, New York.

Salonen, J.T., Kottke, T.E., Jacobs, D.R. Jr, and Hannan, P.J. (1986). Analysis of community-based cardiovascular disease prevention studies—evaluation issues in the North Karelia Project and the Minnesota Heart Health Program. *International Journal of Epidemiology*, **15**, 176.

Schulman, K.A., Berlin, J.A., Harness, W., *et al.* (1999). The effect of race and sex on physicians' recommendations for cardiac catheterization. *New England Journal of Medicine*, **340**, 618.

Schwartz, L.M., Woloshin, S., and Welch, H.G. (1999). Misunderstandings about the effects of race and sex on physicians' referrals for cardiac catheterization. *New England Journal of Medicine*, **341**, 279.

Schwoebel, V., Dauvisis, A.-V., Helynck, B., *et al.* (1992). Community-based evaluation survey of immunizations in Burkina Faso. *Bulletin of the World Health Organization*, **70**, 583.

Scrimshaw, S.C.M. and Hurtado, E. (1987). *Rapid assessment procedures for nutrition and primary health care: anthropological approaches to improving programme effectiveness.* UCLA Latin American Center Publications, Los Angeles, CA.

Sekikawa, A., Eguchi, H., Tominaga, M., *et al.* (1999). Evaluating the reported prevalence of type 2 diabetes mellitus by the Oguni diabetes registry using a two-sample method of capture-recapture. *International Journal of Epidemiology*, **28**, 498.

Selvin, S. (1996). *Statistical analysis of epidemiologic data* (2nd edn). Oxford University Press.

Smith, G.S. (1989) Development of rapid epidemiologic assessment methods to evaluate health status and delivery of health services. *International Journal of Epidemiology*, **18** (Supplement 2), S1.

Smith, P.G. and Morrow, R.H. (1991). *Methods for field trials of interventions against tropical diseases: a 'toolbox'*. Oxford University Press.

Sommer, A., Hussaini, G., Muhilal, T.I., Susanto, D., and Saroso, J.S. (1980). History of nightblindness: a simple tool for xerophthalmia screening. *American Journal of Clinical Nutrition*, **33**, 887.

Susser, M. (1973). *Causal thinking in the health sciences: concepts and strategies in epidemiology*. Oxford University Press, New York.

Tamir, D., Feurstein, A., Brunner, S., Halfon, S.-T., Reshef, A., and Palti, H. (1990). Primary prevention of cardiovascular diseases in childhood: changes in serum total cholesterol, high density lipoprotein, and body mass index after 2 years of intervention in Jerusalem schoolchildren age 7–9 years. *Preventive Medicine*, **19**, 22.

Tollman, S. and Friedman, I. (1994). Community-oriented primary health care—South African legacy. *South African Medical Journal*, **84**, 646.

Trompeter, T. (1992). *Community responsive primary care: a basic guide to planning and needs assessment for community and migrant health.* National Association of Community Health Centers, Washington, DC.

Tunstall-Pedoe, H., Kuulasmaa, K., Mahonen, M., Tolonen, H., Ruokokoski, E., and Amouyel, P. (1999). Contribution of trends in survival and coronary-event rates to changes in coronary heart disease mortality: 10-year results from 37 WHO MONICA project populations. Monitoring trends and determinants in cardiovascular disease. *Lancet*, **353**, 1547.

Turner, A.G., Magnani, R.J., and Shuaib, M. (1996). A not quite as quick but much cleaner alternative to the Expanded Programme on Immunization (EPI) cluster survey design. *International Journal of Epidemiology*, **25**, 198.

Van de Laar, M.J.W., Termorshuizen, F., Slomka, M.J., *et al.* (1998). Prevalence and correlates of herpes simples vitus type 2 infection: evaluation of behavioural risk factors. *International Journal of Epidemiology*, **27**, 127.

Van de Ven, A.H. and Delbecq, A.L. (1972). The nominal group as a research instrument for exploratory health studies. *American Journal of Public Health*, **62**, 337.

Vaughan, J.P. and Morrow, R.H. (ed.) (1989). *Manual of epidemiology for district health management.* World Health Organization, Geneva.

Velzeboer, M.I., Selwyn, B.J., Sargent, F., Pollitt, E., and Delgado, H. (1983*a*). Evaluation of arm circumference as a public health index of protein energy malnutrition in early childhood. *Journal of Tropical Pediatrics*, **29**, 135.

Velzeboer, M.I., Selwyn, B.J., Sargent, F., Pollitt, E., and Delgado, H. (1983*b*). The use of arm circumference in simplified screening for acute malnutrition by minimally-trained health workers. *Journal of Tropical Pediatrics*, **29**, 159.

Venkataswamy, G., Lepkowski, J.M., Ravilla, T., *et al.* (1989). Rapid epidemiologic assessment of cataract blindness. *International Journal of Epidemiology*, **18**, S60.

Von Korff, M. and Parker, R.D. (1980). The dynamics of the prevalence of chronic episodic disease. *Journal of Chronic Diseases*, **33**, 79.

Walter, S.D. and Cook R.J. (1991). A comparison of several point estimators of the odds ratio in a single 2 × 2 contingency table. *Biometrics*, **47**, 795.

Walter, H.J., Hofman, A., Barrett, L.T., *et al.* (1987). Primary prevention of cardiovascular disease among children: three years' results of a randomized intervention trial. In *Cardiovascular risk factors in childhood: epidemiology and prevention* (ed. B.S. Hetzel and G.S. Berenson), p. 161. Elsevier, Amsterdam.

West, S.K., Munoz, B., Turner, V.M., Mmbaga, B.B.O., and Taylor, H.R. (1991) The epidemiology of trachoma in Central Tanzania. *International Journal of Epidemiology*, **20**, 1088.

WHO (World Health Organization) (Division of Epidemiological Surveillance and Health Situation and Trend Analysis) (1993). News from the World Health Organization: rapid evaluation methods in health services. *International Journal of Epidemiology*, **22**, 578.

Wieringa, M.H., Weyler, J.J., Nelen, V.J., *et al.* (1998). Prevalence of respiratory symptoms: marked differences within a small geographical area. *International Journal of Epidemiology*, **27**, 630.

Williams, C.L., Arnold, C.B., and Wynder, E.L. (1977). Primary prevention of chronic disease beginning in childhood. The 'Know Your Body' program: design of study. *Preventive Medicine*, **6**, 344.

Wilson, D.H., Walsh, P.G., Sanchez, I., *et al.* (1999). The epidemiology of hearing impairment in an Australian adult population. *International Journal of Epidemiology*, **28**, 247.

Winkleby, M.A., Ragland, D.R., and Syme, S.L. (1988). Self-reported stressors and hypertension: evidence of an inverse association. *American Journal of Epidemiology*, **127**, 124.

Zocchetti, C., Consonni, D., and Bertazzi, P.A. (1997). Relationship between prevalence rate ratios and odds ratios in cross-sectional studies. *International Journal of Epidemiology*, **26**, 220.

6.4 Principles of outbreak investigation

Kumnuan Ungchusak

Threat of outbreaks

Knowledge of medicine and diseases has increased enormously during the last few decades. With the advance of knowledge, public health services in many countries can implement effective prevention programmes and are able to protect people from many unnecessary illnesses and death. However, people around the world still suffer and die from various known and unknown outbreaks. Some outbreaks are small and involve only a few persons but some affect more than 10 000 individuals (Fig. 1). During 1997, most countries had at least one infectious disease outbreak and several had as many as eight (WHO 1999). Outbreaks can happen anywhere, from a very remote area where no health facility exists to nosocomial outbreaks in a very sophisticated hospital where hundreds of health personnel are employed. It is a challenge for the government and public health professionals of all countries to detect and control these outbreaks as early as possible. Outbreak investigations also provide the opportunity to discover new aetiological agents, to understand factors that promote the spread of the diseases, and at the same time to identify the weaknesses of existing prevention and health programmes. For these reasons, all public health professionals should have the ability to conduct and support outbreak investigations.

This chapter provides a definition and describes the objectives of outbreak investigation, the methods for planning and conducting an investigation, and what needs to be done after the investigation has been completed. For simplicity, this chapter mainly discusses and presents examples of communicable disease investigations in particular. However, the concepts and principles discussed can be applied to non-communicable diseases as well.

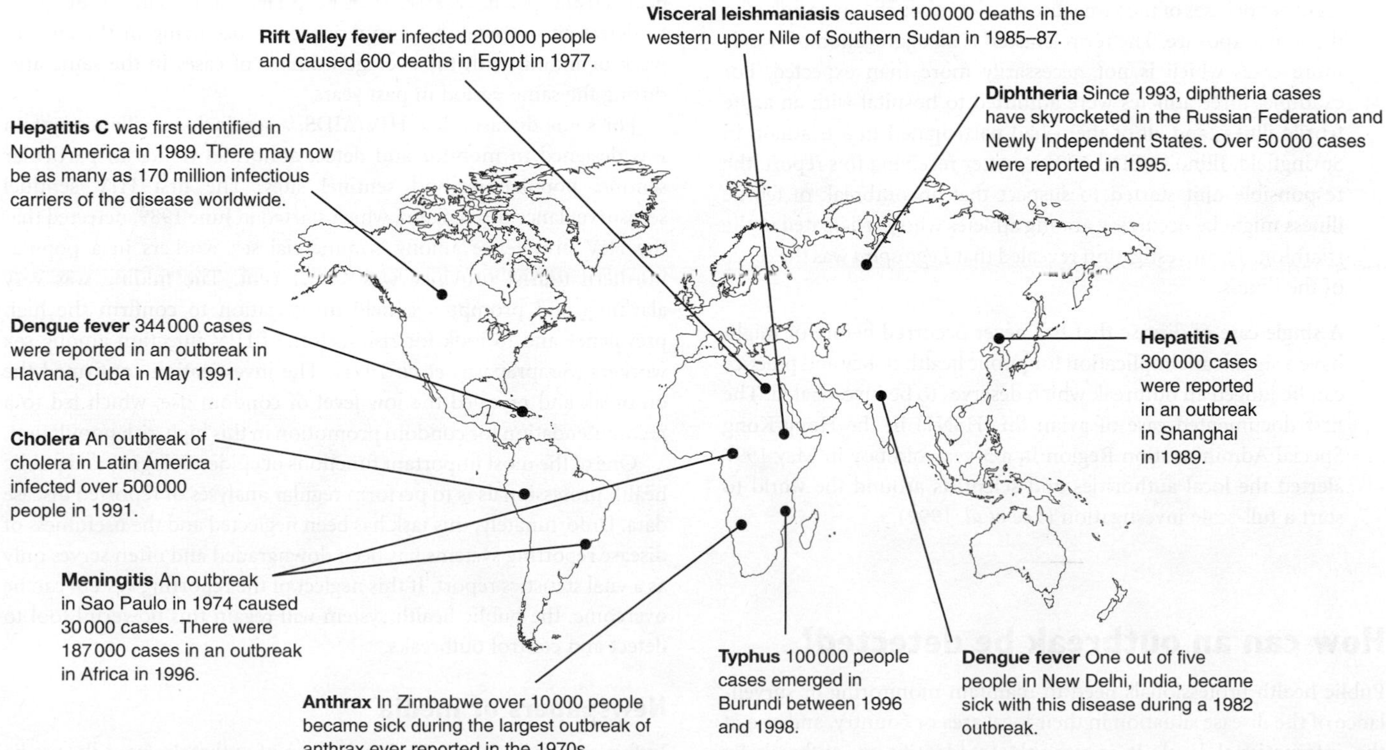

Rift Valley fever infected 200 000 people and caused 600 deaths in Egypt in 1977.
Visceral leishmaniasis caused 100 000 deaths in the western upper Nile of Southern Sudan in 1985–87.
Hepatitis C was first identified in North America in 1989. There may now be as many as 170 million infectious carriers of the disease worldwide.
Diphtheria Since 1993, diphtheria cases have skyrocketed in the Russian Federation and Newly Independent States. Over 50 000 cases were reported in 1995.
Dengue fever 344 000 cases were reported in an outbreak in Havana, Cuba in May 1991.
Hepatitis A 300 000 cases were reported in an outbreak in Shanghai in 1989.
Cholera An outbreak of cholera in Latin America infected over 500 000 people in 1991.
Meningitis An outbreak in Sao Paulo in 1974 caused 30 000 cases. There were 187 000 cases in an outbreak in Africa in 1996.
Typhus 100 000 people cases emerged in Burundi between 1996 and 1998.
Dengue fever One out of five people in New Delhi, India, became sick with this disease during a 1982 outbreak.
Anthrax In Zimbabwe over 10 000 people became sick during the largest outbreak of anthrax ever reported in the 1970s.

Fig. 1 Large disease outbreaks. (Source: WHO 1999.)

What is an outbreak?

The terms outbreak and epidemic can be used interchangeably. But outbreak is more understandable for most people and conveys a greater sense of urgency. Some epidemiologists prefer to use the term epidemic only in a situation that covers a very wide geographical area and involves large populations. For example, it is possible to use the term 'outbreak of HIV' to describe a sharply increasing HIV prevalence rate among commercial sex workers in a city where the normal rate was low in the previous year. But the term 'HIV epidemic' can be used when an abnormally high HIV prevalence is found among sex workers in many cities of the country.

In general, the term outbreak is used for a situation when diseases or health events occur at a greater frequency than normally expected in a specified period and place (Fig. 1).

There is often a misunderstanding that only communicable diseases can cause outbreaks. Non-communicable outbreaks such as mass sociogenic illness are sometimes reported as acute outbreaks of unexplained illness, especially in school settings (CDC 1990, 1996).

Because the criteria for judging an outbreak can be very subjective, it is useful to define the term in a more measurable fashion. The criteria for judging that an outbreak has happened can be one of the following.

1. The occurrence of a greater number of cases or events than normally occur in the same place when compared to the same duration in past years. For example, the epidemic of Kaposi's sarcoma, a manifestation of AIDS, was confirmed in New York when almost 30 cases were reported in 1981, whereas only two or three cases had been reported in previous years (Biggar *et al.* 1988).

2. A cluster of cases of the same disease occurs which can be linked to the same exposure. The term 'cluster' is an aggregation of two or more cases which is not necessarily more than expected. For example, three athletes were admitted to hospital with an acute febrile illness and all of them had participated in a triathlon in Springfield, Illinois (CDC 1998*a*). After receiving this report, the responsible unit started to suspect that an outbreak of febrile illness might be occurring among athletes who participated in the triathlon. The investigation revealed that *Leptospira* was the cause of the illness.

3. A single case of disease that has never occurred before or might have a significant implication for public health policy and practice can be judged an outbreak which deserves to be investigated. The first documented case of avian flu (H5N1) in the Hong Kong Special Administration Region in a 3-year-old boy in May 1997 alerted the local authorities and scientists around the world to start a full-scale investigation (Lee *et al.* 1999).

How can an outbreak be detected?

Public health professionals need to maintain monitoring or surveillance of the disease situation in their local area or country, and also at the international level. It is possible to identify an outbreak by monitoring many sources of information, which will help to detect the abnormal occurrence of disease. Some useful sources are listed below.

Health personnel

Doctors and nurses in a hospital have a good opportunity to observe an abnormal increase in the number of patients with a particular disease or syndrome. An outbreak of suspected mushroom food poisoning in a northern province of Thailand was reported to an epidemiologist during a business telephone conversation with his colleague. The epidemiologist started an investigation and identified the first confirmed outbreak of *Clostridium* botulism food poisoning associated with home-canned bamboo shoots in the country (CDC 1999*a*). Without this personal contact, this outbreak would not have been investigated. Thus, public health authorities should maintain a cordial relationship with doctors and hospital staff both in the governmental and private sectors. Conversely, doctors should report all suspected outbreaks to the local public health authorities.

Laboratory

Every laboratory or network can serve as an excellent source of outbreak notification. The avian flu outbreak in the Hong Kong Special Administrative Region was first discovered by the Influenza Surveillance Network, which reported an abnormal influenza, type A (H5N1) (Lee *et al.* 1999). Without the necessary laboratory capacity, the avian flu might have been overlooked and not triggered a field investigation. A public health professional should communicate regularly with laboratory technicians and vice versa. The laboratory scientists can prevent further spread if they report abnormal findings to the public health authorities regularly and without delay.

Official disease notification systems

Most countries have official systems for notification of cases and deaths from specific diseases from hospitals. The system was designed to detect an outbreak by comparing cases occurring in the current week or month with the average number of cases in the same area during the same period in past years.

For some diseases, like HIV/AIDS, a sentinel surveillance system was designed to monitor and detect abnormal trends in particular sentinel populations and sentinel sites. The first HIV sentinel serosurveillance in Thailand, which started in June 1989, detected that the HIV prevalence among commercial sex workers in a popular northern tourist province was 44 per cent. The finding was very alarming and prompted a field investigation to confirm the high prevalence and to look for risk factors of HIV infection among sex workers (Siraprapasiri *et al.* 1991). The investigation confirmed the outbreak and revealed the low level of condom use, which led to a recommendation for condom promotion in this high-risk population.

One of the most important functions of epidemiologists and public health professionals is to perform regular analyses of reported disease data. Unfortunately, this task has been neglected and the usefulness of disease reporting systems has been downgraded and often serves only as a vital statistics report. If this neglect of the reporting system can be overcome, the public health system will regain this powerful tool to detect and control outbreaks.

Newspapers or media

In fact, public health professionals learn of outbreaks from the media more often than from the official surveillance system. Newspapers receive outbreak news directly from their journalists or people in the community and are able to report them immediately. The Program for Monitoring Emerging Diseases (**ProMED**), the prototype for a communications system that monitors emerging infectious diseases globally and an initiative of the Federation of American Scientists and co-sponsored by the World Health Organization (**WHO**), obtains much of its outbreak news from local or international media. While timeliness is the strength of the media, the validity of the information is often poor and therefore it requires verification.

Village health volunteers

In rural areas where there are no health facilities and communication is limited, village leaders or village health volunteers can often help to recognize an abnormal increase in the numbers of some clinical diseases such as diarrhoea, dysentery, measles, fever, death of unknown aetiology, and so on. For example, the head man in a village of Kachin State in the Union of Myanmar informed the health authorities that seven villagers had died from febrile illness. This information triggered a field investigation, which revealed that malaria was the cause of the outbreak (Dr Myint Win, personal communication, 1999).

Purposes of outbreak investigation

An outbreak investigation can have many purposes as follows.

Controlling the current outbreak

This should be the primary or ultimate goal. If the investigation can start early the findings can guide implementation of appropriate control measures to stop further spread. The avian flu (H5N1) outbreak investigation found a link between infection and illness in chickens and in humans. The same virus was found in both chickens and patients. There were a total of 18 cases and six deaths before the Hong Kong Special Administrative Region decided to kill all 1.5 million chickens in the islands within 3 days to end the outbreak. There have been no cases since (Lee *et al.* 1999). The key to achieving this goal is to eliminate the delay in detecting the outbreak, to start the investigation as soon as possible, and to implement the appropriate preventive steps indicated by the investigation immediately.

Prevention of future outbreaks

Not all investigations start at the beginning or before the peak of the outbreak. The findings or lessons learned from the investigation may be too late to help fully control the current outbreak but they can still contribute to the prevention of future outbreaks. With good investigation, the weaknesses of the prevention programme can be identified. If recommendations are taken seriously, the chance of recurrence of the same outbreak or other diseases that share common risk factors can be reduced.

Research to provide knowledge of the disease

Information about new diseases and their natural history, clinical spectrum, incubation period, and so on, can often be best learned during an outbreak investigation. The most recent outbreak of encephalitis in Malaysia, which continued until the end of April 1999, and resulted in 257 cases and 100 deaths, prompted an international outbreak investigation which resulted in the discovery of a new nipah virus (CDC 1999*b*, *c*). The mode of spread from infected pigs to humans was revealed but there is still much more to be learned.

Evaluation of the effectiveness of prevention programmes

Investigation of an outbreak of disease, which is the target of a public health programme, may reveal weaknesses in that programme. Investigation of an outbreak of vaccine-preventable diseases often identifies populations that have not received the vaccine. For example, the investigation of a measles outbreak that occurred in 1993 in Espindola, a rural community in the Peruvian Andes, revealed that more than a quarter of the 553 residents were affected and that more than 3 per cent of those with measles had died. One year before the outbreak, a national measles campaign targeting children under 15 years of age had been conducted. Although national coverage reported the coverage to be 78 per cent, the investigation found that only 4 per cent of the children in Espindola had actually been vaccinated (Sniadack *et al.* 1999).

Evaluation of the effectiveness of the existing surveillance system

Some aspects of the surveillance system can be evaluated during an outbreak, such as the timeliness, validity, sensitivity, appropriateness of case definitions, and utilization of the surveillance information.

Training health professionals

The Epidemic Intelligence Service of the United States Centers for Diseases Control and Prevention (**CDC**) and 20 Field Epidemiology Training Programs around the world use real outbreaks as an opportunity for training as well as to provide service to investigate the causes and determinants of outbreaks.

Responding to public, political, or legal concern

In many situations, the investigation has to be conducted because the media has publicized the complaints of people to politicians, or even rumours. The main objective for this kind of investigation is to verify the outbreak and diagnosis. If it is groundless, the investigator can supply the media with new information that can end the rumours. Conversely, if it is a true outbreak then the investigator needs to decide what steps need to be taken.

In general, for a real outbreak, many objectives can be achieved fully or at least partially. However, the ultimate goal is to control the current outbreak and to prevent future ones. It is unethical for investigators to compromise this ultimate goal with other goals such as training or non-essential research that does not directly contribute to the control activities.

Components of an investigation team

In this chapter, the term 'investigators' will represent the people who are directly involved in planning and conducting the outbreak investigation from start to finish. In principle, local health professionals at the district or provincial level should take the role of investigators and start the work as soon as possible. For complicated or difficult field investigations, investigators from additional disciplines or even international experts can provide assistance. It is best to form an investigator team with a single principal investigator in charge of the operation. A good investigative team should include the following people.

1. A field epidemiologist who is technically competent to conduct field investigations systematically. The field epidemiologist usually serves as one of the primary investigators and should be involved in all the investigative steps.
2. Disease control people who are experienced in implementing basic disease control measures such as food and environmental sanitation, vector control, vaccination, and so on. If available, an educator who can provide essential knowledge to villagers in clear terms will also be very useful for disease control implementation.
3. Laboratory technicians who are able to provide basic and advanced laboratory support to the investigative team. Laboratory technicians might not need to travel to the field and collect the specimens by themselves except when a special collection procedure is required.
4. Specialists in particular areas; for example, a veterinarian would be very helpful for an outbreak investigation of zoonotic diseases. An entomologist is a key member for an outbreak investigation of vector-borne diseases. A social scientist with expertise in qualitative methods will help identify risk behaviours among affected populations and assess the acceptability of the recommended interventions.
5. Public health administrators, who are good at providing logistic support, mobilizing resources, and providing administrative expertise for the team.
6. Public relations person. In certain conditions when the outbreak has caused panic or has gained the intense attention of the public, the investigative team should recruit or appoint a person to be in charge of public relations and press releases. This person should appropriately reassure and not unduly alarm the public.

In practice, all of these team members are not always available at the subdistrict or district level due to limited human resources. Public health professionals and field epidemiologists need to have basic knowledge of all these relevant disciplines and be able to assume tasks if needed.

Owing to the sudden nature of the field investigation, it is better to establish in advance a list of people who will be on call and ready to join the investigative team once an outbreak has occurred.

Prior to the implementation of an investigation

The principal investigator should consider all of the following issues before initiating a field investigation.

Assessing the existence of the outbreak

No matter how the outbreak news was obtained, the investigator should confirm the validity of the information. The best way is to have direct communication with the responsible local health authority or field staff. It is not unusual for the information to be groundless. Sometimes the outbreak did happen but the media incorrectly quoted the name of the place. The investigator should carefully check with all other possible local health authorities in order not to miss the outbreak.

Gathering the available basic information

If the local health authority or field staff confirms the existence of the outbreak, the investigator should ask for additional information related to the situation and control measures being implemented.

Information related to the disease situation

1. What are the main symptoms and signs of the patients?
2. By whom and how was the diagnosis made, for example using only clinical or also laboratory evidence?
3. How many patients were seen and how many have died?
4. What was the average age of the patients and were there any differences in sex distribution?
5. Where did the patients come from? Are they clustered or scattered?
6. When was the increased number first observed and what is the trend at the moment?

Information related to control and response activities

1. What has already been done in terms of the field investigation and implementation of control activities?
2. Are there any serious constraints to compromise the field investigation and in implementing control measures?
3. Who are the key people responsible for the investigation and control activities?

It is not necessary to gather all of this information before leaving for the field but having it will help the investigator to plan an effective investigation.

Ensuring that clinical specimens and suspected materials were collected

It is absolutely vital to contact the doctors who saw the cases and made the diagnosis to obtain relevant clinical specimens such as serum, blood, and so on, for future laboratory tests. The items to which the cases were exposed, such as food and water, should be collected immediately before anything is destroyed unintentionally. The investigator should contact the local and reference laboratories so that the necessary supplies and equipment can be obtained immediately.

Obtaining permission and adequate support from the local and national authorities

The investigative team should ask the permission of the local health authority, and in some situations a national authority. This will create a sense of shared responsibility and partnership. Most of the time, local authorities are pleased to receive assistance. In a few situations, the local authority might be unhappy having outside people for the field investigation because of the sensitive nature of the problem. The investigator needs to convince local authorities that a thorough and good investigation will benefit their organization more than harm it. The investigator should also request field support from the key authorities such as field staff who will facilitate the fieldwork, providing transportation, medication, and so on.

Field operation plan

The investigator needs to have a short meeting among team members to summarize the situation, set up the objectives of the investigation, divide responsibility among team members, and check the readiness of laboratory and logistical support.

It is also important to plan the duration of the field investigation. The investigative team should stay in the field until all investigation processes such as data collection, analysis, interpretation, and the executive summary have been completed. Leaving the field without accomplishing all these objectives will cause delay in the implementation of control measures. Most outbreak investigations should plan to obtain preliminary results and recommendations within 1 or 2 weeks and no later than a month after the investigation begins. This is to make sure that the findings will be in time to assure control of the current outbreak. Additional studies and subsequent investigations can be done later.

This initial plan usually needs to be revised once the team arrives in the field. A normal practice in the field is that the team members should have a meeting at the end of each day to review and plan specific activities for the next day.

Reviewing current knowledge of the outbreak

The investigator or one of the team members should be assigned to review current knowledge of the outbreak. The *Control of communicable diseases* manual (Chin 2000) is very useful for a quick review of most infectious diseases. Searching the literature from the Internet, using as key words the 'outbreak and name of the disease', is useful to learn about previous studies done in different countries and settings.

The investigation team should not spend too much time preparing a perfect plan because of the urgency of the outbreak, but rather should obtain what is most necessary and start the investigation as soon as possible.

Steps of outbreak investigation

An outbreak investigation is an observational study in nature because the events have already happened. Every outbreak investigation needs to start with a good descriptive study followed by analytical studies whenever possible and necessary. Conclusions about the causes, mechanisms, and determinants of the outbreak need to be based on sound epidemiological, clinical, laboratory, and environmental evidence.

A descriptive study can help to identify the risk population and risk area so that immediate interventions can be directed to the most needy people and area. A good descriptive study can also generate hypotheses about how the outbreak has spread and what factors contributed to the abnormal occurrence of the disease. In theory, hypotheses derived from a descriptive study should be confirmed by further analytical study. In reality, this is not always possible because of many constraints.

It is preferable to translate the methodology for outbreak investigation into steps of action. Gregg (1996) has divided the outbreak investigation process into 10 steps. With a slight modification, this chapter will also divide the investigation process into 10 steps (Box 1). Steps 1 to 4 use descriptive epidemiology to generate basic facts and hypotheses, steps 5 to 7 are processes to test hypotheses and make conclusions, and steps 8 to 10 emphasize the important of communication of the results and follow-up of the recommendations.

Box 1 Ten steps to take in an outbreak investigation

1. Confirm the existence of the outbreak
2. Verify the diagnosis and determine the aetiology of the disease
3. Develop a case definition, start case-finding, and collect information on cases
4. Describe person, place, and time and generate hypotheses
5. Test hypotheses using an analytic study
6. Do necessary environmental or other studies to supplement the epidemiological study
7. Draw conclusions to explain the causes or the determinants of the outbreak based on clinical, laboratory, epidemiological, and environmental evidence
8. Report and recommend appropriate control measures to concerned authorities at the local, national, and, if appropriate, international levels
9. Communicate the findings to educate other public health professionals and the general public
10. Follow-up of the recommendations to assure implementation of control measures

This outline of steps for outbreak investigation does not imply a strict sequence of action. In real outbreak investigation, many steps can happen at the same time depending on the situation.

Step 1: Confirm the existence of an outbreak

The main question is: Is this a true outbreak? Applying the definition of an outbreak outlined above, the investigator should be able to establish or refute the existence of the outbreak. Investigators should review the number of cases with the local health officers or hospital staff and compare it with the number found at the same period recorded in past years.

For example, the outbreak of trichinosis in North Rhine-Westphalia, Germany, was confirmed because there were 52 cases in a 3-month period between November 1998 and January 1999 compared with no more than 10 cases annually during the same time period in the past 10 years (CDC 1999*d*).

Step 2: Verify the diagnosis and aetiology of the disease

If the number of cases fit the case criteria for the outbreak, the next related questions are:

- What is the correct diagnosis and aetiology of the disease?
- What can be done immediately to prevent new cases from occurring?

Knowing the exact diagnosis and aetiology of the disease will help to establish appropriate preventive measures immediately. This will protect susceptible people and allow the team to start education of villagers to avoid the risk factors. For example, many adults in a remote village were sick with fever, muscle and joint pain, rash over the body, and so on. If the diagnosis and aetiology of the disease is unknown, the local public health officials will find it very difficult to educate the public or implement effective preventive programmes. Until the serology of some patients showed sharply rising immunoglobulin M antibodies to dengue virus, control measures to destroy the larvae of the *Aedes* mosquito, the vector of dengue, which breeds in water containers, could not be started.

In many situations, an unknown or unclear diagnosis can cause panic due to rumour. This is demonstrated by an outbreak of pneumonic plague in Surat, India, in 1994 and of encephalitis in Malaysia in 1999, which resulted in a severe panic among local people and foreign tourists. Thus it is very important to obtain the exact diagnosis as rapidly as possible.

Investigators should have basic knowledge of the clinical diagnosis and how to confirm the aetiology of suspected diseases by well-established laboratory techniques. It is recommended that investigators should visit and talk with some patients, review and visualize the signs and symptoms, and hold discussions with the attending doctors. The information from this step will help to develop a case definition to facilitate active case-finding. The information on the aetiology will also help to interpret the findings from the later descriptive study and establish a causal association.

The investigators should also visit the laboratory facilities and ask for either positive or negative results of the testing of specimens. It is not necessary that cases have to be laboratory confirmed, but at least some of the apparent clinical cases or deaths should be confirmed. Once there are some laboratory-confirmed cases, the investigator will find it more reasonable to assume that other cases with the same clinical manifestation in the same period and location are the same disease.

It is unfortunate that specimens from patients are often thrown away when the primary results (either positive or negative) are obtained. The investigators should plan with the doctors and laboratory technicians to do further laboratory investigation on the specific strain, and to establish drug sensitivities, genetic markers, and so on. Many new laboratory technologies, such as serological testing, culture and isolation, and molecular techniques, are very powerful for diagnosis and tracking the connection between cases.

Step 3: Develop an appropriate case definition, start case-finding, and collect information on cases

At this stage, the investigator needs to answer at least three questions.

- Who should be counted as cases?
- Are there more undetected cases in the hospitals and in the community?
- What are the characteristics of cases?

To answer these three questions the investigators must follow these three small steps.

Developing an appropriate case definition

It is important that the investigator should develop a case definition, which will be applied consistently during the investigation. The definition should be sensitive or adequate at the beginning in order to capture all actual cases. A good case definition for investigative purpose should be time and place specific. The case definition should not include any specific suspected exposure that the investigator plans to verify. This would create selection bias when the investigator wants to generate the hypothesis or test the hypothesis in the following steps. Using the information from the previous steps, the investigator can divide the case definition into different levels. For example, in an investigation of leptospirosis among athletes participating in the triathlon in Illinois and Wisconsin in 1998, the following definitions were used (CDC 1998*b*).

1. A suspected case is a triathlon participant who manifests at least two of the following symptoms or signs: chills, headache, myalgia, diarrhoea, eye pain, or red eyes during the period of 21 June to13 August 1999. These criteria were based solely on a set of clinical signs and symptoms and were rather loose.
2. A confirmed case is a suspected case who has laboratory confirmation by serology (an immunoglobulin M ELISA and microagglutination test titre greater than or equal to 400), or a positive tissue immunohistochemical test, or a positive culture of *Leptospira.*

In some instances, the investigator might need to apply a definition of 'probable case'. A probable case is not fully confirmed by specific laboratory testing but has unique clinical or preliminary laboratory test results. The definition of the same disease in different investigations can be slightly different based on the availability of the laboratory support.

Active case-finding

In places where there is a good surveillance system, cases from all hospitals will be reported to the epidemiology unit at the district or provincial level. Investigators can apply the case definition and count the number of cases and review data that are collected on the reporting form. If there are enough cases and basic information on cases has already been gathered then investigators can start to do descriptive epidemiology.

Conversely, if only a few cases have been seen at the health facility, the investigators should plan to search for cases in the community. The investigator has to start a process called active case-finding. The objective of active case-finding is to have enough cases to analyse. At the same time, this case-finding will give a better picture of the magnitude of the outbreak. For example, in the outbreak of leptospirosis among triathlon athletes in Wisconsin and Illinois in 1998, only three cases were reported from the hospital at the beginning. The investigators co-operated with many state health departments by making a telephone call survey and in the end they succeeded in interviewing 1194 athletes. Among them, 110 or 9 per cent had an illness that met the suspected case definition of leptospirosis. The investigators also obtained acute serum from 70 cases, 24 of whom were confirmed as having leptospirosis by both immunoglobulin M and microagglutination tests (WHO 1978).

In the above example, it sounds easy to do active case-finding by telephone interview. However, investigators need to try their best to do active case-finding whenever it is necessary no matter how difficult it is. Very often, the investigators have to visit many hospitals in the outbreak area and review medical records by themselves. Sometimes, they have to search the cases in each village by doing interviews from house to house. This is the real nature of outbreak field investigations and the way people learn epidemiology. This active case-finding in the community will also provide another two benefits as follows.

1. Control measures can be implemented if the aetiology of the disease is known and treatable. During an investigation using active case searching in a village that reported seven deaths from malaria illness in Kachin State in the Union of Myanmar, the investigator found 94 probable cases and 53 microscopically confirmed malaria infections. All of the probable and confirmed cases found by this active process were treated. Without this measures there might be more deaths later on (Dr Myint Win, personal communication, 1999).
2. Rapid environmental assessment can be started during the visit to the affected families or villages. From this direct interview with the cases, the investigators can develop some hypotheses and implement some necessary interventions immediately such as sanitation improvement in food handlers and treatment of water to prevent water-borne outbreaks.

In situations in which the outbreak is not localized but widespread, the investigator might need to use the media to alert the public about the outbreak. People can then avoid suspected exposures and see a health-care provider if they have developed symptoms compatible with the case definition.

Collecting information on cases

For each case, the investigator should collect at least four types of information.

1. Identifying information: name, hospital number, contact person, and address of contact. This additional information will help to avoid duplication of enumerated cases. The investigator can also maintain communication with these cases when more information is needed.
2. Demographic information: age, sex, occupation, religion, ethnicity, area of residence, place of work, and so on. This is important information which will help to determine the characteristics and distribution of cases.
3. Clinical information: the symptoms and signs, the date of onset, the duration of illness, and results of diagnostic procedures. These data will help to confirm that this is a true case, provide the pattern of clinical manifestations, and also the distribution of cases by time.
4. Suspected risk factors: the investigators can ask for a history of exposure to some factors before disease developed. The timing of interest usually is one incubation period if the aetiology is known or suspected. Questions about contacts with other patients who have similar clinical symptoms are also very helpful. If the diagnosis is not known, the investigator might collect this group of information in a qualitative manner.

The investigator should develop a questionnaire as a tool to collect the relevant information from the hospital or during active case searching in the community. In practice, some of the information will not be available or not of good quality. The investigators should indicate all data that are in doubt.

Step 4: Describe the outbreak in person, place, and time, and hypotheses formation

In this step the investigators need to answer the following questions.

- What are the main clinical features?
- Who is the population at risk?
- What are the risk factors?
- What are the most likely explanations of how the outbreak began?

The simple approach is to analyse clinical information from each case and see the distribution of factors in terms of person, place, and time. The analysis should be done using rates rather than absolute numbers. The investigator needs to obtain the denominators from an available source or to estimate them. Using rates, the investigator can compare and determine the populations and areas of highest risk. With the advent of computers, many software programs are available to analyse this data. A popular one is Epi Info which is a public domain software from the American CDC which was designed specifically for field investigations. In the absence of a computer the investigators can still analyse the data manually. Individual questionnaires can be compiled into a line listing, which includes important variables of all cases. With this line listing simple counts can be made. In this way, the investigator will gain knowledge about populations and areas of risk. Resources and control measures can then be directed to the risk populations and risk areas. The enumeration will also produce information for hypothesis formation to explain how and why the outbreak happened.

Clinical manifestation of cases

Signs and symptoms of cases can be analysed in percentages and shown in a summary table. In an outbreak of unknown aetiology, the clinical information will help to differentiate the diagnosis. For an outbreak in which the aetiology is already known, the investigators still need to compare the clinical information found in the investigation with previous knowledge. Any discrepancy found, such as the attack rate, mortality rate, severity, and so on, should be carefully examined because this might indicate that a new strain or different specific host response is occurring. The high mortality rate of approximately 40 per cent in the nipah encephalitis outbreak in Malaysia 1999 (CDC 1999*c*) indicated that this outbreak might not be due to the usual endemic encephalitis.

Index case

The investigators should analyse the characteristics of cases by sex, age, occupation, ethnicity, and so on. At first this can be done by examining the proportion of all cases, but the specific attack rate by age and sex will be more useful for comparisons and hypotheses formation. The rates will provide useful indicators of the possible aetiology of the outbreak. In the Ebola haemorrhagic fever outbreak in Zaire in 1976, all ages and both sexes were affected but females slightly predominated. Age- and sex-specific attack rates indicated that adult females had the highest attack rate. This finding suggested that parenteral injection with unsterilized syringes and needles given during antenatal care in the local hospital was the means of transmission (WHO 1978).

The outbreak of nipah encephalitis in Malaysia in early 1999 was initially thought to be due to Japanese encephalitis alone. However, after careful analysis of the descriptive information, it was clear that the cases were mainly male, adult, working in pig farming, and of

Chinese ethnicity. This descriptive information did not fit the pattern for Japanese encephalitis, which affects mainly children of both sexes with no preference for a particular ethnicity. The investigator then began to suspect other organisms and to hypothesize that working in pig farming increased the risk of becoming ill.

Index and outlier case In infectious diseases, the first case on the epidemic curve or the index case is important because of the possibility that he or she brought the disease into the community. Cases that appear at the very beginning or at the end of the epidemic should also be given careful attention. These cases are called 'outlier cases' and can provide important information about the source and the way in which the disease is spread. Fruit juice from a vendor in a school was suspected as the source of a food poisoning outbreak involving Methomyl, a carbamate insecticide, in a secondary school in Bangkok, Thailand. This hint came from the first case, which was a worker sending ice to the school vendor. He was kindly given a cup of juice by the vendor and became ill without taking any other food items from the school. Without this information, it would have been quite difficult for the investigators to suspect any particular food or drink from the list of eight food items sold that morning. Thus the very first and very last cases in the epidemic curve should be critically appraised. The first case might not be the true index case because of misdiagnosis, an unrelated case to the epidemic, and so on. The late cases may be due to misdiagnosis, being an unrelated case to the epidemic, or a secondary case that had a different exposure than the majority of the cases in the epidemic.

Place

The investigators can calculate the attack rate of cases by different places. These can be place of residence, place of work or place of exposure, and so on. Places with a high attack rate often indicate the source of infection or contamination. A spot map showing the location of cases can give a very good idea of the source as had been demonstrated by Snow in his classical investigation of a cholera outbreak in the Golden Square area of London between August and September 1854 (Snow 1936). In that investigation Snow found most cases clustered around the Broad Street pump. From this information, Snow deduced that the Broad Street pump was probably the primary source of the outbreak.

If cases are scattered in many places, the investigators should explore the secular pattern of the case over time. This will indicate whether the outbreak started in one area and spread to other areas or whether people living in different places had a common exposure.

Time

The aim is to show the occurrence of cases over time and look for a pattern of occurrence. In general, there are two major types of outbreaks, a common source and a propagated source. The way to differentiate these two patterns of outbreak is to draw an epidemic curve which shows the number of cases (on the y axis) over time of onset (on the x axis) (Fig. 2). The epidemic curve of each outbreak will suggest whether the mode of spread is by common source or person to person.

A common source outbreak This kind of outbreak happens when people get the infection by exposure to the same source of infection. For example, a group of people contract hepatitis A infection because they eat the same contaminated food served during a wedding party. A common source outbreak can be divided into a point common source and a continuous common source.

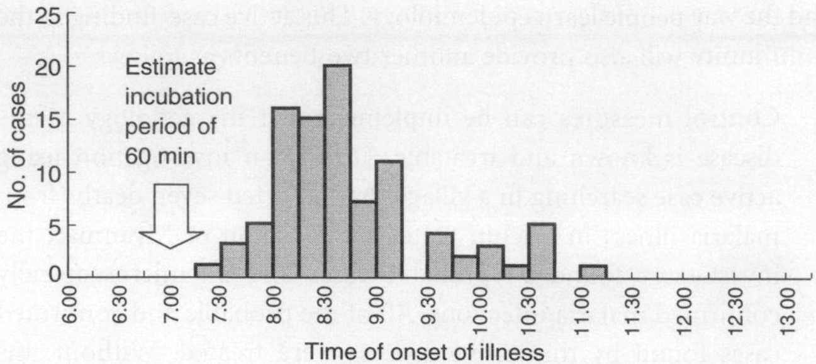

Fig. 2 Epidemic curve of food poisoning in secondary school, Bangkok, Thailand, 1981 (n = 101). (Courtesy of Dr Somsak Wattanasri, Division of Epidemiology, Ministry of Public Health, Thailand.)

1. A point common source outbreak occurs when there is one single source that exists for a very short time and all cases have common exposure to it in that same particular period.
2. A continuous common source outbreak occurs when there is only one source, which provides continuous or intermittent exposure over a longer period.

Epidemic curve of a point common source outbreak The epidemic curve shows a sharp increase of many cases suddenly followed by a rapid decline, though not as rapid as at the beginning of the epidemic. Another criteria to judge a point common source is that the first case and the last case usually happen within one incubation period.

If the aetiology and the knowledge of the incubation period of the disease are known, the investigators can then roughly estimate the probable time of the initial exposure. This can be done by identifying the peak of the epidemic from the curve and counting back on the x axis the equivalent of the incubation period. The investigator can also use the first case and count back on the x axis a duration of the minimum incubation period, which will also give a rough estimate of the time of exposure.

If the aetiology of the disease is not known, but the epidemic curve fits well with a point common source outbreak, the investigator can estimate the average incubation period if he or she knows the time of common exposure. In the outbreak of Methomyl food poisoning in a school, 101 students became ill after eating food in the school around 7.30 a.m.; the average incubation period was estimated to be 60 min using the duration between the time of known exposure to the peak of the epidemic curve as shown in Fig. 2.

Epidemic curve for a continuous common source outbreak The epidemic curve shows an abrupt increase in the number of cases but, instead of having a peak and a decline within one incubation period, new cases persist for a longer time with a plateau shape instead of a peak before decreasing. However, if there are many peaks or irregular jagged curves this suggests an intermittent common source.

A propagated outbreak

This kind of outbreak is caused by a transmission from one person to another person which requires direct contact such as touching, biting, kissing, or sexual activities.

Epidemic curve of propagated source outbreak The epidemic curve shows a slow increase in the number of cases with progressive peaks approximately one incubation period apart. The investigators might observe an abrupt decrease in new cases because everyone has already been infected. The span from the first to the last cases will also last longer than several incubation periods.

The outbreak of measles in 1993 in Espindola, a rural area in Peru, clearly showed a propagated pattern (Fig. 3). The outbreak began following the arrival of a family from Ecuador in July. Two children of this family developed measles during the journey. A welcome party for the family was held, after which 10 people who attended the party developed measles 1 to 2 weeks later. Several of these new measles cases also attended either a baptism or funeral at the local church. During the subsequent week another 11 cases who attended the baptism or funeral developed similar symptoms (Sniadack *et al.* 1999).

Step 5: Testing the hypotheses by analyses

In an outbreak of infectious disease, the investigator needs to answer the following questions.

- What is the aetiology of the disease?
- What is the source of infection?
- What is the pattern of spread?
- What are the risk factors for an individual to get the disease?
- What are the determinants of the outbreak or the factors which when combined together result in the outbreak?

The aetiology of the disease should be derived from the laboratory study. The pattern of spread can be identified by a careful descriptive study as described above. Sometimes, the descriptive study is not as simple as expected and does not give enough clues. The investigator must patiently re-examine the descriptive information, carry out more active case-finding, and reanalyse the data. The investigator also needs to observe directly the place, lifestyle, or behaviour of the case. These additional investigations usually help the investigator to generate some reasonable hypotheses. For example, a cholera outbreak in a home for mentally disabled children persisted over a 1-month period and the epidemic curve showed a pattern of person-to-person spread. After looking into the attack rate in different buildings in the home the investigator found that some buildings had a very high attack rate. When the investigator visited the home he discovered that the building with the high attack rate was very crowded. Two or three children had to share one single bed. The children also bathed in a small room where they were exposed to faeces from other children. With this direct observation, the hypothesis was formulated that crowding promoted the spread of the disease. In this example, the hypothesis was very reasonable and might not need to be tested. Improving the crowded condition was recommended and action was taken immediately.

In another example, the hypothesis needed to be tested by an analytical study design. The most common one is a case–control study. The investigator needed to define the cases and measure the rate of finding the suspected factors found among cases. He or she then compares this with the rate found among appropriately selected controls. The case definition for the analytical study may be more specific than used for descriptive study in order to reduce misclassifying non-cases as cases. Conversely, the controls may also need to be tested to avoid classifying non-apparent cases as controls.

In the outbreak of Methomyl food poisoning among secondary school students described above, the investigator had already identified 101 cases. Because a high percentage of cases had drunk fruit juice, the investigator hypothesized that drinking fruit juice from one of the food vendors in the school was the risk factor. The investigator decided to conduct a case–control study to prove this hypothesis (Table 1). He selected another 107 students without any diarrhoea, nausea, or vomiting from the same class but with the same gender as the controls. The investigator then asked which of the eight food and drink items the cases and controls took that morning. The odds ratio of drinking any of the three fruit juices calculated from this analytical study was three to seven times higher and was statistically significant. This finding established a significant statistical association between drinking fruit juices and becoming ill.

In this same investigation, the investigator also conducted an historical cohort study, which is another type of analytical study. Out of the total 1544 students, he first identified 416 who ate the breakfast in the school. These 416 students were defined as the cohort population and were interviewed for their consumed food and the occurrence of the illness after eating. The attack rate, or incidence, of becoming ill among those who ate each food item was compared with that in those who did not eat. The relative risk could then be calculated as shown in Table 2.

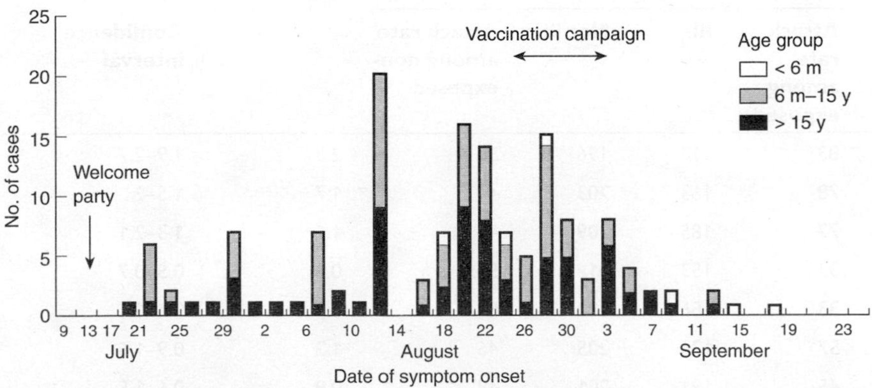

Fig. 3 Measles by date of symptom onset, Espindola, Peru, 1993. (Source: Sniadack *et al.* 1999.)

Table 1 Odds ratios and 95% confidence intervals for specified food items found in a case–control study: Methomyl food poisoning investigation in School A, Bangkok, 7 July 1981

Food item	Cases		Controls		Odds	95% confidence
	Consumed	Did not consume	Consumed	Did not consume	ratio	interval
Fruit juice A	46	55	11	96	7.3	3.3–16.5
Fruit juice B	21	80	7	100	3.7	1.4–10.3
Fruit juice C	13	88	4	103	3.8	1.1–16.8
Syrup	29	72	50	57	0.4	0.2–0.8
Water	9	92	23	84	0.3	0.1–0.8
Noodles	10	91	5	102	2.2	0.6–8.6
Boiled egg in soup	10	91	12	95	0.8	0.3–2.3
Dessert	7	94	9	98	0.8	0.2–2.5

The results of a case–control study and the historical cohort study gave the same conclusion that the source of the outbreak was fruit juice A, B, and C. The historical cohort study took more effort but gave information on the incidence and the relative risk, which better showed the association of exposure and illness.

Step 6: Environmental or other studies to supplement the epidemiological findings

Although an analytical study might be able to confirm the hypothesis, the investigator still needs to find environmental or other evidence to support and explain the epidemiological evidence.

In an outbreak of unknown illness in a rural village of Egypt in which the cases developed severe abdominal pain, persistent vomiting, and generalized weakness, the investigator was able to detect abnormally high blood lead levels among the cases. The analytical study revealed an association between high blood level and eating flour from one mill factory. The mill implicated in the outbreak was visited. Upon arrival at the mill, the investigators noted a lead smelting pot in the corner of the mill. Lead was used by the miller to attach the crosspiece to the grinding stone. Occasionally, the lead would break off and contaminate the flour. The miller reportedly used about 2 kg of lead per year. Analysis of grain from the mill showed no lead; however, lead was found in flour from the surface of the mill stone and in samples of flour after grinding was complete (Abdel-Nasser *et al.* 1996).

Step 7: Establishing the causes of the outbreak

Once the hypothesis has been tested and other necessary studies have been done, the investigators can make their conclusions about the causes of the outbreak. This conclusion is very important because actions should follow. Many restaurants or factories have had to be closed because they were implicated as the source of the outbreak. Outbreak investigations are naturally faced with constraints of time and other uncontrolled conditions, which do not favour a perfect design and methodology. The findings potentially include both random and systemic errors. Before making any conclusion, it is worthwhile for the investigator to examine carefully the weaknesses or limitations of the investigation. In principle, the investigator must identify the cause of the outbreak based on the agreement of the following four pieces of evidence.

Table 2 Relative risk (RR) and 95% confidence intervals for specified food items found in retrospective cohort: Methomyl food poisoning investigation in School A, Bangkok, 7 July 1981

Food item	Exposed			Not exposed			RR	95%
	Ill	Not ill	Attack rate among exposed	Ill	Not ill	Attack rate among non-exposed		Confidence interval
Fruit juice A	90	18	83	112	196	36	2.3	1.9–2.7
Fruit juice B	39	11	78	163	203	44	1.7	1.5–2
Fruit juice C	17	5	77	185	209	47	1.6	1.3–2.1
Tulip soda water	49	96	33	153	118	56.5	0.6	0.5–0.7
Water	16	32	33	186	182	50	0.7	0.4–1
Noodles	20	15	57	176	205	46	1.2	0.9–1.6
Boiled egg in soup	11	13	45	191	201	48	0.9	0.6–1.5
Dessert	2	6	25	200	208	49	0.5	0.1–1.7

Laboratory evidence

The aetiology of the disease has been identified in the patients and in the suspected source of infection. If the investigator cannot identify the aetiology from the suspected source, it is still possible to use some marker to support their conclusions. For example, although a *Vibrio cholerae* type 01 could not be cultured from the drinking water supply of the affected community, the observation of human coliform bacteria in the water helped to indicate that human faeces had really contaminated the water.

Clinical evidence

It is necessary to verify that the clinical manifestations and the incubation period are compatible with the aetiology reported from the laboratory.

Environmental evidence

The examination of the environment should reveal the possibility that the causative factor can pass from the source to the cases. A cooking environment which is dirty or located close to the toilet is convincing evidence for food being contaminated by faeces. Crowding in the bedroom is very convincing evidence for a respiratory tract disease outbreak.

Epidemiological evidence

This epidemiological evidence found in the descriptive and analytical studies should clearly explain the following aspects:

- pattern of spread as described by epidemic curve
- statistical strength of association between exposure and developing the disease
- dose–response relationship, which demonstrates a higher strength of association when the exposure is increasing
- exposure should precede illness.

In the example of the Methomyl food poisoning discussed above, the investigator identified the three fruit juices as the implicated food. In the case–control study (Table 1) cases were many times more likely to have drunk the fruit juice than healthy students. In the retrospective cohort study (Table 2), students who drank either of the three fruit juices were almost twice as likely to become sick as those who did not drink them. Methomyl was identified as the aetiology of this outbreak. It was found in sugar that was used to prepare the implicated fruit juices. Methomyl could produce the clinical signs and symptoms found in the cases and also matched the incubation time of approximately 60 min found in the investigation. Because the food vendor also used Methomyl in her household, it was possible that she accidentally contaminated the sugar with Methomyl since the chemical is colourless.

It is not uncommon to see some disagreement in the evidence from different sources. In this event, the investigator needs to verify the validity of each piece of evidence and discuss the data with people who have expertise in that particular area in order to obtain more information.

Step 8: On-site reporting and recommendations for concerned authorities

The most important step which should lead to a timely response is to report the findings to the responsible individuals both at the local and national levels so that they can take the appropriate action. Keeping this in mind, the investigators need to complete two tasks before leaving the outbreak area.

1. Complete the analysis and data interpretation. Leaving the field without completing these tasks will reduce the sense of urgency necessary to finish the work. Data are easier to retrieve when in the field rather than instructing the field people to send them to the investigative team later.
2. Present the main findings with recommendations. Some findings may be very sensitive because they reflect the weaknesses or mistakes of the health or other authorities. The investigator needs to select the appropriate approach, either formal or informal, with the responsible people. Leaving the field without giving the information that the team obtains from the investigation will do harm to some other people who could be prevented from becoming ill if the information were known. In many urgent situations, the findings and recommendations might be given to the responsible people repeatedly during the outbreak investigation process instead of waiting until the end. The investigators also need to present or communicate the findings and recommendations to the national authorities as soon as possible. The recommendations for action should be based on the findings from the investigation. These might include the following aspects.

What can be done to control this outbreak?

With timely investigation, some interventions can be implemented to stop further spread. In the outbreak of measles in a rural community of Peru, measles vaccine was given to children who were not measles cases aged between 6 months and 15 years regardless of their previous immunization status. Using knowledge about the complication of measles in previous studies, the investigators estimated that the action prevented 87 cases of diarrhoea and 46 cases of pneumonia, and averted five deaths (Sniadeck *et al.* 1999).

How to improve the interventions

Commonly, interventions have to be implemented while the investigation is on going. The investigator should review the measures and give unbiased opinions regarding the appropriateness, the target group, the timing, and the area of implementation. In a cholera outbreak without adequate investigation, some health authorities tried to use mass treatment with tetracycline or doxycycline for all members in the affected community. A careful investigation can help indicate better, more targeted interventions and discourage this kind of mass treatment.

How to prevent future outbreaks

In many instances, the interventions cannot be implemented for the current outbreak but the findings can be used to set up new practices or policies. These recommendations can help prevent future outbreaks. In Thailand the recommendation was made to change Methomyl from a colourless powder to a blue powder following the investigation of food poisoning described above. The Egyptian government, after reviewing the results of the investigation of lead contamination in flour mills, agreed to ban the use of lead in privately owned flour mills.

How to improve the investigation

The investigator should review the performance of the investigation and identify the weaknesses of the methodology or the field operation so that improvements can be made. These might include a more appropriate case definition, a better design, improved laboratory support, a different team composition, less cost, a shorter time course, and so on.

How to improve surveillance

The best time to evaluate the surveillance system is during an outbreak investigation. In most outbreaks, the investigator has to review data from existing surveillance systems. With this direct involvement, the investigator will be able to evaluate the timeliness, completeness, validity of diagnosis, sensitivity of the system, and utilization of the surveillance information.

Step 9: Dissemination of the information

In addition to on-site reporting, the investigator should disseminate the information to educate the public health community and the general public. There may be many other communities that are also prone to a similar outbreak. The information will raise the awareness of health and government authorities to assess their own situation and implement some measures to prevent possible outbreaks. The dissemination of information should be done in a timely manner through weekly or monthly reports. Release of important findings through the mass media is also very useful to educate the public. Before releasing the investigation results through the media, the investigator must make sure that all the facts will be delivered in a constructive manner and will not result in blame to any organization. The investigator should also report the investigation results in an international journal or bulletin such as the *Weekly Epidemiological Record* of the WHO or the *Morbidity and Mortality Weekly Report* of the CDC. This kind of practice is necessary to alert health professionals in other countries and keep them informed of the problem.

Step 10: Follow-up to ensure implementation of control measures

Finally, the investigator should follow-up the investigation by maintaining close communication with the local health authorities. An absence of new cases for at least two incubation periods of the infectious disease under investigation could suggest that the outbreak is subsiding. A good investigator should follow up on the recommendations. An outbreak investigation is a waste of time if good recommendations have not been implemented. The investigator should learn the reasons why the recommendations were or were not implemented. If the recommendations were implemented, the investigator can also learn the impact by observing the trend of the diseases.

Co-operation for international outbreak investigation and preparedness

The world today is especially prone to outbreaks because of frequent cross-border movement, civil war and migration, rapid transportation, international trading, tourism, and so on. An outbreak in one country, therefore, can spread to other countries very easily. An outbreak anywhere in the world must now be treated as a threat to all countries. It is important for each country to build up its capacity for surveillance, outbreak preparedness, and investigation. Besides the CDC Epidemic Intelligence Services, many countries have started training programmes and established a medical detective unit which will be ready to investigate all kind of outbreaks. These training programmes have different names, such as the Field Epidemiology Training Program in about 20 countries, and the Epidemiology European Training Program in the European Community. The WHO has set up an outbreak verification network, a worldwide network of laboratories and reporting sites which collect information on reported and rumoured outbreaks nationally and worldwide. It is a wise investment, and commitment is beginning to be made by international communities to collaborate in information exchange and to help investigate outbreaks together.

Conclusion

Outbreak investigation is an essential function of public health professionals who care for the well being of the community. It is an opportunity to gain new knowledge of diseases and to discover the weaknesses of current public health practices and systems. A good public health professional must always be alert to the possibility of outbreaks. Normal surveillance systems or unofficial sources such as the mass media can be a good source for detection of an outbreak. Before starting the field investigation, the investigator should organize the team, review previous knowledge, prepare the technical and management aspects, and start the investigation as soon as possible. The investigation can be conducted by following the 10 steps outlined above. The investigation usually starts by confirming the existence of the outbreak, verifying the diagnosis, gathering case information, doing descriptive epidemiology, formulating and testing the hypothesis when necessary, doing environmental surveys to supplement epidemiological evidence, and providing timely on-site reporting of the findings with practical recommendations to local and national responsible authorities. Competent outbreak investigation combines sound scientific knowledge and good management skills to resolve the crisis or unexpected situations. It is not enough to understand or memorize these steps. Direct participation in conducting the investigation is needed to gain the necessary skill. A good investigator should be a field-oriented person with good levels of perseverance, scepticism, and common sense. The investigator should not end his or her work with the report but should follow up on the recommendations and continue surveillance of the problem vigorously. In the future more and more joint international investigations will be needed. The rich countries must help the poor build up their epidemiology capacities in order to detect and stop outbreaks before they get out of control. With this co-operation the world will be a safer place amidst the threat of disease outbreaks.

References

Abdel-Nasser, M.A. *et al.* (1996). *Outbreak investigation of an unknown illness in a rural village, Egypt, 1996.* Field Epidemiology Training Programmes, Cairo.

Biggar, R.J. *et al.* (1988). AIDS-related Kaposi's sarcoma in New York City in 1977. *New England Journal of Medicine*, **318**, 252.

CDC (Centers for Disease Control and Prevention) (1990). Mass sociogenic illness in a day-care center, Florida. *Morbidity and Mortality Weekly Report*, **39**, 301–4.

CDC (Centers for Disease Control and Prevention) (1996). Outbreak of unexplained illness in a middle school—Washington, April 1994. *Morbidity and Mortality Weekly Report*, **45**, 6–9.

CDC (Centers for Disease Control and Prevention) (1998*a*). Outbreak of acute febrile illness among athletes participating in triathlons—Wisconsin and Illinois 1998. *Morbidity and Mortality Weekly Report*, **47**, 585–8.

CDC (Centers for Disease Control and Prevention) (1998*b*). Update: leptospirosis and unexplained acute febrile illness among athletes participating in triathlons—Illinois and Wisconsin, 1998. *Morbidity and Mortality Weekly Report*, **47**, 673–6.

CDC (Centers for Disease Control and Prevention) (1999*a*). Foodborne botulism associated with home-canned bamboo shoots—Thailand, 1998. *Morbidity and Mortality Weekly Report*, **48**, 437–9.

CDC (Centers for Disease Control and Prevention) (1999*b*). Outbreak of Hendra-like virus—Malaysia and Singapore, 1998–1999. *Morbidity and Mortality Weekly Report*, **48**, 265–9.

CDC (Centers for Disease Control and Prevention) (1999*c*). Outbreak of nipah Virus—Malaysia and Singapore, 1999. *Morbidity and Mortality Weekly Report*, **48**, 335–7.

CDC (Centers for Disease Control and Prevention) (1999*d*). Trichinellosis outbreaks—North Rhine-Westfalia, Germany, 1998–1999. *Morbidity and Mortality Weekly Report*, **48**, 488–92.

Chin, J. (ed.) (2000). *Control of communicable diseases* (17th edn). American Public Health Association, Washington, DC.

Gregg, M.B. (1996). Conducting a field investigation . In *Field epidemiology* (ed. M.B. Gregg), pp. 44–59. Oxford University Press.

Lee, S.Y., Mak, K.H., and Saw, T.A. (1999). The avian flu (H5N1): one year on. *Public Health and Epidemiology Bulletin*, **8**, 1–8.

Siraprapasiri, T., Thanprasertsuk, S., Rodklay, A., *et al.* (1991). Risk factor for HIV among prostitutes in Chiangmai, Thailand. *AIDS*, **5**, 579–82.

Sniadack, D.H., Moscoso, B., Aguilar, R., *et al.* (1999). Measles epidemiology and outbreak response immunization in a rural community in Peru. *Bulletin of the World Health Organization*, **77**, 545–52.

Snow, J. (1936). *Snow on cholera.* Oxford University Press, London.

WHO (World Health Organization) (1999). *Report on infectious diseases.* WHO/CDS/99.1, p. 39. WHO, Geneva.

WHO (World Health Organization) (1978). Report of an international commission. Ebola haemorrhagic fever in Zaire, 1976. *Bulletin of the World Health Organization*, **56**, 271–90.

6.5 Case–control studies

Noel S. Weiss

In 1971, Herbst *et al.* (1971) reported that the mothers of seven of eight teenage girls diagnosed with clear cell adenocarcinoma of the vagina in Boston during 1966 to 1969 claimed to have taken a synthetic hormone, diethylstilboestrol, while that child was *in utero*. None of the mothers of 32 girls without vaginal adenocarcinoma, matched to the mothers of cases with regard to hospital and date of birth, had taken diethylstilboesterol during the corresponding pregnancy. Within a year, a New York study of five cases and eight girls without vaginal cancer obtained similar results (Greenwald *et al.* 1971). The introduction of prenatal diethylstilboesterol use into obstetric practice in the United States during the 1940s and 1950s, followed by the appearance of this hitherto unseen form of cancer some 20 years later, supported a causal connection between *in utero* exposure to diethylstilboesterol and vaginal adenocarcinoma. The means by which *in utero* diethylstilboesterol exposure might predispose to the occurrence of clear cell vaginal adenocarcinoma was unknown in 1971 (it is now believed that diethylstilboesterol acts by interfering with normal development of the female genital tract, resulting in the persistence into puberty of vaginal adenosis in which adenocarcinoma can arise (Ulfelder and Robboy 1976)). Nonetheless, a causal inference was made at that time by the Food and Drug Administration, which specified pregnancy as a contraindication for diethylstilboesterol use.

The investigation by Herbst *et al.* was a case–control study: a comparison of prior exposures or characteristics of ill people (cases) with those of people at risk for the illness in the population from which the cases arose. Generally, the prior experience of people at risk is estimated from observations on a sample of that population (controls). A difference in the frequency or levels of exposure between cases and controls—that is, an association—may be a reflection of a causal link.

At first glance, the case–control approach appears to proceed backwards, from consequence to potential cause. Nonetheless, if a case–control study enrols cases and controls from the same underlying population at risk of the outcome, and can measure exposure status validly in them, the results obtained will be identical with those from a properly done cohort study. A case–control, cohort, or any other form of non-randomized study does have the potential to identify associations that are not causal, either because of chance or because of the influence of some other factor associated with both exposure and outcome. Even so, the evidence that is provided by well-performed case–control studies can carry great weight when evaluating the validity of a causal hypothesis. Indeed, a number of causal inferences have been based largely on the results of case–control studies. These include, in addition to the diethylstilboesterol–vaginal adenocarcinoma relationship, the connection between aspirin use in children and the development of Reye's syndrome, and the use of absorbent tampons and the incidence of toxic shock syndrome.

One of the criteria used to assess the validity of a causal hypothesis is the strength of the association between exposure and disease, usually as measured by the ratio of the incidence rate in exposed and non-exposed people. In most case–control studies, it is not possible to measure incidence rates in either of these groups. Nonetheless, from the frequency of exposure observed in cases and controls, it is usually possible to estimate closely the ratio of the incidence rates.

To understand how this can be done, consider a cohort study in which exposed and non-exposed people are followed for a certain period of time. The table below summarizes their experience with regard to a particular disease:

Exposed	Yes	No	
Yes	a	b	$a + b$
No	c	d	$c + d$

The cumulative incidence of the disease in exposed and non-exposed people over a given period of follow-up is $a/(a + b)$ and $c/(c + d)$ respectively. The relative risk (RR) is the ratio of these:

$$\mathrm{RR} = \frac{a/(a+b)}{c/(c+d)}.$$

If the incidence of the disease is relatively low during the follow-up period in both exposed and non-exposed people, then a will be small relative to b and c will be small relative to d. Therefore

$$\mathrm{RR} = \frac{a/(a+b)}{c/(c+d)} \approx \frac{a/b}{c/d} = \frac{a/c}{b/d}.$$

In this expression the numerator (a/c) is the odds of exposure in people who develop the disease, the denominator (b/d) is the odds of exposure in people who remain well, and

$$\frac{a/c}{b/d}$$

is the odds ratio (OR). The numerator can be estimated from a sample of cases, while the denominator can be estimated from a sample of non-cases. Neither estimate is influenced by the proportion of cases among the subjects actually chosen for study.

In the following hypothetical example, assume that 100 of 10 000 people exposed to a particular substance or organism developed a disease, in contrast with 300 of 90 000 non-exposed people:

Exposed	Yes	No	
Yes	100	9900	10 000
No	300	89 700	90 000

$$RR = \frac{100/10\,000}{300/90\,000} = 3.00.$$

If a case–control study had been done in this population, in which 50 per cent of cases were included but only 1 per cent of non-cases, the following results would have been obtained:

Exposed	Yes	No
Yes	100 × 0.5 = 50	9900 × 0.01 = 99
No	300 × 0.5 = 150	89 700 × 0.01 = 897

$$RR \approx OR = \frac{50/150}{99/897} = 3.02.$$

In many studies, controls are chosen as they were in the previous example, that is from people who had not developed the disease by the end of the same time period during which other people (the cases) had become ill. In such studies, the less common the disease in both exposed and non-exposed people during the period, the better the odds ratio will estimate the ratio of cumulative incidence. In the example, only 1 per cent and 0.33 per cent of exposed and non-exposed people, respectively, developed the illness, and so the relative cumulative incidence and odds ratio were in close correspondence (3.00 versus 3.02). However, it is also possible to choose controls from people free of disease only until the corresponding cases have been diagnosed; a person can appear in the study first as a control and later as a case. If this approach is used, the odds ratio will be a valid estimate of the ratio of incidence rates (that is, cases divided by person-time at risk) irrespective of the disease frequency (Greenland and Thomas 1982; Pearce 1993).

Retrospective ascertainment of exposure status in cases and controls

Epidemiological studies seek to obtain information on exposures present during an aetiologically relevant period of time. That period varies across aetiological relationships. For example, while excess consumption of alcohol predisposes both to motor vehicle injuries and to cirrhosis of the liver, it does so during considerably different time intervals prior to the occurrence of the injury or the onset of the illness, respectively.

Some case–control studies are nested within cohort studies in which specimens (for example blood or urine) have been obtained prior to diagnosis on all cohort members, but have not yet been analysed for the exposure(s) in question. When these analyses are done on cohort members who developed a particular illness and on controls selected from the cohort, the results obtained cannot have been influenced by events occurring following the diagnosis of the illness. (In order to avoid the possibility of occult illness in cases influencing levels of a suspected aetiological factor, many studies of this type exclude from the analyses specimens obtained within the period prior to diagnosis that might correspond to the duration of the preclinical stage of disease.) Also, among the large majority of case–control studies in which exposure status is not measured until the illness or injury has been diagnosed, some are concerned only with an exposure or characteristic that would have been the same at all times in a person's life. This is true for a genetically determined characteristic such as ABO blood type, or the absence of glutathione transferase M_1 activity (an enzyme that metabolizes several potentially carcinogenic constituents of cigarette smoke). Clearly, these studies are no less valid for having had to measure exposure in retrospect.

However, most case–control studies are required to consider explicitly how best to assess in retrospect subjects' exposure status during one or more possible aetiologically relevant time periods. Possible sources of exposure data include interviews or questionnaires, available records, or physical or laboratory measurements.

Interviews/questionnaires

For many exposures, a subject's memory is an excellent window to the past. A number of important aetiological relationships have been identified through interview-based case–control studies. Generally, study participants will report longer-term and more recent experiences with greater accuracy than shorter-term and more distant ones. Attention to the ways in which questions are asked (Armstrong *et al.* 1992), along with the use of visual aids when appropriate (for example, pictures of medicines, or of containers of household products, and calendars for important life events to enhance recall of the timing of other exposures) will maximize the accuracy of the information received. These efforts, along with the use of the same questions for cases and controls asked in the same way, will also minimize the potential for bias that could result from the subject's or interviewer's awareness of case or control status.

One virtue of exposure ascertainment via interview or questionnaire is that information can be sought for multiple points in the past. It is possible that a given exposure plays an aetiological role only if present at a certain age, for a certain duration, or at a certain time in the past. Because there is often little guidance before a study starts to suggest the most relevant age, length, or recency, key exposures are often elicited throughout much of the subject's lifetime. However, care must be taken not to include exposures that took place after the illness began. An instructive example was provided by Victora *et al.* (1989) in a case–control study of infant death from diarrhoea in relation to type of feeding. These investigators asked mothers whether their child was or was not being breast fed immediately prior to the onset of the fatal illness (mothers of controls were queried about type of feeding prior to a comparable point in time). Mothers were also asked if subsequent to the onset of the illness there had been any changes in type of feeding; following the development of diarrhoea, many children are switched to formula and cow's milk. Relative to infants who were solely breast fed, those who were supplemented with powdered or cow's milk prior to their illness had about four times the risk of diarrhoeal death. However, the authors showed that if one inappropriately considered the feeding method that was present during the illness, about a 13-fold increase in risk associated with supplementation would have been estimated.

Records

Case–control studies have exploited the presence of vital, registry, employment, medical, and pharmacy records, to name a few, as a means of obtaining information on exposures. However, because the information contained in the records will usually have been assembled for purposes other than epidemiological research, it may not provide precisely that information desired by the epidemiologist. For example, a death certificate or an occupational record may state an individual's job, but often not his or her actual exposure to the substance(s) of interest to the study. Or, a pharmacy record will indicate a prescription having been filled, but not necessarily whether the patient took the medication on a given day, or took it at all. This sort of imprecision will impair a study's ability to discern a true association between an exposure and a disease—the greater the imprecision, the greater the impairment. Nonetheless, some very strong associations have been identified through record-based case–control studies. For example, Daling *et al.* (1982) conducted a tumour-registry-based case–control study to test the hypothesis that homosexual men have a relatively high incidence of anal cancer. While registry data do not specify a man's sexual preference, they do contain information regarding his marital status. The investigators found that three times more men with anal cancer than controls (men with a colon or rectal cancer) had never been married. Being single is far from a perfect predictor of homosexuality, of course. Nonetheless, the presence of such a large case–control difference, given the very poor means of gauging the relevant exposure, was a stimulus to conduct interview-based studies that could elicit information regarding sexual history with greater precision. The latter studies showed an exceedingly strong association (odds ratio of 50) (Daling *et al.* 1987).

In case–control studies in which medical records are used to characterize exposure status, care must be taken to restrict the information obtained to that which preceded the case's diagnosis (and the presence of symptoms, if any, that led to the diagnosis). The records of controls must be truncated at similar points in time. Without this safeguard, it is possible that bias will arise because there are systematically more records available to review on cases than controls; the case's illness may have stimulated an enquiry by medical personnel into his or her past, whereas no corresponding enquiry would necessarily have occurred for control subjects.

Physical and laboratory measurements

The recognized limitations of interviews and records in characterizing a variety of potentially relevant exposures have stimulated the conduct of epidemiological studies that use laboratory and other methods of measurement. A woman cannot tell an investigator the level of her reproductive hormones, the concentration of various micronutrients in her blood, or whether her cervix is infected with human papillomavirus, but laboratory tests can. Unfortunately, such tests tell us what these things are only at the time that the specimens have been obtained. For some exposures, there will be a high correlation between the measured level following case and control identification and that present during the aetiologically relevant time period. For example, lead enters and does not leave the dentine of teeth. Therefore, in young school-age children, lead dentine levels are an indicator of cumulative lead exposure, a good portion of which could be relevant to the development of intellectual impairment and other adverse neurological outcomes. In contrast, one would not rely on serum levels of reproductive hormones of postmenopausal cases of breast cancer and controls to indicate what their premenopausal levels were, much less their hormonal status during their very early reproductive years (at which time it is plausible that hormones are exerting their greatest impact on future risk of breast cancer).

Case definition

Ideally, the cases in a case–control study would comprise all (or a representative sample of) members of a defined population who develop a given health outcome during a given period of time. For studies of disease aetiology, that outcome is disease incidence. For studies that seek to determine the efficacy of early disease detection or treatment, the outcome generally is the occurrence of complications of the disease or mortality; such studies have been described in detail elsewhere (Selby 1994; Weiss 1994), and will not be covered any further here.

The population from which cases are to be drawn may be defined geographically, or it may be defined on the basis of other characteristics, such as membership in a prepaid health-care plan or an occupational group. The identification of all newly ill people in a defined population can be facilitated by the presence of a reporting system such as a cancer or malformation registry that seeks to accomplish this identification for other purposes. Occasionally, care for the condition being studied may be centralized, so that it will be necessary to review the records of only one or a few institutions to identify all cases in the population in which those institutions are located. However, in many instances it is not feasible to identify all cases that occur in a given population, and so often case–control studies are based on cases identified from hospital records, or from the records of selected providers from whom patients had sought health care. The study by Herbst *et al.* (1971) of vaginal adenocarcinoma was of this type. Whether or not the cases are derived from a defined population, it is necessary that they be drawn in an unselected manner with regard to exposure status, for example by including in the study all otherwise eligible cases diagnosed or receiving care during a defined time period.

While the goal of a case–control study of aetiology is to enrol incident cases, under some circumstances it may be necessary to enrol prevalent cases at a particular point in time, irrespective of when each one's illness had begun. For some conditions, the date of occurrence may simply not be known. For example, in the absence of very close sero-monitoring, one generally cannot determine when a person acquired an HIV infection. Furthermore, for uncommon diseases of long duration, an incidence series may yield too few cases for meaningful analysis. The disadvantages of using prevalent cases in a case–control study relate in part to the added problems of accurate exposure ascertainment. For prevalent conditions whose date of diagnosis is known, pre-illness exposure information on study subjects must be obtained for more distant points in the past, on average, than would be necessary for an incident series. For prevalent conditions whose date of occurrence is unknown (for example, HIV infection), there will be uncertainty as to the best point in time before which one should elicit exposure information. Also, by studying people remaining alive with a given condition, one is studying at the same time not only aetiological factors, but also those that influence survival from the condition.

Ideally, the criteria used to identify and select individual cases for study should be objective ones of high sensitivity and specificity for the disease. Specificity is of particular concern, since the inadvertent inclusion of people without disease into the case group will generally obscure any true association with exposure. With this in mind, in the case–control study of Reye's syndrome in relation to antecedent analgesic use conducted by the Centers for Disease Control (Hurwitz *et al.* 1985), only cases with a substantial degree of neurological impairment (stage 2 or higher) were included. The use of this criterion minimized the chances that children with diseases other than Reye's syndrome, which generally would have a lesser degree of severity, would be included in the case group. It also was intended to serve as protection against selective misclassification of Reye's syndrome based on knowledge of exposure status, since the hypothesis that aspirin was associated with Reye's syndrome was well known by the time that the study took place. Conceivably, the knowledge that the child had consumed aspirin could have led some doctors to diagnose Reye's syndrome in cases with an atypical illness.

Control definition

Occasionally, the proportion of ill people who have had a specific exposure is so high, unequivocally more than would be expected in the population from which they were derived, that the presence of an association (though not its magnitude) can be surmised from a case series alone (Cummings and Weiss 1998). For example, when it was learned that all cases of a form of pneumonia that was epidemic in Spain in 1981 had ingested adulterated rapeseed oil, a causal inference was drawn, leading to efforts to eliminate further use of that oil. This action was taken before any formal comparison of cases with controls was made (Tabuenca 1981).

However, in the vast majority of instances, an explicit control group is needed to estimate the frequency and degree of exposure that would have taken place among cases in the absence of an exposure–disease association. An ideal control group would be one that consists of individuals:

(1) selected from a population whose distribution of exposure is that of the population from which the cases arose;

(2) who are identical to the cases with respect to their distribution of all characteristics
 (a) that influence the likelihood and/or degree of exposure, and
 (b) that, independent of their relation to exposure, are also related to the occurrence of the illness under study or to its recognition;

(3) in whom the presence of the exposure can be measured accurately and in a manner that is identical to that used for cases.

If the criteria above are not met in a particular study, then selection bias, confounding, or information bias, respectively, will be present.

Minimizing selection bias

If the cases identified in the study are all or a sample of those that occurred in a defined population, one can seek to achieve comparability by choosing as controls people sampled from that same population. For geographically defined populations, a number of different methods of sampling have been used, including random digit dialling of telephone numbers, area sampling, neighbourhood sampling, voters' lists, population registers, motor vehicle licenses, and birth certificates, among others. When cases are members of a prepaid health-care plan who develop an illness or injury, a sample of people who were members of the health plan when the illness or injury occurred can serve as controls. When cases are ill or injured members of an employed population, controls can be selected from that same group of employees.

If cases have not been selected from a definable population at risk for the disease, but rather from people treated for a particular illness at one or a few hospitals or clinics, then selection bias may be introduced if controls are not chosen from people who, had they developed the illness under study, would have received care at these hospitals or clinics, and people who do and do not receive care from these sources differ with regard to their frequency or level of exposure.

Therefore, when cases are chosen from a narrow range of providers of health care, controls are often chosen from other ill people treated by these providers. Such ill controls may also be used if, irrespective of the source of cases, there is no feasible way to sample from the population at large, or if sampling from the population at large would be likely to result in a substantial level of non-response or information bias (see below). For these reasons, in some studies of fatal illness, exposures in people with a given cause of death are compared with exposures in a sample of people who died for other reasons.

However, the choice of ill or deceased controls can itself give rise to selection bias if the illnesses (or causes of death) represented in the control group are in some way associated with the exposure of interest. For example, ill or recently deceased people tend to have been smokers of cigarettes more often than other people (McLaughlin *et al.* 1985), since smoking is associated with a variety of causes of illness and death. Because smoking histories of ill people overstate the cigarette consumption of the population from which the cases arose (even if that population cannot be defined), the odds ratio associated with smoking based on the use of ill people as controls will be spuriously low.

To minimize selection bias related to having chosen ill or deceased controls, an attempt can be made to omit potential controls with conditions known to be related (positively or negatively) to the exposure. For example, in the analysis of a hospital-based case–control study of bladder cancer in relation to prior use of artificial sweeteners, the investigators excluded from their control group people who were admitted to hospital for obesity-related diseases (Silverman *et al.* 1983). They showed that without this restriction, the control group would have a spuriously high proportion of users of artificial sweeteners relative to the population from which their cases actually had come. This approach will succeed to the extent that one judges correctly which conditions truly are exposure-related, and how accurately the presence of those conditions can be determined. For many exposures, this may pose little problem, and judicious exclusion will yield a control group capable of providing an unbiased result. For others, such as cigarette smoking or alcohol drinking, it has been shown that admitting diagnoses or statements of cause of death are incapable of identifying all people with illnesses related to these exposures (McLaughlin *et al.* 1985).

Occasionally, controls are chosen from individuals who are tested for the presence of the disease under study and are found not to have it. For example, people demonstrated to have coronary artery occlusion on coronary angiography have been compared with angiography patients without occlusion with regard to potential risk factors (Thom *et al.* 1992). As another example, the prior use of oral contraceptives was compared between women diagnosed with venous thromboembolism and women seen at the same institution for suspected venous thromboembolism who turned out not to have this condition (Bloemenkamp *et al.* 1999). It may be relatively inexpensive to select controls from people who receive the same diagnostic evaluation as do cases, and it is also possible to achieve case–control comparability with regard to the choice of a health-care provider (and the correlates of that choice). This approach can have an impact on the study's validity if the frequency or degree of exposure differs between otherwise comparable members of a population who do and do not receive the test. It will increase the validity if the disease being investigated is generally asymptomatic, and so would not be detected in the absence of testing. Thus, the relation of the use of oral contraceptives to the incidence of *in situ* cancer of the cervix is best studied in women who have received cervical screening, by comparing oral contraceptive use between cases of *in situ* cancer and women with a negative screen. This is because:

- in most societies, screening is more commonly administered to women who use oral contraceptives than women who do not
- *in situ* cancers are asymptomatic and will not be identified in the absence of cervical screening.

Therefore, if controls are chosen from women in general, who may or may not have received cervical screening, an apparent excess of oral contraceptive users would be present among cases of *in situ* cancer even if no true association were present.

However, the choice of test-negative controls will detract from a study's validity if the large majority of people who develop the disease would soon be diagnosed whether or not the test was administered. There was a controversy in the late 1970s regarding the suitability, in case–control studies of postmenopausal oestrogen use and endometrial cancer, of a control group restricted to women with no evidence of cancer on endometrial biopsy. Among women without endometrial cancer, oestrogen use differs greatly between those who have and have not undergone biopsy, since oestrogen use predisposes to uterine bleeding of non-malignant causes that often leads to endometrial biopsy. Those investigators who believed that there was a great prevalence of occult endometrial cancer in the population suggested that the optimal control group ought to be women undergoing endometrial biopsy and found not to have cancer (Horwitz and Feinstein 1978). However, the majority of investigators believed that no such large pool of prevalent, occult disease existed, and that choosing biopsy-negative controls would lead to a spuriously high estimate of oestrogen use in the population at risk, and thus a spuriously low odds ratio (Shapiro *et al.* 1985).

No matter how controls are defined in a case–control study, selection bias may be introduced to the extent that exposure information is not obtained on all who have been selected to take part. The magnitude of the bias will increase in relation to the frequency of missing data and the degree to which exposure frequencies or levels differ between study subjects on whom exposure status is and is not known. The problem of incomplete ascertainment of exposure on study subjects is particularly common in interview- or questionnaire-based case–control studies. Strategies for minimizing the degree of non-response in case–control studies are discussed in detail elsewhere (Armstrong *et al.* 1992).

Minimizing confounding

Characteristics of confounding variables in case–control studies

Confounding is present when the estimate of the relation between an exposure and disease is distorted by the influence of another factor. In any study design, confounding will occur to the extent that the other factor is both associated with exposure (though not as a result of the exposure) and with the occurrence of the disease or its recognition. In case–control studies alone, a factor may confound even if it is not associated with an altered risk of disease, if the proportions of cases and controls vary across levels or categories of the factor. For example, in a collaborative study of ovarian cancer in relation to use of oral contraceptives (Weiss *et al.* 1981), an attempt was made to identify and interview all incident cases during a several-year period in two American populations. In one of the populations (western Washington State), several controls per case were interviewed, whereas the control-to-case ratio in the other (Utah) was 1.0. Since oral contraceptive use was more common in Washington women than in Utah women, failure to take into account the state of residence in the analysis (for example, by adjustment) would have led to a spuriously high estimate of the frequency of oral contraceptive use in controls relative to that in cases.

Means of controlling for confounding

One straightforward way of preventing confounding is to restrict cases and controls to a single category or level of the potentially confounding variable. For example, in their study of physical activity in relation to primary cardiac arrest, Siscovick *et al.* (1982) excluded people with conditions, such as clinically recognized heart disease, that could both predispose to cardiac arrest and might be expected to alter level of activity. A second way is to obtain information on exposures or characteristics that may differ between cases and controls, and then make statistical adjustments for those that also are found to be related to the exposure/characteristic under investigation (Rothman and Greenland 1998).

Finally, it is possible to match one or more controls to each case's category or level of a potentially confounding factor.

1. It is appropriate to match if the variable is expected to be strongly related to both exposure and to disease. Thus, in a case–control study of breast cancer in relation to use of hair dye, it would make sense to match on gender (if the study had not already been restricted to women) since, in most cultures use of hair dye is more common in women than in men and in the absence of matching the case-to-control ratio would be very uneven between women and men. While confounding by gender could be prevented even without matching by adjustment in the analysis, the statistical precision of the unmatched study would be substantially reduced relative to that of a case–control study having a more similar proportion of female cases and controls.
2. It is appropriate to match if information on possible matching variables can be obtained inexpensively. There are some means of control selection in which information regarding some confounders can be obtained at no cost. For example, from voters' lists or prepaid health plan membership records, it would

generally be possible to choose directly one or more controls who were identical to a given case's age. Conversely, if a population sampling scheme such as random digit dialling were being employed, the age of the respondent would not be known in advance of approaching him or her. Rather than omitting already contacted controls who did not match a particular case's age, the matching can be done much more broadly. Additional control for finer categories of age can be accomplished in the data analysis.

3. It is appropriate to match if information on exposure status cannot be obtained inexpensively. The higher the cost of exposure ascertainment, the greater the incentive to limit the number of control subjects to the number of cases. Case–control differences regarding confounding factors particularly will reduce the statistical power of a study that does not have a surplus of controls. Enriching the group of controls selected with people more similar to the cases with regard to confounding factors (that is, matching) can prevent this loss of statistical power.

In case–control studies of genetic characteristics as possible aetiological factors, some investigators have used a matched design in which a specified type of relative (for example parent, sibling, cousin) is chosen as a control for each case (Yang and Khoury 1997; Witte *et al.* 1999). This approach has the advantage of minimizing potential confounding by other genetic characteristics with which the one of interest is associated. However, it has the disadvantage of excluding a possibly large fraction of cases for whom there is no relative available of the type needed to provide a sample for genetic analysis.

It should be kept in mind that matching alone is not sufficient to eliminate a variable's confounding influence: failure to consider a matching variable in the analysis of the study can lead to a biased result (Rothman and Greenland 1998). Analyses of studies that have matched controls to cases on a given characteristic can adjust for that characteristic as if no matching had taken place. Alternatively, these analyses can explicitly consider cases and controls as matched sets. In the instance of matched case–control pairs and a dichotomous exposure variable, the following table could be constructed.

	Control	
Case	Exposed	Non-exposed
Exposed	*a*	*b*
Non-exposed	*c*	*d*

Only the *b* pairs in which the case was exposed but not the matched control, and the *c* pairs in which the reverse was true, would enter the analysis. The odds ratio would be calculated as *b*/*c*. When there is more than one control per case, the matched odds ratio can be calculated as well (Breslow and Day 1980).

Minimizing information bias

In case–control studies in which information on exposure status is sought via an interview or questionnaire, the chief safeguards against information bias entail asking questions about events that are salient to the respondent, that are framed in an unambiguous way, and that are presented identically to both cases and controls. Employment of these safeguards, however, will not prevent differential accuracy of reporting between cases and controls in all circumstances. Some past exposures/events will simply be more salient to people with an illness, who might have dwelled on possible reasons for its occurrence, than to people without that illness. Other exposures may be viewed as socially undesirable, and there may be a difference between cases and healthy controls in their willingness to admit to them. If the anticipated difference in the quality of information between cases and otherwise appropriate controls is too great, a control group that is less than ideal in other respects may be selected instead so as to minimize the potential for information bias. For example, some studies of prenatal risk factors for a particular congenital malformation that utilize maternal interviews as the source of exposure data have selected as controls infants with other malformations (Rosenberg *et al.* 1983). This control group will provide a more valid result than a control group that consists of infants in general if mothers of malformed and mothers of normal infants report prenatal exposures to a different degree even in the absence of an association, and the exposure in question is not associated with the occurrence of the malformations present in control infants.

Similar reasoning led Daling *et al.* (1987), when conducting their case–control study of anal cancer in relation to a history of anal intercourse, to eschew the geographic population from which their case had arisen as a sampling frame for controls. They feared that interviews that sought information about prior anal intercourse might be more complete among men with cancer than men in the population at large. Thus, they chose as controls men with a cancer of a different site (colon), which they believed was unlikely to have been aetiologically related to prior anal intercourse.

When the exposure under consideration is sufficiently imprecise or is open to subjective interpretation, there may not be any control group that will provide information comparable to that provided by cases. An instructive example comes from a case–control study of Down's syndrome (Stott 1958) conducted shortly before the chromosomal basis for the aetiology of this condition had been learned. The study sought to determine whether emotional 'shocks' during pregnancy might be a risk factor. The author interviewed mothers of children with Down's syndrome with regard to the occurrence of a 'situation or event [that would be] stress- or shock-producing if this would have been its expected effect on an emotionally stable woman'. Identical interviews were administered to mothers of normal children, and also to mothers of retarded children who did not have Down's syndrome. Even though it is not possible that an emotional shock in pregnancy could play any aetiological role in a condition already determined at conception, a far higher proportion of mothers of cases of Down's syndrome reported an emotional shock than did mothers of normal controls (relative risk estimated from the data, 17.0). The use of other retarded children as controls only partially reduced the spuriously high relative risk to a value of 4.3.

When conducting an interview-based study of a rapidly fatal disease, or a disease that impairs a person's ability to provide valid interview data, it is necessary to obtain information from at least some surrogate respondents. Typically, these respondents are close relatives of the cases. In general, for purposes of comparability, similar information ought to be obtained from surrogates of controls, even though the control would be expected to provide more accurate data. Results of case–control studies based on exposure information provided by surrogate respondents need to be interpreted with particular caution. Though by no means present in every instance (Nelson *et al.* 1990), there can be a large difference in the validity of the responses given by case and control surrogates. For example, Greenberg *et al.* (1985) investigated the basis for an apparent strong association between cancer mortality and 'nuclear' work among employees of a naval shipyard which had been found in a comparison of work histories provided by surrogates of men who died from cancer and of those who died of other conditions. They observed that, regarding work in the nuclear part of the industry, surrogates of the cases generally provided information similar to that contained in employment records of the shipyard. In contrast, the surrogates of controls substantially misclassified the nature of their relatives' jobs as not involving radiation. Using the data provided by employment records, which included individual radiation dosimetry (Rinsky *et al.* 1981), little or no association was found between cancer mortality and radiation exposure received at the shipyard.

What was undoubtedly a spuriously negative association was found in a case–control study of lung cancer and passive cigarette smoking that used, for one analysis, information obtained from surrogate respondents (Janerich *et al.* 1990). In this analysis, the relative risk of lung cancer among non-smokers associated with a spouse's having smoked—0.33 (that is, a 67 per cent reduction in risk)—would seem almost certainly due to a spurious minimization or denial of smoking by spouses of cases, who may have feared their habit caused their spouse to develop lung cancer.

Incomparable assessment of exposure status between cases and controls is not confined to interview- or questionnaire-based studies. Most laboratory-based studies seek to prevent this by testing samples blind to case/control status. If feasible, it is desirable to do this blinding as well in studies in which exposure is to be determined from medical or other records. However, there are instances in which the nature of the information available in records has already been influenced by whether the subject is a case or a control. For example, it was found that among 100 infertile women who underwent laparoscopy (Strathy *et al.* 1982), 21 had endometriosis. Only 2 per cent of 200 women undergoing laparoscopy for another indication, tubal ligation, were noted in the records of their procedure to have endometriosis. However, the interpretation of this association is unclear, since the identification and/or recording of endometriosis in cases and controls (women undergoing tubal ligation) may well have been incomparable—only in the infertile women was the laparoscopy expressly done as a diagnostic tool to investigate the possible presence of conditions such as endometriosis.

Estimating the attributable risk from results of case–control studies

Occasionally, a case–control study identifies a large odds ratio relating an exposure and a disease, and for this and other reasons a causal influence of the exposure may be suspected. The decision to seek to limit or eliminate that exposure requires weighing its negative and positive consequences. This weighing must be done in absolute, rather than in relative terms, since the same relative increase (or decrease) in risk is of far greater consequence for common than for rare outcomes. The absolute increase in the risk of disease believed to be due to a dichotomous exposure, sometimes referred to as the 'attributable risk' (AR), can be estimated directly from data gathered in cohort studies or randomized trials as the difference between the incidence among exposed (I_e) and non-exposed people (I_n). The term $I_e - I_n$ can be rewritten as $\mathrm{RR}(I_n) - I_n$, or as $I_n(\mathrm{RR} - 1)$. Since the relative risk can be estimated from the results of a case–control study by means of the odds ratio, the only additional piece of information needed to estimate the attributable risk is an estimate of I_n. For the population in which the study has been conducted, I_n can be estimated if:

(1) the overall incidence (I) of the disease in that population is known or can be approximated;

(2) the frequency of exposure (p_e) in the controls selected for study reasonably reflects that of the population that gave rise to the cases.

Given (1) and (2) above,

$$\begin{aligned} I &= I_e(p_e) + I_n(1 - p_e) \\ &= I_n\mathrm{RR}(p_e) + I_n(1 - p_e) \\ &= I_n[p_e(\mathrm{RR} - 1) + 1], \end{aligned}$$

and so

$$I_n = \frac{I}{p_e(\mathrm{RR} - 1) + 1}.$$

Therefore,

$$\mathrm{AR} = \frac{I(\mathrm{RR} - 1)}{p_e(\mathrm{RR} - 1) + 1} = \frac{I}{p_e + 1/(\mathrm{RR} - 1)}.$$

For example, consider a disease with an incidence rate of 10 per 100 000 per year in a population in which 5 per cent of people have been exposed during a relevant period of time. The following table summarizes data from a case–control study conducted in that population:

Exposed	Cases	Controls	OR
Yes	15%	5%	3.35
No	85%	95%	1

The attributable risk that corresponds to the estimated 3.35-fold increase in risk is

$$\frac{10}{0.05 + 1/(3.35 - 1)} = 20.2 \text{ per } 100\,000 \text{ per year.}$$

From the results of case–control studies that suggest a causal relation, it is also possible to estimate the percentage of exposed people with the disease who developed it because of their exposure, rather than through one or more causal pathways not involving the exposure. This measure, often termed the 'attributable risk per cent' (AR%) among exposed people, is defined as

$$\frac{I_e - I_n}{I_e} \times 100\%.$$

It can be described in terms of the relative risk alone:

$$\mathrm{AR\%} = \frac{I_e}{I_e} - \frac{I_n}{I_e} = 1 - \frac{1}{\mathrm{RR}} = \frac{\mathrm{RR} - 1}{\mathrm{RR}} \times 100\%.$$

Therefore, the results of a case–control study that provide a valid estimate of the relative risk (via the odds ratio) can provide the attributable risk per cent as well, with no additional assumptions or sources of data. It is also possible to estimate the percentage of a disease's occurrence in the population as a whole that resulted from the actions of given exposure. This measure, the 'population attributable risk per cent' (PAR%) or 'aetiological fraction', is simply the attributable risk per cent multiplied by the proportion of cases in that population who were exposed (p_c):

$$PAR\% = AR\% \ (p_c) \times 100\%.$$

In the present example,

$$AR\% = \frac{3.35 - 1}{3.35} = 70.1\%$$

and

$$PAR\% = 70.1\% \ (0.15) = 10.5\%.$$

The role of case–control studies in understanding disease aetiology

Randomized trials will not be able to answer all questions regarding the reasons diseases occur. Many potential disease-causing or disease-preventing exposures cannot be manipulated, either at all—for example, most genetic characteristics—or in any practical way for purposes of a study. For many exposure–disease relationships, either the disease is too uncommon or the induction period is too long to conduct a randomized trial that is not infeasibly large in size or long in duration. Finally, it generally will not be possible to conduct separate randomized trials to measure the impact of all potential types, amounts, and durations of a class of exposure.

Also, it is not possible to rely solely on cohort studies for answers. Just as with randomized trials, the disease outcome being studied may be too rare to allow a cohort approach to be useful. This explains why the aetiologies of vaginal adenocarcinoma and Reye's syndrome, for example, have been evaluated exclusively by case–control studies—these diseases are simply too uncommon for most cohort studies to generate any cases, even in 'exposed' individuals. Prospective cohort studies are also of limited use when the induction period for the exposure–disease relationship is either very short or very long. If the induction period is very short and the exposure status of an individual varies over time, a cohort study would need to assess exposure status repeatedly among cohort members. For this reason, studies of alcohol consumption in relation to the occurrence of injuries typically are case–control in nature (Holcomb 1938). Similarly, unless information on exposure status can be ascertained retrospectively at the time that the cohort is formed, it would not be feasible to initiate a cohort study of a suspected aetiological relation that requires a very long time (perhaps several decades) to manifest itself.

While case–control studies may be of particular value in the evaluation of the aetiology of uncommon diseases, they may have difficulty in obtaining statistically precise results if the frequency of the exposure in the population under study is either extremely common or extremely uncommon (Crombie 1981). Thus, only an association as strong as the one between cigarette smoking and lung cancer could have emerged reliably from case–control studies of several hundred British men conducted in the late 1940s (Doll and Hill 1950), given that well over 90 per cent of that population were cigarette smokers. For very uncommon exposures—for example, occupational exposure to a specific substance suspected of posing a risk to health, or an infrequently prescribed drug—barring a strong observed association based on a large number of subjects, even the best-designed case–control study will usually offer no more than a suggestion of the presence or absence of a relation with regard to the occurrence of a given illness.

References

Armstrong, B.K., White, E., and Sarucci, R. (1992). *Principles of exposure measurement in epidemiology.* Oxford University Press.

Bloemenkamp, K.W.M., Rosendaal, F.R., Buller, H.R., *et al.* (1999). Risk of venous thrombosis with use of current low-dose oral contraceptives is not explained by diagnostic suspicion and referral bias. *Archives of Internal Medicine*, **159**, 65–70.

Breslow, N.E. and Day, N.E. (1980). *Statistical methods in cancer research.* Vol. 1: *The analysis of case–control studies.* Scientific Publication No. 32, IARC, Lyon.

Crombie, I.K. (1981). The limitations of case–control studies in the detection of environmental carcinogens. *Journal of Epidemiology and Community Health*, **35**, 281–7.

Cummings, P. and Weiss, N.S. (1998). Case series and exposure series: the role of studies without controls in providing information about the etiology of injury or disease. *Injury Prevention*, **4**, 34–57.

Daling, J.R., Weiss, N.S., Klopfenstein, L.L., *et al.* (1982). Correlates of homosexual behavior and the incidence of anal cancer. *Journal of the American Medical Association*, **247**, 1988–90.

Daling, J.R., Weiss, N.S., Hislop, T.G., *et al.* (1987). Sexual practices, sexually transmitted diseases, and the incidence of anal cancer. *New England Journal of Medicine*, **317**, 973–7.

Doll, R. and Hill, A.B. (1950). Smoking and carcinoma of the lung. *British Medical Journal*, **2**, 739–48.

Greenberg, E.R., Rosner, B., Nennekens, C., *et al.* (1985). An investigation of bias in a study of nuclear shipyard workers. *American Journal of Epidemiology*, **121**, 301–8.

Greenland, S. and Thomas, D.C. (1982). On the need for the rare disease assumption in case–control studies. *American Journal of Epidemiology*, **116**, 547–53.

Greenwald, P., Barlow, J.J., Nasca, P., *et al.* (1971). Vaginal cancer after maternal treatment with synthetic estrogens. *New England Journal of Medicine*, **285**, 390–3.

Herbst, A.L., Ulfelder, H., and Poskanzer, D.C. (1971). Adenocarcinoma of the vagina: association of maternal stilbestrol therapy with tumor appearance in young women. *New England Journal of Medicine*, **284**, 878–81.

Holcomb, R.L. (1938). Alcohol in relation to traffic accidents. *Journal of the American Medical Association*, **111**, 1076–85.

Horwitz, R.I. and Feinstein, A.R. (1978). Alternative analytic methods for case–control studies of estrogens and endometrial cancer. *New England Journal of Medicine*, **299**, 1089–94.

Hurwitz, E.S., Barren, M.J., Bregman, D., *et al.* (1985). Public Health Service Study on Reye's syndrome and medications. Report of the Pilot Phase. *New England Journal of Medicine*, **313**, 849–57.

Janerich, D.T., Thompson, W.D., Varela, L.R., *et al.* (1990). Lung cancer and exposure to tobacco smoke in the household. *New England Journal of Medicine*, **323**, 632–6.

McLaughlin, J.K., Blot, W.J., Mehl, E.S., *et al.* (1985). Problems in the use of dead controls in case–control studies. II. Effect of excluding certain causes of death. *American Journal of Epidemiology*, **122**, 485–94.

Nelson, L.M., Longstreth, W.T., Koespell, T.D., *et al.* (1990). Proxy respondents in epidemiologic research. *Epidemiology Review*, **12**, 71–86.

Pearce, N. (1993). What does the odds ratio estimate in a case–control study? *International Journal of Epidemiology*, **22**, 1189–92.

Rinsky, R.A., Zumwolde, R.D., Waxweiller, R.J., *et al.* (1981). Cancer mortality at a naval nuclear shipyard. *Lancet*, **1**, 231–5.

Rosenberg, L., Mitchell, A.A., Parsells, J.L., *et al.* (1983). Lack of relation of oral clefts to diazepam use during pregnancy. *New England Journal of Medicine*, **309**, 1282–5.

Rothman, K.J. and Greenland, S. (1998). *Modern epidemiology* (2nd edn). Lippincott-Raven, Philadelphia, PA.

Selby, J.V. (1994). Case control evaluations of treatment and program efficacy. *Epidemiology Review*, **46**, 91–101.

Shapiro, S., Kelly, J.P., Rosenberg, L., *et al.* (1985). Risk of localized and widespread endometrial cancer in relation to recent and discontinued use of conjugated estrogens. *New England Journal of Medicine*, **313**, 969–72.

Silverman, D.T., Hoover, R.N., and Swanson, G.M. (1983). Artificial sweeteners and lower urinary tract cancer: hospital vs. population controls. *American Journal of Epidemiology*, **117**, 326–34.

Siscovick, D.S., Weiss, N.S., Hallstrom, A.P., *et al.* (1982). Physical activity and primary cardiac arrest. *Journal of the American Medical Association*, **248**, 3113–17.

Stott, D.H. (1958). Some psychosomatic aspects of casualty in reproduction. *Journal of Psychosomatic Research*, **3**, 42–55.

Strathy, J.H., Molgaard, C.A., Coulam, C.B., *et al.* (1982). Endometriosis and infertility: A laparoscopic study of endometriosis among fertile and infertile women. *Fertility and Sterility*, **38**, 667–72.

Tabuenca, J.M. (1981). Toxic-allergic syndrome caused by ingestion of rapeseed oil denatured with aniline. *Lancet*, **ii**, 567–8.

Thom, D.H., Grayston, J.T., Siscovick, D.S., *et al.* (1992). Association of prior infection with *Chlamydia pneumoniae* and angiographically demonstrated coronary artery disease. *Journal of the American Medical Association*, **268**, 68–72.

Ulfelder, H. and Robboy, S.J. (1976). The embryologic development of the human vagina. *American Journal of Obstetrics and Gynecology*, **126**, 769–76.

Victora, C.G., Smith, P.G., Vaughn, J.P., *et al.* (1989). Infant feeding and deaths due to diarrhea. *American Journal of Epidemiology*, **129**, 1032–41.

Weiss, N.S. (1994). Application of the case–control method in the evaluation of screening. *Epidemiology Review*, **16**, 102–8.

Weiss, N.S., Lyon, J.L., Liff, J.M., *et al.* (1981). Incidence of ovarian cancer in relation to the use of oral contraceptives. *International Journal of Cancer*, **28**, 669–71.

Witte, J.S., Gauderman, W.J., and Thomas, D.C. (1999). Asymptotic bias and efficiency in case–control studies of candidate genes and gene-environment interactions: basic family designs. *American Journal of Epidemiology*, **149**, 693–705.

Yang, Q. and Khoury, M.J. (1997). Evolving methods in genetic epidemiology. III. Gene–environment interaction in epidemiologic research. *Epidemiology Review*, **19**, 33–43.

6.6 Cohort studies

Manning Feinleib and Norman E. Breslow

Introduction

The cohort study is an observational epidemiological study which, after the manner of an experiment, attempts to study the relationship between a purported cause (exposure) and the subsequent risk of developing disease. As in other observational epidemiological studies, and unlike experimental studies, the suspected causal factor or exposure is not randomly assigned to the study population. However, the cohort study follows the same time direction as an experiment in that the suspected exposure is identified as having or not having occurred in the study population before the occurrence of disease is investigated. Thus, certain biases that may occur in other forms of epidemiological studies can be avoided, specifically those concerned with ascertaining the exposure status of the population. Furthermore, because disease occurrence is identified subsequent to enumeration of exposure groups, this type of study allows direct estimation of the risk of developing disease and how risk varies with time since exposure.

Cohort studies have been given a variety of names including incidence studies, prospective studies, follow-up studies, longitudinal studies, and panel studies, although the latter two terms have more generally been applied to studies involving repeated measurements of the same variables over time. They are similar to the usual scientific experiment in that they proceed from the suspected cause or aetiological agent to the disease outcome with controls or comparison groups selected on the basis of absence of exposure to the putative cause. As a type of observational study, there is no randomization to exposure classes nor is there any attempt to manipulate the exposure. In contrast, case–control studies (also known as case–referent studies and, formerly, as retrospective studies) have no counterpart in experimental science since they work from the outcome event back towards the supposed aetiological factor. Indeed, case–control studies are often viewed conceptually in terms of sampling data from an ongoing (and possibly fictitious) cohort study.

Cohort studies offer the possibility of studying the full range of effects of the suspected aetiological factor. Frequently the suspected aetiological factor is not only related to the occurrence of the disease of primary interest, but may influence the natural history of the disease and may be related to a variety of other health conditions that may not have been suspected at first. A particularly important aspect of cohort studies is that they provide direct estimates of the risk of disease for each exposure group separately. These separate estimates of risk can then be used to estimate a variety of measures of interest to epidemiologists such as the attributable risk, the relative risk, and the aetiological fraction. (These measures of risk are discussed in the section on analysis below and in Table 3.) Although these risks can often be estimated from other types of studies when certain assumptions are made or ancillary information is available, cohort studies permit direct estimates of these measures from the data obtained in the study itself.

The disadvantages of cohort studies are primarily logistic and administrative. Often, relatively large populations have to be followed for long periods of time, thus entailing considerable expense in terms of funding and professional resources. If the disease outcome of interest is rare, the sample sizes required for concurrent studies may be prohibitively large. If the follow-up period is long, which is often the case for chronic diseases, the problem of attrition of the study group due to loss from follow-up, migration, competing causes of death, or gradual deterioration of interest in participation may present serious analytical problems that might negate the value of the overall study. Longitudinal follow-up requires careful attention to maintaining standardized diagnostic methods and criteria. Finally, of course, the longer the study is continued, the more difficult it is to maintain a committed investigative team and stable funding for the project.

In the first part of this chapter we discuss the major methodological aspects of cohort studies: forms of cohort studies, selection of study cohorts, gathering of baseline information, follow-up, and analysis. To illustrate these points we use examples from three studies: a historical cohort study of artificial menopause and breast cancer using available hospital and death certificate information (Feinleib 1968), a prospective cohort study, using mail questionnaires, of cigarette smoking and mortality among British doctors (Doll and Peto 1976), and a prospective cohort study of heart disease in Framingham, Massachusetts, using periodic medical examinations (Kannel *et al.* 1961; Dawber *et al.* 1963). In the second part of the chapter we present the various types of bias that can confound interpretation of cohort studies and suggests ways of identifying, reducing, and/or resolving these biases. In this section examples are drawn from a wider range of studies.

Design of cohort studies

Forms of cohort studies

Cohort studies may take a variety of forms. The key distinction that has been established in the past is based primarily on the availability of data. In prospective (or observational) cohort studies, data on exposure status and disease outcome are not available at the outset of the study: they must be ascertained through the direct efforts of the investigator in the future. In ambispective cohort studies, data on exposure status have been collected in the past and are available from existing records while disease outcome is unknown or incompletely known the investigator is obliged to follow the cohort for subsequent occurrence of the disease. In historical (or non-concurrent) cohort studies, data on exposure status and disease outcome have been collected in the past and are available from existing records, the investigator's efforts are devoted primarily to linking the relevant data files. The basic steps involved in each type of study include selecting the study and comparison groups, obtaining baseline information with regard to exposure and initial health status, and follow-up of the members of the cohort and surveillance for disease outcome.

Selection of the study cohorts

Objectives

There are two approaches to the selection of representative samples of exposed and non-exposed groups to be followed in a cohort study.

1. The identification of a special exposure group defined because of (i) unusual exposure to a suspected causative (aetiological factor), or (ii) unusual lifestyle or work experience.
2. Using a general population sample in which there is heterogeneity of exposure to the suspected aetiological factor.

Where the study group is a special exposure group, it is necessary to find appropriate comparison groups or the means to make comparisons with the general population. When the general population sample is used as a starting point, the various levels of exposure within the study group provide the basis for internal comparisons. Each approach also takes into consideration various logistic constraints, for example accessibility and co-operativeness of the study groups, availability of medical and other records, and anticipated completeness and cost of endpoint surveillance.

Example 1—A historical cohort study of the relation between artificial menopause and breast cancer

Seven case–control studies performed between 1926 and 1962 all reported that artificial menopause (surgical removal of the uterus and/or ovaries) occurred significantly less frequently among breast cancer patients than among a variety of controls. Because the case–control studies did not present information about the extent of surgery (the effect of removal of only the uterus versus removal of the ovaries) or the effects of the age at which the artificial menopause occurred, it was decided to investigate these issues by means of a cohort study. The disadvantage of using a prospective cohort method in elucidating the relation between artificial menopause and breast cancer is that there is a long interval between the gynaecological procedure and the appearance of the disease in appreciable frequency. To reduce this delay it was decided to use the historical cohort approach. The cohorts were selected from the records of two technical hospitals in the Boston area. The study cohorts included all eligible patients seen at these hospitals from 1920 to 1940. Women aged 55 years or younger were eligible for inclusion in the study if they had undergone any of the following procedures as determined from surgical and pathological records: (i) hysterectomy; (ii) unilateral oophorectomy; (iii) bilateral oophorectomy; (iv) radium or X-ray treatment of the ovaries or uterus; (v) cholecystectomy. The last group served as a control cohort.

Certain patients were excluded from the study: (i) women who had a prior mastectomy or a prior breast malignancy or who had undergone castration as part of the treatment for an existing breast tumour; (ii) women treated for pelvic malignancies; (iii) women who had previous removal of their ovaries or a history of natural menopause before the age of 40 years; (iv) women who did not survive their index admission; (v) all who were not residents of Massachusetts at the time of their index procedure. At the final editing of the study abstract forms and the elimination of duplicate records, there were 8387 patients in the study populations. They were subdivided into four 'exposure' categories.

1. Natural menopause—1479 women (including 953 women who underwent cholecystectomy and 526 women who were postmenopausal at the time of the gynaecological procedures for benign conditions).
2. Hysterectomy and bilateral oophorectomy—3241 women (this constitutes the surgically castrated group who were believed to have no residual ovarian activity).
3. Those undergoing hysterectomy and/or unilateral oophorectomy who, as far as could be ascertained from the surgical and pathological records, retained at least one intact ovary—2149 women (referred to as the 'partial surgery' group).
4. Radiation-induced artificial menopause—1518 women.

The partial surgery group constituted a second control cohort and 'sham operations' with which to contrast the women subjected to hysterectomy and bilateral oophorectomy.

It should be noted that it is not possible to relate the actual cohort studies to a clearly definable population. Although in this case adequate records were available for virtually every woman admitted to these hospitals who was eligible for the study, it is not known from what source population these women came. However, it is assumed that the reasons for coming to these particular hospitals were not correlated with both the type of procedure and the subsequent risk of developing breast cancer, i.e. they were not confounding factors (see section on biases below).

Example 2—A prospective cohort study of the relation between cigarette smoking and mortality: the British Doctors Study (Breslow and Day 1987, Appendix IA)

By 1950 several case–control studies had been published and were in agreement in showing that a larger proportion of lung cancer patients had been heavy cigarette smokers and a smaller proportion had been non-smokers than patients with other diseases. Because of the possibility of a variety of biases in these case–control studies, a prospective study was launched in 1951 among the members of the medical profession in the United Kingdom. This group was chosen because it was felt that physicians would respond to mailed questionnaires, would report their smoking histories accurately, and could be followed economically through the death records of the Registrars-General and through the registries of the General Medical Council and the British Medical Association. It was felt that the relation of smoking to health among physicians would be similar to that in the general population. A simple questionnaire was mailed out on 31 October 1951 to 59 600 men and women on the Medical Register.

The replies received from 40 637 doctors (34 445 from men and 6192 from women) were sufficiently complete to be used. From a one-in-ten random sample of the register, it was estimated that this represented answers from 69 per cent of the men and 60 per cent of the women alive at the time of the inquiry. The degree of self-selection in those who replied was assessed in terms of the overall mortality using this one-in-ten sample. The standardized death rate of those who replied was only 63 per cent of the death rate for all doctors in the second year of the inquiry and 85 per cent in the third year. In the fourth to tenth years the proportion varied about an average of 93 per cent and there was no evidence of any regular change with the further passage of years. Evidently the effect of selection did not entirely wear off, but after the third year it had become slight.

Example 3—A prospective cohort study of risk factors for heart disease: the Framingham Heart Study

The Framingham Heart Study is a long-term follow-up study of a sample of adults who lived in the town of Framingham, Massachusetts, in 1950. The first participants were actually examined in 1948 as part of an effort to conduct a demonstration programme in the detection and natural history of cardiovascular diseases. In 1950, however, the study was reconstituted as a long-term epidemiological investigation of coronary heart diseases, and the original voluntary participants were incorporated into a random sample drawn from all adults aged 30 to 60 years living in the town. Of the eligible random sample of 6507 persons, 4469 (68.7 per cent) participated in the examinations. When this number was supplemented with the volunteers, a total cohort of 5209 was obtained. The possible effects of supplementing the cohort to replace the originally selected participants who refused to participate in the reconstituted study are discussed in Example 9 below.

Although it was recognized from the outset that the town of Framingham could be considered neither a random nor a completely representative sample of the United States, the town did have certain characteristics that made it extremely suitable for a long-term epidemiological study. The population of the town was of adequate size (28 000) to provide enough individuals in the desired age range. It was sufficiently compact that the study population could be observed conveniently by means of an examination at a single examining facility, and most of the residents received their hospital care at a single central hospital in the town. Owing in part to a relatively stable economy supported by a diversity of employment opportunities, the population was relatively stable so as to enable adequate follow-up for a long period of time. Both the general community and the medical profession of the town were felt to be co-operative. The town was not believed to be 'grossly atypical in any respect that appeared relevant'.

Since only 68.7 per cent of the eligible random sample participated in the 1950 examinations, it is possible that they might not be representative of the total population. This is a serious concern in all epidemiological studies where participation is voluntary and may be subject to self-selection. In this study it was felt that reasons for not participating were not appreciably related simultaneously to both the characteristics to be studied in the investigation and the risk of developing heart disease (see the section on biases below).

Gathering of baseline information

Objectives

There are multiple objectives to be achieved in gathering baseline information.

1. Valid assessment of the exposure status of the members of the cohort groups.
2. Define the individuals 'at risk'; exclude those individuals with known disease at baseline.
3. Establish a basis for follow-up: obtain identifying data, informed consent, commitment to co-operating in the follow-up (e.g. permission to contact family members and physicians, and to obtain hospital and employment records).
4. Obtain data on important covariates (i.e. other exposures that may be associated with the risk of acquiring the disease) so that adjustments can be made for their contribution to the incidence of disease in analysis (see section on confounding variables below).

Sources of baseline information

Existing records

Baseline information about the cohorts can be obtained from a variety of sources such as available records from hospitals or employment records, interviews of the cohort members or other informants, direct medical and other special examinations, and indirect measures of exposure estimated from investigations of the environment. The availability of written records such as medical or employment records may provide useful information to select and define the cohort. If high-quality records are available, they may permit the study to begin from the point of the recording of the information, thereby adding a considerable period of follow-up time before the actual initiation of the investigation. Studies based on such records with follow-up of patients from such a prior point in time to the present have been given special names such as retrospective cohort studies, non-concurrent cohort studies, and historical prospective studies. There are several other advantages for using previously recorded information. The data are apt to be free from certain biases since they are recorded before any knowledge of the particular study for which they are used. Written records may provide information that is not fully known to the subject, such as details on medical conditions or actual levels of exposure. However, such records may also have certain drawbacks. Records may not be uniformly available for all cohort members. Even when available, the detail and quality of the data in the records are not controllable by the investigator and it is difficult to verify the accuracy of questionable items.

Interviews

One of the more common methods of obtaining information is to interview the cohort members or other informants. A variety of techniques can be used: direct personal interviews, mailed questionnaires, telephone interviews, having the subject complete a questionnaire administered by computer, and using a tape recorder and headphones for asking intimate questions in a crowded setting. When approaches are made to individual cohort members, there are varying rates of response to requests to participate in the study. A wide variety of cohort studies has reported response rates of approximately 65 to 75 per cent for direct interviews. Mail questionnaires, depending on the length of the questionnaire and motivations of the group, often have appreciably lower rates of response. The advantages of interviewing the cohort members include the ability to obtain information on a wide variety of topics. Interviews can provide data on attitudes and permit quite complex questions to be asked with the possibility of probing to ensure accurate recording of responses (such as eliciting histories about diet, exercise, or measures of stress). However, interview data may not always be reliable because the subject may fail to recall information or may not be aware of his or her own habits or history. There is also the possibility that the information may be biased by the subject's knowledge of the aims of the investigation.

Examinations

Medical and other special examinations are necessary to obtain information of which the subject cannot be expected to be aware. Direct examination is often necessitated by the nature of the aetiological factor to be investigated and may be the only way to obtain biologically meaningful information. Subjects often appreciate the availability of an examination, and this may enhance the response rate to certain types of investigations. However, special examinations are usually expensive and require attention to standardization of procedures, training of appropriate observers or laboratory personnel, and quality control across observers and over time. It has also been reported that response rates to medical examinations tend to be biased towards subjects who are relatively free from disease. Direct examination can also be used to validate information obtained from interviews. For example, testing for urinary thiocyanate has been a useful adjunct to smoking studies.

Measure of environment

The fourth type of baseline information is that obtained for each of the groups as a whole, particularly when one is dealing with special exposure groups. Thus it might be appropriate to measure air pollution, exposure to radiation or other toxicological substances, or exposures on the job for an entire group of workers and to apply this measure to each of the individuals in the group. Although this type of information is usually quite useful, particularly when individual measures of exposure cannot be obtained directly, one should be aware that it essentially constitutes 'ecological data', i.e. the measurement of a mean or modal value for a group, which may conceal individual variability within the group.

Example 4—Artificial menopause and breast cancer

All the baseline information for this investigation was obtained from the available surgical and pathological records already filed in the record rooms of two hospitals between 1920 and 1940. The data were felt to be adequate for providing a valid assessment of the exposure status of the members of the cohorts in terms of whether or not they had received the indicated operation. Furthermore, as indicated above, those individuals with known disease could be identified from the available records. In part, the high quality of the records was due to the fact that the hospitals chosen were teaching hospitals for a major medical school, and the records were generally filled out by medical students and interns who provided careful and detailed histories. However, if there was no mention of existing or pre-existing breast cancer, there was no means of confirming this independently of the available records. Likewise, the existence of breast cancer was based solely on the report of the patient to the interviewing physician. Covariates that were available from the hospital records were the age at the time of the index procedure and the parity of the women. Other covariates of possible interest, since they could have been related to both the risk of cancer and the risk of gynaecological procedures, were not available from the records. These included body weight, history of breast feeding, and exposure to diagnostic X-rays.

Example 5–The British Doctors Study

The initial mail questionnaire was intentionally kept short and simple to encourage a high proportion of replies. The doctors were asked to classify themselves into one of three groups: (i) whether they were, at that time, smoking; (ii) whether they had smoked but had given it up; (iii) whether they had never smoked regularly (i.e. had never smoked as much as one cigarette a day, or its equivalent in pipe tobacco, for as long as 1 year). Present smokers and ex-smokers were asked additional questions. The former were asked the age at which they had started smoking, the amount of tobacco that they were currently smoking, and the method by which it was consumed. The ex-smokers were asked similar questions, but relating to the time just before they had given up smoking.

> In a covering letter, the doctors were invited to give any information on their smoking habits or history that might be of interest, but, apart from that, no information was sought on previous changes in habit (other than the amount smoked prior to last giving up, if smoking had been abandoned). The decision to restrict question on amount smoked to current smoking habits was based mainly on the results of [an] earlier case–control study ... [which showed] that the classification of smokers according to the amount that they had most recently smoked gave almost as sharp a differentiation between the groups of patients with and without lung cancer as the use of smoking histories over many years—theoretically more relevant statistics, but clearly based on less accurate data. (Breslow and Day 1987, Appendix IA)

Example 6—The Framingham Heart Study

On the basis of an initial examination and detailed interview, the sample was characterized according to a variety of 'risk factors': blood cholesterol, blood pressure, cigarette smoking status, body mass index, and the presence of a variety of other diseases and conditions. Careful attention was given to standardization of the examination procedures and the structure of the interview.

On the basis of a medical history and examination, an electrocardiogram, and other medical tests, it was found that 82 individuals in the base cohort of 5209 had a cardiovascular event before the baseline examination. Thus the cohort of individuals 'at risk' for the key cardiovascular endpoint of coronary heart disease numbered 5127.

> To establish the basis for follow-up, each of the subjects was advised at the initial interview that it was intended to re-examine

him [or her] at two intervals, and that he [or she] would be approached directly at the appropriate time. The names of a relative, a friend, and the family physician were all recorded so that the subject would be traced in case he [or she] moved during the interval. An abstract of the initial examination was sent to the family physician and the subject was advised by letter as to whether the physician should be consulted or not. The objective of this procedure was to provide some tangible benefit to the subject other than the knowledge of his [or her] contribution to medical science. At the same time, care was taken not to become involved in the medical management of the subjects and to avoid interfering in any way with the relationship between the subject and his [or her] physician. This helped to maintain rapport, not only with the subjects themselves, but with the medical community as well. (Dawber *et al.* 1963)

Follow-up

Objectives

There are multiple objectives to be achieved in follow-up:

- uniform and complete follow-up of all cohort groups
- complete ascertainment of outcome events
- standardized diagnosis of outcome events.

One of the key criteria by which the quality of a longitudinal incidence study can be judged is the extent to which the investigator achieves complete ascertainment of outcome events in all exposure classes. Although a variety of methods are available for follow-up, it is desirable that the follow-up methods be independent of the method used to classify the exposure category in order to ensure uniform ascertainment across all subgroups. Methods of follow-up include correspondence with the subject and other informants, periodic re-examination of the subjects, and indirect surveillance of hospital records and death certificates. (Some countries such as the United Kingdom, the United States, and some Scandinavian countries maintain central death registers which facilitate efficient and complete mortality follow-up.) The duration of follow-up will be governed primarily by the natural history of the disease and the length of the incubation period between exposure and the onset of illness. It is important that the criteria for diagnosis of endpoints be standardized early in the follow-up period. Although criteria for the endpoints may change in the clinical community during the study, it is important that some criteria remain stable over time so that the incidence of cases occurring early in the period of follow-up can be compared with similar cases occurring later on in the observational period. Attention should be paid to criteria to verify the absence as well as the presence of the study endpoints (i.e. to minimize both false-positive and false-negative diagnoses).

Unequal loss of follow-up across different exposure categories presents serious problems in the analysis, and every method possible should be used to ensure uniform surveillance of each group. Because of the possibility of ascertainment bias resulting from knowledge of the exposure class, it is often desirable to have objective endpoint criteria which can be measured by 'blinded' observers. Information used in these criteria should be sought with equal diligence in all exposure classes. This is particularly important when the exposure class is defined by a variable that may lead to different degrees of medical observation, particularly medical examinations that are not under the direct control of the study investigators. For example, if in a study of cardiovascular diseases there is a tendency for participants with high cholesterol levels to receive more frequent electrocardiograms or other examinations by cardiologists, there may be a tendency to diagnose more cardiovascular events, particularly milder events, in this group than in the group with low cholesterol levels. Repeat examination of the subjects, besides providing standardized information on the illnesses under investigation, can often yield additional information about covariates that may be of importance and also allows studies of longitudinal changes in the exposure status.

Example 7—Artificial menopause and breast cancer

All patients in the study were followed from their index admission to 1 December 1961 so that the potential period of observation ranged from 21 to 42 years. The follow-up information was obtained from three sources, of which the first was the hospital records. All information relating to a given patient from any and all admissions to either hospital in the study was located and the data for each patient were then combined into a single record. The second source was the death certificates registered at the Massachusetts Division of Vital Statistics from 1 January 1920 to 31 December 1961. Alphabetical listings of the names of the study patients were compared with those in the index of vital records. Whenever a possible match was obtained, the death certificate was located and the information on the certificate and the identifying data obtained from the hospital chart were compared according to a prescribed set of criteria designed to minimize false matches. Therefore there may have been increased risk of discarding acceptable matches owing to some discrepancies in the available identifying information. All conditions mentioned on the death certificates were coded according to a uniform system. In addition, the underlying cause of death was coded according to the revision of the International Classification of Diseases in use at the State Division of Vital Statistics at the time of the patient's death. Thus direct comparison could be made with published mortality statistics. The third source of follow-up information was the Massachusetts Tumor Registry, a unit of the Bureau of Chronic Disease Control of the Massachusetts Department of Public Health. Since 1927 this registry had recorded all patients diagnosed with, or treated for, malignancies at State or State-aided cancer clinics. Possible matches were obtained according to rules similar to the criteria for death certificate matching. With regard to mortality follow-up, the assumption was made that all patients dying during the study period should be registered at the Division of Vital Statistics. If no death certificate was located, one of three situations may have occurred: (i) the patient was still alive; (ii) before death she had emigrated from the State and was not a resident of Massachusetts at the time of death; (iii) she had died, but no record could be located because of reporting or matching errors (mis-spellings, changes of name, failure to file a death certificate, etc.). From the three sources of information the status of 19 per cent of the women was known as of January 1962. It was noted that those receiving pelvic radiation had slightly more complete follow-up to death than those surgically treated (20 versus 18.9 per cent). This difference was statistically significant but there was no significant difference in completeness of follow-up among the surgically treated groups. The relative success of the follow-up procedure was estimated by comparing the percentages of those in the cohorts known to have died before 1962 with those expected on the basis of published mortality rates and estimated migration rates. It was estimated that the observed deaths would comprise 72.8 per cent of the expected number after allowance for migration.

With the advent of automated data files in hospitals and the creation of national automated databases, including central death registries, follow-up of cohorts such as these should become easier and more complete. Although, as in this study, only a small proportion of the original cohort may be known to have died, if one is confident that those known are nearly all of those who had died and there is no bias for better ascertainment of deaths in one group compared with the other, the results should be valid for mortality endpoints. The British Doctors Study (Example 8) is an illustration of the use of multiple questionnaires, linkage to other files (physician registries), and other forms of contact to ensure that complete follow-up has been attained. It should be noted that the artificial menopause study, using historical records, took less than 3 years to complete, whereas the next two examples of prospective studies took several decades to achieve similar follow-up.

Example 8—The British Doctors Study

The following quotations are from Breslow and Day (1987, Appendix IA).

> During the study, further questionnaires were sent out on three separate occasions to men and on two occasions to women. The purpose was partly to obtain detailed information on smoking habits, in particular giving up smoking, and also to ask additional questions, the relevance of which had emerged during the period of follow-up. Degree of inhalation was asked in these questionnaires, and the use of filter-tipped or plain cigarettes asked in the last questionnaire.
>
> Information about the death of doctors was obtained at first directly from the Registrars-General of the United Kingdom, who provided particulars of every death as referring to a medical practitioner. Later, lists of deaths were obtained from the General Medical Council, and these were complemented by reference to the records of the British Medical Association and other sources at home and abroad. Some deaths came to light in response to the questionnaires. Others were discovered in the course of following up doctors who had not replied to or who had not been sent subsequent questionnaires. Of the 34 440 men studies, 10 072 were known to have died before 1 November 1971, 24 265 were known to have been alive at that date, and 103 (0.3 per cent) were not yet traced.
>
> Many of the 103 untraced doctors were not British, and 67 (65 per cent) were known to have gone abroad. It was felt unlikely that more than about a dozen deaths relevant to the study could have been missed.
>
> Information on the underlying cause of death in the 10 072 doctors known to have died before 1 November 1971 was obtained for the vast majority from the official death certificates. Except for deaths for which lung cancer was mentioned, the certified cause was accepted and (unless otherwise stated) the deaths classified according to the underlying cause. (In only four cases was no evidence of the cause obtainable.) The underlying causes were classified according to the seventh revision of the International Classification of Disease . . . except that a separate category of 'pulmonary heart disease' was created.
>
> Cancer of the lung, including trachea or pleura, was given as the underlying cause of 467 deaths and as a contributory cause in a further 20. For each of the 487 deaths, confirmation of the diagnosis was sought from the doctor who had certified the death and, when necessary, from the consultant to whom the patient had been referred. Information about the nature of the evidence was thus obtained in all but two cases. Doubtful reports were interpreted by an outside consultant, with no knowledge of the patient's smoking history. As a result, carcinoma of the lung was accepted as the underlying cause of 441 deaths and as a contributory cause of 17.

Example 9—The Framingham Heart Study

The key method of follow-up in the Framingham Heart Study was through repeated medical examinations on a 2-year cycle. The greatest loss due to drop-out occurred between the first and second examinations, and those who came in most reluctantly for the initial examination (i.e. towards the end of the recruitment period) seemed to have the highest drop-out rate during the next 30 years. During the first 14 years of follow-up, more than 85 per cent of the participants who were still alive at any examination cycle came in for their examinations. During the subsequent 12 years the examination rates fell to about 80 per cent of the surviving cohort. The chief reasons for non-examination were believed to be the increasing numbers of people who were physically incapacitated or had migrated from the Framingham area.

Indirect follow-up through secondary sources of information was also pursued. The Framingham Union Hospital, the major source of hospital care for the Framingham community, identified each of the Framingham Heart Study participants and notified the study staff of admissions of participants to the hospital. This is particularly important for allowing standardized examination of stroke cases while symptoms of the disease are still present. Mortality follow-up was maintained through regular perusal of vital records at the Town Registrar and following up of obituary notices in newspapers. Mortality follow-up after 30 years was virtually complete with the vital status of less than 2 per cent of the cohort being unknown.

The criteria for diagnosis of cardiovascular and other endpoints investigated in the Framingham Heart Study have been precisely

Table 1 Notation for cohort analysis

$l_j = t_j - t_{j-1}$	Length of *j*th interval, $j = 1, \ldots, J$
N_j	Number of subjects being followed at time t_j
D_j	Number of new disease cases diagnosed in the *j*th interval
T_j	Total observation time for all subjects during the *j*th interval
$D_+ = \Sigma D_j$	Total number of cases
$T_+ = \Sigma T_j$	Total observation time

Table 2 Measures of incidence and risk

Eqn (1)	$I = D_+/T_+$	Average incidence rate over the entire study period
Eqn (2)	$I_j = D_j/T_j$	Average incidence rate over the *j*th interval
Eqn (3)	$CI_j = \sum_{h=1}^{j} I_h l_j$	Cumulative incidence rate to time t_j
Eqn (4)	$CI = CI_J$	Cumulative incidence rate over the entire study period to time t_J
Eqn (5)	$CR = 1 - \exp(-CI)$	Cumulative disease risk over the entire study period (adjusted for intercurrent mortality and loss to follow-up)
Eqn (6)	$CI(t) = \Sigma_{t_j \le t} D_j/N_j$	Cumulative incidence to time *t* (non-parametric estimate)[a]
Eqn (7)	$CR(t) = 1 - \Pi_{\{t_j \le t\}}(1 - D_j/N_j)$	Cumulative risk to time *t* (non-parametric estimate)[a]

[a]Assuming that the intervals are so fine that diagnoses are made only at times t_j.

defined, and the utility of the various sources of information in providing diagnostic information according to the study criteria has been investigated. Throughout the follow-up period the core criteria for the major cardiovascular endpoints have remained fixed and all potential cases are reviewed by a panel of trained medical reviewers.

It should be noted that the rate of disease occurrence in this cohort might have been altered by the subjects' continued participation in the biennial series of examinations. Although no direct advice or treatment was offered to the participants, they were informed through their physicians of abnormal findings such as high blood pressure. If effective preventive measures were instituted in such subjects, then rates of overt cardiovascular diseases would be lowered and would interfere with estimating the 'true' effects of the risk factors. It was felt that during the early period of the study such treatment was not widely offered in this population.

Sampling from the cohort

Substantial reductions in the cost of data collection can often be achieved with little loss of statistical power by limiting the collection of detailed exposure information to judiciously chosen subjects. Such designs are used increasingly in situations, such as studies of HIV, where biological specimens or other information sources have been collected prospectively and preserved for all participants. Conducting biological assays or otherwise processing these data sources for the entire cohort would be prohibitively expensive. Using Prentice's (1986) case–cohort design, the detailed exposure information is ascertained initially for a randomly sampled subcohort that may compromise only a small fraction of the whole. As disease cases occur in other cohort members, detailed exposure information is collected for them also. The major assumption made by this design is that the biological assays, or other detailed exposure measurements, yield the same results on material stored for the cases as they would have yielded had those cases been selected initially as part of the subcohort. An alternative design, known as the nested case–control study, avoids this assumption by sampling a small number of controls for each case at the time of its occurrence and by processing the detailed exposure information for the case and matched controls in the same batch. It is described further in the sequel (see section on the Cox proportional hazards model below). Further substantial improvements in design efficiency are possible by stratifying the subcohort or control samples on the basis of information available for all cohort members.

Data analysis

Grouped data and person-years

If a cohort study has been appropriately designed according to the principles given above, the analysis of the results is relatively straightforward. The first step is to estimate the incidence of the disease of interest for the cohort as a whole and, if the study was designed to make internal comparisons, in the 'exposed' and 'non-exposed' subgroups. If the follow-up period is relatively short and there is little or no loss to follow-up due to death from other conditions, a simple estimate of risk is easily calculated as the number of new (incident) cases diagnosed during the study period divided by the total population at risk at the beginning of the period. Persons who already have the disease at the outset of the study (prevalent cases) are eliminated from the population at risk. For studies of longer duration, however, the risk of disease may change over the course of the study and there may be appreciable losses from the population at risk due to death from other causes, loss from follow-up, or the occurrence of the illness of interest itself. Then it is advantageous to divide the study period into a number of intervals (Fig. 1) and to estimate the incidence rate of disease as outlined in Tables 1 and 2.

Disease risk refers to the probability of developing the disease during the study period (or some subinterval). As a probability it is a dimensionless quantity that must range in value between zero and unity. The incidence rate, however, is a measure of the frequency of the occurrence of disease per unit time relative to the size of the population at risk. Crude incidence is the ratio of the disease risk during a time interval to the length of the interval. Instantaneous incidence, also known as the hazard rate of force or morbidity, measures the rate of diagnosis of new cases per unit time relative to the

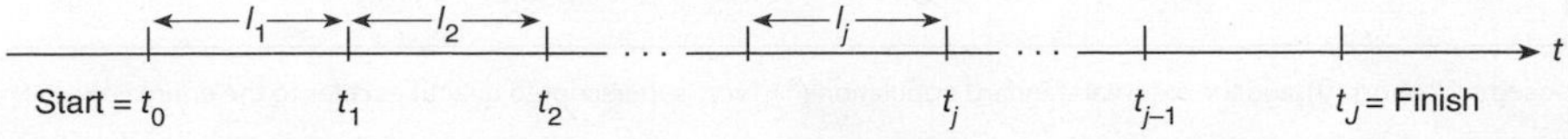

Fig. 1 Division of the study period into *J* time intervals.

size of the disease-free population at risk at time t. The units for incidence rates are t_1 and they have no upper limit quantitatively. Owing to limitations of the available data, it is not possible to estimate precisely the incidence rate at each time t. Instead, estimates are made of the average rates over the study period or over each subinterval by dividing the number of new cases diagnosed in the interval by the total person-years of observation time accumulated during the interval (Table 2, eqns (1) and (2)). Accurate estimation of the person-years denominators requires, for each individual in the study, knowledge of the exact duration of follow-up from the start of the study until diagnosis of the disease of interest, death from a competing cause, or loss from further observation. The contributions from each individual at risk during the jth interval are summed to yield the totals T_j shown in Table 1. If such data are not available, various methods can be used to approximate the person-years of observation. For example, the estimated size of the population at the midpoint of the interval can be multiplied by the interval length.

Another useful measure of disease occurrence, known as the cumulative incidence rate, is obtained by summing the products of incidence rate and interval length over a series of intervals (Table 2, eqns (3) and (4)). The cumulative incidence rate over a specified interval, which is a dimensionless quantity with no upper limit, is related via the exponential function to the disease risk over the interval (eqn (5)). If the disease is rare or the study period is short (so that the cumulative risk is no more than 5 per cent), cumulative incidence and risk are nearly equal. Both can be estimated non-parametrically as a function of time t by choosing the intervals to be so fine that the interval endpoints occur exactly at the times of disease diagnosis (eqns (6) and (7)). Plots of cumulative incidence over time provide a powerful graphic tool for examining the evolution of disease risk in the exposed and non-exposed subgroups. As an example, Fig. 2 shows that breast cancer incidence in a cohort of women treated with radiation for postpartum mastitis paralleled the incidence in the control population until some 16 to 20 years after treatment, but then increased to substantially higher levels.

Although the preceding definitions used time on study as the basic time-scale for estimation of instantaneous incidence, other choices may be more appropriate in some circumstances. The possibilities include age, calendar time, and, for studies where exposure starts

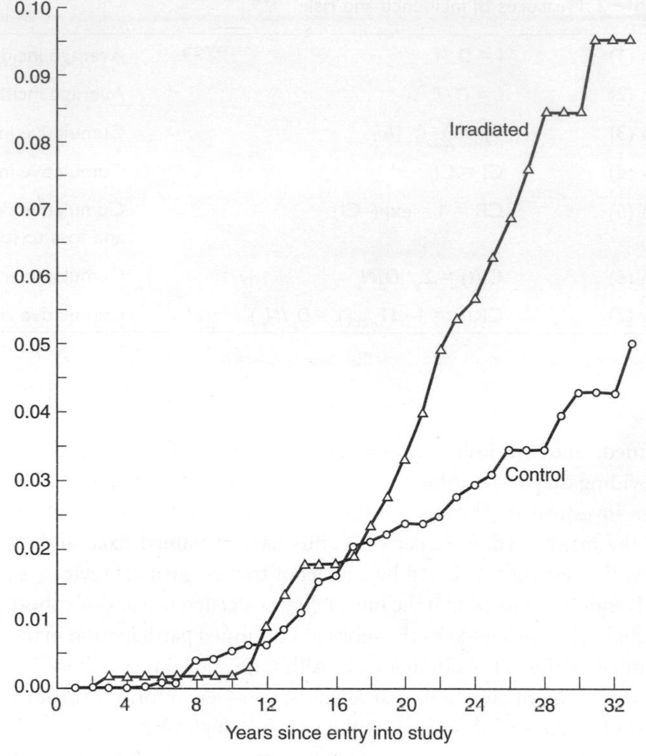

Fig. 2 Cumulative breast cancer morbidity curves for women treated with X-rays for postpartum mastitis (△) and a control group (○), adjusted to the age distribution of the control group. (Source: Shore *et al.* 1977.)

before entry into the study, time since initial exposure. With these other time-scales the population at risk changes due not only to the loss from observation of subjects who die or develop the disease of interest, but also to the entry into the cohort of other subjects depending, for example, on their age or the calendar year at the time that they join the study. All the definitions and formulae continue to apply with these alternative time-scales. More advanced statistical analyses often consider several time-scales simultaneously, using a multidimensional classification of incident cases and person-years

Table 3 Measures of association

Eqn (8)	$SMR = D_+/\Sigma_j T_j I_j^*$	Standardized morbidity ratio
Eqn (9)	$RR_j = I_j^E/I_j^0$	Rate ratio in the jth interval
Eqn (10)	$RD_j = I_j^E - I_j^0$	Rate difference in the jth interval
Eqn (11)	$RR_{MH} = \dfrac{\sum_j D_j^E T_j^0/(T_j^E + T_j^0)}{\sum_j D_j^0 T_j^E/(T_j^E + T_j^0)}$	Mantel–Haenszel summary rate ratio
Eqn (12)	$RD = CR^E - CR^0$	Cumulative risk difference (attributable risk)
Eqn (13)	$RR = CI^E/CI^0$	Relative risk (crude)
Eqn (14)	$AF = \dfrac{CI - CI_0}{CI} = \dfrac{P^E(RR - 1)}{P^E(RR - 1) + 1}$	Aetiological fraction

The superscripts refer to the exposed subcohort (E), the non-exposed subcohort (0), and the external standard population (*). Non-superscripted quantities refer to the entire cohort. P^E denotes the proportion of the population that is exposed.

Table 4 Lung cancer mortality by cumulative radiation exposure among Canadian fluorspar miners

Cumulative WLM	No. of person-years at risk	No. of lung cancer deaths		SMR (O/E ratio)
		Observed	Expected	
0	13 567.8	7	7.00	1.00
1–9	3045.5	3	2.02	1.49
10–239	9510.5	13	7.22	1.80
240–599	5105.5	10	3.87	2.58
600–1979	7107.0	6	1.71	3.51
1980–2039	2415.5	25	1.54	16.23
2040	2889.0	40	1.07	37.38

E, expected; O, observed; SMR, standardized mortality ratio; WLM, working level months of radon daughter exposure.
Data from Committee on the Biological Effects of Ionizing Radiations (1988).

denominators according to age, calendar year, time on study, and other fixed and time-varying factors.

Cohort studies also facilitate the estimation of various measures of association between the exposure of interest and the occurrence of disease. The standardized morbidity ratio (**SMR**) is frequently used in occupational cohort studies to estimate the ratio of cohort rates to standard rates obtained from national health statistics registers or other standard sources. As shown in eqn (8) (Table 3), the SMR is simply the ratio of the number of cases of disease observed to the number of cases expected from the standard rates as applied to the age/time-specific person-years of observation. Dose–response trends may be evident from SMRs that are estimated separately for subcohorts defined by levels of cumulative exposure (Table 4). However, doubts about the comparability of the cohort and the standard population, coupled with the fact that the ratio of SMRs for two or more subcohorts may not adequately summarize the ratios of age/time-specific rates, have led many investigators to discard the SMR in favour of measures of association that do not depend on external rates. The Mantel–Haenszel rate ratio (Table 3, eqn (11)) summarizes the ratios of the age/time-specific rates for the exposed versus the non-exposed members of the cohort. It is closely related to the Mantel–Haenszel relative risk measure that is widely used to summarize tables of exposure/disease odds ratios in case–control studies (see Chapter 6.5). This is the preferred measure of association when, as is often the case, the rate ratios are relatively constant over time but the rate differences are not. The cumulative risk difference (Table 3, eqn (12)), which is also known as the attributable risk or excess risk, provides an absolute measure of the effect of exposure, which is useful for public health workers.

Data from cohort studies can also be used to measure the potential impact of the removal of a suspected aetiological factor. This is measured either in terms of the estimated effect of removal on disease incidence or on the cumulative risk over the study period. The most direct measure of potential impact is known as the aetiological fraction, defined here using risk (Table 3, eqn (13)) rather than incidence. It represents the proportion of all new cases of disease that can be considered to be due to the exposure and therefore that are potentially preventable if the exposure were to be completely removed. Equation (14) shows how it may be represented using two parameters: the proportion P^{E} of the total population with the exposure, and the risk ratio RR^{E}. Although useful for studies of short duration involving a single risk factor, serious conceptual difficulties arise when attempts are made to extend the definition of aetiological fraction for use with multiple interacting risk factors or in situations where a long study period is needed in order to ascertain the temporal aspects of the exposure–disease association.

Example 10—Artificial menopause and breast cancer

Some of the results of this study are shown in Table 5. For the four 'exposure' categories of women who were less than 40 years old at the time of admission into the cohort, 37 cases of breast cancer were discovered to have occurred during the follow-up period. Several difficulties in applying the usual estimates of incidence and risk are readily apparent.

Table 5 Breast cancer in patients with and without artificial menopause

Exposure group	No. in group (N_0)	No. of cases (D_+)	Crude rate (D_+/N_0)	Estimated cumulative risk	Relative risk (RR)
Cholecystectomy	400	6	0.0150	0.0198	1.00
Unilateral oophorectomy	1635	20	0.0122	0.0210	1.06
Hysterectomy and bilateral oophorectomy	1278	6	0.0047	0.0054	0.27
Radiation	468	5	0.0107	0.0106	0.54

1. Because of migration and incompleteness of follow-up, the observed cases are known to be an undercount.
2. The time of onset for each malignancy was not usually known (those ascertained from death certificates did not usually state age at onset).
3. The duration of follow-up for most of the women was not precisely known.

However, by making several assumptions it is possible to obtain some reasonable estimates of the association of breast cancer occurrence with the extent of pelvic surgery. The basic assumption is that whatever inadequacies there were in the follow-up procedures, they occurred uniformly in each of the exposure groups (i.e. the women with natural menopause were no more likely to have migrated than those with surgical menopause), and therefore any cases of breast cancer were equally likely to be ascertained in each group. Another problem is that the frequency with which the various procedures were performed varied considerably during the 21 years of potential admission to the study (for example, pelvic irradiation was more frequent in the 1920s than later). Thus the women in the radiation group tended to have longer potential periods of follow-up than those in the surgical groups. This was handled by examining the specific dates of entry into the study for each woman.

The fourth column of Table 5 gives an estimate of the crude risk of developing breast cancer. For the reasons given above, this is a very poor estimate. The next column gives an estimate of the cumulative incidence rate of breast cancer over the average 30-year follow-up period, which was obtained by estimating the person-years contribution of each woman. Because of the inadequacies in follow-up mentioned above, the estimates shown are undoubtedly lower than the true rates. However, provided that the under-ascertainment was approximately equal in the different exposure groups, there should be less bias in the estimates of relative risk shown in the last column. The cholecystectomy group was considered to be the 'unexposed' or control group. Using eqn (13), the relative risk for the women with unilateral oophorectomy is 1.06, which is not statistically different from the standard group. The relative risk for the women with hysterectomy and bilateral oophorectomy is 0.27, which is significantly less than the standard group. The women receiving irradiation also had a low relative risk for developing breast cancer (0.54), but because this group is small the risk is not statistically significant.

Because of the problems in estimation of the cumulative incidence rates in this study, no attempt was made to obtain estimates of the aetiological fraction.

Example 11—Coronary heart disease and smoking among British doctors

Table 6 shows the numbers of deaths from coronary heart disease and corresponding person-years denominators for smokers and non-smokers observed during the first 10 years of follow-up of the British Doctors Study. The coronary heart disease rates increase markedly with age, but less so for smokers than for non-smokers. Since the rate ratios for smokers versus non-smokers decline sharply with age, whereas the rate differences generally increase, this is an example where neither the Mantel–Haenszel rate ratio nor the cumulative rate difference is very useful in summarizing the age-specific quantities. Either the age-specific rates themselves, or variations in the rate ratios or differences with age, are needed to describe the results of the study adequately. Nevertheless, using the age-specific rates, it can readily be calculated that the cumulative mortality rate in the 35 to 74 years age group is 17.0 per cent for non-smokers and 24.9 per cent for smokers. The corresponding cumulative risks are

$CR^E = 1 - \exp(-0.170) = 15.6$ per cent

and

$CR^0 = 1 - \exp(-0.249) = 22.0$ per cent

for a risk ratio $RR^E = 1.41$ and an attributable risk RD = 6.4 per cent. Assuming that $P^E = 83$ per cent of British doctors were smokers at the beginning of the study period, the aetiological fraction is

$$AF = \frac{0.83 \times 0.41}{(0.83 \times 0.41) + 1} = 25 \text{ per cent.}$$

However, this number should be interpreted cautiously for the reasons mentioned above. The aetiological fraction is much smaller when the coronary heart disease deaths occurring at ages 75 to 84 years are also taken into account. The Mantel–Haenszel rate ratio for the

Table 6 Deaths from coronary heart disease (CHD) among British male doctors

Age group j (years)	**No. of person-years (1000s)**		**No. of CHD deaths**		**CHD rates**[a]		**Rate ratio RR_j**	**Rate difference**[a] **RD_j**
	Non-smokers T_j^0	**Smokers T_j^E**	**Non-smokers D_j^0**	**Smokers D_j^E**	**Non-smokers I_j^0**	**Smokers I_j^E**		
35–44	18.790	52.407	2	32	0.11	0.61	5.73	0.50
45–54	10.673	43.248	12	104	1.12	2.40	2.14	1.28
55–64	5.710	28.612	28	206	4.90	7.20	1.47	2.30
65–74	2.585	12.663	28	186	10.83	14.69	1.36	3.86
75–84	1.462	5.317	31	102	21.20	19.18	0.90	– 2.02
Total	39.220	142.247	101	630	2.58	4.43[b]	1.72	1.85

[a]Per 1000 person-years

[b]Average rates I^0 and I^E over entire age range.

Data from Doll and Hill (1966), as quoted by Breslow and Day (1987).

entire 50-year age span is $RR_{MH} = 1.42$, the attributable risk RD is 3.9 per cent, and the aetiological fraction AF is 9 per cent.

Example 12—The Framingham Heart Study

During the first three decades of its existence, the Framingham Heart Study generated more than 300 publications. Many involved quite sophisticated methodological applications, which are beyond the scope of this chapter.

An example of the relation between the occurrence of coronary heart disease and serum cholesterol based on 6 years of follow-up is shown in Table 7. Data are shown for men who were aged between 40 and 59 years and were free from coronary heart disease at entry. There were 1333 men with measured cholesterol levels and follow-up was complete for 6 years for nearly all of them. These men were classified into tertiles on the basis of their initial serum cholesterol levels as shown in the first column of the table. Person-years of observation were estimated for each tertile based on the assumption that each of the men who developed coronary heart disease was followed on average for half the study period, whereas the other men were followed for the entire 6 years. (It would be better to count those who developed coronary heart disease plus those who died from other causes as contributing 3 years each.) Thus, for example, the average annual incidence for the entire cohort was estimated from eqn (1) as

$$I = \frac{96}{(1333 - 48) \times 6} = 0.0125.$$

The cumulative risks determined from eqn (5) are virtually identical in this instance to the crude risks (number of cases divided by number of persons at risk at the start of the period). The relative risks associated with high cholesterol levels are shown in the next column, where the men with cholesterol levels lower than 210 mg/100 ml are taken as the standard or unexposed group. Men with cholesterol levels between 210 and 244 mg/100 ml have 1.81 times the risk of developing coronary heart disease compared with men with lower cholesterol levels, and men with cholesterol levels above 244 mg/100 ml have risks 3.43 times greater. The attributable risks RD associated with higher cholesterol levels are shown in the last column.

If men could be prevented from having cholesterol levels above 244 mg/100 ml, the potential impact upon the incidence of coronary heart disease can be estimated from the aetiological fraction (eqn (14)). The combined group of men with cholesterol levels below 245 mg/100 ml is considered to be the unexposed groups with a (crude) risk of

$$CR^0 = \frac{16 + 29}{454 + 455} = 0.0495.$$

Then the aetiological factor is

$$AF = \frac{0.0720 - 0.0495}{0.0720} = 0.31,$$

i.e. the risk of coronary heart disease among men could potentially be lowered by 31 per cent if none of them had cholesterol levels over 245 mg/100 ml. A similar calculation showed that if all the men had cholesterol levels below 210 mg/100 ml, the aetiological fraction would be 51 per cent, i.e. half of the cases of coronary heart disease could potentially be prevented. This illustrates the strong dependence of the aetiological fraction on the rather arbitrary specification of the baseline level for a continuous-valued risk factor. Furthermore, since whatever intervention was undertaken to reduce the serum cholesterol levels might have unpredictable effects on the coronary heart disease rates, it is clear that 'potential impact' as used here must be interpreted in terms of statistical association rather than causation.

The Cox proportional hazards model

These examples involve estimation of separate relative risks for each level of a categorical variable relative to a baseline level (RR = 1): cumulative radiation exposure in Example 10, age in Example 11, and serum cholesterol in Example 12. This approach works well when there are sufficient disease cases at each level of exposure to provide stable estimates. For multiple exposures, or for purposes of low-dose extrapolation, it is desirable to model the relative risk as a mathematical function of one or more quantitative exposure variables. In radiation epidemiology, for example, it is common to model the relative risk as a linear function of the radiation dose x:

$$RR(x) = 1 + ax.$$

When there are several exposure variables $x_1, x_2, \ldots$, choice of the log-linear relative risk function implies that the individual exposures have relative risks that multiply:

$$\log RR\,(x_1, x_2, \ldots) = a_1x_1 + a_2x_2 + \ldots.$$

If, for example, exposure to one risk factor doubles the baseline risk while exposure to another triples it, the log-linear model assumes that the joint exposure increases the risk sixfold. Some such modelling assumptions, which must be carefully checked against the data, are needed to make sense of highly multivariate exposure information.

Table 7 Six-year incidence of coronary heart disease according to initial serum cholesterol in men aged 40–59 years

Serum cholesterol (mg/100 ml)	No. in group	No. of cases	Average annual incidence I	Cumulative risk CR	Relative risk RR	Attributable risk RD
<210	455	16	0.0060	0.0352	1.00	0.000
210–244	455	29	0.0107	0.0637	1.81	0.0285
245	423	51	0.0214	0.1207	3.43	0.0855
Total	1333	96	0.0125	0.0720		

Cox (1972) provided a mathematical foundation for relative risk function estimation that revolutionized the statistical approaches to analysis follow-up data collected in both clinical and epidemiological studies. His proportional hazards model assumes that the disease incidence rate at time t for a subpopulation with exposure(s) x is the product of a baseline ($x = 0$) incidence rate $I_0(t)$ multiplied by a parametric relative risk function such as linear or log-linear. The cumulative baseline incidence rate is estimated non-parametrically by a formula that generalizes eqn (6). The parameters (regression coefficients) a in the relative risk function are estimated by comparing the values of the exposure variables for the disease case that occurs at a given time t_j with those of subjects in the risk set of cohort members who are being followed but have not yet developed disease just prior to t_j. The model derives its name from the fact that, in its standard formulation, disease incidence rates for subjects with different exposures are assumed to be in constant proportion (ratio) as a function of time. Important generalizations allow both the exposures and the relative risks associated with them to vary with time. The model led to the realization that costs could be greatly reduced by limiting collection of expensive data items to the disease cases and to a small number of disease-free controls sampled randomly from each of the risk sets. This design, known as the nested case–control study, permits estimation of both the relative risk function and the baseline cumulative incidence rate.

Types of bias and their resolution

In this section the different types of bias that may occur in cohort studies are presented and discussed. Because all the different types of bias are not necessarily present in the same study, we draw examples from additional studies as well as from two of the three studies presented above.

Factors related to the selection of the study population, response rate, collection of information, methodologies used, and analytical strategies employed often introduce biases which, if not anticipated, can lead to incorrect conclusions concerning a possible relationship between an exposure (independent variable) and a disease (outcome variable). Such biases are inherent in all types of epidemiological studies. In this section we shall confine our discussion to the types of biases that affect cohort studies.

There are five broad categories of bias that are operative in cohort studies. These are selection bias, follow-up bias, information bias, confounding bias, and *post hoc* bias. Each of these is discussed separately below. These biases can cause systematic errors, which affect the internal validity of a study. This is in contrast with random errors, which may not affect the internal validity of the study but will reduce the probability of observing a true relationship. A true bias (i.e. a systematic error that is introduced into one group or subgroup to a greater extent than in other subgroups) often leads to the observation of a relationship that is not a true relationship or, vice versa, leads to the conclusion that there is no relationship when, in fact, there is a true relationship between the independent and outcome variables. Errors that occur with equal frequency in all subgroups usually do not affect the validity of a relationship. However, because a certain proportion of the measurements in all the subgroups will be erroneous, the probability of observing a true relationship is diminished and the true magnitude of the relationship may be underestimated.

While internal validity is paramount, it is often important to have external validity in cohort studies as well. External validity refers to the degree to which an association observed in the study populations also holds true in the general population. In order to ensure external validity, the population studies must be representative of the population to which the results of the study will be generalized. In many cohort studies, it is necessary for various reasons to study some subpopulation of the general population. This subpopulation may represent a non-random sample of the general population, such as an occupational group, a group selected from a particular health plan, and so on. If such subpopulations are used, external validity may be reduced.

Selection bias

Selection bias may occur when the group actually studied does not reflect the same distribution of factors (such as age, smoking, race, etc.) as occurs in the general population. This may be because some of the members of the cohort selected originally refuse to participate or, in a non-current cohort study, because records on some individuals are missing or incomplete. Therefore the response rates among the various subgroups invited to participate in the study differ. In some studies particular subgroups may be used for convenience and may not be representative of the general population for other reasons.

Example 13—Effects of volunteering

An example of selective non-response to recruitment was observed and documented in the Framingham studies cited above. It was found that individuals who agreed to participate in these cohort studies were healthier than individuals who did not agree to participate. While this would not affect the internal validity of the study, since the groups to be followed were characterized on the basis of factors present at baseline, it would be likely to reduce the incidence of the disease of interest, particularly in the first few years of the study. Thus the external validity would be diminished, but the internal validity should not be affected for those independent variables defined at baseline. However, because the incidence of disease might be lower in this healthier group that is being followed up, the probability of finding significant relationships would be somewhat diminished. In occupational cohort studies, this type of selection bias has been termed 'the healthy worker effect'.

Example 14—Spectrum of independent variables in study groups

A second problem with selection non-response is associated with the extent to which the population that agrees to participate in the study actually represents the true spectrum of the independent variable.

Early studies of the relationship of dietary cholesterol and saturated fat intake to coronary heart disease in the United States gave inconclusive results. This may have been due, in part, to the fact that very few Americans have dietary cholesterol and saturated fat intakes in the lower ranges, whereas residents of less affluent countries have a higher proportion of individuals with these low levels of intake. If there exists a threshold level of the independent variable necessary to produce disease and the respondents include only individuals with levels of the independent variable that are above the threshold level, then no relationship will be seen between the variable and the disease under study. Thus some of the comparisons of the incidence of coronary heart disease among Americans with higher levels of cholesterol and fat in the diet may not have shown a relationship because the threshold level of dietary fats was below the levels consumed in the study population. Even in situations where there is no threshold level, inclusion of individuals at only one end of the spectrum of the independent variable will reduce the likelihood that a dose–response relationship will be observed. Thus non-response or non-inclusion of participants in the cohort who represent one or the other extreme of the independent variable may affect the internal validity of the study and lead to a false observation that there is no relationship.

Example 15—Presence of incipient disease

Another problem of selection bias occurs when individuals who have incipient disease are included in the cohort. Individuals with the disease of interest should be excluded from the study population at the time of recruitment. However, with many chronic diseases that have a long induction period, such as cancer and heart disease, it is difficult to identify individuals with incipient disease. Their inclusion in the study population may lead to an observation of associations that are, in fact, a result of the disease process rather than a risk factor for the disease.

An association between low cholesterol and risk of cancer has been observed in several cohort studies. The induction period for cancer is probably one or more decades. Individuals who develop cancer in a follow-up period of less than the induction period probably had incipient disease at the time of the formation of the cohort. Thus a low cholesterol level in these individuals may have been a result of the cancer process rather than a risk factor for it.

Example 16—Distribution of covariates

A final example of selection bias occurs when the distribution of covariates that may be related to disease incidence is not equally represented in the study cohorts.

Smoking is related to a number of diseases. In some, it is the probable major cause whereas in others, such as coronary heart disease, it represents only one of several risk factors that increase the probability of developing disease. Thus, if the non-respondents include a higher proportion of smokers than non-smokers, the total incidence of coronary heart disease in the study cohort would be lower than if smokers were appropriately represented in the cohort. However, the effect would be not only to make the observed incidence of coronary heart disease lower in the study population than in the general population, but also to lead to a false estimate of the proportion of coronary heart disease that is associated with smoking (the aetiological fraction). Specifically, the incidence of coronary heart disease among the smokers would be correct, but the proportion of the total numbers of cases that were associated with smoking would be smaller than actually exists because the proportion of smokers in the study population would be lower than in the general population. Thus any estimates of the aetiological fraction of coronary heart disease due to smoking would be too low.

Follow-up bias

One of the major problems in cohort studies is to accomplish the successful follow-up of all members of the cohort. If the loss to follow-up occurs equally in the exposed and unexposed groups, the internal validity should not be affected. Of course, this assumes that the rate of disease occurrence is the same among those lost to follow-up as among those not lost to follow-up within each group. However, if the rate of disease is different among those lost to follow-up, then the internal validity of the study may be affected (i.e. the relationship between exposure and outcome may be changed).

Example 17—Bias resulting from differential incidence in those lost to follow-up

If the rate of lung cancer is higher in those smokers who are lost to follow-up than in those who remain in the study, the observed incidence of lung cancer in those smokers who remain in the study will be lower than the actual incidence of lung cancer in the entire cohort of smokers. The effect will be to observe a lower association between lung cancer and smoking than actually exists (provided that the incidence of lung cancer is the same in non-smokers who were and were not followed). If the lung cancer incidence rate is lower in smokers who are not followed up than in those who are, the reverse effect would occur (i.e. the observed association would be greater than the true association).

Usually the incidence of disease is not known among those lost to follow-up, making it difficult to look for this type of bias. If possible, the occurrence and cause of death should be sought in those who are lost to follow-up. This is easier in the United States now that there is a National Death Registry. If the death rate is similar between those lost and not lost to follow-up within each group, the occurrence of a different incidence of disease in the two groups is less likely.

Another strategy is to compare the known characteristics at baseline of those lost and not lost to follow-up. The more similar the two groups are, the less likely it is that a different incidence of disease occurred in them.

Neither of these strategies guarantees that the incidence was the same in both those followed and those not followed. Therefore the best strategy is to reduce the number lost to follow-up to the lowest level possible.

Example 18–Bias resulting from loss to follow-up of individuals under observation for the independent variable

Another possible source of bias may be observed in studies in which the independent variable is being documented concurrently with the development of the outcome variable, presenting the opportunity for misclassification resulting from loss to follow-up.

In evaluating the relationship between a decline in lung function test results and concurrent levels of exposure to photochemical oxidants at place of residence, a problem arises in considering how to evaluate individuals who have moved from the study area to other areas (Detels *et al.* 1991). In some instances they will have moved to areas with lower levels of exposure to photochemical oxidants and in other instances to areas with higher levels. It is not feasible to maintain constant monitoring for levels of photochemical oxidants in all the areas to which these individuals have moved. If there is indeed a relationship between levels of exposure to photochemical oxidants and decreasing lung test performance, the inclusion in analyses of individuals who have moved to a cleaner area, as if they had remained in the area of high exposure, will lead to misclassification bias and thus to an underestimate of the relationship. However, if individuals who moved to a dirtier area are included, this will lead to misclassification bias with the reverse effect.

Another potential bias is introduced if the individuals who have moved are excluded from the analysis to avoid misclassification bias. Individuals who have moved out of the study area may have done so because of the high level of exposure to photochemical oxidants and their awareness of their declining respiratory ability. This would result in an observed relationship in those not moving that is lower than the true relationship.

While this type of bias is almost impossible to prevent, there are several pieces of information that can assist the investigator in evaluating the magnitude of the bias that may be introduced. Firstly, the investigator may compare lung function test results at baseline among those who remained and those who moved away. Any difference between those retested and those not retested would provide information about the direction, and possibly about the magnitude, of the bias that occurred.

Secondly, it is often possible to send a mail questionnaire to individuals who have moved away from the study area, which should include questions regarding reasons for moving. If it is found, for example, that many of the respondents moved because of the development of respiratory symptoms, the probability of potential bias can be recognized. In addition, the ascertainment of diagnosed respiratory impairment among those not retested would also indicate the presence of bias.

Although there is no completely satisfactory solution to this problem resulting from loss to follow-up, awareness of the potential for bias will enable the investigator to explore various methods to evaluate its effect.

Example 19—Unequal observation

Smoking is associated with a wide range of adverse health outcomes. Any one of these is more likely to result in smokers being seen by a physician, thus increasing the likelihood that the disease of interest may also be diagnosed at that time, i.e. there would be an earlier diagnosis of disease in the smoking individual than in a comparable non-smoking individual who would be less likely to come under medical scrutiny. As a result, there would be an overestimate of the association of the disease of interest with the smoking variable. This overestimate would occur when a crude relative risk analysis (eqn (13)) is used since cohort studies usually have a defined follow-up period. It would also occur when a summary rate ratio based on person-years (eqn (11)) is used since the individual would appear as a case after fewer years of follow-up than would normally occur if he or she were not brought to medical attention as a result of smoking.

Information (misclassification) bias

Information bias occurs when there is an error in the classification of individuals with respect to the outcome variable. This may result from measurement errors, imprecise measurement, and misdiagnosis for whatever reason. Information bias is also termed misclassification bias. If the misclassification occurs equally in all the subgroups of the study population, the internal validity of the study will not be affected, but the precision or probability of being able to demonstrate a true relationship is reduced and the true magnitude of the relationship is likely to be underestimated.

Example 20

If the proportion of cases under- or over-reported in a cohort study of the risk of coronary heart disease is equal among smokers and non-smokers, no change in the observed risk ratio for smoking would occur and the internal validity of the study would be unaffected. However, if the misclassification occurs to a greater extent among either smokers or non-smokers, the observed risk will be altered, thereby affecting the relative risk and incidence difference and, as a result, the internal validity of the study.

Confounding bias

Confounding occurs when other factors that are associated with both the outcome and exposure variables do not have the same distribution in the exposed and unexposed groups. Two common confounders in cohort studies are smoking and age. The risk of disease varies with age for almost all diseases. Likewise, smoking increases the risk of acquiring a wide range of diseases.

Example 21

In a cohort study to determine the risk of coronary heart disease among individuals who drink and do not drink, the prevalence of individuals who smoke is likely to be higher among those who drink than those who do not drink. If one does not take into account the prevalence of smoking in the two groups, there will be a higher incidence of coronary heart disease in the drinking group than in the non-drinking group, which is, in fact, ascribable to smoking rather than to drinking. A false association or non-association also might be observed if the age distributions were not the same in the drinking and non-drinking groups since the incidence of coronary heart disease increases with age.

Confounding bias can result in either an overestimate or an underestimate of the relative risk of an independent variable with disease. Estimates of the effect of confounding variables in a cohort study usually require primarily the use of the investigator's judgement, although the application of specific statistical procedures can help in reducing the effects of recognized confounders (see Chapter 6.10).

Post hoc bias

Another source of potential bias is the use of data from a cohort study to make observations that were not part of the original study intent. Thus interesting relationships that were not originally anticipated are often observed in cohort studies. These findings should be treated as hypotheses that are an appropriate subject for additional studies. Such fortuitous findings should not be considered to have established the validity of a relationship and in no circumstance should the same data be analysed to test hypotheses arising from that data.

Resolution of bias

There are various strategies for reducing the presence of bias in cohort studies. Selection bias can be reduced by careful selection of individuals for inclusion in the study and by making every attempt to characterize differences that may exist between respondents and non-respondents. Although consideration of characteristics that may be more frequent in non-respondents will not eliminate bias, it may permit the investigator to assess the directionality and degree of bias that may have resulted from specific selection procedures. Information bias can be reduced by using well-defined precise measurements and classification criteria for which the sensitivity and specificity have been determined. Follow-up bias can be reduced by intensive follow-up of all study participants and by establishing criteria for follow-up that will assure that all members of the cohort have an equal opportunity for being diagnosed as having the outcome variable. Comparison of the characteristics present at baseline among those lost to follow-up and those successfully followed up may provide information upon which estimates of the nature and degree of bias that may have been introduced through loss to follow-up may be based.

Confounding bias can be reduced in the analysis stage by careful stratification and/or adjustment procedures. However, fine stratification for multiple potential confounders may result in a loss of information, which reduces the likelihood of observing a significant difference. Thus careful consideration should be given to whether proposed adjustment factors are clearly related to the disease outcome. If not, it is usually better not to attempt to restrict the selection of participants or to adjust during analysis. The identification and resolution of bias is primarily a matter of epidemiological judgement. Statistical and analytic techniques designed to reduce bias should be applied only to factors that, in the judgement of the investigators, are potential sources of bias.

We have discussed the major sources of bias in a cohort study. However, this list is far from exhaustive, and additional types of bias will surely be described in the future for which investigators should be alert. More detailed discussions of the problems of cohort studies are given by Kleinbaum *et al.* (1982), Rothman (1986), Breslow and Day (1987), Hennekens and Buring (1987), and Samet and Muñoz (1998).

Summary

Cohort studies are usually the best type of studies for demonstrating the association between an exposure and a disease because it is possible to derive relative and attributable risks and often incidence measures from them. However, they are usually expensive to carry out and large cohorts are required for rare diseases. In addition, there are very significant problems associated with the selection of appropriate groups to be studied and with complete ascertainment of disease occurrence in them. Usually it is necessary to compromise the ideal, thus providing the opportunity for various types of bias to occur that can result in incorrect conclusions. The success of a cohort study often depends on the care of the investigator in recognizing and correcting for these biases.

References

Breslow, N.E. and Day, N.E. (1987). *Statistical methods in cancer research.* Vol. 2: *The design and analysis of cohort studies.* International Agency for Research on Cancer, Lyon.

Committee on the Biological Effects of Ionizing Radiations (1988). In *Health risks of radon and other internally deposited alpha-emitters*, p. 471. National Academy Press, Washington, DC.

Cox, D.R. (1972). Regression models and life tables (with discussion). *Journal of the Royal Statistical Society, Series B*, **34**, 187–220.

Dawber, T.R., Kannel, W.B., and Lyell, L.P. (1963). An approach to longitudinal studies in a community: the Framingham Study. *Annals of the New York Academy of Sciences*, **107**, 539–56.

Detels, R., Tashkin, D.P., Sayre, J.W., *et al.* (1991). The UCLA Population Studies of CORD. X: A cohort study of changes in respiratory function associated with chronic exposure to SO*x*, NO*x*, and hydrocarbons. *American Journal of Public Health*, **81**, 350–9.

Doll, R. and Peto, R. (1976). Mortality and relation to smoking: 20 years' observations on male British doctors. *British Medical Journal*, **ii**, 1525–36.

Feinleib, M. (1968). Breast cancer and artificial menopause: a cohort study. *Journal of the National Cancer Institute*, **41**, 315–29.

Hennekens, C.H. and Buring, J.E. (1987). *Epidemiology in medicine.* Little, Brown, Boston, MA.

Kannel, W.B., Dawber, T.R., Kagan, A., *et al.* (1961). Factors of risk in the development of coronary heart disease—six year follow-up experience. The Framingham Study. *Annals of Internal Medicine*, **55**, 33–50.

Kleinbaum, D.G., Kupper, L.L., and Morgenstern, H. (1982). *Epidemiologic research.* Lifetime Learning, Belmont, CA.

Prentice, R.L. (1986). A case–cohort design for epidemiologic cohort studies and disease prevention trials. *Biometrika*, **73**, 1–12.

Rothman, K. (1986). *Modern epidemiology.* Little, Brown, Boston, MA.

Rothman, K.J. and Greenland, S. (1999). *Modern epidemiology* (2nd edn). Lippincott–Raven, Philadelphia, PA.

Samet, J.M. and Muñoz, A. (ed.) (1998). Cohort studies. *Epidemiologic Reviews*, **20**, 1–136.

Shore, R.E., Hemplemann, L.H., Kowaluk, E., *et al.* (1977). Breast neoplasms in women treated with X-rays for acute postpartum mastitis. *Journal of the National Cancer Institute*, **59**, 813–22.

6.7 Methodology of intervention trials in individuals

Lawrence M. Friedman and Eleanor B. Schron

An intervention trial, or a clinical trial, has been defined in various ways and may be of several kinds. The International Conference on Harmonisation defines a clinical trial as 'any investigation in human subjects intended to discover or verify the clinical, pharmacological, and/or other pharmacodynamic effects of an investigational product (s), and/or to identify any adverse reactions to an investigational product(s), and/or to study absorption, distribution, metabolism, and excretion of an investigational product(s) with the object of ascertaining its safety and/or efficacy' (ICH 1996). This definition has the advantage of applying to all phases of a clinical trial. (This chapter will only address issues relating to the so-called phase III trial. For discussions of phase I and phase II studies, see FDA (1997).) The International Conference on Harmonisation definition has the disadvantage of not including trials of non-pharmacological or non-device interventions (that is, surgical procedures, diet, exercise). More generally, a phase III clinical trial may be defined as 'a prospective study comparing the effects and value of intervention(s) against a control in human beings' (Friedman *et al.* 1998).

Clinical trials are needed because only rarely is the precise pattern or outcome of a disease or condition known. It is not yet possible to identify all of the genetic and environmental factors that lead to disease progression, recovery, and relapse. Also rare is the treatment that is so overwhelmingly successful that even with a vague understanding of the course of the disease, it is possible to say that the treatment is obviously beneficial and has few major adverse effects. More often, the treatment, while useful, is less than perfect. Therefore, in order to determine the true balance of potential benefit and harm from a new treatment or intervention, it is necessary to compare people who have received the treatment with those who have not. Ideally, this comparison will be made in an unbiased objective manner so that, at the end, it is possible to say with reasonable assurance that any difference between those treated and those not treated is due to the treatment.

This chapter can only cover some of the key issues in clinical trials. For more extensive discussions, the reader is referred to any of several textbooks (Pocock 1983; Meinert and Tonascia 1986; Piantadosi 1997; Friedman *et al.* 1998) as well as journals such as *Controlled Clinical Trials* and *Statistics in Medicine.*

Ethical issues in intervention studies

The issue of the ethics of conducting clinical trials has generated considerable discussion and debate. Because interventions may be harmful, as well as helpful, and participants are asked to undergo potential hazards, discomforts, and expenditure of time, the question being addressed in any clinical trial must be important. Knowledge of the answer to the question must be worth these possible harms. In addition, there must be what has been termed 'clinical equipoise' (Freedman 1987). That is, there must be uncertainty as to the usefulness of the intervention among those knowledgeable about the intervention. Individual investigators or doctors may have personal beliefs about the benefits of a new intervention. Those beliefs may prevent them from participating in or entering participants into a clinical trial. The uncertainty in the medical community at large, however, is used to justify the conduct of the trial.

Informed consent of all study participants is essential. The nature of informed consent may differ in different countries and cultures, but the concept of individual choice to join or not join a trial must be universal (CIOMS/WHO 1993; Levine 1993; World Medical Association Declaration of Helsinki 2000). In addition to informed consent at the beginning of a trial, it is sometimes necessary either to modify the consent and/or to alert participants already in a trial to important new information. This can happen, for example, when an adverse effect that is important, but not so serious that a trial must be stopped, is noted. It may also be necessary to reinform participants when one clinical trial of a similar nature or question or intervention is reported while another is ongoing (DHHS 1991).

Selection of the comparison group raises ethical issues. Clinical trials may compare a new or unproven intervention against standard therapy, against no therapy, against a placebo, or in combination with standard therapy against placebo in combination with standard therapy. Whenever the comparison is against no therapy or placebo, the ethics of not treating someone in the best possible way are raised. If indeed there is no good treatment, then it is not a problem. But if a treatment known to be beneficial exists, then a control consisting of no therapy or placebo must be carefully justified. This might be possible if there is no appreciable risk to health or discomfort for the time that effective therapy is withheld (Ellenberg and Temple 2000; Temple and Ellenberg 2000). Often, placebo-controlled trials or trials that have no treatment as the control use both the new intervention and the control (placebo or no treatment) in addition to the best known treatment or standard care. In such trials, the intent of evaluating the new intervention is not to replace an existing one, but to add to it. The ethics of this situation are similar to those where there is no known effective therapy.

Even when there is no known effective therapy, the ethics of using a placebo, and indeed of randomization, have been questioned (Hellman and Hellman 1991). Use of a placebo implies deception. The strictures of abiding by a study protocol reduce a clinician's freedom to do what he or she thinks is in the best interest of the patient. The interests of the individual patient cannot be sacrificed for those of society. Conversely, it has been pointed out that a clinician's views as to the best treatment are often misguided, that hunches about treatment are not particularly helpful to the patient, and that trials can be designed to take into account patient needs (Passamani 1991).

This last point is crucial. Trial design needs to incorporate the highest ethical standards. Whenever there is a potential conflict between the needs of the patient and those of the study, the interests of the patient must take precedence.

Study question

Primary and secondary questions

The most important factor in selection of the study design, population, and outcome measures is the question that is posed. Each intervention study has a primary question that is specified in advance and is used to determine the sample size. As implied by its name, there is typically just one primary question. It is a question that is important to answer and feasible to address. By feasibility is meant the ability to identify and enrol adequate numbers of participants, to employ the intervention in an effective and presumably safe manner, to ensure that there is adequate adherence to the protocol, and to measure the outcome accurately and completely. In addition to the primary question, there may be a variety of secondary questions. Secondary questions may be less important or less feasible to answer. There may be fewer outcomes or the outcomes may be harder to measure. They may be explanatory. That is, they may help the investigator to understand the mechanism of action of the intervention by examining biochemical or physiological processes.

Study outcomes (also termed endpoints or response variables) may be of several sorts. One way of categorizing them is as either discrete or continuous. That is, they may consist of the occurrence of an event, such as a myocardial infarction or survival from cancer, or of a measurement, such as level of blood pressure or number of CD4 lymphocytes. For phase III trials, these outcomes are usually clinically important. That is, they may be fatal or serious non-fatal events, or other clinically meaningful conditions such as alleviation of pain, increased functional status, or change in an important risk factor such as cigarette smoking.

Regardless of the primary outcome, several features pertain (Friedman *et al.* 1998). Firstly, as mentioned above, it must be specified in advance; written in a protocol. Secondly, it must be capable of being assessed in the same way in all participants. Thirdly, it must be capable of unbiased assessment. Fourthly, it must be assessed in all, or almost all, of the participants. As discussed below, significant amounts of missing data can seriously affect the interpretation of the trial.

Surrogate outcomes

Clinical trials can require large numbers of participants, last for years, and be expensive. Trials with a continuous variable as the outcome require fewer participants than do trials with dichotomous outcomes. Also, if the outcome can be assessed before a clinical event has occurred, the study may be shorter in duration. Therefore, there is considerable interest in the use of surrogate outcomes, which are often continuous. A surrogate outcome is one that substitutes for a clinical outcome; it may not, in itself, be important to the participant. An example is blood pressure. Elevated blood pressure is important primarily because it is a risk factor for stroke and heart disease, not because it is generally symptomatic. It has been shown in numerous clinical trials of both diastolic and isolated systolic hypertension that treatment reduces the occurrence of stroke and heart disease (SHEP 1991; Psaty *et al.* 1997; Staessen *et al.* 1997). However, not all methods of reducing blood pressure are without risk. As we do not know all of the potential adverse effects of treatment, for some interventions in some people the risk may outweigh the benefits. This question has arisen with the use of calcium-channel-blocking agents and hypertension (Psaty *et al.* 1997). Similarly, we know that ventricular arrhythmias are associated with increased risk of sudden cardiac death (Bigger 1984). Therefore, for years it made sense to treat people with antiarrhythmic agents to reduce the occurrence of sudden death in those with heart disease and ventricular arrhythmias. Yet, when clinical trials of these agents were conducted, the results were sometimes unfavourable (CAST 1989, 1992; Waldo *et al.* 1995). Ventricular arrhythmia suppression is not a good surrogate for the clinical outcome of sudden cardiac death. Other examples of inadequate surrogate outcomes have been described (Fleming 1995; Fleming and DeMets 1996). Ideal characteristics of a surrogate outcome have been proposed (Prentice 1989), but these are unlikely to be fulfilled. Therefore, judgement as to the usefulness of a surrogate endpoint must be exercised. For phase II studies which do not attempt to address clinical questions, surrogate outcomes are entirely appropriate. For phase III trials, the kinds of issues that must be considered are the extent of correlation between the surrogate and the clinical event of interest, the ease or difficulty (and cost) of obtaining reliable surrogate outcome measurements on all of the participants, the feasibility of obtaining enough participants to conduct a clinical outcome study, the harm of a possibly wrong answer, and the urgency of obtaining an answer. With regard to the possibility of an incorrect answer if a surrogate outcome is used, this may be justified in certain circumstances. For example, if the disease or condition is life-threatening, doctors and patients may require less evidence of clinical benefit and may be less concerned with possible harm from an intervention. The results of a trial with a surrogate outcome may be sufficiently persuasive to allow use of the new intervention. Similarly, in truly life-threatening situations, getting an early answer using a surrogate outcome may outweigh the interest in getting a better, but delayed, answer using a clinical outcome. Early trials in AIDS used surrogate outcomes. At that time, no proven treatments were available.

Efficacy and effectiveness

Intervention studies are sometimes categorized as efficacy trials and effectiveness trials. An efficacy trial attempts to evaluate whether an intervention works under reasonably optimal circumstances. That is, if the active drug is taken as prescribed by essentially all in the intervention group, and if almost no one in the control group takes the active drug, will the drug alter some clinical outcome? An effectiveness trial allows for non-adherence to the assigned treatment; it resembles what is likely to happen in actual clinical practice. Most efficacy trials will be relatively short, as longer trials would have trouble maintaining optimal adherence (Friedman *et al.* 1999).

Studies of equivalency

Sometimes called positive control trials, studies of equivalency address whether the new intervention is as good as an agent known to be worthwhile. It is sometimes difficult to know that an agent is worthwhile. Not all agents proven to be beneficial at some previous time will always be so in all circumstances. This is particularly the case with drugs such as antidepressants (Ellenberg and Temple 2000; Temple and Ellenberg 2000). Therefore, simply showing that a new intervention is no worse than the standard one may not truly prove that the new one is better than placebo. Adding to the complexity is that 'equivalency' must be defined. It is not the same as failing to show a significant difference between the two agents. That could happen simply because the study has an insufficient number of participants, or because participants failed to adhere adequately to the treatments. Because the two agents cannot be shown to be identical (an infinite sample size would be needed), the new intervention must be shown to fall within some predefined boundary that is sufficiently close to the standard therapy. Defining how close will depend on the risks of inappropriately declaring the new agent to be effective and the feasibility of conducting a trial with a large enough sample size.

Clinical significance and statistical significance

An intervention study should have the ability to detect a clinically important difference between groups, if one exists. Conversely, simply showing that a statistically significant difference exists if the outcome is either not clinically meaningful or is so trivial in magnitude as to be unimportant is not worthwhile. Therefore, in determining the question to be posed, and the outcome to be measured, the issue of clinical significance needs to be considered. Factors that enter into the determination are the seriousness and prevalence of the condition or disease, the risks or cost of the intervention, and the usefulness of existing treatments (Friedman 1998).

Interventions versus intervention strategies

Not all interventions need to consist of single treatments. Sometimes, intervention strategies may be tested. For example, in some trials of hypertension treatment, a stepped care approach was used (Hypertension Detection and Follow-up Program Cooperative Group 1979; SHEP 1991). The intent was to see if successful lowering of elevated blood pressure resulted in reduction of stroke or heart disease. If the first antihypertensive agent did not adequately lower the blood pressure, another drug was used or added. At the end of this kind of study, it may not be possible to say that a particular drug is responsible for the observed benefits, but rather a strategy. Sometimes, the strategy may incorporate non-pharmacological as well as pharmacological approaches (for example, diet as well as drug in order to reduce blood pressure).

In trials that compared coronary artery bypass graft surgery against medical therapy (CASS 1983), the comparison was not really coronary artery bypass graft versus medicine. Because, over the follow-up period, a large proportion of the participants in the medical arm received surgery, it was a strategy of early surgery versus surgery later if needed. Yusuf *et al.* (1994) reported 5-, 7-, and 10-year results from an overview of seven trials of coronary artery bypass graft surgery. At 5 years, 25 per cent of the participants assigned to the medical arms had received surgery; at 7 years 33 per cent had done so; at 10 years, 41 per cent had undergone surgery.

These kinds of studies can be important and valid, but the objectives need to be clearly stated. Otherwise, the study may be criticized for not truly making the intended comparisons.

Quality of life and cost-effectiveness

Not all study outcomes need be mortality or major morbidity. Many clinical trials have looked at outcomes such as quality of life or the cost-effectiveness of administering a particular intervention as compared with another.

Health-related quality of life is a multidimensional concept that characterizes an individual's total well being and includes psychological, social, and physical dimensions (Naughton *et al.* 1996). Table 1 shows the kinds of factors generally measured in health-related quality of life instruments.

Cost-effectiveness evaluation may be particularly important when interventions are expensive and where the difference between intervention and control on mortality or major morbidity is small. In a comparison of implantable cardiac defibrillators versus antiarrhythmic drugs, cost-effectiveness was a key secondary outcome. Patients with serious ventricular arrhythmias had a significant reduction in mortality from the defibrillator, but the costs were considerably greater (Larson *et al.* 1997). Hlatky *et al.* (1997) compared quality of life, employment status, and medical care costs during 5 years of follow-up among patients treated with angioplasty or bypass graft surgery. Those in the surgical group had a better quality of life than those in the angioplasty group. Only in a subset of the participants was the cost lower in the angioplasty group.

Though these outcomes are usually secondary ones, they have occasionally been used as the primary outcome in a trial. Croog *et al.* (1986) reported the results of a trial comparing quality of life assessment with two antihypertensive agents. Although the results can

Table 1 Dimensions of health-related quality of life

Primary dimensions
Physical functioning
Psychological functioning
Social functioning
Overall life satisfaction/well being
Perceptions of health status
Additional dimensions
Neuropsychological functioning
Personal productivity
Intimacy and sexual functioning
Sleep disturbance
Pain
Symptoms

Source: Friedman (1998).

be dependent on participant selection and dose, in addition to the characteristics of the agents themselves, this trial did show the value of quality of life assessment as an outcome. Quality of life and psychosocial functioning may also be a key predictor of other outcomes, and are therefore important to measure (Ruberman *et al.* 1984).

Study population

A key part of defining the question to be answered is specifying the kinds of people who will be enrolled in the clinical trial. That is done by means of eligibility criteria, of which there are various sorts (Friedman *et al.* 1998). Firstly, eligible participants must have the potential to benefit from the intervention. That is, they must have the condition that the intervention might affect. Implicit in this is having the degree of severity at a time in the disease process that is modifiable. Also, any change in the condition must be detectable. That is, it cannot be so mild or slowly progressing that to detect a change, the study must be too large or last too long to be feasible. Secondly, participants cannot have known contraindications to the intervention. Thirdly, they should not have other conditions which would make it difficult to detect changes in the condition of interest. An obvious example is someone who has both heart disease and cancer. If a 3-year study of an intervention for the heart disease is planned and the expected survival due to the cancer is less than that, it is unlikely that the person will contribute to answering the question about heart disease. Fourthly, if the study requires participants to return for follow-up visits in order to assess the outcome, people who are unlikely to be able to do so should not be enrolled.

Figure 1 shows how the study participants are derived from the general population. People are excluded at various stages, based on the entry criteria. The final stage indicates that there are identified eligible participants who are not enrolled. This is because participating is strictly voluntary as a result of informed consent. Many people decide that they would prefer not to enrol in the trial.

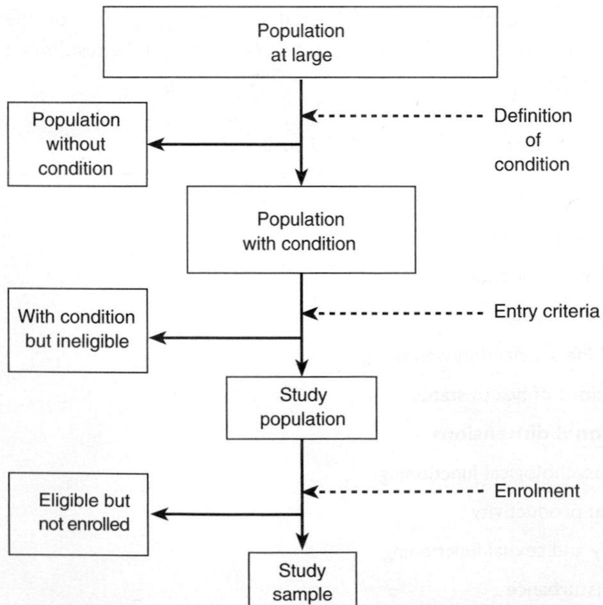

Fig. 1 Relationship of study sample to study population and population at large (those with and without the condition under study). (Source: Friedman *et al.* 1998.)

The issue of who is and who is not enrolled in a trial raises the concepts of validity, generalization, and representativeness (Friedman *et al.* 1998). A properly designed and analysed trial will yield a valid result. That is, it will be possible to say whether or not the intervention is different from or better than the control, in the setting of the kinds of participants who were enrolled.

Depending upon how narrow or broad the study sample is will determine how much the results can be generalized. If the eligibility criteria are highly selective, then the results might only apply to that sort of participant. If the eligibility criteria are broad, with many identifiable kinds of participants, then the results would be more broadly applicable. The reasons for performing one or the other type of study will depend partly on how much is known about the mechanism of action of the intervention. Congestive heart failure may have several aetiologies. If it is known (or surmised) that the intervention only works in heart failure of a non-ischaemic origin, and therefore only such people are enrolled, then the results of the trial would only apply to people with non-ischaemic heart failure. Another reason for a narrowly defined study population might be concern over the risks versus benefits. For example, the first studies of blood pressure reduction were in people with quite elevated pressures (VA 1967, 1970; HDFP 1979). Any benefit from treatment would be easier to find because of the greater likelihood of clinical events in this high-risk group. Also, any adverse effects of the intervention would be more likely to be balanced by the benefits. Not until other trials were conducted in people with lower levels of blood pressure was it possible to say with certainty that such people should be treated. The first studies could not be extrapolated to the lower risk population.

An example of a trial that successfully enrolled a broad population is the Heart Outcomes Prevention Evaluation Study (Heart Outcomes Prevention Evaluation Study Investigators 2000). In that trial, an angiotensin-converting enzyme inhibitor was evaluated in over 9000 participants with either known vascular disease or diabetes plus a risk factor for cardiovascular disease, but without evidence of heart failure. Regardless of the type of patient, the intervention was found to be highly effective in reducing mortality and morbidity.

No clinical trial is truly representative of the population with the condition being studied. Investigators conduct trials in people to whom they have ready access, rather than a random sample of the population. Eligibility criteria exclude some people for study design reasons and not because it is thought that they would not respond to the intervention in the same way as those enrolled. Additionally, there are always differences between volunteers and non-volunteers. If one is rigid, the results would be applied only to people who are identical in all relevant ways to those in the trial. The key word is 'relevant'. Judgement must be used in deciding to whom the results reasonably apply. Are the characteristics of the patient whom one wishes to treat different in respects likely to alter the effect of the intervention as observed in the trial?

Trial designs

Parallel design

In a parallel design study, participants are allocated to intervention or control and stay in that group until the end of the study. Although the typical study has two groups, one intervention and one control, many have more. Thus, there may be more than one intervention group and even more than one control group. When there are only two groups, the comparison is straightforward. When there are more than two groups, the comparisons can become complicated. For example, if there are three groups, two interventions and a control, there can be up to three main comparisons—each intervention against the control and one intervention against the other. This has implications for the overall type I error and therefore for the sample size. Conservatively, one would correct for the number of comparisons, in this case dividing the α level by 3. Instead of requiring a p value of, for instance, 0.05 for significance, each comparison might require a p value of 0.0167. To maintain adequate power to achieve this level of significance, the sample size will need to increase considerably. The possibly lower event rates in the two intervention groups (assuming benefit from the interventions) will also lead to the need for a larger sample size. If only the comparisons of the two interventions against the control are of interest, there is less penalty, and the three-arm design may be more efficient than initiating two individual studies, as the same control group can be used. Even here, as will be seen in the section on sample size, the control group may need to be larger than if there is only one intervention group. Davis *et al.* (1996) have reported on the design of such a study, where four different types of antihypertensive agents are being compared.

Factorial design

If there is an interest in studying more than one intervention at a time, a factorial design study may be more efficient than a parallel design. The simplest factorial design is a two-by-two design. This design will have four groups: treatment A plus treatment B, treatment A plus the control for treatment B, control for treatment A plus treatment B, and control for treatment A plus control for treatment B. The last is the only group that has no exposure to either of the interventions being tested. When this design is analysed, there are two primary analyses. One is treatment A plus treatment B and treatment A plus control for treatment B versus control for treatment A plus treatment B and control for treatment A plus control for treatment B. The other is the two groups with treatment B versus the two groups with control for treatment B. Because the study is designed with adequate power for comparing two groups against another two groups, it is unlikely that there will be adequate power to look at one group against another. This would usually only happen if both interventions show differences, and are additive. An example where this happened is the Second International Study of Infarct Survival (ISIS-2 1988). Factorial designs need not be just two by two. There can be more than two groups for each factor, or even more than two factors. In addition to efficiency, an advantage to the factorial design is that one might derive suggestions of differential effect of treatment in the presence or absence of the other treatment. However, this is also a weakness. If these so-called interactions are present, they may make it difficult to discern an overall effect, particularly if they go in opposite directions (Brittain and Wittes 1989). Examples of successful factorial designs, in addition to the International Study of Infarct Survival studies (1988, 1992), are the Physicians' Health Study (Hennekens and Buring 1989) and the Women's Health Initiative Study Group (1998). Interestingly, for a three-arm parallel design, it is generally thought appropriate to adjust the α level for the number of comparisons. For factorial design, however, the usual practice is not to make such an adjustment.

Cross-over design

In the cross-over design, each participant serves as his or her own control (Friedman *et al.* 1998). In the simplest case, half of the participants would receive intervention followed by control, and the other half the reverse. The major advantage of this design is the smaller sample size. Because each participant is on both intervention and control, half the number of participants are needed. The sample may be even smaller, because the variability is less than in the standard parallel design. There are disadvantages, however. The most obvious one is that the outcomes must be reversible. A cross-over design is not possible if the primary outcome is mortality or a clinical event. A second disadvantage is that there is an assumption of no carry-over effect from one period to the next. If the effect of the intervention persists into the period when the control is being administered, then the apparent effect may be less than the real one. Often, to minimize the likelihood of carry-over, a washout period is inserted between the actual cross-over periods. Unfortunately, it is difficult to prove that a carry-over effect is absent and a participant has truly returned to baseline.

Randomization

The optimal way of allocating intervention or control to clinical trial participants is by means of randomization. Randomization does not guarantee balance in all factors between the groups, but the chances of balance are increased. Unknown as well as known and measured characteristics are likely to be comparable when there is randomization. A properly performed randomization procedure also reduces the opportunity for investigator bias in the allocation of intervention or control. Finally, randomization guarantees that statistical tests of significance will be valid.

Randomization does not require a one-to-one allocation to intervention or control, only that the allocation be unpredictable. Alternative assignment or assignment based on day of the month (for example, odd or even) is predictable, and is not equivalent to randomization. Matching on the basis of important characteristics is also not considered randomization. Flipping an unbiased coin to determine whether a participant is assigned to group A or B can be a valid way of randomizing. In practice, however, tables of random numbers or computer-produced random numbers are more often used.

Randomized studies can, by definition, only have a concurrent control group. That is, a historical control study cannot have randomized allocation. This yields another advantage of randomization, namely that the participants are enrolled in the same time period in both the intervention and control groups. Therefore, temporal trends in care or in the nature of the condition being studied are equal in the two groups.

Randomization procedures

Several procedures for randomly assigning treatments to participants have been developed. The simplest are the fixed allocation procedures. If, for example, 20 participants are needed for a study, a coin may be tossed when each participant is entered. However, the likelihood that the number of participants in the two groups will be different (for instance, 12 to 8 or even more extreme) is about 50 per cent. As the sample size increases, the likelihood of such a large uneven split is reduced. If 100 participants are enrolled, the chance of a 60 to 40 split is only about 5 per cent (Friedman *et al.* 1998).

Blocked randomization is commonly used because of this problem. In blocked randomization, equal numbers of participants in the groups is guaranteed after every several are enrolled. For example, if the block size is four, and the sample size is 12, then after four, eight, and 12 participants are enrolled, there would be equal numbers in treatments A and B. This would be accomplished by specifying that each block of four would have two participants assigned to A and two to B. The order within the block of four would be randomized. Thus, it could be ABAB, AABB, ABBA, BABA, and so on. The hazard with this approach is that if the block size is known to the investigator and the treatments are not completely blinded, the last one of the block (and sometimes the last two) can be predicted. Therefore, often, the block size, as well as the order within the block, is random, and the investigator entering the participants is kept ignorant of the block size.

Another advantage of blocked randomization would be if participant entry criteria are modified partway through a trial. In the absence of blocking, even if at the end of entering all participants there are more or less equal numbers in the groups, there may be imbalance in numbers when only some of the participants have been entered. If, because of lagging participant entry, the eligibility criteria are loosened, different sorts of participants may enrol later during recruitment than enrolled earlier. As a result, the characteristics of the participants in group A may differ from those in group B. With blocked randomization, equal numbers are ensured throughout the enrolment period, and changes in entry criteria would not lead to imbalances between the groups in type of participant.

Stratified randomization is a special kind of blocked randomization. Here, the investigator wishes to ensure that there is balance between group A and B, not only in numbers of participants, but in kind of participant. If, despite the randomization process, there is concern that there will be imbalance between groups for one or two key highly prognostic variables, randomization can be stratified on those variables. Thus, within decades of age, for example, blocked randomization would occur. If sex is also a key variable, there would be blocked randomization within each age–sex category. The problem is that even with only two or three characteristics, each one having two or more factors, the number of strata can rapidly increase (Friedman *et al.* 1998). This can lead to unfilled cells unless many participants are being enrolled. If the sample size is large, randomization will generally lead to good balance, making stratification unnecessary. Therefore, stratified randomization should be done judiciously. If, after the trial is over, it is found that there is a major imbalance in a key factor, an adjusted analysis can be performed. In multicentre trials, randomization is usually done by centre, making the centre one of the important strata. This minimizes the chance that different sorts of participants or different medical practices among centres will confound the results.

In addition to the above fixed randomization procedures, there are various adaptive randomization procedures. In baseline adaptive procedures, the likelihood of randomization to A or B changes in order to reduce imbalances in selected characteristics. In response adaptive procedures, the likelihood or randomization to one or another group changes based on the occurrence of study outcomes. Adaptive randomization procedures are not used as frequently as fixed randomization. For more details of these procedures, see Friedman *et al.* (1998).

Sample size

Clinical trials should be designed with adequate power to answer the question being posed. That is, by the end of the trial, there should be enough events or, in the case of continuous response variable, sufficient precision of the estimate to say with reasonable assurance that the intervention does or does not have the postulated effect. Several factors are considered in the calculation of sample size. For dichotomous outcome studies, these factors are event rate in the control group, expected benefit from the intervention, level of adherence to the intervention, level of adherence to the control regimen, α level, and power. For continuous outcome studies, the mean and variance of the control and intervention groups, plus the level of adherence, α level, and power, would be the relevant variables.

Various references provide formulas for calculating sample size (Lachin 1981; Lakatos 1986; Wu 1988), as does Chapter 6.13. In essence, the factors that lead to the need for larger sample sizes in the dichotomous outcome situation are lower control group event rate, smaller benefit from the intervention (or lesser difference that one wants to detect), smaller α, greater power to detect a real difference (smaller β), and poorer adherence (or greater cross-over). Alpha is commonly selected to be 0.05 (two-sided); power is typically 0.8 to 0.9.

As discussed below, the preferred method of analysis is by 'intention to treat'. This means that, in general, participants remain in the randomization group to which they have been assigned, regardless of their future actions or the degree to which they adhere to the assigned regimen. To the extent that those assigned to the intervention group fail to comply with the intervention, for example by not taking their medication (often called 'drop-out'), the expected benefit from the intervention is reduced. Similarly, to the extent that those assigned to the control group begin taking the intervention (often called 'drop-in'), the control group event rate is altered. The net effect of this non-adherence is a narrowing of the difference between the groups. This, in turn, leads to a larger sample size in order to maintain the same power to detect a real difference. Non-adherence can have an appreciable effect on sample size. A correction factor proposed by Lachin (1981) multiplies the needed sample size by $1/(1 - R_0 - R_1)^2$, where R_0 is the drop-out rate and R_1 is the drop-in rate. Because the factor is squared, the sample size increases rapidly as soon as the combined non-adherence rate goes over 20 per cent. Even a combined non-adherence rate of only 10 per cent means a sample size increase of almost a quarter. More complicated sample size formulas take into account the fact that most non-adherence is not linear, but is often greater earlier in a trial than later (Lakatos 1986; Wu 1988). Another factor sometimes considered in sample size calculations is the estimated time for an intervention to make the postulated biological changes. For example, if cholesterol-lowering drugs act at least partly by reducing arterial plaque, then the time for that process to occur (so-called 'lag time') implies a larger sample size (and a longer study).

As noted in the section above on study question, studies of equivalency may require large sample sizes, depending on what is meant by 'equivalence'. Because the sample size formula contains the difference to be detected in the denominator, if zero difference is planned, the sample size would be infinite. Therefore, one typically specifies a difference δ. If the two treatments show differences less than this, they are considered equal, or at least they have differences that are unimportant. Sample size formulas for such studies are available (Blackwelder and Chang 1984). It should be emphasized that, unlike studies where a difference is being sought, an underpowered study of equivalency will lead to the 'desired' outcome. That is, it will confirm the null hypothesis of no difference. Even more, poor adherence will enhance the likelihood of seeing no difference for either the primary outcome or for adverse effects.

The needed sample size is an estimate because factors such as event rate and adherence are rarely known for certain. It may be prudent, therefore, to be conservative in the assumptions that enter into calculating sample size. The disadvantage of being conservative is that increased size or duration leads to increased cost. Also, entering more people into a trial than is necessary to answer the question may put more people at risk than is appropriate.

Recruitment of participants

A rule of thumb for all phase III clinical trials is that participant recruitment is always more difficult than expected. It is the uncommon clinical trial that finishes enrolment on schedule and the even rarer one that can do so without major recruitment strategy changes. Because recruitment is difficult, it is best to employ multiple strategies and to plan for back-up strategies in advance and to monitor progress closely throughout the enrolment period. Depending on the nature of the study population, back-up strategies would include adding sources of participants (for example, clinics, hospital units) or disseminating information about the trial more widely, to both medical personnel and potential participants. If sufficient resources are available, the strategies might include adding staff whose primary responsibilities involve enhancing enrolment or increasing incentives. The latter raises ethical questions if the incentives are inappropriate in amount or kind. Paying so-called 'finder's fees', for example, would not be acceptable.

If participant enrolment remains slow, several options are available. One approach is to extend the time of enrolment. This has the advantage of not changing other study design factors, but the disadvantages of additional cost and delay in answering the question. A second approach is to accept the smaller sample size. Depending upon how large the shortfall is, the reduced power may not be too great. If the power goes from 90 to 85 per cent or even 80 per cent, that can be acceptable. However, if it falls much below 80 per cent, the study is likely to be underpowered. Some have argued that conducting even underpowered trials is useful, as cumulative meta-analyses of similar trials will yield the answers (Antman *et al.* 1992), but that approach is not recommended here. A third option is to change the entry criteria, so that more people are eligible. Depending on the original criteria, this might be feasible. However, care needs to be taken to make sure that other design assumptions, such as the expected effect of the intervention and the event rate, are not materially changed. In addition, as noted above, a blocked randomization scheme needs to be used to ensure that there is no gross imbalance between groups in participants enrolled before and after the criteria change.

A fourth option is to change the study outcome, so that fewer participants are needed to obtain the same number of events. A study may be originally designed with the outcome of death due to heart disease or non-fatal myocardial infarction. Because of limited resources, some of the other approaches to slow participant accrual are not feasible. It may be decided that the intervention is as likely to affect other important outcomes, such as need for coronary revascularization, as it is to affect myocardial infarction. Adding that event to the primary outcome would increase the event rate considerably, and allow for an answer with fewer participants. In another example, incidence of hypertension may be the outcome in a study looking at prevention of hypertension with weight loss. Instead of using incidence of hypertension as the primary event, mean blood pressure might be used. Going from a dichotomous outcome study to a study using a continuous variable as the outcome will reduce the needed sample size. These sorts of design changes should not be made lightly. They require considerable thought and review. If, because of the changes, the results are not persuasive to the outside community of practising clinicians, there is little point in undertaking them.

Adherence

As discussed in the section above on sample size, adherence (or compliance) on the part of participants is a key factor in clinical trials. It can reduce the power of a trial, and, if truly bad, can make the study results uninterpretable. Therefore, most investigators take steps when planning a study to minimize poor participant adherence. One is to design the study so that the regimen is as simple as possible. For medications, once-daily dosing is preferable to more frequent doses. For lifestyle interventions such as diet or exercise, simpler, more easily remembered programmes are better. Shorter trials have better chances of maintaining good adherence than longer ones. A second method is to select participants who are more likely to adhere. One way is by means of a run-in phase prior to randomization. Unless study participants must be enrolled immediately, for example at the time of an acute event, a run-in period can be used to determine who adheres to the regimen. Potential participants might be given the active medication for several weeks. At the end of that time, only those who took at least 80 per cent (or some other reasonable amount) of the drug would be enrolled. The participants who could not adhere, even over the short term, would not be randomized. This approach has been successfully used in the Physicians' Health Study (PHS 1989; Glynn *et al.* 1994) and the Women's Health Study (Buring and Hennekens 1992). Angiotensin-converting enzyme inhibitors may cause cough in some people. Therefore, to minimize the drop-out rate after randomization, studies of angiotensin-converting enzyme inhibitors have used a short run-in period to exclude those who might not tolerate the drug (Davis 1998). Excluding potential non-adherers on the basis of other demographic or psychosocial factors has been done, but the evidence that it successfully separates good from poor adherers is unclear (Dunbar-Jacob 1998). Educating potential participants about the trial is not only good practice from an informed consent standpoint, but is likely to lead to the enrolment of participants who are better adherers. Being unduly persuasive in enrolling participants may improve the recruitment figures, but it can lead to worse adherence statistics. Because the analysis is done on an intention-to-treat basis, the study is more harmed by someone who drops out after enrolment than by someone who does not enrol.

A variety of techniques to maintain good adherence have been tried. Those that appear to be useful are frequent contact and reminders, providing easy transportation and access to attractive facilities, providing continuity of care, providing special medication dispensers, such as calendar packs, and involving family members, particularly when the intervention is lifestyle change (Schron and Czajkowski 2001). Other techniques include attention to aspects of the trial regimen, such as single-dose formulation for medication, intervention schedules made similar to those in clinical practice, and the use of specially trained personnel.

Adherence monitoring has two purposes. One is to be able to advise participants who are not complying with their regimen on how they might improve. The second is to be able to interpret the results of the trial more accurately. The first requires knowledge of individual adherence; the latter only requires knowing how the groups are performing.

Monitoring individual adherence is important, but there is considerable debate about how accurately it can be done, except for interventions that take place entirely in clinics or hospitals (surgery, vaccine, periodic medication, food feeding studies). Self-reports are simple, but subject to considerable uncertainty. Participants may not remember accurately, and may have a desire to report better adherence than is truly the case. Assessment of activities such as nutritional intake and physical activity are particularly difficult. The use of diaries or other records may help, but still depend on accurate completion by the participant.

For studies involving medication, there are a variety of ways to assess adherence. Pill count is relatively simple, though there are studies that indicate that it over-reports adherence (Rand and Weeks 1998). Participants may forget to return the partially empty containers or may intentionally discard medication that was not taken. Laboratory measures of drug metabolites can be useful, but also may be misleading, as they do not reflect what was ingested long term or show the true pattern of medication usage. Use of special devices that register when a bottle cap is opened has been advocated (Rand and Weeks 1998). Electronic monitoring of this sort can provide a continuous record of dose taking. This probably provides a more accurate measure of adherence, but it is expensive. Even this technique does not prevent a participant from opening the bottle, removing a pill, and then discarding it.

Physiological or biochemical measures that reflect responses to the intervention can be used in some studies. For example, trials of cholesterol-lowering agents which have heart disease as the outcome would periodically measure lipid levels. These are not foolproof indicators of adherence, as individual responses vary, but they are particularly good at demonstrating that on average, after randomization, the intervention group has a different biochemical profile from the control group. One problem with using these sorts of measures as markers of individual adherence is that they may unmask the group to which a participant has been assigned.

Unless one is willing to go to considerable lengths and spend considerable resources, the simple measures of adherence are probably adequate for most purposes. They will certainly indicate gross problems overall, and allow the investigator to conclude, with reasonable assurance, that the intervention was or was not administered satisfactorily, and that there is or is not a difference between the groups in intermediate response variables or biomarkers. For the purposes of individual counselling, the more sophisticated assessments might be more useful than pill count, for example, but whether they are the best uses of limited funds is questionable.

Data monitoring

Data monitoring is an essential part of any clinical trial. If the data become persuasive before the scheduled end of the trial, or if unexpected adverse events occur, the investigator is obligated either to stop the trial or to make necessary design changes. For many trials, the data monitoring function is undertaken by a person or group external to the study investigator structure. For masked studies, this helps to keep the investigator blinded. But more importantly, for all trials, an outside group is less likely to have a bias and less likely to want the study to continue inappropriately because of financial or other reasons. The primary function of this group is to maximize participant safety. Secondarily, it helps ensure the integrity of the trial.

In the process of data monitoring, several kinds of recommendations may be made. Firstly, and most common, would be a recommendation to continue the trial without any change. Secondly, would be a recommendation to modify the protocol in some way. Examples might be changing the participant entry criteria, changing the informed consent to take into consideration important new information, changing the frequency of certain tests to better ensure safety, or even dropping from the study certain types of participants for whom it may no longer be appropriate. Thirdly, there might be reason to recommend extending the trial. This could occur if the participant accrual rate is slower than expected or if the overall event rate is much lower than expected. Fourthly, there might be a recommendation to stop the trial early.

Data monitoring techniques

Regular data monitoring must be performed for ethical reasons. However, this carries a penalty.

> If the null hypothesis, H_0, of no difference between two groups is, in fact, true, and repeated tests of that hypothesis are made at the same level of significance using accumulating data, the probability that, at some time, the test will be called significant by chance alone will be larger than the significance level selected. That is, the rate of incorrectly rejecting the null hypothesis will be larger than what is normally considered to be acceptable. (Friedman *et al.* 1998).

Therefore a variety of stopping boundaries or guidelines have been developed that maintain the overall prespecified α level. Biostatistics references can be consulted for the details of these methods. In essence, the methods fall into three categories: classical sequential, group sequential, and curtailed sampling. In the classical sequential approach (Whitehead 1983), there is no fixed sample size. Participant enrolment and the study end when boundaries for benefit or harm are exceeded. A theoretical advantage of the classical sequential approach is that fewer participants might need to be enrolled than in a fixed sample size design. This design requires study outcomes to occur relatively soon after enrolment, however, so that decisions about enrolment of new participants can be made. As a result, it may have limited usefulness.

The most commonly used monitoring techniques are the group sequential methods. Here, after a group of participants have been enrolled, or after a length of time, the data are examined. In order to conserve the overall α level, the study is not stopped early even if the nominal p value (for example, 0.05) is exceeded. More extreme p values are required for early stopping. An example of such boundaries is that developed by O'Brien and Fleming (1979), which calls for very extreme results early in a study which gradually become less extreme towards the end. If the study goes to the expected end, the significance value is essentially what it would be without any interim monitoring. An approach proposed by Haybittle (1971) and Peto *et al.* (1976) uses a constant extreme value throughout the trial, with the usual p value for significance at the end. Both of these techniques allow the final significance value to be what would be used without monitoring because of the low likelihood of stopping early, given the extreme nature of the boundaries. A modification of these techniques uses what is termed an α spending function (Lan and DeMets 1989). This technique allows for more flexible selection of the times when the data will be monitored.

Another modification of the group sequential methods employs asymmetric boundaries. As noted earlier, for many trials, even those that are not one-sided tests of the hypothesis, it would be inappropriate to continue a trial until the intervention is proven harmful, using the usual p value of 0.05. Therefore, instead of having the monitoring boundary for harm symmetric to the one for benefit, a less extreme monitoring boundary can be developed (DeMets and Ware 1982). Thus, if the one for benefit maintains the overall α at 0.05, the one for harm might maintain it at 0.1, or even less extreme. Even with one-sided tests of hypothesis, an advisory boundary for harm can be implemented, as was the case in the Cardiac Arrhythmia Suppression Trial (Pawitan and Hallstrom 1990).

Curtailed sampling addresses the probability of seeing a significant result if the trial were to continue to its end, given the data at the current time (that is, part way through the trial) (Lan and Wittes 1988). For example, if there is a strongly positive trend with three-quarters of the expected data in hand, one can examine the probabilities of having a statistically significant outcome under various assumptions regarding future data. A reasonable assumption might be that the control group event rate will continue, more or less, as it has been and that the null hypothesis is true. If, under those conditions, the outcome is still significant, there might be reason to stop the study. Conversely, if there is little or no benefit (or a trend towards harm) from the intervention, one might look at how large a benefit would be required from now on to see a significant benefit at the end. If there is little likelihood of that happening, the study might be stopped because continuation would be futile.

Several descriptions of stopping decisions in clinical trials have been published (DeMets *et al.* 1982, 1984; Cairns *et al.* 1991; Friedman *et al.* 1993). These include stopping early for overwhelming benefit, clear harm, or futility. A decision to stop a trial early is irrevocable; therefore, such a decision must be made carefully. Whenever a recommendation is made to stop a study early, factors other than whether or not the monitoring boundaries are crossed need to be considered (Friedman *et al.* 1998). Might the results be due to imbalance in baseline characteristics or to bias in ascertainment of the outcome? Might poor adherence or differential use of concomitant therapy be important? What might be the impact of outcomes other than the primary one on the interpretation of the conclusions? Are there major unexpected adverse effects that need to be considered? How might other ongoing research affect the results? Will the results be persuasive to others? The issues are not just statistical in nature. If they were, there would be little need for a monitoring committee. Instead, an algorithm could be created which would make the decision. But because the decisions depend on a complex interaction of statistics, understanding of the biological mechanism of action of the intervention, knowledge of other research findings, and judgement as to how the results will be received and interpreted, decisions to recommend continuation or stopping are rarely easy and often second-guessed.

Analysis issues

Whom to include

A purpose of assigning intervention or control by means of randomization is to ensure, as far as possible, that there is balance between the groups on both measured and unmeasured factors. Anything that alters that balance, such as removing from analysis some data from some participants, can induce bias. The reason is that it may be difficult to prove that the cause for the exclusion is unrelated to either a key baseline factor or to the intervention or control. Therefore, the general guideline for analysis is called 'intention to treat'. That is, once randomization has taken place, the data from all participants should be included and counted in the group to which they are assigned.

There are several reasons why one would want to withdraw participants or data from the analysis. Firstly, it may be discovered, after enrolment, that a participant is not truly eligible for the trial. Therefore, that person would not contribute meaningfully to answering the question and, in fact, might confuse the issue by providing incorrect information. Also importantly, it might be hazardous for that person to be taking the intervention. Withdrawing such people from the study and the analysis might seem to be straightforward, but often it is not. If the decision that a person is ineligible is made after adverse effects or a clinical event has occurred, it might be viewed as an effort to manipulate the data. Eligibility criteria are commonly subjective and even in blinded trials there may be clues regarding the group to which the participant was assigned. Therefore, if participants are withdrawn from the trial because they are found to be ineligible, it must be done as soon as possible, before any events have occurred or follow-up measurements performed, and without knowledge of the treatment group. If that does not happen, then the best policy is to leave the participant in the study and analyse the data as if he or she is eligible. If it is possibly dangerous for the participant to be on the intervention, that can be discontinued without removing the person from the trial. If the percentage of ineligible people is small, that should not unduly affect the conclusions. If the percentage is large, such that the study integrity might be affected, then there is clearly a larger problem with the conduct of the trial.

A second reason for withdrawal of participants after randomization is poor adherence. As discussed in the sample size section, incomplete adherence to the protocol is best handled by increasing the number of people in the trial. Sometimes, however, it is decided to remove non-adherent participants from the analysis. The argument for doing this is that if they have not taken the intervention, there is no way that they can provide information as to its usefulness. The counter-argument is that lack of adherence may be a reflection of not being able to tolerate one or another of the treatments. Therefore, withdrawing poor adherers leads to an underestimate of the adverse effects. It also biases the analysis because those removed from one group are likely to be different from those removed from the other group. There have been attempts to adjust for non-adherence, but these approaches are questionable.

The classic example of how withdrawing poor adherers from analysis can lead to strange results is from the Coronary Drug Project, a trial of lipid lowering in heart disease patients (CDP 1975). As expected, those assigned to the active medication group who did not take it fared worse than those who did. But those assigned to placebo who did not take the placebo also fared worse than those who did (CDP 1980). This outcome could not be accounted for by measured differences between the adherers and non-adherers. Therefore, unknown confounding factors must have been present, as the difference is not attributable to an inert substance. It is best to include the data from all participants, regardless of level of adherence, in the analysis. If, despite the best efforts of the investigator, adherence is so poor as to compromise the integrity of the trial, then that itself says something about the usefulness of the intervention.

Poor quality or, in the extreme case, missing data is a third reason for withdrawing participants from analysis. Every effort must be made to minimize these. If participants are lost to follow-up, or do not return for key outcome measurements, the data will be missing. To the extent that this constitutes more than a few per cent of the total data, the study is severely impaired. The reason, again, is that there is no assurance that the missing data are independent of the treatment. If participants do not return to the clinic because one of the treatments makes them feel unwell, the data in that group will only be from those who are healthier or better able to tolerate the treatment.

Various statistical methods have been proposed to take into account missing data, but none is perfect (Liang and Zeger 1989; Espeland *et al.* 1992; Proschan *et al.* 2001). In general, they use prior data from the individual or some average from the group to which that individual is assigned to impute the most likely values for the missing data. These techniques can be useful, but as with simply censoring missing data, are limited if the missing data are strongly related to treatment.

The same factors apply to poor-quality data or outliers. Statistical techniques exist for deciding if unusual values are truly outliers (Dixon 1953). Ideally though, all analyses should be performed with and without including the outliers, as there may be important reasons for the apparently strange data that should not be ignored. One practice that is not encouraged is substituting data such as prior measurements from an individual for data that are thought to be incorrect or outlying.

Adjustment procedures

Despite best efforts, study groups may turn out to have imbalances in important factors at baseline. In such cases, it is tempting to adjust for these imbalances. Unless the imbalance is large and the factor is highly correlated with the outcome, however, adjustment is unlikely to make a major difference. Simply showing that there is a statistically significant difference in a baseline covariate is not sufficient reason to adjust on that factor. Conversely, large and potentially important differences may not be statistically significant because of small numbers. Furthermore, there may be several covariates that are imbalanced in a similar direction. Individually, they may not be important, but in the aggregate, they may lead to enough of an imbalance that adjustment is useful. In summary, adjustment for baseline imbalances is legitimate, and should be explored if there are apparent differences. Mostly, this is unnecessary. Certainly, if adjustment converts a non-significant result to a significant one, it needs to be interpreted cautiously.

Conversely, adjustment for post-randomization variables is strongly discouraged. Level of adherence is one example of such a variable. Others might be biomarkers or similar interim measures of the effect of the intervention, as well as concomitant therapy. Because such variables are, or may be related to, the intervention, unlike the baseline factors, adjustment for them can lead to misleading interpretations. Response to an intervention can indicate better prognosis, even in the absence of the intervention (CDP 1980; Anderson *et al.* 1983). Adjustment on such a variable can make an intervention appear beneficial when it is not.

Subgroup analyses

In every clinical trial it is tempting to look at the effects of the intervention in subgroups of participants. This is particularly the case with trials that show no significant difference overall. Even without overall benefit, there might be some subsets that indeed benefit. The problem is that with enough creativity, one can almost always find a group that benefits (and a group that is harmed) from the intervention. Even in trials that have significant overall differences, there is a desire to find the types of participants who benefit the most.

It is generally the case that qualitative interactions are uncommon (Peto 1995). That is, an intervention is unlikely to be beneficial in one subgroup and harmful in another. Conversely, it is quite plausible that there are differential relative effects. Some kinds of people are indeed likely to be helped more than other kinds of people. The problem is that unless the subgroups of interest are specified in advance, it is likely that most of the observed differences are due to chance. The best way of confirming that subgroup differences are real is to examine an independent dataset, usually from another trial of the same question. Somewhat weaker is using independent data from the same trial. This can be done if, during data monitoring, a possible subgroup difference is identified. The data accrued during the remaining period of the trial on participants who have not yet had the event can be confirmatory. Other approaches, such as looking at trends in subgroups defined by continuous variables, especially where there is biological plausibility, can also be used.

As noted, with enough imagination, apparent subgroup differences can be uncovered. 'Fishing', or 'data-dredging' is a natural activity, as unexpected subgroup findings can be important sources of new information and new hypotheses. As opposed to raising new questions, however, conclusions should almost never be drawn from subgroups that are not prespecified. The examples of differences based on signs of the zodiac (ISIS-2 1988) or similar characteristics are cautionary.

Meta-analyses

A separate chapter is devoted to meta-analyses (Chapter 6.12). Therefore, only a brief summary is provided here. Meta-analyses can be important ways of synthesizing data. They enable researchers to incorporate multiple studies of the same question. Because of the added numbers of participants, they provide better estimates of intervention effects in subgroups. They allow one to put together several small studies to see if a larger study should be conducted to address a question more clearly. They do have potential limitations, however. Most important is the effort expended in collecting all of the relevant studies and the judgement that must go into selection of the studies to be combined. Studies that show benefit from an intervention are more likely to be published (Dickerson *et al.* 1987). Therefore, if meta-analyses are not done carefully with clear criteria, biases can be introduced. Another limitation is that only some outcomes can be used. Typically, mortality or major morbidity is the outcome of interest. When deciding on whether or not an intervention is useful, other outcomes, such as adverse effects and quality of life, may be important, but are rarely incorporated into published meta-analyses. The ability to perform meta-analyses easily may lead to several inadequately powered studies yielding an overall statistically significant p value. Examples of probably misleading conclusions from these meta-analyses have been observed, once the single large trial was conducted (LeLorier *et al.* 1997). Any discouragement of the conduct of properly sized trials because of meta-analyses is unfortunate.

Reporting and interpretation

Several guidelines to the proper reporting of clinical trial results have been published (Asilomar Working Group on Recommendations for Reporting of Clinical Trials in the Biomedical Literature 1996; Begg *et al.* 1996). In essence, they call for objective recording of all pertinent aspects. It is recognized that space limitations restrict the amount of information that can be included in a publication. The advent of journal websites, however, allows for the dissemination of supplementary material. Ideally, all of the following should be included in a clinical trial report (Friedman *et al.* 1998).

1. Background and rationale.
2. Specification of the primary question and the response variables used to assess it.
3. Prespecified secondary questions.
4. Nature of the study population, including eligibility criteria, major reasons why people were not entered, and the fact that informed consent was obtained.
5. Sample size calculations and the assumptions used for that calculation.
6. Basic study design features and allocation procedures.
7. Data collection procedures, including efforts to minimize bias, quality control, and event classification.
8. Presentation of key baseline characteristics, by group.
9. Process measures, such as adherence, concomitant therapy usage, performance to procedures, amount of missing or poor quality data, and numbers or participants lost to follow-up.
10. Results for the primary outcome, secondary outcomes (prespecified and other), and adverse events. The statistics and tabulations should reflect the original intent and indicate whether the effects of repeated tests have been taken into account. Confidence intervals, relative risk reduction (or increase), and absolute risk reduction should be presented. Also noted should be where the data were analysed.
11. Adverse effects.
12. Special analyses, such as subgroups, covariate adjustment, and data-derived hypotheses.
13. Interpretation, implications, and conclusions in the context of both study data and information external to the trial.
14. A structured abstract that accurately reflects the body of the paper.

Conclusion

It is not easy to conduct well-designed clinical trials, and there are ethical issues that must be considered. Nevertheless, there is no substitute for good clinical trials in providing important information for clinical use and public health about the possible benefits of interventions. As a result of the development of clinical trial technologies over the past several decades, more clinical decisions are evidence based. Improvements in trial design and analysis are continuing and will have further impact, as will increasing knowledge about genetics, better understanding of disease aetiologies and processes, and pharmacology.

References

Anderson, J.R., Cain, K.C., and Gelber, R.D. (1983). Analysis of survival by tumor response. *Journal of Clinics in Oncology*, **1**, 710–19.

Antman, E.M., Lau, J., Kupelnick, B., *et al.* (1992). A comparison of results of meta-analyses of randomized control trials and recommendations of clinical experts. *Journal of the American Medical Association*, **268**, 240–8.

Asilomar Working Group on Recommendations for Reporting of Clinical Trials in the Biomedical Literature (1996). Checklist of information for inclusion in reports of clinical trials. *Annals of Internal Medicine*, **124**, 741–3.

Begg, C., Cho, M., Eastwood, S., *et al.* (1996). Improving the quality of reporting of randomized controlled trials: the CONSORT statement. *Journal of the American Medical Association*, **276**, 637–9.

Bigger, J.T. Jr (1984). Identification of patients at high risk for sudden cardiac death. *American Journal of Cardiology*, **54**, 3–8D.

Blackwelder, W.C. and Chang, M.A. (1984). Sample size graphs for 'proving the null hypothesis'. *Controlled Clinical Trials*, **5**, 97–105.

Brittain, E. and Wittes, J. (1989). Factorial designs in clinical trials: the effects of non-compliance and subadditivity. *Statistics in Medicine*, **8**, 161–71.

Buring, J.E. and Hennekens, C.H. (1992). The Women's Health Study: summary of the study design. *Journal of Myocardial Ischemia*, **4**, 27–39.

Cairns, J., Cohen, L., Colton, T., *et al.* (1991). Issues in the early termination of the aspirin component of the Physicians' Health Study. *Annals of Epidemiology*, **1**, 395–405.

CASS (Coronary Artery Surgery Study) Principal Investigators and their Associates (1983). Coronary Artery Surgery Study (CASS): a randomized trial of coronary artery bypass surgery: survival data. *Circulation*, **68**, 939–50.

CAST (Cardiac Arrhythmia Suppression Trial) Investigators (1989). Preliminary report: effect of encainide and flecainide on mortality in a randomized trial of arrhythmia suppression after myocardial infarction. *New England Journal of Medicine*, **321**, 406–12.

CAST (Cardiac Arrhythmia Suppression Trial) II Investigators (1992). Effect of the antiarrhythmic agent moricizine on survival after myocardial infarction. *New England Journal of Medicine*, **327**, 227–33.

CDP (Coronary Drug Project) Research Group (1975). Clofibrate and niacin in coronary heart disease. *Journal of the American Medical Association*, **231**, 360–81.

CDP (Coronary Drug Project) Research Group (1980). Influence of adherence to treatment and response of cholesterol on mortality in the Coronary Drug Project. *New England Journal of Medicine*, **303**, 1038–41.

CIOMS/WHO (Council for International Organizations of Medical Science/World Health Organization) (1993). *International ethical guidelines for biomedical research involving human subjects*. CIOMS/ WHO, Geneva.

Croog, S.H., Levine, S., Testa, M.A., *et al.* (1986). The effects of antihypertensive therapy on the quality of life. *New England Journal of Medicine*, **314**, 1657–64.

Davis, B.R., Cutler, J.A., Gordon, D.J., *et al.* (1996). Rationale and design for the Antihypertensive and Lipid Lowering Treatment to Prevent Heart Attack Trial (ALLHAT). ALLHAT Research Group. *American Journal of Hypertension*, **9**, 342–60.

Davis, C.E. (1998). Prerandomization compliance screening: a statistician's views. In *The handbook of health behavior change* (ed. S.A. Shumaker, E.B. Schron, J.K. Ockene, and W.L. McBee), pp. 485–90. Springer, New York.

DeMets, D.L. and Ware, J.H. (1982). Asymmetric group sequential boundaries for monitoring clinical trials. *Biometrika*, **69**, 661–3.

DeMets, D.L., Williams, G.W., Brown, B.W. Jr, *et al.* (1982). A case report of data monitoring experience: the Nocturnal Oxygen Therapy Trial. *Controlled Clinical Trials*, **3**, 113–24.

DeMets, D.L., Hardy, R., Friedman, L.M., and Lan, K.K.G. (1984). Statistical aspects of early termination in the Beta-Blocker Heart Attack Trial. *Controlled Clinical Trials*, **5**, 362–72.

DHHS (Department of Health and Human Services) (1991). National Institutes of Health (NIH) and Office of Protection from Research Risks (OPRR) Reports. *Protection of human subjects*, Title 45, Code of Federal Regulations Part 46, pp. 4–17 (http://ohrp.osophs.dhhs.gov/ humansubjects/guidance/45cfr46.htm).

Dickerson, K., Chan, S., Chalmers, T.C., *et al.* (1987). Publication bias and clinical trials. *Controlled Clinical Trials*, **8**, 343–53.

Dixon, W.J. (1953). Processing data for outliers. *Biometrics*, **9**, 74–89.

Dunbar-Jacob, J. (1998). Predictors of patient adherence: patient characteristics. In *The handbook of health behavior change* (ed. S.A. Shumaker, E.B. Schron, J.K. Ockene, and W.L. McBee), pp. 491–511. Springer, New York.

Ellenberg, S.S. and Temple, R. (2000). Placebo-controlled trials and active-control trials in the evaluation of new treatments. Part 2: Practical issues and specific cases. *Annals of Internal Medicine*, **133**, 464–70.

Espeland, M.A., Byington, R.P., Hire, D., *et al.* (1992). Analysis strategies for serial multivariate ultrasonographic data that are incomplete. *Statistics in Medicine*, **11**, 1041–56.

FDA (Food and Drug Administration) (1997). Department of Health and Human Services (DHHS). *Federal Register*, 17 December, pp. 66 113–19 (http://www.fda.gov/cder/guidance/1857fnl.pdf).

Fleming, T.R. (1995). Surrogate markers in AIDS and cancer trials. *Statistics in Medicine*, **13**, 1423–35.

Fleming, T.R. and DeMets, D.L. (1996). Surrogate end points in clinical trials: are we being misled? *Annals of Internal Medicine*, **125**, 605–13.

Freedman, B. (1987). Equipoise and the ethics of clinical research. *New England Journal of Medicine*, **317**, 141–5.

Friedman, L. (1998). Clinical significance vs. statistical significance. In *Encyclopedia of biostatistics* (ed. P. Armitage and T. Colton), pp. 676–8. Wiley, Chichester.

Friedman, L.M., Furberg, C.D., and DeMets, D.L. (1998). *Fundamentals of clinical trials* (3rd edn). Springer, New York.

Friedman, L.M., Simons-Morton, D.G., and Cutler, J.A. (1999). Comparative features of primordial, primary, and secondary prevention trials. In *Clinical trials in cardiovascular disease* (ed. C.H. Hennekens). W.B. Saunders, Philadelphia, PA.

Glynn R.J., Buring J.E., Manson J.E., *et al.* (1994). Adherence to aspirin in the prevention of myocardial infarction. *Archives of Internal Medicine*, **154**, 2649–57.

Haybittle, J.L. (1971). Repeated assessment of results in clinical trials of cancer treatment. *British Journal of Radiology*, **44**, 793–7.

Heart Outcomes Prevention Evaluation Study Investigators (2000). Effects of an angiotensin-converting enzyme inhibitor, ramipril, on cardiovascular events in high-risk patients. *New England Journal of Medicine*, **242**, 145–53.

Hellman, S. and Hellman, D.S. (1991). Of mice but not men: problems of the randomized clinical trial. *New England Journal of Medicine*, **324**, 1585–9.

Hennekens, C.H. and Buring, J.E. (1989). Methodologic considerations in the design and conduct of randomized trials: the US Physicians' Health Study. *Controlled Clinical Trials*, **10**, 142S–50S.

Hlatky, M.A., Rogers,W.J., Johnstone, I., *et al.* (1997). Medical care costs and quality of life after randomization to coronary angioplasty or coronary bypass surgery. Bypass Angioplasty Revascularization Investigation (BARI) Investigators. *New England Journal of Medicine*, **336**, 92–9.

Hypertension Detection and Follow-up Program Cooperative Group (1979). Five-year findings of the hypertension detection and follow-up program. I. Reduction in mortality of persons with high blood pressure, including mild hypertension. *Journal of the American Medical Association*, **242**, 2562–71.

ICH (International Conference on Harmonisation) (1996). *Guidance for industry. E6 good clinical practice: consolidated guidance*. April (http:// www.fda.gov/cder/guidance/9595nl.pdf).

ISIS-2 (Second International Study of Infarct Survival) Collaborative Group (1988). Randomised trial of intravenous streptokinase, oral aspirin, both, or neither among 17 187 cases of suspected acute myocardial infarction: ISIS-2. *Lancet*, **ii**, 349–60.

ISIS-3 (Third International Study of Infarct Survival) Collaborative Group (1992). ISIS-3: a randomised comparison of streptokinase vs tissue plasminogen activator vs anistreplase and of aspirin plus heparin vs aspirin alone among 41 299 cases of suspected acute myocardial infarction. *Lancet*, **339**, 753–70.

Lachin, J.M. (1981). Introduction to sample size determination and power analysis for clinical trials. *Controlled Clinical Trials*, **2**, 93–113.

Lakatos, E. (1986). Sample size determination in clinical trials with time-dependent rates of losses and noncompliance. *Controlled Clinical Trials*, **7**, 189–99.

Lan, K.K.G. and DeMets, D.L. (1989). Group sequential procedures: calendar versus information time. *Statistics in Medicine*, **8**, 1191–8.

Lan, K.K.G. and Wittes, J. (1988). The B-value: a tool for monitoring data. *Biometrics*, **44**, 579–85.

Larson, G.C., McAnulty J.H., and Hallstrom A. (1997). Hospitalization charges in the Antiarrhythmics Versus Implantable Defibrillators (AVID) Trial: the AVID economic analysis study. *Circulation*, **96**, 1–77.

LeLorier, J., Gregoire, G., Benhaddad, A., *et al.* (1997). Discrepancies between meta-analyses and subsequent large randomized, controlled trials. *New England Journal of Medicine*, **337**, 536–42.

Levine, R.J. (1993). New international ethical guidelines for research involving human subjects. *Annals of Internal Medicine*, **119**, 339–41.

Liang, K.Y. and Zeger, S.L. (1989). Longitudinal data analysis using generalized linear models. *Biometrika*, **73**, 13–22.

Meinert, C.L. and Tonascia, S. (1986). *Clinical trials design, conduct, and analysis*. Oxford University Press, New York.

Naughton M.J., Shumaker, S.A., Anderson, R., and Czajkowski, S.M. (1996). Psychological aspects of health-related quality of life measurement: tests and scales. In *Quality of life and pharmacoeconomics in clinical trials* (2nd edn) (ed. B. Spilker), pp. 117–53. Lippincott-Raven, Philadelphia, PA.

NIH (National Institutes of Health) (1994). *Women's Health Initiative Study Protocol*.

O'Brien, P.C. and Fleming, T.R. (1979). A multiple testing procedure for clinical trials. *Biometrics*, **35**, 549–56.

Passamani, E. (1991). Clinical trials—are they ethical? *New England Journal of Medicine*, **324**, 1589–92.

Pawitan, Y. and Hallstrom, A. (1990). Statistical interim monitoring of the Cardiac Arrhythmia Suppression Trial. *Statistics in Medicine*, **9**, 1081–90.

Peto, R. (1995). Clinical trials. In *Treatment of cancer* (3rd edn) (ed. P. Price and K. Sikora), pp. 1039–43. Chapman & Hall, London.

Peto, R., Pike, M.C., Armitage, P., *et al.* (1976). Design and analysis of randomized clinical trials requiring prolonged observations of each patient. I. Introduction and design. *British Journal of Cancer*, **34**, 585–612.

PHS (Physicians' Health Study) Steering Committee of the Research Group (1989). Final report on the aspirin component of the ongoing Physicians' Health Study. *New England Journal of Medicine*, **321**, 129–35.

Piantadosi, S. (1997). *Clinical trials. A methodologic perspective.* Wiley, New York.

Pocock, S.J. (1983). *Clinical trials. A practical approach.* Wiley, New York.

Prentice, R.L. (1989). Surrogate endpoints in clinical trials: definition and operational criteria. *Statistics in Medicine*, **8**, 431–40.

Proschan, M.A., McMahon, R.P., Shih, J.H., *et al.* (2001). Sensitivity analysis using an imputation method for missing binary data in clinical trials. *Journal of Statistics Planning and Inference*, in press.

Psaty, B.M., Smith, N.L., Siscovick, D.S., *et al.* (1997). Health outcomes associated with antihypertensive therapies used as first-line agents. A systematic review and meta-analysis. *Journal of the American Medical Association*, **277**, 739–45.

Rand, C.S. and Weeks, K. (1998). Measuring adherence with medication regimens in clinical care and research. In *The handbook of health behavior change* (ed. S.A. Shumaker, E.B. Schron, J.K. Ockene, and W.L. McBee), pp. 114–32. Springer, New York.

Ruberman, W., Weinblatt, E., Goldberg, J.D., *et al.* (1984). Psychosocial influence on mortality after myocardial infarction. *New England Journal of Medicine*, **311**, 552–9.

Schron, E.B. and Czajkowski, S.M. (2001). Clinical trials. In *Compliance in healthcare and research* (ed. L.E. Burke and I.S. Ockene). Futura, New York.

SHEP (Systolic Hypertension in the Elderly Program) Cooperative Research Group (1991). Prevention of stroke by hypertensive drug therapy in older persons with isolated systolic hypertension: final results of the systolic hypertension in the elderly program. *Journal of the American Medical Association*, **265**, 3255–64.

Staessen, J.A., Fagard, R., Thijs, L., *et al.* (1997). Randomised double-blind comparison of placebo and active treatment for older patients with isolated systolic hypertension. *Lancet*, **350**, 757–64.

Temple, R. and Ellenberg, S.S. (2000). Placebo-controlled trials and active-control trials in the evaluation of new treatments. Part 1: Ethical and scientific issues. *Annals of Internal Medicine*, **133**, 455–63.

VA (Veterans Administration) Cooperative Study Group on Antihypertensive Agents (1967). Effects of treatment on morbidity in hypertension: results in patients with diastolic blood pressures averaging 115 through 129 mmHg. *Journal of the American Medical Association*, **202**, 1028–34.

VA (Veterans Administration) Cooperative Study Group on Antihypertensive Agents (1970). Effects of treatment on morbidity in hypertension: II. Results in patients with diastolic blood pressures averaging 90 through 114 mmHg. *Journal of the American Medical Association*, **213**, 1143–52.

Waldo, A.L., Camm, J.A., de Ruyter, H., Friedman, P.L., MacNeil, D.J., and Pitt, B. (1995). Survival with oral D-sotalol in patients with left ventricular dysfunction after myocardial infarction: rationale, design, and methods (the SWORD Trial). *Journal of the American College of Cardiology*, **75**, 1023–27.

Whitehead, J. (1983). *The design and analysis of sequential clinical trials.* Halstead Press, New York.

Women's Health Initiative Study Group (1998). Design of the Women's Health Initiative clinical trial and observation study. *Controlled Clinical Trials*, **19**, 61–109.

World Medical Association Declaration of Helsinki (2000). *Ethical principles for medical research involving human subjects.* http://www.wma.met/e/policy/17-c_e.html

Wu, M. (1988). Sample size for comparison of changes in the presence of right censoring caused by death, withdrawal, and staggered entry. *Controlled Clinical Trials*, **9**, 32–6.

Yusuf, S., Zucker, D., Peduzzi, P., *et al.* (1994). Effect of coronary artery bypass graft surgery on survival: overview of 10-year results from randomised trials by the Coronary Artery Bypass Graft Surgery Trialists Collaboration. *Lancet*, **334**, 563–70.

6.8 Community-based intervention trials in developed countries

H. Hoffmeister and G. B. M. Mensink

Health promotion of large populations

Community health in industrial societies is most affected by a few chronic diseases, in particular cardiovascular diseases, cancer, adult-onset diabetes, arthropathies, and chronic diseases of the respiratory tract, liver, and gastrointestinal tract. These diseases develop over a long period of time without severely influencing a person's quality of life. In the early stages no symptoms appear and the subjective health status is not necessarily altered because the body can compensate for the effects of the disease with physiological and metabolic changes.

Despite the role of age, genetic predisposition, and possible influence of micro-organisms, the risk of developing one of these diseases early in life depends considerably on an individual's health behaviour. Habits like smoking, alcohol abuse, high fat consumption, physical inactivity, incorrect posture, and lack of hygiene are likely to raise risk factor levels (for example, increased blood lipid levels, high blood pressure, overweight, atherosclerotic lesions of blood vessels, musculoskeletal disorders, chronic inflammations, and infections). These risks play an important role in the initiation and progression of severe chronic diseases.

Strategies to enhance the population's health

Preventive medicine uses two approaches to reduce the population's risk of contracting one of these diseases.

Medical or high-risk approach

In this approach members of the medical profession screen for elevated risk factors and primarily treat individuals with high risk. The identification of high-risk individuals, their consequent medical treatment, and repeated advice to change their lifestyle is one way to enhance the individual's health and thereby the health of the population. Several controlled intervention studies and experimental studies have shown significant reductions in risk factors as described below. Successes have been particularly high in the reduction of high blood pressure and in the treatment of hypercholesterolaemia, disorders of carbohydrate metabolism, and subsequent cardiovascular diseases. Currently, several projects are being conducted in which people are screening for prevailing infections, for example *Helicobacter pylori*, hepatitis B and C viruses, and *Chlamydia pneumoniae*, and subsequently given treatment to validate the impact on long-term outcomes like cancer, liver cirrhosis, and cardiovascular disease. The high-risk approach has, however, limitations and disadvantages. The previously mentioned chronic diseases are also prevalent among many people without elevated risk factor levels and early medical indications. Screening, drug treatment, and individual health counselling are expensive and, in addition, serious undesired side-effects of drug treatment have been observed.

Public health approach

The public health approach is directed towards general populations in communities, regions, or whole countries rather than to individuals. It is concerned with creating a healthy lifestyle, convincing the population to avoid health risks, and teaching skills to lower or avoid drug abuse and medical consumption and to cope with crucial life events. This public approach tries to enhance the knowledge about risky and preferable health behaviour as well as to change unhealthy attitudes and beliefs. If necessary it may also aim to change the community environment. It is the public health answer in the fight against widespread diseases and the promotion of the population's health. Various uncontrolled activities and programmes are carried out in communities, on a regional and state level, using different ways to increase health knowledge and to influence attitudes and health behaviour of community inhabitants. While it can be assumed that none of these activities have adverse effects, it is not clear whether they really work. Sufficient knowledge about the most effective intervention strategies is missing and often the cost-effectiveness has not been taken into account appropriately.

Determining the impact of community intervention

Scientific evidence is needed to demonstrate that the community approach to promote public health is broadly effective. The different aspects and elements of underlying theories (such as social cognition theory and persuasive communication theory) must be tested in appropriate studies and evaluated with respect to their health impact. The evaluation should also be used as a feedback for the development of lifestyle intervention methods. This is a difficult and expensive scientific task. These aspects of community health are so complex that it is difficult to find a general definition or an agreement about a set of indicators to measure them appropriately. Changes in knowledge—for instance about the unhealthy effects of smoking; good dental hygiene; or attitudes, beliefs, and health behaviour (such as jogging, safer sex, or increased vegetable consumption)—can be observed early by 'process evaluation'. Such changes, however, do not provide certainty of health improvement. The process of determining the physically measurable outcomes of intervention is complicated by the fact that there will be a time delay in changes in risk factor levels and disease prevalence. Changes in morbidity and mortality rates are usually not detectable until several years later.

During the last 25 years a few large community-oriented intervention studies have been conducted in the United States and Europe (Table 1). The objective of these studies was to reduce the occurrence of cardiovascular diseases and other chronic diseases in large populations by means of primary prevention. These studies represent a logical consequence of the modern understanding of non-communicable disease patterns and their development in industrial societies. Nevertheless, these cardiovascular disease intervention studies report only minor changes in indicators of risk, morbidity, and mortality. In addition, the outcomes are inconsistent although intervention measures were more or less similar. Even the well-designed studies, performed with massive intervention effort, show only limited success. The somewhat disappointing results are not necessarily due to a general failure of community-based interventions. Methodological difficulties in design or analysis, of which the researchers were originally unaware, may account for the lack of success. This can be derived from a meta-analysis conducted with published cardiovascular intervention studies, fulfilling the criteria of comparability (Sellers *et al.* 1997). To a certain extent the variability in outcome can be subscribed to different evaluation characteristics like

Table 1 Major community trials on cardiovascular disease prevention

Study details		**Net risk factor changes**		
North Karelia Project (Vartiainen et al. 1994)		*After 20 years*	*Men (%)*	*Women (%)*
Start	1972	Cholesterol	4.0	–1.4
		Smoking	–14.0	–2.7
Duration	10 years intervention	SBP	–0.7	–3.3
		DBP	2.1	–1.0
Population	180 000 inhabitants, aged 25–59 years			
Intervention	Comprehensive community intervention Reduction of cardiovascular risk factors			
Design	One intervention, one (later two) reference group(s)			
Evaluation	Three (later five) independent samples			
Results	After 20 years declining risk factors still observed; initially stronger decline in total mortality, but after 15 years similar to rest of Finland			
Coronary Risk Factor Study (CORIS) (Rossouw et al. 1993)		*After 4 years*	*Men (%)*	*Women (%)*
Start	1979	Cholesterol		
		L	–1.4	–0.6
Duration	4 years intervention	H	1.5	1.5
		Smoking		
Population	11 700 white persons, aged 15–64 years	L	1.8	–17.4
		H	1.7	–22.9
Intervention	Comprehensive community intervention	SBP		
	Small mass media and interpersonal (high intensity) intervention	L	–2.0	–2.4
		H	1.9	–1.1
	Reduce cholesterol, BP, smoking, stress	DBP		
	Increase physical activity	L	–4.3	–3.7
		H	–5.2	–3.2
Design	Two intervention groups (one low intensity, one high intensity intervention), one reference group	BMI		
		L	–0.4	–2.0
		H	–0.4	–1.2
Evaluation	Independent and cohort samples before and after intervention, surveys at 4-year intervals			
Results	Low-intensity intervention achieves as much reduction of risk factors as high-intensity intervention After 12 years the low-intensity intervention town still had a significantly better risk profile (Steyn et al. 1997) The risk profile of the high-intervention town was similar to that of the reference town			

Study details		**Net risk factor changes**		
Stanford Five City Project (Farquhar *et al.* 1990)		*After 6 years*	*Cohort (%)*	*Independent (%)*
Start	1980	Cholesterol	−2	−2
		Smoking	−13	0
Duration	5 years intervention	SBP	−4	−4
		DBP	−5	−5
Population	122 800 people, aged 12–74 years	BMI	0	−2
		Pulse rate	−3	−3
Intervention	Comprehensive community intervention Reduce cholesterol, BP, smoking, weight; increase physical activity			
Design	Two intervention groups, two reference groups, one for mortality and morbidity trend monitoring, based on Three Communities Study			
Evaluation	2-year distances independent and cohort samples			
Results	Reduction in some risk factors and total mortality risk score (−15%); not significant in independent samples			
Minnesota Heart Health Program (Luepker *et al.* 1994)		*After 7 years*	*Cohort (%)*	*Independent (%)*
Start	1980	Cholesterol	1.4	0.5
		Smoking		
Duration	5–6 years intervention	Men	9.5	−1.2
		Women	3.2	−12.1
Population	231 000 adults	SBP	1.1	0.7
		DBP	0.8	−0.3
Intervention	Improve health behaviour	BMI	0.1	−1.2
	Reduce cholesterol by 7 mg/dl, BP by 2 mmHg, smoking by 3%	PA	9.4	6.3
	Increase physical activity by 50 kcal/day	Risk score	3.4	2.8
	Reduce cardiovascular disease morbidity and mortality by 15%			
Design	Three intervention groups, three reference groups matched on size, type, and distance from Minneapolis			
Evaluation	Independent and cohort samples			
Results	Not successful in reducing risk factors more than favourable secular trends No significant reduction of coronary heart disease and stroke morbidity and mortality among 30–74 years age group after 10 years (Luepker *et al.* 1996)			
Pawtucket Heart Health Study (Carleton *et al.* 1995)		*After 8.5 years*	*Cohort (%)*	*Independent (%)*
Start	1981	Cholesterol	−0.7	0.1
		Smoking	−4.1	0.9
Duration	7 years intervention	SBP	0.5	−2.1
		DBP	−0.9	1.6
Population	42 000 people, aged 18–64 years	BMI	0	0.8
		Risk score	−25.6	−21.7
Intervention	Community activation			
Design	One intervention group, one reference group			
Evaluation	Formative and process evaluation, six biennal household surveys			
Results	Small non-significant reductions in cholesterol and BP Not successful in maintaining cardiovascular disease risk reduction			

Study details		**Net risk factor changes**		
German Cardiovascular Prevention Study (Hoffmeister *et al.* 1996)		*After 7 years*	*Men (%)*	*Women (%)*
Start	1984	Cholesterol	–1.9	–1.8
		Smoking	–9.7	–1.8
Duration	7 years intervention	SBP	–1.6	–2.4
		DBP	–1.6	–2.3
		BMI	0.4	–0.3
Population	500 000 people target population, aged 25–69 years			
Intervention	Comprehensive community intervention Reduce cholesterol by 3.5%, BP by 1.5%, smoking by 7.5%, BMI by 1%, mortality by 8%			
Design	Six intervention groups (pooled representative for Germany), one reference group (total of Germany)			
Evaluation	Three independent samples			
Results	Significant reductions of risk factors except BMI, risk score lowered Total and cardiovascular mortality in the pooled intervention regions was not significantly reduced compared with the reference, after 7 years			
Kilkenny Health Project (Shelley *et al.* 1995)		*After 8 years*	*Men (%)*	*Women (%)*
Start	1985	Cholesterol	5.8	–0.7
		Smoking	6.2	–8.8
Duration	8 years intervention	SBP	0	–0.7
		DBP	7.2	2.4
Population	70 000 people	BMI	–2.2	–3.5
Intervention	Comprehensive community intervention			
Design	One intervention group, one reference group			
Evaluation	Independent samples			
Results	Not successful owing to similar changes in risk factor levels in the intervention and reference communities			

Net change = [(level intervention last year/level intervention first year) – (level reference last year/level reference first year)] × 100.

Significance levels are not provided because the studies used different statistical tests, making a direct comparison difficult.

BMI, body mass index; BP, blood pressure; DBP, diastolic blood pressure; H, high-intensity intervention; L, low-intensity intervention; PA, physical activity; SBP, systolic blood pressure.

length of follow-up time, response rates, matching of intervention and reference population, and adjustment for covariates.

In a minor way, the variability of the study results in this meta-analysis was explained by differences in intervention measures. A major critical point for these intervention studies may be that the effects on risk factors are still too weak, thus explaining the lack of impact of these studies concerning morbidity and mortality. Furthermore, even if results are promising after the first phase of intervention, long-term compliance is necessary to achieve substantial effects on disease endpoints. The efforts to achieve prolonged changes in health behaviour may have been insufficient. More understanding of which interventions work and research on the most effective and efficient ways to change the population's health behaviour—especially in the fields of smoking cessation, promoting healthy eating habits (and provision of high-quality foods), and enhancing physical activity in the general population—will help to improve the outcome of future interventions.

In recent years some well-conducted community intervention studies have shown the advantages of this approach. For example, projects concerning HIV infection/AIDS prevention have been successful, at least in Western community intervention projects, in limiting the epidemic (CDC 1999).

The dietary supplementation of communities in general or of high-risk regions with deficiencies in trace elements, minerals, or vitamins is also a possibility. In the 1970s for example, the World Health Organization (**WHO**) and other national health boards recommended the fluoridation of drinking water. Studies conducted in several countries showed lower rates of dental caries after supplementation of fluoride in drinking water compared with reference areas. Partly because of perceived unwanted side-effects, enforced supplementation of this kind is unacceptable in many countries. However, fluoride supplements for treatment in childhood, nutrient-enriched products in regions suffering from micronutrient deficiencies (such as iodine-enriched salt in Western Europe, and selenium-enriched bread in Finland), and folate supplements to be taken before and during pregnancy are commonly available and can be recommended in community health promotion programmes.

Particularly in developing countries, community-based nutrition intervention projects can be successful in the fight against malnutrition, if the underlying problem is identified and understood, and goals and objectives are clearly set. The impact is enhanced if the project concentrates on specific target group like pregnant or breast-feeding mothers.

The final evaluation of an intervention trial should not only focus on health outcome variables but should also include issues such as social and structural characteristics of the intervention communities which strongly determine the outcome of intervention. The intensity and density of the intervention should be optimized to meet the specific goals. The study design should also guarantee enough statistical power to evaluate the achievement of these goals. It is important that the natural variation in health indicators within the observed communities should be estimated before initiation of the trial. The main concerns in the design and the evaluation of community intervention trials are discussed below.

Rationale of community intervention trials

Health promotion within the structure of local communities or regions seems to be a good strategy to reduce common diseases. It is hypothesized that this approach has advantages compared with both individual treatment and to large national programmes (which often lack components that fit the individual). In this context several statements have to be considered.

1. Most people in a community need greater and more specific knowledge about health issues before they are likely to change unhealthy behaviour. In addition, widespread attitudes and beliefs incongruent with evidence-based knowledge have to be corrected.
2. A change to a healthier lifestyle is beneficial, not only for people at high risk but also for all inhabitants of a community. It may also improve life quality and satisfaction.
3. In Western societies most adults have one or more elevated risk factors for cardiovascular (and other chronic) diseases. A reduction of their risk factor levels is likely to have a large impact on the health status of populations.
4. Programmes and activities to promote health in relation to particular disease outcomes will not only reduce the risk for the intended diseases but may also affect many other disease outcomes. For example, healthy lifestyle campaigns directed towards smoking cessation, increased vegetable consumption, and physical activity are useful in preventing many non-communicable diseases (such as cardiovascular diseases, major forms of cancer, adult-onset diabetes, and the chronic diseases of the respiratory and gastrointestinal tract).
5. An action centre implemented in the community which initiates, conducts, and co-ordinates health-oriented programmes is an important tool to improve the health status of a community.
6. Structures already existing within communities such as schools, sports grounds, clubs, and health facilities, and community leaders will facilitate health promotion and preventive measures and make them more cost-effective compared with health promotion solely focused on individuals.
7. An individual is usually influenced by the community in which he or she lives. Health-improving activities within the community will encourage personal involvement in health-related issues.
8. A wider acceptance of health programmes and projects supported by local opinion leaders will enhance confidence in the benefits of such activities and will make it easier for individuals to accept and use them.

Objectives of community intervention trials

The typical conditions of social life and the environment in a community often determine the objectives and the likelihood for success of community intervention. The overall health in such a community is influenced by many aspects such as knowledge, awareness, and behaviour of the individuals, health facilities and provisions within the communities (health-oriented activity groups, hospitals, sports grounds, local media, and so on), and the specific risk profile of the community (regional eating habits and leisure time behaviour, mean risk factor levels, specific morbidity and mortality). Since these aspects interact with each other, the community intervention measures should try to influence all relevant aspects to improve health.

Within the observed community a positive preventive atmosphere has to be created. This process of change in particular health aspects should be studied in intervention trials (in subsequent time periods). In community intervention trials, this 'process evaluation' was seldom used, although it could give a deeper insight into the influences of intervention on the process and determinants of health changes. This cannot be obtained sufficiently solely from measuring the outcome. The achievement of the objectives can be observed by specific outcome measurements, which reflect the changes of various health aspects (Fig. 1).

Improvement of health knowledge, attitudes, and behaviour

Instead of concentrating on an individual's behaviour, community intervention is concerned with the manipulation of health knowledge, health attitudes, and health behaviour in whole communities. Thus, an important goal of community intervention is to achieve a favourable change in these health aspects in the whole population or large groups within the population.

A primary target of community intervention studies is a verifiable improvement of health knowledge in the community which should be maintained for a long period of time. This does not guarantee improved health, but it supports all the other efforts to achieve better health behaviour. A change in health knowledge within the community is one of the earliest detectable effects of community intervention. Health-oriented lessons in schools are very effective in this respect. They may not only influence the children but also their families.

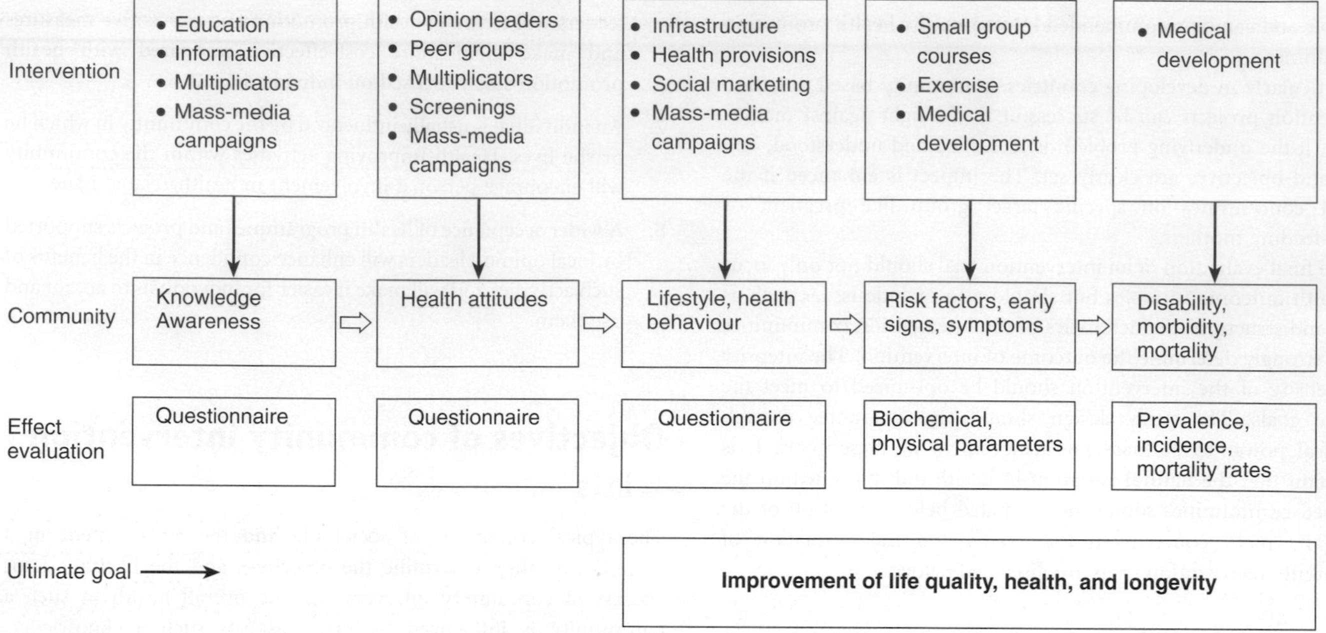

Fig. 1 Elements, pathways, and outcomes of community intervention.

Changes in attitudes and beliefs are further aims of community intervention. Attitudes and beliefs are not always in accordance with the prevailing knowledge. Although many attitudes may be based on particular knowledge, this is not a necessary condition for health attitudes and beliefs. A community may have developed certain health attitudes (like 'too much coffee is bad for your heart') without knowing why the behaviour is unhealthy (it may increase serum cholesterol levels). On the contrary, an increase in knowledge does not always change a person's attitude. Although a certain behaviour (like smoking) may be generally accepted as harmful, it is not necessarily regarded as a risk for oneself ('My grandfather smoked his whole life and lived until 90'). Changes in attitudes and beliefs can also be observed as early effects in intervention populations.

The objective which is most difficult to achieve via intervention actions and programmes is to gain significant influence on the health behaviour of a large part of the community. Although a change in knowledge and attitude is possible, past experience of community intervention trials shows that changes in behaviour with high impact on health (such as smoking, nutritional habits, and physical activity) are difficult to achieve and are even more difficult to maintain over a long period of time.

Changes in behaviour are difficult to achieve even in communities with a well-established infrastructure to enhance and maintain health. This becomes obvious by looking at smoking behaviour. The majority of people are aware that smoking is the most dangerous single health risk of industrialized societies. Even so, a large number of people in these societies smoke. This discrepancy between health knowledge and attitudes was also observed in a study among German schoolchildren. All of the children who smoked on a regular basis knew about the main diseases caused by smoking. But despite this knowledge, 20 per cent of them wanted to continue smoking. The 80 per cent saying that they would like to stop or reduce smoking are more susceptible to programmes, courses, and other community activities concerning smoking cessation.

Societal conditions

An improvement of health knowledge, attitudes, and beliefs does not inevitably lead to changes in behaviour. These changes are likely to occur if the community's health infrastructure is appropriate (that is, enough health-related information sources, courses to stop smoking or other drug consumption, availability of fresh vegetables, low-fat foods, sports grounds, and so on). An improvement in an insufficient infrastructure should be an additional target of intervention. Societal characteristics of a community should therefore be analysed and taken into account before starting a community intervention project. In Germany, there has been a strong growth in self-help groups during the last 30 years. This was initiated by so-called coronary heart groups for patients after myocardial infarction. They started lifelong endurance training and organized healthy lifestyle programmes. Local groups are now concerned with cardiovascular prevention, primary prevention therapies against rheumatic disease, therapies for diabetes, and rehabilitation of specific cancers—these groups meet regularly in many communities. A validation of the effectiveness and efficiency of these forms of community intervention has not been performed.

Risk factors, early signs, and symptoms

Altered behaviour should lead to a measurable change in physical risk factors. Changes in risk factors like obesity, high blood pressure, hypercholesterolaemia, specific liver enzyme levels (as indicators of alcohol abuse), and high resting heart rate (as an indicator of poor physical fitness) can give important indications of the success of intervention. Achieving favourable changes in risk factors is the most common and verifiable goal of community intervention. It is assumed that a favourable change of risk levels or of early signs and symptoms of diseases will improve the health of a population. A community intervention trial is needed to prove this assumption.

The interdependency of risk factor changes, and sometimes contrasting impacts on different disease outcomes, complicates the determination of overall success. An improvement of certain risk factors may induce an undesirable trend in others. Several studies observed an increase in body mass index among people who stopped smoking. Measures to reduce a risk factor may not be beneficial for the prevention of all kinds of disease. Individuals with high levels of cardiovascular risk factors have an increased risk of developing coronary heart disease and premature death. Replacing a high amount of saturated fatty acids by polyunsaturated fatty acids in the diet leads to lowered serum cholesterol levels. This is a favourable change concerning the development of atherosclerosis and cardiovascular diseases, but some studies suggest that there may be an increased risk of specific cancers among individuals who have consumed a high amount of polyunsaturated fatty acids (Hursting *et al.* 1990; Staessen *et al.* 1997; Veierod *et al.* 1997).

It is observed in many studies that people consuming moderate amounts of alcohol have a lower risk for cardiovascular disease than teetotallers and heavy drinkers. This observation is biologically plausible because alcohol intake enhances serum high-density lipoprotein cholesterol and lowers the risk for thrombosis. Even total mortality rates are lower in moderate drinkers compared with teetotallers or heavy drinkers (Hoffmeister *et al.* 1999; Liao *et al.* 2000), although alcohol consumption increases the risk for certain cancers, liver diseases, some other diseases, and traffic accidents. An intervention which recommends total abstinence may therefore not be appropriate. It is possible that societies with very restricted alcohol rules suffer more from alcoholism than those with a liberal attitude.

Several hypotheses about causal links between certain risk factors and the development of disease have been proposed but many could not be confirmed. Therefore, the objective should not be to achieve solely a reduction of risk factor levels. For example, at present, there is a controversy among health scientists whether a high intake of antioxidants (such as tocopherol, vitamin C, provitamin A, and selenium) has a preventive effect on cancer and cardiovascular diseases. As long as convincing evidence for a causal link is missing, it is not regarded as necessary to adapt current recommendations.

Morbidity and mortality rates

The promotion of a healthy lifestyles and improvement of risk factor levels is just one necessary step on the way to increasing health. The final success of a community intervention programme must be analysed on the basis of changes in disability, morbidity, and mortality rates. At the community level, these outcomes are usually measured by prevalence rates, incidence rates, lost years of life, mean age at onset of disease, or mean age at death from a specific disease. Improvement of the quality of life may be measured as well as the average years of disease-free life of a population. Not only are changes in specific mortality rates important but also changes in morbidity rates and premature disabilities. These outcomes are often overlooked in the evaluation of community trials, although they can largely contribute to the healthy life expectancy.

In addition, the intervention should have a positive impact on total mortality. A successful reduction of coronary heart disease mortality through intervention should, for example, not be accompanied by higher cancer mortality rates. A real improvement of health can only be ascertained if total mortality rates are decreased and life expectancy is improved.

Most chronic diseases occur at older ages. To reach older people through community intervention, and to have an essential influence on the morbidity and mortality of very old people, seems impossible. For example, high mortality rates of cardiovascular diseases occurring at old age in a society are not alarming but, on the contrary, provide an indication of superior health status and medical care in this society. Health promotion cannot prevent all diseases and will not lead to immortality. The purpose of the intervention measures is to reduce the occurrence of diseases and deaths early in life. In the Western world this means a reduction of mortality and morbidity before reaching the age of 70 to 80 years. Thus this should be a criterion to measure the success of intervention, which is possible in a well-designed trial.

Early estimate of mortality outcome: the multiple logistic function

As mentioned above, the final evaluation of success of community trials should be based on the changes in premature morbidity and mortality of the disease(s) of interest as well as total mortality. In practice, this can only be evaluated after a long time period in which the detectable changes in disease rates will occur. Changes in risk factor levels will occur much earlier. For example, the elevated risk of smoking on lung cancer will remain for about 10 to 20 years after smoking cessation (for cardiovascular disease, the risk will drop faster). Consequently, most researchers want to summarize risk factor changes to predict changes in morbidity or mortality in the long term. Project financers and politicians in public health are also eager for an early estimate of the success of the intervention programme.

A classical tool to summarize the changes in risk factor levels is the 'multiple logistic function'. Such a function weighs the changes in major risk factors according to their importance as contributors to mortality risk. The weighting factors are derived from multiple logistic regressions of longitudinal mortality data. Multiple logistic functions are used by many epidemiologists to estimate mortality risk from early measured risk factors.

Although these functions are widely used for summary evaluation of risk factor changes, it is important to be careful when applying them. The estimated weights (from a different population) may not reflect the impact of risk factors on mortality in the observed population. The logistic model does not consider follow-up time and censoring (owing to unfinished observation times for drop-outs and individuals still alive). Basically, a multiplicative effect of risk factors is assumed which is not appropriate, for instance, for all coronary heart disease risk factors. Inclusion of new risk factors will therefore change the estimates of the others. The estimated function is likely to be more a reflection of the model than of the data. More recent multiple logistic functions are based on more sophisticated proportional hazard models (Cox and Oakes 1984).

Intervention in communities

The development of chronic diseases early in life may result from unhealthy behaviour patterns and unfavourable life conditions. A major fraction of the population shows such behaviours. Therefore, health promotion and disease prevention programmes try to manipulate this behaviour and try to establish structures which support a healthy lifestyle.

Local communities as the field of intervention activities

Local communities play a key role in the realization of intervention measures. They form the field in which most events of social life take place. They provide the structures and institutions for daily life. For example, the local media are effective instruments for spreading health-related information. Churches, schools, sports clubs, self-help groups, and other organizations with regular meetings are important institutions for creating a positive intervention climate and for establishing norms and reinforcing them frequently. The health system and the food distribution system can also be used for the purposes of health promotion.

Available health structures, information resources, and people and groups with influence and credibility within the community are important tools for reaching the objectives in community intervention trials. They will provide the conditions by which a larger population can be exposed to messages about healthy lifestyle, become involved in health topics, and experience the advantages of improved health behaviour. Different methods of communication, education, and advertising concerning health issues can be used to achieve improvements in health knowledge, attitudes, and behaviour.

Theories and frameworks focused on community intervention trials

Intervention methods and activities in community studies should have a theoretical foundation. Social science research has provided profound experience about the psychological and sociological mechanisms by which new norms in daily life can be achieved and propagated, new fashions can be created, and more involvement in health issues can be generated. Different social theories and frameworks attempt to explain individual behaviour as well as trends and fashions within populations. All of these general behaviour theories can be applied to issues relevant for health. They should be used to define a set of measurements in a community intervention study. Important points and elements applicable to community intervention are listed in Fig. 2.

One of the earliest and most often applied theories is the 'social cognition theory' formerly known as 'social learning theory' (Bandura 1986). The focal point of this theory is that changes of behaviour can be achieved through intensive exposure to important models (ideals or archetypes, such as pop stars or sport stars). Self-efficacy (including self-esteem, self-regard, self-respect, self-confidence, competence, and effective functioning) and group efficacy play an important role in changes of behaviour. It is influenced by personal, observed, or otherwise transferred experiences. Furthermore, according to this theory, for maintenance of a newly adapted behaviour, a supportive social setting and the development of skills are needed.

To adopt this framework for health purposes, opinion leaders in a community (for example, the mayor, the medical professionals, a local sport star) should be involved in intervention management. They should convincingly and repeatedly appeal to the public to stop smoking, eat less fat, be more physically active, and so on. In addition, skills training should be organized within communities.

The 'theory on reasoned action', which became the 'theory of planned behaviour', analyses and predicts behaviour, and was mainly developed by Ajzen and Fishbein and extended by Ajzen and Madden (1986). This framework applied to health promotion, concentrates on establishing the credibility of people distributing information about health issues, favourable lifestyle, and disease prevention measures. The theory suggests that individuals pass through a series of steps from awareness, attitudes, and knowledge acquisition through to motivation and skill development, and finally take action to change behaviour. The prevailing subjective norms in the community have a high impact on the health behaviour of its members. Perceived behaviour control is the ability to cope with difficulties by adapting to positive behaviour. To sustain adapted behaviour, skills of self-management have to be learned. The theory can be used in community intervention trials by regularly distributing information about healthy lifestyle in the media (such as local press and television) whilst ensuring high credibility.

'Persuasive communication' campaigns (McGuire 1984) try to convince individuals to take more responsibility for their own health maintenance. Based on psychological theories concerning communication, attitudes, and behaviour, a seven-step procedure is proposed.

1. Reviewing the realities.
2. Axiological analysis.
3. Surveying the sociocultural situation.
4. Mapping the mental matrix.
5. Teasing out the target themes.
6. Construction of the communication.
7. Evaluating the effectiveness.

The sixth step is the crucial one, because it is the practical application. It uses a communication set containing aspects such as credibility, attractiveness, and power. Elements mediating the communication, such as exposure, skill acquisition, and motivation, are also implemented in this framework.

The 'precede–proceed model' (Green and Kreuter 1991) for educational intervention is a framework to plan and administer health education programmes. It begins with five phases: social, epidemiological, behavioural/environmental, educational/organization, and administration/policy diagnosis. This is followed by implementation, process, impact, and outcome evaluation. This plan of action covers the multidimensionality of health and its large number of collaborators.

'Social market theories' analyse the needs of a target population (Kotler and Clarke 1987). Based on these needs adequate products can be offered and costs and benefits for the provider and consumer can be estimated. Preventive health services are products for which the audience has to be defined, messages have to be developed, and the most effective channels for acceptance selected. These theories combine and apply elements of the theories and frameworks discussed above.

Study design

The community intervention study has by its very nature a quasi-experimental design. It is experimental in the sense that the observer manipulates the intervention community with public health pro-

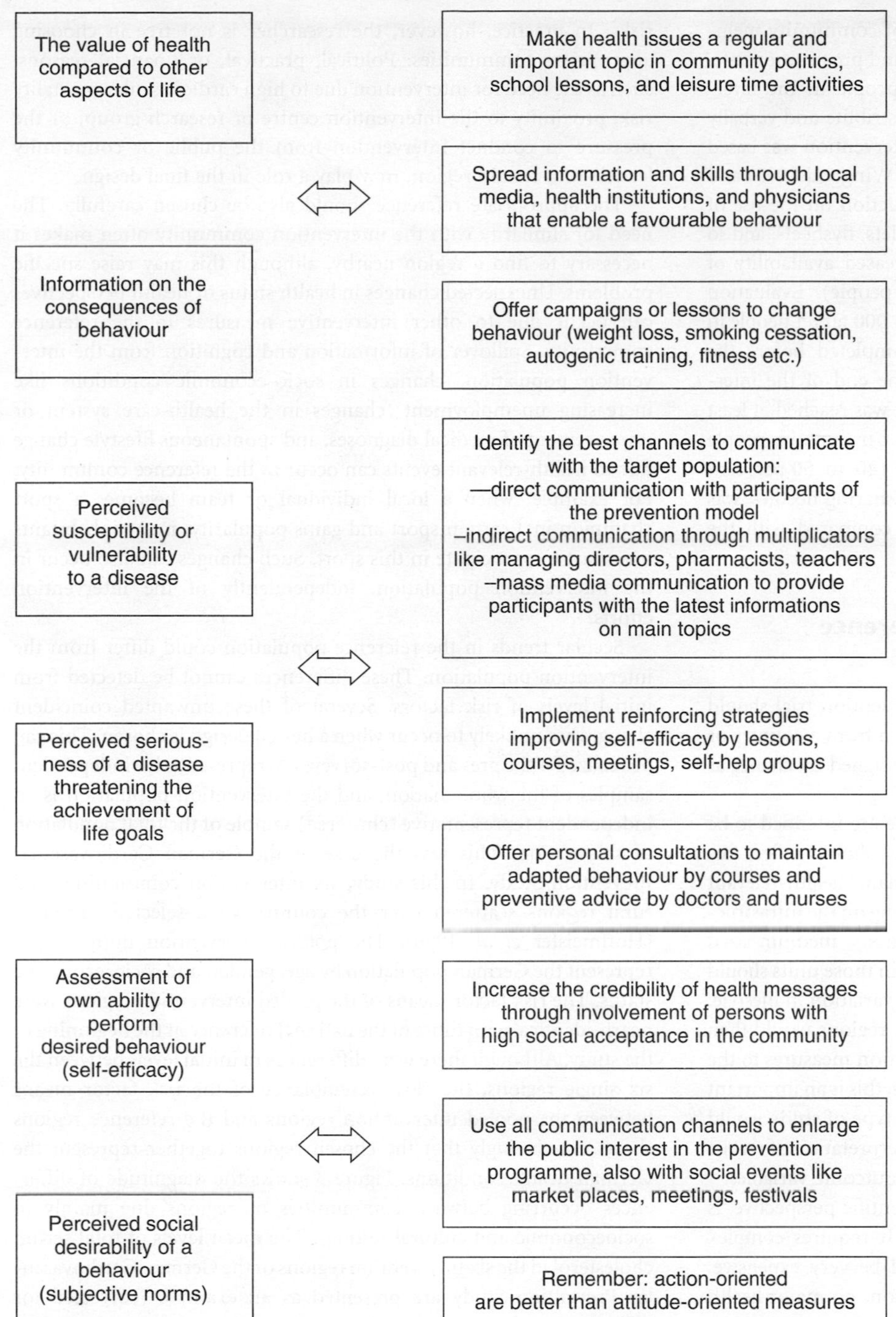

Fig. 2 Focus points for influencing behaviour and elements of intervention.

grammes and observes the changes in the population against a reference (without such manipulation). It is quasi-experimental in so far as the observer cannot control for every exposure or health-related change in the intervention or in the reference community.

A well-chosen study design can partly prevent unwanted confounding exposures and will control more efficiently for unknown or unexpected influences on the population's health. Observing several intervention versus reference communities which are spread over the region of interest is one way of ruling out initial inequalities and lowering the chance of unexpected confounding trends between intervention and reference areas. This can also be achieved by taking 'embedded' intervention communities out of a larger region which may serve as a reference.

Most of the intervention studies listed in Table 1 follow a design comparing intervention with reference communities. A similar design was also used in the successful Centers for Disease Control and AIDS Community Demonstration Projects in the United States. To each of five intervention communities spread over the United States, a reference community was matched by density of community members at risk, availability and use of illegal drugs, and prostitution rate. During 4 years of intervention, around 1000 people in the intervention regions were recruited and trained to distribute and verbally reinforce prevention messages and materials. Intervention was based on behaviour change theories (DiClemente and Wingood 1995) and provided basic AIDS-related information, instruction on the use of condoms, 'small-media' materials (booklets, leaflets, flysheets, and so on) about the role model's progress, and increased availability of condoms and bleach kits (for needle-sharing people). Evaluation was conducted by anonymous interviews with 15 000 target people in 10 cross-sectional waves. Two waves were completed before the implementation of intervention activities. At the end of the intervention, more than half of the target population was reached at least once. A statistically significant increase by 74 per cent in people carrying condoms and safer sexual behaviour (40 to 50 per cent higher), as well as increased bleach use in those sharing needles, was observed in the intervention communities as compared with the reference communities.

The choice of intervention and reference population

Theoretically, the design for a community intervention trial should include a group of communities randomly chosen from a country or region of interest. The chosen units should be assigned by chance as intervention or reference units.

If the findings of an intervention programme are intended to be applied to a larger population in the future, they should reflect this population. The units must represent the main health-relevant differences within the country or region. Depending on the infrastructure of the country it should include rural regions, medium-sized towns, and parts of large towns. Inhabitants within those units should reflect the variety of socio-economic groups and variation in lifestyle. The samples of these intervention and reference regions would then allow generalization of the outcomes of intervention measures to the total population. From a health policy perspective, this is an important aspect of a community intervention study. This type of study would have the additional advantage of avoiding misinterpretation of results due to unknown secular trends and variance of outcome variables.

Such a design, although desirable from a scientific perspective, is often not feasible for many practical reasons. It requires complex organization and logistical support, and would be very expensive. After a long period of intervention and evaluation, no major health impact might be visible and cost-effectiveness might be unfavourable.

Therefore, in most conducted trials, one or only a few regions were taken as intervention and reference areas. Table 1 shows the main characteristics of the major cardiovascular disease community intervention studies. The number of selected communities, size of intervention populations, intervention and observation period, and other typical issues are described. In most of the community intervention trials conducted, between one and three cities or parts of cities were chosen as intervention units and one or two as reference cities.

In such a situation, it is even more important to ensure that the reference community resembles the intervention community as closely as possible. Both regions should be identical with respect to sociodemographic structure, initial risk factor levels, and mortality risks. In practice, however, the researcher is not free in choosing appropriate communities. Political, practical, or financial reasons, such as the need for intervention due to high cardiovascular mortality risk, proximity to the intervention centre or research group, or the pressure to conduct intervention from the public or community leaders of a certain region, may play a role in the final design.

The appropriate reference should also be chosen carefully. The need for similarity with the intervention community often makes it necessary to find a region nearby, although this may raise specific problems. Unexpected changes in health status or health perspectives can occur due to other interventive measures in the reference community. Spillover of information and cognition from the intervention population, changes in socio-economic conditions like increasing unemployment, changes in the health-care system or improvement of medical diagnoses, and spontaneous lifestyle change due to health-relevant events can occur in the reference community. For example, when a local individual or team becomes a sport champion in a certain sport and gains popularity, many inhabitants may start to participate in this sport. Such changes can also occur in the intervention population, independently of the intervention efforts.

Secular trends in the reference population could differ from the intervention population. These differences cannot be detected from initial levels of risk factors. Several of these unwanted coincident changes are unlikely to occur when a nested design is chosen. This can be realized if the pre- and post-surveys are representative independent samples of the whole nation, and the intervention population is an independent representative (clustered) sample of the total population of this nation. This was the case in the German Cardiovascular Prevention Study. In this study, six intervention communities and rural regions scattered over the country were selected (Table 1) (Hoffmeister *et al.* 1996). The pooled intervention units closely represent the German population by age, gender, and socio-economic status. The risk factor means of the pooled intervention regions were nearly identical with those of the national reference at the beginning of the study. Although there were differences in initial levels between the six single regions, the close resemblance of the risk factor means between the pooled intervention regions and the reference regions shows convincingly that the chosen regions together represent the German health conditions. Figure 3 shows the magnitude of differences occurring between communities or regions due mainly to socioeconomic and cultural settings. The mean levels of total serum cholesterol in the six intervention regions of the German Cardiovascular Prevention Study are presented as an example (corrected for differences in age and gender distribution). The figure also shows that the intervention had a delayed impact for this risk factor. Often the financial aspects of such a widespread reference will force projects to use a different reference design. National representative surveys, however, can also be used as national health surveys.

Survey sampling

Population surveys should be conducted before, during (often at midterm), and after the intervention programme. An additional survey, some years after the end of intervention measures, could provide insight into the endurance and implementation of improved health behaviour. The surveys should preferably be independent samples with the same age and socio-economic distributions. Ideally,

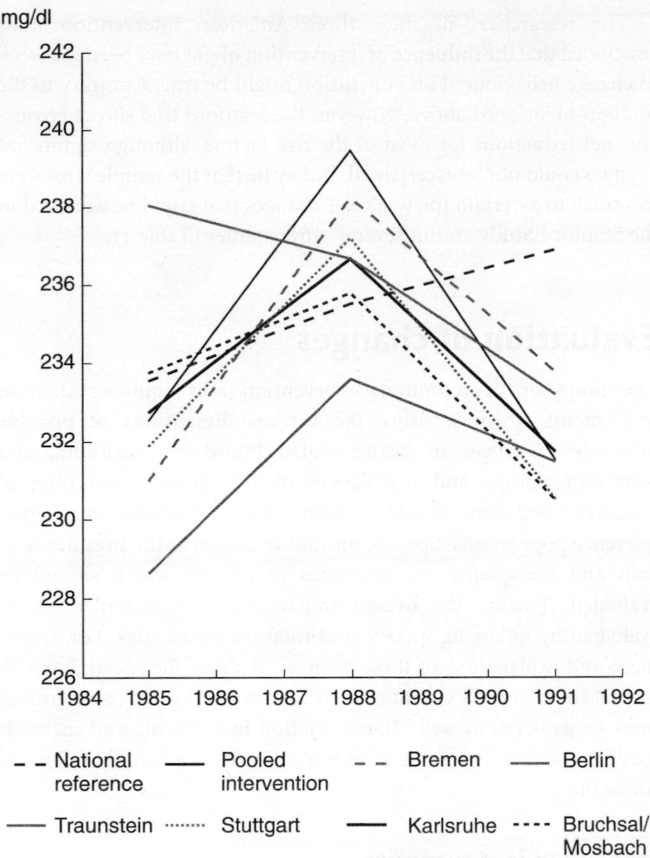

Fig. 3 Changes in mean total serum cholesterol values (German Cardiovascular Prevention Study study, 1984 to 1992).

the samples for both intervention and reference communities should be random, representative, or stratified samples of the community. In a situation where intervention programmes focus on certain risk groups (age, ethnic, or socio-economic factors), it might be more effective to restrict the sample to this target population. Usually community intervention is directed towards the whole population but the disease of interest is only restricted to a certain group (for example, 40- to 60-year age groups for coronary heart disease). Even so, it would be appropriate to sample just this group.

The researcher should make a great effort to achieve maximal response rates in the survey samples. To avoid a substantial bias, the response rate should be at least 70 per cent. Non-respondents can differ considerably from (primary) respondents in health behaviour and sensitivity to health intervention programmes. For a valid evaluation of the intervention-related changes it is important to achieve a high response rate. Non-respondents should be contacted repeatedly to persuade them to participate in the surveys. At the very least, minimal information about non-respondents should be gathered, for instance through a short questionnaire. This should provide some information about the difference between non-respondents and participants.

The attempts to enlarge the response rate should be equal in both the intervention and the reference communities. If response rates between the intervention and reference communities differ considerably, this response bias could have major consequences for evaluation of the intervention trial. In the German national health surveys, for example, the smoking prevalence among spontaneous respondents (first 50 per cent of the sample) was 1 to 2 per cent lower than in the next 20 per cent of respondents. Fortunately, the non-respondents did report no higher smoking prevalence in a short questionnaire.

The use of a cohort sample may have a serious impact on observed risk changes, which possibly restricts the intervention evaluation. Repeated screenings are powerful intervention measures themselves. They induce a strong version of the 'Hawthorne effect'. People, being aware that they are under study, are likely to change their behaviour in a positive way. Thus the screening effect of the cohort survey can affect health behaviour of the participants independent of the intervention programme or could make them react differently to the intervention programme. Therefore, an unbiased estimate of the impact of intervention on the total community is not possible.

In contrast with cross-sectional independent samples, cohort samples may provide information about the people who are susceptible to intervention. In this way, a better evaluation of the intervention programme is possible because the subpopulations which have responded to intervention can be identified. It may also give information about the parts of the intervention programme which were most effective. Ideally, a cohort sample is drawn in combination with independent cross-sectional samples, and so the advantages of both designs can be used.

An attempt to minimize the effect of repeated screenings among cohorts was made in the Minnesota Heart Health Study (Luepker *et al.* 1994) by repeating the surveys for half of the cohort after 2 years and for the other half after 4 years (midterm samples). Finally, the complete cohort sample was remeasured after 7 years of intervention. Whether this really eliminates a cohort screening effect, however, is not clear. This study additionally included independent cross-sectional samples.

Problems with secular trends

For several risk factors as well as for specific morbidity and mortality rates, a gradual upward or downward trend over long periods of time (decades) occurs in various countries and regions. This phenomenon is referred to as the secular trend.

Health behaviours, for example smoking prevalences, will also follow trends, although they have rarely been documented. The outcome variables in community intervention trials therefore have to be controlled for such trends. An intervention programme has to be successful in modifying these secular trends in a favourable direction. An intervention effect will be validated by comparing it with the secular trend estimated from the reference communities. In the German Cardiovascular Prevention Study Study, risk factor changes of the six pooled intervention regions were corrected for the national secular trends by using the entire nation as the reference population. The magnitude of a secular trend in a large population can be seen from the reference trend in Fig. 3.

In the case of small communities a good estimate of secular trends may be a problem. An observer should have carefully gathered information about secular trends in lifestyle and risk factors that he or she wants to modify before the initiation of the intervention programme. If there is already a very sharp decline in their levels, it will be difficult to modify this change additionally by intervention.

In the North Karelia Project (Table 1), the Finnish North Karelia region was chosen as an intervention area because it had the highest cardiovascular mortality rates worldwide at the beginning of the study. Public awareness and concern about this fact might have had an influence on lifestyle and health behaviour changes of the North Karelian inhabitants. This already initiated favourable secular trend cannot be separated from the intervention effects. In North Karelia the favourable trend in risk factors as well as in cardiovascular morbidity and mortality rates continued several years after the intervention measures had stopped. The initial occurrence of cardiovascular diseases was lower in the reference region. It is assumed that the decreasing secular trend in the reference region (Kuopio) was less pronounced. In addition to an intervention effect, differences in secular trends in the outcome variables (risk factors, cardiovascular morbidity, and mortality rates) observed between North Karelia and Kuopio may therefore partly explain the final study results.

Nevertheless, a population being aware of its high cardiovascular disease risk might be highly susceptible to health issues and intervention. Thus, it is possible that the intervention mainly induced the downward trends. The design of this project does not allow for relying on a single explanation, although from a public health view the study was very successful.

In the Kilkenny Heart Project (Shelley *et al.* 1995), the strong secular changes and probably a certain 'contamination' of the reference community by the intervention project resulted in similar risk factor reductions in both the intervention and reference counties.

In contrast with a multi-community intervention trial or a nested intervention trial, a study based on only one or two matched intervention–reference pairs should be matched for more criteria than described above. The paired communities should have the same starting levels of risk factors, morbidity, and mortality rates. If these parameters differ initially, it is an indication for inequalities concerning lifestyle and living conditions between those communities. These differences also could be caused by varying secular trends. Trends (for example, in mortality rates) should ideally be observed in both intervention and reference regions over several years before starting an intervention to achieve an impression of the grade of congruence of the matched communities.

Efforts to detect weak intervention effects

Unexpected or unknown inequalities between the communities can be responsible for different variances and trends in the outcome parameters. These circumstances, together with the limited population size of the units, make it difficult to draw conclusions and to detect the real intervention effects.

The three major community intervention trials in the United States—the Stanford Five City Project (Farquhar *et al.* 1990), the Minnesota Heart Health Program (Luepker *et al.* 1994), and the Pawtucket Heart Health Study (Carleton *et al.* 1995)—did not observe homogeneous and substantial net reductions of risk factors (Table 1), although significant changes occurred for single risk factors in selected sex or age groups. The change in total cardiovascular risk score did not differ significantly between the intervention and reference populations in these trials except for the cohort sample in the Stanford Five City Project. However, even small risk factor reductions conducted in large populations are likely to contribute substantially to the community health.

The researchers in these three American intervention trials concluded that the influence of intervention might have been too weak to change behaviour. This conclusion might be true. Contrary to the findings mentioned above, however, the Stanford trial shows favourable net reductions for most of the risk factors, although significant changes could not be ascertained. It may be that the sample sizes were too small to ascertain the weak net changes that could be achieved in the Stanford Study and in several other studies (Table 1).

Evaluation of changes

The complexity of community intervention trials requires evaluation instruments which measure the various dimensions of possible influences. Changes in health-related knowledge, attitudes, and behaviour, means and prevalences of risk factors, and physical symptoms and signs should be followed in the intervention versus reference populations. Specific morbidity as well as the prevalence of pain and life quality are outcomes of interest which should be evaluated. Finally, the overall impact of intervention must be evaluated by following specific and total mortality rates. For assessment and explanation of these changes, data on the social environmental and economic conditions (societal evaluation) in communities must be gathered as well. The evaluation instruments and methods used in community intervention trials are discussed in the following subsection.

Interview instruments

The main instrument to measure health-related knowledge, attitudes, and behaviour, as well as subjective levels of symptoms, signs, diseases, and quality of life in population samples, is the questionnaire. Widely used and validated scales and question blocks from epidemiological and social science research are available for intervention trials. Self- or interviewer-instructed questionnaires are useful to measure the following issues and many others in a standardized, reliable, and valid way. Interactive computer questionnaires with integrated quality, plausibility, and validity checks are often used.

The following parameters are assessable through questionnaire:

- smoking
- drinking (including alcohol consumption)
- food consumption and eating behaviour (with food frequency lists, food protocol, 24-hour recall, and diet history questionnaires)
- sport or physical activity
- prevalence of chronic diseases, symptoms, signs, and pain
- medication use
- subjective health status and life quality
- frequency of doctor visits or visits to health institutions
- occupation and social status.

Analytical procedures

Physical and biochemical parameters can be measured with high precision and accuracy. Following the principles of good laboratory practice, analytical procedures or measurements will normally result in methodological errors in the range of 2 to 5 per cent. Changes achieved through intervention programmes thus can be determined in representative population samples. The expected changes should be pinpointed at the beginning of the trial. These expected differences should be used for calculating the sample size sufficient to confirm statistical significance of the observed differences.

The physical measurements should be performed under the highest quality standards for preanalytical and analytical procedures. Specially trained people should perform the sampling, storage, and transport of blood and other materials in order to minimize differences in method. Altering procedures of blood sampling (such as using the sitting versus the lying position), for example, would lead to unacceptable variation. Since considerable seasonal differences of risk factor levels and behaviour (for example, cholesterol level, nutrition, and physical activity) can occur, the intervention and reference should be sampled during the same time of the year. Clinical analyses should be performed in a central laboratory with internal and external quality controls. In this way methodological differences between laboratories are reduced. A field investigator could systematically measure too high blood pressure values due to his personality ('Rosenthal effect'), so this should be checked and interviewers should be rotated regularly from the intervention to reference samples.

Morbidity and mortality estimates

Despite the generally large populations in intervention studies, objective and complete assessment of disease events by standardized medical examinations is difficult to achieve. Only frequently occurring and strictly defined diseases like ischaemic heart disease can be assessed sufficiently well. A continuous registration might be the ideal way to measure morbidity rates. This has, however, not been done in community trials. Morbidity data can also be gathered from practising doctors or from hospitals in the communities. This has to be done with careful monitoring of completeness and comparability of the data.

During morbidity and mortality evaluation, it is also important to ensure that availability of medical services and medical treatment do not differ between intervention and reference populations. Although the impact of curative measures like bypass surgery, programmes for early detection of certain cancers (breast, cervix, colon, and so on) on morbidity and mortality rates is controversial, it seems likely that improved medical treatment has a positive influence on morbidity and mortality.

Mortality evaluation

Every intervention trial should evaluate disease-specific mortality and total mortality rates. Since deaths from certain diseases and even from all causes are rare events, long observation times and large communities are necessary. As with risk factor changes, the expected reduction in mortality by intervention has to be pinpointed at the start of the study to estimate the necessary community size. In most intervention trials, the total number of mortality cases in the intervention and reference populations are counted and cumulative mortality rates during the study time (extended with a certain period after intervention) are compared. Causes of death can be ascertained from death certificates, hospital records, and interviews with relatives. In the German Cardiovascular Prevention Study the official national and regional (age-adjusted) mortality rates from the Federal Statistical Office have been used.

As can be seen from Table 1, no convincing intervention effect could be observed on mortality for most trials. This may be due to insufficient influence on risk factors and health behaviour by intervention activities as well as uncontrolled secular trends. Problems in evaluating mortality rates can also arise because of different developments in the population structure between intervention and reference regions. Thus, not only the mortality cases but also the drop-out and drop-in rates have to be considered. The denominator, which means the living part of population in communities and their movements, has to be estimated carefully.

Statistical procedures

The mean levels (or prevalence rates) of outcome variables of the independently drawn samples represent the initial and final health status in the intervention and reference population. In intervention trials with more than two surveys, the additional measurements during intervention time can give insight in the process of intervention-induced changes.

The statistical analysis procedures normally derive their statistical power from the number of individuals within the survey samples. The community is the unit of intervention, but changes in response to the intervention programme can only be measured by looking at individuals. This apparently paradoxical situation for the evaluation process limits the use of usual statistical procedures to measure the changes. Furthermore, the evaluator has to correct for the initial differences between the intervention and reference groups.

The classical way to measure intervention effects is by the use of simple formulas for net changes. Figure 4 shows the imaginary risk factor level in the intervention community (I_0) and in the reference (R_0). At the end of the intervention period, the level was changed in the intervention community (I_1) and reference (R_1). In this example a reduction in the intervention community ($I_1 - I_0$) was achieved whereas the level increased in the reference ($R_1 - R_0$). The net change is often expressed as the percentage change in the intervention community minus the percentage change in the reference (formula (a)) which can be rewritten as a subtraction of ratios ($I_1/I_0 - R_1/R_0$). Variations of this formula have been used in literature ((b) and (c)) to measure net changes. The second formula has the advantage that it allows a direct estimation of confidence intervals because it is defined as a ratio of ratios. The third formula gives the relative change divided by the baseline level in the reference which is assumed to be the baseline for the total population.

The general procedures used to calculate the net changes in intervention communities assume that baseline differences are still the same at the final measurement in the absence of an intervention programme (Fig. 4). This assumption, however, is not very realistic and will be the exception when health changes within communities are considered. Initial differences between community levels can cause complications for the evaluation. If initially measured levels differ between the observed communities, this can partly be due to chance and it is likely that effects similar to a 'regression to the mean' will occur: strong differences due to chance at a first measurement are likely to become smaller at the second measurement. Moreover, an initial high risk-factor level could motivate individuals within the

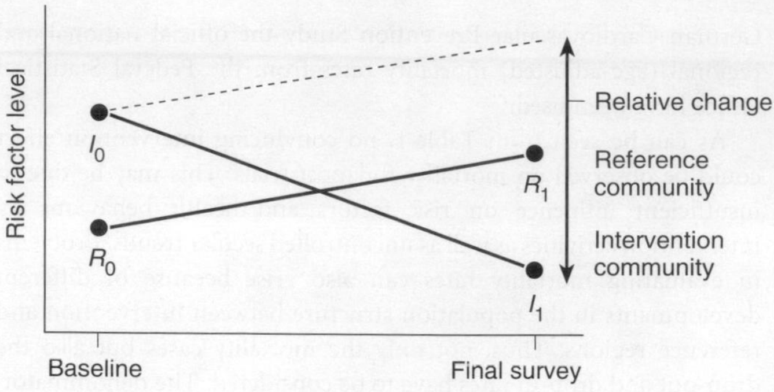

(a) Net change = $\dfrac{I_1-I_0}{I_0} - \dfrac{R_1-R_0}{R_0}$ (percentage change in intervention minus percentage change in reference)

$$\Rightarrow \left[\frac{I_1}{I_0}-1\right] - \left[\frac{R_1}{R_0}-1\right] \Rightarrow \frac{I_1}{I_0} - \frac{R_1}{R_0}$$

Multiplicative proposal[1]

(b) Net change = $\dfrac{(I_1/I_0)}{(R_1/R_0)} - 1 \Rightarrow \dfrac{I_1 \times R_0}{I_0 \times R_1} - 1$

note: (a) can be written as $\dfrac{1}{R_0} \times \dfrac{I_1(R_0-I_0)R_1}{I_0}$

(b) can be written as $\dfrac{1}{R_1} \times \dfrac{I_1(R_0-I_0)R_1}{I_0}$; so (a) = $\dfrac{R_1}{R_0}$ (b)

Proposal where reference serves as base level

(c) Net change = $\dfrac{(I_1-I_0)-(R_1-R_0)}{R_0} \Rightarrow \dfrac{(I_1-I_0-R_1)}{R_0} + 1$

[1]The addition of '−1' makes the direction of the net changes comparable to the other formulas.

Fig. 4 Formulas to calculate net changes on the basis of community levels.

community to change their lifestyle independently of the intervention programme.

In addition, the possible occurrence of a 'ceiling effect' has to be considered: individuals (or parts of communities) with high risk-factor levels may have reached their upper limits. A rising secular trend for this group will stagnate. The evaluation analyses would then over- or underestimate the potential of an intervention measure depending on the occurrence of such an effect in the intervention or reference community. In Fig. 5 a possible ceiling effect is graphically presented. The level of a certain risk factor at baseline in the reference (R_0) rises further during the intervention period and reaches its biological upper limit (R_1). The observed net changes ($I_1 - I_0$ versus $R_1 - R_0$) give an underestimation of the 'true' intervention effect which would be observed when no ceiling effect occurred. A larger effect would be measured if, for instance, the reference were to start at a lower baseline level. It is possible to argue that such an effect is a part of natural circumstances and an intervention should be successful in altering such 'natural' trends. However, this example illustrates how difficult it may be to detect intervention-based changes in reality. On the contrary, a very healthy population can hardly be improved in their risk factor levels due to a similar effect. Multiple samples between the start and the endpoint of the intervention, and the use of multivariate statistical models, can be used to correct for such effects.

An example of a multivariate model to estimate the effect of intervention on various risk factor changes is given in Fig. 6. Such a

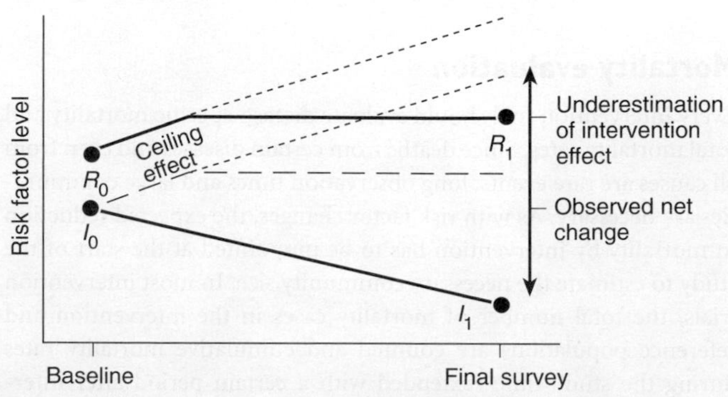

Fig. 5 Biased estimate of intervention net change due to 'ceiling effect'.

Y = age + community + $time_1$ + $time_2$ + (community × $time_1$) + (community × $time_2$)

where

Y =	in linear regression: continuous risk factor like systolic BP, cholesterol
	in logistic regression: dichotomous (like smoking, hypertension)
age =	age of individual in years at time of observation
community =	intervention or reference
$time_1$ =	sample at midtime or other sample
$time_2$ =	final sample (after intervention) or other

The interaction terms (multiplicative terms of community × $time_1$ and community × $time_2$) represent the intervention effect at midtime and after the intervention period.

Fig. 6 Multivariate regression model to estimate intervention effects (Hoffmeister *et al.* 1996).

model allows correction for different time trends and omits variance problems. Additional corrections for within-community correlations have been proposed by Murray *et al.* (1994). Significant risk factor changes in the German Cardiovascular Prevention Study (using the model in Fig. 5) were so evident that no further refinement was considered necessary. Further community intervention research should, however, concentrate on stronger methods to improve health behaviour and to reduce risk factor levels in large populations rather than to refine the statistical handling to detect weak effects.

Conclusion

Various concepts to influence a population's health behaviour and risk have been developed. The effectiveness of such strategies for primary prevention in large populations can be tested with local community intervention trials. The outcome of important community intervention trials has been described and discussed in this chapter with respect to their design. Such trials raise specific design problems (such as choice of intervention and reference, sampling, and secular trends), because the intervention is conducted and changes are measured at a community level and not at an individual level.

The success of prevention programmes can be measured from changes in health behaviour, risk factor levels, morbidity and mortality of specific diseases (diseases of interest), and total mortality. Process evaluation can give information about how such changes were achieved. For the final evaluation of intervention effects specific statistical methods are available.

References

Ajzen, I. and Madden, T.J. (1986). Prediction of goal directed behaviour, attitudes, intentions and perceived behavioural control. *Journal of Experimental Social Psychology*, **22**, 414–53.

Bandura, A. (1986). *Social foundation of thought and action*. Prentice-Hall, Englewood Cliffs, NJ.

Carleton, R.A., Lasater, T.M., Assaf, A.R., Feldman, H.A., and McKinlay, S. (1995). The Pawtucket Heart Health Program: community changes in cardiovascular risk factors and projected disease risk. *American Journal of Public Health*, **85**, 777–85.

CDC (Centers for Disease Control and Prevention) AIDS Community Demonstration Projects Research Group (1999). Community-level HIV intervention in 5 cities: final outcome data from the CDC AIDS Community Demonstration Projects. *American Journal of Public Health*, **89**, 336–45.

Cox, D.R. and Oakes, D. (1984). *Analysis of survival data*. Chapman & Hall, New York.

DiClemente, R.J. and Wingood, G.M. (1995). A randomized trial of an HIV sexual risk-reduction intervention for young African-American women. *Journal of the American Medical Association*, **274**, 1271–6.

Farquhar, J.W., Fortmann, S.P., Flora, J.A., *et al.* (1990). Effects of communitywide education on cardiovascular disease risk factors, the Stanford Five-City Project. *Journal of the American Medical Association*, **264**, 359–65.

Green, L. and Kreuter, M. (1991). *Health promotion planning: an educational and environmental approach* (2nd edn). Mayfield Publishing, Palo Alto, CA.

Hoffmeister, H., Mensink, G.B.M., Stolzenberg, H., *et al.* (1996). Reduction of coronary heart disease risk factors in the German Cardiovascular Prevention Study. *Preventive Medicine*, **25**, 135–45.

Hoffmeister, H., Schelp, F.-P., Mensink, G.B.M., Dietz, E., and Bohning, D. (1999). The relationship between alcohol consumption, health indicators and mortality in the German population. *International Journal of Epidemiology*, **28**, 1066–72.

Hursting, S.D., Thornquist, M., and Henderson, M.M. (1990). Types of dietary fat and the incidence of cancer at five sites. *Preventive Medicine*, **19**, 242–53.

Kotler, P. and Clarke, R.N. (1987). *Marketing for health care organizations*. Prentice-Hall, Englewood Cliffs, NJ.

Liao, Y., McGee, D.L., Cao, G., and Cooper, R.S. (2000). Alcohol intake and mortality: findings from the National Health Interview Surveys (1988 and 1990). *American Journal of Epidemiology*, **151**, 651–9.

Luepker, R.V., Murray, D.M., Jacobs, D.R., *et al.* (1994). Community education for cardiovascular disease prevention: risk factor changes in the Minnesota Heart Health Program. *American Journal of Public Health*, **84**, 1383–93.

Luepker, R.V., Rastam, L., Hannan, P.J., *et al.* (1996). Community education for cardiovascular disease prevention: morbidity and mortality results from the Minnesota Heart Health Program. *American Journal of Epidemiology*, **144**, 351–62.

McGuire, W.J. (1984). Public communication as a strategy for inducing health promotion behavioural change. *Preventive Medicine*, **13**, 299–319.

Murray, D.M., Hannan, P.J., Jacobs, D.R., *et al.* (1994). Assessing intervention effects in the Minnesota Heart Health Program. *American Journal of Epidemiology*, **139**, 91–103.

Rossouw, J.E., Jooste, P.L., Chalton, D.O., *et al.* (1993). Community-based intervention: the Coronary Risk Factor Study (CORIS). *International Journal of Epidemiology*, **22**, 428–38.

Sellers, D.E., Crawford, S.L., Bullock, K., and McKinlay, J.B. (1997). Understanding the variability in the effectiveness of community heart health programs: a meta-analysis. *Social Science and Medicine*, **44**, 1325–39.

Shelley, E., Daly, L., Collins, C., *et al.* (1995). Cardiovascular risk factor changes in the Kilkenny Health Project. A community health promotion programme. *European Heart Journal*, **16**, 752–60.

Staessen, L., De Bacquer, D., De Henauw, S., De Backer, G., and Van Peteghem, C. (1997). Relation between fat intake and mortality: an ecological analysis in Belgium. *European Journal of Cancer Prevention*, **6**, 374–81.

Steyn, K., Steyn, M., Swanepoel, A.S.P., *et al.* (1997). Twelve-year results of the Coronary Risk Factor Study (CORIS). *International Journal of Epidemiology*, **25**, 964–71.

Vartiainen, E., Puska, P., Jousilahti, P., Korhonen, H.J., Tuomilehto, J., and Nissinen, A. (1994). Twenty-year trends in coronary risk factors in North Karelia and in other areas of Finland. *International Journal of Epidemiology*, **23**, 495–504.

Veierod, M.B., Thelle, D.S., and Laake, P. (1997). Diet and risk of cutaneous malignant melanoma: a prospective study of 50,757 Norwegian men and women. *International Journal of Cancer*, **71**, 600–4.

6.9 Community-based intervention trials in developing countries

Zunyou Wu

Introduction

Well-designed randomized community-based intervention trials are recognized as the gold standard for the evaluation of public health interventions. Community-based intervention trials can provide reliable data on the efficacy and cost-effectiveness of control strategies. Community-based strategies to prevent disease and promote health status often use lifestyle interventions that reflect community norms. Such strategies were first used in developed countries for reducing risk factors for cardiovascular diseases (Puska *et al.* 1983; Farquhar *et al.* 1985). In the 1970s and early 1980s, community-based intervention trials were almost exclusively used to target chronic diseases and risk factors for such diseases (Puska *et al.* 1983; Farquhar *et al.* 1985; COMMIT Research Group 1991, 1995; Dietrich *et al.* 1992; Greenberg *et al.* 1994; Luepker *et al.* 1994; Carleton *et al.* 1995; Winkley *et al.* 1996).

Community-based interventions have only recently been used in developing countries. They can, however, provide a sound basis for developing health policy and allocating resources. Community-based trials can be used to control infectious diseases that remain a major public health problem in developing countries.

In the late 1980s and early 1990s, community-based intervention trials in developing countries mainly focused on infectious diseases in children, such as pneumonia (Bang *et al.* 1990; Pandey *et al.* 1991), acute respiratory tract infection (Lye *et al.* 1996), diarrhoea (Chen and Liu 1991), childhood mortality (Bang *et al.* 1990; Tielsch and West 1990; Pandey *et al.* 1991, West *et al.* 1991), and maternal mortality (Fauveau *et al.* 1991). They were also used to increase immunization coverage (Desgrees du Loû *et al.* 1995; Brugha and Kevany 1996) and to reduce risk factors for chronic diseases, such as cardiovascular diseases (Yan *et al.* 1992; Fang *et al.* 1999) and cancer (Osborne *et al.* 1997).

Since AIDS was first reported in 1981, HIV, the infection that causes AIDS, has spread rapidly, particularly in developing countries. The Joint United Nations Program on HIV/AIDS (**UNAIDS**) and the World Health Organization (**WHO**) estimated that about 5.3 million new HIV infections occurred during 2000, of which over 95 per cent were in developing countries (UNAIDS/WHO 2000). Though combined antiretroviral therapy has greatly reduced the mortality from AIDS in most developed countries, the cost is beyond the financial resources of developing counties.

A vaccine for preventing primary HIV infection is still not available. Thus, health education, behavioural intervention, and treatment of sexually transmitted diseases remain key prevention and intervention measures for controlling the HIV/AIDS epidemic in the developing world. To find cost-efficient strategies and measures to combat this pandemic, the WHO has advocated complementing behavioural interventions with improved treatment services for the classic sexually transmitted diseases such as gonorrhoea, syphilis, chancroid, and *Chlamydia* infection. To test the hypothesis that the treatment of bacterial sexually transmitted diseases is a cost-effective health intervention strategy for developing countries to control the epidemic of HIV/AIDS (Over and Piot 1993; World Bank 1993), a landmark study was conducted in the Mwanza Region of Tanzania to evaluate the impact of a community approach using improved sexually transmitted disease treatment to slow the HIV epidemic (Grosskurth *et al.* 1995*a*,*b*; Hayes *et al.* 1995). The study demonstrated that improved treatment for sexually transmitted diseases in the early stages of the HIV epidemic could have a great impact on reducing the incidence of HIV infection. This has provided an impetus for more community-based intervention trials to evaluate strategies for the control of sexually transmitted diseases and/or HIV infection in developing countries.

In the past 5 to 10 years, community-based intervention trials have been widely used in different settings, targeting a broad range of public health issues in developing countries. A community intervention trial was used to evaluate the impact of increased face-washing frequency on the prevalence of trachoma among children in Kongwa, Tanzania (West *et al.* 1995), and whether face-to-face education outreach for attendants at pharmacies increased the sale of oral rehydration salts for cases of diarrhoea in children (Ross-Degnan *et al.* 1996). Smith *et al.* (1996) used a community approach in Kenya to evaluate the effectiveness of treating chronic suppurative otitis media among schoolchildren using dry mopping with topical and systemic antibiotics and topical steroids compared with using dry mopping alone. Chavasse *et al.* used a community approach to evaluate whether fly control reduced the incidence of diarrhoea among children in Pakistan (Chavasse *et al.* 1999).

Similarly, Emerson *et al.* (1999) evaluated the effect of fly control on trachoma and diarrhoea incidence in Gambia using a community intervention trial study design. Morrow *et al.* (1999) evaluated the impact of peer education on increasing exclusive breast feeding to reduce diarrhoea among children.

Du *et al.* (1999) also used a trial to evaluate the effectiveness of the World AIDS Campaign among the general public in Beijing in 1997. Wu (1998) used a trial to promote condom use among female sex workers in entertainment establishments in three counties in Yunnan Province. Wu *et al.* (1999) used a community strategy to prevent initiation of drug use among adolescents and young adults in border areas between Myanmar and China.

Community intervention trials have been used to evaluate the effects of maternal dietary supplements in rural Gambia on birth weight and perinatal mortality (Ceesay *et al.* 1997), the effects of low-dose supplementation with vitamin A or β-carotene on mortality related to pregnancy in Nepal (West *et al.* 1999), and the effects of foods cooked in an iron pot compared with foods cooked in an aluminium pot on iron status and growth of young children in Ethiopia (Adish *et al.* 1999). A stroke prevention trial that involved seven cities in China may be the largest community intervention trial reported from developing countries so far (Fang *et al.* 1999).

Community-based intervention trials conducted in developing countries have influenced clinical and public health practice not only in developing countries but also in the industrialized world. The Mwanza sexually transmitted disease intervention trial demonstrated that improved control of sexually transmitted diseases could reduce the incidence of HIV infection at the early stage of an HIV/AIDS epidemic (Hayes *et al.* 1995, 1997). The result emphasizes the importance of promoting sexually transmitted disease syndromic management for controlling the HIV/AIDS epidemic, particularly in countries in which it is still in the early stages and in which transmission is mainly through sexual intercourse. The Kenya study showed that dry mopping with topical and systemic antibiotics and topical steroids to treat children with chronic suppurative otitis media was much better than dry mopping alone (Smith *et al.* 1996). The Ethiopian study indicated that cooking food in an iron pot is better than in an aluminium pot for reducing the rate of anaemia and for improving the growth of children (Adish *et al.* 1999).

Community-based intervention trials are often complicated and expensive. Owing to the scarcity of resources available in developing countries, designing community-based intervention trials is different than designing the same studies in developed countries. This chapter reviews community-based intervention trials in developing countries. Table 1 summarizes selected community-based intervention trials targeting a broad range of public health issues in developing countries. The chapter will discuss study design, intervention activities, measurement issues, and interpretation of results of community-based intervention trials in developing countries.

Design

Designing community-based intervention trials is more complicated than designing intervention trials at the individual level. Launching community-based intervention trials in developing countries is even more difficult than doing them in developed countries because background information is usually not available. In addition, infrastructures often do not exist, particularly in rural areas where public health interventions are most needed.

Selection of study sites

The first stage of any study is to select an appropriate site for launching a trial. Several issues need to be considered.

Firstly, study sites must have a reasonably high incidence and prevalence of the events of interest. A high incidence is important to increase the cost-efficiency of study and to reduce the duration of the trial. In developing countries, disease incidences are frequently high. In the rural Tanzania sexually transmitted disease study, the average prevalence of syphilis was 7.9 per cent for men and 9.5 per cent for women in the intervention communities and 7.8 per cent for men and 8.8 per cent for women in the comparison communities. The average prevalence of HIV antibody seropositivity was 3.4 per cent for men and 4.1 per cent for women in the intervention communities and 4.1 per cent for men and 4.7 per cent for women in the comparison communities at baseline (Grosskurth *et al.* 1995*a*). In the Rakai (Uganda) sexually transmitted disease study, the average prevalence of syphilis was 10.7 per cent for men and 10.5 per cent for women in the intervention communities, and 9.1 per cent for men and 9.7 per cent for women in the comparison communities. The average prevalence of HIV antibody seropositivity was 14.7 per cent for men and 19.6 per cent for women in the intervention communities, and 13.6 per cent for men and 18.5 per cent for women in the comparison communities at baseline (Wawer *et al.* 1998). In the Hubei diarrhoea study, the incidence of diarrhoea among children was 3.1 episodes per child-year in the intervention communities and 3.3 episodes per child-year in the comparison communities at baseline (Chen and Liu 1991). In the Gambia study, the prevalence of active trachoma at baseline was betweem 8.8 and 12.2 per cent during the wet season, and between 16 and 18 per cent during the dry season (Emerson *et al.* 1999). In the study of the effect of home-based neonatal care on neonatal mortality in rural India, the neonatal rate was 62 per 1000 live births at baseline (Bang *et al.* 1999). In the stroke prevention study in China, the prevalences of hypertension and heart disease were 36.6 per cent and 10.3 to 11.4 per cent respectively, and the incidence of stroke was 233 per 100 000 population at baseline (Fang *et al.* 1999).

Secondly, existing resources, when available, should be used as much as possible, otherwise the intervention will be expensive and will not be sustainable when the trial is completed. In the Nepal study of community-based antimicrobial treatment of pneumonia, indigenous community health workers were exclusively relied on to deliver the intervention (Pandey *et al.* 1991). In an Indian study to reduce pneumonia mortality and total childhood mortality, village health workers and traditional birth attendants were used (Bang *et al.* 1990). In the Tanzania study of the impact of face-washing on trachoma among children, the village structure was utilized for carrying out the study (West *et al.* 1995). In the community drug prevention study in China, schools, families, communities, and health service infrastructures were all used (Wu *et al.* 1999). In the neonatal mortality study in rural India, village women with 5 to 10 years of school education who were willing to work were selected as village health workers to deliver the intervention (Bang *et al.* 1999).

Thirdly, study sites should be representative of most communities affected by the diseases of interest in the country. This is important because the intervention strategies and measures being tested in the trial should be expanded to other regions, or even to the whole country or several countries if they are successful. In the stroke prevention study, the cities of Harbin, Changchun, Beijing, Zhenzhou, Shanghai, Changsha, and Yinchuan were chosen. The seven cities were representative of urban China in terms of geographic location, city size, and prevalence of risk factors and incidence of stroke (Fang *et al.* 1999).

Table 1 Summary of selected community-based intervention trials conducted in developing countries

Hypothesis and targeted outcome	Location	Participants	Study design	Interventions	Results
Hypothesis: mass education about childhood pneumonia and case management of pneumonia by village health workers and birth attendants reduces pneumonia mortality and total childhood mortality *Outcome*: (1) pneumonia-specific childhood mortality; (2) infant mortality; (3) total under-5 mortality (Bang *et al.* 1990)	Gadchiroli, India	102 villages with 58 villages (6176 children aged 0–4 years) in the intervention area and 44 villages (3947 children aged 0–4 years) in the control area	Community-based intervention trial Intervention unit: village Non-random allocation was used. The intervention and control areas were a continuous area except for 'buffer' zone of a few villages A census was carried out to prepare a population register and a list of children under 5 by VHWs before the study. All births and deaths of children under 5 years were recorded by VHWs. In addition, a house-to-house survey was conducted every 6 months by the VHW from another village to detect missed births and deaths. Also, a morbidity study was carried out in 43 villages (25 in intervention and 18 in control areas)	43 of 200 village volunteers were trained as part-time VHWs. Each worker had on average 2000 people in 2.4 villages to look after Mass health education about childhood pneumonia, case management of pneumonia, and training of traditional birth attendants for better maternity and neonatal care were implemented in intervention areas Primary health care and immunization, including measles vaccine, were provided in both intervention and control areas	Case-fatality rate was 0.8% in the intervention compared with 13.5% in the control areas The pneumonia-specific childhood mortality, infant mortality, and total under-5 mortality were significantly lower in the intervention than in the control area (8.1 vs 17.5, 89 vs 121, and 28.5 vs 40.7 per 1000, respectively)
Hypothesis: improved drinking water reduces acute diarrhoea among children *Outcome*: acute diarrhoea (Chen and Liu 1991)	Hubei Province, China	46 villages with 622 children under 5 participated in the study	Community intervention Intervention unit: village Randomization was used Episodes of diarrhoea were reported by mothers Incidences of diarrhoea were compared between intervention and control group at baseline (1986), in 1987 and in 1988	A comprehensive education programme was carried out in intervention villages, including lectures, discussion groups, fliers, word-of-mouth, posters, training both mothers and children to wash hands before eating and after using the toilet, to cut nails regularly, and supplying deep well water for drinking use.	The incidence of diarrhoea among children under 5 years dropped from 3.1 episodes per child-year in 1986 to 1.3 episodes per child-year in 1987 to 0.7 episodes per child-year in 1988 in the intervention group, but dropped from 3.3 episodes per child-year in 1986 to 1.8 episodes per child-year in 1987 to 1.4 episodes per child-year in 1988 in the control group Significant differences were observed between intervention and control groups after the initiation of the intervention

Hypothesis and targeted outcome	Location	Participants	Study design	Interventions	Results
Hypothesis: community members could manage childhood pneumonia, and thus reduce the total under-5 mortality *Outcome*: total mortality for children under 5 years (Pandey *et al.* 1991)	Jumla, western Nepal	The study involved 18 of Jumla's 30 subdistricts, consisting of 115 villages with under-5 population 13 404 children under 5 were involved in the study	Non-randomized controlled trial Intervention unit: subdistrict Subdistricts were similar in socio-economic, ethnic, and health characteristics; all lacked routine child-health services. Deliberate allocation of subdistricts to early versus later intervention was used. By month 13 the entire population was included in the treatment and there was no longer an untreated group of children A household census of children aged under 5 in the 18 subdistricts was done at the start of the study, and all subsequent births and childhood deaths were registered throughout the subsequent 36 months by a set of 115 village-based enumerators.	One member of the village was selected for every 1000 population. They were trained in the WHO strategy of pneumonia case management, which focuses on pneumonia control, and stresses case detection, treatment, and education of mothers about warning signs Programme focused on active case detection. Trained health workers spent 50% of their time visiting 10–15 households every day, and completed a round of target households (about 160) under their responsibility every 2 weeks. It allowed them to continue their regular farming activities. During home visits, workers actively sought out and treated cases of pneumonia in children under 5. Increasing emphasis was placed on maternal education. Referral of children to hospital was not practical since no other health services were available	28% reduction in the risk of death from all causes by the third year of services, with the greatest benefit among infants Carry-out effect was observed in the reduction of deaths due to diarrhoea and measles
Hypothesis: intake vitamin A to reduce preschool child mortality *Outcome*: preschool child mortality (West *et al.* 1991)	Nepal	28 630 children aged 6 to 72 months participated in the study	Community-based intervention trial Intervention unit: ward Double-masked, placebo-controlled, randomized Administrative wards were randomized into intervention (vitamin A) and control (placebo) groups Preschool child mortality was compared between intervention and control groups	Supplement of vitamin A to children in intervention group, placebo in control group	The relative risk of death in vitamin A supplemented group was 0.7 compared to the control group, i.e. 30% reduction in mortality. The reduction was observed in both sexes, at all age groups, and throughout year

Hypothesis and targeted outcome	Location	Participants	Study design	Interventions	Results
Hypothesis: improved maternity care reduces maternal mortality *Outcome*: maternal mortality (Fauveau *et al.* 1991)	Matlab, Bangladesh	In the intervention area, the population size was 47 808 with 10 260 women aged 15–44 years In the control area, the population size was 51 468 with 11 564 women aged 15–44 years	Community-based intervention No random allocation of treatment The effect of programme was evaluated by comparison of direct obstetric maternal mortality between the intervention area with trained midwives services and the control area without midwives	Nurse-midwives were recruited and posted in each outpost of the intervention area Midwives carried out antenatal visits to the pregnant women, assessed risks of complications antenatally, attended as many home deliveries as possible, treated arising complications at the onset before they became too severe, organized referrals and accompanied the patient to the central clinic, and visited as many new mothers as possible within 48 h of delivery	Maternal morality ratios from obstetric complications were similar in both areas during the 3 years preceding the start of the study. During the following 3 years, the ratio was significantly lower in the intervention areas than in the control areas (1.4 vs 3.8 per 1000 live births)
Hypothesis: promotion of healthy behaviour reduces blood pressure among hypertensives *Outcome*: level of blood pressure, cigarette smoking rate (Yan *et al.* 1991)	East District, Beijing, China	All residents aged 15 or above in East District, Beijing, were the target population. The total population was 39 765	Community-based intervention trial Randomization was used Intervention unit: cluster Street clusters were randomized into intervention and control groups After 2 years of intervention, 10% of hypertension patients in the intervention and control groups were randomly selected to evaluate the effectiveness of programme	In the intervention group, health promotion programmes were implemented, including cigarette smoking control, low salt intake, moderate exercise, management of hypertension patients in the community, and surveillance In control group, only surveillance was carried out	After 2 years of the intervention, cigarette smoking rates among hypertension patients dropped 8.37% in the intervention group from 1989 to 1991, but dropped 0.83% in the control group during the same period SBP controlled under 160 mmHg increased from 46.7% in 1989 to 75.7% in 1991 in the intervention group, and decreased from 52.7 to 50% in the control group during the same period DBP controlled under 95 mmHg increased from 53.3% in 1989 to 81.1% in 1991 in the intervention group, and decreased from 52.8 to 50.9% in the control group during the same period

Hypothesis and targeted outcome	Location	Participants	Study design	Interventions	Results
Hypothesis: immunization with three doses of inactivated hepatitis A vaccine reduces clinical hepatitis A among schoolchildren *Outcome*: clinical case of hepatitis A (Innis *et al.* 1994)	Thailand	A total of 40 119 children, aged 1 to 16 years, attending 148 primary schools were involved in the study	Double-blind randomized controlled trial stratified by community Intervention unit: individual child Randomization was used to assign participants to receive either the hepatitis A vaccine or the control vaccine. A block size of 10 participants (i.e. 5 vaccine recipients and 5 control recipients) was used to balance assignment by grade within a school Cases of hepatitis A were identified by evaluating school absences of 2 or more days	Students assigned to the intervention group received hepatitis A vaccine at months 0, 1, and 12. Students assigned to the control group received hepatitis B vaccine following the same scheme	40 cases of hepatitis A were identified during the controlled trial with two in the intervention group and 38 in the control group (2/19 037 vs 38/19 120)
Hypothesis: immunizations reduce childhood mortality *Outcome*: childhood mortality (Desgrees du Loû *et al.* 1995)	Bandafassi, Senegal	Parents who have children of immunization age	Community-based intervention Self-controlled Mortality rates were compared 6 years before and 6 years after the introduction of immunization	Introduce immunization where there had previously been no regular immunization	Neonatal mortality declined 31% Mortality reduced by 20% for children aged 1 to 8 months, and by 48% for children aged 9 to 59 months Reduced mortality positively associated with coverage in villages after the initial national campaign

Hypothesis and targeted outcome	Location	Participants	Study design	Interventions	Results
Hypothesis: increased face-washing behaviour reduces trachoma among children *Outcome*: trachoma prevalence, clean faces (West *et al.* 1995)	Kongwa, Tanzania	All children in the six villages in Kongwa are targeted A sample of children, i.e. 1417, were randomly selected for follow-up	Community-based randomized trial Intervention unit: village Six villages were matched in three pairs. Villages were matched for: maternal education, baseline prevalence of clean faces in young children and baseline prevalence of trachoma status Random allocation was performed in each of the pairs. One of each pair would receive mass treatment followed by the health education campaign (intervention) and the other would receive mass treatment alone (control) Cohort follow-up Trachoma status and facial cleanliness were assessed at baseline and at 2, 6, and 12 months of follow-up	Mass treatment of every member of village was carried out in all 6 villages In addition, a community-based participatory hygiene intervention programme was implemented to promote face-washing of the young children in the three intervention villages. Neighbourhood meetings to build consensus for increasing face-washing as an important approach to trachoma control were reinforced by school plays, seminars with the traditional healers, and meetings with other village groups The intervention activities were intensively carried out for 1 month during and after the mass treatment	Children in the intervention group were 60% more likely to have clean faces than those in the control group The odds ratio of having severe trachoma in the intervention villages was 0.6 compared with the control villages
Hypothesis: home visits by non-health workers increases the immunization rate *Outcome*: immunization rate (Brugha and Kevany 1996)	Urban area of Ghana	Parents of children aged 12–18 months in Nkawkaw (town 1), Kwahu Praso (town 2), and Akwasiho (town 3) in eastern region of Ghana	Randomized controlled trial (in town 1 only) Intervention unit: cluster Contiguous clusters were paired and one of each pair of clusters was randomly chosen for intervention or control. Thirty clusters each were allocated into intervention and control groups During the study period of July 1991 to February 1992, the intervention clusters received home visits and advice about immunizations, but the control did not. At the end of the follow-up	Regular immunization was available in all three towns O-level graduates were trained as interviewers Interviewers advised each of the parents to bring their children to the next clinic for immunization if their children had not completed the immunization schedule. A nurse visit occurred if a child failed to complete the schedule following the referral made by the interviewer at the home visit In town 2, children were immunized at the home visit	In town 1, immunization coverage rose by 26.5 to 86% during the intervention, compared with a 6.0% rise in the control group in the same period In town 2, coverage increased from 38% to 91%

Hypothesis and targeted outcome	Location	Participants	Study design	Interventions	Results
			visit, the control clusters were given advice to bring their children for immunizations	No special effort was given to town 3 since 37 out of 39 children were already immunized	
Hypothesis: dry mopping with topical and systemic antibiotics and topical steroids has a better outcome in treating chronic suppurative otitis media (CSOM) than dry mopping alone *Outcome*: (1) resolution otorrhoea; (2) healing tympanic membranes (Smith *et al.* 1996)	Kiambu district, Kenya	524 children with CSOM, aged 5–15, from 145 primary schools in Kiambu district were involved in the study	Community-based intervention trial Intervention unit: cluster Schools were randomly assigned treatments in clusters of five in a ratio of 2 to dry mopping alone (201 children), 2 to dry mopping with topical and systemic antibiotics and topical steroids (221 children), and 1 to no specific treatment Resolution of otorrhoea and healing of tympanic membranes were assessed at 8, 12, and 16 weeks after induction	In one group, children received dry mopping with antibiotics In the second group, children received dry mopping alone In the third group, children received no specific treatment	51% of the children in the group that received dry mopping with antibiotics had resolved otorrhoea compared with 22% of those who received dry mopping alone and 22% of the controls Healing of the tympanic membranes were 15% in the dry mopping plus antibiotics group, 13% in the dry mopping alone groups, and 13% in the control group
Hypothesis: face-to-face educational outreach for attendants at pharmacies increased the sale of ORS for cases of diarrhoea in children *Outcome*: (1) sales of ORS at pharmacies; (2) communication with customers at pharmacies (Ross-Degnan *et al.* 1996)	Kenya and Indonesia	194 private pharmacies were involved in the study, 107 pharmacies in Kenya, and 87 in Indonesia	Community-based intervention trial Intervention unit: pharmacy In Kenya, before-and-after comparison group design was used In Indonesia, a randomized controlled design was used Sales of ORS, sales of antidiarrhoeal agents, and history-taking and advice to continue fluids and food were measured and compared before and after in Kenya, and between intervention and control in Indonesia	Brief one-on-one meetings between diarrhoea programme educators and pharmacists/owners, followed by small group training sessions with all counter attendants working in the pharmacies	There was a significant increase in knowledge about diarrhoea and its treatment among counter attendants in Kenya where these changes were measured. Sales of ORS increased by an average of 30% in Kenya compared to before the intervention, and 21% in Indonesia compared to the control. Increased communication in both countries was observed

Hypothesis and targeted outcome	Location	Participants	Study design	Interventions	Results
Hypothesis: improved management of ARTI at the community level reduces severe ARTI *Outcome*: reduction of (1) incidence of ARTI and (2) proportion of severe ARTI among children under 5 years (Lye *et al.* 1996)	Pasir Mas, Machang and Pasir Puteh districts, Malaysia	Children under 5 years	Community-based controlled intervention Intervention unit: district Randomization with only two study units 25 villages in one district were selected as intervention villages and another 25 villages in two other districts were selected as the control Incidence of ARTI and proportion of severe ARTI were monitored every 2 weeks over a 62-week period in both intervention and control groups	In the intervention group, training on case management of ARTI was given to health personnel, including hospital medical officers, medical and health officers, medical assistants, public health nursing sisters, public health nurses, assistant nurses, and community nurses-cum-mid-wives who are at the most peripheral level of the health services. Health education was also carried out targeting mothers on how to recognize signs and symptoms of moderate and severe ARTI, and advice on what to do for children managed at home; fast breathing and/or difficulty in breathing was an indication of pneumonia, and the child was advised to be brought to the clinic or hospital. Illustrated billboards, pamphlets, videos, and person-to-person talks were used to disseminate messages	The reduction in incidence between the baseline and at the end of surveillance was significantly higher for the intervention area compared to the control area (2.3 to 0% for intervention and 3.2–2.4% for control, $p < 0.05$). The proportion of severe ARTI in the intervention area was significantly lower than in the control area ($p < 0.05$)
Hypothesis: improved STD treatment services reduces the spread of HIV infection *Outcome*: (1) incidence of HIV infection; (2) prevalence of syphilis; (3) symptomatic urethritis (Grosskurth *et al.* 1995*a*,*b*; Hayes *et al.* 1995; Mayaud *et al.* 1997)	Mwanza, Tanzania	A total of 12 534 adults aged 15–54 were enrolled at baseline 12 communities were matched in six pairs	Community-based intervention trial Intervention unit: community Random allocation of the community was performed within matched pairs A cohort study design was used to determine incidence of HIV infection	The intervention had five components: (a) establishment of a reference clinic; (b) training of health-care providers; (c) supply of effective drugs; (d) regular supervision; (e) health education in the target communities to encourage individuals with STD symptoms to seek treatment early	Over 2 years of follow-up, the proportion of seroconversion were 48 of 4149 (1.2%) in the intervention communities compared with 82 of 4400 (1.9%) in the comparison communities. The HIV incidence was consistently lower in the intervention communities in all six matched pairs. The improved STD services reduced HIV incidence by about 40% The prevalence of syphilis was 6.2% in both intervention and control groups at baseline, but was 5% in the intervention and 7% in the control group at follow-up. The prevalence of symptomatic urethritis was reduced by 50% in intervention group compared with the control group

Hypothesis and targeted outcome	Location	Participants	Study design	Interventions	Results
Hypothesis: comprehensive education increases knowledge of and attitudes towards STDs/AIDS and condoms, and increases condom use with clients among sex workers *Outcome*: (1) consistent condom use; (2) knowledge of STD/AIDS; (3) knowledge of condoms preventing STDs/HIV (Wu 1998)	Yunnan, China	Female sex workers in 30 entertainment establishments in Chengjiang, 34 establishments in Ruili and 23 establishments in Longchuan were involved in the study	Community intervention Intervention unit: entertainment establishment Non-random allocation, self-comparison (before and after control)	Comprehensive intervention activities including lectures, discussions, women's talk (a few sex workers, one being a trained peer, talking freely about sex), playing video cassettes and tape cassettes, distribution of educational folders and condoms Before and after comparison was used	After the 3-month intervention, knowledge of the three main transmission routes for HIV increased from 18 to 98% in Chengjiang, 44 to 88% in Ruili, and 0 to 59% in Longchuan. Knowledge that the use of condoms reduced the risk of STDs/HIV infection increased from 58 to 99% in Chengjiang, 55 to 91% in Ruili, and 55 to 90% in Longchuan. Condom use during the last incident of sexual intercourse increased from 54 to 89% in Chengjiang, 69 to 91% in Ruili, and 59 to 61% in Longchuan. Condom use during the last three incidents of sexual intercourse increased from 31 to 77% in Chengjiang, from 51 to 75% in Ruili and from 39 to 41% in Longchuan
Hypothesis: improved STD treatment services reduces the spread of HIV infection *Outcome*: (1) incidence of HIV infection; (2) prevalence of STDs (Wawer *et al.* 1998; Wawer *et al.* 1999)	Rakai, Uganda	5834 subjects were enrolled in intervention communities and 5784 were enrolled in control communities	Community-based intervention trial Intervention unit: cluster Random allocation of the community was performed without matching A cohort study design was used to determine incidence of HIV infection	Community-level control of STDs through home-based, mass treatment strategy, i.e. all consenting adults were given directly observed STD therapy at home every 10 months irrespective of laboratory test results or the presence of symptoms	The incidence of HIV infection was 1.5 per 100 person-years in both intervention and control groups In pregnant women, the follow-up prevalence of trichomoniasis, bacterial vaginosis, gonorrhoea, and *Chlamydia* infection were significantly lower in the intervention group than in the control group. No difference was observed on incidence of HIV infection in pregnant women

Hypothesis and targeted outcome	Location	Participants	Study design	Interventions	Results
Hypothesis: controlling flies reduces the incidence of diarrhoea among children *Outcome*: diarrhoea incidence (Chavasse *et al.* 1999)	Peshawar, Pakistan	Six study villages and two control villages The study was from 1995 to 1997. At any one time, about 500 children were being followed up Newborn infants were recruited and children reaching their fifth birthday were released from the study	Community-based intervention trial Intervention unit: village Randomization was used Six study villages were randomly assigned into two groups of three. Flies were controlled with insecticide in three villages in group A in 1995 but not in 1996, and in three villages in group B in 1996 but not in 1995. Another two villages were selected as the control group Diarrhoea incidence was monitored through mothers' reports for all children under 5 years of age in the six villages in groups A and B during weekly interviews by a health worker Fly density was monitored by use of sticky fly-papers	Flies were controlled with insecticide in villages in group A in 1995 but not in 1996, in villages in group B in 1996 but not in 1995	Incidence of diarrhoea was lower in the sprayed villages than in the unsprayed villages in both 1995 (mean episode per child-year 6.3 vs 7.1) and 1996 (4.4 vs 6.5), with a reduction in incidence of 23% At times other than the fly season, there was no evidence of a difference in diarrhoea morbidity between sprayed and unsprayed villages
Hypothesis: peer education increases exclusive breast feeding, thus reduces diarrhoea among children *Primary outcome*: exclusive breastfeeding *Secondary outcomes*: (1) duration of breast feeding; (2) episode of diarrhoea in first 3 months; and (3) maternal satisfaction with counselling (Morrow *et al.* 1999)	Mexico City	Pregnant women in 39 clusters in San Pedro Martir 170 pregnant women were identified, 12 refused, 28 were ineligible and excluded 130 participated	Community-based randomized controlled trial Intervention unit: cluster 13 clusters in six-visit group; 13 clusters in three-visit group; and 13 clusters in control group Cohort follow-up Five follow-up interviews were scheduled for all study mothers at 2, 3, and 6 weeks, and at 2 and 3 months postpartum to record infant-feeding practices in the previous week Study duration was 22 months	Home-based peer counselling Three women were trained through 1 week of classes, 2 months in lactation clinics and with a mother-to-mother support group, 1 day of observation and demonstration by visiting experts, and 6 months of practice in a neighbourhood before the intervention trial In the six-visit group, mothers were visited in mid and late pregnancy, in the first week and weeks 2, 4, and 8 postpartum. In the three-visit group, mothers were visited in late pregnancy, in the first week, and week 2 postpartum. Control group mothers with lactation problems were referred to their own doctors	Exclusive breast feeding was 67% in the six-visit group, 50% in the three-visit, and 12% in the control group at 3 months postpartum Infants in intervention groups had a lower rate of diarrhoea than the control group, 12% vs 26%

Hypothesis and targeted outcome	Location	Participants	Study design	Interventions	Results
Hypothesis: community-based intervention reduces incidence of drug use among adolescents *Outcome*: incidence of drug use (Wu *et al.* 1999)	Yunnan, China	All villagers in 38 villages, with 19 villages and 10 schools in the intervention group, and 19 villages and nine schools in the control group	Community-based intervention trial Intervention unit: village Non-random location was used Villages were matched in group for prevalence of drug use, and the number of drug users documented in 1996 Community, family, school, and clinic approaches were used Incidence of onset of drug use was compared before and after between the intervention and control groups	Training workshops, playing of videos, competition games, entertainment, application of agriculture technology, poverty alleviation, etc., were implemented by departments of health, education, entertainment, and sciences and technology in the intervention villages and schools from March 1997 to October 1998	The incidence of drug use declined from 3.54% to 1.88% in the intervention area (reduction of 1.66%) and from 2.13% to 1.5% in the control area (reduction of 0.63%), an attributable reduction of 103% Knowledge of transmission routes and prevention measures was greater in the intervention group (36.6%) than in the control group (5.3%) after the intervention
Hypothesis: small media (leaflets, fliers, stickers, letters to families, posters, and so on) and person-to-person communication is better than mass media in correcting misconceptions about AIDS *Outcome*: knowledge and attitude about AIDS (Du *et al.* 1999)	Beijing, China	All residents in Beijing	Community-based controlled intervention Intervention unit: street cluster Non-random allocation. Two districts were selected as intervention communities using small media and personal communication. The rest of the residents in Beijing were exposed to a mass media AIDS campaign as the control Knowledge and attitudes about AIDS were assessed by two cross-sectional surveys using a random sampling scheme interviewing a sample of subjects in the intervention and control group before and after the campaign	In the intervention group, comprehensive strategies were used, such as workshops, group discussion, person-to-person talks, exhibitions, posters, fliers, and letters besides the mass media campaign on radio and television, and in newspapers In the control group, only radio, newspapers, and television were used for the campaign	Knowledge of the three HIV transmission routes and at least three prevention methods among the general public increased from 65.9 and 73.9% to 80.5 and 78.4%, respectively, in the control communities ($p < 0.01$, $p < 0.05$), while they changed from 83 and 92.4% to 84 and 92.2%, respectively, in the intervention communities. Knowledge of non-transmission routes among the general public did not change in the control communities but increased significantly in the intervention communities ($p < 0.01$)

Hypothesis and targeted outcome	Location	Participants	Study design	Interventions	Results
Hypothesis: the incidence of stroke is expected to be reduced by 25% over 3.5 years of intervention with multiple risk factors *Outcome*: incidence of stroke (Fang *et al.* 1999)	Seven cities in China (Harbin, Changchun, Beijing, Zhengzhou, Shanghai, Changsha, Yinchuan)	18 786 subjects (⩾ 35 years old) were recruited in the intervention and 18 876 in the control cohort	Community-based controlled intervention Intervention unit: geographic community with about 10 000 population Non-random allocation. Two communities were selected: one close to the collaborating hospital was assigned to the intervention and the other assigned to the control in each of seven cities Level of blood pressure, prevalence of hypertension, heart disease, diabetes, current smoking, and current drinking were assessed at baseline and follow-up. Cumulative incidence of stroke was compared between the intervention and control group over 3.5 years	In the intervention group subjects with hypertension, heart disease, or diabetes were managed through the provision of health education to the full community. Subjects with hypertension and diabetes or heart diseases were visited every 2 weeks, subjects with hypertension only were visited every 4 weeks, subjects with borderline hypertension were visited every 8 weeks. Education was mainly information dissemination using door-to-door leaflets, posters, and stickers. Contents included risk factors for stroke and how to reduce these risk factors by modifying personal behaviours In the control group, nothing was done except the surveys	The baseline annual incidence of stroke was 229 and 237 per 100 000 population for the intervention and control groups, respectively. The 3.5-year cumulative incidence was 0.93% in the intervention and 1.34% in the control groups (RR = 0.69, 95% confidence interval 0.57–0.84)
Hypothesis: home-based neonatal care, including management of sepsis (septicaemia, meningitis, pneumonia), would reduce the neonatal mortality rate by at least 25% in 3 years *Outcome*: (1) neonatal mortality rate; (2) infant mortality rate; and (3) perinatal mortality rate (Bang *et al.* 1999)	Gadichiroli district, Maharashtra state, India	Pregnant women, grandmothers, and neonates	Community-based controlled intervention Intervention unit: village Non-random allocation. 39 villages for the intervention and 47 villages for the control groups. They are contiguous Stepwise introduction of interventions and coverage was used. In the first year, female VHWs collected detailed data from the third trimester to 28 days after birth in order to estimate the natural incidence of neonatal morbidity and need for care, and to plan further interventions. In the second year, female VHWs were trained in home-based management of neonatal illness and the intervention took place. Education of mother and grandmother was introduced in the third year.	In the intervention group: trained VHWs provided diagnoses and management of neonatal health issues including prevention of birth asphyxia, temperature maintenance in winter, encouraging mothers to start breast feeding in the first hour after birth and to continue exclusive breast feeding, prevention of superficial infection, and early detection and treatment of sepsis. Health education of pregnant women and grandmothers was actively implemented in the third year	Neonatal mortality decreased from 62 per 1000 at baseline to 25 per 1000 in year 3 in the intervention area, but remained almost the same in the control area (57.7 per 1000 at baseline and 59.6 per 1000 in year 3) The infant mortality rate decreased from 75.5 per 1000 at baseline to 38.8 per 1000 in year 3 in the intervention area but changed only slightly in the control area (77.1 per 1000 at baseline and 74.9 per 1000 in year 3) The perinatal mortality rate decreased from 68.3 per 1000 at baseline to 47.8 per 1000 in year 3 in the intervention area but increased from 64.9 per 1000 at baseline to 91.5 per 1000 in year 3 in the control area

Hypothesis and targeted outcome	Location	Participants	Study design	Interventions	Results
			Mortality rate was compared between before and after the intervention between the two groups		
Hypothesis: fly control decreases the prevalence of trachoma as well as childhood diarrhoea *Outcome*: incidence of trachoma and childhood diarrhoea (Emerson *et al.* 1999)	Sanjal area, Gambia	Residents in four villages in Sanjal, Gambia	Community-based controlled intervention Intervention unit: village cluster Non-random allocation. Two pairs of villages were selected from 23 available small villages. One village from each pair was arbitrarily assigned to the intervention and the other acted as a control with one pair for the wet season and another pair for the dry season Incidence of trachoma and childhood diarrhoea were compared between the intervention and control villages in both wet and dry seasons	In the intervention group, flies were controlled by ultra-low-volume application of 0.175% volume to volume deltamethrin within and up to 20 m outside each village In the control group, flies were controlled by an 'attack' phase of spraying every 2 days for 2 weeks, followed by a 'maintenance' phase of spraying twice weekly in the wet season, and once weekly in the dry season	There was no difference in community prevalence of active trachoma at baseline in either village pairs (wet season intervention 8.8% vs control 12.2%; dry season 18% vs 16%). The prevalence of trachoma was lower in the intervention than control villages in both seasons after the 3 month intervention (wet season 3.7% in the intervention group vs 13.7% in the control, $p = 0.04$; dry season 10% in the intervention group vs 18.9% in the control, $p = 0.09$)
Hypothesis: cooking food in iron pots reduces iron deficiency anaemia among children *Outcome*: (1) change of haemoglobin concentration; (2) weight and length of children (Adish *et al.* 1999)	Tigray, Ethiopia	Children aged 2–5 years	Community-based controlled intervention Intervention unit: household Randomization was used for household allocation. 407 households were selected for the study. One child from each household was recruited for cohort follow-up Haemoglobin concentration, weight, and length of children were assessed and compared at baseline and at 3-month and 12-month follow-ups between the intervention and control groups	In the intervention group, each household received one 2-litre iron pot for cooking food; in the control each received one 2-litre aluminium pot for cooking food	The average haemoglobin concentration increased 1.7 g/dl in the intervention group compared with 0.4 g/dl in the control over 12 months. The mean differences between the groups in weight and length gain in 12 months (adjusted for baseline weight or length) were 0.1 kg (95% CI 0.1–0.3) and 0.6 cm (0.1–10)

ARTI, acute respiratory tract infection; CI, confidence intervals; CSOM, chronic suppurative otitis media; DBP, diastolic blood pressure; ORS, oral rehydration salts; RR, relative risk; SBP, systolic blood pressure; STD, sexually transmitted disease; VHW, village health worker.

Qualitative study of communities

Communities vary within regions and across regions. Usually little background information about study communities is available in developing countries. It is essential to understand the community fully, to ensure the success of community-based intervention trials. Thus, collecting information about administrative structures and cultural characteristics is necessary before carrying out the trial.

Several methods can be used to collect existing information and obtain essential additional information. Firstly, it is important to interview key informants in the community. Key informants include community administrative leaders, community religious leaders, opinion leaders, and a sample of other residents. This method has been widely used in many studies. In a community-based prevention of reproductive tract infections among rural women, extensive interviews of key informants was carried out in communities (Fang *et al.* 1999; Yin *et al.* 1999). Secondly, focus group discussion can be used to collect information quickly. This method was used before designing intervention activities for the drug prevention trial in China (Wu *et al.* 1999), the condom promotion trial among female sex workers in China (Wu 1998), and the reproductive tract infection prevention trial in China (Fang *et al.* 1999; Yin *et al.* 1999). The third method is on-site observation. This method was also used in promoting condom use among female sex workers in China (Wu 1998) and in the reproductive tract infection prevention study (Fang *et al.* 1999; Yin *et al.* 1999) in China. Often these qualitative methods are used jointly with other methods.

How much effort should be put into a qualitative study prior to a trial varies from study to study depending on how complex the proposed intervention is, how complex the communities involved in the trial are, how much background information already exists, the prior experience of the person directing the trial, and how much money is available for the study. For the trial promoting exclusive breast feeding, only a rapid ethnographic study of infant feeding was employed before the intervention trial was initiated (Morrow *et al.* 1999).

Community consultation

Different communities include different subgroups of people. Each subgroup has its own characteristics, interests, and needs. Comprehensive consultation with different subgroups is very important for developing effective intervention work plans. In the drug prevention study in China, a wide range of people were consulted, including government leaders in different government sectors, such as education, health, public security, culture and entertainment, agriculture technology, ethnic group management, and poverty alleviation, as well as community leaders, youth leaders, women leaders, student leaders, teachers, village health workers, and drug users (Wu *et al.* 1999).

There is no rule for determining how much community consultation is needed. It depends on the complexity of the proposed intervention and the complexity of the community. The same targeted intervention may require different intensities of community consultation depending on the characteristics of the communities. In the study promoting consistent condom use among female sex workers, the extent of community consultation differed between study sites (Wu 1998). In Chengjiang County, comprehensive consultation was sought from officials from all government sectors involved in entertainment management as well as from establishment owners and the sex workers themselves. In Ruili and Longchuan counties, in which the investigators had had extensive prior experience, only local health officials, establishment owners, and sex workers themselves were consulted.

Consultation is not only important for developing appropriate and effective intervention strategies and work plans but also to provide the opportunity for local community members to learn skills, and to identify barriers for promoting changes in the community. Even more important, by being consulted, community leaders and members perceive that they are respected by the investigators, that they share the ownership of the project, and therefore that they share the responsibility for the success of the project.

Often people in the community think that they work for the investigators and not for themselves or for their community. This perception occurs because they are usually paid or partly paid by the project or by project director, and they are told what the problems are and how to solve them. This perception is counterproductive, particularly for sustaining the changes after the trial is closed. It is important to promote the perception that the project is the community's project, that it will benefit the community, and that everyone has a responsibility to participate. One way to do so is to involve the target community in the design, implementation, and evaluation of the project.

Sample size

The sample size, in terms of the intervention units in community-based prevention trials, is usually much smaller than in trials conducted at the individual level. This is because the sampling units are communities, not individual people. The small sample size affects not only the study power, but also the comparability between intervention and comparison groups whether or not randomization is used.

To obtain a similar study population size (that is, number of participants), the investigator may choose either a small number of communities which have large populations, or a large number of communities which have smaller populations. If communities are homogeneous, either is acceptable for archiving comparability between intervention and control groups. If communities are heterogeneous, a larger number of small communities should be considered. In the community intervention trails listed in Table 1, the number of communities involved varied. Most studies involved 10 to 50 communities or clusters as study units. Some only had one unit and some had more than 200 units. In the Mauritius non-communicable disease prevention study, it was not feasible to use a control area in the small island, and therefore only one unit was used (Dowse *et al.* 1995). Emerson *et al.* (1999) used two pairs of villages to study control of trachoma and diarrhoea in Gambia. In the trial of hepatitis A inactivated vaccine, 148 primary schools were used. A block size of 10 participants was used to balance assignment by grade within a school (Innis *et al.* 1994). In the study to promote exclusive breast feeding in San Pedro Martir, 39 clusters with two to four city blocks each were used as randomization units (Morrow *et al.* 1999). Adish *et al.* (1999) used 407 households to evaluate the impact of foods cooked in iron pots with that of food cooked in aluminium pots on iron-deficiency anaemia among children in Ethiopia.

The control group

In principle, the control group is very important in community intervention trials to separate the impact of the intervention from other factors that might affect the trial. Sometimes rates before the intervention may serve as a control. However, when the intervention period is long, perhaps a few years, many other changes may have occurred which may affect disease rates. Furthermore, under very rare circumstances, it is unethical to have a control group.

In 1987, the Senegal government introduced immunization programmes into Bandafassi, an isolated area that previously had had no regular immunization programme. Since immunizations were the only change introduced into the area during this period, it was possible to assess the impact of immunization on childhood mortality by comparing mortality rates before and after the immunization programme was introduced. Desgrees du Loû *et al.* (1995) found that after the introduction of immunization the neonatal mortality declined 31 per cent, the mortality rate for children between 1 and 8 months of age declined by 20 per cent, and the mortality rate for children between 9 and 59 months declined by 48 per cent. The study also demonstrated that the decline in childhood mortality was greater in villages that maintained a higher coverage after the initial campaign, whereas mortality increased again in villages where the coverage declined.

In the early 1990s, the Thai government launched a national AIDS campaign, promoting condom use and implementing a '100 per cent condom' policy in all brothels. It is not ethically acceptable to set up a parallel control group since condom use was already known to be effective in reducing sexual transmission of HIV (Pinkerton and Abramson 1997; Ngugi *et al.* 1998; Phoolcharoen 1998; Phoolcharoen *et al.* 1998). After condom promotion was implemented nationwide, the incidence and prevalence of sexually transmitted diseases declined dramatically, accompanied by a decline in HIV infections (Wongkhomthong *et al.* 1995; UNAIDS 1998).

Before and after comparisons can sometimes provide solid evidence of the effectiveness of an intervention programme, particularly when the study period is short. In the study promoting consistent condom use with clients among female sex workers in China, identifying a control group was almost impossible since sex workers move around quickly (Wu 1998). Interchange between the intervention and control groups would increase use of the intervention by the control and reduce the apparent difference between them. This could result in an incorrect conclusion that condom promotion had no effect. However, a significant beneficial impact was documented during the period following the 3-month intervention. Knowledge of the three main transmission routes of HIV rose from 18 to 98 per cent in Chengjiang, from 44 to 88 per cent in Ruili, and from 0 to 59 per cent in Longchuan. Knowledge that condom use reduced the risk of sexually transmitted disease/HIV infection rose from 58 to 99 per cent in Chengjiang, from 55 to 91 per cent in Ruili, and from 55 to 90 per cent in Longchuan. Condom use for the last three incidents of sexual intercourse rose from 31 to 77 per cent in Chengjiang, from 51 to 75 per cent in Ruili, and from 39 to 41 per cent in Longchuan. These changes were unlikely to have been due to factors other than the intervention itself.

To evaluate the World AIDS Campaign comparing the effectiveness of mass media alone with mass media plus small media (leaflets, fliers, stickers, letters to families in the community, posters, and so on), both a parallel control group and a before–after control were used and both confirmed changes within 2 months after the intervention had begun (Du *et al.* 1999).

Often the results of trials using the pre-/post-study design are difficult to interpret. Concurrent controls usually provide a more valid comparison. This design was almost exclusively used in community-based intervention trials launched in developing countries that have been published over the last few years. In the Mwanza study of the impact of improved sexually transmitted disease treatment on the HIV epidemic, six pair-matched comparison communities were used (Grosskurth *et al.* 1995*b*; Hayes *et al.* 1995). The six comparison communities were similar to intervention communities at baseline regarding the baseline prevalence of HIV and syphilis. They were also similar with respect to most of the measured risk factors (Grosskurth *et al.* 1995*a*,*b*). In the Rakai sexually transmitted disease Control for AIDS Prevention Study, 10 community clusters were randomized with five assigned to intervention and five to control groups (Wawer *et al.* 1999).

Concurrent control groups were also used in the community trials to reduce childhood mortality rates (Bang *et al.* 1990; Pandey *et al.* 1991), the evaluation of the effect of maternity care on infant mortality (Fauveau *et al.* 1991; Ronsmans *et al.* 1997), the assessment of the impact of face-washing on trachoma prevalence (West *et al.* 1995), the impact of maximizing immunization coverage (Brugha and Kevany 1996), the impact of increasing HIV/AIDS-related knowledge to change attitudes and increase safer sex practices (Ronsmans *et al.* 1997), the use of the syndromic management of sexually transmitted diseases in pharmacies (Garcia *et al.* 1998), the effect of promoting exclusive breast feeding (Morrow *et al.* 1999), the prevention of iron-deficiency anaemia (Adish *et al.* 1999), the prevention of drug initiation (Wu *et al.* 1999), and stroke prevention (Fang *et al.* 1999) in developing countries.

The randomized community trial to evaluate the impact of fly control on the incidence of childhood diarrhoea in Pakistan offered a unique example of different control groups (Chavasse *et al.* 1999). The study consisted of three areas: area A, area B, and a control area. Area A was sprayed in 1995, not sprayed in 1996, and traps were set in 1997. Area B was not sprayed in 1995, it was sprayed in 1996, and no traps were set in 1997. The control area was not sprayed from 1995 to 1997. Areas A and B were switched to control areas in 1995 and in 1996.

Randomization and matching

The randomized controlled trial study design is more frequently used in the evaluation of the impact of a health intervention than before. Unmeasured confounding factors are expected to be equally distributed in the intervention and comparison groups by random allocation of communities into the two groups. Unbiased effect-estimates and valid confidence intervals can, therefore, be obtained. It is believed that this design is usually better than using comparison before and after the introduction of the intervention.

When a community intervention trial design is chosen, the unit for randomization is the community or cluster rather than the individual. Usually the number of units for randomization in community intervention trial studies is small. To avoid biases, nonetheless, randomization is as important in studies of communities as it is in studies of individuals.

When the number of communities is very small, randomization is less likely to achieve comparability between intervention and control groups (Rothman and Greenland 1998). When only a few communities are available for the study, random assignment to treatment and control groups is difficult to perform to achieve the comparability between the two arms. If only two study communities are studied, no matter how well researchers do randomization, incomparability between intervention and control will likely remain.

Given a small number of units for study, and substantial variation in the outcome variables and some major risk factors, pairwise matching of communities is often used in community trials. The rationale for matching is to improve power in randomized studies. However, if matching variables are not strongly associated with the outcome, matching actually reduces study power through loss of degrees of freedom with a small number of experimental units (Martin *et al.* 1993).

In the study of the effect of face-washing on trachoma, three paired villages were matched on maternal education level, baseline prevalence of clean faces in young children, and trachoma status. Within each pair, one village was randomized to the intervention and the other to the control group (West *et al.* 1995). In the Mwanza study, matching was used because there were variations in HIV prevalence and incidence in different parts of the study region (Hayes *et al.* 1995). Communities were matched on roadside, lakeshore, or rural location, geographic area, and pre-existing level of sexually transmitted diseases based on clinic records at the health centre. Randomization was performed within each matched pair.

When study communities are similar in prevalence and incidence of events and related key risk factors, matching is not necessary. In this situation, randomization can be directly performed without matching. For example, in the Rakai sexually transmitted disease prevention trial, matching was not used because of the homogeneous character of the study communities (Garcia *et al.* 1998; Wawer *et al.* 1999).

In certain circumstances, neither paired matching nor randomization of intervention units is possible. For example, in the drug prevention study in China, 19 intervention villages were matched to 19 comparison villages to achieve approximately equal prevalence and incidences of drug use at baseline (Wu *et al.* 1999). Because of the need to ensure that the control villages were not 'contaminated' by receiving intervention messages from the intervention villages, the intervention and control villages were separated by a mountain range.

Sometimes matching is not feasible either because data on outcomes of interest and risk factors among study communities are not available, or the number of units is too small to permit effective matching. In the study to maximize immunization coverage through home visits in Ghana, only three towns were selected as study units. Neither randomization nor matching was performed (Brugha and Kevany 1996).

When a community intervention programme includes education, particularly through mass media, as part of the intervention, randomization is not feasible for several reasons even though the number of communities is relatively large. Firstly, contamination is a major problem. The mass media usually covers relatively large areas. To avoid contamination, intervention communities must be separated from the control communities. Secondly, acceptability of research by the community is sometimes an issue. In some developing countries, communities do not accept the concept of 'research' or 'study' nor do they understand the need for controls. They often only support community programmes or projects that they believe will be beneficial, or at least potentially beneficial to their communities. Randomization may give the community the perception that they are only being used as guinea pigs. Thirdly, randomization may not be logistically feasible. Finally, many poor countries believe that the expense of having control communities is not cost-effective. In these situations it is important to educate the government in the need for controls. In a community-based intervention trial to reduce childhood mortality from pneumonia, a total of 102 villages were involved (Bang *et al.* 1990). The interventions included mass education about childhood pneumonia and case-management of pneumonia by village health workers and traditional birth attendants. In the study, 58 villages in one area were assigned to the intervention group and 44 villages in another area were treated as the control group. The intervention and control areas were, however, continuous areas except for a small 'buffer' zone of a few villages. In this example, given the geographic proximity of the intervention and control communities and the wide coverage by the mass media, researchers had to choose randomization without using mass media, or use the mass media but not have a control area.

Cohort versus repeated cross-sectional samples

To evaluate the impact of community trials, either a cohort study design or a repeated cross-sectional survey design can be used, or both can be used simultaneously. Results based solely on a cohort may not be representative of the target population. Even if the population of interest was those who reside in the community continuously during the intervention, the cohort sample is usually a self-selected subset of that group who are willing to be followed up. Therefore, it is probably not representative of the entire target population. Conducting both cohort and repeated cross-sectional surveys may be an ideal way to evaluate impact of intervention. It is expensive and often not logistically possible. Thus, either cohort or repeated cross-sectional surveys have been used almost exclusively in all community-based interventions conducted in developing countries.

The decision to choose either a cohort study, or repeated cross-sectional surveys, depends on the characteristics of the outcome variable, the information-collecting system available at the study sites, and the amount of funds available for the study. Sometimes a cohort study makes more sense and is the only choice. In other situations, only a serial cross-sectional study is feasible.

In the two studies of reducing childhood mortality (Bang *et al.* 1990; Pandey *et al.* 1991), a cohort study design was used. In the India study (Bang *et al.* 1990), a census was carried out before the study. All births and deaths of children under 5 years were recorded by village health workers in each village. In the Nepal study (Pandey *et al.* 1991), a similar method was employed. A household census of children under 5 years old was done at the start of the study, and all subsequent births and childhood deaths were registered throughout the subsequent 36 months.

A cohort study design was also used in the two landmark sexually transmitted disease intervention studies (Hayes *et al.* 1995; Grosskurth *et al.* 1995*b*; Wawer *et al.* 1998, 1999). In the Tanzania study (Grosskurth *et al.* 1995*b*; Hayes *et al.* 1995), the incidence of HIV infection in the intervention and comparison communities was assessed during the 2-year follow-up. A cohort of 12 000 adults aged 15 to 54 years was recruited. A random sample of 1000 from each group was selected, regardless of HIV status at baseline. Nested case–control studies were carried out within the cohort at baseline and follow-up. In the Rakai study (Wawer *et al.* 1998, 1999), an 'open' cohort study design was used. Home visits were conducted in both the 28 communities in the intervention group and the 28 communities in the comparison group. Subjects aged 15 to 59 years were enrolled for follow-up every 9 to 10 months.

In the study of the impact of HIV testing and counselling upon changes in condom use and sexual behaviours among men attending sexually transmitted disease clinics, a cohort design was used (Bentley *et al.* 1998). Subjects were followed-up at 3-month intervals. In the trachoma study (West *et al.* 1995), children's trachoma status and facial cleanliness were observed at baseline and at 2, 6, and 12 months after intervention. In the study of peer counselling to promote exclusive breast feeding, the cohort study design was also used (Morrow *et al.* 1999). All study mothers were followed-up at 2, 4, and 6 weeks and at 2 and 3 months postpartum to record infant-feeding practices in the previous week and whether the infant had experienced diarrhoea since the last interview.

In the two HIV/AIDS-related education studies, repeated cross-sectional surveys were used to assess the impact of the intervention programme (Pauw *et al.* 1996; Du *et al.* 1999). Knowledge was assessed at baseline and after the education intervention programme had been implemented.

In some situations, the cohort study design is almost impossible to use. For example, the repeated cross-sectional study design was the only feasible choice in the study of promoting condom use (Wu 1998) as sex workers move frequently and are difficult to follow up.

Sometimes a retrospective cohort can be reconstructed in repeated cross-sectional surveys. In the prevention of drug use intervention study in China (Wu *et al.* 1999), the incidence of drug use among adolescents and young adults was estimated based on a reconstructed retrospective cohort derived from repeated cross-sectional surveys. This was possible because there was very little migration in or out of the villages and the village leader was responsible for recording any that did occur.

Intervention activities

Types of intervention

The content of community interventions can include changes in public policy, the environment, community norms, and personal behaviours at both the individual and community levels. In broad terms, intervention programmes can be grouped into four types:

- individual-level programmes, such as self-study manuals, one-to-one communication or counselling, and peer education programmes
- mass media campaigns such as radio and television advertisement or newspaper stories
- public policy changes, such as mandated non-smoking areas in public places and syndromic management of sexually transmitted diseases at clinics
- group interventions such as educational programmes in schools or with informal groups such as support organizations of drug users or sex workers.

Often community-wide interventions include programmes of each type. Choosing which types of interventions to use should be determined by the characteristics of the communities, the diseases of interest, and other factors. Usually, individually targeted intensive interventions may be of limited use in community trials because participation in these kinds of programmes is low, and thus the population-level impact will be small. Generally, a combined approach is more likely to be effective than one which uses only one approach.

Usually, well-designed mass media campaigns are effective for increasing basic knowledge but not effective for correcting misconceptions (Du *et al.* 1999). Public policy change probably is the most cost-efficient way to make an impact. For example, the '100 per cent condom' policy for brothel-based prostitutes in Thailand reduced the incidence and prevalence of sexually transmitted diseases dramatically (Wongkhomthong *et al.* 1995; UNAIDS 1998). But even this approach was combined with mass education on the threat of HIV and the efficacy of condoms.

Intensity of intervention

Often a community health intervention trial can be designed, funded, and implemented in a place where other health-related programmes may already be under way with public and/or private sponsorship in both experimental and control communities. Thus, many community intervention trials may be testing only an incremental increase in the general level of health promotion in intervention communities, not the effectiveness of the intervention alone. Therefore, any community intervention programme must be sufficiently potent to be 'heard' beyond the background noise of ongoing health promotion activities. Thus, an intervention programme should direct resources towards interventions that are relatively unique and not available in control communities.

In order to prevent epidemics of childhood diseases such as measles and polio, a high immunization coverage must be achieved. When the immunization coverage for measles reaches above 80 per cent, an epidemic of measles among children is less likely to occur when an index case is introduced. Conversely, if the coverage is less than 50 per cent, the epidemic is more likely to occur if an index case is introduced. Similarly, the intensity of an intervention must reach a certain level, otherwise the intervention programme will not be able to produce a change. For example, when a needle exchange programme was introduced in Vancouver City, the epidemic of HIV infection among injecting drug users still took off (Strathdee *et al.* 1997; Schechter *et al.* 1999). Additional research indicated that the availability of the needles and syringes in the exchange programmes was insufficient for stopping the transmission of HIV among injecting drug users.

In the study to promote exclusive breast feeding in San Pedro Martir, Mexico City, two intervention groups with different counselling frequencies, six visits and three visits, were compared with a control group that had no intervention (Morrow *et al.* 1999). Infants were followed up until 3 months of age to assess the effect of the peer education programme on promoting exclusive breast feeding and on the incidence of diarrhoea among children. Exclusive breast feeding was achieved in 67 per cent in the six-visit group, 50 per cent in the three-visit group, and 12 per cent in the control group.

In the study promoting condom use among female sex workers in China (Wu 1998), six on-site education and condom promotion programmes were given at all three study sites. However, one of the study sites was not able to provide sexual health-care services, including sexually transmitted disease diagnosis and treatment, to sex workers. Sex workers at that study site had a lower increase in knowledge and a lower increase in consistent condom use rate with clients, compared with the other two sites.

How much intervention is less than enough, how much is just enough, and how much is more than enough varies depending on such variables as the nature of the intervention, the characteristics of the target population, and the cultural characteristics of the society. Thus, no guidelines can be formulated to cover all circumstances.

Sustainability of intervention

The sustainability of an intervention is one of most important issues in conducting community-based interventions in developing countries. Several factors affect sustainability. Firstly, the cost of intervention—the cheaper the intervention is, the more sustainable the programme will be. In the Mwanza sexually transmitted disease study, during the 2 years of follow-up, 11 632 cases of sexually transmitted diseases were treated in the intervention health units; 252 HIV infections were averted each year in the intervention group compared with control group. The average per capita cost was US$0.39. It was estimated that the average cost per disability-adjusted life year saved was US$10, ranging from US$2.51 to US$47.86. The estimated cost-effectiveness of the intervention (that is, improved treatment services for sexually transmitted diseases) compared favourably with the cost of childhood immunization programs (US$12 to US$17 per disability-adjusted life year) (Gilson *et al.* 1997). Such intervention programmes may be affordable for developing countries.

Secondly, the simpler the intervention is, the more sustainable the programme will be. In a study on reducing childhood mortality in Nepal (Pandey *et al.* 1991), the intervention programme focused on active case detection. Every day each health worker visited 10 to 15 households with children under 5 years old, most within a 30 minute walk of the worker's home. Workers completed a round of the target households (about 160) under their responsibility every 2 weeks. The intervention occupied about half each worker's time and allowed the continuation of regular farming activities. In the Mwanza sexually transmitted disease study, the intervention had five components: establishment of a reference clinic, training of health-care providers, ensuring a constant supply of effective drugs, and regular supervision and health education in the target communities to encourage individuals with sexually transmitted disease symptoms to seek treatment early (Mayaud *et al.* 1997). In the Rakai sexually transmitted disease study, because of the lack of a clinical infrastructure in the study areas and the high prevalence of sexually transmitted diseases in the communities, a mass treatment strategy was used and all consenting adults were given directly observed sexually transmitted disease therapy in their home every 10 months, irrespective of laboratory test results or the presence of symptoms (Wawer *et al.* 1999). These strategies would be possible for many developing countries.

Thirdly, the higher the proportion of people in the community covered by the intervention, the more likely the programme will be sustained. In the Rakai sexually transmitted disease study, all consenting adults were given treatment (Wawer *et al.* 1999). In the neonatal care and management study, coverage with the intervention increased from 75.1 per cent in 1995–1996, to 85.2 per cent in 1996–1997, and to 93.3 per cent in 1997–1998 (Bang *et al.* 1999).

Fourthly, the higher the intensity of the intervention, the less likely the programme will be sustained because maintaining high intensity is usually expensive, difficult, and often results in 'burn-out' of both workers and participants. However, if the intensity is not high enough, the programme may not be able to produce changes.

If the programme itself can generate profits, the sustainability of the programme is likely. From July 1998 to August 1999, condom vending machines were installed in communities for condom social marketing in Shenzhen City, Guangdong Province, where many migrants live. The price of a single condom was 1 Yuan Chinese Renminbi (equivalent to US$0.12) and was therefore affordable for everyone in the community. Taking into account the staff salaries, the base price of condoms, and the cost of the vending machines for the 8-month period, the profits generated from condoms bought from the vending machines was estimated at 100 per cent (Wu 1999).

Measurement

The overall aim of a community-based intervention programme is to reduce morbidity and/or mortality. For most community intervention trials conducted in developing countries, either morbidity or mortality is used as the outcome variable to evaluate the impact of the intervention.

In the two diarrhoea control studies, the reported incidence of diarrhoea among children under 5 years old was used as the outcome measure to assess the effectiveness of the intervention (Chen and Liu 1991; Chavasse *et al.* 1999). In the breast-feeding study, both the prevalence of exclusive breast feeding and the incidence of diarrhoea among children were used to evaluate the impact of the intervention (Morrow *et al.* 1999). In the two sexually transmitted disease studies conducted in Africa, the incidence of sexually transmitted diseases and HIV infection were used to evaluate intervention effects (Hayes 1995; Grosskurth *et al.* 1995*b*; Mayaud *et al.* 1997; Mawer *et al.* 1998; Mawer *et al.* 1999).

In the childhood mortality study in Nepal (Pandey *et al.* 1991) and India (Bang *et al.* 1990), mortality was used as the outcome variable. In the study of the reduction of maternal mortality, mortality was again chosen as an outcome measurement (Fauveau *et al.* 1991; Ronsmans *et al.* 1997).

Direct measures of outcome variables, such as disease incidence or mortality, provide valid data to assess the effectiveness of an intervention programme. However, determining them is often expensive. The high cost of individual-level measurements may limit the number of surveys that can be done and thus the statistical power of the evaluation. The high cost of measuring incidence often precludes long-term monitoring for late effects, which can be important since the time lag between programme implementation and individual-level effects is often uncertain and may be long. Serial cross-sectional surveys are also expensive but are usually less expensive than incidence studies.

Because of these problems, other measures are often used as surrogate markers for morbidity. Examples of the surrogate or intermediate outcomes that are measured in a variety of behavioural intervention studies include knowledge, attitudes, beliefs, intentions, behavioural skills, and behaviours. In two community-based HIV/AIDS education interventions, knowledge, sexual behaviours, and condom use behaviours were used as outcome variables to assess the impact of the interventions (Pauw *et al.* 1996; Bentley *et al.* 1998).

Interpretation

Interpretation of results is sometimes difficult. Interpretation must be made especially cautiously when no control group is used. In the Matlab study of maternal mortality in Bangladesh (Fauveau *et al.* 1991), it was concluded that maternal mortality was significantly lower in areas with maternal/child health-care and family planning programmes than in the control area. About 6 years later, continued observation indicated that there was no difference between the maternal/child health-care and family planning programmes and comparison areas (Ronsmans *et al.* 1997). The authors thus concluded that the introduction of the maternity-care programme coincided with declining trends in direct obstetric mortality in the areas covered by the programme although it is also possible that the effectiveness of the intervention declined.

There were two landmark community-based intervention trials, both undertaken in Africa, to determine what impact sexually transmitted disease prevention and control might have on HIV infection rates. The first, in Mwanza, Tanzania, focused on enhanced syndromic diagnosis and treatment of symptomatic sexually transmitted diseases (Grosskurth *et al.* 1995*b*). The second, in Rakai, Uganda, focused on treatment of all members of the intervention communities regardless of the presence of symptoms (Wawer *et al.* 1999). Both studies used a randomized study design. The Mwanza study revealed a 38 per cent reduction in HIV incidence in the communities that received the intervention, compared with control communities, but no difference was found in terms of sexually transmitted disease incidence. However, the Rakai study did not find any difference in terms of HIV infection between the intervention and control areas, although the prevalence of syphilis and trichomoniasis was significantly lower in the intervention area than in the control area. Among pregnant women, the prevalence of trichomoniasis, bacterial vaginosis, gonorrhoea, and *Chlamydia* infection were significantly lower in the intervention group than in the control group. How does one interpret the conflicting results from these two community intervention trial studies? There are three possibilities. Either one of the two study results is invalid or both are invalid or both are valid. One rational interpretation for the discrepancy between the two findings is that control of sexually transmitted diseases has an impact on reducing HIV incidence only when the epidemic is in the early stage. Once the prevalence of HIV has reached a threshold level, resulting in a high probability of sex with an HIV-infected partner, the role of sexually transmitted diseases may be reduced (Hitchcock and Fransen 1999).

Conclusion

Community intervention trials are increasingly being used in developing countries and cover an expanding range of public health issues, including infectious diseases, neonatal mortality, malnutrition, and unhealthy behaviours, as well as chronic diseases such as cardiovascular diseases. One advantage of conducting community intervention trials in developing countries is the usually high prevalence or incidence of events that makes such trials more cost-efficient. More importantly, they often address urgent preventable health problems in these countries.

However, it is often more challenging to implement community intervention trials in developing countries because of the lack of background information, lack of infrastructure, and lack of trained and experienced resource personnel. Several criteria need to be considered before beginning community intervention trials in developing countries. Study sites should have a reasonably high incidence of the health events of interest. A qualitative study of the social and cultural characteristics of the community may need to be conducted. Community consultation should be carried out before finalizing the intervention plan. Local resources should be used for the intervention. The type of intervention and the intensity of the intervention must be considered acceptable to the communities. Simplicity, affordability, and sustainability of intervention strategies should always be emphasized. Community interventions have been demonstrated to be effective in developing countries but more trials are needed for the many public health problems still affecting developing countries.

References

Adish, A.A., Esrey, S.A., Gyorkos, T.W., Jean-Baptiste, J., and Rojhani, A. (1999). Effect of consumption of food cooked in iron pots on iron status and growth of young children: a randomized trial. *Lancet*, **353**, 712–16.

Bang, A.T., Bang, R.A., Tale, O., *et al.* (1990). Reduction in pneumonia mortality and total childhood mortality by means of community-based intervention trial in Gadchiroli, India. *Lancet*, **336**, 201–6.

Bang, A.T., Bang, R.A., Baitule, S.B., Reddy, M.H., and Deshmukh, M.D. (1999). Effect of home-based neonatal care and management of sepsis on neonatal mortality: field trial in rural India. *Lancet*, **354**, 1955–61.

Bentley, M.E., Spratt, K., Shepherd, M.E., *et al.* (1998). HIV testing and counseling among men attending sexually transmitted disease clinics in Pune, India: changes in condom use and sexual behavioral over time. *AIDS*, **12**, 1869–77.

Brugha, R.F. and Kevany, J.P. (1996). Maximizing immunization coverage through home visits: a controlled trial in a urban area of Ghana. *Bulletin of the World Health Organisation*, **74**, 517–24.

Carleton, R.A., Lasater, T.M., Assaf, A.R., Feldman, H.A., and McKinlay, S. (1995). The Pawtucket Heart Health Program: community changes in cardiovascular risk factors and projected disease risk. *American Journal of Public Health*, **85**, 777–85.

Ceesay, S.M., Prentice, A.M., Cole, T.J., *et al.* (1997). Effect on birth weight and perinatal mortality of maternal dietary supplements in rural Gambia: 5 year randomized control trial. *British Medical Journal*, **315**, 786–90.

Chavasse, D.C., Shier, R.P., Murphy, O.A., Huttly, S.R.A., Cousens, S.N., and Akhtar, T. (1999). Impact of fly control on childhood diarrhea in Pakistan: community-randomized trial. *Lancet*, **353**, 22–5.

Chen, S.K. and Liu, X.X. (1991). Efficiency evaluation of combined intervention measures with improving drinking water first to prevent infantile acute diarrhea. *Chinese Journal of Epidemiology*, **12**, 289–91.

COMMIT (Community Intervention Trial for Smoking Cessation) Research Group (1991). Community Intervention Trial for Smoking Cessation (COMMIT): summary of design and intervention. *Journal of National Cancer Institute*, **83**, 1620–28.

COMMIT (Community Intervention Trial for Smoking Cessation) Research Group (1995). Community Intervention Trial for Smoking Cessation (COMMIT): I. Cohort results from a Four-Year Community Intervention. *American Journal of Public Health*, **85**, 183–92.

Desgrees du Loû, A., Pison, G., and Aaby, P. (1995). Role of immunizations in the recent decline in childhood mortality and the changes in the female/male mortality ratio in Rural Senegal. *American Journal of Epidemiology*, **142**, 643–52.

Dietrich, A.J., O'Connor, G.T., Keller, A., Carney, P.A., Levy, D., and Whaley, F.S. (1992). Cancer: improving early detection and prevention. A community practice randomized trial. *British Medical Journal*, **304**, 687–91.

Dowse, G.K., Gareeboo, H.G., Alberti, K.G.M.M., *et al.* (1995). Changes in population cholesterol concentrations and other cardiovascular risk factor levels after five year of the non-communicable disease intervention program in Mauritius. *British Medical Journal*, **311**, 1255–9.

Du, H., Wu, Z., Jia, P.Q., Qiao, L., Liu, H., and Wang, T. (1999). Comparison of effectiveness of mass media with small media and personal communication in the World AIDS Campaign in Beijing in 1997–1998. *Chinese Journal of Prevention and Control STD and AIDS*, **5**, 1–4.

Emerson, P.M., Lindsay, S.W., Walraven, G.E.L., *et al.* (1999). Effect of fly control on trachoma and diarrhea. *Lancet*, **353**, 1401–3.

Fang, X.H., Kronmal, R.A., and Li, S.C. (1999*a*). Prevention of stroke in urban China: a community-based intervention trial. *Stroke*, **30**, 495–501.

Fang, J., Wu, Z., Duan, L., *et al.* (1999*b*). Qualitative study of reproductive tract infection among rural women in Ruili City, Yunnan Province. *Chinese Rural Health Service Administration*, **19**, 49–51.

Farquhar, J.W., Fortmann, S.P., Maccoby, N., *et al.* (1977). Community education for cardiovascular health. *Lancet*, **i**, 1192–5.

Farquhar, J.W., Fortmann, S.T., Flora, J.A., *et al.* (1985). The Stanford Five-City Project: design and methods. *American Journal of Epidemiology*, **122**, 323–34.

Fauveau, V., Stewart, K., Khan, S.A., and Chakraborty, J. (1991). Effect on mortality of community-based maternity-care program in rural Bangladesh. *Lancet*, **338**, 1183–6.

Ford, K., Wirawan, D.N., Fajans, P., Meliawan, P., MacDonald, K., and Thorpe, L. (1996). Behavioral intervention for reduction of sexually transmitted disease/HIV transmission among female commercial sex workers and clients in Bali, Indonesia. *AIDS*, **10**, 213–22.

Garcia, P.J., Gotuzzo, E., Hughes, J.P., and Holmes, K.K. (1998). Syndromic management of STDs in pharmacies: evaluation and randomized intervention trial. *Sexually Transmitted Infections*, **74** (Supplement 1), S153–8.

Gilson, L., Mkanje, R., Grosskurth, H., *et al.* (1997). Cost-effectiveness of improved treatment services for sexually transmitted diseases in preventing HIV-1 infection in Mwanza Region, Tanzania. *Lancet*, **350**, 1183–6.

Greenberg, R.A., Strecher, V.J., Bauman, K.K., *et al.* (1994). Evaluation of a home-based intervention program to reduce infant passive smoking and lower respiratory illness. *Journal of Behavioral Medicine*, **17**, 273–90.

Grosskurth, H., Mosha, F., Todd, J., *et al.* (1995*a*). A community trial of the impact of improved sexually transmitted disease treatment on the HIV epidemic in rural Tanzania: 2. Baseline survey results. *AIDS*, **9**, 927–34.

Grosskurth, H., Mosha, F., Todd, J., *et al.* (1995*b*). Impact of improved treatment of sexually transmitted diseases on HIV infection in rural Tanzania: randomized controlled trial. *Lancet*, **346**, 530–6.

Hayes, R., Mosha, F., Nicoll, A., *et al.* (1995). A community trial of the impact of improved sexually transmitted disease treatment on the HIV epidemic in rural Tanzania: 1. Design. *AIDS*, **9**, 919–26.

Hayes, R., Wawer, M., Gray, R., Whitworth, J., Grosskurth, H., Mabey, D., and HIV/STD Trials Workshop Group. (1997). Randomised trials of STD treatment for HIV prevention: report of an international workshop. *Genitourinary Medicine*, **73**, 432–43.

Hitchcock, P. and Fransen, L. (1999). Preventing HIV infection: lessons form Mwanza and Rakai. *Lancet*, **353**, 513–15.

Innis, B.L., Snitbhan, R., Kunasol, P., *et al.* (1994). Protection against hepatitis A by an inactivated vaccine. *Journal of American Medical Association*, **271**, 1328–34.

Kevany, J.P. and Brugha, R.F. (1996). Maximizing immunization coverage through home visits: a controlled trial in an urban area of Ghana. *Bulletin of the World Health Organization*, **75**, 517–24.

Luepker, R.V., Murray, D.M., Jacobs, D.R., *et al.* (1994). Community education for cardiovascular diseases prevention: risk factor changes in the Minnesota Heart Health Program. *American Journal of Public Health*, **84**, 1383–93.

Lye, M.S., Nair, R.C., Stat, M., Choo, K.E., Kaur, H., and Lai, K.P.F. (1996). Acute respiratory tract infection: a community-based intervention study in Malaysia. *Journal of Tropical Pediatrics*, **42**, 138–43.

Martin, D.C., Diehr, P., Perrin, E.B., *et al.* (1993). The effect of matching on the power of randomized community intervention studies. *Statistics in Medicine*, **12**, 29–38.

Mayaud, P., Mosha, F., Todd, J., *et al.* (1997). Improved treatment services significantly reduce the prevalence of sexually transmitted diseases in rural Tanzania: results of a randomized control trial. *AIDS*, **11**, 1873–80.

Morrow, A.L., Guerrero, M.L., Shults, J., *et al.* (1999). Efficacy of home-based peer counseling to promote exclusive breastfeeding: a randomized controlled trial. *Lancet*, **353**, 1226–31.

Ngugi, E.N., Plummer, F.A., Simonsen, J.N., *et al.* (1998). Prevention of transmission of human immunodeficincy virus in Africa: effectiveness of condom promotion and health education among prostitutes. *Lancet*, **ii**, 887–90.

Osborne, M., Boyle, P., and Lipkin, M. (1997). Cancer prevention. *Lancet*, **349** (Supplement II), 27–30.

Over, M. and Piot, P. (1993). HIV infection and sexually transmitted diseases. In *Disease control priorities in developing countries* (ed. D.T. Jamison, W.H. Mosley, A.R. Measham, and J.L. Bodadilla), pp. 455–527. Oxford University Press.

Pandey, M.R., Daulaire, N.M.P., Starbuck, R.S., Houston, R.M., and McPherson, K. (1991). Reduction in total under-five mortality in western Nepal through community-based antimicrobial treatment of pneumonia. *Lancet*, **338**, 993–7.

Pauw, J., Ferrie, J., Villegas, R.R., Martinez, J.M., Gorter, A., and Egger, M. (1996). A controlled HIV/AIDS-related health education programme Managua, Nicaragua. *AIDS*, **10**, 537–44.

Phoolcharoen, W. (1998). HIV/AIDS prevention in Thailand: success and challenges. *Science*, **280**, 1873–4.

Phoolcharoen, W., Ungchusak, K., Sittitrai, W., and Brown, T. (1998). Thailand: Lessons from a strong national response to HIV/AIDS. *AIDS*, **12** (Supplement B), S123–35.

Pinkerton, S.D. and Abramson, P.R. (1997). Effectiveness of condoms in preventing HIV transmission. *Social Science and Medicine*, **44**, 1303–12.

Puska, P., Salonen, J.T., Nissinen, A., *et al.* (1983). Change in risk factors for coronary heart disease during 10 years of a community intervention programme (North Karelia project). *British Medical Journal*, **287**, 1840–4.

Ronsmans, C., Vanneste, A.M., Chakraborty, J., and van Ginneken, J. (1997). Decline in maternal mortality in Matlab, Bangladesh: a cautionary tale. *Lancet*, **350**, 1810–14.

Ross-Degnan, D., Soumerai, S.B., Goel, P.K., *et al.* (1996). The impact of face-to-face educational outreach on diarrhea treatment in pharmacies. *Health Policy and Planning*, **11**, 308–18.

Rothman, K.J. and Greenland, S. (1998). *Modern epidemiology* (2nd edn). Lippincott–Raven, Philadelphia, PA.

Schechter, M.T., Strathdee, S.A., Cornelisse, P.G.A., *et al.* (1999). Do needle exchange programmes increase the spread of HIV among injection drug users? An investigation of the Vancouver outbreak. *AIDS*, **13**, F45–F51.

Smith, A.W., Hatcher, J., Mackenzie, I.J., *et al.* (1996). Randomized controlled trial of treatment of chronic supporative otitis media in Kenyan schoolchildren. *Lancet*, **348**, 1128–33.

Strathdee, S.A., Patrick, D.M., Currie, S.L., *et al.* (1997). Needle exchange is not enough: lessons from the Vancouver injecting drug use study. *AIDS*, **11**, F59–F65.

Tielsch, J.M. and West, K.P. (1990). Cost and efficiency consideration in community-based trials of vitamin A in developing countries. *Statistics in Medicine*, **9**, 35–43.

UNAIDS (United Nations Program on HIV/AIDS) (1998). *Relationships of HIV and STD declines in Thailand to behavioral change, a synthesis of existing studies.* UNAIDS Best Practice Collection Key Material. UNAIDS, Geneva.

UNAIDS/WHO (United Nations Program on HIV/AIDS and the World Health Organization (2000). *AIDS epidemic update: December 2000.* UNAIDS/WHO, Geneva.

Wawer, M.J., Gray, R.H., Sewankambo, N.K., *et al.* (1998). A randomized, community trial of intensive sexually transmitted disease control for AIDS prevention, Rakai, Uganda. *AIDS*, **12**, 1211–25.

Wawer, M.J., Sewankambo, N.K., Serwadda, D., *et al.* (1999). Control of sexually transmitted diseases for AIDS prevention in Uganda: a randomized community trial. *Lancet*, **353**, 525–35.

West, K.P. Jr, Pokhrel, R.P., Katz, J., *et al.* (1991). Efficacy of vitamin A in reducing preschool child mortality in Nepal. *Lancet*, **338**, 67–71.

West, S., Munoz, B., Lynch, M., *et al.* (1995). Impact of face-washing on trachoma in Kongwa, Tanzania. *Lancet*, **345**, 155–8.

West, K.P. Jr, Katz, J., Khatry, S.K., *et al.* (1999). Double blind, cluster randomized trial of low dose supplementation with vitamin A or β carotene on mortality related to pregnancy in Nepal. *British Medical Journal*, **318**, 570–5.

Winkley, M.A., Taylor, C.B., Jatulis, D., and Fortmann, S.P. (1996). The long-term effects of a cardiovascular disease prevention trial: the Stanford Five-City Project. *American Journal of Public Health*, **86**, 1773–9.

Wongkhomthong, S., Kaime-Atterhog, W., and Ono, K. (1995). *AIDS in the developing world: a case study of Thailand.* ASEAN Institute for Health Development, Mahidol University, Thailand.

World Bank (1993). *World development report 1993: investing in health.* Oxford University Press, New York.

Wu, Z. (1998). *Final Report for the World Bank: intervention on female prostitutes in Yunnan.* Chinese Academy of Preventive Medicine, Beijing.

Wu, Z. (1999). *Sustainability of condom vending machine in condom marketing in Shenzhen, Guangdong province.* Ministry of Health, People's Republic of China.

Wu, Z., Zhang, J.P., Detels, R., *et al.* (1999). Community-based program on prevention of drug use and HIV transmission in Yunnan, China. Presented at 5th International Congress on AIDS in Asia and the Pacific.

Yan, D.Y., Jin, Y.Q., Yang, Y., *et al.* (1992). Primary analysis on hypertension community control in East City of Beijing. *Chinese Journal of Epidemiology*, **13**, 348–50.

Yin, H.P., Ji, G.P., Wu, Z., Liu, M.R., and Ning, X.W. (1999). Qualitative study of KAP about RTI/STD/AIDS among MCH providers and their clients. *Chinese Rural Health Service Administration*, **19**, 52–4.

6.10 Concepts of validity in epidemiological research

Sander Greenland

Some of the major validity concepts in epidemiological research are outlined in this chapter. The contents are organized into three main sections: validity in prediction problems, validity in causal inference, and special validity problems in case–control and retrospective cohort studies. Familiarity with the basics of epidemiological study design and a number of terms of epidemiological theory, amongst them risk, competing risk, average risk, population at risk, and rate, are assumed. A number of textbooks provide more background and depth than can be given here. Among them, Checkoway *et al.* (1989), Walker (1991), Kelsey *et al.* (1996), and Chapters 1 to 11 of Rothman and Greenland (1998) provide epidemiological treatments, while Breslow and Day (1980, 1987), Clayton and Hills (1993), and Chapters 12 to 21 of Rothman and Greenland (1998) focus on statistical details.

Despite similarities, there is considerable diversity and conflict amongst the classification schemes and terminologies employed in various textbooks. This diversity reflects that there is no unique way of classifying validity conditions, biases, and errors. It follows that the classification schemes employed here and elsewhere should not be regarded as anything more than convenient frameworks for organizing discussions of study validity and epidemiological inference.

Several important study designs, including prevalence studies and ecological studies, are not discussed in this chapter. Such studies require consideration of the above validity conditions and also require special considerations of their own. Further details of these and other designs can be found in the general textbooks cited above. For a review of the special problems of ecological studies, see Greenland and Robins (1994) and Morgenstern (1998). Meta-analytic methods are discussed by Greenland (1994, 1998*a*).

Also not covered are a number of central problems of epidemiological inference, including choice of effect measures and interpretation of statistics. Critical discussions of effect measures are given by Greenland (1987), Greenland and Robins (1988), Greenland *et al.* (1986, 1991), and Chapter 4 of Rothman and Greenland (1998). Oakes (1990) and Barnett (1999) provide introductions to competing schools of statistical inference. They discuss shortcomings of the prevailing approaches to statistics and alternative approaches as well; see also Berger and Berry (1988), Goodman and Royall (1988), and Greenland (1998*b*). Rubin (1991) contrasts different statistical approaches to causal inference, and Greenland *et al.* (1999*a*) provide an introduction to graphical methods in causal inference. Poole (1987*a*, *b*), Goodman (1992, 1993, 1999), Greenland (1990, 1993*b*), and Chapter 12 of Rothman and Greenland (1998) discuss the use and misuse of statistical inference in epidemiological research.

Inference and validity

Epidemiological inference is the process of drawing inferences from epidemiological data, such as prediction of disease patterns or identification of causes of diseases or epidemics. These inferences must often be made without the benefits of direct experimental evidence or established theory about disease aetiology. Consider the problem of predicting the risk and incubation (induction) time for AIDS among people infected with HIV-1. Unlike an experiment, in which the exposure is administered by the investigator, the date of HIV-1 infection cannot be accurately estimated in most cases; furthermore, the mechanism by which 'silent' HIV-1 infection progresses to AIDS is not known with certainty. Nevertheless, some prediction must be made from the available data in order to prepare effectively for future health-care needs.

As another example, consider the problem of estimating how much excess risk of coronary heart disease (if any) is produced by coffee drinking. Unlike an experimental exposure, coffee drinking is self-selected; it appears that people who use coffee are more likely to smoke than non-users and probably tend to differ in many other behaviours as well (Greenland 1993*a*). As a result, even if coffee use is harmless, we should not expect to observe the same pattern of heart disease in users and non-users. Thus small coffee effects should be very difficult to disentangle from the effects of other behaviours. Nevertheless, because of the high prevalence of coffee use and the high incidence of heart disease, determination of the effect of coffee on heart disease risk may be of considerable public health importance.

In both these examples, and in general, inferences will depend on evaluating the validity of the available studies, or the degree to which the studies meet basic logical criteria for absence of bias. In each section of this chapter major concepts of validity in epidemiological research as applied in three settings—prediction from one population to another, causal inference from cohort studies, and causal inference from case–control and retrospective cohort studies—are outlined and illustrated. Parallel aspects of each application will be emphasized. In particular, each problem requires consideration of comparison validity, follow-up validity, specification validity, and measurement validity. Case–control studies require the additional consideration of case- and control-selection validity, and are often subject to additional sources of measurement error beyond those occurring in prospective cohort studies. Similar problems arise in retrospective cohort studies.

Validity in prediction problems

The following prediction problem will be used to illustrate the basic concepts of validity in epidemiological inference. A health clinic for homosexual men is about to begin enrolling HIV-l-negative men in an unrestricted programme that will involve retesting each participant for HIV-1 antibodies at 6-month intervals. It can be expected that, in the course of the programme, many participants will seroconvert to positive HIV-1 status. Such participants will invariably ask difficult questions, such as: What are my chances of developing AIDS over the next 5 years? How many years do I have before I develop AIDS? In attempting to answer these questions, it will be convenient to refer to such participants (that is, those who seroconvert) as the target cohort. Even though membership of this cohort is not determined in advance, it will be the target of our predictions. It will also be convenient to refer to the time from HIV-1 infection until the onset of clinical AIDS as the AIDS incubation time. Reasonable answers could be provided to a participant's questions if it were possible to predict AIDS incubation times accurately, although we would also have to estimate the time elapsed between infection and the first positive test.

There might be someone who responds to the questions posed above with the following anecdote: 'I've known several men just like the ones in this cohort, and they all developed AIDS within 5 years after a positive HIV-1 test'. No trained scientist would conclude from this anecdote that all or most of the target cohort will develop AIDS within 5 years of seroconversion. One reason is that the men in the anecdote cannot be 'just like' men in our cohort in every respect: they may have been older or younger when they were infected; they may have experienced a greater degree of stress following their infection; they may have been heavier smokers, drinkers, or drug users, and so on. In other words, we know that the anecdotal men and their postinfection life events could not have been exactly the same as the men in our target cohort with respect to all factors that affect AIDS incubation time, including measured, unmeasured, and unknown factors. Furthermore, it may be that some or all of the men referred to in the anecdote had been infected long before they were first tested, so that (unlike men in our target cohort) the time from their first positive test to AIDS onset was much shorter than the time from seroconversion to AIDS onset.

Any reasonable predictions must be based on observing the distribution of AIDS incubation times in another cohort. Suppose that we obtain data from a study of homosexual men who underwent regular HIV-1 testing, and then assemble from these data a study cohort of men who were observed to seroconvert. Suppose also that most of these men were followed for at least 5 years after seroconversion. It cannot be expected that any member of this study is going to be 'just like' any member of our target cohort in every respect. Nevertheless, if it was possible to identify no difference between the two cohorts with respect to factors that affect incubation time, it might be argued that the study cohort could serve as a point of reference for predicting incubation times in the target cohort. Thus, henceforth the study cohort shall be referred to as our reference cohort. Note that our reference and target cohorts may have originated from different populations; for example, the clinic generating the target cohort could be in New York, but the study that generated the reference cohort may have been in San Francisco. For both the target and reference cohorts, the actual times of HIV-1 infection will have to be imputed, based on the dates of the last negative and the first positive tests.

Suppose that our statistical analysis of data from the reference cohort produces estimates of 0.05, 0.25, and 0.45 for the average risk of contracting AIDS within 2, 5, and 8 years of HIV-1 infection. What conditions would be sufficient to guarantee the validity of these figures as estimates or predictions of the proportion of the target cohort that would develop AIDS within 2, 5, and 8 years of infection? If by 'valid' we mean that any discrepancy between our predictions and the true target proportions is purely random (unpredictable in principle), the following conditions would be sufficient.

- Comparison validity (*C*). The distribution of incubation times in the target cohort will be approximately the same as the distribution in the reference cohort.
- Follow-up validity (*F*). Within the reference cohort, the risk of censoring (that is, follow-up ended by an event other than AIDS) is not associated with risk of AIDS.
- Specification validity (*Sp*). The distribution of incubation times in the reference cohort can be closely approximated by the statistical model used to compute the estimates. For example, if one employs a log-normal distribution to model the distribution of incubation times in the reference cohort, this model should be approximately correct.
- Measurement validity (*M*). All measurements of variables used in the analysis closely approximate the true values of the variables. In particular, each imputed time of HIV-1 infection closely approximates the true infection time, and each reported time of AIDS onset closely approximates a clinical event defined as AIDS onset.

The first condition concerns the external validity of making predictions about the target cohort based on the reference cohort. The remaining conditions concern the internal validity of the predictions as estimates of average risk in the reference cohort. The following sections will explore the meaning of these conditions in prediction problems.

Comparison validity

Comparison validity is probably the easiest condition to describe, although it is difficult to evaluate. Intuitively, it simply means that the distribution of incubation times in the target cohort could be almost perfectly predicted from the distribution of incubation times in the reference cohort, if the incubation times were observed without error and there was no loss to follow-up. Other ways of stating this condition are that the two cohorts are comparable or exchangeable with respect to incubation times, or that the AIDS experience of the target cohort can be predicted from the experience of the reference cohort.

Confounding

If the two cohorts are not comparable, some or all of our risk estimates for the target cohort based on the reference cohort will be biased as a result. This bias is sometimes called confounding. There has been much research on methods for identifying and adjusting for such bias (see the textbooks cited above). (The term 'bias' is here used in the informal epidemiological sense, and corresponds to the formal statistical concept of inconsistency.)

To evaluate comparison validity, we must investigate whether the two cohorts differ on any factors that influence incubation time. If so, we cannot reasonably expect the incubation time distributions of the two cohorts to be comparable. A factor responsible for some or all of the confounding in an estimate is called a confounder or confounding variable, the estimate is said to be confounded by the factor, and the factor is said to confound the estimate.

To illustrate these concepts, suppose that men infected at younger ages tend to have longer incubation times and that the members of the reference cohort are on average younger than members of the target cohort. If there were no other differences to counterbalance this age difference, we should then expect that members of the reference cohort will on average have longer incubation times than members of the target cohort. Consequently, unadjusted predictions of risk for the target cohort derived from the reference cohort would be biased (confounded) by age in a downward direction. In other words, age would be a confounder for estimating risk in the target cohort, and confounding by age would result in underestimation of the proportion of men in the target cohort who will develop AIDS within 5 years.

Suppose that it is possible to compute the age at infection of men in the reference cohort, and that within 1-year strata of age, for instance, the target and reference cohorts had virtually identical distributions of incubation times. The age-specific estimates of risk derived from the reference cohort would then be free of age confounding and so could be used as unconfounded estimates of age-specific risk for men in the target cohort. Also, if we wished to construct unconfounded estimates of average risk in the entire target cohort, we could do so via the technique of age standardization.

To illustrate, let P_x denote our estimate of the average risk of AIDS within 5 years of infection among members of the reference cohort who become infected at age x. Let W_x denote the proportion of men in the target cohort who are infected at age x. Then the estimated average risk of AIDS within 5 years of infection, standardized to the target cohort's age distribution, is simply the average of the age-specific reference estimates P_x, weighted by the age distribution (at infection) of the target cohort; algebraically, this average is the sum of the products W_xP_x over all ages and is denoted by $\Sigma_x W_xP_x$. Considered as an estimate of the overall proportion of the target cohort that will develop AIDS within 5 years of HIV-1 infection, the standardized proportion $\Sigma_x W_xP_x$, will be free of age confounding.

The preceding illustration brings forth an important and often overlooked point: when employing standardization to adjust for potential biases, the choice of standard distribution should never be considered arbitrary. In fact, the standard distribution should always be taken from the target cohort or the population about which inferences will be made. If inferences are to be made about several different groups, it may be necessary to compute several different standardized estimates.

Methods for removing bias in estimates by taking account of variables responsible for some or all of the bias are known as adjustment or covariate control methods. Standardization is perhaps the oldest and simplest example of such a method; methods based on multivariate models, which are discussed below, are more complex.

Unmeasured confounders

If all confounders were measured accurately, comparison validity could be achieved simply by adjusting for these confounders (although various technical problems might arise when attempting to do so). Nevertheless, in any non-randomized study we would ordinarily be able to think of a number of possible confounders that had not been measured or had been measured only in a very poor fashion. In such cases, it may still be possible to predict the direction of uncontrolled confounding by examining the manner in which people were selected into the target and reference cohorts from the population at large. If the cohorts are derived from populations with different distributions of predictors of the outcome, or the predictors themselves are associated with admission differentially across the cohorts, these predictors will become confounders in the analysis.

To illustrate this approach, suppose that HIV-1 infection via an intravenous route (for example through needle sharing) leads to shorter incubation times than HIV-1 infection through sexual activity. Suppose also that the reference cohort had excluded all or most intravenous drug users, whereas the target cohort was non-selective in this regard. Then incubation times in the target cohort will on average be shorter than times in the reference cohort owing to the presence of intravenously infected people in the target cohort. Thus we should expect the results from the reference cohort to underestimate average risks of AIDS onset in the target cohort.

Random sampling and confounding

Suppose, for the moment, that our reference cohort had been formed by taking a random sample of the target cohort. Can predictions about the target made from such a random sample still be confounded? With the above definition of confounding, the answer is yes. To see this, note for example that by chance alone men in our sample reference cohort could be younger on average than the total target; this age difference would in turn downwardly bias the unadjusted risk predictions if men had longer incubation times at younger ages.

Nevertheless, random sampling can help to ensure that the distribution of the reference cohort is not too far from the distribution of the target cohort. In essence, the probability of severe confounding can be made as small as necessary by increasing the sample size. Furthermore, if random sampling is used, any confounding left after adjustment will be accounted for by the standard errors of the estimates, provided that the correct statistical model is used to compute the estimates and standard errors. The latter condition is examined below under the section on specification validity.

Follow-up validity

In any cohort study covering an extended period of risk, subjects will be followed for different lengths of time. Some subjects will be lost to follow-up before the study ends. Others will be removed from the study by an event that precludes AIDS onset, which in this setting is death before AIDS onset from fatal accidents, fatal myocardial infarctions, and so on. Because subjects come under study at different times, those who are not lost to follow-up or who die before developing AIDS will still have had different lengths of follow-up when the study ends; traditionally, a subject still under follow-up at study end is said to have been 'withdrawn from study' at the time of study end.

Suppose that we wish to estimate the average risk of AIDS onset within 5 years of infection. The data from a member of the reference cohort who is not observed to develop AIDS but is also not followed for the full 5 years from infection are said to be censored for the outcome of interest (AIDS within 5 years of infection). Consider, for example, a subject killed in a car crash 2 years after infection but before contracting AIDS: the incubation time of this subject was censored at 2 years of follow-up.

Follow-up validity means that over any span of follow-up time, risk of censoring is unassociated with risk of the outcome of interest. In our example, follow-up validity means that over any span of time following infection, risk of censoring (loss, withdrawal, or death before AIDS) is unassociated with risk of AIDS. All common methods for estimating risk from situations in which censoring occurs (for example person-years, life table, and Kaplan–Meier methods) are based on the assumption of follow-up validity. Given follow-up validity, it can be expected that, at any time t after infection, the distribution of incubation times will be the same for subjects lost or withdrawn at t and subjects whose follow-up continues beyond t.

Violations of follow-up validity can result in biased predictions of risk; such violations are referred to as follow-up bias or biased censoring. To illustrate, suppose that younger reference subjects tend to have longer incubation times (that is, lower risks) and are lost to follow-up at a higher rate than older reference subjects. In other words, lower-risk subjects are lost at a higher rate than higher-risk subjects. Then, after enough time, the average risk of AIDS in the observed portion of the reference cohort will tend to be overestimated, that is, higher than the average risk occurring in the full reference cohort (as the latter includes both censored and uncensored subject experience).

The follow-up bias in the last illustration would not affect the age-specific estimates of risk (where age refers to age at infection). Consequently, the age bias in follow-up would not produce bias in age-standardized estimates of risk. More generally, if follow-up bias can be traced to a particular variable that is a predictor of both the outcome of interest and censoring, bias in the estimates can be removed by adjusting for that variable. Thus, some forms of follow-up bias can be dealt with in the same manner as confounding.

Specification validity

All statistical techniques, including so-called 'distribution-free' or 'non-parametric' methods, as well as basic contingency table methods, are derived by assuming the validity of a sampling model or error distribution. A common example is the binomial model, which is discussed in all the textbooks cited in the introduction. For parametric methods, the sampling model is a mathematical formula that expresses the probability of observing the various possible data patterns as a function of certain unknown constants (parameters). Although the parameters of this model may be unknown, the mathematical form of this model incorporates only known or purely random aspects of the data-generation process; unknown systematic aspects of this process (such as most follow-up and selection biases) will not be accounted for by the model.

All parametric statistical techniques also assume a structural model, which is a mathematical formula that expresses the parameters of the sampling model as a function of study variables. A common example is the logistic model (Breslow and Day 1980; Checkoway *et al.* 1989; Kelsey *et al.* 1996; Rothman and Greenland 1998). The structural model is most often incorporated into the sampling model, and the combination is referred to as the statistical model. An estimate can be said to have specification validity if it is derived using a statistical model that is correct or nearly so.

If either the sampling model or the structural model used for analysis is incorrect, the resulting estimates may be biased. Such bias is sometimes called specification bias, while the use of an incorrect model is known as model mis-specification or specification error. Even when mis-specification does not lead to bias, it can lead to invalidity of statistical tests and confidence intervals.

The true structural relation among the study variables is almost never known in studies of human disease. Furthermore, in the absence of random sampling and randomization, the true sampling process (that is, the exact process leading people to enter and stay in the study groups) will also be unknown. It follows that we should ordinarily expect some degree of specification error in an epidemiological analysis. Minimizing such error largely consists of contrasting the statistical model against the data and against any available information about the processes that generated the data (McCullagh and Nelder 1989), such as prior information on demographic patterns of incidence.

Many statistical techniques in epidemiology are based on assuming some type of logistic model. Examples include all the popular adjusted odds ratios, such as the Woolf, maximum likelihood, and Mantel–Haenszel estimates, as well as tests for odds ratio heterogeneity. Classical 'indirect' adjustment of rates and other comparisons of standardized morbidity ratios depend on similar multiplicative models for their validity (Breslow and Day 1987).

The degree of bias in traditional epidemiological analysis methods when the model assumptions fail has not been extensively studied. A few traditional methods, such as directly standardized comparisons and the Mantel–Haenszel test, remain valid under a wide variety of structural models. In addition, risk regression has been extended to situations involving more general models than assumed in classical theory (Breslow and Day 1987; Hastie and Tibshirani 1990). Leamer (1978) and White (1993) give more details on the effects of specification error in multiple regression problems, while Maldonado and Greenland (1994) and Greenland and Maldonado (1994) examine the implications of specification error in epidemiology.

Measurement validity

An estimate from a study can be said to have measurement validity if it suffers from no bias due to errors in measuring the study variables. Unfortunately there are sources of measurement error in nearly all studies, and nearly all sources of measurement error will contribute to bias in estimates. Thus evaluation of measurement validity primarily focuses on identifying sources of measurement error and attempting to deduce the direction and magnitude of bias produced by these sources.

To aid in the task of identifying sources of measurement error, it may be useful to classify such errors according to their source. Errors from specific sources can then be further classified according to characteristics that are predictive of the direction of the bias they produce. One classification scheme divides errors into three major categories, according to their source:

- procedural error, arising from mistakes or defects in measurement procedures
- proxy-variable error, arising from using a 'proxy' variable as a substitute for an actual variable of interest
- construct error, arising from ambiguities in the definition of the variables.

Regardless of their source, errors can be divided into two basic types, differential and non-differential, according to whether the direction or magnitude of error depends on the true values of the study variables. Two different sources of error may be classified as dependent or independent, according to whether or not the direction or magnitude of the error from one source depends on the direction or magnitude of the error from the other source. Finally, errors in continuous measurements can be factored into systematic and random components. As described in the following subsections, these classifications have important implications for bias.

Procedural error

Procedural error is the most straightforward to imagine. It includes errors in recall when variables are measured through retrospective interview (for example, mistakes in remembering all medications taken during pregnancy). It also includes coding errors, errors in calibration of instruments, and all other errors in which the target of measurement is well defined and the attempts at measurement are direct but the method of measurement is faulty. In our example, one target of measurement is HIV-1 antibody presence in blood. All available tests for antibody presence are subject to error (false negatives and false positives), and these errors can be considered to be procedural errors of measurement.

Proxy-variable error

Proxy-variable error is distinguished from procedural error in that use of proxies necessitates imputation and hence virtually guarantees that there will be measurement error. In our example, we must impute the time of HIV-1 infection. For instance, we might take as a proxy the infection time computed as 6 weeks before the mid-point between the last negative test and the first positive test for HIV-1 antibodies. Even if our HIV-1 tests are perfect, this measurement incorporates error if (as is certainly the case) time of infection does not always occur 6 weeks before the mid-point between the last negative and first positive tests.

Construct error

Construct error is often overlooked, although it may be a major source of error. Consider our example in which the ultimate target of measurement is the time between HIV-1 infection and onset of AIDS. Before attempting to measure this time span, the events that mark the beginning and end of the span must be unambiguously defined. While it may be reasonable to think of HIV-1 infection as a point event, the same cannot be said of AIDS onset. Symptoms and signs may gradually accumulate, and then it is only by convention that some point in time is declared the start of the disease. If this convention cannot be translated into reasonably precise clinical criteria for diagnosing the onset of AIDS, the construct of incubation time (the time span between infection and AIDS onset) will not be well defined let alone accurately measurable. In such situations it may be left to various clinicians to improvise answers to the question of time of AIDS onset, and this will introduce another source of extraneous variation into the final 'measurement' of incubation time.

Differential and non-differential error

Errors in measuring a variable are said to be differential when the direction or magnitude of the errors tend to vary across the true values of other variables. Suppose, for example, that recall of drug use during pregnancy is enhanced among mothers of children with birth defects. Then a retrospective interview about drug use during pregnancy will yield results with differential error, since false-negative error will occur more frequently among mothers whose children have no birth defects.

Another type of differential error occurs in the measurement of continuous variables when the distribution of errors varies with the true value of the variable. Suppose, for example, that women more accurately recall the date of a recent cervical smear test (Papanicolaou or Pap test) than the date of a more distant test. Then a retrospective interview to determine length of time since a woman's last cervical smear test would tend to suffer from larger errors when measuring longer times.

Errors in measuring a variable are said to be non-differential with respect to another variable if the magnitudes of errors do not tend to vary with the true values of the other variable. Measurements are usually assumed to be non-differential if neither the subject nor the person taking the measurement knows the values of other variables. For example, if drug use during pregnancy is measured by examining prepartum prescription records for the mother, it would ordinarily be assumed that the error will be non-differential with respect to birth defects discovered postnatally. Nevertheless, such 'blind' assessments will not guarantee non-differential error if the measurement scale is not as fine as the scale of the original variable (Flegal *et al.* 1991; Wacholder *et al.* 1991) or if there is a third uncontrolled variable that affects both the measurement and the other study variables.

Dependent and independent error

Errors in measuring two variables are said to be dependent if the direction or magnitude of the errors made in measuring one of the variables is associated with the direction or magnitude of the errors made in measuring the other variable. If there is no association of errors, the errors are said to be independent.

In our example, errors in measuring age at HIV-1 infection and AIDS incubation time are dependent. Our measure of incubation time is equal to our measure of age at AIDS onset minus our measure of age at infection; hence overestimation of age at infection will contribute to underestimation of incubation time, and underestimation of age at infection will contribute to overestimation of incubation time. In contrast, in the same example it is plausible that the errors in measuring age at infection and age at onset are independent.

Misclassification and bias towards the null

Measurement of a binary (dichotomous) variable is called better than random if, regardless of the true value, the probability that the measurement yields the true value is higher than the probability that it does not. In other words, the measurement is better than random if it is more likely to be correct than incorrect, no matter what the true value is. Given two binary variables, better-than random measurements with independent non-differential errors cannot inflate or reverse the association observed between the variables. In other words, any bias produced by independent non-differential error in better-than-random measurements can only be towards the null value of the association (which is 1 for a relative risk measure) and not beyond.

If either variable has more than two levels, then (contrary to assertions in most pre-1990 literature) the preceding conditions are not sufficient to guarantee that the resulting bias will only be towards the null and not beyond (Dosemeci *et al.* 1990). Despite this insufficiency, knowing that errors are independent and non-differential can increase the plausibility that any resulting bias is towards the null. For further discussions of sufficient conditions for error to produce bias towards the null, see Dosemeci *et al.* (1991), Flegal *et al.* (1991), Wacholder *et al.* (1991), and Weinberg *et al.* (1994).

There is one important situation in which the assumption of independent non-differential measurement error and hence bias towards the null have particularly high plausibility: in a double-blind clinical trial with a dichotomous treatment and outcome, successful blinding of treatment status during outcome evaluation should lead to independence and non-differentiality of treatment and outcome measurement errors. Successful blinding thus helps to ensure (although it does not guarantee) that any bias produced by measurement error contributes to underestimation of treatment effects.

Systematic and random components of error

For well-defined measurement procedures on continuous variables, measurement errors can be subdivided into systematic and random components. The systematic component (sometimes called the bias of the measurement) measures the degree to which the procedure tends to underestimate or overestimate the true value on repeated application. The random component is the residual error left after subtracting the systematic component from the total error.

To illustrate, suppose that in our study HIV-1 infection time was unrelated to time of antibody testing and that the average time of HIV-1 seroconversion was 8 weeks after infection. Then, even if one used a perfect HIV-1 test, a procedure that estimated infection time as 6 weeks before the mid-point between the last negative and first positive test would on average yield an estimated infection time that was 2 weeks later than the true time. Thus the systematic component of the error of this procedure would be +2 weeks. Since AIDS incubation time is AIDS onset time minus HIV-1 infection time, use of this procedure would add –2 weeks (that is, a 2-week underestimation) to the systematic component of error in estimating incubation time.

Each of the components of an error, systematic and random, may be differential (that is, may vary with other variable values) or non-differential, and may or may not be independent of the error components in other variables. We shall not explore the consequences of the numerous possibilities. However, one important (but semantically confusing) fact is that, for certain quantities, independent and non-differential systematic components of error will not harm measurement validity in that they will produce no bias in estimation.

To illustrate, suppose that in our example we wish to estimate the degree to which AIDS incubation time depends on age at HIV-1 infection. Suppose also that the systematic components of the measurements of incubation time and age of infection are –2 weeks and +2 weeks (as above), and do not vary with true incubation time or age at measurement (that is, the systematic components are non-differential). Then the systematic components, being equal, will cancel out when we compute differences in incubation time and differences in age at infection. Since only these differences are used to estimate the association, the observed dependence of incubation time on age at infection will not be affected by the systematic components of error (although it may be biased by the random components of error).

Summary of example

The example of this section provides an illustration of the most common threats to the validity of predictions. The unadjusted estimates of AIDS risk may be confounded if the target and reference cohorts differ in composition, and may also be biased by losses to follow-up or use of an incorrect statistical model. Finally, our predictions are likely to be compromised by errors in measurements. These sources of error should be borne in mind in any attempt to predict AIDS incidence.

Validity in causal inference

Concepts of valid prediction are applicable in evaluating studies of causation; comparison validity, follow-up validity, specification validity, and measurement validity must each be considered. In fact, as argued below, problems of causal inference can be viewed as a special type of prediction problem, namely prediction of what would happen (or what would have happened) to a population if certain characteristics of the population were (or had been) altered.

To illustrate validity issues in causal inference, we shall consider the hypothesis that coffee drinking causes acute myocardial infarction. This hypothesis can be operationally interpreted in a number of ways.

1. *There are people for whom the consumption of coffee results in their experiencing a myocardial infarction sooner than they might have, had they avoided coffee.*

While this hypothesis is appealingly precise, it offers little practical guidance to an epidemiological researcher. The problem lies in our inability to recognize an individual whose myocardial infarction was caused by coffee drinking. It is quite possible that myocardial infarctions precipitated by coffee use are clinically and pathologically indistinguishable from myocardial infarctions due to other causes. If so, the prospect of finding convincing physiological evidence concerning the hypothesis is not good.

This impasse could be overcome by examining a related epidemiological hypothesis, that is, a hypothesis that refers to the distribution of disease in populations. One of many such hypotheses is as follows.

2. *Among five-cup-a-day coffee drinkers, cessation of coffee use will lower the frequency of myocardial infarction.*

This form not only involves a population (five-cup-a-day coffee drinkers) but also asserts that a mass action (coffee cessation) will reduce the frequency of the study disease. Thus the form of the hypothesis immediately suggests a strong test of the hypothesis: conduct a randomized intervention trial to examine the impact of coffee cessation on myocardial infarction frequency. This solution has some profound practical limitations, not least of which would be persuading anyone to give up or take up coffee drinking to test a speculative hypothesis.

Having ruled out intervention, we might consider an observational cohort study. In this case our epidemiological hypothesis should refer to natural conditions, rather than intervention. One such hypothesis is as follows.

3. *Among five-cup-a-day coffee drinkers, coffee use has elevated the frequency of myocardial infarction.*

There have been a number of conflicting cohort and case–control studies of coffee and myocardial infarction. The present discussion will be confined to the issues arising in the analysis of a single study. For a review of issues arising in the analysis of multiple studies (meta-analysis) using the coffee–myocardial infarction literature as an example, see Greenland (1994, 1998*a*); additional discussion of the coffee–myocardial infarction literature may be found in Greenland (1993*a*).

Consider a cohort study of coffee and first myocardial infarction. At baseline, a cohort of people with no history of myocardial infarction is assembled and classified into subcohorts according to coffee use (for example never-drinkers, ex-drinkers, occasional drinkers, one-cup-a-day drinkers, two-cup-a-day drinkers, and so on). Other variables are measured as well: age, sex, smoking habits, blood pressure, and serum cholesterol. Suppose that at the end of 10 years of monitoring this cohort for myocardial infarction events, we compare the five-cup-a-day and never-drinker subcohorts, and obtain an unadjusted estimate of 1.22 for the ratio of the person–time incidence rates of first myocardial infarction among five-cup-a-day drinkers and never-drinkers (with 95 per cent confidence limits of 1.00 and 1.49). In other words, it appears that the rate of first myocardial infarction among five-cup-a-day drinkers was 1.22 times higher than the rate among never-drinkers. (Hereafter, myocardial infarction means first myocardial infarction, risk means average risk, and rate means person–time incidence rate.)

The estimated rate ratio of 1.22 may not seem large. Nevertheless, if it accurately reflects the impact of coffee use on the five-cup-a-day subcohort, this estimate implies that people drinking five cups a day at baseline suffered a 22 per cent increase in their myocardial infarction rate as a result of their coffee use. Given the high frequency of both coffee use and myocardial infarction in many populations, this could represent a substantial health impact. Therefore a careful evaluation of the validity of the estimate should be performed.

As in the previous AIDS example, we can proceed by examining a series of conditions sufficient for validity of the estimate as a measure of coffee effect.

- Comparison validity (*C*). If the members of the five-cup-a-day subcohort had instead never drunk coffee, their distribution of myocardial infarction events over time would have been approximately the same as the distribution among the never-drinkers.
- Follow-up validity (*F*). Within each subcohort, the risk of censoring (that is, follow-up ended by an event other than myocardial infarction) is not associated with the risk of myocardial infarction.
- Specification validity (*Sp*). The distribution of myocardial infarction events over time in the subcohorts can be closely approximated by the statistical model on which the estimates are based.
- Measurement validity (*M*). All measurements of variables used in the analysis closely approximate the true values of the variables.

These four conditions are sometimes called internal validity conditions because they pertain only to estimating effects within the study cohort rather than to generalizing results to other cohorts. They are sufficient but not necessary for validity, in that certain violations of the conditions will not produce bias in the effect estimate (although most violations will produce some bias). The meaning of these conditions for an observational cohort study of a causal hypothesis is explored in the following sections. An important phenomenon known as effect modification, which is relevant to both internal validity and generalizability, is also discussed.

Comparison validity

In our example, comparison validity simply means that the distribution of myocardial infarctions among never-drinkers accurately predicts what would have happened in the coffee-drinking groups had the members of these groups never drunk coffee. Another way of stating condition *C* is that the five-cup-a-day and never-drinker subcohorts would be comparable or exchangeable with respect to myocardial infarction times if no one had ever drunk coffee.

Despite its simplicity, note that the comparison validity condition depends on the hypothesis of interest in a very precise way. In particular, the research hypothesis (hypothesis 3 above) is a statement about the impact of coffee among five-cup-a-day drinkers. Thus this subcohort is the target cohort, while never-drinkers serve as the reference cohort for making predictions about this target.

To illustrate further the correspondence between comparison validity and the hypothesis at issue, suppose for the moment that our research hypothesis was as follows.

4. *Among never-drinkers, five-cup-a-day coffee use would elevate the frequency of myocardial infarction.*

In examining this hypothesis, the never-drinkers would be the target cohort and the coffee drinkers would be the reference cohort. Thus the comparison validity condition would have to be replaced by a condition such as *C′*.

- *C′*. If the never-drinkers had drunk five cups of coffee per day, their distribution of myocardial infarctions would have been approximately the same as the distribution among five-cup-a-day drinkers.

Other ways of stating condition *C′* are that the five-cup-a-day and never-drinker subcohorts would be comparable or exchangeable with respect to myocardial infarction times if everyone had been five-cup-a-day drinkers, and that the myocardial infarction experience of five-cup-a-day drinkers accurately predicts what would have happened to the never-drinkers if the latter had drunk five cups a day.

Confounding

Failure to meet condition *C* results in a biased estimate of the effect of five-cup-a-day coffee drinking on five-cup-a-day drinkers, a condition sometimes referred to as confounding of the estimate. Similarly, failure to meet condition *C′* results in a biased estimate of the effect that five-cup-a-day drinking would have had on never-drinkers.

To evaluate comparison validity, it is necessary to check whether the subcohorts differed at baseline on any factors that influence myocardial infarction time. If so, it should not be expected that the myocardial infarction distributions of the subcohorts were comparable, even if the subcohorts had the same level of coffee use. In other words, it should not be expected that condition *C* (or *C′*) would hold. If condition *C* failed, our estimates would suffer from confounding. This is so, regardless of whether adjustment appeared to change the association of coffee use and myocardial infarction (Greenland *et al.* 1999*b*).

In our example, it is important to note that several studies have found a positive association between cigarette smoking (an established risk factor for myocardial infarction) and coffee use (Greenland 1998*a*). It also seems plausible that a person habituated to a stimulant such as nicotine would be attracted to coffee use as well. Thus we should expect to see a higher prevalence of smoking among coffee users in our study.

Suppose then that, in our cohort, smoking is more prevalent among five-cup-a-day subjects than never-drinkers. This elevated smoking prevalence should have led to elevated myocardial infarction rates among five-cup-a-day drinkers, even if coffee had no effect. More generally, we should expect the myocardial infarction rate among never-drinkers to underestimate the myocardial infarction rate that five-cup-a-day drinkers would have had if they had never drunk coffee. The result would be an inflated estimate of the impact of coffee on the myocardial infarction rate of five-cup-a-day drinkers. Similarly, we should expect the myocardial infarction rate among five-cup-a-day drinkers to overestimate the myocardial infarction rate that never-drinkers would have had if they had drunk five cups a day.

Adjustment for measured confounders

As in the prediction problem, the data can be stratified on potential confounders with the objective of creating strata within which confounding is minimal or absent. We can also employ standardization to remove confounding from estimates of overall effect. Again, some care in the selection of the standard is required.

To illustrate, let R_{xz} denote the estimated rate of myocardial infarction among cohort members who drank *x* cups of coffee per day and smoked *z* cigarettes per day at baseline, with R_{0z} denoting the estimated rate among never-drinkers. Let W_{xz} denote the proportion of person-time among *x*-cup-per-day drinkers that was contributed by *z*-cigarette-per-day smokers. Finally, let R_{xc} be the crude (unadjusted) rate observed among cohort members who drank *x* cups per day at baseline, with R_{0c} denoting the estimated crude rate among never-drinkers.

Suppose that any change in coffee-use patterns would have negligible impact on the person–time distribution of smoking in the cohort. The predicted (that is, expected) rate among five-cup-a-day drinkers had they never drunk coffee, adjusted for confounding by smoking, is the average of the smoking-specific estimates from the never-drinker (reference) subcohort weighted by the smoking distribution of the five-cup-per-day (target) cohort. Algebraically, this average is the following sum (over *z*):

$$\Sigma_z W_{5z} R_{0z}.$$

This sum is commonly termed the rate in the never-drinkers standardized to the distribution of smoking among five-cup-a-day drinkers. Such terminology obscures the fact that the sum is a prediction about the five-cup-a-day drinkers, not the never-drinkers.

Given the last computation, a smoking-standardized estimate of the increase in myocardial infarction rate produced by coffee drinking among five-cup-per-day drinkers is the rate ratio standardized to the five-cup-per-day smoking distribution:

$$\Sigma_z W_{5z} R_{5z} / \Sigma_z W_{5z} R_{0z}.$$

This formula reveals a property common to a simple standardized rate ratio: the same weights W_{xz} must be used in the numerator and denominator sums. Some insight into this formula can be obtained by noting that the crude rate R_{5c} among the five-cup-a-day drinkers is equal to

$$\Sigma_z W_{5z} R_{5z}$$

so that the standardized rate ratio can be rewritten as

$$R_{5c} / \Sigma_z W_{5z} R_{0z}.$$

This version shows that the ratio is a classical observed (crude) over expected ratio, or standardized morbidity ratio.

Another standardized rate ratio is

$$\Sigma_z W_{0z} R_{5z} / \Sigma_z W_{0z} R_{0z}.$$

This differs from the previous standardized ratio in that the weights are taken from the never-drinkers (W_{0z}) instead of five-cup-a-day drinkers (W_{5z}). Insight into this formula can be obtained by noting that the numerator sum is simply a prediction (expectation) of what would have happened to the never-drinkers if they had been five-cup-a-day drinkers, while the denominator sum is equal to the crude rate R_{0c}, among never-drinkers. Thus the last standardized ratio is a smoking-standardized estimate of the increase in the myocardial infarction rate that five-cup-a-day drinking would have produced among the never-drinkers.

Standardization is appealingly simple in both justification and computation. Unfortunately, if the number of cases occurring within the confounder categories tends to be small (under five or so), the technique will be subject to various technical problems including possible bias. These problems can be avoided by broadening confounder categories or by not adjusting for some of the measured confounders. Unfortunately, both these strategies are likely to result in incomplete control of confounding. To avoid having to adopt these strategies, many researchers attempt to control confounding by using a multivariate model. This remedy has problems of its own, some of which are addressed in the section on specification validity below.

Another problem is that standardized procedures (as well as typical modelling procedures) take no account of potential exposure effects on the adjustment variables or their distribution. Thus, in the above example, to justify use of the fixed weights W_{xz} the dubious assumption had to be invoked that changes in coffee use would only negligibly affect the smoking distribution. This issue is briefly discussed in the section on intermediate variables below.

Unmeasured confounders

Among the possible confounders not measured in our hypothetical study are diet and exercise. Suppose that 'health conscious' subjects who exercise regularly and eat low-fat diets also avoid coffee. The result will be a concentration of these lower-risk subjects among coffee non-users and a consequent overestimation of coffee's effect on risk.

Confounding by unmeasured confounders can sometimes be minimized by controlling variables along pathways of the confounders' effect. For example, if exercise and low-fat diet lowered myocardial infarction risk only by lowering serum cholesterol and blood pressure, control of serum cholesterol and blood pressure would remove confounding by exercise and dietary fat. Unfortunately, such control may also generate bias if the controlled variables are intermediates between our study variable and our outcome variable.

If external information is available to indicate the relationship in our study between an unmeasured confounder and the study variables, an indirect method to adjust for the confounder can be used (Schlesselman 1978; Flanders and Khoury 1990). If external information is unreliable or unavailable, it is still possible to examine the sensitivity of our results to unmeasured confounding (Cornfield *et al.* 1959; Flanders and Khoury 1990; Rosenbaum 1995; Chapter 19 in Rothman and Greenland 1998).

Randomization and confounding

Suppose, for the moment, that the level of coffee use in our cohort had been randomly assigned and that the participants diligently consumed only their assigned amount of coffee. Could our estimates of coffee effects from such a randomized trial still be confounded? By our earlier definition of confounding, the answer is yes. To see this, note for example that by chance alone the five-cup-a-day drinkers could be older on average than the never-drinkers; this difference would in turn result in an upward bias in the unadjusted estimate of the effect of five cups a day, since age is an important risk factor for myocardial infarction.

Nevertheless, randomization can help to ensure that the distributions of confounders in the different exposure groups are not too far apart. In essence, the probability of severe confounding can be made as small as necessary by increasing the size of the randomized groups. Furthermore, if randomization is used and subjects comply with their assigned treatments, any confounding left after adjustment will be accounted for by the standard errors of the estimates, provided that the correct statistical model is used to compute the effect estimates and their standard errors (Robins 1988; Greenland 1990).

Intermediate variables

In effect estimation, it is important to take care to distinguish intermediate variables from confounding variables. Intermediate variables represent steps in the causal pathway from the study exposure to the outcome event. The distinction is essential, for control of intermediate variables can increase the bias of estimates.

To illustrate, suppose that coffee use affects serum cholesterol levels (as suggested by the results of Curb *et al.* 1986). Then, given that serum cholesterol affects myocardial infarction risk, serum cholesterol is an intermediate variable for the study of coffee effects on this risk. Now suppose that we stratify our cohort data on serum cholesterol levels. Some coffee drinkers will be in elevated cholesterol categories because of coffee use and so will be at elevated myocardial infarction risk because of coffee effects, yet these subjects will be compared with never-drinkers in the same stratum who are also at elevated risk due to their elevated cholesterol. Therefore the effect of coffee on myocardial infarction risk via the cholesterol pathway will not be apparent within the cholesterol strata, and so cholesterol adjustment will contribute to underestimation of the coffee effect on myocardial infarction risk. Analogously, if coffee affected myocardial infarction risk by elevating blood pressure, blood pressure adjustment will contribute to underestimation of the coffee effect. Such underestimation can be termed overadjustment bias.

Intermediate variables may also be confounders and thus present the investigator with a severe dilemma. Consider that most of the variation in serum cholesterol levels is not due to coffee use and that much (perhaps most) of the association between coffee use and cholesterol is not due to coffee effects, but rather to factors associated with both coffee and cholesterol (such as exercise and dietary fat). This means that serum cholesterol may also be viewed as a confounder for the coffee–myocardial infarction study and that estimates unadjusted for serum cholesterol will be biased unless they are also adjusted for the factors contributing to the coffee–cholesterol association.

Suppose that a variable is both an intermediate and a confounder. It will usually be impossible to determine how much of the change in the effect estimate produced by adjusting for the variable is due to introduction of overadjustment bias and how much is due to removal of confounding. Nevertheless, a qualitative assessment may be possible in some situations. For example, if we know that the effects of coffee on serum cholesterol are weak and that most of the association between coffee and serum cholesterol is due to confounding of this association by uncontrolled factors (such as exercise and diet), we can conclude that the cholesterol-adjusted estimate is the less biased of the two. Alternatively, if we have accurately measured all the factors that confound the coffee–cholesterol association, we can control these factors instead of cholesterol to obtain an estimate free of both overadjustment bias and confounding by cholesterol. Finally, if we have multiple measurements of coffee use and cholesterol over time, techniques are available that adjust for the confounding effects of cholesterol but do not introduce overadjustment (Robins and Greenland 1994).

Direct and indirect effects

Often, we may wish to estimate how much of the effect under study is indirect relative to an intermediate variable (in the sense of being transmitted through the intermediate), or how much of the effect is direct relative to the intermediate (not mediated by the intermediate). For example, we might wish to estimate how much of coffee's effect on myocardial infarction risk is due to its effect on serum cholesterol, or how much is due to coffee effects through pathways not involving cholesterol.

One common approach to this problem is to adjust the coffee–myocardial infarction association for serum cholesterol level via ordinary stratification or regression methods and then use the resulting estimate as the estimate of the direct coffee effect. This procedure is potentially biased as it may introduce new confounding by determinants of serum cholesterol, even if these determinants did not confound the total (unadjusted) association (Robins and Greenland 1992). However, given sufficient data, it is possible to obtain separate estimates for direct and indirect effects using special stratification or modelling techniques (Robins and Greenland 1994).

Follow-up validity

In our example, follow-up validity means that follow-up is valid within every subcohort being compared. In other words, over any span of time during follow-up, myocardial infarction risk within a subcohort is unassociated with censoring risk in the subcohort. Given follow-up validity, we can expect that, at any follow-up time *t*, the myocardial infarction rates in a subcohort will be the same for subjects lost or withdrawn at *t* and subjects whose follow-up continues beyond *t*.

In fact, we should expect follow-up to be biased by cigarette smoking: smoking is associated with mortality from myocardial infarction and from many other causes; the association of smoking with socioeconomic status might also produce an association between smoking and loss to follow-up. The result would be elevated censoring among high-risk (smoking) subjects. As a consequence, unadjusted estimates of myocardial infarction risks will underestimate those risks in the complete subcohorts (as the latter includes both censored and uncensored subject experience). If the degree of underestimation varies across subcohorts, bias in the relative risk estimates will result.

In fact, the degree of underestimation should vary in this example because of the variation in smoking prevalence across subcohorts. Nevertheless, variation in smoking prevalence is not necessary for smoking-related censoring to produce biased estimates of absolute effect. For example, if smoking-related censoring produced a uniform 15 per cent underestimation of the myocardial infarction rate in each subcohort, all rate differences would also be underestimated by 15 per cent.

Analogous to control of confounding, any bias produced by smoking's association with myocardial infarction and censoring can be removed by smoking adjustment. As before, if adjustment is by standardization, the standard distribution should be chosen from the target subcohort.

Some authors classify follow-up bias as a form of confounding because the same correction methods can sometimes be applied. Nevertheless, the two phenomena are reversed with respect to the causal ordering of the third variable responsible for the bias: confounding arises from an association of the study exposure (coffee use) with other exposures (such as smoking) that affect outcome risk; in contrast, follow-up bias arises from an association between the risk of the study outcome (myocardial infarction) and risks of other end-points (such as other-cause mortality or loss to follow-up) that are affected by exposure. Furthermore, certain forms of follow-up bias cannot be removed by adjustment. These problems are discussed in the statistics literature under the topic of dependent competing risks; see Kalbfleisch and Prentice (1980) and Slud and Byar (1988) for discussions of this issue.

Some authors (Kelsey *et al.* 1996) classify follow-up bias as a form of selection bias. Here, we reserve the latter term for a special problem of case–control studies (discussed below).

Specification validity

As noted above, the use of a statistical method based on an incorrect model (specification error) can lead to bias in estimates and improper performance of statistical tests and interval estimates. All statistical techniques, including non-parametric methods, must assume some sort of model for the process generating the data; however, in the absence of randomization or random sampling, it will rarely be possible to identify a 'correct' sampling model. In addition, structural assumptions are rarely (if ever) exactly satisfied. Thus some specification error should be expected. As before, minimization of specification error must rely on checking the model against the data and against background information about the processes generating the data.

Recall that the unadjusted rate ratio estimate for five-cup-a-day versus never-drinkers is 1.22 in the present example, with 95 per cent confidence limits of 1.00 and 1.49, and a p value of 0.05. Suppose that these figures were obtained by the person–time methods given in textbooks such as Breslow and Day (1987) or Rothman and Greenland (1998). These methods are based on a binomial sampling model for the number of cases who drank five cups a day at baseline, given the combined (total) number of cases among five-cup-a-day and never-drinkers. In our example, the validity of this model depends on the assumption that the myocardial infarction rate remains constant within subcohorts over the follow-up period. It follows that the model and hence the statistics given earlier cannot be valid in our example; the subcohort members grow older over the follow-up period, and hence the myocardial infarction rates must increase with follow-up time.

The invalidity just noted can be rectified by stratifying either on follow-up time or the variable responsible for the change in rates over follow-up time (here, age). The stratification need only be fine enough to ensure that the myocardial infarction rate change within strata is negligible over follow-up. As noted above, however, smoking and perhaps other factors responsible for confounding or follow-up bias must also be adjusted for. If we stratify finely enough to remove all the bias from these sources, the resulting estimates would be undefined or so unstable that they would tell us nothing about the association of coffee and myocardial infarction.

The standard solution to such problems is to compute adjusted estimates using regression models. These are structural models representing a set of assumptions (usually rather strong ones) about the joint effects of the study variables. Such models allow estimates and tests to be extracted from what would otherwise be hopelessly sparse data, at a cost of a greater risk of bias arising from violations of the assumptions underlying the models (Robins and Greenland 1986). For further details of cohort modelling, see Breslow and Day (1987), Checkoway *et al.* (1989), Hosmer and Lemeshow (1989), Clayton and Hills (1993), Kelsey *et al.* (1996), or Rothman and Greenland (1998).

Measurement validity

Unlike sex, the continuous variables of coffee use, cigarette use, blood pressure, cholesterol, and age are time-dependent covariates. With the exception of age (whose value at any time can be computed from birth date), this fact adds considerable complexity to measuring these variables and estimating their effects.

Consider that we cannot reasonably expect a single baseline measurement, no matter how accurate, to summarize adequately a subject's entire history of coffee drinking, smoking, blood pressure, or cholesterol. Even if the effect of a subject's history could be largely captured by using a single summary number (for example total number of cigarettes smoked), the baseline measurement may well be a poor proxy for this ideal and unknown summary. For these reasons, we should expect proxy-variable errors to be very large in our example.

Proxy-variable error in the study variables

The degree of proxy-variable error in measuring the study variables depends on the exact definitions of the variables that we wish to study. In turn, this definition should reflect the hypothesized effect that we wish to study. To illustrate, consider the following acute-effect hypothesis.

1. *Drinking a cup of coffee produces an immediate rise in short-term myocardial infarction risk. In other words, coffee consumption is an acute risk factor.*

This hypothesis does not exclude the possibility that coffee use also elevates long-term risk of myocardial infarction, perhaps through some other mechanism; it simply does not address the issue of chronic effects.

One way to examine the hypothesis would be to compare the myocardial infarction rates among person-days in which one, two, three, and so on cups were drunk with the rate among person-days in which no coffee was drunk (adjusting for confounding and follow-up bias). If we had only baseline data, baseline daily consumption would have to serve as the proxy for consumption on every day of follow-up. This would probably be a poor proxy for daily consumption at later follow-up times where more outcome events occur. A 'standard' analysis, which only examines the association of baseline coffee use with myocardial infarction rates, is equivalent to an analysis that uses baseline consumption as a proxy for consumption on all later days.

Thus, estimates from a standard analysis would suffer large bias if considered as estimates of acute coffee effect.

The proxy-variable error in this example could easily be differential with respect to the outcome: person-days accumulate more rapidly in early follow-up, where the error from using baseline consumption as the proxy is relatively low; in contrast, myocardial infarction events accumulate more rapidly in later follow-up, where the error is probably higher. This difference in accumulation illustrates an important general point: errors in variables can be differential, even if the variables are measured before the outcome event. Such phenomena occur when errors are associated with risk factors for the outcome; in our example, the error is associated with follow-up time and hence age. In turn, such associations are likely to occur when measurements are based on proxy variables.

Suppose now that we examine the following chronic-effect hypothesis.

2. *Each cup of coffee drunk eventually results in a long-term elevation of myocardial infarction risk.*

This hypothesis was suggested by reports that coffee drinking produces a rise in serum lipid levels (Curb *et al.* 1986); it does not address the issue of acute effects. One way to examine the hypothesis would be to compare the myocardial infarction rates among person-months with different cumulative doses of coffee (perhaps using a lag period in calculating dose; for example, one might ignore the most recent month of consumption). If we had only baseline data, however, baseline daily consumption would have to be used to construct a proxy for cumulative consumption at every month of follow-up. This construction could be done in several different ways. For example, we could estimate subjects' cumulative doses up to a particular date by multiplying their baseline daily consumption by the number of days that they had lived between age 18 and the date in question. This estimate assumes that coffee drinking began at age 18 and the baseline daily consumption is the average daily consumption since that age. We should expect considerable error in such a crude measure of cumulative consumption.

The degree of bias in estimating chronic effects could be quite different from the degree of bias in estimating acute effects. Furthermore, as discussed below, the errors in each proxy will make it virtually impossible to discriminate between acute and chronic effects.

Measurement error and confounding

If a variable is measured with error, estimates adjusted for the variable as measured will still be somewhat confounded by the variable. This residual confounding arises because measurement error prevents construction of strata that are internally homogeneous with respect to the true confounding variable (Greenland 1980).

To illustrate, consider baseline daily cigarette consumption. This variable can be considered a proxy for consumption on each day of follow-up or can be used to construct an estimate of cumulative consumption (analogous to the cumulative coffee variable discussed above). Suppose that we stratify the data on a cumulative smoking index constructed from the baseline smoking measurement. Within any stratum of the index, there would remain a broad range of cumulative cigarette consumption. For example, two subjects who were age 40 and smoked one pack a day at baseline would receive the same value for the smoking index and so end up in the same stratum. However, if one of them stopped smoking immediately after baseline, while the other continued to smoke a pack a day, after 10 years of follow-up the former subject would have 10 less pack-years of cigarette consumption than the continuing smoker.

Suppose now that cumulative cigarette consumption is positively associated with cumulative coffee consumption. Then, even within strata of the smoking index, we should expect subjects with high coffee consumption to exhibit elevated myocardial infarction rates simply by virtue of having higher levels of cigarette consumption. As a consequence, the estimate of coffee effect adjusted for the smoking index would still be confounded by cumulative cigarette consumption.

In some cases a study variable may appear to have an effect (or no effect) only because of poor measurement of an apparently unimportant confounder. This can occur, for example, when an important confounding variable is measured with a large amount of non-differential error. Such an error would ordinarily reduce the apparent association of the variable with the exposure, and would also make the variable appear to be a weak risk factor, perhaps weaker than the study exposure. This in turn would make the variable appear to be only weakly confounding, in that adjustment for the variable as measured would produce little change in the result. However, this appearance would be deceptive because adjustment for the variable as measured would eliminate little of the actual confounding by the variable.

As an example, suppose that coronary proneness of personality was measured only by the baseline yes/no question: Do you consider yourself a hard-driving person? Such a crude measure of the original construct would be unlikely to show more than a weak association with either coffee use or myocardial infarction, and adjusting for it would produce little change in our estimate of coffee effect. Suppose, however, that coronary-prone personalities have an elevated preference for coffee. Such a phenomenon would lead to a concentration of coronary-prone people (and hence a spuriously elevated myocardial infarction rate) among coffee drinkers, even after stratification on response to the above question.

One would ordinarily expect adjustment for a non-differentially misclassified confounder to produce an estimate lying somewhere between the crude (unadjusted) estimate and the estimate adjusted for the true values of the confounder (Greenland 1980). Unfortunately, if the true confounder has more than two levels, it is possible for adjustment by the misclassified confounder to be more biased than the crude estimate (Brenner 1993). It is also possible for adjustment by factors that affect misclassification to worsen bias (Greenland and Robins 1985).

Measurement error and separation of effects

Measurement errors can severely reduce our ability to separate different effects of the study variable because of their impact on the effectiveness of adjustment procedures. Suppose in our example that we wished to estimate the relative strength of acute and chronic coffee effects. To do so we must take account of the fact that acute and chronic effects will be confounded. When examining acute effects, person-days with high coffee consumption will occur most frequently among people with high cumulative coffee consumption. As a consequence, if cumulative coffee consumption is a risk factor, it will be a confounder for estimating the acute effects of coffee consumption. By similar arguments, if coffee consumption has acute effects, these will confound estimates of the chronic effects of cumulative consumption.

Unfortunately, both cumulative and daily consumption are measured with considerable error. As a result, any effect observed for one may be wholly or partially due to the other, even if the other has little or no apparent effect.

Repeated measures

One costly but effective method for reducing the degree of proxy-variable error in measuring time-dependent variables is to take repeated (serial) measurements over the follow-up period and ask subjects to report their prebaseline history of such variables at the baseline interview. In our example, subjects could be asked about their age at first use and level of consumption at different ages for coffee and cigarettes; they could then be recontacted every year or two to assess their current consumption. Of course, not all subjects may be willing to co-operate with such active follow-up, but the penalties of some extra loss may be far outweighed by the benefit of improved measurement accuracy.

Errors in assessing incidence

An important form of measurement error in assessing incidence is misdiagnosis of the outcome event. In the AIDS example, a false-positive diagnosis of AIDS would result in underestimation of incubation time, while a false-negative diagnosis would result in overestimation. In the present example, false-positive errors would result in overestimation of myocardial infarction rates, while false-negative errors would result in underestimation. These errors will be of particular concern when the study depends on existing surveillance systems or records for detection of outcome events.

There are special cases in which the errors will induce little or no bias in estimates (Poole 1985), provided the errors have little effect on the person-time observed. If the only form of misdiagnosis is false-negative error, the proportion of outcome events missed in this fashion is the same across cohorts, and there is no follow-up bias, then the relative risk estimates will not be distorted by the underdiagnosis. Suppose in our example that all recorded myocardial infarction events are true myocardial infarctions, but that in each subcohort 10 per cent of myocardial infarctions are missed. The myocardial infarction rates in each subcohort will then be underestimated by 10 per cent; nevertheless, if we consider any two of these rates, say R_0 and R_5, the observed rate ratio will be

$$\frac{0.9R_5}{0.9R_0} = \frac{R_5}{R_0}$$

which is undistorted by the underdiagnosis of myocardial infarction. Nonetheless, if coffee primarily induced 'silent' myocardial infarctions and these were the most frequently undiagnosed events, the coffee effect would be underestimated.

In an analogous fashion, if the only form of misdiagnosis is false-positive error, the rate of false positives is the same across cohorts, and there is no follow-up bias, then rate differences will not be distorted by the overdiagnosis. Suppose that the rate of false positives in our example is R_f in all subcohorts; then if we consider any two true rates, say R_0 and R_5, the observed rate difference will be

$$(R_5 + R_f) - (R_0 + R_f) = R_5 - R_0$$

which is undistorted by the overdiagnosis of myocardial infarction. However, if there is non-differential underdiagnosis of myocardial infarction, as is probably the case in our example, the rate difference will be underestimated.

Effect-measure modification (heterogeneity of effect)

Estimation of effects usually requires consideration of effect-measure modification, which is also known as effect modification, effect variation, or heterogeneity of effect. As an example, suppose that drinking five cups of coffee a day elevated the myocardial infarction rate of men in our cohort by a factor of 1.40 (that is, a 40 per cent increase), but elevated the myocardial infarction rate of women by a factor of only 1.10 (a 10 per cent increase). This situation would be termed modification (or variation or heterogeneity) of the rate ratio by sex, and sex would be called a modifier of the coffee–myocardial infarction rate ratio.

As another example, suppose that drinking five cups of coffee a day elevated the myocardial infarction rate in men in our cohort by a factor of 400 cases per 100 000 person-years but elevated the rate in women by a factor of only 40 cases per 100 000 person-years. This situation would be termed modification of the rate difference by sex, and sex would be called a modifier of the coffee–myocardial infarction rate difference.

As a final example, suppose that drinking five cups of coffee per day elevated the myocardial infarction rate in our cohort by a factor of 1.22 in both men and women. This situation would be termed homogeneity of the rate ratios across sex.

Effect modification and homogeneity are not absolute properties of an effect but instead are properties of the way that the effect is measured. For example, suppose that drinking five cups of coffee per day elevated the myocardial infarction rate in men from 1000 cases per 100 000 person-years to 1220 cases per 100 000 person-years, but elevated the rate in women from 400 cases per 100 000 person-years to 488 cases per 100 000 person-years. Then the sex-specific rate ratios would both be 1.22, homogeneous across sex. In contrast, the sex-specific rate differences would be 220 cases per 100 000 person-years for males and 88 cases per 100 000 person-years for females, and so are heterogeneous or 'modified' by sex. Examples such as this show that one should not equate effect modification with biological concepts of interaction such as synergy or antagonism (Rothman and Greenland 1998, Chapter 18).

Effect modification can be analysed by stratifying the data on the potential effect modifier under study, estimating the effect within each stratum, and comparing the estimates across strata. There are several potential problems with this approach. The number of subjects in each stratum may be too small to produce stable estimates of stratum-specific effects, particularly after adjustment for confounder effects. Estimates may fluctuate wildly from stratum to stratum owing to random error. A related problem is that statistical tests for heterogeneity in stratified data have extremely low power in many situations, and therefore are likely to miss much if not most of the heterogeneity when used with conventional significance levels (such as 0.05). Finally, the amount of bias from confounding, measurement error, and other sources may vary from stratum to stratum, in which case the observed pattern of modification will be biased (Greenland 1980).

Effect-measure modification and generalizability

Suppose that we succeed in obtaining approximately unbiased estimates from our study. We can then confront issues of generalizability (external validity) of our results. For example, we can ask whether they accurately reflect the effect of coffee on myocardial infarction rates in a new target cohort. We can view such a question as a prediction problem in which the objective is to predict the strength of coffee effects in the new target cohort. From this perspective, generalizability of an effect estimate involves just one validity issue in addition to those discussed so far, namely confounding of the predicted effect by effect modifiers.

Suppose that the rate increase (in cases per 100 000 person-years) produced by coffee use is 400 for males and 40 for females among five-cup-a-day drinkers in both our study cohort and the new target. If our study cohort is 70 per cent male while the new target is only 30 per cent male, the average increase among five-cup-a-day drinkers in our study cohort would be $0.7 \times 400 + 0.3 \times 40 = 292$, whereas the average increase in the new target would be only $0.3 \times 400 + 0.7 \times 40 = 148$. Thus, any valid estimate of the average increase in our study cohort will tend to overestimate greatly the average increase in the new target. In other words, modification of coffee's effect by sex confounds the prediction of its effect in the new target. This bias can be avoided by making only sex-specific predictions of effect or by standardizing the study results to the sex distribution of the new target population.

Summary of example

The example used in this section provides an illustration of the most common threats to the validity of effect estimates from cohort studies. The unadjusted estimates of coffee effect on myocardial infarction will be confounded by many variables (such as smoking), and there will be follow-up bias. As a result, the number of variables that must be controlled is too large to allow adequate control using only stratification. The true functional dependence of myocardial infarction rates on coffee and the confounder is unknown, so that estimates based on multivariate models are likely to be biased. Even if this bias is unimportant, our estimates will remain confounded because of our inability to measure the key confounders accurately. Finally, our inability to summarize coffee consumption accurately would further bias our estimates, making it impossible to separate acute and chronic effects of coffee use reliably.

Given that there are several sources of bias of unknown magnitude and different directions, it would appear that no conclusions about coffee effect could be drawn from a study like the one described above, other than that coffee does not appear to have a large effect. This type of result—inconclusive, other than to rule out very large effects—is common in thorough epidemiological analyses of observational data. In particular, inconclusive results are common when the data being analysed were collected for purposes other than to address the hypothesis at issue, for such data often lack accurate measurements of key variables.

Validity in case–control and retrospective cohort studies

Case–control studies

The practical difficulties of cohort studies have led to extensive development of case–control study designs. The distinguishing feature of such designs is that sampling is intentionally based on the outcome of individuals.

In a population-based or population-initiated case–control study, one first identifies a population at risk of the outcome of interest, which is to be studied over a specified period of time or risk period. As in a cohort study, one attempts to ascertain outcome events in the population at risk. Nevertheless, unlike a cohort study, one selects people experiencing the outcome event (cases) and a 'control' sample of the entire population at risk for ascertainment of exposure and covariate status.

In a case-initiated case–control study, one starts by identifying a source of study cases (for example a hospital emergency room is a source of myocardial infarction cases). One then attempts to identify a population at risk such that the source of cases provides a random or complete sample of all cases occurring in this population. Study cases recruited from the source occur over a risk period; controls are selected in order to ascertain the distribution of exposure in the population at risk over that period.

Case–control studies may also begin with an existing series of controls (Greenland 1985). Regardless of how a case–control study is initiated, evaluation of validity must ultimately refer to a population at risk that represents the target of inference for the study.

Relative risk estimation in case–control studies

The control sample may or may not be selected in a manner that excludes cases. If people who become cases over the risk period are ineligible for inclusion in the control group (as in traditional case–control designs), a 'rare-disease' assumption may be needed to estimate relative risks from the case–control data. In contrast, if people who become cases over the risk period are also eligible for inclusion in the control group (as in newer case–control designs), the rare-disease assumption can be discarded. These points are discussed in more detail in the textbooks cited above.

The basics of case–control estimation will be illustrated with the following example. We wish to study the effect of coffee drinking on rates of first myocardial infarction and we have selected a population for study (for example, all residents aged 40 to 64 in a particular town) over a 1-year risk period. At any point during the risk period, the population at risk comprises people in this selected population who have not yet had a myocardial infarction.

Suppose that the average number of never-drinkers in the population at risk was 20 000 over the risk period, the average number of five-cup-a-day drinkers was 10 000, there were 120 first myocardial infarctions among never-drinkers, and there were 90 first myocardial infarctions among five-cup-a-day drinkers. Then, if one observed the entire population without error, the estimated rates among never-drinkers and five-cup-a-day drinkers would be

$$\frac{120}{200\,000 \text{ person-years}}$$

and

$$\frac{90}{10\,000 \text{ person-years}}.$$

Thus, if we observed the entire population, the estimated rate ratio would be

$$\frac{90/10\,000 \text{ person-years}}{120/20\,000 \text{ person-years}} = \frac{90/120}{10\,000/20\,000} = 1.50.$$

This estimate depends on only two figures: the relative prevalence of five-cup-a-day versus never-drinkers among cases (90/120), and the relative prevalence in the person-years at risk (10 000/ 20 000). These two relative prevalences are often called the case exposure odds and the population exposure odds.

The first relative prevalence (numerator) could be estimated by interviewing an unbiased sample of all the new myocardial infarction cases that occur over the risk period, and the second relative prevalence (denominator) could be estimated by interviewing an unbiased sample of the population at risk over the risk period. The ratio of relative prevalences from the case- and control-sample interviews would then be an unbiased estimate of the population rate ratio of 1.50. This estimate is called the sample odds ratio.

Three points about the preceding argument should be carefully noted. Firstly, no rare-disease assumption was made. Secondly, the control sample of the population at risk was accumulated over the entire risk period (rather than at the end of the risk period); such sampling is called density sampling (Chapter 7 in Rothman and Greenland 1998) or risk-set sampling (Breslow and Day 1987). Thirdly, because of the density sampling, someone may be selected for the control sample, and yet have a myocardial infarction later in the risk period and become part of the case sample as well. Methods for carrying out density sampling can be found in the textbooks cited above.

Validity conditions in case–control studies

The primary advantages of case–control studies are their short time frame and the large reduction in the number of subjects needed to achieve the same statistical power as a cohort study. The primary disadvantage is that more conditions must be met to ensure their validity (in addition to the four listed in the cohort study example).

Suppose that our case–control study data yield an unadjusted rate-ratio estimate (odds ratio) of 1.50, with 95 per cent confidence limits of 1.00 and 2.25. The following series of conditions would be sufficient for the validity of this figure as an estimate of the effect of drinking five cups of coffee a day (versus none) on the myocardial infarction rate.

- Comparison validity (*C*). If five-cup-a-day drinkers in the population at risk had instead drunk no coffee, their distribution of myocardial infarction events over time would have been approximately the same as the distribution among never-drinkers.
- Follow-up validity (*F*). Within each subpopulation defined by coffee use, censoring risk (that is, population membership ended by an event other than myocardial infarction, such as emigration or death from another cause) is not associated with myocardial infarction risk.
- Specification validity (*Sp*). The distribution of myocardial infarction events over time in the subpopulations can be closely approximated by the statistical model on which the estimates are based.
- Measurement validity (*M*). All measurements of variables used in the analysis closely approximate the true values of the variables.
- Selection validity (*Se*). This has two components:
  - (a) case-selection validity: if one studies only a subset of the myocardial infarction cases occurring in the population over the risk period (for example, because of failure to detect all cases), this subset provides unbiased estimates of the prevalence of different levels of coffee use among all cases occurring in the population over the risk period
  - (b) control-selection validity: the control sample provides unbiased estimates of the prevalences of different levels of coffee use in the population at risk over the risk period.

Issues of comparison validity, follow-up validity, specification validity, effect modification, and generalizability in case–control studies parallel those in follow-up studies, and so will not be discussed here. Case–control studies are vulnerable to certain problems of measurement error that are less severe or do not exist in prospective cohort studies. These problems are discussed first, and then selection validity and modelling are examined. Finally, analogous issues in retrospective cohort studies are briefly discussed.

Retrospective ascertainment

A special class of measurement errors arises from retrospective ascertainment of time-dependent variables when attempting to measure past values of the variables. Retrospective ascertainment must be based on individual memories, existing records of past values, or some combination of the two. Therefore such ascertainment usually suffers from faulty recall, missing or mistaken records, or lack of direct measurements in existing records.

Retrospective ascertainment may be an important component of a cohort study. For example, the cohort study of coffee and myocardial infarction discussed above could have been improved by asking subjects about their coffee use and smoking prior to the start of follow-up. This information would allow one to construct better cumulative indices than could be constructed from baseline consumption alone, although the resulting indices would still incorporate error due to faulty recall.

Unless records of past measurements are available for all subjects, measurements on cases and controls must be made after the time period under study since subjects are not selected for study until after that period. Thus, unlike cohort studies, most case–control studies of time-dependent variables depend on retrospective ascertainment. Considering our example, there may be much more error in determining daily coffee consumption 10 years before interview than 1 month before interview; it might then be expected that case–control studies are more accurate for studying acute effects than for studying chronic effects. Nonetheless, if acute and chronic effects are heavily confounded, the elevated inaccuracies of long-term recall will make it impossible to disentangle short-term from long-term effects. As illustrated above, this confounding can arise in a cohort study. In a cohort study such confounding can be minimized by taking repeated measurements. In contrast, such confounding would be unavoidable in a case–control study based on recall, even if detailed longitudinal histories were requested from the subjects.

The preceding observations should be tempered by noting that some case–control studies have access to exposure measurements of the same quality as found in cohort studies, and that the exposure measurements in some cohort studies may be no better than those used in some case–control studies. For example, a cohort study in which measurements are derived by abstracting routine medical records would suffer from no less measurement error than a case–control study in which measurements are derived by abstracting the same records.

Outcome-affected measurements

One common potential problem in case–control studies is outcome-affected recall, often termed recall bias. These terms refer to the differential measurement error that originates when the outcome event affects recall of past events. Examples arise in case–control studies of birth defects, for instance. If the trauma of having an affected child either enhances recall of prenatal exposures among case mothers or increases the frequency of false-positive reports among case mothers, estimates of relative risk will be upwardly biased by effects of the outcome on case recall (although this bias may be counterbalanced by other biases, such as recall bias among controls (Drews and Greenland 1990)).

One method commonly proposed for preventing bias due to outcome-affected recall is to restrict controls to a group believed to have recall similar to the cases. Unfortunately, one usually cannot tell to what degree this restricted selection corrects the bias from outcome-affected recall. Even more unfortunately, one usually cannot tell if the selection bias produced by such restriction is worse than the recall bias one is attempting to correct (Swan *et al.* 1992; Drews *et al.* 1993).

A problem similar to outcome-affected recall can occur when the outcome event affects a psychological or physiological measurement. This is of particular concern in case–control studies of nutrient levels and chronic disease. For example, if colon cancer leads to a drop in serum retinol levels, the relative risk for the effect of serum retinol will be underestimated if serum retinol is measured after the cancer develops. Errors of this type can be viewed as proxy-variable errors in which the post-outcome value is a poor proxy for the pre-outcome value of interest.

Selection validity

Selection validity is straightforward to understand but can be extraordinarily difficult to verify. A violation of the selection validity conditions is known as selection bias. Many case–control designs and field methods are devoted to avoiding such bias (Schlesselman 1982; Kelsey *et al.* 1996; Chapter 7 in Rothman and Greenland 1998).

In some instances it may be possible to identify a factor or factors that affect the chance of selection into the study. If in such instances we have accurate measurements of one of these factors, we can stratify on (or otherwise adjust for) the factor and thereby remove the selection bias due to the factor. Because of this possibility, some authors classify selection bias as a form of confounding. Nevertheless, there are some forms of selection bias that cannot be removed by adjustment. These points will be illustrated in the following subsections.

Case-selection validity

Unbiased selection of a case series can be best assured if one can identify every case that occurs in the population at risk over the risk period. This requires a surveillance system for the outcome of interest, such as a population-based disease registry. In our coffee–myocardial infarction example, we would probably have to construct a myocardial infarction surveillance system from existing resources, such as emergency room admission records, ambulance service records, and paramedic records.

Even if all cases of interest can be identified, selection bias may arise from failure to obtain information on all of the cases. In our example, many cases would be dead before interview was possible. For such cases, there are only two alternatives: attempt to obtain information from some other source, such as next of kin or coworkers, or exclude such cases from the study. The first alternative increases measurement error in the study. The second alternative will introduce bias if coffee affects risk of fatal and non-fatal myocardial infarction differently, or if coffee affects risk of myocardial infarction survivorship. To illustrate, suppose that coffee drinking reduced one's chance of reaching the hospital alive when a myocardial infarction occurred. Then the prevalence of coffee use among myocardial infarction survivors would under-represent the prevalence among all myocardial infarction cases. Underestimation of the rate ratio would result if fatal myocardial infarction cases were excluded from the study.

It might seem possible to remove the case-selection bias in this example by redefining the study outcome as non-fatal myocardial infarction. This does not remove the bias, however; it only leads to its reclassification as a bias due to differential censoring (here classified as a form of follow-up bias). In a study of non-fatal myocardial infarction, fatal myocardial infarction is a censoring event associated with risk of non-fatal myocardial infarction; if fatal myocardial infarction is also associated with coffee use, the result will be underestimation of the rate ratio for non-fatal myocardial infarction. More generally, it is usually not possible to remove bias by placing restrictions on admissible outcomes.

Unfortunately, exclusion is the only alternative for cases that refuse to participate or cannot be located. In our example, if such cases tend to be heavier coffee users than others, underestimation of the rate ratio would result. However, suppose that, within levels of cigarette use, such cases were no different from other cases with respect to coffee use. Then adjustment for smoking would remove the selection bias induced by refusals and failures to locate cases. (Of course, such adjustment would require accurate smoking measurement, which is a problem in itself.)

Bias that arises from failure to detect certain cases is sometimes called detection bias. If our surveillance system used only hospital admissions, many out-of-hospital myocardial infarction deaths would be excluded, and a detection bias of the sort described above could result.

Control-selection validity

Unbiased selection of a control group can best be assured if one can potentially identify every member of the population at risk at every time during the risk period. In such a situation one could select controls with one of many available probability sampling techniques, using the entire population at risk as the sampling frame. Unfortunately, such situations are exceptional.

Many studies attempt to approximate the ideal sampling situation through use of existing population lists. An example is control selection by random digit dialling; here, the list (of residential telephone numbers) is not used directly but nevertheless serves as a partial enumeration of the population at risk. This list excludes people without telephone numbers. In our example, if people without telephones drink less coffee than people with telephones, a control group selected by random digit dialling would over-represent coffee use in the population at risk. The result would be underestimation of the rate ratio.

One could redefine the population at risk in the previous example so that the telephone-related selection bias did not exist by restricting the study to people with telephones. This would require excluding people without telephones from the case series. The resulting relative risk estimate would suffer no selection bias. The only important penalty from this restriction is that the resulting estimate might apply only to the population of people with telephones, which is a problem of generalizability rather than a problem of selection validity. In a similar fashion, it is often possible to prevent confounding or selection bias by placing restrictions on the population at risk (and hence the control group). In such instances, however, one must take care to apply the same restrictions to the case series and avoid using restrictions based on events that occur after exposure (Chapter 7 in Rothman and Greenland 1998; Poole 1999).

Even if all members of the population at risk can be identified, selection bias may arise from failure to obtain information on all people selected as controls. The implications are the reverse of those for case-selection bias. In our example, if controls who refuse to participate or cannot be located tend to be heavier coffee users than other controls, overestimation of the rate ratio would result. This should be contrasted with the underestimation that results from the same tendency among cases.

More generally, one might expect an association of selection probabilities with the study variable to be in the same direction for both cases and controls. If so, the resulting case-selection and control-selection biases would be in opposite directions and so, to some extent, they would cancel one another out, although not completely. To illustrate, suppose that among cases the proportions who refuse to participate are 0.05 for five-cup-a-day drinkers and 0.02 for never-drinkers, and among controls the analogous proportions are 0.20 and 0.10. These refusals will result in the odds of five-cup-a-day versus never-drinkers among cases being underestimated by a factor of 0.95/0.98 = 0.97; this in turn results in a 3 per cent underestimation of the rate ratio. Among controls, the odds will be underestimated by a factor of 0.80/0.90 = 0.89; this results in a 1/0.89 = 1.12, or a 12 per cent overestimation of the rate ratio. The net selection bias in the rate-ratio estimate will then be 0.97/0.89 = 1.09, or 9 per cent overestimation.

For further discussions of control-selection validity, see the textbooks cited above, and also Schlesselman (1982), Savitz and Pearce (1988), Swan *et al.* (1992), and Wacholder *et al.* (1992).

Matching

In cohort studies, matching refers to selection of exposure subcohorts in a manner that forces the matched factors to have similar distributions across the subcohorts. If the matched factors are accurately measured and the proportion lost to follow-up does not depend on the matched factors, cohort matching can prevent confounding by the matched factors, although there are statistical reasons to control the matched factors in the analysis (Weinberg 1985).

In case–control studies, matching refers to selection of subjects in a manner that forces the distribution of certain factors to be similar in cases and controls. Because the population at risk is not changed by case–control matching, such matching does not prevent confounding by the matched factors. In fact, it is now widely recognized that case–control matching is a form of selection bias that can be removed by adjusting for the matching factor; to the extent the factor has been closely matched and accurately measured, this adjustment also controls for confounding by the factor (Rothman and Greenland 1998, Chapter 10).

As an example, suppose that our population at risk is half male, that the men tend to drink less coffee than the women, and that about 75 per cent of our cases are men. Unbiased control selection should yield about 50 per cent men in the control group. However, if we matched controls to cases on sex, about 75 per cent of our controls would be men. Since men drink less coffee than women and men would be over-represented in the matched control group, the matched control group would under-represent coffee use in the population at risk. Note, however, that matching does not affect the sex-specific prevalence of coffee use among controls, and so the sex-specific and sex-adjusted estimates would be unaffected by matching. In other words, the selection bias produced by matching could be removed by adjustment for the matching factor.

The conclusion to be drawn is that matching can necessitate control of the matching factors. Thus, in order to avoid increasing the number of factors requiring control unnecessarily, one should limit matching to factors for which control would probably be necessary anyway. In particular, matching is usually best limited to known strong confounders, such as age and sex in the above example (Schlesselman 1982; Rothman and Greenland 1998, Chapter 10).

More generally, the primary theoretical value of matching is that it can sometimes reduce the variance of adjusted estimators. However, there are circumstances in which matching can facilitate control selection and so is justified on practical grounds. For example, neighbourhood controls may be far easier to obtain than unmatched general population controls. In addition, although neighbourhood matching would necessitate use of a matched analysis method, the neighbourhood-matched results would incorporate some control of confounding by factors associated with neighbourhood (such as socio-economic status and air pollution).

Special control groups

It is not unusual for investigators to select a special control group that is clearly not representative of the population at risk if they can argue that (a) the group will adequately reflect the distribution of the study factor in the population at risk; or (b) that the selection bias in the control group is of the same magnitude of (and so will cancel with) the selection bias in the case group. The first rationale is common in case–control studies of mortality in which people dying of other selected causes of death are used as controls; in such studies, selection validity can be assured only if the control causes of death are unrelated to the study factor. The second rationale is common in studies using hospital cases and controls; in particular, selection validity can be assured in such studies if the control conditions are unrelated to the study factor, and the study disease and the control conditions have proportional exposure-specific rates of hospital admission (Schlesselman 1982).

Selection into a special control group usually requires membership in a small and highly select subset of the population at risk. Thus use of a special control group requires careful scrutiny for mechanisms by which the study factor may influence entry into the subset. See Schlesselman (1982) and Kelsey *et al.* (1996) for discussions of practical issues in evaluating special control groups, and Rothman and Greenland (1998) for validity principles in mortality case–control studies (so-called proportionate mortality studies).

Case–control modelling

The most popular model for case–control analysis is the logistic model. Details of logistic modeling for case–control analysis are covered in many textbooks including Breslow and Day (1980), Schlesselman (1982), Hosmer and Lemeshow (1989), Clayton and Hills (1993), Kelsey *et al.* (1996), and Rothman and Greenland (1998, Chapter 21).

One important aspect of case–control modelling is that matched factors require special treatment. For example, suppose that matching is done on age in 5-year categories and age is associated with the study exposure. To control for the selection bias produced by matching, one must either employ conditional logistic regression with age as a stratifying factor, or else enter indicator variables for each age-matching category into an ordinary logistic regression (the latter strategy has the drawback of requiring about 10 or more subjects per age stratum to produce valid estimates). Simply entering age into the model as a continuous variable may not adequately control for the matching-induced bias (Rothman and Greenland 1998, Chapter 21).

Summary of example

The example in this section provides an illustration of the most common threats to validity in case–control studies (beyond those already discussed for cohort studies). After adjustments for possible confounding and follow-up bias (along the lines described for the cohort study), there may still be irremediable selection bias, especially if we use only select case groups (for example myocardial infarction survivors) or control groups (for example hospital controls). In addition, retrospective ascertainment will lead to greater measurement error than prospective ascertainment, and some of this additional error may be differential.

Given the even greater number of potential biases of unknown magnitude and different directions, it would appear that (as in the cohort example) no conclusions about coffee effect could be drawn from a study like the one described above, other than that coffee does not have a large effect. Again, this is a common result in thorough epidemiological analyses of observational data.

Retrospective cohort studies

Two major types of cohort studies can be distinguished depending on whether members of the study cohort are identified before or after the follow-up period under study. Studies in which all members are identified before their follow-up period are called concurrent or prospective cohort studies, while studies in which all members are identified after their follow-up period are called historical or retrospective cohort studies. Like case–control studies, retrospective cohort studies often require special consideration of retrospective ascertainment and selection validity.

In particular, retrospective cohort studies that obtain exposure or covariate histories from post-event reconstructions are vulnerable to bias from outcome-affected measurements. Suppose, for example, that a study of cancer incidence at an industrial facility had to rely on company personnel to determine the location and nature of various exposures in the plant during the relevant exposure periods. If these personnel were aware of the locations at which cases worked (as when a publicized 'cluster' of cases has occurred), biased exposure assessment could result. Such problems can also occur in a prospective cohort study if exposure or covariate histories are based on post-event reconstructions.

Retrospective cohort studies can also suffer from selection biases analogous to those found in case–control studies. Suppose, for example, that a retrospective cohort study relied on company records to identify members of the cohort of plant employees. If retention of an employee's records (and hence identification of the employee as a cohort member) were associated with both the exposure and outcome status of the employee, the exposure–outcome association observed in the incomplete study cohort could poorly represent the exposure–outcome association in the complete cohort of plant employees.

Conclusion

Uncertainty about validity conditions is responsible for most of the inconclusiveness inherent in epidemiological studies. This inconclusiveness can be partially overcome when multiple complementary studies are conducted, that is, when new studies are conducted under conditions that effectively limit bias from one or more of the sources present in earlier studies. Ideally, after enough complementary studies have been conducted, each known or suspected source of bias will have been rendered unimportant in at least one study. If at this point all the study results appear consistent with one another (which is not the case for coffee and myocardial infarction, although the studies of smoking and lung cancer provide a good example), the epidemiological community may reach some consensus about the existence and strength of an effect.

Even in such ideal situations, however, one should bear in mind that consistency is not validity. For example, there may be some unsuspected source of bias present in all the studies, so that they are all consistently biased in the same direction. Alternatively, all the known sources of bias may be in the same direction, so that all the studies remain biased in the same direction if no one study eliminates all known sources of bias. For these and other reasons, many authors warn that all causal inferences should be considered tentative, at least if drawn from observational epidemiological data alone (Rothman 1988; Rothman and Greenland 1998, Chapter 2).

References

Barnett, V. (1999). *Comparative statistical inference* (3rd edn). Wiley, New York.

Berger, J.O. and Berry, D.A. (1988). Statistical analysis and the illusion of objectivity. *American Scientist*, **76**, 159–65.

Brenner, H. (1993). Bias due to nondifferential misclassification of a polytomous confounder. *Journal of Clinical Epidemiology*, **46**, 57–63.

Breslow, N.E. and Day, N.E. (1980). *Statistical methods in cancer research. I: The analysis of case control studies.* IARC, Lyon.

Breslow, N.E. and Day, N.E. (1987). *Statistical methods in cancer research. II: The analysis of cohort data.* IARC, Lyon.

Checkoway, H., Pearce, N., and Crawford-Brown, D. (1989). *Research methods in occupational epidemiology.* Oxford University Press, New York.

Clayton, D. and Hills, M. (1993). *Statistical models in epidemiology.* Oxford University Press, New York.

Cornfield, J., Haenszel, W.H., Hammond, E.C., *et al.* (1959). Smoking and lung cancer: recent evidence and a discussion of some questions. *Journal of the National Cancer Institute*, **22**, 173–203 (Appendix A).

Curb, J.D., Reed, D.M., Kautz, J.A., *et al.* (1986). Coffee, caffeine, and serum cholesterol in Japanese men in Hawaii. *American Journal of Epidemiology*, **123**, 648–55.

Dosemeci, M., Wacholder, S., and Lubin, J.H. (1990). Does nondifferential misclassification of exposure always bias a true effect towards the null value? *American Journal of Epidemiology*, **132**, 746–8.

Dosemeci, M., Wacholder, S., and Lubin, J.H. (1991). The authors clarify and reply. *American Journal of Epidemiology*, **134**, 441–2.

Drews, C.D. and Greenland, S. (1990). The impact of differential recall on the results of case–control studies. *International Journal of Epidemiology*, **19**, 1107–12.

Drews, C., Greenland, S., and Flanders, W.D. (1993). The use of restricted controls to prevent recall bias in case–control studies of reproductive outcomes. *Annals of Epidemiology*, **3**, 86–92.

Flanders, W.D. and Khoury, M.J. (1990). Indirect assessment of confounding: graphic description and limits on effects of adjusting for covariates. *Epidemiology*, **1**, 239–46.

Flegal, K.M., Keyl, P.M., and Nieto, E.J. (1991). Differential misclassification arising from nondifferential errors in exposure measurement. *American Journal of Epidemiology*, **134**, 1233–44.

Goodman, S.N. (1992). A comment on replication, *P*-values and evidence. *Statistics in Medicine*, **11**, 875–9.

Goodman, S.N. (1993). *P*-values, hypothesis tests, and likelihood: implications for epidemiology of a neglected historical debate. *American Journal of Epidemiology*, **137**, 485–96.

Goodman, S.N. (1999). Toward evidence-based medical statistics. I: The *P* value fallacy. *Annals of Internal Medicine*, **130**, 995–1021.

Goodman, S.N. and Royall, R.M. (1988). Evidence and scientific research. *American Journal of Public Health*, **78**, 1568–74.

Greenland, S. (1980). The effect of misclassification in the presence of covariates. *American Journal of Epidemiology*, **112**, 564–9.

Greenland, S. (1985). Control initiated case–control studies. *International Journal of Epidemiology*, **14**, 130–4.

Greenland, S. (1987). Interpretation and choice of effect measures in epidemiologic analyses. *American Journal of Epidemiology*, **125**, 761–8.

Greenland, S. (1990). Randomization, statistics, and causal inference. *Epidemiology*, **1**, 421–9.

Greenland, S. (1993*a*). A meta-analysis of coffee, myocardial infarction, and coronary death. *Epidemiology*, **4**, 366–74.

Greenland, S. (1993*b*). Summarization, smoothing, and inference. *Scandinavian Journal of Social Medicine*, **21**, 421–9.

Greenland, S. (1994). A critical look at some popular meta-analytic methods. *American Journal of Epidemiology*, **140**, 290–6.

Greenland, S. (1998*a*). Meta-Analysis. In *Modern epidemiology* (ed. K.J. Rothman and S. Greenland), (2nd edn). Lippincott-Raven, Philadelphia, PA.

Greenland, S. (1998*b*). Probability logic and probabilistic induction. *Epidemiology*, **9**, 322–32.

Greenland, S. and Maldonado, G. (1994). The interpretation of multiplicative model parameters as standardized parameters. *Statistics in Medicine*, **13**, 989–99.

Greenland, S. and Robins, J.M. (1985). Confounding and misclassification. *American Journal of Epidemiology*, **122**, 495–506.

Greenland, S. and Robins, J.M. (1988). Conceptual problems in the definition and interpretation of attributable fractions. *American Journal of Epidemiology*, **128**, 1185–97.

Greenland, S. and Robins, J.M. (1994). Ecologic studies: biases, misconceptions, and counterexamples. *American Journal of Epidemiology*, **139**, 747–60.

Greenland, S., Schlesselman, J.J., and Criqui, M.H. (1986). The fallacy of employing standardized regression coefficients and correlations as measures of effect. *American Journal of Epidemiology*, **123**, 203–8.

Greenland, S., Maclure, M., Schlesselman, J.J., *et al.* (1991). Standardized coefficients: a further critique and a review of alternatives. *Epidemiology*, **2**, 387–92.

Greenland, S., Pearl, J., and Robins, J.M. (1999*a*). Causal diagrams for epidemiologic research. *Epidemiology*, **10**, 37–48.

Greenland, S., Robins, J.M., and Pearl, J. (1999*b*). Confounding and collapsibility in causal inference. *Statistical Science*, **14**, 29–46.

Hastie, T. and Tibshirani, R. (1990). *Generalized additive models*. Chapman & Hall, New York.

Hosmer, D.W. and Lemeshow S. (1989). *Applied logistic regression*. Wiley, New York.

Kalbfleisch, J.D. and Prentice, R.L. (1980). *The statistical analysis of failure-time data*. Wiley, New York.

Kelsey, J.L, Whittemore, A.S., Evans, A.S., and Thompson, W.D. (1996). *Methods in observational epidemiology* (2nd edn). Oxford University Press, New York.

Leamer, E.E. (1978). *Specification searches*. Wiley, New York.

McCullagh, P. and Nelder, J.A. (1989). *Generalized linear models*, (2nd edn). Chapman & Hall, New York.

Maldonado, G. and Greenland, S. (1994). A comparison of the performance of model-based confidence intervals when the correct model form is unknown. *Epidemiology*, **5**, 171–82.

Morgenstern, H. (1998). Ecologic studies. In *Modern epidemiology* (ed. K.J. Rothman, and S. Greenland), (2nd edn). Lippincott-Raven, Philadelphia, PA.

Oakes, M. (1990). *Statistical inference*. Epidemiology Resources, Chestnut Hill, MA.

Poole, C. (1985). Exceptions to the rule about nondifferential misclassification (abstract). *American Journal of Epidemiology*, **122**, 508.

Poole, C. (1987*a*). Beyond the confidence interval. *American Journal of Public Health*, **77**, 197–9.

Poole, C. (1987*b*). Confidence intervals exclude nothing. *American Journal of Public Health*, **77**, 492–3.

Poole, C. (1999). Controls who experienced hypothetical causal intermediates should not be excluded from case–control studies. *American Journal of Epidemiology*, **150**, 547–51.

Robins, J.M. (1988). Confidence intervals for causal parameters. *Statistics in Medicine*, **7**, 773–85.

Robins, J.M. and Greenland, S. (1986). The role of model selection in causal inference from nonexperimental data. *American Journal of Epidemiology*, **123**, 392–402.

Robins, J.M. and Greenland, S. (1992). Identifiability and exchangeability for direct and indirect effects. *Epidemiology*, **3**, 143–55.

Robins, J.M. and Greenland, S. (1994). Adjusting for differential rates of prophylaxis therapy for PCP in high-versus low-dose AZT treatment arms in an AIDS randomized trial. *Journal of the American Statistical Association*, **90**, 737–49.

Rosenbaum, P.R. (1995). *Observational studies*. Springer-Verlag, New York.

Rothman, K.J. (1988). *Causal inference*. Epidemiology Resources, Chestnut Hill, MA.

Rothman, K.J. and Greenland, S. (1998). *Modern epidemiology* (2nd edn). J.B. Lippincott, Philadelphia, PA.

Rubin, D.R. (1991). Practical implications of modes of statistical inference for causal effects, and the critical role of the assignment mechanism. *Biometrics*, **47**, 1213–34.

Savitz, D.A. and Pearce, N. (1988). Control selection with incomplete case ascertainment. *American Journal of Epidemiology*, **127**, 1109–17.

Schlesselman, J.J. (1978). Assessing the effects of confounding variables. *American Journal of Epidemiology*, **108**, 3–8.

Schlesselman, J.J. (1982). *Case-control studies: design, conduct, analysis*. Oxford University Press, New York.

Slud, E. and Byar, D. (1988). How dependent causes of death can make risk factors appear protective. *Biometrics*, **44**, 265–70.

Swan, S.H., Shaw, G.R., and Schulman, J. (1992). Reporting and selection bias in case–control studies of congenital malformations. *Epidemiology*, **3**, 356–63.

Wacholder, S., Dosemeci, M., and Lubin, J.H. (1991). Blind assignment of exposure does not always prevent differential misclassification. *American Journal of Epidemiology*, **134**, 433–7.

Wacholder, S., M.L., McLaughlin, J.K., Silverman, D.T., and Mandel, J.S. (1992). Selection of controls in case–control studies. *American Journal of Epidemiology*, **135**, 1019–50.

Walker, A.M. (1991). *Observation and inference: an introduction to the methods of epidemiology*. Epidemiology Resources, Chestnut Hill, MA.

Weinberg, C.R. (1985). On pooling across strata when frequency matching has been followed in a cohort study. *Biometrics*, **41**, 103–16.

Weinberg, C.R., Umbach, D., and Greenland, S. (1994). When will non-differential misclassification preserve the direction of the trend? *American Journal of Epidemiology*, **140**, 565–71.

White, H. (1993). *Estimation, inference, and specification analysis*. Cambridge University Press, New York.

6.11 Causation and causal inference

Kenneth J. Rothman and Sander Greenland

In *The Magic Years*, Fraiberg (1959) characterized every toddler as a scientist, busily fulfilling an earnest mission to develop a logical structure for the strange objects and events that make up the world that he or she inhabits. To survive successfully requires a useful theoretical scheme to relate the myriad events that are encountered. As a youngster, each person develops and tests an inventory of causal explanations that brings meaning to the events that are perceived and ultimately leads to increasing power to control those events.

Parents can attest to the delight that children take in forming causal hypotheses and then meticulously testing them, often through exasperating repetitions that are motivated mainly by the joy of understanding. At a certain age, a child will, when entering a new room, search for a wall switch to operate the electric light. Upon finding one, the child will switch it on and off repeatedly to test the discovery beyond any reasonable doubt. Experiments such as those designed to examine the effect of gravity on free-falling liquids are usually conducted with careful attention, varying the initial conditions in subtle ways and reducing extraneous influences whenever possible by conducting the experiments safely removed from parental interference. The fruit of such scientific labours is a working knowledge of the essential system of causal relations that enables each of us to navigate our complex world.

A general model of causation

If everyone begins life as a scientist, creating his or her own inventory of causal explanations for the empirical world, everyone also begins life as a pragmatic philosopher, developing a general causal theory that some events or states of nature are causes with specific effects or effects with specific causes. Without a general theory of causation, there would be no skeleton on which to hang the substance of the many specific causal theories that one needs to survive. Unfortunately, the concepts of causation that are established early in life are too rudimentary to serve well as the basis for scientific theories. We need to develop a more refined set of concepts that can serve as a common starting point in discussions of causal theories.

Concept of sufficient cause and component causes

To begin, we need to define cause. We can define a cause of a specific disease event as an antecedent event, condition, or characteristic that was necessary for the occurrence of the disease at the moment it occurred, given that other conditions are fixed. In other words, a cause of a disease event is an event, condition, or characteristic that preceded the disease event and without which the disease event would not have occurred at all or until some later time. In this definition it may be that no specific event, condition, or characteristic is sufficient by itself to produce disease. This definition, then, does not define a complete causal mechanism, but only a component of it.

A common characteristic of the concept of causation that we develop early in life is the assumption of a one-to-one correspondence between the observed cause and effect. Each cause is seen as necessary and sufficient in itself to produce the effect. Thus, the flick of a light switch appears to be the singular cause that makes the lights go on. There are less evident causes, however, that also operate to produce the effect: the need for an unspent bulb in the light fixture, wiring from the switch to the bulb, and voltage to produce a current when the circuit is closed. To achieve the effect of turning on the light, each of these is equally as important as moving the switch, because absence of any of these components of the causal constellation will prevent the effect.

For many people, the roots of early causal thinking persist and become manifest in attempts to find single causes as explanations for observed phenomena. Nevertheless, experience and reflection should easily persuade us that the cause of any effect must consist of a constellation of components that act in concert (Mill 1843). A 'sufficient cause', which means a complete causal mechanism, can be defined as a set of minimal conditions and events that inevitably produce disease; 'minimal' implies that all of the conditions or events are necessary. In disease aetiology, the completion of a sufficient cause may be considered equivalent to the onset of disease. (Onset here refers to the onset of the earliest stage of the disease process, rather than the onset of signs or symptoms.) For biological effects, most and sometimes all of the components of a sufficient cause are unknown (Rothman 1976).

For example, smoking is a cause of lung cancer, but by itself it is not a sufficient cause. Firstly, the term smoking is too imprecise to be used in a causal description. One must specify the type of smoke, whether it is filtered or unfiltered, the manner and frequency of inhalation, and the onset and duration of smoking. More importantly, smoking, even defined explicitly, will not cause cancer in everyone. So who are those who are 'susceptible' to the effects of smoking? Or, to put it in other terms, what are the other components of the causal constellation that act with smoking to produce lung cancer?

When causal components remain unknown, one may be inclined to assign an equal risk to all individuals whose status for some components is known and identical. Thus, men who are heavy cigarette smokers are said to have approximately a 10 per cent lifetime risk of developing lung cancer. Some interpret this statement to mean that all men would be subject to a 10 per cent probability of lung cancer if they were to become heavy smokers, as if the outcome, aside from smoking, were purely a matter of chance. In contrast, we view the assignment of equal risks as reflecting nothing more than assigning to everyone within a specific category, in this case male heavy smokers, the average of the individual risks for people in that category. In the classical view, these risks are either 1 or 0, depending on whether or not the individual will or will not get lung cancer.

We cannot measure the individual risks, and assigning the average value to everyone in the category reflects nothing more than our ignorance about the determinants of lung cancer that interact with cigarette smoke. It is apparent from epidemiological data that some people can engage in chain smoking for many decades without developing lung cancer. Others are or will become 'primed' by unknown circumstances and need only to add cigarette smoke to the nearly sufficient constellation of causes to initiate lung cancer. In our ignorance of these hidden causal components, the best we can do in assessing risk is to classify people according to measured causal risk indicators and then assign the average risk observed within a class to people within the class. As knowledge expands, the risk estimates assigned to people will depart from the average according to the presence or absence of other factors that affect the risk.

For example, we now know that smokers with substantial asbestos exposure are at higher risk of lung cancer than those who lack asbestos exposure. Consequently, with adequate data we could assign different risks to heavy smokers based on their asbestos exposure. Within categories of asbestos exposure, the average risks would be assigned to all heavy smokers until other risk factors are identified.

Figure 1 provides a schematic diagram of sufficient causes in a hypothetical individual. Each constellation of component causes represented in Fig. 1 is minimally sufficient to produce the disease, that is there are no redundant or extraneous component causes—each one is a necessary part of that specific causal mechanism. Component causes may play a role in one, two, or all three of the causal mechanisms pictured.

Figure 1 does not depict aspects of the causal process such as prevention, sequence of action, dose, and other complexities. These aspects of the causal process can be accommodated in the model by an appropriate definition of each causal component. Thus, if the outcome is lung cancer and factor E represents cigarette smoking, it could be defined more explicitly as smoking at least two packs a day of unfiltered cigarettes for at least 20 years. If the outcome is smallpox, which is completely prevented by immunization, factor U could represent 'unimmunized'. More generally, the preventive effects of a factor C can be represented by placing its complement 'no C' within sufficient causes.

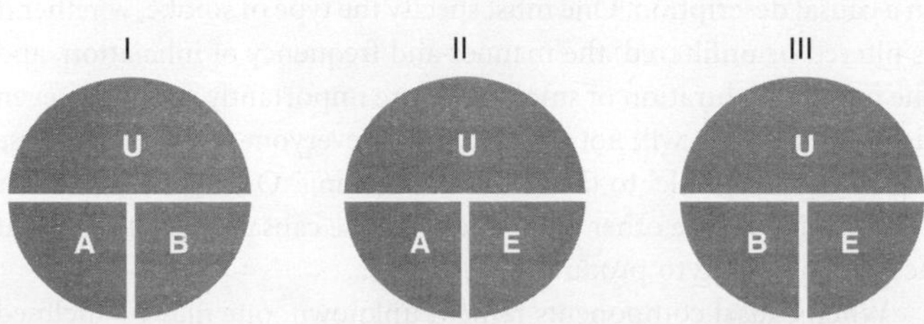

Fig. 1 Three sufficient causes of a disease.

Strength of causes

The causal model exemplified by Fig. 1 can facilitate an understanding of some key concepts such as 'strength of effect' and 'interaction'. As an illustration of strength of effect, Table 1 displays the frequency of the eight possible patterns for exposure to A, B, and E in two hypothetical populations. Suppose that U is always present (ubiquitous) and Fig. 1 represents all the sufficient causes capable of acting for each individual in each population. Here and throughout this chapter we will assume that 'disease' refers to a non-recurrent event, such as death or first occurrence of a disease. Under these assumptions, the response of each individual under the exposure pattern in a given row can be found under the response column.

The proportion acquiring a disease in any subpopulation (the incidence proportion) can be found simply by multiplying the number at each exposure pattern by the response for that pattern, summing these products to get the total number of disease cases in the subpopulation, and dividing this total by the population size. If exposure A is unmeasured, the pattern of these incidence proportions in population 1 would be those in Table 2.

As an example of how the proportions in Table 2 were calculated, let us review how the incidence proportion among people with B present, but E absent was calculated. There were 100 people with A present, B present, and E absent, all of whom became cases, because A and B are sufficient to produce the disease in combination with the background causes. There were 900 people with A absent, B present, and E absent, none of whom became cases, because they did not have a sufficient cause. Thus, among all 1000 people with B present and E absent, there were 100 cases, giving a proportion of 0.10.

It is evident from Table 2 that for population 1, E is a much stronger determinant of incidence than B. This difference is reflected in the fact that the presence of E increases the incidence by 0.9, whereas the presence of B increases incidence by only 0.1.

Table 3 shows the analogous results for population 2. Although the members of this population have exactly the same causal mechanisms

Table 1 Exposure frequencies for three component causes in two hypothetical populations according to the possible combinations of the component causes

Exposures			Response (outcome)	Frequency of exposure pattern	
A	B	E		Population 1	Population 2
1	1	1	1	100	900
1	1	0	1	100	900
1	0	1	1	900	100
1	0	0	0	900	100
0	1	1	1	900	100
0	1	0	0	900	100
0	0	1	0	100	900
0	0	0	0	100	900

Table 2 Pattern of incidence proportions for component causes B and E in hypothetical population 1 assuming that component cause A is unmeasured

	B 1, E 1	B 1, E 0	B 0, E 1	B 0, E 0
Cases	1000	100	900	0
Total	1000	1000	1000	1000
Proportion	1.00	0.10	0.90	0.00

operating within them as do the members of population 1, the relative strengths of E and B are reversed; B is now a much stronger determinant of incidence than E. This is so despite the fact that the crude proportions of members with A, B, and E are exactly 50 per cent in both populations and even though within each population, A, B, and E have no association with one another.

One key difference between populations 1 and 2 is that the condition under which E acts as a necessary and sufficient cause—the presence of A or B, but not both—is common in population 1 but rare in population 2. In population 1, 3600 people or 90 per cent of the total have A or B but not both and the incidence proportion for E merely reflects this percentage. In contrast, only 400 people or 10 per cent of the total in population 2 have A or B but not both. This difference in the frequency of necessary and sufficient conditions for E to cause the disease explains the difference in the strength of the effect of E for the two populations. A similar explanation applies to the different strength of effect for factor B in the two populations.

We will call the condition necessary and sufficient for a factor to produce disease the causal complement of the factor. Thus, the condition 'A or B but not both' is the causal complement of E in the above example. This example shows that the strength of a factor's effect on a population depends on the relative prevalence of its causal complement. This dependence of the effects of a specific component cause on the prevalence of its causal complement has nothing to do with the biological mechanism of the component's action, since the component is an equal partner in each mechanism in which it appears. Nevertheless, a factor is a strong cause if its causal complement is common. Conversely, a factor with a rare causal complement will appear to be a weak cause.

The strength of a cause may have tremendous public health significance, but it may have little biological significance. The reason is that given a specific causal mechanism, any of the component causes can be either strong or weak. The identities of the components of a sufficient cause is part of the biology of causation, whereas the strength of a cause is a relative phenomenon that depends on the time- and place-specific distribution of component causes in a population. Over

Table 3 Pattern of incidence proportions for component causes B and E in hypothetical population 2 assuming that component cause A is unmeasured

	B 1, E 1	B 1, E 0	B 0, E 1	B 0, E 0
Cases	1000	900	100	0
Total	1000	1000	1000	1000
Proportion	1.00	0.90	0.10	0.00

a span of time, the strength of individual causal risk factors within a specific causal mechanism for a given disease may change, because the prevalence of specific component causes in various mechanisms may also change. The causal mechanisms in which these components act could remain unchanged, however.

The preceding discussion has focused on the absolute increase in incidence (often referred to as 'risk difference') as the measure of the strength of effect. More commonly, a ratio measure is used. The arguments we have just given also apply to ratio measures. The magnitude of such measures depends profoundly on the prevalence of complements to the factor under study. In addition, however, ratio measures depend on the prevalences of components of sufficient causes in which the factor does not participate. Thus, in the above example, the prevalence of A will affect the apparent strength of E, as measured by the ratio of incidence proportions, not only through completion of sufficient cause II (in which A is complementary to E), but also through completion of sufficient cause I (in which E does not participate). The net impact can be observed by comparing the incidence ratios for E when B = 1: in population 1 this ratio is 0.90/0.10 = 9, whereas in population 2 this ratio is only 1.00/0.90 = 1.1.

Interactions between causes

Two component causes acting in the same sufficient cause may be thought of as interacting biologically to produce disease. Indeed, one may define biological interaction as the participation of two component causes in the same sufficient cause. Such interaction is also known as causal co-action or joint action. The joint action of the two component causes does not have to be simultaneous action: one component cause could act many years before the other, but it would have to leave some effect that interacts with the later component.

For example, suppose a traumatic injury to the head leads to a permanent disturbance in equilibrium. Many years later, the faulty equilibrium may lead to a fall while walking on an icy path, causing a broken hip. The causal mechanism for the broken hip includes the traumatic injury to the head as a component cause, along with its consequence of a disturbed equilibrium. The causal mechanism also includes the walk along the icy path. These two component causes have interacted with one another, although their time of action is many years apart. They also would interact with the other component causes, such as the type of footwear, the absence of a handhold, and any other conditions that were necessary to the causal mechanism of the fall and the broken hip that resulted.

The degree of observable interaction between two specific component causes depends on how many different sufficient causes produce disease and the proportion of cases that occur through sufficient causes in which the two component causes both play some role. For example, in Fig. 2, suppose that G were only a hypothetical substance that did not actually exist. Consequently, no disease would occur from sufficient cause II, because it depends on an action by G and factors B and F would act only through the distinct mechanisms represented by sufficient causes I and III. Thus, B and F would be biologically independent. Now suppose that C disappears from the environment and is completely replaced by G. Factors B and F will then act together in the mechanism represented by sufficient cause II and, thus, will be found to interact biologically. Thus, the extent of biological interaction between two factors is dependent on the relative prevalence of other factors.

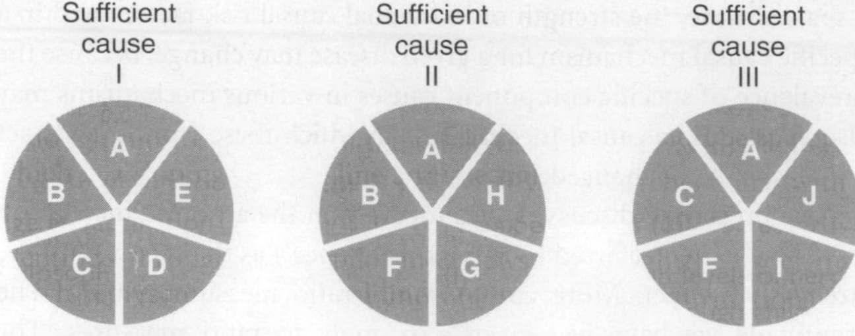

Fig. 2 Three sufficient causes of a disease.

Proportion of disease due to specific causes

In Fig. 1, assuming that the three sufficient causes in the diagram are the only ones operating, what fraction of disease is caused by U? The answer is all of it; without U, there is no disease. U is considered a 'necessary cause'. What fraction is due to E? E causes disease through two mechanisms, II and III, and all disease arising through either of these two mechanisms is due to E. This is not to say that all disease is due to U alone or that a fraction of disease is due to E alone; no component cause acts alone. It is understood that these factors interact with others in producing disease.

A widely discussed but unpublished paper from the 1970s, written by scientists at the National Institutes of Health, proposed that as much as 40 per cent of cancer is attributable to occupational exposures. Many scientists thought that this fraction was unacceptably high and argued against this claim (Higginson 1980; Ephron 1984). One of the arguments used in rebuttal was as follows: x per cent of cancer is caused by smoking, y per cent by diet, z per cent by alcohol, and so on; when all these percentages are added up, only a small percentage, much less than 40 per cent, is left for occupational causes. This rebuttal is fallacious, because it is based on the naive view that every case of disease has a single cause. In fact, since diet and smoking and asbestos and other factors interact with one another and with genetic factors to cause cancer, each case of cancer could be attributed to many separate component causes.

There is a tendency to think that the sum of the fractions of disease attributable to each of the causes of the disease should be 100 per cent. For example, in their widely cited work *The Causes of Cancer*, Doll and Peto (1981) created a table (Table 20) giving their estimates of the fraction of all cancers caused by various agents; the total for the fractions was nearly 100 per cent. Although they acknowledged that any case could be caused by more than one agent, which would mean that the attributable fractions would not sum to 100 per cent, they referred to this situation as a 'difficulty' and an 'anomaly'. It is, however, neither a difficulty nor an anomaly, but simply a consequence of allowing for the fact that no event has a single agent as the cause. The fraction of disease that can be attributed to each of the causes of disease in all the causal mechanisms actually has no upper limit; for cancer or any disease, the total of the fraction of disease attributable to all the component causes of all the causal mechanisms that produce it is not 100 per cent but infinity. Only the fraction of disease attributable to a single component cause cannot exceed 100 per cent.

A single cause or category of causes that is present in every sufficient cause of disease will have an attributable fraction of 100 per cent. Much publicity attended the pronouncement in 1960 that as much as 90 per cent of cancer is environmentally caused (Higginson 1960). Since 'environment' can be thought of as an all-embracing category that represents non-genetic causes, which must be present to some extent in every sufficient cause, it is clear on a priori grounds that 100 per cent of any disease is environmentally caused. Thus, Higginson's (1960) estimate of 90 per cent was an underestimate.

Similarly, one can show that 100 per cent of any disease is inherited. MacMahon (1968) cited the example given by Hogben (1933) of yellow shanks, a trait occurring in certain genetic strains of fowl fed on yellow corn. Both the right set of genes and the yellow corn diet are necessary to produce yellow shanks. A farmer with several strains of fowl, feeding them all only yellow corn, would consider yellow shanks to be a genetic condition, since only one strain would acquire yellow shanks, despite all strains having the same diet. A different farmer, who owned only the strain liable to get yellow shanks, but who fed some of the birds yellow corn and others white corn, would consider yellow shanks to be an environmentally determined condition because it depends on diet. In reality, yellow shanks is determined by both genes and the environment; there is no reasonable way to allocate a portion of the causation to either genes or the environment. Similarly, every case of every disease has some environmental and some genetic component causes and, therefore, every case can be attributed both to genes and to the environment. No paradox exists as long as it is understood that the fractions of disease attributable to genes and to the environment overlap with one another.

Many researchers have spent considerable effort in developing heritability indices, which are supposed to measure the fraction of disease that is inherited. Unfortunately, these indices only assess the relative role of environmental and genetic causes of disease in a particular setting. For example, some genetic causes may be necessary components of every causal mechanism. If everyone in a population has an identical set of the genes that cause disease, however, their effect is not included in heritability indices, despite the fact that having these genes is a cause of the disease. The two farmers in the example above would offer very different values for the heritability of yellow shanks, despite the fact that the condition is always 100 per cent dependent on having certain genes.

If all genetic factors that determine disease are taken into account, whether or not they vary within populations, then 100 per cent of disease can be said to be inherited. Analogously, 100 per cent of any disease is environmentally caused, even those diseases that we often consider purely genetic. Phenylketonuria, for example, is considered by many to be purely genetic. Nonetheless, the mental retardation that it may cause can be successfully prevented by appropriate dietary intervention.

The treatment for phenylketonuria illustrates the interaction of genes and the environment to cause a disease commonly thought to be purely genetic. What about an apparently purely environmental disease such as 'killed in an automobile accident'? It is easy to conceive of genetic traits that lead to psychiatric problems such as alcoholism, which in turn lead to drunk driving and consequent fatality. Consider another more extreme environmental example, 'killed by lightning'. Again, partially heritable psychiatric conditions can influence whether someone will take shelter during a lightning storm. The argument may be stretched on this example, but the point that every case of disease has both genetic and environmental causes is theoretically defensible and has important implications for research.

Induction period

The diagram of causes in Fig. 2 also provides a model for conceptualizing the induction period, which may be defined as the period of time from causal action until disease initiation. If, in sufficient cause I, the sequence of action of the causes is A, B, C, D, and E and we are studying the effect of B, which, let us assume, acts at a narrowly defined point in time, we do not observe the occurrence of disease immediately after B acts. Disease occurs only after the sequence is completed, so there will be a delay while C, D, and, finally, E act. When E acts, disease occurs. The interval between the action of B and the disease occurrence is the induction time for the effect of B.

In the example given earlier of an equilibrium disorder leading to a later fall and hip injury, the induction time between the occurrence of the equilibrium disorder and the later hip injury might be very long. In an individual instance, we would not know the exact length of an induction period, since we cannot be sure of the causal mechanism that produces disease in an individual instance, nor when all the relevant component causes acted. We can characterize the induction period relating the action of a component cause to the occurrence of disease in general, however, by accumulating data for many individuals. A clear example of a lengthy induction time is the cause–effect relation between exposure of a female fetus to diethylstilboestrol and the subsequent development of adenocarcinoma of the vagina. The cancer occurs generally between the ages of 15 and 30 years. Since exposure to diethylstilboestrol occurs before birth, there is an induction time of 15 to 30 years for the carcinogenic action of diethylstilboestrol. During this time, other causes presumably are operating; some evidence suggests that hormonal action during adolescence may be part of the mechanism (Rothman 1981).

It is incorrect to characterize a disease itself as having a lengthy or brief induction time. The induction time can be conceptualized only in relation to a specific component cause. Thus, we say that the induction time relating diethylstilboestrol to clear cell carcinoma of the vagina is 15 to 30 years, but we cannot say that 15 to 30 years is the induction time for clear cell carcinoma in general. Since each component cause in any causal mechanism can act at a time different from the other component causes, each can have its own induction time. For the component cause that acts last, the induction time equals zero. If another component cause of clear cell carcinoma of the vagina that acts during adolescence were identified, it would have a much shorter induction time for its carcinogenic action than diethylstilboestrol. Thus, induction time characterizes a specific cause–effect pair rather than just the effect.

In carcinogenesis, the terms initiator and promoter have been used to refer to component causes of cancer that act early and late, respectively, in the causal mechanism. Cancer itself has often been characterized as a disease process with a long induction time. This characterization is a misconception, however, because any late-acting component in the causal process, such as a promoter, will have a short induction time. Indeed, by definition the induction time will always be zero for at least one component cause, the last to act.

Disease, once initiated, will not necessarily be apparent. The time interval between disease occurrence and detection has been termed the latent period (Rothman 1981), although others have used this term interchangeably with induction period. The latent period can be reduced by improved methods of disease detection. Conversely, the induction period cannot be reduced by early detection of disease, since disease occurrence marks the end of the induction period. Earlier detection of disease, however, may reduce the apparent induction period (the time between causal action and disease detection), since the time when disease is detected, as a practical matter, is usually used to mark the time of disease occurrence. Thus, diseases such as slow-growing cancers may appear to have long induction periods with respect to many causes because they have long latent periods. The latent period, unlike the induction period, is a characteristic of the disease and the detection effort applied to the person with the disease.

Although it is not possible to reduce the induction period proper by earlier detection of disease, it may be possible to observe intermediate stages of a causal mechanism. The increased interest in biomarkers, such as DNA adducts, is an example of attempting to focus on causes more proximal to the disease occurrence. Biomarkers reflect the effects of earlier-acting agents on the organism.

Some agents may have a causal action by shortening the induction time of other agents. Suppose that exposure to factor A leads to epilepsy after an interval of 10 years, on average. It may be that exposure to a drug, B, would shorten this interval to 2 years. Is B acting as a catalyst or as a cause of epilepsy? The answer is both: a catalyst is a cause. Without B the occurrence of epilepsy comes 8 years later than it comes with B, so we can say that B causes the onset of the early epilepsy. It is not sufficient to argue that the epilepsy would have occurred anyway. Firstly, it would not have occurred at that time and the time of occurrence is part of our definition of an event. Secondly, epilepsy will occur later only if the individual survives an additional 8 years, which is not certain. Agent B not only determines when the epilepsy occurs, it can determine whether it occurs. Thus, we should call any agent that acts as a catalyst of a causal mechanism, speeding up an induction period for other agents, as a cause in its own right. Similarly, any agent that postpones the onset of an event, drawing out the induction period for another agent, is a preventive. It should not be too surprising to equate postponement to prevention: we routinely use such an equation when we employ the euphemism that we prevent death, which actually can only be postponed. What we prevent is death at a given time, in favour of death at a later time.

Generality of the model

The main utility of this model of sufficient causes and their components lies in its ability to provide a general but practical conceptual framework for causal problems. The attempt to make the proportion of disease attributable to various component causes add to 100 per cent is an example of a fallacy that is exposed by the model: the model makes it clear that, because of interactions, there is no upper limit to the sum of these proportions. The epidemiological evaluation of interactions themselves can be clarified with the help of the model.

How could the model accommodate varying doses of a component cause? Since the model appears to deal qualitatively with the action of component causes, it might seem that dose variability cannot be taken into account. But this view is overly pessimistic. To account for dose variability, one need only to postulate a set of sufficient causes, each of which contains as a component a different dose of the agent in question. Small doses might require a larger or rarer set of complementary causes to complete a sufficient cause than that required by large doses (Rothman 1976). In this way the model could account for the phenomenon of a shorter induction period accompanying larger doses of exposure, because there would be a smaller set of complementary components needed to complete the sufficient cause.

Those who believe that chance must play a role in any complex mechanism might object to the intricacy of this deterministic model. A probabilistic (stochastic) model could be invoked to describe a dose–response relation, for example, without the need for a multitude of different causal mechanisms; the model would simply relate the dose of the exposure to the probability of the effect occurring. For those who believe that virtually all events contain some element of chance, deterministic causal models may seem to misrepresent reality. Nevertheless, the deterministic model presented here can accommodate classical 'chance', but it does so by reinterpreting chance as deterministic events beyond the current limits of knowledge or observability.

For example, the outcome of a flip of a coin is usually considered a chance event. In classical physics, however, the outcome can in theory be determined completely by the application of physical laws and a sufficient description of the starting conditions. To put it in terms more familiar to epidemiologists, consider the explanation for why an individual acquires lung cancer. One hundred years ago, when little was known about the aetiology of lung cancer, a scientist might have said that it was a matter of chance. Nowadays we might say that the risk depends on how much the individual smokes, how much asbestos and radon the individual has been exposed to, and so on. One might then ask, for an individual who has smoked a specific amount and has a specified amount of exposure to all the other known risk factors, what determines if this individual will get lung cancer? Today's answer might well be that it is a matter of chance. We can explain much more of the variability in lung cancer occurrence nowadays than we formerly could, by taking into account specific factors known to cause it, but at the limits of our knowledge we ascribe the remaining variability to what we call chance. In this view, chance is seen as a catch-all term for our ignorance about causal explanations.

We have so far ignored more subtle considerations of sources of unpredictability in events, such as transcomputably complex deterministic behaviour, chaotic behaviour (in which even the slightest uncertainty about initial conditions leads to vast uncertainty about outcomes), and quantum-mechanical uncertainty. In each of these situations, a random (stochastic) model component may be essential for any useful modelling effort. Such components can be introduced in the above conceptual model by treating unmeasured component causes in the model as random events, so that the causal model based on components of sufficient causes can have a random element.

Philosophy of scientific inference

Causal inference may be viewed as a special case of the more general process of scientific reasoning. The literature on this topic is too vast for us to review, but we will provide a brief overview of certain points relevant to epidemiology, at the risk of some oversimplification.

Modern science began to emerge around the sixteenth and seventeenth centuries, when the knowledge demands of emerging technologies (such as artillery and transoceanic navigation) stimulated inquiry into the origins of knowledge. An early codification of the scientific method was Bacon's *Novum Organum* (1620), which presented an inductivist view of science. In this philosophy, scientific reasoning is said to depend on making generalizations or inductions from observations to general laws of nature; the observations are said to induce the formulation of a natural law in the mind of the scientist. Thus, an inductivist would have said that Jenner's observation of a lack of smallpox among milkmaids induced in his mind the theory that cowpox (common among milkmaids) conferred immunity to smallpox. Inductivist philosophy reached a pinnacle of sorts in the canons of John Stuart Mill (1843), which evolved into inferential criteria that are still in use today.

Inductivist philosophy was a great step forward from the medieval scholasticism that preceded it, for at least it demanded that a scientist make careful observations of people and nature, rather than appeal to faith, ancient texts, or authorities. Nonetheless, by the eighteenth century, the Scottish philosopher David Hume (1739) had described a disturbing deficiency in inductivism: an inductive argument carried no logical force; instead, such an argument represented nothing more than an assumption that certain events would in the future follow in the same pattern as they had in the past. Thus, to argue that cowpox caused immunity to smallpox because no one got smallpox after having cowpox corresponded to an unjustified assumption that the pattern observed so far (no smallpox after cowpox) will continue into the future. Hume (1739) pointed out that, even for the most reasonable sounding of such assumptions, there was no logic or force of necessity behind the inductive argument.

Of central concern to Hume (1739) was the issue of causal inference and failure of induction to provide a foundation for it.

> Thus not only our reason fails us in the discovery of the ultimate connexion of causes and effects, but even after experience has inform'd us of their constant conjunction, 'tis impossible for us to satisfy ourselves by our reason, why we shou'd extend that experience beyond those particular instances, which have fallen under our observation. We suppose, but are never able to prove, that there must be a resemblance betwixt those objects, of which we have had experience, and those which lie beyond the reach of our discovery. (Hume 1739)

In other words, no number of repetitions of a particular sequence of events, such as the appearance of a light after flipping a switch, can establish a causal connection between the action of the switch and the turning on of the light. No matter how many times the light comes on after the switch has been pressed, the possibility of coincidental occurrence cannot be ruled out. Hume (1739) pointed out that observers cannot perceive causal connections, but only a series of events. Russell (1945) illustrated this point with the example of two accurate clocks that perpetually chime on the hour, with one keeping time slightly ahead of the other; although one invariably chimes before the other, there is no causal connection from one to the other. Thus, assigning a causal interpretation to the pattern of events cannot be a logical extension of our observations, since the events might be occurring together only by coincidence or because of a shared earlier cause.

Causal inference based on mere coincidence of events constitute a logical fallacy known as *post hoc ergo propter hoc* (Latin for 'after this therefore on account of this'). This fallacy is exemplified by the inference that the crowing of a rooster is necessary for the sun to rise because sunrise is always preceded by the crowing.

The *post hoc* fallacy is a special case of a more general logical fallacy known as the 'fallacy of affirming the consequent'. This fallacy of confirmation takes the following general form: 'We know that if H is true, B must be true and we know that B is true therefore H must be true'. This fallacy is used routinely by scientists in interpreting data. It is used, for example, when one argues as follows: 'if sewer service causes heart disease, then heart disease rates should be highest where sewer service is available; heart disease rates are indeed highest where sewer service is available therefore, sewer service causes heart disease'. There, H is the hypothesis 'sewer service causes heart disease' and B is the observation 'heart disease rates are highest where sewer service is available'. The argument is of course logically unsound, as demonstrated by the fact that we can imagine many ways in which the premises could be true but the conclusion false, for example economic development could lead to both sewer service and elevated heart disease rates, without any effect of sewer service on heart disease.

Russell (1939) summarized the fallacy this way:

> 'If *p*, then *q*; now *q* is true therefore *p* is true.' E.g., 'If pigs have wings, then some winged animals are good to eat; now some winged animals are good to eat therefore pigs have wings.' This form of inference is called 'scientific method.'

Russell was not alone in his lament of the illogicality of scientific reasoning as ordinarily practised. Many philosophers and scientists from Hume's time onward attempted to set out a firm logical basis for scientific reasoning. Perhaps none has attracted more attention from epidemiologists than the philosopher Karl Popper.

Popper addressed Hume's problem by asserting that scientific hypotheses can never be proven or established as true in any logical sense. Instead, Popper observed that scientific statements can simply be found to be consistent with observation. Since it is possible for an observation to be consistent with several hypotheses that themselves may be mutually inconsistent, consistency between a hypothesis and observation is no proof of the hypothesis. In contrast, a valid observation that is inconsistent with a hypothesis implies that the hypothesis as stated is false and so refutes the hypothesis. If you wring the rooster's neck before it crows and the sun still rises, you have disproved that the rooster's crowing is a necessary cause of sunrise. Or consider a hypothetical research programme to ascertain the boiling point of water (Magee 1985). A scientist who boils water in an open flask and repeatedly measures the boiling point at 100°C will never, no matter how many confirmatory repetitions are involved, prove that 100°C is always the boiling point. Conversely, merely one attempt to boil the water in a closed flask or at high altitude will refute the proposition that water always boils at 100°C.

According to Popper (1968), science advances by a process of elimination that he called conjecture and refutation. Scientists form hypotheses based on intuition, conjecture, and previous experience. Good scientists use deductive logic to infer predictions from the hypothesis, and then compare observations with the predictions. Hypotheses whose predictions agree with observations are confirmed only in the sense that they can continue to be used as explanations of natural phenomena. At any time, however, they may be refuted by further observations and replaced by other hypotheses that better explain the observations. This view of scientific inference is sometimes called refutationism or falsificationism.

Refutationists consider induction to be a psychological crutch: repeated observations did not in fact induce the formulation of a natural law, but only the belief that such a law has been found. For a refutationist, only the psychological comfort that induction provides explains why it still has its advocates.

One way to rescue the concept of induction from the stigma of pure delusion is to resurrect it as a psychological phenomenon, as Hume (1739) and Popper (1968) claimed it was, but one that plays a legitimate role in hypothesis formation. The philosophy of conjecture and refutation places no constraints on the origin of conjectures. Even delusions are permitted as hypotheses and, therefore, inductively inspired hypotheses, however psychological, are valid starting points for scientific evaluation. This concession does not admit a logical role for induction in confirming scientific hypotheses, but it allows the process of induction to play a part, along with imagination, in the scientific cycle of conjecture and refutation.

The philosophy of conjecture and refutation has profound implications for the methodology of science. The popular concept of a scientist doggedly assembling evidence to support a favourite thesis is objectionable from the standpoint of refutationist philosophy, because it encourages scientists to consider their own pet theories as their intellectual property, to be confirmed, proven, and, when all the evidence is in, cast in stone and defended as natural law. Such attitudes hinder critical evaluation, interchange, and progress. The approach of conjecture and refutation, in contrast, encourages scientists to consider multiple hypotheses and to seek crucial tests that decide between competing hypotheses by falsifying one of them. Since falsification of one or more theories is the goal, there is incentive to depersonalize the theories. Criticism levelled at a theory need not be seen as criticism of its proposer. It has been suggested that the reason why certain fields of science advance rapidly while others languish is that the rapidly advancing fields are propelled by scientists who are busy constructing and testing competing hypotheses the other fields, in contrast, 'are sick by comparison, because they have forgotten the necessity for alternative hypotheses and disproof' (Platt 1964).

Some twentieth century philosophers of science, most notably Kuhn, have emphasized the role of the scientific community in determining the validity of scientific theories. These critics of the conjecture and refutation model have suggested that the refutation of a theory involves making a choice. Every observation is itself dependent on theories.

For example, observing the moons of Jupiter through a telescope seems to us like a direct observation, but only because the theory of optics on which the telescope is based is so well accepted. When confronted with a refuting observation, a scientist faces the choice of rejecting either the validity of the theory being tested or the validity of the scientific infrastructure of the theories on which the refuting observation is based. Observations that are falsifying instances of theories may at times be treated as 'anomalies', tolerated without falsifying the theory in the hope that the anomalies may eventually be explained. An epidemiological example is the observation that shallow-inhaling smokers had higher lung cancer rates than deep-inhaling smokers. This anomaly was eventually explained when it was noted that smoking-associated lung tumours tend to occur high in the lung, where shallowly inhaled smoke tars tend to be deposited (Wald 1985).

In other instances, anomalies may eventually lead to the overthrow of current scientific doctrine, just as Newtonian mechanics was discarded (remaining only as a first-order approximation) in favour of relativity theory. Kuhn (1962) claimed that in every branch of science the prevailing scientific viewpoint, which he termed 'normal science', occasionally undergoes major shifts that amount to scientific revolutions. These revolutions signal a decision of the scientific community to discard the scientific infrastructure rather than to falsify a new hypothesis that cannot easily be grafted onto it. Kuhn (1962) and others have argued that the consensus of the scientific community determines what is considered accepted and what is considered refuted.

Kuhn's critics characterized this description of science as one of an irrational process, 'a matter for mob psychology' (Lakatos 1970). Those who cling to a belief in a rational structure for science consider Kuhn's vision to be a regrettably real description of much of what passes for scientific activity, but not prescriptive for any good science.

The philosophical debate about Kuhn's description of science hinges on whether he meant to describe only what has happened historically in science or instead meant to describe what ought to happen, an issue about which he has not been completely clear.

> Are Kuhn's remarks about scientific development . . . to be read as descriptions or prescriptions? The answer, of course, is that they should be read in both ways at once. If I have a theory of how and why science works, it must necessarily have implications for the way in which scientists should behave if their enterprise is to flourish. (Kuhn 1970)

The idea that science is a sociological process, whether considered descriptive or normative, is an interesting thesis. Regardless of the answer, we suspect that most epidemiologists (and most scientists) will continue to function as if the following classical view of the goal of science is correct: the ultimate goal of scientific inference is to capture some objective truths and any theory of inference should ideally be evaluated by how well it leads us to these truths.

Those holding the objective view of scientific truth nevertheless concede that our knowledge of these truths will always be tentative. For refutationists this tentativeness has an asymmetric quality: we may know a theory is false because it consistently fails the tests we put it through, but we cannot know that it is true, even if it passes every test we can devise, for it may fail a test as yet undevised. With this view, any theory of inference should ideally be evaluated by how well it leads us to detect errors in our hypotheses and observations.

There is another philosophy of inference that, like refutationism, holds an objective view of scientific truth and a view of knowledge as tentative or uncertain, but which focuses on an evaluation of knowledge rather than truth. Like refutationism, the modern form of this philosophy evolved from the writings of eighteenth century British philosophers, but the focal arguments first appeared in a pivotal essay by Thomas Bayes (1763) and, hence, the philosophy is usually referred to as Bayesianism (Howson and Urbach 1989). Like refutationism, it did not reach a complete expression until after the First World War, most notably in the writings of Ramsey (1931) and DeFinetti (1937) and, like refutationism, it did not begin to appear in epidemiology until the 1970s (Cornfield 1976).

The central problem addressed by Bayesianism is the following. In classical logic, a deductive argument can provide you no information about a scientific hypothesis unless you can be 100 per cent certain about the truth of the premises of the argument. Consider the centrepiece of refutationism, the logical argument called *modus tollens*: 'If H implies B and B is false, then H must be false'. This argument is logically valid, but it does the scientist little of the good claimed by refutationists, because the conclusion follows only on the assumptions that the premises 'H implies B' and 'B is false' are true statements. If these premises are statements about the physical world, we cannot possibly know them to be correct with 100 per cent certainty, since all observations are subject to error. Furthermore, the claim that 'H implies B' will often depend on its own chain of deductions, each with its own premises of which we cannot be certain.

For example, if H is 'television viewing causes homicides' and B is 'homicide rates are highest where televisions are most common', the first premise used in *modus tollens* to test the hypothesis that television viewing causes homicides will be 'if television viewing causes homicides, homicide rates are highest where televisions are most common'. The validity of this premise is doubtful—after all, even if television does cause homicides, homicide rates may be low where televisions are common because of socio-economic advantages in those areas.

Continuing to reason in this fashion, we could arrive at a more pessimistic state than even Hume imagined: not only is induction without logical foundation, but deduction has no scientific utility because we cannot insure the validity of all the premises. The Bayesian answer to this problem is partial, in that it makes a severe demand on the scientist and puts a severe limitation on the results. It says roughly this: If you can assign a degree of certainty or personal probability to the premises of your valid argument, you may use any and all the rules of probability theory to derive a certainty for the conclusion and this certainty will be a logically valid consequence of your original certainties. The catch is that your concluding certainty, or posterior probability, may depend heavily on what you used as initial certainties or prior probabilities. And, if those initial certainties are not the same as those of a colleague, that colleague may very well assign a different certainty to the conclusion than you derived.

Because the posterior probabilities emanating from a Bayesian inference depend on the person supplying the initial certainties and, thus, may vary across individuals, the inferences are said to be subjective. This subjectivity of Bayesian inference is often mistaken for a subjective treatment of truth. Not only is such a view of Bayesianism incorrect, but it is diametrically opposed to Bayesian philosophy. The Bayesian approach represents a constructive attempt to deal with the dilemma that scientific laws and facts should not be treated as known with certainty, yet classical deductive logic yields conclusions only when some law, fact, or connection between is asserted with 100 per cent certainty.

A common criticism of Bayesian philosophy is that it diverts attention away from the classical goals of science, such as the discovery of how the world works, towards psychological states of mind called 'certainties', 'subjective probabilities', or 'degrees of belief' (Popper 1968). This criticism fails, however, to recognize the importance of the scientist's state of mind in determining what theories to test and what tests to apply.

In any research context there will be an unlimited number of hypotheses that could explain an observed phenomenon. Some argue that progress is best aided by severely testing (empirically challenging) those explanations that seem most probable in the light of past research, so that shortcomings of currently 'received' theories can be most rapidly discovered. Indeed, much research in certain fields takes this form, as when theoretical predictions of particle mass are put to ever-more precise tests in physics experiments. This process does not involve a mere improved repetition of past studies. Rather, it involves tests of previously untested but important predictions of the theory.

Probabilities of auxiliary hypotheses are also important in study design and interpretation. Failure of a theory to pass a test can lead to rejection of the theory more rapidly when the auxiliary hypotheses upon which the test depends possess high probability. This observation provides a rationale for preferring population-based to hospital-based case–control studies, because the former have a higher probability of unbiased subject selection.

Even if one disputes the above arguments, most epidemiologists desire some interval estimate or evaluation of the likely range for an effect in the light of available data. This estimate must inevitably be derived in the face of considerable uncertainty about methodological details and various events that led to the available data and can be extremely sensitive to the reasoning used in its derivation. Psychological investigations have found that most people, including scientists, reason poorly in general and especially poorly in the face of uncertainty (Kahnemann *et al.* 1982; Piattelli-Palmarini 1994). Bayesian philosophy provides a methodology for sound reasoning and, in particular, provides many warnings against being overly certain about one's conclusions (Greenland 1998*a,b*).

Such warnings are echoed in refutationist philosophy. As Medawar (1979) put it: 'I cannot give any scientist of any age better advice than this: the intensity of the conviction that a hypothesis is true has no bearing on whether it is true or not'. We would only add that the intensity of a conviction that a hypothesis is false has no bearing on whether it is false or not.

Vigorous debate is a characteristic of modern scientific philosophy, no less in epidemiology than in other areas (Rothman 1988). Perhaps the most important common thread that emerges from the debated philosophies is Hume's legacy that proof is impossible in empirical science. This simple fact is particularly important to epidemiologists, who often face the criticism that proof is impossible in epidemiology, with the implication that it is possible in other scientific disciplines. Such criticism may stem from a belief by some that an experiment can somehow provide proof, whereas the non-experimental nature of much epidemiological work precludes definitive proof. Others hold the view that 'statistical' relations are only suggestive and believe that detailed study of mechanisms within single individuals can reveal cause–effect relations with certainty. Both of these views unfairly devalue epidemiological work.

Regarding the first view, the non-experimental nature of a science does not preclude impressive scientific understanding; presumably geologists and astronomers do not lose sleep over their inability to conduct double-blind randomized trials. Even when they are possible, randomized trials do not provide anything approaching proof—many have only fuelled controversies (Rothman 1985). As for the second view, it overlooks the fact that all relations are suggestive in exactly the manner discussed by Hume: even the most careful and detailed mechanistic dissection of individual events cannot provide more than associations, albeit at a finer level.

All of the fruits of scientific work, in epidemiology or other disciplines, are, at best, only tentative formulations of a description of nature, even when the work itself is carried out without mistakes. The tentativeness of our knowledge does not prevent practical applications, but it should keep us sceptical and critical, not only of everyone else's work, but our own as well.

Causal inference in epidemiology

Biological knowledge about epidemiological hypotheses is often scant, making the hypotheses themselves at times little more than vague statements of causal association between exposure and disease. These vague hypotheses have only vague consequences that can be tested, apart from a simple iteration of the observation. To cope with this vagueness, epidemiologists usually focus on testing the negation of the causal hypothesis, that is, the null hypothesis that the exposure does not have a causal relation to disease. Then, any observed association can potentially refute the hypothesis, subject to the assumption (auxiliary hypothesis) that biases are absent.

Nonetheless, if the causal mechanism is stated specifically enough, epidemiological observations can provide crucial tests of competing non-null causal hypotheses. For example, when toxic shock syndrome was first studied, there were two competing hypotheses about the origin of the toxin. Under one hypothesis, the toxin was a chemical in the tampon, so that women using tampons were exposed to the toxin directly from the tampon. Under the other hypothesis, the tampon acted as a culture medium for staphylococci that produced the toxin. Both hypotheses explained the relation of toxic shock occurrence to tampon use. The two hypotheses, however, lead to opposite predictions about the relation between the frequency of changing tampons and the risk of toxic shock. Under the hypothesis of a chemical intoxication, more frequent changing of the tampon would lead to more exposure to the toxin and possible absorption of a greater overall dose. This hypothesis predicted that women who changed tampons more frequently would have a higher risk than women who changed tampons infrequently. The culture-medium hypothesis predicts that the women who change tampons frequently would have a lower risk than those who leave the tampon in for longer periods, because a short duration of use for each tampon would prevent the staphylococci from multiplying enough to produce a damaging dose of toxin. Thus, epidemiological research examining how the risk of toxic shock relates to the frequency of tampon changing was able to refute one of these theories (the chemical theory was refuted).

Another example of a theory easily tested by epidemiological data related to the finding that women who took replacement oestrogen therapy were at a considerably higher risk of endometrial cancer. Horwitz and Feinstein (1978) conjectured a competing theory to explain the association: they proposed that women taking oestrogen experienced symptoms such as bleeding that induced them to consult a doctor. The resulting diagnostic work-up led to the detection of endometrial cancer in these women. Many epidemiological observations could have been and were used to evaluate these competing hypotheses. The causal theory predicted that the risk of endometrial cancer would tend to increase with increasing use (dose, frequency, and duration) of oestrogens, as for other carcinogenic exposures. Conversely, the detection bias theory predicted that women who had used oestrogens only for a short while would have the greatest risk, since the symptoms related to oestrogen use that led to the medical consultation tend to appear soon after use begins. Because the association of recent oestrogen use and endometrial cancer was the same in both long-term and short-term oestrogen users, the detection bias theory was refuted as an explanation for all but a small fraction of endometrial cancer cases occurring after oestrogen use. (Refutation of the detection bias theory also depended on many other observations. Particularly important was the theory's implication that there must be a large reservoir of undetected endometrial cancer in the typical population of women to account for the much greater rate observed in oestrogen users.)

The endometrial cancer example illustrates a critical point in understanding the process of causal inference in epidemiological studies: many of the hypotheses being evaluated in the interpretation of epidemiological studies are non-causal hypotheses, in the sense of involving no causal connection between the study exposure and the disease. For example, hypotheses that amount to explanations of how specific types of bias could have led to an association between exposure and disease are the usual alternatives to the primary study hypothesis that the epidemiologist needs to consider in drawing inferences. Much of the interpretation of epidemiological studies amounts to the testing of such non-causal explanations for observed associations.

Causal criteria

In practice, how do epidemiologists separate out the causal from the non-causal explanations? Despite philosophical criticisms of inductive inference, inductively oriented causal criteria have commonly been used to make such inferences. If a set of necessary and sufficient causal criteria could be used to distinguish causal from non-causal relations in epidemiological studies, the job of the scientist would be eased considerably. With such criteria, all the concerns about the logic or lack thereof in causal inference could be forgotten: it would only be necessary to consult the check-list of criteria to see if a relation were causal. We know from philosophy that such a set of criteria does not exist. Nevertheless, lists of causal criteria have become popular, possibly because they seem to provide a road map through complicated territory.

A commonly used set of criteria was proposed by Hill (1965); it was an expansion of a set of criteria offered previously in the landmark Surgeon General's report on smoking and health (US Department of Health, Education and Welfare 1964), which in turn were inspired by the inductive canons of Mill (1862). Hill suggested that the following aspects of an association be considered in attempting to distinguish causal from non-causal associations: strength, consistency, specificity, temporality, biological gradient, plausibility, coherence, experimental evidence, and analogy. The popular view that these criteria should be used for causal inference makes it necessary to examine them in detail.

Strength

For Hill and others, the strength of association refers to the magnitude of the ratio of incidence ('relative risk') or some analogous ratio measure. Hill's argument was essentially that strong associations are more likely to be causal than weak associations because, if they could be explained by some other factor, the effect of that factor would have to be even stronger than the observed association and therefore would have become evident. Conversely, weak associations are more likely to be explained by undetected biases. To some extent this is a reasonable argument, but, as Hill himself acknowledged, the fact that an association is weak does not rule out a causal connection. A commonly cited counter-example is the relation between cigarette smoking and cardiovascular disease: one explanation for this relation being weak is that cardiovascular disease is common, making any ratio measure of effect comparatively small compared with ratio measures for diseases that are less common (Rothman and Poole 1988). Nevertheless, cigarette smoking is not seriously doubted as a cause of cardiovascular disease. Another example would be passive smoking and lung cancer, a weak association that few consider to be non-causal.

Counter-examples of strong but non-causal associations are also not hard to find; any study with strong confounding illustrates the phenomenon. For example, consider the strong but non-causal relation between Down's syndrome and birth rank, which is confounded by the relation between Down's syndrome and maternal age. Of course, once the confounding factor is identified, the association is diminished by adjustment for the factor. These examples remind us that a large association is neither necessary nor sufficient for causality, nor is weakness necessary nor sufficient for the absence of causality. In addition to these counter-examples, we have to remember that neither relative risk nor any other measure of association is a biologically consistent feature of an association; rather it is a characteristic of a study population that depends on the relative prevalence of other causes. A strong association serves only to rule out hypotheses that the association is due to some weak unmeasured confounder or some other modest source of bias.

Consistency

Consistency refers to the repeated observation of an association in different populations under different circumstances. Lack of consistency, however, does not rule out a causal association, because some effects are produced by their causes only under unusual circumstances. More precisely, the effect of a causal agent cannot occur unless the complementary component causes act or have already acted to complete a sufficient cause. These conditions will not always be met. Thus, transfusions can cause HIV infection but they do not always do so: the virus must also be present. Tampon use can cause toxic shock syndrome, but only rarely when certain other, perhaps unknown, conditions are met. Consistency is apparent only after all the relevant details of a causal mechanism are understood, which is to say very seldom. Furthermore, even studies of exactly the same phenomena can be expected to differ in their results simply because they differ in their methodologies. Consistency serves only to rule out hypotheses that the association is attributable to some factor that varies across studies.

Specificity

The criterion of specificity requires that a cause lead to a single effect, not multiple effects. This argument has often been advanced to refute causal interpretations of exposures that appear to relate to myriad effects, in particular by those seeking to exonerate smoking as a cause of lung cancer. Unfortunately, the criterion is invalid.

Causes of a given effect cannot be expected to lack other effects on any logical grounds. In fact, everyday experience teaches us repeatedly that single events or conditions may have many effects. Smoking is an excellent example: it leads to many effects in the smoker. The existence of one effect does not detract from the possibility that another effect exists.

Furthermore, specific effects are as liable to be confounded as non-specific effects. Therefore, specificity for an exposure does not result in greater validity for any causal inference regarding the exposure. Hill's discussion of this criterion for inference is replete with reservations, but, even so, the criterion is useless and misleading.

Temporality

Temporality refers to the necessity that the cause precede the effect in time. This criterion is inarguable, in so far as any claimed observation of causation must involve the putative cause C preceding the putative effect D. It does not, however, follow that a reverse time order is evidence against the hypothesis that C can cause D. Rather, observations in which C followed D merely shows that C could not have caused D in these instances; they provide no evidence for or against the hypothesis that C can cause D in those instances in which it precedes D.

Biological gradient

Biological gradient refers to the presence of a monotonic (unidirectional) dose–response curve. We often expect such a monotonic relation to exist. For example, more smoking means more carcinogen exposure and more tissue damage and, hence, more opportunity for carcinogenesis. Some causal associations, however, show a single jump (threshold) rather than a monotonic trend; an example is the association between diethylstilboestrol and adenocarcinoma of the vagina. A possible explanation is that the doses of diethylstilboestrol that were administered were all sufficiently great to produce the maximum effect from diethylstilboestrol. Under this hypothesis, for all those exposed to diethylstilboestrol, the development of disease would depend entirely on other component causes.

The somewhat controversial topic of alcohol consumption and mortality is another example. Death rates are higher among non-drinkers than among moderate drinkers, but ascend to the highest levels for heavy drinkers. There is considerable debate about which parts of the J-shaped dose–response curve are causally related to alcohol consumption and which parts are non-causal artefacts stemming from confounding or other biases. Some studies appear to find only an increasing relation between alcohol consumption and mortality, possibly because the categories of alcohol consumption are too broad to distinguish different rates among moderate drinkers and non-drinkers.

Associations that do show a monotonic trend are not necessarily causal; confounding can result in a gradual relation between a non-causal risk factor and disease if the confounding factor itself demonstrates a biological gradient in its relation with disease. The non-causal relation between birth rank and Down's syndrome mentioned above shows a biological gradient that merely reflects the progressive relation between maternal age and Down's syndrome occurrence.

These issues imply that the existence of a monotonic association is neither necessary nor sufficient for a causal relation. A non-monotonic relation only refutes those causal hypotheses specific enough to predict a monotonic dose–response curve.

Plausibility

Plausibility refers to the biological plausibility of the hypothesis, an important concern but one that may be difficult to judge. Sartwell (1960), emphasizing this point, cited the remarks of Cheever, who was commenting on the aetiology of typhus before its mode of transmission (via body lice) was known.

> It could be no more ridiculous for the stranger who passed the night in the steerage of an emigrant ship to ascribe the typhus, which he there contracted, to the vermin with which bodies of the sick might be infested. An adequate cause, one reasonable in itself, must correct the coincidences of simple experience.

The point is that what was to Cheever an implausible explanation turned out to be the correct explanation, since it was indeed the vermin that caused the typhus infection. Such is the problem with plausibility: it is too often not based on logic or data, but only on prior beliefs.

The Bayesian approach to inference attempts to deal with this problem by requiring that one quantify, on a probability (0–1) scale, the certainty that one has in those prior beliefs, as well as in new hypotheses. This quantification displays the dogmatism or open-mindedness of the analyst in a public fashion, with certainty values near 1 or 0 betraying a strong commitment of the analyst for or against a hypothesis. It can also provide a means of testing those quantified beliefs against new evidence (Howson and Urbach 1989). Nevertheless, the Bayesian approach cannot transform plausibility into an objective causal criterion.

Coherence

Taken from the Surgeon General's report on smoking and health (US Department of Health, Education and Welfare 1964), the term coherence implies that a cause and effect interpretation for an association does not conflict with what is known of the natural history and biology of the disease. The examples Hill (1965) gave for coherence, such as the histopathological effect of smoking on the bronchial epithelium (in reference to the association between smoking and lung cancer) or the difference in lung cancer incidence by sex, could reasonably be considered examples of plausibility as well as coherence; the distinction appears to be a fine one. Hill emphasized that the absence of coherent information, as distinguished, apparently, from the presence of conflicting information, should not be taken as evidence against an association being considered causal. Consequently, at least according to Hill, coherence should not be a criterion for causal inference. Conversely, the presence of conflicting information may indeed refute a hypothesis, but one must always remember that the conflicting information may be mistaken or misinterpreted (Wald 1985).

Experimental evidence

It is not clear what Hill meant by experimental evidence. It might have referred to evidence from laboratory experiments on animals or to evidence from human experiments. Evidence from human experiments, however, is seldom available for most epidemiological research questions and animal evidence relates to different species and usually to levels of exposure very different from those experienced by humans. From Hill's examples, it seems that what he had in mind for experimental evidence was the result of removal of some harmful exposure in an intervention or prevention programme, rather than the results of formal experiments (Susser 1991). The lack of availability of such evidence would at least be a pragmatic difficulty in making this a criterion for inference. Logically, however, experimental evidence is not a criterion but a test of the causal hypothesis, a test that is simply unavailable in most circumstances. It is also not as decisive as often thought. For example, the hypothesis that malaria is caused by swamp gas can be tested by draining swamps to see if the malaria rates in local residents goes down. Indeed, the rates will drop, but not because swamp gas causes malaria.

Analogy

Whatever insight might be derived from analogy is handicapped by the inventive imagination of scientists who can find analogies everywhere. At best, analogy provides a source of more elaborate hypotheses about the associations under study; the absence of such analogies only reflects lack of imagination or experience, not the falsity of the hypothesis.

Conclusion

As is evident, these standards of epidemiological evidence offered by Hill to judge whether an association is causal are saddled with reservations and exceptions. Hill himself was ambivalent about the utility of these 'standards' (he did not use the word criteria in the paper). On the one hand, he asked 'in what circumstances can we pass from this observed *association* to a verdict of *causation*?' (Hill 1965, emphasis in original). Yet, despite speaking of verdicts on causation, he disagreed that any 'hard-and-fast rules of evidence' existed by which to judge causation: 'None of my nine viewpoints [criteria] can bring indisputable evidence for or against the cause-and-effect hypothesis and none can be required as a *sine qua non*' (Hill 1965).

Actually, the fourth viewpoint, temporality, is a *sine qua non* for causality: if the putative cause did not precede the effect, that indeed is indisputable evidence that the observed association is not causal (although this evidence does not rule out causality in other situations, for in other situations the putative cause may precede the effect). Other than this one condition, however, which may be viewed as part of the definition of causation, there is no necessary or sufficient criterion for determining whether an observed association is causal.

This conclusion accords with the views of Hume, Popper, and others that causal inferences cannot attain the certainty of logical deductions. Although some scientists continue to promulgate causal criteria as aids to inference (Susser 1991), others argue that it is actually detrimental to cloud the inferential process by considering check-list criteria (Lanes and Poole 1984). An intermediate refutationist approach seeks to alter the criteria into deductive tests of causal hypotheses (Maclure 1985; Weed 1986).

References

Bacon, F. (1620). *Novum organum*. Joannem Billium, London.

Bayes, T. (1763). An essay towards solving a problem in the doctrine of chances. *Philosophical Transactions of the Royal Society*, **53**, 370–418.

Cornfield, J. (1976). Recent methodological contributions to clinical trials. *American Journal of Epidemiology*, **104**, 408–24.

DeFinetti, B. (1937). Foresight: its logical laws, its subjective sources. Reprinted in *Studies in subjective probability* (ed. H.E. Kyburg and H.E. Smokler). Wiley, New York, 1964.

Doll, R. and Peto, R. (1981). *The causes of cancer*. Oxford University Press, New York.

Ephron, E. (1984). *The apocalyptics. Cancer and the big lie*. Simon and Schuster, New York.

Fraiberg, S. (1959). *The magic years*. Scribner's, New York.

Greenland, S. (1998*a*). Induction versus Popper: substance versus semantics. *International Journal of Epidemiology*, **27**, 543–8.

Greenland, S. (1998*b*). Probability logic and probabilistic induction. *Epidemiology*, **9**, 322–32.

Higginson, J. (1960). Population studies in cancer. *Acta Union Internationale Contra Cancrum*, **16**, 1667–70.

Higginson, J. (1980). Proportion of cancer due to occupation. *Preventive Medicine*, **9**, 180–8.

Hill, A.B. (1965). The environment and disease: association or causation? *Proceedings of the Royal Society of Medicine*, **58**, 295–300.

Hogben, L. (1933). *Nature and nurture*. Williams and Norgate, London.

Horwitz, R.I. and Feinstein, A.R. (1978). Alternative analytic methods for case–control studies of estrogens and endometrial cancer. *New England Journal of Medicine*, **299**, 1089–94.

Howson, C. and Urbach, P. (1989). *Scientific reasoning. The Bayesian approach*. Open Court, LaSalle, IL.

Hume D. (1739). *A treatise of human nature*. Oxford University Press edition, with an Analytical Index by L.A. Selby-Bigge, published 1888. Second edition with text revised and notes by P.H. Nidditch (1978).

Kahnemann, D., Slovic, P., and Tversky, A. (1982). *Judgment under uncertainty heuristics and biases*. Cambridge University Press, New York.

Kuhn, T.S. (1962). *The structure of scientific revolutions* (2nd edn). University of Chicago Press.

Kuhn, T.S. (1970). Reflections on my critics. In *Criticism and the growth of knowledge* (ed. I. Lakatos and A. Musgrave). Cambridge University Press.

Lakatos, I. (1970). Falsification and the methodology of scientific research programmes. In *Criticism and the growth of knowledge* (ed. I. Lakatos and A. Musgrave). Cambridge University Press.

Lanes, S.F. and Poole, C. (1984). 'Truth in packaging?' The unwrapping of epidemiologic research. *Journal of Occupational Medicine*, **26**, 571–4.

Maclure, M. (1985). Popperian refutation in epidemiology. *American Journal of Epidemiology*, **121**, 343–50.

MacMahon, B. (1968). Gene–environment interaction in human disease. *Journal of Psychiatric Research*, **6** (Supplement 1), 393–402.

Magee, B. (1985) *Philosophy and the real world. An introduction to Karl Popper*. Open Court, La Salle, IL.

Medawar, P.B. (1979). *Advice to a young scientist*. Basic Books, New York.

Mill, J.S. (1843). *A system of logic, ratiocinative and inductive*. Parker, Son and Bowin, London.

Piattelli-Palmarini, M. (1994). *Inevitable illusions*. Wiley, New York.

Platt, J.R. (1964). Strong inference. *Science*, **146**, 347–53.

Popper, K.R. (1968). *The logic of scientific discovery*. Harper and Row, New York.

Ramsey, F.P. (1931). Truth and probability. Reprinted in *Studies in subjective probability* (ed. H.E. Kyburg and H.E. Smokler). Wiley, New York, 1964.

Rothman, K.J. (1976). Causes. *American Journal of Epidemiology*, **104**, 587–92.

Rothman, K.J. (1981). Induction and latent periods. *American Journal of Epidemiology*, **114**, 253–9.

Rothman, K.J. (1985). Sleuthing in hospitals. *New England Journal of Medicine*, **313**, 258–60.

Rothman, K.J. (ed.) (1988). *Causal inference*. Epidemiology Resources, Boston, MA.

Rothman, K.J. and Poole, C. (1988). A strengthening programme for weak associations. *International Journal of Epidemiology*, **17** (Supplement), 955–9.

Russell, B. (1939). Dewey's new 'Logic'. In *The philosophy of John Dewey* (ed. P.A. Schlipp). Tudor, New York. Reprinted in *The basic writings of Bertrand Russell* (ed. R.E. Egner and L.E. Dennon). Simon and Schuster, New York, 1961.

Russell, B. (1945). *A history of Western philosophy*, Book III, Chapter XVII. Simon and Schuster, New York.

Sartwell, P. (1960). On the methodology of investigations of etiologic factors in chronic diseases—further comments. *Journal of Chronic Diseases*, **11**, 61–3.

Susser, M. (1991). What is a cause and how do we know one? A grammar for pragmatic epidemiology. *American Journal of Epidemiology*, **133**, 635–48.

US Department of Health, Education and Welfare (1964). *Smoking and health: report of the Advisory Committee to the Surgeon General of the Public Health Service*. US Government Printing Office, Washington, DC.

Wald, N.A. (1985). Smoking. In *Cancer risks and prevention* (ed. M.P. Vessey and M. Gray). Oxford University Press, New York.

Weed, D. (1986). On the logic of causal inference. *American Journal of Epidemiology*, **123**, 965–79.

6.12 Systematic reviews and meta-analysis

Matthias Egger, George Davey Smith, and Jonathan A. C. Sterne

The volume of data that needs to be considered by practitioners and researchers is constantly expanding. In many areas it has become impossible for the individual to read, critically evaluate, and synthesize the state of current knowledge, let alone keep updating this on a regular basis. Reviews have become essential tools for anybody who wants to keep up with the new evidence that is accumulating in his or her field of interest. Reviews are also required to identify areas where the available evidence is insufficient and further studies are required. However, since Mulrow (1987) and Oxman and Guyatt (1988) drew attention to the poor quality of conventional narrative reviews it has become clear these are an unreliable source of information. In response there has, in recent years, been increasing focus on formal methods of systematically reviewing studies, to produce explicitly formulated, reproducible, and up-to-date summaries of the effects of health-care interventions. This is illustrated by the sharp increase in the number of reviews that used formal methods to synthesize evidence (Fig. 1).

This chapter discusses terminology and scope, provides some historical background, and examines the potentials and pitfalls of systematic reviews and meta-analysis.

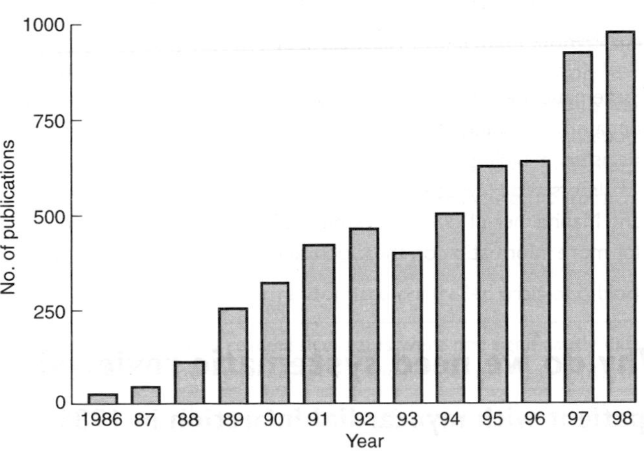

Fig. 1 Number of publications concerning systematic reviews and meta-analysis 1986 to 1998. Results from Medline search using text word and medical subject (MESH) heading 'meta-analysis' and text word 'systematic review'.

Systematic review, overview, or meta-analysis?

A number of terms are used concurrently to describe the process of systematically reviewing and integrating research evidence, including 'systematic review', 'meta-analysis', 'research synthesis', 'overview', and 'pooling'. Chalmers and Altman (1995) defined systematic review as a review that has been prepared using a systematic approach to minimizing biases and random errors which is documented in a materials and methods section. A systematic review may, or may not, include a meta-analysis, which is a statistical analysis of the results from independent studies, which generally aims to produce a single typical estimate of a treatment effect (Huque 1988). The distinction between systematic review and meta-analysis is important because it is always appropriate and desirable to review a body of data systematically, but it may sometimes be inappropriate, or even misleading, to pool results statistically from separate studies (O'Rourke and Detsky 1989).

The scope of meta-analysis

A clear distinction should be made between meta-analysis of randomized controlled trials and meta-analysis of epidemiological studies. Trials of high methodological quality that examined the same intervention in comparable patient groups will provide unbiased estimates of the underlying treatment effect and the variability between trials can confidently be attributed to random variation. Meta-analysis of these trials will provide an equally unbiased estimate of the treatment effect, with an increase in the precision of this estimate. A fundamentally different situation arises in the case of epidemiological studies. As discussed in detail below, due to the effects of confounding and bias, observational studies may produce estimates of associations that deviate from the truth beyond what can be attributed to chance. Combining a set of epidemiological studies will thus often provide spuriously precise, biased estimates of associations. Davis (1992) has written:

Meta-analysis begins with scientific studies, usually performed by academics or government agencies, and sometimes incomplete or disputed. The data from the studies are then run through computer models of bewildering complexity, which produce results of implausible precision.

While systematic reviews have clear advantages over conventional reviews, it is crucial to understand the limitations of meta-analysis and

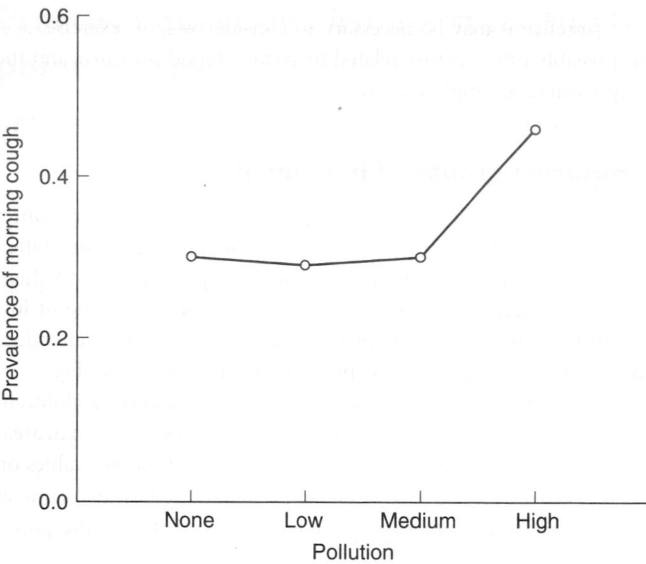

Fig. 6 Prevalence of morning cough in children against pollution level (simulated data).

would be seen if the populations of all such children exposed to these pollution levels could be observed? In other words, is the equivalent population line horizontal?

Information on parents' smoking habits will give a plot of two lines (Fig. 7). There are now several questions.

1. Are the differences between the pollution level groups in the population the same in the two parental smoking groups? That is, are the population lines parallel to each other?
2. Are the population differences between the pollution groups non-zero in either parental smoking group? That is, is either population line non-horizontal?

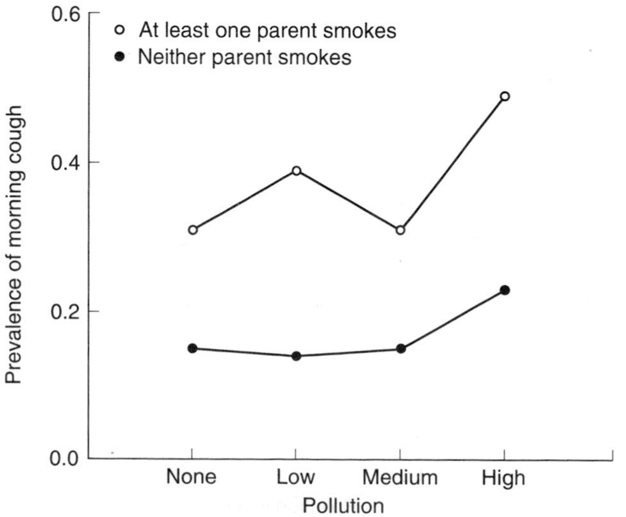

Fig. 7 Prevalence of morning cough in children against pollution level by parents' cigarette smoking habits (simulated data).

3. At a fixed pollution level is there a difference between the parental smoking groups in the population? That is, is there a vertical separation between the population lines?

Proportions: case–control studies

In a study of sudden infant death syndrome various information was collected on all the infants dying in this way in a particular area and period of time—these were the cases. The same information was collected on the same number of randomly selected control children born in the same period and still alive. Such studies are known as case–control or retrospective studies. The latter name arises because the study starts after the event of interest and consists of looking back in time at what preceded the event. The data are given in Table 1.

The question here is: Does the risk of sudden infant death change with the age of the mother? It is not possible to obtain a direct estimate of this risk, which is that of an infant becoming a case (risk = number of cases/number at risk), because the number at risk is not known. However, with some assumptions—mainly that the sampling fraction for the controls (the proportion that the sample is of the population) is the same for all the age groups—it is possible to manage without it. A proxy measure, the proportion P = cases/(cases + controls), is constructed and used to investigate the patterns in the data. These proportions are given in the last row of Table 1. When these proportions are plotted against the midpoint of the mothers' age group (Fig. 8), they show a slightly negative trend with increasing maternal age.

If the controls are known to be 1 per cent of all possible controls (i.e. a sampling fraction of 0.01), the usual estimates of risk would be

$$\frac{17}{17+900} \quad \frac{22}{22+2300} \quad \frac{17}{17+1600} \quad \frac{5}{5+1300}$$

or

$$0.0185 \quad 0.0095 \quad 0.0105 \quad 0.0038.$$

These are much smaller than the proportions but, when plotted, give a line with practically the same shape. The question then becomes: Does the line deviate from the horizontal more than could easily arise by chance if the equivalent population line is horizontal?

Three or more categories of outcome

A study of illness behaviour in women used, as a measure of depression, the number of positive responses to questions on loss of

Table 1 Cases of sudden infant death and controls by mother's age

	Mother's age (years)			
	< 20	**20–**	**25–**	**30+**
Cases	17	22	17	5
Controls	9	23	16	13
Cases and controls	26	45	33	18
P	0.65	0.49	0.52	0.28

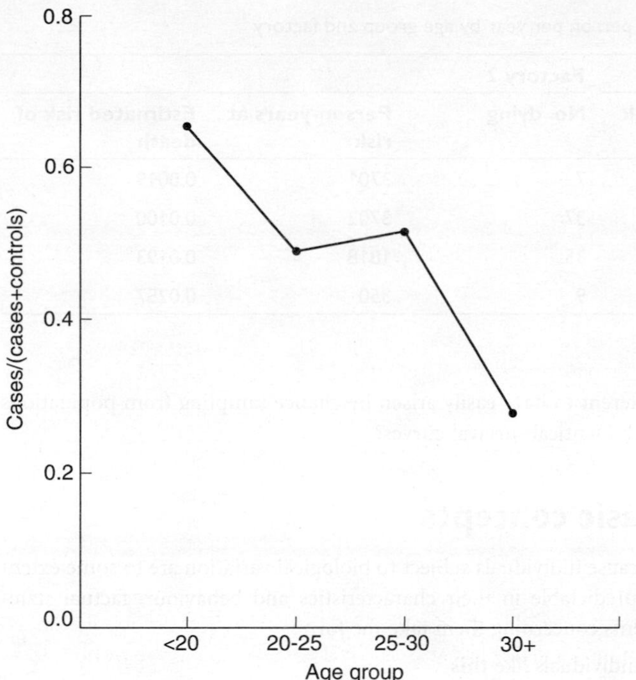

Fig. 8 Cases of sudden infant death as proportions (cases/(cases + controls)) by mother's age group.

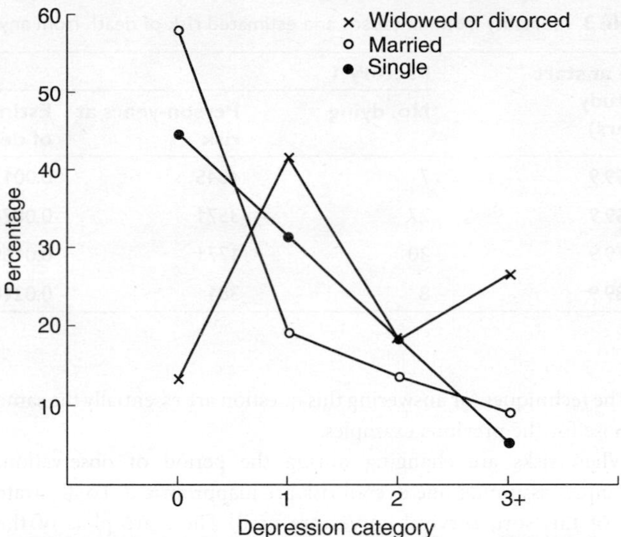

Fig. 9 Percentage of women in each marital status group plotted against depression category.

appetite, 'nerves', depression or irritability, sleeplessness, and undue tiredness. The numbers in the various depression categories and their marital states are given in Table 2. The question is: Does the pattern of depression in women differ according to their marital status?

Statistically, as a deduction from the sample to the population, the question becomes: Is the proportional distribution among the depression categories in the population of all such women the same for each marital status? That is, are the 38 single women distributed among the depression categories in the same proportions, apart from differences that could arise from sampling variation, as the 88 married and the 60 widowed or divorced women? The proportional allocation can be seen more easily if the frequencies are expressed as percentages of the total in that particular marital status group (Table 2).

Figure 9 gives a plot of the percentage frequencies as a separate line for each marital status group. If the proportional allocation to the depression categories were the same, these lines would fall on top of one another. Therefore the question becomes: Are these lines, obtained from a sample, more different than could easily arise by chance if the three equivalent population lines are really identical?

Table 2 Classification of women by marital status and answers to questions related to depression

Marital status	No. of positive responses (%)				
	0	1	2	3 or 4	Total
Single	17 (45)	12 (32)	7 (18)	2 (5)	38 (100)
Married	51 (58)	17 (19)	12 (14)	8 (9)	88 (100)
Widowed or divorced	8 (13)	25 (42)	11 (18)	16 (27)	60 (100)

Survival data

This general title is used to cover data that arise when the interest is in the risk of some event occurring. The event may be death, but it need not be, and survival data techniques are appropriate for comparing the chances of remission for patients on different treatments and other such events.

The first example considered annual mortality in relatively large groups of people. The usual analyses for data of this type assume that all subjects were at risk of the event for the whole of a specified period. However, if someone is lost to observation halfway through the year they have been at risk, as far as the study is concerned, for only half a year. With large numbers and small risks the numbers observed for only part of a period are small, and ignoring the problem does little harm. When the numbers in the groups to be compared are relatively small, the times at risk must be taken into account.

If it can be assumed that, within each group of subjects to be compared, each individual is running the same risk throughout the chosen time period, this is relatively straightforward. The periods of time for which each individual was observed are summed over all the individuals in the group. If the period of time is a year and the times at risk are expressed as fractions of a year, this gives the number of 'person-years at risk' (obviously it may at other times be necessary to use 'woman-years at risk', 'patient-weeks at risk', and so on).

Then the estimate of the annual risk of death (or other event) is simply the ratio of the number of deaths to the number of person-years at risk.

In an occupational health study of cancer, groups of current and ex-workers in two industrial environments were observed for a number of years. The overall mortality is given in Table 3. The initial question is: Is the risk of death from any cause different in the two environments? The estimated risks per person per year are given in Table 3, and Fig. 10 shows the estimated risks plotted against age. The question becomes: Are these lines surprisingly far apart if the equivalent lines in the population represented by this sample of individuals are identical?

Table 3 Mortality from all causes and estimated risk of death from any case per person per year by age group and factory

Age at start of study (years)	Factory 1			Factory 2		
	No. dying	Person-years at risk	Estimated risk of death	No. dying	Person-years at risk	Estimated risk of death
50–59.9	7	4045	0.0017	7	3701	0.0019
60–69.9	27	3571	0.0076	37	3702	0.0100
70–79.9	30	1771	0.0169	35	1818	0.0193
80–89.9	8	381	0.0210	9	350	0.0257

The techniques for answering this question are essentially the same as those for the previous examples.

When risks are changing during the period of observation, techniques assuming one overall risk are inappropriate. To illustrate data of this sort, survival curves are used. These are plots of the percentage in a group still surviving against time elapsed since some defined starting point such as date of entry to the study.

Data of this type arose from a clinical trial comparing radiotherapy with hormone treatment for cancer of the prostate. The question was: Which is the better treatment?

This is not a simple question. The treatment giving the greater chance of survival at 5 years, for example, is not necessarily the treatment that gives the longest life expectancy. It is necessary to look at the relative shapes of the survival curves. During the trial 44 patients received radiotherapy and 48 received hormone treatment. The survival curves for the two groups are shown in Fig. 11.

There is some divergence of the curves and the primary question becomes: Do the curves for the population represented by these samples differ? Or in other words: Are these sample curves too different to have easily arisen by chance sampling from populations with identical survival curves?

Basic concepts

Because individuals subject to biological variation are to some extent unpredictable in their characteristics and behaviour, factual statements concerning them take the form:

- individuals like **this**
- treated like **this**
- tend to respond like **this**.

The **individuals** are the items being observed. They may be patients, tissue samples, rats, or geographical areas. They may even be the same patient observed at different times, for example when a sequence of separate blood samples is taken or results are obtained from a repeatedly administered psychiatric test.

The **individuals like this** make up the population in the statistical sense (i.e. any strictly defined group of individuals). The human

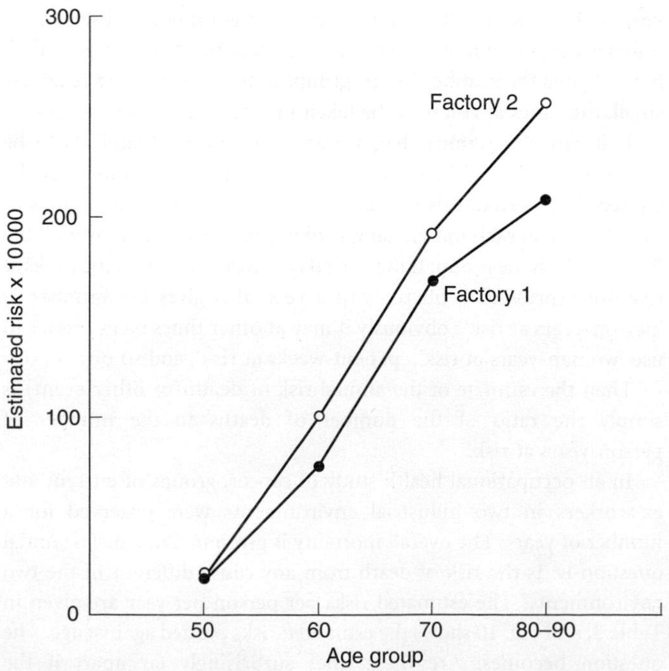

Fig. 10 Estimated risks of death against age by factory.

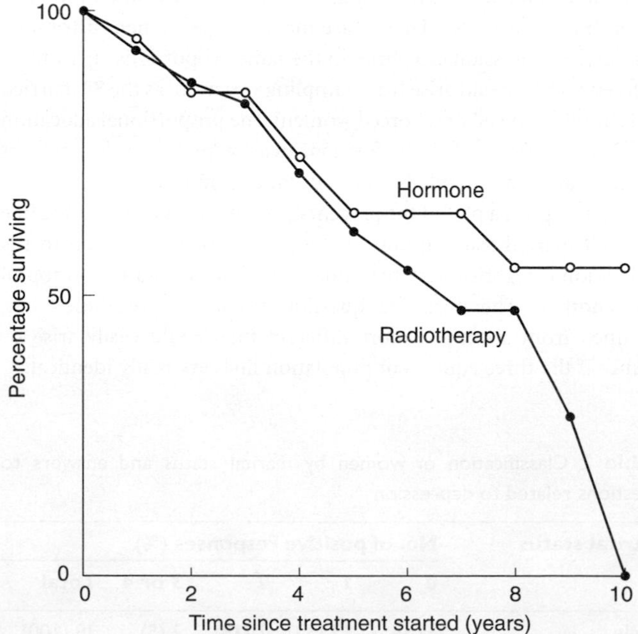

Fig. 11 Survival curves for patients with cancer of the prostate receiving radiotherapy or hormone treatment.

population of a country may be the statistical population of interest, but it will usually be a sample of the general population of all such humans who might exist now or in the future. Researchers in London, United Kingdom, will want to be able to generalize their findings beyond Londoners and will generally wish to conclude that the results apply to all such patients in the United Kingdom now and possibly in the future.

The population should be defined before the study begins, and the sample to represent it chosen accordingly. However, practical circumstances can have a considerable effect on the sampling. This makes it necessary for the researcher to indicate how, and with what qualifications, results from a sample apply to a particular population. In addition, most studies will involve individuals from identifiable subpopulations. For example, studies involving physical characteristics such as lung function which may differ systematically between the sexes require that results are obtained separately for the two samples representing the subpopulations male and female. If that is not done, and the findings in the two samples not shown to be consistent, it is not safe to combine all the data to arrive at a general conclusion.

This implies that if there are two subpopulations which may differ in respects important to the study in question, data must be collected to identify from which subpopulation each individual arose. These subpopulation-defining characteristics or variables (such as sex, age, social class, etc.) are often a nuisance. For example, it is not usually necessary to study how the sexes differ—this is mostly known. It is necessary only in order to confirm that the effects of interest are consistently found in all the subpopulations. If this can be assumed at the beginning, studies can be simplified by restricting them to one sex or one age group, for example, a simplifying option that is always worth considering at the design stage. Generally, however, data must be collected on individuals from a number of subpopulations.

Clinical trials are studies of subjects who have been 'treated' in some way which must be defined and possibly measured, for example as a dose. In most trials two or more groups receiving different treatments will be compared, and so the treatment, type, or dosage may vary from one individual to another. Therefore the treatment is a variable and will be represented in the data collected during the trial by numerical values identifying the type of treatment and/or the dosage.

Observational studies of naturally occurring 'experiments' may be concerned with assessing the effect on individuals of some experience, or exposure to some aspect of the environment. As for a treatment, it is necessary to define and measure the experience or exposure. Again, it must be represented by a variable with numerical values.

To assess the manner in which individuals tend to respond to being treated in some way or undergoing some experience, a variable is required to measure or classify the response. This is the response or outcome variable. Furthermore, because they will vary in a random way even in a homogeneous population in which all are treated identically, these variables are known as random variables. The way in which they vary is described by the distribution of their values in the sample and by inference in the populations.

Univariate, multivariate, and multivariable methods

In *A Dictionary of Statistical Terms* (Marriott 1990) a **variate** is defined to be a 'variable with an associated probability distribution'. This means that only the outcome or y variables are variates since the explanatory or x variables in regression modelling are assumed to be error free by the mathematics even if errors in the x variables are taken into account in the interpretation of the results. That means that any method concerned with a single y variable is univariate even if there are many x variables, as in multilinear regression.

Tukey proposed the term **multivariable** for statistical methods which involved several explanatory or x variables and one outcome variable (the single variate) and where appropriate this is the terminology that will be used here although all the methods covered in this chapter are univariate.

Types of variables

The choice of which analytical approach to use largely depends on the nature of the response variable. There are two main categories—quantitative and qualitative.

Quantitative variables have an obvious associated scale on which distances have a clear interpretation. They can arise in two forms—continuous or discrete. Continuous variables are generally measurements and every value within some sensible range is possible (e.g. serum cholesterol or peak expiratory flow rate). Discrete variables are generally counts where only certain values on the scale are possible (e.g. number of previous heart attacks or number of schistosome eggs in a stool sample).

Qualitative variables are associated with a set of categories. The categories may have a natural ordering as in severity of a condition, category of remission, social class, etc. These are known as ordinal variables and, although they have to be treated as categories, they are usually interpretable as sections of an underlying scale. Categories such as blood group and type of health services contact do not have an order and are termed nominal variables.

Functions of variables

The function of response variables is clear. They provide the yardstick by which the effects of treatment or experience are measured. However, variables are also used to identify the subpopulation to which an individual belongs so that an analysis can assess and allow for differences between subpopulations. They are also used to measure or classify treatment or experience.

There is no obvious general term for these last two classes of variable. They are sometimes called predictor variables because studies are often concerned with how well they predict outcome or response. They may also be referred to as independent or explanatory variables because the analysis is essentially assessing how variations in response or outcome depends or can be explained by differences in their values. The response variable is often referred to as the dependent variable.

Perhaps the simplest terminology of all, following mathematical convention, classes the treatment, exposure, and subpopulation variables, all of which tend to appear on the horizontal axis of graphical plots, as x variables. The response variables generally appear on the vertical axis of such plots and are known as y variables.

Describing data patterns—models

A model, in the statistical sense, is simply an algebraic formula for describing some pattern or structure in variable data. Consider the

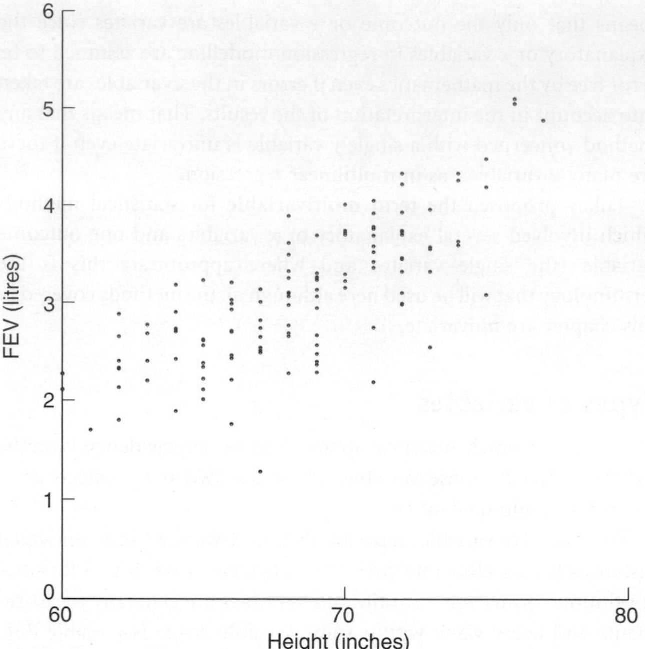

Fig. 12 Forced expiratory volume FEV (l/min) in young adults versus height in inches.

relationship between forced expiratory volume (**FEV**) and height in a sample of students (Fig. 12). There is a tendency for the taller individuals to have larger FEV values. If the individuals are grouped on the height scale (e.g. all individuals with heights between 62 and 64 inches are treated as if they were 63 inches, those between 65 and 67 inched as if they were 66 inches, etc.), the plot becomes a set of separate groups of points (Fig. 13).

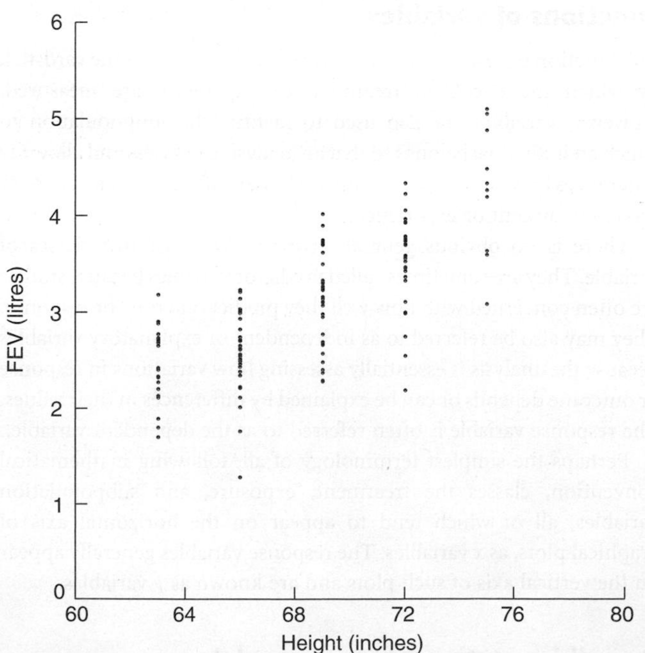

Fig. 13 Forced expiratory volume FEV (l/min) in young adults versus height groups.

There is an array or distribution of FEV values for each height group. These are known as conditional distributions. They are the distributions of FEV values conditional on the individuals concerned all having the same height (or in this case being in the same height group). It can now be seen that the trend in FEV values is a systematic tendency for these conditional distributions to move up as height increases. The distributions overlap, but their centres are located at a generally higher position in the taller height groups. It is not easy to describe the behaviour of the individual points, but it is possible to be reasonably precise about the relative positioning or location of the conditional distributions. The models to describe this sort of pattern have the form

location of distribution = reference value + horizontal position effect.

The behaviour of individual points has to be described in terms of the location of their particular distribution and the way in which they are dispersed or spread about the location. In Fig. 13 the data were grouped to show the conditional distributions, but this is wasteful of information. Some method is needed to describe the trend in the raw data.

The simplest model is a straight-line trend. This model assumes that the height or x variable effect is a steady increase (or decrease) in the FEV or y variable distribution locations, usually represented by the arithmetic mean defined below. That is, for each unit change in height there is the same change in mean FEV at all points on the height axis. The model for this is

mean FEV = reference value + (change/unit height) × height.

This is known as a regression line model. In more general terms it becomes

$$y = a + bx$$

which is the equation representing a straight line on a plot of y against x (in this case FEV against height). This is shown diagrammatically in Fig. 14 where a, which is the height of the line when $x = 0$, is known as the intercept and b, the slope of the line, is called the regression coefficient. FEV at zero height makes no practical sense but it makes the algebra simpler to represent the regression line by

FEV = intercept + b × height.

Finding the 'best' straight line to describe a trend means estimating the appropriate intercept and slope; this is known as fitting the regression line. In theory, any values of a and b are possible, and so the possibilities are infinite. The problem is to define what is the 'best' line to describe a set of data and then to deduce the values of a and b that give this 'best' line as functions of the data values.

In practice the 'best' fitting line is defined by the **principle of least squares.** This principle can be illustrated by considering a general line on a scatter diagram with a and b unspecified (Fig. 15). Each point deviates from the line (in the y direction) by some amount. The principle of least squares states that the 'best' line is the one that makes the 'sum of all the deviations squared' as small as possible. This means that a and b must be chosen to make the sum of all d^2 a minimum. Using this principle it is possible mathematically to deduce standard formulae which can be used to calculate the appropriate a and b for any set of data.

Before we discuss further how models are defined and used, it is necessary to consider how to define and measure the important

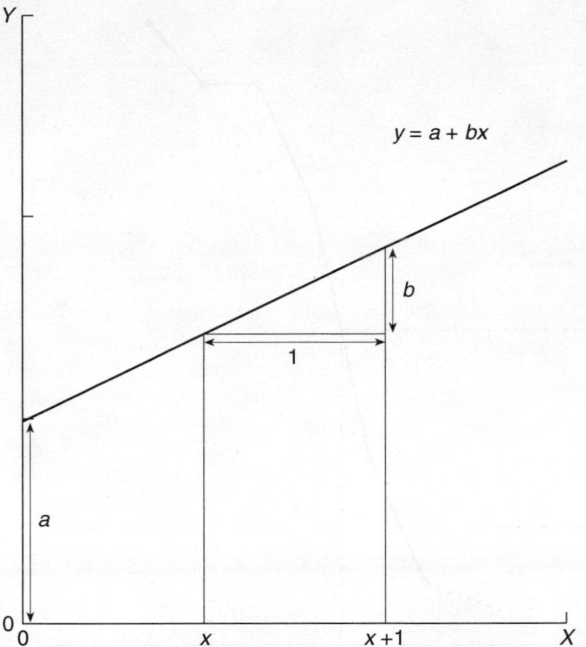

Fig. 14 Diagrammatic representation of the straight-line regression model $y = a + bx$.

characteristics of the distributions whose relative positioning they are used to describe and test.

The characteristics of distributions

The characteristics of the distributions represented by the arrays of points in Fig. 13 are not at all clear. Their location can be judged to some extent, but how the individuals are dispersed about the central

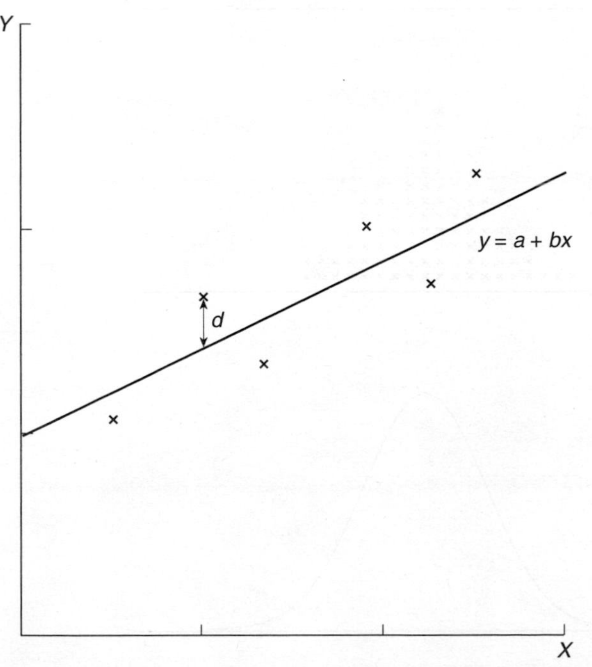

Fig. 15 Deviations of data points from the model $y = a + bx$.

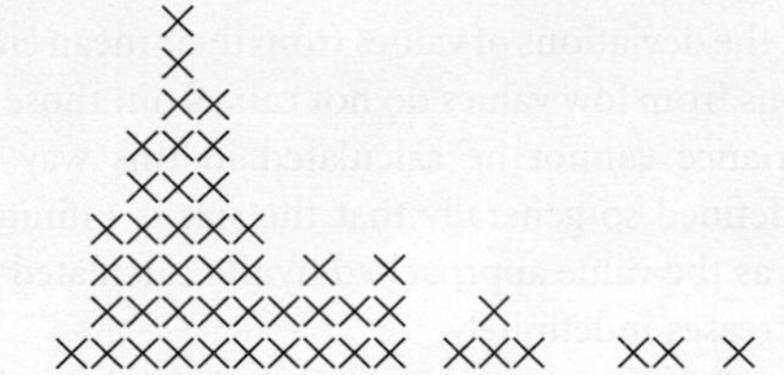

Fig. 16 Representing a sample of values as a histogram.

location cannot be seen so easily. Single distributions are better displayed as histograms.

To represent a sample as a histogram the scale is divided into intervals of equal length and the points within an interval are drawn on top of one another as shown in Fig. 16. Points falling where two intervals join could go in either, but for graphical techniques it does not really matter. Usually they are allocated to the higher interval.

The shape is somewhat 'ragged' but one can see, in addition to its location and spread, that the distribution is rather asymmetrical. There is a longer 'tail' on the high-value or positive side. Such distributions are called **skew**, and since skewness can affect the analysis some method is needed to detect and measure it. There are specific measures of skewness, but they are rarely necessary in practice. Graphical techniques are usually adequate to detect whether it is present to an extent that matters. Conversely, location and dispersion require precise measures and on occasion a complete numerical specification of the distribution is required, for which centiles are used.

Measures of location

There are three commonly used measures of location: the arithmetic mean, the median, and the mode.

The **arithmetic mean** is the sum of all the values in a distribution or a sample divided by the number of values. It is by far the most useful measure of location and is usually referred to simply as the mean. For a sample it is

mean = sum of all values/number of values.

The **median** is the variable value such that half of the values in a distribution are above it and half are below. It is easy to find and useful for simple descriptions of asymmetrical distributions. However, it is not very easy to handle in more complex analyses.

The **mode** is the value in a distribution which occurs most frequently. It is of occasional use for describing single distributions.

Measures of dispersion

There are a multitude of measures of dispersion in the literature, but only a few are commonly used.

The **range** is the distance, on the scale of measurement, between the highest and lowest values. It is occasionally used for describing the spread of small samples. Obviously, as sample sizes increase, the range will automatically increase and, since it depends on the least characteristic pair of individuals in the sample, its usefulness is limited.

The **variance** is a direct measure of spread about the arithmetic mean. For a sample it is defined as

$$\frac{\text{sum for all values of (value} - \text{mean value)}^2}{\text{number of values} - 1}$$

Notice that 'squaring' the deviations of values from their mean ensures that negative deviations from low values do not cancel out those from high values. The variance cannot be calculated in this way for a population (usually defined so generally that the size is infinite). In this case, it is defined as the value approached by the calculated value as the sample size increases indefinitely.

Because the variance is an average squared deviation it is not in the original units of the variable in question. For this reason its square root, the **standard deviation (SD)**, is frequently more useful. This gives quite an accurate measure of how far from the mean individuals are likely to occur in a given distribution. Unless a distribution is very asymmetrical, individuals more than 3 SDs from the mean will occur only very rarely; most individuals (approximately 95 per cent) will fall within 2 SDs of the mean.

Centiles

Centiles are points on the variable scale that exceed a specified percentage of the distribution. Consider a sample of 10 systolic blood pressure values with the distribution shown in Table 4. Ten per cent (one value) of the sample is below 110 mmHg and therefore that is the 10th centile. Seven values (70 per cent) are below 130 mmHg and so that is the 70th centile, and so on. However, this approach only gives the centiles that occur at the ends of the intervals. Considering the sample as a representative of a much larger population, it is possible to go a little further by plotting the cumulative frequency, as a percentage, against the upper ends of the intervals (Fig. 17). It is far from smooth, but various centiles can be deduced by estimating where the 'curve' reaches the equivalent height on the per cent cumulative frequency scale. This method estimates the 50th centile, which is the median, as 125 mmHg. For more precise estimates a smooth curve could be drawn through the points. Alternatively, assumptions about the shape of the population curve can be made and the appropriate estimates deduced mathematically. To understand this process it is necessary to consider in detail how sample distributions and their characteristics relate to those of the population.

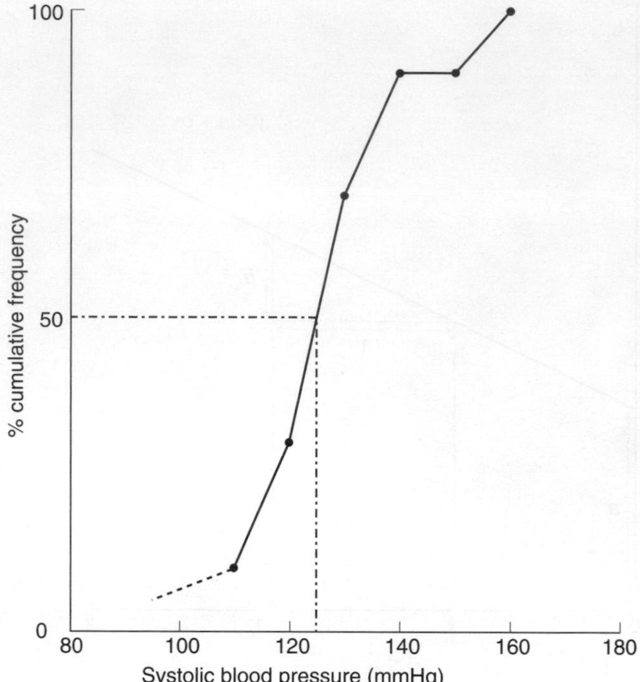

Fig. 17 Cumulative frequency plot of a sample of systolic blood pressure values.

Inferring the truth—sample to population

Distributions

Consider a sequence of histograms obtained from larger and larger samples of an infinite population (Fig. 18). As the sample size increases, the distribution becomes smoother with a more clearly defined shape. As the sample size is increased indefinitely (with the vertical scale reduced appropriately), the shape tends to a smooth curve. For many biological variables this will be close to a symmetrical 'bell-shaped' distribution known as the normal distribution, which can be defined in precise mathematical terms.

Table 4 Frequency distribution of a sample of 10 adult males according to their systolic blood pressures

Systolic blood pressure (mmHg)	Frequency of values	Cumulative total
From 100 to just under 110	1	1
From 110 to just under 120	2	3
From 120 to just under 130	4	7
From 130 to just under 140	2	9
From 140 to just under 150	0	9
From 150 to just under 160	1	10

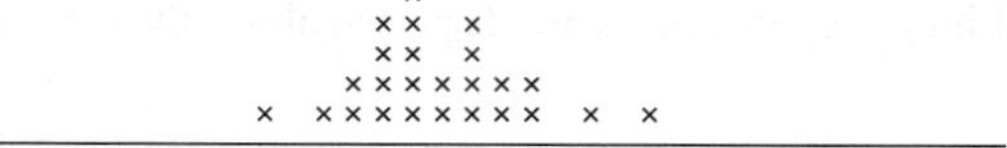

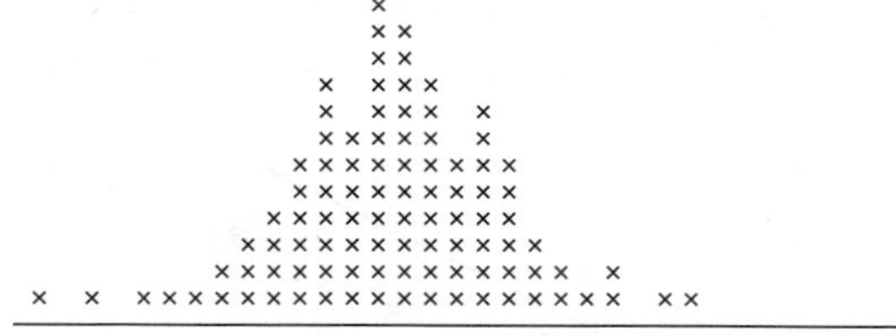

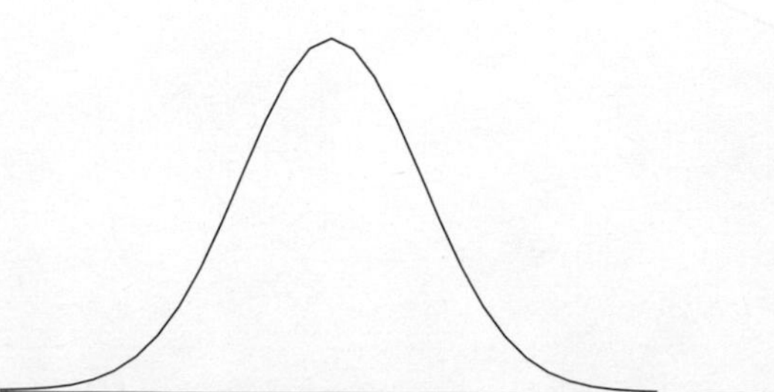

Fig. 18 Histograms from samples of increasing size approaching a smooth population curve.

Probabilities

In the sample of 10 systolic blood pressures (Table 4), two out of ten were in the range 110 to 120 mmHg. Therefore the proportion of the sample between 110 and 120 mmHg is 2/10 = 0.2. If the names of the 10 individuals were written on pieces of paper which were mixed up in a hat, and then one was picked at random, the probability that it was an individual in the range 110 to 120 would be 2/10 (0.2). There are two of the sort required and ten in total.

The probability of selecting an individual with a systolic blood pressure less than 100 mmHg from this 'hat' is 0/10, i.e. zero or impossible. The probability selecting an individual with a pressure less than 180 mmHg is 10/10, i.e. 1.0 or certain. Notice that 120 is the 30th centile and the probability of an individual below 120 is 0.3 or 30 per cent. The probability of an individual below the 15th centile is 0.15 or 15 per cent, and so on.

From the probability of selecting an individual below a particular point it is possible to deduce the probability of an individual on or above that point. Three of the ten individuals are below 120, which gives the probability of such an individual as 0.3. Seven of the ten are greater than or equal to 120, i.e. a probability of 0.7. Thus probability (value $\geqslant$ 120) is

$$\frac{\text{number} \geqslant 120}{\text{total number}} = \frac{10 - (\text{number} < 12)}{\text{total number}} = \frac{10-3}{10}$$

$= 7/10$ or $(10 - 3)/10$.

The probability of an individual being greater than or equal to some value is 1 minus the probability of being less than that value:

$p(\text{value} \geqslant 120) = 1 - p(\text{value} < 120)$.

For example

$p(< 110) = 1/10 = 0.1,$

$p(\geqslant 110) = 9/10 = 1 - p(< 110) = 0.9,$

and so on.

As sample sizes increase and the histogram approaches the smooth population curve, the numbers become indefinitely large. However, the area above an interval and beneath the curve is in the same ratio to the total areas as the number in that interval to the total number. In practice, population distributions are scaled so the curve encloses an area exactly equal to unity. This means that the area above any interval is the proportion of individuals with values in that interval. This in turn is the probability that an individual picked at random has a value in that particular interval. Therefore, if the area of the population distribution between the two values 110 and 120 is 0.15, the population having a systolic blood pressure between 110 and 120 is 0.15 (Fig. 19).

The probability that an individual selected at random has a value greater than 150 is the area A under the curve from 150 upwards. Since $A = 0.1$, this means that 10 per cent of the population will have systolic blood pressures of 150 or above.

The area below 150 is $1 - A$, so that the probability of an individual below 150 is $1 - A = 0.9$. This means that the remaining 90 per cent of individuals have systolic blood pressures below 150. Consequently 150 is the 90th centile of the population distribution.

The centiles of the population can be obtained as long as there is some way of obtaining the areas under the population distribution

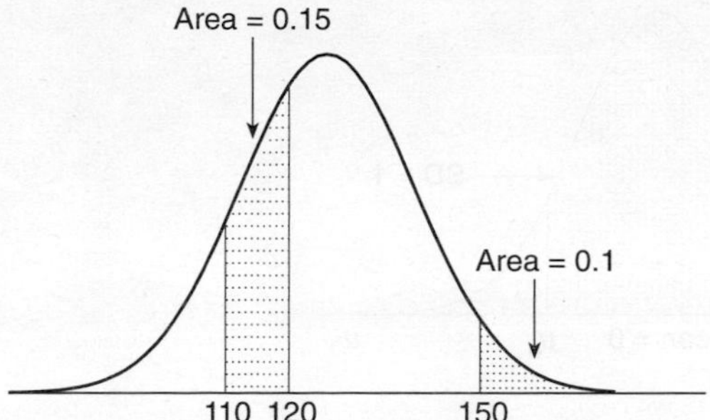

Fig. 19 Areas of the population distribution as probabilities.

curve. If we represent the 10th centile of the variable y as $y_{0.1}$ the area below $y_{0.1}$ is 0.1, the area below $y_{0.2}$ is 0.2, and so on.

The normal distribution

For various reasons random variables that appear to follow a normal distribution are common in nature—for example, human height, haemoglobin levels, systolic blood pressure, etc. Others can be made to follow a normal distribution by a transformation of their scale. Possibly even more important is the fact that, for all but the smallest samples, averages are themselves random variables from approximately normal distributions whatever the distributions of the original values. Because of this and its amiable mathematical nature, the normal distribution holds a central place in statistical theory and practice.

The theoretical normal distribution is completely specified by its mean and variance. The distribution is symmetrical about the mean and areas beneath the curve can be obtained mathematically. For example, it is known that if the variable is y, the 2.5th centile is

$y_{0.025} = \text{mean} - 1.96 \text{ SD}.$

This implies that in a normal distribution only 2.5 per cent of the individuals will be more than 1.96 SDs below the mean. Similarly, only 2.5 per cent will be more than 1.96 SDs above it. Combining these, it further implies that the range of values

mean − 1.96 SD to mean + 1.96 SD

will include 95 per cent of individuals in the population and exclude only 5 per cent.

The normal distribution is so useful that the percentage cumulative frequencies for the standard distribution, which has a mean of zero and variance of unity, have been widely tabulated (Lindley and Miller 1964) and are easily calculated with most statistical software (e.g. Minitab, Stata, GLIM, and Excel). The equivalent values for a normal variable with any mean and variance can be deduced from these.

The tabulated values are the areas under the mathematically defined population distribution curve below the given values of the standard normal variable u, say, as in Fig. 20. The area P_0 in Fig. 20 is the percentage cumulative frequency at u_0 which is the probability of a value below u_0, i.e.

$p(\text{value} < u_0) = P_0.$

The probability of a value at or above u_0 is

$p(\text{value} < u_0) = 1 - P_0$

and the probability of a value between u_0 and u_1 is

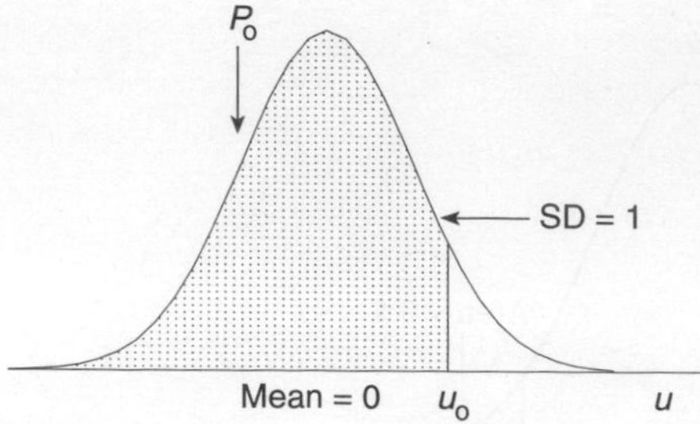

Fig. 20 Probabilities and the standardized normal distribution curve.

$p(u_0 < \text{value} < u_1) = P_1 - P_0$

where P_1 is the area under the curve below u_1.

The variable u is effectively the number of SDs that a value is from the mean. Equivalent probabilities for variables with a different mean and variance are deduced by calculating how many SDs each value is from its mean and treating these as values of u.

For example, suppose that systolic blood pressure in adult males is normally distributed with mean 130 and SD 1.5 to calculate the probability of an individual value less than 160 mmHg, note that it is 30 mmHg (i.e.2 SDs) above the mean. This implies that

$p(\text{value} < 160) = p(u < 2).$

Since from tables

$p(u < 2) = 0.977,$

it can be deduced that

$p(\text{value} < 160) = 0.977$

and the required probability is 97.7 per cent. These techniques allow the probabilities of individual sample values to be deduced if the population distribution is known.

However, the problem is really in the opposite direction. The need is to deduce the population characteristics from the sample values. A method is required to assess how close sample values such as the mean are to the unknown population equivalents. This is done by considering how the values of a sample estimate might vary if further samples were taken from the same population. Each sample will differ and estimates from them will vary.

Estimation and sampling distributions

It is simplest to start by considering how the sample mean varies in a sequence of samples all taken the same way from the same population. The result can be generalized to any estimate (e.g. a regression coefficient, a difference between means, etc.) calculated from a sample. Suppose that a sequence of samples of four values ($n = 4$) is taken from the systolic blood pressure (SBP) distribution and the mean is calculated for each. These sample means will themselves have a distribution which, because it can only arise as a result of repeated sampling, is known as a **sampling distribution**. In this distribution of means, samples with all values at one extreme of the population distribution will be rare. As a result the sample means will be more tightly clustered about the population mean than are the individual observations. In addition, as long as the sampling was properly random, the mean of the sampling distribution will be the same as the population mean. Because of this, the sample mean is said to be an unbiased estimate of the population mean. It can be shown that if the sampling is repeated indefinitely, the sampling distribution of the mean will tend to a smooth curve with the same mean as the population of individual values but a smaller standard deviation. In fact, it can be shown mathematically that this standard deviation of the mean is

$$\text{SD (mean SBP)} = \frac{\text{SD(SBP)}}{\sqrt{(\text{sample size } n)}}.$$

Therefore for samples of size 4 and SD = 15,

$\text{SD (mean SBP)} = 15/\sqrt{4} = 15/2 = 7.5$

and the spread of the sampling distribution for this mean is half the spread of the population distribution of the individual systolic blood pressure values.

It should be remembered that the complete sampling distribution exists only in theory. In practice there is only a single sample mean which is one observation from the distribution. The narrower the spread of this distribution, the nearer the single value available is likely to be to the truth. This spread, represented by the standard deviation of the sampling distribution, indicates how precise a single sample mean is as an estimate. It indicates the likely error in the estimate. Largely because of this the standard deviations of sampling distributions are almost universally referred to as standard errors (**SEs**):

$$\text{SE (mean)} = \text{SD (mean)} = \text{SD (original variable)}/\sqrt{n}.$$

Thus the standard error of a mean (or of any other estimate) indicates its precision as an estimate. For samples of 100 values ($n = 100$), the sample means would have had a standard deviation of 15/10 or 1.5, which is a very small spread. The estimate can be made as precise as required by increasing the sample size.

Therefore the standard error of a sample mean is

$$\begin{aligned}\text{SE (mean)} &= \text{SD (original variable)}/\sqrt{\text{sample size}} \\ &= \text{SD}/\sqrt{n}\end{aligned} \quad (1)$$

which can be deduced mathematically by the application of some fairly general rules. The same techniques can be used to deduce the standard errors of regression coefficients, differences between means, and so on. In fact, appropriate standard errors can be obtained for any value calculated from a sample.

Confidence intervals

Although the estimate is chosen as the 'best guess' at the population value, it will not usually be exactly right. In practice the standard error and the estimate are used to obtain a range of values defining an interval on the original variable scale which will contain the unknown population value with some chosen probability.

Fortunately, for reasonably large samples ($n > 30$) and some fairly mild assumptions, the sampling distributions of many common estimates are close to normal. This means, for example, that the sample value will only fall outside the range

true value − 1.96 SE to true value + 1.96 SE

for 5 per cent of such samples. With some algebra it follows that the interval

estimate − 1.96 SE to estimate + 1.96 SE

will include the true population value in 95 per cent of such samples. This means that one can be 95 per cent confident that an interval calculated in this way will include the true population value. Other confidence intervals, such as 99 per cent, are obtained by taking the appropriate centile of the standard normal distribution instead of 1.96.

These calculations need the population standard deviation of the original variable. Since this is rarely known, it is necessary to use the sample value as an estimate. This does not matter very much for large samples, but it may if the sample size falls below about around 30. As a result for small samples the standard normal distribution cannot be used. It is necessary to use what is known as the *t* distribution. The centiles of the normal distribution, such as $u_{0.975} = 1.96$, have to be replaced by the equivalent centiles of the *t* distribution appropriate to the sample size. Nonetheless the appropriate 97.5 centiles are all close to 2. These centiles are commonly denoted by $t_{f,\,0.975}$, where *f* is known as the degrees of freedom and represents the amount of information available to estimate the population standard deviation used in the calculation of the standard error. The degrees of freedom are invariably the total sample size minus the number of values estimated from the sample. It can be seen from tables (e.g. Lindley and Miller (1964) or statistical programs such as GLIM) that

$$t_{20,\,0.975} = 2.09$$

$$t_{30,\,0.975} = 2.04$$

$$t_{40,\,0.975} = 2.02$$

$$t_{60,\,0.975} = 2.00$$

and only when the degrees of freedom approaches 500 do the 97.5 centiles of the two distributions become the same to two decimal places:

$$t_{473,\,0.975} = 1.96 = u_{0.975}.$$

However, for most practical purposes, once there are more than 60 degrees of freedom, the *t* distribution can be assumed to be the same as the normal distribution.

Sample sizes for estimation

The sample size for an estimation is determined by the precision required. The usual approach to defining precision is to stipulate that there should be a high probability (often 95 per cent) that the estimate is close to the true value. 'Close' is usually defined as within some small percentage such as 5 per cent of the correct value. Clearly, this means that the approximate size of the value being estimated must be known.

Consider the problem of estimating a population mean from a sample. Ninety-five per cent of means from unbiased samples will be within 1.96 SEs of the true value. This implies that if 1.96 × SE is less than 5 per cent of the true value, the precision will be as specified.

If *M* represents the value to be estimated, the sample will be large enough if

$$1.96 \times \mathrm{SD}/\sqrt{n} \leqslant 0.05 \times M$$

i.e.

$$n \geqslant (1.96)^2 \times \mathrm{SD}^2/(0.05 \times M)^2. \qquad (2)$$

With this sample size one can be 95 per cent confident that the estimate will be within 5 per cent of the true value.

Example To estimate the mean systolic blood pressure for men between 30 and 60 years old to within 5 per cent with 95 per cent confidence. It is known from previous work that the true value *M* is about 150 mmHg and that the SD is about 15. Using eqn (2), this means that the sample size needs to be

$$n \geqslant (1.96 \times 15)^2/(0.05 \times 150)^2 = 16.$$

This is very small, so that 5 per cent is not a very stringent requirement in this context. Requiring a higher degree of precision, for example that the estimate must be accurate to 1 per cent, implies a sample size of

$$n \geqslant (1.96 \times 15)^2/(0.01 \times 150)^2 = 385.$$

Significance tests

The probability that a sample 95 per cent confidence interval will not contain the true population value is less than or equal to 5 per cent. This means that, for any hypothetical population value, it is possible to judge whether the sample estimate is surprisingly far from it by seeing whether it falls outside the 95 per cent confidence interval. If a value hypothesized for the population falls outside this interval, then the probability of the sample giving this interval and hence the estimate, assuming that the hypothesized population value is correct, is less than 5 per cent. Therefore

$$p(\text{estimate}|\text{population value}) \leqslant 0.05$$

or as it is frequently written $p < 0.05$.

A significance test is a procedure which can be used, assuming that the hypothesis to be tested is true, to calculate the probability *p* of sample values occurring as far or further from those expected as those actually observed. Some value, called a test statistic, which has a known sampling distribution is calculated from the sample. This is frequently the number of standard errors that an estimate is from the population value expected from the hypothesis. The *p* value can then be obtained from the sampling distribution of the test statistic. If *p* is less than 5 per cent, the sample value is taken as evidence significant at the 5 per cent level that the hypothesis is untrue.

In 5 per cent of tests using a 5 per cent significance level, surprising values of the test statistic will occur even though the hypothesis is correct. This error—concluding that a hypothesis is not true when it is—is known as a type I error. Therefore if a test uses a 5 per cent level of significance, there will be a 5 per cent risk in using the test of a type I error. Notice that the risk may be set as required in a test by altering the level of significance to be used. Finally, there is a risk that even when the hypothesis is false, samples may be obtained which produce unsurprising values of the test statistic. This leads to the error of accepting as true a hypothesis which is actually false. This is a type II error. The size of sample needed to give a reliable test of some hypothesis must take both types of error into account. Sample size calculations for significance testing are discussed in a later section.

There is a close relationship between confidence interval calculations and significance tests. Any hypothesis that predicts a population value can be tested by inspecting whether the value falls inside the appropriate confidence interval. Using the 99 per cent confidence interval this is equivalent to $p < 0.01$.

Suppose that a study is estimating the population mean systolic blood pressure for adult males. For a moderately large sample ($n > 30$) with mean 120 mmHg and standard error 2.0, the 95 per cent confidence interval is

$120 \pm 1.96 \times 2.0$ or 116.1–123.9.

The probability of results as extreme as 120 if the true value is 130 is less than 5 per cent since 130 is well outside the interval. The estimated 120 mmHg is significantly different from 130 mmHg at the 5 per cent level because it is surprisingly far from the population value of 130 ($p < 0.05$). It is reasonably clear that the sample is from a population with a lower mean value than 130 mmHg. However, it must be remembered that, by definition, 5 per cent of the confidence intervals will exclude the true value. This is a type I error as discussed above. If this system is used in making decisions, they will be wrong 5 per cent of the time.

Although the use of confidence intervals is quite sufficient, it is common to calculate the p values directly. As implied above, this is most frequently done by calculating, as a test statistic, how many standard errors separate the estimate and the hypothetical value:

$$\frac{\text{estimate} - \text{hypothetical value}}{\text{SE of the estimate}}.$$

What centile this is of the t or standard normal distribution is then determined from tables which for a given value of the variable give the probability of values below it, say P.

The probability of values equal to or above that obtained is then $1 - P$, which is the probability of surprisingly high values. Surprisingly low values will also be possible, and so the probability of values as surprising as that observed will be twice $1 - P$ or

$p = 2(1 - P)$.

These are the basic concepts of statistics. It is now necessary to consider how these techniques are used to answer practical questions from real data.

Types of analyses

Measured outcomes

Simple regression

Figure 21 shows some data on chromosome abnormalities and blood lead levels from female workers in a battery factory. The research question was: Does lead exposure damage chromosomes?

If it is assumed that current lead levels in the blood reflect overall exposure, the question can be expressed as: In the population of all such subjects as these, is the number of chromosome abnormalities higher, on average, in those with high blood lead levels than it is in those with low levels? This is the same as asking: Is the trend in these points sufficiently non-horizontal to indicate a real trend in the population?

To answer the question it is necessary to fit the least-squares regression line and test whether the sample regression coefficient is consistent with a true value of zero. Alternatively, it is simply necessary to show that a non-zero trend model fits the data significantly better than a horizontal-line model to demonstrate that the apparent trend is unlikely to be due to chance.

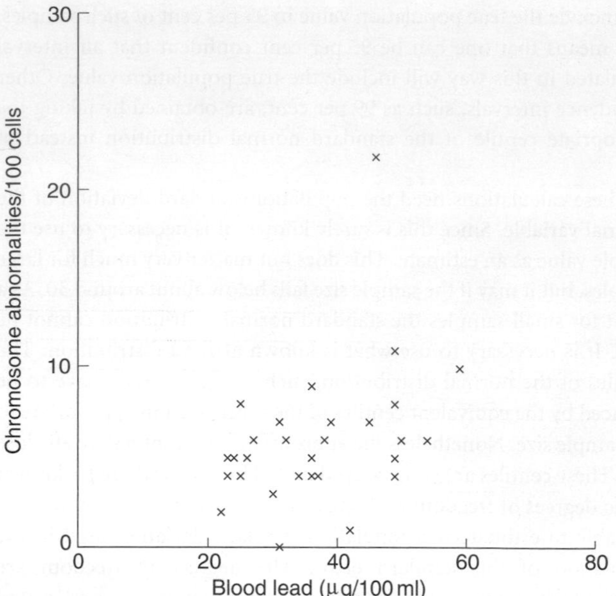

Fig. 21 Chromosome abnormalities per 100 cells and blood lead levels. (Source: Forni and Sciame 1975.)

To demonstrate how a regression line is fitted, a number of algebraic definitions are needed. The variance of a set of values has already been introduced as

sum for all values = (value – mean value)^2/(number of values – 1)

which for values of a variable y becomes

$$\text{sum } (y - \bar{y})^2/(n - 1) \tag{3}$$

where $\bar{y}$ (pronounced y bar) is the conventional abbreviation for the mean of a sample of y values. The sum of squared deviations construction is so common in statistical calculations that it is convenient to have a special notation. In this chapter we shall use

$Syy = \text{sum } (y - \bar{y})^2$.

Although it will not be used here many statistical texts use Σ to denote summation. In that notation the above becomes

$$Syy = \sum (y - \bar{y}^2). \tag{4}$$

For an x variable, the equivalent is

$$Sxx = \text{sum } (x - \bar{x})^2. \tag{5}$$

and finally

$$Sxy = \text{sum } (y - \bar{y})(x - \bar{x}). \tag{6}$$

The sum of squared deviations minimized when we fit a regression line is essentially Sdd, but it is more often called the residual sum of squares (**RSS**) or Sr.

In general

Sr = sum (y – value predicted by the model)^2

which, for a simple regression line, becomes

Sr = sum (y – height of line)^2.

Now, to fit the regression line of the form

$y = a + bx$

to describe the trend in chromosome abnormalities as blood lead increases means choosing the most appropriate values for a and b. The principle of least squares means that a and b are required to make the sum of the squared deviations Sr a minimum. For this line the residual sum of squares is

$$Sr = \text{sum } (y - a - bx)^2. \quad (7)$$

It can be shown mathematically that this is a minimum when the slope

$$b = Sxy/Sxx \quad (8)$$

and the intercept

$$a = \bar{y} - b\bar{x}. \quad (9)$$

The minimum value of Sr when a and b take these values is

$$Sr = Syy - Sxy^2/Sxx. \quad (10)$$

The residual sum of squares is the basic measure of how well a model, in this case $y = a + bx$, fits the data. If points are widely scattered about the line, Sr will be large, indicating a bad fit. If the points fall more or less on a straight line, Sr will be small, indicating that a straight-line model fits the data well.

The variance of the deviations about the line is called the residual variance and is denoted by

$$s^2 = Sr/(n - 2) \quad (11)$$

where $n - 2$ is the number of degrees of freedom and is the amount of information available to estimate the residual variance. This is the number of observations (or points on the plot) minus the number of parameters in the model that need to be estimated. Here it was necessary to estimate two parameters — the intercept and the slope. The residual variance can be used to calculate the standard error of b which is

$$SE(b) = \sqrt{(s^2/Sxx)}. \quad (12)$$

For the data on women battery factory workers, where y is the number of chromosome abnormalities per 100 cells and x is the blood lead level in μg/100 ml, the values required in the analysis to fit a simple regression line are

$n = 30 \quad \bar{y} = 5.97 \quad \bar{x} = 36.37$

with

$Syy = 432.97 \quad Sxx = 3302.96 \quad Sxy = 460.37.$

Therefore the estimates of a and b are

$a = \bar{y} - b\bar{x} = 5.97 - 0.14 \times 36.37 = 0.90$

$b = Sxy/Sxx = 460.37/3302.96 = 0.14.$

From eqn (10)

$Sr = 432.97 - 460.37^2/3302.96 = 368.80$

so that

$s^2 = Sr/(n - 2) = 368.80/28 = 13.17$

and

$SE(b) = \sqrt{(s^2/Sxx)} = 0.06.$

Therefore the line giving the 'best' representation of the apparent trend in the least-squares sense is

$\text{ABS} = 0.90 + 0.14 \times \text{BL}$

where ABS denotes chromosome abnormalities and BL denotes blood lead levels. If it is assumed that the sampling distribution of b is sufficiently near normal, the 95 per cent confidence interval for the 'true' value of the slope is

$0.14 - 1.96\ (0.06)$ to $0.14 + 1.96\ (0.06)$

or

0.02 to 0.16.

Since this does not include zero it is a reasonably strong indication that the population trend is not zero, i.e.the observed trend is significantly different from a population value of zero at the 5 per cent level. A sample regression slope could not easily occur this far from zero by chance ($p < 0.05$).

The significance test of the zero slope hypothesis is performed by calculating how many standard errors the slope 0.14 is from the expected zero, i.e.

$$\frac{\text{observed slope} - \text{expected slope}}{\text{SE (slope)}} = \frac{0.14 - 0}{0.06} = 2.33$$

which is well above 1.96, as the confidence interval also showed. Therefore there is strong evidence of a trend in the population represented by this sample. Higher numbers of chromosome abnormalities will be found in those individuals who have higher blood lead levels.

There was one 'outlying' individual with 22 abnormalities on the plot. If the results had been less conclusive, it might have been wise to repeat the analysis excluding this individual. Her effect on the analysis could then be assessed and the interpretation modified appropriately, but it is not really necessary here. Note that the t distribution should be used for samples this size. The t distribution centile equivalent to the standard normal 1.96 for 28 degrees of freedom is 2.05 (about 5 per cent higher), but even if the t value is used the conclusions are exactly the same.

It is is still unclear whether these results really mean that lead in the blood damages chromosomes. Partly for this reason it is customary to describe significant trends as indicating only a real 'association' between the variables, in order to make it clear that the existence of a trend in the population in no way proves a 'causal relationship'. This single finding must be added to the whole body of knowledge on the subject before conclusions can be carried that far.

Apart from tests of the assumptions that the population line is straight and not a curve, that there is a similar residual variance at all x values, and that the underlying distribution is normal, this analysis is complete.

In fact, since any trend is indicative of the relationship—in this case between lead exposure and chromosome abnormalities—whether or not it is straight hardly matters. Whether the residuals have a normal distribution is more crucial since inferences from confidence intervals and significance tests all assume that they do. How to test these assumptions will be discussed later. Meanwhile it is useful to consider how this analysis can be approached and in a more general way applicable to most common problems. In some circumstances the question cannot be phrased so that it becomes a test of a single parameter. In such cases the question has to be expressed as a comparison of different models.

In the lead data example used above, the equivalent model comparison is between a model of the form

$y = a + bx$

which is a sloping straight line and the model

$y = a$

which represents a horizontal line.

If there is a significant trend, the second model will fit the data significantly worse than the first. How well a model describes data is measured by the residual sum of squares—the smaller *Sr*, the better the fit. Comparisons of the fits of two models are made by comparing their residual sums of squares.

As should be clear from this example, the more parameters there are in a model, the smaller the residual sum of squares *Sr* can be made. Choosing the intercept and the slope, two parameters for a sloping line, makes it possible to fit the model closer to the data points than when the fitting process is restricted to choosing one parameter (e.g. the intercept for a horizontal line). For the model

$y = a + bx$

the residual sum of squares is

$Sr = 368.75$

and the residual variance is

$s^2 = 13.17.$

For the horizontal-line model when the intercept (height of the line) is simply the mean of *y*, the residual sum of squares is

$Sr = 433.0,$

i.e. an increase of 64.25.

The increase has one degree of freedom associated with it since one parameter has been dropped from the more complicated model. On the hypothesis that the trend is a chance event in this particular sample, 64.25 is a further estimate of the residual variance. This means that if the hypothesis is true, $64.25/s^2$ should be about 1.0 since it is the ratio of two estimates of the same variance; the value in this example is $64.25/13.17 = 4.88$.

The numerator, which is the increase in *Sr* resulting from simplifying the model, has one degree of freedom. The denominator, which is the residual variance from the most complicated model, has $n - 2 = 28$ degrees of freedom. If the 'no-trend' hypothesis is true, this variance ratio can be shown to have a sampling distribution with a

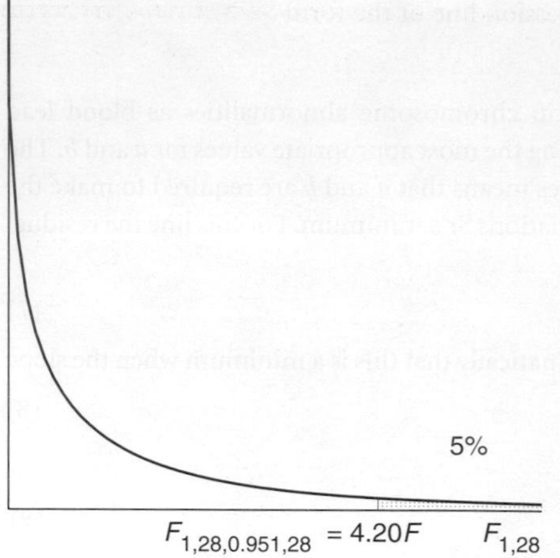

Fig. 22 *F* distribution with 1 and 28 degrees of freedom.

particular mathematical form called the *F* distribution (in this case with 1 and 28 degrees of freedom). By applying what is known as an *F* test, this can be used to assess how surprising an observed variance ratio is.

The *F* distribution of 1 and 28 degrees of freedom is illustrated in Fig. 22. The 95th centile of the *F* distribution is 4.20, and less than 5 per cent of *F* values calculated in this way from a sample should occur this far above 1.0. This implies that the value 4.88 is surprisingly large ($p < 0.05$) if the population has no trend. It suggests that the horizontal-line model is incorrect. Surprisingly low values can occur, but they have little meaning. If anything, they imply that the model fits the data surprisingly well given the amount of variation present. Generally, they are treated as insignificant.

The interpretation of this analysis is that it is either necessary to assume a freak sample or that the non-zero trend model was necessary to describe this data. In practice it would be taken as reasonably strong evidence that there was a trend in the population. The estimated regression coefficient with a confidence interval should then be obtained to demonstrate the magnitude of the effect.

This model comparison approach to the analysis is best presented in tabular form, giving what is known as an 'analysis of variance' (although it is actually an analysis of residual sums of squares). The analysis is given in Table 5 where the residual sum of squares from model 1 is S_1 and the mean square MS is the sum of squares divided by the degrees of freedom for a model.

Table 5 Analysis of variance to test for a linear trend in chromosome abnormalities by blood lead (BL) levels

Model		SS	DF	MS	F
1	Intercept and trend on BL: sloping line	$S_1 = 368.75$	28	$S_2 = 13.17$	
2	Intercept, but no trend: horizontal line	$S_2 = 433.00$	29		
(2 – 1)	Due to trend	64.25	1	64.25	$F_{1,28} = 64.25/13.17 = 4.88$

SS, sum of squares; DF, degrees of freedom; MS, mean sum of squares.

To construct such analysis of variance tables it is only necessary to obtain the residual sum of squares for the two models. A test of the parameters omitted when model 1 is changed to the simpler model 2 is then immediately available as

$$F_{1,28} = (S_2 - S_1)/s^2. \qquad (13)$$

Since all that is needed for this approach is the residual sum of squares for each model, it is not even necessary to fit them. In practice they are fitted because it is necessary to know the likely magnitudes of the effects, not just whether they exist or not.

Non-linear regression

In a given analysis a straight-line trend may well be inadequate, and a curved-line trend might fit the data better. To test this, a model representing a curved trend is fitted and the fit is compared with that of a straight-line model. The simplest model for a curved trend is known as a quadratic and takes the form

$$y = a + bx + cx^2.$$

In the lead data example, this is equivalent to

$$\text{ABS} = \text{intercept} + b\text{BL} + c\text{BL}^2$$

where ABS and BL denote for chromosome abnormalities and blood lead levels respectively. The model is fitted exactly as before with a, b, and c chosen so that the residual sum of squares is minimized.

The formulae are rather more complicated than for the straight-line model; therefore, although this model can be fitted by hand, it is tedious. However, it is very easy to fit with a professionally produced package program on a computer, and it is not necessary to know the formulae in detail.

The hypothesis that there is no curvature in the population can be tested very easily by calculating

$$t = \frac{c - \text{expected } c}{\text{SE}(c)} = \frac{c - 0}{\text{SE}(c)}$$

Since we have fitted three parameters, this has $n - 3$ degrees of freedom where n is the number of data points. The fitted model for the lead data gives

intercept $a = 2.77$

linear coefficient $b = 0.03$

quadratic coefficient $c = 0.0014$ with $\text{SE}(c) = 0.0066$.

Therefore, for the t test of curvature,

$$t = \frac{0.0014 - 0}{0.0066} = 0.2 \text{ with 27 degrees of freedom.}$$

This is very far from the value needed for significance which is a little above 2.0 ($t_{0.975} = 2.05$ on 27 degrees of freedom). Obviously there is little evidence that the population trend is not a straight line.

Comparing two groups

The above analysis of the lead study data looked at the association between chromosome abnormalities and blood lead levels. However, current blood lead level may not reflect long-term exposure. Figure 23 shows a comparison of individuals from lead-free areas in the factory with those exposed to lead in their work. The values for the exposed individuals appear to be slightly higher with a wider spread. To investigate this more precisely, it is necessary to calculate the means and standard deviations for the two groups (Table 6).

Table 6 Chromosome abnormalities (ABS) in female battery factory workers by exposure group (findings when one woman with ABS = 22 was excluded are shown in parentheses)

	Not exposed		Exposed		All	
Number	12	(12)	18	(17)	30	(29)
Mean	4.00	(4.00)	7.28	(6.41)	5.97	(5.41)
SD	1.71	(1.71)	4.36	(2.43)	3.87	(2.44)

The question becomes: 'Are the means surprisingly different?' This is tested by fitting a model of the form

mean ABS = reference value + group effect.

Taking the 'reference value' as the mean for group 1 (not exposed), the group effect is zero for that group and equal to the difference between the two means for group 2. Fitting this model by least squares is exactly the same as allowing each group to have its own mean:

mean ABS = 4.00 + 0 for group 1

mean ABS = 4.00 + (7.28 – 4.00) for group 2.

Each mean minimizes the sum of squared deviations within its own group Syy_1 and Syy_2, say, so that the total residual sum of squares $Sr = Syy_1 + Syy_2$ is a minimum.

The variances for the groups separately are calculated as $Syy_1/(n_1 - 1)$ for group 1 and $Syy_2/(n_2 - 1)$ for group 2. To compare the group means, it is necessary to assume one underlying residual variance. On this assumption both samples contain information on the residual variance, and the information is pooled as the overall residual sum of squares Sr to estimate it. Therefore the pooled estimate of variance is Sr divided by its degrees of freedom.

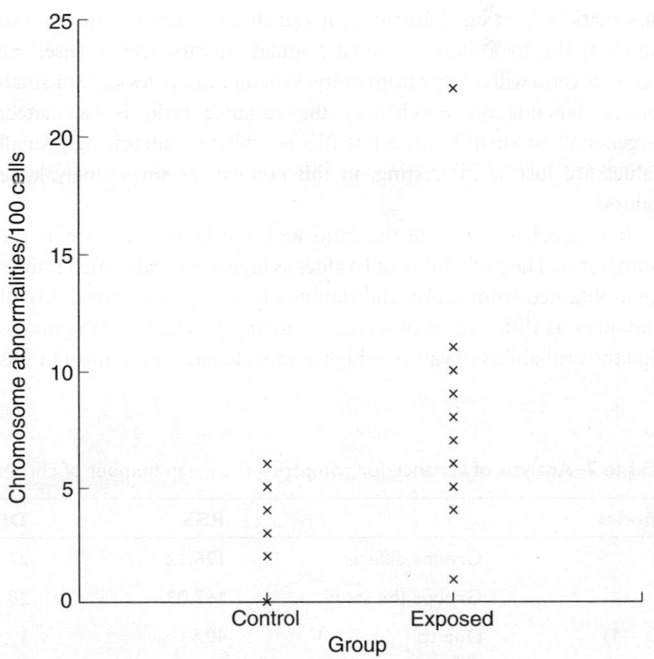

Fig. 23 Chromosome abnormalities and exposure group.

The number of degrees of freedom for the above model is $n_1 + n_2 - 2$ because there are $n_1 + n_2$ values in total and two parameters (the two means) have been estimated. Now

$Syy_1 = 32.00 \quad Syy_2 = 323.61.$

Therefore

$Sr = Syy_1 + Syy_2 = 355.6$

and, since $n_1 = 12$ and $n_2 = 18$,

$$s^2 = Sr/(n_1 + n_2 - 2) = 355.6/28 = 12.7. \quad (14)$$

The difference between the means, which is the group 2 effect since the reference value is the group 1 mean, is

difference = 7.28 – 4.00 = 3.28

which has the standard error

$$\text{SE(difference)} = \sqrt{[s^2(1/n_1 + 1/n_2)]} = \sqrt{[12.7(1/12 + 1/18)]} = 1.33. \quad (15)$$

A significance test of the hypothesis that the population difference is zero is obtained as

$$t = \frac{\text{difference} - \text{hypothesized difference}}{\text{SD (difference)}} = \frac{3.28 - 0}{1.33} = 2.47.$$

The probability of values as far from zero as 2.47 occurring by chance, obtained from tables of the t distribution with 28 degrees of freedom, is about 0.02, and so $p < 0.05$. The difference is significant at the 5 per cent level ($p < 0.05$) on the assumption that the two samples came from populations with identical variances.

However, the two groups actually have very different standard deviations and hence variances (Table 6), and so the assumption should be tested. This is done using a form of the F test. If the population variances are the same, the variances from the two groups are estimating the same thing. In that case their ratio will be an observation from an F distribution and should have a value close to unity. If the hypothesis of equal population variances is false, the variance ratio will deviate from unity. Whether this gives large or small values depends on which way the variance ratio is calculated: large/small or small/large. Since this is arbitrary, surprisingly small values are just as interesting, in this context, as surprisingly large values.

It is usual to calculate the ratio with the larger variance as the numerator. The probability of F values as high as the calculated ratio is then obtained from tables and doubled to give p, the probability of variances as different as observed occurring by chance. This means that the probability of values as high as the calculated ratio must be less than 0.025 for the probability of obtaining variances this different by chance to be less than 0.05.

The SDs of the two groups were 1.71 and 4.36 and so the variance ratio (large/small) is

$$F = (4.36/1.71)^2 = 6.50$$

with 18 – 1 = 17 and 12 – 1 = 11 degrees of freedom. The tables show that only 2.5 per cent of values from the $F_{17,\,11}$ distribution should occur above 3.33. This implies that our variances are significantly different at the 5 per cent level ($p < 0.05$). The assumption of equal variances is clearly unsafe and some corrective action is required.

In these data the difference in the variances is largely due to one very high value of ABS (22) from an individual in the exposed group. If she is removed (Table 6), although the SDs are still different, the F value

$$F_{16,\,11} = (2.43/1.71)^2 = 2.02$$

is less than the 95th centile of $F_{16,\,11}$ which is 2.37. Thus the probability of variances this different by chance is at least $2 \times 0.05 = 0.10$. There is now no real evidence of unequal variances and no reason not to perform the standard analysis.

The residual sum of squares reduces to 126.12 with 27 degrees of freedom and so the residual variance becomes 4.67. The difference between the means is 6.41 – 4.00 = 2.41 and the standard error of this difference is now

$$\text{SE(difference)} = \sqrt{[4.67(1/12 + 1/17)]} = 0.81.$$

The t test becomes $t = 2.41/0.81 = 2.98$, which is in fact even more significant than before because removing the extreme point has reduced the standard error more than it has the difference.

The above analysis in which a single model is fitted is possible and sufficient because the question of interest can be reduced to a test of a single parameter. However, when several groups have to be compared this is not really possible and the model comparison approach is required.

In a model comparison analysis of these data there are two models. The first is the one assuming that the population means are different:

(1) mean ABS = reference value + group effect

where the reference value is the group 1 mean. As before, the residual sum of squares for this model is Syy for group 1 plus Syy for group 2. Calling this S_1, we have

$$S_1 = 126.12$$

(omitting the individual with ABS = 22). The residual variance from this model is $s_2 = 4.67$.

Table 7 Analysis of variance for comparing the mean number of chromosome abnormalities in two groups

Model		RSS	DF	MS	F
1	Groups different	126.12	27	4.67	
2	Groups the same	167.03	28		
(2 – 1)	Due to difference	40.91	1	40.91	$F_{1,27} = 40.91/4.67 = 8.76$

RSS, residual sum of squares; DF, degrees of freedom; MS, mean sum of squares.

Table 8 Mean systolic blood pressure by age in males from a study of the effect of hypertension clinics

	Age group (years)					
	20–29.9	**30–39.9**	**40–49.9**	**50–59.9**	**60+**	**All**
Number	340	303	302	207	288	1440
Mean	141.9	146.0	150.1	149.2	156.9	148.5
SD	20.4	19.9	22.7	21.4	24.7	22.4

The second model, assuming no difference, is

(2) mean ABS = reference value

where the reference value is the overall mean of the two groups estimating the supposedly constant population mean. The residual sum of squares for this model is the value of *Syy* calculated from both groups combined into one sample. Calling this S_2, we have

$S_2 = 167.03$

and the analysis of variance table is as given in Table 7. Since $F_{1,\,27,\,0.99} = 7.68$, this gives a probability of a difference of this magnitude (given the hypothesis of no difference between the populations) of $p < 0.01$. This is the same *p* value as for $t = 2.98$ obtained using the alternative *t* test of the relevant parameter in a single fitted model. In fact, they are the same test in two different forms.

Comparing three or more groups

Consider data from a study designed to assess the effects of well-publicized hypertension clinics on blood pressure levels in the community. There is some evidence that systolic blood pressure increases with age in a non-linear way. For this reason the analyses were performed using age groups rather than exact ages. At the beginning of the study the mean systolic blood pressure for males in the control district which had no clinic was as shown in Table 8.

There is a tendency for the mean value to increase with age (Fig. 24). The SDs are all about the same, and so an assumption of equal variances is reasonable. The appropriate model is

(1) mean SBP = reference value + group effect.

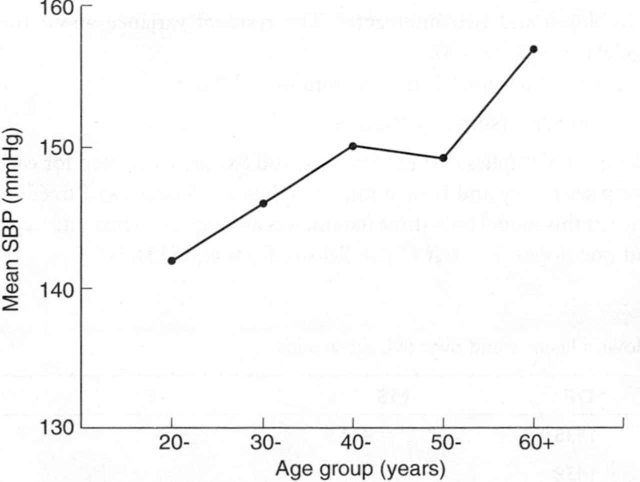

Fig. 24 Mean systolic blood pressure (SBP) by age in males, from a study of hypertension clinics.

Because it simplifies the interpretation of the fitted parameters the group 1 mean (men aged 20–29 years) is taken as the 'reference value'. The 'group effects' are then the differences between the mean of that particular group and the group 1 mean, i.e. the reference value.

The model then has five parameters:

- the reference value (mean for group 1)
- the group 2 effect G_2 (group 2 mean – reference value)
- the group 3 effect G_3 (group 3 mean – reference value)
- the group 4 effect G_4 (group 4 mean – reference value)
- the group 5 effect G_5 (group 5 mean – reference value).

To fit the model, estimates for these five parameters must be obtained as the means and differences implied above with the residual sum of squares *Sr* and hence the standard errors of the parameter estimates. Since the model essentially allows each group to have its own mean, *Sr* is the sum of the *Syys* obtained separately from each group. Calling this S_1 and its degrees of freedom f_1, where

f_1 = (total number of values – number of parameters)

gives

$S_1 = 685\,211$ with $f_1 = (1440 - 5) = 1435$.

Thus the residual variance is

$s^2 = 685\,211/1435 = 477.5$.

The simpler model where differences are assumed to be chance is simply one overall mean:

(2) mean SBP = reference value

with the overall mean as the reference value which represents a single horizontal line. How well this fits the data is measured by the residual sum of squares about the overall mean. This is simply *Syy* from all 1440 individuals treated as one sample, which is $S_2 = 723\,110$. The analysis of variance is given in Table 9.

F values of 19.8 with 4 and 1435 degrees of freedom are extremely unlikely to occur by chance ($p \ll 0.01$). The sample sizes are so large that the small but consistent changes in SBP are highly significant. A linear trend model

(3) mean SBP = intercept + *b*(age),

taking individuals in the same group as having the same age, gives a test of whether the population trend is curved in any way.

When the data are treated as one large sample and a simple regression line is fitted, the residual sum of squares from eqn (10) is

$S_3 = Syy - Sxy^2/Sxx$

and

$S_3 = 688\,123.$

Table 9 Analysis of variance comparing mean systolic blood pressures in five age groups

Model		SS	DF	MS	F
1	Groups different	S_1 = 685 211	1435	s^2 = 477.5	
2	One overall mean	S_2 = 723 110	1439		
(2 – 1)	Due to group differences	$S_2 - S_1$ = 37 899	4	9475	19.8

SS, sum of squares; DF, degrees of freedom; MS, mean sum of squares.

for these data. Since two parameters have been fitted, the number of degrees of freedom is

$1440 - 2 = 1438.$

The analysis of variance is given in Table 10. Since F with 3 and 1435 degrees of freedom needs to exceed 2.60 for significance at the 5 per cent level there is little evidence that a linear trend is not an adequate representation. The estimated slope is

$b = Sxy/Sxx = 0.68$ mmHg/year

and, from eqn (12),

$\mathrm{SE}(b) = 0.08.$

The analysis shows that the means differ significantly and that the way that hey differ is adequately represented by a linear trend. This implies that the slope of the linear trend is significantly non-zero and the direct test is

$t = 0.68/0.08 = 8.5$ $(p < 0.01)$.

Comparing groups allowing for trends

Consider the problem of comparing lung function, in particular FEV, in smokers and non-smokers. The underlying question is: Does smoking affect lung function? It appears that the study simply requires samples of smokers and non-smokers to test whether their respective populations differ. However, for an efficient analysis, the samples need to be as similar as possible in other respects so that, for example, a preponderance of males in the smokers will not bias the comparison. It is possible to avoid this bias by restricting the study to one sex. Unfortunately, this approach cannot be used to avoid bias due to such things as height. Some height differences will inevitably occur. It is possible to ensure that the groups have the same range of heights, which avoids the problem of systematic bias. Nonetheless, the variation in lung function is increased as a result of height differences. This decreases the sensitivity with which group differences can be detected.

Quantitative variables interfering with group comparisons in this way are known as covariates, and analyses involving them are known as analyses of covariance. The analysis of covariance uses regression techniques to deduce from the data in this example whether FEV changes with height in the same way for both groups and, if it does, what FEV differences would be seen between smokers and non-smokers if they all had the same height. Four main circumstances can arise as illustrated in Fig. 25.

The biases illustrated in Fig. 25 can be avoided by designing the study to keep the height distributions of the groups similar. In practice, it is more important to remove the variation due to covariate differences in order to increase the sensitivity with which the analysis estimates and tests the group differences.

If the trend lines in two groups are parallel, the groups differ by the same amount at all heights. As long as both groups have the same range of height it is possible to predict how they will differ without specifying a height. To investigate this it is necessary to compare the fit of parallel and non-parallel models. Assuming straight-line trends, an assumption that would need testing in practice, the models are as follows.

1. Non-parallel:

mean FEV = group intercept + group slope × height

(i.e. each group has its own slope and intercept).

2. Parallel:

mean FEV = group intercept + common slope × height

(i.e. each group has its own intercept, but the same slope).

If there are $n = n_1 + n_2$ points in total, the residual sum of squares for model 1 is

S_1 = sum for both groups of $(Syy - Sxy^2/Sxx)$

with $n - 4$ degrees of freedom because four parameters have been fitted (two slopes and two intercepts). The residual variance about this model is $s^2 = S_1/(n-4)$.

The residual sum of squares from model 2 is

S_2 = sum Syy – (sum Sxy)^2/sum Sxx

where 'sum' implies that the Syy, Sxx, and Sxy are calculated for each group separately and then summed. S_2 has $n - 3$ degrees of freedom since in this model only three parameters are required (two intercepts and one slope). The test of parallelism, from eqn (13), is

Table 10 Analysis of variance testing whether mean systolic blood pressure follows a linear trend over five age groups

Model		SS	DF	MS	F
1	Groups different (any trend)	685 211	1435	s^2 = 477.5	
3	Linear trend	688 123	1438		
(3 – 1)	Due to non-linearity	2912	3	970.7	2.03

SS, sum of squares; DF, degrees of freedom; MS, mean sum of squares.

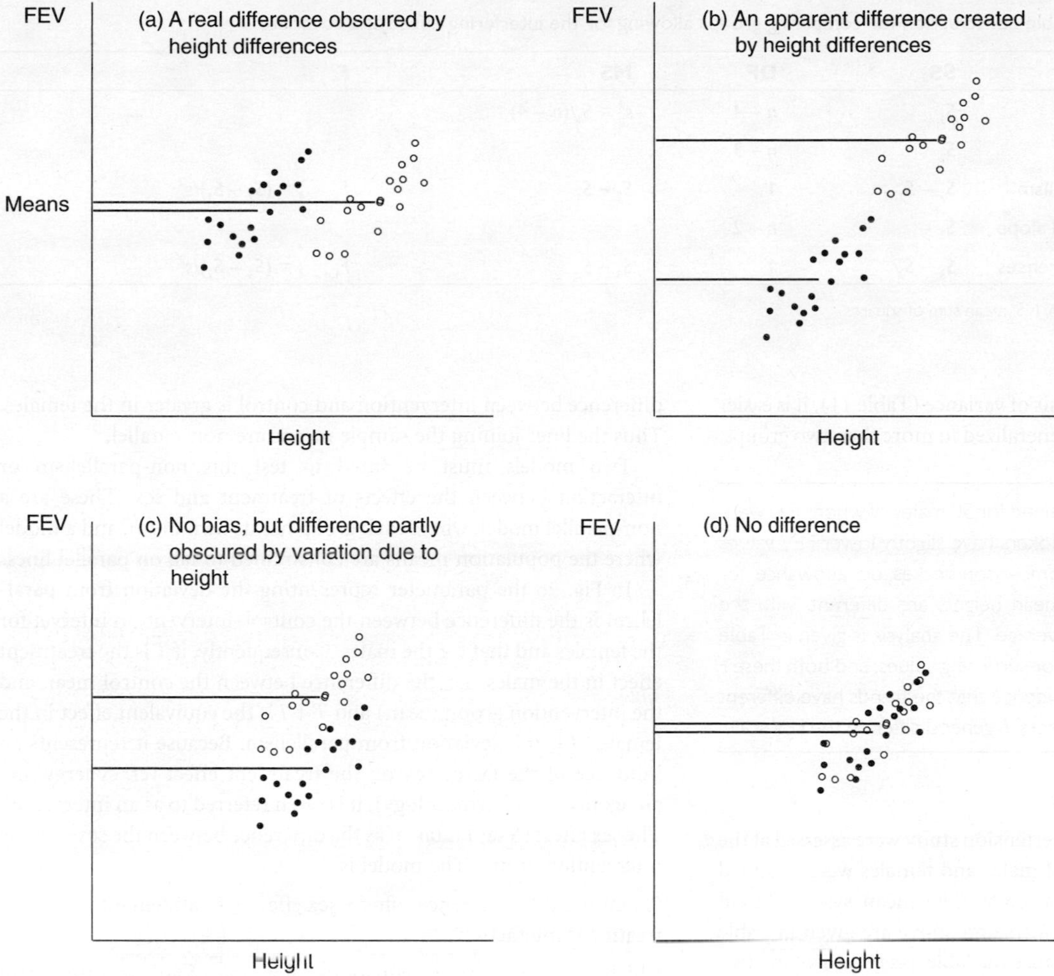

Fig. 25 Two-group scatter diagrams to illustrate the ways in which a covariate may influence a group comparison.

$F_{1,\, n-4} = (S_2 - S_1)/s^2$

which is compared with the appropriate F distribution centile.

If it seems reasonable to accept that the population trends are parallel, the estimated slope is, from eqn (8),

$b = \text{sum } Sxy/\text{sum } Sxx$

and, from eqn (12),

$\text{SE}(b) = \sqrt{(s^2/\text{sum } Sxx)}$.

The group difference allowing for height is then constant for all heights and most easily calculated as the difference between the intercepts, i.e.

mean FEV difference − slope × mean height difference.

Although the algebra is beyond the scope of this text, it can be shown that the variance of this is

$\text{var(diff)} = s^2[1/n_1 + 1/n_2 + (\text{mean height difference}^2/\text{sum } Sxx)]$

from which we can obtain

$\text{SE(diff)} = \sqrt{[\text{var(diff)}]}$

which gives us a t test of the group difference allowing for height.

For more complex situations with several groups and possibly more than one covariate, the group differences are more easily tested by model comparison. Considering the single covariate case to avoid excessive complications, a third model is fitted assuming that all intercepts and slopes are the same in the population. This means that only one intercept and one slope need to be estimated. To fit them the groups are ignored and all the data combined as one. The model is as follows.

3. Coincident trend lines:

mean FEV = intercept + slope × height.

The residual sum of squares from this model is

$S_3 = Syy \text{ all data} - (Sxy \text{ all data})^2/Sxx \text{ all data}$

with $n-2$ degrees of freedom. The test for group differences is again an F test performed by obtaining the difference between the Sr for the two models and dividing by the residual variance obtained from the most complex model, in this case model 1, as in eqn (13):

$F_{1,\, n-4} = (S_3 - S_2)/s^2$.

Table 11 Analysis of covariance table construction for comparing groups allowing for the interfering effect of a covariate

Model		SS	DF	MS	F
1	Non-parallel	S_1	$n - 4$	$s^2 = S_1/(n - 4)$	
2	Parallel	S_2	$n - 3$		
(2 – 1)	Due to non-parallelism	$S_2 - S_1$	1	$S_2 - S_1$	$F_{1,n-4} = (S_2 - S_1)/s^2$
3	Same intercept and slope	S_3	$n - 2$		
(3 – 2)	Due to group differences	$S_3 - S_2$	1	$S_3 - S_2$	$F_{1,n-4} = (S_3 - S_2)/s^2$

SS, sum of squares; DF, degrees of freedom; MS, mean sum of squares.

When this is expressed as an analysis of variance (Table 11), it is easier to see how this approach may be generalized to more than two groups.

Example Mean FEV values were obtained for 50 males of whom five were regular smokers (Table 12). The smokers have slightly lower FEV values than the non-smokers, but the comparison makes no allowance for differences in height. In fact, the mean heights are different, with the smokers being slightly shorter on average. The analysis is given in Table 13. Since *F* values will exceed unity for surprising values, and both these *F* values are less than 1, there is no evidence that the trends have different slopes or the smokers and non-smokers in general differ on the FEV scale.

Groups in a cross-classification

The effects of intervention in a hypertension study were assessed at the end of a 5-year period. Samples of males and females were obtained from the control and intervention areas. The mean systolic blood pressure values for those aged 60 years and above are given in Table 14. This is a 2 × 2 classification because the table has two rows and two columns. The groups are defined by the categorical variables 'sex' in one direction and 'treatment' in the other. For historical reasons, variables used to classify individuals are known as factors, and their values—the actual categories—are known as levels.

To assess the effects of intervention it is necessary to investigate whether the difference between the intervention and control areas is the same in both sexes. If it is, an overall estimate of the effect using data from both sexes is required. This must then be tested against zero to assess whether the hypothetical population of such individuals treated in this way would show a non-zero effect. If the effects are different for the two sexes, they have to be estimated and tested for each sex separately.

Figure 26 shows that the intervention means are well below those of the equivalent control groups. The females have consistently higher values than the males, and there is a slight suggestion that the difference between intervention and control is greater in the females. Thus the lines joining the sample means are non-parallel.

Table 12 Mean FEV values for 50 males by smoking behaviour together with mean height in inches

	Non-smokers	Smokers
Number	45	5
Mean FEV (l/min)	3.34	3.23
SD	2.33	2.83
Mean height (inches)	70.6	69.0

Two models must be fitted to test this non-parallelism or interaction between the effects of treatment and sex. These are a non-parallel model, where each group has its own mean, and a model where the population means are constrained to fall on parallel lines.

In Fig. 26 the parameter representing the deviation from parallelism is the difference between the control–intervention interval for the females and that for the males. Consequently, if T is the treatment effect in the males (i.e. the difference between the control mean and the intervention group mean) and $T + I$ is the equivalent effect in the females, I is the deviation from parallelism. Because it represents an influence of the factor sex on the treatment effect (cf. synergy and antagonism in pharmacology), it is often referred to as an interaction. The sex effect (S say) is taken as the difference between the sexes in the intervention group. The model is

(1) mean SBP = reference value + sex effect + treatment effect + sex × treatment interaction

which represent four equations for the four sex–treatment combinations:

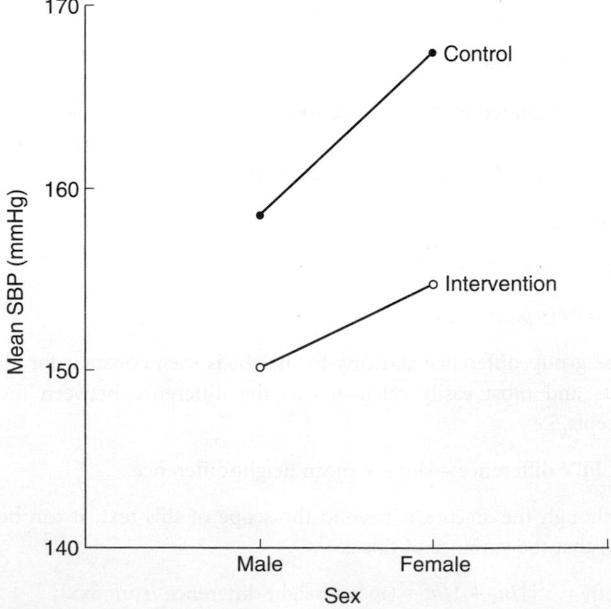

Fig. 26 Mean systolic blood pressure (SBP) by sex and treatment group from a study of hypertension.

Table 13 Analysis of covariance comparing FEV in cigarette smokers and non-smokers allowing for height differences

Model		SS	DF	MS	F
1	Non-parallel trends with height	12.91	46	$s^2 = 0.28$	
2	Parallel trends	12.99	47		
(2 – 1)	Due to non-parallelism	0.08	1	0.08	$F \ll 1$
3	Same intercept	13.03	48		
(3 – 2)	Due to group differences	0.04	1	0.04	$F \ll 1$

SS, sum of squares; DF, degrees of freedom; MS, mean sum of squares.

male intervention mean = rv

male control mean = $rv + T$

female intervention mean = $rv + S$

female control mean = $rv + S + T + I$.

The estimate of the interaction can be calculated using

$\hat{I}$ = (control mean – intervention mean) females – (control mean – intervention mean) males

which, when the data are substituted, gives

$(167.4 - 154.7) - (158.5 - 150.1) = 12.7 - 8.4 = 4.3.$

The Sr from this model is

S_1 = sum of Syy from the four groups = 488 486.2

with $n - 4$ degrees of freedom, where n is the total number of subjects in all four groups and four is subtracted because four parameters need to be estimated. Therefore the residual variance is

$s^2 = S_1/(n-4) = 488\,486.2/893 = 547.0$

which can be used to obtain a standard error for $\hat{I}$:

$$\mathrm{SE}(\hat{I}) = \sqrt{[s^2(1/n_1 + 1/n_2 + 1/n_3 + 1/n_4)]} = 3.16.$$

Therefore a test of the hypothesis that the true deviation from parallelism is zero is

$$t = (\hat{I} - 0)/SE(\hat{I}) = 4.3/3.16 = 1.36.$$

Since there are 893 degrees of freedom, the t distribution is almost the same as the standard normal distribution (Fig. 20). This means that the value would have to exceed 1.96 for significance at the 5 per cent level. Since it does not, there is little evidence of an interaction. The effect of intervention, if any, is the same for both sexes.

The parallel-line model is

(2) mean SBP = reference value + sex effect + treatment effect.

Unfortunately, no simple formula for Sr can be obtained from this model and the analysis cannot easily be done without a statistical package on a computer. When there are only two treatment groups a technique due to Yates (described very thoroughly by Snedecor and Cochran 1967), which uses averages of the mean differences weighted according to the group sizes, can be applied. However, it is laborious and not very general. The Sr from this model, S_2 say, will have $n - 3$ degrees of freedom. The three fitted parameters will be the reference mean, the average difference between the sexes, and one treatment effect averaged over both sexes. The effects can be tested using

t = estimate/SE(estimate)

or, for the generality required for comparing several groups, by fitting models without them. To test the treatment effect it is necessary to fit

(3) mean SBP = rv + sex effect

with $Sr = S_3$ and $n - 2$ degrees of freedom. The F test for the treatment effect is

$$F_{1,n-4} = (S_3 - S_2)/s^2.$$

Exactly the same procedure can be used to test the sex effect. The full analysis of variance is given in Table 15.

Example The actual analysis for the systolic blood pressure data is given in Table 16. Since the 95th centile $F_{1,893}$ is 3.84, there is no evidence of interaction. The other two F values are highly significant, indicating that the differences between both the treatment groups and the sexes are highly significant ($p < 0.001$). The treatment effect is estimated using model 2 and was found to be 10.6 with SE 1.58. This means that, all else being equal, individuals receiving the second treatment (the intervention) will be on average 10.6 mmHg below the control group. The approximate 95 per cent confidence interval for the 'true' effect of intervention is estimate ± 2 SE which gives –13.76 to –7.44. The 'true' difference between the sexes is estimated in a similar way, showing females to be higher on average by 6.5 mmHg with an approximate 95 per cent confidence interval of 6.5 ± 1.57 mmHg.

Table 14 Mean systolic blood pressures by sex and intervention group of subjects in a hypertension study

	Area	
	Control	**Intervention**
Male		
Number	200	223
Mean	158.5	150.1
SD	24.2	21.0
Female		
Number	191	283
Mean	167.4	154.7
SD	27.5	21.5

Table 15 Analysis of variance comparing means in a two-way classification

Model		SS	DF	MS	F
1	With interaction	S_1	$n-4$	$s^2 = S_1/(n-4)$	
2	No interaction	S_2	$n-3$		
(2 – 1)	Due to interaction	$S_2 - S_2$	1	$S_2 - S_1$	$F_{1,\,n-4} = (S_2 - S_1)/s^2$
3	No treatment effect	S_3	$n-2$		
(3 – 2)	Due to treatment	$S_3 - S_2$	1	$S_3 - S_2$	$F_{1,\,n-4} = (S_3 - S_2)/s^2$
4	No sex effect	S_4		$n-2$	
(4 – 2)	Due to sex	$S_4 – S_2$	1	$S_4 - S_2$	$F_{1,\,n-4} = (S_4 - S_2)/s^2$

SS, sum of squares; DF, degrees of freedom; MS, mean sum of squares.

Table 16 Analysis of variance comparing mean systolic blood pressure in groups classified by sex and treatment

Model		SS	DF	MS	F
1	With interaction	488 486.2	893	$s^2 = 547.0$	
2	No interaction	489 499.2	894		
(2 – 1)	Due to interaction	1013.0	1	1013.0	$F_{1,\,893} = 1.85$
3	No treatment effect	514 316.2	895		
(3 – 2)	Due to treatment	24 817.0	1	24 817.0	$F_{1,\,893} = 45.4$
4	No sex effect	498 866.2	895		
(4 – 2)	Due to sex	9367.0	1	9367.0	$F_{1,\,893} = 17.1$

SS, sum of squares; DF, degrees of freedom; MS, mean sum of squares.

The general principles of the above analyses apply to much more complicated situations. A study design may lead to cross-classifications with many more than two factors. Any of the factors may have more than two levels. As well as a cross-classification, there may be one or more covariates to allow for in the analysis. Even so, the pattern of the analysis is more or less the same. A computer can be used to obtain the appropriate residual sums of squares together with estimated parameters representing the group differences of interest and their standard errors.

Repeated or paired measurements

Repeated observations are made on the same subjects when changes over time are of interest. In addition, subjects may be matched in pairs or larger groups to increase the precision of an investigation.

An important reason for performing analyses using covariates or interfering factors is to explain and remove some of the variation observed in the response variable and thus increase the precision of the analysis. In comparisons of a treatment with a control the main source of variation is between the individuals within the groups. There may be a clear difference between the means of the control and treatment groups, but the degree of overlap among individual values may well mean that the observed difference cannot be distinguished from possible chance effects.

In certain circumstances it is possible to use each individual as his or her own control or, as in studies of twins, there may be a very well-defined pairing. This means that the part of the response unique to the individual (or the pair) appears in both the control and the treatment measurement and cancels out when the difference is calculated. As Fig. 27 shows, the consistent way in which the lines joining paired points slope upwards gives a much stronger impression of a genuine treatment effect than the points alone.

The questions dictating which models need to be fitted and compared are as follows.

- Is the effect of treatment the same for all subjects? That is, are the population lines parallel?

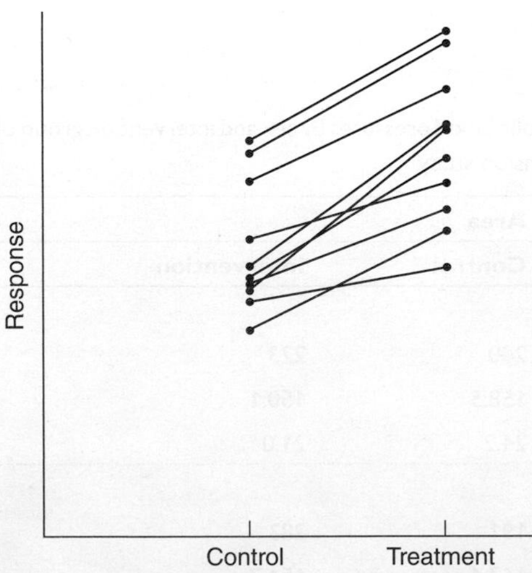

Fig. 27 Paired observations plotted against treatment category.

Table 17 Analysis of variance for paired measurements

Model		SS	DF	MS	F
1	Parallel lines	S_1	$n - 1$	s^2	
2	Horizontal lines	S_2	n		
(2 – 1)	Due to non-parallelism	$S_2 - S_1$	1	$S_2 - S_1$	$F_{1,\, n-1} = (S_2 - S_1)/s^2$

SS, sum of squares; DF, degrees of freedom; MS, mean sum of squares.

- Assuming the effect is the same for all is it non-zero? That is, are the population lines non-horizontal?

The first question cannot be answered if, as is usual, there is only one measurement for each subject within a group. In a non-parallel-line model every pair of points has its own line which fits them exactly and there are no deviations. This means there is no information about the underlying variation, and therefore inferences cannot be made about the population. To address this particular question, it is necessary to replicate some of the measurements.

To answer the second question, it is necessary to fit a set of parallel lines to the pairs of points. The model is

(1) mean $Y = rv$ + subject effect + treatment effect

where the 'treatment effect' is actually the mean of the differences between treatment and control. The subject effects represent the height of the lines in Fig. 27. It is not necessary to estimate these effects—they are included in the model to keep them out of the residual sum of squares and hence reduce the residual variance. There are $2n$ points from n subjects; the model requires n parameters for the subjects and one parameter for the treatment group difference. Thus the residual sum of squares S_1 has $2n - (n + 1) = n - 1$ degrees of freedom.

The model appropriate to the hypothesis that the treatment has no effect is

(2) mean $Y = rv$ + subject effect

which is simply a set of horizontal lines. The model requires one parameter for each subject, and so the residual sum of squares S_2 has $2n - n = n$ degrees of freedom. The analysis of variance is given in Table 17.

This is a very simple example. In practice, there may well be subpopulations such as sex represented in the sample, and it will be necessary to check that effects are the same in each. There will frequently be more than two treatment groups. The model comparison approach can be extended quite simply to handle both situations. However, it does need quite sophisticated computing facilities.

In this simplest of cases, the test of the treatment effect can be expressed as what is known as the paired t test. Denoting the treatment–control difference for each subject by d, we have

treatment effect = mean d

Table 18 Means of paired blood pressure readings

	First reading	Second reading
Number	10	10
Mean	157.6	152.1
SD	17.0	17.0

and the test of the estimate against zero is

$$t = \text{mean } d/\sqrt{(s_d^{\,2}/n)}$$

where s_d is the standard deviation of the n differences.

Example In an investigation of the accuracy of blood pressure measurements, two measurements of systolic blood pressure were taken about 5 minutes apart. These replicated readings ought to differ in a purely random way unless the process of measurement affects the value. The comparison here is not between two treatments, but between the first and second reading. The mean values are given in Table 18. If these are treated as two independent groups the apparent decrease is far from significant.

Table 19 gives the analysis of variance obtained by fitting the models with subject parameters to take account of the pairing. The F value on 1 and 9 degrees of freedom for testing the effect is 4.55. The 95th centile of this F distribution is $F_{1,\,9,\,0.95} = 5.12$ and the 90th centile is 3.35; hence it can be deduced that $0.05 < p \ll 0.10$. The model with a reading effect fits better, but not startlingly so. The evidence is ambiguous. It is probably necessary to repeat the investigation with a larger sample before coming to a conclusion as to the existence or otherwise of a reading effect.

Treating the analysis as a straight paired t test the mean difference is

$d = 5.55$(1st – 2nd reading)

and the residual sum of squares of the differences about their mean is

$Sdd = 598.6$

with 9 degrees of freedom. Therefore the variance of the differences is

$s_d^{\,2} = 598.6/9 = 66.5$

and

$$t = \frac{d}{\text{SE}(d)} = \frac{5.5}{\sqrt{66.5/10}} = 2.13.$$

This must be compared with the 97.5th centile of the t distribution with 9 degrees of freedom which is 2.26. Thus, as for the F test, p obtained in this way is greater than 0.05. In fact, this t value is the square root of the above F value ($2.26^2 = 5.12$), illustrating that in this case F and t are effectively the same test and will always produce the same answer.

Sample size calculations for comparing means

Sample sizes for significance tests of means are calculated in much the same way as they are for estimation with one extra complication (see the section on sample sizes for estimation). The probability of accepting an incorrect hypothesis (i.e. a type II error) must be taken into account. Since the standard error of the test statistic is a function of the sample size n and the residual variance, which must be known or estimated, the calculation amounts to solving for n

Table 19 Analysis of variance to test for a change over time in duplicate systolic blood pressure readings

Model		SS	DF	MS	F
1	Reading effect	299.3	9	33.25	
2	No reading effect	450.5	10		
(2 – 1)	Due to reading effect	151.2	1	151.2	$F_{1,9} = 4.55$

SS, sum of squares; DF, degrees of freedom; MS, mean sum of squares.

$$\frac{\text{smallest interesting value of the test statistic} - \text{value expected if hypothesis true}}{\text{SE of test statistic}} \geq Za + Zb.$$

The values Za and Zb are centiles of the standard normal distribution which are determined by the size of the type I and type II errors considered acceptable. The t distribution might be more appropriate. However, since the t distribution centiles can be determined only if the degrees of freedom, and hence the sample size, are known, the argument becomes circular. It is simpler to use the normal distribution and remember that the calculated sample sizes may be slightly smaller than is necessary.

Za will usually be 1.96 for a type I error of 5 per cent. Demanding an 80 per cent chance of detecting when the hypothesis is false, which implies a type II error of 20 per cent, means that Zb must be taken as 0.84, the 80th centile of the standard normal distribution.

For a paired t test, as above, the expected difference, given the usual hypothesis of no effect, is zero. If the smallest interesting difference is D, a 5 per cent significance level is to be used ($Za = 1.96$), and if an 80 per cent chance of detecting a real difference as large as D is required ($Zb = 0.84$), then the sample size n (the number of pairs) must satisfy

$$\frac{(D-0)}{s_d/\sqrt{n}} \geq 1.96 + 0.84.$$

Note that D is assumed positive, which makes no difference and simplifies the calculations. This requires that

$$n \geqslant (1.96 + 0.84)^2 \times (2s_d^{\,2}/D^2).$$

Example Suppose that it is important to detect a difference of 5 mmHg between paired blood pressure measurements. With type I and II errors of 5 and 20 per cent, this requires a sample size of

$$n \geqslant (1.96 + 0.84)^2 \times 2 \times 66.5/25 = 41.7.$$

Thus at least 42 pairs of measurements are required.

If two independent groups are to be compared, the calculations are similar except that the form of the standard error becomes that given in eqn (14). If D is the smallest interesting difference, the sample size is obtained by solving

$$\frac{D-0}{\sqrt{s^2(1/n_1 + 1/n_2)}} \geq Za + Zb$$

for n_1 and n_2. Since analyses are most efficient if the sample sizes are equal, if we assume that $n_1 = n_2 = n$ the number in each group must satisfy

$$n \geqslant (Za + Zb)^2\, 2s^2/D^2.$$

Example In a study to assess the effect of jogging on systolic blood pressure, two independent groups, one consisting of joggers and one of non-joggers, are compared. The appropriate test statistic is the difference between the means. This is known as a two-group t test. If D is set at 5 mmHg, the two error levels I and II are taken as 5 per cent and 20 per cent respectively, and the residual variance taken from previous studies is 225, the number in each group must be

$$n \geqslant (1.96 + 0.84)^2 \times 2 \times 225/25 = 141.1,$$

i.e. 142 subjects are required in each group.

The analyses in the preceding sections cover most of the situations that arise in practice when responses are measured.

Qualitative responses—two-category outcomes

Maximum likelihood estimation

Exactly the same questions arise for qualitative as for quantitative responses, and the same general approach is used as described above. However, there are a few essential differences which must be discussed.

Typically, two-category outcomes arise when the effects of some treatment or experience are judged according to whether an individual responds or not, has a symptom or not, and so on. The outcome variables are responses with the values **no** or **yes**. It is conventional to represent such variables numerically as 0 and 1. Clearly, such variables cannot have normal distributions and the principle of least squares cannot be used, but apart from this the conceptual approach to the analysis is identical with that for measured outcome variables.

In general, the underlying distribution is taken as binomial and, instead of mean values, it is the proportions of individuals in each category that are of interest. In the population these proportions are the probabilities or 'risks' of individuals picked at random belonging to the specified category. An algebraic model is needed to describe how the 'risk' of an individual being in category 1 (responding, having a symptom, etc.) changes from one group to another or according to values of some measured x variable or covariate.

To fit these models (i.e. to estimate the parameters) the 'maximum likelihood principle' is used instead of the least-squares approach. Essentially this means assuming not only that the sample obtained is not unusual, but also that it is the most likely sample to occur. Once the form of the conditional distributions is determined—in this case binomial—the probability of the sample can be calculated for any algebraic model describing the pattern in the population 'risks', for example population risk = some function of $(a + bx) = g(a + bx)$.

The likelihood or probability of the sample is then a more complex function involving $g(a + bx)$ and the data values. The values of the parameters a and b are chosen to maximize this probability or likelihood. Apart from this difference the process follows much the same lines as the least-squares approach.

To illustrate the analysis of this type of data, consider several groups of similar men exposed to differing levels of pollution classified according to whether they have a persistent cough or not. If there is a positive relationship, the proportion with cough will start close to some minimum (it cannot go below zero) for low pollution levels, start to rise at some point, and then level off as it approaches some upper limit (it cannot exceed 1.0) for high levels of pollution. This produces an S-shaped or sigmoid curve which is characteristic of data where the response variable is constrained between two limits—in this case 0 and 1. From a sample it may appear that there is some sort of relationship even when there is none. The curve may be a chance deviation from a horizontal line. A test is needed to assess whether there really is an effect of exposure on the risk of response. This is obtained by using an algebraic model to describe the curve. The parameters representing how increasing the dose affects response can then be estimated and tested.

If subpopulations are represented in the sample, it will be necessary to compare two or more such dose–response curves. For example, the effect of pollution on respiratory symptoms might have to be assessed using a sample containing smokers and non-smokers. Smokers might well have a consistently higher risk. It is necessary to allow for this when assessing the apparent dose–response relationship. There will be two sigmoid curves representing how risk changes with pollution, one for each of the smoking effects while assessing the effect of pollution. At the tails of such curves the risks are very close to 0 or 1. Small changes in these may be, proportionally, very important. It is necessary to take into account that a change in risk from 0.01 to 0.02 (1 to 2 per cent) is in fact a doubling of the risk, while the same absolute change in the middle of the curve, say 0.50 to 0.51 (50 to 51 per cent), is a relatively trivial proportional change in risk.

In practice this is allowed for by converting the values to the logistic or log(odds) scale. Using the variable y, values for the proportion with cough, i.e. p(cough), are calculated as

$$y = \log\{p(\text{cough})/[(1 - p(\text{cough})]\}$$

where the logarithmic function is the natural logarithm to the base e, and the function $p/(1 - p)$ is known as the odds. Therefore

if $p(\text{cough}) = 0.01$, then $y = \log(0.01/0.99) = -4.6$

if $p(\text{cough}) = 0.50$, then $y = \log(0.5/0.5) = 0.0$

if $p(\text{cough}) = 0.99$, then $y = \log(0.99/0.01) = +4.6$.

This pulls the lower tail of the curve down and pushes the upper tail up with an overall effect of straightening the sigmoid curves.

The order of points on the curve is unchanged by moving from the p to the y scale. An increase on the logistic scale automatically implies an increase on the risk scale.

Transforming proportions to the logistic scale

$$y = \log[p/(1 - p)]$$

turns a sigmoid curve into a straight line. The reverse transformation

$$p = 1/[1 - \exp(-y)]$$

turns a straight line into a sigmoid curve. The exponential function is the antilogarithm for logarithms to the base e. This means that trends in proportions can be assessed and compared by fitting straight-line models

$$y = a + bx$$

on the logistic scale. Specific risks can be estimated or compared using the reverse transformation.

All the analyses of the section on measured outcomes can be applied to proportions using this approach. Any proportion can be considered as a point on a sigmoid curve and the same approach can be used for comparing two or more groups, possibly in some cross-classification, at the same time as allowing for the effects of covariates.

However, because maximum likelihood and not least squares is used to fit the models, the residual sum of squares cannot be used to indicate how well a model fits the data. It is necessary to use what Nelder and Wedderburn (1972) have called the 'deviance', which is defined as

$$\text{deviance} = -2 \times \log\ (\text{likelihood})$$

where the 'likelihood' is the probability of the sample for the given model.

The analysis of variance to compare two models produces a ratio that is an observation from an F distribution if the two models fit the data equally well. In the analysis of deviance for qualitative response variables, the difference between two deviances is, approximately, an observation from a distribution known as the χ^2 distribution. This distribution is widely used, and so values from it can be calculated in most general statistical software packages, and tables (Lindley and Miller 1964) are available from which centiles and p values can be obtained.

Unfortunately, most practical problems involving proportions can be handled only with the aid of a computer and a good statistical package. The analysis can only be performed by hand if the problem is greatly simplified. The following sections cover the general approaches first and then indicate how simpler analyses can be performed at the cost of a few assumptions.

Comparing two groups allowing for a covariate

Table 20 gives some simulated data on the prevalence of cough in children exposed to different levels in pollution. The proportions increase steadily with increasing pollution and they may well arise from the tails of sigmoid curves.

The questions are as follows.

1. Is the effect of pollution the same in both groups? That is, on the logistic scale are the equivalent population lines parallel?

Table 20 Prevalence (number at risk) of children with cough by pollution level and smoking in the home (simulated data).

Smoking in the home	SO_2 pollution level		
	Low (100 μg/m³)	Medium (200 μg/m³)	High (300 μg/m³)
No	0.05 (37)	0.20 (25)	0.33 (12)
Yes	0.09 (32)	0.29 (28)	0.53 (17)

If parallelism can be assumed:

2. Is there an effect of pollution? That is, are the equivalent population lines non-horizontal?
3. Is there an effect of exposure to smoking? That is, are the equivalent population lines separated vertically?

For this analysis it is necessary to fit the following models (*rv* is the reference value which is the predicted proportion for the low pollution/non-smoking reference group transformed to a value on the logistic scale).

1. **Non-parallel**—a different pollution effect in each smoking group:

$y = rv$ + smoking effect + smoking group pollution effect.

2. **Parallel**:

$y = rv$ + smoking effect + pollution effect.

3. **Horizontal**—no pollution effect:

$y = rv$ + smoking effect.

4. **Coincident lines**—no smoking effect:

$y = rv$ + pollution effect.

The analysis was performed using a computer and the statistical package GLIM (Francis *et al.* 1993). Other packages such as BMD-P (Dixon 1981), Egret (Statistics and Epidemiology Research Corporation and Cytel Software Corporation 1992), and Stata (Stata Corporation 1993) can be used to perform the same analyses but, in many cases, not so easily. GLIM requires as input the numbers at risk and the numbers responding (i.e. those with symptoms) for each cell of the two-way table (Table 20) to fit the models and obtain their deviances. From these, the analyses of deviance in Table 21 can be constructed.

From line (2 – 1), there is no evidence of non-parallelism. The difference between the two deviances gives a χ^2 value of 0.04 which is trivial compared with the 95th centile of the χ^2 distribution with one degree of freedom, which is 3.84. Whatever the association, it is the same whether or not the child is exposed to cigarette smoking in the home.

From line (3 – 2), omitting the pollution effect from the parallel-line model gives a much worse fitting model. Values as large as the χ^2 value testing the slope of the pollution trend against zero (i.e. 17.2) should occur by chance in less than 0.1 per cent of such investigations. The 99.9th centile of the χ^2 distribution on one degree of freedom is only 10.83. These simulated data very strongly indicate that there is an association at these levels between increasing pollution levels and increasing risk of having a symptom.

The effect of smoking in the home is not so clear. The smoking effect, i.e. the separation of the two lines, appears to be no more than could easily occur by chance. The χ^2 value of 1.94 on one degree of freedom is well below the 3.84 required for significance.

The parallel-line model (2) is adequate to describe these data and it provides estimates of the effects. On the logistic scale, the model is

$y = a + smk + b \times \text{pollution}$

where a is the intercept for the non-smoking group, the smoking effect smk is the vertical separation of the lines, and b is the slope or regression coefficient of the pollution trends. The computed analysis gives estimates with approximate standards errors as

$a = -3.87$ SE(a) = 0.69

$smk = 0.61$ SE(smk) = 0.44

$b = 0.0113$ SE(b) = 0.0029.

The pollution effect can be tested by comparing b with zero using the standardized normal distribution

$u = 0.0113/0.0029 = 3.90$ (cf. 1.96).

This gives an equally significant result to that of the χ^2 test. They are essentially two ways of doing the same thing using different assumptions.

The test of the smoking effect, 0.61/0.44 = 1.39, is consistent with this χ^2 result, i.e. well below 1.96. The confidence interval, which therefore includes zero, is

$0.61 \pm 1.96 \times 0.44$ or -0.25 to 1.47.

This shows that the data are consistent with quite large values, up to 1.47. In such circumstances it is wise to investigate what the effects on the logistic scale mean in terms of estimated risks.

Taking pollution as 100 μg/m^3, the low category on the logistic scale, the model predicts that for the non-smoking (ns) group

$y_{ns} = -3.87 + 0.0113 \times 100 = -2.74$

Table 21 Analysis of deviance for comparing prevalences of respiratory symptoms in children classified by exposure to air pollution and cigarette smoking

Model		Deviance	DF	Approximate χ^2
1	Different pollution effects Non-parallel	0.40	2	
2	Identical effects Parallel	0.44	3	
(2 – 1)	Due to different effects	0.04	1	0.04 (cf. $\chi^2_{1,0.95} = 3.84$)
3	No pollution effect Horizontal	17.64	4	
(3 – 2)	Due to pollution effect	17.20	1	17.20 ($p < 0.01$)
4	No smoking effect Coincident lines	2.38	4	
(4 – 2)	Due to smoking effects	1.94	1	1.94 (not significant)

DF, degrees of freedom.

and for the smoking (s) group

$y_s = -8.87 + 0.61 + 0.0113 \times 100 = -2.13.$

If $y = \log[p/(1-p)]$, then

$p = 1/[1 + \exp(-y)]$

so that

$p_{ns} = 1/[1 + \exp(+2.74)] = 0.061$

and

$p_s = 1/[1 + \exp(+2.13)] = 0.106.$

This means that the estimated risks of having the symptom 'cough' are 6.1 per cent for non-smokers and 10.6 per cent for smokers. Although it does not reach significance in this dataset, the effect of exposure to smoking is estimated as an increase in risk of 4.5 per cent. The risk of 6.1 per cent has nearly doubled on going from children who are not exposed to smoking to those who are. If this were to represent a real effect, it would obviously be important.

The ratio of the two risks is known as the relative risk, i.e. the risk of those exposed relative to the risk of those not exposed. This is calculated as

relative risk = 0.106/0.061 = 1.74

which is nearly 2, indicating that the risk is nearly doubled by exposure to pollution.

An approximation of the relative risk is provided by the odds ratio which, for the smoking factor, is

$$\frac{p_s/(1-p_s)}{p_{ns}/(1-p_{ns})}.$$

Because the analysis uses the logistic scale, this is in fact

$\exp(smk) = \exp(0.61) = 1.84$

which is rather larger than the relative risk. Nonetheless, for small risks (about 5 per cent or less), the odds ratio is a good approximation to the relative risk.

There are a number of tests specifically designed for comparing such estimates of relative risk with the value expected (1.0) if the true risks are identical (for further discussion of this topic see Chapter 6.12). Apart from slightly differing assumptions, they are effectively the same test as that derived from the model comparison in the analysis of deviance. In addition, fitting and comparing models has allowed the use of all the data from several pollution groups. The model comparison approach is much more general. It can be extended to cover very complicated datasets and it allows estimates of all the various effects to be obtained in a relatively straightforward way.

Approximate confidence intervals for the estimates of risk and relative risk can be obtained from the parallel-line model. However, this can only be done indirectly by first calculating the confidence limits on the logistic scale as

estimate $\pm$ 1.96 standard error (estimate)

and then converting the limits of the confidence interval back to the risk scale. The predicted y value for the smoking group is

$y = a + b \times 100.$

The standard error of y, SE(y), which is the square root of the sampling variance of y, is a function of the sampling variances of a and b with what is known as their covariance. The interdependence of estimates has not been discussed, but this must be taken into account when standard errors of functions of estimates are required. For a full discussion see Armitage and Berry (1987). All that is needed are the covariances of the estimates and these are readily obtained during computer analysis. For $y = a + bx$ the variance var(y) of y is then calculated using

$\mathrm{var}(y) = \mathrm{var}(a) + 2x \times \mathrm{covariance}\ (a, b) + x^2 \times \mathrm{var}(b).$

For this analysis, the computer produced the values

$\mathrm{var}(y) = 0.48$

$\mathrm{var}(b) = 8.3 \times 10^{-6}$

$\mathrm{cov}(a, b) = -0.0017$

Therefore

$\mathrm{var}(y) = 0.48 + 200\ (-0.0017) + 100^2 \times 10^{-6} \times 8.30 = 0.22$

and

$\mathrm{SE}(y) = \sqrt{[\mathrm{var}(y)]} = 0.47.$

Therefore the 95 per cent confidence interval for y in the non-smoking group is

$-2.74 \pm 1.96 \times 0.47$ or -3.66 to -1.82.

Converting back to the risks scale, the equivalent confidence interval for the risk in this group is 0.025 to 0.139. In the group exposed to smoking the equivalent figures are 10.6 per cent for the best estimate of risk with a confidence interval of 5.0 to 21.3 per cent. This gives an estimated relative risk of 10.6/6.1 = 1.75.

It is not simple to obtain a confidence interval for the true relative risk, but is quite straightforward for the odds ratio. On the logistic scale, the effect of smoking is $0.61 \pm 1.96 \times 0.44$ or -0.25 to 1.47. The odds ratio is estimated as exp(0.61), and the approximate confidence limits are exp(−0.25) to exp(1.47), i.e. 0.77 to 4.35.

The data are reasonably consistent with a true odds ratio as low as 0.77 (i.e. the non-smoking group having a lower risk than the smoking group) or as high as 4.35 (i.e. the group exposed to smoking having a risk of more than four times that of those not exposed). Since this range includes 1, it means that the odds ratio is not significantly different from 1.

The conclusions from these simulated data are first that there is strong evidence of a pollution effect—going from low to medium to high pollution in these individuals at least doubles and then trebles the risk in both the smoking and non-smoking groups. Secondly, there is some suggestion that a larger study might identify an important effect of exposure to smoking, since these results are not inconsistent with a fourfold increase in risk of cough in those exposed to smoking compared with those not so exposed.

Comparing two proportions

If data are available only for the high pollution group as in Table 22, the problem reduces to comparing two proportions. The prevalence of cough is 4/12 or 33.3 per cent in the non-smoking homes and 9/17 or 52.9 per cent in the smoking homes. The question is: Are these two proportions more different than could easily occur by chance?

The hypothesis to test is that there is a single 'true' risk which is the same for both groups and that the differences arose by chance. This

Table 22 Numbers of children with cough according to whether they were exposed to smoking in the home[a]

Cough	Smoking in the home		Total
	No	Yes	
Yes	4 (5.4)	9 (7.6)	13
No	8 (6.6)	8 (9.4)	16
Total	12	17	29

[a]The numbers expected if there was no association between exposure and risk of cough are given in parentheses.

single risk, assuming the hypothesis true, is best estimated by using all the data, that is by 13/29 = 44.8 per cent.

This means that, in studies like this, on average 44.8 per cent of each group would be expected to fall in the cough category. On this basis the expected numbers can be calculated for each cell of the table: 5.4 is 44.8 per cent of 12, 7.6 is 44.8 per cent of 17, etc. The problem becomes one of assessing whether the cell frequencies are surprisingly far from those expected. For each cell the measure of the difference between the observed and expected frequencies is taken as

$$\frac{(\text{observed frequency} - \text{expected frequency})^2}{\text{expected frequency}}$$

or, more simply, using an abbreviated notation

$(O - E)^2/E.$

The summation of this over all the cells of the table gives a measure of how the table as a whole deviates from what would be expected if the hypothesis were true, i.e.

sum for all cells of $(O - E)^2/E$

which can be shown to have a χ^2 distribution on one degree of freedom. This is because the analysis is essentially comparing a model with two different proportions or parameters with a model with one proportion or parameter. Measures of the difference between these two models have one degree of freedom. In this case

$$\chi^2 = (4-5.4)^2/5.4 + (9-7.6)^2/7.6 + (8-6.6)^2/6.6 + (8-9.4)^2/9.4 = 1.09$$

which is a long way from significance at the 5 per cent level (cf. 3.84).

Practical problems rarely reduce to the comparison of two proportions without gross simplification. Nonetheless, a number of alternatives to this test have been developed over the years. There is also much discussion as to which is right. Fortunately, it rarely matters. Yates (1934) pointed out that sum$(O-E)^2/E$ was more nearly a χ^2 variable if the test was slightly modified by subtracting 0.5 from the frequencies on the diagonal with the largest product (in this case the 8,9 diagonal). This is probably the most sensible test to use in this context. When only small numbers are available, a test known as Fisher's exact test is more precise.

Fisher's test calculates the exact probability of this or more surprising tables occurring given the marginal totals and the hypothesis. It therefore gives p values directly. Those requiring the algebraic details should consult Armitage and Berry (1987). A number of statistical packages (e.g. Epi-Info (Dean *et al.* 1994) and StatXact (Mehta and Patel 1992)) provide a facility for performing Fisher's exact test for 2 × 2 tables.

Sample sizes for comparing proportions

The exact solution to this problem leads to a very complicated formula (Casagrande *et al.* 1978). This has been implemented in the menu-driven sample-size calculation system Sample (Andrews and Swan 1994) using the macro facility in GLIM (Francis *et al.* 1993). However, for most practical purposes it will be sufficient to use a calculation analogous to that for comparing means. The sample sizes obtained will be slightly smaller than optimum, but this can be regarded as an increase in the risk of a type II error. If this matters, the risk can be set lower and the calculations repeated. The calculations are based on expressing the χ^2 test above in the form

$$\frac{\text{estimate} - \text{expected value}}{\text{SE (estimate)}}$$

where the estimate is the difference between two proportions; the expected value is usually zero. The test statistic is

$$\frac{r_1/n_1 - r_2/n_2}{\sqrt{p(1-p)(1/n_1 - 1/n_2)}}$$

where $p = (r_1 + r_2)/(n_1 + n_2)$. This has a sampling distribution close to normal even for quite small proportions and values of n_1 and n_2. This means that the statistic can be tested against 1.96 for a 5 per cent significance level. As for comparing means, it is efficient to keep the groups the same size. The number in each group must then satisfy

$$\frac{D}{\sqrt{p(1-p)(2/n)}} \geq Za = Zb$$

where D is the smallest difference of interest, and Za and Zb are centiles of the standard normal distribution determined by the choice of what risks of type I and II errors are acceptable. In this calculation p is taken as the average of the two proportions expected if the hypothesis is false. The number must satisfy:

$n \geqslant (Za + Zb)^2 \times 2\, p(1 - p)/D^2.$

Example What sample size is needed to detect a difference in the prevalence of respiratory symptoms between children in two towns with differing air pollution levels? If the prevalence is about 20 per cent and the smallest interesting difference is 5 per cent, $p = 0.20 + 0.05/2 = 0.225$. If the acceptable risks of type I and II errors are 5 per cent and 20 per cent respectively, the number in each group must satisfy

$n \geqslant (1.96 + 0.84)^2 \times 2 \times 0.225(1 - 0.225)/(0.05)^2$

which gives $n \geqslant 1093.7$. Thus 1094 subjects are needed in each group and 2188 in total.

This and the earlier section on sample size for comparing means give a simplified guide to sample-size calculations. Lachin (1981) gives a very comprehensive guide, and the Sample system (Andrews and Swan 1994) provides a conveniently automated approach for most practical problems.

Repeated observations

An individual can be classified as having or not having a symptom several times during a course of treatment. This produces an analysis problem analogous to that of repeated measurements. Using a subject parameter in the model allows it to be analysed in much the same way,

Table 23 Distribution of subjects according to errors made on their regimen before and after provision of a patient-held treatment record

Before record	After record	
	Errors	No errors
Errors	4	4
No errors	0	2

employing an analysis of deviance instead of the analysis of variance. Odds ratio estimates for risks before and after some treatment or exposure can then be obtained as the square root of the equivalent estimate as described in the section above on comparing two groups allowing for a covariate. In practice, a modified form of model fitting is used for this type of data which also arises in the matched case–control studies discussed below and in Chapter 6.12. A comprehensive discussion of the model fitting approach in this context is given by Breslow and Day (1980), and the method of analysis with the computer package GLIM is fully described in the *GLIM4 Manual* (Francis *et al.* 1993).

In the simplest case analogous to the paired t test problem a technique known as McNemar's test can be used.

Example using McNemar's test Geriatric patients in the community often have complex drug regimens to follow. Table 23 gives some data from a study to assess whether a specially designed patient-held treatment record affects the error rate when the patients are questioned on their regimen.

It is possible to analyse these data using a model-fitting approach, but in this simple case it is not necessary. On the hypothesis that the subjects are equally likely to make errors before and after, as many should improve as become worse. This means that those who changed should be equally divided between the two types of change possible.

In these data four changed—they all became better at identifying their drug dosages. The probability of a result as surprising as this if there was only a 50 per cent chance of improving is required. This is exactly the same as the probability of getting 'heads' in all four tosses of a coin, which is $0.5 \times 0.5 \times 0.5 \times 0.5 = 0.0625$. An equally surprising result would have been all four becoming worse, which is the equivalent of four 'tails'. Since this also has the probability $p = 0.0625$, the probability of a result this surprising is $p = 0.0625 \times 2 = 0.125$. Therefore, although the result seems interesting, the probability of such extreme results is certainly not less than 0.05. If the effect was genuinely of this magnitude, a larger sample would be needed to show it as significant.

Comparing proportions from separate samples: case–control or retrospective studies

If cases with a particular disease or condition and controls are not matched to have the same values of potentially interfering factors (such as age and sex), the data from case–control studies are analysed in exactly the same way, using the model-fitting approach, as any other set of proportions taking the ratio of cases to cases plus controls as the proportions. Odds ratios, assessing the effects on risk of factors in the model, are obtained from the fitted model as described above.

If the cases and controls have been matched in some way according to factors that might be related to the risk of becoming a case, then the correct analysis is more complicated. Further discussion may be found in Breslow and Day (1980), Schlesselman (1982), and Francis *et al.* (1993).

More than two categories of outcome

Categorical outcomes arise when individuals can respond to treatment or experience in several ways not easily measured. For example, a treatment for Hodgkin's disease can be assessed according to whether the patients 'died', 'got worse', 'stayed the same', or 'showed signs of remission'. The clinician's overall classification is preferred in this case to a single measure of well being such as white cell count.

It is always possible to combine some of the categories so that there are only two, for example 'no remission' and 'remission'. This permits the response to be treated as a proportion and allows the use of the methods described in the previous section. In practice this is often the most sensible thing to do, although it wastes information. Alternatively, some way must be found for describing responses in many categories by models.

Consider data from a trial comparing two treatments (A and B) for Hodgkin's disease. The outcomes, assessed after a fixed period of treatment, were 'no response or died', 'partial remission', and 'complete remission'. The results are given in Table 24.

It is necessary to compare how the two groups are distributed among the response categories. This is best done by plotting the frequencies against the remission category for each of the treatment groups. Joining the points within each treatment group makes the diagram easier to interpret (Fig. 28). The true responses are represented on the horizontal axis. However, if the frequencies on the y axis are considered as the response variable, the pattern to be described by an algebraic model has exactly the same form as discussed in previous sections for means and proportions. The y variable in this context is a 'count' or frequency. It is usual to assume that they arise from a theoretical distribution called the Poisson distribution.

Table 24 Distribution of Hodgkin's disease patients by treatment and remission category[a]

Treatment	Remission category			Total
	1. None/died	2. Partial remission	3. Complete remission	
A	16 (40)	9 (23)	15 (37)	40 (100)
B	11 (24)	4 (9)	31 (67)	46 (100)

[a] Treatment group percentages are given in parentheses.

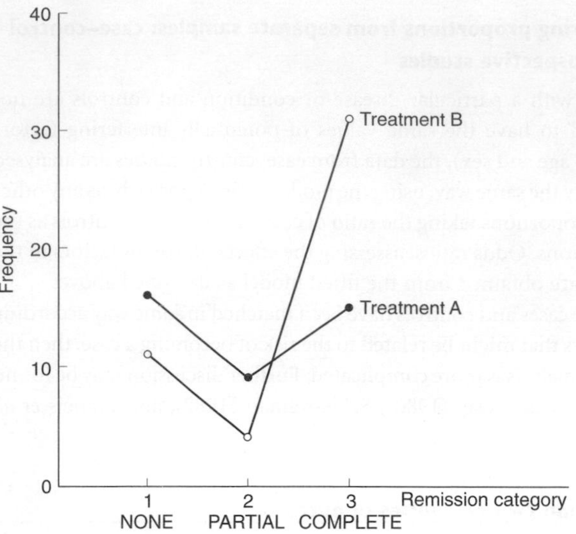

Fig. 28 Frequency of Hodgkin's disease patients versus remission category by treatment group. (Source: British National Lymphoma Investigation 1975.)

For proportions obtained from counts in two categories of response, it was necessary to use the logistic scale to fit the models. For frequencies it is necessary to use another scale, and the most useful and appropriate is the logarithmic scale. This is logical because changes in frequencies seen when moving to groups at higher risk are likely to be proportional. On the frequency scale, distances representing the same proportional difference will change with the frequency. On the log(frequency) scale these distances will stay constant which means that constant proportional effects will give parallel-line models. For this reason this analysis has come to be known as 'log linear modelling'.

Notice that if there had been many more subjects in treatment group A the frequencies would all be larger. The A line would have been much higher than the B line, even if the treatments were equally effective. Because of this it is the parallelism of the lines, not their separation, that is the main interest.

To test whether there are significant differences in the shapes of the distributions it is necessary to compare models with and without interaction parameters. Because the height of the lines does not matter, it is not necessary to treat it as a random variable and waste information estimating some 'true' height. This is avoided by forcing the model-fitting process to choose estimates for the 'height' parameters so the model fits or predicts the observed total frequencies exactly.

Apart from the use of the log scale, since the constraints on the models and the interaction are the model parameters of prime interest, the analysis is much the same as for proportions. Maximum likelihood and analysis of deviance are used to produce approximate χ^2 tests of the interaction parameters quantifying the hypothesis of interest.

Comparing two groups with three outcomes

The models to be compared are as follows.

1. **Non-parallel:**

$y = rv$ + treatment effect + remission category effect + treatment $\times$ remission category interaction.

2. **Parallel:**

$y = rv$ + treatment effect + remission category effect.

Model 1 requires six parameters. Since there are only six points it will fit the data exactly and there are no degrees of freedom and no deviance. A computer analysis gave the deviance from the parallel-line model as 8.17 on two degrees of freedom and so the analysis of deviance is as in Table 25.

Since the 95th centile of the χ^2 distribution with two degrees of freedom is 5.99, the outcome distributions of the two treatment groups are significantly different ($p < 0.05$). It only remains to make quantitative statements about how the 'relative risk' of ending up in the various remission categories varies according to treatment using the estimated frequencies from the non-parallel model and the treatment group totals. In this simple case, this gives estimates of risk equal to the percentages in Table 24.

This approach easily extends to more complex problems, for example if initial severity subgroups had to be taken into account.

Comparing frequencies in a two-way classification

If the data are as simple as in the above example, the frequencies can be compared directly with a χ^2 test using expected frequencies calculated assuming the hypothesis to be tested as true (Table 26).

On the hypothesis that the treatments are equally effective, 31.4, 15.1, and 53.5 per cent of individuals would be expected to fall into the three response categories whatever the treatment (Table 26). This means that 31.4 per cent of the 40 patients receiving treatment A are expected to fall into response category 1:

$$\frac{31.4}{100} \times 40 = \frac{27}{86} \times 40 = 12.6.$$

Similarly, 15.1 per cent of 13 = 6 patients are expected to fall into category 2, and so on.

As when comparing two proportions, the test of whether the frequencies are surprisingly far from those expected on the hypothesis of equally effective treatments is

$\chi^2 = \text{sum } (O - E)^2/E = 8.03.$

This is not quite the same as the analysis of deviance χ^2 value because the analyses make slightly different assumptions. However, the conclusion is much the same and, unless 5 per cent is inappropriately regarded as a 'magic' cut-off point, these two approaches will usually lead to the same conclusions.

Table 25 Analysis of deviance comparing the frequency distribution of Hodgkin's disease patients among three remission categories for two treatment groups

Model		Deviance	DF	χ^2
1	Non-parallel	7	0	
2	Parallel	8.17	2	
(2 – 1)	Due to non-parallelism	8.17	2	8.17

DF, degrees of freedom.

Table 26 Distribution of Hodgkin's disease patients by treatments and remission category[a]

	Response			Total
	Category 1	Category 2	Category 3	
A	16 (12.6)	9 (60)	15 (21.4)	40
B	11(14.4)	4(7.0)	31(24.6)	46
Total	27	13	46	86
Percentage	31.4	15.1	53.5	100

[a]The frequencies expected assuming equally effective treatments are given in parentheses.

Survival or event data

These data arise when individuals observed over time are at risk of some event. The event may be death, menarche, coronary heart attack, and so on. After death or menarche, the individual is no longer at risk—the event cannot occur again. A coronary heart attack could in fact be the first of many, but if observation of the subject is discontinued after the event it can be treated as terminal and standard analyses can be used.

If these data consist of numbers dying in a cohort observed for a fixed period, the analysis is simply a comparison of proportions. The techniques of the earlier section on qualitative two-category responses will usually suffice. Annual mortality rates from different geographical areas can be analysed in this way, treating them as proportions, but there may be complications as discussed by Pocock *et al.* (1981). Nonetheless, the analysis of mortality data of this sort by a model-fitting approach avoids the use of standardizing techniques whereby mortality figures were traditionally adjusted for age and sex effects before group comparisons were made, notably using standardized mortality ratios. Such adjustments make possibly unwarranted and certainly untested assumptions about the effects of age and sex being the same in all the groups to be compared, and for that reason must be used with care. Standardization methods are well covered by Armitage and Berry (1987).

When the individuals are at risk of the event for varying periods of time, the problem cannot easily be considered as an analysis of proportions. There are two main types of problem. In the first it is assumed that the risk is constant over time within the groups to be compared. In the second case the risk changes with time. The remaining discussion will be restricted to these two types of survival data.

Constant risks

The risk per unit time for an individual in a group observed for varying lengths of time can be estimated from the number experiencing the event by dividing the number of deaths by the accumulated time at risk. The modelling approach to analysing such data requires that the number of deaths in each group is taken as the response variable and the accumulated time at risk used as a covariate.

In the occupational health study data in Table 27 the deaths were classified according to factory and age at the start of the observation period. The table also gives the total person-years at risk (**PYR**) within each group. Since the response variable is a count, the appropriate analysis requires using the number of deaths as a Poisson response variable and fitting the models on the logarithmic scale.

The questions to be answered are: Is the effect of age the same in both factories? If it is: Are the risks, allowing for age, different in the two factories? The models required to answer these questions are as follows.

1. **Non-parallel age trends**:

$y = \log(\mathrm{PYR}) + rv +$ factory effect + factory-specific slope $\times$ age

If straight-line age trends are assumed the models are as follows.

2. **Parallel age trends**:

$y = \log(\mathrm{PYR}) + rv +$ factory effect + slope $\times$ age.

3. **No factory effect**:

$y = \log(\mathrm{PYR}) + rv +$ slope $\times$ age.

4. **No age effect** (for completeness):

$y = \log(\mathrm{PYR}) + rv +$ factory effect.

When these models are fitted, the analysis of deviance in Table 28 is obtained.

The 95th centile of the χ^2 distribution with one degree of freedom is 3.84 and values less than this could well occur by chance. Obviously the age effect producing a χ^2 value of 89.19 is very marked and real. The factory effect gives a χ^2 of 1.73 which does not appear to indicate much. However, the initial deviance of 12.70 on four degrees of freedom indicates that the first model is a long way from the data points. The linear age trends do not fit the data well, and so the subsequent analysis must be treated with caution. In fact fitting an age-squared term to allow for curvature gives a much smaller

Table 27 Number of deaths by age group and factory from a study of occupational mortality

Age at start of study (years)	Number of deaths	
	Factory 1	Factory 2
50–59.9	7 (4045)	7 (3701)
60–69.9	27 (3571)	37 (3702)
70–79.9	30 (1777)	35 (1818)
80–89.9	8 (381)	9 (350)

[a]Person-years at risk are given in parentheses.

Table 28 Analysis of deviance comparing mortality in two factories allowing for different age structures

Model		Deviance	DF	χ^2
1	Non-parallel linear age trends	12.70	4	
2	Parallel trends	12.71	5	
(2 – 1)	Due to non-parallelism	0.01	1	0.01
3	No factory effect	14.44	6	
(3 – 2)	Due to factory effect	1.73	1	1.73
4	No age effect	101.90	6	
(4 – 2)	Due to age effect	89.19	1	89.19

DF, degrees of freedom.

deviance. The model with such a term, but assuming a zero difference between the two factories,

5. $y = \log(\text{PYR}) + rv + b \times \text{age} + c \times \text{age}^2$

fits the data well with a deviance of 2.09 on five degrees of freedom. Therefore there is very little evidence of a factory effect.

Observed and expected deaths

In simple cases a hypothesis can be used to deduce the number of deaths expected and these can then be used to calculate $(O - E)^2/E$ for appropriate groups. This is then used to obtain a simple χ^2 test. In the above example the hypothesis to be tested was that the risks were equal in the two factories. The risk for each age group per person-year is calculated as

sum of deaths/sum of PYRs.

The expected deaths in each factory are obtained from this multiplied by the appropriate PYR. For the 50-year-olds in factory 1, this gives

$$\text{expected deaths} = 4045 \times \frac{7+7}{4045+3701} = 4045 \times 0.0018 = 7.3.$$

Similarly, for factory 2

expected deaths = $3701 \times 0.0018 = 6.7$

and so on for all age groups.

The overall χ^2 to test the hypothesis of no factory effect on risk is the sum of the eight $(O - E)^2/E$ values:

$$\frac{(7-7.3)^2}{7.3} + \frac{(7-6.7)^2}{6.7}$$

$$+\frac{(27-31.4)^2}{31.4} + \frac{(37-32.6)^2}{32.6}$$

$$+\frac{(30-32.1)^2}{32.1} + \frac{(35-32.9)^2}{32.9}$$

$$+\frac{(8-8.9)^2}{8.9} + \frac{(9-8.1)^2}{8.1}$$

$$= 1.70.$$

This has four degrees of freedom because there were eight observations and to calculate the χ^2 value it was necessary to estimate four parameters (the risks for the four age groups). The conclusions are the same, but this approach is impossibly tedious if there are many more than two groups to compare. The modelling approach is almost inevitable for a thorough analysis which estimates the magnitude of the various effects.

Changing risks—survival curves

For each individual, data of this type will consist of the length of time observed and the reason that he or she was lost to observation. The period of observation may start at birth, diagnosis, start of treatment, or some other appropriate point in time. An individual who dies, has some other terminal event, or drops out during the the study is then lost to observation. When a study is concluded, observation stops on the survivors.

Life-table survival curves are used to investigate survival in a group of individuals observed for differing periods of time. The survival curve is a plot of the percentage of individuals surviving against time elapsed from diagnosis, or other appropriate points. The life-table calculations to obtain these percentages from individuals observed for varying lengths of time are moderately simple, but not obvious.

Consider a number of subjects entering and leaving a trial at different times as shown in Fig. 29. Using time since entry as the

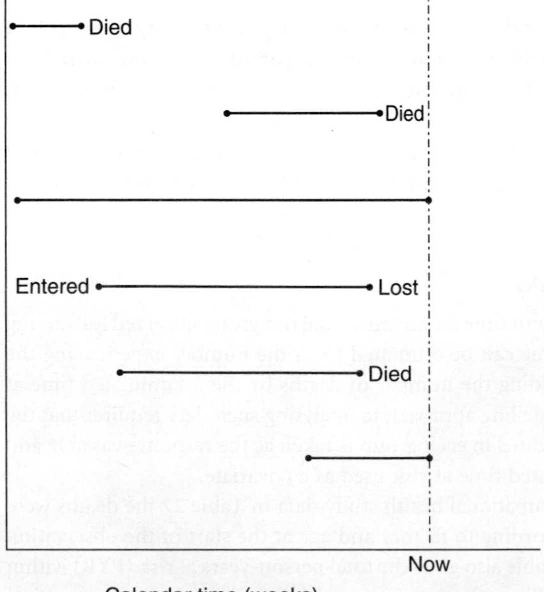

Fig. 29 Observation periods of subjects in a trial.

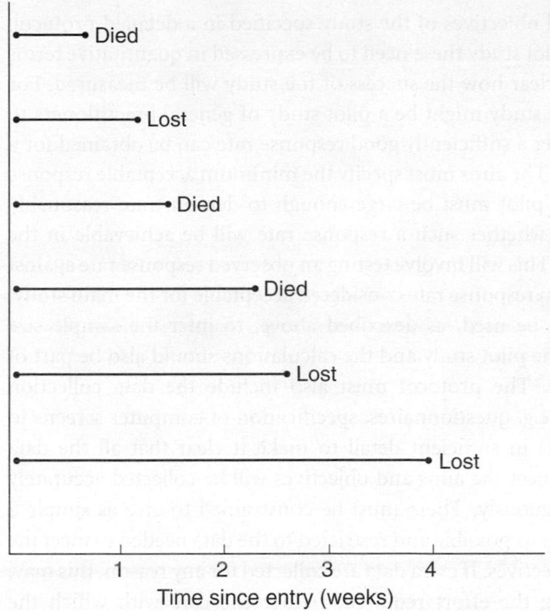

Fig. 30 Observation periods of subjects in a trial from time of entry.

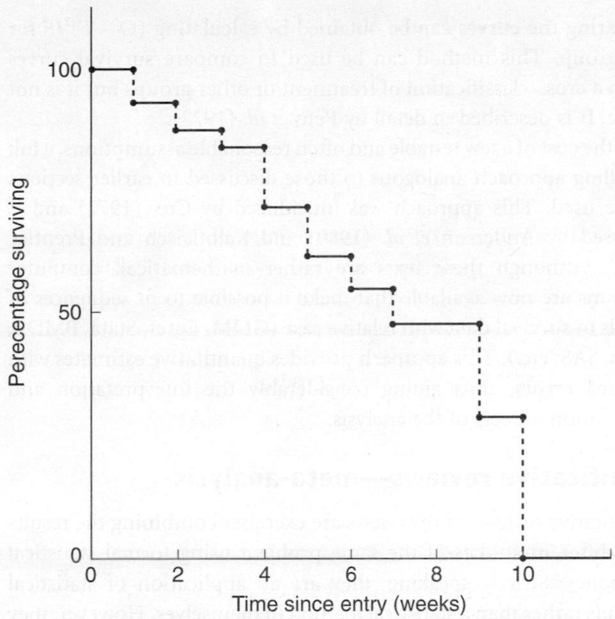

Fig. 31 Life-table survival curve for the radiotherapy group in a trial of treatments for cancer of the prostate.

horizontal scale gives a modified plot (Fig. 30) from which the number of subjects at risk and dying in each week since entry can be seen. In the first week after entry six subjects were at risk and one had died. This gives an estimated death rate of 0.17 and hence a survival rate of 0.83. In week 2 four were at risk all the time, one was at risk for half a week, and one died, giving a death rate of 1/4.5 = 0.22 and a survival rate for individuals reaching the second week of 0.78.

The chance of an individual surviving the second week, which requires that he or she survives both the first and the second weeks, is $0.83 \times 0.78 = 0.65$. This is the estimated cumulative survival rate. Plotting it against time from treatment gives the survival curve. Conventionally, individuals lost in any interval are treated as having been at risk for half the interval.

The life-table for cancer of the prostate patients in the radiotherapy group of a trial comparing radiotherapy and hormone treatments is given in Table 29. The adjusted number at risk is the number entering the interval minus half the number lost to observation during it. Plotting the percentage surviving S against the upper end of the time intervals gives the survival curve shown in Fig. 31. It is not appropriate to draw a smooth curve through the points since such curves give a spurious impression of accuracy.

Comparisons of a small number of survival curves can be made by hand using what is known as the 'log rank' test. On the hypothesis of no difference between two curves, the number of deaths expected in each group can be calculated. A χ^2 test on one degree of freedom

Table 29 Life-table for patients with cancer of the prostate in the radiotherapy group of a clinical trial

Time since entry (years)	Number died	Number at risk	Number lost	Adjusted number at risk	Estimated probability of Death	Estimated probability of Survival	Estimated proportion of survivors at end of interval
0–1	3	44	3	42.5	0.071	0.929	0.929
1–2	2	38	10	33.0	0.061	0.939	0.873
2–3	1	26	3	24.5	0.041	0.959	0.837
3–4	3	22	3	20.5	0.146	0.854	0.715
4–5	2	16	4	14.0	0.143	0.857	0.613
5–6	1	10	1	9.5	0.105	0.895	0.548
6–7	1	8	1	7.5	0.133	0.867	0.475
7–8	0	6	3	4.5	0.000	1.000	0.475
8–9	1	3	1	2.5	0.400	0.600	0.085
9–10	1	1	0	1.0	1.000	0.000	0.000

comparing the curves can be obtained by calculating $(O - E)^2/E$ for each group. This method can be used to compare survival curves within a cross-classification of treatment or other groups but it is not simple. It is described in detail by Peto *et al.* (1977).

At the cost of a few testable and often reasonable assumptions, a full modelling approach analogous to those discussed in earlier sections can be used. This approach was introduced by Cox (1972) and is discussed by Anderson *et al.* (1980) and Kalbfleisch and Prentice (1980). Although these texts are rather mathematical, computer programs are now available that make it possible to fit sequences of models to survival data with relative ease (GLIM, Egret, Stata, BMDP, S-plus, SAS, etc.). This approach provides quantitative estimates with standard errors, thus aiding considerably the interpretation and presentation aspects of the analysis.

Quantitative reviews—meta-analysis

Quantitative reviews or overviews are exercises combining the results from different studies of the same problem using formal statistical techniques. Strictly speaking, they are an application of statistical methods rather than a statistical method in themselves. However, they have become of increasing importance in making the best use of the results from several clinical trials assessing the same treatment and for combining observational studies investigating factors associated with a particular outcome. Consequently it would be remiss to neglect them in a discussion of statistical methods in public health. A good overview can be found in *The Handbook of Research Synthesis* (Cooper and Hedges 1994) and a good discussion of the role and use of meta-analysis is given by Pocock and Thompson (1991*a*), and the same authors give a clear account of the methods and assumptions involved in a paper entitled 'Can meta-analysis be trusted?' (Pocock and Thompson 1991*b*). Other useful general texts include Mosteller and Colditz (1996) and Normand (1999). Parmar *et al.* (1998) give, with examples, some useful techniques for extracting from published papers the results needed for an effective meta-analysis.

Effectively the statistical methods involved are the same as those discussed above using 'study', i.e. the study from which each part of the overall dataset was obtained, as a factor. If differences between exposed and unexposed, or treated and untreated, are not systematically different from one study, or category of studies, to the next, then it will be appropriate to obtain a single combined estimate of the effect of interest. This is done by calculating an overall pooled estimate of the effect of exposure or treatment using the results from the separate studies weighted appropriately to take their size into account. This will give a more precise estimate of the true effect. If the raw data can be obtained, such weighting is done automatically in a routine regression analysis. If the data are in the form of means, explicit weighting is required according to the numbers of observations involved. Data in the form of proportions or 2×2 tables can be combined using logistic regression. In the simpler cases a procedure known as the Mantel–Haenszel test, described fully by Schlesselman (1982), can be used. This and other techniques are available in a user-defined facility in Stata called Metan (Bradburn *et al.* 1998). A good example of an overview meta-analysis of the benefits of diuretics in pregnancy is given by Collins *et al.* (1985).

Design, data management, and analysis

Although surveys and other epidemiological studies may appear simple, it is easy to perform them ineffectively. The design stage needs the aims and objectives of the study specified in a detailed protocol. Even for a pilot study these need to be expressed in quantitative terms so that it is clear how the success of the study will be measured. For example, the study might be a pilot study of general practitioners to assess whether a sufficiently good response rate can be obtained for a major study. The aims must specify the minimum acceptable response rate and the pilot must be large enough to demonstrate reasonably conclusively whether such a response rate will be achievable in the larger study. This will involve testing an observed response rate against the minimum response rate considered acceptable for the main study. The test can be used, as described above, to infer the sample size needed for the pilot study and the calculations should also be part of the protocol. The protocol must also include the data collection documents (e.g. questionnaires, specification of computer screens to be used, etc.) in sufficient detail to make it clear that all the data required to meet the aims and objectives will be collected accurately and unambiguously. These must be constrained to give as simple a data structure as possible and restricted to the data needed to meet the aims and objectives. If extra data are collected for any reason, this may, by increasing the effort required, reduce the care with which the important information is recorded and may complicate the data-management system required, absorbing time and resources. The data will be wasted if they are not analysed, and, if analysed, they will effectively reduce the confidence that can be put in all positive findings. The last disadvantage arises because the more analyses performed the greater is the chance that a type I error (i.e. a false-positive finding) will occur. These are more important points than they might seem because most studies suffer from collecting too much data and very few indeed suffer from collecting too little. Finally, the protocol should have a section clarifying the analysis strategy and methodology to be used so that the needs of the analysis, in terms of data content and structure, and its appropriateness are given careful thought early in the design stage.

Data management can range from the relatively trivial (e.g. a survey where a single questionnaire is completed by an easily accessible sample of individuals and entered into the computer in a format immediately readable by the statistical packages to be used in the analysis) to the potentially very complex systems required for multicentre longitudinal studies following subjects recruited continuously and followed up for long periods. However, even the simplest case entry to the computer may introduce errors in the data, and systems of checking and verifying the process (e.g. double-entry verification) need to be employed. It is tempting to use routine commercial database packages for storing data from epidemiological studies, but there are dangers in this. Unless the package is like Epi-Info (Dean *et al.* 1994), which was specifically designed for such studies, it will be unlikely to include good data entry checking facilities. It may also, by tempting the user into using the 'electronic filing cabinet' facilities, lead to data being collected in a form that is quite inappropriate for statistical analysis (e.g. free-text responses, alphabetic variables potentially misspelt, individual subject data spread over an unpredictable number of separate records, etc.). There may be circumstances where all of these may be necessary, but they complicate the data management and analysis considerably and where possible they should be avoided. Statistical packages generally require what are known as 'flat' files where there are a fixed (i.e. constant) number of variable values for each individual study unit and the variable that each value represents is deducible from its position in the individual record. For example, the third value in every record may be a 1 or 2 indicating the individual's gender (1 for male, 2 for female), the 15th value their systolic blood pressure on entry to the study, and so on. Any system of data collection and storage must be designed so that the data can be converted into this form or the statistical analysis will become extremely difficult to organize and very time consuming.

The analysis will vary considerably according to the nature of the study. However, there are a few general principles which should guide the analysis strategy so that a process starting with possibly hundreds of variable values for each subject converges to a few appropriate and justifiable conclusions relevant to the aims and objectives of the study. Most analyses will be concerned with assessing whether some outcome (e.g. death, recovery, etc.) is systematically affected by some explanatory variable (e.g. exposure, treatment, etc.). This will generally require an analysis involving the comparison of regression models. A strategy is needed for deciding how to handle both outcome and explanatory variables in the analysis. The study protocol should have identified the outcome variable or variables to be studied in order to meet the aims. However, when several outcomes have been identified, as is often the case, it is necessary to identify which is of primary importance and how to deal with them overall. In most cases the best strategy is to identify the primary outcome variable and pursue the analysis right through with that. Other outcome variables should then be analysed on the same lines and the results of those analyses used in support of the conclusions that emerged from the main analysis. In this way the type I and type II errors can be considered as confined largely to the tests and decisions involved in the main analysis. The explanatory variables frequently generate an even larger problem. In many studies, even when experienced statisticians have been thoroughly involved in the design, information is collected on very large numbers of potential explanatory or *x* variables. Some of these will be of primary importance to the aims of the study (for example, the treatment in a clinical trial or the exposure of interest in an observational study). Others will be variables known to have an effect on the outcome of interest, such as age and sex in a study of blood pressure. In addition, there will probably be a number of variables which it was thought might affect outcome and hence have effects which could, by confounding, bias the estimation of the effects of interest. Estimating these confounding effects may even be a subsidiary part of the aims and objectives of the study.

A strategy for coping with large numbers of explanatory variables which is usually effective is to group them into three categories. The first includes such essential variables as those that must be present in the final analysis—the intervention, exposure variables implied by the study aims, and the confounding variables generally agreed to have an effect on the outcome under consideration whose effects cannot safely be assumed zero. The second category should contain the possibly interesting *x* variables whose effects could be assumed zero, in this study at least, if an analysis including the first category variables showed them to be unable to contribute any further explanatory effect on variation in the outcome variable. The third category, which in good studies would generally be empty, is for the variables on which information was collected just in case they might have an effect or because they seemed interesting and the marginal cost of collecting them had appeared very small to the questionnaire designer. Once collected, these variables should be included in the analysis or their collection will have been futile.

The overall strategy is first to assess, possibly in groups, whether variables from the third category contribute anything to explaining variation in the outcome variable after all variables in the first category, and possibly those in the second, have been taken into account. Only those third-category variables with a clear association with outcome in these analyses should be considered further. The remainder can be ignored in subsequent analyses and the finding reported as evidence that they appear not to have independent effects on outcome. Secondly, the effects of second-category variables need to be investigated systematically to assess which of them contribute anything to explain variation, beyond that contributed by the first-category variables and any from the third category that could not be ignored.

By this stage a modelling analysis should have focused on a manageable set of *x* variables whose independent effects, separately and combined, can be assessed from a single model. At this point, if not earlier, consideration should be given to investigating the possibility of interactions, or effect modifications as they are termed in the epidemiological literature. Until they have been assessed and shown to be negligible, any inferences concerning individual effects are based on an untested assumption that all interactions are zero. If significant interactions are found, the situation becomes quite complicated. For example, if the effect of treatment, say, is different in males from that found in females, this needs to be allowed for in all further analyses. The efficient way is to keep that interaction term in the model. In more complex situations with several interactions involving gender it may be easier, especially in the interpretation and presentation, to perform separate analyses for males and females. Comparing the results, identifying where they are similar and where different, is then a relatively clear way of presenting the results of a complex analysis of a complex dataset.

If it is assumed that interactions can be ignored or are taken into account appropriately, the remainder of the analysis is a process of testing the main effects of interest and obtaining their estimates and confidence limits for a clear presentation identifying the nature and import of the findings, focused clearly on those of most importance for the aims of the study.

In practice it is usually a good idea to develop the analysis system (i.e. stored sequences of commands for the chosen statistical package) on part of the data following the above strategy from beginning to end. This enables all the unforeseen pitfalls in the computing and analysis sequence to be identified early enough for solutions to be found before the full dataset is ready for analysis. The final analysis can then be completed quickly and efficiently as soon as the dataset is complete and results can be obtained while the data are young.

Conclusion

Obviously special problems require special techniques which cannot be discussed here. Nonetheless, the range of problems discussed and the appropriate analytical approaches cover the major part of statistical activity in public health research and epidemiology. With reasonable computing facilities, most practical problems can be tackled using these methods. More detailed texts covering most of the material presented here from a more traditional point of view are Armitage and Berry (1987), Altman (1991), and Bland (1987). In addition Clayton and Hills (1993) cover most of the methodology in this chapter and more from a slightly different, and helpful, perspective in their excellent text *Statistical Models in Epidemiology*. Finally, *A Dictionary of Statistical Terms* (Marriott 1990) and the excellent *Encyclopedia of Biostatistics* (Armitage and Colton 1998) provide clear explanations of all relevant statistical terms and methods.

References

Altman, D.G. (1991). *Practical statistics for medical research.* Chapman & Hall, London.

Anderson, S., Auquier, A., Hauck, W., Oakes, D., Vandaele, W., and Weisberg, H.I. (1980). *Statistical methods for comparative studies.* Wiley, New York.

Andrews, N.J. and Swan, A.V. (1994). A sample size investigation system using GLIM4. *GLIM Newsletter*, **23**, 4–11.

Armitage, P. (1960). *Sequential medical trials.* Blackwell Scientific, Oxford.

Armitage, P. and Berry, G. (1987). *Statistical methods in medical research.* Blackwell Scientific, Oxford.

Armitage, P. and Colton, T. (1998). *Encyclopedia of biostatistics*, Volumes 1–6. Wiley, Chichester.

Bland, M. (1987). *An introduction to medical statistics.* Oxford University Press.

Bradburn, M.J., Deeks, J.J., and Altman, D.A. (1998). Metan—an alternative meta-analysis command. *Stata Technical Bulletin*, **44**, 4–15.

Breslow, N.E. and Day, N.E. (1980). *Statistical methods in cancer research.* Vol. 1: *The analysis of case–control studies.* IARC Scientific Publication 32, International Agency for Research on Cancer, Lyon.

British National Lymphoma Investigation (1975). Value of prednisone in combination chemotherapy of stage IV Hodgkin's disease. *British Medical Journal*, **iii**, 413.

Casagrande, J.T., Pike, M.C., and Smith, P.G. (1978). An improved approximate formula for calculating sample sizes for comparing two binomial distributions. *Biometrics*, **34**, 483.

Clayton, D. and Hills, M. (1993). *Statistical models in epidemiology.* Oxford University Press.

Collins, R., Yusuf, S., and Peto, R. (1985). Overview of randomised trials in pregnancy. *British Medical Journal*, **290**, 17–22.

Cooper, H. and Hedges, L.V. (1994). *The handbook of research synthesis.* Sage, Thousand Oaks, CA.

Cox, D.R. (1972). Regression models and life tables (with discussion). *Journal of the Royal Statistical Society B*, **34**, 187.

Dean, A.G., Dean, J.A., Coulombier, D., *et al.* (1994). *Epi Info, Version 6.* Centers for Disease Control and Prevention, Atlanta, GA.

Dixon, W.J. (ed.) (1981). *BMDP statistical software.* University of California Press, Berkeley, CA.

Forni, A. and Sciame, A. (1975). Chromosome and biochemical studies in women occupationally exposed to lead. *Archives of Environmental Health*, **35**, 139.

Francis, B., Green, M., and Payne, C. (ed.) (1993). *The GLIM System Release 4 Manual.* Oxford University Press.

Kalbfleisch, J. and Prentice, R.L. (1980). *The statistical analysis of failure time data.* Wiley, New York.

Lachin, J.M. (1981). Introduction to sample size determination and power analysis for clinical trials. *Clinical Trials*, **1**, 93.

Lindley, D.V. and Miller, J.C.P. (1964). *Cambridge elementary statistical tables.* Cambridge University Press.

Marriott, F.H.C. (1990) *A dictionary of statistical terms.* Longmans, Harlow.

Mehta, C. and Patel, N. (1992). *StatXact.* Cambridge.

Mosteller, F. and Colditz, G.A. (1996). Understanding research synthesis (meta-analysis). *Annual Review of Public Health*, **17**, 1–23.

Nelder, J.A. and Wedderburn, R.W.M. (1972). Generalised linear models. *Journal of the Royal Statistical Society A*, **135**, 370.

Normand, S.L.T. (1999). Meta-analysis: formulating, evaluation, combining, and reporting. *Statistics in Medicine*, **18**, 321–60

Parmar, M.K.B., Torri, V., and Stewart, L. (1998). Extracting summary statistics to perform meta-analyses of the published literature for survival endpoints. *Statistics in Medicine*, **17**, 2815–34.

Peto, R., Pike, M.C., Armitage, P., *et al.* (1977). Design and analysis of randomised clinical trials requiring prolonged observation of each patient. II: Analysis and examples. *British Journal of Cancer*, **35**, 1.

Pocock, S.J. (1983). *Clinical trials—a practical approach.* Wiley, Chichester.

Pocock, S.J. and Thompson, S.G. (1991*a*). The role of meta-analyses in clinical and epidemiological research. In *Coronary heart disease epidemiology: from aetiology to public health* (ed. M. Marmot and P. Elliott). Oxford University Press.

Pocock, S.J. and Thompson, S.G. (1991*b*). Can meta-analysis be trusted? *Lancet*, **338**, 1127–30.

Pocock, S.J., Shaper, A.G., Cook, D.G., *et al.* (1980). British Regional Heart Study—geographical variation in cardiovascular mortality and the role of water quality. *British Medical Journal*, **280**, 1243.

Pocock, S.J., Cook, D.G., and Beresford, S.A.A. (1981). Regression of area mortality rates on explanatory variables: what weighting is appropriate. *Journal of Applied Statistics*, **30**, 286.

Ryan, T.A., Joiner, B.L., and Ryan, B.F. (1981). *Minitab reference manual.* Minitab Project, Pennsylvania.

Schlesselman, J.J. (1982) *Case–control studies—design, conduct, analysis.* Oxford University Press.

Snedecor, G.W. and Cochran, W.G. (1967). *Statistical methods* (6th edn). Iowa State University Press, Ames, IA.

SPSS (1990). *SPSS.* Chicago, IL.

Stata Corporation (1993). *Stata reference manual. Release 3.1* (6th edn). Stata Corporation, College Station, TX.

Statistics and Epidemiology Research Corporation and Cytel Software Corporation (1992). *Egret.* Seattle, WA.

Whitehead, J. (1992). *The design and analysis of sequential clinical trials.* Ellis Horwood, London.

Yates, F. (1934). Contingency tables involving smaller numbers and the χ^2 test. *Journal of the Royal Statistical Society*, **1** (Supplement), 217.

6.14 Mathematical models of transmission and control

Roy Anderson and D. James Nokes

Introduction

The aim of this chapter is to show how simple mathematical models of the transmission of infectious agents within human communities can help to aid the interpretation of observed epidemiological trends, to guide the collection of data towards further understanding, and to help in the design of programmes for the control of infection and disease. A central theme is to improve understanding of the interplay between the variables that determine the typical course of infection within an individual and the variables that control the pattern of infection and disease within communities of people. This theme hinges on an understanding of the basic similarities and differences between different infections in terms of the number of population variables (and consequent equations) needed for a sensible characterization of the system, the typical relations between the various rate parameters (such as birth, death, recovery, and transmission rates), and the form of expression that captures the essence of the transmission process.

Model construction, whether mathematical, verbal, or diagrammatic, is in principle the conceptual reduction of a complex biological or population-based process into a more simple idealized and easily understandable sequence of events. Consequently, the use of mathematical modelling as a descriptive and interpretative tool is a very common exercise in scientific study. Its use, therefore, in epidemiological study should not be viewed as intrinsically difficult or beyond the comprehension of those trained in medical or biological disciplines. The reductionist approach, inherent in model construction, which helps to define processes clearly and identify the most important components of a system, is employed in many areas of public health research and practice. The following situations, for example, are all likely to involve, at the very least, the implicit use of models to simplify and aid understanding: the assessment of the cause and severity of sporadic epidemics of *Salmonella* or hepatitis A virus food poisoning or Legionnaires' disease; the cost-effectiveness analysis of various measures used to combat an infection within a hospital, within a community, countrywide, or globally; or the identification of the factors that control the maintenance of an endemic infection within a community.

Most epidemiological problems, by definition, are concerned with the study of populations and so involve quantitative scores of, for example, abundances and rates of spread. Thus it is invariably necessary to convert any descriptive model of process into a more formal mathematical framework so that we work with numbers and not words. The use of a more formal structure enables us to incorporate quantitative estimates of abundances or rates, derived from experiment or field observations, into the model and to make predictions of the likely behaviour of the system under varying conditions, particularly when we are concerned with the introduction or alteration of measures to control infection or disease.

It is the step of translation from verbal or diagrammatic description into a formal mathematical framework that arouses the deepest suspicions amongst medical or public health workers. Quite naturally this response is in part a consequence of the use of, what is to many, a strange symbolism to describe familiar verbal or conceptual identities. It must be remembered, however, that mathematics is the most precise language we have available for scientific study and once a problem is formulated in mathematical terms many techniques are available to pursue the logical consequences of the stated assumptions. The clear and unambiguous statement of assumptions is of course a particular attribute of mathematical, as opposed to verbal, description. Excessive use of symbolism or formal methods of analysis can confuse as opposed to clarify and it must be admitted that some sections of the mathematical epidemiological literature have drifted from their original moorings and sail free from the constraints of data or relevance. But to jump from this observation to the belief that mathematical models have nothing to contribute in practice to the design of public health programmes is a mistake. Sensibly used, mathematical models are no more and no less than tools for thinking about things in a precise way.

The second area of suspicion, aside from symbolism, concerns simplification. A frequent criticism of mathematical work in epidemiology is that model formulation involves too many simplifying assumptions despite known biological complexity. This is often true, and needs to be remedied, but it is in part a consequence of the infancy of the discipline and, in some cases, a result of inadequate quantitative understanding of a particular problem. There are, however, two important counter-arguments to the criticism of simplification. Firstly and most importantly, it is often the case in biological study that a few processes dominate the generation of observed pattern despite the fact that many more can, to a lesser degree, influence the outcome. The identification of the dominant processes is an important facet of model construction and, what is termed, sensitivity analysis. The second point concerns scientific method. The process of understanding the consequences of a series of simple assumptions and building upon this by slowly adding complexity is directly analogous to the laboratory scientist's approach of carefully controlling most variables and allowing a few to vary in a planned design. Carefully building complexity on a simple framework can greatly facilitate our understanding of the major factors that influence or control a particular process or pattern.

The chapter is organized as follows. The second section following this introduction provides a brief review of the historical development of mathematical epidemiology and outlines the types of infection that will be considered in latter sections. The third section addresses the problems of model construction, design, and application. The fourth section examines the major concepts in quantitative epidemiology that have been derived from mathematical study, such as threshold host densities for the persistence of an infection, the basic reproductive rate, and herd immunity. In the fifth section methods are explored by which to obtain some of the basic epidemiological parameters from empirical observation. The sixth section turns to applied problems and considers the use of models in the design of control strategies for infection and disease, and the final section is reserved for concluding thoughts. Throughout, mathematical details are kept to a bare minimum and the reader interested in technical details of model construction and analysis is referred to papers in specialist journals.

Historical perspective

The application of mathematics to the study of infectious disease appears to have been initiated by Daniel Bernoulli in 1760 when he used a mathematical method to evaluate the effectiveness of the techniques of variolation against smallpox (Bernoulli 1760). Further interest did not occur until the middle of the nineteenth century when, in 1840, William Farr effectively fitted a normal curve to smoothed quarterly data on deaths from smallpox in England and Wales over the period 1837 to 1839 (Farr 1840). This empirical approach was further developed by John Brownlee (1906) who considered in detail the 'geometry' of epidemic curves. The origins of modern mathematical epidemiology owe much to the work of Hamer, Ross, Soper, Kermack, and McKendrick who, in different ways, began to formulate specific theories about the transmission of infectious disease in simple but precise mathematical statements and to investigate the properties of the resulting models (Ross 1911; Kermack and McKendrick 1927; Soper 1929). The work of Hamer (1906), Ross (1911), Soper (1929), and Kermack and McKendrick (1927) led to one of the cornerstones of modern mathematical epidemiology via the hypothesis that the course of an epidemic depends on the rate of contact between susceptible and infectious individuals. This led to the so-called 'mass-action' principle in which the net rate of spread of infection is assumed to be proportional to the density of susceptible people multiplied by the density of infectious individuals. In turn this principle generated the celebrated threshold theory according to which the introduction of a few infectious individuals into a community of susceptibles will not give rise to an epidemic outbreak unless the density or number of susceptibles is above a certain critical value (see the review by Fine (1993)).

Since these early beginnings the growth in the literature has been very rapid and reviews have been published by Bailey (1975), Becker (1979), Anderson and May (1985*c*, 1991), Dietz (1987), and Scott and Smith (1994). In more recent work there has been an emphasis on the application of control theory to epidemic models (Wickwire 1977), the study of the spatial spread of the disease (Cliff *et al.* 1993), the investigation of the mechanisms underlying recurrent epidemic behaviour (Anderson and May 1982), the importance of heterogeneity in transmission (Anderson and May 1985*a*), the formulation of stochastic (probabilistic) models (Ball 1983), the formulation of models for indirectly transmitted infections with complex lifecycles (Anderson and May 1985*b*; Rogers 1988), the study of sexually transmitted infections such as gonorrhoea and HIV (Hethcote and Yorke 1984; Anderson *et al.* 1986; May and Anderson 1987), and the development of models for infectious agent transmission in developing countries with positive net human population growth rates (Anderson *et al.* 1988; McLean and Anderson 1988*a*,*b*). Such theoretical work is beginning to play a role in the formulation of public health policy (Babad *et al.* 1995) and the design of control programmes (Nokes and Anderson 1991) but there is a need in future work for greater emphasis on data-oriented studies that link theory with observation.

In the following sections we attempt to give a flavour of recent work and to distil the major conclusions that have emerged in particular areas. We have deliberately chosen to concentrate on directly transmitted viral and bacterial infections that constitute the major infectious diseases of children in developed countries and, as a consequence of the recent pandemic of AIDS, sexually transmitted infections. Our reasons are simply that the mathematical models are more highly developed in these fields by comparison with others (e.g. vector-borne infections), that theory has close contact with empirical epidemiological data in these areas, and that model structure is somewhat simpler than for other infections such as metazoan parasites.

Model construction

Definition of terms

Epidemiology

Epidemiology as a subject is concerned with the study of the 'behaviour' of an infection or disease within a population or populations of hosts (= humans). 'Behaviour' refers to observed patterns such as the incidence (the rate at which new cases arise or are reported) of infection or disease. Examples of 'behaviour' are epidemics (a rise and subsequent fall in incidence) and endemicity (the stable maintenance of infection within the human community). The aim of the discipline is to determine the underlying processes and understand the interactions between them, that generate observed patterns (e.g. the rate of spread of infection and the pattern of susceptibility to infection). Epidemiology is a quantitative discipline that draws on statistical techniques for parameter estimation and mathematical methods for delineating the dynamic changes that occur through time, across age classes, or over different spatial locations. The discipline also makes use of modern molecular (e.g. DNA probes and polymerase chain reaction) and immunological (measures of the abundances of antibodies specific to an infectious agent's antigens) techniques for the detection and quantification of current and past infection or disease.

Populations

The definition and description of the host and parasite populations is of obvious importance in epidemiological studies. A population is an assemblage of organisms of the same species (or genetic type etc.) which occupy a defined point or points in the plane created by the dimensions of space and time. The basic unit of such populations is the individual organism (i.e. parasite or human host). Populations may be divided (= stratified) into a series of categories or classes, the members of which possess a unifying character or characters such as age, sex, or their stage of development. Such subdivisions may be made on spatial or temporal criteria to distinguish a local population from a larger assemblage. The boundaries in space, time, and genetic constitution between different populations are often vague, but it is important to define what constitutes the 'study population' as clearly as possible.

The natural history of infection

Mathematical models are often used to depict the rate of spread or transmission of an infectious agent through a defined human community. For their formulation three broad classes of information are required.

1. The modes and rates of transmission of the agent.
2. The typical course of events within an individual following infection.
3. The demographic and social characteristics of the human community.

The mode of transmission (i.e. direct, indirect, horizontal, vertical, etc.) is of obvious importance (Table 1), but if there is more than one route the relative efficiency of each in determining overall transmission must be understood. When considering microparasitic infections (e.g. viruses, bacteria, and protozoa that multiply directly within the host) it is generally not possible to measure the pathogen abundance within the host (i.e. the burden or intensity of infection). However, following invasion it is important to obtain quantitative information on the typical durations of the latent and infectious periods of the infection and the incubation period of the disease it induces. As depicted in Fig. 1, the latent period is defined as the average period of time from the point of infection to the point when an individual becomes infectious to others, the infectious period denotes the average period over which an infected person is infectious to others, and the incubation period defines the average period from infection to the appearance of symptoms of disease. In practice all these periods are variable between individuals, depending on factors such as the size of the inoculum of the infectious agent that initiates infection, the genetic background of host and parasite, past experience of infections, and the nutritional status of the host. The use of an average is an economy of thought and where knowledge permits models should be based on distributed latent and infectious periods. In some instances the infectious period may be influenced by patient management practices such as the confinement of an infected person once symptoms of infection are diagnosed (e.g. measles and tuberculosis).

There are instances in the case of viral and bacterial infections when a knowledge of pathogen abundance within blood, excretions, secretions, and other tissues or organs of the host can be of importance in determining the infectivity of an infected person to susceptible contacts. A good example is provided by HIV-1. Current evidence suggests that the infectiousness of an infected person varies greatly over the long and variable incubation period of the disease AIDS that the virus induces (Fig. 2). It is believed on the basis of recorded fluctuations in HIV antigenaemia that a short period of high infectiousness occurs shortly after infection, followed by a long period of low to negligible infectiousness (perhaps many years) before infectiousness again increases as the infected patient develops symptoms of AIDS (Anderson and May 1988). In these cases rather complex models are required to mirror the natural history of infection (Anderson 1988).

The human immune response to infection, its ability to confer protection against reinfection, and the duration of this protection have important implications for model construction. For the majority of childhood viral infections the assumption of lifelong immunity following recovery appears to be correct. However, as one moves up a scale of parasite structural (antigenic) complexity from viruses to bacteria to protozoa in general the duration of acquired immunity

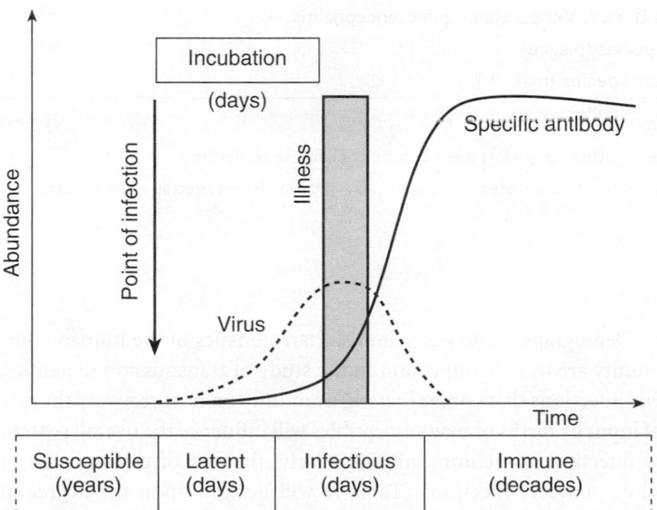

Fig. 1 Schematic representation of the typical time-course of an acute viral or bacterial infection in a host individual and the corresponding progression through infection classes (note the different time durations within each of these classes). (Source: Nokes and Anderson 1988.)

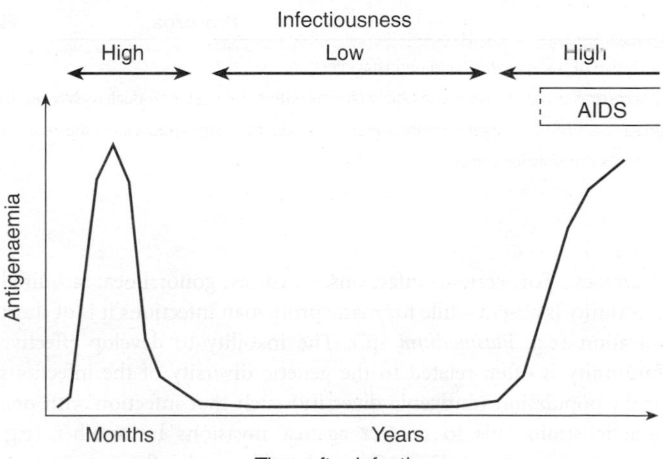

Fig. 2 Possible changes in HIV-1 concentration in the blood of an infected individual (antigenaemia) and in the associated degree of infectiousness during the long incubation period of AIDS

Table 1 Epidemiological classification of infectious diseases of public health importance in developed countries

Mode of transmission	Type of parasite	Examples (diseases or agents)
VERTICAL[a]	Micro[b]	
	Viruses	Rubella, hepatitis B, cytomegalovirus, retroviruses
	Protozoa	*Toxoplasma gondii*
HORIZONTAL		
Direct		
Close contact	Micro	
	Viruses	Measles, mumps, rubella, Epstein–Barr virus, herpes simplex-1, respiratory syncytial virus, influenza-2, varicella, common cold
	Bacteria	Diphtheria, pertussis, bacterial meningitis
	Macro[c]	
	Nematodes	*Enterobius vermicularis* (pinworm)
Environmental	Micro	
	Viruses	Hepatitis A, polio, Coxsackie
	Bacteria	Tetanus, *Shigella*, *Salmonella*, typhoid, cholera, Legionnaires' disease
	Protozoa	*Giardia intestinalis*, amoebiasis
	Macro	
	Nematodes	Pinworm
Sexual	Micro	
	Viruses	Hepatitis B, HIV, herpes simplex-2, cytomegalovirus
	Bacteria	*Neisseria gonorrhoeae*, syphilis
	Protozoa	*Trichomonas vaginalis*
Not direct		
Via other host species (zoonoses)	Micro	
	Virus	Rabies
	Protozoa	*Toxoplasma gondii*
	Macro	
	Nematodes	*Toxocara species*
	Cestodes	*Taenia solium*, *T. saginata*, *Echinococcus granulosus* (hydatid)
Vector-borne[d]	Micro	
	Viruses	Hepatitis B, HIV, Venezuelan equine encephalitis
	Bacteria	*Yersinia* species (plague)
	Protozoa	*Plasmodium* species (malaria)

[a]Inclusive of transplacental and perinatal infection.

[b]Microparasites are those that multiply directly within the host individual, usually resulting in acute infections and subsequent durable immunity to reinfection.

[c]Macroparasites are larger parasites whose reproductive stages pass out of the host. Infection intensity is thus a process of accumulation, and can be measured as worm burden.

[d]Needle transmission is included.

decreases. For certain infections, such as gonorrhoea, acquired immunity is absent while for many protozoan infections it is of short duration (e.g. *Plasmodium* sp.). The inability to develop effective immunity is often related to the genetic diversity of the infectious agent population (antigenic diversity) such that infection with one genetic strain fails to protect against invasions by another (e.g. *Neisseria gonorrhoea*, *Neisseria meningitidis*, and influenza viruses). The question of immunity can be complicated by a degree of cross-immunity (non-specific in character) resulting from infection by dissimilar organisms (e.g. many bacterial infections of the respiratory tract).

Demographic and behavioural characteristics of the human community are usually important in the study of transmission dynamics. For infections that confer lifelong immunity on host recovery the rate of input by births of new susceptibles will influence the overall pattern of infection in a community. Similarly, the rate of transmission of 'close contact' infections (Table 1) will depend upon the degree of mixing between individuals and the density and age distribution of susceptibles and those infected. Heterogeneity in behaviour within a community is of particular importance in the study of sexually transmitted infections since rates of sexual partner change vary greatly between individuals (Johnson *et al.* 1992, 1994). More generally, heterogeneity in any behaviour, whether sexual or social mixing, must be captured in model formulation.

It will be clear from the preceding comments that much quantitative detail about the natural history of infection must be understood for accurate model formulation. In many instances such detail is not available, but model formulation can greatly facilitate our knowledge of what needs to be understood to define the transmission dynamics of a given infection. With respect to many childhood viral and bacterial infections, such as measles, rubella, mumps, pertussis, and diphtheria, a great deal is understood about the natural history and, hence, much of the work on mathematical models has focused on those infections. Their direct route of transmission, their tendency to induce lifelong immunity, plus, in most cases, the availability of serological or virological techniques to detect past or current infection facilitates the acquisition of quantitative data.

Units of measurement

The unit of measurement employed in epidemiological study depends on the type of infection. The most basic unit is that of the individual parasite. As already discussed, in most cases this unit is not a practicable option for microparasitic organisms due to difficulties in detection and quantification (however, advances in molecular biology and biochemistry are generating new techniques which may be of value in the near future). As such, the most useful unit is that of the infected host which allows the human community to be stratified on the basis of whether individuals are susceptible, infected but not yet infectious (= latent or pre-patent), infectious, and recovered (= immune in the case of many viral infections). Infection may be detected directly (e.g. DNA probes, virus, or bacterial culture) or indirectly by the presence of antibodies specific to pathogen antigens (serological and salivary tests). Seropositivity does not necessarily discriminate between infected and recovered individuals, but for many viral and bacterial infections serological surveys of a population, perhaps stratified by age, sex, and other variables carried out longitudinally (through time via cohort monitoring) or horizontally (across age classes) provide a key measure of transmission and the broad epidemiological characteristics of the infection.

What models describe

At any point in time a population may be classified by the density or number of susceptible, infected, and immune individuals. With the passing of time and concomitantly as individuals age, people may move from one infection class to the next. As such, with the recruitment of new susceptibles by birth and, in some cases, the loss of

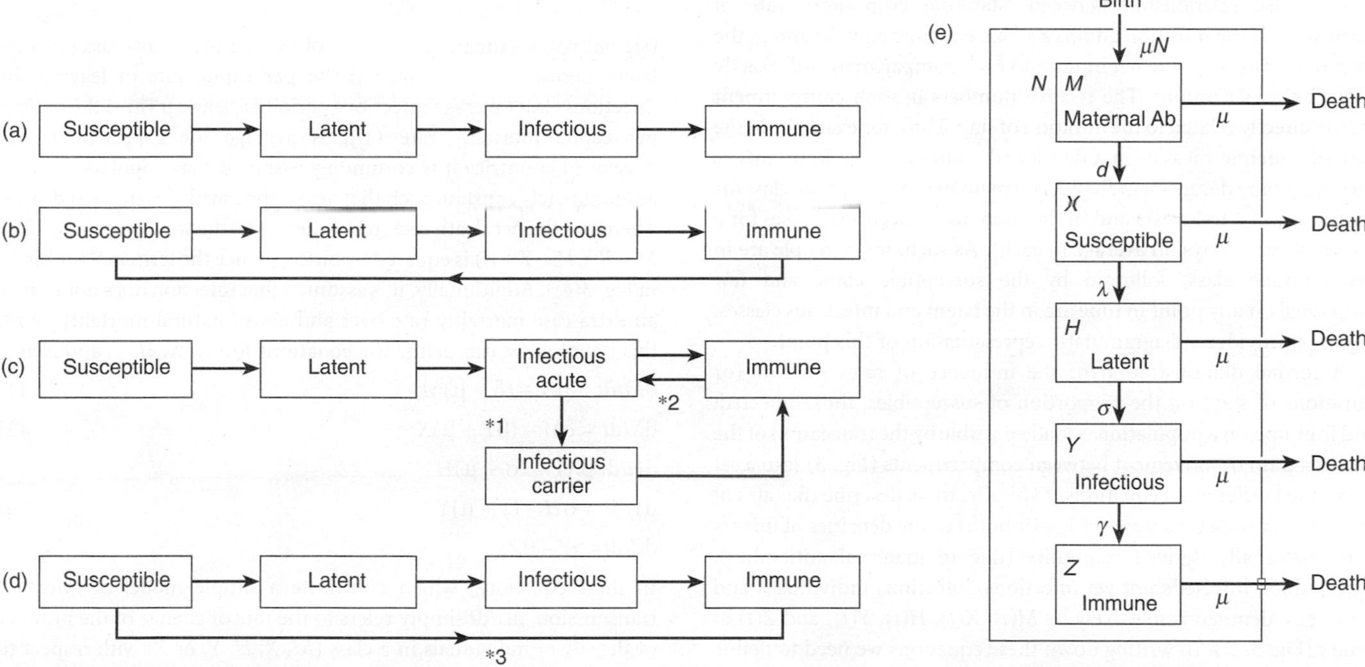

Fig. 3 Flow diagrams used to describe the movement of individuals within populations compartmentalized according to infection status to particular parasitic agents. (a) Simple model for infections inducing lasting immunity (e.g. measles, mumps, rubella, yellow fever, and poliomyelitis) or (b) in which immunity is transient and individuals subsequently return to the susceptible pool (e.g. *Neisseria gonorrhoea*, typhoid, cholera, *Trichomonas vaginalis*). (c) Many infections persist within the host for long periods of time, during which the infected individual may remain infectious (1), as is the case for carriers of hepatitis B virus, gonorrhoea, *Salmonella typhi*, and *Treponema pallidum* (syphilis), chronic tuberculosis patients, or during recrudescence of herpes viruses and malaria. The epidemiological importance of this characteristic is that it enables the perpetuation of such infections in low density communities (see discussion of the mass-action principle in the text). For other infections immunity is defence against disease but not asymptomatic reinfection (2) from which new infectious individuals arise (e.g. *Haemophilis influenzae* and *Neisseria meningitidis*). (d) Vaccination (3) has the effect of transferring individuals directly from the susceptible to the immune class. (e) More detailed description of the transmission dynamics of an acute microparasitic infection which explicitly accounts for births and deaths in the population. All neonates are born possessing maternally derived protective antibody. The net birth rate is assumed to equal the sum of the net death rates for each subpopulation (compartment), that is, births = μN, where $N = M + X + H + Y + Z$ = constant population size. The per capita rates defining movement between infection classes are described in the text.

immunity, the population structure is a dynamic process with individuals flowing from one class to the next. Mathematical models of transmission attempt to capture the dynamic nature of these changes in the form of difference (discrete time steps) or differential (continuous time) equations (Scott and Smith (1994) give a simple introduction). With respect to microparasitic infections where the population is stratified or compartmentalized by infection status, the resulting models are often referred to as compartmental models. The types and numbers of compartments will depend upon the type of infectious agent and the details of its natural or life history. A number of examples are recorded in Fig. 3 in the form of flow diagrams. These diagrams form a useful intermediary step between biological comprehension and mathematical formulation.

Population rates of flow

Following the introduction of an infection into a stable population the number or density of individuals within the various infection compartments will depend on the rates of flow between compartments such as infection and recovery rates. The size of a population in a specific compartment will depend on the magnitude of those rates that determine the entry and duration of stay. In general, the shorter the duration of stay (the higher the rate of leaving) in a particular compartment the smaller the size of the population in that category (the inverse relationship between 'standing crop' and 'rate of turnover'). If the infection attains a stable endemic equilibrium in the human community, the net input into each compartment will exactly balance the net output. The relative numbers in each compartment will be directly related to the duration of stay. Thus, for example, in the case of endemic measles in a developed country where immunity is lifelong (many decades), individuals remain in the susceptible class for an average of 4 to 5 years and in the latent and infectious classes for a few days (say 7 days on average in each). As such, most people are in the immune class, followed by the susceptible class, and few individuals at any point in time are in the latent and infectious classes. Figure 4 provides a diagrammatic representation of this point.

A formal demonstration of the influence of rates of flow (or durations of stay) on the proportion of susceptibles, those infected, and immunes in a population is made possible by the translation of the flow diagram of movement between compartments (Fig. 3) into a set of coupled differential equations. Typically, these describe the rates of change with respect to time (or age or both) of the densities of infants with maternally derived immunity (due to maternal antibodies), susceptibles, infecteds not yet infectious, infectious individuals, and immunes, denoted respectively by $M(t)$, $X(t)$, $H(t)$, $Y(t)$, and $Z(t)$ at time t (Fig. 3(e)). In writing down these equations we need to define the rates of flow between compartments by a series of symbols. For example, in common notation δ (delta) defines the loss of maternally derived immunity, i.e. the average per person rate of loss of passive protection. The absolute rate of loss from or movement out of class M (Fig. 3) requires that the per capita rate (i.e. person/unit of time) be multiplied by the size of the M subpopulation, that is δM (which has units of persons/unit of time). If δ is the per capita rate of movement out of class M then the average duration of maternally derived immunity is $1/\delta$. These principles apply to the other rate terms shown in Fig. 3(e). Hence, using conventional symbols, β (beta) is the transmission coefficient that defines the probability of contact and infection transfer between a susceptible and infectious person, σ (sigma) defines the per capita rate of leaving the latent class (average latent period $1/\sigma$), γ (gamma) the per capita rate of leaving the infectious class (average infectious period $1/\gamma$), and μ (mu) the natural per capita mortality rate ($1/\mu$ is average life expectancy). For developed countries it is commonly assumed that population size is approximately constant such that net births exactly balance net deaths. Therefore the net death rate, μN (where N is the total population size $M + X + H + Y + Z$) is equated by births (hence the term mN for births in Fig. 3(e)). Additionally, it is assumed that infection does not induce an extra case mortality rate over and above natural mortality. With this notation we can define the equations for M, X, H, Y, and Z as

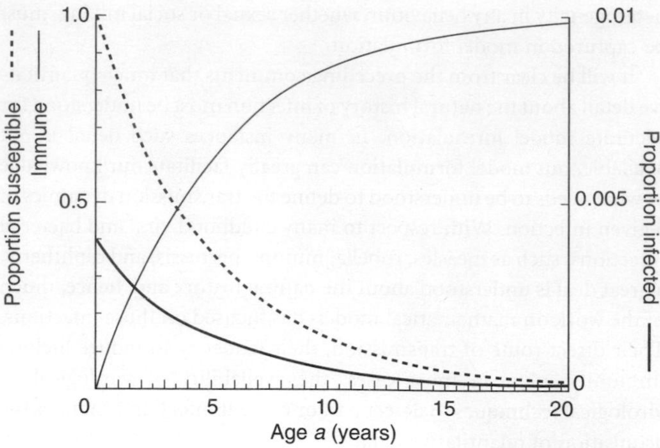

Fig. 4 The proportions of a population who are in the susceptible, infected (either latent or infectious), and immune classes for a typical childhood viral infection. In this example, which is based on measles, the force of infection, λ = 0.2 per year (corresponding to an average age at infection of 5 years) and the rate of movement from the latent class, σ, and recovery from infectiousness, γ, is 52 per year (corresponding to an average duration of stay in each of these infected classes of 1 week). Note that the proportion of the population in the infected classes is always much less than that in the susceptible or the immune classes (Fig. 1).

$$dM/dt = \mu N - (\delta + \mu)M \quad (1)$$

$$dX/dt = \delta M - (\beta Y + \mu)X \quad (2)$$

$$dH/dt\ \beta XY - (\sigma + \mu)H \quad (3)$$

$$dY/dt = \sigma H - (\gamma + \mu)Y \quad (4)$$

$$dZ/dt = \gamma Y - \mu Z. \quad (5)$$

In these equations, which constitute a simple model of infection transmission, $d\square/dt$ simply refers to the rate of change of the number or density of individuals in a class (M, X, H, Y, or Z) with respect to (over) time. The right-hand side of each of these equations then expresses precisely what the rate of change is. For a simple introduction to the definition, manipulation, and interpretation of such differential equations in the epidemiological context, the reader is referred to Scott and Smith (1994). The major assumptions incorporated in the above equations are that the net rate of infection βXY is proportional to the density of susceptibles multiplied by the density of infectious individuals, that individuals leave each compartment at a constant per capita rate (other than for the susceptible class, X, (see below)) because it is assumed that the per person rates δ, μ, σ, and γ, do not change over time, and that net births exactly balance net deaths (reasonably accurate for developed countries). To explore what these assumptions imply in terms of the dynamics of transmission and the numbers or proportions of individuals in each class we need to solve these equations either analytically to obtain explicitly expressions for $M(t)$, $X(t)$, $H(t)$, $Y(t)$, and $Z(t)$ in terms of the rate parameters and the variable time (t) or numerically to generate projections of changes in the numbers in each compartment through time (Scott and Smith 1994). In the case of simple models we can often obtain exact analytical solutions as is the case for the equation for $M(t)$ in the model defined by eqns (1) to (5). The solution gives us the number of infants with maternally derived protection at time t, $M(t)$:

$$M(t) = \{(\mu N)/(\mu + \delta)[1 - e^{-(\mu+\delta)}t]\} + M(0)e^{-(\mu-\delta)}t \tag{6}$$

where $M(0)$ is the number protected at time $t = 0$.

More generally, the complexity of the life histories of many infections makes analytical solution difficult or impossible and numerical methods are required. Modern computers make light work of very complex systems of equations describing disease transmission and many software packages are available for the solution of sets of differential equations and now for model making. Nevertheless, in these cases some general analytical insights can be obtained by examining the equilibrium properties of the model which is done by setting the time derivatives (i.e. the d/dt) equal to zero, that is such that there are assumed to be no further changes in the number of individuals within each infection class because the flows into and out of any one category are equal. These equations can then be solved to determine the numbers at equilibrium (i.e. at stable endemicity) in each class (referred to as M^*, X^*, H^*, Y^*, and Z^*). For example, in the simple model of eqns (1) to (5) by simple algebraic manipulation we obtain

$$M^* = \mu N/(\delta + \mu) \tag{7}$$

$$X^* = (\sigma + \mu)(\gamma + \mu)/\beta\sigma \tag{8}$$

$$H^* = (\gamma + \mu)Y^*/\sigma \tag{9}$$

$$Y^* = (\delta M^* - \mu X^*)/\beta X^* \tag{10}$$

$$Z^* = \gamma Y^*/\mu \tag{11}$$

where N is the constant representing the total population size. These equilibrium solutions illustrate how the various rate parameters that determine flow between compartments influence the numbers of individuals in each compartment when the infection is at an endemic steady state. For example, based upon the assumptions in our model for an acute childhood infection (eqns (1)–(5)), we can suggest that at endemic equilibrium the number or density of individuals in the maternal antibody class, M^*, is directly dependent upon the net rate of births (where births equal deaths, μN) and inversely related to the rate of loss from the class ($\delta + \mu$) (where $1/(\delta + \mu)$ is the average duration in the maternal antibody protected class).

Parameter estimation

The preceding section provided a clear illustration of the numerous parameters that are necessary to define even the simplest model of direct transmission within a human community. To make the best use of a model it is desirable to have available estimates for each of the parameters for a given infection. Some, such as the demographic rates of birth and mortality and total population size, can be easily obtained via national census databases (usually finely stratified by age and sex in developed countries). Others, such as the average latent and infectious periods, must be determined either by clinical studies of the course of infection in individual patients (e.g. measures of change in viral abundance during the course of infection) or by detailed household studies of case-to-case transmission. Statistical methodology plays an important role in this instance since, as noted earlier, latent, infectious, and incubation periods are rarely constant from one individual to the next. Statistical estimation procedures have been developed to help derive summary statistics of these distributions (e.g. means and variances) (Bailey 1975).

Invariably, the most difficult parameter to estimate is the transmission coefficient β (see eqn (2)), which is a measure of the rate of contact between members of a population plus the likelihood of infection resulting from contact. In some cases, such as certain sexually transmitted infections (e.g. gonorrhoea), direct estimates can be obtained via contact tracing methods (Hethcote and Yorke 1984). More commonly, indirect methods must be employed, often themselves based on model formulation and analysis. A simple example employs the model defined in the previous section by eqns (1) to (5). We can define the component βY of the transmission term as the per capita rate at which susceptibles (X) acquire infection. This rate is commonly referred to as the 'force of infection' and denoted by the symbol λ (lambda). Analysis of the model reveals that the average age at which an individual typically acquires infection, A, is approximately related to the force of infection by the expression

$$A \approxeq 1/\lambda. \tag{12}$$

Hence if we can estimate A from an age-stratified serological profile or from age-defined case-notification records (Box 1) we can, via eqn (12), estimate λ. More generally, this rate often varies with age and more complex methods of estimation must be employed given good age-stratified serological data (see Grenfell and Anderson 1985). Put in simple terms, if the proportion susceptible at age $a + 1$ is $x(a + 1)$ then the force of infection over the age interval $a \rightarrow a + 1$ (defined per unit of age) is simply

$$\lambda = -\ln[x(a + 1)/x(a)]. \tag{13}$$

With serological data finely stratified by age, under the assumption that the infection confers lifelong immunity upon recovery, eqn (13) can be used to estimate how λ changes with age in a given community. For most childhood viral and bacterial infections λ is a function of age, changing from low values in infant classes to high in child to young teenage classes back to low in adult age classes (Fig. 5). This is thought to reflect patterns of intimate contact via attendance at school and play activities.

Further complications may arise if rates of contact or transmission vary through time, perhaps due to seasonal factors such as the aggregation and dispersal of children at term and school holiday periods (Yorke *et al.* 1979; Anderson 1982; Bolker and Grenfell 1993). The problems of parameter estimation are considered in more detail in a later section.

Concepts in quantitative epidemiology

The incidence of infection and disease

Transmission by direct contact and the law of mass action

When close contact between infectious and susceptible individuals is necessary for transmission, the number of new cases in a population which arise in a unit of time (i.e. incidence of infection) is often

Box 1 Surveillance profiles

Two infections (i) and (ii) are at endemic equilibrium (i.e. roughly constant incidence in time) in a stationary host population (i.e. births are equal to deaths). The changes, with time or increasing age, in the proportion of the population that has experienced each infection may be estimated from longitudinal cohort or horizontal cross-sectional surveys (serological or case notifications) of individuals from birth to life expectancy L.

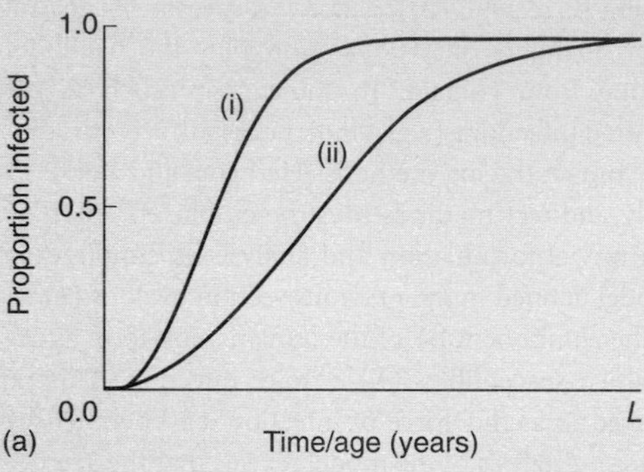

The steeper profile of (i) compared with (ii) is an indication that the basic reproductive potential R_0 of infection (i) exceeds that for infection (ii) such that

R_0(i) R_0(ii).

Assume that each infection induces lifelong immunity; then, from the above profiles, changes with age/time in the proportion x susceptible to each infection are as shown in figure (b)

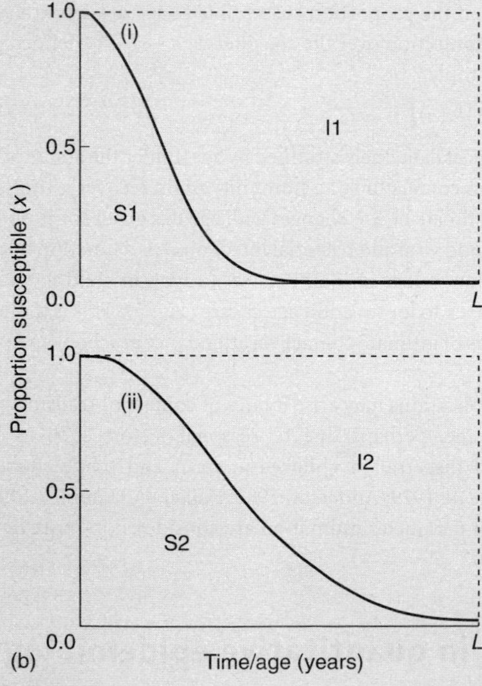

The (equilibrium) proportion of the total population susceptible to infection (i) is

x^*(i) = area S1/(area S1 area I1)

and for infection (ii) it is

x^*(ii) area S2/(area S2 area I2).

Note that the equilibrium proportion susceptible to infection (i) (with the higher reproductive rate) is smaller than that for infection (ii) (with a lower rate of reproduction), i.e.

$x^*(\text{i}) < x^*(\text{ii})$.

The relationship between these two epidemiological parameters may be usefully expressed as

$R_0(\text{i}) = 1/x^*(\text{i})$

and

$R_0(\text{ii}) = 1/x^*(\text{ii})$.

Summing the proportion susceptible, $x(a)$, in the above graphs for each age class from age 0 years (time 0) to L years, we can determine the average age at infection, A:

$x(a) = x(0) + x(1) + x(2) + \ldots + x(L) = A = S$

from which it can be seen that

$A(\text{i}) < A(\text{ii})$.

Note also that

$R_0(\text{i}) = L/A(\text{i}) = L/S1$

and

$R_0(\text{ii}) = L/A(\text{ii}) = L/S2$.

(See also eqns (12) and (13), and Anderson and May (1983), for estimation of the force of infection from surveillance profiles.)

Summary examples

Assume infection (i) is measles and infection (ii) is rubella in the United Kingdom with average lifespan L of 75 years. If S1 = 5 and S2 = 10, then $A(\text{i})$ = 5 years and $A(\text{ii})$ = 10 years, and

$x^*(\text{i}) = 5/75 = 0.066'$ $x^*(\text{ii}) = 10/75 = 0.133'$.

Therefore

$R_0(\text{i}) = 1/0.066' = 15$

or

$R_0(\text{i}) = 75/5 = 15$

and

$R_0(\text{ii}) = 1/0.133' = 7.5$

or

$R_0(\text{ii}) = 75/10 = 7.5$.

The implications of this difference in the basic reproductive rate of infection to the proportion of the population that must be vaccinated in order to eradicate each infection can be seen in Fig. 11.

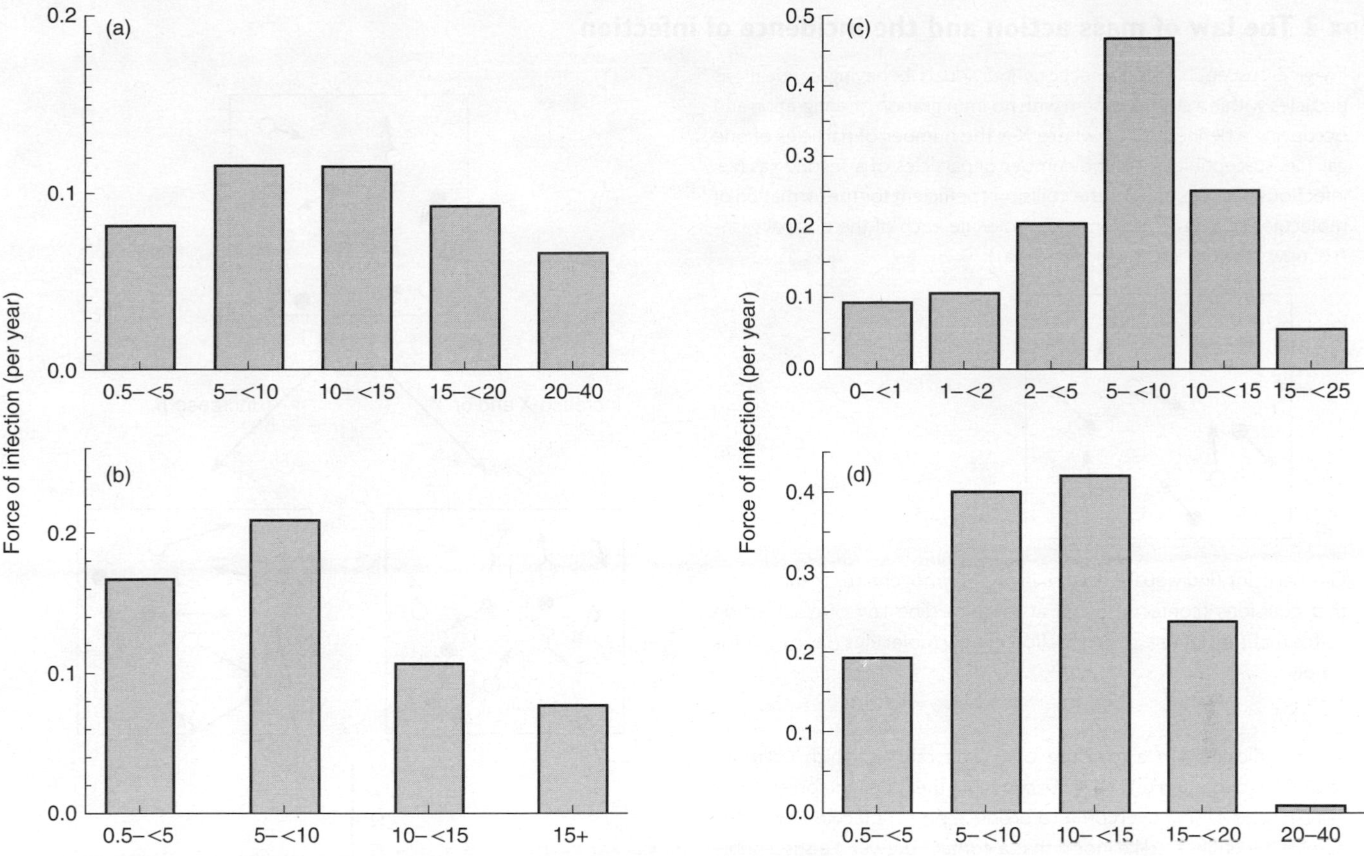

Fig. 5 Examples of the age-dependent nature of the per susceptible rate of transmission for common childhood viral and bacterial infections. Graphs (a) and (b) derive from horizontal cross-sectional serological surveys in the United Kingdom, of rubella (Nokes *et al.* 1986) and mumps (Anderson *et al.* 1987) respectively. Graphs (c) and (d) provide estimates based on case-notification data for England and Wales for whooping cough (Anderson and May 1985*b*) and measles (Grenfell and Anderson 1985) respectively.

assumed to be approximately given by the density (or number) of susceptibles, X, multiplied by the density (or number) of infectious persons, Y, multiplied by the probability of an effective (infectious) contact between an infectious person and a susceptible, β (i.e. βXY). This relationship is commonly referred to as the 'law of mass action' by analogy with particles colliding within an ideal gas system (Box 2). The basic assumption implicit in this concept is that the population mixes in a random manner (often referred to as homogeneous mixing). The term βXY which describes net transmission is the major non-linear expression in most compartmental models of directly transmitted viral and bacterial infections. It is, of course, a crude approximation of what actually occurs in human communities and more realistic refinements of this assumption are discussed in later sections. However, it provides a convenient point of departure for model construction and analysis.

The transmission coefficient β

The probability of transmission, β, is made up of two components, namely the rate at which contacts occur between susceptible and infectious persons and the likelihood that transmission will result from a contact. Consequently β is dependent on sociological and behavioural factors within the host population (i.e. rate of mixing) and the biological properties that determine the infectiousness of an infected person and the susceptibility of an uninfected individual. These biological properties involve factors such as the virulence of the infectious agent and the genetic background plus the nutritional status of the human host.

Incidence estimates

The incidence of infection, I, can be measured by direct observation of new cases, such as notifications of measles or pertussis. Unfortunately, however, measures of incidence tell us nothing about the respective densities of susceptibles or infectious people, nor the magnitude of the transmission coefficient β. It is common practice in epidemiology for I to be expressed as the number of cases per unit of population (usually 100 000 people in a defined class, such as age or sex) over a defined period of time such as 1 year (e.g. 5/100 000 per annum). Such measures are often referred to as attack rates (**AR**). However, they are a rather poor measure of the intensity of transmission within a population since they take no account of the proportion of the community (or age or sex class) that is susceptible to infection (Box 3). A better measure of the rate at which susceptibles acquire infection is provided by a parameter termed 'the force of infection' commonly denoted by the symbol λ. It simply defines the probability that a susceptible individual will acquire infection over a short period of time (i.e. a per susceptible (= per capita) rate of infection) and, in the terminology of the mass-action principle, is defined as $\lambda = \beta Y$. Here β might be thought of as the force of infection for one infectious person

Box 2 The law of mass action and the incidence of infection

Imagine susceptible and infectious individuals behaving as ideal gas particles within a closed system with no immigration or emigration and occupying a defined space, where X is the number of particles of one gas (i.e. susceptibles), Y is the number of particles of a second gas (i.e. infectious people), and β is the collision coefficient for the formation of molecules of a new gas from one molecule each of the original gases (i.e. new cases of infection) (figure (a)).

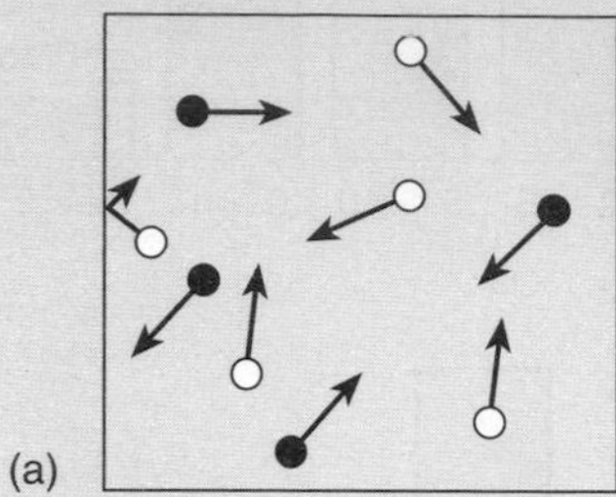

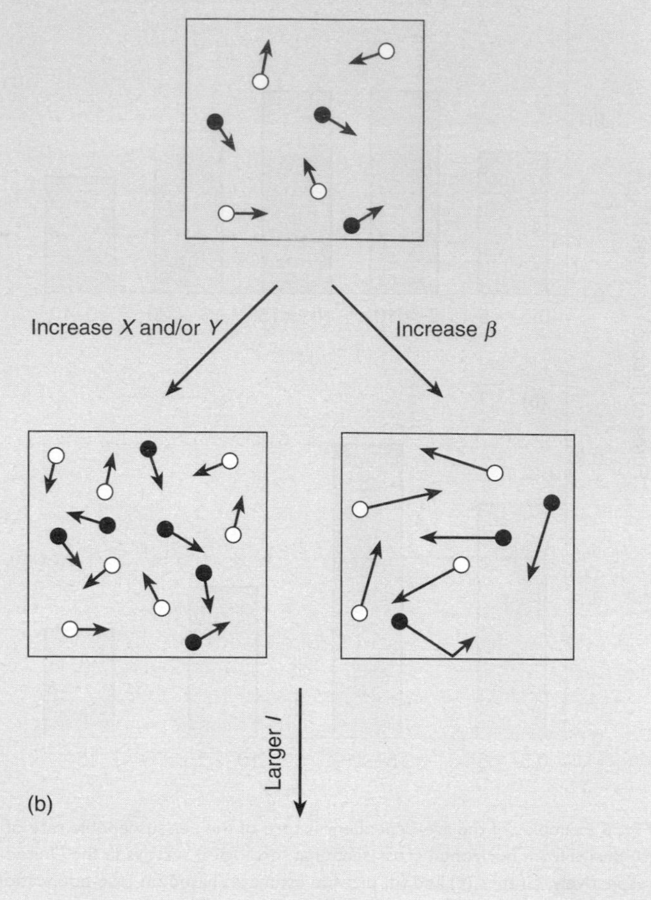

Gas particles (individuals) are mixing in a homogeneous manner such that collisions (contacts) occur at random. The law of mass action states that the net rate of production of new molecules (i.e. cases), I, is simply

$$I = \beta XY.$$

The coefficient β is a measure of (i) the rate at which collisions (contacts) occur and (ii) the probability that the repellent forces of the gas particles can be overcome to produce new molecules, or, in the case of infection, the likelihood that a contact between a susceptible and an infectious person results in the transmission of infection. Under these assumptions, the incidence of infection will be increased by larger numbers (or densities) of infectious and susceptible persons and/or high probabilities (β) of transmission (figure (b)).

in a community. Estimates of this rate λ can be derived from age-stratified serological profiles or case notifications (Anderson and May 1983, 1991; Grenfell and Anderson 1985) (Fig. 5).

Validity of the mass-action principle

Despite the simplicity of the notion of homogeneous mixing implicit in the mass-action principle of transmission, the predictions of simple compartmental models based on this assumption often mirror observed epidemiological patterns surprisingly well (Anderson and May 1982). In part, this is a consequence of increased travel, movement, and mixing within many societies in developed countries. Measles epidemics, for example, are often synchronous in England and Wales, with a clear distinction in all parts of these regions between years of high incidence and years of low incidence (Fig. 6). However, the less able an infection is to spread through a particular population (lower R_0, see below) then the more important are slight deviations from homogeneous mixing, resulting in a lower degree of synchrony of epidemics in a country (Fig. 7). The assumption is most appropriate for infections which are spread by close contact between individuals such as respiratory infections transmitted by contaminated droplets and nasopharyngeal secretions. In such cases, the survival of the infectious agent in the external environment is of very short duration (i.e. minutes). As such, there is no significant reservoir of infectious stages to maintain transmission in the absence of infectious persons.

Many kinds of heterogeneities can invalidate the mass-action principle and much attention in recent years has been devoted to their inclusion in compartmental models. The major sources are heterogeneities arising from age-related factors, that determine contact and mixing patterns (i.e. 'who mixes with whom') and spatial factors such as differences in population densities in urban and rural areas of a country (Anderson and May 1984, 1991; May and Anderson 1984). Such sources of heterogeneity are very important in the design of control policies based, for example, on mass vaccination and models have been developed to assess their impact.

Heterogeneity in behaviour is of particular importance in the study of sexually transmitted infections such as gonorrhoea and HIV. One of the major determinants of the rate of spread of such infections is the distribution of the rate of sexual-partner change within a defined community (Fig. 8). These distributions are typically highly heterogeneous in character (i.e. the variance in the rate of partner change is much greater in value than the mean rate of partner change) where most people have few different sexual partners in a lifetime (or over a defined period of time) and a few have very many. The activities of individuals in the 'tail' of the distribution (the highly sexually active)

Box 3 Interpreting attack rates

Care should be exercised when interpreting attack rates in the absence of information on the proportion of individuals within the population who are immune as a result of previous infection (assuming we are considering an infection such as measles that induces lasting immunity on recovery). A simple illustrative example is given below based on case notification for measles.

Age (years)	Attack rate per head of population in that age class	Percentage immune in the age class	Modified attack rate based on infection per head of the susceptible population
2	180/100 000	10	180/90 000
10	20/100 000	90	180/90 000

At a first glance at column 2, the attack rate suggests that infants aged 2 years have a much greater chance of acquiring infection than children aged 10 years. However, if we adjust the denominator of the attack rate from per head of population in that age class to per head of susceptible population in the age class, we see from the fourth column that the rate of infection is identical in both age classes.

are clearly important for the persistence and spread of infection since those with many partners are both more likely to acquire infection and more likely to transmit it to others.

Simple theory based on compartmental models of the transmission of infections such as gonorrhoea and HIV assumes that the net rate at which infection is spread in, for example, a male homosexual community is determined by the proportion of infectious persons

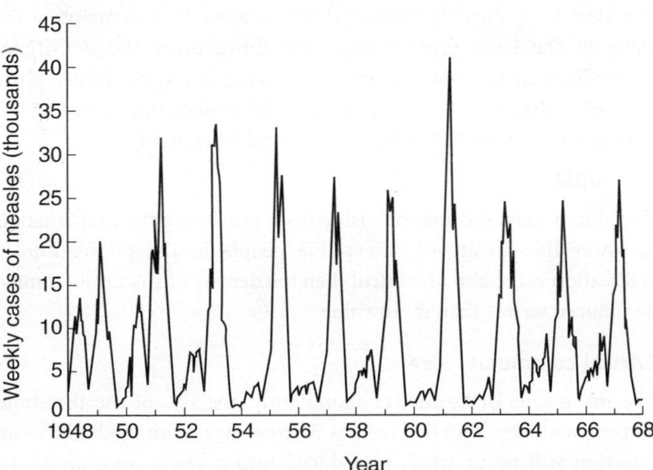

Fig. 6 The number of cases of measles reported each week in England and Wales between 1948 and 1968. (Source: Office of Population Census and Surveys, London.)

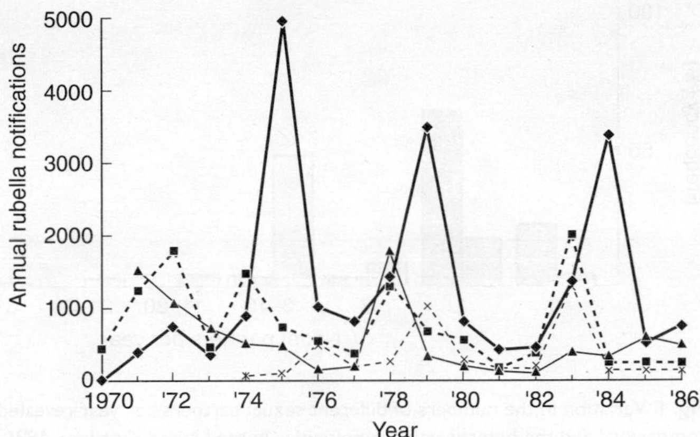

Fig. 7 Annual rubella case notifications reported by four city health authorities in England: Leeds (♦), Bristol (■), Manchester (▲), and Newcastle (×). The dominant interepidemic period is roughly 4 to 5 years with peak incidence often slightly out of phase between cities (compare with Fig. 6). (Source: Communicable Disease Surveillance Centre, London.)

(Y/N where N is the total size of the sexually active population) multiplied by the density of susceptibles (X) multiplied by a transmission coefficient β. This coefficient is defined as the probability that a sexual contact (per partner) results in transmission, B, multiplied by the effective rate of sexual-partner change, c (which determines contacts). If the population mixed homogeneously, this effective rate would simply be the mean rate of sexual-partner change, m. When great heterogeneity in rates of partner change is present within a population the effective rate must be defined in terms of this variability as well as the mean rate of activity. If we assume that the population is divided into classes with different rates of partner change and that partners are chosen (from any class) in proportion to their representation in the population multiplied by the rate of partner change in each group (an assumption of 'proportional mixing' (Anderson *et al.* 1986; May and Anderson 1987; Garnett *et al.* 1992; Gupta and Anderson 1992)), then the effective rate of partner change, c, is given by

$$c = m + (s^2/m) \tag{14}$$

where m is the mean rate of partner change and s^2 is the variance in the rate. The importance of variability in contact is clear from this simple equation. For example, suppose the mean rate per year is unity but the variance is five times greater. If we assumed that homogeneous mixing occurred our estimate of the effective rate would be 1, but if we take account of heterogeneity the effective rate is six times as large. The influence of the small proportion of highly sexually active individuals on the overall transmission rate is very significant.

Transmission thresholds and the basic reproductive rate of infection

The basic reproductive rate of infection R_0

A key measure of the transmissibility of an infectious agent is provided by a parameter termed the basic reproductive rate (or, also in the literature, basic reproduction number or ratio) and denoted by the symbol R_0. It measures the average number of secondary cases of infection generated by one primary case in a susceptible population.

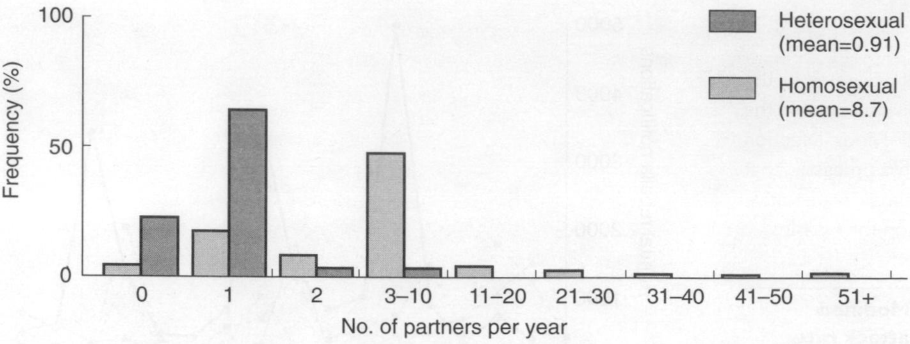

Fig. 8 Variation in the numbers of different sexual partners per year revealed from surveys of the male homosexual and the heterosexual communities in the United Kingdom, 1986 (Anderson 1988). The skewed distribution observed in each instance (an indication that although the majority of individuals have few partners, a few have very many), and the mean rate of sexual-partner change (indicated), are both of significance to the perpetuation and rate of spread of sexually transmitted diseases in the community.

Its value is defined by the number of susceptibles present with which the primary case can come into contact (X) multiplied by the length of time the primary case is infectious to others, D, multiplied by the transmission coefficient, β (rate of effective mixing):

$$R_0 = \beta XD. \tag{15}$$

Note that R_0 is a dimensionless quantity (i.e. the units of measurement cancel out) that defines the potential to produce secondary cases (in a totally susceptible population) per generation time (i.e. the average duration of the infection).

The basic reproductive rate is of major epidemiological significance since the condition $R_0 = 1$ defines a transmission threshold below which the generation of secondary cases is insufficient to maintain the infection within the human community. For values above unity the infection will trigger an epidemic and, with a continual input of susceptibles, will result in endemic persistence. A further quantity of interest is the effective reproductive rate R which defines the generation of secondary cases in a population which contains susceptibles and immunes (as opposed to just susceptible individuals). If the prevalence or incidence of infection is stable through time, the effective reproductive rate R must equal unity in value a situation in which each primary case gives rise, on average, to a single secondary infectious individual.

Factors that influence R_0

The simple expression $R_0 = \beta XD$ (appropriate for directly transmitted infections under the mass-action assumption) provides a framework for assessing how different epidemiological factors influence transmission success. Clearly, high transmission coefficients, long periods of infectiousness, and high densities of susceptibles enhance the generation of secondary cases. Note that its value depends not only on the properties that define the course of infection in an individual (i.e. the duration of infectiousness, D), but also on attributes of the host population such as the density of susceptibles, X, and the component of β that determines the rate of contact or mixing. A good example of the influence of population level characteristics is provided by the rate of transmission of the measles virus in urban centres in developed and developing countries. The more rapid rise in the proportion of children who have experienced infection, with age, in developing countries by comparison with developed regions is in part a consequence of higher population densities and poorer living conditions (McLean and Anderson 1988*a*).

Principles of control

The threshold condition for persistence of an infection, defined by $R_0 = 1$, captures the essence of the problem of control. To eradicate an infection we must reduce the value of the basic reproductive rate below unity. Similarly, to reduce incidence the value of R_0 must be reduced below the level that pertains prior to the introduction of control measures. Reductions can be achieved by reducing the infectious period D by, for example, the isolation of infectious persons (perhaps recognized by clinical symptoms of disease), reducing the number or density of susceptibles, usually by immunization, and by altering the social and behavioural factors that determine transmission such as improving living conditions to reduce overcrowding (in the case of sexually transmitted infections, education can serve to reduce rates of sexual-partner change or promote the use of condoms to lower the probability of transmission).

The threshold density of susceptibles

It is clear from the definition of R_0 given above that to maintain the value of the basic reproductive rate above unity the density of susceptibles in the population must exceed a critical value. More precisely, this critical level X_T is (for the mass-action assumption) obtained by setting $R_0 = 1$ in eqn (15) and rearranging:

$$X_T = 1/\beta D. \tag{16}$$

The aim of mass vaccination, aside from protecting the individual, is to lower the density of susceptible people in the population. If eradication is the aim of control then the density of susceptibles must be reduced to less than X_T in value.

Critical community size

The magnitude of R_0 and, concomitantly, the size of the threshold density of susceptibles determines whether or not an epidemic of an infection will occur when introduced into a given community. In practice, however, for infections that induce lasting immunity in those who recover, the long-term endemic persistence of infection will depend on the renewal of the supply of susceptibles by new births or, to a lesser extent, by immigration. As such, the net birth rate in a community, which is itself dependent on the total population size (or density), will influence the likelihood of persistence. There is, therefore, a critical community size for the endemic persistence of a given infection. In certain island communities, immigration of susceptibles and infectious individuals may also play a role in the long-term persistence of a given infection (Black 1966; Anderson and May 1986, 1991). These factors are of growing significance as rates of population movement increase as a result of, for example, improved air transport services. Table 2 provides an example of the relationship between community size and the likelihood of the endemic persistence of the measles virus.

The concepts of a threshold density of susceptibles and a critical community size are most relevant for directly transmitted viral and bacterial infections that induce lasting (= lifelong) immunity. The production of long-lived infective stages or the use of vectors (such as mosquitoes) lessen the importance of the human population density for the persistence of an infection. In the case of sexually transmitted infections, simple models suggest that there is no critical density of susceptibles for persistence since the magnitude of R_0 can be approximately given by

$$R_0 = BcD \tag{17}$$

where c is the effective rate of sexual-partner change, D is the average duration of infectiousness, and B is the transmission probability per partner contact (Anderson *et al.* 1986). This is simple to arrive at theoretically. If, as stated earlier, the incidence of cases of a sexually transmitted disease is defined as

$$I = BcXY/N \tag{18}$$

then following the introduction of a single infectious person ($Y = 1$), infectious over a period D, into a totally susceptible population ($N = X$), the number of secondary cases will be represented by eqn (17).

The dependence upon the number of susceptibles is lost. Biologically this is more difficult to grasp, but it does seem reasonable that the rate of sexual-partner change should be more important to the potential for spread of a sexually transmitted disease than the number of susceptibles in the population.

Table 2 Island community size and endemic persistence of measles

	Population size (units of 100 000)	Percentage of months in which no cases were reported
Hawai	5.50	0
Fiji	3.46	36
Iceland	1.60	39
Samoa	1.18	72
Solomon	1.10	68
Fr. Polynesia	0.75	92
New Caledonia	0.68	68
Guam	0.63	20
Tonga	0.57	88
New Hebrides	0.52	70
Gilbert and Ellice	0.40	85
Greenland	0.28	76
Bermuda	0.41	49
Faroe	0.34	68
Cook	0.16	94
Niue	0.05	95
Nauru	0.03	95
St Helena	0.05	96
Falkland	0.02	100

Source: Anderson (1982*b*).

Regulation of infection within human communities

The regulation (i.e. modulation or control) of the incidence or prevalence of a particular infection within a human community is largely determined by the level of herd immunity (i.e. the proportion of the population immune to infection) and the net rate of input of new susceptible individuals. A simple example serves to illustrate this point. Consider a closed population with no inflow or outflow of susceptible, infected, or immune individuals. If the densities of susceptibles, infecteds, and immunes at time t are defined by $X(t)$, $Y(t)$, and $Z(t)$ respectively, then under the mass-action assumption of transmission the rates of change in the densities with respect to time can be captured by three coupled differential equations:

$$\mathrm{d}X/\mathrm{d}t = -\beta XY \tag{19}$$

$$\mathrm{d}Y/\mathrm{d}t = \beta XY - \gamma Y \tag{20}$$

$$\mathrm{d}Z/\mathrm{d}t = \gamma Y. \tag{21}$$

It is assumed here that there is no latent period of infection (individuals are infectious once infected), that the average duration of infectiousness is given by $D = 1/\gamma$ where γ is the rate of recovery from infection, that immunity is lifelong, and that no losses occur due to mortality. If we start with a totally susceptible population and introduce a few infecteds, the occurrence of an epidemic will depend upon the magnitude of the basic reproductive rate R_0 ($R_0 = \beta XD$) and, concomitantly, whether or not the density of susceptibles exceeds the critical threshold value X_T ($X_T = 1/\beta D$) (Fig. 9). Assuming that R_0 is greater than unity then an epidemic will occur, but as time progresses the density of susceptibles will decline ($X \rightarrow Y \rightarrow Z$) until the effective reproductive rate R is less than unity (i.e. susceptible numbers fall below the threshold X_T) and the infection dies out.

For the persistence of the infection one of two things must happen. Firstly, suppose susceptibles are continually introduced into the population at a net rate bN where b is the per capita birth rate and that natural mortalities occur in each class at a per capita rate μ. For simplicity we further assume that net births exactly balance net deaths ($bN = \mu N$) to maintain the total population at a constant size. With these assumptions and provided that $R_0 \geqslant 1$, we find that the infection persists in the population (Fig. 10(a)) with an endemic equilibrium density of susceptibles again equal to X_T and equilibrium densities of infecteds, Y and immunes, Z, given by

$$Y^* = [\mu/(\mu + \gamma)](N - X_T) \tag{22}$$

$$Z^* = (\gamma/\mu)Y^*. \tag{23}$$

Secondly, suppose that there are no new births and no mortality but that immunity is of short duration such that individuals leave the immune class Z to regain the susceptible class X at a per capita rate α

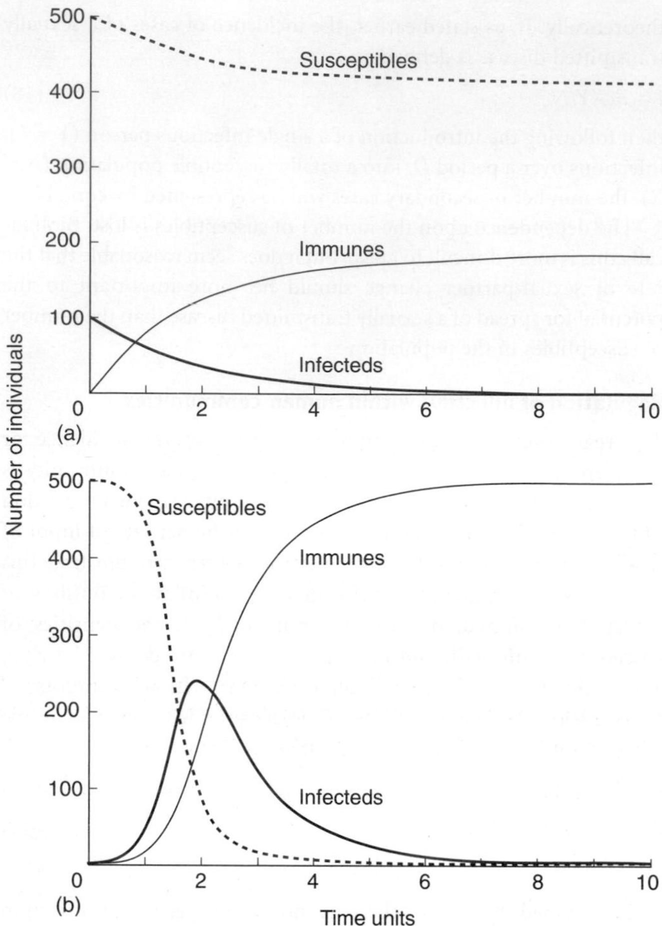

Fig. 9 Conditions for an epidemic. (a) Host density (susceptibles) below the threshold level (at time 0, $X = 500$, $Y = 100$, $Z = 0$, $\beta = 0.0001$, $\gamma = 1$, $R_0 = 0.005$, XT 10000). (b) Host density above the threshold level (at time 0, $X = 500$, $Y = 1$, $Z = 0$, $\beta = 0.01$, $\gamma = 1$, $R_0 = 5$, $XT = 100$).

(alpha) where $1/\alpha$ is the average duration of immunity. We again find that the infection can persist (Fig. 10(b)) (provided that $R_0 \geqslant 1$) with equilibrium densities of infecteds and immunes of

$$Y^* = [\alpha/(\alpha + \gamma)](N - X_T) \tag{24}$$

$$Z^* = (\gamma/\alpha)Y^*. \tag{25}$$

Note that the faster the loss of immunity (α large) the higher the equilibrium density of infecteds and the lower Z^*.

These two examples show how the net input of susceptibles and the degree of herd immunity (as controlled by the duration of immunity to reinfection following recovery) influence the likelihood that an infection will persist endemically after the initial epidemic has swept through a susceptible population following the introduction of an infection. In these simple models of the transmission of direct-contact infections, the density of infecteds tends to exhibit oscillatory behaviour after the introduction of infection due to the rise and fall in the density of susceptibles taking the effective reproductive rate above and below unity in value. These oscillations are seen to damp down, settling to the equilibrium values given analytically (e.g. eqns (22)–(25)). This propensity to exhibit oscillatory behaviour is more apparent if the infection is of short duration such that infection prevalence is sensitive to the availability of susceptibles and induces long-lasting immunity since it takes some time, under these circumstances, for new births or loss of immunity to replenish the supply of susceptibles such that R is again above unity in value. Maintenance of these oscillations over the longer period would require a force to be applied periodically—in reality this might derive from seasonal changes in mixing rates as a result of school opening and closing. In Fig. 10 it should be noted that the numbers infected, Y, are always increasing when susceptibles, X, exceed the threshold X_T (thus $R < 1$) and are always on the decrease when $X < X_T$ (when $R < 1$). Hence, infection is being driven by the availability of susceptibles.

Other factors that can promote long-term persistence include the production of infective stages that are able to survive for long periods

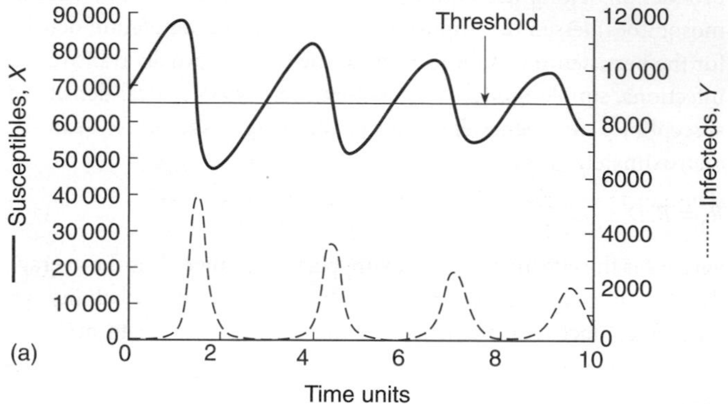

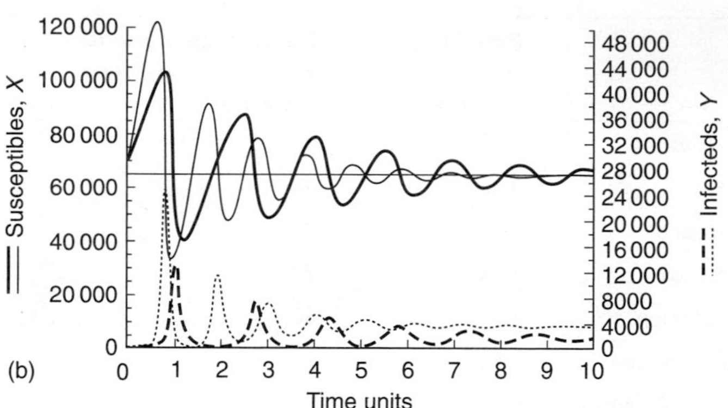

Fig. 10 Conditions for the persistence of an infection in a community. In each case solid curves represent susceptible numbers and dashed lines are infected. (a) Renewal of susceptibles by births (initial conditions: $X = 70\,000$, $Y = 1$, $Z = 930\,000$, $\beta = 0.0004$, $\gamma = 26$, $\mu = 0.02$, $\alpha = 0$, $R_0 = \beta N/(\mu + \gamma) \approxeq 15$, $X = 65\,050$). Notice that the numbers of susceptibles oscillates above and below the threshold susceptible number, X_T (marked) and that each epidemic starts when susceptible numbers exceed the threshold, X_T, and subsequently decays as susceptibles fall below the threshold, X_T. Oscillations of X and Y (and Z, not shown) gradually damp over time towards the predicted equilibrium values X^*, Y^*, and Z^* (see text).
(b) Renewal of susceptibles through waning immunity, at rate α of 0.05 (thick lines) or 0.1 (thin lines) (corresponding average durations of immunity are 20 and 10 units of time respectively) (other initial settings as for (a) above except for no mortality, i.e. $\mu = 0$). Notice that for the two different rates of loss of immunity the equilibrium susceptible numbers are the same ($X^* = X_T$) since waning immunity has no impact on R_0. However, a higher rate of loss of immunity does result in an increase in numbers of infecteds at equilibrium, Y^*.

in the external environment, sexual transmission, vertical transmission, from mother to unborn offspring, vector transmission, and the carrier state in which some individuals (for genetic or other reasons) atypically harbour the infection for long periods of time (see Table 1 and Fig. 3 for examples).

Herd immunity and mass vaccination

When an infection is persisting endemically in a community such that the net rate at which new cases of infection arise is approximately equal to the net rate at which individuals recover and acquire immunity, the effective reproductive rate R is equal to unity in value. This is known as endemic equilibrium. In practice, for many common viral and bacterial infections the incidence of infection fluctuates both on seasonal and longer-term cycles. The effective reproductive rate therefore fluctuates below and above unity in value as the incidence and density of susceptibles change (see Figs 6 and 10). However, the average value over a series of incidence cycles (both seasonal and longer term) will be approximately equal to unity in the absence of control intervention or changing social and demographic patterns. The effective reproductive rate is reduced below the basic reproductive rate in relation to the fraction of contacts that are with susceptible individuals $x = X/N$, i.e. by the simple equation

$$R = R_0 x. \tag{26}$$

At equilibrium when R is on average unity, the proportion susceptible represents a threshold, x^*, below which infection rates would decline (see Fig. 10). Thus from eqn (26) we see that at equilibrium this proportion susceptible x^* is equal to the reciprocal of the basic reproductive rate R_0 (i.e. $R_0 \approx 1/x^*$). The magnitude of x^* (and therefore R_0) can be determined from cross-sectional serological surveys given data on the age structure of the population. If x_i is the proportion susceptible in age class i and pi is the proportion of the population in the same age class then

$$x* = \sum_{i=1}^{n} x_i p_i \tag{27}$$

in a population with n age classes. This assumes that the serological profile is unchanging over time (Box 1).

To block transmission and eliminate an infection it is necessary to raise the level of herd immunity by mass vaccination such that the magnitude of the effective reproductive rate is less than unity in value. If x^* is the threshold susceptible proportion then $1 - x^*$, which we call p_c, represents the herd immunity threshold. Vaccinating a proportion of the population $p > p_c$ will lead to elimination of the infection. Therefore this quantity is a critical level for mass vaccination and since, from eqn (26), $x^* = 1/R_0$, p_c may be related to the basic reproductive rate in the following way:

$$p_c = 1 - 1/R_0. \tag{28}$$

The relationship between p_c and R_0 is depicted diagrammatically in Fig. 11: the larger the magnitude of the infection's transmission potential (as measured by R_0) the greater the proportion of the population that must be immunized to block transmission. Note that it is not necessary to vaccinate everyone in the community to prevent the spread of infection. The principle of herd immunity implies the indirect protection of the individual conferred by the protection

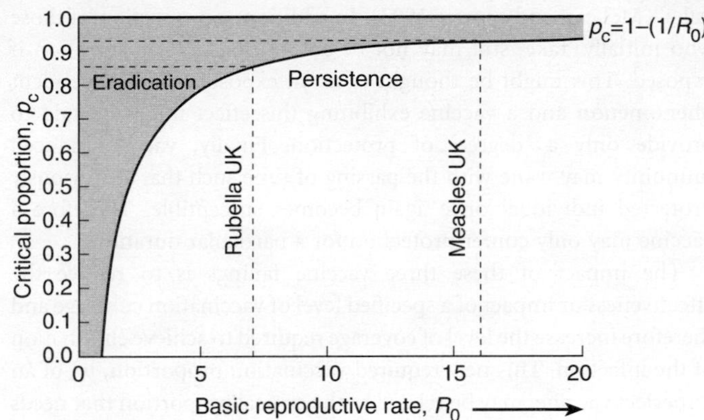

Fig. 11 Relationship between the proportion of the population vaccinated at or near birth and the likelihood of an infection persisting or, alternatively, being eliminated. Infectious agents with high basic reproductive rates in defined communities will be more difficult to control by mass vaccination as illustrated by the example of measles and rubella in the United Kingdom. (Source: Nokes and Anderson 1988.)

(= vaccination) of the population. The mechanism underlying this concept is that of the critical density of susceptibles required to maintain the magnitude of the reproductive rate above unity in value.

Age at vaccination

In general, immunization programmes are introduced by focusing on cohorts of children such that the level of immunization coverage is built up over many years of routine vaccination, that is as children pass some age gateway. In these circumstances, p_c of eqn (28) must be interpreted as the proportion of each cohort vaccinated as soon after birth as is practically feasible, taking account of the need to immunize after the decay in maternally derived specific antibody. For most viral infections the average duration of protection against infection provided by maternal antibodies is approximately 6 months. Clearly, it will take many years of cohort immunization to achieve the desired level of artificially induced herd immunity. A further complication is that it is often the case that the average age at vaccination is higher than what is epidemiologically ideal, resulting from the desire to link vaccination with a delivery opportunity (such as first attendance at school) or variation in the age of delivery resulting perhaps from inefficiency in the co-ordination system or motivation of the population. In this case, simple mathematical models suggest that the level of vaccination coverage required to eradicate the infection under a policy which vaccinates (with a vaccine with 100 per cent efficacy) at an average age of V years is

$$p > [1 + (V/L)]/[1 + (A/L)] \tag{29}$$

where L is human life expectancy and A is the average age at which the infection was acquired prior to the introduction of vaccination (Anderson and May 1983). It is clear from this expression that transmission cannot be interrupted unless the average age at vaccination, V, is less than the average age at infection, A, prior to control.

Imperfect vaccines

Various forms of vaccine failure can be specified. At the time of delivery only a proportion of individuals may respond by generating protective immunity postimmunization. This has been called vaccine 'take' (McLean and Blower 1993). In addition, a proportion of those who initially 'take' still may not be able to fend off an infection if exposed. This might be thought of as an exposure–dose-dependent phenomenon and a vaccine exhibiting this effect might be said to provide only a 'degree' of protection. Finally, vaccine-induced immunity may wane with the passing of time such that a previously protected individual once again becomes susceptible. Therefore a vaccine may only confer protection for a particular duration.

The impact of these three vaccine failings is to reduce the effectiveness or impact of a specified level of vaccination coverage and therefore increase the level of coverage required to achieve elimination of the infection. This new required vaccination proportion, $p^\wedge$, of an imperfect vaccine, may be related to the critical proportion that needs to be effectively vaccinated for elimination, p_c, in the form

$$p^\wedge = p_c/\varphi \tag{30}$$

where φ is the effective vaccine efficacy defined as

$$\varphi = \omega_1\omega_2\,[\mu/(\mu + \omega_3)] \tag{31}$$

(McLean and Blower 1993). Here ω_1 is 'take', ω_2 is 'degree', $1/\omega_3$ is 'duration' (i.e. ω_3 is the rate of waning vaccine-induced immunity), and μ is the death rate. The effects of 'take' and 'degree' are clearly going to be in direct proportion to their magnitude. For example, if a vaccine is being used to interrupt transmission of an infection with an R_0 value of 10 (for which, from eqn (28), the critical proportion to be effectively immunized, p_c, is 0.9) but only 90 per cent of those vaccinated respond (i.e. $\omega_1 = 0.9$), then the new proportion needing to be vaccinated is 0.9/0.9 = 1.0, i.e. 100 per cent coverage. The effect of a vaccine waning over time is less obvious but may be seen from Fig. 12. Here vaccine impact *f* due to the waning immunity effect (for a vaccine which has perfect 'take' and 'degree') is related to the rate of loss of vaccine-induced immunity, expressed as the time taken for 10 per cent of those vaccinated to lose protection. We can see from this graph that even a slight waning of immunity may cause a very significant reduction in the impact of a vaccine, for example if 10 per cent of those effectively vaccinated at birth lose their immunity by age 30 years vaccine impact is reduced by 20 per cent (i.e. $\varphi = 0.8$ from Fig. 12) and in our above example of an infection with R_0 = 10, 100 per cent vaccination in infants would not be sufficient to eliminate transmission.

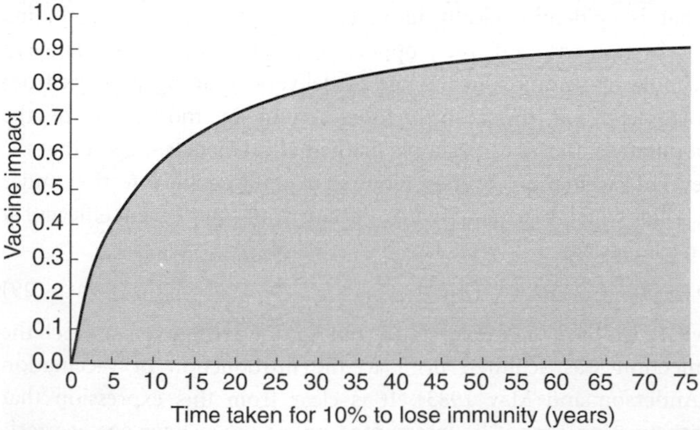

Fig. 12 The impact of an imperfect vaccine. The time taken for 10 per cent of individuals to lose their immunity after vaccination is related to the impact of a vaccine, $\varphi = \mu/(\mu + \omega)$ (the vaccine is assumed to have perfect 'take' and 'degree'). Here, the proportion whose immunity has waned in τ years, p_τ, is related to the rate of loss of immunity by the expression $p_\tau = \exp(-\omega\tau)$.

As a final note of caution, the components that make up the term vaccine impact, φ, have a compounding effect since they are multiplied by one another. Thus even if each individually is of little significance, the compounded effect on impact may still be very significant.

The prevalence of infection and the basic reproductive rate

A further epidemiological feature arising from the existence of a critical density of susceptibles to maintain infection concerns the relationship between the magnitude of the basic reproductive rate and the prevalence of infection in a population in which the infectious agent persists endemically. As depicted in Fig. 13 simple models predict that the relationship is non-linear such that a marked reduction in the endemic prevalence or incidence will only occur as the transmission potential is reduced to an extent where it approaches the threshold level $R_0 = 1$. The practical implication is that we should not expect the decline in the incidence of infection induced by mass vaccination to be directly proportional to the level of vaccination coverage. The greatest changes are predicted to occur when coverage attains high levels.

Interepidemic period *T*

Many viral and bacterial infections that induce lasting immunity to reinfection and which have high transmission potentials (R_0 large) tend to exhibit oscillatory fluctuations in incidence. A good example is that of measles which in the United Kingdom prior to mass

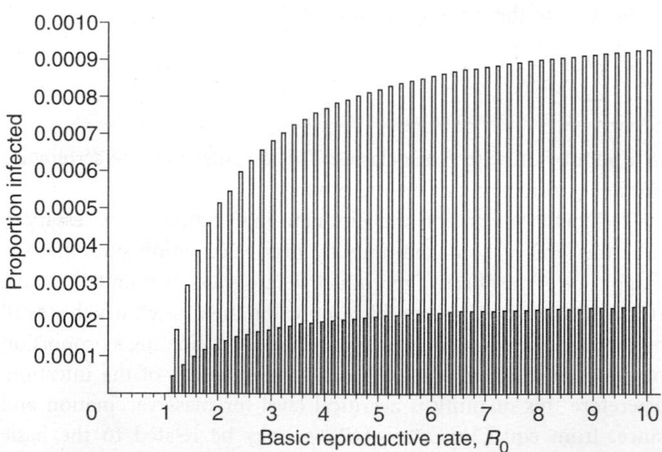

Fig. 13 Predicted changes in the equilibrium proportion of a population infected (i.e. the stable endemic prevalence of an infection) as the transmission potential of the microparasitic agent varies. For infections where there is no loss of immunity, the level of the plateau of prevalence is dependent upon the rate of input of new susceptibles (i.e. the birth rate, *b*) and the duration of infectiousness, $1/\gamma$. In the figure, b = 1/75 per year and γ = 52 per year (i.e. a 1-week infectious period) (closed bars) or γ = 13 per year (i.e. a 4-week period) (open bars). An important point to observe is that the greatest changes in the proportion infected occur over the first few increments of R_0 (irrespective of the magnitude of *b* or γ.)

vaccination oscillated on a seasonal basis (owing to the aggregation and desegregation of children for school term and holiday periods) and a longer-term 2-year cycle with years of high incidence separated by years of low incidence (Anderson *et al.* 1984) (Fig. 6). Time-series analyses reveal that these longer-term cycles for infection such as measles, mumps, rubella, and pertussis are not due to chance fluctuations but arise as a result of the dynamic interaction between the net rates of acquisition of infection and immunity on recovery.

Simple models based on the mass-action assumption suggest that the interepidemic period, T, of the longer-term cycles is determined by the generation time of the infection, k, defined as the sum of the latent and infectious periods and the transmission potential of the infection inversely measured by the average age at infection, A, where

$$T = 2\pi(AK)^{1/2}. \quad (32)$$

This simple prediction matches well the observation for a variety of common childhood infections prior to mass vaccination (i.e. the 2-year cycles of measles, the 3-year cycles of mumps, the 4- to 5-year cycles of rubella, and the 3- to 4-year cycles of pertussis). Non-seasonal oscillation arises as a consequence of the exhaustion of a supply of susceptibles, as an epidemic passes through a population, plus the time lag that arises before new births replenish the pool to trigger the next epidemic. As such the interepidemic period is also influenced by the birth rate of the community (which influences the average age of infection, A, in eqn (32)). For example, in developing countries such as Kenya with high birth rates, measles tends to cycle on a 1-year time scale in urban centres as opposed to the 2-year cycle in the United Kingdom prior to control (McLean and Anderson 1988*b*).

Parameter estimation

Survey data

Survey data on the incidence or prevalence of infection (past or current) can be obtained in a variety of ways. Longitudinal (= through time) data can be acquired by monitoring a cohort of people through time and recording infection as it occurs. Horizontal (= one point in time) – cross-sectional (= across age and sex classes) can be acquired by a survey at one point in time or over a short interval of time, by the examination of different age classes within the population. Such surveys are of most use when based on serological examinations to determine the proportion of individuals in a given age class who have antibodies specific to the antigens of a particular infectious agent. These cross-sectional serological profiles reflect the proportion in each age class who have, at some time in the past, experienced infection. Case-notification data stratified by age and sex, and recorded over a set interval of time such as 1 year, can be accumulated to indicate what proportion of the cases occurs by any given age. This may then be used to infer changes in the proportion who experience infection as a function of age. Such data are clearly less reliable than serological information since they are dependent on a lack of bias in reporting efficiency by age class. Bias is to be expected if the seriousness of the disease induced by infection changes with age (e.g. rubella in women and mumps in men) or where the incidence of subclinical (i.e. undetectable) infections is age dependent.

An alternative to the use of serum for the detection of specific antibodies to infectious agents is saliva. More specifically, when looking for systemic antibodies (e.g. immunoglobulin G and M) the fluid which collects around the gums and under the tongue (as distinct from salivary gland secretions) is rich in serum antibodies. This is known as gingivocrevicular exudate or secretion. The disadvantage of using salivary fluid for antibody detection is the low concentration of immunoglobulin it contains relative to serum. Immunoglobulin G in whole saliva is approximately 1000-fold less concentrated than in serum, although in crevicular fluid it may only be five-fold more dilute (Mortimer and Parry 1991). In recent years highly sensitive assays have been developed to overcome the dilution problems and, accompanied by developments in devices for the collection of crevicular fluid samples, have now been successfully employed in the detection of antibodies to a variety of infections, including measles, rubella, and mumps (Perry *et al.* 1993; Brown *et al.* 1994) human parvovirus, and hepatitis B virus (core antibodies) (Parry *et al.* 1989), and HIV (Holmstrom *et al.* 1990; Behets *et al.* 1991; Van Den Akker *et al.* 1992).

The advantages of using saliva over serum are numerous and associated largely with the collection procedure. For example, sampling is non-invasive and is more acceptable which will assist in response level, the collection process is easier and can be carried out by non-technical personnel, and there is lower risk to both subject and investigator (Mortimer and Parry 1991). Surveys based on saliva collection offer great potential in the fields of epidemiology and surveillance, including the measurement of population immunity in the evaluation of the impact of vaccination programmes of infection prevalence in assessing the rate of spread of infections, such as HIV, through communities. The opportunity for longitudinal surveillance will be beneficial to studies of spatial and temporal patterns of disease spread and salivary diagnosis will become increasingly useful in outbreak investigation and control.

When conducting surveys a number of points should be borne in mind. Firstly, sample sizes should be as large as practically possible, finely stratified by age (preferably infants to elderly people). How large will depend upon what we wish the accuracy or power (see Sokal and Rohlf 1981) of subsequent analyses to be, but 25 to 50 per yearly age class is a rough working estimate. Secondly, the incidence of infection may oscillate on a seasonal or longer-term basis. As such, it is good practice to carry out surveys that span epidemic and interepidemic years. Thirdly, systematic changes through time may occur in a given population due to social, behavioural, economic, or other changes. Examples include the observed reduction in the incidence of hepatitis A in northern European countries over the past few decades due to improved standards of hygiene and the rise in the incidence of gonorrhoea in certain developed countries during the 1960s and 1970s due to changes in sexual behaviour (e.g. increased rates of sexual-partner change). Basic reproductive rates and rates of infection may therefore change through time irrespective of the impact of control measures.

The basic reproductive rate of infection

Estimating individually the component parameters that determine the magnitude of the basic reproductive rate, R_0, is fraught with many problems. In the case of directly transmitted viral and bacterial infections, we require a knowledge of the transmission coefficient, β, the density of susceptibles, X, and the average duration of infectiousness. In practice it is often easier to use indirect methods to arrive at estimates of R_0 employing serological data finely stratified by age. As discussed earlier, the rate of decay with age in the proportion susceptible to infection provides measures of the age-dependent forces of infection ($\lambda(a)$). These in turn can be used to obtain an estimate of the average age, A, at which an individual typically acquires infection. Mathematical models can be used to define a relationship between the magnitude of R_0 and the average age at infection. In the simplest case the relationship is of the form

$$R_0 = Q/A \qquad (33)$$

where Q denotes the reciprocal of the net birth rate of the community. In developed countries where net births are approximately equal to net deaths the quality Q is equal to the average life expectancy (from birth) L (Anderson and May 1985*a*). More generally, if maternally derived antibodies provide protection for an average of F years R_0 is related to A by the expression

$$R_0 = Q/(A - F). \qquad (34)$$

A simple example of the use of this equation is provided by the transmission of the measles virus in the United Kingdom prior to the introduction of mass vaccination. In this case the values of A, L, and F were 5 years, 75 years, and 0.5 years respectively, leading to an R_0 estimate of between 16 and 17. The inverse relationship between R_0 and A makes good intuitive sense—infections with high transmission potentials will tend to have low average ages at infection and vice versa. These notions are depicted diagrammatically in Box 1, and Table 3 lists some estimates of R_0, A, L, and the critical level of vaccination coverage to block transmission, p_c, for a variety of common infectious agents in defined localities.

An alternative method to that outlined above is based on the prediction of simple models that the magnitude of R_0 is related to the fraction of the population susceptible to infection, x^* when the infection has attained its endemic equilibrium. The relationship is simply

$$R_0 = 1/x^* \qquad (35)$$

and arises from the fact that at equilibrium the effective reproductive rate is equal to unity in value (see eqn 26). Note that eqns (33) and (35) imply that the average age at infection, A, is inversely related to the equilibrium fraction of susceptibles in a population, x^* required to ensure each primary case gives rise on average to at least one secondary case (Box 1). In general, however, the method based on estimating the average age at infection is the better one given good age-stratified serological data.

Latent and infectious periods

Two sources of data are available to estimate latent and infectious periods. The first derives from clinical, virological, and immunological

Table 3 Epidemiological parameters for a variety of childhood infections in developed countries in the absence of mass vaccination

Infection	Average age at infection A (years)	Location and date	Data type	Life expectancy L (years)	R_0[a]	p_c (%)
Measles	5.0	England & Wales, 1948–68	Case notifications	70	15.6	94
	5.5	USA, large families, 1957	Serology	70	14.0	93
	8.0	USA, small families, 1957	Serology	70	9.3	89
Whooping cough	4.5	England & Wales, 1944–78[b]	Case notifications	70	17.5	94
	4.9	USA, urban, 1908–17	Case notifications	60	13.6	93
	6.5	USA, rural, 1908–17	Case notifications	60	10.0	90
Chickenpox	8.6	USA, urban, 1913–17	Case notifications	60	7.4	86
	6.8	USA, urban, 1943	Case notifications	70	11.1	91
Mumps	7.0	UK, urban, 1977	Serology	75	11.5	91
	5.7	Netherlands, urban, 1980	Serology	75	14.4	93
	9.9	USA, urban, 1943	Case notifications	70	7.4	86
Diphtheria	10.4	USA, 1912–28	Case notifications	60	6.1	84
Rubella	10.8	England, urban, 1980–84[c]	Serology	75	7.3	86
	10.2	GDR, 1972	Serology	70	7.2	86
Scarlet fever	8.0	USA, urban, 1908–17	Case notifications	60	8.0	88
	12.3	USA, rural, 1918–19	Case notifications	60	5.1	80

Parameter definitions given in text (data from a variety of sources).

[a] $R_0 = L/(A - F)$ where F is duration of maternally derived protection, assumed to last for 6 months in all cases. Note that no consideration of age-dependent forces of infection is given (see text).

[b] Encroaches on to vaccination era.

[c] Male serology—only females vaccinated under selective immunization policy.

studies of the course of infection in individual patients. For some common microparasitic infections, the presence of the infectious agent in host tissues, excretions, and secretions can be directly assessed. Durations of antigenaemia in body fluids and secretions or of infective particles in specific cells will, in many instances, reflect the period over which an infected person is infectious to others (although this is, of course, not always the case as, for example, with the latent herpesviruses).

Alternatively, statistical methods can be employed in the study of transmission within small groups of individuals. The classic data on measles, collected by Hope Simpson (1952) in the Cirencester area of England during the years 1946 to 1952, record the distribution of the observed time interval between two cases of measles in 219 families with two children under the age of 15 years. The bulk of these observations represent case-to-case transmissions within a family. However, in a small number of families, where the observed interval is only a few days it may be assumed that these cases are double primaries, both children having been simultaneously infected from some outside source. Statistical methods, based on chain binomial models, can be used to derive estimates of the latent, infectious, and incubation periods (Bailey 1973). A rough guide to these periods for various common viral and bacterial infections is presented in Table 4. Some of these estimates are based on detailed analyses of case to case data while others are more speculative.

Sexually transmitted infections

Rather different problems in parameter estimation, to those outlined above, are presented by sexually transmitted infections. By way of an illustration and given the topicality of the infection, we focus on HIV.

The characteristics of most sexually transmitted diseases cause their epidemiology to differ from that of common childhood viral and bacterial infections. Firstly, the rate at which new infections are produced does not appear to be closely correlated with population density. Secondly, the carrier phenomenon in which certain individuals harbour asymptomatic infection is often important. Thirdly, many sexually transmitted diseases induce little or no acquired immunity on recovery. Fourthly, net transmission depends on the degree of heterogeneity in sexual activity prevailing in the population and the degree to which individuals in one sexual activity class (perhaps defined in terms of the rate of sexual-partner change) mix with those in the same and in different classes (i.e. 'who has sex with whom').

The basic reproductive rate, R_0, in its simplest form is determined by the transmission probability, B, multiplied by the effective rate of sexual-partner change, c, multiplied by the average duration of infectiousness, D. Heterogeneity in sexual activity is a major influence on the magnitude of transmission success. Recent national surveys of sexual attitudes and lifestyles suggest that most people have few different sexual partners and a few have many (Anderson and May 1988; ACSF 1992; Johnson *et al.* 1994). The distributions of reported numbers of sex partners per defined period of time therefore tend to be skewed with a long right-hand tail where a few individuals report many partners (Fig. 14). As pointed out earlier, under these circumstances the variance in partner numbers, s^2, is much greater in value than the mean, m, and the effective rate of sexual partner change, c, is defined as $c = m + (s^2/m)$ (as in eqn 14). It follows that those with high rates of sexual partner change play a disproportionate role (relative to their proportional representation in a community) in the spread of infection. In the case of HIV each component of R_0 is difficult to measure due to the sensitivity and the practical difficulties associated with the study of sexual behaviour and the long and variable incubation period of the disease AIDS induced by the infection. Over the long incubation period infectiousness appears to vary widely for an individual and between individuals.

As a consequence some indirect measure of transmission potential is required. Mathematical models of transmission suggest that the doubling time t_d (the average time over which the number of cases of infection doubles) of an epidemic of HIV in a defined risk group (e.g. male homosexuals), during the early stages of the epidemic, is related to the magnitude of R_0 by the equation

$$t_d = D\ln(2)/(R_0 - 1) \quad (36)$$

where D denotes the average duration of infectiousness. Current estimates of the incubation period of HIV suggest a mean period of

Table 4 Average duration of infection classes for a variety of microparasites

Infectious disease	Latent period $1/\sigma$ (days)	Infectious period $1/\gamma$ (days)	Incubation period[a] (days)
Measles	6–9	6–7	11–14
Chickenpox	8–12	10–11	13–17
Rubella	7–14	11–12	16–20
Hepatitis A	13–17	19–22	30–37
Mumps	12–18	4–8	12–26
Polio	1–3	14–20	7–12
Smallpox	8–11	2–3	10–12
Influenza	1–3	2–3	1–3
Scarlet fever	1–2	14–21	2–3
Whooping cough	6–7	21–23	7–10
Diphtheria	2–5	14–21	2–5

[a]Time to appearance of symptoms.

Source: Anderson (1982*b*).

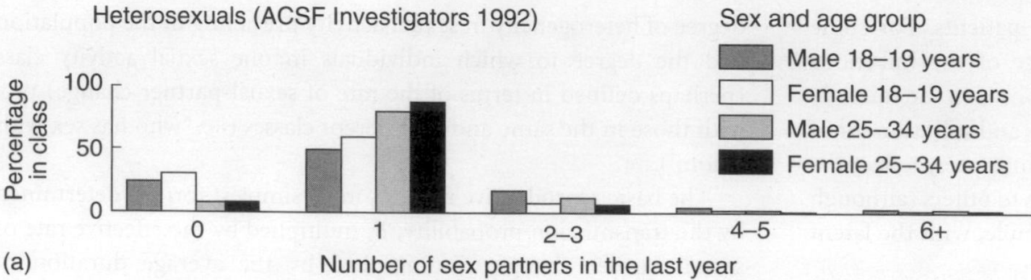

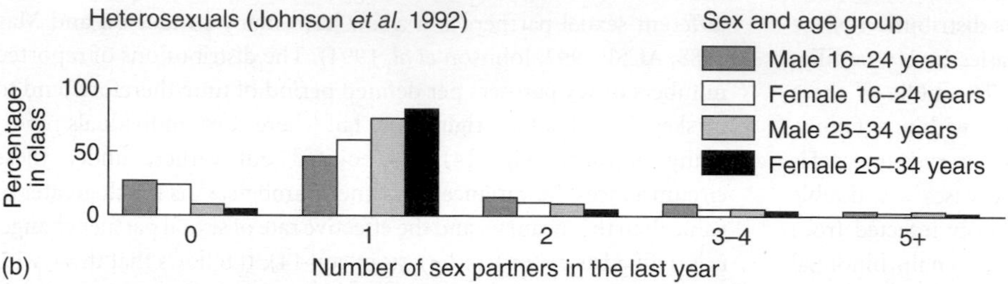

Fig. 14 Frequency distributions of the reported number of different sexual partners over the past year in two surveys in (a) France (ACSF 1992) and (b) Britain (Johnson *et al.* 1992) of sexual attitudes and lifestyles, stratified by age and sex. The similarities in the results of the two surveys are striking.

approximately 8 years. It is probable that the average infectious period is much shorter perhaps of the order of 2 years or so (however, this is uncertain at present; see Anderson and May 1988). If we assume the value of D lies between 2 and 6 years eqn (32) gives estimates of R_0 in the range of 2.7 to 6, given an observed doubling time of around 10 months in male homosexual communities in the United States during the early 1980s (May and Anderson 1987). Of course, this method of estimation is very crude, but it provides a rough guide to the degree to which sexual habits must change in order to reduce the magnitude of R_0 below unity in value (i.e. by a factor of 3 to 6).

More generally, certain of the parameters that determine the magnitude of R_0 may vary between the sexes. This is certainly the case for gonorrhoea (Hethcote and Yorke 1984) and it may be true for HIV. In these circumstances, when considering transmission via heterosexual contact, the basic reproductive rate adopts the form

$$R_0 = (B_1 B_2 c_1 c_2 D_1 D_2) \qquad (37)$$

where the subscripts 1 and 2 denote males and females respectively.

Further complications arise in the definition of the case reproductive number, R_0, when we take into account the pattern of mixing between different strata of the sexually active population. For example, in light of the data presented in Fig. 14 concerning heterogeneity in reported rates of sexual partner acquisition per year in France and Britain, it seems sensible to stratify the population by the rate of sexual partner change into low-, medium-, and high-'activity' classes. The magnitude of any epidemics of a sexually transmitted disease and the endemic level of infection in a community will depend on the degree to which the small number of people with high rates of sexual-partner change mix with the medium- and low-activity classes. If mixing is random across activity classes the infection will be widely disseminated in the community. However, if mixing is highly assortative (i.e. like with like) the infection will tend to be restricted to the small proportion of individuals in the high-activity class (the so-called 'core' group) with a few cases in the other classes. The prevailing pattern of mixing is therefore of great importance in determining the prevalence of an sexually transmitted disease and the degree to which it is disseminated in a defined community. Recent studies of mixing patterns based on contact tracing via sexually transmitted disease clinics suggest that mixing is more assortative than random in character (Garnett and Anderson 1993). Once mixing is taken into account it is necessary to redefine transmission success in terms of the number of secondary cases of infection in group i generated by contact with infectives in group j, R_{0ij}, where

$$R_{0ij} = p_{ij} BcD. \qquad (38)$$

Here p_{ij} is the probability that a susceptible in group i has a sexual contact with someone in group j.

Again, more generally, the population is structured by other variables such as age, ethnicity, area of residence, and educational attainment. Here again, behavioural studies suggest a degree of assortative mixing with respect to the choice of sexual partner—except in contact with commercial sex workers.

Models and the design of control programmes

Mathematical models can be of help in defining the targets for a control programme, in interpreting observed epidemiological changes under the impact of control, and in discriminating between different approaches (Nokes and Anderson 1987, 1988, 1991, 1992, 1993; Garnett *et al.* 1992; Gupta and Anderson 1992). In this section we consider two themes, namely, the design of mass vaccination programmes to control childhood viral and bacterial infections and education to induce changes in sexual behaviour to control sexually transmitted diseases.

Impact of mass vaccination

In practical terms, the level of vaccination coverage in a given community or country is determined by a variety of economic and logistical factors (developing countries) or motivational and legislative issues (industrialized countries). However, models can define the ideal goal of a given programme. We have already outlined the relationship between the critical level of vaccination coverage required to block transmission, *pc* and various epidemiological (R_0), demographic (net birth rate and life expectancy, *Q* and *L*), and logistical (*V*, the average age at vaccination) parameters (see eqns (28) and (29) and Table 3) and vaccine properties (see eqns (30) and (31)). In many instances, the high transmission potentials of common childhood viral and bacterial infections imply very high levels of infant vaccination coverage if transmission is to be interrupted. If vaccine efficacy is less than 100 per cent (e.g. the current pertussis vaccines), then problems may arise in attaining these targets even if legislation enforces vaccination of all children before entry to school (as in the United States). Models emphasize the point that to obtain the best effects very high levels of coverage should be aimed at with vaccination at as young an age as is practically feasible given the complications presented by the presence of maternally derived antibodies in infants.

Aside from defining targets for vaccination coverage, models can assist in interpreting the impact of a given programme on epidemiological parameters such as the incidence of infection, the average age at infection, and the interepidemic period. In a later part of this section we consider the principles underlying an alternative approach to mass vaccine intervention, that of pulsed immunization across age cohorts, which has recently met with such success in controlling polio and measles in Central and South America.

Incidence of infection

Immunization has the direct effect of reducing the number of cases of infection as a result of the protection of the vaccinated individuals ($X \rightarrow Z$, see Fig. 3(d)). Since this reduces the number of infectious persons in the vaccinated population, an indirect effect is a reduction in the net rate of transmission of the virus or bacterium. This is the principle of herd immunity, where susceptibles gain protection from the vaccinated proportion of the population. Provided the infection is able to persist endemically (i.e. the level of coverage is less than that required for eradication), models suggest that the equilibrium proportion of susceptibles in the population will remain constant irrespective of the level of coverage below the critical point for eradication. This prediction is illustrated diagrammatically in Fig. 15. The level of coverage simply reduces the proportion of seropositive individuals who have acquired immunity via infection as opposed to via vaccination. As mentioned earlier (see Fig. 13) the manner in which the incidence declines as the level of coverage rises is non-linear in form with the most dramatic reductions occurring as the proportion vaccinated approaches the critical point for the interruption of transmission. As the level of coverage approaches the critical point the proportion of immune persons who possess vaccine-induced immunity approaches unity.

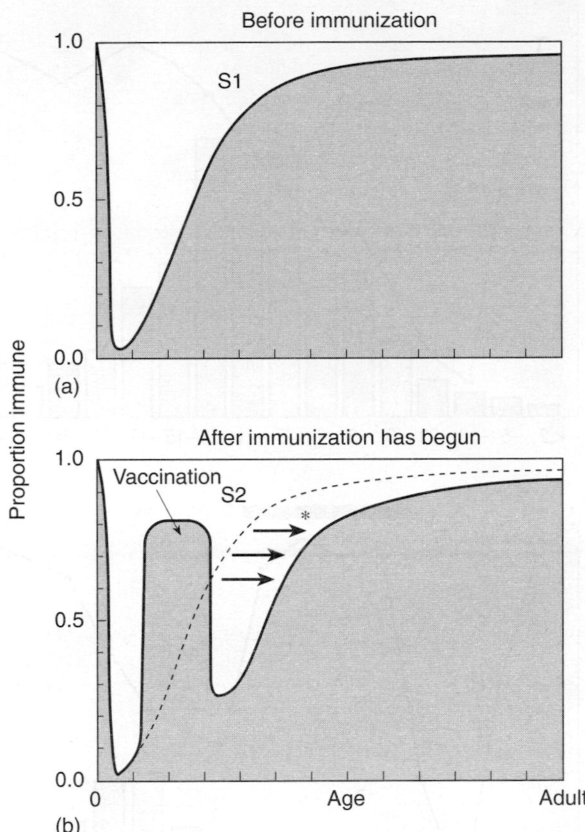

Fig. 15 Diagrammatic representation of the predicted impact of mass immunization (against a typical childhood viral or bacterial infection) on the age distribution of susceptibility in a population. Before immunization (a) there is a 'valley' of susceptibles (S1) in the young age classes. Attempts to fill in this valley by vaccination (b) reduces the rate of transmission of the infection thus lowering the probability of unvaccinated individuals being infected. As a consequence there is an upward shift in the ages of susceptibles (*) from that pertaining before vaccination (dotted line). Two points are important: (i) the number or proportion of susceptibles after immunization has begun (area S2) is roughly unchanged from that which existed before immunization (area S1) and (ii) the average age of susceptibles increases. (Source: Nokes and Anderson 1988.)

The average age at infection

As a direct result of reducing the net rate of transmission, vaccination acts to increase the average age at which susceptibles acquire infection over that pertaining prior to control (i.e. by reducing the probability of coming into contact with an infectious person). Observation now bears out the expectation of an increased average age of susceptibles and of infection as a result of mass vaccination programmes. The example in Fig. 16 shows the prevaccination (1982) serological profile (or distribution of susceptibles by age) for rubella in Finland (Fig. 16(a)) and the profile (for males only) in 1986, 4 years after mass infant measles, mumps, and rubella (**MMR**) vaccine was introduced (Fig. 16(b)) (Ukkonen and Von Bonsdorf 1988). The similarity with Fig. 15 is striking. Also shown in Fig. 16 is the changing distribution of diagnosed rubella cases, with a marked increase in the average age. Later we discuss how this change in the age distribution of the incidence of infection can influence the incidence of disease arising

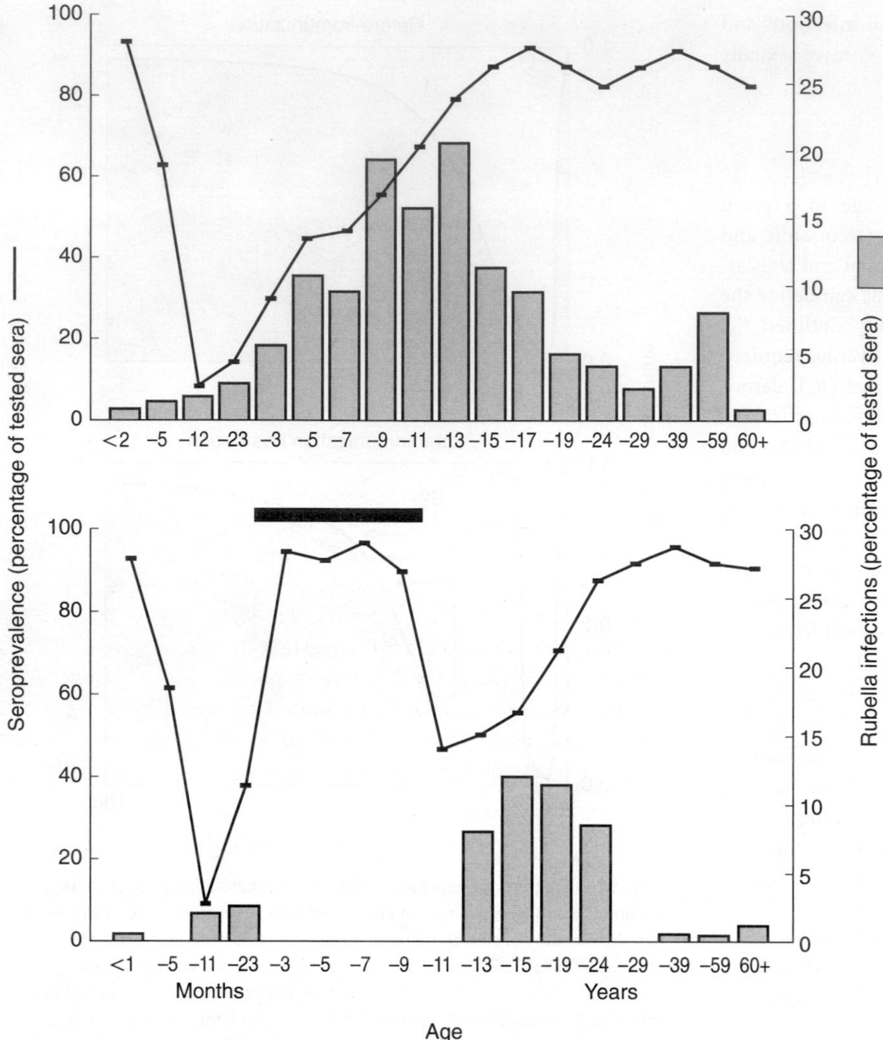

Fig. 16 The observed impact of mass immunization against rubella in Finland (Ukkonen and Von Bonsdorf 1988). (a) The prevaccination (1982) age seroprevalence of specific rubella antibodies (line) with the age distribution of diagnosed cases (bars). (b) Four years after mass infant MMR vaccination was introduced with the age range affected shown by the solid bar (data for males only) (other details as for (a)). (Source: Nokes and Anderson 1993.)

from infection if older people differ in their vulnerability to complications and concomitant morbidity when compared with younger people.

Interepidemic period

Simple models also predicted that a reduction in the transmission rate in a vaccinated population will act to lengthen the interepidemic period over that pertaining prior to control (Anderson and May 1983). This may be shown easily using our model in Fig. 10 if a proportion of all individuals entering the population are vaccinated at the time of birth (starting from time unit 5 onwards), resulting in an increase in the time taken for susceptibles to build up to threshold numbers and, hence, an increase in the interval between epidemics (Fig. 17). This pattern has been observed in various vaccinated communities (Fig. 18).

Cautionary notes

The changes in epidemiological patterns of infection induced by vaccination are not always beneficial. An increased interepidemic period, for example, can induce complacency in the community with respect to the need to maintain high levels of vaccination coverage. Motivating parents to ensure that their children are vaccinated during long periods of low incidence (the troughs in the epidemic cycle) can be problematic particularly if there is some small but measurable risk associated with vaccination. At the start of a mass immunization programme the probability of serious disease arising from vaccination is usually orders of magnitude smaller than the risk of serious disease arising from natural infection. As the point of eradication is approached, the relative magnitudes of these two probabilities must inevitably be reversed. The optimum strategy for the individual (not to be vaccinated) therefore becomes at odds with the needs of society (to maintain her immunity) (Nokes and Anderson 1991). This issue—

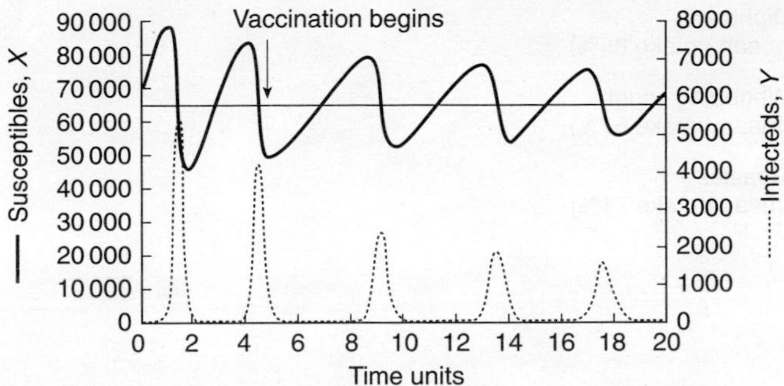

Fig. 17 Predicted impact of vaccination on the interepidemic period. Vaccination of 50 per cent of all births was introduced at time 5 into the model given in Fig. 10 (with the same initial settings).

which was central to the decline in the uptake of pertussis vaccine in the United Kingdom during the mid to late 1970s—can be overcome by legislation to enforce vaccination (as in the United States), but its final resolution is only achieved by global eradication of the disease agent so that routine vaccination can cease.

Other problems concern doubts over the role played by exposure to natural infection in boosting vaccine-induced immunity and, in some cases, worries over the duration of protection provided by vaccination. If enough is understood about these problems mathematical models could be used to decide whether or not to revaccinate a proportion of the immunized population and, if so, what is the best age to revaccinate. Similarly, recent evidence for measles suggests that passive immunity in infants of mothers whose own protection was vaccine derived wanes more rapidly than in infants whose mothers were naturally infected (Markowitz *et al.* 1996). The consequences of this are that, on the one hand, infants become susceptible to infection at an earlier age than was previously the case, but, on the other hand, it may allow for the lowering of the age of vaccine delivery. The merits of this latter issue could well be addressed using mathematical models.

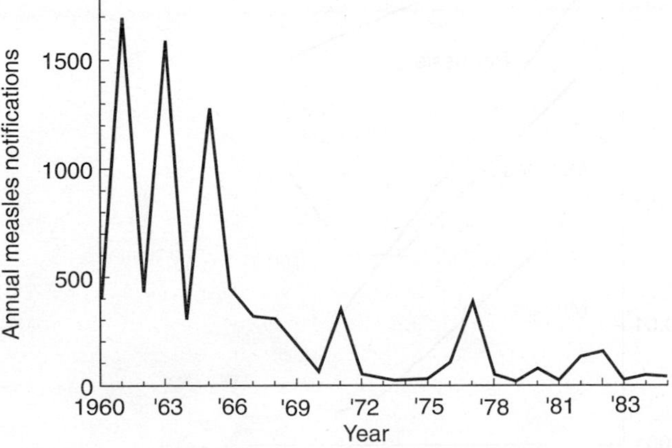

Fig. 18 Annual measles notifications for the city of Oxford, England, for the period 1960 to 1985. The introduction of measles vaccination in 1966 has resulted in a significant increase in the period between epidemics. (Source: Office of Population Census and Surveys, London.)

Variation in vaccine uptake

Ideally, vaccination coverage should be high and constant both through time and in different regions of a country. In practice, however, this is rarely the case. With respect to time, once incidence is reduced to a low level, problems can arise in stimulating public health workers to maintain coverage at high levels. More importantly, after introduction, most immunization programmes show a slow increase in rates of coverage. This obviously results in a delay in experiencing the full benefits and must be recognized in assessing the impact of a given policy. It takes many decades before the full benefits of a cohort immunization programme are manifest. Model simulations of the impact of such programmes on the incidence of infection and disease clearly illustrate this point (Anderson and May 1983, 1985*a,c*). Of greater concern, however, is the variation in vaccine uptake in different regions of a country. Levels of vaccine coverage for sentinel antigens (measles, diphtheria 3, and pertussis 3) in the United Kingdom, for example, varied widely between different regions in the late 1980s (Fig. 19), a problem which has been greatly diminished as a result of improved vaccine programme co-ordination. To block transmission countrywide effectively it is necessary to ensure that the targets laid out in Table 3 are attained in each area. Otherwise, pockets of infection in regions of low uptake will continue to trigger small epidemics in other areas. The upsurge of mumps in certain states in the United States in the late 1980s (Wharton *et al.* 1988) is an example of the potential hazards of spatial variation in vaccine uptake.

Non-uniformity in human population density

Non-uniformity in the spatial distribution of humans, with some people living in dense aggregates and others living in isolated or small groups, can lead to heterogeneity in transmission rates. Models suggest that this can result in the transmission potential of an infection (R_0) being greater on average than suggested by estimation procedures which assume spatial homogeneity (Anderson and May 1984; May and Anderson 1984). Under these circumstances, theory suggests that the optimal solution appears to involve 'targeting' vaccination coverage in relation to group size with dense groups receiving the highest levels of coverage. The optimal programme is defined as that minimizing the total, communitywide number of immunizations needed for elimination or for a defined level of control. This strategy reduces the overall proportion that must be vaccinated to block transmission, compared with that estimated on the assumption of spatial homogeneity. This conclusion has practical significance for the control of infections such as measles and pertussis in some developing countries, where rural–urban differences in population density tend to be much more marked than in developed countries (Anderson and May 1991). It is probable that in many regions of Africa and Asia, diseases such as measles cannot persist endemically in rural areas without frequent movement of people between low-density (rural) and high-density (urban) populations. Under these circumstances, transmission might be blocked in both regions by high levels of mass immunization in the urban centres alone.

Age-dependent factors

Analyses of case-notification records and serological profiles suggest that, for many common infections (measles, rubella, and pertussis), the per capita rate of infection ($\lambda(a)$) depends on the ages of

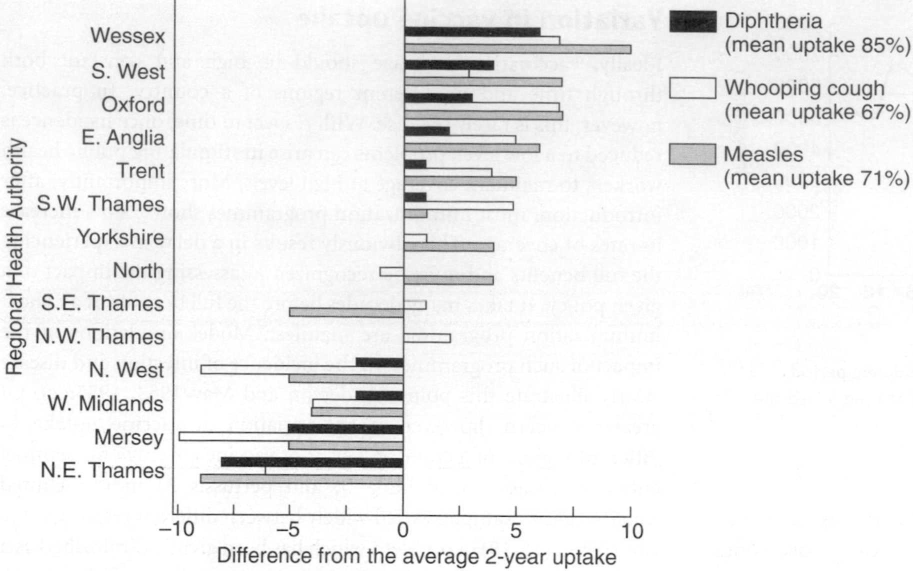

Fig. 19 Regional variation in immunization uptake for sentinel agents in England, 1986. (Source: Nokes and Anderson 1988.)

susceptible individuals, changing from a low level in the 0- to 5-year age classes, via a high level in the 5- to 15-year age classes, back to a lower level in the adult age classes (Fig. 5). This is of interest both because it reflects behavioural attributes of human communities and because of its impact on the predicted level of vaccination required to eliminate transmission. The high levels of the force of infection in the 5- to 15-year-old classes are thought to arise as a consequence of frequent and intimate contacts within school environments (Anderson and May 1985*c*; Nokes *et al.* 1986; Anderson *et al.* 1987). Theoretical studies which take account of age dependence in the force of infection predict somewhat lower rates of vaccination than those arrived at under the simple mass-action assumption (Table 3). However, it should be emphasized that the values listed in Table 3 provide a good first approximation of the targets to be obtained in a vaccination programme. The reason why the observed age-related changes in the force of infection influence the predicted level of coverage relates to the tendency for mass vaccination to shift the age distribution of susceptibility (Figs 15 and 16). Susceptibles who avoid infection and vaccination may move from an age class with a high force of infection into an older class with a lower rate.

Does mass vaccination always reduce disease incidence?

The risk of complications arising from infection is often dependent upon the age at which exposure occurs. The newborn are particularly vulnerable due to their immunological immaturity and are therefore more likely to suffer morbidity and even mortality (Fig. 20). Protection by maternally derived antibody moderates the risk during this time of great vulnerability but, in developing countries, factors such as malnutrition and high incidences of secondary 'opportunist' infections can result in high mortality rates as a result of infant and childhood viral and bacterial infection. In general where the risk of serious disease is higher in the young than old people, mass vaccination will always act to reduce the incidence of disease.

In developed countries case fatalities are much less common and the greatest problem is morbidity and the risk of serious disease. Of particular concern are infections where the risk of severe complications increases with age (Fig. 21). Whether this trend is important depends on the quantitative details of such factors as how risk changes with age, the average age at which the vaccine is administered, the average age at infection, and how the rate (or force) of infection changes with age prior to the introduction of immunization (Knox 1980; Anderson and May 1983, 1985*a*; Anderson *et al.* 1987; Nokes and Anderson 1991) (Fig. 21).

Rubella and mumps are clear examples because of the risk of congenital rubella syndrome in infants born to mothers who

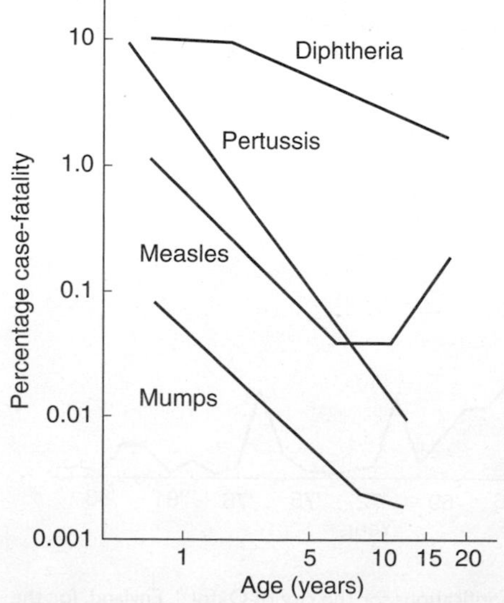

Fig. 20 Age-dependent mortality associated with infection from a variety of childhood viruses and bacteria. (Source: MIMS 1987.)

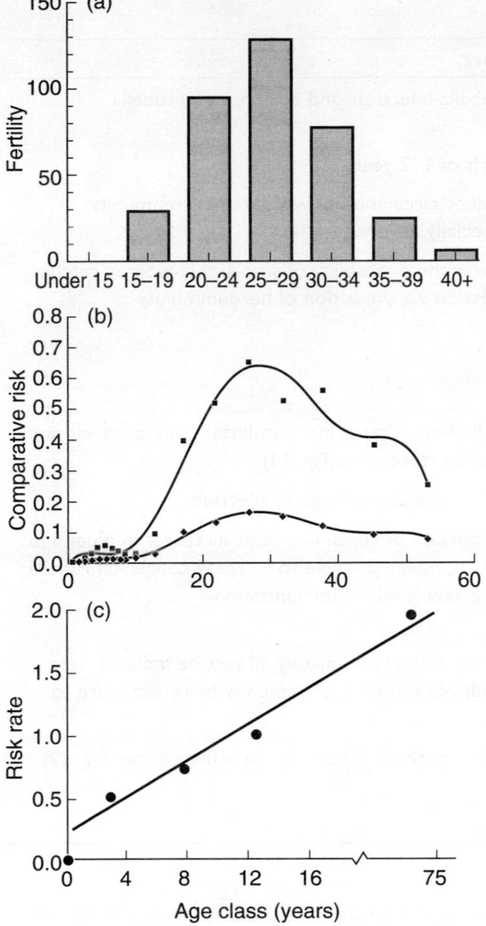

Fig. 21 Age-dependent risk of complications from infection: (a) the likelihood of fetal transmission of rubella virus with concomitant risk of congenital rubella syndrome is directly related to age-specific fertility of women (data for England and Wales 1985 from OPCS Monitor FMI 86/2) (b) changes in the risk of complications from mumps infection in the United Kingdom relative to age and sex. In addition to meningitis and encephalitis, males (■) may suffer orchitis (data from Anderson *et al.* 1987). Note here that the term comparative risk, refers to the risk compared with other age classes. (c) Measles encephalitis per 100 000 cases in the United States. (Source: Anderson and May 1983.)

contracted rubella in their first trimester of pregnancy and the occurrence of orchitis and the associated risk of sterility in post-pubertal males plus infection of the central nervous system following mumps infection. The crux of the problem relates to how mass vaccination changes the age profile of the incidence of infection. Any level of coverage will reduce the incidence of infection but by increasing the average age at which those still susceptible acquire infection certain levels of coverage may increase the incidence of disease. The important question is whether the increase in the proportion of cases in older people will result in an increase in the absolute numbers of cases of serious disease.

This problem has resulted in the adoption of different vaccination programmes against rubella (to control congenital rubella syndrome) in different countries (Table 5). Until the introduction of MMR vaccine in the United Kingdom in 1988, girls only were vaccinated at an average age of around 12 years, so as to allow rubella virus to circulate in males and young females and create naturally acquired immunity in the early years. By contrast, it has always been the case in the United States for both boys and girls to be vaccinated at around 2 years of age, with the aim of blocking rubella virus transmission. Mathematical models predict that the United States policy is best if very high levels of vaccination (80 to 85 per cent of each yearly cohort) can be achieved at a young age, while the United Kingdom policy is better if this cannot be guaranteed (Fig. 22). A mixed policy is predicted to be of additional benefit over the selective policy alone if moderate to high levels of vaccine uptake among boys and girls can be achieved at a young age (60 per cent) (Anderson and Grenfell 1986).

The process of using mathematical models to evaluate the impact of a particular mass vaccination policy in a community is detailed in Box 4, in this case for mumps. At the time of the introduction of MMR infant vaccination in the United Kingdom in November 1988 such studies as these suggested that provided moderate to high levels of coverage (60–65 per cent) could be achieved then the change in policy was unlikely to increase the incidence of serious disease (Anderson *et al.* 1987). Following the implementation of the MMR vaccine, coverage rose from the level of uptake for measles vaccine at the time of around 70 per cent by age 2 years (the level of update for measles vaccine at the time) to 90 per cent within the space of 2 years. Thoughts have now turned to the required strategy for elimination of these three infections and use is being made of mathematical models to explore the possible options, such as a two-dose schedule (Babad *et al.* 1995). For rubella, and specifically for the issue of when to remove the selective arm of the vaccination strategy, we now have the example from the Scandinavian countries to guide our policy. Data from Finland, for example, clearly show the need to continue schoolgirl vaccination until the cohorts with high-level immunity through infant vaccination span the entire high-fertility age groups. Note that this concurs with predictions made prior to the observations becoming available (Nokes and Anderson 1987).

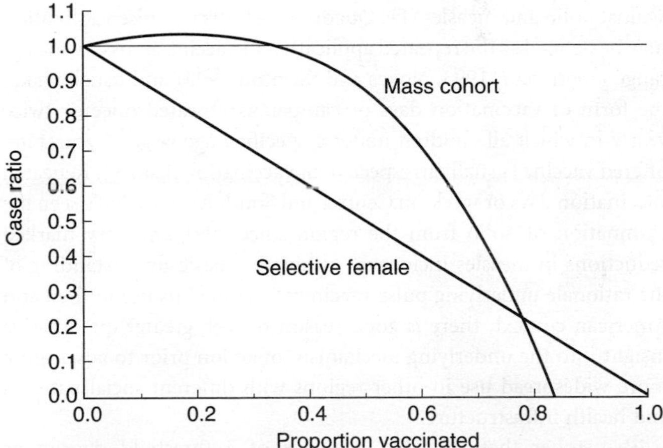

Fig. 22 Effectiveness of different rubella immunization programmes. Changes in the predicted case ratio (i.e. the average number of rubella infections in pregnant women after the introduction of immunization divided by average prevaccination number) under increasing levels of coverage for two types of policy, namely, selective immunization of girls of average age 12 years or mass vaccination of children (aged 2 years). Low to medium levels of uptake favour adoption of a selective immunization programme compared with mass vaccination which has the undesirable effect of increasing the average age at infection.

Table 5 Strategies of rubella immunization

	Selective		Mass cohort	
Aim	Eliminate congenital rubella, not rubella infection		Eliminate rubella infection, and so congenital rubella	
Age at vaccination	Prepubertal girls (10–15 years)		Boys and girls of 1–2 years	
Philosophy	(i)	Build upon levels of herd immunity attained through childhood	(i)	Reduce circulation of wild virus in community, especially children
	(ii)	Reduce the proportion of susceptible women of childbearing age	(ii)	Lower the probability of susceptible women catching infection via the action of herd immunity
	(ii)	Allow continued circulation of virus in male and young female segments of the population		
Overall incidence of infection	Very little impact at any level of coverage		(i)	Reduction in cases in a non-linear manner as vaccine level increases (see Fig. 13)
			(ii)	Increase in average age at infection
Other concerns	(i)	Cannot eradicate congenital rubella unless 100 per cent of women 'at risk' are immune (via infection in childhhod or immunization)	(i)	Proportion of remaining cases increases in older age classes, hence possible to increase congenital rubella at certain levels of immunization
	(ii)	Herd immunity largely natural with continued re-exposure to infection and boosting of antibody response	(ii)	Herd immunity ultimately all vaccine induced. Less solid? No boosting of immunity by re-exposure to virus
Which policy?	Suitable for lower levels of vaccination coverage (see Fig. 22)		Suitable if high levels of uptake can be achieved (see Fig. 22)	
Country (as example)	UK		USA	

The strategy of pulse vaccination

The use of the alternative strategy of pulse vaccination as a method of control of childhood vaccine-preventable diseases has gained prominence in the early 1990s largely as a result of success in the Americas against polio and measles (De Quadros *et al.* 1991). Pulse vaccination may be defined as the repeated application of vaccine across a wide age range (Agur *et al.* 1993; Nokes and Swinton 1995) and usually takes the form of vaccination days or campaigns repeated once or twice yearly in which all children under a specified age (e.g. 15 years) are offered vaccine (usually irrespective of vaccination history). Repeated vaccination days or weeks in Central and South America have seen the elimination of polio from the region since 1991 and very marked reductions in measles incidence. Although a basic understanding of the rationale underlying pulse vaccination guided its use in the Latin American context, there is good reason to seek greater quantitative insight into the underlying mechanism of action prior to advocating more widespread use in other regions with different social patterns and health infrastructure.

Remember that it is the presence of a threshold density or proportion of susceptibles in a population which enables endemic persistence of acute vaccine-preventable infections (i.e. infections requiring close contact to effect transmission and which develop lasting immunity following recovery). Vaccination of a fraction of an endemic proportion susceptible lowers the effective reproductive rate below unity and incidence declines (this may be quite a considerable reduction if a pulse is administered across a wide age range). Lowering the number of infectious persons in the population results in a lowering of the force of infection acting upon susceptibles. In turn fewer infections leads to a build-up once more in susceptible numbers to the threshold level. The principle behind pulse vaccination rests upon these simple conditions. The aim of repeatedly pulsing is to maintain susceptible numbers below the threshold density or fraction and thereby maintain a continual decline in incidence (i.e. by maintaining $R < 1$). In practical quantitative terms we are interested in the timing of successive pulses to achieve this objective.

The interpulse interval depends upon three factors: what fraction of the population are susceptible at endemic equilibrium, how much of this susceptible population is immunized as a result of the campaign, and how rapidly are susceptibles replenished after a campaign. Translating these into epidemiological terms, we note that the proportion of the susceptible population vaccinated in a single pulse is $p'x^*$ where p' is the vaccination coverage and x^* is the endemic fraction susceptible (related to the basic reproductive rate in the form $x^* = 1/R_0$). In addition, if the total population is approximately constant in size, then, ignoring any further infection, the rate of replenishment of susceptibles by births is equal to the death rate, $\mu = 1/L$ (where L is life expectancy at birth). Therefore the minimum time taken after pulsing to recover the equilibrium fraction, i.e. the interpulse period T_v, is

$$T_v = p'x^*L \tag{39}$$

and, since $x^* = 1/R_0 = A/L$, we obtain

$$T_v = p'A \tag{40}$$

(Agur *et al.* 1993). This gives the common-sense result that if all susceptibles were to be immunized by a pulse of vaccine, i.e. $p' = 1.0$, then the time taken to recover the threshold fraction would be

Box 4 Epidemiology and control of mumps virus infection

Incidence of infection

Mumps is typical of the childhood viral infections with peak incidence in the young age classes and relatively few cases occurring in adulthood (figure (a)).

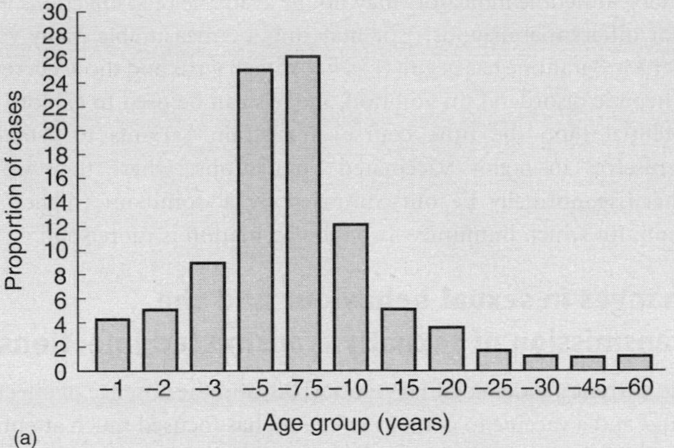

(a)

Information of this sort, obtained from age-specific case notification data or age-serological profiles, is used to derive age-dependent rates of transmission as shown in Fig. 5(b) in the main text.

Incidence of disease

Various types of complications are associated with mumps virus infection (figure (b)). In the prevaccination era mumps was the most common cause of viral meningitis in the United Kingdom, and is also a significant cause of encephalitis and, in postpubertal males, of orchitis.

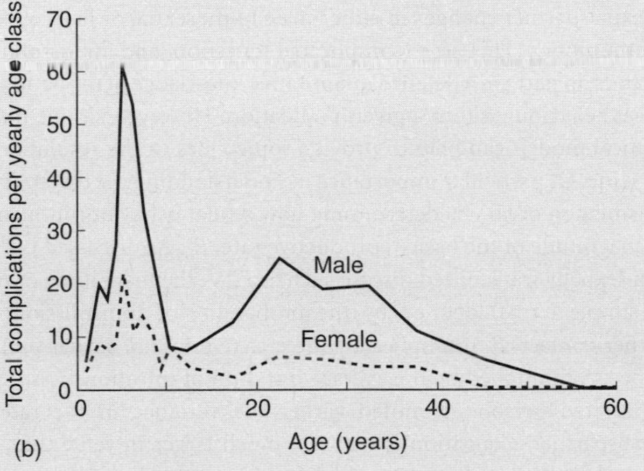

(b)

Scaling these age-complication data by the proportion of cases of infection in the corresponding age classes (shown above), it is possible to drive the relative risk of complications from infection, as shown in Fig. 21(b) in the main text. What becomes apparent from these data analyses is that, although fewest cases of infection occur in the older age classes, there remain substantial numbers of cases of complications, such that infection in older persons runs a considerably greater risk of resulting in complications when compared with infection in the young.

Mass vaccination and the incidence of infection

Figure (c) shows the predicted numbers of cases of mumps infection across a wide range of age classes, through time, before and after the introduction of a programme of mass cohort immunization (60 per cent of 2-year-olds). The force of infection is assumed to remain constant with age at 0.15 per year (corresponding to an average age at infection before immunization of 6.7 years). The epidemic peaks in the prevaccine period show the majority of cases occurring in the youngest age classes. Subsequent to the initiation of immunization two changes should be noted: (a) the obvious and expected decline in infection incidence (particularly in the young), and (b) an increase in the age at which the remaining cases occur, indicated by the wave of infections migrating, in time, into the older age classes. The implications of this shift in the age distribution of cases on the incidence of disease are addressed below.

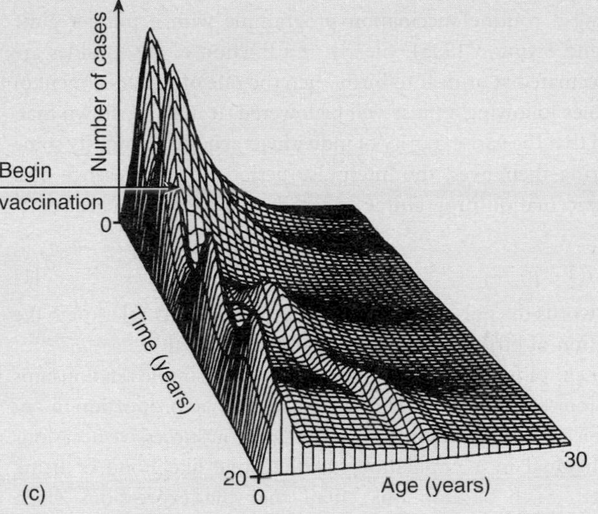

(c)

Mass vaccination and the incidence of disease

The effect of a rise in the proportion of cases in the older age classes (predicted above) on the incidence of complications is dependent upon two things: (a) the level of cohort immunization that can be attained, and (b) the age-dependent nature of the risk of complications seen in Fig. 21. Simulations that help to unravel this problem are shown in figure (d) (adapted from Anderson *et al.* 1987), recording the change in the predicted risk ratio (i.e. the average number of complications after immunization has begun divided by the average number of complications occurring before) over various levels of childhood immunization (note that the risk ratio is unity for no benefit from immunization). Obviously there is little benefit to be obtained by vaccination at less than 60 per cent, and indeed vaccination at anything less than 70 per cent is potentially hazardous when considering orchitis alone. Such a phenomenon is a direct result of the combination of increased average age at infection and of the risk of complications with age.

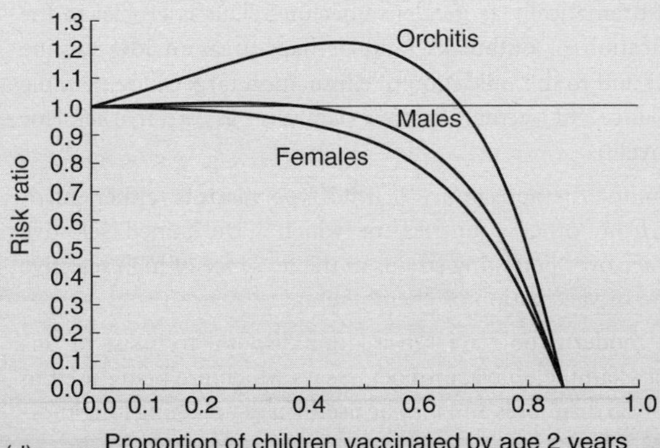

(d)

equivalent to the average age at infection. The higher the average age at infection, that is the lower the transmission potential of the infection, the higher the endemic fraction susceptible and the consequent increase in the permitted interval between pulses. An observation from this analysis is that it is possible to eliminate an infection using a pulse vaccination proportion, p', which is less than the critical level of coverage predicted to be required for a continuous immunization process. The reason for this is that by vaccinating repeatedly across an age range, some individuals will receive multiple opportunities to receive the vaccine and there is therefore a build-up of vaccine-induced immunity with increasing age.

One complication that ought to be considered is the effect of combining a routine vaccination programme with a pulse regime (Nokes and Swinton 1995). Clearly, if a fraction of susceptibles are being vaccinated at or near to birth, then the rate of replenishment of susceptibles following a pulse will be lowered. It may be shown that, provided that the vast majority of individuals acquire immunity some time during their lives, the interpulse period in the presence of a routine vaccination programme in which a proportion p are vaccinated is

$$T_v = p'A/(1-p). \tag{41}$$

In other words the pulse interval is lengthened in direct relation to the new fraction of births which are susceptible, $(1-p)$.

Major simplifying assumptions underlie these simple relationships for the interpulse period. It is assumed that a proportion p' of susceptibles of any age are vaccinated and that on successive occasions each individual in a population has the same likelihood of being vaccinated. Such assumptions entail that the expressions given provide simple guidelines to aid understanding. Models of greater complexity are required which expand upon these ideas to give more practical guidelines (Nokes and Swinton 1995).

Monitoring the impact of control programmes

There is an ever-growing need to establish a co-ordinated surveillance programme to monitor the impact of control programmes against microparasitic infections (Nokes and Cutts 1993). The needs include the following.

1. To establish the impact of a specified control programme on a particular outcome variable, such as incidence of infection. This is of increasing importance as control programmes near their goals of elimination, where indicators of process, such as vaccination coverage, simply do not relate well enough to outcome.
2. To establish the accuracy of outcome indicators, such as notifications of infectious disease, the efficiency of which commonly fall off dramatically as incidence declines. This is crucial to the identification of outbreaks (and perhaps areas of low vaccine uptake) and to the validation of elimination targets, for example surveillance of acute flaccid paralysis as a marker for poliomyelitis.
3. To monitor the appearance of wild-type variants, either introduced from other countries, or which have gained selective advantage over persisting strains in the presence of high selective pressure of vaccination or chemotherapy.

Various modern tools are now at our disposal to assist in this process. For example, saliva antibody assays which are being used to confirm clinical diagnoses and may be useful in establishing longitudinal surveillance systems and molecular probes by which to identify the origins of strains in infection outbreaks and the arrival of variants able to circulate in the presence of high-level vaccine-associated immunity.

Mathematical models also have a role to play in this area of epidemiology. They facilitate the assessment of the impact of mass vaccination programmes through their predictive capability, where suitable outcome indicators may not be available (e.g. infections with poor differential diagnosis) or may only be measurable many years after a programme has begun (e.g. hepatitis B virus and the occurrence of hepatic disorders). In addition, models can be used to explore the potential (and the time course) for strain variants to establish themselves in highly vaccinated populations, where they would otherwise normally be out-competed by a dominant (higher R_0) strain, for which immunity through vaccination is more solid.

Changes in sexual behaviour and the transmission of sexually transmitted infections

The current pandemic of HIV and AIDS, and the absence of effective drugs and a vaccine to combat infection, has focused much attention in recent years on how to induce changes in sexual behaviour via education and media publicity campaigns to slow the spread of infection. The most important behaviour relevant to the rate of spread is the distribution of the rates of acquiring new sexual partners within a defined population (Fig. 8). A major characteristic of this behaviour is the heterogeneity between individuals within a given community. A central question in this problem is whether it is best to aim health educational programmes at the whole population, with the aim of reducing average rates of sexual-partner change or whether it is best to target education at high-risk groups such as those with very high rates of sexual-partner change (in either male homosexual or heterosexual communities). This is a complicated question and its resolution depends, in part, on a detailed quantitative knowledge of the pattern of sexual behaviour within a given population. However, simple mathematical models can help to provide some clues to the resolution of this issue. Of particular importance in understanding the dynamics of transmission of HIV is determining how sexual behaviour influences the magnitude of the basic reproductive rate, R_0. As discussed earlier, for a sexually transmitted disease such as HIV, the magnitude of R_0 is (in simple terms) defined by the probability of transmission per partner contact, B, multiplied by the effective rate of sexual-partner change, c, multiplied by the average duration of infectiousness, D, of an infected person. As noted earlier the variance in the rate of sexual-partner acquisition is typically much larger in value than the mean and, hence, those with high rates of partner change play a disproportionate role (relative to their proportional representation within a sexually active population) in the spread of infection (Fig. 14). This simple theoretical result suggests that greater benefit is to be gained (in terms of reducing R_0) by targeting education at those with higher than average rates of sexual-partner change. In practice the identification of such individuals is problematic in the absence of detailed survey data that relate this behaviour to other characteristics. The surveys of sexual behaviour that have been completed to date show a strong age dependency (with young adults having the highest rates of sexual-partner change) but little else of help in identifying correlates (ACSF 1992; Johnson *et al.* 1992). However, attendees at sexually transmitted disease clinics are an important target group, since sexually transmitted diseases other than HIV are more frequently present among those with high rates of partner change. Small changes in behaviour in the highly sexually active are likely to have a major impact on the prevalence of sexually transmitted diseases in a community.

Conclusion

We have glossed over much detail and ignored many complications in model formulation and analysis in this chapter. The interested reader is therefore urged to consult the source references. Our aim has been to define, as simply as possible, the central concepts underpinning the study of the transmission dynamics of infectious diseases and the major conclusions that have emerged from the development and analysis of mathematical models of transmission and control.

The recent convergence of mathematical theory and observation in epidemiology has created a powerful set of tools for the study of the population biology of infectious disease agents. At present the potential value of these techniques is not widely appreciated by public health scientists and medical personnel. Many people have rightly criticized models that pursue the mathematics for its own sake, making only perfunctory attempts to relate the findings to epidemiological data. But there is a converse danger which is less widely understood. The complexities of the course of infection within an individual and its spread between people are such that years of clinical experience and the most refined intuition will not always yield reliable insights into the factors that control the transmission dynamics of a given infectious agent and how these are influenced by perturbations introduced by control measures. Moreover, insensitive use of a computer will not always help in understanding these problems, for if a computer is given inappropriate instruction it will usually give inappropriate answers. What is needed, in our view, is increased collaboration between epidemiologists and mathematicians, with the models being founded on data (and with their predictions being tested against available facts) and with verbal hypotheses being founded on clear mathematical statements of the assumptions. We hope that the contents of this chapter stimulate interest in this goal.

References

ACSF (1992). AIDS and sexual behaviour in France. *Nature*, **360**, 407–9.

Agur, Z., Cojocaru, L., Mazor, G., Anderson, R.M., and Danon, Y.L. (1993). Pulse mass measles vaccination across age cohorts. *Proceedings of the National Academy of Sciences of the United States of America*, **90**, 11698–702.

Anderson, R.M. (1982). Directly transmitted viral and bacterial infections of man. In *Population dynamics of infectious diseases—theory and applications* (ed. R.M. Anderson), pp. 1–37. Chapman & Hall, London.

Anderson, R.M. (1988). Epidemiology of HIV infection: variable incubation plus infectious periods and heterogeneity in sexual activity. *Journal of the Royal Statistical Society, Series A*, **151**, 66–93.

Anderson, R.M. and Grenfell, B.T. (1986). Quantitative investigation of different vaccination policies for the control of congenital rubella syndrome (CRS) in the U.K. *Journal of Hygiene (Cambridge)*, **96**, 305–33.

Anderson, R.M. and May, R.M. (1982). Directly transmitted infectious diseases: control by vaccination. *Science*, **215**, 1053–60.

Anderson, R.M. and May, R.M. (1983). Vaccination against rubella and measles: quantitative investigations of different policies. *Journal of Hygiene (Cambridge)*, **90**, 259–325.

Anderson, R.M. and May, R.M. (1984). Spatial, temporal and genetic heteogeneity in host populations and the design of immunization programmes. *IMA Journal of Mathematics Applied in Medicine and Biology*, **1**, 233–66.

Anderson, R.M. and May, R.M. (1985*a*). Age-related changes in the rate of disease transmission: implications for the design of vaccination programmes. *Journal of Hygiene (Cambridge)*, **94**, 365–436.

Anderson, R.M. and May, R.M. (1985*b*). Herd immunity to helminth infection and implications for parasite control. *Nature*, **315**, 493–6.

Anderson, R.M. and May, R.M. (1985*c*). Vaccination and herd immunity to infectious diseases. *Nature*, **318**, 323–9.

Anderson, R.M. and May, R.M. (1986). The invasion, persistence and spread of infectious diseases within animal and plant communities. *Philosophical Transactions of the Royal Society of London*, **314**, 533–70.

Anderson, R.M. and May, R.M. (1988). Epidemiological parameters of HIV transmission. *Nature*, **333**, 514–22.

Anderson, R.M. and May, R.M. (1991). *Infectious diseases of humans: dynamics and control.* Oxford University Press.

Anderson, R.M., Grenfell, B.T., and May, R.M. (1984). Oscillatory fluctuations in the incidence of infectious disease and the impact of vaccination: time series analysis. *Journal of Hygiene (Cambridge)*, **93**, 587–608.

Anderson, R.M., Medley, G.F., May, R.M., and Johnson, A.M. (1986). A preliminary study of the transmission dynamics of the human immunodeficiency virus (HIV), the causative agent of AIDS. *IMA Journal of Mathematics Applied in Medicine and Biology*, **3**, 229–63.

Anderson, R.M., Crombie, J.A., and Grenfell, B.T. (1987). The epidemiology of mumps in the UK: a preliminary study of virus transmission, herd immunity and the potential effect of immunization. *Epidemiology and Infection*, **99**, 65–84.

Anderson, R.M., May, R.M., and McLean, A.R. (1988). Possible demographic consequences of AIDS in developing countries. *Nature*, **332**, 228–34.

Babad, H.R., Nokes, D.J., Gay, N.J., Miller, E., Morgan-Capner, P., and Anderson, R.M. (1995). Predicting the impact of measles vaccination in England and Wales: model validation and analysis of policy options. *Epidemiology and Infection*, **114**, 319–44.

Bailey, N.T.J. (1973). Estimation of parameters from epidemic models. In *Mathematical theory of the dynamics of biological populations* (ed. M.S. Bartlett and R.W. Hiorns), p. 253. Academic Press, London.

Bailey, N.T.J. (1975). *The mathematical theory of infectious diseases and its implications*. Griffin, London.

Ball, F. (1983). The threshold behaviour of epidemic models. *Journal of Applied Probability*, **20**, 227–41.

Becker, N. (1979). The uses of epidemic models. *Biometrics*, **35**, 295–305.

Behets, F.M., Edidi, B., Quinn, T.C., *et al.* (1991). Detection of salivary HIV-1-specific IgG antibodies in high risk populations in Zaire. *Journal of Acquired Immune Deficiency Syndromes*, **4**, 183–7.

Bernoulli, D. (1760). Essai d'une nouvelle analyse de la mortalité causée pour la verole et des avantages de l'incubation pour la prevenir. *Memoires Mathematiques et Physiques de l'Academie Royale des Sciences (Paris)*, **1**, 1–45.

Black, F.L. (1966). Measles endemicity in insular populations: critical community size and its evolutionary implications. *Journal of Theoretical Biology*, **2**, 207–11.

Bolker, B.M. and Grenfell, B.T. (1993). Chaos and biological complexity in measles dynamics. *Philosophical Transactions of the Royal Society of London. B Biological Sciences*, **251**, 75–81.

Brown, D.W.G., Ramsay, M.E.B., Richards, A.F., and Miller, E. (1994). Salivary diagnosis of measles: a study of notified cases in the UK, 1991–3. *British Medical Journal*, **308**, 1015–17.

Brownlee, J. (1906). Statistical studies in immunity: the theory of an epidemic. *Proceedings of the Royal Society of Edinburgh*, **26**, 484–521.

Cliff, A., Haggett, P., and Smallman-Raynor, M. (1993). *Measles: an historical geography*. Blackwell Scientific, Oxford.

De Quadros, C.A., Andrus, J.K., Olive, J.-M., *et al.* (1991). Eradication of poliomyelitis: progress in the Americas. *Pediatric Infectious Disease Journal*, **10**, 222–9.

Dietz, K. (1987). Mathematical models for the control of malaria. In *Malaria* (ed. W.H. Wensdorfe and J.A. MacGregor), p. 1087. Churchill Livingstone, Edinburgh.

Farr, W. (1840). *Progress of epidemics. Second Report of the Registrar General of England and Wales*, pp. 91–8. HMSO, London.

Fine, P.E.M. (1993). Herd immunity: history, theory, practice. *Epidemiologic Reviews*, **15**, 265–302.

Garnett, G.P. and Anderson, R.M. (1993). Contact tracing and the estimation of sexual mixing patterns: the epidemiology of gonococcal infections. *Sexually Transmitted Diseases*, **20**, 181–91.

Garnett, G.P., Swinton, J., Brunham, R.C., and Anderson, R.M. (1992). Gonococcal infection, infertility and population growth: II. The influence of heterogeneity in sexual behaviour. *IMA Journal of Mathematics Applied in Medicine and Biology*, **9**, 127–44.

Grenfell, B.T. and Anderson, R.M. (1985). The estimation of age-related rates of infection from case notifications and serological data. *Journal of Hygiene*, **95**, 419–36.

Gupta, S. and Anderson, R.M. (1992). Sex, AIDS and mathematics. *New Scientist*, 12 September, pp. 34–8.

Hamer, W.H. (1906). Epidemic disease in England. *Lancet*, **i**, 733–9.

Hethcote, H.W. and Yorke, J.A. (1984). Gonorrhoea: transmission dynamics and control. *Lecture Notes in Biomathematics*, **56**, 1–105.

Holmstrom, P., Syrjanen, S., Laine, P., Valle, S.-L., and Suni, J. (1990). HIV antibodies in whole saliva detected by ELISA and Western blot assays. *Journal of Medical Virology*, **30**, 245–8.

Hope Simpson, R.E. (1952). Infectiousness of communicable diseases in the household. *Lancet*, **i**, 1145–55.

Johnson, A.M., Wadsworth, J., Wellings, K., Bradshaw, S., and Field, J. (1992). Sexual lifestyles and HIV risk. *Nature*, **360**, 410–12.

Johnson, A.M., Wadsworth, J., Wellings, K., Field, J., and Bradshaw, S. (1994). *Sexual attitudes and lifestyles*. Blackwell Scientific, Oxford.

Kermack, W.O. and McKendrick, A.G. (1927). A contribution to the mathematical theory of epidemics. *Proceedings of the Royal Society of London, Series A*, **115**, 700–21.

Knox, E.G. (1980). Strategy for rubella vaccination. *International Journal of Epidemiology*, **9**, 13–23.

McLean, A.R. and Anderson, R.M. (1988*a*). Measles in developing countries. Part II. The predicted impact of mass vaccination. *Epidemiology and Infection*, **100**, 419–42.

McLean, A.R. and Anderson, R.M. (1988*b*). Measles in developing countries. Part I. Epidemiological parameters and patterns. *Epidemiology and Infection*, **100**, 111–33.

McLean, A.R. and Blower, S. (1993). Impefect vaccines and herd immunity to HIV. *Proceedings of the Royal Society London B*, **253**, 9–13.

Markowitz, L.E., Albrecht, P., Rhodes, P., *et al.* (1996). Changing levels of measles antibody titers in women and children in the United States: impact on response to vaccination. *Pediatrics*, **97**, 53–8.

May, R.M. and Anderson, R.M. (1984). Spatial heterogeneity and the design of immunization programs. *Mathematical Biosciences*, **72**, 83–111.

May, R.M. and Anderson, R.M. (1987). The transmission dynamics of HIV infection. *Nature*, **326**, 137–42.

Mortimer, P.P. and Parry, J.V. (1991). Non-invasive virological diagnosis: are saliva and urine specimens adequate substitutes for blood? *Reviews in Medical Virology*, **1**, 73–8.

Nokes, D.J. and Anderson, R.M. (1987). Rubella vaccination policy: a note of caution. *Lancet*, **i**, 1441–2.

Nokes, D.J. and Anderson, R.M. (1988). The use of mathematical models in the epidemiological study of infectious diseases and in the design of mass immunization programmes. *Epidemiology and Infection*, **101**, 1–20.

Nokes, D.J. and Anderson, R.M. (1991). Vaccine safety versus vaccine efficacy in mass immunization programmes. *Lancet*, **338**, 1309–12.

Nokes, D.J. and Anderson, R.M. (1992). Mathematical models of infectious agent transmission and the impact of mass vaccination. *Reviews in Medical Microbiology*, **3**, 187–95.

Nokes, D.J. and Anderson, R.M. (1993). Application of mathematical models to the design of immunization strategies. *Reviews in Medical Microbiology*, **4**, 1–7.

Nokes, D.J. and Cutts, F.T. (1993). Immunizations in the developing world: strategic challenges. *Transactions of the Royal Society of Tropical Medicine and Hygiene*, **87**, 353–4, 398.

Nokes, D.J. and Swinton, J. (1995). The control of childhood infection by pulse vaccination: an epidemiological approach. *IMA Journal of Mathematics Applied in Medicine and Biology*, **12**, 29–53.

Nokes, D.J., Anderson, R.M. and Anderson, M.J. (1986). Rubella epidemiology in south-east England. *Journal of Hygiene (Cambridge)*, **96**, 291–304.

Parry, J.V., Perry, K.R., Panday, S., and Mortimer, P.P. (1989). Diagnosis of hepatitis A and B by testing saliva. *Journal of Medical Virology*, **28**, 255–60.

Perry, K.R., Brown, D.W.G., Parry, J.V., Panday, S., Pipkin, C., and Richards, A. (1993). Detection of measles, mumps and rubella antibodies in saliva using antibody capture radioimmunoassay. *Journal of Medical Virology*, **40**, 235–40.

Rogers, D.J. (1988). A general model for the African trypanosomiases. *Parasitology*, **97**, 193.

Ross, R. (1911). *The prevention of malaria* (2nd edn). Murray, London.

Scott, M.E. and Smith, G. (ed.) (1994). *Parasitic and infectious diseases epidemiology and ecology* (1st edn). Academic Press, London.

Sokal, R.R. and Rohlf, F.J. (1981). *Biometry* (2nd edn). W.H. Freeman, San Francisco, CA.

Soper, M.A. (1929). Interpretation of periodicity in disease prevalence. *Journal of the Royal Statistical Society A*, **92**, 34–61.

Ukkonen, P. and Von Bonsdorf, C.-H. (1988). Rubella immunity and morbidity: effects of vaccination in Finland. *Scandinavian Journal of Infectious Diseases*, **20**, 255–9.

Van Den Akker, R., Van Den Hoek, J.A.R., Van Den Akker, *et al.* (1992). Detection of HIV antibodies in saliva as a tool for epidemiological studies. *AIDS*, **6**, 953–7.

Wharton, M., Cochi, S.L., Hutcheson, R.H., Bistowish, J.M., and Shaffner, W. (1988). A large outbreak of mumps in the post vaccine era. *Journal of Infectious Diseases*, **158**, 1253–60.

Wickwire, K. (1977). Mathematical models for the control of pests and infectious diseases: a survey. *Theoretical Population Biology*, **11**, 182–238.

Yorke, J.A., Nathanson, N., Pianigiani, G., and Martin, J. (1979). Seasonality and the requirements for perpetuation and eradication of viruses in populations. *American Journal of Epidemiology*, **109**, 103–23.

6.15 Microcomputers, the Internet, and epidemiology

Ralph R. Frerichs and Beatrice J. Selwyn

Introduction

Epidemiology is, by definition, a quantitative science, using numbers to study disease patterns in populations and devise control strategies. As the complexity of epidemic profiles has increased, so has the need for analytic methods to address time and space relationships associated with diseases. Epidemiology, as a discipline, has responded with an identity that is separate from other fields such as medicine, statistics, or health services research (Rothman and Greenland 1998). Mainframe computers have long served epidemiology and helped mould the evolving discipline. Yet, starting in the mid-1970s, a new form of computing was under way, allowing individuals to program their analyses on personal computers, rather than on large institutional machines. At first, microcomputers were merely tools for word processing, graphics, and record maintenance. Eventually, they became the instrument of choice for communication and analysis (Frerichs and Selwyn 1991). The movement from mainframe computers to microcomputers is part of an evolving trend towards individual empowerment, with contemporary epidemiologists being able to conduct population-based research without expensive large computers and extensive teams of investigators. Enormous information resources are also being availed to individuals by microcomputers, through connections to the World Wide Web (or Internet). Timely information and rapid communication are characteristic of the Internet, providing new opportunities for epidemiology. The additional empowerment that microcomputers and the Internet create has also allowed scientists in developing countries to analyse and present findings quickly, thereby enriching our understanding of worldwide disease occurrence.

In the following sections, we will first describe computing hardware, software, and Internet linkage of use to epidemiologists. Next, we will present five applications of microcomputer and Internet use in epidemiology: the John Snow site (subject-specific reference website), Supercourse (education website), the immunization information system (service site), years of potential life lost calculations, and disease modelling with STELLA. Other applications have been presented in earlier editions of this book, including the use of microcomputers for conducting case–control studies, cohort studies, and understanding misclassification (Frerichs and Selwyn 1991), and for medical record studies, rapid surveys, and vaccine effectiveness studies using available data, surveillance, telecommunication, and distance learning (Frerichs and Selwyn 1997). The final section of this chapter concludes with a view of the future.

Hardware and software

Computers have undergone considerable miniaturization over the years, and now come in various shapes and sizes. The link between computers and the Internet has also created new categories of machines and new ways of conducting epidemiological research. In this section we shall first describe the hardware, or physical components of computers and related devices, and then address software uses for epidemiologists.

Computer hardware

Microcomputers now range in size from desktop machines to miniature equipment. The brain of the computer is a series of small silicon chips that are mounted on a board in the unit. The chips are the microprocessor that understand and process a series of binary numbers with values of either 1 or 0. Such binary digits are termed **bits** and are the basic units of a computer. All communication with the microcomputer has to be translated into bits before the computer can work with the information. The bits are combined to create numerical, alphabetical, and graphic characters termed **bytes**. An example of a byte is the letter Q, which in bits is written as 10101001. Usually eight bits are needed by the computer to create one character or byte. Computers typically process more than one byte at a time, which partially defines their speed. A 32-bit computer processes four characters at a time, while a 64-bit computer can process eight characters at a time. To process information, the computer must first load data into memory, measured in kilobytes (termed K or 1000 bytes) or megabytes (termed MB or 1 million bytes). A single-lined typed page has 2500 to 3000 characters. Hence a computer would need to have at least 3 K of memory to hold a single page. Even the smallest handheld computers now have 512 000 bytes of memory (512 K), enough to hold about 170 pages of data. Larger microcomputers now often have 128 000 000 bytes of memory (128 MB), enough to hold over 42 000 pages of typed text or data. Besides data, computer memories must also hold sizeable software programs. As a result, the actual number of pages that can be loaded in memory at one time varies greatly.

Perhaps the smallest computers are those that look like thickened credit cards. Such cards with 512 K of memory are being sold commercially as personal data managers, but also have potential as sources of medical records, important for persons who want access to their own medical information (Glagola 1998). Other investigators have used watch-sized computers to obtain medical data in care facilities (Overdyk *et al.* 1999). Palm-sized computers, now with 2 to

8 MB of memory, some featuring wireless access to the Internet, have become very popular as personal information managers. They also are being used for near real-time epidemiological research, with subjects recording data on events shortly after they occur (McKay 1999). Book-sized computers with a touch screen and no keyboard are being used for distributing electronic books and reference material, and are very helpful for conducting interviews or medical chart reviews. As portable and desktop microcomputers have been in widespread use for more than a decade, inexpensive used models are now available for researchers in even the poorest countries.

Other hardware

Besides the computer, three items commonly used by epidemiologist are storage devices, modems, and computer image projectors. Storage devices are used to store text, figures, sound, and video in digital form as bits or 0,1 codes. Text requires the least amount of storage space, while video requires the most. The recordable **CD-RW** (compact disc—read, write) and **DVD** (digital videodisc) will soon become common for storing and retrieving such extensive information. The former contains about 600 to 1400 MB of information, while the latter holds 4000 to 6000 MB of information. Both permit reading and writing of data. As the denser DVD becomes widely available, the storage potential for epidemiological data will increase dramatically, both for books and other reference material, and for sound and sight documentation of field activities.

Modems (**mod**ulator–**dem**odulator machines) convert digital data used by computers to analogue signals used by telephones and then back to a digital form for use by another computer. Such devices link computers to many sites, and support data transmission, electronic mail, facsimile transmission, and downloading of audio or video files from the Internet to personal computers. Usually, modems are either voiceband with transmission across telephone lines typically used for sound, or broadband with transmission across cable lines, high-speed telephone lines, or via satellite, featuring much wider communication channels.

Computer image projectors are gradually replacing slide projectors as the device of choice for presenting instructional material or research findings. Coupled with computer and graphics software, such projectors encourage the production of many more slides than would typically be produced with photographic slides or transparencies, thereby adding intermediate logic steps that frequently are left out of formal presentations. This adds to the clarity of the talk. When adding sound speakers, the projector can also transmit voice, thereby bringing another dimension to professional or educational presentations.

Software

Computer programs that control the functions of hardware and direct its operation are termed software. Such programs fall into many categories, but we will mention only those of greatest use.

Word-processing is the most common application of microcomputers for epidemiologists. These programs are often used to create research proposals, design questionnaires, prepare lecture notes, write reports, and prepare manuscripts for publication. Besides presenting text in various formats and type styles, such software offers many editing and proof-reading functions, including electronic dictionaries, thesauri, and grammar guides. In addition, some feature speech recognition, allowing text entry by voice rather than by keyboard and typing.

Data-management programs are important to epidemiologists for the rapid transformation of raw data into useful information for unravelling disease aetiology, assisting administrators, or formulating public policy. Data are rearranged as information (i.e. rates, indices, etc.), and then presented in tables or graphs for printing or perhaps for display on monitor screens.

Statistical programs are essential to epidemiologists, many of whom have had extensive courses in statistics as well as epidemiology. At times, statisticians and epidemiologist hold different views of how data should be analysed, including such fundamental issues as the use of significance tests versus confidence intervals, or multivariate analyses with stepwise algorithms rather than conceptual algorithms based on biological hypotheses (Rothman and Greenland 1998). With excellent statistical software available, epidemiologists are often able to do their own form of analysis, as is increasingly requested by epidemiological and public health journals.

Spreadsheet programs are among the most useful for epidemiologists. The term 'spreadsheet' comes from the practice of accountants who spread large sheets of paper on a table to look at columns and rows of financial data. These programs divide the computer screen into a series of columns and rows with individual cells containing data, text, or formulae, which relate one cell to another. When a cell entry is changed, it may affect the numerical or text values in many other cells, depending on how the variables are related. Among many uses, spreadsheets are employed to create tables and graphs, to model disease processes, and to understand the consequences of factors such as selection and misclassification bias (Frerichs and Selwyn 1991).

Graphics software is included with most spreadsheet software, but is are available in free-standing graphics programs. The intent of such programs is to visualize relationships to enhance understanding, for publication in books or journals, or for presentations in classroom or professional settings. Word-based and image-based perceptions may vary dramatically, depending on the concepts being expressed or the cognitive setting (Ware 1999). Graphics programs are especially useful in verbal settings, and help greatly to make major points in written presentations.

Project-management software is important for epidemiologists who are involved in project scheduling or management, keeping track of money, resources, and time. Progress reports emanating from the software can then be sent to funding or other accountable agencies. Project-management software allows investigators to separate proposed studies into various components and estimate both the order of completion and the time and resources necessary for finishing each component. Items such as unexpected sick days, reductions in funds, or the availability of extra interviewers can quickly be entered into the program to determine the most efficient course to take. Often the results are presented as time lines.

Special interest software

Perhaps the most useful software programs for the practising epidemiologist are Epi Info and Epi Map, developed by the Centers for Disease Control and Prevention (**CDC**) and distributed free via the Internet by both CDC and the World Health Organization (**WHO**) (Harbage and Dean 1999). The Epi Info program was originally intended for outbreak investigations, but has been used around the world in a wide variety of epidemiological studies (Dean 1999). The software is employed to design interview or examination schedules, manage data, and perform various statistical analyses common to epidemiology. Epi Map is intended for computer mapping, producing publishable maps from geographic boundary files and data values entered directly from the keyboard, supplied in Epi Info, or obtained from a database management program (Dean 1999). The data for the maps may be counts, rates, or other numerical values. The values in the maps can be represented as shading or colour patterns for each geographic entity. They can also be presented as dot maps with dots proportional in number to the values placed in each geographic area. Finally, the program can produces cartograms with size of the area increased or decreased depending on the number of events or persons in the area.

The Internet

Description

The Internet, or World Wide Web, is making important changes in the way epidemiology functions. The Web is a complex of networks that connect computers around the world. Two components make up the Internet. The first performs storage and retrieval of information and is characterized by a series of servers—microcomputers with special software and information to be shared with other people. The second component is the client browser, or program on the user's microcomputer that handles both the display of information and recognition of data or text files moving in and out of the local machine. With both servers and clients around the world and a network that links them together, information, including text, graphics, sound, and video, is easily shared with millions of users (Nielsen 1999).

To use the Internet, a person must have a microcomputer or other computing device, a browser, a connection via telephone or cable modem, satellite, or short-distance communication links, and a uniform resource locator (**URL**) that provides the address to be visited. For example, the URL for the Department of Epidemiology at the University of California at Los Angeles (**UCLA**) is http://www.ph.ucla.edu/epi/. The address has three components. The first is http://, which states that the file to be viewed is a hypertext document to be recognized by the browser. The second component is the institution, www.ph.ucla.edu/epi/, or the Department of Epidemiology at the UCLA School of Public Health. The third component is the initial file to be opened. When this is not stated, as is the case in our example, the computer automatically looks for index.html, an introductory file that is located in the server directory.

With information flowing from the World Wide Web to personal computers, a crucial element is the attachment to the Internet, sometimes referred to as the pipeline. Like oil or water pipelines, the larger the pipe, the greater the volume flowing per unit time. With the Internet, the volume flow is information, stored and transmitted in various formats. With small files consisting mainly of text, telephone modems that transmit voiceband work very well with no observable delays in information access. However, with large files consisting of complex graphics, or perhaps sound or video, the modem pipelines are too small and the information takes a long time to be transmitted. Larger pipelines—termed broadband—have been created, but are not yet widely available in wealthier countries, and certainly are scarce to non-existent in the developing world. With such broadband transmission, sound, video, and cinematic files become as transmittable as text files with conventional telephone modems.

Functions

Surveillance

To respond effectively to communicable disease outbreaks, governing agencies need an effective disease surveillance system. Feedback is vital for control programs so that local health workers can use information that is tallied and summarized at the national or international level. Such feedback is increasingly provided by epidemiological Internet sites with tables and graphs showing time trends, progress towards targets, and control efforts (Anonymous 2000). Such a data bank and accompanying feedback system was established for rabies by the WHO in 1998. National rabies reference laboratories throughout the world have direct on-line access to all national data for a given period of time, along with rabies prevalence, diagnosis, treatment, and vaccine production (Anonymous 1998). The global monitoring of influenza was also established as a goal of the WHO. Using the Web to provide access to influenza activity, the WHO was able to provide real-time epidemiological information to a broad public health and medical audience (Flahault *et al.* 1998). A similar Web-based surveillance program for a wide variety of infectious diseases is being established in the WHO Regional Office for Europe, with broad-ranging access to graphical and tabular data (Anonymous 1999). Finally, the CDC, in collaboration with the United States Department of Agriculture (**USDA**), has established a genetic identification network for microbial agents in food-poisoning outbreaks (Ranson and Kaplan 1998). Most state laboratories are participating via the Internet by collecting and quickly analysing samples from sick people and submitting the findings to CDC. At the same time, the USDA and the CDC are analysing data from suspected foods, and then comparing their findings with those of the state laboratories. Because food-borne outbreaks often cross state and international lines, such a broad surveillance programme using the Web makes outbreak tracking much more effective.

Information

The Internet has become the equivalent of a great library, with information available on a wide variety of topics, both current and historical. A milestone was reached at the start of 2000 when the number of Web pages was announced to have reached 1 billion (Clark 2000). Many epidemiology and public health journals are now on the Internet, including *Journal of the American Medical Association*, *The Lancet*, and the *New England Journal of Medicine* (Fernandez *et al.* 1999). A partial list of publications of interest to epidemiologists is shown in Table 1. Epidemiology manuals and books are also available on the Web for both reading and printing, as will be described further in the section on applications below (Joffres and La Porte 1998). Finally, the Internet will increasingly have available audio and video recordings of oral presentations from professional meetings or symposiums. To encourage such activities, the *New England Journal of Medicine* recently issued an editorial policy that an oral presentation

Table 1 Internet addresses of selected on-line journals and publications

Title	Address
British Medical Journal	http://www.bmj.com/
Bulletin of the World Health Organization	http://www.who.org/bulletin/
Emerging Infectious Diseases	http://www.cdc.gov/ncidod/eid/
Epidemiology	http://www.epidem.com/
International Journal of Epidemiology	http://ije.oupjournals.org/
Journal of the American Medical Association	http://jama.ama-assn.org
Morbidity and Mortality Weekly Report	http://www.cdc.gov/mmwr/
New England Journal of Medicine	http://www.nejm.org
The Lancet	http://www.thelancet.com
Weekly Epidemiological Record	http://www.who.int/wer/

on the Web would not be considered a prior publication, and thus would still be eligible for written publication (Kassirer 1999).

Research

The first wave of Internet applications focused on providing timely information. More recently, however, investigators have started to consider how the Internet might be used for research purposes. Wilcox (1999) has suggested that when research articles are published, the questionnaire, interview schedule, or examination form be made available on the Web. He further opined that doing so would improve the quality of data-collection instruments. Some have suggested that Internet users might serve as a population for research investigations, providing a fast mechanism for administering medical surveys (Houston and Fiore 1998). Unfortunately, little was presented on the considerable biasing factors that might influence the findings. Still others demonstrated that a cohort of trained asthmatic patients could be induced with an Internet-based telemonitoring system to perform spirometric self-testing at home (Finkelstein *et al.* 2000). Finally, the Internet is increasingly being used to recruit patients into clinical trials, relying on disease-specific websites, on-line enrolment forms, and e-mail (Larkin 1998).

Service

As broadband coverage increases, providers are able to use both telephone and video to provide consultation services via the Internet. One such program in Spain is attempting to provide supplementary home social and health services for the elderly, disabled, and chronically ill (Valero *et al.* 1999). Another group in rural Canada is linking medical experts at central sites with patients and practitioners at remote locations (Watanabe *et al.* 1999). Finally, investigators in London have conducted supplementary psychiatric consultations using interactive television and broadband connection to support a primary care mental health team (McLaren *et al.* 1999).

Education

With the use of interactive audio and video, the Internet has increasingly been used for distance education and supplementation of conventional education. In Germany, videoconferencing has been carried out with low-cost personal computers (Klutke *et al.* 1999). In over 220 sites in Europe, oncologists were provided with clinical continuing education by panels of experts using the Internet among other communication channels (Geraghty and Young 1999). Finally, the Internet in the United States is being used to broadcast lectures at professional meetings including interviews on topics such as HIV/AIDS, bioterrorism, and prostate cancer.

Applications

Epidemiologists are using microcomputers in many ways. We present below five examples that are relevant to epidemiology, featuring the Internet and different types of software. The applications were selected to demonstrate variation in approach and method, showing uses in a wide variety of economic and developmental settings.

John Snow site

John Snow (1813–1848) is widely known among epidemiologists for his demonstration in London of the spread of cholera by faecal contamination, and among anaesthesiologists for his early clinical use of ether and chloroform. Of necessity, the description of his life and work fills only a few pages in introductory epidemiology texts (Gordis 1996). Moreover, Snow's seminal work, *On the Mode of Communication of Cholera* (Snow 1855), is no longer in print and thus is not readily available to those wanting additional detail. Potentially unavailable as well are two maps Snow used in 1854, one for describing cholera cases attributed to the Broad Street pump outbreak and the other for the grand experiment in which some London residents received contaminated drinking water and others did not. All this information, together with additional details of his life, has now been included in a website on John Snow, as shown in Fig. 1 (Frerichs 2000). The site features three unique components: (a) pages with text, figures, and photographs, (b) lectures with sound and animation, and (c) a geographic information system for London in the nineteenth century.

Pages

Websites are usually comprised of a series of pages, linked together by the click of a mouse key. Links are usually within the site of the host server, but are sometimes with related sites that someone else has created in another server. In the John Snow site, some of the pages address his early life, others his education, and still others his professional work that garnered the admiration of epidemiologists. These pages can be viewed with a regular telephone modem using voiceband transmission. Pages also present photographs, showing current pictures of historical structures, including a tour of his homes, the Broad Street area, and a pub that was named in his honour. Other pages present the text and maps of his 1855 book, while still others are linked to sites that provide additional reference material on people or events in his life.

Lectures

Three lectures are presented on John Snow which use sound and animated graphics, the pace of which is controlled by the user. These lectures require a broadband connection. Conventional slide presentations convey static images in a fixed manner. Animated slides are more dynamic. The viewer of such slides steps through the logic of a

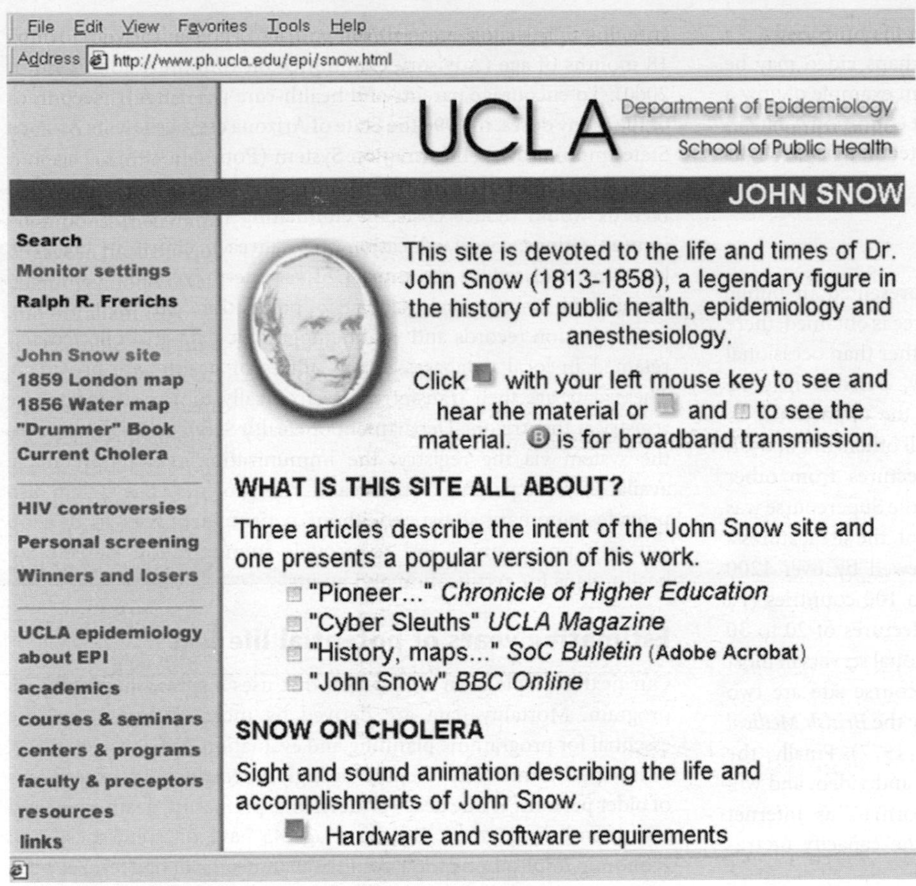

Fig. 1 Example of a subject-specific reference website for epidemiology.

problem in a systematic manner, adding one line, set of words, or symbols until the main point is made. The experience is similar to having an instructor write notes and draw pictures on a blackboard, different from transparencies or slides that show everything at once. The first animated lecture in the Snow site tells of his early life and views of cholera, the second focuses on the 1854 Broad Street pump outbreak, and the third on the 1854 grand experiment, which classified households by disease and exposure to contaminated water. Lectures enriched by sound and animation, such as these, will increasingly be used for education purposes. However, because graphic and sound files are much larger than text files, users will need to have a broadband pipeline to receive them.

Geographic information system

In 1857, a year before the death of John Snow, a map of London was published by James Reynolds. During the following years, the map was annually reissued, updated to reflect changes in the community (Jarman 1859). The 1859 version of the map is included in the John Snow website, featured as a geographic information system (**GIS**) to reference events in Snow's career and in London during his lifetime (1813–1858). Because they are complex images with colour and much detail, moderate-sized maps are too large as files to be viewed in detail on the Internet, even with a broadband connection. Thus the historical map was divided into levels, with each level having smaller sections but greater resolution. The 1859 map has 22 rows and 33 columns, showing 712 quarter-mile-square cells (15 cells were combined in the title). As shown in Fig. 2, the map is divided into six levels, with each level being a subdivision of the earlier level. The lowest level is information linked to a quarter-mile square or cell. If there is relevant matter in the cell, the location is marked and a page is attached which provides additional data, both as text and figures (including slices from the more detailed *Ordnance Survey Maps* of 1864 to 1873). With time, historians and on-site collaborators will add

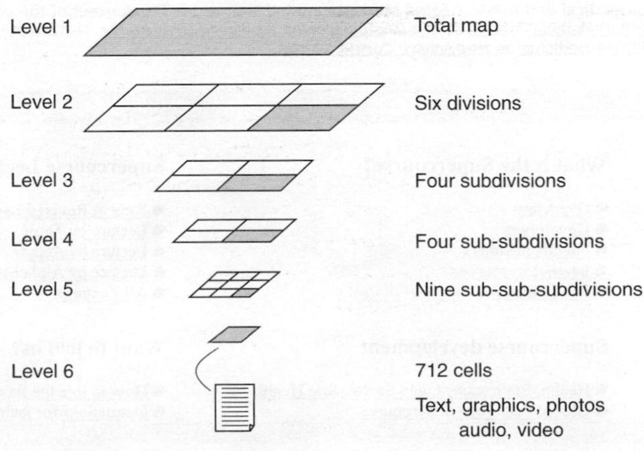

Fig. 2 Geographic information system for 1859 map of London.

text and current photographs to the respective cells. Subsequently, if a talented voice or actor is found, sound and perhaps video may be added as well. Thus, the 1859 map GIS serves as an example of how a network of geographic cells can be used to present educational data in space and time, and be made available for interested people throughout the world via the Internet.

Supercourse

Formal education in epidemiology is usually presented in public health or medical schools. However, once the degree is obtained, there are few opportunities for continuing education other than occasional sessions at professional meetings. Alternatively, persons may be working in public health settings but not have the opportunity to attend an academic epidemiology programme. Still others might want to supplement their existing education with lectures from other institutions or other faculty. For all such persons, the Supercourse was created on the World Wide Web (Fig. 3). At present, the site features a library of about 80 lectures prepared and reviewed by over 1200 epidemiologists and statisticians from more than 100 countries (La Porte *et al.* 2000). The material is presented as lectures of 20 to 30 slides, and can be accessed from more than 20 regional servers in most areas of the world. Also available at the Supercourse site are two textbooks on statistics and epidemiology issued by the *British Medical Journal* (Coggon 1977; Swinscow and Campbell 1977). Finally, the course developers are experimenting with sound and video, and will probably present lectures in more advanced formats as Internet pipelines expand for individual users beyond the capacity of traditional telephone modems.

Immunization information system

In the United States, children typically receive 16 doses of six vaccines (hepatitis B; diphtheria, tetanus and pertussis; *Haemophilus influenzae* type B; poliomyelitis; measles, mumps, and rubella; varicella) before 18 months of age (Advisory Committee on Immunization Practices 2000). To encourage parents and health-care providers to keep track of the many doses, in 1996 the State of Arizona established the Arizona State Immunization Information System (Popavich 1996). The state officials postulated that such a system of automated immunization records would reduce costs by eliminating the need for duplicate immunizations, target education and outreach efforts in high-risk locations, and reduce the impact of vaccine-preventable childhood diseases in the general paediatric population. In their system, immunization records and vital demographic data are collected and retained in local databases in the offices of health-care providers. These data are then transferred electronically to a central database registry at the Arizona Department of Health Services. By linking into the system via the registry, the immunization records are made available to the parents or the health-care provider. The system also provides summary statistics without patient identifiers to develop outreach programmes and to provide immunization statistics to health plans for certification and audits.

Estimating years of potential life lost

Our next example is an application that uses a spreadsheet software program. Mortality data are derived by most countries, and are essential for programme planning and evaluation. Yet as societies age, cause-specific mortality rates increasingly reflect the death experiences of older persons. While death is inevitable, premature death is not and can often be prevented. Deaths at age 45 have different social and economic implications for a country than deaths at age 85. Yet both ages of death are given the same weight or importance when comparing mortality rates. Over two decades ago, Romeder and McWhinnie (1977) proposed a premature mortality indicator that tallied lost years rather than lost lives. This measure was subsequently adopted by several nations, including the United States, which

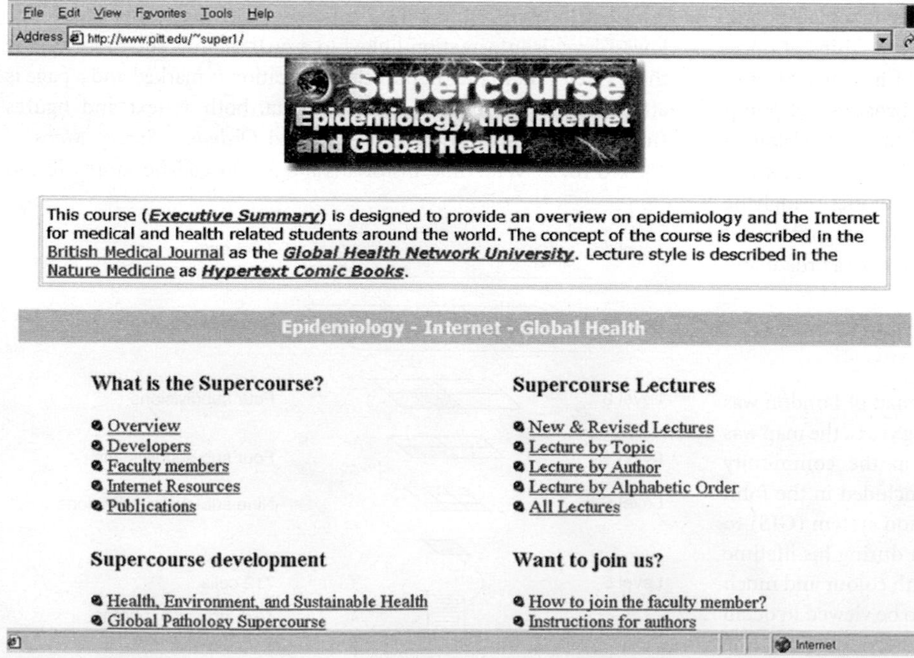

Fig. 3 Example of an educational website for epidemiology.

currently reports years of potential life lost (**YPLL**) before age 75 for the most common causes of death (Kramarow *et al.* 1999). However, epidemiologists and health planners may find that the presentation of YPLL rates in summary tables is not to their liking—they may want information on death categories that are not listed, or different age cut-offs, or with age groups weighted to reflect their economic or social importance. To this end, we will briefly describe the concept and formulae, and then show a spreadsheet program that provides useful estimates of YPLL using published population data and mortality rates.

Information on dates of birth and death are used to derive age-specific death rates as shown in part A of Fig. 4. A death is counted as a single event, but tallied by age of death. While a goal of society might be to avoid early or premature deaths, a cut-off point needs to be established to define premature death. If being able to live to at least 65 years is the goal, then years lost due to premature death before age 65 would be tallied as shown in part B of Fig. 4. If the goal is life to at least age 75 or even 85 years, then years lost due to an earlier death would be tallied as shown in parts C and D respectively of Fig. 4. Death among persons older than the cut-off point would not be included as potential lost years.

In the United States, deaths rates are regularly presented per 100 000 population by age group as under 1 year, 1 to 4 years, 5 to 14 years, continuing to 75 to 84 years and 85 years and older. The formulae for estimating years of potential life lost before ages 65, 75, and 85 are presented below, along with a weighting factor that estimates the value of people in the age group to the society.

Estimated YPLL before age 65 is given by

$$\widehat{\text{YPLL}}_{65} = \sum_{i=<1}^{55-64}\left(z_i w_i n_i \frac{r_i}{100\,000}\right) 100\,000 \Big/ \sum_{i=<1}^{55-64} n_i$$

where i denotes eight age categories (< 1 year; 1–4 years; 5–14 years; 15–24 years; 25–34 years; 35–44 years; 45–54 years; 55–64 years), z_i is the number of years of potential life lost per ith age category (64.5 for < 1; 62 for 1–4; 55 for 5–14; 45 for 15–24; 35 for 25–34; 25–35 to 44; 15 for 45–54; 5 for 55–64), w_i is the value weight for the age category (always 1.0 in this example), n_i is the number of people in the population in the ith age group, and r_i is the rate numerator per 100 000 for age group i that is listed in published mortality reports.

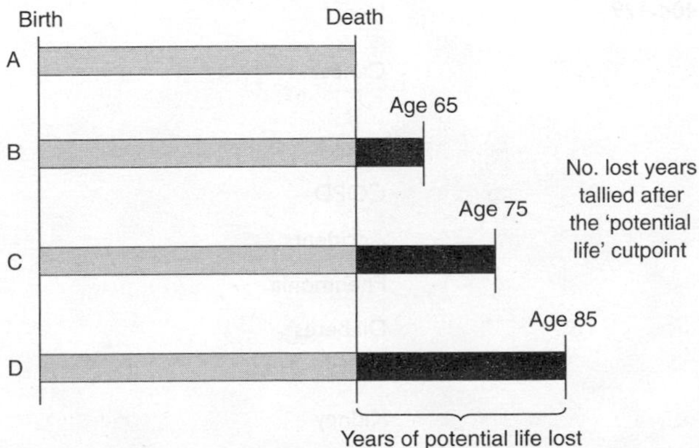

Fig. 4 Varying forms of years of potential life lost.

Estimated YPLL before age 75 is given by

$$\widehat{\text{YPLL}}_{75} = \sum_{i=<1}^{65-74}\left(z_i w_i n_i \frac{r_i}{100\,000}\right) 100\,000 \Big/ \sum_{i=<1}^{65-74} n_i$$

where i denotes nine age categories (< 1 year; 1–4 years; 5–14 years; 15–24 years; 25–34 years; 35–44 years; 45–54 years; 55–64 years; 65–74 years), z_i is the number of years of potential life lost per age category (74.5 for < 1; 72 for 1–4; 65 for 5–14; 55 for 15–24; 45 for 25–34; 35 for 35–44; 25 for 45–54; 15 for 55–64; 5 for 65–74), and w_i, n_i, and r_i are as previously defined.

Estimated YPLL before age 85 is given by

$$\widehat{\text{YPLL}}_{85} = \sum_{i=<1}^{75-84}\left(z_i w_i n_i \frac{r_i}{100\,000}\right) 100\,000 \Big/ \sum_{i=<1}^{75-84} n_i$$

where i denotes 10 age categories (< 1 year; 1–4 years; 5–14 years; 15–24 years; 25–34 years; 35–44 years; 45–54 years; 55–64 years; 65–74 years; 75–84 years), z_i is the number of years of potential life lost per age category (84.5 for < 1; 82 for 1–4; 75 for 5–14; 65 for 15–24; 55 for 25–34; 45 for 35–44; 35 for 45–54; 25 for 55–64; 15 for 65–74; 5 for 67–84), and w_i, n_i, and r_i are as previously defined.

Spreadsheet program

The formulae are entered into a computer spreadsheet program, as shown in Table 2 where calculations are presented for deaths due to diseases of the heart in 1997 in the United States. The top six rows of the spreadsheet are filled with text or numbers, while rows 7 to 10 contain formulae that calculate the components of the YPLL index. The specific formulae are shown in the lower section of Table 2, where rows 7 to 10 are repeated.

To illustrate the calculations of YPLL we will use United States mortality data from 1997 for the top 10 causes of death (Hoyert *et al.* 1999), as shown in Table 3. In our resultant graphs we will use the abbreviated term for each cause of death, rather than the more extensive terms presented in Table 3 by title and ICD code.

The National Center of Health Statistics of the United States derives the years of potential life lost before age 75 for selected causes, including eight of the top 10 death categories. The estimated YPLL_{75} derived using eqn (2) underestimated the actual YPLL_{75} by 3.7 per cent for diseases of the heart, 3.5 per cent for cancer, 4.6 per cent for stroke, 6.9 per cent for chronic obstructive pulmonary disease, 5.8 per cent for pneumonia and influenza, 3.8 per cent for diabetes, 3.8 per cent for suicide, and 2.6 per cent for diseases of the liver. Thus the values presented here should be viewed as estimates, not exact calculations.

The mortality rates for the top 10 causes of death are shown in Fig. 5(a), presented in the same order as in Table 3 from highest to lowest. When viewed by premature death, the rankings differ considerably. For YPLL before age 65 (Fig. 5(b)), cancer is ranked highest, followed by accidents, heart, and suicide. For YPLL before age 75 Fig. 5(c) or before age 85 Fig. 5(d), the rankings remain similar but attenuated. Thus it is evident that, at least in the United States, the age of the cut-off point for YPLL derivations makes a difference in the rankings of the burden of the disease, although these are more similar than the dramatic differences when compared with mortality rates. The choice of cut-off point is left to the reader, although each can be derived on a microcomputer using a spreadsheet software program.

Table 2 Spreadsheet of YPLL for diseases of heart using United States Mortality Data, 1997

	A B	C	D	…	L	M	N	O	P	Q
1		**Age group**								
2		**< 1 year**	**1–4 years**	…	**75–84 years**	**85+ years**	**Sum**	**Age cutpoint**	**Population**	**Rate per 100 000**
3	*Population*	*3 796 593*	*15 353 002*	…	*11 705 713*	*3 871 348*	*267 636 072*			
4	*Value weight*	*1.0*	*1.0*	…	*1.0*	*1.0*				
5	*Heart*									
6	*Rate*	*16.4*	*1.4*	…	*1943.6*	*6198.9*				
7	*Est. no*	*622.6*	*214.9*	…	*227 512.2*	*239 981.0*				
8	*YPLL < 65*	*40 160.4*	*13 326.4*	…			*1 425 104*	*< 65*	*233 560 458*	*610*
9	*YPLL < 75*	*46 386.8*	*15 475.8*	…	*1 137 561.2*		*3 322 414*	*< 75*	*252 059 009*	*1318*
10	*YPLL < 85*						*7 054 404*	*< 85*	*263 764 723*	*2675*
	Spreadsheet formulae									
7	*Est no*	*C$3/100000*C6*	*D$3/100000*D6…*		*L$3/100000*L6*	*M$3/100000*M6*				
8	*YPLL < 65*	*(65-0.5)*C$4*C$7*	*(65-3)*D$4*D$7…*				*@SUM(C8.L8)*	*< 65*	*@SUM(C3-J4)*	*N8*100000/P8*
9	*YPLL < 75*	*(75-0.5)*C$4*C$7*	*(75-3)*D$4*D$7…*				*@SUM(C9.L9)*	*< 75*	*@SUM(C3-K4)*	*N9*100000/P9*
10	*YPLL < 85*	*(85-0.5)*C$4*C$7*	*(75-3)*D$4*D$7…*		*(85-80)*L$4*L$7*		*@SUM(C10.L10)*	*< 85*	*@SUM(C3-L4)*	*N10*100000/P10*

Systems approach to epidemiology

Epidemiologists often develop causal webs for describing disease aetiology, or for considering possible prevention and control programmes. Given this orientation, aspects of systems theory are a natural adjunct to the discipline. Modelling software, now available on the microcomputer, offers a useful tool for considering problems from a systems perspective. The dynamics of epidemics, heart disease patterns, and other diseases or events can be modelled using such systems software. The programs allow one to set up the initial conditions and then alter values to see the effect on patterns of disease. Furthermore, models can introduce prevention strategies to determine the effect on disease outcomes. As models are not real, they are not an end in themselves. Instead, modelling should be viewed as a tool to help epidemiologists understand the dynamic and often complex aspects of disease occurrence.

Systems thinking is natural to epidemiology. The traditional aetiological model of agent, host, and environment is essentially a systems model of disease occurrence. A system is defined as a group of interacting, interrelated, or interdependent components that form a complex and unified whole (Anderson and Johnson 1997). The whole has a purpose to it—something that is being accomplished. This purpose may not be readily apparent to an observer, but there is an organizing and driving force among the parts or variables of the system. The behaviour of the system is derived from the relationships of the variables within the system boundaries. The variables may be tangible (like people and viruses) or intangible (like values and feelings). The parts are arranged in a specific way. Changing the arrangement changes the behaviour of the system. To illustrate systems thinking, we will present two models of viral diseases: the common cold and yellow fever. The first involves a microbe that is

Table 3 Top 10 causes of death, United States, 1997

Cause of death	ICD-9 code[a]	Abbreviation
Diseases of the heart	390–398, 402, 404-429	Heart
Malignant neoplasms, including neoplasms of lymphatic and haematopoietic tissues	140–208	Cancer
Cerebrovascular diseases	430–438	Stroke
Chronic obstructive pulmonary diseases and allied conditions	490–496	COPD
Accidents and adverse effects	E800–E949	Accidents
Pneumonia and influenza	480–487	Pneumonia
Diabetes mellitus	250	Diabetes
Suicide	E950–E959	Suicide
Nephritis, nephrotic syndrome, and nephrosis	580–589	Kidney
Chronic liver disease and cirrhosis	571	Liver

[a] *International Classification of Diseases, Ninth Revision.*

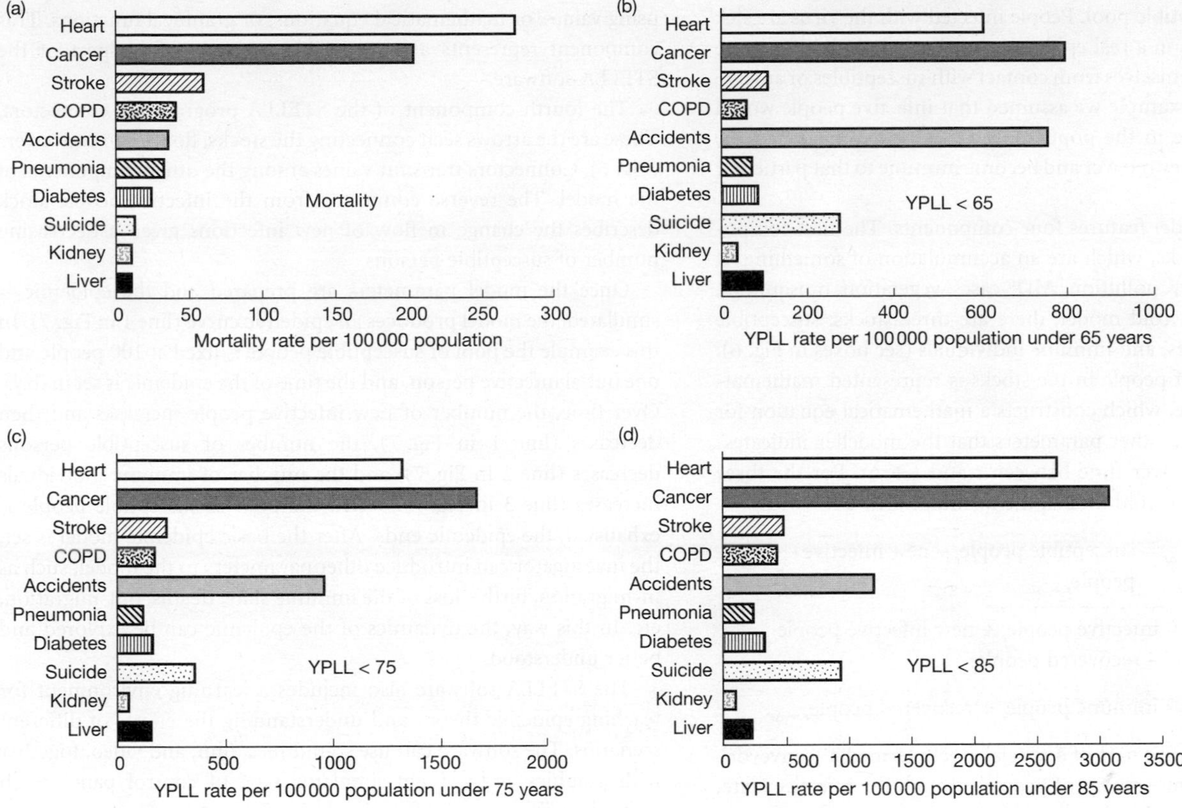

Fig. 5 (a) Mortality rates and (b), (c), (d) estimated YPLL for varying age cut-off points for the top 10 causes of death, United States, 1997.

transmitted directly from person to person through respiratory excretions, while the second is an agent transmitted indirectly via a mosquito vector. Models of both diseases are run on microcomputers.

For simple diseases such as the common cold, people can be categorized as susceptibles, infectives, and immunes. In an open population with persons moving in and out, the relationship between susceptible and infective people is reinforcing, such that as the number of susceptibles increases, so does the number of infective people. In a closed population, where there are no replacements for the pool of susceptibles, there is a reciprocal relationship between susceptible and infective persons. As the number of people entering the infective category increases, the pool of susceptibles decreases, creating feedback that will end the epidemic or outbreak once the pool of susceptible people is depleted.

STELLA is a software program for modelling epidemics on the microcomputer (Richmond 1997; STELLA Research Software 2000). To create a model, the system needs first to be conceptualized. Typically, the process involves identifying the epidemiological links between agents and hosts as they function in their environment. Specifically, the process involves a statement of purpose, the list of component variables, decisions about the time frame and systems boundaries to use, a picture of the behaviour that is to be explained, establishment of the feedback loops that exist among the variables, and creating and then testing the model (Albin 1997). Once operational, the model is used to experiment with various prevention and control strategies.

Common cold

The goal of the first simulation is to identify and understand the relationships that produce an epidemic curve of the common cold. Of course, the ultimate purpose is to decide where public health officials might intervene in the epidemic process. Rather than asking, 'What are all the factors that influence an epidemic of the common cold?', the systems thinker asks, 'How does an epidemic actually evolve?' Thus, this approach uses operational thinking by asking how people and disease agents interact to produce epidemics. To employ the STELLA software, the user must first introduce the components of the model. The program then converts the components to differential equations and proceeds with the modelling process. The user can introduce mathematical parameters, equations, or graphs to define the dynamics of the system. The components of the STELLA software used to computerize the model will be described in detail.

The propagated epidemic of a common cold begins with the introduction of the virus into a pool of 100 susceptible people who are exposed to one infective person. The model assumes homogeneous mingling of infected people with susceptible persons. For the virus to be transmitted, a susceptible individual must first be exposed to an infective person. In the current model, the probability of such exposure in the population being studied is 10 per cent. Once exposure to an infective person has occurred, the virus still may not be transmitted. The transmission rate for the common cold model is assumed to be 25 per cent among exposed people. The rate at which new infections occurs depends on exposure and dose factors, and on the size of the susceptible pool. People infected with the virus are sick for several days, and in a real epidemic may be so sick that for some days they remove themselves from contact with susceptibles or anyone else. In this simple example we assumed that infective people would continue to circulate in the population. Once people have had the respiratory illness, they recover and become immune to that particular virus.

The STELLA model features four components. The first component is boxes or stocks, which are an accumulation of something. It can be people, money, pollution, AIDS cases, vegetation, mosquitoes, etc. In the common cold model, there are three stocks: susceptible people, infective cases, and immune individuals (see boxes in Fig. 6). The accumulation of people in the stocks is represented mathematically by the software, which constructs a mathematical equation for each stock (given the other parameters that the modeller indicates) showing the change over time between t and $t + \Delta t$. For the three stocks in the common cold model, the formulae are

$$\text{susceptible people}_{t+\Delta t} = \text{susceptible people}_t - \text{new infective people}_{t+\Delta t}$$

$$\text{infective people}_{t+\Delta t} = \text{infective people}_t + \text{new infective people}_{t+\Delta t} - \text{recovered people}_{t+\Delta t}$$

$$\text{immune people}_{t+\Delta t} = \text{immune people}_t + \text{recovered people}_{t+\Delta t}.$$

The infective people are part of a special stock, termed a 'conveyor', that serves to delay movement of people through the infective state, giving them time to be ill before they move to recovery. In this case we used a median duration of 3 days. People enter the infective state, ride along the conveyor for 3 days, and then get off by recovering to the immune state (Fig. 6).

The second component describes the dynamics of the system, presented in STELLA by the flow. In the common cold model shown in Fig. 6, flow is illustrated with double-lined arrows as the rate of new infections and the rate of recovery. Regulator valves in the centre of the flow lines alter the flow, depending on factors such as exposure, transmission, and recovery rates. Stocks and flows work together to generate the epidemic.

The third component of the STELLA model is the converter, represented by a circle. In the common cold epidemic model, converters are the exposure rate and the transmission rate (Fig. 6). Converters change the input to the output, or in this instance convert susceptible persons into infective people. Converters can be defined using values, or mathematical equations, or graphical functions. This component represents a very flexible and powerful aspect of the STELLA software.

The fourth component of the STELLA program are connectors. These are the arrows seen connecting the stocks, flows, and converters (Fig. 6). Connectors transmit values among the other components of the model. The reverse connector from the infective people stock describes the change in flow of new infections given a decreasing number of susceptible persons.

Once the model parameters are prepared and the epidemic is simulated, the model produces an epidemic curve (line 1 in Fig. 7). In this example the pool of susceptible people is fixed at 100 people and one initial infective person, and the time of the epidemic is set in days. Over time, the number of new infective people increases and then decreases (line 1 in Fig. 7), the number of susceptible persons decreases (line 2 in Fig. 7), and the number of immune individuals increases (line 3 in Fig. 7). When the pool of susceptible people is exhausted, the epidemic ends. After the basic epidemic model is set, the investigator can introduce other parameters to the model, such as in-migration, births, loss of the immune state, deaths, out-migration, etc. In this way, the dynamics of the epidemic can be explored and better understood.

The STELLA software also includes a learning environment for teaching epidemic theory and understanding the effects of different scenarios. The software can use sound files, film, and video, together with graphics and a flight-simulator type of control panel. Such technology is very useful for stimulating interest among novice users, thereby helping to develop systems-oriented thinking skills.

Yellow fever

The modelling process can become quite complex, especially with a disease such as yellow fever which features mosquito and human interactions. The dynamics of the mosquito population are modelled separately from the human population and then linked together to generate a yellow fever epidemic (Fig. 8). The model, based on the work of Albin (1997), starts with the mosquito population becoming infected with the yellow fever virus. The success of the epidemic depends on the number of infectious mosquitoes and on the probability of infected mosquitoes biting susceptible humans. If they bite immune humans, no infection results. Once humans become infected they serve as the pool for reinfecting the mosquito population. Humans can die from yellow fever or they can recover and

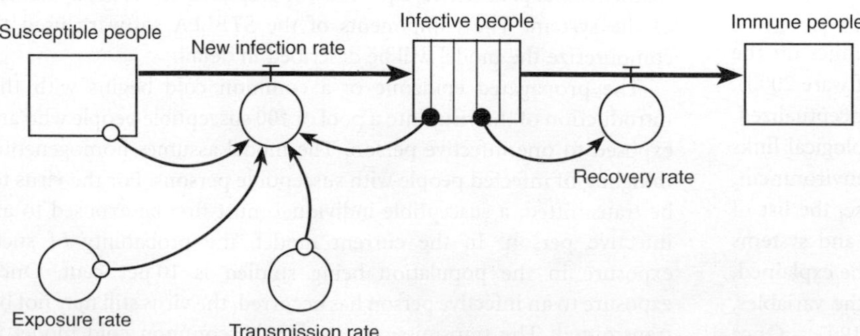

Fig. 6 Epidemic model of the common cold created using STELLA.

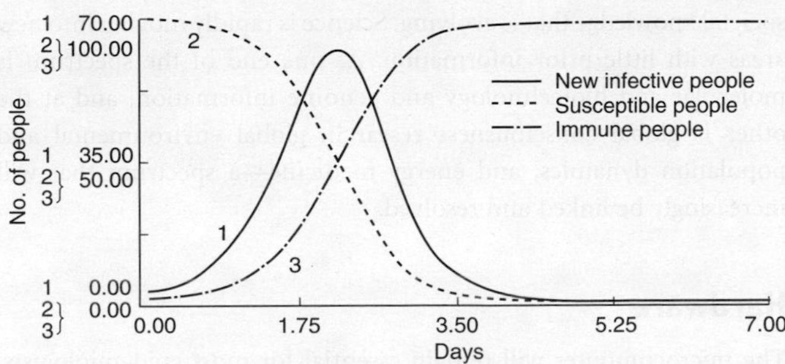

Fig. 7 Graph of epidemic model of cold created using STELLA.

retain lifelong immunity. Such a complex epidemic is especially useful in an educational setting in which students consider how humans interact with the environment and are able to try different approaches to control activities. The yellow fever model is available on the Internet (Systems Dynamics in Education Project 2000), and offers a useful teaching exercise for understanding epidemics (Glass-Husain 1993).

While epidemic models are interesting examples of systems theory, various other public health problems and biological processes have also been modelled with the STELLA software. These include models for diabetes and drug addiction, and for a number of non-physical variables such as attitudes, values, etc. Also available is a health behaviour model of cigarette smoking. Each relies on the same four components (i.e. stock, flow, converter, connecter) to create a complex system, and then uses the power of the microcomputer to simulate a dynamic system.

View of the future

By definition, the future is always left to the imagination. With this thought in mind, we will generate mental images of the trends and directions that computers, software, and the Internet will take. In the preceding sections of this chapter, we have tried to avoid mentioning specific computers or software because of the rapid changes that are taking place, fostering obsolescence every few years. Instead we tried to focus on general categories of hardware and software that will remain available in the future. Finally, we described five applications of epidemiological importance using current computing and Internet technology, some of which would not have been possible in earlier years. In this concluding section, we will look into the future, first with some general comments and then thoughts specific to hardware, software, and the Internet.

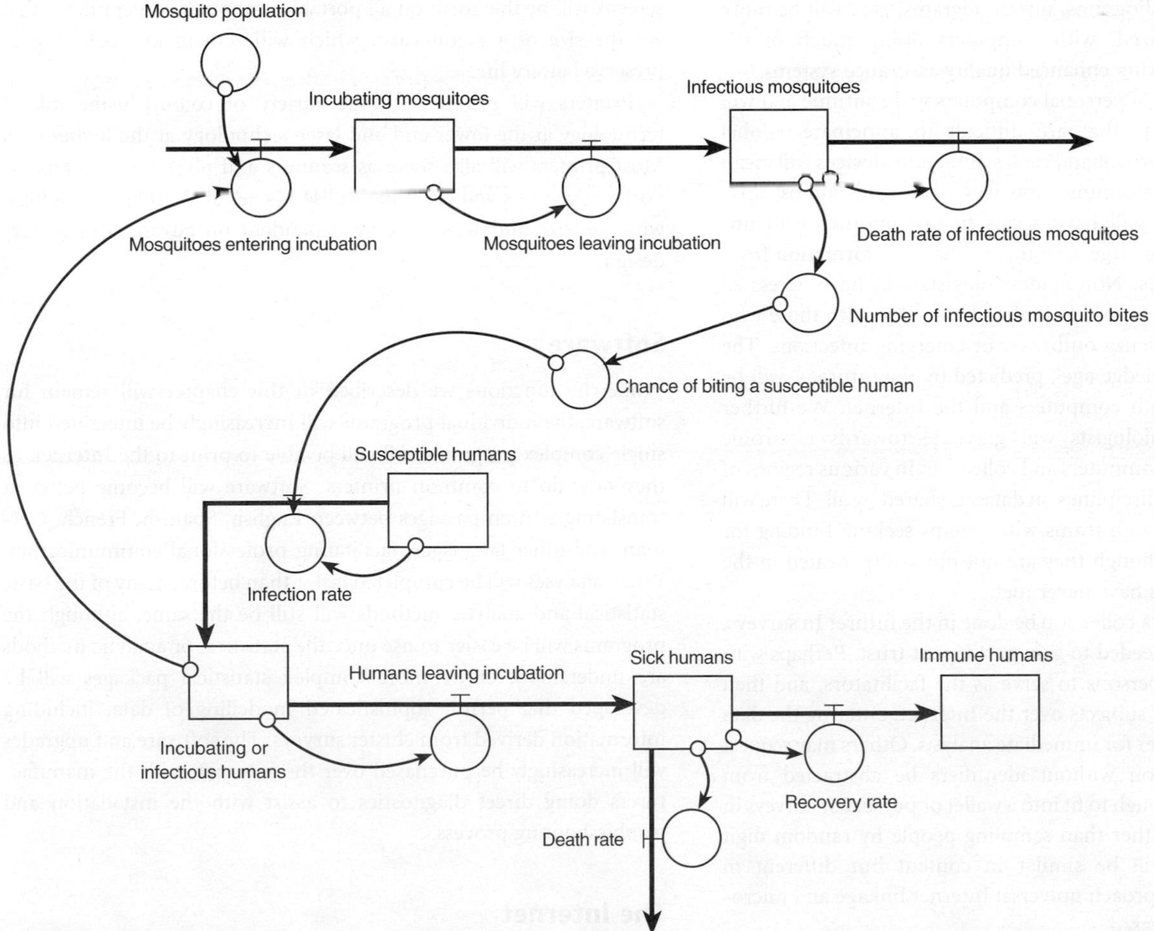

Fig. 8 Epidemic model of yellow fever created using STELLA.

Computer technology is increasing in speed and complexity faster than most people appreciate. At present, computers are said to be doubling in speed every 12 months (Kurzweil 1999), while the total amount of information available in the world is doubling every 18 months or less (Petersen 1998). Software programs are now capable of recognizing continuous human speech with a vocabulary of about 60 000 words and accuracy levels similar to those of skilled human typists (Kurzweil 1999). Technology is advancing to the point where devices a billionth of a meter in size (a nanometer) will soon hold about 4 gigabits (a billion bits) or more (Petersen 1998). Developers are working on holographic memory devices that could replace hard disks, yet store more than 10 gigabytes of data on something the size of a sugar cube. Also under development are optical integrated circuits that would be 1000 times faster than current silicon chips (Petersen 1998). Before the next edition of this book arrives, such items should be appearing in the marketplace.

What this means to epidemiologists is that they will have access to smaller, lighter, and more powerful computers with the ability to store very large databases and to process and analyse data much faster than is now possible. In addition, information will potentially be garnered by microprocessors that store medical data, including patient records, in medical institutions and provider offices. Ethical issues will be debated and resolved, providing epidemiologists with access to vast amounts of data containing unique but non-personal identifiers. Many measurements of biological and medical information, such as DNA typing, electrocardiograms, ultrasonograms, etc., will be more accurate and standardized, with computers doing much of the measurement and featuring enhanced quality assurance systems.

The interconnection of personal computers will continue and will have far-reaching effects that are difficult to anticipate. Global networks connected by broadband cables or satellite devices will mean almost instantaneous communication with colleagues almost anywhere. Epidemiologists will have access to one another with unprecedented ease, and to large amounts of shared information from past and current studies. Non-epidemiologists will have access to some of the same information, as is already the case with those who check the status of influenza outbreaks or emerging infections. The emergence of the 'knowledge age', predicted by the futurists, will be greatly facilitated by both computers and the Internet. We further anticipate that epidemiologists will gravitate towards electronic research, working with computers and colleagues in various regions of the world with assorted disciplines on datasets shared by all. There will probably be virtual research teams with groups seeking funding for research projects even though they are not physically located in the same place, and perhaps have never met.

How will primary data collection be done in the future? In surveys, often a friendly face is needed to gain participant trust. Perhaps with time we will use local persons to serve as the facilitators, and then conduct interviews with subjects over the Internet, entering the data directly into the computer for immediate analysis. Others may request that medical information without identifiers be abstracted from patients' cards, small enough to fit into a wallet or purse. For surveys in the developed world, rather than sampling people by random digit dialling, the process will be similar in content but different in procedure as nations approach universal Internet linkage and microcomputer access is increased.

Epidemiologists will need more powerful computers and more systems software packages to be able to model and analyse the complex societal knowledge that is evolving. Science is rapidly moving into new areas with little prior information. At one end of the spectrum is molecular and biotechnology and genome information, and at the other is global consciousness research, global environmental and population dynamics, and energy medicine—a spectrum that will increasingly be linked and resolved.

Hardware

The microcomputer will remain essential for most epidemiologists, both for research and for information sharing and retrieval. The next generation of desktop microcomputers will have 512 megabytes (space for 512 million typed characters) of random access memory, a 400 000-megabyte (40-gigabyte) hard disk drive, which will serve as a holding area for 1000 gigabytes of erasable optical storage, a 1-gigabyte DVD disk drive, and a 17-inch flat liquid crystal display monitor with 1280 × 1024 pixel screen resolution, having the ability to create thousands of on-screen colours with flicker-free images. Broadband modems or satellite linkages will become routine. A microphone will be attached to the computer for dictating and converting oral words to written words. Both a page scanner and electronic pencil will be common for entry of book chapters, journal articles, photographs, and hand-written notes. Portable or notebook computers will also be more powerful, although not as powerful as desktop machines. Colour screens will be the norm on all portable computers except those that are the size of a credit card, which will remain monochrome to preserve battery life.

Printers will produce a wide variety of colours using ink-jet technology at the lower end and laser technology at the higher end. Most printers will also serve as scanners and photocopiers. Finally, portable printers will continue to use ink-jet or thermal technology, with the size and weight being dependent on advances in battery design.

Software

While the functions we described in this chapter will remain for software, the individual programs will increasingly be integrated into single complex programs. All will be able to print to the Internet, as they now do to common printers. Software will become better at translating written passages between English, Spanish, French, German, and other languages, facilitating professional communication. While analyses will be completed faster than before, many of the basic statistical and analytic methods will still be the same, although the programs will be easier to use once the statistical or analytic methods are understood. Other more complex statistical packages will be developed that permit sophisticated modelling of data, including information derived from cluster surveys. The software and upgrades will increasingly be purchased over the Internet, with the manufacturers doing direct diagnostics to assist with the installation and troubleshooting process.

The Internet

The broad trend towards individual empowerment will continue over time. Electronic mail has already replaced the telephone and regular mail service for many people. Using the Internet, more individuals will have personal sites that describe their experiences or life in pages, slide and sound exhibits, and video shows. A similar trend will occur with epidemiologists, although their sites will focus more on professional output, including articles and oral presentations.

Internet courses will continue to evolve from the slide shows that are now common, to animated slides and sound, and eventually to video. The video will expand in two forms. The first is real-time presentations similar to current videoconferencing, which allows for interactive questions and answers, and the second is stored videos, available for viewing at any time. Students will increasingly use logic branches to study issues and concepts, with answers and guidance provided at each branch for both right and wrong answers. Books will continue to be important, as will class notes. However, they will be distributed via the Internet either for local printing and viewing or as files for electronic books. Class notes will downloaded as files and printed by the student. In developing countries, much will depend on the cost of satellite transmission, possibly subsidized by more prosperous nations as a component of foreign assistance. In such a setting the educational process will be greatly enhanced for those able to incur the cost.

Course lectures will be routinely recorded and made available as Internet files for downloading as compressed files for use in portable players. Thus those who need repetition, or just more time, will be able to individualize the educational experience. Finally, the distinction between home and office will become less apparent, as contact and communication occurs over the Internet rather than in person.

Conclusions

Over the years, the fundamental concepts of epidemiology have served the profession well. We continue to honour the reasoning of Dr John Snow, who more than 150 years ago was able to identify the aetiological mechanism for cholera, 25 years before the agent was actually identified. Yet we often overlook the many erroneous paths that have been travelled, and the inefficiency of some epidemiological research. To this end, microcomputers and the Internet bring additional tools to epidemiology, stimulating new approaches that promote the advancement of science. Such advancement by public health professionals in various international settings is what fulfils the promise of technology for individual empowerment.

References

Advisory Committee on Immunization Practices (2000). Recommended childhood immunization schedule—United States, 2000. *Morbidity and Mortality Weekly Report*, **49**, 35–38, 47.

Albin, S. (1997). *Building a system dynamics model: Part 1—conceptualization. Systems dynamics in education project.* MIT Systems Dynamics Group, Boston, MA.

Anderson, V. and Johnson, L. (1997). *Systems thinking basics: from concepts to causal loops.* Pegasus Communications, Boston, MA.

Anonymous (1998). RABNET—strengthening international surveillance of human and animal rabies. *Weekly Epidemiological Record*, **73**, 254–5.

Anonymous (1999). Web-based surveillance data system (CISID): WHO European Region. *Weekly Epidemiological Record*, **74**, 427–8.

Anonymous (2000). An integrated approach to communicable disease surveillance. *Weekly Epidemiological Record*, **75**, 1–7.

Clark, D. (2000). Inktomi promises improved searches for customers after study of the Web. *Wall Street Journal*, 18 January 2000.

Coggon, D., Rose, G., and Barker, D.J.P. (1997). *Epidemiology for the uninitiated* (4th edn). (http://www.bmj.com/epidem/epid.html). BMJ Publishing, London.

Dean, A.G. (1999). Epi Info and Epi Map: current status and plans for Epi Info 2000. *Journal of Public Health Management and Practice*, **5**, 54–7.

Fernandez, E., Sobreques, J., and Schiaffino, A. (1999). Epidemiology and public health journals on the Internet. *Journal of Epidemiology and Community Health*, **53**, 510–12.

Finkelstein, J., Cabrera, M.R., and Hripcsak, G. (2000). Internet-based home asthma telemonitoring: can patients handle the technology? *Chest*, **117**, 148–55.

Flahault, A., Dias-ferrao, V., Chaberty, P., Esteves, K., Valleron, A.J., and Lavanchy, D. (1998). FluNet as a tool for global monitoring of influenza on the Web. *Journal of the American Medical Association*, **280**, 1330–2.

Frerichs, R. (2000). John Snow site. (http://www.ph.ucla.edu/epi/snow.html). University of California at Los Angeles.

Frerichs, R.R. and Selwyn, B.J. (1991). Microcomputer applications in epidemiology. In *Oxford textbook of public health* (2nd edn) (ed. W.W. Holland, R. Detels, and E.G. Knox), pp. 271–84. Oxford University Press.

Frerichs, R.R. and Selwyn, B.J. (1997). Microcomputers and epidemiology. In *Oxford textbook of public health* (3rd edn) (ed. R. Detels, W.W. Holland, J. McEwen, and G.S. Omenn), pp. 721–33. Oxford University Press.

Geraghty, J.G. and Young, H.L. (1999). Continuing medical education by satellite: implications for oncology education. *European Journal of Cancer Care*, **8**, 48–50.

Glagola, M.J. (1998). Access control for electronic patient records. *Radiological Management*, **20**, 44–50.

Glass-Husain, W. (1993). *Teaching system dynamics: looking at epidemics. Systems Dynamics in Education Project. Road Maps (D-4243).* (http// sysdyn.mit. edu/road-maps/rm). MIT Systems Dynamics Group, Boston, MA.

Gordis, L. (2000). *Epidemiology* (2nd edn). W.B. Saunders, Philadelphia, PA.

Harbage, B. and Dean A.G. (1999). Distribution of Epi Info software: an evaluation using the Internet. *American Journal of Preventive Medicine*, **16**, 314–17.

Houston, J.D. and Fiore, D.C. (1998). Online medical surveys: using the Internet as a research tool. *MD Computing*, **15**, 116–20.

Hoyert, D.L., Kochanek, K.D., and Murphy, S.L. (1999). Deaths: final data for 1997. *National Vital Statistics Reports*, **47**.

Jarman, R. (1859). *Reynolds map of modern London, divided into quarter mile sections.* James Reynolds, London.

Joffres, M.R. and La Porte, R.E. (1998). Bringing epidemiology manuals and books onto the Internet through Epilink. *American Journal of Epidemiology*, **147**, 325–9.

Kassirer, I.P. (1999). Posting presentations at medical meetings on the Internet. *New England Journal of Medicine*, **340**, 803.

Klutke, P.J., Baruffaldi, F., Mattioli, P. Toni, A., and Englmeier, K.H. (1999). Guidelines for multipoint videoconferencing using low-cost, PC-based equipment. *Journal of Telemedicine and Telecare*, **5**, 198–202.

Kramarow, E., Lentzner, H., Rooks, R., Weeks, J., and Saydah, S. (1999). *Health and aging chartbook. Health United States, 1999.* National Center for Health Statistics, Hyattsville, MD.

Kurzweil, R. (1999). *The age of spiritual machines when computers exceed human intelligence.* Penguin Putnam, New York.

Larkin, M. (1998). Where to find clinical trials on the Web. *Lancet*, **351**, 1140.

LaPorte, R.E, Sekikawa, A., and Aaron, D.J. (2000). *The Supercourse.* (http://www.pitt.edu/∽super1/). University of Pittsburgh.

McKay, J.R. (1999). Studies of factors in relapse to alcohol, drug and nicotine use: a critical review of methodologies and findings. *Journal of the Study of Alcohol*, **60**, 566–76.

McLaren, P., Mohammedali, A., Riley, A., and Gaughran, F. (1999). Integrating interactive television-based psychiatric consultation into an urban community mental health service. *Journal of Telemedicine and Telecare*, **5** (Supplement 1), S100–2.

Nielsen, J. (1999). *Designing web usability: the practice of simplicity*. New Riders, Indianapolis, IN.

Overdyk, F.J., Haynes, G.R., and Arvanitis, P.J. (1999). Patient-borne memory device facilitates 'point of care' data access. *MD Computing*, **6**, 60–3.

Petersen, J. (1998). *The road to 2015: profiles of the future*. Arlington Institute, Arlington, VA.

Popavich, N. (1996). Pilot projects start with managed care plans. *ASIIS Interface*, **2**, 1–2.

Ranson, G. and Kaplan, B. (1998). USDA uses PulseNet for food safety. *Journal of the American Veterinary Medical Association*, **213**, 1107.

Richmond, B., Peterson, S., and Soderquist, C. (1997). *STELLA: an introduction to systems thinking*. High Performance Systems, Hanover, NH.

Romeder, J.-M. and McWhinnie, J.R. (1977). Potential years of life lost between ages 1 and 70: an indicator of premature mortality for health planning. *International Journal of Epidemiology*, **6**, 143–51.

Rothman, K.J. and Greenland, S. (1998). *Modern epidemiology* (2nd edn). Lippincott–Raven, Philadelphia, PA.

Snow, J. (1855). *On the mode of communication of cholera*, (2nd edn). John Churchill, London.

STELLA Research Software (2000). http://www.hps-inc.com. High Performance Systems, Hanover, NH.

Swinscow, T.D.V. and Campbell, M.J. (1977). *Statistics at square one* (9th edn). (http://www.bmj.com/ collections/statsbk/index.shtml). BMJ Publishing, London.

Systems Dynamics in Education Project (2000). *Road maps— a self-study guide to learning system dynamics.* (http//sysdyn. mit. edu/road-maps/). MIT Systems Dynamics Group, Boston, MA.

Valero, M.A., Arredondo, M.T., del Nogal, F., Rodriguez, J.M., and Torres, D. (1999). Using cable television networks for interactive home telemedicine services. *Journal of Telemedicine and Telecare*, **5** (Supplement 1), S91–2.

Ware, C. (1999). *Information visualization: perception for design*. Morgan Kaufmann, San Francisco, CA.

Watanabe, M. Jennett, P., and Watson, M. (1999). The effect of information technology on the physician workforce and health care in isolated communities: the Canadian picture. *Journal of Telemedicine and Telecare*, **5** (Supplement 2), S11–19.

Wilcox, A.J. (1999). The quest for better questionnaires. *American Journal of Epidemiology*, **150**, 1261–2.

6.16 Public health surveillance

Ruth L. Berkelman, Donna F. Stroup, and James W. Buehler

Public health surveillance is the epidemiological foundation for modern public health. Surveillance data resulting from the continuous monitoring of the occurrence of a disease or condition, such as AIDS or lead poisoning, underlie what public health actions are taken and reflect whether these actions are effective. The term 'surveillance' is derived from the French word meaning 'to watch over' and, as applied to public health, means the close monitoring of the occurrence of selected health conditions in the population. Although surveillance methods were originally developed as part of efforts to control infectious diseases, basic concepts of surveillance have been applied to all areas of public health. Public health surveillance has been expanded to include not only information on diseases, injuries, and other conditions but also information such as the prevalence of risk factors, both personal and environmental.

Definition

In 1963 Langmuir defined disease surveillance as 'the continued watchfulness over the distribution and trends of incidence through the systematic collection, consolidation, and evaluation of morbidity and mortality reports and other relevant data' together with timely and regular dissemination to those who 'need to know' (Langmuir 1963). In 1968 the 21st World Health Assembly described surveillance as the systematic collection and use of epidemiological information for the planning, implementation, and assessment of disease control; in short, surveillance implied 'information for action' (WHO 1968). The role and concept of public health surveillance continue to evolve as the scope of surveillance broadens and as increasingly sophisticated methods are applied (Thacker *et al.* 1989; Thacker and Stroup 1994).

Surveillance should begin when there exists or is likely to occur a public health problem for which programmes for prevention and control of a health event have been or may need to be initiated. A critical component of the definition of surveillance is that surveillance systems include the ongoing collection, analysis, and use of health data. Thus, health information systems (for example, registration of births and deaths, routine abstraction of hospital records, health surveys in a population) that are general and not linked to specific prevention and control programmes do not, by themselves, constitute surveillance. However, data collected from ongoing health information systems may be useful for surveillance when systematically analysed and applied on a timely basis.

History

The idea of collecting data, analysing them, and considering a reasonable response stems from Hippocrates (Eylenbosch and Noah 1988). When writing on disease occurrence, Hippocrates made a distinction between the steady state, the endemic state, and the abrupt change in incidence—the epidemic. Possibly, the first public health action that can be attributed to surveillance occurred in the 1300s when public health authorities in a port near the Republic of Venice prevented passengers from coming ashore during the time of epidemic bubonic plague in Europe. The first Bill of Mortality was issued in London in 1532 as a consequence of fear of a plague epidemic. John Graunt's treatise *Natural and Political Observations on the Bills of Mortality* published in 1662 is generally recognized as one of the first documents to describe use of numerical methods for monitoring public health. In 1776 Johann Peter Frank advocated a more extensive monitoring of health in Germany that would support public health efforts related to the health of schoolchildren, prevention of injuries, maternal and child health, and public water and sewage disposal.

William Farr is recognized as the founder of the modern concept of surveillance. As Superintendent of the Statistical Department of the General Registrar's Office in Great Britain from 1839 to 1879, he collected, analysed, and interpreted vital statistics and disseminated the information in weekly, quarterly, and annual reports. He did not stop with publication of official reports, but regularly contributed papers to medical journals and even used the public press to achieve effective action (Langmuir 1976). Thus, he took the responsibility of seeing that action was taken on the basis of his analyses.

In the nineteenth century, Farr's efforts at health monitoring were extended by Edwin Chadwick, who investigated the relationship between environmental conditions and disease. Chadwick was followed by Louis Rene Villerme, who analysed the relation between poverty and mortality in Paris. In the United States, Lemuel Shattuck also published data that related deaths, infant and maternal mortality, and infectious diseases to living conditions. He further recommended standardized nomenclature for cause of disease and death, and the collection of health data that included sex, age, locality, and other demographic factors. The first international list of causes of death was developed in 1893 (Eylenbosch and Noah 1988).

Increasingly, elements of surveillance were applied to aid in detecting epidemics and in preventing and controlling infectious diseases. In 1899 the United Kingdom began compulsory notification of selected infectious diseases. National morbidity data collection on plague, smallpox, and yellow fever was initiated in 1878 in the United

States, and by 1925 all states were reporting weekly to the United States Public Health Service on the occurrence of selected diseases. In a public health context, the term surveillance was increasingly applied to programmes of reporting selected infectious diseases in a population, with less emphasis on its application to quarantine of individuals (Langmuir 1963; Thacker and Gregg 1996).

Similar reporting activities were occurring in Europe at about the same time. In 1907 the Office International d'Hygiene Publique, predominantly composed of European member states, was created (WHO 1958). The office was to disseminate information in a monthly bulletin on the occurrence of selected diseases, most notably cholera, plague, and yellow fever. In the succeeding decades, other diseases were recommended for surveillance in step with the International Sanitary Regulations. However, many of the morbidity and mortality reporting systems were not systematic and were still largely developed for long-term archival functions.

Since the early 1950s, the critical importance of surveillance to public health efforts has been demonstrated frequently. In 1955 acute poliomyelitis among recipients of the poliomyelitis vaccine in the United States threatened national vaccination programmes that had just begun. In collaboration with state health departments, the American Centers for Disease Control (**CDC**) developed an intensive national surveillance system, and at one point a daily report was being issued regarding poliomyelitis cases. The surveillance data assisted epidemiologists in demonstrating that the problem was limited to a single manufacturer of the vaccine and allowed the vaccination programme to continue with a resulting dramatic decline in cases of acute poliomyelitis in the United States in successive years (Langmuir 1963). During the worldwide malaria control programme, surveillance was used to determine areas of continued transmission and to focus spraying efforts, as well as to document those areas without malaria (Raska 1966). With the subsequent decline in malaria control efforts, surveillance data have documented the re-emergence of malaria in many areas of the world. In so doing, these data have contributed to renewed interest in malaria control at the end of the twentieth century.

Surveillance was also the foundation for the successful global campaign to eradicate smallpox. When the campaign began in 1967, efforts were focused on achieving a high vaccination level in countries with endemic smallpox; however, it was soon evident that a programme based on surveillance to target vaccinations in limited areas would be more efficient. Smallpox reporting sources, usually medical facilities, were contacted on a routine basis, and thus a reporting network was firmly established in most countries. In addition, other reporting sources were often established, including markets, schools, police, agricultural extension workers, and others. In 1973, as the goal of eradication neared, a systematic house-to-house search for cases was established in India and subsequently used widely in Pakistan and Bangladesh (Henderson 1976). Well-designed surveillance systems for data collection, tabulation, and routine feedback were vital to the success of the programme.

In 1981, shortly after the disease later named AIDS was recognized, national surveillance was begun in the United States and other countries. Even before the aetiological agent, HIV, was identified, surveillance data contributed to identifying modes of transmission, population groups at risk for infection, and, equally important, population groups not at risk for infection. These data have been instrumental in directing public health resources to programmes, preventing further spread of HIV, and averting widespread public hysteria (Jaffe *et al.* 1983).

The need for a strong infrastructure for surveillance systems is currently being re-emphasized not only as countries face the emergence and re-emergence of infectious diseases (Berkelman *et al.* 1994; Heymann and Rodier 1998) but also as a result of the increasing threat of biological terrorism (Henderson 1999). Plans for detecting terrorist events include strengthening current surveillance systems as well as establishing new ones, such as surveillance of emergency calls for medical assistance, and admissions of patients to intensive care units for respiratory conditions.

The potential usefulness of surveillance as a public health tool to address problems beyond infectious disease was emphasized in 1968 when the 21st World Health Assembly recommended the application of surveillance principles to a wider scope of problems, including cancer, atherosclerosis, and social problems such as drug addiction (WHO 1968). Many of the principles of surveillance traditionally applied to acute infectious diseases have also been applied to chronic diseases and conditions, although some differences in surveillance techniques have been observed (Thacker *et al.* 1995) (Table 1). Even though chronic diseases may have long latency periods, trends in their incidence may change relatively quickly, and surveillance can play a key role in detecting these changes when effective interventions are applied (Berkelman and Buehler 1990).

In addition to the increased scope of health problems under surveillance, the methods of surveillance have expanded from general disease notification systems to include survey techniques, sentinel health-provider systems, and other approaches to data collection (Thacker and Berkelman 1988; Thacker and Stroup 1994). Beyond disease notification, an ideal surveillance system would provide analyses of risk factors for disease and injury.

The assimilation of computers into the workplace has made possible more efficient data collection as well as more rapid and sophisticated analyses (Dean *et al.* 1998). In the United States, all state health departments are linked to the CDC by computer for the routine collection and dissemination of selected data on notifiable health conditions (CDC 1991). In developing countries, computers are increasingly being used with epidemiological programmes for analysis and mapping (Frerichs 1991; Dean *et al.* 1993). Geographical information systems are also in widespread use.

The explosive development of technology will include the development of high-capacity storage devices, expansion of the capabilities of the internet, use of local- and wide-area networks for entry of surveillance data at multiple computers simultaneously, and development of new programming tools, video and computer integration, and voice and pen input. Integration of systems, including data standards, is needed to allow maximal use of these advancements (Morris *et al.* 1996).

Purposes of surveillance

A surveillance system should be designed to meet the needs of a prevention and control programme (Table 2). These needs usually include a description of the temporal and geographical trends in the occurrence of a health event in a particular population. Most importantly, surveillance systems should identify changes in disease occurrence. The data should be useful for substantiating patterns of both endemic and epidemic disease.

Table 1 Acute and chronic disease surveillance

	Common characteristics	Acute disease surveillance	Chronic disease surveillance
Purpose	Monitor trends. Describe problem and estimate health burden. Direct/evaluate programmes for prevention and control	Emphasis on weekly or monthly variations to detect outbreaks	Emphasis on year-to-year trends
Data	Regular	Reliance on notification by health-care providers/laboratories	Greater use of existing databases (e.g. vital statistics, hospital discharges)
Data analysis	Descriptive statistics for time, place, person	Emphasis often on case counts	Emphasis usually on rates
Data dissemination	Regular; frequency reflects data collection. Audience targeted	More frequent	Less frequent

The role of surveillance in guiding public health programmes is illustrated by the first major national disease control activity initiated by the CDC—the Malaria Eradication Programme. Surveys in the mid-1930s had established malaria to be an endemic problem deeply rooted in the south-eastern part of the United States. An extensive chlorophenothane (DDT) spraying programme was launched after the Second World War, and surveillance was instituted in 1947. Data from this surveillance system established rapidly that endemic malaria had essentially disappeared, probably even before the DDT programme was under way (Langmuir 1963). In this case, surveillance was used as the basis for dismantling a public health programme and redirecting public health resources to problems of higher priority.

However, the need for surveillance may continue for a disease even when prevention and control programmes are cut back, particularly for infectious diseases such as tuberculosis, dengue fever, or malaria whose incidence may change quickly. Generally, the more quickly re-emergence of a disease is detected, the more quickly and efficiently it can be controlled (CDC 1992*a*; PAHO 1994).

Surveillance data are also useful for evaluating the effectiveness of prevention and control programmes (CDC 1992*b*) and of regulations or laws modified or initiated to address public health concerns (for example safety of food and water, alcohol-related motor vehicle injuries). Monitoring of changes in the incidence of the disease or condition is necessary, and monitoring associated risk factors (food and water sanitation, self-reports of drinking and driving) may also be useful. The rapid decline in morbidity from many infectious diseases in certain populations has been related directly to vaccination campaigns that were conducted as a result of surveillance data on disease incidence. Direct correlation of a single intervention to a specific disease outcome may be difficult when the aetiology of the disease is multifactorial, but the impact of an intervention on disease outcome, including its incidence and severity, remains the ultimate test of policy.

Table 2 Purposes of public health surveillance

To define public health priorities
To characterize disease patterns by time, place, and person
To detect epidemics
To suggest hypotheses
To identify cases for epidemiological research
To evaluate prevention and control programmes
To facilitate planning, including projection of future trends and health-care needs

Assessment of the burden of disease, including its incidence (that is, the number of people newly affected each year) and its current and projected prevalence (that is, the number of people affected by the disease at any point in time), is essential to planning public health programmes. For example, in the 1980s, surveillance for AIDS was critical to the forecasting of the future impact of that disease in the United States (Gail and Brookmeyer 1988; Institute of Medicine 1988). With the ageing of the population, projections of disease prevalence in the elderly are being emphasized (Murray and Lopez 1997).

Surveillance may be initiated to identify risk factors associated with disease and to suggest hypotheses for further investigation; cases identified through surveillance are sometimes used in case–control studies, as in the early studies of toxic shock syndrome and the AIDS epidemic (Shands *et al.* 1980; Jaffe *et al.* 1983). Effective preventive actions were formulated based on such research even before the aetiological agents, a toxigenic strain of *Staphylococcus aureus* and HIV, were discovered.

Establishing a surveillance system

Establishing a surveillance system requires a statement of objectives, definition of the disease or condition under surveillance, and implementation of procedures for collecting, interpreting, and disseminating information. Surveillance systems can be considered as information loops, or cycles, that involve health-care providers, public health agencies, and the public. A weakness in any part of the loop or information chain weakens the entire surveillance process. For example, if public health measures mandate that infectious conditions such as cryptosporidiosis must be reported, the surveillance system will be successful only if laboratories have the capacity to diagnose the infection (Berkelman 1994). Likewise, if the diagnosis on a hospital discharge record is coded incorrectly, surveillance data based on hospital discharge records will reflect the inaccuracies.

The information cycle begins when cases occur and is completed when information about these cases is made available and is used for prevention and control. This process may involve multiple cycles, ranging from the local response to individual cases to the development of national policies based on information aggregated from many cases.

Essential to the completion of the surveillance cycle is the return of information to those who 'need to know' (Langmuir 1963), and thus attention must be directed not only to procedures for collecting data but also to procedures for ensuring that useful information is returned to constituents.

The likelihood that effective interventions can be found, can prevent the occurrence of disease, or can alleviate the course of existing disease is an important consideration in determining whether a surveillance system will be useful. However, even in the absence of a currently effective intervention, surveillance data can indicate the need for legislation (for example, the use of surveillance data on traumatic head injuries to influence legislation regarding mandatory use of bicycle helmets in children) or the need for more resource allocation if a problem poses an increasing health threat (for example, development of a pneumococcal vaccine for children aged under 2 years old becomes more urgent as the incidence of multidrug-resistant pneumococci increases). A surveillance programme is less likely to succeed if no clearly effective control or prevention measures are defined.

Health priorities for surveillance must be continually evaluated as new infections emerge (for example, *Escherichia coli* 0157:H7), the population is exposed to new hazards (for example, new consumer products, environmental contamination), and other health conditions change. Surveillance for both the disease or condition, as well as for associated risk factors and prevention services, should be considered.

Public health surveillance in developing countries: special considerations

Many aspects of public health surveillance are similar for developed and developing countries; these include the steps of system design and the principle of collecting information for action. However, existing data sources and resources for targeted data collection are generally far more limited in developing countries than in developed countries; scarce resources have led to relatively inexpensive and innovative surveillance techniques in many developing countries.

Tracking disease trends (particularly infectious diseases) has been the main reason surveillance systems have been instituted in developing as well as developed countries (Langmuir 1963). Many infectious diseases and other conditions of public health import—diarrhoea, malaria, pneumonia, and malnutrition—occur in settings with only rudimentary health care and few laboratory resources. Diseases are often empirically treated, and lack of definitive diagnosis may hinder surveillance and response efforts. Resources for surveillance that contribute to passive disease notification may result in inadequate data to meet surveillance or other health objectives (Sandiford *et al.* 1992).

Successful surveillance systems have been developed and maintained for targeted conditions; their success is partly dependent on features that include low budget, simplicity of reporting procedures, personal rapport with people in the network, regular feedback, and visible intervention consequent upon reporting specific conditions. For example, surveillance for childhood vaccine-preventable diseases has been conducted in Vellore, India, for more than a decade; every hospital (both government and private) is enrolled and participates in the system (John *et al.* 1998).

Programmes to eradicate polio (and previously smallpox) make extensive use of surveillance to monitor the progress toward reaching their goals (CDC 1999*a*). Eradication programmes must rely on targeted surveillance, which becomes more important (and expensive) as the target disease approaches eradication (Henderson 1998). The resources for targeted surveillance activities, including laboratory support, for an eradication or other specific programme may come from other countries, and may include both public and private donors.

In many developing countries, the process of linking surveillance to objectives highlights the need for mortality data and the absence of vital registration. The most basic health statistics are limited in many developing countries, with death registration inadequate or non-existent. Use of the verbal autopsy, which uses a caretaker interview to determine the cause of death, may assist in following mortality patterns in places without routine death registration (Kaufman *et al.* 1997; Fantahun 1998; Tollman *et al.* 1999). Sensitivity in establishing an accurate cause of death may be lower for some acute febrile conditions such as malaria than for conditions such as maternal causes, injuries, tuberculosis, and AIDS (Chandramohan *et al.* 1998), and different techniques in conducting verbal autopsies may result in quite different sensitivities for specific conditions (Quigley *et al.* 1996).

Other sources of health information may include United Nations International Children's Emergency Fund (**UNICEF**), the World Health Organization (**WHO**), international conferences, non-governmental organizations, and population laboratories (for example, the International Center for Diarrheal Disease Research, Bangladesh). Although health problems are similar in many low-resource settings, relying on data from other countries can create major problems when there are geographical differences in the incidence of the condition. In addition, the health impact associated with certain conditions such as hepatitis B, rotavirus, or malaria may be significantly different in different regions and countries.

The design of surveillance systems must consider such issues as resources available, security, geography, population dispersion and mobility, type of health system, and literacy. Problems (more common but not unique to developing countries) may include limited personnel available for public health, multiple vertical systems, lack of laboratory capacity, and infrastructure and communications constraints (for example, lack of equipment, supplies, or electrical power).

Solutions to address the lack of personnel for public health and prevention have included voluntary systems (using community health workers, traditional birth attendants, or village volunteers). More familiar solutions are public health training programmes designed to meet human resource gaps (Adams and Hirschfeld 1998). Concerns about the cost-effectiveness of short-term training and the lack of applicability of long-term training to academic graduates have resulted in programmes targeting the specific needs of public health agencies. Examples include the Field Epidemiology Training Programs and the Public Health Schools Without Walls (Music and Schultz 1990; Cardenas *et al.* 1998), training programmes that have been initiated in both developed and developing countries.

Concurrently, the increase in availability of computers to analyse and transmit surveillance data and the decrease in the cost of such technology offers increased opportunity for surveillance. Epi Info is a public health computer program designed to assist data management and analysis that is available free and over the internet (Dean 1999); this tool has been used successfully in both developed and developing countries. This program is available in seven languages (English, French, Spanish, Arabic, Russian, Chinese, and Serbo-Croat), and manuals or portions of it have been translated into these languages and Italian, Portuguese, German, Norwegian, Hungarian, Czech, Polish, Romanian, Indonesian, and Farsi. Epi Info and other information systems should be seen as tools to be used to provide data to policy-makers and others to inform decisions which improve health.

Surveillance system objectives

Defining the objectives of a surveillance system depends on what information is needed, who needs it, and how it will be used. Implementing a system will require a balance of competing interests, and a clear statement of objectives will provide a framework for subsequent decisions. For example, the desire to collect detailed information about cases may compete with needs to assess the number of cases rapidly. Thus, if the primary objective is to obtain rapid case counts, less information would be collected about each case to avoid delays in reporting. The objectives of a surveillance system will be shaped by its target population and its constituents, the nature of prevention and control programmes, and the health problem under surveillance.

Target population

A surveillance system seeks to identify health events within a specified population. This population may be defined on the basis of where people live, work, attend school, or use health-care services. Alternatively, the population may be defined on the basis of where health events occur. For example, a surveillance system that monitors newborn health as a measure of prenatal care services would focus on deliveries to women who live within a community and not on women who live elsewhere but deliver in the community's hospitals. In contrast, surveillance of traffic injuries aimed at identifying roadway hazards could include all injuries that occur in a community, regardless of whether affected people are community residents.

Constituents of surveillance systems

Surveillance systems are likely to have many constituents, including health-care providers, public health professionals, researchers at academic health centres, politicians, media reporters, the public, and others with diverse perspectives and uses for surveillance data. Because these diverse needs cannot always be satisfied, the primary or most important constituents should be identified.

Nature of public health programmes

The objectives of surveillance systems will be shaped by the objectives and capabilities of the public health programmes they serve. For example, a programme to eradicate an infectious disease requires intensive surveillance in the final stages of the campaign that emphasizes identification of all people with the disease (Hinman and Hopkins 1998). This strategy was used in the smallpox eradication programme and has also been employed in the poliomyelitis eradication programmes in the Americas (Foege *et al.* 1975; Biellik *et al.* 1992). In contrast, an educational programme to influence behaviour may depend on a surveillance system that describes the practices of a sample of people in a community (Remington *et al.* 1988).

Health problems under surveillance

It is necessary to decide exactly what disease or health problem will be under surveillance, using such criteria as the magnitude of the public health problem (or potential magnitude) as well as the capacity to prevent or control the disease or condition through public health actions. Surveillance may frequently be conducted for any of several points along a spectrum, ranging from exposure to an adverse outcome. It is important to consider which manifestation(s) or stage(s) of a disease should be under surveillance. For example, manifestations of ischaemic heart disease include abnormal diagnostic tests in the absence of symptoms, angina pectoris, acute myocardial infarction, and (sudden) death. If the goal of surveillance is to assess the burden of the disease on health-care systems, a broad definition that encompasses various manifestations may be appropriate. If the purpose is to monitor trends in the disease, a more limited and severe manifestation, such as myocardial infarction, may be the appropriate target for surveillance. If resources are limited, surveillance based on analyses of death certificates may be most feasible; however, interpretation of trends may be complicated by independent trends in the occurrence of the disease, advances in treatment, or changes in coding vital records. Alternatively, attention may be focused on risk factors for cardiovascular disease, such as hypertension, smoking, cholesterol levels, and physical activity (Arnett *et al.* 1998; McQueen 1999). For surveillance of infections carried by animals or arthropods (such as rabies and encephalitis), surveillance of infection in the reservoir host may be as important as surveillance in the human population.

Case definition

The case definition is fundamental to any surveillance system because it is the formal answer to the question of what manifestations of a disease or condition are under surveillance (CDC 1997) (see http://www.cdc.gov/epo/dphsi/casedef). It is both a criterion for determining who is counted and a guide to local health departments for case investigations and follow-up. It ensures that the same measure is used across geographical areas. The case definition must be sufficiently inclusive (sensitive) to identify people who require public health attention but sufficiently exclusive (specific) to avoid unnecessary diversion of that attention. In addition, the case definition must be usable by all people on whom the system depends for case reporting. There is no ideal case definition for any particular disease or condition. The following are two possible case definitions that could be used in conducting surveillance for hepatitis A.

Definition 1

Illness characterized by jaundice, elevated liver enzymes, and serological detection of immunoglobulin M antibodies against hepatitis A. This definition presumes that affected people will have access to health-care services, including diagnostic testing. This approach would exclude people who have an epidemiological and clinical picture consistent with hepatitis A but who lack serological testing. The definition also does not include people with asymptomatic hepatitis A infection. An alternative may be to use a definition that includes all people with a positive test for immunoglobulin M antibodies against the hepatitis A virus. To accommodate these possibilities, the case definition may be subdivided to allow for symptomatic versus asymptomatic cases or for gradations based on certainty of diagnosis (confirmed case, presumptive case, possible case, and so on).

Definition 2

Illness characterized by yellow eyes. This definition is simple and may be appropriate in a setting where hepatitis A transmission has been documented and where there is limited access to diagnostic services, where field staff have little formal training, and where there is an emergent need to assess a population rapidly (for example, a common-source outbreak). With this definition, hepatitis case counts may include some people with jaundice caused by other conditions, but the lack of specificity may not substantially affect the usefulness of the overall information.

Neither of these two definitions or possible variations is inherently better than the other, and each may be appropriate in a given setting. The first definition is more specific but may lack utility in circumstances in which laboratory testing is limited. The second definition would not be appropriate for a population in which the majority of people are immune to hepatitis A, either because of past infection or vaccination.

Thus, the definition must be geared to the circumstances of each surveillance system. The definition must also remain current as conditions change. During the course of the poliomyelitis eradication campaign, different definitions have been used, with a less specific definition needed when cases of poliomyelitis are common. Following successful vaccination campaigns and a large reduction in disease incidence, case definitions for poliomyelitis require more specificity, which in turn requires laboratory confirmation of cases of acute flaccid paralysis (Andrus *et al.* 1992).

A similar range of possible case definitions also exists for surveillance systems that focus on adverse health exposures rather than disease outcomes. For example, in a surveillance system that addresses occupational hazards, exposure to a harmful substance may be monitored by self-report of workers, by company log-books of manufacturing procedures, or by routine measurement of substances in the work environment, on workers' clothing, or in specimens collected from workers. Each of these possible case definitions would require different levels of co-operation from the company or workers, and each may be subject to unique limitations that could bias surveillance.

The flow of information

Although surveillance systems for chronic diseases and other conditions frequently rely on multiple data sources that may be collected primarily for purposes other than public health, many surveillance systems depend on data acquired explicitly for surveillance purposes and rely on a sequential flow of these data through the full surveillance cycle. Each facet of this process should be carefully planned, as described below.

Reporters

People responsible for reporting cases may be all health-care providers in a defined area, selected providers, or people at specific institutions (for example clinics, health-care organizations, laboratories, hospitals, schools, factories, and so on). In addition to communicating case reports, reporters may be responsible for collecting specimens needed by public health agencies for laboratory confirmation or application of molecular epidemiological techniques (for example, determining whether a case of poliomyelitis has been caused by a vaccine strain or a wild-type poliomyelitis virus).

Data collection instruments

The desire to collect detailed information must be tempered by the need to limit data to items that can be reliably and consistently collected over the long term. Forms or other data collection instruments that are too detailed and too complicated will not be welcomed by those on whom the surveillance system must depend. This is independent of whether the forms are computerized, although computerization may make the process more acceptable to reporters. In addition, computerized systems that exist for other purposes (for example patient records) may permit more detailed collection of data without additional burden to the reporter.

In addition to the widespread use of computers in surveillance (Koo and Wetterhall 1996), standards for exchanging information are critical to the future utility of all public health surveillance and information systems. Many coding systems currently used in public health are not compatible with the needs of other organizations. In 1996, the American Congress passed the Health Insurance Portability and Accountability Act to encourage the development of standards for data related to health care (Chute *et al.* 1998). The passage of this legislation has increased the level of activity related to integration of clinical information in the United States.

Timing

Surveillance systems provide data on a regular basis, ranging from daily to annually. Whatever periodicity is used should be specified and adhered to by participants in all phases of the surveillance loop; reporting should occur even when the number of reported cases is zero. To contain an outbreak of meningococcal meningitis, the health department must receive reports of cases quickly (that is, within 24 h) so that necessary control measures may be taken immediately. In contrast, a breast cancer registry evaluating the effectiveness of targeted screening services for breast cancer may collect and analyse data on a quarterly basis or even less frequently. To achieve the objective of the surveillance system, the appropriate timing should be considered as the system is established. With increasing computerization and Internet use, reporting at the time of case identification is becoming a reality.

Aggregation of data

Surveillance data may be in the form of individual patient records or aggregate counts and tabulations. For example, there may be a need at the local level to maintain records on individual people to direct follow-up services. In addition, individual data permit more flexibility of analysis than aggregate data, and computerization has facilitated transfer of case-specific data more easily to a central level.

Data transmission

The mode of data transmission will depend on both the need for timeliness and communications resources. In many health agencies in developed and developing countries, computers are still unavailable and reliance on postage of forms and facsimile transmission is needed. During the 1980s, computers were introduced and increasingly used in surveillance systems, facilitating transmission of data in electronic formats and Internet communications (Valleron *et al.* 1986; CDC 1991; Koo and Wetterhall 1996).

Computerization has also been helpful in transmitting molecular data on isolates of certain pathogens, such as the pulsed field gel electrophoresis patterns of *E. coli* 0157:H7 through Pulse-Net (http://www.cdc.gov/ncidod/dbmd/pulsenet/pulsenet.htm). In addition, computerization may facilitate and enhance regular and personal contact among public health officials, health-care providers, and others who participate in such activities as a closed electronic mail system. The Emerging Infections Network, in which hundreds of infectious disease practitioners participate in the United States, uses an electronic mail conference for on-line discussion when new insights into disease occurrence are needed and allows for close communication between public health officials and health-care providers (Executive Committee of the Emerging Infections Network 1997).

Data management and dissemination

The following issues in data management and dissemination should be considered in planning for storage, analysis, and dissemination of surveillance information.

Updating records

Surveillance data often need to be updated. Information that was initially unattainable may become available, follow-up investigations yield supplemental information, people initially classified as meeting or not meeting a case definition may be reclassified, errors in reporting may be identified and corrected, and duplicate case reports may be recognized and culled. One approach to handling these and other changes is to maintain both provisional and final records, including separate publications for provisional and final data. When analysing trends, it is often useful to compare provisional data in one period of time with provisional data from another point in time, since bias in preliminary data may change when data are updated. Provisional reports may satisfy immediate information needs, whereas final and more delayed reports can accommodate corrections and updates to a reasonable limit and can serve an archival function. Computerization facilitates record updates.

Selecting measures for time and place

A case report may include dates, such as those of the onset of disease, the diagnosis, the report to local health authorities, and the report to regional or national health authorities. Analyses of surveillance data may be based on the date of any of these events. However, if there are, for example, long delays between dates of diagnosis and report, analyses of trends based on date of diagnosis will be unreliable for the most recent periods. Similarly, surveillance data may be tabulated on the basis of the site of occurrence of the health event, the site of diagnosis, or the residence of people reported. The selection of these measures for time and place may also differ for provisional and final surveillance reports. As with other statistical methods, the availability of software aids spatial analysis methods (Dean *et al.* 1991; Biomedware 1994).

Confidentiality

Preventing inappropriate disclosure of surveillance data is essential both to the privacy of people with reported cases of disease and to the trust of participants in the surveillance system. The protection of confidentiality begins with limiting data collection and transmission to a minimum and includes ensuring the physical security of surveillance records, the discretion of surveillance staff, and legal safeguards (Federal Committee on Statistics 1994). To elicit public health surveillance information from the public and from health-care providers, strong laws that assure a careful procedure for maintaining and reporting data are frequently necessary to ensure the privacy of personal information (Gostin and Hadley 1998). Privacy regulations in the United States are currently based on a patchwork of state and local legislation and may lack adequate protection for electronic health information. Recent bills introduced in the American Congress include definitions of protected information and descriptions of disclosures that may occur with or without consent. Sometimes forgotten in the discussion of health information privacy is the concept that use of electronic information systems can often improve the security of data.

Physical protection of records is accomplished by rules of conduct for people involved in the design, development, operation, or maintenance of any surveillance system. For example, confidential records should be kept locked up at all times when not in use. When confidential records are in use, they must be kept out of the sight of people not authorized to work with the records. Except as needed for operational purposes, copies of confidential records should not be made. When confidential surveillance records are in the possession of other agencies, provision should be made for their protection.

Provision of data containing identifiers of individuals or establishments should be held to the minimum number deemed essential to perform public health functions. Categories should be sufficiently broad to avoid inadvertent identification of an individual person or institution. In particular, release of information for small geographical areas must be carefully considered to protect confidentiality (Committee on National Statistics 1993).

Initiating and maintaining participation

Public health agencies depend on the ongoing co-operation of others to identify and report cases in most surveillance systems. Whether reporting is required by law, is voluntary, or is financially rewarded, most reporting still takes time and effort (this may change as information systems play a larger role). Many approaches require contact of public health professionals with the reporting sources; dissemination of reports that document the usefulness of surveillance data are likely to be a key to initiating and maintaining participation in the system. In addition to professional meetings and other personal contacts, electronic mail affords an excellent route of informal communication between public health professionals and health-care providers.

For certain diseases, reporting is often required by law. Although legal mandates may not guarantee reporting, they establish the authority under which health agencies conduct surveillance. In addition, reporting laws and regulations may identify not only those who are required to report cases but also those who may report cases without fear of liability for violation of privacy. Statutes may also protect health agencies from forced disclosure of the identity of people with particular diseases.

Organizational structure

If the surveillance loop of data collection, analysis, interpretation, and feedback is to function as a continuous process, an organizational structure is required. Such a structure depends on the resources available, including the number of personnel and their level of training, the technology available for communication and data management (for example computers), and financial constraints, as well as the number and type of diseases, health conditions, or risk factors under surveillance. In one example of a simple form of reporting, the organizational structure requires health-care providers to report a single disease or health event on a regular basis to a co-ordinating public health authority. A more complex form would include a network of reporting units dealing concurrently with problems related to many diseases. In any case, the structure must allow data to be gathered from various sources and evaluated by epidemiologists in time for appropriate action to be taken. These data must be routinely disseminated to a targeted audience and reproduction and telecommunication equipment are minimal requirements.

The structure should provide support for training of key personnel in surveillance through seminars, distance-based learning, or other venues that give field and central staff the opportunity to review procedures and to resolve operational problems. Appropriate technical support, such as provision of diagnostic reagents, laboratory space, and computer equipment, must also be ensured. Finally, the need for regular evaluation of the surveillance systems should be recognized.

Delegating tasks to international, national, regional, and local health authorities should depend on information needs and resources at each level. Particular attention should be directed to the local level because primary responsibility for information collection and public health responsibilities are usually local. Central agencies are responsible for guiding, as well as co-ordinating, data collection procedures; they ensure that surveillance data are collected using standardized methodology such that the data from one geographical area can be reliably compared with data from another area and such that the data can be aggregated into regional or national summaries. Also, because many monitoring efforts for non-infectious conditions (for example, traffic injuries, water pollution, and so on) are often dealt with by governmental agencies other than public health agencies (for example, police authorities, environmental protection agencies), there needs to be effective co-ordination between health authorities and other appropriate authorities; for this purpose, procedures may need to be established to ensure the necessary communication.

Data collection

Public health surveillance data are collected in many ways, depending on the nature of the health event under surveillance, potential methods for identifying the disease, the population involved, the resources available, and the goals of the programme. Some surveillance systems may rely on a single source of data with alternate data sources being used periodically to evaluate or to enhance the completeness of routine surveillance data.

Notification systems

Notifiable disease reporting is the surveillance approach traditionally used by public health programmes. A system of notification is based on laws or regulations by health authorities that require reporting of selected diseases or conditions, usually infectious, to the health department to support and direct prevention and control programmes (Rousch *et al.* 1999). Notification reporting may be instituted at many levels (local, national, and international). Ultimately, under a system of notification, the reporting will be most useful and most accurate for diseases if surveillance is supported and emphasized at a local level. People or institutions with responsibility for reporting to the public health authority often include doctors, other health-care providers, coroners and medical examiners, laboratories, and hospitals. Historically, doctors and other health-care workers such as infection control practitioners have been most important to systems of notification. Reliance on laboratory reporting and on computerized records collected primarily for other reasons is increasing.

In any country, the extent of notification activities depends on the availability of facilities and resources—trained staff, laboratory and other equipment, epidemiological services, and liaison with health-care providers and other key reporters—as well as the health priority of the disease and method of diagnosis (Berkelman *et al.* 1994). Reports are often initiated by health-care providers or other reporting source; for some diseases for which more complete reporting is sought, public health professionals may contact major reporting sources and/or review laboratory or other relevant records to ensure that cases are ascertained. These systems of reporting have been described as passive and active respectively, but the distinctions are not always clear. Data for many surveillance programmes represent a mixture of both reports elicited by public health professionals contacting health-care providers or reviewing records and reports submitted by health-care providers to public health officials without direct solicitation. Computerization of patient and laboratory records should facilitate reporting.

Reporting is generally incomplete for most notifiable diseases (Hinman 1977; Vogt *et al.* 1983). If people are asymptomatic or have only mild symptoms, they will not usually seek health care. Patients and doctors may conceal diseases that carry a social stigma, such as sexually transmitted diseases. Health-care providers may also fail to report because they may be unaware of regulations or because they may treat the symptoms without a complete laboratory investigation. Completeness of reporting may also be significantly influenced by factors such as medical community interest and publicity; the most important is probably the intensity of surveillance efforts, which is closely linked to availability of resources (Davis and Vergeront 1982; Buehler *et al.* 1992). Many incomplete data may serve their purpose, however. Epidemics, as well as general temporal and geographical trends, can be determined as long as the proportion of cases detected remains consistent over time and across geographical areas.

A comparison between cases of viral hepatitis reported by practitioners in private practice and cases reported in a population covered by an insurance plan in Israel demonstrated that, although completeness of reporting by the doctors was only 37 per cent, the distribution of reported cases by season and age was similar to that recorded in the insured population (Brachott and Mosley 1972). However, under-reporting may affect representativeness; a study of under-reporting of acute viral hepatitis in the United States demonstrated that homosexual men with hepatitis B and blood transfusion recipients with non-A non-B hepatitis were less likely to be reported than members of other risk groups (Alter *et al.* 1987). Thus, surveillance data acquired through reports initiated by health-care providers may not accurately reflect the risk for specific populations.

The potential for re-emergence of infectious diseases requires continued vigilance and capacity to respond, even though the control programme may not be a high public health priority (for example, plague). As new infectious agents are recognized, the need to expand the surveillance system to control these agents effectively has been recognized in many countries. Furthermore, as international travel and commerce facilitate the rapid spread of pathogens from one part of the globe to another, the need for improved international communicable disease surveillance has become apparent (Institute of Medicine 1992; Heymann and Rodier 1998).

Although infectious conditions have dominated the list of notifiable diseases in most countries, other diseases and conditions may also have to be reported. Adverse drug reactions, occupational injuries, poisonings, and specified malignancies, among others, may be required to be reported, particularly in developed countries (Faich *et al.* 1987; DeBock 1988; Freund *et al.* 1989; Koo and Wetterhall 1996).

In settings where the infrastructure does not exist to support accurate case reporting systems yet there is a need to assess the impact of a disease on morbidity, an alternative and potentially simple and rapid approach is to survey hospitals periodically for the number of admissions attributed to a particular condition (DeCock *et al.* 1989). Another crude but inexpensive surveillance system for diseases with high morbidity rates and for which notification may not be appropriate (for example, gastrointestinal illnesses or influenza) may be based on absenteeism from schools or industry, depending on the ages of the affected populations.

Health-care provider networks

Networks of health-care providers have been organized in recent years, primarily to gather information on selected health events. Most have been organized by practising doctors on a voluntary basis; in many European countries, these networks have formed firm relationships with both public health authorities and academic centres, and often form the basis for morbidity surveillance (Valleron *et al.* 1986).

The strengths of sentinel provider systems include the commitment of the participants, the possibility of collecting longitudinal data, the flexibility of the system to address a changing set of conditions, and the ability to gain information on all patient-provider encounters, regardless of severity of illness. The most severe limitation of this type of system is that the population served by these doctors may not be representative of the general population. In addition, the illness must be fairly common to provide representative incidence data from a small sample of doctor contacts.

Example

A voluntary network of general practitioners in Belgium was initiated in 1978 (Stroobant *et al.* 1988). Practitioners were selected who were representative of Belgian general practitioners according to age and sex and who were geographically distributed to ensure coverage of the country. Participants report weekly and the results are sent to the participants on a quarterly basis. The list of health problems has included selected vaccine-preventable diseases, respiratory conditions, and suicide attempts, with some health problems such as mumps and measles reported continuously and others on a less frequent basis. A high level of participation has been documented, with the degree of form completion and continuity of reporting as criteria for assessment. The network has been evaluated in terms of its possible biases, such as non-participation of practitioners and difficulties in estimating the population at risk for the health problems under study; methods have been developed to reduce these biases (Lobet *et al.* 1987).

Example

The British Paediatric Surveillance Unit (**BPSU**) (http://bpsu.rcpch.ac.uk) was initiated in 1986 through the collaboration of several agencies: the British Paediatric Society, the Public Health Laboratory Service Communicable Disease Surveillance Centre, and the Department of Epidemiology at the University of London. The BPSU has also added collaborators from specialty groups such as orthopaedics, rheumatology, and dermatology. The BPSU has enabled paediatricians to participate in the surveillance of infections and infection-related conditions and in studies of uncommon disorders. It also provides a mechanism by which new diseases can be detected quickly and monitored. The reporting system involves the mailing of a monthly card which contains the disorders currently being surveyed. Examples of conditions under surveillance have included HIV infection and AIDS, insulin-dependent diabetes mellitus, acute flaccid paralysis, and new variant Creutzfeldt–Jakob disease in children.

Example

In 1979 the Ministry of Public Health in China and the Chinese Academy of Preventive Medicine initiated a sentinel network of surveillance sites to address the need for more timely and representative data (Cheng 1992; Yang 1992). Data from county and provincial epidemic prevention stations are reported to the Chinese Academy of Preventive Medicine. The entire surveillance system consists of five components: the National Notifiable Diseases Reporting System, disease-specific surveillance systems for endemic areas, mortality statistics, natality statistics, and a sentinel surveillance system for approximately 35 infectious diseases, births, deaths, vaccinations, and risk factors. Data are analysed monthly, and a report is distributed to health officials in more than 3000 counties. The data have been used to develop prevention programmes (Zhang 1990), detect changes in infectious agents (Shen *et al.* 1984), and influence policy affecting communities (Yang *et al.* 1997).

Laboratory surveillance

Surveillance of routinely collected laboratory reports has been particularly useful for certain infectious conditions. For instance, in the United States, reporting from many public health laboratories is automated (Bean *et al.* 1992). In England and Wales nearly all microbiology laboratories report positive identifications of specified infections each week to the Communicable Disease Surveillance Centre. The advantages of the laboratory reporting system are its specificity, its flexibility in adding new diseases, its rapidity, and the amount of detail about the infectious agent that can be provided. Reports indicate trends or the appearance of rare infections originating from a common source that could not be identified by a single laboratory. One disadvantage is that the number of people from whom specimens are tested is usually not reported. In addition, the people tested may not be representative of the population at risk. For some infections, such as toxic shock syndrome, there is no laboratory test, and for many common illnesses a specimen may not be taken (for example influenza).

Nosocomial infection surveillance is often based on review of laboratory records by an infection control nurse or other designated staff (Brachman 1982). In 1970 in the United States, the National Nosocomial Infection Study was initiated to monitor the frequency and trends of nosocomial infection in American hospitals. Approximately 160 hospitals participate in what is now a voluntary national surveillance system, with microbiology studies reported on 90 per cent of infected patients (Gaynes *et al.* 1991). A network of laboratories of different medical centres around the world has been established to conduct surveillance of antibiotic resistance for various pathogens (Stelling and O'Brien 1997).

In addition, the use of molecular tools to enhance surveillance of pathogens is growing in many countries. PulseNet serves as a American network of public health laboratories that performs DNA 'fingerprinting' on bacteria that may be foodborne. The network permits rapid comparison of these 'fingerprint' patterns through an electronic database, for example, similar pulsed field gel electrophoresis patterns of *E. coli* 0157:H7 bacteria isolated from ill people suggest that the bacteria come from a common source, for example, a widely distributed contaminated food product (http://www.cdc.gov/ncidod/dbmd/pulsenet/pulsenet.htm).

Disease registries

Registries are comprehensive longitudinal listings of people with particular conditions. They often include detailed information about diagnostic classification, treatment, and outcome. Registries were initially established primarily for epidemiological research on individual diseases or conditions to develop aetiological hypotheses and to identify cases for further research (Weddell 1973). Registries have also been used to ensure the provision of appropriate care and to evaluate changing patterns of medical care; unlike other disease information systems, they cut across the different levels of severity of illness and may provide information over time about individual people. Recently, the value of registries for monitoring disease incidence and its distribution, as well as for evaluating the effectiveness of targeted screening programmes, has been more widely recognized.

To focus on selected diseases or conditions, registries often develop a constituency that promotes participation and reporting. Most registries rely on numerous sources of data for case detection including, but not limited to, hospitals, laboratories, and death records; few registries rely primarily on doctor notification. Public health professionals probably have the most experience with cancer registries and registries for congenital malformations.

Population-based cancer registries generally have relied on multiple sources of data, including most importantly clinical pathology laboratories and hospital diagnoses (Parkin 1988). Death certification is also important, and other records such as those from oncology or radiotherapy units are also useful where available. There has been increasing adherence to internationally recognized standards and the resulting data are used to compare the incidence of cancer in different geographical locations and distinct ethnic groups (Raymond 1997). In the United States, several population-based registries have been developed that conduct surveillance for cancer, and the national Co-ordinating Council for Cancer Surveillance was organized in 1995 to facilitate a collaborative approach among the involved organizations and to ensure maximal efficiency (Swan *et al.* 1998). In contrast, in many developing areas of the world, population-based surveillance systems are not feasible (Parkin 1986), but surveillance in selected institutions or laboratories may still be useful.

Surveillance for birth defects was first initiated in many parts of the world in response to the thalidomide tragedy; registries were established to provide reliable baseline rates for specific birth defects and to detect increases in the prevalence of birth defects as a means of rapidly identifying human teratogens (Kallen *et al.* 1984; Holtzman and Khoury 1986). The CDC has conducted birth defects surveillance in metropolitan Atlanta since 1967 by using multiple sources of ascertainment of all serious birth defects observed in stillborn and liveborn infants or recognized by signs and symptoms apparent in the first year of life (Edmonds *et al.* 1981; CDC 1993). The birth defects registry system in metropolitan Atlanta has been a valuable resource for monitoring rates of change of specific defects (Yen *et al.* 1992) and for conducting numerous genetic and epidemiological investigations of risk factors for birth defects (Mulinare *et al.* 1988; Erickson 1992). Moreover, the registry serves as a model for other state surveillance systems (Lynberg and Edmonds 1992). A total of 38 states are conducting or are planning birth defects surveillance activities (Erickson 1997). In addition to monitoring birth defect rates and serving as the basis for epidemiological studies, the data from these state registries are used to evaluate the effectiveness of prevention activities and to refer children for health services and early intervention programmes (Edmonds 1997).

Internationally, approximately 30 countries are now conducting birth defects surveillance and are members of international organizations such as the International Clearinghouse for Birth Defects Monitoring Systems (International Clearinghouse for Birth Defects Monitoring Systems 1998) and, for Europe, the EuroCAT (Lechat and Dolk 1993). The International Clearinghouse, for example, conducts a spectrum of surveillance activities that includes monitoring of selected conditions (for example, several birth defects, Down's syndrome, multiple congenital anomalies) and the exchange of 'rumours', cluster information, and findings of still unpublished studies (International Clearinghouse for Birth Defects Monitoring Systems 1998). Additionally, the Clearinghouse promotes collaborative epidemiological studies and the development of new surveillance programmes worldwide.

Health information systems

Surveillance systems often depend on existing health data collection systems; these systems may be either integral to surveillance or serve as an adjunct to surveillance for specific diseases or conditions. Lack of accuracy and specificity in these existing data systems remains a concern, however, and most surveillance systems continue to need an additional data collection system to meet the needs of specific prevention and control programmes (Calle and Khoury 1991).

Data from medical claims records, death certificates, and other existing databases may not contain enough information to define public health priorities for reducing disease incidence. For example, an increase in deaths from cirrhosis, not otherwise specified, may be the result of an infectious agent, alcohol use, or other toxin. The occurrence of bladder cancer may or may not be related to a particular environmental exposure. These data are often most useful as an adjunct to surveillance systems designed more specifically for prevention and control programmes.

Vital records

Mortality statistics serve as the most accessible source of data for comparisons of many health problems. In most developed countries, registration of deaths is compulsory and largely complete. Records include basic demographic information, the cause or causes of death, and other descriptive information about the circumstances of death. In other countries, registration may be conducted only in major cities, or not at all. Verbal autopsies may be used in areas without death registration (Kaufman *et al.* 1997; Chandramohan *et al.* 1998).

In all countries, the accuracy and specificity of many diagnoses are limited, and changes in the use of diagnostic categories and codes over time, together with variation in the quality of information, are limiting factors. For example, a study by the American National Cancer Institute revealed that seven countries in Europe and North America coded the underlying cause of death the same for only 53 per cent of a sample of 1246 death certificates sent to these countries (Percy and Dolman 1978). Despite these limitations, vital statistics, particularly mortality statistics, are used to support many surveillance activities.

Example

Death certificates have been used in maternal mortality surveillance as a source of data to demonstrate progress towards reduction in maternal mortality in association with increased use of prenatal care and other factors. Analyses of death certificates in the United States have highlighted racial differences in mortality rates over time and differences in maternal mortality rates for women aged greater than 35 years. Because maternal mortality rates are often based on number of live births, this surveillance system also depends on birth certificate information (Kaunitz *et al.* 1984).

There is frequently a lengthy interval between death and collection and analysis of death certificates, which may make such vital statistics less useful for surveillance purposes when more current data are needed. However, summary vital data can be rapidly collected. For example, weekly reporting of deaths from 121 American cities to CDC has been integral to the surveillance of influenza epidemics in that country (Choi and Thacker 1981). In addition, automated systems for coding mortality information are both expanding and improving internationally (CDC 1999*b*).

Medical examiner and coroner reports

For a more detailed description of circumstances surrounding deaths (including autopsy reports, toxicology studies, and police reports), medical examiner and coroner records may be useful. In the United States, these reports are most representative of deaths caused by intentional and unintentional injuries and other unnatural causes. These records have been used for surveillance of such conditions as heat-wave-related mortality, sudden unexplained death syndrome in Southeast Asian refugees, and alcohol-related injuries (Jones *et al.* 1982; Berkelman *et al.* 1985; Parrish *et al.* 1987; Koo and Birkhead 1998). Systematic necropsy examinations have also been useful in ascertaining the contribution of tuberculosis to mortality of HIV-infected individuals in West Africa.

Medical care records

Hospital records and other medical care records may be a useful source of information on diagnoses, surgical procedures, and patient demographic characteristics. However, with increases in length and complexity of the medical record, retrieval of information has often been difficult and time-consuming. Although computerization of parts of these records has allowed their use for routine surveillance, a major limitation has often existed when identifiers are not recorded because repeat admissions and discharges by individual patients usually cannot be identified.

Hospital discharge records have been useful for surveillance of many medical care technologies, such as trends in the use of hysterectomies in the United States (particularly by geographical region), in the rate of coronary artery bypass graft procedures by sex and race, and in the assessment of outcome with carotid endarterectomies (Sattin *et al.* 1983; Thacker and Berkelman 1986; Caper 1987; McBean and Gornick 1994). More recently, hospital discharge record systems have been used as an alternative data source to evaluate surveillance data sets.

Relying exclusively on measurements of mortality from death certificates and morbidity from medical records can produce an underestimate of the impact of many diseases or conditions, such as malaria and arthritis, which may not result in contact with a health-care provider. A more complete estimate of the impact of disease has been attempted by including a measure of the loss of healthy life resulting from disability (Murray and Lopez 1997).

Insurance records and workers' compensation claims

Insurance records and workers' compensation claims have been useful for surveillance of injuries and illnesses in specific geographical locales. Because regulations governing completion and submission of forms differ both among and within juridictions, data derived from these systems cannot easily be compared. In addition, the use of medical claims data for surveillance may be limited by the accuracy of diagnostic recording as well as the problem of comparing different health systems (Pollack and Ringen 1992).

The severity of reported injury varies and is influenced by regulations influencing eligibility for workers' compensation, and other legislation related to compensation and medical care, rehabilitation of those injured at work, and the degree of fear of job loss resulting from absence from work. Data from these systems generally provide an underestimate of the actual incidence or prevalence of the health condition under surveillance, the underestimate may be of a considerable degree.

Example

In an evaluation of claims for workers' compensation as an adjunct to an occupational lead surveillance system, the usefulness of claims was demonstrated: the likelihood that a company had a case of lead poisoning strongly correlated with the number of claims against the company (Seligman *et al.* 1986).

Surveys of health behaviour and doctor utilization

Household surveys of the general population, such as the National Health Interview Survey conducted in the United States (http://www.cdc.gov/nchs/nhis.htm) or the General Household Survey in England and Wales (Fraser *et al.* 1978; Twigg 1999), have provided information at the national level on personal health practices such as alcohol use and smoking, disabilities, and doctor encounters. In the People's Republic of China, in addition to mandated information on acute infectious conditions, sentinel sites, known as disease surveillance points, are chosen through a statistical sample of provincial areas. These sites collect data on health events and medical encounters for the entire population within their jurisdiction (Cheng 1992; Yang 1992).

Although national estimates may be gained more efficiently from such surveys, local programmes may benefit from involvement in data collection and the flexibility to adapt data collection to their particular needs. Interview surveys conducted by telephone and in person can obtain personal health-related information with only minor differences in the reported prevalence of various health conditions between the two techniques. In developed countries, where most residences have telephones, telephone interviews have the advantages of lower cost and ease of supervising interviewers (Siegel *et al.* 1991).

Hazard and exposure surveillance

In addition to surveillance of health outcomes, two other types of surveillance are also used: hazard surveillance and exposure surveillance. Hazard surveillance has been defined as the 'assessment of the occurrence of, distribution of, and the secular trends in levels of hazards (toxic chemical agents, physical agents, biomechanical stressors, as well as biological agents) responsible for disease and injury' (Wegman 1992). Exposure surveillance is the monitoring of a population for the presence of an agent or the clinically non-apparent effects of an environmental hazard (for example, lead) or infectious agent (for example, HIV) in people within a population (Weniger *et al.* 1991). These types of surveillance may be complementary. Indeed, the optimal strategy for preventing or reducing the impact of a specific public health problem sometimes dictates the use of all three types of surveillance. For example, although hazard surveillance is an excellent measure available to detect potential health threats and to provide opportunities for primary prevention, exposure and outcome surveillance may provide valuable information for the evaluation of the effectiveness of hazard and exposure-reduction regulations.

Remote sensing and geographical information system technologies are now being used as an adjunct to disease surveillance (Barinaga 1993; Washino and Wood 1994) (see below). A major goal of this approach is the identification of environmental parameters that affect the patterns of disease risk and transmission.

Example

In 1993 the southern Kerio Valley of Kenya experienced the first cases of yellow fever ever recorded in that country. The virus had recently infected the monkey population in the valley, and forest-dwelling mosquitoes were passing the virus from monkeys to people entering the forest. The human population in the area was vaccinated, but the question remained as to whether the inhabitants of the nearby cities also required vaccination. Satellite photographs are being used to determine whether continuous forest corridors to any of the cities exist through which the virus can travel from one monkey population to another.

Analysis of surveillance data

The uses of public health data often derive from a simple analysis of surveillance data according to the basic epidemiological parameters of time, place, and person. Analysis of data over time can reveal trends in disease or injury upon which public health actions or the need for such actions may be evaluated.

The characteristics of the people or groups who develop specific diseases or sustain specific injuries are important in understanding the disease or injury, identifying those at high risk, and targeting intervention efforts. For example, disparities in health (incidence or severity of disease) among members of different population groups highlight the need to identify cultural, economic, or social factors associated with these health problems (Hahn and Stroup 1994).

When combined with appropriate population information, morbidity or mortality rates can be calculated to compare risks of disease and the magnitude of various health problems. Often rates are examined in broad age groups that are selected to reflect the different sets of conditions affecting mortality rates in each group (Doll 1974). Proper analysis of surveillance data can also assist in determining aetiology, setting priorities, determining modes of transmission, risk factors associated with disease, and opportunities for prevention or control, detecting epidemics, monitoring long-term trends, making projections of future disease occurrence, and evaluating effectiveness of interventions.

Typically, public health surveillance data are completed, summarized, and reported over specified time intervals (for example weeks, months, or years). Methods applicable to such time series data can be used to separate true temporal trends in the underlying risk from the random fluctuations, or 'noise'. The surveillance data should be plotted over the time during which they were collected. A clearer picture of this possible trend and of meaningful short-term patterns in these data are more evident if the random day-to-day variation in the number of cases is reduced. Smoothing potentially highlights meaningful patterns in collections of observed data by reducing the level of random noise (Devine and Parrish 1998). More advanced methods for analysis of surveillance data by time includes autoregressive time series techniques (Box and Jenkins 1976), generalized regression methods (Zeger 1988; Singh and Roberts 1992), and Bayesian modelling (Stroup and Thacker 1993). In addition, forecasts may be made by using regression and time series analyses, for example as for the surveillance of influenza (Fig. 1) (Serfling 1963; Choi and Thacker 1981; Lui and Kendal 1987; CDC 1999*c*), or analyses may combine information from several surveillance series (Newhouse *et al.* 1986; Stroup *et al.* 1988). In addition, modern methods (for example, Bayesian techniques) that incorporate information in addition to the data themselves, such as changes in a surveillance case definition or surveillance information from contiguous data (Stroup and Thacker 1993), can be useful when applied to public health surveillance data.

The approach to the prevention and control of disease and injury is often determined by circumstances unique to 'place': the geographical distribution of the disease or of its causative exposures or risk-associated behaviour. The analysis of surveillance data by place has long used dot density maps. As with analysis by time, smoothing approaches can reduce the random noise in maps of surveillance data (Fig. 2) (CDC 1996; Devine and Parrish 1998). Timely and positionally accurate spatial or georeferenced information, in a digital format, is improving the ability to monitor disease occurrence, health inequalities, environmental exposures, and related health risks, and advance hypothesis generation about the associative causation of disease aetiologies and outcomes (Richards *et al.* 1999). For example, from the American Bureau of the Census national digital street and geographical boundary files, or Topologically Integrated Geographic Encoding and Referencing (**TIGER**) system, epidemiologists can translate or geocode street addresses into unique latitude and longitude locations. These locations then can be examined with computationally rigorous spatial statistical data analysis techniques using geographical information systems. New and continually expanding computational opportunities permit dynamic space–time modelling of georeferenced data on the extent, structure, and association of diseases and suspected covariates (Anselin 1998).

Compared with traditional methods of mapping, geographical information systems offers potentially substantive cost savings for local disease surveillance and prevention activities. For example, epidemiologists in local health departments have used geographical

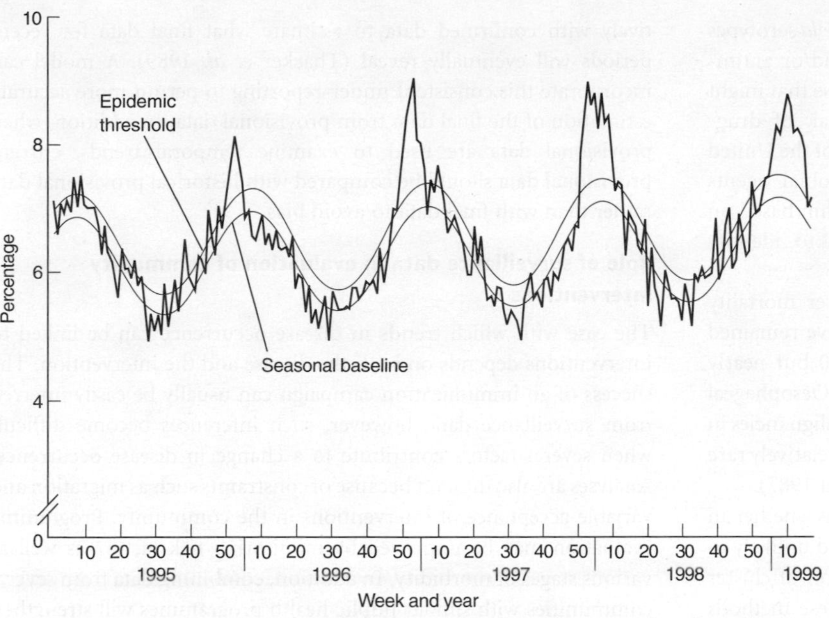

Fig. 1 Pneumonia and influenza mortality for 122 American cities, January 1995 to April 1999 (CDC 1999c).

information systems to design automated early warning surveillance systems for newborns with a known residential potential for elevated exposures to nitrate-nitrogen in drinking water (Boria *et al.* 1999). Other applications have resulted in identifying locations with elevated risks of Lyme disease (Glass *et al.* 1995) and rodent bite and infestation (Childs *et al.* 1998).

Epidemic detection and cluster analysis

Many epidemics are detected by astute health-care providers who note or suspect an increase in disease occurrence often before disease reports are received, assembled, and reviewed by health departments. The ongoing surveillance process between health practitioners and health departments increases the likelihood that providers will contact the health department when they suspect an outbreak or any unusual occurrence of disease.

Surveillance is most likely to detect epidemics in situations where cases, despite their aetiological link, are occurring over a wide geographic area (Cliff *et al.* 1992), over a relatively gradual period (Nobre and Stroup 1994), or among a well-defined subgroup with links among cases (for example, epidemiological links or similar molecular patterns of isolates) that would not be apparent to individual practitioners.

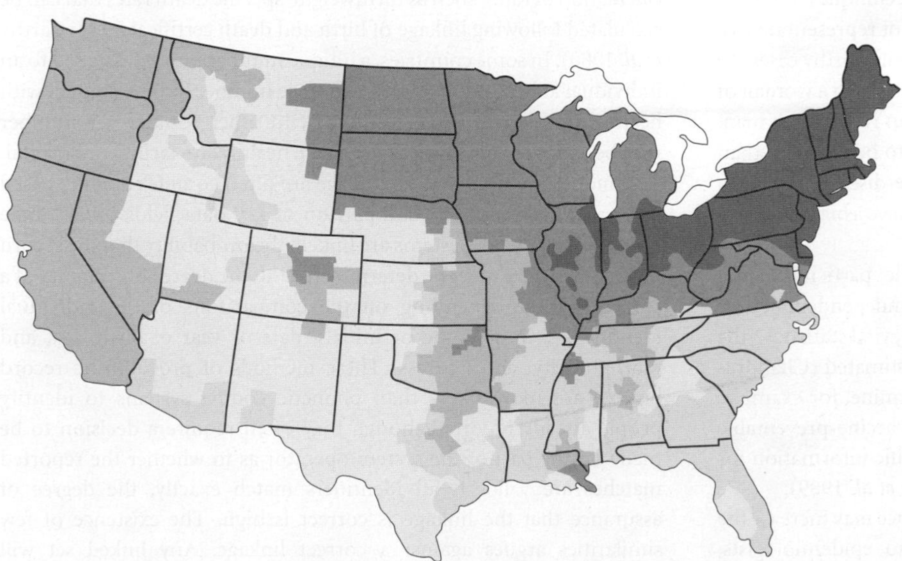

Fig. 2 Smoothed age-specific death rates (per 100 000 population) for age 70, colorectal cancer, white females from death certificates 1988 to 1992 and population data for 1990 (CDC 1996).

For example, laboratory-based surveillance of *Salmonella* serotypes has identified outbreaks in which unusual serotypes and/or antimicrobial patterns identify an outbreak of diarrhoeal disease that might otherwise have gone undetected, such as the outbreak of drug-resistant *Salmonella newport* in a large geographical area of the United States, which originated from animals fed antimicrobial agents (Holmberg *et al.* 1984). In addition, a computer algorithm based on application of cumulative sums has been developed to identify outbreaks of *Salmonella* (Hutwagner *et al.* 1997).

In another example, age-adjusted oesophageal cancer mortality rates in white men and women in the United States have remained fairly steady during the period between 1950 and 1980 but nearly doubled for African-Americans during the same period. Oesophageal cancer has gradually become one of the most common malignancies in African-American men aged below 55 years, while still a relatively rare cancer in white men of a similar age (Blot and Fraumeni 1987).

A frequent concern of the analysis of surveillance data is whether an apparent cluster of health events in time is significant and unlikely to have occurred by chance alone. Although the application of cluster detection methods is growing (CDC 1990), many of these methods require further examination and their use in surveillance remains controversial (Hutwagner *et al.* 1997; Devine and Parrish 1998). Most of these methods involve a comparison of observed incidence with a historical baseline and may involve clustering in time (Wallenstein 1980; Gallus *et al.* 1986; Stroup *et al.* 1993), clustering in space (Cliff and Ord 1981), or clustering in both time and space (Klauber 1975), with the availability of statistical software aiding spatial and other analyses (Dean 1991; Biomedware 1994). For example, a computer algorithm based on application of cumulative sums has been developed and used to identify outbreaks of *Salmonella*. These methods of cluster detection may be most helpful when used as an exploratory analysis to advise more intensive investigations (Besag and Newell 1991).

Statistical limitations of surveillance data

Surveillance data have traditionally had specific characteristics that have made application of standard statistical techniques difficult. Firstly, reporting bias may produce data that are not representative of the population. For example, severe or otherwise noteworthy cases are more likely to be reported than minor illnesses. Rubella in a woman of child-bearing age is more likely to be reported than rubella in a man, and a patient in some clinics may be more likely to be reported than patients seen in other settings, particularly if the disease is socially stigmatizing. Health-care provider networks may have a biased sample of doctors (Lobet *et al.* 1987).

Secondly, under-reporting may be considerable, particularly in a voluntary system of notification. When another independent source of data is available (for example, hospital discharge, vital statistics), the total number of cases actually occurring can be estimated (Chandra-Sekar and Deming 1949; Cormack 1963) to determine, for example, the sensitivity of two systems for detecting vaccine-preventable diseases (Orenstein *et al.* 1986). In addition, specific information for each case may be incompletely reported (Buehler *et al.* 1989).

Provisional data increase the timeliness and hence may increase the usefulness of public health surveillance data to epidemiologists; however, provisional data may differ markedly from final data that have been confirmed. To enhance the usefulness of provisional data for recent periods, epidemiologists may compare these data retrospectively with confirmed data to estimate what final data for recent periods will eventually reveal (Thacker *et al.* 1989). A model can incorporate this consistent under-reporting to permit more accurate estimation of the final data from provisional data. In addition, when provisional data are used to examine temporal trends, current provisional data should be compared with historical provisional data rather than with final data to avoid bias.

Role of surveillance data in evaluation of community interventions

The ease with which trends in disease occurrence can be linked to interventions depends on both the disease and the intervention. The success of an immunization campaign can usually be easily inferred from surveillance data; however, such inferences become difficult when several factors contribute to a change in disease occurrence. Analyses are also difficult because of constraints such as migration and variable acceptance of interventions in the community. Programme evaluation may be improved by monitoring risk factors as well as various stages of morbidity. In addition, combining data from several communities with similar public health programmes will strengthen the assessment of programme effectiveness.

Mathematical models can be used to elucidate the complexities of evaluating community interventions (Stroup and Teutsch 1998). Such models have been used most extensively for infectious diseases. However, models for predicting the decline of mortality rates given changes in risk factors have also been developed for mortality due to cirrhosis using population changes in levels of consumption of alcohol (Skog 1984), for cardiovascular disease using changes in cigarette consumption in a population (Kullback and Cornfield 1976), and for blood lead levels given changes in legislation banning lead from petrol (Annest *et al.* 1983).

Linkage of surveillance data to other information sources

Given the complexity of establishing new data and information systems, there is increasing interest in the combination of existing databases for surveillance purposes. Linkage of datasets has facilitated calculation of rates, such as birthweight-specific death rates that can be calculated following linkage of birth and death certificates (McCarthy *et al.* 1980). In some countries, a unique number may be assigned to an individual at birth to serve as a reference number for any contact with health-care services (Paterson 1988). In other countries, a number may be assigned only for use at a single health-care facility or hospital. Techniques involved in data linkage are often complex and are based on matching records by comparison of key data fields (Newcombe 1988). When record systems are linked, the probability that the record linkage is correct must be determined, with the degree of certainty of a correct linkage depending on the comparisons of the individual identifiers such as name or initials, date or year of birth, sex, and race/ethnicity, and address. These methods of probabilistic record linkage are more likely than phonetic coding systems to identify people already reported though they often require a decision to be made on the part of the system operator as to whether the reported matches are valid. If all identifiers match exactly, the degree of assurance that the linkage is correct is high. The existence of few similarities argues against a correct linkage. Any linked set will normally contain a small number of pairs that should not have been linked and, conversely, will have missed a few pairs that should have been linked. An advantage of probabilistic data matching is that records may frequently be linked even when parts of the identifying information are either incomplete, miscoded, or mispelled.

Dissemination of data

Communication of surveillance data is an essential step in the surveillance chain. The purpose of the communication and the audience targeted must be defined. Appropriate feedback must be given to those providing the data to demonstrate their usefulness and to stimulate further reporting. People providing the data should be credited for their contributions and acknowledged for their provision of accurate and complete data. Public health professionals, policy-makers, or others who may be responsible for taking action or setting the direction of public health programmes in response to surveillance data must receive the information that they need from the surveillance system on a timely basis and in an appropriate format for their use. Web sites are increasingly used by agencies collecting surveillance data as with the CDC's *Morbidity and Mortality Weekly Report* (www.cdc.gov/MMWR) and the WHO's *Weekly Epidemiological Record* (www.who.int/wer).

The data must be provided on a regular basis, with the frequency of surveillance reports dependent on the nature of the surveillance system, the characteristics of the disease process (for example, surveillance reports on measles are required more frequently than reports on cancer), and the public health impact of the disease. For diseases and other health events requiring major policy decisions (for example removal of lead paint from older homes), it may be useful to provide frequent updates to remind policy-makers of the potential for prevention. In general, reports need not be issued at more frequent intervals than the data are collected from reporting sites. Provisional data should be accepted for dissemination, since rapid turn-around of data is usually more important than absolute accuracy and completeness; rarely have provisional data driven major public health decisions in directions different from those that would have been based on final data.

The format for dissemination varies with the target audience, but in any case, the design of the communications should be as creative as possible without losing essential information. A creative design will help to make the information stand apart from other documents and receive greater attention. Most policy-makers and clinicians would prefer to see the data interpreted using graphics accompanied by an abbreviated summary text; in particular, key decision-makers need simple easily understood graphics. The important role that graphs can play in visually decoding large quantities of data has been clearly demonstrated, with graphic displays giving the reader an understanding of large and complex datasets not conveyed easily in other ways (Tukey 1977; Tufte 1983; Pommerenke *et al.* 1994; Cleveland 1985; Dean *et al.* 1998). Computer graphics, in particular, have made the results of data analysis far more useful to private and public policy-makers in their planning and management of health-care resources. However, many epidemiologists and other scientists, including mathematicians projecting the future course of diseases, find the more detailed raw data in tabular format or on electronic media most useful. Comparison with previous years or previous periods (for example, experience of the last 12 months compared with experience of the previous 12 months) is often helpful.

Maps are useful in providing rapid insight into the geographical occurrence of diseases, and there is strong interest in computer mapping and graphic displays. Mapping both absolute counts of disease occurrence and rates of disease for more common conditions may be considered, particularly when geographical areas are quite variable in their population density.

Evaluation of surveillance systems

Surveillance systems should be periodically evaluated to ensure that important public health problems are under surveillance and that useful information for disease prevention and control is collected. An evaluation of a surveillance system should include a review of its objectives, a detailed description of its operation, an assessment of its performance, and recommendations (CDC 1988; Teutsch and Churchill 1994).

The performance of surveillance systems can be judged by using a series of attributes, including sensitivity, timeliness, representativeness, positive predictive value, acceptability, flexibility, simplicity, and costs. The importance of individual attributes will vary among systems, and efforts to improve on a system's performance on one attribute may compete with efforts to improve its performance on another. Thus the evaluation of surveillance systems should not focus solely on the extent to which each attribute is achieved but rather on the attainment of the appropriate balance of attributes. The ultimate impact of improvements in surveillance should be assessed in terms of improvements in health (Thacker *et al.* 1986).

Sensitivity

The sensitivity of a surveillance system can be judged by its completeness of case reporting. If all people with the condition under surveillance in the target population are detected by a surveillance system, then its sensitivity is 100 per cent. Sensitivity of surveillance systems can be measured by comparing routinely collected case reports with data obtained by special case-finding methods. For example, the sensitivity of AIDS surveillance has been assessed through detailed review of death certificates and various hospital records, such as laboratory data, patient log-books, and computerized discharge diagnoses (Chamberland *et al.* 1985; Rosenblum *et al.* 1992).

Timeliness

Timeliness refers to the entire surveillance cycle, ranging from how quickly cases are reported to the distribution of surveillance reports. The assessment of timeliness is dependent on the condition (for example, the assesment of timeliness would be quite different for meningitis than for cancer). Electronic communication has the capacity to improve timeliness significantly.

Representativeness

Representativeness is a measure of how well reported cases in a population reflect all cases that actually occurred in the population. This comparison often requires independent surveillance, which ascertains as many cases as possible in the population for a given time period (Klaucke 1994). Surveillance reporting is rarely complete, and cases that are reported may differ from unreported cases in terms of demographic characteristics, site or use of health-care services, or risk exposures (Alter *et al.* 1987). Representativeness of surveillance data is also affected by the quality of descriptive data that accompany case reports. Incomplete or incorrect data on surveillance forms limit representativeness.

Positive predictive value

People with reported cases of disease may not actually have the disease in question. This may reflect incorrect diagnoses (false positives), a lack of specificity in the case definition, or errors in the interpretation of the case definition. If all people reported as cases had the disease in question, then the positive predictive value would be 100 per cent. Positive predictive value depends both on the specificity of diagnostic tests and the case definition and on the prevalence of the condition under surveillance. Evaluation of the positive predictive value is difficult and requires a careful review of cases detected through routine methods. For example, hospital-based stroke surveillance based on readily available admission diagnoses was found to include a substantial proportion of people without cerebrovascular disease when more stringent diagnostic criteria were applied (Barker *et al.* 1984).

The concept of positive predictive value can be extended to the detection of epidemics in a surveillance system. If change in disease occurrence is used as an indicator to trigger investigations, then a high frequency of 'false alarms' would indicate a low predictive value for epidemic detection.

Acceptability

Surveillance systems depend on the co-operation of many people over a long period. If procedures are easy to follow and useful information is returned to participants, then acceptability is likely to remain high. Other factors, including protection of confidentiality of individual cases, may also be critical to the acceptability of surveillance systems.

Flexibility

The circumstances under which surveillance systems operate are subject to change, ranging from logistical constraints to information needs; surveillance systems should have sufficient flexibility to accommodate these changes. For example, surveillance for AIDS has been ongoing during a period of rapid evolution in the understanding of the disease, during the introduction of a diagnostic test for HIV infection, and during changing diagnostic and treatment practices as a once rare disease has become more common. Surveillance for AIDS has been flexible as demonstrated by revisions to the case definition in the 1980s and early 1990s (CDC 1992*c*).

Simplicity

Simplicity is desirable throughout the entire cycle in surveillance systems and is closely tied to other attributes such as acceptability, flexibility, and costs.

Costs

Surveillance systems incur costs in time, equipment, and supplies, which may be difficult to judge relative to their public health value. Evaluation of the costs and benefits of aggressive versus less aggressive case-finding methods in surveillance of selected notifiable diseases has yielded different conclusions that vary according to specific local circumstances (Hinds *et al.* 1985; Vogt *et al.* 1986). A description of the time requirements and costs of a surveillance system is useful for its evaluation (Hinds *et al.* 1985; Vogt *et al.* 1986; Stroobant *et al.* 1988; Morris *et al.* 1996).

The evaluation of a surveillance system should conclude with an assessment of its structure and usefulness, considering its mix of attributes in relation to its objectives. Recommendations should state whether the system should be continued and what specific changes, if any, should be made.

Conclusion

Public health surveillance has historically galvanized prevention and control programmes ranging from smallpox eradication and immunization campaigns for childhood diseases to programmes to prevent HIV infection and AIDS. Surveillance has also taken on increased visibility and importance in evaluating and directing prevention and control efforts for non-infectious diseases and conditions. Surveillance systems represent information loops, with data flowing from local to central agencies and back. Surveillance provides a stimulus to keep prevention and control activities moving rapidly and in the right direction, guiding the response to individual cases as well as public policy.

Effective public health interventions depend upon a continuing and reliable source of information. The data must be timely and representative of the population; they must be analysed and interpreted with feedback to the reporters and dissemination to those formulating and implementing public health policy. Resources necessary for the maintenance of the surveillance systems and for their regular evaluation should be allocated, balancing needs for data to direct prevention activities with needs for resources to implement those activities.

References

Adams, O.B. and Hirschfeld, M. (1998). Human resources for health. *World Health Statistics Quarterly*, **51**, 28–32.

Alter, M.J., Mares, A., Hadler, S.C., and Maynard, J.E. (1987). The effect of underreporting on the apparent incidence and epidemiology of acute viral hepatitis. *American Journal of Epidemiology*, **125**, 133–9.

Andrus, J.K., de Quadros, C., Oliver, J.M., and Hull, H.F. (1992). Screening of cases of acute flaccid paralysis for poliomyelitis eradication: ways to improve specificity. *Bulletin of the World Health Organization*, **70**, 591–6.

Annest, J.L., Pirkle, J.L., Makuc, D., *et al.* (1983). Chronological trend in blood lead levels between 1976 and 1980. *New England Journal of Medicine*, **308**, 1373–7.

Anselin, L. (1998). Exploratory spatial data analysis in a geocomputational environment. In *Geocomputation, a primer* (ed. P. Longley, S. Brooks, R. McDonnell, and M. MacMillan), pp. 77–94. Wiley, New York.

Arnett, D.K., Sprafka J.M., McGovern P.G., *et al.* (1998) Trends in cigarette smoking: the Minnesota Heart Survey, 1980 through 1992. *American Journal of Public Health*, **88**, 1230–3.

Barinaga, M. (1993). Satellite data rocket disease control efforts into orbit. *Science*, **261**, 31–2.

Barker, W.H., Feldt, K.S., and Feibel, J. (1984). Assessment of hospital admission surveillance of stroke in a metropolitan community. *Journal of Chronic Diseases*, **37**, 609–15.

Bean, N.H., Martin, S.M., and Bradford, H. Jr (1992). PHLIS: an electronic system for reporting public health data from remote sites. *American Journal of Public Health*, **82**, 1273–6.

Berkelman, R.L. (1994). Emerging infectious diseases in the United States, 1993. *Journal of Infectious Diseases*, **170**, 272–7.

Berkelman, R.L. and Buehler, J.W. (1990). Public health surveillance of noninfectious chronic diseases: the potential to detect rapid change in disease burden. *International Journal of Epidemiology*, **19**, 628–35.

Berkelman, R.L., Herndon, J.L., Callaway, J.L., *et al.* (1985). A surveillance system for alcohol- and drug-related fatal injuries. *American Journal of Preventive Medicine*, **1**, 21–8.

Berkelman, R.L., Bryan, R.T., Osterholm, M.T., LeDuc, J.W., and Hughes, J.M. (1994). Infectious disease surveillance: a crumbling foundation. *Science*, **264**, 368–70.

Besag, J. and Newell, J. (1991). The detection of clusters in rare diseases. *Journal of the Royal Statistical Society*, **154**, 143–55.

Biellik, R.J., Bueno, H., Olive, J.-M., *et al.* (1992). Poliomyelitis case confirmation: characteristics for use by national eradication programmes. *Bulletin of the World Health Organization*, **70**, 79–84.

Biomedware (1994). *Statistical sortware for the clustering of health events.* Biomedware, Ann Arbor, MI.

Blot, W.J. and Fraumeni, J.F., Jr (1987). Trends in oesophageal cancer mortality among US blacks and whites. *American Journal of Public Health*, **77**, 296–8.

Boria, W., Berke, R., Clark, M., and Reisenweber, G.M. (1999). Public notification to families with newborns at risk of methemoglobinemia from drinking water exposure, Clymer, New York, 1996–1998. *Journal of Public Health Management and Practice*, **5**, 37–8.

Box, G. and Jenkins, G. (1976). *Time series analysis: forecasting and control.* Holden-Day, Oakland, CA.

Brachman, P.S. (1982). Surveillance. In *Bacterial infections of humans* (ed. A.S. Evans and H.H. Feldman), pp. 49–61. Plenum Medical, New York.

Brachott, D. and Mosley, J.W. (1972). Viral hepatitis in Israel: the effect of canvassing physicians on notifications and the apparent epidemiological pattern. *Bulletin of the World Health Organization*, **46**, 457–64.

Buehler, J.W., Stroup, D.F., Klaucke, D.N., *et al.* (1989). The reporting of race and ethnicity in the National Notifiable Diseases Surveillance System. *Public Health Reports*, **104**, 457–65.

Buehler, J.W., Berkelman, R.L., and Stehr-Green, J.K. (1992). The completeness of AIDS surveillance. *Journal of Acquired Immune Deficiency Syndrome*, **5**, 257–64.

Calle, E.E. and Khoury, M.J. (1991). Completeness of the discharge diagnoses as a measure of birth defects recorded in the hospital birth record. *American Journal of Epidemiology*, **134**, 69–77.

Caper, P. (1987). The epidemiologic surveillance of medical care. *American Journal of Public Health*, **77**, 669–70.

Cardenas, V., Sanchez, C., De la Hoz, F., *et al.* (1998) Colombia Field Epidemiology Training Program. *American Journal of Public Health*, **88**, 1404–5.

CDC (Centers for Disease Control) (1988). Guidelines for evaluating surveillance systems. *Morbidity and Mortality Weekly Report*, **37** (S-5).

CDC (Centers for Disease Control) (1990). Guidelines for investigating clusters of health events. *Morbidity and Mortality Weekly Report*, **39** (RR-11).

CDC (Centers for Disease Control) (1991). National electronic telecommunications system for surveillance—United States, 1990–1991. *Morbidity and Mortality Weekly Report*, **40**, 502–3.

CDC (Centers for Disease Control) (1992*a*). Meeting the challenge of multidrug-resistant tuberculosis: summary of a conference. *Morbidity and Mortality Weekly Report*, **41** (RR-11), 49–57.

CDC (Centers for Disease Control) (1992*b*). A framework for assessing the effectiveness of disease and injury prevention. *Morbidity and Mortality Weekly Report*, **41** (RR-3).

CDC (Centers for Disease Control) (1992*c*). 1993 revised classification system for HIV infection and expanded surveillance case definition for AIDS among adolescents and adults. *Morbidity and Mortality Weekly Report*, **41** (RR-17).

CDC (Centers for Disease Control) (1993). Surveillance for and comparison of birth defect prevalences in two geographic areas—United States, 1983–88. CDC Surveillance Summaries, 19 March 1993. *Morbidity and Mortality Weekly Report*, **42** (SS-1).

CDC (Centers for Disease Control) (1996). *Atlas of United States Mortality.* DHHS publication number 97-1015, US Department of Health and Human Services, Hyattsville, MD.

CDC (Centers for Disease Control) (1997). Case definitions for infectious conditions under public health surveillance. *Morbidity and Mortality Weekly Report*, **46** (RR-10).

CDC (Centers for Disease Control and Prevention) (1999*a*). *Proceedings of the international effort on automating mortality statistics.* US Department of Health and Human Services, Public Health Service, Washington, DC.

CDC (Centers for Disease Control and Prevention) (1999*b*). Progress toward global poliomyelitis eradication—1997–1998. *Morbidity and Mortality Weekly Report*, **48**, 416–21.

CDC (Centers for Disease Control and Prevention) (1999*c*). Update: influenza activity—United States and worldwide, 1998–1999 season, and composition of the 1999–2000 influenza vaccine. *Morbidity and Mortality Weekly Report*, **48**, 374–8.

Chamberland, M.E., Allen, J.R., Monroe, J.M., *et al.* (1985). Acquired immunodeficiency syndrome in New York City: evaluation of an active surveillance system. *Journal of the American Medical Association*, **254**, 383–7.

Chandramohan, D., Maude, G.H., Rodrigues, L.D., and Hayes, R.J. (1998). Verbal autopsies for adult deaths:their development and validation in a multi-centre study. *Tropical Medicine and International Health*, **3**, 436–46.

Chandra-Sekar, C. and Deming, W.E. (1949). On a method for estimating birth and death rates and the extent of registration. *Journal of the American Statistical Association*, **44**, 101–15.

Cheng, C.M. (1992). Disease surveillance in China. In *Proceedings of the 1992 International Symposium on Public Health Surveillance* (ed. S. E Wetterhall). *Morbidity and Mortality Weekly Report*, **41** (Supplement), 111–22.

Childs, J.E., McLafferty, S.L., Ramses, A., *et al.* (1998). Epidemiology of rodent bites and prediction of rat infestation in New York City. *Amercan Journal of Epidemiology*, **148**, 78–87.

Choi, K. and Thacker, S.B. (1981). An evaluation of influenza mortality surveillance, 1962–1979. I. Time series forecasts of expected pneumonia and influenza deaths. *American Journal of Epidemiology*, **113**, 215–26.

Chute, C.G., Cohn S.P., Campbell, J.R., *et al.* (1998) A framework for comprehensive health terminology systems in the United States: development guidelines, criteria for selection and public policy implications. *Journal of the American Medical Informatics Association*, **5**, 503–10.

Cleveland, W.S. (1985). *The elements of graphing data.* Bell Telephone Laboratories, Murray Hill, NJ.

Cliff, A.D. and Ord, J.K. (1981). *Spatial processes, models, and application.* Pion, London.

Cliff, A.D., Haggett, P, and Stroup, D.F. (1992). The geographical structure of measles epidemics in the northeastern United States. *American Journal of Epidemiology*, **136**, 592–602.

College of American Pathologists (1999). SNOMED RT and READ Codes to be combined in an international terminology of health. Joint development agreement by the College of American Pathologists and United Kingdom's Secretary of State for Health. Press release, March 1999 (available at http://.www.cap.org/html/public/snomed intl.html).

Committee on National Statistics, Commission on Behavioral and Social Sciences and Education, National Research Council, and Social Science Research Council (1993). *Private lives and public policies: confidentiality and accessibility of government statistics.* National Academy Press, Washington, DC.

Cormack, R.M. (1963). The statistics of capture–recapture. *Ocean Marine Biology Annual Review*, **6**, 455–506.

Davis, J.P. and Vergeront, J.M. (1982). The effect of publicity on the reporting of toxic-shock syndrome in Wisconsin. *Journal of Infectious Diseases*, **145**, 449–57.

Dean, A.G. (1999). Epi Info and Epi Map: Current status and plans for Epi Info 2000. *Journal of Public Health Management and Practice*, **5**, 54–7.

Dean, A.G., Dean, J.A., Burton, A.H.,and Dicker, R.C. (1991). Epi Info: a general purpose microcomputer program for public health information systems. *American Journal of Preventive Medicine*, **7**, 178–82.

Dean, A.G., Dean, J.A., Burton, J.H., ***et al.*** (1993). *Epi Info, Version 6*. A word processing, database and statistics program for epidemiology on microcomputers (computer program). Centers for Disease Control and Prevention, Atlanta, GA.

Dean, A.G., Shah, S.P., and Churchill, J.E. (1998). DoEpi. Computer-assisted instruction in epidemiology and computing and a framework for creating new exercises. *American Journal of Preventive Medicine*, **14**, 367–71.

De Bock, A. (1988). Surveillance for accidents at work. In *Surveillance in health and disease* (ed. W.J. Eylenbosch and D. Noah), pp. 191–201. Oxford University Press, New York.

DeCock, K.M., Odehouri, K., Moreau, J., ***et al.*** (1989). Rapid emergence of AIDS in Abidjan, Ivory Coast. *Lancet*, **334**, 408–11.

Devine, O. and Parrish, R.G. (1998) Monitoring the health of a population. In *Statistics in public health* (ed. D.S. Stroup and S.M. Teutsch), pp. 59–91. Oxford University Press, New York.

Doll, R. (1974). Surveillance and monitoring. *International Journal of Epidemiology*, **3**, 305–14.

Edmonds, L.D. (1997). Birth defects surveillance at the state and local level. *Teratology*, **56**, 5–7.

Edmonds, L.D., Layde, P.M., James, L.M., ***et al.*** (1981). Congenital malformations surveillance: two American systems. *International Journal of Epidemiology*, **10**, 247–52.

Erickson, J.D. (1992). Teratology data from the Atlanta birth defects case control study. *Teratology*, **43**, 41–51.

Erickson, J.D. (1997). Introduction: birth defects surveillance in the United States. *Teratology*, **56**, 1–4.

Executive Committee of the Infectious Diseases Society of America Emerging Infections Network (1997). Emerging Infections Network: a new venture for the Infectious Diseases Society of America. *Clinical Infectious Diseases*, **25**, 34–6.

Eylenbosch, W.J. and Noah, N.D (ed.) (1988). *Surveillance in health and disease.* Oxford University Press.

Faich, G.A., Knapp, D., Dreis, M., and Turner, W. (1987). National adverse drug reaction surveillance: 1985. *Journal of the American Medical Association*, **257**, 2068–70.

Fantahun, M. (1998) Patterns of childhood mortality in three districts of north Gondar Administrative Zone. A community-based study using the verbal autopsy method. *Ethiopian Medical Journal*, **36**, 71–81.

Federal Committee on Statistics (1994). *Private lives and public policies.* US Department of Health and Human Services, Washington, DC.

Foege, W.H., Millar, J.D., and Henderson, D.A. (1975). Smallpox eradication in West and Central Africa. *Bulletin of the World Heath Organization*, **52**, 209–22.

Fraser, P, Beral, V., and Chilvers, C. (1978). Monitoring disease in England and Wales: methods applicable to routine data-collecting systems. *Journal of Epidemiology and Community Health*, **32**, 294–302.

Frerichs, R.R. (1991). Epidemiologic surveillance in developing countries. *Annual Reviews in Public Health*, **12**, 80–257.

Freund, E., Seligman, P.J., Chorba, T.L., ***et al.*** (1989). Mandatory reporting of occupational diseases by clinicians. *Journal of the American Medical Association*, **262**, 3041–4.

Gail, M.H. and Brookmeyer, R. (1988). Methods for projecting course of acquired immunodeficiency syndrome epidemic. *Journal of the National Cancer Institute*, **80**, 900–11.

Gallus, G., Mandelli, C., Marchi, M., and Radaelli, G. (1986). On surveillance methods for congenital malformations. *Statistics in Medicine*, **5**, 565–71.

Gaynes, R.P., Culver, D.H., Emori, T.G., ***et al.*** (1991). The national nosocomial infections surveillance system: plans for the 1990s and beyond. *American Journal of Medicine*, **91**, 116S–20S.

Glass, G.E., Schwartz, B.S., Morgan, M.M., III, Johnson, D.T., Noy, P.M., and Israel, P. (1995). Environmental risk factors for Lyme disease identified with geographic information systems. *American Journal of Public Health*, **88**, 1019–21.

Gostin, L.O. and Hadley, J. (1998). Health service research: public benefits, personal privacy, and proprietary interests. *Annals of Internal Medicine*, **129**, 833–5.

Hahn, R.A. and Stroup, D.F. (1994). Race and ethnicity in public health surveillance: criteria for the scientific use of social categories. *Public Health Reports*, **109**, 7–15.

Henderson, D.A. (1976). Surveillance of smallpox. *International Journal of Epidemiology*, **5**, 19–28.

Henderson, D.A. (1998) Eradication: lessons learned from the past. *Bulletin of the World Health Organization,* **76** (Supplement 2), 17–21.

Henderson, D.A. (1999). The looming threat of bioterrorism. *Science*, **283**, 1279–82.

Heymann, D.L. and Rodier, G.R. (1998) Global surveillance of communicable diseases. *Emerging Infectious Diseases*, **4**, 362–5.

Hinds, M.W., Skaggs, J.W., and Bergeisen, G.H. (1985). Benefit cost analysis of active surveillance of primary care physicians for hepatitis A. *American Journal of Public Health*, **75**, 176–7.

Hinman, A.R. (1977). Analysis, interpretation, use and dissemination of surveillance information. *Pan American Health Organization Bulletin*, **11**, 338–43.

Hinman, A.R. and Hopkins, D.R. (1998). Lessons from previous eradication programs. In *The eradication of infectious diseases* (ed. W.R. Dowdle and D.R. Hopkins), pp 19–32. Wiley, New York.

Holmberg, S.D., Osterholm, M.T., Senger, K.A., and Cohen, M.L. (1984). Drug-resistant *Salmonella* from animals fed antimicrobials. *New England Journal of Medicine*, **311**, 617–22.

Holtzman, N.A. and Khoury, M.J. (1986). Monitoring for congenital malformations. *Annual Review of Public Health*, **7**, 237–66.

Hutwagner, L.C., Maloney, E.K., Bean, N.H., Slutsker, L.K., and Martin, S.M. (1997) Using laboratory-based surveillance data for prevention: an algorithm for detecting *Salmonella* outbreaks. *Emerging Infectious Diseases*, **3** (www.cdc.gov/ncidod/eid/vol3no3/hutwagnr.htm).

Institute of Medicine (1988). *Approaches to modeling disease spread and impact. Report of a workshop on mathematical modeling of the spread of human immunodeficiency virus and the demographic impact of acquired immune deficiency syndrome, 15–17 October 1987.* National Academy Press, Washington, DC.

Institute of Medicine (1992). *Emerging infections: microbial threats to health in the United States.* National Academy Press, Washington, DC.

International Clearinghouse for Birth Defects Monitoring Systems (1998). *Annual report 1998.* International Centre for Birth Defects, Rome.

Jaffe, H.W., Choi, K., Thomas, P.A., ***et al.*** (1983). National case control study of Kaposi's sarcoma and *Pneumocystis carinii* pneumonia in homosexual men: epidemiologic results. *Annals of Internal Medicine*, **99**, 293–8.

John, T.J., Samuel, R., Balraj, V., and John, R. (1998). Disease surveillance at district level: a model for developing countries. *Lancet*, **352**, 58–61.

Jones, T.S., Liang, A.P., Kilbourne, E.M., ***et al.*** (1982). Morbidity and mortality associated with the July 1980 heat wave in St Louis and Kansas City, Missouri. *Journal of the American Medical Association*, **247**, 3327–31.

Kallen, B., Hay, S., and Klinberg, M. (1984). Birth defects monitoring systems: accomplishments and goals. In *Issues and reviews in teratology* (ed. H. Kalter), Volume 2, pp. 1–22. Plenum, New York.

Kaufman, J.S., Asuzu, M.C., Rotimi C.N., Johnson, O.O., Owoaje, E.E., and Cooper, R.S. (1997). The absence of adult mortality data for sub-Saharan Africa: a practical solution. *Bulletin of the World Health Organization*, **75**, 389–95.

Kaunitz, A.M., Rochat, R.W., Hughes, J.M., *et al.* (1984). Maternal mortality surveillance, 1974–1978. *Centers for Disease Control Surveillance Summaries*, **33**, 5SS–8SS.

Klauber, M..R. (1975). Space–time clustering tests for more than two samples. *Biometrics*, **31**, 719–26.

Klaucke, D.N. (1994). Evaluating public health surveillance. In *Principles and practice of public health surveillance* (ed. S.M. Teutsch and R.E. Churchill), pp. 158–74. Oxford University Press.

Koo, D. and Birkhead, G.S. (1998). Prospects and challenges in implementing firearm-related injury surveillance in the United States. Not a flash in the pan. *American Journal of Preventive Medicine*, **15** (Supplement 3), 120–4.

Koo, D. and Wetterhall, S.F. (1996). Historical and current status of the National Notifiable Diseases Surveillance System. *Journal of Public Health Managment and Practice*, **2**, 4–10.

Kullback, S. and Cornfield, J. (1976). An information theoretic contingency table analysis of the Dorn study of smoking and mortality. *Computers and Biomedical Research*, **9**, 409–37.

Langmuir, A.D. (1963). The surveillance of communicable diseases of national importance. *New England Journal of Medicine*, **268**, 182–92.

Langmuir, A.D. (1976). William Farr: founder of modern concepts of surveillance. *International Journal of Epidemiology*, **5**, 13–18.

Lechat, M.F. and Dolk, H. (1993). Registries of congenital anomalies: EuroCAT. *Environmental Health Perspectives*, **101** (Supplement 2), 153–7.

Lobet, M.P., Stroobant, A., Mertens, R., *et al.* (1987). Tool for validation of the network of sentinel general practitioners in the Belgian health care system. *International Journal of Epidemiology*, **16**, 612–18.

Lui, K.J. and Kendal, A.T. (1987). Impact of influenza epidemics on mortality in the United States from October 1972 to May 1985. *American Journal of Public Health*, **77**, 712–16.

Lynberg, M.C. and Edmonds, L.D. (1992). Surveillance of birth defects. In *Public health surveillance* (ed. W. Halperin, E.L. Baker, and R.R. Monson), pp. 157–77. Van Nostrand Reinhold, New York.

McBean A.M. and Gornick, M. (1994). Differences by race in the rates of procedures performed in hospitals for Medicare beneficiaries. *Health Care Financing Review*, **15**, 77–90.

McCarthy, B.J., Terry, J., Rochat, R.W., *et al.* (1980). The under-registration of neonatal deaths: Georgia, 1974–1977. *American Journal of Public Health*, **70**, 977–82.

McQueen, D.V. (1999) A world behaving badly: the global challenge for behavioral surveillance. *American Journal of Public Health*, **89**, 1312–14.

Morris, G., Snider, D., and Katz, M. (1996) Integrating public health informatics and surveillance systems in the United States. *American Journal of Epidemiology*, **2**, 24–7.

Mulinare, J., Cordero, J.F, Erickson, J.D., and Berry, R.J. (1988). Periconceptional use of multivitamins and the occurrence of neural tube defects. *Journal of the American Medical Association*, **260**, 3141–5.

Murray, C.J.L. and Lopez, A.D. (1997). Global burden of disease study. *Lancet*, **349**, 1269–76, 1347–52, 1436–42, 1498–504.

Music, S.I. and Schultz, M.G. (1990). Field epidemiology and training programs: new international health resources. *Journal of the American Medical Association*, **263**, 3309–11.

Newcombe, H.B. (1988). *Handbook of record linkage.* Oxford University Press.

Newhouse, V.F., Choi, K., D'Angelo, L.J., *et al.* (1986). Analysis of social and environmental factors affecting the occurrence of Rocky Mountain spotted fever in Georgia, 1961–75. *Public Health Reports*, **101**, 419–28.

Nobre, F.F. and Stroup, D.F. (1994). A monitoring system to detect pattern changes in public health surveillance data. *International Journal of Epidemiology*, **23**, 408–18.

Orenstein, W.A., Bart, S.W., Bart, K.J., *et al.* (1996). Epidemiology of rubella and its complications. In *Vaccinating against brain syndromes: the campaign against measles and rubella* (ed. E.M. Grunberg, C. Louis, and S.E. Goldson), pp. 49–69. Oxford University Press, New York.

PAHO (Pan American Health Organization) (1994). Dengue fever in Costa Rica and Panama. *Epidemiological Bulletin*, **15**, 9–10.

Parkin, D.M. (ed.) (1986). *Cancer occurrence in developing countries.* International Agency for Research on Cancer, Lyon.

Parkin, D. (1988). Surveillance of cancer. In *Surveillance in health and disease* (ed. W.J. Eylenbosch and N.D. Noah), pp. 143–65. Oxford University Press.

Parrish, R.G., Tuckcr, M., Ing, R., and Encarnacion, C. (1987). Sudden unexplained death syndrome in southeast Asian refugees: a review of CDC surveillance. *Centers for Disease Control Surveillance Summaries*, **36**, 43–53.

Paterson, J.G. (1988). Surveillance systems from hospital data. In *Surveillance in health and disease* (ed. W.J. Eylenbosch and N.D. Noah), pp. 49–61. Oxford University Press.

Percy, C. and Dolman, A. (1978). Comparison of the coding of death certificates related to cancer in seven countries. *Public Health Reports*, **93**, 335–50.

Pollack, E.S. and Ringen, K. (1992). Risk of hospitalization for specific nonwork-related conditions among laborers and their families. *American Journal of Industrial Medicine*, **23**, 417–25.

Pommerenke, F.A., Miller, R.W., Srivastava, S., and Ackermann, S.P. (1994). Targeting cancer control: the state cancer control map and data program. *American Journal of Public Health*, **84**, 1479–82.

Quigley, M.A., Armstrong Schellenberg, J.R., and Snow, R.W. 1996. Algorithms for verbal autopsies: a validation study in Kenyan children. *Bulletin of the World Health Organization*, **74**, 147–54.

Raska, K. (1966). National and international surveillance of communicable diseases. *World Health Organization Chronicle*, **20**, 315–21.

Raymond, L. (1997). Techniques of registration. In *Cancer incidence in five continents* (ed. D.M. Parkin, S.L. Whelan, J. Ferlay, and J. Young), Volume 7. IARC, Lyon.

Remington, P.L.S., Smith, M.Y., Williamson, D.F., *et al.* (1988). Design, characteristics and usefulness of state-based behavioral risk factor surveillance: 1981–1987. *Public Health Reports*, **103**, 366–75.

Richards, T.B., Henriques, W.D., Croner, C.M., Brown, C.K., Saccenti, J.C., and Berry, P.J. (1999). Toward a GIS sampling frame for surveys of local health departments and local boards of health. *Public Health Management and Practice*, **5**, 65–75.

Rosenblum, L., Buehler, J.W., Morgan, M.W., *et al.* (1992). Completeness of AIDS case reporting, 1988: a multisite collaborative surveillance project. *American Journal of Public Health*, **82**, 1495–9.

Rousch, S., Birkhead, G., Koo, D., Cobb, A., and Fleming, D. (1999). Mandatory reporting of diseases and conditions by health care professionals and laboratories. *Journal of the American Medical Association*, **282**, 164–70.

Sandiford, P., Annett, H., and Cibulskis, R. (1992). What can information systems do for primary health care? An international perspective. *Social Science and Medicine*, **34**, 1077–87.

Sattin, R.W., Rubin, G.L., and Hughes, J.M. (1983). Hysterectomy among women of reproductive age, United States, update for 1979–1980. *Centers for Disease Control Surveillance Summaries*, **32**, 1SS–7SS.

Seligman, P.J., Halperin, W.E., Mullan, R.J., and Frazier, T.M. (1986). Occupational lead poisoning in Ohio: surveillance using worker's compensation data. *American Journal of Public Health*, **76**, 1299–1302.

Serfling, R.E. (1963). Methods for current statistical analysis of excess pneumonia-influenza deaths. *Public Health Reports*, **78**, 494–506.

Shands, K.N., Schmid, G.P., Dan, B.B., *et al.* (1980). Toxic-shock syndrome in menstruating women: association with tampon use and *Staphylococcus aureus* and clinical features in 52 cases. *New England Journal of Medicine*, **303**, 1430–42.

Shen, F.Z., Shou, P.J., and Zhao, G.F. (1984). Influenza surveillance in Shanghai. *Chinese Medical Journal*, **97**, 339–4.

Siegel, P.Z., Brackbill, R.M., Frazier, E.L., *et al.* (1991). Behavioral risk factor surveillance, 1986–1990. *CDC Surveillance Summaries, Morbidity and Mortality Weekly Report*, **40** (SS-4), 1–23.

Singh, A. and Roberts, G. (1992). State space modeling of cross-classified time series of counts. *International Statistical Review*, **60**, 321–35.

Skog, O. (1984). The risk function for liver cirrhosis from lifetime alcohol consumption. *Journal of Studies on Alcohol*, **45**, 199–208.

Stelling, J.M. and O'Brien, T.F. (1997) Surveillance of antimicrobial resistance: The WHONET program. *Clinical Infectious Diseases*, **24** (Supplement 1), S157–68.

Stroobant, A.W., Van Casteren, V., and Thiers, G. (1988). Surveillance systems from primary care data: surveillance through a network of sentinel general practitioners. In *Surveillance in health and disease* (ed. W.J. Eylenbosch and N.D. Noah), pp. 62–74. Oxford University Press.

Stroup, D.F. and Teutsch, S.M. (ed.) (1998). *Statistics in public health: quantitative approaches to public health problems.* Oxford University Press, New York.

Stroup, D.F. and Thacker, S.B. (1993). A Bayesian approach to the detection of aberrations in public health surveillance data. *American Journal of Epidemiology*, **4**, 435–43.

Stroup, D.F., Thacker, S.B., and Herndon, J.L (1988). Application of multiple time series analysis to the estimation of pneumonia and influenza mortality by age: 1962–1983. *Statistics in Medicine*, **7**, 1045–59.

Stroup, D.F, Wharton, M., Kafadar, K., and Dean, A.G. (1993). An evaluation of a method for detecting aberrations in public health surveillance data. *American Journal of Epidemiology*, **137**, 373–80.

Swan, J., Wingo, P., Clive R., *et al.* (1998). Cancer surveillance in the U.S.: can we have a national system? *Cancer*, **83**, 9.

Teutsch, S.M. and Churchill, R.E. (ed.) (1994). *Principles and practice of public health surveillance.* Oxford University Press, New York.

Thacker, S.B. and Berkelman, R.L. (1986). Surveillance of medical technologies. *Journal of Public Health Policy*, **7**, 363–77.

Thacker, S.B. and Berkelman, R.L. (1988). Public health surveillance in the United States. *Epidemiologic Reviews*, **10**, 164–90.

Thacker, S.B. and Stroup, D.F. (1994). Future directions of comprehensive public health surveillance and health information systems in the United States. *American Journal of Epidemiology*, **140**, 383–97.

Thacker, S.B. and Gregg, M.B. (1996). Implementing the concepts of William Farr: the contributions of Alexander D. Langmuir to public health surveillance and communications. *American Journal of Epidemiology*, **144**, 523–8.

Thacker, S.B., Redmon, S., Rothenberg, R.B., *et al.* (1986). A controlled trial of disease surveillance strategies. *American Journal of Preventive Medicine*, **2**, 345–50.

Thacker, S.B., Berkelman, R.L., and Stroup, D.F. (1989). The science of public health surveillance. *Journal of Public Policy*, **10**, 187–203.

Thacker, S.B., Stroup, D.F., Rothenberg, R.B., and Brownson, R.C. (1995). Public health surveillance for chronic conditions: a scientific basis for decisions. *Statistics in Medicine*, **14**, 629–41.

Tollman, S.M., Kahn K, Garenne, M., and Gear, J.S. (1999). Reversal in mortality trends: evidence from the Agincourt field site, South Africa, 1992–1995. *AIDS* **13**, 1091–7.

Tufte, E.R. (1983). *The visual display of quantitative information.* Graphics Press, Cheshire, CT.

Tukey, J.W. (1977). *Exploratory data analysis.* Addison-Wesley, Reading, MA.

Twigg, L. (1999). Choosing a national survey to investigate smoking behavior: making comparisons between the General Household Survey, the British Household Panel Survey and the Health Survey for England. *Journal of Public Health Medicine*, **21**, 14–21.

Valleron, A.J., Bouvet, E., Garnerin, P., *et al.* (1986). Computer network for the surveillance of' communicable diseases: the French experiment. *American Journal of Public Health*, **76**, 1289–92.

Vogt, R.L., LaRue, D., Klaucke, D.N., and Jillson, D.A. (1983). Comparison of active and passive surveillance systems of primary care providers for hepatitis, measles, rubella and salmonellosis in Vermont. *American Journal of Public Health*, **73**, 795–7.

Vogt, R.L., Clark, S.W., and Kappel, S. (1986). Evaluation of the state surveillance system using hospital discharge diagnoses, 1982–1983. *American Journal of Epidemiology*, **123**, 197–8.

Wallenstein, S. (1980). A test for detection of clustering over time. *American Journal of Epidemiology*, **111**, 367–72.

Washino, R.K. and Wood, B.L. (1994). Application of remote sensing to arthropod vector surveillance and control. *American Journal of Tropical Health and Hygiene*, **50** (Supplement 6), 134–44.

Weddell, J.M. (1973). Registers and registries: a review. *International Journal of Epidemiology*, **2**, 221–8.

Wegman, D.H. (1992). Hazard surveillance. In *Public health surveillance* (ed. W. Halperin and E.L. Baker Jr), pp. 62–75. Van Nostrand Reinhold, New York.

Weniger, B.G., Limpakarnjanarat, K., Ungchusak, K., *et al.* (1991). The epidemiology of HIV infections and AIDS in Thailand. *AIDS*, **5** (Supplement 2), 271–85.

WHO (World Health Organization) (1958). *The first ten years of the World Health Organization.* WHO, Geneva.

WHO (World Health Organization) (1968). *Report of the technical discussions at the 21st World Health assembly on 'National and global surveillance of communicable diseases'.* WHO, Geneva.

Yang, G. (1992). Selection of DSP points in second stage and their representation. *Chinese Journal of Epidemiology*, **13**, 197–201.

Yang, G.H., Stroup, D.F., and Thacker, S.B. (1997). National public health surveillance in China: implications for public health in China and the United States. *Biomedical and Environmental Sciences*, **10**, 1013–19.

Yen, H., Khoury, M.J., Erickson, J.D., *et al.* (1992). The changing epidemiology of neural tube defects in the United States. *American Journal of Diseases in Children*, **146**, 857–61.

Zeger, S. (1988). A regression model for time series of counts. *Biometrika*, **75**, 621–9.

Zhang, K.X. (1990). Forecast of the incidence of encaphalitis B in Liao Ning province. *Chinese Journal of Epidemiology*, **1**, 67.

7

Social science techniques

7.1 Sociological and psychological investigations

Myfanwy Morgan, John Spicer, and Margaret Reid

Introduction

Sociology and psychology share a number of common interests and areas of study in the public health field. These include issues relating to the psychosocial environment as causes of disease, help-seeking behaviours and adherence with treatment, lifestyle changes and effective health promotion interventions, ageing, disability and mental illness, and the measurement of health status and quality of life. However, each discipline is characterized by its own perspectives and concepts, and by differences in their focus and explanations. Whereas psychology is primarily concerned with the personality, motivations, and behaviours of individuals, sociology focuses on the characteristics of social groupings and the wider socio-economic and political structures within which they are embedded.

This chapter describes the theoretical perspectives and methods of investigation that characterize sociological and psychological studies in the health field. Each section also has examples of the applications of these disciplines to particular areas of public health; topics relating to the sociology part are chronic illness, ethnicity, and the professions, and those relating to psychology are coronary heart disease and condom usage.

Sociological investigations

Medical sociology as a specialized field of sociological enquiry has partly developed alongside public health medicine. Both disciplines have brought their particular expertise to examine such issues as the causes and distribution of ill health and the organization and provision of care, often working in multidisciplinary teams. Sociology and public health medicine frequently trace the origins of their common interests in the role of economic, social, political, and cultural factors in health and disease patterns to the nineteenth-century struggles of physicians and public health reformers like Virchov in Germany, Chadwick in the United Kingdom, Shattuck in the United States, and Coronel in The Netherlands. The development by social scientists and public health specialists of systematic studies to examine the social distribution and causes of non-infectious conditions (such as lung cancer, bronchitis and coronary heart disease), as well as questions relating to the organization and provision of health services, dates from the late 1940s in both Britain and the United States (Hoffer and Schuler 1948; Pearce and Crocker 1949). This was encouraged by changing patterns of disease, increasing concerns about the social conditions and health of populations, and developments in social science survey techniques.

The period of rapid growth of medical sociology started in the 1950s in the United States and about a decade later in the United Kingdom. The founding of an international journal, *Social Science and Medicine*, which forms a marker in the development of the discipline, occurred in 1966. However, from the early 1960s the paths of sociology and public health medicine began to diverge, reflecting their separate concerns and disciplinary developments. During this period medical sociology was increasingly critical of the assumptions and limitations of the biomedical model. For example, sociologists drew attention to the wider societal determinants of individual behaviours such as smoking, diet, and non-uptake of services, and were critical of what was viewed as a 'victim blaming' stance and overly individualistic approaches to health promotion (McKinlay 1975). They also promoted the rights of consumers/patients to make choices and be listened to in relation to the provision of medical care, highlighted areas of potential disagreement and conflicts between professionals and patients (Bloor and Horobin 1975; Oakley 1980), and drew attention to the adverse effects of long-term care in institutions run on custodial lines on patients' self-concept and behaviours (Goffman 1961; Wing and Brown 1970).

From the late 1970s, sociology and public health medicine experienced a new phase of shared interests. This largely reflected the adoption by public health of a broader social model of the causes of ill health and appropriate interventions, as exemplified by the development of what is often referred to as the New Public Health (Ashton and Seymour 1988; Martin and McQueen 1989). This is an approach that sees many contemporary health problems as social rather than individual problems, and therefore requires healthy public policies (in terms of housing, the environment, food policies, and so on) to support the promotion of health. The move towards a more social and participative model of health care was also encouraged by broader changes in society. This includes the greater importance attached to local communities having a voice in determining local needs and priorities, and to patients being afforded a more active role in treatment choices and in assessing the outcomes of health care.

The rate of growth of medical sociology (or what is now appropriately termed the sociology of health and illness) has varied between countries. However, currently there is considerable activity across different parts of the world. For example, the first three issues of *Social Science and Medicine* in 2000 (Volume 50, numbers 1 to 3) contained 33 papers that were distributed geographically (based on the location of the first author) as follows: Western Europe (13 of which 11 from United Kingdom), North America (11), Southeast Asia and Pacific Rim (five), Africa (three), and South America (one). Many of the topics covered are similar across these areas, although research takes account of particular local circumstances, cultural beliefs, and characteristics of health systems.

Research undertaken by sociologists in the health field ranges from empiricist quantitative surveys, to more sociologically informed analyses of health and care issues, to research which is primarily concerned with developing new sociological theories and explanations. Similarly, sociologists may often employ quantitative methods of investigation and undertake large-scale surveys or participate in randomized controlled trials, as well as conducting more in-depth studies using qualitative methods of data collection and analysis. While acknowledging the considerable overlap and collaboration between the disciplines of public health medicine and sociology, this section nevertheless focuses on what is distinctive about sociological investigations in terms of their perspectives, the methods of investigation employed, and the questions addressed.

Sociological perspectives

The broad conceptual framework for sociological investigations comprises theories of the nature and workings of society. However, sociology is characterized by a range of theories rather than a single unified approach. These theories influence ways of 'seeing' the social world and inform the questions asked about particular aspects of health, medicine, and health care and the types of explanations given, as well as influencing the methods of research.

Sociological theories can be broadly divided into structural and social action theories. Structural theories emphasize the characteristics and operation of the broad structures of society, which are viewed as comprising an external social reality that shapes prevailing beliefs, values, and behaviours of social groups. In contrast, social action theories acknowledge the existence of multiple realities, and are concerned with the individual's subjective perception of their social world and actions on the basis of meanings. However, each of these broad theoretical perspectives comprises distinct sociological traditions that differ in their focus and explanations of the nature and workings of society. This diversity forms an important strength of sociological investigations in public health as in other fields of enquiry. Moreover, all sociological research involves a theoretical position, albeit this is often implicit. Thus although sociological research in the field of health and medicine has a strong empirical tradition, it is always based on some assumptions regarding the nature of social reality which in turn influences the questions posed and how evidence is collected, analysed, understood, and used. As Alderson (1998) observes, 'hypotheses are explicit, but when theories are implicit their power to clarify or to confuse, and to reveal or obscure new insights, can work unnoticed'.

Structural theories

Structural theories share a common focus on the structure of society and its institutions, and regard society as constraining and shaping the beliefs, values, and patterns of behaviour of social groups. They also emphasize the objective nature of social phenomena and the possibility of applying positivist methods in their study (see section on sociological methods). However, structural theories differ in their view of the nature of society and the relationships between groups. They can be broadly divided into consensual theories that assume a consensus of values and goals which forms the basis of social solidarity and co-operation (and is therefore compatible with a fairly medicocentric approach), and conflict theories that emphasize the struggle for advantage between different groups in society.

Consensual theories, most notably that of functionalism, played an important role in the early development of sociology. Particularly influential was Talcott Parsons (1902–1979), who undertook a theoretical analysis of society from a functionalist perspective and applied this to the question of how society contains the potentially disruptive effects of illness (Parsons 1951). Parsons regarded illness as dysfunctional for the smooth running of society because sick people are not able to fulfil their normal social roles (work roles, familial roles, community activities, and so on). Parsons thus depicted illness as a social as well as a biological phenomenon. He identified the mechanisms evolved by society to manage and control the amount of illness in society as being achieved through the special status and role assigned to sick people (the 'sick role') and the complementary role for doctors. Specific expectations of the sick person are identified as the need to seek professional help (in relation to the nature and severity of the illness) and to co-operate with the doctor. Privileges are the granting of exemption from performance of normal duties and responsibilities relative to the nature and severity of the illness (such as time off work), and being viewed as in need of care. Reciprocal expectations of doctors include the need to apply a high degree of knowledge and skill to problems of illness, to act for the welfare of the patient rather than their own self-interest, to be objective and emotionally detached, and to be guided by the rules of professional conduct. These expectations of both doctor and patient both ensure that the patient is restored to health and hence normal role performance as quickly as possible, and also that the privileges of the sick role are not abused through inappropriate entry or malingering.

Parsons' theory has been criticized for not being applicable to chronic illness and for being ethnocentric. However, his ideas extended the view of illness from a purely biological state to the social sphere and have since been widely employed. For example, the ambivalent responses often displayed by the public and medical staff to conditions such as alcoholism, overdoses, and AIDS can be explained by their unwillingness to view such conditions purely as sickness requiring treatment and therefore to grant such people the privileges of the sick role. Instead, there is a tendency to ascribe notions of responsibility and thus of punishment to such patients and possibly to their close relatives (Pollack *et al.* 1992). Similarly, issues regarding the appropriate expectations of family members following major illness, and the adverse effects on recovery of placing them in a dependent sick role, are of relevance for successful rehabilitation.

Whereas functionalist theory with its emphasis on explaining social stability was influential in the early development of sociology, by the late 1960s it had been largely replaced by conflict theories which were more in keeping with the tenor and mood of the times. Marxist theory (historical materialism) focused on the question of how social change happens. Karl Marx (1818–1883) depicted society as progressing through a series of stages and revolutionary transformations based on the development of systems of production. In brief, the economic infrastructure was seen as determining the dominant social relations and major institutions of society, including its political structures, laws, and ideology, with the basic social division in modern capitalist society being on class lines. The relationship between the owners and the propertyless workers, the proletariat, was depicted as an antagonistic and exploitative one, sustained by the inequality in power and resources.

Materialist theories were influential in the health field during the 1970s and early 1980s, especially in relation to analyses of the social causes and distribution of disease. This political economy framework shifted the focus for understanding inequalities in health from the activities of the individual and the institution of medicine, to the effects of inequalities in income and the organization of work in capitalist economies. Rates of ill health among workers and their families was partly attributed to physical health risks associated with work, including exposure to toxic substances and risks of accidents and injury, and reflected the contradiction that exists between the pursuit of health and the pursuit of profit (Doyal 1981). Similarly, the stresses associated with workers' lack of autonomy and situation of alienation in the sphere of production was viewed as a cause of psychological health risks (Schwalbe and Staples 1986). Workers' lack of satisfaction in the sphere of production was also seen as encouraging the pursuit of satisfaction in the sphere of consumption, thus leading to high rates of cigarette smoking and other behaviours harmful to health (Navarro 1982).

Historical materialism is now in decline as a general theory, reflecting both the decline of communism and the restructuring of capitalism. However, it has drawn attention to sectional interests and social conflict as a routine feature of modern societies, and to power and domination as a means through which social integration and the consent of subordinate groups may be secured. This emphasis on conflict and competing interests was associated in the health field with the demystifying of medicine and an emphasis on its iatrogenic effects (Illich 1977), and assessments of the limited contribution of medicine to the decline in mortality rates (Powles 1973). In terms of the doctor–patient relationship there was a new emphasis on the conflicts that may occur between doctor and patient, given their differing interests and knowledge (Freidson 1970). Studies of health policies also demonstrated the effects of competing interests, with different coalitions occurring in relation to different issues (for example, restrictions on tobacco sales or controls on environmental pollution, and so on) (Calnan 1984). A further change was the emergence of feminist analyses which regard gender relations rather than class relations as generating fundamental inequalities and oppression (Jagger and Rothenberg 1984). This focused attention on gender issues in relation to health and health care, and particularly the effects on health of women's domestic position and labour force participation. In addition, greater attention has been paid in the United Kingdom to the significance of ethnicity for health and health care following the recording of self-assessed ethnicity in the 1991 census, while issues of race and ethnicity had traditionally received greater attention in the United States.

Whereas consensual and conflict theories were developed to explain the nature and workings of industrial society, new challenges for sociological theory have been presented by the recent period of rapid and extensive social change leading to a 'postmodern' era. This process has been likened to the industrial revolution, in that it involves the transformation of the major institutions of society and permeates all aspects of everyday life and self-identity. Movement into an era of postmodernity is driven by a process of 'globalization', which involves changes in the economic, technological, and social spheres. This includes the deregulation of markets and economic liberalization, the diffusion of technology and increased speed of communications, increased regionalization, greater involvement of the state in intergovernmental business, and the development of a global culture which crosses divides of time and space. Such changes weaken traditional institutions (including traditional structures of the family and the character of work) and the powerful collective identities that went with them. As a result society is becoming more fragmented, heterogeneous, and 'individualized', with society forming a collection of factions competing for power and resources (Giddens 1991, 1994; Beck 1992). For example, in contrast to the traditional emphasis on social class as a major social division, there is much debate as to whether social class continues to be a meaningful category or can be viewed as just one of several patterns of power and inequality (Savage and Miles 1994). Increased emphasis is therefore now given in the health field, as in other branches of sociology, to the variety of social groupings, defined by age, gender, and ethnicity, as well as socio-economic circumstances. However, it is argued that such groupings, although of relevance for people, are no longer the units that determine individual experience. Instead the heterogeneity of social life is emphasized, with individuals no longer primarily defined in terms of occupation and class but seen as constructing 'self-identities' through consumption and lifestyle which form the major cleavage in contemporary society (Baumann 1987). However, Higgs and Scambler (1998) caution that postmodern perspectives give insufficient attention to the continuing significance of class, including the salience of an excluded underclass and an inconspicuous ruling/capitalist class.

Social action theories

Social action theories are based on a fundamentally different view of the social world from structural theories. The latter take a realist perspective and regard the world as having an existence independent of our perception of it. The object of social science (as with the natural sciences) is therefore to establish the truth about how the social world operates. In contrast, social action theories regard the social world as consisting of a series of representations. Their aim is therefore to understand subjective meanings, and they regard social action as a product of how individuals interpret the world and interact with others on the basis of these meanings. They also emphasize the fluidity that exists, with individuals having the ability to select, interpret, and bestow meaning upon their interactions with others. However, self-direction is seen as always limited by the actions and expectations of others, with the result that individuals engage in processes of 'negotiation, impression management and meaning creation' (Fine 1993).

The social action perspective had its origins in the writings of Max Weber (1864–1920), George Herbert Mead (1863–1931), Husserl (1890–1938), and Schutz (1899–1959). However, its rise to prominence occurred in the 1960s and 1970s and it is now extremely influential within the health field. Like other perspectives, it encompasses different theoretical positions, most notably those of symbolic interactionism, phenomenology, ethnomethodology, and social constructionism. These traditions although all emphasizing the subjective nature of the social world, nevertheless differ in their origins and underlying philosophical assumptions, and give differing accounts of the ways in which social actors make social life. Symbolic interactionism, for example, developed from the work of Mead (1934). This theoretical approach argues that human social conduct has a symbolic character, and what permits human beings to interact and form relationships and society is their ability to understand one another's gestures and responses. Symbolic interactionism also emphasizes the importance of learning about the culture or subculture of the people under study and therefore frequently uses observation and ethnographic analysis. Phenomenology, which developed from the writings of Schutz (1962, 1964), is primarily concerned with interaction between individuals (for example, between doctor and patient) or within small groups, which is regarded as being governed by a principle of reciprocity of perspectives. This involves assumptions about what each person makes about the other and the means by which social actors construct intersubjective understandings. According to Schutz this is achieved through possession of a common stock of knowledge which is constantly modified and refined on the basis of our experiences and interactions.

Interpretive studies in the health field are sometimes theoretically grounded in a particular sociological tradition. However, much qualitative research is more generally based on the assumptions of a social action approach, in terms of an emphasis on uncovering subjective meanings and the acceptance of multiple realities. A major area of study in the health field has been the meanings held by lay people and the reasons for their actions, with such research often serving to render intelligible what appeared irrational based on a medical perspective. An example is research undertaken to explain the high levels of patient non-compliance. Quantitative studies indicate that on average 40 to 50 per cent of patients treated for chronic conditions are non-compliant with drug regimes. This phenomenon was traditionally viewed in terms of a framework of patient 'default', and attributed to patient's lack of medical knowledge, problems of forgetting, and the complexity of drug regimes. Responses mainly involved giving patients more medical information, providing drug counters and other aids to remembering, simplifying drug regimes, and improving doctors' communication skills. In contrast, qualitative studies informed by a social action approach acknowledged the existence of multiple realities and explored patients' own meanings and the reasons for their actions. For example, Donovan and Blake (1992) conducted open interviews with 54 patients attending a rheumatology clinic and also observed consultations. Altogether one-half of these respondents were considered to be non-compliant, with common reasons being worries about side-effects, worries about becoming dependent on the drugs or that their bodies would become tolerant, and worries that the drugs would lose their effectiveness. They noted that rather than 'defaulting',

> [p]atients carried out their cost–benefit analyses in theory and many put them into practice. Some would decide that the risks outweighed the benefits of the drugs.... In most cases, however, drugs would be taken 'on trial' for whatever period seemed most appropriate to patients. (Donovan and Blake 1992)

Patients' medication use was thus more adequately described as 'reasoned decision-making' rather than as 'non-compliance'. Similar findings across a wide range of conditions and treatments have led to an emphasis on the more active involvement of patients in the consultation. This requires giving greater priority to patients' beliefs, preferences, and co-operation through patient-centred consultations and achieving a 'concordance' between doctor and patient in relation to treatment decisions (Chewning and Sleath 1996). The question has thus been raised of whether the term 'patient', which portrays passivity, compliance, and an unequal relationship between the user of health-care services and the provider, is still an appropriate term (Neuberger and Tallis 1999).

Other examples of research that stems from this notion of the more active participating 'patient', and makes intelligible what are viewed in medical terms as 'inappropriate' patient behaviours, include qualitative research examining 'problems' of the uptake or non-uptake of medical services and preventive measures (Kai 1996; Cornford and Morgan 1999), studies of lay definitions of 'health' (Williams 1983), lay images of disease and of persons 'at risk' (Davison *et al.* 1991), and the meanings of stigmatizing illness (Scambler and Hopkins 1986). There has been much less emphasis on the study of professionals' beliefs and practices, although an interpretive perspective and qualitative methods are increasingly employed in organizational evaluations to elicit the perspectives of different stakeholders (see section on professionals perspectives).

So far this section has focused on approaches that may be characterized as subtle realist, and which emphasize subjectivity and the existence of multiple realities (Pope and Mays 2000). However, another sociological tradition adopts an extreme relativist position (radical relativism or 'antirealist') and holds that social and human reality are mind-created (or socially constructed realities) and not merely mind-shaped and created through interaction. This tradition is thus based on the assumption that it is not possible to have any knowledge of a phenomenon apart from our own experience of it, and all accounts are regarded as of equal status and validity. This approach is exemplified by the writings of Michel Foucault (1926–1984). A major strand of Foucault's work is his constructionist analysis of the history of medical ideas in France (Foucault 1976). This involved charting the change from speculatively based medicine of the eighteenth century to the scientifically based medicine of the nineteenth. Foucault explained this change in terms of the emergence of a new 'clinical gaze' or way of seeing the patient's body, rather than forming the result of reasoned development and progress. For example, developments in pathological anatomy and the invention of the stethoscope with the opportunities they offered for viewing the internal workings of the body are regarded as giving rise to a change in the reality of disease. This involved a shift from the galenic humoral theory in which disease is seen as a disturbance in the body's balance towards the belief in the solid invariate reality of the body, and the status of a disease as a 'thing' separated from the self and how the individual feels. Disease entities therefore form products of social reasoning and social practices rather than something 'real'. To call a set of symptoms 'bronchitis' or 'coronary heart disease' does not therefore mean that a disease entity exists independently of social context, but is how medical science, in a given time and place with the aid of laboratory tests and theories, has come to define it. All knowledge is therefore contingent, with medical belief systems, like other belief systems, being created as a result of reasonings that are socially imbued. Moreover, Foucault suggests that the way the body is seen, described, and constructed might be called 'political anatomy'. It is political because changes in the way the body is viewed are based on certain mechanisms of power and wider changes in society. This approach therefore involves the study of language and texts as forms of discourse, which help to create and reproduce systems of social meaning (Tonkiss 1998).

A major critique of radical constructionist (and postmodernist) approaches is that if all knowledge is regarded as socially relative, we have no standards by which to judge the merits of different types of treatment or technological intervention. Indeed, Bury (1986) questions whether in this context the constructionist view itself can have any validity. For example, data showing a relationship between social class and health would be seen from a radical constructionist perspective as merely the effects of particular epidemiological techniques, rather than as something 'real' requiring social action. An extreme relativist position therefore means that research cannot derive any unequivocal insights relevant to action, and as a result commands little support among applied health service researchers. Nevertheless, this perspective is important in drawing attention to ways in which interpretations and responses to the sick body can be viewed as fabrications of powerful discourses rather than discoveries of 'truths', and as such has been particularly influential in relation to feminist analyses of the body as a key site of oppression. For example, the construction of disease categories (e.g. hysteria) and assumptions about women's bodies can be viewed as maintaining gender relations and reinforcing traditional roles (Shuttleworth 1990). Similarly, definitions of childbirth as a 'medical problem' and associated discourses in terms of risk and clinical safety are viewed as supporting the control of childbirth by the medical profession (Kitzinger 1992).

Structure and agency

A recent development in sociological theory is an attempt to overcome traditional theoretical divisions, and to bring together notions of structure with a social action perspective. Key theoretical approaches are Giddens' (1984) theory of structuration and Bhaskar's (1989) critical realism.

The attempt to link structure and agency in the health field is illustrated by the proposals of Popay *et al.* (1998*b*) for future research on inequalities in health. They argue that the existing quantitative work in this field consists mainly of unidimensional explanations within 'risk factor' epidemiology and do not encompass the full complexity of social processes. Conversely, qualitative studies of individual behaviours (although emphasizing beliefs and actions) tend to be divorced from context, in terms of the structures of power and control in which individuals are embedded. Popay *et al.* argue that future research should take account of material conditions in terms of the places people inhabit (for example, run-down area of large city, suburban housing area, local health services and recreational facilities, and so on), to explore the ways in which structures affect the dynamics of everyday life. Examples of questions to be addressed, include 'How do individuals living in the most materially disadvantaged areas of society make sense of and act upon their environments, with what consequences for their health and those they care for?' and 'What is the relationship between material risk, individual experience and action at the individual or group level?' Popay *et al.* explain that:

> [a]ttention to the meanings people attach to their experience of places and how this shapes social action could provide a missing link in our understanding of the causes of inequalities in health. In particular, the articulation of these meanings—which we refer to as lay knowledge—in narrative form could provide invaluable insights into the dynamic relationships between human agency and wider social structures that underpin inequalities in health. (Popay *et al.* 1998*b*)

Sociological theory and medical sociology

This section has drawn attention to the diversity of perspectives within sociology and identified some of the current debates. The latter includes the changes in society associated with movement into an era of postmodernity, differing assumptions regarding relativism as exemplified by interpretive and radical constructionist approaches, and attempts to link agency and structure. These developments, together with the increasing prominence of interpretive approaches and qualitative methods, are reflected in work within the health field and provide new insights in relation to both clinical and public health issues as illustrated in subsequent sections (see section on areas of sociological investigation).

For sociologists working in the health field, the distinction between sociology of medicine and sociology in medicine still holds. The former comprises sociologists whose main interest is to advance theoretical knowledge through research in the field of health and illness. The latter comprises sociologists primarily concerned with addressing medical or health service issues, who in the United Kingdom are mainly located in departments of public health or other medical departments. A recent change has been the increasing emphasis on work that may be classified as sociology of medicine. This has stemmed particularly from research that is now referred to as the sociology of the body, which brings together developments in Foucauldian, postmodernist, and feminist analyses, and addresses such issues as sociology's replication of the mind/body dualism, the influence of the Foucauldian reconceptualization of power, and the conditions of life in postmodernity. One aspect of the latter is the possibility of controlling the body (through drugs, transplants, and so on) in ways that were never possible in the past, but which also raise new issues about what the body actually is. Other issues are concerns with the shaping of the body through lifestyle choices, physical interventions and cultural expectations, the lived body in terms of chronic illness, and political dimensions of the regulation and control of bodies in relation to for example reproduction, death, and the provision of physical capital (Nettleton 1995).

Sociology in medicine also continues as a strong tradition and applies sociological theories and insights to public health issues. Sociologists engaged in this activity sometimes employ quantitative methods, specializing particularly in survey research. Such studies conform closely to epidemiological work, especially in relation to research examining the distribution and explanations of social inequalities in health. However, increasingly sociologists in medicine apply an interpretive perspective and employ qualitative methods to examine clinical and public health issues, particularly in relation to the perspectives and evaluations of patients and consumers. This framework and methodology, although differing from the assumptions and methods of epidemiological research, is now accorded official recognition and acceptance. This is reflected in the recent acknowledgement by medical journals of the contribution of this approach to the understanding of health-care and health services issues (Black 1994).

Sociological methods

Sociological investigations employ a range of methods which can be classified as belonging to two main research traditions, those of quantitative and qualitative research. Each is derived from a set of philosophical assumptions, with issues around qualitative research being more debated and discussed than for the former. The logic of each tradition does not apply to the other, although it is common for novice researchers to ask inappropriate questions of qualitative research, which derive from the quantitative tradition. This section therefore defines the key features of these traditions and how they contribute to the understanding of public health. It pays particular attention to qualitative methods, however, as its logic and techniques are less familiar to epidemiologists and other clinical scientists, and involve a radical departure from the assumptions and methods of the scientific model that form the basis of quantitative research.

Quantitative research

Quantitative methods derive from a positivist philosophy, of which a key element is the view that social phenomena are objective and external to the individual and thus take the form of social 'facts'. It will be suggested later in the chapter that there is a move in the sociology of health and illness towards greater use of qualitative methods, but it remains the case that there is a solid contribution to public health by social scientists using quantitative techniques.

The model for quantitative research derives from laboratory-based science. Key features include the assumption that there is no relationship between the researcher and the researched, that the 'social facts' remain constant over the study period, and that the well-conducted study will have high reliability (repeatability) and validity. Taken out of the laboratory context, this set of assumptions provides difficulties for researchers in the public health and social science fields who wish to carry out good quality research in a social environment. The problems hold true for many different methods, including designing randomized controlled trials, which although 'classically' designed to test drug treatments are sometimes employed to evaluate the introduction of a new form of service. Thus, among other things, researchers pay special attention to problems associated with reliability and validity, and issues of bias in the data collection.

Data employed in a quantitative study derives from a number of sources. Some may be drawn from 'secondary' sources; for example using routinely collected hospital statistics, government surveys, and census data. Social scientists, however, are commonly involved in the collection of primary data using a variety of methods, such as randomized controlled trials, health needs assessments, and large-scale surveys. Sociologists bring to such research a knowledge of the meanings and significance of concepts such as social class, gender, ethnicity, and age, which are of value in examining and interpreting health inequalities, variations in uptake of services, or variations in the incidence of particular disease conditions between males and females. Sociology has also contributed other concepts and interpretations in studying the social determinants of health and health outcomes, including relative (and absolute) poverty and social exclusion, social networks and support, lay beliefs about health and illness behaviours, and the possible effects of occupational/social mobility and diagnostic decision-making on observed patterns of disease.

The quantitative tradition is based upon the scientific method, which is distinct along a number of dimensions to qualitative methods, as set out on Table 1. Studies using quantitative methods require the research question to be predefined, so that the study tests a precise hypothesis or set of research questions. It is also essential at this stage to define the variables, such as social class or 'working women', since these variables have to be translated into categories that can be incorporated into the study design (for example, the questionnaires) and which have meaning for the study. Thus to operationalize the category of 'working women' in a study of the effects of pregnancy on women in paid employment, the researchers would have to decide where to set cut-offs for hours worked per week (for example, up to 10 h/week, 11 to 20 h/week, and so on), or to simplify matters,

Table 1 Quantitative and qualitative research

	Quantitative	Qualitative
View of the world	Social reality exists as objective, measurable phenomena, external to the individual (positivism)	Social reality is subjectively interpreted and experienced (interpretive)
Logic of enquiry	Deductive based on testing formal hypotheses to establish causal relationships	Inductive reasoning with understanding of social processes derived from data
Research design	Quantitative, with sample selection, data collection and analyses based on scientific procedures and ensuring repeatbility and generalizable results	Qualitative, based on detailed study of social processes of groups of interest to elicit interpretations and responses
Validity	Corresponds to an objective reality	Corresponds to subjective reality; other terms include trustworthiness credibility, plausability

perhaps to make the distinction between women working full or part time. The appropriate definition of key variables is crucial to the success of the study. For example, researchers may wish to draw up their categories in the knowledge that 17.5 h is defined as half-time employment, and that a category of 11 to 20 h would cut across this important distinction. By limiting the study to working women the researchers should be aware that they will miss the inclusion of various categories of women who carry out unpaid work (housewives, women working unpaid in the family business, and so on) but for whom the health impact may be similar to those with paid work.

Setting out the research questions and defining the independent variables are critical stages in the research process, and these allow no second chances if poorly defined. Thus in order to carry out a quantitative study, the researcher(s) must be familiar with the field of study. For example, it is important to be aware of all the options that are available to the subject responding to the questionnaire, since lack of fit between the subject's preference and the options set out in the questionnaire decreases the validity of the study. It is normal to pilot any questionnaire, sometimes twice, to ascertain the validity of the questions.

Most quantitative research in this field requires collecting 'primary' data using a self-completed or interview-administered questionnaire. The questionnaire is a central part of the researcher's armoury in the maintenance of reliability since all respondents will receive the same questionnaire and the same letter of introduction. As importantly, the measurement (for example, alcohol consumption, attitudes towards pain) should work in a consistent way with each individual. If the questionnaire is interviewer administered, the researcher should be trained to check that all procedures are systematically carried out with all respondents to reduce possible biases within the data collection. Questions are generally precoded and allow only a limited range of responses, while some studies also incorporate prevalidated measures including psychometric tests (for example, measuring anxiety or depression) and other measures relating to social support, quality of life, health status, and so on (Bowling 1991).

Questionnaires vary along several continuums. They may be sent through the post (self-administered), or carried out with a trained interviewer administering the schedule (for example, on the doorstep or in the shopping mall, or, increasingly, by telephone). The method selected will depend in part upon the research issue, intended sample size, and funding available. All approaches have their benefits and disadvantages. Response rates may vary depending on the approach, the group being questioned, and their interest in the topic. With the increasing number of studies being carried out, some health service staff and patients are in a danger of being over-researched. It is therefore important to make the questionnaire clearly laid out, as brief as possible, and of interest to the respondents to increase the possibility of a high response rate (issues of questionnaire wording, sequencing, appearance, and enhancing the response rate are dealt with clearly by McColl *et al.* (1998)). Sampling is a complex issue; researchers often wish to gain a representative sample of a population (since total population sampling is usually out of the question) but there are a number of routes to achievement of the most appropriate sample, which are discussed by Arber (1993) among others.

The key to the success of quantitative research is the ascertainment of statistical relationships between variables. Analysis may be complex, and requires statistical knowledge, although computer packages such as Minitab and the Statistical Package for the Social Sciences (**SPSS**) can aid the process. However, the choice of statistical tests is affected by the distribution of the data and it is important that social scientists either become statistically literate and/or work with statisticians.

Quantitative research in sociology thus conforms to the broader principles of scientific research shared by public health and other clinical sciences. It assumes that there is an objective reality which can be measured, and that studies are reliable (repeatable) and valid. Many public health issues have been tackled with the survey approach uniting sociologist and epidemiologist. Sociologists have less often become involved with other quantitative approaches such as case–control or cohort studies. It is increasingly common, however, for those designing randomized controlled trials to acknowledge the importance of measuring 'consumer satisfaction' or 'professionals views' of the intervention and to co-opt a sociologist onto the project (for example, Tucker *et al.* 1996; Turnbull *et al.* 1996). While this is not ideal, it does ensure that randomized controlled trials include these concepts in their design, as well as incorporating prevalidated measures of health outcome based on health status or quality of life measures.

Qualitative research

Qualitative research is the methodological tradition used more often by interpretist or social action perspectives described above. These methods have a long tradition in sociology and characterized many of the early sociological studies undertaken in the United States in the 1940s, as well as forming the general methodology of anthropological research. However, acknowledgement of the legitimacy of the approach in the medical field is more recent. A series of articles published in the *British Medical Journal* in the summer of 1994 (subsequently published as an edited collection (Mays and Pope 1996)) could be seen as a marker of acceptance. More generally, with a broadening definition of public health to include topics such as social exclusion, social networks, and other social determinants of health, has come recognition of the contribution of subjective experience to health planning and policy. Today qualitative methods are frequently employed in clinical and health services research, and in a wide range of community health studies and health needs and health impact assessments. These approaches, where the respondent's beliefs and experiences are prioritized, are appropriate where there is a gap in the existing literature and where a new line of thinking needs to be established. This may relate to an understudied group or population, or where there is a need to develop a greater in-depth understanding of an issue.

There are several main sociological traditions that have an affinity with qualitative research, and are separated by subtle differences in analysis and emphasis. Whilst it is not appropriate in this chapter to provide an in-depth discussion of the methodological approaches associated with each tradition, the key features of qualitative research will be discussed.

Qualitative methods

Qualitative approaches are most commonly field based and include interviews, focus groups, and observational work—'words and actions' (Lofland and Lofland 1995). Secondary source analysis may also be included, such as library-based research drawing upon discourse analysis, and historical and documentary research. Finally, action-based methods in terms of process evaluation and action research are now considered valuable contributions to public health research.

Qualitative research (contrary to the assumptions of quantitative methods) acknowledges that there is always an interaction between the researcher and the researched. Researchers in this tradition are trained to be more reflexive about their role, reflecting critically upon the ways in which interaction with the respondents/field situation may influence the data collected. Researchers continue to debate the extent to which commonality between researcher and researched may enhance data collection. Some have argued that shared gender (for example, woman researcher/woman respondent) is highly influential in establishing trust between the two (Oakley 1981). Others have suggested that the supremacy of gender should not be assumed and that other factors, for example, 'ethnicity', may be more important than gender to some respondents (Douglas 1992). The essence is that these potential influences are acknowledged and discussed as they may ultimately affect the nature of the interview and the data collected as a result.

Interviews

Interviews are a central tool of the qualitative researcher, although it is important to be wary of the increasing use of the term 'interview' to describe a questionnaire-designed study in which the interviewer has talked the respondent through the schedule. It should also be noted that the key to identifying a qualitative study is the data analysis, which for a qualitative study would usually be in the form of thematic analysis from interview transcripts.

Interviews in qualitative research may take a number of forms, although most often used is the semi-structured (or semi-standardized) interview. In this form of interview the researcher starts with a list of topics and questions to be asked at every interview (often identified through earlier pilot interviews), although the order may alter and the researcher may probe for more information and follow-up a line of thinking with a respondent. At the other end of the 'structure' continuum is the non-standardized or unstructured interview, representing what Lofland and Lofland (1995) call 'the guided conversation'. This form of interview gives considerable flexibility in terms of the range and order in which issues are discussed, and is particularly useful as a strategy for investigating new subjects where respondents' views are unknown.

Interviews in qualitative research are usually tape-recorded and subsequently transcribed. The process is lengthy; interviews may last from 30 min to 2 or 3 h with a respondent but it may take as long as 5 to 10 h to transcribe and check the transcription. This process contributes to the perception of qualitative research as slow and time-consuming. Analysis (see below) is also a lengthy process.

Personal interviews are the most common method of data collection in qualitative research and have been employed with increasing frequency to study a wide range of issues of importance to public health. These include charting the meaning of illness (Kelly 1992), analysing the ways in which low-income families construct their daily diet (Dowler and Calvert 1995), and examining what individuals think about risk (Hart and Flowers 1996).

Brief mention has already been made of the sample in qualitative research. Numbers involved in interview studies are usually relatively small compared with sample sizes associated with quantitative studies. Indeed, the underlying assumptions of sampling is quite different, with the aim being to sample in such a way as to achieve a good representation of those characteristics thought to be important for the study. There are different sampling techniques, including purposive or systematic sampling, which is the deliberate choice of respondents, subjects, or setting to represent a wide range of opinion or experience (for example, one might take a consecutive sample of attenders at a clinic or a general practice). Theoretical sampling is based on a previously developed hypothesis or theory (for example religion is an important factor, so sampling would take place with attention to religious affiliation). A third type of sampling, 'snowball' sampling, is used when the individuals under study are difficult to access through normal routes (for example, studying homeless individuals) and respondents may therefore introduce other potential respondents.

Focus groups

Focus groups form an alternative to the personal interview. They have been employed by sociologists since the 1950s, but became known primarily as the tool of market researchers where they were used to carry out rapid checks on public attitudes (for example, in relation to consumer goods or political attitudes). However, focus groups have recently achieved a new status as a valid research tool (Barbour and Kitzinger 1999). The method brings together a group of individuals (usually six to eight), often selected with reference to age, gender, and other criteria, to discuss a series of topics, using the group or collective interaction to produce insights. Focus groups are regarded as having particular application for studying, among other things, ethnic groups, sensitive topics (Kitzinger 1994; Kitzinger and Farquer 1999), and organizational change (Barbour 1999). They have also found a niche as a research tool for investigating consumer views, as demonstrated in studies by Schwarz *et al.* (2000), Lanza and Ericsson (2000), French and Chopra (1999), Lansbury (2000), and Williams and Clark (2000). In all these examples, and especially the first two, focus groups are seen to provide valuable data for use in the development of health policy. Several of these studies also served as a first stage in the development of a larger study to generate hypotheses based on informants' insights. For example, Lanza and Ericsson's consumer-led focus groups on clinical guidelines preceded a survey on the topic.

With a skilled facilitator (who may use a number of techniques to encourage participation from group members), focus groups can provide rich data and elicit not only the views and experiences of group members but also areas where conflicts may arise and disagreements are expressed. The importance of trust has already been raised in relation to interviews and it is equally true here. Respondents are invited to participate in a focus group, sometimes with a small payment as an inducement. To facilitate free discussion and communication during the short time of the group, the researcher must establish trust between himself or herself and members of the group, emphasizing the confidential nature of the study and ensuring that individuals understand the purpose of the group (Cunningham-Burley *et al.* 1999).

Focus groups suffer from a number of drawbacks, including the evident 'self-selection' of individuals who may be willing to turn up to discuss their views and beliefs with a series of strangers. Many who feel marginal or who lack confidence may simply not respond to the invitation, or be reluctant to express their views, leaving the group dominated by the 'socially included' in society. One way to avoid this difficulty is to use an existing group as the basis for the focus group, such as a group of pensioners, mother and toddlers, or a support group who meet regularly and who are familiar with each other (Kitzinger 1994). However, it is important that 'gatekeepers' do not select individuals seen to be appropriate for the exercise.

Observation

As Hammersley and Atkinson (1997) note, 'all social researchers are participant observers'. All qualitative researchers may use observation as an adjunct to other methods of data collection, for example, when visiting an interviewee in their home or their work place, the 'observant' interviewer would note the context of the interviewee's life. However, participant observation (or observation, since not all researchers have the opportunity to become actively participant in the social context under enquiry) is a specific method with its own logic and rules. Participant observation is based on the structured observation of social life as it occurs; or, to put it more formally, 'participant observation refers to the process in which an investigator establishes and sustains a many-sided and relatively long-term relationship with a human association in its natural setting for the purpose of developing a scientific understanding of that association' (Lofland and Lofland 1995).

Researchers using this method are based within the context under study, spending as much time as possible becoming familiar with the lives of the respondents. Research using this method is often described as ethnographic. Ethnographic research is traditionally concerned with the study of culture and cultural meanings, although Hammersley and Atkinson (1997) emphasize the looseness of definition of the term 'ethnography'. In keeping with its anthropological origins, there is a strong emphasis on first-hand field study, that is, research involving considerable periods based in social contexts and settings, and involving informal interviews, discussions, and observation. Ethnographic methods relating to public health issues have been usefully employed to understand students training to be health professionals (Atkinson 1981), working-class family life in London (Cornwell 1984), and the culture of drug takers (McKeganey and Barnard 1992). Part of the process of establishing credibility with the researched group is learning through rigorous observation as well as informal interviews what the important values are of the group. As with other methods, the researcher sets out to gain the trust of the researched. Thus McKeganey and Barnard (1992) spent a year 'in the field' in their ethnographic study of street-workers in Glasgow. Pavis and Cunningham-Burley (1999), exploring street culture among young people in East Lothian, reported 70 h of participant observation.

Observational data collected in the form of field-notes (as in anthropology) is often accompanied by additional data collected through interviews and possibly questionnaires. Thus Pope (1991), in her study which examines the process by which hospital waiting lists are created and maintained, reports a range of methods, although the data collected through observation are key to her analysis and explanation of the waiting list phenomenon. In such situations the researcher often does not know in advance the area and issues to focus upon, and therefore progressive focusing takes place. Thus after reviewing the initial field-notes, the researcher may decide to 'focus down' on specific areas of investigation. Although observational studies provide valuable data on actions tied to particular situations and circumstance, they have the drawback of being labour intensive and expensive.

Action research

The term 'action research' is normally attributed to Lewin (1946) who defined action research as 'a way of generating knowledge about a social system while, at the same time, attempting to change it'. Meyer (2000) brings out its particular qualities, and describes action research as 'a style of research rather than a specific method', and one which contributes simultaneously to social science and social change. Three key features of action research are identified as its participatory character (requires participants to perceive a need for change and be willing to play an active part in the research and change process), its democracy (requires participants to be seen as equals with the researcher and to be consulted on the action process and methods of evaluation which is negotiated with participants), and its contribution to both social science knowledge and local change (the former requires that the report is presented with considerable contextual detail to aid generalization).

An action research approach is most common in community work. However, it has also been employed in identifying problems in clinical practice, helping to develop potential solutions, and facilitating change within the health services, especially by members of the nursing profession (Titchen and Binnie 1993; East and Robinson 1994). East and Robinson (1994) have described a 2-year action research project that aimed to facilitate the management of change in a district general hospital. The study brought out clearly the differing agendas of the participants both within the hospital (demonstrated by a case study of the nurses' experience of change at ward level) and those of the clinical nursing staff and the general managers. Similarly, a study by the Royal College of Physicians in England is exploring the roles of clinicians, clinical audit staff, and managers in implementing clinical audit and ways of overcoming organizational barriers to audit (Berger 1998).

Action research is not tied to a particular methodology and may use a number of different methods to capture the process of change and to evaluate the nature of any changes that have occurred. However, it generally employs qualitative methods with data collected through interviews and observation as well as documentary sources. There is a move towards stressing the value of documenting the experience of change, and many of the more exciting action research projects in nursing, education, and social work have incorporated this element.

Mixed designs

A 'mixed method' study design is increasingly common and viewed as desirable, with each method drawing out distinct features of the issue under study. Thus a questionnaire study may identify the spread of views on an issue, while an additional set of interviews with a sample of subjects might provide a greater understanding of why different views are held. The concept of 'triangulation' is often used in this respect, with the researchers using multiple and different methods which may involve a mix of interviews, observation, and routine data to approach the same issue. Triangulation is a form of validation in research, with the assumption that the emergent findings using one method will support those achieved from another method in corroborating an overall interpretation. However, the way in which methodologies from different traditions actually combine together as a form of validation is still debated.

Data analysis and validity

> The question is not whether the data are biased but to what extent [the researcher has] rendered transparent the processes by which data have been collected, analysed and presented. (Popay *et al.* 1998*a*)

Data analyses are an on-going feature of qualitative research, bound up with the collection and processing of the data from the study. The iterative process of data collection and hypothesis testing is explicit in 'grounded theory' but is essentially part of all qualitative methods. The raw material for qualitative researchers is words; as 'data' these can be in the form of transcriptions from (tape-recorded) interviews or focus groups, notes written by the researcher(s) from interviews and field-notes in which they have recorded their fieldwork experiences, and occasionally diaries kept by the respondents themselves.

From early on in the study, the researcher will begin to think about concepts that seem important, useful, or in some way to provide insight into the respondent's experiences. At the beginning of analysis, the researcher will identify a set of codes or categories, which derive from the data. Some of the codes may be practical (for example, family relations, descriptions of heart attack, contact with general practitioner), but others may be more abstract such as 'independence', 'coping strategies', 'bad days', and so on. Within an extended set of codes it may be appropriate to construct subdivisions, such as dividing up the types of 'coping strategies' or different types of communication with the general practitioner, if the data provide examples of such divisions. There is no hard-and-fast rule about coding the data, some preferring quite complex systems and others starting with quite a broad basic framework. The important—and distinctive—feature of most qualitative research is that the data suggest the codes, rather than the researchers working to a prior hypothesis of what they wish to examine. The researcher will then apply this coding system to all the transcripts, either by hand, or by using one of a number of computer packages available to aid this process. These packages can be time-consuming to master but generally help the next stage of the analysis, which is to develop themes from the codes. These themes may be based around one or more codes; thus one theme in a study of patients with heart disease could be the different ways in which patients manage their medication taking. Much research rests at this point in the analysis and remains quite 'literal', reporting at a fairly concrete level of what the data have shown. However, many qualitative researchers will try to create some kind of 'higher-order' theory from their research and to draw out at a more abstract level of meaning from the data. Thus in our example, the researchers may look at notions of patients' independence and patient strategies to remain self-monitoring of their condition. Similarly in a study of the experiences of relatives of critically ill patients, Walters (1995) summarized the findings into four themes or sets of concepts, 'making sense', 'plain talk', 'being with', and 'seeing'. At an even higher level of abstraction one could see whether these concepts might apply to other conditions and situations. By so doing, it creates opportunities for the research to achieve greater generalizability, that is, generalizability at a theoretical level.

Grounded theory as a form of analysis was developed and elaborated in the 1960s by Glaser and Strauss (1965, 1967). At that time it was proposed as a form of analysis in which data analysed inductively in a rigorous manner resulted in the production of substantive and formal theoretical statements. It is fair to say that since then the term has been widely misused and that even its original proponents themselves do not agree about the process (see Melia's thoughtful discussion of the varying approaches to grounded theory (Melia 1997)). Grounded theory essentially refers to theory which has been 'worked up' from an iterative process, reviewing the data to derive hypotheses which are then tested in the field, repeating the process with revised hypotheses until the theory is seen to be supported fully within the data. Although many researchers report that they use this method, true grounded theory demands a commitment to data analysis and time in the field that is beyond the limit of many researchers.

The issue of validity in qualitative research most sharply distinguishes these methods from quantitative research. The assessment of the quality of qualitative research remains the focus of debate (Hammersley 1990; Murphy *et al.* 1998) and views of those within the field diverge. Some dislike the term 'validity' with its connotations of 'being able to establish the truth of any research beyond all possible doubt', and prefer to suggest that the way in which the soundness of study should be assessed is by using concepts of plausibility, credibility, trustworthiness, and the nature of generalizations made from the data. Ways of establishing 'validity' are difficult to summarize succinctly, and are subject to debate over form as well as terminology (Murphy *et al.* 1998; Seale 1999). Clarity of exposition of method is the key. However, the increasing publication of qualitative research in journal article form with their assigned word limits makes it difficult to provide a full description and reflection on the methods employed.

Areas of sociological investigation

The sociology of health and illness covers a wide and diverse range of topics. For example, a recent textbook covers the following topics: social construction of medical knowledge, lay perceptions of health and illness, the experience of health and illness, the sociology of the body, interactions between patients and health-care providers, and the patterning of health and illness in relation to social class, gender, race and ethnicity, and other social groupings, and the social organization of both formal and informal health care (Nettleton 1995). A number of authors have attempted to classify the concerns of sociology based on some organizing principle. A useful example is Turner's (1987) level of analysis approach. He argues that a comprehensive sociology of health and illness must involve the study of health and illness at three levels: the 'individual' level (which examines perceptions of health and illness), the 'social' level (which examines the social creation of disease categories and health-care organizations), and the 'societal' level (which examines health-care systems within the political context).

This section provides examples of the application of sociological perspectives and methods of investigation in relation to three areas—chronic illness and disability, ethnicity and health, and professionals' perspectives. The aim is not to provide a comprehensive review of these topics, but rather to illustrate the ways in which different perspectives and approaches focus attention on different issues and types of explanations, and to demonstrate the range of sociological concerns and methods of research.

Chronic illness and disability

The social dimensions of chronic illness and disability have formed a major area of study by public health specialists and sociologists from the late 1960s. This reflects the increasing prevalence of chronic disease and the opportunities such conditions offer for examining the social aspects of sickness. Research by sociologists has involved both collaborative studies with public health colleagues concerned with the conceptualization and measurement of 'disability', and qualitative research to investigate individuals' personal experiences and strategies in relation to chronic illness.

Conceptualization and assessment of 'disability'

An early stream of sociological research examined the consequences of chronic illness for both patients and families (Blaxter 1976). In addition, social scientists collaborated with clinicians and public health specialists in assessing the prevalence of disability in the population and needs of disabled people (Jefferys *et al.* 1969). These bodies of research informed the development of the World Health Organization's (**WHO**) model of the consequences of chronic illness—Classification of Impairment, Disabilities, and Handicaps (WHO 1980). This model provided a consistent terminology in the field and formally acknowledged that the consequences of chronic illness may extend from the medical to the social sphere. The WHO model distinguished three categories: (a) individual impairment, in terms of abnormality in the structure or function of the body whether through disease or trauma; (b) disability in everyday life (that is, restriction in ability to perform tasks, especially those associated with everyday life and self-care activities); (c) the experience of handicap, which refers to the disadvantage for a given individual, arising out of impairment and disability, that limits or prevents the fulfilment of a role that is normal (such as handicap in relation to work, education, or social activities). Impairments often lead directly to disability and may in turn place an individual at a disadvantage (handicap) in one or more spheres of life. However, the WHO model recognized that an impairment may not cause any disability (for example, severe facial scar, or controlled epilepsy) but nevertheless lead to considerable disadvantage or 'handicap', reflecting the societal meanings of the condition and consequent feelings of 'stigma' and shame.

The WHO model provided a framework for community-based studies undertaken by sociologists and others to examine the impacts of disability, including research examining the ways in which material and social circumstances may mediate the relationship between impairment, disability, and handicap (Locker 1983; Patrick and Peach 1989). Policies relating to the planning and provision of social care, community services, and financial benefits for people with disabling conditions also led to considerable emphasis on the measurement of the prevalence and severity of 'disability' and the conduct of national and local community-based studies. However, over time official definitions and measures of disability have increasingly broadened and now define greater numbers of people as 'disabled', thus underlining the social construction of this category (Martin *et al.* 1988).

The dominance of the WHO model has recently been challenged by the emergence of a 'disability movement' and the writings of academic disability theorists. These groups adopt a radical sociopolitical perspective derived from a conflict model, and criticize the WHO framework for being an overly 'medical' (or individualistic) model, as it locates the 'problem' of disability in terms of individual impairment (Oliver 1996). In contrast they depict disability as a social phenomenon, arising from material and cultural forces that effectively 'dis-able' people. As Barnes (1991) explains:

> In our view, it is society which disables physically impaired people. Disability is something imposed on top of our impairments, by the way we are unnecessarily isolated and excluded from full participation in society. Disabled people are therefore an oppressed group in society.

The social model thus regards disability as socially created and the product of the ways in which society is organized and its exclusionary practices, rather than the product of individual disabilities. For example, the built environment generally assumes that people can climb stairs, see instructions, and take extended steps on buses. The social model of disability therefore provides a radically different perspective to the traditional framework in emphasizing the need for social action rather than individual interventions. The former includes the achievement of improved rights, greater social acceptance, and changes in the material and social conditions of life that increase independence and opportunities for participating in the mainstream of society. The social model also requires that the measurement of disability should focus on the extent to which environments are disabling, rather than the assessment of individual's functional abilities (Abberley 1992).

Bury (1996, 1997), a medical sociologist who has written extensively in the field of disability and chronic illness, has drawn attention to what he regards as an overemphasis of the social model on the societal determinants of disability, with insufficient attention given to the varying experiences of people with different types of impairments and the significance of their underlying medical condition. For example, pain and associated activity restrictions may form an important aspect of some people's experience of chronic illness. French (1993) (herself part of the group of disabled disability theorists) also observes that there can be limits to the extent to which restrictions may be removed through social measures (such as the problems she experiences in interaction as a consequence of being blind). The social model has also been criticized for treating disabled people as a socially homogeneous group, with little attention given to the social meanings and effects of gender, ethnicity, and other social characteristics (Lonsdale 1990).

Despite such criticisms, the social barrier model has been important in directing attention to the importance of environmental barriers in limiting activity and participation. This model also raises issues of the control of professionals over what is regarded as a dependent and devalued client group, through defining the problems of this group in their own (medical) terms. Social barriers theorists thus challenge the goal of medicine in terms of achieving 'normality', and instead emphasize the need for greater acceptance of diversity and for the involvement of disabled people themselves in determining policies and priorities (Oliver 1996). The social model also stresses the importance of individual autonomy and choice, rather than seeing disabled people as passive recipients of services, and emphasizes the need for greater acceptance of the ordinary needs of disabled people in terms of medical care, social activities and family life, and so on.

The social model of disability is increasingly reflected in work regulations, building regulations, and other public, health, and social policies (Campbell and Oliver 1996). This conceptualization is also informing a revision of the WHO International Classification of Impairments, Disabilities, and Handicaps (**ICIDH-2**) which is described as providing a synthesis of the medical and social approaches to disablement in terms of a 'biopsychosocial' model (Bickenbach *et al.* 1999). This new model conceptualizes each dimension of disablement (impairments, activity limitations, and participation restrictions) as an interaction between intrinsic features of the individual and that person's social and physical environment. It also accords each dimension equal significance as representing different and independent facets of disablement, and recognizes that each requires different social responses or interventions.

This analysis of formal models of disability thus illustrates the ways in which accounts are often partial, and emphasizes different aspects of social reality. It also demonstrates the way in which the dominant framework serves to influence the nature of health/social policies, the formulation of research questions, and associated measurement issues.

Individual meanings and experiences

An interpretive perspective has informed a second strand of sociological research. This has involved in-depth interview-based studies of the meanings of chronic illness and disability for individuals, and the ways in which such meanings are constructed, negotiated, and transmitted, and often reconstructed through the course of illness. Early work focused on the crisis created by major disability. Examples include Davis' classic study of childhood polio, entitled *Passage Through Crisis* (Davis 1963), Scott's study of how people learn to be 'blind people' (Scott 1969), and Voysey's study of parental experiences of children with disabilities and the problems of coping with uncertainty (Voysey 1975). More recently, a number of studies have provided a temporal framework to take account of the emergent character of chronic illness, and followed the pathway from the initial disruption of illness, to the process of explanation and legitimation, treatment, and adaptation.

A key concept describing the impact of chronic illness is Bury's (1982) notion of 'biographical disruption' that derived from his in-depth study of people with rheumatoid arthritis. Biographical disruption recognizes that the onset of chronic illness represents an assault both on the person's physical self and on his or her self-identity. This occurs at two levels of meaning. One is the consequence for the individual of the onset of disruptive symptoms on everyday life at home or work. Studies of specific disorders such as multiple sclerosis (Robinson 1988), diabetes (Kelleher 1988), and ulcerative colitis (Kelly 1992) demonstrate how symptoms disrupt the flow of normal everyday life and introduce considerable uncertainty into it. Patients therefore expend considerable effort in managing their symptoms and limiting their practical consequences. For example, Kelly's (1992) study of ulcerative colitis sufferers drew attention to their problems of the unpredictability of symptoms, especially diarrhoea, who may therefore manage this by avoiding eating and drinking in public. Similarly, people with epilepsy try to avoid stress and other situations that increase risks of a fit. More generally, people seek to establish a way of life with symptoms or disability, often involving changes in daily activities and making tasks more manageable, while still leading valued lives. A second level of biographical disruption arises from the symbolic significance of chronic illness in terms of its implications for self-identity. For example, disfigurement and deformity associated with skin conditions and arthritis can have a major impact on self-identity, especially for women given the cultural value placed on attractiveness (Londsdale 1990). In addition, many conditions including epilepsy, mental illness, and cancer of the bowel are surrounded by negative social meanings or 'stigma', and result in feelings of shame and fears of avoidance and exclusion. In-depth studies of people with particular chronic conditions (Macdonald 1988; Scambler 1989; Pinder 1990) have identified a number of strategies that people may adopt to avoid or minimize these negative social responses in interaction with others. Sufferers also need to come to terms and 'make sense' of their condition. An in-depth study by Williams (1984) of 30 arthritis sufferers indicated that this was achieved through a process of what he termed 'narrative reconstruction'. This involves people making sense of the onset of their illness through reorganizing their own biography. Williams suggests that this process enables people to reconstruct a sense of order from the fragmentation produced by chronic illness, and also notes that clinical explanations are often inadequate for this purpose.

The success of the individual's adaptation to chronic conditions is demonstrated by a recent survey that indicated that 54 per cent of people with serious disabilities reported that they experience a good or excellent quality of life (Albrecht and Devlieger 1999). Factors associated with such positive assessments were identified as people's ability to understand their condition, take control, and introduce order and predictability. Successful adaptation may be enhanced by an individual's ability to mobilize supportive social ties and material resources (Locker 1983; Morgan *et al.* 1984), although the effects of these social circumstances have been given relatively little attention.

For the future, Kelly and Field (1998) suggest that chronic illness identities may become less coercive and constraining than at present, with the development of a more fluid and open society in the postmodern world, a greater tolerance of difference, and a kind of relativism in the aesthetics of appearance. Moreover, the continually changing and uncertain nature of postmodern society means that chronic illness may become just one more burden an individual has to contend with rather than a central aspect of identity. Another important change is the increasing challenge to the hegemony of medicine and the greater range of discourses available to draw on in making sense of chronic illness. These include those associated with various types of alternative and complementary medicine, local and national self-help organizations, and entertainment and the mass media. Complementing these changing patterns of social life are advances in effective drug regimes and surgery, which may increasingly help to limit and contain the disruption and discontinuity associated with chronic illness.

Ethnicity and health

In the 1970s sociologists in the United States carried out small-scale studies of different ethnic groups (for example, Jewish and Italian immigrants) and demonstrated the way in which concepts such as pain, illness, and health experiences were culturally created and expressed (Zola 1975). The inclusion of 'race' as a variable in sociological and epidemiological research remains important in the United States, and represents a key form of stratification within the society. In the United Kingdom by contrast, research has concentrated on the majority culture. Until the 1980s very little social and biomedical research acknowledged the ethnic diversity of the United Kingdom population or explored issues such as health status in relation to ethnicity. By the 1980s, sociologists began to investigate the health experiences of different ethnic groups, with this research generally being qualitative, small scale, and in-depth. Within the most recent decades, large-scale surveys have also contributed considerably to the knowledge of the health patterning of specific ethnic groups (Marmot *et al.* 1984; Balarajan and Balusu 1990; Nazroo 1997), with the last of these notably bringing a sociological awareness to the investigation at this level of ethnicity and health by introducing concepts such as poverty and socio-economic status, and discussion about the relevance of formal measure of class to ethnic minority groups.

As with disability research (see above), the emerging literature on ethnicity and health contains a number of highly debated topics, with researchers disagreeing on terminology, focus, and approach. This section can only briefly identify the key issues, note the areas of contention, and identify ways in which sociology can contribute to the further development of studies of ethnicity and health. What is evident is that sociological research has played a major role in the understanding of factors affecting the health of ethnic minorities within the United Kingdom, and also that a large research agenda remains to be developed.

Definitions

Terminology in this sensitive area is important, ethnocentric, and ever changing. As a concept ethnicity—in theory—can be applied to members of any group since it may be understood as 'cultural practices and outlooks that distinguish a given community of people' (Giddens 1989; Smaje 1995). In reality, however, the study of ethnicity in the United Kingdom generally refers to specific groups, not usually (as in the earlier American research) to Jewish, Italian, or Irish groups (although there are exceptions), but most frequently to the more recent migrated 'black' ethnic minorities. The largest groups among the latter are South Asian (Indian, Pakistani, Bangladeshi), African-Caribbean (previously termed 'West Indian', then 'Afro-Caribbean'), and Chinese, together constituting about 5 per cent of the United Kingdom population.

Problems exist in the allocation of individuals to ethnic groups. Previously, this has been crudely undertaken in the United Kingdom using country of birth of the individual (and their parents). Only in 1991 did the United Kingdom census include a question on self-assessed ethnicity. However, this classification, which identified eight main 'ethnic' groups, was problematic in a number of respects, including the mixture of ethnic and racial categories and an assumed homogeneity within the 'white' group (represented by a single category to include people from Cyprus, Turkey, the Republic of Ireland, and other areas). Considerable numbers of people also allocated themselves to 'other' categories. More generally, the approach to ethnic classification adopted and the categories identified serves to construct official meanings of ethnicity. As Bhopal (1997) observes, the variations in definitions employed make cross-national and intercountry comparisons difficult.

Descriptive studies

Social action theory underlies much of the early qualitative research carried out with ethnic minority groups. Research studies have described the cultural beliefs, experiences, and lifestyles of individuals and groups from ethnic minorities now established in the United Kingdom. To take a few examples, Homans (1983) studied food choice among young pregnant Asian women living in Britain, exploring amongst other issues notions of 'hot' and 'cold' foods. Work by other female researchers identified aspects of South Asian life that had previously remained hidden. This includes research by Currer (1986) and by Fenton and Sadik-Sangster (1996) on mental health concerns of women of South Asian origin. These studies highlighted the culturally specific nature of diagnoses and challenged psychological research, which suggested (using psychological tests) that the rates of psychological distress and psychiatric admissions were lower for those of South Asian origin compared with the white population. More recently, Bradby (1997) carried out research with young South Asian women in Glasgow to investigate their understanding about diet and foods, prompted by concerns about the role of diet in the higher incidence of coronary heart disease among South Asians. Bradby spent time during the research period visiting and informally talking to her respondents as well as carrying out formal interviews. Her research demonstrates the value of a qualitative approach in exploring strongly held cultural beliefs. Bradby proposed that there was a conceptual division in her sample's perception of food groups, between what was seen as 'our foods' (a systemic or Ayurvedic model of food which is based on assessing the merit of different foods in terms of an equilibrium), and 'their foods' (the Western-based model which breaks foods down into their components such as proteins, vitamins, and so on) and which judges the value of foods on this basis. Bradby argues that health promotion activities need to take into account cultural understanding of such beliefs to be effective in influencing behaviours and practices. Overall, the importance of these studies lies in their attempt to understand and respect different cultural groups and to explain behaviours previously hidden or misinterpreted. Researchers have tended, however, to underline the differences in culture rather than to explore the similarities.

The issue of racism within the health services is a very difficult area to research, for as Pearson (1989) notes, less favourable treatment 'is not demonstrated through hard outcome measures or performance indicators'. Observational data and interviews with midwives contributed to Bowler's (1993) analysis of the stereotyping of Asian women attending for maternity care in a United Kingdom hospital. Midwives comments in interviews, but as importantly as revealed through observational work, reflected their views that Asian women lacked communication skills and were not 'compliant' in attending for care. Their behaviour in hospital (for example in labour) was also interpreted as being antisocial. The negative stereotypes that became attached to Asian women indicated a lack of understanding of cultural variation and resulted in women receiving less helpful care.

Quantitative approaches

A second strand of research has employed quantitative techniques and has been underpinned by a structuralist approach, although it is difficult to trace the precise theoretical origins of some work. In the 1980s and early 1990s there were a number of localized small-scale studies focusing upon the uptake of certain services, such as the maternity services, mental health services, and the relationship between maternal and child health (Smaje 1995). Findings from these studies were difficult to combine to gain a wider overview of ethnic health, since projects varied in their definitions of ethnicity and in the groups researched (or ignored), and offered little in the way of explanations for perceived variations.

Several larger-scale epidemiological surveys provide a broad overview of ethnic minority health. Marmot *et al.* (1984) reviewed the mortality of ethnic minorities compared with that of the white population in the Immigrant Mortality Study of the Office of Population Census and Study (**OPCS**), and Balarajan and Bulusu (1990) provided an analysis of mortality as part of the OPCS Mortality and Geography study among foreign-born residents of England and Wales, 1979 to 1983. Both studies were methodologically flawed (Smaje 1995) but have been seen as useful contributions to the dialogue about the health status of ethnic groups. A more complex picture of morbidity emerged from Nazroo's (1997) national survey of the ethnic minorities (5196 respondents) with a comparison sample of the white population (2867 respondents). This study demonstrated considerable ill health among ethnic minority men and women. One-third reported 'fair or poor' health, a fifth reported a long-standing illness, and one-sixth reported that their performance of moderately exerting activities was curtailed by poor health. Overall, Pakistanis and Bangladeshis had the worst reported health, and these groups also reported the highest rates of heart disease. In this study health status was investigated both for differences and similarities between ethnic groups, with the author noting that the Chinese, Indian, and African-Asians experienced better health than other minority groups. Furthermore, Nazroo highlighted the important contribution of socio-economic status as a predictor of health. This and other work (Amin and Oppenheim 1992; Jones 1992) challenges the accepted link between ethnicity and poor health status by emphasizing the significance of the intervening variable of low socio-economic status. Many ethnic minorities live in considerable poverty for a number of reasons, including difficulty of gaining higher-grade employment, poor working conditions, and poorer-grade housing in both the private and local authority markets. However, some studies have failed to include any measures that might pick up deprivation status, instead accounting for poor health solely by the variable 'ethnicity'.

Certain key messages emerge for any social or biomedical researcher. The complexities of research on ethnic minority groups in the United Kingdom are beginning to be understood and it now seems that much of the earlier work, particularly in the quantitative tradition, was simplistic and naive. More recent research and debate, often by sociologists, have suggested that there is a large research agenda still to be tackled. Douglas (1998), for example, has argued that interest in the United Kingdom has focused mainly on the largest of the groups, those of South Asian origin, often to the neglect of other minorities, for example, the Chinese and Vietnamese, African-Caribbean, and other smaller groups (including refugees). Research has also focused upon selected issues, for example, heart disease, 'Asian rickets', and the haemoglobinopathies, and ignored other conditions such as cancer.

It has also been argued, with powerful examples supporting the thesis, that the study of ethnic health is incomplete unless comparisons are drawn between 'ethnic' health status and that of the white population (Bhopal 1997; Nazroo 1997). Previously, many studies simply reported on the health of a specific ethnic group with no attempt to compare the findings with those for white groups whose health status may be similar, worse, or better. Furthermore, it is important to draw out similarities between the health of white and ethnic minority groups since these are as revealing as the differences. It has also been noted that when comparisons are made with the white population the assumption is always that the white population formed the 'norm' against which other ethnic groups should be compared. Moreover, the assumption of homogeneity within a single ethnic group has been shown to be misleading with differences associated with varying socio-economic circumstances, length of migration, and intergenerational changes, whilst the heterogeneity of the white population has also seldom been researched.

Finally, a research agenda for those adopting a qualitative approach to work in this field relates to questions concerning the quality of health care experienced by ethnic minority men and women, as well as how major common conditions are perceived, acted upon, and managed within ethnic minority families. More broadly, studies of social networks and of family life of ethnic minority groups would contribute considerably to the understanding of ethnic minority determinants of health.

Professional perspectives

Sociological work on health professionals dates back many years, when a rather academic debate existed about the structure and role of 'professions'. Early analyses were shaped by functionalist theories, later becoming replaced by a number of 'structuralist' critiques. These were generally directly towards all professions in a discussion of 'professionalism', a device by which certain groups achieve control over occupational standing and expertise in society. More specifically, sociologists directed their attention to analysing the medical profession which held a high and, some would argue, overvalued position in society (Freidson 1970; Johnson 1972; Illich 1977). Central issues in this literature included an examination of how medicine maintained its status and autonomy in society and its dominance over other professions, such as nursing (Freidson 1970). As Annandale (1998) observed, Freidson's writing 'captured the collective imagination of a generation of sociologists'. However, not all agreed with Freidson's analysis, and McKinlay and Stoeckle (1988) took the controversial view that today doctors sell their labour power on the market in the same way as any other worker. However, the general tenor of this debate was not to see members of the medical profession as members of the proletariat, but rather as a group that had until recently managed to maintain considerable power in society, manifest in their degree of self-governance. Studies published in the form of monographs described aspects of the self-monitoring process by the members of the medical profession, including Atkinson's (1981) study of medical education and Bosk's (1981) study of the management of medical errors.

The extent to which political developments have more recently curtailed medical power is an interesting question, and one that brings out the relevance of what may originally have been seen to be an intellectual exercise. Freidson (1994) himself acknowledges the challenges to the profession but feels that medicine is still attempting to police itself. In the United Kingdom this occurs through the General Medical Council, although recent 'scandals' relating to professional practice have resulted in questions about the effective fulfilment of this role, and in future there is likely to be considerably more public scrutiny of the medical profession.

Most importantly, in the United Kingdom over the last decades there has developed within the National Health Service (**NHS**) a new culture in which managerialism, rather than professionalism, is the dominant discourse. The rise of general management within the NHS and the construction of a series of institutions of clinical governance (for example, the National Institute for Clinical Excellence) have curtailed the autonomy of the medical profession. Social scientists continue to chart the changes over the past decade and have noted that the claim of the medical profession to rely upon 'clinical judgement' as the basis for self-governance is threatened by evidence-based medicine which has 'achieved the status of official policy in the NHS' (Harrison and Pollitt 1995).

Health professionals—a social action perspective

Continued, and some would argue continual, change within the health services in the United Kingdom means that traditional hierarchies are no longer fixed, and health professionals are at times asked to play dual roles, such as clinician and manager (Owens and Petch 1995). These circumstances have led a number of sociologists to investigate—using a social action perspective—the manner in which health professionals negotiate their work, create and maintain professional boundaries, and respond to change. This approach, whilst overtly often fairly atheoretical, ultimately derives from seminal work carried out in the 1960s and 1970s by researchers interested in understanding how professional groups interacted within the organization of the hospital. For example, Strauss *et al.* (1963) studied, among other things, the 'negotiated order' of hospital life, looking behind what was taken for granted about professional work and the division of labour, while Mechanic (1962) wrote perceptively about the informal power of lower participants of organizations. Research on the health service now takes a similar approach, examining not the formal roles of health professionals but rather looking at what lies 'behind' the new policies and changing roles of health service staff. Examples relate to a wide range of topics, including the study of medical professionals involved in management roles (Harrison and Pollitt 1995; Wilcocks 1999), and issues of interprofessional collaboration and conflict (Owens *et al.* 1995).

Work on this topic is important, since constant reorganization within the health service is accompanied by shifting roles and occupational boundaries, and a social action approach allows the research to 'unpack' the social context in some detail. For example, in a study using a mix of quantitative and qualitative methods, Fenwick *et al.* (1998) were able to uncover concerns held by the study general practitioners over new midwife-led schemes introduced into the community as a result of the policy document *Changing Childbirth* (Department of Health 1993). Many of the general practitioners questioned reported that they saw their pregnant patients fewer times during the pregnancy, and the majority were concerned that the midwives were not offering an informed choice to the women or were even dissuading them from visiting their general practitioner. Interviews with a sample of the practitioners also revealed the importance that they attached to their maternity work. The study suggests, as others have done (Cheyne *et al.* 1995), that changes in the organization of health services may often be accompanied by a redrawing of professional boundaries and tasks. The ensuing difficulties and conflicts may well inhibit the overall success of these high-level policy changes and deserve to be studied in considerable detail as a guide to successful policy changes in the future.

Professional views of official policy also provide another area where the social action approach has been applied. Challenging the view that the application of policies is a non-problematic exercise, the sociologist attempts to understand what these policies mean to professionals by asking such questions as, 'What do they understand by the policy?', 'Do they agree with it?', and 'How may it affect work routines?' In a study of maternity hospital policy, Beeken and Waterston (1992) investigated the attitudes of hospital and community midwives and health visitors towards breast feeding in a Newcastle hospital by sending the staff a postal questionnaire (92 per cent responded). Although the majority of staff reported that hospital policies were intended to facilitate breast feeding (for example through rooming-in) the researchers found that some nurses reported opinions about breast feeding which were at variance with hospital policy. For example, 47 per cent disagreed or strongly disagreed with the statement that 'Milk company advertising should be banned in the antenatal clinic' and over a quarter disagreed with the statement that 'Healthy babies are breast-fed babies'.

Other examples that strikingly demonstrate the gulf between official policy and the views of the rank and file workers include Williams and Calnan's (1994) study of general practitioners' views about health promotion surrounding coronary heart disease. In face-to-face interviews the general practitioners reported considerable ambivalence towards the efficacy of behavioural choice, noting also time constraints in carrying out health promotion activities and the difficulties of identifying individuals at risk. They also reported that whilst they recognized that prevention was important they found health promotion 'tedious, dull, and boring', and had little time or interest to attend to this aspect of their work.

Relatively little research has examined the agency of professionals and the ways in which they may attempt to maintain control within their working situation, and this is an area that would benefit from greater study. More generally, considerable attention has been paid to the consumer as a recipient of health care, as a respondent in the research process, and as a patient whose views are increasingly worthy of attention, but the voice of health professionals is less heard. Health professionals are key players in health service research (for example, in randomized controlled trials, health promotion campaigns); they are routinely expected to help recruit patients, implement interventions, and facilitate and interpret such research. However, ways in which the research may have an impact on their workload or the intervention may affect their working practices is little explored, and very little research has examined the complexities of the work situation of professionals and the uncertainties associated with their redefined roles.

Future directions

Medical sociology has traditionally worked closely with public health and clinical specialists, and this is likely to continue, with such issues as the social causes and distribution of disease, the organization and provision of medical care, and the development and implementation of preventive programmes, all having important social aspects and dimensions. The contributions of sociology to these areas arises both from its techniques of enquiry (particularly the application of qualitative methods), and its body of knowledge concerning the nature and influences of social factors and processes which operate both at a micro-level and in terms of broader social structures. However, it is increasingly difficult to determine precise disciplinary boundaries, as sociology, psychology, and public health medicine each draw on concepts and explanations developed in the other disciplines in addressing public health issues, and over time these become part of the accepted wisdom in the field. For example, the sociological distinction between disease and patients' experience of illness is now commonplace and subjective health status measures are employed routinely in assessing the outcome of medical care. Similarly, effective health education is also accepted to require not merely the provision of health advice but also to address people's personal beliefs and take account of the situation and context of their lives. More generally, whereas qualitative methods were traditionally largely confined to sociologists and anthropologists, they are increasingly employed by public health doctors and other medical specialists to investigate the perceptions and experiences of patients and health professionals.

Areas of specialization are influenced by prevailing concerns in the health field and priorities for research funding, and therefore vary over time and between countries. However, current trends suggest that in the United Kingdom issues of social inequalities in health, in terms not only of socio-economic position but also the effects of ethnicity and gender, will form important foci of research and collaboration between sociologists and public health doctors, as will issues of community priorities and rationing, and assessments of the quality and acceptability of health care. In addition, assessment of the quality of qualitative research and requirements for synthesizing qualitative studies and producing systematic reviews are likely to receive increased attention.

Medical sociology has traditionally had an applied focus (especially in the United Kingdom) and this is likely to continue. However, increasingly this subfield is also characterized by greater emphasis on theoretical concerns and developments. Indeed, Turner (1992) suggests that the sociology of health and illness has the potential to 'become the leading edge of contemporary sociological theory'. This is because the body, which is central to health and illness, is forming an important dimension of sociological debates and raises in acute form issues of the relationship between body and mind, culture and nature, and self and society. Such developments in the theoretical basis of the discipline will provide new insights and concepts that may later be applied to questions posed by clinicians, public health specialists, and policy makers. Thus future work in sociology in medicine is likely to be strengthened by developments both in theory and method.

Psychological investigations

Throughout its history of over a century the discipline of psychology has included health issues within its ambit of research and practice.

Not surprisingly, most attention has been paid to mental health. The present chapter, however, focuses on psychology's contributions to the realm of physical health, illness, and disease. Prior to the 1960s, the most notable contribution of psychologists to public health investigations was the development of psychosomatic theories of disease. In the 1960s psychological variables and measures began to appear in large-scale epidemiological studies. For example, at this time the prospective Framingham Heart Study included assessment of type A behaviour (excessive aggression, ambition, competitiveness, and time urgency), and subsequently showed that the attribute significantly increased the risk of coronary heart disease in men and women (Haynes *et al.* 1980). This type of research became known as behavioural or psychosocial epidemiology, explicitly recognizing psychological contributions to the broad epidemiological picture and to public health issues (Kaplan *et al.* 1990).

The following decade saw the emergence of the fields known as behavioural medicine, behavioural health, and health psychology (Matarazzo 1980). Definitions of the first two vary, but broadly refer respectively to the integrated contributions of the behavioural and biomedical sciences to the diagnosis, treatment, and rehabilitation of the sick, and to the maintenance of health and prevention of sickness in the healthy. Within this multidisciplinary framework, health psychology has been defined conventionally as the

> educational, scientific and professional contributions of the discipline of psychology to the promotion and maintenance of health, the prevention and treatment of illness, the identification of etiologic and diagnostic correlates of health, illness, and related dysfunction, and the improvement of the health care system and health policy formation. (Matarazzo 1980)

In the last 20 years behavioural medicine, behavioural health, and especially health psychology have developed at an extraordinary pace. Professional societies, research institutes, specialist journals, textbooks, training courses, conferences, and positions in universities and health agencies have proliferated in many countries (Jansen and Weinman 1991). In Europe alone the development of health psychology has recently prompted a Health Psychology 2000 report by a special Task Force of the European Federation of Professional Psychologists' Associations (Marks *et al.* 1998). Not surprisingly health psychologists have so far focused their attentions mainly on the health problems of developed countries, conducting extensive research on chronic diseases such as coronary heart disease and cancer, and on risk factors such as a high-fat diet and a sedentary lifestyle. However, some interest is now emerging among health psychologists into the health issues faced by developing countries such as malnutrition and family planning (Aboud 1998).

The extreme diversity and proliferation of psychologists' contributions to investigations of health in recent times means that this chapter can only provide a broad outline of their methodological approaches, and a few selected examples of substantive findings. The next section outlines the characteristic ways in which psychologists formulate theory about health phenomena. Following this, some of their distinctive approaches to research design, measurement, and statistical analysis are discussed.

Psychological theory

Authors of texts in health psychology and behavioural medicine conventionally characterize their fields as theoretically located in the 'biopsychosocial model' (Schneiderman and Tapp 1985; Taylor 1995). The model, which is attributed to Engel (1977), envisages health and illness as the product of the complex interactions of biological, psychological, and social processes. It is usually contrasted with the biomedical model, which is seen as reductionistic and focused on illness and disease rather than health. The term 'biopsychosocial' is regarded not just as a shorthand way of signalling the need to take account of three different types of variables, but more importantly as a reminder that such variables are to be seen as comprising systems. From this perspective, explanations and interventions need to be conceptualized at the system level of the individual and of the social systems in which he or she is embedded rather than at the level of the variable. For example, a biopsychosocial account of healthy dietary practices cannot be reduced to nutritional components, but must incorporate relevant cognitive, emotional and behavioural attributes of the individual, and the social and cultural forces that shape them. This would be a commonplace observation to a medical anthropologist or sociologist, but is a much-needed reminder to psychologists who, by virtue of their disciplinary focus, tend towards individualistic if not reductionistic explanations.

The biopsychosocial model has been promoted by health psychology and behavioural medicine, with until recently surprisingly little critical reflection. McLaren (1998) has suggested that the biopsychosocial model is not a model at all, and provides no real theoretical force or constraint. Even those who believe that the biopsychosocial model has something to offer as a general guide question whether psychologists are actually heeding its messages. Thus concerns have been raised that in practice psychologists in the health field continue to study variables rather than systems, decontextualizing and fragmenting individuals, and then trying to reassemble them with statistical analysis (Spicer and Chamberlain 1996; Ogden 1997; Spicer 1997). A more radical response has been to reject the biopsychosocial model, on the grounds that any natural systems approach based on quantitative analysis of variables cannot capture the meanings and contexts of health-related experience. Instead, qualitative paradigms and methods are needed to interpret the discourses and narratives of people's health worlds (Murray and Chamberlain 1998, 1999).

Perhaps not surprisingly in a new and rapidly growing area, the theoretical foundations of health psychology and behavioural medicine have yet to settle. The biopsychosocial model has at least served a useful rhetorical function in helping psychologists establish an identity in the health arena. But the serious questions as to its theoretical and methodological implications, and its ideological relationship with the biomedical model, are only beginning to be addressed. Given the extreme diversity of the issues embraced by health psychology and behavioural medicine, it seems unlikely that a single foundation will be found. More likely a variety of theories and methods will be adopted depending on the question at hand, though the vexed question of amalgamating findings from disparate approaches remains (Buchanan 1992).

Despite creaking foundations, there is no shortage of theories in health psychology which address public health concerns. Two examples of influential theories will give the flavour of psychological theorizing in this area: the health belief model and the transactional theory of stress and coping. Health behaviours are seen as any actions taken to prevent or detect disease or to improve well being (Conner and Norman 1996). As such, they encompass such activities as dietary control, physical exercise, visiting health professionals, and adhering to prescribed medications. The predominant strategy for attempting to uncover the determinants of health behaviours in psychology has been to devise so-called social cognition models. These theoretical models assume that the most important determinants of social behaviours such as those concerning health are to be found in people's cognitions: their rational cost–benefit analyses of whether or not to engage in the behaviour. One of the earliest and most influential social cognitive models was the health belief model (Becker 1974; Sheeran and Abraham 1996). This envisages the decision to engage in smoking, for example, as a function of the individual's perceived susceptibility to and the severity of the health consequences of smoking, as well as the perceived benefits and barriers relating to the behaviour. The model also includes general motivations concerning health, triggers to action, and background demographic, personality, and social factors, but the cognitive variables are seen as the key determinants. As Conner and Norman (1998) note in a helpful review of the health belief model and other social cognitive models, the model has been tested on a diverse range of health behaviours including smoking, alcohol use, dietary practices, exercise, health screening activities, contraceptive use, compliance with medical regimens, and visits to health professionals. Meta-analyses of these studies suggest that many health behaviours can be consistently predicted by each of the health belief model cognitions, most successfully with perceived barriers, followed by susceptibility, benefits, and severity. No single component of the model, however, predicts more than 4 per cent of variance in health behaviour so, even when considered overall, the health belief model provides a limited capacity for predicting health behaviours.

The partial success of the health belief model is not surprising given its limitations. The broad limitations, discussed by Conner and Norman (1998), are worth noting here because they are often voiced as criticisms of theories in health psychology generally. A first limitation is the small set of constructs included in the model. Conner and Norman (1998) highlight in particular the absence of personal control and perceived social pressure as important determinants of health behaviours. More generally, the concern is often expressed that psychological theories of health are too circumscribed. To be comprehensible and testable, theories have to be selective, but not to the extent of omitting important constructs. A second limitation is the lack of a theoretical account that explains how the cognitions are connected with each other and with behaviour. Without such an explanation, the model is little more than a list of constructs, which provides a weak basis for interventions. The third limitation is the variety of ways in which investigators have measured the health belief model cognitions—a latitude which can be partially explained by the lack of theory clearly specifying the constructs and their relationships. This loose linkage between constructs and measures is a concern which frequently surfaces in health psychology. Finally, the health belief model and many other theories in health psychology have been criticized for their failure to capture process. Giving up smoking, for example, is clearly a multistage process involving reflection, planning, execution, and maintenance. Cognitions are undoubtedly relevant at each stage and across each transition, but determining which and when particular cognitions are important requires a theory which goes beyond the static simplicity of the health belief model. Some other theories of health behaviour that avoid some of these limitations are discussed in the applications section below.

A very different approach to theorizing in health psychology can be found in Lazarus's theory of stress and coping (Lazarus and Folkman 1984), though it did not originate in this field. The concept of stress has loomed large in the health arena for many years, and Lazarus's psychological theory has provided one of the most sophisticated and influential explanatory accounts. The theory is transactional in the sense that it attempts to characterize the continual transactions between person and environment, focusing on those defined as stressful. Interpretations of events and situations are given a central role in the model via the concept of appraisal. Primary appraisal refers to the person's evaluation of whether they are confronting a demand on their resources and, if so, whether the demand constitutes a threat of harm, loss, or challenge. Secondary appraisal refers to a person's evaluation of their ability to cope with the demand using personal or environmental resources. Coping strategies are the actual steps taken by the individual to deal with the demand and, in Lazarus's scheme, are categorized into problem-focused and emotion-focused strategies. The former address the problem itself, while the latter deal with the emotions generated by the problem. These categories are further subdivided into eight specific strategies or 'ways of coping' such as confrontive coping, distancing, self-control, and seeking social support. Stressful experiences are those where demands on resources are not met, either in prospect or following ineffective attempts at coping.

The complexity and sophistication of Lazarus's theory emerge in two ways. Firstly, the demand–primary appraisal–secondary appraisal–coping–outcome dynamic is not a simple linear sequence. These processes interweave and involve transformations such as reappraisals and anticipatory coping manoeuvres. Secondly, the ways in which these dynamics unfold depend on a range of idiosyncratic factors such as personality attributes (including available and preferred ways of coping), beliefs, and commitments concerning the situation, personal skills and capabilities, and the availability of environmental resources and constraints. In more recent discussions, Lazarus (1991) has elaborated the theory still further, most notably highlighting the key role of emotions. Such a brief description does scant justice to this theory, but at least its complexity should be apparent.

Lazarus's theory has generated enormous debate and has informed extensive research in the health field (Bartlett 1998). However, it is striking that virtually none of this research constitutes a test of the theory as such. Instead, investigators continue to choose particular variables (appraisals of life events, particular coping strategies such as denial, stress-prone personality traits such as type A behaviour, or social support) and attempt to link them individually to health and disease states. In so doing, they lose the transactional force of the theory as well as many of its other strengths.

Lazarus (1990) has called for more longitudinal research to expose the links between stress, coping, and health. But, as Bartlett (1998) argues, the problems of testing the theory run much deeper. The psychological methods needed to capture the dynamic complexities of this or any similar theory have yet to be developed. Ironically the research designs and particular methods used by most health psychologists are best suited to testing the type of theories of which they are most critical—piecemeal static models of limited scope. From one perspective this is deeply problematic, but the tension between theory and method can also be seen as a force which will drive the development of both.

Psychological methods

Most of the methodological strategies adopted by psychologists working in public health research are not distinctive to their discipline. The use of cross-sectional and prospective surveys, programme evaluations, randomized control trials, probability sampling strategies, interviews and questionnaires, and statistical analysis is common to a variety of researchers in public health. In fact, this sharing of methods across disciplines is increasing as public health researchers attempt to incorporate elusive psychological and social phenomena such as stress, lifestyle, and quality of life (Daly *et al.* 1997). Within health psychology, the growing interest in qualitative methods noted above is producing a convergence of approaches with those developed by sociologists and anthropologists (Murray and Chamberlain 1999).

This extensive sharing of methods makes it unnecessary and inappropriate to repeat discussions contained in this and other chapters. Instead, this section highlights and illustrates some methodological strategies that are particularly characteristic of psychologists' investigations of health. These encompass using laboratory experiments to test causal hypotheses about health-related behaviour, enhancing the quality of psychological measurement, and using multivariate statistical techniques, especially those designed to test complex causal models of health determinants and consequences.

Laboratory experiments

Since its inception in the late nineteenth century, psychology has made extensive use of laboratory experiments to evaluate causal hypotheses about behaviour and mental life. The logic of experimentation is the same as that for randomized controlled trials, but the laboratory setting permits greater control of extraneous variables. In essence, an independent variable is manipulated under controlled conditions to test whether a dependent variable varies in a way consistent with a causal hypothesis. Control strategies are primarily aimed at preventing the operation of confounding variables. These mask the true relationship between the independent and dependent variables by virtue of their relationships with both. Confounds may be controlled by holding them constant or by the use of some balancing strategy such as matching or random allocation of participants to experimental conditions. Such control strategies help to ensure that the effects of any manipulations of the independent variable are not confounded with variations in experimental procedure, or with differences in individual characteristics such as age, personality, and experience. Experimental designs can become very complex according to the number of independent and dependent variables, and the ways in which participants are exposed to experimental conditions (Keppel 1991; Kirk 1995). However, the fundamental logic of manipulation and control remains throughout.

An example from the cardiovascular disease literature shows these ideas in action. The reactivity hypothesis suggests that risk of coronary heart disease and hypertension may be increased in people who consistently over-react physiologically to psychological stress (Turner 1994). Many experimental studies have tried to elucidate the nature of the stressors that might elicit reactivity and the characteristics of reactors. In one such study (Brown and Smith 1992) husband and wife couples were randomly allocated to one of two laboratory tasks: a general discussion or a competitive argument in which the 'winner' received the chance of a monetary reward. During these activities blood pressure, hostile behaviours, and anger experiences were recorded in a standardized form. Results showed that during the argument, but not the discussion, husbands exhibited notable increases in blood pressure and anger, whereas wives did not. It was concluded that striving for interpersonal control may induce blood-pressure reactivity, but that this process is moderated by spouse status. The authors then discussed the implications of the results for psychological interventions to reduce reactivity and disease risk.

Since the laboratory experiment is generally seen as a powerful way to demonstrate causal processes, it is tempting to accept results and interpretations uncritically, especially when the design and analyses are complex. However, the application of the strategies of manipulation and control to human experience raises many questions and difficulties, both technical and ethical. There is a considerable literature on the subtle ways in which experimenters and participants can unwittingly introduce biases that can confound results (Rosenthal 1994). Even when these are controlled, the question remains as to whether all participants construe their experiences in the same way and in the way intended by the experimenter (Harré 1993). Even more fundamental is the 'identity problem': the question of whether complex psychological processes such as interpersonal control can be induced or simulated in a laboratory in ways which retain their meanings in everyday life (Greenwood 1989). Without some reassurance as to the ecological validity of psychological laboratory results, implications for the understanding and enhancement of health cannot be legitimately drawn. Despite the many challenges, psychological laboratory investigations have an important role to play in elucidating psychological aspects of health, especially when the results are incorporated with those from other research strategies. In the case of the reactivity hypothesis, for example, the importance of psychological control is becoming apparent from a range of epidemiological, ambulatory, and laboratory studies of blood-pressure reactivity (Steptoe 1998).

Enhancing the quality of psychological measurement

Psychologists make use of a wide range of measurement instruments to investigate public health concerns. Johnston and Johnston (1998) have recently provided a comprehensive overview of these measures, and other more detailed guides are also available (McDowell and Newell 1987; Bowling 1991, 1995; Cohen *et al.* 1995; Johnston *et al.* 1995). As Johnston and Johnston (1998) note, measurements are taken in a variety of modes: self-reports in interviews and questionnaires, observations of behaviour, physiological assessment, and health-care records. The attributes measured are extremely diverse and include appraisals of stressors, health, and illness, health-related behaviours such as exercise and adherence to medication, emotional precursors and consequences of illness, personality factors, coping strategies, communication processes between patients and health-care providers, and social resources.

Whatever the nature of the measuring instruments, their quality is assessed using well-established principles of psychometric theory (Nunnally and Bernstein 1994; Anastasi and Urbina 1997). These distinguish between various types of reliability (consistency) and validity (accuracy) and provide a statistical basis for assessing the quality of life measures. For example, the WHO Quality of Life Assessment Instrument-100 measures 24 facets of quality of life using four questionnaire items for each. A recent report on the reliability and validity of the WHO Quality of Life-100 (WHO Quality of Life Group 1998) provides correlational data which demonstrate the internal consistency or homogeneity of the 24 subscales. It also addresses the factorial validity of the 24 facet scores, showing that they cluster into four domains rather than the six which had been suggested initially. Discriminant validity of the items is demonstrated by their ability to distinguish between healthy and unhealthy respondents, and construct validity of the facets and domains is shown by the pattern of correlations between these scores and those on an overall quality of life subscale.

Distinguishing and assessing multiple types of reliability and validity can provide a comprehensive evaluation of measurement quality, but such information can be difficult to integrate for a particular measure. The multitrait–multimethod strategy (Campbell and Fiske 1959) has helped investigators to combine data on some types of validity. The problem of integrating reliability data, which may reflect measurement error due to different times of administration, different observers, or heterogeneous items, has also been addressed by Cronbach's generalizability theory (Cronbach *et al.* 1972; Shavelson *et al.* 1989). This allows the investigator to quantify different sources of error within one analytic framework, and then to estimate how the quality of the measuring instrument would be affected by manipulation of particular sources. Streiner and Norman (1995) provide a helpful and detailed introduction to this approach in a health context using the Objective Structured Clinical Examination as an example. Despite being available for some years in the psychological literature, neither the multitrait–multimethod technique nor generalizability theory have made much impact in public health research. They are demanding in terms of both study design and analysis. However, the gains they offer in developing and assessing effective measuring instruments are more than sufficient to warrant their wider use.

Enhancing the quality of psychological measurement can also be achieved by elucidating the psychological and social processes that occur during the measurement process. How well does the structure of a scale requiring a respondent to rate their intention to exercise mesh with their cognitive schemas? What are the best ways to recover memories of past events such as seeking medical care? Does the use of a standardized interview on health problems disrupt normal social processes and undermine the participant's ability to provide the interviewer with accurate information? These and similar questions have received increasing attention from psychologists and other social scientists in recent years (Hipler *et al.* 1987; Tanur 1991; Abraham and Hampson 1996).

Ostrom (1987), for example, raises the worrying concern that continuous rating scales do not map onto respondents' cognitive representations since, according to cognitive theory, the latter have an all-or-none categorical form. Accordingly, respondents are obliged to decompose the scale into categories which may be highly idiosyncratic. Thus, respondents' apparently simple and comparable ratings may hide individual cognitive processes that make the aggregation of ratings highly questionable. Turning to memory, Loftus *et al.* (1991) report a series of studies on patients' recall of visits to health professionals where they found that respondents systematically underestimated their total number of visits, but overestimated the frequency with which they had undergone a specific procedure. They use these findings to reflect on the relative merits of asking questions with different time frames, and of guiding respondents' recall backwards or forwards along a time line. As a final example, Suchman and Jordan (1991) provide an incisive exploration of the tensions between the interview seen as a standardized instrument of assessment and as a conversation, partly using data from the National Health Interview Survey in the United States. They explore the conventional proposition that the validity of interview data requires shared understandings among the researcher, the interviewer, and the interviewee. However, they argue that these shared meanings depend on the availability of conversational resources that 'routinely mediate uncertainties of relevance and interpretation' (Suchman and Jordan 1991). These resources are inevitably suppressed to some degree, they argue, by the scripted nature of the interview, and accordingly validity is threatened. Researchers are clearly aware of this problem in general, and make use of devices such as clarifying definitions and probes to ensure that the meanings of questions and responses are standardized. However, the concern remains that this approach is guided by an overly simple view of the social dynamics of interviews, especially their capacity for suppressing responses.

It should be stressed that cognitive and social research on the processes underlying psychological measurement in the health context has not progressed very far. Although there is no shortage of relevant theory and findings within cognitive and social psychology, research which explicitly brings them to bear on measurement issues is limited and has so far raised more questions than answers or clear recommendations. It seems reasonable to suggest that this type of research is a potentially important contribution that psychologists can make to the enhancement of measurement and thus to the overall quality of research in public health.

Multivariate statistical techniques

Multivariate statistical techniques play a central role in psychological research in all fields including health. A variety of excellent texts are available (Grimm and Yarnold 1995; Tabachnick and Fidell 1996), and psychologists contribute to the development of the techniques in journals such as *Psychological Methods* and the *Journal of Multivariate Analysis*. Techniques such as multiple and logistic regression, discriminant analysis, and log-linear analysis enable the estimation and testing of hypothesized effects while statistically holding constant any measured confounding variables. The particular technique selected depends partly on the assumptions that the analyst is prepared to make about their data, especially the level of measurement which has been achieved. Although statistical control of confounds is less effective than experimental control, it provides a powerful analytic tool when experimentation is impossible or inappropriate: a common situation in psychological analyses of health.

A notable development in this area is the increasing application of structural equation modelling using programs such as LISREL, AMOS, and EQS (Hayduk 1996; Tabachnick and Fidell 1996). Structural equation models are an extension of path analysis (Klem 1995), which is in turn an elaboration of regression analysis. They enable the analyst to estimate and test complex networks of relationships including causal chains, reciprocal relationships, and feedback loops. A particular model can be assessed using one powerful and efficient analysis, as opposed to the piecemeal decomposition of relationships required by earlier techniques. Furthermore, structural equation models allow the analyst to incorporate multiple measures (indicators) of any construct (latent variable), and to build estimates of measurement error into the analysis. Thus a structural equation model analysis is able to test simultaneously a causal model and a measurement model using extensions of regression and factor analysis. Again, this contrasts with traditional approaches which treat statistical evaluation of measures and of causal relationships as two separate steps.

Structural equation models are very useful for the evaluation of competing models since they provide helpful indices of fit between the theoretical model and the data. For example, Hall *et al.* (1998) used LISREL to compare two models that sought to explain why sicker patients report less satisfaction with their medical care. The simpler model envisaged the dissatisfaction to be directly attributable to patients' generalized negativity, while the more complex model hypothesized that the dissatisfaction effect was mediated by negative interactions with doctors. Health status and doctor–patient communication were assessed with multiple measures and satisfaction with a single measure in two samples. The analyses showed that generally the simple model provided a better fit to the data, though there was some slight evidence of mediation in one of the samples. This example illustrates the simultaneous analysis of a causal and measurement model, but structural equation models can also be used to analyse one or the other in isolation. The structural equation model analysis of a measurement model is known as confirmatory factor analysis. For example, in their evaluation of the WHO Quality of Life-100 described above, the WHO Quality of Life Group (1998) conducted a confirmatory factor analysis using the EQS program to test whether the facets clustered into one, four, or six domains. As noted above, the four-domain model provided the best fit to the data according to this structural equation model analysis.

The analysis of structural equation models can be daunting to the novice, though the availability of good introductory texts and the increasing friendliness of computer programs is helping to reduce this problem. Regardless of this, the technique will inevitably become widely used in public health research since multiple measures are often needed to capture the complexity of health-related phenomena, and theoretical accounts of their relationships are becoming increasingly complex. Complexity in the theoretical and measurement domains will have to be matched by a corresponding sophistication of statistical analysis.

Areas of psychological investigation

In the last 20 to 30 years, psychologists have applied their theories and methods to a wide range of problems in the public health arena. The contents of any standard text in health psychology (for example DiMatteo 1991; Taylor 1995) reveal investigations of the following:

- why people do or do not engage in healthy behaviours such as exercise and safe sex
- the psychological precursors and consequences of many diseases such as cardiovascular diseases, cancer, and diabetes
- patients' interpretation of physical symptoms
- patients' engagement with health professionals
- how patients cope with pain and chronic conditions
- the psychological problems faced by health professionals
- the psychological aspects of terminal illness and bereavement.

In turn these investigations increasingly inform primary, secondary, and tertiary interventions aimed at improving public health. This section provides discussion of just two examples of psychological investigations: psychological precursors of coronary heart disease and psychological determinants of condom usage. These illustrate psychological approaches to predicting disease and promoting health, respectively. They also exemplify different psychological foci: personality and the social environment in the former and cognitive processes in the latter. Conversely, the two examples have in common an extensive research base so that it is possible to discuss patterns of findings rather than isolated studies.

Psychological risk factors for coronary heart disease

The aetiology of coronary heart disease has been a major focus of attention for psychologists because of the disease's major impact on morbidity and mortality in developed countries, and the clear implication of antecedent behavioural factors. A comprehensive review of psychological risk factors for coronary heart disease was undertaken in the mid-1990s as part of a larger review of behavioural research in cardiovascular, lung, and blood health and disease by the National Heart, Lung, and Blood Institute Task Force (NHLBI Task Force 1998). The report distinguishes between lifestyle factors, such as smoking, exercise, and diet; individual characteristics such as personality and physiological reactivity to stress; and psychosocial variables such as socio-economic status, social support, and occupational stress. Since the role of lifestyle factors in cardiovascular diseases is discussed elsewhere (Chapter 9.1), this section illustrates psychological research with examples from the latter two categories.

Research on individual psychological characteristics and coronary heart disease has been dominated by the type A behaviour pattern: a profile of excessive competitiveness, sense of urgency, ambition, and hostility. There have been many accounts of the history of the type A behaviour pattern and its association with coronary heart disease (Strube 1991) which tend to highlight similar themes. The first is the complexity of the pattern originally described by the cardiologists Freidman and Rosenman in the 1960s (Freidman and Rosenman 1974), and the rapidity with which this was simplified by other investigators. Whereas the type A behaviour pattern was conceived as a complex pattern of person–environment interaction, it quickly became treated as a personality trait. This development was not unrelated to the proliferation of self-report measures of the pattern which were unable to evaluate the key behavioural components (for example, vocal mannerisms, posture, and conversational style) which Friedman and Rosenman assessed with their structured interview. As a result, analyses of the links between the type A behaviour pattern and coronary heart disease have been beset with problems of shifting definitions and of measures which are not highly correlated with each other.

A second theme is the changing pattern of results from epidemiological studies. Two major prospective studies in the 1970s—the Western Collaborative Study and the Framingham Study—reported that the type A behaviour pattern doubled the risk of coronary heart disease independently of established risk factors. However, major studies in the following decade, notably the Multiple Risk Factor Intervention Trial, failed to find any association between the type A behaviour pattern and coronary heart disease using various different measures of the pattern. Despite these mixed findings, meta-analyses have demonstrated a statistically reliable association (Booth-Kewley and Friedman 1987; Matthews 1988). Explanations for the variability in results include the use of different measures and study designs, the health and socio-economic status of the study populations, and the increasing prevalence of the pattern. It is also possible that the effect of the type A behaviour pattern may depend on the specific coronary heart disease endpoint. Spicer *et al.* (1996) and others have suggested, for example, that the type A behaviour pattern may increase the risk of non-fatal coronary events, but decrease the risk of fatal events.

Another possible explanation has led to the main theme in current research on coronary-prone behaviour. This is the proposal that only some components of the type A behaviour pattern confer coronary risk, and that the most potent of these is hostility. Research in this area has broadened beyond the type A behaviour pattern emphasis on hostile behaviour to include affective aspects such as anger, and cognitive aspects such as cynicism and mistrust of others. An impressive array of evidence now shows a consistent link between hostility, broadly defined, and coronary heart disease (Siegman and Smith 1994; Miller *et al.* 1996). This epidemiological linkage is given further credibility by evidence showing that hostility is reliably associated with variables which might mediate coronary risk such as smoking, lipid levels, poor social support, and physiological hyperreactivity (Siegman and Smith 1994). Hostility levels might also provide a partial explanation of the well-established inverse association between socio-economic status and risk of coronary heart disease.

Although research on type A behaviour pattern/hostility has dominated the study of coronary-prone behaviour, other psychological characteristics have also received attention. Booth-Kewley and Friedman's (1987) meta-analysis highlighted a strong association between depression and coronary risk. The National Heart, Lung, and Blood Institute Task Force report (NHLBI Task Force 1998) also gives prominence to depression as a coronary risk factor, noting further that it increases the risk of future coronary heart disease events in myocardial infarction patients, regardless of their severity status. Of related interest is a body of literature on 'vital exhaustion', which the report describes as a 'mental state characterized by unusual fatigue, a feeling of being dejected or defeated, and increased irritability'. This state is interesting, not only because of its demonstrated association with coronary risk, but also because of its resonances with the findings on depression and anger. Theoretical attempts to link type A behaviour, anger, and depression have been made (Price 1983), but the theory as a whole has received little empirical attention.

Psychological risk factors for coronary heart disease have also been sought in the environment. Two noteworthy examples of this type of research are investigations of job strain and poor social support. Job strain is generated by occupations that are highly demanding but offer little latitude for decision-making and control in general. Schnall *et al.* (1994) have reviewed studies on the association between job strain and coronary heart disease, and found supporting evidence. That said, the association is not always present, most notably in a more recent prospective study of patients undergoing diagnostic testing for coronary heart disease where job strain was not related to coronary heart disease prevalence or to subsequent morbidity or mortality (Hlatky *et al.* 1995).

An extensive literature has developed on the health effects of social isolation and poor social support (House *et al.* 1988). Isolation is evaluated in terms of the degree of social contact and the individual's experience via partners, friends, relatives, and organizations. In contrast, support refers to individuals' perceptions of what social resources they can call on when necessary. Many different sorts of support have been distinguished, such as material, emotional, and informational support, and a variety of support measures have been developed. The review by House *et al.* (1988) provides compelling evidence of a reliable association between poor social resources and health, especially between social isolation and all-cause mortality. More recently Shumaker and Czajkowski (1994) have brought together the evidence relating to poor social resources and cardiovascular disease and again documented consistent associations. The effects of social resources on health may be most obviously explained in terms of social influences on health-related behaviours such as diet, health checks, and adherence to medications. In addition, there is growing evidence to suggest that social resources may also benefit physiological functions such as blood pressure (Uchino *et al.* 1996).

The foregoing is no more than a limited sample of the enormous literature on psychological risk factors for coronary heart disease. Only a few major epidemiological topics have been highlighted, and hardly any mention has been made of the numerous experimental and animal studies aimed at elucidating risk mediation, or of the intervention literature. Nonetheless, even the limited research reviewed constitutes a substantial contribution. After their extremely comprehensive review, the National Heart, Lung, and Blood Institute Task Force prefaced its 1998 report with the conclusions:

> Behavioral research has contributed significantly to the understanding of disease risk and the progression and clinical manifestations of disease. Effective modification of individuals' behavior and/or psychosocial environments can potentially reduce disease risk, ameliorate the burdens of illness, and promote recovery and rehabilitation. (NHLBI Task Force 1998)

Psychological determinants of condom usage

An earlier section introduced the theme of health behaviours and the use of social cognitive models to uncover their psychological determinants. This section provides a brief account of two models that have superseded the health belief model discussed above, an account which draws in particular on the reviews of Conner and Norman (1996, 1998). More specifically, it summarizes some results from research that have applied these models to the problem of condom usage. This particular health behaviour is important in the context of both unwanted pregnancy and sexually transmitted diseases such as HIV. As Conner and Norman (1998) note, condom usage is still worryingly low despite extensive public health messages. For example, they cite figures from the General Household Surveys in the United Kingdom indicating that usage among 16- to 24-year-olds increased from 6 per cent in 1983 to only 12 per cent in 1991.

One of the most influential social cognitive models is the theory of planned behaviour (Ajzen 1991), which has been applied to a wide range of behaviours inside and outside the health field. According to the theory, a behaviour such as using a condom is most directly determined by how strongly the individual intends to carry out the behaviour, and by the degree to which they perceive the act as within their control. Intentions themselves are influenced not only by perceived control, but also by attitudes and so-called 'subjective norms'. In this context, attitudes refer to what the person believes about the outcomes of using a condom in conjunction with the value they attach to those outcomes. Subjective norms refer to the person's beliefs about whether significant others would prefer him or her to engage in the behaviour, and the strength of the person's motive to comply with this preference. Other more indirect behavioural determinants are also proposed, but the key factors are attitudes, subjective norms, and perceived control, which mainly influence behaviour via intentions. According to this model, people's decision to use a condom is thus strongly determined by their motives, beliefs, and evaluations with respect to their capacity to act, the outcomes of their action, and the views of salient others.

Another social cognitive model of interest is derived from protection motivation theory (Rogers 1983). This envisages the decision to use a condom as immediately determined by the person's motivation to protect his or her health, which is influenced by appraisals of both the threats and rewards associated with not engaging in the behaviour, and the issues surrounding the actual performance of the behaviour. As Conner and Norman (1998) note, these appraisals are conceptually similar to Lazarus's notions of primary and secondary appraisal that were discussed in the earlier section on theory. Of particular interest in the latter set of appraisals is the notion of efficacy. This encompasses response efficacy, the sense that a behaviour will be effective in protecting health, and self-efficacy, the belief that the person is capable of carrying out the behaviour. People's beliefs about efficacy seem to play a critical role in determining their health behaviours. Conner and Norman (1998) show how the construct plays a key role in a variety of social cognitive models including protection motivation theory, and review evidence from correlational and intervention studies which support its importance.

Turning to the evidence on relationships between social cognitions and condom usage, Sheeran *et al.* (1999) have recently published a meta-analysis of 121 studies that have used social cognitive models, notably those summarized above, or at least elements of them. These studies are of heterosexuals from a variety of countries, just over a third of whom are university students. The analysis provides average correlations (weighted by sample size) between social cognitive model elements and condom usage. Interestingly, there appeared to be few differences between the pattern of correlations found in cross-sectional studies and in prospective designs. Since the latter studies, although only 15 per cent of the total, provide the most rigorous test of social cognitive model hypotheses, the following figures are taken from this subset. As the theory of planned behaviour suggests, the most powerful correlate is the intention to use a condom as indexed by an average correlation of 0.46. This is particularly striking when compared with the correlation of 0.39 for previous use. It is a truism that past behaviour tends to be a strong predictor of its recurrence, but intention appears to be a stronger determinant. The next-strongest correlations were for attitudes towards condoms and so-called descriptive norms (beliefs about the views and behaviours of others regarding condom use): $r = 0.33$ in both cases. Self-efficacy is then correlated 0.24 with usage, at about the same level as age (–0.23).

There are other statistically significant though weak correlations between cognitive factors and condom usage. The correlations presented here are sufficient, however, to support the effectiveness of the social cognitive model approach. It is worth highlighting that in the full analysis the effects of intentions, attitudes, norms, and self-efficacy are notably stronger than those of knowledge about the risks of not using condoms, or of gender or socio-economic status. This evidential emphasis on attitudes, motives, and beliefs has clear implications for health-promotion programmes and especially the need to move beyond the provision of information (Bennett and Murphy 1997).

Future directions

In the words of the Health Psychology 2000 report (Marks *et al.* 1998): 'The mission of professional health psychology is to promote and maintain wellbeing through the application of psychological theory, methods and research, taking into account the economic, political, social, and cultural context'. As with most mission statements, it is hard to disagree with such lofty and desirable ambitions. In the context of public health, psychologists encounter various enablements and constraints in trying to achieve this mission. Returning to the biopsychosocial model, psychologists are well placed to play various 'bridging' roles across the three levels of analysis. Their social psychological accounts of attitudes and decision-making in individuals are needed to inform population-level interventions aimed at enhancing health. Psychophysiology, which has a long history in psychology, helps to explain how individual behaviour can result in disease processes. Furthermore, psychological analyses are also needed to help to explain the impact of social forces on biological processes. In attempting to work within this biopsychosocial perspective, psychologists have a wide range of theories and methods to draw on, as exemplified in this chapter. Moreover, since they are interested in behaviour and behaviour change, they are used to seeking effective explanations and interventions.

The main constraints that psychologists face in developing their contributions to public health are implied by the phrase above 'taking into account the economic, political, social and cultural context'. Most health psychologists are not trained or used to thinking in these terms. Some progress may be made by extending the training of health psychologists into other disciplines and by their participation in multidisciplinary teams (Marks *et al.* 1998). But 'taking into account' ultimately requires theoretical work that spans the multiple levels of analysis found in the public health domain. So, although psychologists have the potential to help build the bridges described above, they face the major theoretical challenge of locating their explanations of individual behaviour in its multiple contexts. An increasing number of psychologists, notably qualitative researchers, are engaging with this fundamental problem, and reflecting on their ideological role in the health arena (Murray and Chamberlain 1999). In their short history health psychology and behavioural medicine have already made extensive contributions to public health. This will no doubt continue, but the potential for even more fundamental contributions remains to be developed.

References

Abberley, P. (1992). Counting us out: a discussion of the OPCS disability surveys. *Disability, Handicap and Society*, **7**, 139–55.

Aboud, F.E. (1998). *Health psychology in global perspective*. Sage, Thousand Oaks, CA.

Abraham, C.S. and Hampson, S.E. (1996). Special issue on controversy and method in the interpretation of verbal reports in health psychology research. *Psychology and Health*, **11**.

Ajzen, I. (1991). The theory of planned behaviour. *Organizational Behaviour and Human Decision Processes*, **50**, 179–211.

Albrecht, G.L. and Devlieger, P.J. (1999). The disability paradox: high quality life against all odds. *Social Science and Medicine*, **48**, 977–88.

Alderson, P. (1998) The importance of theories in health care. *British Medical Journal*, **317**, 1007–10.

Amin, K. and Oppenheim, C. (1992). *Poverty in black and white*. Child Poverty Action Group/Runnymede Trust, London.

Anastasi, A. and Urbina, S. (1997). *Psychological testing* (7th edn). Prentice-Hall, Englewood Cliffs, NJ.

Annandale, E. (1998). *The sociology of health and medicine: a critical introduction*. Polity Press, Cambridge.

Arber, S. (1993). *Designing samples*. In *Researching social life* (ed. N. Gilbert). Sage, London.

Ashton, J. and Seymour, H. (1988). *The new public health*. Open University Press, Buckingham.

Atkinson, P. (1981). *The clinical experience. The construction and reconstruction of medical reality*. Gower, London.

Balarajan, R. and Bulusu, L. (1990). Mortality among immigrants in England and Wales 1979–1983. In *Mortality and geography: a review in the mid-1980s* (ed. M. Britton), Vol. 9. OPCS, London.

Barbour, R. (1999). Are focus groups an appropriate tool for studying organisational change? In *Developing focus group research* (ed. R. Barbour and J. Kitzinger). Sage, London.

Barbour, R. and Kitzinger, J. (ed.) (1999). *Developing focus group research*. Sage, London.

Barnes, C. (1991). *Disabled people in Britain and discrimination*. Hurst, London.

Bartlett, D. (1998). *Stress: perspectives and processes*. Open University Press, Buckingham.

Baumann, Z. (1987). *Legislators and interpreters: on modernity, postmodernity and intellectuals*. Polity Press, Cambridge.

Beck, U. (1992). *Risk society: towards a new modernity*. Sage, London.

Becker, M.H. (1974). The health belief model and sick role behavior. *Health Education Monographs*, **2**, 409–19.

Beeken, S. and Waterston, T. (1992). Health service support for breastfeeding—are we practising what we preach? *British Medical Journal*, **305**, 285–7.

Bennett, P. and Murphy, S. (1997). *Psychology and health promotion*. Open University Press, Buckingham.

Berger, A. (1998). Why doesn't audit work? *British Medical Journal*, **316**, 875–6.

Bhaskhar, R. (1989). *A philosophical critique of the contemporary human sciences*. Harvester Wheatsheaf, Hemel Hempstead.

Bhopal, R. (1997). Is research into ethnicity and health racist, unsound or important science? *British Medical Journal*, **314**, 1751–6.

Bickenbach, J.E., Chatterji, S., Badley, E.M., and Ustun, T.B. (1999). Models of disablement, universalism and the international classification of impairments, disabilities and handicaps. *Social Science and Medicine*, **48**, 1173–87.

Black, N. (1994). Why we need qualitative research (editorial). *Journal of Epidemiology and Community Health*, **48**, 425–6.

Blaxter, M. (1976). *The meaning of disability*. Heinemann, London.

Bloor, M. and Horobin, G. (1975). Conflict and conflict resolution in doctor–patient interactions. In *A sociology of medical practice* (ed. C. Cox and A. Mead). Collier Macmillan, London.

Booth-Kewley, S. and Friedman, H.S. (1987). Psychological predictors of heart disease: a quantitative review. *Psychological Bulletin*, **101**, 343–62.

Bosk, C.L. (1981). *Forgive and remember. Managing medical failure*. University of Chicago Press, London.

Bowler, I. (1993). 'They're not the same as us': midwives stereotypes of South Asian descent maternity patients. *Sociology of Health and Illness*, **15**, 157–78.

Bowling, A. (1991). *Measuring health*. Open University Press, Buckingham.

Bowling, A. (1995). *Measuring disease*. Open University Press, Buckingham.

Bradby, H. (1997). Health, eating and heart attacks: Glaswegian Punjabi women's thinking about everyday food. In *Food, health and identity* (ed. P. Caplan), pp. 213–33. Routledge, London.

Brown, P.C. and Smith, T.W. (1992). Social influence, marriage and the heart: cardiovascular consequences of interpersonal control in husbands and wives. *Health Psychology*, **11**, 88–96.

Buchanan, D. (1992). An uneasy alliance: combining qualitative and quantitative research methods. *Health Education Quarterly*, **19**, 117–35.

Bury, M. (1986). Social constructionism and the development of medical sociology. *Sociology of Health and Illness*, **8**, 137–69.

Bury, M. (1996). Defining and researching disability: challenges and responses. In *Exploring the divide: illness and disability* (ed. C. Barnes and G. Mercer). Disability Press, Leeds.

Bury, M. (ed.) (1997). Chronic illness and disability. In *Health and illness in a changing society*. Routledge, London.

Calnan, M. (1984). The politics of health: the case of smoking control. *Journal of Social Policy*, **13**, 279.

Campbell, D.T. and Fiske, D.W. (1959). Convergent and discriminant validation by the multitrait-multimethod matrix. *Psychological Bulletin*, **56**, 81–105.

Campbell, J. and Oliver, M. (1996). *Disability politics: understanding our past, changing our future*. Routledge, London.

Chewning, B. and Sleath, B. (1996). Medication decision-making and management: a client-centred model. *Social Science and Medicine*, **42**, 389–98.

Cheyne, H., Turnbull, D., Lunan, C.B., Reid., M., and Greer, I.A. (1995). Working alongside a mid-wife led unit; what do obstetricians think? *British Journal of Obstetrics and Gynaecology*, **102**, 485–7.

Cohen, S., Kessler, R.C., and Gordon, L.U. (1995). *Measuring stress: a guide for health and social scientists*. Oxford University Press.

Conner, M. and Norman, P. (ed.) (1996). *Predicting health behaviour*. Open University Press, Buckingham.

Conner, M. and Norman, P. (1998). Health behavior. In *Comprehensive clinical psychology* (ed. D. Johnston and M. Johnston), Vol. 8, *Health psychology*, pp. 1–37. Elsevier, Oxford.

Cornford, C. and Morgan, M. (1999) Elderly peoples' beliefs about influenza vaccination. *British Journal of General Practice*, **49**, 519–21.

Cornwell, J. (1984). *Hard earned lives*. Tavistock Press, London.

Cronbach, L.J., Gleser, G.C., Nanda, H., and Rajaratnam, N. (1972). *The dependability of behavioral measurements: theory of generalizability of scores and profiles*. Wiley, New York.

Cunningham-Burley, S., Kerr, A., and Pavis, S. (1999). Theorising subjects and subject matter in focus group research. In *Developing focus group research* (ed. R. Barbour, and J. Kitzinger), pp. 186–99. Sage, New York.

Currer, C. (1986). Concepts of mental well- and ill-being: the case of Pathan mothers in Britain. In *Concepts of health and illness* (ed. C. Currer and M. Stacey). Berg, Leamington Spa.

Daly, J., Kellehear, A., and Gliksman, M. (1997). *The public health researcher: a methodological guide*. Oxford University Press.

Davis, F. (1963). *Passage through crisis: polio victims and their families*. Bobbs-Merrill, Indianapolis, IN.

Davison, C., Davey Smith, G., and Frankel, S. (1991). Lay epidemiology and the prevention paradox: the implications of coronary candidacy for health education. *Sociology of Health and Illness*, **13**, 1–19.

Department of Health (1993). *Changing childbirth, Parts 1 and 2. Report of the Expert Maternity Group*. HMSO, London.

DiMatteo, M.R. (1991). *The psychology of health, illness, and medical care*. Wadsworth, Belmont, CA.

Donovan, J.L. and Blake, D.R. (1992). Patient non-compliance: deviance or reasoned decision-making? *Social Science and Medicine*, **34**, 507–13.

Douglas, J. (1992). Black womens' health matters: putting black women on the research agenda. In *Women's health matters* (ed. H. Roberts), pp. 33–45. Routledge, London.

Douglas, J. (1998). Meeting the health needs of women from black and ethnic minority communities. In *Women and health services* (ed. L. Doyal). Open University Press, Buckingham.

Dowler, E. and Calvert, C. (1995). *Nutrition and diet in lone-parent families in London*. Family Policy Studies Centre, London.

Doyal, L. (1981). *The political economy of health*. Pluto Press, London.

East, L. and Robinson, J. (1994). Changes in process; bringing about change in health care through action research. *Journal of Clinical Nursing*, **3**, 57–61.

Engel, G.L. (1977). The need for a new medical model: a challenge for biomedicine. *Science*, **196**, 129–36.

Fenton, S. and Sadiq-Sangster, A. (1996). Culture, relativism and the expression of mental distress: South Asian women in Britain. *Sociology of Health and Illness*, **2**, 66–85.

Fenwick, N., Morgan, M., McKenzie, C., and Wolf, C. (1998). General practitioners' attitudes to the development of midwifery group practices. *British Journal of General Practice*, **48**, 1395–8.

Fine, G. (1993). The sad demise, mysterious disappearance, and glorious triumph of symbolic interactionism. *Annual Review of Sociology*, **19**, 61–87.

Foucault, M. (1976). *The birth of the clinic: an archaeology of medical perception*. Tavistock Press, London.

Freidman, M. and Rosenman, R.H. (1974). *Type A behaviour and your heart*. Wildwood House, London.

Freidson, E. (1970). *The profession of medicine*. University of Chicago Press.

Freidson, E. (1994). *Professionalism reborn*. Polity Press, Cambridge.

French, S. (1993). Disability, impairment or something in-between? In *Disabling barriers—enabling environments* (ed. J. Swain, V. Finkelstein, S. French, and M. Oliver) Sage, London.

French, N.K. and Chopra, R.V. (1999). Parent perspectives on the roles of paraprofessionals. *Journal of the Association for Persons with Severe Handicaps*, **24**, 259–72.

Giddens, A. (1984). *The constitution of society*. Polity Press, Cambridge.

Giddens, A. (1989). *Sociology*. Polity Press, London.

Giddens, A. (1991). *Modernity and self-identity*. Polity Press, Cambridge.

Giddens, A. (1994). *Beyond left and right: the future of radical politics*. Polity Press, Cambridge.

Glazer, N. and Strauss, A. (1965). *Awareness of dying*. Aldine, Chicago, IL.

Glazer, N. and Strauss, A. (1967). *The discovery of grounded theory*. Aldine, Chicago, IL.

Goffman, E. (1961). *Asylums*. Penguin, Harmondsworth.

Greenwood, J.D. (1989). *Explanation and experiment in social psychological science*. Springer-Verlag, New York.

Grimm, L.G. and Yarnold, P.R. (ed.) (1995). *Reading and understanding multivariate statistics*. American Psychological Association, Washington, DC.

Hall, J.A., Milburn, M.A., Roter, D.L., and Daltroy, L.H. (1998). Why are sicker patients less satisfied with their medical care? Tests of two explanatory models. *Health Psychology*, **17**, 70–5.

Hamilton, D. (1994). Traditions, preferences and postures in applied qualitative research. In *Handbook of qualitative research* (ed. N. Denzin and Y. Lincoln). Sage, London.

Hammersley, M. (1990). *Reading ethnographic research*. Longman, London.

Hammersley, M. and Atkinson, P. (1997). *Ethnography, principles in practice*. Routledge, London.

Harré, R. (1993). *Social being* (2nd edn). Basil Blackwell, Oxford.

Harrison, S. and Pollitt, C. (1995). *Controlling health professionals; the future of work and organisation within the NHS* (2nd edn). Open University Press, Buckingham.

Hart, E. and Bond, M. (1995). *Action research for health and social care*. Open University Press, Buckingham.

Hart, G. and Flowers, P. (1996). Recent developments in the sociology of HIV risk behaviour. *Risk, Decision and Policy*, **1**, 153–65.

Hayduk, L.A. (1996). *LISREL issues, debates and strategies*. Johns Hopkins University Press, Baltimore, MD.

Haynes, S.G., Feinleib, M., and Kannel, W.B. (1980). The relationship of psychosocial factors to coronary heart disease in the Framingham study. *American Journal of Epidemiology*, **111**, 37–58.

Higgs, P. and Scambler, G. (1998) Explaining health inequalities: how useful are concepts of social class? In *Modernity, medicine and health: medical sociology towards 2000* (ed. G. Scambler and P Higgs). Routledge, London.

Hipler, H-J., Schwarz, N., and Sudman, S. (ed.) (1987). *Social information processing and survey methodology*. Springer-Verlag, New York.

Hlatky, M.A., Lam, L.C., Lee, K.L., *et al.* (1995). Job strain and the prevalence and outcome of coronary artery disease. *Circulation*, **92**, 327–33.

Hoffer, C.R. and Schuler E.A. (1948). Measurement of health needs and health care. *American Sociological Review*, **13**, 719–24.

Homans, H. (1983). 'A question of balance': Asian and British women's perceptions of food during pregnancy. In *The sociology of food and eating—essays in the social significance of food* (ed. A. Murcott). Gower, Aldershot.

House, J.S., Landis, K.R., and Umberson, D. (1988). Social relationships and health. *Science*, **241**, 540–5.

Illich, I. (1977). *Limits to medicine. Medical nemesis: the expropriation of health*. Penguin, Harmondsworth.

Jagger, A. and Rothenberg, P. (1984). *Feminist frameworks*. McGraw-Hill, New York.

Jansen, M.A. and Weinman, J. (ed.) (1991). *The international development of health psychology*. Harwood, Philadelphia, PA.

Jefferys, M., Nullard, J.B., Hyman, M., and Warren, M.D. (1969). A set of tests for measuring motor impairment in prevalence studies. *Journal of Chronic Diseases*, **28**, 303–9.

Johnson, T. (1972). *Professions and power*. Macmillan, London.

Johnston, M. and Johnston, D.W. (1998). Assessment and measurement issues. In *Comprehensive clinical psychology*, (ed. D. Johnston and M. Johnston), Vol. 8, *Health psychology*, pp. 113–35. Elsevier, Oxford.

Johnston, M., Wright, S., and Weinman, J. (1995). *Measures in health psychology: a user's portfolio*. NFER-Nelson, Windsor.

Jones, T. (1992). *Britain's ethnic minorities*. Policy Studies Institute, London.

Kai, J. (1996). What worries parents when their pre-school children are acutely ill, and why: a qualitative study. *British Medical Journal*, **313**, 983–6.

Kaplan, R.M., Sallis, J.F., and Patterson, T.L. (1990). *Health and human behavior*. McGraw-Hill, New York.

Kelleher, D. (1988). Coming to terms with diabetes: coping strategies and non-compliance. In *Living with chronic illness* (ed. R. Anderson and M. Bury), pp. 136–55. Unwin-Hyman, London.

Kelly, M.P. (1992). *Colitis*. Routledge, London.

Kelly, M.P. and Field, D. (1998). Conceptualising chronic illness. In *Sociological perspectives on health, illness and health care* (ed. D. Field and S. Taylor). Blackwell Science, Oxford.

Keppel, G. (1991). *Design and analysis: a researcher's handbook* (3rd edn). Prentice-Hall, Englewood Cliffs, NJ.

Kirk, R.E. (1995). *Experimental design: procedures for the behavioral sciences* (3rd edn). Brooks/Cole, Pacific Grove, CA.

Kitzinger, S. (1992). Birth and violence against women: generating hypotheses from women's accounts of unhappiness after childbirth. In *Women's health matters* (ed. H. Roberts). Routledge, London.

Kitzinger, J. (1994). The methodology of focus groups: the importance of interaction between research participants. *Sociology of Health and Illness*, **116**, 103–21.

Kitzinger, J. and Farquer, C. (1999). The analytical potential of 'sensitive moments' in focus group discussions. In *Developing focus group research* (ed. R. Barbour and J. Kitzinger). Sage, London.

Klem, L. (1995). Path analysis. In *Reading and understanding multivariate statistics* (ed. L.G. Grimm and P.R. Yarnold), pp. 65–97. American Psychological Association, Washington, D.C.

Lansbury, H. (2000). Chronic pain management: a qualitative study of elderly people's preferred coping strategies and barriers to management. *Disability and Rehabilitation*, **22**, 2–14.

Lanza, M.L. and Ericsson, A. (2000). Consumer contributions in developing clinical practice guidelines. *Journal of Nursing Care Quality*, **14**, 33–40.

Lazarus, R.S. (1990). Stress, coping and illness. In *Personality and disease* (ed. H.S. Freeman), pp. 97–120. Wiley, New York.

Lazarus, R.S. (1991). *Emotion and adaptation.* Oxford University Press, New York.

Lazarus, R.S. and Folkman, S. (1984). *Stress, appraisal and coping.* Springer, New York.

Lewin, K. (1946). Action research and minority problems. *Journal of Social Issues*, **2**, 34–46.

Locker, D. (1983). *Disability and disadvantage: the consequences of chronic illness.* Tavistock Press, London.

Lofland, J. and Lofland, L. (1995). *Analysing social settings.* Wadsworth, London.

Loftus, E.L., Smith, K.D., Klinger, M.R., and Fiedler, J. (1991). Memory and mismemory for health events. In *Questions about questions: inquiries into the cognitive bases of surveys* (ed. J.M. Tanur), pp. 102–37. Russell Sage Foundation, New York.

Lonsdale, S. (1990). *Women and disability: the experience of physical disability among women.* Macmillan, London.

McColl, E., Jacoby, A., Thomas, L., *et al.* (1998). Designing and using patient and staff questionnaires. In *Health services research methods* (ed. N. Black, J. Brazier, R. Fitzpatrick, and B. Reeves). BMJ Books, London.

Macdonald, L. (1988). The experience of stigma: living with rectal cancer. In *Living with chronic illness: the experience of patients and their families* (ed. R. Anderson and M. Bury). Unwin-Hyman, London.

McDowell, I. and Newell, C. (1987). *Measuring health: a guide to rating scales and questionnaires.* Oxford University Press.

McKeganey, N. and Barnard, M. (1992). *AIDS, drugs and sexual risk.* Open University Press, Buckingham.

McKinlay, J. and Stoeckle, J. (1988). Corporatisation and the social transformation of doctoring. *International Journal of Health Services*, **18**, 191–205.

McLaren, N. (1998). A critical review of the biopsychosocial model. *Australian and New Zealand Journal of Psychiatry*, **32**, 86–92.

Marks, D.F., Bruecher-Albers, C., Donker, F.J., *et al.* (1998). Health Psychology 2000: the development of professional health psychology; EFPPA Task Force on Health Psychology final report. *Journal of Health Psychology*, **3**, 149–60.

Marmot, M., Adelstein, A., and Bulusu, L. (1984). *Immigrant mortality in England and Wales 1970–1978.* OPCS Studies on Population and Medical Subjects, No. 47, HMSO, London.

Martin, D. and McQueen, D. (ed.) (1989). *Readings for a new public health.* Edinburgh University Press.

Martin, J., Mettzer, H., and Elliot, D. (1988). *The prevalence of disability among adults.* HMSO, London.

Matarazzo, J.D. (1980). Behavioral health and behavioral medicine: frontiers for a new health psychology. *American Psychologist*, **35**, 807–17.

Matthews, K.A. (1988). Coronary heart disease and type A behaviors: update on and alternative to the Booth-Kewley and Friedman (1987) quantitative review. *Psychological Bulletin*, **104**, 373–80.

Mead, G.H. (1934). *Mind, self and society from the standpoint of social behaviourism.* University of Chicago Press.

Mechanic, D. (1962). Sources of power of lower participants in complex organisations. *Administration Science Quarterly*, **7**, 349–64.

Melia, K. (1997). Producing 'plausible stories': interviewing student nurses. In *Context and method in qualitative research* (ed. G. Miller and R. Dingwall). Sage, London.

Meyer, J. (2000). Using qualitative methods in health related action research. *British Medical Journal*, **320**, 178–81.

Miller, T.Q., Smith, T.W., Turner, C.W., Guijarro, M.L., and Hallet, A.J. (1996). A meta-analytic review of research on hostility and physical health. *Psychological Bulletin*, **119**, 322–48.

Morgan, M., Patrick, D.L., and Charlton, J.R. (1984). Social networks and psychosocial support among disabled people. *Social Science and Medicine*, **19**, 489–99.

Murphy, E., Dingwall, R., Greatbatch, D., Parker, S., and Watkson, P. (1998). Qualitative research methods in health technology assessment; a review of the literature. *Health Technology Assessment*, **2**.

Murray, M. and Chamberlain, K. (1998). Special issue. Qualitative research. *Journal of Health Psychology*, **3**.

Murray, M. and Chamberlain, K. (1999). *Qualitative health psychology: theories and methods.* Sage, London.

Navarro, V. (1982). The labor process and health. *International Journal of Health Services*, **12**, 5.

Nazroo, J.Y. (1997). *The health of Britain's ethnic minorities. Findings from a national survey.* Policy Studies Institute, London.

Nettleton, S. (1995). *The sociology of health and illness.* Polity Press, Cambridge.

Neuberger, J. and Tallis, R. (1999). Do we need a new word for patients? *British Medical Journal*, **318**, 1756–7.

NHLBI (National Heart, Lung, and Blood Institute) Task Force (1998). *Behavioral research in cardiovascular, lung, and blood health.* National Institutes of Health, Bethesda, MD.

Nunnally, J.C. and Bernstein, I.H. (1994). *Psychometric theory* (3rd edn). McGraw-Hill, New York.

Oakley, A. (1980). *Women confined: towards a sociology of childbirth.* Martin Robertson, Oxford.

Oakley, A. (1981). Interviewing women; a contradiction in terms. In *Doing feminist research* (ed. H. Roberts). Routlege and Kegan Paul, London.

Ogden, J. (1997). The rhetoric and reality of psychosocial theories of health: a challenge to biomedicine? *Journal of Health Psychology*, **2**, 21–9.

Oliver, M. (1996). *Understanding disability: from theory to practice.* Macmillan, London.

Ostrom, T.M. (1987). Bipolar survey items: an information processing perspective. In *Social information processing and survey methodology* (ed. H.-J. Hipler, N. Schwarz, and S. Sudman), pp. 71–85. Springer-Verlag, New York.

Owens, P. and Petch, H. (1995). Professionals and management. In *Interprofessional issues in community and primary health care* (ed. P. Owens, J. Carrier, and J. Horder), pp. 37–55. Macmillan, London.

Owens, P., Carrier, J., and Horder, J. (1995). *Interprofessional issues in community and primary health care.* Macmillan, London.

Parsons, T. (1951). *The social system.* Free Press, New York.

Patrick, D.L. and Peach, H. (1989). *Disablement in the community.* Oxford University Press.

Pavis, S. and Cunningham-Burley, S. (1999). Male youth street culture; understanding the context of health-related behaviours. *Health Education Research: Theory and Practice*, **14**, 583–96.

Pearce I.H. and Crocker L.H. (1949). *The Peckham experiment.* Allen and Unwin, London.

Pearson, M. (1989). Sociology of race and health. In *Ethnic factors in health and disease* (ed. J. Cruickshank and D. Beevers). Wright, Sevenoaks.

Pinder, R. (1990). *The management of chronic illness: patient and doctor perspectives on Parkinson's disease.* Macmillan, London.

Pollack, M., Poucheler, G., and Pierret, J. (1992). *AIDS: a problem for sociological research.* Sage, London.

Popay, J., Rogers, A., and Williams, G. (1998*a*). Rationale and standards for the systematic review of qualitative literature in health services research. *Qualitative Health Research*, **8**, 341–51.

Popay, J., Williams, G., Thomas, C., and Gatrell, T. (1998*b*). Theorising inequalities in health: the place of lay knowledge. *Sociology of Health and Illness*, **20**, 619–44.

Pope, C. (1991). Trouble in store: some thoughts on the management of waiting lists. *Sociology of Health and Illness*, **13**, 194–212.

Pope, C. and Mays, N. (ed.) (2000). *Qualitative research in health care* (2nd edn). BMJ Books, London.

Powles, J. (1973). On the limitations of modern medicine. *Science, Medicine and Management*, **1**, 1–30.

Price, V.A. (1983). *Type A behavior pattern: a model for research and practice.* Academic Press, New York.

Robinson, I. (1988). Reconstructing lives: renegotiating the meaning of multiple sclerosis. In *Living with chronic illness* (ed. R. Anderson and M. Bury), pp. 43–66. Unwin-Hyman, London.

Rogers R.W. (1983). Cognitive and physiological processes in fear appeals and attitude change: a revised theory of protection motivation. In *Social psychophysiology: a sourcebook* (ed. J.T. Cacioppo and R.A. Petty), pp. 153–76. Guilford, New York.

Rosenthal, R. (1994). Interpersonal expectancy effects: a 30-year perspective. *Current Directions in Psychological Science*, **3**, 176–9.

Savage, M. and Miles, A. (1994). *The remaking of the British working class.* Routlege, London.

Scambler, G. (1989). *Epilepsy.* Routledge, London.

Scambler, G. and Hopkins, R. (1986). Being epileptic: coming to terms with stigma. *Sociology of Health and Illness*, **8**, 26–43.

Schnall, P.L., Landsbergis, P.A., and Baker, D. (1994). Job strain and cardiovascular disease. *Annual Review of Public Health*, **15**, 381–411.

Schneiderman, N. and Tapp, J.T. (ed.) (1985). *Behavioral medicine: the biomedical approach.* Lawrence Erlbaum, Hillsdale, NJ.

Schutz, A. (1962). *Collected papers*, Vol. 1. Martinus Nijhoff, The Hague.

Schutz, A. (1964). *Collected papers*, Vol. 2. Martinus Nijhoff, The Hague.

Schwalbe, M.L. and Staples, C.L. (1986). Class position, work experience and health. *International Journal of Health Services*, **16**, 583.

Schwartz, M., Landis, S.E., Rowe, J.E, Janes, C.L., and Pullman, N. (2000). Using focus groups to assess primary care patients' satisfaction. *Evaluation and the Health Professions*, **23**, 58–71.

Scott, R. (1969). *The making of blind men.* Russell Sage Foundation, New York.

Seale, C. (1999). Quality in qualitative research. *Qualitative Enquiry*, **5**, 465–78.

Shavelson, R.J., Webb, N.M., and Rowley, G.L. (1989). Generalizability theory. *American Psychologist*, **44**, 922–32.

Sheeran, P. and Abraham, C. (1996). The health belief model. In *Predicting health behaviour* (ed. M. Conner and P. Norman), pp. 23–61. Open University Press, Buckingham.

Sheeran, P., Abraham, C., and Orbell, S. (1999). Psychosocial correlates of heterosexual condom use: a meta-analysis. *Psychological Bulletin*, **125**, 90–132.

Shumaker, S.A. and Czajkowski, S.M. (ed.) (1994). *Social support and cardiovascular disease.* Plenum, New York.

Shuttleworth, S. (1990). Female circulation: medical discourse and popular advertising in the mid-Victorian era. In *Body/politics: women and discourses of science* (ed. M. Jacobus, E.F. Keller, and S. Shuttleworth). Routlege, London.

Siegman, A.W. and Smith, T.W. (1994). *Anger, hostility, and the heart.* Lawrence Erlbaum, Hillsdale, NJ.

Smaje, C. (1995). *Health, 'race' and ethnicity; making sense of the evidence.* King's Fund Institute, London.

Spicer, J. (1997). Systems analysis of stress and coping: a testing proposition. *Journal of Health Psychology*, **2**, 167–70.

Spicer, J. and Chamberlain, K. (1996). Developing psychosocial theory in health psychology: problems and prospects. *Journal of Health Psychology*, **1**, 161–71.

Spicer, J., Jackson, R., and Scragg, R. (1996). Type A behaviour, social contact and coronary death. *Psychology and Health*, **11**, 733–43.

Steptoe, A. (1998). Psychophysiological bases of disease. In *Comprehensive clinical psychology* (ed. D. Johnston and M. Johnston). Vol. 8, *Health psychology*, pp. 39–78. Elsevier, Oxford.

Strauss, A., *et al.* (1963). The hospital and its negotiated order. In *The hospital in modern society* (ed. E. Freidson). Free Press, New York.

Streiner, D.L. and Norman, G.R. (1995). *Health measurement scales: a practical guide to their development and use* (2nd edn). Oxford University Press.

Strube, M.J. (ed.) (1991). *Type A behavior.* Sage, Newbury Park, CA.

Suchman, L. and Jordan, B. (1991). Validity and the collaborative construction of meaning in face-to-face surveys. In *Questions about questions: inquiries into the cognitive bases of surveys* (ed. J.M. Tanur), pp. 241–67. Russell Sage Foundation, New York.

Tabachnick, B.G. and Fidell, L.S. (1996). *Using multivariate statistics* (3rd edn). Harper Collins, New York.

Tanur, J.M. (ed.) (1991). *Questions about questions: inquiries into the cognitive bases of surveys.* Russell Sage Foundation, New York.

Taylor, S.E. (1995). *Health psychology* (3rd edn). McGraw-Hill, New York.

Titchen, A. and Binnie, A. (1993). Research partnershsips: collaborative action research in nursing. *Journal of Advanced Nursing*, **18**, 858–65.

Tonkiss, F. (1998). Analysing discourse. In *Researching society and culture* (ed. C. Seale). Sage, London.

Tucker, J., Hall, M.H., Howie, P.W., *et al.* (1996). Should obstetricians see women with normal pregnancies? A multi-centre randomised controlled trial of routine antenatal care by general practitioners and midwives compared with shared care led by obstetricians. *British Medical Journal*, **312**, 554–9.

Turnbull, D., Holmes, A., Shields, N., *et al.* (1996). Randomised, controlled trial of efficacy of midwife-managed care. *Lancet*, **348**, 213–18.

Turner, B.S. (1987). *Medical power and social knowledge.* Sage, London.

Turner, B.S. (1992). *Regulating bodies; essays in medical sociology.* Routledge, London.

Turner, J.R. (1994). *Cardiovascular reactivity and stress.* Plenum, New York.

Uchino, B.N., Cacioppo, J.T., and Kiecolt-Glaser, J.K. (1996). The relationship between social support and physiological processes: a review with emphasis on underlying mechanisms and implications for health. *Psychological Bulletin*, **119**, 488–531.

Voysey, M. (1975). *A constant burden: the reconstitution of family life.* Routledge and Kegan Paul, London.

Walters, A.J. (1995). A hermaneutic study of the experiences of relatively of critically ill patients. *Journal of Advanced Nursing*, **22**, 998–1005.

WHO (World Health Organization) (1980). *International classification of impairments, disabilities and handicaps.* WHO, Geneva.

WHO (World Health Organization) Quality of Life Group (1998). The World Health Organization quality of life assessment (WHOQOL): development and general psychometric properties. *Social Science and Medicine*, **46**, 1569–85.

Wilcocks, S. (1999). Clinical management and cultural diversity: the cultural context of doctor involvement in the managerial process. *Health Services Management Research*, **12**, 212–16.

Williams, R.G.A. (1983). Concepts of health and illness: an analysis of lay logic. *Sociology*, **17**, 182–205.

Williams, G. (1984). The genesis of chronic illness: narrative reconstruction. *Sociology of Health and Illness*, **6**, 175–200.

Williams, S. and Calnan, M. (1994). Perspectives on prevention: the views of General Practitioners. *Sociology of Health and Illness*, **16**, 372–93.

Williams, R.D. and Clark, A.J. (2000). A qualitative study of women's hysterectomy experience. *Journal of Women's Health and Gender-based Medicine*, **9**, S15–25.

Wing, J.K. and Brown, G.W. (1970). *Institutionalism and schizophrenia.* Oxford University Press.

Zola, I. (1975). Culture and symptoms: an analysis of patients' presenting complaints. In *A sociology of medical practice* (ed. C. Cox and A. Mead). Collier-Macmillan, London.

7.2 Demography and public health

Emily Grundy

Introduction

The health and health-care needs of a population cannot be measured or met without a knowledge of its size and characteristics. Demography is concerned with this essential 'numbering of the people' and with understanding population dynamics—how populations change in response to the interplay between fertility, mortality, and migration. This understanding is a prerequisite for making the forecasts about future population size and structure which should underpin health-care planning. Analysis of both the present and the future necessitates a review of the past. The number of very old people in a population, for example, depends on the number of births eight or nine decades earlier and risks of death at successive ages throughout the intervening period. The proportion of very old people depends partly on this numerator but more importantly on the denominator (the size of the population as a whole)—itself a function of reproductive behaviour, mortality, and net migration from yesterday back through time. The number of births in a population depends not just on current patterns of family building, but also on the number of women 'at risk' of reproduction—itself a function of past trends in fertility and mortality. Similarly, the number of deaths (and their distribution by cause) is strongly influenced by age structure. For this reason, although life expectancy at birth in the developed world is some 13 years longer than in the less developed world (78 and 65 years respectively), crude death rates—deaths per 1000 population of all ages—are very similar (eight and nine) (World Bank 1999).

Formal or pure demography is largely concerned with answering questions about how populations change and how these changes can be measured. The broader field of population studies embraces the questions of why these changes occur, and with what consequences.

A major theme of this work is the complex interrelationship between population change and human health. This chapter presents information on demographic methods and data sources in the context of their application to health and population issues.

Global issues

There are currently very substantial differences between regions of the world in population characteristics and trends and predominant public health issues. As illustrated in Fig. 1, the size of the world's population is growing at an unprecedented rate and was estimated to comprise some 6 billion people in October 1999 (UNFPA 1999). While it took an estimated 123 years (from 1804 to 1927) for the world to increase its population from 1 to 2 billion, the increase from 5 to 6 billion was achieved in a tenth of the time (1987 to 1999) (UN 1999). Most of this growth has been in the developing world where currently about 98 per cent of world population increase takes place (Population Reference Bureau 1999; UNFPA 1999). In many countries of sub-Saharan Africa, 40 per cent or more of the population is aged 15 or under and the total population is expected to have more than doubled in size between 1985 and 2015 (Bulatao and Stephens 1992). By contrast, many European countries are expected to experience real falls in population size between 1998 and 2050, by which latter date approaching a quarter of their populations will be aged 65 or more (US Bureau of the Census 1992; UNFPA 1999). These differences in age structure, and associated variations in levels of fertility and mortality, are illustrated for regions of the world in Table 1. Clearly these variations have enormous implications for the health and health-care priorities of the populations concerned. In the developing countries of the world a third of all deaths occur among infants and children aged under 5 years; deaths of those aged 65 or more account for a slightly lower proportion. In the developed world, by contrast, deaths of elderly people aged 65 or more account for 72 per cent of the total and those of children under 5 less than 3 per cent (Fig. 2). As a result, as shown in Fig. 3, only 2 per cent of the world's deaths among those under 5 years of age occur in the populations of developed regions, compared with 42 per cent of the world's deaths in elderly age groups.

Closely related to these age variations (and differences in the level of mortality) are differences in the cause structure of death (Preston 1976*a*). Communicable diseases, maternal and perinatal conditions, and nutritional deficiencies account for 35 per cent of all deaths in low- and middle-income countries compared with only 6 per cent of deaths in high-income states. Conversely, non-communicable diseases are responsible for 54 per cent of deaths in low- and middle-income countries but 87 per cent in high-income ones (WHO 1999). While in parts of the world reproductive health, including family planning and measures to reduce the spread of HIV/AIDS, present the most pressing public health problem, in many developed countries concerns about the growing proportion of old—particularly very old—people and the possible implications of recent changes in family systems predominate.

The watershed that separates populations with high fertility, relatively high mortality, young age structures, and rapid growth from those with low vital rates, older age structures, and slow or no growth is conceptualized as the demographic transition. Identifying and explaining this and the associated profound changes, termed the epidemiological and health transitions, has been described as the

Table 1 Age structure, fertility, and life expectancy: world regions and selected countries, 1998 or 1999

Region	Percentage aged		Total fertility rate	Life expectancy at birth
	< 15	⩾ 65		
Africa	43	3	5.3	52
Sub-Saharan Africa	45	3	5.7	49
Northern Africa	36	4	3.3	66
Asia	31	6	2.7	67
India	34	5	3.2	64
China	26	7	1.8	72
Japan	15	17	1.5	80
Latin America and Caribbean	32	5	2.7	69
North America	21	13	2.0	77
USA	22	13	2.1	76
Europe	18	15	1.4	78
Italy	14	18	1.2	79
Spain	15	17	1.2	78
Poland	20	12	1.5	77
UK	19	16	1.7	77
Australia	21	13	1.8	80
World	30	7	2.8	63

Source: US Bureau of the Census, international database.

central preoccupation of modern demography (Demeny 1972). Before turning to the causes, progress, and consequences of these transformations, the basic methods and materials of demographic analysis must be considered and the issue of population dynamics—how populations change—must be addressed.

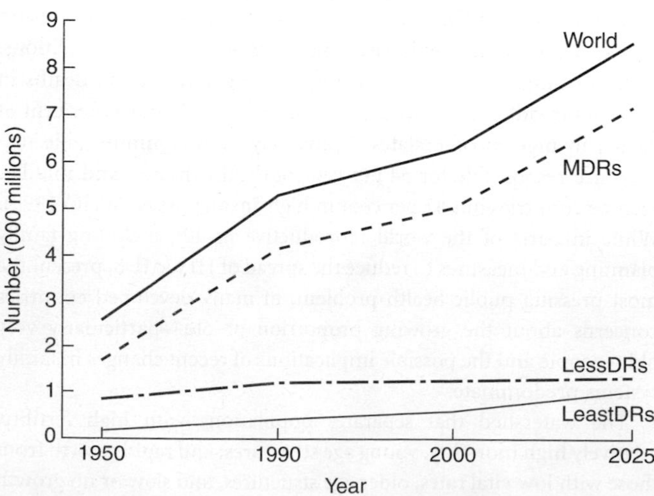

Fig. 1 World population data and projections: 1950 to 2025. (Data from WHO 1992*a*; UN 1999.)

Demographic data and methods of analysis

In the seventeenth century John Graunt, a London merchant, used data from the London Bills of Mortality to devise an early life table. This pioneering work has led to him being dubbed the 'father of modern demography' (Smith and Kayfitz 1977). However, Graunt was seriously handicapped by the fact that, although he had information on numbers of deaths, he lacked data on the population at risk and could not compute death rates. Essentially all demographic analysis requires data both on the population 'stock' and on 'flows' in and out—births, deaths, and migration. The traditional sources of information on the former are population censuses and, for the latter, vital registration systems.

Population censuses

Head counts of the population, generally for military or tax purposes, have an ancient history but the first 'modern' censuses were undertaken in Scandinavia in the eighteenth century. In England and Wales the first census was undertaken in 1801, although a question on age was not included until 1841. During the nineteenth century censuses spread throughout Europe and are now almost universal. As well as basic questions about age, sex, marital status, and place of residence, data on other characteristics such as employment, education, and housing are often collected. The United Nations, which has done much to ensure that a minimum of roughly comparable questions are included in as many countries as possible, recommends that censuses be conducted at least decennially in years ending in 0 or 1. Recommendations about particular topics are also sometimes made; in the 1990–1991 round, for example, disability was emphasized and questions on this were included in a number of countries, including the United Kingdom.

Censuses have many strengths and are generally the only source of data for small areas or small population subgroups. Although primarily a tool for collecting data on population 'stock', censuses have also been used as ways of finding out about vital events, which is particularly useful if other data sources are sparse. In the 1911 and 1971 British censuses, for example, detailed fertility histories were collected from married women. Many countries use censuses to provide data on recent internal migration (through questions on place of residence one or more years earlier) and on immigration (through questions on country of birth and/or date of entry for those born elsewhere). Indirect estimation techniques developed by Brass (1975) and others mean that data from simple questions on number of children who have died, widowhood, and orphanhood included in some developing countries can be used to assess mortality levels (UN 1983). Taking a census requires not only a reasonable administrative infrastructure, but also the co-operation of the population to be enumerated. Some countries, including Germany and The Netherlands, have given up taking censuses because the latter is lacking.

Against the strengths of censuses must be set the huge costs of collecting and processing census data and the major problems involved in ensuring it is of reasonable quality. When censuses are taken, difficulties arising from errors and omissions are common, even in developed countries with a long history of census taking.

Young geographically mobile adults, members of minority ethnic groups, infants, and the very old are the groups most likely to be under-enumerated. In the 1991 British census, for example, an estimated 1.2 million people were missed, including 10 per cent of males in their twenties and 8 per cent of those aged 85 or more (Heady *et al.* 1994). Groups such as seasonal migrants (including students), naval and military personnel, and people temporarily away from

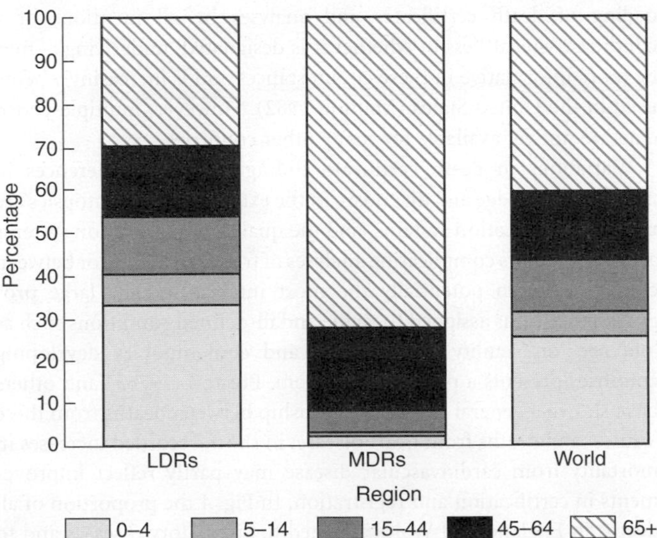

Fig. 2 Distribution of deaths by age group in less developed and more developed regions, 1990. (Data from WHO 1992*a*.)

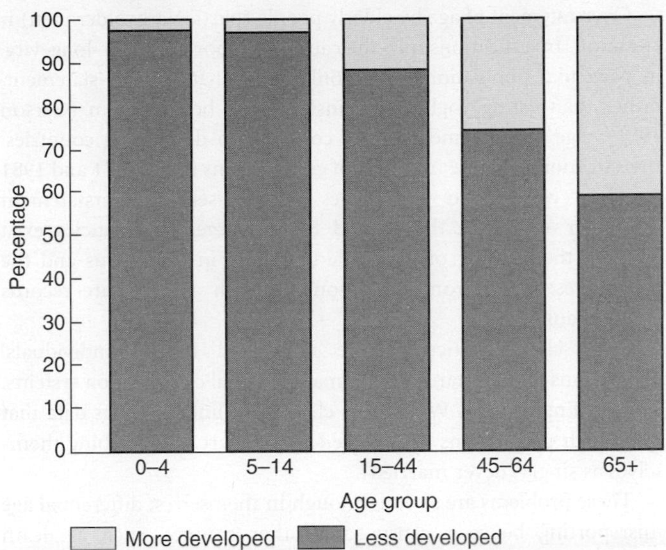

Fig. 3 Distribution of deaths (%) between more and less developed regions by age, 1990. (Data source: WHO 1992*a*.)

home present particular problems. Not only are they more likely to be missed, but a decision has to be made about whether they should be assigned to their place of usual or legal residence (assuming it can be determined), or counted as belonging to the place of enumeration. The former system is termed *de jure*, the latter *de facto*. The issue of assigning people to some place of usual residence is important as often resources are distributed on the basis of population size and characteristics. Moreover, it is essential to try and ensure that demographic events recorded in one system (vital registration) are attributed to the population actually 'at risk' of experiencing them. In the developed world, for example, most deaths occur in hospitals which may draw patients from a wide area. If no attempt is made to assign these decedents to the region or locality where they lived prior to hospital admission, areas including large hospitals will appear to have very high mortality rates while in others recorded mortality will be artificially low.

Assessment of the extent of under-enumeration is usually achieved through census validation surveys (surveys of a sample of census addresses in which intensive efforts are made to contact non-respondents and to check information supplied by respondents) and comparisons with population estimates from other data sources. Ensuring near-complete enumeration is only part of the problem; the quality of the data collected is also a major concern.

Age misreporting is one of the most serious problems that must be estimated and allowed for in analyses of census and similar data. In many populations, people may not always know their exact age and some approximation is reported or made by an enumerator. 'Heaping' on ages ending in 0 or 5 is a common result. Heaping can be detected by looking at the age distribution and applying various tests of consistency and such data are normally adjusted before publication. More serious problems arise when reported age is based on other characteristics, such as marital status, number of children, or grandparent status, as clearly any analysis of, for example, age at first marriage will be biased.

Overstatement of age by elderly people (particularly older men) is common. Investigations into the causes of reported 'super-longevity' in particular populations commonly show that age mis-statement, rather than eating yoghurt for instance, lie behind them (Garson 1991). Age overstatement is not confined to developing countries. Investigations into the numbers of centenarians in the 1971 and 1981 Censuses in England and Wales showed serious overstatement (Thatcher 1992). In the United States, large discrepancies exist between the number of very elderly people in the census and the number estimated from other sources, such as Medicare records (Kestenbaum 1992).

Other characteristics may be 'mis-stated' because individuals' perceptions of their status do not match official classification systems. Thus in England and Wales, it is clear from linked census data that quite high proportions of divorced men revert to describing themselves as single (never married).

These problems are serious enough in themselves; differential age misreporting between census and other sources, such as death certificates, present a further difficulty. Numerator–denominator discrepancies may introduce serious bias into the analysis of mortality at advanced ages, or by characteristics such as occupationally defined social class or marital status (Fox and Goldblatt 1982).

Vital registration

Data on demographic events are needed, as well as data on population characteristics. In the developed world these data are usually drawn from vital registration systems—the compulsory registration of births, marriages, and deaths. In some countries, principally Scandinavian, which maintain population registers, details of geographical moves are also recorded.

Compulsory registration of births and deaths was established in most European countries during the nineteenth century. In England and Wales, for example, civil registration was introduced in 1837. Subsequent improvements to the system included those following the 1874 Births and Deaths Registration Act which made parents legally responsible for registering births and required attending doctors to supply information on cause of death. Other revisions have since been made, for example the inclusion of firstly the mother's and later the father's age on the confidential section of birth certificates. Most developed countries now have well-established registration systems with complete, or very near complete, coverage. In the developing world, however, many people have no need for certificates of birth or marriage. Consequently, vital registration systems are frequently seriously incomplete or non-existent, although there are some exceptions and some countries, including India and China, which have sample registration systems for selected areas. By 1998 half the countries of the world had registration systems with at least 90 per cent complete registration. However, as many of the world's most populous countries are in the other half, over all fewer than a quarter of vital events worldwide are thought to be recorded (World Bank 1999). Even in well-established systems, the fact that registration is undertaken primarily for administrative reasons may mean that demographically relevant details are not recorded. In England and Wales, for example, the number of legitimate children previously borne by the mother is recorded on the confidential section of the birth certificate. Previous births outside marriage, now of growing significance, are not recorded and so true parity cannot be measured from registration data.

The quality of the information supplied and coded is very important. No one registers his or her own death and the information obtained from proxy informants (relatives or, quite frequently, undertakers) about details such as last occupation may be inaccurate. Age, however, is thought to be more reliably recorded on death certificates than in censuses (at least in developed countries), presumably because it is more often checked against other records.

Cause of death

Death certificates are the major source of information on cause of death. In developed countries cause of death is generally certified by a doctor and coded according to the International Classification of Diseases (**ICD**). There is substantial scope for error and inconsistency at the various stages involved in assigning cause of death. The ICD, which originated from work undertaken by the nineteenth century British medical statistician, William Farr, is now in its tenth revision; each revision has been associated with changes particularly affecting certain causes of death (Alderson 1981). Changes in coding instructions have also been made from time to time (Ashley and Devis 1992). 'Fashions' and national preferences also seem to influence assignment of cause of death, as illustrated in a number of classic papers in which case studies of deaths were distributed to doctors in different countries. Place of death may also be important. In Britain an apparent rise in respiratory disease mortality among elderly people in the 1950s and 1960s was found on investigation largely to reflect the increased proportion of deaths occurring in hospital. The junior hospital doctors who filled out the death certificates were much more likely than family doctors to ascribe the deaths of elderly people to bronchopneumonia (OPCS 1981). Changes over time, and variations between countries, in the use of autopsies also affect cause of death assignment.

Elderly people, now the vast majority of decedents in developed countries, are more likely than the young to suffer multiple pathologies and the number of conditions recorded on death certificates has been increasing, although it varies between countries (Alderson 1981; Ashley and Devis 1992). Choice of one over another as the 'true' underlying cause of death is bound to be partially arbitrary. Multiple coding of death certificates and analyses by all mentions of a condition—regardless of whether it is designated 'underlying'—may be more informative in these circumstances and is increasingly being used in the United States (Manton 1982). However, multiple-coded data are not yet available for many other countries.

Variations in death certificate coding reflecting differences in medical knowledge and diagnosis, in the extent to which autopsies are used, in classification systems, and the quality of registration systems are major factors complicating analyses of trends over time or between countries—often potentially the most interesting. The large proportion of deaths assigned to vague and ill-defined conditions such as 'old age' or 'senility' in historical and contemporary developing countries presents a particular problem. Preston (1976*a*) and others have shown a general inverse relationship between deaths from these 'causes' and deaths from heart disease; in short, recorded increases in mortality from cardiovascular disease may partly reflect improvements in certification and registration. In Fig. 4 the proportion of all deaths in England and Wales assigned to circulatory diseases and to ill-defined causes is shown for age groups over 65 from 1911–1915 to 1997. It can be seen that large proportions of deaths among the very old were assigned to ill-defined groups early in the century and that

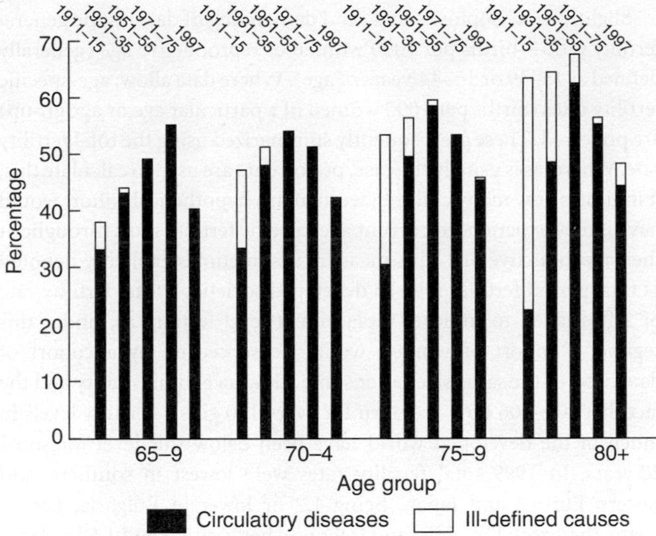

Fig. 4 Percentage of all deaths due to circulatory diseases and ill-defined causes, age groups 65–69 to 80+, England and Wales, 1911–1915 to 1997. (Data from ONS 1998.)

declines in this proportion were associated with increases in the proportion attributed to circulatory diseases.

In countries which lack adequate certification and registration systems, data on deaths by cause are seriously limited. To compensate for this, attempts have been made to develop protocols for collecting information from lay informants which can be used to assign cause of death (Garenne and Fontaine 1990; Snow *et al.* 1992). However, although this approach has been useful in a number of small-scale investigations of population subgroups, its widespread application would be extremely costly.

Other data sources

Sample surveys now represent a major addition or, in some cases an alternative, to conventional demographic data sources. Most developed countries have a range of government-sponsored surveys which provide far more detailed information on, for example, health-related behaviour, family building strategies, or reasons for migration than it would be possible to collect in a census. In the developing world, where other data sources are scarce, surveys of various kinds often present the best source of data on basic demographic parameters. Data quality is potentially much better in a survey than a census, as it is more likely that well-trained interviewers can be used. The World Fertility Survey, an international population research programme launched in 1972 to determine fertility levels throughout the world, and its successor, the Demographic and Health Survey Programme, have been particularly valuable in providing data for a range of countries, including many lacking adequate vital registration systems. Other approaches to data capture include multiround surveys, in which respondents are asked about events since last contact, and dual-record systems which involve two independent data collection systems (one often a multiround survey), the results of which are then combined. This method allows some estimation of missed events to be made, but is expensive. These approaches are described in more detail in most standard demographic textbooks (Shryock *et al.* 1976; Newell 1988; Pollard *et al.* 1990; Hinde 1998).

The raw materials of demography relate to individuals' most personal experiences—sexual activity, family formation, birth control, reproduction, marital breakdown, illness, and death. All of these experiences occur in a social framework which attaches value to some of these behaviours and stigmatizes others. Not surprisingly, respondents in censuses and surveys may be reluctant to disclose non-marital pregnancies, illegal abortions, illegal migration, or deaths of relatives from AIDS. Concealment has also been the policy of some national governments which have treated demographic data as official secrets.

As well as allowing for these personal and political factors, the enormous potential complications arising from people's uncertainties about age or other 'basic' characteristics, uncertain recollections of prior events, and the vast scope for administrative errors of various kinds have to be considered. In this context the demographer's traditional obsession with data quality becomes understandable. Very real current questions turn on issues of data quality. In the United States, for example, death rates for African-Americans are higher than those for white people until the age of 75 years or so when they appear to 'cross over'. This has been interpreted as an effect of selective survival and the differential health challenges faced by black and white Americans. As these challenges are greater on average for black than white people it is argued that only the most healthy black people survive to old age and so their mortality thereafter is lower than that of white people (Markides and Keith 1995). However, detailed investigation, including matching with other sources of information on age, has shown that this 'cross-over' is almost certainly an artefactual result of differences between ethnic groups in the extent of age misreporting in censuses and on death certificates. Age mis-statement in the census is worse among African-Americans, many of whom were born in the Southern States which did not have birth registration systems until 1920. As a result late age mortality rates in this group have been underestimated (Elo and Preston 1994).

The statistics produced in series like the United Nations demographic yearbooks have their origins in what is or has been done by millions of people, mediated by what is said about these events and experiences, further filtered by how this is recorded, processed, and analysed. Some assessment of data quality is given in the foreword to the United Nations demographic yearbooks, but sometimes users may pay insufficient attention to this. Apart from this series, and a range of other United Nations publications (UNFPA 1998; UN 1999), a number of other organizations produce international reference works. These include the World Health Organization (**WHO**), which produces the *World Health Statistics Annual* (WHO 1998) and other publications, the World Bank (World Bank 1999), and the United States Census Bureau for International Research (US Bureau of the Census 1992). The United Nations regional directorates, the Organization for Economic Co-operation and Development (**OECD**), the Council of Europe, and Eurostat (Eurostat 1998) also produce very helpful series and 'one-off' compilations for particular regions.

Analysis of demographic data

A standard array of techniques and measures forms the basis of much demographic analysis, the most common of which are described briefly below. Further detail is supplied in a number of textbooks (Shryock *et al.* 1976; Newell 1988; Pollard *et al.* 1990; Hinde 1998). Analysis involves not just the application of a particular technique, but decisions about what units of analysis to use and how to group them. A major distinction of the latter type is between period and cohort analysis. Period analysis deals with events of a particular time period (for example, mortality rates from 1995 to 1999) while cohort analyses follow the experience of individuals through time. Cohorts in this sense are defined as groups of people who have experienced the same significant event at the same time. Thus birth cohorts comprise people born in a particular year or group of years and marriage cohorts those marrying at a particular time. Other important events, such as leaving school, divorce, or retirement, may also be used to define a cohort. The health status of individuals at one point in time is clearly likely to be influenced by past exposures and environments, including experiences very early in life (Barker 1992). For this reason cohort and 'life-course' approaches to analysing mortality and other indicators of population health have an intuitive appeal.

Birth cohort and time period are two of the dimensions which locate people in time; the third is age. Duration effects (such as duration of marriage or length of exposure to a particular pathogen) may also be important. Models in which age, period, and cohort effects are considered separately have been used in mortality analyses, but less so in analyses of reproductive behaviour (Hobcraft *et al.* 1982). Cohort effects may be substantial and, unless allowed for, may mask relationships between, for example, age and various risks or patterns of behaviour. Differences in the smoking behaviour of cohorts, for example, have a major effect on the relationships between age and smoking-related disease observed at different periods.

Other decisions about whether to use individuals, families, households, or geographical areas as units of analysis are often constrained by data availability. Until relatively recently, for example, most census data were only available as aggregate tabulations. The growing availability of microdata—individual-level information—has greatly extended the scope of demographic analysis. Other innovations include the development of sample record linkage systems, such as the Office of National Statistics Longitudinal Study in England and Wales (Fox and Goldblatt 1982). In these datasets individuals' census records are linked with their vital registration records so numerator–denominator biases in, for example, the analysis of mortality are avoided.

Measurement of fertility

Fertility means the child-bearing performance of a woman, couple, or population. Generally only live births are included. The term fecundity, by contrast, is used to refer to the physiological capability of producing a live-born child. Confusingly, in the French-speaking world the meaning of these terms is reversed, so *fécundité* in French means fertility in English. A rough idea of fertility may be gained from using census or survey data to calculate child–woman ratios: the ratio of 0- to 4-year-olds to women aged 15 to 49 years. However, the survival of infants (and their mothers) affects these ratios, so they are generally only used if no other data are available.

The simplest measure of fertility commonly used is the crude birth rate—the number of births in a particular year per 1000 population. As the denominator of this includes those not 'at risk' of giving birth (men and women outside the reproductive age groups), it is really a ratio rather than a rate. Crude birth rates are influenced by the age structure of the population, but less seriously than crude death rates. In the late 1990s crude birth rates ranged from 10 per 1000 in parts of Europe to 41 per 1000 in sub-Saharan Africa.

Slightly more sophisticated (and demanding of data) is the general fertility ratio—births per 1000 women of reproductive age (generally defined as 15–49 or 15–44 years of age). Where data allow, age-specific fertility rates (births per 1000 women of a particular age or age group) are preferred. These are frequently summarized using the total fertility rate. Where, as is usually the case, period data are used to calculate this, it indicates how many children women in a hypothetical cohort would have if they experienced current age-specific fertility rates throughout their reproductive life. This measure is sometimes explicitly denoted as total period fertility rate. In developed societies a total fertility rate of 2.1 is taken to indicate replacement level fertility as, under this regime, a cohort of women would be succeeded by a cohort of daughters of the same size (after some allowance for mortality and the fact that 105–106 boys are born for every 100 girls). Fertility levels in much of the developed world have been below this level for some 20 years. In 1999 total fertility rates were lowest in southern and eastern Europe and Japan, being 1.2 or lower in Bulgaria, Latvia, Spain, the Czech Republic, and Italy, and between 1.2 and 1.5 in a large number of other countries including Germany, Greece, Russia, Japan, Poland, and Sweden. Total fertility rates are highest in sub-Saharan Africa; in 1999 Niger, Oman, Ethiopia, and Uganda had estimated total fertility rates close to, or above, 7.

One difficulty with the total fertility rate, particularly as a tool for examining trends during periods of change, is that it is affected by changes in the 'tempo' rather than the 'quantum' of child bearing. If women start delaying their fertility but 'catch up' later, there will be a divergence between cohort and period measures, as the latter will be based partly on the behaviour of earlier cohorts whose timing of births was different (Cooper 1991). Similarly, if women have children earlier, total fertility rates will rise, even if eventual family sizes remain unchanged. Crises of various kinds may also produce large tempo effects. In many central and eastern European states fertility rates have fallen precipitously since 1990, but couples may 'make up' these births if conditions improve. For this reason, many statistical offices have used cohort measures of fertility as the basis for projections rather than period ones. Although apparently a technical matter, considerable controversy surrounds this issue, particularly in France where it has inspired front-page articles in *Le Monde* and acrimonious resignations of demographers. This reflects a long-standing French pronatalist tradition and concern about low fertility. In this context it is vital to know whether recent trends in fertility, as measured by total fertility rates, are partly an artefactual result of changes in the timing of births or whether they really indicate a change in final family size.

More sophisticated measures of fertility include parity progression ratios. These indicate the probability of proceeding from one birth to another (for example, what proportion of mothers with two children progress to having a third). Parity progression ratios are normally calculated for cohorts who have completed, or nearly completed, their child bearing. However, it is also possible to use data on births by birth order to derive period, rather than cohort, progression ratios (Feeney and Yu 1987). Summary information on measures of fertility and reproduction are summarized in Boxes 1 and 2.

Marriage patterns have a major influence on fertility, and upsurges and downturns in marriage are associated with lagged upsurges and downturns in births. Where possible, demographers have often preferred to calculate age-specific marital fertility rates (and total fertility rates and other measures) on the grounds that the unmarried population is not 'at risk' (or at very reduced risk) of child bearing.

Box 1 Fertility measures

Definitions

Fertility: the child-bearing performance of individuals, couples, or populations.

Fecundity: the physiological capability of producing a live birth.

Parity: the number of children previously born alive (or sometimes number of previous confinements) to a woman or couple. Nulliparous women are those who have borne no children.

Measures

Crude birth rate (CBR): the ratio of births in a year (other specified period) to the average population in the same year/period (mid-year population), expressed per 1000.

$$\text{CBR} = \frac{\text{number of births}}{\text{mid-year population}} \times 1000.$$

General fertility rate (GFR): births to women aged 15–44/49 in a year/period per 1000 women aged 15–44/49 in the same period.

$$\text{GFR} = \frac{\text{number of births to women 15–44/49}}{\text{mid-year population of women aged 15-44/49}} \times 1000.$$

Age-specific fertility rate (ASFR): number of births to women aged x (or x to $x + n$) per 1000 women aged x (or x to $x + n$) where n is the length of an age interval. ASFRs are frequently calculated for 5-year age groups from 15–19 to 40–44 or 45–49.

$$\text{ASFR} = \frac{\text{number of births to women aged } x}{\text{mid-year population of women aged } x} \times 1000.$$

Total (period) fertility rate (TFR/TPFR): the sum of the age-specific fertility rates for all reproductive age groups for a particular period (usually a year), conventionally expressed per woman. The TFR indicates how many children a woman would have if throughout her reproductive life, she had children at the age-specific rates prevalent in the specified year or period.

$$\text{TFR} = \sum_{x=15}^{45-49} fx$$

where fx is the age-specific fertility rate at age x. If rates for age groups, rather than single years, are used then the sum of the age-specific rates must be multiplied by the number of single ages included in the group (usually 5).

$$\text{TFR} = 5 \times \sum_{x=15-19}^{45-49} fx.$$

Parity progression ratio: the probability of a women of parity x progressing to parity $x + 1$.

Sources: various; see Pressat and Wilson (1985) which provides a valuable guide to demographic terms and issues.

Changes in marital fertility indicative of deliberate attempts to limit family size are regarded as one of the defining features of the fertility 'transition' (see below) and so distinguishing these from changes due to variations in the 'at risk' (married population) has been particularly emphasized. However, in a growing number of populations, rises in non-marital child bearing mean that restricting analyses to marital fertility is no longer appropriate.

Box 2 Reproduction ratios

Measures

Gross reproduction rate (GRR): the sum of the age-specific female fertility rates (births of daughters), for all reproductive age groups for a particular period (usually a year) conventionally expressed per woman. The GRR indicates how many daughters a woman would have if, throughout her reproductive life, she had children at the age-specific rates prevalent in the specified year of period. The GRR can be calculated either by summing female age-specific fertility rates (relating to births of daughters rather than all births) or using the formula

$$\text{GRR} = \text{TFR} \times \text{proportion of female births}.$$

The proportion of female births can be taken as 0.488 (100/205) in the absence of more detailed information.

Net reproduction rate (NRR): the average number of daughters that would be borne, according to specified rates of mortality and of bearing daughters, by a woman subject through life to these rates. The NRR employs the same fertility data as the GRR, but also takes into account the effects of mortality. An NRR of 1.0 indicates that a population's fertility and mortality levels would result in exact replacement of mothers by daughters.

Reproduction rates

In the long term, populations will grow if mothers replace themselves with one or more (surviving) daughters and decline if they fail to achieve this. Theoretically, it would also be possible to measure the replacement of fathers by sons, but in practice the difficulties involved in obtaining paternity data make this unfeasible. Reproduction rates thus relate only to female fertility—that is, births of daughters. The gross reproduction rate is derived in exactly the same way as the total fertility rate except that age-specific birth rates based only on births of daughters are used in the calculation. The net reproduction rate makes an allowance for mortality—specifically the chance that a daughter will survive to the age her mother was when she was born. The net reproduction rate cannot be calculated unless both age-specific fertility and mortality data are available (although it can be approximated using the gross reproduction rate and appropriate life table survival data). Changes in either fertility or mortality (or both) will mean a divergence between period measures (based on the experience of a hypothetical cohort) and the experiences of real cohorts.

Measurement of mortality

As for fertility, the simplest measure of mortality is the crude mortality rate, deaths per 1000 population. However, as noted above, this is strongly influenced by age structure, and age- and sex-specific rates, or measures based on them, which are much preferred if data are available to calculate them. As in epidemiology, both direct and indirect standardization are sometimes used to make comparisons between populations with different age and sex structures. Standardized mortality ratios, which are frequently used to compare, for example, mortality in different regions of countries, are calculated using indirect standardization. This involves selecting a set of 'standard' age-specific mortality rates, for example those for a national population, and applying these to the numbers of people in the relevant age groups in the subpopulation of interest, for example the population of a particular region. This yields an 'expected' number of deaths—the number of deaths there would be in the subpopulation if age-specific death rates were the same as those in the standard population. The ratio of observed to expected deaths, conventionally multiplied by 100, gives the standardized mortality ratio. Thus, for example, a standardized mortality ratio of 124 indicates that mortality in the subpopulation is 24 per cent higher than in the standard population, allowing for age differences. Standardized mortality ratios are useful summary measures of differences in mortality, but they give no indication of the level of mortality.

Age-specific death rates are calculated using the numbers of deaths at age x (or between ages x and $x + n$) in a particular year as the numerator and the mid-year population of the same age as the denominator. The rate derived is conventionally expressed per 1000 or per 100 000 population. In this calculation, the mid-year population is used as a measure of the average population at risk on the assumption that deaths are evenly distributed throughout the year. However, for some age groups, notably infants, this assumption is invalid. In developed countries deaths in the first 3 days of life may account for half or more of all deaths in the first year of life. Moreover, information on the size of population aged less than 1 year normally comes from birth data (as in nine out of ten years relevant census data will not be available). For these reasons live births in a particular year are conventionally used as the denominator of the infant mortality rate while deaths to infants aged less than 1 year constitute the numerator. Some infants dying in a given year will have been born in the previous year and some born in the year in question will die the following year. This can cause distortions if there are large annual fluctuations in numbers of births (or infant deaths) and often 3-year averages are preferred.

Infant mortality rates were very high in some parts of historical Europe (300 or even 400 deaths per 1000 live births in regions of Russia and Germany at the end of the nineteenth century (van de Walle 1986)). In England and Wales, where declines in infant mortality came later than declines in other age groups, the infant mortality rate at the start of the twentieth century stood at some 140 infant deaths per 1000 live births and a third of all deaths occurred among those under 5 years of age. Infant mortality in contemporary developed countries is now extremely low—fewer than five infant deaths per 1000 live births in Sweden, Norway, Finland, and Singapore. There have also been huge falls in infant mortality in much of the developing world, but rates remain high—well over 100 deaths per 1000 live births in parts of sub-Saharan Africa.

Variations on this kind of scale have a very substantial demographic impact. Infant mortality has also attracted particular research interest because of hypothesized and observed links with fertility behaviour and as an indicator of public health standards and conditions. Particularly in this latter context, perinatal, early and late neonatal and postneonatal mortality rates are often distinguished where data allow (Box 3). A further refinement is to try and distinguish 'endogenous' mortality (from congenital malfunctions and birth trauma) from 'exogenous' causes which are more amenable to intervention.

Box 3 Mortality measures

Measures

Crude death rate: the ratio of deaths in a year (other specified period) to average population in the same year/period (mid-year population), expressed per 1000.

$$\text{CDR} = \frac{\text{number of deaths}}{\text{mid-year population}} \times 1000.$$

Age-specific mortality rate(ASMR): number of deaths to persons aged x (or x to $x + n$) per 1000 persons aged x (or to $x + n$).

$$\text{ASMR} = \frac{\text{deaths to persons aged } x}{\text{mid-year population of persons aged } x} \times 1000.$$

Standardized mortality ratio (SMR): the ratio (× 100) of observed to expected deaths in a study population. Expected deaths are calculated by applying a set of standard age-specific mortality rates to the age distribution of the study population. Standardized ratios are only useful for comparisons. They have no intrinsic meaning.

$$\text{SMR} = 100\,\frac{\Sigma r_i = \text{observed}}{\Sigma n_i P_i = \text{expected}}.$$

Infant mortality rate (IMR):

$$\text{IMR} = \frac{\text{number of deaths to infants aged} <1 \text{ year in year } x}{\text{number of live births in year } x} \times 1000.$$

This is sometimes decomposed into neonatal mortality rates (deaths of live born infants during the first 4 weeks) and postneonatal mortality (from 4 to 52 weeks). The perinatal mortality rate measures late fetal deaths (stillbirths) and early neonatal deaths relative to live births.

Perintal mortality rate =

$$\frac{\text{stillbirths} + \text{deaths under 1 week}}{\text{stillbirths} + \text{livebirths}} \times 1000$$

Stillbirths used to refer to deaths of fetuses of 28 or more weeks gestation; however, an earlier threshold of 24 weeks is now more generally used.

Life tables

Life-table analysis is a core demographic technique and life tables provide one of the most powerful tools for analysing mortality and other non-renewable processes.

Life tables are derived from age-specific mortality rates and show the probability of dying (and surviving) between specified ages. They also allow the calculation of various other indicators, including expectation of life. If complete data on the mortality of a birth cohort are available, then a cohort life table may be constructed. However, the use of cohort life tables is obviously only possible retrospectively. More commonly period mortality rates, based on mortality rates at a particular time, are calculated. These life tables show death (and survival) probabilities for a hypothetical cohort with an arbitrary radix (number of babies at the beginning) usually set to 10 000, 100 000 or some other multiple of 100.

Specific notation is used in life-table analysis; this is summarized in Box 4. The basis of the table is a set of probabilities of dying, ${}_nq_x$, where x refers to age at the start of an interval whose length is specified by n. Thus ${}_5q_{50}$ refers to the probability of someone alive at 50 dying between age 50 and age 55. The complement of ${}_nq_x$—the probability of surviving—is denoted ${}_np_x$. The (hypothetical) number of survivors at each age is given by l_x; thus l_0 equals the radix (of 100 000) and l_{75} the number of survivors at age 75. The number of person years lived in an interval (${}_nL_x$) and the total number of person years lived after a particular age (T_x) are often not shown in published tables but are steps on the way to the calculation of e_x, life expectancy at age x.

This indicator of survival is very frequently used and provides a measure of the level of mortality which is very largely independent of the age structure of the population. This makes it more useful than either a standardized mortality ratio (which gives no indication of level) or a crude death rate (which is strongly influenced by age structure). Life expectancy either at birth (e_0) or further life expectancy at a particular age, say 65 (e_{65}), is calculated by dividing total person-years lived after age 0 or 65 (T_0 or T_{65}) and dividing it by the number of survivors aged 0 (l_0) or 65 (l_{65}). Methods of calculation are given in all standard textbooks. The level of infant mortality is a powerful influence on e_0 (as so many potential person-years are lost through an infant death). In high mortality populations e_0—mean age at death—varies substantially from the median age at death. In Mozambique and Sierra Leone, for example, median age at death in 1990 was only 2, compared with an average (mean) life expectancy of 43 and 38 respectively. In low-mortality populations the correspondence between the two is much closer; in Sweden and Japan in 1990 life expectancy at birth and median age at death were both 78 (World Bank 1993).

Model life tables

Patterns of age-specific death rates show certain similarities whatever the level of mortality. Death rates tend to be higher in infancy than later childhood and rise with age from around the age of puberty. Because of the tendency for death rates at one age to be associated with death rates at other ages in a given population, it is possible to derive hypothetical schedules, called model life tables, describing variations in mortality by age and sex, normally in terms of a limited number of parameters which allow for particular features of the mortality pattern of the population considered. Model life tables are derived from empirical data from countries where these are available. They are extremely useful aids for the estimation of mortality by age in populations with defective data. They are also used (in conjunction with fertility data) to show the outcomes of particular fertility and mortality regimes on, for example, population age structure. All demographic texts give further details of their derivation and application.

Box 4 Life-table measures and notation

x = age attained last birthday

l_x = *number of survivors at age x*, so l_{65} is the number of people alive at age 65 in the hypothetical life-table population

l_0 = the radix of the life table (hypothetical number of babies), usually 100 000

${}_nq_x$ = *probability of dying between age x and x + n*, so ${}_4q_1$ is the probability of dying between age 1 and 5 years for a person aged 1

${}_nP_x$ = *probability of surviving between ages x and x + n*, so ${}_{20}P_{65}$ is the probability of surviving from age 65 to 85 years for a person aged 65

${}_nD_x$ = *number of deaths between age x and x + n*

${}_nL_x$ = *number of person years lived between x and x + n*

T_x = *total number of person years lived after age x*

e^0_{0x} = *expectation of life at age x*, so e^0_0 is expectation of life at birth

Other applications of life table analysis

Life tables are an essential part of much demographic analysis (including, for example, making population projections) and are widely used to analyse events other than death. The oft-quoted figure that one in three marriages in England and Wales will end in divorce is based on life-table analysis of age- and duration-specific divorce probabilities in the mid-1980s (Haskey 1988); more recent work suggests a higher proportion. Life-table methods are also used to measure contraceptive use failure rates and contraceptive use discontinuation rates.

Multiple decrement life tables allow 'decrements' from more than one event—for example different causes of death. Cause elimination life tables are also used to identify the 'pure' severity of a particular cause of death. Multistate models allow analysis of a range of transitions, particularly those where re-entries into a particular state, such as being married or living in a certain region, are possible. These more sophisticated applications require more detailed data.

Measurement of migration

In many countries migration is the predominant influence on the spatial distribution of the population. In the developing and newly industrialized world, recent rural to urban migration has resulted in the phenomenal growth of cities, often lacking the infrastructure to meet the needs of the expanding population for basic services such as sanitation and power. In Brazil, for example, three-quarters of the population in 1991 lived in urban areas and 36 per cent of the total population were in cities with more than a million inhabitants. In 1965 the equivalent proportions were 56 and 24 per cent respectively (World Bank 1993).

In the older developed world, by contrast, urbanization has been succeeded by 'counter-urbanization' involving migration from cities to suburbs or beyond. One result has been a growing concentration of those unable to move (the old and disadvantaged) in inner-city areas.

Measuring migration represents particular difficulties. Some of these arise from problems of definition. The classical definition of internal migration is 'a permanent or semi-permanent move across an administrative boundary' (UN 1970). Use of this definition excludes the large volume of movement which takes place within administrative areas—often termed residential mobility—although in many contexts knowing about this may be very important. Use of this definition also means that the extent of migration recorded depends partly on the size of administrative area considered. In a country divided into many small areas a move of over 5 km will count as migration, while in countries divided into few larger ones a move of over 500 km may not. This means that international comparison of internal migration rates is potentially misleading. Even the distinction between international (between country) and internal (within country) migration may be problematic if boundaries are contested or changing. The temporal dimension to migration presents further difficulties. What constitutes permanent or semi-permanent and how should groups such as seasonal migrants be treated?

The reason for defining migration as a move over a boundary is largely a pragmatic one. Often only moves of this kind are recorded; moreover this is the form of data required by the primary users—local administrations. For research purposes, however, analyses of all moves (preferably with an indication of distance moved) may often be preferred. Some countries have registration systems ('population registers') in which changes of address or moves between districts are recorded (although with varying completeness and immediacy). More commonly censuses are used to find out about migration. Questions on usual address 1 or 5 years ago allow the proportion of movers in the population to be measured (except for those aged less than 1 or 5 years). These data also allow gross flows—inflows and outflows—between pairs of areas to be measured. Moves, as opposed to movers, are not, however, directly measured as someone moving several times in the reference period cannot be distinguished from someone moving only once. Those leaving an address and later returning to it cannot be identified either. This means that the length of the reference period used is important; the proportion of migrants in the 5 years preceding a census will not equal five times the proportion moving in 1 year before the same census.

In the absence of direct census data, estimates of migration can be made indirectly using the 'balancing equation' referred to below. Differences in the size of a population at two points in time (censuses) not accounted for by natural increase or depletion must be due to migration (or errors in the data). If good vital registration data are available, then both births and deaths can be taken into account. If they are lacking, then the survival of groups enumerated in the first of a pair of censuses must be estimated from a life table and the number of expected survivors compared with the number enumerated in the second census (obviously ageing must be allowed for, so the number of 20- to 29-year-olds in the first census will be compared with 30- to 39-year-olds 10 years later). These methods only allow estimation of net migration (balance between in-migration and out-migration). Their major weakness lies in the fact that the residual population balance assumed to be due to migration may in fact reflect differences in the quality of the two censuses considered or errors in the estimates of survival used.

Survey data are also used to measure migration and potentially provide illuminating information on the reasons for, and consequences of, migration. However, as migration over long distances is a relatively rare event, even large samples may yield relatively few such migrants. A similar problem besets samples of international travellers, such as the United Kingdom International Passenger Survey, designed to estimate flows of international migrants through port or border surveys. Tourists and business travellers comprise the vast bulk of people entering or leaving so surveys are an inefficient way of identifying immigrants and emigrants. Unfortunately, other data are often lacking as legal and administrative record systems are frequently concerned with citizenship and right of abode rather than international migration *per se* (and virtually never with emigration).

At the local level, migration flows may be the predominant influence on population size. Migrants differ from non-migrants so migration has a potentially strong impact on population structure and characteristics. Migration also has a role in determining exposures to new infections. The stresses of migration on the migrant, on those left behind, and possibly on those in the area of destination also indicate that migration is an important element to take account of in health planning. However, both the quality and the timeliness of routinely available migration data may make this difficult.

Population projections

Population projections represent one of the most widely used outputs of demographic analysis. Strictly speaking, a projection simply represents the outcome of applying various assumptions about future fertility, mortality and migration and so differs from a forecast, which implies prediction. However, projections are often treated as forecasts and the degree of uncertainty inherent in them is not always sufficiently acknowledged. The most common method of projection is the component method, based on the balancing equation

$$P_t = P_0 + B - D + I - E$$

where P_t is the population at an end of period, P_0 is the population at the beginning of a period, and B, D, I, and E represent births, deaths, immigrations, and emigrations during the same period (that is, net migration). Population subgroups may be similarly defined in terms of entries and exits. Entry to the population aged 75 to 84 years is through ageing (passage from 74 to 75); exit is through further ageing (84 to 85) or death. Although very straightforward, this simple accounting equation is an important one, both methodologically and as a formal reminder of the need to consider past as well as current events.

When making projections, assumptions are made about the three components of change—births, deaths, and migration—and applied to age and sex groups within the initial population to give a projection of future size and structure. To a large extent assumptions are based on recent trends together with other information on, for example, survey data on fertility intentions or (sometimes) models of change in particular causes of death. Forecasting fertility is generally regarded as the most problematic area of population projection; projections of the future population size of the United Kingdom varied widely during the period 1955–1974 when birth rates first rose and then fell. Recently greater attention has also been paid to the errors that have been made in forecasting mortality in developed countries. This has little effect on age groups in which survival is high, but can have quite substantial impacts on forecasts of the number of elderly people (Murphy 1995). At the subnational level migration is an important, and sometimes quite volatile, element which is difficult to predict, especially by those in central statistical offices lacking local knowledge.

International migration is also difficult to deal with because it is affected by policies and events outside the country for which the projection is being made and is often a sensitive political issue. Patterns may vary hugely—witness recent mass movements of refugees. Within the larger countries of Europe, Switzerland has the highest proportion of 'foreign' residents—19 per cent in 1997—and 60 per cent of Swiss population growth in the past 15 years has been due to net immigration. In 1993 over two-thirds of (net) immigrants came from former Yugoslavia (UN ECE 1994; Council of Europe 1999). In many other Western European countries, particularly Germany and the United Kingdom, rates of immigration increased during the 1980s and, as in Switzerland, have contributed significantly to population growth (Coleman and Chandola 1999).

Population dynamics

Any population comprises those who have made an entry and not yet exited. When whole populations of defined geographical areas are considered, the only means of entry are birth or immigration and the only means of exit are death or emigration.

Analyses of multiple transitions are rather more complex. The married population, for example, comprises those who have married and not yet died or been widowed or divorced. While being born, dying, or passing from one age to another are unrepeatable events, multiple entries and exits to the state of being married are possible, necessitating the use of multistate models.

Of the three demographic determinants of population size, structure, and growth, fertility is nearly always of much greater importance than either mortality or migration. Every birth represents not just an addition to the current generation of children, but also potentially an exponentially increasing augmentation in the size of future generations. Death carries no such promise of future return, at least in this world. The third demographic determinant—migration—is generally not of significant magnitude to have a major impact on national populations, although there are exceptions. At the subnational level, however, migration may have a very important effect.

For social and biological reasons fertility, mortality, and migration have interactive effects. Decreases in mortality among those with reproductive potential, for example, influence not just the size of the age group affected at the time, but also the size of succeeding generations. Werner (1987) has estimated that, had the 1841 female birth cohort in England and Wales suffered only negligible mortality before the age of 45 years, children born to the cohort would have averaged nearly five per woman as compared with the three per woman (in the original birth cohort) actually achieved.

Declines in male mortality, particularly in populations where large age differences between spouses are common and remarriage of widows is rare, will similarly tend to increase fertility by effectively increasing the proportion of women of reproductive age who are still married. Conversely, reductions in fertility clearly reduce the risk of maternal mortality and may have further positive effects on the survival of mothers, infants, or both. Child bearing at very young ages (under 18 years of age) or old ages (over 35 years of age) and short birth intervals (less than 18 months) all have particular risks (Hobcraft 1991), so a reduction in fertility involving less early or late child bearing and longer birth intervals will have particular benefits. Average age at motherhood also influences rates of population growth. The average age of mothers at the birth of their daughters is termed the mean length of a generation and is generally around 29 years. A shorter interval will mean more rapid generational succession (and so faster population growth), while a longer one will have the opposite effect.

Migration has an effect on both the other demographic parameters because migrants differ from the general population. International migrants are generally young and in good health and often may move from relatively high fertility populations to low fertility populations. As a result immigrants may serve to (temporarily) 'rejuvenate' the host population and, at least initially, have higher fertility and lower mortality. In the United Kingdom, for example, in the mid-1980s the total fertility rate for women born in Bangladesh or Pakistan was 5.6, compared with 2.9 for women born in India and 1.8 in the population as a whole (Shaw 1988). In England and Wales, age-standardized mortality ratios for most immigrant groups are below 100 (that is, below average) although the Irish and Scots have above-average mortality. Standardized mortality ratios have also been shown to be raised among second-generation Irish in England, in contrast with the more usual pattern whereby migrant groups in time take on the mortality and morbidity characteristics of the host population (Balarajan and Bulusu 1990).

For these reasons the demographic characteristics of population subgroups largely comprising immigrants and their immediate descendants may vary substantially from those of the population as a whole. The length of the interval since the main period of migration is also important. In Great Britain in 1995 to 1997, for example, over 40 per cent of the population of Bangladeshi origin was aged under 15 and only 5 per cent were aged 60 or over. This reflects both the relatively high fertility of British women born in Bangladesh, but also the fact that half of all immigrants from Bangladesh had migrated since 1975 (Schuman 1999).

Population growth

Population growth is obviously a function of the balance of births and deaths and the extent of net migration. Changes in the size of a population produced by the surplus (or deficit) of births over deaths are termed natural increase (or decrease). A common indicator of growth is the crude rate of natural increase—the difference between the crude birth rate (annual births per 1000 population) and the crude death rate (annual deaths per 1000 population). If net migration is zero, this will be the same as the growth rate of the population—the overall annual change in the population divided by the population size—(conventionally expressed as a percentage). Many populations in Europe have had fertility rates below the level required for long-term replacement for 20 years or more, yet in most cases births still outnumber deaths (exceptions are Italy, Germany, and Sweden) (Council of Europe 1998). This apparent paradox largely reflects the fact that the number of births is a function of the number of potential mothers, as well as of their fertility patterns. If the former is increasing so too may the numbers of births, even if women have fewer children each.

The young age structures of many populations in the developing world mean that these populations have a huge built-in potential for growth. Most sub-Saharan African populations are expected to double in size between 1995 and 2015, despite the devastating impact of HIV/AIDS mortality (UN 1999). Population momentum is the measure which gives the ratio of the ultimate size a given population would achieve to current population size if fertility were to fall immediately to replacement level.

Intrinsic rate of natural increase: stable population theory

Early in the twentieth century Lotka (1907) demonstrated mathematically that a population closed to migration and subject to unchanging age-specific fertility and mortality rates for a long period would eventually have a fixed age structure (in which the proportion in each age group remained unchanged) and would grow at a constant rate. This type of population is called a stable population. The fixed age structure of a stable population is independent of the initial age structure—two very different populations subject to the same unchanging rates for a long period would eventually assume the same structure. A particular variant of a stable population is a stationary population—one in which birth and death rates are constant and in balance and so population growth is zero. The L_x column of the life table is an example of a stationary population. The number of births is fixed (the radix) and the age distribution is also fixed. In non-stationary stable populations the age structure is also fixed but the size of every age group is growing at the same constant rate as the overall population and the number of births. This is called the intrinsic rate of natural increase and is a function of the net reproduction rate and the mean length of a generation (approximated by the mean age of child bearing). Non-stationary stable populations can be calculated by adjusting the L_x values of a particular life table to allow for the intrinsic rate of growth. These are often published in conjunction with model life tables to show the effects of particular (unchanging) fertility and mortality regimes (Coale and Guo 1989).

Although stable and stationary populations are theoretical constructs, real populations at various times have met the model requirements closely enough to allow stable population theory to be used to develop methods for indirectly estimating fertility and mortality in populations lacking adequate directly derived data. Stable population models are also widely used for insurance, pension, and personnel planning.

Age structure

One of the most important results of the work of Lotka and his successors (Coale 1957) was to show theoretically that fertility is the predominant influence on age structure. This has also been demonstrated empirically (Carrier 1962). High fertility populations such as those of contemporary developing countries (Fig. 5) have a pyramid shape with each successive cohort being larger than its predecessor. 'Old' populations, such as that of England and Wales (Fig. 6), are more rectangular in structure with a gradual tapering at the top. This difference is the result of sustained downward trends in fertility which reduce the proportion of children in more recently born cohorts in the population and so lead to a corresponding increase in the proportion of older people (survivors of larger cohorts). Historically, and apparently paradoxically, improvements in mortality in those populations which now have high proportions of old people in fact served to offset the trend towards population ageing, as they chiefly benefited the young—and led to increases in the proportions surviving to have children themselves. Population pyramids graphically illustrate both the future and the past of populations. The structure of the Russian, Estonian, and Ukrainian populations, for example, shows the legacy of high male mortality in the Second World War, and high mortality in both sexes during the collectivist period. Wars and other crises affect births as well as deaths. The 1998 populations of Russia and the Ukraine show severe indentations at age 50 to 54 years, reflecting low fertility and high numbers of infant deaths during the period of collectivization, famine, and purges in the 1930s, and further indentation around age 45 years reflecting low fertility during the Second World War (Velkoff and Kinsella 1993). Bulges in population pyramids due to high numbers of births have 'echo' effects when members of large cohorts themselves have children.

Although fertility has the greatest potential impact on age structure and population growth, in some circumstances mortality may become a more important influence. Many populations in developed countries now have fertility at or below the level required for long-term replacement, average expectations of life at birth of 75 years or more, and near universal survival to the end of the (female) reproductive span. In these demographic conditions, further improvements in

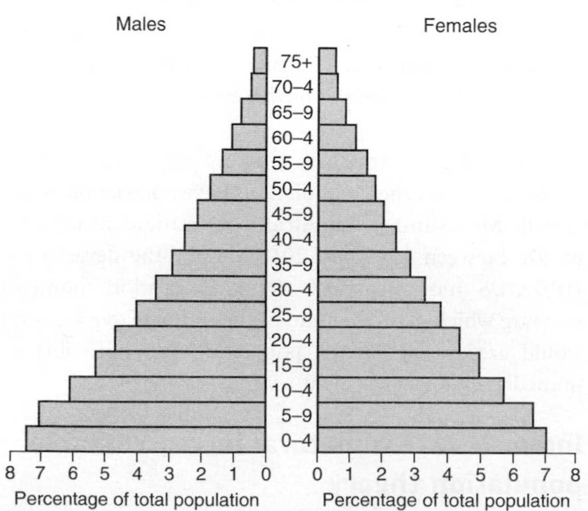

Fig. 5 Population pyramids for a less developed country (Egypt, 1992). (Source: *United Nations Demographic Yearbook* 1994.)

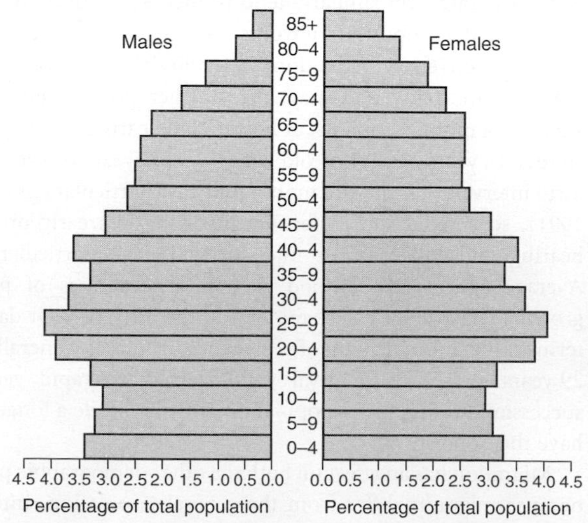

Fig. 6 Population pyramids for developed countries (England and Wales, 1991). (Source: *United Nations Demographic Yearbook* 1994.)

Table 2 Life table estimates of survivorship in England and Wales, 1970 to 1972 and 1994 to 1996

Percentage surviving at age	Males		Females	
	1970–72	1994–96	1970–72	1994–96
5	97.7	99.2	98.2	99.4
25	96.4	98.3	97.6	99.0
45	95.8	95.4	95.4	97.5
65	70.4	81.2	82.4	88.2
85	11.4	22.0	27.2	39.6

Source: OPCS/ONS Mortality Statistics, DHI No. 24 (1992) and No. 29 (1998).

mortality have the greatest impact at old ages and further population ageing occurs from the apex, rather than, or as well as from, the base of the population pyramid. Mortality changes are now the main motor of the further ageing of the populations of a number of developed countries with already old age structures (Preston *et al.* 1989). Recent changes in mortality at older ages have been quite substantial in a number of developed countries. Table 2 shows life-table survivorship based on period mortality data from England and Wales in the early 1970s and mid-1990s. The mortality rates of the latter period imply survival to age 85 years for 40 per cent of women. Moreover, changes in survivorship between the two periods were greater at older ages than at younger, and mortality at young ages is now so low that there is little scope for demographically important further change.

Population ageing is now a major issue in the developed world and a subdiscipline of demography focusing on the demography of ageing has emerged. Population ageing is also rising high on the agenda in a number of recently industrialized and some developing countries. In these latter populations the pace of demographic change has been much faster than occurred historically in the Western world. As a result, the pace of population ageing has also accelerated. The proportion of the Japanese population aged 65 years of age or over increased from 7 per cent in 1970 to nearly 16 per cent in 1997. In France a similar increase took 130 years to achieve. The origins of these age structure changes lie in the demographic transition.

The demographic transition

Towards the end of the nineteenth century (earlier in France) both birth and death rates started falling in a number of Western countries. Long-term trends in fertility and in the proportion of women in certain age groups ever married in England and Wales are shown in Table 3. It can be seen that between 1871–1875 and 1911–1915 the total fertility rate dropped from 4.8 to 2.8; by the early 1930s it was below replacement level, a development which was viewed with alarm and led to the first Royal Commission on Population. Although modern methods of contraception were lacking, it was clear that this huge drop in fertility was the result of the deliberate limitation of family size. Half of all couples married in the 1870s had six or more children compared with 12 per cent of couples married in 1911/1915 (Coleman and Salt 1992). Expectation of life at birth meanwhile increased by some 15 years between the end of the nineteenth century and the early 1930s. Gains were greatest at young ages and greater for women than for men.

Scholars attempting to understand these profound changes sought to relate changes in demographic regimes to changes in the economic and social environment and so originated the theory of the demographic transition. The 'classical' view propounded by Notestein (1945) and others was that in 'traditional' societies fertility and mortality are both high and roughly in balance. Change is driven by

Table 3 Long term trends in fertility (TFRs) and marriage (percentage of 20–24 and 35–39 year old women ever-married), England and Wales

Years	TFR	Percentage of women in age group ever-married		
		Year	20–24	35–39
1871–75	4.8			
1901–05	3.5	1901	27	80
1921–25	2.4	1921	27	80
1931–35	1.8	1931		
1951–55	2.2	1951	48	87
1961–65	2.8	1961	58	90
1971–75	2.1	1971	60	93
1981–85	1.8	1981	46	94
1991	1.8	1991	25	90
1998	1.7	1997	14	86

Sources: OPCS (1987); Coleman and Salt (1992); ONS (1999*a,b*).

One result of growing scientific knowledge is the greater potential importance of public policy and education. Historical research suggests that in the nineteenth century differences in child mortality by level of mother's education or standard of living were slight, while in contemporary developing countries they are marked. Countries such as Sri Lanka which have vigorously pursued public health programmes and achieved high levels of education, have attained particularly marked gains in life expectancy. In the developed world differentials in health-related behaviour are also strongly associated with income and education. In England, for example, some 40 per cent of men in households headed by an unskilled worker smoke cigarettes, compared with 12 per cent of men from professional groups (Prescott-Clarke and Primatesta 1997). It has also been argued that societal factors—such as the extent of income inequalities and degree of social cohesion—may account for some of the differences between developed countries in the overall level of mortality (Wilkinson 1996).

The process of the epidemiological transition (or at least the initial phases) is now complete or under way in much of the world. Non-communicable causes of death now predominate not just in the developed world, but also in Latin America and East and Southeast Asia and are projected to become increasingly important elsewhere.

Gender differentials

Changes in gender differentials in mortality are a major component of the epidemiological transition. Figure 7 shows sex ratios in mortality rates by age for England and Wales in 1901 and 1997. It can be seen that the extent of female advantage was considerably greater in 1997 and most marked in young adulthood and late middle age. Although the former peak is more pronounced, the latter (and continuing differential in old age) is much more important demographically, as death rates are much higher at these older ages. In north-western European populations, such as those in England and Wales, The Netherlands, Denmark, Sweden, Norway, and Switzerland, about half the gender difference in life expectancy at birth is due to differences among those aged 65 years or more. In much of Eastern Europe, where sex differentials in mortality are greatest, the age pattern is rather different. Countries such as Hungary and Poland show a smaller decline from the 20- to 24-year-old peak in sex ratios of mortality and a greater proportion of the overall difference in life expectancy at birth is due to gender differences among 35- to 44-year-olds than is the case in Western Europe (UN Secretariat 1988; Velkoff and Kinsella 1993).

In all developed and the great majority of developing countries, female life expectancy is now greater than male (Fig. 8), but there is considerable variation in the extent of this difference. Low-mortality countries generally have larger sex differences in life expectancies than high-mortality populations, reflecting the association between falls in mortality and an increasing female advantage. Waldron (1985), in a review of this topic, pointed to changes in the intrahousehold allocation of resources, declines in causes of death specifically or primarily affecting women (such as maternal mortality and respiratory tuberculosis), gender differences in health-related behaviour and in exposure to occupational hazards, and the possibly greater

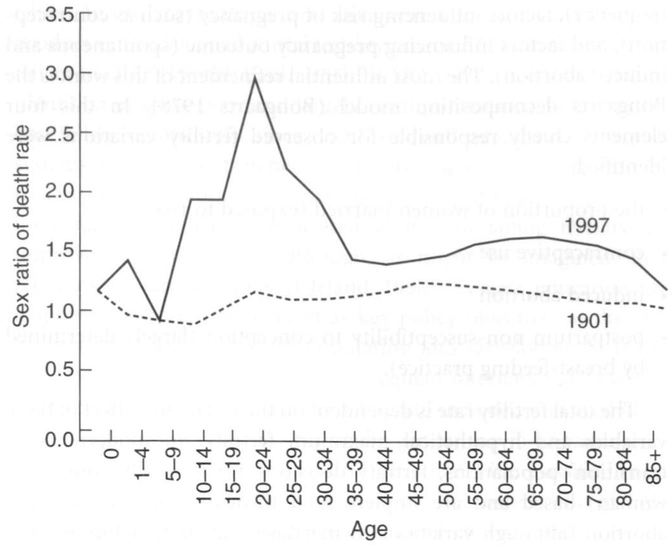

Fig. 7 Sex ratios of death rates (males/females) by age in England and Wales, 1901 and 1997. (Data from UN 1988; ONS 1997.)

susceptibility of men to stresses associated with socio-economic changes, as causal factors.

In a few developing countries, such as Bangladesh, Pakistan, and Iran, the female advantage in mortality is either very slight or non-existent. The low status of females and consequent inequitable distribution of resources is partly thought to account for this. A more

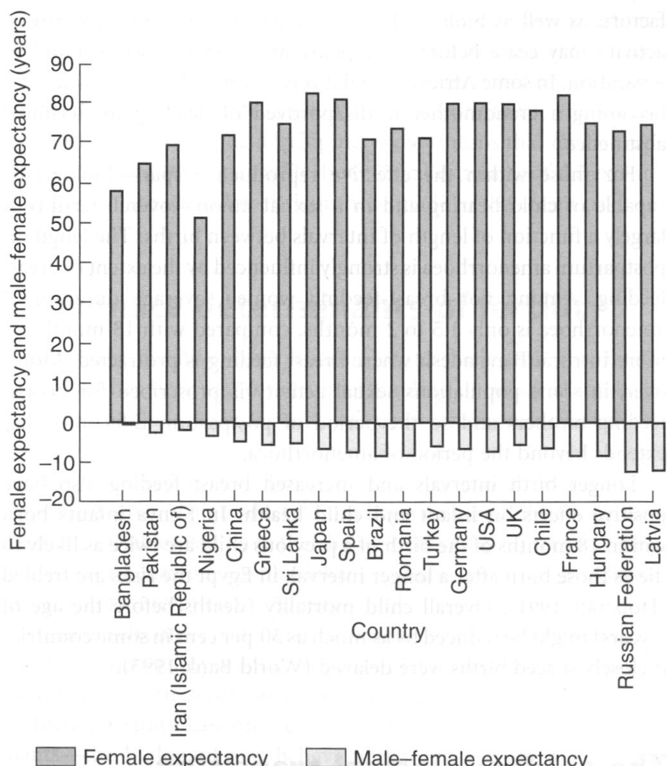

Fig. 8 Female life expectancy at birth (e_0) and male disadvantage in e_0, selected countries, 1995–2000. (Data from UN 1999.)

extreme example of discrimination against females—female infanticide—has been alleged to account for the biologically implausible sex ratio of infants and children in China. This allegation is highly controversial and may reflect girls being 'hidden' from officials by couples anxious for the chance of having a son (Zeng *et al.* 1993). While the extent of sex-selective infanticide is disputed, recent trends in sex ratios at birth in countries with strong preferences for male offspring and small families, such as China and the Republic of Korea, are clearly indicative of sex-selective abortion. The future demographic and social implications of this are a growing area of concern (Zeng *et al.* 1993; Coale and Bannister 1999).

In Western developed countries a large proportion of the sex differential in life expectancy at birth is due to differences in ischaemic heart disease (well over a third in Britain, Sweden, and Finland), lung cancer (5 to 15 per cent), and accidents and violence (10 to 20 per cent) (UN Secretariat 1988). The twentieth-century epidemic of smoking and attendant smoking-related diseases is undoubtedly a major cause of gender differences in death. In some populations, including England, Wales, Italy, and the United States, there are recent signs of a reduction in the extent of female advantage in life expectancy (Kinsella and Gist 1998; UN Secretariat 1988). This may partially reflect the narrowing of differentials in exposure to tobacco as cohorts including larger proportions of female smokers reach later life. In the United States, age-adjusted death rates from respiratory cancer increased by over 400 per cent for white females aged 65 years or more between 1960 and 1986, while among white males the increase was 115 per cent (Furner *et al.* 1993). However, in other countries with very high overall life expectancy such as Japan, France, and Germany, gains in female longevity continue to outpace those of males.

Particularly in Eastern Europe, alcohol is also a factor contributing to gender differentials in mortality. As discussed further below, in contrast to the experience of many Western developed nations, male mortality has stagnated or deteriorated in much of Eastern Europe in recent decades; in Russia the crude death rate increased by over a third between 1989 and 1993 (Shapiro 1994) and male life expectancy at birth dropped to 56 in 1994 (WHO 1998). In the former Soviet Union, however, there was a sharp drop in mortality, particularly among men, in 1986 to 1987 (unfortunately, since reversed). This has been attributed to measures introduced in May 1985 to reduce alcohol consumption (Virganskaya and Dmitriev 1992).

Gender differences in mortality are generally discussed in terms of female advantage. However, this advantage has some negative consequences. The elderly population in nearly all countries of the world is predominantly female. In some populations, notably those of the former Soviet Union, the legacy of heavy male war-related mortality, together with the general trend towards differential mortality, has resulted in a particular preponderance of females in elderly age groups. Widowhood is consequently high. Other populations with very different demographic patterns but with large age differences between spouses, notably Bangladesh, also have high proportions of widows. Apart from the economic and social disadvantages which often result from widowhood, older women experience more disability than older men and spend proportionately less of their life free of disability (Robine *et al.* 1998). This seems to reflect women's greater risk of disability from musculoskeletal disorders and (related) longer survival than men after onset of disability (Manton *et al.* 1995).

As a result of population ageing, the epidemiological transition, and recent declines in mortality rates at older ages, the issue of measuring and assessing trends in morbidity, and their relationship with mortality, is now a topic of major concern.

Recent trends in mortality

In much of the developed world rapid gains in life expectancy in the first half of the twentieth century were followed by a period of stagnation in adult male mortality rates in the 1950s or 1960s. It was assumed by some analysts of the period that further major falls in mortality were unlikely, either because endogenous mortality rates from degenerative diseases were inextricably associated with urbanization or industrialization, or because life expectancy was close to biological limits (Bourgeois-Pichat 1952). However, during the 1970s both male and female mortality began to fall again in many developed countries (excluding Eastern Europe). These gains were greatest in older age groups (where the scope for further reduction was greatest). As a result, changes in death rates at older ages have come to play an increasingly important role in both population ageing and in overall mortality change. Myers (1995), in a detailed examination of changes in six developed countries, found that in five of them the proportion of overall life expectancy increase in the 1980s, due to gains among those aged 65 years or more, was over 40 per cent for males and nearly 60 per cent for females. Table 4 shows that in Japan 48 per cent of the female and 31 per cent of the male gain in life expectancy at birth during 1985 to 1990 was due to falls in mortality among those aged 75 or over. In 1955 to 1960, by contrast, half of female and two-thirds of male gains were due to falls in child mortality, while changes among those aged 65 years or over had no or a negative effect on life expectancy. Improvements in the mortality of older people have been just as, or more, evident among the 'older old' as among those in their sixties or seventies (Manton and Vaupel 1995). Indeed painstaking analyses of verified and corrected data show remarkable falls in mortality at very advanced ages leading to an 'explosion' of centenarians (Thatcher 1999). In England and Wales, for example, there were some 5523 centenarians in 1996 compared with about 100 in 1911 (the total population over this period increased by 44 per cent).

Recent gains in life expectancy in many developing countries have also been substantial. Between 1978 and 1998 average life expectancy at birth increased by 10 years or more in Bangladesh, India, and Indonesia (WHO 1999). In other regions, however, recent changes have been less benign. Since 1990, mortality has increased in over 30 countries of the world (World Bank 1999). In Russia and other 'transition' countries of the former USSR levels of mortality have stagnated or deteriorated reflecting the collapse of previous support systems, extensive alcohol abuse, and resurgence of infectious diseases, including diphtheria. Even more grim is the situation in those parts of sub-Saharan Africa most severely affected by the HIV/AIDS epidemic.

In the nine African countries with an adult HIV prevalence of 10 per cent or more, average life expectancy in 1995 to 2000 is estimated to be 48 years, compared with the 58 years that would have been expected in the absence of AIDS (UN 1999). In Botswana a quarter of the adult population has HIV/AIDS. Such high rates of morbidity and premature mortality have enormous social and economic implications for the well being of future, as well as current, generations. In the 19 African countries considered in a recent United States Agency for International Development study (USAID 1997), an estimated 16 per cent of the population under 15 years of age—up to 40 million children—will be orphaned by AIDS in 2010.

Table 4 Contribution of mortality reduction in each broad age group to the increase in life expectancy, Japan 1955–1990

	Life expectancy (years)		Contribution of mortality reduction in each age group (%)				
	At beginning of period	Gain by end of period	0–14	15–39	40–64	65–74	75+
Males							
1955–60	63.6	1.7	65	27	16	0	−8
1965–70	67.7	1.6	38	9	28	15	14
1975–80	71.7	1.6	20	15	25	24	16
1985–90	74.7	1.1	9	10	30	20	31
Females							
1955–60	67.7	2.4	53	26	21	5	-6
1965–70	72.9	1.7	28	11	24	17	20
1975–80	76.9	1.9	13	10	25	23	29
1985–90	80.5	1.4	7	5	20	21	48

Source: Kono (1994).

Disability-free or healthy life expectancy

Ruzicka and Kane (1990) are among those who have argued that one important consequence of the epidemiological transition has been a decline in the usefulness of conventional indicators of the health of a population, such as life expectancy and cause-specific mortality. Many of the most common chronic conditions reported by the growing proportions of older people, such as musculoskeletal and sensory impairments, may have serious implications for health status but are not directly life-threatening and do not feature as prominent recorded causes of death. If, as some have argued, recent reductions in mortality are due partly to the prolongation of the process of dying rather than an extension of healthy life, then life expectancy may be becoming a less valid summary indicator of a population's health. In response to these concerns, increasing attention has been paid to disaggregating life expectancy into 'healthy' and 'unhealthy' or 'disabled' components. Estimates of healthy life expectancy now exist for over 30 countries and an international network has been established to promote standard methodologies and harmonization of data (Robine *et al.* 1992). Most existing estimates have been derived from cross-sectional morbidity or disability prevalence data used in conjunction with age-specific mortality data. More sophisticated (and data-demanding) multistate approaches which allow transitions both to and from disabled states have also been pursued (Rogers *et al.* 1990). One result of this work has been to demonstrate formally the greater disability experienced by women.

A slightly different approach to the measurement of population health has been adopted by the World Bank which, together with the WHO, has developed the disability-adjusted life year as a way of quantifying the full loss of healthy life (World Bank 1993). This ambitious exercise involved calculating the years of life lost by each death (defined as the difference between actual age of death and expectation of life at that age in a low-mortality population) and then making a further adjustment to allow for disability according to duration of the condition, with a weighting for severity. The disability data used in this project were drawn from community surveys and expert opinion and both deaths and disability were cause-specified (a process also involving the use of expert opinion where other data were lacking).

Further development of this approach is in progress and doubtless revisions of some of the detailed results may be suggested as other data become available. However, the estimation of disability-adjusted life year data represents a major step forward in the assessment of the burden of disease in the world's diverse population. As can be seen in Figs 9 and 10, this measure graphically illustrates the different problems faced by various world regions. In parts of the developing world, notably sub-Saharan Africa, loss of disability-adjusted life years is greatest among the young. In the developed market economies, by contrast, the health of the older population represents the major public health challenge.

Implications of recent demographic trends

In the developed world there have been substantial variations in post-transition fertility levels and trends. Many developed countries experienced a post-Second World War 'baby boom' during the 1950s and early 1960s. In Britain this peaked in 1964 when the total fertility rate reached 2.9. The baby boom was more pronounced in the United States where the total fertility rate in the late 1950s exceeded 3.6. Japan, by contrast, had a very short baby boom (1947 to 1949). The baby boom was followed by a 'baby bust' period in which fertility declined to very low levels in the 1970s. In most North and European countries fertility rates continued to fall in the 1970s but have since stabilized. Recent falls in fertility have been most pronounced in southern and eastern Europe (and in Ireland) and in general, northern European fertility levels are now higher than southern European ones. Fertility rates in the United States are slightly higher, being close to replacement level rather than below it. Although there have been recent increases in the population of women remaining childless in some developed countries, more important demographically has been the shift towards smaller families. In Portugal, for example, a third of all births in 1965 were to mothers who already had at least three children; by 1995 only 5 per cent of births were fourth or higher order (Council of Europe 1999). The reasons for these recent trends and for the very

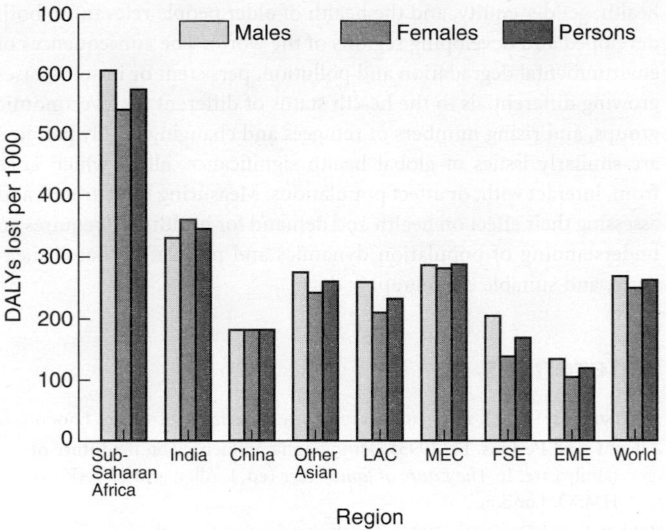

Fig. 9 Disability-adjusted life years lost per 1000 population by world region, 1991. (Data source: World Bank 1993.)

low fertility now prevalent in much of the developed world remain a matter of lively debate. Economic changes, including the increased labour force participation of women, attitudinal shifts, and advances in the availability of effective birth control have all been proposed as predominant influences. All are probably important, and all may have interactive effects (Becker 1981; Murphy 1993).

The very low fertility in most of Europe and the rest of the developed world (including Japan and the newly-industrialized Southeast Asian nations), the continued ageing of the population, and recent changes in patterns of family organization have raised concerns in a number of countries about the implications of these demographic trends (Allen and Perkins 1995). On the one hand, a group deemed to have substantial support needs (the old) is growing, while on the other, it is feared that the ability or willingness of younger generations to meet these needs may be diminishing.

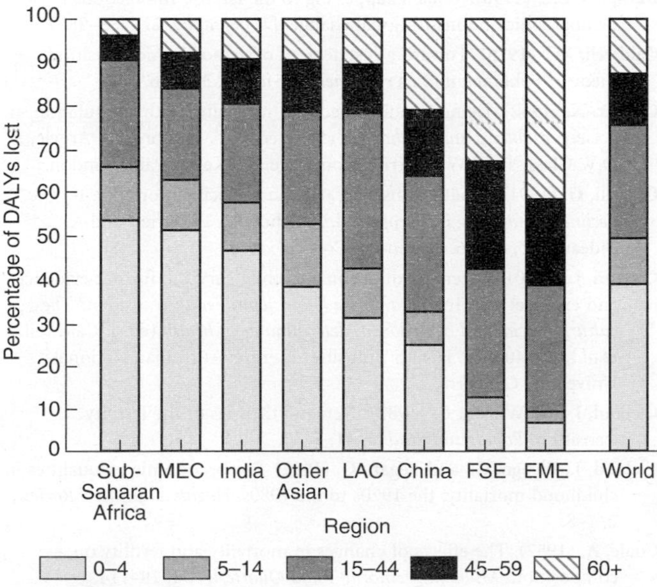

Fig. 10 Distribution of disability-adjusted life years lost by age group and world region, 1991. (Data source: World Bank 1993.)

Currently, and even more so in the recent past, the elderly populations of some developed countries, particularly in north-west Europe, include large proportions who lack children. In Ireland in the late 1970s, for example, a third of elderly people were childless—a legacy of the extreme variant of the European marriage system which prevailed until relatively recently. In the short term, many developed countries will see decreases in the proportion of childless old people (as the parents of the baby boom attain elder status). Moreover, the recent narrowing of sex differentials in mortality observed in some countries has resulted in a delay in the age of widowhood and increase in the proportion of older women still married. Increases in the extent of childlessness and celibacy among postwar birth cohorts and rises in divorce, however, suggest a rather different long-term future. In a number of European countries, a fifth of those born in 1955 are projected to remain childless; in later cohorts this proportion may be even higher (Roussel 1994). In the United States some 60 per cent of recently contracted marriages may end in divorce and 45 per cent of children will experience the break up of their parents' marriage by the age of 18 years (Bumpass 1990). In Britain current divorce rates imply that over 40 per cent of marriages will end this way (Haskey 1996). Rates of entry into marriage are also diminishing; in Britain and a number of other countries first partnerships are now more often formed through cohabitation than by formal marriage (Kiernan 1999).

In a number of European countries over a quarter, or even half, of all births now occur outside marriage. A large proportion of these (particularly in Scandinavia) are born to couples who have not legally formalized their union rather than to single parents. Union breakdown (divorce) is still the major cause of lone parenthood. Lone parent families now account for 10 per cent or more of all families with children in many parts of Europe.

In Britain the most recent estimates show that in 1991 nearly a fifth of dependent children lived in lone-parent families, compared with fewer than 8 per cent in 1971. In some areas of London lone-parent families account for over 40 per cent of all families with dependent children (Haskey 1994). In the United States, the proportion of children living in mother-only families increased from 8 per cent in 1960 to 23 per cent in 1992 (Da Vanzo and Rahman 1993). Such families suffer a number of disadvantages, many of which may have implications for the health of the children raised in them.

Increases in divorce, lone parenthood, and the participation of married women in the labour force are frequently cited as constraints on the availability of younger generations to provide support for their elders. While the evidence to support these hypothesized relationships is rather weaker than often assumed (Sundström 1994), recent changes in patterns of family formation and dissolution have been interpreted by some as indicative of a major reorientation from familial to individual goals and aspirations representing a 'second demographic transition' or 'cultural shift' (van da Kaa 1987; Inglehart 1990). If so, this has far-reaching implications for inter- and intragenerational patterns of support, including socialization and rearing of children and support for older people.

Demographic changes in fertility and mortality patterns determine not only the 'macro' composition and size of populations but also kinship patterns and the proportion of life spent in certain types of familial relationship. Lower fertility implies a reduced 'supply' of children, siblings, cousins, aunts, uncles, nephews, and nieces. Lower mortality, however, means an increase in the availability of older-generation relatives and an increase in the shared life enjoyed by adult children and their parents and grandparents. In Britain today half of all 50-year-olds still have a surviving parent and three-quarters of adults are members of families including at least three living generations linked in direct descent (Grundy *et al.* 1999).

Whether recent changes in partnership, parenthood, and household characteristics (including large increases in the proportions living alone) represent a second demographic transition (van da Kaa 1987) or the continuation of changes attendant on the first one (Bumpass 1990) is still a matter of debate. If current low levels of fertility persist, the populations of more developed countries will start to decline in size in the twenty-first century, unless negative natural increase is offset by immigration. In most developed countries, between 10 and 18 per cent of the population are aged 65 years or over, and 4 to 7 per cent are aged 75 years or over. In the early decades of this century those over 65 years of age will account for nearly a quarter—and those over 75 years of age 10 per cent or more—of most European populations. In Japan, projections suggest that over 15 per cent of the population will be aged at least 75 years (and 27 per cent at least 65 years old) by the year 2025. Even if the health status of the older population improves over time (owing to improvements in the health legacy of later cohorts), the impact of these demographic changes on demand for health care, particularly long-term care, is likely to be substantial.

The transition to lower fertility now seems to have been initiated in most of the world. However, fertility levels are still high, the population young, and population growth rapid in regions of the developing world particularly sub-Saharan Africa. Despite fears that the pace of decline in infant and child mortality might have slowed in the 1980s, research based principally on the Demographic and Health Survey Programme suggests that this was not the case and that in Northern Africa, Latin America, and Asia the pace of decline continued or increased during the 1980s and 1990s (Cleland *et al.* 1992; UNFPA 1998).

Continuing improvement in both child and adult mortality is projected for the developing world. Particularly in sub-Saharan Africa, these projections have been revised downwards to take account of AIDS. In the nine African countries with the highest seroprevalence rates, average life expectancy at birth in 2010 to 2015 is projected to reach only 47 years, instead of 64 years in the absence of AIDS—a loss of 17 years (UN 1999).

One result of the differing demographic trends in developed and developing countries is the decreasing demographic significance of the former. In 1950 a third of the world's population lived in more developed regions, by 1990 this proportion had fallen to 23 per cent, and by 2200 it is projected to be only 10 per cent (UN 1999). Among the many consequences of this shift is an increase in the potential impact of migration from less to more developed countries on the latter.

While there are major differences in demographic indicators and the composition of the population, there is perhaps less divergence in trends between the less and more developed world than has been the case in earlier periods. Moreover, a number of population-related issues are now firmly established as areas of global concern. The ICPD programme of action included recommendations on reproductive health, gender equity, and the health of older people relevant to both developed and developing regions of the world. The consequences of environmental degradation and pollution, persistent or in some cases growing differentials in the health status of different socio-economic groups, and rising numbers of refugees and changing family patterns are similarly issues of global health significance, all of which arise from, interact with, or affect populations. Measuring these trends and assessing their effect on health and demand for health care requires an understanding of population dynamics and population-based measures, and suitable demographic data.

References

Alderson, M. (1981). *International mortality statistics.* Macmillan, London.

Allen, I. and Perkins, E. (1995) Demographic influences on the future of family care. In *The future of family care* (ed. I. Allen and E. Perkins). HMSO, London.

Ashley, J. and Devis, T. (1992). Death certification from the point of view of the epidemiologist. *Population Trends*, **67**, 22–8.

Balarajan, R. and Bulusu, L. (1990). Mortality among immigrants in England and Wales, 1979–83. In *Mortality and geography: a review in the mid 1980s* (ed. M. Britton), pp. 103–21. HMSO, London.

Barker, D.J.P. (1992). *Fetal and infant origins of adult diseases.* BMJ Publications, London.

Becker, G.S. (1981). *A treatise on the family.* Harvard University Press, Cambridge, MA.

Bongaarts, J. (1978). A framework for analysing the proximate determinants of fertility. *Population and Development Review*, **4**, 105–32.

Bourgeois-Pichat, J. (1952). Essai sur la mortalité 'biologique' de l'homme *Population*, **3**, 381–94.

Brass, W. (1975). *Methods for estimating fertility and mortality from limited and defective data.* University of North Carolina, Laboratories for Population Statistics, Chapel Hill, NC.

Bulatao, R.A. and Stephens, P.W. (1992). *Global estimates and projections of mortality by cause, 1970–2015.* World Bank Policy Research Working Papers (Population Health and Nutrition), WPS1007. World Bank, Washington, DC.

Bumpass, L.L. (1990). What's happening to the family? Interactions between demographic and institutional change. *Demography*, **27**, 483–98.

Caldwell, J.C. (1976). Toward a restatement of demographic transition theory. *Population and Development Review*, **2**, 321–66.

Carrier, N. (1962). Demographic aspects of the ageing of the population. In *Society, problems and methods of study* (ed. A.T. Welford, M. Argyle, D.V. Glass, and J.W. Morris). Routledge and Kegan Paul, London.

Casselli, G. (1991). Health transition and cause specific mortality. In *The decline of mortality in Europe* (ed. R. Schofield, D. Reher, and A. Bideau), pp. 68–96. Clarendon Press, Oxford.

Cleland, J. (1990). Maternal education and child survival: further evidence and explanations. In *What do we know about health transition? The cultural, social and behavioural determinants of health* (ed. J. Caldwell *et al.*), pp. 400–19. Health Transition Centre, Australian National University, Canberra.

Cleland, J. and Wilson, C. (1987). Demand theories of the fertility transition. *Population Studies*, **41**, 5–30.

Cleland, J., Bicego, G., and Fegan, G. (1992). Socioeconomic inequalities in childhood mortality: the 1970s to the 1980s. *Health Transition Review*, **2**, 1–8.

Coale, A. (1957). The effects of changes in mortality and fertility on age composition. *Milbank Memorial Fund Quarterly*, **34**, 79–114.

Coale, A. (1973). The demographic transition. In *International Population Conference 1973.* International Union for the Scientific Study of Population, Liège.

Coale, A. and Bannister, J. (1999). Five decades of missing females in China. *Demography*, **31**, 459–79.

Coale, A. and Guo, G. (1989). Revised regional model life tables at very low levels of mortality, *Population Index*, **55**, 613–43.

Coale, A. and Guo, G. (1990). New regional model life tables at high expectation of life (addendum to 1989 paper). *Population Index*, **56**, 27–41.

Coleman, D. and Chandola, T. (1999). Britain's place in Europe's population. In *Changing Britain: families and households in the 1990s* (ed. S. McRae), pp. 37–67. Oxford University Press.

Coleman, D. and Salt, J. (1992). *The British population: patterns, trends and processes.* Oxford University Press.

Cooper, J. (1991). The divergence between period and cohort measures of fertility. *Population Trends*, **63**, 19–21.

Council of Europe (1998). *Recent demographic developments in Europe.* Council of Europe Publishing, Strasbourg.

Da Vanzo, J. and Rahman, M.O. (1993). American families: trends and correlates. *Population Index*, **59**, 350–86.

Davis, K. and Blake, J. (1956). Social structure and fertility: an analytic framework. *Economic Development and Cultural Change*, **4**, 211–35.

Demeny, P. (1972). Early fertility decline in Austria-Hungary: a lesson on demographic transition. In *Population and social change* (ed. D.V. Glass and R. Revelle), pp. 153–72. Edward Arnold, London.

Dyson, T. and Murphy, M. (1985). The onset of demographic transition. *Population and Development Review*, **11**, 299–340.

Elo, I.T. and Preston, S.H. (1994). Examining African-American mortality from incomplete data. *Demography*, **31**, 427–58.

Eurostat (1998). *Demographic statistics 1981.* Eurostat, Luxembourg.

Feeney, G. and Yu, J. (1987). Period parity progression measures of fertility in China. *Population Studies*, **41**, 77–102.

Fox, A.J. and Goldblatt, P.O. (1982). *Longitudinal study: socio-demographic mortality differentials.* HMSO, London.

Furner, S.E., Maurer, J., and Rosenberg, H. (1993) Mortality. In *Health data on older Americans United States, 1992* (ed. J.F. Van Nostrand, S.E. Furner, and R. Suzman), pp. 77–112. Vital Health Statistics 3(27). National Center for Health Statistics, US Department of Health and Human Services, Hyattsville, MD.

Garenne, M. and Fontaine, O. (1990). Assessing probable causes of death using a standardized questionnaire: a study in rural Senegal. In *Measurement and analysis of mortality: new approaches* (ed. J. Vallin, S. D'Souza, and A. Palloni), pp. 123–42. Clarendon Press, Oxford.

Garson, L.K. (1991). The centenarian question: old age mortality in the Soviet Union 1897–1970. *Population Studies*, **45**, 265–78.

Grundy, E.M.D. (1996). Ageing in Europe. In *Europe's population in the 1990s* (ed. D. Coleman). Oxford University Press.

Grundy, E., Murphy, M., and Shelton, N. (1999). Looking beyond the household: intergenerational perspectives on living kin and contacts with kin in Great Britain. *Population Trends*, **97**, 19–27.

Haskey, J. (1988). Trends in marriage and divorce and cohort analyses of the proportion of marriages ending in divorce. *Population Trends*, **54**, 34–7.

Haskey, J. (1990). The ethnic minority populations of Great Britain: estimates by ethnic group and country of birth. *Population Trends*, **60**, 35–8.

Haskey, J. (1994). Estimated numbers of one parent families and their prevalence in Great Britain in 1991. *Population Trends*, **78**, 5–19.

Haskey, J. (1996). The proportion of married couples who divorce: past patterns and current prospects. *Population Trends*, **83**, 25–36.

Heady, P., Smith, S., and Avery, V. (1994). *1991 census validation survey: coverage report.* HMSO, London.

Hinde, A. (1998). *Demographic methods.* Edward Arnold, London.

Hobcraft, J. (1991). Child spacing and child mortality. Paper presented at the DHS World Conference, Washington DC, 5–7 August. Results summarized in DHS World Conference Executive Summary (December 1991, Ann K. Blanc). DHS, Columbia, MD.

Hobcraft, J., Menken, J., and Preston, S. (1982). Age, period and cohort effects in demography: a review. *Population Index*, **48**, 4–43.

Inglehart, R. (1990). *Culture shift in advanced industrial society.* Princeton University Press.

Kestenbaum, B. (1992). A description of the extreme aged population based on improved Medicare enrolment data. *Demography*, **29**, 411–26.

Kiernan, K. (1999). Cohabitation in western Europe. *Population Trends*, **96**, 25–32.

Kinsella, K. and Gist, Y. (1998). *Gender and aging—international brief.* IB/98–2. US Bureau of the Census, Washington, DC.

Knodel, J. and van de Walle, E. (1979). Lessons from the past: policy implications of historical fertility studies. *Population and Development Review*, **5**, 217–45.

Kono, S. (1994). Demography and population ageing in Japan. In *Ageing in Japan.* JARC, Tokyo.

Lotka, A. (1907). Relation between birth and death rates. *Science*, **26**, 21–2.

Manton, K.G. (1982). Changing concepts of morbidity and mortality in the elderly population. *Milbank Memorial Fund Quarterly, Health and Society*, **60**, 183–244.

Manton K.G. and Vaupel, J.W. (1995). Survival after the age of 80 in the United States, Sweden, France, England and Japan. *New England Journal of Medicine*, **333**, 1232–5.

Markides, K.S. and Keith, V.M. (1995). Race, aging and health in the United States. *Reviews in Clinical Gerontology*, **5**, 339–45.

Menken, J. (1989). Proximate determinants of fertility and mortality: a review of recent findings. In *Demography as an interdiscipline* (ed. J.H. Stycos). Transaction Publishers, New Brunswick, NJ.

Murphy, M. (1993). The contraceptive pill and women's employment as factors in fertility change in Britain 1963–1980: a challenge to the conventional view. *Population Studies*, **47**, 221–44.

Murphy, M.J. (1995). Methods for forecasting mortality and their performance. *Reviews in Clinical Gerontology*, **5**, 217–27.

Myers, G. (1995). Comparative study of mortality trends among older persons in developed countries. In *Health and mortality among elderly populations* (ed. G. Casselli and A. Lopez). Clarendon Press, Oxford.

Newell, C. (1988). *Methods and models in demography.* Belhaven Press, London.

Notestein, F.W. (1945). Population: the long view. In *Food for the world* (ed. T.W. Schulz), pp. 36–57. University of Chicago Press.

Omran, A.R. (1971). The epidemiologic transition: a theory of the epidemiology of population change. *Milbank Memorial Fund Quarterly*, **49**, 509–38.

ONS (Office for National Statistics) (1998). *Mortality statistics—cause.* Series DH2. HMSO, London.

ONS (Office of National Statistics) (1999*a*). Table 1.6 *Population Trends*, p. 97. HMSO, London.

ONS (Office of National Statistics) (1999*b*). *Marriage and divorce statistics.* Series FM2. HMSO, London.

ONS (Office of National Statistics) (1999*c*). *Mortality statistics—general.* Series DH1. HMSO, London.

OPCS (Office of Population Censuses and Surveys) (1981). *Trends in respiratory mortality 1951–1971.* Series DHI No.7. HMSO, London.

OPCS (Office of Population Censuses and Surveys) (1987). *Birth statistics 1837–1983.* Series FM1 No.13. HMSO, London.

OPCS (Office of Population Censuses and Surveys) (1992). *1990 mortality statistics.* Series DH1. HMSO, London.

Pollard, A.H., Yusuf, F., and Pollard, G.N. (1990). *Demographic techniques* (3rd edn). Pergamon Press, Sydney.

Population Reference Bureau (1999). *World Population Data Sheet.* Population Reference Bureau, New York.

Prescott-Clarke, P. and Primatesta, P. (1997). *Health survey for England 1995* Vol. 1: *Findings*. HMSO, London.

Pressat, R. and Wilson, C. (1985). *The dictionary of demography*. Basil Blackwell, Oxford.

Preston, S.H. (1976*a*). *Mortality patterns in national populations*. Academic Press, New York.

Preston, S.H. (1976*b*). The changing relation between mortality and level of economic development. *Population Studies*, **29**, 231–48.

Preston, S.H., Himes, C.L., and Eggers, M. (1989). Demographic conditions responsible for population aging. *Demography*, **26**, 691–704.

Robine, J.M., Blanchet, M., and Dowd, J.E. (ed.) (1992). *Health expectancy: First Workshop of the Healthy Life Expectancy Network (REVES)*. HMSO, London.

Robine, J.M., Mormiche, P., and Sermet, C. (1998). Examination of the causes and of the mechanisms of the increase in disability-free life expectancy. *Journal of Aging and Health*, **10**, 171–91.

Rogers, A., Rogers, R.G., and Belanger, A. (1990). Longer life but worse health? Measurement and dynamics. *Gerontologist*, **30**, 640–9.

Roussel, L. (1994). Fertility and family. In *European Population Conference Proceedings*, Vol. I. UN Economic Commission for Europe/Council of Europe/UN Population Fund. United Nations, New York.

Ruzicka, L. and Kane, P. (1990). Health transition: the course of morbidity and mortality. In *What we know about health transition: the cultural, social and behavioural determinants of health*, Vol. 1 (ed. J. Caldwell *et al.*), pp. 1–26. Health Transition Centre, Australian National University, Canberra.

Schuman, J. (1999). The ethnic minority populations of Great Britain—latest estimates. *Population Trends*, **96**, 33–43.

Shapiro, J. (1994). The Russian mortality crisis and its causes. In *Russian economic reform in jeopardy* (ed. A. Aslund). Pinter, London.

Shaw, C. (1988). Components of growth in the ethnic minority population. *Population Trends*, **52**, 26–30.

Shryock, H.S., Siegel, J.S., and Stockwell, E.G. (1976). *The methods and materials of demography* (abridged edition). Academic Press, New York.

Smith, D. and Keyfitz, N. (ed.) (1977). *Mathematical demography: selected papers*. Springer-Verlag, New York.

Snow R.W., Armstrong, J.R., Forest, D., *et al.* (1992). Childhood deaths in Africa: uses and limitations of verbal autopsies. *Lancet*, **340**, 351–5.

Sundström, G. (1994). Care by families: an overview of trends. In *Caring for frail elderly people*. OECD, Paris.

Thatcher, A.R. (1992). Trends in numbers and mortality at high ages in England and Wales. *Population Studies*, **46**, 411–26.

Thatcher, R. (1999). The demography of centenarians in England and Wales. *Population Trends*, **96**, 5–12.

UN (United Nations) (1970). *Methods of measuring internal migration*. Population Studies, No. 47. UN, New York.

UN (United Nations) (1983). *Indirect techniques for demographic estimation, Manual X*. UN, New York.

UN (United Nations) (1991). *World population prospects 1990*. UN, New York.

UN (United Nations) (1993). *World population prospects: the 1992 revision*. UN, New York.

UN (United Nations) (1995). *Population and development*. Volume 1: *Programme of action adopted at the International Conference on Population and Development, Cairo, 5–13 September 1994*. UN, New York.

UN (United Nations) (1999). *World population prospects: the 1998 revision*. UN, New York.

UNECE (United Nations Economic Commission for Europe) (1994). *International migration bulletin No. 5*. UNECE, Geneva.

UNECE/UNFPA (United Nations Economic Commission for Europe and United Nations Population Fund) (1992). *Changing population age structures: demographic and economic consequences and implications*. UN, Geneva.

UNFPA (United Nations Population Fund) (1994). *Population: putting people first*. UN DPI/1519/SOC/CON. UN, New York.

UNFPA (United Nations Population Fund) (1998). *The state of world population 1998*. UNFPA, New York.

UNFPA (United Nations Population Fund) (1999). *The state of world population 1999*. UNFPA, New York.

United Nations Secretariat (1988). *Sex differentials in life expectancy and mortality in developed countries: an analysis by age groups and causes of death from recent and historical data*. Population Bulletin of the United Nations No. 25. UN, New York.

US Agency for International Development (1997). *Children on the brink: strategies to support children isolated by HIV/AIDS*. Executive report. USAID, Washington DC.

US Bureau of the Census (1992). *An aging world II*. *International Population Reports*, pp. 25, 92–3. US Government Printing Office, Washington, DC.

van da Kaa, D.J. (1987). Europe's second demographic transition. *Population Bulletin*, **42**.

van de Walle, F. (1986). Infant mortality and the European demographic transition. In *The decline of fertility in Europe* (ed. A.J. Coale and S.C. Watkins), pp. 201–33. Princeton University Press.

Velkoff, V.A. and Kinsella, K. (1993). *Ageing in Eastern Europe and the former Soviet Union*. US Bureau of the Census, Center for International Research. US Government Printing Office, Washington, DC.

Virganskaya, I.M. and Dmitriev, V.I. (1992). Some problems of medicodemographic development in the former USSR. *World Health Statistics Quarterly*, **46**, 4–13.

Waldron, I. (1985). What do we know about causes of sex differences in mortality? A review of the literature. *Population Bulletin of the United Nations*, **18**.

Werner, B. (1987). Fertility statistics from birth registrations in England and Wales 1837–1987. *Population Trends*, **48**, 4–10.

WHO (World Health Organization) (1992*a*). *Global health situation and projections, estimates*. Division of Epidemiological Surveillance and Health Situation and Trend Assessment, WHO, Geneva.

WHO (World Health Organization) (1992*b*). *World health statistics annual*. WHO, Geneva.

WHO (World Health Organization) (1998). *World health statistics annual*. WHO, Geneva.

WHO (World Health Organization) (1999). *The world health report 1999*. WHO, Geneva.

Wilkinson, R.G. (1996). *Unhealthy societies: the afflications of inequality*. Routledge, London.

Woods, R.I., Watterson, P.A., and Woodward, J.H. (1989). The causes of rapid infant mortality decline in England and Wales, 1861–1921 (Part II). *Population Studies*, **43**, 113–32.

World Bank (1993). *World development report 1993: investing in health, world development indicators*. Oxford University Press, New York.

World Bank (1999). *World development indicators 1999*. World Bank, Washington, DC.

Wrigley, E.A. and Schofield, R.S. (1981). *The population history of England 1541–1871: a reconstruction*. Edward Arnold, London.

Zeng, Y., Tu, P., Gu, B., Xu, Y., Li, B., and Li, Y. (1993). Causes and implications of the recent increase in the reported sex ratio at birth in China. *Population and Development Review*, **19**, 283–302.

7.3 Health promotion, health education, and the public health

Keith Tones

Overview

Most health and medical professionals will have formed some opinion about the nature and pretensions of health education and health promotion. It would, however, not be surprising if there were some confusion about the precise interpretation of these two interrelated concepts since they can have a multitude of meanings and underlying philosophies. This chapter aims to clarify these conceptual uncertainties.

Furthermore, even those who have only the most sketchy acquaintance with health education and health promotion will quite reasonably ask whether the increasing importance attached to health promotion is justified by results and will probably raise the issue of its evidence base. Since it is now accepted that medical interventions should be subjected to such scrutiny, it is quite legitimate to expect health promotion to provide answers to such questions. This chapter is not a comprehensive text on evaluation. Nonetheless, some consideration will be given to the important matter of effectiveness and efficiency. Indeed, it will be asserted that the inherent complexity of programmes designed to influence individual behaviour and social systems requires an evaluation strategy that is substantially different from those espoused in assessing the effectiveness of medical interventions—whether at the individual or population level. In short, it will be argued that a different research paradigm is needed for the appraisal of health promotion together with a new 'gold standard' for the assessment of excellence. Analysis of the various psychological, social, and environmental influences on human behaviour in health and illness—which is one of the main purposes of this chapter—should also offer valuable insights into what it means to develop an effective intervention. It should also generate more thoughtful and realistic consideration of what health promotion might be expected to achieve.

Accordingly, this chapter aims to illuminate the contribution which human behaviour makes to health and illness. More particularly, the author will consider how health might be promoted and disease prevented by the judicious application of educational strategies. Prior to this, some brief consideration will be given to the part played by health education in the new health promotion 'movement' and how it might contribute to the public health.

Having examined the social, psychological, and environmental factors which typically influence people's health and illness behaviours, strategies and tactics which might be adopted to influence health choices will be described. This will involve a macrolevel analysis of how communities come to adopt new ideas and practices. It will also include a more detailed and individual focus on the principles of effective communication and provide guidelines for the educational process.

Finally, key features of the systematic design of community-wide health promotion programmes will be discussed. This will incorporate a review of the potential and limitations of key settings and strategies such as mass media, school, and the workplace. Reference will also be made to the importance of skilful use of appropriate educational methods and techniques—and, in accordance with the commitment to give some thought to the question of efficiency, some final remarks will be devoted to the thorny issue of evaluation.

Health promotion—an essentially contested concept

A full discussion of the nature of health promotion and its relationship with health education cannot be entertained here and a more complete analysis is provided by Tones and Tilford (1994). It is important to note firstly that the concept of health promotion is essentially contested: it has a variety of meanings and is thus used to describe a number of different activities—many of which may be based on different philosophies. From the early 1980s, as the concept of health promotion acquired wider currency, several different individuals and organizations provided their own definitions and selectively interpreted the term so that it matched their own agendas, philosophies, and construction of reality. Quite frequently this interpretation was explicitly or implicitly compared with the 'outmoded' or 'ineffectual' activities of health education. For instance, some people argued that health promotion should primarily be concerned with the achievement of 'wellness' (or even 'high level wellness').

A number of influential publications by the United States Department of Health, Education and Welfare (1978, 1979) and the Department of Health and Human Services (1980) contrasted health promotion with 'health protection' and 'preventive health services'. Health promotion was primarily viewed as primary prevention and defined mainly in terms of individual lifestyle change. Emphasis was also placed on the importance of stating precise objectives.

Still others confused ideology with strategy and characterized health promotion in terms of the use of vigorous—and sometimes frenetic—media-centred programmes. The more sophisticated of these approaches drew on social marketing theory for support, making the false assumption that 'marketing health' was no different from marketing commercial products.

Rather depressingly, many professionals merely substituted 'health promotion' for the particular variety of health education they had been accustomed to practice. This has led to such anomalous and even oxymoronic notions that individuals should be empowered so that they would comply with medical recommendations.

Health promotion and the health field concept

It would be entirely logical to define health promotion as any planned measure designed to improve health. The appropriateness of the measures would be determined by careful analysis of the major determinants of health. In fact, one of the more important influences on the development of health promotion was a simple model popularized by the Lalonde Report on the health of Canadians (Lalonde 1974) and described as the 'health field concept'. This simple 'map of health territory' asserts that there are four main 'inputs' to individual health:

- genetic predisposition
- the health services
- individual behaviours and lifestyle
- environmental circumstances.

Health promotion is typically involved with three of these inputs: it is concerned to promote health by seeking to influence lifestyle, health services, and, above all, environment. Apart from some passing consideration for genetic counselling, the 'inherited' aspects of health receive little attention. It is also worth noting that, in the health field analysis, the curative services are largely excluded from the health service input. This might seem somewhat churlish since the experience of disease certainly militates against what most people would consider to be health. However, the exclusion has less to do with absent mindedness or malevolence than with a desire to make the already complex concept of health promotion more manageable.

It is, however, quite clear that the health field concept has led to an increasing acceptance that environmental circumstances constitute the most important of all the 'inputs' to health. The notion of environment refers to far more than the physical circumstances in which people live, work, and play but incorporate social, economic, and cultural dimensions (Wilkinson and Marmot 1998). Health promotion is, therefore, not concerned only with the physical environment but also with the cultural and socio-economic circumstances which substantially determine health status. Figure 1 summarizes the major determinants of health and illness.

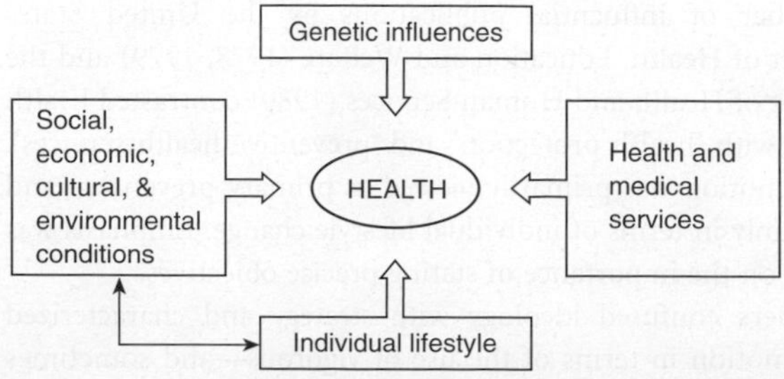

Fig. 1 The health field concept.

Clearly, the various environmental influences may be health promoting or health damaging. Higher socio-economic status is generally health promoting: lower socio-economic status generally militates against good health. Major inequalities lead to feelings of helplessness and hopelessness; social exclusion tends to reduce the potential for good health while social support is almost universally health enhancing. Productive employment fosters good health while unemployment is pathogenic.

Furthermore, although attempts to change cultural values and beliefs are problematic, the health-damaging effects of some cultures are a major concern for health promotion. For example, the culture associated with poverty is a major health hazard, as are those practices associated with the general oppression of women together with more specific manifestations such as genital mutilation.

Health education and the ascendancy of prevention

Before considering further the role of health promotion in influencing people's health choices, it may be helpful to provide a reminder of certain historical circumstances which contributed to the emergence of health education—which is, in many respects, the predecessor of health promotion proper.

Over a period of some 150 years, there occurred in 'developed' countries what might be described as a rise, fall, and resurrection of public health. During this time three phenomena having special significance for health education and health promotion were recorded. Firstly, there was a substantial improvement in the health of the population (as measured by increased life expectancy and a reduction in premature death); secondly, there was a general rise in living standards; thirdly, the status, power, and cost of curative medicine were significantly enhanced. Health education has figured at various stages in this 'public health career', if not in a lead then at least in a supportive role.

Some form of education (or, more accurately, 'propaganda') was present in the great days of the first public health movement in the nineteenth century. Typically, this took the form of pamphleteering and, what would now be called 'advocacy', for the implementation of various social and sanitary reforms. Health education, however, emerged as a professional activity some time later and its emergence paralleled an increasing disillusion with what many considered to be the failure of curative medicine to fulfil its early promise. It is beyond the scope of this chapter to discuss the well-rehearsed arguments about the limitations of modern medicine, though these might, however, be caricatured as follows.

1. Despite substantial developments in theoretical understanding and access to increasingly sophisticated technologies, medicine failed to acquire the 'magic bullets' capable of curing the 'new generation' of chronic degenerative disease.
2. The disappointing lack of success in curing disease had, nonetheless, been accompanied by both increasing lay expectations of medicine—and by dramatically escalating cost. Moreover, curative pretensions were associated with an unacceptable level of iatrogenic disease and, arguably, with a diminution of medicine's traditional caring function.

3. Accordingly, it was asserted, that what might not be cured should be prevented. Furthermore, since human behaviour is intimately implicated in the aetiology and management of preventable disease, prevention could be achieved by the deployment of appropriate behaviour change strategies.
4. Education was, therefore, appropriated by preventive medicine in order to persuade people to adopt lifestyles and behaviours that would prevent and simultaneously save money for an increasingly budget-conscious health service.

Health education, then, became closely involved with preventive medicine. Its twofold task was to prevent disease at primary, secondary, and tertiary levels and to promote the proper use of medical services. In order to achieve these goals, it was expected to cajole or coerce people into adopting lifestyles which, according to contemporary epidemiological wisdom, would prevent the onset of any given disease. People should also be persuaded to use appropriate screening services to detect precursor deviations from normality and asymptomatic disease. They should also learn how to deal with signs and symptoms in an approved fashion, for example by presenting treatable conditions to a medical practitioner at an early stage while accommodating to 'trivial' or self-limiting conditions and/or subscribing to sensible self-medication.

In addition to its secondary prevention function, health education also had a role in tertiary prevention. This would include such measures as fostering compliance with medication in order to prevent relapse and helping people readjust to normal life after having experienced some disabling condition.

The values and practices associated with the form of health education described above, constitute what is typically described as a 'preventive medical model'. Figure 2 summarizes its major components, and these might usefully be compared with the health field concept described in Fig. 1.

Health promotion: the contribution of the World Health Organization

The preventive model described above has been subjected to sharp criticism for a number of reasons. While the importance of preventing disease has not been challenged, the traditional preventive approach to health education is considered to be of very limited effectiveness. Moreover, its ideological foundation—the values and assumptions about people and society on which it is based—are considered to be inappropriate to a modern democratic society. Accordingly, the present chapter adopts the definition of health promotion developed by the World Health Organization (**WHO**) in its 'Health for All' movement, of which health promotion could legitimately be called the 'militant wing'. It subscribes to the original conceptualization (WHO 1984) and to the philosophy embodied in the seminal Ottawa Charter (WHO 1986).

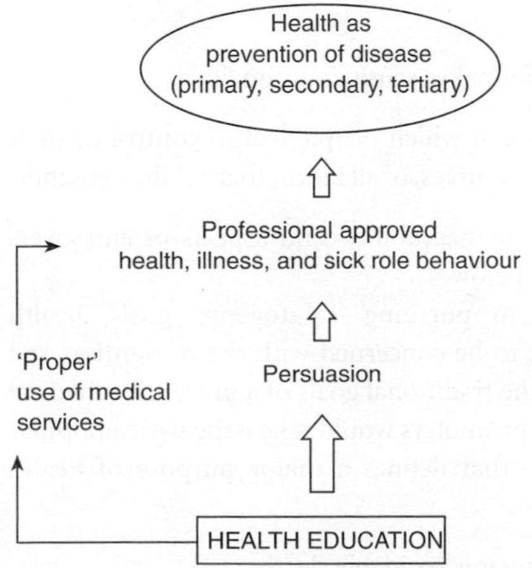

Fig. 2 A preventive model of health education.

The ideology and values of health promotion

Four major principles encapsulate WHO's ideological stance as follows.

1. Health is a positive state; it is an essential commodity which people need in order to achieve a socially and economically productive life.
2. Health is not just an individual responsibility. To seek to cajole individuals into taking responsibility for their own health while ignoring the social and environmental determinants of health is fundamentally unethical.
3. Substantial progress in health promotion depends on achieving equity and rectifying inequalities in health within and between nations.
4. The success of health promotion depends on the achievement of individual and community empowerment.

A holistic perspective

The holistic definition of health enshrined in the WHO's constitution still underpins current philosophy. It asserts that health is concerned with well being and not merely the absence of disease. Its purpose is to make it possible for people to achieve socially and economically productive lives. While the definition has been criticized as vague and unworkable, the reality of its existence and importance is regularly recognized by health promotion workers who have to deal with the complexities of society and human behaviours and their multifaceted influences on the clients they are seeking to help. This holistic dimension is powerfully illustrated by a recent article in the *British Journal of General Practice* (Sweeney 1998). In this, Sweeney cites Cassell's (1991) holistic formulation of 'personhood' which:

> include(s) personality and character; a past with life experiences that provide a context for illness; a family with ties that may be positive or negative; a cultural background; a variety of roles and relationships; a body and a self-image of that body; a secret life of fears, desires, hopes, and fantasies; a perceived future and... a transcendental dimension (that is some sort of life of the spirit, however that is expressed). . . . [E]ach aspect of personhood is susceptible to injury and damage, and ...this injury is what causes suffering. . . . Suffering can occur in relation to any aspect of a person and it occurs when the person perceives his or her impending destruction or disintegration. The sort of injuries that cause suffering are the death and suffering of loved ones,

powerlessness, helplessness, hopelessness, the loss of a life's work, deep betrayal, isolation, homelessness, memory failure, unremitting fear, and physical agony.

The pursuit of equity

The importance of equity for the promotion of health is now almost part of conventional wisdom. The primacy given by the WHO to the achievement of equity has recently been reiterated and re-emphasized in the visionary strategy *Health for All in the Twenty-first Century* (WHO 1998*a*). It asserts that: 'Equity underpins the concept of Health for All'. This is essentially 'a call for social justice' and 'requires the removal of unfair and unjustified differences between individuals and groups'.

Empowerment

The 'empowerment' of communities and individuals figures prominently in WHO's lexicon of health promotion principles. Indeed, the capacity of individuals to gain control over their lives and their health is often cited as the single most important goal of health promotion. Apart from acquiring control at an individual level, people should become actively involved in fostering the health of their communities. Additionally, as part of the related process of demedicalization, there should be a shift in the balance of power between doctors and other health professionals and their clients. Co-operation and empowered patient choice should replace the traditional emphasis on 'compliance'. Concern for human dignity, quality of life, and quality of care should be central to the delivery of health services.

The Ottawa Charter

The Ottawa Charter occupies a particularly important role in the development of the principles and practice of health promotion. It embodies the ideological commitments discussed above but also incorporates five key strategies consistent with the ideology. These have been reaffirmed in the Jakarta Declaration (WHO 1997) which, in turn, contributed to the first World Health Assembly resolution on health promotion (WHO 1998*c*). These 'essential strategies for success' are as follows:

- build healthy public policy
- create supportive environments
- strengthen community action
- develop personal skills
- reorient health services.

Further observations will be made about these strategies when the proposed 'empowerment model' of health education and health promotion is reviewed.

An empowerment model of health promotion

So far, some of the limitations of the narrow individualistic focus of the preventive model of health promotion have been discussed. Whilst considering these criticisms, the features of an expanded approach that is consistent with the principles of health promotion will be outlined. The requirements of such an approach are summarized in Fig. 3.

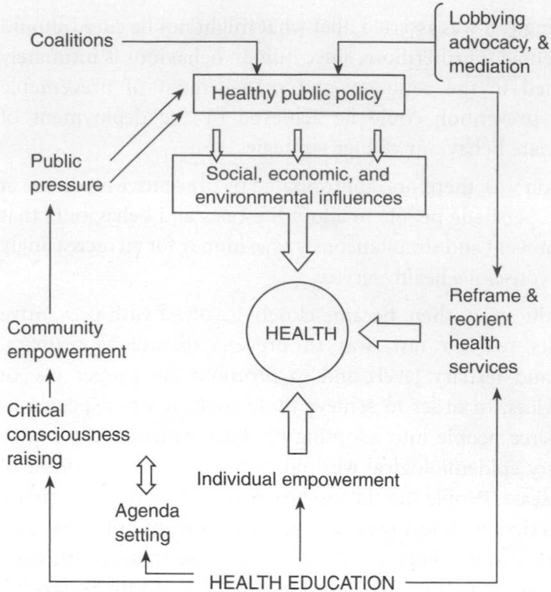

Fig. 3 An empowerment model.

The interpretation of health

The empowerment model acknowledges that health has both 'positive'/holistic dimensions whilst being simultaneously substantially concerned with the prevention and management of disease.

Despite the dangers of empty and naïve philosophizing about 'positive health', it is important to make two points. Firstly, it is possible to devise 'positive'/holistic conceptualizations that can be operationalized and measured; secondly, there is frequently a substantial relationship between such conceptualizations and the preventive goals of medicine. One such formulation is of particular value, both because it meets this two-point criterion and because of its relationship with health promotion's empowerment imperative. This conceptualization has been defined by Antonovsky (1979, 1996) as 'salutogenesis'. Central to this concept is the 'sense of coherence' which has three main components.

- Comprehensibility: 'to have confidence that sense and order can be made of situations'.
- Meaningfulness: that 'life makes sense emotionally'.
- Manageability: the extent to which people feel in control of their lives and have adequate resources, of all kinds, to meet life demands.

The relationship between 'manageability' and aspects of empowerment are further explored below.

Whatever its interest in pursuing 'salutogenic' goals, health promotion must continue to be concerned with the prevention and management of disease—the traditional goals of a preventive medical model. Indeed, few health promoters would take issue with a popular definition of 'health gain' that defines a major purpose of health services as follows.

- Adding years to life: reducing avoidable deaths.
- Adding health to life: reducing disease and disability.

- Adding life to years: enhancing quality of life.

Although prevention is of prime concern to health promotion, it is important to note that there is a major distinction between the philosophy, strategies, and methods used in the model of health promotion adopted here and the traditional 'victim-blaming' approach. At the heart of this distinction is the principle of individual and community participation. For instance, if general practitioners view disease as solely due to patient stupidity, ignorance, or perverseness, and continue to treat them in a paternalistic fashion and demand compliance with 'doctors' orders', then they are not acting in accordance with the principles of health promotion. Indeed, the notion of 'compliance' or 'adherence' is intrinsically incompatible with these principles (Tones 1998).

Building healthy public policy

The pre-eminence given by the Ottawa Charter to 'building healthy public policy' is a central feature of the model of health promotion defined in Fig. 3. Just as the nineteenth-century public health movement owed its success to legislative, economic, and engineering measures, it has been argued that these same measures should be deployed to address current health problems (and in developing countries, to continue to address some nineteenth-century problems). Problems such as pollution and environmental degradation may have had a different character in the twentieth century but they are still problems. As noted above, the problems of poverty and inequity still continue, albeit in the guise of relative disadvantage. Accordingly, if the principles of health promotion are to be taken seriously, then what is rather glibly called the 'political will' must be harnessed to the task of tackling unhealthy social and environmental circumstances and by implementing appropriate health policies. Recent publications by the United Kingdom Department of Health have acknowledged the importance of seriously engaging with policy issues (Department of Health 1999*b*) and, in particular, with policies designed to reduce health inequalities (Department of Health 1999*a*). Although they attract greater publicity, macrolevel strategies (such as the implementation of tobacco advertising bans) are just one category of policy addressed by health promotion. Equally important are policies at the microlevel (for example, the establishment in hospitals of 'baby-friendly' policies designed to provide an environment in which the choice of breast rather than bottle feeding becomes the easy choice). The Ottawa Charter identified three related activities designed to facilitate the development of healthy public policy: lobbying, advocacy (lobbying on behalf of the relatively powerless), and mediation (negotiation designed to mediate between the often competing interests of, for instance, commercial and health interests).

The contribution of health education

'Political' action designed to build healthy public policy is of major importance. Without seeking to undermine the importance of such action, the position adopted here is that the success of strategies such as lobbying and advocacy will be severely constrained—or even impossible—without a major commitment to health education.

Indeed it is possible to distil the essence of health promotion into the following simple formula:

$$\text{health promotion} = \text{health education} \times \text{healthy public policy.}$$

Without policy measures to provide a supportive environment, the potential for successful health education may be considerably reduced—even at the level of the educational encounter between health professional and patient. Conversely, the implementation of controversial or otherwise 'difficult' policy decisions will be impossible without the kind of public pressure which can only result from effective 'consciousness raising' health education. Figure 3 shows this synergistic relationship between health education and the construction of healthy public policy as well as health education's role in influencing individual health choices.

Empowering individual health choices

One of the major functions of a 'revitalized' health education is that of influencing individual health choices. However, its purpose and techniques differ quite fundamentally from the more traditional preventive approach discussed above. The emphasis is less on persuasion and more on support. The goal is not manipulation and compliance but one of empowerment through building self-confidence and the provision of skills: also, 'making the healthy choice the easier choice'. The meanings of some of these terms of empowerment will be made more explicit when the psychological and social determinants of health-related behaviours are examined below.

The proper use of services

As may also be observed from Fig. 3, health education is still concerned with promoting the appropriate use of health services—although what is or is not 'appropriate' may be open to debate. One of the most important functions of health education is to expand the horizons of service users and providers. It seeks to broaden or even reframe the definition of health services, and raise awareness of the substantial role which various organizations and services, such as transport and housing, have to play in enhancing public health. Of particular importance is the assertion that the consideration of health implications should be a routine element in the development and implementation of every organizational or service policy.

Simultaneously, health education should also maintain its traditional function of helping to provide those communication and educational skills which professionals and lay people need to provide effective health education for their colleagues, clients, and the public at large.

Critical consciousness raising and community empowerment

Although a redefinition of the meaning of health services may be quite novel, an even more radical health education function appears in Fig. 3. This is directly congruent with the Ottawa Charter's exhortation to 'build healthy public policy'. As noted above, the creation of new health policy is frequently a task of large proportions, especially in the face of counter-pressures from the various vested interests which are sometimes described as the 'anti-health lobby'. It was also observed that only the concerted force of public pressure (and perhaps the ballot box) might be sufficient to bring about substantial policy change, for example to influence levels of unemployment or deal with the health problems associated with poverty. For this reason, one of the essential functions of health education is not merely to bring health issues to the attention of the public (a process sometimes known as 'agenda setting'), but rather to generate the kind of indignant concern which is encapsulated in Freire's (1974) term 'critical consciousness raising'.

Enhanced consciousness about social issues may be necessary for community action but it is frequently insufficient. It must be supplemented by that mix of beliefs, attitudes, and competences which contribute to an 'active empowered community'. Accordingly, one of health education's major supportive functions is to create a sense of community, foster social support, and provide the variety of skills needed if individuals and their community are to influence the policy-making process and make a positive contribution to public health.

Some of these educational goals might seem as grandiose and unattainable as some of the visions of positive health or well being. However, if these are the stepping stones leading not only to salutogenic but also to preventive outcomes, then the aims and pretensions must be operationalized and translated into precise objectives to guide health promotion practice, and provide a series of indicators to judge the success or failure of interventions.

To begin this 'translation' process, a technical analysis of health education describing key features of human behaviour in health and illness will be outlined, thus providing guidelines for improving communication between client and health professional and/or enhancing the design and implementation of health education programmes. However, it is appropriate to emphasize that this detailed focus on health education is partial in that no similar analysis is provided for the strategies and activities involved in policy development and implementation, which is beyond the scope of this chapter.

Health education: a technology

The discussion of health education so far has been fundamentally ideological, in terms of what the purpose of health education should or should not be. The simple preventive model has been challenged, the general principles of health promotion have been espoused, and an empowerment model has been endorsed. However, it is also important to consider health education as a technical activity—as a set of procedures designed to achieve whatever goals have been generated by ideological preference. These often conflicting goals have one thing in common: they aim to influence decision-making and behaviour. Indeed, a technical definition of health education is not difficult to provide and for the purposes of this chapter the following is proposed. Health education is any intentional activity which is designed to achieve health or illness-related learning, that is, some relatively permanent change in an individual's capability or disposition. Effective health education may thus produce changes in knowledge and understanding or ways of thinking, it may influence or clarify values, it may bring about some shift in belief or attitude, it may facilitate the acquisition of skills, and it may even effect changes in behaviour or lifestyle.

Before specifying the requirements for efficient communication and effective education, it is important to understand how constructs such as those in the above definition can be applied in a social context and interact to influence behaviour. For example, it is important to know how knowledge relates to practice, how beliefs influence attitudes, and which skills are necessary for empowered decision-making. Therefore the next section considers the factors influencing health choices and the broader question of human behaviour in health and illness.

Human behaviour in health and illness

Health and illness: a career-line perspective

The purpose of health education is to promote learning and influence the kinds of choices that individuals make when they are healthy or ill. From the perspective of the medical practitioner, the choices which are habitually made leave a lot to be desired—frequently being characterized as neither logical nor rational. While this is not necessarily true, the frustrations of health workers may be understood by briefly considering what conventional research wisdom illustrates about the major influences on individuals' progress from health to illness and ideally the return to their former health status. This process is embodied in the 'sickness career'.

In formulating the idea of the sickness career, it is important to acknowledge the relevance of three concepts from medical sociology: the notions of 'health behaviour', 'illness behaviour', and the 'sick role'. Health behaviour refers to any activities which individuals might undertake while believing they are healthy in order to minimize the likelihood of future disease—for instance by adopting a healthy lifestyle or taking steps to detect asymptomatic disease. In other words, appropriate health behaviour should result in primary prevention.

Conversely, illness behaviour refers to those activities undertaken by individuals in response to symptom experience. It typically includes mental debate about the significance and seriousness of those symptoms, lay consultation, decisions about action (including self-medication), and possibly contact with health professionals. The adoption of appropriate illness behaviour should, therefore, result in the attainment of secondary prevention goals.

The notion of the sick role was developed to describe the behaviours of those people—typically in Western societies—whose contact with health professionals resulted in the legitimation of their illness status. Conferment of the sick role involves both rights and duties. Patients have the right to claim exemption from normal activities, such as work, and they can also expect help from other people, especially medical practitioners. Conversely, patients are expected to make every effort to get better and are duty bound to comply with medical advice.

Depending on the nature and stage of the disease, conformity to the sick role may result in either secondary or tertiary preventive gains. For instance, compliance with prescribed medication should reverse the disease process and/or prevent more serious consequences; compliance with recommendations for rehabilitation should result in patients relinquishing the sick role and viewing themselves as healthy even though they have some residual disability or functional impairment.

Kasl and Cobb (1966) provide a seminal review of these various concepts which are integral to the 'sickness career': this is summarized in Fig. 4.

When considering the progress of a hypothetical individual along the sickness career, it is important to observe that there is usually a major discrepancy between the subjective world of this 'actor' and the relatively objective reality represented by medical diagnosis and the

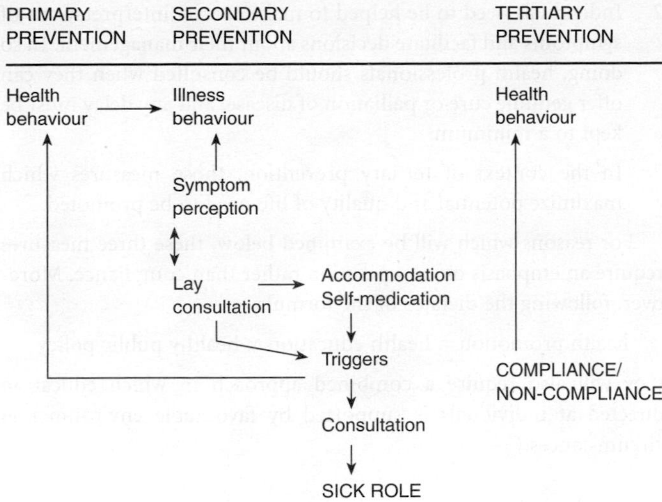

Fig. 4 A sickness career.

logical and rational analyses and recommendations made by health educators. Sometimes there is also a substantial gap between people's knowledge of what healthy living entails and their actual health practices—just as there may be a hiatus between the information presented by health practitioners and their clients' compliance with this medically approved advice. Some indication of the extent to which individuals adopt appropriate health behaviour is provided by a recent survey of the health and lifestyle of a national sample of British men and women (Blaxter 1990). Around 15 per cent of the sample were practising healthy behaviours in four key areas: smoking, alcohol consumption, diet, and exercise (though it was reported that 'only about 5 per cent had totally 'unhealthy' lives in those respects). It is also important to note from this study that interpretations of the meaning of health and the values attached to these varied widely; notions such as quality of life and well being exist in the world of lay interpretations of health and it would be unwise to ignore these when making judgements about 'prudent lifestyles'. In short, 'objective' prescriptions of health behaviour are always paralleled by 'subjective' interpretations of healthy behaviour.

It thus seems quite likely that the hypothetical individual's health behaviour will not please health professionals. What might be expected of the individual's illness behaviour as he or she moves further along the 'sickness career'? At the risk of lapsing into caricature, a summary of research results in this area is prudent. At any time, a substantial majority of people will be experiencing symptoms. If illness were the same thing as disease experience, then most people would appear to be ill most of the time. It would be useful to repeat the results of Wadsworth *et al.*'s (1971) survey of 1000 randomly selected people in two London boroughs. This research discovered only 49 individuals who had not experienced at least one painful or distressing symptom during the previous 14 days. Conversely, when asked to rate their health in general, a very different situation was revealed. Thirty-five per cent of this apparently diseased and distressed population considered that they were in 'perfect health'. A further 34 per cent rated their health as 'good', while only 21 per cent and 10 per cent respectively believed that they were in 'fair' or 'poor' health.

The process of symptom perception is not a routine physiological activity. It is, in fact, similar to the process involved in interpreting an educational message. Attention is paid to the stimulus in question and an active attempt is made to decipher its meaning. A hypothesis is entertained about symptom significance and a decision is made on the basis of sensory evidence. As with, for instance, the interpretation of a message on a poster, symptom perception can be accurate or inaccurate; it can be biased by expectation, prejudice, and wishful thinking. Moreover, as is known from instances of mass psychogenic illness and so-called 'medical students' disease', symptoms can be illusory; bodily symptoms may be either invented or grossly misinterpreted.

Symptom perception has a well-recognized social and even ethnic dimension. Zola's (1973) classic research into illness behaviour demonstrated consistent differences between American-Italian, Irish, and Anglo-Saxon responses to symptoms presented at outpatient clinics at an ear, nose, and throat hospital and at an eye hospital. For example, 'Italians had significantly more complaints of greater variety, and in more places than did the Irish . . . Italians [claimed] that the symptoms interfered with their general mode of living and the Irish just as vehemently [denied] any such interference.' Moreover, Italians much more often considered that pain constituted a major part of their problem.

Zola described the process of translating symptom into action rather elegantly: 'Virtually every day of our lives we are subject to a vast array of bodily discomforts. Only an infinitesimal amount of these get to a physician. Neither the mere presence nor the obviousness of symptoms, neither the medical seriousness nor objective discomfort, seems to differentiate those episodes which do and do not get professional treatment'.

In Wadsworth *et al.*'s (1971) survey, 188 symptomatic individuals took no action while 562 of the 1000 sample took 'non-medical' action. As Zola observed, only a relative minority of individuals actually consult a health professional. Furthermore, the majority of those consulting present with minor conditions and those with serious or potentially life-threatening conditions are equally well represented outside treatment.

Of those who are symptomatic but do not seek a professional consultation, a majority either just accommodate to the symptoms or employ self-medication. At all events, the process of lay referral is widespread. Indeed Freidson (1961, 1970) posited the existence of a lay referral system which involves a network of 'potential consultants from the intimate confines of the nuclear family through successively more select, distant and authoritative laymen until the "professional" is reached.' Freidson also asserted that the likelihood of individuals utilizing any given health service depended on two interacting variables:

- the density of the social network
- the extent to which the values and beliefs of the members of that network were congruent with those of the professional practitioner.

For instance, if a particular community was characterized by an 'extended lay referral system' of close friends and family—and if that community considered that medical treatment was the appropriate way to treat any given symptom—then there was a high likelihood that the individual would yield to interpersonal and social pressure and report rapidly to the local doctor.

Zola is also responsible for pointing out that accommodation to symptoms—perhaps after a long delay incorporating lay consultation—can break down and result in a possibly reluctant consultation. He noted what he called 'non-physiological patterns of triggers to the decision to seek medical aid':

- the occurrence of an interpersonal crisis
- perceived interference (by the symptoms) with social or personal relations
- sanctioning (approval or pressure from some significant other person
- perceived interference with vocational or physical activity.

Zola also noted a further—and somewhat different—trigger which he called 'temporalizing of symptomatology'. He illustrated this phenomenon by describing the way in which patients from an 'Anglo-Saxon' background would set external time criteria for action—such as, 'If it isn't better in 3 days, or 1 week, or 6 months, then I'll take care of it.' The relevance of temporalizing for the problem of delay in presenting potentially treatable and serious conditions is self-evident.

The latter part of the 'sickness career' is what happens once patients embark on their consultations. Firstly, it is not uncommon for people not to present all of their symptoms—including those of greatest concern. People tend to accumulate symptoms like money in a savings bank until there is a sufficient balance to justify a visit to their doctor. Alternatively, it might merely be an excuse to seek counselling for a personal or social problem unrelated to any of the symptoms presented.

Unfortunately, despite a fairly common tendency, at least in United Kingdom, to be generally satisfied with their doctor, around 40 to 50 per cent of patients will be dissatisfied with their most recent consultation and, more significantly, some 40 to 50 per cent will not comply with the advice they receive. Assuming that the advice they received was sound, this statistic should be a cause for concern, implying as it does that approximately half of the professional resources used during the consultation is wasted. As noted above, an emphasis on compliance is incompatible with the goals of health promotion (Tones 1998). Moreover, given the figures mentioned above, it is manifestly inefficient. The preferred approach—co-operation, consultation, negotiation, and participation—can hardly fail to produce better results.

The purpose of this review of the sickness career is to highlight the complexities and uncertainties associated with human behaviour in health and illness. Unless health practitioners have insight into these complexities and what often appear to be merely irrational decisions, they cannot hope to deliver efficient health education; their health promotion strategies will be fundamentally flawed. The remainder of this chapter examines the psychological, social, and environmental factors which govern health-related decisions. It will also outline how healthy choices can be facilitated through effective communication and education. Firstly, a summary of the implications for public health of the facts embodied in the sickness career is as follows.

1. Health behaviour needs to be influenced in such a way that individuals are empowered to adopt lifestyles and make choices which contribute to the primary prevention of disease, while at the same time maximizing their quality of life and their own subjective health goals.
2. Individuals need to be helped to make correct interpretations of symptoms and facilitate decisions about their management. In so doing, health professionals should be consulted when they can offer genuine cure or palliation of disease, and any delay must be kept to a minimum.
3. In the context of tertiary prevention, those measures which maximize potential and quality of life need to be promoted.

For reasons which will be examined below, these three measures require an emphasis on co-operation rather than compliance. Moreover, following the dictates of the formula

$$\text{health promotion} = \text{health education} \times \text{healthy public policy}$$

they will also require a combined approach in which education directed at individuals is supported by favourable environmental circumstances.

Understanding health choices

Ideological models and technical models

At the beginning of this chapter, models of health promotion that embody the ideological positions and value judgements underlying different preferred modes of working were discussed. This section now turns to a consideration of what might be termed 'technical models', that is, models which provide an explanation of constructs and factors that might be used to achieve the goals implicit or explicit in the ideological models. Figure 5 shows the relationship between these two kinds of model and how both of these, in turn, influence practice.

The health action model

The health action model provides a good example of a technical model. While it is used here to show how the preferred empowerment model might be translated into practice, it could equally well provide a similar service for a preventive model.

Common sense tells us that it is important to have some understanding of the factors which influence human behaviour in health and illness before it is possible to develop efficient health promotion programmes. Many people (either consciously or intuitively) subscribe to a simple but outmoded notion embodied in the so-called 'KAP' formula. This formula asserts that the mere provision of knowledge (K) is insufficient to persuade individuals to adopt sound health practices (P). An intermediate stage must be supplied which involves the development of attitudes (A) favourable to the adoption of the approved healthy practices. While it is undeniable that

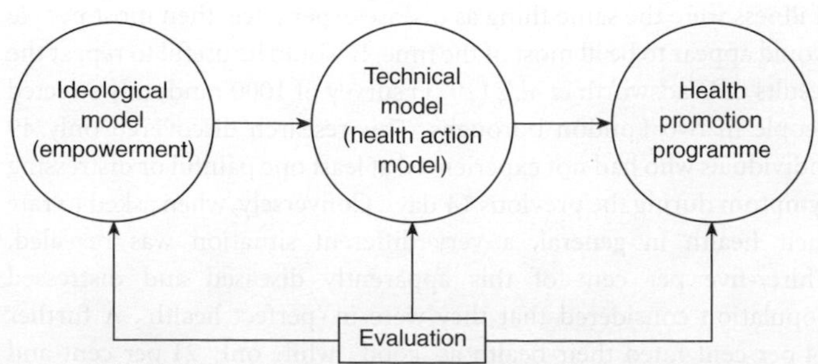

Fig. 5 Health promotion models and programme evaluation.

failure to make healthy choices cannot typically be attributed to lack of knowledge, the notion of attitude is itself oversimplistic and limited. Reality is much more complex and a more sophisticated conceptualization than the KAP formula must be found.

There is a plethora of more complex theories and models which seek to explain human decision-making—both in general and in relation to health and illness. In this chapter, the health action model will be used as an explanatory framework since it was originally developed to provide theoretical guidelines for health education programmes (Tones 1979). It was subsequently updated to take account of the emerging concept of health promotion (Tones 1987; Tones and Tilford 1994).

The main features of the health action model are summarized in Fig. 6. It shows how an individual's intention to undertake any given health action is influenced by three main systems: a set of beliefs, a cluster of motivational factors, and various normative pressures. More importantly, before intention can be translated into practice, a variety of facilitating factors must be in place. These may comprise additional knowledge or key skills. Furthermore, the environment itself must be favourable if the healthy choice is to be the easy choice. As observed above, one of the primary goals of health promotion is the construction of healthy public policy to create supportive environments which reduce the impediments to healthy decision-making. The importance of these different systems are now elaborated in turn.

The importance of health beliefs

Influencing health beliefs is a main concern of health education. A belief is a subjective probability judgement which describes the extent to which an individual considers a particular circumstance or relationship is true. For example in the context of current public health concerns, one of the main tasks of education would be to convince people that the following examples of medically received wisdom are indeed true:

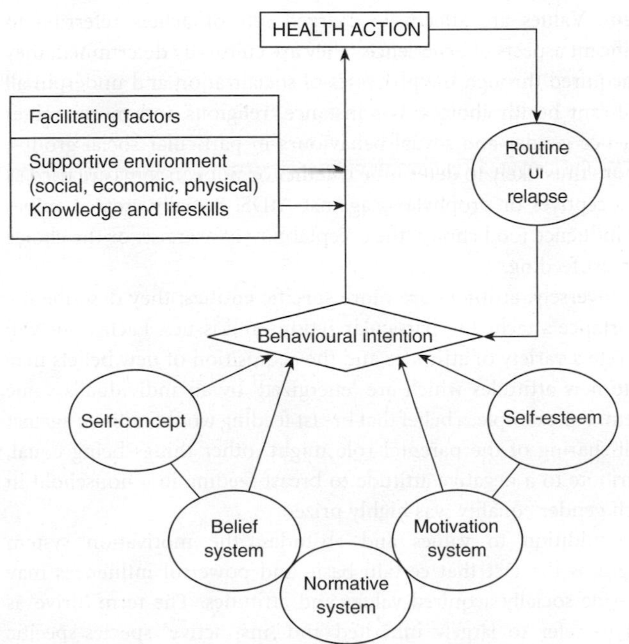

Fig. 6 Health action model.

- HIV is transmitted by the exchange of body fluids
- AIDS is a fatal disease
- intravenous drug users are susceptible to infection
- smoking is related to a number of serious diseases
- immunization will protect against a variety of specific childhood diseases
- having a mammogram will involve only minor discomfort and provide peace of mind.

The importance of beliefs is not merely limited to an individualistic preventive model. In pursuit of healthy public policy, it would be hoped that the population might be persuaded to accept that:

- poverty and unemployment are inextricably associated with preventable death and disease
- a ban on tobacco advertising will contribute to improvements in public health
- government is reluctant to take action against unhealthy commercial interests; writing a protest letter to a member of parliament might well contribute to a change in policy.

The importance of several of the beliefs listed above may be illustrated by reference to a well-known model of some historical importance which was originally developed to explain why people did or, more significantly, did not use medical services. The model in question is the health belief model (for a discussion see Becker 1984) which posits that individuals will not take appropriate health actions unless:

- they believe that they are susceptible to a given disease
- they consider that the disease is serious
- they accept that the recommended preventive measures will actually be effective
- they believe that undertaking the recommended action will not incur excessive costs or disadvantages.

If these conditions prevail, the probability of action will be enhanced but some trigger (for example similar to those ascribed to Zola above) may also be needed.

A comprehensive review of the important but complex subject of health beliefs is not possible here. However, three further kinds of belief should receive some brief consideration if we are to gain a more complete insight into the requirements of behaviour change strategies. They are beliefs about the causes of disease, beliefs derived from perceptions of risk and beliefs about 'affect'.

It would seem self-evident that one of the tasks of education is to ensure that disease causation or the nature of the risk factors associated with diseases should be properly understood. It is perhaps less obvious how these causal beliefs (sometimes termed 'causal attributions' or 'theories of illness') might indirectly influence health decisions. Let us consider the role of beliefs in promoting early diagnosis of skin cancer.

Before seeking medical help, individuals must be aware of the potential implications of the symptom they are experiencing: they must believe that this might be cancer. The chances of seeking help will also be increased if they believe they are susceptible to skin cancer—perhaps as a result of having accepted that their particular skin type is at increased risk of damage from exposure to the sun.

Conversely, action may well be inhibited by the long-recognized phenomenon of 'cancerophobia', that is, an unrealistic level of fear about the disease which, in turn, derives from a number of subordinate beliefs. One of these is the belief that treatment is (a) generally ineffective because cancer is essentially incurable, and (b) painful and distressing.

It is frequently difficult to provide an educational 'treatment' for pessimism about cancer—largely due to a failure to recognize root causes which include inappropriate causal attributions, that is, believing 'myths' about the nature and origin of cancers. It is necessary to probe further before structuring an educational programme. If this is done, then it will be seen that people will have a variety of 'theories' about the causes of cancer. For example, a 'retribution' theory describes a conviction that cancer is a kind of punishment visited on the individual for past sins and moral transgressions. Conversely, the 'seed and trigger theory' infers that everybody has cancer within them in a dormant form, like a seed, merely waiting for some event (almost any event—a knock, stress at work, family upset) to trigger it.

Of equal importance is the fact that many people consider that cancer is one single undifferentiated disease. Thus, if people know that in some cases treatment usually seems to fail—and believe that all cancers are the same—then pessimism is a logical outcome. The educational task (preferably carried out in the school setting) is thus one of providing appropriate biological understanding. Figure 7 summarizes this cluster of interacting beliefs and motivational elements.

Returning briefly to the health belief model, the concept of susceptibility needs a rather more critical analysis than it usually receives. It certainly seems to make sense that those at risk of disease or other negative consequences must believe that they are susceptible to those consequences before they will be inclined to take preventive action. However, it is not only important to understand why people may not accept the level of risk to which they are exposed (for example because of a tendency to overestimate the likelihood of the unlikely and underestimate the real frequency of quite common threats), it is also important to acknowledge that many people actively seek risk. These 'risk takers' would not be keen to undertake the behaviour in question unless they believed they were susceptible to possible negative consequences. Various explanations have been advanced for the motivational effect of risk taking: these include a sensation-seeking personality trait, a hypothesized 'addiction' to endorphins, and a desire to demonstrate control (arguably, a healthy trait). Lyng (1990) described the attractions of a particular form of exercising control as 'edgework', and noted that a prerequisite for the satisfaction experienced in exerting control in hazardous circumstances (such as sky-diving) was the belief that there was a 'clearly observable threat to one's physical or mental well-being or one's sense of an ordered existence . . . in which the individual's failure to meet the challenge at hand will result in death or, at the very least, debilitating injury'.

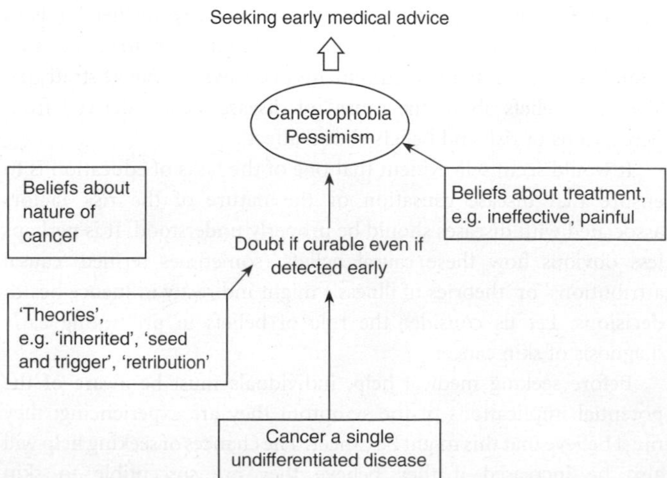

Fig. 7 Hierarchy of beliefs about cancer.

The third example of the need to take account of a key belief in order to develop appropriate educational methods concerns 'affect'. Affect refers to various motivational states or feelings. Beliefs about affect might in certain circumstances materially influence an individual's intention to adopt a particular health-related behaviour. For instance, Marsh and Matheson's (1983) national survey of British smoking attitudes and behaviour demonstrated that one of the more significant determinants of individuals' intention to give up smoking was whether or not they believed that they would be able to cope with the negative affect of withdrawal or relinquish the positive affect associated with emotional and 'physiological' gratification derived from their habit.

Similarly, Davis (1992) has suggested that the main reason militating against the rehabilitation of 'addicts' is not so much the physiological aspects of addiction and withdrawal but the belief that they are addicted.

Values, attitudes, and feelings

In addition to a belief system, Fig. 6 incorporates a motivation system—a complex of different affective elements. These affective elements ultimately determine an individual's intention of adopting a particular course of action.

Individuals' values form an important part of the motivation system. Values are affectively charged sets of beliefs referring to significant aspects of experience. They are culturally determined; they are acquired through the processes of socialization and underpin all significant health choices. For instance, religious and moral values influence gender and sexual behaviours in particular social groups; they are thus likely to determine whether or not condoms are used as contraceptives or prophylaxis against AIDS. Socially created values may influence food choice, the acceptability of exercise, or the choice of breast feeding.

Conversely, attitudes are more specific entities: they describe the importance attached to particular actions and issues. Each value will generate a variety of attitudes and the acquisition of new beliefs may create new attitudes which are 'energized' by an individual's value system. For example, a belief that breast feeding would militate against a full sharing of the parental role might, other things being equal, contribute to a negative attitude to breast feeding in a household in which gender equality was highly prized.

In addition to values and attitudes, the motivation system recognizes the fact that certain basic and powerful influences may over-ride socially acquired values and attitudes. The term 'drive' is used to refer to largely inherited and 'instinctive' species-specific motivational factors such as hunger, sex, and pain. It is also used here to describe acquired motivators having drive-like qualities such as those arguably ascribed to the addictive state. The importance of drives in determining behaviours is self-evident. A teenager might, for example, believe in her susceptibility to an unwanted pregnancy, accept the benefits of condom use, and have acquired the skills needed to use them. However, even if she also has a well-developed moral sense, her values and attitudes may succumb to the imperative of sexual passion.

Frequently there may be no obvious drive influencing intention to act but, nonetheless, the presence of certain emotional states may signify the existence of motivational factors derived from drives. Guilt and anxiety in this context may thus be viewed as a fractionated or 'diluted' versions of pain or fear. Everyday experience confirms the importance of such emotional states in determining action. Indeed, as will be argued, the problem of maintaining post-decisional healthy behaviours—and of managing relapse—is one of the more difficult tasks facing health professionals.

Before considering the third major set of influences on behavioural intention—the normative system—it is important to emphasize the interaction of these various systems. As argued above, sets of beliefs which are congruent with people's value systems create positive attitudes and intentions. Conversely, values and attitudes frequently influence beliefs. 'Autistic thinking' (believing what it is comfortable to believe) is a common phenomenon and people often resolutely refuse to accept apparently rational arguments about, for instance, the hazards of smoking because to do so would create too much uncomfortable dissonance. Indeed 'wish fulfilment' and defensive avoidance may typically lead to selective attention and biased perception causing people to misinterpret verbal messages and ignore or even 'fail to see' threatening posters.

The normative system

The normative system needs little explanation: despite our own beliefs and personal preferences, our intentions may be influenced for good or ill by other people. The normative system subdivides these social influences into general social norms and the more direct impact of significant others (that is, individuals or groups of individuals having special significance such as spouse, family, or peer group). General social norms conveyed via the mass media will have less impact than observations of normal practices in the individual's own community which, in turn, will exert less pressure than direct interpersonal interaction with those close to us.

What is less obvious is the separate but interrelated function of belief and motivation. Firstly, the intention to act is affected by beliefs about social norms and anticipation of how significant others are likely to react to intended actions. Secondly, these beliefs will only influence intentions if the reaction of other people is valued and/or we are motivated to comply with their wishes (real or imagined) or feel it is important to conform to social norms. For example, a person's intention to adhere to recommended alcohol limits will depend not only on the belief that a friend would approve but also on a desire to please that friend.

Again, whether or not an individual decides to wear protective headgear while cycling could be influenced not merely by a belief that very few people appear to wear crash helmets but also by the extent to which that individual is prepared to tolerate the possible ridicule which might result from deviating from normal practice.

The lay referral system, which features in the normative system in Fig. 6, has already been discussed in the context of a 'sickness career'. This concept provides a useful explanation of the ways in which normative pressures in a given type of community might influence use or non-use of particular health services.

Empowering health choices and providing support

Several references have already been made to empowerment. Not only is this an ideologically indispensable condition for health promotion, it is also an essential element within that cluster of psychosocial and environmental variables which determine whether or not individuals adopt behaviours leading to primary, secondary, or tertiary outcomes. It has also been argued that concepts such as empowerment must be operationalized if precise and measurable objectives are to be developed in health promotion. This will now be attempted as this next section identifies and reviews the ways in which environmental circumstances and related factors may enable or inhibit empowered choices.

Personality, self-empowerment, and health choices

Although the relevance of a sensation-seeking trait has been mentioned, personality—the relatively enduring cluster of personal traits and attributes which can provide a holistic profile of any given individual—is not considered to be a particularly useful concept in helping to explain human behaviour in health and illness, at least not in terms of potential application to the design of health education programmes. Although such personality traits as hypochondriasis or emotional stability may have an important bearing on individual health, there is little evidence that these factors materially influence the adoption of healthy lifestyles. Conversely, there is one cluster of characteristics which is considered to be highly relevant to health promotion—both ideologically and technically. It involves two complementary attributes: self-esteem and locus of control.

The dichotomy between the belief and motivation systems in the health action model is important in order to explain the relationship between locus of control and self-esteem. In addition to specific beliefs about, for example, the costs and benefits of adopting a course of action, each individual has a complex set of beliefs about the self. The sum total of these beliefs forms what is often defined as 'self-concept'. As with any other belief or belief system, self-concept describes the extent to which any given person accepts that he or she truly possesses a number of attributes—positive or negative. Hence self-concept may be realistic or unrealistic. Self-concept also includes beliefs about the body or physical appearance—that is, body image.

Self-esteem is a complementary feature of the self-concept and is one of the most important and powerful values in the motivation system. It refers to the extent to which the individual values the attributes which make up the self-concept. Just as people formulate attitudes to any aspect of their world in accordance with their value system, they also develop attitudes to themselves. The sum of these attitudes defines their self-esteem.

The central relevance of self-esteem for healthy decision-making may be readily summarized. At one level of reasoning, a quite common-sense assertion can be made: presumably if people possess a good measure of self-worth, they are more likely to respond to the exhortation of preventive medicine to 'look after themselves'. Again, the acquisition of self-esteem (based on a realistic self-concept and taking account of the rights of others) can be confidently identified as one of the less illusory and contentious goals of 'positive' mental health promotion.

More specifically, the possession of self-esteem has been associated with a tendency to have the courage of one's convictions (and hence an increased capacity to resist social pressure to do unhealthy things). It has also been suggested that people having higher self-esteem are more able to handle threat in a productive manner. For instance, in response to fear-arousing educational messages, those having high self-esteem are more likely to be able to cope with threat rather than resort to defensive avoidance behaviours.

Furthermore, it also seems likely that people enjoying high self-esteem will experience greater dissonance when acting in a manner inconsistent with their beliefs and values. For instance, an individual having high self-esteem, and who also values health, would feel considerably more uncomfortable knowing that he or she were overweight than someone having a lower level of self-worth. Dissonance is one of those emotional states incorporated in the motivation system. It is, perhaps, not quite as uncomfortable as guilt, embarrassment, or anxiety but, nonetheless, one prefers to avoid it if at all possible.

It should not, however, be assumed that high self-esteem necessarily provides an antidote to unhealthy behaviour. For example, it seems likely that 'self-affirmation' and celebration of a particular self-image may be one of the many apparently contradictory factors contributing to young people's determination to smoke—despite their awareness of the associated risks (Denscombe 2001).

Empowerment and the notion of control

Self-esteem has many sources—such as the way people have been treated in their childhoods and the way that peers react. Self-esteem also seems to be closely related to the extent to which people feel in control of their lives. Beliefs about control are central to health promotion's ideological goal of active and empowered people and communities; however, there are different types and degrees of beliefs about control, some of which are briefly considered.

Reference was made above to attributional beliefs: that is, how one explains the nature and causes of disease and illness. One particular application of attribution theory centres on how people explain the various vicissitudes which they experience during their lives. Of special importance is the extent to which they explain what happens to them in terms of their own agency rather than the agency of other people or mere fate.

The notion of perceived locus of control is perhaps the most widely known of the psychological constructs associated with beliefs about control. Rotter (1966) defined the essence of this concept in a seminal article which argued that people could be differentiated according to the extent to which they believed that their lives were controlled by chance or powerful others rather than by their own efforts. Although people are normally distributed on this trait, those who largely consider they are influenced by external forces are considered to have an external locus of control. Conversely, those who have confidence that whatever happens to them—pleasant or unpleasant—is substantially within their domain of influence are said to have a predominantly internal locus of control. Shakespeare recognized the importance of this construct when he observed

> Men at some time are masters of their fates:
> The fault, dear Brutus, is not in our stars,
> But in ourselves, that we are underlings.
>
> *Julius Caesar*, Act I, Scene 2.

A more complete review is not appropriate here. However, the development of scales for health-related locus of control has resulted in research demonstrating that there is indeed an association between internality and the likelihood of making healthy choices (Wallston and Wallston 1978; Tones 1992).

Conversely, it seems fairly clear from the work of Seligman (1975) and others that the state of 'learned helplessness', which derives from a belief that events are not influenced in any way by individual action, is both intrinsically unhealthy and militates against decision-making of any kind. Indeed, the importance currently attached to combating social exclusion is substantially determined by its contribution to the debilitating states of hopelessness, helplessness, and alienation.

Two further situations in which beliefs about control can have a positive influence will be mentioned here. Firstly, the feeling of control which results from receiving information, involvement in decision-making, and the acquisition of competences to influence events (aversive or otherwise) can enhance not only the likelihood of making healthy decisions but also the achievement of therapeutic outcomes (Egbert *et al.* 1964; Langer and Rodin 1976). The second situation relates to an especially relevant and practically applicable aspect of control described as self-efficacy.

The construct of self-efficacy is associated with Bandura (1977, 1986). People who have self-efficacy expectations believe that they are capable of performing a particular activity. Whereas locus of control is a generalized trait, self-efficacy is specific. For example, while someone might believe that she is generally not in control of her life, she might be persuaded that she could actually come for her mammogram and leave her children in the crèche—thoughtfully provided by the health centre. Conversely, another person might feel generally in charge of his life but, because of a belief that he could not cope with the loss of affect associated with giving up smoking, would be convinced that he would not be able to make that particular healthy choice. So, following one simple formulation, people must not only believe that a health decision is beneficial and worthwhile, they must also believe they are capable of implementing it. Accordingly, influencing self-efficacy beliefs must be accorded a high priority.

Facilitating decision-making: the provision of support

One of the more illuminating components of social learning theory—with which Bandura (1977, 1986) was closely associated—was the concept of reciprocal determinism. This states that there is a reciprocal relationship between human action and environmental circumstances. On the one hand, most people can exert some degree of influence on their environment; on the other hand, people do not operate in a vacuum and must take account of these environmental constraints and limitations which can act as barriers to free choice.

As noted above in the health action model, health promotion is not only concerned with influencing beliefs, motivation, and intention to act: it has a responsibility to do all it can to ensure that intention is translated into practice. Accordingly, Fig. 6 reveals the necessity to facilitate choice by taking account of a number of factors which can either increase the likelihood of sustained healthy behaviours or act as barriers to their attainment. The first, and arguably the most significant, of these factors is the environment.

The environment can be viewed at a macrolevel in terms of the broad range of circumstances addressed in the earlier discussion of health promotion. The major physical and socio-economic aspects of the social system require the application of healthy public policy at various levels 'to make the healthy choice the easy choice'. The importance of this cannot be overestimated but needs no further consideration here.

Conversely, following the principle of reciprocal determinism, the significance of what could be termed the microenvironment needs to be emphasized. That is, the immediate social and physical circumstances which can influence health choices. For example, the intimate environment of the home can serve to trigger smoking and must be actively managed in order to facilitate smoking cessation. Conversely, the availability of social support can help individuals succeed in their determination to change their behaviour. A substantial literature on the health benefits of social support has accumulated in recent years (Gottlieb and McLeroy 1992; Mittelmark 1999), although a detailed review is beyond the scope of this chapter. It is sufficient to comment here on the importance of, for instance, a general practitioner arranging supportive social environments for patients. The spouse and family of a patient might be involved in the discussion of how best to support that family member's behaviour change programme. Or a 'buddy system' might be introduced into a self-help group: participants in a smoking clinic might, for example, be asked to maintain contact with each other between meetings in order to support their mutual resolve to quit smoking.

Providing skills and preventing relapse

One of the points emphasized in the health action model is the importance of providing the knowledge and skills which people need to ensure that any given health action will materialize and be sustained. Knowledge is clearly important. For example, intention to co-operate with medication will not happen unless the patient knows when and how much medication is to be taken. Less obviously, perhaps, is the need for skills acquisition. It is important to record at this point, contrary to what has often been written in health education curriculum guides, that empowerment requires more than the provision of decision-making skills. Such skills should be restricted to the cognitive functions involved in the systematic scanning of alternative courses of action together with clarification of key personal values. They are an important component in the empowerment process, but genuine voluntary decision-making will typically require such capabilities as psychomotor competences—such as dexterity in the use of a condom or the efficient practice of first aid techniques. They will also include social interaction skills. An intention to communicate assertively with a partner about safer-sex practices will fail unless verbal and non-verbal skills have been practised to a high level of proficiency.

Sustaining behaviours which involve loss of gratification or some degree of initial discomfort is one of the most difficult of the tasks which health education seeks to facilitate. In addition to managing the microenvironment—as indicated above—training in the use of 'self-regulatory' skills will usually be required. For instance, the difficulties intrinsic to the control of 'addictive behaviours' have been well documented. Accordingly, a variety of techniques associated with behaviour modification approaches have been evolved to help people monitor their behaviours and environmental circumstances, avoid temptation, and discover substitute gratifications and rewards for successful maintenance of the healthy activities they have chosen to adopt.

Figure 8 provides an overview of the social, environmental, and psychological dynamics of the process of empowerment.

So far in this chapter, a map has been provided on which to plot the multitude of psychological, social, and environmental determinants of any particular health or illness-related behaviour in the form of the health action model. It is therefore a good opportunity to revisit the evaluation question and to ask to what extent this discussion of these psychosocial and environmental factors might have increased the sophistication of our thinking on matters of measurement. These very factors can provide a number of intermediate indicators of effectiveness and efficiency. Both preventive and empowerment goals will require evidence of successful learning such as the acquisition of relevant beliefs, clarification of values, shifts in attitudes, and adoption of skilled behaviours. Bearing in mind the importance of the environment, evidence that policies have been successfully initiated and implemented should be identified. For instance, the following intermediate indicators would provide partial and proximal measures of longer-term success: the number of no smoking areas provided in a workplace, ready availability of condom machines, and the provision of a responsive user-friendly service in an outpatient clinic.

The important matter of evaluation will receive more detailed discussion below.

Behaviour change: influencing health choices

The communication process: lessons from failure

Successful learning is at the heart of the successful health promotion enterprise and the educational encounter. Learning is not possible, however, without efficient communication.

There is no universally agreed definition of communication—although effective communication is believed to be a universally good

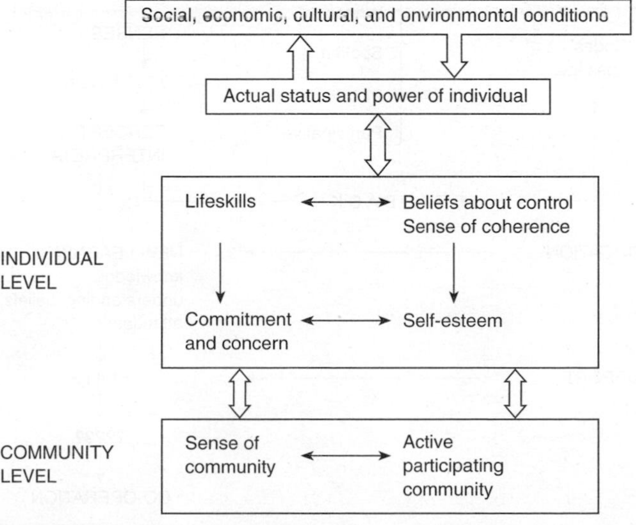

Fig. 8 The dynamics of empowerment.

thing. However, the term is often used in two different senses in the context of health promotion. Occasionally it is used to describe the whole process of influencing behaviour change. Communication failure, according to this conceptualization, would describe failure to change lifestyle or comply with recommended advice. Alternatively, use of the term communication may be restricted to the provision of information. This narrower definition is employed here and the process is described in Fig. 9.

Communication consists of the transmission of messages from a given source to an audience which may comprise one or more individuals. In the classic research situations described below, the communicators are health professionals—usually doctors—while the audience consists of patients or clients. Effective communication occurs when the audience's interpretation of the message matches that of the communicator.

Given the difficulties people frequently experience in interpreting communications, the notion of 'coding' is highly appropriate. This code may be symbolic, pictorial, or participatory. A symbolic message would normally be in either spoken or written form. Alternatively or additionally some pictorial presentation may be used, for example in the form of a visual aid. Less commonly—and often in educational settings—the audience may be invited to participate actively for the sake of more effective communication. For example, role play might be used to convey emotional impact.

When people respond successfully to a communication, the message must first reach their senses: they must be able to see and hear it. Secondly, the message must attract and sustain their attention. Thirdly, it must be correctly interpreted—a process involving perception.

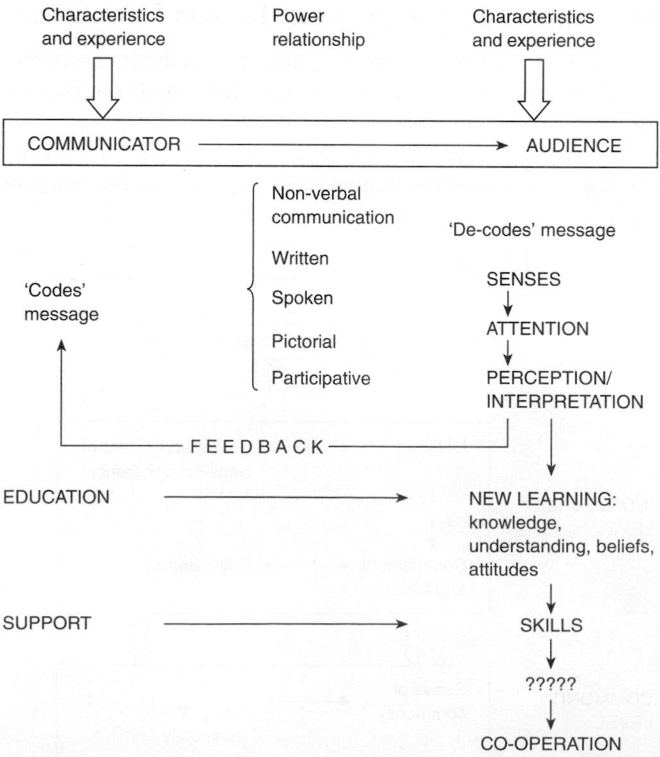

Fig. 9 The process of communication and education.

The feedback loop shown in Fig. 9 is an essential feature of the communication process. Communication cannot be successful unless communicators check the effectiveness of the process during and/or immediately after the interaction by asking questions or noting non-verbal reactions.

It is also clear from Fig. 9 that the communication process is materially affected by the expectations, emotional state, and other characteristics of both source and audience. For instance, patients' anxiety may well result in their selectively attending to a particular message or misperceiving it. The ways in which certain attributes of doctors might affect the consultation will be considered below.

Figure 9 includes an important feature of the communication process—non-verbal communication. In many instances, aspects of non-verbal communication, such as facial expression, tone of voice, or posture, may be more important than the spoken word—particularly in conveying attitudes and feelings. Moreover, it is often through non-verbal communication that communicator and audience exchange impressions about their characteristics. Of course, the roles of audience and communicator will reciprocate in accordance with the ebb and flow of conversation. The doctor will ask a question and the patient, in responding to it, then becomes the communicator—and the doctor has the task of decoding the resulting message.

Compliance and the sick role

In a classic analysis, Parsons (1951) specified a 'proper role' for doctor and patient in Western society. Sociologically, his stance was 'functionalist': he argued that the peculiar relationship between doctor and patient existed because it was functional in that it met an important social need. As mentioned above, patients are accorded certain privileges when their 'sickness status' has been legitimized by the medical profession. They are excused normal duties but are expected to make every effort to get better and resume the role of healthy person by complying assiduously with medical advice.

However, this parsonian perspective has been challenged as oversimplistic and idealistic. Freidson (1970) argued that the interaction between practitioner and patient is characterized by conflict rather than compliance. On the basis of the author's review of research in this area, both points of view seem to obtain in real life. On the one hand, patients frequently disagree with their doctors and do not comply with advice; on the other hand, they tend to be reluctant to engage in a process of negotiation and bargaining for fear of being labelled 'bad patients'.

The justification for the Parsonian view of the unequal distribution of power between patient and doctor (and, more generally, between medicine and society in general) is quite simple. The doctor assumes power in the best interest of the patient since there is a 'competence gap' between health professional and client resulting from the complex and esoteric body of knowledge which the doctor acquires through a long process of training and socialization. In the words of DiMatteo and Di Nicola (1982), 'The disparity in power and control carves an emotional chasm between physician and patient—a chasm that is bridged only by the physician's altruism and orientation to serving people'.

Clearly there is an alternative view which applies to the process of professionalization. Following George Bernard Shaw's observation (1911) that the 'professions are a conspiracy against the laity' (*The Doctor's Dilemma*, Act I), doctors seek to maintain this imbalance in power and resort to mystification in a purely self-seeking way. Moreover, from a health promotion perspective, there are major practical disadvantages inherent in patients' adoption of a sick role. Firstly, primary prevention requires people to look after themselves and adopt a prudent lifestyle. They must make everyday decisions and cannot merely comply with a simple medical prescription. Secondly, in so far as there is no simple cure for the majority of contemporary diseases, and a good deal of uncertainty surrounds the very notion of risk factors, co-operation rather than compliance is an absolute necessity. Furthermore, the notion of 'affective neutrality' embodied in the traditional prescription for the relationship between doctors (and professions allied to medicine) and their patients actively militates against the requirements for effective education and counselling. It is not possible to maintain emotional distance whilst simultaneously displaying respect, empathy, and genuineness: for example, Zola's (1986) description of the 'language of endearment, familiarity and/or belittlement' which characterizes a 'top–down' approach to communication is completely at odds with the need to encourage client and patient to be assertive and take responsibility for their own health.

A disparity of power is not only bad for patients, it is also bad for doctors. Apart from the high non-compliance rate, doctors who wish to be empathic and encourage patients to be assertive may find it extremely difficult to cast off their heavy burden of legitimate authority because patients may not let them do so. The solution from a health promotion perspective is not difficult to formulate—although not at all easy to implement in practice. On the one hand, all health practitioners can be trained in counselling skills—provided that they are convinced of the benefits of relinquishing some of the less productive aspects of their professional socialization. On the other hand, the general public should be sufficiently well educated about health and illness that they will not only be able to make reasoned decisions about their health and illness behaviour but they will also have a more realistic appreciation of what medicine can achieve.

This general education about health and the health services is entirely congruent with the WHO's desire to reverse the process of medicalization and achieve a reorientation of health services. It is an integral part of the ideology of health promotion. Also, when increasing concern is being shown about escalating cost—and an associated need for some sort of 'rationing'—an educated public will not only be more consumer-oriented but should also be more willing and able to make democratic decisions through the ballot box about the kind of health service it wants. Furthermore, the very notion of compliance is alien to health promotion's axiomatic allegiance to participation and co-operation.

Factors associated with failure in communication and education

There has been a good deal of research into communication failure. A substantial proportion of this research has focused on the doctor–patient encounter. The reasons for this partiality are not absolutely clear: it may not necessarily be because doctors are worse communicators than other professionals but rather that the outcome of failure may be more dramatic. Most doctors have exposed themselves to scrutiny in this way. Nevertheless, the results of this research highlight the requirements of effective educational interventions. The distinction between communication and education is often unclear in the research literature on failure, and typically includes examples of both unsuccessful communication and unsuccessful education (defined as a failure to promote health or illness-related learning).

An extensive literature review is not appropriate here. However, an outline of some key research findings is provided below. Ley (1990) provides a more detailed review.

As observed in the 'sickness career', there appears to be a good deal of dissatisfaction with medical communications and a high level of non-compliance. Ley (1990) reviewed 33 different investigations into the levels of patient dissatisfaction with communication: this ranged from 5 to 82 per cent with a mean rate of around 37 per cent. Ley also summarized four reviews of compliance in the late 1970s and noted their mean non-compliance rates for four areas: medication, clinic attendance, diet, and 'miscellaneous'. The average non-compliance across all of these studies was around 46 per cent.

As Pascoe (1983) cogently demonstrates, the notion of patient dissatisfaction is rather vague: it has been used here merely to describe the extent to which patients like or dislike the communication they have received from medical practitioners. However, it is clear that the relationship between non-compliance and dissatisfaction is tenuous. Indeed, Ley found a correlation of only +0.26 between these two variables. People's failure to follow advice must be explained in some other way.

One factor which would logically militate against compliance is misperception of the message communicated by the health professional. Tuckett *et al.* (1985), after researching doctor–patient interactions in 1000 consultations in primary care, provide valuable insights not only into patient misperception and misinterpretation of communications but also into two other important areas directly relevant to education. They demonstrated not only a high level of misinterpretation of messages but also a not insubstantial 'lack of commitment' by patients to courses of action which they had understood. They also checked the extent to which patients had forgotten what their doctor had told them. There were, in all, some 34 per cent of consultations in which the patient either 'did not remember or make sense 'correctly' or was not 'committed' to key points.

The extent to which patients actually forget the information they have been given is a matter of some debate. Ley (1990), in his comprehensive literature review, reported that the mean percentage of information recalled by patients after their medical consultations was approximately 60 per cent in hospital patients and 65 per cent in general practice patients. In other words patients appear to forget about 40 per cent of what they have been told. Conversely, Tuckett *et al.* (1985) found only 10 per cent of consultations after which the patient was unable to recall key points correctly. Moreover, they ascribed some of this memory deficit to the fact that patients were not committed to the advice offered. So, according to Tuckett *et al.*, factors other than memory failure must account for failure to comply with medical advice.

Explaining non-compliance

In providing a cogent explanation for non-compliance, there are three sets of key actors involved. Firstly, there is the doctor or health professional; secondly, there is the patient, client, or learner; thirdly, there is what might be described as lay opinion which will include not only the lay referral system mentioned above, but a kind of background noise of information coming from the mass media and other educational agencies, formal or informal. It is therefore wrong to consider non-compliance as merely patient failure. Indeed, one further example of Ley's (1990) rigorous literature review is an intriguing analysis of what he calls 'non-compliance by health care professionals with rules for good patient care'. He examined 19 research studies into the activities of psychologists, pharmacists, nurses, dentists, emergency medical technicians, and medical practitioners. The mean proportion of professionals not complying with recommended practice was about 60 per cent—rather higher than patients' failure rate.

Compliance will not happen if communication fails, that is if the message does not reach the senses, if patients do not pay attention, and if they misinterpret the message. At the next stage, that of influencing client learning and behaviour, further consideration is needed of Tuckett *et al.*'s (1985) comments on the lack of commitment to doctors' advice which many patients demonstrated in their research. What does this lack of commitment mean?

Lack of commitment is best understand in terms of attitude theory: the patient has a negative attitude to the course of action recommended by the doctor. This negative attitude may be understood by reference to key beliefs. One of these beliefs will be similar to the notion of self-efficacy. For instance, although patients might accept that a recommended course of action—such as a period of bed rest—will be beneficial, if they know that bed rest is incompatible with environmental circumstances and domestic duties, then there will inevitably be a lack of commitment and co-operation. Educational programmes must include environmental analysis and support.

The health action model is useful to explain a second reason for a possible lack of commitment to action, a point emphasized by Tuckett *et al.* The majority of patients consulting a doctor or nurse will already have made their own diagnosis of their presenting problem and will probably have identified beforehand the kind of prescription needed—for instance, some form of medication. Failure to confirm the patients' expectations is likely to be a cause for dissatisfaction and, possibly, non-co-operation. More significant though is the reason why patients make their diagnosis in the first place. The explanation frequently derives from patients' causal attributions and what Tuckett *et al.* preferred to call 'theories of disease'. An example will serve to clarify this observation.

Consider the case of a patient who presents with a rash on his leg. The doctor diagnoses a self-limiting allergic condition of no great significance and prescribes an emollient cream. Later, at interview, it becomes clear that the patient was not committed to the recommended advice although he had understood it thoroughly and had complete recall of key points. The reason for the non-compliance followed a self-diagnosis which had its roots in a dimly formed association of the complaint with phlebitis—which in turn had a kind of metaphorical association with the bite of a flea and the resultant association with a blood disorder. This latter was described in terms of the blood being 'too rich'—due to too rich a diet. The rash was symptomatic of this underlying disorder. Accordingly, the patient is reluctant to comply with the doctor's recommended treatment and this leads him to formulate his own treatment plan. His own (very logical) preferred remedy would have been a medicine to 'cleanse the blood'; medication was his treatment of choice though he would have accepted a recommended change in diet—even if he had been unwilling to cope with the loss of gratification. The patient duly makes some marginal dietary changes—such as cutting down sugar intake. The disorder, as predicted by the general practitioner, was indeed self-limiting and the rash duly disappeared—thus confirming the patient's diagnosis and his theory of illness.

The educational implication of incidents such as this is made abundantly clear by Tuckett *et al.*: if they want to reduce non-compliance, practitioners must first explore patients' theories of illness—a process involving negotiation and co-operation rather than prescription and compliance.

In the context of patients' beliefs, a number of beliefs identified in the health action model are applicable to the arena of compliance with medical advice. These will not be repeated here but the various health belief models are highly relevant. The probabilities of co-operation will be substantially increased to the extent that patients accept their own (or their children's) susceptibility to a medical condition, rate it as serious, and believe that the prescribed measures will be effective without at the same time entailing too many costs—in terms of such barriers to action as inconvenience, discomfort, loss of money, and so on.

Before leaving the question of non-cooperation, it is worth recalling that aspect of the health action model which was concerned with facilitating the translation of intention into practice. Assuming that a patient is committed to the advice provided and believes that the recommended action is manageable in his or her social and environmental circumstances, then it is essential to ensure as far as possible that those circumstances are in fact conducive to compliance. For this reason, the educational encounter should include, where necessary, the provision of any skills needed by the patient together with the requisite environmental and social support.

The various constructs and processes described in Fig. 9 can now be translated into a more detailed set of guidelines for an educational consultation. Firstly, however, it is important to consider a key issue which has a bearing on both the question of empowerment—which is central to the practice of health promotion—and also the whole matter of patient co-operation.

Characteristics of the health promoter

Patient commitment may depend on whether patients prefer to believe their doctors or would rather rely on their own theories of illness and the lay referral system from which they derive. There is a kind of credibility clash between professional and lay referents.

The characteristics of the health promoter are of particular importance in the educational process and it has long been recognized in communication and attitude theory that there are at least two varieties of credibility. One of these has been described as 'legitimate' or 'expert' authority: credibility is thus bestowed on a person who is perceived to have a high level of relevant (and often technical) expertise—especially if supported by some formal status conferred by state institutions. Doctors would be included in this category.

Conversely, lay people are often accorded a kind of 'referent' authority despite their lack of formal status; indeed, their status will derive from their very membership of the lay community. Rogers and Shoemaker (1971) coined the word 'homophily' to explain the way in which referent authority operates. This principle states that members of a social group are most likely to be influenced by 'opinion leaders' who embody the norms of that particular community and are perceived to share those characteristics of community members which are deemed to be important.

According to this principle, all professionals whose social group and background are, by definition, different from their clients' social milieu, will find it difficult to influence anyone from a different social class or ethnic group. While clients might accept the doctor's superior knowledge about illness—provided that it does not conflict with lay wisdom and everyday experience—they will be reluctant to believe that doctors can really appreciate the problems their patients face as, for example, an unemployed single parent living in a slum. Advice will therefore be treated with a degree of scepticism.

However, and very significantly, the principle of homophily also states that it is possible for people from different circumstances to have credibility provided that they also have empathy. Since empathy is a recognized social interaction skill, it can be taught. Indeed, any health promoter working face to face with clients—either singly or in a group setting—needs a repertoire of social interaction skills. Central to the socially skilled response is the capacity to interpret correctly key aspects of the client's mental state by appropriate use of questioning and sensitivity to non-verbal communication. The successful communicator and educator should be capable of responding flexibly to the perceived needs of the client: they need to provide 'different strokes for different folks'. Key components of the skilled response and the mental set underlying those skills is what has often been called the 'holy trinity' of counselling: respect, empathy, and genuineness. Though empathy is a social skill which can be learned, respect and genuineness are less easily acquired. Indeed, it has been argued that respect and genuine interest in a client cannot be faked; they will usually be detected by the client—probably as a result of 'non-verbal leakage'. The implications for effective education are that health professionals must have a genuine interest in their clients and possess a variety of communication and social interaction skills.

In the context of the interaction between doctor and patient, there is strong evidence that patient satisfaction is associated with a liking for the doctor's interpersonal skills—even if this is only described in terms of 'perceived friendliness'. It also seems likely that many doctors lack the flexibility of response associated with a socially skilled performance. Indeed, it is all too easy for professionals to caricature clients in the educational or caring setting.

Byrne and Long (1976), in an important British study, made a distinction between 'doctor centred' and 'patient-centred' modes of social interaction in the consultation. The former approach focused primarily on gathering information—by questioning, probing, and analysing. Conversely, the patient-centred approach demonstrated key features of the skilful educational encounter and was characterized by various 'micro skills': active listening, providing the patient with a breathing space in which to think and speak, asking 'open' clarifying questions rather than closed questions requiring merely the answer 'yes' or 'no', and empathic reflection of patients' concerns and feelings. Byrne and Long also described an important tendency for doctors to use only one interaction style with a variety of different patients: the antithesis of providing different strokes for different folks.

As noted above, Tuckett *et al.* (1985) urged practitioners to explore patients' theories of illness if they wished to maximize co-operation with their advice. The patient-centred techniques presented above are exactly those needed to investigate client theories, perceptions, beliefs, and attitudes. Although the most frequently cited reason for doctors not undertaking health education is lack of time, it is very likely that investment in a patient-centred educational approach will pay dividends in reducing the problem of non-compliance.

Tuckett *et al.* also noted that patients had an irritating tendency to expect doctors magically to divine their uncertainties, anxieties, and concerns. If and when they failed to do so, patient satisfaction plummeted. The researchers asked these patients why they did not question their doctors or, if they were not committed to the advice offered, why they did not explain their doubts or even challenge the doctor's point of view. Their answers revealed a decidedly low level of empowerment.

1. Sixty per cent of the respondents identified questions which they would have liked to have asked the doctor—but did not do so; they gave a total of 104 reasons for staying silent.

2. Thirty-three per cent of respondents had doubts which, again, they did not express; they gave 44 reasons for keeping quiet. Most of these various reasons reflected the nature of the 'power relationship' between doctor and patient. They included the following specific statements:

   - 'felt hurried'
   - 'frightened of a bad reaction from doctor'
   - 'frightened doctor will think less well of patient'
   - 'felt it was not up to the patient to ask/mention'.

Tuckett *et al.* examined in some detail the level of patient participation in the consultation and recorded this level of involvement with reference to what they identified as five key 'consultation tasks'. Two of these tasks concerned patients' theories of illness and the extent to which they expressed doubts about doctors' advice. Forty-four per cent of patients showed 'no sign' of expressing doubts; 73 per cent made no attempt at all to explain their ideas about their symptoms and the underlying illness.

The context of the general public's need for health education within the arena of general health promotion initiatives serves as an introduction to the next section which provides a wider perspective on influencing health and illness decisions. Certain aspects of mounting community-wide programmes in a number of different settings and contexts will be discussed. Specific educational techniques will then be considered, many of which will be relevant to the needs of effective communication and education in the encounters between health professionals and patients. However, before tackling this issue, it would be useful to assess the insights made so far into the issue of assessing effectiveness and efficiency.

The need to use intermediate indicators of success by measuring patients' or clients' beliefs, attitudes, and skills has been identified. An extra dimension has been added in the form of so-called 'process evaluation'. If, for example, doctors' social interaction skills influence patients' beliefs and attitudes, and increase the likelihood of their co-operating with recommended advice, then it is reasonable to assess these. Assessing the extent to which health professionals exhibit an appropriate level of such skills as an intermediate indicator of not only patient adherence to a prescribed regime but also as a marker on the route to longer-term reductions in mortality and morbidity would be very useful. Accordingly, an evaluation of this 'process' can provide a valuable 'quality audit' of practitioner performance.

Influencing behaviour: strategies, settings, and contexts

Before discussing specific communication techniques and the educational methods needed to influence behaviours in the specific milieu of primary care, an overview will be provided at the macrolevel of key settings and contexts for the 'delivery' of health education. Firstly, a few important generalizations can usefully be made about how social systems or 'communities' tend to change.

Change at the macrolevel: the adoption of innovations

One of the most useful reviews of community-level change is provided by communication of innovations theory (Rogers and Shoemaker 1971; Rogers 1995). It generalizes from seven major research traditions and illuminates the process whereby 'an idea, practice, or object perceived as new by an individual' comes to be adopted (or rejected) by a community or, more precisely, a social system. The social system is typically geographically defined but may be 'relational', for instance a 'community' of doctors within a particular region.

A number of generalizations may be made about the communication of innovations and these are concerned with five phenomena:

- rate of adoption
- nature of the social system
- characteristics of potential adopters
- characteristics of change agents
- characteristics of the innovation.

Firstly, it is salutary to note that the rate of adoption of new practices is characteristically slow. Additionally and irrespective of the time taken, the process is described by an 'S-shaped' curve which demonstrates the fact that the rate of change is initially slow, gathers momentum, and then tails off. This fact has in turn been ascribed to different adopter attributes. So-called 'innovators' (amounting to perhaps 2.5 per cent of the population) seize on the innovation eagerly; they are followed by a category of 'early adopters' (arguably 13.5 per cent of the population) who are then followed by an 'early' and 'late majority' who account for 68 per cent of the whole group. Finally a collection of some 16 per cent die-hard 'laggards' bring up the rear. These findings reflect only a situation in which the innovation is sufficiently attractive to create social change.

These observations show that expectations of rapid change in response to public communication exercises are unrealistic. They also have implications for the continuous monitoring of the effect of such communications. There are more significant implications to be drawn from the remaining three phenomena under consideration.

The rate of adoption of an innovation will be influenced by the characteristics of the social system itself. It is argued that a 'traditional' community will always take longer to adopt an innovation than a more modern 'cosmopolitan' population. Of greater significance is the importance of taking account of the community's 'felt needs'. For instance, if a given social group recognizes that it has a particular need and discovers a remedy, change will be relatively rapid and will not involve any interference from external 'change agents'. If those change agents manage to supply the solution to a problem which the members of a community have identified, again the innovation will be relatively speedy. Conversely, an attempt to impose an externally generated solution on a community which does not believe it has a problem is doomed to failure. If, however, a sensitive community development programme is employed, the community worker/health educator may gradually raise the level of 'critical consciousness' of a community such that it becomes aware of a need which it has not yet articulated. Subsequently, the effective educator or community worker will act as a facilitator, provide support, and work as an advocate to meet the newly awakened need.

The importance of credibility and the principle of 'homophily' is paramount. Like the doctor, teacher, or nurse, the community worker must possess the social skills associated with communicating respect, empathy, and genuineness. They must enlist the support of community 'opinion leaders' and others who already enjoy credibility in the eyes of the people.

Table 1 summarizes the relationship between perceptions of need and the origin of the innovation.

Finally, it is important to consider the real and perceived attributes of the innovation itself. Ideally, it should have a number of characteristics as follows.

1. It should be seen to be simple rather than complex.
2. People should believe it can be readily tried and the beneficial effects should be observable sooner rather than later.
3. Importantly, the innovation should be compatible with existing culture and norms and should have a fairly clear advantage compared with current practice.
4. It should not appear to incur any substantial costs—financial or otherwise.

It is a salutary exercise to check the public's perception of any given health promotion measure—such as condom use or the adoption of vigorous cardioprotective exercise—in relation to the costs and benefits involved and the other perceived features of the proposed innovation.

Mass media: limitations and potential

Some of the broader strategies and settings in which health promotion fosters the adoption of health and illness related innovations can be usefully considered. The strategic use of mass media will be the first subject for discussion.

One of the most confident assertions emerging from communication of innovations theory is that interpersonal channels of communication are more effective than mass media publicity when it

Table 1 Community participation and adoption of innovations

Level of community participation	Anticipated rate of adoption of the innovation
Community spontaneously recognizes it has a problem	Very rapid change
Community identifies solution to problem	
External agency considers that community has a problem	Very slow—or never!
Prescribes solution	

comes to persuading communities to change their practices. Since mass media are not merely frequently employed in health promotion but are often viewed as a panacea, it is important to provide a brief summary of the capabilities of this highly important strategy for public education.

Firstly, by definition, the mass media have the potential for reaching a mass audience, therefore influencing a very large numbers of individuals 'at a stroke'. Secondly, the mass media mediate the educational message using such channels as television or the printed word. Because of the mediated nature of the message, there is no possibility for receiving immediate feedback from the audience—and, as argued above, immediate feedback is a prerequisite for effective communication. Therefore mass media cannot provide 'different strokes for different folks'; nor is it possible for producers and presenters to react creatively to the many different audience responses to the message. Lazarsfeld and Merton (1948) identified three major conditions in which mass media were most likely to effect a given population substantially. These were described as 'monopolization', 'canalization', and 'supplementation'. Thus, mass media would not be influential unless:

- the recipient of the media messages lived in relative social isolation or was not exposed to counter-messages
- they canalized or built on already existing motivation
- they were used to supplement and support other initiatives such as interpersonal education and/or policy developments.

Therefore, in the absence of these circumstances, the mass media are unlikely to be effective in changing attitudes and behaviours—particularly where these involve some loss of gratification or are perceived to result in discomfort or major inconvenience. Furthermore, the mass media cannot teach complex skills or provide understanding of complex issues. However, the mass media can very successfully raise awareness and reinforce other initiatives.

There are many different types of media; therefore the generalizations listed below should be treated with caution. For a more comprehensive account of the complex theoretical and practical dimensions of mass media, see MacShane (1979), Salmon (1989), Backer *et al.* (1992), and Tones and Tilford (1994).

Generalizations about mass media use in health promotion

1. Different mass media can achieve different effects.
2. There is a major difference between the persuasive use of mass media and 'documentaries' or 'educational broadcasting'.
3. Various incidental effects of media (for example, the portrayal of alcohol use in soap operas) may have a negative influence on health. 'Healthy public policy' is needed to regulate any demonstrably harmful effects.
4. Persuasive advertising will generally have a minimal effect on beliefs, attitudes, and behaviour—especially when the particular behaviour involves a loss of gratification, inconvenience, or discomfort.
5. Mass media have a limited potential for teaching complex concepts or providing psychomotor or social interaction skills.
6. Mass media can have a valuable 'climate setting' role and be extremely effective in 'agenda setting' or 'critical consciousness raising' (Tones 1996).

The substantial amount of research into social marketing in general and the use of mass media for health promotion in particular allows a number of specific observations and recommendations to be made.

1. More effective campaigns use multiple media.
2. More effective campaigns use mass media as part of community-wide programmes to support other activities—in school, primary care, and so on.
3. More effective campaigns are co-ordinated with direct service delivery—for example information 'hotlines' and support services.
4. More effective campaigns involve key power figures and groups in mass media organizations and government.
5. Role models should be carefully selected: it is essential to ensure that the target group identifies with the models selected and that they continue to retain their appeal and credibility.
6. Consultative collaboration should be used as part of a broad health promotion strategy in order to influence media policy and thus mitigate any negative effects of the portrayal of health matters in the media.
7. Campaigns should emphasize positive behaviour change rather than negative consequences, and current rewards rather than the avoidance of distant negative consequences.
8. Any anxiety-provoking media messages should be accompanied by mechanisms for reducing that anxiety.
9. More effective campaigns use educational messages in entertainment contexts.
10. Campaign timing is very important.
11. Repetition of a single (simple) message is more likely to create an impact.
12. Campaigns should use key marketing principles such as 'audience segmentation', setting modest and realistic goals, 'formative evaluation', and message 'pretesting'.
13. Audience segmentation is likely to be more productive if it is based on psychographics as part of the pretesting strategy (for example exploration of beliefs and values using qualitative research techniques) rather than demographics (broader focus on such variables as social class using quantitative techniques).
14. A good deal of thought and effort should be devoted to 'media advocacy' using 'creative epidemiology'.
15. Health promotion should, wherever possible, get value for money by generating newsworthy stories which create unpaid advertising.

The main function of the mass media is to support general community-wide initiatives which centre on interpersonal education techniques supported by 'healthy public policy'. Accordingly, a brief review of the various key settings and contexts in which these interpersonal methods typically operate is provided.

Key settings and contexts for health promotion

Health promotion may be employed in a number of settings and contexts: for example, in schools, local authority institutions, youth clubs, workplaces, pharmacies, and by the various health and medical services. Two principles will guide the discussion which follows. The first of these emphasizes the importance of a 'healthy alliance' between the various delivery systems; and the second makes the common sense assertion that each particular context and setting has its own strengths and peculiar potential for promoting health and its own limitations.

The concept of intersectoral collaboration figures prominently in the WHO's formulation of health promotion practice. Synergistic effects will result from collaboration towards the goals of health promotion. At the time of writing the notion of a 'healthy alliance' is enjoying a degree of popularity in the United Kingdom in the form of 'Health Action Zones' and 'Healthy Living Centres'. These initiatives are, in the words of the recent White Paper on the health of the nation (Department of Health 1999*b*), designed to 'build local capability' and 'regenerate health in communities'. Collaboration between key agencies—especially the National Health Service (**NHS**), local government, and primary health care—is seen as essential in tackling the social determinants of disease.

Two kinds of collaborative endeavour are worth noting. The first is often described in relation to a notional 'health career'. For example, it is helpful to construct a 'smoking career' as a basis for devising a coherent programme of smoking education. The smoking career identifies the progress made by individuals who at some point are recruited to smoking as 'experimental smokers', become 'regular smokers', and subsequently either give up their habit (thus swelling the ranks of 'ex-smokers') or continue along their career as regular and probably dissonant smokers concerned at their increased risk of tobacco-related disease or premature death.

A number of important influences on the smoking career have been identified. These include the extent to which parents 'model' smoking by their example or encourage it by their *laissez-faire* attitude or positive approval. They also include peer group example and the various psychological and social needs which lead to young people exposing themselves to the pressures of one peer group rather than another. They include the normative pressures of the workplace and the general background 'noise' provided by mass media.

Macrofactors such as socio-economic status exert a continuing and, typically, mediating effect. People who are from unskilled manual occupations have a higher level of smoking than those who work in management or the professions. Even more substantial rates of smoking are apparent in the unemployed or those who experience some other form of social deprivation.

A more detailed analysis of the smoking career is beyond the scope of this chapter; however, the significance of a career-line analysis for the systematic planning of health promotion programmes is clear. If the tendency to adopt and sustain smoking results from the combined and cumulative effects of socialization and a variety of environmental circumstances, then health promotion not only needs to take account of these various pressures but must also develop a competing programme. Such a programme should also have a cumulative effect by ensuring that a variety of agencies, formal and informal, operate in a compatible and synergistic fashion so that the school programme builds on initiatives undertaken in primary care, setting the scene for later mass media campaigns and efforts in the workplace and wider community.

The second kind of synergistic programme is cross-sectional rather than longitudinal. It concerns the establishment of 'healthy alliances' and intersectoral collaboration. Collaboration between those providing health education, who are seeking to influence people's behaviours, must be supplemented by supportive healthy public policy if the maximal synergistic effect is to be achieved. This principle is important in a number of crucial health promotion settings which could contribute to the general collaborative effort. The WHO notes in the Jakarta Declaration (WHO 1997) the importance of its 'settings for health' approach:

> There is now clear evidence that . . . particular settings offer practical opportunities for the implementation of comprehensive strategies. These include mega-cities, islands, cities, municipalities, local communities, markets, schools, the workplace, and health care facilities.

The review which follows is necessarily brief but a more complete treatment of health promotion settings and strategies can be found in Bracht (1999), Green and Kreuter (1999), Glanz *et al.* (1997), Whitehead and Tones (1991), and Tones and Tilford (1994).

The workplace

The workplace has been viewed as an important location for health promotion for many years in the United States although there are signs that its popularity has increased in recent years in Europe. In this context, reference will be made to the two themes which recur in this review:

- the advantages and limitations of any given setting for establishing health promotion programmes
- the importance of incorporating complementary health policy.

All settings contribute to health whether or not they have a health promotion policy, and that influence may be good or bad. For instance, a workplace which has poor safety procedures, creates stress in the workforce through poor staff relationships, regularly threatens redundancy, and offers only unhealthy food in smoke-clouded canteens is obviously contributing negative effects to health.

The workplace offers a great opportunity for health educators to gain access to a large proportion of the adult population (in the United Kingdom, some 26 million people) in a well-defined and, ideally, supportive setting.

Conversely, there are certain problematic aspects to be taken into account. The organizational goals of the workplace are fundamentally different from the goals of health promoters. Indeed, the sole purpose of the commercial sector is to maximize profit. Fortunately, though, managers seem to be increasingly convinced that health promotion in their workplaces will actually increase profit. The rationale is as follows: a health promotion programme as part of workers' welfare provision enhances the public image of the company; it enhances staff morale and reduces turnover and its associated retraining costs; sickness absence rates should decline; productivity should improve. Moreover, in countries like the United States where the national health system is dominated by private health insurance, those costs should be dramatically reduced. There is a good deal of evidence that these managerial perceptions are justified.

In the United Kingdom, the public sector employs a substantial proportion of the workforce—and the profit motive is perhaps less significant. The NHS provides a particular apposite example of such a workforce—and it is a matter of some interest that one of the more important requirements of the WHO's 'Health-Promoting Hospital' initiative is that health service institutions and organizations develop an 'exemplary' occupational health service incorporating health education, empowerment, and supportive health-promoting policy.

For any health promotion programme to be completely effective, it must be fully incorporated into the everyday working of a given organization. Even if the resources were available, outside health professionals should not be expected to provide a direct service. However, although an occupational health service might be an obvious candidate for the health promotion task, provision can be patchy—especially in small industries and organizations. This fact leads to the second of the two themes mentioned above: the policy imperative.

Policy is important at two levels. The possible lack of a proper occupational health service has implications for macrolevel policy in terms of financial support, legislation, and nurse training. At the local level, the importance of policy has been thoroughly emphasized. For many years it has been acknowledged that blaming accidents on workers' carelessness or failure to take proper precautions is a classic example of victim blaming, and there has been a corresponding improvement in safety legislation and environmental protection schemes. More recently, a good deal of progress has been made in the adoption and implementation of health policy in areas related to other aspects of lifestyle: smoking policies are now commonplace, alcohol policies are being increasingly implemented, and a start is being made in providing healthy eating and, less frequently, exercise facilities.

The health-promoting school

The school is conventionally regarded as an obvious place for teaching about health and the emergence of any particular health concern is likely to lead to the somewhat aggrieved question, 'What are the schools doing about it?'

The issue of designing and implementing health education curricula in schools has a long pedigree. It has a substantial theoretical and practical base, and an associated extensive literature. A wide variety of teaching materials, curriculum planning guides, and training initiatives have been launched. Some further insights into this sophisticated world are provided by Ryder and Campbell (1988) and Nutbeam *et al.* (1991).

The major advantage for ensuring a sound health promotion presence in the school curriculum is the fact that young people spend a long time in this setting—in the United Kingdom, some 15 000 hours *in toto*. Moreover, schoolchildren are at a relatively early point in their health career. Logically, there is a prime opportunity for influencing attitudes and behaviours at a formative stage.

Much more important, however, is the possibility for schools to provide horizontal rather than vertical health education programmes. One of the major implications of the kind of analysis conducted in the health action model is a need to take a sophisticated look at the factors contributing to health and illness behaviours. Quite basic attributes and competences, such as self-esteem, locus of control, or the possession of various 'lifeskills', will influence all kinds of health decision. Accordingly, rather than focusing on current epidemiological priorities—and professionally defined health problems—the focus should be on root causes and solutions. This point has been more extensively argued elsewhere (Tones 1993*b*), but it is clear that a broad 'horizontal' programme of school-based personal, social, and health education will lay a proper foundation for empowered decision-making. This will be both more productive and economical than concentrating solely on 'vertical' programmes such as accident prevention or cancer education.

One of the recent features of school health education has been the formal acknowledgement of a need to ensure that health teaching is consistent with the general life of the school. The existence of a 'hidden curriculum' has always been acknowledged by general theory and practice in education. It has been part of the conventional wisdom of the school sector that the school's 'ethos' can have substantial effects for good or ill. The relatively recent accentuation of this phenomenon in the health context characterizes contemporary definitions of the 'health-promoting school'. Following this principle, it is important that schools should deliberately formulate policies which will complement teaching: nutrition education should not take place in a setting where only unhealthy snacks and school meals are on offer. Exhortations about self-worth will have relatively little impact in an ambience where only the academically outstanding appear to be valued.

The health-promoting hospital

Reference has already been made to the health-promoting hospital initiative which represents the most significant recent setting in which attempts are being made to ensure that 'healthy public policy' supports other health endeavours. In this context treatment features prominently although education is increasingly assuming a higher profile. The origin of the health-promoting hospital was the Healthy Cities movement and its 'ratification' was the Budapest Declaration (WHO 1991). The main features of hospitals subscribing to the principles of the Budapest Declaration are summarized as follows.

1. The health-promoting hospital has an integrated policy for promoting positive health for patients, staff, and visitors covering all aspects of the hospital environment and the transactions occurring within it.
2. The health-promoting hospital should be seen as part of the local community it serves and should maintain active links and alliances with community groups and agencies.
3. The health-promoting hospital should have a model occupational health service which provides an example of good practice for other workplaces.
4. The health-promoting hospital is characterized not only by effective communication and good patient education; it strives to empower the patients in its care.

The pedigree and rationale of these four principles are self-explanatory. However, the notion of positive health emphasized by the Budapest Declaration and the empowerment question do merit a little further elaboration. The concept of positive health is by no means clearly articulated but is closely associated with the condition of empowerment. Macleod Clark's (1993) distinction between 'sick' nursing and 'health' nursing is clearly germane to this debate. The evolutionary or perhaps revolutionary move from 'sick nursing' behaviours, which are 'dominating, generalized, prescriptive, reassuring, directive' to 'health nursing' would be entirely consistent with the goals of a health promoting hospital. Macleod Clark's description of 'health nursing' is also congruent with the recommendation for effective doctor–patient consultations. Unlike 'sick nursing', it involves the processes of 'collaboration, negotiation, facilitation, the provision of support, and the individualization of communication'.

This accentuation of empowerment in the hospital setting is indeed intriguing, bearing in mind that the hospital has traditionally provided a classic example of 'total institutions'. According to Taylor (1979), a hospital is one of the few places where an individual forfeits control over virtually every task he or she customarily performs.

Interestingly, the management executive of the British NHS, has apparently taken the notion of the health-promoting hospital very seriously in their publication of guidelines (NHS 1994) and provision of general support. This level of commitment was illustrated by a nursing officer from the Department of Health who cited the results of departmental research into health education and health promotion in nursing in acute areas. She quoted the following extract:

> The data revealed that the ward climate needs to be such that nurses feel valued, supported, autonomous and empowered members of the ward team. This appeared to facilitate health education and health promotion via increasing morale and enabling nurses to support and empower their patients rather than maintain traditional role distinctions and the unequal balance of power inherent in these. (Cited by Weeks 1993)

Community development

The final example of a setting or context considered here is that of community development—like health promotion itself, a complex and often contested concept. It is difficult, in a brief review, to avoid caricature and oversimplification. At one level community development can be viewed as a setting which merely differs from other settings in its informality of approach. However, the most significant feature of the approach is its ideology. Community development should not be confused with so-called 'community-wide' programmes which involve the deployment of the widest possible range of agencies in a common cause—such as the prevention of coronary heart disease. Nor does community development equate with those 'outreach' programmes which deliver services to those members of the community who do not use existing facilities; neither is it synonymous with educational programmes which use community workers to 'get through' to the 'hard-to-reach'. Community development does involve working with those so-called 'resistant' groups in settings characterized typically by urban squalor, disadvantage, and deprivation.

Community development is of particular relevance to health promotion since its ultimate concern is with empowerment and its ideology is best described in terms of an empowerment model—as defined at the beginning of this chapter. The ideological imperative is with remedying disadvantage and achieving a fairer distribution of resources in society. It typically operates by employing community 'change agents' to work with people in relatively small geographical areas. Their task is to help the community identify its 'felt needs'. A successful intervention would raise people's consciousness and concern over their social circumstances; their beliefs and perceptions should change and they should feel more confident in their ability to agitate for social and environmental change; and they would acquire skills to help them to achieve the changes which they have identified as important. In short, they would be empowered. The contribution that a health promoter or community worker might make to such an intervention is summarized in Fig. 10.

Although they do not match this pure and idealized form of community development, many community health projects embody the 'bottom-up' empowering stance of the ideal type. Since they often start with well-recognized public health issues, they may bypass the stage of identifying felt needs though they would consider it essential to consult the community extensively about its perception of need within the somewhat narrower domain of health and prevention.

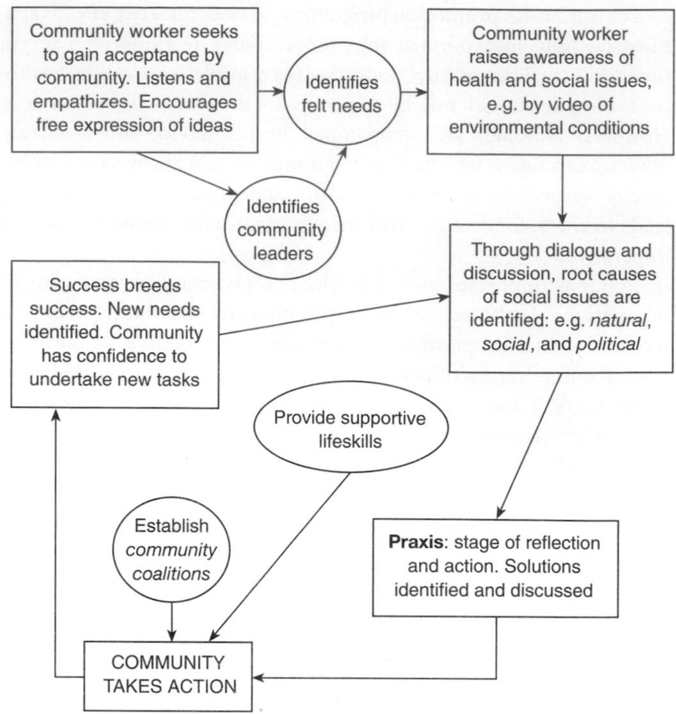

Fig. 10 A process of community development.

Community health projects do not, therefore, attempt to 'colonize' a community with health workers whose purpose is to infiltrate and manipulate networks in order to achieve predetermined goals and meet specific targets imposed in an authoritarian way—as will be clear from the following list of the characteristics of community health projects (derived from Rosenthal 1983):

- firmly based outside health professions
- concerned with addressing inequalities in health and health-care provision
- concerned to promote collective awareness of social causes of ill health
- assert that the monopoly of information about health and ill health by professionals must be challenged both individually and collectively
- activities centre on work with small groups of local people
- projects have a catalyst function in stimulating local health, social, and educational services.

It is important to reaffirm that the use of empowering techniques—whether in the community or a hospital—does not merely serve ideological ends. If successful, the empowering effects of community health projects are more likely to lead to the adoption of medically approved preventive behaviours than competing, disease-focused vertical programmes delivered in a traditional way.

Requirements of systematic programme design

Microlevel analysis would reveal that a variety of specific communication techniques and educational methods are usually used in all of the settings explored above. Before considering the appropriate selection of these methods, the relationship between settings and methods in the context of a systematic approach to designing health promotion programmes is shown in Fig. 11.

Any programme will involve an assessment of need—explicitly or implicitly. Figure 11(a) contrasts 'normative' (that is professionally prescribed) needs with a community's 'felt needs'—and notes that both might be over-ruled by the superior force of political imperatives. At all events a process of prioritizing competing demands must take place. The process of assessing need and the associated resource implications would be typically followed by identification of aims and an analysis of the relative contribution to be made by health policy measures and health education within a variety of different settings. Where a programme involves a synergistic amalgam of both policy and education, programme design and evaluation will be considerably facilitated by the statement of precise and detailed objectives. Since the purpose of health education is to facilitate learning, the educational task would therefore be expressed as 'learning objectives'. Both sets of objectives would be stated in respect of the target group(s) or individuals who will ideally benefit from the programme.

This procedure should be preceded by an educational diagnosis—a process of pretesting designed to determine the relevant characteristics of the target group—including such features as existing practices, levels of knowledge, and attitudes. A picture or profile of the community itself would be developed to illuminate programme planning. This latter analysis would include a review of organizations and institutions that might be useful in enhancing delivery strategies. It should also involve a critical appraisal of socio-economic and other environmental circumstances as a basis for defining clear policy goals. The construction of both kinds of profile should form part of the

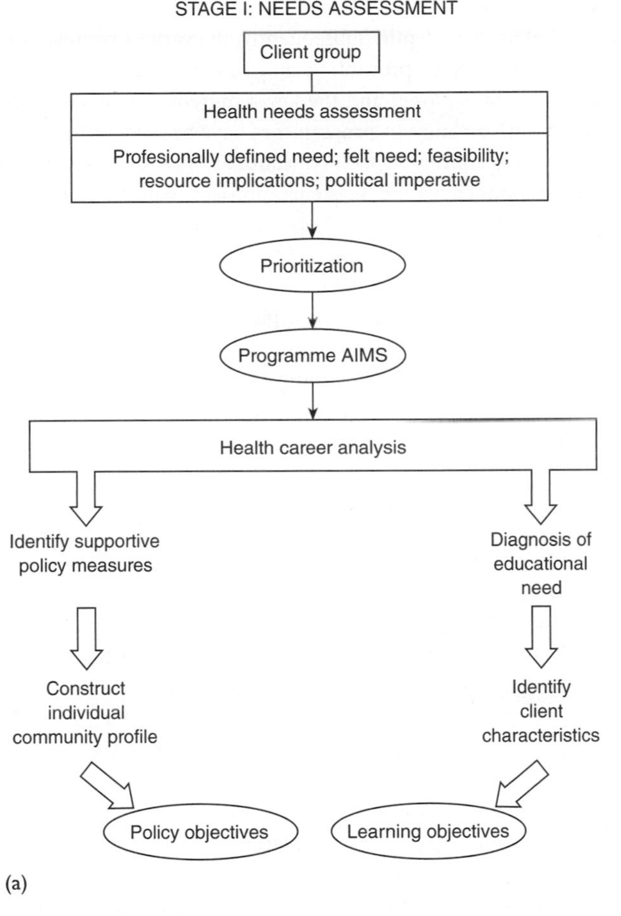

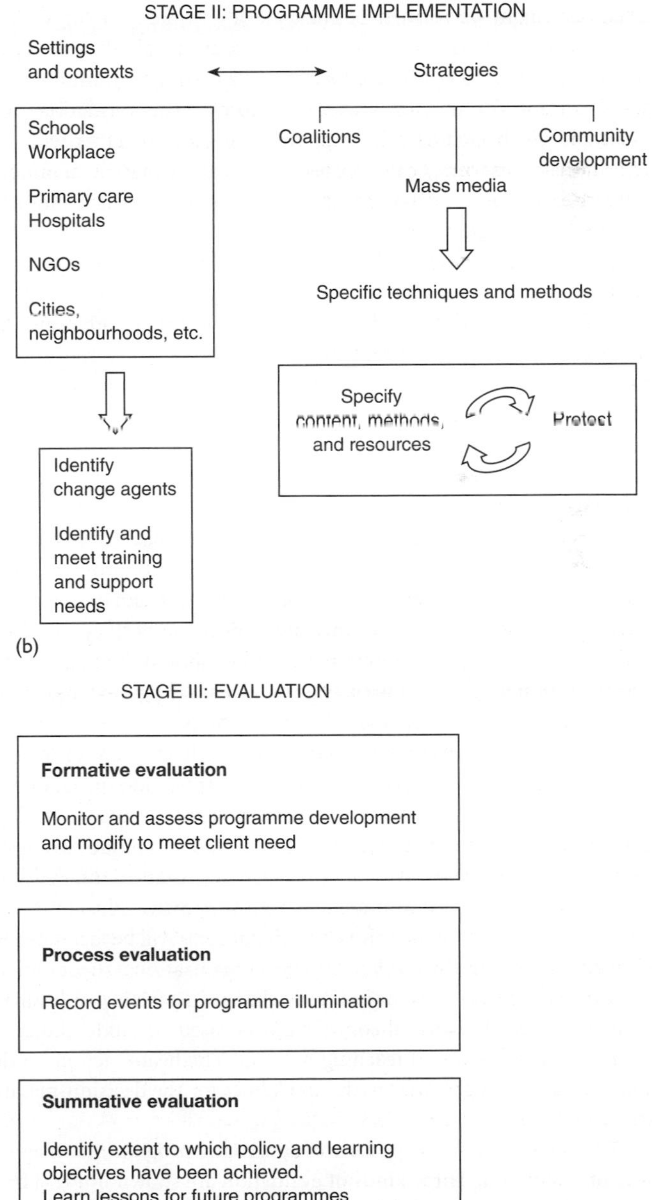

Fig. 11 (a) Programme planning: needs assessment. (b) Programme implementation. (c) Evaluation.

general database on which decisions might be made about health promotion strategies and the methods needed to translate educational and policy objectives into practice.

A 'health career analysis' provides a useful developmental perspective which allows planners to identify the mix of strategies and settings which should maximize the chance of an effective outcome. For instance, the construction of a 'smoking career' would identify important influences on recruitment to smoking, such as family, socio-economic group, community values and social network, school ethos, peer group, and mass media. Accordingly, a programme designed to prevent the adoption of smoking would employ strategies and initiate programmes in settings which would ensure the provision of education, supported by facilitative policies, at the most productive points on the health career.

There should be 'intersectoral collaboration' between the various agencies and institutions contributing at various stages on the health career to maximize their cumulative impact. Simultaneously, 'healthy alliances' might be formed between health workers in the various settings outlined. This kind of alliance is increasingly described as a 'community coalition' (*Health Education Research* 1993), although the term community is used somewhat loosely. The formation of a coalition which includes 'the great and the good' together with key local decision-makers, health professionals, representatives of important organizations, and lay members is likely to provide a powerful impetus for change.

Figure 11(b) describes the implementation stage and also shows how 'change agents' within the various settings and contexts might be identified. These are the potential health educators or advocates for change. The extent to which they have the necessary motivation, knowledge, skills, and competences will vary substantially from context to context therefore they may need training prior to programme implementation. As argued below, evaluation of the success of that training may provide one of a series of 'indirect' indicators of programme efficiency.

Since health-promotion programmes may range from regional campaigns to a single clinical consultation, a series of group sessions within a health promotion clinic in primary care, or an entire school curriculum, their content will vary dramatically in both comprehensiveness and style. Nonetheless, decisions should be made after consideration of the requirements of given settings or modes of delivery but before the specification of methods and the selection of 'adjuvant' learning resources or visual aids such as videos or leaflets. The development of policies rather than education programmes would follow a similar general pattern. Policy objectives would be translated into content, and various tactics and techniques would be employed to achieve implementation. In many instances this developmental process will occur in tandem with supportive education. The achievement of both policy and educational goals will be facilitated by consulting relevant theory. For instance, organizational theory might provide valuable insights for initiating change in a factory or business setting whereas learning theory should be used to guide choice of programme content and teaching method. The health action model outlined above might offer useful guidelines for the decision-making process.

The final stage in the process of systematic programme design is one of evaluation. Three kinds of evaluation are shown in Fig. 11(c): summative, formative, and process. Further reference will be made to these in the final section of this chapter. It is sufficient to note here that summative evaluation assesses programme effectiveness by noting the extent to which learning objectives have been achieved. Formative evaluation monitors progress and, where necessary, supplies guidelines for 'remedial work' and social action. Conversely, process evaluation makes available detailed documentation of the processes and procedures which have taken place during the programme to provide insight into possible reasons for its successes or failures.

Change at the microlevel: selecting methods for facilitating learning and changing behaviours

This chapter has so far considered the general nature and philosophy of health promotion and health education. The relationship between these two complementary procedures and the ways in which people and communities make decisions—and perhaps even change their behaviours—have been considered. The processes of communication and education, and the requirements of successful learning, have also been analysed in some depth. Subsequently, the various contexts and settings in which health promotion and health education typically operate have been explored and the key requirements for designing systematic health promotion programmes have been identified.

This section is concerned with educational methodology which is an integral component within a systems approach to health education. Methods are relatively specific and operate at the micro- rather than the macrolevel of strategic planning. Very similar methods may be used in a variety of the several contexts or settings which were considered above. They may, for example, form part of community development or be used as a supplement to mass media. In their turn, particular audiovisual aids or learning resources might be used as adjuncts to methods. For instance, group discussion may be facilitated by a short trigger video. Conversely, a video used on its own (for example at a display in a health fair) falls into the category of mass media.

There is only one logical justification for using one or more educational methods, and that is to supply the conditions necessary for efficient learning. The logic should be: (a) identify the kind(s) of learning involved in a particular programme; (b) specify the conditions which must be supplied in order to promote the kind of learning identified (that is, a 'relatively permanent change in capability or disposition'); (c) select the educational method(s) which are most suitable for supplying the conditions in question. For instance, if the health education goal is only to produce understanding of the risk factors associated with coronary heart disease, then good question-and-answer technique together with a clear well-programmed explanation supported by an appropriate visual aid and a written leaflet will probably suffice. Indeed, this basic teaching form is usually present in most 'cocktails' of rather more exotic techniques.

However, less traditional methods will usually be needed to achieve the particular goals of health promotion. For example, 'experiential' learning would be considered a better tactic for influencing beliefs and attitudes, and equipping learners with skills. Experiential learning was mentioned above in the context of the discussion of alternative modes of 'coding' messages in the communication process (for a more complete review, see Tones (1993*a*)). Health education is more than the mere provision of information: it involves the skilful selection and practice of particular techniques, of which some specific examples are offered below.

Experiential learning and skills training

Despite the etymology of the word 'doctor', it is relatively uncommon to use the term 'teaching' in a health context. Nonetheless, since teaching involves the efficient promotion of learning, this is exactly what is happening in any successful educational encounter. Moreover, teaching should not be equated with a didactic presentation of information by an expert source. Teaching involves deliberately engineering opportunities for learning—which includes such activities as explaining or counselling but which may well consist of providing experiences for the learner.

In this example of a drugs course, a group of adolescents are required to work in pairs. They are given a pack of different cards which separately depict different types of information about drugs. The pack includes a card which only has the word 'legal' or 'illegal' printed on it. Another card describes the effects of an unnamed drug. A further card describes the effects of an unnamed drug on the user. Yet another card includes a description of a 'typical' hypothetical user. The two young people then proceed to match a set of, perhaps, 12 commonly used drugs with the various attributes on the cards.

Clearly, a teacher could have told them the facts (which would have seemed boring) or given them a list to read later (which they may or may not have done). Conversely, the experiential expedient ensures participation and attention. They are not expected to remember the information but are given a list of the correct matches once they have completed their problem-solving task. Furthermore, because coffee, alcohol, and cigarette smoking are included in the list of drugs they begin to learn something about the socially constructed definition of substances.

The next procedure might be to take nine drugs cards and arrange them in some kind of priority order in respect of their seriousness and social acceptability. The cards now become a learning resource for triggering debate and discussion to help the learners clarify their opinions and values about drug misuse as part of the process of facilitating decision-making.

Role play is a commonly used method in health education which illustrates the principles of experiential learning. It is part of the broader methodological category of simulation and gaming. Its peculiar strengths derive from the opportunities which it provides for problem solving and attitude change. For example, trainee town planners (an important group of health promoters) might be provided with a detailed but fictitious case study of a mental health dispute. This could represent the not uncommon 'not-in-my-backyard' syndrome in which local residents are angered by the potential siting of a half-way house for the mentally ill in their neighbourhood. The participants are then required to act out various roles: the mental health worker, the local councillor, the angry local resident, the local general practitioner, and so on. Ideally, the exercise should not only provide good insights into this kind of problem but may also generate a more positive attitude to the half-way house and even influence beliefs, concerns, and general attitudes relating to mental illness itself.

Turning to the question of skills training, this cannot be acquired by merely providing information. For example, consider the learning requirements of teaching young people first aid procedures as part of a harm minimization strategy in drug education. They will not only have to see these procedures properly modelled by a competent practitioner, but will also need to practice the procedures and receive rapid feedback so that they can correct their errors and internalize correct responses.

The requirements of learning social interaction skills are less obvious. For instance as part of a series of health promotion 'clinics' designed to reduce coronary heart disease risk, it is clear that the group members' commitment to follow 'sensible drinking' guidelines requires the support of appropriate social interaction skills—as noted in Fig. 6. They need to acquire competences in refusing an alcoholic drink in the difficult context of a 'round-buying' culture. They might readily learn four rules of verbal assertiveness (be clear in your own mind what you want to say; state your position; state your reason; acknowledge the other person's position or feelings). However, in order to apply these rules in a real-life scenario, they will need to learn not only what to say but also how to say it. They will need social skills and they would be provided by following the kind of techniques which would be used to teach cardiopulmonary resuscitation skills: demonstration and modelling followed by repetition, feedback, correction of errors, and reinforcement of good practice. Accordingly they will have to practice four rules of non-verbal assertive behaviour: using an appropriate tone of voice, correct eye contact, facial expression consistent with verbal message, and proper body language. Practice followed by consolidation through role play should consolidate the newly learned competence.

Learning in groups

This discussion of educational methodology will conclude with a brief review of the two most common situations in the health-care context: the face-to-face consultation and group teaching session. Any specific method might be 'nested' within another method. For instance, group work on mental health promotion would typically include a practice of skills element in which individuals learn techniques of relaxation. This discussion will focus on some of the key features of group work *per se*—and will use the example of an antenatal class to exemplify these.

This review of group work is necessarily brief. Even the definition of 'group' creates problems. However, for the purposes of this discussion, the group is considered as a kind of mini-community involving a relatively small aggregate of people sharing a peculiar complex of interpersonal interactions and dynamics.

The most obvious comparative advantage of group teaching is its potential for quite intensive interpersonal interaction. At the simplest level, it is possible to involve every group member in the learning task, gain immediate feedback about the current state of participants' learning, and provide the 'different strokes' referred to above. While intensity of interaction over a given period of time will be greater in the one-to-one circumstance, there are two extra dimensions in the group. The first of these is the expertise and experience of other (lay) members; the second is the often very powerful effect of group norms.

Assuming that the subject of the antenatal class is infant feeding, three major factors appear to influence intention to breast or bottle feed. Therefore it is logical to focus this discussion on these factors. Breast feeding is typically influenced by (a) beliefs about the benefits of the practice for the baby's health, (b) beliefs about its costs in respect of inconvenience, and (c), more importantly, the embarrassment factor. Accordingly, although some explanation by a group leader (for example, a midwife) will be necessary at some stage, the main thrust of the class should be to allow the mothers to explore the beliefs and values they share about feeding babies—especially in relation to the three factors listed above. In this context, beliefs and attitudes may change as other group members' views and experiences are discussed.

Complementary learning experiences may also be built into the class. A nursing mother might serve as a credible communicator and could 'model' breast feeding. Moreover, as breast feeding is clearly a psychomotor skill, an opportunity must be provided, at a later support stage, to practise that skill—probably in the confines of a health-promoting hospital ward.

The activities of the antenatal class are entirely consistent with an empowerment approach: the goal is to help women make a choice of breast or bottle feeding. Conversely, group dynamics might be deliberately exploited by zealous health educators determined to instil the desirability of breast feeding. The best example of this is the work of Lewin (1943) and later Bond (1958) who employed the so-called 'group discussion-decision' technique. Lewin demonstrated that this method was superior to a lecture in persuading housewives to change their family's diet (not surprising perhaps) and also (more surprising) better than face-to-face advice from a dietitian. The effect, it has been argued, is due to two factors: firstly, the effect of individual group member's commitment (possibly in public) to a particular course of action; secondly, the impact of group pressure. Clearly, the method can misfire dramatically if the group norm swings against the outcome which the group leader is seeking to manipulate.

As a final observation in this discussion of the value of group methods, the necessity of the group leader/facilitator having both a knowledge of group dynamics and those social interaction skills needed to manage the learning experiences of the participants should be reiterated.

One-to-one encounters: the consultation

In this final consideration of methodology, an attempt will be made to integrate earlier observations about the complementary—and, to some extent, consecutive—processes of communication and education. Figure 12 summarizes the key features of these processes.

Although the processes described in Fig. 12 are applicable to a greater or lesser extent to all educational methods, the dyadic encounter between doctor/health worker and client epitomizes these.

The principles of effective communication are that in order to ensure that clients correctly interpret the communication, the communicator must check clients' existing knowledge, beliefs, and attitudes (in an empathic manner) and 'encode' the message in an appropriate format. Particular care must be taken with non-verbal communication. The communicator must try to ensure that, where

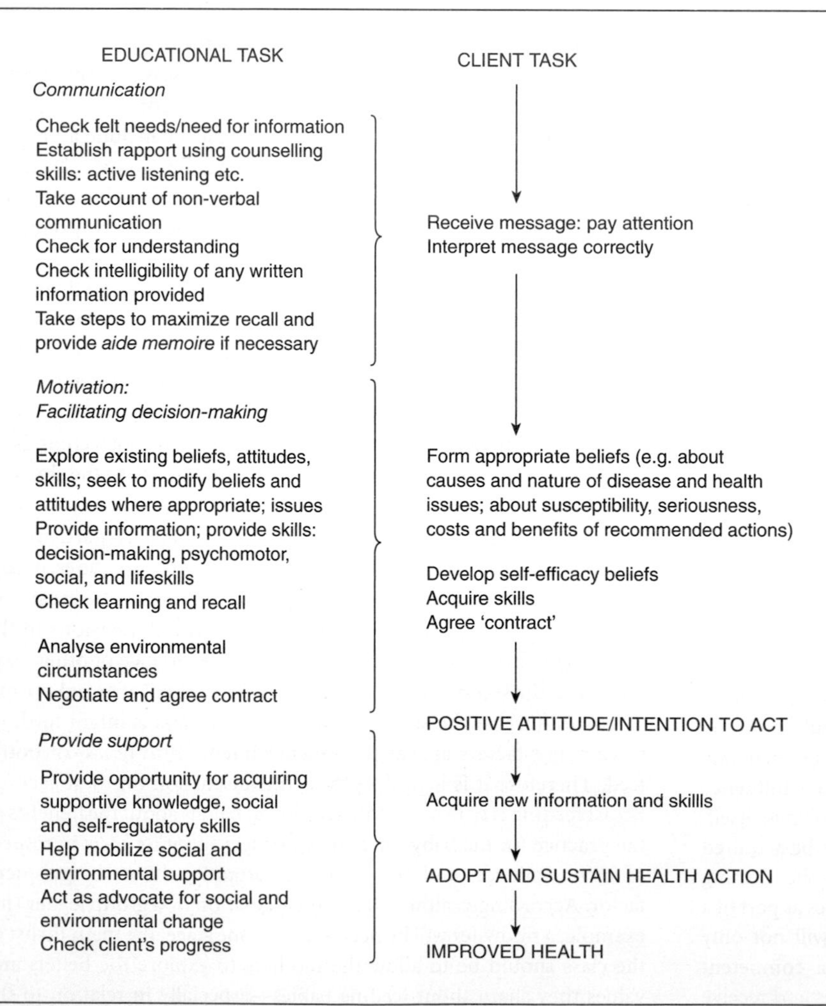

Fig. 12 Health promotion and the consultation.

necessary, messages are remembered and, above all, check that they have been correctly interpreted and understood.

The requirement for the teacher/health educator to ensure client recall features twice in Fig. 12. Firstly, steps must be taken to minimize forgetting of important information at the initial stage of communication. Secondly, in terms of motivating and facilitating client choice, it is important to check learning and recall. By definition, learning involves change; and change is stored in the memory as discussed below.

Remembering and forgetting

In an earlier reference to the importance of forgetting in the context of communication failure, two different viewpoints were discussed. On the one hand, Tuckett *et al.* (1985) considered that the inability to recall information made an insignificant contribution to patient lack of commitment to recommended actions. On the other hand, Ley (1990) apparently demonstrated that patients forgot about 40 per cent of the information provided. How can these seemingly conflicting observations be reconciled?

Human information processing systems have a limited capacity. People can, therefore, recall only a limited amount of data at any one time. Indeed, Miller (1956) argued convincingly that the actual amount which could be handled was 'seven plus or minus two' bits of information. It is, thus, not surprising that a substantial proportion of certain kinds of information will be forgotten. It is equally clear that the amount remembered may be enhanced by the use of various mnemonics and Ley (1990) advised doctors to employ a variety of such devices to optimize patient recall. These memory-enhancing techniques included simple repetition of items of information, emphasizing especially important items, and using 'explicit categorization'. This latter technique involves the practitioner providing a kind of advance warning of the number of pieces of information that should be remembered. For instance a doctor might say: 'I am, first of all, going to tell you the results of the tests you had last week; I will then tell you what is wrong with you; we will next discuss the implications of this . . .' and so on. There is reliable evidence that the adoption of these rather mechanical measures are effective in increasing the amount which patients can recall after the consultation.

Another tradition of psychological research does not focus on the quantitative aspects of forgetting but rather seeks to describe and explain qualitative changes. Forgetting does not merely consist of data loss; it involves a process of active reconstruction. Just as the process of perception is no mere photographic phenomenon but consists of an energetic striving to make sense of the world, the process of remembering incorporates 'effort after meaning' and interpretation. People reconstruct their imperfect memories until they make sense. In doing so they often fail to remember what actually happened but recall what they expected to happen and/or would have liked to have happened. Doctors have often been surprised and alarmed at patients' spurious recollections of earlier consultations and their firm conviction about the reality of diagnoses which were never made and advice never given.

Whether considering the quantitative or the qualitative aspects of memory, there is one consistent finding of paramount significance: people will have more complete and accurate recall if the information provided can be assimilated into existing understanding. Two observations may thus be made: firstly, a population which has received general health education should have superior recall; secondly, the highly recommended 'counselling' practice of exploring clients' theories and beliefs will not only diminish attitudinal barriers but should also result in better understanding and consequently a diminished chance of forgetting important information.

Even if recommendations for healthy actions have been provided in an insightful and meaningful fashion, people will still have difficulty in recalling detailed lists of data—no matter how useful. One solution is to employ mnemonics, or more simply, an appropriate written leaflet (preassessed for its 'readability').

Persuasion or empowerment?

From the educational process described in Fig. 12, a key element in the checklist centres on the motivation of the learner and the facilitation of decision-making. Two principles of health promotion are being illustrated in operational form: firstly, that health promotion is concerned to empower rather than to coerce; secondly, that healthy choices are more likely to result from making the healthy choice the easy choice than from the deployment of attitude change techniques.

Motivation is obviously an essential precursor to action but should be achieved in the following way:

- ensuring access to necessary information
- checking clients' beliefs, attitudes, skills—that is, their learning readiness
- remedying information deficit, influencing beliefs, and providing skills
- conducting a thorough analysis of environmental and situational factors which might militate against client choice
- establishing a 'contract' with the client.

The central role of beliefs and other psychosocial factors in motivating people to adopt health behaviours is discussed earlier in this chapter. Nonetheless, the interaction between environmental analysis, skills acquisition, and self-efficacy beliefs deserves further emphasis. Individuals must believe that they are actually capable of undertaking recommended actions before they will invest time and effort into complying with these recommendations. Since persuasion and exhortation alone are unlikely to convince the doubtful, some or all of the following procedures will be needed. Firstly, the practitioner and the client—in counselling mode—must critically examine the social and environmental circumstances in which the client will have to undertake the proposed behaviour. Assuming that the client has already been motivated as a result of previous exploration of values and beliefs, necessary skills must be provided. These might include psychomotor competences such as the skills needed to exercise safely and beneficially after myocardial infarction. They might include cooking and even shopping skills to support a healthier diet. Social interaction skills will frequently be essential—perhaps to help a parent cope with a troublesome adolescent.

If behaviours have been modelled by a credible communicator (as described in the earlier observations on group teaching) and skills have been acquired, clients may come to believe that they might actually achieve the goal they desire. People must, however, be reasonably convinced that environmental conditions are not so negative that, even with skills, they are bound to fail. The result of this interaction should be a 'contract' accepted by both health educator and learner. The contract may actually be in written form—in which case it may serve not only to enhance commitment but might also provide a useful reminder.

Situational support and the problem of relapse

As shown in Fig. 12, the final phase of the one-to-one educational consultation involves the provision of support. It is assumed that, if things have gone according to plan, the contract will have resulted in the client adopting the specific healthy behaviours. As their contribution to contracting, health professionals will do whatever is feasible to engineer actual changes in the environment as well as giving clients the skills they need to manage situational barriers to action. Clearly, there are limits to what even the most dynamic health worker can achieve—although a commitment to health promotion implies the adoption of an advocacy role which involves pressing for policies which reduce unhealthy social circumstances. At the macrolevel, lobbying and advocacy must involve the professional body as a whole. At the very least, health workers can usually marshal social support even if they are unable, as individuals, to have much effect on major environmental problems. Again, at a more immediate and practical level, there have been a number of examples of a primary health-care team holding 'benefits clinics' in which advice is provided on how to claim financial support.

In the discussion of the health action model above, those 'drive-like' states which are sometimes described as 'addictions' were mentioned. People seeking to make a change in their lifestyle, which involves an attempt to control such drives or some significant loss of gratification, frequently fail to achieve their aspirations. This matter of relapse has important implications for the educational encounter and a so-called transtheoretical model developed by DiClemente and Prochaska (1982) is of particular relevance. The model describes how individuals frequently move through a series of stages before finally committing themselves to a sustained change in health-related behaviours. It provides a useful insight, for example, into the ways in which heavy smokers might move round a cyclical trajectory before they eventually succeed in giving up smoking. According to the model (Prochaska 1992; Prochaska and DiClemente 1986) they may move through five stages of change. The first three are called precontemplation, contemplation, and action. Some clients will move onto the fourth stage, 'maintenance', while many others will find themselves in the fifth 'relapse' stage. The assumption is made that while many may fail and return to the contemplation stage, many will eventually succeed in moving on to the maintenance stage.

A system of 'motivational interviewing' or counselling has been based on Prochaska and DiCelemente's analysis (Rollnick *et al.* 1992). The success of the counselling approach will, however, undoubtedly be enhanced if clients can acquire a number of self-regulatory skills which would minimize the likelihood of relapse. This kind of skill is discussed later in the chapter. Self-regulation is a significant notion within the general body of theory known as 'behaviour modification': a full discussion of the theory and practice of behaviour modification is beyond the scope of this chapter (Kanfer and Karoly 1972; Watson and Tharp 1989).

These skills are designed to help people to gain control over the various powerful drives and emotions which are inconsistent with their values and attitudes. Briefly, self-regulation normally consists of monitoring the reciprocal relationship between environment and behaviours. People are helped to monitor and record their actions—for instance noting the circumstances which trigger their smoking and the degree of pleasure or relief they gain from any particular cigarette. They are taught to monitor any gaps between the goals they have set themselves and their actions. They learn how to control their environment in order to avoid temptation and break well-established unhealthy routines. They are helped to identify substitute gratifications—for instance acquiring relaxation skills as an alternative to smoking as a stress management device. Finally, clients are encouraged to consolidate healthy behaviours by rewarding themselves for achieving their targets.

Education and communication skills

The purpose of this chapter is to explore the complexities of human behaviour in health and illness, and to examine the contribution which health education might make to broader health promotion programmes. The difficulties involved in influencing behaviour are demonstrated, and a framework for effective action in various settings and contexts is also provided. A wide range of methods are available for those who seek to undertake the complementary tasks of communication and education. Consideration of the detailed techniques which are required in the various interpersonal encounters between health and education workers, and their different client groups, leads to the conclusion that a high level of skill is needed to influence and support health choices. While demystification is both possible and desirable, effectiveness and efficiency cannot be expected without competence.

Success in health promotion: assessing effectiveness

A rationale for evaluation

The assessment of success in health promotion and health education has already been mentioned; for a thorough treatment of evaluation see Green and Lewis (1986), Sarvela and McDermott (1993), and Tones and Tilford (1994). In order to acquire more detailed insight into the levels of success which have been recorded for different kinds of health education intervention, readers might usefully consult the extensive 14-volume review provided by the International Union of Health for Health Promotion and Education (1994). However, given the increasing demands for 'proof' of the effectiveness of health promotion at a time when resources for traditional medical interventions are failing to meet demand, it would be remiss not to give some consideration to this issue. However, at the outset it must be made clear that merely to ask whether or not health promotion works is a naive question. We do not, for instance, usually ask whether politics works. And yet to ask whether health promotion works is a question of a similar level of generality. People may well ask whether health services are successful but most serious researchers would consider that question as ingenuous. They would at least expect to know which services were to be investigated and require further specification of client groups, situations, and attendant circumstances.

Therefore, bearing in mind that the term 'evaluation' refers to the process of measuring the extent to which certain valued outcomes have been achieved, it is important to be clear about what success means for those concerned with health promotion. At one level, this is not difficult to specify. For example, in the United Kingdom, evidence that programmes had achieved greater equity might be looked for in the progress towards slaying William Beveridge's 'five giants': 'disease, idleness, ignorance, squalor and want'. Such broad goals are not only remarkably difficult to achieve but are also too general to be used as indicators of success.

Before giving further consideration to the selection of more appropriate indicators of health promotion success, it is worth recalling the main reasons for evaluating any given programme.

Efficacy, effectiveness, and efficiency

Three broad criteria are typically used in defining programme success: efficacy, effectiveness, and efficiency. The term 'efficacy' is used here in accordance with Brook and Lohr's (1985) distinction: 'Efficacy refers to the probability of benefit to individuals in a defined population . . . *under ideal conditions of use*' (emphasis added). Effectiveness simply refers to the extent to which a programme has achieved its goals. The distinction is important to note and, although Brook and Lohr were considering general health service research, it is especially apposite to health promotion since it is rare to find programmes operating under ideal circumstances—as noted below in relation to the discussion of type 3 error. For instance, a particular alcohol education intervention might need supportive fiscal policy to reduce consumer demand for alcohol. The need for a long-term programme involving parental modelling and effective teaching in primary school might be specified as a prerequisite for work with adolescents. Ideally, the adolescents should have received a properly structured course of assertiveness training before exploring their values and attitudes about alcohol, which should have provided them with the understanding and competences needed to refuse offers of alcohol at a party as part of their particular role as 'designated driver'. However, such conditions rarely obtain, so even if educators are convinced that such a programme would achieve its stated goal, only four school sessions are normally devoted to alcohol—a much more limited situation than the ideal.

The matter of 'efficiency' leads into the domain of relative effectiveness. Efficiency describes the extent to which a given programme has achieved its goals by comparison with some alternative or competing intervention. For instance, if a course of medication could lower population cholesterol levels more quickly and completely than dietary change, it would be a more efficient strategy. Also, it could be that consistent and repeated price increases on cigarettes might be superior to education as a strategy for reducing tobacco consumption. Or, if health education delivered by the primary health-care team could substantially lower the prevalence of smoking in girls, it would be a more efficient procedure than building smoking education programmes into schools. If it was possible to show that using a 'group discussion-decision' method with a practice nurse leader resulted in higher adoption and maintenance of the practice of breast feeding than authoritative advice from a general practitioner, then the group work should be judged to be the method of choice.

On cost-effectiveness

One of the most important criteria for appraising the efficiency of programme interventions is by calculating the relative financial costs of competing interventions (cost-effectiveness analysis). Conversely, 'cost–benefit analysis' not only states the costs in monetary terms but also seeks to place a price tag on the benefits to be accrued from the programme. A calculation of the cost per given benefit is then possible (typically expressed as a cost–benefit ratio). On the one hand, there is quite firm evidence that health promotion can achieve results which demonstrate not only cost-effectiveness but also commendable cost–benefit ratios. On the other hand, cost-effectiveness can be a double-edged weapon. A brief elaboration of these assertions will be provided but it is important to note that cost is by no means always used as a criterion for action. Mooney (1977), for instance, convincingly demonstrated the truth of this observation when he showed that the cost for a variety of preventive measures ranged from £50 per life saved for stillbirth screening to £20 million per life saved for alterations to high-rise flats following the collapse of the Ronan Point tower block in London due to a gas explosion.

Returning to evidence of financially sound interventions, as long ago as 1974, Green showed how a specific health education programme resulted in a saving of $7.81 per dollar invested in a hypertension screening and education programme. He also demonstrated that using group discussion techniques to educate asthmatic patients about the best means of controlling their condition notched up a cost–benefit ratio of 1 to 5 (Green 1974).

More recently, a British study of the effectiveness of family planning services (Laing 1982) identified conservative benefit to cost ratios of 1.3 to 1 for preventing 'typical unplanned pregnancies', a ratio of 4.5 to 1 for preventing pregnancies among mothers of three or more children, and a ratio of 5.3 to 1 for unplanned premarital conceptions. As the author put it, 'for every £100 spend on family planning services, the public sector can expect a benefit of £130, £450 and £530 respectively'.

In relation to smoking education programmes, Townsend (1986) argued that if a hypothetical mass media programme were to result in 1000 people giving up smoking permanently, 10 000 giving up temporarily, 2000 cutting down, and 15 000 seriously considering giving up, then 2991 life years would be saved at a cost of £84 per life. This is admittedly a hypothetical example, but Phillips and Prowle (1993) offered a more tangible analysis of benefits by calculating the costs and benefits of the 'Heartbeat Wales' programme. They were unable to ascribe cause and effect precisely; however, on a 'pessimistic worst case' assumption that the programme had only a 10 per cent impact rate on the actual decline in smoking in Wales over a 4-year period (1985 to 1989), they estimated that the 'net cost per working life year saved . . . worked out at approximately £64'.

Finally, recent studies in the United Kingdom have demonstrated the efficiency of general practitioners providing advice to stop smoking in accordance with quite stringent economic criteria. For a budget of £1 million, a relatively straightforward and simple intervention has been calculated to 'notch up' some 59 888 quality-adjusted life years compared with, for example, a much lower figure for breast screening (302 quality-adjusted life years). Again, it is generally considered that hip replacement is a highly efficient and appropriate surgical procedure yet it costs £750 per quality-adjusted life year compared with £167 for general practitioner-provided smoking-related advice (Godfrey *et al.* 1989).

Despite this positive evidence of effectiveness, economic indicators of success should be treated with caution. Even allowing for 'discounting'—the process whereby future costs are considered less important than current costs—it seems likely that really effective health promotion, which defers death and generates a large elderly population, will in the final analysis increase the already substantial medical costs involved in treating very old people as well as increasing the pensions and benefits cost to the nation. Perhaps the most useful approach to this dilemma is to follow the recommendations made by Cohen (1981). Prevention (and health promotion) should be treated as a 'merit good', that is, something which satisfies a 'merit want'. According to Musgrave (1959; cited by Cohen 1981), merit wants are 'so meritorious that their satisfaction is provided for through the public budget over and above what is provided for through the market and paid for by private buyers'. Clearly, such a view has special significance at this time in the development of thinking about health services and the market place. At all events, health promotion can demonstrate its capacity to satisfy quite stringent measures of efficiency. However, the indicators of effectiveness and efficiency which are most appropriate for those seeking to evaluate success need to be examined more critically.

Epidemiological indicators

Health promotion has different goals—including that of empowerment—although the orientation of this chapter is towards the prevention of disease. Even so, a major principle underlying the evaluation of health promotion initiatives is that traditional epidemiological indicators are inappropriate—and even behavioural outcomes may not be the most useful way of appraising general efficacy.

This assertion might seem a little surprising. After all, if health promotion has a useful contribution to make to achieving preventive outcomes, is it not reasonable to assess success in terms of reductions in mortality and morbidity? There are two main reasons for not doing so. Firstly, there is often some degree of uncertainty associated with the postulated links between particular behaviours and specific disease outcomes—at any rate on a population basis. It would therefore be unreasonable to claim that health promotion has been ineffective if it has influenced lifestyle but, despite this, the changes in behaviour had not led to a reduction in disease. For instance, given the uncertainty associated with postulated links between saturated fat consumption and breast cancer, it would be unwise to measure the success of dietary interventions in terms of a decline in breast cancer mortality. Indeed, given the fact that risk factors for many diseases may fail to explain a substantial amount of the variance in mortality and morbidity, a cause-and-effect relationship between behaviour change and 'medical' outcome would not be expected to occur. If epidemiological research has failed to demonstrate any link between behaviours and 'medical' outcome, then it is completely unethical to use health promotion strategies to change those behaviours. Epidemiological indicators should provide justification for undertaking health promotion; they should not be used to assess its effectiveness.

At first glance, it might be argued that failure to establish clear epidemiological links casts doubts on the wisdom of undertaking behaviour change programmes. This is manifestly untrue: in the example provided above, dietary changes which were of unproven benefit for preventing cancer of breast might well be effective in preventing other disorders. Moreover, even if behaviour changes were insufficient on their own to achieve a given preventive outcome, it may well be a necessary component in a broader programme of interventions.

The importance of intermediate indicators

Even lifestyle changes or other behavioural indicators may not be appropriate indicators of the success of health promotion. While in some instances, it would be reasonable to expect to see a change in behaviour after a particular educational intervention (for example, a school-based smoking programme might, if properly conducted, delay the onset of smoking in school pupils), in other cases, behavioural outcomes would not be feasible. One such instance is provided by programmes where a particular educational input could not be expected to influence a given outcome for many years. For instance, a successful cancer education programme which effectively teaches children about the nature of cancers in such a way as to contribute to a reduction in cancerophobia could not be expected to have an impact on a woman's utilization of mammography screening until the girls in question had reached middle age.

An even more important reason for using intermediate indicators derives from the fact that decisions about health or illness are multiply determined. Health education is not at all like a medication. Even a relatively straightforward face-to-face consultation between nurse and patient is much more complex and sophisticated than administering pills and potions. Health decisions are not the result of a simple linear progression from provision of knowledge through attitude change to the adoption of healthy practices. Accordingly one single input—simple or complex—is unlikely to achieve a desired output. Consider the case of one of the more simple educational interventions—a mass media 'commercial' seeking to influence dietary practices. At the very least, the following chain of events must take place before a successful outcome might be achieved. The target audience would need to be adequately exposed to the message and become aware of its existence, they would need to interpret and understand it correctly, they would need to believe it and assess its personal relevance, they would typically consider the possible costs and benefits involved in undertaking the changes in diet recommended by the programme, and they would then assess the likelihood of their having the expertise and stamina needed to make those changes. If these several steps have been successfully negotiated and if the audience has not been antagonized or made anxious by the message, a positive attitude to adopting a healthy diet might result. Before that attitude can be translated into practice, the client group will need a variety of skills and additional knowledge, and they must be able to find the healthy products and be able to afford them. This process can be simplified into the following sequence: awareness → knowledge → beliefs → attitudes → support → action. If we assign hypothetical probabilities to each stage being satisfactorily negotiated (expressed as a percentage of the population achieving the requisite goal) then the likelihood of success in terms of behaviour change might be depicted as follows:

awareness → knowledge → beliefs/attitudes → support → action
30 per cent × 85 per cent × 31 per cent × 40 per cent ≈ 3 per cent.

This 'formula' is based on 30 per cent of the audience having become aware of the message, 85 per cent of that particular group understanding it, 31 per cent of the 85 per cent believing it and being committed to the recommended action, but only 40 per cent having appropriately supportive environmental and social circumstances. The result (quite creditable if judged by the standards of commercial advertising) is an approximate 3 per cent change in behaviour. These figures are not completely hypothetical. The percentages for awareness, knowledge, and beliefs/attitudes are based on the average figures expected for well-pretested cancer education materials (Romano 1984). The assumption that 40 per cent of those exposed to the media programme will receive the necessary social, environmental, and educational support they need is hypothetical—and probably somewhat optimistic.

To improve effectiveness, the mass media input would need to be complemented by a variety of different educational interventions. These would be designed to achieve different learning outcomes and be delivered over a period of time in a variety of contexts and settings. Ideally, the educational programme would be supplemented by appropriate healthy public policy. Accordingly, it makes sense to assess each of these inputs separately; for example, understanding of the nutritional information on which dietary decisions are based might best be provided in schools and assessed there. Empowerment-related beliefs and attitudes could also be supplied in the personal and social education programme within the school and/or in the works canteen—and supported by effective food labelling in the supermarket.

Indirect indicators

Occasionally, even intermediate indicators may not be necessary for valid appraisal of effectiveness of inputs. For instance, health practitioners may need to assess the efficiency of a communication skills course provided for nurses in general practice. Assuming that the course is sound, the trainees will become more skilled in educating their clients. Their new skill will, in turn, ultimately be reflected in more effective work with patients. In the longer term, they and the course they have completed may contribute to clients' behaviour change—and may even have some small impact on the prevalence of disease.

Clearly, important decisions have to be made about which particular intermediate and indirect indicators to select. These decisions can only be based on good-quality theories derived from research. Following remarks made above about the relevance of epidemiological indicators, it is not surprising that the evaluation designs which have been traditionally associated with medical research are frequently not relevant to the needs of health promoters seeking to enhance the quality of their programmes.

Research design: key issues

As has been shown, health promotion programmes should not be seen as 'one-shot' activities: they require complex, cumulative, and sophisticated subprogrammes. For this and other reasons, traditional epidemiological research designs are frequently inappropriate for evaluating health promotion work. Furthermore, a quantitative approach to the analysis and description of research results will often be less useful than qualitative measures.

The randomized controlled trial has been and still is the 'gold standard' for rigorously assessing the effectiveness of certain kinds of intervention. Recent observations have been made by the Executive Director of the Welsh Health Planning Forum about the limited extent to which a whole range of currently accepted health-care initiatives may be said to be of proven value—using the 'gold standard'. According to his so-called 'health gain rhomboid' (Warner 1989), only some 20 per cent of these initiatives are of proven effectiveness, 20 per cent have been shown to lead to a proven reduction in health gain, while equal proportions either 'appear unpromising' or have 'uncertain effects'. He cites Brook and Lohr (1985) to support his claim that only 20 per cent have been evaluated by randomized controlled trial.

The equivalent of the randomized controlled trial in behavioural sciences and education is the 'true experimental design' which employs techniques of randomization and uses one or more control groups. These designs probably have to be somewhat more sophisticated than the randomized controlled trial because of the more complex nature of the inputs. For instance, an educational programme would not only involve recording whether or not an input had been provided but also would typically assess the extent to which a number of objectives had been achieved. Evaluation tools of this kind are readily available but there has been increasing doubt about the value of using experimental designs. Indeed, prevailing evaluation practices in education were challenged by Hamilton *et al.* (1977) in an important publication revealingly entitled *Beyond the Numbers Game*. More recently—and with specific reference to health promotion—a WHO Working Group has accepted the kinds of reservations that have been expressed about the randomized control trial by many working in education and the social sciences. Conclusion 4 of the Working Group's Report states:

> The use of randomized control trials to evaluate health promotion initiatives is, in most cases inappropriate, misleading and unnecessarily expensive. (WHO 1998*b*)

For present purposes, only four issues associated with the randomized controlled trial or true experimental design will be noted as follows.

1. For the kind of community-wide intervention which is likely to maximize the impact of a health promotion programme, it is virtually impossible to identify a valid control or comparison area. This is partly for ethical reasons (as with certain medical randomized controlled trials): if it is reasonably clear that communities will benefit from the intervention, it is unethical to withhold it. More importantly, perhaps, it is virtually impossible to avoid 'contamination' of the comparison area since the programme in the experimental area is likely to trigger similar enterprises in the proposed control community—a fact clearly demonstrated by the Heartbeat Wales coronary heart disease prevention programme (Nutbeam *et al.* 1993).

2. It is a fundamental error to equate a 'medical' with an educational initiative. The presence of human volition introduces a substantial degree of uncertainty into the proceedings and requires a complex and sophisticated programme completely unlike the administration of medication or a surgical procedure.

3. It is not only important to know that a given intervention has achieved success (or failure) but it is imperative to discover why the initiative might have been effective or ineffective. In short, even when an experimental design is feasible, process evaluation (see comments on evaluation in relation to Fig. 11) will also be needed. For example, if a group teaching session conducted by a practice nurse was more successful in increasing patients' commitment to take exercise than one-to-one sessions in which the doctor was the key educator, it would be valuable to know exactly why this might have been the case. The '5Ws + H formula' could beneficially be applied: Who did What to Whom, When and Where—and How? This could only be assessed in practice by observing and recording what actually happened in these sessions.

4. Most importantly, it is critical to move beyond process evaluation and concentrate on formative evaluation. The illumination provided by formative evaluation does not merely provide insight into what has happened but uses that insight progressively in order to enhance programme effectiveness in the 'here and now'. Accordingly, it is at the heart of action research—and after all, health promotion is the militant wing of public health! Ideally, both the action dimension and the underlying research process should incorporate maximal community/client participation.

A tale of three errors

It is useful to consider three major threats to the validity of evaluations of health promotion programmes. These are often expressed in terms of three different kinds of error: types 1, 2, and 3. Greatest attention is typically paid to the first of these while the third type is commonly ignored.

Type 1 error occurs when claims of success or failure are unjustified—typically due to a lack of adequate controls. The randomized controlled trial/true experimental design is the supreme antidote to type 1 error. Type 2 error occurs when the inadequacy of the research design results in failure to recognize changes that have actually occurred—often because insufficiently sensitive measuring devices were used or because of a failure to use the right indicators. Type 3 error is of particular importance to health promotion. Briefly, type 3 error occurs when an inadequate programme is judged as a failure—without acknowledging the reality of its inadequacy. The problem is not so much one of drawing the wrong conclusions about the effectiveness of an intervention. Rather, it involves inappropriate generalization from that failure—for instance when an effectiveness review of a particular kind of initiative, such as programmes designed to reduce unwanted pregnancies, is judged on the basis of a sample of deeply flawed, even inept, interventions. Accordingly, the problem is not so much one of research but rather one of ineptitude in programme design. Sidell *et al.* (1997) provide a cautionary tale of a health-promotion programme that employed an inefficient technique (casual distribution of leaflets to air passengers flying to torrid climates) to achieve an unattainable outcome (change in pattern of holiday sunbathing). The authors used a randomized controlled trial to assess the impact of this ineffectual initiative and discovered that there had been no change in (reported) behaviour. Decades of research and practice in the use of mass media, as outlined above in the relevant section, would have cautioned against such a wasteful use of time and resources. Green and Tones (1999) and Tones (2000) provide further discussion of this tale of three errors.

The qualitative dimension

Qualitative research techniques are essential to efficient illuminative evaluation and are often considered to be alien to the allegedly more rigorous methods associated with randomized controlled trials. Only brief observations can be made here about qualitative methodology but, given its importance in health promotion and the degree of controversy associated with its use, it may be helpful to provide the following summary.

1. Qualitative methods should be an integral part of the 'pretesting' stage of programmes. They are used for assessing learning readiness and needs, providing rich insights into underlying reasons for people's health-related actions, and formulating hypotheses and testing theory.
2. Formative evaluation monitors the progress of groups and individuals by providing a series of assessments which are then used to modify educational inputs to maximize the chance of success. Although quantitative techniques might be used, qualitative methods are better able to provide readily applicable information about not only the nature and extent of change in the clients but also about attendant circumstances—such as the characteristics and effect of a group leader or health educator.
3. Summative evaluation records the effect of the whole intervention—typically by administering some form of 'post-test' and comparing the results of this with a 'pretest'. Traditionally, a true or quasi-experimental design would be employed to allow health promoters to claim credit for any apparent changes in the target group. For the reasons discussed above, the use of the randomized controlled trial should be the exception rather than the rule. However, where this particular design is deemed appropriate, it should routinely be accompanied by qualitative methods in the interest of gaining illumination.
4. Qualitative methods do not have to sacrifice the rigour associated with quantitative approaches; indeed, validity and reliability can be achieved through the use of appropriate techniques. Of particular importance is the technique of 'triangulation' which, for example, pools information from a variety of different sources in order to assemble multifaceted 'evidence' on which to base decision-making.

Can health promotion be effective?

There are three major reasons for conducting programme evaluations.

1. To assess programme effectiveness and efficiency.
2. To use the results of evaluation research to improve the programme, to build better theory, and to add to the general body of health promotion knowledge and thus improve the general quality of decision-making about programme design.
3. To respond to various 'political imperatives'.

These political imperatives are well known among health promoters. Frequently the initiation of research and the reporting of results are driven largely by the need to gain future funding and/or ensure the survival of a programme. Alternatively, research might be commissioned with the often covert purpose of accumulating evidence in order to close down a programme of work. Contradictory results may, in both instances, be 'massaged' or even suppressed. Furthermore, many programmes have been launched over the years in spite of evidence that they were unlikely to be effective; clearly, in this latter instance, there are implicit, even concealed, effectiveness outcomes having little to do with the programme itself. If performance indicators for such interventions were ever to be made public, then they would be of a political nature. For example, a logically appropriate measure of success might be an acceptable percentage increase in government popularity in the opinion polls.

Health promotion is the concern of health promoters rather than political outcomes and, although this chapter has not assembled a comprehensive and detailed review of effectiveness studies, it should hopefully be clear from the incidental examples provided that there is quite consistent evidence that health promotion can frequently be effective when the right conditions have been met. It is important to note that this does not happen too often and it might be legitimate to speculate about the degree of success which might be achieved if programmes were to incorporate all we know about good practice. For example, much more impressive results should be expected where a synergistic input of both education and healthy public policy is provided.

However, there is a caveat: if people are genuinely empowered, their choice may not reflect the prevailing concerns of medicine. But, this risk is worth taking since empowered people will mostly be more rather than less inclined to adopt medically approved actions—and if the principles of empowerment have been properly operationalized, more rather than less success will be experienced.

This chapter concludes by reporting three different perspectives on success—each of which provide valid evidence of health promotion's potential effectiveness. The first relates to traditional preventive goals but refers to a situation in which policy measures and education are inextricably linked. Warner (1981) makes the following observation (in a United States context):

> In the absence of the antismoking campaign, adult per capita cigarette consumption in 1987 would have been an estimated 78–89 per cent higher than the level actually experienced . . . [As a result,] an estimated 789 200 Americans avoided or postponed smoking-related deaths and gained an average of 21 additional years of life expectancy each.

In the second example, a school- and community-based health education programme in South Carolina demonstrated specific relationships between input and output. It showed rather conclusively that, compared with three comparison counties, statistically significant reductions occurred in adolescent pregnancy rates (Vincent *et al.* 1987). According to the researchers, the target county showed a 'remarkably sustained decline . . . not observed in comparison counties' whose unwanted pregnancy rates increased during the same period.

The final example is drawn from a study by Durrant (1993). It reports the result of using creative arts in the setting of a general practitioner practice (Tones and Green 1999). It used qualitative methodology to describe what appears to be clear gains in empowerment by patient participants. It also provides a few hints and suggestions about possible longer-term health gains. The first component of the triangulation procedure is a general practitioner's perceptions of the impact of the programme:

> We have seen people grow in confidence, make important decisions, get on better with their families, have more patience with their children, make friends, and grow as people.

A second component is provided by the evidence of a community worker associated with the venture:

> As they gain confidence in the sessions, they take this out onto the street, and this is seen in their daily lives. They feel they can apply for jobs they thought they never could have applied for, moved to better houses, taken on the council about the poll tax or the water meters, or allowances. We have people here now who wouldn't think twice about making a banner and campaigning outside the Town Hall to save local amenities.

Both of the above perceptions of the situation are corroborated and 'fleshed out' by more detailed explanations and justifications for the observations. Clearly though, additional evidence would help to strengthen conclusions about the empowering effects of creative arts. Discussion with patients themselves provides a third 'triangulated' component. Two examples provide further illumination and serve as a suitable conclusion to this chapter:

> I found a new self, one that I didn't think was there. People said my paintings were good, and I went home thinking something good about myself for a change, that I was worth something. I've always been a nervous character and I haven't had a lot of faith in myself and what I could achieve. Suddenly I could do something that other people recognized was good, and it made me feel great, and that's lasted. (Mrs Black)

> [T]he sense of satisfaction that the arts work gave me, made me value me for the first time. This made me able to do things—only on a small front—like make decisions that I would've taken ages to make. Because I could see something I had created, it makes me think I can do things in my life, that before I had no control over. I haven't changed the world, but I'm doing little things for me, like writing to shops to complain, to the bus station about the lack of buses, things like that. (Mrs Red)

References

Antonovsky, A. (1979). *Health, stress and coping: new perspectives on mental and physical wellbeing.* Jossey-Bass, San Francisco, CA.

Antonovsky, A. (1996). The salutogenic model as a theory to guide health promotion. *Health Promotion International*, **11**, 11–18.

Backer, T.E., Rogers, E.M., and Sopory, P. (1992). *Designing health communication campaigns: what works?* Sage, Newbury Park, CA.

Bandura, A. (1977). Self-efficacy: toward a unifying theory of behavioural change. *Psychological Review*, **64**, 191–215.

Bandura, A. (1986). *Social foundations of thought and action: a social cognitive theory.* Prentice-Hall, Englewood Cliffs, NJ.

Becker, M.H. (ed.) (1984). *The health belief model and personal health behavior.* C.B. Slack, Thorofare, NJ.

Blaxter, M. (1990). *Health and lifestyles.* Tavistock Press, London.

Bond, B.W. (1958). A study in health education methods. *International Journal of Health Education*, **1**, 41–6.

Bracht, N. (ed.) (1999). *Health promotion at the community level: new advances* (2nd edn). Sage, Newbury Park, CA.

Brook, R. and Lohr, K. (1985). Efficiency, effectiveness, variations and quality. *Medical Care*, **23**, 710–22.

Byrne, P.S. and Long, B.E.L. (1976). *Doctors talking to patients.* HMSO, London.

Cassell, E.J. (1991). *The nature of suffering and the goals of medicine.* Oxford University Press.

Cohen, D. (1981). *Prevention as a merit good.* Health Economics Research Unit, University of Aberdeen.

Davis, J.B. (1992). *The myth of addiction.* Harwood, Switzerland.

Denscombe, M. (2001). Uncertain identities and health-risking behaviour: the case of young people and smoking in late modernity. *British Journal of Sociology*, **52**, 157–77.

Department of Health (1999*a*). *Reducing health inequalities: an action report.* HMSO, London.

Department of Health (1999*b*). *Saving lives: our healthier nation.* HMSO, London.

DiClemente, C.C. and Prochaska, J.O. (1982). Self change and therapy change of smoking behaviour: a comparison of processes of change in cessation and maintenance. *Addictive Behaviours*, **7**, 133–42.

DiMatteo, M.R. and Di Nicola, D.D. (1982). *Achieving patient compliance: the psychology of the medical practitioner's role.* Pergamon, New York.

Durrant, K. (1993). The creative arts and the promotion of health in community settings. Unpublished M.Sc. dissertation, Leeds Metropolitan University.

Egbert, J., Battit, G.E., Welch, C.E., and Bartlett, M.K. (1964). Reduction of post operative pain by encouragement and instruction of patients. *New England Journal of Medicine*, **270**, 825–7.

Freidson, E. (1961). *Patients' views of medical practice.* Russell Sage Foundation, New York.

Freidson, E. (1970). *The profession of medicine.* Dodd, Mead, New York.

Freire, P. (1974). *Education and the practice of freedom.* Writers and Readers Publishing Cooperative, London (originally published in Portuguese, 1967).

Glanz, K., Lewis, F.M., and Rimer, B.K. (ed.) (1997). *Health behavior and health education: theory, research and practice* (2nd edn). Jossey-Bass, San Francisco, CA.

Godfrey, C., Hardman, G., and Maynard, A. (1989) *Priorities for health promotion: an economic approach.* Discussion Paper 59. Centre for Health Economics, University of York.

Gottlieb, N. and McLeroy, K.R. (1992). Social health. In *Health promotion in the workplace* (2nd edn) (ed. M.P. O'Donnell). Delmar Publishing, New York.

Green, J. and Tones, B.K. (1999). Towards a secure evidence base for health promotion. *Journal of Public Health Medicine*, **21**, 133–9.

Green, L.W. (1974). Toward cost-benefit evaluation of health education: some concepts, methods and examples. *Health Education Monographs*, **2**, 34–64.

Green, L.W. and Kreuter, M.W. (1999). *Health promotion planning: an educational and ecological approach* (3rd edn). Mayfield, Palo Alto, CA.

Green, L.W. and Lewis, F.M. (1986). *Measurement and evaluation in health education and health promotion.* Mayfield, Palo Alto, CA.

Hamilton, D., *et al.* (ed.) (1977). *Beyond the numbers game: a reader in educational evaluation.* Macmillan, London.

Health Education Research: Theory and Practice (1993). Special issue on community coalitions. *Health Education Research: Theory and Practice*, **8**.

International Union for Health Promotion and Education (1994). *Improvement of the effectiveness of health education and health promotion: a series of publications and a database.* IUHPE Regional Office for Europe, Utrecht.

Kanfer, F.H. and Karoly, P. (1972). Self-control: a behavioristic excursion into the lion's den. *Behavior Therapy*, **3**, 398–416.

Kasl, S.V. and Cobb, S. (1966). Health behavior, illness behavior and sick role behavior. *Archives of Environmental Health*, **12**, 246–66.

Laing, W.A. (1982). *Family planning: the benefits and the costs.* Policy Studies Institute, London.

Lalonde, M. (1974). *A new perspective on the health of Canadians.* Government of Canada, Ottawa.

Langer, E.J. and Rodin, J. (1976). The effects of enhanced personal responsibility for the aged. *Journal of Personality and Social Psychology*, **34**, 191–8.

Lazarsfeld, P.F. and Merton, R.K. (1975). Mass communication, popular taste and organized social action. In *Mass communications* (ed. W. Schramm), pp. 492–512. University of Illinois Press, Urbana, IL.

Lewin, K. (1953). Forces behind food habits and methods of change. *Bulletin of the National Research Council*, **108**, 35–65.

Ley, P. (1990). *Communicating with patients.* Chapman & Hall, London.

Lyng, S. (1990). Edgework: a social psychological analysis of voluntary risk taking. *American Journal of Sociology*, **95**, 851–86.

Macleod Clark, J. (1993). From sick nursing to health nursing: evolution or revolution? In *Research in health promotion and nursing* (ed. J. Wilson-Barnett and J. Macleod Clark). Macmillan, London.

MacShane, D. (1979). *Using the media.* Pluto Press, London.

Marsh, A. and Matheson, J. (1983). *Smoking attitudes and behaviour.* HMSO, London.

Miller, G. (1956). The magical number seven, plus or minus two: some limits on our capacity for processing information. *Psychological Review*, **63**, 81–7.

Mittelmark, M. (1999). Editorial. *Health Education Research*, **14**.

Mooney, G.H. (1977). *The valuation of human life.* Macmillan, London.

Musgrave, R. (1959). *The theory of public finance.* McGraw-Hill, London.

NHS (National Health Service) Management Executive (1994). *Health promoting hospitals: a guidance document.* HMSO, London.

Nutbeam, D., Haglund, B., Farley, P., and Tilgren, P. (1991). *Youth health promotion: from theory to practice in school and community.* Forbes, London.

Nutbeam, D., Smith, C., Murphy, S., and Catford, J. (1993). Maintaining evaluation designs in long term community based halth promotion programmes: Heartbeat Wales case study. *Journal of Epidemiology and Community Health*, **47**, 127–33.

Parsons, T. (1951). *The social system.* Free Press, New York.

Pascoe, G.C. (1983). Patient satisfaction in primary health care: a literature review and analysis. *Evaluation and Programme Planning*, **6**, 185–210.

Phillips, C.J. and Prowle, M.J. (1993). Economics of a reduction in smoking: case study from Heartbeat Wales. *Journal of Epidemiology and Community Health*, **47**, 215–23.

Prochaska, J.O. (1992). What causes people to change from unhealthy to health enhancing behaviour? In *Preventing cancers* (ed. T. Heller, L. Bailey, and S. Pattison). Open University Press, Buckingham.

Prochaska, J.O. and Di Clemente, C. (1986). Toward a comprehensive model of change. In *Treating addictive behaviors: processes of change* (ed. W.R. Miller and N. Heather). Plenum, New York.

Rogers, E.M. (1995). *Diffusion of innovations* (4th edn). Free Press, New York.

Rogers, E.M. and Shoemaker, F.F. (1971). *Communication of innovations.* Free Press, New York.

Rollnick, S., Heather, N., and Bell, A. (1992). Negotiating behaviour change in medical settings: the development of brief motivational interviewing. *Journal of Mental Health*, **1**, 25–37.

Romano, R. (1984). *Pretesting in health communications.* National Cancer Institute, Bethesda, MD.

Rosenthal, H. (1983). Neighbourhood health projects: some new approaches to health and community work in parts of the United Kingdom. *Community Development Journal*, **13**, 122–31.

Rotter, J.B. (1966). Generalised expectancies for internal versus external control of reinforcement. *Psychological Monographs*, **80**, 1–28.

Ryder, J. and Campbell, L. (1988). *Balancing acts in personal, social and health education.* Routledge, London.

Salmon, C.T. (ed.) (1989). *Information campaigns: balancing social values and social change.* Sage, Newbury Park, CA.

Sarvela, P.D. and McDermott, R.J. (1993). *Health education evaluation and measurement: a practitioner's perspective.* Brown and Benchmark, Madison, WI.

Seligman, M.E.P. (1975). *Helplessness: on depression, development and death.* W.H. Freeman, New York.

Sidell, M., Jones, L., Katz, J., and Peberdy, A. (1997). *Debates and dilemmas in promoting health.* Macmillan/Open University Press, London.

Sweeney, B. (1998). The place of the humanities in the education of a doctor. *British Journal of General Practice*, **48**, 998–1102.

Taylor, S.E. (1979). Hospital patient behavior: reactance, helplessness, or control? *Journal of Social Issues*, **35**, 156–84.

Tones, B.K. (1979). Past achievement, future success. In *Health education: perspectives and choices* (ed. I. Sutherland). Allen and Unwin, London.

Tones, B.K. (1987). Devising strategies for preventing drug misuse: the role of the health action model. *Health Education Research*, **2**, 305–18.

Tones, B.K. (1992). Health promotion, empowerment and the concept of control. In *Health education: politics and practice* (ed. D. Colquhoun). Deakin University Press, Victoria, Australia.

Tones, B.K. (1993*a*). Changing theory and practice: trends in methods, strategies and settings in health education. *Health Education Journal*, **52**, 126–39.

Tones, B.K. (1993*b*). The importance of horizontal programmes in health education. *Health Education Research*, **8**, 455–9.

Tones, B.K. (1996). Models of mass media: hypoderemic, aerosol or agent provocateur? *Drugs: Education, Prevention and Policy*, **3**, 29–37.

Tones, B.K. (1998). Health promotion: empowering choice. In *Adherence to treatment in medical conditions* (ed. L.B. Myers and K. Midence). Harwood, Amsterdam.

Tones, B.K. (2000). Evaluating health promotion: a tale of three errors. *Patient Education and Counseling*, **39**, 227–36.

Tones, B.K. and Green, J. (1999). *A case study of Withymoor Village surgery: a health hive*. Health Promotion Design, 42 Moseley Wood Lane, Leeds, UK.

Tones, B.K. and Tilford, S. (1994). *Health education: effectiveness, efficiency and equity*. Chapman & Hall, London.

Townsend, J. (1986). Cost effectiveness. In *Smoking control: strategies and evaluation* (ed. J. Crofton and M. Wood). Health Education Council, London.

Tuckett, D., Boulton, M., Olson, C., and Williams, A. (1985). *Meetings between experts*. Tavistock Press, London.

United States Department of Health, Education and Welfare (1978). *Disease prevention and health promotion*. Washington, DC.

United States Department of Health Education and Welfare (1979). *Healthy people*. Washington, DC.

United States Department of Health and Human Services (1980). *Promoting health, preventing disease: objectives for the nation*. Washington, DC.

Vincent, M.L., Clearie, A.F., and Schlucter, M.D. (1987). Reducing adolescent pregnancy through school and community based education. *Journal of the American Medical Association*, **257**, 3382–6.

Wadsworth, M., Butterfield, W.J.H., and Blaney, R. (1971). *Health and sickness: the choice of treatment*. Tavistock Press, London.

Wallston, K.A. and Wallston, B.S. (ed.) (1978). Health locus of control. *Health Education Monographs*, **6**.

Warner, K.E. (1981). Effects of the antismoking campaign: an update. *American Journal of Public Health*, **79**, 144–51.

Warner, M.W. (1989). Present needs and future context: forces for change in health care in the United Kingdom. In *Health care systems in Canada and the United Kingdom* (ed. K. Lee). Keele University Press.

Watson, D.L. and Tharp, R.G. (1989). *Self-directed behavior: self-modification for personal adjustment*. Brooks/Cole, Pacific Grove, CA.

Weeks, V. (1993). The Department of Health view. In *Promoting health: is there a role for hospital staff?* (ed. A. Gatherer, A. McBride, and Z. Moorwood). Health of the Nation Unit, Oxford Regional Health Authority.

Whitehead, M. and Tones, B.K. (1991). *Avoiding the pitfalls*. Health Education Authority, London.

Wilkinson, R. and Marmot, M. (ed.) (1998). *The social determinants of health: the solid facts*. WHO, Centre for Urban Health, Copenhagen.

WHO (World Health Organization) (1984). *Health promotion: a discussion document on the concepts and principles*. WHO Regional Office for Europe, Copenhagen.

WHO (World Health Organization) (1986). *Ottawa Charter for Health Promotion: an international conference on health promotion*. WHO Regional Office for Europe, Copenhagen.

WHO (World Health Organization) (1991). *Budapest Declaration on Health Promoting Hospitals*. WHO Business Meeting, Budapest, Hungary, 31 May to 1 June. WHO, Geneva.

WHO (World Health Organization) (1997). *The Jakarta Declaration on leading health promotion into the 21st century*. WHO, Geneva.

WHO (World Health Organization) (1998*a*). *Health for all in the twenty first century*. WHO, Geneva.

WHO (World Health Organization) (1998*b*). *Health promotion evaluation, recommendations to policymakers*. WHO, Copenhagen.

WHO (World Health Organization) (1998*c*). *Resolution WHA42.44 on health promotion to the fifty first World Health Assembly*. WHO, Geneva.

Zola, I.K. (1973). Pathways to the doctor—from person to patient. *Social Science and Medicine*, **7**, 67–89.

Zola, I.K. (1986). Illness behaviour—a political analysis. In *Illness behavior: a multidisciplinary model* (ed. S. McHugh and T.M. Vallis). Plenum, New York.

7.4 Community assessment of behaviour

Donald E. Morisky

In 1988, the Institute of Medicine of the National Academy of Science published *The Future of Public Health*, a report that continues to stimulate interest and discussion on the core functions of public health. In this landmark report, the Institute of Medicine recommended a shift from the traditional clinical service functions of health agencies (Walker 1989; Scutchfield *et al.* 1997). The report sought to define new boundaries of public health by identifying three core functions of public health—assessment, policy development, and assurance—functions that are comparable with those generally ascribed to the medical care system: diagnosis and treatment. Assessment is the analogue of diagnosis, except that the diagnosis or problem assessment is made for a community or a population. Also, assurance is analogous to treatment in that it implies that the required remedies or intervention strategies are put into place. Finally, policy development is an intermediate role of collectively deciding which remedies or intervention techniques are most appropriate and tailored for the problems identified. These core functions broadly describe what public health does as opposed to its definition. The first of these core functions, assessment, will be addressed in detail in this chapter.

This chapter focuses on the process of community health assessment and improvement, including the conceptualization of community factors that influence health and health behaviour. In addition, the variety of approaches and techniques employed in conducting a needs analysis are described. *Healthy People 2010* is used as an example of a comprehensive data assessment technique, in which goals and objectives are identified and quantified. The dependence of national and state data-gathering systems provides a solid basis for the establishment of national objectives (US Department of Health and Human Services 2000).

In order to develop and implement community-based programmes that address the social and psychological determinants of health-related behaviours, a solid theoretical and conceptual framework is required. This chapter identifies several psychosocial and sociostructural/environmental theories which have guided programme implementation and evaluation. A set of examples is presented as to how investigators and communities have employed needs analysis techniques in the development of their intervention strategies. Also, examples of how communities have benefited from scientifically validated behavioural, environmental, and psychosocial assessment of determinants of major health concerns are presented. Finally, a detailed overview of the needs assessment processes in a large-scale community HIV/sexually transmitted disease prevention programme in the Philippines is presented.

Community health assessment is a dynamic process undertaken by an investigative team of health professionals to identify the health needs of the community, resulting in prioritizing health concerns and collaborative action planning. Both quantitative and qualitative assessment procedures are employed in gathering the necessary information specific to the target population. The quantitative assessment provides the numerical indicators, along with its statistical parameters; qualitative assessment involves descriptive information that supplements and complements these statistical data. Quantitative assessment provides answers to who and how much; qualitative assessment provides answers to the why and how.

What makes a community?

Traditionally, a community has been thought of as a geographical area with specific boundaries, such as census tracts, 'zip' or postal code areas, a neighbourhood, city, county, or state. However, in the context of community health, 'community' is defined as a group of individuals sharing a common characteristic. Communities can be defined by location, race, ethnicity, age, work site, interest in particular problems or situation in life, health concern, or common bonds (Glasgow *et al.* 1997; VanEenwyk 1997; Han *et al.* 1999). Examples of communities include the individuals residing in the city of Los Angeles (location), the Asian community (race), the Hispanic community (ethnicity), senior citizens (age), the hotel industry (occupation), the homeless (specific population), individuals on public assistance (particular outcome), patients with hypertension (health concern), or church members (common bond). A community may be as small as a group of students in a particular class or as large as all the individuals who make up an entire nation.

Community health, which is a component of the field of public health, includes both private and public (government) efforts of individuals, groups, and organizations to promote, protect, and preserve the health of those in the community. Community health is the sum of all governmental and non-governmental efforts. Community health includes personal health, which is made up of individual actions and decision-making activities that affect the health of an individual or his or her immediate family members. These activities may be preventive or curative in nature but seldom do not primarily affect the behaviours of others. Choosing not to smoke, to engage in physical exercise, to wear a seat belt regularly, and to visit the doctor are all examples of personal health decisions (Pinder 1994).

Community health activities are those that are aimed at protecting or improving the health of a population or a community. Maintenance of accurate vital health statistics (birth and death records), sanitation services to protect the food and water supply, and participating in fund-raising activities for a voluntary health organization are all examples of community health activities (McKenzie *et al.* 1999).

Psychosocial and behavioural determinants of health

There are a number of factors that affect the health of a community, and for this reason, the health status of each community is quite different. These factors may be physical, social, and/or cultural. They also include the ability of the community to organize and work together as well as the individual behaviour of individuals in the community. Physical factors include the influences of geography, such as the climate and altitude. In tropical countries where warm humid temperatures and rain prevail throughout the year, parasitic and infectious diseases are a leading community health concern. Other physical factors include the quality of our environment, community size and population density, and industrial development. Industrial development, like size, can have either positive or negative effects on the health status of a community. Industrial development provides a community with increased resources for community health programmes but may also bring with it environmental pollution and occupational illnesses. Communities that experience rapid industrial development need to regulate the manner in which industries obtain raw materials, discharge byproducts, dispose of wastes, treat and protect their employees, and clean up environmental accidents. Unfortunately, many policy regulations are often passed only after these communities have suffered significant reductions in the quality of their life and health (American Thoracic Society 1996).

Social and cultural factors are also important in the health of a community. Social factors include those interactions that arise from individuals or groups within a community. For example, individuals who live in urban communities, where life is fast-paced, experience higher rates of stress-related illnesses than those who live in rural communities, where life is more leisurely. Conversely, the health-related resources in rural areas may not be equivalent to the urban areas. Cultural factors arise from guidelines (both explicit and implicit) that individuals 'inherit' from being a part of a particular society. These guidelines tell them how to view the world and how to behave in relation to other people, to supernatural forces, and to the natural environment.

The beliefs, traditions, and prejudices of community members can also affect the health of a community. The beliefs of those in a community about such specific health behaviours as exercise and smoking can influence policy makers on whether or not they will spend money on hiking trails or no smoking legislation (Moskowitz *et al.* 1999). The traditions of specific ethnic groups can influence the types of foods, restaurants, and services available in a community. Prejudice in one specific ethnic or racial group against another can result in acts of violence and crime. Racial and ethnic disparities will continue to put certain groups at greater risks.

National as well as local economies can affect the health of a community through reductions in health and social services. An economic downturn means that lower tax revenues will be available for programmes including public assistance and community health care. This occurs because revenue shortfalls cause agencies to experience budget cuts. With less money, communities often must alter their eligibility requirements, thereby restricting aid to only the most needy individuals.

Individuals in political office, either nationally or locally, can also improve or jeopardize the health of their community by the decisions they make (Lemen 1999). Generally, the argument is over greater or lesser governmental participation in health issues. For example, in the United States, there has been a long-standing discussion on the extent to which the government should involve itself in health care. Historically, Democrats have been in favour of such action while Republicans have been against it. However, as the cost of health care has continued to grow. Both sides now see the need for some type of increased regulation (Levin-Epstein 1999).

Religion also plays a major role in the health of a community (Ellison and Levin 1998). A number of religious organizations have taken a position on health care, such as limiting the type of medical treatment their members can receive. Some do not permit immunizations; others do not permit their members to be treated by a doctor. Still others prohibit certain foods. Some religious communities actively address moral and ethical issues such as abortion, premarital intercourse, and homosexuality (Sheard 2000).

The influence of social norms can be positive or negative and can change over time. Cigarette smoking is an excellent example. During the 1940s, 1950s, and 1960s, it was quite socially acceptable to smoke in most settings. In fact, in 1960, 53 per cent of American men and 32 per cent of American women smoked. Thus, in 1960 it was socially acceptable to be a smoker, especially if you were male. In 1994 those percentages had dropped to 28 per cent for males and 23 per cent for females, in most public places it has become socially unacceptable to smoke (Montazeri and McEwen 1997). The current lawsuit in the United States against tobacco companies by both the state attorneys general and private citizens provide further evidence that smoking is no longer socially acceptable (Novotny and Siegel 1996; Balbach and Glantz 1998).

Unlike smoking, alcohol consumption represents a continuing negative social norm in America, especially on college campuses. The normal expectation seems to be that drinking is fun, and certainly everyone wants to have fun. Despite the fact that most college students are below the legal age limit to drink alcohol, still 80 to 90 per cent of college students drink (Clements 1999). In 1997, the Harvard School of Public Health College Alcohol Study resurveyed colleges that participated in a 1993 study. The findings revealed little change in binge drinking: a slight decrease in percentage of binge drinkers and slight increases in percentages of abstainers and frequent binge drinkers (Wechsler *et al.* 1998).

Finally, socio-economic status has perhaps the most significant effect on health. In the United States and Western Europe, the gap in health status and mortality between those with and without economic power and social resources continues to widen. Those in the community with the lowest socio-economic status also have the poorest health and the most difficulty in gaining access to health care, primarily due to lack of health insurance in the United States. The point of entry into the health-care system for most Americans is the family doctor or the family health maintenance organization. The economically disadvantaged seldom have a family doctor. For these individuals, the point of entry is the local hospital emergency room. It is therefore not surprising that individuals with incomes below the federal poverty level have death rates twice as high as those with incomes above the poverty level (Amler and Dull 1987).

Conceptualizing the needs of the target population

In order to establish a useful and effective programme for a specific target population, programme planners must determine the needs and wants of these individuals. This procedural assessment technique is referred to as a needs assessment or analysis. Similar terms, such as social diagnosis, epidemiological diagnosis, behavioural diagnosis, educational and administrative diagnosis (Green and Kreuter 1999), and community analysis/community diagnosis are also found in the literature (Dignam and Carr 1992). The purpose of the needs assessment is to determine whether the needs of the target population are being met. This information is part of the six steps in the development and conceptualization of a health promotion/disease prevention programme. These steps consist of the following:

- needs assessment
- problem(s) identification
- setting goals and objectives
- intervention development
- programme implementation
- programme evaluation.

Identifying needs

Needs assessment is the process of evaluating the problems and solutions identified for a specific target population. The population can be as small as a clinical study involving patients with hypertension (Morisky *et al.* 1983; Ward *et al.* 2000), a community of individuals sharing a similar cardiovascular disease, breast cancer, or sexually transmitted disease concerns (Ward *et al.* 1982; Morisky *et al.* 1989; Tiglao *et al.* 1996), or a national sample of mothers with children under 2 years of age to assess breast-feeding practices (Morisky *et al.* 1992). Assessing needs moves beyond the information gathering of need identification, requiring evaluative judgments about problems and their solutions. McKillip (1987) identifies three models of needs assessment: the discrepancy model, the marketing model, and the decision-making model. The most popular assessment procedure is the discrepancy or gap model, in which one identifies desirable performance standards. These performance expectations are indicators of what ought to be. For example, health counsellors may be asked about performance standards on risk behaviour knowledge among programme participants, health maintenance organizations may be asked about member participation in smoking cessation programmes, or a county health department may be asked about the completion of care of patients with active tuberculosis. Once the performance standard has been defined, the next step in the analysis is performance measurement. Actual outcomes are determined for the target population on each of the performance dimensions. This is most often done by surveys, although additional needs assessment techniques are conducted, including resource inventory, social indicator analyses, utilization of services, and structured group assessment techniques.

Survey techniques

Surveys are a popular method of gathering information on needs. They provide a flexible means of assessing the expectations both of subgroups of the target population and of other audiences to the need analysis. Surveys can generate a great deal of information; they can probe knowledge, attitudes, beliefs, and opinions as well as measure behaviours and population characteristics. Surveys, however, have the potential to be expensive and complex. Three survey methods are usually considered for needs assessment: face-to-face interviews, telephone interviews, and mailed surveys.

Face-to-face interviews

The face-to-face interview allows for in-depth, person-to-person exchanges. It is the most appropriate of all survey techniques for the developmentally disabled but it is also the most expensive. Blinson *et al.* (1996) have estimated the cost per completed interview varied over time, ranging from a low of $US48 during the height of survey activity to $US243. The average cost per completed interview overall was $US113. Several factors contributed to the overall costs of interviews, including the economy of the community, the number of call-backs made, and local environmental conditions. Additional issues to consider in personal interviews include the question format, consisting of the use or rankings versus ratings, controlling for social desirability of responses, and readability. Use of coding of open-ended responses is also an important consideration. Pilot testing of the instrument can identify potential responses to open-ended questions, thereby eliminating their need. In cases where open-ended questions are required, the interviewer should be trained to record responses verbatim. These responses are then subjected to content analysis, in which independent investigators categorize responses into specific dimensions. For example, in a community household survey, adults ever diagnosed with high blood pressure, were previously on medication and had stopped their medication were asked 'Why did you stop taking your medication?' The questionnaire identified seven categorical answers and one 'other' response. These 'other' responses were categorized into doctor-related responses or patient-centred responses (Levine *et al.* 1982). It should be remembered that the 'other category' should contain the fewest proportion of responses.

Telephone interviews

This technique has become a very popular method for conducting a survey, particularly in areas having a high ratio of telephones to households. It is estimated that in the United States, approximately 98 per cent of households have a telephone (Anderson *et al.* 1998). With the advent of random-digit dialling and computer-assisted telephone dialling (Slade *et al.* 1995), easy techniques have been identified for drawing representative samples. However, telephone surveys also have certain drawbacks, including multiple call-backs for individuals not home, difficulties associated with the impersonal nature of phone contact, and distractions of the respondent. Visual aids cannot be used, so the interviewer must be able to convey verbally all information regarding response choices and skip patterns. Despite these cautions, telephone surveys tend to be the method of choice for relatively short surveys. Response rates are generally higher in telephone surveys compared with face-to-face interview—as high as 90 per cent for telephone surveys compared with as low as 54 per cent for personal interviews (Templeton *et al.* 1997).

Mailed surveys

A mailed survey is perhaps the most difficult assessment procedure with respect to getting participants to complete all items in the survey. Also, response rates are generally poorest among mailed surveys. Furthermore, it is impossible to follow-up on certain questions and there is no opportunity to probe on answers to highly salient issues. In all survey techniques, it is important for the researcher to assess the potential causes of non-response and the differences between the observed values in the sample compared with what may have been gained if the sample was complete, particularly when the response rate is low (Asch *et al.* 1997).

Validation of response

Valid assessment of personal health risk behaviours has always been a challenge to investigators. Gerbert *et al.* (1999) describe a study to determine if primary care patients' disclosures of potentially stigmatizing behaviours would be affected by (a) their expectation about whether or not their doctor would see their disclosures, and (b) the assessment method. A questionnaire assessing HIV, alcohol, drug, domestic violence, tobacco, oral health, and seatbelt risks was completed by 1952 primary care patients; half were told their responses would be seen by the researcher and their doctor and half were told that their responses would be seen by the researcher only. Patients were randomly assigned to one of five assessment methods: written, face-to-face, audio-based, computer-based, or video-based. The results of the study indicated that, across all risk areas, patients did not disclose differently whether or not they believed their doctor would see their disclosures. Technologically advanced assessment methods (audio, computer, and video) produced greater risk disclosure (4 to 8 per cent greater) than traditional methods in three of seven risk areas. These findings suggest patients are not less willing to disclose health risks to a research assistant knowing that this information would be shared with their doctor and that a number of assessment methods can effectively elicit patient disclosure. Potentially small increases in risk disclosure must be weighed against other factors, such as cost and convenience, in determining which method(s) to use in different health-care settings.

Different assessment techniques may also result in less socially desirable or biased responses. It is well known that many individuals are quite embarrassed when questioned about their sexual behaviour. Liu *et al.* (1998) used an innovative technique to assess drug use and sexual behaviours among rural populations in China. Sensitive questions related to these behaviours were administered using a tape recorder, earphones, and an answer sheet that did not include the text. It is not known exactly how much this technique improved the validity of the assessment, but researchers identified high response rates and high completion rates of sensitive questions.

Resources inventory

Resource inventories describe the services available to a target population and reveal gaps and limitations in the service. A resource inventory may indicate underutilized services and may assist agencies and funding organizations to avoid launching services and programmes where there is already a great deal of competition. However, by itself, a resource inventory cannot indicate need. The collection of service information by type of provider and service will make the resource inventory most useful. Ward *et al.* (1982) described the community assessment technique utilized to identify community resources related to the control of high blood pressure in East Baltimore. Hypertension-related resources were direct (hospitals, clinics, doctor's offices, pharmacies, dental offices) as well as indirect (churches, recreation centres, social service offices, schools, and work sites). A 'windshield' survey was conducted to enumerate all hypertension-related resources within a 21-census tract area comprising a health-planning district. While most of the direct services were included in the programme implementation, several indirect services, particularly churches, recreation centres, and barber (beauty) shops, proved to be important players in the programme. Without the complete identification and enumeration of hypertension-related resources in the community, the programme would not have been as effective (Levine *et al.* 1982, 1983; Bone *et al.* 1984).

Social indicator analysis

Social indicators are aggregate statistical measures that depict important aspects of a social situation and of underlying historical trends and developments. Through synthetic estimation procedures, characteristics of subgroups can be estimated from data concerning a larger group. Risk factors are social indicators that predict undesirable outcomes such as infections, injuries, or hospital admissions. Census and other national indicators, such as the Health Examination Survey or the Health and Nutrition Examination Survey in the United States are some examples. These social indicators are generally available only for large groups of individuals and are often tied to a specific geographical area.

Social indicators describe population distributions, for example, ethnicity, age, or place of residence. They describe government expenditures and other inputs, such as the number of doctors per 100 000 population. They measure social concerns such as quality of life, crime rates, and unemployment. Social indicators are often considered 'objective' or 'hard data'. Finally, they reveal problems rather than solutions in a needs assessment.

Health service utilization

Examining solutions to problems involves estimating how much use will be made of the solutions. Development of a service or programme that will be used is important to all need analysis models. Few agencies or governmental units can afford to fund services that are not utilized. Use analysis is based on comparative expectations; patterns of utilization for one group may indicate patterns for another. Use can be redirected from the experience of current programmes or programmes offered to a similar population. Use can also be compared among subgroups or the target population. Statistical indicators used to define utilization include rates, ratios, and other indices such as incidence and prevalence.

Rates of infection, admissions, or services provided are basic to use analysis. A rate is a fraction, with a numerator and a denominator. The numerator comes from agency records and the denominator from the service or target population. The numerator is the number of individuals served or number of services provided; the denominator is the number eligible in the population. Because numerators are based on agency records, they are usually easier to compute than denominators. Rates apply in many areas. The incidence of a disease is the rate of new cases (numerator) occurring in a defined time period (usually 1 year) divided by the population at risk (denominator) and multiplied by some base. An infection rate is the number of individuals diagnosed with the disease divided by the number of individuals exposed and multiplied by some base. A use ratio compares two services (for example, abortions to births), characteristics of the populations (for example, number of infected men to number of infected women), or some measure of services to number of individuals served (for example, faculty to student ratios). A third assessment of use compares the fit between use and expectations. If the index is positive, use exceeds expectations; if it is negative, use falls short of expectations. Researchers often refer to this as a percentage of unmet need.

Structured group assessment

Perhaps the simplest method of needs assessment is to assemble a group of experts and concerned individuals and charge them with identifying the needs of the population served by the organization or agency. Using their knowledge and experience with the population and the services available, a need analysis committee can identify problems and their solutions. Structured groups provide a supplement and alternative approach to the need assessment techniques previously reviewed. One of the most popular structured processes is the focus group, which has been widely used in marketing to assess consumers' reactions to products or packaging (Moore 1987). They can be used in need assessment to explore the acceptability and accessibility of proposed solutions, or to test hypotheses generated from other social indicator or use analysis. Most often, the focus group is used to explore issues in which little information is known or to identify content areas of a proposed questionnaire. Baldwin *et al.* (1999) describe a multisite study to determine the HIV/AIDS prevention needs of Native American out-of-treatment drug users. The investigators conducted a series of focus groups at each of their four study sites to assess various community needs. Results, many of which would not have been identified through individual surveys, indicated that group members strongly recommended direct involvement of key members of the Native American community in conducting outreach and intervention activities, involving Native American people as the sources of information, and utilizing local and tribally relevant forms of delivering the message.

Focus groups serve both as an alternative and as a supplement to survey techniques.

Nominal process groups also involve structured group processes but unlike focus groups, which are generally comprised of homogeneous members having a commonly shared concern, nominal process groups involve heterogeneous groups representing a wide variety of concerns, some shared and some unshared. It is this heterogeneity of the population that is instrumental in defining important needs in the community. Gilmore (1977) presents a detailed description of the nominal process group, including community representation, seating of group members around a table, a 'round-robin' approach to maximize participation, silent listing of concerns, individual ranking, group ranking, prioritizing, and final selection of key concerns.

A Delphi panel is another technique used to assess social conditions and is used primarily if face-to-face interviews are not practical (Linstone and Turoff 1975). It is particularly useful when accurate, quantitative data are non-existent or where judgemental descriptive information is invaluable. A group of experts in a given topic respond to a series or rounds of questionnaires to be analysed by a single individual. Generally, the initial questionnaire is constructed in a suggestive open-ended format, so as not to restrict creative responses. Successive questionnaires, however, attempt to refine and synthesize information gathered by ranking and prioritizing opinions. The Delphi technique has been applied to a number of research issues including technological forecasting, programme development, and policy analysis. Kar (1990) has used this technique in the identification and ranking of social indicators for primary health care.

According to Judd (1972), there are three distinguishing characteristics of the Delphi process. The first is anonymity of response, which is accomplished through the use of mailed questionnaires and avoiding face-to-face interactions. Modern communication technology, such as anonymous e-mail addresses, has greatly facilitated the Delphi process and allowed an international level of participation. A second feature is multiple interactions, that is, the opportunity for respondents to revise their opinions. Finally, participants are provided with summary feedback of group responses from the previous round of questionnaires. This process facilitates a convergence of the distribution of responses expressed in terms of descriptive statistics.

After this discussion of the different types of assessment techniques, together with their strengths and limitations, this section will move on to the application of these various methods in the assessment of national health objectives for the nation.

Healthy People: objectives for the nation

For over two decades, the American Department of Health and Human Services has used health promotion and disease prevention objectives to improve the health of the American people. The first set of national health objectives was published in 1979 in *Healthy People: The Surgeon General's Report on Health Promotion and Disease Prevention* (US Department of Health, Education, and Welfare 1979). Five challenging goals were set to reduce mortality among four different age groups. Through the combined efforts of public health agencies across the nation, most national targets were achieved. A new set of goals and target objectives were identified for the *Healthy People 2000* document, which significantly expanded the 1990 objectives. Major objectives in this document are delineated far more extensively according to demographic and socio-economic dimensions of risk. For example, major goals and objectives addressed the importance of reducing health disparities and increasing the span of healthy life for Americans. The process of formulating these objectives was based on maximum participation and consensus building among experts, professionals, and national advocacy organizations. The draft document was sent out to over 3000 organizations around the country for comment and review. The Institute of Medicine of the National Academy of Sciences carried out a series of eight regional hearings on behalf of a consortium of 300 national membership organizations, the state health departments, and the federal Office of Disease Prevention and Health Promotion. At these regional hearings, local community leaders and professionals from all sectors provided testimony on issues that needed to be addressed (Stoto *et al.* 1990).

The *Healthy People 2010* document reflects the evolution of public health during the previous decade. New preventive therapies, vaccines, pharmaceuticals, and computerized systems have had a tremendous impact on medicine and public health practice. New partnerships are being defined between public health departments and health-care delivery organizations. Simultaneously, demographic changes reflecting an older and more racially diverse population in the United States have created new demands on the health-care system. Development of the year 2010 objectives began as early as 1996, where the stakeholders of year 2000 objectives attended a consortium meeting entitled, 'Building the prevention agenda for 2010: lessons learned'. This meeting was complemented by numerous focus groups where consortium members discussed the current framework, goals, and objectives to assess the improvements needed to make the 2010 agenda relevant to the first decade of the twenty-first century.

In developing the leading health indicators for 2010, the American Department of Health and Human Services convened a working group of 22 members representing the Office of Public Health and Science and the Department of Health and Human Services. The potential uses of leading health indicators, the criteria to be applied in its selection, and examples of each were documented in a background report. The criteria for these indicators included the following:

- audience interpretability (generally understood, relevant, and salient to the general public)
- population applicability (reflects an issue that applies in important ways to the diverse national population)
- problem impact (addresses a problem of substantial impact, such as increased morbidity, mortality and/or economic costs)
- linked to objectives (must be linked to one or more of the 2010 objectives)
- representative (reflect the state of the nation or a particular subregion)
- measurable (one for which data can be anticipated from an established data source on a regular basis)
- multilevel trackability (one for which data can be anticipated at multiple levels and for multiple groups—such as national, state, and country levels, as well as by age, gender and ethnicity)
- sensitivity to change (over a reasonably short period of time)
- profile balance (the indicators should reflect a balance among targets that does not overemphasize any one group or condition)
- relevance to policy and individual action (the set of indicators should be useful in directing public and operational initiatives, that is, changes reported in the status of a measure from one period to the next should offer lessons to the policy domain that are readily interpretable).

Input from the public was critical in developing the leading health indicators. Community and citizen participation was maximized in the finalization of the goals and objectives of *Healthy People 2010* by placing a draft copy on the internet and soliciting public comment. As a result of this dynamic and interactive process, leading health indicators have been identified which address important issues to diverse national populations. Each indicator is linked to one or more of the 2010 objectives and is quantified from an established data source on a regular basis. However, conspicuously missing from the 2010 objectives is a separate section dedicated to surveillance and data systems. Table 1 identifies the two broad goals for community health: (a) to increase the quality as well as the years of healthy life; (b) to

Table 1 *Healthy People 2010*: goals and priority areas for objective setting

Promote healthy behaviours	Promote healthy and safe communities	Improve systems for personal and public health	Prevent and reduce diseases and disorders
1. Physical activity and fitness 2. Nutrition 3. Tobacco use	4. Educational and community-based programmes	10. Access to quality health services	16. Arthritis, osteoporosis, and chronic back conditions
	5. Environmental health	11. Family planning	17. Cancer
	6. Food safety	12. Maternal, infant, and child health	18. Diabetes
	7. Injury/violence prevention	13. Medical product safety	19. Disability and secondary conditions
	8. Occupational safety and health	14. Public health infrastructure	20. Heart disease and stroke
	9. Oral health	15. Health communication	21. HIV
			22. Immunization and infectious diseases
			23. Mental health and mental disorders
			24. Respiratory diseases
			25. Sexually transmitted diseases
			26. Substance abuse

eliminate disparities in health status, health risks, and use of preventive interventions among population groups. In order to reach these goals, over 360 objectives and a number of subobjectives were developed and organized as part of 26 priority areas. These areas consist of promoting healthy behaviours, promoting healthy and safe communities, improving systems for personal and public health, and preventing and reducing diseases and disorders.

The proposed framework for *Healthy People 2010* revolves around the vision 'healthy people in healthy communities'. This concept is based on the idea that health improvement begins at home with what people do, individually, in families and communities to promote physical, mental, and social health. Schools, worksites, community programmes, religious institutions, voluntary organizations, senior citizen centres, and other organizations can deliver preventive health messages.

Surveillance and data sources

Public health surveillance is the systematic collection, analysis, interpretation, dissemination, and use of health information (see Chapter 6.16). Surveillance data systems provide information on morbidity, mortality, and disability from acute and chronic conditions, injuries, personal, environmental, and occupational risk factors associated with illness and premature death, and preventive and treatment services and costs. This information is used to understand the health status of the population and to plan, implement, describe, and evaluate public health programmes that control and prevent adverse health events. To be of maximum usefulness, public health data must be reasonably accurate, timely, and available in a usable form.

Numerous data sources have been identified in which surveillance information is obtained. These include the national vital statistics system, national hospital discharge data, the Health and Nutrition Examination Survey, the National Health Interview Survey, and the Behavioral Risk Factor Surveillance System, amongst others. These national data sources provide annual, continuous, and periodic measures for three or more of the 365 objectives for the year 2010. The American Public Health Service plays an important role in the development and conduct of surveillance and data collection. American Public Health Service activities include the collection and analyses of health information at the national, regional, and, when possible, state and local levels. They also assist the states and local agencies in conducting public health surveillance and evaluation of data by providing standards, definitions, methods, computer software, training, and co-ordination.

Although the American Public Health Service takes the leading role in national public health data collection activities, it is only one partner within the larger structure necessary to collect national public health data. The national vital statistics system obtains information on births, deaths, marriages, and divorces from all 50 states, New York City, the District of Columbia, Puerto Rico, the American Virgin Islands, and Guam. Programmes in each state collect vital information from many sources in local communities, including medical examiners, coroners, hospitals, and justices of the peace. Other data collection systems are based on sample surveys and depend upon the participation of thousands of private citizens nationwide. For example, the National Health Interview Survey is a continuing nationwide sample survey in which data are collected through personal household interviews. In 1987, the personal and demographic characteristics, illnesses, chronic and acute conditions, use of health resources, and other health topics were collected for approximately 123 000 individuals (NCHS 1989). In order to determine the frequency and predictors of receipt of HIV test results, over 19 000 adults were interviewed in 1994 and 1995 for the American National Health Interview Survey. Investigators used predictive modelling to determine factors independently associated with decreased likelihood of receiving HIV test results. The results indicated that an estimated 2.3 million of the 17.5 million people tested annually for HIV infection did not receive their test results (Tao *et al.* 1999).

Theoretical models used in community-based research

Needs analysis/assessment of the target population is the indespensable condition in the conceptualization, development, design, implementation, and evaluation of community-based programmes. Without this component, investigators would not know what particular determinants are responsible for the health-related risk-taking behaviours of their targeted populations. These determinants can be broadly categorized into internal cognitive factors (such as levels of knowledge, attitudes, beliefs, values, and predispositions) and external factors (such as access, availability, and affordability of health services, social norms, and environmental reinforcements). Health promotion and disease prevention planners know their populations and have ideas about what determines client behaviours as well as their strengths and needs as individuals and as a community.

This 'hands-on' knowledge about what works is termed 'informal theory'. Whether implicit or explicit, some form of theory generally provides the foundation of prevention interventions. Formal theory is made up of principles and methods about prevention and behaviour change that have already proven useful in some areas of disease prevention and behaviour change. Theories can give programme planners a framework for establishing the rationale guiding specific intervention approaches, or help to explain aspects of risk-taking behaviour when working with a new population. Using theories to design prevention interventions can help improve programmes, saving valuable time and resources (Valdiserri 1989).

Role of theory in behavioural assessment

Theory is one of many tools that can have a significant influence on the planning of intervention programmes, based on the assessment and interpretation of needs analysis data. Many may claim that behavioural assessment is atheoretical, merely collecting data on risk factors and causes of disease. The underlying theoretical assumptions of collecting data on risk factors that have been causally linked to or associated with major diseases have rarely been examined. However, without a theoretical or conceptual framework guiding the collection of factors, determinants, and indicators of risk, an inappropriate intervention programme may be set in place, resulting in null or negative effects.

Theories generally begin their focus on the individual's psychological process, such as attitudes and beliefs, then go into theories emphasizing social relationships, and end with structural factors to explain human behaviour. Many of the theories discussed below are used in combination with other theories, such as cognitive theories, social influence approaches, and sociostructural/environmental theories working together to address personal beliefs and attitudes as well as external influences on behaviours, such as peer influences and health provider reinforcement, and access, availability, and affordability of health services. This combination of approaches provides a strong foundation for effective programme planning and implementation. The problem of AIDS as a global epidemic concern is used as an example in each of the theoretical perspectives.

The health belief model

The health belief model, social cognitive theory, and the theory of reasoned action are examples of intrapsychic theories directed towards individual perceptions. The health belief model, developed in the 1950s (Hochbaum 1956, 1959), holds that health behaviour is a function of individual's sociodemographic characteristics, knowledge, and attitudes. Catania *et al.* (1990) have conceptualized components of this model into their AIDS risk reduction model with application to the behaviour of condom use for HIV prevention. According to this model, a person must hold the following beliefs in order to be able to change behaviour:

- perceived susceptibility to a particular health problem ('Am I at risk for AIDS?')
- perceived seriousness of the condition ('How serious is AIDS' or 'How hard would my life be if I got AIDS?')
- belief in the effectiveness of the new behaviour ('If I use condoms, then I will not get AIDS')
- cues to action (witnessing the death or illness of a close friend or relative due to AIDS)
- perceived benefits of preventive action ('If I start using condoms, I can avoid HIV infection')
- barriers to taking action ('I don't like using condoms').

In this value-expectancy model, promoting action to change one's behaviour includes changing individual personal beliefs. Individuals weigh the benefits against the perceived costs and barriers to change. For change to occur, benefits must outweigh costs. With respect to HIV, interventions often target perception of risk, beliefs in severity of AIDS ('there is no cure'), beliefs in effectiveness of condom use, and benefits of condom use or delaying onset of sexual relations.

Social cognitive theory

Social cognitive theory or social learning theory states that new behaviours are learned either by modelling the behaviour of others or by direct experience. Social learning theory focuses on the important roles played by vicarious, symbolic, and self-regulatory processes in psychological functioning and looks at human behaviour as a continuous interaction between cognitive, behavioural, and environmental determinants (Bandura 1977). Central tenets of the social cognitive theory are self-efficacy—the belief in the ability to implement the necessary behaviour ('I know I can insist on condom use with my partner')—and outcome expectancies—beliefs about outcomes such as the belief that using condoms correctly will prevent HIV infection.

Programmes built on social cognitive theory integrate information and attitudinal change to enhance motivation and reinforcement of risk reduction skills and self-efficacy. Specifically, activities focus on the experience people have in talking to their partners about sex and condom use, the positive and negative beliefs about adopting condom use, and the types of environmental barriers to risk reduction. A meta-analysis of HIV risk-reduction interventions that used social cognitive theory in controlled experimental trials found that 12 published interventions with mostly uninfected individuals all obtained positive changes in risk behaviour (Greenberg 1996).

Theory of reasoned action

Ajzen and Fishbein (1975) popularized the theory of reasoned action in the mid-1960s. This theory is based on the assumptions that individuals are usually quite rational and make systematic use of the information available to them. People consider the implications of their actions in a given context at a given time before they decide to engage or not engage in a given behaviour, and that most actions of social relevance are under volitional control (Ajzen and Fishbein 1975). The theory of reasoned action is conceptually similar to the health belief model but adds the construct of behavioural intention as a determinant of health behaviour. Both theories focus on perceived susceptibility, perceived benefits, and constraints to changing behaviour. The theory of reasoned action specifically focuses on the role of personal intention in determining whether a behaviour will occur. A person's intention is a function of two basic determinants:

- attitude (towards the behaviour)
- 'subjective norms' (that is, social influence).

'Normative' beliefs play a central role in the theory, and generally focus on what an individual believes other people, especially influential people, would expect him or her to do. For example, for a person to start using condoms, his or her attitude might be 'Having sex with condoms is just as good as having sex without condoms' and subjective norms (or the normative belief) could be 'Most of my peers are using condoms; they would expect me to do so as well.' Interventions using this theory to guide activities focus on attitudes about risk reduction, response to social norms, and intentions to change risky behaviours.

Stages of change model

The stages of change model (sometimes called the transtheoretical model), developed early in the 1990s specifically for smoking cessation by Prochaska and colleagues (Prochaska and DiClemente 1992; Prochaska *et al.* 1992), posits six stages that individuals or groups pass through when changing behaviour: precontemplation, contemplation, preparation, action, maintenance, and relapse. With respect to condom use behaviour, the stages could be described as follows.

1. Has not considered using condoms (precontemplation).
2. Recognizes the need to use condoms (contemplation).
3. Thinking about using condoms in the next months (preparation).
4. Using condoms consistently for less than 6 months (action).
5. Using condoms consistently for 6 months or more (maintenance).

6. Slipping-up with respect to condom use (relapse).

In order for an intervention to be successful it must target the appropriate stage of the individual or group, for example raising awareness between stages 1 and 2. Groups and individuals pass through all stages, but do not necessarily move in a linear fashion (Prochaska and DiClemente 1992). As with previous theories, the stages of change model emphasizes the importance of cognitive processes and uses Bandura's concept of self-efficacy. Movement between stages depends on cognitive–behavioural processes.

Diffusion of innovation model

The diffusion of innovation model provides an understanding of how new ideas or behaviours are introduced and become accepted by a community. People in the same community adopt new behaviours at different rates and respond to different methods of intervention (Rogers 1983). The diffusion of innovation model provides a useful framework for examining the adoption of a new behaviour. This model categorizes individual behaviour change into five stages: awareness, interest, persuasion, decision, and adoption. Individuals pass through these stages and adopt new behaviours at different rates. The model classifies these different rates of change by dividing the population into five groups: innovators, early adopters, early majority, late majority, and laggards. When a new behaviour is introduced into a population, the cumulative curve follows an S-shaped pattern, as more individuals reach the fifth stage and adopt or internalize the new behaviour.

The diffusion of innovation theory is closely linked to the stages of change model of behaviour change. Both the diffusion of innovation theory and the stages of change models are based on the assumption that individuals pass through several stages before successfully achieving behaviour change. The major distinction between these two models is that the stages of change model limits examination of behaviour change to the individual level, while diffusion of innovation goes beyond the individual to describe behaviour change in a population. The stages of change model explains the process of behaviour change, from not being aware of the negative effects of a behaviour, to maintaining safer behaviours. The stages of change model has traditionally been used to analyse the cessation of addictive behaviour from a psychological perspective. However, if the stages of change model is expanded and viewed from a community/public health perspective, the two models appear to have many shared components. Figure 1 presents the comparative features of these two theoretical constructs and potential linkages of stages of behavioural change in the models.

Community assessment of HIV/AIDS in the Philippines

Asia has been identified as the next epidemic zone for AIDS in the world, following sub-Saharan Africa. The countries in Asia with the highest estimate of HIV/AIDS are India, Thailand, Cambodia, Myanmar, and Vietnam (UNAIDS 2000). However, there is considerable variability with respect to the number of reported cases within Asia. For example, as of January 2000, the Philippines, with an estimated population of 75 million, reports a total of 1336 AIDS documented cases. The estimated number of HIV-infected people amounts to 40 000. In contrast, Thailand with a population of approximately 61 million reports over 70 000 cases as of 1997 and an estimated 800 000 people infected with HIV. Sentinel surveillance involving serological testing of high-risk populations has been conducted in each of these countries. However, in the Philippines, seroprevalence assessment has been discontinued in two regions and replaced with behavioural sentinel surveillance assessments owing to the small numbers of high-risk groups and very low seropositivity rates. There are a number of reasons speculated by researchers for the significantly lower infection rate in the Philippines, including the lack of a viral pool, very low levels of injectible drug use, geographical dispersion of the population in an archipelago of over 7100 islands compared with one contiguous country, low number of weekly sexual partners among commercial sex workers, and the presence of government-sponsored social hygiene clinics throughout the country.

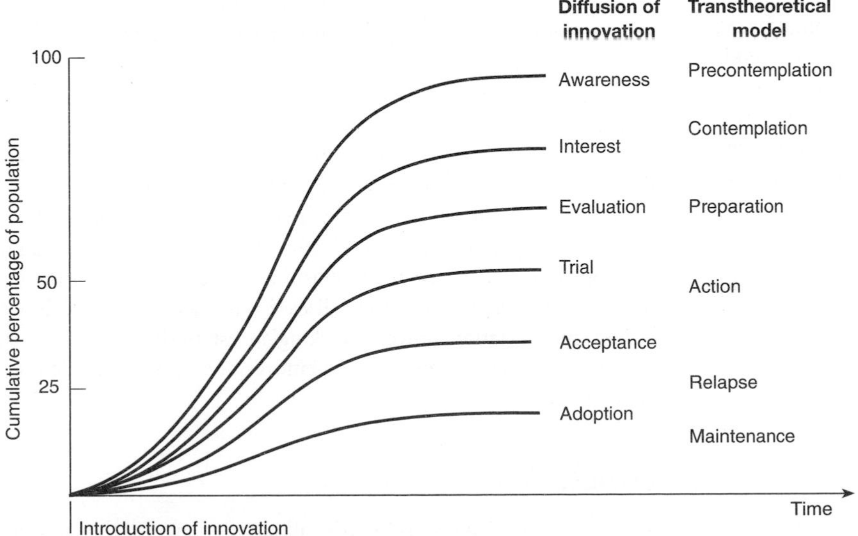

Fig. 1 An integrative model of diffusion of innovation and the transtheorectical model.

In 1994, a community behaviour assessment was conducted in four communities in the southern Philippines, as part of a 4-year National Institute of Allergy and Infectious Diseases funded research on behavioural interventions in support of HIV/AIDS prevention (Morisky *et al.* 1995). The study was undertaken in areas where many of the high-risk workers are employed and where interventions focusing on behavioural aspects of HIV/AIDS prevention were not adequately developed. The behavioural assessment conducted during the first year of the research study served as a basis for the development and conceptualization of targeted educational interventions directed towards managers and supervisors of commercial business establishments (such as bars, night clubs, karaoke clubs, and so on) and their female employees, also known as guest relation officers. Table 2 identifies the various needs assessment strategies conducted in each locality, beginning with a situational analysis of the community. This assessment procedure provides invaluable information on the resources related to AIDS prevention in the community, including existing services provided by governmental and non-governmental agencies. The social hygiene clinic, under the City Health Department, provides weekly clinic examinations for all guest relation officers. The City Health Department requires that all employees of bars, night clubs, karaoke centres, and massage parlours be registered in the local social hygiene clinic and undergo weekly examinations. The social hygiene clinic is staffed with a doctor, nurse/midwife, and medical technologist. All guest relation officers attend the same weekly schedule according to the type of establishment. Unobtrusive observations were conducted in each social hygiene clinic in order to assess registration/attendance procedures, interpersonal communication techniques between client and staff, and opportunities for educational interventions in the clinic during examination waiting time. Independent focus group discussions were conducted for guest relation officers and their managers or supervisors of the various establishments to assess knowledge of HIV/AIDS, attitudes regarding AIDS prevention, satisfaction with social hygiene clinic visits, condom use behaviour, and the role of the manager/supervisor in reinforcement of safe sexual behaviours (Tiglao *et al.* 1996). Retrospective record reviews of all currently registered guest relation officers were conducted in each clinic to provide baseline data on clinic attendance, and the results of the clinic examination. Structured personal interviews were held with both managers/supervisors and guest relation officers. Finally, continued monitoring of weekly social hygiene clinic attendance by the guest relation officers and examination results provided ongoing assessment information. Social hygiene clinic attendance was conceptualized as a ratio of number of weeks attended during the month and the number of weeks actually worked during that month. This measure quantifies clinic attendance based on 'at-risk behaviour'.

Table 2 Community assessment techniques: HIV/AIDS prevention in the Philippines

Clinical observations
Record review of STD rates in SHC
Exit interviews with SHC clients
Focus group discussions with GROs and managers
Personal interviews with GROs and managers

GRO, guest relations officer (sex worker); SHC, social hygiene clinic; STD, sexually transmitted diseases.

The needs assessment was instrumental in identifying educational and organizational behaviour change strategies to be tested using a quasi-experimental design in the four communities. It was apparent that the managers/supervisors of the establishments played a critical role in the reinforcement of AIDS-related knowledge, attitudes, and safe sexual behaviours. It was also identified in the interviews that a small group of guest relation officers were interested in being trained in HIV prevention techniques to serve as peer educators in their respective establishment. Consequently, from this broad community assessment, a four-group quasi-experimental design was implemented in the four study sites, consisting of a peer education strategy, manager/supervisor training, the combination of peer educator and manager training, and a standard control site.

Programme monitoring is an essential ingredient in ongoing community assessment. Both process assessments (documentation that activities took place, such as training programmes, distribution of educational materials) and formative evaluation assessments (reviewing clinic records for completion, ensuring completion of interviews, monitoring attendance) are critical to the success of the programme. Process assessment is not evaluative in the sense that it provides information as to whether or not the outcome was successful or unsuccessful, it only provides information that the activity or intervention took place. However, this type of assessment is of major importance because if at the end of the programme no effect is found, then a question remains over whether the programme was implemented as originally conceptualized. Documenting the time, place, and amount provides an audit trail in which the investigator can assess critical links in the chain of events that make a programme successful. Formative assessment is evaluative in the sense that data collection instruments are assessed immediately in order to ensure that information is recorded accurately and whether or not changes in impact (knowledge, attitudes, or beliefs) are being noted as a result of the intervention activities. If this is found not to be true, then the programme manager needs to modify the intervention activities, such as making group sessions more convenient so as to maximize attendance or provide child care to participants who cannot otherwise attend because of household responsibilities.

Predictors of appointment-keeping behaviour included knowledge of HIV transmission, self-efficacy in communication skills, and positive reinforcement from establishment managers (Sneed and Morisky 1998). Guest relation officers were more than twice as likely to report consistent use of condoms if managers made these available at the establishment, in the presence of an establishment rule concerning the use of condoms with customers, and if they had ever attended an educational seminar on AIDS prevention. The significance of an organizational policy regarding safe sexual practices among guest relation officers is evidenced by the lower rate of sexually transmitted diseases among establishments having an educational policy. The sexually transmitted disease rate was 40 per cent lower among guest relation officers working in establishments in which educational policy was enacted and enforced (3.5 per 100 clinic visits versus 4.9; $p < 0.001$).

Conclusion

Behavioural assessment is a critical component in the conceptualization and design of community-based intervention programmes. It is often identified as one of the most important aspects of public health surveillance. As indicated in this chapter, surveillance is at the centre of an epidemiological approach to public health and community assessment of behavioural indicators occupies a key role in the social science concerns of public health. Regardless of the perspective, the perceived need is clear for systematic information relating to the mission of public health to promote, protect, and preserve the health of the public. If progress is to continue in meeting the goals and objectives for the nation in 2010, particularly with respect to the improvement of quality of life for all and removal of health disparities, the most scientifically valid and culturally appropriate techniques must be employed for community assessment. New partnerships are being realized between data collectors, data analysers, and data users as well as between governmental and non-governmental organizations. The challenge to these partnerships is to refine these data surveillance techniques in order to provide the most accurate, valid, and useful indicators resulting from community behavioural assessment. Once this is accomplished, the findings need to be translated into treatment and prevention interventions that can be incorporated into community health delivery systems.

References

Ajzen, I. and Fishbein, M. (1975). *Belief, attitute, intention, and behaviour: an introduction to theory and research.* Addison-Wesley, Reading, MA.

American Thoracic Society (1996). Health effects of outdoor air pollution. Committee of the Environmental and Occupational Health Assembly of the American Thoracic Society. *American Journal of Respiratory and Critical Care Medicine*, **153**, 3–50.

Amler, R.W. and Dull, H.B. (1987). *Closing the gap: the burden of unnecessary illness.* Oxford University Press, New York.

Anderson, J.E., Nelson, D.E., and Wilson, R.W. (1998). Telephone coverage and measurement of health risk indicators: data from the National Health Interview Survey. *American Journal of Public Health*, **88**, 1392–5.

Asch, D.A., Jedrziewski, M.K., and Christakis, N.A. (1997). Response rates to mail surveys published in medical journals. *Journal of Clinical Epidemiology*, **50**, 1129–36.

Balbach, E.D. and Glantz, S.A. (1998). Tobacco control advocates must demand high-quality media campaigns: the California experience. *Tobacco Control*, **7**, 397–408.

Baldwin, J.A., Trotter, R.T., II, Martinez, D., Stevens, S.J., John, D., and Brems, C. (1999). HIV/AIDS risks among Native American drug users: key findings from focus group interviews and implications for intervention strategies. *AIDS Education and Prevention*, **11**, 279–92.

Bandura, A. (1977). Self-efficacy: toward a unifying theory of behavioral change. *Psychological Review*, **84**, 191–215.

Blinson, K., Dignan, M., Michielutte, R., and Wells, H.B. (1966). The cost of conducting face-to-face household interviews in a rural, Native American population. The North Carolina Native American Cervical Cancer Prevention Project. *Cancer*, **78**, 1587–91

Bone, L.R., Levine, D.M., Parry, R.E., Morisky, D.E., and Green, L.W. (1984). Update on the factors associated with high blood pressure compliance. *Maryland State Medical Journal*, **33**, 201–4.

Catania, J.A., Kegeles, S.M., and Coates, T.J. (1990). Toward an understanding of risk behavior: an AIDS risk reduction model. *Health Education Quarterly*, **17**, 53–72.

Clements, R. (1999). Prevalence of alcohol-use disorders and alcohol-related problems in a college student sample. *Journal of American College Health*, **48**, 111–18.

Dignam, N.B. and Carr, P.A. (1992). *Program planning for health education and health promotion.* Lea and Febiger, Philadelphia, PA.

Ellison, C.G. and Levin, J.S. (1998). The religion–health connection: evidence, theory, and future directions. *Health Education and Behavior*, **25**, 700–20.

Gerbert, B., Bronstone, A., Pantilat, S., McPhee, S., Allerton, M., and Moe, J. (1999). When asked, patients tell: disclosure of sensitive health-risk behaviors. *Medical Care*, **37**, 104–11.

Gilmore, G.D. (1977). Needs assessment processes for community health education. *International Journal of Health Education*, **21**, 164–73.

Glasgow, R.E., Cummings, K.M., and Hyland, A. (1997). Relationship of worksite smoking policy to changes in employee tobacco use: findings from COMMIT. Community Intervention Trial for Smoking Cessation. *Tobacco Control*, **6**, S44–8.

Green, L.W. and Kreuter, M.W. (1999). *Health promotion planning: an educational and ecological approach* (3rd edn). Mayfield, Mountain View, CA.

Greenberg, J. (1996). *AIDS education: interventions in multicultural settings* (ed. I. Schenker and G. Saber-Friedman). Plenum Press, New York.

Han, B., Small, B.J., and Haley, W.E. (1999). The effects of race, gender, and education on the structure of self-rated health among community-dwelling older adults. *Annals of the New York Academy of Sciences*, **896**, 442–7.

Hochbaum, G.M. (1956). Why people seek diagnostic X-rays. *Public Health Reports*, **71**, 377–80.

Hochbaum, G.M. (1959). *Public participation in medical screening programs: a social-psychological study.* Public Health Service, Washington, DC.

Judd, R.C. (1972). Use of Delphi methods in higher education. *Technological Forecasting and Social Change*, **4**, 173–86.

Kar, S.B. (1990). Primary health care: implications for the medical profession and education. *Academic Medicine*, **65**, 301–6.

Lemen, R.A. (1999). Role of government in occupational and environmental health. *International Journal of Occupational and Environmental Health*, **5**, 283–6.

Levine, D.M., Morisky, D.E., and Bone, L.R. (1982). Data based planning for educational interventions through hypertension control programs for urban and rural populations in Maryland. *Public Health Reports*, **97**, 107–12.

Levine, D.M., Bone, L.R., Steinwachs, D.M., Parry, R.E., Morisky, D.E., and Sadler, J.S. (1983). The physician's role in improving patient outcome in high blood pressure control. *Maryland State Medical Journal*, **32**, 291–3.

Levin-Epstein, M. (1999). Problem of uninsured returns to center stage. Democrats, Republicans offer differing solutions. *Hospital Outlook*, **2**, 6–7, 9.

Linstone, H.A. and Turoff, M. (1975). *The Delphi method: techniques and applications.* Addison-Wesley, Reading, MA.

Liu, H., Xie, J., Yu, W., *et al.* (1998). A study of sexual behavior among rural residents of China. *Journal of Acquired Immune Deficiency Syndromes and Human Retrovirology*, **19**, 80–8.

McKenzie, J.F., Ringer, R.R., and Kotecki J.E. (1999). *An introduction to community health* (3rd edn). Jones and Bartlett, Sudbury, MA.

McKillip, J. (1987). *Need analysis: tools for the human services and education.* Sage, Beverly Hills, CA.

Montazeri, A. and McEwen, J. (1997). Effective communication: perception of two anti-smoking advertisements. *Patient Education and Counseling*, **30**, 29–35.

Moore, C.M. (1987). *Group techniques to generate, develop, and select ideas.* Sage, Newbury Park, CA.

Morisky, D.E., Levine, D.M., Green, L.W., Shapiro, S., Russell, R.P., and Smith, C.R. (1983). Five-year blood pressure control and mortality following health education for hypertensive patients. *American Journal of Public Health*, **73**, 153–62.

Morisky, D.E., Fox, S.A., Murata, P.J., and Stein, J.A. (1989). The role of needs assessment in designing a community-based mammography education program for urban women. *Health Education Research*, **4**, 469–78.

Morisky, D.E., Chaudhury, A.S., Kar, S.B., and Chen, K.R. (1992). Knowledge and attitudes concerning breastfeeding and immigration practices in Pakistan. Presented at the Annual Meeting of the American Public Health Association, Washington, DC.

Morisky, D.E., Detels, R., Tiglao, T., *et al.* (1995). Behavioral research in support of HIV/AIDS prevention in the Philippines. Presented at the Annual Meeting of the American Public Health Association, Washington, DC.

Moskowitz, J.M., Lin, Z., and Hudes, E.S. (1999). The impact of California's smoking ordinances on worksite smoking policy and exposure to environmental tobacco smoke. *American Journal of Health Promotion*, **13**, 278–81

NCHS (National Center for Health Statistics) (1989). *Health, United States, 1988*. US Department of Health and Human Services, Hyattsville, MD.

Novotny, T.E. and Siegel, M.B. (1996). California's tobacco control saga. *Health Affairs*, **15**, 58–72.

Pinder, L. (1994). Medicine for the twenty-first century: challenges in personal and public health promotion. *American Journal of Preventive Medicine*, **10**, 39–41.

Prochaska, J.O. and DiClemente, C.C. (1992). Stages of change in the modification of problem behaviors. *Progress in Behavior Modification*, **28**, 183–218.

Prochaska, J.O., DiClemente, C.C., and Norcross, J.C. (1992). In search of how people change. *American Psychologist*, **47**, 1102–14.

Rogers, E.M. (1983). *Diffusion of innovations* (3rd edn). Free Press, New York.

Scutchfield, F.D., Hiltabiddle, S.E., Rawding, N., and Violante, T. (1997). Compliance with the recommendations of the Institute of medicine report, *The Future of Public Health*: a survey of local health departments. *Journal of Public Health Policy*, **18**, 155–66.

Sheard, A. (2000). Bible's stance on homosexuality. Bible shows no understanding of homosexual orientation as mutually supportive and affirming. *British Medical Journal*, **320**, 514–15.

Slade, G.D., Brennan, D., and Spencer, A.J. (1995). Methodological aspects of a computer-assisted telephone interview survey of oral health. *Australian Dental Journal*, **40**, 306–10.

Sneed, C.D. and Morisky, D.E. (1998). Applying the theory of reasoned action to condom use among sex workers. *Social Behavior and Personality*, **26**, 317–28.

Stoto M.A., Behrens R., and Rosemont C. (ed.) (1990). *Healthy people 2000: citizens chart the course.* National Academy Press, Washington, DC.

Tao, G., Branson, B.M., Kassler, W.J., and Cohen, R.A. (1999). Rates of receiving HIV test results: data from the US National Health Interview Survey for 1994 and 1995. *Journal of Acquired Immune Deficiency Syndromes*, **22**, 395–400.

Templeton, L., Deehan, A., Taylor, C., Drummond, C., and Strang, J. (1997). Surveying general practitioners: does a low response rate matter? *British Journal of General Practice*, **47**, 91–4.

Tiglao, T., Morisky, D.E., Tempongko, S., Baltazar, J., and Detels, R. (1996). A community participation action research approach to HIV/AIDS prevention among sex workers. *Promotion and Education*, **3**, 25–8.

UNAIDS (2000). *UNAIDS report 2000: regional statistics and features.* UNAIDS website: http://www.unaids.org/hivaidsinfo/statistics/june98/fact_sheets/.

US Department of Health and Human Services (2000). *Healthy People 2010.* US Government Printing Office, Pittsburgh, PA.

US Department of Health, Education, and Welfare (1979). *Healthy people: the Surgeon General's report on health promotion and disease prevention.* US Government Printing Office, Washington, DC.

Valdiserri, R.O. (1989). *Preventing AIDS: the design of effective programs.* Rutgers University Press, New York.

VanEenwyk, J. (1997). Approaches to community concerns: applied public health. *Public Health*, **111**, 405–10.

Walker, B., Jr (1989). The future of public health: the Institute of Medicine's 1988 report. *Journal of Public Health Policy*, **10**, 19–31.

Ward, W.B., Levine, D.M., Morisky, D.E., *et al.* (1982). Controlling high blood in inner city Baltimore through community health education. In *Perspectives on community health education* (ed. R.W. Carlow). Third Party Publishing, Oakland, CA.

Ward, H.J., Morisky, D.E., Lees, N.B., and Fong, R. (2000). A clinic and community-based approach to hypertension control for an underserved minority population: design and methods. *American Journal of Hypertension*, **13**, 177–83.

Wechsler, H., Dowdall, G.W., Maenner, G., Gledhill-Hoyt, J., and Lee, H. (1998). Changes in binge drinking and related problems among American college students between 1993 and 1997. Results of the Harvard School of Public Health College Alcohol Study. *Journal of American College Health*, **47**, 57–68.

7.5 Health economics and public health

M. Christopher Auld, Cam Donaldson, Craig Mitton, and Phil Shackley

Introduction

Economics is the science of choice. In public health, such choice can take place at two levels: for governments or other health purchasers, between different health-care and public health programmes, or, for an individual, in terms of how health is 'traded' against other goods in life. The former level of choice requires economic evaluation and the latter requires an understanding of the contribution of economics to the analysis of how individuals respond to changes in health policy or to changes in the (perceived) prevalence of disease.

In the following section, some basic concepts from micro-economics, which underlie all economic theories of choice, are defined. These are 'rational choice theory', 'opportunity cost', and 'production'. Following this, the focus will be on what most public health practitioners probably perceive as the main contribution of health economics: the use of economic evaluation in appraising interventions. The third section begins with an introduction to the main techniques of economic evaluation. In the fourth section, a list of costs and benefits, which should be considered for inclusion in economic evaluations, is provided. Principles of measurement and valuation of costs are then outlined in the fifth section. In the sixth section, concentration is on valuing the benefits of health care. In the seventh section, following presentations of economic evaluation methods, a priority setting framework for use by health (care) purchasers, known as programme budgeting and marginal analysis, is outlined. The remainder of the chapter focuses on the growing contribution of economics to analysing how individuals respond to public health and health promotion policies. Individuals, either implicitly or explicitly, weigh up the costs and benefits of their actions, some of which affect health. Any policy aimed at influencing health will, therefore, change these costs and benefits. Therefore, the eighth section extends the opportunity cost concept to a model of consumer behaviour, and demonstrates the usefulness of this framework for predicting the effects of public health policies. The conclusion summarizes the contribution of economics to evaluating public health practice and policy, and includes a checklist for measurement and valuation of costs and benefits in economic evaluation.

Key concepts in micro-economics

Economics is most famously defined as 'the science which studies human behaviour as a relationship between ends and scarce means which have alternate uses' (Robbins 1935). In shorter form, economics is about choice: starting with the premise that individuals have ends (for instance, comfort, health, social status, and pleasure) and limited resources to achieve those ends, economics seeks to make positive statements regarding how social systems work and make normative statements regarding which policies can be expected to make people better off.

Rational choice theory

Economists typically model behaviour as resulting from rational choices on the part of individuals. It is important to emphasize that 'rational' in this context is a piece of technical jargon only loosely related to its more common meaning. In economics, individuals are rational if they are aware of and can rank the options available to them and have consistent beliefs about the way the world works. The ranking itself can be utterly irrational in the common use of the word: for instance, crack addicts can be perfectly rational in the economic sense, even if economists and everyone else agrees that their behaviour is perfectly irrational in the everyday sense. See Becker and Murphy (1988) for an analysis of rational choice in the context of addictive goods.

What is meant by a 'consistent ranking of outcomes?' Suppose there are three outcomes of interest, A, B, and C. Loosely, the individual is said to have rational or consistent preferences over these outcomes if it is the case that (a) they can state they either prefer one outcome to another, or they are indifferent between the two outcomes, and (b) if A is preferred to B and B is preferred to C, then it is not the case that C is preferred to A. These are minimal requirements to allow a model to make predictions about what a person will choose in a given situation. They are further required to make normative statements about various policies: if preferences cycle (that is, C is preferred to A in the example above), then we cannot say what outcome makes the person better off.

If it is the case that a person is rational in the above sense, then, as an analytical convenience, it is possible to assign numbers to various outcomes such that the ranking of the numbers captures the individual's subjective ranking of outcomes: if A is preferred to B, then the number attached to A is higher than the number attached to B. See Mas-Colell *et al.* (1995) for an extensive discussion.

Any such assignment of numbers to outcomes is called a utility function. Since the most preferred outcome available in a given situation will be the one selected, and since, by construction, that outcome will have the highest utility, the decision can be recast as one of maximizing utility subject to whatever constraints the individual faces. The tool 'utility function' is therefore fundamental to economic analysis.

Opportunity costs and constraints

The key concept of cost in economics is opportunity cost: the value of the next best alternative forgone. Suppose, for instance, that you have an afternoon off and have narrowed your selection of what to do with it to either reading a novel or gardening. The opportunity cost of reading the novel is the forgone opportunity to garden, and vice versa. The observation that whenever a decision is made, regardless of the context, an opportunity cost is incurred leads to both the labelling of economics as 'the dismal science' and Milton Friedman's pithy truism, 'there is no such thing as a free lunch'. For instance, if a millionaire donates funds to build a new wing on a hospital, the economist will tend to be the curmudgeonly person at the back of the room pointing out the opportunity cost of the new wing was an increase in the nursing staff, which may have better served patients. Notice that the economist's notion of costs is not necessarily even related to money, as in the novel/gardening example above.

Since costs are defined in terms of forgone opportunities, in order to evaluate interventions and make predictions about behaviour, it is important to specify what options are available to the decision-maker. Given the assumption of rationality and the useful device of a utility function to represent a given individual's rational preferences over the domains of interest, if the set of choices available are also specified it is possible to predict a choice and aid the evaluation of options. The content of economic analysis is in the implications arising from the different choices available either to individuals or social decision-makers. For example, at the level of programme evaluation, by using resources to meet one need, opportunities to use these resources in other programmes are forgone. Therefore, to ensure the most efficient use of resources, it is necessary to know the resources consumed (that is, costs), and benefits produced, by each programme. Only then is it possible to choose that combination of programmes which maximizes benefits to the community.

Production

In addition to analysing individual behaviour using the above concepts, another useful tool of economics involves analysis of the decisions of governments, non-profit agencies, firms, and individuals which produce some output using a variety of inputs. For instance, an automotive firm uses labour, machinery, land, and time to produce cars. A hospital might use doctors, nurses, and machines to 'produce' health in patients, and individuals might use time and market goods to 'produce' their own health (for instance, by buying and using an exercise machine).

The basic tools in production theory can be illustrated with an example. Consider a hospital which produces health, H, using only physicians, P, and nurses, N. We can write the relationship between health produced and the inputs as a function $H = H(P, N)$. If the hospital can hire nurses for WN dollars and can hire physicians for WP dollars per unit of time, the hospital's payroll for that unit of time will total $C = WPP + WNN$. To produce the most health for any given budget C, the hospital must solve the following problem:

$\max_{P,\,N} H(P, N)$

subject to

$W_N N + W_P P = C.$

The solution gives the number of nurses and physicians hired to make patients as healthy as possible for a given budget. Notice that the economic logic here is based on opportunity cost; the hospital should keep hiring nurses up until the point where the opportunity cost of another nurse, in terms of the health that forgone physician services would provide, is just equal to the health benefits the marginal nurse provides. The problem above is illustrated in Fig. 1. The iso-cost line represents all combinations of nurses and physicians which can be afforded; being on the line represents the limits of affordability. The iso-quant curve, $H()$, represents different quantities of 'health' which can be produced by different combinations of physicians and nurses. The reason it is this shape is because as fewer and fewer nurses are employed, it would take more and more physicians to ensure the same level of production, and vice versa. Theoretically, there are an infinite number of iso-quants in the diagram, although they are not allowed to cross each other. Given that costs cannot exceed the limits set by the iso-cost curve shown, the highest level of output which can be achieved is at the point (N^*, P^*). Any other point either costs more money (C is higher) or is associated with lower output of health. This point is also cost-effective in that a given amount of health is achieved at least cost, thus providing the basis for one of the economic evaluation techniques discussed in the following section.

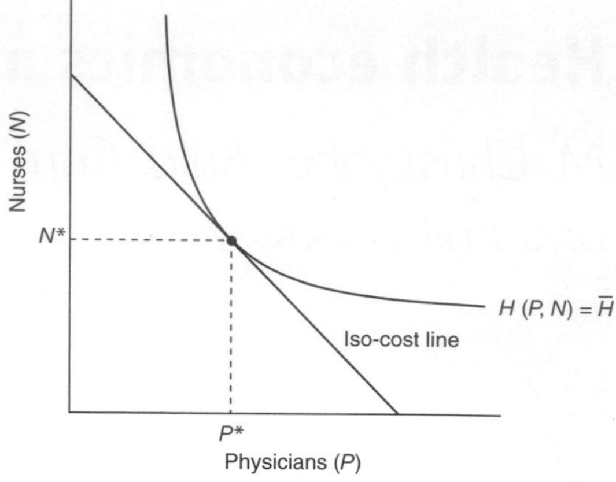

Fig. 1 Maximizing production.

This model of a hospital is very simple and is used to illustrate how economists view both organizations and individuals as 'producing' outcomes of interest given available resources. Having outlined the basic methods of analysis employed by micro-economists in thinking about health-related matters, it is possible to consider how these concepts are used in economic evaluation and in evaluating behavioural responses to public health policies.

Techniques of economic appraisal for programme evaluation

Following on from the above concepts, there are three related economic appraisal techniques; cost–benefit analysis, cost-effectiveness analysis, and cost–utility analysis. Each technique has advantages and difficulties associated with it. However, as Mooney (1989) has said: 'ease cannot be allowed to dictate use; it is a question of what is best for which question'. Therefore, which technique to use should be determined by the question to be addressed in a given evaluation.

Table 1 Questions of allocative and technical efficiency

Allocative efficiency questions	Technical efficiency questions
Surgery for tonsillectomy versus outpatient clinics for asthmatics	Day surgery versus inpatient stay for tonsillectomy
	Local versus hospital-based clinics for asthmatics

Principally, economic evaluation is useful in addressing two levels of question—about allocative and technical efficiency. With allocative efficiency, all health-care programmes have to compete with each other for more (or fewer) resources. Concern is with how many of the scarce resources to allocate to each programme. Thus, in Table 1, surgery for tonsillectomy and outpatient clinics for asthmatics would compete with each other for more (or fewer) resources.

With technical efficiency, concern is more about how best to deliver a programme or to achieve a given objective. The resources already allocated to the programme are taken as given. Therefore, in the cases outlined in Table 1, technical efficiency questions would address how best to deliver surgery for tonsillectomy and how best to provide asthma clinics.

Generally, with allocative efficiency, one group of patients/clients will gain at the expense of another group. With technical efficiency, the same group will be treated, but the question is how. The distinction is important, although it often becomes blurred in practice.

Cost–benefit analysis

Cost benefit analysis is used to address allocative efficiency questions, such as:

- Is it worth allocating resources to achieving this goal?
- How much more or how much less of society's resources should be allocated to achieving this goal or to this type of health care?

Thus, cost–benefit analysis can appear to involve looking at one health-care programme in isolation (although the alternative of doing nothing, or current practice, is always implied). Looking at one programme alone, cost–benefit analysis addresses the question of whether its benefits are greater or less than its opportunity costs. Looking at several competing projects, comparisons are made on the basis of the costs and benefits of each. If not all projects can be funded, the combination that maximizes benefits should be chosen. In both cases, costs and benefits still need to be known.

In principle, answers to the above questions require all costs and benefits to be valued in a commensurate unit (such as money). If everything is measured in one unit, comparisons are straightforward. The valuation of benefits in money terms is the most obvious distinguishing characteristic of cost–benefit analysis. Conceptually, cost–benefit analysis has a very wide range of applicability as, with everything valued in commensurate terms, it could be used to compare health-care objectives with each other or with those arising in other sectors of the economy.

In practice, however, the monetary valuation of benefits in cost–benefit analysis is difficult. How can a value be placed on the saving of life or the relief of suffering? Health improvements are traditionally valued in money terms by using one of two approaches: the human capital approach and the willingness to pay approach. Each of these is reviewed in the section below on measurement and valuation of benefits.

Not surprisingly, ideal cost–benefit analyses are rare in the field of health care, despite the name being included in the titles of many articles. In many cost–benefit analyses, the cost of a new intervention is often assessed against 'benefits' measured in terms of cost savings. However, this clearly involves only a comparison of costs. No consideration is given to the difficult issue of valuing health improvements and other benefits in monetary terms (Birch and Donaldson 1987). Two exceptions are recent evaluations of public health measures of reducing food-borne risk and water fluoridation (Donaldson *et al.* 1996; Shackley and Dixon 2000).

Despite problems of valuing benefits, cost–benefit analysis remains a useful tool, particularly in setting out a decision-making problem. By identifying the costs and benefits associated with different health-care programmes and valuing what can be valued, one can explicitly observe the trade-offs between tangible and intangible costs and benefits resulting from a decision to implement, or not to implement, a health-care programme. A good example of this is the work on costs and benefits of introducing child-proofing of drug containers in the United Kingdom in the early 1970s. In 1971 a decision was taken not to introduce such child-proofing on the basis of its cost (£500 000 per annum at the time). Using conservative estimates, Gould (1971) showed that without child-proofing there would be 16 000 hospital admissions per annum at a cost of £30 per admission, resulting in costs of £480 000 per annum. Thus, the extra cost of child-proofing was £20 000 per annum. If only 20 lives could be saved by child-proofing, the decision not to child-proof would imply that the life of a child was worth less than £1000 per annum.

Such trade-offs would almost certainly have remained implicit in the absence of cost–benefit analysis, thereby not allowing them to be subjected to the same degree of scrutiny. In the absence of such scrutiny, important aspects of efficiency may not be recognized. Cost–benefit analysis, by analysing who receives benefits and bears costs, also opens up important issues of the distribution (or equity) of health and health care which would have remained uncovered. Thus, although economics is often criticized for ignoring equity, it can actually highlight such issues. By quantifying some values and making others explicit, cost–benefit analysis can be a very useful decision-making aid. This 'balance sheet' approach to cost–benefit analysis has been outlined in more detail by McIntosh *et al.* (1999). It also forms the basis of the more practical form of economic evaluation, programme budgeting and marginal analysis (see below). Because decisions about what types of health care to provide cannot be avoided, subjecting decisions to the systematic framework that cost–benefit analysis provides, despite its imperfections, is useful. In the absence of cost–benefit analysis, values would remain implicit and, perhaps, be more prone to error. Avoiding the analysis does not avoid the need for a decision to be made.

Cost-effectiveness analysis

Cost-effectiveness analysis is the most common form of economic evaluation in health care because of its relative simplicity. Its use does not require benefits to be valued in money terms. Cost-effectiveness analysis deals with technical efficiency and seeks to answer the following question. Given that it has been decided that a goal is to be achieved, what is the best way of doing so or what is the best way of spending a given budget? (Remember the point of tangency in Fig. 1.) Thus, cost-effectiveness analysis always involves comparison of at least two options with the same goal.

Cost-effectiveness analysis can take two main forms. In the first, if the health outcomes of the alternatives to be compared are known to be equivalent, only cost differences need be analysed. The least costly alternative is obviously most efficient as resources are saved which can be put to some other beneficial use without reducing the health outcomes of the client group being studied (Russell *et al.* 1977). This is often referred to as cost-minimization analysis.

In the second form of cost-effectiveness analysis, alternatives may differ in terms of cost and effect. A ratio is produced for each alternative in which the numerator is cost and the denominator is the health effect under consideration. Health effects are measures of final outcome: they might be life years saved, heart attacks prevented, or improved physical function. The cost-effectiveness ratio produced for each alternative is a measure of cost per unit of health effect. The alternative with the lowest cost-effectiveness ratio is best. Within a given budget, more health can be produced by implementing this alternative. For example, Doessel (1978) used a cost per life year saved ratio in comparing alternatives for the treatment of chronic renal failure.

The phrase 'within a given budget' is of crucial importance. Often authors produce a ratio of extra costs per extra unit of health effect of a new intervention over current treatment, and call their analysis an 'incremental cost-effectiveness analysis' (Boyle *et al.* 1983; Kristiansen *et al.* 1991; Mark *et al.* 1995; Johannesson *et al.* 1997). However, such studies are not cost-effectiveness analyses. Some judgement is required as to whether such extra costs are worth incurring, that is whether more resources should be allocated to that area of care. The resources to meet these extra costs will inevitably come from some other health-care programme (that is, either from another group of patients within the budget or from another budget altogether). This takes us back to broader comparisons, which is the role of cost–benefit analysis, not cost-effectiveness analysis.

Another limitation of cost-effectiveness analysis is the use of natural measures of outcome. For example, in evaluating different treatments for chronic renal failure, enhanced (or maintained) quality of life can be as important an outcome as improving life expectancy. Therefore, to use 'life years gained' as the outcome in a cost-effectiveness ratio will mean that other important aspects of outcome are missed. Also, one should be careful with outcome measures such as cholesterol reduction, blood pressure, and, even more so, cases detected. This is because the relationship between these and final outcome (that is, health) may be either unclear or not constant across different cases. Nevertheless, to reiterate, cost-effectiveness analysis is very useful for addressing issues of technical efficiency.

Cost–utility analysis

Cost–utility analysis lies somewhere between cost-effectiveness analysis and cost–benefit analysis. It can be used to assess not only technical efficiency, but also allocative efficiency within the health-care sector. The basic outcome in cost–utility analysis is 'healthy years'. The difference between cost–utility analysis and cost-effectiveness analysis is that years of life in states less than 'full health' (for example, disability) can be converted to healthy years by the use of various techniques. To date, the most common forms of conversion are quality-adjusted life years and healthy years equivalents (Williams 1985; Torrance 1986; Mehrez and Gafni 1989; Gafni and Zylak 1990). Again, each of these techniques, and their challenges, is reviewed in the section below on measurement and valuation of benefits.

Cost–utility analysis may be seen as an improvement on cost-effectiveness analysis as it attempts to combine more than one outcome measure. Cost–utility analysis can also be seen as an improvement on cost–benefit analysis as it permits comparisons of programmes within the health sector without the need to place monetary values on their benefits. However, this advantage is limited when non-health benefits and non-health-care costs enter into analyses. So far, quality-adjusted life years and healthy years equivalents do not consider non-health aspects of benefit (for example, utility from process, such as the care environment in long-term care). Likewise, cost–utility analysis can address allocative efficiency within health services if health-care costs only are included. Once non-health benefits and non-health-care costs are included, a broader framework (cost–benefit analysis) is likely to be required for analysis of allocative efficiency (Gerard and Mooney 1993).

However, cost–utility analysis is valuable when quality of life is an important outcome. In particular, cost–utility analysis is important where there is the possibility that either one alternative evaluated is better than others in terms of effects on survival but worse in terms of quality of life, or one alternative is better than others in terms of some aspects of quality of life but worse in terms of other aspects.

Identification of costs and benefits

The principles of identifying costs and benefits in cost–benefit analysis, cost-effectiveness analysis, and cost–utility analysis are essentially the same for each type, although including a broader range of societal costs is likely to lead one towards a cost–benefit analysis. Identification of relevant costs and benefits involves a listing of all items of resource use and aspects of well being affected by the project, that is, in a comparison of the situations with and without the programme. This ensures that attention is paid to both tangible and intangible costs and benefits. The process of measurement involves the estimation of amounts of resources used and benefits produced by programmes in naturally occurring units. For instance, staffing resources would be measured in terms of time. The final step involves monetary valuation or estimation of quality-adjusted life years/healthy years equivalents where possible.

The principles relating to identification are fivefold: to be aware of the question that is being asked, to keep the principle of opportunity cost in mind when identifying costs and benefits, what this implies in terms of categorizing what is a cost and what is a benefit, how far and how wide the analysis should go, and double counting.

What question is being asked?

As in any research task, it is important to be aware of the exact nature of the question that is being asked before setting out to collect data in detail. Drummond and Mooney (1983) demonstrate this by reference to a particular example. In one study, the answers to a question about the cost of a delivery in a Scottish maternity unit were £540, £510, and £210 (Gray and Steele 1979). The point is that each of the answers is appropriate, depending on the question being asked. To demonstrate, consider the following questions and answers.

- What is the current health service unit cost of a delivery in a Scottish maternity unit? Answer: £540.
- If we wanted to increase the number of deliveries in Scottish specialist maternity units, assuming that the number of beds is increased, what would be the extra health service unit cost per delivery? Answer: £510.
- If we wanted to increase the number of deliveries in Scottish specialist maternity units, assuming that the number of beds is fixed, what would be the extra health service cost per delivery? Answer: £210.

The first cost is simply an average, calculated by dividing the total cost of a unit by the number of deliveries. The other two costs are marginal or incremental, which relate to changes in either the size of maternity units or the number of deliveries that can be undertaken within a unit that remains constant in size. Most often, questions relating to economic evaluation are of the latter type, that is 'Should we do more or less of this?' Obviously, it is important to consider marginal costs and benefits. The concept of marginal cost is discussed in more detail below. The important point to remember at this stage is that when the question posed is, 'What does X cost?', the reply should be 'Why do you want to know?'

Identifying opportunity costs

In keeping with the concept of cost introduced above, items to be identified for inclusion in the cost side of an economic evaluation are any resources that have an opportunity cost as a result of being used in the health-care programmes under consideration. This may seem self-evident, but it is not always followed. Instead, analysts sometimes classify any negative effect of a health-care programme as costs and positive effects as benefits. Alchian (1972) has noted this erroneous tendency.

It is the resources used as inputs to health-care interventions that have opportunity costs. Such costs are often measured in terms of money, but what we are really concerned with is the benefits of an intervention compared with the benefits we could obtain if that money could be used in another (the next best) activity. Sometimes cost is used to mean burden, but the two are not synonymous in economic evaluation. This means that, beyond resource use, adverse effects of health care on people's well being should not be counted as costs.

For example, anxiety is often counted as a cost (even though it is rarely valued). An example of this has been provided by Buhaug *et al.* (1989). However, anxiety *per se* does not have an opportunity cost—it is not a resource that could be used in some other beneficial activity. This is not to say that anxiety should be ignored; it has a negative effect on well being and should be counted on the benefit side. Assuming all other effects on well being to be equivalent, if two programmes differ in terms of anxiety and cost, then if one is less costly and incurs less anxiety, it will be more efficient than the other. If one programme is more costly and incurs less anxiety, then a judgement has to be made as to whether the reduction in anxiety is worth the cost incurred. This issue has been the subject of debate in the *Medical Journal of Australia* (Gerard *et al.* 1990; Stanford 1990). How to measure such effects on well being is part of the subject matter of the section below on the measurement and valuation of benefits.

Practically, all negative effects on well being resulting from a health-care programme should be netted out on the benefit side in a cost–benefit analysis, the effectiveness side in a cost-effectiveness analysis, and the utility side in a cost–utility analysis. (Strictly, given that cost-effectiveness analysis may use only one-dimensional measures of outcome, this cannot be done if positive and negative effects are in different dimensions.) Likewise, cost savings should be handled as negative costs and netted out on the cost side. In effect, they are savings in resource inputs. This is the only way of ensuring that improvements in well being, on one side, are compared with their resource (or opportunity) costs on the other. Costs will then reflect resource use, which is correct, as it is resources that have opportunity costs.

Categorizing costs and benefits

General guidance as to what costs should be included in an economic evaluation is given in Table 2. All the costs listed relate to resources used. The list is not exhaustive. Neither is it appropriate to include the full range of costs listed in Table 2 in every evaluation. Costs included will depend on the objectives and context of the evaluation. Hence, Table 2 serves as a checklist. Listing costs in this way represents an attempt to ensure that items that are difficult to measure receive as much prominence as easily measurable items.

Health-care resource costs are often classified under four main headings: staffing, consumables, overheads, and capital. The most obvious health-care resource cost is that of professional staff time, which usually forms the largest part of the running costs of any programme. Consumable items are those with a limited life which are used by (or on behalf of) the patient, such as drugs and medical/surgical supplies.

Less obvious costs are overheads, which are often referred to as non-patient-related costs. Overhead costs are those shared by more than one programme. The most common examples are in hospitals where administration, management, heating, lighting, laundry, linen,

Table 2 Identification of costs for inclusion in economic evaluations

Health-care resources
Staffing
Consumables
Overheads
Capital
Other related services
Community services
Ambulance services
Voluntary services
Costs incurred by clients and their families
Inputs to treatment
Out-of-pocket expenses
Time lost from work
Costs borne externally to health and welfare services

and cleaning services are provided centrally. The problem is to determine how much of these costs to allocate to the health-care programme being evaluated.

It may be thought that one small programme has no overall effect on such costs, thus presenting an appealing argument for ignoring them. For example, having one less ward is unlikely to change the total financial costs of administration in a large general hospital. However, in the absence of the programme, if people working in centralized departments could have spent their time on some other beneficial activity, there will be an opportunity cost of the programme. This opportunity cost should be valued. Therefore, although the health-care programme sometimes does not add to financial costs, it may still have opportunity costs which should be counted. This demonstrates that accounting costs and economic costs are not the same.

Time-scale is also important here. In the short term, admission of some extra patients may have little impact on staff costs (that is, most costs remain fixed). A fixed cost is a cost that does not vary with activity. In the long run, however, most costs vary with the introduction of the programme. For example, the admission of a large number of patients over time may lead to the employment of extra staff or existing staff working extra hours. What was a fixed cost in one context (that is, the short term) is now a variable cost in another context (that is, the longer term). It is variable opportunity costs (that is, those that change as activity changes) that should be counted in any particular costing context.

Capital items include land and buildings as well as major items of equipment. It may be thought that these items have already been paid for and so should not be included as a cost. This argument is true only when such capital has no alternative beneficial uses (that is, no opportunity cost). If there is an alternative use, there is an opportunity cost which should be valued in some way. Likewise, even if equipment has no obvious and immediate alternative use, perhaps it could be sold and the proceeds used in another beneficial activity. Again, this opportunity cost should be counted. In addition, time-scale is important here. The opportunity costs of many capital items may be fixed in the short run but variable in the longer term.

The cost of other related services includes the staffing, supplies, capital, equipment, and overhead costs associated with community, ambulance, and voluntary services. Clients and families too are often used to provide care (for example, informal care at home) and also incur out-of-pocket expenses, such as transport costs. As described above, the principle of opportunity cost should be invoked when deciding on which of these to cost and to what extent. None of these resources are necessarily 'free' in that their use is likely to incur an opportunity cost. If so, they should be counted in an economic evaluation.

All these costs are usually called the direct costs of a health-care programme (Drummond *et al.* 1997). Indirect costs of a programme are secondary costs related to paid and unpaid productive activities. Productive activities are those arising from participation in the labour force and from housework. Indirect costs arise because treatment could require confinement to hospital or one's home. This can result in a temporary loss to the community from reduced productive activity. The danger in including such costs is that they may have occurred anyway because of the patient's illness, and so the actual treatment itself does not add to opportunity costs. Thus it is the cost of inputs to treatment that are relevant and not the cost of the patient's illness. The benefit of earlier return to work is a welfare (or well-being) gain to society, which, as already established, should be dealt with on the benefit and not the cost side of an analysis.

Benefits for inclusion in economic evaluations are listed in Table 3. This follows directly from the discussion of identifying opportunity costs, including negative as well as positive health effects and negative as well as positive effects in non-health-related well being. The inclusion of production gains is more controversial, not only because of problems with the human capital approach (see below), but also because it is unclear whether including such gains in addition to other benefits (such as quality-adjusted life years, healthy years equivalents, and willingness to pay) involves double counting, that is respondents may have already considered effects on productive activity when giving quality-adjusted life year, healthy years equivalent, or willingness to pay values (Gold *et al.* 1996).

How far and how wide should we go?

There comes a time when we have to evaluate our own activities, that is, evaluate the evaluation. Part of this process involves the decision about how extra pieces of information will affect the evaluation. Some costs may not be included in an evaluation, particularly those that are small and difficult to collect. The decision about which costs to include may also depend on the viewpoint of the policy-makers. Often health-care providers and funders are interested only in costs to the health-care system. In other situations, such as evaluation of community care options, it is obviously relevant to examine costs incurred by informal carers or caregivers, such as family and friends. From an economic perspective, the study would ideally take a societal perspective, including as broad a range of costs as possible—although, as pointed out above, once the study goes beyond considerations of health-care (or certainly, public sector) resources and health benefits, it will usually take the form of a cost–benefit analysis.

Another common problem here is how far in the future to look. This is a particular problem for preventive programmes. For instance, breast cancer screening may detect breast cancer at an early stage and therefore lengthen life compared with no screening; however, people who survive may develop other conditions in the future. Should the future costs and benefits of treating these (unrelated) conditions be included?

One argument for not including such costs and benefits is that the decision about whether or not to treat a future condition may be separate from the one being taken now and should be based on the

Table 3 Identification of benefits for inclusion in economic evaluations

Positive
Health gains (e.g. life years gained)
Non-health-related effects on well being (e.g. information, reassurance)
Production gains
Negative
Health deterioration (e.g. side-effects, anxiety)
Non-health-related effects on well being
Production losses not incurred during treatment

costs and benefits of alternative ways of treating the future disease. If the future costs and benefits of treating heart failure make breast cancer screening less efficient than not screening, should we no longer offer screening? With the hope of living longer, people may say 'Give me screening but don't treat me if I get heart failure in the future', a perfectly rational and reasonable response, and one that would involve an efficient use of resources.

However, analysts should be careful in evaluating preventive programmes, since life tables are often used to estimate survival owing to the lack of ability to follow-up patients over a number of years. These tables permit approximation of survival given certain characteristics, such as age and medical history, and take into account the possibility of such future adverse events as heart failure and the effects (in terms of life years) of treatment for these adverse events. In principle, the costs of treating future conditions should be included in such cases (Meltzer 1997). In practice, however, there are no cost equivalents to data on life tables. This often makes the estimation of future costs difficult. Despite this, discounting (see the section below on the measurement and valuation of costs) of such future costs to present values often reduces their significance dramatically (Bush *et al.* 1973). Therefore, the best approximation may be to use life tables for survival and to ignore future costs of treating other conditions. As a word of caution, the nearer in time such future costs arise and the more directly related they are to the preventive activity evaluated, the more important it becomes to make some attempt to estimate their magnitude (Meltzer 1997).

Double counting

As well as the problems on the benefit side referred to above, one should be careful to avoid counting the same cost twice. For instance, assume that the aim of a hypothetical economic evaluation is to compare the costs of general practitioners/family doctors versus hospital doctors for minor surgery. For each of these, it may seem appropriate to count the fee paid to doctors and cost the amount of time taken to carry out the procedure separately and then add the two together to obtain a total cost. However, to count costs in such a way would constitute an example of double counting, as the fee paid to doctors already accounts for time spent on their activities.

Measurement and valuation of costs

After identification comes measurement. In costing, this involves measuring resource used in naturally occurring units. Thus, from Table 4, staffing costs will often be measured in units of time, whilst other items of resource use are measured in various other units (for example grams of drugs and number of diagnostic tests ordered).

The cost of any item used in a health-care programme is made up of the unit cost of the item multiplied by the quantity used. The stage of measurement is important as it involves explicit registration of quantities of items used by programmes being evaluated. Quantities of items used are often more relevant to readers of a report than are expressions of the product of price and quantity, particularly if the reader is from another country or another region of the same country. This is because price and quantity data may vary within and between countries. Costings in which the price and quantity of each item used are expressed separately as well as after they have been multiplied together are more useful. Both prices and quantities can then be adjusted to suit other situations.

Many elements of valuing health-care costs are straightforward. For instance, we have already said that staffing costs represent the largest component of health-care costs. Referring to Table 4 again, it is usual to value such costs using wage rates or salaries plus other labour costs. However, although such a procedure may seem straightforward, it is not always advisable simply to accept such monetary figures at face value (see the subsection below on unthinking acceptance of market values). Despite this, market prices are generally accepted as first approximations to the unit cost of most other items within consumable, overhead, and capital categories. Community services, ambulance services, and family/patient expenses should be costed in the same way as health service resources. It should be noted that using patients' and families' leisure time also has an opportunity cost. This is difficult to measure. Transport studies have estimated the value of

Table 4 Measurement and valuation of costs

Resource use	How measured	Basis of valuation
Health services		
Staffing	Time (e.g. hours, months, years)	Wage rates/salaries plus other labour costs
Consumables	Units/amounts consumed	Market prices
Overheads	Units/amounts consumed	Wages rates plus other labour costs/market prices (allocated)
Capital	Units/amounts consumed	Market prices/conversion costs/official valuer's estimate
Other related services		
Community services	Units/amounts consumed	Market prices/conversion costs/official valuer's estimate
Ambulance services	Units/amounts consumed	Market prices/conversion costs/official valuer's estimate
Voluntary services	Units/amounts consumed	Imputed values for staff costs
Clients and their families		
Inputs to treatment	Hours	Wages rates plus other labour costs/imputed values
Expenses	Units/amounts consumed	Market prices/actual expenses
Time lost from work	Hours/days/weeks/years	Wages rates plus other labour costs/imputed values

leisure time to be 25 per cent of the local average gross wage rate per hour (Harrison 1974), although a more recent study, specific to health care, has estimated different weights for different types of unpaid activities forgone (Torgerson *et al.* 1994).

In finding a monetary value (never mind how good a value) to place on a resource, the greatest problems arise in areas of voluntary care and time lost from housework. No readily available market values exist for such occupations and therefore in most cases a value is imputed from an analogous market. For instance, the wage rate for auxiliary nursing staff has been used to cost inputs by volunteers into respite services for mentally handicapped adults (Gerard 1990). Sometimes it is difficult to find truly analogous markets. For instance, it is difficult to cost housework because of its irregular and long hours, which make it untypical of other occupations. In many cases, average female labour costs may be a more accurate reflection of the opportunity cost of housework.

Despite appearing relatively straightforward, there are a number of principles and pitfalls to take into account in the measurement and valuation of health-care costs. These are addressed in the following subsections.

Counting costs in a base year

An obvious but important point about valuation of health-care costs is that they should be counted in a base year, that is, adjusted so as to eliminate the effects of inflation. This should be done because 'real' resource use is what is to be measured. If the general inflation rate is running at 5 per cent per annum, in a year's time £105 will purchase the same amount of resources as £100 now. The costs of £100 now and £105 occurring in a year's time are equivalent in real terms (that is, in terms of the real amounts of resources that they can fund), although their 'nominal' monetary values do not show this to be the case. This is a particular problem when costs of alternative programmes are spread in different proportions across different years, as in the hypothetical example in Table 5. Here, surgical and drug therapy are alternative treatments for a hypothetical condition. Assume that each has the same effects but different cost streams, with the inflation rate at 5 per cent per annum. Thus, a cost of £1050 occurring in a year's time is equivalent to £1000 now (that is, £1050/1.05), and £1102.5 occurring in two years' time is also equivalent to £1000 now (£1102.5/1.05^2). Use of unadjusted costs would result in the conclusion that surgery is more efficient (that is, less costly and equally effective) than drug therapy. However, the costs of drug therapy appear to be higher only because of inflation. After adjusting costs for the rate of inflation (by adjusting costs to year 0 prices), the two therapies are shown to be equally efficient.

Discounting

As stated in the previous subsection, not all costs and benefits of health-care programmes occur at the same point in time. The most obvious example is in prevention, where costs are incurred early for the achievement of health benefit later.

The question is, should costs (and benefits) occurring at different points in time be given equal weighting? Most economists would say that they should not. This is because individuals in a society display a tendency to prefer to put off costs to the future rather than pay them now. This 'time preference' arises because of the opportunity cost that would arise by allocating funds to paying costs now rather than later and not having those funds available to pursue some other beneficial activity in the meantime. Thus discounting is simply an opportunity cost concept applied over time. This myopia partly accounts for the existence of interest rates (that is, these rates partly reflect the opportunity cost of not being able to use the resources in an alternative way in the meantime).

Other common reasons to explain discounting are diminishing marginal utility of wealth and health. Diminishing marginal utility of wealth refers to the principle that as societies become wealthier over time, the value of an extra £1 in the future is less than the value of an extra £1 now. Likewise, as health improves over time, the value of an extra unit of health improvement in the future is less than that now. At the margin, money and health are worth less over time and therefore future gains and losses in money and health should be discounted.

In summary, a cost arising in the future impinges less than an equivalent cost arising now. As a result, future costs should be discounted (that is, given less weighting) in order to reflect this. Similarly, people prefer to have benefits sooner rather than later, and so future benefits should also be discounted.

Extending the example given in Table 5 to Table 6, those costs occurring now (that is, in year 0) are not discounted. Those occurring in years 1 and 2 are discounted. In this example, year 1 and year 2 costs have been discounted back to present values by multiplying the original cost in each year (that is, £1000) by a discount factor. Usually, discount factors and present values do not have to be calculated as they are often already available in tables, such as that in the Appendix below which provides a list of discount factors and present values annually from 0 to 50 years at a discount rate of 5 per cent. Some government publications and textbooks contain tables of discount factors at various discount rates (HM Treasury 1982; Drummond *et al.* 1997). The calculation of the discounted costs of our hypothetical drug treatment in years 1 and 2 is explained in the Appendix. From Table 6 it can be seen that, after adjusting for inflation and discounting, drug therapy is now less costly (and therefore more efficient) than surgery.

Table 5 Adjusting costs to base year

Alternatives	**Costs arising (£ per person per annum)**			
	Year 0	**Year 1**	**Year 2**	**Total**
Surgery	3000	–	–	3000
Drug (unadjusted for inflation)	1000	1050	1102.5	3152.5
Drug (adjusted to year 0 prices)	1000	1000	1000	3000

Table 6 Hypothetical example of discounting

Alternatives	Costs arising (£ per person per annum)			
	Year 0	Year 1	Year 2	Total
Surgery	3000			3000
Drug (unadjusted for inflation)	1000	1050	1102.5	3152.5
Drug (adjusted to year 0 prices)	1000	1000	1000	3000
Drug (discounted)	1000	952[a]	907[a]	2859

[a]See Appendix.

In reality, society's exact discount rate is not known. It is difficult to observe a rate. Should it be the rate on long-term government bonds or based on some other interest rates (or average of rates) prevailing in the economy? Drummond *et al.* (1997) recommend a choice of discount rate that is consistent with the following features: it should be consistent with economic theory (between 2 and 10 per cent), include government recommended rates (from 5 to 10 per cent), and be consistent with other published studies and with current practice (from 3 to 10 per cent, but usually 5 per cent). The recommended rates are different in different countries. Given such variation in recommended rates, it is best to test the sensitivity of one's results to variations in the discount rate.

Marginal or incremental costing

Often decisions relating to health-care programmes are not about whether to introduce a programme but, rather, whether to have slightly more or slightly less of a programme. For example, the question may be 'Should we change the screening interval for mammography from 3 years to 1 year?' rather than 'Should we have a mammography screening programme at all?'

It follows that it is important to calculate the marginal rather than the average costs of a programme. The marginal cost is the cost incurred or saved from producing one unit more or one unit less of a programme, whereas average cost represents the total cost of the programme divided by total units produced up to the point at which the calculation is made. There is no a priori reason to assume that both costs will be equivalent unless total costs rise at a constant rate as the programme is expanded. For instance, although it may cost £25 000 per annum on average to care for an elderly person in hospital, it is unlikely that this amount would be saved if one person less were admitted or that £25 000 would be added to total annual costs if one person more were admitted. This is because certain costs, such as heating, lighting, and some staffing costs, remain fixed and will not vary with small changes in patient load.

To illustrate the principles of opportunity cost and the margin within the context of screening, consider the alternatives for a programme aimed at reducing heart disease in a group of 200 000 men aged 40 to 49 years. One alternative is to promote healthy eating in the population in combination with general practitioner screening for high cholesterol levels (serum concentration 6.0 to 7.9 mmol/l), followed by dietary treatment for those in the relevant range; we shall refer to this as the combined approach. An alternative is to use population promotion of healthy eating on its own; we shall refer to this as the population approach.

It is assumed that health gain can be measured adequately in terms of healthy years. Table 7 shows that the total cost of the combined approach has been estimated at about £40 038 000 with a total benefit of 4200 healthy years, at an average cost of £9530 for each healthy year gained. Whether this represents a reasonable investment is open to question. The question is put beyond doubt, however, when the marginal costs are examined. The second row of data shows that the population approach alone would have yielded 3800 healthy years anyway, at a cost of £38 000 or £10 for each healthy year gained. The additional 400 healthy years are gained by the combined approach at an additional cost of £40 million, a marginal (or, more accurately, incremental) cost of £100 000 for each healthy year gained. The marginal cost for each healthy year gained by the combined programme is over 10 times its average cost (thus highlighting the danger of looking at simple averages and hence the importance of marginal analysis). Reorganization of health-care resources to permit the addition of screening and dietary treatment would presumably be judged as not worthwhile. The opportunity cost is too great or, in plainer language, the resources could be better spent on some other health-producing activity, although, strictly, it is policy-makers, not economists, who should make the judgement.

Table 7 Costs and benefits of strategies to reduce cholesterol

Strategy	(1) Total cost (£)	(2) Total benefit (healthy years)	(3) Added cost (£)	(4) Added benefit (healthy years)	(5) Average cost per healthy year ((1)/(2)) (£)	(6) Marginal cost per healthy year ((3)/(4)) (£)
No action	0	0	0	0		
Population	38 000	3800	38 000	3800	10	10
Combined	40 038 000	4200	40 000 000	400	9530	100 000

Source: Kristiansen *et al.* (1991).

Patient-based versus per diem costs

Ideally, when comparing two groups of patients consuming alternative types of health care, one would like to follow through each individual's consumption of health-care and other resources. Each individual's consumption of resources could then be separately valued and a cost per patient calculated.

Valuing opportunity costs is straightforward in some situations (for example, when nursing is done on a one-to-one basis). Such costing is difficult in other situations because of the problem of joint costing. This problem arises when several patients consume a common resource simultaneously and no rule exists as to how to divide the cost between each individual. For example, a nurse may be providing direct care to one patient on a hospital ward whilst supervising several others. In such circumstances, the cost of the nurse's time cannot be allocated other than arbitrarily.

As a last resort, in such cases it is easier to calculate the per diem cost, or cost per bed day, of providing a particular service and multiply this by the length of stay or lengths of use by the patients concerned. For instance, the cost per bed day per annum of a hospital would be calculated by dividing the total cost per annum of running the hospital by the number of bed days per annum used in the hospital.

The problem with using hospital average costs per bed day is that they may not reflect actual resource use by the client group in question if calculated at too general a level. A cost per bed day that is calculated on the basis of that hospital's entire caseload is unlikely to be representative of the cost per bed day for specific conditions; a day in intensive care would be credited with the same cost as a day spent in a postnatal ward. Therefore it is advisable to isolate costs per bed day for the specialties that are of interest. This procedure still requires considerable research effort. For non-hospital or non-institutional settings, such as home nursing or outpatient clinics, similar techniques can be used to calculate a cost per visit. For each study patient, the number of visits would then be multiplied by the cost per visit.

Overhead costs

Overhead costs are costs shared by more than one programme but, unlike joint costs, can be divided amongst programmes in an apparently sensible way. The most common example arises in a hospital environment where services such as administration, management, heating, lighting, laundry, linen, and cleaning services are provided centrally. The problem for the analyst is to determine how much of the costs of these departments to allocate to the programme being evaluated. Whether one decides to allocate such costs at all will depend on the scale of incremental change considered in the analysis (see the subsection above on marginal or incremental costing).

The solution to this problem is to ensure that overhead costs are allocated to programmes within the hospital on a reasonable basis, that is, they should represent differences between overhead opportunity costs with and without the existence of the patients concerned. Examples of simple methods of allocation are listed in Table 8. Sometimes these will suffice, although details of more sophisticated overhead allocation mechanisms can be found elsewhere (Drummond *et al.* 1997).

Costing capital

The costs of capital assets, such as land, buildings, and equipment, usually arise at a single point in time, usually at the inception of the programme being evaluated. Despite this, such capital assets are used over time, and at any point in time an asset may be resold for an amount that will be less than its initial cost and that will decrease as time goes by (except for the special case of property in 'boom' periods, which makes no difference to the general approach to dealing with capital costs). Thus, despite an initial one-off outlay, the opportunity costs of capital assets are spread over time. This is accounted for by spreading the opportunity cost of capital assets over the number of years of their life judged relevant in each particular circumstance.

The most common method of doing this is to calculate an 'equivalent annual cost'. Using this method the initial outlay on a capital asset is converted to an annual sum which, when paid over a number of years (usually an estimated or known life of the asset), would add up to the initial value of the capital asset plus the opportunity cost of resources tied up with the asset (because, for example, they could have earned a certain rate of interest if invested). This principle is best understood by relating it to the principle of a mortgage on a house, whereby the cost of the house plus interest charges are reflected in a series of annual (or monthly) equivalent mortgage repayments. As with discount factors and present values, equivalent annual costs do not have to be separately calculated as they are readily available in tables, such as that in the Appendix to this chapter. This table displays the equivalent annual costs of £1 discounted at a rate of 5 per cent for payback periods of 0 to 50 years. An example of a conversion of a capital cost to an equivalent annual cost is also provided in the Appendix.

One further problem with costing is in determining a cost for some capital items which can then be converted to an equivalent annual cost. This is not a problem for items for which actual (and recent) purchase prices are available. Problems arise with land and buildings that already exist at the start of the programme and may have been paid for many years before the programme commenced. Such items should be costed if their use by the health-care programme prevents their use in some other beneficial activity. The most common ways of

Table 8 Simple methods of allocating overhead costs

Department	Method of allocation
Heating, lighting, cleaning	(Square metres taken up by the programme) divided by (square metres taken up by whole hospital) multiplied by (department cost)
Laundry, linen	(Number of requisitions from the programme) divided by (the number of requisitions from the whole hospital) multiplied by (departmental cost)
Administration, management	(Number of cases admitted to the programme) divided by (number of cases admitted to the hospital) multiplied by (departmental cost)

costing such items are to obtain an estimate of the price that the item would attract if made available on the open market, to obtain an estimated cost of replacing the item, or to obtain an estimate of the rental or lease value of the item.

Unthinking acceptance of market values

Economists are often criticized for using market values as a reflection of true opportunity cost. However, such values are often used only as baselines, and adjustments can be made as required. For instance, the readiness of economists to impute values for the unpaid labour of volunteers and home-makers demonstrates that market values are not always accepted at face value (Donaldson *et al.* 1986; Donaldson and Gregson 1989). Market values would clearly result in the assignment of zero costs to inputs to care by volunteers and home-makers, despite the fact that these resources have opportunity costs.

One should also be wary of values arising for resources for which markets do exist. For instance, owing to rigidities in modern markets the cost of a doctor is greater than the cost of a nurse. Therefore, other things being equal, a doctor-oriented health-care programme will appear to be more costly than a nurse-oriented alternative. However, if a shortage of nurses and a glut of doctors existed, it may be that investment in the nurse-oriented programme would impose a greater opportunity cost than investment in the doctor-oriented programme. This is because the nurse-oriented programme may attract nurses from other health-care specialties, potentially sacrificing benefits to other patients. Alternatively, owing to the glut of doctors, the doctor-oriented programme may involve little opportunity cost to patients in other specialties if doctors can be recruited from the dole queue.

Sometimes it is necessary to attempt to work back to what a market value would have been in the absence of some imposed distortion. For instance, taxes imposed on certain commodities bear no relation to their opportunity cost and often distort the true costs of such commodities. These examples demonstrate that, at first glance, market values should be used only as indicators of cost and that analysts should realize that they may not represent true opportunity costs.

Sensitivity analysis

Inevitably, a costing exercise will be subject to some degree of uncertainty. Where one has not been able to estimate costs accurately, some assumptions may have been made about possible values that such costs could take. Sensitivity analysis is useful in such situations as it involves testing the sensitivity of the results (or conclusions) of an evaluation to variations in variables about which one is uncertain. Readers of a report or article can then judge which assumptions, and thus results, are more appropriate to their local situation. A sensitivity analysis can also indicate where further research is needed to obtain a more accurate estimate of a variable which is critical to the end result.

As an example of sensitivity analysis, Hundley *et al.* (1995) examined the extra cost of introducing a midwives' unit rather than a consultant-led labour ward in intrapartum care. The baseline extra cost of the midwives' unit was estimated to be £40.71, which would add about 10 per cent to the total costs of delivery. However, there were uncertainties over capital costs and midwife staff costs. For the former, it was unclear whether the conversion of rooms for the midwives' unit would have occurred anyway. Deducting this from the baseline results in an extra cost of £36.89. Similarly, some geographical areas would not require the upgrading of midwives which was required in the study location. This would result in an extra cost of £25.01. Combining both these assumptions resulted in an extra cost of £21.19 for the midwives' unit. The midwives' unit would break even only if no extra staff were required as well as no upgrading of existing staff, an unlikely scenario.

The most probable candidates for sensitivity analysis in a costing exercise are production effects, items that have been excluded because of difficulty of collecting data, imputed values, the discount rate, and the lengths of life for capital items. In some cases assumptions about the possible values that a variable can take are arbitrary. On other occasions it may be possible to base a sensitivity analysis on the confidence limits of a statistical estimate of a variable. The effect of such extreme values on results could be tested using upper and lower confidence limits as extreme values. For example, in studying the effects of the use of prophylactic antibiotics on wound infections in Caesarean sections, Mugford *et al.* (1989) estimated costs based on assumptions that the odds of infection would be reduced by either 70 or 50 per cent (the approximate limits of the 95 per cent confidence interval of the odds ratio).

These principles also apply to estimates of benefits. The analyst may be unsure about estimates of life years gained or quality of life. If so, the sensitivity of results to variation in such estimates should be tested. The methods of estimating such benefits will now be examined.

Measurement and valuation of benefits

Associated with each evaluative technique are particular methods for measuring and valuing benefits. Each of these methods is summarized in Table 9. The crudest measures of benefit are those used in cost-effectiveness analysis, where benefits are measured in terms of one-dimensional natural units. In cost–utility analysis, benefits are measured not in physical units, but in terms of healthy years. Healthy years are represented by a single utility-based health index, which incorporates effects on both quantity and quality of life. The most common measure is the quality-adjusted life year, of which there are two distinct forms—generic and condition-specific. As the names suggest, the former are applicable over a large range of interventions and conditions, while the latter are applied to specific conditions. In recent years an alternative to quality-adjusted life years, the healthy years equivalent, has been developed (Mehrez and Gafni 1989). The most comprehensive (but also the most technically difficult) form of benefit measurement occurs in cost–benefit analysis, where benefits are measured in monetary terms. The two principal methods for doing this are the human capital approach and willingness to pay.

Measures used in cost-effectiveness analysis

As outlined above, cost-effectiveness analysis is the simplest form of economic evaluation in health care. In its simplest form, in which costs only are compared, it is necessary to know that the outcomes of alternatives are equivalent or that the less costly alternative is no less beneficial. In such situations it does not matter if outcomes are one-dimensional or multidimensional. For example, in a study comparing different methods of providing long-term care for elderly

Table 9 Identification and measurement of benefits in economic evaluation

Evaluative technique	Benefits	Unit of measurement
Cost-effectiveness analysis	Quantity of life or quality of life	Life years gained
		Natural units: pain reduction; cases detected; activities of daily living; cholesterol reduction
Cost–utility analysis	Quantity and quality of life	Healthy years: quality-adjusted life years (generic or condition-specific); healthy years equivalents
Cost–benefit analysis	Quantity and quality of life (possibly including some non-health aspects)	Money: human capital; willingness to pay

people, no differences in survival and activities of daily living were found between the alternatives (Bond *et al.* 1989). In view of this, a subsequent study focusing on cost-effectiveness was able to concentrate on cost differences only (Donaldson and Bond 1991).

However, in situations in which cost-effectiveness ratios are used, the outcome (or benefit) is always one-dimensional. The appropriate measure depends upon the programme being compared. For programmes whose major effect is to extend life, life years gained would generally be used. In contrast, if the major effect of the programmes is to improve quality of life rather than quantity of life, then some other measure would be more appropriate. For example, in comparing programmes for the prevention of coronary heart disease, unit reductions in serum cholesterol might be an appropriate measure. Similarly, if two antenatal screening programmes are being compared, cases detected might be chosen. Concentration on such narrow measures of benefit, however, may mean that other important benefits are overlooked. Consider an example in which dialysis is compared with transplantation for the treatment of chronic renal failure. In general, quality of life following a successful transplant will be higher than quality of life associated with dialysis (Klarman *et al.* 1968; Doessel 1978). However, if life years gained is chosen as the measure of outcome, these effects on quality of life cannot be incorporated explicitly into the evaluation.

Generic quality-adjusted life years

Generic quality-adjusted life years are typically derived from multi-attribute utility scales, which are instruments for estimating health state values. The five most widely used multi-attribute utility scales are the quality of well being scale (Kaplan *et al.* 1976), Rosser's disability/distress classification (Rosser and Kind 1978), the 15-dimensional measure of health-related quality of life (Sintonen and Pekurinen 1993), the health utility index versions 1, 2, and 3 (Torrance *et al.* 1995), and the Euroqol EQ-5D (Euroqol Group 1990). Of these, perhaps the most widely used is the EQ-5D which was developed by a multidisciplinary group of researchers in five different countries (Euroqol Group 1990). The five dimensions of the EQ-5D are mobility, self-care, usual activities, pain/discomfort, and anxiety/depression. Each dimension has three levels, thus enabling the EQ-5D to define 243 different health states (see Table 10 for the dimensions and their levels). The inclusion of two extra health states, unconscious and dead, means that there are 245 possible health state descriptions.

The EQ-5D is designed to be administered in the form of a self-completed questionnaire. Subjects are asked to define their own health state in terms of the five dimensions and their levels and then asked to mark on a visual analogue scale how good or bad they think their current health is. The visual analogue scale is presented as a vertical line on a page divided into 100 equal intervals and with the endpoints marked 'worst imaginable health state' and 'best imaginable health state'. The visual analogue scale values are interpreted as the health state weights.

A number of commentators have argued that visual analogue scale values are a poor indicator of individuals' strength of preference (Loomes and McKenzie 1989; Nord 1991). In view of this criticism the developers of the Euroqol employed the time trade-off technique (see next subsection) to generate a tariff of quality of life weights for each EQ-5D health state (Dolan 1997). The tariff was based on health state values elicited in a large-scale survey undertaken in the United Kingdom by the Measurement and Valuation of Health Group at the University of York (Measurement and Valuation of Health Group

Table 10 Dimensions of the Euroqol EQ-5D

Mobility
I have no problems in walking about
I have some problems in walking about
I am confined to bed
Self-care
I have no problems with self-care
I have some problems washing or dressing myself
I am unable to wash or dress myself
Usual activities (e.g. work, study, housework, family or leisure activities)
I have no problems with performing my usual activities
I have some problems with performing my usual activities
I am unable to perform my usual activities
Pain/discomfort
I have no pain or discomfort
I have moderate pain or discomfort
I have extreme pain or discomfort
Anxiety/depression
I am not anxious or depressed
I am moderately anxious or depressed
I am extremely anxious or depressed

1994). The tariff allows each of the EQ-5D health states (identifiable by a unique five-digit number corresponding to the levels for each of the five dimensions) to be converted into a score which can be used as the quality adjustment weight in the calculation of quality-adjusted life years. The best health state (that is, 11111) is assigned a value of 1.0 and death is assigned a value of 0. The remaining health states are assigned positive or negative scores depending upon whether they are valued as being better or worse than death respectively. It should be noted that different tariffs are available for different socio-economic groups.

In order to illustrate the calculation of quality-adjusted life years using an EQ-5D tariff, consider the following simple example of an individual with varicose veins facing two alternative treatments—compression hosiery or sclerotherapy—and whose remaining life expectancy is 10 years (note that neither treatment affects life expectancy). Table 11 presents the EQ-5D health states that the individual can expect to experience for the rest of their life under each treatment regimen. For compression hosiery, the total expected quality-adjusted life years is 5.65, while sclerotherapy is expected to yield 6.54 quality-adjusted life years. The expected quality-adjusted life year gain from sclerotherapy compared with compression hosiery is simply 6.54 – 5.65 = 0.89 quality-adjusted life years. If the cost of sclerotherapy over and above the cost of compression hosiery is, for instance, £2000, then the cost per quality-adjusted life year gained from sclerotherapy is £2000/0.89 = £2247. It should be noted that the above example does not include any adjustment for the differential timing of the benefits from each treatment. If account is to be taken of this then each of the tariff weights should be adjusted by an appropriate discount factor (see section on discounting above).

The Euroqol EQ-5D has been criticized for being too simplistic and insensitive to changes in health status (Gafni and Birch 1993). However, a recent review of the literature pertaining to the five main multi-attribute utility scales concluded that on the basis of a number of factors, such as practicality, reliability, and various dimensions of validity, the EQ-5D and the health utility index should be the scales of choice (Brazier *et al.* 1999).

Condition-specific quality-adjusted life years and healthy years equivalents

The main difference between condition-specific and generic quality-adjusted life years lies in the way in which health states are described to subjects. With condition-specific quality-adjusted life years the health-state descriptions focus on the characteristics of the condition being evaluated. This is in contrast with generic quality-adjusted life years where the health-state descriptions are more general.

There are two main methods of generating condition-specific quality-adjusted life years: standard gamble and time trade-off. The standard gamble is based directly on the axioms of standard utility theory; it is the classic method of measuring preferences under uncertainty. The technique can be used to measure health-state preferences for chronic and temporary health states. The discussion here focuses on the use of the technique to calculate quality-adjusted life years for a chronic health state preferred to death. For details of how the standard gamble can be applied to temporary health states and health states not preferred to death see, for example, Froberg and Kane (1989) or Torrance (1986).

An example of the standard gamble framework for a chronic health state preferred to death is shown in Fig. 2. To measure preferences for health state i, subjects are asked to choose between two alternatives. One offers the certain outcome of remaining in the chronic health state for the rest of one's life, whilst the other is a gamble representing a treatment with two possible outcomes. These outcomes are (a) return to full health for the rest of one's life (with an associated probability P of occurring), and (b) immediate death (which has a probability of occurrence of $1 - P$). The probability P of a successful outcome is varied by an iterative process until the subject is indifferent (that is, cannot choose) between the gamble and the certainty. The probability

Table 11 Calculation of quality-adjusted life years

Years of remaining life	Compression hosiery		Sclerotherapy	
	EQ-5D health state	Tariff (quality of life) score	EQ-5D health state	Tariff (quality of life) score
1	12111	0.82	12111	0.82
2	12111	0.82	12111	0.82
3	22111	0.75	12111	0.82
4	22111	0.75	12111	0.82
5	22211	0.71	12121	0.69
6	22221	0.59	12121	0.69
7	22221	0.59	22121	0.69
8	22222	0.52	22221	0.59
9	22223	0.08	22222	0.52
10	22323	0.02	22223	0.08
11	Dead	0.00	Dead	0.00
Total		5.65		6.54

P^* at which the subject is indifferent is used to calculate the utility value of the health state as follows. The outcomes 'return to full health' and 'death' are assigned utility values of unity and zero respectively. At the indifference probability P, the value (measured in terms of expected utility) of the two alternatives is equal, yielding the following simple equation:

$$U\text{ (state } i) = P^*U \text{ (full health)} + (1 - P^*)\, U \text{ (death)}.$$

Because the utility from full health equals 1.0 and the utility from death equals 0.0, this equation can be reduced to

$$U\text{ (state } i) = P^*.$$

Therefore, for the case of a chronic health state preferred to death, the utility of the health state is simply P (the indifference probability). The utility of the health state can then be used to calculate the number of quality-adjusted life years from the treatment in a similar way to that described for generic quality-adjusted life years.

Time trade-off was developed by Torrance *et al.* (1972) as a substitute for the standard gamble technique. The intention was to develop a technique specifically for use in health care, which gave the same (or similar) values as the standard gamble but which was easier for subjects to understand. Two important differences between time trade-off and the standard gamble should be noted. Firstly, time trade-off does not have an axiomatic foundation; secondly, subjects are asked to choose between two certain alternatives rather than between a certain outcome and a gamble. Like the standard gamble, time trade-off can be used to elicit health-state preferences for chronic and temporary health states that may or may not be preferred to death. An example of a time trade-off framework for a chronic health state preferred to death is shown in Fig. 3. Preferences for health state i are established by eliciting from subjects the number of years in full health (Z years) that is equivalent to spending the rest of their life (T years) in the chronic health state. The value Z^* at which the subject is indifferent between the two alternatives is used to calculate the value of the health state as follows. Full health is assigned a value of unity and death a value of zero. It is assumed that individuals have a value function of the form $V = h_1T$, where h is the preference value for health state i ($0 < h_1, < 1$) and T is remaining years of life.

A value function assigns a real number to each possible outcome in a choice problem under certainty. Utility functions are appropriate for uncertain choices.

At Z^*, the value functions of the two alternatives are equal, yielding the following equation:

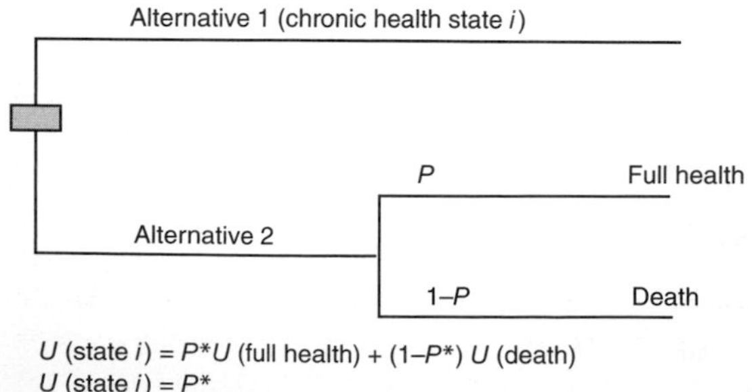

Fig. 2 Standard gamble for a chronic health state preferred to death.

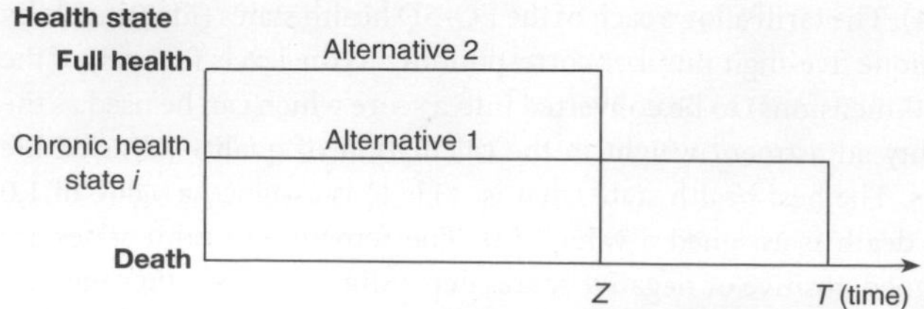

Fig. 3 Time trade-off for a chronic health state preferred to death.

$$V \text{ (alternative 1)} = V \text{ (alternative 2)}, h_1T = 1.0 \times Z^*.$$

Therefore, the preference value for the chronic health state i is $h_1 = Z^*/T$. The value of the health state can be used to calculate the number of quality-adjusted life years from the treatment in the same way as described above for generic quality-adjusted life years.

Although the authors have, for purposes of exposition, shown how values for chronic health states are derived, there are examples in the literature, using the same basic principles, of the derivation of values for temporary health states (Johnston *et al.* 1998).

In recent years an alternative to quality-adjusted life years has been developed—the healthy years equivalent (Mehrez and Gafni 1989). Like quality-adjusted life years, healthy years equivalents combine quantity and quality of life into a single measure. The definition of a healthy years equivalent for a chronic health state is as follows (for a more general definition see Mehrez and Gafni (1989)). Let Q represent the chronic health state of an individual and T the individual's remaining years of life. Let $U(Q, T)$ be the utility function of the individual, which describes the utility of being in health state Q for T years followed immediately by death. Let Q^* represent full health and H^* the healthy years equivalent of (Q, T). The problem is defined as follows: find H^*' such that $U(Q^*, H^*) = U(Q, T)$. The main difference between quality-adjusted life years and healthy years equivalents is that, in calculating the former, the utility weight of a health state is multiplied by the time spent in the health state. The utility weight is based on individual preferences but the duration is not. The algorithm for calculating healthy years equivalents allows individuals to express their preferences for both the health state and the duration.

There is controversy within health economics as to the added value of healthy years equivalents over quality-adjusted life years and the reader is referred to articles by the critics (Buckingham 1993; Culyer and Wagstaff 1993; Johannesson *et al.* 1993; Loomes 1995) and the advocates (Gafni *et al.* 1993; Mehrez and Gafni 1993) of healthy years equivalents.

Monetary measures

In recent years the most common method of measuring health-care benefits in cost–benefit analysis has been willingness to pay. However, the application of willingness to pay to health care is a relatively recent phenomenon, and for many years the dominant measurement technique was the human capital method.

Under the human capital approach, health improvements are valued in terms of future productive worth to society from individuals being able to return to (paid and unpaid) work following the health improvement. Productive worth tends to be proxied by future earnings potential. This immediately raises questions about how to deal with women, elderly people, and the unemployed (Avorn 1984). Furthermore, if a truly societal perspective is to be taken in an economic evaluation, it may be that, in economies with substantial amounts of unemployment, there is little opportunity cost in losing a worker due to premature retirement or death. As many workers can be replaced, preventing their loss may add little to overall productivity. This has led to controversy over whether or not to include only production losses incurred during the period of replacing a worker in economic evaluations (Koopmanschap *et al.* 1995; Johannesson and Karlsson 1997).

It is generally acknowledged that willingness to pay is a more theoretically correct measure of benefit in that it captures in one measure notions of human capital as well as other benefits of health care. The principle of willingness to pay is very simple—the utility that an individual gains from something is valued by the maximum amount that he or she would be willing to pay for that something. The technique of willingness to pay is often criticized for attempting to assign a monetary value to things that are considered by many to be incommensurate with monetary valuation (for example, the environment, human life, and so on). However, it has to be remembered that such valuations are being made anyway. These valuations arise from the implicit judgements of decision-makers. What is important is not the unit of value *per se*, but rather the notion of sacrifice embodied in the technique. In economics, something only has value if an individual is prepared to sacrifice something in order to acquire it. In valuing a health-care programme, it is difficult to ask respondents what services they would give up to have more of that programme. It is easier to ask individuals to state the maximum amount that they would be willing to pay for more of the programme and for some possible alternative uses of those resources. Thus it is largely for convenience of comparison that money is the chosen numeraire.

One advantage of willingness to pay over other measures of benefit discussed so far is that it provides the opportunity for individuals to value other potential benefits of health care beyond just health gain. The value of a health-care intervention can be measured by the maximum amount individuals are prepared to pay for the intervention. Exactly how much individuals are willing to pay will partly depend on the perceived benefits to them of the intervention. One of the assumptions of quality-adjusted life years and healthy years equivalents is that the only benefit from health care is improvement in health-related quality of life. However, there is evidence that this is not always the case (Berwick and Weinstein 1985; Mooney and Lange 1993; Donaldson and Shackley 1997). Other possible sources of benefit might include the provision of information (for example, from screening), dignity (for example, in long-term care), and the process of care (for example, invasive versus non-invasive interventions).

Depending upon the context of the evaluation, there are a number of different ways in which individuals can be asked to imagine they have to pay. These include out-of-pocket payments (Miedzybrodzka *et al.* 1994), one-off extra taxation payments (Olsen and Donaldson 1998), and payments for insurance (Gafni 1991).

There are also a number of different ways of asking willingness to pay questions. These include payment card questions in which subjects are presented with a series of prompts from which to select a value, open-ended questions in which respondents are asked to state their maximum willingness to pay without prompting, and closed-ended questions in which each respondent is presented with a willingness to pay value and asked to indicate whether or not they would be prepared to pay that value. Each method has its advantages and disadvantages, and there is no overall consensus as to which is the best method (Johannesson and Jonsson 1991).

The willingness to pay technique is not without its problems. A frequent criticism is that it is inevitably a function of ability to pay, which, it is argued, could have implications for equity. There are, however, ways of dealing with this (Donaldson 1999). This is similar to the weighting of quality-adjusted life years to reflect concerns other than health gain, such as severity of illness (Nord *et al.* 1999).

The use of cost per quality-adjusted life year data in health-care decision-making

So far, this chapter has focused on the measurement and valuation of benefits *per se*. However, it is also important to consider how the different measures of benefit can be used in practice to aid decision-making. In particular, it is useful to discuss the practical applications of cost per quality-adjusted life year and willingness to pay data.

Cost per quality-adjusted life year ratios have two principal applications. The first is to compare alternative interventions for the same condition. Here, the intervention with the lowest cost per quality-adjusted life year ratio is the most technically efficient. This is simply an extension of cost-effectiveness analysis.

The second (and more problematic) use of cost per quality-adjusted life year ratios is to help judge relative priorities across different programmes in health care. Cost per quality-adjusted life year ratios can be calculated for a wide variety of disparate interventions, ranging from general practice advice to give up smoking, chiropody, and so on, to renal dialysis and heart transplantation. Because the measure of outcome is the same for all interventions, across programme comparisons can be made. It is possible to construct cost per quality-adjusted life year league tables in which interventions are ranked in terms of increasing cost per quality-adjusted life year ratios, that is, decreasing relative efficiency. Indeed, such an exercise has been carried out in the state of Oregon in the United States, although not without problems (Dixon and Welch 1991; Tengs 1996). Quality-adjusted life year league tables have been criticized on a number of grounds, and great care should be taken in their construction and interpretation (Gerard and Mooney 1993; Birch and Gafni 1994). Among the many potential problems of quality-adjusted life year league tables, the following are particularly worthy of note. The most serious problem is that each item in the league table has a different comparator. The cost per quality-adjusted life year gained of programme A may have been produced by comparing programme A with programme B. However, if B is inefficient to begin with, A may also be inefficient.

The use of ratios in league tables also hides the fact that programmes of various sizes are being compared. Thus a small programme C, which is further down the table, could be combined with a programme D, which is higher up, to produce more quality-adjusted life years than a larger programme E in the middle.

With respect to transferability of cost per quality-adjusted life year league tables across locations, on the cost side, different locations will tend to have different cost structures and therefore different marginal costs of expansion and contraction. On the benefit side, the capacity of individuals in one location to benefit from a particular intervention will tend to be different from that of individuals in another location, thus leading to different levels of quality-adjusted life years gained. Because of this potential for variations at the margin between locations, it is likely that a cost per quality-adjusted life year league table used in one location will not be applicable to other locations. Ideally, therefore, if (and it is a big 'if') cost per quality-adjusted life year league tables are to be used for priority setting, they should be locally based. The correct application of a crude locally based league table is preferable to the misapplication of a more sophisticated league table from another location.

Using willingness to pay data in health-care decision-making

A recent example of using willingness to pay to aid priority setting was an evaluation of public sector health-care programmes in northern Norway (Olsen and Donaldson 1998). Members of the public were asked their willingness to pay in extra taxation for each of the following: the introduction of a helicopter ambulance service to serve remote communities, an expansion in the number of heart operations performed, and an expansion in the number of hip operations performed. Subjects were presented with detailed descriptions of the programmes and were told that only one could be implemented. They were also asked to state the reasons for their willingness to pay responses.

The use of willingness to pay is not restricted to issues of allocative efficiency—it can also be used to address narrower questions. A recent example of this is the study by Donaldson *et al.* (1998) in which the relative benefits of two alternative locations for delivery of a baby were evaluated. Using the results from a recently completed randomized trial (Hundley *et al.* 1994), pregnant women were given descriptions of care in midwife-managed units and in traditional labour wards. They were asked for their preference for one over the other and then were asked about their maximum willingness to pay to have their preferred rather than their less preferred option. The results displayed a clear preference for the midwife-managed unit. Despite the usefulness of such a result, there are limitations as to how these data can be used. The midwife-managed unit was also more costly than the labour ward (Hundley *et al.* 1995). Thus the more beneficial new form of care (the midwife unit) would also be more costly. This may imply the allocation of more resources to maternity care in order to achieve more benefit.

However, those resources would have to come from some other (presumably beneficial) use. Ideally, values would also be required for this alternative use (as in the case of the northern Norway study described above). In studies which find that total willingness to pay elicited from users of a programme is greater than the programme cost, it may be tempting to conclude that such a programme is worthwhile. However, the opportunity cost context is one where resources for such a programme will have to come from some other use. The decision to invest in the programme is really a community decision. To reiterate, when using willingness to pay values to aid priority setting (particularly in a publicly financed health-care system), the relative values of members of the community are of importance (see the northern Norway example above), and not the absolute values of users. The willingness to pay values of users indicate the strength of preference of the users for the services being evaluated and are still useful in that context. For instance, such values could indicate that the preferences of a minority group are particularly strong. If this strength of preference is not sufficient to outweigh that of the majority, such values may still indicate to the decision-maker that providing both types of care evaluated is the fairest option. However, it should be remembered that providing such choice may come at a substantial cost.

Programme budgeting and marginal analysis

Health-care decision-makers cannot conduct full-scale economic evaluations for every decision which they have to make. However, they are still faced with situations of scarcity of resources, whereby they do not have enough resources to meet all of the claims of those resources. The question then is whether the principles outlined above can at least be used as a framework for a more pragmatic evaluatory process to support health-care priority setting in 'day-to-day' contexts. One such framework is programme budgeting and marginal analysis. This economic approach to needs assessment has been used in several care settings in the United Kingdom, Australia, New Zealand, and Canada (Mooney 1984; Donaldson and Farrar 1993; Cohen 1994; Ruta *et al.* 1996; Peacock and Edwards 1997; Scott *et al.* 1998; Mitton *et al.* 1999).

The overall aim of programme budgeting and marginal analysis is to provide assistance to health authority managers in directing resources in a manner in which the impact of health care on the health needs of the local population is maximized (Donaldson and Mooney 1991). In principle, programme budgeting and marginal analysis allows this to happen by addressing both technical and allocative efficiency (Mooney *et al.* 1994). Furthermore, by permitting the analysis of who receives resources, programme budgeting and marginal analysis also allows issues of equity to be addressed (Mooney *et al.* 1986; Viney *et al.* 1995). Its starting point is to examine how resources are currently spent before focusing on marginal health gains and costs of changes in that spend, through comparison within or across programmes of care (Donaldson and Farrar 1993).

The first component of programme budgeting and marginal analysis, programme budgeting, is a means for describing the pattern of spending within health authorities and its distribution between groups in the population (Gold *et al.* 1997), with emphasis not on inputs and activities, but rather on how these inputs and activities contribute to improving the health status of individuals (Pole 1974; Wiseman *et al.* 1998). A five-step approach for conducting programme budgeting and marginal analysis has been reported (Donaldson *et al.* 1995), and can be summarized as in Table 12.

The first step is to identify the programme of interest and determine the total resources available for the programme. The programme budget can classify expenditure by programme (that is, disease group), by service inputs grouped by sector of care (that is, primary care, acute care), or by other means such as population demographics (Pole 1974; Mooney 1977; Miller *et al.* 1997). The next step is to describe the current pattern of activity and spending for the programmes and subprogrammes, using data available through an information system or by collecting data prospectively. The programme budget allows for comparison of the allocation of resources over time (Mooney *et al.* 1986) or with the allocation of resources in other regions (Craig *et al.* 1995; Miller *et al.* 1997), and also can indicate particular areas for marginal analysis by making the resource

Table 12 Five-step approach to a budgeting and marginal analysis programme

1. What is the total amount of resources available?
2. How are these resources currently spent (and how does this pattern of spending fit with activity and objectives)?
3. What is our 'wish list' in terms of services which are the main candidates for receiving more resources or for being introduced (and what are the costs and benefits of these expansions/introductions)?

4a. Can any services which are currently in receipt of funding be provided to the same level of effectiveness but with less resources (thus becoming more technically efficient), so allowing some of the items on the wish list to be implemented?

4b. If improvements in technical efficiency are not possible, are there any services which should receive less resources because they provide only a small amount of effectiveness per £ spent relative to something on the wish list (thus minimizing opportunity costs)?

5. Evaluation of the impact of changes and consideration of potential trade-offs with equity

allocation process more explicit (Cohen 1995; Twaddle and Walker 1995).

Following this, decisions can be made as to which services are candidates for expansion and which services are candidates for reduction. At this third step, marginal analysis begins, and planning groups are often convened. This panel might consist of doctors, other clinical professionals, health authority managers, patients, and other interest groups (Cohen 1995). In the fourth step, scenarios which involve increases and reductions in spending can be presented to the panel, who can then make priority lists of which services should be expanded or reduced. The key at this point is in focusing on marginal benefits per unit of resource spent, thus alleviating the need to assess total needs and overall benefits. Proposed expansions in services can be funded in one of two ways:

- by providing some services at the same level of effectiveness, but at less cost (that is, technical efficiency improvements)

or, if this cannot be done,

- by taking resources from some areas of effective care, only if, at the margin, they provide less effectiveness per unit of resource spent than the proposed expansion (that is, improving allocative efficiency).

Thus, at this stage, the proposed options (expansions and contractions) have to be evaluated. Local data can be supplemented with evidence on effectiveness and cost-effectiveness from the literature (Donaldson and Farrar 1993; Cohen 1995). These results can also be used in conjunction with other means, such as needs assessments, review of local and national policy, other consumer/public views, and other health professional views, to determine priorities (Cohen 1995; Craig *et al.* 1995; Miller *et al.* 1995; Ruta *et al.* 1996). Finally, health authority decision-makers have to decide whether resource shifts will actually follow the recommendations of the planning group, and specifically address whether any trade-off with equity results from the potential increases in efficiency (Mooney *et al.* 1993).

Such planning mechanisms can be used either within programmes of care (for example, maternity care) or across programmes of care. The former is known as 'micro programme budgeting and marginal analysis' while the latter is known as 'macro programme budgeting and marginal analysis'. The technique has also been applied at the level of primary care, where groups of general practitioners are given budgetary responsibility for organizing and purchasing primary, secondary, and tertiary services for their registered population (Scott *et al.* 1998). Such activity could be known as 'meso programme budgeting and marginal analysis'.

The major challenge with such a framework is that it is data hungry. While costing data may be available at the local level, it is more difficult to obtain data on the benefits of alternatives of care. Programme budgeting and marginal analysis deals with this real problem by obtaining judgements from expert panels, and supplementing this information with available evidence from the literature. Ultimately, no matter how few data exist, decisions still have to be made. As such, this pragmatic approach to programme budgeting and marginal analysis has been suggested (Scott *et al.* 1999), using a combination of expert opinion and the literature on the benefit side, and locally available data with estimations where required, supplemented by economic evaluations from the literature, on the cost side. Overall, programme budgeting and marginal analysis can serve to inform complex decisions by highlighting, in an explicit manner, the relationship between the costs and benefits of a particular action. International experience to date suggests that this economic pragmatic approach can be an important part of the priority-setting process.

Micro-economic analysis of public health policy: more theory and some examples

Activity in the use of economics in assessing behavioural changes as a result of public health and health-promotion policies is growing. Before illustrating this with examples from the literature, it is important to outline, in more detail, the 'canonical model of the consumer', a cornerstone of micro-economic analysis.

A model of consumer behaviour

This model simply extends the notion of opportunity cost, introduced above. It may appear to be quite technical to non-economists, but it is useful in analysing the behavioural responses of individuals to public health and health promotion interventions. The theory is introduced here in the context of utilization of dental care.

Assume individual A has Y dollars to spend on visits to the dentist, V, and all other goods, G, measured in dollars. The cost of purchasing other goods and the cost of dental visits cannot then exceed Y, so we can express the set of options available to the individual as $Y \geqslant pV + G$, where p is the price of a visit to the dentist. This formula is called a budget constraint; it gives the choices available as a function of the prices and incomes of the decision-maker. If the person is rational in the earlier economic sense, we also know their behaviour can be analysed as prices and incomes change by examining the properties of the constrained optimization programme:

$\max_{D,\ G} U(D, G)$

subject to

$pD + G \geqslant Y,$

where $U(\ldots)$ is the utility function representing the individual's tastes over dentist visits and other goods.

Figure 4 displays a graphical representation of the person's utility maximization problem. The budget constraint in (G, V) space is the straight line in the diagram. Where it meets the V axis, the consumer is spending all of his or her money on dental visits, and, where it meets the G axis, all money is spent on other goods. Moving away from the origin, the axes represent increasing amounts of visits and other goods. Points above the budget constraint cost more than Y, points below the constraint cost less than Y, and points on the constraint cost exactly Y. The most preferred combination of visits and other goods, V^* and G^* respectively, can be found by finding the (V, G) pair which is both affordable (does not cost more than Y) and associated with the highest level of utility, denoted by the 'indifference curves' U in Fig. 4. The indifference curve is this shape because it is assumed that, as more and more dental visits are consumed, they are worth less and less to the consumer, and therefore he or she would give up less of other goods for each increment in dental visits. This is known as diminishing marginal utility. Within (G, V) space there is an infinite number of indifference curves. These curves are not allowed to cross each other, otherwise the analysis would not make any sense.

Those to the northeast of U would represent higher levels of utility whilst those to the southwest would represent lower levels of utility. The preferred point is denoted E in Fig. 4; any other point is either not affordable or puts the consumer on a lower level curve, which would be a less preferred combination.

The solutions to this problem reveal the relationship between other goods and dental visits as functions of the parameters of price and income. The function giving dental visits as a function of price, conditional on income, $D(p, Y)$, is called the demand curve for dental visits. Notice that the opportunity cost of one more dental visit is p units of other goods, and that the cost of one more unit of other goods is $1/p$ units of dental visits. For example, if the price of a dental visit is £50, then one visit costs £50 worth of other goods, and £1 spent on other goods has an opportunity cost of 1/50 of a dental visit.

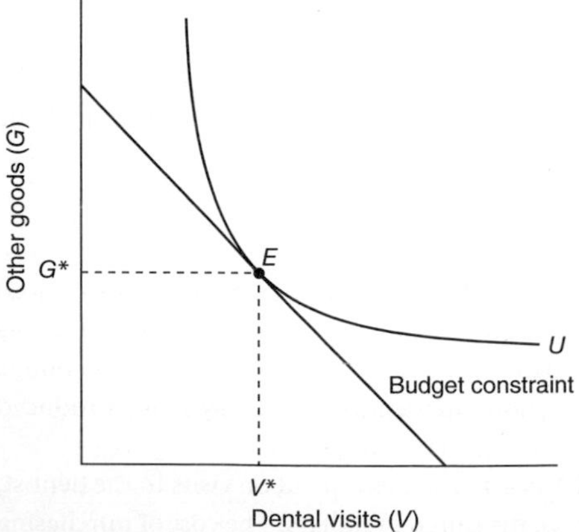

Fig. 4 Indifference curves and budget constraints.

Generally, it is possible to determine the opportunity cost of a marginal change in one of the choice variables by computing the derivative of the constraint at the current choice; since the constraint here is linear, opportunity costs are the same regardless of where on the budget constraint they are calculated.

More generally, constraints need not be financial, and the constraint need not be linear. Consider a simple model of social choice over how much health care to provide. Suppose society can allocate its resources to produce either health care, HC, or food, F. The results generalize easily to an arbitrary number of goods. Producing more health care comes at the cost of producing less food, and as more and more health care is produced each successive unit treats fewer and fewer serious cases, since people will tend to 'pick the lowest hanging apples first' (that is, recalling the notion of diminishing marginal utility, it is assumed that the patients who need treatment the most will get it first). Hence, the opportunity cost of producing an extra unit of health care increases as we produce more and more health care, so the constraint can only be written as some non-linear function. Imagine that social preferences can be treated like individual preferences and can be summarized by a utility function $U(HC, F)$, it is possible to compute the socially preferred production of health care and food related to a given constraint. Although Arrow's famous Impossibility Theorem implies such an exercise, it is at best dubious. (For a detailed explanation see Mas-Colell *et al.* (1995)).

It would then be possible to examine how changes in the economy which move the constraint about would affect optimal provision of health care; for instance, a technological improvement might make more of both food and health care available.

Grossman's model

The analytical underpinnings of many models in health economics are based on Grossman's (1972*a*,*b*) research, which in turn extended earlier work on the allocation of time within households by Becker (1965). The application of this model in empirical studies has paralleled similar efforts in epidemiology. Grossman's model combines the simple analyses of consumers and of firms discussed above: individuals are assumed to have preferences over their own state of health and other desired outcomes (such as, for instance, spending time with their children or reading books). Grossman places individuals with such preferences in a dynamic world in which they can sell their time in labour markets, use both time and money to 'produce' both health and other outcomes with various combinations of time and money, and are subject to the biological process of ageing. Notice that individuals are explicitly assumed to be willing to trade off their health status for other goals; the question is not whether they do so, but how changes in incentives change how much health they trade off for other life goals.

The model yields a rich set of interesting results. In Grossman's framework, for instance, time of death is determined by the individual's choices; a given individual who chooses to invest more time and money to keep themselves healthy will tend to live longer, and the choice to invest more in health is itself determined by the person's preferences and resources available. The model predicts that rising labour market incomes will yield greater health investment and thus lower morbidity and mortality at any age. This view, that it is an individual's own behaviour that leads to observed health outcomes, and that that behaviour is affected by factors such as labour market opportunities, meshes with a large body of empirical research documenting the importance of 'lifestyle' and income as predictors of health and the perhaps surprisingly small impacts of changes in the provision of health care itself (McKeown 1976; Newhouse and Friedlander 1980; Brook *et al.* 1983; Berger and Leigh 1988). Grossman's model also suggests that health, education, labour market outcomes, and the health-care system form a system with a variety of interacting causal effects, and thus that analysis of how to increase the efficacy of the health-care system or other interventions aimed to increase health must consider the complex interactions jointly to determine outcomes.

Demand for safety and the curious effects of airbags

One theme stressed in the discussion above is the importance of considering how policy changes will tend to change the incentives individuals face and therefore individuals' behaviour. Consider the effects of a policy which forces consumers to purchase cars in which they are less likely to be seriously harmed or killed in the event of an accident. Such systems include mandatory passive restraint systems (such as airbags), collapsible steering columns, or side-impact reinforcements. Common sense suggests that such policies will necessarily reduce traffic fatalities, but the economics of the situation suggest that we must consider, in addition to the technical and engineering aspects of the situation, how behaviour will change in order to estimate how much fatalities can be expected to be reduced. Common sense may also be mistaken; it is possible that legislation of this sort may actually increase fatalities.

An individual can choose to drive slowly or at speed, to drive with much attention or carelessly, to talk on a mobile phone while driving or not, to drive while under the influence of alcohol or not, and many other choices which affect the likelihood of a collision. For simplicity, all of these choices can be grouped together into one category called 'intensity', with higher values of intensity representing actions tending to produce greater injury probabilities. Also assume that, if the probability of an accident is constant, people would prefer more intensity; they would rather get where they are going sooner and with less time and effort exerted to avoid accidents.

It is now possible to cast the situation as an economic model. Individuals can be considered to have preferences over our index 'intensity' and over safety, with more of both being preferred outcomes. For a given driver in a given car in a given city, we can associate a level of intensity, I, with a probability of being hurt in accident, $P = P(I \mid \Phi)$, where Φ is a set of parameters reflecting the characteristics of the car, driving conditions in the city, and so forth. The individual can be modelled as choosing the optimal trade-off between intensity and safety, subject to the constraint that increases in speed will reduce safety, in the same manner as the optimal trade-off between dental visits and other goods is modelled above, subject to the constraint that more money spent on dental visits will reduce money available for other goods.

Solving the utility maximization problem generates predicted driver behaviour as a function of the factors placed in Φ. How can changes in these factors affect behaviour? Suppose, for instance, that the driver has airbags fitted in his car. In this model, the probability of being hurt in an accident decreases for any given level of I. Since individuals like both intensity and safety, this shift out of the constraint will tend to cause a change in behaviour such that both intensity and safety increase; the driver goes faster and uses less care, but not by enough to outweigh the increased safety the airbag confers. Therefore there would be fewer driver fatalities but more accidents and more injuries amongst bicyclists and pedestrians. The 'common-sense' answer is at best misleading; whether mandatory safety systems are good policy depends not only on their engineering efficacy and cost, but also on how strongly drivers will change their behaviour in response to those systems.

This idea, often called 'risk homeostasis' or 'risk offsetting', was introduced by Peltzman (1975) and has been employed in a number of settings. Peltzman's empirical analysis suggested that the mandatory safety improvements imposed on manufacturers in the late 1960s had an alarming effect; the ensuing decrease in driver fatalities was completely offset by an increase in third-party fatalities. Other studies have found that safety legislation tends to reduce fatality rates on net, but that the effect is lower than it would have been in the absence of risk offsetting behaviour (Lave *et al.* 1977, 1996; Graham 1984). The concept has been investigated in a variety of other settings, for instance child-resistant bottle caps (Viscusi 1984), workplace safety regulation (Viscusi 1979), and mattress flamability standards (Linneman 1980).

Economic epidemiology

As a final example of economic analysis in health settings, a brief survey of the nascent field of economic epidemiology is presented. Economic epidemiology is distinguished by an emphasis on endogenous individual behaviour in the context of infectious disease. Specifically, this field examines how individuals will change their risky behaviour during the course of an epidemic and how that change in behaviour will, in turn, affect the spread of disease.

To underscore the importance of behavioural considerations, consider an individual who is at risk of contracting a sexually transmitted disease. Suppose that this individual has S randomly matched partners per year, and that the probability of contracting the disease P can be approximated as a linear equation in S, $P = \beta S$, where β is a transmission coefficient that depends on the biology of the disease and the proportion of partnerships with infected individuals. Suppose that a partially effective vaccine is made available such that the probability of transmission per partner is decreased. Will this vaccine reduce the probability that this individual becomes infected?

Holding the number of partners constant, the vaccine must reduce the probability the individual becomes infected. But the individual will generally change his behaviour if vaccinated; much like the driver in the previous section who drove faster in a car equipped with an airbag, this individual at risk of disease will take more risk (have more partners) when vaccinated. If this behaviour is incorporated into the analysis, we can write $S = S(\beta)$, such that $S(\beta)$ represents a sort of 'demand curve' for partners as a function of risk of transmission. Differentiating $P = \beta S(\beta)$ with respect to β shows that the vaccine will only reduce this individual's probability of becoming infected if it is the case that a 1 per cent decrease in the transmission coefficient produces less than 1 per cent increase in number of partners. The possibility cannot then be ruled out that introducing the vaccine into the population will spur rather than retard the spread of disease.

Epidemiological models of disease spread, which incorporate economic behavioural models, include those of Auld (1996), Kremer

(1996), and Geoffard and Philipson (1996). One important result of these studies includes the notion that the hazard rate from susceptibility to infection may be decreasing in the proportion of the population infected; as more people become infected, those who are still susceptible face more incentive to reduce or cease engagement in risky behaviour. A possibly counterintuitive result is the theoretical possibility of 'fatalism', an increase in risk per partner producing increases in risky behaviour. This result will tend to hold for very high-risk individuals who may have lower incentive to avoid risky behaviour as the risk per partner rises since they may believe it is likely they have already been infected. Auld's (1997) empirical analysis showed that a sample of gay men in San Francisco reduced their number of partnerships per 6-month period by about 17 per cent on average in response to a 10 per cent increase in the proportion of the (gay) population infected with HIV/AIDS. Other empirical analysis of behaviour in an epidemiological context includes the result that 'assortive matching'—the tendency for infected individuals to match with other infected individuals, and vice versa—reduces HIV positivity/AIDS incidence by 25 to 40 per cent relative to the standard epidemiological assumption of random matching across infection states (Dow and Philipson 1996, Philipson and Dow 1998) and Ahitiv *et al.*'s (1996) result that condom use is an increasing function of local AIDS prevalence. See Philipson (1999) for a comprehensive review of recent work in economic epidemiology.

Table 13 Checklist for economic evaluation of health care

1. What economic question is being asked?
2. What are the alternatives being evaluated?
3. What changes in service provision are being considered'?
4. From whose viewpoint(s) are costs and benefits being estimated?
5. What resources are used by each of the programmes to be evaluated?
6. Which of these resources incur true opportunity costs?
7. Which groups in society bear the burden of the cost of these resources: health services, insurance companies, clients, or clients' families?
8. What are the benefits and who receives these benefits?
9. Are there any production effects associated with client participation in the programme?
10. Are there any costs identified which would have no impact on the result of the evaluation or whose collection requires too much research effort relative to their potential impact?
11. Can results be expressed in terms of quantities of resources used as well as their prices?
12. Do readily available market values exist for the items (staffing, consumable, overhead, capital) costed? It not, from where can imputed values be obtained?
13. Are costs and benefits spread over a number of years, thus raising the importance of
    - counting costs in a base year?
    - discounting?
14. What is the decision context with respect to marginal costs/benefits? Are we talking about the introduction of a totally new programme, the expansion of an existing programme, or a comparison of a new with an expanded programme?
15. Can patient-based costing be carried out? If not, how can accurate per diem costs be obtained?
16. What are the appropriate mechanisms for the allocation of overhead costs to the programmes?
17. What is the appropriate length of life to apply to capital assets used in the programmes?
18. Do market values accurately reflect opportunity costs?
19. Has sensitivity analysis been carried out? The most likely candidates for sensitivity analysis are
    - production effects
    - items excluded because of the effort required to collect data
    - imputed values
    - estimates of future benefits and costs
    - discount rate
    - length of life of capital items
20. What is the appropriate measure of benefit? This will depend on
    - the question being asked
    - whether benefits are multiple or singular (and include more than just health gain)
    - whether it is thought that the more beneficial treatment will cost more

Table 14 Discount factors, equivalent annual costs, and present values of £1 per year for a discount rate of 5% (base date is year 0)

Year	Discount factor (present value of £1)	Equivalent annual cost of £1	Present value of £1 per year
1	0.9524	1.0500	0.952
2	0.9070	0.5378	1.859
3	0.8638	0.3672	2.723
4	0.8227	0.3820	3.516
5	0.7835	0.2310	4.329
6	0.7462	0.1970	5.076
7	0.7107	0.1728	5.786
8	0.6768	0.1547	6.463
9	0.6446	0.1407	7.108
10	0.6139	0.1295	7.722
11	0.5847	0.1204	8.306
12	0.5568	0.1128	8.863
13	0.5303	0.1065	9.394
14	0.5051	0.1010	9.899
15	0.4810	0.0963	10.380
16	0.4581	0.0923	10.838
17	0.4363	0.0887	11.274
18	0.4155	0.0855	11.690
19	0.3957	0.0827	12.086
20	0.3769	0.0802	12.462
21	0.3589	0.0780	12.821
22	0.3418	0.0760	12.163
23	0.3256	0.0741	13.489
24	0.3101	0.0725	13.799
25	0.2953	0.0710	14.094
26	0.2812	0.0696	14.375
27	0.2678	0.0683	14.643
28	0.2551	0.0671	14.898
29	0.2429	0.0660	15.141
30	0.2314	0.0651	15.372
31	0.2204	0.0641	15.593
32	0.2099	0.0633	15.803
33	0.1999	0.0625	16.003
34	0.1904	0.0618	16.193
35	0.1813	0.0611	16.374
36	0.1727	0.0604	16.547
37	0.1644	0.0598	16.711
38	0.1566	0.0593	16.838
39	0.1491	0.0588	17.017
40	0.1420	0.0583	17.159
41	0.1353	0.0578	17.294
42	0.1288	0.0574	17.423
43	0.1227	0.0570	17.546
44	0.1169	0.0566	17.663
45	0.1113	0.0563	17.774
46	0.1060	0.0559	17.880
47	0.1009	0.0556	17.981
48	0.0961	0.0553	18.077
49	0.0916	0.0550	18.169
50	0.0872	0.0548	18.256

Conclusion

The aim of this chapter has been to provide an introduction to how economics methods can be used to assess the impacts of public health policy.

This has been done at the level of the individual, weighing up costs and benefits to themselves of particular courses of action. The main insights of the economics approach here are to highlight that:

- individuals may be prepared to trade off health against other 'goods' in life
- the introduction of a public health policy may change the 'incentives' which individuals face, causing them to behave in ways which reduce the overall effectiveness of the original policy
- in modelling the spread of disease, it is important to consider the costs and benefits faced by individuals with respect to decisions on whether or not to participate in 'hazardous' activities.

A further aim of the chapter has been to provide a step-by-step guide to the principles of costing and measurement of benefits in the economic evaluation of public health programmes, and to use simple examples to illustrate how some of the concepts can be applied. It is important to follow such principles in order to render such work relevant to the decision contexts of economic evaluation.

As a result of providing a general overview, not all the principles outlined in this chapter will be applicable to every evaluation undertaken. For instance, one would not apply the principle of discounting to an evaluation of health-care alternatives whose costs and effects occur over a period of only a few months. However, it is important to use the principles outlined here as a guideline for which costs and benefits should be valued and how this is to be done. The guideline comprises the questions listed in Table 13 above. These questions should be addressed in advance of an evaluation. The answers to each of them will very much determine the nature of the exercise carried out. However, it is also important to refer to the checklist whilst an evaluation is ongoing and once it has been completed.

The task may seem daunting and often is. However, answering each of these questions will render any evaluation not only easier in the long run but also relevant to the decision-making context in which it is to be applied. In the 'day-to-day' world of decision-making, where full economic evaluations cannot always be undertaken, a more practical framework to apply might be that of programme budgeting and marginal analysis. The basic framework (or questions to be asked) which follows from this approach is detailed in Table 12. Because of the number of questions to be asked and the detailed nature of many exercises in costing and benefit estimation, it is recommended that an economist be involved in any health services evaluation, particularly in the design stage. If people are to use the techniques of economic evaluation then they ought to be fully understood. It is hoped that this chapter has shed some light on such understanding.

Appendix: discounting

The figure £2859 (from Table 6) comprises:

$1000 + (1000 \times 1/1.05) + (1000 \times 1/1.05^2)$
$= 1000 + (1000 \times 0.95240) + (1000) \times (0.9070)$

where 0.954 and 0.9070 are discount factors. In general

$D_n = 1/(1 + r)_n$

where D_n is the discount factor, r is the discount rate, and n is the number of years ahead. In the example in Table 6 the discount rate r is 0.05 (or 5 per cent). Discount factors are obtainable directly from tables such as Table 14 above, which provides a list of discount factors annually from 1 to 50 years into the future at a discount rate of 5 per cent. The first two values in the column headed 'discount factor' are 0.9524 and 0.9070. This is because we are interested in discount factors 1 and 2 years from year 0 (which is now).

Present values

An alternative way of arriving at £2859 would be as follows:

$£2859 = 1000 \times (1 + 1.8594).$

The sum of our discount factors (0.9524 + 0.9070) is 1.8594, which is the present value of £1 expended in years 1 and 2. Thus, if annual costs are all equal, calculation of discounted costs can be speeded up by calculating the present value of the sum of the discount factors and multiplying the present value by the annual amount expended (in this case £1000). In Table 14, 1.8594 is the second value in the column headed 'present value of £1 per year'. This is because we are looking up to 2 years from year 0.

Equivalent annual costs

Let us assume that our surgical and drug interventions in Tables 5 and 6 each incurred capital costs of £100 per patient and that the capital assets are costed only for the duration of each programme. From Table 14, it can be seen that three annual payments of 37 pence (that is, 36.72 pence rounded up) discounted at 5 per cent would sum to £1. Therefore three annual payments of £37 discounted at 5 per cent would sum to £100, that is

$$\frac{37}{(1.05)} + \frac{37}{(1.05)^2} + \frac{37}{(1.05)^3} = 100.$$

In this example, as capital costs are equivalent in each treatment regimen, their inclusion makes no difference to the final result that drug therapy is more efficient.

References

Ahitiv, A., Hotz, J., and Philipson, T. (1996). Is AIDS self-limiting? Evidence on the prevalence elasticity of the demand for condoms. *Journal of Human Resources*, **31**, 869–98.

Alchian, A.A. (1972). Cost. In *International encyclopaedia of the social sciences* (ed. D. Stills), Volume 3. Macmillan, London.

Auld, M.C. (1996). *Choices, beliefs, and infectious disease dynamics*. Queen's University Institute of Economic Research, Discussion paper 938. Queen's University, Ontario.

Auld, M.C. (1997). *Behavioral response to the AIDS epidemic: structural estimates from panel data*. University of Calgary.

Avorn, J. (1984). Benefit and cost analysis in geriatric care: turning age discrimination into health policy. *New England Journal of Medicine*, **310**, 1294–300.

Becker, G.S. (1965). A theory of the allocation of time. *Economic Journal*, **75**, 493–517.

Becker, G. and Murphy, K. (1988). A theory of rational addiction. *Journal of Political Economy*, **96**, 675–700.

Berger, M. and Leigh, J. (1988). The effect of alcohol use on wages. *Applied Economics*, **20**, 1343–51.

Berwick, D.M. and Weinstein, M.C. (1985). What do patients value? Willingness to pay for ultrasound in normal pregnancy? *Medical Care*, **23**, 881–93.

Birch, S. and Donaldson, C. (1987). Applications of cost benefit analysis to health care: departures from welfare economic theory. *Journal of Health Economics*, **6**, 211–25.

Birch, S. and Gafni, A. (1994). Cost-effectiveness ratios: in a league of their own. *Health Policy*, **28**, 133–41.

Bond, J., Gregson, B.A., and Atkinson, A. (1989). Measurement of outcomes within a multicentred randomized controlled trial in the evaluation of the experimental NHS nursing homes. *Age and Ageing*, **18**, 292–302.

Boyle, M.H., Torrance, G.W. Sinclair, J.C., and Horwood, S.P. (1983). Economic evaluation of neonatal intensive care of very-low-birthweight infants. *New England Journal of Medicine*, **308**, 1330–7.

Brazier, J., Deverill, M., Green, C., Harper, R., and Booth, A. (1999). A review of the use of health status measures in economic evaluation. *Health Technology Assessment*, **3**.

Brook, R.H., Ware, J.E., Rogers, W.H., ***et al.*** (1983). Does free care improve adult's health? Results from a randomized controlled trial. *New England Journal of Medicine*, **309**, 1426–34.

Buckingham, K. (1993). A note on HYE (healthy years equivalent). *Journal of Health Economics*, **11**, 301–9.

Buhaug, H., Skjeldstad, F.E., Backe, B., and Dalen, B. (1989). Cost effectiveness of testing for chlamydial infections in asymptomatic women. *Medical Care*, **27**, 833–41.

Bush, J.W., Chen, M.M., and Patrick, D.L. (1973). Health status index in cost-effectiveness: analysis of a PKU program. In *Health status indexes* (ed. R.L. Berg). Hospital and Educational Research Trust, Chicago.

Cohen, D. (1994). Marginal analysis in practice: an alternative to needs assessment for contracting health care. *British Medical Journal*, **309**, 781–5.

Cohen, D. (1995). Messages from Mid Glamorgan: a multi-programme experiment with marginal analysis. *Health Policy*, **33**, 147–55.

Craig, N., Parkin, D., and Gerard, K. (1995). Clearing the fog on the Tyne: programme budgeting in Newcastle and North Tyneside Health Authority. *Health Policy*, **33**, 107–25.

Culyer, A.J. and Wagstaff, A. (1993). QALYs and HYEs. *Journal of Health Economics*, **11**, 311–23.

Dixon, J. and Welch, H.G. (1991). Priority setting: lessons from Oregon. *Lancet*, **337**, 891–4.

Doessel, D.P. (1978). Economic analysis and end stage renal disease: an Australian study. *Economic Analysis and Policy*, **8**, 21–36.

Dolan, P. (1997). Modelling valuations for Euroqol health states. *Medical Care*, **35**, 1095–108.

Donaldson, C. (1999). Valuing the benefits of publicly-provided health care: Does 'ability to pay' preclude the use of 'willingness to pay'? *Social Science and Medicine*, **49**, 551–63.

Donaldson, C. and Bond, J. (1991). Cost of continuing-care facilities in the evaluation of experimental National Health Service nursing homes. *Age and Ageing*, **20**, 160–8.

Donaldson, C. and Farrar, S. (1993). Needs assessment: developing an economic approach. *Health Policy*, **25**, 95–108.

Donaldson, C. and Gregson, B. (1989). Prolonging life at home: what is the cost? *Community Medicine*, **11**, 200–9.

Donaldson, C. and Mooney, G. (1991). Needs assessment, priority setting, and contracts for health care: an economic view. *British Medical Journal*, **303**, 1529–30.

Donaldson, C. and Shackley, P. (1997). Does 'process utility' exist? a case study of willingness to pay for laparoscopic cholecystectomy. *Social Science and Medicine*, **44**, 699–707.

Donaldson, C., Wright, K., and Maynard, A. (1986). Determining value for money in day hospital care for the elderly. *Age and Ageing*, **15**, 1–7.

Donaldson, C., Walker, A., and Craig, N. (1995). *Programme budgeting and marginal analysis: a handbook for applying economics in health care purchasing.* Scottish Forum for Public Health Medicine, Glasgow.

Donaldson, C., Mapp, T., Ryan, M., and Curtin, K. (1996). Estimating the economic benefits of avoiding food-borne risk: is 'willingness to pay' feasible? *Epidemiology and Infection*, **116**, 285–94.

Donaldson, C., Hundley, V., and Mapp, T. (1998). Willingness to pay: A method for measuring preferences for maternity care? *Birth*, **25**, 33–40.

Dow, W. and Philipson, T. (1996). An empirical investigation of the implications of assortive matching on the incidence of HIV. *Journal of Health Economics*, **15**, 735–49.

Drummond, M. and Mooney, G. (1983). *Essentials of health economics.* Northern Health Economics, Aberdeen.

Drummond, M., O'Brien, B., Stoddart, G., and Torrance, G. (1997). *Methods for the economic evaluation of health care programmes.* Oxford University Press.

Euroqol Group (1990). Euroqol—a new facility for the measurement of health-related quality of life. *Health Policy*, **16**, 199–208.

Froberg, D.G. and Kane, R.L. (1989). Methodology for measuring health-state preferences—II. Scaling methods. *Journal of Clinical Epidemiology*, **42**, 459–71.

Gafni, A. (1991). Willingness to pay as a measure of benefits: relevant questions in the context of public decision making about health care programmes. *Medical Care*, **29**, 1246–52.

Gafni, A. and Birch, S. (1993). Searching for a common currency: critical appraisal of the scientific basis underlying European harmonization of the measurement of Health Related Quality of Life (Euroqol). *Health Policy*, **23**, 219–28.

Gafni, A. and Zylak, C.J. (1990). Ionic versus non-ionic contrast media: a burden or a bargain? *Canadian Medical Association Journal*, **143**, 475–8.

Gafni, A., Birch, S., and Mehrez, A. (1993). Economics, health and health economics: HYEs versus QALYs. *Journal of Health Economics*, **11**, 325–39.

Geoffard, P. and Philipson, T. (1996). Rational epidemics and their public control. *International Economic Review*, **37**, 603–24.

Gerard, K. (1990). Economic evaluation of respite care for children with a mental handicap: a preliminary analysis of problems. *Mental Handicap*, **18**, 150–5.

Gerard, K. and Mooney, G. (1993). QALY league tables: handle with care. *Health Economics*, **2**, 59–64.

Gerard, K., Salkeld, G., and Hall, J. (1990). Counting the costs of mammography screening: first year results from the Sydney study. *Medical Journal of Australia*, **152**, 466–71.

Gold, M.R., Siegel, J.E., Russell, L.B., and Weinstein, M. (1996). *Cost effectiveness in health and medicine.* Oxford University Press.

Gold, L., Raftery, J., and Soderlund, N. (1997). *Costing diseases at DHA level: a standardised approach?* Health Economists' Study Group, York.

Gould, D. (1971). A groundling's notebook. *New Scientist*, **51**, 217.

Graham, J.D. (1984). Technology, behaviour, and safety: an empirical study of automobile occupant-protection regulation. *Policy Science*, **74**, 141–51.

Gray, A.M. and Steele, R. (1979). *The identification of the costs of maternity care: a programme approach to health service expenditure.* Health Economics Research Unit. Discussion paper 03/79. University of Aberdeen.

Grossman, M. (1972*a*). On the concept of health capital and the demand for health. *Journal of Political Economy*, **80**, 223–55.

Grossman, M. (1972*b*). *The demand for health: a theoretical and empirical investigation.* Occasional paper 119. Columbia, New York.

Harrison, A.J. (1974). *The economics of transport appraisal.* Wiley, New York.

HM Treasury (1982). *Investment appraisal in the public sector.* HMSO, London.

Hundley, V., Cruickshank, F., Lang, G., *et al.* (1994). Midwife managed delivery unit: a randomised controlled comparison with consultant led care. *British Medical Journal*, **309**, 1400–4.

Hundley, V., Donaldson, C., Lang, G.D., *et al.* (1995). Costs of intrapartum care in a midwife managed delivery unit and a consultant led labour ward. *Midwifery*, **11**, 103–9.

Johannesson, M. and Jonsson, B. (1991). Economic evaluation in health care: is there a role for cost-benefit analysis? *Health Policy*, **17**, 1–23.

Johannesson, M. and Karlsson, G. (1997). The friction cost method: a comment. *Journal of Health Economics*, **16**, 249–55.

Johannesson, M., Pliskin, J.S., and Weinstein, M.C. (1993). Are healthy years equivalents an improvement over quality adjusted life years? *Medical Decision Making*, **13**, 281–6.

Johannesson, M., Jonsson, B., Kjekshus, J., *et al.* (1997). Cost effectiveness of simvastatin treatment to lower cholesterol levels in patients with coronary heart disease. *New England Journal of Medicine*, **336**, 332–6.

Johnston, K., Brown, J., Gerard, K., O'Hanlon, M., and Morton, A. (1998). Valuing temporary and chronic health states associated with breast screening. *Social Science and Medicine*, **47**, 213–22.

Kaplan, R.M., Bush, J.W., and Berry, C.C. (1976). Health status: types of validity and the index of well-being. *Health Services Research*, **11**, 478–507.

Klarman, H.F., Francis, J.O., and Rosenthal, C.D. (1968). Cost-effectiveness analysis applied to the treatment of chronic renal disease. *Medical Care*, **6**, 48–54.

Koopmanschap, M.A., Rutten, F.F.H., van Ineveld, B.M., *et al.* (1995). The friction cost method for measuring the indrect costs of disease. *Journal of Health Economics*, **14**, 171–89.

Kremer, M. (1996). Integrating behavioral choice into epidemiological models of the AIDS epidemic. *Quarterly Journal of Economics*, **111**, 549–73.

Kristiansen, I.S., Egen, A.E., and Thelle, D.S. (1991). Cost effectiveness of incremental programmes for lowering serum cholesterol concentration: is individual intervention worthwhile? *British Medical Journal*, **302**, 1119–22.

Lave, C., Elias, P., and Robertson, L.S. (1977). A critical analysis of Peltzman's 'The effects of automobile safety regulation'. *Journal of Economic Issues*, **11**, 587.

Linneman, P. (1980). The effects of consumer safety standards: the 1973 mattress flammability standard. *Journal of Law and Economics*, **23**, 461–79.

Loomes, G. (1995). The myth of the HYE. *Journal of Health Economics*, **14**, 1–8.

Loomes, G. and McKenzie, L. (1989). The use of QALYs in health care decision making. *Social Science and Medicine*, **28**, 299–308.

McIntosh, E., Donaldson, C., and Ryan, M. (1999). Recent advances in the methods of cost-benefit analysis in health care: matching the art to the science. *Pharmaco-Economics*, **15**, 357–67.

McKeown, T. (1976). *The rise of modern populations.* Academic Press, New York.

Mark, D.B., Hlatky, M.A., Califf, R.M., *et al.* (1995). Cost-effectiveness of thrombolytic therapy with tissue plasminogen activator as compared with streptokinase for acute myocardial infarction. *New England Journal of Medicine*, **332**, 1418–24.

Mas-Colell, A., Whinston, M., and Green, J. (1995). *Microeconomic theory.* Oxford University Press.

Measurement and Valuation of Health Group (1994). *The measurement and valuation of health: first report on the main survey.* Centre for Health Economics, University of York.

Mehrez, A. and Gafni, A. (1989). Quality adjusted life years, utility theory, and healthy years equivalents. *Medical Decision Making*, **9**, 142–9.

Mehrez, A. and Gafni, A. (1993). Healthy years equivalents versus quality adjusted life years: in pursuit of progress. *Medical Decision Making*, **13**, 287–92.

Meltzer, D. (1997). *Accounting for future costs in medical cost-effectiveness analysis.* Working paper 5946. National Bureau of Economic Research, Cambridge, MA.

Miedzybrodzka, Z., Shackley, P., Donaldson, C., and Abdalla, M. (1994). Counting the benefits of screening: a pilot study of willingness to pay for cystic fibrosis carrier screening. *Journal of Medical Screening*, **1**, 82–3.

Miller, P., Parkin, D., Lewis, D., and Gerard, K. (1995). *Final report of the project 'Developing programme budgeting and marginal analysis in purchasing organisations'.* University of Newcastle upon Tyne.

Miller, P., Parkin, D., Craig, N., Lewis, D., and Gerard, K. (1997). Less fog on the Tyne? Programme budgeting in Newcastle and North Tyneside. *Health Policy*, **40**, 217–29.

Mitton, C., Donaldson, D., and Dean, S. (1999). Developing a framework for priority setting in regionalised settings: the role of economics. Presented at the Canadian Health Economics Research Association, 17–19 August, Edmonton, Alberta.

Mooney, G. (1977). Programme budgeting in an area health board. *Hospital and Health Services Review*, November, 379–84.

Mooney, G. (1984). Program budgeting: an aid to planning and priority setting in health care. *Effective Health Care*, **2**, 65–8.

Mooney, G.H. (1989). Economic evaluation: the Australian road to health service efficiency. In *Health care evaluation. Report of the National Health Care Evaluations Workshop*. Public Health Association of Australia, Canberra.

Mooney, G. and Lange, M. (1993). Antenatal screening: what constitutes 'benefit'? *Social Science and Medicine*, **37**, 873–8.

Mooney, G., Russell, E., and Weir, R. (1986). *Choices for health care: a practical introduction to the economics of health provision.* Macmillan, London.

Mooney, G., Gerard, K., Donaldson, C., and Farrar, S. (1993). *Priority setting in purchasing: some practical guidelines.* Research paper no. 6. National Association of Health Authorities and Trusts, Birmingham.

Mooney, G., Jan, S., and Seymour, J. (1994). The NSW health outcomes initiative and economic analysis. *Australian Journal of Public Health*, **18**, 244–8.

Mugford, M., Kingston, J., and Chalmers, I. (1989). Reducing the incidence of infections after Caesarean section: implications of prophylaxis with antibiotics for hospital resources. *British Medical Journal*, **299**, 1003–6.

Newhouse, J.P. and Friedlander, L.J. (1980). The relationship between medical resources and measures of health: some additional evidence. *Journal of Human Resources*, **15**, 200–18.

Nord E. (1991). The validity of a visual analogue scale in determining social utility weights for health states. *International Journal of Health Planning and Management*, **6**, 234–42.

Nord, E., Pinto, J.L., Richardson, J., *et al.* (1999). Incorporating societal concerns for fairness in numerical valuations of health programmes. *Health Economics*, **8**, 25–40.

Olsen, J.A. and Donaldson, C. (1998). Helicopters, hearts and hips: using willingness to pay to set priorities for public sector health care programmes. *Social Science and Medicine*, **46**, 1–12.

Parsonage, M. and Neuberger, H. (1992). Discounting and health benefits. *Health Economics*, **1**, 71–5.

Peacock, S. and Edwards, D. (1997). *Setting priorities in South Australian community health: the mental health program budget.* Center for Health Program Evaluation, Monash University, Melbourne.

Peltzman, S. (1975). The effects of automobile safety regulation. *Journal of Political Economy*, **83**, 677–725.

Philipson, T. (1999). Economic epidemiology and infectious diseases. In *Handbook of health economics* (ed. J.P. Newhouse and A.J. Culyer). North-Holland, Amsterdam.

Philipson, T. and Dow, W. (1998). Infectious disease transmission and infection-dependent matching. *Mathematical Biosciences*, **148**, 161–80.

Pole, J. (1974). Programs, priorities and budgets. *British Journal of Preventive and Social Medicine*, **28**, 191–5.

Robbins, L. (1935). *The nature and significance of economic science.* Macmillan, London.

Robertson, L.S. (1996). Reducing death on the road: the effects of minimum safety standards, publicized crash tests, seat belts, and alcohol. *American Journal of Public Health*, **86**, 31.

Rosser, R. and Kind, P. (1978). A scale of valuations of states of illness: is there a social consensus? *International Journal of Epidemiology*, **7**, 347–58.

Russell, I.T., Devlin, B., Fell, M., *et al.* (1977). Day case surgery for hernias and haemorrhoids: a clinical, social and economic evaluation. *Lancet*, **i**, 844–7.

Ruta, D., Donaldson, C., and Gilray, I. (1996). Economics, public health and health care purchasing: the Tayside experience of programme budgeting and marginal analysis. *Journal of Health Service Research and Policy*, **1**, 185–93.

Scott, A., Currie, N., and Donaldson, C. (1998). Evaluating innovation in general practice: a pragmatic framework using programme budgeting and marginal analysis. *Family Practice*, **15**, 216–22.

Scott, A., Donaldson, C., and Scott, S. (1999) Program budgeting and marginal analysis: pragmatism and policy (editorial). *Journal of Health Services Research and Policy*, **4**, 1–2.

Shackley, P. and Dixon, S. (2000). Using contingent valuation to elicit public preferences for water fluoridation. *Applied Economics*, **32**, 777–87.

Sintonen, H. and Pekurinen, M. (1993). A fifteen-dimensional measure of health-related quality of life (15D) and its applications. In *Quality of life assessment: key issues in the 1990s* (ed. S.R. Wallner and R.M. Rosser), pp. 185–95. Kluwer, Dordrecht.

Stanford, M. (1990). Counting the costs of mammography screening: first year results from the Sydney study. *Medical Journal of Australia*, **153**, 175.

Tengs, T.O. (1996) An evaluation of Oregon's Medicaid rationing algorithms. *Health Economics*, **5**, 171–82.

Torgerson, D., Donaldson, C., and Reid, D. (1994). Private versus social opportunity cost of time: valuing time in the demand for health care. *Health Economics*, **3**, 149–55.

Torrance, G.W. (1986). Measurement of health state utilities for economic appraisal: a review. *Journal of Health Economics*, **5**, 1–30.

Torrance, G.W., Thomas, W.H., and Sackett, D.L. (1972). A utility maximization model for evaluation of health care programmes. *Health Services Research*, **7**, 118–33.

Torrance, G.W., Furlong, W., Feeny, D., and Boyle, M. (1995). Multi-attribute preference functions. Health utilities index. *Pharmacoeconomics*, **7**, 503–20.

Twaddle, S. and Walker, A. (1995). Programme budgeting and marginal analysis: application within programmes to assist purchasing in Greater Glasgow Health Board. *Health Policy*, **33**, 91–105.

Viney, R., Haas, M., and Mooney, G. (1995). Program budgeting and marginal analysis: a guide to resource allocation. *NSW Public Health Bulletin*, **6**, 29–32.

Viscusi, K. (1979). The impact of occupational health and safety regulation. *Bell Journal of Economics*, **10**, 117–40.

Viscusi, K. (1984). The Lulling effect: the impact of child-resistant packaging on aspirin and analgesic ingestions. *American Economic Review*, **74**, 324–7.

Williams, A. (1985). Economics of coronary artery bypass grafting. *British Medical Journal*, **291**, 326–9.

Wiseman, V., Mooney, G., and Stephenson, J. (1998). *An economic approach to priority setting in health care.* University of Sydney.

7.6 Cost-effectiveness analysis: concepts and applications*

Dean T. Jamison

Many of the world's poorest countries spend less than $10 per person per year on health services. High-income countries spend thousands of dollars per year. Yet across this entire expenditure range of several orders of magnitude questions arise about value gained for money spent on health. Most poor countries suffer huge burdens from some mix of childhood infection, malaria, maternal deaths, tuberculosis, and HIV/AIDS. Highly effective interventions exist to address most (but not all) of these conditions. If a few additional dollars per year were available, misspending those dollars on interventions offering relatively little health gain for the money would entail lost opportunities to postpone many deaths and prevent much serious disability. High-income countries also face choices: Could an improved mix of interventions reduce overall costs (or at least their rate of growth) while maintaining existing levels of health? Which of the effective but usually costly new interventions emerging from the research and development pipeline should public or private insurance plans cover?

Therefore concern with value for money (or cost-effectiveness) spans income levels. Neither is the issue one principally for the private sector, for non-governmental organizations, or for the public sector. Each has a potential interest. Analysts have responded to this interest over a period of several decades and produced a substantial literature on both methods and results. Thus the purpose of this chapter is to introduce the reader to this literature.

The chapter begins with a brief discussion of background and terminology, and then describes methods of cost-effectiveness analysis (**CEA**). It illustrates use of these methods with an application that provides a sense of results and one way that they can be used. We are all used to hearing statements of the sort 'prevention is more cost-effective than cure' or 'tertiary facilities are not cost-effective in low-income countries'. The application section includes discussion of the cost-effectiveness generalizations that would support or undermine such propositions. More frequently, analysts use CEA to assess options for dealing with a particular problem—options involving scale of intervention or choice of technique. Discussion in this chapter covers these issues as well.

Background

CEA in health comprises one part of a very much larger literature on project appraisal, i.e. on assessment of the economic desirability of alternative 'projects' from a social perspective. Antecedent to such analyses is assessment of whether the project should be financed by the public sector (or by the decision-maker using the analysis). The perspective of this chapter is, for the most part, that of a public-sector decision-maker responsible for a broad range of preventive and curative health services. Barr (1993) reviews arguments, mostly around insurance market failure, for including personal clinical services for the entire population in what is to be publicly financed. Musgrove (1995) discusses related issues. Table 1 lists three approaches to the economic appraisal of projects or interventions and indicates their realm of applicability.

Cost-minimization analysis examines the costs of alternative approaches to achieving a quite specific objective, for example the cost per infant death averted or new HIV infection averted. The purpose is to identify the least-cost method of achieving the objective and to see how both cost and choice of technique vary as the magnitude of the objective varies. For example, if one had very modest goals with respect to the prevention of HIV infection, the least-cost approach might very well be blood screening in hospitals; more substantial goals would entail addition of more costly programmes—treatment of sexually transmitted diseases, condom use, etc.—to achieve the goal at minimum total cost. Note that in this example, as will often be the case, the average cost per HIV infection averted will rise as the target number of infections averted rises. Cost-minimization analysis has the virtues of specificity and of ease of communication concerning results. The disadvantage becomes apparent if there is a need to compare the attractiveness of efforts to reduce infant mortality rate with those to avert HIV infections: costs can be compared but outcomes remain incommensurable.

Cost–benefit analysis, in contrast, allows comparison of projects (or interventions or investments) across the entire economy. It does so by placing monetary values on outcomes as well as inputs. Kilowatt-hours of electricity can be compared with kilograms of rice by multiplying each by its price to obtain a total value. However, the simple word 'price' conceals vast complexities, particularly when used to measure social benefits. There is an extensive literature on the theoretical methods as well as applications in different contexts of monetary valuation of benefits or costs when markets are distorted or incomplete. Stern and Ferreira (1997, pp. 567–9) provide a brief overview of these issues and of related issues concerning the distribution of costs and benefits. Benefits and costs occur over time—with benefits usually following costs—and alternative figures of merit (e.g. present value of net benefits or the internal rate-of-return) generate orderings of outcomes by desirability. Squire (1989) and Layard and Glaister (1994) provide excellent overviews of the methods of cost–benefit analysis and the related literature.

* Parts of this chapter are revised and updated from Jamison (1993).

Table 1 Choice of economic appraisal techniques

Economic appraisal technique	Applicable for assessing			
	Options to achieve a specific objective	**Options throughout the health sector**	**Options inside and outside the health sector**	**Intrinsic value**
1 Cost-minimization analysis	Yes	No	No	No
2 Cost-effectiveness analysis (sometimes called cost-utility analysis)	Yes	Yes	No	No
3 Cost–benefit analysis	Yes	Yes	Yes	Yes

Practical difficulties associated with monetary valuation of benefits often lead analysts to utilize the much simpler methods of cost minimization (with the concomitant limits on applicability of the results). In addition to practical difficulties there is the more fundamental problem, in assessing health intervention options, of placing dollar value on human life (or other health outcomes). Sometimes this can be non-controversial, as when Levin *et al.* (1993) use labour productivity increases associated with reducing anaemia to derive benefit measures to weigh against the costs of anaemia control. Their findings—of high dollar benefits relative to dollar costs—can either be compared with findings for interventions in other sectors or, more importantly, to assess intrinsic value: if benefits exceed costs the intervention is worth doing (ignoring possible public-sector fiscal constraints). If one can overcome practical and other problems with cost–benefit analysis, its results have the virtue of standing alone in the sense of indicating intervention desirability independently of comparison with alternatives.

In the health sector, CEA lies between cost-minimization analysis and cost–benefit analysis (Table 1). CEA rests on a non-financial metric designed to allow comparisons across the health sector. The concept most typically used is that of the quality-adjusted life-year (**QALY**), which can be measured in many ways, but which then allows costs per QALY gained to be compared for interventions addressing a broad range of problems (by assigning, for example, a QALY value both to an HIV infection averted and to an infant death averted). However, even focusing analysis to within the health sector cannot be completely done by CEA. Some interventions which may be undertaken principally for health reasons, such as reducing ambient air pollution, have other outcomes—in this case reduced pollution-related corrosion and the amenity value of clean air. These outcomes elude the QALY metric but must be explicitly listed as inputs to the decision-making process.

This chapter focuses on CEA. That said, work on cost minimization will often in practice prove essential to CEA. Likewise, empirical observations of what societies appear to be prepared to pay for a QALY, or more frequently to avert a death (which can be converted to QALYs), have increasingly been undertaken. Jones-Lee (1994) reports on 27 valuations of a 'statistical life' of which he categorizes 16 as 'more reliable'. While 10 of the 16 studies estimated a value of over £1 000 000 for a statistical life, one estimate fell under £250 000. These (or other) estimates of the value of a statistical life allow CEAs to be immediately translated into cost–benefit analyses. From experience it can be suggested that an explicit valuation of human life for cost–benefit analysis usually generates reactions that distract from a discussion of improving efficiency of resource allocation in the health sector. The interested reader is referred to Viscusi (1993), Jones-Lee (1994), Tolley *et al.* (1994), and Pauly (1995) for valuable reviews of the monetary valuation of health outcomes.

Part of the value of undertaking CEA lies in the ability to formulate generalizations—or to indicate their inapplicability. Doing so requires care and consistency concerning the definitions that underlie the generalizations, and in this chapter attempts to be quite explicit. Table 2 provides a number of definitions and distinctions that will be used later in the chapter. Perhaps the central point to note in Table 2 is the distinction between 'interventions' *per se* and the 'instruments of policy' that can encourage (or discourage) intervention or intended behaviour change. Although most CEAs concern intervention, some concern instruments of policy (Wells 1999). More is needed concerning the latter, which, after all, is what policy can do to change behaviour. In this context it will be important to consider the potential fungibility of resources if the policy instrument consists of direct investment. Lower-level decision-makers may redirect previously allocated resources away from activities that a higher-level authority is seeking to encourage by funding it (Devarajan *et al.* 1997).

CEAs in the literature vary substantially in their underlying methodologies and assumptions, and therefore comparisons are frequently difficult. Yet without being able to compare substantial numbers of interventions—a point to which we shall return—the relative attractiveness of individual interventions remains uncertain and generalizations are difficult or impossible. To define best practice in methods and to provide a template for comparative studies, the United States Public Health Service convened a major review panel in 1993. Gold *et al.* (1996) reported its conclusions. Discussion in this chapter for the most part follows the United States Public Health Service guidelines. More extensive and technical discussion of the theory and methods of CEA than is appropriate for this chapter is provided by Garber *et al.* (1996) and Garber (2000), and the interested reader is referred to these reviews.

Assessing the cost-effectiveness of intervention

This section contains a discussion of general issues associated with choosing interventions, i.e. with criteria for cost-effective choice. The nature of the instruments open to government to promote cost-effective intervention have been outlined in Table 2. The purpose is

Table 2 Definition of terms

1. **Intervention**

The term 'intervention' is used in this chapter to denote actions taken by or for individuals to reduce the risk, duration, or severity of an adverse health condition. Interventions are the proximal cause of deliberate changes in risks, duration, or severity. Instruments of policy (see below) encourage, discourage, or undertake interventions. Stopping smoking, for example, is an intervention that an individual can take to reduce risk from a range of diseases; taxing tobacco products is a potential instrument of government policy to encourage this intervention. Interventions are divided into those that are 'public health' and those that are 'clinical'

1.1 **Public health interventions** are sought of or directed toward entire populations or population subgroups; this chapter divides public health interventions into five broad categories: change of personal behaviour, control of environmental hazards, immunization, mass chemoprophylaxis, and screening and referral

1.2 **Clinical interventions** are provided at facilities, usually to individuals. This chapter divides clinical interventions into those that can be provided at the clinic (community, private, work- based, or school-based), at a district hospital, or at a referral hospital.

2. **Objectives of intervention**

In this chapter, the objectives of intervention are structured into five categories[a]

2.1 **Primary prevention** aims to reduce the risk of a condition occurring by lowering the level of risk factors or instituting policies to forestall their emergence (the latter is sometimes referred to as 'primordial prevention')

2.2 **Secondary prevention** aims to reduce the duration or severity of a condition or physiological risk factor in order to forestall its leading to more adverse consequences

2.3 **Cure** of a condition aims to remove its cause and restore function to the status quo ante.

2.4 **Rehabilitation** aims to restore (or partially restore) physical, psychological, or social function resulting from a previous or chronic condition

2.5 **Palliation** aims to reduce pain and suffering from a condition for which no means of cure or rehabilitation is currently available (this may range from the use of aspirin for headaches to the use of opiates to control terminal cancer pain)

3. **Instruments of policy**

These are the activities that can (potentially) be undertaken by governments or other entities that wish to encourage or discourage interventions, or, importantly, to expand the menu of potential intervention. Five major instruments or policy are distinguished

3.1 Use of **information, education, and communication** seeks to improve the knowledge of individuals (and service providers) about the consequences of their choices

3.2 Use of **taxes and subsidies** on commodities, services, and pollutants seeks to effect appropriate behavioural responses

3.3 Use of **regulation and legislation** seeks to limit availability of certain commodities, to curtail certain practices, and to define the rules governing finance and provision of health services

3.4 Use of **direct expenditures** seeks to provide (or finance provision of) selected interventions (e.g. immunizations), to provide infrastructure (e.g. medical schools) that facilitates provision of a range of interventions, or altering infrastructure that influences behaviour (e.g. installing speed bumps or removing the handle of the Broad Street pump)

3.5 Undertaking **research and development** (or encouraging them through subsidies) is an instrument central to the goal of expanding the range of interventions available and reducing their cost.

[a]The *Dictionary of Epidemiology* (Last 1988) provides a helpful discussion of different types of prevention but, interestingly, has no entries for 'cure' or 'rehabilitation'. Their term 'tertiary prevention', which is not used here, seems to encompass both 'rehabilitation' and 'palliation', as we define those terms.

not to provide an account of the (many) methodological issues associated with economic assessment of intervention options; rather, it is simply to describe the basic concepts being applied, raise a few particular issues, and refer the reader to the relevant literature. In addition to the comprehensive work for the United States Public Health Service previously mentioned, valuable additional background can be found in Weinstein and Stason (1977), Drummond (1987*a,b*) Johannesson and Weinstein (1993), Sloan and Conover (1995), Weinstein (1995), and Drummond *et al.* (1997).

As previously indicated it is useful to consider two distinct uses for CEA. One is to inform broad policy generalizations and the other is to help assess the relative attractiveness of changes in the scale of implementation of an intervention or in the technique for addressing a specific problem. In either case the analyst must specify a base case and define the intervention as a change from that base. For policy generalizations it will typically be useful to include consideration of large changes; for addressing specific problems more modest increments will be typical. The natural base case for dealing with specific problems will usually be the status quo, and what is to be considered as 'given' for the purpose of analysis will usually be substantial (although dependent on time frame). Establishing a base case for policy generalizations is less obvious. Guidelines being developed at the World Health Organization (**WHO**) (Murray *et al.* 1999) suggest using the '...null set of related interventions.' Substantial practical difficulties are likely to be associated with ascertaining the consequences of no intervention, and the utility to policy-makers of trying to imagine a starting point so different from their own may be limited. In most cases a more natural approach will be to identify base cases close to current reality for policy-makers in a number of paradigmatic circumstances. Incremental cost-effectiveness assessments from those bases will then provide more naturally interpretable information. In this context it will often prove important to consider explicitly the effects of doing less than is being done in the base case, thereby generating negative costs and negative effects. Such 'negative intervention' may often prove highly cost-effective.

Outcome measurement: QALYs

A critical choice in applications of economic analysis to resource allocation is that of whether to value outcomes because of their economic benefits or because of some more proximal effectiveness measure (Table 1). To provide a clearer sense of the context for CEA it is worth a brief additional discussion of approaches to monetary valuation of health outcomes. To a lesser extent some of these points also relate to cost analysis. When there are good markets for products, benefits can be assessed in monetary terms by using market prices (i.e. willingness of consumers to pay) to value benefits as well as to value costs. Even when willingness-to-pay valuation cannot be assessed directly because of lack of market prices, as is typically true in the health sector, questions in surveys are increasingly being used to elicit information about hypothetical willingness to pay (or contingent valuation). Briscoe and de Ferranti (1988) indicate the potential for contingent valuation in water projects, and there are early applications in education (Jamison and Lumsden 1975, Table 2). Pervasive problems of consumer ignorance of effectiveness of intervention and a widespread tendency for individuals systematically to underestimate risks (Weinstein 1989) suggest that willingness-to-pay assessments will need to be used with caution when applied to health. An alternative approach—sometimes called the human capital approach—is to view health investments as instrumental to improving economic productivity; thus estimates of the effect of a health intervention on productivity provide a lower bound to total benefits. One example comes from assessing the effect on the productivity of rubber plantation workers of correcting iron deficiencies (Basta *et al.* 1979; Levin *et al.* 1993); other examples come from assessment of the effect on economic productivity of malaria control efforts. It is worth noting that both the willingness-to-pay and the human capital approaches inevitably imply different values to be attached to the life of different individuals of the same age in the same country—and even greater variation across countries. Phelps and Mushlin (1991), Johanneson and Meltzer (1998), Bleichrodt and Quiggen (1999), and Garber (2000) further discuss the close relation (and sometimes equivalence) between cost-effectiveness and cost–benefit analyses.

More typically, however, outcomes will be assessed in deaths or disability averted, rather than dollars, and the task is to come up with some measure for making such an assessment that allows comparisons across the health sector (i.e. that allows CEA), even if intersectoral comparisons (cost–benefit analyses) remain infeasible or subject to excessive ethical debate. There is now a valuable literature on how effectiveness measures to aggregate the disability-, morbidity-, and premature-mortality-averting effects of interventions across the health sector might be constructed and applied (Zeckhauser and Shepard 1976; Kaplan and Bush 1982; Barnum 1987; Feachem *et al.* 1992; Fox-Rushby and Hanson 2001). Such measures, in addition to providing the effectiveness measures for CEAs, can be used with epidemiological information to assess the burden of disease in a population, as has been done for the major regions of the world by Murray *et al.* (1994) (most recently updated in WHO (2000)).

Table 3 sets forth the characteristics of the main approaches to disability weighting that serve as the core of effectiveness measurement. Stouthard *et al.* (1997) provide a clear exposition of methods for disability weighting with an informative application for The Netherlands. From a practical perspective, the use of ratings based on expert judgement is probably the best that can now be done if the purpose of the analysis is to compare interventions across the sector; however, as Preston (1991) has noted, these measures must be used with care. It is also worth noting that the construction of QALYs requires value judgements, although they are less subject to controversy than is explicit valuation of human life. (Even measures involving mortality only, such as numbers of deaths averted, while they appear to be value-free, if used to measure intervention effectiveness or disease burden, rest on strong value judgements. Minimally, a mortality based measure rests on the implicit value judgement that disability is not a concern.)

A workable measure for effectiveness for most CEAs will be QALYs gained. The QALY gain associated with averting a death at a given age is, simply, the life expectancy at that age (in the local environment), with life-years gained in the future discounted back to the present (typically at a discount rate of 3 per cent per annum). Unhealthy life-years are given lower weights than healthy ones, depending on the degree of disability (assessed by one of the rating procedures listed in Table 3); therefore the effectiveness of interventions to address morbidity or disability can be measured in terms that allow comparison with interventions that delay mortality. The QALY measures now used are particular forms of the more general concept introduced by Zeckhauser and Shepard (1976). Garber and Phelps (1997) provide the basic theoretical underpinnings for CEAs in health that adjust life-years for quality; in particular, they point to conditions allowing a dollar value to be assigned to a QALY so that, if desired, a CEA can be directly reinterpreted as a cost–benefit analysis.

Timing of outcomes can be dealt with through discounting. Johannesson (1992) provides a general discussion of discounting healthy life-years, and Cropper *et al.* (1992) report empirical assessments of time preference for saving lives. Most analysts value years of healthy life at all ages equally; however, this assumption can be readily relaxed to give greater weight to those age groups likely, say, to have more dependants (Musgrove 1991). The variant of the QALY known as the 'disability-adjusted life-year' (**DALY**) does weight different age groups differently. DALYs have been used for disease burden assessment and CEA in a number of recent World Bank and WHO documents (World Bank 1993; Murray *et al.* 1994; WHO 1996, 2000). An overview is given in Chapter 2.9. Sensitivity analyses were undertaken in the initially published disease burden assessment using DALYs (Murray *et al.* 1994) and it was concluded that results were insensitive to age weights over a broad range.

In principle, QALYs can also be weighted to reflect how equitably they are distributed in ways that are standard in project evaluation outside the health sector (Squire 1989). Wagstaff (1994) provides a valuable overview of this possibility (but concludes that a more general approach, not involving QALYs, would be preferable).

An important outcome of publicly financed intervention, which is usually neglected in the CEA literature, is the contribution to reducing

Table 3 Alternative approaches to measuring outcomes[a]

Approach to measurement	Cost of implementation	Possible bias	Example or application
Mortality			
Deaths averted	Very low	Highly biased against conditions involving disability; equally weights death in very old age and in middle age	Assessment of priorities in child survival (Walsh and Warren 1979)
Years of potential life lost	Very low	Highly biased against conditions involving disability	Regularly used by CDC to assess burden of disease in the United States (MMWR 1992)
Quality-of-life adjusted life-years (QALYs)[b]			
Expert ratings assessment	Low	Unrepresentative experts	Ghana Health Assessment Project Team (1981)
Survey-based	Medium	NA	Rosser scale (Rosser and Kind 1978); European quality-of-life assessments (EuroQol Group 1990)
Risk trade-offs	High	Questionable relevance of artificial gambles	Various quality-of-life assessments (Tan-Torres 1990)
Quantity-of-life trade-offs			
Individual length vs. quality of life	Medium/high	Probably low for patient-level decision-making	Various quality-of-life assessments (Tan-Torres 1990)
Across individuals	Medium	Probably low bias for social decision-making	Vaccine development study (Institute of Medicine 1986; Nord 1991)
Calibration of pre-existing condition-specific studies	Medium	Probably low	Cairns and Johnston (1991)

CDC, Centers for Disease Control and Prevention; NA, not applicable.

[a]This table does not review approaches to measuring the economic benefits of changes in health status. Such measures—based, for example, on willingness to pay for reductions in the probability of adverse outcomes or an assessment of health-related determinants of labour productivity (human capital)—allow conclusions to be drawn about the inherent attractiveness of particular health interventions relative to their cost, not simply by comparison with other interventions. Tolley *et al.* (1994) and Pauly (1995) provide valuable overviews of this literature, which is briefly discussed in the text.

[b]Each of the methods for quality of life measurement—ratings, risk trade-offs, quantity-of-life trade-offs, and calibrations—can be undertaken by different groups, possibly with different results. The groups can be of 'experts', respondents to a survey, or, in a clinical setting, potential patients. See Fallowfield (1990) for a general discussion of these matters.

financial risk for households. A tuberculosis intervention and measles immunization may, in the relevant age range, have costs per QALY that are close, but the greater costs of treatment and income loss associated with tuberculosis would entail much greater risk protection from the former. A significance evaluation of the Medicare program in the United States (Skinner and McClellan 2000) explicitly examined this issue. More will need to be done in the future.

Costs

Costs of inputs are generally assessed at market prices. However, this simple observation masks much complexity, both conceptually and in practice. Luce *et al.* (1996) provide a valuable overview of these issues in the specific context of CEA for health. Several important issues are highlighted below, but the interested reader is referred to Luce *et al.* (1996) for a more thorough treatment.

Tradeable and non-tradeable inputs

Costs for some inputs into health care (e.g. semiskilled labour) may be lower in developing countries. These costs are typically for inputs that cannot be traded internationally, and their existence undermines attempts to estimate costs that are not simply country specific. Squire (1989) provides a general discussion of approaches to dealing with tradeables in project analysis through the use of 'shadow prices'. His recommendations are more relevant to country-specific assessments than to cross-national comparisons.

The working conclusion of this chapter is that considerations of cost variability between high- and low-income countries are of minimal significance (relative to other uncertainties)for tradeables (e.g. non-patented drugs, most equipment, and high-level manpower). Real costs for facilities and lower-level manpower do vary across countries, leading some analysts to conclude that costs are most usefully expressed as fractions of local per capita income—a method that assumes that essentially no health sector inputs are internationally tradeable. The CEA for cancer interventions developed by Barnum and Greenberg (1993) is an example of an attempt to divide costs into those for traded goods and those for non-tradeables. Their assessments suggest that local costs will often be important and that those who attempt to assess the cost-effectiveness of intervention in a country-specific context should pay close attention to this issue unless there is a free market for foreign exchange and the costs of non-tradeables are similar to those of the comparator country. It is a matter of judgement about the extent to which costing of non-tradeables undermines efforts to form generalizations across countries. My own view is that such generalizations are both useful and possible, but that they are best done within groups of countries with broadly similar income levels.

Patient and home provider time

Another important issue in cost analysis concerns assessment of the amount and value of time required of patients or caretakers. Attention to time costs is important both for improving cost analyses and because behavioural response to the availability of an intervention may be sensitive to time requirements. The importance of mothers' time, in particular for compliance with child survival interventions, has been stressed by Leslie (1989). These time costs are potentially difficult to value (Briscoe and de Ferranti 1988) and are often neglected. The United States Public Health Service provides recommendations for subsequent work that would help to redress this omission (Gold *et al.* 1996). A related issue concerns treatment of costs that will ensue from intervention success. For example, Levin *et al.* (1993) point out that substantial food costs can result from micronutrient supplementation or parasite control—appetites improve. The existence of such costs suggests the importance, in these cases, of broadening the definition of the intervention.

Joint costs

A final issue concerning cost analysis is that of joint costs, i.e. the situation where several interventions are essentially made available with a (partially) common set of inputs. Over (1988) provides an extended discussion in the context of immunization. Some authors handle this in part by defining interventions in terms of natural packages; for example, Jamison *et al.* (1993) consider the preventive intervention for poliomyelitis to be diphtheria–pertussis–tetanus vaccine plus poliomyelitis immunization, and to assess the cost-effectiveness of that package, because poliomyelitis immunization would usually be given with the other vaccines. In many cases, however, such packaging would become too unwieldy, and in these cases analysts should note where joint costs would need to be considered in country-specific applications.

Other issues

Thus, for comparisons across interventions, CEAs use the common metric of dollar cost per QALY gained, with the understanding that

Table 4 Factors influencing variation in cost effectiveness

Influencing factor	Important examples
Epidemiological environment	
Prevalence of condition	Screening and referral programs for leprosy and for cervical and breast cancer
Incidence of condition	BCG immunization for tuberculosis; preventive measures for many injuries
Case-fatality rate	Measles immunization; oral rehydration therapy for diarrhoea
Transmission dynamics of infectious conditions	Treatment of sexually transmitted diseases in core versus non-core groups; vector control for malaria, dengue
Existence of competing risks or synergisms	Measles vaccination results in amplification of cost-effectiveness by strengthening individuals in a general way. Among the very young or elderly, competing risks reduce the cost-effectiveness of some targeted interventions
Individual characteristics	
Age	Cancer treatment: more cost-effective for younger patients
Tendency to compliance	Tuberculosis chemotherapy; antihypertensive medication
Tendency to self-refer	Sexually transmitted diseases control
Levels of risk factors	High levels of hypertension and hyperlipidaemia enhance intervention cost-effectiveness of preventive measures for heart disease
Individual variation in values	Attitude toward disability relative to risk of death; can lead to individual differences in intervention value
System characteristics	
Local costs of non-traded inputs to health-care system	Real costs of care-intensive interventions (such as hospitalization to ensure compliance with tuberculosis chemotherapy) are low where wages are low because most health-care personnel are relatively immobile internationally
Generalized systemic competence	Case management of dengue haemorrhagic fever: high cost and low effectiveness in unsophisticated systems. Cost per QALY at the margin of some interventions in a system with high level of professionalism and capacity may be much lower than in less well-developed systems
Discount rate	Hepatitis B immunization: where discount rates are high, interventions with pay-offs well into the future become relatively less attractive, and age of the patient becomes a less significant determinant of cost-effectiveness

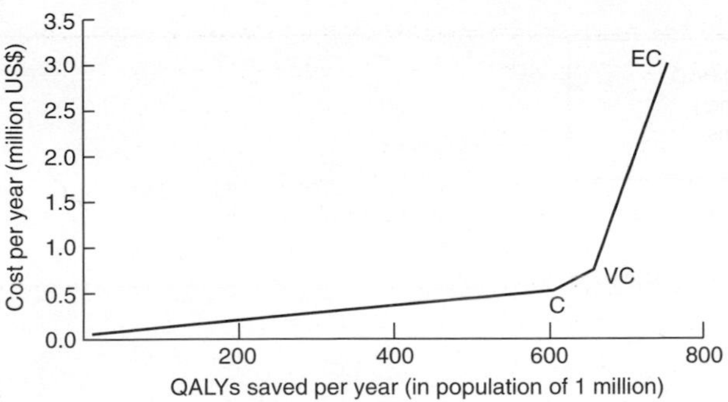

Fig. 1 Increasing cost per QALY associated with more complete control of dengue.

incremental costs and cost-effectiveness will probably vary across locales (even after controlling for intervention quality) because of differences in individuals, in epidemiological conditions, in delivery system characteristics, in the initial degree of penetration of the intervention into the population, and in the range of available alternatives. Table 4 lists many important factors that lead to variation in incremental cost-effectiveness, and, to the extent that interventions are first applied where their cost-effectiveness is highest, these factors collectively will lead to rising costs per QALY with increased application of an intervention. Figure 1 illustrates this for control of dengue; up to a point, improved case management is most cost-effective, but beyond that point chemical and then environmental strategies of vector control must be introduced if a higher level of control for dengue is to be sought.

Intervention specificity and targeting

The phenomenon of rising costs per QALY comes up implicitly in many analyses; the cause of the phenomenon is, frequently, the lack of intervention specificity and, also frequently, the need for costly targeting, case-finding, or compliance monitoring. Intervention specificity refers to what fraction of intervention recipients would benefit assuming that the intervention is applied exactly to the individuals to whom it should be applied. Specificity will be influenced by such factors as 'prevalence of the condition', 'incidence of condition', and 'levels of risk factors' (Table 4). For example, many countries specify that BCG vaccination for tuberculosis be applied to all newborns, but it is a benefit, *ex post*, only to that tiny fraction of children who would have died in childhood from miliary tuberculosis without it. In contrast, tuberculosis chemotherapy for sputum positives, although costly, will not be applied unless necessary—it is highly specific. Initially targeting BCG or other interventions to populations at highest risk, although inevitably at some cost, will maximize cost-effectiveness while simultaneously advancing equity objectives (Mosley and Jolly 1987). Although the incremental cost per QALY gained by expanding coverage may be rising, sufficient resource availability may justify expansion.

To continue the tuberculosis example, patients who seek care, and who are then compliant with the treatment regimen, cost less than those for whom active case-finding is required or who require careful monitoring for compliance. All these factors lead to another reason for rising costs per incremental QALY gained. To take another example, oral rehydration therapy in the hospital or clinic setting is highly cost-effective; it will only be used for severe cases of diarrhoea, and it is likely to be applied effectively by qualified medical personnel. However, when oral rehydration therapy is taken to the community, cost-effectiveness declines substantially both because of a decrease in intervention specificity (mild cases will be treated unnecessarily) and because home treatment will be applied less effectively than hospital treatment in severe cases.

These points are relatively obvious, but there is often an optimistic bias towards assessing cost-effectiveness under assumptions of favourable targeting and compliance costs and of favourable intervention specificity. One might expect, as previously noted, rising marginal costs and decreasing marginal effectiveness as interventions are extended through populations; these combine to dilute cost-effectiveness. Thus, favourable case cost-effectiveness estimates can be real, but their margin of applicability may be limited. In principle, it is desirable to acquire some sense of the responsiveness of intervention cost-effectiveness to a range of parameters, particularly the extent of application of the intervention. In practice, sensitivity analysis is sometimes possible but often difficult—and comparisons are then made for 'representative' estimates of incremental cost-effectiveness to provide general guidance to decision-makers. When there are great differences in the incremental cost-effectiveness of different interventions—as this chapter concludes there to be—this 'general guidance' can suggest important redirections of policy.

Fixed costs

When an intervention requires large fixed costs, total programme costs need to be weighed against total effects; simple assessment of marginal cost and effectiveness fails to suffice. The fixed costs involved in (to take several examples) investing in major facilities, mounting a media-based health education programme, or devising regulations and procedures can be substantial. Fixed costs need not be financial; managerial or political attention to a problem may have an important fixed-cost element. When fixed cost may be important, understanding the total burden of disease is necessary for estimating potential total intervention effects. By the same token CEAs will need to include consideration of large increments in intervention. (Examples include Barnum *et al.* (1980) for analysis of simultaneous scaling up of multiple child survival interventions or Watts and Kumaranayake (1999) for a brief discussion of scaling up AIDS control interventions in Africa.)

Disease burden assessment needs can be combined with CEA in an explicit way to help evaluate where there might be large payoffs to research and development investments or to focused political or managerial attention on reallocation of interventions. This requires an analysis, essentially, of whether a major disease burden persists mainly because of a lack of knowledge about the disease and its determinants, a lack of tools, or failure to use the existing tools efficiently. Of course, more than one factor is likely in each case. Where possible, this analysis can be quantitative. Figure 2 illustrates an analytical approach applied recently (WHO 1996). By using data on the efficacy of the available cost-effective interventions and consulting the judgement of field experts on the proportion of the population receiving effective interventions, it is possible to estimate the following.

- What portion of the potential burden of each disease or condition is now being averted.

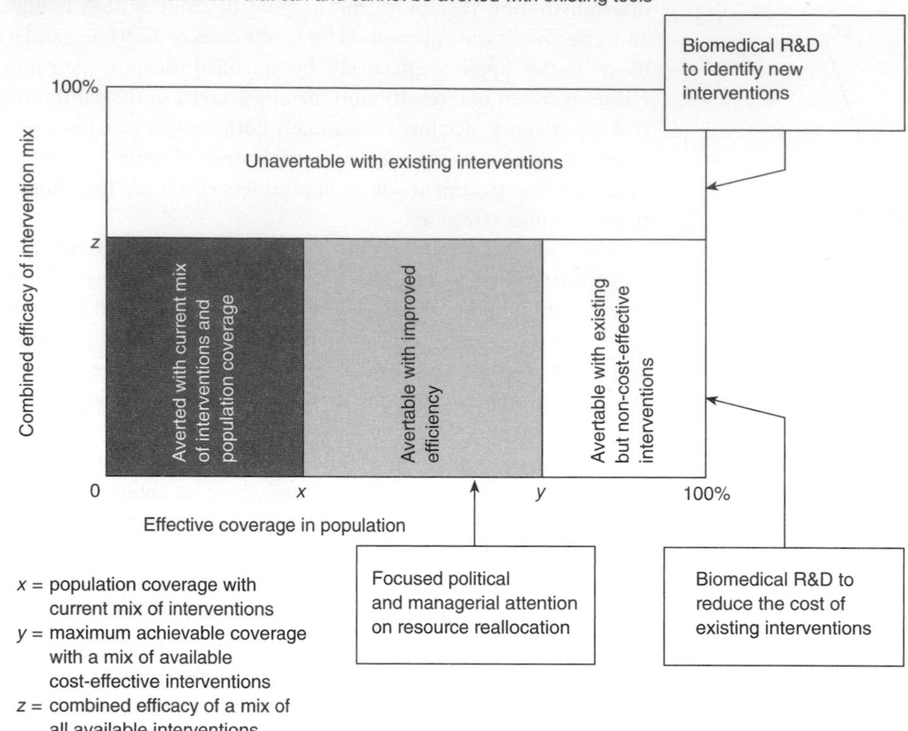

Fig. 2 Analysing the burden of a health problem to identify control and research needs: R&D, research and development.

- What could be averted now with better use of existing cost-effective interventions.
- What could be averted now, but only with interventions that are not cost-effective.
- What cannot be averted with existing interventions but would require new ones.

The analysis is intended to identify where the greatest needs lie, and thereby guide assessment of priorities for different major fixed commitments such as research and development or political attention. The unit of currency employed for this analysis is, once again, the QALY. While such analyses are not intended to suggest that some spurious precision can be achieved in the analysis of need, they do indicate a sense of the approximate distribution of the effort required.

The area of the rectangle in Fig. 2 represents the total estimated disease burden (in QALYs) from a given condition (e.g. diarrhoeal disease), under the counterfactual assumption that current explicit control interventions were not being applied. The horizontal axis represents the extent to which effective treatment is reaching the population, i.e. how far into the population a mix of interventions is penetrating. The vertical axis represents the combined efficacy of this mix. The subdivisions within that square represent different portions of the burden: that which is being averted now by the existing mix of cost-effective interventions among the people that the intervention is reaching, that which could be averted if the existing interventions were used more efficiently, that which could be averted with existing tools, but not cost-effectively, and that which could not be averted with existing interventions. Calculations of the relative share occupied by each subdivision can help to spell out the priorities. For example, where it is calculated that a large portion of the total burden of a certain disease cannot be averted with the existing cost-effective tools, there is a strong case for research and development to develop new ones (if the disease burden is sufficiently large). Where it is calculated that a large fraction of the burden could be averted if existing tools were used more efficiently, and the absolute disease burden is large, there is a strong case for political and managerial attention to achieve fuller employment of available cost-effective interventions. Meltzer (2001) and Kremer (2001) provide valuable discussions of assessing the cost-effectiveness of research and development investments in health.

Non-health outcomes of health interventions

An additional problem in applications concerns interventions that have outcomes outside the health sector. Table 5 lists a number of important examples. Obviously, CEA applied to health outcomes only will understate the overall value of these interventions. While cost–benefit analysis would solve this problem, applicability may be difficult for the reasons previously discussed. Under these circumstances a clear listing of costs, probable health effects, and non-health effects will at least inform the analysis.

Perhaps the clearest examples are the control of smoking, the promotion of breast feeding, and environmental improvements. Limitation of smoking markedly reduces risk for lung cancer, ischaemic heart disease, and chronic obstructive pulmonary disease;

Table 5 Selected interventions with multiple outcomes

Intervention	Outcome		
	Main health outcome	**Secondary health outcome**	**Non-health outcomes**
Provision of water supplies and sanitation	Control of diarrhoeal diseases	Control of skin, respiratory, and helminthic infections	Saving of household time; welfare improvements
Provision of soap	Control of diarrhoeal diseases	Control of skin, respiratory, and helminthic infections	Welfare improvements
Reduction of vehicle speed limits	Reduced severity and incidence of crash-related injuries		Reduction in property damage from vehicle crashes; energy conservation; time costs
Control of smoking	Reduced incidence of lung cancer, heart disease, and chronic obstructive pulmonary disease	Reduced incidence of minor cancers; reduction in burn injuries	Welfare loss for current addicts, welfare gain for non-smokers; freeing of land and labour for uses other than tobacco production
Vector control	Reduced incidence of vector-borne diseases		Improved welfare when vectors, such as mosquitoes, are nuisances
Female education	Reduced child mortality rates	Improved child growth; improved adult health	Higher levels of female productivity and earnings; improved congruence between actual and desired fertility levels
Breast feeding	Improved child growth through improved nutrient availability and protection against diarrhoea	Protection of child against infectious disease; postponement of next pregnancy; possible long-term cognitive benefits to child	Savings in costs of infant formula and bottles; time costs for mother
Family planning services	Reduced child mortality	Reduced maternal morbidity and mortality	Economic and welfare gains from improved control of level and timing of fertility

The discussion of outcome measurement in the text points to the importance of financial risk reduction as an important outcome of intervention that needs to be more explicitly included in CEA

outside the health sector it reduces (at least to some extent) property damage from fire and frees productive resources for alternative use. Likewise, breast feeding has multiple health effects: it enhances child immunity, reduces exposure to infection, provides balanced nutrition, and, by suppressing ovulation, postpones the next pregnancy (Anderson 1990). However, the cost of breast feeding includes, like many health-promoting interventions, substantial amounts of mothers' time, which is not easily valued in terms, say, of wages forgone (Leslie 1992). Finally, whereas environmental interventions have beneficial health consequences, their main objectives may lie outside the health sector; World Bank (1992) provides a comprehensive discussion.

Thus when interventions for health have a range of non-health outcomes, assessment of the attractiveness of these interventions should, ideally, quantitatively aggregate intervention effects along multiple dimensions. Likewise, for clinical intervention there will frequently be joint costs (associated, for one example, with the availability of diagnostic facilities in a district hospital); again, in country-specific application, these matters can be assessed more quantitatively than they can be in a general overview.

The purpose of this section has been to introduce concepts without attempting to provide a detailed discussion of methods. In the next section an extended example of application of CEA is provided both to convey broad substantive lessons and to indicate how CEA has now become a working tool of the health policy analyst. A number of valuable handbooks on methods exist and, as indicated earlier, this chapter is in the spirit of the United States Public Health Services recommendations. Box 1 encapsulates that perspective.

An application: the World Bank Health Sector Priorities Review

In this section we summarize the findings of 25 condition-specific analyses, principally relevant to low- and middle-income countries, which were undertaken for the World Bank's Health Sector Priorities Review (**HSPR**) (Jamison *et al.* 1993). Earlier in this chapter it was noted that dividing interventions into two broad categories—public health and clinical—was conducive to discussing policy trade-offs and this section is so divided. (Table 2 defined what is included in each of these categories.) First we deal with public health interventions, and then with clinical interventions. Unless otherwise specified, the assessments are of incremental cost-effectiveness from an implicitly defined typical starting point, and they are designed to reach

Box 1 United States Public Health Service recommendations on cost-effectiveness analysis

In 1993 the United States Public Health Service convened a Panel on Cost-Effectiveness in Health and Medicine. The Public Health Service asked the Panel to assess the current state of the art of CEA in health and to provide recommendations for the conduct of future studies. Gold *et al.* (1996) bring together the Panel's conclusions, and their Appendix A provides a summary of recommendations. The following extracts provide the highlights of that summary.

Purpose of CEA

CEA evaluates a given health intervention through the use of a 'cost-effectiveness ratio.' In this ratio, all health effects of the intervention (relative to a stated alternative) are captured in the denominator, and changes in resource use (relative to the alternative) are captured in the numerator and valued in monetary terms.

- CEA is an aid to decision-making, not a complete procedure for making resource allocation decisions in health and medicine, because it cannot incorporate all the values relevant to such decisions.

Costs

- The major categories of resource use that should be reflected in the numerator of a cost-effectiveness ratio include costs of health-care services, costs of patient time expended for the intervention, costs associated with care-giving (paid or unpaid), other costs associated with illness such as child care or travel expenses, and costs associated with non-health impacts of the intervention (e.g. on the education system or the environment).
- Time spent seeking care or undergoing an intervention is a resource and a component of the intervention. It should be valued in monetary terms and incorporated in the numerator of a cost-effectiveness ratio. For individuals in the labour force, wages are generally an acceptable measure of time costs.
- In aggregating resource costs across time, CEAs should be conducted in constant dollars that remove general price inflation.
- 'Transfer payments' (e.g. cash transfers from tax payers to welfare recipients) associated with a health intervention redistribute resources from one individual to another. While administrative costs associated with such transfers are included in the numerator of a cost-effectiveness ratio, the transfers themselves are not, as by definition, their impact on the transferer and the recipient cancel out.

Outcome measurement

- Incorporation of morbidity and mortality consequences into a single measure should be accomplished using QALYs. In general, as lives saved or extended by an intervention will not be in perfect health, a saved life-year will count as less than one full QALY.
- In general, community preferences for health states are the appropriate ones for use. If distinct subgroup preferences are identified that will markedly affect a cost-effectiveness ratio, the study should provide this information and conduct sensitivity analyses that reflect this difference.
- The health-related quality of life of those whose lives have been saved or extended by a health intervention may be influenced by characteristics such as age, gender, or race. This may affect the analysis in ways that are ethically problematic. In these instances, sensitivity analyses should be conducted to indicate explicitly how the results are affected by these characteristics.

Discounting

- Costs and health outcomes should be discounted to present value with the shadow-price-of-capital approach to evaluating public investments. This rate (often termed the social rate of time preference) can be approximated by the real rate of return on long-term government bonds, and a real riskless discount rate of 3 per cent is now appropriate. Because of the large number of previous CEAs that have adhered to a discount rate of 5 per cent, analysts should perform sensitivity analyses using 5 per cent. The discount rate should be subject to review, and possible revision, over time in light of significant changes in the underlying economic data.
- Costs and health outcomes should be discounted at the same rate.

Uncertainty

- At a minimum, univariate (one-way) sensitivity analyses should be conducted in order to determine where uncertainty or lack of agreement about some key parameter's value could have substantial impact on the CEA's conclusions.
- Where possible, where parameter uncertainty is a major concern, a reasonable confidence interval should be estimated based on either statistical methods or simulation.

generalizable conclusions rather than to inform decision-making in a specific context. The need for manageability constrained the range of conditions covered; Jamison (1993, pp. 3–4, 6) discusses selection criteria and outcomes for what was viewed as an initial effort. The HSPR reached a number of substantive conclusions and these are discussed to give a sense of the input CEA can make to informing policy.

Five strategies of public health intervention

Public health interventions were organized into five separate strategies in the HSPR: those designed to change personal behaviour, to control environmental hazards, to immunize, to provide mass chemoprophylaxis, and to establish mechanisms for screening and referral. In reviewing health policies, or intervention alternatives, it will often be useful to do so within each of these five broad strategies because of commonalities of logistics, policy instruments, and approaches within each. (This is true despite the frequently great diversity of conditions to be addressed within any one intervention strategy.)

Before turning to the summary of findings, the issue of joint costs (and multiple outcomes) of interventions in light of conclusions from the HSPR are discussed. The analysis upon which the HSPR was based was structured by diseases (or adverse health conditions more generally), and the issues addressed in the individual analyses thus concern the nature, cost, and effectiveness of the interventions available for dealing with each condition. In many cases, of course, any given intervention will address multiple conditions and, indeed, may well have important effects outside the health sector altogether.

Looking across findings of the individual chapters in the HSPR, it is clear that multiple effects and joint cost problems complicate the task of assessing cost-effectiveness in many important instances; that said, it is more generally true that these problems are relatively minor or can be dealt with by reasonable approximations and simplifications in the analysis.

A few general conclusions on each public health approach emerged from the HSPR.

Personal behaviour change

Some personal behaviour changes that are favourable for health outcomes tend to occur naturally as incomes rise; these include, at least for many cultures, improved hygienic behaviours, increased energy intake and quality in the diet, and decreased crowding. Improvements in these behaviours are typically important for the pre-epidemiological transition diseases and can often be affected by educational interventions even though the main force driving improvements—income increases—is beyond the domain of health policy.

Other behaviours are likely either to be less dependent on income levels (e.g. breast-feeding behaviour, sexual practices) or to be adversely influenced by income increases, at least for a period of time (e.g. dietary excess, sedentary lifestyle, smoking, alcohol consumption). Most of these are risk behaviours for post-transition conditions. Although the natural course of development may well improve these behaviours, the HSPR found scope for affordable government policy to influence them. Regulatory policies and, in particular, taxation policies for tobacco, alcohol, and fatty meats show great promise for inducing behavioural change and, currently, are very much underused. Education of elites and the public are complementary instruments, not least because they generate the political will and popular support for regulation and taxation. The extremely high cost-effectiveness of smoking control makes it, perhaps, the top priority for governmental action.

Environmental hazards control

Rising incomes help with improving water supply and sanitation, which are likely to be important in the prevention of a broad range of infectious and parasitic diseases. Specific investments in water supply and sanitation are unlikely because of high costs to be justified in terms of health benefits alone. However, vector control is at least marginally cost-effective for a number of conditions (malaria, onchocerciasis, dengue) in some environments. Industrialization introduces new hazards into the environment (lead, mercury, etc.) that can produce severe lifetime disability if not effectively controlled. Cleaner fuels and improvements in ventilation of indoor fireplaces and cookstoves can substantially reduce risks for chronic obstructive pulmonary disease; and occupational and transport safety measures are important in many specific instances. In principle, protective measures can be delivered through environmental intervention; water fluoridation for the prevention of caries is one example. Another problem is lead toxicity resulting from excess use of lead-based paints and combustion of gasoline with high lead content. Some research (reviewed by Pollitt (1990)) indicates that lead toxicity may be far more important than previously thought as a determinant of slow development and impaired mental functioning.

Immunization, mass chemoprophylaxis, and screening

Interventions that can be characterized under the headings immunization, mass chemoprophylaxis, and screening all share certain common characteristics: they involve the direct administration or application of a specific technical intervention to individuals on a one-by-one basis, they are directed to certain target populations, and the coverage of the target population is important to produce the desired effect. Technically, each of these intervention strategies is highly efficacious when correctly applied to a compliant subject, but their actual effectiveness in developing country settings is strongly conditioned by the local administrative, managerial, and logistical capabilities, as well as by traditional cultural constraints.

Most immunization interventions are highly cost-effective, and many of them address highly prevalent conditions. Measles and tetanus vaccination appear particularly cost-effective and worthy of relatively greater attention within immunization programmes. Far more could be efficiently spent on immunization than is now being spent and, even though costs of delivery tend to rise as more marginal populations are reached, extending immunization programmes to virtually universal coverage is likely to prove both cost-effective and a practical way of significantly improving the health of the poor.

One particularly promising application of mass chemoprophylaxis is the administration of antihelminthic medication and micronutrient supplements to school-age children. Here, cost-effectiveness appears quite high for conditions that, although of extremely high prevalence, have only recently been seen to be of substantial importance for intellectual and physical development. A programme of chemoprophylaxis for school-age children could, like the Expanded Programme on Immunization for younger children, be expected to serve as the starting point for an ultimately much expanded capacity to deal with the health needs of this age group.

Perhaps the most significant cancers for which treatment may be cost-effective (breast, cervical) are those for which early screening and referral are important; therefore, as non-communicable diseases become increasingly significant, this strategy will become increasingly relevant. The emerging strategies for the treatment of acute respiratory infections in children all rely heavily on community-based programmes for early detection and quick referral; with increased experience, improvements in the capacity for cost-effective screening and referral programmes can be expected to develop.

Clinical interventions

Facilities to provide clinical intervention vary continuously in size, in the degree of complexity (and range) of the conditions that they address, in the sophistication of their facilities and equipment, and in the training and skill of their staff. Nonetheless, for conducting comparable CEAs it is useful to use generally accepted terminology in categorizing facilities into three groups (clinic level, district hospitals, and referral hospitals), while recognizing that this categorization involves much simplification and that the appropriate classification structure will vary substantially from country to country. Table 6 indicates (in a very general way), for each of these three levels of facility, examples of the kinds of interventions they might address and

Table 6 Clinical intervention: level of facility and mode of intervention

Level of clinical facility	Typical conditions addressed	Intervention mode			
		Diagnostic	Therapeutic		
			Medical	Surgical	Physical or psychological therapy
Clinic (private, community, and school and work based)	Minor trauma; simple injections; support of population-based interventions; uncomplicated childbirth; family planning	Clinical	Short list of essential drugs (about 20)	Sutures	Important potential role for supervising physical therapy
District hospital	Complicated childbirth fractures and burns; complicated infections; cataract; hernia; appendectomy; diabetes, hypertension, and similarly complex condition	Clinical; basic laboratory; basic radiological facilities	Long list of essential drugs (about 200)	Capacity to deal with abdominal surgery, many fractures, Caesarean sections, and some rehabilitative surgery	Design and management of more complex regimens of physical and psychological therapy
Referral hospital	More complicated medical and surgical conditions	More advanced laboratory and radiological facilities	As above, but also specialized drugs and chemo- and radiotherapy	As above but also capacity for more complicated surgery of head and chest	Support capacity for district hospitals

the capacity such a facility might have for primary modes of diagnostic and therapeutic intervention.

One lesson that emerged from this HPSR is that currently CEA is severely constrained by the paucity of data relating to the effect and cost of clinical interventions in low- and middle-income environments. In the absence of such analyses, it is perhaps natural for developing countries to import, to the extent that resources permit, the methods of case management used or being developed in high-income countries. Of course, the key phrase here is, 'to the extent that resources permit.' Available resources permit the import of high-cost interventions for only a tiny proportion of a developing country's population. In order to extend access to services for the rapidly emerging epidemic of AIDS as well as for the impending epidemic of non-communicable disease, radically lower cost methods of case management will need to be developed from the rich range of technologies and procedures that now exist, or that are coming into being. Several additional observations can be made.

- Curative care for tuberculosis and the sexually transmitted diseases appears to be extremely cost-effective; further, such care is not now being provided to anything like the extent it should be, given the high burden of morbidity and mortality resulting from these conditions. The surgical treatment of cataracts is also highly cost-effective.
- The extremely diverse range of clinical interventions of moderate cost-effectiveness (medical management of angina or diabetes are examples as is surgical management of cervical cancer) suggests that country-specific analyses of these conditions are required and that facilities capable of competently handling diverse conditions will need to be developed.
- The cost is sufficiently high for some clinical interventions to imply that, even if they are effective (as is the case with coronary artery bypass grafting to deal with angina), their marginal cost-effectiveness (in this case relative to medical management) is so poor that their use should be actively discouraged until other more cost-effective interventions can be delivered to their appropriate potential.
- Control of pain from terminal cancer could benefit perhaps 1.5 million individuals annually at acceptable costs; current legislation and standard practices greatly limit what is done in relation to what potentially could be done.
- Rehabilitation (in particular from leprosy, poliomyelitis, and injury) shows promise of being extremely cost-effective, but very little attention has been accorded to rehabilitation and little is known about how best to provide services on a population basis or what might be expected in terms of effectiveness and cost.

Again, as with the discussion of public health interventions, one theme that emerges from this review of clinical intervention cost-effectiveness is that of complexity and diversity. Many interventions are clearly not cost-effective, and public policy should make every effort to discourage their use. However, the available evidence does suggest that a broad range of interventions, addressing a similarly broad range of conditions, will prove cost-effective. Many of these interventions are not now being used to anything like the extent that they should be. Likewise, much of what is currently undertaken by the clinical system is misdirected (towards interventions of low cost-effectiveness) or simply inefficiently used. The redirection of substantial resources from interventions of low cost-effectiveness towards those with very high cost-effectiveness is clearly possible; a central task of health policy must be to design implementation strategies and government policy instruments that can promote these potential efficiency gains.

Table 7 Intervention cost-effectiveness by objective

Cost per QALY	Number[a]	Primary prevention	Secondary prevention	Cure	Rehabilitation	Palliation
< $25	22	10	8	5	0	0
$25–$75	6	2	4	0	0	0
$75–$250	13	4	6	0	2	1
$250–$1000	2	2	0	0	0	0
> $1000	9	2	5	1	3	2
Total	52	20	23	6	5	3

[a]The total number of interventions does not equal the number of objectives, as some interventions have multiple objectives.

Source: Jamison (1993) (on pp. 3, 4, and 6 Jamison discusses the process for selecting conditions to be included and lists major excluded topics).

Lessons from the Health Sector Priorities Review

Five very broad conclusions can be drawn from the HSPR—one methodological and the other four substantive. The methodological conclusion is that it is feasible, on a broad scale, systematically to assess intervention cost-effectiveness in the health sector in a way that can provide broad policy guidance. The effort required is substantial, but results that allow broad intrasectoral assessment of intervention priorities can be obtained.

One substantive conclusion is that the available evidence points to great variation, across interventions, in marginal cost-effectiveness. Tables 7 and 8 summarize this evidence by grouping interventions into ranges of marginal cost per QALY for different intervention objectives (Table 7) and for different public health and clinical approaches (Table 8). The challenge ahead is that of designing and implementing instruments of government policy that will greatly expand use of the interventions in the first several rows of these tables while decreasing use of interventions, like many of those in the last row of the tables, that provide very little value for money.

Garber and Phelps (1997) calculate that under a reasonable range of assumptions it will make economic sense to pay for QALYs up to a cost of about twice the level of per capita income; this leads to a second substantive conclusion from Tables 7 and 8, which is that, in many countries, quite a broad array of specific additional intervention is likely to prove attractive by any reasonable economic standard. (Such intervention could be financed either by reallocation from non-cost-effective interventions within the health sector or from resources outside the sector.)

The third substantive conclusion concerns the extent to which public health as opposed to clinical strategies tend to be more cost-effective and the extent to which seeking primary preventive objectives will tend to be more cost-effective than seeking other objectives (see Table 2 for relevant definitions). Again, Tables 7 and 8 summarize material in ways that allow these questions to be addressed. Although there are some patterns (in particular, primary prevention via immunization accounts for many highly cost-effective interventions), in general it can be concluded that there is no particularly strong general tendency for primary prevention or public health interventions to have superior cost-effectiveness.

The fourth substantive conclusion from the HSPR is that few cost-effective interventions in low- and middle-income countries require more specialized facilities than those available at district hospitals. Thus, even though one cannot argue, in general, in favour of prevention over cure or public health over clinical intervention, one can, at least tentatively, conclude that district hospitals and lower-level facilities potentially offer almost all attractive interventions. A strong caveat here is that relatively few surgical interventions were assessed. Many of the more cost-effective surgical interventions can be done in a district hospital, but some may require referral facilities.

Table 8 Intervention cost-effectiveness by public health and clinical approaches

Cost per QALY	Public health						Clinical	
(US$)	Environmental	Mass chemo-prophylaxis	Immunization	Screening and referral	Behaviour change	Primary care	District hospital	Referral hospital
< 25	1	6	5	0	3	4	3	1
25–75	0	1	1	0	2	1	1	1
75–250	2	0	1	0	2	8	3	0
250–1000	0	0	0	1	1	0	0	0
> 1000	0	0	0	0	0	2	1	4
Total	3	7	7	1	8	15	8	6

Source: Jamison (1993) (on pp. 3, 4, and 6 Jamison discusses the process for selecting conditions to be included and lists major excluded topics).

Conclusions

Multiple methods can provide decision-makers with insights into resource allocation in health; for example, cost-minimization analysis, CEA, and cost–benefit analysis. Methods for undertaking these analyses are now mature, although controversy continues on specific points. Extensive efforts over many years have yielded a large harvest of results. Among the methods in use, CEA appears most relevant for many purposes, but little additional effort may be required to recast results in terms of cost-minimization or cost–benefit analyses. In short, CEA and its relatives have been tested as working tools for the analyst.

That said, much remains to be done that goes beyond specific individual applications, important as those remain. Parallel analyses of a broad array of interventions provide information more than in proportion to the number of interventions. Much of what has caught political attention in CEA has resulted from these larger efforts, although only few exist. Further investment in large comparative studies (taking a number of paradigmatic environments as the base case) will both generate valuable insights directly and serve as solid starting points for more tailored country-specific efforts.

Notes

1. An example of negative intervention may be useful. Many countries now place individuals with severe mental illness in specialized mental hospitals that provide very long-term (and hence expensive) care. An increasingly advocated alternative would be short-term inpatient care in general hospitals combined with long-term medical management on an outpatient basis. Scaling back or closing mental hospitals would gain dollars, possibly at the cost of QALYs. From the perspective of a national decision-maker, assessing the cost-effectiveness of closing down existing facilities is likely to prove more salient than would an exercise that hypothesizes no intervention as the base case and concludes that the health system should have avoided building mental hospitals in the first place. The widespread existence of mental hospitals for long-term care makes generic analysis of the desirability of closing them down valuable (perhaps for several paradigmatic environments).

2. Most procedures for measuring QALYs result in an interval scale of measurement, i.e. a scale unique up to an affine transformation. That is, if q_1 is a utility function resulting from the measurement process, then q_2 will equally well represent that measurement process if $q_2 = a + bq_1$, $b > 0$. Incremental CEA utilizing interval scales will preserve cost-effectiveness ratios under permissible transformations of the utility function. Any attempt at assessing cost-effectiveness in a more absolute way (e.g. not with respect to a stated starting point) will require a scale of measurement that is stronger in the sense that it will need to be unique up to a similarity transformation ($q_2 = bq_1$, $b > 0$) if cost-effectiveness ratios are to be preserved. Such a scale, which has a natural zero that interval scales lack, is called a ratio scale. Use of QALYs or DALYs to measure burden of disease also requires a ratio scale of measurement. The existing literature on utility measurement in health lacks an axiomatic formulation of the conditions under which such a scale will exist and, until such a formulation is undertaken, the theoretical foundation for disease burden measurement will remain shaky. Krantz *et al.* (1971) give a thorough discussion of measurement theory, including a discussion of conditions under which two differently established interval scales on a set of outcomes can be used to generate an underlying ratio scale. These are conditions that indicate when, in the health context, utility measures generated by the time–trade-off method and the standard gamble method on the same set of outcomes would suffice to identify a ratio scale.

3. Existing disease burden studies (and CEAs) discount life-years lost from the life expectancy at the age of death to the present. For reasonable discount rates, this implies that the QALY or DALY loss associated with a death just after birth lies within 20 to 30 per cent of the loss associated with a death at age 20. This ratio differs substantially from the factor of 2 to 4 that has been obtained in the limited number of empirical assessments reported, such as Institute of Medicine (1986). At the same time, deaths before birth are treated as having no loss—at patent variation with human reaction and social willingness to pay to avert late fetal death. This issue is quantitatively important in that there are about 4 million stillbirths annually (2 million of which are in the 12 hours before the expected time of birth). A conceptual approach to dealing with these two problems, and a related complete recalculation of the global burden of disease, appears in Jamison *et al.* (2002). See also Musgrove (1991).

4. Garber (2000) discusses the question of what cost to assign pharmaceuticals (or devices) that are covered by patent. Patents confer temporary monopolies on the patent holders that allow prices to be set at levels often far above the marginal cost of production and packaging. This provides incentives for new product development. If a CEA uses the market price (i.e. monopoly price) of a patented drug as its measure of cost, clearly it cannot properly be considered an incremental CEA. Garber argues that if the CEA is undertaken from a consumer perspective, the practical approach will nonetheless be to use market prices (or whatever price can be negotiated by an influential purchaser) for costs. Pharmaceutical companies often adopt 'tiered' pricing regimes that result in lower prices in low-income countries. This will be profit-maximizing from the company's perspective and will result in patented drug prices in developing countries being much closer to the marginal cost of production, thereby attenuating the problem that Garber raises. For this reason CEAs from a low-income country perspective should not treat patented drugs as tradeables.

5. Practical work in CEA often devotes substantial effort to defining and structuring the set of alternatives (Garber 2000, pp. 193–6). One result will often be to demonstrate that one or more alternatives are in some sense dominated by other alternatives under consideration. Which techniques should be chosen early (i.e. under very tight budget constraints) and which ones should be added later can be assessed. Finally, only in the context of considering closely related options can the attractiveness of a more costly but better technique be assessed. An example comes from an analysis of the attractiveness of coronary artery bypass grafts (**CABG**) in Brazil (Briscoe 1990), which concluded that CABG for disease in the left main coronary artery was a 'good buy' because the cost per QALY was only about 25 per cent of Brazil's

GDP per capita. However, this was the cost per QALY of CABG relative to doing nothing. Medical management and (now) angioplasty are less costly but nonetheless effective alternatives to CABG. The right way to think about CABG is in terms of how much more it would cost than one of these alternatives and how many more QALYs it would buy. It is likely that considered as incremental to alternatives the cost per QALY for CABG would be far higher than the original estimate. Thus the cost-effectiveness of any one intervention can be highly sensitive to the range of alternatives being considered.

6. The extent to which environmental interventions are justified on health grounds varies. While some discussions of air quality, for example, place importance on the amenity value of clean air, others emphasize health consequences. A particularly important example of the need to consider non-health outcomes, in the context of very poor environments, concerns improving water supplies (from the collection of surface water, say, to wells serving a community). Unclean and inadequate water supplies undoubtedly contribute substantially to risks of diarrhoeal and other diseases which kill millions of people every year. Increased quantities of cleaner water will have important health benefits. However, improving water supplies is very costly, and in most circumstances would appear to be non-cost-effective relative to public health or clinical interventions to reduce child mortality; that is, they would appear non-cost-effective if there were no other benefits. Other benefits include time savings (usually for women) in fetching water and the amenity value (beyond the sanitary value) of the cleaner bodies, clothing, and dwellings that improved water supplies facilitate. A cost–benefit analysis, if it were feasible, would place a monetary value on all benefits that would allow combining them. If a cost–benefit analysis cannot be done in an acceptable way, can CEA help to inform decisions? This is probably best done through sensitivity analysis. If all the non-health benefits can be given monetary values, one can calculate the dollar value per QALY that would be required for a satisfactory rate of return to the investment in water supplies. A high value would suggest that the water supply intervention was unattractive. Alternatively, one can calculate the cost of the intervention that would make the cost per QALY of improved water competitive with alternatives for reducing child mortality. If the calculated cost is much less than the actual cost, this would suggest that primary justification for the water-supply investment should be for its other benefits, not its health benefits, even if the other benefits cannot be valued in monetary terms.

7. In many ways the World Bank review is very much in the spirit of several previous reviews (Walsh and Warren 1979, 1986; Ghana Health Assessment Project Team 1981; Walsh 1988). These reviews provide assessments of priorities for the control of communicable childhood diseases in developing countries. The World Bank's effort in 1993 involved more extensive use of economic analysis and covered a much broader range of conditions. Other recent work in this comparative spirit, but emphasizing effectiveness, includes Amler and Dull (1987) and the United States Department of Health and Human Services (1991), which reviewed a broad range of preventive intervention policies for the United States, and, more for clinical preventive services, the United States Preventive Services Task Force (1989) review of the effectiveness of 169 interventions. The state of Oregon in the United States rank ordered over 700 interventions, using cost-effectiveness and other criteria, for the purpose of rationing limited public resources to provide health care for the poor; Strosberg *et al.* (1992) discuss many facets of the Oregon Plan. Patel (1989) reviewed estimates of cost and effectiveness for a range of health interventions for UNICEF, and Jha *et al.* (1998) assessed the relative cost-effectiveness of 40 potentially important interventions in the West African context. The Harvard 'life-saving' project assessed cost per life saved of several hundred preventive options (Tengs *et al.* 1995; Tengs 1996). Udvarhelyi *et al.* (1992) provide a comprehensive review of medical cost-effectiveness and cost–benefit studies from the perspective of their methodological adequacy. All these approaches to the analytic evaluation of health practices fall within the general area of CEA.

8. Once somewhat comparable cost-effectiveness assessments are available for a range of interventions, analyses focusing on only a limited set of interventions can be put into the context provided by existing studies. For example, careful analysis for the sub-Saharan Africa context of malaria control (Goodman *et al.* 1999) and HIV-1 transmission interruption (Kumarayake and Watts 2000) both benefit from and contribute to an increasing understanding of intervention cost-effectiveness in Africa.

9. Health-care expenditures of over $1000 billion in 1997 for the 270 million people of the United States well exceeded the GNP of China ($924 billion) with a population at the time of 1.24 billion. It was over triple the combined GNPs of all the World Bank member countries of sub-Saharan Africa, which have a total population of about 630 million and a combined GNP of only about $323 billion.

10. A separate line of evidence, albeit only suggestive, for inefficiency resulting from variation in marginal cost-effectiveness is the very high degree of observed variation in procedure frequency in somewhat similar environments (Sanders *et al.* 1989).

11. Details are provided in Jamison (1993, Annex tables 1A–3 to 1A–6).

References

Amler, R.W. and Dull, H.B. (ed.) (1987). *Closing the gap: the burden of unnecessary illness.* Oxford University Press, New York.

Anderson, M.A. (1990). Nature and magnitude of the problem of suboptimal breastfeeding practices. Presented at the International Policymakers Conference on Breastfeeding, Florence..

Barnum, H. (1987). Evaluating healthy days of life gained from health projects. *Social Science and Medicine*, **24**, 833–41.

Barnum, H. and Greenberg, E.R. (1993). Cancers. In *Disease control priorities in developing countries* (ed. D.T. Jamison, W.H. Mosley, A.R. Measham, and J.L. Bobadilla), pp. 529–60. Oxford University Press for the World Bank.

Barnum, H, Barlow, R., Fajardo, L., and Pradilla, A. (1980). *A resource allocation model for child survival.* Oeldeschlager, Gunn and Hain, Cambridge, MA.

Barr, N. (1993). *The economics of the welfare state* (2nd edn). Stanford University Press.

Basta, S.S., Soekirman, D.K., and Scrimshaw, N.S. (1979). Iron deficiency anemia and the productivity of adult males in Indonesia. *American Journal of Clinical Nutrition*, **32**, 916–25.

Bleichrodt, H. and Quiggen, J. (1999). Life-cycle preferences over consumption and health. When is cost-effectiveness analysis equivalent to cost–benefit analysis? *Journal of Health Economics*, **18**, 681–708.

Briscoe, J. (1990). *Brazil: the new challenge of adult health*. World Bank, Washington, DC.

Briscoe, J. and de Ferranti, D. (1988). *Water for rural communities*. World Bank, Washington, DC.

Cairns, J. and Johnston, K. (1991). *Condition-specific outcome measures as an alternative to across-programme QALYs*. Health Economics Unit, University of Aberdeen.

Cropper, M.L., Aydede, S.K., and Portney, PR. (1992). Rates of time preference for saving lives. *American Economic Review*, **82**, 469–72.

Devarajan, S., Squire, L., and Sutchiwart-Naruput, S. (1997). Beyond rate of return: reorienting project appraisal. *World Bank Research Observer*, **12**, 35–46.

Drummond, M.F. (ed.) (1987*a*). *Economic appraisal of health technology in the European Community*. Oxford University Press.

Drummond, M.F. (1987*b*). Methods for economic appraisal of health technology. In *Economic appraisal of health technology in the European Community* (ed. M.F. Drummond). Oxford University Press.

Drummond, M.F., O'Brien, B.J., Stoddart, G.L., and Torrance, G.W. (1997). *Methods for the economic evaluation of health care programs* (2nd edn). Oxford University Press.

EuroQol Group (1990). EuroQol—a new facility for the measurement of health-related quality of life. *Health Policy*, **16**, 199–208.

Fallowfield, L. (1990). *The quality of life*. Souvenir Press, London.

Feachem, R.G.A., Kjellstrom, T., Murray, C.J.L., Over, M., and Phillips, M.A. (1992). *The health of adults in the developing world*. Oxford University Press, New York.

Fox-Rushby, J.A. and Hanson, K. (2001). Calculating and presenting disability-adjusted life years in cost-effectiveness analysis. *Health Policy and Planning*, **16**, 326–31.

Garber, A.M. (2000). Advances in CE analysis. In *Handbook of health economics* (ed. J.P. Newhouse and A.J. Culyer), pp. 181–221. Elsevier, Amsterdam.

Garber, A.M. and Phelps, C.E. (1997). Economic foundations of cost-effectiveness analysis. *Journal of Health Economics*, **16**, 1–31.

Garber, A.M., Weinstein, M.C., Torrance, G.W., and Kamlet, M.S. (1996). Theoretical foundations of cost-effectiveness analysis. In *Cost-effectiveness in health and medicine* (ed. M.R. Gold, J.E. Siegel, L.B. Russell, and M.C. Weinstein), pp. 25–53. Oxford University Press, New York.

Ghana Health Assessment Project Team (1981). Quantitative method of assessing the health impact of different diseases in less developed countries. *International Journal of Epidemiology*, **10**, 73–80.

Gold, M.R., Siegel, J.E., Russell, L.B., and Weinstein, M.C. (ed.) (1996). *Cost-effectiveness in health and medicine*. Oxford University Press, New York.

Goodman, C.A., Coleman, P.G., and Mills, A.J. (1999). Cost-effectiveness of malaria control in sub-Saharan Africa. *Lancet*, **354**, 378–85.

Institute of Medicine (1986). *New vaccine development, establishing priorities*, Vols 1 and 2. National Academy Press, Washington, DC.

Jamison, D.T. (1993). Disease control priorities in developing countries: an overview. In *Disease control priorities in developing countries* (ed. D.T. Jamison, W.H. Mosley, A.R. Measham, and J.L. Bobadilla), pp. 3–34. Oxford University Press for the World Bank.

Jamison, D.T. and Lumsden, K.G. (1975). Television and efficiency in higher education. *Management Science*, **21**, 920–30.

Jamison, D.T., Mosley, W.H., Measham, A.R., and Bobadilla, J.L. (ed.) (1993). *Disease control priorities in developing countries*. Oxford University Press for the World Bank.

Jamison, D.T., Jamison, J., Bobadilla, J.L., and Zupan, J. (2002). A recalculation of the global burden of disease: estimates are highly sensitive to assumptions about events around the time of birth. In preparation.

Jha, P., Bangura, O., and Ransom, K. (1998). The cost-effectiveness of forty health interventions in Guinea. *Health Policy and Planning*, **13**, 249–62.

Johannesson, M. (1992). On the discounting of gained life-years in cost-effectiveness analysis. *International Journal of Technology Assessment in Health Care*, **8**, 359–64.

Johannesson, M. and Meltzer, D. (1998). Some reflections on cost-effectiveness analysis. *Health Economics*, **7**, 1–7.

Johannesson, M. and Weinstein, M.C. (1993). On the decision rules of cost-effectiveness analysis. *Journal of Health Economics*, **12**, 459–67.

Jones-Lee, M.W. (1994). Safety and the saving of life, the economics of safety and physical risk. In *Cost–benefit analysis* (ed. R. Layard and S. Glaister), pp. 290–318. Cambridge University Press.

Kaplan, R.M. and Bush, J. (1982). Health-related quality of life measurement for evaluation research and policy analysis. *Health Psychology*, **2**, 61–80.

Krantz, D.H., Luce, D.R., Suppes, P., and Tversky, A. (1971). *Foundations of measurement*. Vol. I, *Additive and polynomial representations*. Academic Press, New York.

Kremer, M. (2001). Public policies to stimulate development of vaccines and drugs for neglected diseases. Department of Economics, Harvard University.

Kumaranayake, L. and Watts, C. (2000). Economic costs of HIV/AIDS prevention activities in sub-Saharan Africa. *AIDS*, **14** (Supplement 3), S239–52.

Last, J.M. (ed.) (1988). *A dictionary of epidemiology* (2nd edn). Oxford University Press, New York, for the International Epidemiological Association.

Layard, R. and Glaister, S. (1994). Introduction. In *Cost–benefit analysis* (ed. R. Layard and S. Glaister), pp. 1–56. Cambridge University Press.

Leslie, J. (1989). Women's time: a factor in the use of child survival technologies? *Health Policy and Planning*, **4**, 1–16.

Leslie, J. (1992). Women's time and the use of health services. *IDS Bulletin*, **23**, 4–7.

Levin, H.M., Pollitt, E., Galloway, R., and McGuire, J. (1993). Micronutrient deficiency disorders. In *Disease control priorities in developing countries* (ed. D.T. Jamison, W.H. Mosley, A.R. Measham, and J.L. Bobadilla), pp. 421–54. Oxford University Press for the World Bank.

Luce, B.R., Manning, W.G., Siegel, J.E., and Lipscomb, J. (1996). Estimating costs in cost-effectiveness analysis. In *Cost-effectiveness in health and medicine* (ed. M.R. Gold, L.B. Russell, J.E. Siegel, and M.C. Weinstein), pp. 176–213. Oxford University Press, New York.

Meltzer, D. (2001). Addressing uncertainty in medical cost-effectiveness analysis. Implications of expected utility maximization for methods to perform sensitivity analysis and the use of cost-effectiveness to set priorities for research. *Journal of Health Economics*, **20**, 109–29.

MMWR (1992). Years of potential life lost before ages 65 and 85—United States, 1989–1990. *Morbidity and Mortality Weekly Report*, **41**, 313–15.

Mosley, W.H. and Jolly, R. (1987). Health policy and program options, compensating for the negative effects of economic adjustment. In *Adjustment with a human face* (ed. G.A. Cornea, R. Jolly, and F. Stewart). Clarendon Press, Oxford.

Murray, C.J., Evans, D., Acharya, A., and Baltussen, R. (1999). *Development of WHO guidelines on generalised cost-effectiveness analysis*. GPE Discussion Paper 4, WHO, Geneva.

Murray, C. J., Jamison, D.T., and Lopez, A.D. (1994). The global burden of disease in 1990: summary results, sensitivity analysis and future directions. *Bulletin of the World Health Organization*, **72**, 495–509.

Musgrove, P. (1991). *The burden of death at different ages: assumptions, parameters and values*. Occasional Paper 12, Latin America and the

Caribbean Regional Office, Human Resources Division, Technical Department, World Bank, Washington, DC.

Musgrove, P. (1995). Cost-effectiveness and the socialization of health care. *Journal of Health Policy*, **32**, 111–23.

Nord, E. (1991). The relevance of QALYs in prioritizing between different patients. Presented at the 12th Nordic HESG meeting, Copenhagen.

Over, M. (1988). *Cost-effective integration of immunization and basic health services in developing countries: the problem of joint costs.* Working Paper 23, World Bank, Washington, DC.

Patel, M.S. (1989). *Eliminating social distance between North and South: cost-effective goals for the 1990s.* Staff Working Paper 5, UNICEF, New York.

Pauly, M.V. (1995). Valuing health care benefits in money terms. In *Valuing health care: costs, benefits, and effectiveness of pharmaceuticals and other medical technologies* (ed. F.A. Sloan), pp. 99–124. Cambridge University Press.

Phelps, C.E. and Mushlin, A.I. (1991). On the (near) equivalence of cost-effectiveness and cost–benefit analysis. *International Journal of Technology Assessment in Health Care*, **7**, 12–21.

Pollitt, E. (1990). *Malnutrition and infection in the classroom.* UNESCO, Paris.

Preston, S.H. (1991). Health indexes and health sector planning. Presented at the Workshop on the Policy and Planning Implications of the Epidemiological Transition in Developing Countries, National Research Council, Washington, DC.

Rosser, R.M. and Kind, P. (1978). A scale of valuations of states of illness, is there a social consensus? *International Journal of Epidemiology*, **7**, 347–58.

Sanders, D., Coulter, A., and McPherson, K. (1989). *Variation in hospital admission rates: a review of the literature.* Paper 79, Kings Fund, London.

Skinner, J. and McClellan, M. (2000). *The incidence of Medicaid.* Working paper, National Bureau of Economic Research, New York.

Sloan, F.A. and Conover, C.J. (1995). The use of cost-effectiveness/cost-benefit analysis in actual decision making, current status and prospects. In *Valuing health care, costs, benefits, and effectiveness of pharmaceuticals and other medical technologies* (ed. F.A. Sloan), pp. 207–32. Cambridge University Press.

Squire, L. (1989). Project evaluation in theory and practice. In *Handbook of development economics*, Vol. 2 (ed. H.B. Chenery and T.N. Srinivasan). North-Holland, Amsterdam.

Stern, N. and Ferreira, F. (1997). The World Bank as intellectual actor. In *The World Bank: its first half century*. Vol. 2, *Perspectives* (ed. D. Kapur, J.P. Lewis, and R. Webb), pp. 523–609. Brookings Institution, Washington, DC.

Strosberg, M.A., Weiner, J.M., Baker, R., Fein, I.A. (ed.) (1992). *Rationing America's medical care: the Oregon Plan and beyond.* Brookings Institution, Washington, DC.

Stouthard, M.E., *et al.* (1997). *Disability weights for diseases in The Netherlands.* Department of Public Health, Erasmus University, Rotterdam.

Tan-Torres, T. (1990). *Comparison of different methods of eliciting utilities for outcome states in leprosy.* Clinical Epidemiology Unit, Department of Medicine, University of the Philippines, Manila.

Tengs, T.O. (1996). Enormous variation in the cost-effectiveness of prevention: implications for public policy. *Public Health*, **2**, 13–17.

Tengs, T.O., Adams, M.E., and Pliskin, J.S. (1995). Five-hundred life-saving interventions and their cost-effectiveness. *Risk Analysis*, **15**, 369–90.

Tolley, G., Kenkel, D., and Fabian, R. (ed.) (1994). *Valuing health for policy: an economic approach.* University of Chicago Press.

Udvarhelyi, I.S., Colvitz, G.A., Rai, A., and Epstein, A.M. (1992). Cost-effectiveness and cost–benefit analyses in the medical literature. *Annals of Internal Medicine*, **116**, 238–44.

USDHHS (US Department of Health and Human Services) (1991). *Healthy people 2000: national health promotion and disease prevention objectives.* US Government Printing Office, Washington, DC.

US Preventive Services Task Force (Chairman, R.S. Lawrence) (1989). *Guide to clinical preventive services.* Williams & Wilkins, Baltimore, MD.

Vicusi, W.K. (1993). The value of risks to life and health. *Journal of Economic Literature*, **31**, 1912–46.

Wagstaff, A. (1994). Health care, QALYs and the equity–efficiency tradeoff. In *Cost–benefit analysis* (ed. R. Layard and S. Glaister), pp. 428–47. Cambridge University Press.

Walsh, J.A. (1988). *Establishing health priorities in the developing world.* Adams, Boston, MA, for the United Nations Development Program.

Walsh, J.A. and Warren, K.S. (1979). Selective primary health care—an interim strategy for disease control in developing countries. *New England Journal of Medicine*, **301**, 967–74.

Walsh, J.A. and Warren, K.S. (ed.) (1986). *Strategies for primary health care: technologies appropriate for the control of disease in the developing world.* University of Chicago Press.

Watts, C. and Kumaranayake, L. (1999). Thinking big: scaling up HIV-1 interventions in sub-Saharan Africa. *Lancet*, **354**, 1492.

Weinstein, M.C. (1995). From cost-effectiveness ratios to resource allocation: where to draw the line? In *Valuing health care: costs, benefits, and effectiveness of pharmaceuticals and other medical technologies* (ed. F.A. Sloan), pp. 77–97. Cambridge University Press.

Weinstein, M.C. and Stason, W.B. (1977). Foundations of cost-effectiveness analysis for health and medical practices. *New England Journal of Medicine*, **296**, 716–21.

Weinstein, N.D. (1989). Optimistic biases about personal risks. *Science*, **246**, 1232–33.

Wells, K.B. (1999). The design of partners in care: evaluating the cost-effectiveness of improving care for depression in primary care. *Social Psychiatry and Psychiatric Epidemiology*, **34**, 20–9.

WHO (1996). *Investing in health research and development.* Report of the Ad Hoc Committee on Health Research Relating to Future Intervention Options. Document TDR/Gen/96.1, WHO, Geneva.

WHO (2000). *World health report 2000. Health systems: improving performance.* WHO, Geneva.

World Bank (1992). *World development report 1992. Development and the environment.* World Bank, Washington, DC.

World Bank (1993). *World development report 1993 Investing in health.* World Bank, Washington, DC.

Zeckhauser, R. and Shepard, D. (1976). Where now for saving lives? *Law and Contemporary Problems*, **40**, 5–45.

7.7 Management and public health

David J. Hunter

> To be sure, the fundamental task of management remains the same: to make people capable of joint performance through common goals, common values, the right structures, and the training and development they need to perform and to respond to change. (Drucker 1990)

If, as the management specialist Peter Drucker claims, 'management world-wide has become the new social function' (Drucker 1990) then this has profound implications for all organizations whether in the business or service sectors. Regardless of whether organizations exist for profit or are non-profit, the responsibilities of the managers running them are essentially the same. They include defining strategy and goals, developing people, measuring performance, and marketing the organization's services. But this is not to suggest that there are universal ways of managing, or that what works in the private sector must also apply to the public sector. As will be shown, simplistic assumptions about management are not helpful in the context of health care. Arguably, the sector has already endured through successive waves of reform the passing fashions of management consultants with little evidence of sustained success.

Within the health sector, there has been a global revolution in the organization of health services. Management has been held up as the principal instrument through which the supply-side objectives of the reforms can be achieved as well as those which seek to shift the emphasis in health policy away from an exclusive concentration on health services and towards the notion of health in its wider sense. In both these spheres public health is seen as having a critical contribution to make to the management task.

The relationship between management, planning, and public health has been a long-standing, and at times difficult, one. In modern health-care systems, public health needs management more than ever but this reliance, not always recognized or accepted, often causes offence or a feeling of unease because it is regarded in some quarters as leading to unacceptable compromise in respect of the scientific knowledge-based bedrock of the specialty of public health medicine. There is no equivalent science of managing since management is contingent upon particular circumstances and contexts and has no universal application. Hardly surprising, therefore, that considerable ambivalence exists in the relationship between public health and management.

The tension set up by the public health medicine ethos of rational scientific inquiry on the one hand and the management ethos of making change happen on the other can be entirely healthy and creative since the excesses of one can be tempered by those of the other. For instance, sometimes management is about achieving change for which there exists no (or incomplete) evidence that it is the right thing to do or will even work. Conversely, public health specialists have been variously accused of not acting on the results of their scientific enquiries, or of taking too long to complete these when the need for action is pressing, and of being managerially weak or incompetent especially when it comes to the need for political skills in winning support for a particular line of action. The consequence has often been a failure to implement policies or to manage change effectively.

But the relevance of management 'science' and planning for public health can only be established if they are seen to contribute to public health's primary purpose of improving the health of populations. Recent developments in management in many health-care systems around the world which have undergone, are undergoing, or can expect to undergo reform create particular difficulties for public health. During the late 1980s and for most of the 1990s, these centred on market models aimed at improving efficiency through competition, and directed towards the needs and preferences of individual consumers or users of services rather than the needs of communities or populations. Despite a move in the late 1990s away from market-style mechanisms to more collaborative forms of working with a stress on partnerships, the tension between meeting the needs of populations on the one hand and those (plus demands and wants) of the individual on the other poses a special challenge to public health practitioners and managers charged with the task of finding an acceptable balance between them.

Debates about priority-setting or rationing are especially acute at the interface between the individual as consumer and as citizen.

Against this broad context, this chapter is organized into four sections. The first section reviews the notion of management and the management process in general terms. The second considers the evolution of management in the context of health policy and health sector reform in recent years. The third section looks critically at the relationship between public health and management and develops the points made in the two preceding sections. A final section attempts to pull the arguments together and looks ahead to a new synthesis between public health and management in the context of global developments in health-care systems. The implications of these developments for management education, training, and development for public health, and the need for change in these, are considered.

Management and the management process

What is management?

Management is often thought of as a bag of techniques or tools and as a set of particular skills with which those undertaking management need to be equipped. These skills cover planning, financing, personnel, marketing, and contracting. While important, they are not a substitute for the 'softer' dimensions of management that stress the importance of essential principles and core values. All too often these cultural aspects are given insufficient attention or are ignored altogether. The 'hard' and 'soft' sides of management must go hand in hand, with prior attention being given to principles and values.

Management thus has four dimensions:

- the culture, principles, and values of management
- the structure of management
- the techniques employed by managers
- the setting, or infrastructure, of management.

Each of these dimensions is considered briefly in turn.

The culture of management

The culture of management is made up of the attitudes and values that help set a pattern of behaviour for actions and opinions. What managers do may be more or less the same in different organizations and countries; how they do it may be quite different. The most important principles and values are as follows.

1. Management is about people—its task is to make people capable of performing jointly, to make their strengths effective and their weaknesses irrelevant.
2. Management is about securing commitment to shared values—its primary task is to think through, set, and exemplify those objectives, values, and goals to which all those working in organizations subscribe.
3. Management is about developing staff—its task is to provide continuous training and development for all members of the workforce.
4. Management is about achieving results—in a hospital, for instance, results are healed or comforted patients.

Traditional notions of management or administration, particularly in respect of public services, placed the stress on a number of core values such as honesty, fairness, prevention of distortion, inequity, bias, and abuse of office. These values emphasized process controls rather than output controls. In other words, due process was arguably more important than the outputs to be expected from the managerial/administrative arrangements in place. How the job was done was as, or more, important than the results from it.

Conceptions of management since the late 1980s have progressively placed the emphasis on ends rather than means, even if these might be achieved at the expense of guarantees of honesty, neutrality, and fair dealing. It assumes a culture of (public service) honesty as given. In loosening up management, and blurring the division between public and private sectors, in keeping with the latest fashion for public–private partnerships, the extent to which the new management is likely to induce corrosion in terms of the traditional values listed above remains to be tested. Something of a watershed was reached in Britain in 1994 when the issue of corporate governance rose to the top of the health policy agenda in the midst of enquiries by the House of Commons Public Accounts Committee into allegations of fraud and corruption in the British National Health Service (**NHS**), particularly in the period since the 1991 reforms (NHS Executive 1994). The next section returns to this issue of the new management.

Management structure

The structure of management refers to the way organizations are designed. They range from tight bureaucratic structures, with clear command and control relationships and strict rules (that is, closed systems), to loose networks with a large degree of discretionary decision-making (that is, open systems). In between, variants such as project-based and matrix structures may be found. Current notions of management favour increasing individuals' opportunities to make *ad hoc* decisions, that is, empowering them by loosening up the rules and processes to be followed, while at the same time tightening the control of results. Individuals, organizations, and systems are held accountable for the choices and decisions they make in this loose–tight arrangement—one that is loose about means, tight about ends.

In a political context, and most health-care systems find themselves in one to a greater or lesser degree, the purity of the management response can become contaminated by higher level political factors which cannot be ignored. So, even if it makes managerial sense to be tight about ends and loose about means, political reality may dictate the precise opposite, or may even result in abandoning the loose–tight distinction in favour of a tight–tight regime. Governments favouring a centralized, command-and-control system of policy-making and implementation, in order to deliver on their election promises and because they may genuinely, if somewhat naively, believe it is the way to effect change, are vulnerable to such distortions.

Management techniques

Management techniques amount to a bag of tools that managers should master and a range of competencies with which they need to be familiar to be effective. These include in no particular order:

- communication skills (consultation, negotiation, and conflict management)
- management by objectives
- human resource management
- economics, finance, and accounting
- (strategic) planning and marketing
- project management
- quality assurance.

To be able to participate in needs assessment and issues concerning clinical effectiveness and health outcomes, which constitute a major component of the management challenge in health care, health-care managers also need knowledge about public health.

Setting

The setting in which the manager operates is made up of the physical infrastructure such as buildings and technology (especially information technology). These matters are beyond the scope of this chapter and are not considered further.

Models of management

There are four 'world-views', or doctrines, about the management of organizations (Moore 1996) as follows:

- traditional bureaucracy—with an emphasis on clear structure, hierarchical chains of command, clear accountability for performance
- new public management—with an emphasis on making organizations more like firms operating in markets through the introduction of competition to improve performance (Hood 1991)
- 'Japanese' organization model or 'clan'—'solidarity' model of organization in which a sense of identity with, and pride in, the organization itself is the main source of motivation
- professionalism—shares the 'Japanese' model's assumption that people work better when they are trusted and their performance is not closely monitored; the sense of identity is with the profession rather than with the organization, or possibly dual loyalty to both exists.

The central point about these world-views, or doctrines, is that management is not a purely technical enterprise. Ideas, culture, and ideologies make a real difference.

Within many health-care systems undergoing reform, there has been a shift from models of traditional bureaucracy and professionalism to a model of new public management where the emphasis is on encouraging public bureaucracies to mimic some of the 'successful' features of private sector management practices. These include government and public services steering more and rowing less, being mission-driven rather than rule bound, and being more responsive to the customer and to quality (Osborne and Gaebler 1993).

Although some of the competitive elements of new public management are out of favour with health-care reformers in the late 1990s who are talking the language of partnership and joined-up management, much of the ethos, and many of the principles, of new public management remain alive. For instance, the focus on managing for outcomes and on insisting that professionals be managed and held to account for their practices and the resources they consume continues to hold sway among policy-makers.

While elements of new public management thinking seem entirely appropriate for particular aspects of health-care activities, some commentators believe that it is misleading to regard it as a generic solution for every management design problem within the health sector or, indeed, elsewhere in the public sector (Stewart 1998; Hunter 1999). In particular, it is a mistake to overlook the professional nature of the majority of any health-care system's work. Other management models may be more appropriate in the conduct of professional work. Later sections return to the limitations of a new public management approach in health care.

It cannot be said that a science or profession of management exists (see below) but a number of attributes can be identified which collectively attempt to define public management and its distinctive features. These are that it should

- be close to the citizen and customer
- be able to learn from a changing environment and apply that learning
- be capable of using that learning to determine strategy and policy direction
- work through political processes that steer management action
- devolve responsibility and sharpen accountability
- continually review performance.

Public management possessing these attributes is concerned with survival and with being adaptable. It stresses multiple objectives, teamwork, high trust relationships, and sharing information. It requires skilled managers who can operate appropriately in situations of extreme political uncertainty, ambiguity, and continuous change. Most health-care systems, and the function of public health within them, possess these features in abundance.

A key issue when considering management in a health-care context is the extent to which health-care organizations, whether publicly funded or not, and their management can be regarded as unique or at least different from other types of organizations, in particular from industrial or business organizations. Shortell and Kaluzny (1983) believe they are different and list the key differences as follows:

- defining and measuring output are difficult
- the work involved is felt to be more highly variable and complex than in other organizations
- more of the work is of an emergency and non-deferrable nature
- the work permits little tolerance for ambiguity or error
- the work activities are highly interdependent, requiring a high degree of co-ordination among diverse professional groups
- the work involves an extremely high degree of specialization
- organizational participants are highly professional, and this primary loyalty belongs to the profession rather than to the organization
- there exists little effective organizational or managerial control over the group most responsible for generating work and expenditure: clinicians
- in many health-care organizations, particularly hospitals, there exist dual lines of authority, which create problems of co-ordination and accountability, and confusion of roles.

The uniqueness of health-care organizations can be overstated, especially if this implies that little can be done to improve managerial performance in the face of deep-seated and unique impediments. Yet, as Shortell and Kaluzny acknowledge, health-care organizations may at least be unusual, if not unique, in their possession of the above characteristics in combination: 'It is the confluence of professional, technological, and task attributes that makes the management of health-care organizations particularly challenging'.

The independence of professionals from managerial control is less of a problem in situations where output is readily defined and measured. It is a rather different situation, as in health-care systems, when clear performance criteria do not exist and yet external bodies hold the organization responsible for the activities of the relatively independent group of professionals. Public health doctors stand somewhere in the middle of this complex of centripetal and centrifugal forces and are often placed in the position of trying to secure an effective accommodation between the requirements of the managerial domain on the one hand and those of the professional domain on the other. Indeed, it is this continuous struggle between these two domains which lies at the heart of successive reorganizations of health-care systems around the world, particularly those witnessed in European and Australasian countries over the past 10 years or so. This argument is developed further below in the light of the 'cult of managerialism' which has become a universal feature of virtually all health-care systems.

The managerial role

The literature on management is rich and diverse. A brief synopsis is offered of key developments in the conception of management and organizations. Classical theorists, such as Taylor (1911), viewed organizations in strictly rational, formal, and closed-system terms. They sought to formulate universal principles which would apply in all circumstances. These principles of scientific management consisted of:

- programming the job
- choosing the right person to match the job
- training the person to do the job.

Weber (1978) took these rational principles further in terms of developing the ideal bureaucratic organization governed by a set of five clear rules and requirements:

- the organization is guided by explicit specific procedures for governing activities
- activities are distributed among office holders
- offices are arranged in a hierarchical authority structure
- candidates are selected on the basis of their technical competence
- officials carry out their functions in an impersonal fashion.

The aim was to apply the rules in such a way as to ensure uniformity of practice and standards, and impersonality in the fair and equitable application of the rules and standards. Managerial initiative and creativity (sometimes referred to as entrepreneurial flair) were seen to be stifled by such rigidities. Moreover, the formal organization was seen as the 'one best way' to structure an organization and it made no allowance for the informal organization which existed alongside the formal organization and was often responsible for what actually happened in practice. Whereas the formal organization was regarded as rational and functional, the informal organization was seen as irrational and dysfunctional.

The closed-system rational model of organization with its principles of management has been powerful in terms of its influence on successive generations of managers and on writers about management. It still lies at the heart of some conceptions of operations research and management. While possessing severe limitations, which natural or organic system theories have challenged, most health-care organizations are organized and managed to some degree along bureaucratic lines. The natural or open-system approach developed as a reaction against the rigidities and other limitations of the rational, closed-system approach.

The rational model of management is based on three stages which are considered to be necessary in the realization of a rationally calculated decision:

- the decision-maker considers all of the alternative courses of action that are open
- her or she identifies and evaluates all of the consequences which would flow from the adoption of each alternative
- he or she selects that alternative the public consequences of which would be preferable in terms of his or her most valued ends.

Above all, a rational decision entails clarity and agreement about goals and objectives, and a search for the best possible means of attaining them. The development, and application, of management techniques like cost–benefit analysis, programme planning budgeting, management by objectives, operational research, corporate planning, and zero-based budgeting illustrate the successive attempts by reformers to find ways to bring decision-making more in line with the rational model.

Although these and other techniques, usually offered by management consultants and economists, are intended to enable a rational choice to be made among a range of alternatives, in fact few of the techniques make an impact on actual decisions for the simple reason that the demands of rational analysis are in practice too great despite the sincerest efforts to achieve it.

A rational model, as Allison (1971) has suggested, presupposes the existence of a consensus within an organization among decision-makers. The greater the degree of rationality in a decision process, the greater the emphasis on consensus, harmony, a corporate approach to decision-making, and 'technical' criteria for the evaluation of proposals. Allison's rational actor model sees choices in any field of decision-making as being clearly defined and based on rational assessments of public desires—it is merely a matter of fulfilling well-defined goals in an optimal manner. Decisions taken within the framework of the rational actor model reflect a single, coherent, and consistent set of calculations about particular problems. The possibility of organizational and political complications fouling the smooth-running machine simply do not enter into the model's orbit, largely because rational models are normative and prescriptive rather than descriptive.

Although of limited value in illuminating how managers operate and decisions are taken, and although inclined to obscure rather than to reveal, an appreciation of rationality can provide further understanding of the management process. The structure of most organizations, including health-care systems, is largely derived from rational theories. Moreover, these theories underlie the public language in which politicians and policy-makers must argue and provide the legitimation of their bargains from whatever motives and interests these result. Similarly, managers may make decisions by doing deals but they would still be obliged to argue in the language of a rational model of the organization's interests. Adherence to a rational paradigm remains strong, if only symbolically.

But, in the end, a rational model is flawed because it assumes a unitary view of organizational and managerial relationships and that all those making decisions identify with, and share in, a common superordinate goal. In the case of health services such a goal could be the welfare of patients. Tensions, or clashes of interest, between stakeholders are perceived as irrational and are defined as 'technical' problems—for example, a failure in communication, poor information, incomplete analysis, and so on. The unitary perspective denies the existence of sectional interests and is therefore unable to account for the activities and influence of such interests. To do so, a pluralist perspective is required which acknowledges the coexistence of various groups each with its own objectives and interests to pursue.

Not until the late 1950s did the balance begin to shift as a result of a series of studies which sought to focus rather more attention on possible impediments to the efficiency and effectiveness of management and organizational structures. Rational structures of decision-making and managerial control as the primary determinants of organizational life were challenged on the grounds that the empirical evidence from a variety of studies did not support this view of how organizations worked in practice. 'Scientific management' was shown to be severely defective in its explanatory power.

The growth and maturation of the social sciences in the late 1950s marked a new departure in organization and management studies. It was led by Crozier (1964), Simon (1957), March and Simon (1958), Burns and Stalker (1961), and Vickers (1968). These and other studies all attached importance to the existence of alternative systems of management, one appropriate to relatively stable technological and market conditions (the 'mechanistic' system of management articulated by Burns and Stalker), and the other to situations in which technology and market factors were changing fairly rapidly (the 'organic' system of management). They also demonstrated the importance of concepts like 'bounded rationality', 'satisficing', and 'appreciative judgement' in governing the actions of managers since there were cognitive limits on rationality which lead to the adoption of devices to assist the decision-making process. In the 1960s, an important book appeared—*Psychiatric Ideologies and Institutions* (Strauss *et al.* 1964). This introduced the concept of 'negotiated order' within organizations whereby the various stakeholders in large psychiatric hospitals had quite different ideas about the appropriate management and care of patients. There had to be some accommodation among these and this was achieved through a process of negotiation. There was a recognition that organizations comprise disparate decentralized units in which the actors perform with different perspectives and priorities, and decisions are made by much pulling and hauling among them and not by a single rational choice.

In later studies of organization and management, the role of politics and power was seen as critically important in the achievement of goals (Bachrach and Baratz 1962, 1963, 1970; Pfeffer 1981, 1992). For Pfeffer, problems of implementation and management failure are 'problems in developing political will and expertise—the desire to accomplish something, even against opposition, and the knowledge and skills that make it possible to do so' (Pfeffer 1992). Accomplishing change in organizations requires more than an ability to solve technical or analytical problems. Because change threatens the status quo or a group of stakeholders (possibly more than one), it becomes essential to understand organizational politics if one is to manage change effectively and steer it in the desired direction. Pfeffer warns against ignoring the social realities of power and influence. Unless and until we come to terms with these, then organizational and managerial paralysis, that is, the failure to mobilize sufficient political support to take action, will become more evident. In place of implementing decisions, managers will spend endless amounts of time and energy on the decision-making process.

The concern with understanding organizational politics and power centred, as noted above, on the problem of implementation. Pressman and Wildavsky (1972), in a classic study of the issue, raised awareness of the importance of implementation as an area for study, especially in the context of policy-making. Implementation is not a passive process, faithfully enacting a policy. It inevitably reformulates the policy at the same time. Pfeffer (1992) argues that implementation is becoming more difficult because:

- changing social norms and greater interdependence within organizations have made traditional, formal authority less effective than it once was
- developing a common vision is increasingly difficult in organizations comprised of heterogeneous members.

Pfeffer maintains that managing power is an essential requirement in the achievement of desired goals. A number of steps are involved as follows (Pfeffer 1992).

1. Decide what your goals are, what you are trying to accomplish.
2. Diagnose patterns of dependence and interdependence: which individuals are influential and important in achieving your goal?
3. What are their points of view likely to be? How will they feel about what you are trying to do?
4. What are their power bases? Which of them is more influential in the decision?
5. What are your bases of power and influence? What bases of influence can you develop to gain more control over the situation?
6. Which of the various strategies and tactics for exercising power seem most appropriate and are likely to be effective, given the situation you confront?
7. Based on the above, choose a course of action to get something done.

These steps, and the whole issue of learning how to manage with power, are especially important in respect of public health when so much of what happens requires an ability to influence (not control) the behaviour of others, to change the course of events, to overcome resistance and non-compliance, and to get people to do things that they would not otherwise do. There are implications for the education and development of those working in public health which are taken up in the final section of this chapter. The converse is also true, namely the problems of performance and effectiveness are problems of power and politics—power imbalances, powerlessness, and the inability of some groups to get their ideas or suggestions taken seriously. These problems are likely to occur in the health-care settings in which performance outcomes are often difficult to assess, especially at the total organizational level, and in which results are likely to be long term.

Studies such as those mentioned above began to show how complex and variegated organizations are. Their management is similarly complex and multifaceted. Organizations were described as ambiguous, contained competing groups, subscribed to vague objectives, and appeared to be pursuing different goals simultaneously. In such settings, policies and decisions were not marked out through formal organizational and managerial structures but were agreed in *ad hoc* fashion through an unending process of discussion, bargaining, and negotiation between the relevant stakeholders. What occurs in practice in organizations can therefore best be described as a 'continuous bargaining–learning process' (Cyert and March 1963).

This convergence of studies of how organizations and managers operated in practice which appeared in the late 1950s and early 1960s was eclipsed through the 1970s and 1980s, although may be making a comeback at the start of the 21st century. Whereas there had been a drawing away from the conception of organization and management embodied in scientific management or Weberian bureaucracy, with important exceptions, like Mintzberg's studies of managerial work, the 1970s and 1980s saw a rekindling of interest in the principles of bureaucracy and scientific management.

As the earlier discussion in this section demonstrated, the management structure of industrial and business organizations was held up as a model for public sector services, like health, to adopt and, in extreme instances, mimic. Simplistic, almost naive notions about how organizations functioned pervaded the 'new rationalism' which permeated government in the United Kingdom and elsewhere from the 1970s on. Such notions were to some extent a reaction against the studies of organizations which sought to demonstrate how diverse, pluralistic, and multilayered they in fact were. But insights of this type were uncomfortable and unsettling for managers and policy-makers intent on the achievement of clear goals and objectives. The undermining of the scientific management school of thought with its comfortable certainties about the nature of organization and management was bound to result in a backlash and a nostalgic harking back to a simpler explanation. This may largely be responsible for what Burns (1994) has called 'the recrudescence of the hard-line managerialism which has manifested itself in recent years first in America and then in Britain and Europe'. This hard-line managerialism has been to the fore in health-care reform in developed countries in recent years. Developing countries are being attracted to similar solutions (Collins *et al.* 1994). These issues are explored further in the next section following a summary of the argument so far.

Summary

If health-care management cannot be said to be unique, although contingency theorists might argue that it is, there is no disputing its distinctiveness or the differences it displays. But there is no general all-purpose science of management. Nevertheless, certain theories and concepts over the years have influenced in powerful ways the conception and practice of management. In particular, the theory of scientific management, and related notions of rational decision-making, have been a major influence on the design of management systems. The weakness of scientific management lies in the evidence that managers in practice do not behave according to the theory. To understand how they operate it is necessary to turn to the behavioural sciences and to apply concepts like politics, power, and bargaining. These have revolutionized the understanding of management and the context in which managers operate. Yet, rational theories of management continue to inform the public face of management. They legitimize actions even if they are not the primary determinants of them.

The new rationalism and health

As mentioned above, during the 1970s, a 'cult of managerialism', which remains evident some 30 years later, swept through government in a number of countries. It was directed towards improving the performance of public services which were seen to be overadministered and undermanaged. Allegedly, public services like health had weakly articulated goals and, where they existed, ineffective means of achieving them. The industrial and business sector was used as a source of ideas and practical ways forward. There was also a new-found enthusiasm for the mechanistic and rationalistic approaches to management which had been discredited in the 1960s by studies of how organizations and managers in fact operated. Notions of comprehensive rational planning and command and control mechanisms for running organizations were prevalent in the 1970s as politicians wrestled to contain public expenditure and improve the performance of public services. The 1974 reorganization of the British NHS was a model example of these concepts and ideas being put into practice on a grand scale (Hunter 1980).

By the 1980s, the political climate had shifted dramatically. Not only were public services being accused of poor management but their very existence was being challenged. The prevailing political ideology was unequivocal in its opposition to monopoly public services and actively sought ways of privatizing them, or parts of them, as a means of containing costs and improving performance through the principle of competition and markets.

These developments have been described by Hood (1991) as constituting 'the new public management'. As a movement, the new public management has caught the imagination of governments worldwide. It constitutes a kind of managerial pandemic reinforced by the World Bank's endorsement of it (World Bank 1993). The new public management, argued Hood, 'is one of the most striking international trends in public administration' (Hood 1991). Its rise is linked with four other administrative trends occurring at the same time:

- attempts to slow down or reverse government growth in public spending
- the shift towards privatization and quasi-privatization and away from core government institutions
- the development of automation, particularly in information technology, in the production and distribution of public services
- the development of a more international agenda, increasingly focused on general issues of public management, policy design, decision styles, and intergovernmental co-operation.

New public management, as Hood describes it, is a loose shorthand label for a set of broadly similar doctrines which dominated the management reform agenda in many of the Organization for Economic Co-operation and Development countries from the late 1970s (Pollitt 1990). It sought to replace 'old' public management which, with its complex bureaucratic structures and centralizing ethos, had failed spectacularly to improve the performance of services. Some observers saw new public management as nothing more than 'a gratuitous and philistine destruction of more than a century's work in developing a distinctive public service ethic and culture' (Hood 1991). Moreover, a contradiction was seen to lie at the heart of new public management thinking. Despite talk of the need for innovation and flexibility, this was to be relieved through a series of instruments, notably purchaser–provider separations, contracts, and targets, all of which are more than capable of limiting both innovation and flexibility (Stewart 1998).

New public management has seven doctrinal components (adapted from Hood (1991)):

- hands-on professional management in the public sector
- standard setting, performance measurement, and target setting, particularly where professionals are involved
- emphasis on output controls linked to resource allocation
- the disaggregation or 'unbundling' of previously monolithic units into provider/producer functions, and the introduction of contracting
- the shift to competition as the key to cutting costs and raising standards
- stress on private-sector management style and a move away from the public service ethic—this includes the introduction of marketing and public relations techniques
- discipline and parsimony in resource use—cost cutting, doing more with less, controlling labour union demands.

New public management derived its theoretical origins from two sources: the new institutional economics and business-type managerialism. The former helped to generate a set of related reform doctrines built on notions of contestability, user choice, transparency, and incentive structures. Such doctrines were markedly different from traditional notions with their emphasis on orderly hierarchies and the elimination of overlap. The business-type managerialism was merely the latest in a succession of waves of this type which began in the 1970s and were described earlier. It was in the tradition of the scientific management movement, also described above, although it underwent a facelift and image change, and in the process acquired a new jargon. Central to this type of managerialism was a set of common beliefs: professional management (a) was generic and portable, (b) was paramount over technical expertise, (c) required high discretionary power to achieve results, and (d) was central and indispensable to better organizational performance.

There is no single accepted explanation for the considerable appeal of new public management. It would appear to be a response to global socio-economic changes with an abhorrence of 'statist' and uniform approaches in public policy and a perception that public services seem to be run more for the convenience of those providing them rather than those paying for and using them. Part of the appeal is that it cuts across party lines and can be seen to be politically neutral.

An emphasis on health sector reform adopting a particular managerial approach based on new public management principles has been encouraged by the World Bank (1993). The thrust of the World Bank's approach has been to promote diversity and competition. A system of 'managed competition' is seen to offer a number of advantages although its limitations and disadvantages are acknowledged in passing. Managed competition or care pursues cost-effective health spending, universal insurance coverage, and cost containment through tightly regulated competition among companies that provide a specified package of health care for a fixed annual fee. Evaluations of it show mixed results but Light (1994, 1999) regards competing managed care systems as unlikely to tackle the great health-care needs of the twenty-first century and the diseases of chronicity and preventable morbidities.

The World Bank claims that the encouragement of competition in the delivery of health services coupled with effective regulation would increase the effectiveness of health spending. But would it? The transaction costs associated with competitive systems are high and may outweigh any benefits which may be forthcoming (Evans 1997). The evidence that competition in health care leads to gains that are not eliminated by other factors does not exist (Maynard 1993).

Growing concern among centre-left governments elected in the latter half of the 1990s that the application of market-style mechanisms may have resulted in various dysfunctional aspects in organizational design and management practice, notably greater fragmentation and rising management costs, have resulted in new waves of reform aimed at acknowledging that connected problems require 'joined-up' solutions. Therefore, and this is crucial, without abandoning all aspects of new public management thinking, governments have sought to modify some of its market-style features. Arguably, this has given rise to emerging tensions over the style of management that is most appropriate for the health-care enterprise.

Critics of new public management accuse it of being all hype and no substance (Rhodes 1995; Stewart 1998). Scratch away the trendy jargon and fashionable packaging and a fairly orthodox approach to management is all too evident. The language spoken may have changed but beneath it all the old problems and weaknesses remain. Other critics claim that new public management has simply led to a rapid growth of managers without evidence of effectiveness in terms either of lowering costs or improving health.

Wider criticisms of new public management centre on the inappropriate importation of business sector practices into a public service culture. In particular, especially in health care, notions of competition and markets are viewed as anathema and as ultimately leading to the destruction of a public service ethos. The idea that a pure market is possible in health care is akin to the naivety of those who subscribe to the 'scientific management' school of thought with its simplistic beliefs about rationality and human behaviour. Understanding how markets actually work and the concept of market failure echo the work on 'negotiated order' by Strauss *et al.* (1964) described above. If organizations are political constructs in which various interests jostle for supremacy, then markets can be similarly manipulated and subject to the interplay of power between stakeholders. Managers, therefore, need to understand the nature of organizations from such a behavioural perspective if they are going to succeed in moving them closer to agreed goals.

As Handy (1994) has written, 'the acceptance of paradox as a feature of our life is the first step towards living with it and managing it'. Whereas Handy, rather like Taylor and his theory of 'scientific management', and Weber with his theory of 'rational bureaucracy', used to think that paradoxes were the visible signs of an imperfect world which demanded to be eradicated, he no longer believes in the possibility of perfection: 'Paradox I now see to be inevitable, endemic and perpetual. The more turbulent the time, the more complex the world, the more the paradoxes' (Handy 1994). While it may be possible and desirable to minimize the inconsistencies and understand the puzzles in the paradoxes it is not possible to solve them completely. In the final analysis, 'paradoxes are like the weather, something to be lived with, not solved, the worst aspects mitigated, the best enjoyed and used as clues to the way forward. Paradox has to be *accepted*, coped with and made sense of ...' (Handy 1994). It does not have to be resolved—only managed.

What does this mean for managing and planning for health? The buzz-words in the management literature, many of them far from new but dusted down because they resonate with the spirit of the times, are complexity, paradox, ambiguity, and uncertainty. Chaos theory and complexity science have replaced comprehensive rational theory as offering more accurate explanations of how the management task has changed and of what is required to achieve sustainable change (Zimmerman 1999). Successful organizations and managers live with paradox. Organizations have to be planned and yet remain flexible, be differentiated and integrated at the same time, be small in some ways but large in others, be centralized some of the time and decentralized for most of it. Whereas managers used to believe that their task was to choose between such opposites, the task is in fact one of reaching an accommodation between them. It is all a matter of balance and of constantly adjusting and fine-tuning it.

Organic open systems of management, which Burns and Stalker (1961) and others wrote about in the early 1960s, were back in vogue in the late 1990s, albeit sitting uneasily alongside notions of new public management which remained popular. However, the terms post-Fordist, postbureaucratic, and postmodernist are used to distinguish such forms from their mechanistic counterparts described by Taylor and Weber (Hoggett 1991). In Handy's words (Handy 1994):

> The organisations of the future may not be readily recognisable as such. When intelligence is the primary asset the organisation becomes more like a collection of project groups, some fairly permanent, some temporary, some in alliance with other parties.

In such a context there are clear limits to management—it is not a panacea for organizational pathologies and social ills. It is possible that we are living through a time called the edge of chaos—a time of turbulence, creativity, and transition out of which a new order may materialize and gel.

Management: science or liberal art?

As a consequence of the foregoing distillation of theories of organization and management over the past 90 years or so, it is hardly surprising that establishing an integrated management 'science' in the conventional sense is regarded as highly improbable (Whitley 1988). The low degree of standardization of intellectual objects and concepts in the management sciences is exacerbated by the difficulty in separating them from managerial practices. Management researchers, as Whitley affirms, have not been able to isolate general phenomena and processes which could reasonably be claimed to underlie managerial practices. As the preceding discussion has demonstrated, this is a reflection of 'the necessarily contingent, contextual and relatively unstable nature of managerial tasks and activities' (Whitley 1988). It is a conclusion shared by Kotter (1982) in his study of 15 general managers. He states that the data from his sample show a complexity 'which often makes many managerial textbook concepts seem woefully inadequate'. Even the general managers themselves had difficulty understanding the level of complexity. Management at this senior level looks far more like an art than a science although patterns of behaviour can be discerned.

Management is not independent of the phenomena it seeks to control, influence, or manipulate. It is in fact part of these phenomena. Indeed, these phenomena largely shape and define management and the particular management style adopted. When these get out of step and lack congruence, as may be happening in health-care services where a particular conception of management borrowed from the industrial sector is overlaid on to a professional organization, then cognitive dissonance is likely to occur as well as attempts to temper that particular management style (Lloyd *et al.* 1999). To this extent, management is a dynamic activity able to adapt to its environment. Where management cannot adapt, it is likely to be recast or overturned through a reorganization, or through a series of individual acts against particular managers.

Drucker (1990) claims that management is a liberal art:

> 'liberal' because it deals with the fundamentals of knowledge, self-knowledge, wisdom, and leadership, 'art' because it is practice and application. Managers draw on all the knowledge and insights of the humanities and the social sciences.

For this reason, management cannot be called a science. For Drucker, because management deals with people and their values, it is a humanity.

In short, management is not a distinct activity or function which can be studied in isolation from the context in which it occurs. The notion of a generic management which can be applied to any organizational setting is therefore suspect and ignores the subtle interaction between management and its particular locus. Standardized skills of the type to be found in medicine and law, and other professions, do not exist and therefore are not subject to 'scientification'. Attempts to establish a general 'science of managing' are doomed to failure since managing is not a standardized activity but is highly context-specific. As Kotter (1982) argues:

> if 'professional management' means the ability to manage nearly anything well by relying on universal principles and skills and not on detailed knowledge of the specific business involved and close relationships with specific people involved in that business, then *not one* of the effective executives in this study was a 'professional manager'.

Nor did Kotter's managers operate in a well-organized, proactive, and reflective way. Yet their seeming 'irrationality' and disorganization worked.

Planning for health

Notions of planning and strategy have mostly tended to follow management fads and fashions. So, in the 1960s and 1970s when concepts of management tended to be of the command-and-control top-down variety, concepts of planning were similarly of a centralized, synoptic rationality type. The subsequent failure of comprehensive rational planning was accounted for by its adherence to a definition of comprehensiveness in a world that lacks any comprehensive political power or institutions. In challenging the somewhat mechanistic and simplistic view of strategy underpinning comprehensive rational planning, Mintzberg's (1990) notion of strategy as a result of a myriad of decisions and not the logical or inevitable outcome of economic and technical rationality is akin to the bureaucratic politics view of organizational life most ably illuminated by Allison (1971). Mintzberg (1988) defines strategy as what organizations actually achieve and not just what they intend to achieve: 'Defining strategy as a plan in advance of taking action is not sufficient'.

In understanding health planning it is therefore necessary to move away from the corporate planning models prevalent in the 1960s and 1970s in a number of countries, with their emphasis on synoptic rationality, and to look at what managers actually do by way of planning. A distinction, paralleling 'closed' and 'open' systems of management, can be made between planned strategy on the one hand and emergent strategy on the other. McKevitt (1992) describes the distinction as follows:

> *Planned strategy* emphasises direction and control of the organisation and it is thus more suited to a predictable external environment. *Emergent strategy* ... puts the emphasis on organisational learning whereby corrective action can be taken to alter strategic direction and to experiment, adapt and review the original decision in the context of changing circumstances.

Arguably, it was the failure of the rational comprehensive model of planning prevalent in many health-care systems that led to widespread disillusionment with health planning of any description and eventually to the various reform moves in the 1980s and into the 1990s with their emphasis on decentralized market-type solutions.

Public health was directly involved in these various developments since the notion of planning, whatever interpretation of it was adopted, was seen as essential in addressing the dilemma of rising demand for health care coupled with finite resources. Some form of priority-setting that was transparent and equitable was regarded as essential. Through the 1970s and early 1980s, planners, many of them with a public health qualification, struggled to develop a robust planning framework for health services. Their efforts were always doomed to failure because, rather like the adherents to the theory of 'scientific management', they failed (or forgot) to acknowledge that to secure effective change it is necessary to acquire ownership for it from those affected by it. It cannot be imposed from above, at least not if it is to be implemented successfully.

For Barnard (1991), the failure of rational central planning in the British NHS paved the way for 'the school of thought which in many countries enjoyed ascendancy during the past decade [with its] reaffirmation of the superiority of markets and price mechanisms as the means of satisfying human wants'. Managed competition and devolved management replaced the corporate rationalist approach. The health-care reforms of the 1970s were seen to be overly cumbersome and bureaucratic, and to belong to an outmoded rationalist tradition based on Taylorism and his theory of 'scientific management'. Failure, in Barnard's (1977) view, was virtually guaranteed since

- there is no simple product or range of products in the health service which would allow rationalization in the interests of efficiency
- consumer behaviour is difficult to understand in the health-care context
- conflicting local interests make consultation and collaboration laborious
- the dominant feature of health-care delivery is one which involves concentrating on relieving present problems and not on the provision or attainment of a desirable state of affairs some time in the future, that is, 'the urgent' forever drives out 'the important'.

Many of these factors remain current. Rathwell (1987) concludes his study of strategic planning in the British NHS by cataloguing the reasons for its failure. Chief among these is the separation between management and planning. There is a failure to connect the two. As a consequence, planning is viewed as a highly prescriptive function not keyed into the real world. Management is in practice little more than administration.

With the move in many countries in the late 1980s and early 1990s towards notions of managed markets and a separation of purchaser–provider responsibilities to permit the creation of competition, the planning function passed to the purchaser organization. The separation of roles was seen as desirable because, whereas planners in integrated organizations had been regarded as victims of provider capture, under the new arrangements operational responsibilities would pass to providers leaving purchasers free to think and act strategically. The greater clarity of functions was heralded as an important opportunity for public health because its skills would be central to the purchasing task. The emphasis on health gain and the need to demonstrate that medical investments were effective in improving health status gave public health a new lease on life. But the difficulties arising from making the purchaser–provider split work, and the long-term nature of issues associated with effectiveness and outcomes, have rather blunted public health's ability to make a significant impact. However, before pursuing these matters in the context of equipping public health practitioners with appropriate management skills, it is necessary first to reflect upon the nature of management in public health. Before doing so, a summary of the discussion thus far is in order.

Summary

The purpose of this section has been to describe in general terms the evolution of theories of management, planning, and organization and to show how these have impacted upon public management and health-care services. In offering this overview of developments in management, it can be seen that a general science of management is not possible or meaningful because the practice of management cannot be isolated from the context in which it is practised.

The next section adopts a narrower focus and, on the basis of the above discussion on evolving notions of management, examines the specific relationship between management, planning, and public health, and the application of management and planning to public health.

Management and public health

Biomedical systems operate very differently from management systems and are able to subscribe to scientific principles of thought and action, and cause and effect. Perhaps it is their training for this world which makes clinicians, including public health specialists, ill-equipped for a management role, especially of the type studied by Kotter (1982), and described in the previous section. Whereas they may be searching illusively for an understanding of their managerial role rooted in a science of management, in fact what is required is a quite different conception of the management task. Unlike medicine, the nature of managerial skills is not clearly established, nor are they standardized to the same extent. Practitioner-controlled knowledge does not exist in management as it does in medicine. As has been shown in the preceding discussion concerning changing theories and conceptions of management, managerial skills deal with much more variable, contingent, and unstable phenomena which include managerial practices themselves. Management's interdependence with the very realities it is seeking to control or influence shapes it.

The tension between bureaucratic and professional models of control is mentioned in the introduction. In the last section, attempts to subdue professional autonomy, if not curtail it, through managerial reform are described. The history of health-care reform globally has been one marked by border skirmishes between managers and professions, notably the medical profession. At the core of the management revolution in health care has been the view that doctors must increasingly accept managerial responsibility as well as be managed themselves by non-medical professional managers. In the United Kingdom, the arrival of general management in 1984 heralded a new era of difficult relations between the medical profession and the new breed of general managers. No longer is the medical profession responsible for what happens, and does not happen, in health policy. Bureaucratic politics have eroded the medical profession's authority (Morone 1993).

It seems that Sir Roy Griffiths, architect of general management in the NHS, was not altogether happy with this outcome. As he argued in a lecture 7 years after the introduction of general management, he never intended his report to be confrontational with the professions (Griffiths 1991). He understood general management 'as shorthand for the introduction of an effective management process. I did not intend that the result should be yet another profession in the NHS to work in parallel with other professions'.

Even in America, the land of market-led medicine, the medical profession's freedom is strictly curtailed through a variety of management decrees and controls. As Morone puts it, 'control over health policy had passed from providers and legislators to the health bureaucracy' (Morone 1993). The managed care movement has evolved to monitor in detail the ways in which doctors operate. What was once deemed specialized knowledge is now subject to protocols and guidelines. Professional models of organization are progressively being transformed into managerial ones. The micromanagement of medical work is in evidence in many health-care systems in Europe and Australasia. It is occurring through an emphasis on evidence-based medicine and on concepts like clinical governance which are intended to improve clinicians' performance by encouraging them to manage their work more effectively. Much of the thinking underlying clinical government includes managerial notions like leadership, creating development plans, clarifying accountability, and so on. These various developments have led to intense debate among sociologists about the extent to which medicine has become 'deprofessionalized' and 'proletarianized' (Hafferty and McKinlay 1993).

Public health specialists occupy a halfway position between the worlds of management and professionalism. They are therefore partially exempt from the power play between medicine and management because they subscribe to a population-based approach to health care and are generally more sympathetic than many of their clinical colleagues to a managerial perspective on matters like planning and priority-setting. For their part, managers are generally more concerned about the collective, that is, about the total population within a locality, and the principle of solidarity.

But if the frontier between medicine and management is shifting perceptibly towards managers as a result of health systems reforms, and related developments in the areas of medical audit and clinical effectiveness, does this not work to the advantage of public health and those who practise it? Or do public health specialists feel threatened by, or oppose, the tighter managerial grip on the grounds that it can operate to compromise their independence and freedom as professionals to speak out and can exert inappropriate pressure to produce quick results (Griffiths and Hunter 1999)?

The specialty of public health medicine is itself ambivalent in its response to these questions. Indeed, there are clear divisions of opinion between those who believe public health must be an active part of the management system with a place at the top table and those who wish public health to remain detached in order to preserve its independence and professional integrity.

Part of the dilemma for public health and its uneasy relationship with management may lie in the model of management which many health-care systems have imported, and only marginally adapted, from the industrial and business sector. As mentioned in the previous section, recent years in virtually all areas of public policy have witnessed a recrudescence of hard-line managerialism. It runs counter to professional conceptions of management which have more in common with post-Fordist notions. These are now fashionable and may offer a means of resolving the tension between bureaucratic and professional models of managerial control. Rather than polarizing these which recent health systems reforms have tended to do, unintentionally or not, the issue may in fact be one of finding a new synthesis in which traditional collegiate forms of professional organization are in fact precisely those needed in order to achieve team working, initiative, and collaboration among a range of diverse skills on the basis that complex problems demand complex solutions (Hunter 1999). As Handy (1994) puts it, 'organizations will be flatter, more flexible and more dispersed'. More importantly, he continues:

> The old language of management no longer seems appropriate. It never was appropriate in some quarters. Professional organisations, doctors, architects, lawyers, academics have never used the word manager, except to apply it to the more routine service functions—the office-manager, catering-manager. The reason was not just a perverse snobbery but an instinctive recognition that professionals have always worked on the principle of the doughnut. This was necessary because every assignment was slightly different; flexibility and discretion had to be built in.

The doughnut principle (see Handy 1994) requires an inside-out doughnut, one with the hole on the outside and the dough in the middle. Organizations have realized that they have their essential core, a core of necessary jobs and necessary people, a core which is surrounded by an open flexible space which they fill with flexible workers and flexible supply contracts. The strategic issue for organizations is to decide what activities and which people to put in which space.

Arguably, public health has been derailed because it has been forced to conform to an inappropriate 'scientific management' model whereas in fact its own professional instincts might have served it better had it not had to conform to a mechanistic model of management—the 'old' management imported from much, though by no means all, of the business sector, and some of which lingers under the guise of new public management. Yet, public health's roots in a scientific medical model of health and disease may have contributed to the dilemma confronting it. Though severely limited in its ability to describe or modify organizational life, scientific management at least resonated with the scientific tradition underpinning public health medicine from which it derived its legitimacy and credibility. Behavioural approaches to management sit uneasily with the scientific tradition. While the 'new' (public) management (see above) with its emphasis on outcomes may come closer to public health's concerns, its simultaneous focus on markets and individuals as consumers runs counter to public health's values and responsibilities.

A new managerial paradigm

Public health has flirted with management and in its innocence has been drawn to an inappropriate model which negates the intrinsic strengths of the specialty itself. These strengths derive from its roots in the profession of medicine. In this and other professions, collegiate forms of working operate in place of hierarchy and rigid levels of management. In such a context management is founded on trust whereas the managerialism prevalent in many health services in recent years, and evident in much new public management thinking, is founded on distrust. Performance management is centred on providing proof of performance and on individuals and organizations answering for what they fail to do. Concepts like 'chain of command' and 'centralization versus decentralization' are essentially about exercising control.

In contrast with these mechanistic notions, network structures represent a paradigm shift and derive from the flatter doughnut-configured organizations which have emerged in the 1990s. Flexible organic structures look set to replace rigid, inflexible bureaucratic structures. Given the rapid pace of change, the revolution in knowledge and its transmission via the information superhighway, organizational structures which are not extremely adaptable and open to the environment will simply not survive. Structures, and the management systems operating them, will need to be more transitory and *ad hoc* at all levels—operational, strategic, and administrative (Mintzberg 1980).

Network organizations, which function according to the doughnut principle in so far as they possess a central core surrounded by a constellation of project teams which exist for the duration of particular tasks and are then reformed, will survive. Such structures are flexible and fast moving because they can change quickly as the environment changes. They can also better tap external expertise and knowledge rather than attempt to provide it all in-house.

Without seeing the disappearance entirely of the traditional bureaucratic type of organization in health services, it is likely that network organizational structures will become more widespread. Developments in health services such as the purchaser–provider separation, management by contract, managed competition, integrated care/clinical pathways, and so on, will most likely encourage the network organization. The idea is not especially new. Writing in the early 1970s about the loss of the stable state and about what might replace it, Schon (1973) defined the roles of the network manager. Such a person was required in order to allow organizations to be continually redesigned 'without flying apart at the seams' (Schon 1973).

In network organizations a new set of roles becomes necessary. They are essential to the design, creation, negotiation, and management of networks. Schon (1973) identifies six roles:

- systems negotiator
- 'underground' manager—maintains and operates informal networks
- manoeuvrer—operates on a project basis
- broker
- network manager—oversees official networks of activities
- facilitator.

These roles are difficult and demand high personal credibility for their successful execution. They are often performed by those who exist on the margins of organizations. As will be suggested in the next section, public health's management function is perhaps best understood by drawing parallels between the expectations of it and the notion of network management described by Schon.

If there is a congruence between the new managerial paradigm described above which is emerging in public services like health care and professional forms of organization, then public health may, or could, be at the leading edge of developments in management. In reshaping the management roles they assume, public health specialists are in fact part of a broader shift taking place in the nature and definition of management in health care. From attempts in the 1970s, 1980s, and early 1990s to strengthen management in order to control professionals, there is evidence of a shift towards different managerial forms in which professionals potentially have a great deal to offer. This movement seems wholly in keeping with the general management function as Griffiths perceived it in his 1991 Audit Commission lecture (Griffiths 1991).

Summary

The tension between bureaucratic and professional models of control lies at the core of public health's uneasy relationship with management. Arguably, it may not be management *per se* which is the problem but rather the type of management to which public health is expected to confirm or contribute. At the same time, notions of management with a behavioural bias can pose problems for a discipline whose origins lie in a scientific rational model of disease and illness. Yet, of all those practising medicine, only public health specialists appear to be pivotally placed to marry professional collegiate forms of managing with network management. But before this can happen, public health needs to rid itself of the clutter of outmoded and inappropriate management constructs which have tended to limit its impact over the past 20 years or so. It also needs to acknowledge the importance of a public health management role.

Perhaps the future lies in a synthesis of public health's traditional professional ethos combined with a grounding in the newer, emerging notions of management. Such a synthesis may be termed public health management. The next and final section considers what is understood by public health management and how it can be brought to life.

Public health and management: towards a synthesis

Improving the health of populations is a challenge confronting all countries in both the developed and developing worlds. Health-care reform has been a catalyst in the long-running debate about how best to improve health because of a renewed emphasis on health as distinct from health care. The twin specialisms, or professions, at the centre of these concerns are public health and management.

As health care has become more complex a false antithesis has emerged between public health and health services management. Whereas public health specialists have generally looked outwards towards society and the health needs of the population, health services managers have tended to focus inwards on the organization, and particularly on the financially demanding secondary and tertiary care sectors. The shift towards a primary-care-led health-care delivery system is forcing a rethink. At the same time, many public health practitioners believe that they have become overidentified with health-care services. Indeed, this dilemma has become more acute with the growing emphasis on clinical governance and evidence-based medicine all of which appear fairly dependent on public health practitioner involvement (Wylie *et al.* 1999).

The notion of public health management is an attempt to bring together public health's planning and management skills but to give them a higher profile and recast them in the light of the discussion in preceding sections on the changing conceptions of management and planning. The concept involves mobilizing society's resources, including the specific resources of the health service sector, to improve the health of populations (Alderslade and Hunter 1992, 1994; Hunter 1993; Richardson *et al.* 1994; Hunter 1998).

The objective of health improvement has a long history among public health practitioners. The discipline of public health medicine has had twin intellectual approaches—knowledge and action—which have gone together. In practice, there has been a tension between knowledge and action, with many practitioners in public health focusing on knowledge rather than action. Public health management seeks to integrate the two approaches so that public health knowledge can be harnessed to action through the deployment of appropriate management and planning skills. These skills are rooted in an open systems approach to management, drawing on related notions of negotiated order and network management described above.

To this end, public health management demands skills other than those generally to be found in public health. Those working in today's public health function are expected to respond to the multisectoral nature of health problems and serve a variety of agencies. Working in a multisectoral arena to develop healthy alliances is akin to the marginal position desired by network managers and discussed by Schon (1973).

These are heavy demands requiring well-honed political and managerial skills in addition to the traditional scientific skills associated with public health. It is a particularly difficult synthesis to achieve not because of the range of skills required but because they come from two quite distinct paradigms. The traditional basis of public health medicine belongs to the positivist biomedical view of scientific enquiry, whereas the political and managerial skills base comes from an intuitive contextual orientation grounded in how organizations work. The tradition is sociological and anthropological rather than biomedical. This may explain why public health specialists often find 'scientific management' theories more immediately appealing than theories of a less 'rational' and more behavioural persuasion where uncertainty, complexity, paradox, and ambiguity figure prominently.

Public health management is, like public health itself, a multidisciplinary activity. Clear implications flow from this for the direction and type of training in public health medicine and in related areas which have a public health focus.

There is a need for public health doctors, non-medical public health specialists, and managers to find an intellectual focus for joint working since each group has a vital contribution to make to the superordinate goal of improved health. Failure to find this can only result in further interprofessional rivalry and a lack of co-ordinated working. Public health management demands knowledge and management skills of the highest order. Public health managers must be able to adopt a strategic approach and be able to describe and understand the health experience of populations and analyse the factors affecting health. To achieve change, skills in leadership and political action are necessary; managers have to operate in a multiprofessional multiagency environment and be able to achieve multisectoral change. Operating on the margins of their own organizations becomes a prerequisite.

In taking forward this multisectoral approach and health agenda, a number of key processes are involved:

- building alliances and networks with non-health service organizations; relationships will be based on influence rather than on direction and control
- market management: having a strategic framework based on health improvement, the capacity to work within alliances, possessing good market-relevant information
- attention needs to be given to organizational fitness for purpose; it means moving away from functional departments and towards a blending of skills in task forces and in project-managed initiatives—such a team approach will be looser and more fluid than conventional functional departments with their often lengthy hierarchies and multiple layers of management.

Training implications

Moving forward in respect of these processes has implications for management training and development for practitioners of public health management. Certain competencies and qualities are critical although little empirical work has been carried out to identify these in practice-based contexts. An Australian study (Lloyd 1994) identified 'key figure' attributes for the effective public health manager as being the following:

> charisma, commitment, drive, and an ability to function in a loosely regulated environment while at the same time dealing with bureaucratic processes.

These qualities are regarded as central in attempts to foster fundamental change in the direction of health services towards measurable health gain. There is growing acceptance of the need for political and management skills. A former Chief Medical Office in England, Sir Kenneth Calman, believes that (Calman 1993):

> The practical implications of public health are an art and require special skills in themselves. Skills need emphasising and include both management and political skills in the communication of ideas and complex public health issues.

Developing the catalogue of competencies further, Lloyd (1994) reports on the need for competencies relevant to the leadership of complex work groups—communication skills, interpersonal skills, understanding of organizational behaviour, intellect, analytical skills, planning skills, accounting skills, and an understanding of how the system works.

Management education has been a perennial issue for public health. But it needs to be less concerned with theoretical approaches and the prevailing bureaucratic and economic rationalist model of health management and focused instead on social organization, behavioural approaches, and interpersonal skills. This type of management training is weak or non-existent and yet, as can be seen from the preceding sections of this chapter, it is crucial. A frequent criticism of management training for public health doctors has been its largely mechanistic nature. Curricula have mostly remained rooted in conventional approaches and management practices applicable to operating in a bureaucratic organization, or in administrative practices, and in a mainly theoretical approach to management. They are based, not surprisingly, on conservative individualistic principles and reflect the ideology of scientific reductionism emphasizing such activities as organizational delegation, industrial-style negotiation, policy interpretation, and information dissemination. Such processes tend to assume and reinforce the established tradition of élitist management and top-down hierarchical control. As Lloyd (1994) concludes:

> It reflects a fundamentally authoritarian, and hence limited, appreciation of what the management role can encompass, as well as having minimal significance in terms of influencing the health of the population.

In contrast, the challenges posed by the new public health demand an approach to management education that emphasizes the dynamic dimension of the learning organization and of managing change (Forster *et al.* 1994). Management principles derived from conventional health bureaucracies are no longer relevant or appropriate. With organizations being re-engineered, delayered, and right-sized, they are flatter. Managers achieve results through enabling, facilitating, and delegating and not through an exclusive or predominant focus on top-down hierarchical command-and-control mechanisms. They need to work in teams and across professional and organizational boundaries. As an American management expert on leadership, Bennis, has put it, great achievements, particularly in the complex modern world, can only be collective: 'none of us is as smart as all of us' (Bennis 1998). The competencies needed for team work centre on building networks and deploying political skills such as networking and manoeuvring to maximize the influence that can be brought to bear on a given problem.

Thompson (1990) makes a similar case when he argues that students of health-care management are not being adequately equipped with a comprehensive range of knowledge and the skills to apply it to real problems. He laments the failure of organization and management research to influence the direction of management (Hunter 1988). The impact of most of the findings from management research appear to be on management itself but not on the community being served and how management affects it.

Conclusion

The rise of management in health-care systems is a global phenomenon and has been much in evidence over the past 25 years or so. Central to all managerial reforms has been a technocratic faith in improved management and in its capacity to resolve deep-seated, and essentially political, problems. A principal feature of the evolution of management in health-care systems has been the struggle between doctors and managers, whether played out overtly or covertly.

The so-called 'new rationalism' of the 1970s and early 1980s has re-emerged in a new guise in the 1990s, albeit with a slightly different focus. This is known as the 'new public management' and it is largely a reaction to the perceived failures of what might be called old public management or a traditional public administration approach to public sector management. Part of the search for different management models was fuelled by a loss of faith in comprehensive, or synoptic, rational planning led from central government.

But whatever the perceived failures of old public management, new public management is also flawed. In particular, markets and medicine do not mix well. Markets are of limited utility in health-care systems governed by principles of:

- equity or social justice
- access to care at time of need
- comprehensive coverage.

Market failure cannot be dismissed as being of no consequence. Even the World Bank, a supporter of markets, acknowledges this. However, although new public management may not offer a wholly satisfactory or stable basis for managing health care, its disciplines have, possibly unwittingly, loosened up sclerotic structures and conventions and paved the way for a possible paradigm shift in respect of how health policy and management is conceived of and conducted. Public health is critical to these developments but the training for it will require modification in respect of management skills.

In the achievement of health policy goals, particular management skills and competencies are desirable as well as an orientation that requires that public health and general management progressively overlap and move closer together. They already share a common policy and management agenda, including the following elements:

- a focus on health and not just health care
- a focus on outcomes and improvements in health status
- achieving a balance between collective and individual actions.

Given the description in this chapter of health-care systems as political systems where a plurality of interests hold power, there are implications for public health and management. Public health cannot achieve change unless it is prepared to embrace management. Scientific detachment and political innocence alone will achieve little. At the same time, a set of core values and principles is vital if managers are to gain confidence to manage. The paradigm shift, therefore, posits that management and public health are inseparable in the creation and implementation of a change agenda in health care and that this should be reflected in the management education and development that those involved in public health receive.

References

Alderslade, R. and Hunter, D.J. (1992). Forward march. *Health Service Journal*, **19**, 22–3.

Alderslade, R. and Hunter, D.J. (1994). Outward bound. *Health Service Journal*, **27**, 22–4.

Allison, G.T. (1971). *Essence of decision.* Little, Brown, Boston, MA.

Bachrach, P. and Baratz, M.S. (1962). The two faces of power. *American Political Science Review*, **56**, 947–52.

Bachrach, P. and Baratz, M.S. (1963). Decisions and non-decisions: an analytical framework. *American Political Science Review*, **57**, 632–42.

Bachrach, P. and Baratz, M.S. (1970). *Power and poverty.* Oxford University Press, New York.

Barnard, K. (1977). Promises, patients and politics: the conflicts of the NHS. In *Conflicts in the National Health Service* (ed. K. Barnard and K. Lee), pp. 13–25. Croom Helm, London.

Barnard, K. (1991). Trends in health care: beyond market economics? A reflection on 40 years past and 10 years future. In *New directions in managing health care* (ed. R. Bengoa and D.J. Hunter), pp. 133–40. World Health Organization and Nuffield Institute for Health Services Studies, Leeds.

Bennis, W. (1998). *Organising genius: the secrets of creative collaborations.* Nicholas Brealey, New York.

Burns, T. (1994). Preface. In *The management of innovation* (3rd edn) (T. Burns and G.M. Stalker), pp. vii–xx. Oxford University Press.

Burns, T. and Stalker, G.M. (1961). *The management of innovation.* Tavistock Press, London.

Calman, K. (1993). The scientific basis of public health. Address to the Annual Conference of the Faculty of Public Health Medicine, Glasgow, 27 June.

Collins, C., Green, A., and Hunter, D.J. (1994). International transfers of NHS reforms: problems and issues. *Lancet*, **344**, 248–50.

Crozier, M. (1964). *The bureaucratic phenomenon.* Chicago University Press.

Cyert, R.M. and March, J.G. (1963). *A behavioural theory of the firm.* Prentice-Hall, Englewood Cliffs, NJ.

Drucker, P. (1990). *The new realities.* Mandarin, London.

Evans, R.G. (1997). Health care reforms: who's selling the market, and why? *Journal of Public Health Medicine*, **19**, 45–9.

Forster, D.P., Acquilla, S., Halpin, J., Hill, P., Watson, H., and Watson, A. (1994). Public health medicine training and the NHS changes. *Public Health*, **108**, 457–62.

Griffiths, R. (1991). *Seven years of progress: general management in the NHS.* Audit Commission Management Lectures No 3. Audit Commission, London.

Griffiths, S. and Hunter, D.J. (ed.) (1999). *Perspectives in public health.* Radcliffe Medical Press, Oxford.

Hafferty, F.W. and McKinlay, J.B. (ed.) (1993). *The changing medical profession: an international perspective.* Oxford University Press, New York.

Handy, C. (1994). *The empty raincoat.* Hutchinson, London.

Hoggett, P. (1991). A new management in the public sector? *Policy and Politics*, **19**, 243–56.

Hood, C. (1991). A public management for all seasons. *Public Administration*, **69**, 3–19.

Hunter, D.J. (1980). *Coping with uncertainty: policy and politics in the National Health Service.* Research Studies Press/Wiley, Chichester.

Hunter, D.J. (1988). The impact of research on restructuring the British NHS. *Journal of Health Administration Education*, **6**, 537–53.

Hunter, D.J. (1993). Public health management: implication for training. *HFA 2000 News*, **23**, 5–7.

Hunter, D.J. (1998). Editorial: public health management. *Journal of Epidemiology and Community Health*, **52**, 226–8.

Hunter, D.J. (1999). *Managing for health: implementing the new agenda.* Institute for Public Policy Research, London.

Kotter, J.P. (1982). *The general manager.* Free Press, New York.

Light, D.W. (1994). Managed care: false and real solutions. *Lancet*, **344**, 1197–9.

Light, D.W. (1999). The sociological character of health care markets. In *Handbook of social studies in health and medicine* (ed. G.L. Albrecht, R. Fitzpatrick, and S.C. Scrimshaw). Sage, London.

Lloyd, P. (1994). Management competencies in health for all: new public health settings. *Journal of Health Administration Education*, **12**, 187–207.

Lloyd, P., Braithwaite, J., and Southon, G. (1999). Empowerment and the performance of health services. *Journal of Management in Medicine*, **13**, 83–94.

McKevitt, D. (1992). Strategic management in public services. In *Rediscovering public services management* (ed. L. Willcocks and J. Harrow), pp. 33–49. McGraw-Hill, London.

March, J.G. and Simon, H. (1958). *Organisations.* Wiley, New York.

Maynard, A. (1993). Creating competition in the NHS: is it possible? Will it work? In *Managing the internal market* (ed. I. Tilley), pp. 58–68. Chapman, London.

Mintzberg, H. (1980). Structure in 5s: a synthesis of the research on organisation design. *Management in Science*, **226**, 332.

Mintzberg, H. (1988). Opening up the definition of strategy. In *The strategy process: concepts, contexts and cases* (ed. J.B. Quinn *et al.*). Prentice-Hall, Englewood Cliffs, NJ.

Mintzberg, H. (1990). *Mintzberg on management.* Free Press, London.

Moore, M. (1996). *Public sector reform: downsizing, restructuring, improving programme.* Forum on Health Sector Reform. Discussion Paper No. 7. WHO, Geneva.

Morone, J.A. (1993). The health care bureaucracy: small changes, big consequences. *Journal of Health Politics, Policy and Law*, **18**, 723–39.

NHS (National Health Service) Executive (1994). *Corporate governance in the NHS Code of Conduct. Code of accountability.* Department of Health, London.

Osborne, D. and Gaebler, T. (1993). *Reconvening government.* Plume, London.

Pfeffer, J. (1981). *Power in organisations.* Pitman, Massachusetts.

Pfeffer, J. (1992). *Managing with power.* Harvard Business School Press, Cambridge, MA.

Pollitt, C. (1990) *Managerialism and the public services: the Anglo-American experience.* Basil Blackwell, Oxford.

Pressman, J.L. and Wildavsky, A. (1972). *Implementation.* University of California Press, Berkeley, CA.

Rathwell, T. (1987). *Strategic planning in the health sector.* Croom Helm, London.

Rhodes, R.A.W. (1995). Foreword: governance in the hollow state. In *Rethinking public policy-making* (ed. M. Blunden and M. Dando), pp. 1–6. Sage, London.

Richardson, A., Duggan, M., and Hunter, D.J. (1994). *Adapting to new tasks: the role of public health physicians in purchasing health care.* Nuffield Institute for Health, Leeds.

Schon, D. (1973). *Beyond the stable state.* Penguin, Harmondsworth.

Shortell, S.M. and Kaluzny, A.D. (ed.) (1983). *Health care management: a text in organisation theory and behaviour.* Wiley, New York.

Simon, H. (1957). *Administrative behaviour.* Free Press, New York.

Stewart, J. (1998). Advance or retreat: from the traditions of public administration to the new public management and beyond. *Public Policy and Administration*, **13**, 27.

Strauss, A., Schutzman, L., Butcher, R., Elrich, D., and Sabatini, M. (1964). *Psychiatric ideologies and institutions.* Free Press, New York.

Taylor, F.W. (1911). *Principles of scientific management.* Harper, New York.

Thompson, D. (1990). Organisation studies: time for change. *Health Services Management*, **3**, 270–2.

Vickers, G. (1968). *The art of judgement.* Methuen, London.

Weber, M. (1978). *The Protestant ethic and the spirit of capitalism.* Basic Books, New York.

Whitley, R. (1988). The management sciences and managerial skills. *Organisation Studies*, **9**, 47–68.

World Bank (1993). *World development report: investing in health.* Oxford University Press, New York.

Wylie, I., Griffiths, S., and Hunter, D.J. (1999). Everywhere and nowhere—a Socratic dialogue on the new public health. *British Medical Journal*, **319**, 839–40.

Zimmerman, B. (1999). Complexity science: a route through hard times and uncertainty. *Health Forum Journal*, **42**, 42–6, 69.

7.8 Problems, politics, and processes: public health sciences and policy in developed countries

Peter Davis

The stature and significance of the public health sciences derive almost entirely from their application. In the same way that the knowledge and expertise of the clinician make sense only in the service of patient care, so the claims of public health carry weight in proportion to their direct and effective application in policy and practice. Public health is necessarily an applied discipline. The mandate is clear; in keeping with other developed countries, it has been estimated that nine preventable conditions are responsible for over half the deaths in the United States, while less than 5 per cent of health spending is formally devoted to prevention (Atwood *et al.* 1997). The potential for preventive action is obviously substantial.

Despite its importance to public health, however, this link between action and knowledge has received relatively limited attention in the discipline (Brownson *et al.* 1997). Essentially, the primary interface between the public health sciences and policy has no clear signposts and lacks a plausible and authoritative academic rationale. This gap in the academic framework of public health partly reflects the predominantly technical ethos of pubic health, particularly given the centrality of disciplines like epidemiology and biostatistics. Just as important, however, is the highly problematic nature of the knowledge–policy link in the public arena. The parallel with the clinician—knowledge in the service of care—breaks down at this point. It is not as easy to translate public health knowledge into policy as it usually is to apply clinical knowledge in the practice setting. Action in the public arena inevitably raises ethical, technical, and political issues of a complexity and intractability that are not usually faced in clinical medicine (de Leeuw 1993).

The focus of this chapter is on identifying the key parameters of the link between the public health sciences and policy, formulating a pertinent framework for addressing this all-important connection, and suggesting a series of guidelines for future academic work and public health practice in this area. While many examples will be drawn from the areas of disease prevention and health promotion, it should be noted that structural change involving the social and economic determinants of health remain part of the public health brief as envisaged here.

For the purposes of this chapter public policy in health refers to the set of principles that guide the decision-making of governments in the health sector. The field of interest extends beyond the health-care system and includes non-governmental as well as state actors. The principal focus, furthermore, is on the policy system—the overall institutional pattern within which policies are made—and, within that system, on the policy-making process (Spasoff 1999).

Translating knowledge into action

The problematic nature of the knowledge–action link can be discussed at a number of levels. In one sense this is a quite generic issue about the relationship between science and policy with a bearing upon the work of a wide range of scientists whose research might be used to inform policy (Jasanoff 1990). A second set of issues—again of a more generic kind—are those of special relevance to disciplines with a public policy brief. These concern the role of government, and the ethics and justification for administrative intervention (Gillroy and Wade 1992). Finally, there are the group of issues that are more specific to the public health sciences dealing, firstly, with their disciplinary base and, secondly, with their translation into policy and effective implementation in practice (Beaglehole 1990).

Science and policy

The traditional concept of the role of the scientist has been as of a 'dispassionate creator of knowledge'. Under this view science is value free, its findings are of universal application, and scientists are expected to retain a position of objectivity, keeping their personal prejudices at a distance from their work and avoiding public controversy. To an important extent these prescriptions for personal behaviour serve to insulate scientific work from extraneous dispute, thus focusing argument and controversy on matters of common scientific discourse to which agreed methodologies and data can be brought to bear. This is the conventional view of the laboratory sciences.

Beyond this, however, these prescriptions for the scientific role are quite understandable given the very real uncertainty there is about the interpretation of scientific findings once they come to be applied in the public arena. In the paradigmatic scientific research setting, findings are generated under carefully controlled—frequently experimental laboratory—conditions. These conditions are not replicated in the real world where they are applied. Nevertheless, it is in these 'real world' circumstances that the carefully nurtured aura of value neutrality is breached because at this point scientific application touches upon the frequently competing interests of different groups in the community (Greenberg 1992).

There are two broad institutional and personal responses to this conundrum at the policy interface; Jasanoff (1990) has referred to them as research science and regulatory science respectively. According to the first, and most common, perspective, scientists retain a conventional interpretation of their role, concentrate on the generation rather than the application of knowledge, and allocate to their citizen role any broader responsibilities in the public arena (Rothman and Poole 1985). This does not mean that their work may not have major consequences for public well being, nor does it mean that their perspective as scientists does not influence their worldview. It is just that the two domains are effectively kept separate (Stallones 1982).

For a growing number of scientists, however, their work is not restricted to the research setting and the generation of knowledge. These scientists are required—as part of their work role—to interpret and apply scientific knowledge in judicial and regulatory environments. Under these conditions the norms of science are brought hard up against the public reality of controversy, of popular and judicial review, and of political and policy imperatives. While many of the core issues remain technical in character, they are debated in a relatively politicized and contentious environment (Fletcher 1997). Nevertheless, institutional arrangements of varying effectiveness have been developed to manage the interface between science and its application to regulatory issues. There are lessons to be drawn here for public health, which features as one of the central institutional strands in the emergence of regulatory science (for example, in environmental protection, occupational safety and health, and vigilance over pharmaceuticals).

The role of the public sector

An important stimulus to the growth of the regulatory function to which science is increasingly contributing has been the burgeoning of the public sector in all the advanced economies. This expansion has been both qualitative—for example, the extension into new regulatory arenas such as environmental protection—and quantitative, with the steady growth in traditional areas of concern such as health, education, and superannuation. This has occurred despite concerted attempts across the developed world by governments of all political colours to reduce taxes and to contain the size of the state sector.

What explains this growth? In particular, is there any theoretical rationale that can guide us in a normative or prescriptive sense in judging the appropriateness of state activity? Since much of this activity calls upon the professional and academic contribution of various disciplines in the natural and 'policy' sciences, how is it best to judge the boundaries for work of this kind?

In simple explanatory terms the growth of the public sector can be accounted for by resort to a number of theories, including demographic change, democratic values and political competition, the rise of social democracy, bureaucratic expansionism, and warfare, among others. Such theories may help to account for the variable size of the public sector in different countries and over time, for example. On their own, however, they do not provide an analytical framework within which to view the role of the state when judging the appropriateness of administrative intervention (for instance, for any specific episode of policy-making).

A central analytical insight in this context is to see public policy as principally, if not exclusively, concerned with collective action problems; according to this perspective administrative intervention of this kind—that is, public policy—is concerned with finding ways of synthesizing a 'public interest' from individual wants and needs. In other words, the role of public policy is to co-ordinate potentially disparate individuals towards co-operative solutions for problems that they face jointly but are unable to solve separately (Gillroy and Wade 1992).

The key economic concept that applies here is that of 'market failure'. This means that market conditions for a good or service are such that they fail under normal circumstances to reach a level that is socially desirable. There are two principal circumstances or mechanisms at play—externalities and public goods. In the case of the first, the actions of individuals far from being solely of private significance—such as a simple purchase in the market—bear in an important way upon the collective welfare of others. Examples in the instance of public health might be passive smoking, infectious disease, or environmental pollution. In each of these cases there is a potentially adverse effect on the well being of others that results from the private actions of an individual. Although the minimization of these adverse effects—such as epidemic infection or air pollution—is likely to be the desired outcome for a great majority of citizens, their uncoordinated efforts cannot achieve this, and any private market is likely to underprovide such services. The role of public policy is to overcome this 'collective action' problem by regulation and by other forms of administrative intervention.

In the case of public goods, market circumstances are such that the provision of certain kinds of goods and services is both 'non-excludable' (difficult or impossible to exclude people from their use) and non-rival (use by one person does not restrict use by another). Thus, a health promotion campaign cannot exclude people nor can it charge people for 'using' it. Furthermore, use by one person (that is, exposure to the campaign) does not restrict use by another, nor does it limit the potential benefit that might be had by all from such an initiative. Under these circumstances it is difficult for the private market—which relies on charging individuals for services received—to provide such goods.

The fact that negative externalities exist, or that certain services—so-called public goods—will not be provided under normal market circumstances, does not necessarily mean that administrative intervention will follow. Nor does it dictate the level and extent of such intervention. These are determined by wider social values and by the balance of political forces. Nevertheless, such analytical criteria indicate areas where public policy might best be directed—so-called collective action problems—if it is going to make the maximum and most effective difference to achieving desired social outcomes (Lane 1993).

The case of public health

In considering the relationship between the public health sciences and policy there are two principal matters at issue. Firstly, are the disciplines typically used in the production of public health knowledge such that the results of such work have a high probability of being translated into feasible and effective public policy? Secondly, what special attempts have to be made to ensure that once usable public health knowledge is available, it is shepherded through the policy process and effectively implemented?

Despite the long involvement of public health researchers and practitioners in social action and despite their reliance on at least a rudimentary level of knowledge about social and political context, the active participation of the social and policy sciences in public health work is of fairly recent origin (Mechanic 1995). The core public health sciences have been of a more technical kind, principally epidemiology and biostatistics, together with related clinical and laboratory disciplines. Such a narrow disciplinary base has, however, come to be seen as unsustainable—for two reasons. Firstly, it is now increasingly appreciated that the traditional interventions of disease prevention need to be adequately contextualized if they are to be delivered effectively (Schmid *et al.* 1995). The effectiveness, as opposed to the efficacy, of such interventions is not something that can just be left to simple improvisation in the field. Secondly, with the growing salience of the chronic and non-communicable diseases in the developed countries, issues of health promotion are now much more important, and these have brought with them an irreducibly and strongly behavioural dimension to the public health sciences (O'Neill and Pederson 1992).

On both these grounds, therefore, if the true value of public health knowledge and expertise is to be realized, then the way in which public health researchers and practitioners conceptualize problems has to be informed and shaped by the social and behavioural sciences (Snider and Satcher 1997). Thus, to take an example in the area of disease prevention, it might be perfectly understandable within a conventional view of science to advocate, for instance, a particular immunization schedule for the prevention of childhood infectious diseases on the grounds of its technical superiority. But from the point of view of effective delivery, it is important to take account also of 'contextual' matters, such as the adequacy of information and recall systems, ease of practitioner use, and patient acceptability. For public health practice, what counts is going to be the level of uptake, particularly among hard-to-reach groups. These features, while considered contextual within a conventional view of science, become part of the disciplinary core for an applied enterprise like the public health sciences (Holtgrave *et al.* 1997).

Similarly, but much more starkly, with issues of health promotion, smoking behaviour, alcohol consumption, and contraceptive use, for example, are all culturally sanctioned activities that have to be placed in their broader social and behavioural context if practitioners and policy-makers are to have any chance of advancing the cause of health-promoting change. Furthermore, moving into the context of the wider institutional environment—for example, related industries and cultural systems—the canvas of public health is a broad one (Milio 1988). Indeed, there is a strong argument for saying that social structural and wider sociopolitical forces need to be taken into account if effective and sustained public health advances are to be achieved at a societal level (McKinlay 1993).

Given this commitment to intervene in the real world in order to improve health outcomes—both at the individual and the societal level—public policy becomes the primary mechanism by which the potential of public health knowledge and skills can be released and translated into effective action (Lomas 1990). Thus an understanding of political context, the policy process, and implementation and delivery is crucial to good public health practice (Williams-Crowe and Aultman 1994). An essential condition for an easy and natural linkage to policy is, as has already been argued, an appropriate conceptualization of public health problems. But while an essential contributory factor, a firm disciplinary grounding of this kind is not on its own a sufficient condition for good policy work. What is also required is an alertness to political context and a sound appreciation of the policy process. These three elements—problem definition, political context, and policy process—are the foundations of the framework to be outlined here. Each requires a substantial contribution from the social sciences, particularly sociology and political science.

Articulating a framework

A number of models have been suggested for framing the knowledge–policy interface in public health. The focus of Lee *et al.* (1997) for example, was on health policy in the United States. In this context they drew up a framework consisting of three formal stages of policy development—problem identification and agenda setting, policy adoption, and policy implementation—and went on to identify key cultural and institutional factors shaping health policy in the American setting. Richmond and Kotelchuck (1991), by contrast, provided a stronger linkage with the scientific foundations of public health. They saw an essential component of effective health promotion and disease prevention as being the knowledge base, along with political will and social strategy. Brownson *et al.* (1997) suggested four factors as important to policy development and implementation in public health—identification of health risks and preventive options, intervention development, policy development, and policy enactment and assurance.

These models have a lot in common. They all identify a series of stages or components that appear to be important preconditions for the translation of public health potential into action. In general, they also see both technical factors (for example, knowledge base) and issues of power as being significant determinants of success. Furthermore, for all of the models the policy process itself is seen as central and as encompassing a series of identifiable and distinct stages that need to be traversed if a successful outcome is to be achieved. Finally, the effective implementation and delivery of a policy or a programme are seen as intrinsic to the model—and not outside it—and therefore as essential to success.

These are the core components that will feature at the heart of the analytical framework to be outlined here. Firstly, this chapter will suggest that the essential starting point for any successful translation of public health potential into action is an adequate and appropriate definition of the problem in hand. By this is meant an adequate knowledge base, a professional consensus on both the definition of, and the likely solution to, the problem in hand, an acceptable ethical and philosophical base for intervention, and the appropriate intellectual and conceptual linkages to the policy process. Secondly, an essential precondition for effective public health action is a favourable political climate. It is the very nature of public policy that it requires the mobilization of support and the transfer of resources. This cannot be done without the appropriate political alignment of forces. This is a function of power and the garnering of support. Nor is this a matter of achieving the necessary alignment at just one point in time, for instance, to secure a particular decision. The entire policy process—the third component to the analytical framework—remains hostage to the balance of power, right through to implementation, delivery, and evaluation. Clearly 'process' and 'power' are intertwined, but this third element to the framework—policy process—can be understood as an analytically distinct dimension in which institutional, managerial, and other instrumental mechanisms are the principal focus.

Defining the 'problem'

At its simplest level, the issue of problem definition can be stated as one of professional consensus. The issue is whether there is a professional consensus on both the importance of the problem and the best method for its resolution. Thus, the issue of tobacco control has had almost unanimous support among public health professionals as a principal focus of policy attention, at least since the 1970s. The mechanisms of disease causation and its aetiology have been well established and are beyond scientific dispute: it is a major cause of death, it is a discretionary rather than a central life activity, and it appears to be highly preventable. Contrast this with alcohol control. The excessive consumption of alcohol is implicated in a wide range of problem areas. Yet its control has been a point of some controversy among public health professionals, particularly since evidence has revealed some beneficial health effects of moderate consumption for some groups. This lack of consensus has related to the target outcome for policy (alcohol consumption levels, road traffic accident rates, mortality from cirrhosis of the liver), the importance of alcohol *vis-à-vis* other areas of public health concern, and the mechanisms for intervention (price, availability, consumption control, harm reduction). Furthermore, there have been competing public health, commercial, and social definitions of the significance of alcohol. Besides which, in considering alcohol as a product, while obviously discretionary, it remains intertwined with many core life activities (like eating and socializing), thus making it a more difficult area to isolate and modify through normal policy mechanisms.

Clearly, therefore, problem definition is crucial. In essence, an issue that lacks clarity of definition and professional consensus has little chance of progressing up the policy agenda. Nevertheless the issue of problem definition goes well beyond the simple achievement of scientific consensus. It is the object of this section to canvass these broader dimensions of the issue.

Scientific parameters

In the conventional view of science, disinterested investigators apply standard and accepted methodologies to data deployed in carefully controlled experimental settings. In the course of this work they generate empirical results that contribute incrementally to the advancement of knowledge. This view of science as a set of practices and procedures is allied to an epistemological perspective that sees the scientific enterprise as one that discovers objective facts and laws of universal application.

Yet, to an important extent, science is not just a set of practices and procedures; it is a living social enterprise. This relates not only to the preconditions for scientific productivity—adequate resources, functioning teams, institutional support, collegial networks, and reward systems—but even to the determination of 'facts' and the forging of consensus around scientific findings (Latour 1987). In the case of health research funds, for example, the allocation of resources seems to have more to do with the established hierarchies of science, political imperatives, and commercial potential than with public health significance. Thus the disciplines of public health, particularly the behavioural and social sciences, have generally been the 'Cinderella' of health research funding.

Even more fundamental to the scientific enterprise are sociological insights that get to the heart of scientific thinking itself. According to this perspective, scientific thought should be seen as a representation of observed reality rather than as an objective and invariant analytical system (Kuhn 1970). Thus, amendments to such systems may take on more the characteristic of a change in beliefs than just an alteration in analytical categories. This is particularly pertinent to much public health research that has increasingly revolved around risk factor epidemiology, to the detriment of attention to broader social structural and contextual forces (Pearce 1996). These contrasting analytical tendencies represent scientific preferences and belief systems about social reality, and have a long history going back to the early theoretical disputes of mid-nineteenth century public health between contagion and miasma (Tesh 1988).

The influence of social context is very much more apparent once attention is moved away from the cloistered environment of the research setting and towards the arena of application—that is, using Jasanoff's (1990) distinction, from research science to regulatory science. This terrain is clearly a contested one. Science, the state, and a range of interest groups vie to define key public health 'problems', interpreting evidence, weighing alternatives, and attempting to shape the agenda (Spector and Kitsuse 1987). For example, the tobacco industry has been particularly active in trying to influence the debate on passive smoking effects, in much the same way as the pharmaceutical industry has across a wide range of scientific arenas. The stakes are high and the traditional mechanisms of peer review and of open, dispassionate debate are not necessarily a match for successfully arbitrating deeply entrenched ideological differences, whether these derive from political, scientific, or commercial preferences (Greenberg 1992).

An important development in generating professional consensus has been the emergence of the evidence-based medicine movement and the growing use of reviews, meta-analyses, and consensus conferences (Lomas 1991). These devices, together with more deliberate strategies for achieving professional consensus, such as pilot studies, formal hearings, tribunals, and commissions of inquiry, increase opportunities for canvassing alternative evidence and interpretations. A particularly interesting development has been the emergence of formally designated centres for the assessment of health technology across a number of countries. Criteria for the assessment of health technology have been developed and the field has become rapidly professionalized, with an emerging consensus on procedures and key findings.

The development of the evidence-based medicine movement has done much to systematize the search for agreed criteria of evidence (Muir Gray 1997). To the traditional criteria for establishing causal linkage have been added an adjudication on levels of evidence from published studies, and a sophisticated discussion about the methodological strengths and weaknesses of different research designs. It is these more conventional hallmarks of scientific work, together with agreement on their theoretical underpinnings and wider significance, that provide the preconditions for professional consensus on any given public health problem.

Definition and importance

One useful outcome of the 'sociology of science' approach outlined in the previous section is the highlighting of the importance of certain core, definitional activities in making sense of a problem area for the professional community of interest. Thus, 'cot death' or sudden infant death syndrome, framed a potentially esoteric issue—unexplained infant deaths—in such a way that it became more meaningful within policy, clinical, scientific, and even popular discourse. In a similar fashion, the framing of public health questions in terms of risk behaviours sets the context for a specific group of scientific, and consequential policy, activities. For example, alcohol abuse considered at the clinical level leads to a focus on personality and biological predisposition; at the population level, by contrast, issues of availability and consumption patterns come into focus (Jeffery 1989). A similar argument applies with a preference for certain methodological techniques and research designs emphasizing conventional criteria of rigour; in these instances, approaches that use qualitative research techniques and that try to understand the perspective of key stakeholders may be overlooked (O'Neill and Pederson 1992).

Other broader definitional processes may be at work in the emergence of key public health problems to policy prominence. Feminists have argued, for example, that issues of importance of special interest to women, for instance, domestic violence and menstruation, are not given high priority, a point that may be reiterated for other areas that are of interest to less powerful groups, such as minority ethnic groups and the elderly. Thus, there are social parameters to problem selection and definition that may influence the course of scientific progress and the availability of relevant information for policy formulation (Mechanic 1993).

The likelihood that an issue will be defined as an important and relevant one has much to do with the wider policy process. Political salience, public visibility, personal immediacy, perception of threat—all these are likely to contribute to an issue surmounting the threshold of policy relevance (Rochefort and Cobb 1993). But what about criteria within the professional community—is there agreement at this level on the relative importance of public health issues?

Impact on the heath of the community is clearly a key criterion of importance. Methodologies such as the burden of disease have been significant in establishing a sense of priority among broad competing areas of public health concern (Murray and Lopez 1996). Within these broader categories, the population attributable risk is a marker of significance (Northridge 1995). Where the proportion of a population exposed to a particular risk is high (for instance, a fifth) and where the relative impact of that risk is also high (for instance, a factor of 3) then the argument for public health action in the case of a relatively common disease or disorder can be said to be a strong one.

The scale of the health problem at issue is clearly a precondition for action. Another essential criterion is modifiability or tractability. Although this dimension has not been quantified in a standardized way across problem areas, for the purposes of assessing public health importance it has to be addressed. A judgement has to be made as to whether there are established and tractable mechanisms for intervention that are effective. Other criteria that need to be considered are those of cost-effectiveness and impact on the existing shape of health inequalities. There are a range of methods for prioritizing health problems, risk factors, and interventions in order to select preferred strategies (Spasoff 1999).

To summarize, in order to reach the desired threshold of importance as a basis for professional consensus, a public health issue has to meet a number of criteria. It has to be seen to have a major health impact, the key risk factors should be highly modifiable, its cost should be within the bounds of other comparable interventions, and the proposed action should either reduce, or at the very least not exacerbate, health inequalities. Any such initiative should also meet ethical criteria and norms of social acceptability.

Policy linkages

In attempting to transcend the knowledge–action gap an essential feature of successful problem definition is the identification of clear links to the policy process. The conceptualization of a public health issue should be such that the indications for policy intervention are reasonably clear. On its own, for example, the ground-breaking work of Doll and Hill (1950; 1964) in identifying the link between smoking and lung cancer was not sufficient to direct attention to a series of feasible policy options. Nor was it intended to do so. This was core scientific work of immense humanitarian significance, and yet the translation of that essential technical breakthrough into action on any substantial scale had to await further analysis that addressed the contextual and institutional determinants of smoking behaviour. Neither moral exhortation nor simple prohibition were going to be either feasible or effective policy instruments. Thus a conceptualization of the smoking–lung cancer link that brought in wider policy-relevant variables was a crucial precursor to successful policy-making and eventual action (Davis 1994).

As this example suggests, the translation of knowledge into action may require additional analytical and empirical work in order to bridge the conceptual gap between core technical disciplines, such as epidemiology and risk assessment, on the one hand and the policy arena on the other (Levenstein 1996). This is an argument not for altering or diminishing the contribution of basic technical work, but for augmenting it with closely allied behavioural and social science perspectives. In this sense this is both a traditional call for multidisciplinary research, as well as a plea for academic teamwork within the public health sciences. What is needed is a careful sequencing of academic work such that, once the key findings of the more technical disciplines and the basic sciences are established, these results can be rapidly relayed to those in health promotion and policy development (Hersey *et al.* 1996). This happens too infrequently.

In some areas of technical work the links into effective delivery are already well established. This is the well-worn path of regulatory science, as in environmental health and occupational health and safety. In these areas technical findings are incorporated into established regulatory systems in a relatively straightforward and uncontentious manner. It is the expansion of these regulatory frameworks into new fields that sanction individual behaviours, such as smoking, alcohol consumption, and contraceptive use, where serious controversy is likely to arise. An important role can be played in these areas by the 'expert committee' helping to negotiate the science–policy interface (Berridge and Stanton 1999).

There are two approaches to capturing greater policy sensitivity in the conventional public health framework. The model that prevails in disease prevention initiatives and conventional regulatory science is one of augmentation; that is, adding to an existing scientific endeavour analytical perspectives that are closer to the policy process (Hinman 1997). These are arenas in which a more traditional model of disease is dominant and the function here is a bridging one between science and policy. Health promotion, by contrast, provides an alternative paradigm—a more multidimensional model of health—and in this perspective the behavioural and social science factors are quite central to problem definition (Snider and Satcher 1997). In these fields an alternative to the multidisciplinary teamwork model is one in which the approach is interdisciplinary, and co-operation across disciplines occurs at the conceptual and policy level. To an important extent science is policy under this approach.

Regardless of the particular model, the message is that the translation of public health knowledge into effective action requires a conceptualization of the behavioural and social sciences that can establish the key links to the policy process (Rutten 1995). In particular, as Link and Phelan (1995) argue, it is important to identify what puts people 'at risk of risks', and this requires the analysis of social conditions as fundamental causes of disease (the epidemiological expression of this insight is presented by Rose 1985).

Managing power relations

Perhaps the least understood dimension to the interface between scientific knowledge on the one hand and policy intervention on the other is that of power. For the public health practitioner there is almost something distasteful, even underhand, about acknowledging the role that power and political position might play in achieving what appear to be self-evidently laudable and highly noble public objectives (such as saving lives and preventing illness and disease). Yet, this is the reality of the field of public policy; support must be mobilized, resources transferred, regulations instituted, programmes established, and administrative interventions sustained and carried through to successful completion (Williams-Crowe and Aultman 1994). At every point, issues of power, position, and politics are crucial.

One fundamental weakness for public health is that it lacks a powerful, united, and consistent political constituency. This is partly because some of the greatest achievements of public health are nearly invisible; death, disease, and injury averted are hard to relate to and quantify (Remington 1990). Furthermore, there are no major, cohesive and articulate constituencies that recognize and openly acknowledge the benefit they derive from public health initiatives (apart from those they employ), and there are many groups whose interests may be affronted by energetic public health action. Therefore, on political grounds alone, policy initiatives in public health are difficult to mount and sustain.

This being the case, an understanding of the political context for public health action is an essential precondition to policy formation. Tobacco control is an instance where a professional consensus on the case for intervention is not in question and where a relatively sophisticated and policy-relevant conceptualization of the issue has been developed. Yet, formidable obstacles to progress in this area remain because of the powerful constituency against regulatory and policy change that is nurtured by the tobacco companies. The issue of political feasibility has to be addressed right across the spectrum of public health action.

The distribution of power

One of the central concerns of political theory in the area of policy formulation and implementation is the configuration of power. If power is defined as the ability to achieve one's goals even against the opposition of others, then the distribution of power is crucial to any understanding of the policy process. While such an understanding may have a rationale in political theory, it will—just as importantly for the present discussion—have a basis in empirical case studies and an operational significance for policy-making in public health (Lewis and Considine 1999).

At the risk of oversimplification, there are broadly two theories on the configuration of power: (a) pluralism, which stresses the dispersion of power, and (b) the structural interest model, which emphasizes the relative concentration of power. Behind these two models of the distribution of power lie entire theoretical systems and views of the way in which the world works. The pluralist theory derives from a perspective on society and the distribution of power that is benign and optimistic. According to this model, society is relatively egalitarian and the threshold for entry into the policy arena is low. Thus, almost any group can enter the policy process, and those groups that do enter the policy arena on any given issue are more or less evenly balanced in power and resources. The classic expression of this model remains Dahl's *Who Governs? Democracy and Power in an American City* (Dahl 1961) and the theory perhaps best exemplifies the role of interest groups in the relatively fluid system of government in the United States, particularly at the level of community politics.

The structural interest model, by contrast, posits a relative concentration of power in the hands either of a few key groups or of an élite (Duckett 1984). According to this view of power the real decisions and interactions take place at a relatively rarified level in the power hierarchy and frequently at times and places that are largely invisible to the public. While multiple interest groups may be present and apparent, the real work of politics and strategic choice comes down to a few key players with the power to influence the final outcome. In its most public form this model is most consistent with the corporatist decision-making processes of relatively structured societies with highly institutionalized systems of power-broking, frequently organized around the state and its bureaucracy (Lembruch and Schmitter 1982). Examples here would be some European countries and Asian countries such as Japan. Another version of this theory sees such processes as being less formally recognized and institutionalized, and more the outcome of the positional power of key agencies that routinely exercise influence in decision-making. An early outline of this view in the health field is Alford's *Health Care Politics: Ideological and Interest Group Barriers to Reform* (Alford 1975).

The pluralist model has a good deal of empirical plausibility in the health sector. Crucially, the sector is heavily populated with interest groups. Thus, almost every health condition has its own voluntary association and mutual support group, many communities are organized to lobby for local services, there are the major charities, and, finally, provider and supplier groups are all well organized and active. More than almost any other sector, health is characterized by a myriad of groups who lobby and act in a very public way, to an important extent because health is publicly funded in most countries. Debates about the allocation of public resources are highly visible and politicized.

Another feature that has until recently underscored the pluralistic nature of the health sector has been the relatively static quality of health system arrangements, at least until the 1980s (Klein 1990). Essentially the central architectural features of most health systems had remained largely unchanged for decades, and change, to the extent that it occurred, took place in an incremental fashion. Thus, in a period of reasonably steady economic growth, increments of service took place at the margins, and frequently these incremental changes resulted from the activities of one group or another advocating for a particular service or policy. This contrasted with the large-scale, systemic, and structural changes more characteristic of health-care policy in the 1980s and 1990s (Ham 1997).

While a pluralist model may best reflect the public face of debate and incremental change in the health sector, the realities of power for major decisions and for the backdrop to the 'small' decisions accord far more to the structural interest model. Thus, in major issues of health system change, the medical profession is a key veto group. Similarly, health insurance, medical suppliers, and pharmaceutical interests constitute a formidable force in the politics of health. Thus for major health service issues it would seem that the state, the medical profession, and, in some countries, health insurers and business, are the key players in shaping the course of policy-making (Bergthold 1988).

What of public health issues? Again, there is evidence for both of these perspectives. At the community level, and in the case of conditions for which there is no obvious commercial interest, a pluralistic model would seem to be the relevant one. In many instances groups are trying to achieve incremental change over a reasonably long period of time with uncertain policy pathways and endpoints. Thus, actions to address diabetes or asthma are constrained more by the intractability of the problem—including broader structural determinants—than any direct opposition by affected groups. Similarly, there are some issues where the policy problem is more one of gaining public support than addressing the interests of any well-organized groups (road traffic accidents, for example) (de Leeuw and Polman 1995).

One example of a public health issue where a pluralist model seems particularly appropriate is that of community water fluoridation. The adjustment of fluoride levels in central water supplies has been shown to be a safe and effective public health measure for preventing tooth decay for over 50 years (Ripa 1993). And yet, once the technical health issues have become secondary to wider political considerations of safety and individual rights, adoption of this measure has been slow. Crucial in the decision to fluoridate community water supplies have been the media, the nature of formal decision-making processes, consumer and wider social movements, the role of public agencies and key health professional organizations, and other community variables (Frazier 1984).

Nevertheless, for some of the 'big' issues of public health, structural interests are at the heart of the political arena. The major example in this regard is tobacco control, where controls on advertising, price increases, and the creation of smoke-free environments, have all been opposed by the industry. Similarly, the alcohol and food industries have been very active in other areas of public health concerned with diet and alcohol consumption. The public health task is made very much more difficult in these circumstances since a single, powerful opponent can work at a number of levels of the policy process to block public health initiatives.

Issue definition and agenda setting

A central element of the political context to policy is the ability of different groups to shape the definition of key issues and to set the agenda (Kindgon 1995). This occurs within a framework of values and wider economic and social forces that set the environment and provide the openings for policy initiatives (Burris 1997). For example, the United States is unique among the advanced Western democracies in the limited role it accords the state in the funding, organization, and delivery of health care. This represents a particular historical tradition, the values of individualism, and a special combination of economic interests—such as health insurers—and social groups (a large, affluent middle class able to afford private insurance), together with a federal political system characterized by weak party alignment (Lee *et al.* 1997). This particular set of environmental forces places major constraints on the range and characteristics of possible health reform initiatives that have any chance of being comsidered for the policy agenda in the United States.

Therefore, there are certain larger forces that shape the structure of opportunities and possibilities for policy. Within these parameters, however, issue definition and agenda setting are crucial to determining the initiation of the policy process, and these are to an important extent reflective of, and contributory to, the structure of power. Essentially, groups that are able to get issues defined in a way favourable to their interests, and that can then go on to lodge those issues in a prominent place on the formal policy agenda, are in a strong position to get their own way in the policy-making process.

Again, as in the case of the distribution of power, there are two broad tendencies in the study of issue definition and agenda setting. According to the pluralistic model, advocacy groups initiate issues from outside the formal institutional framework. Such advocates articulate an issue or grievance, identify solutions, and attempt to expand support for their case, culminating, if successful, in their cause entering the formal, institutional agenda (Cobb and Elder 1983). There are many examples of this kind in the health sector, with groups championing local causes or particular services, attempting to establish coalitions of support, and working through the media towards building the momentum for formal recognition of the issue in the policy process. Examples of this are the siting of local facilities, the provision of a new technology or service, or the recognition of some new public health or environmental hazard. In the public health field the building of public momentum behind a tobacco control agenda is a classic example of social mobilization and coalition building (Sato 1999).

An alternative model derives from the structural interest model and emphasizes the élite and relatively closed nature of decision-making in many instances. For certain key power groups the quickest and surest way to achieving a desired position on the institutional agenda with a view to some policy initiative is through relatively private avenues of influence rather than by public campaign. This may be partly because the issues at stake are rather technical and do not have a broad constituency—for example, screening practices in primary care (Florin 1998). In other cases, this route is preferred because it is a way of achieving policy success without attracting public opposition. For example, nearly every provider group in the health field has its own statute governing matters such as qualifications, recruitment, regulation, discipline, and so on.

There is unlikely to be a broad public interest in these matters and many such issues are relatively technical and uncontentious. Yet, the question of the quality of health practice and the methods by which, for instance, the medical profession goes about dealing with patient complaints and professional competence are potentially of wide interest and generate recurrent public unease and dissatisfaction (Stacey 1992). Similarly, powerful commercial lobbies would far rather deal with key issues in private where their influence can be exerted to its maximum and decisions can be shielded from potentially disruptive public scrutiny. In other circumstances, where such issues are already in the public domain—or where governments need to feel the pressure of public opinion—such interest groups are also adept at building and nurturing public support for their position.

A gap in both these models is a failure to allow for initiatives that may emanate not from interest groups, large or small, but from within the apparatus of government itself. Governments and bureaucracies, albeit frequently on the prompting of interest groups, initiate issue definition and agenda-setting exercises to try to set the climate for administrative intervention (Robins and Backstrom 1994). To some extent this can be seen as an acknowledgement that an issue is on the formal, institutional agenda. For example, tobacco control legislation may be under consideration after a long public campaign started externally to formal institutional structures, and the public heath bureaucracy may see it as timely to maintain a climate of public support (Sato 1999). In other instances, initiatives may derive from other parts of the bureaucracy, such as the finance ministry, or some official watchdog agency, or even from the executive or legislative arms of government.

Aside from positional power and influence in issue definition and agenda setting, a key dimension that advocacy groups, lobbyists, and governmental and bureaucratic agencies have to consider is the cultural salience and relevance to core values of their problem focus. Issue definition is not merely a function of positional influence, size, resources, and institutional and environmental opportunity—although these all help and are essential preconditions for successful agenda setting. Centrality to core values and culturally salient concerns and symbols are crucial as well. For example, certain social groups and conditions are stigmatized, while others are highly valued. Thus, causes associated with mental health struggle, while those associated with the ailments of children thrive (Nelson 1984).

The resolution of many key public health issues turns on the particular value framework within which they are viewed by the public. Whether it be the fencing of private swimming pools, gun control, or restrictions on smoking and drinking, a primary aspect of the public definition of these issues is whether they are seen as matters of health and safety or controversies impinging on the expression of individual rights (Burris 1997). For advocacy groups, lobbyists, and governmental agencies involved in these controversies, positioning of the issue in relation to these two value complexes becomes crucial and much energy is devoted to presenting the issue in the appropriate light (Chapman and Lupton 1994). Again, certain groups are greatly advantaged because of their material resources (which enables them to run public relations campaigns), their access to the media, or relevant cultural assets (such as positive public image, high social status), and these can become crucial in issue definition and agenda setting. Thus, an important stage in the campaign for greater tobacco control in many countries has been the advent of both the medical profession and key charity groups, such as the cancer societies. This has both lifted the public perception of the cause and its legitimacy, and at the same time detracted from the relative standing of its opponents, at a critical juncture in the development of the issue and its passage onto the formal, institutional agenda.

Apart from the philosophical battle between health and safety definitions on the one hand and individual rights on the other, there have been other polarities in the coloration of public policy issues concerned with individual well being. One important tussle has been that between legal and public health definitions. The issue of HIV and AIDS remains an area in which public health concepts, and a framework of human rights, are in contest with more punitive policies deriving from the law and the criminal justice system (Kirp and Bayer 1992). There are many other areas of fluidity where groups are attempting to negotiate new definitions. Thus, groups with varying disabilities—physical, mental, intellectual, vision—have sought to redefine their condition from that of dependent patients in treatment to a human rights perspective as clients in partnership with service agencies (Scotch 1989). Pharmaceutical companies, by contrast, are moving in the opposite direction (Payer 1992). They are attempting to convert an ever-expanding range of life conditions into treatable ailments, a process called 'medicalization' by sociologists (Conrad 1992). More broadly, this touches upon competing clinical and public health definitions of issues, where treatment philosophies compete with prevention in issue definition (for example, treatment for alcohol dependency versus public policy initiatives to reduce alcohol-related harm) (Remington 1990).

The question of issue definition and agenda setting, therefore, relates to power, both in its positional and in its cultural and ideological sense. Issues that are defined by influential groups and that are able to claim salience to core cultural values have a much greater chance of being seen favourably by the public and by those in decision-making positions. This, in turn, gives them a much better chance of entering the formal institutional agenda.

Negotiating the policy process

The question of power relations has been discussed to this point as a characteristic of the environment external to the policy process. As will be evident in the discussion that follows, the negotiation of positional power and influence remains central to the passage of policy. Nevertheless, the emphasis in this section will be on the policy process as an institutional framework in which policies are formulated, decisions made, policy instruments selected, and programmes delivered. Clearly, this is a somewhat formalistic approach, and one that is adopted only for the purposes of exposition. In practice, problem definition, political context, and the policy process are inextricably intertwined, although exerting varying influences at different stages of the policy cycle.

The institutional framework

An analysis of power can tend to emphasize the raw ingredients of group relations and positional influence. Power can be seen as a force that emanates from the brute facts of material resources and privileged social position. Thus the emphasis in the previous section is on advocacy groups, lobbyists, and governmental agencies as actors in a dynamic field of power relations. Such an approach emphasizes the role of actors with distinct interests and capabilities. Yet, the interaction of these agencies, and to some extent their source of power, is shaped by institutions. In other words, the patterns of interaction between agencies are shaped, though not ultimately determined, by relatively established rules and processes that are socially sanctioned and often legally enshrined (Goodin 1996) (for a health application, see Immergut (1992)).

In the case of the policy process there is a clear organizational context through which policy issues are channelled. Principally, this represents the formal structures of government for a health application (Howlett and Ramesh 1995). In the case of the advanced Western democracies this means understanding the respective roles of the different arms of government—executive and legislature—and of the bureaucracy. For example, a very important distinction has to be drawn between the differing policy capacities of the executive and the legislature, respectively. The executive arm of government is in a position to formulate and carry out policy, but it cannot on its own necessarily secure political legitimacy, full financial support (where this is taxpayer funded), or legal sanction (for instance, a change in the law). These are functions of the legislature. Crucially, it is important for the purposes of political symbolism that key policy changes are publicly debated and passed through the legislature.

However, the opportunities for legislatures to play an active role in policy formulation and development are limited. This is partly because in most parliamentary systems there is a close relationship between the political alignment of the executive and the majority of the legislature. It is also partly because of the relatively technical nature of most policy issues in the modern state. Such is the technical nature of many issues that individual legislators cannot be expected to have the resources or the background to command the policy agenda on the myriad of matters that come before them. A combination of the resources of the bureaucracy at the command of the executive, together with strong party allegiances in most parliamentary systems, means that the legislature plays little active role in policy formulation. Nevertheless, individual members can raise issues publicly in the debating chamber and they do scrutinize policy proposals and monitor programme implementation in the committee room.

In presidential systems the separation of powers between the executive and the legislature means that the support of the majority in the house cannot be taken for granted, and hence there is more room for negotiation and bargaining. A further distinction needs also to be drawn between federal and unitary systems of government. The capacity for making consistent and coherent policy is much more difficult in federal systems because of the distinct sets of responsibilities and jurisdictions at national and state levels. This means that there is a frequent requirement for negotiation and considerable opportunity for jurisdictional disputes. If we add to its presidential and federal nature the lack of party discipline in the American system, then consistent, coherent, and long-term policy development would seem to be difficult indeed (Steinmo and Watts 1995).

Leichter (1991) compared these fundamental differences in political structures for the United States and Great Britain across a number of major health promotion issues (smoking, alcohol, road safety, and HIV/AIDS). While the unitary nature of the British political system encouraged clarity and decisiveness in policy-making, it did not necessarily lead either to greater creativity or to the 'right' result (as judged from a conventional public health perspective). Indeed, the multiple nature of the American political system meant that, while federal initiatives on health promotion might be blocked at the centre, experimentation with a diversity of interventions could take place at the level of the individual state. While clarity, coherence, and decisiveness might not have been apparent in the American context, creativity, inventiveness, diversity, and local ownership were.

In many respects the key element of the institutional framework for the purposes of policy-making is the bureaucracy. While, symbolically speaking, the legislature is important for imparting public support to policy proposals, and while the executive plays a central role as the embodiment of political leadership, appointed officials largely drive the detail of policy formulation. In principle they are answerable to elected politicians in the executive arm of government, but there is a limit to the extent to which generalist politicians can effectively maintain scrutiny over specialist advisers and bureaucrats supposedly at their command.

This being the case, the structure of the bureaucracy itself becomes a key factor in the policy process. In the case of the health bureaucracy, officials usually retain a host of formal committees and informal advisory groups in order both to nurture links with key constituencies in the sector and to maintain competency and intelligence in a range of policy and technical areas. Beyond this there are important distinctions to be made within the health bureaucracy—functionally between public health and health care, for example, and operationally between policy advice and service delivery. Apart from the health ministry there are other sections of the bureaucracy that are important to health policy-making. For example, the finance ministry will typically set the fiscal parameters for health funding, the transport ministry will be important for certain public health campaigns, education and environmental health for others, and the police and judiciary for still others. Any attempt to negotiate the policy process requires a full understanding of these organizational intricacies. Indeed, most public health initiatives require intersectoral allegiances and partnerships of this kind for their success.

Policy formulation

If, as argued above, policy formulation and development does not take place in the legislature—the most public and symbolically important debating forum in the advanced Western democracies—then where does it occur? It is at this point that the institutional and agency approaches to policy meet. There is an institutional framework—part public, part invisible—that sets the context for policy formulation, but these institutional settings have to be populated by active agencies and individuals motivated by the desire to achieve certain policy goals (Howlett and Ramesh 1995).

In this connection a new terminology has been developed that combines the organizational apparatus of institutions with the active and instrumental characteristics of advocacy groups, lobbyists, and official agencies. Thus analysts have identified policy networks as being sets of individuals and groups with an interest in a particular policy issue which they wish to advance. Members of networks are in regular interaction on their common issues of interest, although the regularity and coherence may vary greatly. In some areas, where interests are well defined and of long standing, the issue networks that have formed are highly integrated and stable. In some instances such networks are so small, stable, and predictable that they have been termed 'iron triangles', referring to their longevity and intractability (Jordan 1986). To take a public health example, such an iron triangle would typically include the public health bureaucracy representing the interests of the state, the industry or interest being regulated (such as the tobacco or alcohol industry), and an advocacy coalition (of health and related consumer groups).

The concept of an 'iron triangle' is relevant to the discussion of power and its distribution; this particular form of policy network derives from a structural interest configuration of power. Clearly, power and influence are concentrated in this set of circumstances, and policy debates are promoted in a highly stylized and predictable fashion. Nothing much will change until, and unless, there is some significant shift in the balance of power (for instance, a change of government, or an international event, or a new ally to the coalition). An alternative set of interacting relationships to that based on the structural interest model is the issue network, an association based on a wide range of loosely connected groups. This follows a more pluralistic concept of power distribution. Issue networks are perhaps more common in the health arena, since the health sector exhibits such a wide range of issues around which local and small special interest groups can coalesce.

Policy networks as defined here—ranging from the cohesive and predictable sets of actors to broader and looser associations—provide the framework of allegiances, interest, and ideology that help to define the parameters within which policy is formulated. Debates, public and private, take place among the principal actors, and these debates in turn help to shape the progress of policy (Read 1992). Another important contributor to these debates is the policy community. While policy networks refer to associations of actors in relatively frequent and predictable interaction over key policy areas in which they have strong and potentially conflicting interests, policy communities have their basis in a common area of expertise. The participants in policy communities may have markedly different perceptions of their policy area, but they enjoy a sufficiently common intellectual base as to permit a community of discourse on that policy. Thus there is a constant exchange of information, setting the context for policy formation.

At its most public the policy community is displayed in academic conferences, the writings of journalists, and books, speeches, and articles. This is generally the arena in which public health scientists can most clearly see their role, that is, contributing to debates among those with a level of expertise in a public health issue. These communities have played a crucial role in preparing the ground for policy development in a number of fields. Most recently the advent of HIV/AIDS as a new and unheralded public health challenge precipitated a widening debate among those with a basic understanding of the area. Thus, gay activists, public health bureaucrats, and academics helped to define the nature of the problem area and the range of potential policy options. This was preparatory to the entry of the issue on the formal institutional agenda and its progress in the policy development process through to implementation (for the New Zealand case, see Lindberg and McMorland (1996)).

Decision-making

The decision-making process is at the heart of public policy. The intensity of interest in a policy area is in direct proportion to the desire for or against change in the existing policy settings. In the case of policy networks of the iron-triangle type, the routinized and predictable nature of these relationships, and the carefully balanced nature of power that they reflect, suggest there is little possibility of change in these cases. To the extent that change does occur in these circumstances, it will be of a relatively major and systemic kind. In the case of issue networks, however, a change in policy settings is more likely, but will be of a more minor variety.

These alternative scenarios indicate two broad types of decision-making process (Walt 1994). In the first instance decisions revolve around issues for which the stakes are high and that require a relatively major mobilization of power and resources. Decisions of this kind are strategic and may have long-term consequences since they change long-standing and stable sets of arrangements. A recent instance has been the rash of health system restructuring that has afflicted most of the advanced economies, prompted by financial stress and ideological challenge. Long-established sets of relationships and assumptions were disrupted by the introduction of a range of new funding and structural arrangements (Ham 1997). In the public health area the introduction of tobacco control initiatives across a number of countries broke an apparent long-standing policy deadlock.

Major and strategic decisions of this kind have also been linked to an idealized rational model of the policy-making process. In principle, policy change, if it is to be mounted, needs to be synoptic and all embracing, if it is properly to co-ordinate all aspects of the issue under consideration. In this sense rational decision-making takes into account longer-term strategic objectives (Alexander 1986). Nevertheless, the concept of rational decision-making is probably better considered a normative one, that is, a desirable objective, rather than providing an accurate description of actual decision-making processes.

At the other end of the spectrum are decisions taken at the margins of the system and involving less central policy goals. These are usually promoted by smaller interests operating within looser, issue-type networks. They do not require the major mobilization of power and resources, and their focus is shorter term and less strategic. In the health system, and indeed any policy sector, most decisions are of this type. They involve bargaining and compromise, and the achievement of relatively small-scale amendments to existing policy settings (Lindblom 1965).

It has been argued that this style of decision-making—the incremental model—is both a better description of the policy process as it is, and a reasonable guide as to how policy should be conducted. There are two reasons why incremental decisions are likely to be the norm. Firstly, there is the inertia of existing arrangements and power relations, such that it is more likely both to achieve agreement and to secure a shift in resources at the margin, and in smaller scale, than in a major and thorough-going fashion. Secondly, the incremental model follows much more closely the traditional way in which bureaucracies work, and it is officials who usually have a determining role in setting the policy agenda.

Most decisions in the health sector are of the incremental type. There are few decisions that are of the major strategic kind, for example population funding equalization or comprehensive tobacco control. The typical decision is one that lies at the margins, for example the extension of an existing service, a new service opened in a small way, a shift in enforcement of current tobacco control legislation, or extending infectious disease control initiatives to a new arena. The problem with such a style of decision-making is that, while it may accurately describe the way in which the great majority of decisions are made, it does little to maintain or ensure the overall coherence of policy. Thus a series of incremental decisions, each clearly justified in its own light as achieving a limited objective, may in the aggregate actually undermine larger policy goals. For example, incremental public health initiatives, while improving health overall, may at the same time deepen social inequalities in health.

It is this concern—with the larger impact of disjointed and uncoordinated incremental decisions—that has fuelled the rational model of decision-making. While decisions may not usually or normally be made in full consideration of their strategic significance, this concept of decision-making is one that is held up by many policy analysts as a desirable *modus operandi* (Hogwood and Gunn 1984). Realistically this rational strategic approach is likely to occur only in circumstances where decision-makers are provided with a relatively unconstrained and simple set of policy circumstances, for example a major opportunity for political change. As an ideal, this model remains attractive to those involved in public health policy-making, at least as an organizational tool for policy appraisal. Nevertheless, the most effective policy approach is likely to be 'mixed scanning', involving a mix of rational planning and incremental adjustment (Etzioni 1967).

Implementation and delivery

Decision-making lies at the heart of the policy process since it alone can precipitate a formal change in policy settings. However, it should be noted that a decision not to alter an existing policy may be just as important as a decision to institute changes formally (Bachrach and Baratz 1963). Thus, the decision not to prosecute a tobacco company that is transgressing existing legislation, for example, has nearly as much effective force as a decision to change the legislation in a more liberal direction. In other circumstances, the ability to prevent an issue coming to decision can be a victory of great strategic importance. For example, the ability of the tobacco industry for years to prevent full consideration of voluntary codes of conduct in a formal decision-making process, which in many circumstances were likely to go against them, was vital in maintaining sponsorship and advertising under existing codes.

In most cases, however, effective decision-making does entail change to existing policy settings. This is usually the desired outcome in much public health policy since typically the promotion of public health objectives involves some modification to a status quo that is dominated by economic and individualistic values (Burris 1997). This being so, the key to policy success is the implementation process. Traditionally, this part of the policy cycle was viewed as relatively unproblematic, being seen as principally an administrative function. However, a series of studies revealed that the objectives of many programmes—agreed and sanctioned in formal policy—were not being achieved in practice. The assumption of ready and straightforward implementation was not fulfilled. From this insight into the incompleteness of traditional models of the policy process sprung the study of implementation and a closer assessment of policy design and policy instruments (Pressman and Wildavsky 1984).

It is perhaps remarkable that the implementation process was ever considered to be an administrative formality. Indeed, the surprise is rather that policies are implemented as intended or even at all, such are the formidable obstacles to moving from formal policy prescription to actual social and behavioural change. The nature of the problems that policy is addressing are usually complex, multifaceted, and sometimes quite intractable. The greatest likelihood of implementation success is in circumstances where the policy has relatively simple technical features, represents a relatively marginal change to the status quo, is implemented by a single agency, has a clear single objective, and is of short duration. It also helps if the policy does not upset powerful interest groups and has relatively low visibility with the public (Walt 1994).

In the political science literature two broad schools of thought about the implementation process have been identified (Mazmanian and Sabatier 1989). For those coming from a more conventional model of the administrative apparatus, successful implementation was seen as issuing in a relatively linear and hierarchical fashion from the source of policy and power, namely from 'above'. An alternative approach to this conventional administrative model was one that emphasized the active participation of other non-bureaucratic actors and saw implementation as less linear and hierarchical; this reflected a more interactive process from 'below' characterized by bargaining among the affected parties.

There are a number of fairly clear preconditions for effective implementation, the principal being the political climate. Before anything can happen, the required political resources must be available; that is, legitimacy, effective administrative apparatus, and relative policy consensus. However, financial, managerial, and technical resources must be available over and above this. Without the required financial support, a policy cannot progress, or can only be implemented incompletely. Finally, management competency and technical capacity are required to secure an effective outcome (Grindle and Thomas 1991).

An important consideration in determining the particular style of implementation is policy content; that is, the type of policy being addressed and kinds of instruments being brought to bear. Thus, one question that has to be asked is whether the policy is addressing an issue of distribution (providing a new service or extending an existing one), redistribution (moving resources from one group to another), or regulation (Palmer and Short 1989). A second set of issues concerns the kinds of policy instrument likely to be considered; that is, market mechanisms, or voluntary, family, and community endeavours, or administrative initiatives such as regulation or directive provision of services (Linder and Peters 1989).

Most public health initiatives are fundamentally regulatory in thrust since they frequently require changes in behaviour and activity relevant to health outcomes. Conversely, most health-care questions are distributive in their implications since they usually involve decisions to introduce or extend the delivery of services to key population groups. The public funding of health care frequently raises redistributive questions, since such resources are generally allocated disproportionately to more needy groups with poorer material circumstances, such as the young, the elderly, and the poor.

Again, many public health matters naturally lend themselves to the deployment of regulatory policy instruments and/or the direct provision of services. Typically, a public health initiative requires change to existing patterns of behaviour or activities. Frequently this involves some regulatory or administrative intervention and usually this can only be delivered and enforced by an officially sanctioned agency of the state. A striking departure from this tradition was the almost universal reliance on non-statutory mechanisms in the response to HIV/AIDS across the developed world (Kirp and Bayer 1992). Indeed, non-governmental organizations are playing an increasingly important role as partners in public health initiatives (Walt 1994).

Three scenarios for knowledge in action

The framework developed in this chapter has been organized around three strands of deliberation. In the first instance it has been argued that for any public health initiative to occur it requires a clear definition of the problem to be addressed in a manner that makes it susceptible to policy intervention. This requires an embedding of the issue within an action-oriented social science framework. Secondly, even where there is a clear definition and a solid professional consensus around that definition, the political climate has to be favourable to its progression onto the policy agenda. Finally, an issue, once well defined and favoured by the political environment, has to pass through a relatively well-established set of processes if it is to be implemented effectively.

Stated in this fashion, the picture is of a relatively orderly and linear progression from problem formulation, through the garnering of political support, to policy development and implementation. Clearly, this is an overly rationalistic representation of what is usually a far more complex and disordered process. Indeed, one authority sees these three strands of interest operating as three relatively independent streams (Kindgon 1995). Thus, there are at any time a number of 'problems' awaiting policy solution, some of them of long standing, others being relatively new and potentially urgent. Then, there is an established distribution of power and a range of interest groups focused on policy questions which, when taken together, provide a series of political opportunities for administrative action. Finally, there is a range of policy solutions and settings either in position or in process that are available in the immediate political culture and institutional environment.

The conventional view of translating knowledge into action is to see it as a progression from problem definition through advocacy and political support to policy outcome. There are a number of areas where this model applies. Thus, the advent of HIV/AIDS presented a novel problem that could not be ignored and for which there were no clear policy precedents. Problem definition proceeded to policy development at a reasonably low political threshold, only requiring high-level political support once a series of relatively unprecedented policy options were proposed.

Many public health problems, however, are of long standing and do not offer any clear-cut technical solutions. Furthermore, there is frequently a political readiness to deal with these issues; examples include teenage pregnancy, youth suicide, mental health, and poor diet. Still more intractable are issues of health inequalities and social determinants of health (Marmot and Wilkinson 1999). These are problems in search of the right policy prescription. The mobilization of political resources will still be required in these circumstances, but the principal requirement is a feasible policy option.

Finally, there are those public health problems about which a clear problem definition and policy options have emerged, but that await the correct political climate. For example, according to Berridge (1999) passive smoking was a 'scientific fact waiting to emerge'. The public acceptability of passive smoking was shaped by a complex number of factors, only one of which was the scientific evidence. It was consistent with a growing individualistic and environmental ethos, giving medical and scientific legitimacy to a position that had originated from a moral, and then a personal rights, issue.

Each of these three scenarios requires a slightly different approach to the knowledge–action link. In the case of new problems, or existing problems about which there is new knowledge, the definitional process and its links into feasible policy options is a key step, as exemplified in the case of HIV/AIDS. In the case of long-standing problems for which the balance of power is not a crucial consideration, the development of feasible policy options is the essential prerequisite to moving the issue along to some resolution. Finally, where a problem is clearly defined and feasible, and well-established policy options are available, the issue of political climate is salient. This can either be nurtured through advocacy and lobbying or has to await a significant shift in the balance of power at the level of the formal political process.

Conclusion

Traditionally, disciplines of a more technical kind like epidemiology, biostatistics, and a range of laboratory sciences have been at the core of public health. It is through the application of this expertise that some of the most startling breakthroughs in prevention have been achieved. Increasingly, however, as public health has moved from the more conventional issues of disease prevention to include those of health promotion, and as the awareness of larger policy questions has impinged on public health practice, so the salience of the policy process has become more marked. This chapter has outlined a framework for the analysis of the interface between the public health sciences and the policy process. It has argued that a consideration of policy should permeate the 'basic sciences' of public health—in the sense that the conceptualization of fundamental public health issues should be permeated by the social sciences in order to facilitate links to policy. The approach should be one that is interdisciplinary with the social sciences at a conceptual level. Furthermore, once the move is made into the application of this core public health expertise, the political climate and the policy process are both crucial determinants of effective translation of knowledge into effective public health practice.

References

Alexander, E. (1986). *Approaches to planning: introducing current planning theories, concepts and issues.* Gordon and Breach, New York.

Alford, R. (1975). *Health care politics. ideological and interest group barriers to reform.* University of Chicago Press.

Atwood, K., Colditz, G.A., and Kawachi, I. (1997). From public health science to prevention policy: placing science in its social and political contexts. *American Journal of Public Health*, **87**, 1603–6.

Bachrach, P. and Baratz, M.S. (1963). Decisions and nondecisions: an analytical framework. *American Political Science Review*, **57**, 1947–52.

Beaglehole, R. (1990). Epidemiology and health policy: how do we stop the band playing? *New Zealand Medical Journal*, **103**, 323–5.

Bergthold, L.A. (1988). Purchasing power: business and health policy change in Massachusetts. *Journal of Health Politics*, **13**, 425–51.

Berridge, V. (1999). Passive smoking and its pre-history in Britain: policy speaks to science? *Social Science and Medicine*, **49**, 1183–96.

Berridge, V. and Stanton, J. (1999). Science and policy: historical insights. *Social Science and Medicine*, **49**, 1133–8.

Brownson, R.C., Newschaffer, C.J., and Ali-Abarghoui, F. (1997). Policy research for disease prevention: challenges and practical recommendations. *American Journal of Public Health*, **87**, 735–9.

Burris, S. (1997). The invisibility of public health: population-level measures in a politics of market individualism. *American Journal of Public Health*, **87**, 1607–10.

Chapman, C. and Lupton, D. (1994). *The fight for public health. Principles and practice of media advocacy.* BMJ Publishing, London.

Cobb, R.W. and Elder, C. (1983). *Participation in American politics: the dynamics of agenda-building.* Johns Hopkins University Press, Baltimore, MD.

Conrad, P. (1992). Medicalization and social control. *Annual Review of Sociology*, **18**, 209–32.

Dahl, R. (1961). *Who governs? Democracy and power in an American city.* Yale University Press, New Haven, CT.

Davis, P. (1994). A sociocultural critique of transition theory. In *Social dimensions of health and disease. New Zealand persectives* (ed. J. Spicer, A. Trlin, and J.A. Walton), pp. 162–75. Dunmore Press, Palmerston, New Zealand.

de Leeuw, E. (1993). Health policy, epidemiology and power: the interest web. *Health Promotion International*, **8**, 9–52.

de Leeuw, E. and Polman, L. (1995). Health policy making: the Dutch experience. *Social Science and Medicine*, **40**, 331–8.

Doll, R. and Hill, A.B. (1950). Smoking and carcinoma of the lung. *British Medical Journal*, **September 30**, 739–48.

Doll, R. and Hill, A.B. (1964). Mortality in relation to smoking: ten years' observations of British doctors. *British Medical Journal*, **1**, 1399–410.

Duckett, S. (1984). Structural interests and Australian health policy. *Social Science and Medicine*, **16**, 959–66.

Etzioni, A. (1967). Mixed-scanning: a 'third' approach to decision-making. *Public Administration Review*, **27**, 385–92.

Fletcher, S.W. (1997). Whither scientific deliberation in health policy recommendations? Alice in the wonderland of breast-cancer screening. *New England Journal of Medicine*, **336**, 1180–3.

Florin, D. (1998). Influencing national policy; public health medicine and coronary heart disease. *Journal of Public Health Medicine*, **20**, 80–5.

Frazier, P.J. (1984). Public and professional adoption of selected methods to prevent dental decay. In *Social sciences and dentistry: a critical bibliography* (ed. L.K. Cohen and P.S. Bryant), pp. 84–144. Quintessence Publishing, London.

Gillroy, J.M. and Wade, M. (ed.) (1992). *The moral dimensions of public policy choice. Beyond the market paradigm.* University of Pittsburgh Press.

Goodin, R.E. (ed.) (1996). *The theory of institutional design.* Cambridge University Press, New York.

Greenberg, M. (1992). Impediments to basing government health policies on science in the United States. *Social Science and Medicine*, **35**, 531–40.

Grindle, M. and Thomas, J. (1991). *Public policies and policy change.* Johns Hopkins University Press, Baltimore, MD.

Ham, C. (ed.) (1997). *Health care reform. Learning from international experience.* Open University Press, Buckingham.

Hersey, J.C., Collins, J.W. Gershon, R., and Owen, B. (1996). Methodologic issues in intervention research—health care. *American Journal of Industrial Medicine*, **29**, 412–17.

Hinman, A.R. (1997). Quantitative policy analysis and public health policy: a macro and micro view. *American Journal of Preventive Medicine*, **13**, 6–11.

Hogwood, B.W. and Gunn, L.A. (1984). *Policy analysis for the real world.* Oxford University Press.

Holtgrave, D.R., Doll, L.S. and Harrison, J. (1997). Influence of behavioral and social science on public health policymaking. *American Psychology*, **52**, 167–73.

Howlett, M. and Ramesh, M. (1995). *Studying public policy. Policy cycles and policy subsystems.* Oxford University Press.

Immergut, E.M. (1992). *Health politics: interests and institutions in Western Europe.* Cambridge University Press.

Jasanoff, S. (1990). *The fifth branch. Science advisers as policymakers.* Harvard University Press, Cambridge, MA.

Jeffery, R.W. (1989). Risk behaviors and health: contrasting individual and population perspectives. *American Psychology*, **44**, 1194–202.

Jordan, A.G. (1986). Iron triangles, woolly corporatism and elastic nets: Images of the policy process. *Journal of Public Policy*, **1**, 95–123.

Kindgon, J.W. (1995). *Agendas, alternatives, and public policies.* Little, Brown, Boston.

Kirp, D.L. and Bayer, R. (ed.) (1992). *AIDS in the industrialized democracies. Passions, politics, and policies.* Rutgers University Press, New Brunswick, NJ.

Klein, R. (1990). Research, policy, and the National Health Service. *Journal of Health Politics, Policy and Law*, **15**, 504–23.

Kuhn, T.S. (1970). *The structure of scientific revolutions.* University of Chicago Press.

Lane, J.-E. (1993). *The public sector. Concepts, models and approaches.* Sage, London.

Latour, B. (1987). *Science in action. How to follow scientists and engineers through society.* Open University Press, Buckingham.

Lee, P. R., Benjamin, A.D. and Weber, M.A. (1997). Policies and strategies for health in the United States. In *Oxford textbook of public health* (3rd edn) (ed. R. Detels, W.W. Holland, J. McEwen, and G.S. Omenn), pp. 297–321. Oxford University Press.

Leichter, H.M. (1991). *Free to be foolish. Politics and health promotion in the United States and Great Britain.* Princeton University Press, Princeton.

Lembruch, G. and Schmitter, P. (1982). *Patterns of corporatist policy-making.* Sage, Beverly Hills.

Levenstein, C. (1996). Policy implications of intervention research: research on the social context for intervention. *American Journal of Industrial Medicine*, **29**, 358–61.

Lewis, J. M. and Considine, M. (1999). Medicine, economics and agenda-setting. *Social Science and Medicine*, **48**, 393–405.

Lindberg, W. and McMorland, J. (1996). 'From grassroots to business suits': the gay community response to AIDS. In *Intimate details and vital statistics. AIDS, sexuality and the social order in New Zealand* (ed. P. Davis), pp. 102–19. Auckland University Press.

Lindblom, C. (1965). *The intelligence of democracy: decision making through mutual adjustment.* Free Press, New York.

Linder, S.H. and Peters, G.B. (1989). Instruments of government: perceptions and contexts. *Journal of Public Policy*, **9**, 35–58.

Link, B.G. and Phelan, J. (1995). Social conditions as fundamental causes of disease. *Journal of Health and Social Behavior*, Special Issue, 80–94.

Lomas, J. (1990). Finding audiences, changing beliefs: the structure of research use in Canadian health policy. *Journal of Health Politics, Policy and Law*, **15**, 525–42.

Lomas, J. (1991). Words without action? The production, dissemination, and impact of consensus recommendations. *Annual Review of Public Health*, **12**, 41–65.

McKinlay, J.B. (1993). The promotion of health through planned sociopolitical change: challenges for research and policy. *Social Science and Medicine*, **36**, 109–17.

Marmot, M. and Wilkinson, R.G. (ed.) (1999). *Social determinants of health.* Oxford University Press.

Mazmanian, D.A. and Sabatier, P.A. (1989). *Implementation and public policy.* University Press of America, Lanham, MD.

Mechanic, D. (1993). Social research in health and the American sociopolitical context: the changing fortunes of medical sociology. *Social Science and Medicine*, **36**, 95–102.

Mechanic, D. (1995). Emerging trends in the application of the social sciences to health and medicine. *Social Science and Medicine*, **40**, 1491–6.

Milio, N. (1988). Making healthy public policy; developing the science by learning the art: an ecological framework for policy studies. *Health Promotion*, **2**, 263–74.

Muir Gray, J.A.M. (1997). *Evidence-based healthcare: how to make health policy and management decisions.* Churchill Livingstone, New York.

Murray, C.J.L. and Lopez, A.D. (1996). Evidence-based health policy—lessons from the Global Burden of Disease. *Science*, **274**, 740–3.

Nelson, B.J. (1984). *Making an issue of child abuse.* Chicago University Press.

Northridge, M. (1995). Annotation: public health methods: attributable risk as a link between causality and public health action. *American Journal of Public Health*, **85**, 1202–4.

O'Neill, M. and Pederson, A.P. (1992). Building a methods bridge between public policy analysis and health public policy. *Canadian Journal of Public Health*, **83** (Supplement 1), S25–30.

Palmer, G. and Short, S. (1989). *Health care and public policy.* Macmillan, Melbourne.

Payer, L. (1992). *Disease mongers. How doctors, drug companies and insurers are making you sick.* Wiley, New York.

Pearce, N. (1996).Traditional epidemiology, modern epidemiology, and public health. *American Journal of Public Health*, **86**, 678–83.

Pressman, J.L. and Wildavsky, A.B. (1984). *Implementation: how great expectations in Washington are dashed in Oakland.* University of California Press, Berkeley, CA.

Read, M. (1992). Policy networks and issue networks: the politics of smoking. In *Policy networks in British government* (ed. D. and R. Rhodes Marsh). Clarendon Press, Oxford.

Remington, R.D. (1990). From preventive policy to preventive practice. *Preventive Medicine*, **19**, 105–13.

Richmond, J.B. and Kotelchuck, M. (1991). Co-ordination and development of strategies and policy for public health promotion in the United States. In *Oxford textbook of public health* (ed. W.E. Holland, R. Detels, and G. Knox). Oxford University Press.

Ripa, L.W. (1993). A half-century of community water fluoridation in the United States: review and commentary. *Journal of Public Health Dentistry*, **53**, 17–44.

Robins, L. and Backstrom, C. (1994). The role of state health departments in formulating policy: a survey on the case of AIDS. *American Journal of Public Health*, **84**, 905–9.

Rochefort, D.A. and Cobb, R.W. (1993). Problem definition, agenda access, and policy choice. *Policy Studies Journal*, **21**, 56–71.

Rose, G. (1985). Sick individuals and sick populations. *International Journal of Epidemiology*, **14**, 32–8.

Rothman, K.J. and Poole, C. (1985). Science and policy making. *American Journal of Public Health*, **75**, 340–1.

Rutten, A. (1995). The implementation of health promotion: a new structural perspective. *Social Science and Medicine*, **41**, 1627–37.

Sato, H. (1999). The advocacy coalition framework and the policy process analysis: The case of smoking control in Japan. *Policy Studies Journal*, **27**, 28–44.

Schmid, T.J., Pratt, M., and Howze, E. (1995). Policy as intervention: environmental and policy approaches to the prevention of cardiovascular disease. *American Journal of Public Health*, **85**, 1207–11.

Scotch, R. (1989). Politics and policy in the history of the disability rights movement. *Milbank Quarterly*, **67**, 380–400.

Snider, D.E. and Satcher, D. (1997). Behavioural and social sciences at the Centers for Disease Control and Prevention. *American Psychology*, **52**, 140–2.

Spasoff, R.A. (1999). *Epidemiological methods for health policy.* Oxford University Press, New York.

Spector, M. and Kitsuse, J.I. (1987). *Constructing social problems.* Aldine de Gruyter, New York.

Stacey, M. (1992). *Regulating British medicine: the General Medical Council.* Wiley, Chichester.

Stallones, R.A. (1982). Epidemiology and public policy: pro- and anti-biotic. *American Journal of Epidemiology*, **115**, 485–91.

Steinmo, S. and Watts, J. (1995). It's the institutions, stupid! Why comprehensive national health insurance always fails in America. *Journal of Health Politics, Policy and Law*, **20**, 329–71.

Tesh, S. (1988). *Hidden arguments: political ideology and disease prevention policy.* Rutgers University Press, New Brunswick, NJ.

Walt, G. (1994). *Health policy. An introduction to process and power.* Zed Books, London.

Williams-Crowe, S.M. and Aultman, T.V. (1994). State health agencies and the legislative policy process. *Public Health Reports*, **109**, 361–7.

7.9 Public health sciences and policy in developing countries

Prayura Kunasol, Khanchit Limpakarnjanarat, and Prasert Thongcharoen

Introduction

Developing countries are those countries with a low average income as well as a low gross national product compared with the 'developed countries'. A shortage of resources prevails in these countries in terms of both national socio-economic development budget and infrastructure, especially in health-care delivery systems and trained human resources. Most developing countries suffer additionally from poverty, political instability, social unrest, and security problems that command the majority of their national budgets. The share of the total budget remaining for health is very small, usually less than 5 per cent, which is a small proportion compared with the developed world (World Bank 1993). Thus, they are often dependent on external support. The limited financial resources result in poor environmental sanitation and high morbidity and mortality from those preventable communicable diseases that have been eliminated from developed countries (Murray and Lopez 1996).

An appropriate health-care delivery system should follow good health planning resulting from a well-formulated public health policy. A shortage of capable health planning personnel leads to inappropriate national health policy development. In the developing countries, the major concern among policy-makers has been curative services (Doherty *et al.* 1999) to alleviate suffering from the major diseases prevalent in the locality. Thus, priorities are for hospitals to serve the immediate needs of sick patients instead of preventive services that are more cost-effective and impact on a greater proportion of the population. Furthermore, limited knowledge and technologies to ascertain health problems often leads to inappropriate health decisions by leaders. Public health sciences should be the basis for the formulation of public health policy but there is a lack of well-trained health personnel and experts in health planning.

The need to incorporate public health research into the formulation of public health policy in developing countries has to be recognized by policy-makers, especially politicians. Advocacy for appropriate health policy decisions by politicians should be carried out by knowledgeable public health experts. Strategies for public health policy formulation involve active participation by the key stakeholders including:

- health providers both in the curative and preventive fields
- resource-allocating authorities (e.g. budget bureaux, civil servant commissions, national economic and social development boards)
- intended recipients of the policy
- representatives of the general population, including the mass media and both local and national politicians.

Priorities in health have to be agreed upon by the majority of the stakeholders before specific policies can be accepted and implemented as a national plan. However, public health policy in developing countries evolves according to existing health problems and changes over time and in different situations.

Public health sciences used in policy formulation include epidemiology, biostatistics, clinical sciences, microbiology, immunology, behavioural sciences, public health administration, and health economics. The majority of these sciences are normally found in schools of public health but not all developing countries have schools of public health. Even in those developing countries where the training institutions for public health exist, they are rarely used to assist in the development of policy formulation and health administration. The design and implementation of health-care delivery systems, particularly primary health care, should be based on public health science principles to ensure their effectiveness in resolving health problems prevalent in the community. The availability of public health sciences, however, is dependent on the existence of training facilities for public health personnel. A shortage of financial support, as well as a lack of training facilities for public health personnel, limits the ability to utilize public health sciences for health policy formulation. Although there is less need for public health sciences for long-standing well-understood major acute infectious diseases, policy formulation and public health intervention are usually less complicated. However, utilization of the public health sciences is essential for dealing with the emerging and re-emerging diseases, and the rapidly increasing prevalence of non-communicable diseases. Development of public health sciences is therefore essential for developing countries to prevent continuing human and economic loss due to unabated health problems.

Developing countries with limited resources need to formulate those health policies that are most cost-effective. Surveillance can identify priority diseases but the use of public health sciences is essential to design effective public health surveillance systems for the early detection of health problems. Effective intervention measures can be implemented based on surveillance. Surveillance systems are also needed to evaluate the effectiveness of health-care delivery systems. Thus, public health sciences are major tools for policy-makers to plan and implement appropriate cost-effective health programmes.

In developing countries, academic institutions have greater access to public health sciences and technology than public health workers since most scientific books are written in English or one of the European languages which few health workers understand. The language barrier may therefore prevent public health workers from learning new technologies and health strategies. The involvement of local health personnel in pilot projects and clinical trials may assist them to learn new developments in health sciences and technology. Networking among research and academic institutions in developed and developing countries can also update the knowledge of the latest technologies of health workers in the public health sciences. The development of an international epidemiological surveillance system, proposed during the Twenty-first World Health Assembly in 1968, was a major step to encourage health workers to utilize public health sciences in planning and monitoring health-care delivery systems in developing countries.

The application of public health sciences and policy in developing countries can be classified into three groups according to the type of health problem and the strategies applied to resolve them.

1. Policies developed in response to immediate health problems confronting the community, for example malaria, yaws, and rabies.
2. Policies developed from existing knowledge, which are recommended by international organizations to address specific health problems, for example the smallpox and poliomyelitis eradication programmes, the Expanded Program on Immunization, the Control of Diarrhoeal Diseases programme, and the Acute Respiratory Infection Control programme.
3. Control of specific diseases policies which are derived from national scientific research, for example AIDS, hepatitis B, hepatitis A, Japanese B encephalitis, and measles.

These three categories demonstrate how health sciences have contributed to public health policy development in developing countries.

Public health policy developed in response to immediate health problems

A developing country in the 1950s (Thailand) experienced an outbreak of acute haemorrhagic fever resulting in high morbidity and case fatality. There was limited knowledge about the natural history of the disease. Initially, public health policy focused on establishing treatment facilities in the affected areas. The policy was then modified, focusing more on learning about the disease by seeking international support in the 1960s. The intervention strategy for acute haemorrhagic fever subsequently emphasized vector control mainly by insecticides, initially followed by larval control (Bang and Tonn 1993). This is a demonstration of the evolution of policies for disease control in developing countries as public health knowledge increases in which the natural history of health problems are not well established initially and which have limited resources. Public health policy has to be formulated according to the prevailing situation, and will concentrate initially on providing immediate relief by setting up treatment facilities, followed by organization of scientific studies of the disease with assistance from international communities such as the World Health Organization (**WHO**), and subsequently by initiating effective control strategies. This is currently true for developing countries suffering from newly recognized, emerging, and re-emerging diseases.

Poliomyelitis is another example of an infectious disease that developing countries have had to face in which the initial response was to establish clinical facilities to cope with the disease. Improvement of environmental sanitation resulting in an older age at exposure to poliomyelitis, coupled with a decreasing infant mortality rate, resulted in a large outbreak of acute poliomyelitis in Thailand in 1952. There were more than 300 cases of poliomyelitis treated in Bangkok, which required special treatment facilities such as iron lungs. The King of Thailand himself donated a special fund for treatment and rehabilitation in response to the poliomyelitis epidemic. After the major outbreak in Bangkok, the disease spread throughout the country to other urban and rural areas. The outcomes of disease were not just limited to transient illness and mortality but also included disability, resulting in economic and social problems for families, the community, and health service providers. The foundation for the crippled, also under royal patronage, requested that the government consider oral poliomyelitis vaccination as a public health policy for preventing the disease. This resulted in a request from the Ministry of Public Health to the WHO in 1965 for an epidemiological study on the disease burden caused by poliomyelitis in Thailand and appropriate intervention measures which could be undertaken, including the feasibility of using the oral poliomyelitis vaccine. The last case of poliomyelitis was reported in Thailand in 1997. It is anticipated that poliomyelitis will be declared as eradicated in Thailand by the first few years of the twenty-first century. This example also demonstrates the evolution of policy formulation from a problem based on a knowledge-based response acquired with assistance from an international technical organization.

Rabies is a major health problem for developing countries. Treatment requires postexposure vaccination for people exposed to the animal reservoir, especially stray dogs. The disease has a 100 per cent case fatality rate once established, thus it is potentially a major health problem. The public health policy in Thailand was to provide postexposure vaccination against rabies free of charge using government funds. For religious reasons, a policy for control of the dog population by killing stray dogs was not generally accepted and thus lacked community support. Formulation of health policy towards rabies control in this situation was based on public perception and sensitivity of the community rather than on scientific knowledge and was not cost-effective. A better approach was to vaccinate both domestic and stray dogs, including those living in temple precincts. This policy gradually gained the co-operation and support of the public.

As late as 1988, Thailand and the rest of Asia were considered to be relatively free of HIV infection. However, that year, an explosive epidemic of HIV began among injecting drug users that ultimately spread to all levels of society. Thai officials moved from complacency to action despite controversy about the potential effect on the tourist industry during the 'Visit Thailand Year'. The government realized that the country could not sustain its high growth in national income in the face of a huge HIV epidemic. The negative effects of uncontrolled HIV/AIDS on tourism, foreign investment, and remittances from Thai nationals working abroad were also recognized. The government decided to launch a policy to control the HIV epidemic by establishing a national AIDS prevention and control committee chaired by the prime minister. Screening of donated blood was established and expanded very quickly nationwide with the provision of reagents for HIV testing. A multisectoral co-ordinated planning and budgeting of HIV/AIDS-related activities among 14 ministries, international funding agencies, and local sources of support. The Thai strategy led to a broad consensus on the importance of taking action. To monitor the epidemic, Thailand established a comprehensive national HIV surveillance system in 1989. Increased spending for the prevention of HIV spread was initiated in 1991. Based on the experience gained from the sexually transmitted disease control programme, condom promotion became the basis of the HIV/AIDS control strategy. The government decided to mandate and enforce a policy of 100 per cent condom use in commercial sex establishments. The immediate impact was increased condom use in brothels and a continued decrease in sexually transmitted disease incidence. The prime minister's office also launched a national campaign through the mass media to promote changes in the sexual behaviour of the population. Recent surveys have demonstrated that there have been changes in sexual behaviour in Thailand since the campaign was initiated (Nelson *et al.* 1996).

Policies developed from existing knowledge recommended by international organizations

Poliomyelitis eradication programme

As stated above, poliomyelitis has been a public health problem in developing countries. Much has been learned about the disease in the past two decades which has made eradication possible. Humans are the only reservoir, and a highly effective vaccine is available. These characteristics make a global policy of poliomyelitis eradication feasible (Ruff 1999). However, global eradication of poliomyelitis requires a global effort to achieve a high coverage of poliomyelitis vaccination (over 90 per cent). This requires the implementation of an intensive surveillance and case investigation system, which needs strong commitment from policy-makers and health-care personnel, including allocation of resources. The WHO made eradication of poliomyelitis a programme priority and implemented a global eradication programme based on surveillance and intensive case finding. Eradication has now been achieved in many countries, both developed and developing alike, and is now found in only a few countries.

The WHO Expanded Programme on Immunization

Immunization has been recognized as one of the most powerful and cost-effective strategies to prevent and control diseases. For this reason, the WHO established the Expanded Programme on Immunization in May 1974. The countries of the South-East Asia region have expressed their commitment to reduce morbidity, disability, and mortality from those diseases for which potent, safe, and cost-effective vaccines are available. The Expanded Programme on Immunization has achieved a decline in all vaccine-preventable diseases. In many countries, this has been achieved through the establishment of vertical programmes to immunize children under 1 year of age systematically. In Thailand, for example, there has been a remarkable decline in many vaccine-preventable diseases, including diphtheria, pertussis, tetanus, measles, and hepatitis B, as well as poliomyelitis.

Following the successful smallpox eradication campaign, which included intensive surveillance, case investigation, and active case-finding, eradication has been proposed for other vaccine-preventable diseases such as poliomyelitis (see above). This policy cannot succeed, however, unless all countries agree to this goal as a health priority. The United Nations International Children's Emergency Fund (**UNICEF**) and the WHO Global Programme for Vaccines and Immunization has now been organized and has adopted a framework which differentiates countries based on their capacities and vaccine needs (Batson 1998) as a basis for further action against vaccine-preventable diseases. Futher control must be based on sound public health science as the smallpox and poliomyelitis eradication programmes were.

The WHO Control of Diarrhoeal Disease programme

The high incidence and mortality from diarrhoeal diseases in infants justifies making control of these diseases a public health priority. Giving simple oral rehydration therapy and promoting breast feeding, based on the results of public health research, has greatly reduced childhood deaths from diarrhoea. A further reduction in morbidity requires national co-operation to improve sanitation, which is a difficult goal to achieve.

The WHO Acute Respiratory Infection Control programme

The Acute Respiratory Infection Control programme has been instituted because acute respiratory infections kill more than 4 million children every year in developing countries, most of which are caused by pneumonia. The WHO has developed simple and effective guidelines for the treatment of pneumonia based on research which has been incorporated into its Integrated Management of Childhood Illness Strategy (IUATLD 1998). Thailand incorporated the strategy into its national programme in 1990. Training of health-care workers and pharmacists and the implementation of the WHO guidelines, as revised by local experts, were instituted nationwide in Thailand. With the implementation of epidemiological surveillance, these rates could be assessed. Since the programme was implemented, there has been a reduction in pneumonia mortality and case-fatality rates and a decline in the inappropriate use of antibiotics.

Policies for the control of specific diseases derived from national scientific research

Only a few descriptive studies of policies derived from national scientific research have been reported from developing countries. Research is only one of many equally legitimate elements to be considered by policy-makers (Trostle *et al.* 1999). A few examples from Thailand will be used here to demonstrate the impact of incorporating research results into policy decision-making and implementation.

Hepatitis B vaccination policy

Public health policy formulated and developed to cope with the hepatitis B problem in Thailand provides an interesting case study. The evolution of public health policy on hepatitis B vaccination began in 1985 when a committee on control and prevention of viral hepatitis was set up by the Ministry of Public Health. The committee recommended vaccination of newborn children with hepatitis B vaccine. The Department of Communicable Disease Control adopted the policy in 1987 and launched the hepatitis B vaccination programme under the Seventh Five-year Public Health Development Plan (1992 to 1996). The rationale behind this was based on several medical and epidemiological studies of hepatitis B carried out by scientists from the Chulalongkorn and Mahidol Universities, the Armed Forces Research Institute of Medical Sciences, and the Ministry of Public Health. The carrier rate of hepatitis B virus was found to be 8 to 10 per cent in the 1980s while the infection rate in the general Thai population was 50 to 75 per cent, a very high endemicity. There were roughly 1 million deliveries every year, of which about 6 to 8 per cent were from hepatitis B carrier mothers resulting in the birth of 30 000 new hepatitis B carriers annually. This group served as a reservoir of hepatitis B virus. The evidence of a strong association between chronic infection of hepatitis B virus and hepatocarcinoma has been well documented. Although both plasma-derived and recombinant DNA hepatitis B vaccines were available, they were very costly.

Several different strategies for a hepatitis B vaccination programme were, therefore, proposed to the Ministry of Public Health with the support of scientific evidence. The evidence included cost-effectiveness analysis as well as operational research to assess the feasibility of an intervention using the existing health-care delivery system. An economic model was designed to compare the strategy of vaccination of all newborn infants without serological screening with other options, that is, vaccinating only newborns from hepatitis B carrier mothers. After reviewing the results of the cost–benefit analysis, the Ministry of Public Health decided to adopt the policy of vaccinating all newborns without screening for the hepatitis B virus carrier status in the mother.

During the period 1988 to 1992, a pilot programme was conducted in two provinces, Chiang Mai and Chonburi, to demonstrate that hepatitis B vaccine could be effectively administered along with other Expanded Program on Immunization vaccines without compromising the success of the existing immunization programme. The results from the pilot study, combined with other immunological studies of hepatitis B vaccination from academic institutes, contributed greatly to the policy of inclusion of hepatitis B vaccine in the existing Expanded Program on Immunization in 1992.

The public health policy on the nationwide hepatitis B vaccination programme was the result of incorporating public health scientific studies, including biomedical, epidemiological, and health economic studies carried out by health scientists in Thai universities, research institutes, and the Ministry of Public Health. The collaboration and exchange of experiences from health institutions and universities played a major role in the public health policy decision to be one of a few countries that included hepatitis B vaccine in the Expanded Program on Immunization programme prior to the WHO recommendation in 1997.

The development of human resources in health contributes to capacity building in health research that allows decision-makers to incorporate scientific research into policy formulation. Policy formulation to fight hepatitis B in many developing countries with a high incidence of hepatitis B, such as Thailand, Indonesia, Kenya, and Cameroon, presented a problem since the cost of vaccine was high, far beyond the capacity of most developing countries to pay. Hepatitis B had to also compete with other health problems prevalent in these countries (Muraskin 1995). The public health policy-makers in those countries needed to employ public health research to convince political bodies and the public that the vaccine programme was feasible, practical, and achievable. The experiences in Thailand, Indonesia, and many developing countries demonstrate that co-operation and collaboration between public health researchers, policy-makers, and politicians is essential for the formulation of effective health policies. The strategy used for the control of hepatitis B can also be applied to other public health problems.

Prevention of HIV transmission from mother to child

After the announcement of the success of the study on zidovudine in preventing HIV transmission from mother to infant in the United States and Europe, many developing countries, including Thailand, became interested. However, the cost of treating the mother for the last two trimesters of pregnancy was perceived as too high to implement. The Thai Ministry of Public Health approved a clinical trial of a short course of zidovudine to determine its efficacy in preventing HIV perinatal transmission. In 1998, the study was completed and published (Shaffer *et al.* 1999). An efficacy of 51 per cent, and the relatively affordable cost of short-term zidovudine treatment of mothers, led the Ministry of Public Health to recommend short-course zidovudine treatment for all HIV-infected mothers in Thailand (Kanshana *et al.* 2000).

Conclusion

Public health sciences and policy development in developing countries have evolved to address existing health problems. Knowledge gained from research needs to be used by public health administrators for effective policy development, especially in developing countries. Developing countries with limited resources need to formulate health policy appropriate to the problems facing them using the most cost-effective strategies. Application of public health sciences to policy formation can be organized into three strategies: (a) policies developed in response to immediate health problems confronting the community; (b) policies developed from existing knowledge recommended by international organizations; (c) policies for the control of specific diseases derived from national scientific research. For each it is important for public health researchers and decision-makers to co-operate in the formulation of health policy. To achieve this goal it is important to provide training for public health professionals, preferably in national schools of public health as well as abroad.

References

Bang, Y.H. and Tonn, R.J. (1993). Vector control and intervention. In *Monograph on dengue/dengue hemorrhagic fever* (ed. P. Thongcharoen). WHO Regional Publication no. 22, SEARO. WHO, Geneva.

Batson, A. (1998). Sustainable introduction of affordable new vaccines: the targeting strategy. *Vaccine*, **16** (Supplement), 593–8.

Doherty, J., McIntyre, D., Bloom, G., and Brijlal, P. (1999). Health expenditure and finance: who gets what? *Bulletin of the World Health Organization*, **77**, 156–8.

IUATLD (International Union Against Tuberculosis and Lung Diseases) (1998). Communique from the International Conference on Acute Respiratory Infections, Canberra, Australia, 7 to 10 July 1997. Acute respiratory infections: the forgotten pandemic. *International Journal of Tuberculous Lung Disease*, **2**, 2–4.

Kanshana, S., Thewanda, D., Teeraratkul, A., *et al.* (2000). Implementing short-course zidovudine to reduce mother–infant HIV transmission in a large pilot program in Thailand. *AIDS*, **14**, 1617–23.

Muraskin, W.A. (1995). *The war against hepatitis B: a history of the international task force on hepatitis B immunization.* University of Pennsylvania Press, Philadelphia, PA.

Murray, C.J.L. and Lopez, A.D. (1996). *Global health statistics: a compendium of incidence, prevalence, and mortality estimates for over 200 conditions.* Harvard University Press, Cambridge, MA.

Nelson, K.E., Beyrer, C., Eiumtrakol, S., Khamboonruang, C., and Celentano, D. (1996). Changes in sexual behavior and a decline in HIV infection among young men in Thailand. *New England Journal of Medicine*, **335**, 297–303.

Ruff, T.A. (1999). Immunization strategies for viral diseases in developing countries. *Review of Medical Virology*, **9**, 121–38.

Shaffer, N., Chuachoowong, R., Mock, P., *et al.* (1999). Short-course zidovudine for perinatal HIV-1 transmission in Bangkok, Thailand: a randomised controlled trial. *Lancet*, **353**, 773–80.

Trostle, J., Branfman, M., and Longer, A. (1999). How do researchers influence decision-makers? Case studies of Mexican policies. *Health Policy Plan*, **14**, 103–14.

World Bank (1993). *World development report 1993: investing in health.* Oxford University Press.

8

Environmental and occupational health sciences

8.1 Environmental and occupational health sciences in public health

Jonathan Samet

Introduction

Overview

Humankind has long been concerned about the environment and health and disease. As early as 500 BC, Hippocrates (Clifton 1752) in *Upon Air, Water, and Situation* wrote of the relevance of the environment to health, commenting on seasons and weather, the siting of cities, and the nature of the water. He further urged consideration of 'the mode in which the inhabitants live, and what are their pursuits, whether they are fond of drinking and eating to excess, and given to indolence, or are fond of exercise and labor'. Across the centuries, this concern for the environment has shifted from very general theories about disease causation by the environment, like miasma, to today's highly focused and mechanistic formulations directed at specific agents or classes of agents and particular diseases. The workplace has been one environment of particular concern, as workplace exposures have been known for centuries to cause potentially avoidable diseases.

The environment has been a maintained focus for public health research and intervention because many disease-causing agents released by human activities may be subject to control, bringing the possibility of health promotion and disease prevention. As a societal 'common good', the quality of the environment is to be preserved for the benefit of all and protected against disease-causing contamination. Over the centuries, governments have attempted to preserve and promote the quality of the environment. In the case of air pollution, for example, civil suits were brought over air pollution even in Roman times, and regulations to control smoke were implemented as early as the 1300s in London (Brimblecombe 1999). Today, complex regulations are in place in many developed countries to limit pollutant emissions into the air from vehicles and stationary sources, like power plants. Regulations are also generally in place to assure the quality of water and the safety of food. Developing countries are also faced with the rising challenge of environmental degradation and workplace hazards as manufacturing moves from the developed to the developing countries. Simultaneously, many of these countries are still attempting to provide basic public health measures, such as safe drinking water and food.

Historically, the workplace environment has been a specific locus for research and regulation. Clinicians have long noted that workers developed diseases caused by their exposures (Raffle *et al.* 1987). Ramazzini, considered as the 'father of occupational medicine', published his seminal treatise on diseases of workers, *De Morbis Artificum Diatriba*, in 1700 (Raffle *et al.* 1987). These sentinel occurrences of disease were often noted because of distinctive clinical features—silicosis and asbestosis, for example—or because of unusual clusters—thoracic malignancy in the radon-exposed miners of Schneeberg and Joachimsthal for example. The working conditions of the Industrial Revolution brought reform attempts in Europe but specific regulations to protect workers against occupational diseases largely happened in the twentieth century (Raffle *et al.* 1987; Rosen 1993).

Throughout the centuries, concern for worker and population health has been motivated by evidence showing the adverse effects of workplace and environmental exposures. This evidence has had multiple sources including the observations of astute clinicians, like Ramazzini, epidemiological investigation, and toxicological investigation. A variety of processes, some quite elaborate and formulaic, have been developed to translate scientific evidence on adverse effects into policy. In the United States and many other countries, both developed and developing, administrative entities have been created for the purpose of protecting the public's health against environmental and occupational agents. In the United States, for example, there are the Environmental Protection Agency, the Nuclear Regulatory Commission, the Mine Safety and Health Administration, and the Occupational Safety and Health Administration. Even with agencies and regulations in place, surveillance remains necessary for programme evaluation and enforcement.

This chapter addresses the scientific methods used in public health to address the adverse effects of occupational and environmental exposures. Chapters that follow cover some of these same topics in greater depth. This chapter provides a general framework for conceptualizing exposures to environmental agents and then covers the general research methods used to generate data on adverse effects, along with the limitations of these methods. Specific methodologies for particular areas are considered. Finally, the processes for translating scientific evidence into policy in these areas are addressed. For those seeking further information, Rom's textbook *Environmental and Occupational Medicine* (Rom 1998) is a leading recent volume; its chapters provide overviews of broad areas and coverage of the public health consequences of some of the most significant environmental and occupational exposures. Textbooks of occupational medicine include those by Raffle *et al.* (1987) and Rom (1998), and the topic of occupational and environmental respiratory diseases is comprehensively addressed in *Occupational and Environmental Respiratory Disease* edited by Balmes *et al.* (1996). Epidemiological research has played a key role in characterizing the effects of occupational and environmental agents. Several books have addressed methods in occupational epidemiology (Monson 1990; Checkoway *et al.* 1989) and selected issues in environmental epidemiology have been addressed (National Research Council 1991*a*; Steenland and Savitz 1997; Lippmann 1999).

These volumes, as for most of the scientific literature, focus on environmental and occupational health in the developed countries of the world. There has been far less attention given to the developing countries, many now facing the dual challenges of the persistent problems of still uncontrolled infectious diseases and rapid industrialization with its consequences for workers specifically and the quality of the environment generally. Additionally, rising populations in many developing countries and the centralization of the population in large 'mega-cities', epitomized by Mexico City with more than 20 million inhabitants, pose environmental problems on a new scale (McMichael 1995).

The world also faces new forms of environmental problems that reflect global environmental change: depletion of the ozone layer by release of freons and other ozone-consuming chlorofluorcarbons and rising concentrations of carbon dioxide and other greenhouse gases. Ozone depletion is of concern because of the increased exposure to cancer-causing ultraviolet radiation that will result. The Earth's atmosphere is warming, in association with the rising concentrations of greenhouse gases; potential health consequences include increased mortality from exposure to extremely hot temperatures, altered patterns of infectious diseases, and altered patterns of exposure to outdoor allergens and combustion-related air pollutants, following increased power generation (McMichael 1995). An introduction to these new problems is provided in *Climate Change and Human Health*, a World Health Organization (**WHO**) report (WHO 1996).

Identifying occupational and environmental risks

Clinical medicine and the research methods of public health have long held interlocking roles in the identification of occupational and environmental agents that threaten the public's health. Clinicians, through the identification of sentinel cases, have often been the first to identify the new occupational diseases. Examples are abundant: vinyl chloride and angiosarcoma of the liver, identified by a surgeon who saw several patients from the same polymerizing unit within the same plant (Creech and Johnson 1974) and asbestos and mesothelioma, identified by a pathologist who accumulated a series of patients (Wagner *et al.* 1960). At the community level, clinicians may also have a role, although public health statistics and surveillance most often provide the initial warnings of risk. The potentially lethal effects of outdoor air pollution were convincingly demonstrated in a series of disasters early in the twentieth century that were associated with obvious excess mortality (American Thoracic Society 1996*a*,*b*; Denison *et al.* 1998). In the London Fog of 1952, a remarkable episode of atmospheric stagnation with extremely high levels of air pollution, there were several thousand excess deaths during the week of the fog (Logan 1953). Sophisticated techniques for time-series analysis can now be applied to large databases to detect far more subtle effects in the surrounding 'noise' from the many other factors that influence mortality counts (Samet and Jaakkola 1999).

While etiological hypotheses derived from clinical observation and review of public health data are still key strategies for identifying harmful agents, an array of toxicological approaches is now available to predict prospectively the risks of new agents. These include comprehensive bioassays involving exposure of animals to the agent with rigorous assessment for disease and evidence of injury at the tissue, cellular, or even molecular level (Clayton and Clayton 1991; Hayes 1994; Fan and Chang 1996; Niesink and de Vries 1996; Hodgson and Levi 1997; Crosby 1998; Rose 1998; Shaw and Chadwick 1998; Marquaedt *et al.* 1999), short-term assays using cellular or other systems, and knowledge of structure–activity relationships. The explosive advances in cellular and molecular biology are certain to bring more sensitive test methods. However, given the large number of new agents coming into production with potential for human exposure, most agents still have no or only limited specific evaluation. Animal bioassays are expensive and extrapolation from animal species to humans may be a source of substantial uncertainty, depending on the agent and the injury of concern.

Epidemiological approaches also have a key role in characterizing risks of both workplace and environmental agents. They provide directly relevant evidence on exposures as they occur in the population, capturing risks at relevant levels of exposure and across the range of human susceptibility. However, epidemiological studies can provide evidence only after exposure has occurred and epidemiological data are particularly powerful for characterizing risks of feasibly and accurately measured exposures with strong effects. Exposure measurement error tends to blunt the sensitivity of epidemiological studies and sufficiently precise and certain data may not be obtained for some agents, particularly those not having a strong effect on risk.

The approach to characterizing the hazard of occupational and environmental agents is now typically multidisciplinary. Toxicologists address uptake, distribution, metabolism, and mechanisms of toxicity; exposure assessment scientists (often referred to as 'exposure assessors') evaluate the distribution and determinants of exposure, and epidemiologists assess the risks to exposed populations. The resulting data may be substantial and in need of synthesis in order to make a determination as to the existence of a hazard. There are a variety of processes used for this purpose, ranging from informal exercise of expert judgement to formal combination and analysis of the data.

Determination of the presence of a hazard is much akin to the judgment that an association between an agent and a disease is causal. The criteria proposed by Hill (1965) or the very similar approach of the 1964 Surgeon General's Report on tobacco (USDHEW 1964) are often used for this purpose. A number of agencies have developed guidelines and general approaches for this purpose as well: the International Agency for Research on Cancer (WHO/IARC 1972), which undertakes a formal quantitative risk assessment, and the United States Environmental Protection Agency (USEPA 1986).

Pathways for policy formulation

For occupational and environmental agents, there are a variety of pathways leading from scientific evidence to policy formulation (Table 1). These pathways and the resulting control strategies may vary by the source of contamination, the medium of exposure, the locus of exposure, and the people exposed; there is also substantial heterogeneity in regulatory approaches comparing countries around the world. In the United States, for example, the Occupational Safety and Health Administration has jurisdiction over workplaces other than mines, which are covered by the Mine Safety and Health Administration. Radiation exposures are regulated by multiple legislative authorities and agencies, which separate occupational

Table 1 Some pathways for translation of epidemiological evidence into policy

Regulatory
Occupational health and safety
Environmental quality
Drug safety
Public health recommendations
Vaccination
Diet
Smoking
Legal system
Cause of injury
Health-care delivery
Practice guidelines
Outcome assessment

exposures, medical exposures, and exposures related to the nuclear industry. Food issues are handled by the Food and Drug Administration and the Environmental Protection Agency covers air quality and drinking water quality through disparate legislative mandates. Risks are not uniformly measured and managed across the range of agencies and exposures.

Risk management policies are intended to assure that exposures convey an acceptable level of risk, whether in the workplace or the general environment (Lowrance 1976). The four elements of quantitative risk assessment, as formulated by the National Research Council of the United States National Academy of Sciences (National Research Council 1983), represent the substrate for decision-making.

- Hazard identification—is there a hazard?
- Dose–response—what is the relationship between exposure or dose and risk?
- Exposure assessment—what is the distribution of exposure?
- Risk characterization—what is the risk to the population?

As a first step, a decision is needed as to whether the exposure poses a hazard. For many policy issues related to environmental and occupational exposures, the evidence comes from numerous and sometimes heterogeneous studies. Synthesis of such data for policy purposes has often been accomplished by expert review and consensus, tabular summary, or application of criteria for causality. These processes have proved effective, particularly for strong associations, but uncertainties in the evidence have sometimes undermined conclusions, particularly if conclusions weighted by policy implications are reached. An example is the epidemiological evidence on passive smoking, which has been the scientific basis for programmes to reduce smoking in public places and repeatedly questioned by the tobacco industry and its consultant scientists (Samet and Wang 2000).

Combining evidence from multiple studies, whether experimental or observational, has proved to be an efficacious approach for synthesis. This combination can be accomplished by meta-analysis, combining summary estimates from individual studies, and pooled analysis, analysing data jointly from individual participants in multiple studies. While the use of meta-analysis has been questioned (Bailar 1997), properly conducted meta-analyses have yielded useful and sometimes unexpected findings. Pooled analysis is a more powerful approach, offering the possibility of controlling confounding, and exploring effect modification or interaction at the individual level, but requiring the effect of creating the pooled data set for analysis. This approach was used, for example, in pooling the data from 68 000 participants in 11 cohort studies of underground miners in order to develop a risk model for radon and lung cancer (Lubin *et al.* 1994). The pooling yielded unequivocal evidence that radon caused lung cancer, even in non-smokers, and provided a relatively precise characterization of the exposure–response relationship. The array of alternative approaches for synthesis, ranging from expert opinion to quantitative summary, has not been rigorously evaluated, but more recent approaches, involving a systematic evaluation and quantitative summary of data seem preferable.

An understanding of the dose–response or exposure–response relationship is essential for advancing risk management policies that imply an assured and acceptable level of risk. Different dose–response curves, having differing implications for population risk and risk management strategies, may be biologically plausible (Fig. 1). A dose–response curve without a threshold indicates that any level of exposure conveys some risk, while the presence of a threshold indicates a level that might direct the level at which a standard should be set. A margin of safety could be incorporated into an exposure standard by using a 'safety factor' to place a standard for concentration or exposure at some point higher than the threshold. The dose–response relationship might also be non-linear (Fig. 1).

To complete the characterization of population risk, information is also needed on the distribution of exposure (Fig. 2), including its shape and span, and the extent of the population exposed to high-end or unacceptable levels. To protect the public's health, risk management strategies may need to address both the typical exposures, which drive overall risk to the population, and the upper-end exposures, which place some individuals at unacceptable risk. By combining the exposure distribution and the dose–response relationship, overall risk can be characterized and the implications of alternative control strategies evaluated. Regardless of the specific control approach, risk management should be implicitly or explicitly based in evidence on risk formulated in this fashion.

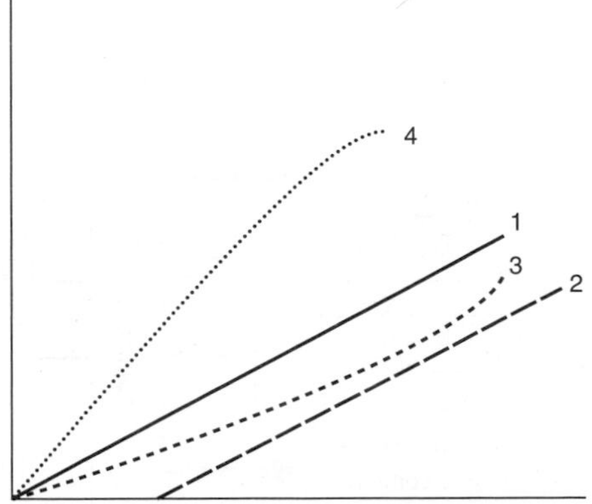

Fig. 1 Examples of dose–response models used for carcinogens: 1, linear non-threshold mode; 2, linear threshold model; 3, sublinear non-threshold model; 4, supralinear non-threshold model (Samet and Burke 1998).

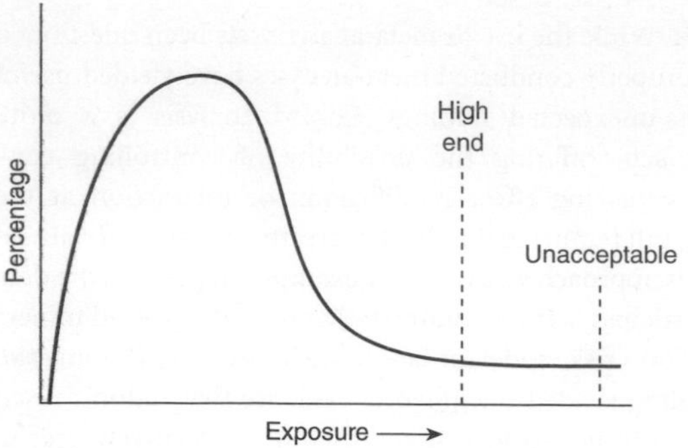

Fig. 2 Characterization of the distribution of exposure, including its shape and span, and the extent of the population exposed to high-end or unacceptable levels.

Exposures to occupational and environmental agents

Overview

Agents present in the general environment and occupational settings cause injury when exposure, that is, contact with the agent, takes place. This section sets out a general framework for considering exogenous exposures that affect health. In its 1991 report, *Human Exposure Assessment for Airborne Pollutants* (National Research Council 1991*b*), the American National Research Council offered a useful general framework for conceptualizing the paths from contaminant sources to health effects (Fig. 3). Pollutant sources contaminate the key media by which exposures arise: air, water, soil, and food. For some types of agents, the exposure occurs through physical contact, rather than through some medium of transmission: ionizing and non-ionizing radiation and heat, for example. The contaminated medium may transport the agent over long distances or the contaminant may be concentrated within the food supply, as may occur with mercury in fish which consume mercury-containing plants. For some exposures, for example, lead, multiple media may be relevant. In some countries, lead exposures come from lead introduced into water from pipes, from foods and beverages contaminated with lead from pottery made with lead-containing glazes, and from airborne lead from fuel combustion in motor vehicles.

In measuring or estimating exposures, whether for the purpose of monitoring compliance with exposure limits or for the purposes of research, the exposure indicators used should be appropriate to the adverse health effect of concern. Selection of the proper indicators should be guided by an understanding at the mechanistic level of the time course over which the exposure causes injury. For example, cumulative exposure may be most relevant to cancer risk while exposures to transient, high levels of irritants may produce lung irritation or asthma. Thus, lung cancer risk in radon-exposed miners can be estimated using cumulative exposure or exposures during past time windows (National Research Council 1998) while even transient exposure to toluene di-isocyanate may result in asthma (Banks 1998). For many agents, there may be uncertainty as to the relevant time frame over which exposures should be estimated and feasibility and instrumentation characteristics may be over-riding concerns for the measurement strategy.

Definitions

The terms concentration, exposure, and dose are conceptually distinct, although often blurred together in the context of public health research. Concentration refers to the amount of material present in the medium; the level of chloroform in drinking water or the mass of respirable particles in a given volume of outdoor air, for

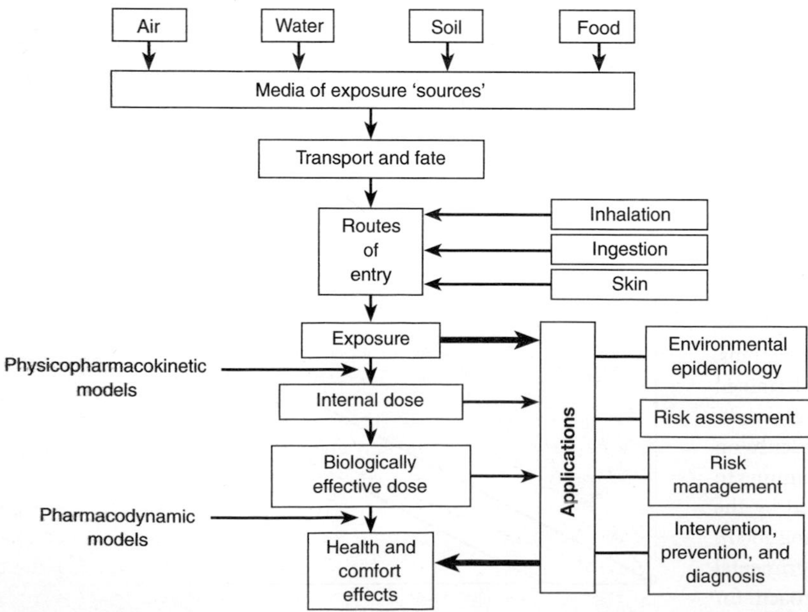

Fig. 3 Representation of the pathways from sources and media of exposure to health effects. (Adapted from National Research Council 1991*b*.)

example. Concentrations are often limited by regulation and consequently measurement data may be available that have been made for compliance purposes. Such data may be useful for research purposes as well. Exposure can be defined as the contact of pollutant with a susceptible surface of the body, which for air pollutants includes the eyes, nose, mouth and throat, the airways, and the skin (National Research Council 1991*b*). Exposure generally has the units of concentration and time and is estimated as the product of the concentration of material and the amount of time spent in contact with the material. The exposure of an individual over time can be characterized as a concentration–time function or an exposure–time function. Depending on the type of health effects and the underlying mechanism, it may be appropriate to formulate exposure as average exposure over a specified time period, or as cumulative exposure over the lifetime or for a relevant period. The relevant exposure metric depends on the underlying biological mechanisms leading from exposure to health effect. For cancer, for example, cumulative exposure may be the most relevant indicator of risk.

For public health purposes, both individual exposures and the distribution of the population's exposures are of interest. For any particular individual, exposure should be sufficiently low so as not to exceed a threshold of acceptability of the associated risk; for the population, the distribution should not convey an overall level of risk that is judged unacceptable. Risk assessment is used for estimating risk at the population level.

Dose refers to the amount of material that is absorbed or deposited in the body. There are a variety of dose measures: total dose, potential dose, internal dose, and biologically effective dose. Total dose refers to the total amount of material received from all contaminated media; potential dose is the amount of material that could be absorbed, if absorption were complete; and internal dose is the material actually absorbed in body tissue. Biologically effective dose refers to the amount of material actually reaching the biological site of action, such as a particular organ, cell, chromosome, or gene, depending on the level of definition. Before an agent can cause damage at the site of action, a metabolic step may be necessary that produces a toxic metabolite. Pharmacokinetic models describe the relationship between dose and biologically effective dose.

Framework for assessment of exposure

For both research purposes and for public health protection, estimates of exposure and dose for environmental agents may be needed. The conceptual framework provided by Fig. 3 can be used for this purpose. Any strategy needs to consider the media of exposure and the activities associated with exposure, factors associated with the level of exposure, the relationship between exposure and dose, and the host determinants of biologically effective dose. The concept of the microenvironment has been developed for exposure assessment for air pollutants, particularly indoor air pollutants. A microenvironment is a space where the concentrations of the pollutants of interest are sufficiently homogeneous for the purposes of exposure assessment.

Indoor exposure to radon is a useful example for applying the framework provided in Fig. 1 (National Research Council 1998). Radon concentrations vary in different indoor environments and are typically higher in residences than in workplaces or public places. At any given level of exposure, greater physical activity increases the amount of radio-activity inhaled and hence the dose of radiation reaching the target cells in the lung. The relationship between exposure and dose may be further influenced by the presence of a chronic lung disease or the changes in the lung that occur with smoking. Concentration is a widely used surrogate for exposure and dose, particularly for those environmental agents for which concentrations are routinely measured. However, concentration may be a poor surrogate for some agents, depending on the complexity of the links from concentration to exposure to dose.

Biomarkers

The general term 'biomarker' refers to a measurement of an indicator of susceptibility, exposure or dose, or response that is made in a biological material—blood, saliva, cells, tissues, or urine, for example (Hulka *et al.* 1990; National Research Council 1991*b*). For exposure or dose, biomarkers have been developed with the expectation of obtaining indicators that may provide a more accurate assessment of risk and that will not be subject to the error that frequently affects estimates made using epidemiological approaches.

A biomarker of exposure is an exogenous substance or its metabolite, the product of an interaction between xenobiotic agent and a target molecule in the body which can be measured in some compartment of the human body including tissues, cells, fluids, or expired air (National Research Council 1989). There is a continuum of biomarkers from indicators of exposure to early signs of health effects. Biomarkers are surrogates for exposure or dose; the relationship of the biomarker to exposure may be physiologically complex and variable among individuals. There are many well-known examples of biomarkers of exposure that are now proving useful not only for research purposes but also for tracking exposures of population or worker groups. For involuntary exposure of nonsmokers to cigarette smoke, for example, levels of nicotine or cotinine can be measured in body fluids, providing a highly specific and valid marker of exposure (Benowitz 1999; Samet and Wang 2000). Adducts of carcinogens bound to DNA in white blood cells can also be measured; adducts of the polycyclic aromatic hydrocarbon carcinogen, benzo[*a*]pyrene, have been associated with exposure to outdoor air pollution (Perera *et al.* 1992) and to cigarette smoke (Crawford *et al.* 1994).

Some biomarkers can be measured at little expense and without use of invasive methods. The level of carbon monoxide in an exhaled breath sample is a potentially useful indicator of dose for exposures to this gas in urban settings or from active smoking. Other biomarkers require collection of blood or some other biological sample. With present technological capabilities, markers of genetic risk can be assessed on buccal tissue cells obtained by scraping and then smearing the scraped material onto a slide.

Environmental exposure assessment

For air contaminants, exposure assessment approaches can be divided broadly into direct and indirect assessment methods; this same broad scheme has general applicability. In direct assessments of exposure, a measurement is made for each individual. For example, for measuring exposure to an air pollutant, each individual carries a personal monitor which registers the encountered concentrations continuously or integrated over a given time-period. Measurement of a biomarker would also constitute a direct measure of exposure. In indirect assessment, exposure for individuals is estimated using a model-based approach. For example, exposure to air pollutants is often estimated using the microenvironmental model, which considers each microenvironment where time is spent, the concentration of the contaminant in the microenvironment, and the amount of time spent in each. The total cumulative (integrated) exposure E_{tot} of an individual can be estimated by multiplying the pollution concentration C_{ij} in each microenvironment by the time T_{ij} spent in that environment and summing the time-weighted concentrations:

$$E_{tot} = \Sigma C_{ij} T_{ij}.$$

Concentrations in the microenvironments might be obtained by measurement or by a model-based approach. Similarly, the T_{ij} might be documented using a time–activity questionnaire or inferred from a model.

For some environmental contaminants, exposures may occur through multiple environmental media. Exposures to polycyclic aromatic hydrocarbons may result from contact with air contaminated by vehicle emissions or industrial point sources, such as steel mills or power plants, and from ingestion of cooked foods. The relative contributions of sources and media to total personal exposure depend on the strengths of the sources and individual behaviour, including patterns of food cooking and consumption and time activity (Lioy *et al.* 1988; Butler *et al.* 1993). In a study of 10 homes in one industrial American town, food ingestion was found to be the predominant pathway for exposure to benzo[*a*]pyrene, even though industrial sources of emissions were present (Butler *et al.* 1993). Over a 2-week interval, both outdoor and indoor air samples were collected over a 24-h period for 2 weeks. Food samples were collected from family meals each day, and two samples of water and one sample of soil were taken for analysis for benzo[*a*]pyrene. In addition, one person within each household completed daily questionnaires on time spent on various activities (Lioy and Waldman 1990). Water and soil were found to be minor pathways for exposure to benzo[*a*]pyrene, while air and food were the most significant sources of exposure. A comparison of the levels of benzo[*a*]pyrene in air and food indicated food ingestion as the predominant exposure source.

Exposures to lead may also take place through multiple media: (a) inhalation of air contaminated by emissions from vehicles burning leaded gasoline; (b) consumption of water contaminated by leaching from lead pipes; (c) ingestion of lead-containing foods and debris, including house dust and flakes of lead paint (Centers for Disease Control and Prevention 1991; National Research Council 1993; Breen and Stroup 1995; Howson *et al.* 1996). The relative contributions of the three routes of exposure vary around the world. In many countries, leaded gasoline is no longer used, diminishing the contribution of inhalation. In some countries, traditional pottery made with lead-containing glaze remains a strong source of lead exposure, particularly if used for food storage. In the United States, many older housing units in inner cities have been repeatedly painted inside with lead-containing paints. In assessing exposure to lead, the design strategy would need to consider each of the potential routes of exposure. Blood lead level has long been used as a biomarker of exposure or dose, while more recently X-ray fluorescence for measurement of bone lead has been developed as a tool to measure cumulative exposure. An understanding of the sources contributing to total personal exposure to environmental agents is relevant not only to research but to the implementation of control programmes, which should target the strongest and most readily remediable sources.

Occupational exposure assessment

For research purposes, the health effects of workplace exposures have typically been investigated for two broad purposes: (a) determination of whether an industry, occupation, or specific agent increases disease risk, and (b) assessment of the exposure–response relationship between the level of exposure and risk. A range of strategies may be used to classify exposures of worker groups (Table 2) (Checkoway *et al.* 1989). At the simplest level, employment in a particular occupation or industry may serve as the exposure indicator. Far more complex approaches may be used, including detailed workplace monitoring and biomarkers. Strategies for developing quantitative or semi-quantitative exposure measures may draw on historical records of concentrations of agents of interest in the workplace, complemented by measurements at the time of the study (Stewart *et al.* 1991). Gaps in the historical database may weaken this approach.

The discipline of industrial hygiene has long been concerned with measuring exposures of workers and assuring that the exposures are within acceptable limits. Before the early twentieth century, however, the health of workers was of little concern to the public. During the eighteenth and nineteenth centuries, a few occupational diseases were identified and in the early 1900s, public awareness and concern for workers' health was engendered when Alice Hamilton, a physician, first presented strong evidence that toxins caused disease and then proposed the means for preventing such illnesses. The public's increased awareness of occupational hazards led to new legislation for workers' compensation and a 'renaissance' period for industrial hygiene and occupational medicine.

The American Industrial Hygiene Association was formed in 1939, when professional interest in industrial hygiene had grown considerably. Industrial hygiene is now defined in *Patty's Industrial Hygiene and Toxicology* series (Clayton and Clayton 1991) as follows:

> that science and art devoted to the recognition, evaluation, and control of those environmental factors or stresses, arising in or from the work place, which may cause sickness, impaired health and well-being, or significant discomfort and inefficiency among workers or among the citizens of the community.

The industrial hygienist is trained to evaluate exposure and safety issues in the workplace, including measurement of exposures to the most common agents. The measurement approach is guided, in principle, by the microenvironmental model, and attention is focused on workplace environments or worker groups anticipated to have similar exposure levels. The diversity of workplace environments and

Table 2 Types of exposure data in occupational epidemiology studies

Type of data	Approximation to dose
Quantified personal measurements	Best
Quantified area- or job-specific data	
Ordinally ranked jobs or tasks	
Duration of employment in the industry at large	
Ever employed in the industry	Worst

Data from Checkoway *et al.* (1989).

worker groups necessitates a broad training background that may include various fields such as engineering, biology, chemistry, and physics, along with additional specialized study and extensive experience. Frequently, measurements made by industrial hygienists are a component of data used to estimate exposures and the contemporary research team addressing an occupational exposure will almost always include an industrial hygienist.

Workplace measurements of exposure agents and other industrial hygiene data are most often collected for compliance purposes. This approach to exposure monitoring may, however, be affected by bias, particularly if directed at those people or work areas where standards are most likely to be exceeded. Additionally, if used for retrospective exposure assessment, gaps in the historical record are inevitable and changing measurement methods and operations technology over time may further complicate exposure reconstruction.

Another widely used approach is the job–exposure matrix, using jobs held as a surrogate for the exposures that were likely to have been sustained. The typical job–exposure matrix is a cross-tabulation of various exposure indicators and job factors that can be systematically linked to estimate the risk of exposure in an individual worker or to create an exposure profile. Simple matrices may include major job categories (e.g. two-digit codes from the International Standard Classification of Occupations) and dichotomous exposure status categories. More complex matrices may include specific job titles (e.g. four-digit codes from the International Standard Classification of Occupations) and tasks, ordinal levels of exposure for a given job title or task, years of employment, and calendar year of exposure. Job–exposure matrices can be designed for population-based, industry-based, or company-specific studies. While experts are needed to develop the matrices, this approach does not require experts to evaluate each individual employee and standardized modules have been developed (Stewart and Stewart 1994; Stewart *et al.* 1996; Stewart *et al.* 1998). The job–exposure matrix approach is a more economically feasible method of exposure assessment, particularly for larger cohort studies, when direct measurements of exposure are not available. This method also avoids the possibility of differential information bias from interviews since exposures are not directly addressed and it is unlikely that self-reporting of job history will differ by interviewer or respondent.

Standardized job–exposure matrices were proposed several decades ago, as a wave of occupational cohort studies was initiated. Hoar *et al.* (1980) developed a system for linking jobs to potential exposures to occupational carcinogens. This general approach was refined by Siemiatycki (1991) who tailored the approach for a large population-based case–control study of occupational risk factors for cancer in Montreal. The principles underlying the approach are generally relevant. The method involves a highly detailed coding of exposures by trained industrial hygiene experts, using data from interviews and other sources. This approach utilizes information on job histories and tasks to estimate exposures, rather than relying on self-reported exposures and recall. Table 3 summarizes the steps for the individual exposure assessment method. The method is dynamic and can add new information concerning exposures, but it is resource intensive and costly.

Job–exposure matrices have continued to evolve and to incorporate increasingly complex algorithms. With data available from the National Occupational Hazard Survey, the National Institute for Occupational Safety and Health designed a computerized matrix specifically to incorporate these data for exposure assessment (Sieber *et al.* 1991). The National Cancer Institute has developed a computer-assisted telephone interview, a computer program that facilitates interviews for the collection of exposure information through traditional work history questions and additional job-specific questions formulated by industrial hygienists (Stewart and Stewart 1994; Stewart *et al.* 1996). Responses to the questions prompt branching of questions to more specific exposure-related experiences related to the specific job. If more information is needed, an industrial hygienist can review a work history and formulate additional questions for the interviewer to follow up with the worker. This mechanism for interaction between the industrial hygienist and the worker is unique since data collection and exposure assessment are traditionally separate processes.

However, there are disadvantages to using the job–exposure matrix approach, with the main problem being non-differential exposure misclassification which is unavoidable due to the heterogeneity of exposures for given job titles and tasks, particularly across industries and over time. This problem may be particularly severe in population-based exploratory studies, in which hundreds of job titles may be grouped into a few dozen categories. More accurate job–exposure matrices can be developed for specific companies or work sites (Goldberg *et al.* 1993) by using more specific job codes to minimize grouping of job titles and tasks without creating an unmanageable

Table 3 Individual exposure assessment method

Steps	External collaborators	Sources
Develop list of likely exposure substances	Industrial hygienists, chemists, engineers	
Develop self-administered questionnaire		
Develop and administer detailed semi-structured questionnaire	Industrial hygienists, chemists, engineers	
Collect data sources for coding of exposures		Interviews, employers, consultants, bibliographic sources (technical handbooks, industrial directories, journals, monographs)
Train experts on coding procedures	Industrial hygienists, chemists	
Code questionnaires: degree of certainty, route of contact, concentration, frequency	Additional coders	

Data from Siemiatycki (1991).

number of categories. Another drawback of job–exposure matrices is inadequate and incomplete accounting of work histories. Gaps may be impossible to avoid and records or recall may introduce errors. In industrial hygienist based systems, validity of exposure assignments will also depend on the knowledge of the expert and familiarity with the local occupations and industries.

Exposure measures

For research and regulatory purposes, exposure measures should appropriately reflect the biological relationships between exposures and disease risks. Exposures can be characterized with diverse metrics (Table 4). The relevance of these metrics to health effects depends on the process by which the agent causes injury and the relationship of that process to the eventual development of disease. For chronic obstructive pulmonary disease, for example, risk depends on the total amount smoked (USDHHS 1984), while for asthma induced by toluene di-isocyanate, transient exposures, not necessarily at high levels, may lead to sensitization (Banks 1998). Exposure assessment strategies or standards and guidelines for exposures should be reflective to the extent possible of the exposure metric which best fits with biological understanding.

Table 4 Exposure metrics in environmental epidemiology

Cumulative exposure
Exposure during a susceptibility window
Recent exposure
Time since first exposure
Age at first exposure
Exposure rate
Peak exposure
Exposure above threshold

Adverse health effects of environmental and occupational agents

Overview

Health, as defined by the WHO, is a holistic concept that includes not only the absence of disease but achieving a state of well being (WHO 1946). While historically, research and control strategies have been directed at disease and disease prevention, a far broader range of adverse effects are relevant to health, broadly defined. In fact, contemporary research on occupational and environmental agents may be directed at effects of environmental exposures on mood, functioning, and quality of life. Using biomarkers, it is possible to identify evidence of injury consequent to environmental exposures; however, the implications of elevated levels of biomarkers for future disease risks may be more uncertain. For example, workers in occupations involving exposure to benzo[*a*]pyrene have elevated levels of adducts of benzo[*a*]pyrene in the DNA of their white cells, in comparison with unexposed individuals (Schulte *et al.* 1993). While these adducts are a useful indicator of exposure and internal dose, their implications for future cancer risk are uncertain. The continued evolution of toxicological sciences at the molecular and cellular level will probably bring increasingly sensitive biomarkers of injury and of the earliest stages of disease. Using exposure information, it is also possible to predict future risks for some diseases, particularly cancer, for individuals and populations. What level of risk is acceptable and what degree of certainty is needed for decision-making?

Using this information to define the boundaries between adverse and non-adverse levels of effect will be challenging. Deepening mechanistic understanding will be helpful as the models for disease processes become more certain, offering a platform for interpreting the biomarker data. Societies will also be challenged to separate effects that should prompt control from those that may be tolerated. For effects on quality of life, for example, there may be divergent views across stakeholder groups or across governments. There may be greater willingness to tolerate visibly polluting industry in a newly developing country than in the developed and de-industrializing countries. For risk assessments, boundaries of acceptability for risk levels have evolved through application, but with little systematic consideration of societal issues and with little stakeholder involvement (Rodricks 1992).

The issues faced in identifying adverse health effects were recently reviewed by the American Thoracic Society (2000) for the example of air pollution. In setting air quality standards or guidelines, whether for outdoor or indoor air, decision-makers need to interpret an increasingly broad array of evidence on adverse health effects—evidence that spans from molecular-level effects to increased mortality. Even the interpretation of mortality data is not straightforward, as the degree of life-shortening underlying the positive associations found between air pollution levels and daily mortality counts is not well quantified. If these associations reflect only a slight advancement of the timing of death of people with severe, endstage heart and lung disease, they might not be considered adverse. The statement of the American Thoracic Society on these issues is informative, as it separates the roles of scientists and decision-makers in interpreting the evidence; across the spectrum of effects from not adverse to clearly adverse, lines of demarcation should be made on a societal basis.

Health effects of occupational and environmental agents

The range of health effects of occupational and environmental agents is extraordinarily broad, touching on every organ system and many acute and chronic diseases. The health effects may be close to instantaneous, death by asphyxiation from oxides of nitrogen or carbon monoxide inhalation, or follow on a lengthy incubation process during which the disease process completes itself, as in the 30 to 40 years from first exposure to asbestos to the development of mesothelioma. Considering malignancy alone, occupational exposures have been associated with cancers of the skin, brain, nasal sinuses, larynx, lung, gastrointestinal tract, liver, kidney, and bladder, and with leukaemias and other haematological malignancies (Table 5). Considering the respiratory tract, occupational and environmental agents cause and exacerbate acute and chronic obstructive lung diseases, including asthma, and cause specific forms

Table 5 Occupational exposures associated with principal cancers

Cancer	Occupational exposure
Bladder	4-aminobiphenyl, arsenic, auramine, benzidine, magenta, 2-naphthylamine, *O*-toluidine, polycyclic aromatic hydrocarbons
Brain	Arsenic, chromium, polycyclic aromatic hydrocarbons, vinyl chloride
Connective tissue/ sarcoma	Dioxins, phenoxy herbicides
Gastrointestinal	Arsenic, asbestos, chromium, ethylene oxide, ionizing radiation, iron, polycyclic aromatic hydrocarbons
Kidney	Arsenic, chromium, polycyclic aromatic hydrocarbons
Larynx	Asbestos, polycyclic aromatic hydrocarbons, sulphuric acid
Liver	Arsenic, trichloroethylene, vinyl chloride
Lung	Arsenic, asbestos, beryllium, *bis*-chloromethyl ether, cadmium, chlorinated hydrocarbons, chromium, ionizing radiation, iron, mustard gas, nickel, polycyclic aromatic hydrocarbons, silica, sulphuric acid, vinyl chloride
Lymphatic and haematopoietic	Benzene, 1,3-butadiene, chromium, dioxins, ethylene oxide, ionizing radiation, phenoxy herbicides, polycyclic aromatic hydrocarbons, tetrachloroethylene, trichloroethylene
Nasopharyngeal and sinus	Arsenic, chromium, formaldehyde, nickel
Prostate	Arsenic, cadmium, chromium
Skin	Arsenic, chromium, polycyclic aromatic hydrocarbons

Data from Blair and Kazerouni (1997), Boffetta *et al.* (1997), Lynge *et al.* (1997), Vineis and Pirastu (1997), Veys (1996), Monson and Christiani (1997), Hayes (1997), and Rom (1998).

of occupational lung disease such as asbestosis, silicosis, and coal workers' pneumoconiosis (Table 6).

Assessment of health outcomes in studies of occupational and environmental agents needs to be done with rigour to assure high validity and to minimize misclassification. For many health outcomes, standardized approaches for assessment have been developed that should be used whenever possible. The WHO offers standards for classification of deaths, the International Classification of Diseases, that is periodically updated (WHO 1992). Standardized questionnaires and methods for physiological assessment have long been in use for investigating respiratory diseases, for example (Samet 1989). The availability of standardized questionnaires facilitates comparisons across study populations and assures comparability in repeated assessment of outcomes. Use of standardized approaches for physiological measures similarly assures comparability; methods have been proposed and used for lung function testing, blood pressure measurement, and neuropsychological functioning for example.

Table 6 Selected environmental and occupational agents and associated respiratory diseases

Exposure	Disease
Cigarette smoking	Chronic obstructive pulmonary disease
Soy beans	Asthma
Toluene di-isocyanate	Occupational asthma
Coal dust	Coal workers' pneumoconiosis
Asbestos	Asbestosis
Silica	Silicosis
Pigeons	Hypersensitivity pneumonitis
Radon progeny	Lung cancer
Asbestos	Mesothelioma

It is beyond the scope of this chapter to review specific outcome measures in detail. Researchers should be certain to use standardized and accepted approaches, if available.

Study designs for human research

Overview

The observational study designs used to investigate the risks of exposure to environmental and occupational agents follow those used throughout epidemiological research—the cross-sectional study or survey, cohort study, and case–control study—as well as the more recently developed nested designs (Gordis 1996). The ecological study, carried out at the group level, is also used for investigating environmental exposures, particularly if exposures are relatively uniform across population groups. Experimental designs have been used infrequently, although investigations directed at 'natural experiments' of changing exposures have been carried out and trials of preventive agents have also been conducted. For investigation of both occupational and environmental agents, specific designs have been refined so as to best fit with investigational circumstances. The key designs used for occupational and environmental studies are addressed below.

Ecological studies

Ecological studies involve groups, defined typically by geographical location, and time and demographic characteristics, as the unit of analysis. Exposures are inferred for groups of individuals, and the health characteristics of the group are assessed in relation to the inferred exposures. For example, the average annual lung cancer mortality rates for American counties have been examined in relation to the average of radon measurements made in the county (Cohen and Colditz 1994). The feasibility of this design is enhanced by use of data collected routinely for administrative or regulatory purposes, such as air pollution and mortality data. An inherent limitation, often referred to as the 'ecological fallacy', is the assumption that exposure–outcome relationships observed at the group level hold at the individual level. Additionally, confounding may be difficult to control because group-level data on potential confounders are not available and ecological regression models cannot fully adjust for the potential confounders (Robins and Greenland 1989; Stidley and Samet 1993).

Newer hierarchical designs that incorporate individual-level information on potential confounding factors and group-level information on environmental exposures offer the possibility of both controlling confounding and exploring effect modification. For example, Peters *et al.* (1999*a*,*b*) are assessing the effects of air pollution exposure on the respiratory health of children in the Los Angeles area. Twelve communities were selected to provide a gradient of exposure to the air pollutants of interest, particularly ozone. Exposure for individuals is inferred based on measurements made at schools in the communities; these estimates will be refined using information based on individual-level time–activity information.

Ecological studies have long been cast as useful for 'hypothesis generation' and not for hypothesis testing because of the ecological fallacy. Nonetheless, studies of the ecological design have been widely used for testing hypotheses concerning the risks of environmental agents and, in fact, the risks of some environmental exposures, which are relatively uniform across communities, may only be addressed using ecological designs. Time-series designs, inherently ecological, have been widely used for time-varying exposures, such as air pollution, and health outcome measures, such as hospital admission or death counts. In such time-series designs, confounding at the individual level may be of little concern, because personal characteristics do not vary on the time-frame of the analysis and confounding at the ecological level by time-varying factors (e.g. season) can be handled in the analysis.

These ecological designs have been most widely applied to ambient or outdoor air pollution. In fact, some of the most dramatic evidence on the health effects of air pollution came from the well-chronicled air pollution disasters of the twentieth century, like the London Fog of 1952 (Brimblecombe 1999). Readily evident excesses of morbidity and mortality occurred at times of extremely high levels of air pollution. Both cross-sectional and time-series approaches have been used to assess the adverse effects of air pollution. For example, rates of lung cancer mortality have been compared across urban and rural areas to assess urban air pollution as a risk factor for lung cancer (Samet and Cohen 1999) and associations of mortality rates from various causes have been examined with county-level mortality and air pollution data (Lave and Seskin 1977). Small-area analysis, using data from small geographical areas across which exposures can be reasonably assumed to be uniform, has also been applied to air pollution and other environmental agents (Elliott *et al.* 1992*b*).

For example, Elliott *et al.* (1992*a*) explored the risk of lung and larynx cancers associated with exposure to emissions from waste incinerators, using circular areas around 10 incinerator sites as indicators of exposure levels. For each site, two circular geographical bands were defined around the incinerator, with the inner band being 0 to 3 km in radius from the incinerator and the outer band being 3 to 10 km from the site. For their main analysis, Elliott *et al.* pooled together the observed and expected numbers of cancers from the 10 incinerator sites, combining information from the inner and outer bands. Smaller increments of bands within the 10 km were used to analyse for decreasing trend in cancer risk with increasing distance from the sites. Despite having adequate power through pooling of data from multiple sites, no statistically significant excesses in lung and larynx cancers were found either near (0–3 km) or distant from (3–10 km) the incinerators.

More recently, time-series designs have been widely applied, as advances in hardware, software, and statistical methods have facilitated analyses that would not previously have been possible (Diggle *et al.* 1994). Flexible modelling approaches, such as generalized additive models (Hastie and Tibshirani 1990), can be used to control for potential temporal confounding by season or other factors; these models can also handle complex and correlated data structures that may have led to uncontrollable bias with prior modelling approaches. Time-series methods have now been widely applied to air pollution and mortality and morbidity counts, using such morbidity indicators as numbers of hospital admissions or emergency visits. The general approach is to control for potential temporal confounders, such as season or epidemic influenza, using appropriate smoothing so that shorter-term associations of air pollution with mortality can be evaluated (Kelsall *et al.* 1997). Studies of this design, conducted in individual cities throughout the world, have shown that, even at today's levels, air pollution, particularly particulate air pollution, remains associated with morbidity and mortality (American Thoracic Society 1996*a*,*b*; Denison *et al.* 1998; Pope and Dockery 1999).

The time-series approach has now been refined and strengthened by its extension to incorporate multiple locations into a common analysis, whether through meta-analysis or pooled analysis. The Air Pollution and Health: a European Approach Study applies a common analytical approach to data on morbidity and mortality from multiple locations and then combines the city-specific estimates of the effect of air pollution using meta-analysis (Katsouyanni *et al.* 1996). Dominici *et al.* (2000) have developed a bayesian hierarchical modelling approach for combining evidence on the health effects of air pollution across locations. In the National Morbidity, Mortality, and Air Pollution Study carried out in the United States, evidence on the health effects of air pollution has been combined from the largest 90 cities (Fig. 4). Using these methods, it is also possible to explore the factors responsible for any heterogeneity of the effect of air pollution across locations. The general approach should have abundant application to other types of environmental agents.

Cross-sectional studies

The survey remains a widely used, although inherently limited design, for investigating risks of occupational and environmental agents. The design of a survey is usually straightforward, feasibility is generally not a barrier, and costs are typically not high. In a survey, observations concerning exposure and outcome are made at one point in time, although an attempt may be made to capture past exposures and to relate prior exposures to current disease status or other measures. Interpretation of cross-sectional data for causality is consequently

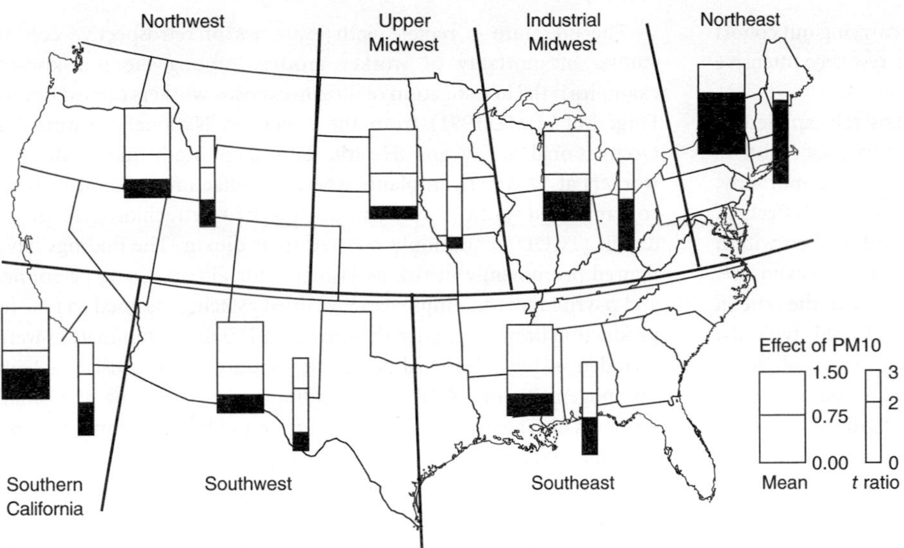

Fig. 4 Map of the United States showing the pooled effect estimate for particulate matter (PM_{10}) at lag – 1 for the 90 cities by seven regions considered in the geographical analysis of the findings of the National Morbidity, Mortality, and Air Pollution Study (Samet *et al.* 2000).

limited, as the temporal relationship between exposure and outcome may be uncertain.

For occupational groups, the cross-sectional study is most often used to characterize the health status of workers and often specifically to assess evidence of injury in organs that are the likely targets of the workplace exposures. For example, a survey might be directed at workers exposed to respiratory irritants or dusts that cause lung disease; the evaluation methods might include a respiratory symptoms questionnaire, lung function testing, chest radiograph, and even a clinical evaluation. Worker rosters, either company or union, can often be used to identify the target population for investigation, thereby minimizing potential bias from participation based on health status. Numerous studies of this type have been carried out, directed for example at asbestosis, silicosis, coal workers' pneumoconiosis, occupational bronchitis, and asthma. In a survey of respiratory diseases in uranium miners, Samet *et al.* (1983) selected the workers with the longest underground employment, using worker records as a sampling frame. The study showed that approximately 10 per cent of the participants, all actively working miners, had radiographic evidence of lung disease consistent with silicosis, and that lung function level decreased with increasing time worked underground.

Cross-sectional designs are also used to study the effects of environmental agents at the community level. In this context, feasibility remains a key rationale for using this approach. Cross-sectional approaches might be used in circumstances where the effects of particular exposures or sources of exposure on community residents are of concern. Thus, cross-sectional studies have been conducted to investigate the effects of heavy metals emitted by a smelters on children living nearby (McMichael *et al.* 1988), of petrochemical emissions on the respiratory health of children living in the Kanawha Valley in the American state of West Virginia (Ware *et al.* 1993), and of the frequency of allergic and respiratory diseases in children in the former eastern and western parts of Germany (von Mutius *et al.* 1994).

Cross-sectional studies have the potential to be informative if valid gradients of exposure can be established. This goal may be met by selecting communities that offer a range of exposure, based on available monitoring information, and making comparisons across communities, or by establishing gradients of exposure within communities. For example, the 24 Cities Study was conducted by investigators at Harvard to address the health effects of acidic air pollution on the health of children (Cunningham *et al.* 1996). The communities were selected based on prior monitoring data to provide a gradient of exposure to acid aerosols. While the outcome data were collected for each child, this design approach is now recognized as hierarchical and may be referred to as 'semi-ecologic' (Kunzli and Tager 1997). While data on outcome and potential confounding and modifying factors have been collected at the individual level, exposure has been estimated at the community level. In the study of West Virginia schoolchildren (Ware *et al.* 1993), exposures within the community were estimated on the basis of monitors for volatile organic compounds that were placed at each of the community's 74 schools.

Cohort studies

The cohort design, involving follow-up of individuals with ascertainment of outcome over time, has a central role in investigating the risks of occupational and environmental agents. The cohort design can be applied either retrospectively, if available data are sufficient for cohort selection, exposure assessment, and outcome characterization, or prospectively, if resources are sufficient for follow-up of a population of adequate size, exposure assessment over time, and outcome tracking. If carried out retrospectively, the design gains in feasibility and efficiency because events that have already taken place are the focus of investigation and, if carried out prospectively, the design affords the opportunity to characterize exposures using the optimal, affordable strategy. Nested designs (the nested case–control and case–cohort studies) offer efficient approaches for carrying out cohort studies, particularly if exposure characterization is resource intensive (Samet and Muñoz 1998).

The retrospective cohort study has been extensively applied to occupational groups, using work records and other types of registries for cohort identification and exposure assessment and mortality, either total or cause-specific, as the primary outcome. The effects of exposure can be assessed by comparison to unexposed workers within the same population, assessment of risks across a gradient of exposure, and comparison to an external reference population, often the general population. The latter design is the most commonly used; typically, standardized mortality rates are calculated to compare observed mortality in the worker group to expected mortality based on the general population. The comparison rates are standardized to the age and other characteristics of the population of interest. The appropriateness of the general population as the comparison group is a matter for judgment, as the worker population may differ in its distributions of potential confounding or modifying factors.

The 'healthy worker effect' refers to one particular form of bias that may result from using the general population as the comparison group (Checkoway *et al.* 1989). The term 'healthy worker effect' was first used in a 1974 article by McMichael *et al.* (1974). Employed people generally tend to be healthier than unemployed people, as illness and disability are barriers to employment. The healthy worker effect is considered to reflect both selection bias, as working people tend to be healthier, and confounding, reflecting risk factor differences between employed and unemployed people. Consequently, comparison of mortality of employed to unemployed people, without an adverse effect of employment on mortality, would tend to find a lower risk of mortality in unemployed people.

Estimates of the magnitude of the healthy worker effect, when there is no hazardous exposure in the workplace, have ranged from about 10 to 30 per cent reduction in the true standardized mortality (Choi 1992). The magnitude of the effect may vary with a number of factors, including time since hire and specific cause of death. It also may diminish over time, tending to reduce with duration of employment as the effect of illness on employment status wanes. The degree of bias may vary by cause, being typically greater for cardiovascular diseases.

The literature is replete with examples of retrospective cohort studies of mortality of worker groups. Among the well-known examples is the investigation of dioxin-exposed workers carried out by Fingerhut *et al.* (1991) from the American National Institute for Occupational Safety and Health. This large study included 5172 workers at 12 American plants where manufactured chemicals were contaminated with the byproduct 2,3,7,8-tetrachlorodibenzo-*p*-dioxin (TCDD), commonly referred to as dioxin. The findings have figured prominently in risk assessments for dioxin. Using personnel and payroll records, employees identified as being assigned to jobs in production or maintenance that involved TCDD contamination were included in the cohort. Although the findings were consistent with carcinogenicity of TCDD, the findings are limited by the small numbers observed for each type of cancer and lack of information on smoking. A summary of the findings is provided in Table 7.

The prospective cohort design has also been extensively used for studies of occupational and environmental agents. By virtue of being carried out prospectively, many aspects of the design can be made optimal. The investigators can implement exposure and outcome assessment strategies that will be as comprehensive as resources will permit, validation studies can be nested within the full cohort study, and potential confounding and modifying factors can be characterized. These strengths have given the prospective cohort study the greatest credibility among the epidemiological study designs, but a modern cohort study of an occupational or environmental agent may require substantial resources and funding, as well as sufficient observation time. The informativeness of the cohort design has also been advanced by new methods for longitudinal analysis that can flexibly model time-varying relationships in the data and accommodate correlated observations over time (Diggle *et al.* 1994; Thomas 1998).

The cohort design may be used on either short or long time-frames in investigating occupational and environmental agents. Short-term designs may be used in the workplace to evaluate changes in health outcome measures across a workshift; changes in lung function or neuropsychological functioning, for example, might be measured and linked to simultaneously measured exposures. For environmental exposures, particularly, air pollution, short-term cohort studies, often

Table 7 Mortality from all cancers and from respiratory cancers (trachea, bronchus, and lung) according to latency period and duration of employment at the plants studied

Duration of employment (years)	All cancers		Respiratory cancer	
	Deaths observed	Standardized mortality rate	Deaths observed	Standardized mortality rate
< 5	71	120	19	96
5 to < 10	21	104	3	46
10 to < 15	18	89	7	105
15 to < 20	23	91	7	81
20 to < 25	34	134	12	133
25 to < 30	31	116	18	180[a]
$\geqslant 30$	54	135	19	126
Overall	252	116	85	112

[a] $p < 0.05$.

Data from Fingerhut *et al.* (1991).

termed 'panel' studies, may be used to track variation in physiological measures and symptoms in relation to variation in exposure. Potentially susceptible groups are often investigated with the goals of enhancing the sensitivity of the investigation to detecting effects and of obtaining evidence relevant to protecting their health. For example, panel studies of air pollution often involve people with asthma or chronic obstructive pulmonary disease. Ostro *et al.* (1994) included adults with asthma in two panel studies on respiratory morbidity and indoor and outdoor air pollution. Exposure to indoor air pollution (that is, combustion from gas or wood stoves and fireplaces, and environmental tobacco smoke) was assessed from daily diary recordings by the panel of 164 asthmatics, as well as the occurrence of several respiratory symptoms (Ostro *et al.* 1994). In the study on outdoor air pollution, 207 subjects recorded respiratory symptoms in a daily diary, while exposure data were obtained from air monitoring for daily levels of several ambient air pollutants, including hydrogen ion, fine particulates, nitrates, and sulphates (Ostro *et al.* 1991).

Longer-term prospective cohort studies may be needed to address the chronic effects of environmental and occupational agents on health status and disease risk. Such studies have been carried out, for example, to address the effect of air pollution on mortality (Dockery *et al.* 1993), lead exposure on neuropsychological development (Needleman and Gatsonis 1990; Baghurst *et al.* 1992; Tong *et al.* 1998), and coal dust on lung function change (Attfield and Wagner 1998). The hallmark use of the prospective cohort study is for unique exposures, such as the atomic bomb survivors or Chernobyl victims.

The Port Pirie study of lead-exposed children illustrates the strength of the design with its incorporation of repeated measures of blood lead, the exposure measure, and of neuropsychological functioning, the outcome measure (Fig. 5) (Tong *et al.* 1998). The Port Pirie cohort consisted of 537 children born to women living near a lead smelter. Maternal blood lead levels were measured antenatally and at delivery, while children's blood lead levels were measured at delivery from the umbilical cord, at 6 and 15 months, and then annually from age 2 to 7 years (McMichael *et al.* 1988; Tong *et al.* 1998). Additional factors and qualitative measures of outcomes were assessed through interviews of the mother at the time of each blood sample collection. Neuropsychological development of the children was quantitatively evaluated using a number of behavioural and cognitive assessments, including intelligence tests, at various ages. The most recent assessment of this cohort at ages 11 to 13 years showed increased frequency of behavioural and emotional problems associated with higher lifetime blood lead exposure.

The prospective cohort design may be strengthened and made more efficient by using an intermediate marker of the outcome of interest, rather than waiting for the final outcome itself (Muñoz and Gange 1998). For example, rate of decline of lung function may be measured as the primary outcome measure, rather than awaiting for the development of clinically evident lung disease or death from lung disease. The rate of decline of lung function could be determined in a prospective cohort study by repetitively measuring lung function and estimating its change over follow-up. Studies of such intermediate markers are most properly carried out with the prospective cohort approach.

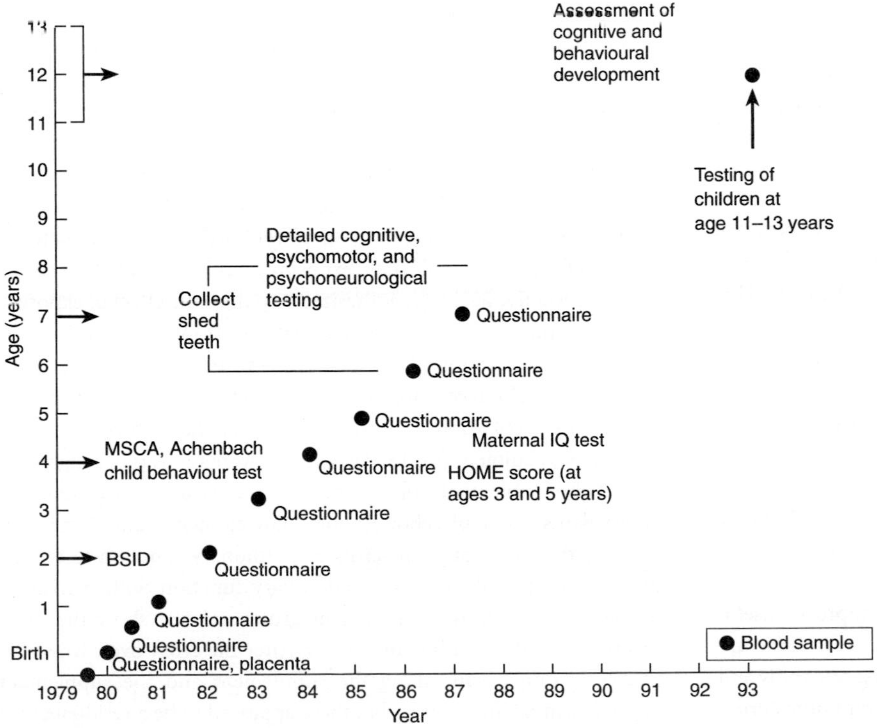

Fig. 5 Research design of the Port Pirie Cohort Study: BSID, Bayley Scales of Infant Development; HOME, Home Observation for Measurement of the Environment; MSCA, McCarthy Scales of Children's Abilities (Tong *et al.* 1998).

Case–control studies

The case–control design has been used extensively to characterize occupational and environmental causes of cancer, but much less frequently for other diseases. The design has proved particularly useful for cancer, as there is often a lengthy period from the time of first exposure until excess risk is manifest. The utility of the case–control method for studying environmental exposures was well documented by the early studies of cigarette smoking and lung cancer (Doll and Hill 1950; Wynder and Graham 1950), which provided convincing evidence linking smoking to lung cancer. The case–control design has now been used to explore occupational and environmental causes of most of the predominant types of cancer. The cases and controls themselves are the principal source of information on exposure. Some exposure misclassification is unavoidable as a result, as study participants may be asked to supply a profile of environmental and occupational exposures across their lifetimes. For some exposures, such as urban air pollution, it may be possible to only obtain information on surrogates, such as place of residence, and some exposures, such as diet, are unavoidably reported with misclassification. Conversely, increasingly sophisticated data collection approaches, like the job–exposure matrices, are enhancing the quality of the information that can be obtained from case–control studies.

Hybrid approaches such as the nested case–control and case–cohort studies, have features of the case–control and cohort designs. In a nested case–control study, the cases constitute those people within the full cohort developing the outcome of interest during follow-up; the controls are selected, typically with matching, from those people at risk when the cases developed the outcome. This design is often used if exposure assessment is resource intensive or based in biomarker measurement; efficiency is gained because exposures are not calculated for the full cohort. With sampling of a sufficient number of controls, estimates of effect from a nested case–control study and a full cohort study are comparable (Breslow *et al.* 1982). The nested case–control approach has been used frequently for occupational cohorts, for which comprehensive exposure estimation may be quite complex. For example, Samet *et al.* (1989) carried out a case–control study of exposure to radon progeny and lung cancer risk, involving 65 cases and 230 controls, selected from a full cohort of 3469 miners. This approach was used because exposure estimation involved lengthy review of individual work histories and matching against extensive databases on levels of radon progeny in mines. Findings were similar when analyses for the full cohort were completed (Samet *et al.* 1991).

In the case–cohort design, a sample of the cohort is drawn at the start of follow-up and exposures are characterized for these people and those cohort members who subsequently develop disease (Prentice 1986). This design has not yet had widespread application to environmental and occupational exposures.

The case–crossover design is a recently proposed approach useful for studying acute events associated with brief exposures (Maclure 1991). It is a variant of the case–control study involving cases only and comparison of exposures during the biologically-relevant time period for the outcome and a comparison time period. In effect, the case–crossover design enhances study efficiency by having each case serve as his or her own control, thereby eliminating potential confounding by such personal characteristics as age, gender, and socio-economic status. Analysis is generally self-matched using conditional logistic regression modelling.

The design has application to time-varying environmental exposures, such as air pollution. A representative application is to investigate the short-term association of air pollution with mortality; relevant case exposures are postulated to occur shortly before the time of death and control exposures can be estimated at times just prior to or even after time of death. In one such study in Philadelphia by Neas *et al.* (1999), the case exposures occurred in the '48-hour period ending at midnight on the day of death' and the control exposures occurred 1, 2, and 3 weeks before and after the case exposure period. In another study by Lee and Schwartz (1999) in Seoul, Korea, the date of death was the case exposure period, and the dates 1 or 2 weeks prior to and after date of death were the control exposure periods (that is, the same day of the week as the day of death). The Philadelphia study confirmed the results of earlier Poisson regression analysis of the same data, showing a positive association between total suspended particulates and daily mortality. The Seoul study found an association of premature death with sulphur dioxide levels, a finding that persisted with various analytical approaches.

Intervention studies

In intervention studies, the investigator controls the exposure status of study participants. The randomized clinical trial, which has the central elements of randomization to control and comparison arms, is generally used to evaluate the efficacy of therapeutic regimens, including drug therapies. A key strength of the randomized clinical trial is control of selection bias and confounding through randomization. The design has potential application to occupational and environmental exposures in evaluating interventions to reduce disease risk, although few such trials have been carried out. The use of randomized trials is distinct from studies based around regulatory and programmatic interventions to reduce exposures, which may afford an opportunity to evaluate the consequences of reducing exposures.

Randomized controlled trials have been carried out to evaluate the effects of reduced pollution exposures and also the effects of chemopreventive agents hypothesized to reduce the effect of exposure to occupational and environmental agents. For example, Romieu *et al.* (1998) used a randomized trial combined with a cross-over design to examine the effect of antioxidant supplementation on respiratory function of street workers in Mexico City, who have chronically high exposures to ambient ozone. Participants were randomly assigned to take daily supplements of vitamins E and C and β-carotene, all antioxidants, or a placebo. Results showed significant differences between the two groups in terms of pulmonary function tests. The placebo group had decreased pulmonary function with increasing ozone levels, while the supplement group did not show the same inverse association with ozone levels. After the cross-over, when the placebo group began taking the supplement and the supplement group began taking the placebo, there appeared to be a residual effect of the antioxidants. In this second phase of the study, Romieu *et al.* found that the placebo group had decreases in pulmonary function that were less pronounced than the decrements found before the cross-over.

Toxicological approaches

Overview

Numerous new chemicals and other potentially toxic agents are introduced regularly into the workplace and general environments. Each of these agents cannot feasibly be evaluated using epidemiological approaches; in fact, only a minority of the disease-causing agents to which people are exposed have been evaluated using epidemiological data. The science of toxicology has emerged over recent decades as a complementary approach to observational studies for characterizing the risks of environmental and occupational agents. The approaches of toxicology include characterization of structure–activity relationships to predict potential toxicity, description of the uptake, metabolism, and distribution of agents, and short- and long-term assays. Toxicological evaluation holds the promise of predicting the potential for injury and increased human disease risk before agents are introduced and exposures occur. However, the large volume of new agents poses a challenge even for toxicological approaches, and validity of assay systems for predicting human disease remains a key uncertainty.

Human toxicology studies

In a study design sometimes referred to as a 'clinical study', human volunteers may be exposed to agents under carefully controlled concentrations at levels that are judged a priori to have no potential long-term consequences. The laboratory setting affords the opportunity to characterize the effects of experimentally manipulated exposures, rather than the often complex circumstances of exposure in the community setting. Additionally, more rigorous and invasive assessment of outcomes is possible in the experimental setting and the outcomes evaluated are often directed at biomarkers of injury. The findings of clinical studies may be useful for bridging from laboratory models to the population.

This design has been extensively used for studying the health effects of inhaled agents: carbon monoxide, ozone, nitrogen oxides, particles, and even some occupational agents, like cotton dust. For ozone, for example, protocols have involved exposures of up to 8 h with intermittent exercise to increase the dose of ozone reaching the lung (American Thoracic Society 1996*a*,*b*). These studies have shown replicable decline of lung function across the exposure interval and a spectrum of susceptibility. The exposure protocols have been coupled in some investigations with bronchoscopy to collect lung tissue and fluid specimens. This invasive assessment has shown the earliest changes in the lung's tissues following exposure to ozone and provided insights into the mechanisms by which ozone affects lung function.

Interpreting evidence on environmental and occupational agents

Overview

Research on environmental and occupational agents is inherently application oriented, serving to provide evidence that drives interventions to protect human health. Given the sometimes sweeping societal implications of such evidence, rigorous review and criticism by stakeholders is inevitable. Even evidence that is seemingly definitive, like the findings on smoking and lung cancer, have not escaped criticism; for decades, the tobacco industry has questioned the scientific findings on active smoking and disease, and more recently on passive smoking, even as reviewing scientific authorities designated active and passive smoking as causing disease. Several themes almost inevitably emerge in current considerations of evidence on occupational and environmental agents:

- the existence of toxicity at low levels of exposure—often referred to as 'weak effects'
- confounding as an explanation for association between the agent of concern and the outcome
- the form of the relationship between exposure and risk
- the presence of particularly susceptible groups within the population.

These cross-cutting issues are addressed below.

'Small' or 'weak' effects

For many agents, exposures to the general population occur at levels at which biological understanding suggests that increases of risk should be relatively small. Nonetheless, if exposure is common, the public health burden, that is, the attributable risk, may still be substantial. Examples of such agents and associated risks include exposure to environmental tobacco smoke in the workplace and lung cancer risk, and residential exposure to radon and lung cancer risk. Both these exposures are widespread; smoking is still allowed in many workplaces and radon is ubiquitous in indoor environments. While only a small percentage of the population may have exposures that lead to unacceptable individual risk, the pattern of exposure for the population may lead to unacceptable risk at the population level.

Critics of epidemiological research on such agents are often dismissive, setting aside the findings as only 'weak effects' without acknowledging the basis for public health concern. The argument is often made that for relative risk values below some arbitrary threshold, perhaps 2 to 3, epidemiological findings have little validity as sources of bias, particularly as confounding may have resulted in the observed effect and that epidemiological methods cannot adequately account for such bias. These general arguments, championed by critics of epidemiological research and of its use in risk assessment, may hold as limitations of specific studies, but the arguments have no general merit. Properly designed studies anticipate potential confounding and other forms of bias and populations of sufficient size can be studied to assure that power is adequate for effects in a range of interest, even if below relative risks of 2 or 3.

Concerns about toxicity at low levels of exposure may not readily be set aside by toxicological investigations, which require large sample sizes at exposures associated with lower levels of risk, as do epidemiological studies. Knowledge of underlying mechanisms of injury may address the plausibility of increased risk at lower levels of exposure. For example, in the instance of indoor radon, the Biological Effects of Ionizing Radiation VI Committee of the American National Research Council (National Research Council 1998) concluded that indoor radon increased lung cancer risk, even at lower levels of exposure. This conclusion was based on an understanding of the mechanism by which the responsible form of radiation, α particles, causes injury to genetic material in cells.

Measurement error for both exposure and outcome is often raised as a further limitation to studies of environmental agents, particularly at exposures associated with small effects. Feasibility often leads to the use of surrogate measures of exposure, such as the presence of a smoker in the home as an indicator for exposure to environmental tobacco smoke, in place of directly measured exposure or dose. Outcome measures may also be subject to misclassification, as inevitably occurs, for example, with the cause of death listed on death certificates. In general, the structure of errors in outcomes and exposures, particularly if random, tend to reduce associations, implying that observed effects may underestimate actual effects. In the example of outdoor air pollution, critics questioned the association of particulate air pollution with mortality, proposing that measurement error in exposures contributed to the positive associations (Lipfert 1997*a*,*b*; Lipfert and Wyzga 1997). However, a detailed assessment of the problem indicated that measurement error arising from using centrally located monitors in place of personal exposure would generally reduce associations, not increase them (Zeger *et al.* 1999).

Confounding

Risks for many disease are multifactorial and the results of research on occupational and environmental agents may be biased if the effects of other factors, also associated with disease risk, are not properly taken into account. Confounding arises if the occupational or environmental agent of concern is associated with another factor, which itself increases risk for the outcome of interest (Rothman and Greenland 1997). Confounding is typically addressed as a study is designed and potential confounding factors are listed so that necessary data can be collected; and in analysis, using adjustment and modelling to control for the effect of confounding.

Critics of observational studies often raise the possibility that observed effects represent uncontrolled confounding, sometimes offering lengthy lists of 'potential confounders' or proposing that there are unknown factors which have led to biased risk estimates through confounding. The adequacy of adjustment methods may also be questioned. For example, in passive smoking and disease, critics have repeatedly proposed many potential confounders for associations of environmental tobacco smoke with respiratory diseases in children, lung cancer, and coronary heart disease (Lee 1986, 1987, 1988, 1992; Lee *et al.* 1986; Witorsch and Witorsch 1989). Some of the proposed confounders have not met one of the conditions for confounding—an independent association with the outcome of interest.

While there may be legitimate concern for uncontrolled confounding, epidemiological judgement may appropriately set aside confounding as an explanation for association of an occupational or environmental agent with disease risk. Persistence of the association with analytical control for confounding, consistency across studies having differing patterns of potential confounding, and the presence of a dose–response relation with the exposure of interest weigh against confounding as the explanation for association. Arguments for unknown and uncontrolled X factors should be set aside as non-scientific and indicative of subjective bias against real evidence in hand.

Form of the relationship between exposure and risk

For policy development, the form of the relationship between exposure (or dose) and risk is almost inevitably critical to decision-making. Exposure–response curves of different configurations carry substantially different implications for risk management (Fig. 1). The linear no-threshold relationship, widely assumed for carcinogenesis, implies that any exposure carries some risk and that no 'safe' level of exposure can be found. This type of relationship has been generally assumed for ionizing radiation, with some support from experimental and observational research. Yet, heated debate continues on its application to radiation and to chemical carcinogenesis generally. Some have proposed that low levels of exposure even convey reduced risk, a phenomenon referred to as 'hormesis'. The existence of a threshold offers the possibility of reducing exposures to a risk-free range, while some curvilinear relationships imply higher risks at lower doses. The form of the exposure–response relationship is also critical in extrapolating risks observed at higher levels of exposure, often in occupational settings, to lower levels of exposure, often those received by the general population.

Susceptibility

For many occupational and environmental agents, exposure does not necessarily lead to the development of disease. Even heavy cigarette smokers do not all develop a tobacco-related disease, such as lung cancer or chronic obstructive pulmonary disease. For many occupational and environmental agents, there is likely to be a wide range of susceptibility in the population, reflecting not only genetic factors but characteristics of the exposed person, such as having a chronic disease like asthma. For public health protection, an understanding of the range of susceptibility and its determinants is essential as a basis for providing adequate protection to all exposed people. The current extraordinary pace at which understanding of the genetic basis of disease is evolving offers the prospect of soon identifying genetic determinants of susceptibility for some occupational and environmental agents. New technology, such as chip arrays, should facilitate the exploration of gene–environment interactions at a depth and pace that seemed out of reach only a few years ago (National Institute of Environmental Health Sciences 1999).

For some exposures, the presence of an underlying chronic disease may heighten susceptibility. For inhaled pollutants, the underlying increased responsiveness of the airways of asthmatics may heighten their susceptibility. Even within people having asthma, there is a range of susceptibility spanning those with lesser and greater degrees of underlying airways responsiveness. Age has also been considered as a determinant of susceptibility for many agents, with infants, young children, and the elderly considered at risk. The developing organs and evolving host defences of infants are considered to underlie their susceptibility while the failing host defences and high prevalence rates of chronic diseases render the elderly vulnerable to environmental pollutants.

During this century, research will probably identify the genetic basis of susceptibility to many environmental agents. The complete sequencing of the human genome is now a reality. The potential has already been shown in a few specific examples. For the development of the chronic lung disease, berylliosis, in beryllium-exposed workers, greatly increased risk has been demonstrated in workers having a specific immune response genotype (Kreiss *et al.* 1994). For lung cancer in cigarette smokers, multiple genes have been explored that determine the rate at which carcinogens in tobacco smoke are metabolized, as have genes that determine the efficacy of DNA repair processes (Wang and Samet 1997). Already, much has been written on the challenges that will be faced when susceptible individuals can be identified with certainty (Khoury 1996, 1997).

Summary

Occupational and environmental agents remain a threat to public health worldwide. For many agents, for example those long associated with occupational diseases, the scientific evidence on causation has long been adequate and emphasis has shifted to prevention and surveillance. For many other agents, for example pollutants in the general environment, controversy remains concerning the magnitude of the risk to populations and competing interests among stakeholders may impede policy formulation. Additionally, each of the many exposures in the occupational and general environments cannot be fully investigated. The scale of environmental problems is also shifting. While there are still hazardous exposures in many long-studied microenvironments like the home or workplace, regional problems from urbanization and large point sources are increasingly frequent and some problems are now at the global scale.

In response to the maintained need for scientific evidence on the health risks of occupational and environmental agents, research methods have continued to evolve in their sophistication and informativeness. There are now well-documented research methods for carrying out studies of many types of agents and health effects. The epidemiological approaches have been refined and joined with increasingly sophisticated exposure assessment strategies. Toxicological science contributes a foundation of mechanistic understanding and biomarkers offer the possibility of linking findings in the laboratory and population. For policy-making purposes, there are model approaches for synthesizing information, often involving multidisciplinary teams of scientists. Examples from the United States include committees of the National Research Council of the National Academy of Sciences and the Environmental Protection Agency's formulaic process for setting outdoor air quality standards.

However, these approaches require funding and the availability of knowledgeable scientists who can contribute in the policy-making process. Funding is also needed to develop the base of evidence on the agent(s). These approaches may have lesser applicability in developing countries, which nonetheless face equivalent or even greater risks from occupational and environmental agents. New models are needed that will serve the needs of developed and developing countries alike; perhaps, new global technologies for communication and information transfer will prove useful for this purpose.

References

American Thoracic Society (2000). ATS statement: what constitutes an adverse health effect of air pollution. *American Journal of Respiratory and Critical Care Medicine*, **161**, 665–73.

American Thoracic Society and Committee of the Environmental and Occupational Health Assembly (1996*a*). Health effects of outdoor air pollution. Part 1. *American Journal of Respiratory and Critical Care Medicine*, **153**, 3–50.

American Thoracic Society, Committee of the Environmental and Occupational Health Assembly, Bascom, R., Bromberg, P.A., Costa, D.A., *et al.* (1996*b*). Health effects of outdoor air pollution. Part 2. *American Journal of Respiratory and Critical Care Medicine*, **153**, 477–98.

Attfield, M.D. and Wagner, G.R. (1998). Respiratory disease in coal miners. In *Environmental and occupational medicine* (ed. W.N. Rom), (3rd edn), pp. 413–33. Lippincott-Raven, Philadelphia, PA.

Baghurst, P.A., McMichael, A.J., Wigg, N.R., *et al.* (1992). Environmental exposure to lead and children's intelligence at the age of seven years. The Port Pirie Cohort Study. *New England Journal of Medicine*, **327**, 1279–84.

Bailar, J.C., III (1997). The promise and problems of meta-analysis. *New England Journal of Medicine*, **337**, 559–61.

Balmes, J., Harber, P., and Schenker, M.B. (1996). *Occupational and environmental respiratory disease.* Mosby, St Louis, MO.

Banks, D.E. (1998). Respiratory effects of isocyanates. In *Environmental and occupational medicine* (ed. W.N. Rom), (3rd edn), pp. 537–63. Lippincott-Raven, Philadelphia, PA

Benowitz, N.L. (1999). Biomarkers of environmental tobacco smoke. *Environmental Health Perspectives*, **107**, 349–55.

Blair, A. and Kazerouni, N. (1997). Reactive chemicals and cancer. *Cancer Causes and Control*, **8**, 473–90.

Boffetta, P., Jourenkova, N., and Gustavsson, P. (1997). Cancer risk from occupational and environmental exposure to polycyclic aromatic hydrocarbons. *Cancer Causes and Control*, **8**, 444–72.

Breen, J.J. and Stroup, C.R. (1995). *Lead poisoning: exposure, abatement, regulation.* CRC Lewis, Boca Raton, FL.

Breslow, N.E., Lubin, J.H., and Marek, P. (1982). *Multiplicative models and the analysis of cohort data.* 50. US National Institutes of Health, Bethesda, MD.

Brimblecombe, P. (1999). Air pollution and health history. In *Air pollution and health* (ed. S.T. Holgate, J.M. Samet, H.S. Koren, and R.L. Maynard), pp. 5–18. Academic Press, San Diego, CA.

Butler, J.P., Post, G.B., Lioy, P.J., Waldman, J.M., and Greenberg, A. (1993). Assessment of carcinogenic risk from personal exposure to benzo(a)pyrene in the Total Human Environmental Exposure Study (THEES). *Journal of Air Waste Management Association*, **43**, 970–7.

Centers for Disease Control and Prevention (1991). *Preventing lead poisoning in young children.* United States Department of Health and Human Services, Washington, DC.

Checkoway, H., Pearce, N.E., and Crawford, D.J. (1989). *Research methods in occupational epidemiology.* Oxford University Press, New York.

Choi, B.C.K. (1992). Definition, sources, magnitude, effect modifiers, and strategies of reduction of the healthy worker effect. *Journal of Occupational Medicine*, **34**, 979–88.

Clayton, G.D. and Clayton, F.E. (1991). *Patty's industrial hygiene and toxicology* (4th edn). Wiley, New York.

Clifton, F. (trans.) (1752). *Upon air, water, and situation; upon epidemical diseases; and upon prognosticks, in acute cases especially* (orig. Hippocrates) (2nd edn). Lockyer Davis, London.

Cohen, B.L. and Colditz, G.A. (1994). Tests of the linear–no threshold theory for lung cancer induced by exposure to radon. *Environmental Research*, **64**, 65–89.

Crawford, F.G., Mayer, J., Santella, R.M., *et al.* (1994). Biomarkers of environmental tobacco smoke in preschool children and their mothers. *Journal of the National Cancer Institute*, **86**, 1398–402.

Creech, J.L., Jr and Johnson, M.N. (1974). Angiosarcoma of liver in the manufacture of polyvinyl chloride. *Journal of Occupational Medicine*, **74**, 150–1.

Crosby, D.G. (1998). *Environmental toxicology and chemistry*. Oxford University Press, New York.

Cunningham, J., O'Connor, G.T., Dockery, D.W., and Speizer, F.E. (1996). Environmental tobacco smoke, wheezing, and asthma in children in 24 communities. *Respiratory and Critical Care Medicine*, **153**, 218–24.

Denison, D., Mallick, B., and Smith, A. (1998). Automatic bayesian curve fitting. *Journal of the Royal Statistics Society Series B*, **60**, 333–50.

Diggle, P.J., Liang, K.Y., and Zeger, S.L. (1994). *Analysis of longitudinal data*. Oxford University Press, New York.

Dockery, D.W., Pope, C.A. III, Xu, X., *et al.* (1993). An association between air pollution and mortality in six United States cities. *New England Journal of Medicine*, **329**, 1753–9.

Doll, R. and Hill, A.B. (1950). A study of the aetiology of carcinoma of the lung. *British Medical Journal*, **2**, 740–8.

Dominici, F., Samet, J., Xu, J., and Zeger, S. (2000). Combining evidence on air pollution and daily mortality from the largest 20 United States cities: a hierarchical modeling strategy. *Journal of the Royal Statistics Society, Series C*, **163**, 263–302

Elliott, P., Hills, M., Beresford, J., *et al.* (1992*a*). Incidence of cancers of the larynx and lung near incinerators of waste solvents and oils in Great Britain. *Lancet*, **339**, 854–8.

Elliott, P., Kleinschmidt, I., and Westlake, A.J. (1992*b*). Use of routine data in studies of point sources of environmental pollution. In *Geographical and environmental epidemiology: methods for small-area studies* (ed. P. Elliott, J. Cuzick, D. English, and R.Stern). Oxford University Press.

Fan, A.M. and Chang, L.W. (1996). *Toxicology and risk assessment. principles, methods, and applications.* Marcel Dekker, New York.

Fingerhut, M.A., Halperin, W.E., Marlow, D.A., *et al.* (1991). Cancer mortality in workers exposed to 2,3,7,8-tetrachlorodibenzo-*p*-dioxin. *New England Journal of Medicine*, **324**, 212–18.

Goldberg, M., Kromhout, H., Guenel, P., *et al.* (1993). Job exposure matrices in industry. *International Journal of Epidemiology*, **22**, S10–15

Gordis, L. (1996). *Epidemiology*. W.B. Saunders, Philadelphia, PA

Hastie, T.J. and Tibshirani, R.J. (1990). *Generalized additive models*. Chapman and Hall, New York.

Hayes, A.W. (1994). *Principles and methods of toxicology* (3rd edn). Raven Press, New York.

Hayes, R.B. (1997). The carcinogenicity of metals in humans. *Cancer Causes and Control*, **8**, 371–85.

Hill, A.B. (1965). The environment and disease: association or causation? *Proceedings of the Royal Society of Medicine*, **58**, 295–300.

Hoar, S.K., Morrison, A.S., Cole, P., and Silverman, D.T. (1980). An occupation and exposure linkage system for the study of occupational carcinogenesis. *Journal of Occupational Medicine*, **22**, 722–6.

Hodgson, E. and Levi, P.E. (1997). *A textbook of modern toxicology* (2nd edn). Appleton and Lange, Stamford, CT.

Howson, C.P., Hernandez-Avila, M., and Rall, D.P. (1996). *Lead in the Americas: a call for action*. National Institute of Public Health, Mexico.

Hulka, B.S., Wilcosky, T.C., and Griffith, J.D. (1990). *Biological markers in epidemiology*. Oxford University Press, New York.

Katsouyanni, K., Schwartz, J., Spix, C., *et al.* (1996). Short-term effects of air pollution on health: a European approach using epidemiologic time series data: the APHEA protocol. *Journal of Epidemiology and Community Health*, **50**, S12–18.

Kelsall, J.E., Samet, J.M., Zeger, S.L., and Xu, J. (1997). Air pollution and mortality in Philadelphia 1974–1988. *American Journal of Epidemiology*, **146**, 750–62.

Khoury, M.J. (1996). From genes to public health: the applications of genetic technology in disease prevention. Genetics Working Group. *American Journal of Public Health*, **86**, 1717–22.

Khoury, M.J. (1997). Genetic epidemiology and the future of disease prevention and public health. *Epidemiology Review*, **19**, 175–80.

Kreiss, K., Miller, F., Newman, L.S., Ojo-Amaize, E.A., Rossman, M.D., and Saltini, C. (1994). Chronic beryllium disease—from the workplace to cellular immunology, molecular immunogenetics, and back. *Clinics in Immunology and Immunopathology*, **71**, 123–9.

Kunzli, N. and Tager, I.B. (1997). The semi-individual study in air pollution epidemiology: a valid design as compared to ecologic studies. *Environmental Health Perspectives*, **105**, 1078–83.

Lave, L.B. and Seskin, E.P. (1977). *Air pollution and human health*. Johns Hopkins University Press, Baltimore, MD.

Lee, P.N. (1986). Passive smoking. *British Journal of Cancer*, **54**, 1019–21.

Lee, P.N. (1987). Passive smoking and lung cancer association: a result of bias? *Human Toxicology*, **87**, 517–24.

Lee, P.N. (1988). *Misclassification of smoking habits and passive smoking*. Springer Verlag, Berlin.

Lee, P.N. (1992) *Environmental tobacco smoke and mortality*. Karger, Basel.

Lee, J.T. and Schwartz, J. (1999). Reanalysis of the effects of air pollution on daily mortality in Seoul, Korea: a case–crossover design. *Environmental Health Perspectives*, **107**, 633–6.

Lee, P.N., Chamberlain, J., and Alderson, M.R. (1986). Relationship of passive smoking to risk of lung cancer and other smoking-associated diseases. *British Journal of Cancer*, **54**, 97–105.

Lioy, P.J. and Waldman, J.M. (1990). The personal, indoor and outdoor concentrations of PM-10 measured in an industrial community during the winter. *Atmosphere and Environment*, **24B**, 57–66.

Lioy, P.L., Waldman, J.M., Greenberg, A., Harkov, R., and Pietarinen, C. (1988). The Total Human Environmental Exposure Study (THEES) to benzo(a)pyrene: comparison of the inhalation and food pathways. *Archives of Environmental Health*, **43**, 304–12.

Lipfert, F.W. (1997*a*). Air pollution and human health: perspectives for the 1990s and beyond. *Risk Analysis*, **17**, 137–46.

Lipfert, F. (1997*b*). Clean air skepticism. *Science*, **278**, 19–20.

Lipfert, F.W. and Wyzga, R.E. (1997). Air pollution and mortality: the implications of uncertainties in regression modeling and exposure measurement. *Journal of Air Waste Management Association*, **47**, 517–23.

Lippmann, M. (1999). *Environmental toxicants: human exposures and their health effects* (2nd edn). Van Nostrand–Reinhold, New York.

Logan, W.P.D. (1953). Mortality in the London fog incident 1952. *Lancet*, **i**, 336–8.

Lowrance, W.W. (1976). *Of acceptable risk: science and the determination of safety*. William Kaufmann, Los Altos, CA.

Lubin, J.H., Boice, J.D. Jr, Edling, C., *et al.* (1994). *Radon and lung cancer risk: a joint analysis of 11 underground miners studies*. United States Department of Health and Human Services, Public Health Service, National Institutes of Health, Bethesda, MD.

Lynge, E., Anttila, A., and Hemminki, K. (1997). Organic solvents and cancer. *Cancer Causes and Control*, **8**, 406–19.

Maclure, M. (1991). The case–crossover design: A method for studying the transient effects of risk of acute events. *American Journal of Epidemiology*, **133**, 144–53.

McMichael, A.J. (1995). *Planetary overload: global environmental change and the health of the human species* (Canto edn). Cambridge University Press, New York.

McMichael, A.J., Spirtas, R., and Kupper, L.L. (1974). An epidemiologic study of mortality within a cohort of rubber workers 1964–72. *Journal of Occupational Medicine*, **16**, 458–64.

McMichael, A.J., Baghurst, P.A., Wigg, N.R., Vimpani, G.V., Robertson, E.F., and Roberts, R.J. (1988). Port Pirie Cohort Study: environmental exposure to lead and children's abilities at the age of four years. *New England Journal of Medicine*, **88**, 468–75.

Marquardt, H., McClellan, R.O., and Schafer, S. (1999). *Toxicology*. Academic Press, London.

Monson, R.R. (1990). *Occupational epidemiology* (2nd edn). CRC Press, Boca Raton, FL.

Monson, R.R. and Christiani, D.C. (1997). Summary of the evidence: occupation and environment and cancer. *Cancer Causes and Control*, **8**, 529–31.

Muñoz, A. and Gange, S.J. (1998). Methodological issues for biomarkers and intermediate outcomes in cohort studies. *Epidemiology Review*, **20**, 29–42.

National Institute for Environmental Health Sciences (1999). Environmental Genome Project website. http://www.niehs.nih.gov/envgenom/home.htm.

National Research Council and Committee on the Institutional Means for Assessment of Risks to Public Health (1983). *Risk assessment in the federal government: managing the process.* National Academy Press, Washington, DC.

National Research Council (1989). *Biologic markers in pulmonary toxicology.* National Academy Press, Washington, DC.

National Research Council and Committee on Environmental Epidemiology (1991*a*). *Environmental epidemiology.* Volume 1. *Public health and hazardous wastes.* National Academy Press, Washington, DC.

National Research Council and Committee on Advances in Assessing Human Exposure to Airborne Pollutants (1991*b*). *Human exposure assessment for airborne pollutants: advances and opportunities.* National Academy Press, Washington, DC.

National Research Council (1993). *Measuring lead exposure in infants, children, and other sensitive populations.* National Academy Press, Washington, DC.

National Research Council, Committee on Health Risks of Exposure to Radon, Board on Radiation Effects Research and Commission on Life Sciences (1998). *Health effects of exposure to radon (BEIR VI).* National Academy Press, Washington, DC.

Neas, L.M., Schwartz, J., and Dockery, D. (1999). A case–crossover analysis of air pollution and mortality in Philadelphia. *Environmental Health Perspectives*, **107**, 629–31.

Needleman, H.L. and Gatsonis, C.A. (1990). Low-level lead exposure and the IQ of children. A meta-analysis of modern studies. *Journal of the American Medical Association*, **263**, 673–8.

Niesink, R.J. and de Vries, J. (1996). *Toxicology: principles and applications.* CRC Press, Boca Raton, FL.

Ostro, B.D., Lipsett, M.J., Wiener, M.B., and Selner, J.C. (1991). Asthmatic responses to airborne acid aerosols. *American Journal of Public Health*, **81**, 694–702.

Ostro, B.D., Lipsett, M.J., Mann, J.K., Wiener, M.B., and Selner, J. (1994). Indoor air pollution and asthma. Results from a panel study. *American Journal of Respiratory and Critical Care Medicine*, **149**, 1400–6.

Perera, F.P., Hemminki, K., Gryzbowska, E., *et al.* (1992). Molecular and genetic damage in humans from environmental pollution in Poland. *Nature*, **360**, 256–8.

Peters, J.M., Avol, E., Navidi, W., *et al.* (1999*a*). A study of 12 Southern California communities with differing levels and types of air pollution. I. Prevalence of respiratory morbidity. *American Journal of Respiratory and Critical Care Medicine*, **159**, 760–767.

Peters, J.M., Avol, E., Gauderman, W.J., *et al.* (1999*b*). A study of 12 Southern California communities with differing levels and types of air pollution. II. Effects on pulmonary function. *American Journal of Respiratory and Critical Care Medicine*, **159**, 768–75.

Pope, C.A., III and Dockery, D.W. (1999). Epidemiology of particle effects. In *Air pollution and health* (ed. S.T. Holgate, J.M. Samet, H.S. Koren, and R.L. Maynard), pp. 673–705. Academic Press, San Diego, CA.

Prentice, R.L. (1986). A case–cohort design for epidemiologic cohort studies and disease prevention trials. *Biometrika*, **73**, 1–11.

Raffle, P.A.B., Lee, W.R., McCallum, R.I., and Murray, R. (1987). *Hunter's diseases of occupations.* Little, Brown, Boston, MA.

Robins, J.M. and Greenland, S. (1989). Estimability and estimation of excess and etiologic fractions. *Statistics and Medicine*, **8**, 845–59.

Rodricks, J.V. (1992). *Calculated risks. Understanding the toxicity and human health risks of chemicals in our environment.* Cambridge University Press.

Rom, W.N. (1998). *Environmental and occupational medicine* (3rd edn). Lippincott-Raven, Philadelphia, PA

Romieu, I., Meneses, F., Ramirez, M., *et al.* (1998). Antioxidant supplementation and respiratory functions among workers exposed to high levels of ozone. *American Journal of Respiratory and Critical Care Medicine*, **158**, 226–32.

Rose, R. (1998). *Environmental toxicology: current developments.* Gordon and Breach Science, Amsterdam.

Rosen, G. (1993). *A history of public health.* Johns Hopkins University Press, Baltimore, MD.

Rothman, K. and Greenland, S. (1997). *Modern epidemiology* (2nd edn). Lippincott–Raven, Hagerstown, MD.

Samet, J.M. (1989). Definitions and methodology in COPD research. In *Clinical epidemiology of chronic obstructive lung disease* (ed. M. Hensley and N. Saunders), pp. 1–22. Marcel Dekker, New York.

Samet, J.M. and Burke, T.A. (1998). Epidemiology and risk assessment. In *Applied epidemiology: theory to practice* (ed. R.C. Brownson and D.B. Petitti), pp. 137–75. Oxford University Press, New York.

Samet, J.M. and Cohen, A.J. (1999). Air pollution and lung cancer. In *Air pollution and health* (ed. S.T. Holgate, J.M. Samet, H.S. Koren, and R.L. Maynard), pp. 841–64. Academic Press, San Diego, CA.

Samet, J.M. and Jaakkola, J.J.K. (1999). The epidemiologic approach to investigating outdoor air pollution. In *Air pollution and health* (ed. S.T. Holgate, J.M. Samet, H.S. Koren, and R.L. Maynard), pp. 431–60. Academic Press, San Diego, CA.

Samet, J.M. and Muñoz, A. (1998). Evolution of the cohort study. *Epidemiology Review*, **20**, 1–14.

Samet, J.M. and Wang, S.S. (2000). Environmental tobacco smoke. In *Environmental toxicants: human exposures and their health effects* (ed. M. Lippmann), (2nd edn), pp. 319–75. Van Nostrand–Reinhold, New York.

Samet, J.M., Young, R.A., Morgan, M.V., Humble, C.G., Epler, G.R., and McCloud, T.C. (1983). Prevalence survey of respiratory abnormalities in New Mexico uranium miners. *Health Physics*, **46**, 361–70.

Samet, J.M., Pathak, D.R., Morgan, M.V., Marbury, M.C., and Key, C.R. (1989). Radon progeny exposure and lung cancer risk in New Mexico uranium miners: a case–control study. *Health Physics*, **56**, 415–21.

Samet, J.M., Pathak, D.R., Morgan, M.V., Key, C.R., and Valdivia, A.A. (1991). Lung cancer mortality and exposure to radon decay products in a cohort of New Mexico underground uranium miners. *Health Physics*, **61**, 745–52.

Samet, J.M., Zeger, S.L., Dominici, F., *et al.* (2000). *Morbidity and mortality from air pollution in the United States: the National Morbidity, Mortality, and Air Pollution Study (NMMAPS).* Health Effects Institute, Cambridge, MA.

Schulte, P.A. and Perera, F.P. (1993). *Molecular epidemiology: principles and practices.* Academic Press, New York.

Shaw, I.C. and Chadwick, J. (1998). *Principles of environmental toxicology.* Taylor and Francis, London.

Sieber, W.K., Jr, Sundin, D.S., Frazier, T.M., and Robinson, C.F. (1991). Development, use, and availability of a job exposure matrix based on national occupational hazard survey data. *American Journal of Industrial Medicine*, **20**, 163–74.

Siemiatycki, J. (1991). *Risk factors for cancer in the workplace.* CRC Press, Boston, MA.

Steenland, K. and Savitz, D. (1997). *Topics in environmental epidemiology.* Oxford University Press, New York.

Stewart, P.A. and Stewart, W.F. (1994). Occupational case–control studies: II. Recommendations for exposure assessment. *American Journal of Industrial Medicine*, **26**, 313–26.

Stewart, P.A., Blair, A., Dosemeci, M., and Gomez, M. (1991). Collection of exposure data for retrospective occupational epidemiologic studies. *Applied Occupational and Environmental Hygiene*, **6**, 280–9.

Stewart, P.A., Stewart, W.F., Heineman, E.F., Dosemeci, M., Linet, M., and Inskip, P.D. (1996). A novel approach to data collection in a case–control study of cancer and occupational exposures. *International Journal of Epidemiology*, **25**, 744–52.

Stewart, P.A., Stewart, W.F., Siemiatycki, J., Heineman, E.F., and Dosemeci, M. (1998). Questionnaires for collecting detailed occupational information for community-based case control studies. *American Industrial Hygiene Association Journal*, **59**, 39–44.

Stidley, C.A. and Samet, J.M. (1993). A review of ecologic studies of lung cancer and indoor radon. *Health Physics*, **93**, 234–51.

Thomas, D. (1998). New techniques for the analysis of cohort studies. *Epidemiology Review*, **20**, 122–34.

Tong, S., Baghurst, P.A., Sawyer, M.G., Burns, J., and McMichael, A.J. (1998). Declining blood lead levels and changes in cognitive function during childhood. The Port Pirie Study. *Journal of the American Medical Association*, **280**, 1915–19.

USDHEW (United States Department of Health Education and Welfare) (1964). *Smoking and health.* Report of the Advisory Committee to the Surgeon General. DHEW Publication No. PHS 1103. US Government Printing Office, Washington, DC.

USDHHS (United States Department of Health and Human Services) (1984). *The health consequences of smoking—chronic obstructive lung disease. A report of the Surgeon General.* US Government Printing Office, Washington, DC.

USEPA (United States Environmental Protection Agency) (1986). Guidelines for carcinogen risk assessment. *Federal Register*, **51**, 33992–4003.

USEPA (United States Environmental Protection Agency) (1992). *Guidelines for exposure assessment.* EPA/600Z-92/001 FRL-4129–5. Office of Health and Environmental Assessment, Washington, DC.

Veys, C.A. (1996). ABC of work related disorders: occupational cancers. *British Medical Journal*, **313**, 615–19.

Vineis, P. and Pirastu, R. (1997). Aromatic amines and cancer. *Cancer Causes and Control*, **8**, 346–55.

von Mutius, E., Martinez, F.D., Fritzsch, C., Nicolai, T., Roell, G., and Thiemann, H.H. (1994). Prevalence of asthma and atopy in two areas of West and East Germany. *American Journal of Respiratory and Critical Care Medicine*, **149**, 358–64.

Wagner, J.C., Sleggs, C.A., and Marchand, P. (1960). Diffuse pleural mesothelioma and asbestos exposure in the north western cape province. *British Journal of Industrial Medicine*, **17**, 260–71.

Wang, S.S. and Samet, J.M. (1997). Tobacco smoking and cancer—the promise of molecular epidemiology. *Salud Publica de Mexico*, **39**, 331–45.

Ware, J.H., Spengler, J.D., Neas, L.M., *et al.* (1993). Respiratory and irritant health effects of ambient volatile organic compounds: the Kanawha County Health Study. *American Journal of Epidemiology*, **137**, 1287–301.

Witorsch, R.J. and Witorsch, P. (1989). A critical analysis of the relationship between parental smoking and pulmonary performance in children. *Offentliche Gesundheitswesen*, **51**, 78–83.

WHO (World Health Organization) (1946). *Constitution of the World Health Organization.* WHO, New York.

WHO (World Health Organization) and International Agency for Research on Cancer (IARC) (1972). *IARC monographs on the evaluation of carcinogenic risk to chemicals to man.* 1. International Agency for Research on Cancer, Geneva.

WHO (World Health Organization) (1992). *ICD 10: International statistical classification of diseases and related health problems* (10th edn). WHO, Geneva.

WHO (World Health Organization) and McMichael, A.J., Haines, A., Slooff, R., and Kovats, S. (ed.) (1996). *Climate change and human health.* WHO, Geneva.

Wynder, E.L. and Graham, E.A. (1950). Tobacco smoking as a possible etiologic factor in bronchiogenic carcinoma. A study of six hundred and eighty-four proved cases. *Journal of the American Medical Association*, **143**, 329–36.

Zeger, S., Thomas, D., Dominici, F., *et al.* (1999). *Exposure measurement error in time-series studies of air pollution: concepts and consequences.* Johns Hopkins University, Baltimore, MD.

8.2 Toxicology and environmental health: applications and interventions in public health

Bernard D. Goldstein and Michael Greenberg

Introduction

In recent decades we have witnessed a public outcry against pollution of the environment that parallels the force of the Sanitary Revolution of the mid-nineteenth century. New national and international governmental organizations reflect the political potency of this public concern. The chemical, electronics, and petroleum industries, whose previously steady growth had greatly accelerated following the Second World War, are now forced to consider factors other than utility and cost in the development of new products and the marketing of old ones. Substantial societal investments have been made in the developed countries to clean up old environmental pollution problems and to prevent new ones. Government departments that made and tested weapons of mass destruction now spend large portions of their budgets on cleaning up contamination and destroying their weapons. As with the Sanitary Revolution, part of the rationale has been a developing understanding of the relationship of a foul environment to human ill health, part is simply a human revulsion to dirty air, tainted water, and a blighted natural environment. Moreover, we have come to recognize that sustainable development of the Earth's resources is not possible under the related threats of population growth and environmental degradation.

As we develop more understanding of the Earth, its ecosystems, and the pathways of chemical exposure, problems once thought to be limited to the natural environment have been shown to pose risks to human health, for example contamination of drinking water by hazardous waste dumps. The most substantial long-range threat to human health posed by environmental chemicals is the alteration of the Earth's atmosphere. Chlorofluorocarbons (**CFCs**) and other compounds are producing a decrease in the levels of stratospheric ozone, which prevents shorter-range ultraviolet light rays from penetrating to the Earth's surface, a protective mantle that has been present through much of evolution. The implications of climatic alterations, such as the greenhouse effect caused primarily by increased fossil fuel use and by agricultural practices, are potentially dire. Together, the secondary effects of the alteration of our global climate could be disastrous to human health, and could include major changes in the range and habitat of disease vectors, severe flooding, and famine from crop failure (McMichael 1994).

The global climate issue illustrates five points that are pertinent to this chapter.

1. Understanding the effects of chemicals is crucial to environmental health.
2. The system in which chemicals act, whether the human body or planet Earth, is a closed one with only limited response, repair, and regenerative potential.
3. The effects of chemical and physical agents on health are often delayed and indirect, but nonetheless disastrous.
4. Local, national, and international control efforts have tended to be most effective when dealing with a single pollutant in a single medium directly producing overt effects, and least effective when dealing with complex chemical mixtures, with pollutants that cross traditional air, water, soil, and food boundaries, and with effects that are delayed or indirect.
5. A complex set of formal and informal policy processes need to be considered and employed to reduce the risk.

In this chapter we focus on the science of toxicology as it relates to environmental health. We also consider some of the interfaces between environmental health sciences and public policy. Toxicology is the science of poisons (Amdur *et al.* 1991). Knowledge about poisons extends back to the beginning of history as humans became aware of the toxicity of natural food components. The Bible contains injunctions concerning poisons, including how to avoid them. Greek and Roman history gives evidence of the use of poisons as an instrument of statecraft, an approach that was extended in the Middle Ages with such notable practitioners as the Borgias. Toxicologists tend to view Paracelcus, a seventeenth-century alchemist and a bit of a charlatan, as their ancestor, crediting him with the first law of toxicology—that the dose makes the poison (Gallo and Doull 1991). There are two other major maxims that underlie modern toxicology: that chemicals have specific biological effects, and that humans are members of the animal kingdom.

This chapter discusses 'laws' and general concepts of toxicology pertinent to understanding how a chemical or physical agent acts in a biological system. The focus is on the biological response, rather than on the intrinsic property of the agent, although the latter is briefly reviewed (Plaa 1991). This chapter is restricted to human health, although many of the concepts are applicable to ecological health as well.

Laws of toxicology

The dose makes the poison

Central to toxicology is the exploration of how dose is related to response. As a generalization, there are two types of dose–response curves (Fig. 1). One is an S-shaped curve that is characterized by having at lowest doses no observed effect and, as the dose increases, the gradual development of an increasing response. This is followed by a linear phase of increase in response in relation to dose and, eventually, a dose level at which no further increase in response is observed. Of particular pertinence to environmental toxicology is that this curve presumes that there is a threshold level below which no harm whatsoever is to be expected. There is an ample scientific base for the existence of thresholds for specific effects (Aldridge 1986). For example, if undiluted sulphuric acid is splashed on the skin it is capable of producing a severe burn. Yet one drop of pure sulphuric acid in a bathtub of water is sufficiently dilute to be entirely without effect. Thresholds for an adverse effect will differ among individuals based upon a variety of circumstances, some of which are genetically determined and others may represent stages of life or specific circumstances. In the example of sulphuric acid on the skin, there are genetically determined differences in susceptibility related to the protective presence of skin hair, babies will be more susceptible than adults, and skin that is already cut will be at particular risk. This S-type dose–response curve is assumed to fit all toxic effects except those that are produced by direct reaction with genetic material.

The second general type of dose–response curve has no apparent threshold dose. It covers those endpoints caused by persistent changes in the genes. This occurs in cancers, in which a so-called somatic mutation occurring in a single cell results in a clone of cancer cell progeny. Similarly, germ-like mutations can occur in the DNA of cells involved in reproduction. The genetic code can be considered as bits of information strung on a line in such a way that alteration of one single bit of information can have a profound effect on the overall meaning. It is believed that a single change in DNA can alter the genetic code in such a way to lead to a mutated cell. It therefore follows that any single molecule of a chemical compound, or packet of energy of a physical agent, such as ionizing radiation, that can alter DNA is theoretically capable of causing a persistent mutation. If the chemical adduct or other change in DNA is not repaired by cellular enzymes, each molecule or ionizing ray theoretically has the possibility of changing a normal cell to a cancerous cell. The resultant dose–response curve starts at a single molecule, that is, it has no threshold below which the risk is zero (Fig. 1). There is no absolutely safe dose. In this highly simplified scheme, the shape of the curve is linearly

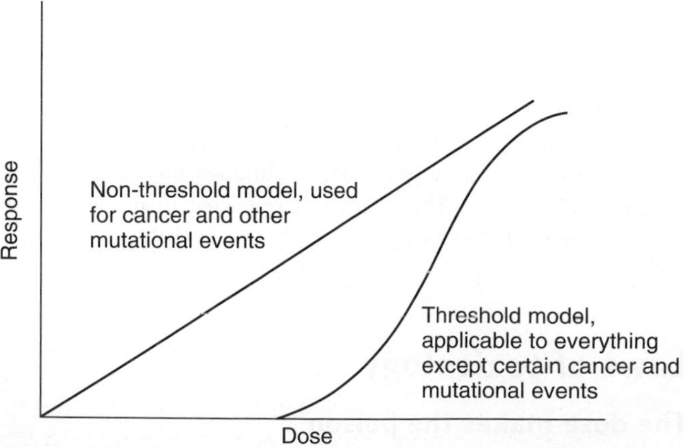

Fig. 1 Dose–response curves.

related to dose. The result is that the risk of two molecules of a DNA-altering chemical causing a mutation is twice that of one molecule. Eventually, the dose level is sufficiently high that it results in dead cells. As dead cells do not reproduce, they cannot be the basis for cancer or for inherited abnormalities. Note also that relatively few chemicals are capable of directly altering the DNA of a living cell. Further, the risk of any one molecule actually causing cancer is infinitesimally small—despite the immense number of carcinogenic molecules in the smoke of one cigarette, only a minority of cigarette smokers ever develop cancer. Yet the assumption that the risk is not zero has a major impact on communicating to the public about cancer risk from chemical and physical carcinogens. Industry has often claimed that a threshold exists for carcinogens and for a few chemical mechanistically based toxicological research has substantiated that claim. The prudent public health approach to known or potential human carcinogens places the burden of proof on an industry making such a claim (see Chapter 8.8).

Specificity

That chemical and physical agents have specific effects has been called the second law of toxicology. The concept is no different from recognizing that possession of a gun does not make one a murder suspect if the victim has been stabbed to death. This principle is well understood by the public in terms of medicine: aspirin will help with your headache but is useless for constipation, while laxatives have the opposite specificity. Nevertheless, various surveys suggest that the selectivity of effects of environmental chemicals is not well understood by the public; many believe that a chemical that can cause cancer in a particular organ can cause cancer and other diseases anywhere in the body.

The specificity of effects is due both to chemistry and to biology. Understanding the relationship between chemical structure and biological effect has been a central core of both pharmacology and toxicology. Structure–activity relationships (**SAR**) are often used to design a chemical with a specific effect that might be useful as a therapeutic agent. Also, SAR is used to predict whether a new chemical being readied for manufacture might be of potential harm. While SAR is a useful tool, the predictive value is too limited to be used without recourse to additional testing of a potentially toxic agent. For example, one methyl group separates toluene from benzene, only the latter causing bone marrow damage and leukaemia; ethanol from methanol, the latter causing acute acidosis and blindness; and η-hexane from either η-heptane or η-pentane, with only hexane being responsible for peripheral nerve damage. These differences reflect specificity in the formation of toxic metabolites and in interaction with biological receptors.

Chemical structure is also an important determinant of the specific characteristic of environmental persistence. There is substantial scientific and public concern about agents that accumulate in the human body or in the general environment. Many such compounds have already been banned or severely restricted (e.g. dichlorodiphenyltrichloroethane (DDT) and polychlorinated biphenyls (PCBs)). There is a consensus that development or use of additional persistent and accumulative agents should be avoided, particularly as standard toxicological approaches cannot predict all untoward effects and it can be decades before reversal of the environmental effects of a persistent organic compound is possible. Sometimes, non-persistent compounds may be precursors of persistent agents, such as dioxins and dibenzofurans often produced in the incineration of chlorine containing wastes. The possibility that such compounds subtly alter oestrogenic hormone function has become a matter of intense interest (Colborn *et al.* 1993).

Specificity of effects is also conferred by the susceptibility of biological processes that lead certain cells to be more of a target to environmental agents. For example, haemoglobin, the iron-containing protein in red blood cells, is responsible for the delivery of oxygen to the tissues in the body. Significant toxicity can occur through several specific mechanisms. Oxidation of the reduced ferrous form to the ferric form of iron in the haemoglobin impairs the ability to carry and release oxygen in the tissues. Various chemical agents oxidize intracellular iron, including nitrites that are common contaminants of well water in agricultural communities. Carbon monoxide, an otherwise relatively inert gas, sufficiently resembles oxygen so that it can bind to the oxygen combining site of haemoglobin, thereby displacing oxygen. There are many other examples in which a normal body process is disrupted by an exogenous chemical through oxidation, covalent addition, or fitting into a niche designed through evolution to accommodate an internal chemical that it superficially resembles.

Humans are animals

That humans are animals is the third law of toxicology. The conceptual foundation for extrapolating findings in animals to expected effects in humans is a central facet of modern toxicology. The basic principles of cell and organ function are common to all of biology. All cells must obtain energy, build internal structures, and release waste. Specificity of toxic effects is relatively similar across mammals. In other words, a kidney poison in one species is likely to be a kidney poison in another, although there are exceptions. However, dose–response considerations often vary substantially, reflecting differences in adsorption, distribution, metabolism, excretion, function, and target organ susceptibility among species. Understanding the factors responsible for interspecies differences greatly facilitates extrapolation from animals to humans. Once elucidated, the role of different absorption rates, metabolism or other factors can be taken into account, often through a mathematical approximation called physiologically based pharmacokinetics (Frantz *et al.* 1994).

Human pathways of exogenous chemicals

A central focus of toxicological science is the assessment of the pathways taken by a chemical from its entrance into the body until its eventual excretion. This process is usually divided into four related processes of absorption, distribution, metabolism, and excretion (Gallo *et al.* 1987).

Absorption

Absorption of a chemical into the body occurs through the mouth, respiratory tract, and skin. Depending upon the specific chemical, the route of exposure can have major implications to absorption into the body and the resultant toxicity. For example, almost 100 per cent of inhaled lead particles are absorbed into the circulation as compared with a much smaller per cent of ingested lead. Internal factors can affect absorption, particularly from the gastrointestinal tract. For example, iron and calcium deficiencies, which are common in children in inner city areas where lead is prevalent, both produce an increase in absorption of ingested lead. The milieu of the exposure agent can also have an effect on its bioavailability. For example, the rate at which benzene in gasoline is absorbed through the skin is increased by the addition of oxygenated components to the gasoline mixture, and the extent to which dioxin in soil is absorbed through the gastrointestinal tract differs many hundred-fold depending upon the source of the contaminated soil (Umbreit *et al.* 1986).

Often, a single route of absorption is dominant. Nevertheless, in many instances more than one route is important. For example, exposure due to contamination of well water through a leaky underground storage tank is usually thought of solely in terms of water intake. However, depending upon the height of the water table there may be evaporation into the basement producing inhalation exposure, and during showering there is likely to be both inhalation and transdermal absorption.

Distribution

Distribution of the chemical, once inside the body, occurs through different pathways. In part this distribution depends upon the route of absorption. Most compounds absorbed in the gastrointestinal tract go directly to the liver and may go no farther, while inhaled agents first go to the lung or other parts of the respiratory tract. Distribution also depends upon the chemical and physical properties of the agents. Small particles tend to be distributed deep within the respiratory tract, while larger particles wind up in the nose or upper respiratory tract. Chemicals that are poorly soluble in water, for example oils, usually distribute within fatty tissues, and only certain types of compounds can penetrate from the blood to the brain. Distribution will often depend upon organ-specific factors. For example, the high levels of iodine in the thyroid are due to a specific thyroid pump for the uptake of iodine needed for the synthesis of thyroid hormones.

Metabolism

Metabolism in the narrowest sense of the term refers to alteration of chemicals by the body (Kato *et al.* 1989). The major metabolic function of the body is to alter food into energy or structural materials. Most foods and other exogenous chemicals are metabolized in the liver. All organs have metabolic capability, often related both to organ function and to susceptibility to toxic agents. Understanding the specifics of the enzyme and enzyme families responsible for metabolism within cell types is important to the question of why chemicals have specific effects in specific organs.

Metabolism is often divided into two phases. Phase I reactions usually involve oxidation, reduction, or hydrolysis and often result in converting exogenous chemicals into substances capable of being converted by phase II enzymes into conjugates that can be excreted from the body, or into building blocks useful for synthesis of body components. The major family of enzymes involved in phase I reactions are cytochrome P-450 containing mono-oxygenases, of which there are multiple forms with varying degrees of specificity.

Metabolism of foreign substances is often protective, converting unwanted absorbed materials into chemical forms that are readily excretable. Thus, a fat-soluble agent can be converted into more water-soluble agents capable of being excreted in the bile or the urine. At times, metabolism is central to toxicity through the conversion of relatively inactive compounds into harmful agents (Guengerich and Liebler 1985). A variety of compounds ranging from polycyclic organic hydrocarbon components of soot to the leukaemogen benzene require metabolic activation to become carcinogenic. In the case of benzene, about 50 per cent of the body burden is exhaled unmetabolized and about 50 per cent is metabolized into potentially toxic metabolites. Slowing benzene metabolism leads to an increase in the relative amount exhaled rather than metabolized and a decrease in bone marrow toxicity. In contrast, speeding up benzene metabolism increases its toxicity (Snyder *et al.* 1993). For example, alcohol induces an increase in the specific cytochrome P-450 responsible for benzene metabolism and has been shown to potentiate benzene toxicity.

Excretion

Excretion from the body can occur through a variety of routes. These include the gastrointestinal tract for unabsorbed ingested components, and the urine for water soluble agents of appropriate molecular weight and charge. The urinary excretion rate can be substantially affected by the state of body hydration. Agents metabolized in the liver are often excreted through the biliary tract. Significant loss of volatile compounds can occur through the respiratory tract, as noted above for benzene. Other routes of excretion include sweat and lactation, the latter unfortunately putting the infant at risk when mothers' milk contains toxic agents.

Susceptibility

One of the more difficult problems in toxicology is to understand the basis for differences in human susceptibility to environmental insults (Grandjean 1995). In some individuals cigarette smoking will cause death at a relatively young age due to lung and other cancers, chronic lung disease, or cardiovascular disease, while other individuals with the same or greater smoking history will survive with relatively minimal damage until much older. A partial explanation is that certain environmental toxins act to speed up the effects of impacts that would have occurred later in life due to genetic or other environmental causes. For example, someone who would have died of a heart attack at age 70 due to an inherited tendency to cholesterol accumulation in their arteries coupled with a high cholesterol intake in the diet, may have a heart attack at age 55 because of the added insult of cigarette smoking. Increasing asthma rates among African-Americans has become a major public health issue in the United States, with many possible factors contributing to susceptibility currently under consideration. Understanding the interaction of genetic and environmental factors in human disease will be greatly abetted by current research on the human genome. While a genetic basis for most diseases will be discernible, it must be emphasized that the inherited factors will usually be necessary but not sufficient to lead to disease. Except for certain childhood disorders, environmental factors will usually determine whether and when the genetically determined disease will become manifest (see Chapter 2.4).

The known causes of increased human susceptibility to a specific level of a noxious environmental agent fit into four classes: increased uptake into the body increased delivery of the agent or its metabolite to the target organ increased susceptibility of the target organ to damage and increased susceptibility of the individual to a given level of target tissue damage. Increased absorption of an air pollutant may simply represent the difference between sitting on a park bench and jogging in the park. The tragic finding of two dead children in the back seat of a snowbound car with the motor left running, while the adults in the front seat are only unconscious, is due primarily to the greater respiratory rate per body size in the children, leading to a greater uptake of carbon monoxide (Plunkett *et al.* 1992). Genetically determined differences in certain enzymes are well known to affect the rate of metabolism of certain drugs and environmental agents significantly, both detoxification of a noxious compound and activation to a noxious form. For example, acetylation, a common metabolic process, occurs at a relatively fast or slow rate depending upon common variants of the responsible gene and enzyme. Other key metabolic enzymes can have their activity altered by dietary components, alcohol, therapeutic drugs, or previous exposure to the noxious agent. Target organs also may react differently to a given level of an environmental agent or its metabolite. As examples, one in seven black males in the United States has an inherited variant of the enzyme glucose-6-phosphate dehydrogenase that protects against malaria but leaves the red blood cells at particular risk to oxidizing drugs, and there are individuals who are at high risk of sunlight-induced skin cancer because they are lacking certain enzymes capable of repairing the DNA damage caused by ultraviolet light. Lastly, individuals may be more susceptible to harm from an environmental toxin not because their target organ response is greater, but because the effect of a loss of function is more deleterious. For example, cigarette smokers have no more, and perhaps even less, lung responsiveness to inhalation of the air pollutant ozone. This is presumably because the increased mucus in the airways of smokers acts to scrub out the ozone before it reaches the lung cell surface. Yet, because cigarette smokers have so much less overall respiratory capability than do non-smokers, a relatively small ozone-induced additional loss of respiratory capability may have more of an impact on the actual functioning of a smoker than of a non-smoker. Similarly, the loss of lung and other organ reserve with ageing will make an elderly individual more susceptible than a younger adult to an identical toxic effect in an organ.

The special problem of mixtures

Except in special circumstances, human exposure to potentially toxic chemical and physical agents occurs as part of a mixture. We are genetically well programmed to deal with mixtures—most foodstuffs contain an enormous variety of chemicals. However, the science of toxicology, and the regulation of chemicals, has generally focused on individual chemicals rather than the broad mix of agents that are present in contaminated air or water, or in such common consumer products as gasoline.

An example of the problem posed by this approach is the recent change in the automotive fuel mixture in the United States to include oxygenates such as methyl tert-butyl ether (**MTBE**). Many people are complaining about non-specific symptoms related to the addition of MTBE to gasoline. These clinical complaints are not well supported by the information in the toxicology database. However, the relevant toxicological database is almost totally restricted to studies of MTBE alone, rather than MTBE in gasoline.

The issue of how to predict the effect of mixtures is not confined solely to a single exposure matrix. As described above, ingestion of alcohol alters the level of metabolic enzymes responsible for the activation or inactivation of a variety of drugs and environmental chemicals. Many other food constituents have such effects, often in different directions from each other. An unexpected finding of the effect of alcohol consumption on the metabolism of a drug was traced to a natural component of grapefruit juice used to dilute the alcohol given to the study participants (Bailey *et al.* 1994).

Most studies of mixtures have found that the effects are additive in that they are predictable by summing up the effects of the individual components of the mixture. This is particularly true when agents have similar effects. At times, the interaction is synergistic. For example, the lung cancer incidence due to cigarette smoking plus occupational asbestos exposure is far greater than should be expected due to the sum of the risks (Selikoff *et al.* 1968). Antagonism also occurs; for example, exposure to toluene plus benzene leads to less benzene toxicity to the bone marrow than if the exposure were to benzene alone (Andrews *et al.* 1977). This is believed to be due to both agents being metabolized by the same metabolic machinery. Benzene is converted into a bone marrow toxin while toluene is converted into a harmless agent. If there is sufficient toluene available to tie up the metabolic machinery, benzene metabolism will be slowed and a less toxic metabolite will be formed. Note that no interaction between toluene and benzene occurs when exposure levels are relatively low as there is then sufficient metabolic machinery to handle both of these compounds independently. Potentiation also occurs when one agent (e.g. alcohol) that has no effect itself increases the effect of another agent.

In view of the almost infinite number of potential combinations of exogenous chemical and physical agents, studying them all is impossible. Two approaches have been developed to deal with this problem. One is to study those combinations to which humans are likely to be exposed, for example gasoline. The other is to focus on understanding the mechanism of toxicity of the individual components so as to predict interactive effects.

The interface between toxicological science and public policy

Toxicology is relied on as a way of protecting the public and the general environment. Toxicology has two important roles: detection of cause and effect relationships linking environmental chemical and physical agents to adverse effects to humans or the environment, and development of techniques capable of preventing these problems. Toxicologists usually approach questions of causation of disease by starting with the chemical or physical agent and studying its effects in laboratory animals or in test tube systems. One of the more exciting aspects of modern toxicology is the possibility of linking subtle biological markers indicative of exposure with biomarkers showing early effects, thereby providing epidemiologists with powerful early warning tools to evaluate cause and effect relationships between environmental exposure and human diseases (National Research Council 1989).

The use of toxicology to test the safety of chemicals

Assessment of the safety of chemicals has evolved into a relatively standardized approach, particularly when considering new chemicals being developed for the market. The starting assumption is that all chemicals have toxic effects. To protect the public and the worker it is necessary to know what specific effect occurs at what dose.

A relatively standardized battery of laboratory tests has been developed to assess chemical toxicity. Although varying greatly in effectiveness and cost, they are of value when used with judgement and with understanding of basic mechanisms of toxicity that govern the ability to predict effects. For certain types of endpoints, such as mutations, there are a variety of apparently effective testing procedures. For other endpoints, such as neurobehavioural effects, we are far less able to predict whether a new agent may have an adverse outcome in humans.

The Ames test for mutagenesis is an example of a short-term test designed specifically to screen for potentially cancer-causing chemicals. By using a bacterial test system that can readily show when a mutation occurs, and coupling that to an actively metabolizing fraction of rodent liver, compounds that are capable of producing mutations can usually be detected (Ames *et al.* 1975). Other short-term tests for mutagenesis depend upon mammalian cells *in vitro* or *in vivo*. The classic long-term test lasts almost 2 years, close to the lifetime of a rat or mouse. The dose chosen is one that is maximally tolerated by the laboratory animal in a 90-day trial. The use of a high dose, well beyond that of usual human exposure, has been controversial. Detractors point out that at high doses the toxicological response mechanisms may differ from that at usual doses, and that cell toxicity may lead to false positive findings, particularly of cancer. Supporters point out the effectiveness to date of detecting potential human carcinogens and the statistical impossibility of finding even a 1 in 1000 cancer risk using only at most a few hundred test animals exposed to usual environmental doses (National Research Council 1993).

Some of these useful animal tests are under attack by animal rights activists, although for most adverse endpoints there are no validated *in vitro* test procedures capable of protecting the public, or for that matter, capable of protecting pets, such as cats and dogs, that have benefited greatly from the development of chemical products that decrease their suffering and prolong their life.

In some cases, laws and governmental regulations specify the toxicological test information necessary, depending upon the type of product, for example pesticides or food additives. In all cases public concern and the activities of toxic tort plaintiffs' lawyers have produced pressure on chemical industries to carry out careful screening of new compounds for adverse effects before they are released to the market. Perhaps 1500 new chemicals pass through the screening process and enter the market each year in the United States.

The role of toxicological information in setting environmental health standards

As discussed below, the setting of environmental health standards depends upon many factors, including legal requirements and political, economic, and social considerations. Certain laws, such as the United States Clean Air Act, require the Administrator of the Environmental Protection Agency to set ambient standards based upon the protection of sensitive populations, but with no consideration of the costs to achieve the standard. Other laws, such as the Toxic

Substances Control Act in the United States, expressly attempt to balance the value to society of new chemical products against the potential risks to human health and the environment from use of these chemicals.

Not surprisingly, there are different levels of toxicological information required by these different laws. As a generalization, chemical agents developed for the marketplace can be considered under four headings: agents clearly intended to have a biological impact in humans, primarily therapeutic drugs or vitamins; agents with more limited biological effects in humans, such as cosmetics that alter skin moisture or food additives aimed at the taste bud; agents for which a biological impact is intended, but not in humans, such as pesticides or herbicides; and chemical agents for which no biological effect is desired, such as paints and window cleaners. Before a new drug can be marketed, the Food and Drug Administration requires extensive animal studies and then carefully controlled trials in humans. In contrast, in the United States premanufacturing notification for a new paint thinner requires little more than identifying the chemical structure and perhaps a few short-term test-tube assays. Usually, the chemical industry is sufficiently concerned about liability issues and the good name of the company so that it will more extensively test a new product before putting it on the market.

Protection factors and weight of evidence

Setting standards for exposure to chemicals has evolved from a rather straightforward arithmetic formulation based upon relatively minimal data in animals to the present day situation where there is often a large body of evidence, including information about humans. As a generalization, the toxicology of the past used a dose–response approach to establish a no observed effect level (**NOEL**) in laboratory animals. The NOEL is in essence the highest tested level below the threshold. Various protection factors, often mislabelled as safety factors (Goldstein 1990), were then applied, usually by dividing the NOEL by factors of 10 each for the greater variability in humans than in inbred laboratory animals, for the possibility that humans were more sensitive than the laboratory species under study, and even for the possibility that there were unobserved effects in the laboratory animals that were pertinent to humans. The resultant level, usually one-hundredth or one-thousandth of the NOEL, was then used to establish the standard. In the United States the new Food Quality Protection Act adds another factor of 10 for the protection of children.

Variants of this protective factor approach still exist, often in the more sophisticated form of a reference dose or benchmark dose. However, particularly in situations where there is a relatively mature database, a more formal approach to the weighing of evidence is often taken. For example, the United States Clean Air Act requires that the Environmental Protection Agency (**EPA**) Administrator sets an ambient standard for each of six major air pollutants: ozone, sulphur dioxide, particulates, nitrogen dioxide, carbon monoxide, and lead. The standard is required to protect sensitive populations from adverse effects with an adequate margin of safety. The law also sets up the Clean Air Scientific Advisory Committee, a seven-member panel that carefully reviews the evidence and makes recommendations to the EPA Administrator, including recommendations concerning the margin of safety. The standards are set without recourse to automatic factors of 10. Rather, the available toxicological and epidemiological evidence is carefully weighed as the basis for the recommendation. Recent recommendations have led to the EPA proposing changes in the ambient standards for ozone and for particulates.

The weight of evidence approach is increasingly used to come to judgement about complex issues. An important example is the classification of potential human carcinogens by the International Agency for Research on Cancer (IARC 1992).

Criteria for evaluating environmental policies

Environmental policies in the United States are neither knee-jerk reactions to mass media coverage of environmental risks, as some claim, nor, as many scientists wish, are they the product of carefully conceived analyses of all the factors that should be considered (Portney 1990; Carlisle and Chechile 1991). Eight criteria for policy formation are described below in the form of questions asked by decision-makers or analysts. The first two are always explicitly considered; the last three are often not considered.

1. Health/safety/environmental protection. This is clearly the first criterion. What risks will the proposed policy decrease? Will it increase any risks? To what certainty are these risks known and predictable from toxicology and epidemiology? In other words, how much uncertainty is there? The greater the uncertainty, the greater the importance of the other seven criteria.
2. Legal/political feasibility. Is the proposed policy consistent with existing legal mandates? Can it be implemented with existing legislative mandates and rules? Does it support national, state, and local political goals? For example, in the United States will the policy be consistent with a political trend toward less government, less interference with private enterprise, transfer of authority from the national government to state and local governments, from government to private enterprise?
3. Reactions from stakeholders. What interest groups are likely to support the proposed policy, oppose the proposed policy? Will elected and agency officials support or oppose it? Can they be persuaded to support it? What will be voter and media reactions?
4. Economic feasibility. Is the policy affordable? Can we prepare an implementation strategy that reaches the ultimate goal in divisible stages? Will the investment of a small amount of money in the initial stages accomplish most of the goals?
5. Benefits/costs. Will the proposed policy yield economic, social, and health benefits that exceed the costs? Are there advantages of using the funds for this purpose rather than another environmental protection policy? Is the proposed approach the least costly or most cost-effective way to obtain the desired benefits?
6. Ethical imperative. Does the proposed policy disproportionately benefit some groups (economic, ethnic, racial, generation, gender) while placing others at greater risk? How will the consent of the most seriously impacted groups be obtained? Does the policy increase the probability of damaging a unique national or cultural resource?
7. Time pressure. What will happen if the policy is deferred for 1, 5, 10, 20, or more years?

8. Flexibility. Is the policy adaptable to advances in science and engineering and changes in the political climate?

The clean-up of nuclear and chemical wastes at the major nuclear weapons sites that are the responsibility of the United States Department of Energy (**DoE**) is a widely publicized illustration of the complex interactions of these eight policy factors (Office of Environmental Management 1995*a*,*b*). We briefly summarize key points and pose an important policy question under each category. Regarding **environmental health and safety** a great deal is known about the toxicological properties of radio-active materials. The high level radio-active wastes and radiological hot spots at the DoE's major sites in Colorado, Idaho, Tennessee, South Carolina, and Washington are clearly dangerous, and plumes of contaminated ground water are another concern. However, the public is buffered from these threats by engineering controls, security, and open space. A goal is to convert the most dangerous materials from liquid to solid forms so that they cannot migrate into the environment. A key policy question is whether every possible gram of radiological and chemical waste be removed even if that entails destroying natural ecological systems that have been undisturbed for decades.

The United States government has **legal requirements and a political system** that oblige it to prevent exposure to the legacy of 50 years of developing, manufacturing, and testing nuclear weapons. Only during the last decade has the security veil at these weapons sites been lifted to the point that other federal agencies, such as the EPA, tribal nations, and state governments, have a legal say in the clean-up and future uses of the sites. The DoE has signed legal agreements with the EPA and states that requires it to meet mandated clean-up objectives. In other words, it can no long act unilaterally. A key policy question is how much of a role other federal agencies, and especially state and local governments, should play in the future of the DoE sites.

Psychological studies show that the word 'nuclear' engenders great fear. **Stakeholders** do not want nuclear facilities, especially waste management facilities, near them. Highly publicized attempts to bury high-level waste in Yucca Mountain have been vehemently opposed by the government and the overwhelming majority of the residents of the State of Nevada. An important policy question is how responsive the federal government should be to these fears of human health effects and economic stigma when it makes location decisions.

The DoE has an environmental management budget of about $6 billion out of a total budget of $16 billion. This is the largest environmental management budget of any government agency in the world. Yet the **economic feasibility** of clean-up of sites to levels desired by the states and local governments is problematic because the DoE's budget is under considerable pressure by the United States Congress and Executive branch. About 70 per cent of the DoE environmental management budget is spent at the five sites in Colorado, Idaho, Tennessee, South Carolina, and Washington. The communities surrounding these sites depend on the DoE to support their economies. In other words, the **costs** are to United States taxpayers as a whole whereas the **benefits** are geographically concentrated in a few locations. How much influence should the economic impact of DoE expenditures have on how the DoE's funds should be spent?

The American government has a **moral obligation**, which is has acknowledged through the DoE, to remediate the nuclear waste sites. However, the issue is how much clean-up needs to occur. Economic analyses estimate costs ranging from $100 to $400 billion over 70 years. The lowest estimate translates into controlling dangerous materials, monitoring, and securing the sites. The most expensive approach requires the removal and/or destruction of nuclear materials and opening them up for public access. Should the American population as a whole commit hundreds of billions of dollars to remediate these sites back to levels that approach their precontamination levels?

Time pressure and **flexibility** are important policy drivers in the case of the DoE's major weapons sites. Some of the radio-active materials will be dangerous for thousands of years. These sites require long-term stewardship. While dangerous material decay, scientists will be developing new methods of destroying and controlling nuclear waste. Should the DoE delay clean-up of radio-active materials while waiting for new technological developments?

Overall, the management of the legacy of nuclear weapons production in the United States illustrates both the important role of toxicology and its complex interactions with other factors that play in policy formation.

Environmental health issues are increasingly international. The ability of humans to affect our planet has increased both because of the increase in our number and the increase in our power to interact with the environment. Many closely connected feedback loops have been demonstrated between our biosphere and our planet, including its atmosphere, climate, and oceans. Destruction of forests in one part of the world can have an impact on the climate for much of the rest of the planet. The loss of the protective effects of stratospheric ozone due to the use of CFC refrigerants is just one example of inadvertent effects of human activities that alter planetary systems so as to adversely affect human health. Our increasing interconnectedness in telecommunications, transportation, and trade also is having a profound impact, both for good and bad. We are now more able to recognize and communicate potential global problems, but we also appear more willing to wrap economic trade issues in the green flag of environmental protectionism. The precautionary principle is an excellent example of a valuable formulation of a principle that is basic to public health, yet is at risk of being distorted for economic and nationalistic purposes.

Developing countries are particularly at risk. In their rush to become modern producers, these countries make economic decisions to produce industrial products cheaply without instituting costly environmental safeguards. In addition, hazardous waste from developed countries may be more cheaply disposed of in developing countries, thus hazardous jobs and hazardous chemicals may be exported by developed countries to developing countries that have less stringent and less costly environmental regulations. Sea-level rise and severe climate events will have greater impact on poorer more densely populated areas without the resources to prevent or respond to the impacts. The lack of environmental health infrastructure and expertise also puts developing nations at risk; at times due to the inability to recognize the hidden threats of policies imposed upon them by the international community. A case in point is the horrific results of arsenic poisoning of village water supplies in Bangladesh in which simple tube wells, used to replace contaminated surface drinking water sources, in many cases tapped into groundwater that was heavily contaminated with arsenic.

Conclusion

Toxicology occupies an important niche between science and public policy. Its major contribution has been to provide tools to policy-makers and the public that have prevented what would have been substantially greater environmental degradation, including adverse human health impacts. As society changes due to new technology and to the challenge of sustainable development in the face of increased human population, the role of toxicology in enlightened public policy will become even more important. However, while toxicological information is critical to decision-making, it is not the sole determinant of policy, particularly when uncertainty exists.

References

Aldridge, W.N. (1986). The biological basis and measurement of thresholds. *Annual Review Pharmacology and Toxicology*, **26**, 39–58.

Amdur, M., Doull, J., and Klaasen, C. (ed.) (1991). *Toxicology* (4th edn). Pergamon Press, New York.

Ames, B., McCann, J., and Yamasaki, E. (1975). Methods for detecting carcinogens and mutagens with the *Salmonella*/mammalian microsome mutagenicity test. *Mutation Research*, **31**, 347–64.

Andrews, L.S., Lee, E.W., Witmer, C.M., Kocsis, J.J., and Snyder, R. (1977). Effects of toluene on the metabolism, disposition, and hemopoietic toxicity of ^{3}H benzene. *Biochemical Pharmacology*, **26**, 293–300.

Bailey, D.G., Arnold, J.M., and Spence, J.D. (1994). Grapefruit juice and drugs. How significant is the interaction? *Clinical Pharmacokinetics*, **26**, 91–8.

Carlisle, S. and Chechile, R. (ed.) (1991). *Environmental decision making: a multidisciplinary perspective.* Van Nostrand–Reinhold, New York.

Colborn, T., vom Saal, F.S., and Soto, A.M. (1993). Developmental effects of endocrine-disrupting chemicals in wildlife and humans. *Environmental Health Perspectives*, **101**, 378–84.

Frantz, S.W., Beatty, P.W., English, J.C., Hundley, S.G., and Wilson, A.G. (1994). The use of pharmacokinetics as an interpretive and predictive tool in chemical toxicology testing and risk assessment: a position paper on the appropriate use of pharmacokinetics in chemical toxicology. *Regulatory Toxicology and Pharmacology*, **19**, 317–37.

Gallo, M. and Doull, J. (1991). History and scope of toxicology. In *Toxicology* (4th edn) (ed. M.O. Amdur, J. Doull, and C.D. Klaasen), pp. 3–11. Pergamon Press, New York.

Gallo, M., Gochfeld, M., and Goldstein, B.D. (1987). Biomedical aspects of environmental toxicology. In *Toxic chemicals, health, and the environment* (ed. by L.B. Lave and A.C. Upton), pp. 170–204. Johns Hopkins University Press, Baltimore, MD.

Goldstein, B.D. (1990). The problem with the margin of safety: toward the concept of protection. *Risk Analysis*, **10**, 7–10.

Grandjean, P. (1995). Individual susceptibility in occupational and environmental toxicology. *Toxicology Letters*, **77**, 105–8.

Guengerich, F.P. and Liebler, D.C. (1985). Enzymatic activation of chemicals to toxic metabolites. *CRC Critical Reviews in Toxicology*, **14**, 259–307.

IARC (International Agency for Research on Cancer) (1992). *Monographs evaluating carcinogenic risk to humans*, Vol. 237. World Health Organization, Geneva.

Kato, R., Estabrook, R.W., and Cayen, M.N. (1989). *Xenobiotic metabolism and disposition.* Taylor and Francis, London.

McMichael, A. (1994). Global environmental change and human health: new challenges to scientist and policy-maker. *Journal of Public Health Policy*, **15**, 407–19.

National Research Council (1989). *Biological markers in reproductive toxicology*, p. 395, National Academy Press, Washington, DC.

National Research Council (1993). Use of the maximum tolerated dose in animal bioassays for carcinogenicity. In *Issues in risk assessment*, pp. 15–186. National Academy Press, Washington, DC.

Office of Environmental Management, US Department of Energy (1995*a*). *Closing the circle on splitting the atom.* Department of Energy, Washington, DC.

Office of Environmental Management, US Department of Energy (1995*b*). *Estimating the Cold War mortgage.* Department of Energy, Washington, DC.

Plaa, G. (1991). Toxic response of the liver. In *Toxicology* (ed. M.O. Amdur, J. Doull, and C.D. Klaasen), pp. 334–53. Pergamon Press, New York.

Plunkett, L.M., Turnbull, D., and Rodricks, J.V. (1992). Differences between adults and children affecting exposure assessment. In *Similarities and differences between children and adults, implications for risk assessment* (ed. P. Guzelian, C. Henry, and S. Olin), pp. 79–94. ILSI Press, Washington, DC.

Portney, P. (ed.) (1990). *Public policies for environmental protection.* Resources for the Future, Washington, DC.

Schuck, P. (1986). *Agent Orange on trial.* Harvard University Press, Cambridge, MA.

Selikoff, I.J., Hammond, E.C., and Churg, J. (1968). Asbestos exposure, smoking, and neoplasia. *Journal of the American Medical Association*, **204**, 106–12.

Snyder, R., Witz, G., and Goldstein, B.D. (1993). The toxicology of benzene. *Environmental Health Perspectives*, **100**, 293–306.

Umbreit, T., Hesse, E., and Gallo, M. (1986). Bioavailability of dioxin in soil from a 2,4,5-T manufacturing site. *Science*, **232**, 497–9.

8.3 Radiological sciences

Arthur C. Upton

Introduction

This chapter reviews the health effects of electromagnetic waves, including ionizing and non-ionizing radiations, accelerated atomic particles, high-intensity ultrasound, and electromagnetic fields. These various forms of energy differ from one another in their biological effects so that each is considered separately in the remarks that follow, beginning with a discussion of the effects of ionizing radiation.

Ionizing radiation

Nature, sources, and environmental levels

Ionizing radiations are those forms of radiation which can deposit enough localized energy in living cells to dislodge electrons from atoms. Such radiations include electromagnetic waves of extremely short wavelength (Fig. 1) and accelerated atomic particles (for example, electrons, protons, neutrons, α particles). Doses of ionizing radiation are measured in terms of energy deposition (Table 1).

Natural sources of ionizing radiation include cosmic rays, radium and other radio-active elements in the Earth's crust, internally deposited ^{40}K, ^{14}C, and other radionuclides present normally in living cells, and inhaled radon and its daughter elements (Table 2). The dose received from cosmic rays can differ appreciably from the value tabulated, depending on one's elevation; that is, it can be twice as high at a mountainous site (for example, Denver) as at sea level, and it is up to two orders of magnitude higher at jet aircraft altitudes (NCRP 1987). Likewise, the dose received from radium may be increased by a factor of 2 or more in regions where the underlying earth is rich in this element (NCRP 1987). In any case, however, the largest dose is usually that received by the bronchial epithelium from inhaled ^{222}Rn, a colourless odourless α-emitting gas formed by the radio-active decay of ^{226}Ra (Table 2); furthermore, depending on the concentration of

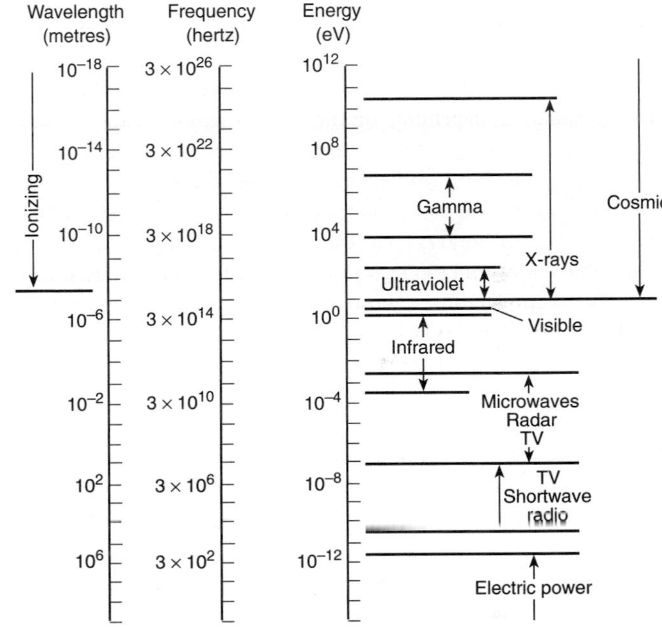

Fig. 1 The electromagnetic spectrum. (Source: Mettler and Upton 1994.)

Table 1 Quantities and dose units of ionizing radiation

Quantity dose	Unit	Definition
Absorbed dose	Gray (Gy)[a]	Energy deposited in tissue (1 J/kg)
Equivalent dose	Sievert (Sv)[b]	Absorbed dose weighted for the ion density (potency) of the radiation
Effective dose	Sievert (Sv)	Equivalent dose weighted for the sensitivity of the exposed organ(s)
Collective effective dose	Person-Sv	Effective dose applied to a population
Committed effective dose	Sievert (Sv)	Cumulative effective dose to be received from a given intake of radio-activity
Radio-activity	Becquerel (Bq)[c]	One disintegration per second

[a] Another unit used for the same purpose is the rad; 1 rad = 100 erg/g = 0.01 Gy.

[b] Another unit used for the same purpose is the rem; 1 rem = 0.01 Sv.

[c] Another unit used for the same purpose is the curie (Ci); 1 Ci = 3.7 × 1010 disintegrations/s = 3.7 × 1010 Bq.

radon in indoor air, the dose from radon and its decay daughters may vary by an order of magnitude or more (NCRP 1984). In cigarette smokers, moreover, even larger doses (up to 0.2 Sv (20 rem) per year) are received by the bronchial epithelium from the polonium (another α-emitting decay product of radium) that is normally present in tobacco smoke (NCRP 1984).

In addition to ionizing radiation from natural sources, people are exposed to radiation from artificial sources as well, the largest being the use of X-rays in medical diagnosis (Table 2). Lesser sources of exposure to manmade radiation include radio-active minerals (for example, ^{238}U, ^{232}Th, ^{40}K, ^{226}Ra) in building materials, phosphate fertilizers, and crushed rock; radiation-emitting components of TV sets, smoke detectors, and other consumer products; radio-active fallout from atomic weapons (for example, ^{137}Cs, ^{90}Sr, ^{89}Sr, ^{14}C, ^{3}H, ^{95}Zr); and nuclear power (for example, ^{3}H, ^{14}C, ^{85}Kr, ^{129}I, ^{137}Cs) (Table 2).

In various occupations, some workers receive additional doses of ionizing radiation, depending on their job assignments and working conditions. The average annual effective dose received occupationally by monitored radiation workers in the United States is less than that received from natural background, and in any given year less than 1 per cent of such workers receive a dose approaching the maximum permissible yearly limit (50 mSv (5 rem)) (NCRP 1989). Substantially larger occupational doses, however, are received by workers in less-developed countries, where adequate facilities, equipment, and safety measures are often lacking (UNSCEAR 1988).

Table 2 Average amounts of ionizing radiation received annually from different sources by a member of the United States population

Source	**Dose**[a]	
	Millisieverts	**Per cent**
Natural		
Radon[b]	2.0	55
Cosmic	0.27	8
Terrestrial	0.28	8
Internal	0.39	11
Total natural	2.94	82
Artificial		
X-ray diagnosis	0.39	11
Nuclear medicine	0.14	4
Consumer products	0.10	3
Occupational	< 0.01	< 0.3
Nuclear fuel cycle	< 0.01	< 0.03
Nuclear fallout	< 0.01	< 0.03
Miscellaneous[c]	< 0.01	< 0.03
Total artificial	0.63	18
Total natural and artificial	3.57	100

[a]Average effective dose to soft tissues.

[b]Average effective dose to bronchial epithelium alone.

[c]Department of Energy facilities, smelters, transportation, and so on.

Adapted from National Academy of Sciences (1990).

Nature and mechanisms of injury

As ionizing radiation penetrates living cells, it collides randomly with atoms and molecules in its path, giving rise to ions and free radicals, which break chemical bonds and cause other molecular alterations that may injure the cells. The spatial distribution of such events along the path of an impinging radiation depends on the energy, mass, and charge of the radiation; X-rays and γ-rays are sparsely ionizing in comparison with charged particles, which typically are densely ionizing.

Although any molecule in the cell may be altered by radiation, DNA is the most critical biological target because of the limited redundancy of the genetic information it contains. A dose of radiation large enough to kill the average dividing cell (2 Sv (200 rem)) causes hundreds of lesions in the cell's DNA molecules (Ward 1988). Most such lesions are reparable, but the complex lesions produced by a densely ionizing radiation (such as a proton or an α particle) are generally less reparable than those produced by a sparsely ionizing radiation (such as an X-ray or a γ-ray) (Goodhead 1988; Ward 1988). For this reason, the relative biological effectiveness of densely ionizing radiations is higher than that of sparsely ionizing radiations for most forms of injury (ICRP 1991).

Any damage to DNA that remains unrepaired or is misrepaired may be expressed in the form of mutations, the frequency of which approximates 10^{-5} to 10^{-6} per locus per sievert (NAS 1990). Because the mutation rate appears to increase as a linear non-threshold function of the dose, it is inferred that traversal of the DNA by a single ionizing particle may, in principle, suffice to cause a mutation (NAS 1990).

Also resulting from radiation damage to the genetic apparatus are changes in chromosome number and structure, the frequency of which increase with the dose in radiation workers and others exposed to ionizing radiation. So well characterized is the dose–response relationship that the frequency of chromosome aberrations in blood lymphocytes can serve as a useful biological dosimeter in radiation accident victims (IAEA 1986).

Radiation damage to genes, chromosomes, and other vital organelles may be lethal to affected cells, especially dividing cells, which are highly radiosensitive as a class (ICRP 1984). Measured in terms of proliferative capacity, the survival of dividing cells tends to decrease exponentially with increasing dose; 1 to 2 Sv (100 to 200 rem) generally suffices to reduce the surviving population by about 50 per cent (Fig. 2).

Although a dose below 0.5 Sv (50 rem) kills too few cells to cause clinically detectable injury in most organs other than those of the embryo, a larger dose may kill enough of the dividing progenitor cells in a tissue to interfere with the orderly replacement of its senescent cells, thereby causing the tissue to undergo atrophy (Fig. 3). The rapidity with which the atrophy ensues will depend in part on the cell population dynamics within the affected tissue; that is, in organs characterized by slow cell turnover, such as the liver and vascular endothelium, the process is typically much slower than in organs characterized by rapid cell turnover, such as the bone marrow, epidermis, and intestinal mucosa (ICRP 1984). In so far as the injury is dependent on the extent to which cell renewal in the exposed tissue is impaired, its severity tends to be reduced by the compensatory proliferation of surviving cells when only a small volume of tissue is

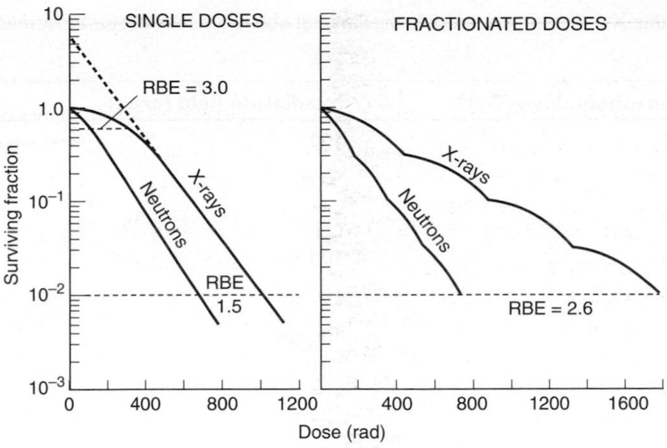

Fig. 2 Typical dose–survival curves for mammalian cells exposed to X-rays and fast neutrons. (From Hall 1988.)

irradiated or when the dose is accumulated gradually over an extended period of time.

Clinical manifestations of acute injury

After its discovery by Roentgen, in 1895, the X-ray was introduced into medical practice so rapidly that radiation injuries began to be encountered almost immediately. The first such injuries were predominantly acute skin reactions on the hands of those working with the early equipment, but within less than a decade many other types of injury also were observed, including the first cancers attributed to radiation (Upton 1986).

The acute effects of radiation encompass a wide variety of reactions (Mettler and Upton 1995), which vary markedly in dose–response relationships, clinical manifestations, timing, and prognosis (Table 3). Such reactions generally result from the severe depletion of progenitor cells in the affected tissues (Fig. 3) and are, consequently, elicited only by doses large enough to kill many such cells. Organs in which cells normally turn over rapidly tend to be the most radiosensitive and the first to exhibit injury. Such a reaction is not elicited unless the dose of radiation exceeds the substantial threshold needed to kill many cells and therefore such reactions are viewed as being non-stochastic (or deterministic) in nature (ICRP 1984); this is different to mutagenic and carcinogenic effects of radiation, which are viewed as stochastic phenomena resulting from random molecular alterations in individual cells that increase in frequency as linear non-threshold functions of the dose (NAS 1990; ICRP 1991).

Radiation injury of normal tissue within or adjoining the treatment field occurs to some degree in most radiotherapy patients, but few persons treated with today's methods experience severe or disabling radiation injuries. By the same token, modern safety practices have all but eliminated injuries from excessive occupational exposure such as were prevalent among early radiation workers. In spite of marked improvements in radiation protection, however, some 285 nuclear reactor accidents (excluding the Chernobyl accident) were reported in various countries between 1945 and 1987, causing more than 1350 persons to be irradiated, 33 of whom were injured fatally (Lushbaugh *et al.* 1987).

Although such accidents have become less frequent, they continue to be reported from time to time, the latest occurring in a processing plant near Tokyo on 30 September 1999, when a critical mass of enriched uranium was produced accidentally, releasing large amounts of radiation. Three workers were injured seriously as a result, and more than 60 others, including seven golfers on a neighbouring course, were exposed to high levels of radiation (Normile 1999). In most such accidents, however, unlike the Chernobyl accident (discussed below), the public was not affected directly.

The Chernobyl accident—the most serious reactor accident to date—released enough radio-activity to require tens of thousands of inhabitants to be evacuated from the surrounding area. This accident, occurring during a reactor test in April 1986, resulted from the improper withdrawal of control rods and inactivation of important safety systems (in violation of the operating rules) which caused the reactor to overheat, explode, and catch fire (UNSCEAR 1988).

The damage to the reactor core and control building allowed large quantities of radiation and radio-active materials to be released during the ensuing 10 days, resulting in radiation sickness and burns in more than 200 emergency personnel and firefighters, 31 of whom were injured fatally. Although the heaviest contamination occurred in the vicinity of the reactor itself and, to a lesser extent, in neighbouring countries of Eastern Europe, the population of the northern hemisphere as a whole is estimated to have received a collective dose commitment of 600 000 person-Sv (60 million person-rem), 70 per cent of which is attributed to ^{137}Cs, 20 per cent to ^{134}Cs, 6 per cent to ^{131}I, and the remainder to various shorter-lived radionuclides (UNSCEAR 1988). Those living in the vicinity of the reactor were given potassium iodide preparations to inhibit the thyroidal uptake of radio-iodine, but infants in a number of areas elsewhere in Eastern Europe are estimated to have received an average of more than 20 mSv (2 rem) to the thyroid gland, largely through ingestion of radio-iodine via cow's milk, and the prevalence of thyroid cancer in such persons has since risen dramatically in Belarus (Astakhova *et al.* 1998) and in the Ukraine (Tronko *et al.* 1999). Organs other than the thyroid typically received only a small fraction of the dose normally accumu-

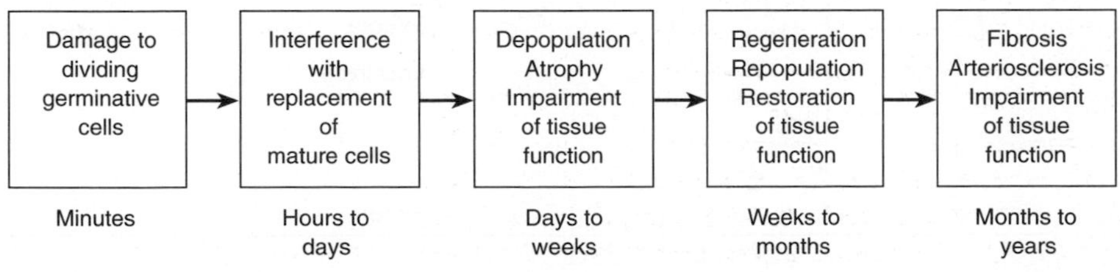

Fig. 3 Characteristic sequence of events in the pathogenesis of non-stochastic effects of ionizing radiation.

Table 3 Approximate threshold doses of conventionally fractionated therapeutic X-radiation for clinically detrimental non-stochastic effects in various tissues

Organ	Injury at 5 years	Threshold dose (Gy)[a]	Irradiation field (area)
Skin	Ulcer, severe fibrosis	55	100 cm^2
Oral mucosa	Ulcer, severe fibrosis	60	50 cm^2
Oesophagus	Ulcer, stricture	60	75 cm^2
Stomach	Ulcer, perforation	45	100 cm^2
Small intestine	Ulcer, stricture	45	100 cm^2
Colon	Ulcer, stricture	45	100 cm^2
Rectum	Ulcer, stricture	55	100 cm^2
Salivary glands	Xerostomia	50	50 cm^2
Liver	Liver failure, ascites	35	Whole
Kidney	Nephrosclerosis	23	Whole
Urinary bladder	Ulcer, contracture	60	Whole
Testes	Permanent sterility	5–15	Whole
Ovary	Permanent sterility	2–3	Whole
Uterus	Necrosis, perforation	$>$ 100	Whole
Vagina	Ulcer, fistula	90	5 cm
Breast, child	Hypoplasia	10	5 cm^2
Breast, adult	Atrophy, necrosis	$>$ 50	Whole
Lung	Pneumonitis, fibrosis	40	Lobe
Capillaries	Telangiectasis, fibrosis	50–60	–
Heart	Pericarditis, pancarditis	40	Whole
Bone, child	Arrested growth	20	10 cm^2
Bone, adult	Necrosis, fracture	60	10 cm^2
Cartilage, child	Arrested growth	10	Whole
Cartilage, adult	Necrosis	60	Whole
CNS (brain)	Necrosis	50	Whole
Spinal cord	Necrosis, transection	50	5 cm^2
Eye	Panophthalmitis, haemorrhage	55	Whole
Cornea	Keratitis	50	Whole
Lens	Cataract	5	Whole
Ear (inner)	Deafness	$>$ 60	Whole
Thyroid	Hypothyroidism	45	Whole
Adrenal	Hypoadrenalism	$>$ 60	Whole
Pituitary	Hypopituitarism	45	Whole
Muscle, child	Hypoplasia	20–30	Whole
Muscle, adult	Atrophy	$>$ 100	Whole
Bone marrow	Hypoplasia	2	Whole
Bone marrow	Hypoplasia, fibrosis	20	Localized
Lymph nodes	Atrophy	33–45	–
Lymphatics	Sclerosis	50	–
Fetus	Death	2	Whole

[a]Dose causing effect in 1 to 5 per cent of exposed persons.

Data from Rubin and Casarett (1972) and ICRP (1984).

lated each year from natural background radiation. In areas outside of Belarus, Russia, and the Ukraine, the highest average effective dose during the first year, received in Bulgaria, is estimated to have approximated 760 μSv, or slightly less than one-third of the average annual effective dose from natural sources (UNSCEAR 1988). Although the dose decreased rapidly with increasing distance from Chernobyl, the accident is estimated to have resulted in a collective dose commitment to the population of the northern hemisphere which is of the order of approximately 600 000 person-Sv (UNSCEAR 1988). Because of the small magnitude of the average dose to a given individual, however, the long-term health effects of the radiation cannot be predicted with certainty. Nevertheless, non-threshold risk models for carcinogenic effects (discussed below) imply that it may cause up to 30 000 additional cancer deaths during the next 70 years, although, with few exceptions, the number of additional cancers in any given country is likely to be too small to be detectable epidemiologically (USDOE 1987).

While less catastrophic than reactor accidents, accidents involving medical and industrial γ-ray sources have been far more numerous, and some have also caused severe injury and loss of life. For example, the improper disposal of a ^{137}Cs source in Goiania, Brazil, in 1987, resulted in the irradiation of dozens of unsuspecting victims, four of whom were injured fatally as a consequence (UNSCEAR 1993).

Although a comprehensive discussion of radiation injuries is beyond the scope of this review, prominent reactions of some of the more radiosensitive tissues are described briefly in the following.

Skin

Owing to the radiosensitivity of cells in the germinal layer of the epidermis, rapid exposure of the skin to a dose of 6 Sv or more produces erythema in the exposed area, which typically appears within a day after exposure, lasts a few hours, and is followed 2 to 4 weeks later by one or more waves of deeper and more prolonged erythema, as well as epilation. If the dose exceeds 10 to 20 Sv, blistering, necrosis, and ulceration may ensue within 2 to 4 weeks, followed by fibrosis of the underlying dermis and vasculature, which may lead to atrophy and a second wave of ulceration months or years later (ICRP 1984).

Bone marrow and lymphoid tissue

Lymphocytes are sufficiently radiosensitive that a dose of 2 to 3 Sv delivered rapidly to the whole body results in a marked depression of the lymphocyte count and immune response within hours (UNSCEAR 1988). Haemopoietic cells in the bone marrow are, likewise, killed in sufficient numbers by a comparable dose that causes profound leucopenia and thrombocytopenia, which develop within 3 to 5 weeks; after a larger dose, such changes may be severe enough to result in fatal infection and/or haemorrhage (Table 4).

Intestine

Stem cells in the epithelium lining the small bowel are also highly radiosensitive; an acute dose of 10 Sv can deplete their numbers sufficiently to cause the overlying intestinal villi to become denuded within days (ICRP 1984; UNSCEAR 1988). If a large enough area of the mucosa is affected, a fulminating and rapidly fatal dysentery-like syndrome results (Table 4).

Gonads

Although mature spermatozoa can survive large doses (> 100 Sv), spermatogonia are so radiosensitive that a dose as low as 0.15 Sv delivered rapidly to both testes will cause oligospermia, and a dose of 2 to 4 Sv will result in permanent sterility. Oocytes, likewise, are radiosensitive: a dose of 1.5 to 2.0 Sv delivered rapidly to both ovaries is sufficient to cause temporary sterility, and a larger dose will result in permanent sterility, depending on the age of the woman at the time of exposure (ICRP 1984).

Respiratory tract

The lung is not a highly radiosensitive organ, but alveolar cells and pulmonary vasculature can be injured sufficiently by rapid exposure to a dose of 6 to 10 Sv to cause acute pneumonitis to develop within the following 1 to 3 months. If a large volume of the lung is affected, the process may terminate in respiratory failure within the ensuing weeks, or in pulmonary fibrosis and cor pulmonale months or years later (ICRP 1984; UNSCEAR 1988).

Lens of the eye

Cells of the anterior epithelium of the lens continue to divide throughout life and are relatively radiosensitive. As a result, acute exposure of the lens to more than 1 Sv may be followed within months by the formation of a microscopic posterior polar opacity, and 2 to 3 Sv received in a single brief exposure (or 5.5 to 14 Sv accumulated over a period of months) may cause a vision-impairing cataract (ICRP 1984).

Other tissues

The tissues mentioned above are generally of higher radiosensitivity than others (Table 3). It is noteworthy, however, that the vulnerability of all tissues is increased when they are in a rapidly growing state (ICRP 1984).

Whole-body radiation injury

If a major part of the body is exposed rapidly to more than 1 Sv, the acute radiation syndrome may result. This syndrome is characterized by an initial prodromal stage involving malaise, anorexia, nausea, and vomiting, an ensuing asymptomatic latent period, a second (main) phase of illness, and finally either recovery or death (Table 4). The main phase of the illness typically takes one of the following four forms, depending on the predominant locus of radiation injury: haematological, gastrointestinal, cerebral, or pulmonary. Another syndrome, termed 'chronic radiation sickness', has been reported in chronically exposed workers of the Mayak nuclear facility and in persons residing down river from the facility who were exposed to radio-active effluents from the plant. The clinical findings in such persons, yet to be reported in other irradiated populations, include varying and persistent leucopenia, thrombocytopenia, arthralgia, asthenia, and various other ill-defined neurological complaints (Kossenko *et al.* 1994).

Localized radiation injury

In contrast to the clinical manifestations of acute whole-body radiation injury, which are often dramatic and prompt, the reaction to sharply localized irradiation, whether from an external radiation source or from an internally deposited radionuclide, tends to evolve slowly and to produce few symptoms unless the volume of tissue irradiated and/or the dose are relatively large (see Table 3).

In this connection, it is noteworthy that although some radio-nuclides (such as tritium, ^{14}C, and ^{137}Cs) tend to be distributed

Table 4 Major forms and features of the acute radiation syndrome

Time after irradiation	Cerebral form (> 50 Sv)	Gastrointestinal form (10–20 Sv)	Haemopoietic form (2–10 Sv)	Pulmonary form (> 6 Sv to lungs)
First day	Nausea Vomiting Diarrhoea Headache Disorientation Ataxia Coma Convulsions Death	Nausea Vomiting Diarrhoea	Nausea Vomiting Diarrhoea	Nausea Vomiting
Second week		Nausea Vomiting Diarrhoea Fever Erythema Prostration Death		
Third to sixth weeks			Weakness Fatigue Anorexia Fever Haemorrhage Epilation Recovery (?) Death (?)	
Second to eighth months				Cough Dyspnoea Fever Chest pain Respiratory failure (?)

systemically and to irradiate the whole body to varying degrees, others are characteristically taken up and concentrated in specific organs, producing injuries that are localized accordingly. Radium and ^{90}Sr, for example, are deposited predominantly in bone and injure skeletal tissues primarily, whereas radio-active iodine concentrates in the thyroid gland, which is the chief site of any resulting injury (Stannard 1988).

Carcinogenic effects

The carcinogenicity of ionizing radiation was first manifested early in the twentieth century by the occurrence of skin cancer and leukaemia in certain radiation workers. It has since been documented extensively by dose-dependent excesses of osteosarcomas and cranial sinus carcinomas in radium dial painters, carcinomas of the respiratory tract in underground hardrock miners, and cancers of many types in atomic bomb survivors, radiotherapy patients, and experimentally irradiated laboratory animals (Upton 1986).

The growths induced by irradiation characteristically take years or decades to appear and exhibit no known features distinguishing them from those induced by other causes. With few exceptions, moreover, their induction has been detectable only after relatively large doses (> 0.5 Sv (50 rem)) and has varied with the type of neoplasm as well as the age and sex of those exposed. In laboratory animals and cultured cells, the carcinogenic effects of radiation have been observed to include initiating effects, promoting effects, and effects on the progression of neoplasia, depending on the experimental conditions in question (NAS 1990). While the molecular mechanisms of these effects remain to be elucidated, the activation of oncogenes and/or the inactivation or loss of tumour suppressor genes appear to be implicated in many, if not all, instances (NAS 1990). The carcinogenic effects of radiation also resemble those of chemical carcinogens in being generally modifiable in similar ways by hormones, nutritional variables, and other modifying factors. In combination with chemical carcinogens the effects of radiation may be additive, synergistic, or mutually antagonistic, depending on the specific chemicals and exposure conditions in question (UNSCEAR 1982, 1986).

Because the existing data do not suffice to describe the dose–incidence relationship unambiguously for any type of neoplasm or to define how long after irradiation the risk of the growth may remain elevated in an exposed population, any risks attributable to low-level irradiation can be estimated only by extrapolation, based on models incorporating assumptions about the relevant parameters (NAS 1990; NCRP 1997).

Various dose–effect models have been used to estimate the risks of low-level irradiation, most of which involve the assumption that the overall risk of cancer increases in proportion with the dose at low dose levels; however, as the carcinogenic potency of X-rays and γ-rays in laboratory animals has been found to be reduced by as much as an order of magnitude when the exposure is prolonged, the risk to humans is generally estimated to increase less steeply with the dose at low doses and dose rates than at high doses and dose rates. Furthermore, as has been emphasized elsewhere (NAS 1990; NCRP 1997), the available data do not exclude the possibility that there may be a threshold in the millisievert dose range, below which the carcinogenicity of radiation is absent altogether. For this reason, the existing estimates cannot be used without caution to predict the risks of cancer that may be attributable to small doses or doses accumulated over weeks, months, or years. The aforementioned uncertainties notwithstanding, models applied to epidemiological data from the atomic bomb survivors and other irradiated populations have nevertheless yielded estimates of the lifetime risks of different forms of cancer that may be attributable to ionizing irradiation (Table 5). In interpreting the estimates, however, it should not be forgotten that they are based on population averages and hence cannot be assumed to apply equally to all individuals. Susceptibility to certain types of cancer (notably cancers of the thyroid and breast) is substantially higher in children than in adults, and susceptibility is also increased in association with certain hereditary disorders, such as retinoblastoma and the naevoid basal cell carcinoma syndrome (Sankaranarayanan and Chakraborty 1995). Although quantitative estimates are, therefore, limited by the aforementioned sources of uncertainty, they are nevertheless judged in some quarters to provide the only rational basis for assessing the extent to which a cancer that arises in a previously irradiated person is attributable to the dose of radiation in question (NIH 1985).

Studies to ascertain whether the rates of cancer and other diseases do, in fact, vary detectably with natural background radiation levels have been inconclusive thus far. A few studies have even suggested an inverse relationship, which has been interpreted by some observers as evidence for the existence of beneficial (or hormetic) effects of low-level irradiation (Luckey 1991); however, such a relationship has not usually persisted after controlling for the effects of confounding variables (NAS 1990; UNSCEAR 1994). That populations residing in areas of elevated natural background radiation have not exhibited significant increases in cancer rates (NAS 1990; UNSCEAR 1994) is

Table 5 Estimated lifetime risks of cancer attributable to 0.1 Sv rapid irradiation

Type or site of cancer	Excess cancer deaths per 100 000	
	Number	Percentage[a]
Stomach	110	18
Lung	85	3
Colon	85	5
Bone marrow (leukaemia)	50	10
Urinary bladder	30	5
Oesophagus	30	10
Breast	20	1
Liver	15	8
Gonads	10	2
Thyroid	8	8
Bone	5	5
Skin	2	2
Remainder	50	1
Total	500	2

[a]Percentage increase in 'background' expectation for a non-irradiated population.
Modified from ICRP (1991) and Puskin and Nelson (1995).

not unexpected, given the low levels of exposure in question; that is, the estimates tabulated above (Table 5) imply that no more than 3 per cent of all cancers in the general population are attributable to natural background radiation. On the other hand, although epidemiological studies of the effects of indoor radon have been inconclusive thus far, owing in part to uncertainties in dosimetry and difficulties in controlling for the influence of smoking and other confounding variables, the data imply that up to 10 per cent of lung cancers in the United States population may conceivably result from residential exposure to radon (NAS 1998). In view of the sizeable magnitude of the presumed risks, guidelines for limiting residential radon concentrations have been recommended in the United States and elsewhere (USEPA 1992).

In occupationally exposed workers, carcinogenic effects of irradiation are no longer readily demonstrable, thanks to modern radiation protection practices, although some cohorts of underground hardrock miners continue to exhibit excessive mortality from lung cancer (NAS 1998). In nuclear workers, likewise, analysis of the pooled data from several large cohorts suggests a dose-dependent excess of leukaemia in this population (Cardis *et al.* 1995) comparable in magnitude with the estimate tabulated above (Table 5). Multiple myeloma and other forms of cancer also have been reported to be increased in frequency in some cohorts of occupationally exposed workers, but such excesses have been observed only inconsistently and are of equivocal significance (Mettler and Upton 1995; NCRP 1997).

Among populations exposed to radio-active fallout, carcinogenic effects on the thyroid gland have been well documented in Marshall Islanders who received large doses to the thyroid in childhood and infancy (possibly up to 20 Gy (2000 rad)) from radio-active iodine, tellurium, and external γ-ray emitters in fallout released by a thermonuclear weapons test at Bikini Atoll in 1954 (Robbins and

Adams 1989). The incidence of thyroid cancer has also been observed to be increased in United States children who resided downwind from the Nevada nuclear weapons test site (Kerber *et al.* 1993) and in children living in areas of Belarus and the Ukraine that were contaminated by radionuclides released in the Chernobyl accident (Astakhova *et al.* 1998; Heidenreich *et al.* 1999).

The occurrence of clusters of leukaemia in children residing in the vicinity of nuclear plants in the United Kingdom has suggested the possibility that such cancers may have resulted from radio-activity released by the plants; however, the releases are estimated to have increased the total radiation dose to such populations by less than 2 per cent, so that other explanations are considered more likely (Doll *et al* 1994). The possibility that the leukaemias in question may have resulted from heritable oncogenic effects caused by occupational irradiation of the fathers of the affected children has also been suggested (Gardner *et al.* 1990); however, this hypothesis is generally discounted for reasons that are discussed below.

Heritable effects

Heritable effects of irradiation, although well documented in other organisms, have yet to be observed in humans. Thus, intensive study of the more than 76 000 children of Japanese atomic bomb survivors, carried out over four decades, has failed to disclose any heritable effects of radiation in this population, as measured by untoward pregnancy outcomes, neonatal deaths, malignancies, balanced chromosomal rearrangements, sex chromosome aneuploids, alterations of serum or erythrocyte protein phenotypes, changes in sex ratio, or disturbances in growth and development (NAS 1990). Estimates of the risks of heritable effects of radiation to future generations must, therefore, rely heavily on extrapolation from findings in laboratory animals.

From the available data, it is inferred that human germ cells are no more radiosensitive than those of the mouse and that the dose required to double the rate of heritable mutations in the human species must be at least 1.0 Sv (NAS 1990). Hence, on the basis of the existing evidence, it is estimated that fewer than 1 per cent of all genetically determined diseases in the human population are attributable to natural background irradiation (Table 6).

The possibility that an excess of leukaemia and non-Hodgkin's lymphoma in young people residing in the village of Seascale, in northern England, was caused by the occupational irradiation of their fathers who worked at the Sellafield nuclear installation, has been suggested by a case–control study (Gardner *et al.* 1990), as noted above. Conflicting with this interpretation, however, are (a) the lack of any comparable excess in larger numbers of children born outside Seascale to fathers who had received similar, or even larger, occupational doses at the same nuclear plant (Wakeford *et al.* 1994*a*), (b) the lack of similar excesses in French (Hill and LaPlanche 1990), Canadian (McLaughlin *et al.* 1993), or Scottish (Kinlen *et al.* 1993) children born to fathers with comparable occupational exposures, (c) the lack of excesses in the children of atomic bomb survivors (Yoshomoto *et al.* 1990), (d) the lack of excesses in United States counties containing nuclear plants (Jablon *et al.* 1991), (e) the fact that the frequency of radiation-induced mutations implied by the interpretation is far higher than established rates (Wakeford *et al.* 1994*b*), and (f) evidence that the mutations causing childhood leukaemia are of a severity likely to interfere with the viability of affected germ cells (Evans 1990). On balance, therefore, the available data fail to support the paternal gonadal irradiation hypothesis (Doll *et al.* 1994). Although interpretation of the observed clusters is complicated by various sources of uncertainty (Ross *et al.* 1999), the possibility of an infectious aetiology for them has been suggested by the occurrence of comparable excesses of childhood leukaemia at other places in the United Kingdom that have experienced similar large influxes of population (Kinlen 1988). By the same token, there is insufficient evidence to conclude that radiation from the Chernobyl accident or other sources is responsible for creating the clusters of childhood leukaemia that have been observed (Alexander and Greaves 1999).

Table 6 Estimated frequencies of heritable disorders attributable to natural background ionizing irradiation[a]

Type of disorder	Prevalence	Contribution from natural background (per million live births)[a]	
		First generation	Radiation equilibrium[b]
Autosomal dominant	180 000	20–100	300
X-linked	400	< 1	< 15
Recessive	2500	< 1	Very slow increase
Chromosomal	4400	< 20	Very slow increase
Congenital defects	20 000–30 000	30	30–300
Other disorders of complex aetiology			
Heart disease	600 000	Not estimated[c]	Not estimated[c]
Cancer	300 000	Not estimated[c]	Not estimated[c]
Selected others	300 000	Not estimated[c]	Not estimated[c]

[a]Values rounded.

[b]Equivalent to ~1 mSv/year, or ~30 mSv/generation (30 years).

[c]Quantitative risk estimates lacking because of uncertainty about the mutational component of the disease(s) indicated.

Based on NAS (1990).

Effects of prenatal irradiation

Throughout prenatal life, radiosensitivity is relatively high, but the effects of a given dose vary markedly depending on the developmental stage of the embryo or fetus at the time of exposure. During the pre-implantation period, the embryo is maximally susceptible to killing by irradiation. Subsequently, during critical stages in organogenesis, it is susceptible to the induction of malformations and other disturbances of development (UNSCEAR 1986), as exemplified by the dose-dependent increase in frequency of mental retardation and the dose-dependent decrease in IQ test scores occurring in atomic bomb survivors who were irradiated between the 8th and 15th weeks (and, to a lesser extent, between the 16th and 25th weeks) after conception (UNSCEAR 1986; NAS 1990).

Susceptibility to the carcinogenic effects of radiation also appears to be relatively high throughout the prenatal period, judging from the association between childhood cancer (including leukaemia) and prenatal exposure to diagnostic X-irradiation (NAS 1990; Doll and Wakeford 1997). This association, although yet to be established as causal in nature, has been observed consistently in many case–control studies and is equally strong in twins (NAS 1990; Doll and Wakeford 1997).

While no excess of childhood cancer has been recorded in prenatally irradiated A-bomb survivors, their numbers were relatively small (Yoshimoto *et al.* 1990). Hence the results of the various case–control studies are interpreted to imply that prenatal irradiation causes a 40 per cent per sievert increase in the risk of leukaemia and other cancers during childhood (UNSCEAR 1988; NAS 1990; Doll and Wakeford 1997).

Prevention

In order to minimize the risks of injury from ionizing radiation, the following principles are recommended as guidelines to be observed in any activities involving exposure to this agent (ICRP 1991): (a) no such activity should be considered justifiable unless it produces a sufficient benefit to those who are exposed, or to society at large, to offset any harm it may cause; (b) in any such activity, the dose and/or likelihood of exposure should be kept as low as is reasonably achievable, all relevant economic and social factors being taken into account; (c) the radiation exposure of individuals resulting from any combination of such activities should be subject to dose limits (Table 7) that are far enough below the thresholds for non-stochastic effects to prevent such effects altogether, and that are also low enough to keep the risks of any resulting stochastic effects (which may have no thresholds) from exceeding socially acceptable levels.

Implicit in these guidelines are the requirements that any facility dealing with ionizing radiation is properly designed, carefully plans and oversees its operating procedures, has in place a well-conceived radiation protection programme, ensures that its workers are adequately trained and supervised, and maintains a well-developed and well-rehearsed emergency preparedness plan, in order to be able to respond promptly and effectively in the event of a malfunction, spill, or other type of radiation accident (Shapiro 1990).

As medical radiographic examinations and indoor radon constitute the most important controllable sources of exposure to ionizing radiation for members of the general public (Table 1), prudent measures to limit irradiation from these sources also are warranted (Upton *et al.* 1990). Other potential risks to human health and the environment calling for increased attention are the millions of cubic feet of radio-active and mixed wastes (mine and mill tailings, spent nuclear fuel, waste from the decommissioning of nuclear power plants, dismantled industrial and medical radiation sources, radioactive pharmaceuticals and reagents, heavy metals, polyaromatic hydrocarbons, and other contaminants) which are present in ever-growing quantities and severely tax existing storage capacities at numerous sites (USDOE 1993). Also, as noted above, there is a widespread and urgent need in less-developed countries for more adequate safeguards to protect occupationally exposed workers and members of the public against excessive exposure to radiation (UNSCEAR 1988).

Table 7 Recommended effective dose limits of ionizing radiation for occupationally exposed workers and members of the public

Occupational exposure[a]	
Annual	50 mSv
Cumulative	age × 10 mSv
Public exposure[a]	
Annual, continuous	1 mSv
Annual, infrequent	5 mSv

[a]Excluding medical and dental exposures.

Data from NCRP (1993).

Non-ionizing radiation

Ultraviolet radiation

Nature, sources, and environmental levels

Ultraviolet radiations (**UVR**) comprise a spectrum (Fig. 1) of electromagnetic waves, subdivided for convenience into three bands: (a) UVA, 400 to 320 nm ('black light'); (b) UVB, 320 to 280 nm; (c) UVC, 280 to 100 nm (which is germicidal). The chief source of UVR for members of the public is sunlight, which varies in intensity with latitude, elevation, and season (AMA 1989). Important manmade sources of high-intensity exposure include sun/tanning lamps, welding arcs, plasma torches, germicidal and black-light lamps, electric arc furnaces, hot-metal operations, mercury vapour lamps, and lasers. Common low-intensity sources include fluorescent lamps and certain laboratory equipment (NIOSH 1972).

Nature and mechanisms of injury

As UVR does not penetrate deeply into human tissues, the injuries it causes are confined chiefly to the skin and eyes. Reactions of the skin to UVR, which are common among fair-skinned people, include sunburn, skin cancers (basal cell and squamous cell carcinomas, and to a lesser extent melanomas), ageing of the skin, solar elastoses, and solar keratoses (English *et al.* 1997). Injuries of the eye include photokeratitis, which may result from brief exposure to a high-intensity UVR source ('welder's flash') or from more prolonged exposure to intense sunlight ('snow blindness'), cortical cataract, and pterygium (Lerman 1988).

The effects of UVR result chiefly from its absorption in DNA with the production of pyrimidine dimers, causing mutational changes in exposed cells. Sensitivity to UVR may be increased by DNA repair defects (for example, xeroderma pigmentosum), by agents (such as caffeine) that inhibit the repair enzymes, and by photosensitizing agents (such as psoralens, sulphonamides, tetracyclines, nalidixic acid, sulphonylureas, thiazides, phenothiazines, furocumarins, and coal tar) which produce UVR-absorbing DNA photoproducts (Harper and Bickers 1989). The carcinogenic action of UVR is mediated primarily through direct effects on the exposed cells, but may involve depression of local immunity as well (Kripke 1988). UVB, although far less intense than UVA in sunlight, plays a more important part in sunburn and skin carcinogenesis (English *et al.* 1997); UVA also, however, contributes to the latter, as well as to tanning, some photosensitivity reactions, ageing of the skin, photokeratitis, and cortical lens opacities (AMA 1989).

Prevention

Excessive exposure to sunlight or other sources of UVR should be avoided, especially by fair-skinned individuals. In addition, protective clothing, UVR screening lotions or creams, and UVR blocking sunglasses should be used for the purpose when necessary. To protect occupationally exposed workers, it is recommended that exposure be limited to 1.0 mW/cm^2 for periods longer than 1000 s and 1000 mW/cm^2 (1.0 J/cm^2) for periods of 1000 s or less (NIOSH 1972; ACGIH 1997).

From an environmental perspective, it is noteworthy that the protective layer of ozone in the stratosphere is being depleted by chlorofluorocarbons and other air pollutants (Rex *et al.* 1997), and that every 1 per cent decrease in ozone is expected to increase the UVR reaching the earth by 1 to 2 per cent, thereby increasing the rates of non-melanotic skin cancer by 2 to 6 per cent (Henriksen *et al.* 1990). The increase in cancer rates is, of course, only one of the adverse effects to be expected; the most serious, perhaps, is the far-reaching impact of increased UVR on vegetation and crop production (Worrest and Grant 1989).

Visible light

Nature, sources, and environmental levels

Visible light consists of electromagnetic waves varying in wavelength from 380 nm (violet) to 760 nm (red) (Fig. 1). Sources of visible light in the environment vary widely in the intensity of their emissions; common high-intensity sources other than the Sun include lasers, electric welding or carbon arcs, and tungsten filament lamps.

Nature and mechanisms of injury

Too bright a light can injure the eye through photochemical reactions in the retina; that is, sustained exposure to intensities exceeding 0.1 mW/cm^2, such as can result from fixating a bright source of light, may produce photochemical blue-light injury, and brief exposure of the retina to intensities exceeding 10 W/cm^2, depending on image size, may cause a retinal burn (Sliney and Wolbarsht 1980). The lens, iris, cornea, and skin also are vulnerable to injury from the thermal effects of laser radiation (Sliney and Wolbarsht 1980). Conversely, too little illumination can also be harmful, causing eyestrain (Huer 1983) and/or seasonal affective disorder (Rosenthal *et al.* 1988).

Prevention

As bright continuously visible light normally elicits an aversion response, which acts to protect the eye against injury, few sources of light are large and bright enough to cause a retinal burn under normal viewing conditions. One must never look directly at a solar eclipse, and in situations involving potential exposure to such high-intensity sources as carbon arcs or lasers, appropriate training, proper design of equipment, and protective eye shields are indicated (Sliney and Wolbarsht 1980; ANSI 1986; ACGIH 1997).

Infrared radiation

Nature, sources, and environmental levels

Infrared radiation (**IR**) consists of electromagnetic waves ranging in wavelength from 7×10^{-5} m to 3×10^{-2} m (Fig. 1). Some such radiation is emitted by all objects with temperatures above absolute zero, but potentially hazardous sources of IR include furnaces, ovens, welding arcs, molten glass, molten metal, and heating lamps.

Nature and mechanisms of injury

The injuries caused by IR are limited chiefly to burns of the skin and cataracts of the lens of the eye. The warning sensation of heat usually prompts aversion in time to prevent the skin from being burned by IR; however, the lens of the eye is vulnerable in lacking both heat-sensing and heat-dissipating ability. As a result, glass blowers, blacksmiths, oven operators, and those working around heating and drying lamps are at risk of IR-induced cataracts (Lydahl 1984).

Prevention

Control of IR hazards requires appropriate shielding of sources, proper training and supervision of potentially exposed persons, and use of protective clothing and goggles. It is also recommended that exposures to IR not exceed 10 mW/cm^2 (ACGIH 1997).

Microwave radiation

Nature, sources, and environmental levels

Microwave and radiofrequency radiation (**MW/RFR**) consists of electromagnetic waves ranging in frequency from about 3 kHz to 300 GHz (Fig. 1). Sources of MW/RFR occur widely in radar, television, radio, cellular phones, and other telecommunications systems, and are also used in various industrial operations (for example, heating, welding, and melting of metals, processing of wood and plastic, high-temperature plasma), household appliances (such as microwave ovens), and medical applications (for example, diathermy and hyperthermy) (ILO 1986).

Nature and mechanisms of injury

The biological effects of MW/RFR have traditionally been regarded as primarily thermal in nature. MW/RFR-induced burns of the skin and other tissues have occasionally resulted from faulty or improperly used household microwave ovens and from the overexposure of patients in whom cutaneous pain and temperature senses that usually warn of impending injury are impaired. Because of the deep penetration of MW/RFR, the cutaneous burns it causes tend to involve dermal and subcutaneous tissues, which heal slowly. Cataracts of the lens of the eye also have been reported to result from high-intensity exposures (> 1.5 kW/m^2) (McRee 1972; Lipman *et al.* 1988), and death from hyperthermia has been encountered in the industrial use of MW/RFR sources (McLaughlin 1957; Roberts and Michaelson 1985). Also well documented is the ability of MW/RFR to interfere with cardiac pacemakers and other medical devices (NCRP 1986).

Although the biological effects of MW/RFR have been attributed primarily to thermal mechanisms in the past, there is growing evidence suggesting the possibility that MW/RFR may elicit some types of effects through non-thermal mechanisms as well. Such effects, which are yet to be documented conclusively, include damage to DNA, impairment of fertility, developmental disturbances, neurobehavioural abnormalities, depression of immunity, stimulation of cell proliferation, and carcinogenic effects in model systems and in humans (NCRP 1986; Tenforde 1998; Elwood 1999; Moulder *et al.* 1999).

Prevention

Proper design and shielding of MW/RFR sources, along with appropriate training and supervision of potentially exposed persons (especially those wearing cardiac pacemakers or other sensitive devices), are indicated. Exposure to MW/RFR power densities exceeding the threshold limit values tabulated (Table 8) may cause detectable heating of tissue and should be avoided (NCRP 1986; ILO 1986; ANSI 1992; ACGIH 1997; ICNIRP 1998).

Extremely low-frequency electromagnetic fields

Nature, sources, and environmental levels

Extremely low-frequency electromagnetic fields (**EMFs**)—that is, time-varying magnetic fields with frequencies below 300 Hz—are present throughout the environment. The largest such fields arise intermittently from solar activity and thunderstorms, during which they may reach intensities on the order of 0.5 T. Far stronger than such naturally occurring EMFs are the localized 50- to 60-Hz fields that are generated by electric power lines, transformers, motors, household appliances, video display tubes (**VDTs**), and various medical devices, notably magnetic resonance imaging (**MRI**) systems (OTA 1989; Tenforde 1992).

For example, the flux density on the ground beneath a 765-kV, 60-Hz power line carrying 1 kA per phase is of the order of 15 T, and close to common household appliances the flux density may range up to 2.5 mT (Tenforde 1992). As the strength of such fields decreases rapidly with distance, however, the average ambient value in the home environment is less than 0.3 T (3 mG). By the same token, while flux densities at video display terminals typically range up to 5 T, those at the location of the operator are generally less than 1 T (Tenforde 1992).

Nature and mechanisms of injury

Extremely low-frequency EMFs induce electrical currents that can alter the properties of cell membranes and exert effects on electrically active tissues (nerves, neuromusculature, retina, heart) and on cardiac pacemakers. Induced current densities under 1 to 10 mA/m^2 produce few, if any, irreversible effects, which is not surprising as similar current densities exist endogenously in many tissues. Induced current densities above 10 mA/m^2, on the other hand, although not genotoxic, reportedly produce various changes in the biochemistry and physiology of cells and tissues (for example, alterations in metabolism, growth rate, melatonin secretion, endocrine activity, and immune response), and current densities above 1 A can cause neural excitation and irreversible effects, such as cardiac fibrillation (Tenforde 1992, 1998).

In addition to the effects produced by strong EMFs, epidemiological data have suggested the possibility of severe effects from long-continued exposure to weaker EMFs; that is, that the risks of leukaemia may be increased by residential exposure to household EMFs in children, that the risks of brain cancer and leukaemia may be increased by occupational exposure to EMFs in utility workers, and that the risks of reproductive disorders may be increased by chronic exposure to EMFs through the operation of VDTs in pregnant women (Bates 1991; Tenforde 1992, 1996; NAS 1996). As yet, however, such epidemiological data are inconclusive, and their interpretation is complicated by uncertainties in exposure assessment and by the lack of established biological mechanisms for the effects in question (NAS 1996; Tenforde 1998). Nevertheless, the fact that such fields have been reported to influence ion transport, melatonin secretion, and tumour promotion in some model systems (Tenforde 1992, 1998) has reinforced public health concern (OTA 1989; NAS 1996).

Prevention

Areas containing EMFs stronger than 0.5 mT, such as exist around transformers, accelerators, MRI systems, and other electric devices, should be posted with warning signs and should be avoided by persons wearing pacemakers. In addition, it is recommended that the strength of any 60-Hz time-varying magnetic field, such as typically exists around an MRI system, should be limited to 1 mT for occupational exposures and to 0.1 mT for those wearing cardiac pacemakers or for continuous exposures involving members of the general public (ACGIH 1997). To minimize the risks, if any, that may be associated with the use of electric blankets, wiring design changes have been

Table 8 Threshold limit values for radiofrequency/microwave radiation

Frequency	Power density[a] (mW/cm^2)	Electric field strength squared[a] (V^2/m^2)	Magnetic field strength squared[a] (A^2/m^2)
30 kHz–3 MHz	100	377 000	2.65
3–30 MHz	$900/f^2$	3770 ($900/f^2$)	900 ($37.7 \times f^2$)
30–100 MHz	1	3770	0.027
100–1000 MHz	$f/100$	3770 ($f/100$)	f (37.7×100)
1–300 GHz	10	37 700	0.265

[a] f denotes frequency in MHz.

Source: ACGIH (1997).

introduced by some manufacturers to cancel the surface 60-Hz EMFs that such blankets would otherwise generate (Tenforde 1992, 1996).

Ultrasound

Nature, sources, and environmental levels

Although often classified for public health purposes with non-ionizing radiation, ultrasound is not a component of the electromagnetic spectrum but actually consists of mechanical vibrations at frequencies above the audible range (that is, above 16 kHz) (NCRP 1983). Sources of high-power low-frequency ultrasound are used widely in science and industry for cleaning, degreasing, plastic welding, liquid extracting, atomizing, homogenizing, and emulsifying operations, as well as in medicine for lithotripsy and other applications. Low-power high-frequency ultrasound is used widely in analytical work and in medical diagnosis (such as ultrasonography).

Nature and mechanisms of injury

The biological effects of ultrasound are similar in mechanism to those of mechanical vibration. High-power low-frequency ultrasound, transmitted through the air or through bodily contact with the generating source, has been observed to cause a variety of effects in occupationally exposed workers, including headache, earache, tinnitus, vertigo, malaise, photophobia, hypercusia, peripheral neuritis, and autonomic polyneuritis. The possibility that it may cause adverse effects on the embryo also has been suggested (NCRP 1983).

Although excessive exposure to high-frequency ultrasound through bodily contact with the source may be expected, in principle, to cause complaints similar to those above, no adverse effects have been observed to result from exposure to high-frequency ultrasound at the low power levels used in medical ultrasonography (NCRP 1983).

Prevention

Protection against injury by ultrasound requires appropriate isolation and insulation of generating sources, as well as proper training and ear protective devices for those working around such sources. Yearly audiometric and neurological examinations of occupationally exposed workers also are recommended (WHO 1982).

Summary and conclusions

The adverse effects on human health caused by different forms of radiant energy are diverse, ranging from rapidly fatal injuries to cancers, birth defects, and hereditary disorders appearing months, years, or decades after exposure. The nature, frequency, and severity of effects depend on the type of radiant energy in question and the particular conditions of exposure. Most such effects are produced only by appreciable levels of exposure and can, therefore, be prevented by keeping any exposure from exceeding relevant thresholds. The genotoxic and carcinogenic effects of ionizing and UVR, in contrast, are presumed to increase in frequency as linear non threshold functions of the dose and therefore not to be entirely preventable without eliminating all exposures to these forms of radiation. As it is not feasible to eliminate exposure to these two forms of radiation completely, protection against their mutagenic and carcinogenic effects requires that exposures to these agents be limited sufficiently to keep any associated risks from exceeding acceptable levels.

To achieve the desired level of protection against each of the different forms of radiation requires knowledge of the relevant exposure–risk relationships, appropriate design and operation of all radiation sources, proper training and supervision of operating personnel, and education of the public in prudent measures for safeguarding health.

These requirements can be met satisfactorily in most situations involving radiation hazards, given the necessary commitment of effort and resources. Unresolved public health problems calling for particular attention at this time, however, include (a) assessment of the risks associated with residential exposure to indoor radon, and of the pertinent remediation strategies, (b) development and implementation of measures for dealing with the hazards posed by the large and growing quantities of radio-active and mixed wastes, (c) assessment of the risks that may be associated with exposure to 60 Hz electromagnetic fields, and (d) further evaluation of atmospheric ozone depletion and its implications for UVR-induced impacts on human health.

References

ACGIH (American Conference of Governmental Industrial Hygienists) (1997). *Threshold limit values and biological exposure indices.* ACGIH, Cincinnati.

Alexander, F.E. and Greaves, M.F. (1999). Ionising radiation and leukaemia potential risks: review based on the workshop held during the 10th Symposium on Molecular Biology of Hematopoiesis and Treatment of Leukemia and Lymphomas at Hamburg, Germany on July 5, 1997. *Leukemia*, **13**, 495–7.

AMA Council on Scientific Affairs (1989). Harmful effects of ultraviolet radiation. *Journal of the American Medical Association*, **262**, 380–4.

ANSI (American National Standards Institute) (1986). *Safe use of lasers.* ANSI, New York.

ANSI (American National Standards Institute) (1992). *IEEE standard for safety levels with respect to human exposure to radiofrequency electromagnetic fields, 3 kHz to 300 GHz (C95.1–1992).* ANSI, New York.

Astakhova, L.N., *et al.* (1998). Chernobyl-related thyroid cancer in children of Belarus: a case–control study. *Radiation Research*, **150**, 340–56.

Bates, M.N. (1991). Extremely low frequency electromagnetic fields and cancer. The epidemiologic evidence. *Environmental Health Perspectives*, **95**, 147–56.

Cardis, E., *et al.* (1995). Effects of low doses and low dose rates of external ionizing radiation: Cancer mortality among nuclear industry workers in three countries. *Radiation Research*, **142**, 117–32.

Doll, R. and Wakeford, R. (1997). Risk of childhood cancer from fetal irradiation. *British Journal of Radiology*, **70**, 130–9.

Doll, R., Evans, N.J., and Darby, S.C. (1994). Paternal exposure not to blame. *Nature*, **367**, 678–80.

Elwood, J.M. (1999). A critical review of epidemiologic studies of radiofrequency exposure and human cancers. *Environmental Health Perspectives*, **107** (Supplement 1), 155–68.

English, D.R., Armstrong, B.K., Kricker, A., and Fleming, C. (1997). Sunlight and cancer. *Cancer Causes and Control*, **8**, 271–83.

Evans, H.J. (1990). Ionizing radiation from nuclear establishments and childhood leukemia—an enigma. *Bioessays*, **12**, 541–9.

Gardner, M.J., Hall, A., Snee, M.P., Downes, S., Powell, C.A., and Terell, J.D. (1990). Results of case–control study of leukaemia and lymphoma among young people near Sellafield nuclear plant in West Cumbria. *British Medical Journal*, **300**, 423–9.

Goodhead, D.J. (1988). Spatial and temporal distribution of energy. *Health Physics*, **55**, 231–40.

Hall, E.J. (1988). *Radiobiology for the radiologist* (3rd edn). J.B. Lippincott, Philadelphia, PA.

Harper, L.C. and Bickers, D.R. (1989). *Photosensitivity diseases. principles of diagnosis and treatment* (2nd edn). B.C. Decker, Toronto.

Heidenreich, W.F., *et al.* (1999). Time trends of thyroid cancer incidence in Belarus after the Chernobyl accident. *Radiation Research*, **181**, 617–25.

Henriksen, T., Dahlback, A., Larsen, S., and Moan, J. (1990). Ultraviolet radiation and skin cancer. Effect of an ozone layer depletion. *Photochemistry and Photobiology*, **51**, 579–82.

Hill, C. and Laplanche, A. (1990). Overall mortality and cancer mortality around French nuclear sites. *Nature*, **347**, 755–7.

Huer, H.H. (1983). Lighting. In *Encyclopedia of occupational health and safety* (ed. L. Parmeggiana), pp. 1225–31. International Labour Office, Geneva.

IAEA (International Atomic Energy Agency) (1986). *Biological dosimetry: chromosomal aberration analysis for dose assessment.* Technical Report No. 260. IAEA, Vienna.

ICNIRP (International Commission on Non-Ionizing Radiation Protection) (1998). Guidelines for limiting exposure to time-varying electric, magnetic, and electromagnetic fields (up to 300 GHz). *Health Physics*, **74**, 494–522.

ICRP (International Commission on Radiological Protection) (1984). Nonstochastic effects of ionizing radiation. ICRP Publication 41. *Annals of the ICRP*, **14**, 1–33.

ICRP (International Commission on Radiological Protection) (1991). 1990 Recommendations of the ICRP. ICRP Publication 60. *Annals of the ICRP*, **21**, 1–3.

ILO (International Labour Office) (1986). *Protection of workers against radiofrequency and microwave radiation: a technical review.* Occupational Safety and Health Series Report No. 57. International Labour Office, Geneva.

Jablon, S., Hrubec, Z., and Boice, J.D., Jr (1991). Cancer in populations living near nuclear facilities. A survey of mortality nationwide and incidence in two areas. *Journal of the American Medical Association*, **265**, 1403–8.

Kerber, R.A., *et al.* (1993). A cohort study of thyroid disease in relation to fallout from nuclear weapons testing. *Journal of the American Medical Association*, **270**, 2076–82.

Kinlen, L.J. (1988). Evidence for an infective cause of childhood leukaemia: comparison of a Scottish New Town with nuclear reprocessing sites in Britain. *Lancet*, **ii**, 1323–7.

Kinlen, L.J., Clarke, K., and Balkwill, A. (1993). Paternal preconceptional radiation exposure in the nuclear industry and leukaemia and non-Hodgkin's lymphoma in young people in Scotland. *British Medical Journal*, **306**, 1153–8.

Kossenko, M.M., Akleyev, A.A., Degteva, M.O., Kosheurov, V.P., and Degtyaryova, R.G. (1994). *Analysis of chronic radiation sickness in the population of the southern Urals.* AFFRI Contract Report 94–1. Armed Forces Radiobiological Research Institute, Springfield, VA.

Kripke, M.L. (1988). Impact of ozone depletion on skin cancers. *Journal of Dermatology and Surgical Oncology*, **14**, 853–7.

Lerman, S. (1988). Ocular phototoxicity (editorial). *New England Journal of Medicine*, **319**, 1475–7.

Lipman, R.M., Tripathi, B.J., and Tripathi, R.C. (1988). Cataracts induced by microwave and ionizing radiation. *Survey of Ophthalmology*, **33**, 200–10.

Luckey, T.D. (1991). *Radiation hormesis.* CRC Press, Boca Raton, FL.

Lushbaugh, C.C., Fry, S.A., and Ricks, R.C. (1987). Nuclear reactor accidents: preparedness and consequences. *British Journal of Radiology*, **60**, 1159–83.

Lydahl, E. (1984). Infrared radiation and cataract. *Acta Ophthalmologica*, **166** (Supplement), 1–63.

McLaughlin, J.R., Clarke, E.A., Nishri, D., and Anderson, T.W. (1993). Childhood leukemia in the vicinity of Canadian nuclear facilities. *Cancer Causes and Control*, **4**, 51–8.

McLaughlin, J.T. (1957). Tissue destruction and death from microwave radiation (radar). *California Medicine*, **86**, 336.

McRee, D.I. (1972). Environmental aspects of microwave radiation. *Environmental Health Perspectives*, **2**, 41–53.

Mettler, F.A. and Upton, A.C. (1995). *Medical effects of ionizing radiation.* Grune and Stratton, New York.

Moulder, J.E., Erdrich, L.S., Malyapa, R.S., Merritt, J., Pickard, W.F., and Vijayalaxmi (1999). Cell phones and cancer. What is the evidence for a connection? *Radiation Research*, **151**, 513–31.

NAS (National Academy of Sciences/National Research Council) (1990). *Health effects of exposure to low levels of ionizing radiation* (BEIR V). National Academy Press, Washington, DC.

NAS (National Academy of Sciences/National Research Council) (1996). *Possible health effects of exposure to residential electric and magnetic fields.* National Academy Press, Washington, DC.

NAS (National Academy of Sciences/National Research Council) (1998). *Health effects of exposure to radon.* National Academy Press, Washington, DC.

NCRP (National Council on Radiation Protection and Measurements) (1983). *Biological effects of ultrasound: mechanisms and clinical implications.* NCRP Report 74. NCRP, Bethesda, MD.

NCRP (National Council on Radiation Protection and Measurements) (1984). *Evaluation of occupational and environmental exposures to radon and radon daughters in the United States.* NCRP Report 78. NCRP, Bethesda, MD.

NCRP (National Council on Radiation Protection and Measurements) (1986). *Biological effects and exposure criteria for radiofrequency electromagnetic fields.* NCRP Report 86. NCRP, Bethesda, MD.

NCRP (National Council on Radiation Protection and Measurements) (1987). *Ionizing radiation exposure of the population of the United States.* NCRP Report 93. NCRP, Bethesda, MD.

NCRP (National Council on Radiation Protection and Measurements) (1989). *Exposure of the U.S. population from occupational radiation.* NCRP Report 101. NCRP, Bethesda, MD.

NCRP (National Council on Radiation Protection and Measurements) (1993). *Limitation of exposure to ionizing radiation.* NCRP Report 116. NCRP, Bethesda, MD.

NCRP (National Council on Radiation Protection and Measurements) (1997). *Uncertainties in fatal risk estimates used in radiation protection.* NCRP Report 126. NCRP, Bethesda, MD.

NIH (National Institutes of Health) (1985). *Report of the NIH Working Group to develop radioepidemiological tables.* NIH Publication No. 85-2748. US Government Printing Office, Washington, DC.

NIOSH (National Institute for Occupational Safety and Health) (1972). *Criteria for a recommended standard: occupational exposure to ultraviolet radiation.* DHEW Publication No. (NIOSH) HSM 73-11009. US Government Printing Office, Washington, DC.

Normile, D. (1999). Nuclear accident: Special treatment set for radiation victim. *Science*, **286**, 207–8.

OTA (Office of Technology Assessment, US Congress) (1989). *Biological effects of power frequency electric and magnetic fields—background paper.* OTA-BP-E-53. US Government Printing Office, Washington, DC.

Puskin, J.S. and Nelson, C.B. (1995). Estimates of radiogenic cancer risks. *Health Physics*, **69**, 93–101.

Rex, M., *et al.* (1997). Prolonged statospheric ozone loss in the 1995–96 Arctic winter. *Nature*, **389**, 835–8.

Robbins, J. and Adams, W. (1989). Radiation effects in the Marshall Islands. In *Radiation and the thyroid* (ed. S. Nagataki), p. 11–24. Excerpta Medica, Tokyo.

Roberts, N.J., Jr and Michaelson, S.M. (1985). Epidemiological studies of human exposures to microwave radiation: a critical review. *International Archives of Occupational and Environmental Health*, **56**, 169–78.

Rosenthal, N.E., Sack, D.A., Skwerer, R.G., Jacobsen, F.M., and Wehr, T.A. (1988). Phototherapy for seasonal affective disorder. *Journal of Biological Rhythms*, **3**, 101–20.

Ross, J.A., Coppes, M.J., and Robison, L.L. (1999). Population density and risk of childhood leukaemia. *Lancet*, **354**, 532.

Rubin, P. and Casarett, G.W. (1972). A direction for clinical radiation pathology: the tolerance dose. In *Frontiers of radiation therapy and oncology* (ed. J.M. Vaeth), pp. 1–16. Karger, Basel, and University Park Press, Baltimore, MD.

Sankaranarayanan, K. and Chakraborty, R. (1995). Cancer predisposition, radiosensitivity and the risk of radiation-induced cancers. I: Background. *Radiation Research*, **143**, 121–43.

Shapiro, J. (1990). *Radiation protection: a guide for scientists and physicians*, (3rd edn). Harvard University Press, Cambridge, MA.

Sliney, D. and Wolbarsht, M. (1980). *Safety with lasers*. Plenum, New York.

Stannard, J.N. (1988). *Radioactivity and health: a history*. US Department of Energy Report, DOE/RL/01830-T59. National Technical Information Services, US Department of Energy, Washington, DC.

Tenforde, T.S. (1992). Biological interactions and potential health effects of extremely-low-frequency magnetic fields from power lines and other common sources. *Annual Review of Public Health*, **13**, 173–96.

Tenforde, T.S. (1996). Interaction of ELF magnetic fields with living systems. In *Handbook of biological effects of electromagnetic fields* (2nd edn) (ed. C. Polk and E. Postow), pp. 185–230. CRC Press, Boca Raton, FL.

Tenforde, T.S. (1998). Electromagnetic fields and carcinogenesis—an analysis of biological mechanisms. In *Wireless phones and health. Scientific progress* (ed. G.L. Carlo), pp. 183–96. Kluwer Academic, Boston, MA.

Tronko, M.D., *et al.* (1999). Thyroid carcinoma in children and adolescents in Ukraine after the Chernobyl nuclear accident: statistical data and clinicomorphologic characteristics. *Cancer*, **86**, 149–56.

UNSCEAR (United Nations Scientific Committee on the Effects of Atomic Radiation) (1982). *Ionizing radiation: sources and biological effects*. Report to the General Assembly, with Annexes. United Nations, New York.

UNSCEAR (United Nations Scientific Committee on the Effects of Atomic Radiation) (1986). *Genetic and somatic effects of ionizing radiation*. Report to the General Assembly, with Annexes. United Nations, New York.

UNSCEAR (United Nations Scientific Committee on the Effects of Atomic Radiation) (1988). *Sources, effects, and risks of ionizing radiation*. Report to the General Assembly, with Annexes. United Nations, New York.

UNSCEAR (United Nations Scientific Committee on the Effects of Atomic Radiation) (1993). *Sources and effects of ionizing radiation*. Report to the General Assembly, with Annexes. United Nations, New York.

UNSCEAR (United Nations Scientific Committee on the Effects of Atomic Radiation) (1994). *Sources and effects of ionizing radiation*. Report to the General Assembly, with Annexes. United Nations, New York.

Upton, A.C. (1986). Historical perspectives on radiation carcinogenesis. In *Radiation carcinogenesis* (ed. A.C. Upton, R.E. Albert, F.J. Burns, and R.E. Shore), pp. 1–10. Elsevier, New York.

Upton, A.C., Shore, R.E., and Harley, N. H. (1990). The health effects of low-level ionizing radiation. *Annual Review of Public Health*, **13**, 127–50.

USDOE (US Department of Energy) (1987). *Health and environmental consequences of the Chernobyl nuclear power plant accident*. DOE/ ER-0332. USDOE, Washington, DC.

USDOE (US Department of Energy) (1993). *US Department of Energy interim mixed waste inventory report: waste streams, treatment capacities and technologies*. DOE/NBM-1100. National Technical Information Services, Springfield, VA.

USEPA (US Environmental Protection Agency) (1992). Technical Support Document for the 1992 Citizen's Guide to Radon. EPA 400-R-92-011. USEPA, Washington, DC.

Wakeford, R., *et al.* (1994*a*). The descriptive statistics and health implications of occupational radiation doses received by men at the Sellafield nuclear installation before the conception of their children. *Journal of Radiological Protection*, **14**, 3–16.

Wakeford, R., *et al.* (1994*b*). The Seascale childhood leukaemia cases—the mutation rates implied by paternal preconceptional radiation doses. *Journal of Radiological Protection*, **14**, 17–24.

Ward, J.F. (1988). DNA damage produced by ioniziong radiation in mammalian cells: identities, mechanisms of formation, and repairability. *Progress in Nucleic Acid Research and Molecular Biology*, **35**, 96–128.

WHO (World Health Organization) (1982). *Ultrasound environmental health criteria*. WHO, Geneva.

Worrest, R.C. and Grant, L.D. (1989). Effects of ultraviolet-B radiation on terrestrial plants and marine organisms. In *Ozone depletion: health and environmental consequences* (ed. R.R. Jones and T. Wigley), pp. 197–206. Wiley, New York.

Yoshimoto, Y., *et al.* (1990). Malignant tumors during the first two decades of life in the offspring of atomic bomb survivors. *American Journal of Human Genetics*, **46**, 1041–52.

8.4 Control of microbial threats: population surveillance, vaccine studies, and the microbiology laboratory

Norman D. Noah

Introduction

Microbiological hazards were until only very recently the foremost causes of death and illness. Even though regulatory priority is now often given to chemical and radiation hazards, they remain serious and are again becoming common causes of ill health. Indeed, since the last edition of this textbook, much has been written on the theme of emerging or resurgent infectious disease. The epidemiological methods used in the investigation of infectious disease are not substantially different from those used in any epidemiological investigation. Nevertheless, there are some investigative techniques that are particularly applicable to infectious diseases. The techniques of surveillance were first used in infectious diseases and the special principles of surveillance as applied to infectious disease are described below in the first part of this chapter. Vaccine trials have many similarities to other epidemiological studies, but nevertheless are sufficiently distinctive to warrant special consideration: they are described in the second part of the chapter. The use of the microbiological laboratory in epidemiological studies of infectious disease, which is crucial to the discipline, is discussed in the third section. The investigation of the host, agent, and environment is described in Chapter 8.5.

Population surveillance

The definition of population surveillance is:

> Continuous analysis, interpretation, and feedback of systematically collected data, generally using methods distinguished by their practicability, uniformity and rapidity, rather than by accuracy or completeness. (Eylenbosch and Noah 1988; Last 1995).

Thus it is a type of observational study (Thacker *et al.* 1983). There are several key words in the definition as provided above which make this the preferred definition. 'Continuous' distinguishes surveillance from a survey. 'Practicability' is the essence of any workable surveillance system. 'Uniformity' ensures that the data can be interpreted sensibly, especially as surveillance is all about trends. 'Rapidity' is important for the system to be useful. And the words 'rather than complete accuracy or completeness' sum up the rough and ready philosophy behind most surveillance systems, which exist primarily for following trends in disease patterns—and for following them quickly. Surveillance essentially is not an academic process, although this does not mean that academic rigour is unnecessary in good practice. However, many of these points need to be qualified and are further discussed later in this section.

The word 'monitoring' should not be used interchangeably with surveillance: it is the ongoing evaluation of a control or management process (Eylenbosch and Noah 1988). The techniques of surveillance are usually necessary for efficient monitoring. Thus monitoring the success or failure of a vaccine policy for a disease will involve surveillance of vaccine use and surveillance of the disease, and possibly include surveillance of side-effects of vaccine and population immunity. Monitoring can become a finely tuned measure in which outcome can be constantly evaluated to adjust the process.

Research is not an essential part of surveillance, although surveillance may facilitate research. Consequently, there has been some discussion about the term 'epidemiological surveillance', and whether 'public health surveillance' is more valid (Thacker and Berkelman 1988).

Types of surveillance

Active and passive surveillance

In passive surveillance the recipient waits for the provider to report. In active surveillance routine checks of the provider are regularly made to ensure uniform and complete reporting. Enhanced surveillance is a term sometimes used to denote a form of active surveillance.

The globally successful smallpox eradication programme used active surveillance; each local health unit was 'coerced, persuaded, and cajoled' to report cases of smallpox each week, intensive further case finding was undertaken when a case was notified, and sources of information other than medical—teachers, schoolchildren, civil, and so on—were used (Henderson 1976). The reporting of a negative return is an important but not an essential part of a surveillance system. For surveillance of very rare diseases, however, completeness becomes more important, and 'negative reporting' becomes essential. Negative reporting has been used most effectively in the surveillance system for rare paediatric diseases, such as Reye's syndrome and Kawasaki disease, run by the British Paediatric Surveillance Unit in Britain (Hall and Glickman 1988).

Sentinel surveillance

Sentinel surveillance is essentially a type of 'sample surveillance' in which reporting sources are situated at various sites covering an area (which may be very large, e.g. a country), and may provide fairly complete reporting within the population covered by each reporting source. This ensures that resources are not wasted in a large unwieldy surveillance system. If the population (total, or age and sex distributions) covered by each reporting centre is known, estimates of the disease or other indicator under surveillance can be made. A good discussion of some of the strengths and weaknesses of a sentinel system based on reporting by general practitioners (**GPs**) can be found in Boussard *et al.* (1996). Systems based on GP reporting are the most common forms of sentinel surveillance and are discussed later in this chapter.

Essentials of a surveillance system

The essential steps in any surveillance system are as follows:

- the collection of data
- the analysis of data
- the interpretation of data
- feedback of information.

These steps are similar to those taken in any scientific process. The collection of data is clearly the basic element of the system, but a failure of any of the other three steps in the process could also lead to failure of the system.

Collection of data

The collection of data has to be systematic, regular, and uniform, and, in infectious diseases particularly, topical and relevant. For collection to be systematic, suppliers of information should understand clearly what needs to be reported, leaving little scope for value judgements in deciding what to report, such as reporting only interesting or rare cases. With infectious disease surveillance, serious infections, rare infections, or those against which a control measure is available or is being planned, tend to be most worthwhile for surveillance.

For clinical reporting case definitions are helpful, especially for new or rare diseases, and even for common and easily recognizable diseases, particularly when they become rare. An early case definition for acquired immune deficiency syndrome (**AIDS**) was essential in the initial surveillance of this infection. Measles is easily recognizable clinically, but a case definition became essential—as indeed did laboratory confirmation of each case notified—when the vaccine campaign in the United States and in England became so successful that the infection became rare.

Case definitions may be rigid, but do not necessarily have to be highly specific. Careful consideration has to be given in individual instances as to whether sensitivity is more important than specificity. It may be important, for example, to choose a high-sensitive low-specific definition to encourage reporting, and then to concentrate on encouraging high specificity as the surveillance system becomes established.

For laboratory reporting, likewise, the criteria for what constitutes an acceptable report need to be understood clearly by the laboratory; for example, isolation of the organism from particular sites, or a fourfold or greater rise in antibody titre, or a single antibody titre above a certain level associated with a clinical feature characteristic of that infection, may all be acceptable, providing reporting is consistent. Nevertheless, in infectious disease there are often difficulties in associating a correctly identified organism with a particular illness, such as isolating an echovirus from a patient with gastroenteritis. In these instances all laboratories should understand clearly whether every such isolation need be reported, or only one where the isolate is considered to contribute to the symptoms (which may involve a value judgement). In the laboratory reporting system run by the Communicable Disease Surveillance Centre in England and Wales, all viral isolates are reported, although there is space on the form for the laboratory to indicate if the isolate is thought not to be relevant to the condition of the patient.

If feedback is to be regular, reporting must also be regular. The *Communicable Disease Report for England and Wales* is produced weekly, and the laboratories report weekly. Regular reporting also helps to maintain discipline and routine, essential ingredients of any surveillance system. The information received from providers must be relevant and topical, otherwise the interest of the participants is rapidly lost and their response will diminish.

Analysis of data

The analysis of data for infectious diseases is similar to that for any other type of epidemiological statistic. The basic principles of analysis by time, place, and person are fundamental.

Time

Analysis by time is necessary if trends are to be discovered from surveillance data. In infectious disease in particular, temporal trends are helpful. In predicting and planning for disease there may be a significant delay between the time of acute illness and the date the infection is diagnosed and then reported. This is generally unavoidable. First, the time of onset of symptoms may be days or weeks before the illness is investigated. There will then be further delays before the disease is diagnosed, and again a delay before it is reported to the surveillance unit. With serological diagnosis, because a rise in antibody occurs only during convalescence, the infection is only confirmed when the patient is better. Even with a weekly reporting system there will be further delay before the infection is finally recorded. The burden of reporting will be increased considerably by asking reporting laboratories to record the date of onset of illness, but the date the first specimen was received in the laboratory is usually readily available and often approximates to the time of acute illness. In the analysis of such data, the interval between this date and the date of reporting may need to be taken into account. Analysing laboratory data by date of first specimen may be less helpful for the immediate detection of changes in incidence. The techniques of analysis by time, and tests for seasonality or periodicity, are outside the scope of this chapter.

Place

The site of the reporting laboratory is normally taken to be the geographical location of the ill person. Except in the best organized of health-care systems, however, this is not always true. In England and Wales, for example, the statutory notifications generally relate to the area of residence of the patient, but the Local Authority to which the infection is notified is not necessarily coterminous with the Health Authority. With laboratory data there are rarely rigid boundaries or catchment areas for hospital or public health laboratories. It may be difficult or impossible to allow for these problems in the analysis of the data, although it may only rarely be necessary to do so.

Analysis by place may show different patterns of infection such as north–south or urban–rural. Generally, national surveillance schemes will point only to broad differences in incidence; for small area differences surveys are usually necessary, except with more sophisticated surveillance systems. Analysis by place is particularly important in outbreak investigations.

Person

Age and sex of cases reported are also important components of a surveillance report. It is possible to conduct a surveillance system based solely on numbers and geographical location, but the sensitivity of the systems will be considerably reduced. Surveillance based on laboratory-reported rubella in England and Wales has shown that, although the incidence in all age groups fell substantially following the introduction of the measles, mumps, and rubella (**MMR**) vaccine in 1989, two epidemics occurred subsequently, one in 1993 and then in 1996 (Fig. 1). However, it was quite clear from surveillance data that the main force of the epidemic fell on adults, especially young adult unvaccinated males (Fig. 2) (Miller *et al.* 1997). Few pregnant women contracted the infection. In an outbreak of hepatitis B caused by a tattooist in one district of England (Limentani *et al.* 1979), a simple analysis of notifications of 'infective jaundice' by time or place would not have uncovered the outbreak. However, analysis of notifications by age and sex revealed an increase in notified cases in males aged 15 to 29 years.

In the laboratory surveillance system in England and Wales, some important and common organisms, such as salmonellas, were reported without the age and sex of the patient, as it would have increased the burden of reporting, collection, and analysis of such data in a pre-computer age to unmanageable levels. Reliance was placed on the ability to detect an increase in a rare Salmonella serotype, or the phage type of a more common serotype. When this occurred, the age and sex of the cases were readily available from the reference laboratory, and often provided some aetiological clues. This relatively crude and insensitive system nevertheless proved valuable, as when an increase in rare *Salmonella ealing* infections proved to be mainly in infants and was subsequently proven to be caused by powdered milk (Rowe *et al.* 1987). In this outbreak the epidemiological evidence was extremely strong while the level of contamination of the milk by the Salmonella was remarkably low.

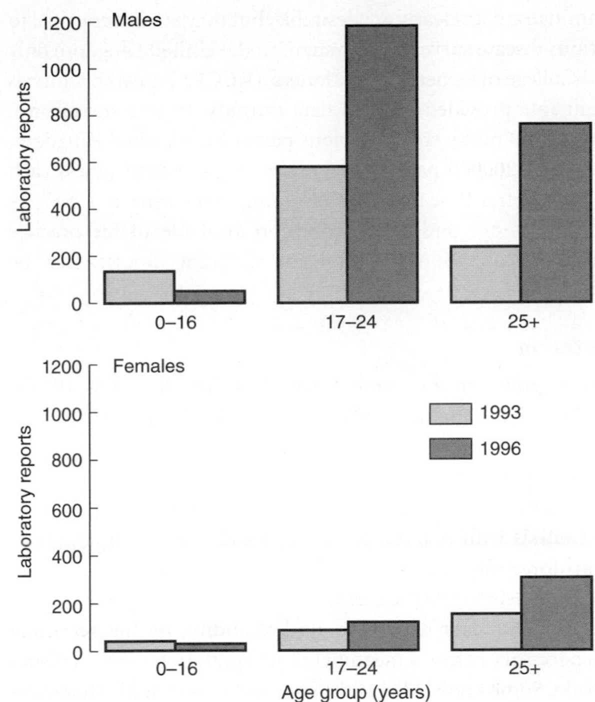

Fig. 2 Rubella: sex and age distribution, laboratory reports 1993 and 1996.

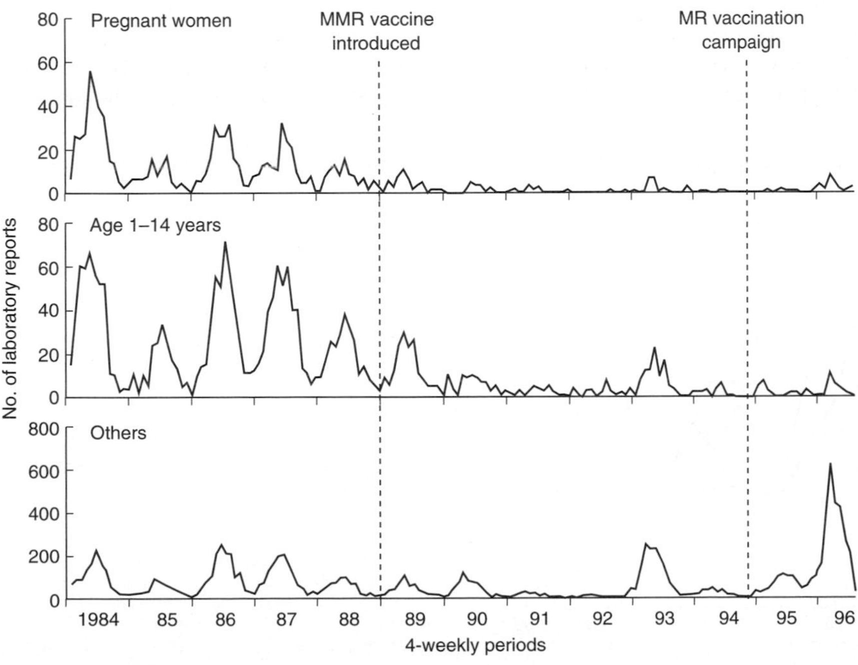

Fig. 1 Rubella: laboratory reports 1984–1996, England and Wales.

Denominator data clearly are desirable, but they are not essential to an infectious disease surveillance system. In the United Kingdom only the Royal College of General Practitioners' (**RCGP**) Research Unit has an in-built rate provided with its data outputs. In this surveillance system, about 40 physicians in various parts of the United Kingdom, covering about 200000 patients, report new episodes of illness each week to the Central Research Unit (Fleming and Crombie 1985). As each GP has an age and sex distribution available of his practice populations, consultation rates for the different illnesses can be calculated.

Interpretation

In the interpretation of surveillance data lies the skill of the epidemiologist. As Langmuir (1976) wrote of William Farr:

> His weekly return was no archive for stale data, but with his facile pen became a literate weapon for effecting change. He presented his analysis with objectivity but then stated his own interpretations forcefully...

In surveillance data a detailed understanding of the reporting system is necessary before a meaningful interpretation of the statistics can be made. Some knowledge of the size and demographic characteristics of the population covered by the surveillance system is also necessary. Every data source carries it own strengths and biases (Moro and McCormick 1988). With each data source, timeliness, completeness, representativeness, and accuracy (Thacker *et al.* 1983) should be considered. To these four qualities should be added that of significance (in its sense of 'importance'). 'Timeliness' may be particularly important with laboratory statistics, where there may sometimes be a considerable delay between disease onset and laboratory diagnosis. Organisms need time to grow in culture, and acute and convalescent samples of sera are needed to demonstrate the fourfold or greater rise in antibody necessary to substantiate a serological diagnosis. Rapid diagnostic methods for identification of an organism and the increasing use of IgM tests, however, have hastened considerably the diagnostic process for some infections. Notifications, although usually made on the basis of a clinical diagnosis, may not always be as prompt as one would expect, and sentinel GP clinical reporting systems tend to be more timely (Tillett and Spencer 1982).

The need for 'completeness' of reporting, particularly of common infections, is often exaggerated. Detection of disease trends by time, place, and person, sufficient for meaningful epidemiological interpretation, is easily feasible with incomplete data. Indeed, striving for completeness may waste resources. For rare diseases, however, or diseases that have become rare following a control programme, completeness grows in importance. Passive surveillance systems rarely achieve completeness; active systems are generally necessary for this.

The 'representativeness' of the data collected needs thought and planning, and the advantages of collecting data from more than one source may provide ways of validating one data source against another. In the surveillance system for infectious diseases in England and Wales conducted by the Communicable Disease Surveillance Centre, for example, the three main sources of data on meningococcal meningitis—hospital, notifications, and laboratory—show similar trends over time (Fig. 3). Source data should be representative for time, place, and person.

The 'significance' of surveillance data should also be evaluated carefully in its interpretation, and this can perhaps be best illustrated diagrammatically, using laboratory reporting of influenza as an example.

If a circumscribed population affected by an outbreak of influenza is represented by the rectangular outline in Fig. 4, the number actually infected will be a proportion of this, represented by the circle (A). However, not all of those infected will have symptoms; those that do belong within circle (B). Only a proportion of these will visit a doctor (C) (whether in hospital or general practice), and progressively smaller proportions will have a specimen sent for examination in a laboratory (D), specimens positive (E), and positive specimens reported to the surveillance unit (F). The biases and variables that occur during these steps also need to be considered. Those with symptomatic infections may be those never previously exposed to the particular influenza variant or subtype, or the very young and the very old, or those with a chronic disability, such as a respiratory condition. Similarly, those who visit a doctor and those whom the doctor investigates may be influenced by several factors, including social

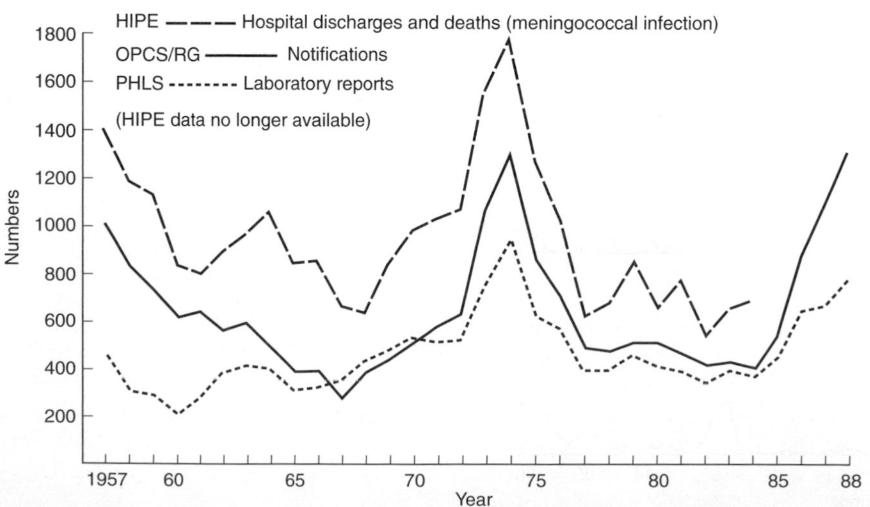

Fig. 3 Acute meningococcal meningitis: three sources of data, England and Wales, 1957–1988.

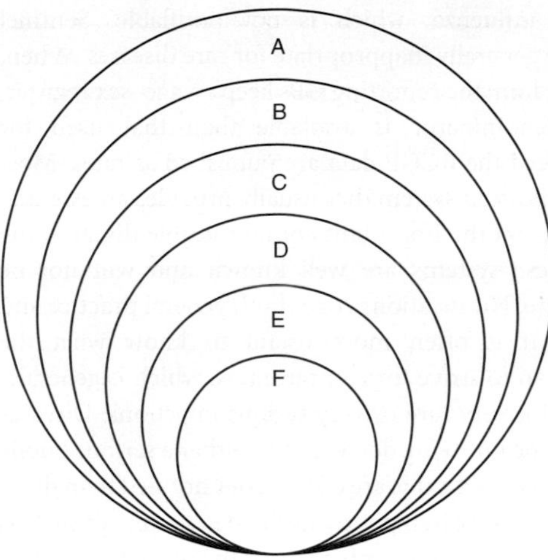

Fig. 4 Stages in the reporting of laboratory infection.

class, age, and severity of disease, and proximity to a laboratory. Laboratory success in its turn will depend on availability and cost of reagents, the interest and expertise of the laboratory, and the age and severity of disease in the patient. Finally, the accuracy, completeness, and timeliness of reporting by the laboratory will be influenced by its motivation, organization, and efficiency, as well as by the usefulness of the surveillance system and the quality and value of its feedback. A similar progression can be worked out for notification, GP, hospital, and death certification data sources (Fig. 5).

The 'accuracy' of the data provided by the laboratory will depend not only on its interest, expertise, and motivation, but also on the clarity of the instructions for reporting provided by the surveillance unit. These include acceptable diagnostic criteria for laboratory data (especially for antibody titre measurements, the levels acceptable to the collection unit should be clarified) and clinical definition for notification and GP data. A Quality Control scheme for participating laboratories is useful, as in the system run by the Public Health Laboratory Service in England and Wales.

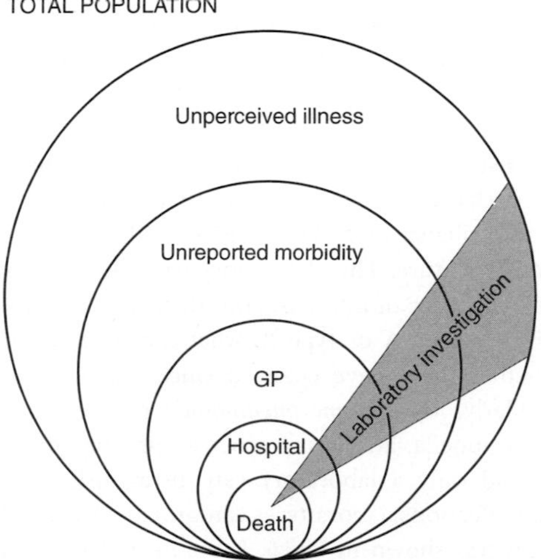

Fig. 5 Stages in the progression of disease.

Dissemination of information and target groups

The logical end, and indeed the purpose of any surveillance system, is the output, and its quality and relevance are critical: not only must it be meaningful and intelligible, but it must also be directed at the appropriate targets, whether they be decision makers or research workers. Moreover, feedback to those who provide the reports has an important motivating role in any surveillance system. Some surveillance and monitoring systems may even improve performance, as in the COVER (cover of vaccination evaluation rapidly) programme in England and Wales. In this surveillance and monitoring system the measurement and publication of performance measures for vaccine coverage in different health districts almost certainly stimulates poorly performing districts to improve (Begg *et al.* 1989).

For infectious disease surveillance systems, weekly or monthly reports are the most appropriate. The ability to adapt to changing patterns of infection—incorporating new diseases of importance, discarding outdated or useless data needs to be in-built. Flexibility to provide urgent information is useful, as for outbreaks, and as methods of communication continue to improve this should make urgent dissemination easier.

The rapid development and availability of electronic methods of storing, analysing, and disseminating data and information have greatly facilitated the practice of surveillance. Powerful microcomputers and electronic networking have allowed data to be transmitted from source to surveillance centre without the use of post and paper—or indeed the tedious completion of surveillance forms. Not only can data be stored in the computers, but pre-programmed statistical analyses of the data can also reveal changes in time, place, or person. Fortunately, the meaningful interpretation of such changes still requires the human element. Finally, the dissemination of information has been revolutionized by the use of electronic methods. In the United Kingdom, the Communicable Disease Surveillance Centre provides rapid information to Health Authorities through its EPINET System. In France, the Minitel System is also effective.

Content and presentation

The summary report should not contain indigestible lists and tables, but easily understood analyses with appropriate evaluation of their significance. Especially for infectious disease, the reports need to be topical and relevant. Thus short summaries of recent trends and changes, together with more detailed reviews of subjects and interests, are important ingredients of a surveillance report, and these can be supplemented by reports of outbreaks and other items of general interest by reporter participants or other contributors.

> A successful report will educate and provide current scientific information for planning, prevention or change. (Eylenbosch and Noah 1988).

Another function necessary for a successful surveillance system is the provision of an information service for individual enquiry. The organization of the surveillance unit and of the data collection system to provide information (as opposed to raw data) is as important a part of any surveillance feedback service as the regular report. For the sporadic inquiry of this type, appropriate interpretation of the information provided is also necessary.

Encouraging regular dialogue between providers, other interested parties, and the central surveillance unit is helpful to fostering a healthy relationship between them and the long-term usefulness of the surveillance system; it can also be regarded as a form of monitoring of the surveillance system.

Ideally, the content and presentation of the output of the surveillance system needs to be adapted so as to be made intelligible to each type of target group; lay politicians and decision makers, for example, might receive a different type of feedback from research workers, and again from the public and media. This is rarely possible with the regular surveillance report, but an information section within the central unit could tailor the response appropriately to the *ad hoc* inquiry. The increasing interest in health by the lay public, media, and politicians makes it essential to provide accurate, relevant, and topical information with skill and flair.

Content of surveillance: sources of data

When discussing the epidemiology of infection, or any other type of disease, it is useful to consider the different stages in the natural history of the disease process (Fig. 5). The figure is similar to that used for laboratory data (Fig. 4). The population again can be represented by the rectangular outline.

Within this population will be a subpopulation who will be infected asymptomatically, or will be immune or carriers. A smaller proportion will develop symptomatic infection, and progressively smaller proportions will have symptomatic unreported infections, visit a doctor, be admitted to hospital, or die. To have a true measure of the total impact of a disease on a population, information at all these levels is needed. In practice it is of course rarely possible, or perhaps necessary, to be so systematic, although information at most levels can often be obtained. Serological surveys will give information on asymptomatic infection or immunity levels, and the taking of appropriate specimens or swabs from persons may detect asymptomatic carriers. Surveillance of predisposition to disease other than that determined by the absence of antibody is more difficult in the field of infectious disease, but surveillance of general functions such as growth, development, and nutritional status of children (Morley 1975; Irwig 1976; Carne 1984) may fall into this category, as will surveillance for infection in certain groups, such as tuberculosis in certain ethnic patients, human immunodeficiency virus (HIV) infection in haemophiliacs and homosexuals, cytomegalovirus infections in the immunosuppressed, or in those subject to certain procedures such as urinary catheterization. Unreported morbidity (Fig. 5) is not usually possible to place under passive surveillance. In a series of surveys conducted by the Office of Population Censuses and Surveys of England and Wales, the General Household Survey, information on unreported morbidity is obtained (Haskey and Birch 1985). Although each survey is finite, the collective information over many surveys constitutes a database suitable for surveillance.

A general practice surveillance system based on a sentinel reporting network was first successfully organized in the United Kingdom by the RCGP in 1966 (Fleming and Crombie 1985), and since then in the Netherlands (Collette 1982) and Belgium (Thiers *et al.* 1979). General practice morbidity data are generally useful for providing information one tier in severity below that of hospital morbidity (Fig. 5). More specifically, in practice they produce information on clinical conditions with very low mortality not covered by notification, such as the common cold, chickenpox, or otitis media. In England and Wales, before mumps and rubella became notifiable in 1988, the RCGP clinical reporting system was an important source of information on these common infections; it remains an important source of information on clinical influenza, which is not notifiable. Sentinel reporting systems are generally inappropriate for rare diseases. When, as in the United Kingdom, the reporting GPs keep an age–sex register, a more accurate denominator is available than that used for notification, and indeed the RCGP data are published as rates. Most countries have a notification system that usually provides an essential source of information on the important communicable diseases; the characteristics of these systems are well known and will not be discussed in detail here. Notifications cover both general practice and hospital morbidity. It is often more useful to know what the notification rate is than to strive for completeness, which is generally only really desirable for very rare or very serious infections. Diseases that are perceived by the notifying doctors to be either a serious public health problem and communicable are often better notified than those that are not. Thus tetanus is often poorly notified in countries such as England and Wales. It must be remembered that the primary objective of a notification system is not for surveillance but to provide an opportunity for local control, for which legal powers are usually available if necessary.

Surveillance systems using hospital admission data clearly only cover a limited, although important, phase in the natural history of an infection. Infections for which hospital data are ideal are those for which patients are usually admitted and admitted once only, and in which the diagnosis can be confirmed. If the hospital reporting system is based on a sample, the disease should not be excessively rare. Meningococcal and other forms of bacterial meningitis are examples of infection that tend to be well documented in hospital data systems. Hospital data, on the other hand, may be available late, months or even years after the event.

Death certification is virtually a universal requirement in most countries. Death certificates are clearly important to any surveillance system, but for infectious diseases their value may be somewhat limited as infections are now less common as a primary cause of death. As infections remain an important cause of morbidity, death certifications need to be supplemented by one or more of the surveillance systems detailed above. They also tend to be too imprecise in deaths attributed to infection.

Other sources of data

Laboratory

Laboratories provide important, perhaps essential, information for the surveillance of infection. Surveillance, supported by laboratory confirmation of clinical cases reported, showed that the malaria epidemics said to be occurring in the malarial southern states of the United States did not exist, and the few cases confirmed microbiologically were imported or relapses (Langmuir 1963). In addition to this 'confirmatory' role in surveillance that laboratories provide, they have an additional 'qualitative' feature. Thus laboratory data cannot only confirm the presence or absence of influenza, but their data can also show whether the virus is type A or type B, what the subtypes or variants are, and whether these have changed since the previous epidemic (Fig. 6). Similarly, *Mycoplasma pneumoniae*, psittacosis, Q fever, several viruses, legionella, and many other agents may cause atypical pneumonia, and only a laboratory can distinguish these successfully. In human infections, laboratories can provide data at all levels of the disease process shown in Fig. 5. Laboratory data often provide information on infection in vectors, animal, other hosts, or the environment, and are especially important with zoonoses.

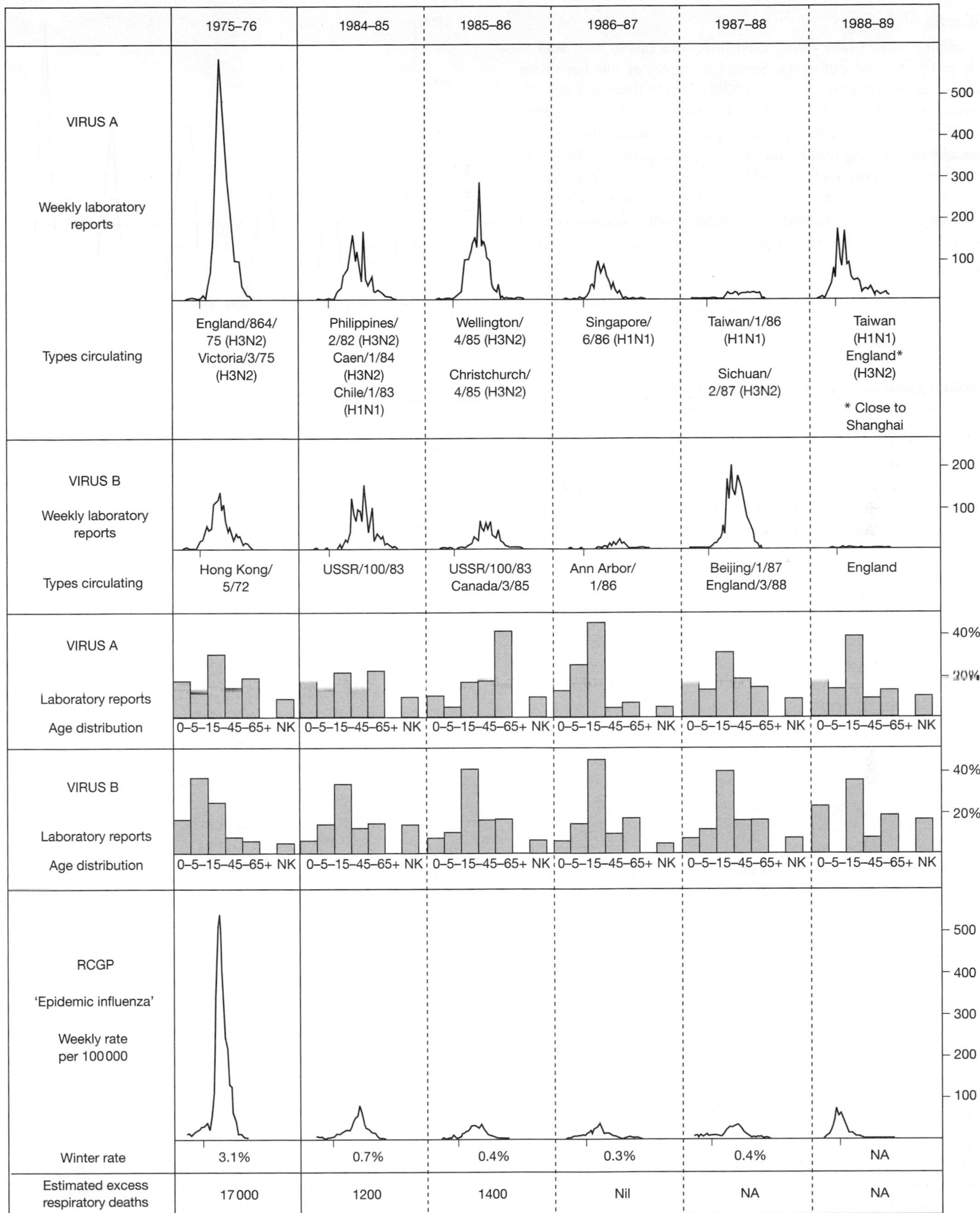

Fig. 6 Influenza surveillance, England and Wales. Indices used in monitoring influenza activity for one major epidemic winter (1975–1976) are compared with five other winters. (Source: *Communicable Disease Report*, **44**, 3–4, 1989.)

Outbreaks

Surveillance of laboratory-diagnosed infections can in itself lead to early recognition of outbreaks. Several examples of this have been reported, especially with salmonellas (Gill *et al.* 1983; Rowe *et al.* 1987; Cowden *et al.* 1989), and with legionellas (Salmon and Bartlett 1995). Surveillance of outbreaks can also provide useful information, especially in assessing trends, and may be particularly worthwhile in countries where more sophisticated sources of data, such as laboratory data on individual infections, may not be available. Outbreak surveillance can be cheap and effective, although it is essentially an insensitive measure of disease trends.

Vaccine utilization

Surveillance of vaccine utilization is an important component of the process of monitoring the effect of vaccine strategy on an infection. In England and Wales the COVER programme fulfils this function (Begg *et al.* 1989) and may have an additional effect in stimulating poorly performing districts to improve coverage. Serological surveillance can provide an indirect measure of the effectiveness of a vaccine strategy (Noah and Fowle 1988).

Sickness absence

Sickness absence records may provide indications of major outbreaks in working populations. Influenza in particular may produce measurable changes in sickness absence. Sickness absence can also be monitored in special groups, such as in boarding schools, and among Post Office workers. Sickness absence is a crude measure of a widespread epidemic, and covers only a selected age group of the population, but can be surprisingly sensitive and can provide an early warning of an epidemic. Only a limited number of countries have this type of information available.

Disease determinants

Biological changes in agent, vector, and the reservoirs of infection can be placed under surveillance. Surveillance of changes in an agent, such as new subtypes or variants of influenza, antibiotic resistance in bacteria, such as the gonococcus and *Staphylococcus*, or protozoa, such as *Plasmodium*, is regularly performed. Surveillance of biological vectors such as ticks and mosquitoes, and of animal reservoirs of infections such as brucellosis and rabies, is an essential component of disease control in many countries.

Susceptibility to infection can be measured by skin testing or serological surveillance. In England and Wales, antibody profiles to current circulating influenza variants and to new variants are regularly performed in small samples of the population to assess the degree of susceptibility to a new variant. The degree of immunity to vaccinatable diseases is also regularly assessed (Morgan-Capner *et al.* 1988). Raska (1971) persuasively argued the use of serum banks and immunological surveys in surveillance.

Other

Other conditions that can be placed under surveillance include abortions, birth defects, injuries, behavioural risk factors, and occupational safety.

Objectives of surveillance

Many of the objectives of surveillance of infectious diseases have already been alluded to in the text and will be summarized here only.

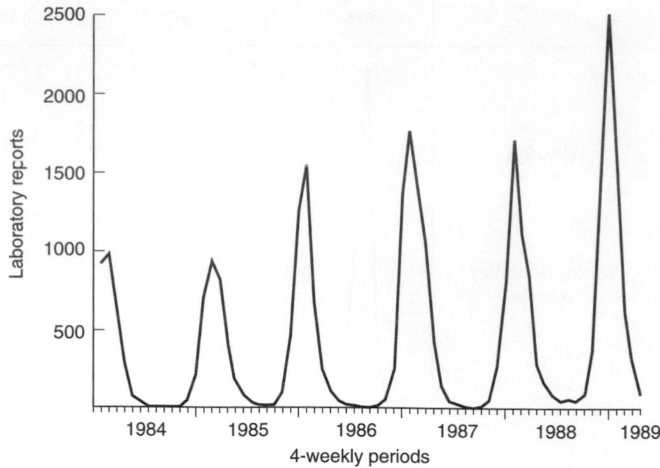

Fig. 7 Laboratory reports of respiratory syncytial virus infections, England and Wales.

The main objectives of infectious disease surveillance are to monitor disease trends in time, place, and person, as illustrated below.

Anticipating changes in incidence

Many infectious diseases follow regular patterns, both seasonal and secular. The respiratory syncytial virus follows a distinct seasonal pattern, causing epidemics every year with the peak incidence, in the Northern Hemisphere, almost invariably shortly after the new year (Fig. 7). Minor variations in this pattern occur (Noah 1989). With some viruses, for example, echovirus, a failure to return to baseline by the end of its yearly cycle signifies that a resurgence will occur the following year (Figs 8 and 9) (Epidemiology Research Laboratory 1975). Some organisms, such as *Mycoplasma pneumoniae,* have long cycles extending over 4 years, but are particularly important as this is a treatable infection and early warning of an epidemic is of practical value (Fig. 10) (Noah 1974; Monto 1974). A review of cyclic variation in infections can be found in Noah (1989).

Early detection of outbreaks

Outbreaks of food poisoning which have been detected only because surveillance revealed an unexpected increase in a salmonella have

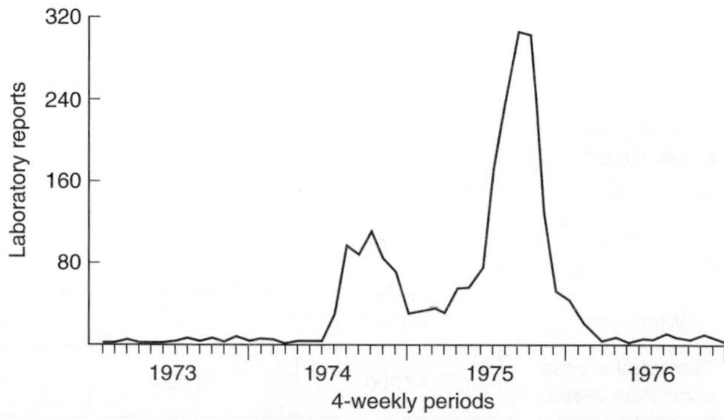

Fig. 8 Laboratory reports of echovirus 19 virus infections, England and Wales.

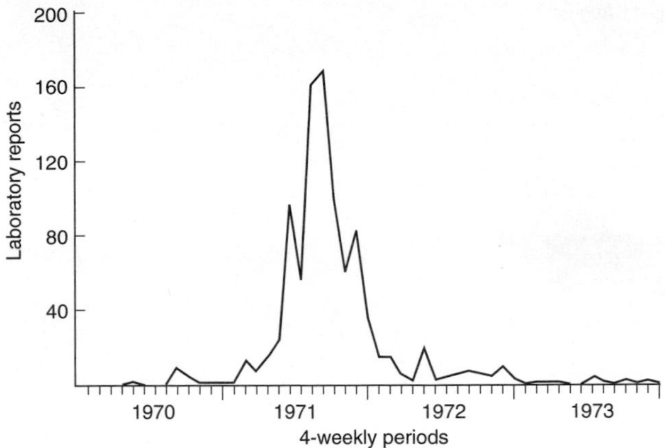

Fig. 9 Laboratory reports of echovirus 4 infections, England and Wales.

already been described, and reports of some of these have been published (Gill *et al.* 1983; Rowe *et al.* 1987; Cowden *et al.* 1989). Occasionally, early detection of a new strain of an organism may lead to premature action which, with hindsight, turns out to have been inappropriate, as with the swine influenza episode (Silverstein 1981). Surveillance may lead to the detection of new infections (e.g. Lyme disease).

In an outbreak of hepatitis caused by a tattooist in England in 1978, surveillance by time alone would not have brought the outbreak to light, but only the characteristic age and sex distribution (young adult males) showed a change (Limentani *et al.* 1979). Analysis of surveillance data by person, time, and place is more likely to reveal changes in pattern than analysis by one of these parameters alone.

Evaluation of effectiveness of preventive measures

Surveillance techniques are used to monitor the effects of a mass vaccination programme. Not only can changes in incidence be measured by time (Hinman *et al.* 1980), but also by person; for example, age changes in measles or mumps (Hinman *et al.* 1980; Cochi *et al.* 1988) have been recorded as a result of mass immunization. There have also been examples of monitoring changes in incidence by place (district) and correlating these changes with vaccination uptake rates (Pollard 1980). Effectiveness of a vaccination programme can also be assessed by serological surveillance (Noah and Fowle 1988). The effect of withdrawing a source of infection, such as a contaminated food, from circulation, can be monitored by surveillance, as with the *Salmonella napoli* outbreak caused by contaminated imported chocolate in England (Gill *et al.* 1983; Fig. 11).

Identification of vulnerable groups

Surveillance can expose vulnerable groups; for example, by revealing ethnic or social differences in tuberculosis incidence. Appropriate action, such as BCG vaccination of neonates in such groups, can be taken. Serological surveillance can also identify susceptibility in particular groups of persons for selective vaccination.

Setting priorities for allocation of resources

From the examples above, it is clear that surveillance programmes can be used to provide information for setting priorities for resource allocation, and hence for planning. This leads to more efficient use of health resources and, although changes cannot always be anticipated in advance, prompt detection of changes can allow redistribution of resources at an early stage. Surveillance can also be useful in uncovering or monitoring changes in health practices, e.g. the increasing rate of Caesarean section in the United States between 1970 and 1988 (Thacker 1994).

Aetiological clues

Infectious disease patterns may help to generate hypotheses for aetiology of chronic diseases. Secular variation compatible with certain infections have been noted with sudden infant death syndrome (Helweg-Larsen *et al.* 1985), insulin-dependent diabetes (Gleason *et al.* 1982), deaths from asthma (Khot and Burn 1984), and anencephalus and spina bifida (Maclean and Macleod 1984).

Setting up a surveillance system

In setting up a surveillance system, all the points discussed above need to be considered. It is important in addition to 'pilot' the system first, or to have a 'trial period' after which necessary adjustments can be made. In practice, as surveillance is essentially an ongoing process, adjustments may be made continually to 'fine tune' the system. Unnecessary extraneous or duplicate reporting should clearly be

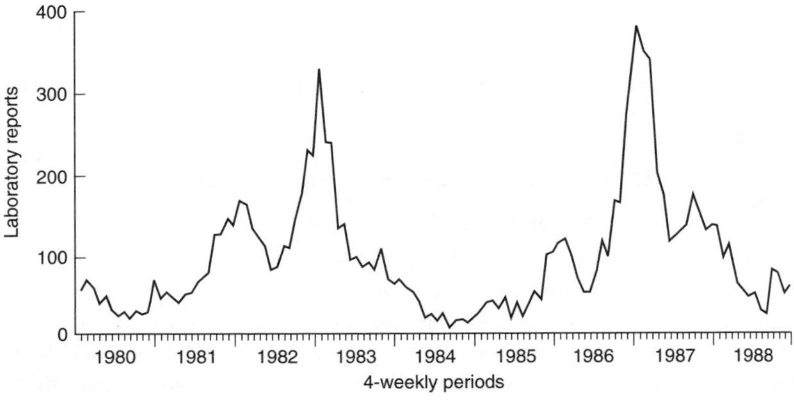

Fig. 10 Laboratory reports of *M. pneumoniae* infections, England and Wales.

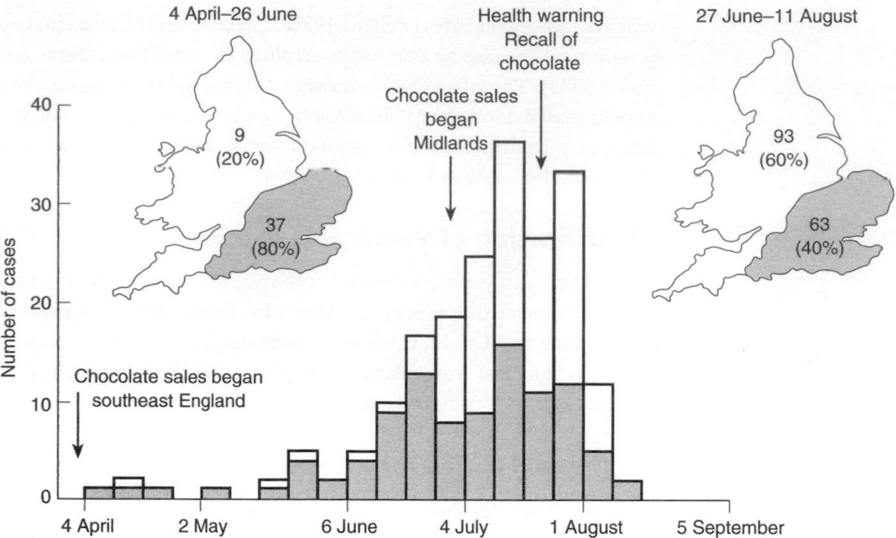

Fig. 11 *S. napoli* outbreak in England and Wales, 1982: distribution of 202 primary household cases.

avoided, and improvements will also need to be made in the methods of flow of the information. Three attributes mentioned by Klaucke (1994) for an efficient surveillance system are simplicity, flexibility, and acceptability. Improving methods for the flow of information to and from the surveillance unit will enhance these three attributes. Electronic methods of reporting, obviating the use of paper, will for example not only simplify the system and reduce the effort involved, but will also increase its acceptability. Moreover, electronic systems make it easier for flexibility to be built-in, so that conditions under surveillance can be added or deleted more easily. The surveillance system should be considered as a network of roads along which the types of consumer product sent can be changed according to need. In England and Wales, when rubella and mumps vaccines were introduced into the routine schedules, the two infections were placed under surveillance using the existing notification network. The laboratory network was used for AIDS, legionnaires' disease, and Lyme disease. Thus, surveillance systems for new conditions were put into operation rapidly, fairly painlessly, and at minimal extra cost.

Acceptability depends on simplicity, and also on the perception by reporters of the importance of the data being collected. Quality of feedback, both in the initial stage of setting-up the system and throughout the operation of the surveillance, clearly affects acceptability.

The technology now available to facilitate surveillance is considerable. Electronic reporting in both directions—reporter to surveillance unit, surveillance unit to reporter and others—is now feasible. Details of the computer technology available are outside the scope of this chapter, and in any case are rapidly changing.

It is now becoming increasingly obvious that 'the links between seemingly far-flung events involving pathogens and their hosts deserve a new kind of scrutiny if we are to deal effectively with emerging and re-emerging infectious diseases' (Fox 1996). The scope of surveillance must increase indefinitely in the next few years so that the effects on infection of changing environments (whether natural or man-made) can be anticipated—and monitored. We need to look not only on human health but on effects on flora and fauna also, because they each affect each other in 'delicate balanced fragility'.

Conclusions

Although considered to be the backbone of public health, surveillance makes use of data gathered for other purposes. Clinical or laboratory diagnoses are generally made for the benefit of the doctor and patient. Thus, surveillance is an efficient way of making use of data that has in effect, 'passed its sell-by date'. '...probably most important, surveillance needs to be used more consistently and thoughtfully by policymakers' (Thacker 1994). It is up to public health physicians and epidemiologists to transform routine statistics into meaningful reliable and timely information so that health policy-makers can be persuaded to act for change—for change is the ultimate goal of surveillance.

Field investigations of vaccines

Vaccines are a time-tested and highly efficient means of controlling many microbial threats. Epidemiological studies are an essential part of the assessment and use of vaccines and may be associated with vaccines in several different ways: (a) in the assessment of the need for a vaccine by undertaking surveillance or surveys; (b) in antibody and field trials to assess the efficacy and safety of the vaccine; (c) in the selection of an appropriate strategy; (d) in the implementation of the vaccine programme. Finally, the use of the vaccine and its effect on the population need to be closely monitored. These logical steps have not always been followed.

Assessment of the need for a vaccine

Morbidity and mortality of disease

The overall morbidity of the infection, and its severity, can (and should normally) be estimated from a surveillance programme. With measles the need for a preventive programme in the United Kingdom was first shown in 1963 (McCarthy and Taylor Robinson 1963). Miller (1964), by studying notifications of measles, was able to estimate the hospital admission rate (1 per cent), the respiratory and otitis media complication rate (6 to 9 per cent), and the neurological complication rate (0.7 per cent). Complication rates like these for an extremely common infection signified a serious health problem. Miller (1978) showed that, although the incidence rates had fallen with the introduction of mass vaccination, these complication rates had changed little with time. Rey (1985) estimated that in France every year 30 people died from measles, 6000 were admitted to hospital, 100 to 200 developed encephalitis, and 10 to 20 subacute sclerosing panencephalitis. Worldwide estimates tend to be cruder but none the less possible; using world health statistics, Cutting (1983) claimed that measles caused 1 to 1.5 million deaths in children in 1981. General practice surveillance systems may also be useful in providing estimates of disease burdens, as for mumps in the United Kingdom (Research Unit of the RCGP 1974). Serological studies are also used to assess the overall impact of an infection on a population, and the vulnerability of a target population. Studies on rubella in 1969 (Cockburn 1969) showed that by adulthood more than 80 per cent of a population had been infected leaving 5 to 15 per cent of pregnant women still susceptible and hence, still vulnerable. In the United States the incidence of clinical rubella in pregnant women was found to vary from 4 to 8 per 10 000 in endemic periods to 20 per 10 000 during epidemics, while subclinical infection could increase by up to threefold (Sever *et al.* 1969; White *et al.* 1969). Sometimes, as in poliomyelitis, crude notification data on the most serious outcomes of poliovirus infection—paralysis and death—can be sufficient to point to a need for a vaccine (Fig. 12). For severe and very rare diseases only a selective vaccine policy can be considered, so these considerations do not apply.

Field studies

Field studies of vaccine efficacy (**VE**) and safety are clearly necessary before a vaccine is licensed for use. Postlicensing studies are also important, but these require a different approach and will be considered separately.

Pre-licensing vaccine trials

The earliest trial (phase 1) of a new vaccine usually involves a small number (usually 20 to 50) of adult volunteers with a low level of risk of acquiring the disease. Antibody is measured and adverse effects are closely monitored. This tests the immunogenicity of the vaccine, following which the dose may be adjusted. Preliminary information on safety is also provided by a phase 1 trial—although limited, this is an important aspect of such a trial.

In the phase 2 trial a larger number of persons, between 100 and 200, constituting a target population is vaccinated. Their risk of acquiring the disease, again, should be low. Efficacy is again estimated by serological testing, and more precise information on dose–response and safety obtained, with some estimates of the rates of the more common side-effects. The number of doses necessary and some preliminary information on contraindications may also become known after a phase 2 trial.

If the phase 2 trial is satisfactory, a large field trial, the phase 3 trial, of perhaps more than 500 high-risk subjects can begin. Vaccine protection is tested against disease acquisition. Questions that need to be answered in a trial like this will include the efficacy of the vaccine, both in degree and duration, the rate of side-effects, both rare and common, the optimum age for giving vaccine, the dose, including how many and at what intervals, and the need for any adjuvants. Further contraindications to the vaccine may become apparent.

VE can be assessed by measuring disease incidence, by serological test, or both. Important considerations in trials based on disease incidence are how much the two groups (case and control) vary in exposure to the infection, and how infection is ascertained in each group.

If, as is generally believed, vaccinated groups tend to consist of those who are of higher social class, and are thus groups which make better use of health services, diseases such as tuberculosis or whooping cough may be less common in them, or less severe, and hence, less likely to be ascertained. While any such disease is more likely to be reported, these confounding factors are unlikely to cancel out each other. Allocation of persons to vaccine or control groups must be random and double blind to minimize the effect of such biases. This is generally known as random individual allocation. Group allocation—class, village, factory—can also be used in vaccine trials; although the control group must also be matched carefully, it is not usually possible to allocate randomly or for the trial to be double blind. Detailed descriptions of how to conduct trials by individual or group allocation are given by Pollock (1966).

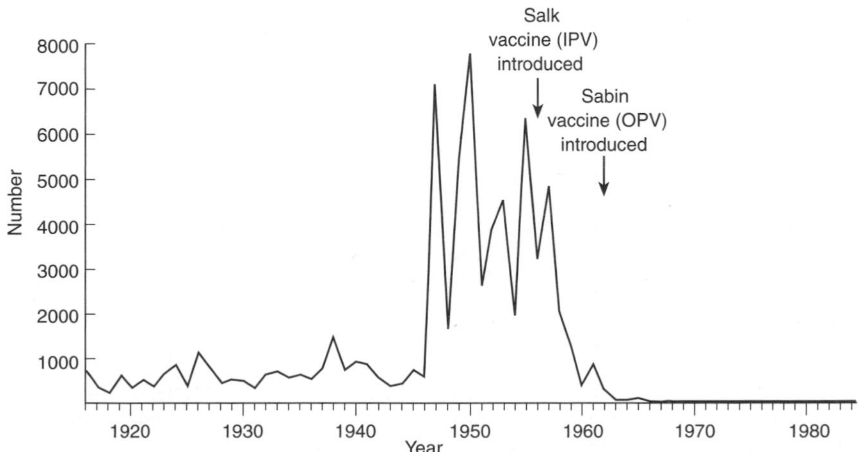

Fig. 12 Poliomyelitis notifications: England and Wales 1919–1983. (Prepared by the Communicable Disease Surveillance Centre.)

The disadvantages of a randomized controlled clinical trial are those of any longitudinal or cohort study: the necessity for large numbers of patients, the expense, the high drop-out rates that occur with long follow-up, and the fact that the vaccine is used under ideal but artificial conditions, the epidemiological equivalent of *in vitro*.

These limitations make postlicensing vaccine trials important (sometimes known as phase 4). Continued assessment, or monitoring, of vaccine use after licensing is mandatory (the equivalent of *in vivo*). Vaccine potency may change, either because of some change at the manufacturing level, or along the chain that gets it to the user, or in storage by the user or as a 'natural' effect with time. The live varicella-zoster vaccine is manufactured to contain 3000 pfu/dose. This is calculated to reach the minimum dose of 1350 pfu by the expiry date, assuming storage under recommended conditions (Arvin 1997). Thus monitoring of vaccines at all levels of the chain is important, especially as vaccines are often used in different climates and different population groups. Rare side-effects may become apparent. In postlicensing trials the populations immunized may be more or less responsive than in the pre-licensing trials on account of a difference in age, social class, or other factors. For these reasons, complacency is unwise after a successful large-scale pre-licensing trial.

Postlicensing monitoring

The success of any vaccine programme will depend on the overall population immunity level achieved. This is a function of efficacy and uptake of vaccine (Noah 1983):

vaccine efficacy × vaccine uptake = population immunity.

The overall immunity level target required will depend on the infectiousness of the disease and on the goals of the vaccine programme, whether it be containment, elimination, or eradication.

VE is at its optimum when the vaccine leaves the manufacturer: factors that may influence efficacy after this include the age of the patient, the site of the injection, the immunological status of the patient, the conditions under which the vaccine has been transported, stored, and made up. In addition, for unknown reasons, the vaccine may not protect some people. Factors influencing the assessment of VE are considered in more detail below.

Vaccine uptake is primarily influenced by the efficiency of the administrative processes in a country or province, but can also be affected by public perception of the vaccine itself (which may be rational or irrational) and of the disease. Generally, a well-organized system for mass vaccination is much more efficient than sporadic vaccination campaigns. Thus, postlicensing studies include not only continuous monitoring of VE, but also of uptake and implementation of the vaccine.

Evaluation of outcome and of side-effects can also be studied.

Assessment of vaccine efficacy

Assessment by incidence

The incidence of the disease in a population after vaccination is compared with that before vaccination. This is a simple and fairly universal undertaking, and is a useful method of assessing the impact of a mass vaccine programme on a population. VE cannot usually be calculated from this method, only the effectiveness of the vaccine programme in broad terms. Moreover, demonstrations of a reduction in incidence following vaccination shows an association that may not be causal, and the well-known rules of Bradford Hill (1971) for assessing causality from association apply. Changing social circumstances, changes in the population, or a natural variation in the incidence of the disease may have caused the change in incidence. In England and Wales scarlet fever declined in both incidence and severity without a vaccine. The use, first, of Salk polio vaccine in 1957, followed by the Sabin vaccine in 1963, reduced the incidence of poliomyelitis to negligible numbers (Fig. 12); however, the introduction of BCG in 1950 had a less than dramatic effect on an already declining disease (Fig. 13). This does not necessarily mean that the BCG vaccine was worthless: a reduction in incidence could have been masked by more complete ascertainment or better diagnosis of cases, and accompanying increase in transmission of or susceptibility to tuberculosis, or a selective decrease in morbidity from a severe but rare form of tuberculosis (e.g. miliary tuberculosis or tuberculosis meningitis), too small to be detected by crude methods. Detailed surveillance would be necessary to detect such changes.

Assessment by immunological testing

Immunological testing includes skin tests, such as tuberculin or Schick, and serological testing. Tuberculin testing, generally using the Heaf or Mantoux tests, is performed to assess a person's immunity before vaccination. It has also been used to assess the quality of different strains of BCG. Schick tests for diphtheria are now performed rarely. The local reaction to smallpox vaccine was used to assess whether or not the vaccine had 'taken'.

Serological testing can be performed using antitoxin (diphtheria and tetanus) or antibody (measles, rubella, etc.) levels. Serological tests first have to be shown to correlate with immunity to disease by disease incidence studies. Studies using such tests can be of two types: seroconversion or seroprevalence (Orenstein *et al.* 1985).

Seroconversion Seroconversion studies are generally used in phases 1 and 2, and sometimes also in phase 3 of pre-licensing trials. They are particularly useful for assessing vaccine response at different ages, as with the measles vaccine, and in different groups of persons; for example, healthy persons and those with immunosuppressive conditions respond differently to pneumococcal vaccine. Seroconversion studies are also useful for assessing VE for rare conditions in which antibody levels have already been shown to correlate with protection,

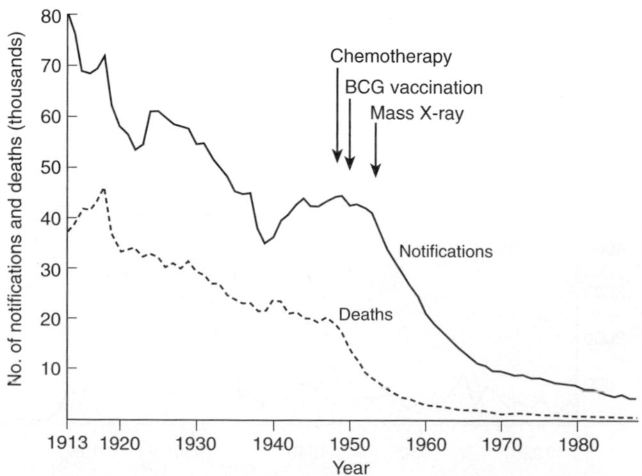

Fig. 13 Respiratory tuberculosis: England and Wales 1913–1988. (Prepared by the Communicable Disease Surveillance Centre.)

as with tetanus, diphtheria, and poliomyelitis. Moreover, seroconversion studies have the advantage that any change in antibody status can be attributed to the vaccine. On the other hand, seroconversion studies require two blood samples and laboratory back up, but these disadvantages can be weighed against the smaller number of subjects that need to be studied. A more serious disadvantage is the absence of a reliable serological test of immunity for some infections, such as whooping cough and meningococcal infections.

Seroconversion studies and incidence studies suffer from the same problems of having a case definition that is too specific (too high an antibody level or too rigorous criteria for diagnosis) thus underestimating efficacy, or one that is too sensitive (too low an antibody level or too loose criteria for diagnosis), which will overestimate efficacy.

Seroprevalence Seroprevalence studies have the advantage of requiring only one blood test but the corresponding disadvantage is relating a 'positive' result to disease or vaccine. Seroprevalence studies can be used to monitor success of the vaccination programme by measuring overall population immunity, which is a function of both efficacy and uptake. Thus, the prevalence of poliovirus antibody in a highly immunized population with no wild virus disease will reflect the efficacy and uptake of the vaccine. The prevalence of rubella antibody in antenatal women or women of childbearing age in a country with a selective rubella vaccine policy (so that the natural epidemics of rubella are virtually unaffected) will measure the overall immunity status of the target group, but it will not easily distinguish how much of this is attributable to natural infection and how much to the success of the vaccine programme (Noah and Fowle 1988). If the expected seroprevalence of rubella antibody in this target group under conditions of natural rubella endemicity is known, then the gain in immunity attributable to vaccination of the target group can be calculated.

With seroprevalence studies the duration of protection can also be evaluated, but Marks *et al.* (1982) pointed out the importance of the timing of immunity measurements since vaccination, and also the age at vaccination. In case–control studies using seroprevalence, these two parameters must be similar in cases and controls; that is, the time lapse between vaccination and testing immunity and the age at vaccination are crucial for matching.

In seroprevalence studies the same caveats apply about sensitivity and specificity of the antitoxin or antibody levels chosen to indicate immunity. In seroprevalence studies the choice of which class of antibody (IgM or IgG) to measure can also be critical.

Seroprevalence studies related to previous vaccination require accurate records of previous vaccination (including timing and number of previous doses of vaccine) for meaningful interpretation (Orenstein *et al.* 1988). Absence of antibody may not always correlate with susceptibility.

Assessment by epidemiological studies

General comments

For epidemiological studies of VE after licensing, a number of general comments need to be made. As with seroprevalence studies, the sensitivity and specificity of the case definition is important, and has always to be a compromise. A highly sensitive case definition will include many spurious cases, leading to a falsely low VE, whereas too specific a case definition will lead to a falsely high VE. Case definition in both control and vaccinated groups should be undertaken with equal vigour, with due awareness of the tendency for case definition to be more specific in the vaccinated group. Exposure in the two groups should be similar; even if vaccinated and control groups have been closely matched by age, sex, social class, and geographical distribution, variations in exposure may still occur. The diagnosis should if possible be made 'blind' (Marks *et al.* 1982). In retrospective studies, ascertainment of vaccination history in the two groups must also be pursued with equal vigour, and again should preferably be done 'blind'. Those with a previous history of the infection should not be included in either group of subjects.

Cohort studies

Outbreak investigations

An outbreak often affords an opportunity to assess VE in a field setting (*in vivo*). The basic steps are to define the cohort under investigation, ascertain all cases according to an acceptable case definition, ascertain vaccination histories in the entire cohort, and calculate attack rates in vaccinated and unvaccinated persons, excluding those with a previous history of disease. For very large cohorts sampling or cluster sampling (Henderson and Sundaresan 1982) can be used. In infections in which most cases occur in fairly well demarcated age groups, the cohort under study will usually exclude those outside these age groups, as well as those too young to have been vaccinated. The optimum age of vaccination can also be ascertained from outbreak studies (Judelsohn *et al.* 1980).

Secondary attack rates in households

Measuring the attack rates in members of a household (secondary cases) following the introduction of an infection by one member of the family (primary case) affords an attractive approach to VE studies because exposures in vaccinated and unvaccinated persons are similar, thus eliminating an important bias in these studies, and also because the denominators (those exposed) can be fairly accurately determined. These types of study, however, need more careful planning than most other postlicensing studies, and they are usually better designed as prospective studies. They also need to be planned to take place during periods of high epidemicity of the infection. Studies on pertussis vaccine in England and Wales, which used secondary attack rates in households, suggested that the vaccines were ineffective (PHLS Whooping Cough Committee and Working Party 1973; PHLS Epidemiological Research Laboratory 1982). This was difficult to believe because the incidence of whooping cough in the country at the time of the first study had been decreasing steadily, and other studies (Noah 1976; Pollard 1980; PHLS Epidemiological Research Laboratory 1982) suggested that the vaccine was effective. The reasons for the failure of the household exposure studies to confirm efficacy were examined by Fine *et al.* (1988); they attributed the apparent lack of VE primarily to the inclusion of retrospectively ascertained cases and of households in which the primary cases constituted a vaccine failure. Secondary attack rates in households have also been used to measure the efficacy of hepatitis A vaccine in preventing secondary cases of the infection (Sagliocca *et al.* 1999)

Cluster sampling (Henderson and Sundaresan 1982) is a modified form of this method of estimating VE. It has the advantage of being cheaper and easier to conduct than a household study, and hence particularly suitable for developing countries, but it is also less rigorous (Orenstein *et al.* 1985).

Retrospective population cohort studies

This type of study depends on the availability of fairly sophisticated disease reporting and vaccination recording systems. For each case of disease ascertained, the vaccination history is verified, and from the number and percentage of those vaccinated in the base population, the attack rates in those vaccinated and unvaccinated can be calculated and VE derived (Noah 1976).

The effectiveness of vaccination, but not its efficacy, can sometimes be checked crudely by observing the correlation between the incidence of disease in separate districts with the vaccination rates in those districts (Sutherland and Fayers 1971; Pollard 1980; Noah and Fowle 1988). Sometimes chance plays a part in affording an opportunity to estimate VE, as in 1970–71 in Texarkana, a city straddling the Texas–Arkansas state line. The Texas side differed from the Arkansas side only in not having a measles vaccine policy, so that during the outbreak of measles, the attack rate (**AR**) in the Texas side of the city was 48.2 per cent compared with 4.2 per cent in the Arkansas side. VE, based on ARs of 105.9 per thousand and 4.3 per thousand in the unimmunized and in the immunized respectively, was 95.9 per cent (Landrigan 1972).

Case–control studies

Case–control studies in vaccination assessments are not common. The design of a case–control vaccine study is similar to that of any other case–control study. Each case of the disease is compared with one or more matched controls without the disease for a history of vaccination against the disease. As in all case–control studies, 'first cases must be representative of all cases in a specified population with respect to the exposure of interest, and controls must be similarly representative of all non-cases in the same specified population. Second information about exposures and other characteristics must be similar in quality for both cases and controls' (Comstock 1994). These specifications are extremely difficult to achieve in vaccine case–control studies. The advantages of a case–control study on the other hand are that it can be done more cheaply, quickly, and with fewer cases than for a cohort study. Moreover, the efficacy of vaccine given many years before can be assessed (Smith 1988) and this approach was used recently in a study in the Gambia to assess the efficacy of three or more doses of trivalent oral polio vaccine (Deming 1992). Nevertheless, bias can occur as the vaccines will not have been administered at random (as, for example, if those of higher SE class have higher vaccination rates but lower expectancy of disease), and the vaccine histories in cases and controls may not be accurate (Smith 1988). The problems that need to be given attention in the design of case–control studies are similar to those in cohort vaccine studies. Comstock (1994) has dealt recently with this subject in some detail and Rodrigues and Smith (1999) have written a useful review of the case–control approach to vaccine evaluation.

The case–control method, nevertheless, lends itself well to BCG efficacy studies (Miceli *et al.* 1988; Smith 1988). First, when the overall incidence of the disease is low, the case–control approach can be used on existing cases of disease to evaluate a vaccine given many years earlier, making it cheaper, quicker, and easier to do than a cohort study. Second, because of the expense of large cohort studies and the time needed to assess the efficacy of BCG, the case–control approach is a more practical one. Third, the difficulty of a 'double-blind' approach to a vaccine such as BCG, and fourth, the large variation (from 100 to 57 per cent) in estimates of efficacy of BCG with randomized controlled trials, underline the disadvantages of the cohort approach in trials of BCG.

Calculation of vaccine efficacy

VE is the ratio of the observed diminution in ARs, that is, the difference in ARs between vaccinated and unvaccinated groups, to the expected AR, in the unvaccinated group. Thus

$$\mathrm{VE} = \frac{\mathrm{AR\ (unvaccinated)} - \mathrm{AR\ (vaccinated)}}{\mathrm{AR\ (unvaccinated)}} \times 100 \text{ per cent}$$

or

$$\mathrm{VE} = (1 - \mathrm{RR}) \times 100 \text{ per cent}$$

where RR is the ratio of AR(vaccinated) to AR(unvaccinated), or relative risk.

In a case–control study, using unmatched controls and odds ratios (OR), results can be arranged as shown in Table 1. Then

$$\mathrm{VE} = (1 - \mathrm{OR}) \times 100 \text{ per cent}$$

where $\mathrm{OR} = ad/bc$.

Refinements of these basic formulae can be found in Orenstein *et al.* (1985) and the impact of various types of bias on VE results is discussed by Orenstein *et al.* (1988).

Monitoring of side-effects of vaccines

Common side-effects

Monitoring side-effects of vaccines begins at the very first phase of vaccine trials, running in parallel with estimations of efficacy. With randomized controlled trials, the evaluation of side-effects after vaccination is fairly straightforward, it being usually sufficient to compare the incidence of any reactions in cases with that in controls. Where it is not practical, possible, or ethical to conduct a placebo-controlled study, some care is necessary in the interpretation of information on side-effects. In uncontrolled cohort studies, local side-effects (such as a stiff or painful arm) can still be evaluated successfully, but other symptoms, such as fever or convulsions that are non-specific to vaccines and may commonly occur from other causes in healthy children, are more difficult to evaluate without a control group. The time between the vaccination and the appearance of a side-effect also needs to be evaluated carefully. In the earliest trials of MMR vaccine meningitis caused by the mumps component was not documented until the subjects were followed up for at least 28 days (Miller *et al.* 1993).

In the early measles vaccine trials in England (Measles Vaccine Committee of the Medical Research Council 1966) 9577 children aged 10 months to 2 years were immunized. Eighteen children developed convulsions, 11 of them between post-vaccination days 6 and 9. Only five convulsions were reported in the control group of 16 327 children, none of them between days 6 and 9. This study established not only

Table 1 Arrangement of results in case–control study

	Case	**Control**
Vaccinated	*a*	*b*
Unvaccinated	*c*	*d*

that convulsions were a real side-effect of measles vaccine, but also that they characteristically occurred during a fixed interval after the vaccine. The need to compare this with the incidence of convulsions after natural disease was also apparent, and they were shown to be at least 10 times more common after the disease than after the vaccine (Miller 1978). This was an extremely important finding in support of the vaccine and illustrates the value of careful epidemiological work in the study of vaccines. In a more recent example (Miller *et al.* 1993), a side-effect of mumps vaccine (aseptic meningitis) was discovered to be more common than expected (1 in 11 000 doses compared with 4 per million) and to be associated with a vaccine derived from a particular strain (Urabe). This was only discovered after the vaccine was licensed. It was subsequently and promptly withdrawn.

Unlike drug trials, the side-effects of a vaccine can sometimes be evaluated not by using a placebo in the control group but by giving a combination of vaccines omitting the vaccine under trial. The side-effects of pertussis vaccine have been investigated by comparing symptoms in the case group after diphtheria–tetanus–pertussis vaccine (**DTP**) with those after DT vaccine in the controls (Pollock *et al.* 1984). Even in this controlled study it was found that adverse publicity to pertussis vaccine led to a reporting bias in the cases given DTP.

Rare side-effects

Various ingenious studies have been set up to investigate the incidence of rare side-effects after vaccination. In Denmark, Melchior (1977) compared the age-specific incidence of infantile spasms during the period when the whooping cough vaccine was given at 5 months, 6 months, and 15 months with that during the period when it was given at 5 weeks, 9 weeks, and 10 months, and found no difference. In England the extremely rare alleged side-effects of serious and permanent (but non-specific) brain damage after whooping cough vaccine (with wildly varying quoted rates of 1 in 50 000 to 1 in a million) were difficult to refute, mainly because of its rarity, and the lack of a recognizable and confirmable syndrome. The publicity engendered by this led to a dramatic fall in the pertussis vaccine uptake rate from about 79 per cent in the early 1970s to 31 per cent in 1975. A carefully controlled case–control study, the National Childhood Encephalopathy Study, was conducted. In this study the presence or absence of a history of recent vaccination was obtained in all cases of 'encephalopathy' reported to the study team and compared with controls. An association was shown between DTP given 3 to 7 days earlier and encephalopathy, but not between DT given at the same time and encephalopathy. It was possible to estimate from this study that the risk of persistent neurological damage in previously healthy children after pertussis vaccine was 1 in 310 000 immunizations, but the 95 per cent confidence limits were very wide, from 1 in 54 000 to 1 in 5.31 million. The reader is referred to the original study (Department of Health and Social Security 1981) for further details of methodology, and to Miller *et al.* (1982) for a balanced review of the whooping cough vaccine controversy.

Other forms of side-effect evaluation include postmarketing surveillance, which may be active or passive (Stetler *et al.* 1987). An active surveillance system is less prone to bias, but is likely to be too expensive and unwieldy; the passive system is more prone to bias, but clearly simpler and cheaper. The record linkage method of post-licensure safety assessment also promises to be a useful and reliable method for the routine surveillance of vaccine safety (Miller *et al.* 1998), as rare side-effects sometimes only become apparent late, often after large well-conducted controlled trials have been successfully completed.

Epidemiological side-effects of vaccination programmes

Mass immunization is mass interference with an ecological process, and inevitably there are side-effects. The most common of these are changes in the age distribution of the infection. The natural cycles of infection are often altered. Usually, if the mass immunization programme involves infants and children, all that this means is a shift of the age distribution to an older age group, without a sustained accompanying increase in incidence in that age group. Outbreaks of rubella and measles in young adults have been reported. This is because if less than ideal coverage occurs or a poor vaccine is used for a mass programme, herd immunity will ensure that fewer people who are susceptible will be exposed to the virus. A group of susceptible persons will then form a 'cohort' who may contract the disease in later life.

In Greece, congenital rubella increased in incidence (Panagiotopoulos *et al.* 1999)—indeed it was reported as an 'epidemic' which occurred in 1993. This was attributed to a sustained poor coverage of less than 50 per cent with MMR vaccine in 1-year-old children. The reported incidence of congenital rubella was 24.6 per 100 000 births in 1993. This was the reported incidence in a single year and the authors did not estimate how much lower than expected was the incidence in the intervening years. Even in this situation it is unlikely that a truly sustained increase in incidence occurred over a long period.

Uptake and implementation of vaccines

> One has to be a stranger in Jerusalem not to realise that public acceptance of an immunisation procedure determines its success or failure. (Cohen 1978)

The need for field studies in vaccines does not cease at efficacy studies. The implementation of the vaccine is as important as its production, and an effective safe vaccine with poor uptake is of hardly greater benefit than no vaccine at all. In recent years this has been recognized and field studies to investigate the factors that influence uptake of vaccines are now common.

Studies on uptake may measure factors associated with social or service conditions. In one study (Jarman *et al.* 1988), social conditions associated with being underprivileged (such as overcrowding, unmarried, or single parents), living in high population density areas, being unskilled, and belonging to certain ethnic groups were found to be linked to low immunization uptake. Reasons given by family (Clarke 1980; Blair *et al.* 1985; Lakhani *et al.* 1987) or by clinic staff (Adjaye 1981; Lakhani *et al.* 1987) for refusal can also be investigated. Single-handed GPs, those aged over 65 years, or those with large list sizes and less than average expenditure on community health services were also associated with low uptake rates (Jarman *et al.* 1988). The efficiency of organization, quality of premises, and adequacy of staffing of three different types of immunization clinic—GP, health centre, and child health clinic—were found to affect compliance (Alberman *et al.*1986).

In another study the provision of individual performance indicators was enough to stimulate GPs to improve rates (Newlands and Davies 1988). Smith *et al.* (1976) noted an interesting phenomenon with an annual influenza vaccination programme in industry: in successive years the uptake of vaccine fell considerably. The reasons for this were fairly complex and were probably associated with the need for giving vaccine yearly, the low incidence of influenza during the periods over which the vaccine was given, and the general perception by the target population that the vaccine was not very effective. The message that emanates from many of these studies, however, is that it is the administrative efficiency of the immunization programme and the motivation of the professionals that are the critical features in improving uptake (Noah 1982; Lakhani *et al.* 1987). Communication strategies can be designed to persuade people to attend (Hingson 1974) and are best used for immunization campaigns.

Evaluation of factors affecting vaccine programmes

The evaluation of the outcome of a vaccine programme can be conducted in several ways. Except with the most successful programmes reasons for non-acceptance of vaccine can be investigated. Reasons for failure/poor uptake may be because of social and professional attitudes to the vaccine, including the effect of the media, or the administrative competence/managerial abilities of those responsible for the programme.

Social and professional attitudes to a vaccine or a vaccine programme may 'make or break' the programme. Tenuous evidence that a vaccine may cause serious side-effects, when given the appropriate publicity, can be enough to reduce uptake considerably. An appropriate label for this phenomenon, for it has occurred more than once, is the 'cry-wolf syndrome'. In the United Kingdom, reports by Kulenkampff *et al.* (1974) of alleged brain damage following the whooping cough vaccine, fuelled by a television programme in the same year, and by 'the writings in the lay press and medical journals and media interviews of a professor who was a 'leading critic of the vaccination policy' (Cherry 1986) led to a catastrophic fall in pertussis vaccine uptake rates from about 79 per cent between 1967 and 1974 to a low of 30 per cent in 1978. Television programmes were found to be especially influential (McKinnon 1979). The controversy had an effect on other routine vaccinations (DT and poliomyelitis), which fortunately was transient and relatively slight. A survey of professional attitudes during the episode (Wilkinson *et al.* 1979) suggested that GPs, clinic doctors, or health visitors were ambivalent towards the pertussis vaccine. Most had noticed an increase in parental concern about the vaccine, which was attributed to 'irresponsible', 'ill-controlled', or 'biased' publicity. Moreover, this phenomenon occurred in the United Kingdom without the often-cited problem of litigation risk in the United States.

Adjaye (1981), however, found that parental attitudes towards immunization were greatly influenced by medical and non-medical members of the health professions, while Berkeley (1983) in a study of attitudes to measles vaccine found that the professionals themselves were unsure about the contraindications to vaccine and to its value. In another study (Guest *et al.* 1986) many professionals offered invalid reasons for failure to give immunization.

Campbell (1983), in analysing reasons for poor uptake of the measles vaccine in Britain, suggested that attitudes and ignorance, a cumbersome policy-making bureaucracy, the absence of legislation (which helped the United States programme) and of a standard record card for each child, and the initiative and motivation required by mothers towards a vaccine given some months after the primary course, were factors that accounted for the unpopularity of measles vaccine in Britain. Encouraging the health professionals to take greater initiative was found to benefit uptake (Carter and Jones 1985). These and other studies (Bussey and Harris 1979; Pugh and Hawker 1986; Lakhani *et al.* 1987) suggested that education of health professionals and an efficient administration with computerized recall and records were important factors in improving uptake rates. In more recent years in Britain, a more efficient system for the administration of vaccination programmes, together with the rapid evaluation of immunization rates (the COVER programme) (Begg *et al.* 1989) have helped considerably in raising MMR vaccine immunization rates to well over 90 per cent. With the computerized COVER programme, districts with poor immunization rates can be targeted. The addition of the mumps and rubella components to the existing measles vaccine has undoubtedly helped also. Indeed this emphasis on efficient administration has since brought the vaccine uptake rates to acceptable levels. In the United States, school immunization laws were also a proven method of improving immunization uptake (Robbins *et al.* 1981), although its value should not be taken for granted in other countries.

Unfortunately, the 'cry-wolf' syndrome has reappeared in Britain to affect measles vaccine uptake. This arose from some weak evidence that Crohn's disease and childhood autism may be associated with measles vaccine (Thompson *et al.* 1995), even though there is good evidence that either association is unlikely (Miller and Waight 1998; Pebody *et al.* 1998; Taylor *et al.* 1999, 2000).

Evaluation of outcome of immunization programmes

The case for long-term serological surveillance of immunization programmes has been forcefully advocated by Evans (1980) and Raska (1971). Evans argued that a surveillance system based on the reporting of disease alone was insufficiently sensitive or specific to monitor a vaccine programme. An individual's history of immunization or disease correlated well with antibody presence in measles and mumps, but less well in rubella and poliomyelitis; moreover, for tetanus natural infection has virtually no bearing on antibody levels.

The reliability of a negative history of disease or immunization was, however, poor for measles, mumps, and rubella. The serological demonstration of satisfactory levels of durable antibody in immunized persons was a more reliable measure of vaccine effectiveness than monitoring the incidence of the disease itself, and absence of antibody in particular communities or specific age groups could identify those who may need protection. Long-term surveillance of immunity after measles vaccination has also been advocated (Anonymous 1976). Serological studies have shown that vaccine failure and not waning vaccine-induced antibody accounted for most of the low or undetectable antibody titres in immunized children, especially those immunized before 13 months of age (Yeager *et al.* 1977).

A study of measles vaccine on the survival pattern of 7- to 35-month-old children in Kasongo, Zaire (Kasongo Project Team 1981) used life-table analysis to evaluate outcome of the vaccination programme in a community with a high measles incidence and measles case-fatality rate. They found that, although the measles vaccine programme undoubtedly reduced the risk of measles death, overall survival was less influenced by measles vaccine after 22 months of age.

Another study found that the success of a vaccine programme against measles, mumps, and rubella using the MMR vaccine was reflected in the virtual disappearance of a common complication of all three infections (encephalitis) in their population of children (Koski-niemi and Vaheri 1989). Improved intellectual performance was an outcome noted in a cohort study in children who had been immunized against pertussis compared with those who had been hospitalized for the disease, even after allowing for social differences in the two groups (Butler *et al.* 1982).

Costing studies of vaccines

Costing studies are important both in assessing the need for a vaccine and in evaluating its efficiency. The detailed methodology of costing studies for infectious disease is considered elsewhere in this book. Costs include costs of the vaccine and its administration. Costs of the vaccine may be influenced by factors as diverse as costs of development and market competition: the price of human-derived hepatitis B vaccine halved when the yeast-derived vaccine began to be marketed. Administration costs will include the cost of the syringe, personnel, accommodation as well as costs of initiating and administering a record and follow-up programme. Benefits include savings on treatment costs, mortality, morbidity, the avoidance of intangibles such as pain and grief, and external benefits (Creese and Henderson 1980). It is debatable whether social benefits of successful intervention should be costed, because the value of such benefits may not be convincing to pragmatic health-care managers. Patrick and Woolley (1981) have pointed out that health managers may fail to be impressed by cost–benefit studies because the costs, which are health costs, have to be weighed against benefits that are usually social. Nevertheless, the benefits of providing supportive cost calculations are an important addition to the valuation of a vaccination programme.

A list of the benefits of immunization, simply and clearly stated, often cannot fail to convince as in one of the earliest such papers (Witte and Axnick 1975) describing the results of 10 years of measles immunization in the United States in terms of lower morbidity and mortality, and improved quality of life (Table 2).

Other studies (Creese and Henderson 1980; Koplan 1985) have amply shown the value for money of measles vaccine in terms of benefit–cost ratios for measles vaccine ranging from 10:1 to 15:1. Cost studies can be successfully performed in general practice (Binnie 1984). In this general practice, over a 20-year period, immunization not only brought about a small financial reward, but also reduced the number of consultations by 40 per cent, even though a home visit was often necessary to immunize a child. Examples of cost–benefit analysis of various immunizations that have demonstrated the benefit of vaccines, and to which the reader is referred for details of methodology, include measles vaccine (Witte and Axnick 1975; Albritton 1978), pertussis vaccine (Koplan *et al.* 1979; Hinman and Koplan 1984, 1985), mumps vaccine (White *et al.* 1985; Koplan and Preblud 1982), poliomyelitis (Fudenberg 1973), pneumococcal vaccine (Patrick and Woolley 1981), and hepatitis B in homosexuals (Adler *et al.* 1983). General articles on cost–benefits of immunization programmes include Creese and Henderson (1980) and Koplan (1985). A formula has been developed for calculating vaccine profitability, defined as the economic yield, positive or negative, obtained per monetary unit invested in a campaign (Carvasco and Lardinois 1987).

Table 2 Benefits of measles immunization over 10 years (United States)

Type of savings	
Cases averted	23 707 000
Lives saved	2400
Cases of retardation averted	7900
Additional years of normal and productive life by preventing premature death and retardation	709 000
School days saved	78 000 000
Physician visits saved	12 182 000
Hospital days saved	1 352 000
Net benefits	$1.3 billion

Source: Witte and Axnick (1975).

Conclusion

This section shows that the methods used in the study of the epidemiology of infection are similar to those used for any other type of disease, but are also sufficiently different to warrant special consideration. This is best illustrated in the section on vaccines. Surveillance, first used in infectious disease, has become an essential technique in public health practice generally. The importance of collaboration between epidemiologists and other scientists, discussed here in relation to the microbiologist, is relevant to any epidemiological specialism.

The epidemiologist and the microbiology laboratory

Close collaboration between infectious disease epidemiologists and microbiologists is essential for effective outbreak investigation and control, for surveillance, and for vaccine use. Moreover, the microbiologist needs the epidemiologist and to have an understanding of epidemiology, as much as the epidemiologist needs the microbiologist and knowledge of microbiology. Microbiology and epidemiology each has strengths and weaknesses that need to be acknowledged; a partnership between the two disciplines is essential in infectious disease epidemiology so that each can complement the other.

Outbreaks often cannot be effectively investigated without the use of epidemiology—in some food poisoning incidents, for example, microbiological technology is still too limited to be able to identify the causal organism in the implicated food or in affected patients. In others, the implicated foods may be unavailable for microbiological testing. Similarly, some outbreak investigations will be unsuccessful without the use of microbiology; in an outbreak of fever and rash in a school in England (McEvoy *et al.* 1987), the epidemiological investigation was considerably hampered by the lack of a microbiological diagnosis. This outbreak is described in more detail below.

For surveillance of infectious disease, notifications based on clinical diagnosis alone, although useful if laboratory support is not available, are often lacking in precision and detail. In epidemiological studies and monitoring of vaccines, microbiological support is also essential for added precision, including for example, evaluating the effect of vaccine on carriage of an organism. Facets of this collaboration between the epidemiologist and the microbiologist (and indeed with other disciplines, such as entomologists and zoologists) are explored in more detail below.

Microbiology for epidemiologists

Infectious disease epidemiologists require sound technical understanding of infection and micro-organisms to perform their work effectively. Knowledge of the ease or difficulty and expense of undertaking laboratory tests is clearly important. An understanding of what the tests mean, and of their sensitivity and specificity is needed for informed interpretation of the results. The epidemiological significance of typing of organisms also has to be understood, as does the meaning of complex antibody tests, e.g. for hepatitis B virus. A working understanding of immunology is also necessary. Some clinical knowledge of infectious disease is essential for the effective recognition and definition of cases, and for their management.

Epidemiology for microbiologists

Microbiologists likewise should have an understanding of the strengths and limitations of epidemiology to be able to work in partnership with epidemiologists. This applies equally both to those microbiologists working in the community and in the hospital. Massive uncoordinated sampling of patients and/or food and the environment can usually be avoided in outbreak investigation. Knowledge of sensitivity and specificity, especially applied to laboratory testing, is essential. For surveillance the importance of routine reporting following clearly defined rules must be recognized.

Aspects of the collaboration between epidemiologist and microbiologist are considered under the subjects of surveillance, outbreaks, and vaccines.

The laboratory in surveillance

Collaboration between microbiologist and epidemiologist undoubtedly leads to more sensitive and more refined surveillance, widening its scope considerably. Notifications of infectious disease, although essential, at best are usually fairly crude indicators of infection.

Confirmation of diagnosis

Clinical diagnoses, normally the basis for notifications, are not always accurate. Clinical malaria in south-eastern United States was shown by laboratory investigation not to be malaria when the Centers for Disease Control was first established in 1941; this early example underlined the importance of the laboratory in surveillance (Langmuir 1963). Rubella is notoriously difficult to diagnose clinically; it is often confused with Fifth disease, for example, and a laboratory surveillance system that includes both rubella virus and parvovirus B19 will distinguish between these. In a successful vaccine programme, as the disease reaches low levels, it is often necessary to confirm each notified case by using the laboratory. Otherwise it is impossible to judge the success of the intervention with any confidence. In the WHO programme for the world eradication of poliomyelitis, the laboratory is essential for confirming the diagnosis even in this easily recognizable and characteristic disease. For WHO to ratify eradication (Wright *et al.* 1991), a country has to continue surveillance with laboratory backup for 3 years before the last confirmed case.

Reaching precision in diagnosis

Most notifiable diseases lack precision, which the laboratory can give. Influenza covers several types, subtypes and variants (Table 3), which are generally indistinguishable clinically. Food poisoning covers not only several different types of infection, but often each of these infections can also be typed or subtyped further. Thus the causes of food poisoning include salmonellas, *Clostridium perfringens*, staphylococci, and *Escherichia coli*. All those organisms can be typed, and the more common salmonellas can be further phage-typed to afford even greater precision in diagnosis. The use of molecular techniques in diagnosis has expanded considerably in recent years and can be used for surveillance as well as outbreak investigation. Antibiotic resistance patterns can also be used for surveillance. Table 3 gives some examples of the precision and detail that surveillance underpinned by the laboratory can provide. Some of this detail is only useful for precision within outbreaks, e.g. phage-typing of staphylococci and *C. perfringens;* others are useful for surveillance—salmonellas, influenza, and meningococcal meningitis.

Increasing the scope of surveillance

There are many infections for which only laboratory surveillance is feasible—these include legionnaires' disease, psittacosis and Q fever, most adenoviral infections, and the enteroviruses (coxsackie A and B, echoviruses). Many of these infections are important public health problems, especially in better-developed countries in which the more traditional epidemic infections found in developing countries have become less common. Most of these infections are important enough to require surveillance to underpin outbreak investigation. Psittacosis and Q fever are zoonoses, and the enteroviruses cause outbreaks of lymphocytic meningitis, Bornholm disease, and other clinical conditions in the autumn season. The environmental sources of legionnaires' disease—mainly water—are well known.

International surveillance

Laboratory diagnosis is important for international surveillance. The spread of *Vibrio cholerae* el Tor across the world has been well-documented (Anonymous 1993). International surveillance of the subtypes and variants of influenza A virus is critical both for documenting spread and for early warning, and for the formulation of vaccines (Gensheimer *et al.* 1999; Snacken *et al.* 1997). Further examples of important infections in which laboratory backup of surveillance plays a key part in control are dengue, HIV-1 and HIV-2, and malaria.

Vectors and reservoirs of infection

The use of the laboratory in tracking the origin and spread of infection in animals and arthropods, as well as in water and soil, is important but will not be discussed here in detail. Influenza virus is of particular interest because of the interchanges and evolution of infection between a variety of animals and humans. The possible origin of new influenza subtypes in the pig and duck populations and its relationship to their agricultural environment of parts of China are still being studied (Webster *et al.* 1992), and the concern caused by avian influenza virus crossing the species barrier from chickens to humans (Snacken *et al.* 1997) was worldwide. The existence of a 'zoonotic pool' for viruses (Morse 1993) clearly justifies close epidemiological and microbiological surveillance to continue for the foreseeable future.

The laboratory in epidemiological investigation of vaccines

Technical microbiological expertise is clearly crucial to the development and preparation of vaccines, and will not be considered further here. The use of the microbiological laboratory will be considered more fully in the section on the field investigation of vaccines in this chapter, so will only be considered in outline.

Table 3 Examples of detail provided by the laboratory

Disease for notification	Laboratory details		
Food poisoning	Salmonellas		
	S. typhimurium	Phage typing	
	S. enteritidis	Phage typing	
	Clostridium		
	C. perfringens	Toxins in faeces	
		Phage typing	
	Staphylococci		
	Staph. aureus	Enterotoxins in food	
	E. coli etc.	O groups	
Influenza	Influenza A	Subtype	Variant
		(e.g. A/Hong Kong)	(e.g. A/Johannesburg/33/94)
	Influenza B		Variant
			(e.g. B/Beijing/184/93)
Meningitis	Bacterial		
	N. meningitidis	Group A, B, C, etc.	Serotyping/sulphonamide
	Strep. pneumoniae		resistance
	H. influenzae		
	etc.		
	Viral		
	Lymphocytic meningitis	Echovirus	
		Coxsackie virus	
Dysentery	Shigella		
	S. sonnei	Types	
	S. flexneri	Types	
	etc.		
	Entamoeba histolytica		
Viral hepatitis	Types A, B, C, D, E, F	Limited typing for type B, but can differentiate between acute infection, 'high-risk' and 'low-risk' carriers, postvaccination state	

In phase 1 and 2 trials, efficacy is usually assessed by measurement of antibody, which requires serological testing. In phase II trials in particular, phasing of vaccine doses will depend on antibody levels found. In field trials (phase 3) microbiology is usually required to confirm diagnosis of cases occurring in both case and control groups, and this may be done by isolation and typing of the organism, or by serology, or both.

As a vaccine programme develops the overall incidence will fall, but cases will continue to occur for some time and microbiological confirmation of diagnosis becomes more important as the incidence diminishes to very low levels. In the present WHO initiative to eradicate poliomyelitis from the world, laboratory facilities worldwide needed strengthening to investigate every reported case of acute flaccid paralysis (Wright *et al.* 1991). Only when every reported case of acute flaccid paralysis proves not to be poliomyelitis over a period of 3 years can there be confidence that eradication has been achieved.

Assessment of vaccine success by serological testing of populations will be described in the section on the field investigations of vaccines.

The laboratory in outbreak investigation

In no other situation is the partnership between microbiologist and epidemiologist more important perhaps than in the investigation of an outbreak. Some outbreaks—such as food-borne outbreaks of small round structured virus infection or hepatitis A—can really only be solved by epidemiological techniques, as the causative organisms cannot easily be detected in food. In others, especially those food-borne outbreaks in which the menu does not offer a choice, so that everyone usually eats everything on offer, the epidemiologist is considerably restricted, and a microbiological solution is often the only hope.

Inevitably, in many outbreaks no foods are available for testing, so that epidemiological analysis is essential. In other outbreaks too many foods are available for microbiological analysis: in a continuing outbreak of gastroenteritis on board ship, investigated by the PHLS Communicable Disease Surveillance Centre, London (O'Mahony *et al.* 1986), no particular meal was obviously at fault. More than 400 food items and ingredients were available for testing and a microbiological approach would have meant that all these had to be tested, without any guarantee of success Careful epidemiological analysis of the outbreak by time, place, and person showed that drinking water was the probable cause of the outbreak, and subsequent investigation of the water tanks revealed a defect through which the water was probably contaminated by sewage outfall from the ship. In other food poisoning outbreaks, the epidemiological proof can be overwhelming, although the level of contamination in the offending food is so low that it is only confidence in the epidemiology that enables the laboratory to persist in ensuring 'microbiological proof'. In an outbreak of *Salmonella ealing* infection caused by powdered infant milk, laboratories sampled more than 4000 unopened milk cartons before the organism was isolated (Rowe *et al.* 1987).

The outbreak of *Streptobacillus moniliformis* infection in a girls' school in rural England illustrated well the need for microbiological and epidemiological expertise (McEvoy *et al.* 1987). Until the microbiological diagnosis was made, the epidemiologists were attempting to analyse a large number of risk factors found in a rural and school environment. When the illness was diagnosed, a review of the literature revealed that one previous outbreak of the infection had been described in Haverhill, Massachusetts (hence the alternative name of Haverhill fever for the illness), and had been attributed to raw milk. The girls in the school had indeed been exposed to raw milk. However, subsequent careful epidemiological analysis showed water to be the cause. An examination of the water supply revealed that water from a pond in the school grounds, which was infested with rodents, was contaminating the school drinking water supply after it had been chlorinated.

Microbiology is useful for confirming foods and other sources of infection in outbreaks, such as water tanks (*Campylobacter*) and cooling towers (*Legionella pneumophila*), birds (psittacosis), and animals (rabies, plague). Increasing precision in microbiological diagnosis—typing of organisms such as phage typing and more recently molecular techniques, as well as typing of toxins—has clearly been useful. In an outbreak of AIDS attributed to a dentist in Florida, molecular typing showed identical patterns in the virus obtained from patients and the primary case, thus confirming beyond reasonable doubt that he had indeed caused the infection in his patients (Hillis and Huelsenbeck 1994).

The epidemiologist can on the other hand aid the microbiologist in giving guidance on the number of patients to test in an outbreak, and the foods or other items that need to be sampled. The pattern of the outbreak is also crucial to its management—in propagated or case-to-case outbreaks, e.g. a salmonella outbreak in a hospital, a planned epidemiological and microbiological approach to both investigation and management is the most efficient option. Point source outbreaks on the other hand tend to create more publicity but are on the whole easier to control. The epidemiologist's role in differentiating between these two types of outbreaks is essential.

The work of the microbiologist in assessing levels of contamination in food is important to management and prevention. Levels of salmonella contamination in eggs have been shown to be extremely low, and the organisms have been discovered in both the white and the yolk, either together or separately (Humphrey *et al.* 1989). This type of information ensures that correct advice on prevention can be given for handling and cooking eggs.

Management issues

In a successful partnership there is always a need for standard operating procedures, which should be drawn up carefully and followed by all participants. These should include protocols for surveillance, covering the reporting of results (when, what, and how) by the laboratory and feedback by the epidemiologists. Standards for laboratory reporting and for epidemiological analysis, and the development and roll-out of new tests as they come into routine use, should be covered. Confidentiality issues on both sides should also be carefully laid down and the appropriate safeguards spelled out.

References

Adjaye, N. (1981). Measles immunization. Some factors affecting non-acceptance of vaccine. *Public Health, London*, **95**, 185.

Adler, M.W., Belsey, E.M., McCutchan, J.A., *et al.* (1983). Should homosexuals be vaccinated against hepatitis B? Cost and benefit assessment. c*British Medical Journal*, **286**, 1621.

Alberman, E., Watson, E., Mitchell, P., *et al.* (1986). The development of performance and cost indicators for preschool immunization. *Archives of Disease in Childhood*, **61**, 251.

Albritton, R.B. (1978). Cost-benefits of measles eradication: effects of a federal intervention. *Policy Analysis*, **4**, 1.

Anonymous (1976). Leading article: vaccination against measles. *Lancet*, **ii**, 132–4.

Anonymous (1993). Cholera—update end of 1993. *Weekly Epidemiological Record*, **69**, 13–20.

Arvin, A.M. (1997). The varicella vaccine. *Current Clinical Topics in Infectious Diseases*, **17**, 110–46.

Begg, N.T., Gill, O.N., and White, J. (1989). COVER (cover of vaccination evaluation rapidly): description of the England and Wales scheme. *Public Health*, **103**, 81.

Berkeley, M.I.K. (1983). *Measles—the effect of attitudes on immunisation*, 41/3, pp. 141–7. Health Bulletin. Scottish Home and Health Department, Edinburgh.

Binnie, G.A.C. (1984). Measles immunization profit and loss in a general practice. *British Medical Journal*, **289**, 1275.

Blair, S., Shave, N., and McKay, J. (1985). Measles matters, but do parents know? *British Medical Journal*, **290**, 623.

Boussard, E., Flahault, A., Vibert, J-F., and Valleron, A.J. (1996). Sentiweb: French communicable disease surveillance on the world-wide web. *British Medical Journal*, **313**, 1381–4.

Bradford Hill, A. (1971). *Principles of medical statistics* (9th edn), Chapter 24. Lancet, London.

Bussey, A.L. and Harris, A.S. (1979). Computers and effectiveness of the measles vaccination campaign in England and Wales. *Community Medicine*, **1**, 29.

Butler, N.R., Golding, J., Haslum, M., *et al.* (1982). Recent findings from the 1970 child health and education study: preliminary communication. *Journal of the Royal Society of Medicine*, **75**, 781.

Campbell, A.G.M. (1983). Measles immunization: why have we failed? *Archives of Disease in Childhood*, **58**, 3.

Came, S. (1984). Place of development surveillance in general practice. *Journal of the Royal Society of Medicine*, **77**, 819.

Carter, H. and Jones, I.O. (1985). Measles immunization: results of a local programme to increase vaccine uptake. *British Medical Journal*, **290**, 1717–19.

Carvasco, J.L. and Lardinois, R. (1987). Formula for calculating vaccine profitability. *Vaccine*, **5**, 123–7.

Cherry, J.D. (1986). The controversy about pertussis vaccine. *Current Clinical Topics in Infectious Diseases*, **7**, 216.

Clarke, S.J. (1980). Whooping cough vaccination: some reasons for non-complction. *Journal of Advanced Nursing*, **5**, 313–19.

Cochi, S.L., Preblud, S.R., and Orenstein, W.A. (1988). Perspectives on the resurgence of mumps in the United States. *American Journal of Diseases of Children*, **142**, 499–507.

Cockburn, W.C. (1969). World aspects of the epidemiology of rubella. *American Journal of Diseases of Children*, **118**, 112.

Cohen, H. (1978). Vaccination against pertussis, yes or no? In *International symposium on pertussis* (ed. C.R. Manclark and J.C. Hill), p. 249. National Institutes of Health, Bethesda, MD.

Collete, B.J.A. (1982). The sentinel practices system in The Netherlands. In *Environmental epidemiology* (ed. P.E. Leaverton), p. 149. Praeger, New York.

Comstock, G.W. (1994) Evaluating vaccination effectiveness and vaccine efficacy by means of case-control studies. *Epidemiologic Reviews*, **16**.

Cowden, J.M., O'Mahoney, M., Bartlett, C.L.R., *et al.* (1989). A national outbreak of *Salmonella typhimurium* DT 124 caused by contaminated salami sticks. *Epidemiology and Infection*, **103**, 219.

Creese, A.L. and Henderson, R.H. (1980). Cost-benefit analysis and immunization programmes in developing countries. *Bulletin of the World Health Organization*, **58**, 491.

Cutting, W.A.M. (1983). Measles immunization. A review. *Journal of Tropical Pediatrics*, **29**, 246–7.

Deming, M., Jaiteh, K.O., Otten, M.W., *et al.* (1992) Epidemic poliomyelitis in the Gambia following the control of poliomyelitis as an endemic disease. 11. Clinical efficacy of trivalent oral polio vaccine. *American Journal of Epidemiology*, **135**, 393–408.

Department of Health and Social Security (1981). *Whooping cough.* Reports from Committee on Safety of Medicines and the Joint Committee on Vaccination and Immunization. HMSO, London.

Epidemiology Research Laboratory (1975). Echovirus 19 this summer? *British Medical Journal*, **ii**, 346.

Evans, A.S. (1980). The need for serologic evaluation of immunization programs. *American Journal of Epidemiology*, **112**, 725.

Eylenbosch, W.J. and Noah, N.D. (ed.) (1988). *Surveillance in health and disease.* Oxford University Press.

Fine, P.E.M., Clarkson, J.A., and Miller, E. (1988). The efficacy of pertussis vaccines under conditions of household exposure. *International Journal of Epidemiology*, **17**, 635.

Fleming, D.M. and Crombie, D.L. (1985). The incidence of common infectious diseases: the weekly returns service of the Royal College of General Practitioners. *Health Trends*, **17**, 13.

Fox, J.L. (1996). ....but new plans for surveillance are still being proposed. *Nature Medicine*, **2**, 733.

Fudenberg, H.H. (1973). Fiscal returns of biomedical research. *Journal of Investigative Dermatology*, **61**, 321.

Gensheimer, K.F., Fukuda, K., Brammer, L., *et al.* (1999). Preparing for pandemic influenza: the need for enhanced surveillance. *Emerging Infectious Diseases*, **5**, 297–9.

Gill, O.N., Bartlett, C.L.R., Sockett, P.N., *et al.* (1983). Outbreak of *Salmonella napoli* infection caused by contaminated chocolate bars. *Lancet*, **i**, 574.

Gleason, R.E., Khan, C.B. Funk, I.B., and Craighead JE. (1982). Seasonal incidence of insulin dependent diabetes (IDDM) in Massachusetts 1964–1973. *International Journal of Epidemiology*, **11**, 39–45.

Guest, M., Horn, J., and Archer, L.N.J. (1986). Why some parents refuse pertussis immunisation. *Practitioner*, **230**, 210.

Hall, S.M. and Glickman, M. (1988). The British paediatric surveillance unit. *Archives of Disease in Childhood*, **63**, 344–346.

Haskey, J.C. and Birch, D. (1985). Statistics from general practice: morbidity and its measurement using practice statistical reports. *Health Trends*, **17**, 32.

Helweg-Larsen, K., Bay, H., and Mac, F. (1985). A statistical analysis of the seasonality in sudden infant death syndrome. *International Journal of Epidemiology*, **14**, 566–574.

Henderson, D.A. (1976). Surveillance of smallpox. *International Journal of Epidemiology*, **5**, 19–28

Henderson, R.H. and Sundaresan, T. (1982). Cluster sampling to assess immunization coverage: a review of experience with a simplified sampling method. *Bulletin of World Health Organization*, **60**, 253–60.

Hillis, D.M. and Huelsenbeck, J.P. (1994) Support for dental HIV transmission. *Nature*, **369**, 24–5.

Hingson, R. (1974). Obtaining optimal attendance at mass immunization programs. *Health Services Reports*, **89**, 53–64.

Hinman, A.R. and Koplan, J.P. (1984). Pertussis and pertussis vaccine. Reanalysis of benefits, risk and costs. *Journal of the American Medical Association*, **251**, 3109–13.

Hinman, A.R. and Koplan, J.P. (1985). Pertussis and pertussis vaccine: further analysis of benefits, risks and costs. *Development in Biological Standardization*, **61**, 429–37.

Hinman, A.R., Brandling-Bennett, A.D., Bernier, R., *et al.* (1980). Current features of measles in the United States: feasibility of measles elimination. *Epidemiologic Reviews*, **2**, 153–70.

Humphrey, T.J., Baskerville, A., Mawer, S., Rowe, B., and Hopper, S. (1989). *Salmonella enteritidis* phage type 4 from the contents of intact eggs: a study involving naturally infected hens. *Epidemiology and Infection*, **103**, 415–23.

Irwig, L.M. (1976). Surveillance in developed countries with particular reference to child growth. *International Journal of Epidemiology*, S57–61.

Jarman, B., Bosanquet, N., Rice, P., *et al.* (1988). Uptake of immunization in district health authorities in England. *British Medical Journal*, **296**, 1775–8.

Judelsohn, R.G., Pleissner, M.L., and O'Mara, D.J. (1980). School-based measles outbreaks: correlation of age at immunization with risk of disease. *American Journal of Public Health*, **70**, 1162–5.

Kasongo Project Team (1981). Influence of measles vaccination on survival pattern of 7–35-month-old children in Kasongo, Zaire. *Lancet*, **i**, 764–7.

Khot, A. and Burn, R. (1984). Seasonal variation and time trends of deaths from asthma in England and Wales (1960–1982). *British Medical Journal*, **289**, 233–4.

Klaucke D.N. (1994) Evaluating public health surveillance. In *Principles and practice of public health surveillance* (ed. S.M. Teutsch and R.E. Churchill). Oxford University Press.

Koplan, J.P. (1985). Benefits, risks and costs of immunization programmes. In *The value of preventive medicine*, Ciba Foundation Symposium 110, pp. 55–680. Pitman, London.

Koplan, J.P. and Preblud, S.R. (1982). A benefit–cost analysis of mumps vaccine. *American Journal of Diseases of Children*, **136**, 362.

Koplan, J.P., Schoenbaum, S.C., Weinstein, M.C., and Fraser, D.W. (1979). Pertussis vaccine—an analysis of benefits, risks and costs. *New England Journal of Medicine*, **301**, 906–11

Kosklniemi, M. and Vaheri, A. (1989). Effect of measles, mumps, rubella vaccination on pattern of encephalitis in children. *Lancet*, **i**, 31–4.

Kulenkampff, M., Schwartzman, J.S., and Wilson, J. (1974). Neurological complications of pertussis inoculation. *Archives of Disease in Childhood*, **49**, 46–9.

Lakhani, A.D.H., Morris, R.W., Morgan, M., Dale, C., and Vaile, M.S. (1987). Measles immunization: feasibility of a 90 per cent target uptake. *Archives of Disease in Childhood*, **62**, 1209.

Landrigan, P.J. (1972). Epidemic measles in a divided city. *Journal of the American Medical Association*, **221**, 567–70.

Langmuir, A.D. (1963). The surveillance of communicable diseases of national importance. *New England Journal of Medicine*, **268**, 182–92.

Langmuir, A.D. (1976). William Farr: founder of modern concepts of surveillance. *International Journal of Epidemiology*, **5**, 13–18.

Last, J.M. (ed.) (1995). *A dictionary of epidemiology* (3rd edn). Oxford University Press.

Limentani, A.E., Elliott, L.M., Noah, N.D., and lambourn, J. (1979). Outbreak of hepatitis B from tattooing. *Lancet*, **ii**, 86–8.

Lynn, R., Nicoll, A., Rahi, J., and Verity, C. (ed.) (1999). *British Paediatric Surveillance Unit annual report 1998/9*. British Paediatric Surveillance Unit, London.

McCarthy, K. and Taylor Robinson, C.H. (1963). Immunization against measles. *British Journal of Clinical Practice*, **17**, 650–9.

McKinnon, J.A. (1979). The impact of the media on whooping cough immunization. *Health Education Journal*, **37**, 198.

Maclean, M.H. and Macleod, A. (1984). Seasonal variation in the frequency of anencephalus and spina bifida births in the UK *Journal of Epidemiology and Community Health*, **38**, 99–102.

Marks, J.S., Hayden, G.F., and Orenstein, W.A. (1982). Methodologic issues in the evaluation of vaccine effectiveness. *American Journal of Epidemiology*, **116**, 510–23.

McEvoy, M.B, Noah, N.D., and Pilsworth, R. (1987). Outbreak of fever caused by *Streptobacillus imoniliformis*. *Lancet*, **ii**, 1361–3.

Measles Vaccine Committee of the Medical Research Council (1966). Vaccination against measles. *British Medical Journal*, **i**, 441–6.

Melchior, J.C. (1977). Infantile spasms and early immunization against whooping cough: Danish survey from 1970 to 1975. *Archives of Disease in Childhood*, **52**, 134–7.

Miceli, I., de Kantor, I., Colalacovo, D., *et al.* (1988). Evaluation of the effectiveness of BCG vaccination using the case-control method in Buenos Aires, Argentina. *International Journal of Epidemiology*, **17**, 629–34.

Miller, C.L. (1978). Severity of notified measles. *British Medical Journal*, **i**, 1253.

Miller, D.L. (1964). Frequency of complications of measles, 1963. *British Medical Journal*, **ii**, 75–8.

Miller, D.L., Alderslade, R., and Ross, E.M. (1982). Whooping cough and whooping cough vaccine: the risks and benefits debate. *Epidemiologic Reviews*, **4**, 1–24.

Miller, E. and Waight, P. (1998). Measles, measles vaccination, and Crohn's disease. *British Medical Journal*, **316**, 1745.

Miller, E., Goldacre, M., Pugh, S., *et al.* (1993) Risk of aseptic meningitis after measles, mumps, and rubella vaccine in UK children. *Lancet*, **341**, 979–82.

Miller, E., Waight, P., Gay, N., *et al.* (1997). The epidemiology of rubella in England and Wales before and after the 1994 measles and rubella campaign. *CDR Review* No. 2, R 26–32.

Miller, E., Waight, P., and Farrington, P. (1998). Safety assessment post-licensure. In *Preclinical and clinical development of new vaccines*. Vol. 95, *Developments in biology standardization* (ed. S. Plotkin, F. Brown, and F. Horaud), pp. 235–43. Karger, Basel.

Monto, A.S. (1974). The Tecumseh study of respiratory illness. *American Journal of Epidemiology*, **100**, 458–68.

Moro, M.L. and McCormick, A. (1988). Surveillance for communicable disease. In *Surveillance in health and disease* (ed. W.J. Eylenbosch and N.D. Noah), p. 166. Oxford University Press.

Morgan-Capner, P., Wright, J., Miller, C.L., *et al.* (1988). Surveillance of antibody to measles, mumps and rubella by age. *British Medical Journal*, **297**, 770–2.

Morley, D. (1975). Nutritional surveillance of young children in developing countries. *International Journal of Epidemiology*, **5**, 51–5.

Morse, S.S. (1993). Examining the origins of emerging viruses. In *Emerging viruses* (ed. S.S. Morse). Oxford University Press, New York.

Newlands, M. and Davies, L. (1988). The use of performance indicators for immunization rates in General Practice. *Public Health*, **102**, 269–73.

Noah, N.D. (1974). *Mycoplasma pneumoniae* infection in the United Kingdom, 1967–1973. *British Medical Journal*, **ii**, 544–6.

Noah, N.D. (1976). Attack rates of notified whooping cough in immunized and unimmunized children. *British Medical Journal*, **i**, 128–9.

Noah, N.D. (1982). Measles eradication policies. *British Medical Journal*, **284**, 99–8.

Noah, N.D. (1983). The strategy of immunization. *Community Medicine*, **5**, 140–7.

Noah, N.D. (1989). Cyclical patterns and predictability in infection. *Epidemiology and Infection*, **102**, 175–90.

Noah, N.D. and Fowle, S.E. (1988). Immunity to rubella in women of childbearing age in the United Kingdom. *British Medical Journal*, **297**, 1301–4.

O'Mahony, M., Noah, N.D., Evans, B., *et al.* (1986) An outbreak of gastroenteritis on a passenger cruise ship. *Journal of Hygiene*, **97**, 229–36.

Orenstein, W.A., Bernier, R.H., Dondero, T., *et al.* (1985). Field evaluation of vaccine efficacy. *Bulletin of the World Health Organization*, **63**, 1055.

Orenstein, W.A., Bernier, R.H., and Hinman, A.R. (1988). Assessing vaccine efficacy in the field. *Epidemiologic Reviews*, **10**, 212–41.

Panagiotopoulos, T., Antoniadou, I., and Valassi-Adam, E. (1999) Increase in congenital rubella occurrence after immunisation in Greece: retrospective survey and systematic review. *British Medical Journal*, **319**, 1462–7.

Patrick, K.M. and Woolley, F.R. (1981). A cost-benefit analysis of immunization for pneurnococcal pneumonia. *Journal of the American Medical Association*, **245**, 473–7.

Pebody, R.G., Paunio, M., and Ruutu, P. (1998). Crohn's disease has not increased in Finland. *British Medical Journal*, **316**, 1745.

PHLS Epidemiological Research Laboratory and 21 Area Health Authorities (1982). Efficacy of pertussis vaccination in England. *British Medical Journal*, **285**, 357–9.

PHLS Whooping Cough Committee and Working Party (1973). Efficacy of whooping cough vaccines used in the United Kingdom before 1968: final report. *British Medical Journal*, **1**, 259–62.

Pollard, R. (1980). Relation between vaccination and notification rates for whooping cough in England and Wales. *Lancet*, **i**, 1180–2.

Pollock, T.M. (1966). *Trials of prophylactic agents for the control of communicable diseases*. Monograph series No. 52. World Health Organization, Geneva.

Pollock, T.M., Miller, E., Mortimer, J.Y., *et al.* (1984). Symptoms after first immunization with DTP and DT vaccine. *Lancet*, **ii**, 146–9.

Pugh, E.J. and Hawker, R. (1986). Measles immunisation: professional knowledge and intention to vaccinate. *Community Medicine*, **8**, 340–7.

Raska, K. (1971). Epidemiological surveillance with particular reference to the use of immunological surveys. *Proceedings of the Royal Society of Medicine*, **64**, 684–8.

Research Unit of the Royal College of General Practitioners (1974). The incidence and complications of mumps. *Journal of the Royal College of General Practitioners*, **24**, 545–51.

Rey, M. (1985). Eradication of measles by widespread vaccination is beneficial and feasible. *Semaine des Hôpitaux de Paris*, **61**, 21–5.

Robbins, K.B., Brandling-Bennett, A.D., and Hinman, A.R. (1981). Low measles incidence: association with enforcement of school immunization laws. *American Journal of Public Health*, **71**, 270–4.

Rodrigues, L.C. and Smith, P.G. (1999) Use of the case-control approach in vaccine evaluation: efficacy and adverse effects. *Epidemiologic Reviews*, **21**, 56–72.

Rowe, B., Hutchinson, D.N., Gilbert, R.J., *et al.* (1987). *Salmonella ealing* infections associated with consumption of infant dried milk. *Lancet*, **ii**, 900–3.

Sagliocca, L., Amoroso, P., Stroffolini, T., *et al.* (1999). Efficacy of hepatitis A vaccine in prevention of secondary hepatitis A infection: a randomised trial. *Lancet*, **353**, 1136–9.

Salmon, R.L. and Bartlett, C.L.R. (1995). European surveillance systems. *Reviews in Medical Microbiology*, **6**, 267–76.

Sever, J.L., Hardy, J.B., Nelson, K.B., *et al.* (1969). Rubella in the collaborative perinatal research study. *American Journal of Diseases of Children*, **118**, 123–32.

Silverstein, A.M. (1981). *Pure politics and impure science: the swine flu qffair.* Johns Hopkins University Press, Baltimore, MD.

Smith, J.W.G., Fletcher, W.B., and Wherry, P.J. (1976). Vaccination in the control of influenza. *Postgraduate Medical Journal*, **52**, 399–404.

Smith, P.G. (1988). Epidemiological methods to evaluate vaccine efficacy. *British Medical Journal*, **44**, 679.

Snacken, R., Kendal, A.P., Haaheim, L.R., and Wood, J.M. (1997). The next influenza pandemic: lessons from Hong Kong. *Emerging Infectious Diseases*, **5**, 195–203.

Stetler, H.C., Mullen, J.R., Brennan, J.P., Livengood, J.R., Orenstein, W.A., and Hinman, A.R. (1987). Monitoring system for adverse events following immunization. *Vaccine*, **5**, 169–74.

Sutherland, I. and Fayers, P.M. (1971). Effect of measles vaccination on incidence of measles in the community. *British Medical Journal*, **1**, 698–702.

Taylor, B., Miller, E., Farrington, C.P., *et al.* (1999). Autism and measles, mumps, and rubella vaccine, no epidemiological evidence for a casual association. *Lancet*, **353**, 2026–9.

Taylor, B., Miller, E., and Farrington, P. (2000). Autism and measles, mumps, and rubella vaccine. *Lancet*, **355**, 409.

Thacker, S.B. (1994) Historical development. In *Principles and practice of public health surveillance.* (ed. S.M. Teutsch and R.E. Churchill). Oxford University Press.

Thacker, S.B. and Berkelman, R.J. (1986). Public health surveillance in the United States. *Epidemiologic Reviews*, **10**, 164–90.

Thacker, S.B., Choi, K., and Brachman, P.S. (1983). The surveillance of infectious diseases. *Journal of American Medical Association*, **249**, 1181–5.

Thiers, G., Maes, R., van Lierde, R., *et al.* (1979). Surveillance van besmettelijke ziekten door een net van peilpraktij ken. *Tijdschrifti voor Geneeskunde*, **12**, 781.

Thompson, N.P., Montgomery, S.M., Pounder, R.E., and Wakefield, A.J. (1995). Is measles vaccination a risk factor for inflammatory bowel disease? *Lancet*, **345**, 1071–4.

Tillett, H.E. and Spencer, I.L. (1982). Influenza surveillance in England and Wales using routine statistics. *Journal of Hygiene*, **88**, 83–94.

Webster R.G., Bean W.J., Gorman O.T, Chambers T.M., and Kawaoka Y. (1992). Evolution and ecology of influenza A viruses. *Microbiological Reviews*, **56**, 152–79.

White, C.C., Koplan, J.P., and Orenstein, W.A. (1985). Benefits, risks and costs of immunization for measles, mumps and rubella. *American Journal of Public Health*, **75**, 739–44.

White, L.R., Sever, J.L., and Alepa, F.P. (1969). Maternal and congenital rubella before 1964: frequency, clinical features, and search for isoimmune phenomena. *Journal of Pediatrics*, **74**, 198–207.

Wilkinson, P., Tylden-Pattenson, L., and Gould, J. (1979). Professional attitudes towards vaccination and immunization within the Leeds Area Health Authority. *Public Health, London*, **93**, 11–15.

Witte, J.J. and Axnick, N.W. (1975). The benefits from 10 years of measles immunization in the United States. *Public Health Report*, **90**, 205–7.

Wright, P.F, Kim-Farley, R.J., de Quadros, C.A., *et al.* (1991). Strategies for the global eradication of poliomyelitis by the year 2000. *New England Journal of Medicine*, **325**, 1774–9.

Yeager, A.S., Davis, J.H., Ross, L.A., *et al.* (1977). Measles immunization. Successes and failures. *Journal of the American Medical Association*, **237**, 347–51.

8.5 The analysis of human exposures to contaminants in the environment

Paul J. Lioy, Amit Roy, and Natalie Freeman

Introduction

The presence of chemical and physical agents in the environments where people live, work, and play may cause illness. Therefore it is essential to develop and employ reliable methods that define the intensity and duration of contact with such agents and assess the likelihood of any cause–effect relationship. The field of exposure analysis and its assessment is associated with epidemiology, risk assessment, and disease intervention and prevention (Lippmann and Lioy 1986; Graham *et al.* 1992; Sexton *et al.* 1992; Jayjock and Hawkins 1993; Ott 1995; Lioy 1999) and the scientists and engineers who conduct these studies now are called exposure analysts (NRC 1985, 1991*b*,*c*) or exposurologists (Ott 1995). The kinds of exposures examined by the exposure analyst are illustrated in Fig. 1. The traditional terms, industrial hygienist and radiation health physicists, refer specifically to those individuals who conduct exposure assessments in the various workplaces and who provided much of the fundamental technical bases for the first sets of field studies.

The exposure measurement techniques may be indirect or direct (NRC 1991*c*). Indirect techniques include sampling locations (microenvironments) where contact may occur with a contaminant, and/or the administration of survey instruments; such as, time/activity questionnaires. Direct techniques include personal monitors worn by individuals, and samples of blood, urine, and other bodily fluids, which permit measurements of exposure and dose for specific individuals.

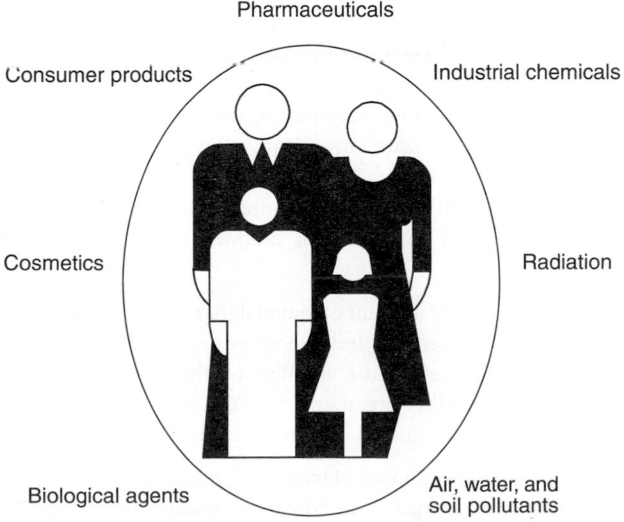

Fig. 1 Types of exposures that may be experienced by the general population.

The measurement of the concentration of physical, chemical, radio-active, and/or biological agents in air, water, food, and so on, and the estimation of human behaviours, using instruments such as time/activity pattern diaries, has led to the development of models that can predict exposure and dose. Currently, it is feasible to trace an agent from its source through pathways into exposed people. Figure 2 illustrates the 'flow' of a contaminant through the points of contact, to the exposure, and to the dose that can appear inside the body. The domain-related scientific and professional disciplines: environmental science, exposure assessment, toxicology, and epidemiology, are also illustrated in Fig. 2.

Format

This chapter describes the features of exposure assessment starting from concepts and theory. The types of exposure measurements and estimates needed for the applications to environmental health will also be illustrated using, in varying detail, information about lead, benzene, trihalomethanes, pesticides, airborne particulate matter, infectious agents, and alternate fuels. Finally, some observations will be made concerning the future of exposure assessment in public health practice.

Basic principles

Over the past 15 years, the theoretical and conceptual bases for exposure assessment have evolved from simple mathematical expressions that consider exposure and dose, to complex mechanistic descriptions of exposure/dose equations and concepts that can describe multiple routes of contact with a toxic agent. The aim, as described by Fig. 2, is to establish a relationship between the release of a toxicant, and a dose that may cause an adverse health outcome (Lioy 1990, 1999; Lioy and Pellizzari 1995).

Some pollutants, such as ozone, are not emitted into the environment but are formed from precursors. In such cases it is necessary to establish a relationship between the release of precursors of the toxicant, the conditions under which the toxicant is formed, and the health effect. The study of the effect of exposure on ecological receptors can have important implications for human health. Ecological effects can have indirect effects on human health, and can also serve

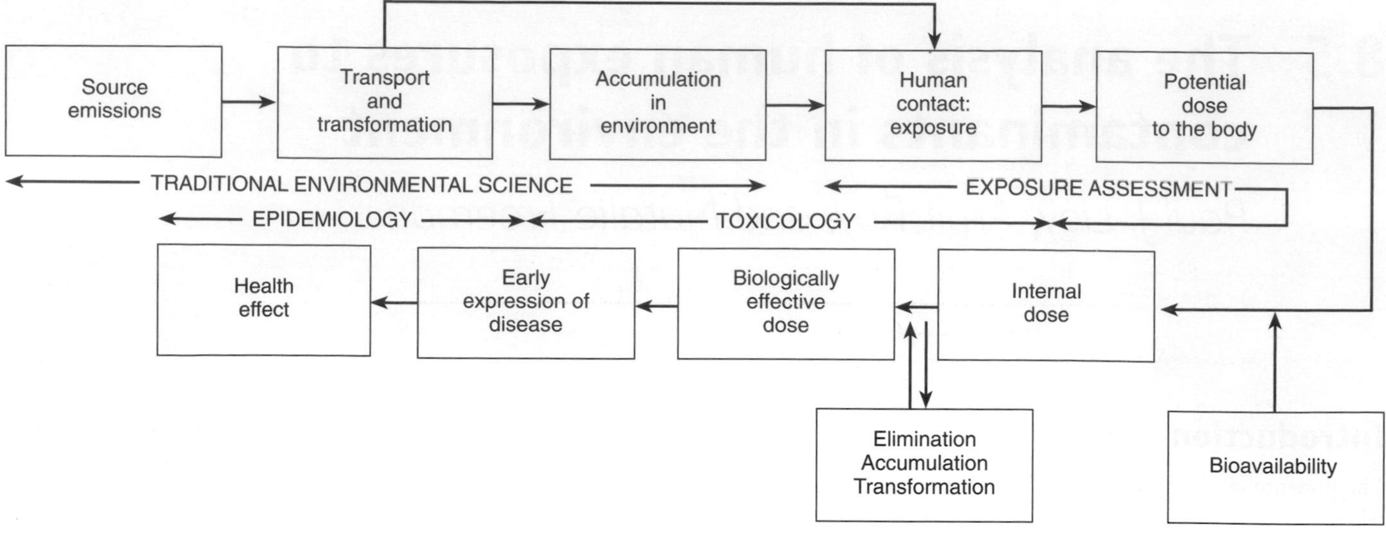

Fig. 2 Continuum for the emission of and exposure to a contaminant and the expression of a health effect. (Source: Lioy 1990.)

as sentinels of human exposure. Ecological effects can also have significant environmental justice implications, because the lives of some tribal and disadvantaged human populations are more closely linked to ecological health than that of the general population.

Exposure to a contaminant is defined as the 'contact at a boundary between a human and the environment at a specific concentration over an interval of time' (NRC 1991*c*). Based on this definition the types of integral or summation equations needed to estimate or describe exposure were identified and are presented in Box 1. The integral equation is an exact expression of an individual's exposure, over the course of time, while the summation provides an approximate representation of exposure. The integral equation requires knowledge of the instantaneous concentration of the toxicant, which is generally available only from modelling studies, whereas the summation requires a knowledge of time-averaged concentrations, which are often available from the application of direct and indirect

Box 1 Equations governing exposure

Exposure

$$E_j = \int_{t_1}^{t_2} C_j(t)\,dt$$

where E_i is the integrated exposure of the *i*th individual to a concentration C_i of a contaminant for time period t_1 to t_2 associated with a biological response.

Microenvironmental increments of exposure

$$\Delta E_{ji} = C_{ji}(\Delta t)\ \Delta t_i$$

where $\Delta E_{j,i}$ is the exposure of person *i* to a contaminant measured over an interval Δt associated with the *j*th activity (or location). These expressions are appropriate for inhalation and dermal exposure, based on which dose can be estimated. For uptake by ingestion, dose is generally estimated directly based upon media concentrations and uptake rate.

measurement techniques. Generalized versions of these equations and concepts can be used to estimate exposures in modelling studies. These can be found in Georgopoulos and Lioy (1994), Ott (1995), and Zartarian *et al.* (1997*b*).

In principle, the uptake of a toxicant can occur via three routes: inhalation, dermal absorption, and ingestion. The definition of exposure provides guidance for the selection of locations for sampling. For the purposes of exposure assessment, any material passing a hypothetical boundary surrounding the body is termed potential dose. Inhaled dose is the amount of toxicant that enters the nose or mouth, dermal dose is the amount that enters the skin, and ingested dose is the amount that enters a hypothetical boundary over the mouth. As suggested by the term potential, the amount of toxicant that actually enters tissue can be significantly lower than the potential dose. These occur at boundaries external to the body; thus, exposure is determined at the points of entry into the body, that is, the nose, mouth, and skin. The data collected can then be used to establish criteria identifying exposure within a population and constructing predictive models (Duan 1982; Ott 1982, 1990; Sexton and Ryan 1988; McKone 1991; Ryan 1991; Georgopoulos *et al.* 1997). Figure 3 illustrates three major routes of uptake: inhalation of airborne agents, ingestion of food and liquids, and skin contact with air, soil, and all types of materials and products.

Once a contaminant has crossed a boundary and entered the body, it is then considered a dose, which is routinely described in one of three ways.

1. Potential dose is the amount of material that enters an hypothetical external boundary around a receptor deposited on a surface, which can potentially cause an effect on the surface or can be transferred to another organ or tissue. The entire mass (100 per cent) is assumed to cause a biological response.

2. Internal dose is the amount of material that actually enters one or more tissues; and target tissue dose is the amount of toxicant that actually reaches sensitive tissue in which the toxic response occurs, or estimated to be available to be absorbed by an organ or tissue or absorbed to a surface and is available to undergo

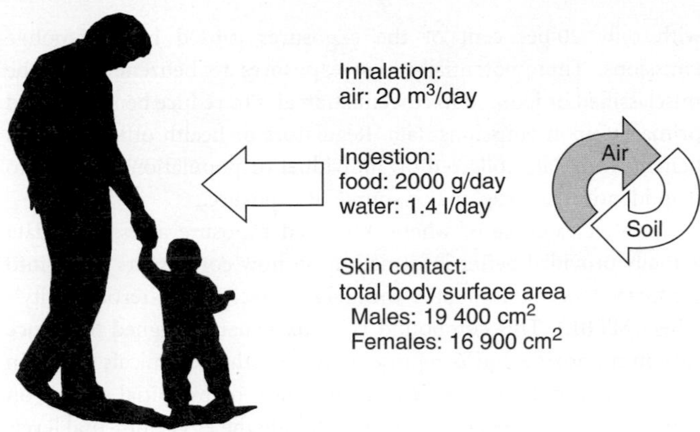

Fig. 3 Routes of exposure. A comprehensive exposure assessment invokes consideration of each possible route through which a chemical can enter the body.

biological processes, which can cause altered physiological function.

3. Biologically effective dose is the amount of target tissue dose required for manifestation of a toxic effect. It is the amount of the contaminant or metabolite that interacts with cellular macromolecules and alters physiological function (Lioy 1990).

The units most frequently encountered when calculating exposure and dose are shown in Table 1.

Biological markers of exposure/dose can be measured in body fluid specimens and then be associated with time of occurrence and/or persistence of the contaminant (NRC 1989*a*). Henderson *et al.* (1992) and Shultc and Perera (1993) published a conceptual framework for describing the persistence of the different types of markers in the body. The general time course of elimination of each type of marker is illustrated in Fig. 4. The results indicate that exhaled parent compounds yield the highest levels of biomarker concentrations relative to exposure concentration. Adducts spend the longest time in the body. The term 'markers of exposure' is currently used to describe most of the above, but in actuality the level of a contaminant or transformed product, present in the body is defined as a dose (NRC 1989*b*, 1992).

Methodologies

The accurate measurement or estimation of exposure requires baseline information about the plausibility of human contact with the contaminant of concern and assists in establishing the data quality objectives for analysing any particular problems. In the selection of the appropriate measurement 'tools', the analyst also needs to account for factors such as the sensitivity and specificity of a technique for each medium or route studied, and ease of sample handling and collection. In some situations simple techniques such as survey instruments are extremely valuable in acquiring semiquantitative data for the characterization exposure (Carpenter and Huston-Stein 1980; USEPA 1988; Lebowitz *et al.* 1989; Robinson *et al.* 1989; Freeman *et al.* 1991, 1997; NRC 1991*c*; Schwab *et al.* 1991; Zartarian *et al.* 1997*b*, 1998). In other cases more complex techniques such as microenvironmental or personal monitors are used to establish the primary route by which human contact occurs with a contaminant (Seifert and Abraham 1983; Akland *et al.* 1985, Spengler *et al.* 1985; Stetter 1986; USEPA 1988; Wallace *et al.* 1988; NRC 1991*c*; Clayton *et al.* 1993; Lioy 1993; Valerio *et al.* 1997; Pellizzari *et al.* 1999). It is important to note, however, that all types of techniques do not have to be employed in a single study. Those selected would depend upon the data quality objectives and the hypotheses being tested for a particular study.

The issue of multimedia contact with contaminants has increased the awareness and the desire to obtain measurements on multiple routes of exposure, and to insure that exposure–response relationships are constructed for the media or routes of greatest concern (McKone 1991; Georgopoulos *et al.* 1997). The data gathered will also improve a manager's ability to prioritizing strategies for intervention and eventual reduction exposure. Experience of exposure analysts with environmental health problems leads to a tacit point: it is not scientifically sound to prejudge which is the most important medium or route of concern for a particular contaminant (Lioy 1990; NRC 1991*c*). Avoiding this pitfall will make it possible to obtain a broader view of a problem and improve the selection of measurement and analytical techniques. In the past, many studies have focused on a limited number of routes, and frequently have led to poorly identified exposures, and eventually selection of inappropriate remedial solutions.

Table 1 Examples of units used to express exposure

Variable	Typical units	
Concentration in media	mg/kg	(food)
	mg/l	(water)
	μg/m^3 and fibres/m^3	(air)
	mg/100 cm^2	(contaminated surface)
	mg/g or per cent	(fraction by weight in consumer products)
Time increments	min, h, day, year, 70 years (lifetime)	
Rate of intake	l/day	
	l/h	
	mg/kg body weight ingested per day (or per meal)	
	mg inhaled per hour	
	minutes	
Quantity available for absorption (potential dose)	mg inhaled, total	
	mg inhaled per kg body weight	
	mg ingested, total	
	mg ingested per kg body weight	
	mg on skin, total	
	mg/cm^2 skin area	
	mg injected or implanted/kg body weight	
Concentration in body tissues	μg/ml blood fibres/ml lung tissue	
Body burden	μg in bone (example)	
Organ dose	mg to liver (example)	

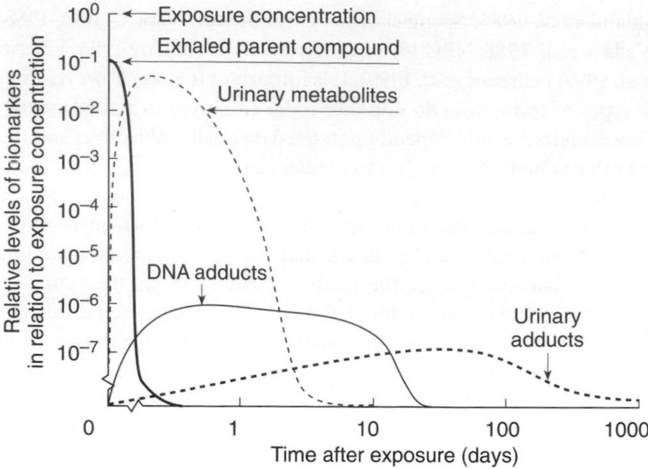

Fig. 4 Hypothetical relationships between different biological markers of exposure and time after a single exposure. (Source: Henderson *et al.* 1992.)

One example of how a poorly designed assessment can lead to misclassification of exposure involves benzene (Wallace 1989). Two pie charts, shown in Fig. 5, apportion benzene exposure within the general population. The first pie chart identifies the emissions of benzene from major environmental sources and has been used in the past to define exposure reduction strategies. The second pie chart identifies the actual benzene exposure experienced by a statistically representative sample of the general population. The clear message from the emissions pie chart is that motor vehicles represent the major source of benzene to the ambient atmosphere and provide the greatest number of opportunities for members of the general population to experience benzene exposures in non-occupational settings. Thus, one is led to believe that the most important source of benzene is the automobile. In contrast, measurements made within personal monitoring studies, also in Fig. 5, have shown that the predominant source contributing to benzene exposure (>50 per cent) is cigarette smoke, with only 20 per cent of the exposures caused by automobile emissions. Thus, potentially high exposures to benzene would be misclassified or ignored in current strategies to reduce benzene based primarily upon emissions data. Regulators or health officials would benefit from data collected on individual or population activities to help identify thc 'truc' major source of exposure.

Another example of where improved exposure assessment data actually provided better information on how commuters come into contact with a contaminant is the fuel additive, methyl-tertiary-butyl-ether (**MTBE**). This compound is an oxygenate designed to reduce carbon monoxide and is representative of other chemicals found in new or reformulated fuels. In this instance, many initial studies on oxygenated fuel were conducted to estimate the environmental levels of MTBE or other hydrocarbons caused by automobile tail pipe emissions. However, experiences of the general public and gasoline station workers with gasoline oxygenated by MTBE at 15 per cent by volume have suggested that the highest exposures to the driver or passengers in an automobile, or garage workers were derived from evaporative emissions released by the engine compartment or gas tank into the interior of a car or in microenvironments adjacent to gasoline service pumps. This is in contrast to the typical tail pipe emissions scenario used in exposure assessments for motor vehicle fuels. Experiments conducted using cars that followed a typical commuter route and then had the gasoline tank filled at some point during the trip are illustrated in Fig. 6. The results showed that the highest exposures to MTBE occurred during a tank refill. The approach used in the study demonstrated the importance of both personal and Microenvironmental analyses in providing insight on what can lead to high exposures to evaporative emissions. Other examples exist for dermal and ingestion exposure; however, the main point is not to demonstrate all misclassifications of exposure that can or have occurred, but to recognize that when you design a study, it must include flexibility to evaluate the possibility that a variety of sources and routes can affect exposure. This will improve the detection of and source apportionment of emissions, and how each affect the intensity of human contact with the contaminants of concern.

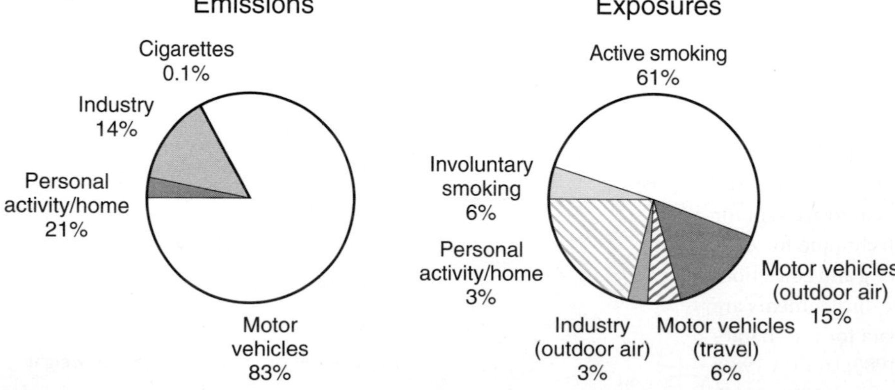

Fig. 5 Benzene emissions versus exposures. 'Personal activity/home' refers to benzene from materials such as paints, adhesives, and marking pens. For individuals who do not actively smoke, the 'active smoking' contribution to exposure is zero, and the other exposure categories increase proportionally. (Source: Wallace 1989.)

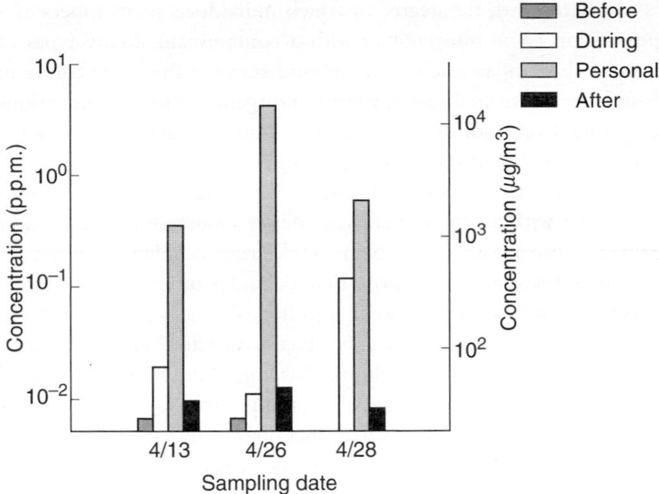

Fig. 6 MTBE exposure samples during commuter refuelling.

Approaches used in exposure analysis

Determination of human contact or the potential contact with a contaminant is not an integral part of traditional environmental quality measurements. Usually there are criteria available for making environmental quality measurements, which establish a statistically representative sampling scheme for determining the areal extent of contamination, and establishing long-term concentration trends within an environmental medium (Ott 1977; Lodge 1989; Lioy 1990; Anderson-Sprecher *et al.* 1994). Unfortunately, these measurements do not provide data that can be used to assess exposure directly. Historically, an assessment of exposure was based primarily on the concentration of a contaminant found in an environmental medium at a single sampling site for a prescribed sampling period. However, little or no information was provided on the duration of contact or the probability of contact with the contaminant by people spending time in the location where the measurements were the being made. More representative historical examples of exposure measurements would be the breathing zone samples collected in occupational settings; however, the concentrations were much higher.

In many cases, environmental quality measurements continue to provide the only data available for calculating exposure–response relationships within various public health-related studies, for example hazardous waste sites and air pollution (USEPA 1989*a*). These data have been used in applications within epidemiology or risk assessment, and have yielded results with a high degree of uncertainty. Also, environmental quality data are rarely collected using strategies that ensure the duration of the measurements is coupled with the relevant biological response time to the presence of a contaminant within the body. As stated previously, the latter point is critical for exposure analysis. All too often environmental quality measurement programmes are based upon a regulatory requirement for determining compliance to a regulation, and/or the limits of detection and collection capacity of a sampler.

The major paradigm shift in framework for exposure analyses, which started at about 1990, has led to the expanded use of personal monitoring and/or microenvironmental monitoring for the development of exposure databases. Both types of monitors are more intrusive than the devices used for monitoring environmental quality as the sample is taken: (a) at or from the individual; (b) in an area occupied by the individual; or (c) from objects used, worn, or eaten by an individual. The samples also require the acquisition of time resolved data on where and how individuals spend their time (Lebowitz 1989; NRC 1991*c*; Freeman *et al.* 1997; Zartarian *et al.* 1997*a*).

A hierarchy of exposure measurements is presented in Table 2, and emphasizes that personal monitoring provides the best data for completing an exposure assessment (NRC 1991*a*). The table should be reviewed with some caution, however, as in some studies even weak metrics of exposure may be adequate for examining the exposure–health effects relationships. The weak metrics are clearly useful in situations where an isolated source significantly affects a specific community, or a major event or episode has caused health effects. In

Table 2 Hierarchy of exposure measurements, estimates, and surrogates

Type of metric		Approximation of human exposure
1.	Quantified personal and biomarker monitoring	Accurate
2.	Quantified area measurements in the vicinity of a person's activities	Accurate to precise
3.	Quantified modelling estimates of contact with contaminates	Precise
4.	Quantified area of ambient measurements in the vicinity of population of concern	Moderate
5.	Surrogates of exposure source use, frequency of contact	Fair
6.	Distance of a source from a residence (other locations) and duration of residence	Fair
7.	Residence or employment in a geographic area in a reasonable proximity to source or	Poor activity
8.	Residence or employment in a defined geographical area containing a major source	Poor

Adapted from NRC (1991*c*).

addition, some techniques currently used for personal exposure could alter a person's usual activity patterns. For instance, personal samplers for particles are usually bulky and cannot be worn comfortably during periods of outdoor and indoor exercise (Lioy 1993). Therefore, based upon needs of a study, it can be safely stated that the exposure analyst has a virtual tool box of techniques to ensure measurements can be used successfully to answer a public health question (Lioy 1992, 1999).

Another component critical to an exposure analysis is the identification of the study population. In contrast to studies on environmental quality, where minimal information is required on the population of concern, examination of exposure requires the selection of either a probability based sample of the general population with possibilities for oversampling of specific subgroups, or a specific subgroup of the population that exhibits characteristics of susceptibility or is potentially at the high end of exposure to a contaminant. The latter is a major challenge because it is difficult a priori to select the high end exposure groups, greater than the 90th percentile (USEPA 1992*a*).

Typical sampling plans based on the general population or populations at risk are illustrated in Table 3. The selection of a susceptible subgroup is more difficult as detailed information is required on the physical or physiological characteristics of interest before selections are made for entry into a study. Some of the major questions that need to be addressed in properly selected susceptible or sensitive individuals are shown in Table 4.

Media and routes of exposure

The preceding discussion generally described the environmental media and routes of entry to the body needed to characterize exposure. Each has been examined over the years to provide information on the magnitude and extent of environmental problems. For exposure assessment there is a special need to know how each medium or route is associated with the degree to which individuals or members of a population come into contact with a contaminant. Many types of sources that impact each medium, and some of the more common issues are shown in Table 5. Clearly, inorganic or organic emissions can come from industrial processes, commercial activities, personal use and activities, disposal activities, and nature.

It is somewhat obvious that the environmental media that can lead to contact with a contaminant include: air, water, soil, and food as people routinely come into contact with these each daily. However, it may be somewhat of a surprise that all routes of entry to the body, except inadvertent or purposeful injection of a biological or chemical contaminant, may be directly or indirectly impacted by a contaminant originally released in one medium. This important point is illustrated in Table 6 for the contaminants lead and pesticides.

Lead can be emitted by sources that directly impact the air, water, soil, and food, then transported to and deposited in another medium, and thereby be made available to indirectly cause exposures via multiple routes of entry to the body. From the standpoint of public health the situation is complicated because there is no easy formula available to determine the route of entry, or to apportion the sources contributing to lead burden. In the case of house dust, lead can be derived from indoor and outdoor sources, and ingestion occurs after dermal adhesion and transfer to the mouth or after the adhesion of the dust to a food or toys (NRC 1993*a*). For pesticide exposures, there is an added source of exposure, as an important way to increase contamination is the direct application of a pesticide to surfaces by a homeowner or resident (this is in addition to any amount derived from the work of a professional exterminator or crop duster) (NRC 1993*b*). However, once in the home there can be re-emission and redistribution of semivolatile pesticides to other surfaces (Gurunathan *et al.* 1998).

The need to complete a source apportionment for lead, pesticides, and other chemicals provides a message for public health officials and the exposure assessor: the obvious answer (source) may not always

Table 3 Summary of sampling for exposure assessment

Sampling design	Condition for most useful application
Haphazard sampling	Only valid when target population and exposure is homogeneous in space and time; hence not generally recommended
Purposive sampling	Target population well defined and homogeneous, so sample-selection bias is not a problem; or specific microenvironmental or personal samples selected for unique value and interest, rather than for making inferences to wider population
Probability sampling	
Simple random sampling	Homogeneous population
Stratified random sampling	Homogeneous population with strata (subregions); might consider strata as domains of study
Systematic sampling	Frequently most useful: trends over time and space must be quantified; can easily be adapted to total exposure
Multistage sampling	Target population large and homogeneous; simple random sampling used to select contiguous groups of population units
Cluster sampling	Economical when population units cluster (e.g. schools of fish); ideally, cluster means are similar in value, but concentrations within clusters should vary widely. Anticipate high end exposures
Double sampling	Must be strong linear relation between variable of interest and less expensive or more easily measured variable

Table 4 Defining high-exposure populations

Data collection methods

Choice of method

- Purposive exposure study
- Applied, or response, epidemiology
- Targeted case–control or cohorts
- Registries
- Reference population surveys
- Complete enumeration

Sampling design

- Representative
- Convenient

Detecting small populations or rare events

Defining subgroups of the population

Cultural characteristics

- Cultural identity
- Heterogeneity within categories
- Sensitive information
- Cultural habits or rituals
- Choice of appropriate indicator

Susceptibility characterizations

- Race
- Gender
- Age
- Disease state
- Population on family genetics
- Occupations (participation or avoidance)

Population

- Mobility
- Estimation of local population size
- Intermarriage
- Assimilation
- Daily living activities
- Proximity to a source or source region
- Observation of any effects

provide the correct way to solve a problem. For instance, a person may live in a residence that has lead-based paint the walls. The first thought would be that the lead paint was the major source of blood lead levels measured in the occupants. If the painted surface is isolated or intact, however, the source that could cause an increase in blood lead may be street dust and/or soil in the neighbourhood. Therefore source apportionment plays a crucial part in linking the point of emission through the route of exposure to an internal or biologically effective dose (previously illustrated in Fig. 2 and Lioy (1999)).

An example of how exposure and risk derived from multiple routes of entry can be underestimated is associated with regulations or public health advisories for potable water supplies. In the 1970s, potential exposures and health risks were based solely on the quantity of the contaminant ingested by drinking the water (USEPA 1980), and the assumed consumption of 2 litres of water per day, which is unusual for

Table 5 Typical sources of contaminants that can be present in various media

Air (outdoor)	
Smelters	Atmosphere reactions
Power plants	Space heating
Petrochemical	Automobiles
Plants	Trucks
Chemical	Transportation
Manufacturing	Water treatment
Paper and pulp	Plants
Cement plants	Autobody repair
Municipal incinerators	Mining operations
Degreasing operations	
Air (indoor)	
Passive smoking	Deodorizers
Household products	Rugs
Indoor combustion	Ventilation system
Disinfectants	Water contaminants
Paint	Paint removers
Water	
Landfills	Domestic waste
Hazardous waste sites	Agriculture
Chemical plants	Agriculture run-off
Pesticides production	Underground storage
Food process industry	Urban street run-off
Sewage treatment	Water system
Septic tank	Sealants
Soil	
Hazardous wastes	Yard clean-up and maintenance
Underground storage tanks	Buried underground
Domestic waste	Storage
Industrial dumping	
Food	
Garden soil	Insufficient food preparation
Agricultural soil	Pesticide residuals
Insufficient food cleaning	Unapproved packaging
Injection	
Contaminated needles and	Contaminated products
objects	Spills and transportation
Contaminated fluids	

Table 6 Routes of entry of contaminants to the body

Contaminant	Medium or pathway	Source
Lead	Outdoor air	Industrial Automobile
	Indoor air	Infiltration of outdoor air
	Outdoor soil	Air deposition Flaking paint Hazardous waste
	Outdoor dust	Air deposition Flaking paint Soil resuspension
	House dust	Tracked dust Paint flaking Air filtration
	Food utensils/ food preparation	Dust deposition Dust contact Pottery/glasses
	Clothing	Surface contact Laundering of clothes
	Water	Water pipes Water supply
	Food	Grown in contaminated soil Preparation
Pesticides	Outdoor air	Spraying of crops or yards
	Indoor air	Spraying of plants Outdoor air filtration
	Outdoor soil	Air deposition Direct spraying of plants/ vegetation
	Outdoor dust	Air deposition Resuspension of soil
	House dust	Indoor spraying Tracked outdoor dust/soil Outdoor air filtration
	Food	Surface deposition Fruit/vegetable contamination
	Food preparation	Surface dust (outdoor/house)
	Water	Run-off from soil Water supply

most members of the general population. Public health advisories on the use of contaminated water supplies, for example wells with water containing contaminants leached from hazardous waste sites, stated that individuals using a particular water supply 'should not drink the water'. If scientists and regulators had seriously considered all the opportunities for contact with potable water prior to estimating the risk, they would have included two other routes of exposure: dermal and inhalation (Brown *et al.* 1984). Only after studies by Andelman (1985), which focused on the shower as a route for inhalation exposure, and Jo *et al.* (1990) and Weisel *et al.* (1993), which demonstrated that significant human exposures to volatile organics occurred via inhalation and the dermal route during showering or bathing, did the public health practice and environmental regulations embrace the concept of total exposure. The results have led to the concept that individuals should 'just not use contaminated water'. According to Jo *et al.* (1990), at least half of an individual's internal dose derived from chloroform found in a public water supply could be from just one 10-min shower per day. Obviously more and varied uses of the water would lead to higher or lower daily internal doses.

The importance of both the dermal and inhalation routes is demonstrated in Fig. 7, for the concentration of chloroform found in exhaled breath after using a swimming pool. Integration of the area under the curve indicates that both routes made similar contributions to an internal dose, even though there is a much slower rate of chloroform accumulation by the dermal route (Georgopoulos *et al.* 1997; Kim and Weisel 1998).

Techniques

The measurement process used to establish the presence of a contaminant in one or more of the above media or routes can become complex and require the application of a variety of techniques. Two primary categories exist for exposure measurements: direct and indirect techniques, Fig. 8 (NRC 1991*c*). These categories correspond to the types of methods being used to collect data or estimate exposure within field studies and modelling simulations respectively. The main differences between these two types of techniques are associated with the proximity of the measurement or estimate of exposure to the individual, and the qualitative or quantitative nature of the information. At present, there is no uniformity in the quality and quantity of techniques available for any category of indirect or direct measurements. In fact, there are major instrumentation needs for each environmental medium and route of exposure. This is not to say that there is a lack of sampling and analytical equipment to measure chemical, physical, and biological agents in various environmental media. However, many have been designed to provide environmental quality measurements rather than human exposure measurements. This is an important point and is substantiated by the fact that many of

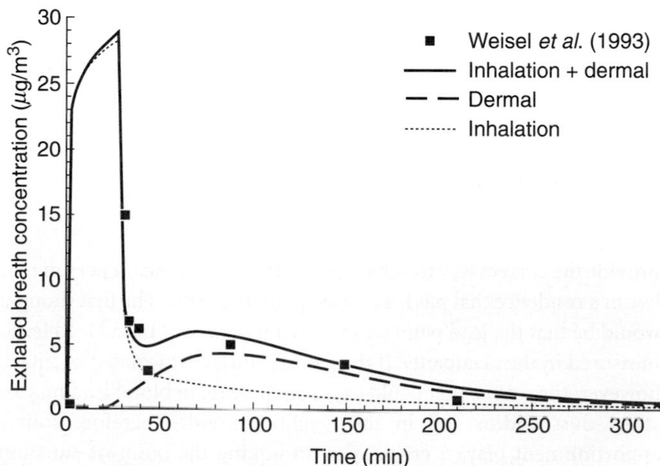

Fig. 7 Exhaled breath concentration of chloroform following inhalation and dermal absorption in a swimming pool (air concentration 100 µg/m³, water concentration 150 µg/l).

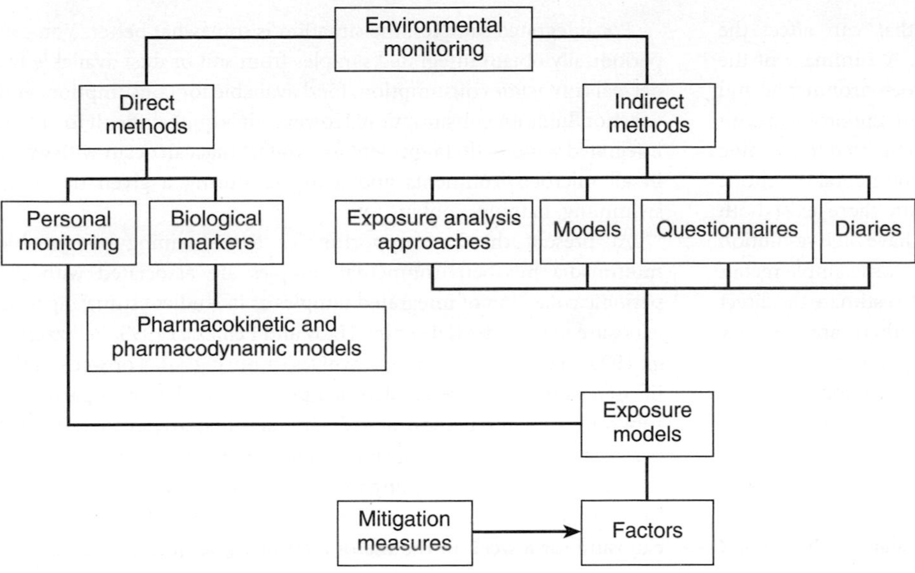

Fig. 8 Possible approaches for analysis of air contaminant exposures. (Source: NRC 1991c.)

the currently available techniques are too bulky to be used in applications requiring either microenvironmental and/or personal measurements (Lioy 1993).

In many cases personal monitors still require optimization for a number of parameters. A list of general technical criteria that must be met to develop these monitors is shown in Table 7 (NRC 1991*c*). It is apparent that the techniques must be compact, and each must have low detection limits and sufficient time resolution in order to obtain human exposures for the chemical(s) under consideration. These three features are difficult to achieve simultaneously in a single device. For example, as an instrument is miniaturized the substrate available for sample collection or the detection volume available for instrumental analyses (e.g. a photocell) is reduced. Consequently, the detection limits will rise and/or the time necessary to collect an adequate sample will increase, which can preclude their use in specific applications, for example low-level short-term exposure or acute exposures or acute exposures. Such incompatibilities can only be eliminated by conducting basic research prior to the development of a sampling programme that will employ a device in any particular application. Sometimes there may be 'off the shelf' devices available for use in an application or study, but the possibilities have been limited for most media and routes of exposure. During the mid-1970s, because of the increased concern about health problems associated with indoor air pollution, technology developed rapidly and microenvironmental and personal air measurements were available for the detection of traditional contaminants (e.g. volatile organics, fine particles, and carbon monoxide). Others are being developed for agents such as microbiological aerosols. Some of the personal monitors are based on passive sampling techniques while other sampling systems use an active pump (Seifert and Abraham 1983; Ryan *et al.* 1986; Samet *et al.* 1987, 1988).

Before the concept of total exposure became a starting point for the design of field studies and risk assessments, the following measurement issue received little attention: How comparable is the data collected by various techniques used across more than one medium or route of entry into the body? Unfortunately, there is no complete answer because of the many different types of physical, chemical, and biological agents that exist and the nature of the emissions, transport,

Table 7 Methods criteria

Factor	Ideal condition
Sensitivity	Detects analytes at levels below those causing adverse health effect; sensitivity 0.1× level of interest; range 0.1–10× level of interest; precision and accuracy ±5%; easy and accurate calibration
Selectivity	No response to similar compounds that might be present simultaneously with the analyte of interest or can differentiate multiple compounds in single device
Rapidity	Short sampling and analysis times compared with biological response time or with significant changes in contaminant concentration; response time 90% in less than 30s; RS232 or equivalent output
Operation	Few complex components to change in the field, quick releases, low noise
Comprehensiveness	Sensitive to all contaminants that could result in a similar adverse health effect
Portability	Sampling and analysis device is rugged and can be worn without modifying the normal behaviour of individual; lower power consumption; battery operated; stabilization time less than 15 min; temperature range −20 to 40°C; humidity range zero to 100%
Cost	Cost of sampling and analysis is not prohibitive; inexpensive; readily available components; few consumables; low maintenance

accumulation, and transformation processes that can affect the occurrence of biologically significant exposures. A summary of the types of techniques employed for collecting microenvironmental and personal samples is shown in Table 8. To illustrate the problem with obtaining comparable measurements Table 8 can be used to examine the situation as it currently exists for microenvironmental monitors. For microenvironmental studies of air pollution there exist both continuous and integrating monitors; the devices have high resolution and low detection limits for specific compounds, for example metals and volatile organics. The data can easily be used to estimate the direct inhalation exposure. However, for other media there are very few comparable techniques available for completing events with even quasi-continuous monitors. In fact, there are no continuous monitors currently available for these sampling media that operate without the constant use of a technician as a personal shadow. For example, take a surface soil sample at every location, he or she came into contact with soil during the day (Hawley 1985). Alternatively, the person would be required to have a trained technician directly shadow his or her movements during the sampling in order to collect the appropriate surface soil samples or provide dermal contact samples similar to those experienced by the subject. In either case the approach is very cumbersome and can lead to many errors.

Table 8 General availability of monitors for measuring exposure

Type/route	Personal	Micro-environmental	Environmental
Inhalation/gases			
C	+	+	+
I	+	+	+
Pesticides			
C	–	+	+
I	+	+	+
Ingestion			
Food			
C	–	–	–
I	+	+	+
Water			
C	–	–	–
I	–	+	+
Soil and dust			
C	–	–	–
I	–	+	+
Dermal			
Water			
C	–	–	–
I	–	+	+
Soil and dust			
C	–	–	–
I	–	+	+

C, continuous monitor; I, integrated monitor; –, not available; +, available.

For integrated samples, the situation is somewhat better. You can periodically obtain integrated samples from soil or dust available for dermal contact or consumption, food available for consumption, and water or fluids for consumption. However, it is quite difficult to obtain integrated samples that represent the contact that can occur with water in all microenvironments and activities during a given day (e.g. swimming, bathing, cooking, etc.).

At present the best opportunities for obtaining comparable multimedia microenvironmental samples are associated with the periodic collection of integrated samples as in studies estimating total exposure in a residential setting (Lioy and Pellizzari 1995; Pellizzari *et al.* 1995). The general concept involves capturing a day or week in the life of a statistical representative sample of a population or particular subgroup of a population at risk. In such a study, an investigator periodically collects a set of short-term samples and/or grab samples over a representative sampling interval. Figure 9 and Table 9 indicate the types of samples that can be collected to estimate a residential exposure for a week in the life of a family. The output from such a measurement study will be a series of microenvironmental samples that are analysed for the chemicals of concern. The data are then used as an input to exposure scenarios to specific environmental contaminants in residential settings. They can also be used to construct total exposure estimates using variants to the summation equations given in Box 1.

One major component of this type of study is the application of questionnaires, which must include a time/activity log that is completed by the members of the household during the time of the field sampling. The data are essential for reducing uncertainties that are inherent with the application of generic exposure scenarios to site- or person-specific assessments.

Table 9 Sampling strategy

Types of samples	Location	Duration
Indoor air	Two high-use rooms	1–7 days
Outdoor air	Breathing zone in yard	1–7 days
Soil	Yard surface	Composited grab
	0–2 cm gridded yard sweep	
	Subsurface	
	0–100 cm gridded dig	
Dust	Flat interior surface	Integrated wipe
	Rugs on interior floor	Integrated vacuum
	Flat exterior walkways	Integrated sweeps
Water	Drinking water	Daily tap water (1 litre)
	Shower water	10–30 min
	Bath water	Daily bath water
Food	Kitchen prepared and consumed meals	1- to 7-day duplicate diet
Activity patterns	Residential actions or events	Daily diary

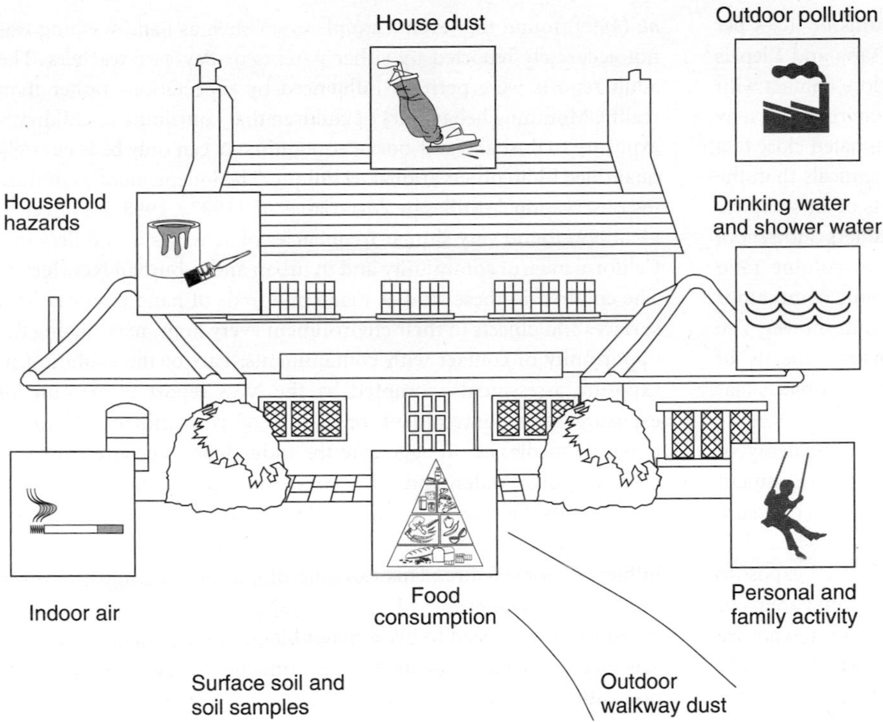

Fig. 9 Types of integrated microenvironmental sentinel for home exposure to metals, pesticides, and/or volatile organics.

Activity logs have become customized to address the exposures that can occur for specific chemicals (Robinson *et al.* 1989; Freeman *et al.* 1991; Schwab *et al.* 1991), in addition to logs that address generic issues on contact with environmental contaminants (e.g. frequency of personal product use and contact with volatile components, frequency, and duration of outdoor activities). For instance, in a study of residential exposure typical questions for a week-long study of chromium exposure would include the following.

1. Were any of the following used in the house today? (a) vacuum; (b) carpet sweeper; (c) broom; (d) dust cloths/mops; (e) wet mops; (f) other house cleaning; (g) laundry.
2. Did you notice any green, yellow, red, or orange deposits or stains on the walls or floors of your home?
3. If you noticed these deposits, were you or members of your family in the room or rooms with these deposits for more than 10 min at a time?

Results obtained by these types of methods can be validated by video records, technician observations, and fluorescent tracer studies (Fenske *et al.* 1991). During the chromium study validation was obtained via observations made by a trained technician.

Although not shown in Fig. 9, a residential microenvironmental study can easily be expanded to include personal monitoring and biological monitoring. Some of the more common are used to measure organic/inorganic chemicals in blood and urine. These samples will provide personal integrated or time series data for the duration of the sampling period (e.g. a day or a week). Biological monitoring data provides baseline information on the residents and can be used to determine if they have been 'truly' in contact with a contaminant. If a residential experiment is repeated one or more times, biological marker data can be valuable in pharmacokinetic model simulations for some contaminants. Follow-up biological monitoring samples can also allow the analyst to establish any incremental changes in dose.

Biological monitoring is currently being used to measure selected heavy metals in blood or urine, volatile organics in blood, and pesticides in blood and urine in studies at hazardous waste sites and within the National Human Exposure Assessment Survey (Pellizzari *et al.* 1995; Pirkle *et al.* 1995). There are also some techniques available for the measurement of metabolites and DNA adducts (Fiserova-Bergerova 1987; Perera *et al.* 1987; NRC 1989*a*,*b*, 1991*c*; Ashley *et al.* 1992). The most notable are associated with the polycyclic aromatic hydrocarbons (Perera 1987). A first-order analysis of the data would be to determine the change in contaminant level for a bodily fluid that could be associated with a change in the type or intensity of exposure that occurred at the residence. A second-order analysis would involve the application of pharmacokinetic models (Gerlowsky and Jain 1983; Caudill and Pirkle 1992).

In 1993, the National Academy of Sciences published a report (NAS 1993) arguing that children are a highly susceptible population for exposure to pesticides. Both in terms of surface-to-volume ratio and physiological function children are different from adults, and may be more susceptible to exposure to environmental contaminants. Their way of interacting with the world is different from adults, and they spend more time on the floor, and take baths rather than showers. Further, infants and toddlers are more likely to mouth objects and exhibit hand-to-mouth behaviours, and have substantially greater food and fluid consumption when expressed as grams or litres per kilogram of body weight than adults (NAS 1993; Tsang and Klepeis 1996, Freeman *et al.* 1997, 1999). Because of their close contact with floors and carpets, the concept of a well-mixed air environment may not be appropriate for the air they breathe. The air inhaled close to a carpet may have very different concentrations of chemicals than the air inhaled 4 or 5 feet from the floor, where the inlets of air samplers are typically placed. The prolonged hot baths of toddlers and school children in combination with the greater surface-to-volume ratio produces potentially greater exposure to volatile organic compounds in water than an adult receives in his or her 5- to 10-min shower. The mouthing behaviours of children become a constant means of incidentally ingesting contaminants on their hands or the objects that they mouth.

In response to the issues raised by the National Academy of Sciences report (NAS 1993), the methods used in exposure assessment have had to change in new directions as interest in children's exposure to environmental contaminants has evolved. Previously, when children were the target population of interest (primarily lead exposure studies), information about the children was obtained from parents or carers. This allowed acquisition of global knowledge about exposure activities such as identifying the microenvironment in which the child spent time or macroactivities such as whether or not the child took a bath or play in a sandbox. The amount of time spent in a microenvironment, submerged in a bath, or in contact with the sand could not effectively be obtained from parents as the parents are often not present with the child, much less timing the events. The temporal information obtained from parents are at best 'guesstimates'.

Collecting information from children also has problems as often the target population is so young that self-reports cannot be obtained. Even children as old as 10 or 12 years have difficulty with concepts of time, and reportage using real-time diaries have not been entirely successful (Schwab *et al.* 1990, 1991). Younger children not only have limited concepts of time, but also may not have the ability to read and complete diaries, or verbally express themselves in response to an interviewer.

Additional problems with understanding children's exposure to environmental contaminants have emerged as the source of exposure has shifted from outdoor and/or indoor air pollutants to water-borne and dust/soil-borne contaminants and the routes of exposure have shifted from inhalation to dermal contact, and dietary and non-dietary ingestion. To understand these sources and routes of exposure information is needed about not only for microenvironments but microactivities, such as, contact with dust and soil, or mouthing objects and fingers (Cohen-Hubel *et al.* 1999; Reed *et al.* 1999). Additional sources of exposure in the child's environment may be the toys the child plays with and mouths (Gurunathan *et al.* 1998). The dynamic character of semivolatile chemicals such as pesticides means that surfaces and objects not directly sprayed may become reservoirs and future sources of exposure. Understanding the potential exposure from these surfaces and objects requires collection of information about microactivities that has seldom been collected.

While parental reportage of time/activity information about their children continues to be used, parental responses are now being supplemented, if not supplanted, by observational methods (Zartarian *et al.* 1997*a*, 1998; Reed *et al.* 1999). Videotaped observations can be used to verify parental responses, quantify use of microenvironments, and collect frequency and duration data about microactivities. Reed *et al.* (1999) found that even a simple event such as hand washing was not accurately reported by either parents or day-care teachers. The adult reports were perhaps influenced by expectations rather than reality. Mouthing behaviours of children that contribute to children's exposure to dust and soil-borne contaminants can only be accurately quantified by an observational technique. The independently conducted observational studies by Zartarian *et al.* (1997*a*, 1998) and Reed *et al.* (1999) found very similar frequencies of activities in toddlers in a Californian farm community and in urban and suburban New Jersey. The children in these studies made hundreds of hand contacts with surfaces and objects in their environment every hour, maximizing the opportunity of contact with contaminants. Part of the evolution in exposure assessment prompted by the NAS report is to think of exposure to a contaminant or family of contaminants from all potential media, i.e. to aggregate the individuals exposure from air, food, soil, dust, water, and other contaminated media. For the child, the 'other media' may be a major pathway, but one for which there are presently few data, and ones for which activities may have a large influence on exposure. This example of children just illustrates the needs of one subgroup of the general population. In the future, investigators will need to fill in major blanks for cultural, gender, and age-specific behaviours that can influence individual or sub-population exposure.

Data analysis and models

Once microenvironmental and/or personal exposure data have been acquired in a field study or estimated by a model there are a number of analyses that can be used to place the data in a form that is helpful for examining a public health issue. The levels of analysis are dependent upon the types and amount of data available from a particular study or a series of companion or comparative studies (USEPA 1989*a*). A parallel issue is the form of the data necessary for the application of interest, for example epidemiology or risk assessment. For instance the data can be reported as exposure using the units of concentration and time ($\mu g/m^3$ per h) or as a time-weighted average ($\mu g/m^3$ per day). Then, depending upon the amount of data available, a distribution of exposure can be constructed and particular statistical quantities calculated from that data. Information that is derived from a distribution of exposures are shown in Fig. 10 (USEPA 1992*a*), and include the mean exposure (50th percentile), the high end exposure, greater than the 90th percentile, the form of the exposure distribution curve, and the worst possible case estimate (bounding estimate) of exposure.

If the database includes information that can be examined across pathways or routes of exposure, the result will be estimates of total exposure across each medium or each route of entry into the body. The data collected that represent a day or week of a family, Table 9, and Fig. 9 can be used to determine the microenvironmental increments to total exposure. Theoretically, an integrated exposure can be derived from microenvironmental exposures by the summation formula found in Box 1.

Risk assessment applications require at least one further level of analysis: a dose calculated from the exposure level. The result can then be used in a risk characterization analysis, and, as stated earlier, these calculations can be in one of three forms: potential, internal, or biologically effective dose. The general form of the equations needed

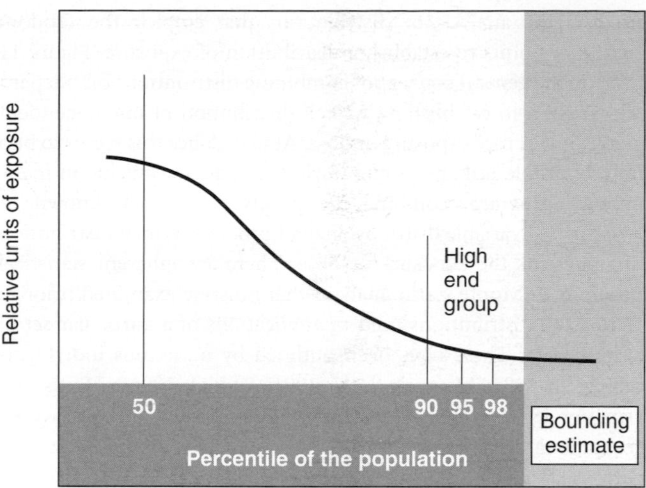

Fig. 10 Major parameters to be determined from a distribution (known/default) of population exposure.

to calculate dose from exposure data are shown in Box 2. Based upon the ancillary information and parameters needed to complete such calculations (e.g. absorption rate) the value most frequently calculated is the potential dose. In rare instances the biologically effective dose can be calculated, but there are large uncertainties in the values used for factors to complete such calculations (e.g. repair rate etc.) (Lioy 1990).

A second reason for calculating a dose from the exposure data is to place units of measurement in a form that are consistent for comparisons among each route of entry. A typical form for dose is micrograms of contaminant per kilogram of body weight per unit of time. The format makes it easier to compare intensity of the contact with the amount that has been deposited within the body for different routes of entry. These data can also be used to determine which of the exposures encountered were at levels that may cause a biological effect.

As shown in Box 2, unless the investigator has acquired biological marker data, the determination of a dose requires information on a series of variables or factors that may only be measurable in detailed exposure assessment studies (USEPA 1989*a*; AIHC 1994). An update on such factors was published by the United States Environmental Protection Agency in 1999 on a CD-ROM. Examples of factors needed to complete dose calculations include breathing rate, skin absorption rate, ingestion rate, internal absorption rate, elimination, and repair rates. Obviously, it is easier to acquire data on breathing or ingestion rate than on organic cellular repair mechanisms. In fact, there are no methods available at the current time that can quantify cellular repair.

A type of data that is not usually available for dose calculations, but could be obtained, is the bioavailability of a contaminant in the matrix that contains it (e.g. soil) (Umbreit *et al.* 1986; Kitsa *et al.* 1992; Ruby *et al.* 1993; Wainman *et al.* 1994; Hamel *et al.* 1998). This value is dependent upon the amount of a contaminant that can be extracted from the matrix (e.g. soil) by bodily fluids found within the digestive system or the lung.

As it is not possible to acquire data routinely in a field study on accumulation or elimination rates, or absorption factors, dose calculations employ what have been conventionally described as generic exposure factors (single values or a distribution of values). Based upon the type of dose calculation the number of exposure factors selected could be minimal or extensive. These are driven by the data quality objectives, the amount of data available, the anticipated variability of the activities affecting the dose, and the types of individual or population characteristics considered to be of importance. Once these types of information have accumulated and the purpose and objectives of the analyses have been established, the analyst can complete either a point estimate of a dose or a distributional estimate of dose.

Point estimates of exposure require the application of an equation similar to those found in Box 2 for each route of exposure and each microenvironment that can lead to an individual having contact with chemicals. For example, selection of ingestion exposure, inhalation exposure, and dermal exposure scenarios can provide an estimate of the potential or, with additional data, an internal dose of a contaminant by completing a calculation similar to that illustrated in Box 3 (USEPA 1989*a*). Results can then be summed for all microenvironments and media to obtain point estimates of exposure for a hypothetical or representative member of the local population. One can also develop a distribution of dose point estimates based upon exposure measurements (e.g. personal monitoring) and/or estimates

Box 2 Generalized equations governing exposure and dose

Integrated exposure

$$E = \int_{t_1}^{t_2} C(t)dt$$

where E is exposure, $C(t)$ is time-variant concentration, and t_1, t_2 are time periods of exposure associated with a specific biological response.

Potential dose

$$D_P = \int_{t_2}^{t_1} C(t)f(t)dt$$

where D_p is the potential dose and $f(t)$ is the contact rate.

Internal dose

$$D_I = \int_{t_1}^{t_2} C(t)f(t)g_{ab}dt$$

where D_I is the internal dose and g_{ab} is the absorption function (e.g. skin, lung membrane, gut).

Target tissue dose

$$D_T = \int_{t_1}^{t_2} C(t)f(t)g_{pk}dt$$

where D_T is the target tissue dose and g_{pk} is the pharmacokinetic model (accounts for absorption, distribution, and elimination processes).

Biologically effective dose

$$D_{BE} = \int_{t_1}^{t_2} f(x)g(ab)p(as,rd,me,el)C(t)dt$$

where p(as,rd,me,el) is a function based on nature of assimilation, repair, elimination, and/or metabolism.

Box 3 Point estimate of potential dose

- Ingestion of chemicals in water or beverages:

$$\text{potential dose} = \frac{CW \times IR \times EF \times ED}{BW \times AT} \text{ mg/kg/day}$$

where CW is the chemical concentration in water, IR is the ingestion rate (l/day), EF is the exposure frequency (days/year), ED is the exposure duration (years), BW is the body weight (kg), and AT is the averaging time (period over which exposure is averaged) (days).

- Chemicals in soil:

$$\text{potential dose} = \frac{CS \times IR \times CF \times FI \times EF \times ED}{BW \times AT} \text{ mg/kg/day}$$

where CS is the chemical concentration in soil (mg/kg), IR is the ingestion rate (mg soil/day), CF is the conversion factor (10^6 kg/mg), FI is the fraction ingested from contaminated source (unitless), EF is the exposure frequency (days/years), ED is the exposure duration (years), BW is the body weight (kg), and AT is the averaging time (period over which exposure is averaged) (days).

- Inhalation of airborne (vapour-phase) chemicals:

$$\text{potential dose} = \frac{CA \times IR \times ET \times EF \times ED}{BW \times AT} \text{ mg/kg/day}$$

where CA is the contaminant concentration in air ($\mu g/m^3$), IR is the inhalation rate (m^3/h), ET is the exposure time (h/day), EF is the exposure frequency (days/year), ED is the exposure duration (years), BW is the body/weight (kg), and AT is the averaging time (period over which exposure is averaged) (days).

- Dermal contact with chemicals in soil:

$$\text{potential dose} = \frac{CS \times CF \times SA \times AF \times ABS \times EF \times ED}{BW \times AT} \text{ mg/kg/day}$$

where CS is the chemical concentration in soil (mg/kg), CF is the conversion factor (10^6 kg/mg), SA is the skin area (cm^2), AF is the soil-to-skin adherence factor (mg/cm^2), ABS is the absorption factor (unitless), EF is the exposure frequency (days/years), ED is the exposure duration (years), BW is the body weight (kg), AT is the averaging time (period over which exposure is averaged) (days).

of exposure using exposure factors characteristic of the population of concern.

There has been a distinct move away from relying exclusively on point estimates of exposure and dose. This is done primarily to reduce the uncertainties that surround identifying a 'most exposed individual' (USEPA 1992*a*), which was frequently described as the person exposed to everything over a lifetime. In fact, exposure assessors are now being encouraged to employ distributional analyses by the frequency distributions of all or selected factors needed to estimate particular exposures or doses. This has led to the use of Monte Carlo techniques for combining the selected distributions of parameters or variables (Rubinstein 1981; Marnicio *et al.* 1991; USEPA 1992*a*, *b*; Hattis and Burmaster 1994). On the surface this appears to be a step forward in the development of exposure/dose data bases especially for risk assessment applications. However, there are some 'land mines' buried in the analysis of distributions that employ the random selection of points to establish a distribution of exposure. Figure 11 illustrates the general concept of combining distributions of independent variables to establish an overall distribution of one dependent variable; in our case exposure or dose. At first glance this seems to be a relatively simple task, as Monte Carlo techniques, available in many computer program, combine the points along each known or approximated variable distribution, and produces a final distribution that represents the exposure or dose. There are inherent statistical limitations to Monte Carlo analyses that must be examined prior to selecting the distributions used in applications of a particular set of exposure data. These have been outlined by numerous individuals (Rubinstein 1981; Marnicio *et al.* 1991; USEPA 1992*a*; Hattis and Burmaster 1994). Beyond the statistical constraints, there are other informational issues that must be evaluated to ensure that the estimates are plausible and realistic. Included is the evaluation of the usefulness of the values combined across distributions to simulate either the high end exposures or low end exposures. An example of a distribution of an exposure factor, fish ingestion, is shown in Fig. 12. It is clear that there is a tendency toward biomodality (AIHC 1994). The shape of the curve indicates different consumption patterns for subgroups of a population. Thus, proper utilization of the data requires knowledge of consumption activities within a potentially affected population.

Evaluations of distributional data must also ascertain whether or not all projected exposures or doses can occur and can they occur for the situation or activity being under investigation. At a minimum sensitivity analyses should be conducted on the tails of the variable distributions used to estimate the exposure/dose. For example, an acute toxin (such as cyanide or ozone) at sufficient concentration to induce a biological response (death or asthma attack respectively) over a short period of time would not logically be coupled with a contact period equivalent to a week or more. An 82-year-old grandparent or unathletic person would not be spending too much time engaging in activities with a high ventilation rate 1.5 m^3/h, when the outdoor ozone concentrations exceed 150 ppb. Finally, a child would not be spending 24 h a day over a 12-year period sitting on the grounds of a

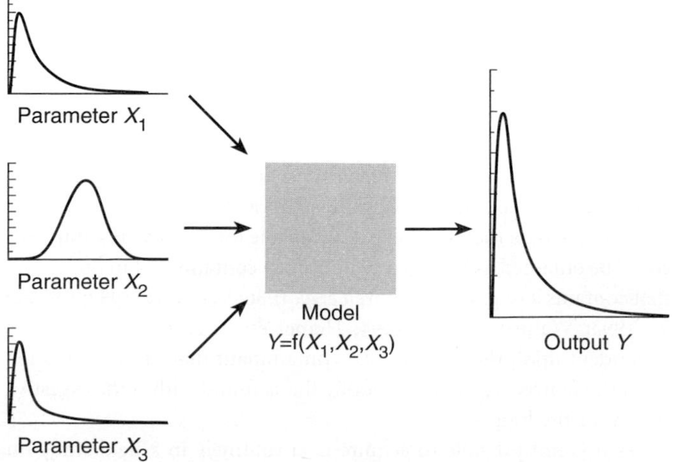

Fig. 11 Representation of Monte Carlo analysis used to construct a dependent variable distribution *Y*.

Min.	Max.	4%	31%	44%	72%	95%
0.4	5.0	0.4	0.8	1.4	2.0	4.0

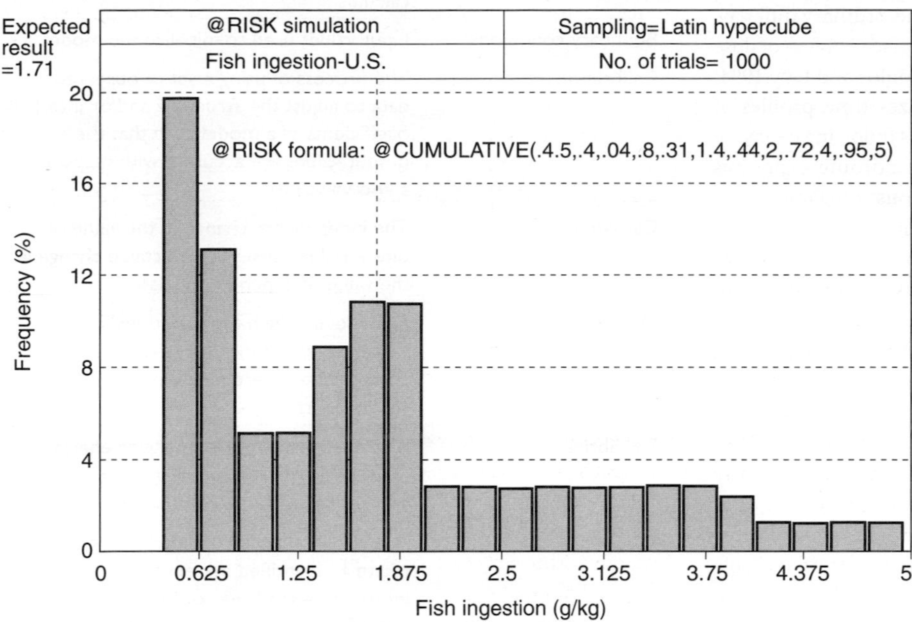

Fig. 12 Distribution of fish ingestion. (Source: AIHC 1994.)

hazardous waste site. These examples may seem somewhat absurd, but if the appropriate constraints are not placed on a distributional analysis of exposure, these types of results and worse could be propagated through a computer program and reported as part of the estimated distribution of exposure or dose.

Although distributional analyses are more likely to be conducted for risk assessments, they are of value in epidemiological studies. A specific case is a comparison of a biological marker data for a contaminant or metabolite with a dose estimated from external exposure measurements. In intervention studies distributional data are of immense value for comparing a point measurement of exposure or dose (individual or affected subgroups) with the values observed and/or estimated for a much larger population (Lioy 1992).

Exposure assessment modelling

Predictions of an exposure or potential dose have been based on emissions, environmental transport and fate modelling (Thibodeaux 1979; Javandel *et al.* 1984; Cohen 1989; Georgopoulos 1990) and population time/location and activity pattern modelling combined with microenvironmental quality modelling (Ott 1980; Duan 1982, 1991; Schwab *et al.* 1991; Pardi 1992; Patrick 1994). This is called a prognostic assessment. Prediction of exposure can also be done based on modelling of biomarker data (Georgopoulos and Lioy 1994), which is called the diagnostic assessment. Whenever possible, both microenvironmental and biomarker data should be used, because these data are from independent sources, and should therefore result in the reduction of overall uncertainty (Roy and Georgopoulos 1998).

It was noted above, in the section on basic principles, that the overarching aim is to relate environmental releases to adverse health effect. Although it is possible to relate exposure with toxic effects, increasingly more direct relationships can be obtained by using potential dose, internal dose, and target tissue dose respectively. Calculation of target tissue dose requires the application of a pharmacokinetic model (sometimes referred to as a toxicokinetic model) that describes the uptake, distribution, metabolism, and elimination the toxicant. Pharmacokinetic models used in exposure assessments are generally compartmental models, which are empirically based, or physiologically based pharmacokinetic (**PBPK**) models that have a mechanistic basis and represent the major tissues of the body as separate compartments, linked by anatomically correct blood flows.

The fraction of an internal dose that reaches the target tissue can be highly dependent upon the route of uptake, and PBPK models, are a natural choice for estimating the target tissue dose for each route of uptake. For example, the fraction of an ingested internal dose that reaches the liver will generally be much greater than that of an inhaled internal dose, which in turn will be greater than that of a internal dermal dose. A further advantage of the PBPK formulation is that it is amenable to interspecies scale-up. This is an important attribute, as ethical and practical reasons generally preclude the intentional dosing of humans with toxic substances. Thus a PBPK model for humans can be developed on the basis of a PBPK model in laboratory animals (Ramsey and Anderson 1984). Moreover, PBPK models can be adapted to reflect the inherent variability in human populations. Model parameters are generally formulated as functions of body weight, and in principle this can be extended to other covariates such as age, height, and sex. Physiologically based models that relate exposure to internal and target tissue dose have been successfully applied to predict doses for a variety of toxicants. Both traditional 'lumped' parameter (ordinary differential equation) formulations as well as 'refined' distributed parameter (partial and ordinary differential equation) schemes, have been used for the inverse problem of dose to exposure medium to reconstruction (Georgopoulos and Lioy 1994; Georgopoulos *et al.* 1994). This approach utilizes time profiles of biomarker concentrations found in excreted fluids following exposure to reconstruct the single and/or multimedia/multiroute exposures experienced by an individual (e.g. simultaneous inhalation and dermal absorption of a volatile organic present in air and water).

A detailed exposure assessment may also require resource-intensive data collection studies or model-based simulations to characterize one or more of the following: source attributes, toxicant properties, geographical domain of influence attributes, population composition/stratification, population time/location pattern and activity patterns, macroenvironmental media properties/concentrations, microenvironmental media properties and concentrations, and the exposure routes and pathways. Consequently, the complexity of the exposure system and the wide range of information requirements necessitate simulation that can describe the exposure to dose or the dose to exposure. Finally, case-specific requirements of available mechanistic information must be available to link each component of the exposure continuum (Fig. 2), and then estimate doses potentially received by a particular population. The overall types of analyses and data needs required to complete an exposure simulation successfully is shown in Table 10 (Patrick 1994).

A general modelling framework can guide the collection and analysis of new data while, on the other hand, the quality and quantity of available data limits the sophistication of any model. Priorities in data collection and model development must be established and the options must be explored for analysing available information and for modelling various components of the exposure system. Components of both single-medium and multimedia environmental and environmental exposure models, such as, for example the Human Exposure Model HEM II (USEPA 1991) used for the assessment of population exposures from air releases, and the STREAM model (Donigian and Mulkey 1992), used for the exposure assessment of pesticide run-off, should be considered in the development and expansion of models.

Microenvironment models should be evaluated prior to their use in assessing exposure for the application under consideration (Ott *et al.* 1988; USEPA 1989*b*). The relative advantages and limitations of stochastic simulation models (such as SHAPE, TRIM, and BEAM), cartesianization, or convolution models, and the most general double covariance models have been summarized elsewhere (Georgopoulos and Lioy 1994). An assumption of log normality for integrated exposures and doses provides a starting step for conducting probabilistic exposure analyses (USEPA 1992*a*); however, such an assumption, combined with the use of the off-the-shelf Monte Carlo simulation software, that typically assume non-correlation among the variables, can lead to erroneous results. Log-normal exposures are usually claimed as a direct result of log normality observed in ambient environmental concentrations; however, deviations to this assumption occur for the impact of isolated strong sources. Exponential concentration probability densities have been shown to apply in such systems. From a practical perspective a two- or three-parameter log-normal distribution is flexible enough to satisfactorily fit the main range of most right-skewed data sets, a reason for its popularity in practice.

Table 10 Exposure modelling: concepts and data

Analytical solution	Method for solving differential equations in a model using classical tools of algebra and calculus
Boundary conditions	Input values used to initialize the model
Calibration	The process of using a set of observed data to adjust the structure and/or internal coefficients of a model such that the output values are accurate with respect to a known value
Causation	The independent change in the value of one variable causes a predictable change in the value of dependent variables
Deterministic model	A model in which the variations in the variables do not include a random component—there is one output for each set of inputs
Equilibrium	A system that is not exchanging energy or matter with its surrounding and is in equilibrium with the surroundings
Model	A theoretical construct attempting to relate an identified system to the data and information available to simulate the system
Numerical solution	Method for solving differential equations using numerical approximation techniques
Sensitivity analysis	The investigation of changes in dependent variable values resulting from changes in values in independent variables and in the posited relationships among variables
Stability	The ability of a numerical integration method to iterate to a solution
Steady state	The case where input to a system is balanced by output; A model in which no variables change for the time period under consideration
Stochastic model	A model in which the variation in one or more variables includes a random component
Verification	Testing of a model following initial calibration to evaluate mode

Adapted from Patrick (1994).

Potential problems are associated with the additional requirements for accuracy of data needed to describe high exposures and doses. It is exactly in that range where assumptions on independence (typical in Monte Carlo simulations) are less valid. One solution in any analysis is to use asymptotic distributions of extremes, such as Gumbel's double-exponential distribution, for the high ends ('distribution tails') of concentration and exposure time.

Practical application of exposure assessment has been mainly driven by generic or 'typical' assumptions (e.g. the person eating large quantities of waste all his or her life). However, as data evolve, management requirements for information obtained from large-scale, comprehensive exposure assessment programmes such as the National Human Exposure Assessment Survey, will be overwhelming by comparison with today's standards for routine exposure data management (Sexton *et al.* 1995). Consequently, state-of-the-art information management tools must be evaluated and used to organize, utilize, and interpret exposure-related data efficiently. These include geographical information systems, interactive scientific visualization systems, distributed relational database management systems, and object-oriented environments for data and model integration.

Exposure probabilities for individuals and populations

Exposure distributions (probability density functions and cumulative distribution functions of exposure) for an individual expresses the probability that an individual will experience a given level of exposure over a specified duration (such as a day, year, or lifetime). The exposure distribution for a population, expresses the probability that a fraction of the population will experience a given level of exposure. Exposure distributions can vary significantly among individuals in a population, resulting in multimodal distributions for a population. For example, the distribution of exposure in a population can be bimodal when a fraction of the population is occupationally exposed at levels much greater than environmental levels experienced by the other fraction of the population. Consequently, population strata need to be characterized to achieve the data quality objectives. Exposure distributions that should be developed include individuals expected to experience the highest long-term exposures, individuals expected to experience the highest short-term exposures, and special or susceptible segments of the population.

As mentioned in the previous section, log-normal distributions of exposures are commonly employed, and they also have been suggested as a 'default' when case-specific information is not available (USEPA 1992*a*). The log-normal distribution possesses many advantageous properties, such as positivity (the probability of a negative exposure is zero), left-skewedness (implying that the average exposure is less than the median exposure), and its mathematical properties are well known as it is closely related to the normal distribution. Multimodal exposure distributions can sometimes be describing by superposition of two or more log-normal distributions. However, its adoption in a particular study should be with caution because log normality of a random variable implies that the randomness in the underlying processes are multiplicative. Other alternatives, such as asymptotic distributions for extreme values (e.g. bi-exponential), could potentially provide more appropriate information for risk analyses.

Attributes related to the potential target population and sensitive subpopulations should include (a) plausible contact patterns with the contaminants for different routes of exposure, (b) spatial population distribution stratification by age, sex , etc., and (c) identification of subgroups of people sharing potentially similar exposure patterns. As stated earlier, identification of time–activity patterns for potentially exposed populations, school children versus adults, men versus women, office workers versus outdoor workers, and so on and of spatial distributions of target population groups are essential for exposure assessments.

Uncertainty analysis

Exposure assessments are inherently uncertain, due to limitations in the precision with which nature can be observed, and due to the randomness inherent in nature. Uncertainty, and the closely related concept of variability, are means of quantifying the lack of knowledge regarding a quantity of interest, which in exposure assessment can be any variable affecting the estimation of exposure. Uncertainty generally refers to a lack of knowledge of a quantity due to limitations in available quantification techniques, whereas variability is a means of representing the lack of knowledge of a quantity due to unavailability of a measurement on the specific instance of the quantity. For example, an exposure assessment involving contaminated soil will be uncertain, because of a lack of knowledge regarding the relevant concentration of contaminant in soil resulting from (a) imprecision in contaminant concentrations measured in soil samples, and (b) variability in measured concentrations in several randomly selected representative samples. The variability in soil concentrations results in uncertainty in exposure assessment because it is not possible a priori to predict the exact concentration in soil that actually causes the exposure. Although it is useful to conceptualize these two sources of uncertainty in exposure assessment, ultimately however, it does not matter whether the lack of knowledge is due to uncertainty or variability, because they are both represented using probability distribution functions, and their effect on the exposure assessment is estimated by propagating the uncertainty through a exposure model in an identical manner. However, it is important to acknowledge explicitly that exposure assessments are inherently uncertain, and therefore exposure assessments should be probabilistic wherever possible. One of the main benefits of conceptualizing uncertainty as arising due to imprecision and variability is the reduction uncertainty by identifying and filling data gaps. The identification of data gaps usually involves a sensitivity analysis to determine the contribution of individual variables to the overall uncertainty in the exposure assessment. Reduction of uncertainty due to imprecision can only be effected by improving instrumentation, whereas it may be possible to reduce the uncertainty in exposure assessments due to variability in underlying factors by stratifying the population from which the samples are drawn (see Table 3). Knowledge of the population probability distribution functions can be used to judge the appropriateness of stratification of the population into smaller groups. For example, bimodal distributions are an indication that there are at least two subpopulations that are more homogeneous. This type of information is important in identifying subgroups by age, sex, race, and so on, and locating susceptible subgroups exposed to a contaminant.

Frequency distributions estimated from frequency distributions can be affected by a small sample size. In some cases only a few data points are available for quantities such as the mean, variance, and distribution. However, a confidence interval may only be calculated when the mean and variance of the distribution are known with certainty (e.g. based on large numbers of samples or data). A small sample size will increase the uncertainty in the mean and the variance. Calculation of tolerance intervals is one method for identifying sources of uncertainty (Mandel 1969).

Uncertainty about the underlying distribution of a variable can limit the application of standard statistical tests. Most tolerance and confidence intervals assume a normal distribution for all measurements. In cases where measurement error dominates the observed variance, this assumption may be reasonable; however, when there is significant interindividual variability, a skewed distribution can result. In this case, tolerance and confidence intervals based on an assumption of normality will not provide valid information error. Thus, it is important to view statistical tests as only one component in determining the accuracy of the exposure data.

Summary

The field of exposure analysis and its application to public health practices provides information and an understanding of the variety of ways an individual or population comes into contact with a contaminant. The approach must be framed within a conceptual framework that can involve multiple disciplines and interdisciplinary studies. Calculations of exposure and dose are data intensive, and often require situation-specific or site-specific data to characterize exposure accurately. Finally, the scientific approaches employed to establish measurement and modelling procedures must consider information on biological mechanisms or health outcomes.

References

AIHC (American Industrial Health Council) (1994). *Exposure Factors Handbook*, Sections 1–7. AIHC, Washington, DC.

Akland, G.G., Hartwell, T.D., Johnson, T.R., and Whitmore, R.W. (1985). Measuring human exposure to carbon monoxide in Washington, DC and Denver, Colorado during the winters of 1982–83. *Environmental Science and Technology*, **19**, 911–18.

Andelman, J.B. (1985). Inhalation exposure in the home to volatile organic contaminants of drinking water. *Science of the Total Environment*, **47**, 443–60.

Anderson-Sprecher, R., Flatman, G.T., and Borgman, L. (1994). Environmental sampling: a brief review. *Journal of Exposure Analysis and Environmental Epidemiology*, **4**, 115–32.

Ashley, D.L., *et al.* (1992). Determining volatile organic compounds in human blood from a large sample population by purse and trap gas chromatography/mass spectrometry. *Analytical Chemistry*, **64**, 1021–9.

Brown, S.H., Bishop, O.R., and Rowan, C.A. (1984). The role of skin absorption as a route of exposure to volatile organic compounds in drinking water. *American Journal of Public Health*, **74**, 479–492.

Carpenter, G.J. and Huston-Stein, A. (1980). Activity, structure and sex-typed behavior in preschool children. *Child Development*, **51**, 862–72.

Caudill, S.P. and Pirkle, J.L. (1992). Effects of measurement error on estimating biological half-life. *Journal of Exposure Analysis and Environmental Epidemiology*, **2**, 463–76.

Clayton, C.A., *et al.* (1993). Particle Total Exposure Assessment Methodology (PTEAM) Study; distribution of aerosol and elemental concentrations in personal, indoors, and outdoor air samples in a southern California community. *Journal of Exposure Analysis and Environmental Epidemiology*, **3**, 220–30.

Cohen, Y. (1989). Multimedia and intermedia transport modeling concepts in environmental monitoring. In: *Intermedia pollutant transport: modeling and field measurements*, (ed. D.T. Allen, I.R. Kaplan, and Y. Cohen). Plenum, New York.

Cohen Hubal, E., Sheldon, L., McCurdy, J., *et al.* (1999). Exposure assessment for children: a review of the factors influencing exposure of children, and the data available to characterize and assess that exposure. *Environmental Health Perspectives*, **108**, 475–86.

Donigian, A.S. and Mulkey, L.A. (1992). STREAM, an exposure assessment methodology for agricultural pesticide runoff. In: *Fate of pesticides and chemicals in the environment*, (ed. J.L. Schnoor). Wiley, New York.

Duan, N. (1982). Models for human exposure to air pollution. *Environment International*, **8**, 305–9.

Duan, N. (1991). Stochastic microenvironment models for air pollution exposure. *Journal of Exposure Analysis and Environmental Epidemiology*, **1**, 235–57.

Fenske, R.A., Curry, P.B., Wandelmaier, F., and Ritter, L. (1991). Development of dermal and respiratory sampling procedures for human exposure to pesticides. *Indoor Environment*, **1**, 11–30.

Fiserova-Bergerova, V. (1987). Development of biological exposure indices (BEIs) and their implementation. *Applied Industrial Hygiene*, **2**, 87–92.

Freeman, N.C.G., Waldman, J., and Lioy, P.J. (1991). Design and evaluation of a location and activity log used for assessing personal exposure to air pollutants. *Journal of Exposure Analysis and Environmental Epidemiology*, **1**, 327–38.

Freeman, N.C.G., Ettinger, A.S., Berry, M., and Rhoads, G.G. (1997). Hygiene and food related behaviors assoicated with blood lead levels of young children from lead contaminated homes. *Journal of Exposure Analysis and Environmental Epidemiology*, **7**, 103–18.

Freeman, N.C.G., Ettinger, A.S., and Rhoads, G.G. (1999). Mouthing and hygiene behaviors of lead-burdened toddlers. *Family and Community Health*, submitted for publication.

Georgopoulos, P.G. (1990). *The EOHSI Compendium of Air Quality Models—1990.* Ozone Research Center Technical Report ORC-TR901101. Environmental and Occupational Health Sciences Institute, Piscataway, NJ.

Georgopoulos, P. and Lioy, P.J. (1994). Conceptual and theoretical aspects of exposure and dose assessment. *Journal of Exposure Analysis and Environmental Epidemiology*, **4**, 253–85.

Georgopoulos, P.G., Roy, A., and Gallo, M. (1994). Reconstruction of using physiologically based pharmacokinetic models. *Journal of Exposure Analysis and Environmental Epidemiology*, **4**, 1–20.

Georgopoulos, P.G., Walia, A., Roy, A., and Lioy, P.J. (1997). An integrated exposure and dose modeling and analysis system: Part 1—formulation and testing of microenvironmental and pharmacokinetic components. *Environmental Science and Technology*, **31**, 17–27.

Gerlowsky, L.E. and Jain, R.K. (1983). Physiologically based pharmacokinetic models: principles and applications. *Journal of Pharmaceutical Sciences*, **72**, 1103–27.

Graham, J., *et al.* (1992). Role of exposure databases in risk assessment. *Archives of Environmental Health*, **47**, 408–21.

Gurunathan, S., *et al.* (1998). Accumulation of chlorpyrifos on residential surfaces and on/in toys accessible to children. *Environmental Health Perspectives*, **106**, 9–16.

Hamel, S.C., Buckley, B., and Lioy, P.J. (1998). Bioaccessibility of metals in soils for different liquid for soil ratios in synthetic gastric fluids. *Environmental Science and Technology*, **32**, 358–62.

Hattis, D.B. and Burmaster, D.E. (1994). Some thoughts on choosing distributions for practical risk analyses. *Risk Analysis*, **14**, 713–30.

Hawley, J.K. (1985). Assessment of health risk from exposure to contaminated soils. *Risk Analysis*, **5**, 282–302.

Henderson, R.F., Bechtold, W.E., and Maples, K.R. (1992). Biological markers as measure of exposure. *Journal of Exposure Analysis and Environmental Epidemiology*, **2** (Supplement 2), 1–14.

Javandel, I., Doughty, C., and Tsang, C.F. (1984). *Groundwater transport: handbook of mathematical models.* Monograph 10, AGU Water Resources, Washington, DC.

Jayjock, M.A. and Hawkins N.C. (1993). A proposal for improving the role of exposure modeling in risk assessment. *American Industrial Hygiene Association Journal*, **54**, 733–41.

Jo, W-K., Weisel, C., and Lioy, P.J. (1990). Routes of exposure and body burden from showering with chlorinated tap water. *Journal of Risk Analysis*, **10**, 575–80.

Kim, H-K. and Weisel, C.P. (1998). Dermal absorption of dichloro-and trichloroacetic acids from chlorinated water. *Journal of Exposure Analysis and Environmental Epidemiology*, **8**, 555–75.

Kitsa, V., *et al.* (1992). Particle size distribution of total and hexavalent chromium in inspirable, thoracic and respirable soils from contaminated sites in New Jersey. *Aerosol Science and Technology*, **17**, 213–29.

Lebowitz, M.D., Quackenboss, J.J., Kollander, M., l'Oczer, M.L., and Colome, S. (1989). Standard questionnaire for estimation of indoor concentrations. *Journal of the Air Pollution Control Association*, **39**, 1411–19.

Lioy, P.J. (1990). The analysis of total human exposure for exposure assessment: a multi-discipline science for examining human contact with contaminants. *Environmental Science and Technology*, **24**, 938–45.

Lioy, P.J. (1992). Exposure analysis and the biological response to a contaminant: a melding necessary for environmental health sciences. *Journal of Exposure Analysis and Environmental Epidemiology*, **2** (Supplement 1), 19–24.

Lioy, P.J. (1993). *Measurement of personal exposure to air pollution: status and needs, measurement challengers in atmospheric chemistry*, pp. 373–92. Advances in Chemistry Series 232. American Chemical Society, Washington, DC.

Lioy, P.J. (1999). Exposure analysis: reflections on its growth and aspirations or its future. *Journal of Exposure Analysis and Environmental Epidemiology*, in press.

Lioy, P.J. and Pellizzari, E. (1995). Conceptual framework for designing a national survey of human exposure. *Journal of Exposure Analysis and Environmental Epidemiology*, **5**, 425–44.

Lioy, P.J., Weisel, C.P., Jo, W-K., Pellizzari, E., and Raymer, J.H. (1994). Microenvironmental and personal measurements of methyl-tertiary butyl ether associated with automobile use activities. *Journal of Exposure Analysis and Environmental Epidemiology*, **4**, 427–41.

Lippmann, M. and Lioy, P.J. (1986). Critical issues in air pollution epidemiology. *Environmental Health Perspectives*, **62**, 243–58.

Lodge, J.P. (1989). *Methods of air sampling and analysis*, (3rd edn). Lewis Publishers, Chelsea, MI.

McKone, T.E. (1991). Human exposure to chemicals from multiple media and through multiple pathways: research overview and comments. *Journal of Risk Analysis*, **11**, 5–10.

Mandel, J. (1969). *The statistical analysis of experimental data*. Wiley, New York

Marnicio, R.J., Hakkinen, P.J., Lutkenhoff, S.D., Hertzberg, R.C., and Moskowitz, P.D. (1991). Risk analysis software and databases: review of Riskware '90 Conference and Exhibition. *Risk Analysis*, **11**, 545–60.

NAS (National Academy of Sciences) (1993). *Pesticides in the diets of infants and children*. National Academy of Sciences, Washington, DC.

NRC (National Research Council) (1985). *Epidemiology of air pollution*. National Academy Press, Washington, DC.

NRC (National Research Council) (1989*a*). *Subcommittee report on biologic markers in pulmonary toxicology*. National Academy Press, Washington, DC.

NRC (National Research Council) (1989*b*). *Report on biologic markers in reproductive toxicology*. Subcommittee on Reproductive and Neurodevelopmental Toxicology Committee on Biological Markers. National Academy Press, Washington, DC.

NRC (National Research Council) (1991*a*). *Environmental epidemiology*, Volume 1: *Public health and hazardous wastes*. National Academy Press, Washington, DC.

NRC (National Research Council) (1991*b*). *Frontiers in assessing human exposures to environmental toxicants*. National Academy Press, Washington, DC.

NRC (National Research Council) (1991*c*). *Human exposure assessment for airborne pollutants: advances and opportunities*. National Academy Press, Washington, DC.

NRC (National Research Council) (1992). *Biologic markers of immunotoxicology*. National Academy Press, Washington, DC.

NRC (National Research Council) (1993*a*). *Measuring lead exposure in infants, children, and other sensitive populations*. National Academy Press, Washington, DC.

NRC (National Research Council) (1993*b*). *Pesticides in the diets of infants and children*. National Academy Press, Washington, DC.

Ott, W. (1977). Development of criteria for siting air monitoring stations. *Journal of the Air Pollution Control Association*, **27**, 543–8.

Ott, W. (1980). *Models of human exposure to air pollution*. Technical Report No. 32. Department of Statistics, Stanford University.

Ott, W. (1982). Concepts of human exposure to air pollution. *Environment International*, **7**, 179–96.

Ott, W.R. (1990). Total human exposure: basic concepts, EPA field studies, and future research needs. *Journal of the Air and Waste Management Association*, **40**, 966–75.

Ott, W.R. (1995). Human exposure assessment: the birth of a new science. *Journal of Exposure Analysis and Environmental Epidemiology*, **5**, 459–72.

Ott, W., Thomas, J., Mage, D., and Wallace, L. (1988). Validation of the Simulation of Human Activity and Pollution Exposure (SHAPE) model using paired days from the Denver, Colorado, carbon monoxide field study. *Atmospheric Environment*, **22**, 2101–13.

Pardi, R.R. (1992). IMES: A system for identifying and evaluation computer models for exposure assessment. *Risk Analysis*, **11**, 319–21.

Patrick, D.R. (1994). *Toxic air pollution handbook*. Van Nostrand Reinhold, New York.

Pellizzari, E., *et al.* (1995). Population-based exposure measurements in EPA Region 5: a phase I field study in support of the National Human Exposure Assessment Survey. *Journal of Exposure Analysis and Environmental Epidemiology*, **5**, 327–58.

Pellizzari, E., *et al.* (1999). Particulate matter and manganese exposures in Toronto, CA. *Atmospheric Environment*, **33**, 721–34.

Perera, F.P., *et al.* (1987). DNA adducts, protein adducts, sister chromatid exchange in cigarette smokers and non-smokers. *Journal of the National Cancer Institute*, **79**, 449–56.

Pirkle, J.L., Needham, L.L., and Sexton, K. (1995). Improving exposure assessments by monitoring human tissue for toxic chemicals. *Journal of Exposure Analysis and Environmental Epidemiology*, **5**, 405–24.

Ramsey, J.C. and Andersen, M.E. (1984). A physiologically based description of the inhalation pharmacokinetics of styrene in rats and humans. *Toxicology and Applied Pharmacology*, **73**, 159–75.

Reed, K.J., Jimenez, M., Lioy, P.J., and Freeman, N.C.G. (1999). Quantification of children's hand and mouthing activities. *Journal of Exposure Analysis and Environmental Epidemiology*, **9**, 513–20.

Robinson, J.P., Wiley, J.A., Piazza, J., and Gerrett, K. (1989). *Activity patterns of California residents and their implications for potential exposure to pollution*. CARB-A6–177–33. California Air Resources Board, Sacramento, CA.

Roy, A. and Georgopoulos, P.G. (1998). Reconstructing week-long exposures to volatile organic compounds using physiologically based pharmacokinetic models. *Journal of Exposure Analysis and Environmental Epidemiology*, **8**, 407–22.

Rubinstein, R.Y. (1981). *Simulation and the Monte Carlo methods*. Wiley, New York.

Ruby, M.V., *et al.* (1993). Development of an *in vitro* screening test to evaluate the 'in vivo' bioaccessibility of ingested mine-waste lead. *Environmental Science and Technology*, **27**, 2870–7.

Ryan, P.B. (1991). An overview of human exposure modeling. *Journal of Exposure Analysis and Environmental Epidemiology*, **1**, 453–74.

Ryan, P.B., Spengler, J.D., and Letz, R. (1986). Estimating personal exposures to NO_2. *Environment International*, **12**, 395–400.

Samet, J.M., Marbury, M.C., and Spengler, J.D. (1987). Health effects of sources of indoor air pollution I. *American Review of Respiratory Disease*, **136**, 1466–87.

Samet, J.M., Marbury, M.C., and Spengler, J.D. (1988). Health effect of sources of indoor air pollution II. *American Review of Respiratory Disease*, **137**, 221–44.

Schwab, M., Spengler, J.D., Ozhaynak, H., and Terblanche, P. (1990). The time/activity component of the Kanawah County health study. In: *Total exposure methodology*, pp. 118–29. Air and Waste Management Association, Pittsburgh, PA.

Schwab, M., Teiblanche, A.P.S., and Spengler, J.D. (1991). Self reported exertion levels on time/activity diaries, application to exposure assessment. *Journal of Exposure Analysis and Environmental Epidemiology*, **1**, 339–56.

Seifert, B. and Abraham, H.J. (1983). Use of passive samplers for the determination of gaseous organic substances in indoor air at low concentration levels. *International Journal of Environmental Analytical Chemistry*, **13**, 237–54.

Sexton, K. and Ryan, P.B. (1988). *Assessment of human exposure to air pollution: methods, measurements and models, air pollution: the automobile and public health*, pp. 207–38. National Academy Press, Washington, DC.

Sexton, K., Seleven, S.G., Wagener, D.K., and Lybarger, J.A. (1992). Estimating human exposure to environmental pollutants: availability and utility of existing databases. *Archives of Environmental Health*, **47**, 398–407.

Sexton, K., Kleffman, D., and Callahan, M.A. (1995). An Introduction to the National Human Exposure Assessment Survey (NHEXAS) and related Phase I field studies. *Journal of Exposure Analysis and Environmental Epidemiology*, **5**, 229–32.

Shulte, P.A. and Perera, E.P. (1993). *Molecular epidemiology*. Academic Press, San Diego, CA.

Spengler, J.D., Treitman, R.D., Tosteson, T.D., Mage, D.T., and Soczek, D.L. (1985) Personal exposures to respirable particulates and implications for air pollution epidemiology. *Environmental Science and Technology*, **19**, 700–7.

Stetter, J.R., Jurs, P.C., and Rose, S.L. (1986). Detection of hazardous gases and vapors. Pattern Recognition Analysis from electrochemical sensor array. *Analytical Chemistry*, **58**, 860–6.

Thibodeaux, L.J. (1979). *Chemodynamics: environmental movement of chemicals in air, water, and soil*. Wiley, New York.

Tsang, A.M. and Klepeis, N.E. (1996). *Descriptive statistics tables from a detailed analysis of the National Human Activity Pattern Survey (NHAPS) data*. US Environmental Protection Agency, Washington, DC.

Umbreit, T.H., Hesse, E.J., and Gallo, M.A. (1986). Bioavailability of dioxin in soil from a 2.4.5-T manufacturing site. *Science*, **232**, 945–7.

USEPA (United States Environmental Protection Agency) (1980). *Federal Register* 79318–79.

USEPA (United States Environmental Protection Agency) (1988). *Total Human Exposure Research Council (THERC). research needs in human exposure: a 5-year comprehensive assessment (1990–1994)*. Office of Research and Development, Washington, DC.

USEPA (United States Environmental Protection Agency) (1989*a*). *Exposure factors handbook*. EPA/600/08–89/043. Office of Health and Environmental Assessment, Washington, DC.

USEPA (United States Environmental Protection Agency) (1989*b*). *Interim on benzene exposure assessment model (BEAM)*. EPA 600/X89/015, Jan. Environmental Measurements and Surveillance Laboratory, Las Vegas, NV.

USEPA (United States Environmental Protection Agency) (1991). *Human exposure model*, II: *User's guide* (Draft). Office of Air Quality Planning and Standards, US Environmental Protection Agency, Washington, DC.

USEPA (United States Environmental Protection Agency) (1992*a*). Guidelines for exposure assessment. *Federal Register* FRL-4129.

USEPA (United States Environmental Protection Agency) (1992*b*). *A Monte Carlo approach to simulating residential occupancy periods and its applications to the general population*. EPA-450/3–92–011. Office of Air Quality Planning and Standards, US Environmental Protection Agency, Washington, DC.

Valerio, F., Pela, M., Lazarotto, A., and Balducci, D. (1997). Prelimlinary evaluation, using passive tubes, of carbon monoxide concentrations in outdoor and indoor air and street shops in Greece. *Atmospheric Environment*, **32**, 2871–6.

Wainman, T., Hazen, R., and Lioy P. (1994). The extractability of CR(VI) from contaminated soil in synthetic sweat. *Journal of Exposure Analysis and Environmental Epidemiology*, **4**, 171–81.

Wallace, L.A. (1989). Major sources of benzene exposure. *Environmental Health Perspectives*, **82**, 165–9.

Wallace, L.A., *et al.* (1988). California TEAM study: breath concentrations and personal air exposures to 26 volatile compounds in air and drinking water of 188 residents of Los Angeles, Antioch and Pittsburgh, California. *Atmospheric Environment*, **22**, 2141–63.

Weisel, C.P., Jo, W-K., and Lioy, P.J. (1993). Utilization of breath analysis for exposure and dose estimates of chloroform. *Journal of Exposure Analysis and Environmental Epidemiology*, **2** (Supplement 1), 55–69.

Zartarian, V.G., Ferguson, A.C., and Leckie, J.O. (1997*a*). Quantified mouthing activity data from a four-child pilot field study. *Journal of Exposure Analysis and Environmental Epidemiology*, **7**, 543–53.

Zartarian, V.G., Ott, W., and Duan, N. (1997*b*). A quantitative definition of exposure and related concepts. *Journal of Exposure Analysis and Environmental Epidemiology*, **7**, 411–38.

Zartarian, V.G., Ferguson, A.C., and Lecke, J.O. (1998). Quantification of mounting activity data from a child pilot study. *Journal of Exposure Analysis and Environmental Epidemiology*, **3**, 543–54.

8.6 Occupational health

David Koh and Jerry Jeyaratnam

Introduction

Occupational health, as defined by a joint committee of the World Health Organization (**WHO**) and the International Labour Organization in 1950, involves the 'promotion and maintenance of the highest degree of physical, mental and social well being of workers in all occupations' (Forsmann 1983). This definition emphasizes the term health rather than disease, and further implies a multidisciplinary responsibility as well as a mechanism for the provision of health services for the working population.

History and development

Historically, the existence of diseases related to work has been documented since antiquity. Imhotep (2780BC) was the chief vizier to the Pharaoh Zoser, the first king of the Third Dynasty of the Old Kingdom. He was also an engineer and architect of the step pyramid at Sakkara, as well as a physician and priest. He described cases of occupational injuries and 'sprain of the vertebrae' among the pyramid builders (Brandt Rauf and Brandt Rauf 1987).

Hippocrates (460–377 BC) emphasized the importance of environmental factors in disease causation in his treatise on *Air, Waters, Places* (Hunter 1969). Both Hippocrates and Galen (AD 130–201) described the diseases of certain occupations, including metallurgists, fullers, tailors, horsemen, farmhands, fishermen, miners, tanners, chemists, and other craftsmen. However, Hippocratic medicine in general did not concern itself with health hazards of occupations. One reason was because of the low social status of the worker. The most hazardous and laborious jobs, for example, mining, were done by the lowest strata of society, such as slaves, prisoners of war, and convicted criminals. The Athenian philosopher Socrates (469–399 BC) offers this description of workers:

> What are called the mechanical arts, carry a social stigma and are rightly dishonored in our cities... Furthermore, the workers at these trades simply have not got the time to perform the offices of friendship or citizenship. Consequently, they are looked upon as bad friends and bad patriots. And in some cities..., it is not legal for a citizen to ply a mechanical trade.

After stagnating for several centuries, occupational health developed further in the Middle Ages. Georgius Agricola (1494–1555), a physician–scholar in the mountains of Silesia and Bohemia wrote extensively on the diseases of miners and smelters of gold and silver. In a 12-volume work, *De Re Metallica,* he described a consumptive lung disease of miners (Hunter 1969).

Paracelsus (1493–1541), a Tyrolean physician, produced a three-volume work *On Miners' Sickness and Other Miners' Diseases*, in which he wrote about pulmonary diseases of miners, diseases of smelters and metallurgists, and diseases caused by mercury (Hunter 1969).

One of the great pioneers in occupational medicine was the Italian physician Bernardino Ramazzini (1633–1714) (Fig. 1). He is often described as the 'Father of Occupational Medicine'. Ramazzini graduated from the University of Parma in 1659, and held the Chairs at Modena (1670) and Padua (1700). His publication *De Morbis Artificum Diatriba*, which appeared in 1700 with a second edition in 1713, was the seminal text in occupational medicine (Felton 1997). He wrote:

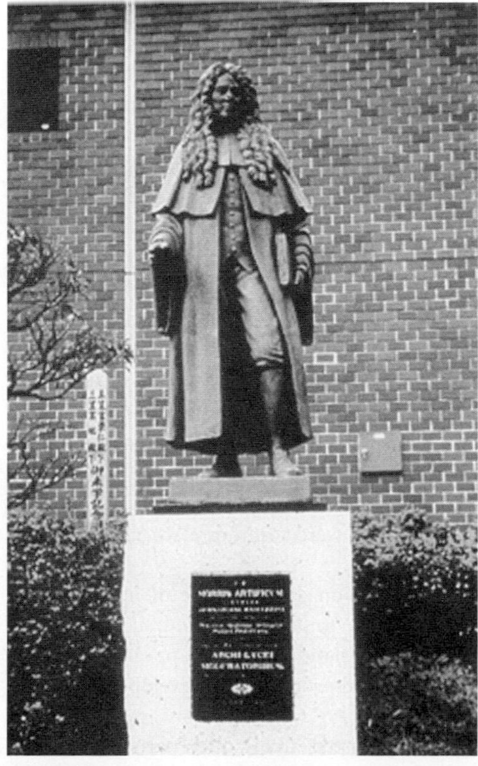

Fig. 1 Bernardino Ramazzini (1633–1714).

> I for one have done all that lay in my power, and have not thought it beneath me to step into workshops of the meaner sort now and again and study the obscure operations of the mechanical arts; all the more that nowadays medicine has been almost entirely converted into a mechanical art, and in the schools they chatter continually about automatism.

One of Ramazzini's most significant aphorisms is the important addition to the teachings of Hippocrates to physicians. Hippocrates taught physicians that 'When you come to a patient's house, you should ask him what sort of pains he has, what caused them, how many days he has been ill, whether the bowels are working and what sort of food he eats.' Following this citation, Ramazzini wrote: 'I may venture to add one more question: What occupation does he follow?'

In his writings, Ramazzini described many occupational illnesses that are still seen today, and furthermore, described the principles for their control. He condemned the lack of ventilation and unsuitable temperatures, he urged labourers in dusty trades to work in spacious, ventilated rooms, he recommended rest intervals in prolonged work and advocated exercise and correct working postures.

The Industrial Revolution and occupational health

The one major event that profoundly influenced and shaped the development of occupational health was the Industrial Revolution in the eighteenth century (Hunter 1969). Dramatic social changes during this period occurred in the Western world. These transformations were related to newly introduced industrial processes. Basically, the change entailed the setting up of factories, which set in motion a variety of social changes to almost resemble a revolution. Formerly, most work was done by craftsmen in rural cottage industries. The industrial revolution resulted in work being carried out in factories in urban centres.

Effects were seen both within the community, as well as in the individual worker. In fact, many consider the most significant health impact of industrialization to be on the community. Family life was disrupted, with men leaving their families and moving to work in new industrial areas. In the industrial areas, health and social problems emerged—such as poor housing and sanitation, alcoholism, prostitution, and poverty. The individual workers too, were victim to the process of industrialization. Inside the factories, individuals were exposed to long hours of work and uncontrolled occupational hazards; and faced the risk of accidents at work. Very often the workers were not familiar with the industrial process and so exposed themselves to greater dangers than necessary. Child labour and apprenticeship of young children were commonplace, and there was an absence of labour legislation.

As problems of industrialization grew, people of influence and political power campaigned to improve working conditions of workers. Occupational health legislation began to appear towards the end of the eighteenth century, and progressively developed to protect the health and rights of workers.

The industrial revolution occurred later in other parts of the world. Japan, in the Far East, experienced a similar phenomenon from the nineteenth century (Tsuchiya 1991).

Even today, some centuries after the Industrial Revolution, we are able to observe the same phenomena in some of the developing nations. Even in the industrialized nations, the very same problems are encountered by migrant workers and other deprived sectors of their society. In the United States, there was a resurgence in child labour in the 1980s, following waves of immigration as well as participation of school children in the service sector (Postol 1993).

In a commentary on prevention in occupational and environmental health, Axelson (1997) noted that throughout history, many examples of rational efforts for prevention can be found. However, he states that 'preventive measures have often been, and still are, neglected or even counteracted for economic reasons.' Thus, some form of legislation is needed to ensure the protection of workers' health.

Development of occupational health legislation

The first environmental cancer was described by Percival Pott over 200 years ago (Doll 1975). This cancer (skin cancer of the scrotum), occurred in chimney sweeps, and was caused by exposure to polycyclic aromatic hydrocarbon compounds in the soot generated by combustion of organic material. This particular cancer could be prevented by improved personal hygiene.

An early piece of legislation in England was the Act for Better Regulations of Chimney Sweeps and their Apprentices 1788. This act stipulated a minimum age of 8 years for chimney sweeps; provided for inspections and hearing of complaints, and required that the master not 'misuse or evil treat' the apprentice. It further stated that the master 'shall at least once in every week, cause the said apprentice to be thoroughly washed and cleansed from soot and dirt', and provided for prosecutions and penalties for violation.

The Health and Morals of Apprentices Act, 1802 (Hunter 1969) applied to apprentices in the cotton and woollen industry. It limited work to a maximum of 12 h a day, and specified that factory walls were to be washed twice a year, and for rooms to be ventilated. This legislation also allowed voluntary factory inspections by visitors.

The Factory Act 1819 set 9 years as a minimum age for the worker, and limited work hours. It extended the law to cover workers other than bound apprentices, but still did not apply to all factories. A later Act in 1833 enforced the appointment of factory inspectors and stated that the age of the worker be certified by a medical person. Other work environments were covered by other legislation, such as the Mines Act 1842, which prohibited women and girls from work in mines, and allowed for government inspection and state interference (Hunter 1969).

Subsequent legislation extended occupational health coverage to all occupations, and many countries today have such comprehensive legislation. However, some countries still retain the Factories Act. One possible reason for this situation is to allow for the allocation and concentration of limited occupational health resources to serve the target population at highest risk, namely, factory workers.

Occupational health legislation has also developed to list requirements for the provision of occupational health services to certain occupations. This has been spelt out in the legislation of some of the more developed countries.

Another recent development of occupational health legislation has been to ensure that employers do not discriminate against applicants and employees with disabilities. One example of this type of legislation is the Disability Discrimination Act 1995 in the United Kingdom (SOM 1997). Employers should also make reasonable accommodations for a known impairment; unless it would cause undue hardship, such as incurring significant difficulty or expense.

Occupational health today

From the humble beginnings outlined above, occupational health has kept pace with developments in society. It remains relevant today. For example, in spite of much improved working conditions compared with two centuries ago, modern day chimney sweeps still experience increased morbidity and mortality. Studies among Scandinavian chimney sweeps show that they have more chest symptoms (Hansen 1990), and have increased mortality from cancers, notably of the lung, bladder, and oesophagus (Evanoff *et al.* 1993).

In 1991, the Commission of the European Communities (1992) conducted a survey of a survey of 12 500 people, representing the national working populations of 12 countries of the European Union. The main findings of the survey are as follows:

- 42 per cent of all workers thought their health was or could be affected by their work
- 40 per cent felt that they ran the risk of an accident at work
- one worker in four was concerned for both his health and his safety
- 27 per cent used potentially dangerous equipment/machinery for more than a quarter of their working hours
- 84 per cent considered industrial accidents and occupational diseases to be common or very common in their country
- 14 per cent of workers reported they have had an industrial accident or occupational disease recognized as such by their competent national body.

Comparable data from the developing and less developed countries are not so easily available. However, it would not be unreasonable to presume that poorer working conditions and greater health risks would be encountered.

As practised today, the cornerstones of occupational health practice are health protection and health promotion of those who work. In many countries, such activities extend beyond the worker to include his or her family members.

Health protection of workers

The protection of the health of the working population is the primary concern of the occupational health practitioner. Occupational injuries and diseases are largely preventable. They unnecessarily affect the health of the working population and have effects on work productivity and on the economic and social well being of workers, their families, and society.

According to recent estimates, the cost of work-related health loss and associated productivity loss may amount to several per cent of the total gross national product of a country. For example, the Health and Safety Executive (**HSE**) in the United Kingdom has estimated that the real costs of personal injury, work accidents, and work-related ill health amount to between 5 and 10 per cent of Britain's gross trading profit (Davies and Teasedale 1994).

In the United States, the total corporate health and safety costs in 1997 were estimated to be $418 billion in direct costs, and over $837 billion in indirect costs (Brady *et al.* 1997).

Assessing the risk of work

Health protection begins with an assessment of risk. Risk assessment is a structured and systematic procedure that is dependent upon the correct identification of hazards and an appropriate estimation of the risks arising from them, with a view to making inter-risk comparisons for purposes of their control of avoidance (HSE 1995). It can be either a qualitative or quantitative process. The reason for risk assessment is to ensure that a valid decision can be made for measures necessary to control exposure to substances hazardous to health arising in the workplace. Such risk assessments in the workplace are legal requirements in many countries.

The expertise, effort, and detail required for risk assessment depends on the nature and degree of risk, and the complexity of the work process. Adequate controls are determined based on several factors: such as the toxicity of substance, numbers exposed, acceptability of risk, the legal requirements, costs, and availability of control measures.

Hazard and risk

There is a distinction between the terms 'hazard' and 'risk'.

A hazard is a substance, agent, or physical situation with a potential for harm in terms of injury or ill health, damage to property, damage to the environment, or a combination of these. Hazards can be physical, chemical, biological, ergonomic, or psychosocial in nature (Table 1). Hazard identification is the process of recognizing that a hazard exists and defining its characteristics.

Risk relates to the likelihood of the harm or undesired event occurring, and the consequences of its occurrence. It is the probability that the substance or agent will cause adverse effects under the conditions of use and/or exposure, and the possible extent of harm. It is thus a function of both exposure to the hazard and the likelihood of harm from the hazard. Extent of risk covers the population that might be affected by the risk, the numbers exposed, and the consequences. Risk assessment is the process of estimating the magnitude of risk, and deciding if the risk is tolerable or acceptable. A tolerable risk may not always be acceptable. It merely refers to a willingness to live with a risk to secure certain benefits, and in the confidence that the risk is being properly controlled (Sadhra and Rampal 1999). The levels of tolerability of risk are different for different countries, and in different working populations and the general public.

Risk assessment process

The process of risk assessment and management should take into account both routine and non-routine activities and conditions, including foreseeable emergency situations. Hazards that are intrinsic to these situations, or generated by such activities should be identified.

Exposed persons should be identified, including non-employees and those who are susceptible and therefore at higher risk because of

Table 1 Types of hazards at the workplace and their health effects

Type of hazard	Examples	Health effect
Physical	Noise	Noise-induced hearing loss
	Local vibration	Traumatic vasospastic disease
Chemical	Various chemicals (e.g. solvents, heavy metals)	Intoxications
		Fibroses
		Cancers
		Allergies
		Nervous system damage
Biological	Bacteria	Infections
	Fungi	Allergies
	Viruses	
Ergonomic	Repetitive work	Musculoskeletal injuries
	Work–rest schedules	Mental stress
		Lowered productivity and work quality
Psychosocial	Organizational stress	Work dissatisfaction
	Conflicts	Burnout
		Depression

illness or other medical conditions. Existing control measures, if any, should be evaluated.

The health risks from the hazards should next be determined and assessed, and a decision made if the risk is acceptable or tolerable. Unacceptable risks should be eliminated or reduced with new or improved control measures, and their effectiveness monitored. If needed, further corrective actions should be implemented. At the same time, workers should be informed of the hazards, risks, and appropriate measures that can be taken to protect themselves.

The steps for risk assessment for chemical, biological, ergonomic, and psychosocial hazards may differ, as illustrated by the following examples. The assessments for chemical or physical exposures are generally more objective and precise than the assessment for psychic stressors.

An example of an initial assessment for a chemical exposure is given in Table 2.

Table 2 An example of an initial assessment for chemical exposure

1.	List substances in the area to be assessed
2.	Determine which are actually used
3.	Obtain suppliers' data sheets
4.	Evaluate data sheets
5.	Inspect places where the substances are handled
6.	Evaluate method of control
7.	Perform environmental monitoring for the chemical if needed

An example of assessment of psychosocial factors

The assessment of psychosocial factors at work is more complex. It may include the evaluation of organizational dysfunction, work conditions, as well as a study of indicators such as sickness absence, staff turnover, and measurement of stress-related illness among employees. The identification of work stressors should review design of tasks, management style, interpersonal relationships, work roles, career concerns, and environmental conditions. Questionnaires to staff can be carried out using validated instruments such as the Occupational Stress Inventory and Occupational Stress Indicator (Wall 1999).

An example of a structured method for an assessment of psychic stressors in the workplace, developed by the Finnish Institute of Occupational Health (Elo 1986), is given in Table 3.

Risk management

Once the degree of risk is assessed, and a decision made that the risk of exposure is unacceptable, some form of control is necessary. There are a wide variety of methods of prevention.

The basic aim of preventive medicine is to prevent the occurrence of disease in an individual or a specific population sector, such as the working population. This is usually achieved by attempts to reduce the risk or contracting a disease. If this is not always possible, another way is by undertaking activities targeted at early detection of disease, namely screening procedures. Customarily several levels of prevention are recognized.

Primary prevention aims to reduce the occurrence of disease by eliminating the cause of disease or reducing exposure to safe levels that prevent it from causing damage, for example banning the use of blue asbestos and reducing noise at its source to levels that do not cause noise-induced deafness.

Table 3 Assessment for psychosocial stressors (Elo 1986)

1.	Responsibility for safety
2.	Responsibility for other people
3.	Responsibility for material values
4.	Solitary work
5.	Burdensome contacts
6.	Repetitiveness
7.	Forced pace
8.	Structural restraints
9.	Demands for attentiveness combined with few stimuli
10.	Demands for precise discriminations
11.	Haste
12.	Demands for complex decision-making
13.	Other factors
14.	Most recent changes in the psychic stress of the work
15.	Overall assessment of psychic stress
16.	Need for corrective measures

Secondary prevention aims to detect situations of early effects of disease before they manifest as clinical symptoms and signs in order take corrective action, for example regular monitoring of blood lead levels among lead exposed workers, regular audiograms among workers exposed to high levels of noise in the work environment.

Tertiary prevention aims to minimize the consequences in persons who already have disease. This activity is largely a curative and rehabilitative procedure and depends on proper and appropriate treatment.

Thus, it is evident that primary and secondary prevention are the major domains of preventive medicine and would thus be the focus of attention in this chapter.

Prevention of occupational diseases

Prevention of occupational disease can take place at various levels, such as at the national level, or at the level of the workplace itself. The main aim is to reduce the occurrence of occupational disease by eliminating the cause or by controlling exposure to safe levels in order to prevent it from causing damage to the health of workers.

Control of new hazards

Animal toxicity studies of chemicals to be used in industry are a reasonable predictor of potential health hazards to humans. On the basis of such studies, legislation in manufacturing nations would control the usage of such chemicals in industrial processes. One limitation is that such controls apply only to the new chemicals that are to be introduced into the market. For instance, it is estimated that only 10 per cent of pesticides in current usage have undergone such toxicological evaluation (Jeyaratnam and Koh 1996).

Control of known hazards

Several countries have legislation to ban the use of substances known to be harmful to human health. At the international level, the United Nations in 1991 compiled a consolidated list of products whose consumption and sale have been banned, withdrawn, severely restricted, or not approved by governments. This publication constitutes a tool that helps governments to keep up to date with regulatory decisions taken by other governments and assists them in considering the scope for eventual regulatory action.

The United Nations Environment Program in 1989 has evolved a procedural mechanism of Prior Informed Consent to inform government of banned agents such that these governments could take appropriate action for their control. The relevant document for this procedure is the *London Guidelines for the Exchange of Information on Chemicals in International Trade*. Chemicals that have been banned or severely restricted in at least five countries have further information made available through Decision Guidance Documents.

At present such documents are available for aldrin, dieldrin, DDT, dinoseb and dinoseb salts, fhroroacetamide, HCH (mixed isomers), polychlorinated biphenyl, polychlorinated terphenyl, polybrominated biphenyl, tris-(2,3-dibromopropyl) phosphate crocidolite, chlordane, chlorodimeform, cyhexatin, heptachlor, and mercury compounds.

By means of such documents, the United Nations system attempts to prevent importing countries from unknowingly using substances banned in countries for health reasons. This type of export of hazardous chemicals also raises an ethical consideration. For instance, is there any justification to manufacture solely for export a chemical banned in the country of manufacture as being hazardous to human health? Surely the answer to this must be a resounding 'No'. Thus the best safeguard would be to ensure that chemicals banned for health reasons in the country of manufacture should not be manufactured solely for export.

At the national level, there may be rules that regulate the import, storage, sale, and transport of legislated substances through a licensing system, for example, for pesticides. Some substances may be subjected to import controls. For instance, in some countries, the use of chlorofluorocarbons and asbestos is limited by a quota system.

Control of hazards at the workplace

Successful prevention of occupational disease could be achieved by controlling exposure to harmful agents to what are considered as safe and permissible levels. This is a form of primary prevention as it is directed at efforts to prevent damage by controlling exposure to safe levels. There are several mechanisms for the control of exposure at the workplace.

Total elimination of the hazard

This method eliminates the health risk completely, and has been used for substances that are carcinogenic, for example asbestos, benzene, or those that can cause serious health effects, such as cadmium. In the United Kingdom, the HSE had regulated that solder should be substituted with solder low in cadmium or cadmium free in the mid-1980s (Mason *et al.* 1999). Other successful examples of total elimination of the hazard include the use of asbestos-free products, benzene free solvents, or solvent-free paints (powdered paints or water-based paints).

Case study 1: Elimination of the hazard from the work process Brazing is a process where a filler metal is melted and allowed to flow into a close fitting joint of two metals. A common filler metal is a copper–zinc–silver–cadmium alloy. Torch brazing was performed in a factory that manufactured compressors. A review of the material safety data sheet of the filler revealed that it contained a significant amount of cadmium. Cadmium is a nephrotoxic agent that is used in the filler metal to reduce its melting point. While cadmium-free alloys are available, these cost more, as a higher silver content is needed to achieve an equivalent melting temperature. Environmental monitoring showed that cadmium in air levels were above the recommended threshold limit values. Biological monitoring of exposed workers showed that a large proportion of exposed workers had blood cadmium values higher than 10 μg/l, the recommended biological exposure index in that country. (Note: the Biological Exposure Index (**BEI**) for cadmium in blood recommended by the American Conference of Governmental Industrial Hygienists (**ACGIH**) is 5 μg/l.) The health risk was found to be unacceptable, and as a result, the brazing alloy used was replaced with a cadmium-free substitute. (Source: Jeyaratnam and Koh 1996.)

Substitution of the hazard

Substitution of the hazard with a less toxic alternative is another feasible option. In the case of operations that use solvents, such as degreasing operations, a less toxic solvent such as 1,1,1-trichloroethane can be used, instead of the more toxic trichloroethylene or tetrachloroethane. Another method could be the substitution of the hazard to a form that reduces risk of exposure.

Case study 2: Substitution of the hazard to a different form to reduce exposure A factory that produced a powdered plastic stabilizer chemical that contained inorganic lead. During statutory medical examinations of the workers, it was found that there was a problem of high lead exposure among its employees. The problem was reduced drastically when the production process was changed so that the end product was in granular form, as compared with the original powdered form. The improvement resulted because granules of lead containing stabilizer were less likely to be airborne, and as a result, airborne contamination was reduced dramatically.

Engineering controls

Designing and redesigning of the process to minimize exposure are some possible control measures. Automation, enclosure, or segregation of a work process, the use of dampeners or mufflers to reduce vibration or noise, reducing the open surface area for the evaporation of volatile toxic agents have been some of the successful measures used. Suppressing the substance by processes such as 'wetting' of dusty operations, or reducing hazardous emissions in the workplace by use of exhaust ventilation are other examples of engineering controls.

Redesign of the workstation or process

Redesign of the workstation to reduce unnecessary and repetitive bending, or to prevent excessive stretching to the limit of the range of movement of the workers, can minimize ergonomic hazards (Fig. 2).

In the case of computer operators, the use of adjustable equipment, the positioning of the workstation to reduce glare, and appropriate work rest pauses can prevent the development of eye strain and musculoskeletal complaints.

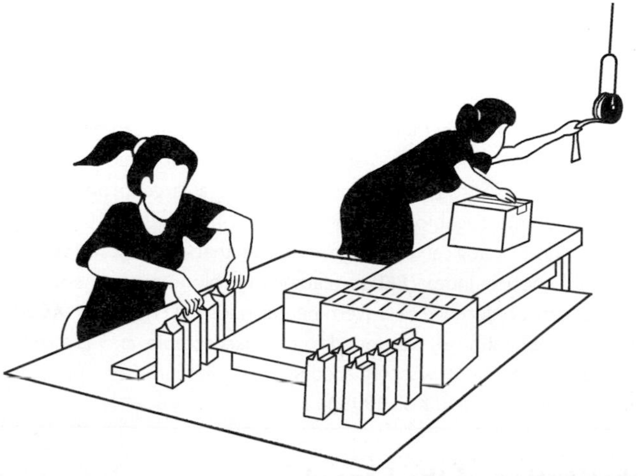

Fig. 2 Ergonomic improvements to this workplace can reduce the risk of musculoskeletal disorders among the workers.

Administrative controls

Administrative controls may be a viable alternative or an additional measure to reduce worker exposure to occupational hazards. This could take the form of job enlargement or job rotation, restriction of hours of work at a hazardous operation, or even temporary job reassignment.

The worker in Fig. 3 is exposed to numerous hazards, such as heat, noise, dust, fumes, and risk of burns and other injuries. In this work situation, his total exposure for the hazardous work conditions can be limited by administratively reducing this particular exposure to an hour or so, during the entire work shift. At other times, the worker is in an air-conditioned and enclosed control room. A better solution would be to automate the process, by use of a robotic arm to feed the oxygen to the furnace.

Education of workers

The training of workers in how to recognize work hazards, how to work safely, and what to do in the event of an emergency or when occupational diseases occur, is another important aspect of prevention. For example, metalworkers are often exposed to skin contact with coolants and soluble oils. Different workers performing the same job can have variable skin contact with coolants, ranging from almost negligible exposure to almost total constant skin contact with the coolants (Wassenius *et al.* 1998). This variation can be explained by differences in hazard awareness, attitude, and practice of safe working techniques in different workers.

Use of personal protective devices

The use of personal protective equipment is often widely practised. It has its merits, a major one being its relative inexpense, and is especially useful for situations of short-term or occasional exposure to occupational hazards. However, protective devices have to be properly selected to be effective against specific hazards, for example, the choice of an appropriate glove for use with a particular solvent. The use of a modern firefighting uniform made of improved thermal protective textile and the inclusion of overpants, resulted in dramatic reductions of thermal injury to firefighters in New York (Prezant *et al.* 1999).

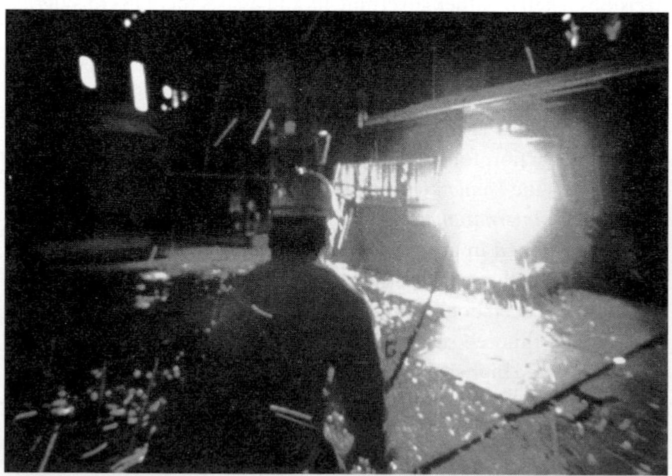

Fig. 3 Worker in an iron and steel mill feeding oxygen to the furnace.

Workers have to be trained to use the equipment correctly and to ensure that it is working effectively, such as respirator fit testing in the use of respirators (Fig. 4). Worker compliance in the use of these devices has to be high, or its protective effects may be less than desired. Finally, protective devices have to be properly maintained and replaced when necessary.

The Occupational Safety and Health Administration (OSHA 1995) stipulates that personal protective equipment should not be used as a substitute for engineering, work practice, and/or administrative controls. Instead, personal protective equipment should be used in conjunction with these controls to provide for employee safety and health in the workplace.

Environmental monitoring

Environmental or ambient monitoring in the workplace is undertaken to measure external exposure to harmful agents. The monitoring is to ensure that exposure is kept within 'permissible levels' so as to prevent the occurrence of disease. The concept of permissible levels assumes that for each substance there is a level of exposure at or below which the exposed worker does not suffer any health impairment.

It must be recognized that permissible levels have their limitations. As such every effort must be made to keep exposure levels as low as possible and the permissible level is a level above which exposure should not occur. This level could also be set for the enforcement of legislation. Furthermore, such levels may be based on incomplete information and previously unsuspected health risks have arisen from substances assumed to be comparatively safe; for example, glycol ethers used in the electronic industry have caused spontaneous abortions.

Permissible levels or occupational exposure limits

Permissible levels, or occupational exposure limits (**OELs**), are standards that are available for many of the common hazards found in workplaces. Standards are available for the commonly encountered physical, as well as chemical hazards. Standards can also be found for some substances of biological origin, including cellulose, some wood, cotton and grain dusts, proteolytic enzymes, and vegetable oil mists.

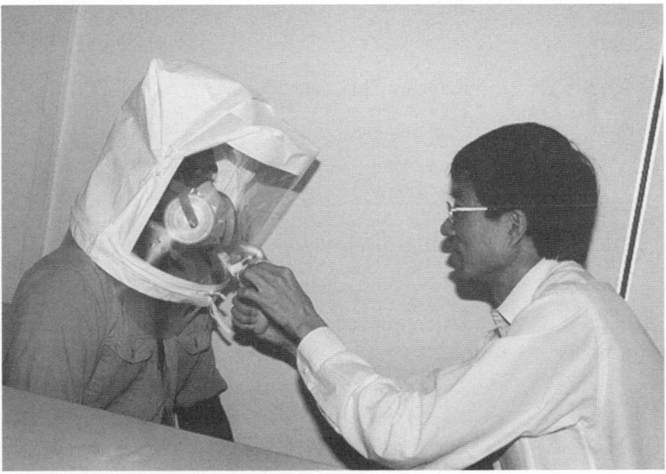

Fig. 4 Fit testing to ensure that the respirator will protect the worker.

Permissible levels are based on the following considerations:

- the physical and chemical properties of substance, including the nature and amount of impurities
- toxicological studies
- available human data.

The use of environmental standards for working conditions depends a great deal on good professional judgement, and hence should be used and interpreted only by trained persons. All standards will have imperfections in their derivation and therefore should have their limitations appreciated by the professionals who utilize them.

The earliest OELs were derived for the chemical industry in the nineteenth century in Germany. These standards were often for acute effects from short-term and very high exposures. With the development of industrial hygiene methods of measuring environmental contaminants and exposures, more and more OELs were developed. Different countries have different exposure limits. The process of standard setting, nomenclature, and applicability would necessarily differ.

For example, different approaches were taken in setting standards in the USSR and the United States in the 1970s (Levy 1999). The USSR standards, which were lower than standards set in the United States at that time, were maximum allowable concentrations that were based on an absence of development of any disease or deviation from normal. In contrast, the United States approach allowed for minor physiological adaptive changes. In addition, the principle in the USSR was that standards should be based entirely on health and not on technological and economic feasibility. In the United States, economic and technological feasibility were important considerations in the development of the standards.

Another consideration would be to take into account the situation for which the standards were set. For example, standards that are set for an 8-h working day would not be applicable for a 12-h workday.

Furthermore, exposure to several hazards simultaneously may occur. In such situations, there may be interactions, with possible synergistic or additive effects. This would then require more stringent control of each individual hazard.

The method of environmental monitoring is also of utmost importance. The choice of the correct collecting devices, sampling strategy, and analysis of the collected samples in accredited laboratories with proper quality control are important considerations that have to be addressed.

Individual variation among exposed persons should also be considered. Age, sex, pre-existing disease, genetic make-up, and social habits, such as smoking; would influence individual susceptibility. Some permissible limits, such as the threshold limit values of the ACGIH, are derived to protect the majority of, but not all exposed persons. Susceptible individuals may still suffer health effects even at levels below the recommended permissible levels. In spite of these preconditions, the sensible use of environmental standards can often result in practical and pragmatic control of many common workplace hazards so that the majority of workers are protected. Supplementary measures, such as biological monitoring, will ensure a safety net to identify workers with excessive body burdens or who have early health impairments.

An example of an environmental standard

One of the best known and widely used of the OELs is the proprietary threshold limit value (**TLV**) system developed by the ACGIH, which will be discussed in some detail.

The concept of 'time-weighted averages' (**TWAs**) and the stated philosophy of protecting 'nearly all workers' (in view of individual variation) are important considerations in the interpretation of the TLVs. TLVs are available for only about several chemicals. TLVs have not been established for a large number of recognized toxic materials.

As stated by the ACGIH, TLVs refer to 'airborne concentrations of substances and represent conditions under which it is believed that nearly all workers may be repeatedly exposed day after day without adverse health effects.' The ACGIH is aware of the wide variation in individuals, due to factors such as age, sex, pre-existing disease, genetic predisposition, and lifestyle habits, such as smoking. This variation would account for a small percentage of workers experiencing discomfort, or even developing illness from some substances at concentrations at or below the TLV.

The TLVs are updated and published annually. They are derived from information from industrial experience, as well as studies in both animal and human populations. The health outcomes of interest vary with different substances. This may range from definite health impairment, to an absence of irritation, narcosis, nuisance; or other forms of stress, as specified.

The ACGIH stresses that the TLVs 'are not fine lines between safe and dangerous concentrations, nor are they a relative index of toxicity.' While serious adverse health effects are not believed likely as a result of exposure to the TLVs, the ACGIH further adds that the 'best practice is to maintain concentrations of all atmospheric contaminants as low as is practical'.

Some definitions

Three categories of TLVs are given. These are to be used for different situations (ACGIH 1999).

1. Threshold limit value time-weighted average (**TLV-TWA**). The TLV-TWA refers to the time-weighted average concentration for an 8-h workday and 40-h workweek. Nearly all workers can be repeatedly exposed to these levels, day after day, without adverse effects. Throughout the workday, excursions above the TLV-TWA are permitted (provided they are below the TLV ceiling), if these are compensated by equivalent excursions below the TLV-TWA. TLVs are not recommended for simple asphyxiants, where the most important consideration is the available oxygen.

2. Threshold limit value short-term exposure limit (**TLV-STEL**). This is a 15-min limit TWA exposure, which should not be exceeded at any time during a workday even if the 8-h TWA is within the TLV-TWA. As defined by the ACGIH, the TLV-STEL is the concentration to which it is believed that 'workers can be exposed continuously for a short period of time without suffering from irritation, chronic or irreversible tissue damage, or narcosis of sufficient degree to increase the likelihood of accidental injury, impair self-rescue, or materially reduce work efficiency,' and provided that the daily TLV-TWA is not exceeded. The STEL supplements the TWA limit for substances with primarily chronic effects, but which also have recognized acute effects.

Table 4 Threshold limit values of selected agents (ACGIH 1999)

Substance	TWA (ppm/mg/m^3)	STEL/C (ppm/mg/m^3)	Notation	TLV basis— critical effects
Acetylene	–	–	–	Asphyxiation
Acetylene tetrabromide	1 ppm	–	–	Irritation, liver
Acrylamide	0.03 mg/m^3	–	Skin, A3	CNS, dermatitis
Asbestos (all forms)	0.1 f/cm^3	–	A1	Asbestosis, cancer
n-Butyl acrylate	2 ppm	–	SEN, A4	Irritation, reproductive
Chlorine	0.5 ppm	1 ppm	A4	Irritation
Chloroacetone	–	C 1 ppm	–	Irritation
Lead chromate				
As Pb	0.05 mg/m^3	–	A2, BEI	Cancer, CNS, reproductive
As Cr	0.012 mg/m^3	–	A2	
Mercury				
Alkyl compounds	0.01 mg/m^3	0.03 mg/m^3	Skin	CNS
Aryl compounds	0.1 mg/m^3	–	Skin	CNS, neuropathy, vision, kidney
Inorganic forms, including metallic Hg	0.025 mg/m^3	–	Skin, A4, BEI	CNS, kidney, neuropathy, vision, reproductive, GI
Welding fumes	5 mg/m^3	–		Metal fume fever, irritation
Wood dust				
Hard wood	1 mg/m^3		A1	Cancer, irritation, mucostasis, dermatitis
Soft wood	5 mg/m^3	10 mg/m^3		Irritation, dermatitis, lung

CNS, central nervous system; GI, gastrointestinal.

3. Threshold limit value ceiling (**TLV-C**). The TLV-C is the concentration that should not be exceeded during any part of the working exposure. For some fast-acting substances, such as irritant gases, the TLV-C might be the only relevant TLV. Environmental measurements for the TLV-C should preferably be instantaneous. In some situations, it is however, permitted to sample over a period not exceeding 15 min.

Notations

Some chemicals with listed TLVs may have a 'skin' or 'sensitizer' notation.

The skin notation highlights the potential significant contribution to the overall exposure by absorption through the cutaneous route, including mucous membranes. Often this occurs via direct skin contact. Workers with impaired skin barrier function, for example from injured or diseased skin, face a higher risk. Important examples of substances with the skin notation include organic solvents and pesticides such as malathion and lindane.

The sensitizer notation refers to the confirmed potential for worker sensitization as a result of dermal contact and/or inhalation exposure. An example of a chemical with a sensitizer notation is n-butyl acrylate, which is both an irritant and a sensitizer. The lack of a sensitizer notation does not necessarily mean that the substance is not a sensitizer.

Carcinogens

The carcinogenic potential of the chemical is denoted by its carcinogenic designation, which ranges from A1 (confirmed human carcinogen), A2 (suspected human carcinogen), A3 (confirmed animal carcinogen with unknown relevance to humans), A4 (not classifiable as a human carcinogen), to A5 (not suspected as a human carcinogen).

Exposures to carcinogens should be kept as low as possible. Many carcinogens act by genotoxic mechanisms, and thus, in theory at least, there may not be a safe level.

The TLVs of some chemicals, with their accompanying notations, are listed in Table 4.

Exposure limits for combined exposures

The toxicity of substances of variable composition, for example, welding fumes (Fig. 5), are dependent on factors such as the welding process and electrodes used, and the particular alloy that is welded. The TLV given, which is based on total particulate concentration, would be adequate only if no toxic elements are present in the welding rod, metal or its coating, and the welding conditions are not conducive to the formation of toxic gases.

Threshold limit values for chemical mixtures can be computed if components in the mixture have either similar toxic effects or independent toxic effects, using the appropriate correction formulas. Details can be found in the TLV and BEI Handbook of the ACGIH.

Exposure limits for physical agents

The threshold limit values for physical agents such as acoustic exposure, electromagnetic radiation, and ergonomic, mechanical, and thermal factors; are also presented.

Different methods of assessment of acoustic exposure are used for different situations, for example, continuous versus impact noise, infrasound and ultrasound. For example, the threshold limit values for noise, measured on the use of the A-weighted network with slow meter response, are as follows (Table 5).

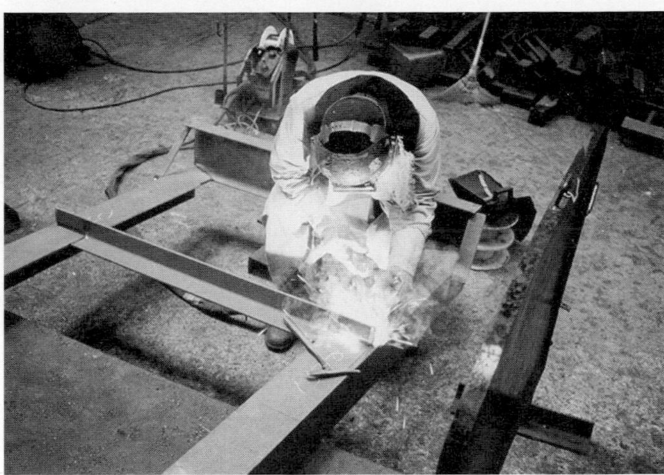

Fig. 5 Welding fumes can contain particulate concentration as well as toxic materials from the welding rod or welded metals.

Personal or area monitoring can also be performed (Figs 6 and 7).

Other considerations

In some instances, other considerations are important. Working and weather conditions (e.g. light or heavy work, indoor or outdoor work, solar load present or absent) are considered in the interpretation of the TLV for heat stress.

Exposures to a combination of factors, such as physical and chemical agents, may result in interaction of these agents, and place added stress on the exposed person. For example, among exposed workers, interactions between physical and psychosocial risk factors can increase the risk of developing work-related musculoskeletal disorders (Devereux *et al.* 1999).

Table 5 Threshold limit values for noise

Duration per day	Sound level (dBA)
24 h	80
16 h	82
8 h	85
4 h	88
2 h	91
1 h	94
30 min	97
15 min	100
7.5 min	103
3.75 min	106
1.88 min	109
0.94 min	112
0.95 min	

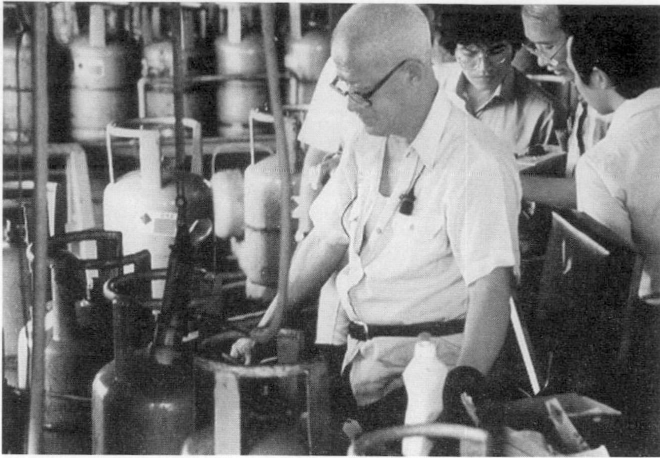

Fig. 6 Personal monitoring for noise exposure.

Pre-employment or pre-placement examinations

Pre-placement/employment medical examinations are undertaken to achieve proper job placement according to the mental and physical capabilities of the worker. By such examination and job placement it is hoped to prevent damage to susceptible workers. It must be recognized that such tests are also undertaken with different objectives, for example: to protect other workers and the general public, for insurance purposes, and to obtain baseline information on fitness.

Education of workers should be given during these assessments. Those who work have a right to know the potential hazards and risks in their work and workplaces. They should be educated on these matters and be given information on how to safeguard their health.

Immunization against diseases that may possibly be contracted on the job, and for which an effective vaccine is available, should also be given. An example is the immunization of health-care personnel exposed to the hepatitis B virus.

There are genetic disorders that can be identified that may make a worker more vulnerable to certain workplace exposures. As an example, people with a deficiency in red cell glucose-6-phosphate dehydrogenase are more susceptible to haemolytic anaemia. As such, persons with this condition are likely to be more susceptible to haemolytic agents. Persons with serum total α_1-antitrypsin deficiency may be considered as susceptible to respiratory irritants (Koh and Jeyaratnam 1998).

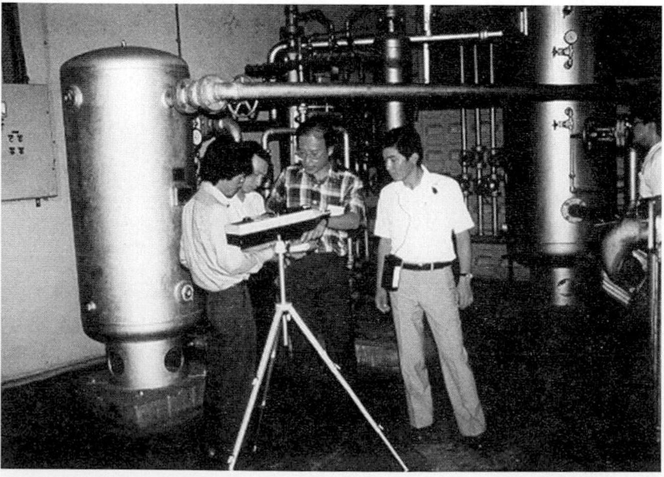

Fig. 7 Area monitoring of noise in the workplace.

Similarly, evidence of other behaviours (e.g. smoking, alcohol consumption) and diseases (e.g. chronic bronchitis, liver, kidney disease), may increase the susceptibility of workers exposed to certain intoxicants.

Biological monitoring of the worker ideally begins at the pre-employment examination stage and can be continued periodically.

Biological monitoring

Biological monitoring complements environmental monitoring in the assessment of health risk in the exposed worker. It is a useful tool in the prevention and management of ill health among workers (Morgan 1997).

One major feature of biological monitoring, as compared with environmental monitoring, is that, for a particular individual, it takes into account exposure from all routes of absorption. As an example, consider the case of workplace exposure to organic solvents. In this instance, skin absorption may be a significant route of entry of the solvent into the body, and ambient environmental air monitoring might be less useful as an indicator of exposure than biological monitoring.

Furthermore, environmental monitoring at the workplace would not account for non-occupational or extra-occupational exposures. A person working in a noisy environment could be additionally exposed to noise in a second job, or as part of the hobby or non-occupational activity of the worker, for instance, reserve military service.

The following case study illustrates how the results of biological monitoring can complement environmental monitoring.

Case study 3: Biological monitoring for carboxyhaemoglobin A worker uses paint stripper in an enclosed workplace, where there are running engines. He can have increased blood carboxyhaemoglobin due to several sources of exposure. Environmental monitoring of carbon monoxide in the poorly ventilated workplace would detect carbon monoxide levels from the exhaust of the running engines. It would not take into consideration the fact that methylene chloride in the paint stripper is metabolized to produce carboxyhaemoglobin. The worker could also be a smoker, and this would further contribute to total carboxyhaemoglobin, which is detected in biological monitoring. (Source: Aw 1995.)

Validation of the biological monitoring marker

A major challenge that has to be addressed is the question of validation. To be useful, an exposure marker must be shown to be able to (in terms of presence and magnitude) reflect accurately past exposure to the agent, and a risk marker should accurately reflect risk of disease outcome. There are many factors to be considered, among which are properties of the biomarker itself, its lifespan and hence the period of exposure reflected, and its stability during collection and processing.

In addition, the importance of understanding intra-individual variability cannot be overemphasized. This variability may be a function of the timing of sample collection, or the sampling procedure itself. Other sources of intra-individual variability could arise from errors in handling, processing, and storing of specimens. Variation in instrumental analysis, such as inherent day to day variation in the assay method, may affect validity of readings. Quality control in the laboratory is important.

Terminology

While some consider any procedure (e.g. periodic radiographs, blood tests, symptom enquiry, etc.) used to monitor exposed workers as biological monitoring, others make a distinction between biological monitoring, and effects monitoring.

Biological monitoring

Biological monitoring refers to the measurement and assessment of workplace agents or their metabolites either in tissues, secreta, excreta, expired air, or any combinations of these to evaluate exposure and health risk compared with an appropriate measure (Aw 1995).

The specific chemical, or its breakdown product, can be measured, to detect the total body burden of the substance. The method of measurement of these substances must be validated and there should be a means to interpret the results obtained in terms of the extent of exposure, and risk to health.

Biological effect monitoring

This refers to the measurement and assessment of early biological effects, of which the relationship to health impairment has not yet been established, in exposed workers to evaluate exposure and/or other health risk compared with an appropriate reference (Zeilhuis and Hendersen 1986). Some examples of include detection of alterations in enzyme levels (e.g. cholinesterase for workers exposed to organophosphorus or carbamate pesticides), or other biochemical changes such as delta aminolaevulinic acid in urine of workers exposed to inorganic lead, or β_2-microglobulin in the urine of cadmium exposed workers.

In the early stages, these changes need not necessarily cause any direct pathological damage to the individual, but rather, reflect situations of excessive exposure. These changes are often reversible on removal of the worker from further exposure.

Health effects monitoring (health surveillance)

Health effects monitoring is 'the periodic physiological or clinical examination of exposed workers with the objective of protecting and preventing occupationally related diseases' (Aw 1995). These examinations detect early clinical effects in exposed workers. Examples of the tests conducted include audiometry for noise-exposed workers, clinical examination for skin lesions in workers exposed to polycyclic aromatic hydrocarbon compounds in tar, pitch, and bitumen, and chest radiographs for workers exposed to pneumoconiosis-producing dusts.

Figure 8 illustrates and summarizes the terminology and levels of prevention that are used in occupational health practice.

An example of a biological exposure limit value

The measurement value obtained by biological monitoring is evaluated as a health risk by comparing it with the corresponding biological exposure limit value. A set of values have been developed by the ACGIH, which include results of biological monitoring as well as biological effects monitoring (ACGIH 1999).

	Primary prevention	Secondary prevention	
Pre-employment Medical examination			
Periodic medical examination	Measurement of intoxicant or metabolite	Early detection of asymptomatic disease	Screening
Biological monitoring	Measurement of health effects	Measurement of health effects	
Molecular biomarkers	? Not proven	? Not proven	

Fig. 8 Summary of terminology and levels of prevention in occupational disease.

The BEI is described as in general representing the 'levels of determinants which are most likely to be observed in specimens collected from a healthy worker who has been exposed to chemicals in the same extent as a worker with inhalation exposure to the TLV' (ACGIH 1999). Exceptions would be made for chemicals for which TLVs are based on non-systemic effects, for example irritation, and for chemicals with significant routes of entry via additional routes of entry (usually percutaneous absorption).

The ACGIH cautions that 'BEIs do not indicate a sharp distinction between hazardous and non-hazardous exposures. Due to biological variability, it is possible for an individual's measurements to exceed the BEI without incurring an increased health risk.' It is further stated that BEIs are not intended for use as a measure of adverse effect or diagnosis of occupational disease. However, if measurements of the individual or group of workers persistently exceed the BEIs, the cause of the excessive values should be investigated, and measures should be taken to reduce the exposure.

BEIs (as used by ACGIH) for some intoxicants are shown in Table 6.

Recent advances in biological monitoring

Technological advances in molecular biology over the last two decades have offered more sophisticated techniques that can be used to study the role of specific exogenous agents and host factors in causing ill health.

These advances have resulted in the development of newer molecular biomarkers of exposure, response, and genetic susceptibility. These include measurements for structural gene damage, gene variation, and gene products in cells and body fluids, for example, oncogenes and tumour suppressor genes, DNA adducts, gene products and genetic polymorphisms, and metabolic phenotypes in environmentally exposed populations (Koh *et al.* 1999).

An understanding of biochemistry and genetics at the molecular level, specific knowledge on metabolism and mechanisms of action, and epidemiology has become increasingly important. This is necessary in order to address the major question of validation and relevance

Table 6 Biological exposure indices (BEIs) of some chemical intoxicants (ACGIH 1999)

Intoxicant	BEI	Source	Sampling time
Carbon monoxide			
Carboxyhaemoglobin	3.5% of haemoglobin	Blood	End of shift
Carbon monoxide	20 ppm	End exhaled air	End of shift
Cadmium and inorganic	5 μg/g creatinine	Urine	Not critical
compounds	5 μg/l	Blood	Not critical
n-Hexane			
2,5-Hexanedione	5 μg/g creatinine	Urine	End of shift
Lead	30 μg/100 ml	Blood	Not critical
Mercury (inorganic)	35 μg/g creatinine	Urine	Pre-shift
	15 μg/l	Blood	End of shift/week
Phenol	250 mg/g creatinine	Urine	End of shift

of these molecular biomarkers. For example, the availability of genetic tests to identify susceptible workers raises issues of ethics, individual privacy, right to work, and the relevance of such tests. Several studies have presented data on the association of environmental measurements and various biomarkers for internal and biologically effective doses, genetic polymorphisms, and early response markers (Table 7).

Given the limitations of individual molecular biomarkers in assessing health risk, and the multifactorial nature of environmental disease, it is likely that a combined approach which examines several of these biomarkers simultaneously, will increase our understanding of the complex issue of disease mechanisms and further refine the process of risk assessment.

Table 7 Examples of molecular biomarkers measured in occupational health studies

Molecular biomarkers	Application	Study population
Exposure marker		
PAH-DNA adduct	Workplace and community exposures and exposure to cigarette smoke, and risk of lung cancer	Foundry workers Coke oven workers General community in industrial areas
Early effect markers		
p53 tumour suppressor gene or its protein product	Specific fingerprint mutation in certain gene codon and risk of liver, breast, lung, and oesophageal cancer	Radon-exposed miners, vinyl chloride monomer workers General population with environmental exposure to aflatoxin B1
H-ras and K-ras gene or its protein product	Increased risk of various cancers, e.g. lung, liver and bladder	Fire-fighters, hazardous waste workers, foundry workers, vinyl chloride monomer workers
Host susceptibility markers		
CYP1A1 polymorphism	Increased risk of lung cancer with exposure to benzo[*a*]pyrene	Foundry workers
NAT2 polymorphism	Increased risk of bladder cancer	Workers exposed to arylamine and hydrazine

Source: Koh *et al.* (1999).

Periodic medical examinations

Periodic medical examinations may be required for some occupational groups in order to effect primary or, failing that, secondary prevention of disease. In many countries, certain categories of employees must undergo statutory periodic medical examination. These examinations are usually for workers exposed to known hazards such as noise, radiation, asbestos, silica, heavy metals, and specific toxic chemicals. In some countries, only properly qualified health personnel, with additional postgraduate training in occupational health, are empowered to perform the examinations, and issue fitness to work certificates. The results of the examinations have to be kept for a specified period of time, and copies sent to the relevant government body.

The objectives of such statutory medical examinations would be to prevent special groups of 'at-risk' workers from developing serious occupational diseases. Regular health examinations, which are specific for the type of hazard the worker is exposed to, are conducted. Workers who are found to show signs of overexposure to any hazard or have early signs of disease can be removed from further exposure. They can be given alternative work until they are fit to return to their former jobs. Furthermore, if signs of overexposure are detected, further control measures can be taken to reduce the exposure and prevent other workers from being similarly affected.

Sometimes, special groups of workers are required to undergo periodic medical examinations for other reasons, such as to certify ongoing fitness to work. Examples of these workers include professional drivers and food handlers.

Notification of occupational diseases

Most countries require the statutory notification of occupational diseases to the government. Notification should be done on the suspicion of occupational disease. The notified case is subsequently investigated and confirmed by the relevant government specialists. Either the employer or health practitioner who sees the worker can notify. In many countries, a list of notifiable occupational diseases is available.

Notification serves as an additional means of control of occupational diseases, undertaken by occupational health and safety professionals in the public sector. It initiates a chain of events, which often includes investigation and confirmation of the index case, and active case finding of other affected persons.

Recommendations for specific preventive measures at the workplace are then prescribed. The authorities would follow up by ensuring that the recommendations have been implemented. If necessary, further evaluation of the effectiveness of the preventive measures can be made.

An example of a notification form is given in Fig. 9 (Ministry of Manpower, Singapore 1999). Figure 10 summarizes the continuum of various means of prevention in occupational health practice.

Tertiary prevention

Tertiary prevention activities are largely curative and rehabilitative procedures. Workers should be removed from further exposure, and the appropriate medical treatment given if indicated. Examples of appropriate treatment include the rendering of first aid promptly after an injury, chelation for severe cases of overexposure to heavy metals, and hyperbaric treatment for cases of compressed air illness.

Disaster planning

Occupational health personnel can also assist in planning for disasters in the workplace and community. Services such as the fire and emergency response services are essential in dealing with disasters at the workplace that may affect the community. As such, planning and practice drills should be done jointly with the relevant local community agencies.

Post-illness or injury evaluation

An evaluation of the health status of the employee returning to work after a prolonged absence from work due to illness or injury is important. The aim is to ensure that the worker has sufficiently recovered from the illness or injury, and that he or she is fit to return to work. The following two issues should be considered.

- Can the worker perform his or her duty without adverse health and safety risks to himself/herself or fellow workers?
- Should he or she return to full-time unrestricted duty, or should some modified, restricted, or alternative duty be given?

Rehabilitation

The rehabilitation of workers is another important aspect of occupational health care. Management, fellow workers, occupational health professionals, and the injured worker have to work together to ensure that suitable alternative duties are provided, and that any work restrictions or physical limitations are understood. There should be clear short- and long-term goals in rehabilitation, and alternative duties should be meaningful and contribute to production (ACOM, ACRM 1987). Sometimes, the use of external rehabilitation resources may be needed.

Worker's compensation

In many countries, workers who are injured at work, or fall ill from hazardous work exposures are eligible for compensation. Employers who carry out economic activities through labour and machines create an environment that may be likely to cause ill health in the employees. Thus employers should be liable for payment of compensation to workers if they are injured or fall sick because of their work.

Legislation concerning employment injury benefits is often called a Workmen's Compensation Act, as in the United States. Employers may be required to insure against their liability under the Act. The workmen's compensation system is designed to minimize litigation and facilitate payment of compensation to injured workers. It is based on a 'no fault' principle. In different countries, certain categories of workers (e.g. domestic helpers) may be excluded.

Other countries may have social insurance to give protection to employment injury victims. The principle of social insurance is that of

TENTH SCHEDULE.

THE FACTORIES ACT.
CHAPTER 104
SECTION 67(1)

NOTICE OF PATIENT SUFFERING FROM INDUSTRIAL DISEASES.

(This notice shall be completed by a registered medical practitioner attending on or called in to visit a patient whom he believes to be suffering from an industrial disease and forwarded to the Chief Inspector of Factories, c/o Department of Industrial Health, Ministry of Manpower, 18 Havelock Road #05–01, Singapore 059764)

Name of Patient	Age	Sex	Race
NRIC/FIN No.	Present Occupation		
Residential Address	Case Summary		
Name and Address of Employer	If patient is deceased state date of last attendance.		

Name of Doctor

Name and Address of Hospital/Clinic

Tel. No. | Doctor's Ref. No.

Diagnosis

Date Signature of Doctor

LIST OF NOTIFIABLE INDUSTRIAL DISEASES

Please tick relevant box

- ☐ ANILINE POISONING
- ☐ ANTHRAX
- ☐ ARSENICAL POISONING
- ☐ ASBESTOSIS
- ☐ BAROTRAUMA
- ☐ BERYLLIUM POISONING
- ☐ BYSSINOSIS
- ☐ CADMIUM POISONING
- ☐ CARBAMATE POISONING
- ☐ CARBON BISULPHIDE POISONING
- ☐ CHROME ULCERATION
- ☐ CHRONIC BENZENE POISONING
- ☐ COMPRESSED AIR ILLNESS
- ☐ CYANIDE POISONING
- ☐ EPITHELIOMATOUS
- ☐ ULCERATION

  (due to tar, pitch, bitumen, mineral oil or paraffin or any compound, product or residue of any such substance)
- ☐ HYDROGEN SULPHIDE POISONING
- ☐ INDUSTRIAL DERMATITIS
- ☐ LEAD POISONING
- ☐ LIVER ANGIOSARCOMA
- ☐ MANGANESE POISONING
- ☐ MERCURIAL POISONING
- ☐ MESOTHELIOMA
- ☐ NOISE INDUCED DEAFNESS
- ☐ OCCUPATIONAL ASTHMA
- ☐ ORGANOPHOSPHATE POISONING
- ☐ PHOSPHORUS POISONING
- ☐ POISONING FROM HALOGEN DERIVATIVES OF HYDROCARBONS
- ☐ REPETITIVE STRAIN DISORDER OF THE UPPER LIMB
- ☐ SILICOSIS
- ☐ TOXIC ANAEMIA
- ☐ TOXIC HEPATITIS

Labour 73-2061-77

NOTE FOR THE REGISTERED MEDICAL PRACTITIONER

All items in this Notification Form must be completed and accompanied by the relevant documents, viz AUDIOGRAM for a Noise Induced Deafness notification and INDUSTRIAL DERMATITIS INVESTIGATION FORM for Industrial Dermatitis notification.

Fig. 9 An example of a notification form for occupational disease.

sharing of risks and pooling financial resources. A social insurance scheme establishes a public channel through a government department or government supervised body, which oversees procedures of screening, determination of award, and payment of benefits.

In the early development of such schemes, only injuries from industrial accidents were covered. This was subsequently enlarged to include occupational diseases. In countries where this is practised, the national legislation would contain a list of those diseases that could be compensated for. The nature of the occupation in relation to each disease may also be prescribed. The worker who suffers from the disease has the advantage of not having to prove that the disease was of occupational origin. Some countries have a more flexible system—any disease that could be shown to be due to an occupation could be considered as compensatable.

Benefits are payable for temporary incapacity or permanent incapacity for workers, and survivors' benefits for those killed at work.

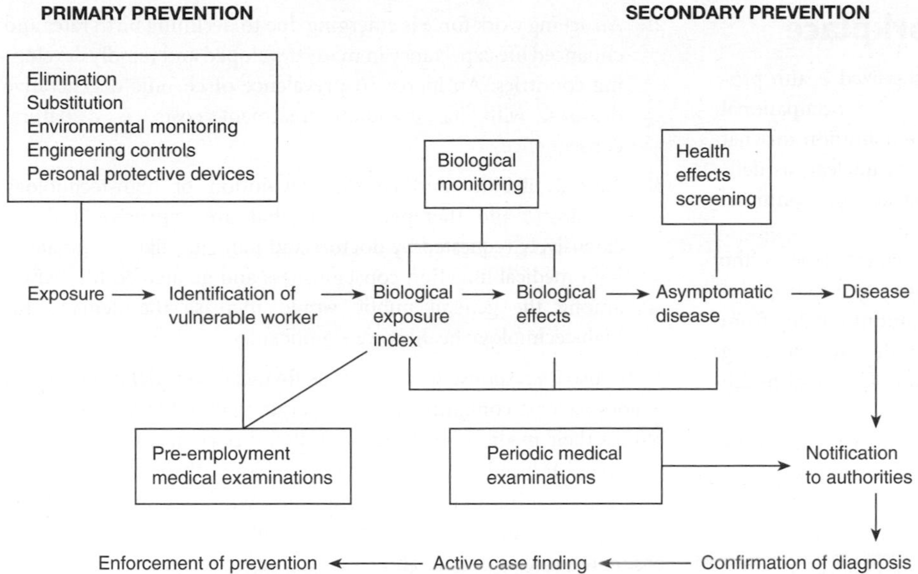

Fig. 10 Continuum of preventive actions in occupational health practice.

Guidelines for the assessment of disability are available in most countries. The final assessments for disability are made when the workers' medical condition has stabilized, and not likely to improve or deteriorate further.

Besides Workmen's Compensation and social insurance schemes, injured workers can sue their employer through common law and claim benefits. This was the only avenue for action in the days before the introduction of Workmen's Compensation schemes. This can be a long process, and the worker has to prove negligence on the part of the employer. In general, workers who have claimed benefits from Workmen's Compensation are not allowed further recourse through this action.

Work-related diseases

The term 'work-related diseases' has been used to describe not only recognized occupational diseases, but also other disorders in which the work environment and performance of work contribute significantly as one of several causative factors (Lesage 1998). These are diseases in which workplace factors may be associated in their occurrence but need not be the only risk factor in each case. Common work-related diseases include: hypertension, ischaemic heart disease, psychosomatic illnesses, musculoskeletal disorders, and chronic non-specific respiratory disease/chronic bronchitis. In these diseases, work may be associated with their causation or may aggravate a pre-existing condition.

In terms of frequency of occurrence, work-related diseases are often more common than pure 'occupational diseases'. While prevention of occupational diseases is possible by the elimination of the workplace hazard, work-related diseases cannot be entirely prevented by only addressing occupational hazards.

Thus, at the workplace, three categories of diseases may be noted in workers.

1. **Occupational diseases**—these are caused by exposure to specific hazards at the workplace. However, in some situations these occupational diseases may also occur among the general community as a consequence of contamination of the environment from the workplace, for example, lead and pesticides. Occupational diseases are cause specific; for example, asbestos causes asbestosis.

2. **Work-related diseases**—these are 'multifactorial' in origin, where factors in the work environment may play a part, together with other risk factors in the development or aggravation of such diseases. These diseases have a complex aetiology.

3. **General diseases affecting the working population**—these are medical conditions prevalent in the community, such as malaria, hereditary haemolytic anaemia, or diabetes mellitus, without a causal relationship with work. The unhealthy worker may not be able to be as productive as his healthy counterpart. Furthermore, work may have a deleterious or aggravating effect on the medical condition.

Table 8 shows the differences between occupational and work-related diseases.

Table 8 Differences between occupational and work-related diseases

Work-related diseases	Occupational diseases
Occur largely in the community	Occur mainly among working population
'Multifactorial' in origin	Cause is specific
Exposure to workplace may be a factor	Exposure to workplace is essential
May be notifiable and compensatable	Notifiable and compensatable

Health promotion at the workplace

Occupational health practitioners have long recognized health promotion to be an integral part of a comprehensive occupational health-care system (ACOM 1983). However, the definition of what really constitutes 'health promotion' is sometimes unclear, as definitions of health promotion differ consequent to the continual evolution of the basic concept of health.

The WHO defines health promotion in its broadest sense as 'the process of enabling people to increase control over, and to improve their health.' Health promotion is seen as a continuum ranging from the treatment of disease, to the prevention of disease, including protection against specific risks, to the promotion of optimal health (WHO 1988).

This definition appears somewhat vague but it does highlight the essence of health promotion. It involves the population as a whole, in the context of their everyday life, rather than focusing on people at risk for specific diseases. Health promotion is, in brief, the social action dimension of health development, other dimensions being biomedical and technological interventions embodied in public health practice (WHO 1991).

It is a process of activating communities, policy-makers, professionals, and the public for health supportive policies, systems, and ways of living. It is manifested by promoting healthy lifestyles and community action for health, and by creating conditions that make it possible to live a healthy life.

Worksite health promotion programmes

Worksite health promotion programmes are common in industrialized countries. Among the developing nations, there is also growing interest in the workplace as a site with great potential for health promotion. Existing occupational health services now face the challenge of adapting to a wider scope of responsibility than its traditional role.

A major reason for the introduction of worksite health promotion programmes is financial in nature. This is especially pressing in the developed countries. As an example, the American health system passes the burden of costs on to the consumer, which would be the employer, as most American companies offer medical benefits as a matter of right to their employees. These medical benefits have become a serious financial burden to the employer in the face of rapidly rising costs of health care. However, the effect of rising health-care costs is now a fairly global concern. There are several reasons for this escalation of health-care costs.

1. There has been a shift in disease profile from communicable diseases to non-communicable diseases. At present, non-communicable diseases are responsible for 70 to 80 per cent of deaths in the developed countries and about 40 per cent in the developing world. The emergent non-communicable diseases are consequent to the successful control of communicable diseases as well as the cultivation of unhealthy lifestyles. In addition, improved life expectancy that follows an enhanced standard of living has led to a rise in chronic degenerative diseases. Curative care for such diseases is limited and expensive, requiring repeated medical consultation and follow-up.
2. An ageing work force is emerging due to declining birth rates and enhanced life expectancy in many developed and rapidly developing countries. An increased prevalence of chronic degenerative diseases, with its attendant treatment costs, is a natural consequence.
3. Easy availability and constant evolution of high-technology diagnostic and therapeutic aids that are expensive, but are extensively requested by doctors and patients alike. A climate of high medical litigation consciousness and greater health literacy among the general public would increase the demand for high-technology health care significantly.

Industry's response to this serious financial consideration is often to adopt a 'cost-containment' policy, arguing that if companies could reduce their medical insurance and disability claims, they would be able to lower health costs and potentially reduce their operating costs. Worksite health promotion programmes, with their goal of keeping employees healthy and reducing medical utilization, are a part of this cost containment policy. Thus the motivating factor here is financial savings, with good health as the means to the end.

The worksite as a setting for health promotion

The increasing interest in worksite health promotion programme is certainly healthy and the workplace has several factors that make it a unique setting for health promotion. Firstly, the workplace is where the worker spends the greater part of their waking hours. The work force also constitutes a captive population and any health promotion programme at the workplace would very likely invite encouraging response. The employer has the luxury of having at their disposal already well-established communications channels. They have existing physical facilities and resources from which they may adapt and expand upon. There is ease of administration and feedback, and the target population identified can be easily followed up. In addition, larger companies have in-house health personnel who can direct and run the programmes. There may be possible savings in health-care dollars as a result, but regardless of financial gain, the employer enjoys the image of being caring, in providing attractive staff welfare schemes.

The worker also benefits significantly. They have the convenience of not needing to expend time and expense in travelling to locations of community-based facilities. In addition, they are part of a homogeneous group that provides strong peer support and influence. They may also enjoy incentives from participating in worksite health promotion programmes (if the company offers any).

Worksite health promotion programmes inevitably leave an impact on society as a whole as well, because workers form a large proportion of the general population. The male worker is often the head of the household, with a strong influence on the family unit. Hence knowledge and benefits obtained from his participation in the programme will also permeate into his family.

Components of worksite health promotion programmes

The nature of the health promotion programmes offered differs greatly among the various companies. There is clearly great breadth and diversity of these worksite health promotion programmes among the companies that do implement them. One reason for this is the large variety of individuals who design and conduct them. Another reason would be the different motivating factors behind the initiation of worksite health promotion programme for each company, for example, cost containment, staff welfare, positive corporate image, and increased productivity. Fielding and Piserchia (1989) reported that 65 per cent of workplaces in America had one or more areas of health promotion activities. Common types of activities included individual health risk assessment, smoking cessation, control and treatment of hypertension, exercise and fitness, weight control, nutrition education, stress management, back problem prevention and care, and of the job accident prevention. Broadly speaking, the components that make up health promotion programmes include medical care, involving early detection and control of conditions that represent illness or are biological precursors to illnesses such as diabetes mellitus or hypertension. Worksite health promotion programme would aim to screen participants using appropriate techniques and subsequently intervene medically if warranted.

Another component would be the modification of high-risk behaviours with known or suspected negative health consequences such as smoking, inactivity, and poor nutrition. Methods to bring about successful behaviour modification include health information, education, counselling, and incentives.

The third component of worksite health promotion programme is overall corporate culture. Healthy behaviour has a better chance of being sustained if it becomes the norm. This would involve initiating company policies such as smoking restrictions, making time and facilities available for exercise and healthy diets, and positive role modelling by top management personnel.

Limitations of workplace health promotion

Despite the exciting possibilities that health promotion holds, it would still be prudent to consider some of the limitations of health promotion at the work place and the problems faced in the planning, implementation, and evaluation of such programmes.

Limitations of prevention and health promotion

Many people automatically assume that prevention is better than cure. However, prevention does have a price, which may sometimes be exorbitant, and is thus not necessarily always better. For illnesses with low prevalence, preventive measures that are directed at large numbers of persons would result in low yields. The costs involved in prevention then would far outweigh the benefits gained in prevention. While it is true that 'a stitch in time saves nine'; this axiom might not apply to every person and every preventive measure (Skrabanek and McCormick 1990). They cautioned that, if the 'one stitch' has to be inserted one hundred times to save one individual from 'nine', it might be unwise to queue for stitching.

The goal of disease prevention, as referred to in most of the worksite health promotion programmes, usually refers to delay, rather than prevention of the disease. This is because many of the target diseases are multifactorial in origin, and while worksite health promotion programmes are mainly directed at the behavioural aspects of lifestyle change, less can be done about the other factors, such as heredity and social class.

Another major limitation to health promotion is the difficulty that exists in arriving at a commonly acceptable and precise definition of health that allows for objective quantification.

Health promotion as a crusade

The zeal for worksite health promotion programmes may sometimes border upon religious fervour, dependent more on faith than facts. This zeal may result in the 'moralization of health' (Conrad 1987*a*), where an individual's character and moral standing are judged on his state of health, based on the premise of individual responsibility for health. This premise is, of course, not true for the diseases of unknown or multifactorial aetiology. In this scenario, 'health deviants' may be stigmatized by their peers for their unhealthy lifestyles, and 'victim-blaming' responses may easily emerge. Employers may blame some workers, such as the high-risk individuals who do not participate in worksite health promotion programmes, for their 'deviant' health behaviour and not doing something about it.

While participation in worksite health promotion programmes may be voluntary, some employees may well be 'coaxed' into participation, and incentives as well as disincentives (such as higher insurance premiums for the overweight and smokers) might be included. Nevertheless, there have been reports (Baun *et al.* 1986; Conrad 1987*b*; Lewis *et al.* 1996) that suggest that worksite health promotion programme participants are relatively 'healthier' and more health conscious that non-participants. This means that to some extent, the worksite health promotion programmes are preaching to the already converted.

A more recent review by Grosch *et al.* (1998) suggested that compared with availability of activities, participation depended less on individual and organizational characteristics. They reported that healthy employees were not consistently more likely to participate in worksite health promotion programme than non-healthy employees.

Conrad (1987*a*) has warned of the expansion of the boundaries of corporate jurisdiction via worksite health promotion programmes. Citing workplace programmes that screen for drugs, HIV/AIDS, or genetic make-up as the more obvious manifestations of this phenomenon, he cautions that worksite health promotion programmes, with their focus on smoking, diet, exercise, and blood pressure are entering the domain of what has been long regarded as private life. This concern might even be extrapolated further, to the (presently unlikely) point of corporate off-site surveillance programmes. One has to be wary of the extension of these boundaries of corporate jurisdiction. At its worst, 'wellness' might become a condition of employment or promotion, which is a type of job discrimination based on lifestyle and health.

Does health promotion really work?

Although there have been some favourable studies to suggest great benefits in health promotion, most authorities would agree that there is a paucity of rigorous scientific proof that addresses this literally multimillion dollar question. Bias in reporting further obscures the truth, as negative results after the input of large sums of money on worksite health promotion programmes, are unlikely to be reported by the persons responsible for the worksite health promotion programmes. Published results may overinflate claims of benefits, and many reports tend to be based on anecdotal evidence or have serious flaws in assumptions, data, or methodology (Warner *et al.* 1988; Conrad *et al.* 1991).

While cost containment may be a primary goal for employers providing worksite health promotion programmes, not all employers would benefit equally from worksite health promotion programmes. An economic model (Patton 1991) suggests that establishments employing highly productive, difficult to replace, and older employees are most likely to benefit. The majority of the economic benefit accrue from productivity gains, while effect on health-care expense, worker mortality, or retiree health expenses are small. The benefits may also appear after a period of time from the start of the worksite health promotion programme. A study of employees at Procter and Gamble (Goetzel *et al.* 1998) showed that in the third year of a worksite health promotion programme, participants had 29 per cent lower health-care costs as compared with non-participants. Overall, recent reviews on worksite health promotion programmes (Anderson and Staufacker 1996; Glanz *et al.* 1996; Heaney and Goetzel 1997; Pelletier 1997) are cautiously optimistic.

Worksite health promotion programmes are often one of the most visible and popular employee benefits. Some employers might use the introduction of worksite health promotion programmes as an excuse for cost shifting and reductions in other health benefit, such as reduced coverage and increased employee cost-sharing for the treatment of illnesses.

Health professionals may be equally quick to jump on the bandwagon of worksite health promotion programmes. As screening activities are often a part of many worksite health promotion programmes, there is certainly the potential of offering costly, profitable and opportunistic screening procedures, many of which have unproven benefits. The Australian College of Occupational Medicine (1983) believes that a conservative approach should be adopted, bearing in mind that no harm should result to the individual. Another requirement for screening procedures is that there should be conclusive evidence that the procedure can alter the natural history of disease in a significant proportion of those screened.

Impact of health promotion on occupational health

As mentioned earlier, occupational health practitioners have long recognized health promotion as an integral part of a comprehensive occupational health-care system. While the main thrust of occupational health is on the identification and control of physical, chemical, biological, and psychosocial hazards in the work environment, the main target of intervention in worksite health promotion programmes is often the individual, rather than the organization or the environment.

Thus there is concern that undue emphasis on worksite health promotion programmes might focus preventive efforts on the worker and divert attention, funding, and action from efforts directed at the work environment—as an example, focusing on individual stress reduction rather than altering a stressful work environment may help people adapt to unhealthy environments. Conrad (1987*b*) commented 'One virtually never hears wellness people discussing occupational disease or hazardous working conditions. Whether they view it as someone else's domain or as simply too downbeat for upbeat wellness programmes is difficult to know. This may in part explain why worksite health promotion has been greeted with scepticism by occupational health veterans.' This diversion of attention from the work environment to the worker and the blurring of the occupational health focus might occur in both management as well as the work force. Care must be taken in implementing worksite health promotion programme to incorporate traditional occupational health concerns into the planning process so that a more complete programme may be developed that truly promotes workplace health in terms of the worker as well as their environment.

Problems of implementation, sustainability, and evaluation

The methodological approaches to health promotion are far less developed and more difficult than the epidemiological methods of planning, implementation, and evaluation of programmes of disease prevention. As an example, even the definition of what constitutes a programme has not been universally accepted (Golaszewski 1992).

There are several reasons for these difficulties. Firstly, there is still lack of knowledge on factors conducive to positive health. Very little research has been undertaken on the determinants of positive health, as it is very difficult to develop measurements of health as opposed to disease. Thus most scientific work has focused on the causes of disease and on its pathogenesis, rather than on positive health.

Secondly, health behaviour is very complex as it is influenced by economic, ecological, social, and political conditions. Thus strategies of health promotion programmes are far broader than those of disease prevention as they involve politics, advertising, health education, advocacy for health and healthy living, economics, community development, and ways to affect changes in peoples' behaviour.

A properly implemented worksite health promotion programme should have written goals or objectives, have person(s) accountable for the achievement of objectives, a budget, and have continuity over time. It should also be a sustainable effort, as compliance with lifestyle changes, a common target of worksite health promotion programmes, has to be sustained to be effective. This may be difficult to achieve. As an example, a review of the literature on the compliance to exercise following worksite health promotion programmes showed that over 50 per cent of participants had dropped out after 6 months (Stoffelmayr *et al.* 1992). This problem of sustainability is a real one for many aspects of worksite health promotion programmes, and requires further research and attention.

Finally, all good worksite health promotion programmes should have evaluation built in as one of their components from the start of the programme. To facilitate proper evaluation, potential evaluators should keep in mind three points.

1. Wherever possible, the evaluator should be independent of the persons who are conducting the health programme in question. This would prevent bias due to vested interest.

2. Proper evaluation requires knowledge of the state-of-the-art on the health problem in question, so that the health evaluator will know what had been done, what can be done, and how it should be done.

3. Design and resources for evaluation should be incorporated into the planning of a health programme. Otherwise, no documentation will be obtained on who was served, how well they were

served, or what changes had occurred from exposure to the programme, which would render subsequent evaluation difficult or impossible.

There are two levels of evaluation that would need to be considered when assessing a programme's effectiveness. These are process and outcome evaluations.

A process evaluation is a quality assessment review of the programme (Koh *et al.* 1994). This concept is not really new in either health care or in health education and promotion. In order to improve programme effectiveness, there is a need to examine continually the processes and skills of personnel who plan and deliver health-related programmes, and the compliance and acceptance of programmes by participants. This is the role of process evaluation. It compares what happened to what is supposed to have happened.

Outcome evaluation seeks to assess the effectiveness of the health programme on the target group (Koh *et al.* 1994). It is concerned predominantly with internal validity, which is the degree to which an outcome can be attributed to a particular intervention, namely did the programme work in this particular setting and did it produce the observed change?

Further development

Health promotion at the workplace is still developing, and much has still to be learnt. The dearth of sound evidence on the merits of worksite health promotion programmes should not be interpreted as a negative assessment of the potential of such programmes, but instead it recommends a healthy scepticism in reading the literature and in the development of a new research-based body of understanding (Warner *et al.* 1988). Pelletier (1997) has more optimistically suggested that 'rather than interpreting the methodological flaws and diversity as inherently negative, we may consider it as indicative of a robust phenomena evident in many types of worksites, with diverse employees, differing interventions, and varying degrees of methodological sophistication'.

Over time, research and development will unravel much concerning the true capabilities and limitations of health promotion in the workplace. It is still worth remembering, however, that the pursuit of health in itself is a worthy goal. Even if nothing else, the incorporation of health promotion into the workplace context will certainly serve to provide a somewhat more balanced perspective of life for the worker.

From occupational health to environmental health

The recent rapid growth in interest in environmental health has created a dilemma as to its identity as a speciality in the field of health. The public interest in environmental health was not matched by a well developed speciality in the health field that could respond to its needs and concerns. Increasingly, occupational health practice today has evolved to encompass environmental health issues as well. This is because of several reasons. Firstly, many sources of pollution originate from the workplace. Secondly, in many other instances, the distinction between the work environment and the home environment may not be clearly defined. This is particularly seen in agriculture and small-scale industries, where a clear demarcation does not exist between the workplace and home.

Furthermore, there are several areas of common ground between occupational and environmental health (Jeyaratnam 1994). A comparison of the factors in the work environment influencing the health of the working population (occupational health) and that of the general environment affecting the health of the community (environmental health), is shown in Table 9. It is evident that there are several areas of similarity between the work environment and the general environment which affect health.

Occupational health practitioners have the necessary skills in clinical medicine, toxicology, hygiene, epidemiology, and preventive health to position themselves for the management of environmental health concerns, as illustrated in the following case study.

Case study 4: From occupational health to environmental health
Villagers living along a river complained of skin disorders a few months after a paper pulp mill was sited upstream from their villages. The residents, who were mainly fishermen and farmers, bathed in the river and used river water for many of their domestic activities. They claimed that pollutants discharged from the paper pulp mill caused the skin disorders. An occupational health team was consulted to resolve the matter. Workplace assessment revealed some occupational health and safety issues that needed to be addressed. The plant utilized modern state-of-the-art technology, with a closed mill system. Monitoring of the effluent from the mill revealed that quality of the discharge was within internationally accepted limits. Examination of a group of the most severely affected villagers revealed that the main skin disorders were fungal infections of the skin, endogenous eczema, and irritant contact dermatitis at specific sites (e.g. from application of topical medicaments, hand dermatitis from use of detergents). A comparison of the existing health records of the village showed no increase in the proportion of cases of skin disorders before and after the paper pulp mill commenced operations. The main health problems were malaria and gastroenteritis. The conclusion was that the villagers' health concerns (with regard to dermatological disorders) were unrelated to the paper pulp mill. However, the mill management provided supplementary community health care through its health-care department, in conjunction with the local health authorities. This gesture was appreciated by the villagers.

Table 9 Comparison of occupational health and environmental health

Occupational health	Environmental health
Hazards in workplace environment	Hazards in community environment
Hazards largely in air	Hazards in air, soil, water, and food
Hazards are physical, chemical, biological, and psychosocial	Hazards are physical, chemical, biological, and psychosocial
Route of exposure: inhalation and dermal	Route of exposure: ingestion, inhalation, and dermal
Exposure period: 8 h/day for working life	Exposure period: lifelong
Exposed population: adults, usually healthy	Exposed population: children, adults, elderly, and sick persons

Conclusion

This chapter has traced the history and development of occupational health and its related legislation. In the practice of occupational health, prevention of work-related and occupational disease is a major objective. The priority in prevention of occupational diseases should be to effect primary prevention. When this fails, secondary prevention activities are undertaken to contain damage. However, health protection is not the only occupational health concern. Health promotion in the working population is another important activity. The workplace is an ideal setting for health promotion activities, and appropriate lifestyle interventions can prevent many of the common causes of morbidity in society. Finally, the practice of occupational health today has extended beyond the domain of the workplace, into the general environment. Hence the term occupational and environmental health might more accurately describe this important aspect of public health.

Further reading

Baxter, P.J., *et al.* (ed.) (2000). *Hunter's diseases of occupations* (9th edn). Arnold, London.

Herzstein, J.A., *et al.* (ed.) (1998). *International occupational and environmental medicine.* Mosby, St Louis, MO.

Rom, W.M. (ed.) (1998). *Environmental and occupational medicine* (3rd edn). Lippincott–Raven, Philadelphia, PA.

Stellman, J.M. (ed.) (1998). *ILO encyclopaedia of occupational safety and health* (4th edn), Vols 1–4. International Labour Organization, Geneva.

References

ACGIH (American Conference of Governmental Industrial Hygienists) (1999). *1999 TLVs and BEIs. Threshold limit values for chemical substances and physical agents. biological exposure indices.* American Conference of Governmental Industrial Hygienists, Cincinnati, OH.

ACOM (Australian College of Occupational Medicine) (1983). *Health promotion in industry.* ACOM, Sydney.

ACOM, ACRM (Australasian College of Occupational Medicine, Australian College of Rehabilitation Medicine) (1987). *Occupational rehabilitation. guidelines on principles and practice.* ACOM, ACRM, Sydney.

Anderson, D.R. and Staufacker, M.J. (1996). The impact of worksite-based health risk appraisal on health-related outcomes: a review of the literature. *American Journal of Health Promotion*, **10**, 499–508.

Aw, T.C. (1995). Biological monitoring. In: *Occupational hygiene* (2nd edn) (ed. J.M. Harrington and K. Gardiner), pp. 276–86. Blackwell Science, Oxford.

Axelson, O. (1997). Some historical notes and remarks on prevention in environmental and occupational health. *International Journal of Occupational Medicine and Environmental Health*, **10**, 339–47.

Baun, W.B., Bernacki, E.J., and Shan, P.T. (1986). A preliminary investigation: Effect of a corporate fitness programme on absenteeism and health care cost. *Journal of Occupational Medicine*, **28**, 18–22.

Brady, W., Bass, J., Royce, M., Anstadt, G., Loeppke, R., and Leopold, R. (1997). Defining total corporate health and safety costs: significance and impact. *Journal of Occupational and Environmental Medicine*, **39**, 224–31.

Brandt Rauf, P.W. and Brandt Rauf, S.I. (1987). History of occupational medicine: Relevance of Imhotep and the Edwin Smith papyrus. *British Journal of Industrial Medicine*, **44**, 68–70.

Cochrane, A.L. and Holland, W.W. (1971). Validation of screening procedures. *British Medical Bulletin*, **27**, 3–8.

Commission of the European Communities (1992). *Europeans and health and safety at work. A survey.* Directorate-General for Employment, Social Affairs and Education. Health and Safety Directorate, Luxembourg.

Conrad, P. (1987*a*). Wellness in the workplace: Potentials and pitfalls of worksite health promotion. *Milbank Quarterly*, **65**, 255–75.

Conrad, P. (1987*b*). Who comes to worksite wellness programmes? *Journal of Occupational Medicine*, **29**, 317–20.

Conrad, K.M., Conrad, K.J., and Walcott-McQuigg, J. (1991). Threats to internal validity in worksite health promotion program research: common problems and possible solutions. *American Journal of Health Promotionion*, **6**, 112–22.

Davies, N.V. and Teasdale, P. (1994). *The costs to the British economy of work accidents and work related ill health.* Health and Safety Executive. HMSO, London.

Devereux, J.J., Buckle, P.W., and Vlachonikolis, I.G. (1999). Interactions between physical and psychosocial risk factors at work increase the risk of back disorders: an epidemiological approach. *Occupational and Environmental Medicine*, **56**, 343–53.

Doll, R. (1975). Pott and the path to prevention. *Archiv fur Geschwulstforschung*, **45**, 521–31.

Elo, A.L. (1986). *Assessment of psychic stress factors at work.* Finnish Institute of Occupational Health, Helsinki.

Evanoff, B.A., Gustavsson, P., and Hogstedt, C. (1993). Mortality and incidence of cancer in a cohort of Swedish chimney sweeps: an extended follow up study. *British Journal of Industrial Medicine*, **50**, 450–9.

Felton, J.S. (1997). The heritage of Bernardino Ramazzini. *Occupational Medicine*, **47**, 167–79.

Fielding, J.E. and Piserchia, P.V. (1989). Frequency of worksite health promotion activities. *American Journal of Public Health*, **79**, 16–20.

Forsmann, S. (1983). Occupational health. In *Encyclopaedia of occupational health and safety* (3rd edn) (ed. L. Parmeggiani), pp. 1491–3, Vol. 2. International Labour Organization, Geneva.

Glanz, K., Sorensen, G., and Farmer, A. (1996). The health impact of worksite nutrition and cholesterol intervention programs. *American Journal of Health Promotion*, **10**, 453–70.

Goetzel, R.Z., Jacobson, B.H., Aldana, S.G., Vardell, K., and Yee, L. (1998) Health care costs of worksite health promotion participants and non-participants. *Journal of Occupational and Environmental Medicine*, **40**, 341–6.

Golaszewski, T. (1992). What is a programme: thoughts on definitions in worksite health promotion. (Editorial) *Journal of Occupational Medicine*, **34**, 162–3.

Grosch, J.W., Alterman, T., Petersen, M.R., and Murphy, L.R. (1998). Worksite health promotion programs in the US: factors associated with availability and participation. *American Journal of Health Promotion*, **13**, 36–45.

Hansen, E.S. (1990). Chest symptoms in chimney sweeps and postmen—a comparative survey. *International Journal of Epidemiology*, **19**, 339–42.

Heaney, C.A. and Goetzel, R.Z. (1997). A review of health-related outcomes of multi-component worksite health promotion programs. *American Journal of Health Promotion*, **11**, 290–307.

HSE (Health and Safety Executive) (1995). *Generic terms and concepts in the assessment and regulation of industrial risks.* HMSO, London.

Hunter, D. (1969). *The diseases of occupations* (4th edn). English Universities Press, London.

Jeyaratnam, J. (1994). Editorial: Occupational and environmental health. *Journal of Occupational Medicine Singapore*, **6**, 1–2.

Jeyaratnam, J. and Koh, D. (ed.) (1996). *Textbook of occupational medicine practice.* World Scientific, Singapore.

Koh, D. and Jeyaratnam, J. (1998). Biomarkers, screening and ethics. *Occupational Medicine*, **48**, 27–30.

Koh, D., Alsagoff, F., and Koh, Y.H. (1994). Health promotion in the workplace. In: *Occupational health in national development* (ed. J. Jeyaratnam and K.S. Chia), pp. 142–63. World Scientific, Singapore.

Koh, D., Seow, A., and Ong, C.N. (1999). New techniques in molecular epidemiology and their relevance to occupational medicine. *Occupational and Environmental Medicine*, **56**, 725–9.

Lesage, M. (1998). Work related diseases and occupational diseases: The ILO International List. In: *Encyclopaedia of occupational safety and health* (4th edn) (ed. J.M. Stellman), Vol. 1, pp. 26.2–26.6. International Labour Office, Geneva.

Levy, L.S. (1999). Standard setting in occupational health. In: *Occupational health risk assessment and management* (ed. S. Sadhra and K.G. Rampal), pp. 118–28. Blackwell Science, Oxford.

Lewis, R.J., Huebner, W.W., and Yarborough, C.M. III (1996). Characteristics of participants and nonparticipants in worksite health promotion. *American Journal of Health Promotion*, **11**, 99–106.

Mason, H.J., *et al.* (1999). Follow up of workers previously exposed to silver solder containing cadmium. *Occupational and Environmental Medicine*, **56**, 553–8.

Ministry of Manpower, Republic of Singapore. (1999). *Notice of patient suffering from industrial diseases.* Department of Industrial Health. http://www.gov.sg/mom/dih/forms.html

Morgan, M.S. (1997). The biological exposure indices: a key component in protecting workers from toxic chemicals. *Environmental Health Perspectives*, **105** (Supplement 1), 105–15.

OSHA (Occupational Safety and Health Administration) (1995). *Personal protective equipment.* US Department of Labor, Washington, DC.

Patton, J.P. (1991). Worksite health promotion: An economic model. *Journal of Occupational Medicine*, **33**, 868–73.

Pelletier, K.R. (1997). Clinical and cost outcomes of multifactorial, cardiovascular risk management interventions in worksites: a comprehensive review and analysis. *Journal of Occupational and Environmental Medicine*, **39**, 1154–69.

Postol, T. (1993). Public health and working children in twentieth-century America: an historical overview. *Journal of Public Health Policy*, **14**, 348–54.

Prezant, D.J., *et al.* (1999). Impact of a modern firefighting protective uniform on the incidence and severity of burn injuries in New York City firefighters. *Journal of Occupational and Environmental Medicine*, **41**, 469–79.

Sadhra, S. and Rampal, K.G. (ed.) (1999). *Occupational health. Risk assessment and management.* Blackwell Science, Oxford.

Skrabanek, P. and McCormick, J. (1990). *Follies and fallacies in medicine.* Prometheus Books, New York.

SOM (Society of Occupational Medicine) (1997). *The Disability Discrimination Act 1995. A guide for occupational physicians.* Society of Occupational Medicine, London.

Stoffelmayr, B.E., Mavis, B.E., Stachnik, T., Robison, J., and Rogers, M. (1992). A programme model to enhance adherence in worksite based fitness programmes. *Journal of Occupational Medicine*, **34**, 156–61.

Tsuchiya, K. (1991). Development of occupational health in Japan. *Sangyo Ika Daigaku Zasshi*, **13**, 191–205.

Wall, L.T. (1999). Auditing stress. *Occupational Medicine*, **49**, 343–4.

Warner, K.E., Wickizer, T.M., Wolfe, R.A., Schilroth, J.E., and Samuelson, M.H. (1988). Economic implications of workplace health promotion programmes: review of the literature. *Journal of Occupational Medicine*, **30**, 106–12.

Wassenius, O., Jarvholm, B., Engstrom, T., Lillienberg, L., and Meding, B. (1998). Variability in the skin exposure of machine operators exposed to cutting fluids. *Scandinavian Journal Work, Environment and Health*, **24**, 125–9.

WHO (World Health Organization) (1988). *Health promotion for working populations.* Technical Report Series 765. WHO, Geneva.

WHO (World Health Organization) (1991). *Action for public health. Health promotion in developing countries.* WHO/HED/91.1. WHO, Geneva.

Zeilhuis, R.L. and Henderson, P.T. (1986). Definitions of monitoring activities and their relevance for the practice of occupational health. *International Archives of Occupational and Environment Health*, **57**, 249–57.

8.7 Ergonomics and public health*

Laura Punnett

Overview

Definition

Ergonomics is the area of scientific research and application concerned with the design of engineered systems and environments to be compatible with human capacities and limitations. According to the International Ergonomics Association, the field 'integrates knowledge derived from the human sciences to match jobs, systems, products and environments to the physical and mental abilities and limitations of people'. Clark and Corlett (1984) wrote that 'ergonomics is the study of human abilities and characteristics which affect the design of equipment, systems and jobs and its aims are to improve efficiency, safety and well-being'.

Tools and systems that are badly designed, or not designed at all, often lead to fatigue, discomfort, injury, or chronic health disorders for the users. A system or device designed according to ergonomic principles should be easier to use, result in less fatigue and ill health, generate fewer errors, be more satisfying to the user, and improve work quality and productivity.

Brief history

Some of the health consequences of poor ergonomic design have been recognized for nearly three centuries, since the work of Ramazzini (1713). In modern times, the professional field was defined in 1949 with the establishment of the Ergonomics Society in the United Kingdom (Murrell 1965). Ergonomics research had begun as early as 1915 in this country with the establishment of the Industrial Fatigue Research Board. Human fatigue was to be prevented through proper allocation of breaks and suitable working hours, and thereby improved efficiency of production would be achieved. During the First World War, the productivity of the British ammunition factories was shown to increase in parallel with a reduction of weekly working hours (Vernon 1921).

Thus the first applications of ergonomics were in the defence industry, in both the United Kingdom and the United States. One important impetus to further development was the nature of the problems encountered during the Second World War with technological change, such as the introduction of new weapons. These new systems were found to perform poorly because of a mismatch between humans and technology. Previous attempts had been made to fit humans to new technology by means of training and information, but neither one could be used to their full capacity with this approach. When knowledge of human capabilities was employed in system design, efficiency and accuracy were vastly improved.

From productivity and safety in military systems, the focus of research and applications in ergonomics has broadened considerably over the years. After the Second World War, the concepts of ergonomics were applied to manufacturing and physically strenuous jobs in other sectors, such as mining and forestry. High aerobic demands and heavy manual handling characterized these jobs, and problems with general fatigue, accidents, and low back pain were widespread.

In modern manufacturing, many such tasks have been mechanized; work reorganization and the use of new technology have reduced aerobic demands in traditionally 'heavy work'. However, these changes have also resulted in increased prevalence of static body positions and repetitive movements, with an accompanying pattern of musculoskeletal problems affecting the neck, shoulder, arm, and hand. Similar problems are encountered in the office environment, especially among people performing data entry work (Punnett and Bergqvist 1997). A substantial minority of the working population still perform physically strenuous jobs, even in developed countries, especially in mining, agriculture, transportation, and construction, and so-called service jobs in health care, food preparation, and cleaning. While the first four sectors are typically male dominated and recognized as hazardous, many employees in the latter jobs are women whose work is perceived as clean and safe, even when it requires a large proportion of their physical capacity.

Since the 1970s, issues such as human–computer interaction and health consequences of poor ergonomics, especially in the occupational setting, have grown in importance. Much more attention is given now than previously to work organization issues ('macro-ergonomics') and prevention of technological system failure, as well as techniques for implementing ergonomic improvements through worker participatory processes.

Geographically, there are some substantial differences in focus within the field. Many American practitioners have a background in engineering rather than in health sciences. The psychological aspects of ergonomics, especially cognitive and sensory perception issues, which are often referred to as 'human factors', dominated research in the United States for many years. Manufacturing systems and consumer issues have received much attention in research from the United Kingdom and Japan. Work physiology has dominated research in the rest of Europe, especially in the Nordic countries, while

* This chapter in the previous edition was written by Dr Åsa Kilbom. The current revision was undertaken with her consent but without her review of specific changes.

Francophone ergonomists emphasize the worker's integrated, subjective experience. These varying emphases reflect differences in scientific traditions, industrial structures, and types of legislation related to occupational injuries.

The advantages of good ergonomics can now be seen in occupational settings, public life, and homes. Reduction of heavy lifting and handling of objects through lifting devices, the introduction of ergonomically designed office furniture and computer keyboards and pointing devices, and the improved design of transportation systems are examples that bear witness to these advances. Much remains to be done, however, to ensure safe, healthy, and productive workplaces, homes, and public spaces.

The 'human–machine' system

In the field of ergonomics, the interaction of the person with the environment has often been conceptualized as the 'human–machine system' (Fig. 1). In this system, the 'machine' presents information to the person, often via one or more displays, the information is perceived by the operator's sensory apparatus (through vision or hearing), and the operator uses his or her cognitive capacity and memory to decide on a suitable response, which is transferred to the 'machine' as a motor activity such as pushing buttons or handling objects. The machine's response involves additional information to the operator, and so on.

Although the first applications were aimed at machines and other technical equipment, in reality humans interact not only with devices but also with the physical and social environment, including with other humans. Now the term most often used is 'human–machine–environment system', and generally with a broader definition. The human operator may interact not only with a machine but also or instead with another human being, who feeds his or her response back via speech, signs (sign interpretation), or touch; alternatively, there may be other responses or inputs from society via road traffic signs, books, or other means. The operator's response can then be via another form of motor activity, such as talking, writing, steering a car, or typing on a keyboard.

One important feature of the human–machine concept is that humans do not perform their actions in isolation, but as part of a system that is in dynamic equilibrium. The aim of the system is to perform efficiently and without mishap, which requires an optimization of the interface between the person and the 'machine' (now a metaphor for any other component of the system). Thus feedback or information must be presented in a way that can be perceived easily and without mistakes, and physical controls must be designed to comply with the person's strength, body dimensions, and natural range of motion. The environment should be conducive to task performance, with attention to temperature, background noise, and psychosocial conditions. Efficiency also implies an optimal allocation of tasks between humans and 'machines', so that each component of the system performs the task for which he, she, or it is best suited (Chapanis 1965; Oborne *et al.* 1993; Mital *et al.* 1994). For example, humans are usually superior to machines in recognition of subtle patterns, decision-making requiring experience, and creativity, while machines are often superior in activities that require both precision and endurance, and/or high repeatability.

This system has traditionally been presented as a closed loop, where deviations from the desired 'state' of the system are corrected. Humans or operators were seen as elements of the system whose task is to respond to the feedback from the 'machine'. The quality of the response depends on their individual physiological, anatomical, sensory, and cognitive capacity. In a complex system with high demands on safety, like a nuclear power plant or chemical processing industry, it is crucial that the operator does not deviate from the desired response to an anticipated situation. Nevertheless, in modern ergonomics it is acknowledged that the individual has a more central role. This 'person-centred' philosophy sees the operator as the one who initiates action, and controls and dominates the system. The human being contributes an ability to anticipate and predict what may happen within the system (Oborne *et al.* 1993), as well as his or her own concepts of the purpose of the system, which may build upon and improve the original design goals (Karasek and Theorell 1990). Training of the power-plant or chemical process operator need not only teach automatic responses to a variety of 'standard' situations but

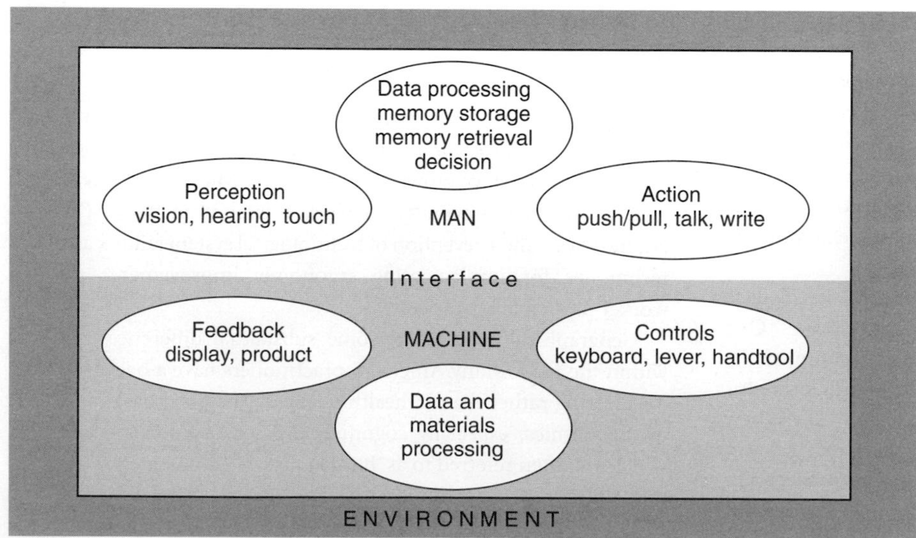

Fig. 1 The human–machine–environment system.

instead may seek to enhance critical thinking and problem-solving skills, while design of the process displays and controls should take account of the operators' knowledge, expectations, and needed information.

Ergonomics as an applied interdisciplinary field

One important characteristic of ergonomics is that it is both a scientific area of research and a practical area of application. Another is that ergonomics is multidisciplinary and requires knowledge in three main areas: (a) anatomy and physiology, (b) psychology, and (c) technology. Although it is impossible to have extensive knowledge in all of these fields, the ergonomist must be able to integrate knowledge from areas other than that of his or her own basic training. In large ergonomic problem-solving projects, a teamwork approach, with representatives of several disciplines with a common ergonomics perspective, is often most successful.

In research, some basic questions have to be tackled separately by psychologists, physiologists, and engineers. However, most ergonomic research is applied to field settings, whether for occupational or consumer problems, and therefore requires a truly multidisciplinary approach. Dialogue among the disciplines is essential to establish common frames of reference. Joint training in ergonomics, where students with varying backgrounds can meet, develop a common outlook, and learn to appreciate the contributions of each other, is key to strengthening multidisciplinary research and problem-solving skills.

The future of ergonomics

In a short period of time, ergonomics has grown to become an important area of scientific research and practical applications. This is especially true for working life, but special ergonomic applications for consumers, for people with physical or mental disabilities and older people, for leisure and sports, and for developing countries are also emerging. Thus ergonomics, through its effects on health, safety, and well being, has a large impact on public health.

The International Ergonomics Association, which was formed by a number of national societies, has issued minimum requirements for training and practical experience in ergonomics, to be fulfilled by those researchers, consultants, and others who wish to be approved as European Ergonomists. Similar requirements have been developed for the United Kingdom, the United States, and Australia. Professional qualifications like these are likely to raise the quality of ergonomics work even further, although there are still geographical and professional differences regarding the areas of expertise considered most important.

Relevant human characteristics

Human capacity for work is a function of body size, strength and fitness, and sensory as well as cognitive capacity. These capacities vary widely by age, between the genders, and among individuals with different hereditary, nutritional, and educational backgrounds. Even within a specific subgroup of the population, individual capacity varies with health, training, and previous experience. Therefore work tasks, as well as tools and other items for use in both occupational and private life, must be designed to fit the capacities of a wide range of people. A strong inverse association exists between the relative capacity available for a task and its duration: the longer time over which a certain demand has to be met, the lower is the relative capacity that can be used without fatigue or injury. Human capacity is seldom taxed up to 100 per cent; the only exceptions are in all-out life-saving operations. More commonly, people use from a small percentage of capacity up to as much as 50 per cent in physically demanding jobs. (No similar estimates are available for sensory or mental capacity, which are more difficult to measure.)

Anthropometry

Workstations, tools, and machines should be designed with enough adjustability to individual differences in body size in order to include virtually all the population as potential users. The most common recommendation is to design workstations and tools to fit the range in body size from the 5th to the 95th percentile of the adult population. Anthropometric data for use in workstation design are available for most parts of the body and for some specific subsets of the population, for example, by gender (Pheasant 1986). Those anthropometric body segments most commonly used for design of workstations and furniture are illustrated in Fig. 2.

There are large variations among ethnic groups in body size, body proportions, and limb length as a proportion of body height. With the increased mobility of population groups around the world, it is no longer acceptable to design workstations only, for instance, for Caucasians in Europe and for the Japanese population in Japan. The wider range of workstation requirements caused by this mixture of population groups must be taken into account. This necessitates the continuous revision of anthropometric data. Unanticipated differences in body size can lead to poor fit of tools, equipment, workstations, gloves, and other personal protective equipment, with resulting increases in biomechanical disadvantage and postural strain.

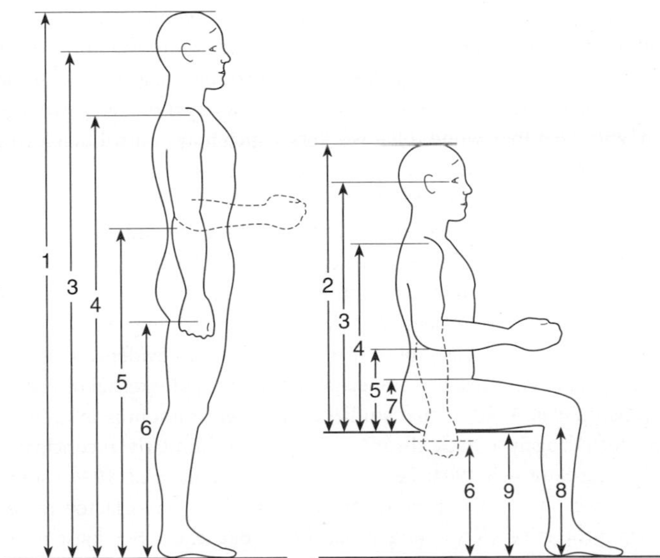

Fig. 2 Commonly used anthropometric measures and their definitions: 1, body height, standing; 2, seated body height; 3, eye height; 4, shoulder height; 5, elbow height; 6, knuckle height; 7, thigh height; 8, seated knee height; 9, seat pan height. (Source: Hansson 1987.)

In addition to the static anthropometric body measures available for workstation and tool design, there is also a need to consider functional or dynamic measures of the human capacity to reach, bend, and stretch (Pheasant 1986). Dynamic anthropometric data can be obtained when subjects are allowed to adopt natural postures and movements to perform a certain task, such as operating hand controls while sitting in a driver cabin. Such measurements are scarce, and the generalizability of the data from one setting to another is uncertain. Usually they have to be collected for each specific work situation.

Physical working capacity

Physical working capabilities relevant for ergonomics include cardiovascular, aerobic, and muscular strength capacity for maximal and submaximal, dynamic, and sustained (static) activity. Most physical capacities demonstrate a peak at around age 20 to 30 years and a gradual decline by about 30 per cent at least to the age of 60 (Åstrand and Rodahl 1986). Women usually have on average a 30 per cent lower maximal aerobic power (expressed in litres of oxygen uptake per minute) than men, and about 30 to 50 per cent lower maximal muscle strength. However, at a given level of relative submaximal exertion, there is no gender difference. The ratio in static strength ranges from 35 to 85 per cent, depending on the tasks and muscles involved (Chaffin *et al.* 1999); it is smaller when men and women have similar industrial experience or athletic training (Messing and Stevenson 1996). There are large interindividual differences in capacity, related to factors such as heredity, physical training, and health status. In all, gender, age, weight, and height together explain only about one-third of the variability in human strength.

Overall, the occupationally active population demonstrates higher capacities than the general population, since the latter includes those too ill to work or otherwise impaired. There are also differences between occupational groups, with higher values usually found in those who perform physically demanding tasks (Åstrand 1967*a*, 1988). This difference appears to be caused mainly by selection, since physically demanding jobs do not usually contain work tasks strenuous enough to introduce a training effect. Moreover, differences between occupations are most obvious in young age groups. In some (but not all) studies, muscle strength shows a larger decrease with age in blue collar than white collar workers, which may be attributable to a combination of musculoskeletal trauma and 'wear and tear' among those performing physically heavy work (Era *et al.* 1992).

Physically fit workers exhibit higher productivity and less fatigue in strenuous jobs than less fit workers (Åstrand 1967*b*). However, it is still an open question whether strong individuals are at a lower risk of musculoskeletal disorders than weaker ones. Among women performing electronics assembly work, there was no evidence that low muscle strength predicted upper-extremity musculoskeletal disorders (Jonsson *et al.* 1988). Other studies of whether or not muscle strength protected against back disorders have been similarly inconclusive (Biering-Sørensen 1984; Leino *et al.* 1987; Kujala *et al.* 1996); some have even shown high muscle force capacity to be a risk factor, rather than protective (Keyserling *et al.* 1980; Barnekow-Bergkvist *et al.* 1998). Stronger muscles are capable of generating higher internal forces, but they do not necessarily greater strength in vulnerable soft tissues such as nerves and spinal discs. Therefore pre-employment strength testing cannot be recommended on a scientific basis as a way of selecting workers unlikely to develop musculoskeletal disorders. Among people in jobs with substantial exposure to ergonomic stressors, individual factors like muscle strength appear to be of less importance for the risk of developing musculoskeletal disorders (Hagberg *et al.* 1995).

Neuromuscular function in precision tasks and the effect of motor control and skill training are areas of rapidly developing research, and these capacities may also become highly relevant to the risk of musculoskeletal disorders.

Sensory perception

Vision, hearing, and touch are primary factors in people's perception of the environment, and thus in their ability to respond appropriately to cues from machines, displays, warning signs, and information received from other sources, including other people. Taste and smell are less important for ergonomics but may be life-saving in toxic environments.

Work with poorly presented sensory information requires an excessively high level of attention, leading to errors, stress, and/or fatigue. In order to enable humans to respond to sensory stimuli without missing information or over-reacting, the contrast between the relevant information and the 'noise' caused by irrelevant visual and hearing stimuli (i.e. the signal-to-noise ratio) must be high. One common example of inadequate signal-to-noise ratio is trying to read texts on computer screens with too little contrast or with bright lights surrounding the screen. In leisure time activities like jogging and cycling, music from earphones can camouflage important safety information from traffic.

Frequently the sensory input from vision is overemphasized in ergonomic design, when sound or touch stimuli might have fulfilled the same purpose. Ergonomics for handicapped individuals has many examples of successful switches from vision to hearing (e.g. traffic signals) and from vision to touch (e.g. Braille).

With advancing age, the sensitivity of the eye to light and of the ear to sound is reduced; therefore the elderly require higher signal-to-noise ratios in order to perceive important information easily and accurately.

Cognitive capacity

In accordance with the human–machine system model, information is perceived through the sensory organs and then processed in the brain, leading to a decision on what action to take. The capacity to process information and make decisions (cognitive capacity) requires short-term (working) memory for processing and long-term memory for storage of relevant experience and knowledge (Kroemer and Grandjean 1997).

Information perception and processing can be improved by presenting information in a form that makes it easy for the brain to code in the short-term memory. Information should be organized in such a way that it is easy to compare and relate to previous training and work experience, and so that it can be stored in the long-term memory and retrieved in a suitable form for use later (Sanders and McCormick 1992).

The capacity for information processing is gradually reduced with age, but it is usually not until the age of around 65 years that a noticeable change occurs (Rabbitt 1991). With increasing age the variation around mean values of cognitive capacities appears to increase, probably because of the training effects of different lifestyles, jobs, and levels of continuing mental exercise (Salthouse 1990; Rabbitt 1991). Neurophysiological and psychological research indicates that it is the brain's 'hardware' (number of brain cells) that declines with age, rather than the 'software' (quality of processing). Even though the memory deteriorates slowly, experience can compensate for reduced capacity, especially in complex decision-making.

Relevant work environment characteristics

Workstation and equipment design

Workstations, equipment, tools, and other objects should be designed in a way that facilitates their use, permits variations in work routines, does not give fatigue, and leads to high efficiency. Common effects of poor workstation design are twisted and bent neck and trunk postures and elevated arms, leading to fatigue, musculoskeletal and other disorders (see below). In the office this applies to the computer and furniture, in industry it applies to machines and tools as well as to supports, and in a kitchen it applies to the layout and the usability of cleaning equipment.

For example, the correct height of a work surface depends on the nature of the task performed (Kroemer and Grandjean 1997). For precision work, the hands must be held relatively close to the eyes to allow sufficient accuracy of visuomotor co-ordination. However, since working with elevated arms is tiring, arm support must be provided. For light manual work with less visual precision, such as on an assembly line, the working area should be close to elbow height (standing or sitting). When lifting or other heavy work is performed, the working height should be even lower (Fig. 3). Frequent changes between sitting, standing, and walking reduce fatigue, and many modern workplaces have work surfaces where the height can be adjusted for both standing and sitting. A minimum requirement is that the height can be adjusted to fit both a tall man and a small woman.

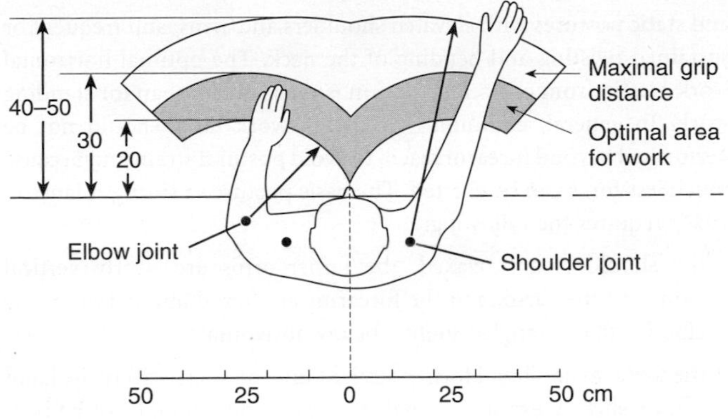

Fig. 4 Optimal work area for the hands in standing work. (Source: Hansson 1987.)

Standing work

The advantage of a standing posture is that the combined mobility of the trunk and arms permits a much larger reach and work area than is possible in the sitting position. Another advantage is that much larger forces can be exerted, especially if the work area is relatively low so that the arms can be held straight and the trunk weight can be used. Conversely, standing work is tiring for the legs, especially for older people and for those with peripheral circulatory problems in the legs. Static standing for at least half the work day is also a risk factor for spontaneous abortion and premature labour among pregnant workers (Gold and Tomich 1994). The horizontal area in front of a standing person that is optimal for arm work is small (Hansson 1987) (Fig. 4). When work is performed standing and walking, it can be made less fatiguing if shoes are changed a few times a day and if the floor is not hard—concrete floors are extremely tiring.

Seated work

Sitting is preferred by most people for prolonged tasks because it is less tiring for the legs. Conversely, in many jobs sitting implies confined

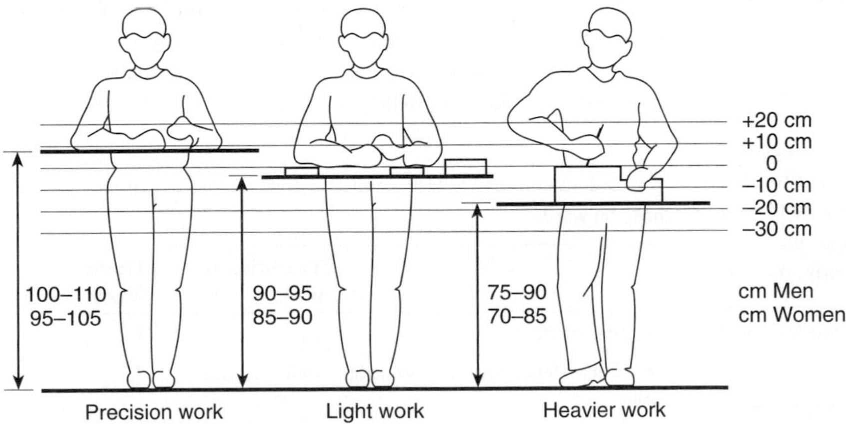

Fig. 3 Recommended height for benches for standing work. The reference line (0) is the height of the elbows above the floor, which averages 1050 mm for men and 98 mm for women in Western populations. (Source: Kroemer and Grandjean 1997.)

and static postures with elevated shoulders and arms, and frequent or sustained twisting and bending of the neck. The optimal horizontal work area in front of a seated person is even smaller than for standing work. In general, commonly occurring work tasks should not be performed beyond forearm reach, to avoid postural strain and because much less force can be exerted. The basic posture in sitting (Hansson 1987) requires the following:

- the shoulders are relaxed, the upper arms are nearly vertical alongside the torso, and the forearms are flexed about 100° at the elbows (that is, angled slightly below horizontal)
- the forearm and hand form a straight line, or alternatively the hand can be slightly extended (angled upward) but should not be bent sideways towards the little finger.

The head posture in seated work is frequently static, especially when fine manual tasks or visually intensive work, such as computer tasks, are performed. The line of vision should be horizontal, or somewhat below horizontal, and the seated workplace must also provide sufficient leg space, because sitting with the trunk twisted to accommodate the legs requires static muscle exertion and is very tiring. For the seated worker, no equipment is more important than a well-padded fully adjustable chair. However, no seated posture—even with good furniture—can be maintained for prolonged periods.

Repetitive work and rest pauses

Lack of recovery time after performance of repetitive work or sustained loading is believed to be an important factor in the aetiology of work-related musculoskeletal disorders, especially of the arm, wrist, and hand. Prolonged repetitive tasks should be avoided by providing frequent breaks and alternative tasks that do not tax the same tissues. Repetitive tasks should not be machine-paced; the individual should be allowed to set his or her own pace and to vary it over the course of the day, as fatigue sets in. Tasks that require precision, force exertion, and speed in combination with repetitiveness imply particularly high risk (Kilbom 1994).

Manual handling

Manual handling of loads—lifting, lowering, holding, carrying, pushing, and pulling—is an important risk factor for low back and other musculoskeletal disorders. The American National Institute of Occupational Safety and Health has developed an equation for estimating the acceptability of a two-handed lift based on the weight of the object, its horizontal distance from the body, the degree of asymmetry, the height of the object, the vertical distance that it is moved, and the frequency of lifting (Waters *et al.* 1993). Although this equation does not apply to all lifting situations, its dissemination has increased awareness about the interactions among these factors in manual handling and how to prioritize them for intervention. Apart from minimizing object weight and distance from the body, manual handling tasks should be designed to eliminate trunk bending and twisting, remove obstructions, provide good coupling of the load and the worker, and eliminate uneven or slippery surfaces.

Case study: Manual handling in nursing (Ljungberg *et al.* 1989) The importance of workstation design, technical lifting aides, and work organization was studied among nursing aides in two hospital geriatric wards. The traditional ward had cramped work spaces, narrow corridors, and small lavatories with room for only one nursing aide to help the patient. Mobile hoists were available but the space was so cramped that they were seldom used. In the modern ward, both corridors and rooms were spacious and about 50 per cent of the beds had motorized overhead hoists for lifting patients. Moreover, the modern ward had a new work organization incorporating 'group-care', in which a senior nurse and two aides shared the responsibility for 12 patients, whereas work at the traditional ward was more like an 'assembly line'.

Patient-handling workload was compared between the two wards. The vertical force in each lifting and carrying manoeuvre, as well as the time for each lift, was measured using wooden shoes instrumented with strain gauges. The work performed in lifting was considerably less in the modern ward, whether expressed as total weight lifted per hour, the duration of each lift, or the proportion of lifts with uneven distribution of weight between right and left leg (Table 1).

It was not possible to distinguish whether the differences in work organization, use and availability of technical aids, or workstation layout most accounted for these large differences; most likely it was a combination of all three. The important point is that physical stresses due to manual handling can be substantially reduced.

Presentation and communication of information

Unfortunately, large-scale accidents bring to public attention the need to present information, in both workplaces and public places, in a way that is easily understandable and compatible with human comprehension (see case studies below). Warning signs must use symbols and icons familiar to people: the colour red signifies something forbidden while green means acceptable or safe to proceed, and the symbol for radio-activity is well known to most. Deficiencies in such conceptual compatibility are especially noteworthy in many computer programs. Movement compatibility implies that there is a concordance between the movement of a control or a lever, and the ensuing movement of a machine or tool—you turn the wheel to the right when you want to make a right turn (Sanders and McCormick 1992). Spatial compatibility reflects human expectations with regard to the relative positioning of displays and controls and the understanding of 'high' versus 'low' measurements; high values are expected to be at the top of, or at the right-handed side of, a display, whereas low values are expected to be represented at the bottom or the left side.

Good quality visual display is important to avoid both fatigue and error. Work at a visual display terminal, especially for prolonged periods, requires that the screen be of high quality with good contrast, no flicker, and adjustable in height (see section on seated work above).

Table 1 Workload in lifting and carrying: comparison of two geriatric hospital wards

	Traditional ward	Modern ward
Number of lifts/h	30	14
Number of lifts/h with asymmetric uplift	14.8	7.5
Cumulated vertical force/h (N)	2880	1660
Average duration of each lift (s)	10.5	4.8
Time for lifting (% of working day)	8.6	1.9

The information on a display or a warning sign (auditory or visual) needs to be coded in a way that accentuates the crucial information, while redundant information is suppressed. Recommendations for the design of warning signs and labels have been given by Lehto (1992). The schematic representation of the very complex London Underground is a good example of a simplified, schematic, yet easily understandable system.

The quality of information processing can be further improved by undivided attention to the task and high motivation. Thus care should be taken when presenting information so that attention is not divided between simultaneous or conflicting demands.

Physical environment

Extremes of temperature and humidity, poor lighting, vibrations, noise, low frequency sound, and slippery or unstable ground conditions can all severely influence working capacity, endurance, and reliability. This is partly because these factors require additional physiological resources in addition to the work task; for instance, heat reduces blood circulation available for working muscles, cold reduces motor precision, and vibrations and slippery ground require extra muscle exertion to stabilize the body. Poor lighting and low frequency background noise impair mental concentration and communication between people. The International Standards Organization has standards on heat and vibration, but their main aim is to prevent ill health; they are not intended for safety purposes or to maintain general well being or productivity.

Work scheduling

Work schedules other than a standard 5-day working week are utilized in hospitals, emergency services, food processing, transportation, communications, steel working, petroleum and paper manufacturing, law enforcement, and other public agencies. In the United States, approximately 16 million people are classified as shiftworkers; up to 45 per cent of the labour force works a designated shift or at least 4 h per week outside of the standard working week (NIOSH 1997). Specific schedules vary tremendously; some have worse consequences than others for fatigue, psychological health, and family and leisure time. Sleep disorders are the most obvious and consistent health consequences. Many shiftworkers also experience gastrointestinal and digestive disorders (Rosa and Colligan 1992). Shiftworkers are at greater risk of coronary heart disease and associated risk factors, including poor diet and tendency to male central obesity, than day workers (Knutsson 1989; Nakamura *et al.* 1997; Tenkanen *et al.* 1998; Steenland 2000). Women with child-care responsibilities often experience additional stress; mental health was worse among female hospital workers who were dissatisfied with their work schedules (Estryn-Behar *et al.* 1990).

Organizational design and management

Work organization—the leadership style (democratic or authoritarian), the hierarchical structure of the organization (flat or high pyramid), the influence of employees on decision-making, the distribution of work tasks among employees, the industrial relations within the organization, the wage/salary negotiating system, the level of technology, and skill utilization—all influence productivity, well being, and health in an organization. These features of the work environment are also referred to as organizational design and management or 'macro-ergonomics' (Hendricks 1986).

The organization of work generates technical constraints on individual workers and thus influences physical load as well as psychological job content and potential 'stress'. Psychological job demands reflect both the physical pace of work and time pressure in processing or responding to information. Decision latitude is based on the worker's decision authority and discretion over skill use, i.e. the ability to control one's own work process and decide which skills to utilize to accomplish the job. According to one widely used model (Karasek and Theorell 1990), high psychological job demands in combination with low decision latitude result in residual job strain and, over time, chronic adverse health effects. This model has proved a powerful predictor of risk of cardiovascular morbidity in numerous countries and industrial sectors; recent research suggests that it is probably also relevant for musculoskeletal disorders, acute occupational injury, and adverse reproductive outcomes related to work demands during pregnancy (see below). The relationship of work organization factors with psychosocial strain has also been demonstrated by intervention studies showing that interventions which increase worker participation in decision-making can resolve strain linked to high levels of demands over which the worker had no control.

Organizations that promote employee initiatives, support development of skills and experience, and let employees exercise choice regarding quality and quantity of work adapt more easily to structural changes in society and appear to maintain a higher level of innovation. The underlying philosophy is that humans not only need bread and clothing for satisfaction and full development; when the above additional demands are met, people can contribute more to the aims of the organization.

The full consequences of work organized along these lines are not yet fully realized; for example, some disadvantages may follow for people with little initiative. Moreover, stress levels may increase above acceptable levels when individuals feel pressured to be as creative and productive as possible. There is no doubt, however, that work organization has a profound influence on productivity and health.

Cost-effectiveness of ergonomic measures in the workplace

Well-designed ergonomic systems often improve efficiency and productivity in industry, both directly and as a result of improved employee health (Simpson 1988; Oxenburgh 1991). In the workplace, productivity, safety, and health may not always be parallel outcomes (Frick 1997). However, there are many situations in which these goals go hand in hand, at least over the longer term.

To evaluate cost-effectiveness, the costs of ergonomic improvements like re-engineering of workstations and tools, introduction of new production methods, and work reorganization can be compared with the past or expected costs of leaving the work system unchanged. Factors that should be balanced against the costs for improvements include high sick-leave rate, compensation claims, staff turnover, and low-quality production such as many rejected products.

Case study: A railway maintenance workshop (Oxenburgh 1991) In a workshop for the maintenance and repair of diesel engines, there were problems with low productivity and unacceptably high injury rates. The workstations required awkward postures because of problems with access, reach, and visibility, and the risk of injury was high because of temporary, makeshift support for engine parts during repair.

A new management style was adopted to encourage worker participation in the change process. Improvements in work systems and practices were introduced via teams of workers and engineers, informed by visits to other workshops, consultants' inputs, and their own experience. Quality control was improved by allowing workers to take responsibility for their work and encouraging customer feedback as to acceptability of the work. The cost for the physical improvements was about 6 per cent of yearly payroll. The injury rate did not decrease, but severity was reduced and injury absenteeism was halved. The productivity gain was very high and throughput of engines increased by 80 per cent. Altogether, the costs of improvements were paid back in 4 months.

Ergonomics and public health

Musculoskeletal disorders

Musculoskeletal disorders are widespread in many countries, with substantial costs and impact on quality of life. In the United States, Canada, and Finland, more people are disabled from working as a result of musculoskeletal disorders than from any other group of diseases (Pope *et al.* 1991; Badley *et al.* 1994; Riihimäki 1995; Rempel and Punnett 1997). Musculoskeletal disorders also constitute a major proportion of all registered and/or compensatable work-related diseases in many countries. Criteria for diagnosis and for evaluating work-relatedness and completeness of reporting vary among countries, making statistical comparisons difficult. However, where record-keeping systems have been developed, musculoskeletal disorders are often the single largest group of conditions, representing a third or more of all registered occupational diseases in the United States, the Nordic countries, and Japan (Pope *et al.* 1991; Vaaranen *et al.* 1994; Bernard 1997). For the Nordic countries in 1991, it was estimated that from 15 to 49 per cent of all musculoskeletal disorders were due to work, and their cost represented approximately 1 per cent of gross national product (Hansen 1993).

Some industries and occupations have musculoskeletal disorder rates up to three or four times higher than the overall frequency. High-risk sectors include nursing facilities, air transportation, mining, food processing, leather tanning, and heavy and light manufacturing of vehicles, furniture, appliances, electrical equipment, electronic products, textiles, clothing, and shoes (Bernard 1997). Upper-extremity musculoskeletal disorders are highly prevalent in manual-intensive occupations such as clerical work, postal service, cleaning, industrial inspection, and packaging (Rempel and Punnett 1997). Back and lower-limb disorders occur disproportionately among truck drivers, warehouse workers, airplane baggage handlers, construction trades, nurses, nursing aides and other patient-care workers, and operators of cranes and other large vehicles (Pope *et al.* 1991).

The work-relatedness of many musculoskeletal disorders has been discussed extensively (Armstrong *et al.* 1993; Bongers *et al.* 1993; Hagberg *et al.* 1995; Scientific Committee for Musculoskeletal Disorders 1996; Bernard 1997; Buckle and Devereaux 1999; Sluiter *et al.* 2000). Both experimental science and epidemiology indicate that job features which increase the risk of work-related musculoskeletal disorders are heavy lifting, repetitive hand motion, static work in which the body is maintained in a fixed posture, vibration, and any of these in combination with each other or with an undesirable psychosocial work environment.

Work-related musculoskeletal disorders cover a wide range of inflammatory and degenerative diseases, including some less well-described states of pain and functional impairment. Clinically, the most common disease entities are tendinitis and related conditions, myalgia, nerve-entrapment syndromes, low back pain, sciatica, and arthrosis. Body regions most commonly involved are the low back, neck, shoulder, forearm, and hand, although recently the lower extremity has received more attention.

Inflammations of tendons and surrounding tissues (tendinitis, peritendinitis, tenosynovitis), especially in the forearm and wrist, elbow, and shoulder, have a high prevalence and incidence in occupations with prolonged periods of repetitive and static work loads (Kurppa *et al.* 1991). Tendon strain accumulates as a function of work pace (the frequency and duration of mechanical loading), the level of muscular effort, and recovery time between exertions (Goldstein *et al.* 1987). Tendon disorders may have an acute or insidious onset, depending on the intensity of the loading. Recovery is usually complete, but some workers develop chronic disorders.

Myalgia, meaning pain and functional impairment of muscles, occurs especially in the shoulder and neck region in occupations with large static demands, when performing precision work with the hands, or in work with the arms elevated (Kilbom *et al.* 1986; Winkel and Westgaard 1992). The forearm muscles may also be affected in hand-intensive tasks (Ranney *et al.* 1995).

Nerve-entrapment syndromes cause pain or other symptoms and loss of sensibility and strength. The most common of these is carpal tunnel syndrome (Hagberg *et al.* 1992; Viikari-Juntura and Silverstein 1999). It occurs in work tasks that require prolonged, repetitive, and forceful gripping or wrist bending, especially if combined with exposure to local vibration. With continued exposure, functional impairment may become permanent.

Degenerative disorders commonly occur in the spine, especially in the neck and low back region, as well as in the hip and knee joints. Such disorders are common in the general population at older ages. However, several factors at work, especially heavy physical work, manual handling of objects, forward bending and twisting of the trunk, and exposure to whole-body vibration (especially while seated) accelerate the degenerative joint process (Riihimäki 1991; Vingård *et al.* 1991; Kirkeskov Jensen and Eenberg 1996). The course of these disorders is chronic, and usually exposure to risk factors at work has lasted for many years before symptoms occur.

In some countries work-related disorders of the upper extremity are referred to as repetition strain injury or cumulative trauma disorders. These terms are intended to convey that the cause is repetitive work or the accumulation of microtrauma over a period of time, but they are clinically imprecise, and sometimes even misleading, since musculoskeletal disorders can also occur as a result of high-intensity exposure for relatively brief periods. It is generally acknowledged that the aetiology of these disorders in the population is multifactorial and may involve risk factors both on and off the job. A more useful term is 'work-related musculoskeletal disorders', which reflects the idea that the work environment contributes substantially to causation in the population, although with varying importance among individuals (WHO 1985). Work-related disorders are thus distinguished from specific 'occupational' disorders where a single factor is both necessary and sufficient to cause the disease (e.g. mesothelioma from asbestos exposure).

Accurate data on the incidence and prevalence of musculoskeletal disorders are difficult to obtain, and the true magnitude is probably underestimated. In addition, regional differences have been noted in the relative frequency of different diagnoses and affected body regions. These may be related to variations in clinical practice, the circumstances under which the disorders were first noted, or the occupational health legislation and compensation systems in each jurisdiction. Nevertheless, there is international agreement that musculoskeletal disorders are a serious problem and that many can be prevented by improved work design.

Acute traumatic injuries in the workplace

Both acute injury and chronic disorders have essentially the same aetiological agents, namely, physical energy transmitted to the human body in doses harmful to tissues. Despite the traditional focus on individual behaviour as the 'cause' of accidents, it is increasingly recognized that factors in the workplace, such as poor machine and tool design and lack of adequate maintenance and care, contribute to many occupational accidents. Instructions and warning signs are often not designed in accordance with ergonomic principles regarding visual perception and information processing. Physical work load is relevant in several ways: fatigue may lead to reduced attention and motor co-ordination, or musculoskeletal trauma may itself manifest as an acute incident (e.g. low back strain) or may lead to an acute episode (e.g. inability to handle a heavy load may result in loss of balance and a slip or fall). The contributions of the physical and psychosocial environment to injury risk have been little studied to date, with a few exceptions (Sundström-Frisk 1984; Moll van Charante and Mulder 1990; Melamed *et al.* 1999). Therefore prevention requires attention to all aspects of ergonomics: technical redesign, information processing demands, physical work environment, and reorganization of work procedures. For these reasons, some have now rejected the term 'accident' altogether, because it implies an unforeseeable or random occurrence, in favour of 'acute injury' or 'incident'—terms more compatible with the public health approach of identifying preventable risk factors.

A high incidence of occupational injuries in industry has been the original impetus for occupational health and safety legislation in many countries. Table 2 summarizes some official statistics on occupational 'accidents' in Sweden (Statistics Sweden 1994). A very large proportion occurred while handling machines, tools, and other technical devices, and much of the cost resulted from relatively long periods of sick-leave for a relatively small number of cases. The two most common 'main events' were 'fall on same level' and 'overexertion of body part', with annual incidence rates of 3.2 and 2.7 per 1000 men and 2.1 and 2.5 per 1000 women respectively.

Although acute injuries are still a major source of mortality and morbidity at work, over the past 10 to 20 years their incidence has been reduced in many Western countries. For example, in Sweden the incidence of reported occupational injuries per 1000 people in the workforce has come down from 40 in 1980 to 16 in 1992 for men and from 11.5 to 7.5 for women over the same period.

Table 2 Distribution and average sick-leave due to cases of reported occupational accidents involving some important 'principal external agencies' (Sweden 1992)

Principal external agency	Percentage of all reported accidents[a]	Average sick-leave days
Hand-held tools and implements	10.9	16
Lifting machines and appliances	14.1	34
Other machines	10.1	29
Construction parts, interior fittings, scaffolding, ladders	21.7	32
Materials, goods, packaging, containers	21.9	29
Chemicals, physical or biological factors	14.9	25

[a] Total number of reported accidents, 67 000.

Cardiovascular and other work-related diseases

The impact of psychosocial 'job strain' on physiological stress response, mental strain, coronary heart disease, hypertension, and other heart disease risk factors is well established (Karasek and Theorell 1990; Kristensen 1996). While estimates of the proportion of heart disease possibly due to 'job strain' vary greatly between studies, perhaps up to 23 per cent of heart disease (over 150 000 deaths per year in the United States) could potentially be prevented if the level of 'job strain' in all jobs was reduced to the average level of all occupations. The economic costs of job stress in general (absenteeism, lost productivity) are difficult to estimate but could be as high as several hundred billion dollars per year in the United States alone (Karasek and Theorell 1990).

For the pregnant worker, physically demanding tasks such as heavy lifting interfere with uteroplacental blood flow and may precipitate uterine contractility later in pregnancy. Such work has been associated with preterm birth (before 37 weeks gestation) and hypertension or pre-eclampsia (Gold and Tomich 1994; Mozurkewich *et al.* 2000). Prolonged standing and shiftwork increase the risk of preterm birth; psychosocial strain is also physiologically relevant (Omer and Everly 1988), although the epidemiology is not conclusive (Hedegaard *et al.* 1996).

Ergonomic applications in transportation systems

Traffic accidents are one of the leading causes of death and disability today. In the United States, traffic injury is second only to cancer in the total financial cost to the community of major disabilities and deaths. Even in some developing countries where infectious disease is still a significant cause of death, traffic injury accounts for a percentage of all deaths similar to that in some highly motorized countries (Trinca *et al.* 1988).

Traffic incidents are often blamed on 'human error'. The car driver 'disregarded' the warning sign, the truck driver stepped on the breaks 'too late', the signal-box attendant 'forgot' the coming train, and so on. What if the warning sign was obscured because of the car design and the position of the sign, the truck driver was just entering a tunnel with sudden (relative) darkness, and the signal-box attendant was tired because of having to work double shifts? Transportation systems can be designed in a way that takes human limitations into consideration, instead of relying on unrealistic instructions, rules, and regulations that do not comply with human capacity.

Traffic incidents have a complex causality, and ergonomics can play an important role for prevention through the design of vehicles and traffic signs, and the engineering of roads and railways. Because of the high speed of movement in traffic, the design of transportation systems has special requirements. Speed places excessive demands on reaction time, short-term memory, and vision of both drivers and pedestrians, although these demands can be moderated by the design of the system (Lay 1986; Ogden 1990).

Reaction time can be reduced by encouraging familiarity, because drivers reset faster to a familiar situation, and by reducing the number of alternatives. For example, unusual intersection layouts and a large number of exits from a roundabout require longer response times.

Short-term memory is crucial for driver performance because most of the driving task relies on information that is never stored in long-term memory. Therefore warning signs should require an immediate response, drivers should be frequently reminded of control information which varies along the road (e.g. speed limits), and the driver should be allowed to respond to one stimulus before the next is imposed.

Of all information required by a vehicle driver, 90 per cent is supplied by vision. As the amount of visual information is almost limitless, the driver must continuously select the most important cues to help in his or her driving. As the data-processing demands increase, the driver tends to be overloaded and to miss some information or to shed part of it. This situation also takes place immediately after a situation of overload. Thus the departure side of an intersection may be relatively more accident prone than the approach side, which also implies that pedestrian crossings and bus stops should not be placed after intersections. Only 1 to 1.5 fixations of vision per second are realistic in driving. Therefore road traffic signs must be separated in time and space and must only be used for the most necessary information. They must be within the field of vision of the driver which, when moving at a certain speed, implies a narrower field both horizontally and vertically than for a stationary observer. Delineation (i.e. markings of road alignment immediately ahead) is especially important at the approach to curves and crests, and for elderly drivers whose visual capacity is often reduced.

The design of the driver cabin directly influences traffic safety by the degree of visibility that it affords to the driver. Cabin design should provide a comfortable seated posture in which the driver can reach all the hand and foot controls and is protected from vibration (Pheasant 1991). Traffic safety is also influenced by circumstances like fatigue, medication, and ill health of the driver, training of drivers and pedestrians, legislation, traffic density, and weather conditions (Ogden 1990; Sanders and McCormick 1992).

Consumer product design

The design of products, implements, and entire systems for use by the general population increasingly involves ergonomics. Some important applications that influence the health or safety of the consumer include the design of furniture and kitchen utensils, floor coverings, handheld tools, and containers. As in the workplace, injuries often happen as a consequence of several factors simultaneously—consider slipping and falling due to a combination of slippery floors and carrying a bulky wobbly object that obscures one's vision. In the kitchen, problems may occur due to unsuitable working heights, poor lighting, and ambiguous labelling of stove controls. Examples of poor ergonomic design of consumer products include carrying purchases in plastic bags with handles which cut into the fingers, trying to open containers that require excessive pinch force, and sorting paper money of different denominations but the same size and colour. In all of these situations, better design would reduce discomfort and fatigue, make the task less time-consuming, and reduce the risk of mistakes.

Devices should be designed to fit the anthropometry, strength, and endurance of the entire population. Information and warning signs must similarly be understandable to populations with large variations in sensory and cognitive capacity, cultural background, and level of schooling. All areas of design must be considered: a product or an implement must be shaped and marked in a way that explains its function, safety devices must be designed without demands on previous training and experience, and size, weight, and grips must fit a wide variety of human body sizes. Therefore design for the public requires even more sophisticated considerations than design for the workplace, where the user population is better defined in terms of physical and psychological capacities and where additional training can be given to selected groups.

This area is becoming increasingly important, partly as a consequence of product liability legislation enacted in many Western countries. The manufacturer of any product can be made economically responsible for a user's injury if it can be demonstrated that deficient design of the product was responsible or that the user could not have been expected to know of the risk. There are also market considerations; since a consumer device is purchased by the end-user, that user (unlike most workers) has the opportunity to choose among available designs, and comfort and ease of use are usually important criteria for the purchaser.

Although usually not described in ergonomic terms, many implements and tools used in sports and leisure time have been developed with an ergonomics approach, emphasizing high levels of achievement and absence of accidents and injuries. Some examples are hand-grip fit in golf clubs and tennis rackets to improve force output and reduce the risk of epicondylitis, and the development of sports shoes to reduce impact forces and periostial and tendon inflammation.

Design for the elderly and for people with physical or mental disability

In recent years there have been advances in design for rehabilitation and for people with physical or mental disabilities, with primary emphasis on compensating for reduced physical capacity such as muscle strength and precision, hearing, vision, and mobility. In the future, more emphasis should also be put on compensating for longer reaction times and reduced cognitive capacity. Computer use, for example, is often out of reach for both people with disabilities and elderly people because of poor visibility, demands on rapid information processing, and the introduction of unfamiliar symbols. In the same way as a handicap may affect only one out of several functional capacities, an elderly person may have most functions well preserved. Therefore there is no need to distinguish between ergonomics for people with physical or mental disabilities and the elderly. In fact, it would make more economic sense if products were designed for use by those with limited abilities, as well as by the more able-bodied (Haigh 1993).

In a recent survey of commercially available products intended for elderly people, it was found that many of them were inappropriate or inadequate to perform the task for which they were intended (Gardner *et al.* 1993). Some did not perform the intended job; others introduced hazards that could have led to serious accidents, but which could have been avoided after simple consumer trials and redesign. One group of ergonomists and designers in Sweden, Ergonomi-Design Gruppen, have successfully designed a range of products for people with disabilities and the elderly (Benktzon 1993). Modification of products such as knives, walking sticks, and cutlery have made people with reduced strength and mobility of the hand or arm more self-sufficient in their everyday life.

The design process is stepwise, starting with thorough documentation of the functional ability of groups with different types of disabilities, preparing a range of test tools, prototype testing, and finally manufacturing. The same approach has been used in the redesign of products for craftsworkers and others with repeated and prolonged use of tools and implements. Small design details can be of vital importance for safety, comfort, and usability. Pliers, screwdrivers, and butcher's knives with improved grip surface and grip diameter, and a coffee pot with its centre of gravity closer to the hand, are other commercial products developed by the group. These all reduce the load on the forearm and hand, improving comfort and decreasing fatigue, and therefore have been widely adopted. Solutions originally created for the elderly or for people with physical or mental disabilities have frequently been found acceptable to a broader range of users (Benktzon 1993).

Public health implications of complex technological environments: two case studies

Disasters in high-tech environments, such as the nuclear power plants in Japan, Chernobyl (Russia), and Three Mile Island (United States), are well known. Such disasters can be ascribed to the combined effects of design defects, conflicts between safety and productivity goals, poor operating and maintenance procedures, and inadequate training (Reason 1990). Ergonomics is central in the causality of many of these accidents because of poor system design, which is not compatible with human capacity and its limitations. The operators or workers involved are often victims, but the reason that these disasters are widely publicized and analysed is that the public—the third party—is exposed to risks without the ability to protect itself. The following two case studies illustrate that serious 'accidents' can and will happen when technical systems have been designed and implemented without ample consideration of human limitations.

Case study: Tram collision In a tram accident in Sweden, 13 people died and 29 were taken to hospital when a tram raced downhill along the track with the brakes disconnected. All those killed or injured were waiting at the next stop, or were pedestrians or car passengers happening to pass further down. The tram had been taken out of service because of a breakdown in the overhead power supply. As the electric power had been cut, the normal electrodynamic brakes did not function and mechanical brakes had automatically taken over. The traffic supervisor in charge of the removal of the tram decided to use the downslope to move the tram further down where the power was intact. However, the mechanical brakes first had to be released, which could be done by a simple handgrip from the outside of each carriage. The intention was to use the mechanical brakes again further down. However, for the mechanical brakes to be functional again they had to be refilled with pressurized air, which could only be done when under electrical power. As a consequence, the tram driver could not stop the tram from racing down the track.

This incident appears to be a typical example of so-called 'human error'. However, the subsequent investigation revealed several errors in the design of the system (Haverikommission 1992). The drivers and supervisors knew that the mechanical brakes must not be released unless the tram was secured by other means, but they did not know why; nor did they know how the brakes were constructed or what the consequences might be of disconnecting the mechanical brakes. Moreover, they had been given no formal training in emergency procedures of this nature. The mechanical brakes had been designed with an external release mechanism that was easily accessible but without any warning signs. This case is an unfortunate example of the combined effects of deficiencies in technical design, training, and emergency procedures that could have been avoided by the application of ergonomic principles.

Case study: Haemodialysis incident In 1983, three patients died and 12 others nearly died while undergoing haemodialysis in a Swedish hospital. The haemodialysis unit fed sterile water to the patients instead of physiological saline. The nurse on duty was charged and later sentenced for negligence, since she had switched off the alarm system of the haemodialysis unit.

In order to understand the sequence of events it is necessary to know the design of the haemodialysis unit alarm panel (Fig. 5). It had six horizontal rows of lamps and switches, for the conductivity (ion concentration) of the haemodialysis fluid, for its temperature, for the level of fluid in the tanks, and for the amount of concentrated saline available

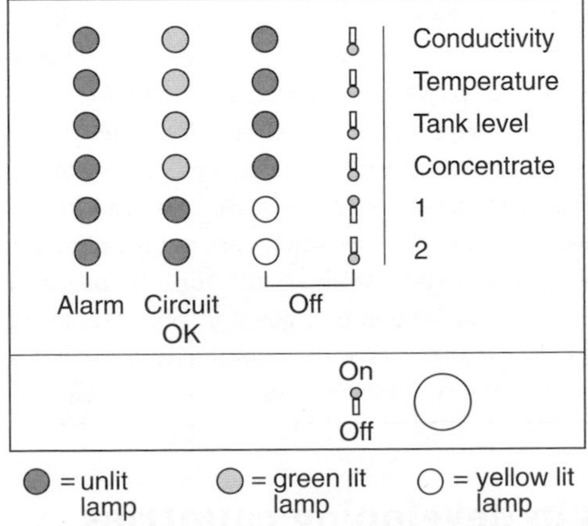

Fig. 5 Control panel of the haemodialysis unit before it was disconnected. (Adapted from Lundberg 1992.)

for diluting with water to create the haemodialysis fluid. Two more rows (1 and 2) were available but not in use. The vertical row of switches was for turning the alarm system on or off, and the first column of lamps (from the right) had yellow warning lamps that were lit when the alarm was in the 'off' position. Since rows 1 and 2 were not in use their alarms had been turned off and therefore the corresponding lamps were lit yellow, i.e. they were constantly indicating a warning. The second vertical column of lamps had green lamps that were lit when the alarm was on and when conductivity, temperature, etc. were within given acceptable levels. The vertical column of lamps to the extreme left had red lamps that were lit when the ion concentration, temperature, tank level, or amount of concentrate were below or above the set 'safe' levels. The main switch at the bottom of the panel was connected to an acoustic alarm that was common for all four alarm functions.

In a retrospective analysis, the most likely series of events was determined as follows (Lundberg 1992). The nurse was experienced in the treatment of haemodialysis patients and with the particular system, which had been in use for several years. Normally the nurses did not have to use the six alarm switches; they had been left on the panel because the unit had needed occasional adjustments by technicians, and the system had to be operational even when one of the circuits was out of function (albeit with intensified surveillance). On the day of the accident, however, the nurse demonstrated the haemodialysis unit to a visitor and explained its function. She noted that the main switch was 'on', i.e. turned up, whereas the four top switches were turned down, i.e. they appeared to be turned off (Fig. 5). Consequently, she turned up the four top switches, believing that she had turned the alarms on. She did not know that the main switch and the other switches had their 'on' and 'off' positions in different directions, and that she was actually disconnecting the alarms. Neither did she know that the emergency stop of the system was disconnected with the same switch. The haemodialysis unit continued working even though the alarms were disconnected. When the concentrated saline solution ran out, it continued with mere distilled water, with disastrous consequences for the patients. The nurse might have been alerted by the fact that the four yellow warning lamps lit up when the alarms were turned off; however, she was used to two of the yellow lights always being on, and said during the trial that she thought they should be on.

Sentencing this duty nurse caused considerable discussion and was widely considered unjust. Obviously the design of the haemodialysis unit, as well as the nurse's understanding of its function, was poor. Insufficient oral information about the system had been provided to the users. Surveillance of the system was done by technicians for whom its function was obvious, but they did not convey their understanding to the nurses operating the system. This case emphasizes the need for unambiguous designs of control panels with consistent markings, for proper training, and for clear written procedures for both routine operation and emergencies. Why then blame only one person? Were not the designers at fault, and the head of the haemodialysis unit for not providing instruction and training? The application of ergonomic principles in the design of this haemodialysis system, as well as for similar surveillance systems used in hospitals, is necessary for the avoidance of 'accidents'.

Ergonomics in developing countries

In developing countries, especially with high rates of unemployment, it is tempting for employers who build up small and middle-sized industries to disregard safety and health (Kogi and Sen 1987). Labour inspectors are scarce and have limited resources, and surveillance of occupational conditions is often lacking. Therefore ergonomics must be promoted not only as a means to improve safety, but also to fulfil other management goals, such as high productivity, and must stem from local initiatives to be effective.

According to Kogi (1991), support from international organizations and states should be organized so as to enable people to identify priority problems and effective solutions using locally available materials and skills. The support should provide for:

- practical advice on how to identify priority problems and how to find solutions
- practical guidance, particularly through 'learning-by-doing', about ways to implement immediate improvements.

The International Labour Organization has developed a training programme targeting entrepreneurs and workers of small and medium-sized enterprises (Louzine 1982) because of the great need for improvements and the scarcity of ergonomists in developing countries. The training programme focuses on the simultaneous improvement of working conditions and productivity, and encourages low-cost voluntary measures using a participatory approach. The following eight themes have been selected for the programme because of their importance for both working conditions and productivity:

- materials storage and handling
- workstation design
- machine safety
- control of hazardous substances
- lighting
- welfare facilities and services
- work premises
- work organization.

During the programme, local examples are used and the participants are encouraged to find practical improvements by means of self-help and sharing of experience. If managers and workers do not see any likelihood of a productivity gain and do not learn to use their own ideas and skills, they will quickly lose interest.

Implementing change

Legislation, standards, and guidelines

National legislation concerning ergonomic factors varies widely between different countries. Traditionally, legislation in occupational health focuses on quantitative data, for example concentrations of chemical substances, or minimum physical dimensions of barriers and guardrails as safety measures. The application of strict quantitative risk assessment in ergonomics has proved controversial for several reasons especially related to the multiplicity of physical risk factors, lack of standardized assessment protocols for each of them, and uncertainties in quantifying the interactions among them for different health outcomes (Viikari-Juntura 1997; Kilbom 1998). At the same time, regulations are desirable because voluntary actions by forward-thinking employers only cover a small proportion of the workforce in any single country, and because those measures generally lag behind technological changes rather than anticipating future health effects.

As an alternative approach, some countries have adopted performance standards based on functional requirements and desired outcomes, for example, that a certain work process must not produce injuries and must comply with safe handling (Kilbom 1995). Such an approach could more feasibly address work organization as well, rather than focusing only on micro-ergonomic issues (Kilbom 1998). Intense effort is under way in the European Community to develop directives relevant for ergonomics (Buckle and Devereaux 1999); some have already been presented for machine work, manual handling (EEC/90/269 Directive), and work at visual display terminals (Dul and de Flaming 1994). In the United States an ergonomics programme standard for prevention of musculoskeletal disorders was proposed by OSHA (1999) but did not stand.

International occupational standards are also continually being developed and refined, but these are usually not legally binding. The International Standardization Organization issues standards complementary to the European Community directives; for example, both whole-body and hand–arm vibration are covered by International Standardization Organization standards. Other examples are the American National Standards Institute proposed standard (2000) on prevention of upper-limb disorders and the American Conference of Government Industrial Hygienists proposal for a threshold limit value on hand activity level.

Large manufacturing or scientific organizations often develop codes of practice or guidelines for the specific area of their activity. These can be made more precise, relating to the conditions at hand at a certain organization, and are therefore useful for the practitioner (Mital and Kilbom 1992; Winkel and Westgaard 1992; Kilbom 1994).

In the public sector, intensification of product liability legislation in many countries has provided better tools for consumers in pursuing safety.

Training

Effective ergonomics programmes in the workplace emphasize engineering controls, especially the ergonomic design of workstations, equipment, tools, and work reorganization, together with a participatory process that engages the workers' knowledge and empowers them to identify and remedy hazards (Hagberg *et al.* 1995). Thus both professional expertise and worker education are required.

In most countries, the labour inspectorate is responsible for the follow-up of ergonomics legislation. Since inspectors are usually poorly trained in ergonomics, this surveillance is often ineffective. In countries with a well-developed occupational health service (e.g. the Nordic countries), physiotherapists and safety engineers are usually well trained in ergonomics and perform valuable work. In the United States, plant nurses frequently provide such services in large companies.

Sometimes the occupational health service is unable to influence sufficiently the development of new workstations—the effort is reactive rather than proactive. For improved ergonomic conditions, both at workplaces and for the public, those responsible for developing technical systems need more training in ergonomics. Thus production engineers, designers, architects, systems engineers (in computing), and personnel managers need more training, which is seldom provided by technical universities. Since few universities provide postgraduate degrees in ergonomics there is so far an unfulfilled need for training, which is even more pronounced in developing countries.

Education of workers to recognize hazards and participate in work redesign processes is essential, although there is little consensus on the specific goals or methods for worker education in occupational health and safety. To be effective, worker education should involve two-way dialogue, value experiential knowledge, recognize the organizational nature of many hazards, and assist workers to develop strategies for corrective action (Wallerstein and Weinger 1992).

Participatory approaches

In recent years it has been proved repeatedly that improvements of ergonomic conditions are most efficiently achieved when all those using a particular system are also involved in its improvement. For example, 'expert' advice from a short-term consultant frequently results in failure if not supported by the experience of those manufacturing or using the product. The knowledge of the consumer or the worker is often unspoken but can be used for product and system improvement in practical trials. The group of people involved in a workplace should include not only the product designer and manufacturing engineer but also the workers, the occupational health staff, those who sell and promote the product, and its users (Gjessing *et al.* 1994; Moir and Buchholz 1996). However, such participatory approaches should not be used to the exclusion of technical expertise, since it is not easy for the worker or consumer to predict new hazards that may arise from a change in design.

Conclusion

The design of tools, equipment, and complex systems to be compatible with human needs, abilities, and expectations is increasingly important in the modern world. Failure to apply these principles impacts negatively on people in their workplaces, in transit, and at home. The necessary knowledge base already exists, although the extent to which it is utilized varies widely among countries and types of applications. Legal requirements appear to be necessary to achieve protection from occupational injury and illness, while market incentives may motivate improved design of many consumer devices.

References

Armstrong, T.J., Buckle, P., Fine, L.J., *et al.* (1993). A conceptual model for work-related neck and upper-limb musculoskeletal disorders. *Scandinavian Journal of Work Environment and Health*, **19**, 73–84.

Åstrand, I. (1967*a*). Aerobic working capacity in men and women in some professions. *Forsvarsmedicin*, **3**, 163–70.

Åstrand, I. (1967*b*). Degree of strain during building work as related to individual aerobic work capacity. *Ergonomics*, **10**, 293–303.

Åstrand, I. (1988). Physical demands in worklife. *Scandinavian Journal of Work Environment and Health*, **14**, 10–13.

Åstrand, P.O. and Rodahl, K. (1986). *Textbook of work physiology.* McGraw-Hill, New York.

Badley, E.M., Rasooly, I., and Webster, G.K. (1994). Relative importance of musculoskeletal disorders as a cause of chronic health problems, disability, and health care utilization: Findings from the 1990 Ontario Health Survey. *Journal of Rheumatology*, **21**, 505–14.

Barnekow-Bergkvist, M., Hedberg, G.E., Janlert, U., *et al.* (1998). Determinants of self-reported neck–shoulder and low back symptoms in a general population. *Spine*, **23**, 235–43.

Benktzon, M. (1993). Designing for our future selves: the Swedish experience. *Applied Ergonomics*, **24**, 19–27.

Bergqvist, U., Wolgast, E., Nilsson, B., and Voss, M. (1995). The influence of VDT work on musculoskeletal disorders. *Ergonomics*, **38**, 754–62.

Bernard, B.P. (ed.) (1997). *Musculoskeletal disorders and workplace factors: a critical review of epidemiologic evidence for work-related musculoskeletal disorders of the neck, upper extremity, and low back.* Department of Health and Human Services, National Institute for Occupational Safety and Health, Cincinnati, OH.

Biering-Sørensen, F. (1984). Physical measurements as risk indicators for low-back trouble over a one-year period. *Spine*, **9**, 106–18.

Bongers, P.M., de Winter, C.R., Kompier, M.A.J., and Hildebrandt, V.H. (1993). Psychosocial factors at work and musculoskeletal disease. *Scandinavian Journal of Work Environment and Health*, **19**, 297–312.

Buckle, P.W. and Devereaux, J. (1999). *Work-related neck and upper limb musculoskeletal disorders*. European Agency for Safety and Health at Work, Luxembourg.

Chaffin, D.B., Andersson, G.B.J., and Martin, B.J. (1999). *Occupational biomechanics* (3rd edn). Wiley, New York.

Chapanis, A. (1965). On the allocation of functions between men and machines. *Occupational Psychology*, **39**, 1–11.

Clark, T.S. and Corlett, E.N. (1984). *The ergonomics of workspaces and machines—a design manual.* Taylor & Francis, London.

Dul, J. and de Flaming, P. (1994). A review of ISO and CEN standards on ergonomics. *Proceedings of the 12th Triennial Congress of the International Ergonomics Association*, pp. 131–3. Human Factors Association of Canada, Toronto.

Era, P., Lyyra, A.L., Viitasalo, J.T., and Heikkinen, E. (1992). Determinants of isometric muscle strength in men of different ages. *European Journal of Applied Physiology*, **64**, 84–91.

Estryn-Behar, M., Kaminski, M., Peigne, E., *et al.* (1990). Stress at work and mental health status among female hospital workers. *British Journal of Industrial Medicine*, **47**, 20–8.

Frick, K. (1997). Can managers see any profit in health and safety? *New Solutions*, **7**, 32–40.

Gardner, L., Powell, L., and Page, M. (1993). An appraisal of a selection of products currently available to older consumers. *Applied Ergonomics*, **24**, 35–9.

Gjessing, G.C., Schoenborn, T.F., and Cohen, A. (1994). *Participatory ergonomic interventions in meatpacking plants.* NIOSH Publication 94–124, Department of Health and Human Services, Cincinnati, OH.

Gold, E.B. and Tomich, E. (1994). Occupational hazards to fertility and pregnancy outcome. *Occupational Medicine*, **9**, 435–69.

Goldstein, S.A., Armstrong, T.J., Chaffin, D.B., *et al.* (1987). Analysis of cumulative strain in tendons and tendon sheaths. *Journal of Biomechanics*, **20**, 1–6.

Grandjean, E. (1988). *Fitting the task to the man. A textbook of occupational ergonomics.* Taylor & Francis, London.

Hagberg, M., Morgenstern, H., and Kelsh, M. (1992). Impact of occupations and job tasks on the prevalence of carpal tunnel syndrome: a review. *Scandinavian Journal of Work Environment and Health*, **18**, 337–45.

Hagberg, M., Hendricks, H., Silverstein, B., Smith, M., Welsh, R., and Carayon, P. (1995). *Work related musculoskeletal disorders (WMSDs): a reference book for prevention.* Taylor & Francis, London.

Haigh, R. (1993). The ageing process: a challenge for design. *Applied Ergonomics*, **24**, 9–14.

Hansen, S.M. (1993). *Arbeidsmiljo og samfundsokonomi.* Nordisk Ministerråd, Nord.

Hansson, J.-E. (1987). Funktionell anatomi, antropometri och biomekanik. In *Människan i arbete* (ed. N. Lundgren, G. Luthman, and K. Elgstrand), pp. 92–118. Almqvist and Wiksell, Stockholm.

Haverikommissionen (1992). *Spårvägnsolycka 1992–03–12.* Report J 1992:1, Swedish Board of Accident Investigation, Stockholm.

Hedegaard, M., Henriksen, T.B., Secher, N.J., Hatch, M.C., and Sabroe, S. (1996). Do stressful life events affect duration of gestation and risk of preterm delivery? *Epidemiology*, **7**, 339–45.

Hendricks, H.W. (1986). Macroergonomics: a conceptual model for integrating human factors with organizational design. In *Proceedings of the human factors in organizational design and management II* (ed. O. Brown and H. Hendricks), pp. 467–77. North-Holland, Amsterdam.

Jonsson, R.G., Persson, I., and Kilbom, A. (1988). Disorders of the cervicobrachial region among female workers in the electronics industry. A two-year follow up. *International Journal of lndustrial Ergonomics*, **3**, 1–12.

Karasek, R.A. and Theorell, T. (1990). *Healthy work. Stress, productivity and the reconstruction of working life.* Basic Books, New York.

Keyserling, W.M., Herrin, G.D., and Chaffin, D.B. (1980). Isometric strength testing as a means of controlling medical incidents on strenuous jobs. *Journal of Occupational Medicine*, **22**, 332–6.

Kilbom, Å. (1994). Repetitive work of the upper extremity: Part 1—Guidelines for the practitioner. Part II—The scientific basis (knowledge base) for the guide. *International Journal of lndustrial Ergonomics*, **14**, 51–86.

Kilbom, Å. (1995). Prevention of musculoskeletal disorders through standards and guidelines: possibilities and limitations. In *From research to prevention* (ed. J. Rantanen, S. Lehtinen, S. Hernberg, *et al.*), pp. 178–86. Finnish Institute of Occupational Health, Helsinki.

Kilbom, Å. (1998). Possibilities of regulatory actions in prevention of musculoskeletal disorders. *Abstracts of PREMUS-ISEOH '98: 3rd International Scientific Conference on Prevention of Work-Related Musculoskeletal Disorders/13th International Symposium on Epidemiology in Occupational Health*, p. 87. Finnish Institute of Occupational Health, Helsinki, Finland.

Kilbom, Å., Persson, J., and Jonsson, B.G. (1986). Disorders of the cervicobrachial region among female workers in the electronics industry. *International Journal of lndustrial Ergonomics*, **1**, 37–47.

Kirkeskov Jensen, L. and Eenberg, W. (1996). Occupation as a risk factor for knee disorders. *Scandinavian Journal of Work Environment and Health*, **22**, 165–75.

Knutsson, A. (1989). Shift work and coronary heart disease. *Scandinavian Journal of Social Medicine*, **44** (Supplement), 1–36.

Kristensen, T.S. (1996). Job stress and cardiovascular disease: a theoretical critical review. *Journal of Occupational Health Psychology*, **1**, 246–60.

Kogi, K. (1991). Participatory training for low-cost improvements in small enterprises in developing countries. In *Participatory ergonomics* (ed. K. Noro and A. Imada), pp. 73–80. Taylor & Francis, London.

Kogi, K. and Sen, R. (1987). Third world ergonomics. *International Reviews of Ergonomics*, **1**, 77–118.

Kroemer, K.H.E. and Grandjean, E. (1997). *Fitting the task to the human: a textbook of occupational ergonomics* (5th edn). Taylor & Francis, London.

Kujala, U.M., Taimela, S., Viljanen, T., *et al.* (1996). Physical loading and performance as predictors of back pain in healthy adults: a 5-year prospective study. *European Journal of Applied Physiology*, **73**, 452–8.

Kurppa, K., Viikari-Juntura, E., Kuosma, E., Huuskonen, M., and Kivi, P. (1991). Incidence of tenosynovitis or peritendinitis and epicondylitis in a meat-processing factory. *Scandinavian Journal of Work Environment and Health*, **17**, 32–7.

Lay, M. (1986). *Handbook of road technology.* Gordon & Breach, London.

Lehto, M. (1992). Designing warning signs and warning labels. Part I: Guidelines for the practitioner. Part II: The scientific basis for the guide. *International Journal of Industrial Ergonomics*, **10**, 78–95.

Leino, P., Aro, S., and Hasan, J. (1987). Trunk muscle function and low back disorders: a ten-year follow-up study. *Journal of Chronic Diseases*, **40**, 289–96.

Ljungberg, A.-S., Kilbom, Å., and Hägg, G. (1989). Occupational lifting by nursing aides and warehouse workers. *Ergonomics*, **32**, 59–78.

Louzine, A. (1982). Improving working conditions in small enterprises in developing countries. *International Labour Review*, **121**, 443–54.

Lundberg, A. (1992). *Dialysmålet–ett öppet såt i svensk rättskipning.* Private report.

Melamed, S., Yekutieli, D., Froom, P., Kristal-Boneh, E., and Ribak, J. (1999). Adverse work and environmental conditions predict occupational injuries. *American Journal of Epidemiology*, **150**, 18–26.

Messing, K. and Stevenson, J. (1996). Women in Procrustean beds: strength testing and the workplace. *Gender, Work and Organization*, **3**, 156–67.

Mital, A. and Kilbom, Å. (1992). Design, selection and use of hand tools to alleviate trauma of the upper extremities. *International Journal of Industrial Ergonomics*, **10**, 1–21.

Mital, A., Motorwala, A., Kulkarni, M., Sinclair, M., and Siemieniuch, C. (1994). Allocation of functions to humans and machines in a manufacturing environment. Part I: Guidelines for the practitioner. *International Journal of Industrial Ergonomics*, **14**, 3–29.

Moir, S. and Buchholz, B.O. (1996). Emerging participatory approaches to ergonomic interventions in the construction industry. *American Journal of Industrial Medicine*, **29**, 425–30.

Moll van Charante, A.W. and Mulder, P.G.H. (1990). Perceptual acuity and the risk of industrial accidents. *American Journal of Epidemiology*, **131**, 652–63.

Mozurkewich, E.L., Luke, B., Avni, M., and Wolf, F.M. (2000). Working conditions and adverse pregnancy outcome: a meta-analysis. *Obstetrics and Gynecology*, **95**, 623–35.

Murrell, K.F.H. (1965). *Ergonomics—man in his working environment.* Chapman & Hall, London.

Nakamura, K., Shimai, S., Kikuchi, S., *et al.* (1997). Shift work and risk factors for coronary heart disease in Japanese blue-collar workers: serum lipids and anthropometric characteristics. *Occupational Medicine*, 47, 142–6.

NIOSH (National Institute for Occupational Safety and Health) (1997). *Plain language about shiftwork.* NIOSH Publication 97-145, Department of Health and Human Services, Cincinnati, OH.

Oborne, D.J., Branton, R., Leal, F, Shipley, P., and Stewart, T (1993). *Person-centred ergonomics. A Brantonian view of human factors.* Taylor & Francis, London.

Ogden, K. (1990). Human factors in traffic engineering. *Institute of Transportation Engineers Journal*, **60**, 41–6.

Omer, H. and Everly, G.S. (1988). Psychological factors in preterm labor: Critical review and theoretical synthesis. *American Journal of Psychiatry*, **145**, 1507–13.

Oxenburgh, M. (1991). *Increasing productivity and profit through health and safety.* CCH Australia, Chicago, IL.

Pheasant, S. (1986). *Bodyspace.* Taylor & Francis, London.

Pheasant, S. (1991). *Ergonomics, work and health.* Macmillan, London.

Pope, M.H., Andersson, G.B.J., Frymoyer, J.W., and Chaffin, D.B. (ed). (1991). *Occupational low back pain: assessment, treatment and prevention.* Mosby–Year Book, St Louis, MO.

Punnett, L. and Bergqvist, U. (1997). *Visual display unit work and upper extremity musculoskeletal disorders. A review of epidemiological findings.* National Institute of Working Life, Solna, Sweden.

Rabbitt, P. (1991). Management of the working population. *Ergonomics*, **34**, 775–90.

Ramazzini, B. (1713). *Diseases of workers.* Reprinted by O & H Press, Thunder Bay, Ontario, 1993.

Ranney, D., Wells, R., and Moore, A. (1995). Upper limb musculoskeletal disorders in highly repetitive industries: precise anatomical physical findings. *Ergonomics*, **38**, 1408–23.

Reason, J. (1990). *Human error.* Cambridge University Press.

Rempel, D.M. and Punnett, L. (1997). Epidemiology of wrist and hand disorders. In *Musculoskeletal disorders in the workplace: principles and practice* (ed. M. Nordin, G.B. Andersson, and M.H. Pope), pp. 421–30. Mosby–Year Book, St. Louis, MO.

Riihimäki, H. (1991). Low-back pain, its origin and risk indicators. *Scandinavian Journal of Work Environment and Health*, **17**, 81–90.

Riihimäki, H. (1995). Back and limb disorders. *Epidemiology of work related diseases* (ed. C. McDonald), pp. 207–38. BMJ Publishing, London.

Rosa, R.R. and Colligan, M.J. (1992). Shift work: health and performance effects. In *Environmental and occupational medicine* (ed. W.N. Rom), pp. 1173–6. Little, Brown, Boston, MA.

Salthouse, T.A. (1990). Influence of experience on age differences in cognitive functioning. *Human Factors*, **32**, 551–69.

Sanders, M. and McCormick, E. (1992). *Human factors in engineering and design.* McGraw-Hill, New York.

Scientific Committee for Musculoskeletal Disorders of the International Commission on Occupational Health (1996). Musculoskeletal disorders: work-related risk factors and prevention. *International Journal of Occupational and Environmental Health*, **2**, 239–46.

Simpson, G. (1988). The economic justification for ergonomics. *International Journal of Industrial Ergonomics*, **2**, 157–63.

Sluiter, J.K., Rest, K.M., and Frings-Dresen, M.H.W. (2000). *Criteria document for evaluation of the work-relatedness of upper extremity musculoskeletal disorders.* SALTSA Joint Programme for Working Life Research in Europe and Academic Medical Center, University of Amsterdam.

Statistics Sweden (SCB) (1994). *Arbetssjukdomar och arbetsolyckor 1992.* Sveriges Officiella Statistik, Stockholm.

Steenland, K. (2000). Shift work, long hours, and cardiovascular disease: a review. *Occupational Medicine*, **15**, 7–17.

Sundström-Frisk, C. (1984). Behavioural control through piece-rate wages. *Journal of Occupational Accidents*, **6**, 49–59.

Tenkanen, L., Sjoblom, T., and Harma, M. (1998). Joint effect of shift work and adverse life-style factors on the risk of coronary heart disease. *Scandinavian Journal of Work Environment and Health*, **24**, 351–7.

Trinca, G., Johnston, I., Campbell, F., *et al.* (1988). *Reducing traffic injury—a global challenge.* Royal Australasian College of Surgeons, Melbourne.

Vaaranen, V., Vasama, M., Toikkanen, J., Jolanki, R., and Kaupinen, T. (1994). *Ammattitauditi 1993 (Occupational diseases in Finland l993).* Institute of Occupational Health, Helsinki.

Vernon, H.M. (1921). *Industrial fatigue and efficiency.* Routledge, London.

Viikari-Juntura, E. (1997). The scientific basis for making guidelines and standards to prevent work-related musculoskeletal disorders. *Ergonomics*, **40**, 1097–117.

Viikari-Juntura, E. and Silverstein, B.A. (1999). Role of physical load factors in carpal tunnel syndrome. *Scandinavian Journal of Work Environment and Health*, **25**, 163–85.

Vingård, E., Hogstedt, C., Alfredsson, L., Fellenius, E., Goldie, I., and Köster, M. (1991). Coxarthrosis and physical work load. *Scandinavian Journal of Work Environment and Health*, **17**, 14–19.

Wallerstein, N. and Weinger, M. (1992). Health and safety education for worker empowerment. *American Journal of Public Health*, **22**, 619–35.

Waters, T.W., Putz-Anderson, V., Garg, A., and Fine, L.J. (1993). Revised NIOSH equation for the design and evaluation of manual lifting tasks. *Ergonomics*, **36**, 749–76.

WHO (World Health Organization) (1985). *Identification and control of work related diseases*, Technical Report Series 714. WHO, Geneva.

Winkel, J. and Westgaard, R. (1992). Occupational and individual risk factors for shoulder–neck complaints. Part I: Guidelines for the practitioner. Part II: The scientific basis (literature review) for the guide. *International Journal of Industrial Ergonomics*, **10**, 79–104.

8.8 Risk assessment and risk management

Gilbert S. Omenn and Elaine M. Faustman

Introduction

Risk assessment as an organized activity of the federal agencies in the United States began in the 1970s. Earlier, the American Conference of Governmental Industrial Hygienists had set threshold limit values for exposures of workers and the Food and Drug Administration (**FDA**) had set acceptable daily intakes for dietary pesticide residues and food additives. In the 'Delaney Clause' of 1958, Congress instructed the FDA to prohibit substances found to cause cancer in animals (or humans, of course) from being used as food additives that could reach humans through the food supply. For some time, it was pragmatic to declare safe any food sources in which standard tests found no evidence of these chemicals (Albert 1994). However, advances in analytical chemistry exposed the fact that 'not detectable' was not the same as 'not present' or 'zero risk'. The agencies had to develop 'tolerance levels' and 'acceptable risk levels'.

In the mid-1970s the United States Environmental Protection Agency (**EPA**) and the FDA issued guidance for estimating risks from low-level exposures to potentially carcinogenic chemicals (Albert 1994). Their guidance set action levels for regulatory attention at estimated risks of one extra cancer over a lifetime of exposure per 100 000 people (EPA, at first) or per million people (FDA and later EPA). These estimated incremental risks represent very conservative acceptable or negligible risk levels. Cancers claim the lives of 230 000 of every million people in the United States. Thus the regulatory agencies seek to prevent an increase from a countable 23 per cent of deaths due to cancers to an estimated risk of 23.0001 per cent. Furthermore, as explained later, these estimates represent worst case or 'upper-bound' estimates, not actuarial counts like the 230 000 cancer deaths per million deaths in the general population. Other countries commonly use a safety factor approach generating, for example an 'acceptable daily intake'.

During the period 1977 to 1980, an Interagency Regulatory Liaison Group was actively engaged in bridging scientific, statutory, and policy considerations with the activities of the EPA and FDA, the Occupational Safety and Health Administration, and the Consumer Product Safety Commission. The White House Office of Science and Technology Policy participated in the scientific discussions supporting risk assessment and risk management (Calkins *et al.* 1980). A framework was developed for identifying potential hazards, characterizing the risks, and managing the risks, usually by reduction of use or reduction of exposures (Table 1).

A National Research Council report *Risk Assessment in the Federal Government: Managing the Process* (National Research Council 1983), subsequently called the *Red Book*, helped the regulatory agencies set in gear a common framework for assessing risks from chemicals. The *Red Book* provided a framework (Table 2) for the hazard identification and

Table 1 Framework for regulatory decision-making about potential hazards and the environment: risk assessment and risk management

1. Identification of hazard
    - Epidemiology
    - Toxicology
    - *In vitro* tests
    - Structure–activity relationships
2. Characterization of risk
    - Potency
    - Exposures
    - Susceptibility
3. Control of risk
    - Information
    - Regulation
    - Substitution

Based on Calkins *et al.* (1980) and Faustman and Omenn (1996).

Table 2 Framework for risk assessment from the *Red Book* (National Research Council 1983)

Hazard identification
Can the agent cause the adverse effect?
Dose–response assessment
What is the relationship between dose and incidence of adverse effects in humans or in animals?
Exposure assessment
What exposures are currently experienced or can be anticipated under various circumstances?
Risk characterization
What is the estimated incidence of the adverse effect in a given population or subpopulation?
What is the nature of the effect?
What is the strength of the evidence?

risk characterization components of the risk assessment/risk management framework in Table 1. A strong research base is an essential aspect (Office of Technology Assessment 1992; Faustman and Omenn 1996; EPA 1996*b*).

The 1990 Amendments to the United States Clean Air Act led to two far-reaching reports. *Science and Judgment in Risk Assessment* (National Research Council 1994) captured the combination of qualitative and quantitative approaches essential to effective assessment of risks. Then the Presidential/Congressional Commission on Risk Assessment and Risk Management (Risk Commission 1997) formulated a comprehensive framework that is being applied widely. The two crucial concepts were putting each environmental problem or issue into public health (and/or ecological) context and proactively engaging the relevant stakeholders from the very beginning of the six-stage process shown in Fig. 1. Particular exposures and potential health effects must be evaluated across sources and exposure pathways and in light of multiple endpoints, not just one chemical, in one environmental medium (air, water, food, products), for one health effect at a time. A similar framework has been utilized by the Health and Safety Executive (**HSE**) Risk Assessment Policy Unit in the United Kingdom (HSE 2000).

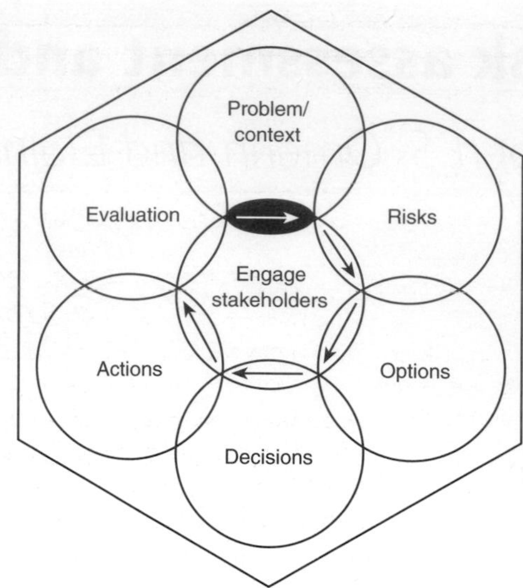

Fig. 1 Environmental health risk management Framework from the United States Commission on Risk Assessment and Risk Management (Omenn Commission). The framework is comprised of six stages: (1) formulate the problem in a broad public health context; (2) analyse the risks; (3) define the options; (4) make sound risk reduction decisions; (5) implement those actions; (6) later evaluate the effectiveness of the actions taken. Interactions with stakeholders are at the centre of the process (Omenn 1996; Risk Commission 1997; Charnley and Omenn 1997; Ohanian *et al.* 1997).

Definitions

Risk assessment is the systematic scientific characterization of potential adverse health effects resulting from human exposures to

Table 3 Major toxic chemical laws in the United States and agency responsible

Environment Protection Agency	
Air pollutants	Clean Air Acts 1970, 1977, 1990
Water pollutants	Federal Water Pollution Control Acts 1972, 1977
Drinking water	Safe Drinking Water Acts 1974, 1996
Pesticides	Fungicides, Insecticides, and Rodenticides Act (FIFRA) 1972
	Food Quality Protection Act (FQPA) 1996
Ocean dumping	Marine Protection, Research and Sanctuaries Act 1972
	Ocean Radioactive Dumping Ban Act 1995
Toxic chemicals	Toxic Substances Controls Act (TSCA) 1976
Hazardous wastes	Resource Conservation and Recovery Act (RCRA) 1976
Abandoned hazardous wastes	Superfund (CERCLA) 1980, 1986
Council for Environmental Quality (now Office of Environmental Policy)	
Environmental impacts	National Environmental Policy Act (NEPA) 1969
Occupational Safety and Health Administration	
Workplace	Occupational Safety and Health (OSH) Act 1970
Food and Drug Administration	
Foods, drugs, and cosmetics	FDC Acts 1906, 1938, 1962, 1977
Consumer Product Safety Commission	
Dangerous consumer products	FDA Modernization Act 1997
Department of Transportation	
Transport of hazard materials	Consumer Product Safety Act 1972
	THM Acts 1975, 1976, 1978, 1979, 1984, 1990 (×2)

hazardous agents or situations. Risk is defined as the probability of an adverse outcome. The term 'hazard' is used by North Americans to refer to intrinsic toxic properties; internationally, this term is defined as the probability of an adverse outcome. This chapter presents risk assessment approaches for both cancer and non-cancer hazards. Analogous approaches can be applied to ecological risks (National Research Council Committee on Risk Assessment Methodology 1993; EPA 1996*a*).

Both qualitative assessment of the nature of effects and strength of the evidence and quantitative estimation of the risk are essential components of the risk characterization (Tables 1 and 2). We emphasize the importance of the phrase 'characterization of risk', as many public health practitioners, environmentalists, and regulators tend to equate risk assessment with quantitative risk assessment, getting a number (or a number with uncertainty bounds), and ignoring crucial information about the strength of the evidence, the nature of the health effect, and the means of avoiding or reversing effects of exposure.

Risk management refers to the process by which policy actions are chosen to deal with hazards identified in the risk assessment/risk characterization process. Risk managers consider the scientific evidence and risk estimates together with statutory, engineering, economic social and political factors in evaluating alternative regulatory options, selecting among the options, and discussing those options with interested parties, the stakeholders.

Risk communication is the challenging process of making risk assessment and risk management information comprehensible to community groups, lawyers, politicians, judges, business people, labour, and environmentalists (Fischhoff *et al.* 1996). Often these people have important inputs for various stages of this process, so listening is a crucial, too often neglected aspect of risk communication. Sometimes the decision makers and stakeholders simply want to know the 'bottom line': Is a substance or a situation 'safe' or not? Others will be interested in knowing why the risk estimates are uncertain and complicated and may be eager to challenge underlying assumptions.

Risk management decisions are reached under diverse statutes in the United States (Table 3) and analogous statutes or regulations in other countries. Some statutes specify reliance on risk alone, while others require a balancing of risks and benefits of the product or activity (Table 4). Risk assessment has provided a valuable framework for priority setting within regulatory and health agencies, in the development process within companies, and in resource allocation in environmental organizations. Similar statutes and regulatory regimes have been developed in many other countries and through such international organizations as the International Programme for Chemical Safety of the World Health Organization (**WHO**). There are significant current efforts toward the harmonization of testing protocols and assessment of risks and standards.

A major challenge for risk assessment, risk communication, and better risk management is to work across disciplines to demonstrate the biological plausibility and clinical significance of the conclusions from epidemiological, lifetime animal, short-term, and structure–activity studies of chemicals thought to have potential adverse effects on human health and the environment. Biomarkers of exposure, effect, or individual susceptibility can link the presence of a chemical in various environmental compartments to specific sites of action in target organs and to host responses (National Research Council 1989*a*,*b*, 1992 *a*,*b*). Mechanistic investigations of the actions of specific chemicals can help us penetrate the black box approach of simply counting tumours in exposed animals. Greater appreciation of the mechanisms and extent of individual variation in susceptibility among humans can help us better protect subgroups of susceptible people and better relate findings in animals to risk estimates in humans. Individual behavioural risk factors and social risk factors are also important. Finally, public and media attitudes toward the local polluters, other responsible parties, and relevant government agencies may be critically important, sometimes leading to what has been labelled 'the outrage factor' by Sandman (1993). Thus, all of the public health sciences are needed for comprehensive risk assessment and risk management (Omenn 1996; Risk Commission 1997).

Table 4 Objectives of risk assessment

1. Balance risks and benefits
Drugs
Pesticides
2. Set target levels of risk
Food contaminants
Water pollutants
3. Set priorities for programme activities
Regulatory agencies
Manufacturers
Environmental/consumer organizations
4. Estimate residual risks and extent of risk reduction after steps are taken to reduce risks

This chapter reviews the status of certain facets of the framework approach and its application to environmental health problems. Details about the contributing scientific fields can be found in Chapters 8.1 to 8.7 and other relevant chapters on epidemiological approaches, risk communication, determinants of health and disease, and public health functions.

Hazard identification: epidemiology, lifetime rodent bioassay, short-term tests, and structure–activity relationships

Epidemiology

The most convincing evidence for human risk is a well-conducted epidemiological study in which a positive association between exposure and disease has been observed (National Research Council 1983). Epidemiological approaches are basically opportunistic. Studies begin either with known or presumed exposures, comparing exposed versus non-exposed individuals, or with known cases, comparing with persons lacking the particular diagnosis. There are important limitations. When the study is exploratory, hypotheses are often weak. Exposure estimates are often crude and retrospective, in particular for conditions with a long latency before clinical manifestations appear, such as cancers. Generally, there are multiple exposures, in particular when a full week or a full lifetime is considered. Lifestyle factors, such as smoking, physical inactivity, and diet, may be important and are difficult to sort out. There is always a trade-off between detailed information on relatively few persons and very limited information on large numbers of persons. Humans are highly outbred, and so the method must consider variation in susceptibility among people who are exposed. Finally, the expression of results (odds ratios, relative risks, and confidence intervals) may be unfamiliar to non-epidemiologists; the caveats self-effacing epidemiologists cite often discourage risk managers (Omenn 1993). Frequently, 'conflicting' studies with results that disagree are not evaluated with respect to size and power of the study to detect the endpoint of interest. To help address these epidemiological challenges, epidemiologists use criteria for evaluating the robustness of associations (Hill 1965).

Epidemiology is in the midst of a transformation. Advances from the human genome project, molecular biomarkers and improved mechanistic hypotheses help epidemiology 'get inside the black box' of statistical associations to gain an understanding that enhances biological plausibility and clinical relevance. 'Molecular epidemiology' is a new phrase that refers to such studies of the molecular events in the causative pathway of human disease. Some hypotheses of causative relationships are being tested with prevention clinical trials. For example, the β-Carotene and Retinol Efficacy Trial (CARET) in the United States and the α-Tocopherol/β-Carotene (ATBC) Trial in Finland, tested the hypothesis arising from observational epidemiology studies that antioxidant vitamins might be chemopreventive agents against the development of lung cancer (and cardiovascular disease) in high-risk populations, namely smokers and asbestos-exposed workers. In these trials, the stunning findings were that not only was there no benefit from the vitamin supplements, but also there were significant increases in lung cancer incidence and in cardiovascular and total mortality (ATBC 1994; Omenn *et al.* 1996; Omenn 1998). These findings have stimulated new laboratory work on the properties and effects of β-carotene. Systematic studies of environmental exposure reduction actions should be considered analogues of such prevention trials.

Many questions arise in the assessment of results from epidemiological studies such as the following.

1. What relative weights should be given to studies with differing results? Should positive results override negative results? Should a study be weighted in accord with its statistical power or its quality? Are there certain kinds of flaws, such as in choice of the control or comparison group, that should make a study be disregarded altogether?
2. What relative weights should be given to the results from different types of epidemiological studies? Should the findings of a prospective study supersede those of a case–control study or case–control findings supersede ecological findings?
3. What statistical significance should be required for results to be considered positive? Should that criterion be different for the primary hypothesis than for correlations that arise from massaging the data afterward?
4. What is the significance of a positive finding in a study in which the route of exposure is different from that under analysis?
5. Should evidence for different types of tumour response be combined (e.g. different tumour sites or benign versus malignant tumours)? What about cancer and non-cancer endpoints?

Lifetime rodent bioassays

Bioassays have been developed as standardized, experimental protocols to identify chemicals capable of causing cancers, birth defects, neurotoxicity, or other toxicity in laboratory animals. Typically, one chemical is tested at a time in rats and mice, both sexes, with 50 animals per dose group and near lifetime exposure to 90, 50, and 10 to 25 per cent of what is determined in preliminary studies to be the maximally tolerated dose. Based on results from 379 long-term carcinogenicity studies, Haseman and Lockhart (1993) concluded that most target sites showed a strong correlation (65 per cent) between males and females, in particular for forestomach, liver, and thyroid tumours; in fact, for efficiency they suggested that bioassays could rely on a combination of male rats and female mice, thereby halving the number of animals required for a lifetime rodent bioassay and assuming that other uses would be found for the female rats and male mice! Estimation and use of the maximally tolerated dose is a vexing problem, not at all resolved by an expert panel (National Research Council Committee on Risk Assessment Methodology 1993) or by others troubled by toxicity or cell proliferation responses at maximal doses that may be not at all be representative of responses at lower doses (Ames and Gold 1990).

Although these bioassays were initially designed for hazard identification, they are now used as the basis for quantitative assessments. Results are extrapolated from high dose to low dose, and then from animals to humans. Such extrapolations have historically required numerous choices, most importantly the choice of dataset, plus assumptions about the dose–response curve from observations in the 10 to 100 per cent range down to 10^{-6} risk estimates at the upper confidence limit or use of a benchmark or reference dose approach (see below). Lifetime bioassays can be enhanced by investigation of mechanisms and assessment of multiple endpoints in the same study (Bucher *et al.* 1996). Based on increasing information about critical mechanistic pathways in cancer, the National Toxicology Program now includes tests in transgenic animal models with sensitized genetic pathways known to be important for human cancers (Tennant *et al.* 1999). These assays (see below) will expedite detection of carcinogens, and can be linked with mechanistically oriented, short-term tests and biomarker and genetic studies in epidemiology. A second initiative is the Environmental Genome Project, aimed at identifying specific genes relevant for a broad range of environmentally induced diseases. Questions from the *Red Book* remain important.

1. Is a positive result from a single animal study sufficient or should positive results from two or more animal studies be required? Should studies be weighted according to their quality and statistical power? Should negative results of similar quality be given less weight?
2. How should evidence of different metabolic pathways or very different metabolic rates between animals and humans be factored into a risk assessment?

Substantial advances in the past decade are discussed later in this chapter.

Short-term tests

Many chemicals in widespread commerce have not been tested adequately for risk assessment purposes (National Research Council 1984; INFORM 1996; EPA 1998*b*). The costs of $1 to $2 million and 3 to 5 years' work per chemical tested are prohibitive in the aggregate. For example, EPA's recent chemical hazard data availability study found that 43 per cent of the United States high production volume chemicals (those produced in excess of 1 million lb/year) have no publicly available studies for any of six basic toxicity endpoints (acute toxicity, chronic toxicity, developmental/reproductive toxicity, genotoxicity/mutagenicity, ecotoxicity, and environmental fate). Only 7 per cent of the high production volume chemicals has a full set of publicly available studies for the six basic endpoints (EPA 1998*b*). The Environmental Defense Fund (1997) book *Toxic Ignorance* has catalysed widespread agreement from international chemical companies to conduct the necessary tests to meet the Organization for Economic Co-operation and Development (**OECD**) requirements for a screening information data system on such high-volume chemicals. Recent public interest in the potential of chemicals to cause endocrine effects has also drawn attention to similar data needs (EPA 1998*a*).

These critical data gaps have sparked renewed interest in devising inexpensive, short-term tests for screening chemicals. Such tests can also yield important information about mechanisms, distinguishing genotoxic from non-genotoxic effects between carcinogens, for example. The *Salmonella* reverse mutation test (Ames test) and certain cytogenetic tests, especially of bone marrow following *in vivo* exposure, seem useful and robust. Nevertheless, progress has been slow and frustrating. Many years have been spent trying to make the mouse lymphoma test and the sister chromatid exchange assay interpretable for risk assessment purposes.

Short-term tests for non-cancer endpoints such as developmental toxicity, reproductive toxicity, neurotoxicity, and immunotoxicity have become available (Atterwill *et al.* 1992; Harris *et al.* 1992; Shelby *et al.* 1993; Whittaker and Faustman 1994; Faustman and Omenn 1996; Lewandowski *et al.* 1999). Mechanistic information from these systems has been applied to risk assessment (Abbott *et al.* 1992; EPA 1994*c*; Leroux *et al.* 1996). A National Toxicology Program Interagency Center for the Evaluation of Alternative Toxicological Methods recently peer reviewed the mouse local lymph node assay for assessing chemicals for their ability to produce allergic contact dermatitis and declared it a valid alternative to currently accepted guinea pig test methods, helping to refine and reduce animal use (NIEHS 1999). This centre is evaluating other tests as alternatives to *in vivo* assays.

A new class of short-term tests utilizes knockout transgenic mouse models (Nebert and Duffy 1997 or Tennant *et al.* 1999). Mutagenic carcinogens can be identified with high sensitivity and specificity using hemizygous *p53*(+/–) mice in which one allele of the *p53* gene has been inactivated. A TG.AC transgenic mouse carrying a *V-Ha-ras* gene construct develops papillomas and malignant tumours in response to mutagenic and non-mutagenic carcinogens and tumour promoters, but not in response to non-carcinogens. It is likely that these animal models will supplant at least part of the two-species, two-sex rodent bioassay in the next decade.

Structure–activity relationships

A chemical's structure, solubility, stability, pH sensitivity, electrophilicity, chemical reactivity, and pathways of metabolism can be important information for hazard identification by inference. Historically, certain key molecular structures have provided regulators with some of the most readily available information on which to assess hazard potential. For example, the majority of the first 14 occupational carcinogens regulated by the Occupational Safety and Health Administration belonged to the aromatic amine chemical class. The EPA Office of Toxic Substances relies on structure–activity relationships (**SARs**) to meet deadlines for responses to premanufacturing notices for new chemicals under the Toxic Substances Control Act (see Table 3). *N*-Nitroso, aromatic amine, amino azo, and phenanthrene structures are alerts to prioritize chemicals for additional evaluation as potential carcinogens. Chemicals with structures related to valproic acid or retinoic acid are suspected as developmental toxicants (Faustman and Omenn 1996).

SARs can be used in assessing the relative toxicity of chemically related compounds. A prominent example was the EPA's reassessment of health risks associated with 2,3,7,8-tetrachlorodibenzo-*p*-dioxin and related chlorinated and brominated dibenzo-*p*-dioxins, dibenzofurans, and planar biphenyls, using toxicity equivalence factors, based on induction of the *Ah* receptor (EPA 1994*b*). The estimated toxicity of environmental mixtures containing these chemicals is the sum of the product of the concentration of each multiplied by its toxicity equivalence factor value. The WHO has organized efforts to reach a consensus on toxicity equivalence factors used for PCBs, PCDDs, and PCDFs for both humans and wildlife (Van den Berg *et al.* 1998).

Integrating hazard identification information

A remarkable collegial effort to relate the findings of short-term tests to the presumed gold standard of the lifetime rodent cancer bioassay result was conducted between 1989 and 1994 under the aegis of the National Toxicology Program and the National Institute of Environmental Health Sciences. For a set of 44 consecutive chemicals entered into the National Toxicology Program lifetime bioassay programme, Tennant *et al.* (1990) predicted the results, based upon knowledge of the structural features of the chemicals, results from short-term tests, and (sometimes) previous bioassay data. In response to their Carcinogen Prediction Challenge, nine other groups of scientists made predictions for the same set of chemicals, based on their own criteria. At the conclusion, an international workshop was held at which the National Toxicology Program lifetime rodent bioassay results for 40 chemicals were revealed: 20 had clear or some evidence of carcinogenicity in one or more of the four species/sex groups of rats and mice, of which 14 were clear positives and nine were positive in more than one organ site (Ashby and Tennant 1994). Tennant *et al.* (1990) correctly predicted 17 of 20 carcinogens and 13 of 20 non-carcinogens; thus, they had a ratio of false positives to false negatives of 2.3, a sensitivity of 0.85 (17 of 20), and a specificity of 0.65 (13 of 20). None of the nine groups did as well; some did no better than chance, using combinations of computerized structural alerts or SARs and results from *in vitro* and *in vivo* tests (Omenn *et al.* 1995). The pattern of results reveals very different approaches to balancing false-negative versus false-positive outcomes, apparently with different implicit 'cut-points'.

Social cost analytical approaches have been published, relying upon short-term tests, lifetime rodent bioassays, or a combination of testing strategies to guide risk management for potentially hazardous chemicals. In the Lave–Omenn value of information model (Lave and Omenn 1986; Lave *et al.* 1988; Omenn and Lave 1988), 'cost-effective' means that the costs of testing plus the social costs of false positives (loss of the economic value of the chemical) and of false negatives (economic value of the disease burden incurred as a result of use of the chemical) are less than the costs of misclassification by simply treating all chemicals as carcinogenic and avoiding exposures to the extent feasible. For example, we might set the cost/consequences of a false negative at $10 million, 10 times the social cost of a false positive, on the average. Then, for the correct prediction of 30 of 40 of the National Toxicology Program results (Tennant *et al.* 1990), the social cost of misclassification would be $7 million for the seven false positives plus $30 million for the three false negatives (Omenn *et al.* 1995). In the Lave–Omenn estimation (Lave and Omenn 1986), if the bioassay were used at $1 million per chemical tested and the true proportion of rodent carcinogens is assumed to be 10 per cent among tested chemicals, the testing ($40 million for 40 chemicals) would have to be 100 per cent accurate just to break even against the alternative of simply calling all chemicals carcinogenic for rodents. Such an alternative practice would require instituting general approaches to minimize exposures. If regulatory decisions could be based on interpretation of far less expensive short-term tests, the margin for cost-effective decision-making would be much greater (Omenn and Lave 1988). Thus, there is considerable incentive to come up with more reliable and more predictive short-term biological and structural approaches.

Risk characterization: dose–response, exposure analysis, variation in susceptibility, and relation of effects in rodents to risk in humans

As noted above, the characterization of risk involves more than quantitative estimation of the risk (with or without uncertainty bounds). Crucial information about the nature of health (and ecological) risks, the strength of the evidence, the feasibility of prevention or treatment of the adverse effects, and the variation of risk in the population cannot be captured in a number; these attributes require careful qualitative and descriptive characterization that can be used in health advisories.

Dose–response

Analyses of dose–response relationships must start with the determination of the critical effect. Many chemicals have more than one adverse effect on health and/or ecological endpoints. The usual practice is to choose the dataset with adverse effects at the lowest levels of exposure, even if not representative, to extrapolate for potential health impacts on humans or ecosystems. Most studies are designed for hazard identification and not risk characterization and hence provide limited quantitative information. Nevertheless, they are used as the basis for quantitative risk estimations for lack of other data. Linearized multistage models for cancer have been used to estimate 'virtually safe doses', generally far below the observable range of our rodent bioassays. For other endpoints a reference dose is developed that is based on low or no effect level determinations, with safety factors driving extrapolation across species to find an acceptably safe exposure level for humans. We continue to use maximally tolerated dose regimens in animals, while awaiting better understanding of the underlying mechanisms, on an organ site by organ site or a chemical by chemical basis.

The fundamental basis of the quantitative relationships between exposure to an agent and the incidence of an adverse response is the dose–response assessment. Approaches for characterizing dose–response include determination of effect levels such as LD_{50} (dose producing 50 per cent lethality), ED_{10} (dose producing an effect in 10 per cent of exposed populations) and no observed adverse effect levels, margins of safety and therapeutic indexes, and various models for extrapolation to very low doses (National Research Council 1983).

For risk assessment purposes, human exposure data for the prediction of human response are usually quite limited. The risk assessor is interested in low environmental exposures of humans, which are way below the observable range of responses from animal assays or from high occupational exposures. Thus, high- to low-dose extrapolation and animal to human risk extrapolation methods comprise major aspects of dose–response assessment.

Threshold approaches

A challenge for risk assessors is the determination of critical adverse effect levels occurring at the lowest exposures. Each endpoint evaluated can have a no effect level (**NOEL**) as well as a no observed adverse effect level (**NOAEL**), lowest observed effect levels, and lowest observed adverse effect level (**LOAEL**). The dose–response curves for these endpoints frequently overlap. New specific responses, such as changes in body weight, can confound interpretation of endpoints, especially developmental toxicity (EPA 1991). EPA endpoint specific guidance documents provide useful information (e.g. EPA 1991). Usually, the critical adverse effect is defined as the significant adverse biological effect that occurs at the lowest exposure level; the NOAEL from that study is then used in quantitative risk evaluation (Barnes and Dourson 1988).

Significance usually refers to both biological and statistical criteria (Faustman *et al.* 1994) and is dependent upon the number of dose levels tested, the number of animals tested at each dose, and the background incidence of the adverse response in the non-exposed control groups. The NOAEL should not be perceived as risk free; NOAELs for continuous endpoints average 5 per cent risk and NOAELs based on quantal endpoints can be associated with a risk of greater than 10 per cent (Allen *et al.* 1994*a*,*b*; Faustman *et al.* 1994).

NOAELs can be used as a basis for risk assessment calculations, such as reference doses or acceptable daily intake values (Lehman and Fitzhugh 1954; Renwick and Walker 1993; Barnes and Dourson 1988). Reference doses (**RfDs**) or reference concentrations (**RfCs**) are estimates of a daily exposure to an agent that is assumed to have no adverse health impact on the human population. Acceptable daily intake (**ADI**) values used by the WHO for pesticides and food additives define the daily intake of a chemical, which, during an entire lifetime, appears to be without appreciable risk on the basis of all known facts (WHO 1962). RfDs and ADI values are typically calculated from NOAEL values by dividing by uncertainty and/or modifying factors (**UF, MF**) (EPA 1991):

$$\mathrm{RfD} = \frac{\mathrm{NOAEL}}{\mathrm{UF} \times \mathrm{MF}}$$

$$\mathrm{ADI} = \frac{\mathrm{NOAEL}}{\mathrm{UF} \times \mathrm{MF}}.$$

These safety factors allow for interspecies (animal to human) and intraspecies (human) variation with default values of 10 each. An additional 10-fold uncertainty factor is used to extrapolate from short-exposure duration studies to a situation more relevant for long-term effects or to account for inadequate numbers of animals or other experimental limitations. The Food Quality Protection Act (1996) now requires the use of an extra 10-fold factor to be protective for children under certain conditions.

If only a LOAEL value is available, then an additional 10-fold factor is used routinely to arrive at a value more comparable with a NOAEL (Goldman 1998; Landrigan and Goldman 1998). MFs can be used to adjust the uncertainty factors if data on mechanisms, pharmacokinetics, or relevance of the animal response to human risk justify such modification (Dourson and Stara 1983; Dourson *et al.* 1985; Dourson and DeRosa 1991). Allen *et al.* (1994*a*) have shown developmental toxicity endpoints that application for the 10-fold factor for LOAEL to NOAEL conversion is too large.

Another way the NOAEL values have been utilized for risk assessment is to evaluate a 'margin of exposure' (**MOE**) or 'margin of safety', based on the ratio of the NOAEL determined in animals (expressed as mg/kg/day) to the intakes or exposure levels for humans. For example, if human exposures are calculated to be via drinking water containing 1 ppm of the chemical, then the exposure for a 50 kg woman would be

$$\frac{(1\ \mathrm{mg/l}) \times (2\ \mathrm{l/day})}{50\ \mathrm{kg}} = 0.04\ \mathrm{mg/kg/day}.$$

If the NOAEL for neurotoxicity is 100 mg/kg/day, then the MOE would be 2500 for the oral exposure route for neurotoxicity from the drinking water. Such a large value is reassuring for public health officials.

Low values of the MOE indicate that the human levels of exposure are close to levels for the NOAEL in animals. There is no factor included in this calculation for differences in human or animal susceptibility or animal to human extrapolation. Thus, MOE values of less than 100 have been used by regulatory agencies as flags for requiring further evaluation.

Some important common human exposures, such as the air pollutants lead, particulates, sulphur oxides, ozone, and carbon monoxide, are so close to LOAELs that regulatory agencies override the margin of safety approach, with considerations of technical feasibility.

The NOAEL approach has been criticized on several points: the NOAEL must, by definition, be one of the experimental doses tested; once identified, the rest of the dose–response curve is often ignored; experiments that test fewer animals often result in higher NOAELs and thus larger reference doses, as well as greater uncertainty; and the NOAEL will vary based on experimental design (Faustman and Bartell 1997).

Because of these limitations, an alternative to the NOAEL approach, the benchmark dose method, was proposed by Crump (1984) and extended by Kimmel and Gaylor (1988). The full dose–response is modelled, and the lower confidence bound for a dose at a specified response level is calculated. Figure 2 shows how a benchmark dose is calculated using a 10 per cent response and a 95 per cent lower confidence bound on dose (LED_{10}). In this case,

$$\mathrm{RfD} = \frac{\mathrm{LED}_{10}}{\mathrm{UF} \times \mathrm{MF}}.$$

Discussion continues on whether the values used for the uncertainty factors and modifying factors for benchmark doses should be the same factors as for the NOAEL or smaller values because of use of the full dose–response curve and of lower confidence bounds on the dose.

The benchmark dose approach has been applied to non-cancer endpoints (Clewell *et al.* 1997; Faustman and Bartell 1997), including specific applications for developmental and reproductive toxicity (Allen *et al.* 1994*a*,*b*; Auton 1994). Benchmark dose values were similar to NOAELs for a wide range of developmental toxicity endpoints. A generalized log logistic dose–response model has advantages in dealing with litter size and intralitter correlations (Allen *et al.* 1994*b*).

The benchmark dose approach has four advantages: it uses the full dose–response curve, as opposed to focusing on a single test dose as in the NOAEL approach; it includes a measure of variability (lower confidence limit on dose associated with upper confidence limit on risk); it uses responses within the experimental range versus extrapolation of responses to low doses not tested experimentally; and it facilitates comparisons of a consistent benchmark response level for RfD calculations across studies and agents (Faustman and Bartell 1997).

Non-threshold approaches

Numerous dose–response curves can be proposed in the low-dose region of the dose–response curve if a threshold assumption is not made. Because risk assessors are frequently interested in postulating exposures that would be associated with very low risks, such as one in a million over a lifetime, they frequently need to extrapolate far below the region of the dose–response curve for which experimentally

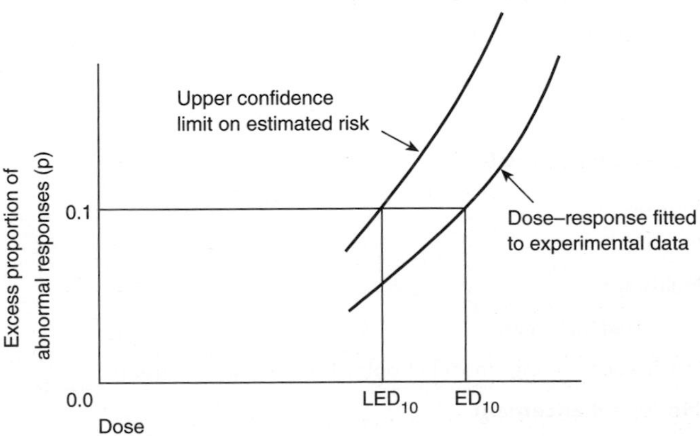

Fig. 2 Illustration of the benchmark dose (BMD) approach. LED_{10} is the lower confidence limit of the dose associated with a 10 per cent incidence of adverse effect. (Based on Kavlock *et al.* 1995.)

observed data are available. Thus, the choice of models for extrapolation has received lots of attention. Two general types of dose–response model exist: statistical or tolerance distribution models and mechanistic models (Krewski and Van Ryzin 1981). Table 5 lists common models that have been used in risk extrapolation.

The distribution models are based on the assumption that each individual has a tolerance level for responding to a test agent. A specific probability distribution is generated for the cumulative dose–response function (Faustman and Omenn 1996).

The mechanistic modelling approach to dose–response relationships tries to take account of the postulated biological mechanisms of response. Radiation research has spawned a series of 'hit models' for cancer modelling, where a 'hit' is defined as a critical cellular event that must occur before a toxic effect is produced. These models assume that an infinitely large number of targets exists (e.g. in the DNA), that the organism's toxic response occurs after only a minimum number of targets has been modified, that a critical biological target is altered if a sufficient number of hits occurs, and that the probability of a hit in the low-dose range of the dose–response curve is proportional to the dose of the toxicant (Brown 1984).

The simplest mechanistic model is the one-hit (one-stage) linear model in which only one hit or critical cellular interaction is required for a cell to be altered. For example, based on somatic mutation theory, a single mutational change could be sufficient for a cell to become neoplastic through a transformational event and dose-independent clonal expansion. The probability statement for these models is

$$P(d) = 1 - \exp(-\lambda d)$$

where λd is the number of hits occurring during a time period. In this theory a single molecule of a genotoxic carcinogen would have a minute but finite chance of causing a mutational event.

Armitage and Doll (1957) developed a multistage model for carcinogenesis based on the hypothesis that a series of ordered stages was required for a cell to undergo mutation, initiation, transformation, and progression to form a tumour. This relationship was generalized by Crump (1980) by maximizing the likelihood function over polynomials so that the probability statement is

$$P(d) = 1 - \exp\,[-\lambda_0 + \lambda d_1 + \lambda d_2 + \ldots + \lambda_1 d^k].$$

If the true value of λ_1 is replaced with $\lambda_1{}^*$ (upper confidence limit of λ_1), then a linearized multistage model can be derived where the expression is dominated by $(\lambda\, d^*)d$ at low doses. The slope $q_1{}^*$ on this confidence interval is used for quantitative cancer assessment. To obtain an upper 95 per cent confidence interval on risk, the $q_1{}^*$ value (Δrisk/Δdose in mg/kg/day) is multiplied by the amount of exposure (mg/kg/day). Thus the upper-bound estimate on risk R is calculated as

$$R = q_1{}^* \text{ risk (mg/kg/day)}^{-1} \times \text{exposure (mg/kg/day)}.$$

This relationship has been used to calculate a 'virtually safe dose', which represents the lower 95 per cent confidence limit on a dose that gives an 'acceptable level' of risk (for example, an upper confidence limit for 10^{-6} excess risk). As both $q_1{}^*$ and 'virtually safe dose' are calculated using 95 per cent confidence intervals, the values are believed to represent conservative estimates.

The EPA has utilized the linearized multistage model to calculate 'unit risk estimates', such as the increased individual lifetime risks of cancer over a 70-year lifespan for a 70-kg human breathing 1 $\mu g/m^3$ of contaminated air or drinking 2 litres of water contaminated at 1 ppm (1 mg/kg/day).

The revised EPA cancer guidelines proposed several alternative approaches (EPA 1996*b*). For example, the lower confidence limit on a benchmark response has been suggested as a point of departure from which linear extrapolation to zero response or application of safety factors could be utilized for cancer risk assessment options depending upon the hypothesized mode of carcinogenic action. Genotoxic and non-genotoxic mechanisms might trigger different quantitative risk assessment approaches for establishing acceptable levels of exposure. Similar methods may be used for non-genotoxic carcinogens and for developmental and other non-cancer toxicants (Page *et al.* 1997; Gaylor *et al.* 1999).

Table 5 Models used in risk extrapolation

Statistical or distribution models
Log-probit
Logit
Weibull
Mechanistic models
One hit
Multihit
Multistage
Linearized multistage
Stochastic two-stage model (Moolgavkar–Venson–Knudson)
Model enhancement
Time-to-tumour response
Physiologically based toxicokinetic models
Biologically based dose–response models

Toxicological enhancements of the models

Table 5 lists three areas of research that have improved the application of models used in risk extrapolation. Physiologically based toxicokinetic modelling generates 'internal effective doses' at target organ sites, rather than relying on single-value external exposure estimates. Biologically based dose–response modelling connects the generalized mechanistic models discussed in the previous section to specific biological processes. Measured rates are incorporated into the mechanistic equations to replace default or computer-generated values. For example, the Moolgavkar–Venson–Knudson model is based on a two-stage model for carcinogenesis; two mutations are required for carcinogenesis, and birth and death rates of cells are modelled through clonal expansion and tumour formation. This model has been applied to human epidemiological data on retinoblastoma and to animal data on kidney and liver tumours in the 2-acetylaminofluorene 'mega mouse' study, bladder cancer in saccharin-exposed rats, rat lung tumours following radiation exposure, rat liver tumours following benzo[*a*]pyrene exposure, and mouse liver tumours following chlordane exposure (Cohen and Ellwein 1990; Moolgavkar and Luebeck 1990; National Research Council Committee on Risk Assessment Methodology 1993). Kohn *et al.* (1993) and Anderson (1983) used physiologically based toxicokinetic and biologically based dose–response information to improve dioxin risk assessment. EPA relied on *Ah* receptor binding in its dioxin risk reassessment (EPA 1994*b*, 2000).

Development of biologically based dose–response models for endpoints other than cancer are limited. Several approaches are being explored in developmental toxicity, utilizing cell cycle kinetics, enzyme activity, litter effects, and cytotoxicity as critical endpoints (Faustman *et al.* 1989, 1999; Shuey *et al.* 1994; Leroux *et al.* 1995; Lewandowski *et al.* 1998; Bartell and Faustman 1998). Unfortunately, there is a lack of specific, quantitative biological information for most toxicants and for most endpoints.

Exposure analysis

Exposure assessment is a crucial element of the risk assessment process, because there is no risk in the absence of exposure. Careful assessment of sources, pathways, environmental transformations, routes of entry, time course of exposure, total exposure from all sources and activities, and translation from ambient levels to target tissue effective dose is essential for exposure assessment. A good example is the work of the Electric Power Research Institute (**EPRI**) on emissions from electric utility boilers (EPRI 1994; Risk Commission 1997; Cullen and Frey 1999). Multiple chemical exposures and chemical–physical–biological agent interactions (Mumtaz *et al.* 1993) and exposure-specific sources of uncertainty (Bailar 1991) still need to be addressed.

The key step in making an exposure assessment is determining what exposure pathways are relevant for the risk scenario under development. The subsequent steps quantitate and sum these pathway-specific exposures for calculation of the overall exposure. The EPA has published guidelines for determining such exposures (EPA 1989*a*,*b*, 1992). Such calculations can include an estimation of total exposures for a specified population, as well as calculation of exposure for highly exposed individuals. The use of a hypothetical maximally exposed individual is no longer favoured in exposure assessment, owing to its extremely conservative assumptions at each step of the estimation. High end exposure estimates and theoretical upper-bound estimates are preferred (Risk Commission 1997).

High end exposure estimates are designed to represent 'a plausible estimate' of exposure of individuals in the upper 90th percentile of the exposure distribution. Theoretical upper-bound estimates are designed to represent exposures at a level that exceeds the exposures experienced by all individuals in the exposure distribution and are calculated by assuming limits for all exposure variables. In contrast, a calculation for individuals exposed at levels near the middle of the exposure distribution is a central estimate. The Risk Commission (1997) recommended use of the high end exposure estimates. A lifetime average daily dose is calculated for illustration in Table 6. In this example an exposure calculation to yield a central estimate and an high end exposure estimate for a potential dioxin exposure from recreational fish is given (EPA 1994 *b*). These estimates differ in the estimates for the amount of fish ingested, the contamination level in the fish, and the frequency of eating meals of recreationally captured fish. Obviously such estimates would differ even more if the full range of potential toxicant containment levels were used. Modelling and utilizing better estimates for the distribution of containment levels is a major focus of exposure assessment research. Subjective uncertainty distributions and Monte Carlo composite analyses of parameter uncertainty are prominent methods, as described elsewhere (National Research Council 1994; Cullen and Frey 1999; Eastman and Omenn 2001). These approaches can provide a reality check which is useful for generating more realistic exposure estimates.

Several endpoint-specific exposure considerations need to be mentioned. In general, estimates of cancer risk use averages over a lifetime. In a few cases, short-term exposure limits are required (for example, ethylene oxide (**EtO**)) and characterization of short, but high levels of exposure are required. In these cases exposures are not averaged over the lifetime. With developmental toxicity it is assumed that a single exposure can be sufficient to produce an adverse developmental effect and there is time-dependent specificity of many adverse developmental outcomes (EPA 1991). In fact, both total exposure (as represented by area under the curve in pharmacokinetic studies) and peak exposures can play significant parts in determining response to developmental toxicants. A recent study with EtO has confirmed that exposure concentration times length of exposure as proposed by Haber's law does not hold for comparing developmental toxicity potencies (Weller *et al.* 1999). Thus, daily doses are used rather than lifetime weighted averages.

By using Monte Carlo based approaches to deal with variability and uncertainty in exposure assessment, EPA is gradually replacing single-point estimates. Finley *et al.* (1994) and Cullen and Frey (1999)

Table 6 Exposure scenarios for dioxin via ingestion of contaminated recreational fish

Central exposure estimate[a]

$$\text{LADD} = \frac{(3 \times 10^{-9}\ \text{mg dioxin/g fish}) \times (150\ \text{g fish/meal}) \times (3\ \text{meals/year}) \times (1.0\ \text{contact/fraction}) \times (70\ \text{years/lifetime})}{(70\ \text{kg body weight}) \times (70\ \text{years/lifetime}) \times (365\ \text{days/year})}$$

$\text{LADD} = 5.3 \times 10^{-11}$ mg/kg/day

High end exposure estimate[b]

$\text{LADD} = 1.2 \times 10^{-9}$ mg/kg/day

LADD, lifetime average daily dose (EPA 1994*d*).

[a]Daily ingestion is calculated using 3 ppt for dioxin level in fish tissue, 150 g of fish consumed per meal, for three meals per year, averaged over 365 days/year. The rate of ingestion for central estimates is 1.2 g of fish per day.

[b]The high end exposure estimate uses 200 g of fish per meal for 10 meals per year and 15 ppt for dioxin contaminant level in the fish tissue based on a study downstream from 104 pulp mills. The rate of ingestion for this high end exposure estimate is 4.1 g of fish per day.

provide useful information and guidance on these probabilistic techniques in exposure assessment. The EPA provides an excellent on-line summary of the available statistical data on factors for human exposure assessment to support such assessments (http://www.epa.gov/ORD/WebPubs/exposure/front.pdf).

An example of the types of specific information available in the handbook (EPA 1997) is given in Table 7 about age-specific tap water intake. The handbook provides data for drinking water, food consumption, soil ingestion, inhalation rates, dermal absorption, product use, and human activity patterns. Such age-specific distributions for soil ingestion rates, inhalation rates, body weights, skin surface area, soil-on-skin adherence, tap water ingestion, fish consumption, residential occupancy, and occupational tenure, can be refined with additional data and can replace point estimates.

The EPA is also dealing with several new issues for exposure assessment as a result of the Food Quality Protection Act of 1996, which required consideration of both aggregate and cumulative exposures. Aggregate exposures refer to the total exposures for a single substance. Good examples are the cross-media exposure analyses that are available for lead and mercury. Cumulative exposures refer to the total exposures to a group of compounds, for example total organophosphate pesticides via all food routes. EPA is developing guidelines for determining not only aggregate and cumulative exposures but also aggregate and cumulative risk estimates. To assess cumulative effects from such exposures EPA is identifying and categorizing pesticides that act by a common mode of action (EPA 1998 *d*; ILSI 1999).

Variation in susceptibility

Both toxicology and epidemiology have been slow to recognize the marked variation in susceptibility among humans and the need to pay attention to outliers. Assay results and toxicokinetic modelling generally utilize means and standard deviations, or even standard errors of the mean, making the range seem smaller. In occupational and environmental medicine, physicians are often asked, 'Why me, Doc?' when they inform the patient that hazards on the job might explain a clinical problem. The EPA and Occupational Safety and Health Administration are expected, under the Clean Air Act and the Occupational Safety and Health Act, to promulgate standards that protect the most susceptible subgroups or individuals in the population. By focusing investigations on the most susceptible individuals, there might be a better chance of elucidating the underlying mechanisms (Omenn *et al.* 1990; Eaton *et al.* 1998). Host factors that influence susceptibility to environmental exposures are several: genetic traits (including sex and age), pre-existing diseases, behavioural traits (including most importantly, smoking), co-existing exposures, medications/vitamins, and protective measures (including respirators, gloves, and other barriers). Genetic studies are of two kinds.

1. Investigations of the effects of chemicals and radiation on the genes and chromosomes, which constitute 'genetic toxicology': tests measure evidence of mutations (Ames test, and adduct formation between chemicals and DNA or between chemicals and proteins), chromosomal aberrations, sister chromatid exchange, DNA repair, and oncogen activation.
2. Ecogenetic studies, identifying inherited variation in susceptibility (predisposition and resistance) to specific exposures, ranging across pharmaceuticals ('pharmacogenetics'), pesticides, inhaled pollutants, foods, food additives, sensory stimuli, allergic and sensitizing agents, and infectious agents.

Variation in susceptibility has been demonstrated for all of these kinds of external agents (Omenn and Motulsky 1978; National Research Council 1993; Nebert 1999). The ecogenetic variation may affect either the biotransformation systems (enzymes that activate or detoxify chemicals) or the sites of action in target issues. Examples of ecogenetic considerations for immune response are seen in humans with beryllium sensitivity. Ethical issues about how such ecogenetic information can be utilized in protecting worker health have been the focus of recent Department of Energy concerns (Bartell *et al.* 2000).

Extrapolation from rodents to humans

Some of the most important scientific advances in the past decade and some of the most promising work for the future provide mechanism-based information for the critical question of relating rodent results to human risks. For all endpoints, it is essential to know more about the similarities and differences across species. Detailed knowledge of molecular mechanisms and cellular and organ system responses can guide us to make better decisions about which chemicals that produce cancers, neurotoxicity, birth defects, or other adverse effects in rodents really represent significant risks of doing the same in humans. Nearly all of our predictions about carcinogenicity risks for humans are based on the results from lifetime rodent bioassays. These

Table 7 Example of exposure factor handbook information: drinking water intake

Age group	Intake(ml/kg per day)		Intake (ml/kg per day)	
	Mean	10th–90th percentiles	Mean	10th–90th percentiles
Infants (<1 year)	302	0–649	43.5	0–101.8
Children (1–10 years)	736	286–1294	35.5	12.5–64.4
Teens (11–19 years)	965	353–1701	18.2	6.5–32.3
Adults (20–64 years)	1366	559–2268	19.9	8.0–33.7
Adults (64+ years)	1459	751–2287	21.8	10.9–34.7
All ages	1193	423–2092	22.6	8.2–39.8

Source: Ershow and Cantor (1989); EPA (1997).

bioassays are hardly themselves a 'gold standard', given their statistical and biological limitations and the observation that congruence of results between rats and mice is only 70 per cent (Lave *et al.* 1988; Haseman and Lockhart 1993). It is unlikely that rodent–human congruence would be higher. EPA's revised cancer risk assessment guidelines (EPA 1996*b*) created a new category of animal carcinogens not likely to be predictive for human cancer risk. As summarized by McClain (1994) and the Risk Commission (1997), we now can cite several rodent carcinogenic responses that are candidates for no similar effect in humans (Table 8).

Briefly, the male rat kidney has been demonstrated to respond with a nephropathy mediated by an α_2-microglobulin for which there is no significant counterpart in humans or in other animals. The EPA action has recognized this distinction. The thyroid and other hormone-dependent tumours in rodents reflect marked species differences in the stimulating and feedback systems; sustained excessive levels of thyroid-stimulating hormone and lack of serum thyroid-binding globulin are the key elements in the hyperplasia and tumours of the rat thyroid. The incidence of spontaneous thyroid follicular cell neoplasia is also much higher in rats in the laboratory (e.g. Fischer 344) and among animals in endemic areas of iodine deficiency where many people have goitres, but thyroid cancer is rarely found in humans at these sites (EPA 1998*c*). Local necrosis and reactive hyperplasia in the bladder and in the forestomach represent responses to high local concentrations of the cytotoxic agent. On the other hand, many chemicals do cause tumours or other adverse effects in other parts of the body when administered (conveniently) by gavage, so the point here applies only to those chemicals whose effects are limited to the local point of application. Lung tumours have occurred with a variety of essentially inert particles, including titanium dioxide and carbon black, when the clearance capacity is markedly exceeded. The mouse liver cancer picture is considerably more complicated, with half a dozen different mechanisms, some of which seem to have definite counterparts in humans. High-dose mechanisms, involving induction of peroxisomes, cytotoxicity, and microsomal enzyme induction, seem much less likely to represent a significant risk in humans.

Information resources

There has been a figurative explosion of toxicology information now available on-line. HazDat can be accessed through the world-wide web by using the following address: http://www.atsdr.cdc.gov/hazdat.html. This database contains information on hazardous substance releases and contaminants, as well as over 160 public health statements from the Agency for Toxic Substances and Disease Registry chemical-specific toxicology profiles. EXTOXNET (http://ace.orst.edu/info/extoxnet/faqs/extoxnet.htm) provides information on the environmental chemistry and toxicology of pesticides, food additives, natural toxicants, and environmental contaminants. It is a product of an *ad hoc* consortium of university toxicologists and environmental chemists.

Other key sources of information for toxicologists are available through large databases such as RTECS, Toxline, and Medline. Scientific publications from the International Agency for Research on Cancer (**IARC**) are useful as is their website at http://depts.washington.edu/irarc/index.html. The EPA provides health hazard information on over 500 chemicals and includes the most current oral RfDs, inhalation RfCs, and carcinogen unit risk estimates (q_1*) on the Integrated Risk Information System (IRIS); however, there are complaints about long lags in updating IRIS information. IRIS can be accessed at http://www.epa.gov/iris/. For Risk Commission documents, use www.riskworld.com.

Table 8 Rodent carcinogenic responses not likely to apply in humans

Tumour site	Illustrative chemical agents
Male rat kidney	D-Limonene, unleaded gasoline
Male bladder	Saccharin, nitrilotriacetic acid
Rat thyroid	Ethyl bis-dithiocarbamate (EBDC) fungicides, goitrogens
Forestomach only (after gavage)	Butyl hydroxyanisole (BHA), propionic acid, ethyl acrylate
Lung	Various particles
Mouse liver	Certain classes of liver carcinogens

Based on Risk Commission (1997), Vol. II, p. 65, and McClain (1994).

Integrating qualitative and quantitative aspects of risk assessment: classification schemes

Qualitative assessment of hazard information should include consideration of the concordance of toxicological findings across species and target organs, of consistency across duplicate experimental conditions, and of adequacy of the experiments to detect the adverse endpoints of interest.

The National Toxicology Program uses several categories in its biennial report on carcinogens. The National Toxicology Program's evaluation guidelines allow for categories of 'known to be human carcinogens,' as well as 'reasonably anticipated to be human carcinogens' where there is limited evidence of carcinogenicity in humans and/or sufficient evidence of carcinogenicity in animals. Sufficient evidence in animals can include dose-related increases in malignant or combined malignant and benign neoplasms in multiple species, tissue sites, and/or by multiple routes of exposure. Also important to the 'sufficient' category are unusual tumours or tumours occurring at an early stage of onset or at different sites.

Similar classifications have been used for both the animal and human evidence categories by the EPA and IARC: sufficient, limited, inadequate, and no evidence (EPA 1994*b*) and sufficient, limited, inadequate, evidence suggesting lack of carcinogenicity, and no evidence (IARC 1994*a*). Table 9 presents IARC's list of human carcinogens, of which 31 are chemical, 18 are pharmaceutical (mostly cancer chemotherapy agents), and 13 are manufacturing processes (IARC 1999). Although differing group number or letter categories are used, striking similarities exist between the EPA and IARC approaches for the overall weight of evidence in carcinogenicity classification schemes. Risk assessment guidelines for carcinogenic substances include relabelled categories described as 'known', 'likely', 'not likely' to be carcinogenic to humans (EPA 1996*b*), and 'cannot evaluate'.

So far we have discussed approaches for evaluating cancer endpoints. Similar weight of evidence approaches for reproductive risk assessment have been proposed. The Institute for Evaluating Health Risks defined an 'evaluative process' by which reproductive and developmental toxicity data can be evaluated consistently and

Table 9 Chemicals and related exposures with sufficient evidence for carcinogenicity in humans

Chemicals	Pharmaceuticals	Manufacturing processes
Aflatoxins	Analgesic mixtures w/phenacetin	Acid mists
Alcoholic beverages	Azathioprine	Aluminium
4-Amino-biphenyl		Auramine
Arsenic and arsenic compounds	Chlornaphazine	
Asbestos	Chlorambucil	Boot and shoe manufacturing
	CCNU (nitrosoureas)	
Benzene	Cyclosporin	Coal gasification
Benzidine	Cyclophosphamide	Coke production
Beryllium and beryllium compounds		
Betel quid with tobacco	Diethylstilbestrol	Furniture/cabinet making
Bis(chloromethyl)ether		
	Melphalan	Haematite (radon)
Cadmium and cadmium compounds	Methoxsalen + UV radiation	
Chloromethyl methyl ether	MOPP (alkylating combinations)	Iron/steel founding
Chromium VI compounds	Myleran	Isopropyl alcohol
Coal tar/pitches		
	Oestrogen (steroidal/non-steroidal)	Magenta
Erionite	Oestrogen (multiple applications)	
Ethylene oxide	Oral contraceptives	Painting
Mineral oils	Tamoxifen	Rubber
Mustard gas	Thiotepa	
	Treosulphan	
2-Naphthylamine		
Nickel and nickel compounds		
Salted fish		
Silica		
Shale oil		
Soot		
Talc with asbestiform fibres		
Tobacco products		
Tobacco smoke		
TCDD(dioxin)		
Vinyl chloride		
Wood dust		

Source: IARC (1999), Table 1, pp. 55–74.

integrated to ascertain their relevance for human health risk assessment (Moore *et al.* 1995).

Ethylene oxide: an example of chemical specific risk assessment

EtO is a colourless gas that is used as a chemical intermediate in the manufacture of industrial products, such as ethylene glycol, polyester fibres, and detergents. EtO is also used as a pesticide fumigant. Over 75 000 hospital workers are exposed via its use as an antimicrobial sterilant. EtO is one of the 25 chemicals of highest production volume in the United States, with over 2.5 million tons produced per year (IARC 1994*b*). There is evidence from animal tests and human exposure studies that EtO is a carcinogen, mutagen, reproductive toxicant, and neurotoxicant. We will focus on an assessment of its carcinogenic effects. EtO has been regulated under the Occupational Safety and Health Administration, Consumer Product Safety Commission, EPA, and FDA statutes (Table 3).

Short-term assay information

EtO has been shown, like many reactive epoxides, to be a direct-acting (genotoxic) mutagen. It has been evaluated in bacterial, plant, *Drosophila* germ cells, and rodent and human cell assays. It causes chromosomal aberrations and point mutations. In fact, EtO is frequently used as a positive control in assays of other potentially mutagenic agents.

Rodent bioassays

All three rodent bioassays conducted with EtO by inhalation found dose related increases in tumours in both rats and mice, both male and female. Increased rates for mononuclear cell leukaemia, peritoneal mesothelioma, mixed brain tumours, alveolar/bronchiolar carcinomas and adenomas, lymphomas, papillary cystadenoma of the harderian gland, uterine adenocarcinomas, and mammary gland tumours were observed (Snellings *et al.* 1984*a,b*). Exposure levels included 0, 10, 33, 50 and 100 ppm for 6 to 7 h/day for 5 days per week for 2 years.

Epidemiology

Published studies of EtO-exposed workers are positive for cancer risk. Of the eight studies of chemical workers exposed to EtO, five found excesses of lymphatic and haematopoietic cancer but only two were significant. The standardized mortality rates for chemical plant workers were approximately nine for stomach and oesophageal cancers and leukaemia (Hogstedt *et al* . 1986). This study, as well as others on chemical plant workers, was complicated by exposure to multiple chemicals besides EtO and by relatively small cohort sizes (700 to 3000 participants). There are four studies of sterilant workers. Studies of 20 000 EtO sterilizer-exposed workers found significant increases in haematopoietic cancers in male workers (Steenland *et al.* 1991); these increases might have been complicated by other exposure factors such as human immunodeficiency infection. The three other smaller studies of sterilant workers showed non-significant increases in lymphatic and haematopoietic cancer. Molecular biomarker studies correlating EtO exposure, levels of hydroxyethyl adducts in haemoglobin, and cancer incidence failed to establish a direct correlation of adducts and cancer but did show a good dose–response relationship for the adducts and EtO exposures (Hagmar *et al.* 1991; Walker *et al.* 1993; Farmer and Shuker 1999; Wu *et al.* 1999).

Qualitative assessment

The EPA has concluded that EtO is a probable human carcinogen (EPA-B2 classification). They determined that there is sufficient animal evidence, but limited to inadequate human evidence, on which to base this qualitative assessment. Because EtO has been shown to have a genotoxic mode of action to produce its carcinogenicity, EPA has used EtO as an example in their revised cancer guidelines (EPA 1999). IARC has upgraded its overall evaluation of EtO from class 2A to class 1 (carcinogenic to humans) based on other data that support its carcinogenicity and mechanisms (IARC 1999).

Exposure assessment

Occupational exposures to EtO are primarily via inhalation. For chemical plant workers, a 7 h/day, 5 days/week, 50 weeks/year exposure scenario is appropriate. An appropriate model of exposure for EtO sterilizer workers in hospitals should include multiple short-term exposure peaks spread throughout the work day, reflecting cycles of EtO sterilizer operation. Both the time-weighted average and short-term exposure limits are believed to be particularly important for genotoxic carcinogens such as EtO, as DNA repair systems are known to be saturable at higher exposure levels.

Kinetics

EtO is rapidly absorbed through the respiratory route and is uniformly distributed throughout the body. The half-life for EtO in humans is approximately 60 min and 12 to 13 min in rats and mice respectively. Two key inactivational pathways have been identified, glutathione conjugation and hydrolysis to ethylene glycol and subsequent metabolism to CO_2. EtO produces both DNA and protein alkylation. At high dose levels EtO is hypothesized to deplete glutathione and produce non-linear dose–effect relationships (Brown *et al.* 1998).

Susceptible populations

Because EtO is a genotoxic carcinogen, individuals with compromised DNA repair pathways would be at greater risk than other individuals. Other susceptible populations include the unborn children of workers. EtO is already a reactive epoxide, not requiring activation; however, it does undergo inactivation via two pathways for which ecogenetic differences could exist.

Quantitative risk assessment and standard setting

The Occupational Safety and Health Administration has used the rodent mesothelioma and leukaemia data to model upper-bound estimates on risk (Snellings *et al.* 1984*a,b*; National Toxicology Program 1987). A q_1* (upper 95 per cent confidence limit on cancer risk) for EtO was set at 3.4×10^{-1}/mg EtO per kg body weight per day based on the EPA's evaluation of the study by Snellings *et al.* (1984*a*) of the incidence of mononuclear cell leukaemia and brain tumours in female rats. The current Occupational Safety and Health Administration time-weighted average for EtO is 1 ppm exposure averaged over an 8-h day. The initially proposed short-term exposure limit value of 5 ppm was not upheld by the courts.

Regulatory risk management/control of exposures

One of the key regulatory needs to improve the safe use of EtO in occupational settings is the establishment of the short-term exposure limit values. Our review of the options supports the establishment of a 15 min exposure limit that must not exceed five times the 8-h time-weighted average. Improved ventilation controls for the EtO sterilization units in hospitals can continue to offer an excellent solution for the safe use of this sterilization process. The Occupational Safety and Health Administration currently provides several recommended engineering options. These include use of non-recirculating exhaust hoods built directly over the sterilizer door, a capture box built over the floor drains for the sterilizers, and extended vacuum purges of the sterilizer chamber with 'door-locked' phases that prevent premature entry.

Substitutes

Few of the alternatives to EtO sterilization are effective or appropriate. Chemical disinfecting (glutaraldehyde is the agent of choice) requires long soaking times (11 h) for comparable levels of sterilization, costs more due to personnel time in processing, and results in alternative exposures. Other less favourable alternatives do not provide adequate sterilization.

Comparing international approaches to carcinogen risk assessment

For many years there has been an information-sharing process aimed at harmonization of chemical testing regimes and clinical trials methodologies, so that data might be accepted in multiple countries that are members of the OECD. The United Nations Conference on the Environment in Rio de Janeiro, Brazil, in 1992 established harmonization of risk assessment as one of its goals, with a co-ordinating role for the International Programme on Chemical Safety. The negotiation in 1994 of the General Agreement on Trade and Tariffs and establishment of a World Trade Organization made harmonization of various aspects of testing, risk assessment, labelling, registration, and standards potentially important elements in trade, not just in regulatory science. Much progress has been achieved for pharmaceuticals (D'Arcy and Harron 1998.)

Moolenaar (1994) summarized the carcinogen risk assessment methodologies used by various countries as a basis for regulatory actions. He tabulated the risk characterization, carcinogen identification, risk extrapolation, and chemical classification schemes of the EPA, the United States Public Health Service, the WHO/IARC, the American Conference of Governmental and Industrial Hygienists, Australia, the European Union, Germany, the Netherlands, Norway, and Sweden. The approach of the EPA to estimate an upper bound to human risk is unique; all other countries estimate human risk values based on the expected incidence of cancer from the exposure under review. The United Kingdom follows a case-by-case approach to risk evaluations for both genotoxic and non-genotoxic carcinogens, with no generic procedures. Denmark, the European Union, the United Kingdom, and the Netherlands all divide carcinogens into genotoxic and non-genotoxic agents and use different extrapolation procedures for each. Norway does not extrapolate data to low doses, using instead the TD_{50} to divide category I carcinogens into tertiles by probable potency. The United Kingdom, the European Union, and The Netherlands all treat non-genotoxic chemical carcinogens as threshold toxicants; a NOAEL and safety factors are used to set acceptable daily intake values. It may be time for the United States to consider applying the benchmark dose method to non-genotoxic carcinogens, instead of the linearized multistage model; towards this goal we are encouraged by the proposals in the EPA's revised cancer guidelines (EPA 1996 *b*).

The OECD countries have a well-established process of comparing economies of member countries for various benchmark parameters. An effort has been initiated to stimulate similar thinking about sentinel measures for comparisons of country performance in environmental protection (Lykke 1992; OECD 1996). The United Nations Conferences in Rio de Janeiro and Kyoto, together with other international forums, have sought an international consensus on the reduction of emissions of global importance (carbon dioxide) and regional importance (sulphur dioxide).

The United States Commission on Risk Assessment and Risk Management (Risk Commission)

The 1990 Clean Air Act Amendments (Title III) established an entirely new program to control 189 named hazardous air pollutants from point sources through promulgation and implementation of technology-based standards. These standards were based on determination of the maximum available control technology for each category of point sources. During the previous 20 years only seven substances had been regulated under this section of the law (vinyl chloride, asbestos, benzene, radionuclides, mercury, arsenic, and beryllium) using chemical-by-chemical, risk-based analyses, largely because of the statutory requirement to determine a no-effect level and then set the standard sufficiently lower to assure an 'ample margin of safety'. For carcinogens, the no-effect level was assumed to be zero. Congress further mandated that EPA determine whether any unacceptable residual risks to health from hazardous air pollutants remain after the maximum available control technology has been implemented.

The National Academy of Sciences was called upon to review the methods used by EPA to determine carcinogenic risks and non-carcinogenic risks, as well. The report *Science and Judgment in Risk Assessment* (National Research Council 1994) reflects the interplay of scientific methods, variability and uncertainty, and social, political, cultural, and economic values. That report was a major input to the Risk Commission mandated by the 1990 Amendments 'to make a full investigation of the policy implications and appropriate uses of risk assessment and risk management under various federal laws to prevent cancer and other chronic human health effects which may result from exposure to hazardous substances'. The Commission operated from 1994 to 1997 and was composed of three members appointed by the President, six by the leaders of the Congress, and one by the National Academy of Sciences, with G.S. Omenn as the chairman.

The Risk Commission made general recommendations about the uses and limitations of risk assessment, uncertainty analysis, economic analysis, peer review, and risk management decision-making, and specific recommendations for the various regulatory agencies and their major programs (Risk Commission 1997). The Commission recognized that it is time to modify the traditional approaches to assessing and reducing risks that have relied upon a chemical-by-chemical, medium-by-medium, risk-by-risk strategy. The output had become too focused on assumption-laden mathematical estimates of small risks associated with exposure to individual chemicals, rather than the overall goal of improved health status through the reduction of significant risks. Thus, the Commission developed the Risk Management Framework shown in Fig. 1. The Framework embraces collaborative and early involvement of stakeholders; requires that a current or potential problem be put into a broader context of public health or ecological health; stimulates identification of the interdependence of multimedia problems; focuses on cumulative risks and on addressing the benefits, costs, and social, cultural, ethical, political, and legal dimensions of the risk reduction options.

The Commission highlighted the importance of mechanisms of toxicity, risks from microbial and radiation exposures (not just from chemicals), use of realistic scenarios in exposure assessments, attention to mixtures of chemicals and multiple interacting exposures. It endorsed extensive modelling of variability in exposures, and expressed reservations about excessive modelling of uncertainty (Goldstein 1995). It supported use of economic analyses, especially cost-effectiveness analysis, but not as the overriding determinant of risk management decisions.

For individual agencies of the United States government, the Commission presented a tiered approach to set priorities for the residual risk mandate on hazardous air pollutants, which will be implemented over the next 10 to 20 years, and recommended that these risks be considered in the context of risks associated with the same pollutants from other sources, other air pollutants (such as the ubiquitous 'criteria air pollutants'—sulphur dioxide, particles, nitrogen dioxide, hydrocarbons, ozone/photochemical oxidants, carbon monoxide, and lead), and other risks to the health of children and adults. Other recommendations addressed early determination of future land use for Superfund site clean-up objectives; comprehensive watershed management approaches for the Clean Water Act; risk assessment improvements adopted in the 1996 Safe Drinking Water Act; streamlined processes for developing permissible exposure limits for air contaminants in the workplace; modification of the 'Delaney Clause' covering food additives to a standard of reasonable certainty of no harm for all population groups, which was adopted in the 1996 Food Quality and Protection Act; endorsed international harmonization of risk assessment and clinical trial protocols for pharmaceuticals and restoration of the authority of the FDA to require scientific evidence to support health claims for dietary supplements; proposed risk-based approaches to priority-setting and budget-making for clean-up of contaminated sites at federal facilities; and urged better control of microbial risks in foods and drinking water. In its reports, the Commission presented numerous examples of stakeholder involvement (volume I) and of risk assessment and risk management outcomes (volume II). These recommendations have had a large influence in the Congress and in federal and state agencies, as well as international forums (HSE 2000).

Comparative analyses of risks and perceptions of risk

This aspect of risk assessment, risk communication, and risk management is so logical that it may be surprising to learn that comparisons of risks are extremely controversial. Public health officials practice comparative risk assessment, at least intuitively, on a routine basis when deciding how to allocate their own time, their staff's time, and other resources. They must make judgements about what and how to advise their local communities about potential and definite risks. They must anticipate the question: 'Compared with what?'

In fact, most people regularly compare risks of alternative activities—in their jobs, in recreational pursuits, in interpersonal interactions, and in investments. Since 1993, members of the United States Congress have pressed for the systematic use by federal regulatory agencies of comparisons of similar and dissimilar risks. The aim is to make the benefits and costs of health, safety, and environmental protection actions more explicit, more comprehensible, and more cost-effective. However, determining how best to conduct comparative risk analyses and do so efficiently has proved difficult, due to the great variety of health and environmental benefits, the uncertainties of dollar estimates of benefits and costs, and the different distributions of benefits and costs across the population.

A new concept, 'environmental justice', has emerged to reflect the ethical guidance that poor, disenfranchised neighbourhoods should be protected as much as well-to-do suburban neighbourhoods (Rios *et al.* 1993; Risk Commission 1997; Institute of Medicine 1999). In fact, the poor may need greater protection due to their coexisting higher risk factors for poor pregnancy outcomes, impaired growth and development, smoking-related cancers, asthma, and lead toxicity, among other health problems. On the other hand, the compelling need to overcome poor rates of prenatal care and childhood immunization, poor housing, lack of education, violence, and joblessness may make hypothetical or long-term estimated risks from chemical pollutant exposures relatively less salient to these communities.

Several formal analyses to compare risks have been developed. One method estimates the contribution of a particular activity or exposure to deaths in the general population, combining reports of actual deaths and estimates of likely or worst-case effects of various risk factors. McGinnis and Foege (1993) compiled the 10 leading reported causes of death for the 2.1 million American deaths in 1990 and then listed the 'real causes of death', beginning with smoking (430 000 excess deaths), then poor diet and physical inactivity, then alcohol (Table 10). The message here is clear: almost one-half of deaths and a higher proportion of premature deaths are caused by preventable risk factors, mostly individual behaviours. They estimated 60 000 deaths per year in the United States from exposure to toxic substances.

Another approach determines the average estimated loss of life expectancy attributable to various causes (Crouch and Wilson 1982). For example, male smokers may lose an estimated 2250 days of life expectancy; persons 20 per cent overweight, 900 days; alcohol users, 130 days; persons of low socio-economic class, 700 days; and those impaired by occupational hazards, 30–300 days. Obviously, these are very rough categories and estimates. A third approach estimates the exposure required to increase the annual death rate by one death per million deaths. Estimates for different exposures include smoking 1.4 cigarettes daily (heart disease and cancers), drinking 0.5 litres of wine daily (cirrhosis of the liver), or eating 40 tablespoons of peanut butter contaminated with aflatoxin daily (liver cancer). Finally, the World Bank and many others are now using disability-adjusted life years (World Bank 1993).

All these approaches have serious limitations because of inadequate information on the variability of the statistics, uncertainty about the size of the population at risk due to specific exposures, complexities of exposures, multiple additional risk factors, and complications aetiology of deaths and disabilities.

Table 10 Causes of death

Listed causes		'Real causes'	
Heart disease	720 000	Tobacco	400 000
Cancers	505 000	Diet/activity patterns	300 000
Cerebrovascular disease	144 000	Alcohol	100 000
'Accidents'	92 000	Microbial agents	90 000
Chronic lung disease	87 000	Toxic agents	60 000
Pneumonia and influenza	80 000	Firearms	35 000
Diabetes mellitus	48 000	Sexual behaviour	30 000
Suicide	31 000	Motor vehicles	25 000
Cirrhosis/liver disease	26 000	Illicit use of drugs	20 000
HIV infection	25 000		
Total US 1990	2 148 000	Total	1 060 000

Based on McGinnis and Foege (1993).

Individuals respond very differently to information about hazardous situations, as do societies. An event that is accepted by one individual may be unacceptable to another (Fischhoff 1981) (see also Chapter 8.9)). Understanding these behavioural responses is critical in developing risk management options. In a classic study, students, League of Women Voters members, active club members, and scientific experts were asked to rank 30 activities or agents in order of their annual contribution to deaths (Slovic *et al.* 1979; Morgan *et al.* 1992)). The lay groups all ranked motorcycles and handguns as high risks and vaccinations, home appliances, power mowers, and football as relatively safe. Club members viewed pesticides, spray cans, and nuclear power as safer than did other lay persons. Students ranked contraceptives and food preservatives as riskier and mountain climbing as safer than did the others. Meanwhile, experts ranked electric power, surgery, swimming, and X-rays as more risky, and nuclear power and police work as less risky, than did lay persons. There are also group differences in perceptions of risk from chemicals among toxicologists according to their work in industry, academia, or government (Neil *et al.* 1994).

Psychological factors such as dread, perceived uncontrollability, and involuntary exposure interact with factors that represent the extent to which a hazard is familiar, observable, and 'essential' (Lowrance 1976; Morgan 1993). Public demand for government regulations often focuses on involuntary exposures and unfamiliar hazards, such as radioactive waste, electromagnetic fields, asbestos insulation, and genetically modified crops and foods. People's perceptions may be related to technical and emotional grounds; Sandman (1993) classified these aspects as 'hazard' and 'outrage' respectively.

A different kind of risk comparison is conducted at the programme planning level across diverse types of risk. The EPA published a landmark review, *Unfinished Business*, in 1987, ranking EPA programmes in priority for more investment, based on the then current funding levels and technical progress. In 1990 EPA's Science Advisory Board followed up with *Reducing Risks* , which categorized the relative risks of cancers, non-cancer endpoints, and various ecological impacts (EPA 1990). Meanwhile, there have been many comparative risk analysis forums or projects in various states. Vermont and Colorado had particularly productive experiences with public involvement. Washington State generated a public process for 'Washington 2010'. A mayoral task force produced 'Seattle's Environmental Priorities', which has guided budget decisions and public understanding. A highly publicized process in California yielded a draft report just before the 1994 state elections, which remained in limbo for many months due to political posturing about environmental justice and social welfare aspects mentioned prominently in the report; its array of high, medium, and low priorities among health and ecological risks has been utilized in state planning. Local governments, faced with unfunded regulatory mandates and limited budgets, are seeking rational and cost-effective options. One approach is the preparation of specific 'community risk profiles (Wernick 1995). Table 11 lists some of the underlying philosophies of regulation.

Economic analyses

The role of economic analysis in regulatory decision-making is controversial and highly political. Public health advocates are generally suspicious that economic analysis places too much emphasis on assigning dollar values to aspects of health and the environment that are difficult, if not impossible, to quantify. Furthermore, the equity implications of policies and regulations may be neglected. For example, if a decision decreases the welfare of the poor and increases the welfare of the wealthy, but the benefit to the wealthy outweighs the loss to the poor (in dollars, not per cent of income), quantitative benefit/cost analyses might show the policy to yield an improvement in aggregate social welfare. Another problem arises from the frequent use of point estimates for benefits and costs. Like the results of risk assessments, economic analyses involve multiple assumptions, choices among data and models, and very substantial uncertainty. As emphasized by the Risk Commission (1997), economic analyses require transparency, peer review, and stakeholder participation just as much as do risk assessments.

In the United States, some statutes (Table 4) require consideration of costs and benefits (pharmaceuticals, pesticides), others explicitly exclude their consideration (Clean Air Act), and others are silent. Morgenstern (1997) concluded that economic analysis so far has played a minor part, primarily because the scientific information on which benefits analyses were based was so weak that the credibility and influence of the economic analyses were undermined.

Table 11 Philosophies of regulation

1. Regulation of only proven human toxicants: 'count the bodies'
2. Best available technology approach: engineering solutions
3. Protect all citizens with equal effectiveness: uniform risk/equal rights
4. Cost-effectiveness or cost-benefit
5. De minimis
6. If any evidence suggests harm, eliminate hazard: 'Delaney' approach; extreme Precautionary Principle

Nevertheless, there is broad agreement that information about the incremental costs and benefits associated with particular options for a regulatory decision can serve the public interest (Arrow *et al.* 1996*a*; Risk Commission 1997). Cost-effectiveness analyses are particularly helpful, as they begin with specification of the public health or ecological regulatory goal (without conversion to monetary values) and then explore and compare the methods of achieving that goal to identify the least costly one. For example, if the health-based goal is to reduce the current ambient ozone standard to 0.10 ppm, cost-effectiveness analysis could be used to help choose among options with different technologies, different costs, and different probabilities of success. Tengs *et al.* (1995) used cost-effectiveness analysis to compare the costs of many different life-saving medical, public health, and environmental regulatory interventions against a common measure, the estimated years of life saved. A similar approach can be used, with fewer assumptions and extrapolations, to assess different means of achieving intermediate regulatory goals. For example, there might be several alternative strategies to reduce automobile exhaust emissions as part of a larger ozone control programme. One might rank the cost of those alternatives per unit of emissions reduced.

Risk communication (see also Chapter 8.9)

Public health agencies and officials regularly engage in communication with the public and with public officials and private sector parties about health risks. It is a primary mission of public health to investigate the causes of health problems and the ways to reduce the incidence and consequences of such problems. Actions must include environmental controls, such as protection of air, water, and food from chemical and microbiological contamination and protection against radioactive exposures in medical care, industry, and the general environment. For inactive (abandoned) hazardous waste sites, the federal Superfund Law requires a public health advisory statement for each of the more than 1300 National Priorities List Sites in the United States. At federal facilities sites, an organized approach has been developed by the United States Department of Energy Environmental Restoration and Waste Management Program, involving local citizens, Indian Nations, and environmental organizations, to deal with the overlapping array of federal and state statutes, regulations, and programmes (Omenn 1994; Boiko *et al.* 1996; van Belle *et al.* 1996).

Actions also must include health education to promote healthy behaviours and reduce unhealthy behaviours—smoking, violence, alcohol and other drug abuse, sexually transmitted diseases, physical inactivity, and social isolation. Clinical preventive services of immunizations, counselling, and screening are important medical contributions to individual patients and public health services are important to the health status of communities. Finally, communication about risks and risk reduction must mobilize public policy in the form of incentives and disincentives for health promotion and against pollution and unhealthy behaviours. In the United States, reports from all Surgeons General since 1979 have sustained a campaign called Healthy People, which embraces health protection, health promotion, and clinical preventive services (Oberle *et al.* 1994). Local communities increasingly take part in that risk communication/health promotion process (Oberle *et al* . 1994). Their knowledge of exposure pathways in the past and of apparent health and ecological effects can redirect the technical assessments. Their view on future uses of contaminated sites can be crucial to deciding how stringent must be the clean up. All of these programmes must be integrated to achieve a reinforcing strategy for disease and injury prevention and for health promotion (Risk Commission 1997; National Research Council 1996).

Conclusions

The scientific community has come a long way in the past 25 years in expanding the science base, in better defining our questions about assumptions and models, and in helping regulators to make risk-based decisions for the protection of human health and the environment. The way ahead should be an acceleration of knowledge from the public health sciences including toxicogenomics (Omenn 2000). We expect important inputs from our constituencies—legislators, regulators, manufacturers, environmentalists, media, and affected communities—throughout the global commons.

References

Abbott, B.D., Harris, M.W., and Birnbaum, L.S. (1992). Comparisons of the effects of TCDD and hydrocortisone on growth factor expression provide insight into their interaction in the embryonic mouse palate. *Teratology*, **45**, 35–53.

Albert, R.E. (1994). Carcinogen risk assessment in the US Environmental Protection Agency. *Critical Reviews in Toxicology*, **24**, 75–85.

Allen, B.C., Kavlock, R.J., Kimmel, C.A., and Faustman, E.M. (1994*a*). Dose response assessments for developmental toxicity II. Comparison of generic benchmark dose estimates with NOAELs. *Fundamental and Applied Toxicology*, **23**, 487–95.

Allen, B.C., Kavlock, R.J., Kimmel, C.A., and Faustman, E.M. (1994*b*). Dose–response assessment for developmental toxicity, III. Statistical models. *Fundamental Applied Toxicology*, **23**, 496–509.

Ames, B.N. and Gold, L.S. (1990). Too many rodent carcinogens: mitogenesis increases mutagenesis. *Science*, **249**, 970–1.

Anderson, E.L. (1983). Quantitative approaches in use to assess cancer risk. *Risk Analysis*, **3**, 277–95.

Armitage, P. and Doll, R. (1957). A two-stage theory of carcinogenesis in relation to the age distribution of human cancer. *British Journal of Cancer*, **11**, 161–9.

Arrow K.J., *et al.* (1996*a*). Is there a role for benefit-cost analysis in environmental, health, and safety regulation? *Science*, **272**, 221–2.

Arrow K.J., *et al.* (1996*b*). Benefit-cost analysis in environmental, health, and safety regulation. A statement of principles.

Ashby, J. and Tennant, R.W. (1994). Prediction of rodent carcinogenicity of 44 chemicals: results. *Mutagenesis*, **9**, 7–15.

ATBC Cancer Prevention Study Group (1994). The effect of vitamin E and beta-carotene on the incidence of lung cancer and other cancers in male smokers. *New England Journal of Medicine*, 33**0**, 1029–35.

Atterwill, C.K., Johnston, H., and Thomas, S.M. (1992). Models for the *in vitro* assessment of neurotoxicity in the nervous system in relation to xenobiotic and neurotrophic factor-mediated events. *Neurotoxicology*, **13**, 39–54.

Auton, T.R. (1994). Calculation of benchmark doses from teratology data. *Regulatory Toxicology and Pharmacology*, **19**, 152–67.

Bailar, J.C., III (1991). Scientific inferences and environmental health problems. *Chance: New Directions for Statistics and Computing*, **4**, 27–38.

Barnes, D.G. and Dourson, M.J. (1988). Reference dose (RfD): description and use in health risk assessment. *Regulatory Toxicology and Pharmacology*, **8**, 471–86.

Barnes, D.G., *et al.* (1995). Benchmark dose workshop. *Regulatory Toxicology and Pharmacology*, **21**, 296–306.

Bartell, S.M. and Faustman, E.M. (1998). Comments on 'An approach for modeling noncancer dose responses with an emphasis on uncertainty' and 'A probabilistic framework for the reference dose (probabilistic RfD)'. *Risk Analysis*, **18**, 663–4.

Bartell, S.M., *et al.* (2000). Risk estimation and value-of-information analysis for three proposed genetic screening programs for chronic beryllium disease prevention. *Risk Analysis*, **20**, 87–99.

Boiko, P.E., *et al.* (1996). Who holds the stakes? A case study of stakeholder identification at two nuclear weapons production sites. *Risk Analysis*, **16**, 237–49.

Brown, C.C. (1984). High-to low-dose extrapolation in animals. In *Assessment and management of chemical risks* (ed. J.V. Rodricks and R.G. Tardiff), pp. 57–79. American Chemical Society, Washington, DC.

Brown, C.D., Asgharian, B., Turner, M.J., and Fennel, T.R. (1998). Ethylene oxide dosimetry in the mouse. *Toxicology and Applied Pharmacology*, **148**, 215–21.

Bucher, J.R., Potter, C.J., Goodman, J.L., Faustman, E.M., and Lucier, G.W. (1996). National Toxicology Program studies: principles of dose selection and applications to mechanistic based risk assessment. *Fundamental Applied Toxicology*, **31**, 1–8.

Calkins, D.R., Dixon, R.L., Gerber, C.R., Zarin, D., and Omenn, G.S. (1980). Identification, characterization, and control of potential human carcinogens: a framework for federal decision-making. *Journal of the National Cancer Institute*, **61**, 169–75.

Charnley, G. and Omenn, G.S. (1997). A summary of the findings and recommendations of the Commission on Risk Assessment and Risk Management (and accompanying papers prepared for the Commission). *Human and Ecological Risk Assessment*, **3**, 701–11.

Clewell, H.J., III, Gentry, P.R., and Gearhart, J.M. (1997). Investigation of the potential impact of benchmark dose and pharmacokinetic modeling in noncancer risk assessment. *Journal of Toxicology and Environmental Health*, **52**, 475–515.

Cohen, S.M. and Ellwein, L.B. (1990). Proliferative and genotoxic cellular effects in 2-acetylaminofluorene bladder and liver carcinogenesis: biological modeling of the ED_{01} study. *Toxicology and Applied Pharmacology*, **104**, 79–93.

Crouch, E.A.C. and Wilson, R. (1982). *Risk/benefit analysis*. Ballinger, Cambridge, MA.

Crump, K.S. (1980). An improved procedure for low-dose carcinogenic risk assessment from animal data. *Journal of Environmental Pathology and Toxicology*, **5**, 675–84.

Crump, K.S. (1984). A new method for determining allowable daily intakes. *Fundamental Applied Toxicology*, **4**, 854–71.

Cullen, A.C. and Frey, H.C. (1999). *Probabilistic techniques in exposure assessment: a handbook for dealing with variability and uncertainty in models and inputs*. Plenum Press, New York.

D'Arcy, P.F. and Harron, D.W.G. (eds). (1998). *Fourth International Conference on Harmonization*. Greystone Books, Northern Ireland.

Dourson, M.L. and DeRosa, C.T. (1991). The use of uncertainty factors in establishing safe levels of exposure. In *Statistics in toxicology* (ed. D. Krewski and C. Franklin), pp. 613–27. Gordon and Breach, New York.

Dourson, M.L. and Stara, J.F. (1983). Regulatory history and experimental support of uncertainty (safety factors). *Regulatory Toxicology and Pharmacology*, **3**, 224–38.

Dourson, M.L., Hertzberg, R.C., Hartung, R., and Blackburn, K. (1985). Novel methods for the estimation of acceptable daily intake.*Toxicology Industrial Health*, **1**, 23–41.

Eaton, D.L., Farin, F., Omiecinski, C.J., and Omenn, G.S. (1998). Genetic susceptibility. In *Environmental and Occupational Medicine* (3rd edn). (ed. W.N. Rom), pp. 209–21. Lippincott-Raven, Philadelphia.

Environmental Defense Fund (1997). *Toxic ignorance*. Environmental Defense Fund, New York.

EPA (1989*a*). *Risk assessment guidance for Superfund. Human health evaluation manual*, Part A. EPA Office of Policy Analysis, Washington, DC.

EPA (1989*b*). *Exposure factors handbook, final report*. EPA Office of Health and Environmental Assessment, Washington, DC.

EPA (1990). *Reducing risk: setting priorities and strategies for environmental protection*. EPA Science Advisory Board, Washington, DC.

EPA (1991). Guidelines for developmental toxicity risk assessment. *Federal Register*, **56**, 63798–826.

EPA (1992). Guidelines for exposure assessment. *Federal Register*, **57**, 22888–938.

EPA (1994*a*). *Guidelines for reproductive toxicity risk assessment*. EPA Office of Research and Development, Washington, DC.

EPA (1994*b*). *Health assessment document for 2,3,7,8-tetrachlorodibenzo-p-dioxin (TCDD) and related compounds*. Vols I–III. EPA Office of Research and Development, Washington, DC.

EPA (1994*c*). *Guidelines for carcinogen risk assessment (draft revisions)*. Office of Health and Environmental Assessment, Exposure Assessment Group, Washington, DC.

EPA (1994*d*). *Estimating exposure to dioxin-like compounds*. Office of Health and Environmental Assessment, Exposure Assessment Group, Washington, DC.

EPA (1996*a*). Proposed guidelines for ecological risk assessment. *Federal Register*, **61**, 47552.

EPA (1996*b*). *Risk assessment guidelines*. EPA Office of Research and Development, Washington, DC.

EPA (1997). *Aggregate exposure. Review document for the Scientific Avisory Panel.* SAP Public Docket, Washington, DC.

EPA (1998*a*). Endocrine disruptor screening program; proposed statement of policy. *Federal Register*, **63**, 71542–71568.

EPA (1998*b*). *Chemical hazard availability study*. EPA Office of Pollution Prevention and Toxics, Washington, DC.

EPA (1998*c*). *Assessment of thyroid follicular cell tumors*. EPA Office of Research and Development, Washington, DC.

EPA (1998*d*). Guidance for identifying pesticides that have a common mechanism of toxicity: notice of availability and solicitation of public comments. *Federal Register*, **63**, 42031–2.

EPA (2000). *Health assessment document for 2,3,7,8-tetrachlorodibenzo-p-dioxin (TCDD) and related compounds*. Office of Research and Development, Washington, DC. (http//www.epa.gov/ncea/dioxin.html)

EPRI (1994). *Electric utility trace substances synthesis report*. Electric Power Research Institute, Palo Alto, CA.

Ershow, A.G. and Cantor, K.P. (1989). *Total water and tapwater intake in the United States: population-based estimates of quantities and sources*, pp. 328–34. Life Sciences Research Office, Federation of American Societies for Experimental Biology, Bethesda, MD.

Farmer, P.B. and Shuker, D.E.G. (1999). What is the significance of increases in background levels of carcinogen-derived protein and DNA adducts? Some considerations for incremental risk assessment. *Mutation Research*, **424**, 275–86.

Faustman, E.M. and Bartell, S.M. (1997). Review of noncancer risk assessment: applications of benchmark dose methods. *Human and Ecological Risk Assessment*, **3**, 893–920.

Faustman, E.M. and Omenn, G.S. (1996). Risk assessment. In *Casarett and Doull's toxicology* (5th ed) (ed. C.D. Klaassen), pp. 75–88. McGraw-Hill, New York.

Faustman, E.M. and Omenn, G.S. (2001). Risk assessment. In *Cassarett and Doull's toxicology. The basic science of poisons* (6th edn) (ed. C. Klaassen). McGraw-Hill, New York.

Faustman, E.M., Allen, B.C., Kavlock, R.J., and Kimmel, C.A. (1994). Dose–response assessment of developmental toxicity: I. Characterization of data base and determination of NOAELs. *Fundamental and Applied Toxicology*, **79**, 229–41.

Faustman, E.M., Wellington, D.G., Smith, W.P., and Kimmel, C.S. (1989). Characterization of a developmental toxicity dose response model. *Environmental Health Perspectives*, **79**, 229–41.

Faustman, E.M., Lewandowski, T.A., Ponce, R.A., and Bartell, S.M. (1999). Biologically based dose–response models for developmental toxicants: lessons from methylmercury. *Inhalation Toxicology*, **11**, 101–14.

Finley, B., Proctor, D., Scott, P., Harrington, N., Paustenbach, D., and Price, P. (1994). Recommended distributions for exposure factors frequently used in health risk assessment. *Risk Analysis*, **14**, 533–53.

Fischhoff, B. (1981). Cost-benefit analysis: an uncertain guide to public policy. *Annals of the New York Academy of Science*, **363**, 173–88.

Fischhoff, B., Bostrom, A., and Quandrei, M.J. (1996). Risk perception and communication. In *Oxford textbook of public health* (3rd edn) (ed. R. Detels, W. Holland, J. McEwen, and G.S. Omenn), pp. 987–1002. Oxford University Press.

Food Quality Protection Act (FQPA) (1996). EPA, Office of Pesticide Programs.

Gaylor, D.W., Kodell, R.L., Chen, J.J., and Krewski, D. (1999). A unified approach to risk assessment for cancer and noncancer endpoints based on benchmark doses and uncertainty/safety factors. *Regulatory Toxicology and Pharmacology*, **29**, 151–7.

Goldman, L.R. (1998). Linking research and policy to ensure children's environmental health. *Environmental Health Perspectives*, **106**, 857–62.

Goldstein, B. (1995). Risk management will not be improved by mandating numerical uncertainty analysis for risk assessment. *University of Cincinnati Law Review*, **63**, 1599–610.

Hagmar, L., *et al.* (1991). An epidemiological study of cancer risk among workers exposed to ethylene oxide using hemoglobin adducts to validate environmental exposure assessments. *International Archives of Occupational and Environmental Health*, **63**, 271–7.

Harris, M.W., *et al.* (1992). Assessment of a short-term reproductive and developmental toxicity screen. *Fundamental and Applied Toxicology*, **19**, 186–96.

Haseman, J.K. and Lockhart, A.M. (1993). Correlations between chemically related site-specific carcinogenic efects in long-term studies in rats and mice. *Environmental Health Perspectives*, **101**, 50–4.

Health and Safety Executive (HSE) (2000). Reducing risks, protecting people. HSE Books, Sudbury, Suffolk. (Discussion document, 1999.)

Hill, A.B. (1965). The environment and disease: Association or causation. *Proceedings of the Royal Society of Medicine*, **58**, 295–300.

Hogstedt, R.J., Aringer, L., and Gustavsson, A. (1986). Epidemiologic support for ethylene oxide as a cancer-causing agent. *Journal of the American Medical Association*, **225**, 1575–8.

IARC (1994*a*). *IARC monographs on the evaluation of carcinogenic risks to humans.* World Health Organization, Lyon.

IARC (1994*b*). Meeting of the IARC working group on some industrial chemicals. *Scandinavian Journal of Work in Environmental Health*, **20**, 227–9.

IARC (1999). *IARC monographs on the evaluation of carcinogenic risks to humans.* World Health Organization, Lyon, France, Vols 1–73 (20 January 1999, update summary). http://193.51.164.11/monoeval/crthall.html

ILSI (1999). *A framework for cumulative risk assessment.* International Life Sciences Institute, Washington, DC.

INFORM (1996). Risks on record: an overview of the Toxic Substances Control Act's substantial risk reporting system with bulletins on selected chemicals. INFORM, New York.

Institute of Medicine (1999). *Toward environmental justice.* National Academy Press, Washington, DC.

Kavlock, R.J., Allen, B.C., Faustman, E.M., and Kimmel, C.A. (1995). Dose response asessments for developmental toxicity. IV: Benchmark doses for fetal weight changes. *Fundamentals of Applied Toxicology*, **26**, 211–22.

Kimmel, C.A. and Gaylor, D.W. (1988). Issues in qualitative and quantitative risk analysis for developmental toxicology. *Risk Analysis*, **8**, 15–20.

Kohn, M.C., *et al.* (1993). A mechanistic model of effects of dioxin on gene expression in the rat liver. *Toxicology and Applied Pharmacology*, **120**, 138–54.

Krewski, D. and Van Ryzin, J. (1981). Dose response models for quantal response toxicity data. In *Statistics and related topics* (ed. M. Csorgo, D.A. Dawson, J.N.K. Rao, and A.K. Seleh), pp. 201–29. North-Holland, Amsterdam.

Landrigan, P.J. and Goldman, L.R. (1998). Report of a panel on the relationship between public exposure to pesticides and cancer. *Cancer*, **83**, 1057–60.

Lave, L.B. and Omenn, G.S. (1986). Cost-effectiveness of short-term tests for carcinogenicity. *Nature*, **334**, 29–34.

Lave, L.B., Ennever, F., Rosenkranz, H.S., and Omenn, G.S. (1988). Information value of the rodent bioassay. *Nature*, **336**, 631–3.

Lehman, A.J. and Fitzhugh, O.G. (1954). 100-fold margin of safety. *Association of the Food and Drug Office United States Quarterly Bulletin*, **18**, 33–5.

Leroux, B.G., Leisenring, W.M., Moolgavkar, S.H., and Faustman, E.M. (1995). A biologically based dose–response model for development. *Risk Analysis*, **16**, 449–58.

Lewandowski, T.A., Bartell, S.M., Pierce, C.H., Ponce, R.A., and Faustman, E.M. (1998). Toxicokinetic and toxicodynamic modeling of the effects of methylmercury on the fetal rat. *The Toxicologist*, **42**, 139.

Lewandowski, T.A., Ponce, R.A., Whittaker, S.G., and Faustman, E.M. (1999). *In vitro* models for evaluating developmental toxicity. In *In vitro toxicology* (ed. S.C. Gad). Raven Press, New York.

Lowrance, W.W. (1976). *Of acceptable risk*, pp. 180. William Kaufmann, Los Altos, CA.

Lykke, E. (1992). *Achieving environmental goals: the concept and practice of environmental performance review.* Pinter, London.

McClain, R.M. (1994). Mechanistic considerations in the regulation and classification of chemical carcinogens. In *Nutritional toxicology* (ed. F.N. Kotsonis, M. Mackey, and J. Hijele), pp. 278–304. Raven Press, New York.

McGinnis, J.M. and Foege, W.H. (1993). Actual causes of death in the United States. *Journal of the American Medical Association*, **270**, 2207–12.

Moolenaar, R.J. (1994). Carcinogen risk assessment: international comparison. *Regulatory Toxicology and Pharmacology*, **20**, 302–36.

Moolgavkar, S.H. and Luebeck, G. (1990). Two-event model for carcinogenesis: biological, mathematical, and statistical considerations. *Risk Analysis*, **10**, 323–41.

Moore, J.A., *et al.* (1995). An evaluative process for assessing human reproductive and developmental toxicity of agents. *Reproductive Toxicology*, **9**, 61–95.

Morgan, G.M. (1993). Risk analysis and management. *Scientific American*, **269**, 32–5, 38–41.

Morgan, M.G., Fischhoff, B., Bostrom, A., Lave, L., and Atman, C.J. (1992). Communicating risk to the public. *Environmental Science and Technology*, **26**, 2048–56.

Morgenstern, R.D. (ed). (1997). *Economic analysis at EPA: assessing regulatory impact.* Johns Hopkins University Press, Baltimore, MD.

Mumtaz, M.M., Sipes, I.G., Clewell, H.J., and Yang, R.S. (1993). Risk assessment of chemical mixtures: biologic and toxicologic issues. *Fundamental and Applied Toxicology*, **21**, 258–69.

National Research Council (1983). *Risk Assessment in the Federal Government: Managing the Process*. National Academy Press, Washington, DC.

National Research Council (1984). *Toxicity testing: strategies to determine needs and priorities*. National Academy Press, Washington, DC.

National Research Council (1989*a*). *Biological markers in pulmonary toxicology*. National Academy Press, Washington, DC.

National Research Council (1989*b*). *Biological markers in reproductive toxicology*. National Academy Press, Washington, DC.

National Research Council (1992*a*). *Biological markers in immunotoxicology* . National Academy Press, Washington, DC.

National Research Council (1992*b*). *Environmental neurotoxicology*. National Academy Press, Washington, DC.

National Research Council (1993). *Pesticides in the diets of infants and children*. National Academy Press, Washington, DC.

National Research Council (1996). *Understanding risk*. National Academy Press, Washington, DC.

National Research Council Committee on Risk Assessment Methodology (CRAM) (1993). *Issues in risk assessment, use of the maximum tolerated dose in animal bioassays for carcinogenicity*. National Academy Press, Washington, DC.

National Research Council Committee on Risk Assessment of Hazardous Air Pollutants (1994). *Science and judgment in risk assessment*. National Academy Press, Washington, DC.

National Toxicology Program (1987). *Toxicology and carcinogenesis studies of ethylene oxide in B6C3F1 mice*. US Department of Health and Human Services, Public Health Service, National Institutes of Health, Research Triangle Park, NC.

Nebert, D.W. (1999). Pharmacogenetics and pharmacogenomics. Why is this relevant to the clinical geneticist? *Clinical Genetics*, **56**, 247–58.

Nebert, D.W. and Duffy, J.J. (1997). How knockout mouse lines will be used to study the role of drug-metabolizing enzymes and their receptors during reproduction, development, and environmental toxicity, cancer and oxidative stress. *Biochemical Pharmacology*, **53**, 249–54.

Neil, N., Malmfors, T., and Slovic, P. (1994). Intuitive toxicology: expert and lay judgments of chemical risks. *Toxicologic Pathology*, **22**, 198–201.

NIEHS (1999). *The murine local lymph node assay: a test method for assessing the allergic contact dermatitis potential of chemicals/compounds*, pp. 14 006–7. Report 99-4494. ICCVAM, Washington, DC.

Oberle, M.W., Baker, E.L., and Magenheim, M.J. (1994). Healthy People 2000 and community health planning. *Annual Review of Public Health*, **15**, 259–75.

Office of Technology Assessment (1992). *Centralized risk assessment research*. National Academy Press, Washington, DC.

Ohanian, E.V., *et al.* (1997). Risk characterization: a bridge in informed decision-making. *Fundamental and Applied Toxicology*, **39**, 81–8.

Omenn, G.S. (1993). Commentary: the role of environmental epidemiology in public policy. *Annals of Epidemiology*, **3**, 319–22.

Omenn, G.S. (1994). Can systematic, integrated risk assessment with full stakeholder participation enhance clean-up at DOE's sites? The 1994 Herbert H.Parker Lecture. In *33rd Hanford Symposium on Health and the Environment . In-situ remediation: scientific basis for current and future technologies* , Part I (ed. G.W. Gee and R. Wing), pp. xv–xxx. Battelle Press, Columbus, OH.

Omenn, G.S. (1996). Putting environmental risks in a public health context. *Public Health Reports*, **111**, 514–16.

Omenn, G.S. (1998). Chemoprevention of lung cancer: the rise and demise of beta-carotene. *Annual Review of Public Health*, **19**, 73–99.

Omenn, G.S. (2000). The genomic era: a crucial role for the public health sciences. *Environmental Health Perspectives*, **108**, 160–1.

Omenn, G.S. and Lave, L.B. (1988). Scientific and cost-effectiveness criteria in selecting batteries of short-term tests. *Mutation Research* , **205**, 41–9.

Omenn, G.S. and Motulsky, A.G. (1978). Ecogenetics: genetic variation in susceptibility to environmental agents. In *Genetic issues in public health and medicine* (ed. B.H. Cohen, A.M. Lilienfeld, and P.C. Huang), pp. 83–111. C.C. Thomas, Springfield, IL.

Omenn, G.S., Omiecinski, C.J., and Eaton, D.E. (1990). Ecogenetics of chemical carcinogens. In *Biotechnology and human genetic predisposition to disease* (ed. C. Cantor, C. Caskey, L. Hood, D. Kamely, and G. Omenn), pp. 81–93. Wiley–Liss, New York.

Omenn, G.S., Stuebbe, S., and Lave, L. (1995). Predictions of rodent carcinogenicity testing results: interpretation in light of the Lave–Omenn value-of-information model. *Molecular Carcinogens*, **14**, 37–45.

Omenn, G.S., *et al.* (1996). Effects of a combination of beta-carotene and vitamin A on lung cancer and cardiovascular disease. *New England Journal of Medicine*, **334**, 1150–5.

Organization for Economic Co-operation and Development (OECD) (1996). Environmental performance reviews. OECD, Paris.

Page, N.P., *et al.* (1997). Implementation of EPA revised cancer assessment guidelines: incorporation of 'mechanistic and pharmacokinetic data.*Fundamental and Applied Toxicology*, **37**, 16–36.

Renwick, A.G. and Walker, R. (1993). An analysis of the risk of exceeding the acceptable or tolerable daily intake. *Regulatory Toxicology and Pharmacology*, **18**, 463–80.

Rios, R., Poje, G.V., and Detels, R. (1993). Susceptibility to environmental pollutants among minorities. *Toxicology and Industrial Health*, **9**, 797–820.

Risk Commission, Presidential/Congressional Commission on Risk Assessment and Risk Management (1997). *A framework for environmental health risk management* (Vol. 1). *Risk assessment and risk management in regulatory decision-making* (Vol. 2). US Government Printing Office, Washington, DC. http:\\www.riskworld.com.

Sandman, P.M. (1993). *Responding to community outrage: strategies for effective risk communication*. American Industrial Hygiene Association, Fairfax, VA.

Shelby, M.D., Bishop, J.B., Mason, J.M., and Tindall, K.R. (1993). Fertility, reproduction and genetic disease: Studies on the mutagenic effects of environmental agents on mammalian germ cells. *Environmental Health Perspectives*, **100**, 283–91.

Shuey, D.L., *et al.* (1994). Biologically based dose–response modeling in developmental toxicology: biochemical and cellular sequelae of 5-fluorouracil exposure in the developing rat. *Toxicology and Applied Pharmacology*, **126**, 129–44.

Slovic, P., Fischhoff, B., Baruch, F., and Lichtenstein, S. (1979). Rating the risks. *Environment*, **21**, 1–20, 36–9.

Snellings, W.M., Weill, C.S., and Maronpot, R.R. (1984*a*). A two-year inhalation study of the carcinogenic potential of ethylene oxide in Fischer 344 rats. *Toxicology and Applied Pharmacology*, **75**, 105–17.

Snellings, W.M., Weill, C.S., and Maronpot, R.R. (1984*b*). A subchronic inhalation study on the toxicologic potential of ethylene oxide in B6C3F1 mice. *Toxicology and Applied Pharmacology*, **76**, 510–18.

Steenland, K., *et al.* (1991). Mortality among workers exposed to ethylene oxide. *New England Journal of Medicine*, **324**, 1402–7.

Tengs, O.T., *et al.* (1995). Five-hundred life-saving interventions and their cost-effectiveness. *Risk Analysis*, **15**, 369–90.

Tennant, R.W., Spalding, J.W., Stasiewicz, S., and Ashby, J. (1990). Prediction of the outcome of rodent carcinogenicity bioassays currently being conducted on 44 chemicals by the National Toxicology Program. *Mutagenesis*, **5**, 3–14.

Tennant, R.W., Stasiewicz, S., Mennear, J., French, J.E., and Spalding, J.W. (1999). Genetically altered mouse models for identifying carcinogens. In *The use of short-and medium-term tests for carcinogens and data on genetic effects in carcinogenic hazard evaluation* (ed. D.B. McGregor, J.M. Rice, and S. Venitt), Vol. 146. IARC Scientific Publications, Lyon.

van Belle, G., Omenn, G.S., Faustman, E.M., Powers, C.W., Moore, J.A., Goldstein, B.D. (1996). Dealing with a lethal legacy. *Washington Public Health*, **14**, 16–21.

Van den Berg, *et al.* (1998) Toxic equivalency factors (TEFs) for PCBs, PCDDs, PCDFs for humans and wildlife. *Environmental Health Perspectives*, **106**, 775–92.

Walker, V.E., Fennell, T.R., Upton, P.B., MacNeela, J.P., and Swenberg, J.A. (1993). Molecular dosimetry of DNA and hemoglobin adducts in mice and rats exposed to ethylene oxide. *Environmental Health Perspectives*, **99**, 11–17.

Weller, E., *et al.* (1999). Dose-rate effects of ethylene oxide exposure on developmental toxicity. *Toxicological Sciences*, **50**, 259–70.

Wernick, I.K. (ed.) (1995). *Community risk profiles: a tool to improve environment and community health.* Rockefeller University, New York.

Whittaker, S.G. and Faustman, E.M. (1994). *In vitro* assays for developmental toxicity. In In vitro *toxicology* (ed. S.C. Gad), pp. 97–122. Raven Press, New York.

WHO (1962). *WHO: Principles in governing consumer safety in relation to pesticide residues.* WHO, Geneva.

World Bank (1993). *World development report: investing in health.* World Bank, Washington, DC.

Wu, K.Y., Ranasinghe, A., Upton, P.B., Walker, V.E., and Swenberg, J.A. (1999). Molecular dosimetry of endogenous and ethylene oxide-induced N7-(2-hydroxyethyl) guanine formation in tissues of rodents. *Carcinogenesis*, **9**, 1787–92.

8.9 Risk perception and communication*

Baruch Fischhoff, Ann Bostrom, and Marilyn Jacobs Quadrel

Introduction

Role of risk perceptions in public health

Many health risks are the result of deliberate decisions by individuals consciously trying to make the best choices for themselves and for those important to them. Some of these choices are private. They include decisions such as whether to wear bicycle helmets and seatbelts, whether to read and follow safety warnings, whether to buy and use condoms, and how to select and cook food. Other choices involve societal issues. They include such decisions as whether to protest the siting of hazardous waste incinerators and half-way houses, whether to vote for fluoridation and 'green' candidates, and whether to support sex education in schools.

In some cases, single choices can have a large effect on health risks (e.g. buying a car with airbags, taking a dangerous job, becoming pregnant). In other cases, the effects of individual choices are small, but can accumulate over multiple decisions (e.g. repeatedly ordering broccoli, wearing a seatbelt, using the escort service in parking garages). In still other cases, choices intended to affect health risks do nothing at all or the opposite of what is expected (e.g. responses to baseless cancer scares, subscription to quack treatments).

In order to make health decisions wisely, individuals need to understand the risks and the benefits associated with alternative courses of action. They also need to understand the limits to their own knowledge and to the advice proffered by various experts. This chapter reviews the research base for systematically describing people's degree of understanding about health-risk issues. Some fundamental topics in designing and evaluating messages for improving that understanding are also considered. Following convention, these pursuits will be called risk perception and risk communication research, respectively.

Role of perceptions about risk perceptions in public health

The fundamental assumption of this chapter is that statements about other people's understanding must be disciplined by systematic data. People can be hurt by inaccuracies in their risk perceptions. They can also be hurt by inaccuracies in what various other people believe about those perceptions. Particularly significant others include doctors, nurses, public health officials, legislators, regulators, and engineers—all of whom have some say in what risks are created, what is communicated about them, and what role laypeople have in determining their own fates.

If their understanding is overestimated, people may be thrust into situations that they are ill-prepared to handle (e.g. choosing among complex medical procedures). If their understanding is underestimated, people may be disenfranchised from decisions that they could and should make. The price of such misperceptions of risk perceptions may be exacted over the long run as well as in individual decisions. The outcomes of health-risk decisions partly determine people's physical and financial resources. Furthermore, the processes by which health-risk decisions are made partly determine people's degree of autonomy in managing their own affairs and in shaping their society.

In addition to citing relevant research results, this chapter will emphasize research methods. One conventional reason for doing so is improving access to material that is scattered over specialist literatures or is part of the implicit knowledge conveyed in professional training. A second conventional reason is to help readers to evaluate the substantive results reported here by giving a feeling for how they were produced.

A less conventional reason is to make the point that method matters. We are routinely struck by the strong statements made about other people's competence to manage risks, solely on the basis of anecdotal observation and intuition. These statements appear directly in pronouncements about, for instance, why people mistrust various technologies or fail to 'eat right'. Such claims appear more subtly in the myriad of health advisories, advertisements, and warnings directed at the public without any systematic evaluation. These practices assume that the communicator knows what people currently know, what they need to learn, what they want to hear, and how they will interpret a message.

Even casual testing with a focus group shows a willingness to have those (smug) assumptions challenged. The research methods presented here show the details that need attention and, conversely, the pitfalls to casual observation. This chapter also shows the limits to such research, in terms of how far current methods can go and how quickly they can get there. It has been our experience that, once the case has been made for conducting behavioural research, it is expected to produce results immediately. That is, of course, a prescription for failure and for undermining the perceived value of future behavioural research. Furthermore, the cumulative attack on public competence can lead to its disenfranchisement and the transfer of authority to technical experts, be they doctors or technology managers. Indeed, some attacks seem designed to effect such a change in the balance of

* Preparation of this chapter was supported by the National Institute of Alcohol Abuse and Alcoholism, the National Institute of Allergies and Infectious Disease, and the National Science Foundation Center for Integrated Assessment of the Human Dimensions of Global Change.

political power. There are those who would just as soon have no research (or ambiguous research) regarding public perceptions of risk so that they can fill the void with their own punditry (Fischhoff *et al.* 1983; Fischhoff 1990; Leiss and Chociolko 1994; Okrent and Pidgeon 1998).

Overview

The next section, on quantitative assessment, treats the most obvious question about laypeople's risk perceptions: Do they understand how large (and how small) various risks are? It begins with representative results regarding the quality of laypeople's quantitative judgements, along with some relevant psychological theory. It continues with issues in survey design, focused on how design choices can affect respondents' apparent competence. Some of these methodological issues reveal substantive aspects of lay risk perceptions.

The following section, on qualitative assessment, shifts the focus from summary estimates of risk to judgements about qualitative features of the events being considered. It begins with the barriers to communication created when experts and laypeople unwittingly use terms differently. For example, when experts tell (or ask) people about the risks of drinking and driving, what do people think is meant regarding the kinds and amounts of 'drinking' and of 'driving'? We then ask how people believe that risks are created and controlled, as a basis for generating and evaluating action options.

The final section provides a general process for developing communications about health risks. That process begins by identifying the information to communicate, based on (a) descriptive study of what recipients know already, and (b) formal analysis of what they need to know in order to make informed decisions. The process continues by selecting an appropriate format for presenting that information. It concludes with an explicit empirical evaluation of the resulting communication, with the process being iterated if the results are wanting. The process is illustrated with examples taken from several case studies, looking at such diverse health risks as those posed by radon, Lyme disease, electromagnetic fields, carotid endarterectomy, and nuclear energy sources in space.

This chapter will not address several issues that belong in a fuller account. These include the roles of emotion, individual differences, culture, and social processes in decisions about risk. This set of restrictions suits the chapter's focus on how individuals think about risks. It may also suit a public health perspective, where it is often necessary to 'treat' populations with information. The success of that effort both depends on and shapes recipients' social and emotional resources for acting on its contents. Good communication can expand the envelope within which people feel that they can understand and act on the facts of risk. Access to missing topics might begin with Jasanoff (1986), Weinstein (1987), Heimer (1988), Krimsky and Plough (1988), National Research Council (1989), Otway and Wynne (1989), Douglas (1992), Krimsky and Golding (1992), Royal Society (1992), Yates (1992), and Leiss and Chociolko (1994).

Quantitative assessment

Estimating the size of risks

A common presenting symptom in experts' complaints about lay decision-making is that 'they (the public) do not realize how small (or large) the risk is'. If that were the case, then the mission of risk communication would be conceptually simple (although still technically challenging)—transmit credible estimates of the magnitude of risks. The need for such communication can be seen in research showing that lay estimates of risk are, indeed, subject to biases (Kahneman *et al.* 1982; Slovic 1987; Weinstein 1987; Stallen and Thomas 1988). Rather less evidence directly implicates these biases in inappropriate risk decisions, or substantiates the idealized notion of people waiting for crisp risk estimates so that they can 'run' decision-making models in their heads. Such estimates are necessary, but not sufficient, for effective decisions. Accurate estimates alone cannot tell people what actions are possible or what goals are worth pursuing. They might not even show what risks are worth worrying about—insofar as there may be nothing to do about large risks, while small risks might be expeditiously handled (Fischhoff *et al.* 1983). Nonetheless, some notion of risk size is needed to begin focusing one's attention.

In one early attempt to evaluate lay estimates of the size of risks, Lichtenstein *et al.* (1978) asked people to estimate the number of deaths in the United States from 30 causes (e.g. botulism, tornadoes, motor vehicle accidents). The 'people' in this study were members of the League of Women Voters and their spouses. Generally, the people in the studies described here have been paid for participation, sometimes drawn from university populations (students and staff) and sometimes recruited through civic groups (e.g. garden clubs, parent–teacher associations, bowling leagues). As a result, they are typically older (and perhaps better motivated) than the proverbial college sophomores of some psychological research. These groups have been found to differ more in *what* they think than in *how* they think, i.e. their respective experiences have created larger differences in specific beliefs than in thought processes. Fuller treatment of sampling issues must await another opportunity.

Lichtenstein *et al.* (1978) used two different response modes, allowing a check for the consistency of responses. One task presented pairs of causes; subjects chose the more frequent and then estimated the ratio of frequencies. The second task asked subjects to estimate the number of deaths in an average year. These subjects were told the answer for one cause, as an anchor, providing an order-of-magnitude feeling for the kinds of answers that were expected; a pretest had found that many subjects lacked a good idea of how many people live or die in the United States in an average year. The study reached several conclusions which have been borne out by subsequent studies (Vlek and Stallen 1981). These concerned internal consistency, anchoring bias, compression, availability bias, and miscalibration of confidence judgements.

Internal consistency

Estimates of relative frequency were quite consistent both within and across response mode. Thus, people seemed to have a moderately well-articulated internal risk scale, which they were able to express even in the unfamiliar response modes used in these studies—in life, they had probably never been asked any question as explicit as these quantitative estimates of risk.

Anchoring bias

Direct estimates were influenced by the anchor that the investigators provided. Subjects told that 50 000 people die annually from vehicle accidents produced estimates two to five times higher than did subjects told that 1000 die from electrocution. Thus, people seem to have less of a feel for absolute frequency, rendering them sensitive to the implicit cues in how questions are asked (Poulton 1989; Hurd 1999; Schwarz 1999).

Compression

Subjects' estimates showed less dispersion than did the statistical estimates. While the statistical estimates varied over six orders of magnitude, the typical subject's estimates ranged over three or four. In this case, the result was overestimation of small frequencies and underestimation of large ones. However, the anchoring bias suggests that this overall pattern might have changed with different procedures, making the compression of estimates the more fundamental result. For example, using an even lower anchor (e.g. the average annual toll of botulism deaths) would have reduced the overestimation of small frequencies and increased the underestimation of large ones. If these responses reflect subjects' actual feeling for the relative size of different risks, then people may have difficulty appreciating the enormous range in the frequencies of life's risks. That would not be surprising, considering how rare it is for media reports or health-care professionals to provide explicit quantitative estimates.

Availability bias

At each level of statistical frequency, some causes of death (e.g. homicide, tornadoes, flood) consistently received higher estimates than others. Additional analyses showed these to be causes that are disproportionately visible (e.g. as reported in the news media, as experienced in subjects' lives). This bias seemed to reflect a special case of a general tendency to estimate the frequency of events by the ease with which they are remembered or imagined—while failing to realize what a fallible index such availability is (Tversky and Kahneman 1973; Kahneman *et al.* 1982). These results are consistent with those in experimental psychology, showing that people are generally quite proficient at tracking how frequently events are observed, but not so good at detecting systematic biases in those observations (Hasher and Zacks 1984; Koriat 1993).

Miscalibration of confidence judgements

In a subsequent study (Fischhoff *et al.* 1977), subjects were asked how confident they were in their ability to choose the more frequent in a pair of causes of death (e.g. tornado, asthma). They tended to be overconfident. For example, they chose correctly only 75 per cent of the time when they were 90 per cent confident of having done so. This result is a special case of the general tendency to be inadequately sensitive to the extent of one's knowledge (Lichtenstein *et al.* 1982; Yates 1989).

Figure 1 shows typical results from such a calibration test. In this case, subjects expressed their confidence in having chosen the correct answer to two alternative questions regarding health risks (e.g. alcohol is (a) a depressant or (b) a stimulant). In the figure, each point reflects the proportion of correct responses associated with answers assigned a particular probability of being correct. Thus, in the lowest curve, subjects were correct about 70 per cent of the time when 100 per cent certain of being correct. The two upper curves reflect a group of middle-class adults and some of their adolescent children, recruited through school organizations. As in other studies of cognitive ability, the judgemental processes of these groups are quite similar (Keating 1988). The third curve reflects at-risk teenagers, recruited from group

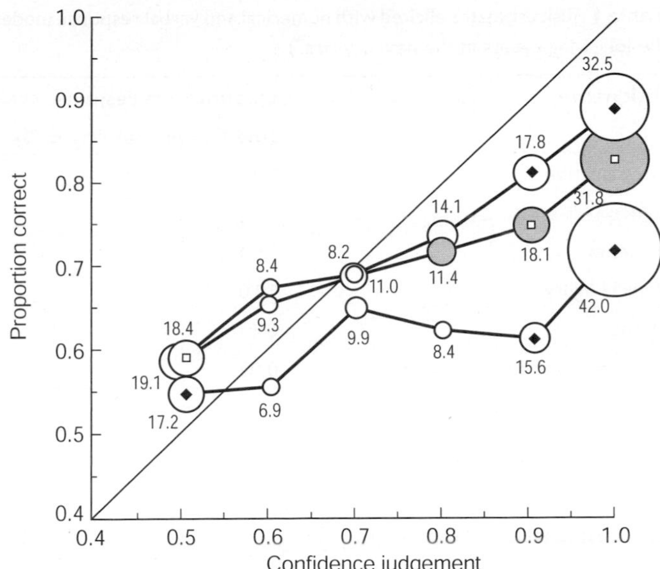

Fig. 1 Calibration curves for adults (top, white: n = 45), not-at-risk teenagers (middle, dark: n = 43), and at-risk teenagers (bottom, white: n = 45). Each point indicates the proportion of correct answers among those in which subjects expressed a particular confidence level. The size of each circle indicates the percentage of answers held with that degree of confidence. (Source: Quadrel 1990.)

homes and treatment centres. They knew less about these risk issues, but were just as confident; indeed, over 40 per cent of their responses indicated complete confidence in the associated answer. One possible explanation of this greater overconfidence is that their personal experiences with risks create an illusion of understanding, leading them to feel inappropriately like experts. A second is that the high-risk teenagers have less ability to think critically about the bases of their beliefs or less willingness to do so. Effective decision-making requires not just having knowledge, but also recognizing the limits to one's understanding.

Response mode problems

One recurrent obstacle to assessing or improving laypeople's estimates of risk is reliance on verbal quantifiers for both communicating and eliciting risk estimates. It is difficult for people to know what experts mean when a risk is described as 'very likely' or 'rare'. It is equally difficult for experts to evaluate lay perceptions expressed in those terms. Such terms mean different things to different people and even to the same person in different contexts (e.g. likely to be fatal versus likely to rain, rare disease versus rare Cubs baseball championship). Such ambiguity has been found even within communities of professionals, such as doctors and intelligence officers (Lichtenstein and Newman 1967; Beyth-Marom 1982; Merz *et al.* 1991). The criticality of such ambiguity depends on how the estimates are used. Sometimes, inferred probabilities of 1 and 10 per cent will lead to the same choice; sometimes they will not. The variability of interpretations should increase with the diversity of individuals and decisions.

Table 1 shows the results of asking a fairly homogeneous group of subjects (undergraduates at an American Ivy League college) to judge seven risks in both quantitative and qualitative terms, with reported statistical rates. The quantitative estimates used a response scale that

Table 1 Risk estimates elicited with numerical and verbal response modes compared with statistical risk estimates ('Please estimate your personal risk to the following events in the next 3 years.')

Risk name	Quantitative response scale (median probability in %)	Verbal response scale		Statistical risk estimate (probability in %)
		Median	Mean	
Electrocution	0.1	1.0	1.67	0.015
Cancer	0.3	2.0	2.09	0.06
Influenza	55.0	5.0	4.72	86.2
Vehicle injury	10.0	3.0	3.38	4.7
Herpes	0.1	1.0	1.73	4.1
HIV virus/sexual transmission	0.02	1.0	1.41	0.2

Source: Linville *et al.* (1993).

explicitly offered probabilities as low as 0.01 per cent (or 1 in 10 000). The qualitative scale used typical labels (converted to interval-scale equivalents in the data analyses: 1, very unlikely; 2, unlikely; 3, somewhat unlikely; 4, somewhat likely; 5, likely; 6, very likely). Comparing the two response scales revealed a non-linear relationship between the two. Specifically, the median probabilities (column 1) associated with the median qualitative estimates (column 2) were as follows: very unlikely, 0.01 per cent; unlikely, 0.5 per cent; somewhat unlikely, 5 per cent; somewhat likely, 25 per cent; likely, 60 per cent; very likely, 96 per cent. Budescu and Wallsten (1995) review the evidence on the predictability of such equivalences across tasks, and what they reveal about experiences with uncertain events.

Lichtenstein *et al.* (1978) provided anchors in order to give subjects a feeling for how to answer. The anchors should have improved subjects' performance by drawing responses to the correct range, within which subjects were drawn to higher or lower values depending on the value of the anchor that they received. Most of the study's conclusions were relatively insensitive to these anchoring effects—except for the critical question of how much people overestimate or underestimate the risks that they face. That depended, in part, on how the question was asked.

Perceived lethality

A study by Fischhoff and MacGregor (1983) provides another example of the dangers of relying on a single response mode. They used four different response modes to ask about the chances of dying, conditional on being afflicted with each of various maladies (in the United States).

1. How many people die out of each 100 000 who contract influenza?
2. How many people died out of the 80 million who caught influenza last year?
3. For each person who dies of influenza, how many have it and survive?
4. Eight hundred people died of influenza last year. How many survived?

Again, there was strong ordinal consistency across response modes, while absolute estimates varied over one to two orders of magnitude. A follow-up study looked for independent evidence of the relative suitability of these different response modes. It found that subjects liked one format much less than the others. They were also least able to remember statistics reported in that format. This was also the format that produced the most discrepant results—estimating the number of survivors for each person who succumbed to a problem.

Perceived invulnerability

Estimating the accuracy of risk estimates requires not only an appropriate response mode, but also a standard against which responses can be compared. The studies described above asked about population risks in situations where credible statistical estimates were available to the investigators. People's performance might be different (and more difficult to evaluate) with risks whose magnitude is less readily calculated. Furthermore, for many decisions, people's understanding of population risks is less relevant than their understanding of personal risks. Unfortunately, personalized risk statistics are usually difficult to come by.

In order to circumvent these problems, some investigators have asked subjects to judge whether they are more or less at risk than others in (more or less) similar circumstances (Svenson 1981; Weinstein 1989; Weinstein and Klein 1996). They find that most people in most situations see themselves as facing less risk than average others; that could, of course, be true for only half a population. A variety of processes could account for such a bias, including both cognitive ones (e.g. the greater availability of the precautions that one takes—than those taken by others) and motivational ones (e.g. wishful thinking). Such an optimism bias could prompt unwanted risk-taking (e.g. because warnings seem more applicable to other people than to oneself). In a direct test of this hypothesis, Quadrel *et al.* (1993) asked subjects to judge the probability of various misfortunes befalling them and several comparison individuals (a close friend, an acquaintance, a parent, a child).

The events involved 'a death or injury requiring hospitalization over the next 5 years', from sources like vehicle accidents, drug addiction, and explosions. Subjects were most likely to see each person's risks similarly, meaning that perceived invulnerability was the exception, rather than the rule. However, when they did make a distinction, they were twice as likely to see themselves as the person facing less risk. This perception of relative personal invulnerability was particularly large for risks seen as under some personal control. Here too, adults and adolescents responded similarly, despite the common belief that teenagers take risks, in part, because of a unique perception of invulnerability (Elkind 1967). A more complicated account is needed to explain the risks that teenagers take and avoid (Schulenberg *et al.* 1997; Arnet 1999).

A log-linear response mode

Figure 2 shows the response mode used in this study. It uses a linear scale for probabilities between 1 and 100 per cent and six cycles of a logarithmic scale for smaller ones. The scale was explained to subjects in groups and introduced with a few examples having obvious and extreme values (e.g. being hit by lightning, catching a cold), in order to help subjects to understand it. Quadrel *et al.* (1993) found similar scale usage, not to mention similar beliefs (as noted above), among groups of middle-class adults, their high-school children, and high-risk teenagers recruited from group homes and treatment centres. The statistical risk estimates of Table 1 were elicited with a variant of this scale. Comparison between columns 1 and 4 allows a quantitative assessment of the accuracy of the risk estimates. Formal analysis might show whether errors of this magnitude would be large enough to influence decisions relying on them (see discussion of value-of-information analysis below).

In Quadrel *et al.*'s administration, the instructions were read aloud to circumvent any problems. However, subsequent studies have just handed out the scales with minimal instructions (Fischhoff and Bruine de Bruin 1999). In a questionnaire study with a random national sample of women, Woloshin *et al.* (1998) found that a log–linear scale was at least as reliable (and well accepted) as four competing response modes (two verbal and two numerical). The limiting factor on the use of such scales may not be the subjects' ability to understand quantitative probabilities, but the clarity of the instructions and their willingness to work. People prefer to receive numerical probabilities, but would rather provide verbal ones (which require less effort and make a weaker commitment) (Erev and Cohen 1990).

The critical question in considering the usefulness of such a response mode is whether the additional information that it provides compensates for the extra demands that it imposes on subjects. For example, does it help to see that the young adults in Table 1 moderately underestimate their risk of herpes infection (over the next 3 years), while moderately overestimating their risk of HIV (although recognizing that it is still very small)? Is it helpful to know that Quadrel *et al.*'s subjects assigned probabilities of less than 1 in 10 million about 10 per cent of the time and probabilities of less than 1 in 10 000 about one-third of the time. Using responses to quantitative scales, Viscusi (1992) has argued that the public-health establishment has more than succeeded in convincing adults of the risks of smoking. If that is the case, then educational efforts should be focused on teenagers or on the risks of addiction. With similar procedures, Black *et al.* (1995) concluded that women in the United States overestimate the risk of breast cancer. If so, then campaigns designed to increase awareness might need to be reconsidered.

The response distributions for these last two studies revealed an anomaly often found with studies using open-ended probability scales (e.g. 'use a number between 0 per cent, meaning impossible, and 100 per cent, meaning certain'). A disproportionate share of responses lay at '50', whereas most responses were much lower. Many of these responses seemed to mean '50–50,' rather than the numeric probability. Such 'blips' seem particularly common when respondents do not know what to say or do not want to think about the event in question—as might be the case with many risks (Fischhoff and Bruine de Bruin 1999). If taken at face value, these 50s inflate group estimates of small risks. If taken as evidence of respondents' discomfort with the question (or epistemic uncertainty), they provide another side to how people deal (or avoid dealing) with risks. Bruine de Bruin (1999) provides further examples of such blips, including ones from technical experts, as well as procedures for recalibrating response distributions that include such expressions of epistemic uncertainty (Gärdenfors and Sahlin 1982).

Realizing the potential of precise response scales requires applying them to precisely defined events. Some years ago, the United States National Weather Service considered abandoning quantitative probability-of-precipitation forecasts because of reported consumer confusion. Murphy *et al.* (1980) discovered that the confusion was actually about the event being predicted. For example, recipients were uncertain whether a 70 per cent chance of rain referred to the portion of the area that would receive rain, the percentage of time that it would rain, the chance of measurable rain at any spot in the area, or that chance at the weather station. (It is the last.) Event ambiguity is treated further below (and by Fischhoff (1994) and Fischhoff *et al.* (1999)). Where the magnitude of risk perceptions matters, we prefer to use quantitative response scales with well-defined events.

Defining risk

These studies provide measures of risk perceptions, if one assumes that people define 'risk' as 'probability of death'. However, observation of scientific practice shows that, even among professionals, 'risk' can have a variety of meanings (Crouch and Wilson 1982;

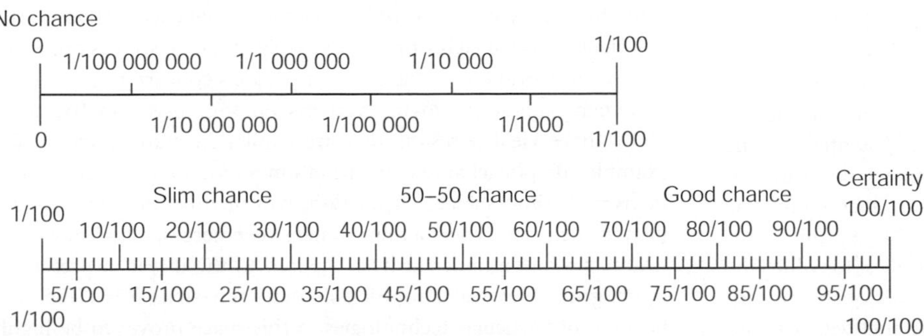

Fig. 2 Log–linear response scale for eliciting probability assessments, facilitating the expression of very small probabilities. (Source: Quadrel *et al.* 1993.)

Fischhoff *et al.* 1984; Royal Society 1992; National Research Council 1996). For some experts, 'risk' equals expected loss of life expectancy; for others, it is expected probability of premature fatality; for still others, it is total number of deaths or deaths per person exposed or per hour of exposure, or loss of ability to work (Starr 1969; Inhaber 1979; Wilson 1979; Kammen and Hassenzahl 1999).

Unwitting use of different definitions can lead to controversy and confusion, insofar as the relative riskiness of different jobs, avocations, technologies, and diseases depends on the choice of definition. Although often left to the conventions of technical experts, the choice of definition is a political/ethical decision that can significantly affect a society's allocation of resources. For example, hazards producing deaths by injury become relatively 'riskier' if one counts the total years lost rather than weighting all deaths equally. That measure of risk places a greater premium on deaths among young people, because more years of life are lost with them. Some of the apparent disagreement between experts and laypeople regarding the magnitude of risks in society seems due to differing definitions of 'risk' (Slovic *et al.* 1979; Vlek and Stallen 1980; Fischhoff *et al.* 1983; National Research Council 1996, 1999).

At times, 'risk' is used as a discrete rather than a continuous descriptor, i.e. an activity or technology is described as being a risk or not being a risk. Conversely, it might be described as being 'safe' or not. Such a shorthand expression naturally conveys rather little information, beyond the summary judgement regarding where the hazard in question falls relative to some threshold. Without further detailed study (using methods like those described here) one could not know what the individual or institution using the phrase meant. The phrase might refer to a general *de minimis* level (reflecting risks that can confidently be treated as not worth worrying about), the invocation of a precautionary principle (reflecting an appraisal of the probability distribution over possible risk levels), or the result of a cost–benefit summary (such that the risk is negligible in the context of the other consequences). Even when people talk in zero-risk terms, they may mean something different than a technical specialist using the same words. When those specialists wish to communicate regarding safety, they bear a particular burden to ensure that their terminology matches that of their audience. Otherwise, their public may feel that a social contract was violated, when they discover what the experts really meant.

Catastrophic potential

One early study asked experts and laypeople to estimate the 'risk of death' faced by society as a whole from 30 activities and technologies (Slovic *et al.* 1979). The experts' judgements were much more highly correlated with statistical estimates of average-year fatalities than were the laypeople's estimates. When laypeople were asked to estimate average-year fatalities, they responded much like the experts. However, when laypeople estimated 'risk of death', they also seemed to consider (what they saw as) the catastrophic potential of the technology (i.e. its ability to cause large numbers of deaths in non-average years). Thus, experts and laypeople agreed about routine death tolls (for which scientific estimates are relatively uncontroversial) and disagreed about the possibility of anomalies (for which the science is typically much weaker). This seemingly reasonable pattern would be obscured by the casual observation that experts and laypeople disagree about 'risk' or by the assumption that any disagreement means that the experts are right and the laypeople are wrong.

Sensing that there was something special about catastrophic potential, some risk experts have suggested that social policy pay special attention to the regulation of hazards carrying that kind of threat. However, one experimental study found that people did not care more for losing many lives in a single incident than for losing the same number of lives in separate incidents (Slovic *et al.* 1984). Rather, catastrophic potential worries people because a technology posing such threats may prove to be out of control, despite its promoters' promises. Such 'surprise potential' is strongly correlated with 'catastrophic potential' in people's judgements; the same is presumably true in scientific estimates (Funtowicz and Ravetz 1990).

When accidents involving large numbers of fatalities are easy to imagine, catastrophic potential can be rated high because of availability, even when estimates of average-year fatalities are relatively low, as was the case for nuclear power in this study.

However, the two features represent rather different ethical bases for distinguishing among risks.

Dimensions of risk

Uncertainty and catastrophic potential are not the only dimensions of risk that might influence how they are judged. Much research and speculation has been devoted to these features of risk (Lowrance 1976; Slovic *et al.* 1980, 1985; Green and Brown 1981; Vlek and Stallen 1981; Cole and Withey 1982), with the set of proposed features running to several dozen (Jenni 1997). This is an unwieldy number of features for a descriptive theory of risk perceptions, a prescriptive guide to risk decisions, or a scheme for predicting public responses to new hazards or hazard-reduction schemes. As a result, various empirical studies have attempted both to test these speculations and to reduce the number of considerations. Most have elaborated on a correlation scheme offered by Fischhoff *et al.* (1978). In it, members of a liberal civic organization rated 30 environmental hazards on nine hypothesized aspects of risk. Factor analysis reduced the mean ratings of nine aspects to two 'dimensions', which accounted for 78 per cent of the variance. Similar patterns were found with students, members of a conservative civic organization, members of a liberal women's organization, and technical risk assessors. Figure 3 shows the factor scores for 30 hazards within the common factor space for these four groups.

Hazards at the high end of the vertical factor (e.g. food colouring, pesticides) tended to be new, unknown, involuntary, and delayed in their effects. High (right-side) scores on the horizontal factor (e.g. nuclear power, commercial aviation) mean that consequences are seen as certain to be fatal, and to affect large numbers of people, should something go wrong. The vertical factor was labelled unknown risk and the horizontal factor dread risk. They might be seen as capturing the cognitive and emotional bases of people's concern respectively.

Other studies, employing variants on this 'psychometric paradigm', have yielded results that are similar in many respects. For example, despite changes in elicitation mode, scaling techniques, items rated, and subject population, two or three dimensions have proved adequate. Where a third dimension emerges, it typically refers to the absolute number of lives exposed to the threat in present or future generations; catastrophic potential has been used as a label. The position of particular technologies in this space proves to be highly robust. Moreover, that position is correlated strongly with various attitudes, including the desired stringency of regulation. Such analyses of mean responses are most suitable for predicting aggregate responses

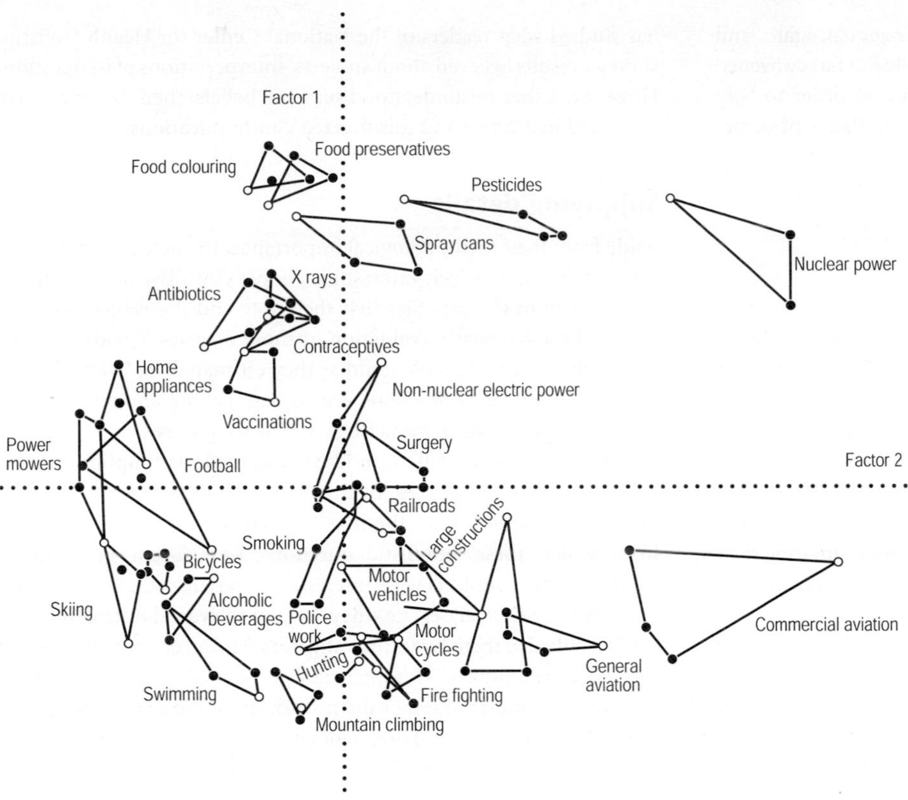

Fig. 3 Location of 30 hazards within the two-factor space obtained from League of Women Voters, student, active club, and expert groups. Respondents evaluated each activity or technology on each of nine features. Ratings were subjected to principal components factor analysis, with a varimax rotation. Connecting lines join or enclose the loci of four group points for each hazard. Open circles represent data from the expert group. Unattached points represent groups that fall within the triangle created by the other three groups. (Source: Slovic *et al.* 1985.)

to hazards. The international and intercultural comparison of such risk spaces has proven to be a fruitful area, with a standard methodology revealing local differences (and similarities) (Kuyper and Vlek 1984; Ënglander *et al.* 1986; Goszczynska *et al.* 1991; Karpowicz-Lazreg and Mullet 1993; Vaughan 1993; Jianguang 1994; Rohrmann 1994).

Risk comparisons

The multidimensional character of risk means that hazards that are similar in many ways may still evoke quite different responses. This fact is neglected in appeals to accept one risk because one accepts another risk that is similar to it in some ways (Fischhoff *et al.* 1981; Crouch and Wilson 1982). The most ambitious of these appeals present elaborate lists of hazards, exposure to which is adjusted so that they pose equivalent statistical risks (e.g. consuming one tablespoonful of peanut butter and living for 50 years at the boundary of a nuclear power plant both create a one-in-a-million risk of premature death). Recognizing that such comparisons are often perceived as self-serving, the Chemical Manufacturers Association commissioned a guide to risk comparisons (Covello *et al.* 1988), which presents many such lists, along with the attached caution (in capital letters): 'Warning! Use of data in this table for risk comparison purposes can damage your credibility'. The guide also offers advice on how to make risk comparisons, if one feels the compulsion, along with examples of more and less acceptable comparisons. Although the advice was derived logically from risk-perception research, it was not tested empirically. In such a test, we found little correlation between the authors' predicted degree of acceptability and that judged by several diverse groups of subjects (Roth *et al.* 1990; MacGregor 1991).

One possible reason for the failure of these predictions is that the manual's authors knew too much (from their own previous research) to produce truly unacceptable comparisons. More important than identifying the specific reasons for this failure is the general cautionary message: because we all have experience in dealing with risks, it is tempting to assume that others share our intuitions. Often, they do not. Effective risk communication requires careful empirical research. A poor risk communication can cause more public health (and economic) damage than the risks that it attempts to describe. One should no more release an untested communication than an untested medical device. The need for research is further magnified when one crosses cultural or national boundaries.

Over the past decade, many risk professionals have recognized the need to have risk priorities, while respecting differences in the definition of risk (Davies 1996). The result has been various forms of risk-ranking exercises, in which groups of citizens debate which risks merit the greatest attention. Participants are allowed (even encouraged) to disagree about which consequences matter. However, staff work attempts to provide a common credible basis for how large and likely those consequences are. Perhaps the most ambitious efforts has been conducted by the United States Environmental Protection

Agency (1993), which has promoted some 50 regional, state, and national exercises. The US National Institutes of Health has convened a director-level Council of Public Representatives, in order to help scientific and lay communities understand one another's priorities (Institute of Medicine 1998).

Qualitative assessment

Event definitions

Scientific estimates of the magnitude of a risk require detailed specification of the conditions under which it is to be observed. For example, a fertility counsellor estimating a woman's risk of an unplanned pregnancy would consider the frequency and timing of intercourse, the kinds of contraceptive used (and the diligence of their application), her physiological condition (and that of her partner), and so on. If laypeople are to make accurate assessments, they require the same level of detail. That is true whether they are estimating risks for their own sake or for the benefit of an investigator studying risk perceptions.

When investigators omit necessary details, they create adverse conditions for subjects. In order to respond correctly, subjects must first guess the question and then know the answer. Consider, for example, the question: 'What is the probability of pregnancy with unprotected sex?' A well-informed subject who understood this to mean a single exposure would be seen as underestimating the risk—by an investigator who intended the question to mean multiple exposures.

Such ambiguous 'events' are common in surveys of public risk perceptions. For example, a National Center for Health Statistics survey (Wilson and Thornberry 1987) question asked: 'How likely do you think it is that a person will get the AIDS virus from sharing plates, forks, or glasses with someone who had AIDS?' Fischhoff (1989*b*) asked a relatively homogeneous group of subjects to answer this question, and then to say what they thought was meant regarding the amount and kind of sharing that it implied. For their responses to be interpretable, subjects must spontaneously assign the same value to each missing detail and investigators must guess what value subjects have chosen. These subjects generally agreed about the kind of sharing (82 per cent interpreted it as sharing during a meal), but not about the frequency (a single occasion, 39 per cent; several occasions 20 per cent; routinely, 28 per cent; uncertain, 12 per cent). Thus, these subjects were answering different questions, rendering their responses ambiguous. In this case, the response mode was also ambiguous (very likely, unlikely, and so on), so that even precise questions would have revealed little. A survey question about the risks of sexual transmission evoked similar disagreement.

Interestingly, all the subjects who reported uncertainty about the frequency and intensity of sharing (or of sexual activity) still made likelihood judgements. If people are willing to respond to survey questions that they do not understand, any relationship between their reported beliefs and behaviours would tend to be blurred. That could, in turn, lead an observer to think, for example, that 'information does not work with teenagers', insofar as their actions seem unrelated to their beliefs. If so, that would be a special case of the general tendency for poor measurement to reduce the power of research designs. An important role of the National Center for Health Statistics study, one of an annual series, is to guide national policy on HIV/AIDS. No one has studied what readers of the National Center for Health Statistics survey's results believed about subjects' interpretations of its question. However, if they misunderstood subjects' beliefs, then they may have produced ineffective and misdirected communications.

Supplying details

Aside from their methodological importance, the details that subjects infer can be substantively interesting. People's intuitive theories of risk are revealed in the variables that they note and the values that they supply. In a systematic evaluation of these theories, Quadrel (1990) asked adolescents to think aloud as they estimated the probability of several deliberately ambiguous events (e.g. having an accident after drinking and driving, contracting AIDS through sex).

These subjects typically wondered (and made assumptions) about a large number of features. In this sense, subjects arguably showed more sophistication than the investigators who created the surveys from which these simplistic questions were taken or adapted. Generally, these subjects were interested in variables that could figure in scientific risk analyses, i.e. they wanted relevant information that had been denied them by the investigators. However, there were some interesting exceptions. Although subjects wanted to know the 'dose' involved with most risks, they did not ask about the amount of sex in a question about the risks of pregnancy or in another question about the risks of HIV transmission. They seemed to believe that an individual either is or is not susceptible to the risk, regardless of the amount of the exposure. In other cases, subjects asked about variables with a less clear connection to risk level (e.g. how well members of the couple knew one another).

In a follow-up study, Quadrel (1990) presented richly specified event descriptions to teenagers drawn from the same populations (school organizations and substance abuse treatment homes). Subjects initially estimated the probability of a risky outcome on the basis of some 12 details. Then, they were asked how knowing each of three additional details would change their estimates. One of those details had been identified as relevant by subjects in the preceding study; two had not. Subjects in this study were much more sensitive to changes in the relevant details than to changes in the irrelevant ones. Thus, at least in these studies, teenagers did not balk at making quantitative judgements regarding complex stimuli. When they did so, they revealed consistent intuitive theories in rather different tasks.

Studies integrating structured and open-ended methods are increasingly being used to get around the limitations of conventional surveys for eliciting beliefs regarding complex or unfamiliar topics (Fischhoff 1991; Schwarz 1996, 1999). These procedures assume that more reactive measurement is needed, if respondents are to understand such topics. They attempt to enrich, rather than bias, responses by offering a neutral mix of competing perspectives and prompts to think more deeply. These methods can also reveal the intuitive theories that respondents invoke, as they construe tasks in personally meaningful ways (McIntyre and West 1992; Gregory *et al.* 1993; Beattie *et al.* 1998; Fischhoff *et al.* 1999; Payne *et al.* 1999). Although groups are sometimes used as a forum for airing issues, the responses that 'count' in these studies are ones made in private by individual participants or in public through collective agreement (as in the risk-ranking exercises). As such they differ from the focus groups popular in market research, in which survey questions, commercial messages, political postures, or consumer products are discussed by groups of laypeople. Focus groups can be very productive in generating otherwise unanticipated perspectives. However, they create rather different situations than those faced by individuals or meaningful groups trying to make sense out of a question, message, or product. Merton (1987), who initially devised focus groups (and, before them, focused interviews) as a technique for uncovering possible hypotheses, has discouraged their use for testing (even those) hypotheses.

Cumulative risk—a case in point

As knowledge accumulates about people's intuitive theories of risk, it will become easier to predict which details subjects know and ignore, as well as which omissions they will notice and rectify. In time, it might become possible to infer the answers to questions that are asked from ones that are not—as well as the inferences that people make from risks that are described explicitly to risks that are not. The invulnerability results reported above show the need for empirical research to discipline extrapolations from one setting to another. Asking people about the risks to other people like themselves is not the same as asking them about their personal risk. Nor can it be assumed that hearing about others' risk levels will lead people to draw personal conclusions.

One common, and seemingly natural, extrapolation is across settings differing in the number of exposures to a risk. Telling people the risk from a single exposure should allow them to infer the risk from the number of exposures they expect to face; asking subjects what risk they expect from one number of exposures should allow one to infer what they expect from other numbers. Unfortunately, for both research and communication, teenagers' insensitivity to the amount of intercourse in determining the risks of pregnancy or HIV transmission proves to be a special case of a general problem. Several reviews (Cvetkovich *et al.* 1975; Morrison 1985) have concluded that between one-third and one-half of sexually active adolescents explain their not using contraceptives with variants of, 'I thought I (or my partner) couldn't get pregnant'. A safe exposure or two might confirm that belief, discouraging behaviour that increased long-term risk.

In another study, Shaklee and Fischhoff (1990) found that adults greatly underestimated the rate at which the risk of contraceptive failure accumulates through repeated exposure—even after eliminating (from the data analysis) the 40 per cent or so of subjects who saw no relationship between risk and exposure. One corollary of this bias is not realizing the extent to which seemingly small differences in annual failure rates (the statistic that is typically reported) can lead to large differences in cumulative risk. Bar-Hillel (1974) and Cohen and Hansel (1958) found underaccumulation in simple clearly described gambles. Wagenaar and Sagaria (1975) found it in estimating cumulative environmental degradation.

After providing practice with a response mode facilitating the expression of small probabilities, Linville *et al.* (1993) asked college students to estimate the probability of HIV transmission from a man to a woman as the result of 1, 10, or 100 cases of protected sex. For one contact, the median estimate was 0.10, a remarkably high value compared with public health estimates (Fineberg 1988; Kaplan 1989). For 100 contacts, the median estimate was 0.25, which is a more reasonable value; however, it is also quite inconsistent with the single-exposure estimate. Assuming their independence, 100 exposures should provide a near-certainty of transmission. Very different pictures of people's risk perceptions would emerge if a study asked just one of these questions. Conversely, risk communicators could achieve quite different effects if they chose to relate the risk of just one exposure or just 100. Communicators might create confusion if they chose to communicate both risks, leaving recipients to reconcile the seeming inconsistency.

Mental models of risk decisions

Each of these studies brought one element of a decision to subjects' attention. A more comprehensive research strategy asks respondents to judge each element in a standard representation of their decision-making situation. Perhaps the most common of such models have an expectancy-value form (Feather 1982). In them, decisions are assumed to be determined by a multiplicative combination of the rated likelihood and (un)desirability of various prespecified consequences. Health belief and theory of reasoned action models fall into this general category. For example, Bauman (1980) had seventh graders evaluate 54 possible consequences of using marijuana, in terms of their importance, likelihood, and valence (i.e. whether each is positive or negative). A 'utility structure index', computed from these three judgements, predicted about 20 per cent of the variance in subjects' reported marijuana usage. Related studies have had similar success in predicting other teenage risk behaviours.

The experience of these studies resembles that of earlier studies of 'clinical judgement', which successfully predicted expert decision-making with multiple regression models applied to experts' ratings of standard variables. Initially, investigators interpreted the regression coefficients as reflecting the weights that people give to different concerns (Hoffman 1960; Hammond *et al.* 1964; Goldberg 1968). However, formal analyses eventually showed that many weighting schemes would produce similar predictions, as long as they contained the same variables (or correlated surrogates) (Wilks 1938; Dawes and Corrigan 1974). The good news in this result is that any linear combination of relevant variables will have some predictive success. The bad news is that it can be very difficult to distinguish alternative models, in terms of their relative accuracy as descriptions of decision-making processes. Thus, linear models can have considerable practical value in predicting choices, while still having limited ability to clarify how choices are made (Camerer 1981; Dawes *et al.* 1989). As a result, linear models provide a sort of cognitive task analysis, identifying the kinds of factors that might be involved in people's choices. Other procedures are needed to clarify the finer structure of how decisions are made.

One such procedure was used by Beyth-Marom *et al.* (1993), who asked teenagers drawn from low-risk settings (e.g. sports teams, service clubs) and their parents to produce possible consequences of several decisions (e.g. deciding to smoke marijuana which was passed around at a party). Some subjects were asked to consider the act of accepting the offer, while others considered the consequences of rejecting it, in order to see whether these formally complementary options would elicit complementary perceptions. In almost all respects, the teenagers and parents responded quite similarly. On average, they produced about six consequences, with a somewhat higher number for accepting the risky offer than for rejecting it (suggesting that the thought of doing something is more evocative than the thought of not doing it). Respondents produced many more bad than good consequences of doing the focal behaviour, but fairly equal numbers for not doing it; thus, avoiding the risk was not as attractive as accepting it was unattractive. Most of the consequences that respondents mentioned were social reactions and personal effects. The social reactions of peers were particularly salient as consequences of rejecting the risk behaviour (e.g. more subjects said 'They will laugh at me if I decline the offer' than 'They will like me if I accept'). The thought of doing a behaviour once and of doing it regularly evoked somewhat different consequences. For example, the social reactions of peers were mentioned more frequently as consequences of 'accepting an offer to smoke marijuana at a party', while decreased mental function was mentioned more frequently for 'using marijuana'. These open-ended questions produced quite different consequences from the ones that appeared in earlier studies which required respondents to evaluate each item in a fixed list (e.g. the proportion of positive consequences was lower here). It would seem difficult to understand lay perceptions, or to improve them, without understanding such details, which seem to require an open-ended approach to emerge. For example, one might waste time and credibility trying to bring adolescents to adult's level of awareness about consequences, something that they already seem to have.

Another study further weakened the degree of imposed task structure by letting teenagers choose three recent difficult decisions in their lives, to be described in their own terms (Fischhoff 1996*a*). These descriptions were coded in terms of their content (what's on teenagers' minds) and structure (how those issues are formulated). Figure 4 shows a moderately well-structured choice about drinking and driving. None of the decisions that the 105 teenagers chose dealt with drinking and driving, although quite a few dealt with drinking. For those decisions that were mentioned, few had an option structure as complicated as that in the simple decision tree of Fig. 4. Rather, most were described in terms of a single option (e.g. whether to go to a party where alcohol would be served).

In a two-option decision, as in Fig. 4, the consequences of the alternative option are logically implied. However, that need not mean that they are intuitively obvious to the decision-maker. Indeed, Beyth-Marom *et al.* (1993) found that the consequences produced for engaging in a risky behaviour were not the mirror image of the consequences of rejecting that opportunity. This asymmetry is also seen in experimental results showing that foregone benefits of decisions, or their opportunity costs are much less visible than their direct costs (Kahneman *et al.* 1991; Thaler 1991). The differential visibility of such consequences can, in turn, be associated with ineffective decision-making. For example, the direct risks of vaccinating one's child loom disproportionately large, relative to the indirect risks of not vaccinating (Harding and Eiser 1984; Ritov and Baron 1990).

We believe that a mix of structured and unstructured studies is needed to piece together a full account of lay decisions—as a prelude to predicting or aiding them. Normative decision theory provides a conceptual framework for determining which topics to study. Descriptive decision theory provides methodological and theoretical tools for pursuing that study. All are imperfect. However, in combination, they can begin to provide the sort of complex descriptions that people's decisions about complex topics deserve. Attention to methodological detail is always critical. Decision variables will explain little if they are measured poorly. People whose behaviour seems unpredictable may lose the respect of observers and, thereby, become the target of manipulation—by others who conclude that this is the only way to get them to behave responsibly (for their own good). In this way, imprecise science (not to mention reliance on anecdotal observation) can undermine civil society.

Mental models of risk processes

Role of mental models

As noted above, people often have flawed intuitive theories of how risks accumulate, not realizing how risks mount up through repeated exposure—and perhaps neglecting the long-term perspective altogether. Such research can improve the communication of quantitative probabilities. Those probabilities are of greatest direct use to individuals who face well-formulated decisions in which quantitative estimates of a health risk (or benefit) play clearly defined roles. For example, a couple explicitly planning their family size need to know the probability of success and of side-effects for whichever contracep-

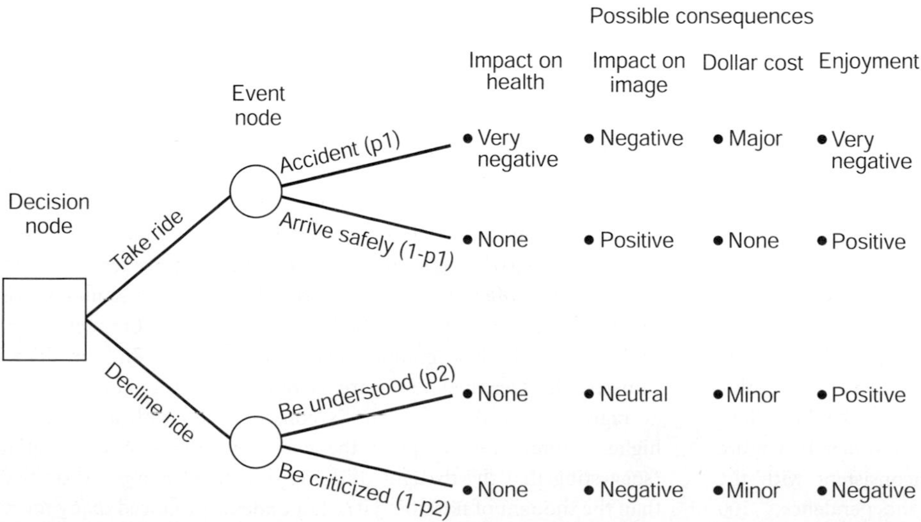

Fig. 4 Decision tree for whether to take or decline a ride from friends who have been drinking. (Source: Fischhoff and Quadrel 1991.)

tive strategies they will consider. Or, a home-owner poised to decide whether to test for radon needs quantitative estimates of the cost and accuracy of tests, the health risks of different radon levels, the cost and efficacy of ways to mitigate radon problems, and so on (Svenson and Fischhoff 1985).

Often, however, people are not poised to decide anything. Rather, they just want to know what the risk is and how it works. Such substantive knowledge is essential for following an issue in the news media, participating in public discussions, feeling competent to make decisions, and generating options among which to decide. In these situations, people's objective is to have intuitive theories that correspond to the main elements of the reigning scientific theories (emphasizing those features relevant to control strategies).

The term 'mental model' is often applied to intuitive theories that are sufficiently well elaborated to generate predictions in diverse circumstances (Galotti 1989). Mental models have a long history in psychology (Craik 1943; Johnson-Laird 1983; Oden 1987), having been used in such diverse settings as uncovering how people understand physical processes (Gentner and Stevens 1983), international tensions (Means and Voss 1985), complex equipment (Rouse and Morris 1986), energy conservation (Kempton 1987), psychological interactions (Furnham 1988), and the effects of drugs (Jungermann *et al.* 1988; Slovic *et al.* 1989).

If these mental models contain critical 'bugs', they can lead to erroneous conclusions, even among people who are otherwise well informed. For example, not knowing that repeated sex increases the associated risks could undermine much other knowledge. Bostrom *et al.* (1992) found that many people know that radon is a colourless odourless radio-active gas. Unfortunately, people also associate radio-activity with permanent contamination. However, this property of (widely publicized) high-level waste is not shared by radon. Not realizing that the relevant radon byproducts have short half-lives, home-owners might not even bother to test (believing that there was nothing that they could do, should a problem be detected). They might also not appreciate the risk in minute concentrations, which release their energy quickly.

Eliciting mental models

In principle, the best way to detect such misconceptions would be to capture people's entire mental model on a topic. Doing so would also identify those correct beliefs upon which communications could be built (and which should be reinforced). The critical methodological threat to capturing mental models is reactivity—changing responses as a result of the elicitation procedure. One wants neither to induce nor to dispel misconceptions, either through leading questions or subtle hints. The interview should neither preclude the expression of unanticipated beliefs nor inadvertently steer subjects around topics (Ericsson and Simon 1980; Galotti 1989; Hendrickx 1991).

Bostrom *et al.* (1992) offer one possible compromise strategy, which has been used for a variety of risks, including HIV/AIDS, other sexually transmitted diseases, vehicle insurance, mammography, Lyme disease, paint stripper, *Cryptosporidium*, and nuclear energy sources in space (Kempton 1991; Maharik and Fischhoff 1992; Fischhoff 1996*b*, 1999*b*; Fischhoff *et al.* 1998; Morgan *et al.*, in press). Their interview protocol begins with very open-ended questions, asking subjects what they know about a topic, then prompting them to consider exposure, effects, and mitigation issues. These basic categories seemed so essential that mentioning them would correct an oversight, rather than introduce a foreign concept. Subjects are asked to elaborate on every topic that they mention, and then to elaborate on those elaborations. Once these minimally structured tasks are exhausted, subjects sort a large stack of diverse photographs according to whether each seems related to the topic, explaining their reasoning as they go. When previously unmentioned beliefs appear at this stage, they are likely to represent latent portions of people's mental models—the sort that might emerge in everyday life if people had cause to consider specific features of their own radon situation. For example, when shown a picture of supermarket produce counter, some respondents told us that plants might become contaminated by taking up radon from the air or soil. Some also inferred that their houseplants would not be so healthy if they had a radon problem.

Once transcribed, interviews are coded into an expert model of the risk. This is a directed network, or influence diagram (Howard 1989; Burns and Clemen 1993), showing the different factors affecting the magnitude of the risk. The expert model is created by iteratively pooling the knowledge of a diverse group of experts, using appropriate elicitation procedures (Fischhoff 1989*a*; Morgan and Henrion 1990; Kammen and Hassenzahl 1999). It might be thought of as an expert's mental model, although it would be impressive for any single expert to have such comprehensive knowledge (e.g. about the factors involved in both lung clearance and building materials emissions). Moreover, laypeople can also be sources of expertise (e.g. about their own behaviour (useful for estimating exposure patterns), about side-effects that have yet to be established in the scientific literature, or about how well equipment actually works).

Figure 5 shows a portion of our influence diagram for radon, focused on reducing the risks in a house with a crawl space. An arrow between nodes indicates that the value of the variable at its head depends on the value of the variable at its tail. Thus, for example, the lungs' particle clearance rate depends on an individual's smoking history. Influence diagrams are convenient ways to display the functional relationships among variables. Their structure allows, in principle, the substitution of quantitative estimates of these relationships and to compute risk levels. Influence diagrams can also be mapped into decision trees, showing the relevance of various facts for decision-making (which can, in turn, provide guidance on the critical question of which are most worth communicating).

Such a model provides a template for characterizing lay mental models in communication-relevant terms. Once mapped into the expert model, lay beliefs can be analysed in terms of their appropriateness, specificity (i.e. level of detail), and focus. For most risks, beliefs can be categorized as pertaining to exposure processes, effects processes (i.e. health and physiology), and mitigation behaviours—the basic components of risk analysis. Other beliefs provide background information, which influences interpreting many of the relations in the diagram (e.g. radon is a gas). In evaluating appropriateness, we characterized beliefs as accurate, erroneous, peripheral (correct, but not relevant), or indiscriminate (too imprecise to be evaluated). Bostrom *et al.* (1992) found that most subjects knew that radon concentrates indoors (92 per cent mentioned), is detectable with a test kit (96 per cent), is a gas (88 per cent), and comes from underground (83 per cent). Most knew that radon causes cancer (63 per cent). However, many also believed erroneously that radon affects plants (58 per cent), contaminates blood (38 per cent), and causes breast cancer (29 per cent). Only two subjects (8 per cent) mentioned that radon decays. (Subjects were drawn from civic groups

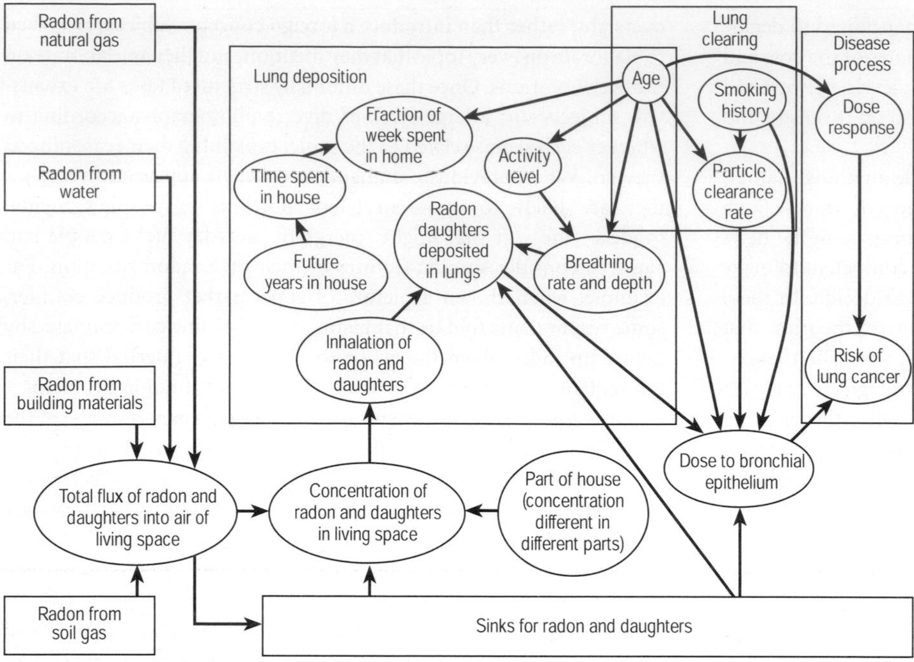

Fig. 5 Expert influence diagram for health effects of radon in a home with a crawl space. This diagram was used as a standard and as an organizing device to characterize the content of lay mental models. (Source: Morgan *et al.* 1992.)

in the Pittsburgh area, which had a moderate degree of radon publicity.) The robustness of these beliefs was examined (and generally confirmed) in subsequent studies using more easily administered structured questionnaires derived from the open-ended interviews.

Creating communications

Selecting information

The first step in designing communications is to select the information that they should contain. In many existing communications, this choice seems arbitrary, reflecting some expert's notion of 'what people ought to know'. Poorly chosen information can have several negative consequences: it can waste recipients' time, it can be seen as wasting their time (indicating insensitivity to their situation), it can take up the place (in the media or school) that could be filled with pertinent information (imposing an opportunity cost), and it can lead them to misunderstand the extent of their knowledge. In addition, recipients may be judged unduly harshly if they are uninterested in information that seems irrelevant to them, but has been deemed significant by the experts. The authors of the Institute of Medicine's important report *Confronting AIDS* (1986) despaired after a survey showed that only 41 per cent of the public knew that AIDS was caused by a virus. Yet, one might ask what role that information could play in any practical decision (as well as what those subjects who answered correctly meant by 'a virus').

The information in a communication should reflect a systematic theoretical perspective, capable of being applied objectively. Below, three candidates are listed for such a perspective, suggested by the research cited above.

Mental model analysis

Communications could attempt to convey a comprehensive picture of the processes creating (and controlling) a risk. Bridging the gap between lay mental models and expert models would require adding missing concepts, correcting mistakes, strengthening correct beliefs, and de-emphasizing peripheral ones. Following the mental model procedure outlined above has several potential advantages: (a) it allows the emergence of lay beliefs that never would have occurred to an expert (e.g. plants are sensitive to radon concentrations); (b) it reduces the chances of omitting critical concepts, by disciplining the experts to define their universe of expertise in terms of the influence diagram; (c) it reduces the clutter created by peripheral information that is routinely included in messages, without much thought to its role; (d) it increases the chances of revealing the terms in which laypeople express their beliefs.

Calibration analysis

Communications could attempt to give recipients the appropriate degree of confidence in their beliefs. They would focus on cases where people confidently hold incorrect beliefs that could lead to inappropriate actions or lack the confidence in correct beliefs needed to act on them. For example, only 45 per cent of the high-risk teenagers in Quadrel's (1990) study knew that having a beer would affect their driving as much as drinking a shot of vodka. However, they were, on average, very confident in their (usually wrong) answers. For this particular question, the adults were just as overconfident as the high-risk youth, whereas the low-risk teenagers judged their chances of a correct response more realistically. Such local misconceptions or 'bugs' can undermine otherwise correct beliefs, and hence deserve focused attention in communications.

Those who provide information have an obligation to communicate how much confidence should be placed in it. For example, Fortney (1988) reported the results of a meta-analysis on all the then available studies of the health effects of oral contraceptives. She concluded, with great confidence, that the effect of contraceptive pill use was somewhere between increasing a woman's life expectancy by 4 days and decreasing it by 80 days (for a non-smoker, using it throughout her reproductive career). Fortney could also say that it was highly unlikely that this forecast would change; the existing research base was so large that no conceivable single additional study could materially change the conclusions. Such an explicit estimation of uncertainty is much more valuable than any verbal summary. Unfortunately, individuals are all too likely to be left guessing at the definitiveness of the studies reported in a typical popular account. Reporting results responsibly is a continuing problem for the scientific community.

Value-of-information analysis

Communications could attempt to provide the pieces of information having the largest possible impact on pending decisions. Value-of-information analysis is the general term for techniques determining the sensitivity of decisions to different information (Raiffa 1968).

Merz (1991) applied value-of-information analysis to a well-specified medical decision—whether to undergo carotid endarterectomy. Both this procedure, which involves scraping out an artery leading to the head, and its alternatives have a variety of possible positive and negative effects. These effects have been the topic of extensive research, providing quantitative risk estimates of varying precision. Merz created a simulated population of patients, varying in their physical conditions and preferences for different health states. He found that knowing about a few, but only a few, of the possible side-effects would change the preferred decision for a significant portion of patients. He argued that communications should focus on these few side-effects; doing so would make better use of patients' limited attention than a laundry lists of possibilities (although none of those should be hidden). He also argued that his procedure could provide an objective criterion for identifying the information that must be transmitted (and understood) in order to ensure medical informed consent.

Between the time that Merz (1991) submitted his dissertation and its defence, the results of a major clinical trial were released. Incorporating them in his model made little difference to its conclusions (Merz *et al.* 1993), i.e. from this perspective, information produced by the trial had little practical importance for determining the advisability of the surgery. This is not to say that the study did not contribute to the understanding of fundamental physiological processes, or that it might not have produced other results that would have been more useful to patients. However, the results give pause for thought regarding the allocation of research resources. Thus, value-of-information analysis can be used for prioritizing the scientific information to be collected as well as that to be transmitted (Fischhoff 2000). For example, it has been applied to the testing of chemicals for carcinogenicity (National Research Council 1983; Lave and Omenn 1986).

The choice among these approaches would depend on, among other things, how much time is available for communication, how well the decisions are formulated, and what scientific risk information exists. For example, value-of-information analysis might be particularly useful for identifying the focal facts for public service announcements. Calibration analysis may be used to identify surprising facts, of the sort that might both grab recipients' attention and change their behaviour. A mental model analysis might be more suited for the preparation of explanatory brochures or curricula.

Formatting information

Once information has been selected, it must be presented in a comprehensible way. That means taking into account the terms that recipients use for understanding individual concepts and the mental models that they use for integrating those concepts. It also means building on the results of research on text comprehension. That research shows, for example, (a) that comprehension improves when text has a clear structure and especially when that structure conforms to recipients' intuitive representation of a topic, (b) that critical information is more likely to be remembered when it appears at the highest level of a clear hierarchy, and (c) that readers benefit from 'adjunct aids', such as highlighting, advance organizers (showing what to expect), and summaries. Such aids might be better than full text for understanding, retaining, and being able to look up information. Fuller treatment can be found in sources such as Reder (1985), Kintsch (1986), Garnham (1987), Ericsson (1988), and Schriver (1989).

In a given application, several formats may meet these general constraints. Atman *et al.* (1994) created two brochures, using clear but different structures for explaining the risks of radon. One was organized around a decision tree, showing the options facing home-owners, the probabilities of possible consequences, and the associated costs or benefits. The second was organized around a directed network, representing, in effect, a simplified version of the expert model partially depicted in Fig. 5. Both brochures were compared with the widely distributed *Citizen's Guide to Radon* (US Environmental Protection Agency 1989), which was built around a question-and-answer format with little attempt to summarize or impose a general structure. All three brochures substantially increased readers' understanding of the material presented in them. However, the structured brochures did better (and similar) jobs of enabling readers to make inferences about issues that were not mentioned explicitly and to give advice to others who had not read the material. To the Environmental Protection Agency's great credit, its brochure was much more extensively evaluated than the vast majority of public health communications—although without the benefit of these procedures from applied cognitive psychology (Desvousges *et al.* 1989; Smith *et al.* 1995).

Evaluating communications

Effective risk communications can help people to reduce their health risks, or to obtain greater benefits in return for those risks that they take. Ineffective communications can not only fail to do so, but also incur opportunity costs, in the sense of occupying the place (in recipients' lives and society's functions) that could be taken up by more effective communications. Even worse, misdirected communications can prompt wrong decisions by omitting key information or failing to contradict misconceptions, create confusion by prompting inappropriate assumptions or emphasizing irrelevant information, and provoke conflict by eroding recipients' faith in the communicator. By causing undue alarm or complacency, poor communications can have greater public health impact than the risks that they attempt to describe. Because communicators' intuitions about recipients' risk perceptions cannot be trusted, there is no substitute for empirical validation (Fischhoff *et al.* 1983; Fischhoff 1987; Slovic 1987; National Research Council 1989).

The most ambitious evaluations ask whether recipients follow the recommendations given in the communication (Lau *et al.* 1980; Weinstein 1987). However, that standard requires recipients not only to understand the message, but also to accept it as relevant to their personal circumstances. For example, home-owners without the resources to address radon problems might both understand and ignore a communication advocating testing, and women might hear quite clearly what actions an 'expert' recommends for reducing their risk of sexual assault, yet reject the political agenda underlying that advice (Fischhoff 1992). Judging a programme's effectiveness according to its behavioural effects requires great confidence that one knows what is right for others.

A more modest, but ethically simpler, evaluation criterion is to ensure that recipients have understood what a message was trying to say. That necessary condition might prove sufficient if the recommended action is obviously appropriate—once one knows the facts. Unfortunately, formal evaluations seem to be remarkably rare among the myriad of warning labels, health claims and advisories, public service announcements, operating instructions, and so on encountered in everyday life and work (Laughery *et al.* 1994).

Evaluating what people take away from a communication faces the same methodological challenges as measuring their ambient risk perceptions. The evaluator wants to avoid changing people's beliefs through cues embedded in how questions and answers are phrased, restricting the expression of non-expert beliefs, or suppressing the expression of inconsistent beliefs (across questions).

For example, in the course of evaluating its radon risk communications, the Environmental Protection Agency (Desvousges *et al.* 1989) posed the following question: 'What kinds of problems are high levels of radon exposure likely to cause? (a) Minor skin problems; (b) eye irritations; (c) lung cancer.' This question seems to risk inflating subjects' apparent level of understanding in several ways. Subjects who know only that radon causes cancer might deduce that it causes lung cancer. The words 'minor' and 'irritation' might imply that these are not the effects of 'high levels' (of anything). Moreover, there is no way for subjects to express other misconceptions, such as that radon causes breast cancer or other lung problems (which emerged with some frequency in open-ended interviews) (Bostrom *et al.* 1992).

Table 2 summarizes approaches to reader-based evaluation. In principle, open-ended interviews provide the best way to reduce such threats. Performing them to the standards of scientific publication is labour intensive. It involves conducting, transcribing, and coding interviews, with suitable reliability checks (in addition to the effort of producing an expert model and determining explicit communication goals). The stakes riding on many risk communications should justify that investment, considering the costs of dissemination and of the ensuing ineffective choices. Realistically, the necessary time and financial resources will not always be available. In some cases, a few open-ended one-on-one interviews might still provide valuable stepping stones to structured tests suitable for mass administration. Those quizzes will cover the critical topics in the expert model, express questions in terms familiar to subjects, and estimate the prevalence of misconceptions. Even if systematic study is impractical, one-on-one interviews, using think-aloud protocols, can be administered quickly, purely for their heuristic value. It is depressing how often this rudimentary precaution is not taken.

The format of a message conveys priorities. Figure 6 shows the expected inhalation dose of methylene chloride, for individuals performing a common paint-stripping task, in a medium-sized room with moderate ventilation. (Details of the model in general and of this

Table 2 Data collection options for reader-based evaluations of risk communications

	Strengths	Weaknesses
Concurrent		
Think-aloud protocol	Protocols identify specific problems with text content and organization; can produce surprises	Costly and time-consuming; difficult to analyse; samples usually small
Retrospective		
Open-ended	Least reactive—avoids structuring answers for respondents	Coding scheme necessary—data potentially difficult to analyse
Interview	Identifies how reader structures knowledge, is less reactive than most methods	Costly and time-consuming; samples usually small
Short questions, recall	Measures what 'sticks' in readers' minds; can measure how readers assign importance	May not elicit information used in actual decision-making; responses driven by context; difficult to analyse
Problem solving (scenarios)	Elicits decision-making information and strategies	Frames problems for respondents—may be reactive
Closed-ended	Data structured, easier, and less expensive to collect and analyse; large samples more feasible	Potentially reactive—may misrepresent respondents' knowledge and attitudes
Knowledge tests (true/false, multiple choice)	Can verify specific misconceptions and beliefs; data readily comparable	Costly; difficult to design valid questions and response scales

Source: Bostrom *et al.* (1994).

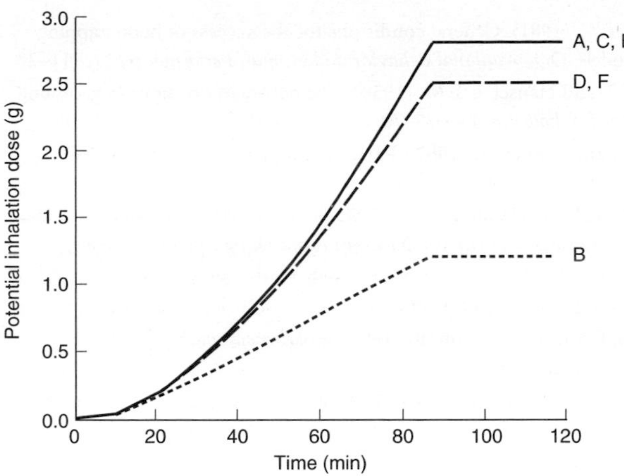

Fig. 6 Inhalation dose of methylene chloride for users of paint strippers who read and follow the first five points on the labels of six products.

specific application are given by Riley *et al.* (1998).) Each curve assumes that users read the first five items on the labels of six different products (taken from the shelves of a local hardware store), and then follow those directions perfectly. Clearly, product B does a much better job than the others for users with these reading habits. That advantage vanishes for users who read only the text emphasized on a label or only the directions (with all labels performing equally poorly). For those (rare?) users who read everything, there is virtually no exposure at all with product A, the labels for B, D, and E produce exposures like those for B in the figure, and products C and F perform no better. Reducing risks to such products requires understanding users' behaviour, reading patterns, and mental models (determining how far they follow the instructions that they read).

Conclusion

Understanding risk perception and risk communication is a complicated business, perhaps as complicated as assessing the magnitude of the risks being considered. A chapter of this length can, at best, indicate the dimensions of this complexity and the directions of plausible solutions. In this treatment, we have emphasized methodological issues because we believe that these topics often seem deceptively simple. Because we ask questions in everyday life, eliciting the beliefs of others may seem straightforward; because we talk every day, it may seem simple to communicate about health risks. Unfortunately, there are many pitfalls to such amateurism, some of which emerge in the research described here. Hints at these problems can be found in those occasions in life where we have misunderstood or been misunderstood, particularly when discussing unfamiliar topics with strangers.

Research on these topics is fortunate in being able to draw on well-developed literatures in such areas as cognitive, health, and social psychology, psycholinguistics, psychophysics, and behavioural decision theory. It is unfortunate in having to face the particularly rigorous demands of assessing and improving complex beliefs about health risks. These often involve unfamiliar topics, surrounded by unusual kinds of uncertainty, for which individuals and groups lack stable vocabularies. Health-risk decisions also raise difficult and potentially threatening trade-offs. Even the most carefully prepared and evaluated communications may not be able to eliminate the anxiety and frustration that such decisions create. However, systematic preparation can keep communications from adding to the problem. At some point in complex decisions, we 'throw up our hands' and go with what seems right. Good risk communications can help people go further into the problem before that happens.

Health-risk decisions are not just about cognitive processes and coolly weighed information. Emotions play a role, as do social

Table 3 Developmental stages in risk management

All we have to do is get the numbers right
All we have to do is tell them the numbers
All we have to do is explain what we mean by the numbers
All we have to do is show them that they have accepted similar risks in the past
All we have to do is show them that it is a good deal for them
All we have to do is treat them nice
All we have to do is make them partners
All of the above

Source: Fischhoff (1995).

Table 4 Conditions for public trust in risk analysis

Scientific conditions
Immediate
Familiarity with specific models
Familiarity with specific inputs
Access to sensitivity analyses
Ability to double-check
Ambient
Familiarity with historical development
Familiarity with underlying science
Familiarity with auxiliary assumptions
Familiarity with analytical perspectives
Social conditions
Immediate
Familiarity with analysts
Recognition by analysis
Reward for participation
Respectful treatment
Ambient
Familiarity with analytical community
Influence on regulatory process
Long-term involvement
Accommodation with process

Source: Fischhoff (1996b).

processes. Nonetheless, it is important to get the cognitive part right, lest people's ability to think their way to decisions be underestimated and underserved. For the resolution of risk issues to hinge on the light of information, rather than the heat of controversy, those managing the risk bear special responsibility to behave in a credible way. If one examines the risks that hit the headlines, it has often been the case that the authorities were slow to realize, or at least acknowledge, that they might be managing a risk that warranted public scrutiny (Fischhoff 1995). Table 3 shows one characterization of the stages that authorities may go through as they gradually (and perhaps begrudgingly) attempt to satisfy their public's desire to understand, and perhaps participate in the control of, a risk. The energies that the public sees iauthorities investing in generating openness partially determine the credibility of the communications that they receive.

Table 4 offers one specification of the conditions that risk specialists must meet in order to secure public trust. It is patterned after the conditions that experts must meet in order to secure one another's trust. It includes both scientific and social conditions, concerning, respectively, the content and the conduct of science. In each domain, there are conditions associated with both each specific case and the general process of analysing risk issues.

References

Arnet, J. (1999). Adolescent storm and stress, reconsidered. *American Psychologist*, **54**, 317–26.

Atman, C.J., Bostrom, A., Fischhoff, B., and Morgan, M.G. (1994). Designing risk communications: completing and correcting mental models of hazardous processes, Part 1. *Risk Analysis*, **14**, 779–88.

Bar-Hillel, M. (1974). Similarity and probability. *Organizational Behavior and Human Performance*, **11**, 277–82.

Bauman, K.E. (1980). *Predicting adolescent drug use: utility structure and marijuana.* Praeger, New York.

Beattie, J., Covey, J., Dolan, P., *et al.* (1998). On the contingent valuation of safety and the safety of contingent valuation. *Journal of Risk and Uncertainty*, **17**, 5–26.

Beyth-Marom, R. (1982). How probable is probable? Numerical translation of verbal probability expressions. *Journal of Forecasting*, **1**, 257–69.

Beyth-Marom, R., Austin, L., Fischhoff, B., Palmgren, C., and Quadrel, M.J. (1993). Perceived consequences of risky behaviors. *Developmental Psychology*, **29**, 549–63.

Black, W.C., Nease, R.F., and Tosteson, A.N.A. (1995). Perceptions of breast cancer risk and screening effectiveness in women younger than 50 years of age. *Journal of the National Cancer Institute*, **8**, 720–31.

Bostrom, A., Fischhoff, B., and Morgan, M.G. (1992). Characterizing mental models of hazardous processes: A methodology and an application to radon. *Journal of Social Issues*, **48**, 85–100.

Bostrom, A., Atman, C.J., Fischhoff, B., and Morgan, M.G. (1994). Evaluating risk comunications: completing and correcting mental models of hazardous processes. Part 2. *Risk Analysis*, **14**, 789–98.

Bruine de Bruin, W. (1999). People's understanding of probability: 'It's a fifty-fifty chance'. PhD Dissertation, Carnegie–Mellon University.

Budescu, D.F. and Wallsten, T.S. (1995). Processing linguistic probabilities: General principles and empirical evidence. In *Decision making from the perspective of cognitive psychology* (ed. J.R. Busemeyer, R. Hastie, and D.L. Medin). Academic Press, New York.

Burns, W.J. and Clemen, R.T. (1993). Covariance structure models and influence diagrams. *Management Science*, **39**, 816–34.

Camerer, C. (1981). General conditions for the success of bootstrapping models. *Organizational Behavior and Human Performance*, **27**, 411–22.

Cohen, J. and Hansel, C.E.M. (1958). The nature of decisions in gambling. *Acta Psychologica*, **13**, 357–70.

Cole, G. and Withey, S. (1982). Perspectives in risk perceptions. *Risk Analysis*, **1**, 143–63.

Covello, V.T., Sandman, P.M., and Slovic, P. (1988). *Risk communication, risk statistics, and risk comparisons: A manual for plant managers.* Chemical Manufacturers Association, Washington, DC.

Craik, K. (1943). *The nature of explanation.* Cambridge University Press.

Crouch, E.A.C. and Wilson, R. (1982). *Risk/benefit analysis.* Ballinger, Cambridge, MA.

Cvetkovich, G., Grote, B., Bjorseth, A., and Sarkissian, J. (1975). On the psychology of adolescents' use of contraceptives. *Journal of Sex Research*, **11**, 256–70.

Davies, J.C. (ed.) (1996). *Comparing environmental risks.* Resources for the Future, Washington, DC.

Dawes, R.M. and Corrigan, B. (1974). Linear models in decision making. *Psychological Bulletin*, **81**, 95–106.

Dawes, R.M., Faust, D., and Meehl, P. (1989). Clinical versus actuarial judgment. *Science*, **243**, 1668–74.

Desvousges, W.H., Smith, V.K., and Rink III H.H. (1989). *Communicating radon risk effectively: radon testing in Maryland.* EPA 230-03-89-408. US Environmental Protection Agency, Washington, DC.

Douglas, M. (1992). *Risk and blame.* Routledge, London.

Elkind, D. (1967). Egocentrism in adolescence. *Child Development*, **38**, 1025–39.

Ënglander, T., Farago, K., Slovic, P., and Fischhoff, B. (1986). A comparative analysis of risk perception in Hungary and the United States. *Social Behavior*, **1**, 55–6.

Erev, I. and Cohen, B.L. (1990). Verbal versus numerical probabilities: efficiency, biases and the preference paradox. *Organizational Behavior and Human Decision Processes*, **45**, 1–18.

Ericsson, K.A. (1988). Concurrent verbal reports on text comprehension: a review. *Text*, **8**, 295–325.

Ericsson, K.A. and Simon, H.A. (1980). Verbal reports as data. *Psychological Review*, **87**, 215–51.

Feather, N. (ed.) (1982). *Expectancy, incentive and action.* Erlbaum, Hillsdale, NJ.

Fineberg, H.V. (1988). Education to prevent AIDS. *Science*, **239**, 592–6.

Fischhoff, B. (1987). Treating the public with risk communications: A public health perspective. *Science, Technology, and Human Values*, **12**, 13–19.

Fischhoff, B. (1989*a*). Eliciting knowledge for analytical representation. *IEEE Transactions on Systems, Man and Cybernetics*, **13**, 448–61.

Fischhoff, B. (1989*b*). Making decisions about AIDS. In *Primary prevention of AIDS* (ed. V. Mays, G. Albee, and S. Schneider), pp. 168–205. Sage, Newbury Park, CA.

Fischhoff, B. (1990). Psychology and public policy: tool or tool maker? *American Psychologist*, **45**, 57–63.

Fischhoff, B. (1991). Value elicitation: is there anything in there? *American Psychologist*, **46**, 835–47.

Fischhoff, B. (1992). Giving advice: decision theory perspectives on sexual assault. *American Psychologist*, **47**, 577–88.

Fischhoff, B. (1994). What forecasts (seem to) mean. *International Journal of Forecasting*, **10**, 387–403.

Fischhoff, B. (1995). Risk perception and communication unplugged: twenty years of process. *Risk Analysis*, **15**, 137–45.

Fischhoff, B. (1996*a*). The real world: what good is it? *Organizational Behavior and Human Decision Processes*, **65**, 232–48.

Fischhoff, B. (1996*b*). Public values in risk research. *Annals of the American Academy of Political and Social Science*, **545**, 75–84.

Fischhoff, B. (1999). Why (cancer) risk communication can be hard. *Journal of the National Cancer Institute Monographs*, **25**, 7–13.

Fischhoff, B. (2000). Scientific management of science? *Policy Sciences*, **29**, 1–15.

Fischhoff, B. and Bruine de Bruin, W. (1999). Fifty/fifty = 50? *Journal of Behavioral Decision Making*, **12**, 149–63.

Fischhoff, B. and MacGregor, D. (1983). Judged lethality: how much people seem to know depends upon how they are asked. *Risk Analysis*, **3**, 229–36.

Fischhoff, B. and Quadrel, M.J. (1991). Adolescent alcohol decisions. *Alcohol Health and Research World*, **15**, 43–51.

Fischhoff, B., Slovic, P., and Lichtenstein, S. (1977). Knowing with certainty: the appropriateness of extreme confidence. *Journal of Experimental Psychology: Human Perception and Performance*, **3**, 552–64.

Fischhoff, B., Slovic, P., Lichtenstein, S., Read, S., and Combs, B. (1978). How safe is safe enough? A psychometric study of attitudes towards technological risks and benefits. *Policy Sciences*, **8**, 127–52.

Fischhoff, B., Lichtenstein, S., Slovic, P., Derby, S.L., and Keeney, R.L. (1981). *Acceptable risk*. Cambridge University Press, New York.

Fischhoff, B., Slovic, P., and Lichtenstein, S. (1983). The 'public' vs. the 'experts': Perceived vs. actual disagreement about the risks of nuclear power. In *Analysis of actual vs. perceived risks* (ed. V. Covello, G. Flamm, J. Rodericks, and R. Tardiff), pp. 235–49. Plenum Press, New York.

Fischhoff, B., Watson, S., and Hope, C. (1984). Defining risk. *Policy Sciences*, **17**, 123–39.

Fischhoff, B., Downs, J., and Bruine de Bruin, W. (1998). Adolescent vulnerability: A framework for behavioral interventions. *Applied and Preventive Psychology*, **7**, 77–94.

Fischhoff, B., Welch, N., and Frederick, S. (1999). Construal processes in preference elicitation. *Journal of Risk and Uncertainty*, **19**, 139–64.

Fortney, J. (1988). Contraception: a life long perspective. In *Dying for love*. National Council for International Health, Washington, DC.

Funtowicz, S.O. and Ravetz, J.R. (1990). *Uncertainty and quality in science for policy*. Kluwer, Boston, MA.

Furnham, A.F. (1988). *Lay theories*. Pergamon, Oxford.

Galotti, K.M. (1989). Approaches to studying formal and everyday reasoning. *Psychological Bulletin*, **105**, 331–51.

Gärdenfors, P. and Sahlin, N.E. (1982). Unreliable probabilities, risk taking and decision making. *Synthese*, **53**, 361–86.

Garnham, A. (1987). *Mental models as representations of discourse and text*. Halsted Press, New York.

Gentner, D. and Stevens, A.L. (ed.) (1983). *Mental models*. Erlbaum, Hillsdale, NJ.

Goldberg, L.R. (1968). Simple models or simple processes? *American Psychologist*, **23**, 483–96.

Goszczynska, M., Tyszka, T., and Slovic, P. (1991). Risk perception in Poland: A comparison with three other countries. *Journal of Behavioral Decision Making*, **4**, 179–93.

Green, C.H. and Brown, R.A. (1981). *The perception and acceptability of risk*. Duncan of Jordanstone School of Architecture, Dundee.

Gregory, R., Lichtenstein, S., and Slovic, P. (1993) Valuing environmental resources: A constructive approach. *Journal of Risk and Uncertainty*, **7**, 177–97.

Hammond, K.R., Hursch, C.J., and Toddy, F.J. (1964). Analyzing the components of clinical inference. *Psychological Review*, **71**, 438–56.

Harding, C.M. and Eiser, J.R. (1984). Characterizing the perceived risks and benefits of some health issues. *Risk Analysis*, **4**, 131–41.

Hasher, L. and Zacks, R.T. (1984). Automatic processing of fundamental information. *American Psychologist*, **39**, 1372–88.

Heimer, C.A. (1988). Social structure, psychology, and the estimation of risk. *Annual Review of Sociology*, **14**, 491–519.

Hendrickx, L.C.W.P. (1991). How versus how often: the role of scenario information and frequency information in risk judgment and risky decision making. Doctoral Dissertation, Rijksuniversiteit Groningen, The Netherlands.

Hoffman, P.J. (1960). Paramorphic models representation of clinical judgment. *Psychological Bulletin*, **57**, 116–31.

Howard, R.A. (1989). Knowledge maps. *Management Science*, **35**, 903–22.

Hurd, M.D. (1999). Anchoring an acquiesence bias in measuring assets in household surveys. *Journal of Risk and Uncertainty*, **19**, 111–36.

Inhaber, H. (1979). Risk with energy from conventional and non-conventional sources. *Science*, **203**, 718–23.

Institute of Medicine (1986). *Confronting AIDS*. National Academy Press, Washington, DC.

Institute of Medicine (1998). *Scientific opportunities and public needs*. National Academy Press, Washington, DC.

Jasanoff, S. (1986). *Risk management and political culture*. Russell Sage Foundation, New York.

Jenni, K. (1997). Attributes for risk evaluation. PhD Dissertation, Carnegie–Mellon University.

Jianguang, Z. (1994). Environmental hazards in the Chinese public's eyes. *Risk Analysis*, **14**, 163–9.

Johnson-Laird, P.N. (1983). *Mental models*. Cambridge University Press, New York.

Jungermann, H., Schutz, H., and Thüring, M. (1988). Mental models in risk assessment: Informing people about drugs. *Risk Analysis*, **8**, 147–55.

Kahneman, D., Slovic, P., and Tversky, A. (ed.) (1982). *Judgment under uncertainty: heuristics and biases*. Cambridge University Press, New York.

Kahneman, D., Knetsch, J.L., and Thaler, R.H. (1991). The endowment effect, loss aversion,and status quo bias. *Journal of Economic Perspectives*, **5**, 193–206.

Kammen, D. and Hassenzahl, D. (1999). *Should we risk it?* Princeton University Press.

Kaplan, E.H. (1989). What are the risks of risky sex? *Operations Research*, **37**, 198–209.

Karpowicz-Lazreg, C. and Mullet, E. (1993). Societal risk as seen by the French public. *Risk Analysis*, **13**, 253–8.

Keating, D.P. (1988). *Cognitive processes in adolescence*. Ontario Institute for Studies in Education, Toronto.

Kempton, W. (1987). Variation in folk models and consequent behavior. *American Behavioral Scientist*, **31**, 203–18.

Kempton, W. (1991). Lay perspectives on global climate change. *Global Environmental Change*, **1**, 183–208.

Kintsch, W. (1986). Learning from text. *Cognition and Instruction*, **3**, 87–108.

Koriat, A. (1993). How do we know that we know? *Psychological Review*, **100**, 609–39.

Krimsky, S. and Golding, D. (ed.) (1992). *Theories of risk*. Praeger, New York.

Krimsky, S. and Plough, A. (1988). *Environmental hazards*. Auburn House, Dover, MA.

Kuyper, H. and Vlek, C. (1984). Contrasting risk judgements among interest groups. *Acta Psychologica*, **56**, 205–18.

Lau, R., Kaine, R., Berry, S., Ware, J., and Roy, D. (1980). Channeling health: a review of the evaluation of televised health campaigns. *Health Education Quarterly*, **7**, 56–89.

Laughery, K.S., Wogalter, M.S., and Young, S.L. (ed.) (1994). *Human factors perspectives on warnings*. Human Factors and Ergonomics Society, Santa Monica, CA.

Lave, L.B. and Omenn, G.S. (1986). Costs effectiveness of short-term tests for carcinogenicity. *Nature*, **324**, 29–39.

Leiss, W. and Chociolko, C. (1994). *Risk and responsibility.* McGill–Queens University Press, Montreal and Kingston.

Lichtenstein, S. and Newman, J.R. (1967). Empirical scaling of common verbal phrases associated with numerical probabilities. *Psychonomic Science*, **9**, 563–4.

Lichtenstein, S., Slovic, P., Fischhoff, B., Layman, M., and Combs, B. (1978). Judged frequency of lethal events. *Journal of Experimental Psychology: Human Learning and Memory*, **4**, 551–78.

Lichtenstein, S., Fischhoff, B., and Phillips, L.D. (1982). Calibration of probabilities: state of the art to 1980. In *Judgment under uncertainty: heuristics and biases* (ed. D. Kahneman, P. Slovic, and A. Tversky), pp. 306–39. Cambridge University Press, New York.

Linville, P.W., Fischer, G.W., and Fischhoff, B. (1993). AIDS risk perceptions and decision biases. In *The social psychology of HIV infection* (ed. J.B. Pryor and G.D. Reeder), pp. 5–38. Erlbaum, Hillsdale, NJ.

Lowrance, W. (1976). *Of acceptable risk.* Kaufmann, San Francisco, CA.

MacGregor, D. (1991). Worry over technological activities and life concerns. *Risk Analysis*, **11**, 315–25.

McIntyre, S. and West, P. (1992). What does the phrase 'safer sex' mean to you? Understanding among Glaswegian 18 year olds in 1990. *AIDS*, **7**, 121–6.

Maharik, M. and Fischhoff, B. (1992). The risks of nuclear energy sources in space: some activists' perceptions. *Risk Analysis*, **12**, 383–92.

Means, M.L. and Voss, J.F. (1985). Star Wars: a developmental study of expert and novice knowledge studies. *Journal of Memory and Language*, **24**, 746–57.

Merton, R.F. (1987). The focussed interview and focus groups. *Public Opinion Quarterly*, **51**, 550–66.

Merz, J.F. (1991). Toward a standard of disclosure for medical informed consent: Development and demonstration of a decision—analytic methodology. PhD dissertation, Carnegie–Mellon University.

Merz, J., Druzdzel, M., and Mazur, D.J. (1991). Verbal expressions of probability in informed consent litigation. *Medical Decision Making*, **11**, 273–81.

Merz, J., Fischhoff, B., Mazur, D.J., and Fischbeck, P.S. (1993). Decision-analytic approach to developing standards of disclosure for medical informed consent. *Journal of Toxics and Liability*, **15**, 191–215.

Morgan, M.G. and Henrion, M. (1990). *Uncertainty.* Cambridge University Press, New York.

Morgan, M.G., Fischhoff, B., Bostrom, A., Lave, L., and Atman, C.J. (1992). Communicating risk to the public. *Environmental Science and Technology*, **26**, 2048–56.

Morgan, M.G., Fischhoff, B., Bostrom, A., and Atman, C. *Risk communication: the mental model approach.* Cambridge University Press, New York, in press.

Morrison, D.M. (1985). Adolescent contraceptive behavior: a review. *Psychological Bulletin*, **98**, 538–68.

Murphy, A.H., Lichtenstein, S., Fischhoff, B., and Winkler, R.L. (1980). Misinterpretations of precipitation probability forecasts. *Bulletin of the American Meteorological Society*, **61**, 695–701.

National Research Council (1983). *Research needs for human factors.* National Academy Press, Washington, DC.

National Research Council (1989). *Improving risk communication.* National Academy Press, Washington, DC.

National Research Council (1996). *Understanding risk: Informing decisions in a democratic society.* National Academy Press, Washington, DC.

National Research Council (1999). *Toward environmental justice.* National Academy Press, Washington, DC.

Oden, G.C. (1987). Concept, knowledge, and thought. *Annual Review of Psychology*, **38**, 203–27.

Okrent, D. and Pidgeon, N. (ed.) (1998). Risk perception versus risk analysis (Special Issue). *Reliability Engineering and System Safety*, **58**.

Otway, H.J. and Wynne, B. (1989). Risk communication: paradigm and paradox. *Risk Analysis*, **9**, 141–5.

Payne, J.W., Bettman, J.R., and Schkade, D.A. (1999). Measuring constructed preferences: towards a building code. *Journal of Risk and Uncertainty*. **19**, 243–70.

Poulton, E.C. (1989). *Bias in quantifying judgment.* Erlbaum, Hillsdale, NJ.

Quadrel, M.J. (1990). Elicitation of adolescents' risk perceptions: qualitative and quantitative dimensions. PhD dissertation, Carnegie–Mellon University.

Quadrel, M.J., Fischhoff, B., and Davis, W. (1993). Adolescent (in) vulnerability. *American Psychologist*, **48**, 102–16.

Raiffa, H. (1968). *Decision analysis: introductory lectures on choices under uncertainty.* Addison-Wesley, Reading, MA.

Reder, L.M. (1985). Techniques available to author, teacher, and reader to improve retention of main ideas of a chapter. In *Thinking and learning skills.* Vol. 2, *Research and open questions* (ed. S.F. Chipman, J.W. Segal, and R. Glaser), pp. 37–64. Erlbaum, Hillsdale, NJ.

Riley, D., Fischoff, B., Small, M., and Fishbeck, P.S. (2001). Evaluating the effectiveness of risk-reduction strategies for chemical products. *Risk Analysis*, **21**, 357–69.

Ritov, I. and Baron, J. (1990). Status quo and omission bias. Reluctance to vaccinate. *Journal of Behavioral Decision Making*, **3**, 263–77.

Rohrmann, B. (1994). Risk perception of different societal groups: Australian findings and cross-national comparisons. *Australian Journal of Psychology*, **46**, 15–163.

Roth, E., Morgan, G., Fischhoff, B., Lave, L., and Bostrom, A. (1990). What do we know about making risk comparisons? *Risk Analysis*, **10**, 375–87.

Rouse, W.B. and Morris N.M. (1986). On looking into the black box: prospects and limits in the search for mental models. *Psychological Bulletin*, **100**, 399–463.

Royal Society (1992). *Risk analysis, perception and management.* Royal Society, London.

Schriver, K.A. (1989). Evaluating text quality: the continuum from text-focused to reader-focused methods. *IEEE Transactions on Professional Communication*, **32**, 238–55.

Schulenberg, J., Maggs, J., and Hurnelmans, K. (ed.) (1997). *Health risks and developmental transaction during adolescence.* Cambridge University Press, New York.

Schwarz, N. (1996). *Cognition and communication: judgmental biases, research methods and the logic of conversation.* Erlbaum, Hillsdale, NJ.

Schwarz, N. (1999). Self reports. *American Psychologist*, **54**, 93–105.

Shaklee, H. and Fischhoff, B. (1990). The psychology of contraceptive surprises: judging the cumulative risk of contraceptive failure. *Journal of Applied Psychology*, **20**, 385–403.

Slovic, P. (1987). Perceptions of risk. *Science*, **236**, 280–5.

Slovic, P., Fischhoff, B., and Lichtenstein, S. (1979). Rating the risks. *Environment*, **21**, 14–20, 36–9.

Slovic, P., Fischhoff, B., and Lichtenstein, S. (1980). Facts and fears: understanding perceived risk. In *Societal risk assessment: How safe is safe enough?* (ed. R. Schwing and W.A. Albers Jr), pp. 181–214. Plenum Press, New York.

Slovic, P., Fischhoff, B., and Lichtenstein, S. (1984). Behavioral decision theory perspectives on risk and safety. *Acta Psychologica*, **56**, 183–203.

Slovic, P., Fischhoff, B., and Lichtenstein, S. (1985). Characterizing perceived risk. In *Perilous progress: Technology as hazard* (ed. R.W. Kates, C. Hohenemser, and J. Kasperson), pp. 91–123. Westview, Boulder, CO.

Slovic, P., Kraus, N.N., Lappe, H., Letzel, H., and Malmfors, T. (1989). Risk perception of prescription drugs: report on a survey in Sweden. *Pharmaceutical Medicine*, **4**, 43–65.

Smith, V.K., Desvousages W.H., and Payne, J.W. (1995). Do risk information programs promote mitigating behavior? *Journal of Risk and Uncertainty*, **10**, 203–21.

Stallen, P.J.M. and Tomas, A. (1988). Public concerns about industrial hazards. *Risk Analysis*, **8**, 235–45.

Starr, C. (1969). Societal benefit versus technological risk. *Science*, **165**, 1232–8.

Svenson, O. (1981). Are we all less risky and more skillful than our fellow drivers? *Acta Psychologica*, **47**, 143–8.

Svenson, O. and Fischhoff, B. (1985). Levels of environmental decisions. *Journal of Environmental Psychology*, **5**, 55–68.

Thaler, R. (1991). *Quasi-rational economics.* Russell Sage Foundation, New York.

Tversky, A. and Kahneman, D. (1973). Availability: A heuristic for judging frequency and probability. *Cognitive Psychology*, **4**, 207–32.

US Environmental Protection Agency (1989). *A citizen's guide to radon.* US Environmental Protection Agency, Washington, DC.

US Environmental Protection Agency (1993). *A guidebook to comparing risks and setting environmental priorities.* US Environmental Protection Agency, Washington, DC.

Vaughan, E. (1993). Individual and cultural differences in adaptation to environmental risks. *American Psychologist*, **48**, 1–8.

Viscusi, K. (1992). *Smoking: Making the risky decision.* Oxford University Press, New York.

Vlek, C. and Stallen, P.J. (1980). Rational and personal aspects of risk. *Acta Psychologica*, **45**, 273–300.

Vlek, C. and Stallen, P.J. (1981). Judging risks and benefits in the small and in the large. *Organizational Behavior and Human Performance*, **28**, 235–71.

Wagenaar, W.A. and Sagaria, S.D. (1975). Misperception of exponential growth. *Perception and Psychophysics*, **18**, 416–22.

Weinstein, N. (1987). *Taking care: understanding and encouraging self-protective behavior.* Cambridge University Press, New York.

Weinstein, N.D. (1989). Effects of personal experience on self-protective behavior. *Psychological Bulletin*, **105**, 31–50.

Weinstein, N.D. and Klein, W.M. (1996). Unrealistic optimism: present and future. *Journal of Social and Clinical Psychology*, **15**, 1–8.

Wilks, S.S. (1938). Weighting systems for linear functions of correlated variable where there is no dependent variable. *Psychometrika*, **8**, 23–40.

Wilson, R. (1979). Analyzing the risks of everyday life. *Technology Review*, **81**, 40–6.

Wilson, R.W. and Thornberry, O.T. (1987). Knowledge and attitudes about AIDS: provisional data from the National Health Interview Survey, August 10–30 1987. *Advance Data*, No. 146.

Woloshin, S., Schwartz, L.M., Byram, S., Fischhoff, B., and Welch, H.G. (1998). Scales for assessing perceptions of event probability: a validation study. *Medical Decision Making*, **14**, 490–503.

Yates, J.F. (1989). *Judgment and decision making.* Prentice Hall, Englewood Cliffs, NJ.

Yates, J.F. (ed.) (1992). *Risk taking.* Wiley, Chichester.

9

Major health problems

9.1 Cardiovascular diseases

Russell V. Luepker

Introduction

Cardiovascular diseases are the leading cause of death and disability in many industrialized countries and they are increasing in the developing world. The principal cardiovascular diseases are related to atherosclerosis: coronary heart disease, stroke, and peripheral vascular disease. Hypertension, congestive heart failure, rheumatic heart disease, cardiomyopathy, and congenital heart disease are also prevalent. The patterns on distributions of these diseases vary in different regions, however, coronary heart disease is assuming pre-eminence in many areas.

The rise of the cardiovascular diseases is attributed to a number of factors. The gradual reduction and elimination of infectious diseases affecting the young and middle-aged has led to longer lives. The major cardiovascular diseases are chronic conditions which are progressive and affect mainly older populations. Longer life expectancy with increased proportions of older individuals in society has brought chronic diseases, particularly cardiovascular disease, to the forefront. Additionally, atherosclerotic related diseases are associated with affluent lifestyles. The widespread availability of foods containing high-fat animal products in many societies leads directly to elevated blood lipids. Surplus food plus reduction in habitual physical activity results in obesity, which also encourages hyperlipidaemia and hypertension. In countries where affluence is growing, these diseases are found first among the wealthy. However, cardiovascular disease gradually affects all segments of the population as better living conditions prevail.

These shifts have led to changing patterns of cardiovascular diseases worldwide. In many industrialized countries, the rates of cardiovascular disease are rising. In other countries, they are falling. In most developing countries, the rates are rising with greater affluence and less infectious disease.

The substantial prevalence of cardiovascular diseases resulted in widespread application of medical treatments to confront this epidemic. In some countries, 20 to 30 per cent of the adult population is currently under treatment for cardiovascular disease or increased risk of cardiovascular disease. There is a rapid development of high-technology procedures for disease treatment and amelioration. The widespread application of these advanced technologies has led to growing costs of health care, in many cases exceeding the ability of many national health budgets to supply these treatments.

The rise in cardiovascular diseases is a phenomenon of the twentieth century. It threatens to be the leading cause of death and disability worldwide in the twenty-first century. Public health can and does play a leading role in the prevention of these diseases. Because risk factors for these diseases are identifiable and readily modified in healthy individuals at the population level, the sources of this epidemic can be confronted. The elimination of these diseases is possible and is a major public health challenge of the coming period.

Burden of cardiovascular diseases

Mortality

Cardiovascular disease is the leading cause of death in many countries and rising in many others. Figure 1 depicts mortality for cardiovascular disease and all causes in 1995 for men and women aged 35 to 74 in selected countries. Cardiovascular diseases account for more than 50 per cent of the deaths in many countries (American Heart Association 1999). A number of different cardiovascular diseases are commonly implicated (Fig. 2). In the United States, as in many industrialized countries, coronary heart disease accounts for approximately half of the deaths while stroke and other cardiovascular causes provide the remainder. In Sweden, coronary heart disease and stroke are about equal. In Japan, stroke is more common as are other hypertension-related diseases, such as congestive heart failure. In Egypt, infectious cardiac diseases are important causes, however, atherosclerotic diseases are increasing (WHO 1995, 1996; American Heart Association 1999). These differences in distributions of cardiovascular disease mortality are associated with different circumstances in those countries and differing methods of classifying death. They also reflect age distributions of the populations, as the most common cardiovascular diseases are strongly associated with increasing age (Fig. 3).

Although rarely appreciated by clinicians, the majority of cardiovascular disease mortality occurs outside of hospitals as 'sudden' cardiac death (McGovern *et al.* 1996; Tunstall-Pedoe *et al.* 1996). It may occur at home, in a public place, during ambulance transport, or in the hospital emergency room. Even those who reach the hospital alive have high rates of mortality which may approach 100 per cent in some categories (for example myocardial rupture, cardiogenic shock). This mortality is commonly associated with coronary heart disease, but also with congestive heart failure and rheumatic heart disease, as lethal cardiac arrhythmias of sudden onset precede death in these conditions.

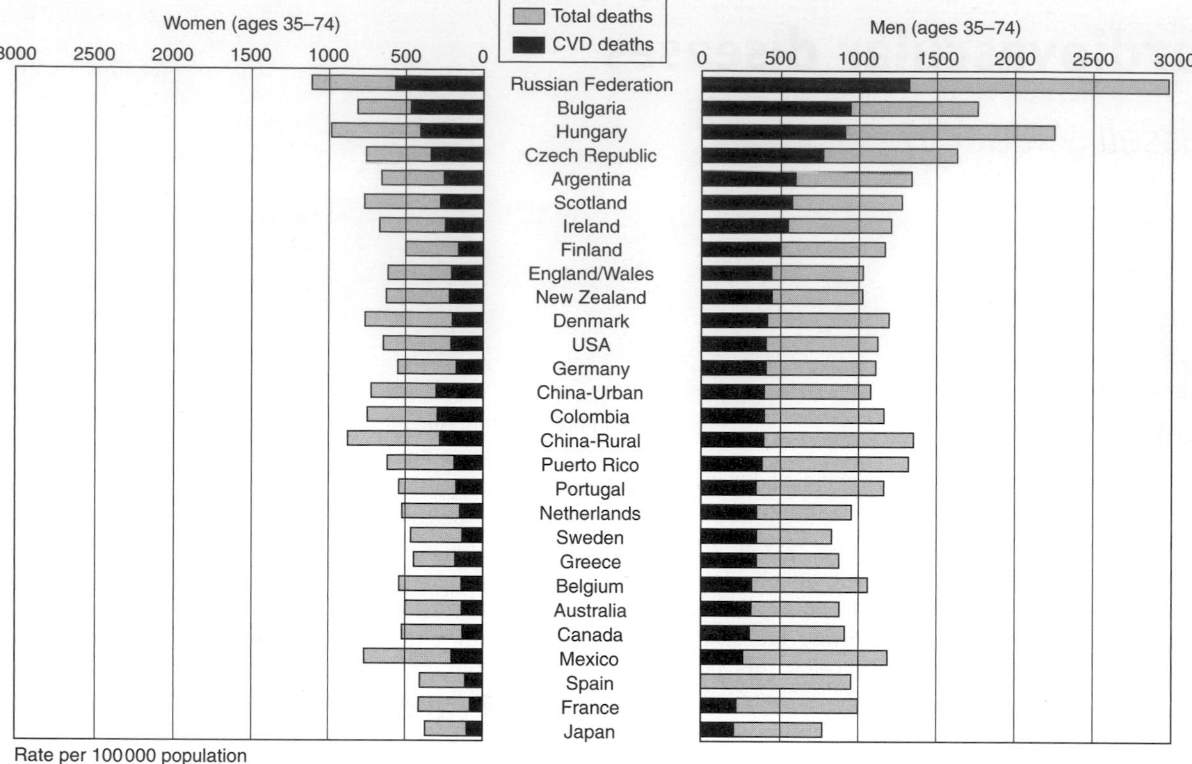

Fig. 1 Death rates per 100 000 population for cardiovascular diseases (CVD) and all causes in selected countries, 1995 (or most recent year available). (Source: American Heart Association 1999.)

Morbidity

While cardiac death is a common outcome of cardiovascular disease, non-fatal disease is also prevalent. As shown in Table 1, cardiovascular disease accounted for 5.8 million hospital admissions with an average length of stay of 5.8 days in the United States in 1995. It also accounts for 52 million visits to the general practitioner. Many of the visits are due to underlying cardiovascular disease, such as angina pectoris or congestive heart failure, or to treatment of risk factors such as hypertension and hyperlipidaemia.

The magnitude of this problem is also shown in Fig. 4 which describes trends in non-fatal and fatal coronary heart disease hospital admissions over time in south-eastern New England in the United States. The rates reflect the age and sex differences in coronary heart disease (Derby *et al.* 2000).

These common diseases now have many high-technology procedures designed to ameliorate the conditions and reduce symptoma-

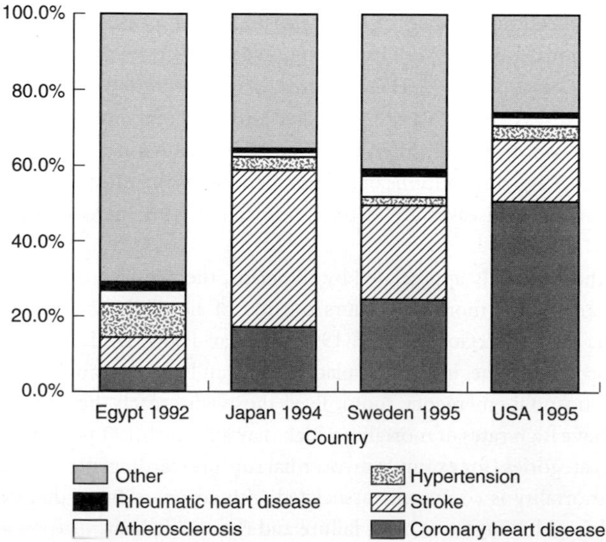

Fig. 2 Cardiovascular disease mortality. (Source: WHO 1995, 1996.)

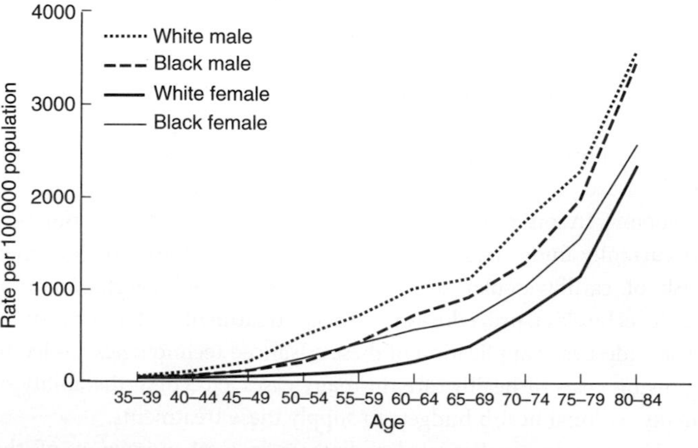

Fig. 3 Death rates per 100 000 population for heart disease by age, race, and sex in the United States, 1996. (Source: NHLBI 1998.)

Table 1 Cardiovascular diseases: number of hospital admissions, general practitioner visits, and deaths from cardiovascular diseases in the United States, 1995

Diagnostic category	ICD-9 codes	Hospital admissions		GP office visits (thousands)	Deaths
		First-listed discharge (thousands)	Length of stay (days)		
Total CVD	390–459, 745–747	5885	5.8	52 209	960 592
Heart disease	390–398, 402, 404–429	4050	5.5	19 738	737 563
Rheumatic heart disease	390–398	18	8.5	420	5147
Hypertensive heart disease	402, 404	122	6.5	683	27 498
Coronary heart disease	410–414	2130	5.3	9941	481 287
Acute myocardial infarction	410	771	6.6	402	218 229
Angina pectoris	413	115	2.8	1849	840
Other CHD	411, 412, 414	1244	4.6	7690	262 218
Diseases of pulmonary circulation	415–417	76	7.6	179	11 978
Pulmonary embolism	415.1	63	8.0	60	9098
Other	415.0, 416–417	13	5.6	119	2880
Acute and subacute endocarditis	421	17	17.3	7	979
Cardiomyopathy	425	34	5.4	395	27 031
Congestive heart failure	428.0	872	6.4	3202	43 010
Atrial fibrillation	427.31	270	4.3	1257	456
Other arrhythmias	426, 427 (except 427.31)	368	4.1	2094	42 376
Other heart diseases	420, 422–424, 428.1 428.9, 429	143	5.3	1560	97 801
Cerebrovascular disease	430–438	926	6.8	2450	157 991

CVD, cardiovascular disease; CHD, coronary heart disease; ICD-9, International Classification of Diseases, Ninth Revision.

Estimates of hospital admissions and general practitioner (GP) visits are subject to sampling variability. Estimates of hospital admissions below 50 000 have a relative standard error of more than 11 per cent. Estimates of GP visits below 588 000 have a relative standard error of more than 30 per cent.

Source: NHLBI (1998).

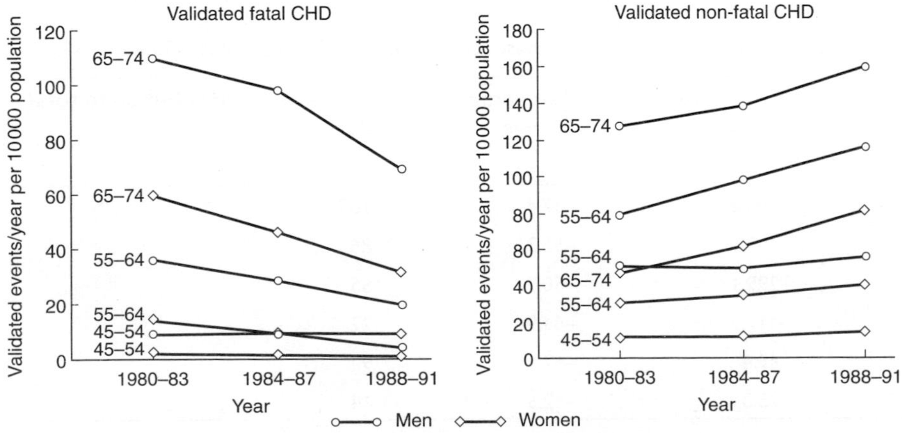

Fig. 4 Total discharges and deaths with International Classification of Diseases Ninth Revision code 410 to 414 in men and women, by age, in southeastern New England, United States, 1980 to 1991. (Adapted from Derby *et al.* 2000.)

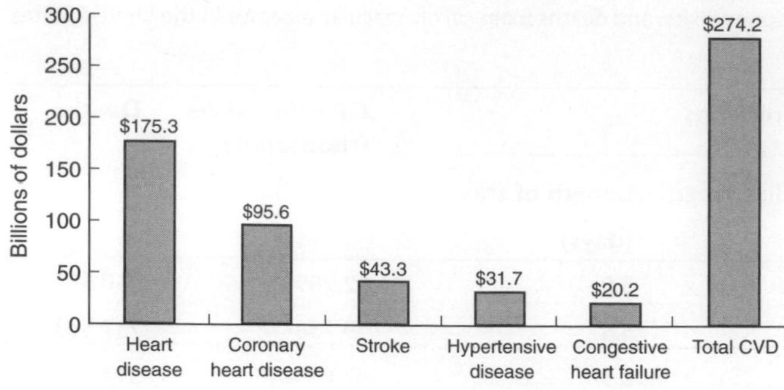

Fig. 5 Estimated direct and indirect costs of cardiovascular diseases (CVD) and stroke in the United States, 1998. (Source: American Heart Association 1999.)

tology. Some can prolong life. These medical procedures and treatments include cardiac surgery, angioplasty, angiography, pacemakers, implanted defibrillators, sophisticated diagnostic testing, and pharmaceuticals. Between the cost of this care and the lost productivity resulting from morbidity and mortality, cardiovascular disease represents an enormous economic burden, as shown in Fig. 5, for the United States in 1998 (American Heart Association 1999).

Disease trends

The epidemic of cardiovascular disease is largely a phenomenon of the twentieth century, and trends within this century are apparent. The Monitoring Trends and Determinants in Cardiovascular Disease (**MONICA**) study demonstrated that coronary heart disease was rising and falling in different nations during the 1980s and 1990s (Fig. 6) (Tunstall-Pedoe *et al.* 1999). A downward trend was noted in the United States with coronary heart disease rates peaking in the mid-1960s and falling substantially since that time (Table 2) (NHLBI 1998). Stroke peaked earlier, declined slowly, and then began a precipitous age-adjusted decline in the 1970s. Non-cardiovascular disease declined somewhat, but accounted for only a small fraction of the lower age-adjusted population mortality. With age-adjusted mortality falling, driven by a decline in cardiovascular disease, the result has been increased longevity in many populations. However, absolute mortality (not adjusted for age) has not fallen significantly, as the disease is pushed into older age groups (Luepker 1994).

Coronary heart disease

A vast body of research enhances the understanding of the aetiology, prevention, and treatment of coronary heart disease (WHO 1982). Important observations are summarized below:

1. Population-based studies show wide differences between countries and groups within those countries (Fig. 1).
2. The differences between populations are strongly related to population levels of established risk factors. These, in turn, are associated with differences in cultural, behavioural, and individual characteristics (Keys 1980).
3. Within populations, lipids, blood pressure, cigarette smoking, and other characteristics are highly predictive of coronary heart disease events in individuals (Dawber *et al.* 1957; Keys 1980; WHO 1982). These risk factors are first evidenced in youth and track into adulthood. That is, high-risk youth are likely to become high-risk adults (Luepker *et al.* 1999).
4. Studies of large-scale migrations from one culture to another demonstrate that an increase in risk factors and coronary heart disease is observed when individuals migrate from a low- to high-risk culture and assume the lifestyle of that new culture (Kagan *et al.* 1974).
5. Population patterns in coronary heart disease are changing rapidly within countries as some rise and some fall (Fig. 6).
6. Changes in coronary heart disease patterns are associated with a reduction in risk characteristics leading to decreased incidence and to improved medical care, leading to increased survival after an initial clinical event (Higgins and Luepker 1989).
7. Clinical trials demonstrate conclusively that a reduction in coronary heart disease mortality and morbidity results from the lowering of traditional risk factors (cholesterol, blood pressure,

Table 2 Age-adjusted death rates[a] and percentage change for all causes of death and cardiovascular disease in the United States (1950 and 1996)

Cause of death	Rate/100 000 population		1950–1996 difference	Percentage change	Percentage contribution to total decline
	1950	1996			
All causes	1446.0	905.2	–540.8	–37.4	100
CVD[b]	841.4	375.9	–465.5	–55.3	86
Heart	587.5	288.4	–299.1	–50.9	55
Stroke	180.7	63.4	–117.3	–64.9	22
Other CVD	73.2	24.1	–49.4	–67.1	9
Non-CVD	604.6	529.3	–75.3	–12.5	14

CVD, cardiovascular disease; CHD, coronary heart disease; ICD-9, International Classification of Diseases, Ninth Revision.

[a]Age-adjusted to the 2000 standard.

[b]Excludes congenital anomalies of the circulatory system.

Source: NHLBI (1998).

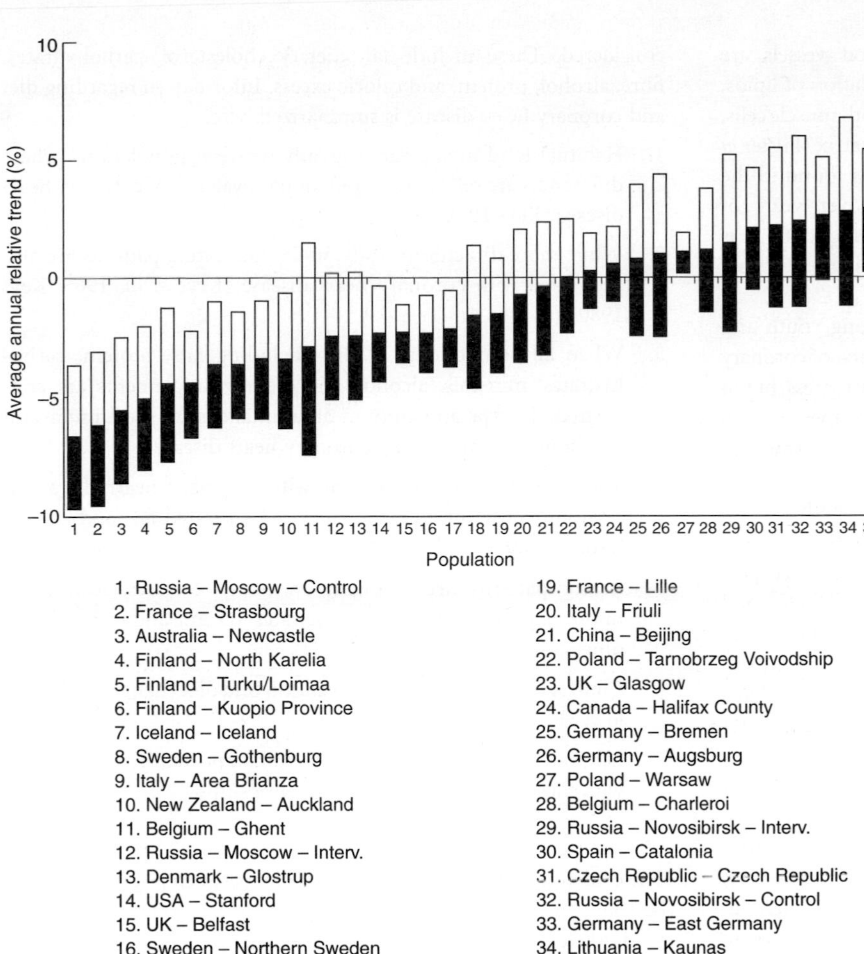

Fig. 6 Trends for coronary events in women (MONICA). (Source: Tunstall-Pedoe *et al.* 1999.)

cigarette smoking) by either behavioural and/or pharmacological methods.

8. The population and trial data are congruent with laboratory and animal studies of atherosclerosis.

Coronary heart disease is the leading cause of adult mortality and a common cause of chronic disability in many countries. Research in coronary heart disease has been comprehensive and diverse including laboratory studies, animal models, clinical studies, population studies, and clinical trials. The evidence from these studies is convergent and implicates population-wide causes for this epidemic. It is apparent that strong cultural and individual factors in the setting of widespread affluence results in elevated risk of the underlying disease atherosclerosis. These influences and risk factors are safely modifiable in individuals and entire populations (WHO 1982; Stone *et al.* 1997; Wood *et al.* 1998*b*; Grundy 1999).

The rationale for disease prevention is found in many observations. Environmental factors encourage population-wide changes in behaviour resulting in mass elevations of risk. As populations live longer, this chronic disease is manifest following prolonged and sustained exposure to risk factors. Widespread genetic susceptibility also plays an important role in the setting of an unfavourable environment. Prevention of coronary heart disease is well founded based on these scientific observations. It begins with primary prevention or prevention of risk factor elevation in the first place (Luepker 1999). It includes identification and reduction of risk in high-risk individuals without manifest disease signs or symptoms. Finally, it rests on the identification of those who continue to be at high risk after coronary heart disease occurs. Well-established population and medical strategies are tested to implement prevention and the epidemic could be controlled with widespread and effective implementation of current knowledge.

Atherosclerosis is the underlying pathology in coronary heart disease. It is a process that affects medium-sized muscular arteries including the coronary, cerebral, and lower extremity vessels. The abdominal and thoracic aorta can also be involved. The lesions of atherosclerosis affecting the internal walls of blood vessels are commonly known as plaques. Plaques are an accumulation of lipids, principally cholesterol esters and free cholesterol, smooth muscle cells, macrophages, T lymphocytes, and connective tissue matrix (Fuster *et al.* 1992*b*; Ross and Fuster 1996). These lesions, when found in the coronary arteries, gradually obstruct blood flow over years of accumulation. They may also act acutely, obstruct blood flow as plaques rupture, and a clot is formed further obstructing blood flow (Fuster *et al.* 1992*a*).

Early lesions of atherosclerosis can be found among youth and young adults when fatty streaks are observed in the intima of coronary arteries (Stary *et al.* 1994, 1995). These fatty streaks may regress, but in populations where coronary heart disease is common, they tend to progress to diffuse intimal thickening and more developed fibrous and calcified plaques (Stary *et al.* 1994, 1995).

Many hypotheses have been advanced to explain the pathogenesis of atherosclerosis (Virchow 1856). The leading hypothesis is the 'response to injury' theory where local factors including hyperlipidaemia, infection, rheological forces, cigarette smoking, diabetes, and others injure the intima of the artery. The response of the arteries to this injury is local plaque formation. Repeated injury increases the size of this lesion (Ross and Glomset 1973). Another theory suggests that a nidus for the lesions is based on aberrant cell growth which initiates the lesion (Benditt and Benditt 1973).

While the usual natural history of atherosclerosis is progression over time, plaques can also regress. In non-human primates, atherosclerotic lesions regress with the reduction of plasma cholesterol levels (Wissler and Vesselinovitch 1976; Clarkson *et al.* 1984). Similarly, humans are observed to have regression in atherosclerotic lesions with lipid lowering by diet, drugs or surgery (Ornish *et al.* 1990; Buchwald *et al.* 1992; Watts *et al.* 1992). Atherosclerotic lesions, while complex and well organized, can regress.

Lesions of coronary atherosclerosis lead to many clinical outcomes, usually in the sixth decade of life or later. Atherosclerosis results in obstruction of blood flow in the coronary arteries with myocardial ischaemia and/or infarction. Angina pectoris or chest pain is related to an imbalance between blood supply and myocardial demands due to narrowed coronary arteries. Other common manifestations include sudden death and heart failure.

Risk factors

There are numerous known risk factors which play a role in the development of atherosclerosis. Risk factors are characteristics discovered initially in prospective epidemiological studies. The aetiological role of risk factors is supported by laboratory experimental data and confirmed with clinical trials in humans. They are characteristics which predict later disease and may play a causal role in the pathological process. These include diet, lipids, obesity, physical inactivity, diabetes, hypertension, tobacco smoking, and others.

Diet

There is substantial evidence to support a causal association of habitual dietary intake with coronary heart disease. Much of that evidence is found in studies comparing populations. However, there is also considerable evidence within populations to suggest the role of individual dietary intake in coronary heart disease morbidity and mortality. Human feeding experiments add evidence as do animal studies. A number of components of habitual diet have been considered. These include fat, dietary cholesterol, carbohydrates, fibre, alcohol, protein, and caloric excess. Information regarding diet and coronary heart disease is summarized here.

1. Habitual food intake varies greatly between populations. These differences are related to population prevalence of coronary heart disease (Keys 1980).
2. While more difficult to study, individual eating patterns are also associated with coronary heart disease (Keys *et al.* 1965; Keys 1980).
3. When all components of diet including fats, protein, carbohydrates, minerals, alcohol, and dietary supplements are considered, the type and amount of fat intake is the most important component in preventing coronary heart disease.
4. The association of dietary fat with coronary heart disease is predominantly through the effects of saturated fats and cholesterol on blood lipids.
5. Eating patterns are changing in many cultures, leading to improving coronary heart disease rates in some and worsening in others.
6. Clinical trials of secondary prevention find diet change effective in lowering coronary heart disease.
7. Laboratory animal studies of non-human primates are congruent with these human diet–disease relationships.

Fat

The evidence is strong for the effect of diet between populations. The best known is the Seven Countries Study which compared habitual food intake in samples from among seven national populations (Keys 1980). This study demonstrated great variability in habitual food intake and a clear association of fatty acids and dietary cholesterol with blood cholesterol levels. Those blood cholesterol levels were a strong predictor of coronary heart disease in initially healthy populations followed more than 25 years (Blackburn and Jacobs 1984).

So central is the association of diet with blood cholesterol level, that many investigators suggest a cholesterol-raising diet is essential for mass expression of coronary heart disease (Blackburn and Jacobs 1984). These conclusions rest on data showing a diet with increased animal fats, specifically saturated fat and cholesterol, is found in populations where disease rates are high. Conversely, populations where these dietary components are low show a decreased incidence of coronary heart disease. Changes in diet seem to precede rising or falling coronary heart disease rates. Such is the case in the United States where diet is changing associated with falling blood cholesterol and coronary heart disease (Table 3). Additional evidence comes from observations in other international studies, where countries such as Japan have elevated levels of blood pressure and cigarette smoking,

Table 3 Nutrient intake in the United States (1978 and 1990)

	1978	1990
Saturated fat (% cal)	13	12
Total fat (% cal)	36	34
Cholesterol (mg/day)	318	291

Source: Johnson *et al.* (1993).

important coronary heart disease risk factors, but fail to manifest high rates of coronary heart disease. The Japanese have lower population levels of blood cholesterol (Keys 1980).

Additional observations on migrating populations show the same conclusions. The Japanese living in Japan have low cholesterol levels and low rates of coronary heart disease. As they move to Hawaii and the United States, they progressively assume the lifestyle of those Westernized cultures and experience elevations in blood cholesterol, obesity, and coronary heart disease rates similar to the local population (Kagan *et al.* 1974). Similar observations have been made among Irish migrants (Kushi *et al.* 1985). Again, the assumption of a high-fat Western diet is associated with increased coronary heart disease.

While the associations between diet and coronary heart disease are very strong in between population comparisons, the data are more conflicting in studies within populations. Here, studies of food intake or eating patterns of individuals modestly predict subsequent disease, if at all. There are several well-recognized reasons for this apparent paradox.

Supportive evidence comes from metabolic ward feeding studies. Here, individuals fed controlled diets of known composition for prolonged periods, show a clear relationship between type and quantity of fat intake and blood cholesterol levels. This relationship is best described by the Keys' formula which relates the intake of saturated fats, polyunsaturated fats, and dietary cholesterol to blood cholesterol levels (Keys *et al.* 1974). The Keys formula is calculated using the formula: $1.35\ (2S - P) + 1.5Z$ where S is the percentage of dietary calories from saturated fatty acids, P is the percentage of dietary calories from polyunsaturated fatty acids, and Z is the square root of dietary cholesterol in mg/1000 kcal (Keys *et al.* 1965). A slight variant of this formula was given by Anderson *et al.* (1979).

Similar associations are described by Hegstad *et al.* (1965). More recent studies have provided increased detail including information on monounsaturated fats, and specific fatty acids including *trans*-fatty acids (Mattson and Grundy 1985; Ascherio *et al.* 1994; Ginsberg *et al.* 1998).

Given clear and consistent associations in between population studies and feeding experiments involving fat, why has such an association not emerged in free living populations? There are several reasons postulated. Among these is the difficulty of measurement of habitual food intake in individuals. While this measure is relatively simple in societies which have little variation in foods, it is particularly difficult in societies where unlimited foods are available and composition is highly variable on a daily basis. Individual data collection, such as 24-h recalls, fail to characterize usual intake adequately (Munger *et al.* 1992). Food frequency approaches which characterize longer periods of time are susceptible to recall bias and difficulty in determining 'average intake' (Feskanich *et al.* 1993).

There are also individual factors in the response to dietary intake. Even when food intake is carefully controlled, the digestion and absorption process may vary between individuals. Thus, two individuals eating the same diet may have a different cholesterol response. Similarly, genetic factors in lipid metabolism may result in differing responses to the same food intake (Jacobs *et al.* 1979).

It is generally acknowledged that a large-scale trial of dietary fat for the primary prevention of coronary heart disease is unlikely to be performed (Gordon 1988). Although coronary heart disease is common in populations, the enormous numbers of individuals needed for randomization, the challenges to effective control of food intake in a free living population, the number of years necessary to accumulate adequate endpoint events, and the cost, precludes such a study. However, there are numerous congruent sources of information that lend strength to the validity of dietary fat recommendations through reduced blood cholesterol and coronary heart disease. Prominent are clinical trials of secondary prevention using diet. Among those are the studies of Ornish *et al.*, who found a beneficial effect of a stringent low-fat diet in patients with known coronary heart disease (Ornish *et al.* 1990). Similar findings were observed by Brown and Page (1958). Supportive evidence may also be found in the consistent observation of the beneficial effects of cholesterol lowering regardless of method. This is widely recognized in trials of secondary prevention of coronary heart disease through lipid lowering (Lipid Research Clinics Program 1984; Buchwald *et al.* 1990; Scandinavian Simvastatin Survival Study 1994; Sacks *et al.* 1996; LIPID Study Group 1998), but also in recent studies of primary prevention with lipid-lowering medications (Shepherd *et al.* 1995; Downs *et al.* 1998).

The recognition that usual food intake is a behaviour strongly related to culture and food availability has resulted in community-based public health strategies to improve dietary intake. The North Karelia and Stanford Three Town Studies were among the first to use public and health professional education about dietary fat to reduce blood cholesterol (Farquhar *et al.* 1977; Puska *et al.* 1995). In both studies, an improved eating pattern with reduced animal fats (saturated fats and cholesterol) resulted in reduced average blood cholesterols in these small communities. Larger studies in medium-sized cities in Europe and the United States showed similar results. Strong favourable secular trends in control communities resulted in modest differences in blood cholesterol levels (GCP Research Group 1988; Farquhar *et al.* 1990; Luepker *et al.* 1994; Carleton *et al.* 1995).

Protein

Comparisons between populations in countries show an ecological correlation between dietary proteins, particularly animal protein and mortality from coronary heart disease. However, there is little evidence that this association is causal. Metabolic ward experiments of men under isocholoric condition, with fat intake held constant while protein intake varied between 5 and 20 per cent of daily calories, found no change in blood cholesterol levels (University of Minnesota, unpublished data). Anitschkow (1983) found that dietary lipids rather than protein resulted in hyperlipidaemia and atherosclerosis in experimental rabbits.

These observations and others suggest that associations observed between populations are the result of animal fat associated with animal protein, rather than the effect of the protein itself. Specifically, consumption of fat from animals and high-fat milk products result in elevated blood cholesterol, rather than their high protein content. In coronary heart disease, it is generally agreed that dietary protein is not a factor in coronary heart disease.

Carbohydrates

A positive association is found between population intake of refined sugars and coronary heart disease. This relationship is confounded by many other dietary components and, importantly, the association of high levels of refined sugars with the usual diet of Westernized industrial countries. In the absence of a plausible biological connection between refined sugars and atherosclerosis, the association may actually be that of the high animal fat intake also found in those societies. However, refined sugars may have other deleterious effects such as dental disease.

Complex carbohydrates are negatively associated with coronary heart disease. Higher intake is found with low coronary heart disease mortality. These are also confounded by fat intake and other dietary factors. There is a plausible biological mechanism by which complex carbohydrates may affect coronary heart disease. Foods which have high levels of carbohydrates, such as fruits and vegetables, also contain fibre including pectins in fruit, bran fibre, and guar gum. These play a role in the absorption of fat and cholesterol in the intestines. Observational studies and clinical trials have demonstrated that increased fibre intake is associated with lower cholesterol levels (Ripsin *et al.* 1992; Jenkins *et al.* 1993). It is important to note that increased fibre intake is best attained by consumption of healthy fruits and vegetables, rather than dietary supplements.

Alcohol

There is a continuing debate regarding the effects of alcohol consumption on cardiovascular disease including coronary heart disease. Several associations are relevant to this issue as follows:

- the association of alcohol consumption with increased blood pressure and the risk of stroke (Criqui 1987)
- the association of alcohol consumption with increased high-density lipoprotein cholesterol and levels of triglycerides (Baraona and Lieber 1979; Gordon *et al.* 1981), both may affect coronary heart disease
- the effect of alcohol on haemostatic factors including fibrinogen, platelet aggregation, and fibrinolysis (Meade *et al.* 1987)
- large doses of alcohol lead to addiction and other severe diseases (Kramer *et al.* 1968). These include cardiovascular diseases such as congestive cardiomyopathy, cardiac arrhythmias, and sudden death (Kuller *et al.* 1989; Regan 1990).

Given these findings, why is there controversy about alcohol intake? It principally stems from epidemiological research which shows moderate intake of alcohol is associated with lower risk of coronary heart disease when compared to non-drinkers (Ferrence *et al.* 1986). Numerous studies support this observation after adjusting for other risk factors and confounders, which stimulates this debate. One controversy focuses on the type of alcoholic beverage containing this benefit. Some have suggested wine is the essential form (Ferrence *et al.* 1986), while others find that other alcoholic beverages such as beer and spirits are equally implicated (Colditz 1990). It is still not certain whether it is the ethanol or some other component in the beverage which has a beneficial effect. Studies of alcohol consumption are also fraught with difficulties. In many, report of consumption is inaccurate with long-term consumption as difficult to ascertain as for other foods. There is also a suggestion that people who are ill eliminate their alcohol consumption as the result of their illness, confusing cause and effect. Finally, there are social factors associated with the intake of certain beverages, particularly the use of wine among the more affluent.

In summary, while there are observational studies associating alcohol intake with lower coronary heart disease rates and plausible biological mechanisms are available, there are also concerns regarding the recommendation of alcoholic beverages as a preventive strategy for coronary heart disease. These rest in the potential for addiction, vehicular accidents, and negative effects on a number of organ systems, including the cardiovascular system.

Vitamins, minerals, and food supplements

Coronary heart disease has many advocates of oral supplements for treatment and prevention. Vitamins, minerals, and other food supplements are promoted as a simple easy way to avoid disease. There are numerous manufacturers who are willing to fulfil this 'need'. However, most of these substances are untested in a rigorous and controlled manner. Among those considered are vitamins C and E, β-carotene, copper, iron, selenium, fish oil, and fibre.

Observational studies show benefit or harm for some (Milner *et al.* 1989; Rimm *et al.* 1993; Stampfer *et al.* 1993; Ascherio and Hunter 1994; Kritchevsky *et al.* 1995; Stampfer and Rimm 1995; Ascherio *et al.* 1999). Very few have been submitted to clinical trials. When this has occurred, either in healthy subjects or those with coronary heart disease, the results have been mixed and the need for more research is recognized (Hennekens *et al.* 1996; Heart Outcomes Prevention Evaluation Study Investigators 2000).

Homocysteine has been evaluated as a risk factor for coronary heart disease. It is a product of methionine metabolism and observational studies consistently show elevated blood homocysteine in association with coronary heart disease (Boushey *et al.* 1995). The exact mechanism for this association is uncertain. Fortunately, supplementation with vitamins B_6, B_{12}, and folate appears to lower homocysteine levels (Osganian *et al.* 1999). The clinical and therapeutic effects of these changes is unknown; recently in the United States, however, folate supplementation was added to many grain products which should result in lower population levels of homocysteine (Boushey *et al.* 1995; Osganian *et al.* 1999).

Blood lipids

The preponderance of population, clinical, and experimental data indicate that blood lipids play a causal role in atherosclerosis and resulting coronary heart disease. Mass elevations in blood lipids appear to be a necessary factor for mass coronary heart disease. The research underlying these statements is summarized below.

1. Mean levels and distributions of blood lipids which vary widely between populations (Pooling Project Research Group 1978; Keys 1980; Stamler *et al.* 1986; Wallace and Anderson 1987) demonstrate a strong graded relationship between levels of total serum or plasma cholesterol and coronary heart disease. The low-density lipoprotein fraction of cholesterol is most atherogenic.

2. High-density lipoprotein cholesterol is inversely related to coronary heart disease. Higher levels are associated with less disease. High-density lipoprotein cholesterol is strongest as a predictor of coronary heart disease in populations where total cholesterol and disease risk is high (Gordon *et al.* 1977; NIH 1993*a*).

3. Although the mechanisms are poorly understood, there is a growing consensus that serum triglycerides, as measured in the fasting state, are associated with coronary heart disease (NIH 1993*a*).

4. Blood cholesterol levels among youth after puberty parallel those of the adult population (Luepker 1999). Those levels among youth track into adulthood (Webber *et al.* 1986).

5. Migration studies demonstrate that blood cholesterol levels rise to the level of the new culture when migrating from a low to a high cholesterol environment (Kagan *et al.* 1974).

6. Blood cholesterol levels continue to be predictive among adults over the age of 65 years, although the relative risk is reduced (Rubin *et al.* 1990; Abbott *et al.* 1997; Aronow and Ahn 1998).
7. Blood cholesterol can be lowered among adults with moderate changes in diet and loss of weight.
8. Clinical trials with lipid-lowering agents among those with moderate to severe blood cholesterol elevations demonstrate reduced coronary heart disease associated with lower cholesterol levels. This occurs both in individuals with coronary heart disease and those without evidence of clinical disease. It is particularly true of the newer statin drugs, but also with other methods (Lipid Research Clinics Program 1984; Buchwald *et al.* 1990; Scandinavian Simvastatin Survival Study 1994; Shepherd *et al.* 1995; Multiple Risk Factor Intervention Trial Research Group 1996; Sacks *et al.* 1996; Downs *et al.* 1998; LIPID Study Group 1998).
9. A progressive fall in blood cholesterol in the United States is associated with changes in the habitual diet during the last 25 years (Johnson *et al.* 1993a).

Population studies of blood lipids consistently show a positive association of mean blood cholesterol with coronary heart disease. As shown in Fig. 7, comparisons between different national groups show a significant association between blood cholesterol levels in health and coronary heart disease events among middle-aged men (Keys 1980). Similarly, data from the Multiple Risk Factor Intervention Trial, where over 356 000 healthy middle-aged men were followed over time, blood cholesterol predicted coronary heart disease outcomes in a progressive and continuous way as shown in Fig. 8 (Stamler *et al.* 1986). This continued gradation of blood cholesterol levels and disease suggest that lower blood cholesterol is better but there is no discrete point at which relative risk is sharply higher. The distributions imply the need for strategies to lower blood cholesterol at the population level, because cholesterol is normally distributed, and most disease events will come from the middle of the distribution, not the high extreme (Blackburn and Jacobs 1984).

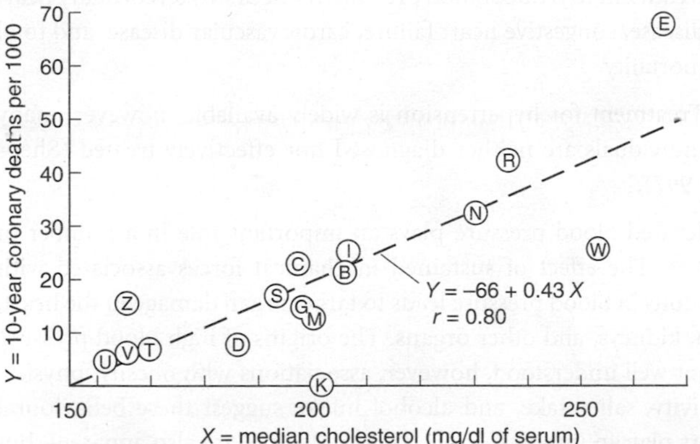

Fig. 7 Coronary heart disease related deaths and cholesterol. Coronary heart disease age-standardized 10-year death rates of the cohorts versus the median serum cholesterol levels (mg/dl) of the cohorts. All men judged free of coronary heart disease at entry. B, Belgrade, Yugoslavia; C, Crevalcore, Italy; D, Dalmatia; E, East Finland; G, Corfu; I, Italian railroad; K, Crete; M, Montegiorgio, Italy; N, Zutphen, The Netherlands; R, American railroad; S, Slavonia; T, Tanushimaru, Japan; U, Ushibuka; V, Velika Krsna, Yugoslavia; W, West Finland; Z, Zrenjanin, Yugoslavia.

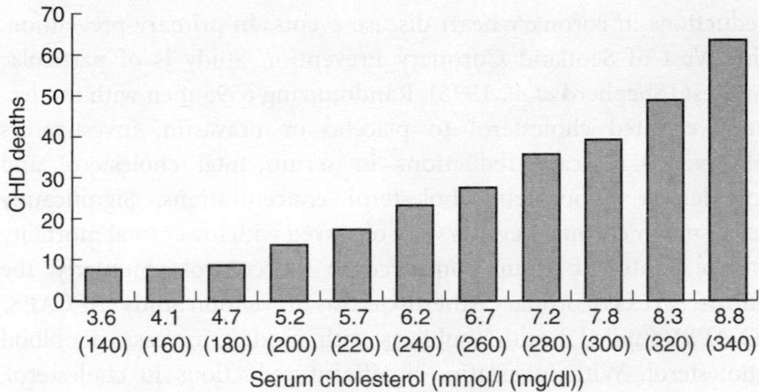

Fig. 8 Coronary heart disease (CHD) related deaths and cholesterol. (Source: Neaton *et al.* 1992.)

Lipids are insoluble in a water medium, namely blood. They are carried as lipoprotein particles in combination with proteins. Total cholesterol is the most widely used blood measure. It represents that chemical entity regardless of the carrier protein. Total cholesterol is commonly divided into three major components based on the density of the particles: low-density lipoprotein cholesterol, high-density lipoprotein cholesterol, and very low-density lipoprotein cholesterol. Each of these fractions is associated with specific protein carrier molecules. Low-density lipoprotein is the largest component of total cholesterol and is the atherogenic fraction. High-density lipoprotein comprises a smaller fraction and is inversely related to coronary heart disease, with higher levels of high-density lipoprotein associated with less disease. The very low-density lipoprotein contains modest amounts of cholesterol, but is the main carrier for triglycerides. Triglycerides are the major entity by which fat is transported and stored in the body.

There is considerable research on subfractions of these lipoproteins and the protein carriers which transport them. While important in research, these subfractions—including lipoprotein A, apolipoprotein E, high-density lipoprotein 2, and high-density lipoprotein 3—and many others are not established measures for clinical use nor are they relevant for public health strategies at this time.

There have been numerous trials designed to lower blood cholesterol or its subfractions. Dietary trials are noted above. However, the majority of trials have been in high-risk individuals by virtue of elevated blood cholesterol or known coronary heart disease. The trials take many years and are costly; however, the results are consistent and clear. The Coronary Drug Project enrolled men between 30 and 64 years old who had a previous myocardial infarction. The nicotinic acid treatment group showed significant lower mortality compared to those on placebo at 15 years after the study began (Canner *et al.* 1986). Similarly, the Lipid Research Clinic Coronary Primary Prevention Trial randomized men with elevated blood cholesterol aged 30 to 59 years to cholestyramine or placebo (Lipid Research Clinics Program 1984). These participants, followed for 7 to 10 years, showed significantly lower cardiovascular disease in the treatment group associated with cholesterol lowering. These and other early trials occurred before the more powerful cholesterol-lowering drugs—the statins. The effects of the early generation of drugs on cholesterol was modest and it is not surprising to find modest effects. Recently, with the use of statins, much larger effects of cholesterol reduction are observed with accompanying greater reductions in coronary heart disease events. In primary prevention, the West of Scotland Coronary Prevention Study is of particular interest (Shepherd *et al.* 1995). Randomizing 6595 men with moderately elevated cholesterol to placebo or pravastin, investigators observed significant reductions in serum total cholesterol and low-density lipoprotein cholesterol concentrations. Significantly fewer major coronary events were observed with lower total mortality in the treatment group compared to the controls. Similarly, the Airforce/Texas Coronary Atherosclerosis Prevention Study (**AFCAPS/TXAPS**) studied healthy subjects with modest increases in blood cholesterol. With lovastatin, significant reductions in cholesterol, coronary events, and all causes of mortality were also observed (Downs *et al.* 1998).

A number of large secondary prevention trials using statin therapy to lower cholesterol have also been completed, including the Scandinavian Simvastatin Survival Study (Scandinavian Simvastatin Survival Study 1994). It demonstrated a significant reduction in all causes of mortality, coronary heart disease mortality, coronary events, and revascularization procedures in patients with known coronary heart disease. The Cholesterol and Recurrent Events trial and the Long-Term Intervention with Fibrostatin in Ischemic Disease trial also demonstrated lipid reductions associated with fewer major coronary events (Sacks *et al.* 1996; LIPID Study Group 1998).

There have also been two important secondary prevention trials with gemfibrozil, a fibric acid derivative. A Finnish trial among men with known coronary heart disease resulted in a significant reduction of coronary events associated with changes in high-density lipoprotein cholesterol and triglycerides. Total cholesterol results were variable (Frick *et al.* 1987). A more recent treatment study of men with average total and low-density lipoprotein cholesterol but low high-density lipoprotein cholesterol with gemfibrozil also produced positive results. High-density lipoprotein cholesterol increased significantly in the treatment group compared to placebo. Coronary events were reduced. Interestingly, serum triglycerides also fell significantly, raising questions about the relative importance of the two lipid effects (Rubins *et al.* 1999).

There is consistent evidence from clinical trials of the benefits of lower total cholesterol and low-density lipoprotein cholesterol. There is also a suggestion that raising high-density lipoprotein cholesterol and lowering triglycerides add to these beneficial effects.

While recognizing that population-wide reductions in blood cholesterol would have great benefits, there are also clinical indicators of elevated blood cholesterol requiring aggressive and pharmacological management. This includes both high-risk individuals who are disease free, as well as in the case of secondary prevention for those who have known coronary heart disease. The Adult Treatment Panel of the United States National Cholesterol Education Program has suggested levels appropriate for further diagnosis and treatment (NIH 1993*a*). These are seen in Table 4. More recently, the European Society of Cardiology made similar recommendations for prevention; however, these recommendations integrate other risk factors (Wood *et al.* 1998*a*).

Table 4 Initial classification based on total cholesterol and high-density lipoprotein cholesterol levels

Cholesterol level	Initial classification
Total cholesterol	
< 200 mg/dl (5.2 mmol/l)	Desirable blood cholesterol
200–239 mg/dl (5.2–6.2 mmol/l)	Borderline to high blood cholesterol
⩾ 240 mg/dl (6.2 mmol/l)	High blood cholesterol
High-density lipoprotein cholesterol	
< 35 mg/dl (0.9 mmol/l)	Low high-density lipoprotein cholesterol

Source: Johnson *et al.* (1993), from the United States National Cholesterol Education Program guidelines.

Blood pressure

Considerable epidemiological, clinical, and experimental data show high blood pressure or hypertension to be a major risk factor for coronary heart disease. Hypertension is also strongly predictive of other diseases including cerebrovascular disease, renal failure, and congestive heart failure. It is also widely recognized that treatment of hypertension to lower blood pressure reduces cardiovascular disease. The problem is common and large portions of the population are exposed or currently under treatment with medication. The important observations about hypertension are as follows.

1. Population studies find a modest relationship between hypertension and coronary heart disease mortality between countries (Keys 1980).
2. Within populations, coronary heart disease is strongly related to both systolic and diastolic blood pressures.
3. Levels of blood pressure among youth track into adulthood (Clarke and Lauer 1985).
4. The primary prevention of hypertension through lifestyle modifications including weight reduction, regular physical activity, decreased sodium intake, and other factors have the potential to reduce the disease burden.
5. For those with fixed hypertension, clinical trials demonstrate that treatment to reduce blood pressure reduces stroke, coronary heart disease, congestive heart failure, cardiovascular disease, and total mortality.
6. Treatment for hypertension is widely available; however, many individuals are neither diagnosed nor effectively treated (Sheps 1997).

Elevated blood pressure plays an important role in a number of diseases. The effect of sustained mechanical forces associated with elevations in blood pressure leads to target organ damage in the heart, brain, kidneys, and other organs. The origins of high blood pressure are not well understood, however, associations with obesity, physical inactivity, salt intake, and alcohol intake suggest these behavioural factors play an important role. Genetic factors are also apparent, but the considerable prevalence of hypertension suggests that these hereditary characteristics are very common in most populations.

As shown in Fig. 9, systolic blood pressure predicts coronary heart disease outcomes between populations in a modest but linear fashion. Many populations worldwide have substantial prevalences of hypertension including the Japanese, Chinese, Africans, and others (over 50 per cent in some adult groups). However, as noted above, the presence of elevated blood cholesterol seem essential for the manifes-

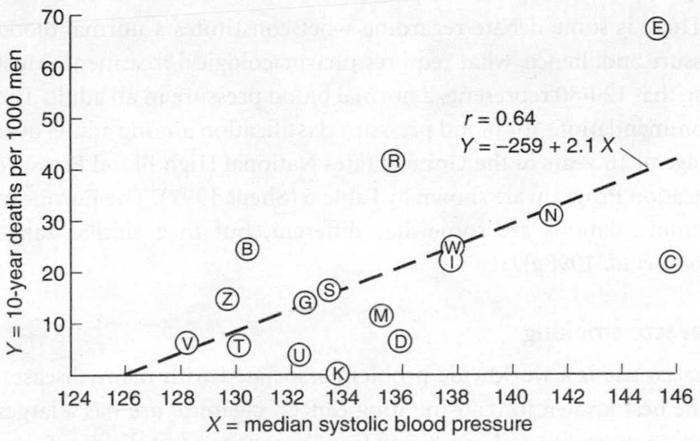

Fig. 9 Coronary heart disease related deaths and systolic blood pressure. The 10-year age-standardized coronary death rates, men without evidence of cardiovascular disease at entry, of the 16 cohorts versus the median systolic blood pressures of those cohorts at entry. B, Belgrade; C, Crevalcore; D, Dalmatia; E, east Finland; G, Corfu; I, Italian railroad; K, Crete; M, Montegiorgio; N, Zutphen; R, American railroad; S, Slavonia; T, Tanushimaru; U, Ushibuka; V, Velika Krsna; W, west Finland; Z, Zrenjanin.

tation of coronary heart disease. For stroke and other sequelae of hypertension, blood lipid elevations do not appear necessary. This is apparent in the Japanese population where stroke is quite common, but coronary heart disease is not.

Within populations, blood pressure is predictive of cardiovascular disease outcomes including coronary heart disease (Kannel *et al.* 1986; Sheps 1997) (Fig. 10). Early studies focused on diastolic blood pressure, but more recently systolic blood pressure, which appears to be more reliably measured, has assumed increasing importance for diagnosis and treatment.

The prevalence of hypertension, regardless of the definition, is substantial. In the United States, between 15 and 20 per cent of adults have high blood pressure by the definition of the National High Blood Pressure Education Program (Sheps 1997). The prevalence of hypertension rises progressively with age and in older age groups, it can affect the majority of the population. In certain racial groups, the prevalence is even higher. Hypertension is a worldwide epidemic.

Table 5 Trends in the awareness, treatment, and control of high blood pressure in adults in the United States (1976–1994)[a]

	NHANES II (1976–80)	NHANES III (phase I) (1988–91)	NHANES III (phase 2) (1991–94)
Awareness	51	73	68
Treatment	31	55	53
Control[b]	10	29	27

NHANES, National Health and Nutrition Examination Survey.

[a]Data are percentage of adults aged 18 to 74 years with systolic blood pressure 140 mmHg or greater, diastolic blood pressure 90 mmHg or greater, or taking antihypertensive medication (Burt *et al.* 1995; NHLBI 1997).

[b]Systolic blood pressure less than 140 mmHg and diastolic blood pressure less than 90 mmHg.

Archives of Internal Medicine (1997), from the United States National High Blood Pressure Evaluation Program.

While hypertension is common, its prevalence has not changed significantly in recent years (McGovern *et al.* 1996). However, in the past 20 years, detection, treatment, and control of high blood pressure has progressively improved. As shown in Table 5, awareness, treatment, and control of blood pressure have substantially increased. In the 1990s, however, there was an apparent levelling of effect in the United States with many still unaware and ineffectively treated (Sheps 1997).

Lifestyle modifications including weight, exercise, and diet offer the potential for preventing hypertension. They have also been found to be effective at lowering moderate hypertension with little risk and minimal cost. Even though lifestyle factors alone may not control high blood pressure, they can reduce the amount of antihypertensive drugs deemed necessary (Neaton *et al.* 1993; Singer *et al.* 1995). Excess body weight is associated with elevation in blood pressure. Weight reduction can reduce blood pressure in obese individuals with hypertension (*Trials of Hypertension Prevention Collaborative Research Group* 1992). Therefore, it is widely recommended that weight reduction is an important part of hypertension control. Weight loss

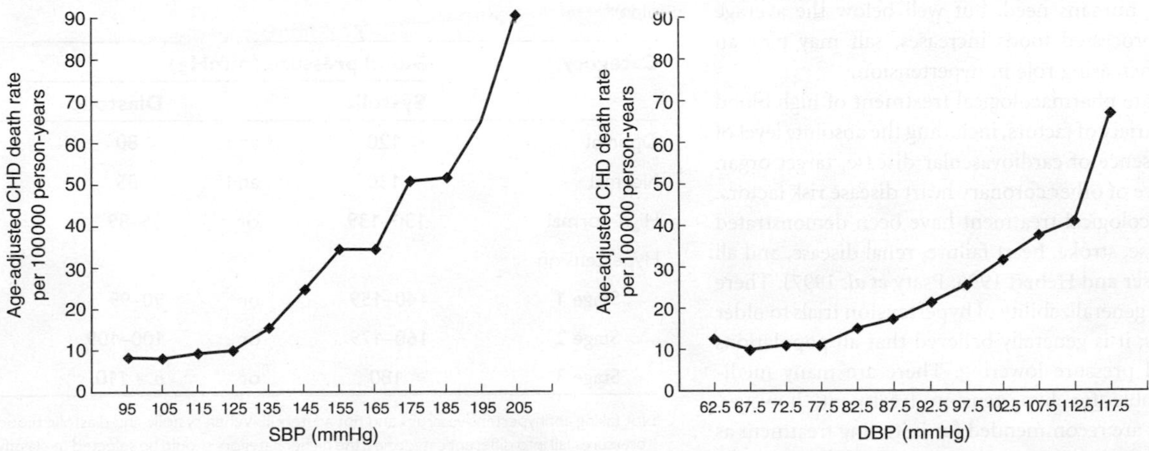

Fig. 10 Coronary heart disease (CHD) and blood pressure. DBP, diastolic blood pressure; SBP, systolic blood pressure. (Source: Neaton *et al.* 1992.)

medications, recently discovered to be associated with heart valve damage and pulmonary hypertension, are not recommended (Connolly *et al.* 1997). Physical inactivity also plays a role in hypertension with unfit individuals having up to 50 per cent increased risk of developing high blood pressure (Blair *et al.* 1984). Moderate physical activity aids in controlling weight and may actually lower blood pressure (NIH 1996). Dietary factors may also play a role in precipitating or reducing hypertension. Alcohol use raises blood pressure. The National High Blood Pressure Education Program recommends no more than 30 ml of ethanol as beer, wine, or whisky per day for men and 15 ml per day for women (Sheps 1997).

Salting of food as a method of preservation is well established over many centuries. However, modern food preservation methods do not require salt and it is mainly an acquired taste. Unfortunately, the human kidney was developed in the setting of low sodium and high potassium diets. Hence, the body is well designed to retain, but not excrete sodium, which it effectively does. The need for sodium is quite small and many times the amount required is consumed in processed food (Blackburn and Prineas 1983).

Salt intake is particularly relevant to hypertension. Population surveys demonstrate strong associations between population blood pressure and salt intake (Gleiberman 1973; Freis 1976; INTERSALT Cooperative Research Group 1988). Migration studies where salt intake is greatly increased among people who migrate from low to high salt cultures is associated with increasing prevalence of hypertension (Joseph *et al.* 1983). Within cultures where associations are more difficult to find, careful measurement results in individual correlations between salt intake and blood pressure (Kesteloot *et al.* 1980).

Clinical studies have found that restriction in salt results in lower blood pressure. Marked sodium depletion, as practised in an earlier era, can even reduce blood pressure among severe hypertensives (Blackburn and Prineas 1983), and sodium restriction enables high blood pressure to be controlled with lower doses of antihypertensive drugs. In some patients, salt restriction may control mild to moderate hypertension without resorting to drugs. Potassium also plays an important role, as increased potassium appears to reduce the blood pressure, enhancing the effects of sodium reduction (Meneely and Battarbee 1976).

Despite widespread information about the role of salt, considerable debate remains. The American National Dietary Goals recommend no more than 6.0 g of sodium chloride daily (Sheps 1997). This remains significantly more than humans need, but well below the average intake. As the use of processed foods increases, salt may play an undiminished or even increasing role in hypertension.

The decision to initiate pharmacological treatment of high blood pressure depends on a variety of factors, including the absolute level of blood pressure, the presence of cardiovascular disease, target organ damage, and the presence of other coronary heart disease risk factors. The benefits of pharmacological treatment have been demonstrated for coronary heart disease, stroke, heart failure, renal disease, and all causes of mortality (Moser and Hebert 1996; Psaty *et al.* 1997). There has been debate over the generalizability of hypertension trials to older adults and other groups; it is generally believed that all populations will benefit from blood pressure lowering. There are many medications currently available for hypertension treatment, however, β-blockers and diuretics are recommended for initiating treatment as they have the longest clinical trial experience and a proven record of reducing morbidity and mortality in clinical trials (Sheps 1997; Psaty *et al.* 1997). Other agents may be required in special circumstances.

There is some debate regarding what constitutes a normal blood pressure and, hence, what requires pharmacological treatment. Most agree that 120/80 represents a normal blood pressure in an adult. The recommendations for blood pressure classification among adults over the age of 18 years of the United States National High Blood Pressure Education Program are shown in Table 6 (Sheps 1997). The European recommendations are somewhat different, but in a similar range (Wood *et al.* 1998*a*).

Cigarette smoking

Tobacco use is a worldwide problem associated with many diseases. While best known for causing lung cancer, cigarette use has a larger effect on mortality and morbidity from coronary heart disease. Some of the salient observations on tobacco use are as follows.

1. Cigarette smoking addicts 20 to 80 per cent of adult men worldwide with a somewhat lower proportion of adult women addicted.
2. Comparisons between populations often find no association between coronary heart disease and the prevalence of cigarette smoking. However, the individual association of cigarette smoking to coronary heart disease is strong.
3. Cigarette smoking is falling in some countries but rising in most, and is a growing epidemic in developing nations.
4. Cigarette smoking begins in youth and gradually increases until it becomes nicotine addiction.
5. The main mechanisms by which cigarette smoking affects coronary heart disease are as a chronic promoter of atherosclerotic lesions and as an acute risk factor increasing sympathetic stimulation and enhancing clotting.
6. While randomized population trials of cigarette use have not been performed, cigarette cessation reduces levels of coronary heart disease mortality.
7. Coronary heart disease is directly related to exposure to tobacco smoke.

Table 6 Classification of blood pressure for adults aged 18 years and older[a]

Category	Blood pressure (mmHg)		
	Systolic		Diastolic
Optimal	< 120	and	< 80
Normal	< 130	and	< 85
High-normal	130–139	or	85–89
Hypertension			
Stage 1	140–159	or	90–99
Stage 2	160–179	or	100–109
Stage 3	⩾ 180	or	*n*> 110

[a]Not taking antihypertensive drugs and not acutely ill. When systolic and diastolic blood pressures fall into different categories, the higher category should be selected to classify the individual's blood pressure status.

Source: *Archives of Internal Medicine* (1997), from the United States National High Blood Pressure Evaluation Program.

8. There is a growing awareness that environmental tobacco smoke or second-hand smoke has a deleterious effect on exposed non-smokers.

Tobacco use through cigarette smoking is one of the major causes of disease and disability in the world. In the United States, there are approximately 47 million adult smokers and it is estimated that 430 000 deaths annually are associated with cigarette smoking (USDHHS 1998*b*). These victims are replaced by the teenagers who begin the smoking habit. In the United States, the direct medical costs of smoking are estimated to be $50 billion/year with similar indirect costs.

Cigarette smoking is linked to the major cardiovascular diseases including myocardial infarction, sudden death, stroke, and peripheral vascular disease (USDHHS 1983, 1997). These associations are found across age, gender, and ethnic groups (USDHHS 1983, 1997; Neaton and Wentworth 1992). The relationship of coronary heart disease mortality to smoking status is shown in Fig. 11. One of the most important findings is the association of cigarette smoking with sudden unexpected death among younger individuals. Similarly, acute myocardial infarction in younger individuals (less than 50 years of age) is very strongly associated with tobacco use (Rosenberg *et al.* 1983; Kannel *et al.* 1984). The interaction of cigarette smoking with other risk factors such as cholesterol, diet, obesity, hypertension, lipids, diabetes, and ECG abnormalities is also well demonstrated (Pooling Project Research Group 1978; Suarez and Barrett-Connor 1984; Williams *et al.* 1986; Multiple Risk Factor Intervention Trial Research Group 1996). Among the strongest pieces of evidence is the observation that continued cigarette smoking after myocardial infarction is predictive of recurrent events and death (Rosenberg *et al.* 1985; Hermanson *et al.* 1988), and those who quit smoking dramatically reduce their chance of a second event or death (Rosenberg *et al.* 1985; Hermanson *et al.* 1988; USDHHS 1990; Kawachi *et al.* 1994).

The mechanisms by which tobacco and the constituents of tobacco smoke affect cardiovascular disease are still debated. Both acute and chronic mechanisms probably contribute. Firstly, there is evidence that smoking plays a direct role in the atherosclerotic process. This is shown by the Pathological Determinants of Atherosclerosis in Youth Study of 1443 autopsies of men and women aged 15 to 34 years who died of trauma (McGill *et al.* 1997). Fatty abdominal and aortic streaks and raised lesions were associated with cigarette use in this otherwise healthy population. This may be the result of injury to the arterial endothelium from smoking (McGill *et al.* 1997; Zimmerman and McGeachie 1987). More acutely, the immediate pharmacological effects of nicotine and carbon monoxide are well known. Platelet adhesion, acute coronary constriction, and tachycardia are commonly cited (Maouad *et al.* 1984; Meade *et al.* 1987). Finally, there is the rapid improvement in patients observed after smoking cessation.

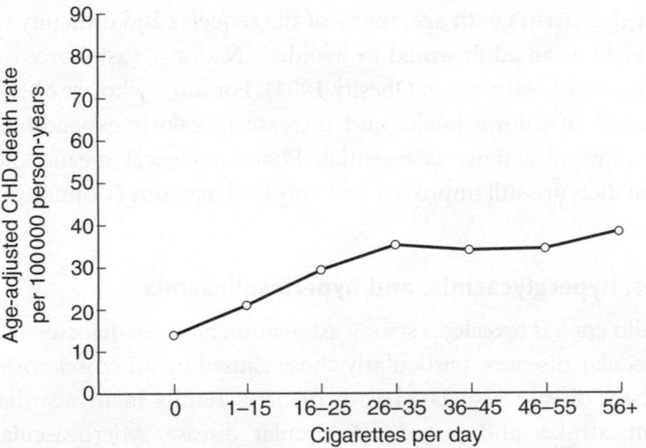

Fig. 11 Cigarette smoking and coronary heart disease (CHD). (Source: Neaton *et al.* 1992.)

In recent years, the focus has shifted to environmental tobacco smoke which affects non-smokers in public and private settings. A number of recent studies suggest consistent and increased relative risk of cardiovascular disease among those exposed to environmental tobacco smoke (Table 7). While it is difficult to measure exposure to environmental tobacco smoke, the consistency of these studies is suggestive and reinforces the effort to control cigarette smoking in public settings (Garland *et al.* 1985; Svendsen *et al.* 1987; Helsing *et al.* 1988; Hole *et al.* 1989; Layard 1995; Tunstall-Pedoe *et al.* 1995; Steenland *et al.* 1996; Kawachi *et al.* 1997).

Trends in cigarette smoking vary by country. While certain countries, such as the United States, have seen significant declines over the past several decades, smoking is static in some countries and rising in others. Of particular concern is the increased marketing of tobacco to countries in the developing world. Similarly, tobacco companies have become more effective at advertising to youth, the source of future smokers.

Programmes to control tobacco use have focused on prevention and cessation. Smoking prevention programmes in the schools have

Table 7 Cohort studies of environmental tobacco smoke and coronary heart disease

Source	Location	Cases/population	Adjusted RR (CI)
Hirayama (1984)	Japan	494/91 540	1.15 (0.93–1.42)
Garland *et al.* (1985)	USA	19/695	2.7 (0.7–10.5)
Svendsen *et al.* (1987)	USA	88/1245	2.2 (0.72–6.92)
Helsing *et al.* (1988)	USA	1358/19 035	M 1.31 (1.05–1.64) F 1.24 (1.10–1.40)
Hole *et al.* (1989)	UK	53/7987	2.01 (1.2–3.4)
Layard (1995)	USA	1389/2916	M 0.97 (0.73–1.28) F 0.99 (0.84–1.16)
Tunstall-Pedoe *et al.* (1995)	UK	70/2278	2.7 (1.3–5.6)
Steenland *et al.* (1996)	USA	3819/309 599	M 1.22 (1.07–1.40) F 1.10 (0.96–1.27)
Kawachi *et al.* (1997)	USA	152/32 046	F 1.91 (1.11–3.28)

CI, confidence interval; F, female; M, male; RR, relative risk.

received considerable attention and met some success (Perry *et al.* 1992). Smoking cessation programmes for older teens are in the testing phase and new programmes are emerging (Sussman *et al.* 1999). Cessation interventions among adults have emphasized behavioural and pharmacological strategies (Fiore *et al.* 1996). These have included nicotine replacement therapy, social support, and skills training/problem solving. In addition, widespread restriction of smoking reduces the societal support for the behaviour.

In summary, cigarette smoking is an addictive behaviour which leads to many health-impairing effects including coronary heart disease. Elimination of cigarette smoking would significantly improve the health of any population.

Overweight and obesity

Excess body weight as fat is increasingly recognized for its importance in the development of cardiovascular diseases. On a population level, overweight and obesity have become common among adults in industrialized countries and the affluent in developing countries. Several important observations include the following.

1. Overweight and obesity are associated with increased mortality.
2. Severe obesity is recognized as an independent risk factor for mortality. Less severe obesity may also be an independent risk factor.
3. Obesity is associated with elevated blood pressure, hyperlipidaemia, diabetes mellitus, and insulin resistance. Reduction in body fat diminishes the level of each of these risk factors.
4. Increasing body weight is a worldwide problem and is the result of excess food in the setting of reduced physical activity.

Obesity is commonly described as excess body fat, however, the exact proportion of fat rendering one overweight or obese is debated. Body mass index, which is weight in kilograms divided by height in meters squared, is a commonly used standard. Expert panels suggest a body mass index above 25 is classified as overweight and above 30 as obese (Eckel and Krauss 1998; USDHHS 1998*a*). More recently, visceral adiposity has been proposed as a better marker for obesity as a predictor of cardiac risk (Freedman 1995). Visceral adiposity is simply measured by the waist to hip ratio, using the circumference of these two sites. Other more complex methods to determine body fat are available but require sophisticated instruments.

Overweight and obesity are an increasing problem in much of the world. As shown in Table 8, both overweight and obesity measured in national surveys have substantially increased in recent years in the United States. Men are more likely to be overweight (body mass index greater than 25 kg/m^2) but women are more likely to be obese (body mass index greater than 30 mg/m^2). Ethnic minorities, such as African Americans and Mexican Americans living in the United States, have similar, if not greater, adiposity.

Table 8 Prevalence of overweight and body mass index levels in the American population (age 20–74 years)

	Overweight (%)		BMI (kg/m^2)	
	1976–80	1988–94	1976–80	1988–94
White men	24.2	32.2	25.5	26.3
White women	24.4	32.6	24.8	25.9
Black men	26.2	33.2	25.5	26.6
Black women	44.5	49.2	27.5	28.3

BMI, body mass index.

Source: Flegal (1996).

The association of obesity with mortality is well established. For the severe or morbidly obese, lifespan is significantly reduced (Sjostrom 1992). For the less severely obese, the debate is that of obesity as an independent risk factor for cardiovascular disease or as one which operates through other known risk factors (Harris *et al.* 1993, 1997; Solomon and Manson 1997). The question is a scientific one rather than one of public health.

Obesity and overweight affects lipoprotein metabolism through higher low-density lipoprotein cholesterol, increased triglycerides, and lower levels of high-density lipoprotein cholesterol. Weight reduction accomplished through diet is associated with significant improvement in lipids (Dattilo and Kris-Etherton 1992). The association of weight and blood pressure is also well established. In the Nurses Health Study, one unit in body mass index was associated with a 12 per cent increase in the risk of hypertension (Huang *et al.* 1998). Other observational studies consistently show this relationship (Dyer and Elliott 1989). Weight loss is well demonstrated to reduce blood pressure. This includes even modest reductions in weight (Stamler *et al.* 1987; Hypertension Prevention Trial Research Group 1990; Wassertheil-Smoller *et al.* 1992; Trials of Hypertension Prevention Collaborative Research Group 1997). In addition, recent research suggests that a diet lower in fat and higher in fruits and vegetables also results in lower blood pressure among the mildly hypertensive (Krauss *et al.* 1998). In each of these studies, weight reduction via diet allows the reduction of antihypertensive medications.

Insulin resistance is the underlying condition associated with adult-onset or type II diabetes. Obesity is a crucial factor in the development of insulin insensitivity and increased interabdominal fat is implicated (Krauss *et al.* 1998). Many suggest that the current epidemic of diabetes is a direct function of increasing obesity. Weight loss can be critical to the control of adult-onset diabetes. Both insulin resistance and hyperglycaemia are significantly reduced when patients lose weight (Paisey *et al.* 1998). This may result in the ability to reduce diabetic therapy.

Clinicians are well aware of the difficulty of obtaining significant and sustained weight loss among patients. Many now suggest that obesity prevention is the best strategy. By reducing the increased adiposity that occurs with age, many of the sequelae and difficulty of losing weight as an adult would be avoided (National Task Force on Prevention and Treatment of Obesity 1994). For those who are obese, both control of calorie intake and increase in calorie expenditure through physical activity is essential. Pharmacological means and starvation diets are still unproven and may be dangerous (Connolly *et al.* 1997).

Diabetes, hyperglycaemia, and hyperinsulinaemia

The insulin era has revealed a strong association between diabetes and cardiovascular diseases, particularly those caused by atherosclerosis. Large vessel disease associated with diabetes results in myocardial infarction, stroke, and peripheral vascular disease. Microvascular disease is associated with retinopathy, renal disease, and cardiomyopathy. In addition to strong associations with known cardiovascular risk factors, diabetes is an independent predictor of disease (Kannel and McGee 1979; Stamler *et al.* 1993). Salient observations regarding diabetes are as follows.

1. Diabetes and hyperglycaemia are strongly related to atherosclerosis.
2. Diabetes and hyperglycaemia are associated with obesity and abnormal lipid patterns.
3. Diabetes is increasing along with obesity in susceptible populations.
4. Control of associated risk factors can reduce the atherosclerotic complications of diabetes.
5. Control of blood glucose in type I diabetics reduces microvascular complications. There is a suggestion of a similar effect among type II diabetes.

The association of clinical diabetes mellitus with coronary heart disease and other atherosclerotic conditions is well documented (West 1978; Pyorala *et al.* 1987) with relative risks at two or three times that for diabetics compared to non-diabetics (Kannel and McGee 1979; Stamler *et al.* 1993). In Fig. 12, the Multiple Risk Factor Intervention Trial data compares diabetics and non-diabetics. It is apparent that diabetes alone in the absence of hypercholesterolaemia, cigarette smoking, and elevated systolic blood pressure results in increased relative risk of cardiovascular disease mortality. The effect of diabetes is magnified when associated with these other risk characteristics.

It was believed that diabetes combined with the use of a high-fat, low-carbohydrate, and low-fibre diet increased vascular complications. It is now clear that the deleterious effects of the disease itself on the endothelium and coagulation abnormality play an important direct role (Carmassi *et al.* 1992; Sowers *et al.* 1994). It was also observed that diabetes is strongly associated with classical risk factors. Diabetics have elevated levels of triglycerides and low-density lipoprotein cholesterol with decreased levels of high-density lipoprotein cholesterol. There is also a high prevalence of obesity and hypertension among diabetics (Knowler *et al.* 1978; Winocour 1992; Schaefer *et al.* 1994; Clarkson *et al.* 1996; Lehto *et al.* 1997).

Cross-cultural comparisons present a more complicated picture. They indicate that factors other than the glucose insulin disorder itself

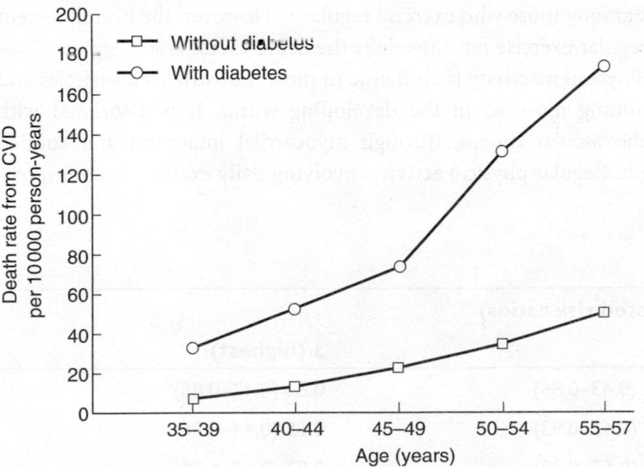

Fig. 12 Cardiovascular disease (CVD) mortality and diabetes. (Source: Stamler *et al.* 1993.)

result in atherosclerosis. Evidence is presented in the apparently low rates of atherosclerosis in diabetic Eastern Jews, Chinese, and south-west American Indians (West 1978; Pyorala *et al.* 1987). The Pima Indians are a classical example of a population exposed to calorie abundance, excessive obesity, and the diabetic phenotype but with little evidence of cardiovascular disease (Knowler *et al.* 1978).

In healthy people, glucose intolerance alone is weak and inconsistently associated with cardiovascular disease risk (Stamler *et al.* 1979; Pyorala *et al.* 1987). However, increased insulin levels were found to predict coronary heart disease in Australia, France, and Finland (Pyorala *et al.* 1987) and it is postulated to be the cause of excess coronary heart disease among Asian immigrants to the United Kingdom (Hughes 1990).

The treatment of diabetes is based on control of blood glucose and treatment of associated risk factors. Lifestyle strategies, weight loss, and physical activity can be effective at reducing blood glucose and controlling the associated risk factors. This is particularly true for type II diabetics. For type I diabetics, insulin for glucose control and control of associated risk factors can reduce diabetic complications.

Pharmacological control of type II diabetes has produced mixed results. The original University Group Diabetes Program reported an increased rate of myocardial infarction with the use of first-generation sulphonylureas in the setting of effective blood glucose control (UGDP 1975). More recent trials with newer oral agents did not observe this complication (UKPDS 1995). The more recent Diabetes Control and Complication Trial studied glucose control in insulin-dependent diabetics. Microvascular complications were significantly reduced (DCCT Research Group 1993). Large vessel disease was also reduced, but the differences were not significant.

The relationship between diabetes, atherosclerosis, and coronary heart disease is well established in people with clinical diabetes living in affluent industrialized cultures. Data from other cultures suggest that other factors are at work. The use of lifestyle strategies, control of other risk factors, and pharmacological measures in diabetes is the standard of care and may reduce cardiovascular complications of this disease.

Physical activity

Physical activity and its opposite, physical inactivity, have assumed increasing importance as risk factors for cardiovascular disease. As society has become more mechanized, a sedentary lifestyle has become the norm. Operating both through other risk factors such as obesity, hypertension, hyperlipidaemia, and diabetes, physical inactivity is associated with cardiovascular disease. However, it is also thought to be independently associated as well. Several important observations regarding physical inactivity include the following.

1. Physical inactivity is associated with acute myocardial infarction and sudden death both for the initial event and recurrent events. Regular activity is associated with reduced events.
2. Physical activity at work is declining.
3. Physical activity in leisure time, while increasing, is still not widespread.
4. Physical inactivity begins with declining exercise among youth as they reach teenage years.
5. Physical inactivity is associated with known risk factors including hyperlipidaemia, hypertension, diabetes mellitus, and obesity. In

addition, physical activity is proposed by some to be an independent risk factor.

6. Systemic and cardiac mechanisms are postulated to explain the observed exercise benefits.

Two of the primary activities of human beings are obtaining and consuming food. Historically, this took considerable physical energy in hunting or farming activities, only a few very affluent were spared from activity. The past two centuries have witnessed a dramatic transition as farming has become more efficient. Mechanized transportation has eliminated the use of physical activity to move from place to place. The workplace has become increasingly mechanized as machines do most or all heavy labour. The result has been a rising tide of physical inactivity (Blackburn and Jacobs 1988).

Much of the information on physical inactivity comes from observational studies. These are hampered by the difficulties of measuring habitual physical activity and the interplay of other risk characteristics in cardiovascular disease outcomes. Meta-analysis by Powell *et al.* of observational studies selected for quality, measurement, and follow-up showed a significant and graded relationship between physical inactivity and the risk of first coronary heart disease event. They calculated a relative risk of 1.9 compared with sedentary individuals (Powell *et al.* 1987). The Multiple Risk Factor Intervention Trial of over 12 000 men demonstrated similar relationships with those with regular leisure time physical activity having lower risk of coronary heart disease and death (Leon *et al.* 1987) (Table 9). Similarly, Paffenbarger *et al.* showed that physical activity after university was more protective than participation in sporting activities during school (Paffenbarger *et al.* 1984). While there are many observational studies, there is general agreement that a primary prevention trial of physical activity is unlikely to be feasible and public health recommendations must come from available data.

There are more data for secondary prevention. Observational studies find that individuals who continue with regular physical activity after myocardial infarction have lower relative risk than those who are sedentary (NIH 1996). These studies are confounded by severity of disease which is associated both with physical inactivity and mortality. Those who are very ill are less likely to exercise and more likely to have increased recurrent events and mortality. For this reason, a number of randomized clinical trials of cardiac rehabilitation after myocardial infarction have been performed. These demonstrate lower mortality associated with exercise, but most studies have been small and underpowered (Wilhelmsen *et al.* 1975; Shaw 1981; Benson *et al.* 1983). A meta-analysis by Oldridge *et al.* of 10 randomized trials found significant improvement associated with cardiac rehabilitation programmes lasting at least 6 weeks (Oldridge *et al.* 1988). The preponderance of published evidence appears to support the benefit of a physical activity programme following acute myocardial infarction (O'Connor *et al.* 1989).

Both observational studies and clinical trials of physical activity have suffered from the lack of well-validated instruments to characterize habitual activity in free living populations. While survey instruments for work and leisure time physical activity are available, they are not ideal.

Physical activity is believed to function through a number of biological and physiological mechanisms. It operates through other cardiovascular risk factors including lipoproteins, carbohydrate metabolism, clotting factors, and obesity. It may result in lower blood pressure and aid in smoking cessation. In addition to its effects on other risk characteristics, physical activity is thought to increase epicardial artery diameter, increase coronary blood flow, and decrease myocardial work and oxygen demand. The heart may work more efficiently and be better able to function under stressful circumstances.

There is considerable debate over public health recommendations for physical activity. Some of the issues include the amount, type, and duration of physical activity needed to obtain beneficial cardiovascular effects. There is also the issue of fitness as an independent factor. Finally, the association of vigorous physical activity with sudden death has increased concerns regarding advice. Considering these factors, several recommendations have emerged in recent years (NIH 1996). These suggest that moderate physical activity such as brisk walking for 30 min on most days of the week is adequate to produce significant benefit in a sedentary society. More vigorous physical activity can be recommended; however, only moderate cardiovascular gains accrue from this addition (NIH 1996). The activity should be of sufficient vigour to increase the heart rate and breathing rate. Regular physical activity will lead to increased fitness; however, much of the association with fitness may be genetically determined rather than the result of training (Blair *et al.* 1989). Nonetheless, observational studies do show that physical fitness is associated with lower rates of cardiovascular disease (Blair *et al.* 1989).

Finally, safety is a crucial consideration in advising physical activity for individuals or public health recommendations. Research has shown an excess risk of sudden death during and shortly after strenuous exercise (Siscovick *et al.* 1984; Mittleman *et al.* 1993). This is a particular issue in those habitually inactive, but there is still excess risk among those who exercise regularly. However, the overall benefit of regular exercise far outweighs the acute excess risk.

Physical inactivity is epidemic in most industrialized societies and becoming more so in the developing world. It is associated with cardiovascular disease through myocardial infarction and sudden death. Regular physical activity involving daily exertion is an import-

Table 9 Mortality and leisure-time physical activity in men

Endpoints	**Tertile of LTPAs (age-adjusted risk ratios)**		
	1 (lowest)	**2**	**3 (highest)**
CHD-related death	1.00	0.63 (0.43–0.86)	0.64 (0.47–0.88)
Sudden death	1.00	0.63 (0.42–0.93)	0.65 (0.44–0.96)
All-cause deaths	1.00	0.71 (0.57–0.88)	0.83 (0.67–1.01)

LTPA, leisure-time physical activity; CHD, coronary heart disease.

Source: Leon *et al.* (1987), from the United States.

ant public health recommendation. The type of physical activity recommended is that which involves large muscle groups for sustained periods of at least 30 min.

Psychosocial factors

Psychosocial factors including personality characteristics and the social environment are popularly believed to play an important role in cardiovascular disease. There are also many professionals who also believe that these factors influence the major diseases of modern life. Despite this widespread belief, it has been difficult to demonstrate causal connections to coronary heart disease or other diseases. This may be due to difficulties in measurement, confounders, or less than convincing biological mechanisms. Nonetheless, emotional states of anger, aggression, fear, anxiety, and depression are associated with physiological changes, which may affect cardiovascular disease. Certain personality types may precipitate or aggravate these factors. There are three major areas that have received the most attention and will be briefly discussed here. They are type A behaviour, hostility, and social support.

Type A behaviour

Type A behaviour is characterized by aggressiveness, competitive drive, preoccupation with deadlines, and time urgency. Historically, it is measured by a structured interview (Friedman and Rosenman 1959). There are also other methods including self-reported inventories and questionnaires. Data in the 1980s found type A behaviour to be associated with coronary heart disease in the Western Collaborative Group Study and the Framingham Study (Rosenman *et al.* 1975; Haynes *et al.* 1980). In the Western Collaborative Group Study a prospective cohort of 3000 men was assessed by the structured interview. The relative risk of fatal and non-fatal coronary heart disease was approximately 2 for type A men. The Framingham Study used a self-administered questionnaire to evaluate type A behaviour. Relative risk for coronary heart disease was similar to that found in the Western Collaborative Group Study (Haynes *et al.* 1980).

Following these initial observations, a number of other studies attempted to replicate these results. A summary of 14 angiography studies found an equal balance of positive and null associations (Dimsdale *et al.* 1981). Several larger prospective studies done in the 1980s failed to confirm earlier findings using either self-administered instruments or the structured interview (Case *et al.* 1985; Cohen and Reed 1985; Shekelle *et al.* 1985*a*, *b*). A reanalysis of the original Western Collaborative Group data also questioned the original results (Ragland and Brand 1988*a*, *b*). Finally, an intervention study was performed to look at behaviour patterns and recurrent coronary heart disease. In this study, performed by the originators of the type A behaviour interview, coronary heart disease outcomes were reduced, but this study has not been replicated (Friedman *et al.* 1984).

Current evidence for type A behaviour is mixed and while there continues to be widespread belief about its importance, there is inadequate evidence to make public health or clinical recommendations regarding its detection and treatment.

Hostility

Initial enthusiasm concerning the findings about type A behaviour led to an attempt to find critical elements accounting for the observed coronary heart disease differences. Early studies in selected groups found an association between hostility and coronary heart disease (Matthews *et al.* 1977; Barefoot *et al.* 1983; Hecker *et al.* 1988). Many studies used parts of the type A behaviour construct. Others used the Minnesota Multi-Phasic Personality Index and its 'Cook Medley Hostility Subscore'. Six prospective studies using the Cook Medley instrument have been published with three positive and three negative findings (Shekelle *et al.* 1983; McCranie *et al.* 1986; Hecker *et al.* 1988; Hearn *et al.* 1988; Leon *et al.* 1988; Barefoot *et al.* 1989).

Recent research suggests that anger or hostility is an acute rather than a chronic risk factor and associated with plaque rupture (Muller *et al.* 1997). This research may provide further insights into this characteristic.

Social support

A number of observational studies find social support or a supportive environment associated with lower coronary heart disease risk. Two Scandinavian studies found a strong relationship between social support and mortality in men (Orth-Gomer and Johnson 1987; Kaplan *et al.* 1988). Disentangling the role of social support from prevalent illness, economic factors, and personality types is difficult. It is apparent that those with a substantial support network, including a supportive spouse, have better coronary heart disease outcomes.

Associated with support, there is increased exploration of environmental factors particularly work situations. Here a number of studies have shown that jobs with high demand and low control of the work environment have a relative risk of about 2 for acute myocardial infarction after controlling for other risk characteristics (Alfredsson *et al.* 1982; Schnall *et al.* 1990). Again, the complex interactions associated with these environments and the response of the individual are likely to play a role, but are difficult to evaluate. Not all humans react similarly to an identical environment.

Acute coronary heart disease risk factors

Most of the risk factors discussed are associated with the underlying disease process, atherosclerosis. If atherosclerosis is prevented, then coronary heart disease as a clinical event is extremely rare. However, since many individuals have atherosclerosis by middle-age or older years, there has been an increasing search for factors which lead to the transition from chronic atherosclerotic disease to acute ischaemia, myocardial infarction, and sudden death. These are sometimes called acute risk factors or triggers.

There were two initial observations leading to these insights. The first related to the pathophysiology of the aortic plaque. While large and obstructing plaques are clearly related to disease, it was also found that small non-obstructive lesions could rupture, form a nidus for clot, and ultimately obstruct the coronary artery. This phenomenon was more likely to result in death than traditional obstructive lesions which were more likely to cause chronic ischaemia and angina pectoris (Fuster *et al.* 1992*a*). The second observation was that of a morning peak in acute myocardial infarction, sudden death, and even stroke. This suggested there were identifiable circumstances associated with disease manifestation (Muller *et al.* 1987; Ridker *et al.* 1990). Further work in this field suggested that sympathetic stimulation with activation of clotting as a potential underlying mechanism. A number of factors were implicated. They included heavy exertion, sexual activity, anger, and other factors (Mittleman *et al.* 1993). Some of the characteristics are modified with aspirin use or β-blockers (Willich *et al.* 1993).

In summary, it is likely that more will be learned about acute risk factors and treatment found to prevent events in individuals with established atherosclerotic disease. This should not be confused with true primary prevention where the atherosclerotic process is prevented.

Other risk factors

In addition to the risk factors described above, there is ongoing research looking for other markers of risk. While classical risk factors explain much or most of the disease relationships, there is still much to learn. Among the most promising areas is that of genetics where markers of coronary heart disease and protential mechanisms will be found.

Congestive heart failure

Congestive heart failure is increasing in prevalence in many areas of the world. Congestive heart failure is a clinical constellation of signs and symptoms resulting from circulatory and neural responses to cardiac dysfunction (Poole-Wilson 1989). This dysfunction usually manifests as inadequate pumping ability by the heart. It can have multiple underlying aetiologies including ischaemic heart disease, hypertension, non-ischaemic cardiomyopathy, infection, diabetes mellitus, and others. Several observations about the population patterns of congestive heart failure are as follows.

1. Population prevalence of congestive heart failure is directly related to the prevalence and types of underlying cardiovascular conditions.
2. Population rates of congestive heart failure vary widely because of the differing definitions and classification systems used to describe cases.
3. Population levels of congestive heart failure are rising as more individuals survive acute myocardial infarction and chronic hypertension.
4. Congestive heart failure is predominantly a disease of older adults and the mortality is substantial.
5. Treatment of congestive heart failure has improved as randomized clinical trials have demonstrated the utility of certain drugs.

Research into congestive heart failure has been hampered by variability in case definition. Symptoms, signs, radiological studies, tests of ventricular performance, and tests of exercise capacity have all been utilized. All methods have limitations and are particularly poor in the classification of mild congestive heart failure (Hlatky *et al.* 1986; Chakko and Gheorghiade 1992). The diagnosis may be commonly confused with obesity-related dyspnoea, poor physical condition, myocardial ischaemia, pulmonary disease, or other conditions.

There are several studies of congestive heart failure incidence. The Framingham Study and the Gothenberg Study are examples of the cohort approach (Eriksson *et al.* 1989; Ho *et al.* 1993). These were able to identify incident cases prospectively and characterize them at the time of diagnosis. Studies in Finland, Holland, and Rochester, Minnesota, are examples of a population approach (Van de Lisdonk *et al.* 1990; Remes *et al.* 1992; Rodeheffer *et al.* 1993). These study types find significant differences in incidence, which ranges from 100 to 500 per 100 000 population per year, and that incidence increases sharply with age.

There are more data available on congestive heart failure prevalence. Rates also vary widely due to differences in methodology and case definition. Observed prevalence in industrialized societies ranges from 300 to 2000 individuals per 100 000 population (unadjusted for age) and 3000 to 13 000 per 100 000 population for those over the age of 65 years (Cowie *et al.* 1997). Of particular interest are the data from the American National Health and Nutrition Examination Survey which show a self-report prevalence of 1.1 per cent for adults aged 25 to 74 years while clinical examination results in a prevalence of approximately 2 per cent (Schocken *et al.* 1992). Congestive heart failure prevalence appears to be rising, largely attributed to increased survival from acute myocardial infarction (Ranofsky 1974; Graves and Gillum 1996).

Mortality from congestive heart failure is substantial with the Framingham Study reporting 5-year survival of 25 per cent for men and 38 per cent for women in an early analysis (Ho *et al.* 1993*b*). Improved survival was observed in the later National Health and Nutrition Examination Survey. Among individuals with congestive heart failure (age greater than 55 years), 61 per cent of women and 28 per cent of men were still alive 15 years later (Schocken *et al.* 1992). However, the validity of congestive heart failure diagnosis on death certificates has been questioned (Cowie *et al.* 1997). Because congestive heart failure is a constellation of science, symptoms, and physiological changes, it is often not considered among the underlying causes of death. For example, in the United Kingdom, congestive heart failure is never used as an underlying cause of death (Cowie *et al.* 1997). In the United States, congestive heart failure is categorized as a cause of death and rose from 10 000 in 1968 to 42 000 deaths in 1993 (USDHHS 1996). It is also a contributing cause of death in many other fatalities (Yusuf *et al.* 1989; Kannel *et al.* 1994).

There are numerous causes of the myocardial dysfunction which underlies congestive heart failure. Hypertensive cardiovascular disease with left ventricular hypertrophy results in a 15-fold greater risk of developing congestive heart failure (Kannel *et al.* 1994). Coronary heart disease, particularly when manifested as myocardial infarction, also leads to increased congestive heart failure with damaged and dysfunctional myocardial muscle. In the Framingham Study, approximately 20 per cent of those who survived myocardial infarction developed heart failure within 5 to 6 years (Kannel 1987). Previously, hypertension was the most common underlying cause of congestive heart failure, but there has been a shift to coronary heart disease as a more common aetiology. Diabetes mellitus with congestive heart failure also increased in prevalence (Ho *et al.* 1993*a*; Levy *et al.* 1996; Davis *et al.* 1997). While these are the major causes of congestive heart failure in industrialized societies, in many nations other diseases play an important role including rheumatic heart disease, cardiomyopathy, and pulmonary heart disease.

As most congestive heart failure is a late consequence of an underlying cardiovascular disease, primary treatment should consist of prevention of that underlying disease whether it is hypertension, coronary heart disease, rheumatic heart disease, or other conditions. If these conditions are adequately controlled, congestive heart failure is uncommon. However, there are currently many individuals with these diseases who have congestive heart failure as the primary cause of their limitation and disability. Traditional treatment with diuretics and digitalis are widely used, however, these have recently been questioned (Cohn 1996). In recent clinical trials, congestive heart failure treated with vasodilators and angiotensin-converting enzyme inhibitors has reduced mortality and increased function, leading to optimism for long-term therapy for congestive heart failure (Cohn *et al.* 1986;

SOLVD Investigators 1991, 1992; Swedberg *et al.* 1992; Johnson *et al.* 1993*b*; Cohn 1996).

Rheumatic fever and heart disease

For centuries, rheumatic fever with resulting rheumatic heart disease was the leading cause of cardiovascular morbidity and mortality worldwide. It continues as an important problem in areas where poverty, overcrowding, malnutrition, and lack of medical care are found (WHO 1984*b*; WHO 1988). Although much less common than previously, it is still a problem even in industrialized countries where outbreaks occur.

Some of the salient observations about rheumatic fever and rheumatic heart disease include the following.

1. Rheumatic heart disease is still common in many developing countries.
2. Outbreaks are observed in developed countries.
3. The origins of rheumatic heart disease are well understood. Throat infections with group A *Streptococcus* can result in acute rheumatic fever with carditis, which may lead to chronic rheumatic heart disease.
4. Primary prevention of rheumatic fever rests in appropriate antibiotic treatment of streptococcal infections.
5. For individuals with a history of rheumatic fever and/or rheumatic heart disease, antibiotic prophylaxis is recommended.

During the 1960s, the incidence of acute rheumatic fever ranged from 23 to 55 per 100 000 urban children aged 2 to 14 years in the United States. Currently, it is less than 2 per 100 000 with a prevalence of rheumatic heart disease of less than 1 per 1000 school-aged children (Dajani 1991). In other parts of the industrialized world, such as Scandinavia, similar low rates are found (WHO 1988). However, in some areas of South America, the prevalence of acute rheumatic fever is significantly higher, ranging from 1 to 10 per cent of school-aged children (PAHO 1970). Similar high rates are seen in areas of Asia and Africa (WHO 1988). The mechanisms by which this infection produces the clinical syndrome of acute rheumatic fever and subsequent rheumatic heart disease is well studied (Catanzaro *et al.* 1954). A group A streptococcal infection of the throat (tonsillopharyngitis) can be followed, in approximately 3 weeks, by an episode of acute rheumatic fever. In outbreak situations, this occurs in up to 3 per cent of those with a throat infection; however, it is usually much lower (Siegel *et al.* 1961). The rheumatic fever attack results in an inflammatory reaction which involves the heart, joints, and/or the central nervous system. Of those with acute rheumatic fever, at least 50 per cent develop some manifestation of carditis, but this proportion rises when more sophisticated diagnostic methods are used (Dajani 1991). The diagnosis of acute rheumatic fever is made principally from the clinical findings using the revised Jones criteria. These include the major manifestations of carditis, polyarthritis, chorea, erythema marginatum, and/or subcutaneous nodules. Other manifestations include arthralgias and fever. Laboratory findings of acute phase reactants including elevated erythrocyte sedimentation rate and C-reactive proteins are common. A positive throat culture for streptococcal antigen and/or increased streptococcal antibody titre aid in making the diagnosis. These criteria may not be sufficiently sensitive in industrialized countries where clinical patterns have changed significantly so that arthritis may be the only presentation. In addition, a significant portion of individuals do not have a symptomatic preceding infection (Wannamaker 1973). Rheumatic fever is most common among youth from age 6 to 15 years with the syndrome rarely observed below the age of 5 years (Bland and Jones 1951).

Rapid antigen tests for the diagnosis of group A streptococcal throat infections are highly specific, but less sensitive. While a positive test suggests the need for treatment, a negative test indicates the need for a throat culture (Dajani *et al.* 1995). Antibody tests can confirm a recent group A streptococcal infection.

Primary prevention of acute rheumatic fever is the recommended approach. Throat cultures should be performed on all patients with tonsillopharyngitis and those with a positive culture for group A streptococcal infections treated (Dajani *et al.* 1995). Antibiotic treatment can effectively prevent acute rheumatic fever even when given up to 9 days from the onset of the infection (Denny *et al.* 1950). The recommended treatment schedule by the American Heart Association is found in Table 10. Treatment can be either oral or by injection.

In individuals with a history of acute rheumatic fever, the likelihood of secondary attacks with additional damage is common, estimated to be approximately 50 per cent of those with streptococcal infections. For this reason, prophylaxis with an antibiotic is widely recommended (Dajani *et al.* 1995).

If group A streptococcal infections are appropriately detected and treated, rheumatic heart disease can be effectively prevented. In those where it is not prevented, life-long valvular heart disease results in diminishing function, and, if left untreated, premature mortality.

Congenital heart disease

Malformations of the heart and cardiovascular system present at birth are among the more common of congenital defects. They are the result of genetic and/or environmental factors. These malformations frequently have significant haemodynamic consequences and may result in severe illness and/or death (Friedman 1997).

Congenital heart disease includes a wide variety of malformations of the cardiovascular system including the septal, heart valve, and great vessels defects. The true incidence of congenital heart disease is difficult to determine but approximates 8 per 1000 live births in the United States (Fyfe and Kline 1990; Friedman 1997). This is probably an underestimate, as much congenital heart disease is not discovered until adulthood, is mild, or is fatal prior to birth. In addition, the 0.8 per cent incidence does not include mitral valve prolapse or non-obstructive bicuspid aortic valves, both of which are common. Males are more likely to have congenital heart disease than females, but the pattern differs by defect type (Samanck 1994).

Genetic transmission plays an important role in congenital heart disease. Family studies find that the offspring of parents with congenital heart disease have an increased malformation incidence ranging from 1.4 to 16.1 per cent (Ferencz 1986). Identical twins are both affected 25 to 30 per cent of the time. However, despite the known genetic clustering and the identification of disorders associated with single genes, it is estimated that only 10 per cent of congenital heart disease has an identifiable genetic origin (Noonan 1978).

Table 10 Primary prevention of rheumatic fever (treatment of streptococcal tonsillopharyngitis)

Agent	Dose	Mode	Duration
Benzathine penicillin G	600 000 units for patients < 60 lb 1200 000 units for patients > 60 lb	Intramuscular	Once
		OR	
Penicillin V (phenoxymethyl penicillin)	250 mg 2–3 times daily	Oral	10 days
For individuals allergic to penicillin			
Erythromycin estolate	20–40 mg/kg per day 2–4 times daily	Oral (maximum 1 g/day)	10 days
		OR	
Erythromycin ethylsuccinate	40 mg/kg per day 2–4 times daily	Oral (maximum 1 g/day)	10 days

Source: Dajani *et al.* (1995), from the United States American Heart Association recommendations.

Maternal infections are estimated to cause 10 per cent of all congenital heart disease. Rubella is commonly implicated when it occurs in the first 2 months of pregnancy with congenital malformations in about 80 per cent of live births. Subclinical Coxsackie and other virus infections are also implicated in congenital heart disease.

There are many exposures associated with increased incidence of congenital heart disease. Acute hypoxia, residence at high altitudes, high carboxyhaemoglobin levels, and cigarette smoking are among potential causes (Alberman and Goldstein 1971). External X-ray exposure is associated with Down's syndrome and other congenital defects (Nora 1971). Metabolic defects including diabetes and phenylketonuria are associated with increases in congenital defects.

Diet- and drug-associated exposures are also implicated. They include the well-known examples of thalidomide and folic acid antagonists. Dextroamphetamines, anticonvulsants, lithium chloride, alcohol, and progesterone/oestrogen are suspected as teratogens acting in the first trimester of pregnancy. Certain pesticides and herbicides are similarly implicated (Zierler 1985).

The overall incidence of congenital heart disease appears to have remained stable although the distribution of defect types may be changing. There are unexplained increases in ventricular septal defect and patent ductus arteriosis. Rubella-related disease is declining, perhaps the result of widespread vaccination for that disease (NHLBI 1979).

The most effective strategy for congenital heart disease is prevention including genetic counselling for families with congenital heart disease, rubella immunization, and avoidance of exposure to known teratogens. Of particular importance are avoidance of alcohol abuse and cigarette smoking.

For many that were born with congenital heart disease, modern medical and surgical techniques can provide palliation, if not a cure. For the most severe cases, heart and heart–lung transplants are assuming increasing importance.

Cardiomyopathy and myocarditis

Cardiomyopathy and myocarditis are a diverse set of diseases that have, as a central feature, pathological involvement of the heart muscle. Congestive heart failure is the frequent outcome of this condition as the heart fails to pump effectively. Cardiomyopathies account for a substantial portion of cardiovascular disease related deaths in developing countries (WHO 1984*a*). However, they are becoming more common in industrialized nations with increasing rates of ischaemic cardiomyopathy.

There are numerous known causes of myopathy as detailed in a recent report by the WHO (Table 11). The WHO advocates that the term cardiomyopathy be reserved for myocardial dysfunction of unknown aetiology; however, it is commonly applied even when the aetiology is known (Richardson *et al.* 1996).

The natural history of cardiomyopathy varies according to the type. Many cases begin with an acute phase where inflammation of the myocardium is common (myocarditis). The widespread use of endomyocardial biopsy has been of some assistance in identifying and classifying myocarditis (Fowles 1985). In many cases, the initial myocarditis is probably undetected because it is mild. There are clinical courses ranging from minimal heart failure to a brief rapid course leading to death. Investigators at the Mayo Clinic in Olmsted

Table 11 Major international causes of cardiomyopathy and myocarditis

Cause	Examples
Inflammatory	Viral, parasitic
Metabolic	Thiamine deficiency, uraemia
Toxic	Cobalt, alcohol
Infiltrative	Amyloidosis, neoplastic
Fibroplastic	Endomyocardial fibrosis
Haematological	Sickle cell anaemia
Hypersensitivity	Penicillin
Genetic	Hypertrophic cardiomyopathy
Acquired	Obesity
Idiopathic	Heat stroke
Physical agents	

Source: Richardson *et al.* (1996).

County, Minnesota, found an incidence of idiopathic dilated cardiomyopathy of 6 per 100 000 person years (Shabeter 1983). Overall prevalence in the United States was 35.3 per 100 000 population (Gillum 1986).

The prevalence of cardiomyopathy appears to be increasing in the United States. However, it is uncertain whether this is an actual increase or improved diagnostic methods and greater clinical sensitivity. For most cases, a specific cause is not known.

Cardiomyopathy is grouped into three major types: (a) dilated, characterized by dilatation of the ventricles and contractual dysfunction with congestive heart failure; (b) hypertrophic, with left ventricular hypertrophy and well-preserved cardiac function; (c) restrictive, with impaired diastolic filling frequently due to scarring of the myocardium of the ventricle. The dilated cardiomyopathy pattern is most commonly observed, although there is considerable overlap between types (Keren and Popp 1992).

Alcohol abuse is the most important cause of cardiomyopathy in the United States accounting for approximately 8 per cent of all cases (Rubin 1979; Okada and Wakafuji 1985). This may operate through a direct toxic effect, thiamine deficiency, or additives such as cobalt in alcoholic beverages. Abstinence may halt or reverse this disease (Regan *et al.* 1977; Rubin 1979; Okada and Wakafuji 1985). Viral infections are a very commonly observed cause of cardiomyopathy. Coxsackie virus, echo virus, influenza, and polio are frequently implicated (Levine 1979). These diseases begin as acute myocarditis and then progress to a chronic condition which results in dilated cardiomyopathy.

Hypertrophic cardiomyopathy is detected by the use of echocardiographic techniques. This condition uncommonly causes difficulty for patients and is usually well managed with medication (Wigle 1988). Chagas' disease is caused by the protozoan *Trypanosoma cruzi*. Beginning as a myocarditis, its clinical manifestations are manifest many years later. The disease is most prevalent in Central and South America with over 20 million thought to be infected with the parasite (Morris *et al.* 1990; Hagar and Rahimtoola 1995). This disease may also be found in non-endemic areas through migration, contaminated blood products, and tourism (Hagar and Rahimtoola 1991). Treatment is available for the acute parasitic infections; however, the cardiomyopathy cannot be directly treated.

Schistosomiasis is a parasitic infection epidemic in the Nile and Yangtze basins. It may involve a majority of the population in certain endemic areas. Chronic pulmonary embolization leads to pulmonary hypertension, right ventricular hypertrophy, and right ventricular heart failure. Direct involvement of the myocardium is rare. New medications can be of assistance in controlling the infection and prevention is the principal strategy employed.

References

Abbott, R.D., Sharp, D.S., Burchfiel, C.M., *et al.* (1997). Cross-sectional and longitudinal changes in total and high-density-lipoprotein cholesterol levels over a 20-year period in elderly men: the Honolulu Heart Program. *Annals of Epidemiology*, **7**, 417–24.

Alberman, E.D. and Goldstein, H. (1971). Possible teratogenic effect of cigarette smoking. *Nature*, **231**, 529–30.

Alfredsson, L., Karasek, R., and Theorell, T. (1982). Myocardial infarction risk and psychosocial work environment: an analysis of the male Swedish working force. *Social Science and Medicine*, **16**, 463–7.

American Heart Association (1999). *Heart and stroke statistical update (1998)*. American Heart Association, Dallas, TX.

Anderson, J.T., Jacobs, D.R., Jr, Foster, N., *et al.* (1979). Scoring systems for evaluating dietary pattern effect on serum cholesterol. *Preventive Medicine*, **8**, 525–37.

Anitschkow, N. (1983). *Experimental atherosclerosis in animals* (ed. E.V. Cowdry), p. 271. Macmillan, New York.

Aronow, W.S. and Ahn, C. (1998). Risk factors for new coronary events in older African-American men and women. *American Journal of Cardiology*, **82**, 902–4.

Ascherio, A. and Hunter, D.J. (1994). Iron and myocardial infarction. *Epidemiology*, **5**, 135–7.

Ascherio, A., Hennekens, C.H., Buring, J.E., Master, C., Stampfer, M.J., and Willett, W.C. (1994). Trans-fatty acids intake and risk of myocardial infarction. *Circulation*, **89**, 94–101.

Ascherio, A., Rimm, E.B., Hernan, M.A., *et al.* (1999). Relation of consumption of vitamin E, vitamin C, and carotenoids to risk for stroke among men in the United States. *Annals of Internal Medicine*, **130**, 963–70.

Baraona, E. and Lieber, C.S. (1979). Effects of ethanol on lipid metabolism. *Journal of Lipid Research*, **20**, 289–315.

Barefoot, J.C., Dahlstrom, W.G., and Williams, R.B. (1983). Hostility, coronary heart disease incidence and total mortality: a 25-year follow-up study of 255 physicians. *Psychosomatic Medicine*, **45**, 59–63.

Barefoot, J.C., Dodge, K.A., Peterson, B.L., Dahlstrom, W.G., and Williams, R.B. (1989). The Cook-Medley hostility scale: item content and ability to predict survival. *Psychosomatic Medicine*, **51**, 46–57.

Benditt, E.P. and Benditt, J.M. (1973). *Evidence for a monoclonal origin of human atherosclerotic plaques*. Proceedings of the National Academy of Sciences of the United States of America, **70**, 1753–6. National Academy of Sciences, Washington, DC.

Benson, D.W., Jr, Benditt, D.G., Anderson, R.W., *et al.* (1983). Cardiac arrest in young, ostensibly healthy patients: clinical, hemodynamic, and electrophysiologic findings. *American Journal of Cardiology*, **51**, 65–9.

Blackburn, H. and Jacobs, D. (1984). Sources of the diet–heart controversy: confusion over population versus individual correlations. *Circulation*, **70**, 775–80.

Blackburn, H. and Jacobs, D.R. (1988). Physical activity and the risk of coronary heart disease (editorial). *New England Journal of Medicine*, **319**, 1217–19.

Blackburn, H. and Prineas, R.J. (1983). Diet and hypertension: anthropology, epidemiology, and public health implications. *Progress in Biochemical Pharmacology*, **19**, 31–79.

Blair, S.N., Kohl, H.W., Paffenbarger, R.S., Jr, Clark, D.G., Cooper, K.H., and Gibbons, L.W. (1989) . Physical fitness and all-cause mortality: a prospective study of healthy men and women. *Journal of the American Medical Association*, **262**, 2395–401.

Blair, S.N., Goodyear, N.N., Gibbons, L.W., and Cooper, K.H. (1984). Physical fitness and incidence of hypertension in healthy normotensive men and women. *Journal of the American Medical Association*, **252**, 487–90.

Bland, E.F. and Jones, T.D. (1951). Rheumatic fever and rheumatic heart disease: a twenty year report on 1000 patients followed since childhood. *Circulation*, **4**, 836–43.

Boushey, C.J., Beresford, S.A., Omenn, G.S., and Motulsky, A.G. (1995). A quantitative assessment of plasma homocysteine as a risk factor for vascular disease. Probable benefits of increasing folic acid intakes. *Journal of the American Medical Association*, **274**, 1049–57.

Brown, H.B. and Page, I.H. (1958). Lowering blood lipid levels by changing food patterns. *Journal of the American Medical Association*, **168**, 1989–95.

Buchwald, H., Varco, R.L., Matts, J.P., *et al.* (1990). Effective lipid modification by partial ileal bypass reduced long-term coronary heart disease mortality and morbidity: five year post-trial follow-up report from POSCH. *New England Journal of Medicine*, **323**, 946–55.

Buchwald, H., Matts, J.P., Fitch, L.L., *et al.* for the Program on the Surgical Control of the Hyperlipidemias (POSCH) Group (1992). Changes in sequential coronary arteriograms and subsequent coronary events. *Journal of the American Medical Association*, **268**, 1429–33.

Burt, V.L., Whelton, P., Roccella, E.J., *et al.* (1995). Prevalence of hypertension in the United States adult population: results from the Third National Health and Nutrition Examination Survey, 1988–1991. *Hypertension*, **25**, 305–13.

Canner, P.L., Berge, K.G., Wenger, N.K., *et al.* (1986). Fifteen year mortality in Coronary Drug Project patients: long-term benefit with niacin. *Journal of the American College of Cardiology*, **8**, 1245–55.

Carleton, R.A., Lasater, T.M., Assaf, A.R., Feldman, H.A., McKinlay, S. and the Pawtucket Heart Health Program Writing Group (1995). The Pawtucket Heart Health Program: community changes in cardiovascular risk factors and projected disease risk. *American Journal of Public Health*, **85**, 777–85.

Carmassi, F., Morale, M., Puccetti, R., *et al.* (1992). Coagulation and fibrinolytic system impairment in insulin dependent diabetes mellitus. *Thrombosis Research*, **67**, 643–54.

Case, R.B., Heller, S.S., Case, N.B., *et al.* (1985). Type A behavior and survival after acute myocardial infarction. *New England Journal of Medicine*, **312**, 737–41.

Catanzaro, F.J., Stetson, C.A., Morris, A.J., *et al.* (1954). Symposium on rheumatic fever and rheumatic heart disease: the role of the streptococcus in the pathogenesis of rheumatic fever. *American Journal of Medicine*, **17**, 749–56.

Chakko, S. and Gheorghiade, M. (1992). Estimating severity of chronic heart failure: A clinical challenge for the 1990s. *American Heart Journal*, **124**, 260–4.

Clarke, W.R. and Lauer, R.M. (1985). Coronary risk factors from childhood to adult life: the Muscatine Study. *Cardiovascular Disease Epidemiology Newsletter*, **37**, 38.

Clarkson, T.B., Bond, M.G., Bullock, B.C., McLaughlin, K.J., and Sawyer, J.K. (1984). A study of atherosclerosis regression in *Macaca mulatta*. V. Changes in abdominal aorta and carotid and coronary arteries from animals with atherosclerosis induced for 38 months and then regressed for 24 or 48 months at plasma cholesterol concentrations of 300 or 200 mg/dl. *Experimental and Molecular Pathology*, **41**, 96–118.

Clarkson, P., Celermajer, D.S., Donald, A.E., *et al.* (1996). Impaired vascular reactivity in insulin-dependent diabetes mellitus is related to disease duration and low density lipoprotein cholesterol levels. *Journal of the American College of Cardiology*, **28**, 573–9.

Cohen, J.B. and Reed, D. (1985). Type A behavior and coronary heart disease among Japanese men in Hawaii. *Journal of Behavioral Medicine*, **8**, 343–52.

Cohn, J.N. (1996). The management of chronic heart failure. *New England Journal of Medicine*, **335**, 490–8.

Cohn, J.N., Archibald, D.G., Ziesche, S., *et al.* (1986). Effect of vasodilator therapy on mortality in chronic congestive heart failure: results of a Veterans Administration Cooperative Study. *New England Journal of Medicine*, **314**, 1547–52.

Colditz, G.A. (1990). A prospective assessment of moderate alcohol intake and major chronic diseases. *Annals of Epidemiology*, **1**, 167–77.

Connolly, H.M., Crary, J.L., McGoon, M.D., *et al.* (1997). Valvular heart disease associated with fenfluramine-phentermine. *New England Journal of Medicine*, **337**, 581–8.

Cowie, M.R., Mosterd, A., Wood, D.A., *et al.* (1997). The epidemiology of heart failure. *European Heart Journal*, **18**, 208–25.

Criqui, M.H. (1987). The roles of alcohol in the epidemiology of cardiovascular diseases. *Acta Medica Scandinavica*, **717** (Supplement), 73–85.

Dajani, A.S. (1991). Current status of nonsupportive complications of group A streptococci. *Pediatric Infectious Disease Journal*, **105**, S25–7.

Dajani, A., Taubert, K., Ferrieri, P., Peter, G., and Shulman, S. (1995). Treatment of acute streptococcal pharyngitis and prevention of rheumatic fever: a statement for health professionals. Committee on Rheumatic Fever, Endocarditis, and Kawasaki Disease of the Council on Cardiovascular Disease in the Young, The American Heart Association. *Pediatrics*, **96**, 758–64.

Dattilo, A.M. and Kris-Etherton, P.M. (1992). Effects of weight reduction on blood lipids and lipoproteins: a meta-analysis. *American Journal of Clinical Nutrition*, **56**, 320–8.

Davis, R.C., Hobbs, F.D.R., McLeod, S., *et al.* (1997). Heart failure prevalence in patients in 'high-risk' groups. *European Heart Journal*, **18**, 597.

Dawber, T.R., Moore, F.E., and Mann, G.V. (1957). Measuring the risk of coronary heart disease in adult population groups: II. Coronary heart disease in the Framingham Study. *American Journal of Public Health*, **47**, 4–24.

DCCT (Diabetes Control and Complications Trial) Research Group (1993). The effect of intensive treatment of diabetes on the development and progression of long-term complications in insulin-dependent diabetes mellitus. *New England Journal of Medicine*, **329**, 977–86.

Denny, F.W., Wannamaker, L.W., Brink, W.R., Rammelkamp, C.H., and Custer, E.A. (1950). Prevention of rheumatic fever: treatment of the preceding streptococcic infection. *Journal of the American Medical Association*, **143**, 151–3.

Derby, C.A., Lapane, K.L., Feldman, H.A., and Carleton, R.A. (2000). Sex-specific trends in validated coronary heart disease rates in Southeastern New England, 1980–1991. *American Journal of Epidemiology*, **151**, 417–29.

Dimsdale, J.E., Gilbert, J., Hutter, A.M., *et al.* (1981). Predicting cardiac morbidity based on risk factors and coronary angiographic findings. *American Journal of Cardiology*, **47**, 73–6.

Downs, J.R., Clearfield, M., Weis, S., *et al.* (1998). Primary prevention of acute coronary events with lovastatin in men and women with average cholesterol levels: results of AFCAPS/TexCAPS. Air Force/Texas Coronary Atherosclerosis Prevention Study. *Journal of the American Medical Association*, **279**, 1615–22.

Dyer, A.R. and Elliott, P. (1989). The INTERSALT Study: relations of body mass index to blood pressure. *Journal of Human Hypertension*, **3**, 299–308.

Eckel, R.H. and Krauss, R.M. (1998). American Heart Association call to action: obesity as a major risk factor for coronary heart disease. *Circulation*, **97**, 2099–100.

Eriksson, H., Svardsudd, K., Larsson, B., *et al.* (1989). Risk factors for heart failure in the general population: the study of men born in 1913. *European Heart Journal*, **10**, 647–56.

Farquhar, J.W., Maccoby, N., Wood, P.D., *et al.* (1977). Community education for cardiovascular health. *Lancet*, **1**, 1192–5.

Farquhar, J.W., Fortmann, S.P., Flora, J.A., *et al.* (1990). Effects of community-wide education on cardiovascular disease risk factors: the Stanford Five-City Project. *Journal of the American Medical Association*, **264**, 359–65.

Ferencz, C. (1986). Offspring of fathers with cardiovascular malformations. *American Heart Journal*, **111**, 1212–13.

Ferrence, R.G., Truscott, S., and Whitehead, P.C. (1986). Drinking and the prevention of coronary heart disease: findings, issues and public health policy. *Journal of Studies on Alcohol*, **47**, 394–408.

Feskanich, D., Rimm, E.B., Giovannucci, E.L., *et al.* (1993). Reproducibility and validity of food intake measurements from a semiquantitative food frequency questionnaire. *Journal of the American Dietetic Association*, **93**, 790–6.

Fiore, M.C., Bailey, W.C., Cohen, S.J., *et al.* (1996). *Smoking cessation.* Clinical practice guideline No. 18. United States Department of Health and Human Services, Public Health Service, Agency for Health Care Policy and Research. AHCPR Publication No. 96–0692.

Flegal, K.M. (1996). Trends in body weight and overweight in the US population. *Nutrition Reviews*, **54**, S97–S100

Fowles, R.E. (1985). Progress of research in cardiomyopathy and myocarditis in the USA. International Symposium on Cardiomyopathy and Myocarditis. *Heart Vessels*, **1**, 5–7.

Freedman, D.S. (1995). Relation of body fat distribution to ischemic heart disease. The National Health and Nutrition Examination Survey I (NHANES I) Epidemiologic Follow-up Study. *American Journal of Epidemiology*, **142**, 53–63.

Freis, E.D. (1976). Salt, volume and the prevention of hypertension. *Circulation*, **53**, 589–95.

Frick, M.H., Elo, O., Haapa, K., *et al.* (1987). Helsinki Heart Study: primary-prevention trial with gemfibrozil in middle-aged men with dyslipidemia. *New England Journal of Medicine*, **317**, 1237–45.

Friedman, W.F. (1997). Congenital heart disease in infancy and childhood. In *Heart disease: a textbook of cardiovascular medicine* (ed. E. Braunwald), (5th edn), pp. 877–962. Saunders, Philadelphia.

Friedman, M. and Rosenman, R.H. (1959). Association of specific overt behavior pattern with blood and cardiovascular findings: blood cholesterol level, blood clotting time, incidence of arcus senilis, and clinical coronary artery disease. *Journal of the American Medical Association*, **169**, 1286–96.

Friedman, M., Thorensen, C.E., Gill, J.J., *et al.* (1984). Alteration of type A behavior and reduction in cardiac recurrences in post-myocardial infarction patients. *American Heart Journal*, **108**, 237–48.

Fuster, V., Badimon, L., Badimon, J., and Chesebro, J. (1992*a*). Mechanisms of disease: the pathogenesis of coronary artery disease and the acute coronary syndromes. *New England Journal of Medicine*, **326**, 310 18.

Fuster, V., Badimon, L., Badimon, J.J., and Chesebro, J.H. (1992*b*). The pathogenesis of coronary artery disease and the acute coronary syndromes. *New England Journal of Medicine*, **326**, 242–50.

Fyfe, D.A. and Kline, C.H. (1990). Fetal echocardiographic diagnosis of congenital heart disease. *Pediatric Clinics of North America*, **37**, 45–67.

Garland, C., Barrett-Connor, E., Suarez, L., Criqui, M.H., and Wingard, D.L. (1985). Effects of passive smoking on ischemic heart disease mortality of non-smokers. *American Journal of Epidemiology*, **121**, 645–50.

GCP Research Group (1988). GCP German Cardiovascular Prevention study. *Design, methods, results*. Program Report. Scientific Institute of the German Medical Association (WIAD), Bonn, Germany.

Gillum, R.F. (1986). Idiopathic cardiomyopathy in the United States, 1970–1982. *American Heart Journal*, **111**, 752–5.

Ginsberg, H.N., Kris-Etherton, P., Dennis, B., *et al.* (1998). Effects of reducing dietary saturated fatty acids on plasma lipids and lipoproteins in healthy subjects: the DELTA Study, protocol 1. *Arteriosclerosis, Thrombosis and Vascular Biology*, **18**, 441–9.

Gleiberman, L. (1973). Blood pressure and dietary salt in human populations. *Ecology of Food Nutrition*, **2**, 143–56.

Gordon T. (1988). The diet–heart idea. *American Journal of Epidemiology*, **127**, 220–5.

Gordon, T., Castelli, W.P., Hjortland, M.C., Kannel, W.B., and Dawber, T.R. (1977). High density lipoprotein as a protective factor against coronary heart disease. The Framingham Study. *American Journal of Medicine*, **62**, 707–14.

Gordon, T., Ernst, N., Fisher, M., and Rifkind, B.M. (1981). Alcohol and high-density lipoprotein cholesterol. *Circulation*, **64**, (Supplement III), 63–7.

Graves, E.J. and Gillum, B.S. (1996). 1994 Summary: National hospital discharge survey: advance data. *National Center for Health Statistics*, **278**, 1–12.

Grundy, S.M. (1999). Primary prevention of coronary heart disease: integrating risk assessment with intervention (review). *Circulation*, **100**, 988–98.

Hagar, J.M. and Rahimtoola, S.H. (1991). Chagas' heart disease in the United States. *New England Journal of Medicine*, **325**, 763–8.

Hagar, J.M. and Rahimtoola, S.H. (1995). Chagas' heart disease. *Current Problems in Cardiology*, **20**, 825–924.

Harris, T.B., Ballard-Barbasch, R., Madans, J., Makuc, D.M., and Feldman, J.J. (1993). Overweight, weight loss, and risk of coronary heart disease in older women. The NHANES I Epidemiologic Follow-up Study. *American Journal of Epidemiology*, **137**, 1318–27.

Harris, T.B., Launer, L.J., Madans, J., and Feldman, J.J. (1997). Cohort study of effect of being overweight and change in weight on risk of coronary heart disease in old age. *British Medical Journal*, **314**, 1791–4.

Haynes, S.G., Feinleib, M., and Kannel, W.B. (1980). The relationship of psychosocial factors to coronary heart disease in the Framingham Study. III. Eight-year incidence of coronary heart disease. *American Journal of Epidemiology*, **111**, 37–58.

Hearn, M.D., Murray, D.M., and Luepker, R.V. (1988). Hostility, coronary heart disease, and total mortality. A 33-year follow-up study of university students. *Journal of Behavioral Medicine*, **12**, 105–21.

Heart Outcomes Prevention Evaluation Study Investigators (2000). Effects of an angiotensin-converting enzyme inhibitor, ramipril, on cardiovascular events in high-risk patients. *New England Journal of Medicine*, **342**, 145–53.

Hecker, M.H.L., Chesney, M.A., Black, G.W., and Frautsch, N. (1988). Coronary prone behaviors in the Western Collaborative Group Study. *Psychosomatic Medicine*, **50**, 153–64.

Hegsted, D.M., McGandy, R.B., Myers, M.L., and Stare, F.J. (1965). Quantitative effects of dietary fat on serum cholesterol in man. *American Journal of Clinical Nutrition*, **17**, 281–95.

Helsing, K.J., Sandler, D.P., Comstock, G.W., and Chee, E. (1988). Heart disease mortality in nonsmokers living with smokers. *American Journal of Epidemiology*, **127**, 915–22.

Hennekens, C.H., Buring, J.E., Manson, J.E., *et al.* (1996). Lack of effect on long-term supplementation with beta carotene on the incidence of malignant neoplasms and cardiovascular disease. *New England Journal of Medicine*, **334**, 1145–9.

Hermanson, B., Omenn, G.S., Kronmal, R.A., *et al.* (1988). Beneficial six-year outcome of smoking cessation in older men and women with coronary artery disease: results from the CASS registry. *New England Journal of Medicine*, **319**, 1365–9.

Higgins, M. and Luepker, R.V. (ed.) (1989). Trends and determinants of coronary heart disease mortality: international comparisons. *International Journal of Epidemiology*, **18** (Supplement 1), S1–S232.

Hirayama, T. (1984). Lung cancer in Japan: Effects of nutrition and passive smoking. In *Lung cancer: causes and prevention* (ed. M. Mizell and P. Correa), pp. 175–95. Verlag Chemie International, New York.

Hlatky, M.A., Fleg, J.L., Hinton, P.C., *et al.* (1986). Physician practice in the management of congestive heart failure. *Journal of the American College of Cardiology*, **8**, 966–70.

Ho, K.K., Pinsky, J.L., Kannel, W.B., and Levy, D. (1993*a*). The epidemiology of heart failure: the Framingham Study. *Journal of the American College of Cardiology*, **22**, 6A–13A.

Ho, K.K., Anderson, K.M., Kannel, W.B., Grossman, W., and Levy, D. (1993*b*). Survival after the onset of congestive heart failure in Framingham Heart Study subjects. *Circulation*, **88**, 107–15.

Hole, D.J., Gillis, C.R., Chopra, C., and Hawthorne, V.M. (1989). Passive smoking and cardiorespiratory health in a general population in the west of Scotland. *British Medical Journal*, **299**, 423–7.

Huang, Z., Willett, W.C., Manson, J.E., *et al.* (1998). Body weight, weight change, and risk for hypertension in women. *Annals of Internal Medicine*, **128**, 81–8.

Hughes, L.O. (1990). Insulin, Indian origin and ischemic heart disease (editorial). *International Journal of Cardiology*, **26**, 1–4.

Hypertension Prevention Trial Research Group (1990). The Hypertension Prevention Trial: three-year effects of dietary changes on blood pressure. *Archives of Internal Medicine*, **150**, 153–62.

INTERSALT Cooperative Research Group (1988). INTERSALT: an international study of electrolyte excretion and blood pressure: results for 24 h urinary sodium and potassium excretion. *British Medical Journal*, **297**, 319–28.

Jacobs, D.R., Anderson, J., and Blackburn, H. (1979). Diet and serum cholesterol: do zero correlations negate the relationships? *American Journal of Epidemiology*, **10**, 77–88.

Jenkins, D.J.A., Wolever, T.M.S., Rao, A.V., *et al.* (1993). Effect on blood lipids of very high intakes of fiber in diets low in saturated fat and cholesterol. *New England Journal of Medicine*, **329**, 21–6.

Johnson, C.L., Rifkind, B.M., Sempos, C.T., *et al.* (1993*a*). Declining serum total cholesterol levels among US adults. *Journal of the American Medical Association*, **269**, 3002–23.

Johnson, G., Carson, P., Francis, G.S., and Cohn, J.N. (1993*b*). Influence of prerandomization (baseline) variables on mortality and on the reduction of mortality by enalapril: Veterans Affairs Cooperative Study on Vasodilator Therapy of Heart Failure (V-HeFT II). *Circulation*, **87**, VI32–VI39.

Joseph, J.G., Prior, I.A.M., Salmond, C.E., and Stanley, D. (1983). Elevation of systolic and diastolic blood pressure associated with migration: the Tokelau Island Migrant Study. *Journal of Chronic Disorders*, **36**, 507–16.

Kagan, A., Harris, B.R., Winkelstein, W., *et al.* (1974). Epidemiologic studies of coronary heart disease and stroke in Japanese men living in Japan, Hawaii and California: demographic, physical, dietary and biochemical characteristics. *Journal of Chronic Disorders*, **27**, 345–64.

Kannel, W.B. (1987). Epidemiology and prevention of cardiac failure: Framingham Study insights. *European Heart Journal*, **8**, 23–6.

Kannel, W.B. and McGee, D.L. (1979). Diabetes and cardiovascular disease. The Framingham Study. *Journal of the American Medical Association*, **241**, 2035–8.

Kannel, W.B., McGee, D.L., and Castelli, W.P. (1984). Latest perspectives on cigarette smoking and cardiovascular disease: the Framingham Study. *Journal of Cardiac Rehabilitation*, **4**, 267–77.

Kannel, W.B., Neaton, J.D., Wentworth, D., *et al.* (1986). Overall and coronary heart disease mortality rates in relation to major risk factors in 325,348 men screened for the MRFIT. Multiple Risk Factor Intervention Trial. *American Heart Journal*, **112**, 825–35.

Kannel, W.B., Ho, K., and Thom, T. (1994). Changing epidemiological features of cardiac failure. *British Heart Journal*, **72**, S3–9.

Kaplan, G.A., Salonen, J.T., Cohen, R.D., Brand, R.J., Syme, S.L., and Puska, P. (1988). Social connections and mortality from all causes and from cardiovascular disease. Prospective evidence from Eastern Finland. *American Journal of Epidemiology*, **128**, 370–80.

Kawachi, I., Colditz, G.A., Stampfer, M.J., *et al.* (1994). Smoking cessation and time course of decreased risks of coronary heart disease in middle-aged women. *Archives of Internal Medicine*, **154**, 169–75.

Kawachi, I., Colditz, G.A., Speizer, F.E., *et al.* (1997). A prospective study of passive smoking and coronary heart disease. *Circulation*, **95**, 2374–9.

Keren, A. and Popp, R.L. (1992). Assignment of patients into the classification of cardiomyopathies. *Circulation*, **86**, 1622–33.

Kesteloot, H., Vuylsteks, M., and Costenoble, A. (1980). Relationship between blood pressure and sodium and potassium intake in a Belgian male population group. In *Epidemiology of arterial blood pressure* (ed. K. Kesteloot and J. Joossens), pp. 345–51. Nijhoff, the Hague.

Keys, A. (ed.) (1980). *Seven countries: a multivariate analysis of death and coronary heart disease.* Harvard University Press, Cambridge, MA.

Keys, A., Anderson, J.T., and Gande, G. (1965). Serum cholesterol response to changes in the diet. *Metabolism*, **14**, 747–87.

Keys, A., Grande, F., and Anderson, J.T. (1974). Bias and misrepresentation revisited—'perspective' on saturated fat. *American Journal of Clinical Nutrition*, **27**, 188–212.

Knowler, W.C., Bennett, P.H., Hammon, R.F., and Miller, M. (1978). Diabetes incidence and prevalence in Pima Indians: A 19-fold greater incidence than in Rochester, MN. *American Journal of Epidemiology*, **108**, 497–505.

Kramer, K., Kuller, L., and Fisher, R. (1968). The increasing mortality attributed to cirrhosis and fatty liver, in Baltimore (1957–1996). *Annals of Internal Medicine*, **69**, 273–82.

Krauss, R.M., Wonston, M., Fletcher, R.N., and Grundy, S.M. (1998). Obesity: impact of cardiovascular disease. *Circulation*, **98**, 1472–6.

Kritchevsky, S.B., Shimakawa, T., Tell, G.S., *et al.* (1995). Dietary antioxidants and carotid artery wall thickness: the ARIC Study. *Circulation*, **92**, 2142–50.

Kuller, L.H., Traven, N.D., Rutan, G.H., Perper, J.A., and Ives, D.G. (1989). Marked decline of coronary heart disease mortality in 35–44-year-old white men in Allegheny County, Pennsylvania. *Circulation*, **80**, 261–6.

Kushi, L.H., Lew, R.A., Stare, F.J., *et al.* (1985). Diet and 20-year mortality from coronary heart disease: the Ireland–Boston Diet–Heart Study. *New England Journal of Medicine*, **312**, 811–18.

Layard, M.W. (1995). Ischemic heart disease and spousal smoking in the National Mortality Followback Survey. *Regulatory Toxicology Pharmacology*, **21**, 180–3.

Lehto, S., Ronnemaa, T., Haffner, S.M., Pyorala, K., Kallio, V., and Laakso, M. (1997). Dyslipidemia and hyperglycemia predict coronary heart disease events in middle-aged patients with NIDDM. *Diabetes*, **48**, 1354–9.

Leon, A.S., Connett, J., Jacobs, D.R. Jr, and Rauramaa, R. (1987). Leisure-time physical activity levels and risk of coronary heart disease and death: the Multiple Risk Factor Intervention Trial. *Journal of the American Medical Association*, **258**, 2388–95.

Leon, G.R., Finn, S.E., Murray, D., and Bailey, J.M. (1988). Inability to predict cardiovascular disease from hostility scores of MMPI items related to type A behavior. *Journal of Consulting and Clinical Psychology*, **56**, 597–600.

Levine, H.D. (1979). Virus myocarditis: a critique of the literature from clinical, electrocardiographic and pathologic standpoints. *American Journal of Medical Sciences*, **277**, 132–43.

Levy, D., Larson, M.G., Vasan, R.S., Kannel, W.B., and Ho, K.K. (1996). The progression from hypertension to congestive heart failure. *Journal of the American Medical Association*, **275**, 1557–62.

Lipid Research Clinics Program (1984). The Lipid Research Clinics Coronary Primary Prevention Trial results: reduction in incidence of coronary heart disease. *Journal of the American Medical Association*, **251**, 351–64.

Long-term Intervention with Pravastatin in Ischaemic Disease (LIPID) Study Group (1998). Prevention of cardiovascular events and death with pravastatin in patients with coronary heart disease and a broad range of initial cholesterol levels. *New England Journal of Medicine*, **339**, 1349–57.

Luepker, R.V. (ed.) (1983). Conference on blood lipids in children. Optimal levels for early prevention of coronary artery disease. *Preventive Medicine*, **12**, 725–905.

Luepker, R.V. (1994). Epidemiology of atherosclerotic diseases in population groups. In *Primer in preventive cardiology* (ed. T.A. Pearson, M.H. Criqui, R.V. Luepker, A. Oberman, and M. Winston), pp. 1–10. American Heart Association, Dallas, TX.

Luepker, R.V. (ed.) (1999). Proceedings from primordial prevention of cardiovascular disease risk factors: an international symposium honoring the career and research of Henry Blackburn, MD. *Preventive Medicine*, **29**.

Luepker, R.V., Murray, D.M., Jacobs, D.R. Jr, *et al.* (1994). Community education for cardiovascular disease prevention: risk factor changes in the Minnesota Heart Health Program. *American Journal of Public Health*, **84**, 1383–93.

Luepker, R.V., Jacobs, D.R., Prineas, R.J., and Sinaiko, A.R. (1999). Secular trends of blood pressure and body size in a multi-ethnic adolescent population: 1986 to 1996. *Journal of Pediatrics*, **134**, 668–74.

McCranie, E.W., Watkins, L.O., Brandsma, J.M., and Sisson, B.D. (1986). Hostility, coronary heart disease (CHD) incidence, and total mortality: lack of an association in a 25-year follow-up study of 478 physicians. *Journal of Behavioral Medicine*, **9**, 119–25.

McGill, H.C., McMahan, C.A., Malcom, G.T., *et al.* for the PDAY Research Group (1997). Effects of serum lipoproteins and smoking on atherosclerosis in young men and women. *Arteriosclerosis and Thrombosis Vascular Biology*, **17**, 95–106.

McGovern, P.G., Pankow, J.S., Shahar, E., *et al.* for the Minnesota Heart Survey Investigators (1996). Recent trends in acute coronary heart disease mortality, morbidity, medical care and risk factors. *New England Journal of Medicine*, **334**, 884–90.

Maouad J., Fernandez F., Barrillon, A., *et al.* (1984). Diffuse or segmental narrowing (spasm) of coronary arteries during smoking demonstrated on angiography. *American Journal of Cardiology*, **53**, 354–5.

Matthews, K.A., Glass, D.C., Rosenman, R.H., *et al.* (1977). Competitive drive, pattern A, and coronary heart disease: a further analysis of some data from the Western Collaborative Group Study. *Journal of Chronic Disorders*, **30**, 489–98.

Mattson, F.H. and Grundy, S.M. (1985). Comparison of effects of dietary saturated, monounsaturated, and polyunsaturated fatty acids on plasma lipids and lipoproteins in man. *Journal of Lipid Research*, **26**, 194–202.

Meade, T.W., Imeson, J., and Stirling, Y. (1987). Effects of changes in smoking and other characteristics on clotting factors and the risk of ischaemic heart disease. *Lancet*, **2**, 986–8.

Meneely, G.R. and Battarbee, H.D. (1976). High sodium-low potassium environment and hypertension. *American Journal of Cardiology*, **38**, 768–85.

Milner, M.R., Gallino, R.A., Leffingwell, A., *et al.* (1989). Usefulness of fish oil supplements in preventing clinical evidence of restenosis after percutaneous transluminal coronary angioplasty. *American Journal of Cardiology*, **64**, 294–9.

Mittleman, M.A., Maclure, M., Tofler, G.H., *et al.* for the Determinants of Myocardial Infarction Onset Study Investigators (1993). Triggering of acute myocardial infarction by heavy physical exertion: protection against triggering of regular exertion. *New England Journal of Medicine*, **329**, 1677–83.

Morris, S.A., Tanowitz, H.B., Wittner, M., and Bilezikian, J.P. (1990). Pathophysiological insights into the cardiomyopathy of Chagas' disease. *Circulation*, **82**, 1900–9.

Moser, M. and Hebert, P.R. (1996). Prevention of disease progression, left ventricular hypertrophy and congestive heart failure in hypertension treatment trials. *Journal of the American College of Cardiology*, **27**, 1214–18.

Muller, J.E., Ludmer, P.L., Willich, S.N., *et al.* (1987). Circadian variation in the frequency of sudden cardiac death. *Circulation*, **75**, 131–8.

Muller, J.E., Kaufmann, P.G., Luepker, R.V., Weisfeldt, M.L., Deedwanis, P.C., and Willerson, J.T. (1997). Mechanisms precipitating acute cardiac events: Review and recommendations of an NHLBI workshop. *Circulation*, **96**, 3233–9.

Multiple Risk Factor Intervention Trial Research Group (1996). Mortality after 16 years for participants randomized to the Multiple Risk Factor Intervention Trial. *Circulation*, **94**, 946–51.

Munger, R.G., Folsom, A.R., Kushi, L.H., Kaye, S.A., and Sellers, T.A. (1992). Dietary assessment of older Iowa women with a food frequency questionnaire: nutrient intake, reproducibility, and comparison with 24-hour dietary recall interviews. *American Journal of Epidemiology*, **136**, 192–200.

National Task Force on Prevention and Treatment of Obesity (1994). Towards prevention of obesity: research directions. *Obesity Research*, **2**, 571–84.

Neaton, J.D. and Wentworth, D. for the Multiple Risk Factor Intervention Trial Research Group (1992). Serum cholesterol, blood pressure, cigarette smoking, and death from coronary heart disease: Overall findings and differences by age for 316 099 white men. *Archives of Internal Medicine*, **152**, 56–64.

Neaton, J.D., Grimm, R.H., Jr, Prineas, R.J., *et al.* (1993). Treatment of mild hypertension study: final results. *Journal of the American Medical Association*, **270**, 713–24.

NHLBI (National Heart, Lung, and Blood Institute) (1978). *Proceedings of the Conference on the Decline in Coronary Heart Disease Mortality*. US Department of Health and Human Services, National Institutes of Health. US Government Printing Office, Washington, DC.

NHLBI (National Heart, Lung, and Blood Institute) (1979). *NHLBI Working Group on Heart Disease Epidemiology Report*. NIH Report 79-1667. US Government Printing Office, Washington, DC.

NHLBI (National Heart, Lung, and Blood Institute) (1997). *The sixth report of the Joint National Commission on Detection, Evaluation and Treatment of High Blood Pressure*. NIH Publication No. 98-4080. National Institutes of Health, Bethesda, MD.

NHLBI (National Heart, Lung, and Blood Institute) (1998). *Morbidity and mortality: 1998 chartbook on cardiovascular, lung, and blood diseases*. National Institutes of Health, Washington, DC.

NIH (National Institutes of Health) (1993*a*). *Second Report of the Expert Panel on Detection, Evaluation, and Treatment of High Blood Cholesterol in Adults*. National Cholesterol Education Program. US Department of Health and Human Services. NIH Publication No. 93–3095. National Institutes of Health, Washington, DC.

NIH (National Institutes of Health) Consensus Conference (1993*b*). Triglyceride, high-density lipoprotein, and coronary heart disease. NIH Consensus Development Panel on Triglyceride, High-Density Lipoprotein, and Coronary Heart Disease. *Journal of the American Medical Association*, **269**, 505–10.

NIH (National Institutes of Health) Consensus Conference (1996). Physical activity and cardiovascular health. *Journal of the American Medical Association*, **276**, 241–6.

Noonan, J. (1978). Twins, conjoined twins and cardiac defects. *American Journal of Diseased Children*, **132**, 17–18.

Nora, J.J. (1971). Etiologic factors in congenital heart diseases. *Pediatric Clinics of North America*, **18**, 1059–74.

O'Connor, G.T., Buring, J.E., Yusuf, S., *et al.* (1989). An overview of randomized trials of rehabilitation with exercise after myocardial infarction. *Circulation*, **80**, 234–44.

Okada, R. and Wakafuji, S. (1985). Myocarditis in autopsy. International Symposium on Cardiomyopathy and Myocarditis. *Heart Vessels*, **1**, 23–9.

Oldridge, N.B., Guyatt, G.H., Fischer, M.E., and Rimm, A.A. (1988). Cardiac rehabilitation after myocardial infarction. Combined experience of randomized clinical trials. *Journal of the American Medical Association*, **260**, 945–50.

Ornish, D., Brown, S.E., Scherwitz, L.W., *et al.* (1990). Can lifestyle changes reverse coronary heart disease? The lifestyle heart trial. *Lancet*, **336**, 129–33.

Orth-Gomer, K. and Johnson, J.V. (1987). Social network interaction and mortality: a six year follow-up study of a random sample of the Swedish population. *Journal of Chronic Disorders*, **40**, 949–57.

Osganian, S.K., Stampfer, M.J., Spiegelman, D., *et al.* (1999). Distribution of and factors associated with serum homocysteine levels in children: Child and Adolescent Trial for Cardiovascular Health. *Journal of the American Medical Association*, **281**, 1189–96.

Paffenbarger, R.S., Jr, Hyde, R.T., Wing, A.L., and Steinmetz, C.H. (1984). A natural history of athleticism and cardiovascular health. *Journal of the American Medical Association*, **252**, 491–5.

PAHO (Pan American Health Organization) (1970). Fourth Meeting of the Working Group on Prevention of Rheumatic Fever, Quito, Ecuador.

Paisey, R.B., Harvey, P., Rice, S., *et al.* (1998). An intensive weight loss programme in established type 2 diabetes and controls: effects on weight and atherosclerosis risk factors at 1 year. *Diabetic Medicine*, **15**, 73 9.

Perry, C.L., Kelder, S.H., Murray, D.M., *et al.* (1992). Community-wide smoking prevention: long-term outcomes of the Minnesota Heart Health Program and the Class of 1989 Study. *American Journal of Public Health*, **82**, 1210–16.

Poole-Wilson, P.A. (1989). Chronic heart failure: cause, pathophysiology, prognosis, clinical manifestations, investigations. In *Disease of the heart* (ed. D.G. Julian, A.J. Camm, K.F. Fox, R.J.C. Hall, and P.A. Poole-Wilson), pp. 24–36. Baillière-Tindall, London.

Pooling Project Research Group (1978). Relationship of blood pressure, serum cholesterol, smoking habit, relative weight, and ECG abnormalities to incidence of major coronary events: final report of the pooling project. *Journal of Chronic Diseases*, **31**, 201–6.

Powell, K.E., Thompson, P.D., Caspersen, C.J., and Kendrick, J.S. (1987). Physical activity and the incidence of coronary heart disease. *Annual Review of Public Health*, **8**, 253–87.

Psaty, B.M., Smith, N.L., Siscovick, D.S., *et al.* (1997). Health outcomes associated with antihypertensive therapies used as first-line agents. A systematic review and meta-analysis. *Journal of the American Medical Association*, **277**, 739–45.

Puska, P., Tuomilehto, J., Nissinen, A., Vartiainen, E. (ed.) (1995). *The North Karelia Project: 20 year results and experiences*. Helsinki University Printing House.

Pyorala, K., Laakso, M., and Uusitupa, M. (1987). Diabetes and atherosclerosis: an epidemiologic view. *Diabetes/Metabolism Review*, **3**, 463–524.

Ragland, D.R. and Brand, R.J. (1988*a*). Coronary heart disease mortality in the Western Collaborative Group Study. Follow-up experience of 22 years. *American Journal of Epidemiology*, **127**, 462–75.

Ragland, D.R. and Brand, R.J. (1988*b*). Type A behavior and mortality from coronary heart disease. *New England Journal of Medicine*, **318**, 65–9.

Ranofsky, A. (1974). *Inpatient utilization of short-stay hospitals by diagnosis: United States, 1971*. Publication no. HRA-75-1767. National Center for Health Statistics, Department of Health Education and Welfare, Washington, DC.

Regan, T.J. (1990). Alcohol and the cardiovascular system. *Journal of the American Medical Association*, **264**, 377–81.

Regan, T.J., Haider, B., Ahmed, S.S., *et al.* (1977). Whisky and the heart. *Cardiovascular Medicine*, **2**, 165.

Remes, J., Reunanen, A., Aromaa, A., and Pyorala, K. (1992). Incidence of heart failure in Eastern Finland: a population-based surveillance study. *European Heart Journal*, **13**, 588–93.

Richardson, P., McKenna, W., Bristow, M., *et al.* (1996). Report of the 1995 World Health Organization/International Society and Federation of Cardiology Task Force on the Definition and Classification of cardiomyopathies. *Circulation*, **93**, 841–2.

Ridker, P.M., Manson, J.E., Buring, J.E., Muller, J.E., and Hennekens, C.H. (1990). Circadian variation of acute myocardial infarction and the effect of low-dose aspirin in a randomized trial of physicians. *Circulation*, **82**, 897–902.

Rimm, E.B., Stampfer, M.J., Ascherio, A., Giovannucci, E., Colditz, G.A., and Willett, W.C. (1993). Vitamin E consumption and the risk of coronary heart disease in men. *New England Journal of Medicine*, **328**, 1450–6.

Ripsin, C.M., Keenan, J.M., Jacobs, D.R., *et al.* (1992). Oat products and lipid-lowering: a meta-analysis. *Journal of the American Medical Association*, **267**, 3317–25.

Rodeheffer, R.J., Jacobsen, S.J., Gersh, B.J., *et al.* (1993). The incidence and prevalence of congestive heart failure in Rochester, Minnesota. *Mayo Clinic Proceedings*, **68**, 1143–50.

Rosenberg, L., Miller, D.R., Kaufman, D.W., *et al.* (1983). Myocardial infarction in women under 50 years of age. *Journal of the American Medical Association*, **250**, 2801–6.

Rosenberg, L., Kaufman, D.W., Helmrich, S.P., *et al.* (1985). The risk of myocardial infarction after quitting smoking in men under 55 years of age. *New England Journal of Medicine*, **313**, 1511–14.

Rosenman, R.H., Brand, R.J., Jenkins, C.D., *et al.* (1975). Coronary heart disease in the Western Collaborative Group Study: final follow-up experience of 8.5 years. *Journal of the American Medical Association*, **233**, 872–7.

Ross, R. and Fuster, V. (1996). The pathogenesis of atherosclerosis. In *Atherosclerosis and coronary artery disease* (ed. V. Fuster, R. Ross, and E.J. Topol), pp. 441–62. Lippincott–Raven, Philadelphia, PA.

Ross, R. and Glomset, J.A. (1973). Atherosclerosis and the arterial smooth muscle cell: proliferation of smooth muscle is a key event in the genesis of the lesions of atherosclerosis. *Science*, **180**, 1332–9.

Rubin, E. (1979). Alcoholic myopathy in heart and skeletal muscle. *New England Journal of Medicine*, **301**, 28–33.

Rubin, S.M., Sidney, S., Black, D.M., Browner, W.S., Hulley, S.B., and Cummings, S.R. (1990). High blood cholesterol in elderly men and the excess risk for coronary heart disease. *Annals of Internal Medicine*, **113**, 916–20.

Rubins, H.B., Robins, S.J., Collins, D., *et al.* (1999). Gemfibrozil for the secondary prevention of coronary heart disease in men with low levels of high-density lipoprotein cholesterol. Veterans Affairs High-Density Lipoprotein Cholesterol Intervention Trial Study Group. *New England Journal of Medicine*, **341**, 410–18.

Sacks, F.M., Pfeffer, M.A., Moye, L.A., *et al.* (1996). The effect of pravastatin on coronary events after myocardial infarction in patients with average cholesterol levels. Cholesterol and Recurrent Events Trial Investigators. *New England Journal of Medicine*, **335**, 1001–9.

Samanck, M. (1994). Boy : girl ratio in children born with different forms of cardiac malformation: a population-based study. *Pediatric Cardiology*, **15**, 53–7.

Scandinavian Simvastatin Survival Study (1994). Randomized trial of cholesterol lowering in 4444 patients with coronary heart disease: the Scandinavian Simvastatin Survival Study (4S). *Lancet*, **344**, 1383–9.

Schaefer, E.J., Lamon-Fava, S., Jenner, J.L., *et al.* (1994). Lipoprotein(a) levels and risk of coronary heart disease in men. The Lipid Research Clinics Coronary Primary Prevention Trial. *Journal of the American Medical Association*, **271**, 999–1003.

Schnall, P.L., Pieper, C., Schwartz, J.E., *et al.* (1990). The relationship between 'job strain' workplace diastolic blood pressure, and left ventricular mass index. Results of a case-control study. *Journal of the American Medical Association*, **263**, 1929–35.

Schocken, D.D., Arrieta, M.I., Leaverton, P.E., and Ross, E.A. (1992). Prevalence and mortality rate of congestive heart failure in the United States. *Journal of the American College of Cardiology*, **20**, 301–6.

Shabeter, R. (1983). Cardiomyopathy: How far have we come in 25 years? How far yet to go? *Journal of the American College of Cardiology*, **1**, 252–63.

Shaw, L.W. (1981). Effects of a prescribed supervised exercise program on mortality and cardiovascular morbidity in patients after myocardial infarction. The National Exercise and Heart Disease Project. *American Journal of Cardiology*, **48**, 39–46.

Shekelle, R.B., Gale, M., Ostfeld, A.M., and Paul, O. (1983). Hostility, risk of coronary heart disease, and mortality. *Psychosomatic Medicine*, **45**, 109–14.

Shekelle, R.B., Hulley, S.B., Neaton, J.D., *et al.* (1985*a*). The MRFIT behavior pattern study. I. Type A behavior and incidence of coronary heart disease. *American Journal of Epidemiology*, **122**, 559–70.

Shekelle, R.B., Gale, M., and Norusis, M. (1985*b*). Type A score (Jenkins Activity Survey) and risk of recurrent coronary heart disease in the Aspirin Myocardial Infarction Study. *American Journal of Cardiology*, **56**, 221–5.

Shepherd, J., Cobbe, S.M., Ford, I., *et al.* for the West of Scotland Coronary Prevention Study Group (1995). Prevention of coronary heart disease with pravastatin in me with hypercholesterolemia. *New England Journal of Medicine*, **333**, 1301–7.

Sheps, S.G. (chair) (1997). Sixth report of the Joint National Committee on Prevention, Detection, Evaluation, and Treatment of High Blood Pressure. *Archives of Internal Medicine*, **157**, 2413–46.

Siegel, A.C., Johnson, E.E., and Stollerman, G.H. (1961). Controlled studies of streptococcal pharyngitis in a pediatric population: 1. factors related to the attack rate of rheumatic fever. *New England Journal of Medicine*, **265**, 559–66.

Singer, D.R., Markandu, N.D., Cappuccio, F.P., Miller, M.A., Sagnella, G.A., and MacGregor, G.A. (1995). Reduction of salt intake during converting enzyme inhibitor treatment compared with addition of a thiazide. *Hypertension*, **25**, 1042–4.

Siscovick, D.S., Weiss, N.S., Fletcher, R.H., and Lasky, T. (1984). The incidence of primary cardiac arrest during vigorous exercise. *New England Journal of Medicine*, **311**, 874–7.

Sjostrom, L.V. (1992). Mortality of severely obese subjects. *American Journal of Clinical Nutrition*, **55**, 516S–23S.

Solomon, C.G. and Manson, J.E. (1997). Obesity and mortality: a review of the epidemiologic data. *American Journal of Clinical Nutrition*, **66**, 1044S–50S.

SOLVD Investigators (1991). Effect of enalapril on survival in patients with reduced left ventricular ejection fractions and congestive heart failure. *New England Journal of Medicine*, **325**, 293–302.

SOLVD Investigators (1992). Effect of enalapril on mortality and the development of heart failure in asymptomatic patients with reduced left ventricle ejection fractions. *New England Journal of Medicine*, **327**, 685–91.

Sowers, J.R., Sowers, P.S., and Peuler, J.D. (1994). Role of insulin resistance and hyperinsulinemia in development of hypertension and atherosclerosis. *Journal of Laboratory and Clinical Medicine*, **123**, 647–52.

Stamler, R., Stamler, J., Lindberg, H.A., *et al.* (1979). Asymptomatic hyperglycemia and coronary heart disease in middle-aged men in two employed populations in Chicago. *Journal of Chronic Disorders*, **32**, 805–15.

Stamler, J., Wentworth, D., and Neaton, J.D. (1986). Is relationship between serum cholesterol and risk of premature death from coronary heart disease continuous and graded? Findings in 356 222 primary screenees of the Multiple Risk Factor Intervention Trial (MRFIT). *Journal of the American Medical Association*, **256**, 2823–8.

Stamler, R., Stamler, J., Grimm, R., *et al.* (1987). Nutritional therapy for high blood pressure. Final report of a four-year randomized controlled trial—The Hypertension Control Program. *Journal of the American Medical Association*, **257**, 1484–91.

Stamler, J., Vaccaro, O., Neaton, J.D., and Wentworth, D. (1993). Diabetes, other risk factors, and 12-year cardiovascular mortality for men screened in the Multiple Risk Factor Intervention Trial. *Diabetes Care*, **16**, 434–44.

Stampfer, M.J. and Rimm, E.B. (1995). Epidemiologic evidence for vitamin E in prevention of cardiovascular disease. *American Journal of Clinical Nutrition*, **62**, 1365S–9S.

Stampfer, M.J., Hennekens, C.H., Manson, J.E., Colditz, G.A., Rosner, B., and Willett, W.C. (1993). Vitamin E consumption and the risk of coronary disease in women. *New England Journal of Medicine*, **328**, 1444–9,

Stary, H.C., Chandler, A.B., Glagov, S., *et al.* (1994). A definition of initial, fatty streak and intermediate lesions of atherosclerosis. A report from the Committee on Vascular Lesions of the Council on Arteriosclerosis, American Heart Association. *Circulation*, **89**, 2462–78.

Stary, H.C., Chandler, A.B., Dinsmore, R.E., *et al.* (1995). A definition of advanced types of atherosclerotic lesions and a histological classification of atherosclerosis. A report from the Committee on Vascular Lesions of the Council on Arteriosclerosis, American Heart Association. *Arteriosclerosis, Thrombosis and Vascular Biology*, **15**, 1512–31.

Steenland, K., Thun, M., Lally, C., *et al.* (1996). Environmental tobacco smoke and coronary heart disease in the American Cancer Society CPS-II cohort. *Circulation*, **94**, 622–8.

Stone, E.J., Pearson, T.A., Fortmann, S.P., and McKinlay, J.B. (1997). Community-based prevention trials: challenges and directions for public health practice, policy, and research. *Annals of Epidemiology*, **S7**, S113–S120.

Suarez, L. and Barrett-Connor, E. (1984). Interaction between cigarette smoking and diabetes mellitus in the prediction of death attributed to cardiovascular disease. *American Journal of Epidemiology*, **120**, 670–5.

Sussman, S., Lichtman, K., Ritt, A., *et al.* (1999). Effects of thirty four adolescent tobacco use and prevention trials on regular users of tobacco products. *Substance Use and Misuse*, **34**, 1469–1503.

Svendsen, K.H., Kuller, L.H., Martin, M.J., and Ockene, J.K. (1987). Effects of passive smoking in the Multiple Risk Intervention Trial. *American Journal of Epidemiology*, **126**, 783–95.

Swedberg, K., Held, P., Kjekshus, J., Rasmussen, K., Ryden, L., and Wedel, H. (1992). Effects of the early administration of enalapril on mortality in patients with acute myocardial infarction. Results of the Cooperative New Scandanian Enalapril Survival Study II (Consensus II). *New England Journal of Medicine*, **327**, 678–84.

Trials of Hypertension Prevention Collaborative Research Group (1992). The effects of nonpharmacologic interventions on blood pressure of persons with high normal levels: results of the Trials of Hypertension Prevention, Phase I. *Journal of the American Medical Association*, **267**, 1213–20.

Trials of Hypertension Prevention Collaborative Research Group (1997). Effects of weight loss and sodium reduction intervention on blood pressure and hypertension incidence in overweight people with high-normal blood pressure: the Trials of Hypertension Prevention, phase II. *Archives of Internal Medicine*, **157**, 657–67.

Tunstall-Pedoe, H., Brown, C.A., Woodward, M., and Travendale, R. (1995). Passive smoking by self report and serum cotinine and the prevalence of respiratory and coronary heart disease in the Scottish Heart Health Study. *Journal of Epidemiology and Community Health*, **49**, 139–43.

Tunstall-Pedoe, H., Morrison, C., Woodward, M., Fitzpatrick, B., and Watt, G. (1996). Sex differences in myocardial infarction and coronary deaths in the Scottish MONICA population of Glasgow 1985 to 1991: presentation, diagnosis, treatment, and 28-day case fatality of 3991 events in men and 1551 events in women. *Circulation*, **93**, 1981–92.

Tunstall-Pedoe, H., Kuulasmaa, K., Mahonen, M., Tolonen, H., Ruokokoski, E., and Amouyel, P. (1999). Contribution of trends in survival and coronary-event rates to changes in coronary heart disease mortality: 10-year results from 37 WHO MONICA project populations: monitoring trends and determinants in cardiovascular disease. *Lancet*, **353**, 1547–57.

UGDP (University Group Diabetes Program) (1975). A study of the effects of hypoglycemic agents on vascular complications in patients with adult onset diabetes. V. Evaluation of phenoformin therapy. *Diabetes*, **24**, 65–184.

UKPDS (United Kingdom Prospective Diabetes Study) Group (1995). UKPDS 13: relative efficacy of randomly allocated diet, sulphonylurea, insulin, or metformin in patients with newly diagnosed non-insulin dependent diabetes followed for three years. *British Medical Journal*, **310**, 83–8.

USDHHS (United States Department of Health and Human Services) (1983). *The health consequences of smoking: cardiovascular disease: a report of the Surgeon General.* DHHS Publication No. PHS-84-50204. USDHHS, Public Health Service, Office of the Assistant Secretary for Health, Office on Smoking and Health, Washington, DC.

USDHHS (United States Department of Health and Human Services) (1990). *The health benefits of smoking cessation: a report of the Surgeon*

General. DHHS Publication No. CDC-90-8416. USDHHS, Centers for Disease Control, Center for Chronic Disease Prevention and Health Promotion, Office on Smoking and Health, Washington, DC.

USDHHS (United States Department of Health and Human Services) (1996). *Data fact sheet. Congestive Heart failure in the United States: a new epidemic.* USDHHS, Public Health Service, National Institutes of Health, National Heart, Lung, and Blood Institute, Washington, DC.

USDHHS (United States Department of Health and Human Services) (1997). *Changes in cigarette-related disease risks and their implication for prevention and control.* NIH Publication No. 97-4213. Monograph 8. USDHHS, Public Health Services, National Institutes of Health, National Cancer Institute, Washington, DC.

USDHHS (United States Department of Health and Human Services) (1998*a*). *Clinical guidelines on the identification, evaluation, and treatment of overweight and obesity in adults: the evidence report.* USDHHS, Public Health Service, National Institutes of Health, National Heart, Lung, and Blood Institute, Washington, DC.

USDHHS (United States Department of Health and Human Services) (1998*b*). *Targeting tobacco use: the nation's leading cause of death: at-a-glance.* Centers for Disease Control and Prevention, Washington, DC.

Van de Lisdonk, E.H., Van den Bosch, W.J.H.M., Huygen, F.J.A., and Lagro-Jansen, A.L.M. (1990). *Diseases in general practice* (in Dutch). Bunge, Utrecht, the Netherlands.

Virchow, R. (1856). Phlogose and thrombose in gefassystem. In *Gesammelte Abdhandlungen zur Wissenschaftlichen Medicin* (ed. R. Virchow), p. 458. Meidinger Sohn, Berlin.

Wallace, R.B. and Anderson, R.A. (1987). Blood lipids, lipid-related measures, and the risk of atherosclerotic cardiovascular disease. *Epidemiologic Reviews*, **9**, 95–119.

Wannamaker, L.W. (1973). The chain that links the heart to the throat. *Circulation*, **48**, 9–18.

Wassertheil-Smoller, S., Oberman, A., Blaufox, M.D., Davis, B., and Langford, H. (1992). The Trial of Antihypertensive Interventions and Management (TAIM) Study. Final results with regard to blood pressure, cardiovascular risk, and quality of life. *American Journal of Hypertension*, **5**, 37–44.

Watts, G.F., Lewis, B., Brunt, J.N., *et al.* (1992). Effects on coronary artery disease of lipid-lowering diet, or diet plus cholestyramine, in the St Thomas' Atherosclerosis Regression Study (STARS). *Lancet*, **339**, 563–9.

Webber, L.S., Cresanta, J.L., Croft, J.B., Srinivasan, S.R., Berenson, G.S. (1986). Transitions of cardiovascular risk from adolescence to young adulthood—the Bogalusa Heart Study: II. Alterations in anthropometric blood pressure and serum lipoprotein variables. *Journal of Chronic Diseases*, **39**, 91–103.

West, K.M. (1978). *Epidemiology of diabetes and its vascular lesions*, pp. 375–402. Elsevier, New York.

WHO (World Health Organization) (1982). *Prevention of coronary heart disease.* Technical Report Series, No. 678. Report of the WHO Expert Committee. WHO, Geneva.

WHO (World Health Organization) (1984*a*). *Cardiomyopathies.*Technical Report Series No. 697. Report of a WHO Expert Committee. WHO, Geneva.

WHO (World Health Organization) (1984*b*). *Intensified program: action to prevent rheumatic fever/rheumatic heart disease.* WHO, Geneva.

WHO (World Health Organization) (1988). *Rheumatic fever and rheumatic heart disease.* Technical Report Series No. 764. WHO, Geneva.

WHO (World Health Organization) (1995). *World health statistics annual.* WHO, Geneva.

WHO (World Health Organization) (1996). *World health statistics annual.* WHO, Geneva.

Wigle, E.D. (1988). Hypertrophic cardiomyopathy 1988. *Modern Concepts in Cardiovascular Disease*, **57**, 1–6.

Wilhelmsen, L., Sanne, H., Elmfeldt, D., Grimby, G., Tibblin, G., and Wedel H. (1975). A controlled trial of physical training after myocardial infarction. Effects on risk factors, nonfatal reinfarction, and death. *Preventive Medicine*, **4**, 491–8.

Williams, R.R., Hasstedt, S.J., Wilson, D.E., *et al.* (1986). Evidence that men with familial hypercholesterolemia can avoid early coronary death: an analysis of 77 gene carriers in four Utah pedigrees. *Journal of the American Medical Association*, **255**, 219–24.

Willich, S.N., Maclure, M., Mittleman, M., Arntz, H.R., and Muller, J.E. (1993). Sudden cardiac death. Support for a role of triggering in causation. *Circulation*, **87**, 1442–50.

Winocour, P.D. (1992). Platelet abnormalities in diabetes mellitus. *Diabetes*, **41**, 26–31.

Wissler, R.W. and Vesselinovitch, D. (1976). Studies of regression of advanced atherosclerosis in experimental animals and man. *Annals of the New York Academy of Sciences*, **275**, 363–78.

Wood, D., De Backer, G., Faergeman, O., Graham, I., Mancia, G., and Pyörälä, K. (1998*a*). Prevention of coronary heart disease in clinical practice. *European Heart Journal*, **19**, 1434–1503.

Wood, D., DeBacker, G., Faergeman, O., Graham, I., Mancia, G., and Pyörälä, K. (1998*b*). Prevention of coronary heart disease in clinical practice. Summary of recommendations of the Second Joint Task Force of European and other Societies on Coronary Prevention. *Journal of Hypertension*, **16**, 1407–14.

Yusuf, S., Thom, T., and Abbott, R.D. (1989). Changes in hypertension treatment and in congestive heart failure mortality in the United States. *Hypertension*, **13**, 174–9.

Zierler, S. (1985). Maternal drugs and congenital heart disease. *Obstetrics and Gynecology*, **65**, 155–65.

Zimmerman, M. and McGeachie, J. (1987). The effect of nicotine on aortic endothelium: a quantitative ultrastructural study. *Atherosclerosis*, **63**, 33–41.

9.2 Neoplasms

Paolo Boffetta, Paul Brennan, and Rodolfo Saracci

Neoplasms include a family of diseases, several hundreds of which can be distinguished in humans by localization, morphology, clinical behaviour, and response to therapy. Whether considered from a biological, clinical, or public health viewpoint, it is the malignant and invasive nature of many of these diseases which is of most importance.

Benign neoplasms represent localized growths of tissue with predominantly normal characteristics: in many cases they cause minor symptoms and are amenable to surgical therapy. Benign tumours, however, can become clinically very important when they occur in organs in which compression is possible and surgery cannot be easily performed (e.g. the brain), and when they produce hormones or other substances with a systemic effect (e.g. adrenaline produced by benign phaeochromocytoma). Relatively little is known about the distribution and causes of most benign neoplasms and, with the exception of benign brain neoplasms, they will not be discussed further in this chapter.

Malignant neoplasms are characterized by progressive growth of tissue with structural and functional differences with respect to the normal tissue. In many cases, the alterations can be so important that it becomes difficult to identify the tissue of origin. A peculiarity of most malignant tumours is the ability to migrate and colonize other organs (process of metastasization) via blood and lymph vessel penetration. The presence and extension of metastases are often the critical factors to determine the success of therapy and the survival of cancer patients.

The pace of growth of malignant neoplasms varies widely, and subclinical neoplasms are often found at autopsy of individuals who have died from other causes. It is assumed that for epithelial neoplasms, 10 or more years elapse between the beginning of the transformation process and the clinical diagnosis. For other types of neoplasms (e.g. sarcomas, lymphomas, leukaemias) this time might be shorter. The long process of carcinogenesis justifies the efforts to develop and apply screening approaches for early detection of subclinical neoplasms in healthy individuals.

At the molecular level, the process of malignant transformation is characterized by alterations in several genes that are responsible for the control of the replication cycle of the cell and other regulatory functions. Many oncogenic genes have been identified, and the distribution of their alterations varies among different neoplasms. However, neoplasms which are morphologically and clinically identical often include different genetic alterations, suggesting that the malignant transformation may result from the accumulation of genetic damage through different pathways.

Most malignant neoplasms arise from epithelial tissues and are defined as carcinomas or cancers. In practice, however, the terms 'malignant neoplasm', 'malignant tumour', and 'cancer' are used interchangeably. Neoplasms are classified according to the International Classification of Diseases—Oncology (WHO 1990) into topographical categories (according to the organ where the neoplasm arises) and morphological categories (according to the characteristics of the cells). More and more often, neoplasms are characterized at the clinical level according to phenotypic aspects (e.g. presence of receptors, production of proteins) and genetic alterations (e.g. mutation in a given gene).

Knowledge about the causes and the possible preventive strategies for malignant neoplasms has greatly advanced during the last century. This has been largely based on the development of cancer epidemiology, which has in turn benefited from the establishment of population-based cancer registries in many areas of the world (see below). In parallel to the identification of the causes of cancer, primary preventive strategies have been developed. Secondary preventive approaches have also been proposed and in some cases their effectiveness has been evaluated. A careful consideration of the achievements of cancer research, however, suggests that the advancements in knowledge about the causes of cancer have not been followed by an equally important reduction in the burden of cancer. Part of this paradox is explained by the long latency occurring between exposure to carcinogens and development of the clinical disease. Changes in exposure to risk factors are therefore not followed immediately by changes in disease occurrence. The main reason for the gap between knowledge and public health action, however, rests with the cultural, societal, and economic aspects of exposure to most carcinogens.

The identification of environmental and genetic determinants of cancer relies on two complementary approaches, the epidemiological and the experimental. The epidemiological approach has produced both general and specific evidence for the role of different types of agents in cancer causation. The evidence of a more general nature derives from the observations of considerable variation (often 10-fold to 100-fold) of the incidence rates of most cancers in different populations, defined according to geographical area. Table 1 reports the ratio of the 80th to the 20th percentile of the ranking of country-specific incidence rates of selected countries, as estimated by Ferlay *et al.* (1998). For all gender-specific rates, the ratio is above 2, and for several it is close to 10. This comparison is based on stable figures, but masks ever larger variations among very-high-risk and very-low-risk areas, which for many neoplasms may reach 100- or even 1000-fold differences. Variations are also shown within countries or according to other characteristics such as ethnic group, religion, or social class. For instance, when contrasted with other religious groups, the Mormons of Utah and the Seventh-Day Adventists of California exhibit low rates for cancers of the respiratory, gastrointestinal, and genital systems. This marked variation in rates according to different axes of exploration is unlikely to be explained chiefly by concomitant genetic variations, and indicates the role of environmental (including lifestyle) determinants.

In addition, the observation of changes of incidence in migrant groups after they have moved to a new living environment suggests a major role of non-genetic factors. Migrants are selected members of a population and they are likely to be in several aspects different from both their population of origin and from the population of the receiving countries. This demands caution when interpreting data from migrant studies, particularly when dealing with minor differences in rates. However, studies like those of Japanese migrants to Hawaii show an assimilation of their cancer incidence rates to the pattern of Caucasians, with the emergence of large differences with respect to the rates in Japan, which appears difficult to explain solely on the basis of selective factors.

Finally, changes in incidence rates in time, particularly when they take place over a few decades are incompatible with a genetic explanation, as changes in the genes of a population pool require much longer intervals. Recorded incidence rates are affected by diagnostic changes and mortality rates are, in addition, affected by changes in treatment effectiveness; however, marked trends like the one for lung cancer (Fig. 1) are most likely to reflect real changes in cancer rates, indicating the operation of environmental factors.

Specific evidence produced by analytical studies (case–control and cohort) has shown the causal role of specific exposures in the aetiology of several malignant neoplasms. One limitation of the epidemiological approach may prove of critical importance in trying to detect comparatively small increases in risk, for example from chemicals polluting the environment. This is that even in the best conditions it is impossible to identify confidently by epidemiological means an increase in risk smaller than perhaps 10 per cent (and serious problems arise in the interpretation of increases below 50 per cent) as the biases inherent in any observational study are of at least this order of magnitude.

Genetic determinants of cancer have also been demonstrated. As discussed below, several inherited conditions carry a very high risk of one or several cancers. High-penetrance genes are identified through

Table 1 Ratio of the 20th and 80th percentile in the ranking of country-specific estimated age-standardized incidence rates of selected cancers

Cancer	Men	Women
Oral cavity	2.8	2.4
Nasopharynx	4.6	7.0
Oesophagus	4.5	8.2
Stomach	3.7	3.0
Colon/rectum	4.9	5.2
Liver	6.3	3.9
Pancreas	4.3	4.3
Lung	8.4	6.4
Melanoma	7.0	8.6
Breast	–	2.7
Cervix	–	3.4
Corpus uteri	–	5.0
Ovary	–	2.2
Prostate	5.3	–
Bladder	3.3	3.1
Kidney	5.1	4.5
Nervous system	6.4	6.1
Non-Hodgkin's lymphoma	2.5	2.7
Leukaemia	2.5	2.7

Data from Ferlay *et al.* (1998).

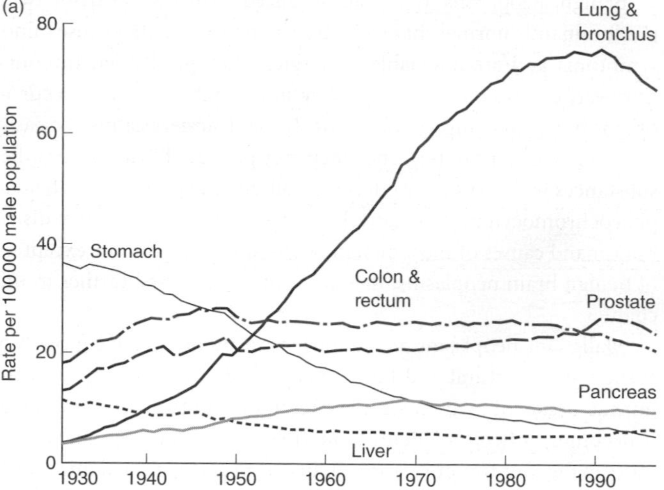

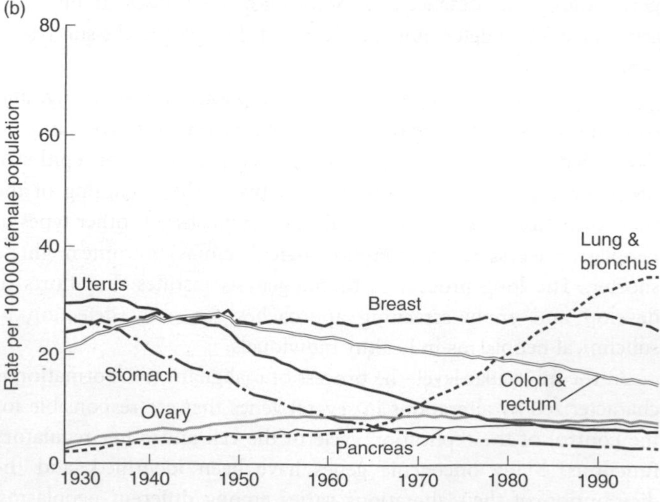

Fig. 1 (a) Age-adjusted cancer death rates, by site, in the United States, 1930 to 1996 for men. (b) Age-adjusted cancer death rates, by site, in the United States, 1930 to 1996 for women. The uterus cancer death rates are for the uterine cervix and uterine corpus combined. (Source: ACS 2000.)

family-based and other linkage studies. These conditions, however, are relatively rare and explain only a small proportion of human cancers. Genetic factors, however, are likely to play an important role in interacting with environmental exposure to determine individual cancer risk.

The experimental approach to identification of carcinogens includes at a more basic level the investigation of mechanisms of carcinogenesis. A result of general relevance has been the demonstration that chemical carcinogens are usually metabolized to reactive molecules with high affinity for electron-rich molecules, like DNA, with which they form combinations ('adducts') (Wild and Pisani 1997). These have been characterized in structure and properties, but the specific, critical lesions directly responsible for the carcinogen-induced malignant transformation have not yet been fully identified. However, there is growing evidence that the action of genotoxic carcinogens, possibly through DNA adduction, results in mutation in proto-oncogenes and tumour suppressor genes (Albertini and Hayes 1997). Not all carcinogens, however, act through DNA damage, and other well-established mechanisms involve non-genotoxic mechanisms, such as enhanced cellular proliferation.

The identification of carcinogens via the laboratory relies on three types of tests: (a) long-term (often lifetime) carcinogenicity tests in experimental animals, most commonly rodents (mice, rats, hamsters); (b) short-term tests assessing the effects of chemical agents on a variety of endpoints belonging to three general classes: DNA damage, mutagenicity, and chromosome damage; (c) mechanistic tests, aimed at identifying the intermediate steps in the compound-specific carcinogenic process.

These tests are valuable to the extent that such effects may reflect underlying events in the carcinogenic process. Indeed, consistent positivity in tests measuring DNA damage, mutagenicity, and chromosomal damage is usually regarded as indicating potential carcinogenicity of the tested agent. Results of laboratory tests constitute useful supporting evidence when adequate epidemiological data for the carcinogenicity of an environmental agent exist (e.g. vinyl chloride), but they become all the more essential when the epidemiological evidence is non-existent or inadequate in quality or in quantity. In the latter case, although no universally accepted criteria exist to translate data automatically from long-term animal tests or short-term tests in terms of cancer risk in humans, an evaluation of the risk can be made on a judgmental basis using all available scientific evidence. This policy has been applied by the International Agency for Research on Cancer (**IARC**) in a systematic programme of evaluation of the carcinogenic risk of chemicals to humans. Within this programme of IARC monographs, agents are classified into group 1 (established human carcinogen), 2A (probable human carcinogens), 2B (possible human carcinogens), and 3 (not classifiable as to carcinogenicity to humans) (IARC 1972–2001). Agents are commonly classified as group 1 when the evidence of their carcinogenicity in humans, derived from epidemiological studies, is considered sufficient, and as group 2A when the evidence in humans is limited and the agent is an experimental carcinogen. Agents in group 2B include mainly experimental carcinogens for which the human evidence is inadequate or non-existent. Between 1972 and 2001, 78 volumes presenting evaluations (and re-evaluations) for 869 chemical, physical and biological agents and groups of agents, as well as exposure circumstances such as occupations, have been published (IARC 1972–2001). A total of 87 agents have been classified as group 1, 63 as group 2A, and 235 as group 2B. The complete list of agents, with their evaluations can be found on the IARC web site (www.iarc.fr).

Principles of primary and secondary cancer prevention

Primary prevention

Many determinants of malignant neoplasms—including ultraviolet radiation, ionizing radiation, tobacco smoking, alcohol drinking, a number of viruses and parasites, and a number of chemicals, industrial processes, and occupational exposures—are sufficiently well established to constitute logical priorities for preventive action. Two more reasons add weight to this priority: some of the agents are responsible for sizeable proportions of the cancers occurring today, and for most agents it is in principle feasible to reduce or even to eliminate exposure completely. If this is taken as the objective of preventive action, some practical points are helpful in guiding such action.

Firstly, none of the data sets allowing a relatively accurate definition of dose (exposure)–response relationships for cancer in humans (such data are available for selected agents, such as tobacco smoking, radon, aflatoxin, and dioxin; Cardis *et al.* 1999) indicate divergence from linearity at low dose, i.e. in the portions of the curves which are of key interest when exposures can be controlled to low levels but, for whatever reason, cannot be completely avoided. From a practical viewpoint, therefore, in assessing the effect of reducing exposure to carcinogens, it is reasonable to build and use a linear dose–response relationship with no threshold.

Secondly, in this formulation, dose means total dose cumulated over time. This implicitly assumes that the carcinogenic effect is equally dependent on the dose rate (dose per unit of time) and on duration of exposure which, multiplied together, give total dose. However, both experimental and epidemiological data indicate that this is not the case. For lifelong exposures in regular smokers, for example, the incidence rate (of lung or bladder cancer in smokers) depends more strongly on duration of exposure, increasing with the fourth power of it, than on dose rate, increasing only with the first or second power of it (Peto 1977). Therefore, for exposures in adult life, and if other biological effects (e.g. genetic) can be excluded, it may be preferable if more people are exposed for shorter periods than fewer people for longer periods.

Furthermore, experimental and epidemiological investigations suggest that the carcinogenic process may be represented as a succession of stages, taking place in the time span from first exposure to a carcinogenic agent to the appearance of clinical cancer (Joint IARC/IPCS/CEC Working Group 1983). In its simplest form, as identified in mouse skin carcinogenesis experiments, the multistage process reduces to two stages: an irreversible 'initiation' stage inducing malignant cells, and a 'promotion' stage which propagates these cells into a malignant growth. A third stage of 'progression', characterized by an increased rate of growth and metastases, as well as an increase in chromosomal changes in the cell, has also been observed. Formal statistical multistage models of carcinogenesis have provided a useful framework to interpret on a common basis of (postulated) mechanism both experimental and epidemiological observations. As the stages are assumed to occur in a specific sequence, some may be described as 'early' and some as 'late'. Epidemiological observations indicate that, for example, smoking has both an early stage effect, as indicated by the existence of a minimum interval of several years before an increase in risk of lung cancer becomes manifest, and a late stage effect, as indicated by the decrease in risk (with respect to non-quitters) soon after stopping smoking. The identification of carcinogens acting mainly at early or late stages would have consequences on the preventive strategies to apply.

The attribution of causality to environmental agents (as done when, for instance, smoking was said to be the cause of some 30 per cent of all cancers; see below) is complicated by the interactive effects of several agents. This is particularly relevant when considering the relative effectiveness of removing (or reducing) exposure to one of two (or more) jointly-acting agents. To illustrate this point, Table 2 presents the results of a large cohort study in insulator workers in the United States and Canada (Hammond *et al.* 1979), classified according to their exposure to asbestos and to their smoking habits. Due to the multiplicative interaction of asbestos and smoking, the group exposed to both agents has the highest lung cancer rates, greatly in excess not only to those not exposed to either agent, but also to those exposed only to asbestos (the excess rate in the latter group is 47.1, while it is 590.3—that is 12.5 times higher—in the group exposed to both agents). Superficially it could be concluded that, since smoking is by far the dominant factor, its removal will correspondingly be far more effective as a preventive measure than asbestos removal. However, this is not true. In fact, if smoking is removed the fraction, or percentage, of the excess rate removed will be

$$[(590.3 - 47.1)/590.3] = 0.92,$$

and if asbestos is removed it will be

$$[(590.3 - 113.13)/590.3] = 0.81.$$

This means that smoking is more effective than asbestos removal, but only by a factor of 0.92/0.81 = 1.14, and not by a factor of 12.5. The result is not surprising if one considers that the bulk of the effect in subjects exposed to both agents is due to their positive interaction (synergism) and thus is removed whichever of the two agents is eliminated. In practical terms, whenever a positive interaction (synergism) occurs between two (or more) hazardous exposures, there is an enlarged possibility of preventive action; the effect of the joint exposure can be attacked in two (or more) ways, each requiring the removal or reduction of one of the exposures; moreover, the larger the size of the interaction relative to the total effect, the more these ways of attack tend to become equal in effectiveness.

It has been mentioned that a number of chemicals, groups of chemicals, and industrial processes have been found, when proper account has been taken of all evidence (laboratory and epidemiological), to be 'probably' carcinogenic for humans, and that a large number of other chemical agents have been demonstrated to be carcinogenic in animals, with no data available in humans ('possible' human carcinogens) (IARC 1999). However, these agents should be considered, for practical purposes, as if they entail a risk of cancer for humans and actions minimizing exposure taken accordingly.

Finally, reducing exposure to carcinogens can be implemented in two major ways: by elimination of the carcinogen or its substitution with a non-carcinogen, or by impeding by various means the contact between the carcinogen and people. Reduction of exposure depends in each case on technical and economic considerations. Generally, however, methods of exposure reduction that minimize the number of decisions involved are to be preferred; for instance, change to an innocuous material in preference to having each user exercise caution in using it.

Table 2 Mortality rate (per 100 000) from lung cancer among American insulator workers, according to exposure to asbestos and smoking

	Asbestos	
	Unexposed	**Exposed**
Smoking		
Unexposed	11.3	58.4
Exposed	122.6	601.6

Data from Hammond *et al.* (1979).

Secondary prevention

Given the limitations still constraining the primary prevention of many cancers, early detection needs to be considered as a secondary and alternative option, based on the reasonable expectation that the earlier the diagnosis and the stage at which a malignancy is discovered, the better the prognosis. This implies that an effective treatment for the disease exists and that the less advanced the cancer at the preclinical stage, the better the scope for treatment, and the better the prognosis. This latter aspect cannot be taken for granted. It is important to keep early detection separate from secondary prevention. The former aspect belongs to the domain of ordinary medical care, while the latter is conducted in asymptomatic populations through large-scale (mass screening) programmes.

Before a screening programme can be adopted on a large scale, a number of requirements need to be fulfilled in addition to the fundamental one (already mentioned) that an effective treatment for the preclinical malignant lesion must be available also on a sufficient scale. These requirements have been extensively discussed in publications specifically addressing the issue of evaluating screening programmes for cancer (Miller 1996).

Any screening test under consideration (i.e. a relatively simple and rapid test aimed at the presumptive identification of preclinical disease) must be capable of correctly identifying cases and non-cases. In other words, both sensitivity and specificity should be high, approaching 100 per cent. While high sensitivity is obviously important, given that the very purpose of screening is to pick up, if possible, all cases of a cancer in its detectable preclinical phase, it is specificity that plays a dominant role in the practical utilization of the test within a defined population, that is in a screening programme. As the prevalence of a preclinical cancer to be screened in well-defined populations is often in the range of 1 to 10 per 1000, if a test is used with a specificity of 95 per cent, then 5 per cent of results will be false-positives. In other words, for every case which will turn out at the diagnostic work-up to be a true cancer (assuming 100 per cent sensitivity), there will be between five and 50 cases falsely identified as such and ultimately found not to be cancers. This situation is likely to prove unacceptable due to too high psychological and economic costs. One solution is an increase in specificity, for example by developing better tests or combinations of tests, or by changing the criterion of positivity of a given test to make it more stringent (this necessarily decreases sensitivity). In addition, one might select populations with relatively high prevalence of the cancer ('high-risk' groups), so as to increase the number of the true positives. Whatever the group on which the programme operates, additional requirements are that the test is safe, easily and rapidly applicable, and broadly acceptable to the population to be examined (e.g. sigmoidoscopy may not be). It has also to be cheap, but what is or is not cheap is better evaluated within a cost-effectiveness analysis of different ways of preventing a cancer case or death, an issue not further discussed here.

If these requirements are met, still nothing is known about the possible net benefit in outcome deriving from the screening programme (in fact, screening test plus diagnostic work-up plus treatment, as applied in a given population). To evaluate benefit, several measures of outcome can be assessed. An early one, useful but not sufficient, is the distribution by stage of the detected cancer cases which, if the programme is ultimately to be beneficial, should be shifted to earlier, less invasive stages of the disease in comparison with the distribution of the cases discovered through ordinary medical care. A second measure of outcome is the survival of cases detected at screening compared with the survival of cases detected through ordinary medical care. This is a superficially attractive but usually equivocal criterion, to the extent that a screening may only advance the time of diagnosis (and therefore the apparent survival time), without postponing the time of death ('lead-time bias'). A final outcome (and the main test of the programme) is the site-specific cancer mortality in the screened population compared with the mortality in the unscreened population.

Correct unbiased comparison of this outcome, and thus unbiased measure of the effect of the screening programme, can only be made within the framework of a randomized controlled trial, in which two groups of subjects are randomly allocated to the screening programme and to no screening (i.e. receiving only the existing medical care system) or to two alternative screening programmes, for instance, entailing different tests or different intervals between periodical examinations. Unfortunately, largely due to pressures to adopt on a large scale screening programmes hoped to be effective, a situation has often arisen where withholding screening to a group has been regarded as unethical, thus preventing the conduct of a proper experiment. Very few randomized trials evaluating the effectiveness of screening programmes are available. Comparisons made through non-randomized experiments (which also are infrequent for the same reason), or through observational studies of what has happened following the introduction of a screening programme in a population, are liable to bias.

Four types of bias are peculiar to the assessment of screening programmes. Firstly, earlier detection only moves forward the time of a patient's diagnosis, without postponing the time of death (lead-time bias): should this be the case the result would only be a longer period of morbidity for the patient. Secondly, because of self-selection, people who elect to receive early detection may be different from those who do not: for instance, they may belong to better educated classes, be generally healthier and health conscious, and this could produce a longer survival independent of any effect of early detection. Thirdly, cancers with longer preclinical phases, which may mean less biological aggressiveness and better prognosis, are more likely to be intercepted by a programme of periodical screening than cancers with a short preclinical phase and a rapid aggressive clinical course (length bias). Finally, because of criteria of positivity adopted to maximize yield of early cases, a number of lesions which in fact would never become malignant growths are included as 'cases', thus falsely improve the survival statistics (overdiagnosis bias).

As observational studies, however, may represent the only source of information to evaluate screening programmes, they need to be carefully considered. Among purely observational situations, one which may provide particularly useful information is that arising when a relatively small, closed population (with no migration in or out) is saturated over a short interval (a few years) with the screening programme to be evaluated. If good ordinary diagnostic and treatment services are available before, during, and after the introduction of the screening, and the mortality rate from the cancer can be regarded as predictable, a clear change in mortality would represent good scientific evidence for effectiveness of the screening programme.

The global burden of neoplasms

The number of new cases of cancer which occurred worldwide in 2000 has been estimated at about 10 100 000 (Table 3) (Ferlay *et al.* 2001). Of these, 5400 000 occurred in men and 4700 000 in women. About 4700 000 cases occurred in developed countries (North America, Japan, Europe including Russia, Australia, and New Zealand) and 5400 000 in developing countries. Among men, lung, stomach, colorectal, prostate, and liver cancers are the most common malignant neoplasms (Fig. 2), while breast, colorectal, cervical, lung, and ovarian cancers are the most common neoplasms among women (Fig. 3).

The number of deaths from cancer was estimated at about 6200 000 in 2000 (Table 3) (Ferlay *et al.* 2001). No global estimates of survival from cancer are available: data from selected cancer registries suggest wide disparities between developed and developing countries for neoplasms with effective but expensive treatment, such as leukaemia, while the gap is narrow for neoplasms without an effective therapy, such as lung cancer (Kosary *et al.* 1995; Sankaranarayanan *et al.* 1998; Berrino *et al.* 1999) (Fig. 4). The overall 5-year survival of cases diagnosed during 1985 to 1989 in European Union countries was 41.0 per cent (Berrino *et al.* 1999).

One complementary approach in assessing the global burden of neoplasms is to estimate the loss in disability-adjusted life years (**DALYs**). This indicator weighs the years of life with disability and adds them to the years lost because of premature death. A recent estimate for 1990 resulted in about 70 000 000 DALYs lost worldwide

Table 3 Estimated number of new cases of cancer (incidence) and of cancer deaths (mortality) in 2000, by gender and geographical area

	Men	Women	Total
Incidence			
Developed countries	2 540 000	2 176 000	4 716 000
Developing countries	2 814 000	2 562 000	5 376 000
Total	5 354 000	4 738 000	10 092 000
Mortality			
Developed countries	1 488 000	1 158 000	2 646 000
Developing countries	2 034 000	1 529 000	3 563 000
Total	3 522 000	2 687 000	6 209 000

Data from Ferlay *et al.* (2001).

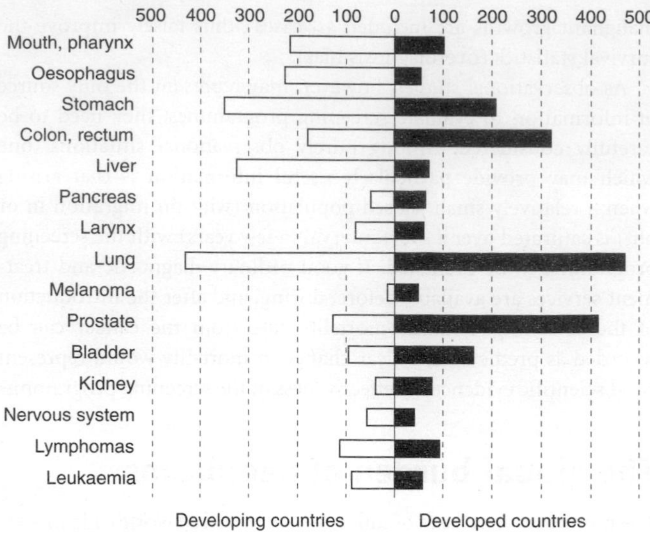

Fig. 2 Estimated number of new cancer cases (× 1000) during 2000 in men. (Source: Ferlay *et al.* 2001.)

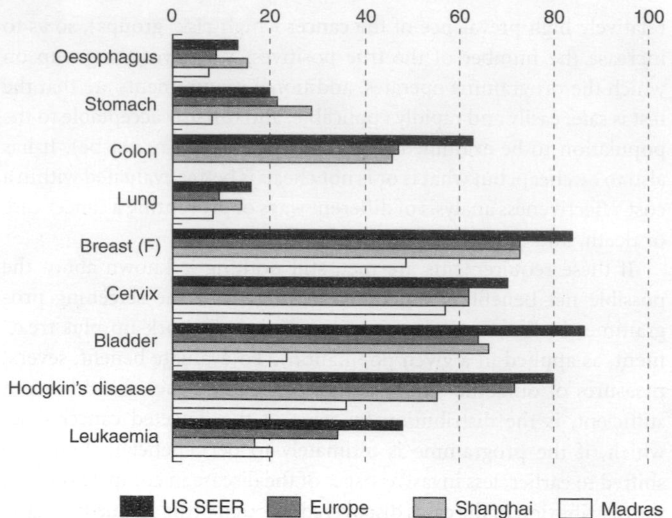

Fig. 4 Five-year relative survival from cancer in selected populations.

because of malignant neoplasms, of which 48 000 000 occurred in developing countries and 22 000 000 occurred in developed countries. Lung cancer was responsible for 8 900 000 DALYs, stomach cancer for 7 700 000, liver cancer for 6 600 000, leukaemia for 4 600 000, and breast cancer for 4 200 000 (Murray and Lopez 1996).

Distribution, causes, and prevention of individual neoplasms

This section includes a systematic review of the descriptive epidemiology of the most important malignant neoplasms. It also includes an overview of the current state of knowledge about the risk factors and the strategies for primary and secondary prevention. A global approach is used which excludes important local aspects of the descriptive epidemiology, aetiology, and prevention of neoplasms. For a more detailed review, the reader is referred to a textbook of cancer epidemiology and prevention edited by Schottenfeld and Fraumeni (1996). All incidence and mortality rates are standardized to the world population.

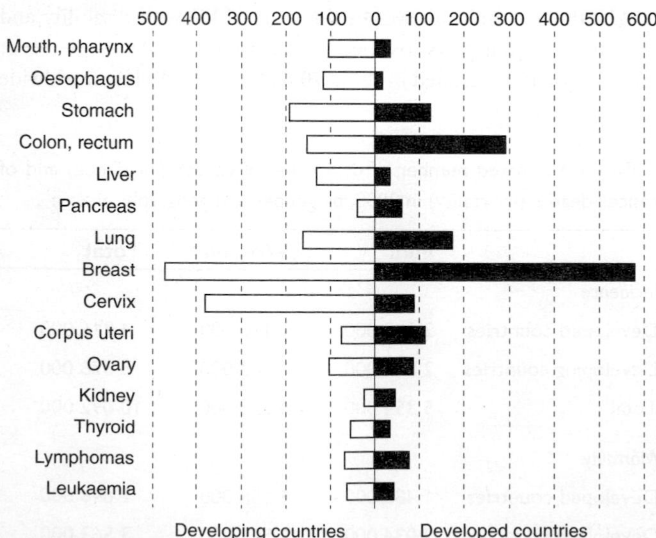

Fig. 3 Estimated number of new cancer cases (× 1000) during 2000 in women. (Source: Ferlay *et al.* 2001.)

Cancer of the oral cavity and pharynx

Tumours of the oral cavity and the pharynx comprise a broad group of different malignant neoplasms. Cancers of the oral cavity, oropharynx (including the tonsil), and hypopharynx are usually considered as a group, because of shared descriptive characteristics and risk factors, while neoplasms arising from the lip, nasopharynx, and salivary glands are treated separately, because of differences in aetiological factors.

An estimated 454 000 new cases of cancers of the oral cavity and pharynx occurred worldwide in 2000, 70 per cent of which were in developing countries (Ferlay *et al.* 2001). The estimated number of deaths is 244 000 (187 000 in developing countries) (Ferlay *et al.* 2001).

Oral cavity, oropharynx, and hypopharynx (Blot *et al.* 1996)

The incidence of cancers of the oral cavity and pharynx varies over 20-fold between high-risk areas (e.g. France, Switzerland, Italy, Spain, India, African-Americans) and low-risk areas (e.g. China, Nordic countries, the United Kingdom). The highest rates in the world among men are recorded in France, those in women are from India. In all populations, rates in men exceed those in women by a factor of 4 to 10. This cancer is very rare before the age of 30 years; above that age, the rate increases logarithmically up to about 60 years of age, after which the rate of increase declines. Incidence rates have increased in Europe and the Americas during the last decades (Coleman *et al.* 1993). When looking at subsites within the oral cavity and the pharynx, cancer of the oropharynx and hypopharynx account for as many or more cases than cancer of the oral cavity in high-risk European populations, while cancers of the tongue, floor of the mouth, and other parts of the oral cavity represent the majority of cases in India and the United States.

Consumption of tobacco smoke is the most important risk factor for cancer of the oral cavity and pharynx (Blot *et al.* 1996). In Western populations, smoking represents the main use of tobacco, and relative risks of oral cancer among smokers, as compared with non-smokers, are of the order of 3 to 10. The risk is higher for heavy smokers, long-term smokers, and smokers of black tobacco or high-tar cigarettes. Cigar and pipe smoking also poses a risk, while stopping smoking is followed by a decrease in risk. In India, chewing of products containing tobacco is the main risk factor for oral cancer, although smoking of cigarettes and 'bidis' (consisting of 0.3 g of tobacco hand-rolled in a dried *tembuzni* leaf) also contribute to the risk. In the United States and Europe, use of tobacco snuff has also been implicated in the genesis of oral cancer.

Consumption of alcoholic beverages increases the risk of oral and pharyngeal cancer (Blot *et al.* 1996). Relative to abstainers and very light drinkers, the risk in heavy drinkers is of the order of 10. While it is clear that all types of alcoholic beverages increase the risk, it is unclear whether there is a quantitative difference in their carcinogenic effect. There is convincing evidence that the effects of tobacco smoking and alcohol drinking are multiplicative, i.e. that the effect of exposure to both is close to the product of their individual effects (Fig. 5). The combined effect of tobacco smoking and alcohol drinking accounts for almost 80 per cent of cancers of the oral cavity and pharynx in Western populations. Similarly, tobacco chewing and smoking and their combination are responsible for a large proportion of these cancers in India.

A diet rich in fruits and vegetables protects from developing cancer of the oral cavity and pharynx in several populations (WCRF 1997). This effect seems to be independent of the effect of tobacco and alcohol. Among the micronutrients that might be implicated in the protective effects exerted by fresh fruits and vegetables are vitamins A, C, E, and B_{12}. A role of β-carotene has been suggested in chemopreventive trials of preneoplastic lesions but not confirmed in trials with clinical cancer as outcome. The role of other dietary factors is unclear, although high consumption of maté, a herbal tea consumed in South America, might also represent a risk factor.

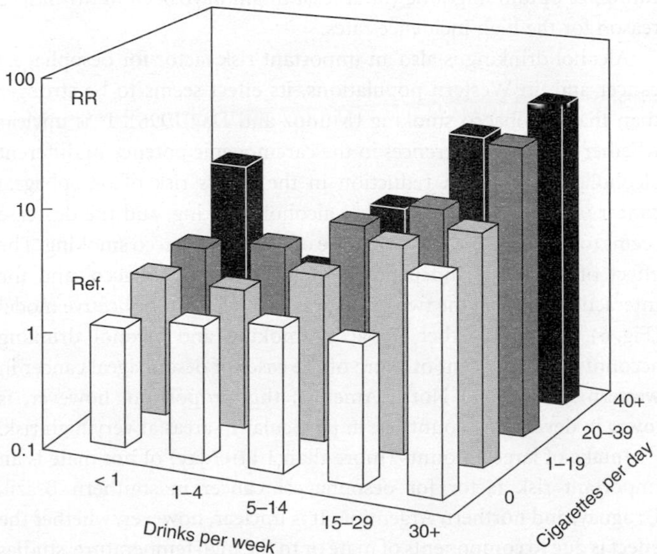

Fig. 5 Risk of oral cancer, tobacco smoking, and alcohol drinking. (Source: Blot *et al.* 1988.)

Human papilloma virus DNA has been frequently detected in preneoplastic and neoplastic lesions of the oral cavity; however, its aetiological role has not yet been fully established (IARC 1995). Other viruses are suspected of playing a role in oral carcinogenesis, including herpes simplex 1 and Epstein–Barr viruses (Blot *et al.* 1996).

Poor oral hygiene and ill-fitting dentures are likely to represent additional risk factors for oral cancer. The use of mouthwash with high alcohol content has also been associated with oral cancer. Several occupations have been sporadically reported to entail an increased risk of oral and pharyngeal cancer. The evidence is somewhat consistent only for employment as a waiter and bartender, probably reflecting an increased consumption of alcohol and tobacco, and for exposure to asbestos.

The role of genetic susceptibility in oral carcinogenesis is probably modest. High-risk families have been reported only occasionally. A role is, however, likely for low-penetrance factors, such as increased sensitivity to mutagens and polymorphism of enzymes implicated in the metabolism of alcohol (alcohol dehydrogenase and aldehyde dehydrogenase).

Lip

The descriptive epidemiology of lip cancer is complicated by misclassification with lesions from adjacent areas of the skin and oral mucosa. This neoplasm is rare in most populations and occurs mainly in the lower lip. The main known causes are solar radiation, smoking of cigarettes, cigars and pipes, and exposure to polycyclic aromatic hydrocarbons. Fishermen and farmers are at increased risk. Infection with herpes simplex virus 1 might also play a role (Blot *et al.* 1996).

Nasopharynx (Yu and Henderson 1996)

The geographical distribution of cancer of the nasopharynx shows high-risk areas in southern China, Southeast Asia, northern Africa, and the Arctic region. Migrant populations from these regions are also at increased risk. It is a rare neoplasm in most Western populations. The male to female ratio is of the order of 2 to 3. In China, the rates are highest in the 45- to 54-year age group, while in low-risk populations a peak is suggested around the age of 20 years.

Infection with Epstein–Barr virus is causally associated with the development of nasopharyngeal carcinoma, although cofactors, which have not been fully understood, are necessary to the virus to exert its action.

Consumption of Chinese-style salted fish, in particular in childhood, has been associated with increased risk of nasopharyngeal cancer, in particular among Cantonese populations from Guangzhou, Hong Kong, and the United States, but also in non-Cantonese populations from southern China and Taiwan. Consumption of other types of salted fish might represent a risk factor in Southeast Asia and the Arctic. Other preserved foods used as weaning food in different areas of China have also been associated to nasopharyngeal cancer: chung choi (a salted root), salted shrimp paste, salted eggs, and preserved fruits. The high rates in northern Africa might be due to consumption of dried mutton, touklia (a spiced mixture of peppers), or harissa (a hot sauce). It is unclear whether the carcinogenic agents in Chinese-style salted fish and other preserved foods are nitrosamines, bacterial mutagens, or other genotoxic substances. Low intake of fresh fruits and vegetables has also been associated with increased risk of nasopharyngeal cancer: in high-risk populations, however, low fruit and vegetable intake is often closely associated with high intake of preserved food, making it difficult to separate the effect of the two factors.

Additional suspected risk factors for nasopharyngeal cancer are occupational exposure to formaldehyde and wood dust, and drinking water rich in nickel, while studies on exposure to fumes and smoke from burning of organic matter, on consumption of Chinese herbal beverages, and on the use of Chinese nasal oil are inconclusive. A moderate association (relative risks of the order of 3 to 5) with tobacco smoking has been detected in several populations. Chronic inflammatory conditions of the ear, nose, and sinuses might act as predisposing factors. Familial aggregation of nasopharyngeal cancer has been shown in China and other high-risk areas: the possible contribution of shared dietary and environmental factors, however, has not been excluded. In addition, there is evidence that certain HLA genotypes increase the risk of this neoplasm. The role of genetic polymorphism to metabolic enzymes is not clear.

Salivary glands

Geographical and temporal comparisons of tumours of the salivary glands are complicated by the inclusion of neoplasms with benign or intermediate clinical behaviour in the series of cases. Incidence rates, however, tend to be low, with high rates (of the order of 2 per 100 000) in Alaska and northern Canada. Men experience higher rates than women, but the ratio rarely exceeds 2. Apart from a role of ionizing radiation, the causes of cancer of the salivary glands are largely unknown: among the suspected causes are low vitamin A intake, hormonal or occupational factors, and infection with Epstein–Barr virus. Tobacco smoking does not seem to play a role (Blot *et al.* 1996).

Prevention

Avoidance of tobacco smoking, chewing, and snuffing and avoidance of excessive alcohol drinking would represent the main preventive measures for cancer of the oral cavity and pharynx. Additional benefits might be obtained from increase in fruit and vegetable intake and improvement of oral hygiene. Avoidance of excessive exposure to solar radiation would represent the main preventive approach for lip cancer. In populations at high risk of nasopharyngeal cancer from China and possibly other countries, avoidance of salted fish and other preserved food, in particular as weaning food, should be recommended.

Oral inspection aimed to identify preneoplastic lesions might be an effective approach for secondary prevention of oral cancer. The inspection can be performed by medically certified professionals, but also, in particular in high-risk areas from developing countries such as India, by specifically trained health workers. Large-scale preventive trials are on-going, that should provide evidence in favour or against this approach (Sankaranarayanan *et al.* 2000).

Cancer of the oesophagus (Muñoz and Day 1996)

There are two main histological types of oesophageal cancer: squamous cell carcinoma and adenocarcinoma. The former occurs mainly in the upper and middle third of the organ, while adenocarcinoma occurs in the lower third. Squamous cell carcinoma is the predominant type in most human populations, in particular in populations at very high risk. In this section, oesophageal cancer is discussed as a whole, although most data refer to squamous cell carcinoma. Peculiar aspects of adenocarcinoma are discussed in below.

The geographical distribution of oesophageal cancer is characterized by very wide variations within relatively small areas. Very high rates (over 50 per 100 000) are recorded in both genders from northern Iran and the provinces of eastern China, Shanxi, Henan, and Jiangsu, in certain areas of Kazakhstan and among men from Zimbabwe. Intermediate rates in men (10 to 50 per 100 000) occur in eastern Africa, southern Brazil, the Caribbean, most of China (with the exception of southern provinces, such as Yunnan, Guizhou, Hunan, and Guangxi), regions of central Asia, northern India, southern Europe, as well as in black Americans. Ethnic factors are suggested by the facts that populations at higher risk in central Asia are of Turkish or Mongolian origin, but not of Caucasian origin, and that black Americans experience in both genders two- to threefold higher rates than white people. In men, rates are two- to 10-fold higher than in women. In many high-risk areas, a decrease in the incidence of oesophageal cancer has occurred during recent decades. The opposite pattern has been shown in low-risk populatons, such as northern Europeans and white people in the United States. In the latter country, the increase was mainly accounted for by an increase of adenocarcinoma of the lower oesophagus (see below), while the incidence of squamous cell carcinoma remained stable.

Tobacco smoking is an important risk factor for oesophageal cancer (Muñoz and Day 1996). The risk in heavy smokers, relative to non-smokers, is of the order of 4 to 8. A linear dose–response relationship has been shown for the duration of smoking and average consumption. Quitting smoking substantially reduces the excess risk. Smoking of black tobacco, high-tar, and hand-rolled cigarettes, as well as of pipe smoking, might exert a stronger effect that smoking of other products. Chewing of tobacco-containing products represents an important risk factor in India and southern Africa, but its role has not been confirmed in central Asia. In the latter region, use (smoking and eating) of opium might be (or at least might have been in the past) a reason for the high incidence rates.

Alcohol drinking is also an important risk factor for oesophageal cancer and, in Western populations, its effect seems to be stronger than that of tobacco smoking (Muñoz and Day 1996). It is unclear whether there are differences in the carcinogenic potency of different alcoholic beverages. A reduction in the excess risk of oesophageal cancer is suggested after quitting alcohol drinking, and the decrease seems to be stronger than in the case of quitting tobacco smoking. The effect of alcohol is independent of the effect of tobacco, and the interaction between the two exposures fits well a multiplicative model (Fig. 6). Taken together, tobacco smoking and alcohol drinking account for 90 per cent or more of the cases of oesophageal cancer in western Europe and North America: this proportion, however, is lower in developing countries, in particular in areas at very high risk.

Intake of large amounts (more than 1 litre/day) of hot maté is an important risk factor for oesophageal cancer in southern Brazil, Uruguay, and northern Argentina. It is unclear, however, whether the effect is due to components of maté or to the high temperature: studies from other areas suggest that intake of hot beverages (e.g. hot tea in Iran, Singapore, and Japan, hot coffee in Puerto Rico, and hot drinks or soups in Hong Kong) increases the risk of oesophagitis and

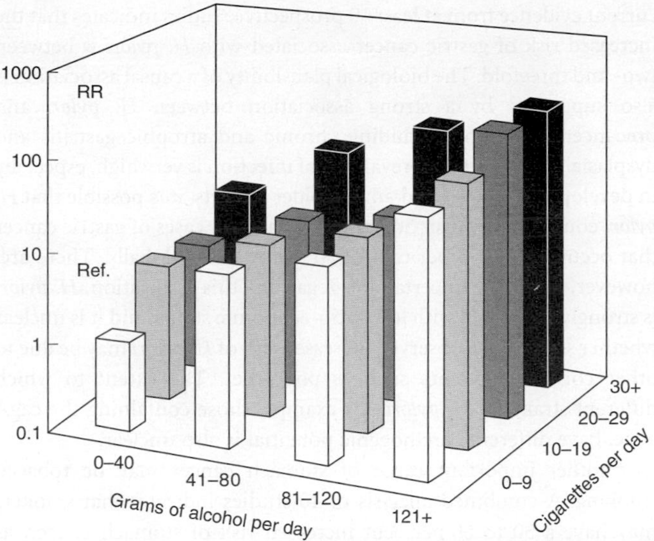

Fig. 6 Risk of oesophageal cancer, tobacco smoking, and alcohol drinking. (Source: Tuyns *et al.* 1977.)

oesophageal cancer, although the evidence is less consistent than in the case of maté.

Dietary factors are likely to play an important role in the aetiology of oesophageal cancer. Reduced intake of fresh fruits and vegetables represents a risk factor. A similar effect has been suggested for low intake of fresh or frozen meat or fish, for low intake of dairy products, and for high intake of barbecued meat. The available data do not allow the full establishment of the potentially preventive role of specific micronutrients from fruits and vegetables, and the results of chemopreventive trials with retinol, riboflavin, vitamin E, zinc, and selenium have failed to show a clear benefit.

In several areas of China, intake of pickled vegetables has been associated with an increased risk of oesophageal cancer. The active carcinogens might be mycotoxins or *N*-nitroso compounds. Mycotoxins, including fumonosin B_1, have also been detected in mouldy corn from high-risk areas in China and southern Africa. In addition, in Japan, eating of bracken fern has been associated with an elevated oesophageal cancer risk. The elucidation of dietary factors implicated in oesophageal carcinogenesis, in particular of the possible role of mycotoxins and *N*-nitroso compounds (including endogenously formed nitrosamines), would represent an important step in the understanding and prevention of this disease.

Among the other environmental agents suspected to cause oesophageal cancer are infection by human papilloma virus, occupational exposure to asbestos, silica, and combustion fumes, and ionizing radiation.

In addition to Barrett's oesophagus (see below), other chronic conditions increase the risk of developing oesophageal cancer. Patients suffering from Plummer–Vinson syndrome, a sideropenic dysphagia due to deficit of iron, riboflavin, and other vitamins, had an increased incidence of oesophageal and hypopharyngeal cancers. Oesophageal cancer risk is also increased among coeliac disease patients, possibly because of nutritional deficiencies.

A familial aggregation of oesophageal cancer has been occasionally shown, with joint segregation of a gene responsible for keratosis palmaris et plantaris (tylosis). Studies of families without the tylosis gene have not provided conclusive evidence of an important role of other high-penetrance genetic susceptibility factors in oesophageal cancer. However, low-penetrance genes, including those encoding for enzymes involved in the metabolism of tobacco and alcohol, may play a role in individual susceptibility to this neoplasm.

Adenocarcinoma

Adenocarcinoma mainly occurs in the lower third of the oesophagus. Its incidence is higher in Western countries, in white people, and in high social class individuals and has sharply increased in the last decades in most Western countries. In countries such as Scotland, it represents the main type of oesophageal cancer. Barrett's oesophagus, a columnar metaplasia of the epithelium, is strongly associated with subsequent development of adenocarcinoma. The main risk factor for Barrett's oesophagus and oesophageal adenocarcinoma is persistent reflux oesophagitis. The associations between adenocarcinoma of the oesophagus and tobacco smoking and alcohol drinking are weak. A protective role of high intake of fruits and vegetables and low intake of salty food has been suggested (Muñoz and Day 1996).

Prevention

Control of tobacco smoking and elevated alcohol drinking remains the main preventive approach in reducing the burden of squamous cell oesophageal cancer in Western populations. Improved diet, in particular increase in consumption of fresh fruits and vegetables, is likely to represent an additional important preventive step. The incomplete understanding of the role of opium derivates, mycotoxins, and other factors complicates the elaboration of preventive strategies in many high-risk regions, although decrease in intake and temperature of maté might be important in South America.

Chemoprevention with micronutrients might represent an additional strategy, although the results of the early trials do not strongly suggest any candidate for population-based actions.

Secondary prevention has been attempted in high-risk areas through endoscopy: also in this case, however, the available evidence does not justify activities at the population level.

Cancer of the stomach

Stomach cancer was the third most frequent cancer worldwide in 2000, accounting for approximately 876 000 new cases or 9 per cent of the global cancer burden (Ferlay *et al.* 2001). High incidence areas, with rates above 25 per 100 000 in men and 15 per 100 000 in women, are found in central and eastern Europe, Portugal, eastern Asia, and parts of South America. The highest observed rates are found in Japan with an incidence rate in 1990 of 78 per 100 000 in men and 33 per 100 000 in women. Low-incidence areas include eastern and northern Africa, North America, and south and Southeast Asia. The rates are approximately twice as high among men as among women and are also two to three times higher among groups with low socio-economic status. Stomach cancer is very rare before the age of 30 years, after which an exponential increase is observed with increasing age.

It has been shown that migrants tend to maintain the high risk of their home country; their offspring tend to acquire a risk closer to their host country. However, the most striking feature of the epidemiology of stomach cancer is the dramatic decline in its incidence which has been observed in most countries over the past 60 years. The decline is apparent for both sexes, although it appears to have occurred earlier in countries which currently have a low risk. This continuous dramatic decline, as well as the results from migrant studies, suggest a strong environmental influence on the disease which is generally believed to be dietary.

Diets high in fruits and vegetables have been consistently shown to have a protective effect against stomach cancer. This evidence appears to be particularly consistent for raw vegetables, citrus fruits, and possibly allium vegetables (onions, leeks, garlic, and so on), with decreased risks of approximately 50 per cent generally being reported. For salted and pickled vegetables, some increased risks have been observed, although the evidence is not conclusive.

Several studies have also examined specific dietary vitamins and minerals. Results from two cohort studies and six of eight case–control studies have shown that consumption of foods with high levels of carotenoid intake are associated with a decreased risk of stomach cancer. Four studies of serum carotenoid levels have also shown a decreased risk with higher levels. Similar consistent results of a decreased risk have also been observed for high vitamin C intake in a number of studies. However, while these may represent real associations it is also possible that carotenoids and vitamin C are simply markers for some other dietary constituent. Results for other dietary vitamins, including vitamin E and retinol, indicate no association. Four intervention trials have also been conducted involving nutrient supplements and stomach cancer. In one of these trials, which was conducted in a Chinese population known to be micronutrient deficient, a combination supplement of β-carotene, vitamin E, and selenium did result in a small (16 per cent) reduced risk of stomach cancer (Blot 1997).

Regarding beverages, no evidence has been found that black tea, coffee, or alcohol influence the risk of stomach cancer. Interestingly, a number of studies of green tea in Japan and China have suggested a protective effect with high levels of consumption. Such an association is biologically plausible, as polyphenol extracts of tea, especially of green tea, are known to have an anticarcinogenic effect in animals.

Worldwide there is a strong and consistent correlation with stomach cancer incidence and high consumption of salt and salted foods. A large number of studies that have examined this relationship have generally found a moderately increased risk of approximately twofold for frequent consumption of salt and salted foods. The relationship is also biologically plausible given that salt may lead to damage of the protective mucosal layer of the stomach. Other methods of food preservation, including curing and smoking foods, have also been found to be weakly associated with stomach cancer, although the evidence is not consistent.

Salting as well as other methods of food preparation, including smoking, curing, and pickling, have become far less common with the advent of refrigeration, both in the home and for industrial storage purposes. The advent in refrigeration has dramatically changed dietary habits in many parts of the world by also ensuring that fresh fruits and vegetables are available for much of the year. While it is not therefore possible to know which dietary agent or agents, if any, are directly responsible for the large decrease in stomach cancer incidence over the last 60 years, it is possible that this has been brought about by a fortuitous side-effect of the invention of refrigeration.

There is now strong evidence that some cases of stomach cancer are caused by infection with the *Helicobacter pylori* bacterium. The current evidence from at least 10 prospective studies indicates that the increased risk of gastric cancer associated with *H. pylori* is between two- and threefold. The biological plausibility of a causal association is also supported by a strong association between *H. pylori* and precancerous lesions, including chronic and atrophic gastritis and dysplasia. Given that the prevalence of infection is very high, especially in developing counties and among older cohorts, it is possible that *H. pylori* could explain over 50 per cent of all new cases of gastric cancer that occur, or over 5 per cent of all cancer cases globally. There are, however, still some uncertainties regarding this association. *H. pylori* is strongly associated with low socio-economic status, and it is unclear whether some of the observed increased risk of *H. pylori* may be due to other correlated factors such as poor diet. The extent to which different strains of *H. pylori*, for example those containing the cagA gene, have different carcinogenic potential is also unclear.

Another important cause of stomach cancer may be tobacco smoking. A combined analysis of 40 studies indicates that smokers may have a 50 to 60 per cent increased risk of stomach cancer, as compared with non-smokers. If this relationship is a truly causal one it would indicate that smoking is responsible for approximately 10 per cent of all cases, or 80 000 cases of stomach cancer annually worldwide.

Primary prevention of stomach cancer by dietary means is feasible by encouraging high-risk populations to increase consumption of fresh fruit and vegetables and decrease consumption of cured meats and salt preserved foods. Prevention may also be feasible through eradication of *H. pylori* infection. *H. pylori* vaccines, which protect against infection but also induce regression of current infection and associated lesions, have been developed in animal models, although a safe and effective vaccine for human populations requires further research. The sequencing of the genome for *H. pylori* is likely to speed up this process. Screening and early detection of stomach cancer have been developed in Japan with the use of X-ray photofluorography to identify possible early lesions, followed by gastroscopy. Screen-detected cases are more likely to be early stage localized disease and are likely to have a greater survival than other cases. The use of gastroscopy for screening and early detection may not, however, be cost-effective in populations outside high-incidence areas.

Cancer of the intestine

Cancer of the intestine is an important human neoplasm, in particular in developed countries. Most cancers of the intestine occur in the large intestine, while cancer of the small intestine is rare in most populations. Of colorectal cancers, approximately two-thirds originate from the colon and one-third from the rectum and the rectosigmoid junction. More than half of the cancers of the colon are located in the sigma and the caecum. Most cancers of the intestine are of adenocarcinoma type, i.e. originate from the glandular cells. Other histological types include carcinoids, sarcomas, and lymphomas.

When taken together, cancers of the colon and rectum accounted in 2000 for an estimated 940 000 new cases and 490 000 deaths worldwide (Ferlay *et al.* 2001). They represent the fourth most frequent malignant disease in terms of incidence and the third for mortality.

Small intestine (Schottenfeld and Islam 1996)

Age-standardized incidence rates of small intestinal cancer are in most populations below one case per 100 000 people in both genders. The highest rates (of the order of 2 per 100 000) are registered among black Americans and the Maori of New Zealand. The neoplasm is more common in men than in women, with a ratio of the order of 1.5 to 3. Its occurrence is correlated with the incidence of colon cancer but not stomach cancer.

Adenocarcinomas account for approximately 50 per cent of neoplasms of the small intestine. They originate mainly in the duodenum and proximal jejunum and are preceded by formation of adenoma. Various hereditary syndromes, such as familial adenomatous polyposis and Peutz–Jeghers syndrome, are characterized by multiple hamartomatous adenomas of the small intestine and, to a less extent, of the colon: these patients carry an increased risk of adenocarcinoma of the small intestine. Similarly, patients with Crohn's disease have a 10-fold increased risk of small intestine adenocarcinoma.

Malignant lymphomas represent about one-quarter of neoplasms of the small intestine: they are mainly of diffuse histiocytic type. Patients with AIDS and coeliac sprue are at increased risk of small cell lymphomas. Carcinoid tumours, which originate from the entero-endocrine (argentaffin) cells, are another important histological type. Limited data are available on the risk factors for this type of neoplasm.

The evidence of a role for environmental factors, such as tobacco smoking and diet, in the genesis of small intestinal neoplasms is at present inconclusive.

Colon (Schottenfeld and Winawer 1996)

The highest rates of colon cancer (around or above 30 per 100 000 in men and 25 per 100 000 in women) are recorded in Oceania (the islands of the Pacific Ocean and neighbouring seas), the United States (in particular among black people), and western Europe. Rates in developing countries are lower (5 to 15 per 100 000). The disease is rare before the age of 45 years, after which the incidence increases exponentially with age. In most populations, rates are higher in men than in women, with a ratio of the order of 1.5; however, given the predominance of women at older ages, the number of cases is similar in the two genders. A small increase in the incidence of colon cancer has been observed during the last decades in most populations, but not in North America, where rates have been stable.

Studies of migrant populations have repeatedly shown that the risk of colon cancer approaches that of the country of adoption within 20 years of residence; the incidence is higher in urban than in rural populations.

The predominant histological type of malignant neoplasms of the colon is the adenocarcinoma. This neoplasm is usually preceded by a polyp, or adenoma, less frequently by a small area of flat mucosa exhibiting various grades of dysplasia. The malignant potential of an adenoma is increased by a surface diameter greater than 1 cm, by villous (rather than tubular) organization, and by severe cellular dysplasia. Carriers of one adenoma larger than 1 cm have a two to four times increased risk of developing colon cancer; this risk is further doubled in carriers of multiple adenomas. On a geographical basis, the prevalence of adenomas detected during colonoscopy closely parallels the incidence of colon cancer.

Many investigations have addressed the possible role of nutrition in colon carcinogenesis (WCRF 1997). Different aspects of diet have been subject to special scrutiny as risk factors for colon cancer: (a) increased total energy intake; (b) a diet rich in animal fat, in particular in meat; (c) high intake of heterocyclic amines and other mutagens formed during the cooking of meat and fish; (d) low intake of vegetable fibres; (e) a diet poor in fresh fruits and vegetables; (f) low intake of antioxidant micronutrients, such as vitamin E, vitamin C, carotenoids, selenium, and zinc. While there is some evidence in favour of a role of each of these aspects of diet in increasing the risk of colon cancer, the interpretation of the data is complicated by their correlation and by the limitations of assessment of dietary factors in observational epidemiology. Two mechanisms have been postulated for the possible carcinogenic role of a diet high in fat and low in fibre: enhancement of conversion of bile acids into mutagens and tumour-promoting agents by the colonic bacterial flora, and formation of oxygen radicals and other lipid peroxidation products (WCRF 1997). While the mechanisms are unknown at present, the strongest evidence indicates a protective effect of a diet low in calories and animal foods, and rich in fruit and vegetables. Following the results of experimental studies, calcium and vitamin D have received attention as potential chemopreventive agents: the available evidence, however, does not consistently suggest a protective effect of dietary or supplemental intake of either agent.

There is growing evidence of an effect of heavy physical activity, both at the workplace and during leisure time, in protecting from colon cancer. This effect seems to be independent of that of diet, although the exact role of different components of energy balance (i.e. excessive intake from diet and insufficient expenditure through physical activity), as well as of adiposity and body composition, is unknown at present.

Several studies have associated tobacco smoking with an increased risk of colonic adenoma. While the studies of colon cancer have not consistently demonstrated a positive association, a modest increased risk following prolonged heavy smoking has been shown in some of the largest prospective studies.

Several large observational studies have provided evidence that regular aspirin intake reduces by 40 to 60 per cent the risk of colorectal cancer as compared with non-use. However, bias and confounding cannot be completely excluded from these studies (IARC 1997*b*).

Patients with ulcerative colitis and Crohn's disease are at increased risk of colon cancer. The overall relative risk has been estimated in the range of 4 to 20, and it is higher for young age at diagnosis, severity of the disease, and presence of dysplasia. The contribution of shared genetic and environmental factors in the genesis of the two inflammatory conditions and of colon cancer is not known. Cholecystectomy has been associated with a moderate (1.5- to twofold) increased risk of right-sided colon cancer, possibly due to continuous secretion of bile. Patients with one cancer of the colon have a double risk to develop a second primary tumour in the colon or rectum, and the risk is greater for early age at first diagnosis. In women, an association has been shown also with cancers of the endometrium, ovary, and breast, possibly due to shared hormonal or dietary factors.

There are several rare hereditary conditions that are characterized by a very high incidence of colon cancer. Familial adenomatous polyposis, due to inherited or *de novo* mutation in the adenomatous polyposis colon gene on chromosome 5, is characterized by a very high number of colonic adenomas and a cumulative incidence of colon or rectal cancer close to 100 per cent by the age of 55 years. Other, more rare, diseases characterized by colonic polyposis, among other features, are Gardner's syndrome, Turcot's syndrome, and juvenile polyposis. All these hereditary conditions, although very serious for the affected patients, account for no more than 1 per cent of colon cancers in the general population.

Two syndromes characterized by hereditary non-polyposis colon cancer, i.e. with increased familial risk of colon cancer in the absence of adenomas, have been described. Lynch syndrome type I is characterized by increased risk of cancer of the proximal (right) colon, and is due to inherited mutation in one of two genes involved in DNA repair. Patients of Lynch syndrome type II also have an increased risk of extracolonic neoplasms, mainly of the endometrium and breast. As a whole, hereditary non-polyposis colon cancer may account for a sizeable proportion of cases of colon cancer in Western populations. In addition to these hereditary conditions, first-degree relatives of colon cancer patients have a two- to threefold increased risk of developing a cancer of the colon or rectum. It is unclear whether the underlying mechanisms are unknown genes at high or moderate penetrance or shared environmental factors.

Rectum (Schottenfeld and Winawer 1996)

The distribution of cancer of the rectum, including the rectosigmoid junction and the anus, parallels the distribution of colon cancer: the highest rates are recorded in Oceania, North America, and central Europe and are of the order of 20 per 100 000 in men and 10 per 100 000 in women. In most populations, incidence rates have been stable in recent decades. The male to female ratio is close to 2.

Most biological and epidemiological features of rectal cancer resemble those described for colon cancer, including the preneoplastic role of adenomas and non-polypoid dysplastic mucosa, the presence of familial syndromes, the increased risk among patients with chronic inflammatory bowel diseases, and the likely protective role of dietary factors and physical activity. In addition, several studies have provided evidence, although not fully consistent, of an association between elevated intake of alcohol, of beer in particular, and increased risk of colorectal adenoma and adenocarcinoma.

Anus (Schottenfeld and Winawer 1996)

The incidence of cancer of the anus is, in most populations, between 0.5 and 1 per 100 000. This neoplasm may occur either in the anal canal or in the perianal region; the predominant histological types are squamous cell carcinoma and transitional cell carcinoma. Women have a higher incidence of cancer of the anus, in particular of the canal, than men.

The epidemiological features of the disease resemble those of sexually transmitted diseases, with an increased incidence among never-married people, men with homosexual preference, and people with an increased number of sexual partners. The disease has also been associated with previous or subsequent history of cancers of the uterine cervix, vagina, vulva, and penis.

Chronic infection with human papilloma virus, in particular types 16 and 18, is the main known risk factor for anal squamous cell carcinoma. Human papilloma virus DNA has been detected both in a high proportion of carcinomas and anal intraepithelial neoplasias, the precursor lesions of invasive cancer.

Other probable risk factors that are likely to interact with human papilloma virus infection are infection with herpes simplex virus, history of anogenital condylomata genital warts, chronic inflammatory conditions such as fistulas, and immunosuppression, including infection with HIV.

Prevention

Increased intake of vegetables and reduced intake of total calories, fat, and meat high in heterocyclic amines, together with increased physical activity, are reasonable suggestions for the primary prevention of colorectal cancer. Control of human papilloma virus infection, possibly via vaccination, would represent the main preventive measure for anal cancer. Chemopreventive strategies cannot be recommended at present.

Surveillance via flexible sigmoidoscopy, involving removal of adenomas, is a recommended secondary preventive measure for people at increased familial risk. An additional approach consists in the detection of occult blood in the faeces. The method suffers from low specificity and, to a lesser extent, low sensitivity, in particular in the ability to detect adenomas. However, trials have shown a reduced mortality from colorectal cancer after annual testing, although this is achieved at a high cost due to an elevated number of false-positive cases. Current recommendations for individuals aged 50 years and over include either annual faecal occult blood testing or flexible sigmoidoscopy every 5 years (Winawer *et al.* 1997).

Cancer of the liver and biliary tract (London and McGlynn 1996)

The descriptive epidemiology of liver cancer is complicated by the large number of secondary tumours of the liver, which are difficult to separate from primary cancers without histological verification. The most common histological type of liver malignant neoplasm is hepatocellular carcinoma; other forms includ childhood tumour hepatoblastoma, and adult tumour cholangiocarcinoma (originating from the intrahepatic biliary ducts) and angiosarcoma (from the intrahepatic blood vessels). Cancers of the extrahepatic biliary ducts are of the adenocarcinoma type. Most liver cancers originate from cirrhotic tissue.

The incidence of liver cancer is high in all developing regions of the world, with the exception of northern Africa and western Asia (Fig. 7). The highest rates (above 40 per 100 000 in men and above 10 per 100 000 in women) are recorded in Thailand, Japan, and certain parts of China. In most industrialized countries, age-standardized rates are below 5 per 100 000 in men and 2.5 per 100 000 in women. Intermediate rates (5 to 10 per 100 000 in men) are observed in areas of southern and central Europe. Rates are two- to threefold higher in men than women, and the difference is stronger in high-incidence than in low-incidence areas. While in developed countries the rates increase linearly with age, in high-risk areas of developing countries a plateau is reached during the fourth decade of age, and rates decrease after the age of 65 years (it is unclear whether this pattern is due to underdiagnosis at older ages). The estimated worldwide number of new cases of liver cancer in 2000 is 560 000, of which more than 80 per cent are from developing countries (54 per cent from China alone) (Ferlay *et al.* 2001). Given the poor survival from this disease, the estimated number of deaths is similar to that of new cases (550 000); liver cancer is the third most frequent cause of neoplastic death in developing countries.

Incidence rates of biliary tract cancer are high (above 3 per 100 000 in men and above 5 per 100 000 in women) in central Europe, South America, Japan, and western Asia. In the United States, rates are higher among people of American-Indian, Hispanic, and Japanese origin than in other groups. Most of the geographical variation is accounted for by cancer of the gallbladder, which represents the

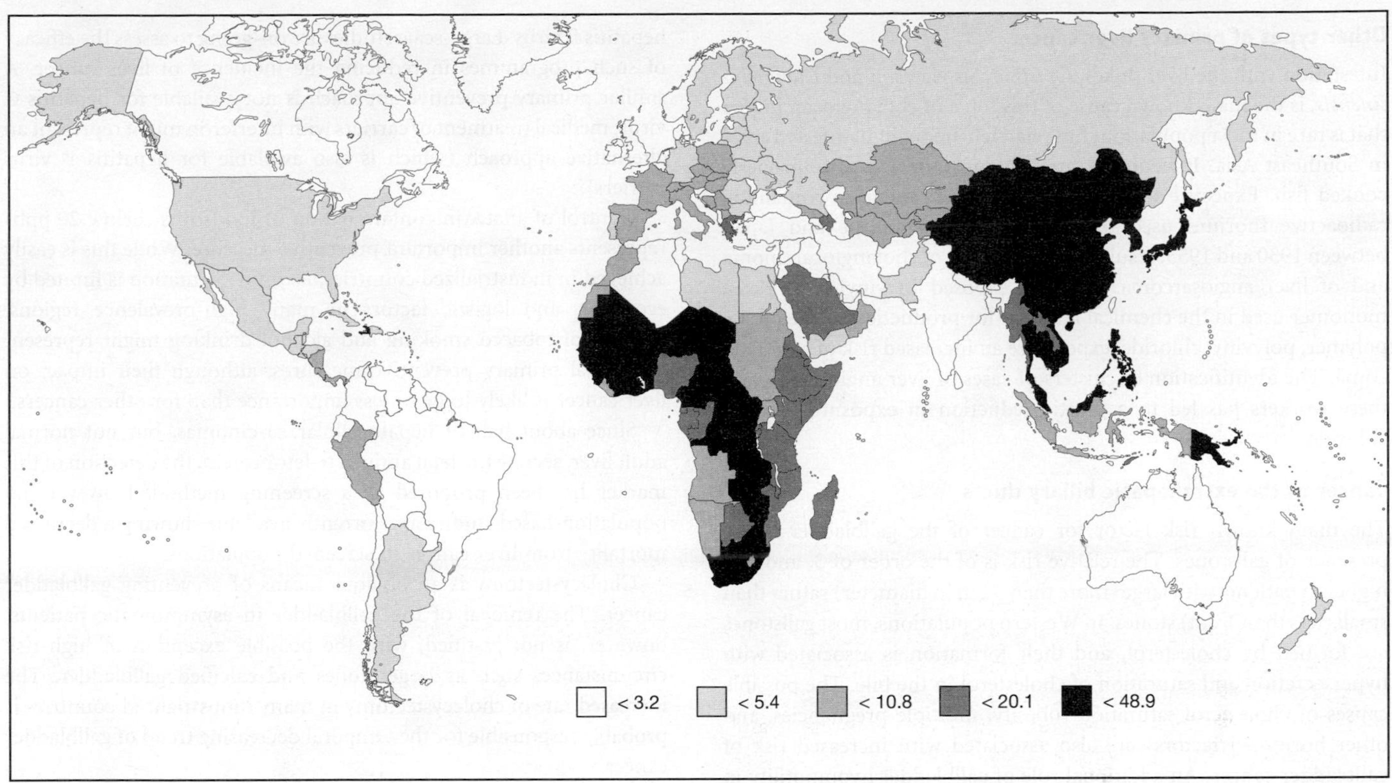

Fig. 7 Incidence of liver cancer: age-standardized rates (worldwide) for men (all ages). (Source: Ferlay *et al.* 2001.)

majority of biliary tract cancers. Rates of gallbladder cancer in women are generally higher than in men, while other biliary tract cancers are slightly more frequent in men: the overall pattern is characterized by female predominance in the occurrence of this neoplasm.

Hepatocellular carcinoma

Chronic infections with hepatitis B and hepatitis C virus are the main causes of hepatocellular carcinoma. The risk increases with early age at infection (in high-risk countries, most hepatitis B virus infections occur perinatally or in early childhood) and the presence of liver cirrhosis. Hepatitis B virus is the main agent in China, Southeast Asia, and Africa, while hepatitis C virus is the predominant virus in Japan and southern Europe. The most frequent routes of hepatitis C virus transmission are parenteral and sexual, perinatal infection being rare. The estimated risk of developing hepatocellular carcinoma among infected subjects, relative to uninfected, ranged between 5 and 50 in different studies. On a global scale, the fraction of liver cancer cases attributable to hepatitis B virus is 60 per cent, and attributable to hepatitis C virus is 24 per cent (Pisani *et al.* 1997).

Ecological studies have shown that the incidence of hepatocellular carcinoma correlates not only with hepatitis B and hepatitis C virus infection, but also with contamination of foodstuff with aflatoxins, a group of mycotoxins produced by the fungi *Aspergillus flavus* and *Aspergillus parasiticus*, which cause liver cancer in many species of experimental animals. Contamination originates mainly from improper storage of cereals, peanuts, and other vegetables and is prevalent in particular in Africa, Southeast Asia, and China. The investigation of the carcinogenic role of aflatoxins in humans has been complicated by the inadequacy of traditional methods of exposure assessment (e.g. questionnaires). During the last decade, however, prospective studies have shown a strong association between biological markers of aflatoxin exposure in serum or urine and risk of subsequent liver cancer. A carcinogenic role of aflatoxins, in particular of aflatoxin B_1, has therefore been confirmed and shown to be independent of that exerted by hepatitis B virus infection.

Alcohol intake increases the risk of hepatocellular carcinoma. The most likely mechanism is through development of liver cirrhosis, although alternative mechanisms such as alteration in activation and detoxification of carcinogens may also play a role. Alcoholic liver cirrhosis is probably the most important risk factor for hepatocellular carcinoma in populations with low prevalence of hepatitis B and hepatitis C virus infection and low exposure to aflatoxins, such as North America and northern Europe. The association between tobacco smoking and hepatocellular carcinoma is not fully consistent, and a possible confounding effect of excessive alcohol intake or infection with hepatitis B and hepatitis C virus has not been completely ruled out. Despite these limitations, the evidence indicates a possible limited effect of tobacco smoking on liver carcinogenesis.

Use of oral contraceptives greatly increases the risk of liver adenomas, and an effect on the risk of hepatocellular carcinoma is plausible, although its magnitude is likely to be small. Case reports have associated the use of anabolic steroids with the development of liver cancer, but the evidence is not conclusive at present. An increase in iron storage in the body is a likely cause of hepatocellular carcinoma: the evidence comes from studies of patients with haemochromatosis or other disorders of iron metabolism. The effect of iron overload seems to be independent of development of cirrhosis and may interact with hepatitis B virus infection.

Other types of primary liver cancer

Infestation with the liver flukes, *Opisthorchis viverrini* and *Clonorchis sinensis*, is the main known cause of this form of cholangiocarcinoma that is rare in most populations but relatively frequent in infested areas in Southeast Asia. Infection occurs via consumption of improperly cooked fish. Exposure to thorotrast, a contrast medium containing radioactive thorium used for angiography in Europe and Japan between 1930 and 1955, resulted in an increase of cholangiocarcinoma and of liver angiosarcoma. Workers exposed to vinyl chloride, a monomer used in the chemical industry for production of the plastic polymer, polyvinyl chloride, experience an increased risk of angiosarcoma. The identification of clusters of cases of liver angiosarcoma in these workers has led to a drastic reduction in exposure to vinyl chloride.

Cancer of the extrahepatic biliary ducts

The main known risk factor for cancer of the gallbladder is the presence of gallstones. The relative risk is of the order of 3, and it is higher in patients with large (more than 3 cm in diameter) rather than small (less than 1 cm) stones. In Western populations, most gallstones are formed by cholesterol, and their formation is associated with hypersecretion and saturation of cholesterol in the bile. The possible causes of cholesterol saturation (obesity, multiple pregnancies, and other hormonal factors) are also associated with increased risk of gallbladder cancer. An additional role of gallbladder hypomotility in stone formation is likely. In Asia, the main types of gallstone are formed by bilirubin salts and have as a risk factor bacterial infection of the biliary system: their association with gallbladder cancer, however, is not clear.

Other suspected risk factors for gallbladder cancer include chronic inflammation; biliary stasis and infection, in particular status of chronic typhoid and paratyphoid carrier; history of gastric resection; reproductive history resulting in increased exposure to endogenous oestrogens and progesterone (early age at menarche, late age at menopause, high parity); obesity; and, possibly, increased energy intake. It is likely that these factors act through gallstone formation, although the available data do not allow a conclusion with respect to their possible role in gallbladder carcinogenesis.

Fewer data are available on risk factors for cancer of extrahepatic biliary ducts. Infestation with the liver flukes causing intrahepatic cholangiocarcinoma, and history of ulcerative colitis are established risk factors but explain only a small proportion of these cancers. Tobacco smoking has been suggested as an additional cause.

Genetic factors are likely to play a role in biliary tract cancer. Patients with hereditary cancer-prone conditions, such as ataxia telangiectasia and hereditary non-polyposis colon cancer, have an increased risk of biliary tract cancer. Furthermore, a familial aggregation has been shown in population-based studies, which might be due to familial predisposition to gallstone formation.

Prevention

The strong role in liver carcinogenesis of infection with hepatitis B virus, a virus for which effective and relatively cheap vaccines are available, suggests that prevention of liver cancer is achievable. In high-prevalence areas, hepatitis B virus vaccination has to be introduced in the perinatal period. In the last decades, many countries from Asia, southern Europe, and, to a lesser extent, Africa have expanded the national childhood vaccination programme to include hepatitis B virus. Large-scale studies are on-going to assess the efficacy of such programmes in reducing the incidence of liver cancer. A similar primary preventive approach is not available for hepatitis C virus; medical treatment of carriers with interferon might represent an alternative approach (which is also available for hepatitis B virus carriers).

Control of aflatoxin contamination of foodstuffs (below 20 ppb) represents another important preventive measure. While this is easily achieved in industrialized countries, its implementation is limited by economic and logistic factors in many high-prevalence regions. Control of tobacco smoking and alcohol drinking might represent additional primary preventive measures, although their impact on liver cancer is likely to be of less importance than for other cancers.

Since about half of hepatocellular carcinomas, but not normal adult liver, secrete the fetal antigen α-fetoprotein, the detection of this marker has been proposed as a screening method. However, no population-based studies are currently available showing a decreased mortality from liver cancer in screened populations.

Cholecystectomy is an obvious means of preventing gallbladder cancer. The removal of the gallbladder in asymptomatic patients, however, is not justified, with the possible exception of high-risk circumstances such as large stones and calcified gallbladder. The increased rate of cholecystectomy in many industrialized countries is probably responsible for the temporal decreasing trend of gallbladder cancer.

Cancer of the pancreas (Anderson *et al.* 1996)

The descriptive epidemiology of pancreatic cancer suffers from geographical and temporal variation in the sensitivity and specificity of clinical diagnosis and in the proportion of histological verification of cases. Even when comparing populations living in the same place at the same time (e.g. different social classes or age groups), differential access to health care might bias the incidence or mortality data.

The great majority of malignant neoplasms of the pancreas originate from the exocrine portion of the organ, which mainly secretes digestive enzymes. They are of the adenocarcinoma type. Rare pancreatic neoplasms include tumours (of uncertain clinical behaviour) of the endocrine portion, which secretes insulin and glucagon, as well as lymphomas and sarcomas.

The highest rates are recorded among black Americans (about 12 per 100 000 in men and 10 per 100 000 in women) and among indigenous populations in Oceania. The lowest rates, which may suffer from underdiagnosis, are recorded in India, Southeast Asia, and northern and central Africa (below 2 per 100 000 in men and 1 per 100 000 in women). In the United States, rates are about 50 to 100 per cent higher in black people as compared with white people living in the same areas. The disease accounts for an estimated 216 000 new cases in 2000, 60 per cent of which occurred in developed countries (Ferlay *et al.* 2001). Given the very poor survival from this disease, mortality rates closely parallel incidence rates. Rates are about 50 per cent higher in men than in women. An increase in incidence and mortality has taken place since the 1970s, in particular in Europe, that can be partly attributed to diagnostic improvements.

The incidence of pancreatic cancer is very low before the age of 40 years and increases logarithmically, without a clear suggestion of a plateau at old age. Urban populations have been reported to have higher rates than rural populations, but this may reflect differences in quality of diagnosis. Migrant studies suggest that first-generation migrants from low- to high-risk areas experience, after 15 or 20 years, rates that are even higher than those of the country of migration, suggesting an important role of environmental exposures occurring late in life.

The best known risk factor for pancreatic cancer is tobacco smoking. The risk in smokers is two- to fivefold higher than that in non-smokers, and a dose–response relationship and a protective effect of quitting smoking have been shown in many populations. The proportion of cases of pancreatic cancer attributable to tobacco smoking has been estimated to be 27 per cent in men and 11 per cent in women (Parkin *et al.* 1994). It is noteworthy that some of the features of the descriptive epidemiology of pancreatic cancer (i.e. a high incidence among black Americans as compared with a low incidence in Africa, and a higher risk among men and urban residents) can simply be explained by differences in smoking habits.

An increased risk of pancreatic cancer has been suggested for low vegetable and fruit intake (WCRF 1997). For other dietary components, namely cereals and sugar, the evidence is not consistent. Early reports of an association between coffee consumption and pancreatic cancer risk have not been confirmed by larger, more recent investigations. A positive association between alcohol drinking and pancreatic cancer has been reported in some, but not all, studies that have addressed this question. The current evidence is consistent with a possible weak effect of heavy alcohol drinking, in particular among smokers.

Several medical conditions have been studied with respect to their association with subsequent risk of pancreatic cancer. History of pancreatitis increases the risk more than 10 fold, with little difference between the alcoholic and non-alcoholic forms of the disease. An increased risk has also been shown in several studies of diabetic patients; the relative risk is likely to fall in the range of 1.5 to 2. Gastrectomy patients are at three- to fivefold increased risk of pancreatic cancer; the association does not appear to be confounded by tobacco smoking.

A familial history of cancer of the pancreas is present is 8 to 10 per cent of patients, suggesting a possible role for genetic factors. Specific hereditary conditions carrying an increased risk of pancreatic cancer include the Li–Fraumeni syndrome, hereditary non-polyposis colon cancer, and a group of rare hereditary pancreatites that involve deficiency in enzyme metabolism: these conditions are likely to explain only a small proportion of cases in the general population.

There is no effective cure for pancreatic cancer, with the exception of surgery for a small number of patients. Screening methods are not available. Primary prevention is the only available tool for this disease: avoidance of smoking would have a very important effect in reducing the number of cases; an increase in dietary consumption of fruits and vegetables is the other recommended preventive measure.

Cancer of the respiratory tract

Malignant neoplasms are important in all organs of the respiratory tract: the nasal cavity and paranasal sinuses, nasopharynx, larynx, lung (including the trachea and the bronchi), and pleura. Cancer of the nasopharynx is discussed above.

Nasal cavity and paranasal sinuses (Roush 1996)

The incidence of cancer of the nasal cavity and paranasal sinuses (sinonasal cancer) is low in most populations (less than 1.5 per 100 000 in men and less than 1.0 per 100 000 in women). Higher rates are recorded in Japan and certain parts of China and India. In Western populations and Japan, squamous cell carcinoma is the main histological type, followed by adenocarcinoma, and 30 to 80 per cent of the cancers originate from the maxillary sinus. In other countries, other forms of sinonasal cancer are important, such as Burkitt's lymphoma of the maxillary or ethmoid sinus in eastern Africa. Time trends have shown in most populations a stable incidence or a small decline in recent decades.

Occupational exposure to wood dust, in particular to dust of hard woods such as beech and oak, is the main known risk factor for sinonasal cancer: the increase in risk (of the order of five- to 50-fold) is strongest for adenocarcinoma and for cancers originating from the sinuses. It is unclear whether dust from soft woods such as pine and spruce increases the risk. The effect is present after 40 or more years since first exposure and persists after cessation of exposure. An increased risk of sinonasal cancer has been shown among workers in nickel refining and chromate pigment manufacture, but not among workers exposed to these metals in other processes, such as plating and welding. Among other suspected occupational carcinogens are formaldehyde, di-isopropyl sulphate, and dichloroethyl sulphide.

A relatively weak association (relative risks in the range of 2 to 5) has shown between tobacco smoking and sinonasal cancer, in particular squamous cell carcinoma. Presence of recurrent polyps represents a risk factor, and a possible role of chronic sinusitis has been suggested. Exposure to thorotrast, a radioactive contrast agent, represents an additional risk factor. Infection with Epstein–Barr virus is implicated in the origin of Burkitt's lymphoma of the sinuses and possibly in the origin of undifferentiated carcinoma.

Control of occupational exposure to hard wood dust and nickel and chromium compounds, as well as avoidance of tobacco smoking, are the two main preventive measures for sinonasal cancer.

Larynx (Austin and Reynolds 1996)

More than 90 per cent of cancers of the larynx are squamous cell carcinomas, and the majority originate from the supraglottic and glottic regions of the organs. The incidence in men is high (10 per 100 000 or more) in southern and central Europe, southern Brazil, Uruguay, and Argentina and among black Americans, while the lowest rates (less than 1 per 100 000) are recorded in Southeast Asia and central Africa. The incidence in women is below 1 per 100 000 in most populations. Rates have not changed markedly during the last two decades. An estimated 140 000 new cases occurred worldwide in 2000, of which 140 000 were among men (Ferlay *et al.* 2001).

Most cases of laryngeal cancer in Western countries (up to 80 per cent in high-risk areas) are attributable to tobacco smoking, alcohol drinking, and the interaction between these two factors. The effect of tobacco, with risks in smokers of the order of 10 relative to non-smokers, seems to be stronger for glottic than supraglottic neoplasms. Studies in several populations have shown a dose–response relationship and a beneficial effect of quitting smoking. Smoking black tobacco cigarettes entails a stronger risk than smoking blond tobacco cigarettes. Studies from India have also reported an effect of chewing tobacco-containing products. The effect of alcohol is stronger for supraglottic tumours than for tumours at other sites; however, it is not clear whether different alcoholic beverages exert a different carcinogenic effect.

A protective effect is probably exerted by high intake of fruits and vegetables, although the evidence regarding specific micronutrients, such as carotenoids and vitamin C, is inadequate to draw a conclusion. It has been suggested in studies from Brazil and Uruguay that maté drinking is a risk factor. Data concerning a possible effect of other foods are not consistent.

Occupational exposure to mists of strong inorganic acids, in particular of sulphuric acid, is an established risk factor for laryngeal cancer. A possible effect has been suggested for other occupational exposures, including nickel, asbestos, and ionizing radiation, but the evidence is not conclusive at present.

Laryngeal papillomatosis is a condition characterized by multiple benign tumours, called papillomas, that are caused by infection with human papilloma virus types 6 and 11, the same types causing genital condylomata acuminata. Infection in children occurs in both genders from vertical infection during delivery; infection in adults is prevalent in men and may occur via orogenital sexual contact. Papillomatosis patients have an increased risk of laryngeal cancer; however, studies aimed at assessing the presence of human papilloma virus DNA have not yet provided conclusive evidence of a higher prevalence of infection in cases of laryngeal cancer than in controls. Another virus for which a causal role has been postulated in laryngeal cancer is herpes simplex virus type 1.

There is no evidence of strong genetic factors in laryngeal carcinogenesis; however, polymorphism for enzymes implicated in the metabolism of alcohol and tobacco, such as glutathione-5-transferase and alcohol dehydrogenase, are likely to represent weak susceptibility factors, with relative risks of the order of 1.5 to 2.

Survival from laryngeal cancer is relatively common (5-year survival rates are of the order of 65 per cent in developed countries and 40 per cent in developing countries) (Sankaranarayanan *et al.* 1998; Berrino *et al.* 1999). These patients are at very high risk of developing a second primary tumour in the oral cavity, pharynx, and lung. While shared risk factors are likely to play an important role, it is plausible that host susceptibility factors are also partially responsible. For example, an increased sensitivity to mutagens has been shown in lymphocytes of laryngeal cancer patients, in particular those with multiple tumours, as compared with controls (Spitz *et al.* 1997).

Control of tobacco smoking and excessive alcohol drinking, possibly together with an increased intake of fruits and vegetables, would prevent the majority of cases of laryngeal cancer (as well as of a number of other cancers) in most populations. Control of exposure to known and suspected occupational carcinogens is an important measure for exposed workers. No screening methods are currently available for laryngeal cancer.

Lung (Blot and Fraumeni 1996)

Lung cancer was a rare disease until the beginning of the twentieth century. Since then, its occurrence has increased rapidly and this neoplasm has become the most frequent malignant neoplasm among men in most countries, and represents the most important cause of neoplastic death worldwide. It accounts for an estimated 901 000 new cases each year among men and 337 000 among women (Ferlay *et al.* 2001). Survival from lung cancer is poor (5 to 10 per cent at 5 years).

In both men and women, the incidence of lung cancer is low before the age of 40 years, and increases up to the age of 70 or 75. The geographical and temporal patterns of lung cancer incidence are to a large extent determined by consumption of tobacco. An increase in tobacco consumption is paralleled some 20 years later by an increase in the incidence of lung cancer, and a decrease in consumption is followed by a decrease in incidence.

The highest incidence rates (more than 100 per 100 000) are recorded among black people from New Orleans, the United States, and Maori from New Zealand (Parkin *et al.* 1997). In some central and eastern European countries, very high mortality rates, with further increasing temporal trends, are reported. On the contrary, mortality rates have started to decline among men from the United States and northern Europe. The lowest incidence rates are reported from Africa and southern Asia (Parkin *et al.* 1997).

Rates in women are high in the United States, Canada, Denmark, and the United Kingdom, and low in countries such as France, Japan, and Spain, in which the prevalence of smoking in women increased only recently. The lowest rates (less than 3 cases per 100 000 people) are recorded in Africa and India. China is a notable exception, with relatively high rates recorded among women (e.g. 37 per 100 000 in Tianjin during 1988 to 1992; Parkin *et al.* 1997), despite a low prevalence of smoking.

The main histological types of lung cancer are squamous cell carcinoma, small cell carcinoma, adenocarcinoma, and large cell carcinoma. Over the last 20 years, the proportion of squamous cell carcinomas, which used to be the predominant type, has decreased and an increase of adenocarcinomas has taken place in both genders. Despite some minor differences, the main risk factors for lung cancer affect all histological types.

A carcinogenic effect of tobacco smoke on the lung has been demonstrated in the 1950s and has been recognized by public health and regulatory authorities since the mid-1960s (USDHHS 1982). The risk of lung cancer among smokers relative to the risk among never-smokers is of the order of 8 to 15 in men and 2 to 10 in women. This overall risk reflects the contribution of the different aspects of tobacco smoking: average consumption, duration of smoking, time since quitting, age at start, type of tobacco product, and inhalation pattern, with duration being the dominant factor. As compared with continuous smokers, the excess risk decreases in ex-smokers after approximately 5 years since quitting, but a small excess risk is likely to persist in long-term quitters throughout life. The risk of lung cancer is lower among smokers of low-tar and low-nicotine cigarettes than among other smokers, and in non-inhalers as compared with inhalers. A protective effect has also been observed among long-term smokers of filtered cigarettes compared with smokers of unfiltered cigarettes. Smokers of black (air-cured) tobacco cigarettes are at a two- to threefold higher risk of lung cancer than smokers of blond (flue-cured) tobacco cigarettes. A causal association with lung cancer has been shown also for consumption of cigars, cigarillos, pipe, bidis, and water pipe.

An association has been shown in many studies between exposure to passive smoke and lung cancer risk in non-smokers. The magnitude of the risk among non-smokers exposed to passive smoke is of the order 15 to 20 per cent (Hackshaw *et al.* 1997).

There is convincing evidence that a diet rich in vegetables and fruits exerts a protective effect against lung cancer (WCRF 1997). Subjects in the categories at highest consumption experience 10 to 50 per cent of the risk of lung cancer of subjects in the categories at lowest consumption. Despite the many risk estimates for intake of other foods, such as cereals, pulses, meat, eggs, milk, and dairy products, the evidence is inadequate to allow a judgement regarding the evidence of a carcinogenic or a protective effect (WCRF 1997).

Several studies have suggested positive associations between total and saturated fat intake and lung cancer risk, and the effect seems to be independent of that of tobacco consumption (WCRF 1997). A large number of studies have reported a reduced risk of lung cancer for high intake of β-carotene (IARC 1998*a*). Similar results have been obtained in studies based on measurement of β-carotene in prospectively collected sera (WCRF 1997). This evidence of a protective effect has been challenged by the results of intervention trials of β-carotene supplementation (IARC 1998*a*). In two of the studies, which included smokers and workers exposed to asbestos, an increase in the incidence of lung cancer was observed in the treated groups: in the other studies, no difference was found between the treated and the control groups. The difference in the results of observational studies and preventive trials can be explained either by a confounding effect by other dietary components in observational studies, or by a paradox effect of β-carotene at very high, non-physiological doses, in particular among smokers.

There is a suggestion from observational studies that high intake of vitamin C, vitamin E, and selenium protects against lung cancer. The evidence regarding other micronutrients is inconclusive at present (WCRF 1997). The available data suggest a small increase in the risk of lung cancer from alcohol drinking, which does not appear to be fully explained by tobacco smoking (WCRF 1997). Furthermore, there is quite consistent evidence that reduced body mass index (usually below 22) is associated with an increased risk of lung cancer; and a certain degree of protection from regular physical activity has been shown in most relevant studies, after adjustment for tobacco smoking (WCRF 1997).

A positive familial history of lung cancer has been found to be a risk factor in several studies. Segregation analyses suggest that inheritance of a major gene, in conjunction with tobacco smoking, might account for 50 to 80 per cent of cases diagnosed below the age of 60 years (Yang *et al.* 1999). In addition, low-penetrance genes involved in the metabolism of tobacco carcinogens might influence individual susceptibility to lung cancer.

Studies of atomic bomb survivors and patients treated with radiotherapy indicate that they are at increased risk of lung cancer (National Research Council 1988). Although the magnitude of the increased risk is moderate (relative risk of the order of 1.5 to 2 for cumulative exposure in excess of 1 Gy), the number of extra cases of lung cancer exceeds that of other neoplasms. Underground miners exposed to radio-active radon and its decay products have been found to be at increased risk of lung cancer. The main concern for lung cancer risk from radon and its decay products, however, comes from residential rather than occupational exposure. A meta-analysis of the eight most informative studies of lung cancer risk from residential exposure resulted in a pooled relative risk of 1.14 (95 per cent confidence interval 1.0 to 1.3) at 150 Bq/m^3 of exposure (Lubin and Boice 1997).

The risk of lung cancer is increased among workers employed in several industries and occupations. For several of these high-risk workplaces, the agent (or agents) responsible for the increased risk have been identified. In other cases, the identification of the relevant carcinogens has not yet taken place (see section below on occupational and environmental agents for details). Occupational agents are responsible for an estimated 5 to 10 per cent of lung cancers in industrialized countries.

Patients with pulmonary tuberculosis are at increased risk of lung cancer; it is not clear whether the excess risk is due to the chronic inflammatory status of the lung parenchyma or to the specific action of the *Mycobacterium*. Chronic exposure to high levels of fibres and dusts might result in lung fibrosis (e.g. silicosis and asbestosis), a condition which entails a great increase in the risk of lung cancer. Chronic respiratory diseases (chronic bronchitis, emphysema, and asthma) have also been associated with lung cancer risk.

There is abundant evidence that lung cancer rates are higher in cities than in rural settings (Speizer and Samet 1994). Although this pattern might result from confounding by other factors, notably tobacco smoking, diet, and occupational exposures, the combined evidence from analytical studies suggests that urban air pollution might be a true risk factor for lung cancer; although the excess risk is unlikely to be larger than 50 per cent.

Two important sources of indoor exposure to potential lung carcinogens are the use of coal-burning heating devices without proper exhaust emission (e.g. the use of kang in northeastern China) and high-temperature cooking, in particular when using unrefined vegetable oils such as rapeseed oil (common in several parts of China). Indoor levels of benzo-(a)-pyrene have been reported to be very high in such exposure circumstances (Smith and Liu 1994). Indoor air pollution is probably a major cause of lung cancer in Chinese women, who experience very high lung cancer rates despite a low prevalence of smoking (Smith and Liu 1994).

Control of tobacco smoking remains the key strategy for the prevention of lung cancer. Reduction in exposure to occupational and environmental carcinogens (in particular indoor pollution and radon), as well as increase in consumption of fruits and vegetables are additional preventive opportunities. No screening approaches are effective to reduce lung cancer mortality.

Pleural mesothelioma (Blot and Fraumeni 1996)

Mesothelioma is the most important primary tumour of the pleura. It can also originate from the peritoneum and the pericardium. Mesotheliomas were considered very rare tumours, until large series of cases were reported in the 1960s among workers exposed to asbestos mining and manufacturing. The descriptive epidemiology of pleural tumours, and mesothelioma in particular, is complicated by geographical and temporal differences in diagnostic accuracy: although underdiagnosis is likely to occur when no information is available on exposure to asbestos, the opposite phenomenon may take place when the doctor or pathologist is aware of past asbestos exposure. In most industrialized countries, the incidence of pleural mesothelioma is of the order of 1 to 1.5 per 100 000 in men and around 0.5 per 100 000 in women. Lower rates are reported from developing countries, where underdiagnosis might be a particularly serious problem. In areas with a high prevalence of occupational exposure to asbestos such as shipbuilding and mining centres, the rates might be as high as 5 per 100 000 in men and 4 per 100 000 in women.

A steep increase in the mortality or incidence rates of mesothelioma has taken place in most industrialized countries since the 1950s. This trend is mainly due to a cohort effect, since individuals heavily exposed to asbestos (those born since 1900) have reached the age of development of mesothelioma. The highest exposures were experienced in the United States by those born around 1910, while in Europe exposure was high also in later cohorts. As a consequence, the increasing trend in mesothelioma occurrence is likely to disappear in the United States, while it will continue until about 2020 in most European countries.

Asbestos is the main known risk factor for mesothelioma. All types of asbestos cause mesothelioma, although the potency of chrysotile appears to be less than that of amphiboles. A distinct feature of the carcinogenic potency of asbestos on the pleura is the importance of time since first exposure: the rate appears to increase with the third power of time since first exposure, with few cases developing within the first 20 years and no apparent decline even after 45 or more years. Circumstances of high non-occupational exposure to asbestos (e.g. spouses of asbestos workers laundering work clothes) have been linked to an increased risk of mesothelioma. The data are inadequate to assess the risk of low-level environmental exposure, although the presence of a small excess risk is plausible.

Environmental exposure to erionite, a naturally occurring mineral fibre, has been linked to high mesothelioma risk in rural areas of Cappadocia, Turkey. The evidence of an effect of other mineral fibres (e.g. fibre glass, ceramic fibres) on the pleura is inadequate. Exposure to asbestos or other mineral fibres is not obvious in a proportion of cases of mesothelioma (40 to 50 per cent in men and 60 to 80 per cent in women): although some of these cases might be due to unrecognized occupational or environmental exposure to asbestos, it is likely that a fraction of cases not related to fibre exposure exists. A role of diet (increased risk among subjects with low fruit and vegetable intake) has been suggested in two case–control studies. Simian virus 40 has been found in a high proportion of tumour samples in various series of cases of mesothelioma, but its aetiological role is still unclear.

Control of occupational exposure to asbestos, in particular to amphiboles, is the main preventive action to reduce the number of mesothelioma cases. This has taken place in the mining and manufacturing industries in many countries: workers at highest risk are today those in the construction industry, mainly in demolition and maintenance. Control of asbestos exposure is deficient in many developing countries. Control of tobacco smoking is not effective to reduce mesothelioma risk; however, given the carcinogenic effect of asbestos also on the lung, and its interaction with tobacco smoking, smoking avoidance and cessation programmes should be incorporated in the surveillance of workers with past asbestos exposure.

Neoplasms of the bone and soft tissue (Miller *et al.* 1996)

Bone cancer

Three main histological types represent the majority of cases of bone cancer: osteosarcoma (originating from the bone tissue and representing 30 to 50 per cent of all bone neoplasms), chondrosarcoma (from the cartilage, 20 to 30 per cent), and Ewing's sarcoma (possibly from primitive nervous tissue, 10 to 20 per cent). Several other rare types (e.g. chordoma, fibrosarcoma, giant cell tumours) comprise some 10 to 20 per cent of all bone cancers. Ewing's sarcoma occurs during the second and third decades of life; the incidence of osteosarcoma is bimodal with peaks between the age of 10 and 30 years, and after age 60, while the incidence of chondrosarcoma resembles that of many cancers with a steady increase throughout life. Rates of all major histological types are higher in men than in women, but in most populations the ratio is of the order of 1.5. There are limited geographical differences in bone cancer incidence, with rates ranging between 1 and 3 per 100 000 in men and between 0.5 and 2 per 100 000 in women.

Ionizing radiation is the best known risk factor for bone cancer. The risk is increased two- to threefold in groups of adult patients undergoing radiotherapy for cancer, as compared with other patients; the relative risk is high among radiotherapy-treated children, in particular among those with inherited mutation in the retinoblastoma gene, suggesting an interaction with genetic susceptibility. The excess risk, however, is apparent only among patients receiving high radiation doses, and studies of populations exposed to lower doses, such as patients treated for benign conditions or atomic bomb survivors, did not show an increased risk. Studies of workers and patients exposed to high doses of radium isotopes also confirmed the role of ionizing radiation in bone carcinogenesis.

Despite the strong relative risks, the number of cases of bone cancer due to ionizing radiation in the general population is small, but few data are available on other risk factors. A role of alkylating agents used in cancer chemotherapy seems likely, while the evidence implying viral infections, traumas, and medical implants is inadequate to reach a conclusion.

Patients with Paget's disease (osteitis deformans, a disease characterized by multiple localized areas of destruction of bone followed by repair) have a high incidence of osteosarcoma and chondrosarcoma; this disease is likely to be responsible for a substantial proportion of cases above the age of 60 years. An hereditary component of Paget's disease is suggested, and unknown environmental factors are likely to play a role in its aetiology. The risk of bone cancer is also increased in other rare syndromes of bone malformation. Bone cancer is one of the neoplasms appearing in the Li–Fraumeni syndrome, caused by an inherited mutation in the p53 gene. Familial aggregation of bone cancer occurs also outside well-defined inherited conditions, suggesting an important role of still unknown genetic factors.

The causes of Ewing's sarcoma are largely unknown. It is not associated with ionizing radiation and it does not appear to aggregate in families.

Primary prevention of bone cancer is hampered by the limited knowledge about its causes and mechanisms. No secondary prevention strategies are available.

Soft-tissue sarcomas (Zahm *et al.* 1996)

Sarcomas originate from the mesenchyma in the space between the organs and within any organ. Sarcomas from the organs are classified within the neoplasms of that organ (e.g. liver angiosarcoma), while those originating from subcutaneous and intervisceral connective tissue are classified in the heterogeneous group of soft-tissue sarcomas. Fibrosarcoma (originating from fibrocytes of the connective tissue), leiomyosarcoma (from smooth muscle cells), and liposarcoma (from fat cells) are common types of soft-tissue sarcomas in most populations. The recent epidemic of AIDS has produced in several populations a sharp increase in the occurrence of Kaposi's sarcoma, a sarcoma from blood vessel cells. Without considering Kaposi's sarcoma (that is discussed below), the incidence of soft-tissue sarcoma presents limited geographical variations, with age-adjusted incidence rates ranging from 1 to 3 per 100 000 in men and from 0.5 to 2 to 100 000 in women. Rates are slightly lower in Asia, and higher in western Europe and North America. An increasing trend in incidence is suggested in industrialized countries, which is not explained by the increasing incidence of Kaposi's sarcoma.

Ionizing radiation is a known risk factor for soft-tissue sarcomas: all types of sarcomas have been reported among patients treated with radiotherapy, the most frequent being malignant fibrous hystiocytoma. In addition, cancer chemotherapy seems to exert an effect independent of that of radiotherapy. A viral agent (e.g. cytomegalovirus, Epstein–Barr virus) has been hypothesized for non-AIDS related Kaposi's sarcoma and for other soft-tissue sarcomas, but no conclusions can be reached at present.

Several occupational exposures have been linked to an increased risk of soft-tissue sarcoma, including in particular phenoxy herbicides and chlorinated hydrocarbon insecticides. For none of these chemicals the evidence of a carcinogenic effect is consistent, with the possible exception of 2,3,7,8-tetrachlorodibenzo-*p*-dioxin, for which a two- to threefold relative risk has been reported in studies of manufacturers and sprayers of contaminated herbicides and of populations exposed during industrial accidents, but not among Vietnam veterans who were also exposed to contaminated herbicides. There is no consistent evidence of an association with dietary factors, traumas, tobacco smoking, and use of smokeless tobacco products.

Transplant patients receiving immunosuppressive therapy as well as patients with primary immunodeficiency syndromes have an increased risk of soft-tissue sarcomas. The occurrence of these neoplasms is also increased in patients with the Li–Fraumeni syndrome, neurofibromatosis type 1, and other rare familial cancer syndromes. Benign tumours in the connective tissue (lipomas, fibromas, and so on) are common and usually do not transform into their malignant counterparts.

Cancer of the skin

There are four main types of skin cancer: squamous cell carcinoma, arising from the epidermal cells; basal cell carcinoma, from basal cells forming sebaceous glands; melanoma, arising from melanocytes; and Kaposi's sarcoma, arising from endothelial cells. Squamous cell carcinoma and basal cell carcinoma share pathological, clinical, and aetiological features, and are often combined under the definition of non-melanocytic skin cancer.

Non-melanocytic skin cancer (Scotto *et al.* 1996)

Given the simplified diagnostic and therapeutic procedures (often treated in outpatient clinics and general practitioner offices) of most non-melanocytic skin cancers, reporting of cases to registries is frequently incomplete, and many cancer registries do not attempt to provide incidence figures. The very good prognosis (a more than 95 per cent survival rate in most populations) makes mortality figures useless to estimate incidence. Population-based data incidence derive therefore from *ad hoc* surveys. A survey conducted in the United States in the late 1970s estimated an age-adjusted incidence rate of squamous cell carcinoma of 68 per 100 000 in white men and 24 per 100 000 in white women; corresponding figures for basal cell carcinoma were 258 and 155 per 100 000. Rates in black people were about 100 times lower than in white people, and squamous cell carcinoma predominates. The comparison with a similar survey conducted in the early 1970s revealed a 4 to 5 per cent increase in the incidence of basal cell carcinoma per year, which can be attributed, at least in part, to improved diagnostic and surveillance procedures. Squamous cell carcinoma rates increased little during the same period. Rates in white people approximate those of all other malignant neoplasms combined. Even higher rates have been recorded in Ireland and among white people living in countries with high solar exposure, such as Australia and South Africa, while black populations have consistently low rates.

The risk of non-melanocytic skin cancer is very low before the age of 20 years, and then increases logarithmically up to about 60 years of age, after which it decelerates. Between 75 and 90 per cent of both squamous and basal cell carcinomas in white people are localized on the face, head, and neck. In black people, the lower extremities are the most frequent location of squamous cell carcinoma.

Solar radiation is the main known risk factor for non-melanocytic skin cancer. For squamous cell carcinoma, the cumulative dose of ultraviolet radiation, disregarding dose rate, appears to be the predominant risk factor, while for basal cell carcinoma sun exposure and sunburning during childhood are the main determinants of subsequent risk. The effect of solar radiation has been shown following occupational, recreational, and involuntary exposure. The strongest association concerns ultraviolet radiation B, with a wavelength in the range 290 to 320 nm. A strong excess of skin cancer has also been shown in psoriasis patients treated with psoralen in combination with ultraviolet radiation A. Solar keratosis is a precursor lesion of squamous cell carcinoma of the skin (not of basal cell carcinoma); it occurs in those areas of the skin exposed to solar radiation. The cumulative progression rate of keratosis to carcinoma (usually through a phase of carcinoma *in situ*, or Bowen's disease) is of the order of 5 per cent. Skin pigmentation is a modifying factor of the carcinogenic effect of ultraviolet radiation, with people with light pigmentation having the greatest risk.

An excess risk of non-melanocytic skin cancer has been shown following exposure to ionizing radiation (in studies of medical personnel, uranium miners, radiotherapy patients, and atomic bomb survivors): the shape of the dose–response curve appears to be linear without threshold. Exposure to arsenic and its inorganic compounds has been linked to an excess of skin cancer in people exposed occupationally, from drinking water or from drugs used in the past. Mixtures of polycyclic aromatic hydrocarbons (coal tar, tar pitch, soot, creosote, lubricating and cutting oils) are also carcinogenic to the skin: an excess of non-melanocytic cancer has been shown in classical occupational epidemiological studies among workers such as chimney sweeps, machine operators, and roofers.

Skin cancer occurs in Asian countries as a consequence of burn scars produced by traditional heating devices kept in close contact to the skin: kangri in Kashmir, India, kairo in some areas of Japan, and kang in northern China. It is possible that polycyclic aromatic hydrocarbons released by the burning material interact with heat in causing the cancer. Other types of ulcer and scar, not related to heat, also predispose to skin cancer: they include for example chronic skin inflammation and infection by biological agents such as tuberculosis and leprosy.

Immunodeficiency increases the risk of squamous cell carcinoma of the skin, as it has been shown in patients treated with immunosuppressive drugs following renal transplant or other conditions. Xeroderma pigmentosum and the naevoid basal cell carcinoma syndrome are rare hereditary conditions characterized by a very high incidence of skin cancer. In the former syndrome, the mechanism is a reduced capacity to repair damage to DNA. The action of immunodeficiency and genetic predisposition may be via an enhancement of the carcinogenic effect of ultraviolet and ionizing radiation, since the neoplasms occur on parts of the body exposed to the sun.

Avoidance of sun exposure, in particular during the middle of the day, is the primary preventive measure to reduce the incidence of skin cancer. There is no adequate evidence of a protective effect of sunscreens, possibly because use of sunscreens is associated with increased exposure to the sun. The possible benefit in reducing skin cancer risk, however, should be balanced against possible beneficial effects of ultraviolet radiation in promoting vitamin D metabolism. Control of occupational skin carcinogens has taken place in many industries, although high exposure circumstances may still take place in developing countries. Avoidance of drinking water with a high arsenic level should be a priority in contaminated areas. Secondary prevention can be achieved by regular skin examination, in particular for high-risk individuals: however, there is a lack of controlled trials on skin cancer screening.

Malignant melanoma (Armstrong and English 1996)

Malignant melanomas occur most frequently on the trunk in men and on the lower limbs in women. While pathologists distinguish several histological types of melanoma, these are likely to represent different stages of the same condition. A special type of melanoma, however, is the rare lentigo malignant melanoma, which occurs on the head and neck, in areas with sun damage.

An estimated 133 000 new cases of malignant melanoma occurred worldwide in 2000 (Ferlay *et al.* 2001). The incidence is highest (of the order of 25 per 100 000) in Australia; it ranges between 5 and 10 per 100 000 in other parts of Oceania, North America, and northern and western Europe, and is below 5 per 1 000 000 in the other regions of the world. In general, the incidence is low in dark-skinned populations. In many white populations, there has been a sharp increase in incidence (3 to 7 per cent per year) during the last decades; this pattern was not observed in non-white populations. Although part of this trend might be explained by increasing awareness and improved diagnosis, it is likely that it largely reflects a true phenomenon. Studies of migrants have shown an increased risk following migration to a country with a sunny climate, such as Israel, South Africa, and Australia. Age at migration is an important determinant of risk, since people who migrated before the age of 10 years retain a risk similar to the risk of the country of origin, while other migrants approach the risk of the host country. The incidence of melanoma is very low before the age of 20 years, and increases linearly with age thereafter, thus showing a higher incidence in young adulthood than many other tumours. The increase with age is steeper for melanomas arising on the face, while the incidence of those on other parts of the body declines after middle age. Overall, there is little difference in risk between men and women, but during reproductive ages the incidence is higher among women.

There is strong evidence of a carcinogenic role of ultraviolet radiation in determining malignant melanoma. Intermittent exposure to the sun seems to play a more important role than total cumulative exposure. However, genetic or other factors, including 'ability to tan' may modify the dose–response relationship between sun exposure and melanoma risk. According to this model, the risk in poor tanners would be mainly determined by cumulative exposure while intermittency would be the main factor for good tanners. In most available studies, the relative risk among subjects in the highest category of usual or recreational exposure to the sun or history of sunburns was 2 to 6, as compared with subjects in the lowest category.

The evidence of an increased risk of melanoma following exposure to fluorescent lamps and other artificial sources of ultraviolet radiation is inadequate.

Colour of hair and eyes, and skin complexion, have been found in many studies to be risk factors for melanoma. Colour of hair seems to be the main predictor of risk, with relative risks in the range of 1.5 to 2 for blond hair and 2 to 4 for red hair as compared with dark or brown hair. Freckling is likely to be an additional risk factor. Skin response to sun exposure and propensity to burn (or poor ability to tan) have also been associated with melanoma risk, with a relative risk mainly in the range of 1.5 to 4. However, pale complexion and propensity to burn are strongly correlated, and the available data are inadequate to separate these two factors completely.

Presence of a high number of naevi is the strongest known risk factor for melanoma. Assessment of the number and type of naevi is not straightforward, and misclassification is likely to affect studies on naevi and melanoma. The relative risk is of the order of 10 for the category at highest number of naevi. Naevi are likely precursors for melanoma. Their number depends on sun exposure, in particular intermittent exposure and sunburns: exposure in childhood is more important than exposure in adulthood. In subjects with familial melanoma, large atypical naevi, referred to as dysplastic naevi, might be found. Individuals with dysplastic naevi and familial melanoma have a very high risk of melanoma. In subjects without familial melanoma, presence of dysplastic naevi seems to be a risk factor independent of number of total naevi.

The number of atypical naevi and the risk of melanoma are increased among immunosuppressed patients. There is no clear evidence of a role of any other risk factor, including dietary factors and exogenous hormones, in the aetiology of melanoma. There is a two- to fivefold increased risk of melanoma in subjects with an affected relative, which seems independent of exposure to solar radiation. Several putative high-risk genes have been proposed to explain the increased familial risk.

Avoidance of solar exposure, especially in childhood, is the only primary preventive measure that can be recommended at present. Use of sunscreen does not protect against melanoma risk. Early diagnosis, in particular of thin lesions, is associated with better survival; screening via medical examination is justified in high-risk individuals, defined according to familial history, type of skin, and reaction to solar radiation.

Kaposi's sarcoma

This form of slowly progressing cutaneous sarcoma was rare before the appearance of the HIV epidemic. The incidence of non-HIV-related Kaposi's sarcoma was highest in the Mediterranean basin and in Africa. No risk factors have been identified, although the lesion is more frequent in rural than in urban areas. Subjects (in particular of homosexual preference) infected with HIV have a high risk of Kaposi's sarcoma. A virus, denominated Kaposi's sarcoma herpes virus or human herpes virus 8, has been identified in HIV-positive cases (IARC 1996). The same virus has been detected in most analysed cases of non-HIV-related sarcoma and is likely to play a causal role in the development of most or all of Kaposi's sarcoma cases. The transmission of the herpes virus in HIV-infected individuals is likely to be via sexual contact: mode of transmission and cofactors in non-HIV individuals are unknown.

Cancer of the breast (Henderson *et al.* 1996)

Over 90 per cent of the neoplasms of the breast originate from the ductal epithelium, while a minority originates from the lobular epithelium. Survival from breast cancer has slowly increased in developed countries, where it now approaches 80 per cent at 5 years. It is unclear how much of the improvement is due to screening as compared with improved treatment. Survival in developing countries remains poor, of the order of 40 to 60 per cent (Sankaranarayanan *et al.* 1998).

Breast cancer is the most common cancer among women worldwide: the estimated number of new cases in 2000 was 579 000 in developed countries and 471 000 in developing countries (Ferlay *et al.* 2001). It is also the most important cause of neoplastic deaths among women, causing an estimated 373 000 deaths worldwide in 2000 (Ferlay *et al.* 2001). The incidence of breast cancer is low (less than 20 per 100 000) in most countries from sub-Saharan Africa, in China, and in other countries of east Asia, except Japan. The highest rates (70 to 90 per 100 000) are recorded in North America, Australia, and northern and western Europe, as well as in Brazil and Argentina. It is important to note that the incidence of breast cancer has grown rapidly during the last decades in many developing countries: for example in Arabic countries breast cancer was a rare disease until the 1970s, and it has now become the most frequent female neoplasm, with rates of the order of 30 per 100 000. In developed countries, incidence rates have slowly increased during recent decades, while mortality rates have remained fairly stable. The incidence increases linearly with age up to menopause, after which a further increase is less marked (developed countries) or almost absent (developing countries) (Fig. 8). Women from high social class have consistently higher rates than women from low social class, the difference being of the order of 30 to 50 per cent.

The cumulative number of regular ovulatory cycles increase the risk of breast cancer. Ecological and analytical studies have shown an increased risk for early age at menarche and late age at menopause. The risk doubles for a difference of 5 years in age at menarche and of 10 years in age at menopause. Similarly, artificial menopause exerts a protective effect.

Pregnancy increases the risk of breast cancer in the short term, probably because of increases in the level of free oestrogens during the first trimester. This effect is particularly strong at first pregnancy. In

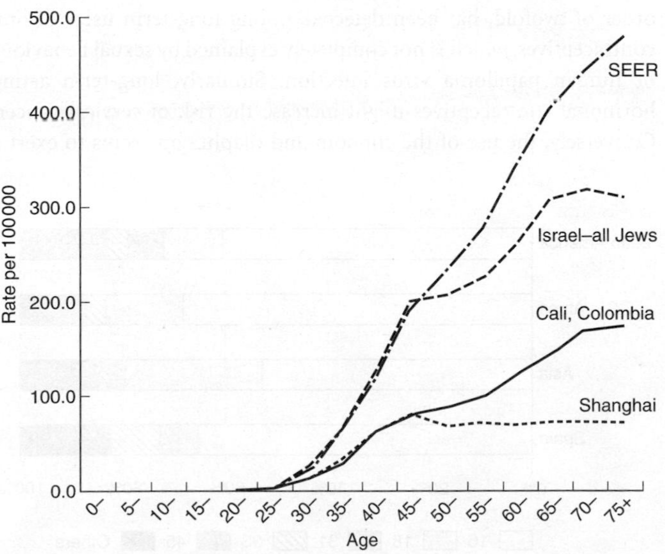

Fig. 8 Age-specific incidence rates of breast cancer in selected populations in the early 1990s.

the long run, however, pregnancy has a beneficial effect, since parous women have a higher level of prolactin and a lower level of sex hormone-binding globulin than nulliparous women. These two effects result in a protective role of early age at first pregnancy (and a small residual protective effect of additional pregnancies) and in an increased risk of women with late first pregnancy. A protective effect of lactation has been shown in several populations, which is probably attributable to the suppression of the ovulatory function caused by nursing. Furthermore, long-term use of hormone replacement therapy carries also an increased risk of breast cancer.

The combined evidence from reproductive factors indicates an important role of oestrogens in breast carcinogenesis. However, a direct assessment of the role of oestrogens can be made in prospective studies containing measurement of hormones made in prospectively collected biological samples and few results are currently available from such studies.

Women suffering from the two most common benign breast diseases, fibrocystic disease and fibroadenoma carry a two- to threefold increased risk of breast cancer. It is likely, however, that the lesions are not preneoplastic conditions, rather that epithelial proliferation, linked to hormonal alterations, is a feature they share with breast cancer.

A familial history of breast cancer in the mother or in a sister is associated with a two- to threefold increased risk of the disease. This role of familial history is likely to result from low-penetrance genes associated with hormonal metabolism and regulation, in particular several of the genes associated with steroid metabolism are polymorphic; and there is some evidence of an increased risk of breast cancer associated with polymorphisms of genes involved in hormone metabolism. In addition, breast cancer risk is greatly increased in carriers of mutations of several high-penetrance genes, in particular BRCA1, BRCA2, and p53. Although the cumulative lifetime risk in carriers of these genes might be as high as 80 per cent, they are rare in most populations and explain only a small fraction (2 to 5 per cent) of total cases. However, there are exceptions such as Ashkenazi Jews, among whom high-risk BRCA1 or BRCA2 mutations are responsible for an estimated 12 per cent of breast cancers.

Although a role of nutrition in breast cancer risk is strongly suggested by international comparisons, the combined evidence from epidemiological studies is only suggestive of a protective role exerted by high intake of fruits and vegetables, while the evidence is inconclusive for other dietary components, including intake of total fat, saturated fat and fibres, and total energy intake. Similarly, results on micronutrients have been elusive, although there is growing evidence of a protective role played by phyto-oestrogens. Hormonal level and nutritional factors during the intrauterine period and childhood are also likely to be important in breast carcinogenesis.

Many lifestyle factors have been investigated as possible causes of breast cancer. An increased risk with increasing weight has been consistently reported among women older than 60 years, but not among younger women. Drinking of three of more alcoholic drinks per day carries an increased risk of the order of 50 to 70 per cent. It is likely that both overweight and heavy alcohol drinking act on breast cancer risk through mechanisms involving hormonal level or metabolism. Tobacco smoking does not carry an increased risk of breast cancer. Studies of occupational factors and of exposure to organochlorine pesticides have failed to provide consistent evidence of an aetiological role.

About 1 per cent of all cases of breast cancer occur in men. The incidence provides limited evidence of geographical variations, with no clear correlation with incidence in women. Conditions involving high oestrogen level, such as gynaecomastia and sex chromatin positivity, are risk factors for breast cancer in men, as is high weight in youth.

Primary prevention of breast cancer has been attempted via nutritional intervention, involving reduction of energy intake, reduction of proportion of calories from fat, and increase in fruit and vegetable consumption. No evidence of efficacy has been produced so far. Tamoxifen, an anti-oestrogen drug used in chemotherapy, has shown a chemopreventive action against breast cancer, although the magnitude of the protection is uncertain. Conversely, tamoxifen increases the risk of endometrial cancer.

The most suitable approach for breast cancer control is secondary prevention through mammography. The effectiveness of screening by mammography in women older than 50 years has been demonstrated, and programmes have been established in various countries. The effectiveness of mammography in women younger than 50 years is not demonstrated. The benefit of other screening approaches, such as physical examination and self-examination, is not known (Moss 1999).

Cancer of the female genital organs

The female genital organs comprise the ovaries and their annexes, the uterus, the vagina, and the external genitals. The uterus is composed of two parts, the cervix and the corpus, which have very distinct physiological and pathological features. Cancers of the cervix and corpus of the uterus are different histologically, clinically, and aetiologically. However, the distinction between cervix and corpus is often neglected in records used for epidemiological purposes, such as death certificates. Today in Europe and North America, most cancers of the uterus without further specification are likely to be cancer of the corpus. This, however, may not have been the case in the past and in other countries, which complicates temporal and geographical comparisons.

Uterine cervix (Schiffman *et al.* 1996)

Cervical cancer is a major public health problem in many developing countries. Incidence rates are high (20 to 40 per 100 000) in sub-Saharan African and Latin American countries, as well as in India and southern Asia. In China, the Middle East, northern Africa, and developed countries, rates are of the order of 5 to 15 per 100 000. This results in a number of cases each year in excess of 471 000, 80 per cent of which occur in developing countries, where it represents the second most common female neoplasm after breast cancer (Ferlay *et al.* 2001). The number of estimated cancer deaths in developing countries (194 000 in 2000) exceeds that from breast cancer. Incidence and mortality rates have decreased steadily in developed countries, but an upturn has been observed among young women. Few data on temporal trends are available from developing countries, but incidence has likely decreased during recent decades. In high-risk countries, rates increase up to the age of 60 years, while in developed countries there is little increase above the age of 40. In most countries, cervical cancer hits preferentially women of lower education and social class.

Most cervical cancers originate from the area of squamous metaplasia called the transformation zone, which is adjacent to the junction between the columnar epithelium of endometrial origin and the keratinizing epithelium of vaginal origin. Most invasive cancers are squamous cell carcinomas or mixed adenosquamous tumours. Invasive carcinoma is preceded by inflammatory and condylomatous atypia, mild dysplasia (also called cervical intraepithelial neoplasia of grade 1), moderate dysplasia (cervical intraepithelial neoplasia grade 2), severe dysplasia and carcinoma *in situ* (which together represent cervical intraepithelial neoplasia grade 3). Atypia and cervical intraepithelial neoplasia grade 1 represent benign alterations due to infection with human papilloma virus, while cervical intraepithelial neoplasia grade 2 and 3 represent steps towards the malignant transformation.

Chronic infection with human papilloma virus is a necessary cause of cervical cancer. Using sensitive molecular techniques, virtually all tumours are positive for the virus, while the prevalence in non-diseased women represents 5 to 40 per cent in the different populations. Different types of human papilloma virus exist, and those associated with cervical cancer are mainly types 16, 18, 31, and 45. In particular, human papilloma virus 16 is a main carcinogen in many populations, while the distribution of other types varies by geographical region (Fig. 9). Differences in prevalence of human papilloma virus infection explain much of the descriptive epidemiology of cervical cancer (geographical patterns, high risk in low social class, and so on). The host response to human papilloma virus infection is important in determining its possible carcinogenic effect; immunosuppression, as present in transplanted patients and HIV-infected individuals, increases the risk of dysplasia and carcinoma *in situ*.

Sexual characteristics of women (early age at first sexual intercourse and high number of sexual partners, in particular before the age of 20 years) and of their male partners (high number of sexual partners, presence of genital diseases, and contact with prostitutes) have been found to be risk factors for cervical cancer in many populations. They mainly reflect an increased likelihood of human papilloma virus infection, in particular at a young age.

Studies of infection with other agents, in particular *Chlamydia* and herpes simplex 2, have failed to provide consistent evidence of an effect independent of human papilloma virus. An increased risk, of the order of twofold, has been detected among long-term users of oral contraceptives, which is not completely explained by sexual behaviour or human papilloma virus infection. Similarly, long-term acting hormonal contraceptives might increase the risk of cervical cancer. Conversely, the use of the condom and diaphragm seems to exert a

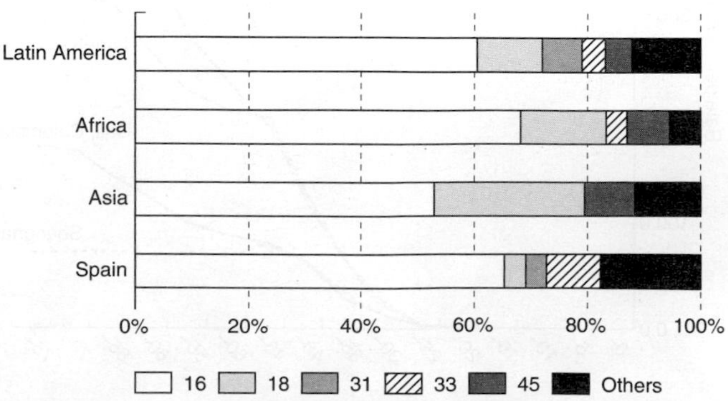

Fig. 9 Prevalence of human papilloma virus types in cases of cervical cancer, by region. (Source: N. Muñoz, personal communication.)

protective effect, possibly via prevention from human papilloma virus infection.

The carcinogenic effect of tobacco smoking that was suggested by early studies has not been confirmed once human papilloma virus infection was taken into account. A possible protective effect of a diet rich in fruits and vegetables has been suggested in several studies, an effect that might be due to increased intake of carotenoids or folate.

Cytological examination of exfoliated cervical cells (the Papanicolaou smear test) is effective in identifying precursor lesions, resulting in a decrease in incidence of and mortality from invasive cancer. The benefit is of the order of a two- to fourfold decreased incidence. There is no conclusive evidence, however, regarding the optimal timing of the test. Cytological smears are not applicable, however, in countries with limited availability of cytologists and pathologists, as in many countries with a high prevalence of human papilloma virus infection and a high incidence of invasive cancer. Alternative approaches for secondary prevention have therefore been proposed, including visual inspection of the cervix with possible enhancement of precursor lesions by acetic acid. Use of human papilloma virus testing as a screening method, either as a first choice for general application or as the triage method of inconclusive cytological diagnoses, is also under trial. The primary method for prevention of cervical cancer, however, would be human papilloma virus vaccination. Several vaccines are currently under development; this work is complicated by the geographical variations in the distribution of human papilloma virus types.

Uterine corpus (Grady and Ernster 1996)

Cancer of the endometrium is the main malignant neoplasm of the uterine corpus, while sarcomas, originating from the muscular tissue, are relatively rare. The descriptive epidemiology of cancer of the uterine corpus is complicated by the large proportion of hysterectomized women in industrialized countries (up to 30 per cent in some birth cohorts of women from the United States). The number of new cases occurring in 2000 worldwide was estimated of the order of 189 000, of which 60 per cent occur in developed countries. The number of cancer deaths is of the order of 45 000 (Ferlay *et al.* 2001). Rates are relatively high (10 to 15 per 100 000) in Europe, North America, Brazil, and Argentina, as well as in Australia, while they are below 5 per 100 000 in most African countries and in southern and eastern Asia. In high-risk countries, the incidence increases up to 60 years of age, and is stable or declines above that age. In the United States, the incidence is higher in white people as compared with black people, while the opposite applies to mortality. The incidence of endometrial cancer is declining in developed countries; few data on trends are available from other countries.

Nulliparity, infertility, and late age at menopause are associated with a two- to threefold increased risk of endometrial cancer. The evidence regarding other reproductive factors is less consistent. Elevated levels of endogenous oestrogens (e.g. in the case of oestrogen-secreting tumours and polycystic ovarian syndrome) are associated with an increased risk of endometrial cancer. However, studies of blood oestrogen level were inconclusive.

An increased risk of endometrial cancer was reported in the 1970s following the use of sequential oral contraceptives. Conversely, combined contraceptives reduce the risk of endometrial cancer by about 50 per cent. Use of oestrogen replacement therapy is associated with a twofold increase in risk of endometrial cancer. The strength of the association depends on the dose and the duration of use; the relative risk is in excess of 5 for 5 or more years of use of products with 1.25 mg or more of conjugated oestrogen. Addition of progestin to oestrogen replacement therapy may protect from the increased risk of endometrial cancer, but it may also reduce the beneficial effects of oestrogens on cardiovascular disease and osteoporosis. An increased risk of endometrial cancer has also been shown among breast cancer patients treated with tamoxifen: it is unclear at present whether in non-high-risk women the protective effect of tamoxifen on breast cancer outweighs the increased risk of endometrial cancer.

An increased risk of endometrial cancer has been consistently reported among obese and fat women as compared with lean women; the magnitude of the relative risk between the top and the bottom quartile of distribution of weight or body mass is of the order of 2, but it can be as high as 5 for the most obese individuals. An increased risk has also been reported among women with diabetes, which does not seem to be fully explained by increased weight in these patients. A decreased risk of endometrial cancer, of the order of 50 per cent, has been reported among smokers in many populations: this result has been attributed to an anti-oestrogenic activity of smoking. The results of studies of diet and endometrial cancer have been somewhat inconsistent: a possible increased risk may occur following low intake of fruits and vegetables and high intake of saturated fat. Several other potential risk factors have been addressed, including alcohol drinking, hypertension, and history of gallbladder disease, without conclusive evidence of a causal association.

Although changes in the composition of oral contraceptives and oestrogen replacement drugs have probably contributed to the prevention of endometrial cancer in the last decades, no strategy for primary prevention exists, beside the recommendation to reduce weight. Secondary prevention through endometrial cytological sampling has been proposed, but there is no evidence of a benefit of screening asymptomatic women.

Ovary (Weiss *et al.* 1996)

Most malignant neoplasms of the ovary originate from the coelomic epithelium; less frequent tumours originate from the germ cells (dysgerminomas and teratomas) and the follicular cells (granulosa cell tumours). The estimated number of new cases worldwide in 2000 was 192 000, that of deaths was 114 000 (Ferlay *et al.* 2001). High incidence rates (of the order of 10 to 12 per 100 000) are found in western and northern Europe and in North America; the lowest rates (below 3 per 100 000) are from China and central Africa. The rates increase up to about the age of 60 years, after which they remain stable. In high-risk countries the rates have remained stable in recent decades.

Pregnancy protects against ovarian cancer, probably through reduction in secretion of gonadotropins. The reduction in risk is of the order of 30 to 60 per cent for three or more pregnancies as compared with none. The same mechanism can be invoked to explain the protective effect exerted by breast feeding which, however, has not been consistently found in all studies. Similarly, the use of oral contraceptives has been consistently shown to protect from ovarian cancer: each year of use carries approximately a 10 per cent decrease in risk. On the contrary, there is no consistent evidence that use of hormonal replacement therapy has an effect on ovarian cancer risk.

The role of hormonal factors in ovarian cancer is unclear; a reduction in risk has been shown following hysterectomy, which might be due to removal of subclinical tumours. A similar reduction in risk, however, has been observed following tubal ligation. The risk of germ cell tumours is increased in girls and young women exposed to exogenous hormones *in utero*.

An increased risk of ovarian cancer has been reported in relation to high body mass (relative risk of the order of 2 in the highest versus the lowest group), although the evidence is not fully consistent. Similarly, an effect of pregestational body weight of mothers has been shown for germ cell ovarian cancers.

The evidence regarding an effect of diet on ovarian cancer risk is largely inconsistent. A possible protective effect of a diet rich in fruits and vegetables has been suggested. Atomic bomb survivors have an increased risk of ovarian cancer, as have women exposed to irradiation following benign pelvic conditions: an effect of exposure to low-level ionizing radiation, however, has not been shown. Early suggestions of an increased risk of ovarian cancer among women exposed to asbestos are now interpreted as resulting from misclassification of peritoneal mesotheliomas. A possible association has been suggested between perineal use of talc and ovarian cancer risk.

The prevention of ovarian cancer is currently hampered by the limited knowledge of its causes and the lack of availability of early diagnostic techniques.

Vagina and vulva (Daling and Sherman 1996)

The incidence of vaginal and vulvar cancers ranges between 0.5 and 2.5 per 100 000: high rates are reported from Europe and North America, while low rates are recorded in eastern Asia. The incidence of vulvar cancer is about three times that of vaginal cancer. They are mainly squamous cell carcinomas; rare types are melanoma, sarcoma, and clear cell adenocarcinoma. Their incidence increases exponentially through life.

Infection with human papilloma virus is the best known risk factor for these cancers, with a relative risk of 10 or greater. Human papilloma virus 16 is the most commonly reported type. Other sexually transmitted diseases have been reported more frequently among cases of vulvar cancer than controls: they include syphilis, infection with herpes simplex type 2, and lymphogranuloma venereum. The evidence, however, is based on few studies that have not controlled for concomitant human papilloma virus infection. Similarly, the associations reported with early age at first intercourse and number of sexual partners might simply reflect human papilloma virus infection.

Pelvic irradiation for cervical cancer or other diseases is another risk factor for vaginal and vulvar cancers. The occurrence of these neoplasms is associated with the presence of other cancers in the anogenital tract; this phenomenon might be explained by human papilloma virus infection at several sites. An association between tobacco smoking and vulvar and vaginal cancers has been suggested in a few studies, which did not control for human papilloma virus infection.

Clear cell adenocarcinoma of the vagina is a rare tumour occurring in girls and young women, mainly following *in utero* exposure to diethylstilboestrol, a synthetic oestrogen used between 1940 and 1970 in several countries. An increased risk of the order of twofold has also been reported for squamous cell carcinoma of the vagina and cervix.

Control of human papilloma virus infection is likely to be an important primary preventive measure for these as well as other anogenital cancers. Screening through visual inspection of high-risk women is recommended.

Cancer of the male genital organs

Prostate (Ross and Schottenfeld 1996)

Cancer of the prostate shows considerable geographical variability. It is the most common malignant neoplasm in men from North America, where the incidence is as high as 100 per 100 000. In other developed countries, the incidence is of the order of 20 to 40 per 100 000, and in most developing countries it is below 30 per 100 000, and it can be as low as 5 per 100 000 in southern and eastern Asia. The estimated number of new cases occurring worldwide in 2000 is about 543 000 (Ferlay *et al.* 2001). Mortality rates show less variability among regions, suggesting that the number of non-fatal cases diagnosed in different countries varies depending on screening and other diagnostic procedures. The estimated number of deaths is 204 000, of which two-thirds occur in developed countries. The incidence of prostate cancer increased slowly during the last decades in most populations; in the United States and Canada, a very rapid increase has been observed since the mid-1980s. Mortality has also been increasing in most countries, although in the last year a decline has been shown in North America. The disease is more common in African-Americans than in European Americans. In most countries, it is more common among affluent groups of the population.

Increased testosterone level in serum has been reported as a risk factor for prostate cancer in several retrospective studies. However, these results might be due to altered hormonal level related to the development of the tumour. The available prospective studies failed to provide convincing evidence of an increased risk linked to increased levels of testosterone or other sexual hormones. Similarly, an increased risk of prostate cancer was reported in retrospective studies following a history of benign prostatic hypertrophy, but no excess risk was found in prospective studies. If an association exists between prostatic hypertrophy and cancer, it could be due to shared aetiological factors or to a common pathological process.

Carriers of BRCA1 and BRCA2 mutations have a four- to fivefold increased risk of prostate cancer. Generally, a history of prostate cancer in first-degree relatives carries a two- to threefold increased risk of developing the same neoplasm. Similar associations, of smaller magnitude, are also suggested for a family history of breast and colon cancers.

It has been shown in several populations that the risk of the disease increases with the number of sexual partners and number of encounters with prostitutes, and with previous history of syphilis and gonorrhoea. Serological studies of human papilloma viruses 16 and 18 have shown an increased risk among positive subjects. It is not clear at present, however, whether syphilis and human papilloma virus are causal factors or markers of infection with other sexually transmitted agents. A possible increased risk following vasectomy has been reported in some studies: other investigations, however, have failed to confirm this association, and no conclusions can be drawn at present.

A possible protective role of high intake of vegetables has been shown in several studies; high intake of meat, dairy products, total fat, and saturated fat might represent a risk factor. The evidence concerning other dietary factors, including fruit intake and intake of specific micronutrients, is inconclusive at present, with the possible exceptions of lycopene, a retinoid present in particular in tomatoes which has been found to be associated with a reduced risk in several studies, and calcium which has been associated with an elevated risk. There is also a suggestion of an increased risk among individuals with elevated serum levels of insulin-like growth factor 1. An increased risk of the disease has been repeatedly reported among subjects with a high weight or body mass.

The wide geographical variability of prostate cancer strongly suggests that environmental factors probably related to diet and other lifestyle factors, such as physical activity, are the main determinants of the disease. Primary prevention, however, is hampered by the fragmentary knowledge of its precise causes. Secondary prevention has been proposed, based on digital rectal examination and measurement of prostate-specific antigen. There is no evidence from controlled trials that either procedure decreases the mortality from prostate cancer. Despite this lack of evidence, these procedures, in particular the prostate-specific antigen testing, have gained popularity in many countries, and are most likely the cause of the steep increase in number of diagnosed cased since the mid-1980s in North America. It is unclear whether the decrease in mortality reported since the mid-1990s in the United States can be attributed to a beneficial effect of unplanned use of prostate-specific antigen testing.

Testis (Schottenfeld 1996)

Some 95 per cent of malignant neoplasms of the testes arise from the germinal tissue. About half of the germinal neoplasms are seminomas, while the remaining comprise teratomas and a variety of rare lesions. Testicular cancer is common at a young age, and its incidence decreases after the age of 30 years (Fig. 10). Teratomas and other non-seminomatous neoplasms predominate before the age of 15 years, after which most tumours are seminomas. Incidence rates are high (3 per 100 000 or more) in the northern part of South America and western Europe, and are low (1 per 100 000 or less) in most of Africa and in eastern and southern Asia. In the United States, rates are higher in European Americans than in African Americans. The global number of new cases in 2000 has been estimated at 49 000, that of deaths at 8700. The incidence has increased in most countries during the last decades, with evidence of a birth cohort effect. In many

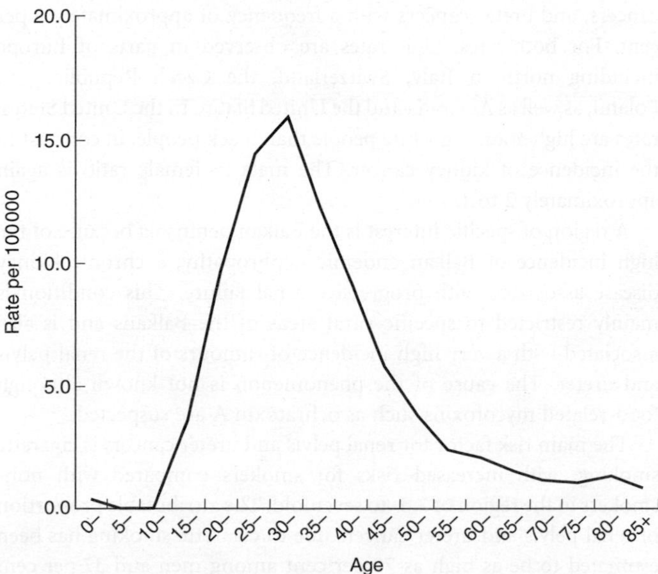

Fig. 10 Age-specific incidence rates of testicular cancer in white Americans, 1988 to 1992. (Source: Parkin *et al.* 1997.)

countries, the risk is higher in the more affluent groups of the population.

Cryptorchism is the best known cause of testicular cancer. The relative risk is of the order of 3 to 10; this risk factor might be responsible for up to 10 per cent of all cases of testicular cancer. The risk is lower when orchiopexy is performed before the age of 10 years than at older ages. This finding suggests that micro-environmental factors might be responsible for the development of cancer in the undescended testis. Several rare diseases in gonadal differentiation, including Klinefelter's syndrome, increase the risk of non-germinal tumours of the testis. Familial aggregation has also been shown for different types of testicular cancer.

Exposure to elevated oestrogen levels during pregnancy, from either endogenous or exogenous origin, might be a risk factor for testicular cancer, although the evidence of an association is not fully consistent among studies.

The limited knowledge about the causes of testicular cancer makes it difficult to devise effective preventive strategies, with the exception of early surgical treatment of cryptorchism.

Penis (Wideroff and Schottenfeld 1996)

Cancer of the penis comprises mainly squamous cell carcinomas, which are commonly preceded by intraepithelial lesions, including Queyrat's erythroplasia and Bowen's disease. The neoplasm in more common (rates of the order of 2 to 4 per 100 000) in Latin America and in south and Southeast Asia, and is rare (0.5 to 1 per 100 000) in North America and Europe. In developed countries, incidence declined during the last decades.

Chronic infection with human papilloma virus is the most important risk factor for penile cancer: the proportion of positive cases is of the order of 90 per cent. Human papilloma virus type 16 is the most frequently found, followed by types 18, 31, 33, and 35. Although the distribution of penile cancer and penile intraepithelial neoplasia parallels the distribution of the corresponding cervical lesions in women, the incidence is generally lower, suggesting differences in either tissue susceptibility or in the role played by cofactors.

A decreased risk of penile cancer has been reported among circumcised men, in particular among those operated on in infancy. The most likely explanation of this effect is a protection against human papilloma virus infection; however, the available studies do not clearly exclude a possible confounding effect of low-risk sexual behaviour. Furthermore, a high risk of penile cancer (relative risk of the order of 10 to 30) has been found among men with phimosis, in particular when it is associated with balanoposthitis (inflammation of the glans penis and prepuce).

Patients treated with oral 8-methoxypsoralen and ultraviolet A radiation for psoriasis or other skin disorders are at increased risk of penile and scrotal cancer, with a relative risk of the order of 50. The carcinogenic effect is attributable to the combination therapy rather than to the skin disease.

Prevention of human papilloma virus infection through vaccination would be the most important preventive measure for penile cancer. Human papilloma virus testing might be used for screening of high-risk individuals. A beneficial effect of circumcision remains unproven. Prevention of exposure to ultraviolet radiation of the genitals might also be beneficial.

Cancer of the urinary organs

The urinary organs comprise the kidneys (renal parenchyma), renal pelvis, ureter, urinary bladder, and urethra. The majority of urinary cancers occur within the bulk of the kidney (renal parenchyma) and bladder. Cancers of the renal pelvis, ureter, and urethra are much rarer and less well studied and are, for statistical purposes, often grouped under kidney cancers. However, these tumours are histologically more similar to those of the bladder than the renal parenchyma, and their aetiology is also likely to be more similar to the aetiology of bladder cancer.

Kidney (McLaughlin *et al.* 1996)

Worldwide, there were approximately 189 000 kidney cancers in 2000, two-thirds of which occurred in developed countries (Ferlay *et al.* 2001). The vast majority of cancers which arise in the renal parenchyma are adenocarcinomas, although nephroblastoma (Wilms' tumour) occurs in children. The highest incidence of renal cell cancers are observed in the Czech Republic, with rates of approximately 15 per 100 000 in men and 7.5 per 100 000 in women. High rates are also observed in parts of Italy and Poland, and among some black populations of the United States. Conversely, rates up to 10 times lower are reported in most Asian and African populations and some, but not all, South American populations. The incidence in males is approximately twice that among females in most populations. The incidence of kidney cancer increases logarithmically from the age of 30 years and plateaus around the age of 60. Strong increasing trends in kidney cancer are occurring among all Caucasian populations and in Japan. Some of the most steep increases are observed among black Americans. It is unlikely that these increasing trends can be explained by increasing detection of presymptomatic tumours and are instead likely to reflect real increases in the number of new cases.

Cigarette smoking has been consistently observed to be a moderate risk factor for kidney cancer, with increased risks compared with never smokers of the order of 1.2 to 2.3. A number of studies have also demonstrated a dose–response relationship with increasing consumption, with risks for heavy smokers ranging from 2.0 to 3.0. The risk appears to decline with increasing years of smoking cessation. Population attributable risk estimates indicate that cigarette smoking, both past and present, is responsible for between 27 and 37 per cent of kidney cancer cases among men, and between 10 and 24 per cent of cases among women. Approximately half of this attributable risk is due to current smoking.

Obesity has been consistently linked with kidney cancer, especially among women, with less consistent and weaker results among men. The mechanism by which obesity causes kidney cancer is unclear, although hormonal changes such as increased levels of endogenous oestrogens may be responsible. Other correlates of obesity, such as hypertension and lack of physical exercise, have not been found to explain this relationship. The population attributable risk of kidney cancer associated with excess weight (defined as being in one of the last three quartiles of body mass index) has been estimated to be over 40 per cent in women and 5 per cent in men.

A history of hypertension has also been linked to kidney cancer, although the strength of this relationship has generally been greatly reduced after adjustment for use of diuretics and other antihypertensive drugs. These findings suggest that use of medications may be the primary risk factor and not hypertension *per se*. Both diuretic and non-diuretic antihypertensive medications have been linked to kidney cancer, with supportive evidence from animal studies. However, identifying whether the real risk is due to the hypertensive state or due to antihypertensive medication has not so far been possible. Whichever of the two is the real risk factor, it is likely to account for a substantial proportion of cases. The attributable risk of reported hypertension or treatment with antihypertensive drugs has been estimated to be 21 per cent overall, and 39 per cent among women.

High protein consumption from meat and dairy products has been associated with chronic renal conditions that may predispose to kidney cancer, and has been weakly associated with an increased risk of kidney cancer of between 30 and 70 per cent, although the evidence is inconsistent. A possible protective effect has also been identified in a number of studies for high consumption of vegetables.

An excess risk of renal cell cancer has been observed in a variety of occupations with exposure to polycyclic aromatic hydrocarbons such as coke and coal oven workers, fire-fighters, and asphalt and tar workers. Excess risks have also been reported for occupations with exposure to gasoline and other petroleum products such as oil refinery workers and petrol station attendants. Exposure to organic solvents and in particular to chlorinated liphatic hydrocarbons has also been suggested as a risk factor in occupations including dry-cleaning and printing. Overall however, the evidence for associations with specific occupational exposures is still inconclusive.

The main avoidable causes of kidney cancer are cigarette smoking and excess body weight, which together account for up to 50 per cent of all cases. Primary prevention in reducing cigarette smoking and obesity are therefore the clearest strategies for reducing the incidence of the disease. A substantial proportion of cases are also likely to be related to hypertension although further information on whether the true risk factor is the disease or the treatment is required in order to clarify implications for prevention.

Renal pelvis and ureter (McLaughlin *et al.* 1996)

Renal pelvis and ureter cancers are mainly transitional cell carcinomas as opposed to adenocarcinomas of the kidney. Renal pelvis cancers occur with approximately 10 per cent of the frequency of renal cell cancers, and ureter cancers with a frequency of approximately 5 per cent. For both sites, high rates are observed in parts of Europe including northern Italy, Switzerland, the Czech Republic, and Poland, as well as Australia and the United States. In the United States, rates are higher among white people than black people, in contrast to the incidence of kidney cancer. The male to female ratio is again approximately 2 to 1.

A region of specific interest is the Balkan peninsula because of the high incidence of Balkan endemic nephropathy, a chronic kidney disease associated with progressive renal failure. This condition is mainly restricted to specific rural areas of the Balkans and is also associated with a very high incidence of tumours of the renal pelvis and ureter. The cause of the phenomenon is not known although food-related mycotoxins such as ochratoxin A are suspected.

The main risk factor for renal pelvis and ureter cancers is cigarette smoking, with increased risks for smokers compared with non-smokers in the region of 2.5- to sevenfold. The attributable proportion of renal pelvis and ureter cancers due to cigarette smoking has been estimated to be as high as 70 per cent among men and 37 per cent among women.

A consistent relationship has also been observed between use of phenacytic containing drugs and cancer of the renal pelvis, with relative risks varying from 2.4-fold to over 12-fold (IARC 1987), and also some evidence of a dose–response relationship. Because of concern over links between nephropathy and phenacetin use, it has been removed from analgesics in most industrialized countries, starting in the late 1960s.

Because of the high proportion of renal pelvic and ureter tumours caused by cigarette smoking, especially current smoking, encouraging current smokers to give up will probably result in a substantial reduction in the number of cases.

Bladder (Silverman *et al.* 1996)

Bladder cancer accounts for approximately two-thirds of all urinary tract cancers with 336 000 cases worldwide in 2000, approximately 50 per cent of which occurred in developed countries (Ferlay *et al.* 2001). The male to female ratio of 3 to 1 is higher than for kidney cancer. The vast majority of bladder cancers are transitional cell carcinomas, with the exception of bladder cancers related to schistosomiasis infection, which are mainly squamous cell carcimonas. High bladder cancer rates are observed throughout southern and western Europe, Scandinavia, the United States, and Australia, although also in Israel, Egypt, and Uruguay. These high rates generally reflect those countries with high levels of cigarette smoking in the past, with the exception of Egypt where most cases are related to infection with *Schistosoma*. Bladder cancer incidence is either rising moderately or is steady in most developed countries, probably reflecting past cohort effects in tobacco consumption.

The most important risk factor for bladder cancer is cigarette smoking and is thought to account for approximately 66 per cent of new male cases and 30 per cent of female cases in industrialized populations. It is likely that smokers of black tobacco are at a higher risk than smokers of blond tobacco and this may explain some of the disparity observed in European incidence rates and also the high incidence observed in Uruguay. The risk associated with smoking is likely to be due to aromatic amines present in cigarette smoke, including benzidine, 4-aminobiphenyl, naphthylamine, and 4-chloro-*O*-toluidine. Bladder cancer risk increases approximately linearly with duration of smoking, reaching a fivefold risk after 5 years. A substantial decrease in risk of bladder cancer is observed within several years for those who gave up smoking, implying a late stage effect in the carcinogenic process.

A high risk of bladder cancer has also been reported among industries which involve exposure to aromatic amines, in particular 2-naphthylamine and benzidine, including the rubber and dyestuff industries. Other occupations which may increase the risk of bladder cancer include leather workers, painters, and drivers, possibly because of exposure to a variety of chemicals including polycyclic aromatic hydrocarbons, polychlorinated biphenyls, formaldehyde, and solvents. The uncertainty surrounding these occupations is again partly due to the difficulty of measuring past exposure to specific chemical agents.

Investigations of diet have provided evidence of decreased risks associated with fruits and vegetable intake, and also some inconsistent evidence of an increased risk associated with coffee consumption. Reasons for the lack of consistency of this latter exposure include the small sample size of many studies and the possibility of residual confounding from other risk factors including cigarette smoking.

The enzyme *N*-acetyl transferase 2 is involved in the detoxification of various bladder carcinogens including arylamines. Its gene includes a dominant mutation which results in slow metabolization and in higher risk of bladder cancer.

Similar to the renal pelvis, a consistent relationship has been observed between use of phenacytic containing drugs and bladder cancer, with relative risks varying from 2.4-fold to over sixfold (IARC 1987). Cyclophosphamide, an alkylating agent which has been used to treat both malignant and non-malignant diseases has also been linked to bladder cancer. Studies based on cohorts of cancer patients indicate an increase in risk of approximately fivefold associated with cyclophosphamide therapy, with higher risks among heavily exposed subjects.

Schistosoma infection is prevalent throughout Africa and is associated with an increased risk of approximately fivefold. Cases associated with *Schistosoma* infection are mainly of the squamous cell type. They are responsible for an estimated 10 per cent of bladder cancer cases in the developing world, and about 3 per cent of cases overall. Some studies have reported an increased risk with history of repeated urinary tract infection among both men and women. Bladder infection was more strongly associated with squamous cell bladder cancer. This relationship, however, needs to be confirmed in further studies.

Regarding prevention, avoidance of cigarette smoking is the most effective public health measure against bladder cancer. Approximately 60 per cent of bladder cancer cases are due to smoking, at least half of which· could be prevented by smoking cessation among current smokers. Prevention of *Schistosoma* infection through avoidance of contaminated waters is important in endemic areas. No effective screening approach is available for bladder cancer.

Cancer of the nervous organs

Eye

Neoplasms of the eye are rare: the incidence is below 1 per 100 000 in all regions of the world, with the exception of central and southern Africa. The main histological types are squamous cell carcinoma, arising from the conjunctiva; retinoblastoma, which arises in children and is relatively common in Africa; and uveal melanoma, which is the main adult type outside Africa. Solar radiation is a cause of conjunctiva carcinoma and uveal melanoma. About 50 per cent of cases of retinoblastoma are caused by an inherited mutation in the Rb gene.

Nervous system (Preston-Martin and Mack 1996)

Over 90 per cent of nervous system neoplasms arise from the brain and the cranial meninges. Data on the descriptive epidemiology of neoplasms of the nervous system are difficult to interpret because of inconsistent inclusion of benign tumours in different series of cases.

Gliomas arise from the glial cells and are classified pathologically as astrocytomas (low grade) and glioblastomas (high grade). They represent 40 to 60 per cent of primary tumours of the brain and cranial meninges, are predominantly malignant, and are more common in men. Meningiomas arise from the cranial meninges and represent 20 to 35 per cent of brain neoplasms, while schwannomas (or neurilemmomas) arise from the Schwann cells of the nerve sheath (mainly of the eight cranial acoustic nerves) and represent 5 to 10 per cent of all brain neoplasms. These two latter types are mainly benign. Rare types of nervous system neoplasms include pituitary adenomas, childhood primary neuroectodermal tumours (also called medulloblastoma), and tumours of the spine and the peripheral nerves.

The incidence of brain tumours is slightly higher in men than in women; the male to female ratio is approximately 1.5 for gliomas and 0.6 for meningiomas. There is a 10-fold geographical variability in the incidence of brain neoplasms; rates in men are above 6 per 100 000 in most countries from the Americas, Europe, and Oceania, and are below 2 per 100 000 in most African countries and in China. In the United States, rates of gliomas are 30 to 50 per cent higher in white people than in other ethnic groups, while rates of meningiomas are higher in black people. The incidence of gliomas tends to be higher among people from high socio-economic groups.

During the last decades, incidence and mortality from brain tumours have increased in most developed countries. For example, during 1973 to 1987 incidence increased in the United States by 23 per cent and mortality by 9 per cent. However, it is likely that part, if not all, of the increase is due to changes in diagnostic and reporting procedures.

Ionizing radiation is the only established environmental risk factor for brain tumours. It causes all three major types of central nervous system tumours, but the association is stronger for meningioma and schwannoma than for glioma. The evidence comes mainly from studies of atomic bomb survivors and of patients given X-ray therapy in the head and neck region. Head trauma has been suggested as a risk factor for meningioma, and acoustic trauma (as in the case of jobs with exposure to loud noise) as a risk factor for acoustic schwannoma. *N*-nitroso compounds, in particular nitrosoureas, are potent experimental brain carcinogens, but the evidence of an aetiological role in humans is inconclusive.

Tumours of the central nervous system occur frequently in rare congenital syndromes, such as neurofibromatosis types 1 and 2, von Hippel–Lindau syndrome, and Li–Fraumeni syndrome.

The very limited knowledge about the aetiology of tumours of the central nervous system offers scarce resources for an effective preventive strategy.

Cancer of the endocrine glands

Thyroid (Ron 1996)

An estimated 71 000 new cases of thyroid cancer occurred in 2000 among women, and 33 000 among men (Ferlay *et al.* 2001). In most areas of the world, the incidence among women is in the range 2 to 5 per 100 000, that in men is between 1 and 2 per 100 000. High-risk areas (incidence over 5 per 100 000 in women) include Central America, Japan, and the Pacific Islands. International comparisons, however, are complicated by possible differences in diagnostic procedures. The most common thyroid neoplasm (50 to 80 per cent of the total) is papillary carcinoma, followed by follicular carcinoma (10 to 40 per cent) and medullary carcinoma (5 to 15 per cent). The incidence of thyroid cancer is very low before the age of 15 years, above which it increases linearly with age, resulting in relatively high rates in young adulthood. In certain populations (e.g. the United States), the incidence in women declines after the age of 50.

Survival from thyroid cancer is very good (a 78 per cent 5-year survival rate in Europe in the early 1990s), resulting in low mortality rates (below 1.2 per 100 000 in women and 0.6 per 100 000 in men in most countries).

In most countries, incidence rates have been stable or have been slowly increasing (less than 1 per cent per year) during the last decades; mortality rates have steadily declined, probably because of improved treatment.

Ionizing radiation during childhood is the main established risk factor for thyroid cancer. The carcinogenic effect seems greater for exposure before the age of 5 years than between 5 and 15 years of age. The pooled analysis of studies of individuals irradiated in childhood for medical conditions and atomic bomb survivors resulted in a summary excess relative risk of 7.7 (95 per cent confidence interval 2.1 to 29) per Gray, and an excess absolute risk of 4.4 (95 per cent confidence interval 1.9 to 10) per 10 000 person years Gray (Ron *et al.* 1995). An effect of external exposure during adulthood is not established. Several studies have been published on adults exposed to iodine-131 for medical purposes. Although these studies suggest an increased risk, their interpretation is complicated by the fact that these patients were treated because of thyroid diseases. Iodine-131 was the main exposure resulting from the accident of the Chernobyl nuclear reactor in 1986; since then, an increased incidence of thyroid cancer has been reported among children living in the contaminated areas of Belarus and Ukraine. Although part of the excess might be due to increased medical surveillance, it is likely that it also reflects a true phenomenon. Studies of occupational exposure to low-level ionizing radiation, typically in the nuclear industry, have failed to show an increased incidence of thyroid cancer.

The higher incidence of thyroid cancer in women as compared with men and the age-specific rates in women suggest a role of reproductive factors in the development of the disease. A number of studies have shown a moderately increased risk (relative risk of the order of 1.5) in women with more pregnancies and in women with a history of miscarriage. The exact role of hormonal and reproductive factors, however, in unclear. Elevated levels of thyroid-stimulating hormones are associated with thyroid growth and possibly thyroid cancer. The evidence of an association between iodine deficiency (and presence of endemic goitre) and thyroid cancer is equivocal; studies from central and southern Europe support such an association, but is not confirmed in studies from northern Europe and North America. It is possible that iodine deficiency increases the risk of follicular thyroid cancer, while the papillary type is linked to an iodine-rich diet. An increased risk of thyroid cancer has been associated in many studies to a history of thyroid nodules: some of the nodules, however, might represent preneoplastic lesions.

A strong genetic component has been shown for medullary carcinoma: about 20 per cent of these neoplasms are associated with an autosomal dominant gene with penetrance close to 100 per cent. It can also be associated with other endocrine neoplasms within the multiple endocrine neoplasia syndromes. Familial factors also play a role in papillary carcinoma. Among the genes associated with thyroid cancer are the ret proto-oncogene (for papillary and medullary carcinomas) and the APC gene for papillary carcinoma.

A possible role of dietary factors in thyroid carcinogenesis has been addressed in many studies. High intake of vegetables, in particular cruciferous vegetables, might protect against the disease, possibly through interference with iodine metabolism. The evidence regarding other dietary factors is inconclusive.

The prospects for prevention of thyroid cancer are complicated by the limited understanding of its aetiology, with the exception of relatively rare high-risk conditions, such as childhood exposure to ionizing radiation and high-risk families.

Endocrine glands

Malignant neoplasms of endocrine glands other than the thyroid are rare in most populations. The incidence rates range between 0.1 and

1 per 100 000 people. About two-thirds of these neoplasms arise from the adrenal gland. About one-third of these tumours are carcinomas, and the remaining proportion shows different histological patterns.

Genetic susceptibility plays a relatively important role for this group of neoplasms: in particular, adrenocortical carcinoma is found in cases of Li–Fraumeni syndrome, and malignant phaeochromocytoma is found in multiple endocrine neoplasia type 2 and the von Hippel–Lindau syndromes. Tobacco smoking has been associated with an increased risk of adrenal cancer in a few studies. The evidence for a carcinogenic role of other factors is inconclusive.

Neoplasms of the lymphatic and haematopoietic organs

The term lymphoma encompasses a diverse group of neoplasms which originate from the cells of the lymphopoietic system. Traditionally, two main groups of lymphomas have been distinguished including Hodgkin's disease, characterized by large polynuclear cells named after Reed and Sternberg, and a diverse group of other lymphomas, defined as non-Hodgkin's lymphomas. The complexity of lymphomas is reflected by the various classifications that have been used to separate different subtypes. The most recent classification system, the Revised European American Lymphoma classification and its adaptation by the World Health Organization (**WHO**) represents an effort to reach a wide medical consensus to allocate all lymphoma cases in clear categories. Neoplasms are divided between B- and T-cell lymphocytes, with over 20 different clinicopathological entities. Importantly, this classification incorporates all lymphoproliferative diseases, including multiple myeloma, B-cell acute lymphoblastic leukaemia, Burkitt's lymphoma, and Hodgkin's disease. Given that the Revised European American Lymphoma classification has only been in use for a number of years, it is necessary to discuss the characteristics of lymphomas and leukaemias under the traditional groups of Hodgkin's disease, non-Hodgkin's lymphoma, multiple myeloma, and leukaemia.

Hodgkin's disease (Mueller 1996)

The incidence of Hodgkin's disease varies from low-incidence populations, with rates lower than 1 per 100 000, including areas of southern and eastern Asia and of sub-Saharan Africa, to high-incidence populations, with rates of the order of 3 per 100 000 found in the United States, in certain European regions such as Italy, and in Jews in Israel. The incidence in men is consistently higher than in women with a ratio of between 1.5 and 2. The incidence has been relatively stable over time and may even be declining. The age of onset of Hodgkin's disease shows a bimodal distribution in developed populations with a first peak between the age of 15 and 35 years and a second peak after the age of 60. In developing countries the first peak tends to be observed during childhood. This bimodal distribution may suggest that the category of Hodgkin's disease includes at least two different entities.

Viral infections play an important role in the aetiology of Hodgkin's disease. Its onset may be related to decreased or delayed exposure to infectious agents during childhood, as indicated by its association with having fewer siblings, living in single-family houses, and early birth order.

Epstein–Barr virus infection is associated with a large proportion, and potentially all, of Hodgkin's disease cases, although its aetiological role remains to be fully established. Epstein–Barr virus is, however, ubiquitous throughout the world with 80 to 100 per cent of individuals being infected by the age of 30 (IARC 1997*a*). In developing countries infection occurs earlier in life, whereas in developed countries infection is often delayed until adolescence. The Epstein–Barr virus genome is present in about 50 per cent of the Reed–Sternberg cells of cases, and another Epstein–Barr virus-related condition, infectious mononucleosis, is associated with a moderately elevated risk of subsequent development of Hodgkin's disease. Sero-epidemiological studies indicate that patients with Hodgkin's disease can be distinguished by an altered antibody profile to Epstein–Barr virus. All of this evidence taken together argues against Epstein–Barr virus simply being a passenger virus, and for a causal association in the development of the disease.

There is only limited evidence of other possible risk factors for Hodgkin's disease. Employment in the wood and chemical industries may entail an increased risk of Hodgkin's disease although the responsible carcinogens, if any, have not been identified.

Non-Hodgkin's lymphoma (Scherr and Mueller 1996)

The incidence of non-Hodgkin's lymphoma is consistently higher than the incidence of Hodgkin's disease. High rates of over 10 per 100 000 are reported from the United States, Australia, western Europe, and from Israel and the Middle East, while low rates of less than 5 per 100 000 are reported from southern and eastern Asia and parts of Africa. Men have a 1.5 to twofold higher incidence than women. There is a strong geographical variation of incidence rates for some lymphoma subgroups. For example, Burkitt's lymphoma is common among children in eastern Africa, and adult T-cell leukaemia/lymphoma is increased in southern Japan and parts of Africa. Conversely, the trend of non Hodgkin's lymphoma shows a steady increase with age in most populations. Exceptions are the populations in which a specific type of lymphoma predominates, such as Burkitt's lymphoma in children.

A striking feature of the epidemiology of non-Hodgkin's lymphoma is the consistently increasing incidence which has been observed in all developed countries. The rate of increase for non-Hodgkin's lymphoma has been approximately 4 per cent per year in most populations where accurate data are available, indicating a doubling of incidence every 20 years. The reasons for the increase in non-Hodgkin's lymphoma incidence have been widely discussed and it is possible that improvement in diagnostic procedures explains part of it, particularly in the elderly. However, it is now accepted that the trend also reflects a real increase in the number of cases, the cause of which is not known.

The current knowledge of potential risk factors for non-Hodgkin's lymphoma is limited. However, there is strong evidence that altered immunological function, either immunostimulation or immunosuppression, entails an increased risk of non-Hodgkin's lymphoma. For example, immunosuppressed renal transplant patients have a risk 30 times higher for developing lymphoma compared with the general population. Lymphomas that develop in immunosuppressed patients share common characteristics. They are generally high-grade B-cell lymphomas and are more likely to be extranodal and of worse prognosis. Lymphomas have also been reported for a variety of other conditions which are either autoimmune in nature, or require immunosuppressive treatment, including rheumatoid arthritis and Sjögren's syndrome.

Infectious agents associated with non-Hodgkin's lymphoma include HIV, human T-cell lymphotropic virus 1, and Epstein–Barr virus. Hepatitis C virus, human T-cell lymphotropic virus 2, and human herpes viruses 6 and 8 have also been linked to the development of non-Hodgkin's lymphoma. In addition, infection with *H. pylori* is a risk factor for gastric lymphoma.

Epstein–Barr virus is particularly prominent in lymphomas developing in immunosuppressed patients, and also in Burkitt's lymphomas. The relationship with other forms of lymphoma is, however, unclear. Regarding HIV, non-Hodgkin's lymphoma is 60 times more frequent among patients with AIDS than in the general population (IARC 1996). About 3 per cent of the patients with AIDS develop a non-Hodgkin's lymphoma, which represents a small contribution to the overall incidence of non-Hodgkin's lymphoma, except in populations with a high HIV prevalence such as regions of sub-Saharan Africa. The AIDS-related lymphomas tend to be high-grade B-cell lymphomas.

Human T-cell lymphotropic virus 1, and possibly type 2, appear to be associated with the rare adult T-cell leukaemia/lymphoma, a disease entity with strong geographical clustering in Japan, the Caribbean, and parts of Africa. Transmission of the human T-cell lymphotropic virus is similar to that of HIV, involving vertical (mother-to-child) transmission, sexual contact, or blood transfusion.

A familial aggregation is present for both non-Hodgkin's lymphoma and Hodgkin's disease: the risk of non-Hodgkin's lymphoma among first-degree relatives of cases has been reported of the order of 1.5 to 4. However, the risk seems higher for siblings of the same sex, suggesting a role of shared environmental factors rather than genetics. Highly penetrant genetic predisposition to lymphomas is not very common but include ataxia telangiectasia, Wiskott–Aldrich syndrome, and hypogammaglobulinaemia. Approximately 25 per cent of the patients with rare forms of genetic immunodeficiency will develop a lymphoma.

The increasing recreational exposure to ultraviolet radiation in some populations and the decrease in the atmospheric ozone layer have been related to the observed increase in the incidence of non-Hodgkin's lymphoma. This hypothesis is supported by cancer registry data which show a strong link between non-Hodgkin's lymphoma and skin cancers, including the frequent occurrence of non-Hodgkin's lymphoma both before and after skin cancer in the same individual. The hypothesis that exposure to ultraviolet light also causes lymphoma has not been proven but it is biologically plausible as there is experimental evidence showing that ultraviolet light radiation produces systemic suppressive effects on the immune system.

Exposure to pesticides has been associated with non-Hodgkin's lymphoma risk in studies conducted both on manufacturing workers and applicators in agriculture. The results, however, are not very compelling, with the possible exception of phenoxy herbicides and chlorophenols. This effect might be due to contamination with dioxin. Farming as an occupation has also been weakly associated with non-Hodgkin's lymphoma risk. It is not clear whether this risk, if present, is accounted for by exposure to ultraviolet radiation, pesticides, or animal viruses. Organic solvents represent another group of chemicals whose association with non-Hodgkin's lymphoma risk has been widely investigated. Only for tetracholorethylene, however, is the evidence somewhat consistent.

Multiple myeloma

Multiple myeloma is a malignancy of the plasma cells with a variable manifestation. High-incidence areas of around 4 per 100 000 include North America, western Europe, and Oceania. Low rates of around 1 to 2 per 100 000 are reported in most of Asia, although part of this may be due to underdiagnosis. Within the United States, black people have approximately double the incidence rate of white people, with the incidence approaching 10 per 100 000 in some areas. Whether this increase among black Americans is due to genetic or environmental effects is unknown. In most populations incidence rates are higher in men although the ratio is usually less than 2. Multiple myeloma rates are very rare among young adults although the incidence increases exponentially from the age of 30 years and plateaus after 60 years of age. It also appears that the incidence of myeloma is increasing, although these trends are difficult to judge and may be due to diagnostic artefacts.

The only established risk factor for multiple myeloma is monoclonal gammopathy of unknown significance, an asymptomatic non-malignant disorder involving proliferation of plasma cells. The increased risk associated with monoclonal gammopathy of unknown significance appears to be of the order of 10-fold, although the lifetime absolute risk is still relatively low (less than 5 per cent). Other conditions have also been reported to be associated with myeloma including rheumatoid arthritis and allergies, although the evidence is inconclusive.

Ionizing radiation has also been reported to be associated with myeloma although results are again inconsistent. Occupational groups which have been reported to have higher myeloma rates include painters and farmers, which might be due to exposure to benzene, other solvents, and pesticides.

Leukaemia

Leukaemias arise in one of the types of white blood cells. They may arise in lymphoblasts, which are lymphoid cells in the early stage of development, resulting in a rapid onset illness termed acute lymphoblastic leukaemia. Alternatively, when the neoplasm involves mature cells, it is termed chronic lymphocytic leukaemia and is usually more sedate. Leukaemias may also be granulocytic in origin, occurring in either young myeloblast cells resulting in acute myeloid leukaemia, or in the mature granulocytes resulting in chronic myeloid leukaemia. There also exist several rarer varieties including monocytic and hairy cell leukaemias.

Acute lymphoblastic leukaemia is the most common childhood cancer, while over 80 per cent of lymphoid leukaemias occurring in adulthood are chronic lymphocytic leukaemia. Incidence rates for chronic lymphocytic leukaemia are difficult to interpret because it is often diagnosed incidentally, or in the course of evaluating other conditions. Differences in medical care may therefore substantially bias incidence data. Bearing this possible ascertainment bias in mind, the highest rates of lymphoid leukaemias are observed in areas of Canada, the United States, western Europe, and Oceania, and are lower in South America the Caribbean, Asia, and Africa. Rates tend to be lower in females although the ratio is usually less than 2. Some increases in leukaemia over time have been reported although the extent to which these represent real increases in incidence is unclear. Some increasing incidence trends have been reported for both chronic myeloid leukaemia and acute myeloid leukaemia, although these are not consistent and may simply reflect changes in diagnostic practices.

Although the cause of most leukaemias is not known, there does exist consistent evidence for two factors, namely ionizing radiation and occupational benzene exposure. Leukaemia was the first cancer to be linked to ionizing radiation after the atomic bombings in Hiroshima and Nagasaki, and clear excesses have been observed for acute lymphoblastic leukaemia, acute myeloid leukaemia, and chronic myeloid leukaemia, but not for chronic lymphocytic leukaemia. Cohorts of patients who have received radiotherapy for both malignant and non-malignant conditions have also been found to be at an increased risk of leukaemia, usually myeloid. Whether there is any increased risk of leukaemia from other sources, including low-level diagnostic radiation, occupational exposure in the nuclear industry for workers and their offspring, or nuclear test explosions, is more contentious. Part of the problem lies in extrapolating from high acute doses experienced in particular circumstances like atomic bomb exposures in Japan, to small or chronic exposures in other instances. There is no consistent evidence that exposure to electromagnetic fields is associated with leukaemia risk.

Some leukaemias are also induced by therapy for a prior malignancy, most notably Hodgkin's disease. Such patients have a 20- to 40-fold increased risk of leukaemia, most of which are acute myeloid leukaemia. The risk appears to be related to chemotherapy including alkylating agents (in particular mechlorethamine, Oncovin, procarbazine, and prednisone combination therapy). The effect is greater when patients are treated with both chemotherapy and radiotherapy, although whether an independent effect exists for radiotherapy is unclear. Other chemotherapy regimes which appear to be associated with acute myeloid leukaemia are those which contain the epipodophyllotoxin drugs teniposide and etoposide.

Occupational benzene exposure is also a recognized cause of leukaemia, in particular for acute myeloid leukaemia. An increased risk of between three- and fivefold has been observed in several occupational cohorts of benzene-exposed workers, including workers in rubber manufacturing, petrol refinery, and printing. Tobacco smoking is a suspected cause of leukaemia.

Prevention

The limited knowledge of the causes of lymphatic and haematopoietic neoplasms limits the opportunity for prevention. Avoidance of known risk factors (e.g. unnecessary radiation exposure, benzene) is likely to result in the prevention of a small proportion of these neoplasms in most populations.

Overview of the causes of human cancer

Figure 11 presents the results of a recent review of the contribution of known causes of cancer in the United States (Harvard Center for Cancer Prevention 1996). This picture broadly applies to other developed countries, while no systematic estimate has been proposed for developing countries. These results, however, are subject to many uncertainties and should be interpreted as approximations.

Tobacco smoking

Tobacco smoking is the main single cause of human cancer worldwide (Chapter 10.1). It is a cause of cancers of the lung, larynx, oral cavity, pharynx, oesophagus, pancreas, kidney, and bladder. It is also a suspected cause of cancers of the nasal cavity and stomach, and of leukaemia. Tobacco smoking has been estimated to cause approximately 30 per cent of all human cancers (Doll and Peto 1981; Harvard Center for Cancer Prevention 1996). However, a detailed review of the number of cancers attributable to tobacco smoking in 1985, which was based on very strict criteria for attribution of cases, resulted in a lower estimate, of the order of 15 per cent, corresponding to about 1 100 000 new cases per year (Parkin *et al.* 1994). This figure should be considered a conservative estimate, and the actual proportion of cancers is likely to be higher. The estimates by Parkin and colleagues were 25 per cent in men and 4 per cent in women and, in both genders, they were 16 per cent in developed countries and 10 per cent in developing countries. The low attributable risk in women (and, to a less extent, in developing countries) is due to the low consumption of tobacco in past decades: the recent upward trend that has taken place among women and in many developing countries will obviously result in a much greater numbers of cancer in the future.

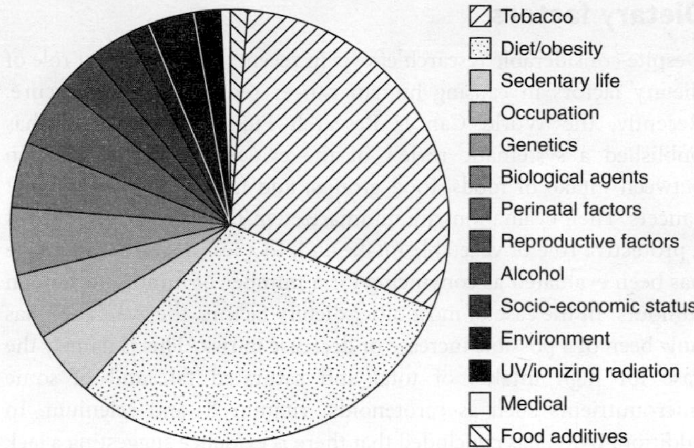

Fig. 11 Proportion of neoplasms attributable to established causes in the United States. (Source: Harvard Center for Cancer Prevention 1996.)

A benefit of quitting tobacco smoking in adulthood has been shown for all major cancers causally associated with the habit. This result emphasizes the need to devise antismoking strategies that address avoidance of the habit among the young as well as reduction of smoking and quitting among adults. In fact, the decline in tobacco consumption that has taken place during the last 20 years among men in North America and several European countries, and which has resulted in decreased incidence of and mortality from lung cancer, has resulted primarily from the increase in quitting at middle age. The great challenge for the control of tobacco-related cancer, however, lies today in developing countries, in particular in China and the other Asian countries: the largest increase in tobacco-related cancers has been forecasted in this region of the world (Peto *et al.* 1999). Despite growing efforts from medical and public health institutions and the growing involvement of non-governmental organizations, the fight against the spread of tobacco smoking among women and in developing countries remains the biggest and most difficult challenge of cancer prevention in the next decades.

Use of smokeless tobacco products has been associated with increased risk of head and neck cancer. Chewing of tobacco-containing products is particularly prevalent in southern Asia, where it represents a major carcinogenic factor.

Dietary factors

Despite considerable research efforts in recent years, the exact role of dietary factors in causing human cancer remains largely obscure. Recently, the World Cancer Research Fund (WCRF 1997) has published a systematic review of the evidence of an association between intake of foods, food groups, and nutrients, and different cancers. Their evaluations are summarized in Table 4. The evidence of a protective role of vegetable intake and, to a less degree, fruit intake has been evaluated as convincing for a number of important human tumours. In the case of most other dietary factors, the evaluation has only been of a possible increase or decrease in risk. This is namely the case for high intakes of total and saturated fat, and of some micronutrients such as carotenoids, vitamin E, and selenium. In addition, IARC has concluded that there is evidence suggesting a lack of cancer-preventive activity for preformed vitamin A (IARC 1998*b*) and for β-carotene when used at high doses (IARC 1998*a*). Despite the limitations of the current understanding of the role of diet in human cancer, systematic reviews have been consistent in suggesting that dietary factors are responsible for about one-third of human cancers, at least in developed countries (Doll and Peto 1981; Harvard Center for Cancer Prevention 1996). The only justified dietary recommendation for cancer prevention is to increase the consumption of vegetables and fruits. A reduction in total caloric intake, however, would contribute to a decrease in obesity, which is also an established risk factor for human cancer (see below).

Obesity and physical exercise

Obesity increases the risk of endometrial cancer and probably the risk of postmenopausal breast cancer and kidney cancer (WCRF 1997). An association is possible also for gallbladder and colon cancer. It is likely that obesity exerts a carcinogenic effect in conjunction with other factors such as insulin resistance, low physical activity, and menopausal status. The magnitude of the excess risk is not very high (for most cancers the relative risk ranges between 1.5 and 2 for body weight higher than 35 per cent above the ideal weight); the attributable risk might be large because of the high prevalence of overweight people. Although no detailed assessments of the risk of cancer attributable to obesity worldwide are available, obesity represents an important target for preventive strategies.

Increased workplace or recreational physical activity decreased the risk of colon cancer and possibly the risk of lung and breast cancer (WCRF 1997). The relative risk of colon cancer for regular versus no activity is of the order of 2. Increasing physical activity should be part of any comprehensive cancer prevention strategy.

Alcohol

Alcohol drinking increases the risk of cancers of the oral cavity, pharynx, larynx, oesophagus, and liver. An association is probable in the case of colon, rectal, and breast cancer (IARC 1988; WCRF 1997). For all cancer sites, risk is a function of the amount of alcohol consumed. Alcohol drinking and tobacco smoking show an interactive effect on the risk of cancers of the head and neck. The evidence of a different effect of various alcoholic beverages is inconclusive at present. Although no systematic review of attributable risks to alcohol drinking is available, it has been estimated to account for 4 to 5 per cent of total cancers (Fig. 11).

Infectious agents

There is growing evidence that chronic infection with some viruses, bacteria, and parasites represents a major carcinogenic factor for humans, in particular in developing countries. A number of infectious agents have been evaluated within the IARC monograph programme (Table 5), and the evidence of a causal association has been classified as sufficient for several of them. Pisani *et al.* (1997) provided global estimates of the number of cases of cancer attributable to biological agents. Their estimate for 1990 is 1 454 000 cases, or 15.6 per cent of total cancers. hepatitis B and hepatitis C virus related liver cancer, human papilloma virus related cervical cancer, and *Helicobacter*-related stomach cancer each provide approximately 30 per cent of the total. Because of the high prevalence of hepatitis B, hepatitis C, and human papilloma virus in developing countries, the estimate of the attributable risk is higher in this part of the world (20.8 per cent of total cancer versus 9.1 per cent in developed countries).

Use of safe, effective, and cheap vaccines represents the best preventive strategy for cancers caused by viruses. Unfortunately, only hepatitis B virus infection can be effectively prevented today. Chronic infection with *H. pylori* can be prevented by antibiotic treatment and sanitation measures, and changes in dietary practices (e.g. avoidance of raw fish) can prevent infection by carcinogenic parasites.

Occupational and environmental agents

IARC have classified approximately 25 occupational and environmental agents, groups of agents, and mixtures as carcinogenic (IARC 1972–2001). Another 20 compounds are classified as probable carcinogens (Table 6). While some (e.g. mustard gas) represent today a historic curiosity, exposure is still widespread for carcinogens such as asbestos, coal tar, arsenic, and silica. Estimates of the global burden of occupational and environmental cancer result in figures of the order of 4 to 5 per cent (Doll and Peto 1981; Harvard Center for Cancer Prevention 1996). It should be stressed, however, that these cancers concentrate among exposed subjects (mainly male blue-collar workers), among whom they may represent up to 20 per cent of total cancers (Boffetta *et al.* 1995). Furthermore, unlike lifestyle factors, exposure is involuntary and can largely be avoided. In fact, reduction of exposure to occupational and environmental carcinogens has taken place in industrialized countries during recent decades. Efforts should be made to avoid exposure also in developing countries.

The available evidence suggests, in most populations, a small role of purely environmental sources of exposure to carcinogens (air, water, soil pollution). Global estimates are of the order of 1 per cent or less of total cancers. This is in contrast with public perception, which often identifies environmental pollution as a major cause of human cancer. It should be stressed, however, that in selected areas (e.g. residence near asbestos processing plants or in areas with drinking water contaminated by arsenic), environmental exposure to carcinogens may represent an important cancer hazard.

Reproductive factors

The evidence of a carcinogenic effect of reproductive factors is strongest for breast cancer: early age at menarche, late age at first pregnancy, and late age at menopause are all associated with a 1.5- to twofold increased risk (Harvard Center for Cancer Prevention 1996). In addition, nulliparity increases the risk of ovarian and possibly

Table 4 Assessment of associations between dietary factors and human cancer (WCRF 1997)

Factor (high intake)	Oral cavity and pharynx	Oesophagus	Lung	Stomach	Pancreas	Liver	Colon and rectum	Breast	Ovary	Cervix	Endometrium	Prostate	Kidney	Bladder
Starch				–Po			+ Po							
Fibre				–In	–Po		–Po	–Po						
Sugar					+ In		+ Po							
Total fat			+ Po				+ Po	+ Po	+ In		+ In	+ Po		+ In
Saturated fat			+ Po				+ Po	+ Po	+ In		+ Po	+ Po		
Cholesterol			+ Po		+ Po			= Pr			+ In			
Animal protein								+ In						
Carotenoids		–Po	–Pr	–Po			–Po	–Po	–In	–Po	–In			–In
Vitamin C	–Po	–Po	–Po	–Pr	–Po		–In	–In		–Po		= Po		–In
Retinol			= Po	= Po				= Po		= Po				–In
Vitamin E			–Po	= Po			–In	= Po		–Po				
Folate							–In			= Po				
Selenium			–Po	–In		- In	= Po							
Iron						+ In	+ In							
Vitamin D							–In							
Calcium							= Po							
Allium compounds				–Po										
Cereals							–In							
Whole grain cereals				–Po										
Refined cereals		+ Po												
Vegetables	–Co	–Co	–Co	–Co	–Pr	–Po	–Co	–Pr	–Po	–Po	–Po	–Po	–Po	–Pr
Fruits	–Co	–Co	–Co	–Co	–Pr			–Pr	–Po	–Po	–Po			–Pr
Meat					+ Po		+ Pr	+ Po				+ Po	+ Po	
Eggs					+ In		+ Po		+ In				= Po	= Po
Fish							= Po	–In	–In					
Milk and dairy products												+ Po	+ Po	
Coffee				+ Pr	= Pr		–In	= Co				= Po	= Pr	+ Po
Maté	+ Po	+ Po												
Black tea				= Pr				= Po					= Pr	=Pr
Green tea				–Po										

+, Increased risk; –, decreased risk; =, no relationship.

Co, convincing evidence of an association; In, insufficient evidence to assess the association; Po, possible association; Pr, probable association.

Table 5 Assessment of associations between infections and human cancer

	Evidence	Target organs[a]	IARC monograph volume
Viruses			
Hepatitis B virus	S	Liver	59
Hepatitis C virus	S	Liver	59
Hepatitis D virus	I	Liver	59
Human papilloma virus types 16, 18	S	Cervix, anus, penis	64
Human papilloma virus types 31, 33	L	(Cervix)	64
Human papilloma virus, other types	I		64
Human immunodeficiency virus 1	S	Kaposi's sarcoma, non-Hodgkin's lymphoma	67
Human immunodeficiency virus 2	I		67
Human T-cell lymphotrophic virus I	S	Adult T-cell leukaemia/ lymphoma	67
Human T-cell lymphotrophic virus II	I		67
Epstein–Barr virus	S	Burkitt's lymphoma, Hodgkin's disease, nasopharynx	70
Human herpes virus 8	L	(Kaposi's sarcoma)	70
Bacterium			
Helicobacter pylori	S	Stomach	61
Parasites			
Schistosoma haematobium	S	Bladder	61
Schistosoma japonicum	L	(Liver, stomach)	61
Schistosoma mansoni	I		61
Opistorchis viverrini	S	Liver	61
Opistorchis felineus	I		61
Clonorchis sinensis	L	Liver	61

I, inadequate; L, limited; S, sufficient.

[a]Established target organs with no parentheses; suspected target organs in parentheses.

Data from IARC 1994*a* (Vol. 59), 1994*b* (Vol. 61), 1995 (Vol. 64), 1996 (Vol. 67), and 1997*a* (Vol. 70).

Table 6 Occupational agents, classified by the IARC monographs programme as carcinogenic to humans

Agents, mixture, circumstance	Main industry, use
Agents, groups of agents	
4-Aminobiphenyl	Pigment
Arsenic and arsenic compounds	Glass, metal, pesticide
Asbestos	Insulation, filter, textile
Benzene	Chemical, solvent
Benzidine	Pigment
Beryllium and beryllium compounds	Aerospace
Bis(chloromethyl)ether and chloromethyl methyl ether	Chemical intermediate
Cadmium and cadmium compounds	Dye/pigment
Chromium[VI] compounds	Metal plating, dye/pigment
Dioxin	Chemical
Ethylene oxide	Sterilant
2-Naphthylamine	Pigment
Nickel compounds	Metallurgy, alloy, catalyst
α- and γ-radiation	Medical
Radon and its decay products	Mining
Silica, crystalline	Stone cutting, mining, glass, paper
Talc containing asbestiform fibres	Paper, paints
Vinyl chloride	Plastics
Mixtures	
Coal-tar pitches	Construction, electrode
Coal-tars	Fuel
Mineral oils, untreated	Metal
Soots	Pigment
Wood dust	Wood
Exposure circumstances	
Aluminium production	
Coal gasification[a]	
Coke production	
Haematite mining (underground) with exposure to radon	
Iron and steel founding	
Painter (occupational exposure)	

[a]Production of gas from distillation of coal.

endometrial cancer. The evidence regarding other types of cancer is inadequate. No detailed estimates are available of the contribution of reproductive factors to the global burden of cancer. Some authors have, however, proposed figures of the order of 3 per cent (Harvard Center for Cancer Prevention 1996).

Perinatal and growth factors

Excess energy intake early in life is possibly associated with breast and colon cancer. The role of attained height, growth factors, and other factors such as insulin resistance or sensitivity in this association is unclear. In addition, high birth weight is possibly associated with an increased risk of breast and prostate cancer. The implications of these findings for preventive strategies will be clarified by a more detailed understanding of the underlying carcinogenic mechanisms (Harvard Center for Cancer Prevention 1996).

Ionizing and non-ionizing radiation

Ionizing radiation causes acute lymphoblastic leukaemia, acute myeloid leukaemia, chronic myeloid leukaemia, and breast, lung, and thyroid cancer. Bone, rectal, and brain cancer may develop following prolonged therapeutic exposure. There is evidence of a linear dose–response relationship between radiation dose and cancer risk. However, levels at which people are commonly exposed to man-made radiation in most countries carry little risk and the main exposure is to natural radiation, including indoor radon. The estimates of the global contribution of ionizing radiation to human cancer are in the range of 1 to 3 per cent (Harvard Center for Cancer Prevention 1996).

Solar (ultraviolet) radiation is carcinogenic to the skin, and it might increase the risk of other neoplasms such as non-Hodgkin's lymphoma because of immunosuppression. Over 90 per cent of skin neoplasms are attributable to sunlight; because of the low fatality of non-melanocytic skin cancer, solar radiation is responsible for only 1 to 2 per cent of total cancer deaths (Harvard Center for Cancer Prevention 1996). Avoidance of sun exposure, in particular during childhood, is an important cancer preventive behaviour. The evidence of a carcinogenic effect of other types of non-ionizing radiation, in particular electric and magnetic fields, is inconclusive.

Medical procedures and drugs

The drugs that may cause or prevent cancer fall into several groups. Many cancer chemotherapy drugs are active on the DNA, in order to block the replication of cancer cells. This, however, might result in damage to normal cells, including cancer transformation. The main neoplasm associated with chemotherapy treatment is leukaemia, although also the risk of solid tumours might be increased. A second group of carcinogenic drugs includes immunosuppressive agents, notably used in transplanted patients. Non-Hodgkin's lymphoma is the main neoplasm caused by these drugs. Replacement oestrogen therapy used in the past to treat menopausal symptoms increases the risk of endometrial cancer. Current hormone therapies include a progestin, which inhibits endometrial growth. It is unclear whether combined replacement therapies are associated with an increased risk of cancer. Oral contraceptives reduce the risk of ovarian and endometrial cancer, although it probably increases the risk of liver cancer. Phenacetin-containing analgesics increase the risk of cancer of the renal pelvis.

No precise estimates are available for the global contribution of drug use to human cancer. It is unlikely, however, that they represent more than 1 per cent in developed countries. Furthermore, the benefits of therapies are usually much greater than the potential cancer risk.

Table 7 European code against cancer

Certain cancers may be avoided and general health improved if you adopt a healthier lifestyle
1. Do not smoke. Smokers, stop as quickly as possible and do not smoke in the presence of others. If you do not smoke, do not try it
2. If you drink alcohol, whether beer, wine, or spirits, moderate your consumption
3. Increase your daily intake of vegetables and fresh fruits. Eat cereals with a high fibre content frequently
4. Avoid becoming overweight, increase physical activity, and limit intake of fatty foods
5. Avoid excessive exposure to the sun and avoid sunburn especially in children
6. Apply strictly regulations aimed at preventing any exposure to known cancer-causing substances. Follow all health and safety instructions on substances which may cause cancer
More cancers may be cured if detected early
7. See your doctor if you notice a lump, a sore which does not heal (including in the mouth), a mole which changes in shape, size, or colour, or any abnormal bleeding
8. See your doctor if you have persistent problems, such as a persistent cough, persistent hoarseness, a change in bowel or urinary habits or an unexplained weight loss
For women
9. Have a cervical smear regularly. Participate in organized screening programmes for cervical cancer
10. Check your breasts regularly. Participate in organized mammographic screening programmes if you are over 50 years of age

Use of ionizing radiation for diagnostic purposes is likely to carry a small risk of cancer, which has been demonstrated only for childhood leukaemia following intrauterine exposure. Radiotherapy increases the risk of cancer in the irradiated organs. There is no clear evidence of an increased cancer risk following other medical procedures, including mammography and surgical implants.

Genetic factors

A number of inherited mutations of a high-penetrance cancer gene increases dramatically the risk of some neoplasms (see sections on specific neoplasms). However, these are rare conditions in most populations and the number of cases attributable to them is rather small.

Familial aggregation has been shown for most types of cancers, in non-carriers of known high-penetrance genes. This is notably the case for cancers of the breast, colon, prostate, and lung. The relative risk is of the order of 2 to 4, and is higher for cases diagnosed at a young age. Although some of the aggregation can be explained by shared risk factors among family members, it is plausible that a true genetic component exists for most human cancers. This takes the form of an increased susceptibility to exogenous carcinogens. The knowledge of low-penetrance genes responsible for such susceptibility is still very limited, although research has currently focused on genes encoding for metabolic enzymes, DNA repair, and hormone receptors. Current estimates of the global contribution of genetic factors to human cancer are in the range of 5 to 10 per cent, of which less than 1 per cent is attributable to high-penetrance genes.

Conclusion

Neoplasms are a group of diverse diseases with complex distributions in human populations and with different aetiological factors. Current knowledge of the causes of human neoplasms and the development of control strategies have led to the elaboration of lists of recommendations for their prevention (Table 7). A comprehensive strategy for cancer control might lead to the avoidance of a sizeable proportion, possibly up to one-half of human cancers (Sikora 1999). However, such a strategy would imply major cultural, societal, and economic changes. More modest objectives for cancer prevention should focus on the neoplasms and the exposures that are prevalent in any given population. For example, vaccination of children against hepatitis B virus is likely to be the most cost-effective cancer prevention action in many countries of Africa and Asia.

Neoplasms will continue to be a major source of human disease and death. Considerable efforts are made in the public and private domains to develop effective therapeutic approaches. Even if major discoveries in the clinical management of cancer patients are accomplished in the near future, the changes will mainly affect the affluent parts of the world. Prevention of the known causes of cancer remains the most promising approach in reducing the consequences of cancer, in particular in countries with limited resources. Control of tobacco smoking and of smokeless tobacco products, increased consumption of fruits and vegetables, avoidance of obesity, moderation in alcohol intake, increased physical activity, avoidance of exposure to solar radiation, and control of known and suspected occupational carcinogens are the main approaches to reduce the burden of human neoplasms.

References

ACS (American Cancer Society) (2000). *Cancer facts and figures 2000*. American Cancer Society, Atlanta, GA.

Albertini, R.J. and Hayes, R.B. (1997). Somatic cell mutations in cancer epidemiology. In *Applicaton of biomarkers in cancer epidemiology*. IARC Scientific Publications No. 142 (ed. P. Toniolo, P. Boffetta, D.E.G.

Shuker, N. Rothman, B. Hulka, and N. Pearce), pp. 159–84. International Agency for Research on Cancer, Lyon.

Anderson, K.E., Potter, J.D., and Mack, T.M. (1996). Pancreatic cancer. In *Cancer epidemiology and prevention* (ed. D. Schottenfeld and J.F. Fraumeni Jr), (2nd edn), pp. 725–71. Oxford University Press, New York.

Armstrong, B.K. and English, D.R. (1996). Cutaneous malignant melanoma. In *Cancer epidemiology and prevention* (ed. D. Schottenfeld and J.F. Fraumeni Jr) (2nd edn), pp. 1282–312. Oxford University Press, New York.

Austin, D.F. and Reynolds, P. (1996). Laryngeal cancer. In *Cancer epidemiology and prevention* (ed. D. Schottenfeld and J.F. Fraumeni, Jr.) (2nd edn), pp. 619–36. Oxford University Press, New York.

Berrino, F., Capocaccia, R., Estève, J., *et al.* (ed.) (1999). *Survival of cancer patients in Europe: the EUROCARE-2 study*. IARC Scientific Publications No. 151. International Agency for Research on Cancer, Lyon.

Blot, W.J. (1997). Vitamin/mineral supplementation and cancer risk: international chemoprevention trials. *Proceedings of the Society of Experimental Biology and Medicine*, **216**, 291–6.

Blot, W.J. and Fraumeni, J.F., Jr (1996). Cancers of the lung and pleura. In *Cancer epidemiology and prevention* (ed. D. Schottenfeld and J.F. Fraumeni Jr) (2nd edn), pp. 637–65. Oxford University Press, New York.

Blot, W.J., McLaughlin, J.K., Winn, D.M., *et al.* (1988). Smoking and drinking in relation to oral and pharyngeal cancer. *Cancer Research*, **48**, 3282–7.

Blot, W.J., McLaughlin, J.K., Devesa, S.S., and Fraumeni, J.F. Jr (1996). Cancers of the oral cavity and pharynx. In *Cancer epidemiology and prevention* (ed. D. Schottenfeld and J.F. Fraumeni Jr) (2nd edn), pp. 666–80. Oxford University Press, New York.

Boffetta, P., Kogevinas, M., Simonato, L., Wilbourn, J., and Saracci, R. (1995). Current perspectives on occupational cancer risks. *International Journal of Occupational and Environmental Health*, **1**, 315–25.

Cardis, E., Zeise, L., Schwarz, N., and Moolgavkar, S. (1999). Review of specific examples of QEP. In *Quantitative estimation and prediction of human cancer risks* (ed. S. Moolgavkar, D. Krewski, L. Zeise, E. Cardis, and H. Møller), pp. 239–304. IARC Scientific Publications No. 131. International Agency for Research on Cancer, Lyon.

Coleman, M., Estève, J., Damiecki, P., Arslan, A., and Renard, H. (1993). *Trends in cancer incidence and mortality*. IARC Scientific Publications No. 121. International Agency for Research on Cancer, Lyon.

Daling, J.R. and Sherman, K.J. (1996). Cancers of the vulva and vagina. In *Cancer epidemiology and prevention* (ed. D. Schottenfeld and J.F. Fraumeni Jr) (2nd edn) pp. 1117–29. Oxford University Press, New York.

Doll, R. and Peto, R. (1981). *The causes of cancer*. Oxford University Press.

Ferlay, J., Parkin, D.M., and Pisani, P. (1998). *Cancer incidence and mortality worldwide* (Globocan I software). International Agency for Research on Cancer, Lyon.

Ferlay, J., Bray, F., Pisani, P., and Parkin, D.M. (2001). *Globocan 2000: cancer incidence, mortality and prevalence worldwide.* IARC Cancer Base No. 5. International Agency for Research on Cancer, Lyon.

Grady, D. and Ernster, V.L. (1996). Endometrial cancer. In *Cancer epidemiology and prevention* (ed. D. Schottenfeld and J.F. Fraumeni Jr) (2nd edn), pp. 1058–89. Oxford University Press, New York.

Hackshaw, A.K., Law, M.R., and Wald, N.J. (1997). The accumulated evidence on lung cancer and environmental tobacco smoke. *British Medical Journal*, **315**, 980–8.

Hammond, E.C., Selikoff, I.J., and Seidman, H. (1979). Asbestos exposure, cigarette smoking and death rates. *Annals of the New York Academy of Science*, **330**, 473–90.

Harvard Center for Cancer Prevention (1996). Harvard report on cancer prevention. Vol. 1: Causes of human cancer. *Cancer Causes Control*, **7**, S3–58.

Henderson, B.E., Pike, M.C., Bernstein, L., and Ross, R.K. (1996). Breast cancer. In *Cancer epidemiology and prevention* (ed. D. Schottenfeld and J.F. Fraumeni Jr) (2nd edn), pp. 1022–39. Oxford University Press, New York.

IARC (International Agency for Research on Cancer) (1972–2001). *IARC monographs on the evaluation of carcinogenic risks to humans*, Vols 1–78. IARC, Lyon.

IARC (International Agency for Research on Cancer) (1987). *Overall evaluations of carcinogenicity: an updating of IARC Monographs Volumes 1 to 42.* IARC Monographs on the Evaluation of the Carcinogenic Risk of Chemicals to Humans, Supplement 7. IARC, Lyon.

IARC (International Agency for Research on Cancer) (1988). *Alcohol drinking. IARc monographs on the evaluation of carcinogenic risks to humans*, Vol. 44. IARC, Lyon.

IARC (International Agency for Research on Cancer) (1994*a*). *Hepatitis viruses. IARC monographs on the evaluation of carcinogenic risks to humans*, Vol. 59. IARC, Lyon.

IARC (International Agency for Research on Cancer) (1994*b*). *Schistosomes, liver flukes and Helicobacter pylori. IARC monographs on the evaluation of carcinogenic risks to humans*, Vol. 61. IARC, Lyon.

IARC (International Agency for Research on Cancer) (1995). *Human papilloma viruses. IARC monographs on the evaluation of carcinogenic risks to humans*, Vol. 64. IARC, Lyon.

IARC (International Agency for Research on Cancer) (1996). *Human immunodeficiency viruses and human T-cell lymphotropic viruses. IARC monographs on the evaluation of carcinogenic risks to humans*, Vol. 67. IARC, Lyon.

IARC (International Agency for Research on Cancer) (1997*a*). *Epstein–Barr virus and Kaposi's sarcoma herpesvirus/human herpesvirus 8. IARC monographs on the evaluation of carcinogenic risks to humans*, Vol. 70. IARC, Lyon.

IARC (International Agency for Research on Cancer) (1997*b*). *Non-steroidal anti-inflammatory drugs. IARC handbooks of cancer prevention*, Vol. 1. IARC, Lyon.

IARC (International Agency for Research on Cancer) (1998*a*). *Carotenoids IARC handbooks of cancer prevention*, Vol. 2. IARC, Lyon.

IARC (International Agency for Research on Cancer) (1998*b*). *Vitamin A. IARC handbooks of cancer prevention*, Vol. 3. IARC, Lyon.

IARC (International Agency for Research on Cancer) (1999). *Surgical implants and other foreign bodies. IARC monographs on the evaluation of carcinogenic risks to humans*, Vol. 74. IARC, Lyon.

Joint IARC/IPCS/CEC Working Group (1983). *Approaches to classifying chemical carcinogens according to mechanism of action.* International Agency for Research on Cancer (IARC) Internal Technical Report No. 83/001. IARC, Lyon.

Kosary, C.L., Ries, L.A.G., Miller, B.A., Hankey, B.F., Harras, A., and Edwards, B.K. (ed.) (1995). *SEER cancer statistics review, 1973–1992: tables and graphs.* NIH Publication No. 96–2789. National Cancer Institute, Bethesda, MD.

London, W.T. and McGlynn, K.A. (1996). Liver cancer. In *Cancer epidemiology and prevention* (ed. D. Schottenfeld and J.F. Fraumeni Jr) (2nd edn), pp. 772–93. Oxford University Press, New York.

Lubin, J.H. and Boice, J.D., Jr (1997). Lung cancer risk from residential radon: meta-analysis of eight epidemiologic studies. *Journal of the National Cancer Institute*, **89**, 49–57.

McLaughlin, J.K., Blot, W.J., Devesa, S.S., and Fraumeni, J.F., Jr (1996). Renal cancer. In *Cancer epidemiology and prevention* (ed. D. Schottenfeld and J.F. Fraumeni Jr) (2nd edn), pp. 1142–55. Oxford University Press, New York.

Miller, A.B. (1996). Fundamental issues in screening for cancer. In *Cancer epidemiology and prevention* (ed. D. Schottenfeld and J.F. Fraumeni Jr) (2nd edn), pp. 1433–52. Oxford University Press, New York.

Miller, R.W., Boice, J.D., Jr, and Curtis, R.E. (1996). Bone cancer. In *Cancer epidemiology and prevention* (ed. D. Schottenfeld and J.F. Fraumeni Jr) (2nd edn), pp. 971–83. Oxford University Press, New York.

Moss, S.M. (1999). Breast cancer. In *Cancer screening: theory and practice* (ed. B.S. Kramer, J.K. Gohagan, and P.C. Prorok), pp. 143–70. Marcel Dekker, New York.

Mueller, N.E. (1996). Hodgkin's disease. In *Cancer epidemiology and prevention* (ed. D. Schottenfeld and J.F. Fraumeni Jr) (2nd edn), pp. 893–919. Oxford University Press, New York.

Muñoz, N. and Day, N.E. (1996). Esophageal cancer. In *Cancer epidemiology and prevention* (ed. D. Schottenfeld and J.F. Fraumeni Jr) (2nd edn), pp. 681–706. Oxford University Press, New York.

Murray, C.J.L. and Lopez, A.D. (ed.) (1996). *The global burden of disease.* Harvard School of Public Health, Boston, MA.

National Research Council (1988). Committee on the Biological Effects of Ionizing Radiations. *Health risks of radon and other internally deposited alpha-emitters.* National Academy of Sciences, Washington, DC.

Parkin, D.M., Pisani, P., Lopez, A.D., and Masuyer, E. (1994). At least one in seven cases of cancer is caused by smoking: global estimates for 1985. *International Journal of Cancer*, **59**, 494–504.

Parkin, D.M., Whelan, S.L., Ferlay, J., Raymond, L., and Young, J. (ed.) (1997). *Cancer incidence in five continents*, Vol. VII. International Agency for Research on Cancer (IARC) Scientific Publications No. 143. IARC, Lyon.

Peto, R. (1977). Epidemiology, multistage models and short-term mutagenicity tests. In *Origins of human cancer* (ed. H.H. Hiatt, J.D. Watson, and J.A. Winsten), pp. 1403–28. Cold Spring Harbor Laboratory, Cold Spring Harbor, NY.

Peto, R., Chen, Z.M., and Boreham, J. (1999). Tobacco—the growing epidemic. *Nature Medicine*, **5**, 15–17.

Pisani, P., Parkin, D.M., Muñoz, N., and Ferlay, J. (1997). Cancer and infection: estimates of the attributable fraction in 1990. *Cancer Epidemiology, Biomarkers and Prevention*, **6**, 387–400.

Preston-Martin, S. and Mack, W.J. (1996). Neoplasms of the nervous system. In *Cancer epidemiology and prevention* (ed. D. Schottenfeld and J.F. Fraumeni Jr) (2nd edn), pp. 1231–81. Oxford University Press, New York.

Ron, E. (1996). Thyroid cancer. In *Cancer epidemiology and prevention* (ed. D. Schottenfeld and J.F. Fraumeni Jr) (2nd edn), pp. 1000–21. Oxford University Press, New York.

Ron, E., Lubin, J.H., Shore, R.E., *et al.* (1995). Thyroid cancer after exposure to external radiation: a pooled analysis of seven studies. *Radiation Research*, **141**, 259–77.

Ross, R.K. and Schottenfeld, D. (1996). Prostate cancer. In *Cancer epidemiology and prevention* (ed. D. Schottenfeld and J.F. Fraumeni Jr) (2nd edn), pp. 1180–206. Oxford University Press, New York.

Roush, G.C. (1996). Cancers of the nasal cavity and paranasal sinuses. In *Cancer epidemiology and prevention* (ed. D. Schottenfeld and J.F. Fraumeni Jr) (2nd edn), pp. 587–602. Oxford University Press, New York.

Sankaranarayanan, R., Black, R.J., and Parkin, D.M. (ed.) (1998). *Cancer survival in developing countries.* International Agency for Research on Cancer Scientific Publications No. 145. IARC, Lyon.

Sankaranarayanan, R., Mathew, B., Jacob, B.J., *et al.* (2000). Early findings from a community-based, cluster-randomized, controlled oral cancer screening trial in Kerala, India. *Cancer*, **88**, 664–73.

Scherr, P.A. and Mueller, N.E. (1996). Non-Hodgkin's lymphomas. In *Cancer epidemiology and prevention* (ed. D. Schottenfeld and J.F. Fraumeni Jr) (2nd edn), pp. 920–454. Oxford University Press, New York.

Schiffman, M.H., Brinton, L.A., Devesa, S.S., and Fraumeni, J.F., Jr (1996). Cervical cancer. In *Cancer epidemiology and prevention* (ed. D. Schottenfeld and J.F. Fraumeni Jr) (2nd edn), pp. 1090–116. Oxford University Press, New York.

Schottenfeld, D. (1996). Testicular cancer. In *Cancer epidemiology and prevention* (ed. D. Schottenfeld and J.F. Fraumeni Jr) (2nd edn), pp. 1207–19. Oxford University Press, New York.

Schottenfeld, D. and Fraumeni, J.F., Jr (ed.) (1996). *Cancer epidemiology and prevention* (2nd edn). Oxford University Press, New York.

Schottenfeld, D. and Islam, S.S. (1996). Cancers of the small intestine. In *Cancer epidemiology and prevention* (ed. D. Schottenfeld and J.F. Fraumeni Jr) (2nd edn), pp. 806–12. Oxford University Press, New York.

Schottenfeld, D. and Winawer, S.J. (1996). Cancers of the large intestine. In *Cancer epidemiology and prevention* (ed. D. Schottenfeld and J.F. Fraumeni Jr) (2nd edn), pp. 813–40. Oxford University Press, New York.

Scotto, J., Fears, T.R., Kraemer, K.H., and Fraumeni, J.F., Jr (1996). Nonmelanoma skin cancer. In *Cancer epidemiology and prevention* (ed. D. Schottenfeld and J.F. Fraumeni Jr) (2nd edn), pp. 1313–30. Oxford University Press, New York.

Sikora, K. (1999). Developing a global strategy for cancer. *European Journal of Cancer*, **35**, 1870–7.

Silverman, D.T., Morrison, A.S., and Devesa, S.S. (1996). Bladder cancer. In *Cancer epidemiology and prevention* (ed. D. Schottenfeld and J.F. Fraumeni Jr) (2nd edn), pp. 1156–79. Oxford University Press, New York.

Smith, K.R. and Liu, Y. (1994). Indoor air pollution in developing countries. In *Epidemiology of lung cancer. Lung biology in health disease* (ed. J.M. Samet), Vol. 74, pp. 151–84. Marcel Dekker, New York.

Speizer, F.E. and Samet, J.M. (1994). Air pollution and lung cancer. In *Epidemiology of lung cancer. Lung biology in health disease* (ed. J.M. Samet), Vol. 74, pp. 131–50. Marcel Dekker, New York.

Spitz, M.R., McPherson, R.S., Jiang, H., *et al.* (1997). Correlates of mutagen sensitivity in patients with upper aerodigestive tract cancer. *Cancer Epidemiology, Biomarkers and Prevention*, **6**, 687–92.

Tuyns, A.J., Péquignot, G., and Jensen, O.M. (1977). Le cancer de l'oesophage en Ille-et-Vilaine en fonction des niveaux de consommation d'alcool et de tabac: des risques qui se multiplient. *Bulletin de Cancer*, **64**, 45–60.

USDHHS (United States Department of Health and Human Services) (1982). *The health consequences of smoking—cancer.* USDHHS, Public Health Service, Office on Smoking and Health, Rockville, MD.

WCRF (World Cancer Research Fund) (1997). *Food, nutrition and the prevention of cancer: a global perspective.* WCRF and American Institute for Cancer Research, Washington,DC.

Weiss, N.S., Cook, L.S., Farrow, D.C., and Rosenblatt, K.A. (1996). Ovarian cancer. In *Cancer epidemiology and prevention* (ed. D. Schottenfeld and J.F. Fraumeni Jr) (2nd edn), pp. 1040–57. Oxford University Press, New York.

WHO (World Health Organization) (1990). *International Classification of Diseases for Oncology (ICD-O)* (2nd edn). WHO, Geneva.

Wideroff, L. and Schottenfeld, D. (1996). Penile cancer. In *Cancer epidemiology and prevention* (ed. D. Schottenfeld and J.F. Fraumeni Jr) (2nd edn), pp. 1220–30. Oxford University Press, New York.

Wild, C.P. and Pisani, P. (1997). Carcinogen-DNA and carcinogen-protein adducts in molecular epidemiology. In *Applicaton of biomarkers in cancer epidemiology* (ed. P. Toniolo, P. Boffetta, D.E.G. Shuker, N. Rothman, B. Hulka, and N. Pearce), pp. 143–58. International Agency for Research on Cancer (IARC) Scientific Publications No. 142. IARC, Lyon.

Winawer, S.J., Fletcher, R.H., Miller, L., *et al.* (1997). Colorectal cancer screening: clinical guidelines and rationale. *Gastroenterology*, **112**, 594–642.

Yang, P., Schwartz, A.G., McAllister, A.E., Swanson, G.M., and Aston, C.E. (1999). Lung cancer risk in families of nonsmoking probands: heterogeneity by age at diagnosis. *Genetics and Epidemiology*, **17**, 253–73.

Yu, M.C. and Henderson, B.E. (1996). Nasopharyngeal cancer. In *Cancer epidemiology and prevention* (ed. D. Schottenfeld and J.F. Fraumeni Jr) (2nd edn), pp. 603–18. Oxford University Press, New York.

Zahm, S.H., Tucker, M.A., and Fraumeni, J.F., Jr (1996). Soft tissue sarcomas. In *Cancer epidemiology and prevention* (ed. D. Schottenfeld and J.F. Fraumeni Jr) (2nd edn), pp. 984–99. Oxford University Press, New York.

9.3 Cerebrovascular disease

Heizo Tanaka, Hiroyasu Iso, Tetsuji Yokoyama, Nobuo Yoshiike, and Yoshihiro Kokubo

Cerebrovascular disease ranks third or higher as a cause of death in industrialized countries. It is also a major contributor to disability. For example, in 1995 the Japanese Ministry of Health and Welfare reported that, in Japan, 32.7 per cent of 284 000 elderly people with severe disability were paralysed as the result of a stroke (Ministry of Health and Welfare 1997).

The documentation of functional gain is insufficient, and increased consideration must be given to quality of life for people with low activities of daily living after the attack. In addition, there are some forms of cerebrovascular disease that include progressive dementia.

According to predictions based on secular trends for the leading causes of death over the past 50 to 100 years in the United States and West European countries, stroke will emerge as a more frequent cause of death than ischaemic heart disease in developing countries after infectious and malnutritional diseases are overcome.

Thus stroke continues to be a major cause of death as well as physical and mental disability, and valid information about its epidemiology and prevention is needed in developed and developing countries alike.

Death rates

In this section we present the pattern of mortality from cerebrovascular disease for males and females by country/area over the last 45 years (WHO 1994, 1996, 1998). During this period, the *International Statistical Classification of Diseases, Injuries and Cause of Death* (**ICD**) has been revised five times. As shown in Table 1, the sixth and seventh revisions for 1948 to 1968 (ICD-6 and ICD-7) classified cerebrovascular disease into four categories. Substantial changes were made in the eighth and ninth revisions (ICD-8 and ICD-9). Cerebral embolism and thrombosis (code 332 in ICD-6 and ICD-7) were divided into codes 432, 433, and 434 in ICD-8 and codes 433 and 434 in ICD-9. Transient cerebral ischaemia, code 435 in ICD-8 and ICD-9, replaced spasm of cerebral arteries, code 333 in ICD-6 and ICD-7. Major changes were made in ICD-9 and the current tenth revision (ICD-10). These changes may affect the apparent secular trend in the death rate from cerebrovascular disease in some countries. In fact, there was a remarkable increase in the rate in Japan 1995 (when ICD-10 was introduced) which was entirely due to changes in coding. Thereafter, it tended to decrease as previously (Ministry of Health and Welfare 1999).

According to the Framingham Study (Corwin *et al.* 1982), 40 per cent of 280 decedents with verified stroke had no mention of stroke on the death certificate and 21 per cent of certificates listing stroke were false positives. There was little change in this pattern of error during the 30 years of the study from 1950 to 1980.

Since computed tomography (**CT**) came into widespread use around 1975, the validity of the diagnosis of stroke has rapidly improved in some countries. Before the development of CT, however, the antemortem diagnosis of stroke rested primarily on clinical diagnosis, consisting of history taking and physical examination, rather than on laboratory measurements. If deaths from cerebrovascular disease are considered as a single entity, as was done in this section, the clinical diagnosis appears to be reliable but its accuracy for differentiating the subtypes of stroke is more or less open to question (Tanaka *et al.* 1982).

Crude death rates

Crude death rates must not be cited to make international comparisons or to assess changes with time in a certain population. However, the rates do provide the absolute magnitude of deaths attributed to cerebrovascular disease in a population.

Table 2 shows crude death rates per 100 000 population from cerebrovascular disease in 33 countries/areas for the most recent year in which they were tabulated (WHO 1996, 1998). The rates ranged from 24.1 per 100 000 (Mexico) to 284.3 (Bulgaria) for males and from 27.3 per 100 000 (Mexico) to 347.2 (Russia) for females. Using the reported average rates of 103.3 for males and 130.0 for females, as well as the 1995 world population size estimated by the United Nations (5687 million), the number of people killed annually by cerebrovascular disease can be estimated at 6.6 million.

Age-adjusted death rates

Figures 1 and 2 show secular trends in age-adjusted death rates from cerebrovascular disease for males in selected countries during the period from 1950 to 1995 (WHO 1994, 1996, 1998). (Since the data for females are similar to those for males, they are not presented here.) As shown in Fig. 1, the age-adjusted rates from cerebrovascular disease tended to decrease for this period in the United States and Western Europe, excluding Spain where a slight increasing trend was observed from 1950 to 1979.

Figure 2 illustrates the trends in Argentina, Mauritius, Japan, and some East European countries. Although the Japanese rate was the highest in the world and increased from 1950 to 1964, it tended to decrease after 1965, reaching the level of West European countries in recent years. This declining trend appears to have been accelerated by

Table 1 Cerebrovascular disease codes according to the sixth, seventh, eighth, ninth, and tenth revisions of *International Statistical Classification of Diseases, Injuries and Cause of Death*

ICD-6, ICD-7		ICD-8		ICD-9		ICD-10	
Code	**Title**	**Code**	**Title**	**Code**	**Title**	**Code**	**Title**
330	Subarachnoid haemorrhage	430	Subarachnoid haemorrhage	430	Subarachnoid haemorrhage	160	Subarachnoid haemorrhage
331	Cerebral haemorrhage	431	Cerebral haemorrhage	431	Intracerebral haemorrhage	161	Intracerebral haemorrhage
				432	Other/unspecified intracranial haemorrhage	162	Other non-traumatic intracranial haemorrhage
332	Cerebral embolism and thrombosis	432	Occlusion of precerebral arteries	433	Occlusion/stenosis of precerebral arteries	163	Cerebral infarction
		433	Cerebral thrombosis	434	Occlusion of cerebral arteries	165	Occlusion and stenosis of precerebral arteries, not resulting in cerebral infarction
		434	Cerebral embolism				
						166	Occlusion and stenosis of cerebral arteries, not resulting in cerebral infarction
333	Spasm of cerebral arteries	435	Transient cerebral ischaemia	435	Transient cerebral ischaemia	164	Stroke, not specified as haemorrhage or infarction
334	Other and ill-defined vascular lesions affecting CNS	436	Acute but ill-defined CVD	436	Acute but ill-defined CVD	167	Other cerebrovascular diseases
		437	Generalized ischaemic CVD	437	Other and ill-defined CVD	168	Cerebrovascular disorders in diseases classified elsewhere
		438	Other and ill-defined CVD	438	Late effects of CVD		
						169	Sequelae of cerebrovascular disease

CNS, central nervous system; CVD, cerebrovascular disease.

nationwide community-based control of hypertension and lifestyle modernization associated with a background of high economic growth (Tanaka *et al.* 1982, 1992).

In East European countries, however, the rates tended to increase for the period 1955 to 1984 and to decrease slightly after 1985. Romania, Bulgaria, and Poland showed increasing trends even in the 1990s.

Incidence

Definition and classification of stroke

In incidence studies, stroke is defined as the occurrence of rapidly developing clinical signs of focal or global disturbances of cerebral function which last for more than 24 h or result in death for which there is no apparent cause other than a vascular accident (WHO 1971, 1972, 1973). Transient episodes of cerebral ischaemia are excluded by this definition. An attempt is made to diagnose the anatomical subtype of stroke (subarachnoid haemorrhage, intracerebral haemorrhage, cerebral infarction, and undetermined type) on the basis of clinical symptoms and signs. If CT or magnetic resonance imaging (**MRI**) findings are available in the population under study, they play a decisive role in the diagnosis of stroke subtypes (see below).

Case ascertainment and verification of diagnosis

The setting up of stroke registries is the most appropriate method of data acquisition on morbidity (WHO 1971, 1972, 1973). Any doctor who is called in to see a stroke patient should notify the registry. The sources of notification may be general practitioners, ambulance personnel, the 'telephone alarm service', hospital reception staff, the police, field nurses, medico-legal authorities, and so on according to local circumstances. The patients should also be referred by lay

Table 2 Crude death rates from cerebrovascular disease in selected countries/areas (most recent year)

WHO region	Country/area	Year	Rate per 100 000	
			Male	Female
Africa	Mauritius	1995	97.6	86.5
America	Argentina	1993	77.8	71.3
	Canada	1995	44.9	59.9
	Mexico	1995	24.1	27.3
	USA	1994	47.4	69.8
Europe	Austria	1995	91.4	151.8
	Belgium	1992	80.1	116.2
	Bulgaria[a]	1994	284.3	265.5
	Czech	1995	148.0	201.6
	Denmark	1995	90.3	121.2
	France	1994	63.5	85.8
	Germany	1995	91.2	154.6
	Greece	1995	153.1	210.2
	Hungary	1995	183.7	206.6
	Ireland	1993	75.1	98.3
	Israel	1995	53.9	57.9
	Italy	1993	112.0	147.6
	Netherlands	1995	62.5	97.6
	Poland	1995	68.8	81.4
	Portugal	1995	213.1	258.0
	Romania	1995	229.5	256.2
	Russia[b]	1995	221.6	347.2
	Spain	1994	87.1	122.5
	Sweden	1995	97.0	128.0
	Switzerland[a]	1994	63.2	92.8
	UK	1995	89.2	146.5
Western Pacific	Australia	1994	59.4	84.9
	China, selected[a]			
	Rural areas	1994	109.0	99.9
	Urban areas	1994	137.2	121.5
	Hong Kong	1995	49.7	57.8
	Japan	1994	91.2	102.4
		1998[c]	106.9	113.1
	New Zealand[a]	1993	62.2	98.5
	Singapore	1995	51.2	62.8
Mean			103.3	130.0

[a] WHO (1996).

[b] Data not available for Chechnya.

[c] Ministry of Health and Welfare (1998). The rates in 1994 were used for the calculation of the mean values.

Source: WHO (1998).

personnel in charge of health services in the area. In general, death certificates, social insurance records, and general practitioner records

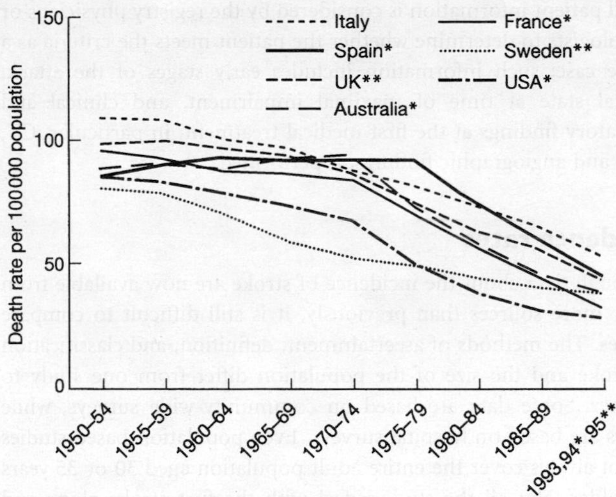

Fig. 1 Secular trends in age-adjusted death rate from cerebrovascular disease in selected countries (United States, West European Countries), males (WHO 1994, 1996, 1998).

are also reviewed periodically. Mass screening examinations or a prevalence study of the total population are the only means of detecting patients who survived stroke but who were not recorded in the documents as described above.

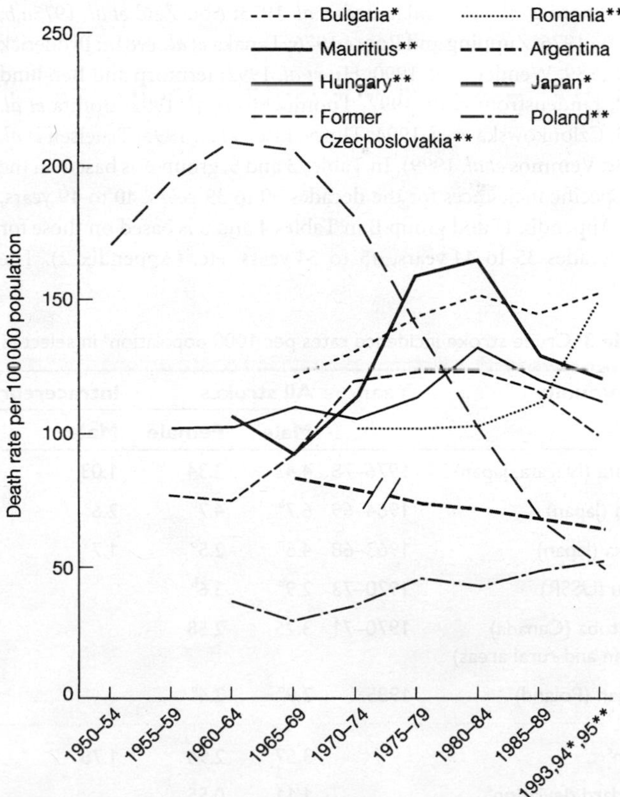

Fig. 2 Secular trends in age-adjusted death rate from cerebrovascular disease in selected countries/areas (Argentina, Japan, Mauritius, East Europe), males (WHO 1994, 1996, 1998).

All patient information is considered by the registry physicians or neurologists to determine whether the patient meets the criteria as a stroke case; such information includes early stages of the attack, clinical state at time of maximal impairment, and clinical and laboratory findings at the first medical treatment, in particular, CT, MRI, and angiographic findings, if performed.

Incidence rates

Although data about the incidence of stroke are now available from many more sources than previously, it is still difficult to compare studies. The methods of ascertainment, definition, and classification of stroke and the size of the population differ from one study to another. Some data are based on community-wide surveys, while others are based on hospital surveys. Even population-based studies do not always cover the entire adult population aged 30 or 35 years and older. Not all the studies deal with the first stroke alone and repeated episodes are often included in the incidence. There are not many reports about the incidence by age, sex, and subtype of stroke. Furthermore, age-specific incidences are shown for the decades 35 to 44 years, 45 to 54 years, etc. in some reports, but for the decades 30 to 39 years, 40 to 49 years, etc. in others. Therefore only available community-based studies on stroke that were performed under conditions comparable with those mentioned in the previous section are reviewed and summarized here.

Tables 3 to 6 present an international comparison of stroke incidence by subtype (Eisenberg *et al.* 1964; Katsuki *et al.* 1964; Parrish *et al.* 1966; Eckstrom *et al.* 1969; Alter *et al.* 1970; Whisnant *et al.* 1971; Matsumoto *et al.* 1973; Melamed *et al.* 1973; Abu-Zeid *et al.* 1975*a*,*b*; Kojima 1976; Zupping and Roose 1976; Tanaka *et al.* 1981*a*; Broderick *et al.* 1989; Wender *et al.* 1990; Hu *et al.* 1992; Jerntorp and Berglund 1992; Lindenstrom *et al.* 1992; Tuomilehto *et al.* 1992; Bonita *et al.* 1993; Czlonkowska *et al.* 1994; Thorvaldsen *et al.* 1995; Truelsen *et al.* 1998*c*; Vemmos *et al.* 1999). In Tables 3 and 5, group A is based on the age-specific incidences for the decades 30 to 39 years, 40 to 49 years, etc. (Appendix 1) and group B in Tables 4 and 6 is based on those for the decades 35 to 44 years, 45 to 54 years, etc. (Appendix 2). The World Health Organization Monitoring Trends and Determinants in Cardiovascular Disease (**WHO MONICA**) Project populations are also included in group B. This project started in the first half of the 1980s to register continuously the occurrence of myocardial infarction and stroke in many populations using a common protocol (Tunstall-Pedoe *et al.* 1988). The incidence rates may be fairly comparable among these MONICA populations.

We estimated the average stroke incidence in the age group 30 years and over using the data reported from several populations (group A, Table 3). The average incidences were as follows: all strokes, 3.57 per 1000 for males and 2.94 per 1000 for females; intracerebral haemorrhage, 1.78 per 1000 for males and 1.12 per 1000 for females; cerebral infarction, 2.44 per 1000 for males and 2.15 per 1000 for females. In group B (Table 4), the average incidence of all strokes in the age group 35 years and over was 4.55 per 1000 for males and 3.36 per 1000 for females. There are few data about subtypes for this group.

The sex- and age-adjusted incidence was computed according to the world 'new' standard population (WHO 1994). The sex- and age-adjusted incidence for people in the age group 30 to 59 years (group A, Table 5) or 35 to 64 years (group B, Table 6) was also computed, because stroke is the most serious health problem in those middle-aged people.

Since mortality rates have declined in some countries (Figs 1 and 2) and a decreasing trend in the incidence of stroke has been observed in some communities, the observation period during which the age-adjusted incidences were compared among studies (Tanaka *et al.* 1981*b*) should be taken into account. In group A (Table 5), both males and females in Akita, Japan (1964–1969), had the highest age-adjusted incidence of intracerebral haemorrhage, cerebral infarction, and all strokes, although there has been a marked decreasing trend in the rates in the population recently (Shimamoto *et al.* 1989).

For males of group B (Table 6), the age-adjusted incidence of all stroke was much higher in non-white people living in Missouri (1964–1965), than in any other population of males. Males aged 35 to 64 years in Fargo–Moorhead (1965–1966), Copenhagen (1976–1988), Shibata (1976–1978), North Karelia (1985–1987), Kuopio (1985–

Table 3 Crude stroke incidence rates per 1000 population[a] in selected communities (group A)

Community	Year	All strokes		Intracerebral haemorrhage		Cerebral infarction		Subarachnoid haemorrhage
		Male	Female	Male	Female	Male	Female	Both sexes
Shibata (Niigata, Japan)	1976–78	4.43	2.34	1.03	0.55	2.61	1.31	0.25
Akita (Japan)	1964–69	6.7[b]	4.7[b]	2.6[b]	1.8[b]	3.0[b]	1.8[b]	
Osaka (Japan)	1963–68	4.5[b]	2.5[b]	1.7[b]	1.0[b]	2.1[b]	1.1[b]	
Tartu (USSR)	1970–73	2.9[b]	3.6[b]			2.3[b]	2.9[b]	0.2[b]
Manitoba (Canada) (urban and rural areas)	1970–71	3.25	2.58					
Poznan (Poland)	1985	2.9[b]	2.4[b]					0.13[b]
Mean[c]		3.57	2.94	1.78	1.12	2.44	2.15	0.19
Standard deviation[c]		1.11	0.55	–	–	0.19	1.06	0.06

[a]30 years old and over.

[b]Estimated from the data in each reference.

[c]Calculated as a mean of each country-specific incidence. If two or more incidence data were available within a country, their average was used as the country-specific incidence.

Table 4 Crude stroke incidence rates per 1000 population[a] in selected communities (group B)

Community	Year	All strokes		Intracerebral haemorrhage		Cerebral infarction		Subarachnoid haemorrhage
		Male	Female	Male	Female	Male	Female	Both sexes
Shibata (Niigata, Japan)	1976–78	5.04	2.63	1.13	0.62	3.02	1.47	0.28
Rochester, MN (USA)	1955–69	4.6[b]	3.8[b]			3.8[b]	2.9[b]	
	1945–54							0.25
Fargo, ND – Moorhead, MN (USA)	1965–66	5.76	5.69					
Mid-Missouri (USA)	1964–65							
White		5.36	4.97					
Non-white		15.07	8.22					
Middlesex, CT (USA)	1957–58		5.2[b]					
Jerusalem	1960–67	3.0[b]	2.4[b]					
Taiwan	1986–90	(3.78)	(2.80)					
Copenhagen	1976–88	(5.7)[b]	(2.9)[b]					
Warsaw	1991–92	(2.8)[b]	(2.6)[b]					
Finland	1983–85							
North Karelia		(3.7)[b]	(2.8)[b]					
Kuopio Province		(4.4)[b]	(3.2)[b]					
Turku/Loimaa		(3.0)[b]	(2.3)[b]					
Auckland (New Zealand)	1991	4.24[b]	4.44[b]					
	1991–93							0.17[b]
Arcadia (Greece)	1994–95	5.02[b]	4.13[b]	0.80[b]	0.44[b]	4.08[b]	3.32[b]	0.12[b]
Mean[c]		4.55	3.36	0.97	0.53	3.63	2.56	0.21
Standard deviation[c]		1.52	1.09	0.23	0.13	0.55	0.97	0.07

[a]35 years old and over.

[b]Estimated from the data in each reference.

[c]Calculated as a mean of each country-specific incidence. If two or more incidence data were available within a country, their average was used as the country-specific incidence.

1987), Kaunas (1985–1987), and Novosibirsk (1985–1987) showed a relatively high incidence (more than 2 per 1000). The age-adjusted incidence of intracerebral haemorrhage for males in the age group of 35 to 64 years was higher in Shibata (1976–1978) than in other areas, and that of cerebral infarction was higher in Rochester (1955–1969).

For females aged 35 to 64 years in group B (Table 6), the age-adjusted incidence of all strokes ranged from 0.45 (Rhein–Neckar region, 1985–1987) to 2.32 (non-white, Missouri, 1964–1965). A relatively high incidence (more than 1 per 1000) was observed in Jerusalem (1960–1967), Beijing (1985–1987), Kaunas (1985–1987), Middlesex (1964–1965), Fargo–Moorhead (1965–1966), Taiwan (1986–199), Kuopio (1985–1987), Novosibirsk (1985–1987), and Mid-Missouri (non-white) (1964–1965) in that order. The incidences of intracerebral haemorrhage in Middlesex (0.49 per 1000 in 1957–1958) and of cerebral infarction in Rochester (0.58 per 1000 in 1955–1969) were the highest among the selected studies.

A relatively high incidence of stroke was observed in the 1940s and 1950s in the United States, which has been one of the countries with the lowest mortality from stroke in the world for the past 50 years and has shown declining trends in the incidence of stroke. This high rate corresponds to the rate for Japan in the 1960s and to the rates for Taiwan, Finland, and Poland in the 1980s. In Rochester, a gradual decrease in the incidence of all strokes very long term has been reported (Table 6).

Prognosis of stroke

The accuracy of long-term prognosis after the onset of stroke in a population depends on the completeness of case ascertainment rather than on follow-up. Some patients may die at home immediately after the attack or during transportation by ambulance. There is a

Table 5 International comparison of incidence of stroke by subtype per 1000 population (group A)

Community	**Year**	**Incidence**					
		Adjusted by sex + age[a]		**Adjusted by age**[a]			
		Both sexes		**Male**		**Female**	
		30+	**30–59**	**30+**	**30–59**	**30+**	**30–59**
All strokes							
Shibata (Niigata, Japan)	1976–78	2.95	0.84	4.20	1.31	1.89	0.38
Akita (Japan)	1964–69	6.41	2.40	7.61	3.24	5.33	1.57
Osaka (Japan)	1963–68	3.24	0.51	4.45	0.69	2.35	0.34
Tartu (USSR)	1970–73	2.84	0.66	3.33	0.88	2.43	0.44
Manitoba (Canada)	1970–71						
Urban area		2.35[b]	0.65[b]	2.69[b]	0.80[b]	2.06[b]	0.50[b]
Rural area							
Poznan (Poland)	1985	2.20	0.99	2.75	1.39	1.70	0.60
Mean[c]		2.90	0.89	3.55	1.20	2.35	0.58
Standard deviation[c]		0.91	0.29	1.28	0.45	0.64	0.14
Intercerebral haemorrhage							
Shibata (Niigata, Japan)	1976–78	0.69	0.31	0.94	0.44	0.46	0.19
Akita (Japan)	1964–69	2.55	1.05	2.91	1.44	2.16	0.67
Osaka (Japan)	1963–68	1.26	0.25	1.64	0.34	0.95	0.16
Tartu (USSR)	1970–73	0.40[d]	0.14[d]				
Manitoba (Canada)	1970–71						
Urban area			0.26		0.22		0.29
Rural area			0.24		0.31		0.19
Mean[c]		0.95	0.29	1.83	0.42	1.19	0.27
Standard deviation[c]		0.78	0.17	–	0.28	–	0.08
Cerebral infarction							
Shibata (Niigata, Japan)	1976–78	1.70	0.23	2.52	0.40	1.03	0.05
Akita (Japan)	1964–69	2.68	0.77	3.52	1.15	1.99	0.41
Osaka (Japan)	1963–68	1.44	0.18	2.10	0.23	0.98	0.12
Tartu (USSR)	1970–73	2.26	0.39	2.62	0.56	1.94	0.21
Manitoba (Canada)	1970–71						
Urban area			0.40		0.53		0.26
Rural area			0.25		0.37		0.14
Mean[c]		2.10	0.36	2.67	0.51	1.64	0.20
Standard deviation[c]		0.23	0.07	0.07	0.10	0.43	0.05
Subarachnoid haemhorrhage							
Shibata (Niigata, Japan)	1976–78	0.23[d]	0.20[d]				
Tartu (USSR)	1970–73	0.20[d]	0.13[d]				
Poznan (Poland)	1985	0.12[d]	0.10[d]				
Mean[c]	0.18	0.14					
Standard deviation[c]	0.06	0.05					

[a]Adjusted to the world 'new' standard population.

[b]Urban and rural area.

[c]Calculated as a mean of each country-specific incidence. If two or more incidence data were available within a country, their average was used as the country-specific incidence.

[d]Age-adjusted incidence.

Table 6 International comparison of incidence of stroke by subtype per 1000 population (group B)

Community	**Year**	**Incidence**					
		Adjusted by sex + age[a]		**Adjusted by age**[a]			
		Male	**Female**	**Male**		**Female**	
		35+	**35–64**	**35+**	**35–64**	**35+**	**35–64**
All strokes							
Shibata (Niigata, Japan)	1976–78	3.53	1.54	5.00	2.29	2.29	0.81
Rochester, MN (USA)	1980–84	(2.41)[b]	(0.88)[b]				
	1975–79	(1.99)[b]	(0.71)[b]				
	1970–74	(2.22)[b]	(0.83)[b]				
	1965–69	(2.58)[b]	(1.18)[b]				
	1960–64	(3.09)[b]	(1.11)[b]				
	1955–59	(3.61)[b]	(1.46)[b]				
	1950–54	(3.84)[b]	(1.31)[b]				
	1945–49	(3.80)[b]	(1.42)[b]				
	1945–54	4.23[b]	1.55[b]				
	1955–69	3.62	1.45	4.55	1.94	2.85	0.98
Fargo, ND–Moorhead, MN (USA)	1965–66	5.15	1.67	5.37	2.04	4.89	1.30
Mid-Missouri (USA)	1964–65						
White		3.23	0.83	3.69	1.05	2.85	0.63
Non-white		7.53	3.66	10.04	5.06	5.50	2.32
Middlesex, CT (USA)	1957–58	4.11	1.38	4.41	1.51	3.82	1.26
Jerusalem (Israel)	1960–67	2.59	1.27	2.96	1.45	2.28	1.09
Taiwan	1986–90	(3.13)	(1.69)	(3.34)	(1.87)	(2.92)	(1.51)
Copenhagen (Denmark)	1976–88	(3.09)	1.50	(4.30)	2.12	(2.12)	0.91
Malmö (Sweden)	1989	(2.09)	(0.73)	(2.56)	(0.92)	(1.69)	(0.54)
Warsaw (Poland)	1991–92	(2.59)	(1.19)	(3.03)	(1.54)	(2.18)	(0.85)
Auckland (New Zealand)	1991			(2.64)	1.14	(2.15)	0.91
	1981			(2.86)	1.12	(2.03)	0.86
Arcadia (Greece)	1994–95	2.40	0.89	2.81	1.08	2.08	0.71
Shanghai (China)	1984–91						
Rural area			0.93		1.12		0.74
Urban area			0.86		0.92		0.79
Rural and urban			0.89		1.02		0.77
WHO MONICA populations							
Beijing (China)	1985 87		1.38		1.60		1.16
Glostrup (Denmark)	1985–87		1.00		1.28		0.73
Kuopio Province (Finland)	1985–87		2.13		2.72		1.56
North Karelia (Finland)	1985–87		1.64		2.32		0.97
Turku/Loima (Finland)	1985–87		1.37		1.91		0.85
Halle County (Germany)	1985–87		0.88		1.14		0.64
Karl Marx Stadt (Germany)	1985–87		0.96		1.18		0.76
Rest of DDR MONICA (Germany)	1985–87		0.76		1.03		0.51
Rhein–Neckar Region (Germany)	1985–87		0.70		0.96		0.45
Friuli (Italy)	1985–87		0.74		0.96		0.53
Kaunas (Lithuania)	1985–87		1.60		2.03		1.20
Warsaw (Poland)	1985–87		0.84		1.14		0.55
Moscow (Russia, control)	1985–87		1.18		1.55		0.82
Moscow (Russia, intervention)	1985–87		1.02		1.33		0.73
Novosibirsk (Russia, intervention)	1985–87		2.06		2.26		1.86
Göteborg (Sweden)	1985–87		0.80		1.05		0.57
Northern Sweden (Sweden)	1985–87		1.23		1.60		0.88
Novi Sad (Yugoslavia)	1985–87		1.27		1.71		0.85

Community	Year	Incidence					
		Adjusted by sex + age[a]		Adjusted by age[a]			
		Male	Female	Male		Female	
		35+	35–64	35+	35–64	35+	35–64
Mean[c]		3.08	1.22	3.72	1.57	2.48	0.93
SD[c]		0.80	0.36	1.14	0.49	0.73	0.31
Cerebral infarction							
Shibata (Niigata, Japan)	1976–78	0.79	0.50	1.07	0.63	0.55	0.36
Rochester, MN (USA)	1945–54	0.41b	0.24b				
Middlesex, CT (USA)	1957–58	1.45	0.47	1.50	0.46	1.39	0.49
Manitoba (Canada)	1970–71						
Urban area			0.35		0.29		0.42
Rural area			0.31		0.42		0.19
Malmö (Sweden)	1989	(0.21)[b]	(0.08)[b]				
Warsaw (Poland)	1991–92						
Arcadia (Greece)	1994–95	0.36	0.19	0.46	0.15	0.30	0.23
Mean[c]		0.57	0.29	1.01	0.40	0.75	0.35
SD[c]		0.34	0.16	0.52	0.20	0.57	0.11
Intracerebral haemorrhage							
Shibata (Niigata, Japan)	1976–78	2.06	0.58	3.05	0.99	1.26	0.20
Rochester, MN (USA)	1945–54	3.29[b]	1.05[b]				
	1955–69	2.84	1.04	3.72	1.51	2.11	0.58
Manitoba (Canada)	1970–71						
Urban area			0.71		0.96		0.47
Rural area			0.62		0.69		0.55
Malmö (Sweden)	1989	(1.11)[b]	(0.45)[b]				
Arcadia (Greece)	1994–95	1.88	0.64	2.25	0.86	1.57	0.42
Mean[c]		1.97	0.67	3.01	1.05	1.65	0.43
SD[c]		0.71	0.20	0.73	0.32	0.43	0.17
Subarachnoid haemorrhage							
Shibata (Niigata, Japan)	1976–78	0.28[b]	0.29[b]				
Rochester, MN (USA)	1945–54	0.24[b]	0.21[b]				
Malmö (Sweden)	1989	(0.08)[b]	(0.08)[b]				
Auckland (New Zealand)	1981–83		0.22				
	1991–93		0.18				
Arcadia (Greece)	1994–95	0.09	0.06				
Mean[c]		0.17	0.17				
SD[c]		0.10	0.10				

( )See Appendix 2 for the age range.

[a]Adjusted to the world 'new' standard population.

[b]Age-adjusted incidence.

[c]Calculated as a mean of each country-specific incidence. If two or more incidence data were available within a country, the average was used as the country-specific incidence. In Rochester, only the incidence data in 1955–69 were used for all-stroke and cerebral infarction, and those in 1945–54 for intracerebral haemorrhage and subarachnoid haemorrhage.

Table 7 Vital prognosis after the onset of first-ever stroke

Study	Stroke subtype	Risk of death (%)		
		1 month	1 year	5 years
Oxfordshire	Cerebral infarction	10	23	52
	Intracerebral haemorrhage	52	62	70
	All strokes	19	31	45
Framingham	Cerebral infarction	15		
	Intracerebral haemorrhage	82		
	All strokes	22		
Rochester	Cerebral infarction	16		
	Intracerebral haemorrhage	58		
	All strokes	23	39	54
Five populations, Japan	Cerebral infarction	9	12	30
	Intracerebral haemorrhage	49	56	64
Ikawa	All strokes		32	61
Moscow	All strokes	37	52	72
Auckland	Subarachnoid haemorrhage	50		
	All strokes[a]	18		
Beijing	Cerebral infarction	13[b]		
	Intracerebral haemorrhage	66[b]		
	Subarachnoid haemorrhage	36[b]		
	All strokes	36[b]		
Shanghai				
Urban area	All strokes (men)	17[c]		
	All strokes (women)	33[c]		
Rural area	All strokes (men)	46[c]		
	All strokes (women)	46[c]		

[a]Excludes subarachnoid haemorrhage.

[b]Risk of death within 3 weeks.

[c]In 1990 and 1991.

possibility that they would be missed from the denominator for the survival rate. Therefore there have been relatively few community-based studies of stroke prognosis. Table 7 shows the cumulative risk of death (1 – survival rate) (Sacco *et al.* 1982; Dyken 1983; Scmidt *et al.* 1988; Kojima *et al.* 1990; Chen *et al.* 1992; Tanaka *et al.* 1992; Dennis *et al.* 1993; Hong *et al.* 1994; Bonita *et al.* 1995; Lauria *et al.* 1995; Truelsen *et al.* 1998*a*), although it is not comparable between studies because of the difference in age composition. Within a study district, risk of death after cerebral infarction appears to be lower than that after cerebral or subarachnoid haemorrhage. A Japanese epidemiological research group sponsored by the National Cardiovascular Center registered all the first-ever stroke patients and followed them prospectively for up to 10 years in five populations in the Osaka, Hiroshima, and Niigata Prefectures (Tanaka *et al.* 1992). As seen in Fig. 3 (survival rates within 5 years), the sex- and age-adjusted vital prognosis of intracerebral haemorrhage and infarction improved between the periods 1965–1974 and 1985–1990. The major contributor to the increase in the survival rates appeared to be the decline in the number of patients with severe stroke as well as improved medical care.

The case-fatality rate is not a satisfactory measure of survival for stroke, a chronic disease, but it may be useful until the survival data are accumulated. According to the Lehigh Valley Recurrent Stroke Study, 9.2 per cent of the 30-day stroke survivors ($n = 662$) were dead at 6 months and the case-fatality rates were 13.1, 21.3, 26.8, and 28.0 per cent at 1, 2, 3, and 4 years respectively (Lai *et al.* 1995). The case-fatality rate was 29.0 per cent (108 of 373) at 12 months in Glasgow, United Kingdom (Muir *et al.* 1996). Prognosis in severe stroke patients who required mechanical ventilation in neurological critical care units was analysed in Heidelberg, Germany, and the 1-year case fatality was reported to be 66.9 per cent (83 of 124) (Steiner *et al.* 1997). Conversely, some studies reported that the case-fatality rate had declined recently. A study from Sweden reported that the decline in stroke fatality rates during the period from 1971 to 1987 appeared to be related to decreases in blood pressure levels and smoking habits (Harmsen *et al.* 1992). According to the Minnesota

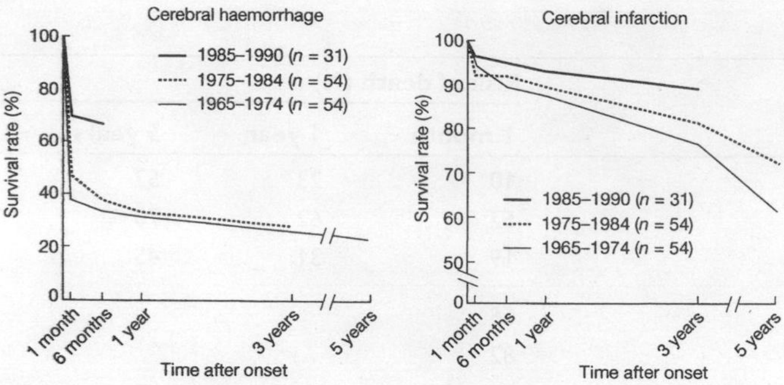

Fig. 3 Sex- and age-adjusted survival curves within 5 years after first-ever stroke determined by the Cox Proportional Hazard Model for five populations in Japan.

Heart Study, age- and sex-adjusted case fatality of hospital admitted patients in the United States improved significantly from 1970 to 1985; the odds ratio of death within 28 days in 1985 versus 1970 was 0.55 and that within 5 years was 0.72. Improved medical care and decreased severity of stroke probably contributed to the gain in survival (McGovern *et al.* 1993).

In the United States in the Lehigh Valley Recurrent Stroke Study (Lai *et al.* 1994), a 13 per cent stroke recurrence rate over an average of 24 months and a 19 per cent rate by the fourth year were observed. Control of hypertension and atrial fibrillation reduced the risk of stroke recurrence after a cerebral infarction. A rate of 14 per cent was observed for 24 months by Hier *et al.* (1991). In Rochester, Minnesota, the recurrence rate was 10 per cent in the first year and 20 per cent by the fifth year (Whisnant *et al.* 1971; Matsumoto *et al.* 1973). The recurrence rate after 1 month was 1.9 per cent of 474 cases in Belluno, Italy (Lauria *et al.* 1995).

Pathology, aetiology, and traditional risk factors for stroke subtypes

Stroke is a complex of subtypes, and includes subarachnoid haemorrhage, intracerebral haemorrhage, embolic infarction, and thrombotic infarction consisting of large-artery occlusive infarction and lacunar infarction. These subtypes may have different pathologies, aetiologies, and risk factors, some of which are similar to those in ischaemic heart disease but some of which are not. The wide use of CT or the recent use of MRI in some developed countries enables reliable diagnosis of stroke subtypes in clinical settings, and the data can be used for epidemiological studies (Walker *et al.* 1981; Foulkes *et al.* 1988; Sankai *et al.* 1991; C.S. Anderson *et al.* 1993; Iso *et al.* 2000).

Subarachnoid haemorrhage

Subarachnoid haemorrhage is defined as haemorrhage in the subarachnoid space, usually caused by the rupture of a saccular aneurysm of large to medium-sized cerebral arteries (diameter, 1–5 mm) or, less commonly, by arteriovenous malformation and other causes. Haemorrhages occurring in the intraparenchymal regions, but demonstrated to be due to aneurysm or arteriovenous malformation, are usually regarded as subarachnoid haemorrhage. Saccular aneurysm is the result of the loss of medial smooth muscle cells along with few proliferations in the intima and a weak adventitia. In addition to hypertension, animal studies indicate that spasms in cerebral arteries may increase haemodynamic stress in vulnerable sites for the development and rupture of saccular aneurysms. Hypertension, smoking, and heavy drinking increase the risk of subarachnoid haemorrhage. The contribution of dyslipidaemia (high or low total cholesterol) and diabetes is minimal in contrast to ischaemic heart disease.

Intracerebral haemorrhage

Intracerebral haemorrhage is defined as haemorrhage in the intraparenchymal regions of the brain not due to aneurysm or arteriovenous malformation. This stroke subtype is usually caused by the rupture of microaneurysms resulting from arterionecrosis (fibrinoid necrosis or lipohyalinosis) of small intracerebral penetrating arterioles (diameter, 100 to 200 μm) of the basal ganglia, thalamus, and brainstem regions. Penetrating arteries are more vulnerable to arterionecrosis through hypertension than small arteries in subcortical regions because they have larger lumens relative to their wall thickness, sustain higher wall stress from blood pressure, and are liable to injury of cell membranes.

The contribution of hypertension to intracerebral haemorrhage is strongest among the stroke subtypes. This means that acute and severe hypertension is likely to cause intracerebral haemorrhage in middle-aged adults, in contrast with ischaemic heart disease, for which low levels of serum total cholesterol are associated with an increased risk of intracerebral haemorrhage (Komachi *et al.* 1977; Kagan *et al.* 1980; Tanaka *et al.* 1982; Iso *et al.* 1989). The increased risk of haemorrhagic stroke with decreased cholesterol concentration was also suggested from recent meta-analysis for 13 cohorts from the People's Republic of China and five from Japan (Eastern Stroke and Coronary Heart Disease Collaborative Research Group 1998). This inverse association may in part be due to the association of low saturated fat and animal protein with the risk of intracerebral haemorrhage (Iso *et al.* 2001).

Considerable evidence suggests that very low serum cholesterol levels accelerate angionecrosis of intracerebral penetrating arteries particularly in the presence of hypertension (Kagan *et al.* 1980; Tanaka *et al.* 1982; Iso *et al.* 1989). In hypertensive rats, a diet-induced increase in serum cholesterol from very low to moderate levels was associated with a reduction in arterionecrosis and strokes. Hypertensive patients with ischaemic cerebral infarction and extracerebral atherosclerosis had higher serum cholesterol levels and less arterionecrosis than hypertensive patients without cerebral infarction. In addition, neonatal rat cardiomyocytes depleted of cholesterol were more prone to anoxia because cholesterol depletion increases permeability and ion fluxes across the membranes of a cardiomyocite, which may lead to cell death. In addition to a possible direct effect on vascular walls, low serum cholesterol levels may prevent atherosclerosis in carotid arteries and large to medium-sized cerebral arteries, which in turn exposes the distal penetrating arteries to higher wall stress and may enhance arterionecrosis in the presence of hypertension.

Heavy drinking also increases the risk of intracerebral haemorrhage due to increased blood pressure levels and reduced platelet aggregation, as it does that of subarachnoid haemorrhage. High serum total cholesterol or glucose intolerance does not affect the risk of intracerebral haemorrhage. The effect of smoking is also minimal.

Embolic infarction

Embolic infarction is regarded as cerebral infarction caused by emboli from extracranial regions. Sources of emboli include ulcerating atherosclerotic plaques in the carotid artery, mural thrombi associated with myocardial infarction (a consequence of surgery for coronary heart disease), atrial fibrillation, valvular heart disease, bacterial endocarditis, and other sources. Some of these sources (carotid plaque and mural thrombosis associated with myocardial infarction and a consequence of surgery for heart disease) are associated with atherosclerosis in origin, and therefore have similar risk factors to those in ischaemic heart disease, but the others are not. This means that risk factors for embolic infarction depend on the sources of emboli.

A close and strong relationship between atrial fibrillation and the subsequent incidence of cerebral infarction (relative risk, 2.6–4.5) was reported by several American and European studies (Wolf *et al.* 1978, 1991; Kannel *et al.* 1982; Benjamin *et al.* 1994). Although this association was identified by some Japanese prospective studies (Tanaka *et al.* 1985; Kitamura *et al.* 1991), the aetiology of atrial fibrillation may differ between the Japanese and Caucasians. According to the Framingham Study (Benjamin *et al.* 1994), most people with atrial fibrillation had suffered from valvular or ischaemic heart disease. In Japanese studies (Tanaka *et al.* 1985; Kitamura *et al.* 1991), however, less than 5 per cent of the subjects with atrial fibrillation at entry had a previous history of valvular disease and the rest (elderly people) had had mild to moderate hypertension for more than 20 years without any heart or atherosclerotic disease. Thus they concluded that atrial fibrillation was mainly due to long-term hypertension, not atherosclerosis.

Large-artery occlusive infarction

Large-artery occlusive infarction is defined as infarction involving the cortical artery regions in the cerebrum and cerebellum (cortex and subcortical areas), presumably caused by *in situ* thrombosis of large or medium-sized cerebral arteries (diameter 1 to 5 mm). This diagnosis is made even when accompanied by infarction of the internal capsule, corona radiata, or basal ganglia on the same side because the occlusion of medium-sized arteries before the branches of small penetrating arteries also cause lacunar infarction. Pathology for this stroke subtype is similar to that for ischaemic heart disease, that is, atherosclerosis in medium-sized arteries, which is characterized by proliferation of intima and medial smooth muscle cells with depositions of lipids and fibrin.

Major risk factors for ischaemic heart disease (high total low-density lipoprotein-cholesterol levels, low high-density lipoprotein-cholesterol levels, glucose intolerance, smoking, hypertension) also increase the risk of this stroke subtype. However, it is not known whether the aetiology is identical between this stroke subtype and ischaemic heart disease.

Lacunar infarction

Lacunar infarction has been defined as one or multiple infarctions involving focal, small, and deep areas such as the internal capsule, corona radiata, basal ganglia, and brainstem, without involvement of the cortex, that are caused by occlusion of small penetrating arteries.

This stroke subtype results from the occlusion of small penetrating arterioles (diameter, 100–200 μm), mostly by arteriosclerosis and sometimes by atherosclerotic plaques in large cerebral arteries in the origin of penetrating arteries. Unlike atherosclerosis, this small-vessel pathology is characterized by the loss of medial smooth muscle cells and degenerative changes of intima with fibrin deposition. During the 'healing process' for these degenerative changes, macrophages infiltrate the intima filled with fat or hemosiderin, and fibroblastic connective tissue replaces fibrinoid material, which causes occlusion of the vascular lumen.

Thus, compared with intracerebral haemorrhage, moderate hypertension with a longer duration, as usually indicated by hypertensive end-organ effects in the electrocardiograms and fundscopic findings, is likely to cause lacunar infarction in the elderly. In addition to hypertension, glucose intolerance also increases the risk of this type of stroke as a microvascular disorder in diabetes, whereas the contribution of dyslipidaemia and smoking is small.

Cultural differences in distribution of stroke subtypes

The distribution of stroke subtypes may differ between Western and Asian countries (Mohr *et al.* 1978; Walker *et al.* 1981; Foulkes *et al.* 1988; Sankai *et al.* 1991; C.S. Anderson *et al.* 1993; Iso *et al.* 2000). As shown in Fig. 4, large-artery occlusive infarction is most common in Western countries, while intracerebral haemorrhage and lacunar infarction is most common in Japan. No large regional difference exists in the proportion of subarachnoid haemorrhage or embolic infarction. However, embolic origins may be mostly atherogenic in Western countries, but not in Japan. Risk factors for total stroke, therefore, depend on the distribution of stroke subtypes.

New risk factors

In the United States, the roughly estimated population-attributable risks for stroke due to hypertension, cigarette smoking, atrial fibrillation, and heavy alcohol drinking are 49.3 per cent, 12.3 per cent, 9.4 per cent, and 4.7 per cent respectively (Gorelick 1994), implying that approximately three-quarters of stroke occurrences can be explained by these traditional risk factors, while the risk factors for one-quarter of those remain to be resolved. Several new risk factors

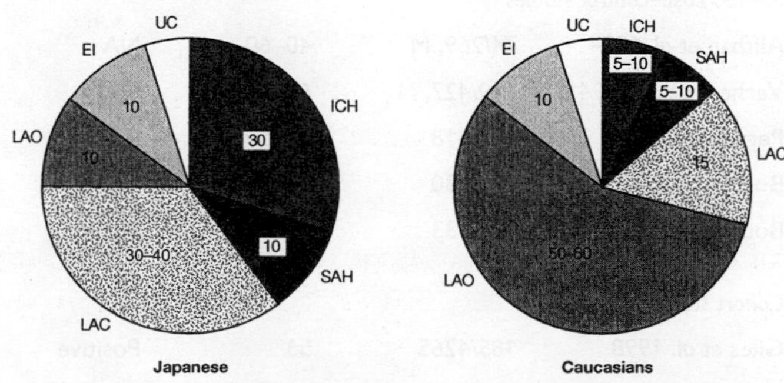

Fig. 4 The proportions of stroke subtypes among Japanese and Caucasians. EI, embolic infarction; ICH, intracerebral haemorrhage; LAC, lacunar infarction; LAO, large artery occlusive infarction; SAH, subarachnoid haemorrhage; US, unclassified stroke.

that have been revealed by recent epidemiological studies may explain considerable parts of them. We briefly refer to these new risk factors in this section.

Homocysteine

We searched the English-language medical literature to find epidemiological studies concerning plasma/serum levels of homocysteine and stroke, and include the papers published during the period 1984 to 1999 in Table 8. Only two of 15 case–control studies reported that homocysteine was not associated with risk of cerebral infarction. Among five nested case–control studies, however, only two studies reported an increased risk of cerebral infarction. All of the three cohort studies observed the positive association.

Table 8 Homocysteine and risk of cerebral infarction

Reference	Number of cases/controls[a]	Age (years)	Results
Case–control studies			
Brattstrom *et al.* 1984	19/17	34–63	Positive
Boers *et al.* 1985	25/40	< 50	Positive
Araki *et al.* 1989	90/45	39–79	Positive
Brattstrom *et al.* 1990	18/46	24–63	Positive
Coull *et al.* 1990	41/31	67/61	Positive
Clarke *et al.* 1991	38/27	< 55	Positive
Brattstrom *et al.* 1992	70/66	38–72	Positive
Dudman *et al.* 1993	51/56	< 61	Positive
Lindgren *et al.* 1995	162/60	51–98	NA
Graham *et al.* 1997	750/800	< 60	Positive
Delport *et al.* 1997	24/24		Positive
Evers *et al.* 1997	125/60		Positive
Yoo *et al.* 1998	78/140	39–82	Positive
Kristensen *et al.* 1999	80/41	18–44	NA
Kittner *et al.* 1999	167/328	15–44	Positive
Nested case–control studies			
Alfthan *et al.* 1994	74/269, M	40–60	NA
Verhoef *et al.* 1994	109/427, M	60	NA
Perry *et al.* 1995	107/118	40–59	Positive
Bots *et al.* 1997	120/630	> 60	NA
Bots *et al.* 1999*b*	120/533	> 55	Positive
Cohort studies			
Giles *et al.* 1998	185/4265	53	Positive
Stehouwer *et al.* 1998	58/878	64–84	Positive
Bostom *et al.* 1999	165/1947	70	Positive

M, males; NA, no association.

[a]For cohort studies, numbers of stroke events along with cohort members.

Beresford and Boushey (1997) reviewed 10 studies, which provided odds ratios or sufficient data to calculate odds ratios of the effect of elevated homocysteine on stroke risk. The summary estimates of the odds ratio of stroke and elevated homocysteine concentration was 2.0 (95 per cent confidence intervals, 1.7–2.4). They also calculated a summary odds ratio based on a change of 5 μmol/l in total homocysteine levels using the seven studies that measured fasting or basal levels of total homocysteine. The combined odds ratio was 1.8 (95 per cent confidence intervals, 1.6–2.0). Biologically plausible mechanisms by which homocysteine might alter the risk of developing atherosclerotic disease include endothelial cell desquamation, oxidation of low-density lipoprotein, monocyte adhesion to the vessel wall, and its direct toxicity to the endothelium. The association of elevated levels of homocysteine with some types of stroke, probably cerebral thrombosis in cortical artery regions, appears to be of the same order as that of other traditional risk factors for stroke, and to be causal.

Diabetes mellitus

Diabetes mellitus has recently become one of the most common diseases in Western countries and Japan. Diabetes mellitus may increase the risk of thromboembolic stroke through multiple and potentially synergistic mechanisms (Wolfe *et al.* 1991), because of acceleration of large-artery atherosclerosis via glycosylation-induced injury, adverse effects on both low-density lipoprotein and high-density lipoprotein cholesterol levels, and plaque formation due to hyperinsulinaemia (Karem 1996).

Patients with diabetes mellitus were found to have excessive risk for cerebral infarction, while the risk of subarachnoid haemorrhage and intracerebral haemorrhage seemed to be unelevated (Abbott *et al.* 1987; Jamrozik *et al.* 1994). The Framingham Study (Wolfe *et al.* 1991) and the American National Health and Nutrition Examination Survey (Kittner *et al.* 1990) showed increased risk of stroke in diabetic patients, while the Rancho Bernardo Study (Barrett-Connor and Khaw 1988) reported a small increased risk of stroke only for women with diabetes mellitus. A Finish prospective study (Tuomilehto *et al.* 1996) demonstrated that diabetes mellitus was the strongest risk factor for stroke in a multivariate analysis. A population-based stroke study in Sweden (6370 stroke events) found that the risk of stroke was 4.1 times higher in diabetic men and 5.8 times higher in diabetic women than in non-diabetic subjects (Stegmayr and Asplund 1995). The Honolulu Heart Study (Abbott *et al.* 1987) observed an increased risk of thrombotic stroke but no increased risk of haemorrhagic stroke for diabetes mellitus among Japanese-American men. The Framingham Study (Kannel and McGee 1979) also showed that the incidence of atherothrombotic stroke (45–74 years) was higher in diabetic than in non-diabetic subjects. A recent case–control study in young adults (15–55 years) reported that the risk of cerebral infarction was 11.6 times higher in diabetic than in non-diabetic subjects (You *et al.* 1997). In conclusion, glucose intolerance or diabetes mellitus appears to be a risk factor for cerebral infarction.

Carotid ultrasonography

Carotid ultrasonography has been used for measuring the intima and media thickness of carotid arteries. The Rotterdam follow-up study showed that an increased common carotid intima and media thickness of carotid arteries was associated with subsequent stroke events (Bots *et al.* 1997, 1999*a*). The Cardiovascular Health Study reported that intima and media thickness of the common and internal carotid arteries was strongly associated with the risk of stroke in asymptomatic older adults (O'Leary *et al.* 1999) In conclusion, increases in intima and media thickness of carotid arteries are directly associated with an increased risk of cerebral infarction, although the relative risk is small. Carotid ultrasonography is difficult to operate and expensive, and it takes a long time (15–30 min) to measure the intima and media thickness of carotid arteries. The standardization of measurement conditions and procedures is essential to reduce measurement error and bias.

Fibrinogen

Plasma fibrinogen is a major determinant of platelet aggregation and blood viscosity. Higher plasma fibrinogen levels are strongly correlated with the development of cerebral infarction as shown in Table 9. All six case–control studies showed plasma fibrinogen was positively associated with the risk of cerebral infarction (Sharma *et al.* 1978; Mistry *et al.* 1990; Qizilbash *et al.* 1991; Resch *et al.* 1992; Beamer *et al.* 1993; Belch *et al.* 1998). Among three cohort studies (Wilhelmsen *et al.* 1984; Welin *et al.* 1987; Smith *et al.* 1997), only one study reported that plasma fibrinogen was not associated with stroke in women. One cross-sectional study reported that plasma fibrinogen was associated with history of stroke subjects (Lee *et al.* 1993). There are several mechanisms whereby fibrinogen could promote atherothrombolism: thrombi formation through hypercoagulable state, acceleration of atherosclerosis, and reduction of blood flow due to high blood or plasma viscosity (Qizilbash *et al.* 1991). In conclusion, plasma fibrinogen is a probable risk factor for cerebral infarction.

Table 9 Fibrinogen and risk of cerebral infarction

Reference	Cases/controls[a]	Age (years)	Results
Case–control studies			
Sharma *et al.* 1978	46/15		Positive
Mistry *et al.* 1990	56/56		Positive
Qizilbash *et al.* 1991	105/232	68	Positive
Resch *et al.* 1992	60/60	64	Positive
Beamer *et al.* 1993	126/84	64	Positive
Belch *et al.* 1998	34/58		Positive
Cohort studies			
Wilhelmsen *et al.* 1984	37/792, M	54	Positive
Welin *et al.* 1987	57/789, M	54	Positive
Smith *et al.* 1997	45/1174	64	Positive
Tracy *et al.* 1999	200/1843, M	> 65	Positive
	242/2575, F	> 65	NA
Cross-sectional study			
Lee *et al.* 1993	320/6783	40–59	Positive

F, females; M, males; NA, no association.

[a]For cohort studies, numbers of stroke events along with cohort members.

Plasminogen activator inhibitor-1 and tissue plasminogen activator

The fibrinolytic factors plasminogen activator inhibitor-1 and tissue plasminogen activator mass concentration were shown to be independent predictors for atherothrombotic events (Hamsten 1993; Meade *et al.* 1993; Lijnen and Collen 1996). While few studies on the relationship between the fibrinolytic variables and stroke were reported, high levels of both tissue plasminogen activator and plasminogen activator inhibitor-1 were observed in patients with a history of stroke (Margaglione *et al.* 1994; Lindgren *et al.* 1996; Carter *et al.* 1998; Kristensen *et al.* 1998; Macko *et al.* 1999), and high levels of tissue plasminogen activator predicted an increased risk of stroke in two prospective studies (Ridker *et al.* 1994; Smith *et al.* 1997). A prospective study showed that tissue plasminogen activator/plasminogen activator inhibitor-1 complex, a novel fibrinolytic marker, was independently associated with the risk of stroke, especially haemorrhagic stroke (Johansson *et al.* 2000). This finding supports the hypothesis that disturbances in fibrinolysis precede stroke attacks. In conclusion, the association of plasminogen activator inhibitor-1 and tissue plasminogen activator with stroke will be a subject worthy to be tested further by cohort or case–control studies.

Genetic factors

If candidate genetic polymorphisms for stroke can be identified, screening for the presence of these alleles may identify a substantial proportion of high-risk individuals. Appropriate monitoring of these individuals, in conjunction with targeted intervention, could then delay or avert the onset of stroke. In this section, we summarize several studies on the relationship between some genetic polymorphisms and stroke. However, the findings of the studies have been contradictory.

Angiotensin-converting enzyme gene

Angiotensin-converting enzyme is the rate-limiting enzyme of the renin–angiotensin system and is known to be involved in vascular remodelling (Morishita *et al.* 1994) and atherosclerosis (Pitt 1994). The angiotensin-converting enzyme gene is located on chromosome 17q23 and consists of 26 exons and 25 introns; insertion (*I*) and deletion (*D*) polymorphisms of 287 base pairs are identified in intron 16. The angiotensin-converting enzyme *D* allele was reported to be associated with elevated plasma angiotensin-converting enzyme levels and angiotensin-converting enzyme activity in a codominant pattern (Rigat *et al.* 1990). As shown in Table 10, the angiotensin-converting enzyme *DD* genotype or *D* allele was found to be associated with cerebrovascular disease in some studies (Markus *et al.* 1995; Margaglione *et al.* 1996; Nakata *et al.* 1997). However, no association was found between angiotensin-converting enzyme *DD* genotype and cerebral infarction in other studies (Sharma *et al.* 1994; Ueda *et al.* 1995; Catto *et al.* 1996). Maeda *et al.* (1996) reported that parental history of stroke was associated with angiotensin-converting enzyme *DD* genotype. Kario *et al.* (1996) observed that hypertensive patients with angiotensin-converting enzyme *D* allele appeared to develop cerebral infarction. A meta-analysis concluded that angiotensin-converting enzyme *D* allele was a modest but independent risk factor

Table 10 Angiotensin-converting enzyme gene and stroke

Reference	Stroke subtype	Cases/controls	Mean age (years)	Genotypes[a]			Associated with
				DD	ID	II	
Case–control studies							
Sharma *et al.* 1994	CI	100/73	67/65	33/23	47/49	20/27	NA
Ueda *et al.* 1995	CVD	488/188	68/65	26/22	56/56	18/22	NA
Markus *et al.* 1995	All CVD	101/137	65/64	36/22	47/52	17/26	
	Lacunar	18		(61)	(28)	(11)	*DD*
	Large vessel	43		(23)	(49)	(23)	
	Uncertain/cardiac	30		(30)	(60)	(10)	
	Tandem	10		(40)	(30)	(30)	
Catto *et al.* 1996	All cases	454/215	74/73	28/29	44/47	28/23	NA
	Primary ICH	48		(35)	(44)	(21)	
	Total anterior circulation CI	242		(28)	(45)	(27)	
	Lacunar infarction	130		(25)	(47)	(29)	
Maeda *et al.* 1996	PHS	27/43	60/59	63/33	19/40	19/28	*DD*
Kario *et al.* 1996	Hypertensive CI	138/104	70/68	25/8	46/53	30/39	*D*
	Hypertensive non-stroke	90	67	(8)	(45)	(47)	*DD*
Doi *et al.* 1997	Thrombotic CI	181/271	< 60	17/11	43/46	40/42	NA
Nakata *et al.* 1997	CI	55/61	66/67	29/11	44/66	27/23	NA
	ICH	38/38	63/63	8/13	45/58	47/30	NA
Agerholm-Larsen *et al.* 1997	CVD (< 50 years)	73/3191	43/43	32/26	44/51	25/23	NA
	CVD (carotid stenosis > 40%)	219/7364	64/61	32/26	44/50	24/24	NA
Cross-sectional studies							
Agerholm-Larsen *et al.* 1997	CVD	160/7233	69/63	24/26	48/50		NA
Margaglione *et al.* 1996	CVD	101/109	64	54/39	37/45		*DD*
Nested case–control study							
Zee *et al.* 1999	Ischaemic stroke	338/338	61/61	34/32	48/47	18/21	NA

CI, cerebral infarction; *D*, angiotensin-converting enzyme *D* allele; *DD*, angiotensin-converting enzyme DD genotype; ICH, intracerebral haemorrhage; ICVD, ischaemic cerebrovascular disease; NA, no association; PHS, parental history of stroke.

[a]The numbers in parentheses are percentages. In some cases percentages may not sum to 100 because of rounding.

for cerebral infarction (Sharma 1998). Conversely, recent cross-sectional and nested case–control studies showed that there was no association between cerebrovascular disease and angiotensin-converting enzyme genotypes (Agerholm-Larsen *et al.* 1997; Zee *et al.* 1999).

Apolipoprotein E gene

The apolipoprotein E ε2 allele is associated with lower, and the ε4 allele with higher serum total and low-density lipoprotein cholesterol levels as compared with the ε3 (Sing and Davignon 1985). As shown in Table 11, the apolipoprotein E ε2 allele was found to be associated with cerebral infarction (Couderc *et al.* 1993), whereas the ε4 allele was found to be associated with cerebral infarction (Margaglione *et al.* 1998; Pedro-Botet *et al.* 1992; Peng *et al.* 1999) and with large-vessel thrombotic stroke (Kessler *et al.* 1997). On the contrary, apolipoprotein E gene polymorphism was shown to be unrelated to either cerebral infarction or haemorrhage in the Japanese population (Nakata *et al.* 1997). A cohort study reported the protective effect of the ε2 allele in an older population (Ferrucci *et al.* 1997), but that apolipoprotein E gene could not be identified as a risk factor for stroke

Table 11 Apolipoprotein E alleles and stroke

Reference	Subject of study	Cases/controls	Average age (years)	Allelles (%)[b]			Associated with
				ε2	ε3	ε4	
Case–control studies							
Mahieux *et al.* 1990	ICVD	59/28	73/72	6/0	84/96	10/4	NA
Pedro-Botet *et al.* 1992	Survived ICVD	100/100	64/64	8/8	73/82	19/11	ε3/ε4
Couderc *et al.* 1993	ICVD	69/68	72/72	7/1	85/93	9/7	ε2
Cona *et al.* 1995	ICVD	104/94	71/72	6/7	82/78[c]	12/15	NA
Hachinski *et al.* 1996	ICVD	85/85	65/65	9/9	77/84	16/12	NA
Kessler *et al.* 1997	Case all	227/225	62/63	9/7	76/81	15/12	NA
	Large-vessel disease	70		7	74	19	ε4
	Lacunar	34		12	71	18	NA
	Cardioembolism	53		10	78	11	NA
	Other	70		8	79	14	NA
Nakata *et al.* 1997	Thrombosis	55/61	66/67	2/6	89/90	9/4	NA
	Intracerebral haemorrhage	38/38	63/63	7/6	86/85	7/9	NA
	Survived ICVD	100/108	66/61	6/8	76/85	18/6	ε4
	ICVD	90/90	63/63	8/11	79/83	13/6	ε3/ε4
Margaglione *et al.* 1998	Case all	322/1126	68/64	9/5	79/85	12/11	ε2
Peng, 1999	Cerebral infarction	201		10	81	9	ε2
Kokubo *et al.* 2000	Atherothrombosis	62		14	72	15	ε2, ε3/ε4
	Lacunar	74		4	88	8	NA
	Unclassified	34		12	88	0	ε2/ε2
	Cardioembolism	31		16	73	11	ε2
	Intracerebral haemorrhage	84		8	78	14	ε2/ε2, ε3/ε4
	Subarachnoid haemorrhage	37		5	74	20	ε4
Cohort studies							
Kuusisto *et al.* 1995	Stroke/cohort members	64/1067	69	5	78	17	NA
Basun *et al.* 1996	Stroke/no stroke	168/956	83/81	11/12[d]	60/56[c]	25/26[d]	NA (> 75 years)
Ferrucci *et al.* 1997	Stroke/no stroke	150/1664	79	9	77	14	ε2 protective (< 80 years)

ICVD, ischaemic cerebrovascular disease; NA, no association, data not shown in the reference.

[a]For cohort studies, numbers of stroke events along with no stroke subjects or cohort members in the parenthesis.

[b]In some cases, percentages may not sum to 100 because of rounding.

[c]Only subjects with ε3/ε3 were included.

[d]Only subjects with ε2 or ε4 heterozygosity were included.

in other populations (Kuusisto *et al.* 1995; Basun *et al.* 1996; Hachinski *et al.* 1996).

Kokubo *et al.* (2000) showed a positive relationship between apolipoprotein E ε2 and the risks of cerebral atherothrombosis and cardioembolism, and intracerebral haemorrhage, and more prominent effect of apolipoprotein E ε2 on the risks in the elderly group than in the middle-aged group. Meanwhile, a positive association of ε4 and the risk of atherothrombotic stroke was shown in the middle-aged group but not in the elderly. Such age-dependent changes in the association of ε2 or ε4 with stroke was also suggested in other studies. Positive associations between ε4 and stroke were detected only in subjects less than 70 years (Pedro-Botet *et al.* 1992; Kessler *et al.* 1997; Margaglione *et al.* 1998; Peng *et al.* 1999). On the contrary, a positive association between ε2 and stroke was found in subjects aged 70 years and over (Couderc *et al.* 1993).

Methylenetetrahydrofolate reductase gene

Elevated levels of plasma/serum homocysteine are probably associated with the risk of carotid artery stenosis and stroke. A common mutation in methylenetetrahydrofolate reductase (**MTHFR**) which is a homocysteine metabolic pathway enzyme was associated with increased homocysteine levels and, thus, an increased risk for cardiovascular disease. Several studies in Western populations demonstrated that the prevalence of homozygous C677T mutation was not significantly higher in controls than in patients with cerebrovascular diseases (Table 12) (Markus *et al.* 1997; Kostulas *et al.* 1998; Salooja *et al.* 1998; Gaustadnes *et al.* 1999; Harmon *et al.* 1999; Press *et al.* 1999; Lalouschek *et al.* 1999*a*,*b*). However, one study in a Japanese population showed that the *V* allele was associated with cerebral infarction (Morita *et al.* 1998).

Table 12 Methylenetetrahydrofolate reductase (**MTHFR**) and β-fibrinogen genes, and stroke (case–control study)

Genetic polymorphism	Reference	Stroke subtype	Cases/controls	Associated with
MTHFR				
T/t	Markus *et al.* 1997	CVD	345/161	NA
T/t	Kostulas *et al.* 1998	CVD	126/70	NA
C677T	Nakata *et al.* 1998	VI, ICH	48, 35/105	NA
C677T	Morita *et al.* 1998	CI	256/325	*V* alelle
C677T	Lalouschek *et al.* 1999*a*	TIA, minor stroke	81/81	NA
C677T	Salooja *et al.* 1998	CVD	271/173	NA
C677T	Harmon *et al.* 1999	VD	174/183	NA
C677T	Lalouschek *et al.* 1999*b*	TIA, minor stroke	96/96	NA
C677T	Press *et al.* 1999	CVD	136/52	NA
C677T	Gaustadnes *et al.* 1999	Thrombosis	403/1084	NA
β-fibrinogen				
Bβ448	Carter *et al.* 1997	CVD	305/197	*1/1* for female
455G/A	Kessler *et al.* 1997	Large-vessel disease	227/225	*AA* genotype
455G/A	Nishiuma *et al.* 1998	Hypertensive CI	85/85	*A* alelle

CI, cerebral infarction; CVD, cerebrovascular disease; ICH, intracerebral haemorrhage; NA, no association; TIA, transient ischaemic attacks.

Fibrinogen gene

High levels of plasma fibrinogen lead to an increased risk of cerebrovascular disease (Wilhelmsen *et al.* 1984; Kannel *et al.* 1987) and peripheral artery disease (Lowe *et al.* 1993). Fibrinogen consists of a glycoprotein comprising pairs of three non-identical polypeptides: Aα, Bβ, and γ chains (Doolittle 1983; Henschen *et al.* 1983). The synthesis of the Bβ chain is considered to be a rate-limiting step in the secretion of fibrinogen from hepatocytes (Yu *et al.* 1984). The 5′ region of the β gene contains binding sites for several *trans*-acting factors, which largely control the expression of the gene (G.M. Anderson *et al.* 1993). Carter *et al.* (1997) reported that fibrinogen Bβ448 *1/1* genotype was associated with cerebral infarction in females but not in males (Table 12). Fibrinogen 455G/A *A* allele was found to be an independent risk factor for cerebral infarction in a Japanse population (Nishiuma *et al.* 1998), whereas no association was observed in a Western population (Kessler *et al.* 1997).

Lifestyle

Diet

Table 13 summarizes the epidemiological studies which reported associations of dietary intake with stroke. Among them, an inverse relation between fat intake and stroke is noteworthy, because it may imply an aetiological difference between stroke and coronary heart disease.

Seven cohort studies on dietary fat and stroke have been reported (Reed 1990; Klag and Whelton 1993; Bronner *et al.* 1995; Gillman *et al.* 1997; Seino *et al.* 1997; Sherwin and Price 1997; Iso *et al.* 2001). Gillman *et al.* (1997) reported the risk of cerebral infarction was inversely related to intakes of fat, saturated fat, and monounsaturated fat that were assessed by the 24-h recall method. Seino *et al.* (1997), who estimated dietary intake of fat by a semi-quantitative food frequency questionnaire, observed the same results as Gillman and his colleagues, but the inverse association did not reach statistical significance. Iso *et al.* (2001) reported an association of a low intake of saturated fat and animal protein with the risk of intracerebral haemorrhage. Four other studies found no relationship between fat or fish oil and stroke.

According to Japanese studies (Tanaka *et al.* 1992; Konishi *et al.* 1993), the Japanese used to have only steamed rice, miso (soybean paste) soup, and salted vegetables every meal during the national privation period before 1950, i.e. high carbohydrate and salt, and extremely low fat and animal protein. The average serum cholesterol was less than 160 mg/dl in males aged 40 to 64 years. The subjects with high blood pressure and low serum cholesterol had a very high risk of stroke, particularly intracerebral haemorrhage and cerebral infarction in penetrating artery regions. Thus, a diet-stroke hypothesis was proposed in Japan: low intake of lipids and low levels of serum cholesterol result in the development of stroke. Epidemiological studies are expected to test the hypothesis.

Although it is well established that diet affects coronary heart disease and its risk factors, data about diet and stroke, particularly the subtypes, are insufficient. Nutritional factors that have cardioprotective effects can be applied to prevention against cerebral thrombosis in cortical artery regions, but not intracerebral haemorrhage and cerebral infarction in perforating artery regions. Additional epidemiological studies on diet and subtypes of stroke should be carried out.

Physical activity

A beneficial effect of increasing physical activity on prevention of stroke remains controversial. The Surgeon General's Report on

Table 13 Inverse association of dietary intake with risk of stroke

	Reference
Food pattern	
Vegetarian	Key *et al.* 1996
	Chang-Claude *et al.* 1992
Western	Klag and Whelton 1993
	Reed 1990
Foods	
Fruits and vegetables	Khaw and Barrett-Connor 1987
	Manson *et al.* 1994
	Acheson and Williams 1983
	Gillman *et al.* 1995
	Vollset and Bjelke 1983
Tea	Keli *et al.* 1996
Milk	Abbott *et al.* 1996
Animal-derived foods	Klag and Whelton 1993
	Reed 1990
Nutrients	
Fat	Gillman *et al.* 1997
	Seino *et al.* 1997
	Klag and Whelton 1993
	Bronner *et al.* 1995
	Sherwin and Price 1997
	Reed 1990
	Iso *et al.* 2001
Protein	Klag and Whelton 1993
	Reed 1990
	Iso *et al.* 2001
Antioxidant vitamins	Ness *et al* 1996
	Manson *et al.* 1993
	Gey *et al.* 1993
Antioxidant minerals	Neve 1996
Other antioxidants	Keli *et al.* 1996
Potassium	Khaw and Barrett-Connor 1987
	Ascherio *et al.* 1998
Calcium	Abbott *et al.* 1996
	Iso *et al.*1999
Vitamin B and folate	Boushey *et al.* 1995
	Blom 1998
	Perry 1999

Physical Activity and Health in 1996 concluded that 'the existing data do not unequivocally support an association between physical activity and risk of stroke' (US Department of Health and Human Services 1996). Although several studies have reported an inverse relationship of leisure-time (Wannamethee and Shaper 1992; Haheim *et al.* 1993; Lindenstrom *et al.* 1993*a*; Shinton and Sagar 1993; Gillum *et al.* 1996; Sacco *et al.* 1998; Agnarsson *et al.* 1999) or on-the-job (Abbott *et al.* 1994; Kiely *et al.* 1994; Nakayama *et al.* 1997; Evenson *et al.* 1999) physical activity to risk of stroke or a U-shaped relationship (Lee and Paffenbarger 1998), others have shown no association between physical activity and stroke (Folsom *et al.* 1990; Harmsen *et al.* 1990; Lindsted *et al.* 1991; Ellekjaer *et al.* 1992; Kiely *et al.* 1994; Nakayama *et al.* 1997; Lee *et al.* 1999; Evenson *et al.* 1999), including several cohort studies (Gillum *et al.* 1996; Nakayama *et al.* 1997; Lee and Paffenbarger 1998; Agnarsson *et al.* 1999; Evenson *et al.* 1999; Lee *et al.* 1999) which were published after the Surgeon General's Report (US Department of Health and Human Services 1996). The reasons for the inconsistent findings may be due to combining different subtypes of stroke, measurement errors of physical activity (Paffenbarger *et al.* 1993), insufficient statistical power to detect the association, and potential confounding factors. The inconsistency may reflect only a weak association between physical activity and stroke (Evenson *et al.* 1999).

A recent large-scale cohort study of 14 575 middle-aged adults in the United States (Evenson *et al.* 1999) identified a weak association of on-the-job physical activity with a reduced incidence of cerebral infarction. However, the United States Physician's Health Study with 533 fatal and non-fatal strokes among 21 823 male physicians (Lee *et al.* 1999) reported that significant associations between frequency of exercise and ischaemic and haemorrhagic strokes disappeared after adjustment for several confounding variables, concluding that the observed inverse association of physical activity with stroke is mediated through beneficial effects on body weight, blood pressure, serum cholesterol, and glucose tolerance.

Alcohol

Although there have been numerous studies investigating the effect of alcohol consumption on the occurrence of stroke, the relationship between alcohol and stroke seems less clear compared to the J-shaped relationship between alcohol consumption and coronary heart disease. Several case–control (Monforte *et al.* 1990; Gill *et al.* 1991; Ben-Shlomo *et al.* 1992; Palomaki and Kaste 1993; Rodgers *et al.* 1993; Beghi *et al.* 1995; Hillbom *et al.* 1995; You *et al.* 1997) and cohort (Iso *et al.* 1995; Kiyohara *et al.* 1995; Wannamethee and Shaper 1996; Ross *et al.* 1997; Yuan *et al.* 1997; Truelsen *et al.* 1998*b*; Hart *et al.* 1999) studies indicated an association of haemorrhagic stroke with habitual or recent heavy drinking of alcoholic beverages. This association was considered to be mediated through acute and chronic effects of alcohol on blood pressure (Wannamethee and Shaper 1996). The protective effect of light to moderate drinking on stroke has not been clearly established (Wannamethee and Shaper 1998) with divergent results from various populations (Gill *et al.* 1991; Lindenstrom *et al.* 1993*b*; Palomaki and Kaste 1993; Rodgers *et al.* 1993; Jamrozik *et al.* 1994; Gronbaek *et al.* 1995; Hansagi *et al.* 1995; Iso *et al.* 1995; Kiyohara *et al.* 1995; Rodriguez *et al.* 1998; Caicoya *et al.* 1999; Sacco *et al.* 1999). This might be partly due to failure to separate ischaemic and haemorrhagic stroke, the use of non-drinkers (including both life-long abstainers and ex-drinkers) as a comparison group (Wannamethee and Shaper 1996, 1998), the possible difference in biological effect amongst beer, wine, and spirits (Truelsen *et al.* 1998*b*), or the possible influence of day-to-day patterns of alcohol consumption (Wannamethee and Shaper 1996). Recent studies, taking into account some of the above-mentioned factors that might distort the study results, found that light to moderate consumption of wine was more strongly associated with lower risk of cerebral infarction (Truelsen *et al.* 1998*b*; Sacco *et al.* 1999) than that of beer and spirits, and that light to moderate alcohol consumption approximately up to 30 g/day was protective against cerebral infarction (Sacco *et al.* 1999; Caicoya *et al.* 1999) or was not beneficial for stroke risk compared with occasional drinking (Wannamethee and Shaper 1996).

As for subarachnoid haemorrhage, a meta-analysis of nine cohort studies and 11 case–control studies concluded that drinking 150 g or more alcohol per week was associated with an increased risk of subarachnoid haemorrhage with a combined odds ratio being 1.5 for case–control studies and a combined relative risk being 4.7 for cohort studies (Teunissen *et al.* 1996).

Smoking

Cigarette smoking is considered to be an established risk factor for stroke (Aldoori and Rahman 1998). A number of case–control studies (Bonita *et al.* 1986; Gill *et al.* 1989; You *et al.* 1993; Howard *et al.* 1998), cohort studies (Abbott *et al.* 1986; Wolf *et al.* 1988; Harmsen *et al.* 1990; Lindenstrom *et al.* 1993*b*; Robbins *et al.* 1994; Wannamethee *et al.* 1995; Haheim *et al.* 1996), and a meta-analysis of 32 separate studies (Shinton and Beevers 1989) have indicated a significantly higher risk in current smokers than in non-smokers for cerebral infarction and subarachnoid haemorrhage (Bonita *et al.* 1986; Longstreth *et al.* 1992; Juvela *et al.* 1993; Teunissen *et al.* 1996). A population-based case–control study in New Zealand found an increased risk of stroke associated with exposure to environmental tobacco smoke among non-smokers and long-term ex-smokers (Bonita *et al.* 1999). A more notable issue regarding an association between smoking and stroke in the public health field might be a potential effect of smoking cessation to reduce the risk of stroke (Abbott *et al.* 1986; Wannamethee *et al.* 1995; Aldoori and Rahman 1998). The Framingham Heart Study clearly showed that smoking cessation reduced the relative risk of stroke to the level of a non-smoker within 5 years after quitting (Wolf *et al.* 1988). A cohort study investigating the effect of stopping smoking in detail (Wannamethee *et al.* 1995) revealed that light smokers (less than 20 cigarettes/day) could revert to the risk level of never smokers, while heavy smokers would retain a more than two-fold risk compared with never smokers even 5 years after quitting, and that the benefit of stopping smoking was greater in hypertensive than in normotensive middle-aged men.

Several studies showed a potential synergistic effect of smoking and oral contraceptive use (Oleckno 1988; Higa and Davanipoor 1991), alcohol consumption (Oleckno 1988), hypertension (Bonita 1986; Bonita *et al.* 1986; Higa and Davanipoor 1991; Haheim *et al.* 1996), and antihypertensive drug use specifically β-blockers (Medical Research Council Working Party 1988; Higa and Davinpoor 1991). Pharmacological treatment of hypertension in smokers with mild hypertension would be less beneficial for reducing the risk of stroke than that in non-smokers with mild hypertension (Medical Research Council Working Party 1988). These findings suggest that all smokers, especially those with hypertension, should be advised that it is not too late to stop smoking for reducing risk of stroke, no matter how long they have been smoking (Gill *et al.* 1991).

Strategies for prevention of stroke

Although the natural history of stroke and stroke subtypes is complex, hypertension is the strongest and most consistent risk factor for stroke as well as a major determinant for stroke prognosis. Therefore, the prevention and control of hypertension is a central strategy for primary, secondary, and tertiary prevention of stroke. Dyslipidaemia, glucose intolerance, and smoking have been less consistent risk factors for total stroke, or have been limited to certain stroke subtypes, and thus the control and prevention of these risk factors is of less importance in the prevention of stroke compared with the prevention of ischaemic heart disease.

Strategies for prevention of stroke are categorized as four modalities: primordial, primary, secondary, and tertiary prevention. Primordial prevention, the early phase of primary prevention, attempts to retard the development of hypertension in the early stage of life including childhood, adolescence, and young adults. Modification of lifestyles including diet (reduced intake of sodium and increased intake of potassium), physical activity (increased physical activity for the control and prevention of overweight), and drinking (reduction of excessive alcohol intake) are major health education activities for primary prevention.

Primary prevention, in a usual form, is the early detection of hypertension through systematic blood pressure screenings and the control of hypertension by either pharmacological or non-pharmacological treatments. Various antihypertensive drugs are available and have been demonstrated as effective for reduction of blood pressure levels in hypertensives. Non-pharmacological treatments such as reduction of sodium intake and alcohol intake, increased potassium intake, increased physical activity, and control of overweight are also effective for reduction of blood pressure levels, and reduce medication requirement for hypertensives.

Secondary prevention is the identification of transient ischaemic attacks to prevent the development of completed stroke. Antithrombotic treatment has been demonstrated to be effective to prevent complete stroke among patients with a history of transient ischaemic attack. However, systematic identification of transient ischaemic attacks is a difficult task in communities. Application of antithrombotic treatment within 12 h of the onset of ischaemic stroke is one of the promising treatments to prevent the complete stroke. If ambulance systems develop to support early antithrombotic treatment, this strategy could be a practical method for secondary prevention.

Tertiary prevention is the rehabilitation for stroke patients to prevent or reduce their disabilities and social handicaps. Tertiary prevention also includes medial and social care for disabled stroke patients to improve or maintain quality of life for themselves and their families. Early physical treatment followed by occupational therapy, verbal therapy, and social support is particularly important to improve prognosis in their activities of daily livings and quality of life for a considerable proportion of stroke patients.

Japan suffers higher mortality from stroke and lower mortality from coronary heart disease than Western countries. To ameliorate the epidemic of stroke, a community-based programme for primordial and primary prevention of stroke was launched in several communities in the 1960s. A recent study in two Japanese communities with different intervention intensity provided evidence on the effect of community hypertension control for stroke prevention (Iso *et al.* 1998).

Community intervention for stroke prevention

There were two agricultural communities (approximately 3000 men and women aged 30 and over in one community and 1500 in the other community with similar age and sex distributions and stable populations over time) in northeastern Japan, 36 miles apart, where mortality from stroke was double that of all Japan. Efforts to control hypertension by systematic blood pressure screening and health education had been widespread in both communities since 1963. However, the fortuitous lack of interest of the government of one community, which started to charge participants for blood pressure screening after 1969, and the retirement of the public health nurse in 1973, caused a difference in penetration of hypertension control efforts. This circumstance permitted the observation of the long-term effect on blood pressure and its clinical sequelae at two levels of intensity of an intervention programme. Furthermore, the full intervention community received continuous government support, systematic education classes for detected hypertensives, and a home broadcasting system for verbal health announcements via a speaker attached to the telephone. The minimal intervention community had no systematic classes or mass-media education.

Approximately 80 per cent of men and 90 per cent of women aged 40 to 69 were screened in both communities in the 1960s. After services were reduced in the reference community, screening rates of general population and hypertensives declined, more in men (to 50 per cent) than in women (to 60 per cent), whereas the full intervention community kept high screening rates. There was a larger decline in stroke incidence for men aged 30 and over in the intervention community (42 per cent in 1970–1975, 53 per cent in 1976–1981, and 75 per cent in 1982–1987) than in the minimal intervention community (5 per cent increase, 20 per cent decrease, and 29 per cent decrease respectively); in women, the decline in stroke incidence was approximately 45 per cent, 50 per cent and 65 per cent respectively in both communities (Fig. 5). Changes in stroke prevalence paralleled those in stroke incidence. Trends in blood pressure levels tended to explain the differential stroke rates in men. The lack of difference in change in stroke rates among women may be because women are more health conscious than men and are more likely to respond to a relatively low programme intensity since the decline in participation in the minimal intervention community in blood pressure screening was not as large in women as men.

Delivery of hypertension control services through intensive, free, community-based screening supplemented by community-based health education and broad citizen support was apparently effective in prevention of stroke.

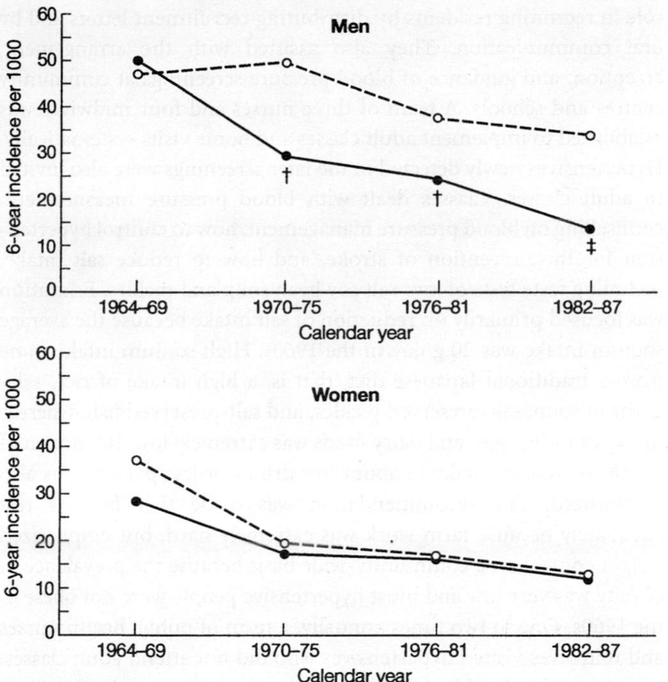

Fig. 5 Sex-specific age-adjusted stroke incidence in the full intervention community (•) and the minimal intervention community (○) for men and women aged 30 years. Difference from the minimal intervention community: †$p < 0.01$, ‡$p < 0.001$. (Source: Iso *et al.* 1998.)

Strategies and organization for hypertension control programme

Realistic strategies and organization for the hypertension control programme in the above study should be mentioned. These activities are similar to those in prevention programmes for ischaemic heart disease in Europe and the United States in terms of multiple strategies and involvement of existing organizations (Tuomilehto *et al.* 1980; Farquhar *et al.* 1990; Luepker *et al.* 1996), but are different in terms of practical approaches and existing resources related to different cultures and environments.

In the full intervention community, the basic strategies for hypertension control included the following:

- systematic blood pressure screening for detection of hypertensives
- referral of high-risk individuals to either of two local clinics when antihypertensive medication was required based on the presence of high blood pressure or end-organ effects in the retinal arterioles or electrocardiogram
- health education for hypertensives at blood pressure screening sites, at adult classes, and via nurse home visits;
- training of volunteers to give health education for dietary improvement
- community-wide media-disseminated education to encourage people to participate in blood pressure screening and to reduce salt intake.

The network and organization for the stroke prevention programme included a local government office, a prefectural health centre, two local clinics, research institutes, and task forces, which held regular meetings to discuss the implementation of the programme. Task forces consisted of public health nurses, midwives, community leaders, and their coworkers from each district of the community. Repeated systematic blood pressure screenings for detection, referral, and follow-up of hypertensives were free of charge. Community leaders and their coworkers, appointed by local government, played a role in recruiting residents by distributing recruitment letters and by oral communication. They also assisted with the arrangement, reception, and guidance of blood pressure screenings at community centres and schools. A team of three nurses and four midwives was established to implement adult classes and home visits systematically. Hypertensives newly detected in the later screenings were also invited to adult classes. Classes dealt with blood pressure measurement, counselling on blood pressure management, how to control hypertension for the prevention of stroke, and how to reduce salt intake, including taste tests of low-salt soy bean soup and pickles. Education was focused primarily on reduction of salt intake because the average sodium intake was 20 g/day in the 1960s. High sodium intake came from a traditional Japanese diet, that is, a high intake of rice, salty soybean soup, salt-preserved pickles, and salt-preserved fish, whereas intake of meat, eggs, and dairy foods was extremely low. Reduction of excessive alcohol intake to about five drinks or less per day was also emphasized. The recommendation was made that farmers rest adequately because farm work was extremely hard, but emphasized weight control on a community-wide basis because the prevalence of obesity was very low and most hypertensive people were not obese in the 1960s. One to two times annually, a team of public health nurses and midwives visited hypertensives who did not attend adult classes, to confirm that a referral had occurred and to offer health education.

Volunteers for diet improvements were trained through annual classes, enhancing knowledge of stroke and practical ways of modifying diet and lifestyle for stroke prevention. These training sessions were instructed by trained nurses, nutritionists, and physicians. The volunteers offered health education to people at blood pressure screenings and at regular public meetings held at local public centres, four or five times a year.

Media dissemination was accomplished by a municipal announcement system transmitted via a speaker attached to each household telephone. This announcement system was used primarily in emergencies, such as fire and earthquake, but also to broadcast health education messages. Individuals could turn the speaker off. The announcement system was used to recruit participants to blood pressure screenings and adult classes a week before and during the events. In addition to this campaign, a regular programme on cardiovascular health was aired for three minutes at 06.30, 12.30, and 18.30 every Thursday. Topics, which were revised monthly, were reduction of salt intake, the importance of balanced diet, proper rest, etc.

Summary

Cerebrovascular disease ranks third or higher as a cause of death in industrialized countries. The age-adjusted death rates from cerebrovascular disease tended to decrease in the United States and Western Europe during the period from 1950 to 1995. Although the Japanese rate was the highest in the world and increased from 1950 to 1964, it tended to decrease after 1965, reaching the level of West European countries in recent years. The estimated international average incidence of all strokes in the age group 30 years and over was 3.57 per 1000 for males and 2.94 per 1000 for females: 1.78 and 1.12 for intracerebral haemorrhage and 2.44 and 2.15 for cerebral infarction. The sex- and age-adjusted vital prognosis of intracerebral haemorrhage and infarction has improved during these three decades because of the decline in the number of patients with severe stroke, improvement of medical care, and a decrease in blood pressure levels. Stroke is a complex of subtypes: subarachnoid haemorrhage, intracerebral haemorrhage, embolic infarction, and thrombotic infarction consisting of large-artery occlusive infarction and lacunar infarction. These subtypes may have different pathologies, aetiologies, and risk factors. Hypertension, smoking, and heavy drinking increase the risk of subarachnoid haemorrhage. The contribution of hypertension to intracerebral haemorrhage is strongest among the stroke subtypes. In addition, low levels of serum total cholesterol and heavy drinking are associated with an increased risk of intracerebral haemorrhage. The risk factors for embolic infarction depend on the proportion of sources of emboli, especially atrial fibrillation. Major risk factors for ischaemic heart disease (high total or low-density lipoprotein-cholesterol levels, low high-density lipoprotein-cholesterol levels, glucose intolerance, smoking, and hypertension) also increase the risk of large-artery occlusive infarction, although it is not known whether the aetiology is identical between infarction and ischaemic heart disease. Moderate hypertension with a longer duration, fundoscopic abnormalities, and glucose intolerance are likely to cause lacunar infarction, whereas the contribution of dyslipidaemia or smoking is small. Approximately three-quarters of stroke occurrences can be explained by traditional risk factors such as hypertension, cigarette smoking, heavy drinking, and atrial fibrillation, while the rest remain to be resolved. Several new risk factors that have been revealed by recent epidemiological studies may explain considerable parts of this latter group. For example, elevated homocysteine or fibrinogen levels and increased carotid intima and media thickness increase the risk of cerebral infarction. Meanwhile, several studies have reported the relationships between stroke and genetic polymorphisms: angiotensin-converting enzyme insertion/deletion, apolipoprotein E gene, MTHFR gene, and fibrinogen gene polymorphisms. The early phase of primary prevention of stroke attempts to stop the development of hypertension in the early stages of life. Modification of lifestyles in diet (reduced intake of sodium), physical activity (increased activity for the control and prevention of overweight), and drinking (reduction of excessive alcohol intake) are major health educational activities for primary prevention. They have been shown to decrease stroke in community intervention trials.

Appendices

Appendix 1 Age-specific stroke incidence rates per 1000 population in selected communities (group A)

Community	Year	Sex	Age-specific incidence (age group)					
			30–39	40–49	50–59	60–69	70–79	80+
All strokes								
Shibata	1976–78	Male	0.26	1.25	3.30	10.42	15.72	27.63
(Niigata, Japan)		Female	0.13	0.22	1.05	3.78	8.01	20.89
		Both sexes	0.20	0.71	2.06	6.72	11.24	23.23
Akita (Japan)	1964–69	Male	0.52	2.25	9.46	18.98	23.03	37.74
		Female	0.31	1.00	4.60	14.04	19.51	34.56
		Both sexes	0.4[a]	1.6[a]	7.0[a]	16.4[a]	21.0[a]	35.7[a]
Osaka (Japan)	1963–68	Male	0	0.85	1.73	11.29	19.92	40.20
		Female	0	0.21	1.11	6.63	11.05	17.11
		Both sexes	0[a]	0.5[a]	1.4[a]	8.8[a]	15.1[a]	25.0[a]
Hisayama	1961–63	Both sexes		1.77	6.34	13.74	20.83	28.85
(Fukuoka, Japan)								
Tartu	1970–73	Male	0.22	0.97	1.97	5.79	15.20	32.4[a]
(Former USSR)		Female	0.03	0.35	1.31	3.72	12.68	28.2[a]
		Both sexes	0.13	0.62	1.58	4.45	13.29	29.3[a]
Manitoba (Canada)	1970–71	Male	0.17	0.65	2.13	5.34	10.41	25.25
		Female	0.23	0.38	1.16	3.33	9.72	21.87
		Both sexes	0.20	0.51	1.63	4.28	9.23	23.39
Poznan (Poland)	1985	Male	0.25	1.10	3.83	5.53	9.64	10.7[a]
		Female	0.15	0.55	1.48	3.47	7.62	9.5[a]
		Both sexes	0.20	0.82	2.59	4.34	8.38	9.8[a]
Oahu (Hawaii, USA)	1969–72	Male			1.46	3.70	1.92	
(Hawaiian Japanese)	1973–76	Male			1.29	2.50	4.78	
	1977–80	Male			0.27	2.24	4.77	0.00
	1981–84	Male				2.38	4.88	6.91
	1985–88	Male				2.37	4.54	8.49
Cerebral haemorrhage								
Shibata	1976–78	Male	0.13	0.42	1.02	2.66	2.84	1.78
(Niigata, Japan)		Female	0.07	0.11	0.49	1.11	1.89	1.43
		Both sexes	0.10	0.26	0.73	1.80	2.28	1.55
Akita (Japan)	1964–69	Male	0.30	1.02	4.06	6.25	9.82	10.65
		Female	0.11	0.64	1.73	4.94	6.33	21.53
		Both sexes	0.20	0.82	2.87	5.56	7.86	17.05

Community	Year	Sex	Age-specific incidence (age group)					
			30–39	40–49	50–59	60–69	70–79	80+
Osaka (Japan)	1963–68	Male	0	0.46	0.80	4.31	8.75	7.50
		Female	0	0.11	0.50	2.46	4.35	7.73
		Both sexes	0	0.27	0.63	3.31	6.36	7.65
Tartu (Former USSR)	1970–73	Both sexes	0.04	0.14	0.33	0.89	1.16	3.5[a]
Manitoba (Canada)	1970–71							
Urban area		Male	0.09	0.29	0.36			
		Female	0.13	0.26	0.64			
		Both sexes	0.11	0.27	0.51			
Rural area		Male	0.12	0.26	0.70			
		Female	0.26	0.06	0.21			
		Both sexes	0.18	0.16	0.45			
Cerebral infarction								
Shibata (Niigata, Japan)	1976–78	Male	0	0.24	1.35	6.25	11.57	22.28
		Female	0	0	0.21	1.84	4.71	16.62
		Both sexes	0	0.11	0.73	3.80	7.58	18.59
Akita (Japan)	1964–69	Male	0	0.60	3.93	9.93	11.00	21.29
		Female	0	0.23	1.38	4.88	11.52	8.42
		Both sexes	0	0.40	2.63	7.29	11.29	12.95
Osaka (Japan)	1963–68	Male	0	0.20	0.69	5.26	8.26	25.70
		Female	0	0	0.50	2.06	6.20	7.06
		Both sexes	0	0.09	0.58	3.53	7.14	13.40
Tartu (Former USSR)	1970–73	Male	0.11	0.51	1.46	4.40	13.49	26.1[a]
		Female	0.03	0.14	0.63	2.70	10.77	26.5[a]
		Both sexes	0.07	0.31	0.98	3.24	11.49	25.4[a]
Manitoba (Canada)	1970–71							
Urban area		Male	0.09	0.35	1.58			
		Female	0.11	0.26	0.55			
		Both sexes	0.10	0.31	1.03			
Rural area		Male	0	0.26	1.18			
		Female	0	0	0.56			
		Both sexes	0	0.13	0.87			
Oahu (Hawaii, USA)	1969–72	Male			1.46	3.70	1.92	
(Hawaiian Japanese)	1973–76	Male			1.29	2.50	4.78	
	1977–80	Male			0.27	2.24	4.77	0.00

Community	Year	Sex	Age-specific incidence (age group)					
			30–39	40–49	50–59	60–69	70–79	80+
	1981–84	Male				2.38	4.88	6.91
	1985–88	Male				2.37	4.54	8.49
Subarachnoid haemorrhage								
Shibata (Niigata, Japan)	1976–78	Both sexes	0.07	0.23	0.38	0.56	0.00	0.00
Tartu (Former USSR)	1970–73	Both sexes	0.02	0.18	0.27	0.30	0.66	0.5[a]
Poznan (Poland)	1985	Male	0.06	0.05	0.21	0.21	0.39	0[a]
		Female	0.04	0.14	0.16	0.15	0.19	0.28[a]
		Both sexes	0.05	0.10	0.18	0.18	0.27	0.20[a]

[a]Estimated from the data in each reference.

Appendix 2 Age-specific stroke incidence rates per 1000 population in selected communities (group B)

Community	Year	Sex	Age-specific incidence (age group)				
			35–44	45–54	55–64	65–74	75+
All strokes							
Shibata (Niigata, Japan)	1976–78	Male	0.51	2.28	5.49	13.80	22.13
		Female	0.18	0.58	2.22	5.12	15.31
		Both sexes	0.34	1.39	3.64	8.90	17.90
Jerusalem (Israel)	1960–67	Male	0.21	1.26	3.93	9.15	10.04
		Female	0.23	0.64	3.20	6.50	9.08
		Both sexes	0.22	0.94	3.49	7.78	9.52
Fargo, ND – Moorhead, MN (USA)	1965–66	Male	0.81	1.91	4.42	11.51	34.94
		Female	0.46	1.45	2.63	10.18	39.08
		Both sexes	0.64	1.68	3.49	10.82	37.16
Mid-Missouri (USA)	1964–65						
White		Male	0	0.26	3.92	7.43	29.27
		Female	0	0	2.55	4.61	26.93
		Both sexes	0	0.13	3.19	5.86	27.92
Nonwhite		Male	0	10.26	7.55	27.78	38.46
		Female	0	7.43	0	19.31	19.11
		Both sexes	0	8.62	3.72	23.16	28.75
Middlesex, CT (USA)	1957–58	Male	0	1.2	4.6	11.9	26.3[a]
		Female	0.2	1.0	3.5	7.2	28.9[a]
		Both sexes	0.1	1.1	4.0	9.4	27.9[a]
Taiwan	1986–90	Male	(0.60)[b]	1.07	5.17	7.90	12.93
		Female	(0)	1.35	4.41	5.53	15.38
		Both sexes	(0.26)	1.22	4.82	6.89	14.17
Copenhagen (Denmark)	1976–88	Male	0.66	1.78	5.18	10.10	(20.37)[c]
		Female	0.41	0.85	1.87	5.45	(10.85)
		Both sexes	0.53[a]	1.3[a]	3.3[a]	7.5[a]	(15)[a]
Malmö (Sweden)	1989	Male	(0.14)[d]	1.13	2.07	7.68	13.3
		Female	(0.06)	0.37	1.62	3.78	11.9
		Both sexes	(0.10)	0.74	1.83	5.46	12.4
Warsaw (Poland)	1991–92	Male	(0.53)[e]	0.98	4.08	7.61	13[a]
		Female	(0.19)	0.96	1.89	4.35	15[a]
		Both sexes	(0.35)	0.97	2.89	5.75	14[a]
Finland	1983–85						

Community	Year	Sex	Age-specific incidence (age group)				
			35–44	45–54	55–64	65–74	75+
North Karelia		Male	0.83	2.58	5.09	9.71	
		Female	0.39	0.70	2.51	8.37	
		Both sexes	0.62[a]	1.7[a]	3.7[a]	8.9[a]	
Kuopio Province		Male	1.27	2.64	5.98	12.48	
		Female	0.65	1.37	3.15	8.79	
		Both sexes	0.98[a]	2.0[a]	4.4[a]	10[a]	
Turku/Loimaa		Male	0.57	1.33	4.42	9.07	
		Female	0.34	0.73	2.12	6.37	
		Both sexes	0.46[a]	1.0[a]	3.1[a]	7.4[a]	
Rochester, MN (USA)	1980–84	Both sexes	(0.10)[d]	1.04	2.09	6.81	13[a]
	1975–79	Both sexes	(0.11)	0.71	1.79	5.61	11[a]
	1970–74	Both sexes	(0.05)	0.65	2.47	5.96	12[a]
	1965–69	Both sexes	(0.07)	1.20	3.14	6.13	13[a]
	1960–64	Both sexes	(0.07)	0.93	3.20	7.83	19[a]
	1955–59	Both sexes	(0.10)	1.08	4.38	8.52	21[a]
	1950–54	Both sexes	(0.10)	1.69	2.99	10.40	23[a]
	1945–49	Both sexes	(0.06)	1.26	4.06	9.95	22[a]
	1945–54	Both sexes	0.34	1.59	3.69	10.81	24.94
	1955–69	Male	0.43	1.58	5.11	10.82	25.04
		Female	0.27	0.71	2.61	6.03	19.88
		Both sexes	0.35	1.10	3.64	7.91	21.56
Auckland (New Zealand)	1991	Male	0.50	1.04	4.23	11.32	20.08[a]
		Female	0.40	0.97	2.56	7.12	21.45[a]
		Both sexes	0.45	1.00	3.39	9.02	20.98[a]
	1991	Male	0.44	0.85	2.76	7.59	11.94[c]
		Female	0.37	0.76	2.05	5.15	11.90[c]
	1981	Male	0.52	1.18	2.14	6.82	16.85[c]
		Female	0.31	0.82	1.88	3.56	13.66[c]
Arcadia (Greece)	1994–95	Male	0.31	1.13	2.40	6.62	17.01[a]
		Female	0.18	0.48	1.96	4.78	13.85[a]
		Both sexes	0.25	0.82	2.18	5.68	15.41[a]
Shanghai (China)							
Rural		Male	0.14	0.66	3.48	9.36	
		Female	0.16	0.75	1.78	6.87	
Urban		Male	0.05	0.39	3.17	8.62	
		Female	0.06	0.48	2.51	7.34	
Rural and urban		Male	0.1	0.50	3.32	8.98	
		Female	0.12	0.61	2.15	7.09	
		Both sexes	0.11	0.56	2.71	7.92	

Community	Year	Sex	Age-specific incidence (age group)				
			35–44	45–54	55–64	65–74	75+
MONICA Project Populations							
Beijing (China)	1985–87	Male	0.18	1.47	4.33		
		Female	0.19	1.03	3.08		
Glostrup (Denmark)	1985–87	Male	0.29	1.45	2.82		
		Female	0.26	0.72	1.57		
Kuopio Province (Finland)	1985–87	Male	0.9	2.40	6.39		
		Female	0.55	1.60	3.31		
North Karelia (Finland)	1985–87	Male	0.97	2.15	4.96		
		Female	0.24	0.93	2.34		
Turku/Loima (Finland)	1985–87	Male	0.54	1.64	4.71		
		Female	0.31	0.70	2.02		
Halle County (Germany)	1985–87	Male	0.23	0.95	3.00		
		Female	0.25	0.60	1.41		
Karl Marx Stadt (Germany)	1985–87	Male	0.27	1.08	2.93		
		Female	0.29	0.54	1.87		
Rest of DDR MONICA (Germany)	1985–87	Male	0.11	0.83	2.93		
		Female	0.22	0.53	1.02		
Rhein–Neckar Region (Germany)	1985–87	Male	0.25	0.85	2.39		
		Female	0.16	0.33	1.11		
Friuli (Italy)	1985–87	Male	0.26	0.89	2.31		
		Female	0.22	0.44	1.19		
Kaunas (Lithuania)	1985–87	Male	0.56	1.96	4.75		
		Female	0.41	1.17	2.64		
Warsaw (Poland)	1985–87	Male	0.35	1.06	2.66		
		Female	0.15	0.51	1.33		
Moscow (control, Russia)	1985–87	Male	0.31	1.63	3.67		
		Female	0.08	0.91	2.03		
Moscow (intervention, Russia)	1985–87	Male	0.21	1.24	3.44		
		Female	0.11	0.57	2.03		
Novosibirsk (intervention, Russia)	1985–87	Male	0.62	2.03	5.50		
		Female	0.36	2.03	4.34		
Göteborg (Sweden)	1985–87	Male	0.28	0.88	2.63		
		Female	0.26	0.48	1.25		
Northern Sweden	1985–87	Male	0.39	1.36	4.09		
		Female	0.33	0.65	2.16		
Novi Sad (Yugoslavia)	1985–87	Male	0.39	1.64	4.15		
		Female	0.23	0.76	2.09		
Cerebral haemorrhage							
Shibata (Niigata, Japan)	1976–78	Male	0.19	0.82	1.19	3.45	2.11
		Female	0.06	0.35	0.91	1.56	1.08
		Both sexes	0.12	0.57	1.03	2.38	1.47
Rochester, MN (USA)	1945–54	Both sexes	0.13	0.24	0.42	1.31	0.96

Community	Year	Sex	Age-specific incidence (age group)				
			35–44	45–54	55–64	65–74	75+
Middlesex, CT (USA)	1957–58	Male	0	0.2	1.6	5.4	7.1[a]
		Female	0	0.4	1.5	2.5	10.3[a]
		Both sexes	0	0.3	1.6	3.8	9.0
Manitoba (Canada)	1970–71						
Urban area		Male	0.11	0.37	0.50		
		Female	0.22	0.42	0.78		
		Both sexes	0.16	0.39	0.65		
Rural area		Male	0.31	0.54	0.46		
		Female	0.13	0.13	0.39		
		Both sexes	0.22	0.33	0.43		
Malmö (Sweden)	1989	Both sexes	(0.02)[d]	0.07	0.19	0.62	1.0a
Arcadia (Greece)	1994–95	Male	0.00	0.17	0.40	1.52	2.26[a]
		Female	0.09	0.19	0.54	0.43	0.91[a]
		Both sexes	0.04	0.18	0.47	0.96	1.57[a]
Cerebral infarction							
Shibata (Niigata, Japan)	1976–78	Male	0	0.70	3.12	8.77	17.91
		Female	0	0.12	0.66	2.34	12.29
		Both sexes	0	0.39	1.73	5.14	14.43
Rochester, MN (USA)	1955–69	Male	0.32	1.18	4.08	8.98	21.05
		Female	0.03	0.36	1.81	1.61	16.33
		Both sexes	0.17	0.72	2.77	6.32	17.86
	1945–54	Both sexes	0.08	1.14	2.66	8.33	21.57
Manitoba (Canada)	1970–71						
Urban area		Male	0.11	0.67	2.84		
		Female	0.15	0.40	1.14		
		Both sexes	0.13	0.52	1.94		
Rural area		Male	0.12	0.47	1.99		
		Female	0	0.33	1.80		
		Both sexes	0.16	0.39	0.65		
Malmö (Sweden)	1989	Both sexes	(0.06)[d]	0.48	1.12	3.46	4.8[a]
Arcadia (Greece)	1994–95	Male	0.23	0.95	1.87	5.01	14.28[a]
		Female	0.09	0.19	1.28	3.50	12.12[a]
		Both sexes	0.17	0.59	1.58	4.23	13.18[a]
Subarachnoid infarction							
Shibata (Niigata, Japan)	1976–78	Both sexes	0.22	0.18	0.56	0.38	0
Rochester, MN (USA)	1945–54	Both sexes	0.13	0.15	0.42	0.37	0.36

Community	Year	Sex	Age-specific incidence (age group)				
			35–44	45–54	55–64	65–74	75+
Malmö (Sweden)	1989	Both sexes	(0.02)[d]	0.15	0.11	0	0.21[a]
Auckland (New Zealand)	1981–83	Male	0.16	0.20	0.13		
		Female	0.22	0.28	0.35		
		Both sexes	0.19	0.24	0.24		
	1991–93	Male	0.04	0.16	0.21		
		Female	0.14	0.28	0.38		
		Both sexes	0.09	0.22	0.29		
Arcadia (Greece)	1994–95	Male	0.08	0.00	0.13	0.09	0.19[a]
		Female	0.00	0.09	0.07	0.43	0.09[a]
		Both sexes	0.04	0.05	0.10	0.26	0.14[a]

[a]Estimated from the data in each reference.

[b]36–44 years.

[c]75–84 years.

[d]0–44 years.

[e]30–44 years.

References

Abbott, R.D., Yin, Y., Reed, D.M., and Yano, K. (1986). Risk of stroke in male cigarette smokers. *New England Journal of Medicine*, **315**, 717–20.

Abbott, R.D., Donahue, R.P., MacMahon, S.W., Reed, D.M., and Yano, K. (1987). Diabetes and the risk of stroke. The Honolulu Heart Program. *Journal of the American Medical Association*, **257**, 949–52.

Abbott, R.D., Rodriguez, B.L., Burchfiel, C.M., and Curb, J.D. (1994). Physical activity in older middle-aged men and reduced risk of stroke: the Honolulu Heart Program. *American Journal of Epidemiology*, **139**, 881–93.

Abbott, R.D., Curb, J.D., Rodriguez, B.L., Sharp, D.S., Burchfield, C.M., and Yano, K. (1996). Effect of dietary calcium and milk consumption on risk of thromboembolic stroke in older middle-aged men. The Honolulu Heart program. *Stroke*, **27**, 813–18.

Abu-Zeid, H.A.H., Choi, N.W., and Nelson, N.A. (1975*a*). Epidemiologic features of cerebrovascular disease in Manitoba: incidence by age, sex and residence, with etiologic implications. *Canadian Medical Association Journal*, **113**, 379–84.

Abu-Zeid, H.A.H., Choi, N.W., Maini, K.K., and Nelson, N.A. (1975*b*). Incidence and epidemiologic features of cerebrovascular disease (stroke) in Manitoba, Canada. *Preventive Medicine*, **4**, 567–78.

Acheson, R.M. and Williams, D.R. (1983). Does consumption of fruit and vegetables protect against stroke? *Lancet*, **i**, 1191–3.

Agerholm-Larsen, B., Tybjaerg-Hansen, A., Frikke-Schmidt, R., Gronholdt, M.L., Jensen, G., and Nordestgaard, B.G. (1997). ACE gene as a risk factor for ischemic cerebrovascular disease. *Annals of Internal Medicine*, **127**, 346–55.

Agnarsson, U., Thorgeirsson, G., Sigvaldason, H., and Sigfusson, N. (1999). Effects of leisure-time physical activity and ventilatory function on risk for stroke in men: the Reykjavik Study. *Annals of Internal Medicine*, **130**, 987–90.

Aldoori, M.I. and Rahman, S.H. (1998). Smoking and stroke: a causative role. Heavy smokers with hypertension benefit most from stopping. *British Medical Journal*, **317**, 962–3.

Alfthan, G., Pekkanen, J., Jauhiainen, M., *et al.* (1994). *AtherosclerosisD, B106*, 9–19.

Alter, M., Christoferson, L., Resch, J., Myers, G., and Ford, J. (1970). Cerebrovascular disease. Frequency and population selectivity in an upper Mid-Western community. *Stroke*, **1**, 454–65.

Anderson, C.S., Jamrozik, K.D., Burvill, P.W., Chakera, T.M.H., Johnson, G.A., and Stewart-Wayne, E.G. (1993). Determining the incidence of different subtypes of stroke: results from the Perth Community Stroke Study, 1989–1990. *Medical Journal of Australia*, **158**, 85–9.

Anderson, G.M., Shaw, A.R., and Shafer, J.A. (1993). Functional characterization of promoter elements involved in regulation of human B beta-fibrinogen expression. Evidence for binding of novel activator and repressor proteins. *Journal of Biological Chemistry*, **268**, 2260–5.

Araki, A., Sako, Y., Fukushima, Y., Matsumoto, M., Asada, T., and Kita, T. (1989). Plasma sulfhydryl-containing amino acids in patients with cerebral infarction and in hypertensive subjects. *Atherosclerosis*, **79**, 139–46.

Ascherio, A., Rimm, E.B., Hernan, M.A. *et al.* (1998). Intake of potassium, magnesium, calcium, and fiber and risk of stroke among US men. *Circulation*, **98**, 1198–1204.

Barrett-Connor, E. and Khaw, K.T. (1988). Diabetes mellitus: an independent risk factor for stroke? *American Journal of Epidemiology*, **128**, 116–23.

Basun, H., Corder, E.H., Guo, Z., *et al.* (1996). Apolipoprotein E polymorphism and stroke in a population sample aged 75 years or more. *Stroke*, **27**, 1310–15.

Beamer, N., Coull, B.M., Sexton, G., de Garmo, P., Knox, R., and Seaman, G. (1993). Fibrinogen and the albumin–globulin ratio in recurring stroke. *Stroke*, **24**, 1133–9.

Beghi, E., Boglium, G., Cosso, P., *et al.* (1995). Stroke and alcohol intake in a hospital population. A case-control study. *Stroke*, **26**, 1691–6.

Belch, J., McLaren, M., Hanslip, J., Hill, A., and Davidson, D. (1998). The white blood cell and plasma fibrinogen in thrombotic stroke. A significant correlation. *International Angiology*, **17**, 120–4.

Benjamin, E.J., Levy, D., Vaziri, S.M., D'Agostino, R.B., Belanger, A.J., and Wolf, P.A. (1994). Independent risk factors for atrial fibrillation in a population-based cohort. The Framingham Heart Study. *Journal of the American Medical Association*, **271**, 840–4.

Ben-Shlomo, Y., Markowe, H., Shipley, M., and Marmot, M.G. (1992). Stroke risk from alcohol consumption using different control groups. *Stroke*, **23**, 1093–8.

Beresford, S.A.A. and Boushey, J.B. (1997). Homocysteine, folic acid, and cardiovascular disease risk. In *Preventive nutrition. The comprehensive guide for health professionals* (ed. A. Bendich and J.D. Rishard), pp. 193–224. Humana Press, New Jersey.

Blom, H.J. (1998). Determinants of plasma homocysteine. *American Journal of Clinical Nutrition*, **67**, 188–9.

Boers, G.L., Smals, A.G., Trijbels, F.J., *et al.* (1985). Heterozygosity for homocystinuria in premature peripheral and cerebral occlusive arterial disease. *New England Journal of Medicine*, **313**, 709–15.

Bonita, R. (1986). Cigarette smoking, hypertension and the risk of subarachnoid hemorrhage: a population-based case-control study. *Stroke*, **17**, 831–5.

Bonita, R., Scragg, R., Stewart, A., Jackson, R., and Beaglehole, R. (1986). Cigarette smoking and risk of premature stroke in men and women. *British Medical Journal*, **293**, 6–8.

Bonita, R., Broad, J.B., and Beaglehole, R. (1993). Changes in stroke incidence and case-fatality in Auckland, New Zealand, 1981–91. *Lancet*, **342**, 1470–3.

Bonita, R., Broad, J.B., Anderson, N.E., and Beaglehole, R. (1995). Approaches to the problems of measuring the incidence of stroke: the Auckland Stroke Study, 1991–1992. *International Journal of Epidemiology*, **24**, 535–42.

Bonita, R., Duncan, J., Truelsen, T., Jackson, RT., and Beaglehole, R. (1999). Passive smoking as well as active smoking increases the risk of acute stroke. *Tobacco Control*, **8**, 156–60.

Bostom, A.G., Rosenberg, I.H., Silbershatz, H., *et al.* (1999). Nonfasting plasma total homocysteine levels and stroke incidence in elderly persons; the Framingham Study. *Annals of Internal Medicine*, **131**, 352–5.

Bots, M.L., Hoes, A.W., Koudstaal, P.J., Hofman, A., and Grobbee, D.E. (1997). Common carotid intima-media thickness and risk of stroke and myocardial infarction: the Rotterdam Study. *Circulation*, **96**, 1432–7.

Bots, M.L., Hoes, A.W., Hofman, A., Witteman, J.C., and Grobbee, D.E. (1999*a*). Cross-sectionally assessed carotid intima-media thickness relates to long-term risk of stroke, coronary heart disease and death as estimated by available risk functions. *Journal of Internal Medicine*, **245**, 269–76.

Bots, M.L., Launer, L.J., Lindemans, J., *et al.* (1999*b*). Homocysteine and short-term risk of myocardial infarction and risk in the elderly: the Rotterdam Study. *Archives of Internal Medicine*, **159**, 38–44.

Boushey, C.J., Beresford, S.A., Omenn, G.S., and Motulsky, A.G. (1995). A quantitative assessment of plasma homocysteine as a risk factor for vascular disease. Probable benefits of increasing folic acid intakes. *Journal of the American Medical Association*, **274**, 1049–57.

Brattstrom, L.E., Hardebo, J.E., and Hultberg, B.L. (1984). Moderate homocysteinemia—a possible risk factor for arteriosclerotic cerebrovascular disease. *Stroke*, **15**, 1012–16.

Brattstrom, L.E., Israelsson, B., Norrving, B., *et al.* (1990). Impaired homocysteine metabolism in early-onset cerebral and peripheral occlusive arterial disease. Effects of pyridoxine and folic acid treatment. *Atherosclerosis*, **81**, 51–60.

Brattstrom, L.E., Lindgren, A., Israelsson, B. (1992). Hyperhomocysteinaemia in stroke: prevalence, cause, and relationships to type of stroke and stroke risk factors. *European Journal of Clinical Investigation*, **22**, 214–21.

Broderick, J.P., Phillips, S.J., Whisnant, J.P., O'Fallon, W.M., and Bergstralh, E.J. (1989). Incidence rates of stroke in the eighties: the end of the decline in stroke? *Stroke*, **20**, 577–82.

Bronner, L.L., Kanter, D.S., and Manson, J.E. (1995). Primary prevention of stroke. *New England Journal of Medicine*, **333**, 1392–1400.

Caicoya, M., Rodriguez, T., Corrales, C., Cuello, R., and Lasheras, C. (1999). Alcohol and stroke: a community case-control study in Asturias, Spain. *Journal of Clinical Epidemiology*, **52**, 677–84.

Carter, A.M., Catto, A.J., Bamford, J.M., and Grant, P.J. (1997). Gender-specific association of the fibrinogen B beta 448 polymorphism, fibrinogen levels, and acute cerebrovascular disease. *Arteriosclerosis, Thrombosis, and Vascular Biology*, **17**, 589–94.

Carter, A.M., Catto, A.J., and Grant, P.J. (1998). Determinants of tPA antigen and associations with coronary artery disease and acute cerebrovascular disease. *Thrombosis and Haemostasis*, **80**, 632–6.

Catto, A., Carter, A.M., Barrett, J.H., *et al.* (1996). Angiotensin-converting enzyme insertion/deletion polymorphism and cerebrovascular disease. *Stroke*, **27**, 435–40.

Chang-Claude, J., Frentzel-Beyme, R., and Eilber, U. (1992). Mortality pattern of German vegetarians after 11 years of follow-up. *Epidemiology*, **3**, 395–401

Chen, D., Roman, G.C., Wu, G.X., *et al.* (1992). Stroke in China (Sino-MONICA-Beijing study) 1984–1986. *Neuroepidemiology*, **11**, 15–23.

Clarke, R., Daly, L., Robinson, *et al.* (1991). Hyperhomocysteinemia: an independent risk factor for vascular disease. *New England Journal of Medicine*, **324**, 1149–55.

Cona *et al.* (1995). *Stroke*, **26**, 2635.

Corwin, L.E., Wolf, P.A., Kannel, W.B., and McNamara, P.M. (1982). Accuracy of death certificate of stroke: the Framingham Study. *Stroke*, **13**, 818–21.

Couderc, R., Mahieux, F., Bailleul, S., Fenelon, G., Mary, R., and Fermanian, J. (1993). Prevalence of apolipoprotein E phenotypes in ischemic cerebrovascular disease. A case–control study. *Stroke*, **24**, 661–4.

Coull, B.M., Malinow, M.R., Beamer, N., Sexton, G., Nordt, F., and de Garmo, P. (1990). Elevated plasma homocyst(e)ine concentration as a possible independent risk factor for stroke. *Stroke*, **21**, 572–6.

Czlonkowska, A., Ryglewicz, D., Weissbein, T., Baranska-Gieruszczak M., and Hier D.B. (1994). A prospective community-based study of stroke in Warsaw, Poland. *Stroke*, **25**, 547–51.

Delport, R., Ubbink, J.B., Vermaak, W.J., Rossouw, H., Becker, P.J., and Joubert, J. (1997). Hyperhomocysteinaemia in black patients with cerebral thrombosis. *Quarterly Journal of Medicine*, **90**, 635–9.

Dennis, M.S., Burn, J.P., Sandercock, P.A., Bamford, J.M., Wade, D.T., and Warlow, C.P. (1993). Long-term survival after first-ever stroke: the Oxfordshire community stroke project. *Stroke*, **24**, 796–800.

Doi, Y., Yoshinari, M., Yoshizumi, H., Ibayashi, S., Wakisaka, M., and Fujishima, M. (1997). Polymorphism of the angiotensin-converting enzyme (ACE) gene in patients with thrombotic brain infarction. *Atherosclerosis*, **132**, 145–50.

Doolittle, R.F. (1983). The structure and evolution of vertebrate fibrinogen. *Annals of the New York Academy of Sciences*, **408**, 13–27.

Dudman, N.P., Wilcken, D.E., Wang, J., Lynch, J.F., Macey, D., and Lundberg, P. (1993). Disordered methionine/homocysteine metabolism in premature vascular disease. Its occurrence, cofactor therapy, and enzymology. *Arteriosclerosis and Thrombosis*, **13**, 1253–60.

Dyken, M.L. (1983). Natural history of ischemic stroke in cerebrovascular disease. In *Butterworth international medical reviews: neurology* (3rd edn) (ed. M.J.G. Harrison and M.L. Dyken), pp. 139–70. Butterworths, London.

Eastern Stroke and Coronary Heart Disease Collaborative Research Group (1998). Blood pressure, cholesterol, and stroke in eastern Asia. *Lancet*, **352**, 1801–7.

Eckstrom, P.T., Brand, F.R., Edlavitch, S.A., and Parrish, H.M. (1969). Epidemiology of stroke in a rural area. Second year of the Mid-Missouri Stroke Survey. *Public Health Report*, **84**, 878–82.

Eisenberg, H., Morrison, J.T., Sullivan, P., and Foote, F.M. (1964). Cerebrovascular accidents. Incidence and survival rates in a defined population Middlesex Country, Connecticut. *Journal of the American Medical Association*, **189**, 883–8.

Ellekjaer, E.F., Wyller, T.B., Sverre, J.M., and Holmen, J. (1992). Lifestyle factors and risk of cerebral infarction. *Stroke*, **23**, 829–34.

Evenson, K.R., Rosamond, W.D., Cai, J., *et al.* (1999). Physical activity and ischemic stroke risk. The atherosclerosis risk in communities study. *Stroke*, **30**, 1333–9.

Evers, S., Koch, H.G., Grotemeyer, K.H., Lange, B., Deufel, T., and Ringelstein, E.B. (1997). Features, symptoms, and neurophysiological findings in stroke associated with hyperhomocysteinemia. *Archives of Neurology*, **54**, 1276–82.

Farquhar, J.W., Fortmann, S.P., Flora, J.A., *et al.* (1990). Effects of community-wide education on cardiovascular disease risk factors: the Stanford Five-City Project. *Journal of the American Medical Association*, **264**, 359–65.

Ferrucci, L., Guralnik, J.M., Pahor, M., *et al.* (1997). Apolipoprotein E ε2 allele and risk of stroke in the older population. *Stroke*, **28**, 2410–16.

Folsom, A.R., Prineas, R.J., Kaye, S.A., and Munger, R.G. (1990). Incidence of hypertension and stroke in relation to body fat distribution and other risk factors in older women. *Stroke*, **21**, 701–6.

Foulkes, M.A., Wolf, P.A., Price, T.R., Mohr, J.P., and Hier, D.B. (1988). The Stroke Data Bank: design, methods, and baseline characteristics. *Stroke*, **19**, 547–54.

Gaustadnes, M., Rudiger, N., Moller, J., Rasmussen, K., Bjerregard Larsen, T., and Ingerslev, J. (1999). Thrombophilic predisposition in stroke and venous thromboembolism in Danish patients. *Blood Coagulation and Fibrinolysis*, **10**, 251–9.

Gey, K.F., Stahelin, H.B., and Eichholzer, M. (1993). Poor plasma status of carotene and vitamin C is associated with higher mortality from ischemic heart disease and stroke; Basel Prospective Study. *Clinical Investigation*, **71**, 3–6.

Giles, W.H., Croft, J.B., Ford, E.S., and Kittner, S.J. (1998). Total homocyst (e)ine concentration and the likelihood of nonfatal stroke: results from the Third National Health and Nutrition Examination survey. *Stroke*, **29**, 2473–7.

Gill, J.S., Shipley, M.J., Tsementzis, S.A., *et al.* (1989). Cigarette smoking. A risk factor for hemorrhagic and nonhemorrhagic stroke. *Archives of Internal Medicine*, **149**, 2053–7.

Gill, J.S., Shipley, M.J., Tsementzis, S.A., *et al.* (1991). Alcohol consumption—a risk factor for hemorrhagic and non-hemorrhagic stroke. *American Journal of Medicine*, **90**, 489–97.

Gillman, M.W., Cupples, L.A., Gagnon, D. *et al.* (1995). Protective effect of fruits and vegetables on development of stroke in men. *Journal of the American Medical Association*, **273**, 1113–17.

Gillman, M.W., Cupples, L.A., Millen, B.E., Ellison, R.C., and Wolf, P.A. (1997). Inverse association of dietary fat with development of ischemic stroke in men. *Journal of the American Medical Association*, **278**, 2145–50.

Gillum, R.F., Mussolino, M.E., and Ingram, D.D. (1996). Physical activity and stroke incidence in women and men. The NHANES I Epidemiologic Follow-up Study. *American Journal of Epidemiology*, **143**, 860–9.

Gorelick, P.B. (1994). Stroke prevention. An opportunity for efficient utilization of health care resources during the coming decade. *Stroke*, **25**, 220–4.

Graham, I.M., Daly, L.E., Refsum, H.M., *et al.* (1997). Plasma homocysteine as a risk factor for vascular disease. The European Concerted Action Project. *Journal of the American Medical Association*, **277**, 1775–81.

Gronbaek, M., Deis, A., Sorensen, T.I., Becker, U., Schnohr, P., and Jensen, G. (1995). Mortality associated with moderate intakes of wine, beer, or spirits. *British Medical Journal*, **310**, 1165–9.

Hachinski, V., Graffagnino, C., Beaudry, M., *et al.* (1996). Lipids and stroke; a paradox resolved. *Archives of Neurology*, **53**, 303–8.

Haheim, L.L., Holme, I., Hjermann, I., and Leren, P. (1993). Risk factors of stroke incidence and mortality: a 12-year follow-up of the Oslo Study. *Stroke*, **24**, 1484–9.

Haheim, L.L., Holme, I., Hjermann, I., and Leren, P. (1996). Smoking habits and risk of fatal stroke: 18 years follow up of the Oslo Study. *Journal of Epidemiology and Community Health*, **50**, 621–4.

Hamsten, A. (1993). The hemostatic system and coronary heart disease. *Thrombosis Research*, **70**, 1–38.

Hansagi, H., Romelsjo, A., Gerhardsson, de Verdier, M., Andreasson, S., and Leifman, A. (1995). Alcohol consumption and stroke mortality: 20-year follow-up of 15,077 men and women. *Stroke*, **26**, 1768–73.

Harmon, D.L., Doyle, R.M., Meleady, R., *et al.* (1999). Genetic analysis of the thermolabile variant of 10-methylenetetrahydrofolate reductase as a risk factor for ischemic stroke. *Arteriosclerosis, Thrombosis, and Vascular Biology*, **19**, 208–11.

Harmsen, P., Rosengren, A., Tsipogianni, A., and Wilhelmsen, L. (1990). Risk factors for stroke in middle-aged men in Goteborg, Sweden. *Stroke*, **21**, 223–9.

Harmsen, P., Tsipogianni, A., and Wilhelmsen, L. (1992). Stroke incidence rates were unchanged, while fatality rate declined, during 1971–1987 in Göteborg, Sweden. *Stroke*, **23**, 1410–15.

Hart, C.L., Smith, G.D., Hole, D.J., and Hawthorne, V.M. (1999). Alcohol consumption and mortality from all causes, coronary heart disease, and stroke: results from a prospective cohort study of Scottish men with 21 years of follow up. *British Medical Journal*, **318**, 1725–9.

Henschen, A., Lottspeich, F., Kehl, M., and Southan, C. (1983). Covalent structure of fibrinogen. *Annals of the New York Academy of Sciences*, **408**, 28–43.

Hier, D.B., Foulkes, M.A., Swiontoniowski, M., *et al.* (1991). Stroke recurrence within 2 years after ischemic infarction. *Stroke*, **22**, 155–61.

Higa, M. and Davanipoor, Z. (1991). Smoking and stroke. *Neuroepidemiology*, **10**, 211–22.

Hillbom, M., Haapaniemi, H., Juvela, S., Palomaki, H., Numminen, H., and Kaste, M. (1995). Recent alcohol consumption, cigarette smoking, and cerebral infarction in young adults. *Stroke*, **26**, 40–5.

Hong, Y., Bots, M.L., Pan, X., Hofman, A., Grobbee, D.E., and Chen, H. (1994). Stroke incidence and mortality in rural and urban Shanghai from 1984 through 1991. Findings from a community-based registry. *Stroke*, **25**, 1165–9.

Howard, G., Wagenknecht, L.E., Cai, J., Cooper, L., Kraut, M.A., and Toole, J.F. (1998). Cigarette smoking and other risk factors for silent cerebral infarction in the general population. *Stroke*, **29**, 913–17.

Hu, H.H., Sheng, W.Y., Chu, F.L., Lan, C.F., and Chiang, B.N. (1992). Incidence of stroke in Taiwan. *Stroke*, **23**, 1237–41.

Iso, H., Jacobs, D.R. Jr, Wentworth, D., Neaton, J.D., and Cohen, J.D. (1989). Serum cholesterol levels and six-year mortality from stroke in 350,977 men screened for the Multiple Risk Factor Intervention Trial. *New England Journal of Medicine*, **320**, 904–10.

Iso, H., Kitamura, A., Shimamoto, T., *et al.* (1995). Alcohol intake and the risk of cardiovascular disease in middle-aged Japanese men. *Stroke*, **26**, 767–73.

Iso, H., Shimamoto, T., Naito, Y., *et al.* (1998). Effects of a long-term hypertension control program on stroke incidence and prevalence in a rural community northeastern Japan. *Stroke*, **29**, 1510–18.

Iso, H., Stampfer, M.J., Manson, J.E., ***et al.*** (1999). prospective study of calcium, potassium, and magnesium intake and risk of stroke in women. *Stroke*, **30**, 1772–9.

Iso, H., Rexrodee, K., Hennekens, C.H., and Manson, J.E. (2000). Application of computer tomography-oriented criteria for stroke subtype classification in a prospective study. *Annals of Epidemiology*, **10**, 81–7.

Iso, H., Stampfer, M.J., Manson, J.E., ***et al.*** (2001). Prospective study of fat and protein intake and risk of intraparenchymal hemorrhage in women. *Circulation*, **103**, 856–63.

Jamrozik, K., Broadhurst, R.J., Anderson, C.S., and Stewart-Wynne, E.G. (1994). The role of lifestyle factors in the etiology of stroke. A population-based case-control study in Perth, Western Australia. *Stroke*, **25**, 51–9.

Jerntorp, P. and Berglund, G. (1992). Stroke registry in Malmo, Sweden. *Stroke*, **23**, 357–61.

Johansson, L., Jansson, J.H., Boman, K., Nilsson, T.K., Stegmayr, B., and Hallmans, G. (2000). Tissue plasminogen activator, plasminogen activator inhibitor-1, and tissue plasminogen activator/plasminogen activator inhibitor-1 complex as risk factors for the development of a first stroke. *Stroke*, **31**, 26–32.

Juvela, S., Hillbom, M., Numminen, H., and Koskinen, P. (1993). Cigarette smoking and alcohol consumption as risk factors for aneurysmal subarachnoid hemorrhage. *Stroke*, **24**, 639–46.

Kagan, A., Popper, J.S., and Phoads, G.G. (1980). Factors related with stroke incidence in Hawiian Japanese men, the Honolulu Heart Study. *Stroke*, **11**, 14–21.

Kannel, W.B. and McGee, D.L. (1979). Diabetes and cardiovascular risk factors: the Framingham study. *Circulation*, **59**, 8–13.

Kannel, W.B., Abbott, R.D., Savage, D.D., and McNamara, P.M. (1982). Epidemiologic features of chronic atrial fibrillation: the Framingham study. *New England Journal of Medicine*, **306**, 1018–22.

Kannel, W.B., Wolf, P.A., Castelli, W.P., and D'Agostino, R.B. (1987). Fibrinogen and risk of cardiovascular disease. The Framingham Study *Journal of the American Medical Association*, **258**, 1183–6.

Karem, J. (1996). Diabetes mellitus. In *Current medical diagnosis and treatment* (ed. L. Tierney, S. McPhee, and M. Papdakis). Appleton and Lange, Stanford.

Kario, K., Kanai, N., Saito, K., Nago, N., Matsuo, T., and Shimada, K. (1996). Ischemic stroke and the gene for angiotensin-converting enzyme in Japanese hypertensives. *Circulation*, **93**, 1630–3.

Katsuki, S., Omae, T., and Hirota, Y. (1964). Epidemiological and clinico-pathological studies on cerebrovascular disease. *Kyushu Journal of Medical Science*, **15**, 127–49.

Keli, S.O., Hertog, M.G., Feskens, E.J., and Kromhout, D. (1996). Dietary flavonoids, antioxidant vitamins, and incidence of stroke: the Zutphen Study. *Annals of Internal Medicine*, **156**, 637–42.

Kessler, C., Spitzer, C., Stauske, D., ***et al.*** (1997). The apolipoprotein E and beta-fibrinogen G/A-455 gene polymorphisms are associated with ischemic stroke involving large-vessel disease. *Arteriosclerosis, Thrombosis, and Vascular Biology*, **17**, 2880–4.

Key, T.J., Thorogood, M., Appleby, P.N., and Burr, M.L. (1996). Dietary habits and mortality in 11 000 vegetarians and health conscious people: results of a 17 year follow up. *British Medical Journal*, **313**, 775–9.

Khaw, K.T. and Barrett-Connor, E. (1987). *New England Journal of Medicine*, **316**, 235–40.

Kiely, D.K., Wolf, P.A., Cupples, L.A., Beiser, A.S., and Kannel, W.B. (1994). Physical activity and stroke risk: the Framingham Study. *American Journal of Epidemiology*, **140**, 608–20.

Kitamura, A., Shimamoto, T., Doi, M., ***et al.*** (1991). Secular trends in prevalence and incidence of atrial fibrillation and associated factors in a Japanese rural population (in Japanese with English abstract). *Japanese Journal of Public Health*, **38**, 98–105.

Kittner, S.J., White, L.R., Losonczy, K.G., Wolf, P.A., and Hebel, J.R. (1990). Black-white differences in stroke incidence in a national sample. The contribution of hypertension and diabetes mellitus. *Journal of the American Medical Association*, **264**, 1267–70.

Kittner, S.J., Giles, W.H., Macko, R.F., ***et al.*** (1999). Homocyst(e)ine and risk of cerebral infarction in a biracial population: the Stroke Prevention in Young Women Study. *Stroke*, **30**, 1554–60.

Kiyohara, Y., Kato, I., Iwamoto, H., Nakayama, K., and Fujishima, M. (1995). The impact of alcohol and hypertension on stroke incidence in a general Japanese population. The Hisayama Study. *Stroke*, **26**, 368–72.

Klag, M.J. and Whelton, P.K. (1993). The decline in stroke mortality. An epidemiologic perspective. *Annals of Epidemiology*, **3**, 571–5.

Kojima, S. (1976). Practical aspects of hypertension and stroke control in a rural population. In *Hypertension and stroke control in the community* (ed. S. Hatano, I. Shigematsu, and T. Strasser), pp. 149–62. WHO, Geneva.

Kojima, S., Omura, T., Wakamatsu, W., ***et al.*** (1990). Prognosis and disability of stroke patients after 5 years in Akita, Japan. *Stroke*, **21**, 72–7.

Kokubo, Y., Chowdhury, A.H., Date, C., Yokoyama, T., Sobue, H., and Tanaka, H. (2000). Age-dependent association of apolipoprotein E genotypes with stroke subtypes in a Japanese rural population. *Stroke*, **31**, 1299–1306.

Komachi, Y., Iida, M., Ozawa, H., ***et al.*** (1977). Risk factors of stroke (in Japanese). *Saishin Igaku*, **32**, 2264–9.

Konishi, M., Iso, H., Komachi, Y., ***et al.*** (1993). Associations of serum total cholesterol different types of stroke, and stenosis distribution of cerebral arteries: the Akita Pathology Study. *Stroke*, **24**, 954–64.

Kostulas, K., Crisby, M., Huang, W.X., ***et al.*** (1998). A methylenetetrahyrofolate reductase gene polymorphism in ischaemic stroke and in carotid artery stenosis. *European Journal of Clinical Investigation*, **28**, 285–9.

Kristensen, B., Malm, J., Nilsson, T.K., Hultdin, J., Carlberg, B., and Olsson, T. (1998). Increased fibrinogen levels and acquired hypofibrinolysis in young adults with ischemic stroke. *Stroke*, **29**, 2261–7.

Kristensen, B., Malm, J., Nilsson, T.K., ***et al.*** (1999). Hyperhomo-cysteinemia and hypofibrinolysis in young adults with ischemic stroke. *Stroke*, **30**, 974–80.

Kuusisto, J., Mykkanen, L., Kervinen, K., Kesaniemi, Y.A., and Laakso, M. (1995). Apolipoprotein E4 phenotype is not an important risk factor for coronary heart disease or stroke in elderly subjects. *Arteriosclerosis, Thrombosis, and Vascular Biology*, **15**, 1280–6.

Lai, S.M., Alter, M., Friday, G., and Sobel, E. (1994). A multifactorial analysis of risk factors for recurrence of ischemic stroke. *Stroke*, **25**, 958–62.

Lai, S.M., Alter, M., Friday, G., and Sobel, E. (1995). Prognosis for survival after an initial stroke. *Stroke*, **26**, 2011–5.

Lalouschek, W., Aull, S., Serles, W., ***et al.*** (1999*a*).C677T MTHFR mutation and factor V Leiden mutation in patients with TIA/minor stroke: a case–control study. *Thrombosis Research*, **93**, 61–9.

Lalouschek, W., Aull, S., Serles, W., ***et al.*** (1999*b*). Genetic and nongenetic factors influencing plasma homocysteine levels in patients with ischemic cerebrovascular disease. *Journal of Laboratory and Clinical Medicine*, **133**, 575–82.

Lauria, G., Gentile, M., Fassetta, G., ***et al.*** (1995). Incidence and prognosis of stroke in the Belluno province, Italy. First-year results of a community-based study. *Stroke*, **26**, 1787–93.

Lee, A.J., Lowe, G.D., Woodward, M., and Tunstall-Pedoe, H. (1993). Fibrinogen in relation to personal history of prevalent hypertension, diabetes, stroke, intermittent claudication, coronary heart disease, and family history: the Scottish Heart Health Study. *British Heart Journal*, **69**, 338–42.

Lee, I.M. and Paffenbarger, R.S., Jr (1998). Physical activity and stroke incidence: the Harvard Alumni Health Study. *Stroke*, **29**, 2049–54.

Lee, I.M., Hennekens, C.H., Berger, K., Buring, J.E., and Manson, J.E. (1999). Exercise and risk of stroke in male physicians. *Stroke*, **30**, 1–6.

Lijnen, H.R. and Collen, D. (1996). Impaired fibrinolysis and the risk for coronary heart disease. *Circulation*, **94**, 2052–4.

Lindenstrom, E., Boysen, G., Nyboe, J., and Appleyard, M. (1992). Stroke incidence in Copenhagen, 1976–1988. *Stroke*, **23**, 28–32.

Lindenstrom, E., Boysen, G., and Nyboe, J. (1993*a*). Lifestyle factors and risk of cerebrovascular disease in women: the Copenhagen City Heart Study. *Stroke*, **24**, 1468–72.

Lindenstrom, E., Boysen, G., and Nyboe, J. (1993*b*). Risk factors for stroke in Copenhagen, Denmark. II. Life-style factors. *Neuroepidemiology*, **12**, 43–50.

Lindgren, A., Brattstrom, L., Norvving, B., Hultberg, B., Andersson, A., and Johansson, B.B. (1995). Plasma homocysteine in the acute and convalescent phases after stroke. *Stroke*, **26**, 795–800.

Lindgren, A., Lindoff, C., Norrving, B., Astedt, B., and Johansson, B.B. (1996). Tissue plasminogen activator and plasminogen activator inhibitor-1 in stroke patients. *Stroke*, **27**, 1066–71.

Lindsted, K.D., Tonstad, S., and Kuzma, J.W. (1991). Self-report of physical activity and patterns of mortality in Seventh-Day Adventist men. *Journal of Clinical Epidemiology*, **44**, 355–64.

Longstreth, W.T. Jr, Nelson, L.M., Koepsell, T.D., and van Belle, G. (1992). Cigarette smoking, alcohol use, and subarachnoid hemorrhage. *Stroke*, **23**, 1242–9.

Lowe, G.D., Fowkes, F.G., Dawes, J., Donnan, P.T., Lennie, S.E., and Housley, E. (1993). Blood viscosity, fibrinogen, and activation of coagulation and leukocytes in peripheral arterial disease and the normal population in the Edinburgh Artery Study. *Circulation*, **87**, 1915–20.

Luepker, R.V., Rastam, L., Hannan, P.J., *et al.* (1996). Community education for cardiovascular disease prevention: morbidity and mortality results from the Minnesota Heart Health Program. *American Journal of Epidemiology*, **144**, 351–62.

McGovern, P.G., Pankow, J.S., Burke, G.L., *et al.* (1993). Trends in survival of hospitalized stroke patients between 1970 and 1985: the Minnesota heart study. *Stroke*, **24**, 1640–8.

Macko, R.F., Kittner, S.J., Epstein, A., *et al.* (1999). Elevated tissue plasminogen activator antigen and stroke risk: the Stroke Prevention in Young Women Study. *Stroke*, **30**, 7–11.

Maeda, Y., Ikeda, U., Ebata, H., *et al.* (1996). Angiotensin-converting enzyme gene polymorphism in hypertensive individuals with a parental history of stroke. *Stroke*, **27**, 1521–3.

Mahieux, F., *et al.* (1990). *Stroke*, **21**, 115.

Manson, J.E., Gaziano, J.M., Jonas, M.A., and Hennekens, C.H. (1993). Antioxidants and cardiovascular disease: a review. *Journal of the American College of Nutrition*, **12**, 426–32.

Manson, J.E., *et al.* (1994). *Circulation*, **103**, 856–63.

Margaglione, M., Di Minno, G., Grandone, E., *et al.* (1994). Abnormally high circulation levels of tissue plasminogen activator and plasminogen activator inhibitor-1 in patients with a history of ischemic stroke. *Arteriosclerosis and Thrombosis*, **14**, 1741–5.

Margaglione, M., Celentano, E., Grandone, E., *et al.* (1996). Deletion polymorphism in the angiotensin-converting enzyme gene in patients with a history of ischemic stroke. *Arteriosclerosis, Thrombosis, and Vascular Biology*, **16**, 304–9.

Margaglione, M., Seripa, D., Gravina, C., *et al.* (1998). Prevalence of apolipoprotein E alleles in healthy subjects and survivors of ischemic stroke: an Italian case–control study. *Stroke*, **29**, 399–403.

Markus, H.S., Barley, J., Lunt, R., *et al.* (1995). Angiotensin-converting enzyme gene deletion polymorphism. A new risk factor for lacunar stroke but not carotid atheroma. *Stroke*, **26**, 1329–33.

Markus, H.S., Ali, N., Swaminatham, R., Sankaralingam, A., Molloy, J., and Powell, J. (1997). A common polymorphism in the methylenetetrahydrofolate reductase gene, homocysteine, and ischemic cerebrovascular disease. *Stroke*, **28**, 1739–43.

Matsumoto, N., Whisnant, J.P., Kurland, L.T., and Okazaki, H. (1973). Natural history of stroke in Rochester, Minnesota, 1955 through 1969: an extension of a previous study, 1945 through 1954. *Stroke*, **4**, 20–9.

Meade, T.W., Ruddock, V., Stirling, Y., Chakrabarti, R., and Miller, G.J. (1993). Fibrinolytic activity, clotting factors, and long-term incidence of ischaemic heart disease in the Northwick Park Heart Study. *Lancet*, **342**, 1076–9.

Medical Research Council Working Party (1988). Stroke and coronary heart disease in mild hypertension: risk factors and the value of treatment. *British Medical Journal*, **296**, 1565–70.

Melamed, E., Cahane, E., Carmon, A., and Lavy S. (1973). Stroke in Jerusalem district, 1960 through 1967: an epidemiological study. *Stroke*, **4**, 465–71.

Ministry of Health and Welfare, Statistics and Information Department (1997). *Report of comprehensive survey of living condition of the people on health and welfare, 1995*, Vol. 1. Health and Welfare Statistics Association, Tokyo.

Ministry of Health and Welfare, Statistics and Information Department (1998). *Vital statistics of Japan*. Health and Welfare Statistics Association, Tokyo.

Ministry of Health and Welfare, Statistics and Information Department (1999). *Vital statistics of Japan*, Vol. 1. Health and Welfare Statistics Association, Tokyo.

Mistry, P., Chawla, K.P., Rai, H.P., and Jaiswal, P. (1990). Plasma fibrinogen levels in stroke. *Journal of Postgraduate Medicine*, **36**, 1–4.

Mohr, J.P., Caplan, L.R., Melski, J.W., *et al.* (1978). The Harvard Cooperative Stroke Registry: a prospective registry. *Neurology*, **28**, 754–62.

Monforte, R., Estruch, R., Graus, F., Nicolas, J.M., and Urbano-Marquez, A. (1990). High ethanol consumption as risk factor for intracerebral hemorrhage in young and middle-aged people. *Stroke*, **21**, 1529–32.

Morishita, R., Gibbons, G.H., Ellison, K.E., *et al.* (1994). Evidence for direct local effect of angiotensin in vascular hypertrophy. *In vivo* gene transfer of angiotensin converting enzyme. *Journal of Clinical Investigation*, **94**, 978–84.

Morita, H., Kurihara, H., Tsubaki, S., *et al.* (1998). Methylenetetrahydrofolate reductase gene polymorphism and ischemic stroke in Japanese. *Arteriosclerosis, Thrombosis, and Vascular Biology*, **18**, 1465–9.

Muir, K.W., Weir, C.J., Murray, G.D., Povey, C., and Lees, K.R. (1996). Comparison of neurological scales and scoring systems for acute stroke prognosis. *Stroke*, **27**, 1817–20.

Nakata, Y., Katsuya, T., Rakugi, H., *et al.* (1997). Polymorphism of angiotensin converting enzyme, angiotensinogen, and apolipoprotein E genes in a Japanese population. *American Journal of Hypertension*, **10**, 1391–5.

Nakata, Y., Katsuya, T., Takami, S., *et al.* (1998). Methylenetetrahydrofolate reductase gene polymorphism: relation to blood pressure and cerebrovascular disease. *American Journal of Hypertension*, **11**, 1019–23.

Nakayama, T., Date, C., Yokoyama, T., Yoshiike, N., Yamaguchi, M., and Tanaka, H. (1997). A 15.5-year follow-up study of stroke in a Japanese provincial city: the Shibata Study. *Stroke*, **28**, 45–52.

Ness, A.R., Powles, J.W., and Khaw, K.T. (1996). Vitamin C and cardiovascular disease: a systematic review. *Journal of Cardiovascular Risk*, **3**, 513–21.

Neve, J. (1996). Selenium as a risk factor for cardiovascular diseases. *Journal of Cardiovascular Risk*, **3**, 42–7.

Nishiuma, S., Kario, K., Yakushijin, K., *et al.* (1998). Genetic variation in the promoter region of the beta-fibrinogen gene is associated with ischemic stroke in a Japanese population. *Blood Coagulation and Fibrinolysis*, **9**, 373–9.

O'Leary, D.H., Polak, J.F., Kronmal, R.A., Manolio, T.A., Burke, G.L., and Wolfson, S.K., Jr (1999). Carotid-artery intima and media thickness as a risk factor for myocardial infarction and stroke in older adults. Cardiovascular Health Study Collaborative Research Group. *New England Journal of Medicine*, **340**, 14–22.

Oleckno, W.A. (1988). The risk of stroke in young adults: an analysis of the contribution of cigarette smoking and alcohol consumption. *Public Health*, **102**, 45–55.

Paffenbarger, R.S. Jr, Blair, S.N., Lee, I.M., and Hyde, R.T. (1993). Measurement of physical activity to assess health effects in free-living populations. *Medicine and Science in Sports and Exercise*, **25**, 60–70.

Palomaki, H. and Kaste, M. (1993). Regular light-to-moderate intake of alcohol and the risk of ischemic stroke. Is there a beneficial effect? *Stroke*, **24**, 1828–32.

Parrish, H.M., Payne, G.H., Allen, W.C., Goldner, J.C., and Sauer, H.I. (1966). Mid-Missouri Stroke Survey, A preliminary report. *Missouri Medicine*, **63**, 816–18.

Pedro-Botet, J., Senti, M., Noges, X., *et al.* (1992). Lipoprotein and apolipoprotein profile in men with ischemic stroke. Role of lipoprotein (a), triglyceride-rich lipoproteins, and apolipoprotein E polymorphism. *Stroke*, **23**, 1556–62.

Peng, D.Q., Zhao, S.P., and Wang, J.L. (1999). Lipoprotein(a) and apolipoprotein E ε4 as independent risk factors for ischemic stroke. *Journal of Cardiovascular Risk*, **6**, 1–6.

Perry, I.J. (1999). Homocysteine, hypertension and stroke. *Journal of Human Hypertension*, **13**, 289–93.

Perry, I.J., Refsum, H., Morris, R.W., Ebrahim, S.B., Ueland, P.M., and Shaper, A.G. (1995). prospective study of serum total homocysteine concentration and risk of stroke in middle-aged British men. *Lancet*, **346**, 1395–8.

Pitt, B. (1994). Angiotensin-converting enzyme inhibitors in patients with coronary atherosclerosis. *American Heart Journal*, **128**, 1328–32.

Press, R.D., Beamer, N., Evans, A., DeLoughery, T.G., and Coull, B.M. (1999). Role of a common mutation in the homocysteine rgulatory enzyme methylenetetrahydrofolate reductase in ischemic stroke. *Diagnostic Molecular Pathology*, **8**, 54–8.

Qizilbash, N., Jones, L., Warlow, C., and Mann, J. (1991). Fibrinogen and lipid concentrations as risk factors for transient ischaemic attacks and minor ischaemic strokes. *British Medical Journal*, **303**, 605–9.

Reed, D.M. (1990). The paradox of high rosk of stroke in populations with low risk of coronary heart disease. *American Journal of Epidemiology*, **131**, 579–88.

Resch, K.L., Ernst, E., Matrai, A., and Paulsen, H.F. (1992). Fibrinogen and viscosity as risk factors for subsequent cardiovascular events in stroke survivors. *Annals of Internal Medicine*, **117**, 371–5.

Ridker, P.M., Hennekens, C.H., Stampfer, M.J., Manson, J.E., and Vaughan, D.E. (1994). Prospective study of endogenous tissue plasminogen activator and risk of stroke. *Lancet*, **343**, 940–3.

Rigat, B., Hubert, C., Alhenc-Gelas, F., Cambien, F., Corvol, P., and Soubrier, F. (1990). An insertion/deletion polymorphism in the angiotensin I-converting enzyme gene accounting for half the variance of serum enzyme levels. *Journal of Clinical Investigation*, **86**, 1343–6.

Robbins, A.S., Manson, J.E., Lee, I.M., Satterfield, S., and Hennekens, C.H. (1994). Cigarette smoking and stroke in a cohort of US male physicians. *Annals of Internal Medicine*, **120**, 458–62.

Rodgers, H., Aitken, P.D., French, J.M., Curless, R.H., Bates, D., and James, O.F. (1993). Alcohol and stroke. A case-control study of drinking habits past and present. *Stroke*, **24**, 1473–7.

Rodriguez A.F., Guallar-Castillon, P., Banegas, B. Jr, Manzano, B.A., and del Rey, C.J. (1998). Consumption of fruit and wine and the decline in cerebrovascular disease mortality in Spain (1975–1993). *Stroke*, **29**, 1556–61.

Ross, R.K., Yuan, J.M., Henderson, B.E., Park, J., Gao, Y.T., and Yu, M.C. (1997). Prospective evaluation of dietary and other predictors of fatal stroke in Shanghai, China. *Circulation*, **96**, 50–5.

Sacco, R.L., Wolf, P.A., Kannel, W.B., and McNamara, P.M. (1982). Survival and recurrence following stroke: the Framingham study. *Stroke*, **13**, 290–5.

Sacco, R.L., Gan, R., Boden-Albala, B., *et al.* (1998). Leisure-time physical activity and ischemic stroke risk: the Northern Manhattan Stroke Study. *Stroke*, **29**, 380–7.

Sacco, R.L., Elkind, M., Boden-Albala, B., *et al.* (1999). The protective effect of moderate alcohol consumption on ischemic stroke. *Journal of the American Medical Association*, **281**, 53–60.

Salooja, N., Catto, A., Carter, A., Tudenham, E.G., and Grant, P.J. (1998). Methylene tetrahydrofolate reductase C677T genotype and stroke. *Clinical and Laboratory Haematology*, **20**, 357–61.

Sankai, T., Miyagaki, T., Iso, H., *et al.* (1991). A population-based study of the proportion by type of stroke determined by computed tomography scan (in Japanese with English abstract). *Japanese Journal of Public Health*, **38**, 901–9.

Scmidt, E.V., Smirnov, V.E., and Ryabova, V.S. (1988). Results of the seven-year prospective study of stroke patients. *Stroke*, **19**, 942–9.

Seino, F., Date, C., Nakayama, T., *et al.* (1997). Dietary lipids and incidence of cerebral infarction in a Japanese rural community. *Journal of Nutritional Science and Vitaminology*, **43**, 83–99.

Sharma, P. (1998). Meta-analysis of the ACE gene in ischaemic stroke. *Journal of Neurology, Neurosurgery and Psychiatry*, **64**, 227–30.

Sharma, P., Carter, N.D., Barley, J., and Brown, M.M. (1994). Molecular approach to assessing the genetic risk of cerebral infarction: deletion polymorphism in the gene encoding angiotensin-1 converting enzyme. *Journal of Human Hypertension*, **8**, 645–8.

Sharma, S.C., Vijayan, G.P., Seth, H.N., and Suri, M.L. (1978). Platelet adhesiveness, plasma fibrinogen, and fibrinolytic activity in young patients with ischaemic stroke. *Journal of Neurology, Neurosurgery, and Psychiatry*, **41**, 118–21.

Sherwin, R. and Price, T.R. (1997). Fat chance: diet and ischemic stroke. *Journal of the American Medical Association*, **278**, 2185–6.

Shimamoto, T., Komachi, Y., Inada, H., *et al.* (1989). Trends for coronary heart disease and stroke and their risk factors in Japan. *Circulation*, **79**, 503–15.

Shinton, R. and Beevers, G. (1989). Meta analysis of relation between cigarette smoking and stroke. *British Medical Journal*, 298, 789–94.

Shinton, R. and Sagar, G. (1993). Lifelong exercise and stroke. *British Medical Journal*, **307**, 231–4.

Sing, C.F. and Davignon, J. (1985). Role of the apolipoprotein E polymorphism in determining normal plasma lipid and lipoprotein variation. *American Journal of Human Genetics*, **37**, 268–85.

Smith, F.B., Lee, A.J., Fowkes, F.J., Price, J.F., Rumley, A., and Lowe, G.D. (1997). Hemostatic factors as predictors of ischemic heart disease and stroke in the Edinburgh Artery Study. *Arteriosclerosis, Thrombosis, and Vascular Biology*, **17**, 3321–5.

Stegmayr, B. and Asplund, K. (1995). Diabetes as a risk factor for stroke. A population perspective. *Diabetologia*, **38**, 1061–8.

Stehouwer, C.D., Weijenberg, M.P., van den Berg, M., Jakobs, C., Feskens, E.J., and Kromhout, D. (1998). Serum homocysteine and risk of coronary heart disease and cerbrovascular disease in elderly men: a 10-year follow-up. *Arteriosclerosis, Thrombosis, and Vascular Biology*, **18**, 1895–1901.

Steiner, T., De Mendoza, G., Georgia, M., Schellinger, P., Holle, R., and Hacke, W. (1997). Prognosis of stroke patients requiring mechanical ventilation in a neurological critical care unit. *Stroke*, **28**, 711–15.

Tanaka, H., Ueda, Y., Date, C., *et al.* (1981*a*). Incidence of stroke in Shibata, Japan: 1976–1978. *Stroke*, **12**, 460–6.

Tanaka, H., Ueda, Y., Tanaka, Y., Date, C., Baba, T., and Hayashi, M. (1981*b*). Supplemental study on incidence of stroke in Shibata, 1976 through 1978: the Shibata Stroke Study. *Osaka City Medical Journal*, **27**, 117–33.

Tanaka, H., Ueda, Y., Hayashi, M., *et al.* (1982). Risk factors for cerebral hemorrhage and cerebral infarction in a Japanese rural community. *Stroke*, **13**, 62–73.

Tanaka, H., Hayashi, M., Date, C., *et al.* (1985). Epidemiologic studies of stroke in Shibata, a Japanese provincial city: preliminary report on risk factors for cerebral infarction. *Stroke*, **16**, 773–80.

Tanaka, H., Yamaguchi, M., Date, C., *et al.* (1992). Nutrition and cardiovascular disease—a brief review of epidemiological studies in Japan. *Nutrition and Health*, **8**, 107–23.

Teunissen, L.L., Rinkel, G.J., Algra, A., and van Gijn, J. (1996). Risk factors for subarachnoid hemorrhage: a systematic review. *Stroke*, **27**, 544–9.

Thorvaldsen, P., Asplund, K., Kuulasmaa, K., Rajakangas, A.M., Schroll, M. (1995). Stroke incidence, case fatality, and mortality in the WHO MONICA project. World Health Organization Monitoring Trends and Determinants in Cardiovascular Disease. *Stroke*, **26**, 361–7.

Tracy, R.P., Arnold, A.M., Ettinger, W., Fried, L., Meilahn, E., and Savage, P. (1999). The relationship of fibrinogen and factors VII and VIII to incident cardiovascular disease and death in the elderly: results from the cardiovascular health study. *Arteriosclerosis, Thrombosis, and Vascular Biology*, **19**, 1776–83.

Truelsen, T., Bonita, R., Duncan, J., Anderson, N.E., and Mee, E. (1998*a*). Changes in subarachnoid hemorrhage mortality, incidence, and case fatality in New Zealand between 1981–1983 and 1991–1993. *Stroke*, **29**, 2298–303.

Truelsen, T., Gronbaek, M., Schnohr, P., and Boysen, G. (1998*b*). Intake of beer, wine, and spirits and risk of stroke: the Copenhagen City Heart Study. *Stroke*, **29**, 2467–72.

Truelsen, T., Bonita, R., Gronbaek, M., Sehnohr, P., and Boysen, G. (1998*c*). Stroke incidence and case fatality in two populations: the Auckland Stroke Study and the Copenhagen City Heart Study. *Neuroepidemiology*, **17**, 132–8.

Tunstall-Pedoe, H., for the WHO MONICA Project Principle Investigators (1988). The World Health Organization MONICA Project (monitoring trends and determinants in cardiovascular disease): a major international collaboration. *Journal of Clinical Epidemiology*, **41**, 105–14.

Tuomilehto, J., Nissinen, A., Salonen, J.T., Kottke, T.E., and Puska, P. (1980). Community programme for control for hypertension in North Karelia, Finland. *Lancet*, **ii**, 900–3.

Tuomilehto, J., Sarti, C., Narva, E.V., *et al.* (1992). The FINMONICA stroke register. Community-based stroke registration and analysis of stroke incidence in Finland, 1983–1985. *American Journal of Epidemiology*, **135**, 1259–70.

Tuomilehto, J., Rastenyte, D., Jousilahti, P., Sarti, C., and Vartiainen, E. (1996). Diabetes mellitus as a risk factor for death from stroke. Prospective study of the middle-aged Finnish population. *Stroke*, **27**, 210–15.

Ueda, S., Weir, C.J., Inglis, G.C., Murray, G.D., Muir, K.W., and Lees, K.R. (1995). Lack of association between angiotensin converting enzyme gene insertion/deletion polymorphism and stroke. *Journal of Hypertension*, **13**, 1597–1601.

US Department of Health and Human Services (1996). *Physical activity and health: a report of the Surgeon General.* CDC, Washington, DC.

Vemmos, K.N., Bots, M.L., Tsibouris, P.K., *et al.* (1999). Stroke incidence and case fatality in southern Greece: the Arcadia stroke registry. *Stroke*, **30**, 363–70.

Verhoef, P., Hennekens, C.H., Malinow, M.R., Kok, F.J., Willett, W.C., and Stampfer, M.J. (1994). A prospective study of plasma homocyst(e)ine and risk of ischemic stroke. *Stroke*, **25**, 1924–30.

Vollset, S.E. and Bjelke, E. (1983). Does consumption of fruit and vegetables protect against stroke? *Lancet*, **ii**, 742.

Walker, A.E., Robins, M., and Weinfeld, F.D. (1981). The National Survey of Stroke: clinical findings. *Stroke*, **119**, 837–9.

Wannamethee, S.G. and Shaper, A.G. (1992). Physical activity and stroke in British middle aged men. *British Medical Journal*, **304**, 597–601.

Wannamethee, S.G. and Shaper, A.G. (1996). Patterns of alcohol intake and risk of stroke in middle-aged British men. *Stroke*, **27**, 1033–9.

Wannamethee, S.G. and Shaper, A.G. (1998). Alcohol, coronary heart disease and stroke: an examination of the J-shaped curve. *Neuroepidemiology*, **17**, 288–95.

Wannamethee, S.G., Shaper, A.G., Whincup, P.H., and Walker, M. (1995). Smoking cessation and the risk of stroke in middle-aged men. *Journal of the American Medical Association*, **274**, 155–60.

Welin, L., Svardsudd, K., Wilhelmsen, L., Larsson, B., and Tibblin, G. (1987). Analysis of risk factors for stroke in a cohort of men born in 1913. *New England Journal of Medicine*, **317**, 521–6.

Wender, M., Lenart-Jankowska, D., Pruchnik, D., and Kowal, P. (1990). Epidemiology of stroke in the Poznan district of Poland. *Stroke*, **21**, 390–3.

Whisnant, J.P., Fitzgibbons, J.P., Kurland, L.T., and Sayre, G.P. (1971). Natural history of stroke in Rochester, Minnesota, 1945 through 1954. *Stroke*, **2**, 11–22.

WHO (World Health Organization) (1971). *Control of stroke and hypertension in the community: report of a WHO meeting, Geneva, February 1971.* WHO, Geneva.

WHO (World Health Organization) (1972). *Community control of stroke and hypertension: report of a WHO meeting, Göteborg, November–December 1971.* WHO, Geneva.

WHO (World Health Organization) (1973). *Control of stroke in the community. Methodological considerations and protocol of WHO Stroke Register.* WHO, Geneva.

WHO (World Health Organization) (1994). *1993 World health statistics annual.* WHO, Geneva.

WHO (World Health Organization) (1996). *1995 World health statistics annual.* WHO, Geneva.

WHO (World Health Organization) (1998). *1996 World health statistics annual.* WHO, Geneva.

Wilhelmsen, L., Svardsudd, K., Korsan-Bengtsen, K., Larsson, B., Welin, L., and Tibblin, G. (1984). Fibrinogen as a risk factor for stroke and myocardial infarction. *New England Journal of Medicine*, **311**, 501–5.

Wolf, P.A., Dawber, T.R., Thomas, H.E., Jr, and Kannel, W.B. (1978). Epidemiologic assessment of chronic atrial fibrillation and risk of stroke: the Framingham Study. *Neurology*, **28**, 973–7.

Wolf, P.A., D'Agostino, R.B., Kannel, W.B., Bonita, R., and Belanger, A.J. (1988). Cigarette smoking as a risk factor for stroke: the Framingham Study. *Journal of the American Medical Association*, **259**, 1025–9.

Wolf, P.A., Abbott, R.D., and Kannel, W.B. (1991). Atrial fibrillation as an independent risk factor for stroke: the Framingham Study. *Stroke*, **22**, 983–8.

Wolfe, J.D., Shapiro, G.G., and Ratner, P.H. (1991). Comparison of albuterol and metaproterenol syrup in the treatment of childhood asthma. *Pediatrics*, **88**, 312–19.

Yoo, J.H., Chung, C.S., and Kang, S.S. (1998). Relation of plasma homocyst (e)ine to cerebral infarction and cerebral atherosclerosis. *Stroke*, **29**, 2478–83.

You, R.X., McNeil, J.J., Hurley, S.F., *et al.* (1993). Smoking as a risk factor for cortical ischaemia presumably due to carotid occlusive disease. *Neuroepidemiology*, **12**, 141–7.

You, R.X., McNeil, J.J., O'Malley, H.M., Davis, S.M., Thrift, A.G., and Donnan, G.A. (1997). Risk factors for stroke due to cerebral infarction in young adults. *Stroke*, **28**, 1913–18.

Yu, S., Sher, B., Kudryk, B., and Redman, C.M. (1984). Fibrinogen precursors: order of assembly of fibrinogen chains. *Journal of Biological Chemistry*, **259**, 10574–81.

Yuan, J.M., Ross, R.K., Gao, Y.T., Henderson, B.E., and Yu, M.C. (1997). Follow up study of moderate alcohol intake and mortality among middle aged men in Shanghai, China. *British Medical Journal*, **314**, 18–23.

Zee, R.Y., Ridker, P.M., Stampfer, M.J., Hennekens, C.H., and Lindpaintner, K. (1999). Prospective evaluation of the angiotensin-converting enzyme insertion/deletion polymorphism and the risk of stroke. *Circulation*, **99**, 340–3.

Zupping, R. and Roose, M. (1976). Epidemiology of cerebrovascular disease in Tartu, Estonia, USSR, 1970 through 1973. *Stroke*, **7**, 187–90.

9.4 Respiratory disease

T. H. Lam and A. J. Hedley

Factors in respiratory disease

Factors that are associated with lung disease but are not readily avoidable include genetic constitution, age, gender, and socio-economic status. Tobacco smoking and environmental air pollution are the principal avoidable causes of morbidity and mortality from the most common and serious chronic lung diseases, lung cancer, and obstructive lung disease. High dietary intake of fresh fruit, including consumption during winter, which raises serum levels of vitamin C, is inversely related to respiratory symptoms and physician-diagnosed bronchitis (Schwartz and Weiss 1990), ventilatory function, and chronic non-specific lung disease (Strachan *et al.* 1991; Meidema *et al.* 1993; Schwartz and Weiss 1994), but the relationship between dietary factors and non-malignant respiratory problems is under-researched and has not attracted adequate attention in public health actions against respiratory disease.

A comprehensive review by the World Cancer Research Fund (1997) concluded that there is convincing evidence that consumption of vegetables and fruits protects against lung cancer and that carotenoids in foods of plant origin are probably protective. Regular physical activity, diets high in vitamins C and E and selenium possibly reduce the risk of lung cancer, and diets high in total fat, saturated fat and cholesterol, and in alcohol, possibly increase risk. Dose–response relationships were observed that show that the relative risk decreases by about 50 per cent as vegetable intake increases from 150 to 400 g/day. A United Kingdom Department of Health Working Group on Diet and Cancer (Department of Health 1998) concluded that the evidence was not strong enough to support causation, but that there is moderately consistent evidence that higher fruit consumption, and weakly consistent evidence that higher vegetable consumption, are associated with lower risks of lung cancer. A plausible mechanism is the antioxidant capacity in protecting against free-radical-induced DNA damage; however, β-carotene and α-tocopherol appear unlikely to be the mediators and the strongly consistent negative association between serum β-carotene and lung cancer has not been confirmed as causal by intervention studies (Omenn *et al.* 1996). The Working Group also warned that there is no evidence that higher fruit and vegetable consumption would mitigate the overwhelming effect of smoking on lung cancer and that smokers with a high consumption of vegetables and fruits are still at high risk of lung cancer.

Derby and Samet (1994) estimated that radon causes 10 per cent of all lung cancer in the United States and 6 per cent in the United Kingdom, but there is still much uncertainty about the role of non-occupational or domestic exposure especially in developing countries. Whereas reduction of radon exposure will certainly lower the risk of lung cancer, it should be noted that the issue of indoor air pollution, including radon emission, is often used by the tobacco industry to confuse or to divert attention away from the issue of passive smoking, which is more readily preventable than radon exposure.

Global respiratory mortality

The *World Development Report 1993* provides a global overview of health status and health systems with special emphasis on developing countries (World Bank 1993). It describes the world pattern of mortality and burden of disease, including respiratory health problems. These data are also presented separately for developed and developing countries. The World Bank (1993) data have been revised by Murray and Lopez (1996, 1997*a*), and hence the results and Tables 1 and 2 supersede the corresponding data in the previous edition of this book (Hedley and Lam 1997).

In 1990, 19 per cent of the 50 million annual deaths in the world were caused by respiratory diseases, including lower respiratory infections (8.5 per cent), chronic obstructive pulmonary disease (**COPD**) (4 per cent), tuberculosis (4 per cent), malignant neoplasms of trachea, bronchus, and lung (2 per cent), all broadly labelled as lung cancer, and asthma (0.3 per cent) and upper respiratory infections (0.1 per cent). After cardiovascular diseases, which accounted for 28 per cent of all deaths, respiratory diseases were the second most common cause of death. If tuberculosis and lung cancer are excluded and reclassified into other categories, respiratory diseases (mainly lower respiratory infections and COPD) would rank third after cardiovascular diseases, infections (including tuberculosis), and parasitic diseases, followed by malignant neoplasms, including lung cancer (Table 1). In 1998, of the 54 million deaths in the World Health Organization (**WHO**) member states, these respiratory diseases accounted for 16 per cent (tuberculosis, 2.8 per cent; lower respiratory infections, 6.4 per cent; upper respiratory infections, 0.1 per cent; lung cancer, 2.3 per cent; COPD, 4.2 per cent; asthma, 0.3 per cent), and still ranked second to cardiovascular diseases (31 per cent) (WHO 1999*a*).

While respiratory diseases in general were the second most common cause of deaths in the developed as well as in the developing countries, the relative importance of the specific diseases in each was different. In developed countries, 12 per cent of the 11 million deaths were the result of respiratory diseases: lung cancer (5 per cent), lower respiratory infections (4 per cent), and COPD (3 per cent). Two of the

Table 1 Deaths caused by respiratory diseases in the world, 1990 (thousands)

	Developing countries[a]				Developed countries[b]			
	Male		Female		Male		Female	
	Ages 0–4	Age 5 and older	Ages 0–4	Age 5 and older	Ages 0–4	Age 5 and older	Ages 0–4	Age 5 and older
Tuberculosis	43	1094	39	746	0	29	0	9
Lower respiratory infections	1328	688	1229	670	12	168	8	196
Upper respiratory infections	14	7	13	6	0	1	0	2
Malignant neoplasms of trachea, bronchus, and lung	0	309	0	113	0	399	0	124
COPD	17	991	23	855	0	206	0	119
Asthma	1	57	1	49	0	13	0	16
All respiratory diseases above	1403	3146	1305	2439	12	816	8	466
Deaths from all causes	6532	14593	6006	12424	126	5441	93	5252
Respiratory/all causes	21%	22%	22%	20%	10%	15%	9%	9%

[a]Developing countries, demographically developing group, including Sub-Saharan Africa, India, China, other Asia and islands, Latin America and the Caribbean, and Middle Eastern crescent regions.

[b]Developed countries, former socialist economies of Europe and established market economies.

Source: Murray and Lopez (1996), Annex Table 6a–i.

three leading respiratory diseases, lung cancer and COPD, are attributable to smoking. In developing countries, 21 per cent of the 40 million deaths were the result of respiratory diseases, including lower respiratory infections (10 per cent), tuberculosis (5 per cent), COPD (5 per cent), and lung cancer (1 per cent). The two leading causes are infections and the next two are smoking related. In developing countries respiratory disease caused a similar proportion of deaths to cardiovascular diseases (23 per cent), whereas cardiovascular diseases caused 48 per cent of all deaths in developed countries.

There were few gender differences in the mortality pattern in those aged up to 4 years in the developed and developing countries. This was true for respiratory infections and asthma from age 5 onwards. In the older age groups, the excess mortality in males caused by lung cancer and COPD in both developed and developing countries can mostly be attributed to smoking. Whereas the total deaths as a result of these two smoking-related diseases were similar to those caused by tuberculosis in developing countries, they were more than 20 times that caused by tuberculosis in developed countries. Therefore, in developing coun-

Table 2 Burden of respiratory diseases in the world (1990) (hundreds of thousands of DALYs lost)

	Developing countries		Developed countries		World	
	Male	Female	Male	Female	Male	Female
Tuberculosis	213.3	166.0	4.1	0.9	217.4	166.9
Lower respiratory infections	563.4	541.7	13.1	10.8	576.5	552.5
Upper respiratory infections	6.3	6.0	0.4	0.4	6.7	6.4
Malignant neoplasms of trachea, bronchus, and lung	31.4	11.5	35.4	10.4	66.8	21.9
COPD	140.9	116.9	22.2	11.4	163.1	128.3
Asthma	50.2	40.2	9.2	8.2	59.4	48.4
All respiratory diseases above	1005.5	882.3	84.4	42.1	1089.9	924.4
Deaths from all causes	6316.5	5865.9	903.8	706.2	7220.3	6572.1
Respiratory/all causes	16%	15%	9%	6%	15%	14%

Developing countries, demographically developing group, including Sub-Saharan Africa, India, China, other Asia and islands, Latin America and the Caribbean, and Middle Eastern crescent regions.

Developed countries, former socialist economies of Europe and established market economies.

Source: Murray and Lopez (1996), Annex Table 9a–i.

tries, tuberculosis and smoking-related diseases are of similar importance in causing respiratory deaths, but smoking-related diseases are the predominant causes in developed countries.

World burden of respiratory diseases

The World Bank and the WHO developed the disability-adjusted life year (**DALY**) to measure the burden of disease (World Bank 1993). The DALY combines healthy life years lost because of premature mortality with those lost as a result of disability. It can be used as a measure of benefits (e.g. the ratio of cost to DALYs gained or the amount needed to gain 1 DALY). The calculation of the DALY is based on the potential years of life lost as a result of a death at a given age, the relative value of a year of healthy life lived at different ages, the discount rate, and the disability weights used to convert life lived with a disability to a common measure with premature death. The updated data (Murray and Lopez 1996, 1997*a*) are presented in Table 2. Throughout the world in 1990, in males and females combined, 201.4 million DALYs (15 per cent) were the result of respiratory diseases. This was less than all injuries (208.6 million DALYs, 15 per cent), and was followed by neuropsychiatric conditions (11 per cent) and cardiovascular diseases (10 per cent).

In developing countries, respiratory diseases were the most important causes of DALYs lost in females, and the second most important in males (second to all injuries), mainly because of lower respiratory infections and tuberculosis. In developed countries, in each gender, respiratory diseases were less important than neuropsychiatric conditions, cardiovascular diseases, and injuries. Lung cancer, lower respiratory infections, and COPD were the main respiratory causes.

Smoking and respiratory deaths in developed countries

Peto *et al.* (1994) have provided a comprehensive estimate of mortality from smoking in developed countries from 1950 to 2000. Details of the problem of respiratory mortality attributed to smoking can be found in Hedley and Lam (1997). In 1990, in developed countries, smoking killed more people than all other causes apart from respiratory diseases; of all deaths caused by smoking, about 43 per cent were respiratory diseases. More than half (54 per cent) of all deaths resulting from respiratory diseases in males and females of all ages were attributed to smoking; the proportions in males and females aged 35 to 69 were 83 per cent and 53 per cent respectively.

From 1975 to 1995, in males, over 90 per cent of the deaths caused by lung cancer, about 70 per cent of those caused by COPD and about 14 per cent of those resulting from other respiratory diseases are attributed to smoking. Both the proportion and number of deaths caused by lung cancer are still increasing slowly because the smoking epidemic has already reached its peak in some countries.

The most striking pattern is seen in females. In 1975, about half of lung cancer, 20 per cent of COPD and 2 per cent of other respiratory disease deaths were attributed to smoking, rising to 72 per cent, 53 per cent, and 7 per cent respectively in 1995. Both the proportion and number of deaths from these causes is increasing sharply because of the increasing trend of smoking in women. There is no sign that the smoking epidemic in women has reached its peak.

The lung cancer death rate is the best indicator of the evolving tobacco epidemic in the developed world. In the European Union, there was a small fall in lung cancer deaths in men from 52.4 per 100 000 in 1985 to 1989 to 49.8 per 100 000 in 1990 to 1994; however, but there is a persistent rise in women during the same period, from 8.9 to 9.6 per 100 000. For truncated rates for men aged 35 to 64 years, the peak was 74.3 per 100 000 in 1980 to 1984, followed by a levelling off and a decline to 68.3 per 100 000 in 1990–94; however, in women, the rate increased more rapidly from 7.7 per 100 000 in 1955 to 1959 to 14.3 in 1990 to 1994 (Levi *et al.* 1999). Female lung cancer rates are still lower in the European Union than in the United States. Breast cancer is still the leading cause of cancer death in women in Europe, but the rate at 35 to 64 years has decreased from 43.0 per 100 000 in 1985 to 1989 to 41.9/100 000 in 1990 to 1994. A more sudden decrease was observed in the United Kingdom (Peto 1998). With the rising trend of lung cancer deaths and decreasing trend of breast cancer deaths, the former will inevitably overtake the position of breast cancer as the top cancer killer in European women early in the twenty-first century. In the United States, from the mid-1980s, lung cancer has killed more women than breast cancer and in Canada this has occurred in the early 1990s with the gap widening.

Both the United Kingdom and United States data show the long delay of several decades, which occurs between the peak of the population smoking prevalence ratios and the peak of lung cancer death rates in men and the benefits that result from the fall in smoking prevalence. Women took up smoking on a large scale much later than men and, therefore, the lung cancer death rates are still rising and the peak of the epidemic will arrive during the next few decades. These patterns of smoking and mortality are now being repeated in developing countries such as China.

Deaths from smoking in developing countries

Smoking killed more people in developed compared with developing countries in the twentieth century but the opposite will be true in the twenty-first century (Peto *et al.* 1994). Estimation of tobacco-attributable mortality in developing countries is more difficult because of the lack of reliable epidemiological data, particularly from large prospective studies. The interaction of smoking and other risk factors for cardiorespiratory diseases, such as cholesterol and air pollution, in developing countries is not clear and should be an important area for further studies. Peto *et al.* (1994) estimated that smoking caused 2 million deaths per year in developed countries and 1 million deaths per year in developing countries in the 1990s, but the deaths in developing countries cannot be reliably broken down by specific diseases as in developed countries. However, smoking causes many more deaths from other diseases than from lung cancer in both developed and developing countries. In the latter, COPD could be more important than coronary heart disease because of the lower cholesterol levels, but cholesterol levels are likely to increase with Westernization.

Apart from China, data from other developing countries are scanty. A simple, cheap, and quick method is needed to estimate the number of deaths due to tobacco. The case–control study method of collecting a history of smoking in a large number of deceased persons from their surviving relatives has great potential. In South Africa, smoking history has to be recorded on the death certificate (Bradshaw *et al.* 1998). In Hong Kong, relatives of deceased persons were successfully interviewed in death registries and the response rate was 94 per cent (Lam *et al.* 1998).

The pattern of smoking and smoking-related mortality, particularly deaths from chronic lung diseases, including tuberculosis, in China is an important warning signal for other developing countries where smoking prevalence is increasing rapidly together with economic developments during the past one to two decades. China has the highest tobacco production and consumption in the world with over 300 million smokers. The main increase in cigarette consumption in China took place only recently and Chinese tobacco mortality will increase substantially if the current smoking pattern persists. Two-thirds of men become smokers before the age of 25 and about half will be killed by tobacco. Of all male deaths at ages 35 to 69, the proportion attributed to tobacco will rise from 12 per cent in 1990 to about 33 per cent in 2030 (Liu *et al.* 1998; Niu *et al.* 1998). Worldwide, tobacco will cause about 10 million deaths a year by 2030, 70 per cent of them in the developing world (Lopez 1998). Unless urgent measures are implemented and the increasing trend of smoking in the developing world is rapidly reversed, the predictions for tobacco-induced health problems are gloomy. Tobacco control measures within developing countries are often weak and ineffective against the aggressive tobacco promotion strategies of the multinational tobacco companies. Successful tobacco control measures in the United States have resulted in faster market expansion of American tobacco companies into Asia and other developing countries to maintain their markets. Tobacco control to prevent this huge impending epidemic in developing countries urgently requires the support of an international public health movement.

Recent international and national actions

Internationally, the WHO (1999*a*) estimated that about 4 million deaths (3.24 million males and 782 000 females) and 49.3 million DALYs (40 million in males and 9.3 in females) in all its member states were attributed to tobacco. The WHO (1998) has published *Guidelines for Controlling and Monitoring the Tobacco Epidemic* and has established the Tobacco Free Initiative, which is a new WHO cabinet project with the express aim of focusing international attention and resources on the global tobacco epidemic. The WHO has also proposed the Framework Convention on Tobacco Control (WHO 1999*b*). This is the first time that the WHO has used its treaty-making powers to promote a global public health movement. A recent World Bank (1999) report also marks the first time an international finance institution, after examining the health and economic questions of tobacco use, has supported measures to reduce the demand for tobacco (see Chapter 10.1).

Nationally, the patterns of tobacco use and control measures of the WHO member states were described in a WHO (1997*a*) global status report. The 1998 United Kingdom White Paper on Tobacco, the first-ever in the country, is a new example of that government's commitment, with expressed budget allocation and targets, to prevent its annual 120 000 tobacco deaths (SCOTH 1998).

Occupational factors and respiratory diseases

Following smoking, occupational factors are the next most preventable causes of respiratory diseases. Occupational factors consist of many different causal agents, which should be considered individually in different work environments. The causal agents or substances are grouped under 'occupational factors' because exposures to them occur predominantly in the work environment. The agents that can cause harm to the respiratory system are classified into dusts (including mineral and organic dusts and particulates), chemicals, biological substances (such as microbiological agents), and physical agents (such as ionizing radiation).

The adverse health effects from occupational factors on the respiratory system range from minor and non-specific symptoms such as cough and phlegm, to fatal and well-defined occupational diseases such as pleural mesothelioma following exposure to asbestos. The effects can also be asymptomatic and recognized only by radiography (such as pleural plaques and fibrosis), lung function tests (such as reduction in forced expiratory volume in 1 s (**FEV1**), the histamine challenge test (to demonstrate increased bronchial hyper-reactivity) and other laboratory tests such as gas transfer. Occupational lung disorders can present as acute responses (such as acute pneumonitis and pulmonary oedema), as a result of acute gassing (poisoning by inhaled toxic gases), acute allergic inflammation (such as acute allergic aveolitis), chronic diseases with a long latency period (such as lung cancer or silicosis), or acute exacerbation of a chronic condition such as asthma. Asthma can also be caused *de novo* by an occupational allergen.

In 1999, the International Labour Office estimated that work-related injuries and diseases kill 1.1 million people annually worldwide, 34 per cent due to cancer, 25 per cent injuries, 21 per cent chronic respiratory diseases, 15 per cent cardiovascular diseases, and 5 per cent others (including pneumoconiosis, nervous and renal disorders). Annually, an estimated 160 million new cases of work-related diseases occur worldwide and respiratory diseases are one of the most common. In 1997, the overall economic losses resulting from work-related diseases and injuries were about 4 per cent of the world's gross national product. Respiratory diseases were responsible for 9 per cent of the costs for work-related injuries and diseases (WHO 1999*c*). It should be noted that the global burden of occupational disease and injuries is certainly underestimated. Data from developed countries are fragmented, and underdiagnosis and under-reporting is much more serious in developing countries. For example, in Latin America, only 1 to 4 per cent of all occupational diseases are reported.

Non-occupational exposures or agents can cause the same respiratory diseases and therefore the question commonly asked is how much of a respiratory health problem can be attributed to occupational exposure. For compensation purposes, occupational lung diseases as the result of exposure to certain agents or associated with a history of working in certain work processes are usually defined or specified in the regulations, so that workers suffering from such diseases are assumed to have derived their diseases solely (or mainly) from their work and are eligible for compensation. There is no requirement to prove that their diseases could not have derived from exposures outside work, even though non-occupational exposure, such as smoking, could be a more important or plausible cause.

Many occupational agents and processes are recognized as occupational causes of lung cancer. Smoking is an independent cause of lung cancer in workers and it can interact with other occupational carcinogens. When there is an interaction of two causal agents, removal of one agent will take away the effect of that agent and the interaction effect of both factors. For example, for a smoker exposed to asbestos, cessation of smoking alone will result in an elimination of 92 per cent of the excess rate, and removal of asbestos alone will result in an elimination of 81 per cent of the excess risk (Harrington and Saracci 1994).

Occupational health practices tend to emphasize occupational carcinogens and ignore smoking, as the latter is not traditionally considered as an occupational factor. The best preventive approach should aim at the removal of both smoking and the known occupational carcinogens. However, measures to remove a carcinogen in the workplace can be difficult, expensive, or even impracticable, for example in developing countries where the worksite situations are the worst. Prevention of smoking, for example by banning smoking and by smoking cessation services, can be more readily implemented and can prevent a large proportion of lung cancer in the workforce, regardless of whether there are exposures to known or unknown occupational lung carcinogens.

Other important respiratory diseases attributable to occupational factors include pneumoconiosis, such as silicosis and asbestosis, occupational asthma, and diseases or syndromes from exposure to organic dusts, such as byssinosis. Workers can present with a whole spectrum of non-specific respiratory symptoms. Whereas chronic non-specific respiratory diseases, including chronic bronchitis, emphysema, and asthma may be common in certain occupational groups exposed to dust or agents inhaled at work, among smokers smoking can be a more important cause than the specific dust or chemicals. Few studies can clarify the independent roles of smoking and a specific dust or chemical and the interaction between the two in cases of pneumoconiosis because most workers affected are smokers. For example, most patients with silicosis are chronic heavy smokers and their lung function shows an obstructive pattern of chronic bronchitis as well as the restrictive pattern due to silica deposition. When the workers claim for compensation the regulations ignore the role of smoking and both the affected workers and their physicians are reluctant to highlight smoking as a probable cause of the health problems for fear of jeopardizing compensation and other claims. Many such patients continue to smoke after receiving compensation and their condition can deteriorate rapidly. Obviously compensation does not improve health *per se*, and pneumoconiosis patients should receive active pulmonary rehabilitation, even if the disease is not curable. Apart from removal from further exposure to the putative occupational agent, smoking cessation should be considered the most important method to improve health and prevent further disability and premature death.

The extent of occupational respiratory disorders is often underestimated by official statistics based on statutory notification or compensation. Special surveys are needed and in the United Kingdom, the Surveillance of Work Related and Occupational Respiratory Diseases project is one good example (Sallie *et al.* 1994).

A new approach is to measure the prevalence of self-reported work-related illness by interviewing a representative sample of the working population. In 1995 in the United Kingdom about 40 000 persons who had ever worked were interviewed in a Labour Force Survey and 7 per cent reported an illness in the last year that was caused or made worse by work (Jones *et al.* 1998). Of the estimated prevalence of 2 million illnesses, lower respiratory disease (mainly asthmatic symptoms) constituted about 10 per cent and ranked third among the most common self-reported work-related disease categories, following musculoskeletal conditions (60 per cent) and stress (25 per cent), whereas pneumoconiosis constituted about 1 per cent. Such an approach based on self-reporting has many limitations but comparison of the results in 1995 with those in a similar survey in 1990 suggests good reliability. It is the only cost-effective method to give a comprehensive estimate of the extent of work-related respiratory problems in the working population as a whole. For an individual worker, an occupational cause claimed by the worker is a good start as this indicates awareness and concern and should prompt the health professionals concerned to discuss the problem and to examine carefully the potential or claimed health risks at work. From a public health perspective, such estimates of occupational health problems in the total population are useful for monitoring the problems and for guiding occupational health promotion strategies.

The principles of primary prevention of occupational respiratory disorders have been discussed by Hedley and Lam (1997) and are not repeated here. Although it is still not clear what would be the interaction effect between smoking and occupational exposure to pneumoconiosis and other specific and non-specific occupational respiratory disorders, the principles and benefits described above for the prevention of lung cancer should apply. Prevention of smoking, including provision of smoking cessation programmes, should be an important part of an occupational health programme to prevent occupational respiratory disorders, including cancer and other health problems.

Since 1997, the International Labour Office and the WHO have jointly started an initiative for the global elimination of silicosis. Elimination is not eradication (as in the case of smallpox) and it implies the possibility of recurrence (Wagner 1998). However, this is the first time that an occupational disease has been targeted for elimination. In more developed countries such as the United States, elimination is a possibility, but in developing countries the situation is likely to get worse before it gets better. The initiative, however, can remind governments, employers, employees, and occupational health professionals that silicosis is preventable and the ultimate target of elimination should be achievable in the not too distant future.

Respiratory health and passive smoking

Passive smoking is the inhalation by non-smoking subjects of the cigarette smoke emitted from the burning end of the cigarette (side-stream smoke) and the smoke inhaled (mainstream smoke) and then exhaled by the active smoker. This mix of tobacco smoke is called environmental tobacco smoke (**ETS**) or second-hand smoke (**SHS**). Concentrations of some carcinogenic and toxic substances are higher in side-stream than mainstream smoke, although ETS is diluted by ambient air.

In the late 1980s, two major reviews in the United States (National Research Council 1986; US Department of Health, Education and Welfare 1986) and one from the United Kingdom (Froggatt 1988) all concluded that ETS causes lung cancer and childhood respiratory illnesses. The conclusions of a comprehensive review from the United States Environmental Protection Agency (USEPA 1992) were the same. The relative risk for lung cancer due to ETS, based on 11 United States studies, was 1.19 (USEPA 1992). The excess risk estimated by the Froggatt Committee (Froggatt 1988) was about 10 to 30 per cent. In a meta-analysis of 37 studies Hackshaw *et al.* (1997) produced a relative risk of 1.24 (95 per cent confidence intervals 1.13 to 1.36). The excess risks were not affected after adjusting for bias and confounding, including confounding due to diet. Their conclusion on lung cancer was accepted by the United Kingdom Scientific Committee on Tobacco and Health (SCOTH 1998), which also reached similar conclusions about the other adverse health effects of ETS, including heart disease and childhood respiratory ill health.

Despite the overwhelming amount of evidence and the unanimous conclusions of many reviews by committees and individual authors that the association between ETS and lung cancer is causal, objections from the tobacco industry and its scientists are still prevalent. A tobacco industry sponsored European Working Group (1996) found a significantly increased risk in its meta-analysis on ETS and lung cancer but then discredited this finding. Their arguments, including misclassification bias, dietary confounding, publication bias, and thresholds were criticized by Smith and Phillips (1996). A recent example is the tobacco industry's misinterpretation of the evidence from a WHO study on the links between passive smoking and lung cancer (Boffetta *et al.* 1998) and this led the WHO to denounce newspaper reports based on the industry's analysis as 'false and misleading' (Bates and Brookes 1999). Barnes and Bero (1998) examined 106 review papers on ETS and concluded that the affiliation with the tobacco industry was the only factor associated with authors concluding that ETS is not harmful.

In children, many reviews by government agencies or committees, non-governmental organizations and individual scientists have concluded that ETS causes respiratory ill health (Royal College of Physicians of London 1992; USEPA 1992; Australian National Health and Medical Research Council 1997; SCOTH 1998). Compared with the issue of ETS and lung cancer, the conclusions about ETS and child health have been subject to much less critique from the tobacco industry and its scientists. On an international level, the 1997 Declaration of the Environmental Leaders of the Eight (**G8**) on Children's Environmental Health stated that children exposed to ETS are more likely to suffer from reduced lung function, lower respiratory tract infections, and respiratory irritations, that asthmatic children are especially at risk and that many of those symptoms lead to increased hospital admission (WHO 1999*d*). This is the first time that ministers of the environment were involved as a group in the passive smoking issue. In response to this declaration, the WHO convened an International Consultation on Environmental Tobacco Smoke and Child Health in January 1999.

The WHO consultation has concluded that ETS is a real and substantial threat to child health and that ETS causes lower respiratory tract infections such as pneumonia and bronchitis, coughing and wheezing, worsening of asthma, and middle ear disease (WHO 1999*d*). About 700 million, or almost half of the world's children are exposed. For lower respiratory illness, during the first year of life, in children whose mothers smoke, the pooled relative risk from over 40 studies was 1.7 (95 per cent confidence intervals 1.6 to 1.9); for paternal smoking alone, the relative risk was 1.3 (95 per cent confidence intervals 1.2 to 1.4). Both asthma and respiratory symptoms are increased in children whose parents smoke, and the pooled relative risks from over 60 studies, for either parent smoking, range from 1.2 to 1.4. The California Environmental Protection Agency (1997) estimated that, each year in the United States, ETS exposure causes: 3000 deaths from lung cancer; 35 000 to 62 000 deaths from ischaemic heart disease; 1900 to 2700 cases of sudden infant death syndrome; 9700 to 18 600 cases of low-birth weight infants; 8000 to 26 000 new cases of asthma in children; exacerbation of asthma in 400 000 to 1 million children; and 150 000 to 300 000 cases of bronchitis or pneumonia children aged 18 months and younger, of which 7500 to 15 000 require hospital admission (Davis 1998).

Passive smoking at work

In the United States EPA (1992) review, no clear conclusion was reached about the adverse health effects of ETS exposure at work. The conclusions about ETS and coronary heart disease from most reviews were based on results predominantly from exposures at home. As for exposure at work, He *et al.* (1994) first reported an association between coronary heart disease and passive smoking at work in Chinese never-smoking women, with a dose–response relationship after adjusting for major risk factors and exposure to passive smoking from the husband. A review of seven studies on passive smoking in the workplace by Wells (1998) concluded that the relative risks for heart disease from passive smoking at work are roughly equal to those from home-based exposures. A meta-analysis by He *et al.* (1999) calculated a relative risk of 1.11 (95 per cent confidence intervals 1.00 to 1.23) for exposure in the workplace.

Although many reviews have concluded that ETS is causally related to lung cancer, few have made specific conclusions about risk estimates for passive smoking at work. The United States Occupational Safety and Health Administration (OSHA 1994) assumed that risk estimates based on residential exposures should accurately reflect occupational risks for most workplaces. Siegel *et al.* (1995) reviewed 10 studies on lung cancer and non-smokers exposed to ETS in the workplace and concluded that these studies support the assumption of a small elevated risk. Using modelling based on nicotine from ETS in office air and salivary cotinine in non-smoking workers, Repace *et al.* (1998) estimated that at the current 28 per cent prevalence of unrestricted smoking in the office workplace, 4000 heart disease deaths and 400 lung cancer deaths occur annually among office workers from passive smoking in the workplace in the United States.

Apart from lung cancer, evidence on the relationship between ETS and respiratory ill health in adults is scarce, in contrast with the huge amount of such evidence in children. In the risk assessment of passive smoking at work, the United Kingdom Health and Safety Commission (HSC 1999) Proposal for an Approved Code of Practice is only based on the two main effects of passive smoking exposure in the workplace: (a) it exacerbates certain diseases, such as asthma and chronic bronchitis; (b) it causes discomfort as it irritates the eyes, nose, throat, and chest, and tobacco smoke has an unpleasant smell. The HSC was not certain about the size and extent of the risk for either cancer or heart disease.

Only a few studies have shown an association between respiratory ill health (other than lung cancer) and ETS exposure in adults. Two of them observed an association for ETS exposure at home in women (Ng *et al.* 1993; Pope and Xu 1993). Wong *et al.* (1999) found a dose–response relationship between respiratory symptoms in non-smoking women and ETS exposure at home after adjusting for outdoor air pollution. White *et al.* (1991) reported that those with ETS exposure at work had more respiratory symptoms but no dose–response relationship was found. Leuenberger *et al.* (1994) reported a significant trend of increasing risk with total ETS exposure at home and at work, but there were no separate data for exposure at work. Although Jaakkola *et al.* (1996) measured ETS at home and at work separately, only the relationship between total exposure and respiratory symptoms was reported.

Smokers are obviously also exposed to passive smoking. Mannino *et al.* (1997) reported that in the United States, 87 per cent of current smokers reported exposure to ETS at home or work, whereas only 20 per cent never-smokers and 23 per cent former smokers were exposed. There are limited data for ETS exposure at home and lung cancer in smokers. Siegel *et al.* (1995) conducted a meta-analysis of six studies that examined lung cancer among smokers (men and women) exposed to ETS at home and the pooled relative risk was 1.3 (95 per cent confidence intervals 1.1 to 1.5). This was consistent with the value of 1.25 in the United States EPA (1992) meta-analysis of seven studies among female smokers exposed to ETS. There is a lack of data on exposure to ETS at work in smokers and no definitive conclusion on the risk of cancer in this group.

In a study on the Hong Kong Police, Lam *et al.* (1999) compared the prevalence of having frequent cough or phlegm among four groups of male officers and the odds ratio adjusted for age, education, marital status, police rank and type of police work, and past occupational dust exposure was 1.00 for never-smokers not exposed to ETS, 1.91 (1.58 to 2.30) for never-smokers exposed to ETS, 2.44 (1.93 to 3.07) for current smokers not exposed to ETS and 4.30 (3.57 to 5.18) for current smokers exposed to ETS ($p < 0.001$). The results were similar after further adjustment for ETS exposure at home.

Only one study has examined the effect on respiratory health before and after legislative prohibition of smoking in the workplace. Eisner *et al.* (1998) found that bar tenders' respiratory symptoms, forced vital capacity (**FVC**) and FEV_1 improved after a decline of self-reported ETS exposure as a result of the smoking ban in California. Stratification by smoking status showed similar results in non-smokers and smokers. The results were also controlled for recent upper respiratory infections. This study has provided important evidence that passive smoking is harmful and that banning smoking can produce immediate benefits on the respiratory health of workers exposed at work.

More research on the effects of ETS exposure, particularly at work in smokers will certainly help to clarify the issue and to support legislative control of smoking in the workplace. The results so far are sufficient to conclude that ETS at work causes ill health in both non-smokers and smokers. Whereas smokers may be convinced that breathing other smokers' smoke is harmful to themselves, the tobacco industry is certain to challenge any legislative restriction of smoking at work and in public places. However, if both non-smoking and smoking employees support restriction or total bans on smoking in their own workplaces, they and their employers can make their own decision to implement control measures to eliminate ETS exposure. Such measures have been adopted in many government and private workplaces in developed countries but progress in developing countries is slow. The only satisfactory smoking areas designed to protect non-smokers are separately ventilated and exhausted areas, but it is likely these areas will be a hazard to smokers. As a comprehensive smoke-free policy always produces better outcomes (Siegel 1995), this is the preferred approach. Strategies to protect non-smokers include education, regulation, legislation, and litigation, but a large number of people continue to be exposed involuntarily to ETS. Education can increase public support for legislation to ban or restrict smoking; however, education alone is usually not effective and legislation is needed. Litigation is being used increasingly in the United States to compensate non-smokers whose health has been adversely affected (Davis 1998) and there have been some well publicized successful cases in the United States, United Kingdom, and Australia. However, such moves are almost unheard of in developing countries.

The recognition of passive smoking as a health hazard is an important milestone in tobacco control in the past two decades in the West, particularly in the United States. The United States OSHA was the first government occupational health agency to propose regulations to ban smoking in work sites except in separately ventilated areas.

A quasi-legal approach using an Approved Code of Practice was proposed in 1999 by the United Kingdom Health and Safety Commission (UKHSC 1999) on passive smoking at work. The code will clarify how the Health and Safety At Work Act of 1974 should be applied to passive smoking as the Act requires 'every employer to ensure, so far as is reasonably practicable, the health, safety and welfare of all his employees' (Bates and Brookes 1999). The Code of Practice does not require a ban on all smoking in all workplaces—only where it is reasonably practicable. It is not aimed to protect customers of restaurants and pubs (or bars), but employers have to do what is reasonably practicable to reduce employees' exposure if they do not ban smoking. If the proposal is approved, the United Kingdom approach would be a useful example for other countries to follow, if legislation for a total ban is not feasible.

Banning smoking in the workplace will encourage smokers to quit smoking. Chapman *et al.* (1999) reviewed 19 studies of the impact of smoke-free workplaces from 1986 to 1996 and showed that 18 studies reported reduction of daily smoking rates and 17 reported reduction of smoking prevalence. The tobacco industry also estimated a big reduction of consumption and a big increase in quitting rate as a result of workplace smoking restriction (Bates and Brookes 1999). Prevention of smoking and passive smoking at work should be an urgent priority in occupational health and public health.

Passive smoking in Asia

The ETS issue is a major problem for the tobacco industry and its efforts to confuse the evidence are well documented (Glantz *et al.* 1996) and will continue to be uncovered. Action against ETS is probably the greatest threat to the expansion of the multinational tobacco companies in Asia and they have gone to great efforts to block it. Whereas the recognition of ETS as a health hazard has prompted strong public health interventions in the West, particularly in the United States, great inertia and barriers to the prevention of passive smoking are common in developing countries. Although scientists in Asia have made significant contributions to the global evidence to support the causal conclusions about ETS, their local evidence has not yet made significant impacts on governments. Most governments, including their environmental and occupational health departments do not consider ETS a high priority (Lam and Hedley 1999). There is slow progress against great barriers and no sign of a major breakthrough in the developing world. Public health workers in developing countries should use the ETS issue, in high profile campaigns, to promote campaigns to protect the health of non-smokers, particularly women and children, and experience and support from the West would be beneficial.

Smoking, passive smoking, and occupational health

Workers who are most exposed to occupational hazards usually come from the lowest socio-economic strata and they have the highest smoking prevalence. This is true in developed countries such as the United States (Stellman *et al.* 1988) and in developed countries such as China (Lam *et al.* 1996). Such workers' excess morbidity and mortality from both exposures is reflected in the highest standardized mortality ratios in the lowest social class in developed countries, such as the United Kingdom, and is the major contributor of poor health in a much larger sector of the working population in developing countries. Occupational health professionals should work closely with tobacco control advocates, target the most vulnerable groups at risk and make the prevention of smoking a top priority. On the other hand many occupational health professionals have been targeted for recruitment by the tobacco industry and become the industry's consultants to speak against the evidence on passive smoking and against tobacco control measures. Such recruitments in Asia have been revealed in internal documents of the industry (Rupp and Billings 1990). Occupational health professionals should be aware of such strategies of the tobacco industry and avoid being inadvertently recruited as the industry's consultants.

The International Commission on Occupational Health (1999) is the most important international organization for occupational health professionals. It has 30 scientific committees and four scientific working groups as of 1 March 1999, but there is none on smoking or passive smoking at work. Under the auspices of the Commission, the International Congress on Occupational Health is the most important international occupational health conference, but smoking and passive smoking have never been given any prime status as topics in plenary sessions, mini-symposia, or other scientific sessions. Unless occupational health professionals change their attitudes about smoking and passive smoking at work and start to tackle these problems seriously, many workers in the new millennium will continue to work in unhealthy smoky workplaces and their health will be seriously affected by both active and passive smoking.

Chronic obstructive pulmonary disease

COPD (ICD9 490–496, excluding 493) is a group of related or overlapping conditions that comprises chronic bronchitis, emphysema, bronchiectasis, bronchial catarrh, and other non-specific obstructive airway diseases. Under different definitions it may be referred to as chronic obstructive lung disease. The prevalence of chronic bronchitis is increasing as the populations of postindustrialized countries age. It may be considerably underdiagnosed in some populations (den Otter *et al.* 1998). Most (75 per cent) mortality from respiratory disease is attributable to COPD, which is the fifth most common cause of death after infectious disease (including respiratory infections), cardiovascular, and malignant and traumatic conditions (WHO 1999*a*).

In the United States, where it is the fourth most common cause of death, COPD is uncommon in those under 40 years of age but the prevalence reaches 10 per cent in 60- to 85-year-olds (Anthonisen 1997). In 1996 it was estimated to be the principal cause of mortality in 100 000 deaths and contributory in many more (Petty and Weinmann 1997).

The strongest risk factor for COPD is smoking (Fletcher *et al.* 1976). It increases the rate of decline of lung function (Camilli *et al.* 1987) and increases the risk of symptoms and premature death (Kuller *et al.* 1989). The global patterns of COPD strongly reflect geographic and demographic patterns of smoking. Future patterns of COPD will be determined by smoking trends and gender differences in rates of increase can be expected in view of the increased prevalence of smoking in women. Among WHO member states the global burden of COPD is estimated at 28.6 million cases, about half of all respiratory diseases, with more than 90 per cent occurring in lower and middle income groups and nearly 60 per cent in China alone (WHO 1999*a*).

In the United Kingdom the pattern of increase and decline in COPD is associated with increases and later declines in smoking in men in the twentieth century (ONS 1997). Other potential causes of chronic respiratory illness and decreased lung function in adult life include birth weight, serious childhood infections, occupational exposures, and ambient air pollution.

Only a minority of all smokers develop COPD (Fletcher *et al.* 1976) and family studies suggest that genetic factors also contribute to its development (Sandford *et al.* 1997). The only established genetic risk factor is homozygosity for the 2 allele of the α_1-antitrypsin gene. Heterozygotes may also be at increased risk. Other genes, including those for α_1-antichymotrypsin and cystic fibrosis membrane regulator and blood groups, and several others have shown a significant association between polymorphisms and COPD (Sandford *et al.* 1997).

The epidemiological evidence for a causal relationship between nutrition and either adverse effects for or protection from asthma and COPD has focused on intake of sodium, *n*-3 fatty acids, antioxidant vitamins, and fresh fruit and vegetables (Smit *et al.* 1999). Although the evidence for a beneficial effect of consuming fish, fruit, and vegetables on both asthma and COPD is increasing the effect of supplementation in subjects with existing asthma remains uncertain. High sodium diets may increase airways reactivity in asthmatics.

The health-care costs of COPD are high with several cost drivers, including frequent hospital admission and long-term oxygen therapy. Other economic costs include years of life lost, disability, and reduced quality of life. In primary care settings in the United Kingdom consultations for COPD are up to four times as frequent as for ischaemic heart disease. In the United States COPD is the third most common cause of hospital admission.

Treatment and rehabilitation may improve both clinical aspects of the disease and quality of life and reduce the overall costs of care. Long-term oxygen therapy is an intervention that improves survival and quality of life in COPD (British Thoracic Society 1997). In patients with acute exacerbations of chronic bronchitis in COPD the use of third line antibiotics increased pharmacy costs but showed a trend towards lower mean total costs (Destache *et al.* 1999). The improved outcomes included reduced failure rate, lower need for hospital admission, and increased remission times. The distress caused by dyspnoea may be associated with a higher prevalence of depression (van Ede *et al.* 1999). Pulmonary rehabilitation may confer substantial benefits in COPD, including improved walking distance and maximal exercise capacity. However, all interventions are likely to be ineffective without smoking cessation and the provision of quitting support services is of paramount public health importance.

Adverse health effects of air pollution

Air quality and sustainable development

The global effects of environmental degradation are now a major public health concern, including the adverse effects of poor-quality indoor and outdoor air. A recent report on health and environment in sustainable development concludes that when assessed in terms of DALYs, environmental factors are associated with almost a quarter of the global burden of disease (WHO 1997*b*). A large proportion of this is attributable to different forms of air pollution. Air pollution is now a problem that affects most human settlements across the planet. In the nineteenth century it typically affected expanding urban areas that arose from the industrial revolution. In the West the principal cause of air pollution in the past has usually been coal, wherever it has been used. Legislation and controls led to cleaner air in many Western industrialized countries, but twentieth-century urban development and the internal combustion engine have been associated with deterioration in air quality. This is now recognized as a hazard for both acute and chronic adverse health effects worldwide.

In many wealthy countries levels of sulphur dioxide and particulates have fallen following clean air legislation and changes in the types of fuels used. On the other hand, concentrations of nitrogen oxides, ozone, ultrafine particulates, and carbon monoxide have risen along with a massive increase in road traffic, particularly diesel-powered vehicles. In developing countries, such as China, both sources of pollution are now present and largely uncontrolled. The growth in vehicular road traffic in Asia must be regarded as still in its early stages so the contribution to pollution from mobile sources will predictably continue to increase for many years.

In addition to escalating numbers of badly adjusted diesel engines the burning of unwashed coal and other high sulphur content fuels has placed many cities, for example those in the Asia Pacific region, among the most polluted in the world. Daily concentrations of pollutants in some cities are similar to those observed in the pollution episodes of London and New York 50 years ago (McMichael and Smith 1999). The London smog was largely generated by domestic coal fires, but in recent years evidence has emerged on the importance in developing countries of indoor pollution from cooking and heating fuels. The combined effects of poor air quality will continue to be a major cause of premature death in developing countries.

In the 1990s the problem of haze in Asia Pacific countries has received international attention. In Malaysia, in the Kelang Valley, satellite imaging reveals haze in association with highways, factories, new housing developments, and agricultural burning. Analysis also suggests that photochemical reactions contribute to the build up of haze in some areas (Samah 1992). Particulate concentrations of over 400 μg/m^3 are typical in haze episodes. In Sumatra, Indonesia, wilful burning of rain forest and scrub in the late 1990s led to disastrous haze episodes lasting for months during the dry season and permeating over large areas of the region, including Singapore and Malaysia. Thousands of additional cases of respiratory and eye problems have been reported, but the overall impact on health, particularly of infants and children, is largely undocumented.

Air pollutants

A wide spectrum of air pollutants are implicated in adverse health effects, although these effects may vary and there is still a lack of evidence and consensus on causal relationships. The principal pollutants of interest can be classified as particulates (either finely divided solids or finely dispersed liquid aerosols), gases, and toxic chemicals such as hydrocarbons.

Comprehensive reviews of particulate and other forms of pollution are given by Holland *et al.* (1979), the American Thoracic Society (1996), and Holgate *et al.* (1999). The characteristics of the four criteria pollutants, respirable suspended particulates, sulphur dioxide, nitrogen dioxide, and ozone together with carbon monoxide, polycyclic hydrocarbons, and volatile organic compounds are summarized by Hedley and Lam (1997).

Factors affecting pollutant levels and exposures

Ambient pollutant levels and the exposure of individuals are affected by rainfall, wind speeds and currents, atmospheric inversion, and human activities. Low wind velocities hinder horizontal dispersion and high pressure and temperature inversions limit vertical dispersion. Local geographical features are also a contributor. Weather patterns result in elevated levels of pollutants because of reduced rain and wind and increased build up of inversion layers in the atmosphere. However, rainfall may increase the exposure of some individuals, because of pollutant laden aerosols resulting from the scouring of the air by raindrops. There are marked seasonal variations in ambient pollutant levels that result from climatic changes. In many Western countries ozone levels are higher in the warm season when mean sunlight levels are highest; however, in tropical or subtropical climates such as Hong Kong ozone levels are highest in the cool dry season when cloud cover is lower (Fig. 1).

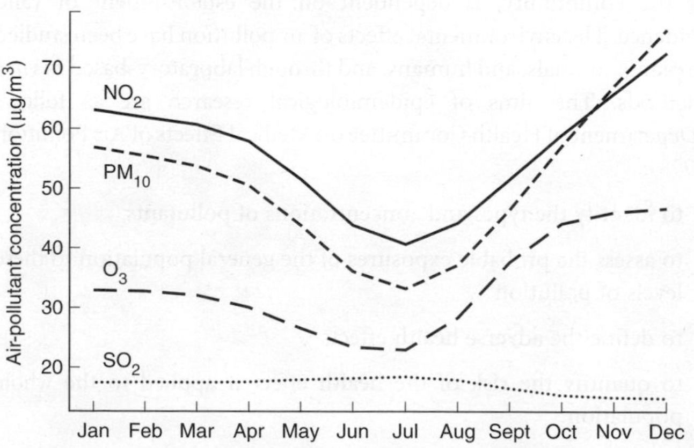

Fig. 1 Hong Kong: smoothed monthly average of air pollutant concentrations.

Assessment of health effects

The current problems in assessment of outdoor air pollution effects on health, and therefore the extent to which epidemiology can support policy-making, can be summarized as follows.

1. Patterns of pollution are heterogeneous between different sites and they cannot be assumed to have the same effects. Examples include the 'reducing' forms of industrial winter smog comprising particulates and sulphur dioxide and 'oxidizing' forms with nitrogen oxides and hydrocarbons and products of photochemical decomposition.

2. Exposure prevalence probably varies markedly within and between different communities and countries.

3. Data from monitoring are strongly influenced by meteorological conditions, including dispersion of pollutants, their concentrations and, therefore, exposures. The interpretation of relationships between pollution and health is confounded because both pollutants and health indices (morbidity, mortality, and health-care utilization) show marked seasonal patterns.

4. The causal relationships between adverse health effects and exposure to specific pollutants or mixtures remain uncertain.

5. Socio-economic factors may confound the interpretation of studies, such as those based on mixed residential and industrial communities, educational attainment, smoking, environmental tobacco smoke, and other indoor pollutants. Housing and nutrition may influence health and confound the interpretation of exposure studies.

6. If poor health or health hazards, or conversely higher income and socio-economic status, are factors in the movement of people away from adverse environments then this will lead to a change in the population of residents and their estimated risks. Such patterns may be difficult to recognize or take account of in ecological studies that involve two or more population groups, but are not based on individual exposures and health records.

Health effects of pollutants

The identification of environmental hazards and their subsequent elimination through social and economic policy, to protect the health of the community, is dependent on the establishment of valid evidence. The environmental effects of air pollution have been studied in plants, animals, and humans, and through laboratory-based *in vitro* methods. The aims of epidemiological research are as follows (Department of Health Committee on Medical Effects of Air Pollution 1998):

- to identify the types and concentrations of pollutants
- to assess the probable exposures of the general population to these levels of pollution
- to define the adverse health effects
- to quantify the risk of the health effect if applied to the whole population.

The possible adverse health effects of air pollution on a population can be represented in the form of a pyramid (Fig. 2).

There are three general groups of evidence from scientific studies.

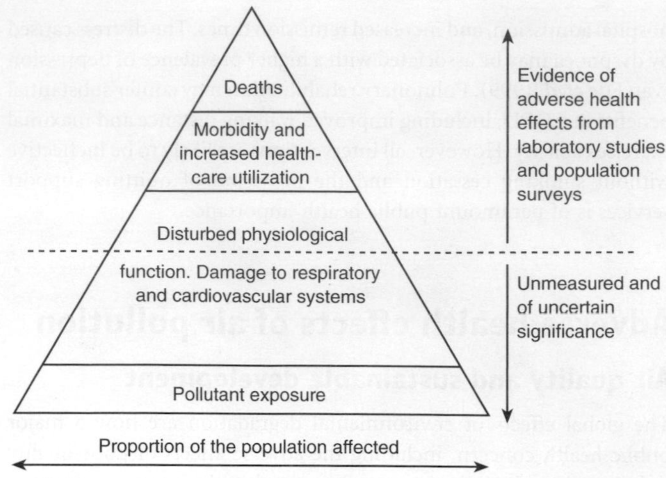

Fig. 2 The population pyramid of air pollution health effects.

- **Experimental**
  Animals
  Humans
  Tissues
- **Observational**
  Time series: acute effects
  Spatial studies
  Cross-sectional: prevalence
  Cohort studies: chronic efects
- **Occupational**
  Surveys of high-risk occupational groups

For example, controlled laboratory experimental work has demonstrated that specific pollutants (i.e. single pollutant exposures) may be associated with inflammatory reactions in tissues; in human volunteers changes in lung function and the development of symptoms such as cough and chest pain have been observed. In animals, genetic factors, genotoxicity, and carcinogenesis can be examined. In humans, controlled studies in volunteers have examined the effects of age, gender, ethnicity, and predisposing existing health problems such as asthma. Special susceptibility to pollutant exposures may be found both in well individuals and those with health problems such as asthma.

The evidence to support public health advocacy for clean air can be drawn from panel studies of patients and epidemiological cross-sectional surveys, and case–control and cohort studies, including cohort-based nested case–control studies. Panel studies are prospective cohort studies but the subjects are not necessarily free of respiratory problems at the start. Usually enquiries form a series of cross-sectional arrays from multiple assessments of the subjects at different points in time. There are relatively few case–control and long-term cohort studies on the health effects of air pollution. Many studies are based on ecological designs in which the health experience of whole populations is examined using routinely collected morbidity and mortality data together with pollutant concentrations. The two types of ecological studies commonly reported are cross-sectional surveys of two or more groups and time-series studies, which use data on daily, weekly, or monthly events such as deaths or hospital admissions. The limitations of these and other epidemiological approaches are summarized by Samet and Jaakkola (1999) and include the so-called ecological fallacy (Last 1995).

Time-series analyses are usually based on large pre-existing databases of, respectively, pollutant concentrations, health-care utilization (such as hospital admissions), and mortality derived from registrations of deaths. These databases are used to estimate variations in daily events such as admissions and deaths within a single population. The advantages of this approach are that it is feasible and relatively inexpensive and time-series analysis can show how short-term distributions of deaths are related to short-term variations in concentrations of pollutants. Therefore it can provide a rapid method of generating evidence on a possible causal relationship between short-term health effects and pollution. Longitudinal time-series analyses, which follow single or multiple populations over time, have several advantages over other types in that they avoid the need to control for common individual-level confounding factors, such as educational attainment, socio-economic status, and smoking prevalence, because these factors are more or less constant from day to day and the population acts as its own control. For example, the frequency of health events in the population being studied on high pollution days is compared with that on lower pollution days (Thurston and Ito 1999). Because they include all members of a population, including those most susceptible to pollution, the results may be the most relevant and generalizable. Their limitations (Thurston and Kinney 1995) include the previously mentioned problem of shared long-term cycles, such as the seasonal variation in both health events and pollutant concentrations.

Daily time-series mortality studies in single populations are now frequently employed by researchers in many countries. McMichael *et al.* (1998), however, have pointed out that time-series analyses, as they are usually performed, cannot distinguish between life shortening due to deaths brought forward (e.g. by days or weeks) by acute effects of pollution in individuals with serious advanced chronic disease and deaths from chronic disease induced by long-term exposure to air pollution. The phenomenon of deaths brought forward, for example due to an episode of pollution, is referred to as harvesting. If this occurs then fewer people would die over the period following the episode. The possible effect of harvesting on mortality estimates remains uncertain. Further studies on variation in daily deaths may help to separate out the acute and chronic effects of pollution. In contrast these conceptual problems may not apply to other non-fatal, outcomes such as hospital admissions and time-series data can contribute to the assessment of health, quality of life, and utilization of services. A schema to represent the possible distribution of deaths from respiratory and cardiovascular disorders due to air pollution has been suggested by the United Kingdom Committee on Medical Effects of Air Pollution (Fig. 3).

Chronic health effects, in terms of incidence and long-term death rates, can best be estimated from long-term cohort studies, in which a large defined group of subjects is followed forward in time with the collection of the best possible information on local pollutant concentrations and individual exposures. Such studies obviously need to be managed over many years; they are inevitably costly and demanding in terms of personnel, expertise, and other facilities. There may also be questions about the generalizability of the findings to other settings because of differences in both prevalent pollutant types and individual exposures. In public health terms the effects of long-term exposure to

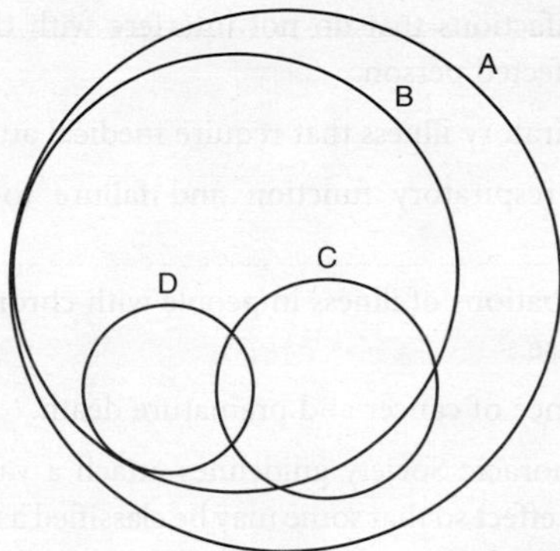

The areas shown are illustrative only and should not be interpreted in any quantitative sense.

A Total deaths occurring in the UK.
B Deaths due to diseases that have been shown to be associated with day-to-day changes in concentrations of particles, e.g. heart attacks and deaths from respiratory disorders.
C Deaths triggered or advanced by day-to-day variations in concentrations of particles.
D Deaths due to diseases caused by chronic exposure to particles.

Fig. 3 Relationship between deaths advanced by exposure to particles and deaths from illness induced by exposure to particles.

air pollution may be more important than that due to brief episodes, for example in terms of person-years of life lost.

In general, although laboratory studies and evidence from occupational exposures in certain types of process workers do provide indications of the toxicity of specific pollutants they do not necessarily allow us to extrapolate the results to estimate the impact of breathing polluted air by the general public. This is at least partly because the different components of general air pollution are more numerous and complex than the pollutants in experimental or occupational exposure. On the other hand even in studies of human populations this complexity of the urban pollutant mixture means that we may not be able to ascribe confidently causality to the observed association between health events, such as admissions and deaths, and variations in concentrations of single specific pollutants such as sulphur dioxide, nitrogen dioxide, respirable suspended particulates (**RSPs**), and ozone. All we may be able to conclude safely is that certain general levels of pollutants of all types and, therefore, their sources are likely to be injurious to health.

Air pollution may cause concern because it degrades the environment and is perceived to impair quality of life, not least because visibility, between ourselves and the horizon, is impaired and the general nature of the environment deteriorates. The visibility index in many Asian cities has been deteriorating markedly during the past 5 years. As judged by letters to newspapers, media reports, and other surveys this undoubtedly has an adverse psychological effect on the community as a whole. Pollutants may cause relatively minor health problems, such as eye or skin irritation, whereas the serious effects of air pollution are associated with lung inflammation and reduced lung function, critical cardiovascular events, and premature death.

The American Thoracic Society (1985) put forward guidelines, on the definition of adverse effects, covering a wide spectrum of measurable or potential adverse health outcomes. They can be summarized on a five-point scale.

1. Irritation and infections that do not interfere with the normal activity of the affected person.
2. Episodes of respiratory illness that require medical attention.
3. Impairment of respiratory function and failure to thrive in children.
4. Increased exacerbations of illness in people with chronic cardiopulmonary disease.
5. Increased incidence of cancer and premature death.

The American Thoracic Society guidelines attach a value judgement to the observed effect so that some may be classified as 'trivial' or 'not medically important'. However, from both a medical and ethical viewpoint it could be argued that it is not justifiable to attach arbitrary values to any adverse effects. This is especially the case if the exposures are involuntary and the impact on quality of life and activities of daily living have not been measured. In terms of health, the wider use of methodology capable of detecting subclinical physiological changes, such as bronchial hyper-reactivity or blood viscosity will continue to redefine levels of impairment. Interventions and long-term epidemiological studies will be needed to determine whether they are associated with permanent harm to the respiratory and cardiovascular systems and premature death.

The measures used to estimate the biological damage of pollution and development of clinical health problems are summarized in Table 3. Laboratory and occupational studies show that air pollution could be harmful, whereas population epidemiological studies are needed to show that pollution is harmful to the health of the public.

Table 3 Health effects and biological markers of response associated with air pollution[a]

Health effect	Biological marker
Excess cardiorespiratory mortality	Deaths from heart or lung disease in excess of number expected; Increased blood viscosity and change in coagulability
Increased health-care utilization	Increased hospital admissions, physician visits, emergency department visits
Asthma exacerbations	Increased health-care consultations and medication use; Decreased lung function
Increased respiratory illness	Increased respiratory infections, episodic symptoms
Increased respiratory symptoms	Cough, phlegm and wheeze
Decreased lung function	Spirometry, peak flow rates, airways resistance
Increased airways reactivity (e.g. bronchial hyper-reactivity)	Altered response to challenge with methacholine, carbachol, histamine, cold air
Lung inflammation	Influx of inflammatory cells, mediators, proteins
Altered host defence	Altered mucociliary clearance, macrophage function, immune response

[a]The clinical or public health significance of some effects are unknown.

Modified from American Thoracic Society (1996).

Mortality from air pollution

The public health effects of environmental air pollution and its changing patterns have been observed worldwide. In the London pollution episode of 1952 the association of high levels of particulates (British Smoke) and sulphur dioxide was associated with 4000 excess deaths (Logan 1953). In a similar episode in 1962 there were only 350 excess deaths (Scott 1963). The difference in pollutants between the two episodes was mainly an 80 per cent reduction in the particulates; however, since then further work has implicated the acid component of particulates.

In addition to the observations on the pattern of mortality in the London smog, there is also the evidence from the winter hazes of New York (1960–1964), total particulate levels in Steubenville, Ohio (1974–1984) and Pennsylvania (1973–1980), and haze in California (1980–1986). Dockery *et al.* (1993) demonstrated the importance of long-term follow-up studies to identify health effects. After adjustment for smoking, occupational exposure, and other factors, the excess risk derived from a mortality rate ratio between cities with the highest and lowest pollution levels in 8000 adults followed for 14 to 16 years in six cities was 26 per cent. Mortality was most strongly associated with levels of fine particulates, including sulphates.

In a pooled analysis (meta-analysis) of nine United States cities and London an increase in PM_{10} of 10 $\mu g/m^3$ was associated with a 3.4 per cent increase in respiratory mortality and 1.8 per cent for cardiovascular deaths (American Thoracic Society 1996). In Birmingham, Alabama, Schwartz (1993) estimated that population exposures to a rise of 100 $\mu g/m^3$ are associated with an 11 per cent excess risk of overall mortality (relative risk is equal to 1.11; 95 per cent confidence intervals 1.02 to 1.20). Because cardiovascular deaths are very common they make the biggest contribution to the overall association between pollution and total mortality.

Positive associations between individual air pollutants and mortality have been demonstrated in time-series analyses in many American, European, and other country studies. In 12 European cities, pooled estimates of the increase in daily mortality per 50 $\mu g/m^3$ increases in concentrations of sulphur dioxide and particulates were 3 per cent and 2 per cent respectively (Katsouannyi *et al.* 1997). Ozone was significantly associated with total mortality in Mexico City (Borja-Aburto *et al.* 1997) (relative risk equals to 1.024 per 200 $\mu g/m^3$ increase in the hourly maximum in ozone). The Air Pollution and Health: a European Approach (**APHEA**) study (Touloumi *et al.* 1996) of four western European cities found a relative risk equal to 1.02 per 50 $\mu g/m^3$ increase in both the hourly and the 8-h ozone concentrations. However, in this APHEA meta-analysis nitrogen dioxide showed no association with mortality. In a London study of air pollution and mortality between 1987 and 1992 (Anderson *et al.* 1996), same day ozone levels were associated with a significant increase in all cause, cardiovascular and respiratory mortality with the effects greater in the warm season and apparently independent of the effects of other pollutants.

In China, in the Dongcheng and Xicheng districts of Beijing, there was a highly significant association between log sulphur dioxide levels and daily deaths, adjusted for temperature and humidity. The strongest effects were for cardiorespiratory disease; chronic bronchitis, COPD (29 per cent), and cor pulmonale (19 per cent). Total mortality risk increased by 11 per cent with doubling of sulphur dioxide concentration (Xu *et al.* 1994).

Cohort studies from the United States have examined, in defined population groups, the relationship between health outcomes and long-term exposures to ambient concentrations of particulates and other pollutants. Two earlier reports (Dockery *et al.* 1993; Pope *et al.* 1995) showed positive associations between long-term concentrations of particles and mortality. The most recent report from the Adventists Health Study of Smog, describes the follow up of a cohort of 6338 non-smoking Californian Seventh Day Adventists from 1977 (Abbey *et al.* 1999). Past smoking and living or working with smokers was controlled for in the analysis. In 1977 to 1992 long-term concentrations of inhalable particles (PM_{10}) and other pollutants, sulphur dioxide, sulphates, nitrogen dioxide, and ozone were related to mortality in males. The statistically significant findings were for all (non-accidental) causes in males for PM_{10} and also for non-malignant respiratory disease and lung cancer in males. In addition, ozone showed an association with lung cancer in males and nitrogen dioxide showed a strong association with lung cancer in both sexes. The investigators adjusted the data for both occupational and indoor sources of air pollutants. The conclusions drawn were that long periods of residence and work in areas of high ambient pollution are associated with increased mortality. However, there are some differences in outcomes between the three cohort studies, and so uncertainties remain about the long-term effects of specific pollutants and their impact on specific health outcomes.

Air pollution, morbidity, and health-care utilization

Since 1980 in North America, Europe, and Asia more than 18 cohort type studies have reported increased risks of adverse health outcomes such as cough, dyspnoea, exacerbation of asthma, upper and lower respiratory infections, and increased use of medication.

Whittemore and Korn (1980) used diaries for asthmatic subjects to record respiratory symptoms on a daily basis. Similar studies have demonstrated associations between air pollution and respiratory symptoms in The Netherlands (Hoek and Brunekreef 1993) and Switzerland (Braun-Fahrlander *et al.* 1992). Another measure employed in the United States is the restricted activity day resulting from respiratory problems associated with particulate concentrations (Ostro and Rothschild 1989). Particulates are associated with local upper respiratory irritation, cough, upper respiratory infections and bronchitis, and lower respiratory tract illness in children in the United States (Ware *et al.* 1986; Dockery *et al.* 1989), Finland (Jaakkola *et al.* 1991), and Hong Kong (Peters *et al.* 1996). In Hong Kong studies of primary school children aged 8 to10 years, living in areas of high and low pollution, have defined the importance of the air pollution hazards together with both active and passive smoking by the children. After adjustment for socio-economic factors, the risks for any cough, phlegm and wheeze symptoms were highest in children (10 per cent) who had ever experimented with cigarettes (odds ratio 1.85; 95 per cent confidence intervals 1.55 to 2.21), followed by those (46 per cent) exposed to smoking in the home (odds ratio 1.15; 95 per cent confidence intervals 1.01–1.30 for exposure to one smoker and odds ratio 1.45; 95 per cent confidence intervals 1.21–1.75 for two or more smokers) followed by the risks attached to living in the most polluted district (odds ratio 1.14; 95 per cent confidence intervals 1.00 –1.29) (Hedley *et al.* 1993). These findings are likely to reflect the situation in many developing urban communities in Southeast Asia.

The urban nature of the hazard is also demonstrated by comparisons of communities living in cities and rural areas. In German studies (Wjst *et al.* 1993; Weiland *et al.* 1994) the 9- to 15-year-olds living close to urban traffic had higher frequencies of asthma-like symptoms, wheezing, and allergic rhinitis. A two- to threefold excess of wheeze, dyspnoea, and rhinitis was found in those living in Pisa compared with the unpolluted Po Delta Valley (Viegi *et al.* 1991). The mean annual total suspended particulate concentrations were three to five times higher in the Pisa urban area.

Emergency department attendances and hospital admissions have been used to estimate the effects of seasonal pollution, such as 'summer haze' and other pollution episodes, and make inferences about the possible importance of specific pollutants. Pope (1989) demonstrated a marked effect on respiratory hospital admissions in Utah Valley following the closure and reopening of a steel mill, which was the principal source of PM_{10}. When 24-h PM_{10} levels exceeded 150 μg/m^3 average admissions for children nearly tripled.

Outdoor exposure to increased levels of nitrogen dioxide was associated with respiratory symptoms and their duration in Switzerland (Braun-Fahrlander *et al.* 1992) and hospital admission for respiratory disease in Birmingham, England (Walters *et al.* 1995). In Germany a time-series study showed a 28 per cent increase in admissions for croup with a daily mean nitrogen dioxide increase of 10 to 70 μg/m^3 (Schwartz *et al.* 1991).

Particulates and sulphur dioxide usually occur together, but there are relatively few data on possible specific effects of sulphur dioxide on health care utilization. In the 1980s, in Vancouver, Bates *et al.* (1990) found emergency room visits were correlated with sulphur dioxide during both winter and summer. Studies in Barcelona and Santander found associations between COPD and relatively low levels of sulphur dioxide. In Hong Kong following the introduction of low sulphur fuels (Peters *et al.* 1996) there was a sharp fall in sulphur dioxide and sulphate in RSP (Fig. 4). Monthly averages for ambient sulphur dioxide in the polluted district ranged from 100 to 140 μg/m^3 for the 6 months before the intervention, falling to less than 20 μg/m^3 following the imposition of fuel regulations. In the same period, total and respirable particulates showed an initial but unsustained decline of 23 per cent and 18 per cent respectively. Sulphate concentrations in respirable suspended particulates showed more stable declines of 47 per cent and 35 per cent in the most and least polluted districts respectively. This was followed by a marked change in the risk of respiratory symptoms between a pair of high and low pollution districts. The between district differences in the prevalence of sore throat or cough, phlegm and wheeze, and doctor consultations for respiratory complaints were reduced, but there was no change in risk attributable to exposure to second-hand smoke for those children who lived in smoking homes. In Paris, Dab *et al.* (1996) found sulphur dioxide to be associated with respiratory admissions but in Amsterdam, Schouten *et al.* (1996) observed a significant negative effect.

Health outcome studies for the effects of pollution on subjects with asthma show marked variation. Bates and Sizto (1987) in Ontario found no association in the 0 to 14 year age group between asthma admissions and ozone or other single pollutants, but a positive

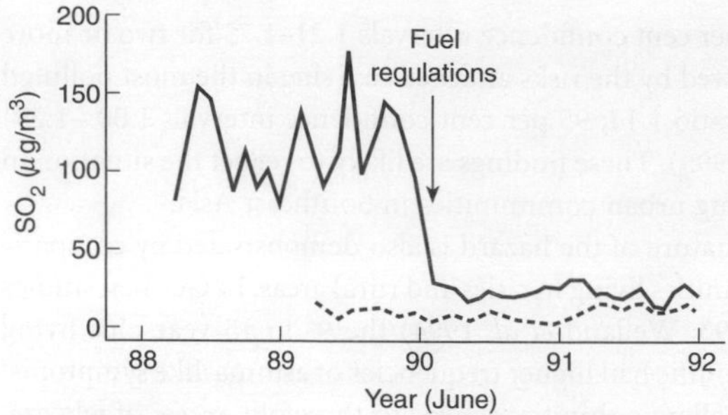

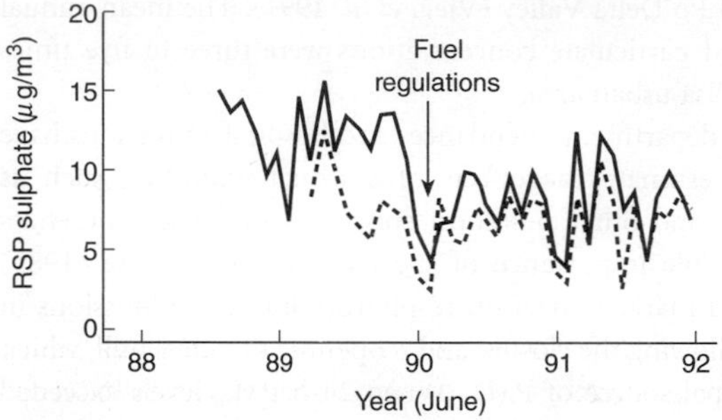

Fig. 4 Trends in air pollution as shown by levels of sulphur dioxide (SO_2) and sulphates in respirable particulates (SO_4 RSP) at monitoring stations in Kwai Tsing (solid line) and in Southern (dotted line) districts measured by the Hong Kong Environmental Protection Department 1988 to 1992, before and after the introduction of regulations restricting the sulphur content of fuels.

relationship for all ages with ozone and sulphates. In southern Ontario air pollution has declined as indicated by the measurement of sulphur dioxide but not ozone, nitrogen dioxide, or coefficient of haze. During the period 1974 to 1983 total respiratory admissions declined 15 per cent, but admissions for asthma rose. However, a consistent summer relationship between sulphates, ozone, temperature, and respiratory admissions was identified independently of asthma. The authors pointed to aerosol sulphates, which explained the highest percentage of the variance in respiratory admissions in summer, but not in winter. They postulated that ozone and sulphates are only indicators of an 'acid summer haze'.

Ito and Thurston (1999) estimated a combined relative risk of 1.18 (95 per cent confidence intervals 1.07 to 1.30) from North American and European studies for asthma admissions associated with an increase in the daily/hourly maximum concentration of ozone of 100 ppb For respiratory admissions in children there is apparently heterogeneity in estimated outcomes across age groups within the same geographical area and in the risks associated with different pollutants. Admission data may vary for many reasons, including local cultural factors and health-care seeking behaviour, the role and efficiency of primary medical care, the nature of the referral system, and the costs of care at all levels. The completeness and quality of the data may also influence findings.

Anderson (1999) has reviewed the health effects of pollution episodes. Major pollution episodes in urban settings have not produced any convincing evidence of exacerbations of asthma in children. These include the 1930 Meuse Valley episode, when those with serious asthmatic problems were mainly older adults. In the 1952 London fog, the general practitioner John Fry noted that asthmatic children in his practice did not become ill (Fry 1953). On the other hand forest fires and volcanic eruptions have caused an increase in deaths and health-care episodes. In a 1987 Californian fire asthma visits increased by 40 per cent and after the Mount St Helens eruption by a factor of 4, but unlike the Californian episode no effect on asthma was observed in the 1994 western Sydney bushfire, which was of similar intensity. In 1991, London experienced a unique high pollution episode with very high levels of nitrogen dioxide reaching an hourly average of 423 ppb All causes of mortality increased for all age groups (relative risk equals to 1.10), together with cardiovascular disease. Admissions of the elderly (65 and above) increased for respiratory disease. However, in children there were no increases in admissions for respiratory diseases overall and only a small non-significant increase for asthma (Anderson *et al.* 1995).

Asthma and wheezing

Burney (1988) has emphasized the need for epidemiological rather than solely clinical and experimental pathophysiological studies as the basis for establishing causation and explaining the current global distribution of asthma. Problems with the definition of asthma complicate the interpretation of prevalence estimates and the apparent differences between surveys.

Asthma is an important cause of ill health in Western developed countries and increasingly in new industrial countries in the developing world but a low prevalence of the disease is found in poor rural communities (Burney 1992). It has been increasing during the last 30 years in terms of estimated incidence, prevalence, and utilization of health care. In the United Kingdom the 30-year increase has been about 50 per cent. These data are drawn from records of national follow-up studies, hospital admissions, use of medication, and registered causes of death.

During the period when asthma has been increasing, industrial and domestic emission of smoke and sulphur dioxide have been declining; particles from diesel exhaust, together with nitrogen oxides and volatile organic compounds have increased during this time. On the other hand, urban concentrations of ozone and nitrogen dioxide have remained relatively stable.

Urban areas have a higher prevalence of asthma and there has been a strong popular view, among the public and media, that this is due to air pollution mainly from mobile sources. However, as Burney (1992) points out air pollution is not the only defining characteristic of urban areas and atopy is generally more common among young people living in more developed environments. This would include those in modern settings in the rural areas of post-industrialized countries. In contrast, there was no association between extremely high domestic particulate concentrations and the prevalence of asthma in children in Papua New Guinea (Anderson 1978).

The United Kingdom Department of Health, Committee on the Medical Effects of Air Pollutants (Department of Health 1995) has reported its conclusions on the association between asthma and air pollution. It stated that:

- there is little or no association between the regional distribution of asthma and air pollution
- comparisons of prevalence between high and low pollution areas have produced inconsistent results

- in the United Kingdom there is no convincing evidence of an urban–rural gradient
- in the United Kingdom and other countries there is a modest relationship between asthma prevalence and local traffic density
- most asthma patients should not be affected by usual ambient levels of pollutants in the United Kingdom
- the observed asthma trends over 30 years are unlikely to be related to changes in non-biological air pollution, excluding spores, fungi, and other allergens.

It has been postulated that population exposure to increasing levels of pollutants such as nitrogen dioxide decrease the threshold of allergen exposure needed to trigger allergic asthma and increase the morbidity associated with existing asthma (Anto and Sunyer 1995). In Barcelona the inhalation of soybean dust originating from the port area, enhanced by temperature inversions, which were also associated with increased concentrations of other pollutants, was associated with outbreaks of asthma. The presence of the inversions initially led to the conclusion that oxides of nitrogen were the principal single cause (Anto *et al.* 1989).

Boezen *et al.* (1999) demonstrated that children who have both bronchial hyper-responsiveness and high concentrations of immunoglobulin E are susceptible to air pollution. In this group the prevalence of lower respiratory symptoms increased significantly by between 32 and 139 per cent for every 100 μg/m^3 increase in particulate matter. The estimated excess risks are quite low but when applied to a population the public health impact would be substantial. The findings provide a possible unifying explanation for individual susceptibility to air pollution but leave unanswered questions about the precise role of allergens in the air during pollution episodes. Furthermore, they do not explain the lack of effect during some severe pollution episodes.

Air pollution and lung function

The impact of air pollution on the general health of the population may be indicated by acute and chronic effects on lung function in both children and adults. All standard measures of lung function, including FEV$_1$, FVC, and peak expiratory flow rate have been shown to be affected by ambient air pollution exposures. In children reductions in lung function have been observed in both well populations and those with a either a past history of wheezing or a medical diagnosis of asthma.

In the United States (Steubenville, Ohio (Dockery *et al.* 1982; Brunekreef *et al.* 1991) and Utah (Pope *et al.* 1992)) and The Netherlands (Hoek *et al.* 1993) exposure to particulates measured as PM$_{10}$ or total suspended particulates (**TSP**) was associated with delayed or lagged reduction in lung function. In children, Dockery *et al.* (1982) found a 2.7 per cent decrease in FEV$_{0.75}$ for a 35-μg/m^3 increase in TSP and in 48 communities across the United States, Schwartz (1989) demonstrated a 6 per cent decrease in FVC with a 100 μg/m^3 increase in TSP. It is postulated that the inhalation of fine particles may lead to an inflammatory response that is followed by later decline in lung function; however, a different mechanism appears to underlie the immediate reduction in lung function seen following ozone exposures (Gold *et al.* 1999).

Age and lifestyle, particularly exercise, which increases ventilation, are associated with variations in exposure and response to pollutants. Young children are particularly active and have high ventilation rates, and in Munich reduced peak expiratory flow rates were observed in 9- to 11-year-old children living in close proximity to dense urban traffic (Wjst *et al.* 1993).

Bronchial hyper-responsiveness, a bronchial constriction response to standardized inhalations of histamine, carbachol, or methacholine, can be measured as a decrease in FEV$_1$. In Norway, exposure to low ambient sulphur dioxide levels in infancy has been related to bronchial hyper-responsiveness in 7- to 13-year-olds (Soyseth *et al.* 1995). In Hong Kong (Tam *et al.* 1994) bronchial responsiveness to a histamine challenge in 8- to10-year-olds varied between districts with contrasting levels of pollution, as did the prevalence of respiratory symptoms (Peters *et al.* 1996). The significance for future health of changes in lung function in children has remained uncertain. Following the introduction of low sulphur fuel regulations in Hong Kong, in the year following the intervention, the prevalence of bronchial hyper-responsiveness declined in both districts, but continued to decline in the second year in the most polluted district (Wong *et al.* 1998).

The observations from investigations such as time-series studies are generally accepted as inputs to environmental risk assessment and management, but major questions about the causal mechanisms remain. Evans and Wolff (1996) explored quantitatively the plausibility of one mechanism that could explain the outcome of cross-sectional studies. Air pollution can accelerate decline in lung function (Xu *et al.* 1991) and lung function (FEV$_1$) is a good predictor of mortality. Evans and Wolff constructed a mathematical model of the chronic effects of continuous exposure to air pollution (1 μg/m^3 per year) for smokers and non-smokers, to estimate the age-specific decline in lung function and loss of life expectancy (Fig. 5). There is an important three-way interaction between smoking and pollution exposure, together with the expected age-related loss of lung function, with about 25 years loss of life expectancy from the combined effect of smoking and pollution. In the model, below the age of 40 the effects of pollution are more readily detected in non-smokers than in smokers. On the basis of their work Evans and Wolff suggest that a figure of 50 000 premature deaths a year is possible due to relatively low levels of ambient particulates.

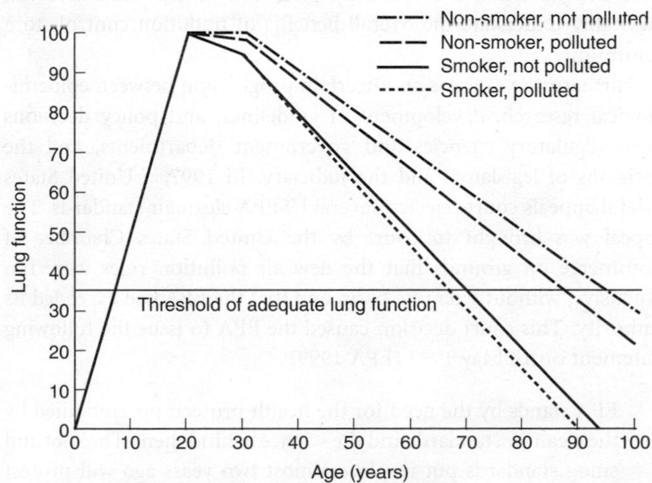

Fig. 5 Schematic diagram of lung function versus age showing loss of life expectancy (LOLE).

Policy-making and prevention

Air-quality guidelines are under revision by the WHO, and many countries are trying to address the problem of both setting and maintaining air quality objectives in their own locality. Local data on health effects are the most suitable, but in the developing world few countries have the resources to generate this information. The current world literature on the health effects of pollution clearly indicates that there are no firm grounds on which to characterize specific levels of individual pollutants as safe. What can be inferred is that both short- and long-term health effects are associated with pollutant mixtures and at levels of individual pollutants that are below current standards. These health effects impact on the current and future health of well populations, including children. Although research designed to explore the possible causal relationship between different pollutant species and health outcomes will continue there is ample evidence to support stringent environmental controls on industrial and mobile sources of pollution. The United Kingdom has set out objectives for further reductions in air pollutants by 2005. A Department of Health Ad Hoc Group on the Economic Appraisal of the Health Effects of Air Pollution (1999) has taken the United Kingdom Committee on Medical Effects of Air Pollution findings on deaths and admissions as the basis for estimating the health-care costs of changes in levels of air pollutants.

The United Kingdom group suggested that the loss of life expectancy incurred when deaths are advanced or 'brought forward' is likely to be not more than a month to a year. Factors used to adjust the valuation of the life foregone include the age of the individuals who die (mostly elderly); the pre-existing quality of life (generally lower because of chronic disease such as COPD). These led inevitably to marked downward adjustments of the estimated willingness to pay to reduce air pollution mortality risks, and much lower than the value attached to road traffic accidents.

Much of the current literature focuses on health events that are represented in the upper part of the population pyramid representing pollution effects such as deaths and hospital admissions. However, surveys of children, a sensitive sentinel group for pollution health effects, show that in many situations pollution is the cause of very high endemic levels of respiratory complaints and use of health services. Cost–benefit analysis based only on more severe outcomes will inevitably understate the overall benefits of pollution controls to a community.

Furthermore, there is an uncertain progression between epidemiological research, development of guidelines, and policy decisions from regulatory agencies and government departments, and the decisions of legislators and the judiciary. In 1997, a United States federal appeals court rejected several USEPA clean air standards. The appeal was brought to court by the United States Chamber of Commerce on grounds that the new air pollution rules were too expensive, without scientific basis, and that the EPA had exceeded its authority. This court decision caused the EPA to issue the following statement on 14 May 1999 (EPA 1999):

> EPA stands by the need for the health protections embodied by the clean air standards and the science behind them. The soot and smog standards put in place almost two years ago will protect the health of 125 million Americans including 35 million children.... If the courts fail to uphold these protective standards, congress must ensure that these protections are preserved for the American people and EPA stands ready to work with them.

The way ahead for effective local legislation will be supported by better evidence on health effects of pollution within countries and regions. But the introduction of environmental controls will require political will, which may only stem from analyses showing that pollution not only harms the health of populations, but the economy as a whole.

Tuberculosis

The changing global situation

Tuberculosis is the most frequent cause of death from any infectious agent. About one-third of the world's population is infected, with about 8 million new cases a year occurring in the mid-1990s, associated with 3 million deaths. Tuberculosis is a leading cause of death in the age group 15 to 44, especially in women, where it is

Table 4 Mortality and DALYs by gender and WHO member states: estimates for 1998

	Deaths (× 1000)	DALYs (× 1000) (%)
World population	5 884 576	5 884 576
Total	53 929	1 382 564
TB both sexes	1498 (2.8%)	28 189 (2.0%)
Males	893 (3.1%)	16 137 (2.2%)
Females	605 (2.4%)	12 052 (1.8%)
High income	18 (0.2%)	142 (0.1%)
Low/middle income	1480 (3.2%)	28 047 (2.2%)
AFR	209 (1%)	5442
AMR		
High income	1	8
Low/middle income	53	1213
EMR	139	3189
EUR		
High income	7	53
Low/middle income	53	853
SEAR		
India	421	7577
Other low/middle income	261	4438
WPR		
High income	10	80
China	259	3878
Other low/ middle income	86	1459

Note that the method of estimation for 1998, as reported in the 1999 World Health Report, is different from that used previously and so earlier reports should not be used for comparison.

WHO Regions: AFR, African; EMR, Eastern Mediterranean; EUR, European; SEAR, South-East Asian; WPR, Western Pacific.

Source: WHO (1999*a*), Annex Tables 2 and 3.

Table 5 Tuberculosis: magnitude of the problem by sex and WHO region: estimates for 1998

	Individuals infected with tuberculosis					
	HIV positive			HIV negative		
	Both sexes	**Male**	**Female**	**Both sexes**	**Male**	**Female**
Deaths (× 1000)						
All member states	365	184	181	1498	893	605
Africa	305	147	158	209	101	108
The Americas						
High income	1	1	0	1	1	0
Low/middle income	13	7	6	53	30	23
Eastern Mediterranean	3	2	1	139	88	51
Europe						
High income	3	2	1	7	4	2
Low/middle income	1	1	0	53	44	9
Southeast Asia						
India	26	18	9	421	281	140
other low and middle income	9	5	4	261	133	128
Western Pacific						
High income	0	0	0	10	7	3
China	3	2	1	259	161	97
Other low/middle income	2	1	1	86	44	42
Incidence (× 1000)						
All member states	619	313	306	7393	4420	2973
Africa	510	246	264	1047	505	543
The Americas						
High income	4	3	1	17	12	6
Low/middle income	22	12	10	378	213	165
Eastern Mediterranean	4	3	2	607	384	223
Europe						
High income	8	5	3	72	48	24
Low/middle income	2	2	0	357	295	62
Southeast Asia						
India	46	31	15	1794	1198	596
Other low/middle income	16	8	8	1146	584	562
Western Pacific						
High income	1	0	0	86	57	29
China	5	3	2	1411	881	530
Other low/middle income	3	2	2	478	243	234
DALYs (× 1000)						
All member states	9032	4365	4667	28 189	16 137	12 052
Africa	7934	3719	4215	5442	2551	2891
The Americas						
High income	7	5	2	8	6	2
Low/middle income	302	159	143	1213	638	575
Eastern Mediterranean	59	37	22	3188	2006	1182
Europe						
High income	20	14	6	53	38	15
Low/middle income	18	15	3	853	732	122
Southeast Asia						
India	476	303	174	7577	4815	2761
other low and middle income	154	78	75	4438	2264	2174
Western Pacific						
High income	2	1	1	80	58	22
China	37	22	15	3878	2286	1592
Other low/middle income	25	13	12	1459	744	715

Source: WHO (1999*a*), Annex Table 10.

responsible for 10 per cent of deaths (Murray and Lopez 1997*b*). Tuberculosis is the cause of about one-third of all AIDS-related deaths in Africa. In 1993, the WHO declared tuberculosis to be a global emergency.

Mortality

The estimates for deaths from tuberculosis in Table 4 (WHO 1999*a*) are for individuals who were HIV negative. The estimated mortality in 1998 was 1.49 million with a range of 1.1 to 2.2 million deaths. Table 5 (also modified from WHO 1999*a*) includes gender-specific estimates for incidence, deaths, and DALYs for HIV-positive and HIV-negative individuals with tuberculosis. An additional 365 000 HIV-positive individuals are estimated to have died from tuberculosis in 1998. Eighty-three per cent of these deaths occurred in Africa, with approximately equal numbers of males and females. Low and middle income groups in the Americas and Southeast Asia, including India contributed 49 000 deaths compared with 9000 from Europe and the whole Western Pacific.

Incidence

The largest numbers of new cases of tuberculosis arise in Southeast Asia (2.9 million), China (1.4 million), and Africa (1.05 million). Forty-nine per cent of African cases are HIV positive. The estimated burden of the disease, expressed as disability adjusted days, is greatest in Southeast Asia, Africa, China, and eastern Mediterranean regions. However, in the Asia Pacific region there is marked variation in reported notifications between both high-income and low-income countries (Table 6) (SEAMIC 1998). Some of these data appear implausible. For example, it seems highly unlikely that a country such as Thailand, with a very high prevalence of HIV infection, would have a tuberculosis notification rate that is less than half of that in Hong Kong where the risk of HIV is still relatively low. On the other hand in three high-income postindustrialized countries or regions, Japan, Singapore, and Hong Kong there is a threefold variation between the highest and lowest notification rates. Given that the information systems supporting notification are relatively well developed these differences are unlikely to be due to under-reporting in Japan and Singapore (Table 6). Many data sources are, however, incomplete (as in, for example, Indonesia and Malaysia for the certification of tuberculosis in deaths), and this raises questions about the validity of the notification data.

Identifying problems in global control of tuberculosis

In the 1980s and 1990s the reverse in the previously established decline of tuberculosis led the WHO to declare the global emergency. The earlier fall in tuberculosis incidence in the nineteenth and twentieth centuries was attributed to improvements in socio-economic conditions and the isolation of infected cases. However, the pattern of disease control this century now describes a U-shaped curve in which the seriousness and complexity of disease is much greater in the second limb of the U (Reichman 1991).

In 1991, The World Health Assembly proposed an effective tuberculosis control strategy with two goals, to be achieved by the year 2000: successful treatment of 85 per cent of cases and detection of 70 per cent. The features of the WHO Directly Observed Therapy Short-course (**DOTS**) strategy were:

- government commitment to tuberculosis control
- case detection focusing on patients with symptoms who self-report to health services
- use of sputum smear microscopy
- standardized administration of the short-course treatment
- direct observation of the chemotherapy for at least 2 months

Table 6 Tuberculosis notifications and mortality in Asia Pacific countries

Country	Year	Population (× 1000)	TB incidence (all forms)	Rate per 100 000	Deaths from tuberculosis											
					Respiratory TB			Rate per 100 000			Other TB			Rate per 100 000		
					T	M	F	T	M	F	T	M	F	T	M	F
Brunei[a]	1996	305 000	140	45.9	3	2	1	1.0	1.2	0.7	3	–	3	1.0	–	2.1
Indonesia[a]	1996	196 263	394 551	201.0	77[c]	50	27	3.0			3[c]	2	1			
Hong Kong[b]	1997	6500	7072	108.8												
Japan[a]	1996	124 709	42 715	34.2	2639	1948	691	2.1	3.2	1.1	219	116	103	0.2	0.2	0.2
Malaysia[a]	1996	21 169	13 539	63.9	430[d]	329	101	2.0	3.0	1.0	143[d]	77	66	0.7	0.7	0.6
Philippines[a]	1994	69 946	118 951	170.1	26 208	17 354	8854	38.2	50.3	26.1	1049	626	423	1.5	1.8	1.2
Singapore[a]	1997	3044	2772	89.3	103	81	22	3.2	5.1	1.3	12	9	3	0.3	0.4	0.1
Thailand[a]	1997	59 788	26 787	44.8	2494	1873	621	4.1	6.2	2.4	1265	934	331	2.1	3.1	1.1
Vietnam[a]	1996	75 355	70 349	93.4	1146[e]						83[e]					

[a]Adapted from SEAMIC Health Statistics 1998, South East Asian Medical Information Center, International Medical Foundation of Japan.

[b]Hong Kong Government Chest Clinic Report 1998.

[c]Based on 10-day sample of discharges from hospital for each quarter.

[d]Medically certified deaths only which comprise 44% of all deaths.

[e]Hospital-based figures only.

- adequate supplies of treatments
- good records and information systems to allow evaluation of treatment results.

The WHO set up a surveillance and monitoring project in 1995 to assess national tuberculosis programmes and to compare regions that had adopted the WHO strategy (DOTS) and those that had not. Raviglione *et al.* (1997) estimated that within those countries that adopted the strategy only 23 per cent of the world population was covered.

Improved delivery of care must focus on early diagnosis and reliable delivery of effective treatments, but in 1998 the WHO identified 22 countries, which accounted for 80 per cent of tuberculosis cases worldwide, of which 16 countries were not making satisfactory progress in the control of the disease (Table 7). Half of those with a poor performance were middle income countries that had the resources but not the political will to tackle the problem (Wise 1998). There is also a wide disparity in funding, in the form of external aid, between different infectious diseases for each patient over the age of 5 years who died from the disease. Tuberculosis is clearly the most underfunded health-care problem in this group (Table 8) (Zumla and Grange 1999).

The failure of tuberculosis controls is exemplified by the problem in the Philippines, which has been estimated to have the highest numbers of cases of tuberculosis per capita in Southeast Asia and is ranked fourth in the world. No progress has been made in two decades, and the situation is complicated by low utilization of services by people with symptoms, high levels of drug resistance (60 per cent for isoniazid), the social stigma attached to the disease, and inability to pay for a full course of treatment (US$75) (Easton 1998).

Tuberculosis is associated with war, famine, social disruption, and poverty, including homelessness, unemployment, imprisonment, and alcoholism. In Russia the incidence and mortality has increased steadily since 1990 with rates of 67.5 per 100 000 and 17.0 per 100 000 respectively since 1996 (Wares and Clowes 1997).

Prospects for the future, in projections of mortality and disability by cause for 1990 to 2020 as part of the Global Burden of Disease Study (Murray and Lopez 1997*c*), indicate that tuberculosis ranked seventh as a cause of death in 1990 and its rank is not predicted to change throughout the 30-year period (Table 9). The projected total number of DALYs attributed to tuberculosis worldwide in 2020 is 42.5 million, of which 42.4 million arise in developing regions (Table 10).

Table 7 Progress in the control of tuberculosis in 22 countries

Slow progress	Afghanistan, Brazil, Ethiopia, India, Indonesia, Iran, Mexico, Myanmar, Nigeria, Pakistan, Philippines, Russian Federation, South Africa, Sudan, Thailand, Uganda
Making progress	Bangladesh, China, Democratic Republic of Congo
Good progress	Peru, Tanzania, Vietnam

Source: adapted from Wise (1998).

Table 8 Resources available in the form of external aid, between different infectious disease groups, for each patient over the age of 5 years who died from the disease

Disease	External aid (US$) for each patient who died
Tuberculosis	8
Malaria	137
Parasitic disease	370
AIDS	925
Leprosy	38 500

Source: adapted from Zumla and Grange (1999).

These current trends are complicated throughout the world by the growing problem of double infection by tuberculosis and HIV. Those developing countries in warm climates will experience the sharpest rises in incidence and this is directly related to the incidence of tuberculosis in the emerging HIV epidemics in Africa, India, and Asian Pacific countries. It will dictate the need for a marked change in priorities and a reallocation of resources from both within and outside of existing services, but the public health priorities are the alleviation of poverty and provision of good quality services to which all those in need have unhindered access.

Many predictions for tuberculosis are pessimistic, but others argue that the tools to implement cost-effective programmes are available. One year of healthy life can be gained for no more than US$3, making tuberculosis intervention one of the most cost-effective interventions in health care (Kochi *et al.* 1997).

Surveillance of tuberculosis

Poor information quality

In many countries, especially those with the highest risks, surveillance and information systems cannot provide information of adequate quality for community diagnoses and monitoring. Surveys on case detection and notification are notoriously unreliable and estimations are largely based on the prevalence of tuberculin reactivity as an indicator of infection by tuberculosis and, by extrapolation, the expected numbers of infected persons who will develop tuberculosis disease (Zumla and Grange 1999).

Incidence and prevalence

The current estimates of the global problem, in terms of both morbidity and mortality of tuberculosis, have been based on a range of clinical and microbiological measures of tuberculosis infection. The principal epidemiological variables used to describe the magnitude, trends, and impact of tuberculosis are:

- incidence (including incidence of smear positive cases)
- prevalence (including prevalence of smear positivity in all cases)
- predicted incidence (including use of skin tests)
- notification rates
- mortality (including case fatality in smear positive and other cases).

Table 9 Changes in ranking for most important causes of death from 1990 to 2020 in baseline scenario

Disorder	Ranking		Change in ranking
	1990	2020 (baseline model)	
Within top 15			
Ischaemic heart disease	1	1	0
Cerebrovascular disease	2	2	0
Lower respiratory infections	3	4	1↓
Diarrhoeal diseases	4	11	7↓
Perinatal disorders	5	16	11↓
Chronic obstructive pulmonary disease	6	3	3↑
Tuberculosis	7	7	0
Measles	8	27	19↓
Road-traffic accidents	9	6	3↑
Trachea, bronchus, and lung cancers	10	5	5↓
Malaria	11	29	18↓
Self-inflicted injuries	12	10	2↑
Cirrhosis of the liver	13	12	1↑
Stomach cancer	14	8	6↑
Diabetes mellitus	15	19	4↓
Outside top 15			
Violence	16	14	2↓
War injuries	20	15	5↑
Liver cancer	21	13	8↑
HIV	30	9	21↑

Source: Murray and Lopez (1997c).

Assessment of the emergent problem depends on the availability of comprehensive, accurate, and continuous information on incidence and mortality. The development and maintenance of surveillance systems is a vital component of any strategy for tuberculosis control and treatment, which in itself is a cost-effective approach to population health. Tuberculosis is a notifiable disease in most countries, but routine audit of the notification of cases is usually lacking and both accuracy and reliability are uncertain. When audit is carried out under-notification is usually identified and improvement occurs when notification procedures are revised and reinforced (Brown *et al.* 1995). Effective notification systems require record linkage between clinical units, pathology laboratories, and pharmacies.

The problem of linking information management with clinical practice requires systems analysis and continuing operations research directed at the chosen solutions. The WHO global tuberculosis programme has started the Global Tuberculosis Research Initiative (McConnell 1998). The aim is to promote operations research and develop the skills and funding to support it. Operations research is need to achieve improvements in surveillance and epidemiology. New approaches are required worldwide for the achievement of these goals in mixed medical economies and between different levels and sectors of health-care systems, which are often complicated by the politics of relationships between government, non-governmental organizations, and health professionals. The first problem to be addressed in tuberculosis control is the quality of information.

Factors influencing global trends in tuberculosis

Ageing communities

Several authors have reported on the rising age of tuberculosis patients in developed countries and a slowing down in the decline of notification rates overall.

To examine long-term trends in tuberculosis, Tocque *et al.* (1998) used a birth cohort analysis approach. They calculated age-specific rates of disease, by different age groups for different birth cohorts, for England and Wales and Hong Kong. In Hong Kong each birth cohort showed a similar pattern of disease by age with rates peaking in the 29- to 39-year age groups and then gradually declining (Fig. 6). Since 1978, regardless of age at that time, all age cohorts showed an increase in tuberculosis rates with age particularly in females. A similar pattern was seen in England and Wales but the peak occurred at an earlier age (less than 25 years) and the pattern of decline with age did not cease until 1984. Life expectancy is increasing steadily, particularly in countries with high or increasing per capita incomes. In the Asia Pacific region this includes the post-industrialized countries or regions of Japan, Taiwan, Singapore, and Hong Kong, but the numbers of elderly are also increasing across many other developing

Table 10 Ten projected leading causes of DALYs in 2020 according to baseline projection

Rank	Worldwide			Developing regions		
	Disease or injury	**DALYs ($\times 10^6$)**	**Cum. %**	**Disease or injury**	**DALYs ($\times 10^6$)**	**Cum. %**
	All causes	1388.8		All causes	1228.3	
1	Ischaemic heart disease	82.3	5.9	Unipolar major depression	68.8	5.6
2	Unipolar major depression	78.7	11.6	Road-traffic accidents	64.4	10.8
3	Road-traffic accidents	71.2	16.7	Ischaemic heart disease	64.3	16.1
4	Cerebrovascular disease	61.4	21.1	COPD	52.7	20.4
5	COPD	57.6	25.3	Cerebrovascular disease	51.5	24.6
6	Lower respiratory infections	42.7	28.4	Tuberculosis	42.4	28.0
7	Tuberculosis	42.5	31.4	Lower respiratory infections	41.1	31.4
8	War injuries	41.3	34.4	War injuries	40.2	34.6
9	Diarrhoeal diseases	37.1	37.1	Diarrhoeal diseases	37.0	37.6
10	HIV	36.3	39.7	HIV	34.0	40.4

Source: Murray and Lopez (1997c), Table 3.

nations. The ageing of communities, therefore, is becoming an important potential factor in the deterioration in control of tuberculosis.

Tobacco

In addition to its contribution to the burden of cancer and heart and respiratory disease, smoking is an importance influence on the risk of tuberculosis mortality.

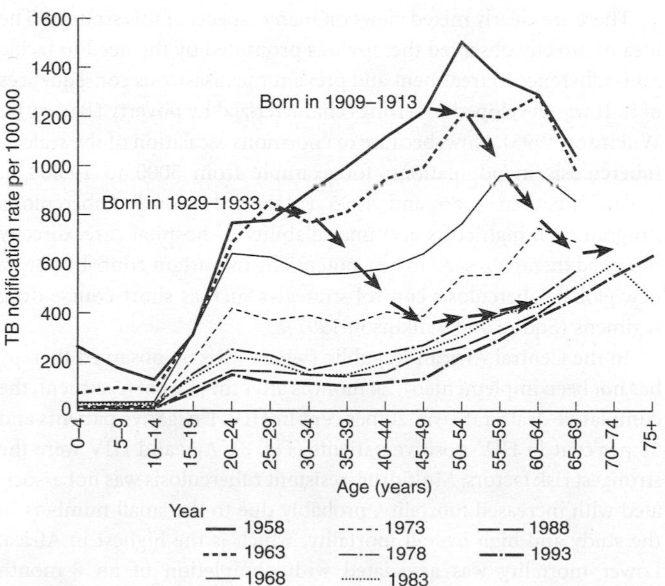

Fig. 6 Age incidence curves for male tuberculosis cases in Hong Kong from 1958 to 1993. The arrows indicate how rates were calculated for two individual birth cohorts as examples of how data were derived to compare age-cohort data between Hong Kong and England and Wales.

In China the smoker to non-smoker tuberculosis mortality ratio for men is 1.17 (rural) and 1.42 (urban) and in women 1.25 and 1.56 respectively (Liu *et al.* 1998), and smoking was estimated to account for 12 per cent of all tuberculosis deaths. A lung that is damaged by smoking may offer a propitious environment for the tuberculosis bacillus (WHO 1999*a*). Because of the high prevalence of smoking in men, in excess of 60 per cent in many Asian countries, tobacco will continue to make an important contribution to the burden of tuberculosis in the twenty-first century.

HIV infection

A new epidemic wave of tuberculosis is following the global increase in HIV with 6 million cases of both HIV and tuberculosis. Seventy-five per cent are estimated to be in Africa (WHO 1994).

In the mid-1990s the prevalence of combined infection with HIV and tuberculosis was about 6 million and HIV was estimated to cause up to half a million new cases of tuberculosis per year (WHO 1996). Information from African countries with reliable information systems (Burundi, Malawi, Tanzania, and Zambia) indicates the impact on their health-care systems from the HIV-related rise in incidence of tuberculosis (WHO 1996). The harm to maternal and child health is particularly serious (Chintu and Zumla 1995); in Zambia, where 25 per cent or more pregnant women are HIV positive, tuberculosis is the principal cause of death in pregnancy (Fylkesnes *et al.* 1997).

Tuberculosis is now a major problem in patients with HIV infection in the United States with an incidence of up to 9000 new cases per year (Markowitz *et al.* 1997). In New York the rate of tuberculosis is four times the national average and associated with nosocomial spread and multidrug-resistant tuberculosis. In London, tuberculosis rates have increased by 35 per cent compared with 15 per cent in England and Wales, but the extent of HIV-associated tuberculosis is uncertain because notification of tuberculosis in HIV is unreliable (Pym *et al.* 1995).

Cost, access to antiretroviral drugs, and adherence to treatment are major obstacles that should be priorities in aid programmes to Africa and in health care for HIV-positive immigrants to Western countries. HIV-related tuberculosis is a barometer for tuberculosis control and highlights weaknesses in its prevention and treatment (Coker and Miller 1997).

Prisons

Prisons have been identified as important reservoirs of tuberculosis, particularly drug-resistant strains, in both Western industrialized and developing countries. Surveys of prisons in New York City, Russia, Azerbaijan, Malawi, and Ethiopa have demonstrated a strong association between tuberculosis and HIV infection in prisoners and both the opportunities for and problems of achieving solutions in these neglected settings (Nyangulu *et al.* 1997; Reyes and Coninx 1997; Coninx *et al.* 1998).

Multidrug-resistant tuberculosis

Poor clinical practice, inadequate supervision and resources, and unethical commercial sales of inappropriate antituberculosis drugs and combinations have all combined to create the problem of drug resistance. The risk of multidrug-resistant tuberculosis, described as the 'Third Epidemic', may become the dominant pattern of tuberculosis spread on several continents, fanning out from countries such as Peru, northern India, Sierra Leone, the Baltic States, and Russia. Outbreaks of drug-resistant tuberculosis, once rare, are now common place and many involve HIV-positive patients. Early outbreaks were associated with high mortality because of failure of recognition and appropriate action. Several outbreaks of multidrug-resistant tuberculosis have occurred in Europe, including nosocomial infections in London and Madrid.

The WHO International Union Against Lung and Tuberculosis Disease global project on Anti-Tuberculosis Drug Resistance and Surveillance 1994 to 1997 in 35 countries found evidence of resistance in all of them, in patients with no previous treatment the prevalence was 9.9 per cent (range 2 to 41 per cent). *Mycobacterium tuberculosis* strains were resistant to one or more drug. High prevalences were found in the former Soviet Union, Asia, Dominican Republic, and Argentina (Pablos-Mendez *et al.* 1998).

Provision of care for tuberculosis and compliance with treatment

Diagnosis

It is estimated that less than half of those with tuberculosis who need medical care are in contact with treatment services. Continuity of care for tuberculosis often breaks down and this represents an additional hazard for community spread of the disease. Diagnosis has always presented problems (Zumla and Grange 1999). The protean manifestations, mimicry of other conditions, validity of tests, including lack of sensitivity (e.g. sputum microscopy) or specificity (chest radiology), and slow procedures (culture) all contribute to the problem.

Nucleic acid technology (polymerase chain reaction and ligase chain reaction) are evolving as potentially useful diagnostic tools. Sequencing of the *M. tuberculosis* genome should also allow development of rapid tests; however, the availability of new technology to those countries that need it most urgently will be limited for many years (Zumla and Grange 1999). Near-patient (as opposed to central laboratory) testing could yield important public health benefits, such as rapid initiation of contact tracing. However, the validity and reliability of such tools in the field will determine their cost-effectiveness. There may also be negative effects on the capture of epidemiological information from central diagnostic facilities, compounding the existing shortfalls in record keeping and notification. Therefore, implementation of these techniques will require their integration with new information technology, for example to enable automatic storage and transmission of results from multiple geographically separate sites (Borriello 1999).

Short-course multiple drug regimens

A wide range of short-course regimens are employed in different countries. Choices are based on past experience and established practice, cost and availability of drugs and evidence for effectiveness in trials. In Hong Kong (Hong Kong Chest Service 1984*a*,*b*) randomized trials of different drug combinations and durations of treatment showed that four-drug regimens were more effective than a three-drug regimen without streptomycin, at preventing relapse at 30 months. Four-drug regimens will contribute to population control of the disease by preventing the development of drug resistance and primary resistance in contacts.

Directly observed therapy

Directly observed therapy has been strongly promoted in the 1990s as the key to the control of tuberculosis in both developing and developed countries. Iseman *et al.* (1993) argued that we cannot afford not to do it and in 1997 the World Bank and the WHO contended that directly observed therapy is the most cost-effective of all health interventions. This revelation, implying a breakthrough in therapeutic management, caused concern and strong arguments that good evidence on the best approaches to implementation of supervised therapy and rigorous evaluation were lacking (Grange and Zumla 1997).

There are clearly mixed views on many aspects of this strategy. The idea of directly observed therapy was prompted by the need to tackle non-adherence to treatment and prevent the disastrous consequences of it. It was developed in settings characterized by poverty (Bayer and Wilkinson 1995). Now, because of enormous escalation of the scale of tuberculosis in populations, for example from 5000 to 19 000 in Malawi between 1985 and 1995 (Malawi National Tuberculosis Programme), high costs and unavailability of hospital care, directly observed therapy is seen to be a potentially important contribution to new global tuberculosis control strategies such as short-course drug regimens (Squire and Wilkinson 1997).

In the Central African Republic (where directly observed therapy has not been implemented), 24 months after the start of treatment, the cumulative death rate was 20 per cent in HIV-1 negative patients and 58 per cent in HIV-positive patients (Fig. 8). Age and HIV were the strongest risk factors. Multidrug-resistant tuberculosis was not associated with increased mortality, probably due to the small numbers in the study and high overall mortality, which is the highest in Africa. Lower mortality was associated with completion of an 8-month treatment plan (Garin *et al.* 1997).

In China the adoption of the WHO DOTS strategy was associated with a cure rate of nearly 90 per cent in new cases and a fall in the treatment failure rate in previously treated cases from 17.6 to 6.2 per cent. Supervision of treatment was provided by village doctors with financial incentives and careful supervision (China Tuberculosis Control Collaboration 1996).

However, a randomized controlled trial of directly observed therapy compared with self-supervised patients showed the equivalence of the two approaches with a trend for better outcomes in the self-supervised group (Zwarenstein *et al.* 1998). The investigators concluded that directly observed therapy is authoritarian, reduces self-reliance, and alienates patients. Flexibility of approach taking into account local conditions is necessary as demonstrated by the success of other approaches in rural Nepal (Jochem *et al.* 1997). The trial carried out by Zwarenstein and colleagues, which included a relatively small number of eligible patients with high treatment interruption rates, was prompted by the high workload imposed by a directly observed therapy programme and its report led to many cautionary statements about advocacy of any one method without adequate testing of its individual components.

Volmink and Garner (1997*a*) argued that it is necessary to develop more reliable reviews of directly observed therapy to support organizations such as the WHO and the World Bank. Without this, rhetoric about directly observed therapy may lead to currently effective programmes being discarded without a thorough evaluation of all the options available. A systematic review of five randomized or pseudo-randomized controlled trials of other preventive or curative strategies for tuberculosis showed that all six interventions tested were effective (Volmink and Garner 1997*b*). The interventions tested that did not include the 'supervised swallowing' procedures of directly observed therapy, were component reminder letters, monetary incentives to patients, health education, intensive supervision of staff and two combinations of these strategies. As all the interventions were effective the findings may indicate a form of Hawthorne effect in which increased overall commitment and intensity and comprehensiveness of interventions yield the desired clinical and public health results. Such an effect can obviously be exploited for benefit, although the precise elements of any one strategy that is responsible for its success may remain unidentified.

The need for a public health approach

Few tuberculosis treatment programmes achieve the aim of 85 per cent adherence and completion of the drug regimen. Inadequate adherence to treatment is very common. This is one of the most serious problems in tuberculosis management and has profound public health implications. Factors that are associated with, or predict, non-adherence have been identified from case studies rather than randomized trials (Table 11). In addition to directly observed therapy and other approaches mentioned previously it is essential that we improve the approach of services to delivering patient communication and education (Table 12). This approach is low cost and extremely effective and in any case should be a mandatory feature of good-quality (i.e. ethical) medical care. It is estimated that 15 to 20 min of patient education yields 2 months of regular attendance without default.

The lessons learned from the New York tuberculosis epidemic demonstrate that even in the West tuberculosis is as much a political and fiscal issue as a medical management problem, and therefore so are the solutions (Coker 1998). In New York, funding for tuberculosis was severely cut in the 1970s. To this was added the internal management problems in tuberculosis services and the growth of

Table 11 Factors associated with non-adherence in the treatment of tuberculosis

Principal problems
Subjective responses of patients, including feeling better and side-effects
Difficult access to health-care facilities
Additional contributing problems
Delay between referrals and appointments
Clinic environments, comfort, cleanliness, refreshments
Duration of treatment
Communication between health professionals and patients
Number of drugs
Side-effects
Cost
Social support

Source: adapted from Cuneo and Snider (1989).

Table 12 Steps to improve adherence and overall effectiveness of programmes

Need for patient-orientated measures to improve compliance	Health-care system response
Education at diagnosis	Provide supervised therapy
One-to-one counselling and communication adjusted to levels of educational attainment and literacy	Use trained outreach workers to provide direct supervision for disadvantaged patients who do not attend clinics
Explanation of changes in treatment regimens	Provide adequate training programmes for health care workers
Services convenient for patients including care at the workplace	Develop services for patients in remote areas
Access to care, including adequate transportation	Recruit volunteers and other non-health personnel to support tuberculosis care
Incentives tailored to patients' personal circumstances	Audit all procedures
High-quality appointments systems, reminders, and fail-safe follow-up methods	Evaluate the cost-effectiveness and acceptability of different programmes
Improve patient autonomy and promote self monitoring and belief in their own actions	
Ensure patients have access to and ownership of information from medical records and other sources	

Source: adapted from Cuneo and Snider (1989).

overcrowding, inequalities, and HIV in high-risk neighbourhoods. Treatment rates dropped to an average of 60 per cent. The response to the crisis cost US$1 billion, but through effective public health action led to a halving of case loads and an 85 per cent reduction in multidrug resistance. Coker recalls the New York City Board of Health slogan of 1915:

> The city can have as much reduction of preventable disease as it wishes to pay for. Public health is purchasable; within natural limitations a city can determine its own death rate.

References

Abbey, D.E., *et al.* (1999). Long term inhalable particles and other air pollutants related to mortality in non-smokers. *American Journal of Respiratory and Critical Care Medicine*, **159**, 373–82.

American Thoracic Society (1985). Guidelines as to what constitutes an adverse respiratory health effect, with special reference to epidemiologic studies of air pollution. *American Review of Respiratory Disease*, **131**, 666–8.

American Thoracic Society/Committee of the Environmental and Occupational Health Assembly of the American Thoracic Society (1996). Health effects of outdoor pollution. *American Journal of Respiratory and Critical Care Medicine*, **153**, 3–5, 477–98.

Anderson, H.R. (1978). Respiratory abnormalities in Papua New Guinea children: the effects of locality and domestic wood-smoke pollution. *International Journal of Epidemiology*, **7**, 63–71.

Anderson, H.R. (1999). Health effects of air pollution episodes. In *Air pollution and health* (ed. S.T. Holgate, J.M. Samet, H.S. Koren, and R.L. Maynard), pp. 461–82. Academic Press, London.

Anderson, H.R., Limb, E.S., Bland, J.M., de Leon, A.P., Strachan, D.P., and Bower, J.S. (1995). Health effects of an air pollution episode in London December 1991. *Thorax*, **50**, 1188–93.

Anderson, H.R., de Leon, A.P., Bland, J.M., Bower, J.S., and Strachan, D.P. (1996). Air pollution and daily mortality in London: 1987–92. *British Medical Journal*, **312**, 665–9.

Anthonisen, N. (1997). Epidemiology and the lung health study. *European Respiratory Review*, **7**, 202–5.

Anto, J.M. and Sunyer, J. (1995). Nitrogen dioxide and allergic asthma: starting to clarify an obscure association. *Lancet*, **345**, 402–3.

Anto, J.M., Sunyer, J., Rodriguez-Roisin, R., Suarez-Cervera, M., and Vazquez, L. (1989). Community outbreaks of asthma associated with inhalation of soybean dust. *New England Journal of Medicine*, **320**, 1097–102.

Australian National Health and Medical Research Council (1997). *The health effects of passive smoking.* Report of the NHMRC Passive Smoking Working Party. Australia Government Publishing Service, Canberra.

Barnes, D.E. and Bero, L.A. (1998). Why review articles on the health effects of passive smoking reach different conclusions. *Journal of the American Medical Association*, **279**, 1566–70.

Bates, C. and Brookes, K. (1999). *New measures to tackle passive smoking in the workplace: question and answers.* UK Action on Smoking and Health. http://www.ash.org.uk/papers/acop.html.

Bates, D.V. and Sizto, R. (1987). Air pollution and hospital admissions in southern Ontario: the acid summer haze effect. *Environmental Research*, **43**, 317–31.

Bates, D.V., Baker-Anderson, M., and Sizto, R. (1990). Asthma attack periodicity: a study of hospital emergency visits in Vancouver. *Environmental Research*, **51**, 51–70.

Bayer, R. and Wilkinson, D. (1995). Directly observed therapy for tuberculosis: history of an idea. *Lancet*, **345**, 1545–8.

Boezen, H.M., *et al.* (1999). Effects of ambient air pollution on upper and lower respiratory symptoms and peak expiratory flow in children. *Lancet*, **353**, 874–8.

Boffetta, P., *et al.* (1998). *European multicentre case-control study of lung cancer in non-smokers.* Technical Report No. 33, International Agency for Research on Cancer, Lyon.

Borja-Aburto, V.H., Loomis, D.P., Bangdiwala, S.L., Shy, C.M., and Rascon-Pacheco, R.A. (1997). Ozone, suspended particulates, and daily mortality in Mexico City. *American Journal of Epidemiology*, **145**, 258–68.

Borriello, S.P. (1999). Near patient microbiological tests. *British Medical Journal*, **319**, 298–301.

Bradshaw, D., Kielkowski, D., and Sitas, F. (1998). New birth and death registration forms—a foundation for the future, a challenge for health workers. *South African Medical Journal*, **88**, 971–4.

Braun-Fahrlander, C., *et al.* (1992). Air pollution and respiratory symptoms in preschool children. *American Review of Respiratory Disease*, **145**, 42–7.

British Thoracic Society/The COPD Guidelines Group of the Standards of Care Committee of British Thoracic Society (1997). BTS guidelines for the management of chronic obstructive pulmonary disease. *Thorax*, **52** (Supplement 5), 1–28.

Brown, J.S., Wells, F., Duckworth, G., Paul, E.A., and Barnes, N.C. (1995). Improving notification rates for tuberculosis. *British Medical Journal*, **310**, 974.

Brunekreef, B., *et al.* (1991). Sensitive subgroups and normal variation in pulmonary function response to air pollution episodes. *Environmental Health Perspectives*, **90**, 189–93.

Burney, P.G. (1992). Asthma. Epidemiology. *British Medical Bulletin*, **48**, 10–22.

Burney, P.G.J. (1988). Why study the epidemiology of asthma? *Thorax*, **43**, 425–8.

Camilli, A.E., Burrows, B., Knudson B., Lyle, S.K., and Lebowitz, M.D. (1987). Longitudinal changes in forced expiratory volume in one second in adults. Effects of smoking and smoking cessation. *American Review of Respiratory Disease*, **135**, 794–9.

Chapman, S., *et al.* (1999). The impact of smoke-free workplaces on declining cigarette consumption in Australia and the United States. *American Journal of Public Health*, **89**, 1018–23.

Chief Medical Officer's Committee on Medical Aspects of Food (1998). *Nutritional aspects of the development of cancer.* HMSO, London.

China Tuberculosis Control Collaboration (1996). Results of directly observed short course chemotherapy in 112 842 Chinese patients with smear-positive tuberculosis. *Lancet*, **347**, 358–62.

Chintu, C. and Zumal, A. (1995). Childhood tuberculosis and infection with the human immunodeficiency virus. *Journal of Royal College of Physicians of London*, **29**, 92–5.

Coker, R. (1998). Lessons from New York's tuberculosis epidemic. *British Medical Journal*, **317**, 616.

Coker, R. and Miller, R. (1997). HIV associated tuberculosis. A barometer for wider tuberculosis control and prevention. *British Medical Journal*, **314**, 1847.

Coninx, R., *et al.* (1998). Drug resistant tuberculosis in prisons in Azerbaijan: case study. *British Medical Journal*, **316**, 1423–5.

Cuneo, W.D. and Snider, D.E., Jr (1989). Enhancing patient compliance with tuberculosis therapy. *Clinics in Chest Medicine*, **10**, 375–80.

Dab, W., *et al.* (1996). Short term respiratory health effects of ambient air pollution: results of the APHEA project in Paris. *Journal of Epidemiology and Community Health*, **50**, S42–6.

Darby, S.C. and Samet, J.M. (1994). Radon. In *Epidemiology of lung cancer* (ed. J.M. Samet), p. 219. Marcel Dekker, New York.

Davis, R.M. (1998). Exposure to environmental tobacco smoke: identifying and protecting those at risk. *Journal of the American Medical Association*, **280**, 1947–9.

den Otter, J.J., van Dijk, B., van Schayck, C.P., Molema, J., and van Weel, C. (1998). How to avoid underdiagnosed asthma/chronic obstructive pulmonary disease? *Journal of Asthma*, **35**, 381–7.

Department of Health (1998). *Nutritional aspects of the development of cancer.* Working Group on Diet and Cancer of the Committee on Medical Aspects of Food and Nutrition Policy. Report on the Health and Social Subjects, No. 48. Department of Health, HMSO, London.

Department of Health/Ad Hoc Group on the Economic Appraisal of the Health Effects of Air Pollution (1999). *Economic appraisal of the health effects of air pollution.* HMSO, London.

Department of Health/Committee on the Medical Effects of Air Pollutants (COMEAP) (1995). *Asthma and outdoor pollution* (Chairman S.T. Holgate). HMSO, London.

Department of Health/Committee on the Medical Effects of Air Pollutants (COMEAP) (1998). *Quantification of the effects of air pollution on health in the United Kingdom.* HMSO, London.

Destache, C.J., Dewan, N., O'Donohue, W.J., Campbell, J.C., and Angelillo, V.A. (1999). Clinical and economic considerations in the treatment of acute exacerbations of chronic bronchitis. *Journal of Antimicrobial Chemotherapy*, **43** (Supplement A), 107–13.

Dockery, D.W., *et al.* (1982). Change in pulmonary function in children associated with air pollution episodes. *Journal of the Air Pollution Control Association*, **32**, 937–42.

Dockery, D.W., *et al.* (1989). Effects of inhalable particles on respiratory health of children. *American Review of Respiratory Disease*, **139**, 587–94.

Dockery, D.W., *et al.* (1993). An association between air pollution and mortality in six US cities. *New England Journal of Medicine*, **329**, 1753–9.

Easton, A. (1998). Tuberculosis controls in Philippines have failed so far. *British Medical Journal*, **317**, 557.

Eisner, M.D., Smith, A.K., and Blanc, P.D. (1998). Bartenders' respiratory health after establishment of smoke-free bars and taverns. *Journal of the American Medical Association*, **280**, 1909–14.

EPA (Environmental Protection Agency) (1999). *Statement of the US EPA on court's decision on clean air rules*, 14 May. www.epa.gov/ttn/oarpg/gen/epastat.pdf.

European Working Group (1996). *Environmental tobacco smoke and lung cancer: an evaluation of the risk.* European Working Group, Tronheim.

Evans, J. and Wolff, S. (1996). Modeling of air pollution impacts: one possible explanation of the observed chronic mortality. In *Particle in our air: concentrations and health effects* (ed. R. Wilson and J.D. Spengler). Harvard University Press, Boston, MA.

Fletcher, C., Peto, R., Tinker, C., and Speizer, F.E. (1976). *The natural history of chronic bronchitis and emphysema.* Oxford University Press.

Froggatt, P. (1988). *Fourth report of the independent scientific committee on smoking and health.* HMSO, London.

Fry, J. (1953). Effects of a severe fog on a general practice. *Lancet*, **i**, 235–3.

Fylkesnes, K., *et al.* (1997). The HIV epidemic in Zambia: socio-demographic prevalence patterns and indications of trends among childbearing women. *AIDS*, **11**, 339–45.

Garin, B., *et al.* (1997). High mortality rates among patients with tuberculosis in Bangui, Central African Republic. *Lancet*, **350**, 1298.

Glantz, S., Slade, J., Bero, L.A., Hanauer, P., and Barnes, D.E. (1996). *The cigarette papers.* University of California Press, Berkeley, CA.

Gold, D.R., *et al.* (1999). Particulate and ozone pollutant effects on the respiratory function of children in southwest Mexico City. *Epidemiology*, **10**, 8–16.

Grange, J.M. and Zumla, A. (1997). Making DOTS succeed. *Lancet*, **350**, 157.

Hackshaw, A.K., Law, M.R., and Wald, N.J. (1997). The accumulated evidence on lung cancer and environmental tobacco smoke. *British Medical Journal*, **315**, 980–8.

Harrington, J.M. and Saracci, R. (1994). Occupational cancer: clinical and epidemiological aspects. In *Hunter's diseases of occupations* (8th edn) (ed. P.A.B. Raffle, P.H. Adams, P.J. Baxter and W.R. Lee), pp. 654–88. Edward Arnold, London.

He, Y., *et al.* (1994). Passive smoking at work as a risk factor for coronary heart disease in Chinese women who have never smoked. *British Medical Journal*, **308**, 380–4.

He, J., *et al.* (1999). Passive smoking and the risk of coronary heart disease—a meta-analysis of epidemologic studies. *New England Journal of Medicine*, **340**, 958–9.

Hedley, A.J. and Lam, T.H. (1997). Respiratory disease. In *Oxford textbook of public health*, Vol. 3 (3rd edn) (ed. R. Detels, W.W. Holland, J. McEwen, and G.S. Omenn), pp. 1081–11. Oxford University Press.

Hedley, A.J., *et al.* (1993). *Air pollution and respiratory health in primary school children in Hong Kong 1989–1992.* Report to Environmental Protection Department, Hong Kong Government. Department of Community Medicine, the University of Hong Kong.

Hoek, G. and Brunekreef, B. (1993). Acute effects of a winter air pollution episode on pulmonary function and respiratory symptoms of children. *Archives of Environmental Health*, **48**, 328–35.

Hoek, G., Brunekreef, B., Kosterink, P., Van den Berg, R., and Hofschreuder, P. (1993). Effect of ambient ozone on peak expiratory flow of exercising children in The Netherlands. *Archives of Environmental Health*, **48**, 27–32.

Holgate, S., Koren, H.S., Samet, J.M., and Maynard, R.L. (ed.) (1999). *Air pollution and health.* Academic Press, London.

Holland, W.W., *et al.* (1979). Health effects of particulate pollution: reappraising the evidence. *American Journal of Epidemiology*, **110**, 525–659.

Hong Kong Chest Service/Tuberculosis Research Centre, Madras/British Medical Research Council (1984*a*). A controlled trial of 2-month, 3 month and 12 month regimens of chemotherapy for sputum smear negative pulmonary tuberculosis: results at 60 months. *American Review of Respiratory Disease*, **130**, 23–8.

Hong Kong Chest Service/Tuberculosis Research Centre, Madras/British Medical Research Council (1984*b*). A controlled trial of 3-month, 4-month, and 6-month regimens of chemotherapy for sputum-smear negative tuberculosis: results at 5 years. *American Review of Respiratory Disease*, **130**, 871–6.

International Commission on Occupational Health (1999). *Membership directory 1999.*

Iseman, M.D., Cohen, D.L., and Sbarbaro, J.A. (1993). Directly observed treatment of tuberculosis. We can't not afford to do it. *New England Journal of Medicine*, **328**, 576–8.

Ito, K. and Thurston, G.D. (1999). Epidemiological studies of ozone exposure effects. In *Air pollution and health* (ed. S.T. Holgate, J.M. Samet, H.S. Koren, and R.L. Maynard), pp. 485–510. Academic Press, London.

Jaakkola, J.J.K., Paunio, M., Virtanen, M., and Heinonen, O.P. (1991). Low level air pollution and upper respiratory infections in children. *American Journal of Public Health*, **81**, 1060–3.

Jaakkola, M.S., Jaakkola, J.J., Becklake, M.R., and Ernst, P. (1996). Effect of passive smoking on the development of respiratory symptoms in young adults: an 8-year longitudinal study. *Journal of Clinical Epidemiology*, **49**, 581–6.

Jochem, K., *et al.* (1997). Tuberculosis control in remote districts of Nepal comparing patient-responsible short-course chemotherapy with long-course treatment. *International Journal of Tuberculosis and Lung Disease*, **1**, 502–8.

Jones, J.R., Hodgson, J.T., Clegg, T.A., and Elliott, R.C. (1998). *Self-reported work-related illness in 1995: results from a household survey.* HSE Books, Sudbury.

Katsouyanni, K., *et al.* (1997). Short term effects of ambient sulphur dioxide and particulate matter on mortality in 12 European cities: results from time series data from the APHEA project. *British Medical Journal*, **314**, 1658–63.

Kochi, A., Nunn, P., Dye, C., and Tayler, E. (1997). Global burden of disease. *Lancet*, **350**, 142.

Kuller, L.H., *et al.* (1989). The epidemiology of pulmonary function and COPD mortality in the Multiple Risk Factor Intervention Trial. *American Review of Respiratory Disease*, **140**, S76–81.

Lam, T.H. and Hedley, A.J. (1999). Environmental tobacco smoke in Asia: slow progress against great barriers. *Journal of the American Medical Association, Southeast Asia*, **15**, 7–9.

Lam, T.H., *et al.* (1996). Smoking and exposure to occupational hazards in 8304 workers in Guangzhou, China. *Occupational Medicine*, **46**, 351–5.

Lam, T.H., Ho, S.Y., Hedley, A.J., and Mak, K.H. (1998). Mentioning smoking as a cause of death on death certificates. *British Medical Journal*, **317**, 1456.

Lam, T.H., *et al.* (1999). Respiratory symptoms and environmental tobacco smoke in police officers in Hong Kong. *The 15th International Scientific Meeting of the International Epidemiological Association, Abstract Book*, Vol. 1, p. 164.

Last, J.M. (1995). *Dictionary of epidemiology* (3rd edn). Oxford University Press.

Leuenberger, P., *et al.* (1994). Passive smoking exposure in adults and chronic respiratory symptoms (SAPALDIA Study). *American Journal of Respiratory and Critical Care Medicine*, **150**, 1222–8.

Levi, F., Lucchini, F., Vecchia, C.L., and Negri, E. (1999). Trends in mortality from cancer in the European Union, 1955–94. *Lancet*, **354**, 742–3.

Liu, B.Q., *et al.* (1998). Emerging tobacco hazards in China: 1. Retrospective proportional mortality study of one million deaths. *British Medical Journal*, **317**, 1399–400.

Logan, W.P.D. (1953) Mortality in the London fog incident 1952. *Lancet,* **i**, 336–8.

Lopez, A.D. (1998). Counting the dead in China. Measuring tobacco's impact in the developing world. *British Medical Journal*, **317**, 1399–400.

McConnell, J. (1998). WHO's tuberculosis research initiative. *Lancet*, **351**, 852.

McMichael, A.J. and Smith, K.R. (1999). Seeking a global perspective on air pollution and health. *Epidemiology*, **10**, 1–4.

McMichael, A.J., Anderson, H.R., Brunekreef, B., and Cohen, A.J. (1998). Inappropriate use of daily mortality analyses to estimate longer term mortality effects of air pollution. *International Journal of Epidemiology*, **27**, 450–3.

Mannino, D.M., Siegel, M., Rose, D., Nkuchia, J., and Etzel, R. (1997). Environmental tobacco smoke exposure in the home and worksite and health effects in adults: results from the 1991 National Health Interview Survey. *Tobacco Control*, **6**, 296–305.

Markowitz, N., *et al.* (1997). Incidence of tuberculosis in the United States among HIV-infected persons. The Pulmonary Complications of HIV Infection Study Group. *Annals of Internal Medicine*, **126**, 123–32.

Meidema, I., Feskens, E.J.M., Heederik, D., and Kromohout, D. (1993). Dietary determinants of long term incidence of chronic non-specific lung diseases. The Zutphen Study. *American Journal of Epidemiology*, **138**, 37–45.

Murray, C.J.L. and Lopez, A.D. (ed.) (1996). *The global burden of disease: a comprehensive assessment of mortality and disability from diseases, injuries, and risk factors in 1990 and projected to 2020*. Harvard University Press, Cambridge, MA.

Murray, C.J.L. and Lopez, A.D. (1997*a*). Mortality by cause for eight regions of the world: Global Burden of Disease Study. *Lancet*, **349**, 1269–76.

Murray, C.J.L. and Lopez, A.D. (1997*b*). Global mortality, disability, and the contribution of risk factors. *Lancet*, **349**, 1436–42.

Murray, C.J.L. and Lopez, A.D. (1997*c*). Alternative projections of mortality and disability by cause 1990–2020: Global Burden of Disease Study. *Lancet*, **349**, 1498–504.

National Research Council (1986). *Environmental tobacco smoke: measuring exposures and assessing health effects*. National Academy Press, Washington, DC.

Ng, T.P., Hui, K.P., and Tan, W.C. (1993). Respiratory symptoms and lung function effects of domestic exposure to tobacco smoke and cooking by gas in non-smoking women in Singapore. *Journal of Epidemiology and Community Health*, **47**, 454–8.

Niu, S.R., *et al.* (1998). Emerging tobacco hazards in China: 2. Early mortality results from a prospective study. *British Medical Journal*, **317**, 1423–4.

Nyangulu, D.S., *et al.* (1997). Tuberculosis in a prison population in Malawi. *Lancet*, **350**, 1284–7.

Omenn, G.S., *et al.* (1996). Effects of a combination of beta carotene and vitamin A on lung cancer and cardiovascular disease. *New England Journal of Medicine*, **334**, 1150–5.

ONS (Office for National Statistics) (1997). *The health of adult Britain 1841–1994*, Vol. 2. Series DS No. 13. HMSO, London.

Ostro, B.D. and Rothschild, S. (1989). Air pollution and acute respiratory morbidity: an observational study of multiple pollutants. *Environmental Research*, **50**, 238–47.

Pablos-Mendez, A., *et al.* (1998). Global surveillance for anti-tuberculosis-drug resistance. *New England Journal of Medicine*, **338**, 1641–9.

Peters, J., *et al.* (1996). Effects of an ambient air pollution intervention and environmental tobacco smoke on children's respiratory health in Hong Kong. *International Journal of Epidemiology*, **25**, 821–8.

Peto, R. (1998). Mortality from breast cancer in UK has decreased suddenly. *British Medical Journal*, **317**, 476–7.

Peto, R., Lopez, A.D., Boreham, J., Thun, M., and Heath, C. Jr (1994). *Mortality from smoking in developed countries 1950–2000. Oxford University Press.*

Petty, T.L. and Weinmann, G.G. (1997). Building a national strategy for the prevention and management of and research in chronic obstructive pulmonary disease: National Heart, Lung and Blood Institute workshop summary. *American Journal of Medical Association*, **277**, 246–53.

Pope, C.A. III (1989). Respiratory disease associated with community air pollution and a steel mill, Utah Valley. *American Journal of Public Health*, **79**, 623–8.

Pope, C.A. and Xu, X. (1993). Passive cigarette smoke, coal heating, and respiratory symptoms of nonsmoking women in China. *Environmental Health Perspective*, **101**, 314–16.

Pope, C.A. III, Schwartz, J., and Ransom, M.R. (1992). Daily mortality and PM_{10} pollution in Utah Valley. *Archives of Environmental Health*, **47**, 211–17.

Pope, C.A. III, *et al.* (1995) Particulate air pollution as a predictor of mortality in a prospective study of US adults. *American Journal of Respiratory and Critical Care Medicine*, **151**, 669–74.

Pym, A.S., Churchill, D.R., Gleissberg, V., and Coker, R.J. (1995). Reasons for increased incidence of tuberculosis. Audit suggests that undernotification is common. *British Medical Journal*, **311**, 570.

Raviglione, M.C., Dye, C., Schmidt, S., and Kochi, A. (1997). Assessment of worldwide tuberculosis control. WHO Global Surveillance and Monitoring Project. *Lancet*, **350**, 1329–30.

Reichman, L.B. (1991). The U-shaped curve of concern. *American Review of Respiratory Disease*, **144**, 741–2.

Repace, J.L., Jinot, J., Bayard, S., Emmons, K., and Hammond, S.K. (1998). Air nicotine and saliva cotinine as indicators of workplace passive smoking exposure and risk. *Risk Analysis*, **18**, 71–83

Reyes, H. and Coninx, R. (1997). Pitfalls of tuberculosis programmes in prisons. *British Medical Journal*, **315**, 1447–50.

Royal College of Physicians of London (1992). *Smoking and the young: a report of a working party of the Royal College of Physician.* Royal College of Physicians, London.

Rupp, J.P. and Billings, D.M. (1990). *Tobacco industry documents. Privileged and confidential attorneys work product, February 14, 1990.* Asia ETS consultant status report. http://www.smokescreen.org/documents.

Sallie, B.A., Ross, D.J., Meredith, S.K., and McDonald, J.C. (1994). SWORD '93 Surveillance of work-related and occupational respiratory disease in the UK. *Occupational Medicine, 44, 177–82.*

Samah, A.A. (1992). Investigation into the haze episodes in the Kelang Valley, Malaysia. In *Association of South East Asian institutions of higher learning seminar proceedings. The role of the ASAIHL in combating health hazards of environmental pollution* (ed. A.J. Hedley *et al.*), pp. 221–7. University of Hong Kong.

Samet, J.M. and Jaakkola, J.J.K. (1999). The epidemiological approach to investigating outdoor air pollution. In *Air pollution and health* (ed. S.T. Holgate, J.M. Samet, H.S. Koren, and R.L. Maynard), pp.431–60. Academic Press, London.

Sandford, A.J., Weir, T.D., and Paré, P.D. (1997). Genetic risk factors for chronic obstructive pulmonary disease. *European Respiratory Journal*, **10**, 1380–91.

Schouten, J.P., Vonk, J.M., and de Graaf, A. (1996). Short term effects of air pollution on emergency hospital admissions for respiratory disease: results of the APHEA project in two major cities in The Netherlands, 1977–89. *Journal of Epidemiology and Community Health*, **50**, S22–9.

Schwartz, J. (1989). Lung function and chronic exposure to air pollution: a cross-sectional analysis of NHANES II. *Environmental Research,* **50**, 309–21.

Schwartz, J. (1993). Air pollution and daily mortality in Birmingham, Alabama. *American Journal of Epidemiology,* **137**, 1136–47.

Schwartz, J. and Weiss, S.T. (1990). Dietary factors and their relationship to respiratory symptoms: NHANES II. *Environmental Research*, **50**, 309–21.

Schwartz, J. and Weiss, S.T. (1994). Relationship between dietary vitamin C intake and pulmonary function in the first national health and nutrition examination survey (NHANES I). *American Journal of Clinical Nutrition*, **59**, 110–14.

Schwartz, J., Spix, C., Wichmann, H.E., and Malin, E. (1991). Air pollution and acute respiratory illness in five German communities. *Environmental Research,* **56**, 1–14.

SCOTH (Scientific Committee on Tobacco and Health) (1998). *Report of the Scientific Committee on Tobacco and Health (SCOTH).* Department of Health. HMSO, London.

Scott, J.A. (1963). The London fog of 1962. *Medical Officer*, **109**, 250–3.

Siegel, M., Husten, C., Merritt, R.K., Giovino, G.A., and Eriksen, M.P. (1995). Effects of separately ventilated smoking lounges on the health of smokers: is this an appropriate public health policy? *Tobacco Control*, **4**, 22–9.

Smit, H.A., Grievink, L., and Tabak, C. (1999). Dietary influences on chronic obstructive lung disease and asthma: a review of the epidemiological evidence. *Proceedings of the Nutrition Society*, **58**, 309–19.

Smith, G.D. and Phillips, A.N. (1996). Passive smoking and health: should we believe Philip Morris's 'experts'? *British Medical Journal*, **313**, 929–33.

South East Asian Medical Information Center/International Medical Foundation of Japan (1998). *SEAMIC Health Statistics*. South East Asian Medical Information Center, Tokyo.

Soyseth, V., *et al.* (1995). Relation of exposure to airway irritants in infancy to prevalence of bronchial hyper-responsiveness in schoolchildren. *Lancet*, **345**, 217–20.

Squire, S.B. and Wilkinson, D. (1997). Strengthening 'DOTS' through community care for tuberculosis. *British Medical Journal*, **315**, 1395–6.

Stationery Office (1998). *Smoking kills: a White Paper on tobacco*. HMSO, London.

Stellman, S.D., Boffetta, P., and Garfinkel, L. (1988). Smoking habits of 800,000 American men and women in relation to their occupations. *American Journal of Industrial Medicine*, **13**, 43–58.

Strachan, D.P., Cox, B.D., Erzinclioglu, S.W., Walters, E.D., and Whichelow, M.J. (1991). Ventilatory function and winter fresh fruit consumption in a random sample of British adults. *Thorax*, **46**, 624–9.

Tam, A.Y.C., *et al.* (1994) Bronchial responsiveness in children exposed to atmospheric pollution in Hong Kong. *Chest*, **106**, 1056–60.

Thurston, G.D. and Ito, K. (1999). Epidemiological studies of ozone exposure effects. In *Air pollution and health* (ed. S.T. Holgate, J.M. Samet, H.S. Koren, and R.L. Maynard), pp. 485–510. Academic Press, London.

Thurston, G.D. and Kinney, P.L. (1995). Air pollution epidemiology: considerations in time series analyses. *Inhalation Toxicology*, **7**, 71–83.

Tocque, K., *et al.* (1998). Long-term trends in tuberculosis. Comparison of age-cohort data between Hong Kong and England and Wales. *American Journal of Respiratory and Critical Care Medicine*, **158**, 484–8.

Touloumi, G., Samoli, E., and Katsouyanni, K. (1996). Daily mortality and 'winter type' air pollution in Athens, Greece—a time series analysis within the APHEA project. *Journal of Epidemiology and Community Health*, **50**, S47–51.

UKHSC (UK Health and Safety Commission) (1999). *Proposal for an approved code of practice on passive smoking at work*. HSE Books, Sudbury.

USCEPA (US California Environmental Protection Agency) (1997). *Health effects of exposure to environmental tobacco smoke*. California Environmental Protection Agency, Office of Environmental Health Hazard Assessment, Sacramento, CA.

USDHEW (US Department of Health, Education and Welfare) (1986). *The health consequences of involuntary smoking. A report of the Surgeon General*. US Department of Health, Education and Welfare, Washington, DC.

USEPA (US Environmental Protection Agency) (1992). *Respiratory health effects of passive smoking: lung cancer and other disorders*. US Environmental Protection Agency, Washington, DC.

USOSHA (US Occupational Safety and Health Administration (1994). Notice of proposed rulemaking; notice of informal public hearing. *Federal Register*, 5 April 5 1994, 29 CFR Parts 1910, 1915, 1926, and 1928.

van Ede, L., Yzermans, C.J., and Brouwer, H.J. (1999). Prevalence of depression in patients with chronic obstructive pulmonary disease: a systematic review. *Thorax*, **54**, 688–92.

Viegi, G., *et al.* (1991). Prevalence rates of respiratory symptoms in Italian general population samples exposed to different levels of air pollution. *Environmental Health Perspective*, **94**, 95–9.

Volmink, J. and Garner, P. (1997*a*). Promoting adherence to tuberculosis treatment. In *Infectious diseases module of the Cochrane database of systematic reviews* (ed. P. Garner *et al.*). Cochrane Library, Update Software, Oxford.

Volmink, J. and Garner, P. (1997*b*). Systematic review of randomised controlled trials of strategies to promote adherence to tuberculosis treatment. *British Medical Journal*, **315**, 1403–6.

Wagner, G.R. (1998). Preventing pneumoconioses and eliminating silicosis: opportunities and illusions. In *Advances in the prevention of occupational respiratory diseases* (ed. K. Chiyotani, Y. Hosoda, and Y. Aizawa), pp. 3–11. Elsevier, Amsterdam.

Walters, S., Phupinyokul, M., and Ayres, J. (1995). Hospital admission rates for asthma and respiratory disease in the West Midlands: their relationship to air pollution levels. *Thorax*, **50**, 948–54.

Ware, J.H., *et al.* (1986). Effects of ambient sulphur oxides and suspended particles on respiratory health of preadolescent children. *American Review of Respiratory Disease*, **133**, 834–42.

Wares, D.F. and Clowes, C.I. (1997). Tuberculosis in Russia. *Lancet*, **350**, 957.

Weiland, S.K., Mundt, K.A., Ruckmann, A., and Keil, A. (1994). Self-reported wheezing and allergic rhinitis in children and traffic density on the street. *Annals of Epidemiology*, **4**, 243–7.

Wells, A.J. (1998). Heart disease from passive smoking in the workplace. *Journal of the American College of Cardiology*, **31**, 1–9.

White, J.R., Froeb, H.F., and Kulik, J.A. (1991). Respiratory illness in nonsmokers chronically exposed to tobacco smoke in the work place. *Chest*, **100**, 39–43.

Whittemore, A.S. and Korn, E.L. (1980). Asthma and air pollution in the Los Angeles area. *American Journal of Public Health*, **70**, 687–96.

WHO (World Health Organization) (1994). *TB—a global emergency. WHO report on the TB epidemic.* WHO, Geneva.

WHO (World Health Organization) (1996). *Tuberculosis in the era of HIV. A deadly partnership.* WHO/TB/96.204. WHO, Geneva.

WHO (World Health Organization) (1997*a*). *Tobacco or health: a global status report.* WHO, Geneva.

WHO (World Health Organization) (1997*b*). *health and environmental in sustainable development. five years after the earth summit.* WHO/EHG/97.8. WHO, Geneva.

WHO (World Health Organization) (1998). *Guidelines for controlling and monitoring the tobacco epidemic.* WHO, Geneva.

WHO (World Health Organization) (1999*a*). *The world health report 1999.* WHO, Geneva.

WHO (World Health Organization) (1999*b*). *The framework convention on tobacco control—a primer.* WHO, Geneva.

WHO (World Health Organization) (1999*c*). *Occupational health: ethically correct, economically sound.* Fact Sheet No. 84. http://www.who.int/inf-fs/en/fact084.html. WHO, Geneva.

WHO (World Health Organization) (1999*d*). *International consultation on environmental tobacco smoke (ETS) and child health, 11–14 January 1999.* NCD/TFI/ETS/99.2. WHO, Geneva.

Wise, J. (1998). WHO identifies 16 countries struggling to control tuberculosis. *British Medical Journal*, **316**, 957.

Wjst, M., *et al.* (1993). Road traffic and adverse effects on respiratory health in children. *British Medical Journal*, **307**, 596–600.

Wong, C.M., *et al.* (1998). Comparison between two districts of the effects of an air pollution intervention on bronchial responsiveness in primary school children in Hong Kong. *Journal of Epidemiology and Community Health*, **52**, 571–8.

Wong, C.M., Hu, Z.G., Lam, T.H., Hedley, A.J., and Peters, J. (1999). Effects of ambient air pollution and environmental tobacco smoke on respiratory health of non-smoking women in Hong Kong. *International Journal of Epidemiology*, **28**, 859–64.

World Bank (1993). *World development report 1993.* Oxford University Press.

World Bank (1999). *Curbing the epidemic governments and the economics of tobacco control.* World Bank, Washington, DC.

World Cancer Research Fund (1997). *Food, nutrition and the prevention of cancer: a global perspective.* World Cancer Research Fund and American Institute for Cancer Research, Washington, DC.

Xu, X.P., Dockery, D.W., and Wang, L.H. (1991). Effects of air pollution on adult pulmonary function. *Archives of Environmental Health*, **46**, 198–206.

Xu, X., Gao, J., Dockery, D.W., and Chen, Y. (1994) Air pollution and daily mortality in residential areas of Beijing, China. *Archives of Environmental Health*, **49**, 216–22.

Zumla, A. and Grange, J.M. (1999). The 'global emergency' of tuberculosis. *Proceedings of the Royal College of Physicians of Edinburgh*, **29**, 104–15.

Zwarenstein, M., Schoeman, J.H., Vundule, C., Lombard, C.J., and Tatley, M. (1998). Randomised controlled trial of self-supervised and directly observed treatment of tuberculosis. *Lancet*, **352**, 1340–3.

9.5 Asthma

Neil Pearce, Jeroen Douwes, and Richard Beasley

Introduction

The word 'asthma' comes from a Greek word meaning 'panting' (Keeney 1964), but reference to asthma can also be found in ancient Egyptian, Hebrew, and Indian medical writings (Unger and Harris 1974; Ellul-Micallef 1976), and asthma has puzzled and confused doctors and patients from the time of Hippocrates to the present day. There were clear observations of patients experiencing attacks of asthma in the second century and evidence of disordered anatomy in the lung as far back as the seventeenth century (Willis 1678). Asthma is often described as an allergic disease and grouped together with other 'allergic' diseases such as rhinitis and eczema, but this assumption is being increasingly questioned. This chapter focuses on asthma, although we occasionally consider studies of rhinitis or eczema in considering the issue of whether asthma is predominantly an allergic disease. We focus on asthma in the general population, but also specifically consider occupational asthma in some instances, since this often provides a useful model in which individual exposures can be better identified (Cullinan and Newman Taylor 1999). Definitions, possible mechanisms, time trends, and population patterns of prevalence are initially considered, followed by evidence regarding primary and secondary causes of asthma. We then discuss the causes of asthma mortality.

Definition

The definition of asthma has become more complex as the understanding of its pathophysiology has increased. However, despite this increased complexity, the basic characteristic features of reversible airflow obstruction by which one recognizes or diagnoses the disease, has changed little over recent years. In this sense, asthma could be regarded as a 'condition' or 'syndrome' rather than a disease (Gergen and Weiss 1995) and it is perhaps most useful to define asthma in terms of the phenomena involved without making any aetiological implications (Gross 1980). The definition initially proposed at the Ciba Foundation Conference in 1959 (Ciba Foundation Guest Symposium 1959) and endorsed by the American Thoracic Society in 1962 (ATS 1962) is that 'asthma is a disease characterized by wide variation over short periods of time in resistance to flow in the airways of the lung'. Although these features receive lesser prominence in some current definitions, as the importance of airways inflammation is appropriately recognized, they still form the basis of the World Health Organization/National Heart, Lung and Blood Institute definition (GINA 1994) of asthma as:

> ... a chronic inflammatory disorder of the airways in which many cells play a role, in particular mast cells, eosinophils and T lymphocytes. In susceptible individuals this inflammation causes recurrent episodes of wheezing, breathlessness, chest tightness and cough, particularly at night and/or in the early morning. These symptoms are usually associated with widespread but variable airflow limitation and are at least partly reversible either spontaneously or with treatment. The inflammation also causes an associated increase in airway responsiveness to a variety of stimuli.

These three components—chronic airways inflammation, reversible airflow obstruction, and enhanced bronchial reactivity—form the basis of current definitions of asthma. They also represent the major pathophysiological events leading to the symptoms of wheezing, breathlessness, chest tightness, cough, and sputum by which doctors clinically diagnose this disorder.

Clinical asthma

There is no single test or pathognomonic feature which defines the presence or absence of asthma. Furthermore, the variability of the condition means that evidence of it may or may not be present on the day, or at the time someone is assessed. Thus, a diagnosis of asthma is made on the basis of combined information from history, physical examination, and respiratory function tests, often over a period of time. Several studies have found the prevalence of doctor-diagnosed asthma to be substantially lower than the prevalence of asthma symptoms in the community (Pearce *et al.* 1993). This is not surprising since a clinical diagnosis of asthma can only be made if a person presents themselves to a doctor; this requires an initial self-assessment of their symptoms (in terms of severity and frequency) as well as access to a doctor once a self-assessment has been made. Several medical consultations may then be required. Thus, diagnosed asthma is a case definition that is dependent not only on morbidity, but also on patient perception of their symptoms, doctor practice, and the availability of health care.

Defining asthma in epidemiological surveys

A major problem of population-based epidemiological surveys of asthma prevalence is the difficulty of defining and diagnosing this condition. This means that comparisons of diagnosed asthma between populations are fraught with difficulty as the differences in diagnostic practice may be as great in magnitude as the real differences in asthma morbidity. It may be possible to address some of these issues by adopting common criteria for asthma diagnosis, and applying these uniformly in prevalence studies. However, for large-scale prevalence studies this is not practical, because of the need for repeated contacts between study participants and doctors.

Thus, asthma prevalence surveys usually focus on self-reported (or parental reported) 'asthma symptoms' rather than diagnosed asthma. Standardized questionnaires on asthma symptoms have therefore become the cornerstone of large studies of the prevalence of asthma (Anderson 1989). This approach allows a large number of participants to be surveyed without great cost, in a short time period. Wheezing, chest tightness, breathlessness, and coughing are all symptoms clinically associated with asthma, but epidemiological studies have shown that wheezing is the most important symptom for the identification of asthma (Lee *et al.* 1983; Gergen *et al.* 1988), and the majority of questionnaires are based on this symptom. However, it is only recently that standardized written and video symptom questionnaires have been developed (see below).

An alternative approach to symptom questionnaires has been to use more 'objective' measures such as bronchial responsiveness testing, either alone or in combination with questionnaires. In particular, it has been suggested that asthma in epidemiological studies should be defined as symptomatic bronchial hyper-responsiveness (Toelle *et al.* 1992). However, although bronchial hyper-responsiveness is clearly related to asthma, and may be involved in many of the pathways by which variable airflow obstruction may occur, variable airflow obstruction may occur independently of bronchial hyper-responsiveness, and vice versa (Pearce *et al.* 1998). Thus, they remain separate phenomena which both involve inflammation of the airways (Chung 1986), and which are both worthy of study in their own right. In fact, available evidence from random population surveys indicates that bronchial hyper-responsiveness (or the combination of bronchial hyper-responsiveness and symptoms) is inferior to symptom questionnaires when compared with the 'gold standard' of a careful clinical diagnosis of asthma (Pekkanen and Pearce 1999). Thus, the method of choice for the first phase of prevalence comparisons is standardized written or video symptom questionnaires (Pearce *et al.* 2000*a*).

Allergy, atopy, and asthma

As noted above, asthma is often described as an allergic disease and grouped together with other 'allergic diseases' such as rhinitis and eczema. This assumption is increasingly being challenged (Pearce *et al.* 1999), and there is growing interest in non-allergic mechanisms for asthma. We therefore first define and discuss allergy and atopy, before considering the evidence that asthma is a predominantly allergic disease. Finally, we discuss non-allergic mechanisms for asthma.

Respiratory allergy

Allergy can be defined as adverse acute or chronic hypersensitivity reactions resulting from immunologic sensitization with production of immunoglobulin E (IgE) against a specific agent (component) or allergen (Schenker *et al.* 1998). Thus, the term 'allergy' refers to symptomatic conditions (asthma, rhinitis, etc.), whereas the term 'sensitization' refers to an individual's immune status assessed by *in vivo* or *in vitro* diagnostic tests. Symptoms can be induced by inhalation of allergens, even at very low concentrations. Individuals who are not sensitized to these allergens will usually not show symptoms even at very high exposure concentrations. Symptoms are caused by inflammatory reactions initiated by allergen-specific IgE antibodies present in the airways, which are only present in substantial amounts in sensitized subjects, and have been produced during a preceding specific immune response to the allergen exposure. Only a proportion of sensitized subjects show symptoms and are thus also allergic. It can take weeks to years between first encounter with an allergen and the development of an allergy.

Allergic asthma is caused by type I IgE-mediated mechanisms in which mast cells, eosinophils, and T lymphocytes play a key role. Exposure to aeroallergens results in specific IgE sensitization in only part of the population (mainly atopic subjects, see below) which can subsequently lead to respiratory symptoms on re-exposure via complex inflammatory mechanisms. Once allergic, a subject can develop symptoms minutes after being exposed. This is known as the early-phase allergic reaction and symptoms develop as a result of mast cell degranulation and release of inflammatory mediators (through allergen–IgE antibody complexes at the surface of the mast cells), causing contraction of bronchial smooth muscle and oedema in the airways. Clinically, this results in a decreased lung function and symptoms of wheeze, shortness of breath, chest tightness, and coughing. During the late phase of the allergic reaction (4 to 8 h after exposure), eosinophil-related inflammatory reactions are particularly important. This reaction is most likely induced by mediators released during the early phase of the allergic reaction and is characterized by the development of a non-specific bronchial hyper-reactivity that can continue to exist for several days. Repeated exposures can result in a more permanent bronchial hyper-reactivity. However, many asthmatics only experience an early phase allergic reaction which is not followed by a late phase reaction, although the reasons for this are unclear.

Atopy

'Atopy' (allergic sensitization) is a common term for type I (IgE-mediated) sensitization and/or type I allergic reactions. In population studies the term 'atopy' is used to indicate the predisposition of individuals to produce increased levels of specific or total IgE after exposure to 'common allergens' such as house dust mite, pet, and various food allergens. In the past, atopy has often been defined on the basis of a family history of asthma, eczema, or other 'allergic diseases'. However, it is now usually assessed by using skin prick tests or specific and/or total serum IgE against common allergens, and it can therefore be defined either in terms of skin prick test positivity or elevated serum IgE levels (Pearce *et al.* 1999). Depending on the definition, 20 to 40 per cent of people living in affluent countries are atopic. In population studies atopy is often associated with an increased risk of airway symptoms associated with conditions such as asthma (Pearce *et al.* 1999). However, in occupational environments subjects may develop specific sensitization and allergies without being atopic.

Aeroallergens

Many macromolecules (particularly proteins) of non-human origin, including those of animals (arthropod proteins, animal danders, proteins in excretia), plants (pollens, latex dust), and micro-organisms (spores of fungi such as *Aspergillus*, *Penicillium*, or from thermophilic bacteria such as *Thermoactinomycetes vulgaris*), can act as allergens by inducing a specific IgE response and provoke allergic reactions in sensitized subjects (Schenker *et al.* 1998). Most studies on indoor allergens report on allergens from house dust mites (particularly *Dermatophagoides pteronyssinus* and *D. farinae*), cats, and dogs. Allergens in the occupational environment can range from cow urinary proteins in farming situations to fungal enzymes in the biotechnology and bakery industry. Low molecular weight allergens such as plicatic acid (in wood dust from western red cedar) and chemical components such as di-isocyanates (e.g. toluene di-isocyanate) can also cause occupational asthma, and although type I allergic reactions are suspected, the specific immunological mechanisms have not yet been resolved (Raulf-Heimsoth and Baur 1998)

Is asthma an allergic disease?

In the last two decades, asthma has increasingly been regarded as an allergic disease involving allergen sensitization (atopy). A theoretical paradigm has evolved in which it is believed that the fundamental aetiological mechanism is that allergen exposure, particularly in infancy, produces atopic sensitization and that continued exposure results in asthma through the development of airways inflammation, which leads to bronchial hyper-responsiveness and reversible airflow obstruction. As Martinez (1997) notes, this paradigm has been used with particular insistence with regards to house dust mite allergens (Peat *et al.* 1996; Platts-Mills *et al.* 1997*b*), but other allergens (cat, cockroach, dog) are also believed to be important. The importance of atopy is most widely accepted for asthma in children, whereas among adults, asthma has traditionally been divided into 'extrinsic' and 'intrinsic' asthma, although this also has been challenged (Burrows *et al.* 1989). It is acknowledged that not all cases of asthma fit this paradigm, for example some occupational causes of asthma do not appear to involve atopy, but these are regarded as interesting minor anomalies that do not threaten the dominant paradigm.

However, a recent systematic review of population-based studies has shown that the proportion of asthma cases that are attributable to atopy (defined as skin prick test positivity) is usually less than half (Pearce *et al.* 1999) (Table 1). Higher estimates (up to two-thirds) can be obtained by using very low cut-off levels of total serum IgE, but these should be interpreted with caustion since such a definition of atopy has limited practical use, and these associations may not always be causal. In this respect, Martinez (1998) questions whether the association of atopy with asthma is entirely causal, on the basis that the development of sensitization after 8 years is not associated with an increased asthma risk, whereas if the association of sensitization and asthma was causal, one would not expect the age at which sensitization occurs to be of major importance.

Non-allergic mechanisms

There is increasing interest in non-allergic mechanisms for asthma. To date there have been few studies of non-allergic mechanisms for asthma in the home environment, due to the difficulties of separating the effects of exposure to allergens (e.g. house dust mite allergen) and other asthma risk factors (e.g. endotoxins) (Michel *et al.* 1991, 1992). However, there have been a large number of studies of non-allergic asthma in the occupational environment, where it is more feasible to identify individual exposures. For instance, in many occupational environments where workers are exposed to organic dust (e.g. farmers, grainworkers, etc.) the majority of asthma and rhinitis cases are non IgE-mediated, and are related to chronic exposure to environmental irritants; only a minority of cases are those of an IgE-based specific antigen–antibody reaction in atopic individuals (Von Essen and Donham 1997). The underlying inflammatory responses are often directed against constituents of bacteria and fungi, but can also be directed against certain plant products. These agents usually interact with specific receptors on inflammatory and other cells. Macrophages and neutrophils (in contrast to eosinophils in allergic respiratory diseases) may be the key inflammatory cells, and the complement system is believed to also be involved. Both mechanisms are part of the immune response to foreign agents (particularly micro-organisms) in order to protect the host from infections.

In the occupational literature, the terms 'asthma' and 'asthma-like disorders' are often used referring to variable airflow limitations with allergic (IgE mediated) and non-allergic underlying mechanisms, respectively. In practice it is not always easy to make a distinction between these disease mechanisms, since the symptoms are often very similar (shortness of breath, wheezing, acute cross shift decrease in lung function, etc.) and the specific pathology is usually unknown or at best only poorly characterized.

Asthma can also be caused by accidental occupational exposures to high concentrations of certain chemicals such as uranium, hexafluoride and ammonia. Peak exposures cause toxic and irritative effects resulting in airway obstruction. These non-allergic forms of asthma that are quite common in the occupational environment are believed to be of little importance in explaining asthma prevalence in the general population; this may in part relate to the lack of recognition of these disorders.

Time trends

It has long been suspected that the prevalence of asthma has been increasing not only in industrialized countries, but also in developing

Table 1 Summary of nine population-based studies in children and seven population-based studies in adults: proportions of asthmatics and non-asthmatics who are atopic and percentage of asthma cases attributable to atopy

	Atopic non-asthmatics (%)	Atopic asthmatics (%)	Pooled relative risk	Cases attributable to atopy (%)
Children	29	58	3.4	38
Adults	24	54	3.7	37

Source: adapted from Pearce *et al.* (1999).

countries (Burr 1987; Anderson 1989; Weitzman *et al.* 1992; Anderson *et al.* 1994; Balfe *et al.* 1996). However, this has been a particularly difficult issue to resolve because of the lack of systematic standardized studies measuring changes in asthma prevalence over time, and some reviewers have argued that the increases in reported prevalence are largely due to increased awareness, labelling, and diagnosis of asthma symptoms (Magnus and Jaakkola 1997). Nevertheless, most studies which have determined the prevalence of asthma symptoms using the same methodology in the same community at different times, have reported that asthma prevalence has increased in recent decades and that the magnitude of the increase has in some cases been substantial (Table 2). Although methodological differences in these studies make it difficult to compare the magnitude of the differences in asthma prevalence between countries, the trend of increasing prevalence amongst populations in countries of widely differing lifestyles and ethnic groups is generally consistent. In some of these studies the prevalence of other 'atopic disorders' has also increased in parallel. For example, Hsieh and Shen (1991) examined the prevalence of allergic disorders in schoolchildren aged 7 to 15 years in Taipei, Taiwan, and found that the prevalence of childhood asthma increased from 1.3 per cent in 1974 to 5.1 per cent in 1985 and 5.8 per cent in 1991. There were similar two- to three-fold increases in the prevalence of allergic rhinitis, eczema, and urticaria, but these occurred after the increase in asthma prevalence.

One of the most informative studies to date is that of Haahtela *et al.* (1990) who analysed the medical examination reports of approximately 900 000 conscripts to the Finnish defence forces from 1966 to 1989, and a proportional but unknown number examined in 1926 to 1961. During 1926 to 1961, the prevalence of asthma recorded at call-up examinations was in the range of 0.02 to 0.08 per cent. However, asthma prevalence increased from 0.29 per cent in 1966 to 1.79 per cent in 1989. The authors concluded that the increase was unlikely to be due to improved diagnostic methods, and that much of the increase was likely to be real. This conclusion was strengthened by a concomitant rise (from 0.12 per cent in 1966 to 0.75 per cent in 1989) in exemptions and discharges due to asthma. This study is consistent with other evidence that the increases in asthma prevalence in industrialized countries appear to have commenced after the Second World War, and particularly in the 1960s and 1970s (Burney *et al.* 1990; Woolcock and Peat 1997).

International prevalence comparisons

The causes of the international increases in the prevalence of asthma are unclear, and are currently a major focus for asthma epidemiology worldwide. An important component of this research process involves standardized international prevalence comparisons (Pearce *et al.* 1997). The key problem in this regard is to gain information on the largest possible number of people in random samples collected in a comparable manner across social groups, regions, and countries. Thus, comparisons of asthma prevalence are increasingly being based on a simple comparison of symptom prevalence in a questionnaire survey in a large number of people (phase I), followed by more intensive testing of factors related to asthma (e.g. bronchial hyperresponsiveness) and risk factors for asthma (skin prick test positivity, serum IgE, and other exposures) in a subsample (phase II). This approach is being used in the international survey of asthma prevalence in adults, the European Community Respiratory Health Survey (**ECRHS**) (Burney *et al.* 1994), and the International Study of Asthma and Allergies in Childhood (**ISAAC**) (Pearce *et al.* 1993; Asher *et al.* 1995).

The European Community Respiratory Health Survey

In each centre of the ECRHS, a representative sample of 3000 adults, aged 20 to 44 years, completed a phase I screening questionnaire seeking information on asthma symptoms and medication use (Burney *et al.* 1994). Individuals answering 'yes' to waking with an attack of shortness of breath, an attack of asthma, or current asthma medications were defined as 'asthmatic'. A random subsample of 600 subjects and an additional sample of up to 150 'asthmatic' individuals were then studied in more detail in phase II, with measurements of skin prick test to common allergens, serum total and specific IgE, bronchial responsiveness to inhaled methacholine, and urine electrolytes, as well as an additional questionnaire on asthma symptoms and medical history, occupation and social status, smoking, the home environment, and the use of medications and medical services. The phase I results (ECRHS 1996) include data from 48 centres, predominantly in Western Europe, with only nine centres from six countries (Algeria, Iceland, India, New Zealand, Australia, and the United States) being from outside Europe. Phase II was conducted in 37 centres in 16 countries (ECRHS 1997).

The International Study of Asthma and Allergies in Childhood

ISAAC (Asher *et al.* 1995) had a similar study design to that of the ECRHS study, with a simple phase I survey and a more in-depth phase II survey. However, the emphasis was on obtaining the maximum possible participation across the world in order to obtain a global overview of asthma prevalence in children (similar to that obtained for cancer in the Cancer Incidence in Five Continents Study; Doll *et al.* 1966). For this reason, phase I (which was conducted in 155 centres in 56 countries) was separated from phase II (which is currently being conducted in a smaller number of centres), and the phase I questionnaire modules were designed to be simple and to require minimal resources to administer. In addition, a video questionnaire involving the audiovisual presentation of clinical signs and symptoms of asthma was developed (Shaw *et al.* 1995) in order to minimize translation problems. The population of interest is schoolchildren aged 6 to 7 years and 13 to 14 years within specified geographical areas. The older age group was chosen to reflect the period when morbidity from asthma is common and to enable the use of self-completed questionnaires. The younger age group was chosen to give a reflection of the early childhood years, and involves parent completion of questionnaires. The phase I findings, involving more than 700 000 children, showed striking international differences in asthma symptom prevalence (ISAAC 1998*a*, *b*). Figure 1 shows the international patterns of 12-month period prevalence of wheezing in 13 to 14 year olds (based on the question 'Have you had wheezing or whistling in the chest *in the last 12 months*?').

What do the ECRHS and ISAAC studies show?

The ISAAC and ECRHS studies provide, for the first time, a picture of global patterns of asthma prevalence, and identify the key phenomena which future research must address and attempt to explain.

Table 2 Changes in asthma prevalence in children and young adults

Country	Period	Asthma prevalence		Reference
		First study	Second study	
Australia	1964–1990	19.1%	46.0%	Robertson *et al.* (1991)
	1982–1992	12.9%	19.3%	Peat *et al.* (1994)
	1987–1992	5.6%	9.3%	Campbell *et al.* (1992), Adams *et al.* (1997)
	1992–1995	9.3%	11.4%	Adams *et al.* (1997)
Canada	1980–1983	3.8%	6.5%	Infante-Rivard *et al.* (1987)
	1980–1990	140/10 000	256/10 000[a]	Manfreda *et al.* (1993)
		125/10 000	254/10 000[b]	
England	1956–1975	1.8%	6.3%	Morrison Smith (1976)
	1966–1990	18.3%	21.8%	Whincup *et al.* (1993)
	1973–1986	2.4%	3.6%	Burney *et al.* (1990)
	1978–1991	11.1%	12.8%	Anderson *et al.* (1994)
England and Wales	1970–1981	11.6%	20.5%[a]	Fleming and Crombie (1987)
		8.8%	15.9%[b]	
Finland	1961–1986	0.1%	1.8%	Haahtela *et al.* (1990)
France	1968–1982	3.3%	5.4%	Perdrizet *et al.* (1987)
Germany	1991/2–1995/6	3.7%	4.1%	Von Mutius *et al.* (1998)
Israel	1986–1990	7.9%	9.6%	Auerbach *et al.* (1993)
Italy	1983–1993/5	2.9%	4.4%	Ciprandi *et al.* (1996)
Japan	1982–1992	3.3%	4.6%	Nishima (1993)
New Zealand	1969–1982	7.1%	13.5%	Mitchell (1983)
	1975–1989	26.2%	34.0%	Shaw *et al.* (1990)
Papua New Guinea	1973–1984	0.0%	0.6%	Dowse *et al.* (1985)
Scotland	1964–1989	10.4%	19.8%	Ninan and Russell (1992)
	1989–1994	19.8%	25.4%	Omran and Russell (1996)
Sweden	1971–1981	1.9%	2.8%	Åberg (1989)
	1979–1999	2.5%	5.7%	Åberg *et al.* (1999)
Tahiti	1979–1984	11.5%	14.3%	Liard *et al.* (1988)
Taiwan	1974–1985	1.3%	5.1%	Hsieh *et al.* (1988)
USA	1964–1983	183/100 000	284/100 000	Yunginger *et al.* (1992)
	1971–1976	4.8%	7.6%	Gergen *et al.* (1988)
	1981–1988	3.1%	4.3%	Weitzman *et al.* (1992)
	1983–1992	9.2%	15.9%	Farber *et al.* (1997)
Wales	1973–1988	4.0%	9.0%	Burr *et al.* (1989)

[a]Men and [b]women, prevalence rates per 10 000 subjects, incidence rates per 100 000 subjects.

Firstly, both studies show a particularly high prevalence of reported asthma symptoms in English-speaking countries (Fig. 1), i.e. the British Isles, New Zealand, Australia, the United States, and Canada (ECRHS 1996; ISAAC 1998*a*). This appears to be unlikely to be entirely due to translation problems, since the same pattern was observed with the ISAAC video questionnaire (ISAAC 1998*a*).

Secondly, the ISAAC survey showed that centres in Latin America also had particularly high symptom prevalence (Fig. 1). This finding is of particular interest in that the Spanish-speaking centres of Latin America showed higher prevalences than Spain itself, in contrast to the general tendency for more affluent countries to have higher prevalence rates.

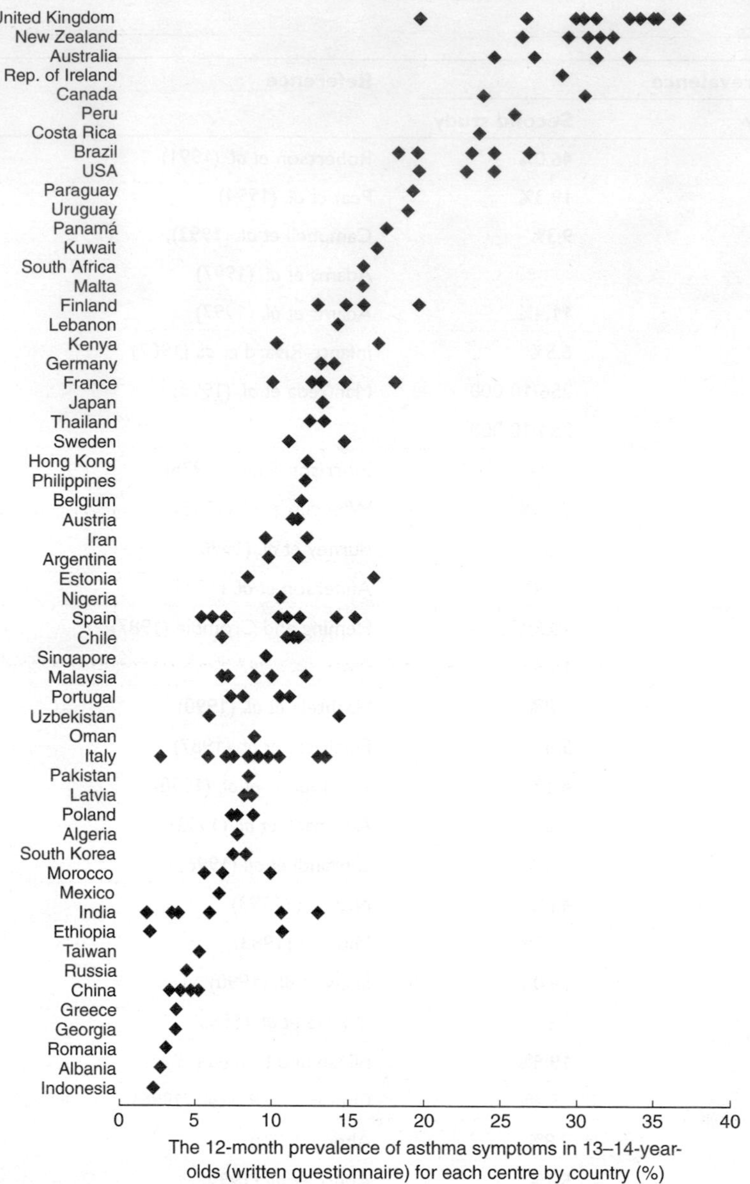

Fig. 1 Wheeze in the previous 12 months for each centre by country ordered according to the mean prevalence for all centres in the country (Source: ISAAC 1998*a*.)

Thirdly, amongst the non-English-speaking European countries, both studies show high asthma prevalence in Western Europe, with lower prevalences in Eastern and Southern Europe. For example, in the ISAAC survey, there is a clear northwest–southeast gradient within Europe, with the highest prevalence in the world being in the United Kingdom, and some of the lowest prevalences in Albania and Greece (ISAAC 1998*a*). The West–East gradient was particularly strong; in particular there was a significantly lower prevalence in the former East Germany than in the former West Germany.

Fourthly, Africa and Asia generally showed relatively low asthma prevalence (Fig. 1). In particular, prevalence was low in developing countries such as China and Indonesia whereas more affluent Asian countries such as Singapore and Japan showed relatively high asthma prevalence rates. Perhaps the most striking contrast is between Hong Kong and Guangzhou which are close geographically, and involve the same language and predominant ethnic group; Hong Kong (the more affluent city) had a 12-month period prevalence of wheeze of 10.1 per cent, compared with 2.0 per cent in Guangzhou (the less affluent city).

Fifthly, in contrast to the asthma findings, the highest prevalences of rhinitis symptoms were reported from centres scattered throughout most regions of the world, including Western Europe, Africa, North America, and South-East Asia; the highest prevalences of eczema were generally in centres of high latitude, including Scandinavia and New Zealand, although there were some notable exceptions including some centres in South America and Africa (Ethiopia). Thus, although the prevalences of these conditions were correlated, the association was not particularly strong and there were numerous centres which had high prevalence for asthma but not for rhinitis and/or eczema, and vice versa. For example, none of the 10 centres with the highest prevalence of rhinitis symptoms (including several centres in France) were represented amongst the highest 10 centres for asthma symptoms, suggesting that the major risk factors are different for these related disorders, or that they involve different latency periods and time trends.

'Established' risk factors

These striking findings from the ISAAC and ECRHS surveys, together with recent studies within Western countries, are challenging established theories of the development of asthma, and facilitating the search for new theoretical paradigms. In this section we review current evidence on 'established' risk factors for asthma. We then consider whether these 'established' risk factors can explain the international patterns and time trends.

Atopy

As noted above, atopy (measured by skin prick test positivity) is a clearly established 'risk factor' for asthma, and there is a strong association within populations, although the proportion of asthma cases that are attributable to atopy is less than half (Pearce *et al.* 1999). Furthermore, although atopy is a 'risk factor' for asthma, it is not a classic environmental 'exposure' (e.g. indoor allergen exposure, smoking, air pollution) which could by itself explain increases in asthma prevalence. Rather it represents a biological response to various exposures (e.g. allergen exposure) which is modified by susceptibility factors (genetic or environmental).

Genetic factors

Asthma appears to be multifactorial in origin and influenced by multiple genes and environmental factors (Panhuysen *et al.* 1995; CSGA 1997). Thus, it is not inherited in the simple Mendelian fashion that is characteristic of single-gene disorders. A particular genetic factor may effect one or more aspects of the complex aetiological process involved in asthma, but whether this genetic potential is expressed will depend on various factors, including whether sufficient exposure to environmental factors occurs. Furthermore, some non-allergic forms of asthma apparently may have no genetic basis at all (Sandford *et al.* 1996). Investigating possible genes for atopy or bronchial hyper-responsiveness), the underlying immunological and physiological components which often characterize clinical asthma is also fraught with difficulties, as control of both IgE production and bronchial hyper-responsiveness are also multifactorial (Zamel *et al.* 1996), and neither is synonymous with asthma.

It is well established that people with a family history of asthma are more likely to develop asthma themselves (Horwood *et al.* 1985), and parental asthma is a stronger predictor of asthma in the offspring than parental atopy (Von Mutius and Nicolai 1996). However, this association is not necessarily due to genetic factors, and could merely reflect similar lifestyles and exposures in family members (Sandford *et al.* 1996). For example one study found that persons whose spouse developed asthma were also more likely to develop asthma (Smith and Knowles 1967), presumably due to common environmental exposures.

Some indication of the possible contribution of genetic factors in asthma is given by studies of twins. For example, Edfors-Lubs (1971) analysed data on 7000 twin pairs from the Swedish Twin Register and found that concordance of asthma in monozygotic twins was greater than in dizygotic twins. However, the concordance was still only 19 per cent, and even this may in part be due to similar environmental exposures in monozygotic twins, including a common intrauterine environment (Godfrey *et al.* 1994). Other large population studies have yielded similar findings, but this may be because these studies have determined asthma on the basis of questionnaires or hospital and pharmacy records, whereas smaller studies with more intensive diagnostic methods have generally yielded higher concordance (Sandford *et al.* 1996).

Attention has particularly focused on chromosomes 5 and 11, both of which may contain genes relevant to asthma and atopy (Doull *et al.* 1996). However, studies investigating linkage to candidate loci have been affected by bias introduced through the methods of acquiring the probands, the broad and variable definitions of atopy, the assumption of a simple Mendelian pattern of inheritance, and the lack of appreciation of antigen-specific factors such as HLA D encoded immune responses. As a result, as with many genetic studies of other major disorders, there have been problems of failing to replicate reported genetic linkage in atopy, for example in the major 'atopy gene' located on 11q13 (Cookson *et al.* 1989, 1993; Morton 1992; Van Herwerden *et al.* 1995).

Demographic factors

There are a variety of demographic factors which are associated with asthma including age (Anderson *et al.* 1992), gender (Anderson *et al.* 1992), and ethnicity (Cunningham *et al.* 1996). Age is the demographic factor which is most strongly related to asthma symptom prevalence with symptoms usually declining at or before the onset of puberty (Balfour-Lynn 1985; Silverman 1995).

The gender differences in asthma prevalence and severity are not large, and asthma is generally an important cause of morbidity in both females and males (Kimbell-Dunn *et al.*, in press). Nevertheless, there is consistent evidence that asthma incidence and prevalence is consistently lower in females than in males before the age of 12 years, whereas during adolescence and adulthood there is evidence of higher incidence and prevalence in females. One possible explanation for the lower incidence and prevalence in females in young children is that the average age of onset in childhood and adolescence may be later in females. For example, Horwood *et al.* (1985) have suggested that much of childhood asthma is a genetically inherited tendency and that the age of expression is later for girls than for boys. Levels of cord blood IgE are lower at birth in girls than in boys (Weeke 1992), indicating a lower risk of the subsequent development of asthma. Some authors have noted that boys have smaller airways relative to lung size than girls, and that this may explain the greater frequency and severity of lower respiratory tract illness in boys, even though infection rates are similar for both sexes (Martinez *et al.* 1988). Alternatively, it is possible that boys have more exposure to factors that increase asthma incidence or duration. Conversely, the relatively higher prevalence (or smaller reduction in prevalence) in females than in males after puberty could be due to hormonal influences on allergic predisposition, airway size, inflammation, and smooth muscle vascular functions (Rubio *et al.* 1988; Redline and Gold 1994). Premenstrual asthma may be especially relevant to the hormonal involvement of asthma since it may not only cause asthma exacerbations but may thereby affect the frequency and duration of asthma symptoms, resulting in an increase in the prevalence of 'current asthma'.

Studies in the 1960s and 1970s (Mitchell and Dawson 1973) suggested that asthma is more common in children in the higher social classes. There has been less evidence of social class differences as the diagnosis of asthma has become more widespread (Littlejohns and MacDonald 1993), even though diagnostic labelling of wheezing in adults differs by social class (Littlejohns *et al.* 1989). However, severe asthma appears to be more common in children in the lower social classes (Mielke *et al.* 1996) and in some disadvantaged ethnic groups (Pomare *et al.* 1992), and low socio-economic status is associated with hospital admissions for asthma (Watson *et al.* 1996) and with reduced lung function in adults (Steinberg and Becklake 1986). This could represent either a greater prevalence of asthma in disadvantaged groups, or increased severity due to environmental factors (e.g. environmental tobacco smoke, nutrition) or inadequate disease management and poor access to health care (Pomare *et al.* 1992; Littlejohn and MacDonald 1993).

Outdoor air pollution

The role of outdoor air pollutants in asthma and other diseases has been extensively studied and debated (Barnes 1994; Bascom *et al.* 1996). 'Conventional' air pollution includes SO_2 and airborne particulates with a size of 10 μm or less which can be inhaled into the lung. More recently, attention has focused on NO_2 as the concentration of this chemical has risen in recent decades due to increasing motor vehicle use. An association between traffic density on residential streets and asthma symptoms has been found in studies in Germany (Duhme *et al.* 1996), Sweden (Pershagen *et al.* 1995), and The Netherlands (Oosterlee *et al.* 1995), but not in the United Kingdom (Livingstone *et al.* 1996). Overall, it is clear that air pollution can provoke exacerbations in pre-existing asthma, but the weight of evidence (Barnes 1994; Bascom *et al.* 1996) does not support a major role for outdoor air pollution as a cause of the initial development of asthma (Pearce *et al.* 1998). Indeed there is a negative association between outdoor air pollution and asthma prevalence at the population level (ISAAC 1998*a*).

Tobacco

Similarly, the evidence for a role of tobacco smoke in asthma is strongest for increases in severity in children who already have asthma (NRC 1986), whereas the evidence for the initial occurrence of asthma (incidence) is much less conclusive (Chen *et al.* 1996). Nevertheless, tobacco exposure, particularly *in utero* and in infancy may enhance sensitization. Overall, it appears that environmental tobacco smoke may be a cofactor provoking attacks of wheezing, rather than an underlying cause of asthma (Strachan and Cook 1998).

Indoor air pollution

Little is currently known about the contribution of indoor air pollutants (other than environmental tobacco smoke) to the incidence and prevalence of asthma. The range of potential pollutants is large, the determinants of ambient levels involve a complex interaction of lifestyle and building factors, and precise measurement of airborne or respirable concentrations is difficult. In addition, indoor air pollution may arise from both indoor and outdoor sources (Brauer *et al.* 1989). Nitrogen dioxide from burning fossil fuels has received by far the most attention (Florey *et al.* 1979; Dodge 1982; Dijkstra *et al.* 1990; Neas *et al.* 1991) while sulphur dioxide from burning sulphur-containing coal or gas, mosquito coil smoke (Koo and Ho 1994), and formaldehyde from wood preparation (Marbury and Kriegler 1991) have also been considered. Particulates from open or closed wood and coal-burning fires have received less attention in developed countries (Osbourne and Honicky 1986; Dockery 1987), but have been studied in developing countries where very high indoor levels have been encountered (Anderson 1974, 1979).

Non-infectious microbial exposure

Indoor exposure to airborne micro-organisms and microbial agents, both in the residential and occupational environment, is widely recognized as a possible cause of acute and chronic non-infectious respiratory diseases such as asthma, rhinitis, bronchitis, and extrinsic allergic alveolitis.

Several population-based studies have suggested that allergic or non-allergic inflammatory reactions to inhaled fungal components, together with reactions to house dust mites, might account for the frequently reported association between living in damp housing conditions and respiratory disorders (Brunekreef *et al.* 1989; Dales *et al.* 1991; Jaakkola *et al.* 1993; Andriessen *et al.* 1998; Peat *et al.* 1998). However, although a role in secondary causation of asthma is likely, it is not clear whether non-infectious microbial exposure plays a role in primary causation.

Several studies have also suggested a role for bacterial exposure and exposure to certain bacterial components such as endotoxins. Studies of Michel *et al.* (1991, 1992) have suggested that in the home environment, endotoxin in house dust may influence the clinical severity of asthma. One cross-sectional study performed in Belgium by the same authors showed that in 69 adult asthma patients the severity of asthma was related to endotoxin levels, but not with mite allergen concentration, measured in their house dust (Michel *et al.* 1996). In a Swedish case–control study (Björnsson *et al.* 1995), asthma-related symptoms were significantly associated not only with house dust mite exposure but also with exposure to bacteria, assessed with a so-called 'non-viable' microscopic counting method.

Occupational exposures

Occupational asthma is 'asthma that is caused, in whole or part, by agents encountered at work' (Burge 1995). Typically, the onset of occupational asthma may occur 1 to 3 years after initial exposure, although some exposures may induce occupational asthma in some workers in less than 1 month (Antó *et al.* 1996). There are now more than 200 known occupational causes of asthma, and asthma is the most common occupational respiratory disease in developed countries (Chan-Yeung 1995). For example, asthma was the most common disease category and accounted for 28 per cent of cases reported to the United Kingdom Surveillance of Work-related and Occupational Respiratory Diseases (**SWORD**) project (Meredith *et al.* 1991). Estimates of the proportion of adult asthma which is thought to be occupational in origin range from 2 to 15 per cent in the United States, 15 per cent in Japan (Chan-Yeung and Malo 1994), 5 per cent in Spain (Kogevinas *et al.* 1996), 2 to 3 per cent in New Zealand (Fishwick *et al.* 1997), and 2 to 6 per cent in the United Kingdom (Meredith and

Nordman 1996). Several studies have shown the importance of avoidance of exposure in occupational asthma (rather than improving asthma management while permitting exposure to continue), but occupational asthma can lead to permanent asthma even after removal from exposure (Burge 1982).

Viruses

Viral infections are a common cause of episodes of wheezing in infancy, predominantly in children with reduced lung function after birth. Most of these children become symptom free after the age of 5 years. A smaller group of children who wheeze as infants will still have wheezing episodes during the early school years. The factors that determine which infants become persistent wheezers are not well understood, but viral infections *per se* are likely to play a minor role (Martinez 1995). Viral infections are also a common cause of exacerbations of asthma and provoke episodes of wheezing in children and adults who already have the condition (Welliver *et al.* 1981; Stenius-Aarniala 1987; Johnston *et al.* 1995). In particular, there is a strong association between viral infections and hospital admission for asthma in both children and adults (Johnston *et al.* 1995).

In children under 5 years of age, respiratory syncytial virus and parainfluenza are the most common pathogens, whereas in older children and adults, rhinovirus and coronavirus which are responsible for the common cold are most commonly implicated (Pattemore *et al.* 1992; Johnston *et al.* 1995; Nicholson *et al.* 1993). Influenza may be associated with particularly severe exacerbations (Pattemore *et al.* 1992) and *Chlamydia pneumoniae* infection has recently been implicated in the pathogenesis of both acute exacerbations and chronic persistent asthma (Allegra *et al.* 1994; Emre *et al.* 1994; Hahn 1996). Viral respiratory tract infections are the most common cause of a severe attack of asthma in childhood, accounting for up to 80 per cent of exacerbations in children (Pattemore *et al.* 1992). They are less commonly associated with exacerbations of asthma in adults (Burney *et al.* 1989), although they may account for up to 40 per cent of severe exacerbations (Beasley *et al.* 1988; Nicholson *et al.* 1993).

House dust mites

Indoor allergens are perhaps the group of risk factors that have received the greatest attention, as a possible major cause of asthma. It is well established that in sensitized asthmatics, allergen exposure can trigger asthma attacks, and that prolonged exposure can lead to the prolongation and exacerbation of symptoms. However, most studies do not show clear associations between house dust mite exposure and symptoms, even when the analysis is restricted to atopic patients (Kuehr *et al.* 1995; Platts-Mills *et al.* 1995; Sporik *et al.* 1999; Vervloet *et al.* 1999), and secondary intervention trials have had mixed results (Gotzsche *et al.* 1998).

However, although there is some evidence for secondary causation, the evidence for primary causation is much weaker. The key study linking allergen exposure in infancy to the subsequent development of asthma is that of Sporik *et al.* (1990) who followed 67 children selected as being at risk because of a family history of atopy. They found an association between der p 1 levels and risk of house dust mite sensitization, but they do not report the findings for overall sensitization. There was an association between exposure to more than 10 μg/g in the first year of life and a history of wheezing, although this association was not statistically significant (odds ratio 2.3, 95 per cent confidence intervals 0.7–7.1, $p = 0.17$). There were marginally non-significant association with 'active wheezing and bronchial hyper-responsiveness' ($p = 0.08$) and with 'receiving medication' ($p = 0.10$). The claim for a primary causal role of house dust mite exposure in the development of asthma largely rests on this study, in which for the findings for asthma itself (rather than specific sensitization) were of marginal statistical significance.

One other longitudinal study by Burr *et al.* (1993) among 453 infants in South Wales with a family history of allergic diseases has been reported. Infants were followed up to the age of 7 years and house dust mite allergen levels in mattress and carpet dust were determined in the first and seventh year of life. The study involved an intervention examining the effect of withholding cow's milk protein during the first 3 months of life and replacing cow's milk with soya milk. No other interventions were employed. Doctor-diagnosed asthma and wheezing at age 7 years was not associated with mite allergen exposure as determined in the first 12 months nor with dust mite levels measured at 7 years of age (odds ratios were not given). Wheezing was also not associated with cat ownership. There were no differences in mite sensitization (determined by skin prick test) at age 7 years between low, moderate, and high mite allergen exposed children was observed (20, 20, and 22 per cent, respectively, when initial exposure was compared, and 19, 19, and 23 per cent when exposure at age 7 years was considered). Withholding cow's milk did not affect the incidence of allergy or wheezing, and it thus seems that the lack of association between house dust mite allergen exposure and asthma symptoms cannot be explained by confounding effects of the intervention.

Cross-sectional studies of asthma prevalence and current allergen exposure also do not show consistent associations. Furthermore, the problem with the interpretation of such studies is that asthma prevalence in a population reflects both asthma incidence and the average duration of the condition. Thus, a factor that prolongs or exacerbates asthma symptoms may thereby increase asthma prevalence even if it has no effect at all on asthma incidence. In any case, most studies in children show negative associations between allergen exposure and current asthma (Pearce *et al.* 2000*b*). However, a major concern in such cross-sectional studies is that allergen avoidance measures may have been adopted as a consequence of developing asthma. This possibility was examined in only a few studies, and these generally found slightly stronger risks when children whose parents had adopted allergen avoidance measures were excluded from the analysis (Verhoeff *et al.* 1995). However, the increase in odds ratios was very small and only noticeable when mite-sensitized cases were compared with non-sensitized controls or non-sensitized cases. Thus, even when allergen avoidance is accounted for, these studies do not suggest that allergen exposure is a major risk factor for childhood asthma.

Other allergens

There are several other indoor and outdoor allergens that have been suggested to be associated with specific atopic sensitization and the development of asthma including cat, dog, cockroach, and *Alternaria* allergens (Platts-Mills *et al.* 1997*a*). However, the evidence for a causal relationship is even weaker than for house dust mite allergens, and many of the studies found no associations or even negative associations between allergen exposure and asthma (Brunekreef *et al.* 1992;

Call *et al.* 1992; Platts-Mills *et al.* 1995). For pets this has often been explained by selection effects, i.e. that families with asthma and/or allergies tend to remove the pet from the home, which in cross-sectional studies may result in a lack of or even negative association (Brunekreef *et al.* 1992).

Recently several studies which have reported a protective effect of pet keeping early in life with regard to the subsequent development of asthma. For example, a recent case–control study in Sweden among 402 children aged between 12 and 13 years showed a strong negative association (odds ratio = 0.34, 95 per cent confidence intervals 0.07 to 0.77) between pet-keeping during the first year of life and asthma (Hesselmar *et al.* 1999). This association remained even after excluding children whose parents had decided against pet-keeping during early childhood because of allergy in the family. In addition, the authors showed that children exposed to cat during the first year of life were less likely to be skin prick test positive to cat allergen at age 12 to 13 years. Similarly, a recent study among 13 932 subjects aged 20 to 44 years from a large number of countries in Europe showed a protective effect of the presence of a dog in the home in childhood on atopy, even after adjusting for family history of allergies (odds ratio = 0.85, 95 per cent confidence intervals 0.77 to 0.94; Svanes *et al.* 1999). Besides other possible reasons such as a potential increased microbial pressure associated with pet ownership that could favour a non-allergic development of the immune system, it could be speculated that pet allergen exposure early in life may induce a specific tolerance which reduces the risk of subsequently becoming allergic or asthmatic. Clearly more studies are needed to elucidate further the role of allergen exposure early in life on the later development of allergies and asthma.

Can the 'established' risk factors explain the international patterns and time trends?

There is little evidence that the 'established' risk factors can account for the global prevalence increases, or the international prevalence patterns that have been observed.

The increases in asthma prevalence cannot be due to genetic factors, since they are occurring too rapidly, and the rapidity of the increases indicates that genetic factors alone are unlikely to account for a substantial proportion of asthma cases (Cullinan and Newman Taylor 1994), although genetic susceptibility to changing environmental exposures may play an important role.

Although the importance of atopy as a marker of asthma risk is well established, in terms of assessing the reasons for the global increases in asthma prevalence, it functions more as a potential intermediate variable which is relevant to the assessment of causal mechanisms, rather than as a primary causal exposure. In fact, standardized comparisons across populations or time periods show only weak and inconsistent associations between the prevalence of asthma and the prevalence of atopy (Pearce *et al.* 1999), and there is no consistent evidence that the increases in prevalence are predominantly occurring through mechanisms involving atopy. In fact, Martinez (1997) has suggested that the consistent associations between atopy and asthma, but the lack of consistent associations between allergen exposure and asthma, occurs because allergen exposure is not, in general, a primary cause of asthma. Rather, asthmatics have a non-specific predisposition to become sensitized to certain aeroallergens, and that this may contribute to the development of asthma symptoms, but sensitization would be the consequence rather than the cause of the asthmatic predisposition. In this situation, exposure to specific allergens, such as house dust mite allergen, would not affect the risk of sensitization or asthma; rather it would merely affect which specific allergens susceptible individuals became sensitized to, and therefore which specific allergens provoked exacerbations in current asthmatics.

The global patterns of asthma prevalence are also inconsistent with the hypothesis that air pollution is a major risk factor for the development of asthma (ISAAC 1998*a*). Regions such as China and Eastern Europe, where there are some of the highest levels of traditional air pollution such as particulate matter and SO_2, generally have lower asthma prevalence than the countries of Western Europe and North America, Australia, and New Zealand which have lower levels of pollution. For example, a study of the prevalence of asthma and atopy in two areas of West and East Germany (von Mutius *et al.* 1994) found that the lifetime prevalence of asthma diagnosed by a doctor, and the prevalence of reported wheezing was similar in the East and West German centres, despite the considerable difference in levels of particulate air pollution. It also appears very unlikely that the international prevalence patterns can be explained by differences in smoking (ISAAC 1998*a*), or in occupational exposures.

Allergen exposure is the risk factor that has perhaps received the most attention as a possible cause of the global increases in prevalence of asthma and allergies. In particular, it has been suggested that increases in indoor allergen exposures, through changes in lifestyle such as wall-to-wall carpeting, cold water washing, greater time spent indoors watching televisions, etc., could account for the global increases in asthma prevalence (Sporik *et al.* 1990; Platts-Mills *et al.* 1997*a*). The only study of English homes at two time points (1979 and 1989) did not demonstrate any change in house dust mite antigen levels (Butland *et al.* 1997), but marked increases have been observed in Australian studies (Peat *et al.* 1994).

The ISAAC (1998*a*) and the ECRHS (1996) studies have consistently found uniformly high levels of asthma prevalence in centres in English-speaking countries, even though there is a wide variation in house dust mite levels across these countries (Martinez 1997). In geographical areas in which house dust mite exposure is very low or absent, including desert regions (Peat *et al.* 1995; Halonen *et al.* 1997) and mountainous regions (Sporik *et al.* 1995), the prevalence of asthma is as high or even higher than that in other areas where house dust mite exposure is high (Martinez 1997). The study of Sporik *et al.* (1995) is particularly interesting in this regard since, in a mite-free environment, asthma prevalence was still high. Although there is weak evidence of lower asthma prevalence in high altitude regions with lower levels of house dust mite antigen (Charpin *et al.* 1988), and some evidence of reduced symptom frequency in asthmatics who move to high altitude regions (Spieksma *et al.* 1971), these studies have recently been reinterpreted with considerable caution (Carswell 1993).

Other available evidence on the association between allergen exposure and the subsequent risk of asthma at the population level is also less than persuasive. For example, Leung *et al.* (1997) reported that asthma prevalence was high in Hong Kong (6.6 per cent for asthma ever), and low in San Bu, China (1.6 per cent), but exposures to house dust mite allergen were similar in Hong Kong and San Bu. Similarly, Fig. 2 shows data from seven Australian surveys in centres

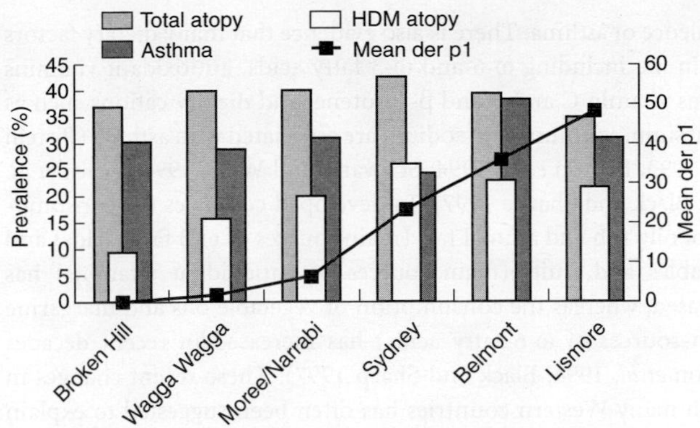

Fig. 2 Mean der p 1 levels and prevalence (per cent) of house dust mite atopy, total atopy, and asthma in six areas of Australia.

with widely differing levels of house dust mite allergen exposure; the overall prevalences of sensitization and asthma were both unrelated to the levels of house dust mite allergen (der p 1) exposure in the six centres. The dominant allergen varied between regions, but there was little overall difference in the prevalence of sensitization or of asthma despite the major differences in der p 1 levels. Similarly, Von Mutius *et al.* (1994) found that asthma was significantly higher in Munich, West Germany (5.9 per cent), than in Leipzig, East Germany (3.9 per cent), and this paralleled the pattern of skin prick test positivity (19.2 per cent and 7.3 per cent). However, house dust mite allergen levels in the East were similar to those in the West (Hirsch *et al.* 1998).

Towards a new paradigm

Thus, for many of the 'established' risk factors there is evidence that exposure causes asthma exacerbations (i.e. secondary causation), but there is little evidence of primary causation, and little evidence that these factors account for the global prevalence increases, or even for a substantial proportion of asthma cases within Western countries. In fact, these risk factors have become 'established' primarily on the basis of clinical studies and case reports of exacerbations in asthma patients. It is natural for doctors and patients to assume that the factors involved in secondary causation may also be important for primary causation. However, in most instances there is little evidence for this hypothesis, and when evidence has been sought (with the possible exception of the study by Sporik *et al.* (1990)) it has usually not been found.

As the 'established' asthma risk factors are increasingly being called into question, epidemiological studies are playing a major role in the search for new theoretical paradigms which are more consistent with the epidemiological evidence and which have greater explanatory power. Recent research has therefore shifted attention from allergens that may cause sensitization and/or provoke asthma attacks, to factors that may 'programme' the initial susceptibility to asthma, through allergic or non-allergic mechanisms.

With regard to allergic mechanisms, it has recently been proposed that the increase in asthma results from a shift in T-cell immunity in infancy and early childhood under influence of certain environmental factors (Holt 1995; Holt *et al.* 1997). Atopy is associated with a specific helper T 2 (T_h2) immune response typified by a production of various cytokines (such as interleukin 4 and 5 and several others) which promote IgE production and infiltration and activation of eosinophils. In contrast, non-atopic subjects mainly show Th1 immunity characterized by production of interferon-γ, that antagonizes the production of IgE antibodies by inhibiting the growth of T_h2 cells (Wierenga *et al.* 1990). Evidence is accumulating that the patterns of T-cell reactivity (T_h1 or T_h2) that determine the atopic/allergic immune responses in adulthood are established during infancy (Prescott *et al.* 1999). During fetal and perinatal life the immune system is strongly skewed in an atopic T_h2 direction (Holt and Macaubas 1997). Several events early in life may contribute to the shift from a mainly T_h2 into a mainly Th1 response. Particularly infections and other microbial exposures have been suggested to be involved (Holt *et al.* 1997; Björkstén 1999). In this regard it has been speculated that a more Westernized lifestyle (as has been adopted by many countries in which a sudden increase in asthma prevalence has been observed) has resulted in a reduced exposure early in life to these 'protecting' agents leading to a persistence of the perinatal T_h2 responses and subsequently in an increased prevalence of atopic diseases such as asthma.

The T_h1– T_h2 theory is consistent with the 'allergen hypothesis' in that it focuses on a role for atopic sensitization and allergen exposure, but it differs from the 'allergen hypothesis' in that it explains the increase in asthma prevalence in terms of an increase in susceptibility to become sensitized (because of reduced exposure to infections, etc.) and subsequently asthmatic (due to allergen exposure) rather than a change in allergen exposure levels.

Alternatively, Martinez (1997) has suggested that asthmatics have a non-specific predisposition to become sensitized to certain aeroallergens, and that this may contribute to the development of asthma symptoms, but that sensitization may be a consequence rather than the cause of the asthmatic predisposition. In particular, they note that the development of sensitization after 8 years of age is not associated with an increased asthma risk (Sherrill *et al.* 1999), whereas if the association of sensitization and asthma was causal, one would not expect the age at which sensitization occurs to be of major importance. Thus, Martinez suggests that sensitization is not important in primary causation (in contrast to the T_h1– T_h2 theory), but is rather the consequence (or a corollary) of having asthma. Thus, susceptible individuals may 'become sensitized' to those aeroallergens that the immune system 'sees' through the airway defence system very early during the process of developing asthma (Martinez 1998), and allergen exposures may primarily determine which allergens that susceptible persons became sensitized to without having any major primary causal role.

Whether or not a T_h1– T_h2 mechanism is involved, it is becoming increasingly clear that the 'package' of changes associated with increasing affluence and Westernization may be contributing to the global increases in asthma prevalence, and that this process involves an increase in asthma susceptibility rather than an increase in exposure to 'established' asthma risk factors. There are several key epidemiological findings that have contributed to this developing paradigm.

Firstly, there is increasing evidence that a small family size is associated with an increased risk of developing asthma (Shaw *et al.* 1994; Moyes *et al.* 1995; Wickens *et al.* 1999*a*). The reasons for this are unclear but the same relationship for atopy has been observed in several studies (Strachan 1989; Von Mutius *et al.* 1994; Matricardi *et al.* 1997; Olesen *et al.* 1997). The most commonly hypothesized explanation is that small family size could reduce infections in infancy and that this could in turn increase the risk of atopy and asthma at older ages (Martinez 1994). However, there is little direct evidence that this explains the family size effect (Wickens *et al.* 1999*a*). Furthermore, it is puzzling why attendance at child care early in life does not also confer a protective effect against asthma, although there is some evidence that early attendance protects against atopy in small families (Krämer *et al.* 1999). Certainly the negative association of asthma and atopy with family size is a major and consistent association which needs to be explained (Strachan 1997). This association is also consistent with international trends towards decreasing family size and increasing asthma prevalence, although changes in family size do not in themselves appear to explain a significant proportion of the asthma prevalence increase (Wickens *et al.* 1999*b*).

Secondly, irrespective of whether or not exposure to infections explains the negative family size association, there is other evidence that certain infections early in life protect against the subsequent development of asthma and atopy. In this respect, measles infections have been found to protect against atopy in Guinea-Bissau (Shaheen *et al.* 1996) and positive tuberculin responses have been found to protect against atopy in Japan (Shirakawa *et al.* 1997), and hepatitis A infections were found to protect against atopy in Italy (Matricardi *et al.* 1997).

Thirdly, it is also possible that medical interventions related to infections, such as immunization (Odent *et al.* 1994; Kemp *et al.* 1997) or antibiotic use (Farooqi and Hopkins 1998; Wickens *et al.* 1999*c*), may contribute to the development of asthma and/or atopy, whether through reducing clinical infections in infancy, or through their direct effects. The evidence for this is equivocal, and not all studies show positive associations, particularly for immunization (Wickens *et al.* 1999), but clearly these hypotheses warrant further investigation along with the possible protective effect of infections. In particular, the study of Farooqi and Hopkins (1998) is of interest since it found an association between antibiotic use in the first 2 years of life and the subsequent development of asthma, which was more marked with broad spectrum antibiotics and was observed irrespective of the indicate for treatment (respiratory tract infection or non-respiratory tract infection).

Fourthly, some recent studies have identified a relatively large size at birth as a risk factor for the subsequent development of asthma in adolescence (Fergusson *et al.* 1998; Leadbitter *et al.* 1999; Gregory *et al.* 1999). The reasons for this are unclear, but fetal growth apparently reflects a number of intrauterine influences, particularly relating to maternal diet and placental function. This is potentially a finding of major importance since anthropometric measures at birth increased during the twentieth century, although once again it is not clear that these trends would explain a significant proportion of the increase in prevalence.

Finally, there is epidemiological evidence that changes in diet may be associated with the increase in asthma. Food production, preferences, and availability have changed dramatically over the past few decades worldwide. In many countries this has resulted in a shift from a traditional diet to a more Westernized diet that differs in fat composition and micronutrient levels. The possible influence of diet (via the mother's diet) may already be important at the prenatal stage, and in the neonatal stage breast feeding may have a protective effect on the development of asthma (Peat and Li 1999). In this respect, the trend in recent decades for the introduction of cow's milk at a very early age to replace breast feeding may have contributed to the higher prevalence of asthma. There is also evidence that many dietary factors later in life including ω-6 and ω-3 fatty acids, antioxidant vitamins such as vitamin C and E and β-carotene, and dietary cations such as magnesium, selenium, and sodium are associated with asthma (Pistelli *et al.* 1993; Britton *et al.* 1994; Schwartz and Weiss 1994; Troisi *et al.* 1995; Black and Sharpe 1997). In developed countries the consumption of oily fish and animal fats (main sources of ω-3 fatty acids) and vegetables and fruits (main sources of antioxidant vitamins) has decreased, whereas the consumption of vegetable oils and margarine (main sources of ω-6 fatty acids) has increased in recent decades (Seaton *et al.* 1994; Black and Sharp 1997). These recent changes in diet in many Western countries has often been suggested to explain the increase in the prevalence of asthma (Seaton *et al.* 1994; Black and Sharp 1997). However, although some experimental evidence is available to support these hypotheses (particularly for the influence of linoleic acid [ω-6 fatty acids] and ω-3 fatty acids (Hwang 1989; Black and Sharp 1997), the evidence in most studies linking diet to asthma prevalence is circumstantial and not all studies show positive associations.

It seems that as a result of this 'package' of changes in the intrauterine and infant environment, we are seeing an increased susceptibility to the development of asthma and/or allergy. Understanding why this increased susceptibility is occurring, and ascertaining which elements of the 'package' of twentieth-century economic development and lifestyle changes are responsible (or whether the entire 'package' is more than the sum of its parts), represents a significant challenge, and a major opportunity, for asthma epidemiologists as we begin the next millenium.

Mortality

Asthma deaths are rare, and asthma prevalence and morbidity are generally of greater concern, and represent a greater population burden of disease, than asthma mortality. In fact, it was once held that 'the asthmatic pants into old age' (Osler 1901). However, asthma deaths do occur, and the patterns of asthma mortality became more complex in the latter half of the twentieth century. There were epidemics of asthma deaths in six countries in the 1960s, and again in New Zealand in the 1970s. These have been superimposed on a more gradual underlying increase in asthma mortality in many countries, which commenced in the 1940s and has been particularly marked in the 1980s, although mortality may be declining during the 1990s. In this section, we commence by briefly considering the long-term time trends in asthma mortality. We then discuss the role of asthma drugs in the mortality epidemics. Following this we consider the possible causes of the gradual rise in asthma mortality which has occurred more recently. Finally, we discuss epidemiological evidence for other risk factors for asthma mortality.

Time trends and the role of β-agonists

Almost all comparative studies of asthma mortality have been confined to the 5 to 34 year age group, because the diagnosis of asthma mortality is more firmly established in this group (Jackson *et al.* 1982; BTA 1984; Sears *et al.* 1986). The effects of changes in diagnostic fashion over time are difficult to quantify, although several attempts have been made by simultaneously examining time trends in other respiratory diseases which could be confused with asthma (Jackson

1993). In general, these exercises have found that changes in diagnostic fashion could not account for the most striking time trends (such as the 1960s mortality epidemics), but it is not possible to exclude changes in diagnostic fashion as an explanation for more gradual changes in asthma mortality (such as the gradual increases in some countries during the 1980s).

Time trends prior to 1960

Figure 3 shows asthma mortality rates per 100 000 person-years in the 5 to 34 year age group in England and Wales, New Zealand, Australia, and the United States during the period 1910 to 1960. The data are shown in 5-year calendar periods because of the small numbers involved for some countries, and the United Kingdom data are not shown for the 1940s, because of possible biases in official statistics for the period of the Second World War (Speizer and Doll 1968). The most striking feature is that asthma mortality was uniformly low, and relatively stable, prior to 1940. The death rate began to increase gradually in the early 1940s, with the rate of increase being greatest in New Zealand and Australia. Mortality declined again in the late 1950s in New Zealand (Beasley *et al.* 1990), England and Wales (Speizer and Doll 1968), but does not appear to have declined in Australia (Baumann and Lee 1990) and the United States (Weiss *et al.* 1993). Comparison of death rates over such an extended period is difficult due to the potential for gradual changes in diagnostic fashion. However, Speizer and Doll (1968) considered that historical asthma mortality data were of acceptable accuracy in the 5 to 34 year age group since death is usually sudden and the method of diagnosis of asthma as a cause of death has remained essentially unchanged during the past 100 years. Furthermore, the time trends for deaths from other obstructive respiratory diseases do not generally suggest that changes in diagnostic fashion are responsible for the gradual increase in mortality from asthma during the 1940s and 1950s (Beasley *et al.* 1990), although this possibility cannot be ruled out (Jackson 1993). However, it is interesting to note that, in the United Kingdom, isoprenaline first became available as a sublingual preparation or as an atomizer spray for use in asthma in 1948 (Beasley *et al.* 1990). Similarly, it is possible that the introduction of corticosteroids in the 1950s may have lead to a decline in mortality (Speizer and Doll 1968).

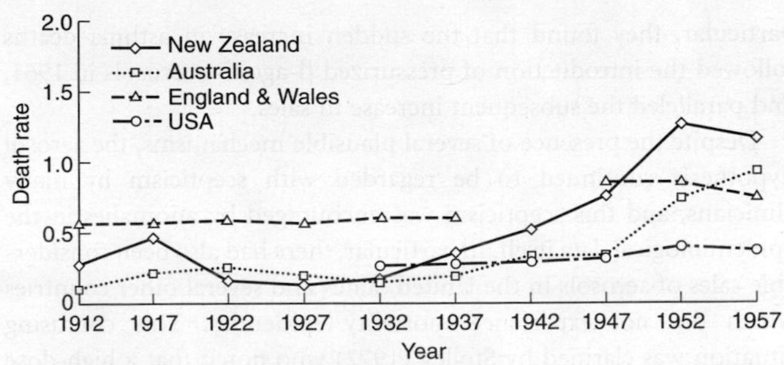

Fig. 3 Asthma mortality in people aged 5 to 34 years in New Zealand, Australia, England and Wales, and the United States during the period 1910 to 1960.

The 1960s mortality epidemics

In contrast to the relatively stable asthma death rates during the first half of the twentieth century, asthma mortality increased dramatically in at least six developed countries in the 1960s, England and Wales, Scotland, Ireland, New Zealand, Australia, and Norway. The time trends are shown in Fig. 4 for three of the epidemic countries (England and Wales, Australia, and New Zealand), and for three countries which did not experience epidemics (the United States, Canada, and Germany). Speizer *et al.* (1968) conducted a detailed examination of the mortality trends in the 5 to 34 year age group in England and Wales. They concluded that the epidemic was real and was not due to changes in death certification, disease classification, or diagnostic practice. They also considered that it was unlikely to be due to a sudden increase in asthma prevalence, but was rather due to an increase in case-fatality due to new methods of treatment. In

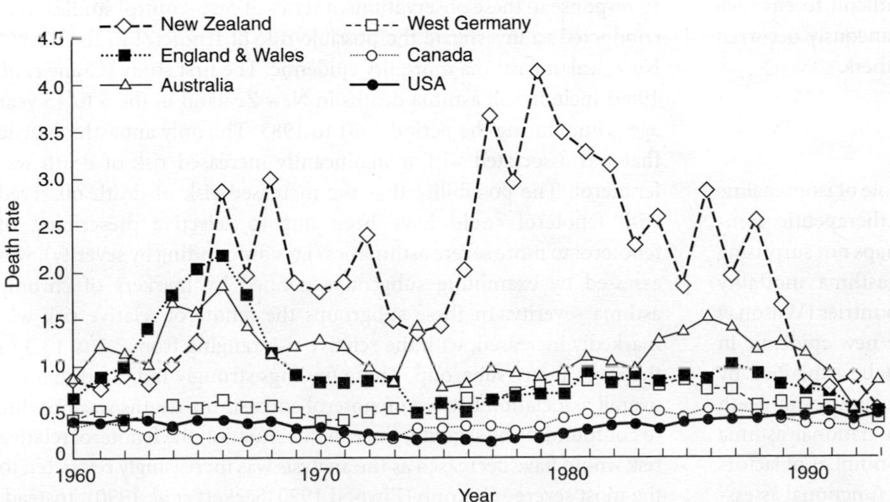

Fig. 4 International patterns of asthma mortality in people aged 5 to 34 years during the period 1960 to 1990.

particular, they found that the sudden increase in asthma deaths followed the introduction of pressurized β-agonist aerosols in 1961, and paralleled the subsequent increase in sales.

Despite the presence of several plausible mechanisms, the aerosol hypothesis continued to be regarded with scepticism by many clinicians, and this scepticism was encouraged by anomalies in the epidemiological data itself. In particular, there had also been considerable sales of aerosols in the United States and several other countries which did not experience mortality epidemics. This confusing situation was clarified by Stolley (1972) who noted that a high-dose formulation of isoprenaline (isoprenaline forte), which contained five times the dose per administration of other isoprenaline aerosols, had only been licensed in eight countries (Anon. 1972). Six of these (England and Wales, Ireland, Scotland, Australia, New Zealand, and Norway) had mortality epidemics which coincided with the introduction of the drug, and in the other two countries (The Netherlands and Belgium) the preparation was introduced relatively late and sales volumes were low. Overall, there was a strong positive correlation internationally between the asthma mortality rate and isoprenaline forte sales in these eight countries, whereas no mortality epidemics occurred in countries in which isoprenaline forte was not licensed, such as Sweden, Canada, West Germany, and the United States (Stolley 1972).

However, by the 1980s, the potential hazards of β-agonist aerosols were disputed in many texts and reviews (Anon. 1979; Benatar 1986; Paterson and Musk 1987; Buist 1988) which argued that the β-agonist theory had been disproved. In fact, very little new evidence has appeared since 1972, with the exception of further analyses conducted by Stolley and Schinnar (1978) which strengthened his original conclusions. The process of 'reinterpretation' of the 1960s epidemic was based on the minor anomalies in the time trend data, which were emphasized, and to some extent exaggerated in subsequent reviews (Stolley and Lasky 1993). In addition, other factors such as delays in seeking medical help began to receive greater emphasis, and it was argued that 'errors of omission are a much more frequent cause of death than errors of commission' (Read 1968). However, delays in starting appropriate treatment can themselves be caused by overtreatment with β-agonists, and acute toxicity is most likely to occur in the presence of such delays. Furthermore, it is very difficult to envisage how (non-drug-induced) delays could have spontaneously occurred and then regressed in some countries but not in others.

The second New Zealand epidemic

Given the reluctance to accept the evidence on the role of isoprenaline forte in the 1960s epidemics, and the resulting therapeutic complacency regarding the safety of β-agonists, it is perhaps not surprising that history repeated itself. In 1976, a second asthma mortality epidemic began in New Zealand, but not in other countries (Wilson *et al.* 1981). Jackson *et al.* (1982) concluded that the new epidemic in New Zealand appeared to be real, and could not be explained by changes in the classification of asthma deaths, inaccuracies in death certification, or changes in diagnostic fashions. A national asthma mortality survey (Sears *et al.* 1985) concluded that a number of factors contributed to asthma deaths including inadequate functional assessment of the severity of asthma, inappropriate drug therapy with over-reliance on β-agonists and underuse of corticosteroids, delay in seeking and in some cases providing medical care, inadequate emergency care, and lack of follow-up after treatment of acute attacks. However, the authors produced no evidence that any of these factors had suddenly increased in 1976 in New Zealand, but not in other countries.

The fenoterol hypothesis

Thus there was no tenable explanation for the second New Zealand mortality epidemic until the fenoterol hypothesis was proposed by Crane *et al.* (1989). An examination of the time trend data (Crane *et al.* 1989) revealed that fenoterol was introduced to New Zealand in April 1976 and that the epidemic began in the same year, with a close parallel between fenoterol sales and asthma deaths in the early years of the epidemic. It was also observed that fenoterol represented less than 5 per cent of the market in most other countries and was not available in the United States. Although fenoterol had a 50 per cent market share in West Germany, β-agonists were generally used less than in New Zealand and the per capita sales of fenoterol were only one-third of those in New Zealand (Beasley *et al.* 1989). Furthermore, although there was no sudden mortality epidemic in West Germany, mortality nearly doubled in the 5 years following the introduction of fenoterol (Beasley *et al.* 1989). A further observation was that fenoterol is dispensed by aerosol in what is effectively a forte preparation at four times the strength of salbutamol (Grant 1990). Finally, a series of laboratory studies found that repeated inhalation of fenoterol resulted in a greater inotropic and chronotropic effect than that of salbutamol, and of isoprenaline (Beasley *et al.* 1991). Fenoterol is relatively long acting and with repeated inhalation over short periods its extrapulmonary effects are cumulative, and greater than those of isoprenaline. The accumulation of extrapulmonary effects with increasing doses over time may be particularly relevant, since patients with severe asthma frequently self-administer large doses of β-agonists (Windom *et al.* 1990). Furthermore, in contrast with salbutamol and terbutaline which are partial agonists at the β-receptors, fenoterol and isoprenaline are full agonists at the β-receptors, thereby resulting in greater maximum extrapulmonary effects (Bremner *et al.* 1996).

Studies of fenoterol and asthma deaths

In response to these observations, a series of case–control studies were conducted to investigate the possible role of fenoterol in the second New Zealand asthma mortality epidemic. The first study (Crane *et al.* 1989) included all asthma deaths in New Zealand in the 5 to 45 year age group during the period 1981 to 1983. The only antiasthma drug that was associated with a significantly increased risk of death was fenoterol. The possibility that the increased risk of death observed with fenoterol could have been due to selective prescribing of fenoterol to more severe asthmatics (i.e. confounding by severity), was assessed by examining subgroups defined by markers of chronic asthma severity. In these subgroups the fenoterol relative risk was markedly increased, with the relative risk ranging from 2.2 to 13.3 in the most severe subgroup. These findings strongly indicated that the overall association between fenoterol and asthma deaths was not due to confounding by severity, since in this situation the fenoterol relative risk would have decreased as the analysis was increasingly restricted to the most severe subgroup (Elwood 1990; Sackett *et al.* 1990). Instead, the opposite pattern was observed. Furthermore, there is little evidence of selective prescribing of fenoterol in the population on which the case–control study was based (Beasley *et al.* 1994).

Table 3 Findings from studies of fenoterol and asthma deaths

	Odds ratio (95% confidence interval)				
	New Zealand				Saskatchewan study
	First study	Second study	Third study		
			Group A	Group B	
Fenoterol	1.6 (1.0–2.3)	2.0 (1.1–3.6)	2.1 (1.4–3.2)	2.7 (1.7–4.1)	4.8 (2.5–9.3)
Salbutamol	0.7(0.5–1.1)	0.7 (0.4–1.2)	0.6 (0.4–1.0)	0.5 (0.4–0.8)	0.9 (0.4–1.7)
Fenoterol only	1.6 (1.0–2.5)	1.9 (1.0–3.7)	2.0 (1.3–3.2)	2.5 (1.6–3.9)	3.7 (1.7–8.0)
Salbutamol only[a]	1.0	1.0	1.0	1.0	1.0

[a]Reference category.

Criticisms were levelled at this case–control study from several sources (O'Donnell *et al.* 1989; Buist *et al.* 1989; Poole *et al.* 1990). The most valid criticism was one that was also noted in the original report (Crane *et al.* 1989), namely that the data for prescribed medicines were obtained from different sources for the cases and controls. This problem was addressed in a second New Zealand case–control study (Pearce *et al.* 1990) of asthma deaths in 5- to 45-year-olds during the period 1977 to 1981 which obtained prescribing information for all cases and controls from routine hospital records, thereby overcoming the potential problem of differential information bias. The overall relative risk of asthma death in patients prescribed inhaled fenoterol was 2.0, and as before, the relative risk again increased markedly when the analysis was restricted to subgroups defined by markers of asthma severity.

A third national case–control study examined the same hypothesis in the same age group during the period 1981 to 1987 (Grainger *et al.* 1991). Two control groups were used in order to address the remaining criticisms which had been made of the previous studies. Whichever control group was used, fenoterol was associated with an increased risk of asthma death, but the alternative control group suggested by critics of the previous studies (Poole *et al.* 1990) actually yielded stronger relative risks than the approach used previously.

A further piece of evidence concerning the role of fenoterol in the second New Zealand epidemic is that, following the warnings about the use of fenoterol by severe asthmatics issued in mid-1989, the mortality rate fell significantly (Pearce *et al.* 1995*a*). However, the strongest evidence in support of the New Zealand findings has come from a Canadian case–control analysis (Spitzer *et al.* 1992) and a cohort analysis of the same data base (Suissa *et al.* 1994), funded by Boehringer Ingelheim, the manufacturer of fenoterol. The fenoterol relative risk was 5.3, with nearly half of the deaths having been prescribed fenoterol compared with 16 per cent of the controls (Pearce and Hensley 1998). Thus the findings were even stronger than those in New Zealand when the studies were analysed in an identical manner (Table 3).

There have been no other formal case–control studies of asthma deaths, but relevant information is provided by two other mortality studies. A review of 30 asthma deaths in Japan (Matsui 1996) yielded findings consistent with those from New Zealand and Saskatchewan (Table 4). This study did not include a control group, and the estimated odds ratio is only based on the fenoterol market share in Japan at the time that the case series of deaths was investigated; nevertheless, it is striking that fenoterol accounted for more than half of the asthma deaths (as in New Zealand and Saskatchewan), at a time when it had only a 18.3 per cent market share. A small cohort study of patients with chronic obstructive pulmonary disease in Germany also found an increased death rate in those prescribed fenoterol compared with those prescribed other β-agonists (Criée *et al.* 1993).

Recent time trends

Until recently, epidemiological studies of asthma mortality had largely concentrated on the causes of the mortality epidemics. These have only occurred with isoprenaline forte and fenoterol, which are high-dose, poorly selective, full β-receptor agonists, with relatively greater cardiac side-effects (Beasley *et al.* 1991). No other β-agonists

Table 4 Proportions of cases (asthma deaths) and controls prescribed fenoterol in case–control studies in New Zealand, Saskatchewan, and Japan

	Total deaths	Cases on fenoterol (%)	Controls on fenoterol (%)	Odds ratio	95% CI
First New Zealand study	117	51.3	40.4	1.6	1.0–2.3
Second New Zealand study	58	51.7	35.7	1.9	1.1–3.4
Third New Zealand study	112	59.8	45.9	1.8	1.2–2.7
Saskatchewan study	44	47.7	15.9	4.8	2.5–9.3
Japanese study	30	53.4	18.3[a]	5.1	2.6–9.9

[a]Market share (this study did not include a formal control group).

have been associated with such epidemics. However, in recent years attention has also focused on the possible causes of the gradual increase in mortality which appears to have occurred in a number of countries during the 1980s (Fig. 4). Although there is still some debate as to whether this increase is occurring (Anderson and Strachan 1991), there does appear to have been a gradual increase in mortality in many countries during the 1980s (Jackson *et al.* 1988), although it now appears that the increase is not being sustained and mortality rates may be declining again (Baumann and Lee 1990; Beasley *et al.* 1997; Campbell *et al.* 1997) (Fig. 4). The causes of the increase and more recent decline are difficult to determine because the changes have been so gradual, and could conceivably be due to changes in diagnostic practice or in the underlying prevalence of asthma. However, it is also possible that the gradual increases in asthma mortality could be due to a class effect of β-agonists. In particular, concern has been raised by several clinical trials which have suggested that regular use of β-agonists could lead to worsening asthma (Sears *et al.* 1990; Van Schayck *et al.* 1991). However, there has been considerable debate as to whether this phenomena is specific to fenoterol or whether it is a class effect of β-agonists, and the extent to which it is dose dependent (Anon. 1990; Lofdahl and Svedmyr 1991; Seale 1991; Burrows and Lebowitz 1992). In fact, a recent randomized cross-over trial of regular versus as-needed salbutamol found less frequent asthma symptoms in the 'regular salbutamol' group (Chapman *et al.* 1994).

Only one epidemiological study has attempted to draw conclusions on the role of a class effect of β-agonists in asthma mortality. This is the case–control study of asthma deaths in Saskatchewan (Spitzer *et al.* 1992) and the related cohort study (Suissa *et al.* 1994) which are discussed above. These reported that, although fenoterol appeared to be especially hazardous, prescription of other β-agonists may also be associated with an increased risk of death. However, a meta-analysis (Mullen *et al.* 1993) shows that the results of Spitzer *et al.* (1992) are significantly different from those reported by other researchers (Strunk *et al.* 1985; Crane *et al.* 1989; Miller and Strunk 1989; Pearce *et al.* 1990; Grainger *et al.* 1991). Thus, the different findings of the Saskatchewan study are probably due to flaws in the study design (Pearce and Hensley 1998).

Other risk factors for asthma mortality

Although most analytical epidemiological studies of asthma deaths have focused on pharmacological risk factors, several case–control studies have examined other risk factors for asthma deaths. These risk factors can be categorized as involving characteristics of the disease (asthma severity), characteristics of the patient (such as psychosocial factors), and environmental exposures.

Asthma severity

Four studies (Rea *et al.* 1986; Ryan *et al.* 1991; Crane *et al.* 1992; Spitzer *et al.* 1992) have examined the association between markers of asthma severity and risk of asthma death in adults (Pearce *et al.* 1995*b*). These have involved three markers of chronic asthma severity: (a) a hospital admission during the previous 12 months; (b) prescription of three or more categories of asthma drugs; (c) prescription of oral corticosteroids. All three markers of chronic asthma severity were associated with an increased risk of subsequent death, but the risk was greatest for patients with a hospital admission for asthma in the previous 12 months. Amongst patients with a recent hospital admission for asthma, the severity marker most strongly associated with an increased risk of death is a previous intensive care admission for asthma (Rea *et al.* 1986), in particular the requirement for mechanical ventilation which has a 5-year mortality rate of up to 20 per cent (Marquette *et al.* 1992).

Characteristics of the asthmatic

Several studies have examined characteristics of the asthmatic which may be associated with an increased risk of death. In particular, Rea *et al.* (1986) have noted that the risk of asthma death in adults is associated with psychosocial problems, and other psychological characteristics of the patient, as well as the underlying severity of the asthma. Similarly, Ryan *et al.* (1991) and Crane *et al.* (1992) have noted an association between asthma deaths and prescription of psychotropic drugs, which is a marker for the existence of psychosocial problems. Strunk *et al.* (1985) have reached similar conclusions in a small study in children which found that various psychosocial factors were associated with an increased risk of asthma death, including, conflicts between the patient's parents and hospital staff regarding medical management; depressive symptoms; and disregard of asthma symptoms.

Analysis of trends in asthma mortality rates within countries often reveals differences between population groups (Sears *et al.* 1985; Sly 1988; Weiss and Wagener 1990; Ehrlich and Bourne 1994). This is illustrated by studies from the United States in which the asthma mortality rates were greater in black people and hispanics (Sly 1988; Weiss and Wagener 1990), and in other socio-economically disadvantaged groups (Weiss *et al.* 1993; McFadden and Warren 1997).

Environmental exposures

Various studies have shown that outdoor air pollution is associated with respiratory mortality (Committee of the Environmental and Occupational Health Assembly of the ATS 1996; Zmirou *et al.* 1998). In the first half of the twentieth century several major air pollution episodes in Europe and the United States have been documented showing large acute effects on mortality (as well as morbidity). Particulate and SO_2 pollution were strongly implicated in the acute mortality associated with these severe pollution episodes (Committee of the Environmental and Occupational Health Assembly of the ATS 1996). People with pre-existing respiratory (or heart) disease were most affected. Epidemiological studies have suggested that even current levels of urban air pollution (particularly fine particulate pollution (PM_{10}), SO_2, O_3, and black smoke) are associated with increases in daily cardiorespiratory mortality (Committee of the Environmental and Occupational Health Assembly of the ATS 1996; Zmirou *et al.* 1998). Particularly subjects with pre-existing respiratory diseases such as asthma seem to have an increased risk. In a review Dockery and Pope (1994) estimated a 3.4 per cent increase in respiratory mortality for each 10 $\mu g/m^3$ increase in PM_{10} and a 1 per cent increase in hospital admissions and emergency departments visits for respiratory complaints and 2 to 3 per cent for asthma.

Another feature which is not evidence from national mortality data is the occurrence of epidemics in discrete locations, associated with environmental exposures. Probably the best studied example is that of the epidemics of life-threatening attacks of asthma (including fatal asthma) in Barcelona in the 1980s, associated with environmental exposure to airborne soybean dust (Antó *et al.* 1986, 1989). Another important example is environmental exposure to *Alternaria* which is one major cause of seasonal episodes of life-threatening asthma (O'Hollaren *et al.* 1991). These studies suggest that repeated environmental exposure to a single organic allergen can lead to recurrent episodes of life-threatening attacks of asthma in a community. While the causative agent may be difficult to identify with general environmental exposures, a wide range of sensitizing agents have been implicated in the occupational setting as causes of severe asthma (Chan-Yeung and Lam 1986).

Seasonal trends in asthma mortality have been observed in a number of countries including the United Kingdom (Khot and Burn 1984), France (Cadet *et al.* 1994), and the United States (Weiss 1990). In each of these countries, asthma mortality in the 5 to 34 year age group is highest in the summer months, in contrast to the older age groups, in which the peak occurs in winter. It is likely that the former trend may relate to reduced access to, or availability of, medical care during the summer holidays, in view of the associated reduction in hospital admission during this period (Khot and Burn 1984; Weiss 1990).

Discussion

What do these epidemiological findings reveal about the major causes of asthma, the global increases in prevalence, and the causes of asthma mortality?

The asthma mortality epidemics reveal problems associated with asthma management, and particularly the potential risks associated with bronchodilator therapy. These epidemics waned after warnings were issued about the safety of isoprenaline forte and fenoterol, and it should be possible to avoid further epidemics by more rigorous investigation of acute and chronic side-effects across a wide dose range, and more careful investigation of the appropriate dose, before further β-agonist asthma drugs are marketed. Attention is now shifting to other aspects of modern medical management of asthma.

The epidemiological findings on prevalence and causes of asthma itself reveal that there are major gaps in current understanding of asthma aetiology. In particular, although atopic sensitization is strongly associated with asthma, it appears to account for less than half of all cases, and there is little evidence that the 'established' environmental asthma risk factors account for international prevalence increases, or even for a substantial proportion of asthma cases within Western countries. This epidemiological evidence not only calls the 'established' risk factors and the predominant atopy paradigm into question; it also identifies associations which any new theory is required to explain. Recent decades have seen decreasing family size, reduced exposure to infections, and increasing size at birth, as well as increasing use of medical interventions such as immunization and antibiotics. It seems that as a result of this 'package' of changes in the intrauterine and infant environment, we are seeing an increased susceptibility to the development of asthma and/or allergy. Understanding why this increased susceptibility is occurring, and ascertaining which elements of the 'package' of twentieth-century economic development and lifestyle changes are responsible (or whether the entire 'package' is more than the sum of its parts), represents a significant challenge, and a major opportunity, for asthma researchers.

References

Åberg, N. (1989). Asthma and allergic rhinitis in Swedish conscripts. *Archives of Disease in Children*, **19**, 59–63.

Åberg, N., Hesselman, B., Åberg, B., and Eriksson, B. (1995). Increase of asthma, allergic rhinitis and eczema in Swedish schoolchildren between 1979 and 1991. *Clinical Experiments in Allergy*, **25**, 815–19.

Adams, R., Ruffin, R., Wakefield, M., *et al.* (1997). Asthma prevalence, morbidity and management practices in South Australia, 1992–1995. *Australia and New Zealand Journal of Medicine*, **27**, 672–9.

Allegra, L., Blasi, F., Centanni, S., *et al.* (1994). Acute exacerbations of asthma in adults, role of *Chlamydia pneumoniae* infection. *European Respiratory Journal*, **7**, 2165–8.

Anderson, H.R. (1974). The epidemiological and allergic features of asthma in the New Guinea Highlands. *Clinical Allergy*, **4**, 171–83.

Anderson, H.R. (1979). Respiratory abnormalities, smoking habits and ventilatory capacity in a highland community in Papua New Guinea, prevalence and effect on mortality. *International Journal of Epidemiology*, **8**, 127–35.

Anderson, H.R. (1989). Is the prevalence of asthma changing? *Archives of Disease in Childhood*, **64**, 172–5.

Anderson, H.R. and Strachan, D.P. (1991). Asthma mortality in England and Wales 1979–1989. *Lancet*, **37**, 1357.

Anderson, H.R., Pottier, A.C., and Strachan, D.P. (1992). Asthma from birth to age 23, incidence and relation to prior and concurrent disease. *Thorax*, **47**, 537–42.

Anderson, H.R., Butland, B.K., and Strachan, D.P. (1994). Trends in prevalence and severity of childhood asthma. *British Medical Journal*, **308**, 1600–4.

Andriessen, J.W., Brunekreef, B., and Roemer, W. (1998). Home dampness and respiratory health status in European children. *Clinical and Experimental Allergy*, **28**, 1191–200.

Anonymous (1972). Asthma deaths: a question answered (editorial). *British Medical Journal*, **ii**, 443–4.

Anonymous (1979). Fatal asthma (editorial). *Lancet*, **ii**, 337–8.

Anonymous (1990). Beta-2 agonists in asthma, relief, prevention, morbidity (editorial). *Lancet*, **336**, 1411–12.

Antó, J.M., Sunyer, J., and the Barcelona Asthma Collaborative Group (1986). A point source asthma outbreak. *Lancet*, **i**, 900–3.

Antó, J.M., Sunyer, J., Rodriguez-Roisin, R., *et al.* (1989). Community outbreaks of asthma associated with inhalation of soybean dust. *New England Journal of Medicine*, **320**, 1097–102.

Antó, J.M., Sunyer, J., and Newman-Taylor, A.J. (1996). Comparison of soybean epidemic asthma and occupational asthma. *Thorax*, **51**, 743–9.

Asher, I., Keil, U., Anderson, H.R., *et al.* (1995). International Study of Asthma and Allergies in Childhood (ISAAC), rationale and methods. *European Respiratory Journal*, **8**, 483–91.

ATS (American Thoracic Society) Committee on Diagnostic Standards (1962). Definitions and classification of chronic bronchitis, asthma and pulmonary emphysema. *American Review of Respiratory Disease*, **85**, 762–8.

Auerbach, I., Springer, C., and Godfrey, S. (1993). Total population survey of the frequency and severity of asthma in 17-year-old boys in an urban area in Israel. *Thorax*, **48**, 139–41.

Balfe, D., Crane, J., Beasley, R., and Pearce, N. (1996). The worldwide increase in the prevalence of asthma in children and young adults. *Continuing Medical Education Journal*, **14**, 433–42.

Balfour-Lynn, L. (1985). Childhood asthma and puberty. *Archives of Disease in Children*, **60**, 231.

Barnes, P.J. (1994). Air pollution and asthma. *Postgraduate Medical Journal*, **70**, 319–25.

Bascom, R., Bromberg, P.A., Costa, D.A., *et al.* (1996). Health effects of outdoor air pollution. *American Journal of Respiratory and Critical Care Medicine*, **153**, 3–50.

Baumann, A. and Lee, S. (1990). Trends in asthma mortality in Australia 1911–1986. *Medical Journal of Australia*, **153**, 366.

Hirsch, T., Range, U., Walther, K.U., *et al.* (1998). Prevalence and determinants of house dust mite allergen in East German homes. *Clinical and Experimental Allergy*, **28**, 956–64.

Holt, P.G. (1995). Environmental factors and primary T-cell sensitization to inhalant allergens in infancy, reappraisal of the role of infections and air pollution. *Pediatric Allergy and Immunology*, **6**, 1–10.

Holt, P.G. and Macaubas, C. (1997). Development of long term tolerance versus sensitization to environmental allergens during the perinatal period. *Current Opinion in Immunology*, **9**, 782–7.

Holt, P.G., Sly, P.D., and Björkstén, B. (1997). Atopic versus infectious diseases in childhood, a question of balance? *Pediatric Allergy and Immunology*, **8**, 53–8.

Horwood, L.J., Fergusson, D.M., and Shannon, F.T. (1985). Social and familial factors in the development of early childhood asthma. *Pediatrics*, 75, 859–68.

Hsieh, K.-H. and Shen, J.-J. (1991). Prevalence of childhood asthma in Taipei, Taiwan and other Asian Pacific countries. *Journal of Asthma*, **25**, 73–82.

Hwang, D. (1989). Essential fatty acids and immune response. *FASEB Journal*, **3**, 2052–61.

Infante-Rivard, C., Sukia, S.E., Roberge, D., and Baumgarten, M. (1987). The changing frequency of childhood asthma. *Journal of Asthma*, **24**, 283–8.

ISAAC Steering Committee (Writing Committee: Beasley, R., Keil, U., Von Mutius, E., Pearce, N.) (1998*a*). Worldwide variation in prevalence of symptoms of asthma, allergic rhinoconjunctivitis and atopic eczema, ISAAC. *Lancet*, **351**, 1225–32.

ISAAC Steering Committee (Writing Committee: Asher, M.I., Anderson, H.R., Stewart, A.W., Crane, J.) (1998*b*). Worldwide variations in the prevalence of asthma symptoms, International Study of Asthma and Allergies in Childhood (ISAAC). *European Respiratory Journal*, **12**, 315–35.

Jaakkola, J.J.K., Jaakkola, N., and Ruotsalainen, R. (1993). Home dampness and molds as determinants of respiratory symptoms and asthma in pre-school children. *Journal of Exposure Analysis and Environmental Epidemiology*, **3**, 129–42.

Jackson, R. (1993). A century of asthma mortality. In *The role of beta agonist therapy in asthma mortality* (ed. R. Beasley and N.E. Pearce), pp. 29–47. CRC Press, New York.

Jackson, R.T., Beaglehole, R., Rea, H.H., *et al.* (1982). Mortality from asthma, a new epidemic in New Zealand. *British Medical Journal*, **285**, 771–4.

Jackson, R., Sears, M.R., Beaglehole, R., *et al.* (1988). International trends in asthma mortality, 1970 to 1985. *Chest*, **94**, 914–18.

Johnston, S.L., Sanderson, G., Pattemore, P.K., *et al.* (1993). Use of polymerase chain reaction for diagnosis of picornavirus infection in subjects with and without respiratory symptoms. *Journal of Clinical Microbiology*, **31**, 111–17.

Johnston, S.L., Pattemore, P.K., Sanderson, G., *et al.* (1995). Community study of role of virus infections in exacerbations of asthma in 9–11 year old children. *British Medical Journal*, **310**, 1225–9.

Johnston, S.L., Pattemore, P.K., Sanderson, G., *et al.* (1996). The relationship between upper respiratory infections and hospital admission for asthma, a time trend analysis. *American Journal of Respiratory and Critical Care Medicine*, **154**, 654–60.

Keeney, E.L. (1964). The history of asthma from Hippocrates to Meltzer. *Journal of Allergy*, **35**, 215–26.

Kemp, T., Pearce, N., Fitzharris, P., *et al.* (1997). Is infant immunisation a risk factor for childhood asthma and allergy? *Epidemiology*, **8**, 678–80.

Khot, A. and Burn, R. (1984). Seasonal variations and time trends of deaths from asthma in England and Wales 1960–82. *British Medical Journal*, **289**, 233–4.

Kimbell-Dunn, M., Pearce, N., Beasley, R. (1999). Asthma. In *Women and health* (ed. M. Goldman and M. Hatch), pp. 724–39. Academic Press, San Diego, CA.

Kogevinas, M., Antó, J.M., Soriano, J.B., *et al.* (1996). The risk of asthma attributable to occupational exposures, a population-based study in Spain. *American Journal of Respiratory and Critical Care Medicine*, **154**, 137–43.

Koo, L.C. and Ho, J.H.-C. (1994). Mosquito coil smoke and respiratory health among Hong Kong Chinese, results of three epidemiological studies. *Indoor Environment*, **3**, 304–10.

Krämer, U., Heinrich, J., Wjst, M., and Wichmann, H.E. (1999). Age of entry to day nursery and allergy in later childhood. *Lancet*, **353**, 450–4.

Kuehr, J., Frischer, T., Meinert, R., *et al.* (1995). Sensitization to mite allergens is a risk factor for early and late onset of asthma and for persistence of asthmatic signs in children. *Journal of Allergy and Clinical Immunology*, **95**, 655–62.

Leadbitter, P., Pearce, N., Cheng, S. *et al.* (1999). The relationship between fetal growth and the development of asthma and atopy in childhood. *Thorax*, **54**, 905–10.

Lee, D.A., Winslow, N.R., Speight, A.N.P., and Hey, E.N. (1983). Prevalence and spectrum of asthma in childhood. *British Medical Journal*, **286**, 1256–8.

Leung, R., Ho, P., Lam, C.K.W., and Lai, C.K.W. (1997). Sensitization to inhaled allergens as a risk factor for asthma and allergic diseases in Chinese population. *Journal of Allergy and Clinical Immunology*, **99**, 594–9.

Liard, R., Chansin, R., Neukirch, F., *et al.* (1988). Prevalence of asthma among teenagers attending school in Tahiti. *Journal of Epidemiology and Community Health*, **42**, 149–51.

Littlejohns, P. and MacDonald, L.D. (1993). The relationship between severe asthma and social class. *Respiratory Medicine*, **87**, 139–43.

Littlejohns, P., Ebrahim, S., and Anderson, H.R. (1989). The prevalence and diagnosis of chronic respiratory symptoms in adults. *British Medical Journal*, **298**, 1556–60.

Livingstone, A.E., Shaddick, G., Grundy, C., and Elliott, P. (1996). Do people living near inner city main roads have more asthma needing treatment? *British Medical Journal*, **312**, 676–7.

Lofdahl, C.-G. and Svedmyr, N. (1991). Beta-agonists—friends or foes? *European Respiratory Journal*, **4**, 1161–5.

McFadden, E.R. and Warren, E.L. (1997). Observations on asthma mortality. *Annals of Internal Medicine*, **127**, 142–7.

Magnus, P. and Jaakkola, J.J.K. (1997). Secular trend in the occurrence of asthma among children and young adults, critical appraisal of repeated cross sectional surveys. *British Medical Journal*, **314**, 1795–9.

Manfreda, J., Becker, A.B., Wang, P.-Z., *et al.* (1993). Trends in physician-diagnosed asthma prevalence in Manitoba between 1980 and 1990. *Chest*, **103**, 151–7.

Marbury, M. and Kriegler, R. (1991). Formaldehyde. In *Indoor air pollution. A health perspective* (ed. J. Samet and J.D. Spengler), pp. 223–51. Johns Hopkins University Press, Baltimore, MD.

Marquette, C.H., Saulnier, F., Leroy, O., *et al.* (1992). Long-term prognosis of near fatal asthma. *American Review of Respiratory Disease*, **146**, 76–81.

Martinez, F.D. (1994). Role of viral infections in the inception of asthma and allergies during childhood, could they be protective? *Thorax*, **49**, 1189–91.

Martinez, F.D. (1995). Viral infetions and the development of asthma. *American Journal of Respiratory and Critical Care Medicine*, **151**, 1644–8.

Martinez, F.D. (1997). Complexities of the genetics of asthma. *American Journal of Respiratory and Critical Care Medicine*, **156**, S117–S122.

Martinez, F.D. (1998). Gene by environment interactions in the development of asthma. *Clinical and Experimental Allergy*, **28**, 21–5.

Martinez, F., Morgan, W.J., Wright, A.L., *et al.* (1988). Diminished lung function as a predisposing factor for wheezing respiratory illness in infants. *New England Journal of Medicine*, **319**, 1112–17.

Matricardi, P.M., Rosmini, F., Ferrigno, L., *et al.* (1997). Cross sectional retrospective study of prevalence of atopy among Italian military students with antibodies against hepatitis A virus. *British Medical Journal*, **314**, 999–1003.

Matsui, T. (1996). Asthma death and β_2-agonists. In *Current advances in pediatric allergy and clinical immunology* (ed. K. Shinomiya), pp. 161–4.Churchill Livingstone, Tokyo.

Meredith, S. and Nordman, H. (1996). Occupational asthma, measures of frequency from four countries. *Thorax*, **51**, 435–40.

Meredith, S.K., Taylor, V.M., and McDonald, J.C. (1991). Occupational respiratory disease in the United Kingdom 1989, a report to the British Thoracic Society and the Society of Occupational Medicine by the SWORD project group. *British Journal of Industrial Medicine*, **48**, 292–8.

Michel, O., Ginanni, R., Duchateau, J., Vertongen, F., Le Bon, B., and Sergysels, R. (1991). Domestic endotoxin exposure and clinical severity of asthma. *Clinical and Experimental Allergy*, **21**, 441–8.

Michel, O., Ginanni, R., Le Bon, B., Content, J., Duchateau, J., and Sergysels, R. (1992). Inflammatory response to acute inhalation of endotoxin in asthmatic patients. *American Review of Respiratory Disease*, **146**, 352–7.

Michel, O., Kips, J., Duchateau, J., *et al.* (1996). Severity of asthma is related to endotoxin in house dust. *American Journal of Respiratory and Critical Care Medicine*, **154**, 1641–6.

Mielke, A., Reitmeir, P., and Wjst, M. (1996). Severity of childhood asthma by socioeconomic status. *International Journal of Epidemiology*, **25**, 388–93.

Miller, D.B. and Strunk, R.C. (1989). Circumstances surrounding the deaths of children due to asthma, a case–control study. *American Journal of Diseases of the Chest*, **143**, 1294–9.

Mitchell, E.A. (1983). Increasing prevalence of asthma in children. *New Zealand Medical Journal*, **96**, 463–4.

Mitchell, R.G. and Dawson, B. (1973). Educational and social characteristics of children with asthma. *Archives of Disease in Childhood*, **48**, 467–71.

Morrison Smith, J. (1976). The prevalence of asthma and wheezing in children. *British Journal of Diseases of the Chest*, **70**, 73–7.

Morton, N.E. (1992). Major loci for atopy? *Clinical and Experimental Allergy*, **22**, 1041–3.

Moyes, C.D., Waldon, J., Dharmalingam, R., *et al.* (1995). Respiratory symptoms and environmental factors in schoolchildren in the Bay of Plenty. *New Zealand Medical Journal*, **108**, 358–61.

Mullen, M., Mullen, B., and Carey, M. (1993). The association between β-agonist use and death from asthma. *Journal of the American Medical Association*, **270**, 1842–5.

Neas, L., Dockery, D., Ware, J., *et al.* (1991). Association of indoor nitrogen dioxide with respiratory symptoms and pulmonary function in children. *American Journal of Epidemiology*, **134**, 204–19.

Nicholson, K.G., Kent, J., and Ireland, C. (1993). Respiratory viruses and exacerbations in adults. *British Medical Journal*, **307**, 982–6.

Ninan, T.K. and Russell, G. (1992). Respiratory symptoms and atopy in Aberdeen schoolchildren: evidence from two surveys 25 years apart. *British Medical Journal*, **304**, 873–5.

Nishima, S. (1993). A study of the prevalence of bronchial asthma in school children in western districts of Japan: comparison between the studies in 1982 and in 1992 with the same methods and same districts. *Arerugi*, **42**, 192–204.

NRC (National Research Council) (1986). *Environmental tobacco smoke, measuring exposures and assessing health effects.* National Academy Press, Washington, DC.

Odent, M.R., Culpin, E.E., and Kimmel, T. (1994). Pertussis vaccination and asthma, is there a link? *Journal of the American Medical Association*, **272**, 592–3.

O'Donnell, T.V., Holst, P., Rea, H.H., and Sears, M.R. (1989). Fenoterol and fatal asthma. *Lancet*, **i**, 1070–1 .

O'Hollaren, M.Y., Yuninger, J.W., Offord, K.P., *et al.* (1991). Exposure to aeroallergen as a possible precipitating factor in respiratory arrest in young patients with asthma. *New England Journal of Medicine*, **324**, 359–63.

Olesen, A.B., Ellingsen, A.R., Olesen, H., *et al.* (1997). Atopic dermatitis and birth factors. *British Medical Journal*, **314**, 1003–8.

Omran, M. and Russell, G. (1996). Continuing increase in respiratory symptoms and atopy in Aberdeen school children. *British Medical Journal*, **312**, 34.

Oosterlee, A., Drijver, M., Lebret, E., and Brunekreef, B. (1995). Chronic respiratory symptoms in children and adults living along streets with high traffic density. *Occupational Environmental Medicine*, **53**, 241–7.

Osbourne, J. and Honicky, R. (1986). Chronic respiratory symptoms in young children and indoor heating with a wood burning stove. *American Review of Respiratory Disease*, **133**, 300 (abstract).

Osler, W. (1901). *The principles and practice of medicine* (4th edn). Pentland, Edinburgh.

Panhuysen, C.I.M., Meyers, D.A., Postma, D.S., and Bleecker, E.R. (1995). The genetics of asthma and atopy. *Allergy*, **50**, 863–9.

Paterson, J.W. and Musk, A.W. (1987). Death in patients with asthma. *Medical Journal of Australia*, **147**, 53–5.

Pattemore, P.K., Johnston, S.L., and Bardin, P.G. (1992). Viruses as precipitants of asthma symptoms, epidemiology. *Clinical and Experimental Allergy*, **22**, 325–36.

Pearce, N.E. and Crane, J. (1993). Epidemiological methods for studying the role of beta agonist therapy in asthma mortality. In *The role of beta agonist therapy in asthma mortality* (ed. R. Beasley and N.E. Pearce), pp. 67–83. CRC Press, New York.

Pearce, N. and Hensley, M.J. (1998). Beta agonists and asthma deaths. *Epidemiologic Reviews*, **20**, 173–86.

Pearce, N.E., Grainger, J., Atkinson, M., *et al.* (1990). Case–control study of prescribed fenoterol and death from asthma in New Zealand 1977–1981. *Thorax*, **45**, 170–5.

Pearce, N.E., Weiland, S., Keil, U., *et al.* (1993). Self-reported prevalence of asthma symptoms in children in Australia, England, Germany and New Zealand, an international comparison using the ISAAC written and video questionnaires. *European Respiratory Journal*, **6**, 1455–61.

Pearce, N., Beasley, R., Crane, J., *et al.* (1995*a*). End of the New Zealand asthma mortality epidemic. *Lancet*, **345**, 41–4.

Pearce, N.E., Beasley, R., Crane, J., and Burgess, C. (1995*b*). Epidemiology of asthma mortality. In *Asthma and rhinitis* (ed. W. Busse and S. Holgate), pp. 58–69 Blackwell Scientific, Oxford.

Pearce, N., Kimbell-Dunn, M., and Beasley, R. (1997). Studying the prevalence and causes of asthma, strategies and methodological issues. *Journal of Epidemiology and Biostatistics*, **2**, 147–59.

Pearce, N., Beasley, R., Burgess, C., and Crane, J. (1998). *Asthma epidemiology, principles and methods.* Oxford University Press, New York.

Pearce, N., Pekkanen, J., and Beasley, R. (1999). How much asthma is really attributable to atopy? *Thorax*, **54**, 268–72.

Pearce, N., Pekkanen, J., and Beasley, R. (2000*a*). Role of bronchial responsiveness testing in asthma prevalence surveys. *Thorax*, **55**, 352–4.

Pearce, N., Douwes, J., and Beasley, R. (2000*b*). Is allergen exposure a major primary cause of asthma? *Thorax*, **55**, 424–51.

Pearce, N., Douwes, J., and Beasley, R. The rise and rise of asthma, a new paradigm for the new millenium? *Journal of Epidemiology Biostatistics*, **5**, 5–16.

Pearce, N., Douwes, J., and Beasley, R. The rise and rise of asthma, a new paradigm for the new millenium? *Journal of Epidemiology Biostatistics*, **5**, 5–16.

Peat, J.K. and Li, J. (1999). Reversing the trend: reducing the prevalence of asthma. *Journal of Allergy And Clinical Immunology*, **103**, 1–10.

Peat, J.K., van der Berg, R.H., Green, W.F., *et al.* (1994). Changing prevalence of asthma in Australian children. *British Medical Journal*, **308**, 1591–6.

Peat, J.K., Toelle, B.G., Gray, E.J., *et al.* (1995). Prevalence and severity of childhood asthma and allergic sensitization in seven climatic regions of New South Wales. *Medical Journal of Australia*, **163**, 22–6.

Peat, J.K., Tovey, E., Toelle, B.G., *et al.* (1996). House dust mite allergens, a major risk factor for childhood asthma in Australia. *American Journal of Respiratory and Critical Care Medicine*, **153**, 141–6.

Peat, J.K., Dickerson, J., and Li, J. (1998). Effects of damp and mould in the home on respiratory health, a review of the literature. *Allergy*, **53**, 120–8.

Pekkanen, J. and Pearce, N. (1999). Defining asthma in epidemiological studies. *European Respiratory Journal*, **14**, 951–7.

Perdrizet, S., Neukirch, F., Cooreman, J., and Liard, R. (1987). Prevalence of asthma in adolescents in various parts of France and its relationship to respiratory allergic manifestations. *Chest*, **91**, 104S–106S.

Pershagen, G., Rylander, E., Norberg, S., *et al.* (1995). Air pollution involving nitrogen dioxin exposure and wheezing bronchitis in children. *International Journal of Epidemiology*, **24**, 1147–53.

Pistelli, R., Forastiere, F., Corbo, G.M., *et al.* (1993). Respiratory symptoms and bronchial responsiveness are related to dietary salt intake and urinary potassium excretion in male children. *European Respiratory Journal*, **6**, 517–22.

Platts-Mills, T.A.E., Sporik, R., Ingram, J.M., and Honsinger, R. (1995). Dog and cat allergens and asthma among school children in Los Alamos, New Mexico, United States, Altitude 7,200 feet. *International Archives of Allergy and Immunology*, **107**, 301–3.

Platts-Mills, T.A.E., Sporik, R.B., Chapman, M.D., and Heymann, P.W. (1997*a*). The role of domestic allergens. In *The rising trends in asthma*, pp. 173–89. Ciba Foundation Symposium 202. Wiley, Chichester.

Platts-Mills, T.A.E., Vervloet, D., Thomas, W.R., Aalberse, R.C., and Chapman, M.D. (1997*b*). Indoor allergens and asthma, Report of the third international workshop. *Journal of Allergy and Clinical Immunology*, **100**, S1–S24.

Pomare, E., Tutengaehe, H., Ramsden, I., *et al.* (1992). Asthma in Maori people. *New Zealand Medical Journal*, **105**, 469–70.

Poole, C., Lanes, S.F., and Walker, A.M. (1990). Fenoterol and fatal asthma. *Lancet*, **i**, 920 .

Prescott, S.L., Macaubas, C., Smallacomb, T., *et al.* (1999). Development of allergen-specific T-cell memory in atopic and normal children. *Lancet*, **353**, 196–200.

Pullan, C.R. and Hey, E.N. (1982). Wheezing, asthma, and pulmonary dysfunction 10 years after infection with respiratory syncytial virus in infancy. *British Medical Journal*, **284**, 1665–9.

Raulf-Heimsoth, M. and Baur, X. (1998). Pathomechanisms and pathophysiology of isocyanate-induced diseases—summary of present knowledge. *American Journal of Industrial Medicine*, **34**, 137–43.

Rea, H.H., Scragg, R., Jackson, R., *et al.* (1986). A case–control study of deaths from asthma. *Thorax*, **41**, 833–9.

Read, J. (1968). The reported increase in mortality from asthma, a clinico-functional analysis. *Medical Journal of Australia*, **i**, 879–91.

Redline, S. and Gold, D. (1994). Challenges in interpreting gender differences in asthma. *American Journal of Respiratory and Critical Care Medicine*, **150**, 1219–21.

Robertson, C., Heycock, E., Bishop, J., *et al.* (1991). Prevalence of asthma in Melbourne schoolchildren: changes over 26 years. *British Medical Journal*, **302**, 1116–18.

Rubio, R.L., Rodriguez, G.B., and Collazo, J.J. (1988). Comparative study of progesterone, estradiol, and cortisol concentrations in asthmatic and non-asthmatic women. *Allergologia et Immunopathologia*, **16**, 263–6.

Ryan, G., Musk, A.W., Perera, D.M., *et al.* (1991). Risk factors for death in patients admitted to hospital with asthma, a follow-up study. *Australian and New Zealand Journal of Medicine*, **21**, 681–5.

Sackett, D.L., Shannon, H.S., and Browman, G.W. (1990). Fenoterol and fatal asthma. *Lancet*, **i**, 46 .

Sandford, A., Weir, T., and Paré, P. (1996). The genetics of asthma. *American Journal of Respiratory and Critical Care Medicine*, **153**, 1749–65.

Schenker, M.B., Christiani, D., Cormier, Y., *et al.* (1998). Respiratory health hazards in agriculture. *American Journal of Respiratory and Critical Care Medicine*, **158** (Supplement), S1–S76.

Schwartz, J. and Weiss, S.T. (1994). Relationship between dietary vitamin C intake and pulmonary function in the first national health and nutrition examination survey (NHANES). *American Journal of Clinical Nutrition*, **59**, 110–14.

Seale, P. (1991). Asthma deaths, where are we now? *Australia and New Zealand Journal of Medicine*, **21**, 678–9.

Sears, M.R., Rea, H.H., Beaglehole, R., *et al.* (1985). Asthma mortality in New Zealand, a two year national study. *New Zealand Medical Journal*, **98**, 271–5.

Sears, M.R., Rea, H.H., de Boer, G., *et al.* (1986). Accuracy of certification of deaths due to asthma, a national study. *American Journal of Epidemiology*, **124**, 1004–11.

Sears, M.R., Taylor, D.R., Print, C.G., *et al.* (1990). Regular inhaled beta-agonist treatment in bronchial asthma. *Lancet*, **336**, 1391–6.

Seaton, A., Godden, D.J., and Brown, K. (1994). Increase in asthma, a more toxic environment or a more susceptible population? *Thorax*, **48**, 171–4.

Shaheen, S.O., Aaby, P., Hall, A.J., *et al.* (1996). Measles and atopy in Guinea-Bissau. *Lancet*, **347**, 1792–6.

Shaw, R.A., Crane, J., O'Donnell, T.V., *et al.* (1990). Increasing asthma prevalence in a rural New Zealand adolescent population, 1975–89. *Archives of Disease in Childhood*, **63**, 1319–23.

Shaw, R., Woodman, K., Crane, J., *et al.* (1994). Risk factors for asthma in Kawerau children. *New Zealand Medical Journal*, **107**, 387–91.

Shaw, R., Woodman, K., Ayson, M., *et al.* (1995). Measuring the prevalence of bronchial hyperresponsiveness in children. *International Journal of Epidemiology*, **24**, 597–602.

Sherrill, D., Stein, R., Kurzius-Spencer, M., and Martinez, F. (1999). On early sensitization to allergens and development of respiratory symptoms. *Clinical and Experimental Allergy*, **29**, 905–11.

Shirakawa, T., Enomoto, T., Shimazu, S., and Hopkin, J.M. (1997). The inverse association between tuberculin responses and atopic disorder. *Science*, **275**, 77–9.

Silverman, M. (1995). Childhood asthma and other wheezing disorders. In *Respiratory medicine* (2nd edn) (ed. R.A.L. Brewis, B. Corrin, G.M. Geddes, and G.J. Gibson), pp. 1239–61. W.B. Saunders, London.

Sly, R.M. (1988). Mortality from asthma 1979–1984 *Journal of Allergy and Clinical Immunology*, **82**, 705–17.

Smith, J.M. and Knowles, L.A. (1967). Epidemiology of asthma and allergic rhinitis. II. In a university-centred community. *American Review of Respiratory Disease*, **92**, 31–8.

Speizer, F.E. and Doll, R. (1968). A century of asthma deaths in young people. *British Medical Journal*, **3**, 245–6.

Speizer, F.E., Doll, R., and Heaf, P. (1968). Observations on recent increase in mortality from asthma. *British Medical Journal*, **i**, 335–9.

Spieksma, F.T.M., Zuidemo, P., and Leupen, H.J. (1971). High altitude and house dust mites. *British Medical Journal*, **1**, 82.

Spitzer, W.O., Suissa, S., Ernst, P., *et al.* (1992). The use of beta-agonists and the risk of death and near death from asthma. *New England Journal of Medicine*, **326**, 501–6.

Sporik, R., Holgate, T., Platts-Mills, T., and Cogswell, J.J. (1990). Exposure to house-dust mite allergen (Der p I) and the development of asthma in childhood. *New England Journal of Medicine*, **323**, 502–7.

Sporik, R., Ingram, J.M., Price, W., *et al.* (1995). Association of asthma with serum IgE and skin test reactivity to allergens among children living at high altitude, tickling the dragon's breath. *American Journal of Respiratory and Critical Care Medicine*, **151**, 1388–92.

Sporik, R., Squillace, S.P., Ingram, J.M., *et al.* (1999). Mite, cat, and cockroach exposure, allergen sensitisation, and asthma in children, a case–control study of three schools. *Thorax*, **54**, 675–80.

Steinberg, M. and Becklake, M.R. (1986). Socio-environmental factors and lung function, a review of the literature. *South African Medical Journal*, **70**, 2704.

Stenius-Aarniala, B. (1987). The role of infection in asthma. *Chest*, **91**, 157S–160S.

Stolley, P.D. (1972). Why the United States was spared an epidemic of deaths due to asthma. *American Review of Respiratory Disease*, **105**, 883–90.

Stolley, P.D. and Lasky, T. (1993). The bellman always rings thrice. *Annals of Internal Medicine*, **118**, 158 .

Stolley, P.D. and Schinnar, R. (1978). Association between asthma mortality and isoproterenol aerosols: a review. *Preventive Medicine*, **7**, 319–38.

Strachan, D.P. (1989). Hay fever, hygiene, and household size. *British Medical Journal*, **299**, 1259–60.

Strachan, D.P. (1997). Allergy and family size, a riddle worth solving. *Clinical and Experimental Allergy*, **27**, 235–6.

Strachan, D.P. and Cook, D.G. (1998). Parental smoking and childhood asthma, longitudinal and case–control studies. *Thorax*, **53**, 204–12.

Strachan, D., Sibbald, B., Weiland, S., *et al.* (1997). Worldwide variations in prevalence of symptoms of allergic rhinoconjunctivitis in children, The International Study of Asthma and Allergies in Childhood (ISAAC). *Paediatric Allergy and Immunology*, **8**, 161–76.

Strunk, R.C., Mrazek, D.A., Wolfson, A., *et al.* (1985). Physiologic and psychological characteristics associated with deaths due to asthma in childhood. *Journal of the American Medical Association*, **254**, 1193–8.

Suissa, S., Ernst, P., Boivin, J.-F., *et al.* (1994) A cohort analysis of excess mortality in asthma and the use of inhaled β-agonists. *American Journal of Review of Respiratory Critical Care Medicine*, **149**, 604–10.

Svanes, C., Jarvis, D., Chinn, S., and Burney, P. (1999). Childhood environment and adult atopy, Results from the European community respiratory health survey. *Journal of Allergy and Clinical Immunology*, **103**, 415–20.

Toelle, B.G., Peat, J.K., Salome, C.M., *et al.* (1992). Toward a definition of asthma for epidemiology. *American Review of Respiratory Disease*, **146**, 633–7.

Troisi, R.J., Willett, W.C., Weiss, S.T., *et al.* (1995). A prospective study of diet and adult-onset asthma. *American Journal of Respiratory and Critical Care Medicine*, **151**, 1401–8.

Unger, L. and Harris, M.C. (1974). Stepping stones in allergy. *Annals of Allergy*, **32**, 214–30.

Van Herwerden, L., Harrap, S.B., Wong, Z.Y.H., *et al.* (1995). Linkage of high-affinity IgE receptor gene with bronchial hyperreactivity, even in absence of atopy. *Lancet*, **346**, 1262–5.

Van Schayck, C.P., Dompeling, E., van Herwaarden, L.A., *et al.* (1991). Bronchodilator treatment in moderate asthma or chronic bronchitis, continuous or on demand? A randomised controlled study. *British Medical Journal*, **303**, 1426–31.

Verhoeff, A.P., Van Strien, R.T., Van Wijnen, J.H., and Brunekreef, B. (1995). Damp housing and childhood respiratory symptoms, the role of sensitization to dust mites and molds. *American Journal of Epidemiology*, **141**, 103–10.

Vervloet, D., Dornelas de Andrade, A., Pascal, L., *et al.* (1999). The prevalence of reported asthma is independent of exposure in house dust mite-sensitized children. E *European Respiratory Journal*, **13**, 983–7.

Von Essen, S.G. and Donham, K.J. (1997). Respiratory diseases related to work in agriculture. In *Safety and health in agriculture, forestry, and fisheries* (ed. R.L. Langley, R.L. McLymore, W.J. Meggs, and G.T. Roberson). Government Institutes, Rockville, Maryland.

Von Mutius, E. and Nicolai, T. (1996). Familial aggregation of asthma in a South Bavarian population. *American Journal of Respiratory and Critical Care Medicine*, **153**, 1266–72.

Von Mutius, E., Martinez, F.D., Fritzsch, C., *et al.* (1994). Skin test reactivity and number of siblings. *British Medical Journal*, **308**, 692–5.

Von Mutius, E., Weiland, S.K., Fritzsch, C., *et al.* (1998). Increasing prevalence of hay fever and atopy among children in Leipzig, East Germany. *Lancet*, **351**, 862–6.

Watson, J.P., Cowen, P., and Lewis, R.A. (1996). The relationships between asthma admission rates, routes of admission, and socioeconomic deprivation. *European Respiratory Journal*, **9**, 2087–93.

Weeke, E. (1992). Epidemiology of allergic diseases in children. *Rhinology*, **30** (Supplement 13), 5–12.

Weiss, K.B. (1990). Seasonal trends in US asthma hospitalizations and mortality. *Journal of the American Medical Association*, **263**, 2323–8.

Weiss, K.B. and Wagener, D.K. (1990). Changing patterns of asthma mortality identifying populations at high risk. *Journal of the American Medical Association*, **264**, 1683–7.

Weiss, K.B., Gergen, P.J., and Wagener, D.K. (1993). Breathing better or wheezing worse? The changing epidemiology of asthma morbidity and mortality. *Annual Review of Public Health*, **14**, 491–513.

Weitzman, M., Gortmaker, S.L., Sobol, A.M., *et al.* (1992). Recent trends in the prevalence and severity of childhood asthma. *Journal of the American Medical Association*, **268**, 2673–7.

Welliver, R.C., Wong, D.T., Sun, M., *et al.* (1981). The development of respiratory syncytial virus-specific IgE and the release of histamine in nasopharyngeal secretions after infection. *New England Journal of Medicine*, **305**, 841–6.

Whincup, P.H., Cook, D.P., Strachan, D.P., and Papacosta, O. (1993). Time trends in respiratory symptoms in childhood over a 24 year period. *Archives of Disease in Childhood*, **68**, 729–34.

Wickens, K., Crane, J., Kemp, T., *et al.* (1999*a*). Family size, infections and asthma in New Zealand children. *Epidemiology*, **10**, 699–705.

Wickens, K., Crane, J., Pearce, N., and Beasley, R. (1999*b*). The magnitude of the effect of smaller family sizes on the increase in the prevalence of asthma in the United Kingdom and New Zealand. *Journal of Allergy and Clinical Immunology*, **104**, 554–8.

Wickens, K., Pearce, N., Crane, J., and Beasley, R. (1999*c*). Antibiotic use in early childhood and the development of asthma. *Clinics in Experimental Allergy*, **29**, 766–71.

Wierenga, E.A., Snoek, M., de Groot, C., *et al.* (1990). Evidence for compartmentalization of functional subsets of $CD2^+$ T lymphocytes in atopic patients. *Journal of Immunology*, **144**, 4651–6.

Willis, T. (1678). *Practice of physick, pharmaceutice rationalis or the operations of medicine in humane bodies*. London.

Wilson, J.D., Sutherland, D.C., and Thomas, A.C. (1981). Has the change to beta-agonists combined with oral theophylline increased cases of fatal asthma. *Lancet*, **i**, 1235–7.

Windom, H., Burgess, C., Crane, J., *et al.* (1990). The self-administration of inhaled beta agonist drugs during severe asthma. *New Zealand Medical Journal*, **103**, 205–7.

Woolcock, A. and Peat, J.K. (1997). *Evidence for the increase in asthma worldwide. The rising trends in asthma*, pp. 122–39. Ciba Foundation Symposium 206. Wiley, Chichester.

Yunginger, J.W., Reed, C.E., O'Connell, J.O., *et al.* (1992). A community-based study of the epidemiology of asthma. *American Review of Respiratory Disease*, **146**, 888–94.

Zamel, N., McClean, P.A., Sandell, P.R., *et al.* (1996). Asthma on Tristan da Cunha, looking for the genetic link. *American Journal of Respiratory and Critical Care Medicine*, **153L**, 1902–6.

Zmirou, D., Schwartz, J., Saez, M., *et al.* (1998). Time series analysis of air pollution and cause-specific mortality. *Epidemiology*, **9**, 495–503.

9.6 Endocrine and metabolic disorders

Basil S. Hetzel, Paul Zimmet, and Ego Seeman

Introduction

Endocrine and metabolic disorders present major public health problems in many parts of the world, including mental retardation resulting from iodine deficiency, diabetic vascular disease, and fractures in the elderly resulting from osteoporosis and calcium loss. Many of these endocrine and metabolic disorders are readily amenable to prevention by public health measures. This chapter provides examples of three major endocrine and metabolic disorders of public health significance.

Iodine deficiency disorders

Basil S. Hetzel

History

Iodine is an essential constituent of the thyroid hormones thyroxine or 3,5,3′,5′ tetra-iodothyronine (T_4), and 3,5,3′ tri-iodothyronine (T_3). The major role of iodine in nutrition arises from the essential role of thyroid hormones in normal growth and development (Stanbury and Hetzel 1980; Hetzel 1989).

The relation of iodine deficiency to enlargement of the thyroid gland, or goitre, was first shown by David Marine who found that hyperplastic changes occurred regularly in the thyroid when the iodine concentration fell below 0.1 per cent (Hetzel 1989). Subsequently, in 1922, Marine and Kimball demonstrated in schoolchildren in Akron, Ohio, that endemic goitre could be both prevented and substantially reduced by administration of small amounts of iodine as potassium iodide in milk given over 10 days twice a year.

Mass prophylaxis of goitre with iodized salt was first introduced in Switzerland and in Michigan in the United States. In Switzerland, the widespread occurrence of a severe form of mental deficiency and deaf mutism (endemic cretinism) was a heavy charge on public funds. However, following the introduction of iodized salt, goitre incidence fell rapidly and new cretins were no longer born. Goitre also disappeared from army recruits (Burgi *et al.* 1990).

A further major development was the administration of injections of iodized oil to people living in inaccessible mountain villages in Papua New Guinea (McCullagh 1963; Buttfield and Hetzel 1967). Subsequently, the prevention of cretinism and stillbirths was demonstrated by the administration of iodized oil before pregnancy in a controlled trial in the Highlands of Papua New Guinea (Pharoah *et al.* 1971). This work opened up the modern concept of the iodine deficiency disorders (**IDD**) resulting from all the effects of iodine deficiency on growth and development, particularly brain development, in an exposed population. Iodine deficiency is now recognized as the most common form of preventable mental defect (Hetzel 1983, 1989).

Although the major prevalence is in developing countries, the problem continues to be very significant in many European countries (France, Italy, Germany, Greece, Poland, Romania, Spain, and Turkey) because of the threat to brain development in the fetus and young infant (Hetzel 1989; Hetzel *et al.* 1990).

The ecology of iodine deficiency

There is a cycle of iodine in nature. Most of the iodine resides in the ocean. It was present during the primordial development of the Earth, but large amounts were leached from the surface soil by glaciation, snow, or rain, and were carried by wind, rivers, and floods into the sea. Iodine occurs in the deeper layers of the soil and is found in oil-well and natural gas effluents. Water from such deep wells can provide a major source for iodine. In general the older an exposed soil surface, the more likely it is to be leached of iodine (Stanbury and Hetzel 1980; Hetzel 1989).

The better known areas to be leached are the mountainous areas of the world. The most severely deficient soils are those of the European Alps, the Himalayas, the Andes, and the vast mountains of China. But iodine deficiency is likely to occur to some extent in all elevated regions subject to glaciation and higher rainfall, with run-off into rivers. More recently it has become clear that iodine deficiency also occurs in flooded river valleys such as the Ganges in India, the Mekong in Vietnam, and the river valleys of China.

Iodine occurs in soil and the sea as iodide. Iodide ions are oxidized by sunlight to elemental iodine which is volatile so that every year some 400 000 tons escape from the surface of the sea. The concentration of iodide in the sea water is about 50 to 60 μg/l; in the air it is approximately 0.7 μg/m^3. The iodine in the atmosphere is returned to the soil by the rain which has concentrations in the range 1.8 to 8.5 μg/l. In this way the cycle is completed.

However, the return of the iodine is slow and small in amount compared with the original loss of iodine, and subsequent repeated flooding ensures the continuity of iodine deficiency in the soil. Hence no 'natural correction' can take place and iodine deficiency persists in the soil indefinitely. All crops grown in these soils will be iodine deficient. As a result human and animal populations which are totally dependent on food grown in such soil become iodine deficient. The iodine content of plants grown in iodine-deficient soils may be as low as 10 μg/kg compared with 1 mg/kg dry weight in plants in a non-iodine-deficient soil. This accounts for the occurrence of severe iodine deficiency in vast populations in Asia who are living within systems of subsistence agriculture in flooded river valleys (India, Bangladesh, Burma, Vietnam, and China).

The physiology of iodine deficiency

The healthy human adult body contains 15 to 20 mg of iodine of which about 70 to 80 per cent is in the thyroid gland. The thyroid weighs only 15 to 25 g so that it has a remarkable concentrating power.

Iodide is rapidly absorbed through the gut. The normal intake and requirement is 100 to 150 μg/day. Excess iodine is excreted by the kidney. The level of excretion correlates well with the level of intake so that it can be used to assess the level of iodine intake (see below).

The thyroid has to trap about 60 μg of iodine per day to maintain an adequate supply of T_4. This is possible because of the very active iodide trapping mechanism which maintains a gradient of 100:1 between the thyroid cell and the extracellular fluid. In iodine deficiency this gradient may exceed 400:1 in order to maintain the output of T_4.

Thyroid secretion is under the control of the pituitary gland through thyroid-stimulating hormone (**TSH**) which is a glycoprotein with a molecular weight of approximately 28 000. There are two subunits—the X subunit has virtually the same structure as other pituitary hormones, and the B subunit is specific for TSH but essentially the same across different species.

The control of TSH secretion is by a 'feedback' mechanism related closely to the level of T_4 in the blood. As the blood T_4 falls, the pituitary TSH secretion is increased to increase thyroid activity, and the output of T_4 into the circulation, and so maintain the necessary level of circulating hormone. If this is not possible because of severe iodine deficiency, the level of T_4 remains lowered and the level of TSH remains elevated. Both these measurements are used for the diagnosis of hypothyroidism due to iodine deficiency at various stages in life, but particularly in the neonate.

Blood thyroid hormones and TSH (the TSH of the pituitary) are determined using radio-immunoassay when known amounts of radio-actively labelled hormones are used and compete with the unknown amount of hormone in the blood in binding to a specific antibody. The technology for these determinations is still advancing and further improvements are being developed (see below).

The development of goitre

The preceding discussion of the production and regulation of thyroid hormones provides the framework for understanding the production of goitre as a result of iodine deficiency (Fig. 1). Although not the only cause, iodine deficiency is the primary cause of goitre. Other factors—'goitrogens' such as thiocyanates can enhance the effect of iodine deficiency—are referred to as secondary factors (Ermans *et al.* 1980).

The basic effect of iodine deficiency is to interfere with the production of thyroid hormones because iodine is an essential constituent of the T_4 and T_3 molecules. The lowering of output from the thyroid leads to a fall in the blood levels of T_4 but some increase in T_3 (the less iodinated hormone is produced preferentially in iodine deficiency).

The fall in the level of T_4 leads to increase in TSH output from the pituitary with increase in uptake of iodide and increased turnover

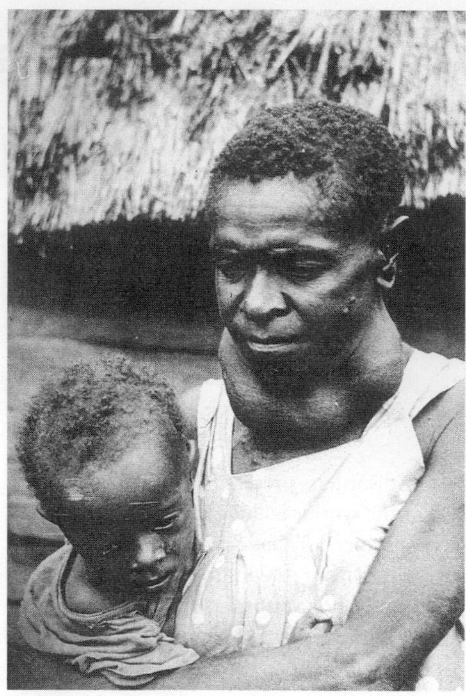

Fig. 1 A mother and child from a New Guinea village who are severely iodine deficient. The mother has a large goitre and the child is also affected. The larger the goitre, the more likely it is that she will have a cretin child. This can be prevented by eliminating the iodine deficiency before the onset of pregnancy.

associated with hyperplasia of the cells of the thyroid follicles. The reserves of colloid containing thyroglobulin are gradually used up, so that the gland has a much more cellular appearance than normal. The size of the gland increases with the formation of a goitre. Enlargement is regarded as significant in the human when the size of the lateral lobes is greater than the terminal phalanx of the thumb of the person examined. More precise measurements can now be made using ultrasound.

Extensive reviews of the global geographic prevalence of goitre have been published (Dunn *et al.* 1986; Hetzel *et al.* 1987; Hetzel 1989; Hetzel and Pandav 1996).

The iodine deficiency disorders

The effects of iodine deficiency on growth and development of a population that can be prevented by correction of iodine deficiency are now denoted by the term IDD. These effects are evident at all stages including particularly the fetus, the neonate, and in infancy, which are the periods of rapid brain growth (Hetzel 1983). The term 'goitre' has been used for many years to describe the effect of iodine deficiency. Goitre is indeed the obvious and familiar feature of iodine deficiency but knowledge has greatly expanded in the last 25 years so that it is not surprising that a new term is needed (Table 1).

The fetus

Iodine deficiency of the fetus is the result of iodine deficiency in the mother. The condition is associated with a greater incidence of stillbirths, spontaneous abortions, and congenital abnormalities, which can be reduced by iodization. The effects are similar to those

Table 1 The spectrum of IDD

Fetus
Abortions
Stillbirths
Congenital anomalies
Increased perinatal mortality
Increased infant mortality
Neurological cretinism
Mental deficiency
Deaf mutism
Spastic diplegia
Squint
Myxoedematous cretinism
Dwarfism
Mental deficiency
Psychomotor defects
Neonate
Neonatal goitre
Neonatal hypothyroidism
Increased susceptibility to nuclear radiation[a]
Child and adolescent
Goitre
Juvenile hypothyroidism
Impaired mental function
Retarded physical development
Increased susceptibility to nuclear radiation[a]
Adult
Goitre with its complications
Hypothyroidism
Impaired mental function
Iodine-induced hyperthyroidism
Increased susceptibility to nuclear radiation[a]

[a]Due to increased uptake of radio-active iodine.

Source: Hetzel *et al.* (1990).

observed with maternal hypothyroidism which can be reduced by thyroid hormone replacement therapy (McMichael *et al.* 1980).

Controlled trials with iodized oil have revealed a significant reduction in recorded fetal and neonatal deaths in the treated group which is consistent with animal evidence indicating the effect of iodine deficiency on fetal survival (Hetzel *et al.* 1990).

A major effect of fetal iodine deficiency is the condition of endemic cretinism which is quite distinct from the condition of sporadic cretinism (Pharoah *et al.* 1980; Hetzel 1989). This condition, which occurs with an iodine intake of below 25 μg/day in contrast to a normal intake of 80 to 150 μg/day, is still widely prevalent, affecting for example up to 10 per cent of the populations living in severely iodine-deficient areas in India, Indonesia, and China. In its most common form, it is characterized by mental deficiency, deaf mutism, and spastic diplegia (Fig. 2); this is referred to as the 'nervous' or neurological type in contrast to the less common 'myxoedematous' type characterized by hypothyroidism with dwarfism.

Apart from its prevalence in Asia and Oceania, cretinism also occurs in Africa (Zaire) and the Andean region of South America

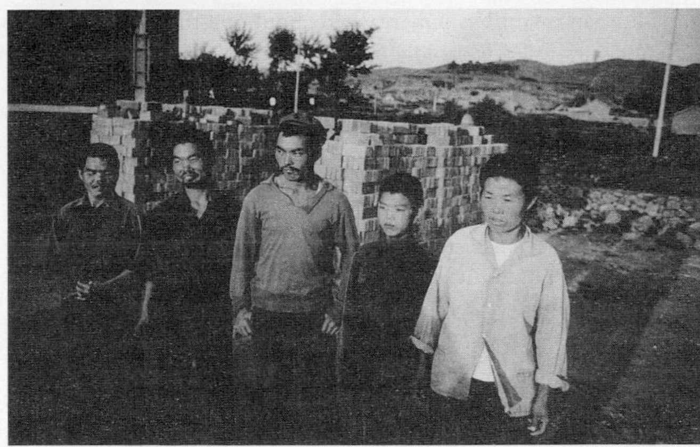

Fig. 2 A mother with her four sons in Chengde, China: three of them (aged 31, 29, and 28 years) are cretins, born before iodized salt was introduced, but the fourth (aged 14) is normal, born after iodized salt became available.

(Ecuador, Peru, Bolivia, and Argentina) (Pharoah *et al.* 1980). In all these situations, with the exception of Zaire, neurological features are predominant. In Zaire the myxoedematous form is more common, probably because of the high intake of cassava (Ermans *et al.* 1980).

There is considerable variation in the clinical manifestations of neurological cretinism which include isolated deaf mutism and mental defect of varying degrees. In China the term 'cretinoid' is used to describe these individuals (Ma *et al.* 1982), which may number five to 10 times those with overt cretinism.

The apparent spontaneous disappearance of endemic cretinism in Italy and Switzerland raised considerable doubts as to the relation of iodine deficiency to the condition. However, a controlled trial in the Western Highlands of Papua New Guinea revealed that endemic cretinism could be prevented by correction of iodine deficiency with iodized oil before pregnancy (Pharoah *et al.* 1971; Pharoah and Connolly 1987).

The value of iodized oil injection in the prevention of endemic cretinism has been confirmed in Zaire and South America. Mass injection programmes have been carried out in New Guinea (1971–1972) and in Zaire, Indonesia, and China. Recent evaluations of these mass programmes in Indonesia and China indicate that endemic cretinism has been prevented where correction of iodine deficiency has been achieved (Hetzel 1989).

The apparent spontaneous disappearance of the condition is now attributed to increase in iodine intake due to dietary diversification as a result of social and economic development affecting more remote rural areas and the use of dietary supplements containing iodine (Burgi *et al.* 1990).

The neonate

An increased perinatal mortality due to iodine deficiency has been shown in Zaire from the results of a controlled trial of iodized oil injections given alternately with a control injection in the latter half of pregnancy (Thilly *et al.* 1986). There was a substantial fall in perinatal and infant mortality with improved birth weight. Low birth weight (whatever the cause) is generally associated with a higher rate of congenital anomalies and higher risk through childhood.

Apart from the question of mortality, the importance of the state of thyroid function in the neonate relates to the fact that at birth the brain of the human infant has only reached about one-third of its full size and continues to grow rapidly until the end of the second year. The thyroid hormone, dependent on an adequate supply of iodine, is essential for normal brain development as has been confirmed by animal studies (Hetzel and Mano 1989; Hetzel *et al.* 1990).

Data on iodine nutrition and neonatal thyroid function in Europe have been published. These data confirm the continuing presence of severe iodine deficiency affecting neonatal thyroid function and hence a threat to early brain development (Delange *et al.* 1986). These data are arousing great concern about iodine deficiency, which is heightened by awareness of the hazard of nuclear radiation following the Chernobyl disaster.

There is similar evidence from neonatal observations in Zaire where rates of chemical hypothyroidism as high as 10 per cent have been found (Ermans *et al.* 1980), as is also found in northern India (Hetzel *et al.* 1987).

These observations indicate a much greater risk of mental defect in severely iodine-deficient populations than is indicated by the presence of classical cretinism. There is a continuing major problem in many European countries such as Italy, Germany, France, and Greece, while Rumania, Bulgaria, and Albania still have very severe iodine deficiency with overt cretinism (Delange *et al.* 1993; Hetzel and Pandav 1996).

The child

Iodine deficiency in children is characteristically associated with goitre. The classification of goitre has been standardized by the World Health Organization (**WHO**) and is discussed below. The goitre rate increases with age so that it reaches a maximum with adolescence. There is a higher prevalence in girls than in boys. Observations of goitre rates in schoolchildren between the ages of 8 to 14 years provide a convenient indication of the presence of iodine deficiency in a community.

In one meta-analysis including 18 studies in which a comparison was made between iodine-deficient children and carefully selected control groups, the mean scores were found to be 13.5 IQ points apart. This meant that the iodine-deficient groups had a mean IQ which was 13.5 points lower than the non-iodine-deficient control group (Bleichrodt and Born 1994). Detailed individual studies demonstrating these defects in Italian and Spanish schoolchildren as well as those from Africa, China, Indonesia, and Papua New Guinea have been published (Delange 1994; Stanbury 1994). There is a serious problem in Europe as well as in many developing countries.

The adult

Iodine administration in the form of iodized salt, iodized bread, or iodized oil have all been demonstrated to be effective in the prevention of goitre in younger adults. Iodine administration may also reduce existing goitre in adults. This is particularly true of iodized oil administration. This obvious effect with the benefits of the correction of hypothyroidism leads to ready acceptance of the measure by people living in iodine-deficient communities.

In northern India a high degree of apathy has been noted in populations living in iodine-deficient areas. This may even affect domestic animals such as dogs. It is apparent that reduced mental function is widely prevalent in iodine-deficient communities with effects on their capacity for initiative and decision-making. This is due to the effect of hypothyroidism on brain function—this condition can be readily reversed by correction of the iodine deficiency (unlike the effects on the fetus and in infancy).

This means that iodine deficiency is a major block to the human and social development of communities living in an iodine-deficient environment. Correction of the iodine deficiency is indicated as a major contribution to development. Increase in physical and mental energy leads to improvements in work output, school learning, and general quality of life. Improved livestock productivity (chickens, cattle, and sheep) is also a major economic benefit.

Magnitude of the problem

The extent of IDD in the world has now been estimated by the WHO (1990). In an estimated at-risk population of 1 billion, in excess of 200 million have goitre and 20 million have some degree of brain damage due to the effects of iodine deficiency in pregnancy. More recently the estimate of the population at risk has been increased to 2.2 billion (WHO 1999).

One review of the problem of IDD in Europe led to an estimate of 140 million (out of a total of 850 million) still at risk of the effects of iodine deficiency, especially on brain development in the fetus and infants over the first 2 years of life. In fact most European countries still have some IDD (Delange *et al.* 1993).

The major regional concentration of population at risk is in Asia which contributes over 1 billion of the world total, with almost half in China (where 40 per cent of the population are at risk) (WHO 1999).

Assessment of iodine status

The assessment of iodine nutritional status is important in relation to public health programmes in which iodine supplementation is carried out. Therefore the problem is one of assessment of a population or group living in an area or region that is suspected to be iodine deficient. The major assessment criteria are as follows:

- thyroid size including the rate of palpable or visible goitre classified according to accepted criteria
- urine iodine excretion
- the determination of the level of blood T_4 or TSH.

Particular attention is now given to TSH levels in the neonate because of the importance of the level of thyroid function for early brain development.

The classification of goitre severity has now been simplified by the WHO (Table 2). There are significant differences in technique between different observers. In general, visible goitre is more readily verified than palpable goitre. Recent observations indicate that

Table 2 Simplified classification of goitre

Grade 0	No palpable or visible goitre
Grade 1	A mass in the neck that is consistent with an enlarged thyroid that is palpable but not visible when the neck is in the normal position. It moves upward in the neck as the subject swallows. Nodular alteration(s) can occur even when the thyroid is not enlarged
Grade 2	A swelling in the neck that is visible when the neck is in a normal position and is consistent with an enlarged thyroid when the neck is palpated

Source: WHO (1994).

palpation of the thyroid overestimates the size of the gland as determined by ultrasonography, particularly in children. For this reason ultrasonography is now replacing palpation when suitable equipment is available (Hetzel and Pandav 1996; Delange 1997).

The determination of urine iodine excretion can be carried out on 24-h samples. However, the difficulties of such collections are usually insurmountable. For this reason determinations can be more conveniently carried out on casual samples from a group of approximately 50 or more subjects. The iodine levels are expressed as micrograms per litre and the range plotted as a histogram. The median level is used as a convenient indicator of the range. It is normally 100 μg/l.

The level of iodine excretion provides a good index of the level of iodine nutrition. The normal requirement for iodine intake is 100 to 150 μg/day increasing to 200 μg/day in pregnancy (Food and Nutrition Board 1989; Delange *et al.* 1993). Improvements in methodology and the availability of modern automated equipment (autoanalyser) are making the analysis of large numbers of samples feasible (WHO 1994). The remedial effects of iodization programmes can also be most conveniently monitored by determination of urine iodine excretion in 50 casual samples from schoolchildren.

The determination of the level of T_4 or TSH provides an indirect measure of iodine nutritional status. The availability of radioimmunoassay methods with automated equipment has greatly assisted this approach, and TSH is now the preferred method because of better stability under tropical conditions and easier methodology. Particular attention should be given to levels of TSH in the neonate as an indication of the risk of brain damage.

In developed countries, where iodine deficiency in humans normally does not exist, all babies born are screened to ensure that they have adequate thyroid hormone levels. These screening programmes use blood from heel pricks of neonates (usually on the fourth postnatal day) spotted onto filter paper which is dried and sent to a regional laboratory. Blood levels of T_4, TSH, or both are measured by immunoassay techniques. The detection rate of neonatal hypothyroidism requiring treatment in the absence of iodine deficiency is about 1 per 3500 babies screened. This rate varies little among developed countries (Burrow 1980).

Neonatal hypothyroid screening has been initiated in several less-developed iodine-deficient regions. As already noted severe biochemical hypothyroidism (T_4 concentrations less than 3 μg/dl) has been reported in up to 10 per cent of neonates in northern India and Zaire (Hetzel *et al.* 1987). It is evident from this and from other reports that, within an iodine-deficient population, serum T_4 levels are lowest at birth and lower in children than in the adult population (Delange *et al.* 1986). In addition, goitrogens such as cassava seem to be much more potent at reducing serum T_4 levels in neonates and children than adults.

To summarize, the most critical evidence for determination of iodine nutrition status comes from measurement of urine excretion of iodine and from the measurement of blood TSH in the neonate. The results of these two determinations indicate the severity of the problem. They can also be used to assess the effectiveness of remedial measures (WHO 2001).

The correction of iodine deficiency

Iodized salt

Since the introduction of iodized salt in Switzerland and the United States, successful programmes have been reported from a number of countries. These include Central and South America (e.g. Guatemala, Colombia), Finland, and Taiwan (Hetzel 1989). However, there has been great difficulty in sustaining these programmes in Central and South America because of political instability. More recently, countries in the former USSR have had major setbacks.

The difficulties in the production and maintenance of quality to the millions that are iodine deficient, especially in Asia, are vividly demonstrated in India, where there was a breakdown in supply. These difficulties have finally led to the adoption of universal salt iodization for India and subsequently to many other countries. This policy includes legislation that makes it illegal for non-iodized salt to be available for human or animal consumption.

In Asia, the cost of iodized salt production and distribution at present is in the range of 2 to 8 American cents per person per year (Hetzel and Pandav 1989). This must be considered cheap in relation to the social benefits described above.

However, there is still the problem of the iodine in the salt actually reaching the iodine-deficient subject. There may be a problem with distribution or preservation of the iodine content—it may be left uncovered or exposed to heat. It should be added after cooking to reduce the loss of iodine.

Potassium iodate is the preferred vehicle over potassium iodide because of its greater stability in the tropical environment (Hetzel 1989). A dose of 20 to 40 mg iodine as potassium iodate per kilogram is recommended to cover losses to ensure an adequate household level (WHO 1996). This assumes a salt intake of 10 g/day; if the level is below this, an appropriate correction can easily be made by increasing the concentration of potassium iodate.

Iodine-induced hyperthyroidism

An increase in incidence of hyperthyroidism has been described following iodized salt programmes in Europe and South America and following the use of iodized bread in Holland and Tasmania (Connolly *et al.* 1970; Stewart *et al.* 1971). A few cases have been noted following iodized oil administration in South America. The condition is easily overlooked in developing countries because of the scattered nature of the population and limited opportunities for observation. Iodine-induced hyperthyroidism occurs widely in Europe because of the persistent prevalence of iodine deficiency in the absence of effective iodization programmes. The condition is largely confined to those over 40 years of age; a smaller proportion of the population in developing countries is affected than in developed countries. Detailed observations are available from the island of Tasmania (Stewart *et al.* 1971; Vidor *et al.* 1973) and, more recently, from Zimbabwe (Todd *et al.* 1995). A review has recently been published.

In Zimbabwe careful investigations revealed that excessive levels of iodine in the salt was the result of faulty mixing at factory level and this had led to the occurrence of iodine-induced hyperthyroidism. This indicates that suitable monitoring procedures for salt and urine iodine are essential to prevent excessive iodine intake and iodine-induced hyperthyroidism. Monitoring is also essential to ensure that the intake is adequate to correct iodine deficiency, which has been a greater problem in Asia and Latin America.

Hyperthyroidism is accompanied by some morbidity and mortality in the older age groups. It is readily controlled with antithyroid drugs, radio-iodine, or subtotal thyroidectomy if it is available. Risk of hyperthyroidism, even with an increase to normal levels of intake, arises because an autonomous thyroid can develop independently of

TSH control, which continues its high rate of secretion in spite of an increase in iodine intake. To reduce iodine-induced hyperthyroidism to a minimum, the median urine iodine level should not exceed 20 μg/dl. Adequate facilities for diagnosis and treatment are required in areas where iodine-induced hyperthyroidism has been detected.

The occurrence of iodine-induced hyperthyroidism with consequent morbidity and mortality is not regarded as a contraindication to iodization programmes (WHO 1996) in view of the enormous benefits that correction of iodine deficiency has for the whole population—particularly the reduction in child mortality, improved child learning, the improved health of women, greater economic productivity, and improved quality of life.

Furthermore, the correction of iodine deficiency prevents the formation of an autonomous thyroid and so prevents the condition of iodine-induced hyperthyroidism with consequent disappearance in subsequent generations. Hence this condition is included as an 'iodine-deficiency disorder' (Table 1).

Iodized oil

Iodized oil by injection or by mouth is singularly appropriate for the isolated village communities so characteristic of mountainous endemic goitre areas. The striking regression of goitre following iodized oil administration ensures general acceptance of the measure (Fig. 3). In a suitable area, the oil (1 ml contains 480 mg iodine) should be administered to all females up to the age of 40 years and all males up to the age of 20 years. A dose of 480 mg will provide coverage for 1 year by mouth and for 2 years by injection (Benmiloud *et al.* 1994).

Iodized milk

This is particularly important for infants receiving formula milk as an alternative to breast feeding. An increase in levels from 5 to 10 μg/dl has been recommended for full-term infants by the International Council for Control of Iodine Deficiency Disorders (**ICCIDD**), and a level of 20 μg/dl has been recommended for premature infants (Delange *et al.* 1993).

Iodized milk has been generally available in the United States, the United Kingdom, and northern Europe, Australia, and New Zealand as a result of the addition of iodophors as disinfectants by the dairy industry. This has been a major factor in the elimination of iodine deficiency in these countries. However, in most countries of southern and eastern Europe this has not occurred and the risk of iodine deficiency continues (Delange *et al.* 1993). Recently, the use of iodophors has been phased out with substantial drop in the level of urine iodine excretion. The possibility of recurrence of iodine deficiency in industrialized countries (e.g. the United States) now exists (Dunn 1998).

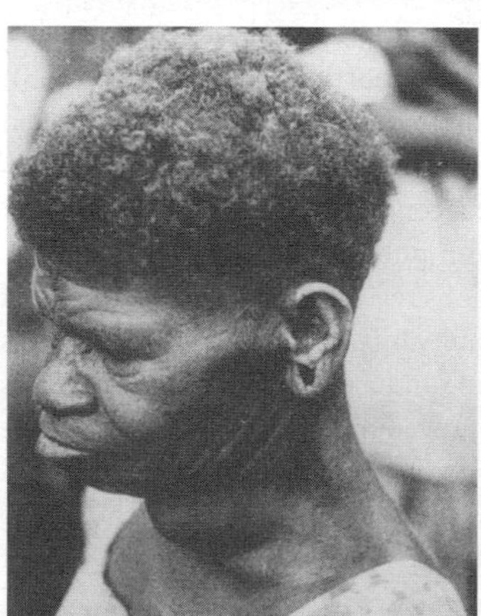

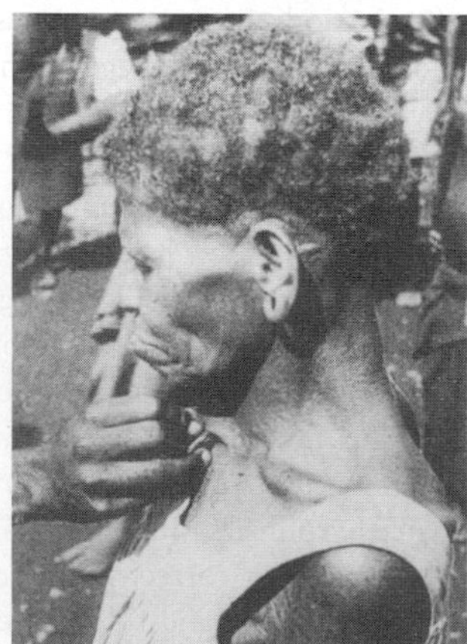

Fig. 3 Subsidence of goitre in a New Guinea woman 3 months after the injection of iodized oil. This is accompanied by a feeling of well being due to a rise in the level of the thyroid hormone in the blood. This makes the injections very popular. (Reproduced from Buttfield and Hetzel 1967.)

The support of the United Nations system

The United Nations system has now recognized IDD as a major international public health problem and adopted a global plan for its elimination by the year 2000 which was proposed by the ICCIDD working in close collaboration with UNICEF and WHO (Hetzel and Pandav 1996). The ICCIDD is an independent expert group of more than 400 professionals in public health, medical and nutritional science, technologists, and planners, drawn from more than 90 countries.

In 1990, the World Health Assembly and the World Summit for Children both accepted the goal of elimination of IDD as a public health problem by the year 2000. These major meetings included government representatives, including heads of state, at the World Summit for Children from 71 countries with a further 88 countries signing the Plan of Action for elimination of IDD as well as other major problems in nutrition and health.

Since 1989 a series of Joint WHO/UNICEF/ICCIDD regional meetings have been held to assist countries with their national programmes for the elimination of IDD. The impact of these meetings has been that governments now realize the importance of iodine deficiency to the future potential of their people. A dramatic example is provided by the government of the People's Republic of China. As is well known, China has a one-child family policy which means that an avoidable hazard like iodine deficiency should be eliminated. In China iodine deficiency is a threat to 40 per cent of the population because of the highly mountainous terrain of China and flooded river valleys—in excess of 400 million people are at risk. In recognition of this massive threat to the Chinese people, the government held a National

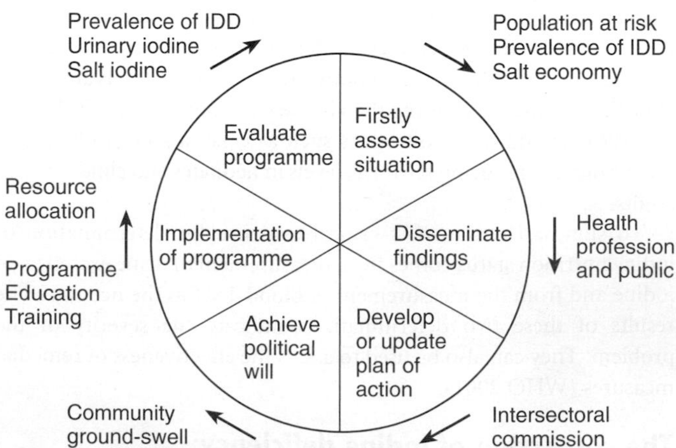

Fig. 4 The 'wheel' represents the continuous 'feedback' process involved in the national IDD control (elimination) programme. All 'actors' in the programme need to understand the whole social process.

Table 3 Current status of household consumption of iodized salt

WHO region	No. of countries with IDD	Percentage of households consuming iodized salt					
		No data	<10%	10%–50%	51%–90%	>90%	Overall[a]
Africa	44	8	6	8	19	3	63
Americas	19	0	0	3	6	10	90
Southeast Asia	9	0	1	2	5	1	70
Eastern Mediterranean	17	5	1	2	6	3	66
Europe	32	10	4	12	4	2	27
Western Pacific	9	0	1	4	3	1	76
Total	130	23	13	31	43	20	68

[a]Total population of each country multiplied by the percentage of households consuming iodized salt. Numbers are then summed for each region and divided by the total regional population.

Source: WHO (1999).

Advocacy Meeting (21–24 September 1993) in the Great Hall of the People, sponsored by the Chinese Premier, Mr Li Peng, under the Chairmanship of Madame Peng Pei-yun of the State Council. The commitment of the government to the elimination of iodine deficiency was emphasized by the Vice-Premier, Mr Zhu Rongyi, to the assembly of provincial delegations led by the provincial governors and the representatives of the international agencies (Hetzel and Pandav 1996).

In Beijing (October 1998) an international workshop was held by the Ministry of Health of China with the ICCIDD. Dramatic progress was reported as indicated by a reduction in mean goitre rate (from 20 to 10 per cent) with normal urine iodine levels. Severe iodine deficiency has persisted in Tibet because of difficulty in the implementation of salt iodization. In other provinces excess of iodine intake was noted in 10 per cent of the population. The need for continuation of monitoring with urine iodine was emphasized at the meeting.

The elimination of IDD at country level

It is now recognized that an effective national programme for the elimination of IDD requires the multisectoral approach as shown in Fig. 4. The 'wheel' must keep turning to maintain an effective programme.

Striking progress with universal salt iodization has now occurred as indicated by the WHO/UNICEF/ICCIDD Report to the 1999 World Health Assembly. Table 3 shows the percentage of households

Table 4 Current status of key elements of IDD control programmes

WHO region	Number of countries						
	Affected by IDD	With national intersectoral co-ordinating body	With plan of action for IDD control	With legislation in place[a]	Monitoring salt quality (process indicators)	Monitoring population status (impact indicators)	With laboratory facilities[b]
Africa	44	35	36	34 (6)	29	24	28
Americas	19	18	18	17	19	19	19
South East Asia	9	9	8	7 (1)	8	7	6
Eastern Mediterranean	17	15	14	14	14	10	11
Europe	32	20	18	20 (3)	17	13	13
Western Pacific	9	8	8	6 (2)	8	6	7
Total	130	105	102	98 (12)	95	79	84
Percentage	100	81	78	75 (9)	73	61	65

[a]The number in parentheses refers to the number of additional countries which have legislation in draft form.

[b]These figures reflect both countries with the capacity for urinary iodine analysis and/or salt iodine levels. However, the standard of laboratories and expertise in each country is very different.

Source: WHO (1999).

consuming iodized salt. Where household data are not available, estimates based on production were used instead. These data show that of 5 billion people living in countries with IDD, 68 per cent now have access to iodized salt. Table 4 shows the status of development of the national programme in the 130 countries affected by IDD. It can be seen that 81 per cent of countries have an intersectoral co-ordinating body and 75 per cent have legislation in place.

Monitoring is now recognized as a key requirement for ensuring the sustainability of IDD control programmes. Table 4 shows the number of countries monitoring both the process indicators (salt) and the outcome indicators (using goitre rates or urine iodine measurements or both) and whether laboratory facilities are available.

The major challenge is not only the achievement of effective salt iodization but its sustainability. In the past a number of countries have achieved effective salt iodization, but in the absence of monitoring, the programmes have lapsed with recurrence of IDD. To this end, the ICCIDD, the WHO, and UNICEF are now offering help to governments with partnership evaluation to assess progress towards the goal and to provide help to overcome any bottlenecks obstructing progress.

Criteria for tracking progress towards the goal of elimination of IDD have been agreed between the ICCIDD, the WHO, and UNICEF (WHO 1994). These include salt iodine (90 per cent effectively iodized) and urine iodine in the normal range (median excretion of 100 to 200 μg/l). The lower level of 100 μg/l is necessary to ensure normal brain development in the fetus and young infant. The higher level of 200 μg/l is designed to minimize the occurrence of iodine-induced hyperthyroidism.

The global partnership

Since 1990 a remarkable global partnership has come together made up of the people and countries with an IDD problem, the international agencies, particularly UNICEF, the WHO, and the ICCIDD, the salt industry from the private sector, and Kiwanis International, a World Service Club of 330 000 members throughout the world which has adopted a fundraising target of US$75 million towards the elimination of IDD by the year 2000 (Hetzel and Pandav 1996). This partnership exists to support countries and governments in their conquest of IDD. This would be the first global triumph in the elimination of a non-infectious disease.

References

Benmiloud, M., Chaouki, M.L., Gutekunst, R., Teichert, H-M., Wood, W.G., and Dunn, J.T. (1994). Oral iodised oil for correcting iodine deficiency: optimal dosing and outcome indicator selection. *Journal of Clinical Endocrinology and Metabolism*, **79**, 20–4.

Bleichrodt, N. and Born, M.P. (1994). A metaanalysis of research on iodine and its relationship to cognitive development. In *The damaged brain of iodine deficiency* (ed. J.B. Stanbury), pp. 195–200. Cognizant Communication Corporation, New York.

Burgi, H., Supersaxo, Z., and Selz, B. (1990). Iodine deficiency diseases in Switzerland one hundred years after Theodor Kocher's survey: a historical review with some new goitre prevalence data. *Acta Endocrinologica*, **123**, 577–90.

Burrow, G.N. (ed.) (1980). *Neonatal thyroid screening*. Raven Press, New York.

Buttfield, I.H. and Hetzel, B.S. (1967). Endemic goitre in Eastern New Guinea with special reference to the use of iodised oil in prophylaxis and treatment. *Bulletin of the World Health Organization*, **36**, 243–62.

Connolly, R.J., Vidor, and Stewart, J.C. (1970). Increase in thyrotoxicosis in endemic goitre area after iodization of bread. *Lancet*, **i**, 500–2.

Delange, F. (1994). The disorders induced by iodine deficiency. *Thyroid*, **4**, 107–27.

Delange, F. (1997). Thyroid volume and urinary iodine in European school children: standardization of values for assessment of iodine deficiency. *Bulletin of the World Health Organization*, **75**, 95–100.

Delange, F., Heidemann, P., Bourdoux, P., and Larsson A. (1986). Regional variations of iodine nutrition and thyroid function during the neonatal period in Europe. *Biology of the Neonate*, **49**, 322–30.

Delange, F., Dunn, J.T., and Glinoer, D. (ed.) (1993). *Iodine deficiency in Europe: a continuing concern*. NATO ASI Series A: Life Sciences, Vol. 241. Plenum Press, New York.

Delange, F.D., de Benoist, B., and Alnwick, D. (1999). Risks of iodine-induced hyperthyroidism after correction of iodine deficiency by iodized salt. *Thyroid*, **9**, 545–56.

Dunn, J.T. (1998). What's happening to our iodine? *Journal of Clinical Endocrinology and Metabolism*, **83**, 3398–400.

Dunn, J.T., Pretell, E.A., and Daza, C.H. (ed.) (1986). *Towards the eradication of endemic goitre, cretinism, and iodine deficiency*. Pan-American Health Organization, Washington, DC.

Ermans, A.M., Moulameko, N.M., Delange, F., and Alhuwalis, R. (ed.) (1980). *Role of cassava in the aetiology of endemic goitre and cretinism*. International Development Research Centre, Ottawa.

Food and Nutrition Board, National Academy of Sciences, National Research Council (1989). *Recommended dietary allowances* (10th edn). Washington, DC.

Hetzel, B.S. (1983). Iodine deficiency disorders (IDD) and their eradication. *Lancet*, **ii**, 1126–9.

Hetzel, B.S. (1989). *The story of iodine deficiency: an international challenge in nutrition*. Oxford University Press.

Hetzel, B.S. and Mano, M. (1989). A review of experimental studies of iodine deficiency during fetal development. *Journal of Nutrition*, **119**, 145–51.

Hetzel, B.S. and Pandav, C.S. (ed.) (1996). *SOS for a billion: the conquest of iodine deficiency disorders* (2nd edn). Oxford University Press.

Hetzel, B.S., Dunn, J.T., and Stanbury, J.B. (ed.) (1987). *The prevention and control of iodine deficiency disorders*. Elsevier, Amsterdam.

Hetzel, B.S., Potter, B.J., and Dulberg, E.M. (1990). The iodine deficiency disorders: nature, pathogenesis and epidemiology. *World Review of Nutrition Dietetics*, **62**, 59–119.

McCullagh, S.F. (1963). The Huon Peninsula endemic. The effectiveness of an intramuscular depot of iodised oil in the control of endemic goitre. *Medical Journal of Australia*, **1**, 769–77.

McMichael, A.J., Potter, J.D., and Hetzel, B.S. (1980). Iodine deficiency, thyroid function, and reproductive failure. In *Endemic goitre and endemic cretinism* (ed. J.B. Stanbury and B.S. Hetzel), pp. 445–60. Wiley, New York.

Ma, T., Lu, T., Tan, U., *et al.* (1982). The present status of endemic goitre and endemic cretinism in China. *Food and Nutrition Bulletin*, **4**, 13–19.

Pharoah, P.O.D. and Connolly, K.J. (1987). A controlled trial of iodinated oil for the prevention of cretinism: a long term follow up. *International Journal of Epidemiology*, **16**, 68–73.

Pharoah, P.O.D., Buttfield, I.H., and Hetzel, B.S. (1971). Neurological damage to the fetus resulting from severe iodine deficiency during pregnancy. *Lancet*, **i**, 308–10.

Pharoah, P.O.D., Delange, F., Fierro-Benitez, R., and Stanbury, J.B. (1980). Endemic cretinism. In *Endemic goitre and endemic cretinism* (ed. J.B. Stanbury and B.S. Hetzel), pp. 395–421. Wiley, New York.

Stanbury, J.B. (ed.) (1994). *The damaged brain of iodine deficiency*. Cognizant Communication Corporation, New York.

Stanbury, J.B. and Hetzel, B.S. (ed.) (1980). *Endemic goitre and endemic cretinism.* Wiley, New York.

Stewart, J.C., Vidor, G.I., Buttfield, I.H., and Hetzel, B.S. (1971). Epidemic thyrotoxicosis in northern Tasmania: studies of clinical features and iodine nutrition. *Australian and New Zealand Journal of Medicine*, **3**, 203–11.

Thilly, C.H., Bourdoux, P.P., Vanderpas, J.B., *et al.* (1986). Neonatal and juvenile hypothyroidism in Central Africa. In *Iodine deficiency disorders and congenital hypothyroidism* (ed. G. Medeiros-Neto, R.M.B. Maciel, and A. Halpern), pp. 26–33. Ache, Brazil.

Todd, C.H., Allain, T., Gomo, Z.A.R., Hasler, J.A., Ndiweni, M., and Oken, E. (1995). Increase in thyrotoxicosis associated with iodine supplements in Zimbabwe. *Lancet*, **346**, 552–3.

Vidor, G.I., Stewart, J.C., Wall, J.R., Wangel, A., and Hetzel, B.S. (1973). Pathogenesis of iodine induced thyrotoxicosis: studies in northern Tasmania. *Journal of Clinical Endocrinology and Metabolism*, **37**, 901.

WHO (World Health Organization) (1990). *Report to 43rd World Health Assembly.* WHO, Geneva.

WHO (World Health Organization) (1993). *Global prevalence of iodine deficiency disorders.* Micronutrient Deficiency Information System (MDIS) working paper no. 1. WHO/UNICEF/ICCIDD, Geneva.

WHO (World Health Organization) (1994). *Indicators for assessing iodine deficiency disorders and their control programmes.* Publication WHO/NUT/94.6. WHO/UNICEF/ICCIDD, Geneva.

WHO (World Health Organization) (1996). *Recommended iodine levels in salt and guidelines for monitoring their adequacy and effectiveness.* Publication WHO/NUT/96.13. WHO/UNICEF/ICCIDD, Geneva.

WHO (World Health Organization) (1999). *Progress towards the elimination of iodine deficiency disorders (IDD).* Publication WHO/NHD/99.4. WHO/UNICEF/ICCIDD, Geneva.

WHO (World Health Organization) (2001). *Assessment of iodine deficiency disorders. A guide for programme managers.* WHO/UNICEF/ICCIDD, Geneva.

The epidemiology of diabetes mellitus

Paul Zimmet

Introduction

Diabetes mellitus affects large numbers of people in a wide range of ethnic groups and at all social and economic levels worldwide. Over 110 million people are reported to suffer from diabetes (WHO 1994) and this is almost certainly an underestimate. Projections suggest that there will be over 230 million diabetics by 2010 (Amos *et al.* 1997) and 300 million by 2025 (King *et al.* 1998), the majority with type 2 diabetes. Thus there is an urgent need for strategies to be implemented to prevent the emerging global epidemic of type 2 diabetes.

Historically, until the latter part of the nineteenth century, the main causes for morbidity and mortality worldwide resulted from epidemics of communicable diseases including typhoid, cholera, smallpox, and influenza (Hennekens and Buring 1987), diseases which are still epidemic in certain developing countries. With industrialization and modernization of societies, major improvements have occurred in housing, sanitation, water supply, and nutrition. These changes, plus the introduction of antibiotics and immunization programmes, radically changed the profile of diseases in developed countries initially, and later in developing countries (Hennekens and Buring 1987; Zimmet *et al.* 1990).

With improvements in public health, mortality from infectious diseases has fallen dramatically (Hennekens and Buring 1987), although recent decades have seen the emergence of devastating communicable diseases such as HIV and the Ebola virus, and the re-emergence of that old public health enemy, tuberculosis (World Health Report 1998). Paradoxically, a marked increase in the prevalence of risk factors for non-communicable diseases, such as type 2 diabetes, cardiovascular disease, hypertension, stroke, and cancer, has occurred and they have become major contributors to morbidity and mortality (Zimmet 1999).

This phenomenon is well illustrated in the Pacific and Indian Ocean islands (Zimmet *et al.* 1990; Zimmet 1995), the site of many of our own epidemiological studies relating to type 2 diabetes and other non-communicable disease. Rapid socio-economic development over the last 40 to 50 years has resulted in a dramatic change of lifestyle from traditional to modern. As the public health aspects of diabetes are so diverse, the main objective of this chapter is to cover aspects relevant to the new classification and diagnostic criteria for diabetes (Alberti and Zimmet 1998) and the prevention of diabetes and its devastating complications.

Impact and cost of diabetes to society

Diabetes is amongst the five leading causes of death by disease in most countries (Finch and Zimmet 1988; WHO 1994). However, mortality statistics greatly underestimate the true diabetes-related mortality, as diabetes is frequently under-reported on death certificates (Finch and Zimmet 1988), a situation that proves a handicap when it comes to creating awareness of diabetes for community public health priorities. Apart from the health impact, the economic cost of diabetes and its complications is enormous, both for health care and for loss of productivity to society (WHO 1994).

While diabetes cost the United States US$20.4 billion in 1987 and US$ 90 billion for 1994, the most recent estimate is around US$100 billion (American Diabetes Association 1998).

Classification of diabetes mellitus—the new recommendations

Diabetes is really a syndrome characterized by hyperglycaemia, but with many causes. The 1985 WHO Study Group classification included a number of clinical classes, of which the two most important were insulin-dependent diabetes mellitus or type 1 diabetes and non-insulin dependent diabetes mellitus or type 2 diabetes, as well as malnutrition-related diabetes, impaired glucose tolerance, and gestational diabetes mellitus (WHO 1985). A revision in classification was long overdue as a result of new data from genetic, epidemiological, and aetiological studies (Zimmet 1995). Considering this global epidemic, the changes proposed for the classification (Fig. 5) and diagnostic criteria for diabetes (Table 5) become very important for global comparisons of incidence and prevalence and monitoring the epidemic. Therefore the recommendations of the 1997 American Diabetes Association report on classification and criteria (American Diabetes Association 1997) followed by the 1998 WHO recommendations (Alberti and Zimmet 1998; WHO 1999) have important implications. The new classification is based on stages of glucose tolerance status with a complementary subclassification according to aetiological type.

Table 5 Aetiological classification of disorders of glycaemia[a]

Type 1
β-cell destruction, usually leading to absolute insulin deficiency
Autoimmune
Idiopathic
Type 2
May range from predominantly insulin resistance with relative insulin deficiency to a predominantly secretory defect with or without insulin resistance
Other specific types
Genetic defects of β-cell function
Genetic defects in insulin action
Diseases of the exocrine pancreas
Endocrinopathies
Drug- or chemical-induced
Infections
Uncommon forms of immune-mediated diabetes
Other genetic syndromes sometimes associated with diabetes
Gestational diabetes[b]

[a]As additional subtypes are discovered it is anticipated that they will be reclassified within their own specific category.

[b]Includes the former categories of gestational impaired glucose tolerance and gestational diabetes.

Source: WHO (1999)

In the new classification, hyperglycaemia, regardless of the underlying cause, can be subcategorized as follows.

- Insulin required for survival (corresponds to the former insulin-dependent diabetes mellitus).
- Insulin required for control, i.e. for metabolic control, not for survival (corresponds to the former insulin-treated non-insulin-dependent diabetes mellitus).
- Does not require insulin, i.e. treatment by non-pharmacological methods or drugs other than insulin (corresponds to non-insulin-dependent diabetes mellitus on diet alone/or coupled with oral agents).
- Impaired glucose tolerance and impaired fasting glycaemia. Impaired glucose tolerance was previously a separate class; it is now categorized as a stage in the natural history of disordered carbohydrate metabolism. Impaired glucose tolerance is coupled with 'impaired fasting glycaemia' (6.1–7.0 mmol/l).

New diagnostic criteria for diabetes

The diagnostic criteria for diabetes have changed on a number of occasions over recent decades (Zimmet 1999). Epidemiological data collected over the last decade led both the WHO and the American Diabetes Association to review and revise the diagnostic criteria (Table 6).

As a result of these epidemiological data, the American Diabetes Association (1997) and the WHO (1999) recommended the following changes:

- the fasting plasma glucose threshold is lowered from 7.8 to 7.0 mmol/l

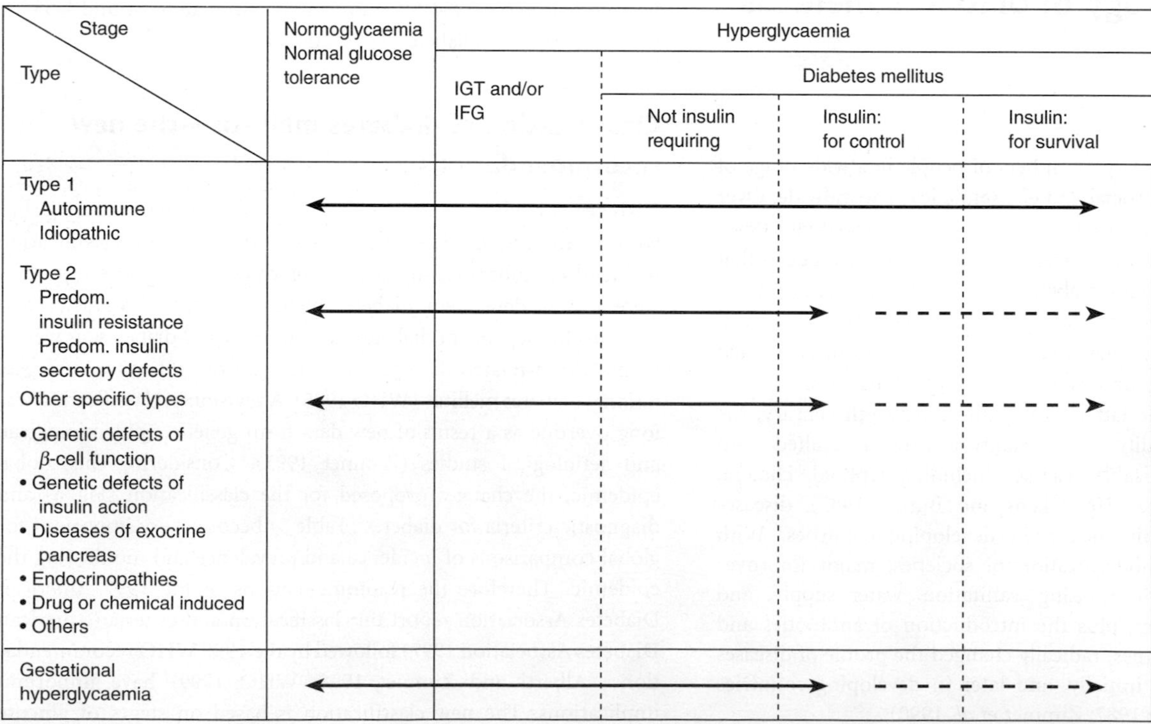

Fig. 5 Disorders of glycaemia: aetiological types and clinical stages. (Data from WHO 1999.)

Table 6 Values for diagnosis of diabetes mellitus and other categories of glucose intolerance

	Glucose concentration (mmol/l (mg/dl))		
	Whole blood (venous)	**Capillary**	**Plasma[a] (venous)**
Diabetes mellitus			
Fasting or	⩾6.1 (⩾110)	⩾6.1 (⩾110)	⩾7.0 (⩾126)
2-h post-glucose load			
or both	⩾10.0 (⩾180)	⩾11.1 (⩾200)	⩾11.1 (⩾200)
Impaired glucose tolerance			
Fasting (if measured)			
and	<6.1 (<110) and	<6.1 (<110) and	<7.0 (<126) and
2-h post-glucose load	⩾6.7 (⩾120)		
<10.0 (<180)	⩾7.8 (⩾140)		
<11.1 (<200)	⩾7.8 (⩾140)		
Impaired fasting glycaemia			
Fasting	⩾5.6 (⩾100) and		
<6.1 (<110)	⩾5.6 (⩾100) and		
<6.1 (<110)	⩾6.1 (⩾110) and		
<7.0 (<126)			
and (if measured)			
2-h post glucose load	<6.7 (<120)	<7.8 (<140)	<7.8 (<140)

[a]Corresponding values for capillary plasma are as follows: for diabetes mellitus, fasting ⩾7.0 (⩾126) and 2-h post-glucose load ⩾12.2 (⩾220); for impaired glucose tolerance, fasting <7.0 (<126) and 2-h post-glucose load ⩾8.9 (⩾160) and <12.2 (<220); for impaired fasting glycaemia, fasting ⩾6.1 (⩾110) and <7.0 (<126) and 2-h post-glucose load (if measured) <8.9 (<160).

For epidemiological or population screening purposes, the fasting value or value 2-h after 75 g of oral glucose may be used alone. For clinical purposes, the diagnosis of diabetes should always be confirmed by repeating the test on another day unless there is unequivocal hyperglycaemia with acute metabolic decompensation or obvious symptoms.

Glucose concentrations should not be determined on serum unless red cells are immediately removed, otherwise glycolysis will result in an unpredictable underestimation of the true concentrations. It should be stressed that glucose preservatives do not totally prevent glycolysis. If whole blood is used, the sample should be kept at 0–4 °C, or centrifuged immediately, or assayed immediately.

Source: WHO (1999)

- impaired fasting glycaemia (fasting plasma glucose 6.1–6.9 mmol/l) is introduced as a new category of intermediate glucose metabolism (named impaired fasting glucose by the American Diabetes Association).

The American Diabetes Association (but not the WHO report) recommended that fasting plasma glucose rather than the oral glucose tolerance test should be the diagnostic test of choice for both clinical and epidemiological purposes. An important question is: What difference will these changes in recommended criteria make to the prevalence of diabetes and the individuals identified as having diabetes? A large number of studies have now been published comparing the old and new criteria. The overall impression is that the oral glucose tolerance test should be retained for the diagnosis of diabetes. Using fasting criteria alone, as recommended by the American Diabetes Association, misses a significant number of people with diabetes. These studies are reviewed in detail elsewhere (Shaw *et al.* 1999*b*).

The impaired glucose tolerance category includes persons whose oral glucose tolerance test is beyond the boundaries of normality by WHO criteria (see below). Impaired glucose tolerance may represent a stage in the natural history of diabetes as these persons are at higher risk than the general population for diabetes (Harris and Zimmet 1992). Subjects with impaired glucose tolerance have a heightened risk of macrovascular disease (Harris and Zimmet 1992) and, because of this and the association with other known cardiovascular disease risk factors including hypertension, dyslipidaemia, and central obesity (Alberti and Zimmet 1998), the diagnosis of impaired glucose tolerance, particularly in otherwise healthy and ambulatory individuals, may have important prognostic implications.

Thus a major question that arises with the American Diabetes Association recommendations (1997) is the value of impaired fasting glycaemia compared with impaired glucose tolerance for predicting future type 2 diabetes. Screening by the American Diabetes Association criteria for impaired fasting glycaemia alone would identify fewer people who subsequently progress to type 2 diabetes than would the oral glucose tolerance test as recommended by WHO (Shaw *et al.* 1999*c*). This latter study demonstrated the higher sensitivity of impaired glucose tolerance over impaired fasting glycaemia for predicting progression to type 2 diabetes. Thus, whilst the new category of impaired fasting glycaemia may broaden and improve our description of states of intermediate glucose metabolism, it should be seen as complementary to rather than a replacement for impaired glucose tolerance.

The American Diabetes Association hoped that their recommendations would simplify the diagnosis of diabetes. However, that has not been the outcome and their recommendations are further clouded by the fact that impaired glucose tolerance is a far better predictor of risk from cardiovascular disease mortality (Davies 1999).

Gestational diabetes mellitus is defined as diabetes first recognized during pregnancy. In the majority of cases, glucose tolerance returns to normal postpartum, but the lifetime risk for impaired glucose tolerance and type 2 diabetes is substantially increased (Alberti and Zimmet 1998). Gestational diabetes mellitus occurs in about 3 per cent of pregnancies in Western nations, but is much higher in high-prevalence communities such as the American Indians and Pacific Islanders (WHO 1994).

The epidemiology of diabetes mellitus

The explosion of interest and activity that has occurred in studies relating to the epidemiology of diabetes over the last two decades has been extraordinary. In his book, *Epidemiology of Diabetes and its Vascular Lesions*, the late Kelly West highlighted the potential for a future epidemic (West 1978) and, in fact, type 2 diabetes has now reached epidemic proportions in many developing nations, as well as in disadvantaged groups in developed countries (Zimmet 1992, 1999). There is every reason to expect that, over the next decade, the epidemic of type 2 diabetes will continue to escalate (Amos *et al.* 1997; Zimmet 1999) so that diabetes and its complications will emerge as one of the major threats to future public health resources worldwide at a huge economic and social cost, particularly in developing countries (Table 7).

Type 1 diabetes

Prevalence and incidence

Type 1 diabetes is a discrete disorder and its pathogenesis involves environmental triggers that may activate autoimmune mechanisms in genetically susceptible individuals leading to progressive loss of pancreatic islet β-cells (Atkinson and Maclaren 1994). Its frequency is low relative to type 2 diabetes, accounting for 10 to 15 per cent of cases of diabetes in European populations. Type 1 diabetes is most common in European populations and is rare in Asians, Native Americans, Pacific Islanders, and black people (Karvonen *et al.* 1993).

In the last 15 years there has been an explosion of publications on the incidence and prevalence of type 1 diabetes as a result of the proliferation of diabetes registers. This initiative has resulted in a vast global network of type 1 diabetes registers and a major international collaboration (WHO Diamond Project Group 1990) covering incidence, prevalence, morbidity, mortality, and molecular epidemiology.

There are far too many reports of prevalence and incidence to summarize in this chapter. However, Fig. 6 provides a view of the incidence of type 1 diabetes in selected countries. There is an almost 60-fold difference between the countries with the highest incidence (Finland) and the lowest (Korea) (Karvonen *et al.* 1993).

Genetic factors in the aetiology of type 1 diabetes

Type 1 diabetes is not directly inherited as a Mendelian trait but is a polygenic disorder (Harrison *et al.* 1999). Predisposition is mediated by different genes that interact in a complex manner with each other and with the environment. Evidence for genetic predisposition comes from twin studies that demonstrate a higher concordance rate for type 1 diabetes in monozygotic twins (25–30 per cent) than in dizygotic twins (5–10 per cent) (Skyler and Marks 1993; Harrison *et al.* 1999). Recent advances in genetic mechanisms are reviewed in detail elsewhere (Bier and Lernmark 1998).

Environmental factors in the aetiology of type 1 diabetes

Viruses There are seasonal trends for type 1 diabetes incidence, with the highest incidence in winter (Warram *et al.* 1994). Also, exposure to a number of viruses has been linked to the development of type 1 diabetes. While the Coxsackie B virus appears to be the most common association, 20 per cent of children with congenital rubella develop type 1 diabetes (Skyler and Marks 1993; Harrison *et al.* 1999). In this latter example, the exposure relates to *in utero* exposure, which is remote from clinical onset, thus raising the issue of other potential *in utero* influences.

Secular trends There has been a marked temporal variation in many populations studied. A rising incidence has been noticed in 35 of 68

Table 7 Estimates of type 1 and 2 diabetes in various regions of the world, 1995–2010 (in thousands)

	1995				2000			2010		
Region	Population	Type 1	Type 2	Total	Type 1	Type 2	Total	Type 1	Type 2	Total
World	5697 038	3539	114 878	118 417	4423	146 804	151 227	5446	215 272	220 718
Africa	731 470	85	7209	7294	142	9270	9412	219	13 933	14 152
Asia	3437 786	1030	61 752	62 782	1608	82 902	84 510	2241	130 056	132 297
North America	296 517	879	12 098	12 977	1019	13 174	14 193	1175	16 360	17 535
Latin America	475 704	309	12 094	12 403	389	15 177	15 566	479	22 062	22 541
Europe	727 787	1155	20 885	22 040	1182	25 325	26 507	1245	31 620	32 865
Oceania	27 774	81	840	921	83	956	1039	87	1241	1328

Source: Amos *et al.* (1997).

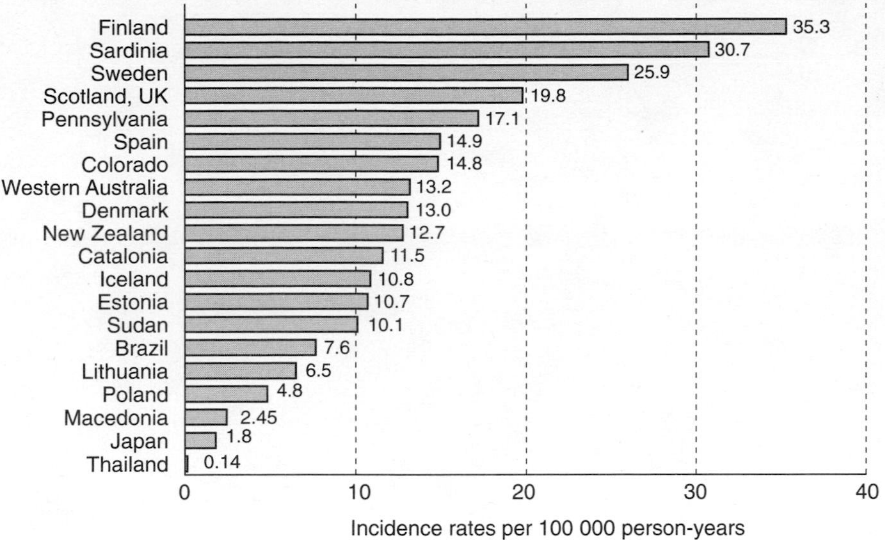

Fig. 6 Incidence of type 1 diabetes from selected countries. (Data from Karvonen *et al.* 1993.)

countries studied (Karvonen *et al.* 1993), while a fluctuating incidence has been recorded in others (Scott *et al.* 1992; Michaelis *et al.* 1993).

Ethnic and migrant studies Studies comparing prevalence and incidence in the same ethnic group provide unique opportunities to unravel the mystery of the putative environmental factors contributing to type 1 diabetes. Type 1 diabetes is uncommon in Asian communities, and very low rates of type 1 diabetes have been confirmed in Korea and China (Karvonen *et al.* 1993), Thailand (Tuchinda *et al.* 1992), and Japan (Karvonen *et al.* 1993). Black Americans have an even lower incidence than Hispanics, but not as low as that recorded in Tanzanians in sub-Saharan Africa (Karvonen *et al.* 1993).

Finland shows the world's highest incidence of type 1 diabetes at 35 in 100 000 (Tuomilehto *et al.* 1992*b*). This is higher than in the other Baltic States (Tuomilehto *et al.* 1992*a*), notably Estonia (Tuomilehto *et al.* 1991), whose populations are linguistically and ethnically very similar to that of Finland but who suffer only a third the incidence. This indicates that environmental factors have a particularly powerful influence on the appearance of type 1 diabetes, and other suggestions relating to environmental risk factors include toxins and nutritional factors. The rodenticide Vacor has also been associated with the development of type 1 diabetes (Tuomilehto *et al.* 1997).

Type 2 diabetes

Prevalence and incidence

Type 2 diabetes constitutes about 85 per cent of all cases of diabetes in developed countries (Zimmet 1999). The diagnosis is usually made after the age of 50 years in Europids, although type 2 diabetes is seen at younger age in high-prevalence populations such as Asian-Indians and Pacific Islanders (Zimmet 1999). In some developing countries, especially those with a high prevalence of diabetes, almost 100 per cent of persons with diabetes fall into this category. There is enormous variation in type 2 diabetes prevalence between populations (King and Rewers 1993; de Courten *et al.* 1997), and exceptionally high rates have been documented in populations who have changed from a traditional to a modern lifestyle, for example up to 40 per cent of adult Native Americans (de Courten *et al.* 1997), Native Canadians (Harris *et al.* 1997), Micronesians, and other Pacific Islanders, and about 20 per cent of adult Australian Aborigines, migrant Asian-Indians, and Mexican-Americans (Zimmet *et al.* 1990; Zimmet 1995). A comparison of age-standardized rates for type 2 diabetes in adults for a number of populations is shown in Fig. 7.

A steady stream of reports on a variety of populations have continued to highlight the explosion of type 2 diabetes in relation to lifestyle change and differences between different ethnic groups (Hamman 1993; King and Rewers 1993; Zimmet 1995). Populations previously free of type 2 diabetes are showing prevalences that are extraordinarily high when compared with developed countries. The reports of a spectacularly high prevalence of type 2 diabetes of over 40 per cent in adults over the age of 40 amongst the Pima Indians of Arizona (Bennett *et al.* 1992) and the Pacific Islanders of Nauru (Zimmet *et al.* 1990) have been followed by studies of related populations. The prevalence rates for a number of other different tribes of Native Americans range from 15 to 41 per cent of adults aged over 45 years, whilst amongst Alaskan Indians, who have had less contact with a Western lifestyle, only 3 per cent of those aged between 45 and 64 years have diabetes. The prevalences in the age range 30 to 64 years in the Pacific Islands of Kiribati and Western Samoa (de Courten *et al.* 1997) are 11 to 16 per cent, and a prevalence of 37 per cent has also been reported in the Melanesians of Papua New Guinea (Dowse *et al.* 1994). At the other end of the scale, very low prevalences of 1 to 2 per cent have been found in parts of Africa and China (Zimmet 1999).

The rates in Europids, both in Europe and North America, come somewhere in the middle of the extremes noted above. Only a few relevant studies have been performed in Europe, and they indicate rates between 5 per cent in the United Kingdom and 13 per cent in Spain (Shaw *et al.* 1999*a*) for those aged over 40 years. In the United States, NHANES II reported that 6 per cent of the Europid population between the ages of 30 and 64 years had type 2 diabetes (Harris *et al.* 1987).

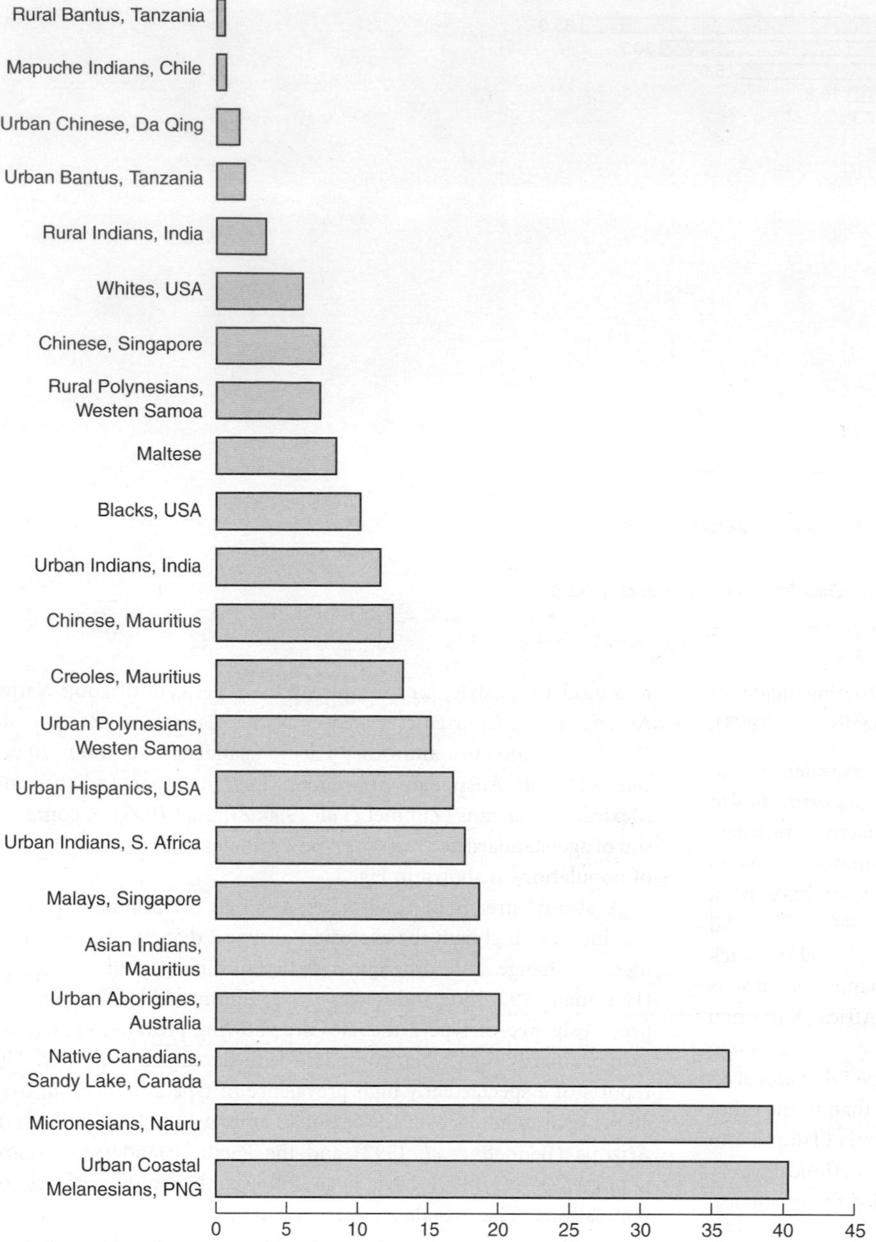

Fig. 7 Prevalence of type 2 diabetes in selected populations (30–64 years) worldwide. Age-standardized against Segi's world population.

A longitudinal epidemiological study in the Indian Ocean island of Mauritius has provided the best gauge of the type 2 diabetes epidemic occurring in large sections of the developing world (Zimmet 1999). As the population, currently 13 000 000, includes people of Asian-Indian, Chinese, and black (Creole) descent, and as these ethnic groups compose nearly two-thirds of the world population, the data from Mauritius provide a microcosm of the global epidemic.

Our previous population-based surveys in Mauritius (1987 and 1992) had shown a high diabetes prevalence. The 1987 prevalence of type 2 diabetes was 10 to 13 per cent in each ethnic group, rising to 20 to 30 per cent in those aged 45 to 74 years. In the most recent study in 1998 (de Courten *et al.* 1999), when 6294 subjects were screened for diabetes with an oral glucose tolerance test, we found a 30 per cent secular increase in diabetes prevalence in the 11 years from 1987. Diabetes now affects close to 20 per cent of the population over 30 years of age. These results, if transposed to parts of India, China, and Africa where modernization and industrialization are occurring, would result in huge increases in the number of cases of type 2 diabetes posing a great public health threat and burden.

Mauritius, apart from revealing a high diabetes prevalence in Asian-Indians and Creoles, showed the highest yet reported prevalence in Chinese (Dowse *et al.* 1990). These results, and evidence that the prevalence of type 2 diabetes doubled between 1984 and 1992 in Singapore's Chinese community (Tan *et al.* 1999), along with high prevalence in Taiwan (Chang *et al.* 1998), provide an alarming indication to the size of the epidemic which could occur in the

People's Republic of China where the overall prevalence of type 2 diabetes was, until recently, believed to be less than 1 per cent (Zimmet 1999). Data are already available that suggest an almost threefold increase in prevalence in certain areas of China within the last two decades (Pan *et al.* 1997). This is highlighted by the data in Fig. 6 comparing the prevalence of diabetes in Chinese populations in China, Singapore, Taiwan, and Mauritius. If China were to experience just half of the current rate of diabetes in Taiwan, the number of individuals with diabetes would increase dramatically from 8 million in 1996 to over 32 million by 2010 (Zimmet 1999).

People from the Indian subcontinent are at especially high risk of type 2 diabetes. Early studies from India reported type 2 diabetes to be relatively rare, but a more recent study in an affluent Indian suburb found diabetes prevalence to be 20 per cent in men aged 45 to 74 years. In a south Indian urban community, two surveys performed 5 years apart showed a 40 per cent rise in diabetes prevalence (Shaw *et al.* 1999*a*). High diabetes rates have now also been found in Asian-Indians in communities located in Pakistan, South Africa, Fiji, and the United Kingdom (Zimmet 1992).

There could be no better rationale for developing primary prevention programmes for diabetes. However, before embarking on intervention activities, it is essential to have a better understanding of both the genetic and environmental determinants of type 2 diabetes.

Genetic factors in the aetiology of type 2 diabetes

Progress in understanding the genetic component of type 2 diabetes, particularly in defining potential candidate genes, has been slow until recently. Family and twin studies, along with the evidence for heightened genetic susceptibility in certain populations and genetic admixture studies (Zimmet 1992), provided firm evidence that the role of the genetic component was very strong. The recent achievements in molecular biology relating to type 2 diabetes have resulted from studying very well defined autosomal dominant forms in extended families with maturity-onset diabetes of the young (Hattersley 1998) and not from the large heterogeneous pool of persons with type 2 diabetes with or without the other components of the metabolic syndrome. There have been some promising results from studies of families with maturity-onset diabetes of the young where associations have been found with the glucokinase and hepatocyte nuclear factor 1α and 4α genes (Yamagata *et al.* 1996*a*,*b*) and with mitochondrial DNA mutations in families with type 2 diabetes and nerve deafness (McCarthy *et al.* 1994; Hattersley 1998).

The new WHO classification (Alberti and Zimmet 1998; WHO 1999) should bring a more rational approach to research by molecular biologists. Apart from the necessity to define diabetes correctly from an epidemiological and therapeutic perspective, the total success of the current thrust to define crucial genes for both type 1 and 2 diabetes depends on correct phenotyping (Zimmet 1999). It is not surprising that most geneticists still regard diabetes as the 'geneticists' nightmare' when clinicians have been asking them to find the diabetes gene(s) while providing samples from poorly defined groups. The search for the type 2 diabetes gene(s) is already difficult enough without this handicap.

While maturity-onset diabetes of the young only accounts for approximately 1 per cent of all type 2 diabetes, the implications for discovering other genes for other forms of diabetes are important. Yet, to find gene(s) associated with any complex disorder such as type 2 diabetes, the task is more formidable. The failure to find a major putative gene for type 2 diabetes despite the advanced stage of the Human Genome Project (Collins 1999) raises many questions over the strategic approach most likely to be successful. Finding the gene(s) has enormous implications not only for screening for 'high-risk' individuals but for targets for potential new therapeutic compounds as well as identifying which individuals are likely to respond to different therapies (Collins 1999). Epidemiologists must continue to play a pivotal role in helping to define the best cohorts for these genetic studies.

Thrifty genes An attempt to explain the high prevalence of obesity and type 2 diabetes in the American Pima Indians, Australian Aborigines, and Pacific Islanders comes through the thrifty gene hypothesis (Neel 1962). The basis for the susceptibility to obesity and type 2 diabetes is unclear, but it could be the result of an evolutionary advantageous thrifty genotype which promoted fat deposition and storage of calories in times of plenty and provided a positive selective advantage during periods of food shortage and starvation (Neel 1962; Dowse and Zimmet 1993). This would have conferred a survival advantage during the regular famines and natural disasters that were interspersed with feast periods (Zimmet 1993), but would result in type 2 diabetes once a sedentary lifestyle and a diet with an excess of energy, simple carbohydrates, and saturated fats were adopted.

Hales and Barker (1992) have suggested that *in utero* factors leading to fetal malnutrition may be the cause of this chronic disease epidemic and they proposed the thrifty phenotype hypothesis. Their proposition is that the causes are entirely environmental and they discount a role for genetic factors. The intellectual exchanges between the proponents of the thrifty genotype and thrifty phenotype hypotheses have become the highlight of many international scientific meetings. The issues challenging the thrifty phenotype have been reviewed in detail by Joseph and Kramer (1996) who listed various direct and indirect pieces of evidence suggesting that the reported association of low birth weight and later type 2 diabetes may be biased rather than causal. They state that 'selection bias, failure to define, measure, and adequately control for the confounding health consequences of social deprivation and inconsistencies in the hypotheses tested and in methods of data analysis and reporting are among the factors that weigh against a causal explanation for the associations observed' (Joseph and Kramer 1996).

While it is clear that the association between low birth weight infants and subsequent type 2 diabetes risk is a true phenomenon, the explanation to explain it is not so simple. There are now strong arguments against an exclusive environmental role and it is likely that genes are also implicated (Zimmet 1999).

Environmental factors in the aetiology of type 2 diabetes

While genetic susceptibility to type 2 diabetes is clearly important, there is strong evidence that the disease is unmasked by environmental factors (Zimmet 1995; de Courten *et al.* 1997). Several environmental risk determinants (Table 8) are associated with an increased risk of type 2 diabetes including nutritional factors, physical activity, central and overall obesity, intrauterine factors, and so on. These are relevant to primary prevention as discussed below and a much more extensive reviews can be found elsewhere (Bennett *et al.* 1992; de Courten *et al.* 1997).

Complications of diabetes

Space limitations prevent a detailed description of the microvascular and macrovascular complications of diabetes which are reviewed in

Table 8 Demographic, behavioural, and environmental risk determinants for type 2 diabetes

Demographic characteristics
Gender
Age
Ethnicity
Modifiable (including behavioural and lifestyle-related) risk factors
Obesity (including distribution and duration of obesity)
Sedentary lifestyle
Nutritional (e.g. high saturated fat, low fibre)
'Westernization', urbanization, industrialization
Intrauterine environment

detail elsewhere (Jarrett 1992; Klein and Moss 1992; Ward 1992; WHO 1994; Hamman 1997; Tuomilehto and Rastenyté 1997). Their main relevance from a public health perspective is the relationship to human suffering and disability, and socio-economic costs through premature morbidity and mortality (Songer 1992; World Bank 1993). For example, the major microvascular complications are diabetic retinopathy, nephropathy, and neuropathy. The extent to which they occur is influenced predominantly by duration of diabetes and degree of metabolic control (WHO 1994). These complications may be apparent at the time of diabetes diagnosis, especially in type 2 diabetes (Harris *et al.* 1992).

Diabetes is the most common cause of adult blindness in developed countries due to retinopathy, cataracts, or glaucoma (Klein and Moss 1992; WHO 1994). Diabetic patients are 17 times more prone to kidney disease, and diabetes is now the leading known cause of endstage renal disease in the United States (WHO 1994). Diabetic neuropathy is probably the most common complication, being present in about 30 to 40 per cent of type 1 and 2 diabetes subjects (WHO 1994).

As for macrovascular disease, atherosclerosis is the most common complication of diabetes among Europids. It accounts for at least two-thirds of deaths (Zimmet and Alberti 1997), a figure that is two to three times greater than that in people without diabetes, and coronary artery disease and cerebrovascular disease are also two to three times more common in diabetics than in non-diabetics (Jarrett 1992). The WHO Multinational Study of Vascular Disease in Diabetics found marked differences in prevalence of macrovascular disease between 14 countries (WHO 1985*b*). The increase in atherosclerosis in diabetics compared with non-diabetics was seen in all populations, even in those where the incidence of atherosclerosis was low, but the prevalence and pattern of microvascular disease were similar between countries.

Numerous epidemiological studies have demonstrated the importance of indices of glycaemic control and the duration of diabetes in determining the prevalence and incidence of diabetic microvascular complications (Zimmet 1999). Subsequent epidemiological data supported this but it required testing in large-scale clinical trials. This happened with the landmark Diabetes Control and Complications Trial (**DCCT**) (1995). The DCCT demonstrated that improved glycaemic control reduces the risk of microvascular complications in type 1 diabetes. However, these findings only applied to type 1 diabetes, and whether these results could be extrapolated to patients with type 2 diabetes awaited confirmation in large trials such as the United Kingdom Prospective Diabetes Study (**UKPDS** 1998*a*). The recently published findings of the UKPDS now provide strong evidence to recommend tight glycaemic control in type 2 diabetes (UKPDS 1998*a*,*b*).

Two-thirds of type 2 diabetes patients die from cardiovascular disease (Zimmet and Alberti 1997). The clustering of type 2 diabetes, a well-documented risk determinant for cardiovascular disease, with the other risk factors including insulin resistance that constitute the metabolic syndrome is now well established (Zimmet 1995). This seems the most likely explanation for this increased cardiovascular disease mortality in type 2 diabetes. Alone, each component of the cluster conveys increased cardiovascular disease risk, but as a combination their effect is cumulative. An important and pivotal study relevant to this cardiovascular disease risk was the randomized clinical trial of cardiovascular intervention, the Scandinavian Simvastatin Survival Study (Pyörälä *et al.* 1997). The use of simvastatin in diabetic subjects with a previous coronary heart disease event resulted in a 55 per cent reduction in the risk of future coronary heart disease events compared with 33 per cent in non-diabetics. The message is now very clear that management should focus not only on tight blood glucose control but also on strategies for the reduction of the other important cardiovascular disease risk factors such as hypertension, dyslipidaemia, and obesity.

Primary prevention of diabetes mellitus

Diabetes is now a major global public health problem, but from a public health perspective type 2 diabetes is by far the most common form, particularly in newly industrialized nations (Zimmet 1999). Prevention of type 1 diabetes is still in an experimental stage (Bier and Lernmark 1998; Harrison *et al.* 1999) and so the major emphasis here will be on prevention of type 2 diabetes.

Prevention of type 1 diabetes

Although type 1 diabetes is probably the most common serious childhood disease, the very low prevalence demands a screening test of high specificity and sensitivity. Furthermore, the test would need to be inexpensive and easy to perform in order to screen a large number of individuals, which would be necessary for the prevention of type 1 diabetes as only 10 to 15 per cent of new cases come from the high-risk group, i.e. first-degree relatives (Bingley *et al.* 1993). Islet cell antibodies, insulin autoantibodies, glutamic acid decarboxylase antibodies, and tyrosine phosphatase antibodies are the markers which have been most commonly used to date (Zimmet *et al.* 1999), but there are major cost and technical limitations to islet cell antibody and insulin antibody assays.

The ability to measure a group of autoantibodies to islet cell constituents, including islet cell antibodies, insulin antibodies, glutamic acid decarboxylase antibodies, and tyrosine phosphatase antibodies, have greatly facilitated the ability to predict future type 1 diabetes (Zimmet 1999). The long preclinical phase of type 1 diabetes provides a window of opportunity for primary prevention with the possibility of a effective screening procedures, and the future availability of immune intervention (Skyler and Marks 1993; Harrison *et al.* 1999). A number of trials are now underway to assess the use of oral nicotinamide, prophylactic parenteral or oral insulin, oral glutamic acid decarboxylase, and intracutaneous bacille Calmette–Guérin (Atkinson and McLaren 1994; Harrison *et al.* 1999), all strategies which may delay or arrest the autoimmune process.

Prevention of type 2 diabetes

Compared with primary prevention of coronary artery disease, virtually no population-based studies of type 2 diabetes have been published yet apart from a major impaired glucose tolerance intervention study from China (Pan *et al.* 1997). The incidence of type 2 diabetes was reduced by a third in the intervention group compared with controls, and this applied equally to non-obese and obese subjects with impaired glucose (Fig. 8). Given the projected epidemic of diabetes in China (Zimmet 1999), the largest population in the world, such a cost-effective intervention provides good news.

However, several population-based studies are currently underway (Diabetes Prevention Program 1999; Eriksson *et al.* 1999). As type 2 diabetes is so heterogeneous, for preventive measures to be fully effective in a community they must be based on knowledge of the risk determinants in that community (Tuomilehto *et al.* 1992*c*). There are sufficient data available to show that type 2 diabetes should be preventable (Zimmet 1999). These data come from a variety of sources, including the impact of lifestyle change on cardiovascular disease risk factors and incidence (Tuomilehto *et al.* 1992*c*), and two studies where indigenous groups at high risk of type 2 diabetes showed improvements in risk factors with traditional diet (O'Dea 1984; Shintani *et al.* 1991) and other lifestyle changes (Dowse *et al.* 1995; Uusitala *et al.* 1996). However, more compelling is the recent report from China where the incidence of progression from impaired glucose tolerance to type 2 diabetes was reduced by over 30 per cent through diet and exercise interventions (Pan *et al.* 1997).

There are two components of the implementation of primary prevention—the population and the high-risk strategies. They are generally complementary (WHO 1994). The population approach may be more appropriate in societies with particularly high genetic susceptibility (in which case the two strategies are effectively the same) (Tuomilehto *et al.* 1992*c*). The high-risk alternative has an advantage for individuals at special high risk for type 2 diabetes, for example first-degree relatives of type 2 diabetes patients, subjects with impaired glucose tolerance or previous gestational diabetes mellitus, and those with the metabolic syndrome, i.e. glucose intolerance, insulin resistance, abdominal obesity, dyslipidaemia, and hypertension (Zimmet 1995).

It is both cost and health effective to use an integrated approach for prevention activities to reduce the common risk factor levels for these non-communicable disease in the community particularly in developing nations (Zimmet 1995). Correction and prevention of obesity, exercise, avoidance of a high-fat diet, and encouraging a high-fibre diet all reduce insulin resistance and reduce the levels of some of the other risk factors for coronary artery disease (Zimmet 1995).

The components necessary for the development of a national diabetes prevention programme form a model for prevention of other non-communicable disease, a model now called the 'Hetzel wheel' (Fig. 9). Prevention programmes should not be commenced without a properly constituted evaluation component, and guidelines for monitoring and evaluation appear in one WHO report (WHO 1994).

To summarize, healthy lifestyle practices such as exercise, appropriate nutrition, maintenance of ideal body weight, smoking cessation, and reduced alcohol consumption targeted at whole communities are also likely to reduce the social and economic burden of type 2 diabetes and other non-communicable disease. The efficacy of primarily non-pharmacological interventions such as those used in the Chinese study of impaired glucose tolerance intervention (Pan *et al.* 1997) provides support for the view that interventions in impaired glucose tolerance subjects should be given a high priority. The American National Institutes of Health have risen to the challenge and funded a major multicentre impaired glucose tolerance intervention to examine the potential for prevention (Diabetes Prevention Program 1998). There may also be a role for pharmacological intervention with biguanides, α-glucosidase inhibitors, and the new therapeutic compounds of the thiozolidodione group. Both approaches are being used in the American study.

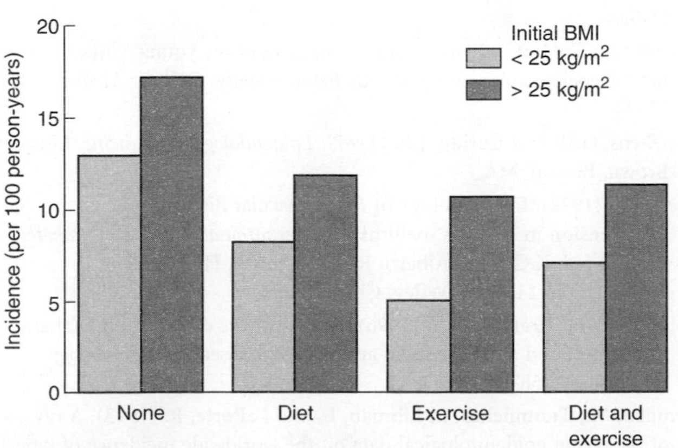

Fig. 8 The effect of diet and exercise in preventing the progression of impaired glucose tolerance to type 2 diabetes in Da Qing, China. (Data from Pan et *al.* 1997.)

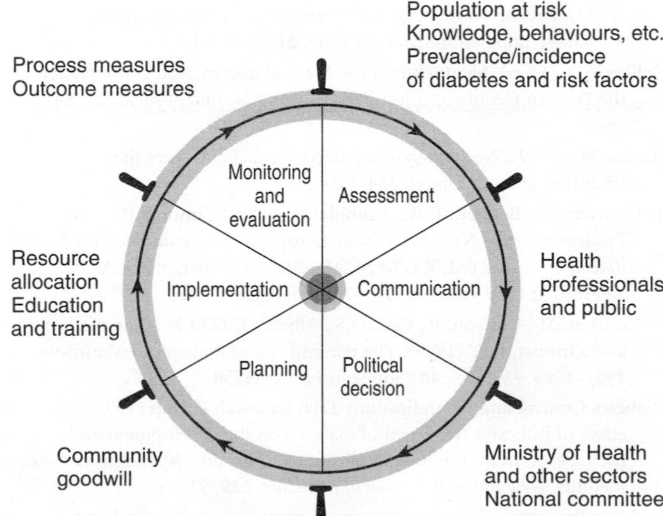

Fig. 9 Control and prevention of diabetes. The components necessary for the development of a national diabetes prevention programme. The 'Hetzel wheel'—these activities form a model for prevention of other non-communicable diseases.

Conclusion

Diabetes is likely to remain a significant threat to public health in the years to come. In the absence of effective interventions for both type 1 and type 2 diabetes, the frequency will escalate worldwide with the main impact being seen in developing nations and in disadvantaged minorities in developed nations (Amos *et al.* 1997; King *et al.* 1998; Zimmet 1999). Thus prevention of diabetes and its microvascular and macrovascular complications is an essential component of future public health strategies for all nations.

References

Alberti, K.G.M.M. and Zimmet, P.Z., for the WHO Consultation Group (1998). Definition, diagnosis and classification of diabetes mellitus and its complications. Part 1: Diagnosis and classification of diabetes mellitus. Provisional report of a WHO consultation. *Diabetic Medicine*, **15**, 539–53.

American Diabetes Association (1997). Report of the Expert Committee on the Diagnosis and Classification of Diabetes Mellitus. *Diabetes Care*, **20**, 1183–97.

American Diabetes Association (1998). Economic consequences of diabetes mellitus in the US in 1997. *Diabetes Care*, **21**, 296–309.

Amos, A., McCarty, D., and Zimmet, P. (1997). The rising global burden of diabetes and its complications: estimates and projections to the year 2010. *Diabetic Medicine*, **14** (Supplement 5), S1–85.

Atkinson, M.A. and Maclaren, N.K. (1994). The pathogenesis of insulin-dependent diabetes mellitus. *New England Journal of Medicine*, **331**, 1428–36.

Bennett, P.H., Bogardus, C., Tuomilehto, J., and Zimmet, P. (1992). Epidemiology and natural history of NIDDM: non-obese and obese. In *International textbook of diabetes mellitus* (ed. K.G.M.M. Alberti, R.A. DeFronzo, H. Keen, and P. Zimmet), pp. 147–76. Wiley, Chichester.

Bier, S. and Lernmark, A. (1998). Diabetes. In *The autoimmune diseases* (ed. N.R. Rose and I.R. MacKay) (3rd edn), pp. 431–57. Academic Press, San Diego, CA.

Bingley, P.J., Bonifacio, E., and Gale, E.A.M. (1993). Can we really predict IDDM? *Diabetes*, **42**, 213–20.

Chang, C.-J., Wu, J.-S., Lu, F.-H., Lee, H.-L., Yang, Y.-C., and Wen, M.-J. (1998). Fasting plasma glucose in screening for diabetes in the Taiwanese population. *Diabetes Care*, **21**, 1856–60.

Collins, F.S. (1999). Shattuck Lecture. Medical and societal consequences of the Human Genome Project. *New England Journal of Medicine*, **341**, 28–37.

Davies, M. (1999). New diagnostic criteria for diabetes—are they doing what they should? *Lancet*, **354**, 610–11.

de Courten, M., Bennett, P.H., Tuomilehto, J., and Zimmet, P. (1997). Epidemiology of NIDDM in Non-Europids. In *International textbook of diabetes mellitus.* (ed. K.G.M.M. Alberti, P. Zimmet, and R.A. DeFronzo) (2nd edn), pp. 143–70. Wiley, Chichester.

de Courten, M., Chitson, P., Cox, H.S., Alberti, K.G.M.M., Tuomilehto, J., and Zimmet, P.Z. (1999). The rise and rise of diabetes in Mauritius 1987–1988. *Diabetes*, **48** (Supplement 1), A1758.

Diabetes Control and Complications Trial Research Group (1993). The effect of intensive treatment of diabetes on the development and progression of long-term complications in insulin-dependent diabetes mellitus. *New England Journal of Medicine*, **329**, 977–86.

Diabetes Prevention Program Research Group (1999). The Diabetes Prevention Program. Design and methods for a clinical trial in the prevention of type 2 diabetes. *Diabetes Care*, **22**, 623–34.

Dowse, G. and Zimmet, P. (1993). The thrifty genotype in non-insulin-dependent diabetes. The hypothesis survives. *British Medical Journal*, **306**, 532–3.

Dowse, G.K., Gareeboo, H., Zimmet, P.Z., *et al.* (1990). High prevalence of NIDDM and impaired glucose intolerance in Indian, Creole and Chinese Mauritians. *Diabetes*, **39**, 390–6.

Dowse, G.K., Spark, R.A., Mavo, B., *et al.* (1994). Extraordinary prevalence of non-insulin-dependent diabetes mellitus and bimodal plasma glucose distribution in the Wanigela people of Papua New Guinea. *Medical Journal of Australia*, **160**, 767–74.

Dowse, G.K., Gareeboo, H., Alberti, K.G.M.M., *et al.* (1995). Changes in population cholesterol concentrations and other cardiovascular risk factor levels after five years of the non-communicable disease intervention programme in Mauritius. *British Medical Journal*, **311**, 1255–59.

Eriksson, J., Lindstrom, J., Valle, T., *et al.* (1999). Prevention of type II diabetes in subjects with impaired glucose tolerance: the Diabetes Prevention Study (DPS) in Finland. *Diabetologia*, **42**, 793–801.

Finch, C.F. and Zimmet, P.Z. (1988). Mortality from diabetes. In *The diabetes annual*, Vol. 4 (ed. K.G.M.M. Alberti and L.P. Krall), pp. 1–16. Elsevier, Amsterdam.

Hales, C.N. and Barker, D.J.P. (1992). Type 2 (non-insulin-dependent) diabetes mellitus: the thrifty phenotype hypothesis. *Diabetologia*, **35**, 595–601

Hamman, R.F. (1993). Genetic and environmental determinants of non-insulin dependent diabetes mellitus (NIDDM). *Diabetes/Metabolism Reviews*, **8**, 287–338.

Hamman, R.F. (1997). Epidemiology of microvascular complications. In *International textbook of diabetes mellitus* (ed. K.G.M.M. Alberti, R.A. DeFronzo, and H. Keen) (2nd edn), pp. 1293–319. Wiley, London.

Harris, M.I. and Zimmet, P. (1992). Classification of diabetes mellitus and other categories of glucose intolerance. In *The international textbook of diabetes mellitus* (ed. H. Keen, R. DeFronzo, K.G.M.M. Alberti, and P. Zimmet), pp. 3–18. Wiley, Chichester.

Harris, M.I., Hadden, W.C., Knowler, W.C., and Bennett, P.H. (1987). Prevalence of diabetes and impaired glucose tolerance and plasma glucose levels in US population aged 20–74 years. *Diabetes*, **36**, 523–34.

Harris, M.I., Klein, R., Welborn, T.A., and Knuiman, M.W. (1992). Onset of NIDDM occurs at least 4–7 years before clinical diagnosis. *Diabetes Care*, **15**, 815–19.

Harris, S.B., Gittelsohn, J., Hanley, A., *et al.* (1997). The prevalence of NIDDM and associated risk factors in native Canadians. *Diabetes Care*, **20**, 185–7.

Harrison, L.C., Kay, T.W.H., Colman, P.G., and Honeyman, M.C. (1999). Type 1 diabetes: from pathogenesis to prevention. In *Diabetes in the new millennium* (ed. J.R. Turtle, T. Kaneko, and S. Osato), pp. 85–100. Endocrinology and Diabetes Research Foundation, University of Sydney.

Hattersley, A.T. (1998). Maturity-onset diabetes of the young: clinical heterogeneity explained by genetic heterogeneity. *Diabetic Medicine*, **15**, 15–24.

Hennekens, G.H. and Buring, J.E. (1987). *Epidemiology in medicine.* Little, Brown, Boston, MA.

Jarrett, R.J. (1992). Epidemiology of macrovascular disease and hypertension in diabetes mellitus. In *International textbook of diabetes mellitus* (ed. K.G.M.M. Alberti, R.A. DeFronzo, H. Keen, and P. Zimmet), pp. 1459–70. Wiley, Chichester.

Joseph, K.S. and Kramer, M.S. (1996). Review of the evidence on fetal and early childhood antecedents of adult chronic disease. *Epidemiology Reviews*, **18**, 158–74.

Karvonen, M., Tuomilehto, J., Libman, I., and LaPorte, R. (1993). A review of the recent epidemiological data on the worldwide incidence of type 1 (insulin-dependent) diabetes mellitus. *Diabetologia*, **36**, 883–92.

King, H. and Rewers, M. (1993). WHO Ad Hoc Diabetes Reporting Group. Global estimates for prevalence of diabetes mellitus and impaired glucose tolerance in adults. *Diabetes Care*, **16**, 157–77.

King, H., Aubert, R.E., and Herman, W.H. (1998) Global burden of diabetes, 1995–2025. Prevalence, numerical estimates and projections. *Diabetes Care*, **21**, 1414–31.

Klein, R. and Moss, S.E. (1992). Visual impairment and diabetes. In *International textbook of diabetes mellitus* (ed. K.G.M.M. Alberti, R.A. DeFronzo, H. Keen, and P. Zimmet), pp. 1373–84. Wiley, Chichester.

McCarthy, M.I., Froguel, P., and Hitman, G.A. (1994). The genetics of non-insulin-dependent diabetes mellitus: tools and aims. *Diabetologia*, **37**, 959–68.

Michaelis, D, Jutzi, E., and Vogt, L. (1993). Epidemiology of insulin-treated diabetes mellitus in the East-German population: differences in long-term trends between incidence and prevalence rates. *Diabete et Metabolisme*, **19**, 110–15.

Neel, J.V. (1962). Diabetes mellitus: a thrifty genotype rendered detrimental by 'progress'? *American Journal of Human Genetics*, **14**, 353–62.

O'Dea, K. (1984). Marked improvement in carbohydrate and lipid metabolism in diabetic Australian Aborigines after temporary reversion to traditional lifestyle. *Diabetes*, **33**, 596–603.

Pan, X., Li, G., Hu, Y., *et al.* (1997). Effect of diet and exercise in preventing NIDDM in people with impaired glucose tolerance: the Da Qing IGT and Diabetes Study. *Diabetes Care*, **20**, 537–44.

Pyorälä, K., Pedersen, T.R., Kjeksus, J., Faergerman, O., Olsson, A.G., and Thorgeirsson, G. (1997). Cholesterol lowering with simvastatin improves prognosis of diabetic patients with coronary heart disease: a subgroup analyses of the Scandinavian Simvastatin Survival Study (4S). *Diabetes Care*, **20**, 614–20.

Scott, R.S., Brown, L.J., Darlow, B.A., Forbes, L.V., and Moore, M.P. (1992). Temporal variation in incidence of IDDM in Canterbury, New Zealand. *Diabetes Care*, **15**, 895–9.

Shaw, J., de Courten, M., and Zimmet, P. (1999*a*). The epidemiology of diabetes: a world-wide problem. In *Diabetes in the new millennium* (ed. J.R. Turtle, T. Kaneko, and S. Osato), pp. 1–9. Endocrinology and Diabetes Research Foundation, University of Sydney.

Shaw, J., de Courten, M., Boyko, E.J., and Zimmet, P. (1999*b*). Impact of new diagnostic criteria for diabetes in different populations. *Diabetes Care*, **22**, 762–6.

Shaw, J. E., Zimmet, P.Z., de Courten, M., *et al.* (1999*c*). Impaired fasting glucose or impaired glucose tolerance. What best predicts future diabetes in Mauritius? *Diabetes Care*, **22**, 399–402.

Shintani, T., Hughes, C.K., Beckham, S., and O'Connor, H.K. (1991). Obesity and cardiovascular risk intervention through the ad libitum feeding of traditional Hawaiian diet. *American Journal of Clinical Nutrition*, **53**, 1647S–51S.

Skyler, J.S. and Marks, J.B. (1993). Immune intervention in type 1 diabetes mellitus. *Diabetes Review*, **1**, 15–42.

Songer, T. (1992). The economic costs of NIDDM. *Diabetes/Metabolism Reviews*, **8**, 389–404.

Tan, C.-E., Emmanuel, S.C., Tan, B.-Y., and Jacob, E. (1999). Prevalence of diabetes and ethnic differences in cardiovascular risk factors. The 1992 Singapore National Health Survey. *Diabetes Care*, **22**, 241–7.

Tuchinda, C., Angsusingha, K., Chaichanwalanakul, K., Likitmaskul, S., and Vannasaeng S. (1992). The epidemiology of insulin dependent diabetes mellitus (IDDM): report from Thailand. *Journal of the Medical Association of Thailand*, **75**, 217–22.

Tuomilehto, J. and Rastenyté, D. (1997). Epidemiology of macrovascular disease and hypertension in diabetes mellitus. In *International textbook of diabetes mellitus* (ed. K.G.M.M. Alberti, P. Zimmet, R.A. DeFronzo, and H. Keen) (2nd edn), pp. 1559–83. Wiley, London.

Tuomilehto, J., Podar, T., Reunanen, A., *et al.* (1991). Comparison of incidence of IDDM in childhood between Estonia and Finland, 1980–1988. *Diabetes Care*, **14**, 982–8.

Tuomilehto, J., Podar, T., Brigis, G., *et al.* (1992*a*). Comparison of the incidence of insulin dependent diabetes mellitus among five Baltic populations during 1983–1988. *International Journal of Epidemiology*, **21**, 518–27.

Tuomilehto, J., Lounamaa, R., Tuomilehto-Wolf, E., *et al.* (1992*b*). Epidemiology of childhood diabetes mellitus in Finland—background of a nationwide study of type 1 (insulin dependent) diabetes mellitus. The Childhood Diabetes in Finland (DiMe) Study Group. *Diabetologia*, **35**, 70–6.

Tuomilehto, J., Knowler, W.C., and Zimmet, P. (1992*c*). Primary prevention of non-insulin-dependent diabetes mellitus. *Diabetes/Metabolism Reviews*, **8**, 339–53.

Tuomilehto, J., Tuomilehto-Wolf, E., Zimmet, P., Alberti, K.G.M.M., and Knowler, W.C. (1997). Primary prevention of diabetes mellitus. In *International textbook of diabetes mellitus* (ed. K.G.M.M. Alberti, P. Zimmet, R.A. DeFronzo, and H. Keen) (2nd edn), pp. 1799–1827. Wiley, Chichester.

UKPDS (UK Prospective Diabetes Study Group) (1998*a*). Intensive blood glucose control with sulphonylureas or insulin compared with conventional treatment and risk of complications in patients with type 2 diabetes (UKPDS 33). *Lancet*, **352**, 837–53.

UKPDS (UK Prospective Diabetes Study Group) (1998*b*). Tight blood pressure control and risk of macrovascular and microvascular complications in type 2 diabetes: UKPDS 38. *British Medical Journal*, **317**, 703–13.

Uusitalo, U., Feskens, E.J.M., Tuomilehto, J., *et al.* (1996). Fall in total cholesterol concentration over five years in association with changes in fatty acid composition of cooking oil in Mauritius: cross sectional survey. *British Medical Journal*, **313**, 1044–6.

Ward, J.D. (1992). Diabetic neuropathy. In *International textbook of diabetes mellitus* (ed. K.G.M.M. Alberti, R.A. DeFronzo, H. Keen, and P. Zimmet), pp. 1385–414. Wiley, Chichester.

Warram, J.H., Rich, S.S., and Krolewski, A.S. (1994). Epidemiology and genetics of diabetes mellitus. In *Joslin's Diabetes Mellitus* (ed. C.R. Kahn and G.C. Weir) (13th edn), pp. 201–15. Lea & Febiger, Philadelphia, PA.

West, K.M. (1978). *Epidemiology of diabetes and its vascular lesions*. Elsevier, New York.

WHO Diamond Project Group (1990). WHO Multinational Project for Childhood Diabetes. *Diabetes Care*, **13**, 1062–8.

WHO (World Health Organization) (1985*a*). *Diabetes mellitus*. WHO Technical Report Series, No. 727. WHO, Geneva.

WHO (World Health Organization) Multinational Study of Vascular Disease in Diabetics (MNSVDD) WHO (1985*b*). Prevalence of small vessel disease in diabetic patients from 14 centers. *Diabetologia*, **28** (Supplement), 615–40.

WHO (World Health Organization) (1994). *Prevention of diabetes mellitus*. WHO Technical Report Series, No. 844. WHO, Geneva.

WHO (World Health Organization) (1999). *Report of a consultation. Definition, diagnosis and classification of diabetes mellitus and its complications. Part 1: Diagnosis and classification of diabetes mellitus.* WHO, Geneva.

World Bank (1993). *World development report 1993: investing in health. World development indicators*. Oxford University Press.

World Health Report (1998). *Life in the 21st century. A vision for all*. WHO, Geneva.

Yamagata, K., Oda, N., Kaisaki, P.J., *et al.* (1996*a*). Mutations in the hepatocyte nuclear factor-1α gene in maturity-onset diabetes of the young (MODY 3). *Nature*, **384**, 455–8.

Yamagata, K., Furuta, H., Oda, N., *et al.* (1996*b*) Mutations in the hepatocyte nuclear factor-4α gene in maturity-onset diabetes of the young (MODY 1). *Nature*, **384**, 458–60.

Zimmet, P. (1992). Challenges in diabetes epidemiology—from West to the rest. *Diabetes Care*, **15**, 232–52.

Zimmet, P. (1993). Hyperinsulinaemia—how innocent a bystander. *Diabetes Care*, **16**, 56–70.

Zimmet, P.Z. (1995). The pathogenesis and prevention of diabetes in adults. *Diabetes Care*, **18**, 1050–64.

Zimmet, P. (1999). Diabetes epidemiology as a trigger to diabetes research. *Diabetologia*, **44**, 499–518.

Zimmet, P. and Alberti, K.G.M.M. (1997). The changing face of macrovascular disease in non-insulin dependent diabetes mellitus in different cultures: an epidemic in progress. *Lancet*, **350** (Supplement 1), S1–S4.

Zimmet, P., Dowse, G., Serjeantson, S., Finch, C., and King, H. (1990). The epidemiology and natural history of NIDDM—lessons from the South Pacific. *Diabetes/ Metabolism Reviews*, **6**, 91–124.

Zimmet, P., Turner, R., McCarty, D., Rowley, M., and Mackay, I. (1999). Crucial points at diagnosis—NIDDM or slow IDDM. *Diabetes Care*, **22**, B59–64.

Osteoporosis: a public health problem

Ego Seeman

Definition

Osteoporosis or bone fragility is characterized by low areal bone mineral density (**BMD**) and microarchitectural deterioration leading to bone fragility (Consensus Development Conference 1993). Fragility conferred by the microarchitectural abnormalities (trabecular thinning, loss of connectedness, cortical thinning, increased intracortical porosity) is unquantified, so that osteoporosis is currently synonymous with 'low' areal BMD.

A WHO panel defined (a) 'normal' areal BMD as values less reduced than 1 standard deviation (**SD**) below the young normal mean, (b) 'low' areal BMD or 'osteopenia' as values between –1 SD and –2.5 SD, and (c) 'osteoporosis' as areal BMD reduced by more than –2.5 SD below the young adult mean (Fig. 10). Severe or 'established' osteoporosis is areal BMD reduced by more than –2.5 SD in the presence of fractures (WHO 1994).

It is misleading to think of osteoporosis in dichotomous terms i.e. having or not having 'osteoporosis', having or not having 'low' areal BMD. Areal BMD is a continuous variable. The lower the areal BMD, the higher is the risk of fracture. The higher the blood pressure, the higher is the risk of stroke (Fig. 11). Areal BMD in patients with fractures and controls overlaps because areal BMD is a measure of risk, not certainty, of fracture (Melton *et al.* 1990).

Osteopenia means mild osteoporosis. It is a radiological term used to alert the doctor to increased fracture risk suggested by radiolucency on radiographs before bone densitometry was available. This term serves no purpose other than suggesting areal BMD is in the lower part of the normal distribution but above the nominal quantitative definition of osteoporosis. 'Established' osteoporosis is also entrenched in the literature and implies that the disease is 'established' after the fracture. This may lead clinicians to withhold treatment unless the fracture is present (the event that treatment should prevent). The disease is bone fragility (osteoporosis, areal BMD lower than –2.5 SD) whether fracture is present or not. The result of the disease of bone fragility is fracture.

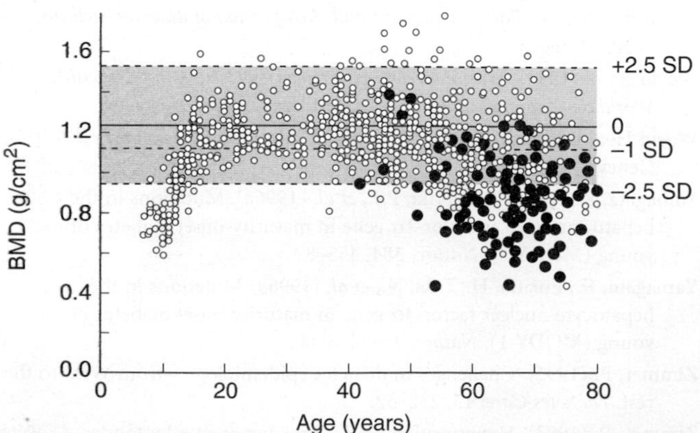

Fig. 10 Areal BMD at the lumbar spine in controls (open circles) and women with spine fractures (solid circles) (see text).

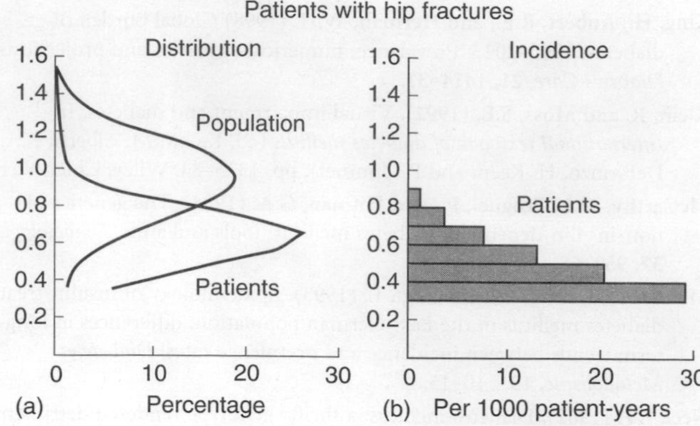

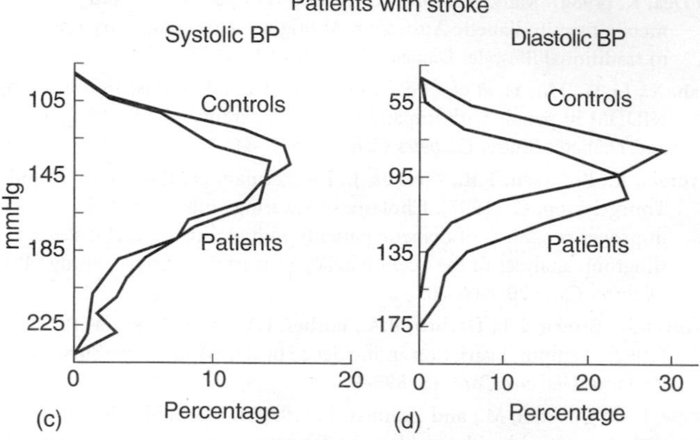

Fig. 11 (a)The lower the areal BMD, the higher is the fracture risk. (b) Areal BMD in patients with fractures and controls overlaps, just as (c) systolic and (d) diastolic blood pressure overlap in patients with stroke and controls. (Modified from Hui *et al.* 1988.)

Epidemiology

Osteoporosis is a public heath problem because of the morbidity, mortality, and financial burden imposed by fractures. The incidence of fracture rises with age and is higher in men than in women before 50 years of age because of trauma. After 50 years of age, bone fragility is responsible for the increasing fracture incidence in women and men. Lifetime fracture risk is 30 per cent in women and 15 per cent in men (Fig. 12) (Cooper and Melton 1992).

Hip fractures

There are over 325 million individuals over 65 years of age in the world. This will increase to over 1500 million by 2050. The increase will be seen particularly in Asia (Fig. 13). The lifetime risk for hip

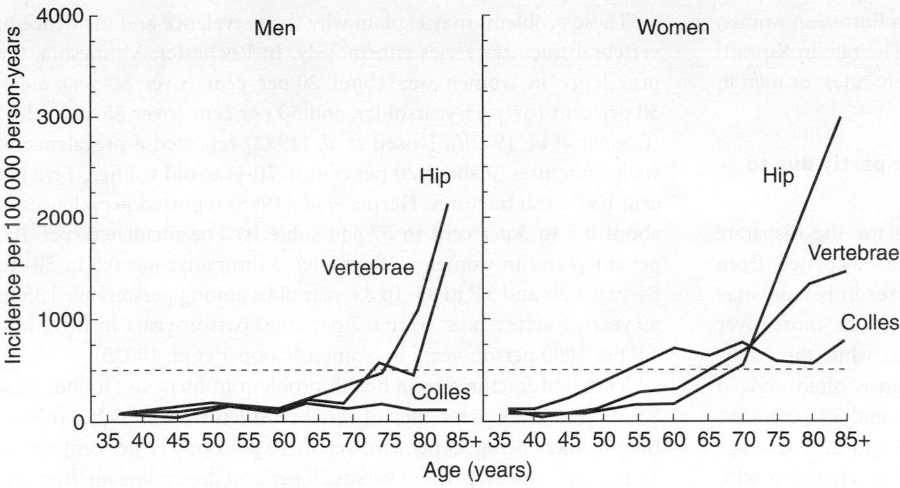

Fig. 12 The age-specific increase in hip, spine, and distal forearm fractures in men and women in Rochester, Minnesota. (Reproduced from Cooper and Melton 1993.)

fracture is 15 per cent in women and 7 per cent in men. In 1990, 30 per cent of the 1.66 million hip fractures worldwide occurred in men. By 2025, the number of hip fractures in men will be similar to the number in women in 1990, a burden compounded by the increases in women in 2025 (Cooper *et al.* 1992*a*). The incidence of hip fracture differs more between countries than between sexes, suggesting that there may be factors other than the menopause responsible for the differing incidence of fracture in women and men.

Barrett *et al.* (1999) estimated the risk of a person aged 65 years suffering a fracture based on data from 583 256 men and 838 507 women. The risks of hip fracture at ages 75, 80, 85, and 90 years were as follows: 2.9, 6.4, 11.2, and 16.3 per cent in white women; 1.1, 2.3,

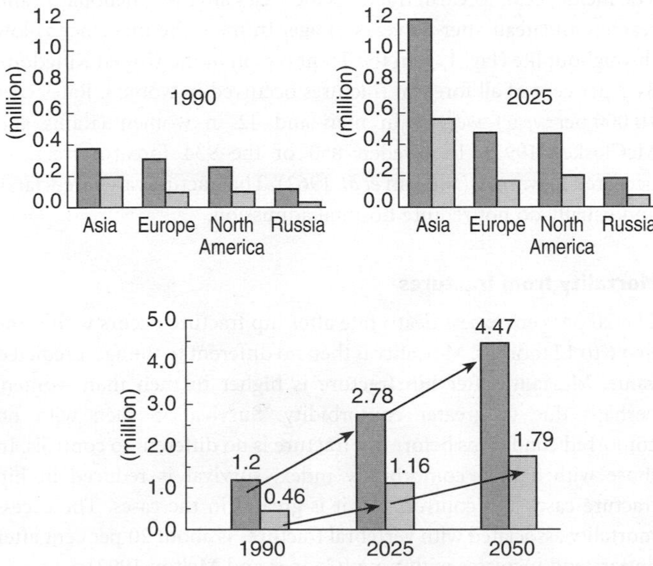

Fig. 13 The expected increase in hip fractures in 2025 will be seen particularly in Asia (upper panels). Thirty per cent of hip fractures occur in men. By 2025, the number of hip fractures in men will be similar to the number in women in 1990 (lower panel). (Modified from Cooper *et al.* 1992*a*.)

3.6, and 5.4 per cent in black women; 1.3, 2.6, 4.1, and 5.5 per cent in white men; 0.9, 1.4, 2.0, and 2.6 per cent in black men. White women had three- to fourfold higher risks than white men and 1.5- to fourfold higher risks than black women.

Kannus *et al.* (1999) reported that the number of hip fractures in patients over 50 years of age admitted to a Finnish hospital between 1970 and 1997 increased from 1857 to 7122. The incidence (per 100 000) increased from 163 to 438 (a 169 per cent rise). Median age at fracture increased from 76 to 82 years in women and from 70 to 76 years in men. After age adjustment, the incidence increased from 292 to 767 in women and from 112 to 233 in men (rises of 60 per cent and 108 per cent respectively). Age-specific incidences rose in all age groups, with greatest increases in older age groups. In contrast, Huusko *et al.* (1999) reported no changes in hip fracture incidence between the period 1982 to 1983 and the period 1992 to 1993. Crude incidences (per 1000 per year) in men and women in 1992 to 1993 were 1.56 and 3.23 and respective incidences were 10.24 and 16.50 in 1982 to 1983. On stratification by age and gender, respective mean annual rates per 1000 in women aged 45 to 54 years, 55 to 64 years, 65 to 74 years, 75 to 84 years, and 85+ years in the two periods were 0.5 versus 0.5, 2.7 versus 1.8, 10.4 versus 8.1, 24.0 versus 24.2, and 3.8 versus 3.9. The authors concluded that there had been a change in the age distribution, not in the age-adjusted incidence, within the last 10 years.

Hagino *et al.* (1999) reported increasing age-specific incidence rates for hip fractures in Japan between 1986 and 1994 (41 to 57 per 100 000 for men and 114 to 145 per 100 000 for women). These rates were similar to those in southern Europe but lower than in white populations in North America and northern Europe. Yan *et al.* (1999) reported 453 hip fractures in 612 170 Chinese aged 50 years or older in 1994. The age-adjusted 1-year cumulative incidence rate was 67 per 100 000 in women and 81 per 100 000 in men, lower than the rates reported in the United States in 1985 (87 and 100 per 100 000 in women and men respectively). The frequency of fracture by bicycle accident was 10 per cent in women and 28 per cent in men.

Memon *et al.* (1998) reported all new hip fracture cases between 1992 and 1995 in Kuwait; rates were 295 per 100 000 in women and

200 per 100 000 in men, similar to that reported in European women and in Asian women living in the United States. The rate in Kuwaiti men is almost equal to that in white American men; rates for men in other Asian countries are half or less.

The differing incidence of hip fracture may be partly due to flawed case ascertainment

Ascertainment errors may be partly responsible for the disparate results (Bacon *et al.* 1996). 'Incidence' is often calculated from discharge records. Failure to identify all cases (e.g. readmissions) may introduce errors. Small sample sizes, particularly in those over 80 years old, may result in an unstable numerator while the population forming the denominator in the calculation is often derived from dated census data. Groupings into 75+, 80+, and 85+ years are often made. Most hip fractures occur at this time and the mean age and distribution within these classifications will be changing with time. Thus the rising incidence may be an artefact of better surveillance. Retrospective analyses may result in underestimates.

Schwartz *et al.* (1999) calculated hip fracture incidence rates from discharge records during the period 1990 to 1992. Rates were lowest in Beijing (45.4 for men, and 39.6 for women) and highest in Reykjavik (141.3 for men, and 274.1 for women). Women had higher rates than men after age 65 years except in Beijing. Review of operating theatre or radiology logs increased the estimated number of hip fractures by 11 per cent. Miscoding increased the number by 1 per cent. When all sources of undercount and overcount were included, final estimates of hip fracture incidence ranged from 15 per cent lower to 89 per cent higher than the original rates based on discharge diagnoses.

If the differing incidences of hip fracture across time, from country to country, and between genders are correct, differences in the incidence of falls, severity of trauma, or bone fragility must be responsible. An increase in the age-specific incidence of falls may be occurring because of a higher prevalence of ill health and use of sedatives, or greater age-related bone loss in persons born more recently, producing greater bone fragility than that seen in persons born earlier.

Irrespective of whether there is a true increase in incidence of hip fracture during the last 20 years, it is clear that the number of hip fractures in the community is increasing because of the increasing number of individuals living into old age. The problem will place an increasing financial burden on the community.

The direct annual costs of hip fractures are £614 million in the United Kingdom, 3.7 billion francs in France, and \$10 billion in the United States (Barrett-Connor 1995). Hospital admission accounts for 44 per cent of these costs. In Switzerland, 50 per cent of the direct costs are incurred in the first 18 days of admission. Thirty per cent of the hospital stay is due to waiting for nursing home availability. About 50 per cent of hip-fracture survivors are discharged to nursing homes. In the United States, \$2 billion of the \$5 billion direct annual costs for long-term care are attributable to nursing home care.

Spine fractures

The epidemiology of spine fractures is less well documented for the the following reasons: (a) about 65 per cent of spine fractures do not reach clinical attention (Cooper *et al.* 1992*c*; Jacobsen *et al.* 1992); (b) the definition of 'deformity' or 'fracture' is unclear (Kanis 1994); (c) most data are prevalence not incidence, and a proportion of the fractures may be due to trauma in youth.

These problems may explain why the prevalence and incidence of vertebral fractures varies enormously. In Rochester, Minnesota, the prevalence in women was about 20 per cent (over 50-year-olds), 30 per cent (over 65-year-olds), and 50 per cent (over 85-year-olds) (Cooper *et al.* 1992*b*). Jensen *et al.* (1982) reported a prevalence of wedge fractures of about 20 per cent in 70-year-old women. Five per cent had crush fractures. Härmä *et al.* (1986) reported prevalences of about 0.5 to 3 per cent in 57 440 subjects. The incidence (per 100 person-years) in women in Rochester, Minnesota, was 0.5 in 50- to 54-year olds and 3.8 in 85- to 89-year olds; among persons aged 35 to 69 years, fracture rates were 0.7 per 1000 person-years in men, and 1.5 per 1000 person-years in women (Cooper *et al.* 1992*b*).

Vertebral fractures are a health problem in men. In Dubbo, New South Wales, the prevalence of vertebral fractures was higher in men than women, being 25 per cent versus 20 per cent, 17 per cent versus 12 per cent, and 27 per cent versus 25 per cent depending on 'fracture' criteria (Jones *et al.* 1994). In the United Kingdom, the prevalence was similar in 15 570 men and women—12 per cent or 20 per cent depending on the criteria used (O'Neill *et al.* 1996). In Korea, the prevalence was 12.5 per cent in men and 20 per cent in women. Elderly men had fewer crush fractures (3.7 per cent) than women (15.3 per cent) (Tsai *et al.* 1996). In Rotterdam, the prevalence in 724 men and 717 women was 8 per cent and 7 per cent respectively (moderate deformities), and 4 per cent and 10 per cent respectively (severe deformities) (Burger *et al.* 1997). In Nebraska, the prevalence in 529 men and 899 women aged 50 to 70 years was 29 per cent in men and 10 per cent in women, and 39 per cent and 45 per cent respectively in 80-year-olds (Davies *et al.* 1996). If vertebral fracture incidence is similar in men and women, the notion of osteoporosis as a disease of women must be discarded. Prospectively derived vertebral fracture incidence data are needed.

Forearm fractures

The incidence of forearm fractures increases after the menopause and reaches a plateau after 60 years of age. In men, the incidence is low throughout life (Fig. 12). In the Trent region in the United Kingdom, 84.2 per cent of all forearm fractures occurred in women. Rates (per 10 000 per year) were 9 in men and 42 in women (Kanis and McCloskey 1992). In Sweden 850 of the 934 forearm fractures occurred in women (Alffram *et al.* 1962). The fractures are rarely fatal, and usually do not require hospital admission.

Mortality from fractures

The 20 per cent excess death rate after hip fracture occurs within the first 6 to 12 months. Mortality is then no different to the age-predicted value. Mortality after hip fracture is higher in men than women, perhaps due to greater comorbidity. Survival in men with no comorbid conditions before hip fracture is no different to controls. In those with a high comorbidity index, survival is reduced in hip fracture cases and controls but it is greater in the cases. The excess mortality associated with vertebral fractures is about 20 per cent after 5 years and increases with time (Cooper and Melton 1992).

Bone density—a surrogate for bone strength

The highest incidence of fractures is 3 to 4 per 100 per year in women aged 80+ in the community reaching 10 to 12 per 100 per year in the highest-risk groups (women in nursing homes, women with very low areal BMD and multiple fractures). Thus neither the occurrence nor the absence of a fracture in an individual provides reliable information regarding causal relationships between a risk factor or treatment and fractures. That is, fractures, the true measure of fragility, cannot be used as an endpoint to study the pathogenesis, prevention, and efficacy treatment of fractures in an individual. This can only be determined in clinical trials.

Areal BMD is a surrogate of bone strength. *In vivo* and *in vitro*, the areal BMD measurement correlates with bone strength and is the best available measure of fracture risk. For a bone mass of 0.6 g/cm, fracture risk (per 1000 person-years) doubles from about 60 to 120 as age increases from 70 to 80 years (Fig. 14). At 70 years, fracture risk increases from 80 to 100 as bone mass decreases from 0.7 to 0.6 g/cm. Age and areal BMD are independent predictors of fracture risk (Hui *et al.* 1988). Age may incorporate factors such as falls and structural changes such as trabecular connectivity.

Bone 'mass' and 'density'—problems in nomenclature

Non-invasive methods measure 'apparent' areal BMD—a mass of mineral contained within an area or volume of tissue, not all of which is bone (Seeman 1997). Bone mass is expressed uncorrected for size (g), or an areal BMD corrected for length and width (g/cm^2) but not depth. Quantitative CT measures mass as a volumetric BMD correcting for length, width, and depth (mg/cm^3). This volumetric BMD measurement is also an 'apparent' density, although the word 'apparent' is omitted from the literature. Quantitative CT is erroneously claimed to be a 'true' density because it is volumetric. Implicit in the context of 'true' is the notion that this volumetric BMD is a better surrogate of bone strength than areal BMD measurements. There is no evidence for this.

'Areal', 'volumetric', and 'apparent' are dropped for convenience, but at the price of understanding. An increase in 'density' occurs through a change in structure within a length, area, or volume of tissue comprised of marrow, fat, cells, and fluid-filled spaces. In a unit of bone tissue, a doubling in the number of trabeculae produces the same increase in density as a doubling of the thickness of existing trabeculae (Fig. 15). The former may be more advantageous biomechanically before menopause, but less so after the menopause because thinner trabeculae may be more susceptible to perforation. Similarly, a doubling of cortical density may be the result of increased endocortical (medullary) or periosteal bone formation. The latter results in a bone more resistant to bending.

The failure to consider the structural basis of changes in 'density' results in serious misunderstanding (Seeman 1997). For example, BMD does not increase in growth; bone size increases. The amount of bone calcium (grams per 100 g fat-free tissue) is established in early intrauterine life and is constant from early in gestation to old age. Peak bone mass is less in women than men because women have smaller bones. Peak volumetric BMD is the same in men and women. These concepts are vital to the understanding of the structural basis of increasing bone 'density' during growth, bone loss during ageing, and the effects of treatment on bone strength.

Changes in bone density during growth and advancing age

Patients with fractures have reduced areal BMD relative to controls because of excessive bone loss or low peak areal BMD. Understanding of the pathogenesis of bone fragility or osteoporosis involves the study of risk and protective factors influencing the skeleton throughout life—during growth, adulthood, and old age.

Growth and peak bone density

Total body calcium increases during growth because the bone size increases. However, the growing bone gains more bone within it (as

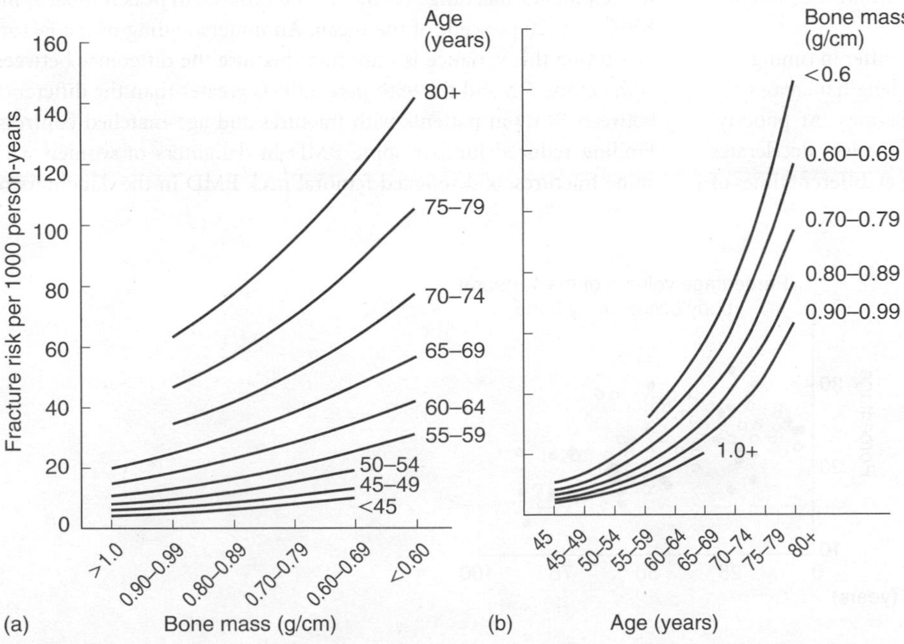

Fig. 14 (a)At any bone mass, fracture risk increased as age increased. (b) For any age, fracture risk increased as bone mass decreases. (Reproduced from Hui *et al.* 1988.)

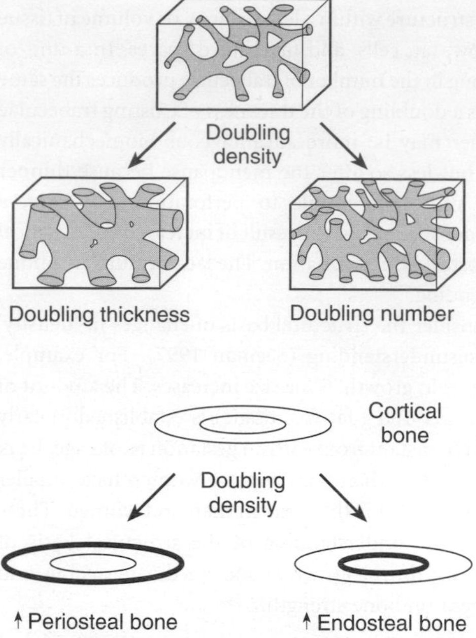

Fig. 15 A doubling in trabecular bone density may be due to doubling of the thickness or number of trabeculae. A doubling of cortical density may be the result of increased endocortical (medullary) or periosteal bone.

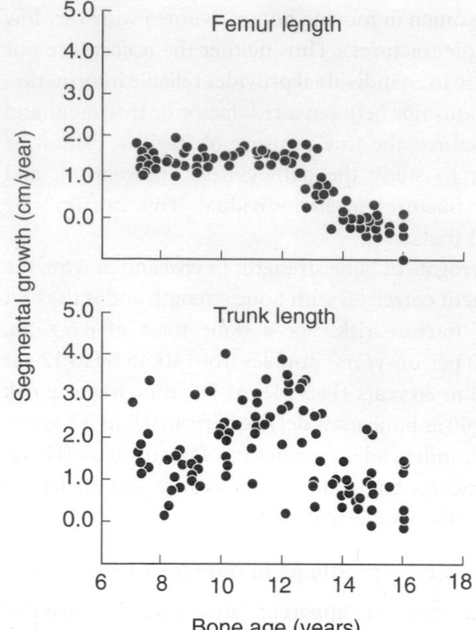

Fig. 17 At puberty, growth of the trunk accelerates while growth of the femur decelerates. (Modified from Tupman 1962.)

cortical thickness increases, as trabeculae are formed at the growth plate and then thicken) so that volumetric BMD is constant before puberty and then increases around puberty as trabeculae thicken further and cortical thickness increases by endocortical contraction, i.e. growth builds a larger skeleton but only a slightly more dense skeleton. Dunnill *et al.* (1967) showed that vertebral size increased from birth to young adulthood and is greater in men than in women. From about 2 years of age, the volume of bone within the vertebral body is constant—'density' is constant (Fig. 16).

Growth of the axial and appendicular skeleton differ in timing and regulation. At the end of the first year of life, trunk length increases at a constant velocity while growth of the legs accelerates. At puberty, growth of the trunk accelerates while growth of the legs decelerates (Tupman *et al.* 1962) (Fig. 17). Diseases occurring at different times of growth may result in site-specific deficits. Regions further from their peak or growing more rapidly may be more severely affected by exposure to disease than regions nearer completion of growth. Thus the effect of a risk factor on the growing skeleton depends on the developmental stage at which exposure occurs as well as the exposure 'dose' (Bass *et al.* 1999).

This heterogeneity in growth and mineral accrual may contribute to the wide normal range for BMD. The variance in peak lumbar spine BMD is ± 20 per cent of the mean. An understanding of the factors explaining this variance is important because the difference between BMD at the 5th and the 95th percentile is greater than the difference between BMD in patients with fractures and age-matched controls. Finding reduced lumbar spine BMD in daughters of women with spine fractures, and reduced femoral neck BMD in the daughters of

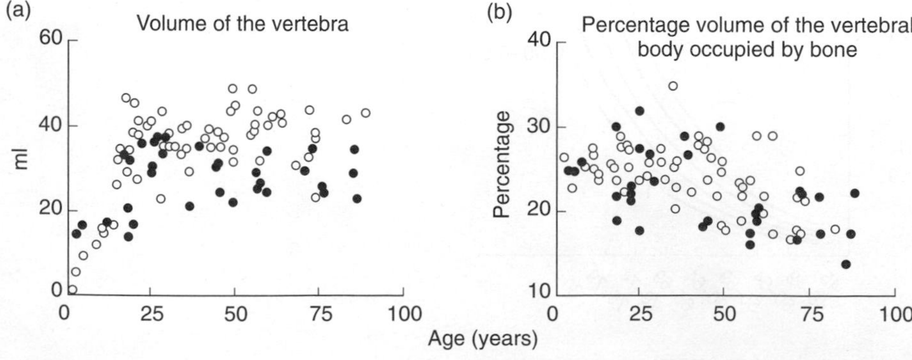

Fig. 16 (a)Vertebral volume increases during growth in females (solid circles) and males (open circles). (b) The volume of bone in vertebral body (bone density) is constant from early life. (Modified from Dunnill *et al.* 1967.)

women with hip fractures, is consistent with the view that a low peak BMD may be a sufficient explanation for the lower BMD found in patients with fractures (Seeman *et al.* 1989, 1994).

Genetics of osteoporosis

About 80 per cent of the variance in areal BMD is explained by genetic factors. Many polymorphisms of candidate genes have been proposed, but few if any reproducible data exist that identify any gene or gene product that accounts for this variance (Seeman 1999). Heritability is the proportion of the total variance (genetic plus environmental) in areal BMD attributable to genetic factors. The statement '80 per cent of areal BMD is genetically determined leaving only 20 per cent to modify' is flawed; heritability is not a constant proportion leaving 20 per cent 'due to' environmental factors that can be changed. The size of the total population variance depends on the factors chosen to describe the trait mean (such as age, gender, height, body composition). If total variance increases due to an increase in the environmental variance, without change in the genetic variance, heritability will decrease. Thus, 'heritability' (a proportion) and 'genetic variance' (an absolute) may give different impressions of the 'strength' of genetic factors.

Areal BMD is not a specific and unambiguous phenotype with identifiable physiological control mechanisms. It is the net result of the modelling and remodelling on the periosteal and endosteal surfaces that give the bone its mass, size, and architecture. Each surface behaves differently during growth and ageing because each is regulated differently. The ambiguity of areal BMD makes this an unsatisfactory phenotype for the identification of the genes that contribute to the regulation of skeletal growth and ageing. No gene, gene product, or gene polymorphism has been reproducibly, and therefore credibly, shown to account for a given proportion of the variance in areal BMD. The data concerning candidate markers such as polymorphisms of the vitamin D receptor, oestrogen receptor, and type 1 collagen genes are inconsistent, perhaps partly because of the questionable value of this phenotype, the use of genetic markers of uncertain biological function, flaws in study design such as small sample sizes, failure to account for confounding, lack of stratification and/or randomization prior to intervention, reliance on statistical adjustment rather than study design, and the use of *post hoc* analyses to infer causation. Distinct morphological structures (trabecular number, thickness, periosteal and endocortical width, cortical thickness) should be quantified by age-, gender-, and race-specific means and variances. Genetic and environmental factors should be sought that explain variance in these structures (Seeman 1999).

Bone loss—an imbalance in bone formation and resorption

After completion of skeletal growth, remodelling occurs at discrete sites throughout the skeleton (basic multicellular units) replacing old with new bone. Osteoclasts resorb a quantum of bone at the basic multicellular units forming a Howship lacuna on the surface of trabecular bone (Fig. 18) (Mosekilde *et al.* 1990). Osteoblasts lay down osteoid which undergoes primary and secondary mineralization.

Bone 'loss' is not only resorptive removal of bone, it is also failure of restoration. This imbalance between bone resorption and bone formation at the basic multicellular units is the structural requirement for bone loss. If the amount of bone removed and replaced is the same, no loss of bone occurs. Bone loss occurs if formation is reduced when resorption is normal and when resorption is increased and formation is either normal or reduced. At the menopause, bone turnover increases—there are more basic multicellular units activated and there is focal imbalance in each. Why bone formation does not 'keep up' is not understood.

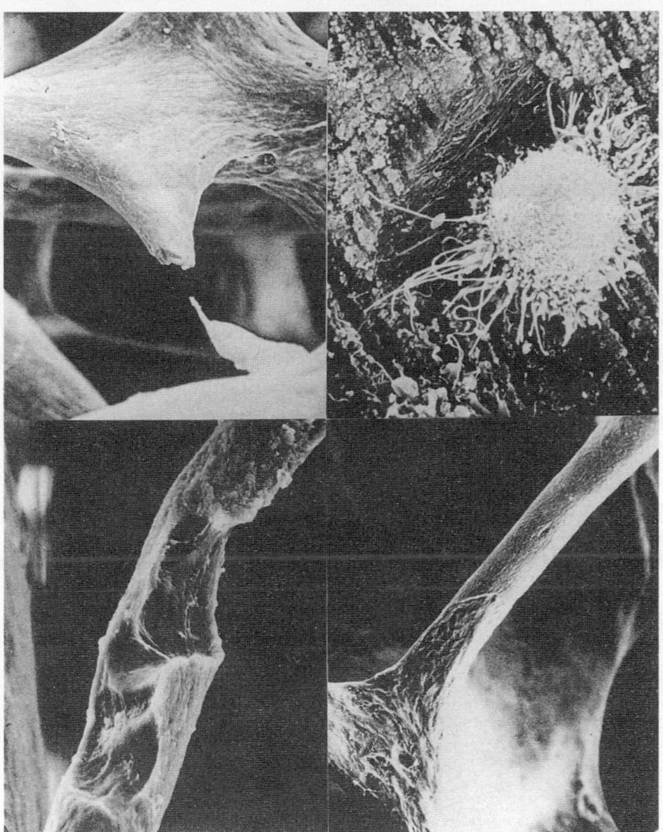

Fig. 18 Electron micrographs showing bone resorption by an osteoclast (upper left), an intact trabeculum (upper right), and a trabeculum undergoing erosion (bottom right) with loss of connectivity (bottom left). (Modified from Mosekilde *et al.* 1993.)

Remodelling occurs on endosteal (endocortical, trabecular, and intracortical) and periosteal surfaces (Parfitt 1994). Trabecular bone loss is more rapid than cortical bone loss because of its greater surface area. Trabecular bone remodelling with imbalance at the basic multicellular units results in thinning, perforation, and loss of trabecular connectivity. Trabecular bone loss contributes progressively less to the overall bone loss because trabeculae disappear and the trabecular surface area for remodelling decreases.

Cortical bone loss is slower and is the net result of endocortical resorption, intracortical bone loss producing porosity, and periosteal bone formation which partly compensates for the endocortical bone resorption and results in increased bone diameter. With advancing age, cortical bone loss accounts for an increasing proportion of the overall bone loss. Continued endocortical bone resorption and increased cortical porosity increase the surface for resorption in cortical bone, 'trabecularizing' cortical bone. Bone loss does not decelerate in old age, it accelerates (Foldes *et al.* 1991; Jones *et al.*

1996). About 70 per cent of the total bone lost during ageing in women is cortical because 80 per cent of the skeleton is cortical bone (Sandor *et al.* 1992).

Gender differences in bone loss

The net amount of total body calcium lost in women is 100 to 150 g more than in men. As men have larger bones, the net loss is 30 to 40 per cent in women but only 10 to 15 per cent in men. The age-related diminution in trabecular bone of the iliac crest in women and men is similar (Fig. 19). Women lose more bone than men because cortical—not trabecular—bone loss is greater (Kalender *et al.* 1989). Cortical bone loss is greater because endocortical resorption is greater in women than in men, and periosteal bone formation is greater in men than in women. The percentage of trabecular surface undergoing resorption increases in women. Trabecular numbers fall due to perforation and loss of connectivity (Fig. 20). Trabecular bone loss in men occurs primarily by reduced bone formation and a fall in trabecular width.

Classification and causes of osteoporosis

Primary and secondary osteoporosis

The most common types of fractures—spine, forearm, and hip—in women and men have no identified cause. They are the morbid event of 'primary' or 'idiopathic' osteoporosis. Postmenopausal (type 1) osteoporosis refers to the occurrence of spine and forearm fractures within the first 20 to 25 years of menopause. Loss of trabecular connectivity associated with the increased bone turnover after the menopause may be responsible for the bone fragility. Senile (type 2) osteoporosis refers to the occurrence of hip fractures in men and women 75 years and older. Age-related loss of both trabecular and cortical bone contribute to bone fragility (Riggs and Melton 1983).

'Secondary' refers to osteoporosis occurring in the setting of an illness or a recognized risk factor for osteoporosis. Illnesses that may be associated with osteoporosis but contribute little to the public health problem of osteoporosis include acromegaly, primary hyperparathyroidism, osteogenesis imperfecta, Cushing's disease, hypo-

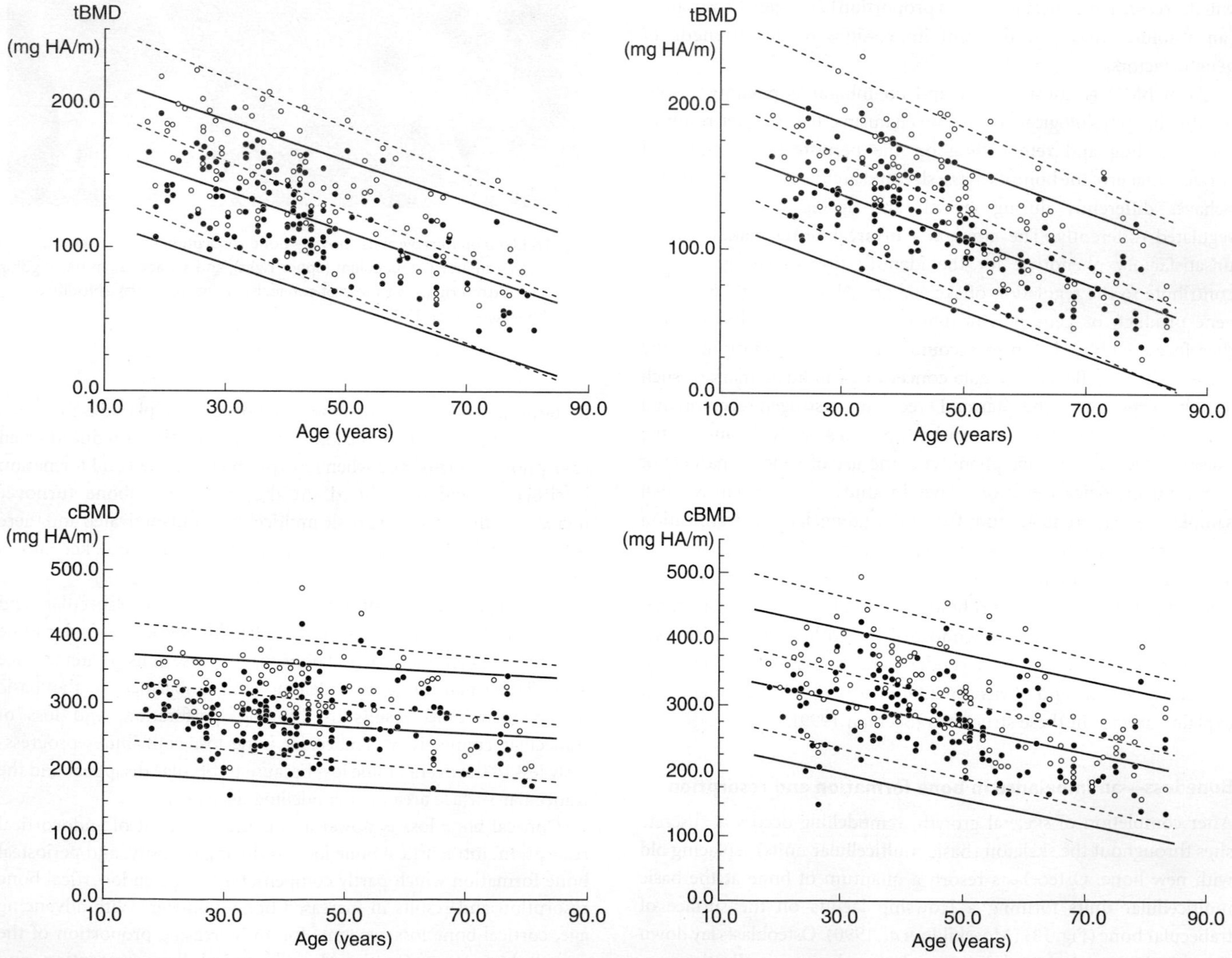

Fig. 19 Upper panels show the similar diminution in vertebral body trabecular bone in men (left) and women (right) by quantitative CT. The diminution in vertebral cortical BMD (lower panels) is less in men (left) than in women (right). (Single energy—open circles, broken regression lines; dual energy—solid circles, continuous regression lines.) (Reproduced from Kalender *et al.* 1989.)

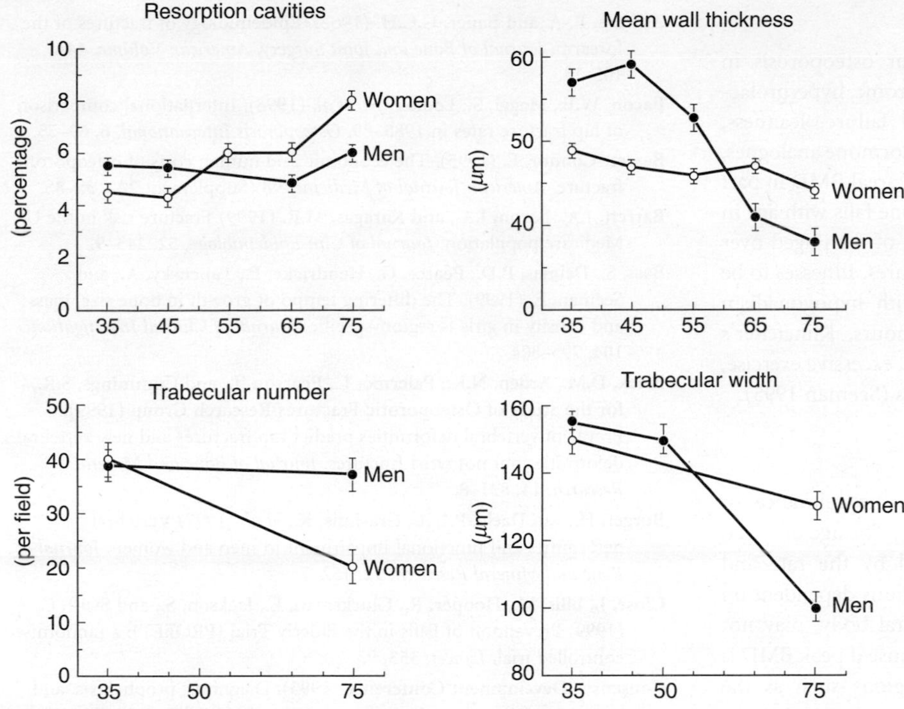

Fig. 20 Bone loss in women occurs by increased resorption, a fall in trabecular number, and loss of connectivity (left upper and lower panels). Bone loss occurs by reduced bone formation (mean wall thickness) and a fall in trabecular width in men (right upper and lower panels). (Modified from Aaron *et al.* 1987.)

pituitarism, and multiple myeloma. Myeloma, malabsorption, primary hyperparathyroidism, and hypogonadism may have no clinical features and must be regarded with a high index of suspicion.

Risk factors for osteoporosis include age, hypogonadism, nulliparity, immobility, Caucasian or Asian race, tobacco use, alcohol abuse, sedentary living, low calcium intake, high caffeine, protein, and salt intakes, low body weight, a family or past history of fractures, small bones, and drugs (corticosteroids, anticonvulsants, cyclosporin, thyroxine, and heparin). Protective factors include black race, osteoarthritis, lactation, multiparity, high calcium intake, exercise, obesity, fluoridated drinking water, exposure to oestrogens, and thiazides.

One of the most important risk fractors for fractures independent of areal BMD or age is the presence of one or more spine fractures. Black *et al.* (1999) reported that the risk of sustaining further spine fractures in the presence of a prevalent spine deformity was 5.4. The risk of hip and of any non-spine fracture was 2.8 and 1.9 respectively in women with baseline deformity. The risk for new spine fractures increased as the number of baseline deformities increased, from 3.2 for one fracture to 10.6 for three or more fractures. Women with most severe deformities had a relative risk of 12.7 for a new deformity.

Risk factors for hip fracture include a maternal history of hip fracture, low body weight, tall stature, previous fractures, hyperthyroidism, inactivity, use of benzodiazepines, anticonvulsants, and caffeine, and reduced muscle strength. The hip fracture incidence (per 1000 per year) was 1.1 (95 per cent confidence intervals, 0.5, 1.6) in women with no more than two risk factors and normal BMD, and 27 (95 per cent confidence intervals, 20, 34) with five or more risk factors and low BMD (Fig. 21) (Cumming *et al.* 1995).

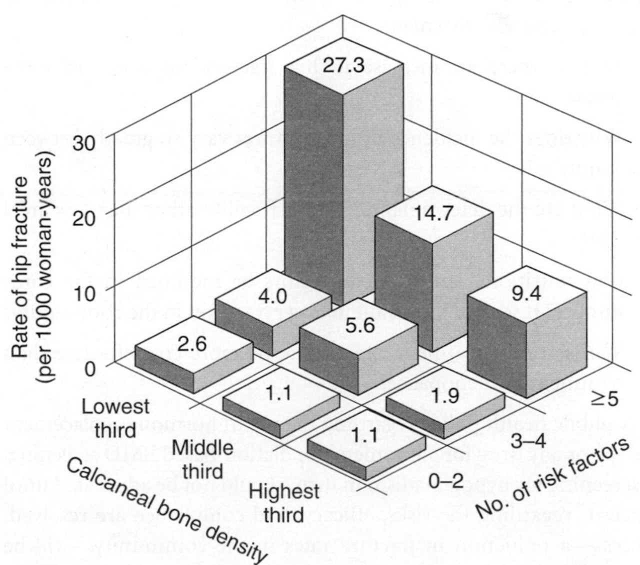

Fig. 21 The incidence of hip fractures (per 1000 women per year) was 1.1 (95 per cent confidence interval: 0.5, 1.6) in women with no more than two risk factors and normal BMD, and 27 (95 per cent confidence interval: 20, 34) in women with five or more risk factors and low BMD. (Reproduced from Cumming *et al.* 1995.)

Hypogonadism

Hypogonadism is an important 'risk factor' for osteoporosis in women and men. Delayed puberty, Kalman's syndrome, hyperprolactinaemia, anorexia nervosa, premature ovarian failure, leanness, tobacco use, use of luteinizing hormone reducing hormone analogues, and excessive exercise are associated with reduced areal BMD in part due to oestrogen deficiency in women. Testosterone falls with age in men. Low testosterone was found in 48 per cent of men aged over 50 years and in 59 per cent of men with hip fractures. Illnesses to be considered in men with fractures associated with hypogonadism include idiopathic hypogonadism, pituitary tumours, Klinefelter's syndrome, hyperprolactinaemia, anorexia nervosa, excessive exercise, haemochromatosis, and exogenous corticosteroids (Seeman 1995).

Conclusion

Reduced regional peak areal BMD establishes the relevance of age-related and sex hormone dependent bone loss. The age of onset, incidence, and type of fracture are determined by the rate and duration of cortical and trabecular bone loss. Regions dependent on trabecular bone for strength, such as the vertebral body, may not tolerate trabecular bone loss following the menopause if peak BMD is reduced. Fragility in predominantly cortical regions such as the proximal femur may emerge later, when age-related bone loss reduces cortical thickness and increases cortical porosity. In the presence of bone fragility, the type of fracture and the age of occurrence of the fracture partly depend on the age-specific pattern of trauma and falls. The mobility of middle age may predispose to spontaneous vertebral fractures, or forearm fractures due to falls defended by the outstretched hand. The poverty of forward movement in the elderly may favour an undefended fall onto the lateral hip region.

From a public health point of view, the problem is hip fractures in both women and men, and vertebral fractures in women, and probably in men. Falls in the elderly are a public health problem and certain questions still remain.

1. Why is there an increase in hip fracture incidence in some countries?
2. Why does the incidence of hip fractures vary so greatly between countries?
3. What are the determinants of bone fragility other than low areal BMD?
4. Can nutritional and lifestyle factors be modified in the community? If so, will this result in fewer fractures in the community?
5. Will starting treatment later in life be more cost-effective than treatment at menopause?

A public health policy regarding the use of hormone replacement therapy or any drug for all women, population-based BMD screening, or screening for hypogonadism in men, should not be advocated until concerns regarding the risks, efficacy, and compliance are resolved. Success—a reduction in fracture rates in the community—will be measured by the epidemiologist.

References

Aaron, J.E., Makins, N.B., and Sagreiy, K. (1987). The microanatomy of trabecular bone loss in normal aging men and women. *Clinical Orthopaedics and Related Research*, **215**, 260–71.

Alffram, P.-A. and Bauer, G.C.H. (1962). Epidemiology of fractures of the forearm. *Journal of Bone and Joint Surgery, American Volume*, **44A**, 105–14.

Bacon, W.E., Maggi, S., Looker, A., *et al.* (1996). International comparison of hip fracture rates in 1988–89. *Osteoporosis International*, **6**, 69–75.

Barrett-Connor, E. (1995). The economic and human costs of osteoporotic fracture. *American Journal of Medicine*, **98** (Supplement 2A), 3S–8S.

Barrett, J.A., Baron, J.A., and Karagas, M.R. (1999) Fracture risk in the US Medicare population. *Journal of Clin Epidemiology*, **52**, 243–9.

Bass, S., Delmas, P.D., Pearce, G., Hendricke, E., Tabensky, A., and Seeman, E. (1999). The differing tempo of growth in bone size, mass and density in girls is region-specific. *Journal of Clinical Investigation*, **104**, 795–804.

Black, D.M., Arden, N.K., Palermo, L., Pearson, J., and Cummings, S.R., for the Study of Osteoporotic Fractures Research Group (1999). Prevalent vertebral deformities predict hip fractures and new vertebral deformities but not wrist fractures. *Journal of Bone and Mineral Research*, **14**, 821–8.

Burger, H., van Daele, P.L.A., Grashuis, K., *et al.* (1997) Vertebral deformities and functional impairment in men and women. *Journal of Bone and Mineral Research*, **12**, 152–7.

Close, J., Ellis, M., Hooper, R., Glucksman, E., Jackson, S., and Swift, C. (1999) Prevention of Falls in the Elderly Trial (PROFET): a randomised controlled trial. *Lancet*, **353**, 93–7.

Consensus Development Conference (1993). Diagnosis, prophylaxis, and treament of osteoporosis. *American Journal of Medicine*, **94**, 646–50.

Cooper, C. and Melton, L.J., III (1992). Epidemiology of osteoporosis. *Trends in Endocrinology and Metabolism*, **3**, 224–9.

Cooper, C., Campion, G., and Melton, L.J., III (1992*a*). Hip fractures in the elderly: a world-wide projection. *Osteoporosis International*, **2**, 285–89.

Cooper, C., Atkinson, E.J., O'Fallon, W.M., and Melton, L.J., III (1992*b*). Incidence of clinically diagnosed vertebral fractures. A population-based study in Rochester, Minnesota, 1985–1989. *Journal of Bone and Mineral Research*, **7**, 221–7.

Cooper, C., Atkinson, E.J., Kotowicz, M., *et al.* (1992*c*). Secular trends in the incidence of postmenopausal osteoporosis. *Calcified Tissue International*, **51**, 100–4.

Cumming, S.R., Nevitt M.C., Browner W.S., *et al.*, **for the Study of Osteoporotic Fractures Research Group** (1995). Risk factors for hip fracture in white women. *New England Journal of Medicine*, **332**, 767–73.

Davies, K.M., Stegman, M.R., Heaney, R.P., and Recker, R.R. (1996). Prevalence and severity of vertebral fracture: the Saunders County Bone Quality Study. *Osteoporosis International*, **2**, 160–5.

Dunnill, M.S., Anderson, J.A., and Whitehead, R. (1967). Quantitative histological studies on age changes in bone. *Journal of Pathology and Bacteriology*, **4**, 275–91.

Foldes, J., Parfitt, A.M., Shin, M-S., Rao, D.S., and Kleerekoper, M. (1991). Structural and geometric changes in iliac bone: relationship to normal aging and osteoporosis. *Journal of Bone and Mineral Research*, **6**, 759–66.

Hagino, H., Yamamoto, K., Ohshiro, H., Nakamura, T., Kishimoto, H., and Nose, T. (1999). Changing incidence of hip, distal radius, and proximal humerus fractures in Tottori Prefecture, Japan. *Bone*, **24**, 265–70.

Härmä, M., Heliövaara, M., Aromaa, A., and Knekt, P. (1986). Thoracic spine compression fractures in Finland.*Clinical Orthopaedics and Related Research*, **205**, 188–94.

Hui, S.L., Slemenda, C.W., and Johnston, C.C., Jr (1988). Age and bone mass as predictors of fracture in a prospective study. *Journal of Clinical Investigation*, **81**, 1804–9.

Huusko, T.M., Karppi, P., Avikainen, V., Kautiainen, H., and Sulkava, R. (1999). The changing picture of hip fractures: dramatic change in age distribution and no change in age-adjusted incidence within 10 years in Central Finland. *Bone*, **24**, 257–9.

Jacobsen, S.J., Cooper, C., Gottlieb, M.S., *et al.* (1992). Hospitalization for vertebral fracture among the aged: a national population-based study, 1986–1989. *Epidemiology*, **3**, 515–18.

Jensen, G.F., Christianson, C., Boese, N.J., *et al.* (1982). Epidemiology of post-menopausal spinal and long bone fractures: a unifying approach to post-menopausal osteoporosis. *Clinical Orthopaedics and Related Research*, **166**, 75–81.

Jones, G., Nguyen, T., Sambrook, P., Kelly, P.J., and Eisman, J.A. (1994). Progessive loss of bone in the femoral neck in elderly people: longitudinal findings from the Dubbo Osteoporosis Epidemiology Study. *British Medical Journal*, **309**, 691–5.

Jones, G., Nguyen, T., Sambrook, P.N., Kelly, P.J., Gilbert, C., and Eisman, J.A. (1996). Symptomatic fracture incidence in elderly men and women: the Dubbo Osteoporosis Epidemiology Study (DOES). *Osteoporosis International*, **4**, 277–82.

Kalender, W.A., Felsenberg, D., Louis, O., *et al.* (1989). Reference values for trabecular and cortical vertebral bone density in single and dual-energy quantitative computed tomography. *European Journal of Radiology*, **9**, 75–80.

Kanis, J.A. (1994). What constitutes evidence for drug efficacy in osteoporosis? *Drugs and Aging*, **3**, 391–9.

Kanis, J.A. and McCloskey, E.V. (1992). Epidemiology of vertebral osteoporosis. *Bone*, **13**, S1–S10.

Kannus, P., Niemi, S., Parkkari, J., Palvanen, M., Vuori, I., and Jorvinen, M. (1999). Hip fractures in Finland between 1970 and 1997 and predictions for the future. *Lancet*, **353**, 802–5.

Maggi, S., Kelsey, J.L., Litvak, J., and Heyse, S.P. (1991). Incidence of hip fractures in the elderly: a cross-national analysis. *Osteoporosis International*, **1**, 232–41.

Melton, L.J., III, Eddy, D.M., and Johnston, C.C., Jr (1990). Screening for osteoporosis. *Annals of Internal Medicine*, **112**, 516–28.

Melton, L.J,. Lane, A.W., Cooper, C., *et al.* (1993). Prevalence and incidence of vertebral deformities. *Osteoporosis International*, **3**, 113–19.

Memon, A., Pospula, W.M., Tantawy, A.Y., Abdul-Ghafar, S., Suresh, A., and Al-Rowaih, A. (1998). Incidence of hip fracture in Kuwait. *International Journal of Epidemiology*, **27**, 860–5.

Mosekilde, L. (1990). Consequences of the remodelling process for vertebral trabecular bone structure: a scanning electron microscopy study (uncoupling of unloaded structures). *Bone and Mineral*, **10**, 13–35.

O'Neill, T.W., Felsenberg, D., Varlow, J., Cooper, C., Kanis, J.A., and Silman, A.J. (1996). The prevalence of vertebral deformity in European men and women: the European Vertebral Osteoporosis Study. *Journal of Bone and Mineral Research*, **11**, 1010–18.

Parfitt, A.M. (1994). Osteonal and hemi-osteonal remodelling: the spatial and temporal framework for signal traffic in adult human bone. *Journal of Cellular Biochemistry*, **55**, 273–86.

Riggs, B.L. and Melton, L.J., III (1983). Evidence for two distinct syndromes of involutional osteoporosis. *American Journal of Medicine*, **75**, 899–901.

Sandor, T., Felsenberg, D., Kalender, W.A., Clain, A., and Brown, E. (1992). Compact and trabecular components of the spine using quantitative computed tomography. *Calcified Tissue International*, **50**, 502–6.

Schwartz, A.V., Kelsey, J.L., Maggi, S., *et al.* (1999) International variation in the incidence of hip fractures: cross-national project on osteoporosis for the World Health Organization program for research on aging.*Osteoporosis International*, **9**, 242–53.

Seeman, E. (1994*a*). Relative contributions of low peak bone mass and bone loss to reduced bone density in osteoporosis. *Osteoporosis International*, **4**, 15–25.

Seeman, E. (1994*b*). Osteoporosis in men. *American Journal of Medicine*, **95**, 22–8.

Seeman, E. (1995). The dilemma of osteoporosis in men. *American Journal of Medicine*, **98** (Supplement 1A), 75S–87S.

Seeman E. (1997). From density to structure: growing up and growing old on the surfaces of bone. *Journal of Bone and Mineral Research*, **12**, 1–13.

Seeman, E. (1999). The genetic determination of the population variants in bone mineral density. In *The aging skeleton* (ed. C. Rosen), pp. 77–94, Academic Press, New York.

Seeman, E., Hopper, J.L., Bach, L.A., Cooper, M., McKay, J., and Jerums, G. (1989). Reduced bone mass in daughters of women with osteoporosis. *New England Journal of Medicine*, **320**, 554–8.

Seeman, E., Hopper, J.L., Tsalamandris, C., and Formica, C. (1994). Bone density in daughters of women with hip fractures. *Journal of Bone and Mineral Research*, **9**, 739–43.

Tsai, K.-S., Twu, S.-J., Chieng, P.-U., Yang, R.-S., and Lee, T.-K. (1996). Prevalence of vertebral fractures in Chinese men and women in urban Taiwanese communities. *Calcified Tissue International*, **59**, 249–53.

Tupman, G.S. (1962). A study of bone growth in normal children and its relationship to skeletal maturation. *Journal of Bone and Joint Surgery, British Volume*, **44B**, 42–67.

WHO (World Health Organization) (1994). *Assessment of fracture risk and its application to screening for postmenopausal osteoporosis*, pp. 1–129. Technical Report Series 843. WHO, Geneva.

Yan, L., Zhou, B., Prentice, A., Wang, X., and Golden, M.H.N. (1999). Epidemiological study of hip fracture in Shenyang, People's Republic of China. *Bone*, **24**, 151–5.

9.7 Public mental health

Peter Tyrer and Freya Tyrer

General background

Public mental health is a concept that has grown in recent years. In the past much of mental health has been in the private domain. We use the word 'private' in all its different meanings, as for many years mental health treatment (as opposed to custodial care) was only available to those with private means, the care of people with mental health problems has generally been a private secretive exercise, and because of the damaging influence of stigma there has been a tendency to keep much of mental illness shrouded in euphemism and understatement so that official statistics are of much less value than in other medical disciplines. However, with the growth of public mental health, a discipline which acknowledges mental health pathology in all settings from the special hospitals for forensic psychiatric patients through to large populations in the community, we are now beginning to obtain a comprehensive picture of mental illness which is immeasurably better than it was 10 years ago. The main disadvantages of private mental health are illustrated by the classical work of the psychoanalyst. The patient (or population with a specific psychiatric disorder) presented to the analyst is assessed and offered flexible, sometimes unlimited, treatment with no agreed measures of outcome (as the intention is for these to be developed by patient and therapist as treatment proceeds), and the outcome, even if positive, is usually of very little help in generalizing to other patients with psychiatric disorders. It adds to the simile to note that the psychoanalyst carries out most of the treatment sitting behind the patient who lies on a couch with little to look at apart from the ceiling. Although this is said to aid treatment, it does not immediately give the impression of improving communication.

However, in the last 10 years, and in particular since the last edition of this textbook, mental health services are being audited and examined in a way which is quite newand which has led to many difficulties. In the United Kingdom, targets in each of the key areas of health were identified at the beginning of this decade, but unfortunately it has to be admitted that there is no satisfactory outcome measure of public mental health that can be easily recorded and which could serve as a yardstick (Anonymous 1992). However, one measure has been selected—prevention of suicide—and although many in the mental health services were unhappy about this being regarded as an index of effectiveness of mental health interventions, it has been of considerable value. The British government set a national target of reducing the death rate from suicide and 'undetermined injury by at least a further sixth (17 per cent) by 2010, from a baseline at 1996' (DoH 1999), and in this regard they appear to have been bolstered by the likely success of their first target—to reduce suicide rates by 15 per cent between 1990 and 2000.

In this chapter we aim to introduce the reader to the wealth and breadth of psychiatric disturbance and to open some of the secret doors that have helped to make the discipline a private one but hindered its public health role. In illustrating the disorders, an epidemiological perspective will be adopted before describing the various interventions that are available and which can generally be described as evidence-based. In the final section we discuss the important question of need in mental health services, both met and unmet, and its implication for the public health physician.

Historical review of mental health service developments in relationship to public health

It is difficult to know to what extent historical developments in mental health are important in understanding the present and future. However, study of the public mental health aspects demonstrate that throughout the centuries there has been an ebb and flow of official attitudes towards mental illness that have affected its practice enormously. At one extreme was total integration of the mentally ill into the rest of the community with no special provision for their care and the belief that such people constitute a common responsibility for the community. This is perhaps best exemplified by mental health care in Ireland a thousand years ago (Robins 1986). At the other extreme is the isolation of the mentally ill from the rest of the community, partly because of stigma and partly because of fear, exemplified by the massive growth of mental hospitals in the United Kingdom in the nineteenth century (Scull 1959).

Although it might be expected that, with increasing knowledge, there would be a steady move towards a more enlightened view of mental illness, the fluctuations of the past do not inspire confidence, and in recent years there has been a strong reaction against the growth of what has become called 'community psychiatry' and the policies of incarceration, or the equivalents in less emotive language, are becoming increasingly attractive again (Coid 1994).

What has altered over the years is the interpretation of mental illness in its sufferers. For centuries there has been a distinction between those mental illnesses which are associated with an apparent loss of reason, the psychoses, from those in which distress is present but reason is maintained and the so-called 'reality-based disorders'. Most of the latter were formally classified under the general heading of 'neurosis', a term which physicians are now taught to ignore as an outdated relic of psychoanalysis (Bayer and Spitzer 1985), but which still has its adherents (Tyrer 1985).

The psychoses have led to fear and loathing in equal measure. The most obvious interpretation of the totally unreasonable behaviour of psychotic disorders is that the person has been possessed, and this has been a common explanation throughout the ages. Supernatural possession is the most common attribution, and whereas innocent possession by alien influences is sometimes inferred on most occasions it is assumed that the devil or other malevolent influences are primarily responsible. There has also been a suspicion that the mad are often clever and devious. This is perhaps expressed most graphically in Shakespeare's comment about Hamlet's madness 'If this be madness, yet there is method in't'. There has also been the suspicion that mad people conspire together as a consequence of supernatural influences, and it is this that has provoked the most fear and consequent retribution; the execution of the witches of Salem in 1692 is a prime example.

Over the course of the past 200 years all forms of mental illness have gradually been brought together as varieties of sickness. Although little treatment was available, such people were cared for as though they were unwell, usually in almshouses or similar places of refuge, and the word 'asylum' developed in this context. However, as the mentally ill became increasingly isolated from other members of the community, the stigma of mental illness increased and integration back into the community became more difficult. Despite this, the period in which mental hospitals grew and isolation of the mentally ill increased was still the most formative in our understanding than any previous period. In the United Kingdom, merely 1046 people with mental illness were treated in hospital settings in 1827, but this had risen to 74 000 by the turn of the century and to a peak of 155 700 by 1959.

The growth of mental hospitals was greatest in countries influenced most by the Industrial Revolution and the consequent growth of large urban conurbations. The famous treatise of Faris and Dunham (1939) showing that schizophrenia was much more prevalent in urban than rural areas was adumbrated nearly a century earlier by Dorothea Dix who correctly inferred that 'there are, in proportion to numbers, more insane in cities than in large towns, and more insane in villages than among the same number of inhabitants dwelling in scattered settlements' (quoted in Porter 1991).

As mental hospitals increased in size and number it was realized that they sometimes created many more problems than they solved and the phenomenon of institutionalization was recognized (Barton 1959). Public opinion, a fickle but extremely important agent of change in psychiatry, steadily turned against mental hospitals which were heavily criticized from both a sociological viewpoint (Goffman 1961) and by the leaders of what became the antipsychiatry movement (Szasz 1960; Laing and Cooper 1964; Laing and Esterson 1970; Foucault 1973). Although the entry psychiatry phase of mental health was only brief, and had much more influence on literature than on psychiatry, it has recurred at various times throughout the history of the subject. In simple form it states that madness is a form of escape from intolerable external pressures—pressures induced by society and the family and not internally (endogenously) produced. It is an attractive hypothesis (hence its appeal in literature) but it has rarely, if ever, shown any value, except indirectly as offering a more humane and understanding approach to people with schizophrenia. Despite this, it continues to attract strong advocates who do not like data to get in the way of a good story, and there continues to be a minority of individuals who believe that schizophrenia and other major mental illness is a consequence of our abnormal society rather than genuine mental illness.

Reasons why public health has historically ignored mental health

Public health medicine has generally had few links with mental health until recently. However, with the growth of the discipline in the nineteenth century it was acknowledged that amidst the epidemics of diseases such as cholera and typhoid, and the need for preventive measures to avoid these (Chadwick 1842), there also needed to be adequate care for the mentally ill. To some extent the growth of mental hospitals followed from a public health policy: people with mental illness were vulnerable and had to be cared for in safe accommodation. The light and airy environment of the country asylums was a much healthier one than the squalor of the inner city.

It was argued that improving the productivity of the population, and spending money for the relief of the poor, led to an improvement in moral and mental behaviour. Early epidemiological studies were confined to the asylums. In 1828, the first statistics were recorded in the United Kingdom of those resident in the asylums and madhouses of the cities by the Lunacy Commissioners. At the General Register Office William Farr carried out the pioneering work in public mental health, and one can regard the birth of public mental health as probably beginning when he published his report on the mortality of the insane (Farr 1864).

In the early twentieth century, public health was preoccupied with preventive medicine and public hygiene and later became involved with surveillance of communicable diseases and the administration of health facilities in different parts of the country. It was not until the late 1950s that an epidemiological approach to public health became dominant again. The data derived from epidemiology informed the local provision and use of resources and this allowed mental illness to be examined in the same way as physical disease. In the early 1950s, most mental health treatment was carried out in asylum settings The peak occupancy was reached in the middle of this decade, but since then has fallen steadily to only a third of its original level. However, this change initially had little impact on public health in general, even though the implications were obvious after the seminal paper of Tooth and Brooke (1961) which predicted a dramatic fall in the resident population of psychiatric institutions.

One of the reasons why mental health did not figure highly on public health agendas was the major difficulty in measuring mental health. However, in the last 25 years there have been major advances in the measurement of mental illness. A large number of questionnaires and rating scales (e.g. the General Health Questionnaire (Goldberg 1972) and the Hospital Anxiety and Depression Scale (Zigmond and Snaith 1983)) have been developed which, despite some limitations, have allowed the symptoms of psychopathology to be measured reliably and accurately in public health settings. Better diagnostic criteria have increased confidence in the two main classification systems—the *International Classification of Diseases* (**ICD**) and the *Diagnostic and Statistical Manual of Mental Disorders* (**DSM**). The latter underwent a major reform in 1980 (American Psychiatric Association 1980) and is mainly responsible for the current groupings. Although the rigidity of these new systems has often been criticized, their introduction was a major advance in the classification of mental illness.

These developments, together with the policies of governments of all political persuasions to transfer the provision of services to the community, has forced mental health onto the agenda of public health. Mental health has developed a public voice with the inception of mental health advocacy organizations such as, in the United Kingdom, MIND, Sane, and the National Schizophrenia Fellowship. However, it is only in the last few years that public health has taken over an overarching role in advising and monitoring those involved in purchasing and providing mental health services. The view that 'epidemiology should derive public health and that public health medicine should be responsible for assessing the health of the population, setting local objectives for health, specifying effective and efficient use of resources and monitoring the achievement of targets', is now public policy (Acheson 1988). Since mental health services account for at least a tenth of the health budgets of virtually all countries, it was not surprising that public health medicine should take a much closer interest in mental health than it had ever done before.

Classification of mental illness

The system of classification of mental disorders has long been a subject of heated debate, disagreement, and criticism, both from within the medical profession and without. The current European classification has evolved over the years through collaboration, research, and debate, involving field trials in over 194 different centres in 55 different countries. The ICD was instituted in Paris in 1900 and has been revised regularly to the current 10th revision (ICD-10), where Chapter V(F) relates to mental and behavioural disorders. The equivalent American classification system (DSM-IV) is roughly similar in its categories to ICD-10 but there are some important discrepancies that hinder interpretation of worldwide epidemiological data. Poor concordance is shown for stress disorders, substance misuse, and some of the anxiety disorders (mainly involving panic) (Andrews *et al.* 1999), and so comparative figures for these diagnoses are questionable where ICD and DSM systems are both included.

Initially, the classifications provided brief thumbnail sketches of clinical concepts. Over the years the definitions of the various syndromes and disorders have become tighter and more rigorous, and both ICD-10 and DSM-IV now provide stricter diagnostic criteria to aid both clinicians and researchers to achieve greater diagnostic agreement. Although it is impossible to do justice to the main psychiatric syndromes in a short chapter, it is important for public health physicians to know the main features of each. Increasingly those with mental illness are being subdivided by diagnosis, and it is important to know something about the relative accuracy and nature of the psychiatric diagnostic process.

The classification of the main disorders is presented in Table 1. In the past, because of the heterogeneity of diagnostic criteria, the apparent incidence and prevalence of certain disorders appeared to vary considerably in different countries. Thus one study, the United States–United Kingdom Diagnostic Project, was able to show that the apparently high levels of schizophrenia in the United States compared with most European countries did not reflect a true difference in prevalence, but rather that different diagnostic criteria were being used for the same illnesses (Cooper *et al.* 1972). These differences are much less now; the International Pilot Study of Schizophrenia demonstrated, using the same criteria, that there were similar rates of schizophrenia in most of the countries in the study (Jablensky *et al.* 1992). This is of particular note since the countries included in the study were so varied (United Kingdom, United States, Taiwan, Switzerland, Russia, Nigeria, Colombia, Czechoslovakia, and Denmark).

Further research into depression showed similar results, namely that the cross-cultural similarities were greater than anticipated. The World Health Organization (**WHO**) collaborative study assessment of depression looked at five centres—Switzerland, Canada, Iran, and Japan (two centres). This study showed that all countries with the exception of Iran (Tehran) had similar rates of depression, and that, despite a degree of variation in presentation, patients from all countries shared a core symptomatology of depressive symptoms (Sartorius *et al.* 1980).

Epidemiology of mental disorders

In an earlier edition of this book, it was emphasized that the backbone of public health strategy is the development and maintenance of an 'accurate, reliable health information system upon which actions can be based' (Detels and Breslow 1986). It has taken some time to develop an appropriate information base for mental disorders, but we have become much closer to it in the last 10 years. The epidemiology of the major mental disorders described in Table 1 is shown in Table 2 and will be described further according to the main groups in ICD-10. However, learning disability (mental retardation) and child disorders are not included in detail here.

The figures taken overall show that mental disorders are surprisingly common, with approximately one in three of the population having had a disorder which is sufficiently severe to warrant a diagnostic label, at least to a trained lay interviewer. However, five out of every seven patients identified in national surveys do not seek or receive any treatment for their disorders (Regier *et al.* 1984, 1998). Nonetheless, the figures from epidemiological surveys are likely to be underestimates, so that what Henderson (2000) calls the 'exaggerated estimate' problem may be incorrect. Only around 80 per cent of people complete epidemiological surveys, and the remaining 20 per cent who are never interviewed are likely to have significantly greater pathology than those who are interviewed.

Organic disorders

This is one of the least satisfactory groups in the classification system, largely because the diagnosis of an organic disorder is based on identification of an organic cause and this is difficult to determine for many conditions until after death. It also includes a very disparate group of conditions, ranging from delirium at one extreme—short-lived episodes associated with confusion and transient psychotic symptoms—through to organic causes of anxiety, depression, personality change, and schizophrenia, and finally to the progressive dementias, which are much more important in public health terms because of their scale. Good epidemiological data are difficult to obtain for most of these, but the dementias are better understood.

Dementia is an acquired global impairment of intellect, memory, and personality occurring in a setting where there is no impairment of consciousness. It is detected first by evidence of increased forgetfulness and personality change. Loss of recent memory is the simplest way of identifying dementia by simple psychological tests; long-term

Table 1 Classification of psychiatric disorders according to ICD-10

Main category	Subcategories	Main features
Organic (F10)	Dementias Delirium Mental disorders due to physical disease Personality or behaviour disorder due to brain disease or injury	Conditions in which brain dysfunction is present and is manifested by disturbances of cognition, mood, perception, or behaviour
Psychoactive substance use (F1)	States of intoxication, harmful use, dependence and withdrawal states and psychosis resulting from use of alcohol, opioids, cannabis, sedatives, cocaine, tobacco, hallucinogens, and other drugs	Includes all mental disorders which are considered to be a direct consequence of drug use and which would not have occurred without consumption of the drug (or drugs)
Schizophrenia, schizotypal and delusional disorders (F2)	Schizophrenia Schizotypal disorder Persistent delusional disorders Acute and transient psychotic disorders Schizoaffective disorders	Conditions in which there are distortions of thinking, perception, and mood not due to an organic condition and which are most prominent in schizophrenia
Mood (affective) disorders (F3)	Manic episodes Depressive episodes Bipolar affective disorder Recurrent depressive disorder Persistent affective disorders	A range of disorders in which disturbance of mood (affect) is the main feature, together with other symptoms which are easily understood in the context of change of mood and activity
Neurotic, stress-related, and somatoform disorders (F4)	Phobic disorder Other anxiety disorders Obsessive–compulsive disorder Stress and adjustment disorders Dissociative and conversion disorders Somatoform disorders	A group of disorders in which certain symptoms, historically recognized as part of 'neurosis', are most marked and which may have a psychological causation
Behavioural syndromes and mental disorders associated with physiological dysfunction and hormone imbalance (F5)	Eating disorders Psychogenic sleep disorders Sexual dysfunctions Mental disorders associated with the puerperium	Disorders in which physiological and hormonal factors may be involved in causation or be prominent in association with the disorder
Disorders of adult personality and behaviour (F6)	Personality disorder Enduring personality change Habit and impulse disorders Gender identity disorders Sexual preference disorders	Conditions of clinical significance in which behaviour patterns tend to be persistent and which are 'the expression of the individual's characteristic lifestyle and mode of relating to self and others'
Mental retardation (F7)	Mild mental retardation Moderate mental retardation Severe mental retardation Profound mental retardation Other types of mental retardation	A condition of 'arrested or incomplete development of the mind' manifest by impairment of skills commonly associated with intelligence
Disorders of psychological development (F8)	Developmental disorders of speech and language Specific developmental disorders of motor function Pervasive developmental disorders (e.g. autism)	Conditions that begin in infancy or childhood, delay in the development of functions related to maturation of the nervous system, and which generally have a steady rather than remitting course
Behavioural and emotional disorders with onset occurring in childhood or adolescence (F9)	Hyperkinetic disorder Conduct disorder Mixed disorder of conduct and emotions Emotional disorder of childhood Disorders of social function (childhood) Tic disorders Other behavioural or emotional disorders	A mixture of disorders in which the only common features are an onset early in life and a fluctuating or unpredictable course

Source: *International Classification of Diseases, 10th Revision*, Chapter 5 (WHO 1992).

Table 2 Annual community prevalence of the main groups of psychiatric disorders

Type of disorder (main ICD-10 classification code)	Annual prevalence[a] (%)	Comment
Any mental disorder	28–29 (30)	Figure lower than might be expected because of extensive comorbidity
Organic mental disorder (mainly dementia) (F0)	Incidence (75–79 years) 2.3 Incidence (80–84 years) 4.6 Incidence (85–89 years) 8.5	Data from Paykel et *al.* (1994)
Substance misuse (F1)	9–11 (5)	Alcohol abuse accounts for 70 per cent of these but there is also strong comorbidity
Schizophrenia (F2)	0.7–1.0	Difficult to determine as schizophrenia is still frequently treated in institutions long term
Any mood disorder (F3)	9.5–11.3 (12)	Includes mixed anxiety–depressive disorder in UK sample
Neurotic or stress disorder (F4)	14	Difficult group to classify as presence of depression complicates classification
Physiological disorder (F5)	2.5–3	Mainly eating disorders
Personality disorder (F6)	9–12	Data from Girolamo and Reich (1993) and Casey (2000)
Bipolar mood disorder	1.2–1.3	This describes the group of conditions in which mania or hypomania is present
Depressive episodes	5–10	
Dysthymic disorder	2.5–5	Equivalent to chronic low-grade depression
Panic disorder	1–2	
Generalized anxiety disorder	3.1 (3)	
Obsessive–compulsive disorder	2.0	
Any phobia	11	
Agoraphobia with panic	3	Age of onset 29 years (Magee *et al.* 1996)
Agoraphobia without panic	2.8	See text for explanation
Simple phobia	9	Age of onset 15 years
Social phobia	8	Age of onset 16 years

[a]United Kingdom figures are given in parentheses.

Data derived from Regier *et al.* (1993), Kessler *et al.* (1994), Meltzer *et al.* (1994), Paykel *et al.* (1994), and Magee *et al.* (1996) from the Epidemiologic Catchment Area Study and National Comorbidity Survey (United States), and the National Psychiatric Morbidity Study (United Kingdom). This includes estimates from surveys in which annual prevalence is not specifically recorded. Lifetime prevalence is preferred by some epidemiologists but there is evidence that these data are inaccurate so they are not included here.

memory is preserved until later in the condition. Two conditions—Alzheimer's disease and vascular dementia—account for most of the dementing illnesses, with normal pressure hydrocephalus, Pick's disease (affecting the frontal lobes initially), Huntington's chorea, AIDS-related dementia, and Creutzfeldt–Jakob disease (with its links to a strain of bovine spongiform encephalopathy) occurring much less frequently. Alcoholic dementia is included among the substance misuse disorders. The incidence of Alzheimer's disease is twice as great as vascular dementia, representing 2.7 per 1000 person-years at risk and vascular dementia 1.2 per 1000 in people over the age of 75 years (Brayne *et al.* 1995*b*). The risk of dementia doubles with each successive 5-year period over the age of 75 years (Paykel *et al.* 1994), and the data indicate that cognitive decline represents a continuum of which dementia is at the extreme (Brayne *et al.* 1995*a*). Vascular dementia is much less age sensitive than Alzheimer's disease (Brayne *et al.* 1995*b*).

Substance misuse

In both ICD-10 and DSM-IV substance misuse is classified according to the main substance involved (e.g. cocaine, amphetamine, alcohol dependence, nicotine, and caffeine). The nature of the misuse (e.g. intoxication, dependence, withdrawal, or psychosis) is then classified separately. Substance misuse has now become recognized as a subspeciality of psychiatry and in some areas there are special drug dependency centres or units. Those with dual diagnosis tend to be seen by general psychiatrists, but this is likely to change (Weaver *et al.* 1999).

Dependence on a drug includes several elements (not all of which need to be present to satisfy the diagnosis): a persistent wish to obtain the drug (drug-seeking behaviour), the development of tolerance with increased use, and the exhibition of a withdrawal syndrome after sudden cessation of the drug. Long-term complications of drug misuse include petty criminality (a large proportion of theft is carried out by addicts), social and occupational decline, and homelessness. There are also the risks of physical disease including hepatitis, oesophageal varices, hepatic cirrhosis, and dementia in clients abusing alcohol, and hepatitis B and C and HIV/AIDS in intravenous drug abusers. Substance misuse problems are growing in most countries of the world and, to date, no public or mental health intervention has had a significant preventive impact.

Schizophrenia

Schizophrenia is a syndromal diagnosis which, despite much interest in recent years, remains an enigma. It was originally described as dementia praecox and although this was later ridiculed when the condition became a 'functional psychosis', it has now been found that there is loss of brain tissue in many sufferers, with the whole brain, amygdala, and hippocampus being smaller than in controls (Lawrie *et al.* 1997). There is still a limited understanding of the aetiology and causal mechanisms involved, which explains why one of our foremost authorities on schizophrenia bleakly concludes that 'as far as defining the clinical boundaries of schizophrenia/dementia praecox are concerned we have not moved very far in the past 100 years' (Johnstone 1999).

Bleuler first coined the term schizophrenia in 1911 to refer to a group of psychoses which were characterized by splitting of mental functions, with delusions and hallucinations secondary to this splitting. Since then the definition of what constitutes schizophrenia has been revised and amended. Affect (the formal psychiatric word for mood), thinking, perception, and behaviour are all impaired in schizophrenia.

The characteristic affect is described as **incongruent** and inappropriate, with individuals laughing in a silly manner when discussing a serious matter. Alternatively, the affect may be **blunted** and the patient appears somewhat unresponsive, demonstrating a limited repertoire of apparent emotions. The patient may be **formally thought disordered** with incoherent illogical thought and lack of understandable associations between thoughts (derailment). This may be mild, making the patient difficult to follow at interview, or severe in which case it may not be possible to understand the patient at all. **Poverty of content of thought** may also be a characteristic feature. The nature of the content of thought may be abnormal, and patients often have delusions. **Delusions** can be varied and include persecutory, grandiose, and referential delusions, as well as more bizarre delusions such as control by external forces, mind reading and insertion, withdrawal, and broadcasting of thoughts. Perception is impaired and auditory hallucinations are common, particularly of voices discussing the patient in the third person, giving a running commentary about what the patient is doing, or giving commands. Other perceptual abnormalities include tactile (or somatic) hallucinations, visual hallucinations, and misperceptions not amounting to hallucinations. The patient's behaviour may exhibit markedly abnormal behaviour because of responses to delusional beliefs or hallucinations, whereas social isolation and self-neglect seem to be more integral features of the underlying disease process.

Patients with schizophrenia are a broad group and have many ways of presenting to psychiatric services. At one end of the spectrum, patients present with predominantly negative symptoms associated with absence of motivation (social withdrawal, apathy, neglect of self-care). At the other end of the spectrum patients show predominantly positive symptoms—hallucinations, delusions, and abnormal behaviours, such as agitation, aggression (which is a serious public and community health issue), and posturing or stereotyped behaviour.

Mood disorders

The classification of mood (or affective) disorders is probably the most complicated and controversial area of classification in psychiatry. These difficulties have largely been removed by recent classifications (ICD-10 and DSM-IV), which use a simpler atheoretical system. Now all mood disorders are classified together under the same rubric of **affective disorders** and largely classified in terms of severity of symptoms and associated disability. The previous separation of psychotic and neurotic depression and the similar separation of reactive and endogenous depression have been abandoned because they have failed to separate homogeneous diagnostic groups. Similarly, individuals with a chronic state of mild depression (dysthymia) are now classified within the affective disorders rather than with patients with personality disorders. Classification is based on symptomatology rather than aetiology.

An affective illness is primarily characterized by the quality of the affect or mood. The distinction is made between unipolar (depression only) and bipolar illnesses (depression and mania at different times). If a patient has an elated mood, this will suggest a diagnosis of hypomania or in more severe cases mania. A lowered mood with predominant feelings of worthlessness, guilt, self-reproach, and pessimism are suggestive of depression. The severity of the condition can further be defined as mild, moderate, or severe, further qualified as bipolar disorder if there has been a previous episode of mania or hypomania, and as a recurrent episode if there have been previous episodes of mania or depression. Dysthymia is a low-grade chronic depressive condition which is relatively common in the population (Table 2) and which shows strong comorbidity with other depressive conditions (sometimes called double depression).

Symptoms of depression include the following:

- insomnia, particularly early morning wakening
- diurnal variation of mood (feeling worse in the morning)
- loss of appetite with weight loss
- loss of libido
- objective evidence of psychomotor retardation.

In addition the mood disorder can be yet further defined by the presence or absence of **psychotic symptoms**—hallucinations and delusions—which in contrast to schizophrenia are usually mood congruent (entirely consistent with the prevailing mood such as delusions of poverty in severe depression).

In severe depression there may be total inactivity (stupor), or the patient expresses nihilistic delusions that they do not exist or that parts of their body have died or stopped working. This is also sometimes described as Cotard's syndrome, and is more prevalent in the elderly (Luque and Berrios 1994).

Neurotic, stress-related, and somatoform disorders

The disorders discussed under this heading fall into a number of different categories but have been grouped together for convenience. This is probably a more heterogeneous group than others, although all these conditions are 'reality-based' in that the symptoms are understandable and based on real experiences, feelings, and events.

These conditions are the most prevalent psychiatric disorders. They include anxiety disorders (generalized anxiety disorder), phobic disorders (agoraphobia, social phobia, and simple phobia), panic disorder, obsessive–compulsive disorder, reactions to acute stress and more prolonged stressors (adjustment disorder), reactions to very severe stress (post-traumatic stress disorder), dissociative (conversion) disorder (formerly called hysteria), and the somatoform disorders, in which the major symptoms are bodily ones. Mixed anxiety–depressive disorder is also included in this group; there are arguments whether this should be a subsyndromal rather than a full mental disorder. The neurotic and stress-related disorders are generally more difficult to classify than other psychiatric disorders, which is illustrated by the high levels of comorbidity shown in Table 2, and the dividing line between normal variation and pathological condition is often very difficult to draw.

The prevalence of any neurotic disorder in the previous week was recorded in a recent United Kingdom study (OPCS 1995) of 10 000 adults in private households (Fig. 1). One in seven had a psychiatric disorder, with mixed anxiety–depressive disorder (7 per cent) and generalized anxiety disorder (3 per cent) being the most common. These disorders were almost twice as common in women (male-to-female ratio of 6 to 11) and had similar prevalence in all age groups between 20 and 60 years of age (Fig. 1).

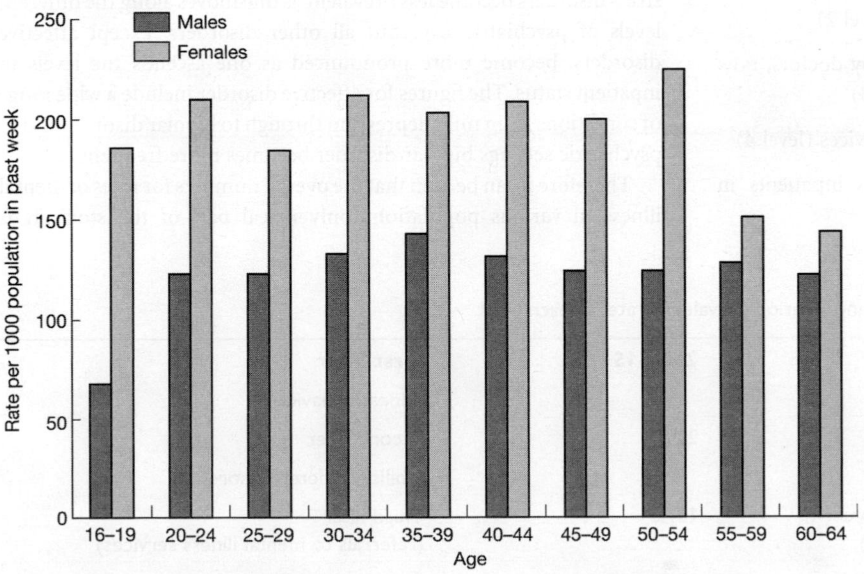

Fig. 1 Prevalence of any neurotic disorder: mixed anxiety and depressive disorder, generalized anxiety disorder, depressive episode, all phobias, and obsessive–compulsive disorder. (Data from OPCS (1995).)

Behavioural syndromes associated with physiological disturbances and physical factors

This is a smaller group comprising eating disorders (mainly anorexia nervosa and bulimia nervosa), sleep disorders, and sexual dysfunction. These are linked to neurotic disorders but have specific physiological consequences (e.g. amenorrhoea in anorexia nervosa) that do not apply to other disorders. Occasionally there are apparent 'epidemics' of eating disorders, particularly in girls' schools.

Personality disorders

It is only in the last 20 years that this concept has been refined sufficiently to stand with other psychiatric diagnoses and the categories of personality disorders have been more rigidly defined. There are numerous definitions of what constitutes a personality disorder but the main characteristics are a persistent abnormality in personal relationships, attitudes, and behaviour that develops early in life and leads to impaired social functioning.

Current psychiatric classifications adopt a categorical system although there is evidence that a dimensional approach is more valid. The main groups are listed in Table 3 in which the ICD-10 and DSM-IV classifications are compared.

The categorical system is not satisfactory because of the degree of overlap (comorbidity) between different diagnoses. Increasingly it is being recognized that three or four clusters—flamboyant (dissocial, histrionic, narcissistic, borderline, and impulsive), odd or eccentric (paranoid, schizoid, and schizotypal), anxious or fearful (anxious, dependent), and obsessive–compulsive (anankastic)—comprise a somewhat better classification system (Tyrer *et al.* 1991; Mulder and Joyce 1997). There is also a dimensional classification which covers the range between normal and severe personality disorder (Tyrer and Johnson 1996). Measuring personality disorder in this way has increased in recent years and has been accentuated by the recognition that some people with severe personality disorder are a threat to the

Table 3 Classification of personality disorder in the international (ICD-10) and American (DSM-IV) systems of classification

ICD-10	DSM- IV
Paranoid	Paranoid
Schizoid	Schizoid
No equivalent	Schizotypal
Dissocial	Antisocial
Emotionally unstable (impulsive and borderline)	Borderline
Histrionic	Histrionic
Anankastic	Obsessive–compulsive
Anxious	Avoidant
Dependent	Dependent
No equivalent	Narcissistic

public mainly because of their propensity for unprovoked violence. In the United Kingdom legislation is proposed that will allow the indefinite detention of those with dangerous severe personality disorder (as yet not formally defined). This has important public health connotations.

Psychiatric services and public mental health

In examining the public health issues in mental illness it is useful to adopt the filter model of Goldberg and Huxley (1980) (Table 4). This helps to explain the importance of the differences between the primary care and secondary care psychiatric services. The five levels are as follows:

- the population as a whole (level 1)
- the total mental morbidity (i.e. those who attend primary care with mental ill health, whether or not it is detected) (level 2)
- the proportion of those identified as mentally ill by doctors, now know as conspicuous psychiatric morbidity (level 3)
- the population being seen by the mental illness services (level 4)
- the relatively small numbers who are treated as inpatients in psychiatric hospitals (level 5).

Goldberg and Huxley separated these five levels by four filters (Table 4) through which patients normally have to pass through before reaching a higher level. However, it is perfectly possible to go directly from level 1 to level 5 (e.g. by presenting as a psychiatric emergency at an accident and emergency department), and in some countries with less co-ordinated health services this form of direct transfer across levels is very common. This is not just a function of whether or not the country is well developed in terms of affluence and productivity; Goldberg and Huxley (1980, pp. 53–5) describe the 'American bypass'—a tendency in the United States for patients to go directly from community to psychiatrist.

The annual period prevalence rates are shown (Table 4) and in epidemiological terms may seem large. However, it is important to understand that many of these cases comprise a low level of illness, and much activity in psychiatric epidemiology is concerned with deciding on the threshold for 'caseness'—a threshold that may be decided more by the procrustean requirements of the classification system than by the need for intervention (Regier *et al.* 1998). It is also important to appreciate that diagnoses within the field of mental illness are much less specific that with physical disorders. Clearly, the diagnosis of diabetes is unequivocal in almost every case, it is associated with disabilities that are clearly secondary to the main disorder (e.g. retinopathy), and it has a fairly predictable time course and outcome. In mental illness we have the difficulties of case identification, problems of classification into homogeneous groups, overlap between disorders with difficulty in deciding which is primary and which is secondary, and unpredictable outcome.

There are some important differences between the annual prevalence of different diagnostic groups in different settings (Fig. 2). It will be noted that by far the largest proportion of patients with psychiatric disorder in the total population (two-thirds of the total) consists of neurotic and stress disorders or personality disorders. Alcohol and drug problems are more common in the community than in those presenting in primary care but, as expected, all other problems are more frequent in primary care within the population. Neurotic and stress disorders become less prevalent as one moves along the different levels of psychiatric care but all other disorders, except affective disorders, become more pronounced as one ascends the levels to inpatient status. The figures for affective disorder include a wide range of conditions from mild depression through to bipolar disorder and in psychiatric settings bipolar disorder becomes more frequent.

Therefore it can be seen that the overall numbers for rates of mental illness in various populations only reveal part of the story. It is

Table 4 Five levels and four filters, with estimates of annual period prevalence rates at each level

Level 1	The community	260–315	First filter (illness behaviour)
Level 2	Total mental morbidity—attenders in primary care	230	Second filter (ability to detect disorder)
Level 3	Mental disorders identified by doctors ('conspicuous psychiatric morbidity')	101.5	Third filter (referrals to mental illness services)
Level 4	Total morbidity—in psychiatric services	23.5	Fourth filter (admission to psychiatric beds)
Level 5	Psychiatric inpatients	5.71	

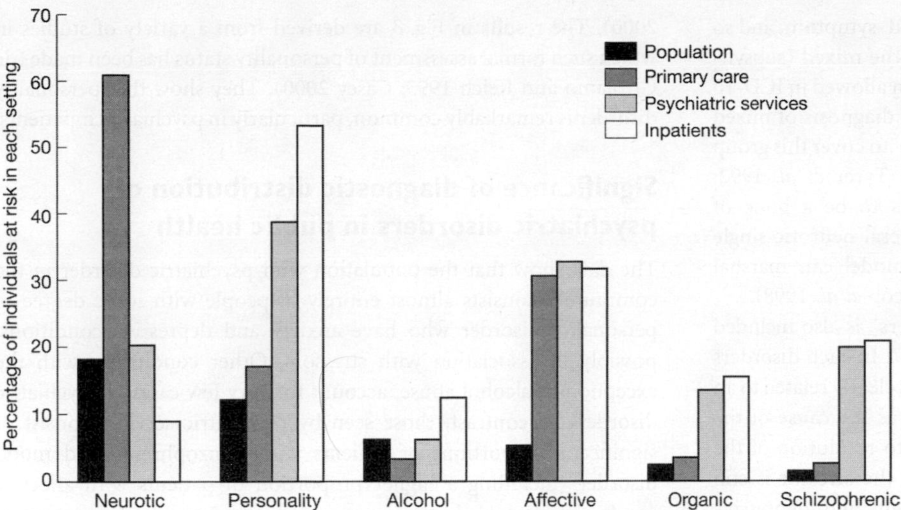

Fig. 2 Differences between the diagnostic distribution of mental disorders in (a) the general population, (b) primary care (conspicuous morbidity) (level 3), (c) psychiatric services (level 4), and (d) psychiatric patients (level 5). Neurotic, neurotic and stress-related disorders; personality, personality disorders; alcohol, alcohol and drug abuse; affective, depressive and manic disorders; organic, organic mental disorders (chiefly dementia); schizophrenic, the group of schizophrenic disorders. (Data from Regier *et al.* (1984), Goldberg and Huxley (1992), and de Girolamo and Reich (1993).)

important to realize that these numbers are not as reliable as those for other disorders because there is great difficulty in separating psychiatric disorders from each other and deciding which is primary. The numbers in Table 2 illustrate one of the problems: the sum of those for individual disorders comes to much more than the total prevalence of mental disorder. This is explained by comorbidity. Thus in the National Comorbidity Survey in the United States, more than half of all lifetime psychiatric disorders in the population occurred in the 14 per cent of the sample who had a history of three or more comorbid disorders (Kessler *et al.* 1994). This suggests that these conditions are not truly comorbid in the original sense of the word—independent conditions occurring at the same time in the same person (Feinstein 1970)—and at least some are intimately associated and therefore consanguid (Tyrer 1996). The problem is that it is impossible to determine the relationship between these disorders through cross-sectional studies. The arguments over whether the conditions should be conjoined or separated is not ultimately a useful issue in clinical practice, but if one of the conditions is a predisposing vulnerability factor or a complication of the other it is important and should be investigated. However, it is only through longitudinal studies that such associations can be determined.

Some of the common examples of comorbidity and the problems it creates refer to four areas: schizophrenia and substance misuse, depression, neurotic and adjustment disorders, and mixtures of mental state and personality disorders. Many of these are referred to as 'dual diagnoses', but there are now so many of these this is becoming a valueless label.

Schizophrenia and substance abuse

This is perhaps the original dual diagnosis (Weaver *et al.* 1999). Abuse of many drugs has been associated with psychotic symptoms that to some extent simulate schizophrenia. The classical example is amphetamine, which can, in acute dosage and also during withdrawal, lead to a paranoid psychotic state that is indistinguishable from paranoid schizophrenia (Connell 1958). Other drugs, notably LSD, have also frequently been implicated in the aetiology of schizophrenia-like psychoses and, more recently, there have also been claims that cannabis can also create a psychotic state although not normally to the extent that it could be regarded as a definitive psychosis (Thomas 1993). Benzodiazepine dependence may also be associated with psychotic disorders after withdrawal (Roberts and Vass 1986). Opioid drugs and cocaine do not create or trigger psychotic disorders.

Cannabis, benzodiazepines, and amphetamines do not create psychotic symptoms in most users, but in those who are vulnerable to developing schizophrenia these drugs may trigger episodes which would not have occurred without the drug exposure. This has important implications in the debate over legalization of cannabis, and we would predict an increase in such dual diagnoses if it were legalized. Diagnostic practice is very difficult when substance misuse is present with schizophrenic symptoms. Clinicians are taught to be parsimonious and to choose only one diagnosis; the outcome is that some diagnose patients who otherwise look identical as having a drug dependence problem whereas others would diagnose schizophrenia.

Mood and adjustment disorders

Mood disorders constitute a separate section in ICD-10, and in this context 'mood' includes the spectrum between depression and mania only. Depression is fairly easy to recognize as a symptom but notoriously difficult to diagnose into homogeneous groups, and in previous classifications the symptom was present in all parts of the diagnostic system. To try and resolve this, all depressive diagnoses are now incorporated in one section in ICD-10. Most of the cases consist of mild and moderate depression which is not associated with any psychotic disorder. However, in most mild mental disorder there are mixed symptoms of anxiety and depression and this apparent 'comorbidity' is difficult to resolve. Anxiety is now officially a 'neurotic' symptom whereas depression is a 'mood' symptom, and so separation has to be achieved unless one adopts the mixed (subsyndromal) diagnosis of mixed anxiety and depression allowed in ICD-10 (WHO 1992). There are some who argue for the diagnosis of mixed syndromes such as the 'general neurotic syndrome' to cover this group of disorders (Tyrer 1985; Andrews *et al.* 1990; Tyrer *et al.* 1992; Sullivan and Kendler 1998), but this continues to be a bone of contention among psychiatrists, as both the general neurotic single model and the two-factor depression–anxiety model can marshal equally convincing arguments in their favour (Jacob *et al.* 1998).

Another category, termed 'adjustment disorders', is also included under the stress disorders in ICD-10 and DSM-IV. In such disorders the patient may be anxious or depressed, but this is clearly related to an obvious psychosocial stressor which is regarded as the cause of the symptoms and which, when removed, will lead to resolution of the clinical problem in most cases. However, while the stressor is still present, the patient will have significant anxiety and depressive symptoms and in many cases this will be recorded through the appropriate diagnostic groupings. However, these are not mental illnesses in any formal sense, because all of us can suffer from adjustment disorders when under conditions of sufficient stress. In symptomatic terms, they are indistinguishable from other forms of anxiety and depression and so are normally included amongst them.

Personality and mental state disorders

Personality disorder has been difficult to diagnose in the past and is regarded in many quarters as a pejorative label. There has also been a tendency to diagnose patients as either having a personality disorder or a mental illness whereas in fact both can exist together as they do not measure the same domain of psychiatric function (Tyrer *et al.* 1991). In old statistics personality disorder usually accounts for only between 2 and 5 per cent of psychiatric disorders but when formal assessments of personality status are made in the populations concerned the proportions increase several-fold (Tyrer and Ferguson 2000). The results in Fig. 3 are derived from a variety of studies in which such formal assessment of personality status has been made (de Girolamo and Reich 1993; Casey 2000). They show that personality disorder is remarkably common, particularly in psychiatric inpatients.

Significance of diagnostic distribution of psychiatric disorders in public health

The data show that the population with psychiatric disorder in the community consists almost entirely of people with some degree of personality disorder who have anxiety and depressive conditions, possibly in association with stressors. Other conditions, with the exception of alcohol abuse, account for very few cases of psychiatric disorder. By contrast, those seen by psychiatric services consist of significant proportions of patients with schizophrenia and mood disorder (including a higher proportion of patients with affective psychosis in which both mania and depression may be present at different time) and a relatively low proportion of those with neurotic and stress-related disorders.

This has to be borne in mind when considering interventions in mental illness. Most of the minor disorders are self-limiting and even if the general practitioner does not have a good detection rate for those who present with mental illness, the amount of distress caused is still relatively small (as what is lost is the more rapid treatment of a condition that will resolve in any case). However, in the psychiatric services there is a greater preponderance of the disorders that need active treatment or have persistent disorders that are extremely difficult to treat (e.g. personality disorder) and the disorder with the greatest disability, schizophrenia, is over 40 times more prevalent in inpatient settings than in the population as a whole.

Because these figures conceal a great deal of variation it is sometimes useful to give the rough limits for the prevalence of each condition within a population. These are shown in Table 5 for a population of 500 000 (including 70 000 over the age of 65 years).

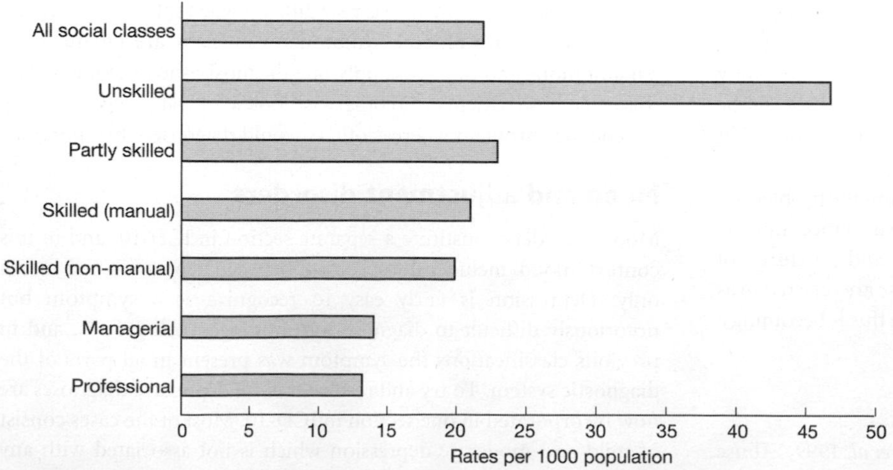

Fig. 3 European standardized mortality rates of suicide and undetermined injury, by social class. Men, aged 20 to 64 years, England and Wales, 1991 to 1993. (Data from Drever and Bunting (1997).)

Table 5 Prevalence of and needs for the main psychiatric disorders in a population of 500 000

Diagnosis	Numerical range[a]	Likely service needs
Neurotic disorder (mainly anxiety disorders)	8000–30 000	Primary care support and counselling; occasionally referral to psychology services; few referred to psychiatrist
Depressive disorders	10 000–25 000	Very similar to neurotic disorders but more referrals to psychiatrists and some inpatient treatment. Contact with accident and emergency departments because of parasuicide (attempted suicide)
Affective (manic–depressive) psychosis	500–2500	Frequent contract with psychiatric and social services and many admissions
Schizophrenia	1000–2500	As for affective psychosis, with even more contact with social services
Dementia	3500	Heavy involvement of social and psychiatric services, particularly in later stages

[a]Variation mainly related to socio-economic deprivation (Jarman 1983) in later stages.

Evidence of public health efficacy of mental health services

Recent shift from mental health of individuals to whole communities with shift of public health into purchasing field

Since the Acheson Report *Public Health in England* highlighted public health medicine's role in reviewing the health of the population, there has been greater awareness of the need to examine mental health as an essential component of population health. As departments of public health in health authorities are now responsible for purchasing mental health services, they need much greater knowledge of the workings of their local mental health provision. The mandatory annual report of the health of the population in the local area also needs to address the mental health of this population. This is a difficult task. Knowledge of whether mental health services are working effectively are seldom possible through official statistics or so-called 'quality indicators' such as waiting times or proportion of attenders to non-attenders. Intimate knowledge of the services is necessary and this can often be boosted by data from patients' organizations or patients themselves, as their levels of satisfaction are better indicators than most others of good functioning services (Shipley *et al.* 2000). Because patients with severe mental illness are often extremely mobile, there is a tendency for disproportionately large numbers to present to psychiatric services in some areas, of which inner cities are the best example. These people do not appear on census figures and therefore their numbers cannot be predicted by sociodeprivation indices such as Jarman scores (Jarman 1983). Some are regarded as 'psychiatric tourists' and may create imbalance in local services (Montgomery and Parshall 1998). These issues need to be considered by public health physicians when planning and funding local services if this is to be done sensitively and appropriately.

Inequalities in health provision are currently high on the political agenda. The recently published *Report of the Independent Inquiry into Inequalities of Health* (Anonymous 1998) focuses on social inequalities and their relationship to health and suicide. It aims to improve 'socioeconomic and living conditions and social cohesions' which will 'have many benefits in addition to their contribution to the prevention of suicide'. In this report young people are targeted, particularly men and the mentally ill. The suicide rate in those in social class 5 is three times greater than in those in social class 1 (Drever and Bunting 1997) (Fig. 3), and so when areas of great social deprivation are found to have higher suicide rates it should not be assumed that they have poor local psychiatric services.

Measuring outcomes in mental health services represents a major challenge to public health as well as an important responsibility. Public health now has to grapple with questions that have bothered the mental health services for years: How is it possible to decide whether a service is providing good or poor care? What targets and outcome measures are available? The need for an easily completed outcome measure (which can also be used as a record of mental health status) has been met to some extent by the development of a Global Assessment of Functioning Scale (Endicott *et al.* 1976) which can be separated into scaled measuring clinical symptoms and social functioning. This is now widely used in the United States and is the fifth axis in DSM-IV (American Psychiatric Association 1994). In the United Kingdom, in response to the *Health of the Nation* initiative, Health of the Nation Outcome Scales have been developed to record outcome in the main areas of change and have commanded wide use (Bebbington *et al.* 1999). The major problem remains that any instrument that is carried out with an unco-operative and psychotic patient cannot be assessed by self-report and the reliability of instruments such as the Global Assessment of Functioning is not particularly good.

Targets for mental health services

In 1992, targets were set for mental illness for the first time, most notably in *The Health of the Nation*, a United Kingdom White Paper setting forward one of the clearest statements on public mental health ever. Like all good public health it emphasizes that the prevention of ill health and promotion of good health is as least as important as treatment of illness in its various forms. Unfortunately, when mental health is considered (and it is a key area) most of the targets evaporate because, to use the words of the document 'there is at present no straightforward and objective way of describing, aggregating and monitoring outcomes of care nor any agreement on clear and reliable measures which could confidently be used as proxies for outcome measures' (Anonymous 1992).

However, there is one unambiguous measure of outcome that is addressed prominently and has been adopted as a major target: suicide. In *The Health of the Nation* (Anonymous 1992) two targets were set: to reduce the overall suicide rate by at least 15 per cent from 11.1 per 100 000 in 1990 to no more than 9.4 per 100 000 population by the year 2000, and to reduce the suicide rate of severely mentally ill people by at least 33 per cent over the same period. Bearing in mind that the suicide rate in the United Kingdom is considerably lower than in most other countries in Europe (Denmark, Finland, Austria, Switzerland, France, and Belgium all have rates greater than 20 per 100 000 population (Moens 1990)), the target appeared to be ambitious but looks likely to be met.

There have been doubts as to whether these targets are achievable by improvements in mental health services (MacDonald 1993), but these are not the only ways they can be achieved. Indeed, the steadily falling suicide rate in older people compared with the rising rate in the young (Charlton *et al.* 1993) means that demographic factors may achieve part of the reduction without any other form of intervention. Suicide is also a good index of priority for mental health services. Almost all mental illness—schizophrenia, affective (manic–depressive) psychosis, substance misuse, learning disability, personality disorder, dementia, panic and anxiety disorders, neurotic, stress and adjustment disorders—have standardized mortality ratio suicide rates that are at least three times greater than expected, and that for psychiatric inpatients exceeds 1000 (Harris and Barraclough 1998).

Doubts still persist; severe mental illness is not defined in any formal classification, and suicide figures can include or exclude many forms of undetermined death that could have an important impact on future figures. Nevertheless, the danger that the figures can be massaged in various ways to achieve the targets unfairly is much less likely with the figures for suicide than any other measure of mental illness. Better measures of outcome in mental illness are urgently needed but the suicide rates have set down a useful yardstick for comparison.

Our Healthier Nation (DoH 1999) was developed as a sequel to *The Health of the Nation* (Anonymous 1992), but with broader targets concentrating on improving health and narrowing the health gap. It stresses the widening of health inequalities in the United Kingdom, and one of its main aims is 'to improve the health of the worst off in society and to narrow the health gap' (DoH 1999).

Improving mental health of populations

All public health physicians are supporters of prevention. If important factors responsible for poor mental health can be identified, these can then be addressed and altered, and if identified correctly, improvement in the mental health of the whole population follows.

Community intervention studies

One of the major problems with severe mental illness is that patients do not present voluntarily to the psychiatric services at an early stage. However, it has often been suggested that if care was available at an earlier stage than at the point of hospital presentation or at the accident and emergency department, better care could be given and unnecessary suffering avoided.

A series of programmes which collectively are often described as 'assertive community treatment', generating from the work of Stein and Test (1980), has demonstrated that such intervention can reduce admission to hospital. Much of this work has been carried out with the severely mentally ill, who account for most of the work of the psychiatric services (Table 3). It has been shown that Stein and Test's model is replicated in the United Kingdom (Muijen *et al.* 1992) and that it is effective. It has also been shown that day hospital care can be a useful substitute for inpatient treatment (Creed *et al.* 1990) and that improving care outside hospital, both by home visiting (Burns *et al.* 1993) and early intervention (Merson *et al.* 1992) can reduce the number and duration of admissions significantly. In the last few years in countries with publicly funded mental health services there has been a growth of multidisciplinary community mental health teams, and these have been shown in a recent systematic review to not only reduce hospital admissions and improve patient satisfaction but also reduce suicide rates (Tyrer *et al.* 1999).

These studies have been carried out by special teams, often created for research purposes, and the findings have not been generalized to services as a whole. However, there is now evidence that those services which have a higher level of community resources do have lower admissions to the country as a whole (Jarman *et al.* 1992). What is much less clear is whether the assertive treatment model is appropriate for all countries and all settings. It has certainly proved to be effective in the United States but here the standard service for state patients is often poor (Lehman and Steinwachs 1998). Where standard services are reasonably competent in administering evidence-based psychiatry, and where there is an existing comprehensive network of services, the apparent gains of assertive community treatment and its rough equivalent, intensive case management, are lost (Holloway and Carson 1998; Thornicroft *et al.* 1998; UK700 Group 1999).

Care programming and care management

For the last 5 years, the care of psychiatrically ill patients has been formalized in a new configuration. The two central elements are care programming and care management. Care programming applies to all individuals seen by the psychiatric service, and extends from a single assessment by a member of the mental health team followed by discharge, to a multidisciplinary arrangement whereby several workers from mental health, social, and voluntary services are all integrated together in providing care. This is too large a range to have much meaning, and the phrase 'discharged into the community under the care programme approach' means the same if the last five words are removed. Care programming overlaps with care management, a term which describes the assessment of needs by social services, who hold the budget for the provision of such needs and therefore prioritize services. The intention is that patients with severe mental illness with complex needs will receive both care programming and care management and ensure that proper allocation of funds is made, whereas those who have less severe needs can be cared for using care programming alone.

There are many aspects of this system which are unsatisfactory and which are difficult to address by purchasers of services. The notion that 'packages of care' can be designed on the basis of needs assessments (see below) is reasonable in principle but impossible to achieve in practice for many people. Needs can change unexpectedly during care and are difficult to anticipate, and many psychiatric patients change their minds and alter their levels of co-operation with treatment..

Care programming and care management are British terms but they are similar to case management in the United States and contain some features that are found in managed care in that country. In October 1994, the supervision register was introduced, owing to concern about the risks created by those with the most severe mental illness and who need the closest supervision. Any patient with severe mental illness who has a significant risk of self-harm, self-neglect, or is dangerous to others, is placed on the register and requires regular reviews.

Unfortunately, all these systems have been introduced without any additional resources and, whilst they may be indicative of good practice and therefore should be followed in any case, the additional bureaucracy involved in their implementation necessitates some additional resources. It is a difficult decision for public health departments involved in commissioning services to decide what level of resources is required and whether or not the implementation of these new arrangements does improve the total mental health of the populations.

Needs assessment

It will be seen from the above account that needs assessment is an essential component of care management and, indeed, of care programming. Although this has a central role in public health strategies, it is important to be aware of its limitations. Needs assessment is ideal for conditions that are well researched, unequivocal in nature, and for which clear guidelines of therapy exist. Thus an elderly person who fractures the neck of a femur has a clear pathway set out for treatment and aftercare that can be easily monitored and costed. The pathway of, for example, a patient admitted with an episode of schizophrenia is very different. Some patients with schizophrenia improve dramatically after a few days and do not have further episodes, whereas other require care almost indefinitely, are unable to look after themselves, and need permanent support and accommodation. The cost of treating the episode for the first group of patients is unlikely to be more than around £1000, whereas treatment for the second group can cost well over £1000 000. Deciding on the relative needs of these individuals, particularly early in treatment, is extraordinarily difficult and often the outcome represents little more than a set of formalized value judgements (Slade 1994).

Stevens and Gabbay (1991), in criticizing much of the literature on needs assessment, emphasize that 'needs' for health care are quite separate from 'wants' and must include the population's ability to benefit from health care and health service interventions. One approach to needs assessment is to consider the prevalence and incidence of mental disorders at both national and local levels and to use this in order to inform the commissioning of mental health services. Unfortunately, this can only be done well when the effectiveness and costs of mental health services and interventions are available. Because most of the information is insufficient, models of service care are often used in order to help purchasers decide which approach is most valuable. Although these can be of use, it is important to realize that they do involve a great deal of guess work. At present it is probably better to use 'proxy measures' such as the Jarman score of the area (Jarman 1984) to predict all the different elements of mental health service required, including the expensive item of bed numbers (Jarman *et al.* 1992).

Service use and effectiveness of intervention

It is useful to discuss interventions in psychiatry in each of the five levels defined by Goldberg and Huxley (1980) (Table 4). Although psychiatric patients can be involved at all of these levels and in different countries there may be much more intervention at one level than another because of the services available. There are still sufficient fundamental differences with the activities at each of the levels to keep them separate.

Level 5: inpatient care

This is the most expensive form of care and in the United Kingdom accounts for 85 per cent of the total costs of psychiatric services. The dramatic reduction in psychiatric inpatient beds in the past 30 years has led to a major shift in the diagnostic representation of inpatients. Organic states (particularly dementias), schizophrenia, and affective psychosis now constitute most of the diagnostic groups admitted to beds for mental illness and there have been significant falls in the proportions of patients admitted with neurotic and stress disorders, and depression (apart from that associated with bipolar affective disorder) (Tyrer *et al.* 1989). When there is greater use of beds than expected, it is usually because there is a lower threshold to the admission of affective disorders in general (Flannigan *et al.* 1994).

There is now a general notion in almost every country that psychiatric admission is not desirable and should be used as an option of last resort. This is because of the perceived perils of institutionalization (the gradation from independence to passive acceptance of a machine-like existence in an impersonal system), stigmatization of admission (the labelling of the victim as permanently 'mad' and alienated from society), and the relatively high cost of inpatient care (around £200 per patient per day), accounting for the disproportionate costs of hospital compared with community services (Merson *et al.* 1996).

In the past some of the dangers of hospital admission have been exaggerated, particularly in the 1960s in which all institutions of society were attacked (Goffman 1961), and they have been reduced by transferring inpatient care from large free-standing mental hospitals into psychiatric units in district general hospitals. It has also been appreciated that institutionalization is not just a consequence of institutions. Patients with psychiatric illness can lose all personal rights, be abused regularly, live in squalor under rigid control, and show all aspects of institutionalized behaviour while living at home with their families. It has also been appreciated that some symptoms that were formerly regarded as a consequence of institutional care, such as posturing, stereotyped behaviour, lack of motivation, and apathy, can be long-term consequences of psychiatric illness, notably schizophrenia, rather than created by the environment.

Nevertheless, public health policy in almost all countries, including developing countries which have never had a significant mental hospital base, has been to promote community care, the results of which are discussed above. However, if additional resources are available beyond those of the personnel in community teams, this can reduce the bed base further. Organizations such as the Richmond Fellowship and St Mungo's Housing Association provide a network of hostels offering varying degrees of independence for up to several years. This can prove invaluable in stabilizing those with psychiatric problems and preventing the cycle of recurring admissions that is common in those who are discharged to substandard accommodation with all its attendant stresses. Other reasons include the reluctance of hospital-based staff to involve themselves in community work (Tyrer 1993) (a reluctance which is in itself another form of institutionalization), poor levels of integration between health and social services in many areas, and restrictions preventing adequate treatment of patients who are non-compliant. Patients who are at risk to themselves or others as a consequence of mental illness can be compulsorily treated, and how this should be done with proper respect for individual rights has long been a subject for debate.

A small number of psychiatric patients are recurrent criminal offenders or are particularly dangerous, and this has led to the development of forensic psychiatry as a separate discipline. Until quite recently forensic psychiatry has been mainly a tertiary referral service which has taken its patients from those who have already been in psychiatric care. Unfortunately, dangerousness and criminal behaviour are extremely difficult to predict. Many such patients have a combination of schizophrenia and personality disorder and may require long periods of detention to protect the public. For this reason special hospitals for the 'criminally insane' have long existed for such patients and, even in the era of community psychiatry, these necessarily have a high threshold for discharge. There is also increasing concern that, with the reduced numbers of psychiatric beds available, mentally ill patients may be diverted to the prison services where they will treated much less appropriately (Gunn *et al.* 1991). To avoid this, there has been a rapid growth of 'court diversion' schemes to assess the psychiatric status of those appearing in court (often for minor offences) so that those who are clearly mentally ill can be transferred to more appropriate care in psychiatric hospitals or other outpatient settings (Joseph 1994).

Forensic psychiatric patients occupy beds for a proportionally longer time, and if there is no appropriate district forensic service with its own bed base the numbers of those in hospital will be greater. Mental health legislation in most countries, largely because of concern for human rights, only has a limited role for compulsory treatments outside hospital, although in the United Kingdom reforms to the Mental Health Act to allow compulsory treatment in the community are likely to be made shortly. Many safeguards would have to be introduced to ensure that this power was not abused, but many countries are now reviewing their mental health legislation because so many more of the seriously mentally ill are being treated outside hospital.

In deciding on the number of beds available in a district, it is important to take into account the levels of social deprivation and particular characteristics of the area. In the United Kingdom Jarman (1983, 1984) has provided an extremely useful set of scores for each district based on their level of social deprivation (underprivileged area scores) which can be used to predict psychiatric admission rates (Jarman *et al.* 1992). However, even these predictions can be distorted by, for example, a small number of homeless mentally ill in the areas concerned. The homeless, because of their extreme levels of social deprivation, absence of contact with statutory services, and reluctance to engage in treatment, account for a disproportionate amount of psychiatric beds used. This is accentuated by the difficulties in finding accommodation once they have been treated and are ready for discharge on clinical grounds. The differences in levels of prevalence of severe mental illness between deprived inner-city areas and affluent rural areas are great and, as yet, inadequately quantified. They need to be borne in mind when extrapolating from data recorded in only one setting. For example, in the county of Buckinghamshire in England, a highly successful community psychiatric service, with a full range of crisis intervention and other services, has been able to reduce hospital admissions dramatically (Falloon and Fadden 1993); such results would be much more difficult to achieve in the inner city.

Level 4: patients attending psychiatric services outside hospital

This group, which can be termed 'extra-cubilar' psychiatry as it does not use hospital beds (Tyrer and Malone 1991), mainly involves outpatient and day care. In the last 20 years there has also been a shift of psychiatric resources towards primary care in the form of liaison psychiatry in general practice. There is now good evidence that a proportion of the severely mentally ill can be treated very effectively as day patients and this may obviate the need for psychiatric admission (Creed *et al.* 1990), but this may not be a realistic option in the less compliant patient. There is also reasonable evidence that the growth of liaison psychiatry in primary care has improved the skills of general practitioners and allowed more patients to continue their episodes of illness entirely in the primary care setting (Tyrer *et al.* 1990*a*). However, the advantage of such liaison still needs to be determined in controlled investigations and to date no impact has been found on psychiatric admission rates (Jackson *et al.* 1993) and the total cost of care is greater because more patients are referred (Goldberg *et al.* 1996).

Levels 2 and 3: hidden and conspicuous psychiatric morbidity in primary care

There has been considerable interest in the impact of educating primary care physicians so that they area able to detect important mental disorders because most psychiatric disorders are seen and assessed initially in primary care. If those disorders that were likely to lead to greater psychiatric morbidity (and progression to higher levels in service terms) and intervene early with effective treatments, this would be a very valuable form of secondary prevention. Evidence that screening psychiatric patients with instruments such as the General Health Questionnaire (Goldberg 1972) improve patient care is largely lacking. There is conflicting evidence from research studies (Johnstone and Goldberg 1976; Hoeper *et al.* 1984) and in ordinary practice this is rarely used. One of the problems is that most of the minor disorders seen in primary care have a favourable outcome which is determined much more by social factors than clinical ones (Huxley and Goldberg 1975) and clinical intervention may have relatively little impact. This may be another area of public health in which screening has failed to live up to its promise and might be replaced by greater input to the population specifically at risk (Holland *et al.* 1994).

More favourable results have been reported in depression, in which the risk of suicide is considerable. The most favourable results have been reported from education programmes aimed at improving the general practitioner's ability to detect significant depression. The most important evidence of the public health value of this approach is a study from the island of Gotland. In Sweden in 1975, the International Committee for the Prevention and Treatment of Depression was founded, with the aim of improving both the understanding and the management of individuals with depressive illnesses. From this evolved the Swedish Committee for the Prevention and Treatment of Depression which was established in 1977 to examine the relationship between postgraduate medical education and depression in the community. In 1982 a study of the incidence of depression was set up in the island of Gotland, off the east coast of Sweden, to investigate the effects of an educational programme for general practitioners. The impact of this programme was evaluated in succeeding years.

The educational programme included lectures and discussions relating to patients with depression, and was aimed at improving the ability of general practitioners to detect and treat cases of depression.

The outcome of the educational programme was most marked in the year after it was given. There was a significant decrease in the number of days spent in hospital because of depressive disorders, a reduction in days of work lost because of depression, and a reduction in the suicide rate by over 50 per cent (Rutz *et al.* 1989). A separate cost–benefit analysis showed that the costs of the educational programme were far outweighed by the benefits shown in terms of health-care savings (Rutz *et al.* 1992*a*). Unfortunately, in subsequent years the suicide rate crept upwards again (Rutz *et al.* 1992*b*) and it had been suggested that continuous education might be necessary to maintain this level of improvement.

There have been some criticisms about this study and the merits of generalizing from its findings. It is far from clear that taking data from this study and using it to make generalizations about medical practice elsewhere in different settings is appropriate as it is unclear to what extent the results of this study represent the unique island environment. There is also little evidence that the intervention has had a long-term effect on suicide rate. To this extent it has had less impact on suicide than other issues that are independent of mental health services. The most marked of these is the replacement of gas containing carbon monoxide (coal gas) by natural gas (containing no carbon monoxide) in the 1960s and this has had a much greater effect on the suicide rate that the Gotland data. Nevertheless the results of this study have encouraged those who feel that mental health services can have an impact on overall suicide rates.

Level 1: psychiatric morbidity in the community

Most people in developed countries with significant psychiatric morbidity present to either the primary care or psychiatric services (Fig. 3).

Only a small number of those at risk might be helped to a greater extent if their problems were detected earlier and appropriate intervention made. One group that could be helped is those patients with schizophrenia who present late in the course of illness because of gradual social withdrawal and severing of links with others in society including health services. There are suggestions from studies of outcome (Johnstone *et al.* 1990) that such late-presenting patients fare particularly badly in terms of outcome and that if they were detected earlier much morbidity could be avoided. However, how this could be done is difficult to contemplate at present.

Prevention

Prevention in psychiatry is more elusive than in other branches of medicine because of the relatively vague and multifactorial aetiology of most mental disorders and this had led to the conclusion that most resources should be directed at those affected by these disorders rather than preventive strategies *per se* (Doll 1983). Its list of achievements is also disappointgly small (Holland and Fitzsimons 1990). However, there have been successes and, increasingly awareness of secondary prevention in particular has created a more optimistic environment. Pardes *et al.* (1989) have identified four areas that need refining before preventative strategies in psychiatry can be implemented more widely: improved psychiatric diagnosis, better epidemiological studies involving longitudinal data linked to health service use, advances in genetics generally and the wider use of genetic counselling in particular, and the potential advantages of biotechnology allowing non-invasive observation of brain function (e.g. positron emission tomography scanning). All these have been improved in the last 10 years and lead us to revise Doll's pessimism.

Primary prevention

By far the most impressive evidence of primary prevention is in the field of mental handicap (now euphemistically termed learning difficulties). Advances in clinical genetics now mean that nearly 40 per cent of the causes of severe mental handicap (Down syndrome, phenylketonuria, tuberose sclerosis, Hurler's syndrome, Lesch–Nyhan syndrome, and Tay–Sachs disease) are caused by identifiable chromosome abnormalities that are potentially preventable (Weatherall 1991). At present, apart from a few special high-risk groups (e.g. Tay–Sachs disease in Ashkenazi Jews) screening before conception is not considered fruitful. The revelation that fragile X syndrome accounts for around 6 per cent of all individuals with mental handicap (Lavoxa *et al.* 1977) has tremendous scope for prevention through general population screening and detection of carriers. Other preventable causes of mental handicap include better obstetric care and supervision of babies with low birth weight (Illsley and Mitchell 1984), the prevention of rubella syndrome by the combined measles–mumps–rubella vaccine (although evidence for this is still awaited) and of neural tube defects by folic acid supplements in pregnancy (MRC Vitamin Study Group 1991). Genetic counselling for most of these disorders is still in its infancy and misleading information or maladroit presentation can create its own morbidity (McGuffin 1994). An important area of public health research is to examine the correct application of this preventative strategy.

Another important example of primary prevention is the introduction of needle-exchange schemes to reduce the transmission of HIV in drug users. There is little doubt that those who use such schemes significantly reduce the risk of developing HIV infection (Stimson *et al.* 1989) but those who avoid such schemes are often most risky in their behaviour. It is also now well established that ready access to illicit drugs and alcohol is probably the single most important precursor of addiction: and if the source of supply is reduced much psychiatric, as well as other morbidity, could be avoided (Royal College of Physicians 1991). Reduction of alcohol use would also be likely to reduce the suicide rate as around a quarter of all those who successfully complete suicide are dependent on alcohol (Barraclough *et al.* 1974). Other potential preventative strategies include the political one of raising the standards of living of all people in the country so that significant social deprivation is reduced to a minimum, which would have a beneficial effect on child psychiatric disorders, personality disorder (particularly of the antisocial type), drug and alcohol abuse, and post-traumatic stress disorders. It might also reduce the incidence of schizophrenia by improving perinatal care in particular (Lewis 1989).

Secondary prevention

There are more opportunities for psychiatric services in secondary prevention, mainly by early intervention to those at risk. For example, reduction of alcohol availability is a political and legal decision that affects alcohol consumption in the whole population, but making those who are at special risk a target for more intensive intervention is more cost-effective and in most cases preferred to general health promotion. In both general practice (Wallace *et al.* 1988) and general hospital admissions (Chick *et al.* 1985) intervention of an educational nature has helped to reduce subsequent alcohol consumption.

However, as with most of these endeavours, the demonstration that reduction can be achieved is rarely followed by generalization from this finding. It is clear that such policies have to be pursued assiduously and persistently in order to be effective. There is considerable argument over whether intervention in children at risk of psychiatric disorder is beneficial or not. Because many such children come from disadvantaged backgrounds it is easy for any such intervention to be nullified by a return to the same cycle of disadvantage. However, Kolvin and his colleagues in particular have argued that children who show behaviour characteristic of maladjustment improve to a significantly greater degree with group therapy (from social workers), behaviour therapy, and what is described as 'nurture work' (support and enrichment from teacher-aides) to a significantly greater degree than a control group of children, and these gains are maintained 3 years after intervention (Kolvin *et al.* 1990).

Affective disorders are common in women of anxious premorbid personality after childbirth and Barnett and Parker (1985) have compared the value of professional psychiatric help to lay support and a control group. The results of this additional support show some evidence that postnatal affective symptoms, particularly anxiety, were reduced in those who received professional help but the findings do not at this stage suggest that such intervention is cost-effective. Like many of these populations it is only secondary intervention that takes place at a late stage (i.e. just before the expression of a psychiatric syndrome) that seems to be effective in preventive terms.

Tertiary prevention

The prevention of disability and relapse in those who already have psychiatric disorder is now part of the standard practice of psychiatry. Unfortunately, it is rarely carried out to its full potential as many psychiatric services, through a combination of limited resources and habitual functioning, are essentially reactive rather than proactive in nature.

Schizophrenia covers a range of conditions that last from a few months to many years, but unfortunately the main effective treatment, antipsychotic drugs, has a high incidence of adverse drug reactions. The acute symptoms, pseudoparkinsonism and akathisia (bodily restlessness), are almost invariably present at some point in treatment, and akathisia in particular is almost impossible to relieve with other drugs such as procyclidine and propranolol which have only a limited effect. In the longer term, the syndrome of tardive dyskinesia is even more disturbing as this syndrome, once developed, is almost impossible to treat and in over a third of patients become permanent irrespective of further antipsychotic drug treatment. Nevertheless, maintenance treatment of schizophrenia by a drug regime is still the preferred option since there is increasing evidence that each relapse and readmission leads to some loss of function which is never regained (Stevens 1982).

However, social measures may also prevent relapse. Combination of maintenance drug treatment and reduction of 'expressed emotion' (interactions of strong emotional content of any type between the schizophrenic patient and others, of whom relatives are usually the most important) is one of the more effective ways of preventing relapse (Leff and Vaughn 1981).

Similarly, long-term antidepressant therapy, including tricyclic antidepressants and mood stabilizers such as lithium and sodium valproate, are all effective in preventing relapse in recurrent depressive and bipolar affective disorders. In general, lithium is preferred for bipolar disorders and antidepressants for persistent (unipolar) disorders. Despite evidence from many studies that such measures are successful, the evidence that their introduction has led to a reduction in relapse in these disorders for the psychiatric population with affective disorders as a whole is not yet available.

Suicide has been referred to early in the context of improved detection of depression. Any preventative measure that reduces the incidence of depression should also reduce suicide rates as approximately 1 in 6 of all depressed patients end their life by suicide (Gunnell and Frankel 1994). If it is possible to reduce the number of fatal means available to commit suicide this may also assist, particularly if the suicidal act is an impulsive one. People in occupations who have ready access to means of successful suicide (e.g. veterinary surgeons, farmers, anaesthetists) have suicide rates of more than twice the average of the general population (Charlton *et al.* 1993). Death by carbon monoxide poisoning through car exhausts is also increasing rapidly (Charlton *et al.* 1993) and has led to initiatives to fit most cars with catalytic converters that reduce the carbon monoxide content of car exhausts.

There is much discussion about the choice of antidepressant drugs in depressed patients. Although there is no doubt that the older antidepressants (mainly tricyclic compounds) are more dangerous in overdose than the newer agents, such as the selective serotonin-reuptake inhibitors (Cassidy and Henry 1987), it is difficult to know how much suicide could be prevented by wider prescription of the newer drugs, since only around 5 per cent of patients committing suicide do so by taking antidepressants alone. Unfortunately, to date there is no successful way of preventing further episodes of parasuicide (attempted suicide) in those seen after completing such an act. The only treatment that has been shown to be effective is a very intensive form of individual and group treatment related to cognitive therapy (Linehan *et al.* 1991), but this is too intensive to be introduced into the National Health Service. Since 1 per cent of patients after an episode of parasuicide commit suicide in the following year and around 20 per cent do so eventually, some way of preventing repetition would be a major gain to public mental health. Shorter forms of Linehan's treatment linked to short treatment booklets have shown initial promise and may present the way forward (Evans *et al.* 1999).

The impact of services in tertiary prevention is also important. Treatments that are effective in preventing relapse are of no value if patients are not maintaining contact with the service. Formal introduction of the care programming approach to psychiatric services in England has not been formally tested apart from one study in which close supervision of vulnerable psychiatric patients by a key worker at regular intervals was more effective than control care in preventing drop out but led to significantly more psychiatric admissions (Tyrer *et al.* 1995). There is a contradiction between these findings and the specific intervention of community mental health teams which have been shown to reduce admissions to hospital and often provide more superior care. The key difference appears to be the presence of a suitably resourced multidisciplinary team that can provide the appropriate skills for patients outside hospitals rather than the common situation in care programming for a single key worker to take most of the clinical responsibility. Under such circumstances it is perhaps not surprising that when the key worker is faced with a deterioration in the patient's condition, admission to hospital becomes more likely.

Conclusion

This chapter illustrates the extensive degree of overlap, and opportunities for collaboration, between the public health and mental health services. There are still large areas that need to be properly developed which, despite the optimism of Caplan (1964), have yielded very little in terms of improving public mental health. It is reasonable to argue that this is partly because so little has been shared between the two disciplines until the last few years.

Public health has a right to decide on how resources are distributed and to ask for targets such as the suicide targets of *Our Healthier Nation* and the satisfaction of the population's needs. Therefore it is right and proper for a public health physician, for example, to question the duties of community psychiatric nurses to ensure that they are addressing these needs with appropriate priority. Community psychiatric nurses have a range of skills and are unable to deploy them all simultaneously (Tyrer *et al.* 1990*b*), and so other professionals, including those from public health, can provide advice based on their relative efficacy and cost, and the needs of the population served.

Simultaneously, public health physicians need to acknowledge the special difficulties of psychiatry. Our failure to achieve good outcome measures in psychiatry is not a consequence of incompetence. Direct measures of psychiatric ill health are now well established but are impractical to apply to whole populations. The search for appropriate proxy measures that could substitute for direct measurement of mental health status continues to preoccupy us greatly and we are making suitable efforts to obtain them. This should not mean that public health should rush into assuming that assessments such as those for needs are necessarily accurate and valid (Stevens and Gabbay 1991; Slade 1994); there is a great deal more to be done before they can be regarded in the same way as visual acuity can be used to measure the success of a treatment policy for cataracts.

Mutual understanding also needs to develop between the different perspectives of public health and mental health professionals. The public health physician has to deal with the health of large numbers and the uniqueness of the individual is relatively unimportant amongst these large numbers. Nevertheless, if a very small number of individuals are receiving care whilst large numbers of equally deserving numbers are not, it is only the person with the wider perspective who will blow the whistle and ask for something to be done. But the public health physician also has to be aware of the difficulties facing the psychiatric services; the idiosyncratic nature of diagnosis with frequent changes from one to the other, varying needs of the psychiatric patient at different times, and the dynamics of interaction between the psychiatric patients and others around about them, including their psychiatric attendants.

So much can be gained by better understanding of the roles of each discipline. On the one hand, public health cannot function as an adequate purchaser of mental health services without an understanding of clinical sensitivities, and on the other the psychiatrist and mental health worker need to have a wider perspective than that of patients under active care. Goldberg and Huxley (1992) sadly conclude at the end of their review of common mental disorders that 'in most countries of the world services for the mentally ill survive on the crumbs left by the banquet of general health care'. Public health can ensure they all eat at the same table.

References

Acheson, D. (1988). *Annual review of the public health.* HMSO, London.

American Psychiatric Association (1980). *Diagnostic and statistical manual of mental disorders* (3rd edn). American Psychiatric Association, Washington, DC.

American Psychiatric Association (1994). *Diagnostic and statistical manual of mental disorders* (4th edn). American Psychiatric Association, Washington, DC.

Andrews, G., Stewart, G., Morris-Yates, A., Holt, P., and Henderson, S. (1990). Evidence for a general neurotic syndrome. *British Journal of Psychiatry*, **157**, 6–12.

Andrews, G., Slade, T., and Peters, L. (1999). Classification in psychiatry: ICD-10 versus DSM-IV. *British Journal of Psychiatry*, **174**, 3–5.

Anonymous (1992). *The health of the nation: a summary of the strategy for health in England.* HMSO, London.

Anonymous (1998). *Report of the independent inquiry into inequalities of health.* HMSO, London.

Barnett, B. and Parker, G. (1985). Professional and non-professional intervention for highly anxious primiparous mothers. *British Journal of Psychiatry*, **146**, 287–93.

Barraclough, B., Bunch, J., Nelson, B., and Sainsbury, P. (1974). A hundred cases of suicide: clinical aspects. *British Journal of Psychiatry*, **125**, 355–73.

Barton, R. (1959) *Institutional neurosis.* John Wright, Bristol.

Bayer, R. and Spitzer, R.L. (1985) Neurosis, psychodynamics and DSM-III: a history of the controversy. *Archives of General Psychiatry*, **42**, 187–96.

Bebbington, P., Brugha, T., Hill, T., Marsden, L., and Window, S. (1999). Validation of the Health of the Nation Outcome Scales. *British Journal of Psychiatry*, **174**, 389–94.

Bleuler, E. (1950). *Dementia praecox or the group of schizophrenias.* International Universities Press, New York.

Brayne, C., Gill, C., Paykel, E.S., Huppert, F., and O'Connor, D.W. (1995*a*). Cognitive decline in an elderly population—a two wave study of change. *Psychological Medicine*, **25**, 673–83.

Brayne, C., Gill, C., Huppert, F.A., ***et al.*** (1995*b*). Incidence of clinically diagnosed subtypes of dementia in an elderly population. Cambridge Project for Later Life. *British Journal of Psychiatry*, **167**, 255–62.

Burns, T., Beadsmoore, A., Bhat, A.V., Oliver, A., and Mathers, C. (1993). A controlled trial of home-based acute psychiatric services. I. Clinical and social outcome. *British Journal of Psychiatry*, **163**, 49–54.

Caplan, G. (1964). *Principles of preventative psychiatry.* Basic Books, New York.

Casey, P. (2000). Epidemiology of personality disorder. In *Personality disorders: diagnosis, management and course* (2nd edn) (ed. P. Tyrer). Butterworth Heinemann, Oxford.

Cassidy, S.L. and Henry, J.A. (1987). Fatal toxicity of antidepressant drugs in overdose. *British Medical Journal*, **295**, 1021–4.

Chadwick, E. (1842). *Report on the sanitary condition of the labouring population of Great Britain.* Edinburgh University Press.

Charlton, J., Kelly, S., Dunnell, K., Evans, B., and Jenkins, R. (1993). Suicide deaths in England and Wales: trends in factors associated with suicide deaths. *Population Trends*, **71**, 34–42.

Chick, J., Lloyd, G., and Crombie, E. (1985). Counselling problem drinkers in medical wards: a controlled study. *British Medical Journal*, **290**, 965–7.

Coid, J. (1994) Failure in community care: psychiatry's dilemma. *British Medical Journal*, **308**, 805–6.

Connell, P.H. (1958). *Amphetamine psychosis.* Oxford University Press.

Cooper, J.E., Kendell, R.E., Gurland, B.J., Sharpe, L., Copeland, J.R.M., and Simon, R. (1972). *Psychiatric diagnosis in New York and London.* Oxford University Press.

Creed, F., Black, D., Anthony, P., Osborn, M., Thomas, P., and Tormenson, B. (1990). Randomised controlled trial of day-patient vs in-patient psychiatric treatment. *British Medical Journal*, **300**, 1033–7.

de Girolamo, G. and Reich, J.H. (1993). *Personality disorders.* WHO, Geneva.

Detels, R. and Breslow, L. (1986). Current scope. In *Oxford textbook of public health: history, determinants, scope, and strategies* (ed. W.W. Holland, R. Detels, and G. Knox), Volume 1. Oxford University Press.

DoH (Department of Health) (1990). *Community care in the next decade and beyond.* HMSO, London.

DoH (Department of Health) (1993). *The Health of the Nation. Key area handbook: mental illness.* HMSO, London.

DoH (Department of Health) (1999). *Our healthier nation. A contract for health.* HMSO, London.

Doll, R. (1983). Prospects for prevention. *British Medical Journal*, **286**, 445–53.

Drever, F. and Bunting, J. (1997). Patterns and trends in male mortality. In *Health inequalities: decennial supplement.* DS Series no. 15. HMSO, London.

Endicott, J., Spitzer, R.L., Fleiss, J.L., and Cohen, J. (1976). The global assessment scale: a procedure for measuring the overall severity of psychiatric disturbance. *Archives of General Psychiatry*, **33**, 766–71.

Evans, K., Tyrer, P., Catalan, J., *et al.* (1999) Manual-assisted cognitive–behaviour therapy (MACT): a randomised controlled trial of a brief intervention with bibliotherapy in the treatment of recurrent deliberate self-harm. *Psychological Medicine*, **29**, 19–25.

Falloon, I.R.H. and Fadden, G. (1993). *Integrated mental health care: a comprehensive community-based approach.* Cambridge University Press.

Faris, R.E.L. and Dunham, H.W. (1939) *Mental disorders in urban areas: an ecological study of schizophrenia and other psychoses.* University of Chicago Press.

Farr, W. (1864). *Letter to the Registrar General on the years 1851–1860. Supplement to the 25th report of the Registrar General.* General Register Office, London.

Feinstein, A. (1970). The pre-therapeutic classification of comorbidity in chronic disease. *Journal of Chronic Diseases*, **23**, 455–62.

Flannigan, C.B., Glover, G.R., Feeney, S.T., Wing, J.K., Bebbington, P. E., and Lewis, S.W. (1994). Inner London collaborative audit of admissions in two health districts. I: Introduction, methods and preliminary findings. *British Journal of Psychiatry*, **165**, 734–42.

Foucault, M. (1973). *Madness and civilisation.* Vintage Books, New York.

Goffman, E. (1961). *Asylums.* Doubleday, New York.

Goldberg, D. (1972). *The detection of psychiatric illness by questionnaire.* Maudsley Monograph 21. Oxford University Press.

Goldberg, D. and Huxley, P. (1980). *Mental illness in the community: the pathway to psychiatric care.* Tavistock Publications, London.

Goldberg, D. and Huxley, P. (1992). *Common mental disorders: a biosocial model.* Tavistock/Routledge, London.

Goldberg, D., Jackson, G., Gater, R., Campbell, M., and Jennett, N. (1996) The treatment of common mental disorders by a community team based in primary care: a cost effectiveness study. *Psychological Medicine*, **26**, 487–92.

Gunn, J., Maden, A., and Swinton, M. (1991). *Mentally disordered prisoners.* Home Office, London.

Gunnell, D. and Frankel, S. (1994). Prevention of suicide: aspirations and evidence. *British Medical Journal*, **308**, 1227–33.

Harris, E.C. and Barraclough, B. (1998). Excess mortality of mental disorder. *British Journal of Psychiatry*, **173**, 11–53.

Henderson, S. (2000). Conclusion: the central issues. In *Unmet need in psychiatry: problems, reources, responses.* Cambridge University Press.

Hoeper, E., Nicz, G., Kessler, L., Burke, J., and Pierce, W. (1984). The usefulness of screening for mental health. *Lancet*, **i**, 33–6.

Holland, W. and Fitzsimons, B. (1990). Public health concerns. How can social psychiatry help? In *The public health impact of mental disorder* (ed. D. Goldberg and D. Tantam), pp. 14–19. Hogrefe and Huber, Toronto.

Holland, W.W., Fitzsimons, B., and O'Brien, M. (1994). 'Back to the future'—public health research into the next century. *Journal of Public Health Medicine*, **16**, 4–10.

Holloway, F. and Carson, J. (1998) Intensive case management for the severely mentally ill: controlled trial. *British Journal of Psychiatry*, **172**, 19–22.

Huxley, P. and Goldberg, D.P. (1975). Social versus clinical prediction in minor psychiatric disorders. *Psychological Medicine*, **5**, 96–102.

Illsley, R. and Mitchell, R.J. (1984). *Low birth weight.* Wiley, Chichester.

Jablensky, A., Sartorius, N., Ernberg, G., *et al.* (1992). Schizophrenia: manifestations, incidence and course in different countries. A World Health Organization ten-country study. *Psychological Medicine*, Supplement 20, 1–97.

Jackson, G., Gater, R., Goldberg, D., Tantam, D., Loftus, L., and Taylor, H. (1993). A new community mental health team based in primary care: a description of the service and the effect on service use in the first year. *British Journal of Psychiatry*, **162**, 375–84.

Jacob, K.S., Everitt, B., Patel, V., Weich, S., Araya, R., and Lewis, G.H. (1998). The comparison of latent variable models of non-psychotic psychiatric morbidity in four culturally diverse populations. *Psychological Medicine*, **28**, 145–52.

Jarman, B. (1983). Identification of underprivileged areas. *British Medical Journal*, **286**, 1705–9.

Jarman, B. (1984). Validation and distribution of scores. *British Medical Journal*, **289**, 1587–92.

Jarman, B., Hirsch, S., White, P., and Driscoll, R. (1992). Predicting psychiatric admission rates. *British Medical Journal*, **304**, 1146–51.

Johnstone, E.C. (1999). Diagnostic issues: concepts of the disorder. In *Schizophrenia: concepts and clinical management* (ed. E.C. Johnstone, M.S. Humphreys, F.H. Lang, S.M. Lawrie, and R. Sandler), p. 38. Cambridge University Press.

Johnstone, A. and Goldberg, D.P. (1976). Psychiatric screening in general practice: a controlled trial. *Lancet*, **i**, 605–8.

Johnstone, E.C., McMillan, J.F., Frith, C.D., Benn, D.K., and Crow, T. (1990). Further investigations of the predictors of outcome following a first schizophrenic episode. *British Journal of Psychiatry*, **157**, 182–9.

Joseph, P.L.A. (1994). Psychiatric assessment at the magistrates' courts. *British Journal of Psychiatry*, **164**, 722–4.

Kessler, R.C., McGonagle, K.A., Zhao, S., *et al.* (1994). Lifetime and 12-month prevalence of DSM-III-R psychiatric disorders in the United States. Results from the National Comorbidity Survey. *Archives of General Psychiatry*, **51**, 8–19.

Kolvin, I., Charles, R., Nicholson, R., Fleeting, M., and Fundudis, T. (1990). Factors in prevention in inner city deprivation. In *Public health impact of mental disorders* (ed. D. Goldberg and D. Tantam), pp. 115–23. Hogrefe and Huber, Toronto.

Laing, R.D. and Cooper, D.G. (1964). *Reason and violence.* Tavistock Publications, London.

Laing, R.D. and Esterson, A. (1970). *Sanity, madness and the family.* Harmondsworth, Penguin.

Lavoxa, R., Ridler, M.A.C., and Bowen-Bravery, M. (1977). An etiological survey of the severely retarded Hertfordshire children who were born between January 1st 1965 and January 31st 1967. *American Journal of Medical Genetics*, **1**, 75–86.

Lawrie, S.M., Abukmei, S., Santosh, C., Chiswick, A., Rimmington J.E., and Best, J.J.K. (1997). Qualitative morphological abnormalities in schizophrenia: an MRI study and systematic literature review. *Schizophrenia Research*, **25**, 155–66.

Leff, J. and Vaughn, C.E. (1981). The role of maintenance therapy and relatives' expressed emotion in relapse of schizophrenia: a two year follow up. *British Journal of Psychiatry*, **139**, 102–4.

Lehman A.F. and Steinwachs, D.M. (1998). Patterns of usual care for schizophrenia: initial results from the Schizophrenia Patient Outcomes Research Team (PORT) Client Survey. *Schizophrenia Bulletin*, **24**, 11–20.

Lewis, S.W. (1989). Congenital risk factors for schizophrenia. *Psychological Medicine*, **19**, 5–13.

Linehan, M.M., Hubert, A.E., Suarez, A., Allmon, D., and Heard, H.L. (1991). Cognitive–behavioral treatment of chronically parasuicidal borderline patients. *Archives of General Psychiatry*, **48**, 1060–4.

Luque, R. and Berrios, G.E. (1994). Cotard's syndrome in the eldery: historical and clinical aspects. *International Journal of Geriatric Psychiatry*, **9**, 957–64.

Macdonald, A. (1993). The myth of suicide prevention by general practitioners. *British Journal of Psychiatry*, **163**, 260.

McGuffin, P. (1994). Genetics. In *Prevention in psychiatry* (ed. E.S. Paykel and R. Jenkins), pp. 32–9. Gaskell, London.

Magee, W.J., Eaton, W.W., Wittchen, H.U., McGonagle, K.A., and Kessler, R.C. (1996). Agoraphobia, simple phobia, and social phobia in the National Comorbidity Survey. *Archives of General Psychiatry*, **53**, 159–68.

Meltzer, H., Gill, B., and Petticrew, M. (1994). *OPCS Surveys of Psychiatric Morbidity in Great Britain. Bulletin 1: The prevalence of psychiatric morbidity among adults aged 16–64, living in private households, in Great Britain*. OPCS, London.

Merson, S., Tyrer, P., Onyett, S., *et al.* (1992). Early intervention in psychiatric emergencies: a controlled clinical trial. *Lancet*, **339**, 1311–14.

Merson, S., Tyrer, P., Carlen, D., and Johnson, A.L. (1996) The cost of treatment of psychiatric emergencies: a comparison of hospital and community services. *Psychological Medicine*, **26**, 727–34.

Moens, G.F.G. (1990). *Aspects of the epidemiology and prevention of suicide*. Leuven University Press.

Montgomery, A.J. and Parshall, A.M. (1998). Implications of urban drift on health care resources in inner London. *Psychiatric Bulletin*, **22**, 494–6.

MRC Vitamin Study Group (1991). Prevention of neural tube defects: results of the Medical Research Council Medical Study Group. *Lancet*, **338**, 131–7.

Muijen, M., Marks, I.M., Connolly, J., and Audini, B. (1992). Home based care and standard hospital care for patients with severe mental illness: a randomised controlled trial. *British Medical Journal*, **304**, 749–54.

Mulder, R.T. and Joyce, P.R. (1997) Temperament and the structure of personality disorder symptoms. *Psychological Medicine*, **27**, 99–106.

OPCS (1995). *OPCS Surveys of Psychiatric Morbidity in Great Britain. Bulletin 1: The prevalence of psychiatric morbidity among adults living in private households: Report 1*. HMSO, London.

Pardes, H., Silverman, M.M., and West, A. (1989). Prevention and the field of mental health: a psychiatric perspective. *Annual Review of Public Health*, **10**, 403–22.

Paykel, E.S., Brayne, C., Huppert, F.A., *et al.* (1994). Incidence of dementia in a population older than 75 years in the United Kingdom. *Archives of General Psychiatry*, **51**, 325–32.

Porter, R. (1991). *The Faber book of madness*, p. 8. Faber and Faber, London.

Regier, D.A., Myers, J.K., Kramer, M., *et al.* (1984). The NIMH Epidemiologic Catchment Area (ECA) Program: historical context, major objectives and study population characteristics. *Archives of General Psychiatry*, **41**, 934–41.

Regier, D.A.., Narrow, W.E., Rae, D.S., *et al.* (1993). The *de facto* US mental and addictive disorders service system: Epidemiologic Catchment Area prospective one-year prevalence rates of disorders and services. *Archives of General Psychiatry*, **50**, 85–94.

Regier, D.A., Kaelber, C.T., Rae, D.S., *et al.* (1998). Limitations of diagnostic instruments for mental disorders: implications for research and policy. *Archives of General Psychiatry*, **55**, 109–15.

Roberts, K. and Vass, N. (1986). Schneiderian first-rank symptoms caused by benzodiazepine withdrawal. *British Journal of Psychiatry*, **148**, 593–4.

Robins, J. (1986). *Fools and mad: a history of the insane in Ireland*. Institute of Public Administration, Dublin.

Royal College of Physicians, Faculty of Public Health Medicine (1991). *Alcohol and the public health*. Macmillan, London.

Rutz, W., von Knorring, L., and Wålinder, J. (1989). Frequency of suicide on Gotland after systematic postgraduate education of general practitioners. *Acta Psychiatrica Scandinavica*, **80**, 151–4.

Rutz, W., Carlsson, P., von Knorring, L., and Wålinder, J. (1992*a*). Cost-benefit analysis of an educational program for general practitioners by the Swedish Committee for the prevention and treatment of depression. *Acta Psychiatrica Scandinavica*, **85**, 457–64.

Rutz, W., von Knorring, F.L., and Wålinder, J. (1992*b*). Long term effects of an educational program for general practitioners given by the Swedish Committee for the Prevention and Treatment of Depression. *Acta Psychiatrica Scandinavica*, **85**, 83–8.

Sartorius, N., Jablensky, A., Gulbinat, W., and Ernberg, G. (1980). WHO collaborative study: assessment of affective disorders. *Psychological Medicine*, **10**, 743–9.

Scull, A. (1959). *Museums of madness: the social organization of insanity in 19th-century England*. Allen Lane, London.

Shipley, K., Hilborn, B., Hansell, A., Tyrer, J., and Tyrer, P. (2000). Patient satisfaction: a valid index of quality of care in a psychiatric service? *Acta Psychiatrica Scandinavica*, **101**, 330–3.

Slade, M. (1994). Needs assessment. *British Journal of Psychiatry*, **165**, 293–6.

Stein, L.I. and Test, M.A. (1980). Alternative to mental hospital treatment. 1: Conceptual model, treatment program and clinical evaluation. *Archives of General Psychiatry*, **36**, 1073–9.

Stevens, J.R. (1982). Neurology and neuropathology of schizophrenia. In *Schizophrenia as a brain disease* (ed. F.A. Henn and H.A. Nasrallah), pp. 112–47. Oxford University Press.

Stevens, A. and Gabbay, J. (1991). Needs assessment needs assessment. *Health Trends*, **23**, 20–3.

Stimson, G.V., Dolan, K., Donoghue, M.C., *et al.* (1989). Syringe exchange schemes: a report and some commentaries. *British Journal of Addiction*, **84**, 1283–90.

Sullivan, P.F. and Kendler, K.S. (1998). Typology of common psychiatric syndromes: an empirical study. *British Journal of Psychiatry*, **173**, 312–19.

Szasz, T. (1960). The myth of mental illness. *American Psychologist*, **15**, 113–18.

Thomas, H. (1993). Psychiatric symptoms in cannabis users. *British Journal of Psychiatry*, **163**, 141–9.

Thornicroft, G., Wykes, T., Holloway, F., *et al.* (1998). From efficacy to effectiveness in community mental health services. PRiSM Psychosis Study 10. *British Journal of Psychiatry*, **173**, 423–7.

Tooth, G.C. and Brooke, E.M. (1961). Trends in the mental hospital population and their effect on future planning. *Lancet*, **i**, 710–13.

Tyrer, P. (1985). The hive system. A model for a psychiatric service. *British Journal of Psychiatry*, **146**, 571–5.

Tyrer, P. (1993). Who is failing the mentally ill? *Lancet*, **341**, 1199–201.

Tyrer, P. (1996) Comorbidity or consanguinity. *British Journal of Psychiatry*, **168**, 669–71.

Tyrer, P. and Ferguson, B. (2000). Classification of personality disorder. In *Personality disorders: diagnosis, management and course* (2nd edn) (ed. P. Tyrer), pp. 13–43. Edward Arnold, London.

Tyrer, P. and Johnson, T. (1996) Establishing the severity of personality disorder. *American Journal of Psychiatry*, **153**, 1593–7.

Tyrer, P. and Malone, S. (1991). Psychiatry without hospital beds: a review of treatment strategies. In *Recent advances in clinical psychiatry* (ed. K. Granville-Grosman), pp. 105–18. Churchill Livingstone, Edinburgh.

Tyrer, P., Turner, R., and Johnson, A.L. (1989). Integrated hospital and community psychiatric services and use of inpatient beds. *British Medical Journal*, **299**, 298–300.

Tyrer, P., Ferguson, B., and Wadsworth, J. (1990*a*). Liaison psychiatry in general practice: the comprehensive collaborative model. *Acta Psychiatrica Scandinavica*, **81**, 359–63.

Tyrer, P., Hawksworth, J., Hobbs, R., and Jackson, D. (1990*b*). The role of the community psychiatric nurse. *British Journal of Hospital Medicine*, **43**, 439–42.

Tyrer, P., Casey, P., and Ferguson, B. (1991). Personality disorder in perspective. *British Journal of Psychiatry*, **159**, 463–71.

Tyrer, P., Seivewright, N., Ferguson, B., and Tyrer, J. (1992). The general neurotic syndrome: a coaxial diagnosis of anxiety, depression and personality disorder. *Acta Psychiatrica Scandinavica*, **85**, 201–6.

Tyrer, P., Morgan, J., Van Horn, E., *et al.* (1995). Randomised controlled study of close monitoring of vulnerable psychiatric patients. *Lancet*, **345**, 756–9.

Tyrer, P., Coid, J., Simmonds, S., Marriott, S., and Joseph, P. (1999) Community mental health team management for those with severe mental illness and disordered personality. In *Schizophrenia module of the Cochrane database of systematic reviews* (ed. C.E. Adams, L. Duggan, J. de Jesus Mari, and P. White). Cochrane Collaboration, Oxford.

UK700 Group (1999). Intensive versus standard case management for severe psychotic illness: a randomised trial. *Lancet*, **353**, 2185–9.

Wallace, P., Cutler, S., and Haines, A. (1988). Randomised controlled trial of general practitioner intervention in patients with excess alcohol consumption. *British Medical Journal*, **297**, 663–8.

Weaver, T., Renton, A., Stimson, G., and Tyrer, P. (1999) Severe mental illness and substance misuse comorbidity: research is needed to inform policy and service development. *British Medical Journal*, **318**, 137–8.

Weatherall, D.J. (1991). *The new genetics and clinical practice*. Oxford University Press.

WHO (1992). *International classification of diseases, 10th revision*. WHO, Geneva.

Zigmond, A.S. and Snaith, R.P. (1983). The Hospital Anxiety and Depression Scale. *Acta Psychiatrica Scandinavica*, **57**, 361–70.

9.8 Dental public health

Stanley Gelbier and Peter G. Robinson

Definition

Under a variety of guises dental public health has come to the fore in developed and developing countries. The British Association for the Study of Community Dentistry defines dental public health as: 'the science and the art of preventing oral diseases, promoting oral health and improving the quality of life through the organized efforts of society'. In the United Kingdom, it has become very sophisticated, there now being a recognized speciality of dental public health. The areas which are perceived to be the business of British consultants and specialists in dental public health include:

- indicators of oral health
- determinants of oral health status
- evaluation of oral health services
- prevention and control of oral disease
- promotion of oral health
- policy and service development and prioritization
- evaluation of technology
- the effectiveness of treatment modalities
- promotion of clinical effectiveness
- evidenced-based commissioning.

Although defining the United Kingdom situation, these areas are of relevance worldwide. They also help to provide cost and clinically effective services.

In order to be prepared to undertake such specialized work, specialist registrars in the United Kingdom undertake a period of education and training. Before entry to the training programme, candidates must possess a fellowship or membership in dental surgery of one of the Royal Surgical Colleges (England, Edinburgh, Glasgow, or Ireland). They also gain a Master of Science degree in dental public health (or its equivalent), either before or during the training period. The training programme takes place under the direction of an established consultant in the specialty. During training they are expected to demonstrate the acquisition of a number of distinctive competencies, which will enable them to undertake their work. These competencies have been divided by the specialty into the eight areas listed below. All have relevance in both developing and developed countries, although the emphasis on particular components will vary according to social factors, the burden of disease, organization of health services, geographical factors, and the economy.

1. **Oral health needs and demands assessment**: description of the determinants of oral disease; identification of determinants amenable to change; understanding the principles of epidemiology and biostatistics in relation to dentistry; derivation of appropriate dental indicators; survey and database design; and data analysis including interpretation of statistics and application of results.
2. **Information technology, commissioning, and evaluation of dental health services**: knowledge of the availability and methods of access to various sources of information within the health service; understanding the contracting processes through which health services are purchased and monitored; contracting and service specification development to meet dental health needs; derivation and measures of oral health improvement and application of appropriate economic analysis.
3. **Promoting oral health**: ability to interpret oral health and dental practice in terms of social relationships and social context; understanding of the principles, methods, and limitations of preventive dentistry and oral health promotion.
4. **Research and development**: identification of appropriate areas for research and development and the application to this of research methodology.
5. **Teaching and training**: at undergraduate and postgraduate level and in multidisciplinary/multiagency settings.
6. **Effective communication**: negotiation; influencing; communication (written, oral, and non-verbal); listening; counselling.
7. **Management**: resource management, control, leadership, planning, conflict management, team work/co-ordination, organization.
8. **Political acumen**: developing policy, political awareness (the art of the possible), evaluating strategy, strategic opportunism.

In the subsequent sections we shall show how some of these areas are used in everyday practice.

The importance of oral health

Oral health is often a low priority for individuals, policy-makers, and public health specialists. In fact, oral health is an important public health problem because oral diseases have significant impacts on individuals and the community, they are widespread, and the two most common diseases—tooth decay (dental caries) and gum (periodontal) diseases—are almost entirely preventable.

The impacts of oral disease range between frank mortality and effects on systemic health and quality of life. Oral diseases also create a considerable burden to both individuals and the community in terms of economic productivity.

Impacts of oral disease

Mortality from oral cancer is related to the site in the mouth and the timing of the diagnosis but 5-year survival is less than 50 per cent. In addition to mortality, oral disease affects other aspects of systemic health. Limited dietary choice and calorific and micronutrient intake are direct consequences of conditions such as xerostomia, poorly fitting dentures, loss of teeth in nursing caries, and oral developmental disorders (Hollister and Weintraub 1993). The role of bacteraemia as a sequel of oral disease and treatment is well known in the aetiology of bacterial endocarditis but periodontal diseases may also be aetiological factors for cardiovascular disease and low birth weight.

Oral diseases also directly affect our quality of life (Slade 1997). Dental pain is very common. As many as one in eight adults in the United States experience toothache over a 6-month period and still more have sore mouths and joint pains (Lipton *et al.* 1993). One in six 8-year-olds in a suburb of London had experienced toothache which had caused them to cry (Shepherd *et al.* 1999). Oral appearance affects our self-esteem, our willingness to interact with others, and influences the judgements other people make about us (Shaw *et al.* 1985; Fiske and Waters 1990). Good dental appearance is regarded as a requirement for some prestigious occupations (Jenny and Proshek 1986).

The economic costs of dental disease are difficult to calculate. As well as the direct costs of disease and treatment, there are indirect costs which might include reduced employment or promotion expectations and opportunities, limitation of academic achievement, and the total societal burden through loss of economic productivity. The direct costs are between 0.2 and 1 per cent of the gross national product in developed countries (van Amerongen *et al.* 1993). The United Kingdom is at the lower end of this range. Yet dentists' fees for treatment within the National Health Service (**NHS**) in England and Wales (population 52 million) for the first 3 months of 1999 were £357 million (equivalent to £1.4 billion per annum) and the figure is rising each year (Dental Practice Board 1999). This sum is all the more surprising when it is considered that only 18 million of the population are registered with an NHS dentist. The cost of treatment provided outside the NHS is not known. An indication of the loss of economic productivity due to dental disease was calculated by Gift *et al.* (1992). In 1989, over 20 million work days and 51 million school hours were lost in the United States due to oral disease and its treatment. These data equate to 1.5 h for each employee annually. Low-income families were more likely to lose time from work and school because of dental disease and so these impacts of oral disease compound the inequalities that already exist in health, income, and educational attainment.

Frequency of oral disease

Oropharyngeal cancers are amongst the 10 most common cancers in the world and their incidence is increasing. The highest reported incidence rates are in India and Sri Lanka where the mouth is the most common site, comprising up to 40 per cent of all cancers. Despite falls in incidence of dental caries over the last three decades, 45 per cent of 5-year-olds in Great Britain have evidence of clinically significant tooth decay (Pitts and Palmer 1995). Periodontal diseases are even more common. More than 80 per cent of adults have inflamed gums (gingivitis) and most have evidence of destruction of the attachment between tooth and bone (periodontitis) (Brown *et al.* 1989; Todd and Lader 1991).

Prevention

Finally, the two most common oral diseases are almost entirely preventable. Clinically significant dental caries occurs only in the presence of excess dietary sugar. Estimates suggest that the incidence of disease could be kept acceptably low at levels of sugar consumption below 10 to 15 kg/person/year (Sheiham 1991). This dietary control of tooth decay can be supplemented by the use of fluorides which demonstrably prevent the disease whether presented in drinking water or in toothpastes. Likewise, the presence of dental plaque is necessary for the most common form of destructive periodontal disease. Targets for oral cleanliness have been calculated which appear to be compatible with freedom from periodontal disease throughout life (Burt *et al.* 1985). Slightly higher levels of plaque might be compatible with acceptably low levels of periodontal disease.

Therefore oral health therefore has a public health significance. This chapter will discuss the features, epidemiology, aetiology, and management of four important oral diseases: dental caries, periodontal diseases, oral cancer, and orofacial trauma. Approaches to oral health promotion in relation to these diseases will be outlined within a common risk factor approach.

Dental caries

Under normal circumstances, there is a chemical equilibrium between the minerals of the tooth and the adjacent oral fluids. The equilibrium is disrupted by acidic metabolites of oral bacteria if there is an excess of dietary sugars. Dental caries is the progressive demineralization of the tooth that results. In the very early stages, the lesion appears as a chalky white spot on the teeth. If the lesion progresses, the surface of the tooth breaks down and there is cavitation. If the caries reaches the underlying dentine, it can spread more readily through the porous and less mineralized tissue toward the pulp. Infection of the pulp may allow the passage of bacteria along the root canals to the alveolar bone.

The direct consequences of this process are destruction of the tooth, pain, and a possible dental abscess. Dentine is sensitive to physical, thermal, and osmotic stimuli. When it is exposed by cavitation there may be transient pain associated with hot or cold drinks or sweet foods. Later, as the pulp becomes inflamed, the discomfort may be spontaneous, exquisitely painful, and of longer duration. In a dental abscess, pressure to the tooth is transmitted to the infected alveolus and the unfortunate person avoids biting or knocking the tooth.

Four factors are necessary for the development of caries: dietary sugars, a susceptible tooth surface, the microflora of dental plaque, and adequate time.

Despite the obvious ethical difficulties of conducting human experimental studies to investigate the role of sugars in the aetiology of dental caries, the evidence implicating them is more than compelling. Rugg-Gunn's (1993) encyclopaedic review classifies this evidence methodologically into human observational studies, human interventional studies, animal experiments, enamel slab experiments, plaque pH studies, and incubation experiments. Dietary sugars are essential if the caries is to be of clinical relevance. The bacteria of dental plaque, particularly *Streptococcus mutans*, metabolize them and so produce acids and use them to form extracellular polysaccharides. The polysaccharides increase the bulk of the plaque, facilitate the adhesion of more bacteria, and restrict the flow of saliva to the tooth surface. With each exposure to sugar the plaque pH falls sharply and rises slowly back to normal levels over the following hours. It follows that caries incidence is related to the frequency of intake of sugars (Gustaffson *et al.* 1954).

The mineral component of the tooth is predominantly calcium and phoshate in the form of hydroxyapatite. At normal pH levels, the hydroxyapatite crystals of tooth are in dynamic equilibrium with these ions in the plaque fluid. At high pH there is remineralization of the tooth, especially in the presence of fluoride. Saliva plays a crucial protective role against caries by simple dilution, by buffering plaque acid, and by acting as a source of minerals and chemical and immunological plaque inhibitory factors. For these reasons dental caries is more frequent in the sites less accessible to the saliva—the pits and fissures of posterior teeth and between these teeth. Caries is also more common in people with restricted salivary flow.

Epidemiology

Caries of the permanent dentition is traditionally measured using an index which records the number of decayed, missing, and filled teeth. A more precise index records the number of surfaces affected and a similar index is used to record the status of the deciduous dentition. Because the index aggregates both disease and treatment experience it is sensitive to the treatment decisions of dentists and so less valid with increasing age. Since each of the categories is equally weighted, it is insensitive to both the severity of the disease and outcomes of treatment. At low levels of caries the number of people 'caries free' (which actually means free from clinical evidence of progressive disease and treatment) may be a more useful community-based measure of disease.

Nonetheless the decayed, missing, and filled teeth index has been used for 60 years and will continue to be used. This does not mean that decayed, missing, and filled teeth index scores of yesteryear are directly comparable with those of today as the criteria for judging a tooth as carious have changed. Although the threshold for diagnosis is usually whether the caries has reached dentine, many previous criteria used a sharp dental probe to determine whether there was cavitation of the tooth (WHO 1979). The criteria now in use in many countries avoid the use of probes to prevent damaging the tooth surface. Consequently, the index is less sensitive and more specific (WHO 1997). However, the dental status of populations is usually summarized by the mean decayed, missing, and filled teeth index of 12-year-old children. Chronological and international comparisons are made with these data.

Although dental caries can be identified in the teeth of skulls found in archaeology, dental caries as it is known today did not emerge until sugar became widely available (Burt 1978). Levels of caries rose during the seventeenth century and reached epidemic proportions in the nineteenth and twentieth centuries. The disease has been exceedingly common in some populations with near universal experience in some generations in many countries. Since systematic data have been collected, the typical pattern has been one of high levels of caries in developed countries associated with exposure to sugars. In the mid-1970s levels in many developed countries began to fall dramatically (Marthaler 1990*a*). In the United Kingdom, the mean decayed, missing, and filled teeth index decreased from 4.8 to 1.2 between 1973 and 1993 and by a similar amount in Australia (4.8 to 1.1) between 1977 and 1993 (Downer 1994; Davies *et al.* 1997).

This fall in caries incidence in developed countries appears to have halted in the early to mid-1980s (Burt 1994; Downer 1994). The mean decayed, missing, and filled teeth index of 5-year-olds in England and Wales fell from 4.0 to 1.8 between 1973 and 1983 but now appears stable at around 1.8. Despite the halted fall there are cohorts of children and young adults who have better oral health than preceding generations. As these cohorts age there will be commensurate improvements in adult oral health.

Data on caries levels aggregated at the national level provide useful information but can mask important trends. The fall in caries incidence has polarized the inequalities in oral health. In times of high disease prevalence nearly everybody had the disease and the inequalities were manifest merely as differences in the number of teeth affected in an individual. With lower disease prevalence a minority of people carry the burden of most of the disease. Half of all 12-year-olds in England and Wales have never had tooth decay of their permanent teeth (Downer 1994). As is the case for most important diseases, in developed countries dental caries and its consequences are increasingly diseases of the poor (Gratrix and Holloway 1994; Watt and Sheiham 1999).

There have been concerns of increasing levels of caries in developing countries although other analysts suggest that there are no major trends (Holm 1990; Manji and Fejerskov 1990; Fejerskov *et al.* 1994). Recent surveys in Africa show that caries levels in 12-year-olds are still relatively low although there are suggestions of increases in some countries. Aggregated national data may mask local variations, and in particular, high caries levels in urban areas. Such trends would reflect economic and cultural trends in the region with the change from traditional starchy foods to greater consumption of refined carbohydrates (Thorpe 1993). Of particular concern is the fact that 90 per cent of the caries in Africa remains untreated.

Traditional treatment

Until the nineteenth century the only useful treatment for dental caries was extraction of the affected tooth. Since then there has been a transition to restorative care in which the infected parts of the tooth are removed and replaced with an inert obdurating filling. During the latter half of the twentieth century technology moved forward, dentists became keen to make use of recent innovations, and patients became willing to pay for them. The result is that operative treatment for adults is increasingly complex and technology intensive. Badly decayed teeth can now be restored with a range of adhesive tooth coloured materials that are either formed in the mouth or prepared in laboratories and then fitted. Originally, missing teeth could only be replaced with removable dentures. Now they can be replaced with bridges which adhere to the remaining teeth or with prostheses supported by osseo-integrated implants which project out through the gingivae.

These treatments provided by dentists might reduce the social impact of dental caries on affected people but play a very minor role in preventing the disease. Dental services explained 3 per cent of the reduction in caries levels in industrialized countries during the 1970s compared with the 65 per cent contribution made by broader socio-economic factors and the availability of fluoride toothpastes (Nadanovsky and Sheiham 1994, 1995).

Implications of changes in caries prevalence

The low incidence of disease experienced in the developed world over the last 15 years has profound implications for the management of dental caries. When the incidence of the disease is low, proportionately more caries affects the accessible occlusal surfaces of the teeth and only simple restorations are needed to treat it (Stamm 1991). The disease also progresses more slowly which allows dentists to defer operative treatment whilst attempting to prevent the spread of the lesion. Many lesions are detected at an earlier stage so that new dental materials can be used in minimally invasive techniques (Elderton 1990).

The lower levels of disease mean that the costs of some dental services might be reduced by reducing the number of interventions and the number of dentists. Increasing the intervals between dental examinations is safe and effective for children and adults with low disease incidence (Riordan 1997). Since most of the restorations required by children are relatively simple, the number and costs of dentists can be reduced by using less highly trained auxiliaries. The reduced burden of disease may allow general dental practitioners to become more involved in health promotion, and to place a greater emphasis on prevention and on quality (Rear 1994). Elderton (1994) has argued for a reduced emphasis on operative technique in dental training so that dentists can become more like physicians working with a range of auxiliaries to obtain the maximum health gain for populations. Conversely, there are still many older people (in this case that means more than around 35 years of age!) who have suffered the ravages of dental caries and its treatment. These people will continue to need and demand increasingly complex treatment for the next 25 years or so (Treasure and Whyman 1995).

Periodontal diseases

Periodontal diseases comprise a range of inflammatory diseases of the periodontium categorized by the position of attachment between gingiva and tooth (Caton 1989). In gingivitis the attachment remains in a healthy position near the cement–enamel junction. Periodontitis is defined by migration of the epithelium which reduces the amount of periodontal ligament and bone supporting the tooth.

Gingivitis is an inflammatory response to plaque. Along with redness and swelling, the gums may bleed on gentle provocation such as cleaning the teeth. Pain is an uncommon feature. Systemic involvement including hormonal changes, skin diseases, and medication use may modify these diseases or cause other gingival changes. The disease is exceedingly common. Bleeding on probing is present in 79 per cent of adults in the United Kingdom and 85 per cent in the United States (Brown *et al.* 1989; Todd and Lader 1991). Erythematous changes are likely to be more frequent.

In periodontitis the loss of periodontal attachment is manifest by deepening of the pockets between the gingivae and teeth and by recession of the gingivae. In severe cases, the supporting structures are so depleted that the teeth become loose. The disease is rarely, if ever, painful unless an acute infection complicates a periodontal pocket ('a lateral periodontal abscess') or if the exposed root surfaces are temperature sensitive.

Sophisticated classificatory systems categorize periodontitis by its age of onset and systemic involvement (Caton 1989), but adult periodontitis is by far the most common form. Its frequency is difficult to assess. The 'burst theories' suggest that there are episodes of localized destructive disease followed by quiescence (Socransky *et al.* 1984). In this case lost periodontal attachment may be the legacy of previous disease and more sophisticated tests are required to detect 'active' disease.

Mild periodontal pocketing is common. For example, it is seen in half or more of adults in the United Kingdom and the United States (Brown *et al.* 1989; Todd and Lader 1991). Evidence of severe periodontitis is much less frequent. Lost attachment or pockets of 6 mm or more (thought to be sufficient to threaten tooth survival) are seen in less than 8 per cent of adults in the United States and the United Kingdom (Miller *et al.* 1987; Todd and Lader 1991). Evidence of the disease is more frequent and severe in countries where tooth cleaning practices are less sophisticated (Loe *et al.* 1986).

One other periodontal disease has public health importance. Acute necrotizing ulcerative gingivitis (Vincent's infection or 'trench-mouth') causes necrosis, ulceration, soreness, and bleeding of the gingivae (Johnson and Engel 1986). The ulcerated papillae may have a grey slough and there may be a characteristic fetor. Lymphadenopathy and mild fever are variable findings. In many developed countries, acute necrotizing ulcerative gingivitis is a disease of young adults. There are no good incidence data, but anecdotally it has become less frequent among some developed populations in recent years. A variant of the disease is associated with HIV infection (Robinson *et al.* 1998). Acute necrotizing ulcerative gingivitis is also seen in African children where it can be progressive in the absence of treatment (Emslie 1963). In severe cases necrosis may extend over adjacent and contiguous tissues to cause gross destruction of oral and facial tissues (known as cancrum oris or noma).

Pathogenesis

The pathogenesis of periodontitis involves the interaction of plaque pathogens with the host's immune system (Genco and Slots 1984). Periodontal destruction occurs directly as a result of pathogenic bacterial components and indirectly via host destructive mechanisms that are part of the immune response to infection (Genco 1990).

Dental plaques are consistently implicated in the aetiology of periodontal diseases. Gingivitis is initiated by plaque and reduced by its mechanical and chemical suppression (Silness and Loe 1964; Loe *et al.* 1965; Loe and Schiott 1970). Plaque is also implicated in periodontitis (Lovdal *et al.* 1958). Plaque pathogens have virulence factors, including endo- and exotoxins, and initiate and enhance alveolar destruction in animal studies (Gibbons and Socransky 1966; Slots and Genco 1984; Holt *et al.* 1988). Progression of periodontal destruction is reduced by controlled oral hygiene (Suomi *et al.* 1971; Axelsson and Lindhe 1978).

Considerable research is devoted to determining which, if any, specific pathogens are responsible for periodontal destruction (the 'specific plaque hypothesis'). Dental plaque is ubiquitous but destructive disease occurs only in a minority of people. Therefore plaque is not sufficient cause for periodontitis, and microbiological research has diverted attention away from the important determinants of periodontal disease susceptibility (Clarke and Hirsch 1995).

Tobacco use is often confounded by poor oral hygiene in periodontal research, but it is now clear that tobacco exerts an independent deleterious effect (Bergstrom 1989; Ismail *et al.* 1990; Stoltenberg *et al.* 1993; Martínez-Canut *et al.* 1995). In addition, periodontal treatment is less effective in smokers (Preber and Bergstrom 1985, 1990). Stress is also a risk factor in periodontal diseases. Greater occupational stress is associated with progression of periodontitis, and acute necrotizing ulcerative gingivitis has been noted among soldiers on difficult postings, students during examination terms, and people with other negative life events (Roth 1951; Giddon *et al.* 1963; Linden *et al.* 1996).

Periodontitis often takes decades to become detectable clinically. Accordingly, it is more common and severe with advanced years because age confounds disease duration (Abdellatif and Burt 1987). Periodontitis is not a consequence of age (Papapanou and Lindhe 1992), it is associated with poor oral hygiene irrespective of age (Suomi *et al.* 1971), and it does not progress in adults with good oral hygiene (Loe *et al.* 1978).

In the last few years, periodontal diseases have been linked to a number of other health problems including cardiovascular diseases, stroke, preterm birth, and low birth weight. A number of authors suggest that periodontal diseases may even be independent risk factors for these diseases. Several reports have focused on the biological plausibility of these associations. Periodontal pathogens may invade endothelial cells or periodontal diseases may provide a burden of endotoxins and cytokines which initiate and exacerbate atherogenesis and thrombus formation (Beck *et al.* 1996; Deshpande *et al.* 1999).

The main epidemiological evidence supporting links between periodontal and other diseases arises from retrospective analysis of cohort data and from case–control studies (Beck *et al.* 1996; Offenbacher *et al.* 1996; Dasanayake 1998). However, there is the potential for misclassification along with other sources of bias in these types of studies. Whilst efforts have been made to control for socio-economic and lifestyle factors, some residual confounding resulting from a failure to account fully for these variables seems inevitable. Specific cardiovascular risk factors such as tobacco use, obesity, and lower serum high-density lipoprotein cholesterol are more common among people with high dental disease experience (Johansson *et al.* 1994). Some of these factors, such as tobacco smoking, are independent risk factors for both cardiovascular and periodontal diseases whereas others may be linked less directly.

This area of research is exciting periodontal researchers. Large-scale cross-sectional, prospective, and intervention studies to evaluate these possible links are underway. In the meantime no firm conclusions can be drawn (Davenport *et al.* 1998; Joshipura *et al.* 1998).

Treatment

For the majority of people the progression of periodontal destruction is compatible with the retention of a natural dentition into old age. Targets for oral cleanliness have been calculated which appear to be compatible with freedom from periodontal disease throughout life or compatible with acceptably low levels of periodontal disease (Burt *et al.*1985).

A significant minority of people (perhaps 5–15 per cent) may loose teeth as a result of periodontal diseases, and considerable effort is spent by dentists and dental hygienists attempting to prevent and treat them. Both the prevention and treatment of periodontal diseases focus on the mechanical removal of plaque. Dental professionals attempt to bring this about by instructing patients in the use of toothbrushes and dental floss. Adjunctive services provided by personal dental services include the removal of calcified plaque (calculus) as it may harbour micro-organisms and provide a mechanical barrier to inhibit effective self-care and planing the surfaces of the roots to remove the superficial layers which might be contaminated with bacterial toxins. In some cases the architecture of the periodontium may be surgically adjusted to excise diseased tissue and allow the entry of toothbrush bristles and dental floss into inaccessible areas. In recent times a technique known as guided tissue regeneration has used membranes of synthetic material to prevent epithelial cells proliferating down the root surface after periodontal surgery. This technique allows modest local gains in attachment between the tooth and the underlying periodontium.

A comprehensive review of professionally administered mechanical oral hygiene practices cast considerable doubts on the effectiveness of most interventions commonly employed to treat periodontal diseases (Frandsen 1986). In general, interventions aimed at improving oral hygiene produce only short-term changes which are not sustained (Kay and Locker 1997). Other procedures to treat periodontal diseases, such as the removal of calculus by scaling and polishing, root planing, and removal of plaque at intervals greater than 4 weeks, may not be effective and are harmful in some circumstances. Fourteen million of these interventions are carried out each year in England and Wales alone.

Oral malignancy

Almost 90 per cent of oral malignancies are squamous cell carcinomas. They may occur on the lip, tongue, gingivae, oral floor, or elsewhere in the mouth. The site is often related to the aetiological factors. Lesions may present as swellings, ulcers, or red or white patches, and many are painless until they become large. Significantly, survival is related to the stage of the disease at presentation. Five-year survival is less than 50 per cent.

Malignant change is often seen in a number of lesions which precede the development of the tumour. These premalignant lesions present as leukoplakias and erythroplakias of unknown origin. Malignant change is also seen, albeit infrequently, in oral lichen planus and hyperplastic candidiasis.

The incidence of oral cancer varies dramatically between and within countries. In England and Wales the incidence is 4.5 per 100 000 which represents approximately 1 per cent of total cancer incidence (OPCS 1994). The highest reported incidence rates are in India and Sri Lanka where the mouth is the most common site and comprises up to 40 per cent of all cancers (Parkin *et al.* 1992). Men are more susceptible than women in almost all populations independent of the effects of tobacco use (Muscat *et al.* 1996).

Variations in the incidence of oral malignancy are largely explained by varying exposure to three major risk factors. Cancer of the lower lip is strongly associated with exposure to sunlight, especially in people with fair skin (Lindquist and Teppo 1978). Tobacco use, whether chewed or smoked, predisposes to intra-oral cancer. The high incidence of oral cancer among southern Asians is largely accounted for by the addition of tobacco to betel quid or *paan* (Johnson and Warnakalasuriya 1993). There are dose–response relationships for the duration of use and type of tobacco inhaled. Alcohol is also an independent aetiological factor and has a synergistic relationship with tobacco use (Rothman and Keller 1972; Blot 1992).

Since oral cancer is predominantly a disease of older people, it is likely that demographic changes, particularly in developing countries, will see an increased incidence of the disease (Swango 1996). However, age-specific incidence rates in developed countries are relatively stable. A reduction in alcohol consumption combined with the reductions in tobacco smoking already evident in some countries has the potential to make sizeable reduction of the burden of these cancers (Macfarlane *et al.* 1996).

Because early intervention determines survival in oral cancer, and because many cases are preceded by premalignant lesions, there is a strong argument for case finding as a method of disease control (Platz *et al.* 1986; Hindle and Nally 1991; Speight *et al.* 1993). Despite the low prevalence of the disease, screening for oral cancer appears to have acceptable validity. Uptake of screening services is greatest when they are offered in workplace settings (Downer 1997).

Dentofacial trauma

Trauma to the teeth is common and frequently causes fracture of the tooth or supporting bone, and bodily movement of the tooth including complete avulsion. In many cases the long-term survival of the tooth is threatened. Since the anterior and most visible teeth are most often involved the result is disfiguring. Approximately one in four teenagers in the United Kingdom have damaged permanent teeth as a result of trauma (Todd and Dodd 1985). The incidence is greatest among young children who have just learnt to walk and among school-age children who may be using bicycles and skateboards (Gelbier 1967). Teenagers and adults who play contact or other vigorous sports are also at risk (Federation Dentaire Internationale 1990). A child's risk of dental trauma is directly related to the distance that the upper teeth protrude in front of the lower teeth (the overjet) (Todd and Dodd 1985). Primary prevention involves wearing a mouthguard during contact sports such as American football, rugby football, hockey, and boxing. Where possible, play areas for young children should have cushioned surfaces.

Aspects of secondary prevention are crucial for traumatized teeth. Deciduous teeth must be monitored in case any infection occurring as a sequel to the trauma threatens the permanent tooth developing beneath it. In permanent teeth, adhesive fillings can be used to protect sensitive fractured teeth and calcium hydroxide dressings may be placed to allow continued root development in immature teeth. However, the most important aspect of secondary prevention is the first aid of teeth which have been knocked out.

Avulsed teeth can be replaced in the socket (Andreasen and Andreasen 1994). Long-term survival rates of avulsed teeth are high, but are greatest if the tooth is replanted within 30 min to prevent drying, if it is stored in an isotonic medium (e.g. milk) in the interim, if the periodontal ligament is not damaged by physical or chemical cleaning, and if the tooth is held in place by a semi-rigid splint for a week. Systemic antibiotic and antitetanus treatments are required.

The effectiveness of this secondary preventive intervention has two public health implications. Informing athletes and their teachers and trainers of these principles can reduce the impact of dentofacial trauma. The need for almost immediate care means that skilled emergency dental services should be available wherever possible. Unfortunately, dentofacial trauma is not limited to office hours.

Oral health promotion

Since oral diseases are brought about by people's behaviours, dentistry has traditionally adopted health education as the central thrust of prevention. Toothbrushing and sugar reduction messages have been repeated in both chairside and public education campaigns. However, dental educators have become disillusioned with the recognition that health education cannot readily change these behaviours which are largely determined by our social and cultural environment. Indeed, health education carries its own dangers of disempowerment and victim-blaming and may increase inequalities in oral health (Labonte and Penfold 1981; Schou and Wight 1994).

Closer examination of the causes of oral disorders reveal the potential value of community-based approaches to maintain oral health by acting on the wider determinants of health. Oral disease is brought about by the consumption of sugars, ineffective oral cleaning, tobacco and alcohol use, limited exposure to fluoride, and stress. The common worldwide trend towards widening inequality in economic, social conditions, and health is because the most important non-communicable diseases are determined by lifestyle factors such as these. Therefore the determinants of oral health are the determinants of health in general, and there are many opportunities for wider social and environmental action to play an invaluable role in promoting oral health. There is an increasing recognition that a 'common-risk factor' approach is fundamental to the integrated approach to oral health promotion (Sheiham 1992). Collective and multidisciplinary action against factors linked to many diseases reduces duplication, saves resources, and improves effectiveness (Grabauskas 1987).

An additional consideration is that preventive strategies which focus on individuals do not appear to be suitable for dental caries and periodontal diseases since as yet there are no effective ways of identifying which individuals are at high risk of developing the diseases (Rose 1985; Johnson 1991*a*,*b*). Whilst individuals at high risk for dental disease cannot be identified with adequate sensitivity and specificity it is possible to identify at-risk populations. In these situations it can be cost-effective to target preventive interventions at people in specific socio-economic groups, attending particular schools, or living in an area with high disease incidence (Burt 1998). However, a strategy of targeted interventions should take place within a common risk factor approach which addresses general health conditions for the whole population. Such an approach will reduce social inequalities and will provide a multiplicity of benefits. It also avoids the limitations inherent in attempting to identify and treat differently those individuals at high risk for disease. Finally, a recognition of the social context in which personal choices are made avoids the social iatrogenesis of describing oral heath in individual terms (Dickson 1995). Dentistry has been quick to adopt approaches which would now be recognized as health promoting. For example, fluoride levels in water supplies were adjusted to prevent dental caries as early as 1945 (Dean *et al.* 1950).

Health promotion, the process of enabling people to take control over and to improve their health, has five broad actions: creating supportive environments, building healthy public policy, strengthening community action, developing personal skills, and reorienting health services (WHO 1984, 1986). Within this approach Sheiham (1995) suggested six policy areas relevant to oral health:

- the use of fluoride

- food and health policies to reduce sugar consumption
- community approaches to improve body hygiene including oral cleaning
- smoking cessation
- policies on reducing accidents
- ensuring access to appropriate preventive care.

This framework will be used in this chapter.

With the growing emphasis on evidence-based health care, oral health promotion must increasingly demonstrate its effectiveness. Recent systematic reviews have aimed to identify oral health promotion practices which yield demonstrable health gains or modified knowledge or behaviours (Brown 1994; Kay and Locker 1996, 1997; Sprod *et al.* 1996). The principle findings were of a paucity of evidence with few reports of well-designed studies in which the intended outcome was health gain. The most robust studies tended to focus on programmes in which the intended outcome was improved knowledge or modification of the behaviours of individuals. Even these studies, which might be termed 'health education', usually involved a relatively short follow-up. The principle finding in meta-analysis was the effectiveness of fluoride to prevent caries (Kay and Locker 1997). A less rigorous approach adopted by Sprod *et al.* (1966) allowed exploration of other avenues of activity and research but still concluded that there was little evaluative literature in relation to the broader issues of health promotion.

One problem of broad strategies to promote health is that they do not lend themselves to current concepts of outcome evaluation (Sprod *et al.* 1996; Health Education Board for Scotland 1996; Stillman-Lowe 1998). The link between environment and oral health is indirect and is often mediated by individual behaviours. It is difficult to construct formal randomized controlled trials for this type of intervention and any health gain may take some time to become measurable. All the effectiveness reviews called for more careful evaluation and for the development of outcome measures more appropriate for oral health promotion. One core concern is the question: 'What is oral health?'

Therefore oral health promotion finds itself at a cross-roads. Broad social and environmental approaches which act at the level of determinants of health and common risk factors for disease offer radical and exciting opportunities to promote health. However, in an increasingly restricted financial climate and with commensurate demands for evidence of effectiveness, proponents of health promotion must act to show how these broader approaches can deliver their promise.

The use of fluoride

The presence of fluoride at the interface between plaque and dental enamel inhibits the development of caries. To be most effective, fluoride should be present both before the teeth start to develop and then continuously throughout life. These findings suggest its effect is derived from a combination of modes of action. Three modes currently receive the most attention: the effect of fluoride on plaque metabolism, the effect of its incorporation during tooth development, and its effect on the dynamics of demineralization and remineralization in exposures which occur after tooth development.

Fluoride is present in dental plaque at concentrations 50 to 100 times higher than in saliva. At these concentrations it can affect the plaque metabolism to prevent the adhesion of plaque to the teeth. As the organisms produce acids, fluoride may be released from the plaque matrix. At these yet higher concentrations it may kill or inhibit acidogenic organisms and so negatively reinforce acid production. The presence of fluoride during dental enamel hydroxyapatite formation may allow its incorporation into the crystal lattice to produce the larger and more stable crystals of fluorapatite which are less soluble. A similar phenomenon occurs during exposure to fluoride after tooth development. The high concentrations of fluoride present in plaque at low pH increases the tendency for enamel to remineralize rather than demineralize. As the minerals precipitate back onto the enamel surface, the available fluoride is incorporated onto the remineralizing enamel as fluorapatite or calcium fluoride, both of which inhibit future demineralization.

Water fluoridation

The beneficial effect of fluoride on dental health was discovered as a consequence of investigations of endemic developmental defects of teeth in Colorado. McKay implicated the water supplies in the aetiology of the staining and pits and discovered that teeth with defects were less susceptible to dental caries than those without (McKay 1933). The staining was shown to be due to fluoride which existed in some of McKay's samples at levels as high as 14 ppm.

Dean *et al.* (1941) went on to demonstrate the inverse relationship between dental caries and the fluoride concentration of drinking water (and the associated fluorosis) in two cross-sectional ecological studies (now called the '21 Cities Studies'). The first intervention trial of fluoridation started in Grand Rapids in 1945 (Dean *et al.* 1950). Since then, similar studies have taken place in many countries including the United Kingdom, the Netherlands, and Australia (Murray *et al.* 1991).

By 1998, approximately 60 countries had reported projects to fluoridate public drinking water supplies. The entire populations of Hong Kong and Singapore receive fluoridated water, 67 per cent of those in Australia, 62 per cent of the United States, and approximately 10 per cent of the United Kingdom.

Where it is possible, fluoridation remains the most cost-effective method of reducing the experience and burden of dental caries. Indeed, it is possibly one of the most cost-effective public health and health promotion measures undertaken in industrialized countries in the last 50 years (Sprod *et al.* 1996). Many of the studies evaluating water fluoridation were conducted in the middle of the twentieth century and lack the scientific rigour of today's standards. A recent systematic review found no randomized controlled trials of water fluoridation (McDonagh *et al.* 2000). Nonetheless, the conclusion was that fluoridation was effective, with a number needed to treat of 6. This figure is relatively high because the incidence of dental caries is relatively low even in the absence of water fluoridation. Fluoridation also prevents the impacts of oral disease by reducing the number of children with toothache and the number who require a general anaesthetic for dental extractions.

Sequential cross-sectional studies show that the maximum benefit occurs in children who have been exposed to fluoridated water since birth (Groeneveld *et al.* 1990). Since the permanent teeth do not begin to erupt until 6 years of age, these data demonstrate that fluoride is beneficial both before and after the teeth erupt. For maximum effect, exposure should be continuous throughout life (Attwood and Blinkhorn 1988). The benefits continue through adulthood (Murray 1971). Long-term exposure also protects against root caries of the teeth of older adults should they become exposed (Burt *et al.* 1986).

There is some evidence that water fluoridation also reduces socio-economic inequalities in caries experience (McDonagh *et al.* 2000). A series of studies conducted in northeast England show that fluoridation is effective across the spectrum of society but more teeth are saved in children from lower socio-economic status families (Carmichael *et al.* 1984, 1989). Several other groups have investigated the nature of this relationship between socio-economic status, fluoridation, and caries (Treasure and Dever 1994). Slade *et al.* (1996) used a range of measures of socio-economic status to show that the presence of fluoride in the drinking water had an additive interaction with socio-economic status in reducing caries experience in 6- and 12-year-olds. In deciduous teeth, fluoridation reduced the difference in caries between rich and poor by the equivalent of one affected tooth surface per child.

The optimal concentration of fluoride in drinking water depends on other exposures to fluoride and on the amount of water drunk. Natural sources of dietary fluoride include tea and the skin and bones of fish (Jenkins and Edgar 1973; Duckworth and Duckworth 1978). Fluoride is also present in foods and beverages processed in areas where the water is fluoridated and there is evidence that it exerts a 'halo effect' which protects people who only receive fluoridated water in this form (Newbrun 1989; Slade *et al.* 1996). However, in many developed countries the largest sources other than that added to the drinking water are from the fluoride added to toothpastes, mouth rinses, and gels.

The amount of fluid drunk is directly related to climactic temperature. Dean *et al.* (1941) originally suggested that the optimal concentration for water fluoridation was 1 ppm (1 mg/l). Since then there has been recognition that living in a warm climate might lead to a high daily dose of fluoride and an awareness that we are exposed to fluoride in other forms. Consequently, lower levels of fluoride are used in warmer climates (US Public Health Service 1962; WHO 1994). For example, the concentration in Hong Kong is 0.5 ppm In Australia, adjusted concentrations vary between 0.6 ppm in Darwin in the subtropical north to 1.1 ppm in Hobart in the more temperate south (Spencer *et al.* 1996).

In many situations fluoridation is the most cost-effective method of administering fluoride. A modest capital investment is required to install the machinery to administer and regulate the addition of fluoride to the drinking water. The whole population is affected and individuals need make no additional effort (such as visiting the dentist) to obtain the benefits. Fluoridation continues to be effective even at the low levels of caries incidence currently seen in the developed world, and the repeated low-dose application achieves the optimal pre- and posteruptive effects. However, fluoridation is less cost-effective in areas without reticulated water supplies serving large populations. In those areas where communities are served by a large number of smaller water supplies other methods of administering fluoride are required.

Fluoride toothpaste

Toothpastes are mixtures of abrasive cleaning agents and refreshing flavourings. They present a good vehicle for the frequent low-dose application of fluoride to increase its availability in dental plaque. Proprietary preparations use a number of agents including sodium fluoride and sodium monofluorophosphate. Stannous fluoride has been used in the past but stained the teeth.

In children, fluoride toothpastes reduce the 2-year incidence of caries by up to 30 per cent (Murray and Naylor 1996) and there is a small additive effect when they are used in areas with water fluoridation (von der Fehr and Moller 1978). Sodium fluoride toothpastes are also effective in preventing caries of the roots of the teeth in older people (Jensen and Kohout 1988).

The effectiveness is primarily related to the concentration of fluoride in the paste up to levels of 2500 ppm (2.5 g of fluoride per kilogram), although most preparations for adults contain approximately 1000 ppm Between 1000 and 2500 ppm each additional 500 ppm provides an additional 6 per cent reduction in caries incidence (Stephen *et al.* 1988). The agent used is less important as long as it is compatible with the abrasive (Holloway and Worthington 1993; Johnson 1993; Stookey *et al.* 1993; Volpe *et al.* 1993). Early fluoride toothpastes used chalk as the abrasive, but this reacted with the fluoride and prevented its release.

In some countries there are special formulations of toothpaste available specifically for children. These toothpastes use lower fluoride concentrations to prevent ingestion of excess fluoride and reduce the risk of dental fluorosis. Again, the effectiveness is related to concentration but preparations containing 500 ppm appear to be similarly effective when compared with conventional preparations (Winter *et al.* 1989).

Therefore toothpastes offer a safe and effective vehicle for the administration of fluoride. The protective effects reported in trials are smaller than those in water fluoridation studies because fluoridation studies usually consider lifetime exposure to fluoride whereas toothpaste trials last for only 2 or 3 years. The addition of fluoride to toothpaste is also compatible with market interests as manufacturers compete to produce the most effective agent. However, the use of fluoride toothpaste has a distinct disadvantage as a broad preventive strategy—it relies on people brushing their teeth. In developed countries, poor oral hygiene and high caries incidence are associated (although not necessarily causally) and so the people who have most to benefit from the use of fluoride toothpastes are less likely to use them frequently. In developing countries, there may not be a tradition of tooth cleaning with toothpastes and Western proprietary brands are likely to be expensive.

Other vehicles for administering fluoride

Other vehicles for administering fluoride can be broadly categorized by whether or not they are taken systemically. Any fluoride taken systemically is liable to have a pre-eruptive effect if it is taken at the correct time. Since systemic fluorides are taken by mouth they are likely to have topical posteruptive effects also.

Fluoridized salt is used by 70 per cent of the population of Switzerland in areas where water fluoridation is not possible (Marthaler 1983). Observational studies of children in that country and in Hungary suggest that the use of salt containing 250 mg fluoride per kilogram has a caries-protective effect, although perhaps not of the same magnitude as that of fluoridated water (Toth 1976; de Crousaz 1985). A controlled study in Colombia demonstrated 48 and 50 per cent reductions in caries incidence (depending on the formulation used) compared with a 60 per cent reduction with water fluoridation (Mejia *et al.* 1976). Therefore fluoridized salt is protective but its use needs to be sustained (Stephen *et al.* 1999).

Fluoride may also be added to milk, school drinking water supplies, and fruit juices. Fluoride was added to the drinking water of schools in the United States for a number of years. Several accidents resulting in acute fluoride poisoning mean that this method is no longer recommended in that country. Early studies using fluoridized milk produced promising results but were flawed. A randomized double-blind trial showed a 43 to 48 per cent reduction in caries after 5 years (Stephen *et al.* 1984). Despite concerns that fluoride added to milk might bind with calcium or proteins to reduce its topical effect (Duff 1981), a number of schemes are being planned in northern England.

One study has tested the effect of fluoridized orange juice. A reduction in caries incidence was observed compared with a group not receiving a drink, but the incidence was also reduced in a group of children receiving a placebo juice without fluoride (Gedalia *et al.* 1981). The use of citrus drinks as a vehicle for fluoride may no longer be recommended because of concerns about the direct erosive effect of the drinks on the teeth.

Dietary fluoride supplements have been used in efforts to duplicate the fluoride intake of drinking water at 1 ppm They usually take the form of sodium fluoride tablets which are sucked or chewed and then swallowed. Early studies of their pre-eruptive effects were flawed by problems of self-selection, lack of controls, and non-blinded examiners, and so failed to distinguish between the effectiveness of the supplements and the confounding effects of patient compliance and other oral-health-related behaviours. Clinical trials of their use after the eruption of the teeth have been more robust and reveal significant preventive effects (DePaola and Lax 1968; Driscoll *et al.* 1978; Stephen and Campbell 1978).

One of the problems of fluoride supplementation is that programmes often rely on the compliance of individuals and their families with an additional health-directed behaviour. Many of the people most susceptible to caries find this new behaviour difficult to adopt. Even in the most compliant individuals, fluoride supplements do not perfectly mimic the effect of water fluoridation since the fluoride is taken as a daily bolus associated with dental fluorosis (Ismail and Bandekar 1999). As a public health measure for children dietary fluoride supplementation is appropriate only for individuals at high risk for dental caries. National bodies in the developed world recommend a number of broadly compatible dosing schedules determined by the age of the child and the fluoride concentration of the drinking water (Riordan 1999). Most schedules for children have been revised downwards in the last 10 years. Dietary fluoride supplements may have some benefit for older people who are more susceptible to root caries in whom there is no risk of fluorosis.

A number of methods of professional application of fluoride have been tried over the years. Gels containing relatively high concentrations of fluoride were applied to the teeth in trays and were effective but only whilst they were being used. Particular care was needed to minimize fluoride ingestion (LeCompte 1987). More cost-effective ways of administering fluoride are usually available.

Safety of fluoride used as a dental public health measure

Fluoride is freely available in the natural world. It is present naturally in almost all fresh groundwaters and is also consumed in some foodstuffs such as fish (especially the skin and bones) and tea. It is difficult to understand how any form of life has evolved and survived unless it was fully able to cope with continuous uptake of fluoride from its environment (Murray *et al.* 1991). Such is the case with humans who thrive in areas where the fluoride concentration of drinking water is several times higher than the therapeutic doses used to prevent dental caries.

In acute poisoning the certain lethal dose is 32 to 64 mg fluoride for each kilogram of body weight and the safely tolerated dose is 6 to 16 mg/kg body weight. In chronic exposures the safely tolerated dose is lower. Approximately 99 per cent of fluoride is stored in the hard tissues and it is there that the signs of chronic toxicity are evident. Skeletal fluorosis manifest as osteosclerosis, calcification of tendons, and exostoses occurs at water fluoride levels over 8 ppm (Srikantia and Siddiqui 1965). Industrial workers exposed to fluoride absorption of 14 to 68 mg/day for 20 years had skeletal fluorosis and gastric diseases. Radiographic changes are not apparent in areas where the water contains fluoride at up to 4 ppm (Morris 1965). If 1 to 2 litres of water are consumed daily, the exposure to fluoride at this concentration would be 8 to 16 mg/day. People in the United Kingdom who drink a lot of tea may take in 8 to 10 mg of fluoride per day (Jenkins and Edgar 1973; Walters *et al.* 1983).

Dental fluorosis is hypomaturation or hypomineralization of the teeth due to chronic ingestion of fluoride. It has a variety of presentations from small white flecks on the tooth to larger white opacities. In the most severe cases large areas of the enamel may be absent. The prevalence and severity of the disease are related to exposure to fluoride, particularly during the third year of life when the crowns of the upper central incisors are being developed. Exposure to fluoride in a number of forms, including drinking water and toothpaste, is associated with dental fluorosis (Hawley *et al.* 1996; Clark and Berkowitz 1997). The link between dietary fluoride supplements and dental fluorosis is particularly strong, and for this reason they are not advised as a public health measure for children in any but the most caries susceptible (Wang *et al.* 1997; Ismail and Bandekar 1999; Riordan 1999). Other strategies to avoid fluorosis involve brushing children's teeth with only a small blob of low-fluoride toothpaste.

Whilst most studies conducted in areas of optimal or near-optimal water fluoridation show some fluorosis, it is infrequently severe (Clark and Berkowitz 1997; Rock and Sabieha 1997). Most cases of fluorosis cannot be noticed by lay people at conversational distance and many young people regard mild fluorosis as more attractive than unaffected teeth (Riordan 1993; Hawley *et al.* 1996).

Fluoride is frequently said to have a number of other adverse effects including cancers and diseases of most other body systems (Royal College of Physicians 1976). Perhaps the most famous claim is that water fluoridation was associated with crude cancer death rates in the 10 largest cities of the United States (Yiamouyannis and Burk 1977). This association was roundly criticized and found to be spurious in two independent analyses accounting for age, sex, and racial differences between the cities (Oldham and Newell 1977; Newbrun 1989).

The literature on the safety of the therapeutic use of fluorides, and in particular water fluoridation, is extensive and not always of the highest quality. However, a number of independent reviews have been and continue to be conducted including those by the Royal College of Physicians in London (1976), the British Department of Health and Social Security (Knox 1985), the Australian National Health and Medical Research Council (1991), WHO (1994), and McDonagh *et al.* (2000).. These reports consistently fail to find associations between water fluoridation and any adverse effects other than dental fluorosis.

There are active antifluoridation lobbies in most developed countries. Such groups tend to be small but very enthusiastic and vociferous with an impact which is often disproportionate to their size or the amount of support they garner. The general arguments given against water fluoridation fall into four main categories. Fluoridation is said to be unsafe, to be ineffective, to constitute mass medication, and to remove the freedom to drink pure water. This very brief review attempts to convey the overwhelming evidence for the effectiveness of water fluoridation in the prevention of caries. As mentioned already, the effectiveness and safety of water fluoridation have been reviewed at a national and international level by several independent bodies and all have supported its continued use. Water supplies are already treated with a number of chemicals to render them fit to drink and so there are precedents for mass medication if it is for the public good. The argument in favour of a 'right' to pure water is more fundamental and emotive. Advocates of fluoridation take a utilitarian view that the sacrifice of this right by the few supports the rights of many to have oral health.

The debate about fluoridation is an interesting one. Antifluoridationists tend to come from relatively healthy middle-class groups. Because children in these groups have the lowest caries experience, they have the least to benefit from the intervention. Unfortunately, the effect of the antifluoridationists is to maintain social inequalities in health. Antifluoridationist arguments are often alarmist and sometimes unorthodox from the viewpoint of scientists. Public debates between pro- and antifluoridationists often end in profluoridationists attempting to refute, in detailed scientific terms, an extensive list of claims. With the current mistrust of science, it can be difficult to make such a position attractive in the face of very emotional arguments. Some proponents of fluoridation avoid open debate with antifluoridationists for this reason.

Diet

Sugars are the major dietary determinant of dental caries experience and are a necessary cause of clinically significant decay. However, evidence that practical health promotion interventions can reduce their intake and so reduce the incidence of caries is lacking (Kay and Locker 1997). Many studies of health education interventions have used self-reported sugar consumption as the primary outcome with the obvious danger of ascertainment bias (Tan *et al.* 1981; Schou 1985). Studies which have measured clinical outcomes have combined health education approaches with the use of fluorides and thus the independent effect of the health education cannot be assessed.

Some of the data which implicate sugars in the aetiology of caries suggest that restriction of dietary sugar is preventive. For example, per capita sugar supplies and caries experience data correlate significantly in simple national ecological comparisons (Sreebny 1982). A children's home in Australia had a dietary regimen with almost no sugar and the children had very low caries levels until they were allowed to make their own food choices at the age of 12 years. Likewise, caries levels fell in parallel with the availability of sugar during the Second World War (Toverud 1957).

Whether these findings can be translated into effective public health strategies remains uncertain. A health-directed food policy seems logical. A common risk factor approach might impact on dental diseases as well as on obesity, diabetes, and cardiovascular diseases. Possible strategies fall within the framework of education, substitution, regulation, pricing, or provision (Sanderson 1984). However, few countries have such policies in place and the resources of health advocates are very limited compared with those of the affluent and powerful lobby of the commercial food industry. Despite these difficulties, it is by operating at this level that public health might have its greatest impact.

As well as approaches aimed at individuals, education can take the form of authoritative dietary guidelines to inform national policies, community initiatives, and caterers. The Committee on Medical Aspects of Food Policy works within the United Kingdom Department of Health and advises the government on food policy relevant to health. Its 1989 the report *Dietary Sugars and Human Disease* focused on 'non-milk extrinsic' sugars by which it meant all sugars other than those taken in fresh fruit or milk (Committee on Medical Aspects of Food Policy 1989). It recommended that the consumption of non-milk extrinsic sugars should be reduced and replaced by fresh fruit, vegetables, and starchy foods. A subsequent report, *Dietary Reference Values for Food Energy and Nutrients for the United Kingdom* set a target for average non-milk extrinsic sugar consumption to constitute no more than 10 per cent of total dietary energy intake, which is approximately 60 g/person/day or 20 kg/year (Committee on Medical Aspects of Food Policy 1991). One important consequence of such an authoritative body making these recommendations has been that numerous other British organizations have followed suit with compatible guidelines.

Dietary sugars can be substituted with artificial sweeteners to reduce caries increments (Frostell *et al.* 1974; Scheinin and Makinen 1975). Sales of sugar-free carbonated drinks in Europe and North America demonstrate the compatibility of this tactic with commercial interests. However, substitution of dietary sugars has only limited potential in oral health promotion. The manufacture of many foodstuffs relies on the bulk and other specific properties of sugars. In addition, some sweeteners have side-effects, and resistance to the extended use of artificial sweeteners persists.

Regulation of advertising and labelling of foods in tandem with the effective use substitution is illustrated by a partnership between dentists and the confectionery industry in Switzerland. The *Zahnfreundlich* (tooth-friendly) logo is used to label non-acidogenic confectionery (Rugg-Gunn 1997). The label is well recognized by children, is commonly seen on confectionery, and is thought to have been effective in reducing levels of decay (Marthaler 1990*b*). Fiscal policies might be used to discourage the manufacture and sale of sugar-containing products. All of the above approaches and direct consumer pressure can be brought to bear on caterers and retail outlets to provide food in a way that makes the healthy choices the easier choices. There are numerous other examples of approaches which may reduce sugars consumption and an exhaustive list is presented by Sheiham (1995).

Oral cleaning

Since plaque is so strongly implicated as a necessary cause of periodontal diseases, it is logical that tooth cleaning should be the cornerstone of their management and prevention. Interventions aimed at improving oral hygiene can be successful and achieve a commensurate reduction in gingival inflammation (Kay and Locker 1997). Interestingly, interventions carried out in dental surgeries have been more effective than school-based interventions. However, most studies have had short follow-up periods and the effectiveness of even the best interventions diminishes with time. Therefore few data show that attempts to improve oral hygiene to prevent destructive disease are effective. Earlier research showing that frequent professional cleaning reduces periodontal destruction had design flaws (Axelsson and Lindhe 1978). Nonetheless, there remains a consensus that the best public health approach to improve periodontal health remains with improved oral hygiene.

The relationship between plaque removal and tooth decay is much more contentious. In Denmark, much preventive dentistry is based on the premise that cleaning the teeth prevents decay. Proponents of this policy cite an uncontrolled study involving both patient education and professional cleaning with a fluoride paste (Carvalho *et al.* 1992). In a carefully designed trial, a similar intervention did not demonstrate any additional preventive effect above a standard preventive programme of fissure sealants and locally applied topical fluoride received by the control groups (Arrow 1997). Sutcliffe's (1996) traditional review considered the effect of research methodology on the observed relationship between oral cleaning and dental caries and concluded that there was 'no unequivocal evidence that good oral cleanliness reduces caries experience'. This area of research is fraught with difficulty. As well as the difficulties of measuring dental disease, studies are susceptible to selection bias, leakage of intervention, and the probable confounding effects between self-reported behaviours, diet, and oral hygiene. Studies where professional cleaning has been effective have used pastes containing fluoride (Ripa 1985; Carvalho *et al.* 1992).

What is known is that brushing with a fluoride toothpaste is effective in preventing caries. Therefore brushing as it is currently practised in most developed countries combats both caries and periodontal diseases and is to be encouraged.

The systematic reviews cited above demonstrated that it is difficult to achieve sustainable changes in oral hygiene behaviour. A recent study of teenagers found good oral hygiene to be associated with not smoking, exercise, healthy eating, managing in school, and having confidence in one's family (Schou 1998). These types of findings invite the common risk factor approach in which oral cleanliness is promoted as both a health-related and health-directed behaviour where cleaning ones teeth makes one feel and look nice and is part of a positive and healthy lifestyle. Toothbrushing is a habit learnt as a young child and therefore is difficult to change later in life (Blinkhorn 1978). This behaviour is often an established routine before the child has seen a dentist, and interventions via health-care workers and social agencies working with young children and their mothers may be useful.

Smoking cessation

The role of smoking in the aetiology of oral cancers and periodontal diseases has already been discussed. Johnson (1997) has listed at 20 oral conditions either directly or indirectly associated with tobacco smoking. In addition to the well-known benefits to cardiovascular and respiratory health, cessation of smoking almost eliminates the increased risk of oral cancer within 5 to 10 years.

Many of the oral conditions, such as stained teeth, receding gums, and altered taste, are readily perceptible to the individual and may encourage or reinforce the desire to stop smoking. The dental team are also often aware of the personal and social circumstances (for example, pregnancy or a new job) that prompt people to give up. Therefore smoking cessation is another area where it is particularly appropriate for dentistry to become integrated into a common risk factor approach (Grabauskas 1987). As clinicians the dental team can be effective in supporting smoking cessation by providing advice (Warnakulasuriya 1984; Raw *et al.* 1998). Indeed, a group of dental practitioners achieved 11 per cent smoking cessation among their patients at 9-month follow-up in dental practices in the United Kingdom (Smith *et al.* 1998).

Prevention of accidents

Several strategies can be used to reduce trauma to teeth. Playground surfaces can be made of impact-absorbing materials which cushion against trauma. Unfortunately, orthodontic treatment of large overjets is complex and prolonged, but can be justified in children of 8 or 9 years to reduce the risk of trauma (Welbury 1996).

The use of mouthguards is compulsory for some sports in some countries. Mouthguards not only prevent dental injuries in sport but also prevent laceration of the facial soft tissues against the teeth (Garon *et al.* 1986; McNutt *et al.* 1989). By absorbing the force of anterior blows they reduce posterior and superior displacement of the mandible. In so doing they reduce the risk of mandibular fracture and may protect the cranial cavity. Mouthguards are usually made of a copolymer of polyvinyl acetate and polyethylene. The most basic type may be obtained prefabricated in a range of sizes. A more sophisticated type may be adapted to fit the mouth, typically by softening it in hot water first. Custom-made devices constructed on models made from impressions of the teeth are the most comfortable and can be made to support the lower teeth and mandible during trauma (Chapman 1985; Stokes *et al.* 1987).

Ensuring access to appropriate preventive care

There has been disillusionment with the prevailing biomedical model of health care. By focusing on the diseases of individuals, it emphasizes the hierarchy of professionals over lay people and treatments rather than prevention. All of these things have taken place with substantial economic and social costs and yet medical care has made a relatively small contribution to health (Illich 1976; McKeown 1976). The biomedical approach distracts attention from the wider social, political, and economic determinants of health. The primary health care approach is a philosophy which recognizes that these determinants are more important than medical interventions (WHO–UNICEF 1978).

Dental services are just as susceptible to the criticisms of the medical model of health care. Just as we know that medical services have limited effect on health, so we are aware that dental treatment has made a relatively small contribution to oral health (Nadanovsky and Sheiham 1994, 1995). Dental services sometimes have the appearance of aiming to provide dental treatment rather than aiming to achieve oral health. Data from the 1970s show that dental services explain 3 per cent of the variation in oral health of 12-year-olds in developed countries compared with the 65 per cent contribution made by broader socio-economic factors. Furthermore, the interventions used in dentistry may also be clinically inappropriate. Dentistry has adopted a surgical approach to treatment with a cycle of placing and replacing fillings. It has long been recognized that the quality of many fillings is not high and that even the decisions to place fillings are idiosyncratic (Elderton 1976; Elderton and Nuttall 1983). Since fillings are often replaced many times over a lifetime, the remaining tooth is increasingly damaged with each new filling.

As well as having little positive impact on oral health, clinical dental services ignore the determinants of disease. With its emphasis on personal behaviour and even with the search for specific periodontal pathogens, clinical dentistry and much dental research actually divert attention from the factors which determine oral health and disease.

Dental services are also costly. National Health Service dentistry costs £1.4 billion per year in England and Wales. Compared with the potential costs of treatment, the resources available are few and are likely to reduce in future. Curative services serve those who can afford them. As well as creating dependence on professionals, the services become focused on those with least health problems.

Since these problems of medical and dental care exist in parallel the same kinds of changes are applicable to both. Twenty years after the introduction of Health for All there are still too few resources, the resources which are available are still poorly allocated, medical staff still congregate around the wealthy people, ordinary people have little control over their own health, and health professionals still do not trust people to make good decisions about their health (Mahler 1981). All of these points apply to dentistry. Worldwide there are people who cannot attend and/or cannot afford dental treatment in its current guise. Even in countries with well-developed socialized systems of dental care, there are major inequalities in oral health (Watt and Sheiham 1999). Dental services are overdue for an evaluation and reorientation. A more holistic practice of dentistry in line with the primary health care approach will also ensure that services are more equitable and appropriate. Such a move will require a challenge to the professional status quo (Dickson 1993).

Whilst realizing the limitations of clinical dentistry, it is important to recognize that it may have a role (as yet undemonstrated in clinical trials) in reducing the psychosocial impacts of oral disease. For this reason it is essential that we generate a greater understanding within dentistry of the nature of oral health. The movement to identify more relevant measures of oral health to assess treatment need and the outcomes of care should be encouraged (Slade 1997). The evidence-based approach, the use of clinical governance, and managed care should provide both the impetus and the means to ensure that only effective and efficient interventions are used.

Dental surgeries are a natural health-related setting for health promotion. Practice-based oral health promotion activities provide an opportunity to increase knowledge and promote self-esteem and empowerment. Their role could be expanded by adopting a common risk factor approach (Croucher 1993). However, practice-based health promotion is only useful for those who attend the services and may exclude those people with the greatest need who do not. In addition, there needs to be a change in emphasis in health education from the elitist prescriptive medical model which ignores the needs of people it serves and so blames 'victims'. Patients should not feel they are being chastised or told to do things. A more effective approach would be a patient-centred model which respects patient autonomy and seeks their active participation in defining their needs (Croucher 1989).

One particular aspect of dentistry in many countries that may need to be revised is the system of payment of fees to dentists for each item of service provided. Fee-per-item service payments encourage dentists to work quickly and have been associated (in the past at least) with overtreatment. This system of payment tends to encourage the curative technical approach to treatment, unless there is a specific fee for prevention. Conversely, whereas salaried dentists have both more time and incentives to emphasize health promotion their productivity is lower (Schou 1993). The potential disadvantages of capitation systems are that they may lead to undertreatment of existing patients and may encourage dentists not to accept patients with high treatment needs (Schoen 1991). Interestingly, there has not been evidence of widespread neglect since the introduction of capitation payments, as long as there is an additional fee for treatments provided (Daley *et al.* 1994).

Other specific changes which could be made to ensure access to dental services can be categorized in the framework used by Penchansky and Thomas (1981). Dental services must be available, accessible, affordable, acceptable, and accommodating.

Clearly people cannot use services that do not exist, and so increasing their availability has a direct effect on service use (O'Mullane and Robinson 1977; Brennan *et al.* 1997). One way of making dental services more available at limited cost is to delegate care to auxiliary staff. With the decreased incidence of dental caries in developed countries, the vast majority of new cavities in children are small and relatively simple to treat. It is therefore not cost-effective to employ highly trained and highly paid dentists to undertake this less demanding and repetitive work. A number of countries including Australia, New Zealand, Canada, and the United Kingdom employ staff with a limited repertoire of treatment options (variously called school dental nurses, dental auxiliaries, and dental therapists) who provide high-quality care at lower cost (Office of the Auditor General Western Australia 1995). Similar data exist for dental hygienists. Dental auxiliary staff work under the supervision of a dentist. By reducing the level of supervision required and expanding the role of ancillary staff the availability of care can be increased whilst limiting costs. Dental hygienists can work independently without reducing either the quality of treatment or patients' satisfaction with it (Perry *et al.* 1997; Freed *et al.* 1997). Likewise, hygienists can be trained to conduct clinical examinations in dental surveys with no compromise to the quality of the data (Kwan *et al.* 1996).

Clearly the expanded use of dental auxiliaries threatens the monopoly on the provision of dental treatment held by dentists. The dental profession is the most constant barrier to the wider use of dental auxiliaries (Riordan 1997). The American Dental Association, for example, has consistently opposed their use since 1975 (Burt and Eklund 1999).

Other characteristics of dental services which limit access were explored in a qualitative investigation of people who did not go to the dentist (Finch *et al.* 1988). The costs of treatment, the need to make an appointment, and the opening hours of dentists all deterred attendance. These obstacles can be reduced by providing subsidized care, arranging services where no appointment is necessary, and where treatment can be provided outside office hours.

Developing countries

Whilst the prevalence of dental caries in many developing countries is still low, other diseases such as oral cancer and dental fluorosis are more common than in most developed countries. Non-industrialized countries also suffer from a shortage of resources including human resources, appropriate technology, and universally available power supplies. Over the last two decades, the additional burden of meeting the costs of the infection control implications of the HIV epidemic have exacerbated any deficiencies in resources (Akpabio 1993).

The traditional curative approach to dental health is limited in any setting but these limitations are more extreme when they are exported to the developing world. The surgical approach to dentistry used in industrialized countries is technology intensive and requires an infrastructure of continuous power and water supply. It involves expensive equipment which is difficult to use and maintain. Dentists, therefore, need to treat patients who can help them recoup their costs. These pressures limit the availability of services and contribute to the inequalities in their provision. Hobdell (1993) has described this situation as 'trying to implement a type of oral health care developed mainly in the last century in another part of the world using equipment and materials developed for use in an entirely different socio-economic and political setting'. Indeed, large parts of the Western model of dental care may be inappropriate in developing countries, including an overemphasis of clinical surveys in health-care planning. Services based on normative assessment limit community participation in health care and ignore the sociodental implications of oral disease. They may also overcomplicate health care. In one notorious example, survey data were used to calculate the periodontal treatment needs of children in Kenya (Manji and Sheiham 1986). Using the WHO model, the treatment proposed would have used the entire dental human resources of Kenya for up to 21 years, allowing for no other care. Services could concentrate on the relatively few conditions which comprise the bulk of oral health problems: toothache (not tooth decay), trauma, oral infections, and neoplasms (Hobdell 1993).

The primary health care approach is still relevant to the provision of dental services in all countries but it is particularly applicable to the developing world. It has five principles: an equitable distribution of services, community involvement in health, a focus on prevention, the use of appropriate technology, and a multisectoral approach. *The Berlin Declaration on Oral Health and Oral Health Services in Deprived Communities* provides comprehensive guidelines for planning, implementing, and evaluating oral health projects within this framework (Mautsch and Sheiham 1995). It was conceived by the Oral Health Alliance, an International network which provides support and information to colleagues working in this field (e-mail: wmautsch@post.klinikum.rwth-aachen.de). Specific examples of activities within this framework are presented below.

Equitable distribution

Tudor Hart's (1971) 'inverse care law' between the availability of services and the need for them also occurs in dentistry. It is particularly extreme in countries where there are wide disparities between rich and poor. In Africa, 80 per cent of the trained professional personnel live and work in affluent neighbourhoods in cities, although the same proportion of the indigenous population live in rural areas (Thorpe 1993). The scope for dental auxiliaries in developing countries may be greater since advocates of their use may not have to compete with the well-established political lobbies of dentists which exist in industrialized nations. Auxiliaries can be used to provide simple but essential treatments to extend the availability of services and reduce inequalities in access (Anumanrajadhon *et al.* 1996).

Models exist for identifying the types of personnel needed for oral health care in deprived communities along with training and evaluation methods (Samarawikrama 1995). Such models consider the frequency of problems, the difficulties encountered in undertaking the different roles, and the identification of the difficulties themselves.

Community development

Community involvement means that people are allowed to take control of their own health, and it is necessary if programmes are to thrive. It is perhaps the most difficult aspect of the primary health care approach since it requires that health professionals must relinquish their traditional hierarchical role. In addition, individuals and communities often regard health as beyond their control and may not regard oral health as a priority. There are isolated examples of wide involvement in oral health. In Brazil, health councils comprised of community representatives, health workers, and civil servants operate at the national, state, and municipal levels. Only in areas where there is a well-organized community have the local health councils been able to implement policy. One council in Porto Alegre identified oral health as a priority. Despite considerable opposition from local dentists and a scarcity of resources, it was able to create an emergency dental service and initiate preventive programmes in schools and health centres (Baldisserrotto 1995).

Focus on prevention

Prevention is universally accepted as an essential component of health care. However, if prevention is to avoid the existing system in which people are passive recipients of information and preventive therapies, it must adopt the principles of health promotion. Examples of a more participative role include the community involvement described in Porto Alegre and the use of individuals from local communities including children in preventive activities.

Appropriate technology

'Appropriate technology' is sometimes taken to mean 'cheap' and 'second rate'. It is neither of these things, but is an approach which recognizes the needs and resources of the local community. The atraumatic restorative technique is a recent development which combines these requirements with new knowledge of the process of dental caries and developments in dental materials science (Frencken *et al.* 1996). It involves removal of decay with hand instruments and filling the cavities with glass ionomer cements. These cements are hand mixed with water on a small pad or slab. Upon insertion, the filling gradually leaks fluoride to prevent secondary disease around the cavity. All the instruments can be carried in a small case and treatment can be provided painlessly without local anaesthesia, at low cost, and without either electricity or expensive dental equipment. Non-dentists can be trained in the technique in a matter of weeks and manuals are available from the World Health Organization (**WHO**). The technique is most suitable for exactly the types of cavities which are found in many developing countries which do not have excessively high caries levels.

Multisectoral approach

We have seen how an effective health strategy might involve a number of departments of both national and local governments, water providers, the educational system, community members, and health-care workers. All of the approaches to health promotion outlined in the second part of this chapter must be integrated. However, integration should mean more than using the resources of other sectors to promote oral health. Such an approach often means that dentists simply get teachers to provide dental health education which carries the risk of not truly involving the other sectors (Mautsch and Sheiham 1995).

Conclusions and future developments in dental public health

The last few years have seen remarkable developments in our understanding of the importance of oral health and its significance as a public health concern. There is a greater knowledge than ever before of the nature of the oral diseases which threaten health (dental caries, periodontal diseases, oral cancer, and dentofacial trauma), the epidemiology of those diseases, and the factors which determine them. Moreover, we are starting to accumulate a body of evidence on the effectiveness of health promotion and treatment strategies. Those strategies include the use of fluoride, food, and health policies to reduce sugars consumption, community approaches to improve body hygiene including oral cleaning, smoking cessation, policies on reducing accidents, and ensuring access to appropriate preventive care. Many of these strategies could work in common with approaches to the promotion of general health.

In keeping with the recognition that clinical services are a minor determinant of health, most of the oral health strategies discussed in this chapter do not involve clinical dental services. There is a developing knowledge of the relative impotence of clinical dentistry to bring about oral health and a greater awareness of its potential harm. The evidence of effectiveness should be used to identify beneficial interventions and should help reorientate dentistry from its traditional curative approach which focuses on the responsibility of clinicians and their individual patients. In so doing we may be able to move toward a more shared responsibility in which all participate.

It is important that all these strands of information are combined. Perhaps most important of all, we need a more universal understanding of what is meant by 'oral health' and its relationship with oral disease. The ways we measure health and the outcomes of interventions will determine not only which interventions we choose but whether we choose to intervene at all.

Future developments in dental public health can be considered in four areas: trends in oral health, the deprofessionalization of dentistry, technological developments, and relationships between oral and general health-care delivery.

Two trends in oral health have been observed. Some countries, particularly developing countries, are experiencing increases in dental caries. The increases are related to the adoption of Western dietary patterns high in sugars. Even if these trends are currently limited to more affluent city dwellers they represent worrying concerns for the future. The increase in treatment needs created by these trends is likely to place an unaffordably high burden on developing economies. To some extent this burden will be moderated by the low levels of perceived need in communities unused to receiving dental treatment. However, if the disability and handicap brought about by oral disease are to be minimized, then appropriate methods of treatment will be required. Numerous examples now exist of dental auxiliaries being used to provide a limited range of treatments in both the developed and developing world. Auxiliaries can be trained quicker to provide care to similar standards to dentists, but at greatly reduced costs. Food and health policies could also be used in countries with rising caries levels to control imports, the production and sale of cariogenic foods and drinks, while encouraging the use of traditional foods.

In many developed countries, the decreased caries incidence witnessed over the last two decades appears to have stabilized in young children. The trend may have stabilized but its effects will continue to change dentistry for decades to come. When coupled with demographic changes, changed attitudes towards oral health and the preservation of teeth seen in developing countries over the last 50 years, this trend produces an interesting pattern. On the one hand there is a growing and ageing group of younger people whose treatment needs will remain lower in terms of volume and complexity than preceding generations. On the other hand, there is a large group of older people who will live for longer and retain many heavily restored teeth for longer. These people will require more care, some of it more complex, than the generations that preceded them. It is difficult to predict whether there will be a net change in the need for dental care or in which direction such a change would be. One likely change will be a greater emphasis on specialization within dentistry. The majority of the young people's needs will comprise simple one surface fillings which could be placed by auxiliaries. However, this change could be offset by the more complex demands of older people seeking dental implants and treatment for root caries and tooth wear which may remain in the domain of specialists.

A dominant political direction over recent years has been the deprofessionalization of dentistry. This trend is manifest in several different forms. In many developed countries, patients are demanding 'rights' as consumers of care. These demands are complemented by the application of marketing theory to dentistry, which places consumer satisfaction as an essential criterion in business success. Thus, patients have been directly and indirectly implicated in moves to regulate the way in which dentists market themselves and have ensured that patient satisfaction is an active concern of dentists. Similar principles are cornerstones of the primary health care approach and the Ottawa Charter for Health Promotion (named community participation and community action, respectively) (WHO–UNICEF 1978; WHO 1986). These activities take public involvement in oral health well beyond clinical dentistry. Even within clinical care, satisfaction is associated with patient compliance and is therefore regarded as an integral part of the process of care rather than just an outcome. Other agencies, such as governments and insurance companies, are increasingly involved in health care. Externally applied measures to minimize the costs of care and increase the accountability of health-care organizations whilst assuring the quality of care all serve to reduce professional power within dentistry.

This trend of deprofessionalization is likely to continue and may help to make oral care more relevant to the needs of the people it serves. Professions resist any tendency to undermine their power. This reaction could present an opportunity for dental public health to facilitate and manage the deprofessionalization of dentistry.

A number of technological developments may also influence oral health and care. The atraumatic restorative technique shows considerable potential for providing simple, inexpensive, and effective treatment for the type of minimal caries seen in developing countries. Because the technique requires minimal training and equipment it will allow services to be provided in relatively small and isolated communities. If the technique is used by partially skilled staff it may also contribute to the deprofessionalization of dentistry in these countries; it will certainly reduce the cost.

In developed countries osseo-integrated implants are increasingly used to support dental prostheses. By providing a stable and retentive base for both single and multiple tooth prostheses, implants show great potential for reducing the handicap brought about by oral disease. One disadvantage is that, for the time being at least, implant treatment demands considerable specialist expertise and is costly. Implants may therefore become a treatment limited to those who can afford them and thus contribute to inequalities in oral health.

Oral health care is becoming increasingly integrated with the delivery of other services. In policy terms greater integration can be seen as part of the multidisciplinary approach enshrined in the Alma-Ata declaration (WHO–UNICEF 1978). There are many examples of integration at the level of clinical service provision. Dental surgeries may be linked with other clinical services in health centres. In some cases dentists invite other types of health-care worker into their practices to provide services. At a broader level of health promotion, integration is particularly compatible with a common risk factor approach to disease. Health educators and health promotors recognize the value of involving other health-care workers, teachers, and other community workers, either as original deliverers or reinforcers of their messages. Oral health also becomes a consideration of local and national governments with debates about fluoridation of water supplies and whether agricultural and fiscal policy are used to promote oral health. It is the role of specialists in dental public health to act as advocates at all these levels.

References

Abdellatif, H.M. and Burt, B.A. (1987). An epidemiological investigation into the relative importance of age and oral hygiene status as determinants of periodontitis. *Journal of Dental Research*, **66**, 13–18.

Akpabio, S.P. (ed.) (1993). Conclusions. In *Promotion of oral health in the African region*, pp. 64–5. Commonwealth Dental Association, London.

Andreasen, J.O. and Andreasen, F.M. (1994). *Textbook and color atlas of traumatic injuries to the teeth.* Munksgaard, Copenhagen.

Anumanrajadhon, T., Rajchagool, S., Nitisiri, P., *et al.* (1996). The community care model of the Intercountry Centre for Oral Health at Chiangmai, Thailand. *International Dental Journal*, **46**, 325–33.

Arrow, P. (1997). Control of occlusal caries in the first permanent molars by oral hygiene. *Community Dentistry and Oral Epidemiology*, **25**, 278–83.

Attwood, D. and Blinkhorn, A.S. (1988). Trends in dental health of ten-year-old children in south-west Scotland after cessation of water fluoridation. *Lancet*, **ii**, 266–7.

Axelsson, P. and Lindhe, J. (1978). Effect of controlled oral hygiene procedures on caries and periodontal disease in adults. *Journal of Clinical Periodontology*, **5**, 133–51.

Baldisserotto, J. (1995). Community participation in a decision making process in a local health council in Porto Alegre City, Brazil. In *Promoting oral health in deprived communities* Mautsch and A. Sheiham), pp. 253–63. Deusche Stiftung fur Internationale Entwicklung, Berlin.

Beck, J., Garcia, R., Heiss, G., Vokonas, P.S., and Offenbacher, S. (1996). Periodontal disease and cardiovascular disease. *Journal of Periodontology*, **67**, 1123–37.

Bergstrom, J. (1989). Cigarette smoking as a risk factor in chronic periodontal disease. *Community Dentistry and Oral Epidemiology*, **17**, 245–7.

Blinkhorn, A.S. (1978). Influence of social norms on toothbrushing behaviour of young children. *Community Dentistry and Oral Epidemiology*, **6**, 222–6.

Blot, W.J. (1992). Alcohol and Cancer. *Cancer Research*, **52** (Supplement), 2119–23.

Brennan, D.S., Carter, K.D., Stewart, J.F., and Spencer, A.J. (1997) *Commonwealth Dental Health Program Evaluation Report 1994–1996.* Australian Institute of Health and Welfare Dental Statistics and Research Unit, Adelaide.

Brown, L. (1994). Research in dental health education and health promotion: a review of the literature. *Health Education Quarterly*, **21**, 83–102.

Brown, L.J., Oliver, R.C., and Loe, H. (1989). Periodontal diseases in the U.S. in 1981: prevalence, severity, extent, and role in tooth mortality. *Journal of Periodontology*, **60**, 363–70.

Burt, B.A. (1978). Influences for change in the dental health status of populations: an historical perspective. *Journal of Public Health Dentistry*, **38**, 272–88.

Burt, B.A. (1994). Trends in caries prevalence in North American children. *International Dental Journal*, **44**, 403–13.

Burt, B.A. (1998). Prevention policies in the light of the changed distribution of dental caries. *Acta Odontologica Scandinavica*, **56**, 179–86.

Burt B.A. and Eklund S.A. (1999). *Dentistry, dental practice, and the community.* W.B. Saunders, Philadelphia, PA.

Burt, B.A., Ismail, A.I., and Eklund, S.A. (1985). Periodontal disease, tooth loss, and oral hygiene among older Americans. *Community Dentistry and Oral Epidemiology*, **13**, 93–6.

Burt, B.A., Ismail, A.I., and Eklund, S.A. (1986). Root caries in an optimally fluoridated and a high-fluoridated community. *Journal of Dental Research*, **65**, 1154–8.

Carmichael, C.L., French, A.D., Rugg-Gunn, A.J., and Furness, J.A. (1984). The relationship between social class and caries experience of five-year old children in Newcastle and Northumberland after twelve years' fluoridation. *Community Dental Health*, **1**, 47–54.

Carmichael, C.L., Rugg-Gunn, A.J., and Ferrell, R.S. (1989). The relationship between fluoridation, social class and caries experience in 5-year-old children in Newcastle and Northumberland in 1987. *British Dental Journal*, **167**, 57–61.

Carvalho, J.C., Thylstrup, A., and Ekstrand, K.R. (1992). Results after 3 years of non-operative occlusal caries treatment of erupting permanent first molars. *Community Dentistry and Oral Epidemiology*, **20**, 187–92.

Caton, J. (1989). Periodontal diagnosis and diagnostic aids. In *World workshop in clinical periodontics* (ed. M. Nevins, W. Becker, and K. Kornman), pp. 11–122. American Academy of Periodontology, Princeton, NJ.

Chapman, P.J. (1985). Prevalence of oro-facial injuries and use of mouthguards in rugby union. *Australian Dental Journal*, **30**, 364–7.

Clark, D.C. and Berkowitz, J. (1997). The influence of various fluoride exposures on the prevalence of esthetic problems resulting from dental fluorosis. *Journal of Public Health Dentistry*, **57**, 144–9.

Clarke, N.G. and Hirsch, R.S. (1995). Personal risk factors for generalized periodontitis. *Journal of Clinical Periodontology*, **22**, 136–45.

Committee on Medical Aspects of Food Policy (1989). *Dietary sugars and human disease.* HMSO, London.

Committee on Medical Aspects of Food Policy (1991). *Dietary reference values for food energy and nutrients for the United Kingdom.* HMSO, London.

Croucher, R. (1989). *The performance gap.* Health Education Authority, London.

Croucher R. (1993). General dental practice, health education, and health promotion: a critical reappraisal. In *Oral health promotion* (ed. L. Schou and A.S. Blinkhorn), pp. 153–66. Oxford University Press.

Daley, F.M., Milsom, K.M., and Lennon, M.A. (1994). The relationship between registration and dental health benefit in 8- and 9-year-old children in Cheshire. *British Dental Journal*, **177**, 416–18.

Dasanayake, A.P. (1998). Poor periodontal health of the pregnant woman as a risk factor for low birthweight. *Annals of Periodontology*, **3**, 206–12.

Davenport, E.S., Williams, C.E., Sterne, J.A., Sivapathasundram, V., Fearne, J.M., and Curtis, M.A. (1998). The East London study of maternal chronic periodontal disease and preterm low birth weight infants: study design and prevalence data. *Annals of Periodontology*, **3**, 213–21.

Davies, M.J., Spencer, A.J., and Slade, G.D. (1997). Trends in dental caries experience of school children in Australia. *Australian Dental Journal*, **42**, 389–94.

de Crousaz, P. (1985). Caries prevalence in children after 12 years of salt fluoridation in a Canton of Switzerland. *Schweizer Monatsschrift für Zahnmedizin*, **95**, 805–15.

Dean, H.T., Jay, P., Arnold, F.A., and Elvove, E. (1941). Domestic water and dental caries II. A study of 2832 white children aged 12- 14 years, of 8 suburban Chicago communities, including Lactobacillus acidophilus studies of 1761 children. *Public Health Reports*, **56**, 761–92.

Dean, H.T., Arnold, F.A. Jr, Jay, P., and Knutson, J.W. (1950). Studies on mass control of dental caries through fluoridation of the public water supply. *Public Health Reports*, **65**, 1403–8.

Dental Practice Board (1999). Data Services Branch. *Gross fees. GDS quarterly statistics*. Dental Practice Board, Eastbourne.

DePaola, P.F. and Lax, M. (1968). The caries-inhibiting effect of acidulated-phosphate chewable tablets: a two-year double blind study. *Journal of the American Dental Association*, **76**, 554–7.

Deshpande, R.G., Khan, M., and Genco, C.A. (1999). Invasion strategies of the oral pathogen *Porphyromonas gingivalis*: implications for cardiovascular disease. *Invasion and Metastasis*, **18**, 57–69.

Dickson, M. (1993). Oral health promotion in developing countries. In *Oral health promotion* (ed. L. Schou and A.S. Blinkhorn), pp. 233–47. Oxford University Press.

Dickson M. (1995). Oral health promotion. In *Promoting oral health in deprived communities* (ed. W. Mautsch and A. Sheiham), pp. 175–86. Deusche Stiftung fur Internationale Entwicklung, Berlin.

Downer, M.C. (1994). Caries prevalence in the United Kingdom. *International Dental Journal*, **44**, 365–70.

Downer M.C. (1997). Oral cancer. In *Community oral health* (ed. C.M. Pine), pp. 89–94. Wright, Oxford.

Driscoll, W.S., Heifetz, S.B., and Korts, D.C. (1978). Effect of chewable fluoride tablets on dental caries in schoolchildren: results after six years of use. *Journal of the American Dental Association*, **97**, 820–4.

Duckworth, C.S. and Duckworth, R. (1978). The ingestion of fluoride in tea. *British Dental Journal*, **145**, 368–70.

Duff, E.J. (1981). Total and ionic fluoride in milk. *Caries Research*, **15**, 406–8.

Elderton, R.J. (1976). The causes of failure of restorations: a literature review. *Journal of Dentistry*, **4**, 257–62.

Elderton R.J. (1990). *Evolution in dental care*. Clinical Press, Bristol.

Elderton, R.J. (1994). The effect of changes in caries prevalence on dental education. *International Dental Journal*, **44**, 445–50.

Elderton, R.J. and Nuttall, N.M. (1983). Variation among dentists in planning treatment. *British Dental Journal*, **154**, 201–6.

Emslie, R.D. (1963). Cancrum oris. *The Dental Practitioner and Dental Record*, **13**, 481–95.

Federation Dentaire Internationale (1990). *Commission of dental products. Working Party No. 7*. FDI World Dental Press, London.

Fejerskov, O., Baelum, V., Luan, W.-M., and Manji, F. (1994). Caries prevalence in Africa and the People's Republic of China. *International Dental Journal*, **44**, 425–33.

Finch, H., Keegar, J., Ward, K., and Sanyal Sen, B. (1988). *Barriers to the receipt of dental care*. British Dental Association, London.

Fiske, J. and Watson, R.M. (1990).The benefit of dental care to an elderly population assessed using a sociodental measure of oral handicap. *British Dental Journal*, **168**, 153–6.

Frandsen, A. (1986). Mechanical oral hygiene practices. In *Dental plaque control measures and oral hygiene practices* (ed. H. Loe and D.V. Kleinman). IRL Press, Oxford.

Freed, J.R., Perry, D.A., and Kushman, J.E. (1997). Aspects of quality of dental hygiene care in supervised and unsupervised practices. *Journal of Public Health Dentistry*, **57**, 68–75.

Frencken, J.E., Pilot, T., Songpaisan, Y., and Phantumvanit, P. (1996). Atraumatic restorative treatment (ART): rationale, technique, and development. *Journal of Public Health Dentistry*, **56**, 135–40.

Frostell, G., Blomlof, L., Blomqvist, T., *et al.* (1974). Substitution of sucrose by lycasin in candy: the Roslagen study. *Acta Odontologica Scandinavica*, **32**, 235–54.

Garon, M.W., Merkle, A., and Wright, J.T. (1986). Mouth protection and oral trauma: a study of adolescent football players. *Journal of the American Dental Association*, **112**, 663–5.

Gedalia, I., Galon, H., Rennert, A., Biderco, I., and Mohr, I. (1981). Effect of a fluoridated citrus beverage on dental caries and on fluoride concentration in the surface enamel of children's teeth. *Caries Research*, **15**, 103–8.

Gelbier, S. (1967). Injured anterior teeth in children. A preliminary discussion. *British Dental Journal*, **123**, 331–5.

Genco, R.J. (1990). Pathogenesis and host responses in periodontal disease. In *Contemporary periodontics* (ed. R.J. Genco, H.M. Goldman, and D.W. Cohen), pp. 184–93. C.V. Mosby, St Louis, MO.

Genco, R.J. and Slots, J. (1984). Host responses in periodontal diseases. *Journal of Dental Research*, **63**, 441–51.

Gibbons, R.J. and Socransky, S.S. (1966). Enhancement of alveolar bone loss in gnotobiotic mice harbouring human gingival bacteria. *Archives of Oral Biology*, **11**, 847–8.

Giddon, D.B., Goldhaber, P., and Dunning, J.M. (1963). Prevalence of reported cases of acute necrotising ulcerative gingivitis in a university population. *Journal of Periodontology*, **34**, 366–71.

Gift, H.C., Reisine, S.T., and Larach, D.C. (1992). The social impact of dental problems and visits. *American Journal of Public Health*, **82**, 1663–8.

Grabauskas, V.J. (1987). Integrated programme for community health in noncommunicable disease (Interhealth). In *The prevention of non-communicable diseases: experiences and prospects* (ed. E. Leparski), pp. 285–310. WHO Regional Office for Europe, Copenhagen.

Gratrix, D. and Holloway, P.J. (1994). Factors of deprivation associated with dental caries in young children. *Community Dental Health*, **11**, 66–70.

Groeneveld, A., Van Eck, A.A.M.L., and Backer Dirks, O. (1990). Fluoride in caries prevention. Is the effect pre- or post-eruptive? *Journal of Dental Research*, **69**, 751–5.

Gustaffson, B.E., Quensel, C.E., and Lanke, L.S. (1954). The Vipeholm dental caries study. The effect of different levels of carbohydrate intake on caries activity in 436 individuals observed for five years. *Acta Odontologica Scandinavica*, **11**, 232–364.

Hawley, G.M., Ellwood, R.P., and Davies, R.M. (1996). Dental caries, fluorosis and the cosmetic implications of different TF scores in 14-year-old adolescents. *Community Dental Health*, **13**, 189–92.

Health Education Board for Scotland (1996). How effective are effectiveness reviews? *Health Education Journal*, **55**, 359–62.

Hindle, I. and Nally, F. (1991). Oral cancer: a comparative study between 1962–67 and 1980–84 in England and Wales. *British Dental Journal*, **170**, 15–19.

Hobdell, M.H. (1993). Essential elements of a primary oral health care model. In *Promotion of oral health in the African region.* (ed. S.P. Akpabio), pp. 99–108. Commonwealth Dental Association, London.

Hollister, M.C. and Weintraub, J.A. (1993). The association of oral status with systemic health, quality of life, and economic productivity. *Journal of Dental Education*, **57**, 901–12.

Holloway, P.J. and Worthington, H.V. (1993). Sodium fluoride or sodium monofluorophosphate? A critical view of a meta-analysis on their relative effectiveness in dentifrices. *American Journal of Dentistry*, **6**, S55–8.

Holm, A.K. (1990) Caries in the preschool child: international trends. *Journal of Dentistry*, **18**, 291–5.

Holt, S.C., Ebersole, J., Felton, J., Brunsvold, M., and Kornman, K.S. (1988). Implantation of *Bacteroides gingivalis* in nonhuman primates initiates progression of periodontitis. *Science*, **239**, 55–7.

Illich, I. (1976). *Limits to medicine.* Penguin, Harmondsworth.

Ismail, A.I. and Bandekar, R.R. (1999). Fluoride supplements and fluorosis: a meta-analysis. *Community Dentistry and Oral Epidemiology*, **27**, 48–56.

Ismail, A.I., Morrison, E.C., Burt, B.A., Caffesse, R.G., and Kavanagh, M.T. (1990). Natural history of periodontal disease in adults: findings from the Tecumseh periodontal disease study, 1959–87. *Journal of Dental Research*, **69**, 430–5.

Jenkins, G.N. and Edgar, W.M. (1973). Some observations on fluoride metabolism in Britain. *Journal of Dental Research*, **52**, 984.

Jenny, J. and Proshek, J.M. (1986). Visibility and prestige of occupations and the importance of dental appearance. *Canadian Dental Association Journal*, **52**, 987–9.

Jensen, M.E. and Kohout, F. (1988). The effect of a fluoridated dentifrice on root and coronal caries in an older adult population. *Journal of the American Dental Association*, **117**, 829–32.

Johansson, I., Tidehag, P., Lundberg, V., and Hallmans, G. (1994). Dental status, diet and cardiovascular risk factors in middle-aged people in northern Sweden. *Community Dentistry and Oral Epidemiology*, **22**, 431–6.

Johnson N.W. (1991*a*). *Risk markers for oral diseases.* Vol. 1, *Dental caries: markers of high and low risk groups and individuals.* Cambridge University Press.

Johnson N.W. (1991*b*). *Risk markers for oral diseases.* Vol. 3, *Periodontal diseases: markers of disease activity and susceptibility.* Cambridge University Press.

Johnson, M.F. (1993). Comparative efficacy of NaF and SMFP dentifrices in caries prevention: a meta-analytic overview. *Caries Research*, **27**, 328–36.

Johnson, N.W. (1997). Oral cancer: practical prevention. *FDI World*, **6**, 6–13.

Johnson, B.D. and Engel, D. (1986). Acute necrotising ulcerative gingivitis. A review of diagnosis, etiology and treatment. *Journal of Periodontology*, **57**, 141–50.

Johnson, N.W. and Warnakalasuriya, K.A.A.S. (1993). Epidemiology and aetiology of oral cancer in the United Kingdom. *Community Dental Health*, **10** (Supplement 1), 13–29.

Joshipura, K.J., Douglass, C.W., and Willett, W.C. (1998). Possible explanations for the tooth loss and cardiovascular disease relationship. *Annals of Periodontology*, **3**, 175–83.

Kay, E.J. and Locker, D. (1996). Is dental health education effective? A systematic review of current evidence. *Community Dentistry and Oral Epidemiology*, **24**, 231–5.

Kay, E.J. and Locker, D. (1997). *Effectiveness of oral health promotion: a review.* Health Education Authority, London.

Knox, E.G. (1985). *Fluoridation of water and cancer: a review of the epidemiological evidence.* HMSO, London.

Kwan, S.Y., Prendergast, M.J., and Williams, S.A. (1996). The diagnostic reliability of clinical dental auxiliaries in caries prevalence surveys—a pilot study. *Community Dental Health*, **13**, 145–9.

Labonte, R. and Penfold, S. (1981) Canadian perspectives in health promotion: a critique. *Health Education*, **4**, 4–9.

Le Compte, E.J. (1987). Clinical aspects of topical fluoride products—risks, benefits and recommendations. *Journal of Dental Research*, **66**, 1066–71.

Linden, G.J., Mullally, B.H., and Freeman, R. (1996) Stress and the progression of periodontal disease. *Journal of Clinical Periodontology*, **23**, 675–80.

Lindquist, C. and Teppo, L. (1978). Epidemiological evaluation of sunlight as a risk factor of lip cancer. *British Journal of Cancer*, **37**, 983–9.

Lipton, J.A., Ship, J.A., and Larach-Robinson, D. (1993). Estimated prevalence of reported orofacial pain in the United States. *Journal of the American Dental Association*, **124**, 115–21.

Loe, H. and Schiott, C.R. (1970). The effect of mouthrinses and the topical application of chlorhexidine on the development of dental plaque and gingivitis in man. *Journal of Periodontal Research*, **5**, 79–83.

Loe, H., Theilade, E., and Jensen, S.B. (1965). Experimental gingivitis in man. *Journal of Periodontology*, **36**, 177–87.

Loe, H., Anerud, A., Boysen, H., and Smith, M. (1978). The natural history of periodontal disease in man. *Journal of Periodontology*, **49**, 607–20.

Loe, H., Anerud, A., Boysen, H., and Morrison, E. (1986). Natural history of periodontal disease in man. Rapid, moderate and no loss of attachment in Sri Lankan laborers 14 to 46 years of age. *Journal of Clinical Periodontology*, **13**, 431–45

Lovdal, A., Arno, A., and Waerhaug, J. (1958). Incidence of clinical manifestations of periodontal disease in light of oral hygiene and calculus formation. *Journal of the American Dental Association*, **56**, 21–33.

McDonagh, M., Whiting, P., Bradley, M., *et al.* (2000). *A systematic review of public water fluoridation.* NHS Centre for Reviews and Dissemination, University of York.

Macfarlane, G.J., Macfarlane, T.V., and Lowenfels, A.B. (1996) The influence of alcohol consumption on worldwide trends in mortality from upper aerodigestive tract cancers in men. *Journal of Epidemiology and Community Health*, **50**, 636–9.

McKay, F.S. (1933). Mottled enamel: the prevention of its further production through a change of water supply at Oakley, Idaho. *Journal of the American Dental Association*, **20**, 1137–49.

McKeown, T. (1976). *The role of medicine. Dream, mirage or nemesis?* The Nuffield Provincial Hospitals Trust, London.

McNutt, T., Shannon, S.W., Wright, J.T., and Feinstein, R.A. (1989). Oral trauma in adolescent athletes. *Paediatric Dentistry*, **11**, 209–13.

Mahler, H. (1981). The meaning of 'Health for All' by the year 2000. *World Health Forum*, **1**, 5–22.

Manji, F. and Fejerskov, O. (1990). Dental caries in developing countries in relation to the appropriate use of fluoride. *Journal of Dental Research*, **69**, 733–41.

Manji, F. and Sheiham, A. (1986). CPITN findings and the manpower implications of periodontal treatment needs for Kenyan children. *Community Dental Health*, **3**, 143–51.

Marthaler, T. (1983). Practical aspects of salt fluoridation. *Schweizer Monatsschrift für Zahnmedizinizinische*, **93**, 1197–214.

Marthaler, T.M. (1990*a*). Caries status in Europe and predictions of future trends. Symposium report. *Caries Research*, **24**, 381–96.

Marthaler, T.M. (1990*b*). Changes in the prevalence of dental caries. How much can be attributed to changes in diet? *Caries Research*, **24**, 212–23.

Martínez-Canut, P., Lorca, A., and Magan, R. (1995). Smoking and periodontal disease severity. *Journal of Clinical Periodontology*, **22**, 743–9.

Mautsch, W. (1995). Multisectoral approach. In *Promotion oral health in deprived Communities* (ed. W. Mautsch and A. Sheiham), pp. 265–82. Zahnmedizinische Entwicklungshilfe, Berlin.

Mautsch, W. and Sheiham, A. (1995). *Promoting oral health in deprived communities.* Zahnmedizinische Entwicklungshilfe, Berlin.

Mejia, D.R., Espinal, F., Velez, H., and Aguirre, S.M. (1976). Use of fluoridated salt in four Columbian communities VIII. *Bol Sanit Panama*, **80**, 205–19.

Miller, A.J., Brunelle, J.A., Carlos, J.P., Brown, L.J., and Loe, H. (1987). *Oral health of United States adults; The national survey of oral health in U.S. employed adults and seniors: 1985–6*. National Institute of Health Publication No. 87–2868. National Institute of Dental Research, Bethesda, MD.

Morris, J.W. (1965). Skeletal fluorosis among Indians of the American South West. *American Journal of Roentgenology, Radium Therapy and Nuclear Medicine*, 608–15.

Murray, J.J. (1971). Adult dental health in fluoride and non-fluoride areas. *British Dental Journal*, **131**, 391–5.

Murray, J.J. and Naylor, M.N. (1996). Fluorides and dental caries. In *Prevention of oral disease* (ed. J.J. Murray), pp. 32–67. Oxford University Press.

Murray, J.J., Rugg-Gunn, A.J., and Jenkins, G.N. (1991). *Fluorides in caries prevention*. Wright, Oxford.

Muscat, J.E., Richie, J.P. Jr, Thompson, S., and Wynder, E.L. (1996) Gender differences in smoking and risk for oral cancer. *Cancer Research*, **56**, 5192–7.

Nadanovsky, P. and Sheiham, A. (1994). The relative contribution of dental services to the changes and geographical variations in caries status of 5- and 12-year-old children in England and Wales in the 1980s. *Community Dental Health*, **11**, 215–23.

Nadanovsky, P. and Sheiham, A. (1995). Relative contribution of dental services to the changes in caries levels of 12-year-old children in 18 industrialized countries in the 1970s and early 1980s. *Community Dentistry and Oral Epidemiology*, **23**, 331–9.

National Health and Medical Research Council (1991). *The effectiveness of water fluoridation*. Commonwealth of Australia, Canberra.

Newbrun, E. (1989). Effectiveness of water fluoridation. *Journal of Public Health Dentistry*, **49**, 279–89.

Offenbacher, S., Katz, V., Fertik, G., *et al.* (1996). Periodontal infection as a possible risk factor for preterm low birth weight. *Journal of Periodontology*, **67**, 1103–13.

Office of the Auditor General Western Australia (1995). *Performance examination: public dental services*. Office of the Auditor General, Perth.

Oldham, P.D. and Newell, D.J. (1977). Fluoridation of water supplies and cancer—a possible association. *Journal of the Royal Statistical Society*, **26**, 125–35.

O'Mullane, D.M. and Robinson, M.E. (1977). The distribution of dentists and the uptake of dental treatment by school children in England and Wales. *Community Dentistry and Oral Epidemiology*, **5**, 156–9.

OPCS (Office of Population Censuses and Surveys) (1994). *Cancer statistics registration* . HMSO, London.

Papapanou, P.N. and Lindhe, J. (1992). Preservation of probing attachment and alveolar bone levels in 2 random population samples. *Journal of Clinical Periodontology*, **19**, 583–8.

Parkin, D.M., Muir, C.S., and Whelan, S.L. (1992). *Cancer incidence in five continents*, Vol. 6. International Agency for Research on Cancer, Lyon.

Penchansky, R. and Thomas, J.W. (1981). The concept of access. Definition and relationship to consumer satisfaction. *Medical Care*, **19**, 127–40.

Perry, D.A., Freed, J.R., and Kushman, J.E. (1997). Characteristics of patients seeking care from independent dental hygienist practices. *Journal of Public Health Dentistry*, **57**, 76.

Pitts, N.B. and Palmer, J.D. (1995). The dental caries experience of 5-year-old children in Great Britain. Surveys coordinated by the British Association for the Study of Community Dentistry. *Community Dental Health*, **12**, 52–8.

Platz H., Fries R., Hudec, M. (1986). *Prognoses of oral cavity carcinomas. Results of a multi-centre retrospective operational study.* Hanser, Munich.

Preber, H. and Bergstrom, J. (1985). The effect of non-surgical treatment on periodontal pockets in smokers and non-smokers. *Journal of Clinical Periodontology*, **13**, 319–23.

Preber, H. and Bergstrom, J. (1990). Effect of cigarette smoking on periodontal healing following surgical therapy. *Journal of Clinical Periodontology*, **17**, 324–8.

Raw, M., McNeill, A., and West, R. (1998). Smoking cessation guidelines for health professionals. A guide to effective smoking cessation interventions for the health care system. *Thorax*, **53**, 1–19.

Rear, S.B. (1994). The effect of changes in caries prevalence on general dental practice. *International Dental Journal*, **44**, 435–8.

Riordan, P.J. (1993). Perceptions of dental fluorosis. *Journal of Dental Research*, **72**, 1268–74.

Riordan, P.J. (1997). Can organised dental care for children be both good and cheap. *Community Dentistry and Oral Epidemiology*, **25**, 119–25.

Riordan, P.J. (1999). Fluoride supplements for young children: an analysis of the literature focusing on benefits and risk. *Community Dentistry and Oral Epidemiology*, **27**, 72–83.

Ripa, L.W. (1985). The roles of prophylaxes and dental prophylaxis pastes in caries prevention In *Clinical uses of fluorides* (ed. S.H.Y. Wei). Lea & Febiger, Philadelphia, PA.

Robinson, P.G., Sheiham, A., Challacombe, S.J., Wren, M.W.D., and Zakrzewska, J.M. (1998). Gingival ulceration in HIV infection. A case series and case control study. *Journal of Clinical Periodontology*, **25**, 260–7.

Rock, W.P. and Sabieha, A.M. (1997).The relationship between reported toothpaste usage in infancy and fluorosis of permanent incisors. *British Dental Journal*, **183**, 165–70.

Rose, G. (1985). Sick individuals and sick populations. *International Journal of Epidemiology*, **14**, 32–8.

Roth, H. (1951). Psychosomatic and nutritional factors related to recurrent necrotizing ulcerative gingivitis. *Journal of the American Dental Association*, **42**, 474–5.

Rothman, K.J. and Keller, A.Z. (1972). The effect of joint exposure to alcohol and tobacco on the risk of cancer of the mouth and pharynx. *Journal of Chronic Disease*, **25**, 14–19.

Royal College of Physicians (1976). *Fluoride, teeth and health.* Royal College of Physicians, London.

Rugg-Gunn A.J. (1993). *Nutrition and dental health.* Oxford University Press.

Rugg-Gunn, A. (1997). Nutrition, dietary guidelines and food policy in oral health. In *Community oral health* (ed. C. Pine), pp. 206–20. Wright, Oxford.

Samarawikrama, D.Y.D. (1995). Appropriate technology, personnel and training. In *Promoting oral health in deprived communities* (ed. W. Mautsch, and A. Sheiham), pp. 347–61. Deusche Stiftungfur Internationale Entwicklung, Berlin.

Sanderson, M.E. (1984). Strategies for implementing NACNE recommendations. *Lancet*, **December 10**, 1352–6.

Scheinin, A. and Makinen, K.K. (1975). Turku sugar studies. I-XXI. *Acta Odontologica Scandinavica*, **33**, 1–349.

Schoen, M.H. (1991). Capitation in dentistry: original concepts and current reality. *Journal of Public Health Policy*, **12**, 199–208.

Schou, L. (1985). Active-involvement principle in dental health education. *Community Dentistry and Oral Epidemiology*, **13**, 128–32.

Schou, L. (1993). Oral health promotion in the workplace In *Oral health promotion* (ed. L. Schou and A.S. Blinkhorn), pp. 189–205. Oxford University Press.

Schou, L. (1998). Behavioural aspects of dental plaque control measures: an oral health promotion perspective. In *European workshop on mechanical plaque control* (ed. N.P. Lang, R. Attstrom, and H. Loe), pp. 287–99. Quintessence, Chicago, IL.

Schou, L. and Wight, C. (1994) Does dental health education affect inequalities in dental health? *Community Dental Health*, **11**, 97–100.

Shaw, W.C., Rees, G., Dawe, M., and Charles, C.R. (1985). The influence of dentofacial appearance on social attractiveness of young adults. *American Journal of Orthodontics*, **87**, 21–6.

Sheiham, A. (1991). Why free sugars consumption should be below 15 kg per person per year in industrialised countries: the dental evidence. *British Dental Journal*, **171**, 63–5.

Sheiham, A. (1992). The role of the dental team in promoting dental health and general health through oral health. *International Dental Journal*, **42**, 223–8.

Sheiham, A. (1995). Development of oral health promotion strategies In *Turning strategy into action* (ed. E. Kay), pp. 9–46. Eden Bianchi Press, Manchester.

Shepherd, M.A., Nadanovsky, P., and Sheiham, A. (1999). The prevalence and impact of dental pain in 8-year-old school children in Harrow, England. *British Dental Journal*, **187**, 38–41.

Silness, J. and Loe, H. (1964). Periodontal disease in pregnancy. II. Correlation between oral hygiene and periodontal condition. *Acta Odontologica Scandinavica*, **22**, 121–35.

Slade, G. D. (1997). *Measuring oral health and quality of life*, University of North Carolina at Chapel Hill.

Slade, G.D., Spencer, A.J., Davies, M.J., and Stewart, J.F. (1996). Influence of exposure to fluoridated water on socioeconomic inequalities in children's caries experience. *Community Dentistry and Oral Epidemiology*, **24**, 89–100.

Slots, J. and Genco, R.J. (1984). Black-pigmented *Bacteroides* species, *Capnocytophaga* species, and *Actinobacillus actinomycetemcomitans* in human periodontal disease: virulence factors in colonization, survival, and tissue destruction. *Journal of Dental Research*, **63**, 412–21.

Smith, S.E., Warnakulasuriya, K.A., Feyerabend, C., Belcher, M., Cooper, D.J., and Johnson, N.W. (1998). A smoking cessation programme conducted through dental practices in the UK. *British Dental Journal*, **185**, 299–303.

Socransky, S.S., Haffajee, A.D., Goodson, J.M., and Lindhe, J. (1984). New concepts of destructive periodontal disease. *Journal of Clinical Periodontology*, **11**, 21–32.

Speight, P.M., Downer, M.C., and Zakrzewska, J.M. (1993). Screening for oral cancer and precancer. Report of a UK working group. *Community Dental Health*, **10** (Supplement 1), 1–89.

Spencer, A.J., Slade, G.D., and Davies, M. (1996). Water fluoridation in Australia. *Community Dental Health*, **13**, 27–37.

Sprod, A., Anderson, R., and Treasure, E.T. (1996). *Effective oral health promotion: literature review.* Health Promotion Wales, Cardiff.

Sreebny, L.M. (1982). Sugar availability, sugar consumption and dental caries. *Community Dentistry and Oral Epidemiology*, **10**, 1–7.

Srikantia, S.G. and Siddiqui, A.H. (1965). Metabolic studies in skeletal fluorosis. *Clinical Science*, **28**, 477–85.

Stamm, J.W. (1991). The epidemiology of permanent tooth caries in the Americas. In *Risk markers for oral diseases.* Vol. 1, *Dental caries: markers of high and low risk groups and individuals* (ed. N.W. Johnson), pp. 132–55. Cambridge University Press.

Stephen, K.W. and Campbell, D. (1978). Caries reduction and cost benefit after 3 years of sucking fluoride tablets daily at school. A double-blind trial. *British Dental Journal*, **144**, 202–6.

Stephen, K.W., Boyle, I.T., and Campbell, D. (1984). Five-year double blind fluoridated milk study in Scotland. *Community Dentistry and Oral Epidemiology*, **12**, 223–9.

Stephen, K.W., Creanor, S.L., Russell, J.I., Burchell, C.K., Huntington, E., and Downie, C.F. (1988). A 3-year oral health dose–response study of sodium monofluorosphosphate dentifrices with and without zinc citrate: anti-caries results. *Community Dentistry and Oral Epidemiology*, **16**, 321–5.

Stephen, K.W., Macpherson, L.M., Gorzo, I., and Gilmour, W.H. (1999). Effect of fluoridated salt intake in infancy: a blind caries and fluorosis study in 8th grade Hungarian pupils. *Community Dentistry and Oral Epidemiology*, **27**, 210–15.

Stillman-Lowe, C. (1998). Effectiveness reviews: progress and problems. In *Designing and evaluating effective oral health promotion* (ed. B. Daly and R.G. Watt), pp. 5–7. Oral Health Promotion Research Group, London.

Stokes, A.N.S., Croft, G.C., and Gee, D. (1987). Comparison of laboratory and intraorally formed mouth protectors. *Endodontic Dentistry and Traumatology*, **3**, 255–8.

Stoltenberg, J.L., Osborn, J.B., Pihlstrom, B.L., *et al.* (1993). Association between cigarette smoking, bacterial pathogens, and periodontal status. *Journal of Periodontology*, **64**, 1225–30.

Stookey, G.K., DePaola, P.F., Featherstone, J.D., *et al.* (1993). A critical review of the relative anticaries efficacy of sodium fluoride and sodium monofluorosphospate dentifrices. *Caries Research*, **27**, 337–60.

Suomi, J.D., Greene, J.C., Vermillion, J.R., Doyle, J., Chang, J.J., and Leatherwood, E.C. (1971). The effect of controlled oral hygiene procedures on the progression of periodontal disease in adults. *Journal of Periodontology*, **42**, 152–60.

Sutcliffe, P. (1996). Oral cleanliness and dental caries. In *Prevention of oral disease* (ed. J.J. Murray), pp. 68–77. Oxford University Press.

Swango, P.A. (1996) Cancers of the oral cavity and pharynx in the United States: an epidemiologic overview. *Journal of Public Health Dentistry*, **56**, 309–18.

Tan, H.H., Ruiter, E., and Verhey, H. (1981). Effect of repeated dental health care education on gingival health, knowledge, attitude, behaviour and perception. *Community Dentistry and Oral Epidemiology*, **9**, 15–21.

Thorpe, S.J. (1993). Oral health status and trends in Africa—a WHO overview. In *Promotion of oral health in the African region* (ed. S.P. Akpabio), pp. 72–6. Commonwealth Dental Association, London.

Todd J.E. and Dodd, T. (1985). *Children's dental health in the United Kingdom 1983.* HMSO, London.

Todd, J.E. and Lader, D. (1991). *Adult dental health 1988 United Kingdom.* OPCS, London.

Toth, K. (1976). A study of 8 years' domestic salt fluoridation for prevention of caries. *Community Dentistry and Oral Epidemiology*, **4**, 106–10.

Toverud, G. (1957). The influence of war and post-war conditions on the teeth of Norwegian schoolchildren. II and III. *Milbank Memorial Fund Quarterly*, **35**, 373–459.

Treasure, E.T. and Dever, J.G. (1994). Relationship of caries with socioeconomic status in 14-year-old children from communities with different fluoride histories. *Community Dentistry and Oral Epidemiology*, **22**, 226–30.

Treasure, E.T. and Whyman, R.A. (1995). Changing patterns of dental disease and the implications for dental practice. *New Zealand Dental Journal*, **91**, 8–11.

Tudor Hart, J. (1971). The inverse care law. *Lancet*, **i**, 405–12.

US Public Health Service (1962). *Public health drinking water standards.* US Government Printing Office, Washington, DC.

van Amerongen B.M., Schutte G.J.B., and Alpherts W.C.J. (1993). *International dental key figures: a dynamic and relational data base analyzing oral health care.* Key Figure, Amsterdam.

Volpe, A.R., Petrone, M.E., and Davies, R.M. (1993). A critical review of the 10 pivotal caries clinical studies used in a recent meta-analysis comparing the anticaries efficacy of sodium fluoride and sodium monofluorophosphate dentifrices. *American Journal of Dentistry*, **6**, S13–42.

von der Fehr, F.R. and Moller, I.J. (1978). Caries-preventive fluoride dentifrices. *Caries Research*, **12**, 31–7.

Walters, M.J., Sherlock, J.C., Evans, W.H., and Read, I. (1983). Dietary intake of fluoride in the United Kingdom and fluoride content of some foodstuffs. *Journal of Science, Food and Agriculture*, **34**, 523–8.

Wang, N.J., Gropen, A.M., and Ogaard, B. (1997). Risk factors associated with fluorosis in a non-fluoridated population in Norway. *Community Dentistry and Oral Epidemiology*, **25**, 396–401.

Warnakulasuriya, K.A.A.S. (1984). Utilization of primary health care workers for the early detection of oral cancer and precancer cases in Sri Lanka. *Bulletin of the World Health Organization*, **62**, 243–50.

Watt, R. and Sheiham, A. (1999). Inequalities in oral health: a review of the evidence and recommendations for action. *British Dental Journal*, **187**, 6–12.

Welbury, R.R. (1996). The prevention of dental trauma. In *The prevention of oral disease* (ed. J.J. Murray), pp. 147–52. Oxford University Press.

WHO (World Health Organization)–UNICEF (1978). *Primary health care, Alma-Ata 1978.* WHO, Geneva.

WHO (World Health Organization) (1979). *A guide to oral health epidemiological investigations.* WHO, Geneva.

WHO (World Health Organization) (1984). *Health promotion: a discussion document on the concepts and principles.* WHO Regional Office for Europe, Copenhagen.

WHO (World Health Organization) (1986). *Ottawa charter for health promotion* . WHO, Geneva.

WHO (World Health Organization) (1994) *Fluorides and oral health.* WHO, Geneva.

WHO (World Health Organization) (1997). *Oral health surveys. basic methods.* WHO, Geneva.

Winter, G.B., Holt, R.D., and Williams, B.F. (1989). Clinical trial of a low fluoride toothpaste for young children. *International Dental Journal*, **39**, 227–35.

Yiamouyannis, J. and Burk, D. (1977) Fluoridation and cancer: age dependence of cancer mortality related to artificial fluoridation. In *Eighth International Society for Fluoride Research Conference.* Society for Fluoride Research, Oxford.

9.9 Musculoskeletal diseases*

Jennifer L. Kelsey and MaryFran Sowers

Introduction

Musculoskeletal diseases are among the most important public health problems. They are common, affect both sexes and all age groups, and are responsible for a substantial amount of impairment and disability. Musculoskeletal disorders range from minor aches and pains to chronic disabling conditions. Although they are occasionally fatal, their main effects are on quality of life and on economic productivity.

Musculoskeletal conditions have been less well studied than other major diseases. This limited attention has probably occurred because musculoskeletal diseases are not usually fatal, they are generally not dramatic because of their gradual onset, and some of the more important musculoskeletal diseases, such as osteoarthritis and osteoporosis, are often considered as inevitable consequences of ageing. In addition, most chronic musculoskeletal conditions do not come to medical attention until they are quite advanced, thus making case ascertainment more difficult in epidemiological studies.

Among the many musculoskeletal conditions that could be considered here, the most common and disabling in adults will be described (osteoarthritis, rheumatoid arthritis, osteoporosis and associated fractures, and back and neck pain), followed by some of the important diseases of adolescence, childhood, and infancy (scoliosis, slipped epiphysis, fractures, and developmental dislocation/dysplasia of the hip).

Magnitude of the problem

Musculoskeletal diseases are a major cause of disability worldwide and place a considerable social and economic burden on all societies (WHO 1992). In the United States, for instance, musculoskeletal problems are the most frequently reported impairment, affecting about 14 per cent of the population (Praemer *et al.* 1999). Table 1 shows that impairment of the back or spine is the most frequent, followed by the lower extremity or hip, and then the upper extremity or shoulder. The prevalence of musculoskeletal impairments increases with age. Among those aged 85 years and older, it is 20 per cent, with impairments of the back or spine and lower extremity or hip accounting for slightly more than half of musculoskeletal impairments. Among impairments, musculoskeletal disorders are the leading cause of days of restricted activity and of days in bed. In Ontario, Canada, musculoskeletal diseases rank first as a cause of long-term health problems and long-term disability, and second as a cause of days of restricted activity (Badley *et al.* 1994).

A survey in the United Kingdom found that 17 per cent of adults report a long-standing musculoskeletal disorder (Bowling 1996). The most important areas of life affected by long-standing disorders of the musculoskeletal system were ability to get around, stand, walk, and go shopping (24 per cent), and to participate in social and leisure time activities (24 per cent). Ability to work was also a major issue (17 per cent), particularly for those of working age. Another study in England (Thompson *et al.* 1974) found that many of the elderly with musculoskeletal diseases live alone. Half of them had difficulties because of stairs, one-third said they would not be able attract attention even in the event of an emergency, 20 per cent were dependent on others for such everyday tasks as taking a bath, doing housework, and getting out of the house.

Acute injuries of the musculoskeletal system, including fractures, dislocations, sprains, and strains, are also common. According to the United States Health Interview Survey (Praemer *et al.* 1999), there are 14.5 musculoskeletal injuries per 100 people per year of sufficient severity to warrant medical care or at least one half day of restricted activity. Among acute conditions, musculoskeletal conditions rank second to respiratory conditions in the frequency with which they are reported.

Musculoskeletal conditions generate substantial health care utilization. About 11 per cent of all hospital admissions in short-stay hospitals in the United States are attributed to musculoskeletal conditions (Praemer *et al.* 1999). Fractures, arthritis, intervertebral disk disorders, and other back problems are responsible for the greatest number of hospital admissions. The population aged 65 years and older accounts for 44 per cent of hospital admissions for

Table 1 Prevalence of musculoskeletal impairments, United States, 1995

Site of impairment	Estimated number of impairments
Back or spine	18 454 000
Lower extremity or hip	13 421 000
Upper extremity or shoulder	4 563 000
All musculoskeletal impairments	36 438 000

Modified from Praemer *et al.* (1999).

* A small portion of the material presented in this chapter has been adapted from Kelsey (1998).

musculoskeletal conditions. Figure 1 shows that among visits to physicians in office-based practice, musculoskeletal conditions rank first, accounting for 17 per cent of all office visits. Fifteen per cent of visits to hospital outpatient departments and 26 per cent of visits to emergency departments are attributable to musculoskeletal conditions. In addition, a significant number of people in the United States use complementary medicine for musculoskeletal problems. In a national sample of adults it was found that 36 per cent of those with back problems, 18 per cent of those with arthritis, and 22 per cent of those with sprains or strains had used unconventional therapy in the past year (Eisenberg *et al.* 1993). In Ontario, Canada, musculoskeletal diseases rank first as a reason for consultations with a health professional and second as a cause of use of both prescription and non-prescription drugs (Badley *et al.* 1994).

Musculoskeletal conditions are also a significant cause of workplace injuries and disability. Among the conditions for which worker disability allowances were granted in the United States in 1992, back disorders ranked sixth, osteoarthritis eighth, and rheumatoid arthritis sixteenth (Social Security Administration 1994, unpublished data).

The monetary cost of musculoskeletal diseases to society is substantial, especially because of the decreased productivity of those affected. The total cost of musculoskeletal diseases in the United States was estimated to be US$215 billion in 1995, with 41 per cent of this amount attributable to direct costs such as for hospital care, physicians and other health care providers, drugs, nursing home care, and administrative costs, and 59 per cent attributable to indirect costs from lost productivity because of morbidity and to a small extent mortality (Praemer *et al.* 1999). Felts and Yelin (1989) reported that costs of musculoskeletal diseases accounted for 1 per cent of the gross national product in the United States. Using somewhat different criteria, Coyte *et al.* (1998) estimated that musculoskeletal diseases cost 25.6 billion Canadian dollars in 1994, or 3.4 per cent of the gross domestic product. Seventy-one per cent of the costs were indirect. Badley (1995) noted that musculoskeletal diseases account for 32 per cent of all chronic disability costs in Canada.

In summary, musculoskeletal conditions have a substantial impact on quality of life in industrialized countries. In the United States, they rank highest among disease groups in the frequency with which they cause impairments and limitation of activity. They rank first in frequency of visits to physicians, and fourth in frequency of hospital admissions and frequency of surgical procedures within hospitals. The costs of musculoskeletal conditions are enormous, including both direct costs for medical care and indirect costs from lost productivity.

Moreover, the enormous societal burden from musculoskeletal diseases is not restricted to industrialized countries with high life expectancies. The limited data that are currently available indicate a large impact of musculoskeletal diseases on the work and personal lives of people in developing countries as well. As in industrialized countries, pain, disability, fatigue, depression, and loss of employment because of musculoskeletal diseases are major problems. For example, the prevalence of rheumatic complaints and of disability from rheumatic complaints in both urban and rural areas of Indonesia is similar to that in Australia (WHO 1992). Work-related problems, many of which could be prevented with proper ergonomic techniques, are particularly common in developing countries (Ahasan *et al.* 1999). In a survey in Thailand, about 50 per cent of female workers in five industries (garment, fertilizer, pharmaceutical, textile, and cigarettes) reported low back symptoms (Chavalitsakulchai and Shahnavaz 1993). Back problems and other musculoskeletal symptoms could often be attributed to modifiable situations, including manual handling of heavy materials, prolonged sitting and standing, awkward work positions, poor machine design and operation, monotonous and repetitive movements, poor work organization, and unsatisfactory work environments. Thus, opportunities already exist to reduce the burden of job-related musculoskeletal disorders in developing countries.

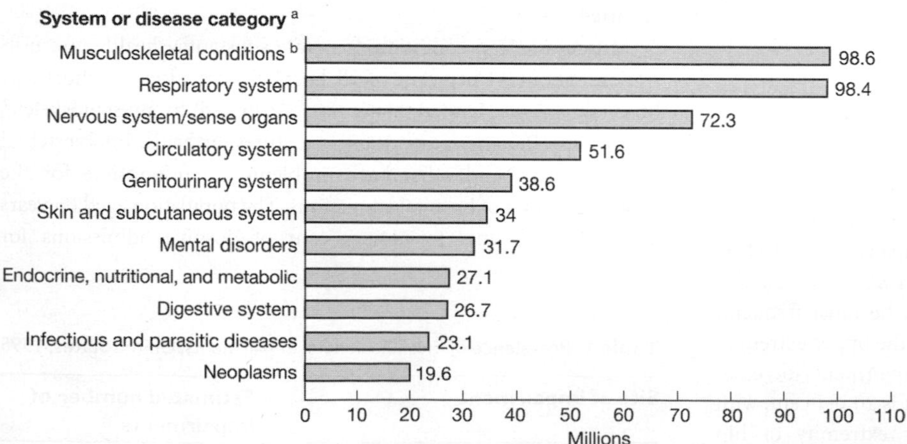

Fig. 1 Estimated number of visits to physicians in office-based practice by category of first-listed diagnosis, United States 1995, National Ambulatory Medical Care Survey. (Source: Praemer *et al.* 1999.)

Some common problems in epidemiological studies of musculoskeletal conditions

Conducting epidemiological studies of musculoskeletal conditions, even in industrialized countries, presents several difficulties not experienced to the same extent in studies of other important chronic diseases such as cancers and coronary heart disease (Kelsey 1982). Firstly, because many musculoskeletal conditions are not fatal, are not necessarily seen in hospitals, have a gradual onset, and often do not even come to medical attention, ascertainment of representative cases for epidemiological study may be difficult. Consequently, many studies of musculoskeletal diseases are based on the experience of particular clinical practices or hospitals. However, cases representative of those occurring in the general population are needed in order to provide an accurate description of disease occurrence, aetiology, and progression in the community. Even if all cases coming to medical attention within a defined geographical area are included in a study, unless the disease under study almost invariably comes to medical attention (such as hip fractures), the factors that bring persons with a given condition to medical attention often cannot be separated from factors that may be related to disease aetiology. For instance, are psychological characteristics of persons seeking care for back pain related to the aetiology of back pain, or are they related to the care-seeking behaviour among those with back pain?

Sometimes a condition for which medical care is virtually always sought, and for which case ascertainment is therefore relatively easy, is used as a surrogate for a disease for which medical care is not necessarily sought. For instance, hip fracture, which is almost always seen in a hospital, has been used as a surrogate for osteoporosis. However, hip fracture depends not only on whether a person has low bone mass, but also on the bone architecture and on whether the person falls and how he or she falls. Thus the risk factors for osteoporosis and hip fracture will overlap, but they will also differ in some respects.

The diagnostic criteria used for a disease may differ from one study to another, making it difficult to compare results. For many of the arthritic disorders, diagnosis is not straightforward. For example, people with arthritis on radiograph may not have symptoms, while people with symptoms do not necessarily show radiographic changes, resulting in an ambiguous case definition of osteoarthritis. Expert committees have established and then periodically revised the criteria for several of the arthritic disorders. When the diagnostic criteria are uniformly applied, this has increased comparability of cases from one study to another. However, the criteria have not always been used uniformly, and since the criteria have changed over time, it is sometimes not possible to examine changes in disease frequency over time. People may say that they have low back pain, but how does a researcher or practitioner know that a person is really in pain if there are no radiographic or other signs? The majority of asymptomatic people have evidence of bulging or protruding intervertebral disks on MRI, so that even MRI may be of limited value without clinical evidence of pathology (Jensen *et al.* 1994). The person may report low back pain only in order to obtain worker's compensation or the person may be truly affected.

Diseases that constitute one end of a continuous distribution, such as osteoporosis and scoliosis, present other problems. To define cases of these conditions, relatively arbitrary cut-off points aimed at classifying individuals as 'diseased' and 'normal' must be employed, but different investigators may chose different cut-off points, thus precluding comparisons from one study to another. In recent years, standard cut-off points have been recommended by committees, so that this situation should improve. Another issue is that it may be difficult to differentiate the aetiology of diseases such as osteoporosis, degenerative disk disease, and osteoarthritis from what is considered normal ageing.

Labels for diseases once considered a single entity may become irrelevant when subcategories of the disease are more clearly delineated. For instance, what was once called 'juvenile rheumatoid arthritis' is now known to be composed of several subtypes, each with its own aetiology. Much information may be lost when several distinct entities are considered as one disease, as exemplified by studies of low back pain that do not consider the contribution of many different disease processes, such as sprains and strains, intervertebral disk herniations, and osteoporosis.

Another concern relates to study design. Cross-sectional studies of the relation between neuromuscular abnormalities and scoliosis, for instance, are difficult to interpret because it is not known whether the neuromuscular abnormalities lead to curvature of the spine or whether curvature of the spine leads to neuromuscular defects. Cross-sectional studies of psychological symptoms and low back pain and of obesity and osteoarthritis present similar difficulties in interpretation. In such situations longitudinal studies, despite their great expense, are needed.

Problems in conducting epidemiological studies of musculoskeletal diseases are magnified considerably in developing countries. Because of shortages of money and human resources, most studies are hospital-based. However, in many developing countries most people do not seek care from a physician or in a hospital unless the disease is quite severe. Instead, inexperienced community nurses often provide care (WHO 1992; Dans *et al.* 1997). In a survey in the Philippines, for instance, it was found that most people with rheumatic complaints who sought treatment were seen by someone other than a physician. Only 23 per cent had seen a general practitioner, and 2 per cent saw a rheumatologist. Care from a physician is frequently not available, accessible, or affordable (Dans *et al.* 1997; Croft 1996). In fact, some countries have no rheumatologists at all (Adebajo 1990). Patriarchal societies may limit access to medical care for women, and relatively few women survive to old age. Consequently, both comparisons of disease frequency in men and women within such countries and comparisons to other countries may be difficult to interpret (Hameed *et al.* 1995; Farooqi and Gibson 1998). In addition, even when affected individuals are seen by qualified medical personnel, the diagnostic criteria vary considerably (Ferraz 1995).

If community surveys are undertaken in developing countries, many difficulties are likely to be encountered. Poor training of personnel, inadequate facilities, limited ability to reach populations for study, a low level of public support, political instability, and bureaucratic rigidity are often encumbrances to epidemiological studies (Ferraz 1995). The diagnostic tests used in such surveys must be simple and inexpensive. If the study is being conducted in a tropical region, reagents and tests used in other geographical areas may not work because of either the heat or the characteristics of the populations being studied. Tests for rheumatoid factor in West Africa are not useful because similar proportions of people with and without rheumatoid arthritis are positive (Adebajo 1990). Rheumatoid nodules are rare in southern Asians with rheumatoid arthritis, suggesting that diagnostic criteria may have to be modified (Hameed *et al.* 1995). In addition, pain, complaints, and manifestations of disability may vary cross-culturally (Croft 1996). Measures of disability often require modification (Adebajo 1990).

It should also be kept in mind that risk factors may be quite different in developing countries. It has been hypothesized, for instance, that osteoporosis may not be such an important cause of fracture in developing countries because high levels of physical activity make bones stronger (Scrimgeour 1992).

Finally, great variation in disease frequency and in risk factor prevalence occur among developing countries, and there is a need for information on specific diseases and risk factors in specific regions. In north Pakistan, for instance, osteoarthritis of the knee is an especially common complaint. Fibromyalgia, low back pain, and soft-tissue rheumatism are next most common, but mainly in the urban poor (Farooqi and Gibson 1989). Thus, not only should one avoid generalizing from one country to another, but frequently one cannot generalize from one part of the same country to another.

Selected musculoskeletal disorders of adults

Osteoarthritis

Osteoarthritis is a condition affecting joints and their constituent parts, including muscle, bone, and cartilage. Increased bone stiffness, increased mineralization of bony tissue around the joint in the form of osteophytes, and loss of cartilage from the joint space are seen. This joint degradation results in pain, loss of mobility, disability, and, increasingly, the need for joint replacement to remediate the pain and loss of mobility. Indeed, osteoarthritis is second only to cardiovascular diseases in the frequency with which it produces severe chronic disability.

The peripheral joints most commonly affected in osteoarthritis are (in descending order of frequency) hands, feet, knees, and hips. Clinically, several subsets of disease are noted based on the pattern of the joint group involvement, such as isolated hip or knee involvement, hand plus knee involvement, or polyarticular involvement.

Estimates of osteoarthritis prevalence have generally used information from two sources: (a) an individual's report of pain, decreased articular movement in the joint, and curtailment of physical functioning; (b) radiographs of the joint. Prevalence estimates depend on case definition (i.e. self-report of symptoms or radiographic appearance) as well as measurement approach (e.g. radiographs of the knees with or without bearing weight). The typical radiographic appearance of the joint includes narrowing of the joint space, subchondral sclerosis, and osteophyte formation, which are assumed to reflect the underlying processes of cartilage loss, bone change, and new bone formation (Kellgren and Lawrence 1963).

In the United States the prevalence of osteoarthritis has been estimated in two national studies: the National Health Examination Survey of 1960 to 62 (hands and feet) and the National Health and Nutrition Survey (**NHANES-I**) of 1971 to 75 (knees and hips). In NHANES-I there was radiographic evidence of osteoarthritis in more than 33 per cent of persons aged 25 to 74 years and more than 70 per cent of persons aged 55 to 74 years (Lawrence *et al.* 1989). NHANES-III has been recently completed. Data on radiographic osteoarthritis of the hands and knees will soon be available.

Many individuals with radiographic evidence of osteoarthritis are asymptomatic. In one American population, only 65 per cent of those older than 55 years of age with radiographic evidence of knee osteoarthritis reported knee pain, and 76 per cent of those with radiographic evidence of hand osteoarthritis reported hand pain (Carman 1989). In women aged 40 to 55 years, 9 per cent had knee osteoarthritis on radiograph and reported pain, 6 per cent had knee osteoarthritis on radiograph in the absence of reported pain, 31 per cent reported knee pain in the absence of radiographic osteoarthritis, and 54 per cent reported no pain and had no radiographic evidence of osteoarthritis in the knee (Lachance *et al.* 2001).

Risk factors

Despite differences in osteoarthritis definitions, several patterns of disease occurrence are evident (Lawrence *et al.* 1989; Lawrence *et al.* 1998). The prevalence of osteoarthritis increases with age, especially after 40 years of age. Almost everyone 65 years or older has at least one joint with a radiographically-defined feature of the disease. Individual joints show the same age-related rise in osteoarthritis prevalence, with the hip showing a later rise than the knee (Lawrence *et al.* 1998). Women are affected more often than men, especially for hand and knee osteoarthritis, and particularly after 50 years of age (Butler *et al.* 1988).

Caucasian populations in developed countries have similar prevalence rates (van Sasse *et al.* 1988), but hip osteoarthritis may be less common in Africa and Asia than in Western countries (Lawrence and Sebo 1980). Knee osteoarthritis shows less geographicalal variation than hip and hand osteoarthritis, possibly reflecting the importance of injury as a cause of knee disease (Lawrence and Sebo 1980).

The aetiology of osteoarthritis is complex and involves modifications in bone, joint, capsule, and muscle and the relation of these elements to each other (Fig. 2). Osteoarthritis appears to be a mechanically driven but chemically-mediated disease process, in which there is attempted (or aberrant) repair (Bleasel and Moskowitz 1995). An evolutionary theory has been put forward to help explain joint distribution (Hutton 1987) based on an understanding that it is a relatively recent evolutionary event that human joints provide pincer

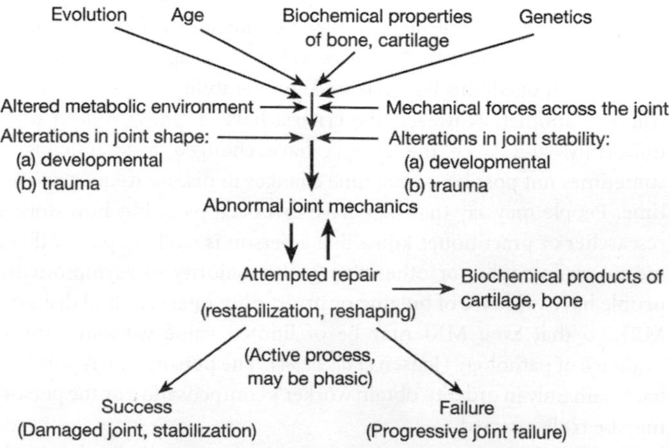

Fig. 2 A schema depicting the aetiology of osteoarthritis.

capability and full weight bearing on the legs. A strong genetic component has been proposed to occur in the biochemical constituents of bone and cartilage that places a person at increased risk. The biology and biochemistry of osteoarthritis is reviewed by Hamerman (1989).

Overweight persons have a higher than expected prevalence of knee osteoarthritis. This is true whether knee osteoarthritis is defined by symptom or radiograph and irrespective of whether the focus is on tibiofemoral (Anderson and Felson 1988; Felson *et al.* 1988) or patellofemoral disease (Manninen *et al.* 1996). The association between obesity and osteoarthritis of the knee is stronger for bilateral than unilateral disease and more marked in women than in men. Prospective data in women suggest that risk for knee osteoarthritis is increased by approximately 15 per cent for each additional kilogram per square metre of body mass index above 27 (Sowers *et al.* 2000). There is prospective evidence that weight loss reduces the risk of subsequent symptomatic knee disease (Felson *et al.* 1992).

The association with weight is weaker or absent for the hip in some studies (Kellgren 1961; Tepper and Hochberg 1993). Symptomatic hip osteoarthritis is more strongly associated with obesity than isolated radiographic disease (Roach *et al.* 1994).

Recent longitudinal studies show that increased weight precedes the occurrence of hand or knee osteoarthritis and is not merely a consequence of it (Carman *et al.* 1994; Manninen *et al.* 1996). For example, Manninen *et al.* found that body mass index was directly and strongly correlated with the risk of developing disabling knee osteoarthritis over a 10-year period. Furthermore, overweight persons with knee osteoarthritis are at higher risk of experiencing progressive disease than persons who are not overweight (Dougados *et al.* 1992).

Weight could act through several mechanisms to contribute to the development of osteoarthritis. Firstly, being overweight increases the amount of force across a weight-bearing joint (Schipplein and Andriacchi 1991). In addition, excess adipose tissue may produce abnormal levels of hormones or growth factors that affect cartilage or underlying bone so as to predispose to osteoarthritis development, although specific metabolic products have not been identified.

Evidence concerning sport and leisure activity as risk factors is conflicting. In part, this conflict may exist because, as a number of studies now indicate, brief applications of physiological loads, in the absence of traumatic twist or torque, stimulate matrix synthesis necessary to maintain cartilage, whereas extended application of loads can lead to cartilage deterioration. Studies of recreational and competitive athletes suggest that regular exercise, including jogging or moderate low-impact running, is not a detectable risk factor for hip and knee osteoarthritis in those with normal joints. However, these activities may increase risk in those with previous joint injuries or developmentally defective joints. Also, individuals who participate in certain other sports such as American football may have an increased risk (Vincelette *et al.* 1972). Prolonged decreased joint use and decreased loading generates changes that make cartilage more vulnerable to injury (Buckwalter *et al.* 1995).

Increased risks of both hip and knee osteoarthritis occur in men and women with jobs that stress the lower limbs. Studies have suggested that knee bending and heavy lifting are associated with radiographic knee osteoarthritis (Felson *et al.* 1991), and that heavy lifting among farmers confers enhanced risk of radiographic hip osteoarthritis (Croft *et al.* 1992). These risks are cumulative and there is evidence of increasing risk with greater number of years spent in such occupations. Hadler *et al.* (1978) showed that women who had worked for many years within the same cotton mill in the United States had patterns of osteoarthritis in the hand that could be directly related to specific tasks performed in the factory.

Persons with osteoarthritis of the knee or hip are more likely to have higher bone mass than others of their age (Sowers *et al.* 1996). Various hypotheses have been proposed to explain a negative association between osteoarthritis and osteoporosis, primarily centred around responses to mechanical forces. It has been hypothesized that stiff subchondral bone, as reflected in greater bone mass, increases cartilage damage with normal joint loading and leads to the development of osteoarthritis (Radin *et al.* 1972). Alternative explanations for the negative association between osteoarthritis and osteoporosis include genetic make-up and differences in response to changing ovarian hormone levels. Also, persons with osteoarthritis may have enhanced osteoblast production and/or a mineralization deposition defect as suggested by the presence of osteophytes and joint space narrowing in hip osteoarthritis (Sowers *et al.* 1999*a*).

Rare inherited diseases of cartilage have been recognized for many years. Also, the familial aggregation of Heberden's nodes (bony protuberances on the margins of distal interphalangeal joints) was first reported many years ago by Stecher (1941). The genetics of the common forms of osteoarthritis are now of considerable interest, as recent studies have suggested that at least 50 per cent of the variability of osteoarthritis in the hands, knees, and hips is accounted for by genetic factors (Cicuttini and Spector 1996; Holderbaum *et al.* 1999). Studies have uncovered rare families with mutations in the collagen 2AI gene whose members express precocious osteoarthritis and varying degrees of chondrodysplasia. Collagen IX mutations have also been implicated. To date these mutations do not appear to influence common forms of osteoarthritis (Holderbaum *et al.* 1999). Current studies are underway to evaluate other candidate genes.

Prevention

Based on current knowledge of risk factors, primary prevention is targeted at avoiding joint trauma, preventing obesity, and modifying occupationally-related joint stress through ergonomic approaches. Techniques for avoiding joint trauma include providing appropriate protection and padding for contact sports and modifying game rules to minimize the kind of contact that is associated with joint trauma (Buckwalter *et al.* 1995). Prompt diagnosis and treatment of earlier joint disease reduces the likelihood of osteoarthritis in these joints.

Some research suggests the importance of developing and maintaining adequate muscle strength as a mechanism to minimize joint stress. Ongoing research and intervention evaluations are aimed at identifying optimal conditioning exercise programmes to enhance musculoskeletal fitness without disease exacerbation of joint damage.

Weight reduction could potentially afford some protection against both the development and progression of osteoarthritis. Reduction of weight has been shown to reduce pain in symptomatic osteoarthritis of the knee (Felson *et al.* 1992).

Therapy can involve the use of analgesics and/or non-steroidal anti-inflammatory drugs to control symptoms of pain, combined with physical and occupational therapy to assure joint range of motion, muscle strength, and an individual's ability to perform activities of daily living. Among those with severe pain and activity limitation, surgery, including joint replacement, is increasingly common. The role of social support is also recognized as important. The use of complementary therapies such as glucosamines and chondroitin sulphate is currently being evaluated in clinical trials.

Rheumatoid arthritis

Rheumatoid arthritis is a chronic inflammatory joint disorder characterized by proliferative synovitis leading to destruction of the articular cartilage and to bony erosions. These typically result in joint deformities. Although symptoms may vary, they typically include pain and stiffness of multiple joints (particularly the small joints of the hands and feet), soft-tissue swelling, increased temperature of affected joints, limitation in range of motion, weakness, fatigue, and loss of endurance.

Rheumatoid arthritis is usually not a fatal disorder, but generally results in substantial chronic disability. The disease is also associated with substantial comorbidity from respiratory and infectious diseases as well as gastrointestinal diseases (Kelsey and Hochberg 1988). Table 2 shows a revised classification for the diagnosis of rheumatoid arthritis published in 1987 by the American College of Rheumatology (**ACR**). Positive classification requires a positive finding for at least four out of the seven criteria (Arnett *et al.* 1988).

The prevalence of rheumatoid arthritis reported from the Rochester (Minnesota) Epidemiology Project (based on the 1987 ACR criteria) is 1 per cent (Gabriel *et al.* 1999), a prevalence consistent with the 0.8 per cent reported in several European populations (Silman and Hochberg 1993). The overall age- and sex-adjusted annual incidence in Rochester, Minnesota, residents aged 35 years and older from 1955 to 1985 was 75.3 per 100 000. There is evidence of a decline in rheumatoid arthritis incidence over the last few decades in both the Unied States and the United Kingdom (Linos *et al.* 1980; Hochberg 1990; Silman and Hochberg 1993; Gabriel *et al.* 1999). As incidence rates have been declining, prevalence has been rising, probably due in part to improved survivorship (Hochberg 1990).

Risk factors

Overall, the incidence is about twice as great in females as males. In Rochester, Minnesota, the annual incidence ranged from 17 per 100 000 in men aged 35 to 44 years to 111 per 100 000 in men aged 75 to 84 years. The incidence was 50 per 100 000 in women aged 35 to 44 years and 123 per 100 000 in women aged 75 to 84 years (Gabriel *et al.* 1999).

Table 2 The 1987 American Rheumatism Association Revised Criteria for the Classification of Rheumatoid Arthritis[a]

Item	Definition
1	Morning stiffness, lasting at least 1 h
2	Arthritis involving at least three joint groups simultaneously
3	Arthritis involving at least one of at least 14 possible areas in the hands or wrists
4	Simultaneous involvement of the same joint areas on both sides of the body
5	Presence of subcutaneous nodules
6	Presence of serum rheumatoid factor
7	Presence of typical radiographic features (juxta-articular osteopenia and/or erosions) on hand and wrist films

[a]Positive classification requires at least four of the seven criteria.

Modified from Amett *et al.* (1988).

Rheumatoid arthritis prevalences are similar in African-Americans and white Americans, but higher prevalences of rheumatoid arthritis have been reported among several Native American tribes (Beasley *et al.* 1973; Harvey *et al.* 1983). Lower prevalences have been reported among some Asian populations (Beasley *et al.* 1983). Asians may also have more mild disease compared with Caucasians (Silman and Hochberg 1993; Lau *et al.* 1996). Reasons for this variation are not known.

The aetiology of rheumatoid arthritis is ill defined. Familial aggregation and a higher concordance rate in monozygotic than in dizygotic twins contribute to the characterization of rheumatoid arthritis as having a substantial heritable component. Genetic studies have focused primarily on autoimmune aspects of the disease, especially the role of the major histocompatibility locus. There is a strong association between rheumatoid arthritis and the class II major histocompatibility antigen HLA DR4, broadly observed across most racial/ethnic groups, and particularly in Caucasians, where the estimate of the relative risk exceeds 4.0 (Ollier and MacGregor 1995). Other work has identified an association with HLA DR1 and the shared epitope (Gregerson *et al.* 1987) between HLA DR1 and HLA DR4 (HLA DR1B1 gene on chromosome 6). The shared epitope is considered a marker for disease severity rather than susceptibility (Weyand *et al.* 1992). Current investigations are also exploring other genetic factors, such as HLA DR3/DR7 and an autoimmunity to type II collagen (Ollier and MacGregor 1995).

While the potential contribution of genetic susceptibility is widely recognized, there remain questions as to the initiating events that give rise to rheumatoid arthritis and its patterns of expression. Infectious agents that have been proposed and/or explored include the Epstein–Barr virus, parvovirus, rubella, and mycoplasma (Alarcón 1995), but no strong evidence exists for an aetiological role for these agents.

Based on early observations of symptom improvement during pregnancy, both hormonal and non-hormonal reproductive factors have been considered. It has been postulated that during pregnancy not only are there alterations in circulating hormone concentrations but that the placenta may also contribute glycoproteins with anti-inflammatory or immunosuppressive properties, particularly in those pregnancies where there are disparities in the mother and fetus HLA antigens (Alarcón 1995).

A role for hormones, including oestrogens, testosterone, and prolactin, has been suggested in both the initiation and the severity of rheumatoid arthritis. Early epidemiological studies reported that oral contraceptives were protective against rheumatoid arthritis (Wingrave 1978). A possible role of oral contraceptives was also suggested by the declining incidence rates among females, but not males, from the period 1960 to 1964 through to 1970 to 1974 (Linos *et al.* 1980). A meta-analysis of epidemiological studies has reported a protective effect (relative risk of ≅ 0.7), with the authors suggesting that the protection was more likely to be associated with progression rather than initiation of rheumatoid arthritis (Spector and Hochberg 1990). This latter suggestion however, does not account for the findings of an apparent shift in the age at onset to older ages. Thus, while a role for exogenous hormonal influence is intriguing, additional studies are needed to evaluate the use of exogenous hormones in the form of replacement therapy as well as contraception. Account must be taken of the selection factors that give rise to their use, as well as to the dose, constitutive hormones, and duration of use.

Prevention

No viable screening or primary prevention measures are available for rheumatoid arthritis. Because of the excess mortality associated with respiratory and infectious diseases, public health interventions should include full utilization of vaccination programmes and the practice of hygienic techniques that limit the opportunity for exposure to infectious agents or transmission of infectious agents. Treatment of rheumatoid arthritis includes the use of analgesics and/or non-steroidal anti-inflammatory drugs to control pain and stiffness, physical therapy to maintain and improve joint range of motion, and occupational therapy to maximize the individual's ability to perform daily activities. Some persons with severe rheumatoid arthritis may be treated with immunosuppressive agents.

Osteoporosis and associated fractures

Osteoporosis has been defined at a Consensus Conference as a disease characterized by low bone mass and microarchitectual deterioration of bone tissue leading to enhanced bone fragility and a consequent increase in fracture risk (Anonymous 1997). Fractures of the hip, vertebrae, and distal radius are particularly common. The World Health Organization (**WHO**) defined osteoporosis as bone mineral density more than 2.5 standard deviations below the mean value of peak bone mass in normal young women (WHO 1994). It has been estimated that, by this definition, 70 per cent of women of age 80 years and older in the United States have osteoporosis in the hip, spine, or distal radius. Almost all women in this age group have bone mass that is below the mean for normal young women (Melton 1995).

Risk factors

Osteoporosis is much more common in females than males. In both females and males, its prevalence increases markedly with age, but the increase in prevalence occurs about 10 years earlier in females than males. Table 3 shows prevalence by age in females. A particularly rapid decrease in bone mass occurs in females in the years immediately following menopause, suggesting that loss of oestrogen is an important aetiological factor in women.

Globally, hip fracture incidence rates are highest in white people in northern European and North American countries, slightly lower in Asians living in economically developed areas such as Hong Kong and the United States, still lower in Hispanics and black people in the United States and in South America, and lowest in less developed areas of Asia such as China and in Africa (Maggi *et al.* 1991; Schwartz *et al.* 1999). In the United States, hip fracture incidence rates are lowest in black people, highest in white people, and intermediate in Asians and Hispanic white people (Villa and Nelson 1996). Although bone mass is highest in black people, there is little difference in the bone mass of white people and Asian-Americans. Thus bone mass cannot be the only factor that explains the differing hip fracture incidence rates in these groups. Bone architecture, fall frequency, and manner of falling are also believed to be important.

Bone mass in later adulthood, when fracture risk is greatest, is a function of bone mass in young adulthood, when bone mass is at its peak, and rate of loss of bone mass after the peak is reached. Numerous family and twin studies have demonstrated a strong genetic component to bone mass in young adulthood. Estimates of the heritability of bone mass range from 45 to 84 per cent, depending on the skeletal site examined (Slemenda *et al.* 1991; Sowers *et al.* 1992). Numerous genes have been considered for their association with bone mass, including the genotypes for the vitamin D receptor, the sex hormone receptor genes, the matrix proteins (such as osteocalcin), and type I collagen genes (Morrison *et al.* 1992; Willing *et al.* 1998; Sowers *et al.* 1999*b*). However, the relative importance of any one gene, particularly that of specific vitamin D receptor genotypes, has been controversial (Eisman 1995; Peacock 1995). Moreover, causative mutations have yet to be identified in any genes, except in a few anecdotal cases (Spotila *et al.* 1994). Although results of studies are not consistent, it appears that such modifiable risk factors as weight, calcium intake, and physical activity also affect premenopausal bone mass but to a lesser extent than heredity (Bonjour and Rizzoli 1996). In some young people, anorexia nervosa and excessive athletic activity contribute to low bone mass. Premenopausal oophorectomy results in loss of bone mass if hormone replacement therapy or another appropriate pharmacological agent is not used.

Other factors known to increase the risk for low bone mass and osteoporotic fractures in postmenopausal women are prolonged immobility, prolonged corticosteroid use, a family history of an osteoporotic fracture, and cigarette smoking (Cumming *et al.* 1997). Established protective factors are hormone replacement therapy (in either the form of oestrogen alone or oestrogen with progestin), certain other pharmaceutical agents (discussed below), obesity, and, to a lesser extent, calcium supplementation. Figure 3 shows that hormone replacement therapy protects against bone loss for as long as it is used, but loss of bone mass continues when replacement hormone use ceases (Christiansen *et al.* 1981). Available evidence indicates that hormone replacement therapy also protects against osteoporotic fractures, but that recent use is again needed for this protection. Higher concentration of endogenous oestrogen around the time of menopause is also associated with a lower rate of bone loss (Cauley *et al.* 1996). Obese postmenopausal women have a reduced risk for low bone mass compared with thin women. On average, thin women have lower oestrogen production, lower concentration of circulating oestrogen, and less mechanical stress on their bones. In addition, fat padding around the hip provides some protection against fracture during a fall. Most randomized trials show a small protective effect of calcium supplementation that is not nearly so great as the protection from hormone replacement therapy (Cumming 1990; Heaney 1996).

Table 3 Percentage of women in Rochester, Minnesota, with bone mineral measurements in the spine, hip, or mid radius more than 2.5 standard deviations below the mean for young normal women

Age group (years)	Percentage
50–59	14.8
60–69	21.6
70–79	38.5
⩾ 80	70.0
Total[a]	30.3

[a]Age-adjusted to the population of white American women aged 50 years and older, 1990.

Modified from Melton (1995).

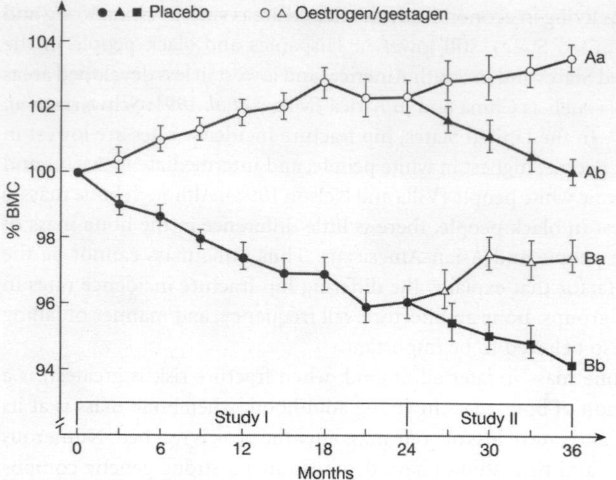

Fig. 3 Bone mineral content (BMC) as a function of time and treatment in 94 (study I) and 77 (study II) women soon after menopause. (Source: Christiansen *et al.* 1981.)

However, a trial of calcium and vitamin D supplementation among institutionalized elderly in France (Chapay *et al.* 1992) showed a 43 per cent decrease in risk for hip fracture. Older postmenopausal women whose dietary calcium intake is very low may be especially likely to benefit from supplemental calcium (Dawson-Hughes *et al.* 1990). Cigarette smoking increases the risk for osteoporosis, probably through a lowering of oestrogen concentration (Seeman 1996). Heredity plays a role in determining postmenopausal bone mass, but its contribution is not nearly so great as for premenopausal bone mass (Sambrook *et al.* 1996).

Most studies report that thiazide diuretics, which decrease urinary calcium excretion, are associated with increased bone mass and decreased hip fracture risk in adults (Cauley *et al.* 1996). Some studies, but not all, have shown an association between low levels of dietary calcium and osteoporosis. Among adults, the amount of dietary calcium consumed during old age may be especially significant (Heaney 1996). Sufficient vitamin D intake would be expected to be necessary for adequate calcium intake, but evidence to date is not consistent. Moderate physical activity probably affords a small amount of protection in adults, but this protective effect is probably lost if a person stops being physically active (Snow *et al.* 1996). Heavy alcohol consumption and caffeine consumption may also increase the risk for low bone mass and for fractures, but data are not consistent. The roles of other dietary constituents are even less certain. At present an area of active investigation is whether phyto-oestrogens protect against loss of bone mass.

In addition to low bone mass, certain architectural and geometric properties of bone affect fracture risk. One such geometric property is hip axis length, which is the distance from the greater trochanter to the inner pelvic rim. Long hip axis length is associated with a higher risk for hip fracture independent of bone mass (Faulkner *et al.* 1993). Differences in hip axis length may explain some of the variation in hip fracture incidence rates among countries and racial groups, since Asians and black people have shorter hip axis length than white people (Villa and Nelson 1996). An architectural property of bone that appears to affect hip fracture risk is the Singh index in the proximal femur (Singh *et al.* 1970). The Singh index ranges from grade VI (normal, all trabecular groups visible) to grade I (marked reduction of even the principal compressive trabeculae). Hip fracture patients have been found to have lower Singh grades, on average, than women of similar age without hip fracture (Peacock *et al.* 1995). It is likely that more geometric and architectural properties of bone that are associated with fracture risk will be identified in the future.

Most fractures of sites other than the spine depend on whether a person falls and how the person falls. Risk factors for falls have been found to be risk factors for hip fracture (Grisso *et al.* 1996). Number of previous falls and a recent increase in the number of falls are both predictive of hip fracture (Schwartz *et al.* 2000). Table 4 shows some host factors associated with falling. The roles of environmental hazards are less well documented (Grisso *et al.* 1996).

How a person falls also affects the likelihood that a fracture will occur. Falling sideways or straight down and landing on the hip or leg, for instance, greatly increase the risk of a hip fracture, while breaking the fall with a hand decreases the risk of hip fracture (but increases risk

Table 4 Host risk factors for falls among the elderly for which the evidence is strong or moderate

Demographic characteristics
Older age
Female sex
Functional level
Limitations in activities of daily living and instrumental activities of daily living
Cane/walker use
History of falls
Gait, balance, strength
slow walking speed
Postural sway
Low lower-extremity strength
Low upper-extremity strength
Impaired reflexes
Sensory
Poor vision
Lower-extremity sensory perception
Chronic illnesses
Parkinson's disease
Other neuromuscular disease
Stroke
Urinary incontinence
Arthritis
Acute illness
Medications, alcohol
Several medications used
Hypnotics
Sedatives
Antidepressants
Antiparkinsonism drugs
Mental status
Cognitive impairment
Depression

Modified from Grisso *et al.* (1990).

of lower forearm fracture) (Hayes *et al.* 1993; Nevitt and Cummings 1993). Thus, not only will the likelihood of fracture depend on how a person falls, but the nature of the fall will also largely determine the skeletal site fractured. Frail women are more likely to fracture their hip or proximal humerus, while more healthy active women are more like to fracture their lower forearm (Kelsey *et al.* 1992; Nevitt and Cummings 1993). Falls from heights or on hard surfaces also increase the risk for fracture (Hayes *et al.* 1993; Nevitt and Cummings 1993).

Prevention

Primary prevention includes trying to achieve high bone mass at young ages by having a diet appropriate in calcium and engaging in sufficient physical activity. Once loss of bone mass has begun, administration of oestrogens with or without progestin will limit further loss of bone mass, but the other benefits and risks of hormone replacement therapy need to be considered as well. Calcium supplementation can provide some protection. Moderate physical activity, such as brisk walking, is often recommended for older people to reduce loss of bone mass, but at most this probably has only a modest beneficial effect.

Two relatively new agents are available to reduce loss of bone mass. The bisphosphonate alendronate has been shown to reduce loss of bone mass in the hip and spine, although not to the same extent as hormone replacement therapy (Hosking *et al.* 1998). However, randomized trials in women have shown that it protects against fracture only in those who already have very low bone mass (Cummings *et al.* 1998). In addition, compliance is a problem because alendronate has to be taken in a rather strict manner to achieve maximal absorption and avoid unpleasant upper gastrointestinal effects (Ettinger *et al.* 1998). The selective oestrogen receptor modulator raloxifene has also been shown to reduce loss of bone mass in the hip and spine in women regardless of their baseline bone mass (Delmas *et al.* 1997; Ettinger *et al.* 1999) although, again, not to the same extent as hormone replacement therapy. However, in the one randomized trial with fracture as an endpoint, raloxifene protected against vertebral fractures but not against non-vertebral fractures, including hip fracture (Ettinger *et al.* 1999). Thus available evidence suggests that neither alendronate nor raloxifene will be useful in the primary prevention of osteoporosis, although both have utility as therapeutic agents.

Screening women in the perimenopausal and early postmenopausal years for high fracture risk by measuring their bone mass with either dual-energy X-ray absorptiometry or single- or dual-photon absorptiometry has achieved some popularity in recent years. However, there are many questions about the usefulness of such screening, such as who should be screened, whether multiple measurement over time are needed, what other information on risk should be obtained along with the measure of bone mass, and what therapy should be used in those with various degrees of low bone mass (Slemenda *et al.* 1996). Ultrasonography, usually of the heel bone, provides information about bone architecture and elasticity as well as bone mineral density, and has been found to predict fracture (Hans *et al.* 1996). Since ultrasound is less expensive and radiation-free compared with other methods of measuring bone mass, it is possible that it will be used more widely for screening in the future. At present, however, there is no consensus that any screening method should be used for healthy women in the general population.

Finally, reducing the frequency and impact of falls among those with osteoporosis is another potential means of reducing the risk of fracture. A randomized trial in a nursing home has shown that wearing protective hip pads substantially reduces the risk of hip fracture (Lauritzen *et al.* 1993), but compliance is a problem.

Low back pain

From 60 to 80 per cent of adults report having had low back pain at some time during their lives (Hult 1954; Walsh *et al.* 1992; Papageorgiou *et al.* 1995). In the United States, 4.6 per cent of workers lose at least one workday during the course of a year, and a total of 10 800 000 workdays are lost annually because of back pain (Guo *et al.* 1999). Fortunately, most episodes of low back pain are of limited duration. A Swedish study, for instance, found that 60 per cent of males in the general population had at some time had low back pain, 16 per cent had been incapacitated for periods ranging from 3 to 6 months, and 4 per cent had been incapacitated for more than 6 months (Hult 1954). The small proportion of cases that become chronic account for most of the cost associated with low back pain. Snook (1982) estimated that 25 per cent of the cases account for 90 per cent of the costs.

As noted above, the category of low back pain consists of a variety of entities with somewhat different aetiologies. However, almost all studies have considered low back pain as a whole, although a few have considered herniated lumbar disk specifically. When risk factors for low back pain as a whole and herniated lumbar disk differ, it will be so noted.

Risk factors

The best predictor of low back pain is a history of low back pain (Papageorgiou *et al.* 1996; Lagerström *et al.* 1998; van Poppel *et al.* 1998). First episodes of low back pain most frequently occur among persons in the age range 20 to 39 years, but the proportion of the population reporting low back pain (either old or new) is relatively uniform across the working years (Biering-Sorenson 1982; Guo *et al.* 1999). Whereas after about age 65 years the prevalence of low back pain decreases in men, prevalence increases in women, probably because of the increasing frequency of vertebral osteoporosis. If only cases seeking medical care or compensation are considered, low back pain is seen more frequently in males than females (Snook 1982; Shelerud 1998), but in surveys in the general population, males and females are affected with approximately equal frequency (Biering-Sorenson 1982; Walsh *et al.* 1992; Papageorgiou *et al.* 1995). Persons in low social classes are more likely to report low back pain than those in higher classes, probably because of their tendency to have jobs requiring heavy physical labour.

People who do heavy manual labour are at increased risk for low back pain (Hales and Bernard 1996). Lifting objects of 11.25 kg or more appears to be particularly detrimental. Specific activities that probably further increase the risk are frequent lifting of heavy objects while bending and twisting the body, holding heavy objects away from the body while lifting, and failing to bend the knees while lifting (Table 5) (Andersson 1981; Kelsey *et al.* 1984*b*). Nursing is one occupation with a particularly high risk for low back pain. Nurses who transfer patients between a bed and a chair, who manually reposition patients, who lift patients in and out of the bath with a hoist, and especially those who must lift in 'save the patient' situations are especially prone to low back pain (Lagerström *et al.* 1998).

Driving of motor vehicles either on or off the job and exposure to whole-body vibration increase the risk for low back pain (Pope *et al.*

Table 5 Estimated relative risk for prolapsed lumbar intervertebral disc associated with lifting more than 11.25 kg on job

Lifting category	Estimated relative risk	95% confidence limits
No lifting while twisting body (reference group)	1.0	Reference group
Lifting while twisting body, knees bent	2.7	0.9–7.9
Lifting while twisting body, knees straight	6.1	1.3–27.9

Modified from Kelsey *et al.* (1984*b*).

1998). Evidence is inconsistent as to whether prolonged sitting or standing in one position confers an increased risk (Hales and Bernard 1996).

Cigarette smoking is associated with an increased risk, probably because of the pressure exerted by frequent coughing or the decreased diffusion of nutrients into the intervertebral disks resulting from smoking (Heliövaara *et al.* 1991). Some studies indicate that tallness is a risk factor for low back pain or specifically sciatica (Heliövaara *et al.* 1991), and that heavy body weight has no, or at most a slight, effect (Hales and Bernard 1996). A narrow spinal canal increases the risk for herniated lumbar disk (Heliövaara *et al.* 1986).

The role of psychological factors in the aetiology of low back pain has been difficult to determine because it is often difficult to separate whether the psychological factors preceded or followed the onset of low back pain. The psychological factor most consistently predictive of low back pain in longitudinal studies is job dissatisfaction (Papageorgiou *et al.* 1997; Krause *et al.* 1998). Other factors reported from longitudinal studies include a high frequency of job problems, psychological job demands, poor social relations at work, work pressure, lack of job control, and monotonous work (Hales and Bernard 1996).

Most low back pain improves without any specific treatment. Predictors of disability from low back pain reported in various studies include previous episodes of low back pain, long duration of pain, a history of past disability and hospital admissions, sciatica and use of analgesia in association with previous low back pain, an onset of pain attributable to trauma, lack of recognition and respect at work, low supervisory support, being unemployed, other disabilities, low educational level, psychological factors, heavy physical demands on the job, dissatisfaction with the job, whether insurance payments are being received, the perception of fault, whether a lawyer has been retained, and heavy body weight (Deyo and Diehl 1988; Cats-Baril and Frymoyer 1991; Hales and Bernard 1996; Wickstrom and Pentti 1998; Müller *et al.* 1999).

Prevention

Various approaches have been used for the primary prevention of low back pain in the workplace. Low back radiographs and medical examinations have not proved useful as predictors of who will develop back pain on the job (Snook 1982). However, careful selection of workers for jobs involving heavy manual work by strength testing may be helpful (Keyserling *et al.* 1980). A randomized trial of an educational programme to reduce back injury in postal workers did not find that the programme reduced the occurrence of back injury, the cost per injury, the time off work per injury, or the rate of repeat injury after return to work (Daltroy *et al.* 1997). Similarly, available evidence suggests that better training in nurses does not result in a decrease in the frequency of low back problems (Lagerström *et al.* 1998). It has been found that training workers to bend their knees while lifting does not reduce the likelihood of low back injuries, in part because of poor compliance (Snook 1982). A better approach may be to redesign jobs to minimize bending and twisting motions while lifting and to reduce the amount of weight that must be lifted (Snook 1988). Redesigning jobs in these ways may also allow injured workers to return to work sooner. Other ways of reducing the frequency of back pain may include smoking cessation, improved physical fitness, moving around from time to time in situations requiring prolonged exposure to one position, vibration dampening, and motor vehicles with good lumbar support and positioning.

To reduce the likelihood of acute back pain progressing to chronic back pain, it is important for those affected to continue their normal activity to the extent that they are able (Malmivaara *et al.* 1995). Also important is return to work after a short period of rest (Nachemson 1983). Upon return to work, however, the worker should avoid activities that may exacerbate the problem, such as heavy lifting or staying in one position for long periods of time.

Back schools have been developed in an attempt to decrease pain and disability through self-involvement and self-reliance (Fish *et al.* 1983). Most back schools teach patients about spinal mechanics so that they can use their backs effectively without pain and damage, try to change attitudes through psychological approaches, and encourage appropriate exercise and physical fitness. There is some evidence to suggest that back schools are quite effective for people with recent onset of low back pain, but not for those with chronic back pain (Lankhurst *et al.* 1983).

Neck pain

Neck pain has been less well studied than low back pain, and, as with low back pain, a variety of conditions can result in neck pain. About 50 to 70 per cent of adults report having experienced neck pain at some time during their lives (Hult 1954; Côté *et al.* 1998*a*).

Risk factors

Some studies report that males and females are affected with approximately equal frequency, while others show a female excess. Chronic neck pain and disability from neck pain occur more frequently in females than males (Bovim *et al.* 1994; Côté *et al.* 1998*a*; Leclerc *et al.* 1999), but males appear to be affected more frequently with herniated cervical intervertebral disk (Kelsey *et al.* 1984*a*). Most neck pain is mild, but about 5 per cent results in disability (Hult 1954; Côté *et al.* 1998*a*). Neck pain occurs most frequently in young adulthood, and there is some evidence that its prevalence decreases with age (Côté 1998*a*; Leclerc *et al.* 1999).

Only a few studies to identify other risk factors for either neck pain in general or herniated cervical intervertebral disk in particular have been undertaken. Prolonged exposure to awkward postures may be associated with mild neck pain. For instance, frequent use of video display terminals with a fixed keyboard height that requires a bent neck can result in neck pain (Yu and Wong 1996). Other risk factors for either general neck pain or herniated cervical disk found in one or more studies include heavy lifting (Kelsey *et al.* 1984*a*; Magnusson *et al.* 1996; Krause *et al.* 1997), cigarette smoking (Kelsey *et al.* 1984*a*; Brage and Bjeredal 1996), driving motor vehicles (Kelsey *et al.* 1984*a*; Krause *et al.* 1997), exposure to whole-body vibration (Kelsey *et al.* 1984*a*; Magnusson *et al.* 1996), psychological distress (Leclerc *et al.* 1999), psychosomatic problems (Leclerc *et al.* 1999), headaches (Leclerc *et al.* 1999), and frequent diving from a board (Kelsey *et al.* 1984*a*). One study found that vehicles in which there were problems in adjusting the seat were particularly detrimental (Krause *et al.* 1997). Repetitive motions, forceful exertions, and constrained positions may increase risk (Hales and Bernard 1996).

Prevention

Little research has been undertaken on predictors of disability from neck pain and on primary prevention. However, it would appear that reduction in the amount of heavy lifting, cigarette smoking, awkward positions (especially at video display terminals), prolonged driving in motor vehicles, and exposure to other sources of whole-body vibration should reduce the incidence of neck pain.

Selected musculoskeletal disorders of children

Scoliosis

The Scoliosis Research Society defines scoliosis as a lateral spinal curve of greater than 10° (Skaggs and Bassett 1996). It is usually associated with rotation of the vertebrae. Only adolescent idiopathic scoliosis will be discussed here. About 2 to 3 per cent of adolescents develop curves of 10° or more before growth ceases, and 2 to 3 per 1000 children develop curves of 30° or more (Shands and Eisberg 1955; Morais *et al.* 1985). Those with large curvature usually develop spinal osteoarthritis in their adult years. Lung and heart complications may also occur. Additional progression of curves sometimes takes place in adults with scoliosis, thus worsening the situation.

Risk factors

The ages at which adolescent idiopathic scoliosis is most frequently diagnosed are 11 to 14 years in girls and 14 to 16 years in boys, the difference in ages reflecting the later onset of the adolescent growth spurt in males. The ratio of female to male cases among the more severe cases seen at surgery is about 5 to 1, but curves of less than 15° are seen with about equal frequency in females and males. Reports from surgical case series indicate that curves occur most frequently at the thoracic level, but school screening programmes that identify mild as well as severe cases have found curves to be most common at the thoracolumbar level (Brooks *et al.* 1975).

The risk for scoliosis in first-degree relatives of cases is about three to four times that in children from the general population (Wynne-Davies 1968). A recent prospective study in a cohort of prepubertal children in Finland free of scoliosis at baseline found several factors that predict the development of scoliosis, including the female sex, trunk asymmetry as indicated by large rip humps on the forward bend test (described below), the degree of thoracic kyphosis, and the degree of lumbar lordosis in boys. Standing height, sitting height, recent increase in sitting height, and early age at gain in sitting height appeared to be risk factors as well, although they did not reach statistical significance (Nissinen *et al.* 1993*a*,*b*). Other reports have also indicated that children who are skeletally more mature at the beginning but not at the end of puberty and children who are taller and thinner than average at the beginning but not at the end of adolescence are at high risk, suggesting that the scoliotic spine grows faster and earlier than the normal spine (Willner 1975; Nissinen *et al.* 1993*b*; Hazebroek-Kampschreur *et al.* 1994). Once girls reach menarche, their risk is considerably reduced (Hazebroek-Kampschreur *et al.* 1994). Other factors that may contribute to the development of scoliosis but for which the evidence is not conclusive are impaired visual and vestibular functioning (Nachemson and Sahlstrand 1977), defects in proprioceptive postural control (Keesen *et al.* 1992), asymmetric muscle activity (Henssge 1968; Alexander and Season 1978), leg-length discrepancies (Nachemson and Sahlstrand 1977), collagen disorders (Francis *et al.* 1977), and abnormalities of the elastic fibre system (Hadley-Miller *et al.* 1994).

Once a curve has developed, several risk factors for progression have been identified, including double curves as opposed to single curves, thoracic curves, larger curves, curves in females, the absence of a sacral tilt, leg-length inequality, early chronological age, and skeletal immaturity (Dickson *et al.* 1980; Lonstein 1988).

Prevention

No means of primary prevention are known. Therefore secondary prevention by screening in schools has become widespread and is in fact required by law in many localities in the United States. The assumption of the screening programme is that if cases of scoliosis are detected early, they can be treated conservatively and surgery can be avoided.

The forward bend test has been used for screening for many years. In the forward bend test, the child's back is examined while the child bends forward from the waist. In scoliosis, the rotation of vertebrae that is often associated with the lateral curvature results in prominent ribs on the concave side of the curve. Accordingly, in this test evidence of a 'rib hump' is considered positive for scoliosis. Nissinen *et al.* (1993*b*) suggest that hump size of 6 mm or greater is the optimal cutoff point for a positive test. In another screening test called moiré topography, a photograph of the back is taken and the degree of topographic asymmetry is measured. Moiré topography has high sensitivity, but because of the large number of false positives it is no longer recommended (Nissinen *et al.* 1993*b*). Recently, the scoliometer, an inclinometer used to measure axial trunk rotation during forward bending (Bunnell 1984), has been introduced as a screening test. Only limited evaluation of the scoliometer has been undertaken to date (Grossman *et al.* 1995; Côté *et al.* 1998*b*). Most school screening programmes use the traditional forward bend test.

School screening programmes identify relatively large numbers of children with possible curvature in their spine. Positive tests are followed by radiographic examination for more definitive diagnosis. Curves of more than 5° are generally monitored by subsequent radiographs every few months. If a curve progresses to 20 to 25° or more, treatment is usually started to prevent further progression. Methods of treatment include exercises, braces, external or internal muscle stimulators, and sometimes surgery.

Despite the widespread acceptance of screening for scoliosis, its effectiveness has been questioned (Williams 1988; United States Preventive Services Task Force 1993*b*; Goldberg *et al.* 1995). Many children screened as positive are not followed up for definitive diagnosis. Many false positives occur even with the forward bend test, resulting in an excess of radiograph examinations and considerable expense and anxiety. A report from a screening programme in Ireland (Goldberg *et al.* 1995) indicates that the positive predictive value of the forward bend test is only 8 per cent, i.e. of every 100 forward bend tests classified as positive, only eight develop clinically significant scoliosis. It is uncertain that school screening programmes have actually caused a reduction in the number of cases of severe curvature that require surgery. There is disagreement about the optimal ages for screening and about whether males should be screened at all. Criteria for referral for diagnosis and treatment need to be better specified, and improved training and evaluation of the nurses who do the screening is needed (Morais *et al.* 1985; Williams 1988). It would be helpful if predictors of progression were better defined. In view of all these uncertainties, the United States Preventive Services Task Force (1993*a*) did not recommend for or against routine screening for scoliosis in adolescents.

Slipped capital femoral epiphysis

In slipped capital femoral epiphysis, the head of the femur is displaced backward and downward off the diaphysis. The actual separation takes place through the layer of hypertrophied cartilage next to the zone of calcified cartilage of the epiphyseal plate. The usual symptoms are pain, stiffness, limp, and a limited range of motion of the hip joint. Slipped epiphysis usually occurs during the adolescent growth spurt, and does not occur once the epiphysis is fused to the shaft of the femur.

The annual incidence of slipped epiphysis has been reported to be 3.4 per 100 000 in the population under age 25 years in Connecticut, United States (Kelsey 1971), 0.7 per 100 000 in New Mexico (Kelsey *et al.* 1970), and to range from 2 to 13 per 100 000 in the age group 7 to 17 years in Gothenburg, Sweden, over a period of several years (Henrikson 1969). In Connecticut and Gothenburg, about 1 in 800 males and 1 in 2000 females will be diagnosed with a slipped epiphysis over the age range at risk (Kelsey 1971; Jerre *et al.* 1996).

Risk factors

Most cases occur between the ages of 10 and 17 years in males and between 8 and 15 years in females. The median age at diagnosis is 13 years for males and 11 years for females (Kelsey 1971; Jerre *et al.* 1996), the earlier age in females corresponding to their earlier onset of puberty. Males are affected more frequently than females, although male to female ratio appears to have decreased over time and varies from one geographical area to another (Hansson *et al.* 1987; Jerre *et al.* 1996; Loder 1996*a*). In males, the left hip is affected about twice as frequently as the right, whereas in females the left and right hips are affected with approximately equal frequency. In both sexes, about 20 to 25 per cent of those with slipped epiphysis have both hips affected (Sorenson 1968; Jerre *et al.* 1996; Loder 1996*a*). Black people are affected with slipped epiphysis two to three times more often than white people (Kelsey 1971). There are several reports that symptoms begin more frequently in spring and summer than in autumn or winter, at least in northern latitudes (Hansson *et al.* 1987; Loder 1996*b*).

A large proportion of children with slipped epiphysis are very overweight. In fact, about half are at or above the 95th percentile for their age (Morscher 1968; Kelsey *et al.* 1972). Children with slipped epiphysis tend to have undergone slower skeletal maturation than average for their age (Sorenson 1968). They tend to be tall for their age at the time of diagnosis, but at maturity their heights are almost normal for their chronological age (Hansson *et al.* 1987). Some familial aggregation of cases has been noted (Rennie 1967).

Most of the established risk factors for slipped epiphysis are related either to a weakening of the epiphyseal plate or to an increase in the shearing stress on the plate. The epiphyseal plate is weaker during periods of rapid growth, such as during the adolescent growth spurt. The growth spurt in males is of greater magnitude and of longer duration than that in females, and the male growth spurt is more likely to have periods of acceleration and deceleration (Acheson 1966). The excess of onset of symptoms in spring and summer may be attributable to more rapid growth in spring and summer (Morscher 1968).

Animal experiments indicate that a deficit of sex hormones relative to growth hormone brings about a widening of the epiphyseal plate and a reduction in the shearing force needed to displace the epiphysis. Oestrogens protect against slipped epiphysis, whereas androgens are protective only in large doses after prolonged exposure, providing another reason for the higher incidence in males than females. Slowly maturing children are exposed for a longer period to high levels of growth hormone relative to sex hormones than are children who mature faster. Tall children also would have a longer exposure to growth hormone relative to sex hormones (Morscher 1968).

During adolescence the epiphyseal plate changes from a horizontal to an oblique plane, so that it becomes more vulnerable to stress from superincumbent weight. Children who are overweight will put more stress on their plate than lighter children. Children with the unusual combination of being overweight and are slow maturers are probably at particularly high risk.

Prevention

Prevention of adolescent obesity is the only known means of reducing the risk for slipped epiphysis. No screening tests are available, but slipped epiphysis should be considered in adolescents who have a limp and hip or knee pain or restriction of motion in the hip. The contralateral hip in children with slipped epiphysis in one hip needs to be carefully monitored, especially if the first slipped epiphysis occurred at an early age (Loder 1996*a*). Early diagnosis is important, as slight displacement treated early by pinning the hip has a favorable prognosis, whereas cases that are diagnosed late and that have severe displacement usually have early onset of osteoarthritis of the hip and permanent disability.

Childhood fractures

Figure 4 indicates that there are two age groups at particularly high risk for fractures: the elderly and children. Fractures in the elderly were considered in the section on osteoporosis. Here, epidemiological and preventive aspects of fractures in children are described.

In the United States, about 1 in 36 persons less than 18 years of age fractures a bone each year (Holbrook *et al.* 1984; Praemer *et al.* 1999). In Wales, 64 per cent of boys and 39 per cent of girls can expect to fracture a bone by 15 years of age (Lyons *et al.* 1999). Most fractures heal quickly in children, and the younger the age, the more rapid the

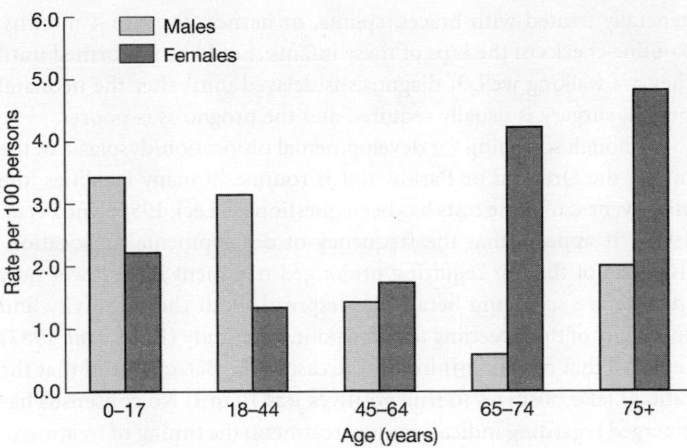

Fig. 4 Average annual rate of persons having fractures, by age and sex, United States, 1992 to 1994, National Health Interview Survey. (Source: Praemer *et al.* 1999.)

healing. However, if the growth plate is involved in the fracture, growth in that bone may be adversely affected. Other rare complications, as in other age groups, are infection, delayed union, nonunion, avascular necrosis, and malunion.

Risk factors

Among children, incidence rates of fracture increase with age until about ages 11 to 14 years in females and until about ages 20 to 24 years in males, and males are at higher risk of fracture throughout childhood (Landin 1983; Worlock and Stower 1986; Cheng *et al.* 1999; Lyons *et al.* 1999). In one study (Cheng *et al.* 1999), the ratio of male to female fracture cases rose from 1.4 to 1 in infancy to 4.9 to 1 in adolescence. Almost all forms of trauma associated with fractures are more common in boys than girls (Landin 1983).

The bones reported to be most frequently fractured in children have varied somewhat from one series to another depending on the sources of cases. The United States Health Interview Survey indicates that the sites most frequently affected are the hand, radius and ulna (especially the distal radius and ulna), carpals, skull and face, clavicle, foot, and humerus (Holbrook *et al.* 1984). Children who have one fracture are at increased risk of having an additional fracture (Landin 1983).

Accidents while playing, sports accidents, and traffic accidents accounted for over half of childhood fractures in a large series from Sweden (Landin 1983). In a series of childhood fracture cases in Wales, sports and leisure-time activities accounted for 36 per cent of fractures, assaults for 3.5 per cent, and road traffic accidents for 1.4 per cent (Lyons *et al.* 1999). Among fractures of specific sites (Landin 1983), fractures of the phalanges of the hands most commonly resulted from contact sports as well as from skating, playing, and fighting. Distal forearm fractures were most often caused by a fall on an outstretched hand; when environmental factors were involved, ball games, bicycle accidents, playground accidents, and skateboard accidents were most common. Carpal and metacarpal fractures tended to result from fighting, falls, bicycle accidents, ball games, skiing, and skating. Fractures of the clavicle were most often the result of falls, ball games, and contact sports. Among foot fractures, the ankle was most frequently involved. Ankle fractures most often resulted from the foot being caught in a bicycle wheel and from falls, but ball games, skateboards, roller skates, mopeds, motorcycle, skiing, skating, cycling, and playing also were responsible for some ankle fractures.

Prevention

Accident prevention is the key to reducing the number of fractures in children, including decreasing the number of sports and recreational injuries, falls, bicycle, motorcycle, and automobile accidents, non-accidental child injuries, and other childhood traumas (Garraway *et al.* 1979; Landin 1983; Lyons *et al.* 1999).

Developmental (congenital) dislocation/dysplasia of the hip

In developmental dislocation/dysplasia of the hip, the head of the femur is displaced completely or partially out of the acetabulum. Because many dislocations tend to occur immediately after birth or occasionally later during the first year of life, the term 'developmental dislocation/dysplasia of the hip' is now frequently used instead of the older term 'congenital dislocation of the hip' (Mooney and Eman 1995). The diagnosis is made shortly after birth in about 80 per cent of cases, while about 20 per cent of the time the diagnosis is made later, especially when the child starts to walk. Available evidence indicates that most of the late-diagnosed cases in fact do develop some time after birth and are not merely cases that were missed close to the time of birth (Mooney and Emans 1995).

Developmental dislocation/dysplasia of the hip includes the following: (a) dislocated hips, which are hips dislocated in a resting position, with the dislocation present at birth; (b) located but unstable or dislocatable hips, which are hips that rest in a located position but are unstable or dislocatable on clinical examination and provocative manoeuvres; (c) dysplastic hips, in which the acetabulum is shallow or dysplastic (Mooney and Emans 1995).

Many hips diagnosed as unstable or dislocatable immediately after birth stabilize during the first few days of life. Hips may become stable so quickly that estimates of prevalence based on examination after the third day of life are less than half of the prevalence estimates at birth (Sharrard 1993). Thus, prevalence estimates are highly dependent on the conditions under which the estimates were made.

These reservations not withstanding, there appears to be considerable variation in the frequency of developmental dislocation/dysplasia of the hip between geographical areas and between racial/ethnic groups. Using data collected before screening for developmental dislocation/dysplasia of the hip at birth became widespread, in most North American and Western European countries and in Australia, New Zealand, and Israel, prevalence rates of around 1 per 1000 to 10 per 1000 births were found. In the Navajo, Apache, and Cree-Ojibwa of North America, the Lapps, and in Hungary, northern Italy, Brittany, and the Faroe Islands, rates from 10 per 1000 to 100 per 1000 births were reported. Conversely, developmental dislocation/dysplasia of the hip was rare in black people in South Africa, the West Indies, and Uganda, and among Chinese living in Hong Kong (reviewed in Kelsey 1982). It must be kept in mind, however, that the nature of the neonatal examination of the infant, the experience of the examiner, the timing of the examination, and the criteria for developmental dislocation/dysplasia of the hip could all affect these figures.

Risk factors

Females are affected about four to six times more frequently than males, possibly because female infants are more susceptible to capsular and ligamentous laxity from the hormones that cause maternal pelvic relaxation during labour (Gunther *et al.* 1993). In the United States, white people are affected more often than black people. In most geographical areas, an excess of cases is diagnosed in children born in late autumn and winter relative to summer (Robinson 1968). First-born children are at higher risk than later children. The ligaments and other tissues in and around the maternal uterus have already been stretched during previous pregnancies, thus allowing more fetal movement in pregnancies after the first (Gunther *et al.* 1993). In unilateral cases, the left hip is affected more frequently than the right, probably because the left hip is positioned against the maternal spine more often than the right hip (Mooney and Emans 1995).

Familial aggregation of developmental dislocation/dysplasia of the hip occurs, and both hereditary and environmental factors are believed to contribute to the familial excess (Record and Edwards 1958; Gunther *et al.* 1993). For a family with one affected parent and one affected child, the risk of an unstable hip in a subsequent child is about 36 per cent (Wynne-Davies 1970). Infants with developmental dislocation/dysplasia of the hip are considerably more likely to have been born by breech delivery than other infants (Robinson 1968; Cyvin 1977; Gunther *et al.* 1993). Possible reasons for the association with breech delivery are that breech position *in utero* limits hip motion and elongates the ligament of the hip joint capsule by persistent upward pressure of the greater trochanter (Jones 1965). Children born by caesarean section are also at elevated risk (Gunther *et al.* 1993). Infants with developmental dislocation/dysplasia of the hip tend to have had longer gestations than other infants (Cyvin 1977).

Prevention

No means of primary prevention of developmental dislocation/dysplasia of the hip are known. However, early detection and treatment of hips with developmental dislocation/dysplasia of the hip is highly important, since without prompt treatment the affected leg may be shorter, the child may limp, surgery may be required, and osteoarthritis of the hip is likely to occur in young adulthood. Accordingly, screening by examining newborn infants for developmental dislocation/dysplasia of the hip is now accepted as a routine procedure.

Two screening tests have generally been used: the Ortolani test and the Barlow test. In the Ortolani test, the hip is placed in flexion and is gently adducted and then abducted. The Ortolani test is considered positive if a palpable jerk and audible click are heard as the head of the femur returns to the acetabulum. Some physicians consider just an audible click to be a positive test. The Barlow test involves exerting gentle downward pressure over the lesser trochanter with the hip in flexion and adduction; an unstable hip will shift from the acetabulum and a sensation similar to the Ortolani sign is produced. When the leg is allowed to abduct, the hip is reduced.

Because many hips noted to be unstable at birth soon become stable spontaneously, these tests are often repeated at around 3 weeks. Infants who are positive by either the Ortolani or Barlow test are generally treated with braces, splints, or harness for 2 to 4 months. Routine checks of the hips of these infants should be performed until they are walking well. If diagnosis is delayed until after the neonatal period, surgery is usually required and the prognosis is poorer.

Although screening for developmental dislocation/dysplasia of the hip by the Ortolani or Barlow test is routine in many localities, the effectiveness of these tests has been questioned (Leck 1986; Knox *et al.* 1987). It appears that the frequency of developmental dislocation/dysplasia of the hip requiring prolonged treatment is no lower now than before screening became widespread. Both the sensitivity and specificity of the screening tests are poor. One study (Knox *et al.* 1987) reported that only one-third of true cases were detected, and that the ratio of false positives to true positives was 10 to 1. No consensus has emerged regarding indications for treatment, the timing of treatment, or the type of splint to be used. It is possible that the screening procedures themselves may bring about hip dislocation (Moore 1989; Jones 1991). These screening tests require experienced examiners (Macnicol 1990), but inexperienced examiners are often used. A better understanding of which hips will spontaneously stabilize would allow more informed decisions to be made about which hips need immediate treatment. There is disagreement about the significance of a soft audible or palpable click without evidence of abnormal movement between the femoral head and acetabulum, and hence there is disagreement about how such infants should be monitored (Fulton and Barer 1984). More studies addressing these issues are needed.

Recently, ultrasound, in which a defined image of the bony and cartilaginous hip can be examined, has become widely available for screening for developmental dislocation/dysplasia of the hip. However, its use as a routine screening test has not been found to be cost-effective, and even its use in high-risk infants is controversial (Hernandez *et al.* 1994; Rosendahl *et al.* 1994; Geitung *et al.* 1996). Some of the problems are that ultrasound is expensive, developmental dislocation/dysplasia of the hip is relatively infrequent, many hips classified as positive on ultrasound develop normally, and cases that develop after the neonatal period will not be detected. It is unclear how an infant with a normal clinical examination but with abnormal ultrasonogram should be treated. Better training is needed to improve the scans and their interpretation (Rosendahl *et al.* 1995). At present, the American Academy of Pediatrics does not have a policy on developmental dislocation/dysplasia of the hip screening.

Conclusion

The impact of musculoskeletal diseases, though substantial now, will probably become much greater over the next several decades. Musculoskeletal diseases are common at all ages, but their greatest impact is on the elderly, among whom they are often associated with severely compromised quality of life and high costs for medical care. In industrialized countries, the ageing of the population is well recognized. In developing countries, the number of people aged 65 years or older is expected to increase by 200 to 400 per cent between 1990 and 2025. Thus, musculoskeletal diseases will account for a significant portion of health care costs in countries throughout the world in the twenty-first century. Identifying feasible prevention strategies and affordable methods of treatment for such ubiquitous diseases of the elderly as osteoarthritis and osteoporosis is thus a high global public health priority. Although some progress has been made in identifying methods of prevention and treatment for osteoporosis through lifestyle changes and pharmaceutical agents, osteoporosis remains a serious problem for many older people, and still better methods need to be developed. Even less is known about means of preventing the development and progression of osteoarthritis, and much more work in this area is clearly needed.

Among people in their working years, osteoarthritis and neck and low back pain are major causes of disability. Some potentially modifiable risk factors have been well established, including injury to joints, cumulative trauma to joints, heavy lifting, and exposure to vibration in the back and neck. However, to date, preventive programmes have done little to reduce the frequency and impact of osteoarthritis and neck and low back pain. For rheumatoid arthritis, another relatively common disease of adults, almost nothing is known about means of primary prevention except for possible risk reduction from the use of oral contraceptives.

For the major musculoskeletal disorders of adults, including osteoarthritis, osteoporosis, low back and neck pain, and rheumatoid arthritis, much more needs to be learned about how to limit the pain and disability among those who are affected. Once people develop osteoarthritis, osteoporosis, rheumatoid arthritis, and, in some instances, back or neck pain, they are likely to be affected for the rest of their lives. Thus, helping people learn how best to cope with these conditions is essential.

Among infants, children, and adolescents, early detection and prompt treatment would appear to offer the best means of reducing the impact of developmental dislocation of the hip, scoliosis, and slipped epiphysis, but many questions have been raised about the effectiveness of existing screening programmes for developmental dislocation of the hip and scoliosis. Prevention of adolescent obesity and of childhood accidents should reduce the frequency of slipped epiphysis and fractures, respectively, if it were possible to modify the lifestyles of children in these respects.

Finally, musculoskeletal disorders are often not given high priority in developing countries, despite the large amount of disability that they cause and their high monetary cost to the community. On the basis of current knowledge, ergonomic improvements and better training in the workplace could be instituted now in many regions. In addition, more information on the most important musculoskeletal problems and risk factors in specific geographical areas is needed if limited funds are to be used wisely. To accomplish this, special surveys must be undertaken. Clinics will need to be established, professional staff and patients educated, and community participation encouraged. Collaboration between epidemiologists in developing and industrialized countries will often be needed to make such surveys successful (Adebajo 1990).

In summary, much remains to be learned about the epidemiology and prevention of this important group of diseases. Better methods of primary, secondary, and tertiary prevention would improve the quality of life of people worldwide and would contribute substantially to increased economic productivity and a reduction in health care costs.

References

Acheson, R.M. (1966). Maturation of the skeleton. In *Human development* (ed. F. Faulkner), pp. 465–500. Saunders, Philadelphia.

Adebajo, A.O. (1990). Rheumatology in the Third World. *Annals of the Rheumatic Diseases*, **49**, 813–16.

Ahasan, M.R., Mohiuddin, G., Vayrynen, S., Ironkannas, H., and Quddus, R. (1999). Work-related problems in metal handling tasks in Bangladesh: obstacles to the development of safety and health measures. *Ergonomics*, **42**, 385–96.

Alarcón, G.S. (1995). Epidemiology of rheumatoid arthritis. *Rheumatic Diseases Clinics of North America*, **21**, 589–604.

Alexander, M.A. and Season, E.H. (1978). Idiopathic scoliosis: an electromyographic study. *Archives of Physical Medicine and Rehabilitation*, **59**, 314–15.

Anderson, J.J. and Felson, D.T. (1988). Factors associated with osteoarthritis of the knee in the first National Health and Nutrition Examination Survey (HANES I). *American Journal of Epidemiology*, **128**, 179–89.

Andersson, G.B.J. (1981). Epidemiologic aspects of low-back pain in industry. *Spine*, **6**, 53–60.

Anonymous (1997). Who are candidates for prevention and treatment for osteoporosis? *Osteoporosis International*, **7**, 1–6.

Arnett, F.C., Edworthy, S.M., Bloch, D.A., *et al.* (1988). The American Rheumatism Association 1987 revised criteria for the classification of rheumatoid arthritis. *Arthritis and Rheumatism*, **31**, 315–24.

Badley, E.M. (1995). The economic burden of musculoskeletal disorders in Canada is similar to that for cancer, and may be higher. *Journal of Rheumatology*, **22**, 204–6.

Badley, E.M., Rasooly, I., and Webster, G.K. (1994). Relative importance of musculoskeletal disorders as a cause of chronic health problems, disability, and health care utilization: findings from the 1990 Ontario Health Survey. *Journal of Rheumatology*, **21**, 505–14.

Beasley, R.P., Wilkens, R.F., and Bennett, P.H. (1973). High prevalence of rheumatoid arthritis in Yakima Indians. *Arthritis and Rheumatism*, **16**, 443–7.

Beasley, R.P., Bennett, P.H., and Lin, C.C. (1983). Low prevalence of rheumatoid arthritis in Chinese: Prevalence survey in a rural community. *Journal of Rheumatology*, **10** (Supplement), 11–15.

Biering-Sorenson, F. (1982). Low back trouble in a general population of 30-, 40-, 50-, and 60-year old men and women. Study design, representativeness, and basic results. *Danish Medical Bulletin*, **29**, 289–99.

Bleasel, J.F. and Moskowitz, R.W. (1995). Osteoarthritis: etiology and specific therapy revisited. In *Osteoarthritic disorders* (ed. K. Kuettner and V. Goldberg), pp. 25–34. AAOS, Rosemont, IL.

Bonjour, J-P. and Rizzoli, R. (1996). Bone acquisition in adolescence. In *Osteoporosis* (ed. R. Marcus, D. Feldman, and J. Kelsey), pp. 465–76. Academic Press, San Diego, CA.

Bovim, G., Schrader, H., and Sand, T. (1994). Neck pain in the general population. *Spine*, **19**, 1307–9.

Bowling, A. (1996). The effects of illness on quality of life: findings from a survey of households in Great Britain. *Journal of Epidemiology and Community Health*, **50**, 149–55.

Brage, S. and Bjerkedal, T. (1996). Musculoskeletal pain and smoking in Norway. *Journal of Epidemiology and Community Health*, **50**, 166–9.

Brooks, H. L., Azen, S. D., Gerberg, E. Brooks, R., and Chen, L. (1975). Scoliosis: a prospective epidemiological study. *Journal of Bone and Joint Surgery, American Volume*, **57A**, 968–72.

Buckwalter, J.A., Lane, N.E., and Gordon, S.L. (1995). Exercise as a cause of osteoarthritis. In *Osteoarthritic disorders* (ed. K. Kuettner and V. Goldberg), pp. 405–17. AAOS, Rosemont, IL.

Bunnell, W.P. (1984). An objective criterion for scoliosis screening. *Spine*, **18**, 1572–80.

Butler, W.J., Hawthorne, V.M., Mikkelsen, W.M., Carman, W.J., Bouthillier, D.L., and Lamphiear, D.E. (1988). Prevalence of radiologically defined osteoarthritis in the finger and wrist joints of adult residents of Tecumseh, Michigan, 1962–65. *Journal of Clinical Epidemiology*, **41**, 467–73.

Carman, W. (1989). Factors associated with pain and osteoarthritis in the Tecumseh Community Health Study. *Seminars in Arthritis and Rheumatism*, **18**, 1–4.

Carman, W.J., Sowers, M.F., Hawthorne, V.M., and Weissfeld, L.A. (1994). Obesity as a risk factor for osteoarthritis of the hand and wrist. A prospective study. *American Journal of Epidemiology*, **139**, 119–29.

Cats-Baril, W.L. and Frymoyer, J.W. (1991). Identifying patients at risk of becoming disabled because of low-back pain. The Vermont Rehabilitation Engineering Center predictive model. *Spine*, **16**, 605–7.

Cauley, J.A., Salamone, L.M., and Lucas, F.L. (1996). Postmenopausal endogenous and exogenous hormones, degree of obesity, thiazide diuretics, and risk of osteoporosis. In *Osteoporosis* (ed. R. Marcus, D. Feldman, and J. Kelsey), pp. 551–76. Academic Press, San Diego, CA.

Chapay, M.C., Arlot, M.E., Duboeuf, F., *et al.* (1992). Vitamin D3 and calcium to prevent hip fractures in elderly women. *New England Journal of Medicine*, **327**, 1637–42.

Chavalitsakulchai, P. and Shahnavaz, H. (1993). Musculoskeletal disorders of female workers and ergonomics problems in five different industries of a developing country. *Journal of Human Ergology (Tokyo)*, **22**, 29–43.

Cheng, J.C.Y., Ng, B.K.W., Ying, S.Y., and Lam, P.K.W. (1999). A 10-year study of the changes in the pattern and treatment of 6,493 fractures. *Journal of Pediatric Orthopaedics*, **19**, 344–50.

Christiansen C., Christensen, M.S., and Transbol, I. (1981). Bone mass in postmenopausal women after withdrawal of oestrogen/gestagen replacement therapy. *Lancet*, **i**, 459–61.

Cicuttini, F.M. and Spector, T.D. (1996). Genetics of osteoarthritis. *Annals of the Rheumatic Diseases*, **55**, 665–7.

Côté, P., Cassidy, J.D., and Carroll, L. (1998*a*). The Saskatchewan Health and Back Pain Survey. The prevalence of neck pain and related disability in Saskatchewan adults. *Spine*, **23**, 1689–98.

Côté, P., Kreitz, B.G., Cassidy, J.D., Dzus, A.K., and Martel, J. (1998*b*). A study of the diagnostic accuracy and reliability of the scoliometer and Adam's forward bend test. *Spine*, **23**, 796–803.

Coyte, P.C., Asche, C.V., Croxford, R., and Chan, B. (1998). The economic cost of musculoskeletal disorders in Canada. *Arthritis Care and Research*, **11**, 315–25.

Croft, P. (1996). The occurrence of osteoarthritis outside Europe. *Annals of the Rheumatic Diseases*, **55**, 661–4.

Croft, P., Coggon, D., Cruddas, M., *et al.* (1992). Osteoarthritis of the hip. An occupational disease in farmers. *British Medical Journal*, **304**, 1269–72.

Cumming, R.G. (1990). Calcium intake and bone mass: a quantitative review of the evidence. *Calcified Tissue International*, **47**, 194–201.

Cumming, R.G., Nevitt, M.C., and Cummings, S.R. (1997). Epidemiology of hip fracture. *Epidemiologic Reviews*, **19**, 244–57.

Cummings, S.R., Black, D.M., Thompson, D.E., *et al.* (1998). Effect of alendronate on risk of fracture in women with low bone density but without vertebral fractures: results from the Fracture Intervention Trial. *Journal of the American Medical Association*, **280**, 2077–82.

Cyvin, K.B. (1977). Congenital dislocation of the hip joint. *Acta Paediatrica Scandinavica*, **263**, 1–67.

Daltroy L.H., Iversen, M.D, Larson, M.G., *et al.* (1997). A controlled trial of an educational program to prevent low back injuries. *New England Journal of Medicine*, **337**, 322–8.

Dans, L.F., Tankeh-Torres, S., Amante, C.M., and Penserga, E.G. (1997). The prevalence of rheumatic diseases in a Filipino urban population: a WHO-ILAR COPCORD Study. *Journal of Rheumatology*, **24**, 1814–19.

Dawson-Hughes, B., Dallal, G.E., Krall, E.A., Sadowski, L., Sahyoun, N., and Tannenbaum, S. (1990). A controlled trial of the effect of calcium supplementation on bone density of postmenopausal women. *New England Journal of Medicine*, **323**, 878–83.

Delmas, P.D., Bjarason, N.H., Mitlak, B.H., *et al.* (1997). Effects of raloxifene on bone mineral density, serum cholesterol concentrations, and uterine endometrium in postmenopausal women. *New England Journal of Medicine*, **337**, 1641–7.

Deyo, R.A. and Diehl, A.K. (1988). Psychosocial predictors of disability in patients with low back pain. *Journal of Rheumatology*, **15**, 1557–64.

Dickson, R.A., Stamper, P., Sharp, A-M., and Harker, P. (1980). School screening for scoliosis: cohort study of clinical course. *British Medical Journal*, **ii**, 265–7.

Dougados, M., Gueguen, A., Nguyen, M., *et al.* (1992). Longitudinal radiologic evaluation of osteoarthritis of the knee. *Journal of Rheumatology*, **19**, 78–83.

Eisenberg, D.M., Kessler, R.C., Foster, C., Norlock, F.E., Calkins, D.R., and Delbanco, T.L. (1993). Unconventional medicine in the United States. *New England Journal of Medicine*, **328**, 246–52.

Eisman, J.A. (1995). Vitamin D receptor gene alleles and osteoporosis: an affirmative view. *Journal of Bone and Mineral Research*, **10**, 1289–93.

Ettinger, B., Pressman, A., Schein, J. Chan, J., Silver, P., and Connolly, N. (1998). Alendronate use among 812 women: prevalence of gastrointestinal complaints, noncompliance with patient instructions, and discontinuation. *Journal of Managed Care Pharmacy*, **4**, 488–92.

Ettinger, B., Black, D.M., Mitlak, B.H., *et al.* (1999). Reduction of vertebral fracture risk in postmenopausal women with osteoporosis treated with raloxifene. Results from a 3-year randomized clinical trial. *Journal of the American Medical Association*, **282**, 637–45.

Farooqi, A. and Gibson, T. (1998). Prevalence of major rheumatic disorders in the adult population of north Pakistan. *British Journal of Rheumatology*, **37**, 491–5.

Faulkner, K.G., Cummings, S.R., Black, D., Palmero, L., Glüer C.-C, and Genant, H.K. (1993). Simple measurement of femoral geometry predicts hip fracture: the Study of Osteoporotic Fractures. *Journal of Bone and Mineral Research*, **8**, 1211–17.

Felson, D.T., Anderson, J.J., Naimark, A., Walker, A.M., Swift, M., and Meenan, R.F. (1988). Obesity and knee osteoarthritis: the Framingham Study. *Annals of Internal Medicine*, **109**, 18–24.

Felson, D.T., Hannan, M.R., Maimark, A., *et al.* (1991). Occupational physical demands, knee bending and knee osteoarthritis. Results from the Framingham Study. *Journal of Rheumatology*, **18**, 1587–92.

Felson, D.T., Zhang, Y., Anthony, J.M., Nalmark, A., and Anderson, J.J. (1992). Weight loss reduces the risk of symptomatic knee osteoarthritis in women: the Framingham Study. *Annals of Internal Medicine*, **116**, 535–9.

Felts, W. and Yelin, E. (1989). The economic impact of the rheumatic diseases in the United States. *Journal of Rheumatology*, **16**, 867–84.

Ferraz, M.B. (1995). Tropical rheumatology. Epidemiology and community studies: Latin America. *Baillières Clinical Rheumatology*, **9**, 1–9.

Fish, J.R., DiMonte, P., and Courington, S.M. (1983). Back schools: past, present, and future. *Clinical Orthopaedics and Related Research*, **179**, 18–23.

Francis, M.J., Smith, R., and Sanderson, M.C. (1977). Collagen abnormalities in idiopathic adolescent scoliosis. *Calcified Tissue Research*, **22** (Supplement), 381–4.

Fulton, M.J. and Barer, M.L. (1984). Screening for congenital dislocation of the hip: an economic appraisal. *Canadian Medical Association Journal*, **130**, 1149–56.

Gabriel, S.E., Crowson, C.S., and O'Fallon, W.M. (1999). The epidemiology of rheumatoid arthritis in Rochester, Minnesota, 1955–1985. *Arthritis and Rheumatism*, **42**, 415–20.

Garraway, W.M., Stauffer, R.N., Kurland, L.T., and O'Fallon, W.M. (1979). Limb fractures in a defined population: frequency and distribution. *Mayo Clinic Proceedings*, **54**, 701–7.

Geitung, J.T., Rosendahl, K., and Sudmann, E. (1996). Cost-effectiveness of ultrasonographic screening for congenital hip dysplasia in newborns. *Skeletal Radiology*, **25**, 251–4.

Goldberg, C.J., Dowling, F.E., Fogarty, E.E., and Moore, D.P. (1995). School scoliosis screening and the United States Preventive Services Task Force. *Spine*, **20**, 1368–74.

Gregerson, P.K., Silver, J., and Winchester, R.J. (1987). The shared epitope hypothesis. An approach to understanding the molecular genetics of susceptibility to rheumatoid arthritis. *Arthritis and Rheumatism*, **30**, 1205–13.

Grisso, J.A., Capezuti, E., and Schwartz, A.V. (1996). Falls as risk factors for fractures. In *Osteoporosis* (ed. R. Marcus, D. Feldman, and J. Kelsey), pp. 599–611. Academic Press, San Diego, CA.

Grossman, T.W., Mazur, J.M., and Cummings, R.J. (1995). An evaluation of the Adams forward bend test and the scoliometer in a scoliosis school screening setting. *Journal of Pediatric Orthopaedics*, **15**, 535–8.

Gunther, A., Smith, S.J., Maynard, P.V., Beaver, M.W., and Chilvers, C.E.D. (1993). A case-control study of congenital hip dislocation. *Public Health*, **107**, 9–18.

Guo, H.-R., Tanaka, S., Halperin, W.E., and Cameron, L.L. (1999). Back pain prevalence in US industry and estimates of lost workdays. *American Journal of Public Health*, **89**, 1029–35.

Hadler, N.M., Gillings, D.B., Imbus, H.R., *et al.* (1978). Hand structure and function in an industrial setting. *Arthritis and Rheumatism*, **21**, 210–20.

Hadley-Miller, N., Mims, B., and Milewicz, D.M. (1994). The potential role of the elastic fiber system in adolescent idiopathic scoliosis. *Journal of Bone and Joint Surgery, American Volume*, **76A**, 1193–206.

Hales, T.R. and Bernard, B.P. (1996). Epidemiology of work-related musculoskeletal disorders. *Orthopedic Clinics of North America*, **27**, 679–709.

Hameed, K., Gibson, T., Kadir, M., Sultana, S., Fatima, Z., and Syed, A. (1995). The prevalence of rheumatoid arthritis in affluent and poor urban communities of Pakistan. *British Journal of Rheumatology*, **34**, 252–6.

Hamerman, D. (1989). The biology of osteoarthritis. *New England Journal of Medicine*, **320**, 1322–30.

Hans, D., Dargent-Molina, P., Schott, A.M., *et al.* (1996). Ultrasonographic heel measurements to predict hip fracture in elderly women: the EPIDOS prospective study. *Lancet*, **348**, 511–14.

Hansson, L.I., Hagglund, G., and Ordeberg, G. (1987). Slipped capital femoral epiphysis in southern Sweden, 1910–1982. *Acta Orthopaedica Scandinavica*, **226**, 1–67.

Harvey, J., Lotze, M., Arnett, F.C., *et al.* (1983). Rheumatoid arthritis in a Chippewa Band: II. Field study with clinical, serologic and HLA-D correlations. *Journal of Rheumatology*, **10**, 28–32.

Hayes, W.C., Myers, E.R., Morris, J.N., Gerhart, T.N., Yett, H.S., and Lipsitz, L.A. (1993). Impact near the hip dominates fracture risk in elderly nursing home residents who fall. *Calcified Tissue International*, **52**, 192–8.

Hazebroek-Kampschreur, A.A.J.M., Hofman, D., Van Dijk, A.P., and Van Linge, B. (1994). Determinants of trunk abnormalities in adolescence. *International Journal of Epidemiology*, **23**, 1242–7.

Heaney, R.P. (1996). Nutrition and risk for osteoporosis. In *Osteoporosis* (ed. R. Marcus, D. Feldman, and J. Kelsey), pp. 483–509. Academic Press, San Diego, CA.

Heliövaara, M., Vanharanta, H., Korpi, J., and Troup, J.D.G. (1986). Herniated lumbar disc syndrome and vertebral canals. *Spine*, **11**, 433–5.

Heliövaara, M., Mäkelä, M., Knekt, P., Ollimpivaara, and Aromaa, A. (1991). Determinants of sciatica and low-back pain. *Spine*, **16**, 608–14.

Henrikson, B. (1969). The incidence of slipped capital femoral epiphysis. *Acta Orthopaedica Scandinavica*, **40**, 365–72.

Henssge, J. (1968). Are the signs of denervation of the muscles of the spine primary or secondary findings in cases of scoliosis. *Journal of Bone and Joint Surgery, British Volume*, **50B**, 882.

Hernandez, R.J., Cornell, R.G., and Hensinger, R.N. (1994). Ultrasound diagnosis of neonatal congenital dislocation of the hip. A decision analysis assessment. *Journal of Bone and Joint Surgery, British Volume*, **76B**, 539–43.

Hochberg, M.C. (1990). Contrasting trends in the incidence and prevalence of rheumatoid arthritis in England and Wales, 1970–1982. *Seminars in Arthritis and Rheumatism*, **19**, 294–302.

Holbrook, T.L., Grazier, K.L., Kelsey, J.L., and Stauffer, R.N. (1984). *The frequency of occurrence, impact and cost of musculoskeletal conditions in the United States*. AAOS, Rosemont, IL.

Holderbaum, D., Haqqi, T.M., and Moskowitz, R.W. (1999). Genetics and osteoarthritis. *Arthritis and Rheumatism*, **42**, 397–405.

Hosking, E., Chilvers, C.E.D., Christiansen, C., *et al.* (1998). Prevention of bone loss with alendronate in postmenopausal women under 60 years of age. *New England Journal of Medicine*, **338**, 485–92.

Hult, L. (1954). Cervical, dorsal, and lumbar spine syndromes. *Acta Orthopaedica Scandinavica*, **17** (Supplement), 1–102.

Hutton, C. (1987). Generalised osteoarthritis: an evolutionary problem? *Lancet*, **i**, 1463–5.

Jensen, M.C., Brant-Zawadzi, M.N., Obuchowski, N., Modic, M.T., Malkasian, D., and Ross, J.S. (1994). Magnetic resonance imaging of the lumbar spine in people without back pain. *New England Journal of Medicine*, **331**, 69–73.

Jerre, R., Karlsson, J., and Henrikson, B. (1996). The incidence of physiolysis of the hip. A population-based study of 175 patients. *Acta Orthopaedica Scandinavica*, **67**, 53–6.

Jones, D.H. (1965). The early diagnosis of congenital dislocation of the hip joint. *British Journal of Clinical Practice*, **19**, 443–9.

Jones, D.A. (1991). Neonatal hip stability and the Barlow test. A study in stillborn babies. *Journal of Bone and Joint Surgery, British Volume*, **73B**, 216–18.

Keessen, W., Crowe, A., and Hearn, M. (1992). Proprioceptive accuracy in idiopathic scoliosis. *Spine*, **17**, 149–55.

Kellgren, J.H. (1961). Osteoarthrosis in patients and populations. *British Medical Journal*, **7**, 1–6.

Kellgren, J.H. and Lawrence, J.S. (1963). *Epidemiology of chronic rheumatism*. F.A. Davis, Philadelphia, PA.

Kelsey, J.L. (1971). Incidence and distribution of slipped capital femoral epiphysis in Connecticut. *Journal of Chronic Diseases*, **23**, 567–87.

Kelsey, J.L. (1982). *Epidemiology of musculoskeletal disorders*. Oxford University Press, New York.

Kelsey, J.L. (1998). Musculoskeletal diseases. In *Maxcy–Rosenau–Last public health and preventive medicine* (ed. R.B. Wallace) (14th edn), pp. 1005–17. Appleton and Lange, Stamford, CT.

Kelsey, J.L. and Hochberg, M.C. (1988). Epidemiology of chronic musculoskeletal disorders. *Annual Reviews of Public Health*, **9**, 379–401.

Kelsey, J.L., Keggi, K.J., and Southwick, W.O. (1970). The incidence and distribution of slipped capital femoral epiphysis in Connecticut and Southwestern United States. *Journal of Bone and Joint Surgery, American Volume*, **52A**, 1203–16.

Kelsey, J.L., Acheson, R.M., and Keggi, K.J. (1972). The body builds of patients with slipped capital femoral epiphysis. *American Journal of Diseases of Children*, **124**, 276–81.

Kelsey, J.L., Githens, P.B., Walter, S.D., *et al.* (1984*a*). An epidemiologic study of acute prolapsed cervical intervertebral disc. *Journal of Bone and Joint Surgery, American Volume*, **66A**, 907–14.

Kelsey, J.L., Githens, P.B., White A.A., III, *et al.* (1984*b*). An epidemiological study of lifting and twisting on the job and risk for acute prolapsed lumbar intervertebral disc. *Journal of Orthopaedic Research*, **2**, 61–6.

Kelsey, J.L., Browner, W.S., Seeley, D.G., Nevitt, M.C., and Cummings, S.R. (1992). Risk factors for fracture of the distal forearm and proximal humerus. *American Journal of Epidemiology*, **135**, 473–89.

Keyserling W.M., Herrin, G.D., and Chaffin, D.B. (1980). Establishing an industrial strength testing program. *American Industrial Hygiene Association Journal*, **41**, 730–6.

Knox, E.G., Armstrong, E.H., and Lancashire, R.J. (1987). Effectiveness of screening for congenital dislocation of the hip. *Journal of Epidemiology and Community Health*, **41**, 283–9.

Krause, N., Ragland, D.R., Greiner, B.A., Fisher, J.M., Holman, B.L., and Selvin, S. (1997). Physical workload and ergonomic factors associated with prevalence of back and neck pain in urban transit operators. *Spine*, **22**, 2117–26.

Krause, N., Ragland, D.R., Fisher, J.M., and Syme, L. (1998). Psychosocial job factors, physical workload, and incidence of work-related spinal injury: a 5-year prospective study of urban transit operators. *Spine*, **23**, 2507–16.

Lachance, L., Sowers, M.F., Jamadar, D., Jannausch, M., Hochberg, M.C., and Crutchfield, M. (2001). The experience of pain and emergent osteoarthritis of the knee. In press.

Lagerström M., Hansson, T., and Hagberg, M. (1998). Work-related low-back problems in nursing. *Scandinavian Journal of Work, Environment and Health*, **24**, 449–64.

Landin, L.A. (1983). Fracture patterns in children. Analysis of 8,682 fractures with special reference to incidence, etiology and secular changes in a Swedish urban population 1950–1979. *Acta Orthopaedica Scandinavica*, **202** (Supplement), 1–109.

Lankhurst, G.J., Van de Stadt, R.J., Vogelaar, T.W., Van de Korst, J.K., and Prevo, A.J.H. (1983). The effect of the Swedish back school on chronic idiopathic low back pain. *Scandinavian Journal of Rehabilitation Medicine*, **15**, 141–5.

Lau, E.M.C., Symmons, D.P.M., and Croft, P. (1996). The epidemiology of hip osteoarthritis and rheumatoid arthritis in the Orient. *Clinical Orthopaedics and Related Research*, **323**, 81–90.

Lauritzen, J.B., Petersen, M.M., and Lund, B. (1993). Effect of external hip protectors on hip fracture. *Lancet*, **341**, 11–13.

Lawrence J.S. and Sebo, M. (1980). The geography of osteoarthritis. In *The aetiopathogenesis of osteoarthrosis* (ed. G. Nuki), pp. 155–83. Pitman, Kent.

Lawrence, R.C., Hochberg, M.C., Kelsey, J.L., *et al.* (1989). Estimates of the prevalence of selected arthritic and musculoskeletal diseases in the United States. *Journal of Rheumatology*, **16**, 427–41.

Lawrence, R.C., Helmick, C.G., Arnett, F.C., *et al.* (1998). Estimates of the prevalence of arthritis and selected musculoskeletal disorders in the United States. *Arthritis and Rheumatism*, **41**, 778–99.

Leck, I. (1986). An epidemiological assessment of neonatal screening for dislocation of the hip. *Journal of the Royal College of Physicians of London*, **20**, 56–62.

Leclerc, A., Niedhammer, I., Landre, M.-F., Ozguler, A., Etore, P., and Pietri-Taleb, F. (1999). One-year predictive factors for various aspects of neck disorders. *Spine*, **24**, 1455–62.

Linos, A., Worthington, J.W., O'Fallon, W.M., and Kurland, L.T. (1980). The epidemiology of rheumatoid arthritis in Rochester, Minnesota: a study of incidence, prevalence and mortality. *American Journal of Epidemiology*, **111**, 87–98.

Loder, R.T. (1996*a*). The demographics of slipped capital femoral epiphysis. An international multicenter study. *Clinical Orthopaedics and Related Research*, **322**, 8–27.

Loder, R.T. (1996*b*). A worldwide study of the seasonal variation of slipped capital femoral epiphysis. *Clinical Orthopaedics and Related Research*, **322**, 28–36.

Lonstein, J.R. (1988). Natural history and school screening for scoliosis. *Orthopedic Clinics of North American*, **19**, 227–37.

Lyons, R.A., Delahunty, A.M., Kraus, D., *et al.* (1999). Children's fractures: a population based study. *Injury Prevention*, **5**, 129–32.

Macnicol, M.F. (1990). Results of a 25-year screening programme for neonatal hip instability. *Journal of Bone and Joint Surgery, British Volume*, **72B**, 1057–60.

Maggi, S., Kelsey, J.L., Litvak, J., and Heyse, S.P. (1991). Incidence of hip fractures in the elderly: a cross-national analysis. *Osteoporosis International*, **1**, 232–41.

Magnusson, M.L., Pope, M.H., Wilder, D.G., and Areskoug, B. (1996). Are occupational drivers at an increased risk for developing musculoskeletal disorders? *Spine*, **21**, 710–17.

Malmivaara, A., Häkkinen, U., Aro, T., *et al.* (1995). The treatment of acute low back pain—bed rest, exercises, or ordinary activity? *New England Journal of Medicine*, **332**, 351–5.

Manninen, P., Riihimaki, H., Heliövaara, M., and Mäkelä, P. (1996). Overweight, gender and knee osteoarthritis. *International Journal of Obesity*, **20**, 595–7.

Melton, L.J., III (1995). How many women have osteoporosis now? *Journal of Bone and Mineral Research*, **10**, 175–7.

Mooney, J.F. and Emans, J.B. (1995). Developmental dislocation of the hip: a clinical overview. *Pediatrics in Review*, **16**, 299–303.

Moore, F.H. (1989). Examining infants' hips – can it do harm? *Journal of Bone and Joint Surgery, British Volume*, **71B**, 4–5.

Morais, T., Bernier, M., and Turcotte, F. (1985). Age- and sex-specific prevalence of scoliosis and the value of school screening programs. *American Journal of Public Health*, **75**, 1377–80.

Morrison, N.A., Yeoman, R., Kelly, P.J., and Eisman, J.A. (1992). Contribution of *trans*-acting factor alleles to normal physiological variability: vitamin D receptor gene polymorphisms and circulating osteocalcin. *Proceedings of the National Academy of Sciences*, **89**, 6665–9.

Morscher, E. (1968). Strength and morphology of growth cartilage under hormonal influence of puberty. *Reconstructive Surgery and Traumatology*, **10**, 3–104.

Müller, C.F., Monrad, T., Biering-Sorensen, F., Darre, E., Deis, A., and Kryger, P. (1999). The influence of previous low back trouble, general health, and working conditions on future sick-listing because of low back trouble. *Spine*, **24**, 1562–70.

Nachemson, A. (1983). Work for all: those with low back pain as well. *Clinical Orthopaedics and Related Research*, **179**, 77–85.

Nachemson, A. and Sahlshand, T. (1977). Etiologic factors in adolescent idiopathic scoliosis. *Spine*, **2**, 176–84.

Nevitt, M.C. and Cummings, S.R. (1993). Type of fall and risk of hip and wrist fractures: the Study of Osteoporotic Fractures. *Journal of the American Geriatrics Society*, **41**, 1226–34.

Nissinen, M., Heliövaara, M., Seitsamo, J., and Poussa, M. (1993*a*). Trunk asymmetry, posture, growth, and risk of scoliosis. A three-year follow-up of Finnish prepubertal school children. *Spine*, **18**, 8–13.

Nissinen, M., Heliövaara, M., Ylikoski, M., and Poussa, M. (1993*b*). Trunk asymmetry and screening for scoliosis: a longitudinal cohort study of pubertal schoolchildren. *Acta Paediatrica Scandinavica*, **82**, 77–82.

Ollier, W.E.R. and MacGregor, A. (1995). Genetic epidemiology of rheumatoid disease. *British Medical Bulletin*, **51**, 267–85.

Papageorgiou A.C., Croft, P.R., Ferry, S., Jayson, M.I.V., and Silman, A.J. (1995). Estimating the prevalence of low back pain in the general population. Evidence from the South Manchester Back Pain Survey. *Spine*, **20**, 1889–94.

Papageorgiou, A.C., Croft, P.R., Thomas, E., Ferry, S., Jayson, M.I.V., and Silman, A.J. (1996). Influence of previous pain experience on the episode incidence of low back pain: results from the South Manchester Back Pain Study. *Pain*, **66**, 181–5.

Papageorgiou, A.C., Macfarlane, G.J., Thomas, E., Croft, P.R., Jayson, M.I.V., and Silman, A.J. (1997). Psychosocial factors in the workplace—do they predict new episodes of low back pain? Evidence from the South Manchester Back Pain Study. *Spine*, **22**, 1137–42.

Peacock, M. (1995). Vitamin D receptor gene alleles and osteoporosis: a contrasting view. *Journal of Bone and Mineral Research*, **10**, 1294–7.

Peacock, M., Turner, C.H., Liu, G. Manatunga, A.K., Timmerman, L., and Johnson, C.C., Jr (1995). Better discrimination of hip fracture using bone density, geometry and architecture. *Osteoporosis International*, **5**, 167–73.

Pope, M.H., Magnusson, M., and Wilder, D.G. (1998). Low back pain and whole body vibration. *Clinical Orthopaedics and Related Research*, **354**, 241–8.

Praemer, A., Furner, S., and Rice, D.P. (1999). *Musculoskeletal conditions in the United States.* AAOS, Rosemont, IL.

Radin, E.L., Paul, I.L., and Rose, R.M. (1972). Role of mechanical factors in pathogenesis of primary osteoarthritis. *Lancet*, **i**, 519–22.

Record, R.C. and Edwards, J.H. (1958). Environmental influences related to the aetiology of congenital dislocation of the hip. *British Journal of Preventive and Social Medicine*, **12**, 8–22.

Rennie, A.M. (1967). Familial slipped capital femoral epiphysis. *Journal of Bone and Joint Surgery, British Volume*, **49B**, 535–9.

Roach, K.E., Persky, V., Miles, T., and Budiman-Mak, E. (1994). Biomechanical aspects of occupation and osteoarthritis of the hip. A case-control study. *Journal of Rheumatology*, **21**, 2334–40.

Robinson, G.W. (1968). Birth characteristics of children with congenital dislocation of the hip. *American Journal of Epidemiology*, **87**, 275–84.

Rosendahl, K., Markestad, T., and Lie, R.T. (1994). Ultrasound screening for developmental dysplasia of the hip in the neonate: the effect on treatment rate and prevalence of late cases. *Pediatrics*, **94**, 47–52.

Rosendahl, K., Aslaksen, A., Lie, R.T., and Markestad. T. (1995). Reliability of ultrasound in the early diagnosis of developmental dysplasia of the hip. *Pediatric Radiology*, **25**, 219–24.

Sambrook, P.N., Kelly, P.J., White, C.P., Morrison, N.A., and Eisman, J.A. (1996). Genetic determinants of bone mass. In *Osteoporosis* (ed. R. Marcus, D. Feldman, and J. Kelsey), pp. 477–82. Academic Press, San Diego, CA.

Schipplein, O.D. and Andriacchi, T.P. (1991). Interaction between active and passive knee stabilizers during level walking. *Journal of Orthopaedic Research*, **9**, 113–19.

Schwartz, A.V. (1999). Epidemiologic aspects of osteoporotic fractures and falls. Ph.D. Dissertation, Stanford University.

Schwartz, A.V., Kelsey, J.L., Maggi, S., *et al.* (1999). International variation in the incidence of hip fractures: cross-national project on osteoporosis for the World Health Organization Program for Research on Aging. *Osteoporosis International*, **9**, 242–53.

Scrimgeour, E.M. (1992). Prevention of fracture of the neck of the femur: evidence from developing countries of the relative unimportance of osteoporosis. *Australia and New Zealand Journal of Medicine*, **22**, 85–6.

Seeman, E. (1996). The effects of tobacco and alcohol use on bone. In *Osteoporosis* (ed. R. Marcus, D. Feldman, and J. Kelsey), pp. 577–97. Academic Press, San Diego, CA.

Shands, A.R. and Eisberg, H.B. (1955). The incidence of scoliosis in the state of Delaware. *Journal of Bone and Joint Surgery, American Volume*, **37A**, 1243–9.

Sharrard, W.J.W. (1993). *Paediatric orthopaedics and fractures*, Vol. 1. Blackwell Scientific, Oxford.

Shelerud, R. (1998). Epidemiology of occupational low back pain. *Occupational Medicine*, **13**, 1–22.

Silman, A.J. and Hochberg, M.C. (1993). *Epidemiology of the rheumatic diseases.* Oxford University Press.

Singh, Y.M., Nagrath, A.R., and Maini, P.S. (1970). Changes in trabecular pattern of the upper end of the femur as an index of osteoporosis. *Journal of Bone and Joint Surgery, American Volume*, **52A**, 457–67.

Skaggs, D.L. and Bassett, G.S. (1996). Adolescent idiopathic scoliosis: an update. *American Family Physician*, **53**, 2327–34.

Slemenda, C.W., Christian, J.C., Williams, C.J., Norton, J.A., and Johnston, C.C., Jr (1991). Genetic determinants of bone mass in adult women: a reevaluation of the twin model and potential importance of gene interaction on heritability estimates. *Journal of Bone and Mineral Research*, **6**, 561–7.

Slemenda, C.W., Johnston, C.C., and Hiu, S.L. (1996). Assessing fracture risk. In *Osteoporosis* (ed. R. Marcus, D. Feldman, and J. Kelsey), pp. 623–33. Academic Press, San Diego, CA.

Snook, S.H. (1982). Low back pain in industry. In *American Academy of Orthopaedic Surgeons Symposium on Low Back Pain* (ed. A.A. White III and S.L. Gordon), pp. 23–38. C.V. Mosby, St Louis, MO.

Snook, S.H. (1988). Approaches to the control of back pain in industry: job design, job placement, and education/training. *Occupational Medicine*, **3**, 45–59.

Snow, C.M., Shaw, J.M., and Matkin, C.C. (1996). Physical activity and risk for osteoporosis. In *Osteoporosis* (ed. R. Marcus, D. Feldman, and J. Kelsey), pp. 511–28. Academic Press, San Diego, CA.

Sorenson, K.H. (1968). Slipped upper femoral epiphysis. *Acta Orthopaedica Scandinavica*, **39**, 499–517.

Sowers, M.F. (1996). Premenopausal reproductive and hormonal characteristics and the risk for osteoporosis. In *Osteoporosis* (ed. R. Marcus, D. Feldman, and J. Kelsey), pp. 529–49. Academic Press, San Diego, CA.

Sowers, M.F., Boehnke, M., Jannausch, M.L., Crutchfield, M., Corton, G., and Burns, T.L. (1992). Familiality and partitioning of variability of femoral neck bone mineral density of women of childbearing age. *Calcified Tissue International*, **50**, 110–14.

Sowers, M.F., Hochberg, M., Crabbe, J.P., Muhich, A., Crutchfield, M., and Updike, S. (1996). Association of bone mineral density and sex hormone levels with osteoarthritis of the hand and knee in premenopausal women. *American Journal of Epidemiology*, **143**, 38–47.

Sowers, M.F., Lachance, L., Jamadar, D., Hochberg, M., Crutchfield, M., and Jannausch, M.L. (1999*a*). The associations of bone mineral density and bone turnover markers with osteoarthritis of the hand and knee in pre- and peri-menopausal women. *Arthritis and Rheumatism*, **42**, 483–8.

Sowers, M.F., Willing, M., Burns, T., *et al.* (1999*b*). Genetic markers, bone mineral density, and serum osteocalcin levels. *Journal of Bone and Mineral Research*, **14**, 1411–19.

Sowers, M.F., Lachance, L., Hochberg, M., and Jamadar, D. (2000). Prevalence of radiographically defined osteoarthritis of the hand and knee in a population of pre- and perimenopausal women. *Osteoarthritis and Cartilage*, **8**, 69–77.

Spector, T.D. and Hochberg, M.C. (1990). The protective effect of oral contraceptives on the development of rheumatoid arthritis. An overview of analytic epidemiologic studies with a meta-analysis. *Journal of Clinical Epidemiology*, **43**, 1221–30.

Spotila, L.D., Colige, A., Sereda, L., *et al.* (1994). Mutation analysis of coding sequences for type I procollagen in individuals with low bone density. *Journal of Bone and Mineral Research*, **9**, 923–32.

Stecher, R.M. (1941). Heberden's nodes. Heredity in hypertrophic arthritis of finger joints. *American Journal of Medical Sciences*, **201**, 801–9.

Tepper, S. and Hochberg, M.C. (1993). Factors associated with hip osteoarthritis. Data from the First National Health and Nutrition Examination Survey (NHANES-I). *American Journal of Epidemiology*, **137**, 1081–8.

Thompson, M., Anderson, M., and Wood, P.N.H. (1974). Locomotor disability—a study of need in an urban community (abstract). *British Journal of Preventive and Social Medicine*, **28**, 70–1.

US Preventive Services Task Force (1993*a*). Screening for adolescent idiopathic scoliosis (policy statement). *Journal of the American Medical Association*, **269**, 2664–6.

US Preventive Services Task Force (1993*b*). Screening for adolescent idiopathic scoliosis. *Journal of the American Medical Association*, **269**, 2667–72.

van Poppel, M.N., Koes, B.W., Deville, W., Smid, T., and Bouter, L.M. (1998). Risk factors for back pain incidence in industry: a prospective study. *Pain*, **77**, 81–6.

van Sasse, J.L.C.M., Vandenbroucke, J.P., van Romunde, L.K.J., and Valkenburg, H.A. (1988). Osteoarthritis and obesity in the general population. A relationship calling for an explanation. *Journal of Rheumatology*, **15**, 1152–8.

Villa, M.L. and Nelson, L. (1996). Race, ethnicity, and osteoporosis. In *Osteoporosis* (ed. R. Marcus, D. Feldman, and J. Kelsey), pp. 435–47. Academic Press, San Diego, CA.

Vincelette, R., Laurin, C.A., and Levesque, H.P. (1972). The footballer's ankle and foot. *Canadian Medical Association Journal*, **107**, 872–4.

Walsh, K., Cruddas, M., and Coggon, D. (1992). Low back pain in eight areas of Britain. *Journal of Epidemiology and Community Health*, **46**, 227–30.

Weyand, C., Hicock, K.C., Conn, D.L., and Goronzy, J.J. (1992). The influence of HLA-DR B1 genes on disease severity in rheumatoid arthritis. *Annals of Internal Medicine*, **117**, 802–6.

WHO (1992). *Rheumatic diseases.* WHO Technical Report Series 816. WHO, Geneva.

WHO (1994). *Assessment of fracture risk and its application to screening for postmenopausal women.* WHO Technical Report Series 843. WHO, Geneva.

Wickstrom, G.J. and Pentti, J. (1998). Occupational factors affecting sick leave attributed to low-back pain. *Scandinavian Journal of Work, Environment and Health*, **24**, 145–52.

Williams, J.L. (1988). Criteria for screening. Are the effects predictable? *Spine*, **13**, 1178–86.

Willing, M., Sowers, M.F., Aron, D., *et al.* (1998). Bone mineral density and it change in white women. Estrogen and vitamin D receptor genotypes and their interaction. *Journal of Bone and Mineral Research*, **13**, 695–705.

Willner, S. (1975). A study of height, weight, and menarche in girls with idiopathic structural scoliosis. *Acta Orthopaedica Scandinavica*, **46**, 71–83.

Wingrave, S.J. (1978). Reduction in incidence of rheumatoid arthritis associated with oral contraceptives. *Lancet*, **1**, 569–71.

Worlock, P. and Stower, M. (1986). Fracture patterns in Nottingham children. *Journal of Pediatric Orthopedics*, **6**, 656–60.

Wynne-Davies, R. (1968). Familial (idiopathic) scoliosis. A family survey. *Journal of Bone and Joint Surgery, British Volume*, **50B**, 24–30.

Wynne-Davies, R. (1970). Acetabular dysplasia and familial joint laxity: two etiological factors in congenital dislocation of the hip. *Journal of Bone and Joint Surgery, British Volume*, **52B**, 704–16.

Yu, I.T.S. and Wong, T.W. (1996). Musculoskeletal problems among VDU workers in a Hong Kong bank. *Occupational Medicine*, **46**, 275–80.

9.10 Public health, epidemiology, and neurological diseases

Walter A. Kukull and James D. Bowen

Introduction

Included in this chapter are brief descriptions of some selected neurological disorders along with a discussion of their general epidemiology. Several themes cut across all of the sections. Case diagnosis is critical to epidemiological study of neurological diseases and disorders. However, diagnosis is difficult for many neurological diseases because specific antemortem biological markers may not exist and clinical diagnosis must be relied on. Variation in clinical criteria can lead to heterogeneity of diagnosed disease. As a case series includes more misclassification of disease diagnoses, the ability to recognize risk factors becomes reduced. Standardization of clinical criteria is one method of limiting the amount of misclassification; in practice, however, standardization is difficult to achieve.

Case ascertainment is a further problem for most epidemiological studies. This addresses the question how were the cases for study detected? If an incidence study must rely on death certificates, it is probably less than optimal for most neurological diseases. The method of identifying and including cases in a case–control study is important because if identification is associated with exposure history, selection bias could result and the findings could then be spurious. Can all identified cases be enrolled in a particular study? Obviously not; many persons decline to participate in studies. Frailty, age, ethnicity, gender, education, and a host of other factors influence participation. An uncontrolled bias may also result if any of these participation factors is systematically related to exposure status. Case-identification methods are critical to cohort studies (and intervention trials) as well. Failure to start with a cohort that is free of the disease of interest will potentially bias results. Lack of sensitivity or specificity in screening or diagnosing disease during follow-up will lead to misestimated incidence and to distorted risk-factor relationships.

Obtaining valid estimates of exposures for analytical risk-factor studies is of great importance. For most neurological diseases exposure determination is complicated by insidious and indeterminate onset of disease, confusing the temporal relationship between exposure and disease. Long-past exposure histories are difficult to construct and validate, especially in diseases that affect memory. Self-report histories and those obtained from proxies are often the basis for risk-factor inference, but may be flawed by distorted recollection or recall bias. Actual records, for example of medication history or occupational exposures, are seldom available. Biological markers of exposure (except for genotype) are difficult to obtain; and some may be affected by disease. Peripheral markers, if available, may not correspond to exposure levels in neuronal tissue. Biopsy may not be feasible or possible and autopsy, while often the gold standard for diagnosis, may reflect cumulative disease processes, leaving the picture additionally confusing.

As one leaves major research institutions or attempts to begin epidemiological research studies in less developed countries, the problems grow in magnitude. Differences in available facilities and local practices are likely the easiest to overcome. Addressing political concerns and suspicions to gain co-operation necessary to begin a study may take additional time and preparation. Case detection, acquisition, and exposure measurement still remain critical but the difficulty in obtaining acceptable levels of each is increased by an order of magnitude.

In the following sections we discuss the current descriptive and analytical research for a number of neurological disorders. We also provide a brief appraisal of the public health burden for these conditions.

Headache

Clinical overview

The pathogenesis of most headaches is poorly understood. Therefore, the nosology of headaches is based on the cause of headaches in those types where the cause is known, and the clinical picture in those in which the cause is unknown. The International Headache Society classification is currently the most commonly used system of classifying headaches (Table 1). It is important to realize that this system is used to classify individual headaches rather than individuals with headaches. Patients may suffer from more than one type of headache, with each day's headache fitting into one of the International Headache Society categories. In fact, most headache patients have more than one type of headache. The International Headache Society classification contains a large number of conditions in which the headaches are symptomatic of neurological or systemic diseases. These include trauma, vascular disorders, disorders of cerebrospinal fluid pressure, infection, neoplasms, toxins, withdrawal states, metabolic disorders, and structural lesions of the head, neck, or cranial nerves. Headaches associated with these conditions are comparatively rare. Idiopathic conditions are far more common and include migraine without aura, migraine with aura, tension-type headaches, and cluster headaches. Because these idiopathic headaches are the overwhelming majority, they have the greatest impact on epidemiological studies.

Table 1 International Headache Society (abbreviated classification of headache)

1	Migraine
	1.1 Migraine without aura
	1.2 Migraine with aura
2	Tension-type headache
3	Cluster headache and chronic paroxysmal hemicrania
4	Miscellaneous headaches unassociated with structural lesion
5	Headache associated with head trauma
6	Headache associated with vascular disorders
7	Headache associated with non-vascular intracranial disorder
8	Headache associated with substances or their withdrawal
9	Headache associated with non-cephalic infection
10	Headache associated with metabolic disorder
11	Headache or facial pain associated with disorder of cranium, neck, eyes, ears, nose, sinuses, teeth, mouth, or other facial or cranial structures
12	Cranial neuralgias, nerve trunk pain, and deafferentation pain
13	Headache not classifiable

Migraine without aura was previously named common migraine. It is an episodic headache that, as its name suggests, has no aura. Some patients experience a vague prodrome for a day or so prior to the onset of the headache. The headache may be unilateral or bilateral. It may change locations during the course of the headache. Some have throbbing pain while others have constant non-throbbing pain. Patients are often overly sensitive to sound (phonophobia) and light (photophobia) or smells. Nausea, vomiting, or diarrhoea may occur. The pain often builds over a few hours. Most last for several hours before slowly subsiding, though some may last for a few days.

Migraine with aura was previously named classic migraine. The identifying feature of this type of headache is the aura. This consists of an alteration of neurological function that usually precedes the headache. The aura most commonly consists of changes in vision with a central area of visual loss surrounded by a rim of shimmering light (the scintillating scotoma). The shimmering may look like flashing or twinkling lights, heat waves, or zigzag lines (fortification spectra). The area of visual abnormality gradually increases in size as the headache attack progresses. Non-visual auras may also occur, including paraesthesias, numbness, weakness, aphasia, or vertigo. Auras usually precede the headache by about 20 min, though the timing may vary. The headache resembles that seen in migraine without aura. It is most commonly, though not always, unilateral. It is most often throbbing and often associated with nausea and vomiting. It typically lasts a few hours. It is episodic and may have a prodrome preceding the headache.

Tension-type headaches are usually bilateral and have a sensation of pressure or a tight band around the head. They are less likely to have a prodrome and less likely to have nausea or vomiting. They do not have auras. They usually last longer than migraine headaches, typically an entire day or even several days. They build up more slowly than migraine headaches.

Cluster headaches are named after their tendency to occur in clusters lasting 2 to 6 months. However, other types of headaches may also occur in clusters and the diagnosis is made based on the characteristics of the headache rather than the clustering. The headache develops abruptly. It usually occurs daily during a cluster and often occurs at the same time of day. The pain is more short-lived than that of other idiopathic headaches and generally subsides within 2 h. It is unilateral and often associated with autonomic changes on the affected side. These include vasodilatation with unilateral flushing, conjunctival injection, nasal drainage, and sweating. Sympathetic dysfunction in the ipsilateral eye (Horner's syndrome) may occur. The pain is more severe than that seen with migraine and patients are often agitated during the attack.

As noted patients often suffer from more than one type of headache. In a single patient, less severe headaches tend to resemble tension-type while more severe ones resemble migraine. There is also a tendency for a patient's headaches to change over time with the headache pattern being classic migraine in youth but more closely matching that of tension-type headaches with time. These headaches may increase in frequency with age and become chronic daily headaches. Some term these headaches transitioned migraine.

Prevalence

Recent studies have assessed the prevalence of headache and migraine in many countries. Most of these studies have used the International Headache Society criteria in some fashion to determine probable diagnosis. Characteristics of the samples selected and analytical designs have differed, sometimes substantially, raising questions of comparability.

Gobel *et al.* (1994) selected a representative sample of 5000 persons from among 30 000 households in Germany. Using International Headache Society criteria, Gobel *et al.* determined that approximately 71 per cent of the subjects reported a history of headache. The lifetime prevalence of migraine was 27.5 per cent. This survey did not rely on use of medical care and so may estimate the underlying lifetime prevalence of both treated and untreated migraine. Lavados and Tenhamm (1997) selected a population sample of approximately 1400 persons in Santiago, Chile, but asked subjects about prevalence of headache within the last year rather than lifetime occurrence. The prevalence of migraine was reported as 7.3 per cent but with a marked gender difference: 2 per cent in males and 12 per cent in females. Merikangas *et al.* (1994) studied the prevalence of headache in persons aged 29 to 30 in Zurich, Switzerland, again using the International Headache Society criteria. Migraine with aura had a 1-year prevalence of 3.3 per cent and migraine without aura showed a 1-year prevalence of 21.3 per cent. These figures are roughly consistent, though somewhat higher than the previous citation; however, some of the increased prevalence may be due to the young adult age group. Francheschi *et al.* (1997) studied an elderly population (mean age 73 years) in Italy to determine whether increasing age would affect reported prevalence. Francheschi *et al.* report that although 18 per cent of subjects admitted to 'troublesome' headaches in the past, only 6 per cent were currently bothered by headache and 1 per cent met criteria for current migraine (per International Headache Society criteria). These results leave the impression that headache problems in young adulthood may not persist into old age. However, in order to evaluate adequately the change in frequency of headache events with age would require a cohort study design instead of a cross-sectional one. O'Brien *et al.* (1994) drew a stratified sample in Canada selecting 2922 subjects for study and conducted a telephone interview based on International Headache Society criteria. The prevalence of migraine was 7.8 per cent in males and 24.9 per cent in females; only about 46 per cent of those with migraine were reported to have ever contacted a physician for their problem. Within women the peak prevalence was seen in the 40- to 44-year age group. Thus, despite the variation in design and case ascertainment methods there may be a gender difference and age-related differences that appear with some consistency in a number of countries.

Osuntokun *et al.* (1992) applied a screening questionnaire to more than 18 000 persons in Nigeria. The questionnaire was not strictly according to the International Headache Society criteria but reportedly showed high sensitivity and specificity when compared to the gold standard neurologist examination for headache. Much lower lifetime prevalence of migraine, 5.3 per cent, was reported in this study than in those primarily comprised of Caucasians. No gender difference was noted, also in contrast to the studies reported above. Stewart *et al.* (1996*a*) compared migraine prevalence in Caucasians, African Americans, and Asian Americans living in the United States. The study involved about 12 000 persons aged 18 to 65 selected from Baltimore County, Maryland, selected by random digit dialling, and interviewed by telephone. Observed prevalence of migraine in Caucasians was 20.4 per cent for women and 8.6 per cent for men; among African Americans, 6.2 per cent in women and 7.2 per cent in men; and among Asian Americans, 9.2 per cent in women and 4.2 per cent in men. Despite obvious geographical and sociodemographic differences, as well as methodological differences between the two studies (Osuntokun *et al.* 1992; Stewart *et al.* 1996*a*), there appears to be a suggestion that susceptibility to migraine may be affected by ethnicity.

Stewart *et al.* (1992) also conducted a large, earlier study of migraine prevalence in about 15 000 persons. Prevalence of migraine was reported as 5.7 per cent for men and 17.6 per cent for women (using standard criteria); lower income was also associated with increased prevalence. These estimates compare favourably with other studies cited above which also included both treated and untreated, self-reported headache. Stewart *et al.* (1995) also conducted a meta-analysis that included 24 population-based studies of migraine. Most of the variation in prevalence estimates, among the studies included, was accounted for by age and gender differences along with case definition. Stewart concluded that after accounting for age, gender, and case definition, migraine prevalence estimates were stable across the studies included in the meta-analysis.

Familial and genetic risks

The influence of genetic constitution on the occurrence of migraine has been investigated principally by studies of familial aggregation and by twin studies. While these classic methods provide general clues concerning whether a genetic component to the disease may exist, their lenses are generally not of sufficient resolution to identify specific genes or linked markers. Progress in molecular genetics is providing remarkable discoveries for many diseases. Preliminary reports of rare mutations in the mitochondrial genome and associations with polymorphic forms of serotonergic and dopaminergic genes and migraine are as yet unsubstantiated, but may be more carefully evaluated and tested in the future (Peroutka 1998).

Two recent twin studies based in the Danish Twin Registry (Gervil *et al.* 1999; Ulrich *et al.* 1999) compared concordance rates of migraine without aura and migraine with aura. Twin pairs with one member affected by a specific type of migraine were selected from the registry. Both monozygotic and dizygotic twins (same sex) were selected for study and the occurrence of migraine was determined by interview and/or examination. The overall lifetime prevalence of migraine with aura for monozygotic and dizygotic twins was 7 per cent, similar to population surveys. The concordance in monozygotic twins was 34 per cent compared to 12 per cent for dizygotic twins. For migraine without aura the pairwise concordance for monozygotic twins was 28 per cent, compared with 18 per cent for dizygotic. This indicates a potential genetic contribution to migraine. But, because there is substantially less than 100 per cent concordance among monozygotic twins, the modifying influence of environmental factors may also be important in migraine aetiology. Ziegler *et al.* (1998) studied monozygotic and dizygotic, female twin pairs, raised together (n = 154) and raised apart (n = 43). This classical twin-study design aimed to tease out the relative contributions of genetic constitution and environmental exposures. Results showed that concordance was higher for monozygotic than dizygotic twins, whether raised together or raised apart. Zeigler *et al.* concluded that about 50 per cent of the variance was explained by genetic factors and the remaining half was due to 'nonshared environmental factors', and measurement error.

Stewart *et al.* (1997*b*) examined familial aggregation in first-degree relatives of migraine probands and first-degree relatives of unaffected control subjects. While some excess of migraine was noted in the relatives of migraine probands, the most pronounced increase was in the relatives of those probands with 'disabling migraine'. Thus, severity appears to be associated with familial risk. Stewart *et al.* concluded that familial factors may account for less than half of migraine cases, but that familial factors, as examined, include both genetic and environmental influences.

Evidence for linkage to a specific susceptibility locus was recently published (Nyholt *et al.* 1998). The analysis was based on three large multigenerational families and it shows linkage on the X-chromosome (Xq). As a potential X-linked dominant, the authors conclude that it may explain an observed excess of migraine in relatives of male probands and that it may also be related to the higher observed prevalence of migraine in females. Nyholt *et al.* acknowledge that much genetic heterogeneity is still likely to exist.

Headache and depression

Breslau and colleagues (Breslau and Davis 1993; Breslau *et al.* 1994) conducted a longitudinal study in 1007 young adults to observe the association between migraine and major depression. They reported a significant threefold increased risk of major depression among those with a history of migraine and also a threefold increased risk for migraine among those with prior depression. This finding raised the possibility that the two disorders may have mechanisms in common. Pine *et al.* (1996) reported a similar longitudinal study that followed 776 persons aged 9 to 18 (in 1983) for up to 9 years. They reported that in subjects with no history of 'chronic impairing headache', those with major depression at baseline had a 10-fold risk of developing such headaches during follow-up. Breslau *et al.* (2000) conducted another study to clarify the association between severe headache or migraine and depression. In this longitudinal study, persons with severe headache experienced approximately a threefold increased risk of first-onset depression but those with major depression at baseline experienced no significantly increased risk of severe headache. However, the previously reported 'bi-directional' association between migraine and depression was replicated.

Stroke and migraine

Data from the Physicians Health Study (Buring *et al.* 1995) and from the National Health and Nutrition Examination Survey (Merikangas *et al.* 1997) support a significantly increased risk of stroke in persons with a history of migraine. Because of the relatively high prevalence of migraine among young women the occurrence of stroke in that population is of some concern. In a World Health Organization case–control study sample Chang *et al.* (1999) reported approximately a threefold increased odds ratio for history of migraine in young women with ischaemic stroke as compared to controls. Tzourio *et al.* (1995) reported a similar level of association in a smaller French study and Mitchell *et al.* (1998) reported a slightly more modest level of association in a study conducted in Australia. Tietjen (2000) cautions that the relationship between migraine and stroke may be complicated by the contribution of additional risk factors, such as cigarette smoking and oral contraceptives, and possibly by genetic factors, as well. Thus, additional study may be needed to describe adequately the true relationship between migraine and stroke.

Costs and public health impact

The estimated 23 million persons with migraines in the United States may miss 150 million work days each year with an associated cost of up to $17 billion (Cady 1999; Hu *et al.* 1999). Many more persons suffer with decreased effectiveness at work than actually miss work days; this results in additional hidden loss of productivity due to migraine (Stewart *et al.* 1996*b*; Schwartz *et al.* 1997). New treatments are relatively effective but only a minority of persons consult physicians for their problem or receive the effective medications (Lipton 1998). Early recognition and treatment of migraine may significantly limit societal and personal costs (Cady 1999).

Traumatic brain injury

Clinical overview

A variety of traumas may afflict the nervous system, including brain, spinal cord, and peripheral nerves. Trauma to the brain is of greatest epidemiological importance. Traumas to the brain may be divided into penetrating or closed head injuries. The damage inflicted by penetrating head injuries varies with the velocity of the penetrating object. Low-velocity injuries such as knives produce less injury than high-velocity objects. High-velocity penetrations like bullets produce more widespread injury since the shock wave of the object projects far beyond the immediate track of the missile. Closed head injuries can lead to brain damage through a variety of mechanisms. Bleeding from tearing of blood vessels may lead to epidural or subdural haematomas with resulting mass effects. The brain may be contused due to the impact, particularly in the inferior frontal and temporal areas which overlie bony protuberances. Cerebral oedema may occur through a number of mechanisms, including injury to blood vessels (vasogenic oedema), injury to cell membranes (cytotoxic oedema), or metabolic changes. Hydrocephalus may develop due to blockage of the routes of normal cerebrospinal fluid flow. Finally, closed head injuries may lead to pathological changes in the brain named diffuse axonal injury. The pathological finding in diffuse axonal injury is the axonal retraction ball. These balls of axonal material occur at the site of axon transection or sites of altered axonal flow which are seen with torsional forces.

The symptoms of focal head injuries are determined by the site of injury. More diffuse injuries lead to altered consciousness or cognitive changes. Altered consciousness ranges from a momentary stun to brief unconsciousness, coma, or persistent vegetative state. Cognitive alterations may be profound but are often mild and difficult to recognize. In subtle cases, neuropsychological testing may be needed to demonstrate the abnormality. Such testing may identify focal changes associated with focal brain injury, but more commonly they find difficulties with attention, concentration, short-term memory, and tasks requiring rapid processing of information.

For mild head injuries, the severity of the injury is usually measured by the degree of post-traumatic amnesia. Amnesia lasting less than 5 min is very mild, less than 1 h is mild, 1 to 24 h is moderate, 1 to 7 days is severe, more than 7 days is very severe, and more than 4 weeks is extremely severe. More severe head injuries are usually classified by the Glasgow Coma Scale. Scores of 13 to 15 are minor, 9 to 12 are moderate, 5 to 8 are severe, and 4 or less are very severe.

Incidence and prevalence

The National Institutes of Health consensus statement (1998) estimated the annual incidence of traumatic brain injury to be 100 per 100 000 persons (in the United States). The prevalence of persons living with impairment resulting from traumatic brain injury may be between 2.5 million and 6.5 million in the United States (National Institutes of Health 1998). Traumatic brain injury accounts for approximately 52 000 deaths each year. The majority of traumatic brain injury incidence is due to vehicular accidents (auto, bicycle, motorcycle) or pedestrian versus vehicle accidents. Violence and assault also contribute substantially. Sports injuries may account for about 3 per cent of traumatic brain injury, but because they tend to be less severe than other types may also be significantly under-reported (National Institutes of Health 1998). Earlier estimates of incidence for the United States, 1970 to 1975, are relatively consistent (Caveness 1979). Ingebrigtsen *et al.* (1998) studied hospital-referred head injury in Norway and reported an annual incidence of 229 per 100 000 population, seemingly greater then the United States estimates. Hillier *et al.* (1997) report an even higher incidence in South Australia of 322 per 100 000. Young adult males predominate as cases in both of these studies and it is estimated that potentially 25 per cent of the annual incidence may require continuing care because of impairment resulting from the injury (Hillier *et al.* 1997). A British study (Moles *et al.* 1999) suggests that ethnicity may modify the risk of traumatic brain injury due to assault, with black males experiencing a two- to threefold predominance in admissions. Of course, findings related to ethnicity may be country specific and associated with a variety of other social and political factors.

The potential for lifelong impact on social and occupational functioning, and years of life lost, is great for traumatic brain injury because the peak incidence occurs among people aged 15 to 24. Traumatic brain injury is about twice as common in males as in females. In this age group, vehicle accidents and violence are the principal causes of traumatic brain injury. Two other age-incidence peaks occur, one among the elderly (75 years and older) and the other among the very young. In these age groups, falls predominate as the immediate cause. Among the very young, a relatively substantial proportion of traumatic brain injury is attributed to assault (National Institutes of Health 1998).

Risk factors

Vehicle accidents

As mentioned above vehicle accidents may account for half of the traumatic brain injury observed in the United States (National Institutes of Health 1998). There are approximately 3 million motor vehicle accidents each year which result in death or severe injury (in the United States) (Murphy *et al.* 2000). For these accidents, well-known risk factors appear to prevail. Consistent with the risk of traumatic brain injury, persons aged 15 to 24 predominate. Alcohol use is an important determinant of motor vehicle accidents and therefore also of traumatic brain injury (National Institutes of Health 1998). Young children typically tend to suffer low-energy type head injury (Berney *et al.* 1994) in household accidents, leading to a more favourable outcome. However, motor vehicle accidents generally result in high-energy accidents and greater morbidity and mortality. Car safety seats for younger children may afford some degree of protection.

Helmets for bicyclists may afford some degree of protection against traumatic brain injury (Rivara *et al.* 1997; Linn *et al.* 1998). A study conducted in British Columbia, Canada (Linn *et al.* 1998), found a fourfold increase in risk of concussion among non-helmet users and a twofold increase in risk of hospital admission. A study in New York found a similar proportion of head injuries among helmeted and non-helmeted child bicyclists (Shafi *et al.* 1998). However, children with helmets were more likely to experience only concussion compared to an excess of skull fractures among non-helmeted children. Rivara *et al.* (1997) studied over 3000 bicycle injuries; roughly half of the bicyclists were wearing helmets at the time of the accident. Overall, about 22 per cent of the cases involved a head injury. Comparing 'serious' injury (injury severity score greater than 8) to less than serious injury, Rivara *et al.* found that younger age and speed increased the risk of a serious injury somewhat, but a fourfold increase in risk was seen if a motor vehicle was involved in the crash. However, risk of 'serious' injury, as defined, was not associated with helmet use. Subjects who experienced neck injury were substantially more likely to die but helmet use did not decrease the risk of neck injury. While this study sounds somewhat negative for helmet use, this may not be the correct interpretation. Collisions involving motor vehicles and bicycles are likely to result in very serious injuries; helmets alone obviously cannot protect against those injuries. In the situation where a bicyclist loses control and crashes, some degree of protection against concussion is likely to be afforded. Among teenagers helmet use may be lower, even when required by law (Puder *et al.* 1999). Thompson and Patterson (1998) summarized studies of bicycle helmets, recommending that they be worn by all competitive and non-competitive riders: 'Helmet use reduces the risk of head injury by 85 per cent, brain injury by 88 per cent and severe brain injury by at least 75 per cent.'

Falls

Among the elderly, falls are one of the more important causes of traumatic brain injury (National Institutes of Health 1998; Luukinen *et al.* 1999). Other neurological conditions such as movement disorders and/or dementia, may make a person more likely to experience falling. Weakness, unsteadiness, certain medications, and other medical conditions may also increase the likelihood of falling. Vision deficits are common in the elderly, due to loss of acuity, glaucoma, macular degeneration, and other causes; poor vision can contribute to falling. Mechanically speaking, elders may be more likely to fall and be injured when surfaces are uneven or slippery, or when they must use a cane or walker. Thus, elders require additional care and help to avoid the serious injury that may result from falls.

The very young are also at increased risk of traumatic brain injury due to falls (National Institutes of Health 1998). They, like the very old, may tend to be unsteady or to use mechanical devices such as walkers or strollers. Unlike their older counterparts, however, 3-year-olds are seldom content to remain still for extended periods: climbing from a shopping cart to visit a toy, exploring a new flight of stairs, or escaping from a crib before nap time is over.

Violence

As much as 20 per cent of traumatic brain injury may be the result of violence, roughly half being due to firearms (National Institutes of Health 1998). The age group at highest risk is 15 to 24 years. While males appear to be more likely to sustain an injury due to violence, women may be more likely to die as a result (Gilthorpe *et al.* 1999). Generally, community violence indicates an increased risk that traumatic brain injury will be involved. Durkin *et al.* (1996) describe the incidence of paediatric, severe non-fatal assault in North Manhattan (New York City) as approximately 60 per 100 000 (about 30 per 100 000 due to firearms). Among adolescents, firearms were the most common method of serious assault and carried more than a 10-fold increased fatality risk. A similar study of general trauma was conducted in Los Angeles County (Demetriades *et al.* 1998). In that study homicides accounted for 45 per cent of traumatic deaths compared to 32 per cent resulting from traffic accidents. The incidence of firearm-related injury or death was 42 per 100 000. The homicide rate varied dramatically by age and ethnic group. Overall it was about 14 per 100 000, but rose to 73 per 100 000 in African-American males and further to 164.2 per 100 000 among 15- to 34-year-old African-American males. While this study speaks to trauma and homicide generally, Lam and MacKersie (1999) states that among children admitted to hospitals 75 per cent are admitted because of trauma and as many as 70 per cent of paediatric trauma deaths are due to head injury. Also, firearms may be involved in a substantial proportion of traumatic brain injury, hence the relevance of these statistics.

Abuse and domestic violence are important causes of traumatic brain injury among women and among children (Jenny *et al.* 1999; Monahan and O'Leary 1999). Monahan and O'Leary estimate that about 35 per cent of the 2 to 3 million women battered each year by their domestic partner sustain traumatic brain injury as a result. The sequelae of these injuries may be difficult to document because they may include behavioural and cognitive deficits as well as the acute physical problems. Abusive head trauma may also be an under-recognized problem among very young children (Jenny *et al.* 1999). So-called 'shaken baby syndrome' and other forms of physical abuse may result in traumatic brain injury as well as in spinal cord injury (1998).

Sports injuries account for a relatively small proportion of serious traumatic brain injury (National Institutes of Health 1998). However, many mild head injuries may go unreported and it is unclear what the long-term risk of such injuries may be. Ferguson *et al.* (1999) suggest that study of mild head injury resulting in postconcussive syndrome may be additionally difficult because of a form of recall bias among the cases based on their expectations of recovery.

Implications for public health

While the actual case fatality rate for traumatic brain injury may be high, that in itself does not describe the major cost. The National Institutes of Health Consensus Statement (1998) estimates that nearly $10 billion are spent annually in the United States for acute and rehabilitative care for new cases. Furthermore, they estimate that lifetime care costs may range from $600 000 to nearly $2 million per person. Personal costs experienced by victims of traumatic brain injury cannot be estimated realistically; lost opportunities for education and employment, changed or foregone personal relationships, and psychological distress may all result from traumatic brain injury (Colantonio *et al.* 1998). Also, as Annegers *et al.* (1998) point out, the risk of seizures following traumatic brain injury is increased up to 17-fold in patients with severe injuries.

The causes of traumatic brain injury are well specified and observable. The challenge remains, however: how can the occurrence of motor vehicle accidents and violence be reduced, thereby dramatically reducing the occurrence of traumatic brain injury?

Back pain

Clinical overview

The many causes of low back pain can be divided according to the anatomical structures involved. Nerve roots may be impinged leading to sciatica. The lumbar plexus or more peripheral nerves may be diseased. The subarachnoid space or meningeal structures may be involved with infection or tumour. Vertebral bodies may be involved with tumours, infections, or fractures. Joints may be affected by a number of diseases, including osteoarthritis, ankylosing spondylitis, or inflammatory diseases. Muscles may be injured or affected by diseases such as myositis. These anatomically based diseases often garner the bulk of medical attention, perhaps because they are more readily defined on testing or because they have treatments which are more frequently successful. However, they constitute a very small portion of back pain cases. By far, the most common cause of low back pain is idiopathic.

The medical history is useful in differentiating some of the types of low back pain. Pain that begins in the low back and radiates in the distribution of a neurological structure is likely due to impingement on that structure. For example, pain radiating down the leg in the distribution of the L5 nerve root is often due to a disk impinging on the nerve root. Back pain following trauma suggests bony disease. Fever or weight loss suggest infectious or neoplastic causes. The physical examination concentrates on focal points of pain, and the examination of relevant neurological pathways.

Tests extend the physical examination. Plain spine radiographs are used to evaluate bone diseases such as trauma, neoplasm, or infection. Better definition may be seen with CT scanning. Scanning with MRI provides the best definition of neurological structures. All of these techniques have a high false-positive rate for identifying causes of low back pain. Electromyography and nerve conduction velocities are used to determine whether damage has occurred to parts of the peripheral nervous system.

Prevalence

Low back pain is one of the most common diseases encountered in general practice, with up to 2 per cent of the population seeking medical care for it each year (Dillane *et al.* 1966). The lifetime prevalence of back pain is very high, ranging from 49 to 70 per cent (Shelerud 1998; Andersson 1999). Prevalence rates vary depending on the manner in which the question is framed. Asking for any history of back pain results in higher rates than asking about pain of specific duration, location, or severity. Only 14 per cent of patients report an episode of back pain lasting at least 2 weeks (Deyo and Twui-Wu 1987).

The point prevalence of low back pain ranges from 12 to 30 per cent (Shelerud 1998; Andersson 1999). In a review of a wide range of neurological disorders, Kurtzke found an annual point prevalence for low back pain of approximately 0.5 per cent with lumbosacral herniated disk disease representing another 0.3 per cent (Kurtzke 1982). The annual incidence of low back pain was approximately 1.5 per cent with lumbosacral herniated disk disease representing another 1.5 per cent (Kurtzke 1982). Surveys more directed towards back pain have higher prevalence rates. Elliott *et al.* (1999), using a community mail survey, found the point prevalence of back pain to be 6 per cent, while Reigo *et al.* (1999) noted an 11 per cent point prevalence for back pain in a population based study. Croft *et al.* (1999) found a 1-year prevalence rate of 34 per cent in men and 37 per cent in women in a prospective study of a population without prior back pain. Again, the rates of back pain vary depending on the duration, location, and severity of the pain.

Many studies of the prevalence of low back pain concentrate on the workforce rather than the general population because of the economic impact of back pain on industry. In a general population sample, Picavet *et al.* (1999) found that the 12-month period prevalence of low back problems for working and non-working men was 44.4 per cent and 45.8 per cent respectively, and for women was 48.2 per cent and 55.0 per cent respectively. Frymoyer *et al.* (1983) reported that about 2 per cent of employees seek medical care each year for low back pain. Behrens *et al.* (1994) noted that back pain related to the work environment (such as repetitive activities, and so on) occurred in 4.5 per cent and that back pain due to a work-related injury occurred in 2.5 per cent of workers. Guo *et al.* (1999) found that 4.6 per cent of workers had back pain for at least 1 week within the past year. Back pain accounts for 20 per cent of compensatable injuries (Klein *et al.* 1984).

Risk factors

There are several demographic and anthropomorphic features associated with low back pain. Those who are 35 to 55 years of age are most commonly affected (Shelerud 1998) but most of these first developed pain in earlier life. In the general population, age has only a modest effect on the 1-year prevalence of back pain, with rates varying from 7.6 to 9.4 per cent across various age ranges in adults (Andersson 1999). In the workforce, however, back pain increases with age (Rossignol *et al.* 1988; van Doorn 1995). Rossignol *et al.* (1988) found that the odds for developing back pain doubled with an increase in age of 23 years. Older workers have longer duration of back pain and more time off from work compared to younger workers (Shelerud 1998). Back pain in the elderly has received relatively less attention, making estimates of prevalence in this age group difficult (Bressler *et al.* 1999). Children also suffer back pain with a lifetime prevalence of 10 per cent in 10-year-olds, 53 per cent in 13-year-olds, and 71 per cent in 15-year-olds (Duggleby and Kumar 1997). In the general population, men and women are equally susceptible to back pain (Shelerud 1998). In the workforce, men predominate, perhaps because more men are in the workforce. There have not been strong associations found between body build, weight, or mild leg length inequality and the development of low back pain (Deyo and Bass 1987; Shelerud 1998). However, some studies suggest that tallness may increase the risk (Shelerud 1998). Those in the highest 20 per cent of body mass index may also be at risk, especially in women (Shelerud 1998; Croft *et al.* 1999). Physical fitness and high levels of physical activity are generally believed to be protective (Cady *et al.* 1979; Shelerud 1998). Lumbar mobility has historically been believed to be protective for back pain, but recent studies have suggested that this is not the case (Shelerud 1998). The association of posture to back pain is also uncertain (Shelerud 1998). An increase in strength was associated with less back pain in some studies, but not in others (Shelerud 1998). Back pain has long been attributed to changes seen on spine radiographs as well as MRI scans. These include degenerative changes, spondylolisthesis, and lumbar stenosis. However, the ability of these changes to predict the development of back pain is poor, in large part because of the high prevalence of these conditions in the asymptomatic population (Shelerud 1998). A family history of back pain carries a relative risk of 2.1 (Rozenberg *et al.* 1998).

Smoking increases the risk of developing low back pain (Deyo and Bass 1987; Frymoyer 1988), but this increase is rather modest (Leboeuf-Yde 1999). Odds ratios in large studies have ranged from insignificant to 3.12, with the majority of studies showing odds ratios of less than 2 (Leboeuf-Yde 1999). Some studies have shown a dose effect (Leboeuf-Yde 1999). Eriksen *et al.* (1999) found that work environment was associated with back pain in smokers but not in non-smokers. It is uncertain whether the association between smoking and back pain reflects a causal relationship or whether smoking serves as a marker for another underlying cause. Previous pregnancy is a risk factor for back pain (Shelerud 1998). Patients with a prior episode of low back pain are at greatly increased risk of recurrence, with the lifetime recurrence reaching as high as 85 per cent (Valkenburg and Haanen 1982).

Patients who are chronically ill with back pain often have emotional factors that interplay with it. Psychological factors such as anxiety, depression, alcoholism, somatization, stress, type A personality, job dissatisfaction, negative body image, a weak ego, and poor drive have been associated with back pain (Anderson 1981; Rozenberg *et al.* 1998; Shelerud 1998). However, it is unknown whether these emotional factors precede the onset of illness or whether they develop as part of the response to the pain (Anderson 1981; Frymoyer *et al.* 1983; Bigos *et al.* 1991). The data regarding psychological factors associated with the work environment and personality profiles such as the Minnesota Multiphasic Personality Inventory are also conflicting (Shelerud 1998). A recent prospective study of transit workers found that psychosocial job factors and physical workload increased the risk of back pain, suggesting that some of the psychosocial factors are contributors to, rather than results of, the condition. The odds ratios were increased for psychological job demands (1.5), job dissatisfaction (1.56), job problems (1.52), and physical labour (3.04) (Krause *et al.* 1998).

Factors associated with employment are often linked with back pain (Devereux *et al.* 1999; Hoogendoorn *et al.* 1999). About two-thirds of back pain cases are related to employment, with one-third occurring in the setting of lifting/twisting and one-third related to falls (Brown 1975). Lifting heavy objects, lifting with twisting movements (Kelsey 1975), and frequent lifting seem to increase injury rates (Kelsey *et al.* 1979). The relative risk of repeated improper lifting may be as high as 7.2 (Rozenberg *et al.* 1998). Driving and jobs that require prolonged sitting also increase the risk of back pain (Kelsey 1975).

Physically demanding work increased the risk of back pain in a number of studies (Shelerud 1998) These studies are difficult to interpret, however, because of the difficulty in accurately quantifying the physical demands of various jobs.

Static work postures such as prolonged sitting, standing, or bending increase the risk of developing back pain (Shelerud 1998). The weight of objects requiring lifting, the frequency of lifting, object bulk, the position from which the object must be lifted, bending, and twisting all increase the risk of occupational back pain (Shelerud 1998).

Vibration, especially in the seated position, seems to increase the risk of back pain (Shelerud 1998). However, most of these jobs also involve prolonged sitting during the operation of motor vehicles.

Public health importance

Back pain is one of the most frequently encountered disorders. The cause of the pain in most cases remains unknown. Though many factors have been associated with back pain, most study designs have been inadequate in determining whether they are a cause or result of the chronic pain. Population-based prospective studies will be needed to determine whether premorbid conditions predict future back pain. The occurrence of back pain, as indicated by the prevalence discussed above, makes it a significant public health concern as well as an important cause of disability.

Epilepsy

Clinical overview

The International League Against Epilepsy classification system for epilepsy (Table 2) (International League Against Epilepsy 1997) is currently the most prominent. Seizures may be classified according to the characteristics of the individual seizure. Location-related seizures (formerly named partial or local seizures) begin in a part of one cerebral hemisphere. The areas of brain initially involved determine the symptoms of location-related seizures. Seizures involving the motor cortex lead to jerking (clonic) movements or stiffening (tonic) movements. Head turning, eye turning, speech arrest, or unusual arm posturing may occur with frontal-lobe seizures. Seizures originating in the parietal region are associated with sensory symptoms including numbness or tingling. Occipital lobe seizures may lead to visual loss, visual hallucinations, or seeing light flashes or colours. Temporal lobe seizures may cause auditory or olfactory hallucinations. The olfactory hallucinations are often unpleasant smells. Unusual abdominal

Table 2 The International League Against Epilepsy classification of epileptic seizures

I	Partial (focal, local) seizures	
	A	Simple partial seizures
	B	Complex partial seizure (with impairment of consciousness)
	C	With impairment of consciousness at onset
	D	Partial seizures evolving to secondarily generalized seizures
II	Generalized seizures	
	A	Absence seizures
	B	Myoclonic seizures
	C	Clonic seizures
	D	Tonic seizures
	E	Tonic–clonic seizures
	F	Atonic seizures
III	Unclassified epileptic seizures	

sensations such as risings or tightness may be noted. Repetitive movements or activities may occasionally be seen with temporal lobe seizures. *Déjà vu* and *jamais vu* may occur. Location-related seizures may (simple partial) or may not (complex partial seizures) be associated with altered consciousness. They may secondarily generalize after a focal onset.

Generalized seizures are those that begin in widespread areas of the brain. The most common type of generalized seizure is noted for muscle stiffening followed by jerking (tonic–clonic). Generalized seizures were formerly called *grand mal* seizures. Absence seizures (formerly *petit mal*) consist of brief episodes of staring and lack of responsiveness. Myoclonic seizures involve brief jerks of muscles rather than repetitive clonic movements. Tonic seizures involve a generalized muscle stiffening. Atonic seizures involve sudden loss of muscle tone.

In addition to the individual types of seizures already noted, there are a number of epileptic syndromes recognized by the International League Against Epilepsy classification. These are distinguished by their age of onset, clinical features, electroencephalographic patterns, and clinical course.

Incidence and prevalence

Aspects of epilepsy epidemiology have been reviewed by a number of contemporary authors, among them: Grunewald and Panayiotopoulos (1993), Senanayake and Roman (1993), Annegers (1994), Gordon (1994), Berg *et al.* (1996), de Bittencourt *et al.* (1996), Duchowny and Harvey (1996), Anderson *et al.* (1997, 1999), Ottman (1997), and Kramer (1999). Below we present several studies that focus on the incidence and prevalence of epilepsy.

Hauser *et al.* (1996) reported the age-adjusted incidence of epilepsy as 44 per 100 000 person-years, based on data from the Rochester Epidemiology Project spanning approximately a 50-year period up to 1980. Reassessment in that same population for 1980 to 1984 yielded a consistent though slightly higher estimate of epilepsy incidence (Zarrelli *et al.* 1999). Importantly, Hauser *et al.* noted that the incidence and prevalence of epilepsy and unprovoked seizures decreased with calendar time among children and increased among the elderly. The prevalence of active epilepsy among those aged 75 or older was reported as 1.5 per cent (as of January 1980). About 1 per cent of persons under age 20 experienced epilepsy; Hauser *et al.* (1996) noted that their prognosis was generally favourable with most achieving control within 2 years. Kramer *et al.* (1998) reported the distribution of different seizure types, among 440 children with two or more unprovoked seizures, attending the paediatric neurology clinic in Tel Aviv. Partial seizures accounted for 52 per cent and primary generalized seizures 33 per cent among children.

Olafsson and Hauser (1999) conducted a survey in rural Iceland determining the prevalence of recurrent unprovoked seizures. Records of primary care physicians and neurologists were used for case identification. The crude age-adjusted prevalence was observed to be 4.8 per 1000 population. Similarly, Beilmann *et al.* (1999) reported on epilepsy in Estonia. The prevalence of 'active epilepsy', as of December 1997, among persons aged 1 month to 19 years was 3.6 per 1000. Beilmann *et al.* concluded that the prevalence of childhood epilepsy in Estonia was similar to that found in other developed countries. However, Beilmann *et al.* included as 'active epilepsy' all those with 'at least one seizure during the last 5 years, regardless of treatment'. Case definition causes concern about the comparability of prevalence proportions obtained. Another example of case definition was presented by Wallace *et al.* (1998), who counted only treated epilepsy for the incidence and prevalence numerators. Treated epilepsy implied specifically that identified cases must be taking antiepileptic medication. Despite this restriction, Wallace *et al.* reported a 1995 prevalence of 5.15 per 1000 persons, rather consistent with other overall estimates. Prevalence increased with age from 3.6 per 1000 in 5- to 9-year-olds to 7.54 per 1000 among those aged 80 to 84. These estimates are considerably higher than those reported by Hauser *et al.* (1996).

Another method of case ascertainment was used by Nicoletti *et al.* (1998, 1999), to study epilepsy and other neurological conditions in Bolivia. For this study a 'door-to-door survey' was conducted; 10 000 persons were screened, approximately 1000 were referred to neurologists, and of those, 112 were determined to have active epilepsy, leading to a prevalence estimate of 11.1 per 1000. In contrast to studies reported above (Hauser *et al.* 1996; Wallace *et al.* 1998), the highest prevalence occurred in the age group 15 to 24 (20.4 per 1000). Regardless of the shift in peak occurrence the prevalence appears dramatically higher than in other studies. Part of the difference may be due to methods; population screening versus clinic-based surveillance. However, the difference between more and less 'developed' countries may also contribute to the disparity.

Mortality

Persons with epilepsy may experience two to three times the risk of death compared to their unaffected counterparts (Cockerell 1996). Sperling *et al.* (1999) examined the relationship between recurrent seizure and risk of death; they compared persons whose seizures had been eliminated by surgery to those with recurrent seizures. The standardized mortality ratio for persons with recurrent seizure was approximately fourfold higher than expected. A longitudinal study conducted in The Netherlands (Shackleton *et al.* 1999) enrolled newly diagnosed epilepsy patients ($n = 1355$) who were followed for a mean of 28 years. Overall, they observed a threefold excess in all cause mortality, and a sevenfold increase among those under age 20. A substantial part of the increased mortality was said to be due to the epilepsy itself. Loiseau *et al.* (1999) studied short-term mortality after first afebrile, provoked, or unprovoked seizure ($n = 804$). After 1 year of follow-up no deaths had occurred among patients with idiopathic seizures. Increased standardized mortality ratios were observed for those with provoked seizures or seizures related to other central nervous system disorders.

Sudden unexplained death in persons with epilepsy (**SUDEP**) (Annegers and Coan 1999) is a substantial risk in younger-aged persons as compared to individuals without epilepsy. Much of the excess risk may be associated with seizure severity, with greater severity leading to greater risk of death (Annegers and Coan 1999). Careful definition of SUDEP is necessary as is attention to methodological detail; early findings may have been the result of selection bias and similar problems (Ficker *et al.* 1998). In a population-based study in Rochester, Minnesota, all persons diagnosed with epilepsy between 1935 and 1994 were followed to determine cause of death. SUDEP rates were compared to the rate of sudden unexplained death in the general population for ages 20 to 40. Although the SUDEP death rate exceeded the expected by 23.7 times, it was still a rare cause of death accounting for only 1.7 per cent of the deaths in the epilepsy cohort. Nilsson *et al.* (1999) investigated SUDEP in Sweden, focusing on risk factors. They found that patients with 50 seizures per year were about 10 times more likely to succumb to SUDEP than patients with two or fewer seizures. Risk of SUDEP was also substantially increased with the number of concomitant antiepileptic drugs, and among those who had frequent medication changes. Compared to the general population the cohort of epilepsy patients experienced an all-cause mortality approximately 3.6 times greater than the general population, with the majority of the excess mortality due to malignant neoplasms; diseases of the circulatory, respiratory, and digestive systems; injury; and poisoning (Nilsson *et al.* 1997). McGugan (1999) provides a current review of SUDEP and notes that young male epileptics with generalized seizures are at greatest risk. The mechanism of death in cases is of course, 'unexplained'; however, many persons have ischaemic damage to the heart even though coronary arteries appear normal (McGugan 1999).

Infectious causes of epilepsy

In developing countries infections are a much more important cause of epilepsy than in the United States and Europe (Senanayake and Roman 1993); overall prevalence of epilepsy may approach 57 per 1000 population. Parasitic, bacterial, and viral infections contribute substantially to this, but hereditary factors, perinatal damage, head trauma, and toxic exposures also play important aetiological roles. From a public health view, the excess risk attributable to many of these exposures is potentially preventable (Senanayake and Roman 1993).

An example of an important infectious risk factor is *Taenia solium* cysticercosis (from pork tapeworm) which can lead to neurocysticercosis. Palacio *et al.* (1998) examined a series of 643 epilepsy patients in Columbia, of whom 376 had serological tests for cysticercus. The prevalence of antibody was 17.5 per cent among late-onset epilepsy patients. Among patients with no CT scan evidence of neurocysticercosis, only 2.7 per cent had antibody. However, a similar study conducted in Honduras (Sanchez *et al.* 1999) raises questions as to the validity of the serology antibody tests in predicting neurocysticercosis. Sanchez *et al.* conclude CT scan findings of neurocycticercosis are necessary for diagnosis. Even though the population is frequently exposed to *T. solium*, as indicated by serology, neurocysticercosis is not always the result. A different view is presented by Bern *et al.* (1999). They combined data from 12 population-based community studies in Peru and showed a seroprevalence of 6 to 24 per cent. The high seroprevalence was presented as evidence for the prevalence of neurocysticercosis. Bern *et al.* estimated a burden of 23 000 to 39 000 symptomatic neurocysticercosis cases in Peru. Extrapolating from these data, Bern *et al.* concluded that cysticercosis is a formidable cause of neurological disease in Latin America. Whether seropositivity is synonymous with neurocysticercosis appears controversial. The common occurrence of the *T. solium* cyst may account for an important fraction of epilepsy in Latin American countries.

Genetics

The rapid progress in mapping the human genome has led to many important findings and will likely continue to do so. The potential contribution of genes to the aetiology of epilepsy has been recently reviewed or commented on by a number of authors, including Berkovic (1997), Ottman (1997), Leppert and Singh (1999), Noebels (1999), Steinlein (1999), and Weissbecker *et al.* (1999).

The gene story in epilepsy is far from complete or clear at this time. There appears to be substantial genetic heterogeneity, and not all findings of association or linkage have been confirmed. There is some degree of consensus, however, that idiopathic generalized epilepsies are likely to have a genetic aetiology (Steinlein 1999). Delgado Escucta *et al.* (1999) points out that approximately half of the prevalent epilepsies in the United States are generalized epilepsies and that, of those cases, juvenile myoclonus epilepsy and childhood absence epilepsy may account for 15 to 45 per cent. Potential gene sites for these two types of epilepsy have been identified on chromosomes 1p, 3p, 6p, 8q, and 15q. Phillips *et al.* (1998) report similar genetic heterogeneity for autosomal dominant frontal-lobe epilepsy with possible sites on 15q and 20q. Plaster *et al.* (1999) report identification of a locus for familial adult myoclonic epilepsy, another idiopathic generalized epilepsy, on chromosome 8q. Xiong *et al.* (1999) conducted a linkage study in two large French-Canadian families with familial partial epilepsy syndrome with variable foci, identifying a locus on 22q. However, they acknowledge that an Australian family with similar phenotype showed no linkage to chromosome 22—again indicating genetic heterogeneity. Lopes-Cendes *et al.* (2000) conducted a genome-wide search for linkage to generalized epilepsy with febrile seizures, and located a linked marker on 2q. However, recognizing that there are multiple phenotypes within the kindred, they also suggest that genetic or environmental factors may modify the effect of the 2q to generalized epilepsy with febrile seizures gene.

Because of the observed phenotypic and genetic heterogeneity, environmental factors may play a role in the expression of disease. Larger epidemiological studies may provide a mechanism for observing that interaction (Ottman and Susser 1992; Ottman *et al.* 1996). Furthermore, genetic epidemiology has been developing rapidly over the past decade, undoubtedly helping to address and clarify the complexities of gene–gene and gene–environment interactions.

Costs and public health burden

The costs of epilepsy are often categorized as direct and indirect (Begley *et al.* 1999, 2000; Beghi *et al.* 2000). The direct costs refer to those specifically involved with epilepsy treatment; the indirect costs include lost work days and unrealized earnings. Begley *et al.* (2000) estimate that the 181 000 new cases of epilepsy in the United States in 1995 will result in a lifetime cost of $11.1 billion. The 2.3 million prevalent cases, in 1995, resulted in an annual cost of $12.5 billion. Begley *et al.* (1999, 2000) estimate that indirect costs may account for 85 per cent of the total and that the largest share of direct costs is attributable to patients with intractable epilepsy. Annegers *et al.* (1999) caution that cost figures for the United States and Europe may derive from different methodologies, thus methods may influence the degree of comparability. With regard to the quality of life reported by persons with epilepsy, Leidy *et al.* (1999) report that seizure frequency is inversely associated with health-related quality of life. Seizure-free individuals report a quality of life similar to the general population; however, more seizures lead to a poorer quality of life, regardless of additional comorbidity and irrespective of gender. Effective seizure control appears to be important in reducing costs as well as increasing patient quality of life.

Dementia

Clinical overview

Dementia presents with a slowly progressive loss of cognitive function. This often begins with trivial forgetfulness, but progresses to more serious cognitive impairment. Behavioural changes may be prominent, including agitation, wandering, personality change, or depression. In late stages, patients may be completely dependent on others. Various definitions of dementia have been used in past research studies, but the *Diagnostic and Statistical Manual of Mental Disorders*, edition IV (**DSM-IV**) is the most commonly used (American Psychiatric Association Task Force 1994). The DSM-IV criteria for dementia require memory impairment and one or more additional cognitive disturbance. These include aphasia (language disturbance), apraxia (impaired ability to carry out motor activities despite intact motor function), agnosia (failure to recognize or identify objects despite intact sensory function), and disturbances in executive functioning (i.e. planning, organizing, sequencing, abstracting). The cognitive deficits must be severe enough to cause significant impairment in social or occupational functioning and represent a significant decline from a previous level of functioning. Dementia must be differentiated from delirium. The causes of dementia are listed in Table 3.

Although Alzheimer's disease is the most common form of dementia, many other disorders must be considered, including drug-induced conditions, alcoholism, stroke, Parkinson's disease, Huntington's disease, subdural haematoma, brain tumours, hydrocephalus, vitamin B_{12} deficiency, hypothyroidism, neurosyphilis, and HIV infection. Criteria for the diagnosis of Alzheimer's disease have been proposed (McKhann *et al.* 1984; American Psychiatric Association Task Force 1994).

Vascular dementia is difficult to differentiate from Alzheimer's disease because of the common association of stroke and Alzheimer's disease in the elderly. The more sophisticated the search for stroke, the more likely strokes will be found. The clinical identification of stroke is surpassed by CT, which is surpassed by MRI. However, the false-positive identification of stroke also increases. Many different criteria have been developed to diagnose vascular dementia (Chui *et al.* 1992; Roman *et al.* 1993; American Psychiatric Association Task Force 1994). Much of the pioneering work in the definition and recognition of vascular dementia can be attributed to Hachinski and colleagues (Hachinski 1983, 1990, 1991, 1994; Wade and Hachinski 1986; Larson *et al.* 1989; Pantoni and Inzitari 1993; Rockwood *et al.* 1999; Rockwood *et al.* 2000).

Recently two additional types of dementia, Lewy body disease (McKeith *et al.* 1992) and frontotemporal dementia (Anonymous 1994), have been separated from Alzheimer's disease based on their clinical presentations and pathology. Lewy body disease presents with cognitive losses. In addition fluctuating cognitive performance, visual hallucinations, and parkinsonism are suggestive of this disease. Memory impairment may not necessarily be prominent in the early stages. Deficits in attention, frontal subcortical skills, and visuospatial ability predominate.

In frontotemporal dementia, changes in behaviour dominate the early course of the disease. These include loss of personal awareness, loss of social graces, disinhibition, overactivity, restlessness, impulsivity, distractibility, hyperorality, withdrawal from social contact, apathy or inertia, and stereotyped or perseverative behaviours. Speech-output changes occur, including progressive reduction of speech, stereotypy of speech, perseveration, and echolalia. Physical signs include early or prominent primitive or 'frontal' reflexes, early incontinence, late akinesia, rigidity, and tremor. Deficits in social comportment, behaviour, judgement, or language are out of proportion to the memory deficit. The memory loss is variable and often appears to be due to lack of concern or effort. Frontal-lobe impairments are notable, including those in abstraction, planning, and self-regulation of behaviour. There are several pathologies that may lead to frontotemporal dementia, including some with dominantly inherited mutations related to the protein tau.

Dementia and Alzheimer's disease

Prevalence and incidence

Evans *et al.* (1989) reported the results of a community study in East Boston. The prevalence estimates for dementia and Alzheimer's disease were based on a complex community-sampling scheme (Beckett and Evans 1994). The results of this study remain controversial but are also widely cited to place an upper bound on potential prevalence of dementia in communities in the United States. Prevalence rose from 3 per cent among those aged 65 to 74 years to 47 per cent in those over 85. Over 80 per cent of the observed dementia cases were classified as Alzheimer's disease. Evans *et al.* later applied the observed rates to census data, projecting that 10.3 million people would have Alzheimer's disease in the year 2050. Recently, a meta-analysis of prevalence studies, worldwide, was conducted (Fratiglioni *et al.* 1999); it was noted that prevalence and incidence rates were geographically consistent except for variation due to methodological differences. Prevalence rose from 0.3 to 1.0 per cent in those aged 60 to 64, to between 43 and 68 per cent in persons aged 95 or older. As a summary figure, prevalence is often reported as 6 to 10 per cent among persons aged 65 or older in North America

Table 3 Causes of dementia

Idiopathic
- Alzheimer's disease
- Frontal–temporal dementia

Focal CNS pathology
- Multi-infarct dementia
- Binswanger's disease
- Multiple sclerosis
- Mass lesions
    - Tumours, multiple sites
    - Tumours, single site
    - Gliomatosis cerebri
    - Abscess
    - Subdural malformation
    - Hydrocephalus

Infections
- AIDS (HIV)
- Chronic meningitis
- Encephalitis
- Progressive multifocal leukoencephalopathy
- Subacute sclerosing panencephalitis
- Syphilis
- Lyme disease
- Prion disease (kuru, Creutzfeldt–Jakob)

Toxins
- Drugs
- Alcohol
- Heavy metals
- Industrial toxins
- Domoic acid

Inherited disease
- Huntington's disease
- Gerstmann–Straussler syndrome
- Porphyria
- Propionic aciduria
- Adult onset lysosomal storage diseases
    - Hexosaminidase
    - Arylsulphatase (MLD)
    - Kuf disease
    - Adrenoleucodystrophy
    - Others
- Myotonic muscular dystrophy
- Down syndrome
- Hereditary ataxias
- Hereditary spastic paraplegias
- Cerebrotendinous xanthomatosis

Systemic disease
- Cardiac
- Pulmonary
- Renal
    - Renal failure
    - Dialysis dementia
- Hepatic
    - Hepatic failure
    - Hepatocerebral degeneration
    - Wilson's disease
- Endocrine
    - Hyper-/hypothyroid
    - Hyper-/hypoparathyroid
    - Hyper-/hypoadrenalism
    - SIADH
- Rheumatological
    - Vasculitis (including SLE)
    - Giant cell arteritis
    - Sarcoid
    - Amyloid
- Neoplastic
    - Metastasis
    - Carcinomatous meningitis
    - Paraneoplastic (limbic encephalitis)

Associated movement disorder
- Huntington's disease
- Parkinsonian diseases
    - Parkinson's disease
    - Progressive supranuclear palsy
    - Postencephalitic dementia
    - Post-traumatic (dementia pugilistica)
    - Diffuse Lewy body disease
- Myoclonus
    - Creutzfeldt–Jakob disease
    - Alzheimer's disease
    - Metabolic derangement
- Other movement disorder
    - Hereditary ataxias
    - Hereditary spastic paraplegia
    - Kuru
    - Wilson's disease
    - Seizures
    - Kuf disease

Deficiency
- Vitamin B_{12} deficiency
- Thiamine
- Niacin (pellagra)

CNS, central nervous system; SIADH, syndrome of inappropriate secretion of antidiuretic hormone; SLE, systemic lupus erythematosus.

(Hendrie 1998). Brookmeyer *et al.* (1998) have estimated that in 1997 there were approximately 2.32 million persons with Alzheimer's disease in the United States; if disease onset could be delayed 2 years there would be 2 million fewer cases in the future.

The substantial burden of dementia prevalence is a function of disease incidence and subsequent survival. Jorm and Jolley (1998) gathered data from 23 studies and produced a meta analysis of dementia incidence. Incidence was estimated for Europe, the United

States, and East Asia; dementia, Alzheimer's disease, and vascular dementia rates were computed. Incidence rates for the United States and Europe were quite similar: 'moderate' dementia incidence rose from 3.6 per 1000 person-years (ages 65 to 69) to 37.7 per 1000 person-years (ages 85 to 89) in Europe, and from 2.4 to 27.5 per 1000 person-years for the same age groups in the United States. The incidence of 'mild' Alzheimer's disease was also computed, and ranged from 2.5 per 1000 person-years (ages 65 to 69) to 46.1 per 1000 person-years (ages 85 to 89), for Europe, compared with 6.1 to 74.5 for the United States, and, 0.7 to 39.7 for East Asia.

Rocca *et al.* (1998) reanalysed dementia and Alzheimer's disease incidence data for 1975 through 1984, based on charted data from the Rochester Epidemiology Project at Mayo Clinic. The results showed dementia incidence overall as 2.2 per 1000 person-years in those aged 65 to 69, rising to 40.8 per 1000 person-years in those aged 90 or more. Similarly for Alzheimer's disease, rates rose from 1.2 to 33.9 per 1000 person-years. Rocca *et al.* noted that annual incidence appeared to stay rather stable during the 1975 to 1984 time interval. After disaggregating the data for the oldest old, Rocca also reported that rates appeared to continue to rise with age after age 84; they also noted that rates were similar for men and women.

The combined analysis of four large ongoing European cohort studies of dementia and Alzheimer's disease was recently reported by Launer *et al.* (1999). Cohorts enrolled in Denmark, France, The Netherlands, and the United Kingdom summed to more than 16 000 members aged 65 or older at enrolment. After a mean follow-up of 2.2 years (comprising approximately 28 600 person-years) the overall incidence of dementia was 14.6 per 1000 person-years, with about two-thirds of these cases due to Alzheimer's disease. Incidence of dementia was 2.5 per 1000 person-years at ages 65 to 69, and rose to 85.6 per 1000 person-years in those aged 90 and older. Similarly Alzheimer's disease rose from 1.2 per 1000 person-years to 63.5 per 1000 person-years across the same age groups. Launer *et al.*'s report is one of the first using data from large cohort studies which are now underway in Europe and in the United States. As more cohort studies begin to report incidence, consistent estimates are likely to emerge.

Although, presumably, the majority of the difference between the rates of dementia and Alzheimer's disease reported above reflect vascular dementia, this cannot be stated with certainty. Despite diagnostic criteria for vascular dementia (Chui *et al.* 1992; Roman *et al.* 1993), this syndrome remains an area of controversy and uncertainty (Nyenhuis and Gorelick 1998; Chui and Gonthier 1999; Gorelick *et al.* 1999; Leys *et al.* 1999; Roman 1999*a*,*b*). Application of the diagnostic criteria has been shown to be difficult and unreliable in practice, even by experienced research investigators (Chui *et al.* 2000). Many of the reliability and validity problems experienced by investigators in classifying a case as 'vascular' or Alzheimer's disease may stem from the mutual exclusion of the two conditions, imposed by the diagnostic criteria. There is growing interest concerning a potential vascular component contributing to dementia in Alzheimer's disease (Brayne *et al.* 1998; Breteler *et al.* 1998; Copeland *et al.* 1999; Di Iorio *et al.* 1999; Goulding *et al.* 1999; Leys *et al.* 1999; Meyer *et al.* 2000).

Because identification of late-stage dementia and Alzheimer's disease holds little hope for treatment applications or for identification of consistent risk factors, interest has begun to focus on early identification of disease. Early forms of pre-Alzheimer's disease or dementia are difficult to distinguish from relatively benign cognitive decline associated with ageing. However, when mild cognitive decline can be identified it appears that perhaps 50 per cent may progress to become dementia (Almkvist *et al.* 1998; Wolf *et al.* 1998; Almkvist and Winblad 1999; Petersen *et al.* 1999; Celsis 2000). Distinguishing between normal persons, those with mild cognitive impairment, and those with incipient dementia/Alzheimer's disease may provide important clues about risk factors and critical periods of exposure prior to disease onset. Reliable and valid distinction may also help to determine whether mild cognitive impairment is a treatable and reversible phenomenon.

Risk (and protective) factors for Alzheimer's disease

Until the mid-1990s most analytical observational studies of Alzheimer's disease were based on a case–control design. In this design, cases of disease were identified and their exposure histories were compared to those of persons without the disease. The design itself is well accepted as a method of study. However, in the case of Alzheimer's disease (and dementia) problems with case ascertainment, case selection, and exposure measurement may have caused at least some results to be biased or spurious. Now, as cohort studies of Alzheimer's disease and dementia are beginning to emerge, findings which were viewed as consistent in case–control studies are being questioned or refuted. One example of this concerns the observation of a potential protective effect for Alzheimer's disease associated with cigarette smoking. A meta-analysis of smoking–Alzheimer's disease studies showed a consistent decreased risk associated with smoking (Lee 1994). The majority of these studies were of the case–control design. When case–control studies rely on cross-sectional samples to obtain cases, they are most likely to encounter those cases with the longest survival after diagnosis (Gordis 1996; MacMahon and Trichopoulos 1996; Rothman and Greenland 1998). Also, when decreased postdiagnosis survival among cases is associated with the exposure of interest (e.g. smoking), a potential spurious excess of exposure among controls may be observed. Wang *et al.* (1999) conducted a cross-sectional and a longitudinal study to observe the smoking–Alzheimer's disease relationship. They found that while mortality between smoking and non-smoking control subjects was rather similar, Alzheimer's disease case smokers had a threefold increase in risk of death as compared to Alzheimer's disease non-smokers. Therefore, because of mortality, smoking would be less common in a cross-sectional sample of Alzheimer's disease cases than among controls. Cohort studies (Launer *et al.* 1999; Merchant *et al.* 1999; Wang *et al.* 1999; Doll *et al.* 2000) where this selection bias is eliminated (essentially) now report either 'no association' or a potential *increased* risk of Alzheimer's disease associated with smoking.

Head trauma (Brayne 1991) has also been shown to be a relatively consistent risk factor for Alzheimer's disease, primarily based on case–control studies. Here, selective recall or recall bias may be more important than the effect of survival, even though risk of death and/or continued cognitive impairment immediately resulting from the injury is substantial (Anonymous 1998). Several recent longitudinal studies now show negligible risk of Alzheimer's disease associated with head injury (Launer *et al.* 1999; Mehta *et al.* 1999; Nee and Lippa 1999), although others still find some potentially increased risk (Tang *et al.* 1996; Schofield *et al.* 1997).

Higher educational level has been proposed as influencing decreased risk of Alzheimer's disease, but the relationship between education and Alzheimer's disease may be quite complex (Gainotti *et al.* 1998; Hendrie 1998; Ott *et al.* 1998; Geerlings *et al.* 1999*a*,*b*; Muller-Spahn and Hock 1999; Stern *et al.* 1999; Hall *et al.* 2000; Munoz *et al.* 2000; Riley *et al.* 2000). Educational level influences a subject's likelihood of participation in epidemiological studies. Educational level influences the diagnostic process, at least in the early stages of disease, because of the individual's ability to respond correctly in testing situations. Education may influence health-care usage and may result in greater income or higher occupational level. The idea that higher education confers greater 'cognitive reserve' to be accessed when disease strikes is tantalizing, though biologically unsubstantiated. Recently an important idea was raised concerning the importance of early life development as increasing susceptibility to Alzheimer's disease (Moceri *et al.* 2000). The biological plausibility for that association has been recently discussed by Alzheimer's disease neuropathologists (Braak *et al.* 1999).

Several 'protective' factors for Alzheimer's disease have been proposed in the past 10 years. These include: anti-inflammatory medications (Breitner 1996; McGeer *et al.* 1996; Stewart *et al.* 1997*a*; Stratman *et al.* 1997; Hendrie 1998; in 't Veld *et al.* 1998; Mortimer 1998; Combs *et al.* 2000), oestrogen replacement therapy (Brenner *et al.* 1994; Haskell *et al.* 1997; Henderson 1997*a*,*b*; Kawas *et al.* 1997; Baldereschi *et al.* 1998; Birge 1998; Yaffe *et al.* 1998; Costa *et al.* 1999; McEwen and Alves 1999; Waring *et al.* 1999; Henderson *et al.* 2000; Mulnard *et al.* 2000; Nourhashemi *et al.* 2000; Slooter *et al.* 1999), and antioxidants such as vitamin C and vitamin E (e.g. Morris *et al.* 1998). While the initial associations appear relatively consistent across studies, designs differ and conclusions are still tentative. Randomized trials for some are either proposed or underway. Results have given no indication that oestrogen replacement therapy is an effective treatment for Alzheimer's disease (Henderson *et al.* 2000; Mulnard *et al.* 2000). That result, however, does not address oestrogen as a preventive measure.

Alzheimer's disease is likely to be heterogeneous both diagnostically and aetiologically. What results in the Alzheimer's disease phenotype may be the sum or product of ageing, environmental factors, genetic constitution, and sociodemographic experiences. Aside from the observable effect of ageing dramatically increasing the risk of dementia and Alzheimer's disease, success in finding environmental risk factors has been limited and potentially related to design and selection factors.

Genetics and Alzheimer's disease

Great progress has been made in the genetics of Alzheimer's disease. However, most of the strict genetic 'causes' of disease have been limited to so-called 'familial' Alzheimer's disease. Familial Alzheimer's disease behaves similarly to an autosomal dominant genetic pattern and tends to affect predominantly persons under 60. Familial Alzheimer's disease, so defined, appears to account for less than 5 per cent of all Alzheimer's disease, but important clues may be gleaned from the study of familial disease that will apply to the more common form (often called sporadic—but it, too, may have undiscovered genetic causes). Several current reviews of Alzheimer's disease genetics include Tanzi *et al.* (1996), Hardy *et al.* (1998), Levy-Lahad *et al.* (1998), Price *et al.* (1998), Tilley *et al.* (1998), Shastry and Giblin (1999), Sisodia (1999), Steiner *et al.* (1999), Tanzi (1999), and St George-Hyslop (2000).

The largest proportion of familial Alzheimer's disease is attributed to mutations in the presenilin 1 gene (chromosome 14) and the next largest known contribution is due to mutations in a homologous gene on chromosome 1, presenilin 2. A very small proportion of cases is due to specific mutations in the amyloid precursor protein gene (chromosome 21). It is abnormal cleavage of the amyloid precursor protein, which results in the formation of amyloid β (1-42) protein. Amyloid β protein aggregates in the brain, forming the characteristic plaques of Alzheimer's disease. Recently very important work has been published concerning identification of enzymes, which cleave the precursor protein abnormally forming the amyloid β 1-42 protein. This work may ultimately help to identify sites for drug intervention, not only for familial but also for non-familial Alzheimer's disease (Hussain *et al.* 1999; Sinha *et al.* 1999; Steiner *et al.* 1999; Vassar *et al.* 1999; Yan *et al.* 1999; Octave *et al.* 2000; Phimister 2000). Perhaps one-quarter to one-half of familial Alzheimer's disease is still of unknown genetic cause (Levy-Lahad *et al.* 1998; Price *et al.* 1998; Shastry and Giblin 1999; Sisodia 1999).

Arguably the strongest and most consistent risk factor for non-familial Alzheimer's disease (other than age) is apolipoprotein E genotype. The association was first described from Allen Roses' laboratory (Corder *et al.* 1993; Saunders *et al.* 1993*a*,*b*; Strittmatter *et al.* 1993; Roses 1994; Roses and Saunders 1994). Apolipoprotein E naturally occurs as three different alleles (ε2, ε3, and ε4) which pair to form one of six genotypes for each individual. Genotypes containing the ε4 allele are associated with increased risk of Alzheimer's disease; homozygous ε4 greatly increased risk (e.g. more than eightfold). Since the initial description of increased risk associated with the ε4 allele, many investigators have observed the association. Discussion of apolipoprotein E genotype is now included in most risk-factor studies of Alzheimer's disease, either as a focus or as a potential confounder/effect-modifier of an association. Farrer *et al.* (1997) provided a meta-analysis of the age and gender effects, and Mayeux *et al.* (1998) later described caveats for the potential value of apolipoprotein E genotype in Alzheimer's disease diagnosis. Despite the huge number of studies including apolipoprotein E genotype relatively little is known concerning how the ε2, ε3, and ε4 alleles actually work to influence the risk of Alzheimer's disease.

Evidence for the effects of other genes on Alzheimer's disease has also been raised. Alpha-2 macroglobulin was first shown as a potential risk factor by Blacker *et al.* (1998), but then a number of other investigators failed to replicate the association (Liao *et al.* 1998; Alvarez *et al.* 1999; Dodel *et al.* 2000; Gibson *et al.* 2000). This association remains controversial. Other genetic associations have been studied but with limited impact to date (Hirano *et al.* 1997; Hutchin *et al.* 1997; Pericak-Vance *et al.* 1997; Ghetti *et al.* 1999; Lilius *et al.* 1999; Meier-Ruge and Bertoni-Freddari 1999; Perry 1999; Roks *et al.* 1999; Shastry and Giblin 1999; Small *et al.* 1999; Bullido *et al.* 2000; Nicoll *et al.* 2000). Progress continues, and there is considerable hope that important genes will be discovered which may provide indications for prevention or therapy.

Peripheral neuropathy

Clinical overview

Though the term peripheral neuropathy may refer to any disease of the peripheral nerves, it is generally used to describe a group of systemic diseases that affect the peripheral nerves rather than focal diseases affecting an isolated nerve. Most of these diseases initially affect longer nerves, with symptoms developing first in the feet and progressing up the legs. There are a few peripheral neuropathies that affect the shorter proximal nerves first. By the time the symptoms have reached the knees, the hands become symptomatic, followed by the anterior trunk and crown of the head. The symptoms that develop depend on the type of nerve fibre involved. Involvement of motor fibres leads to weakness, muscle wasting, and hyporeflexia. If longstanding, motor neuropathies may lead to high arches (pes cavus) or hammer toes. Sensory nerve involvement leads to loss of sensation, distorted sensation (dysaesthesias), or spontaneous unpleasant sensations (paraesthesias). Autonomic neuropathies most commonly lead to postural hypotension but may also include sexual dysfunction, bowel dysfunction, bladder dysfunction, sweating dysfunction, or gastroparesis. The size of the affected nerve fibre can often be suggested by the history, with disease of large fibre causing reflex loss, vibration loss, and joint position loss. Small fibre disease often leads to autonomic dysfunction, dysaesthesias, loss of pain sensation, and loss of temperature sensation.

Electrodiagnostic testing is often performed to diagnose and further classify peripheral neuropathies. Nerve conduction velocities can be used to classify peripheral neuropathies into those that are demyelinating and those that are axonal. Demyelinating neuropathies lead to disproportionate slowing of nerve conduction speeds and increases in latency of responses. Axonal diseases cause disproportional loss of amplitude with relative preservation of conduction speed. Nerve conduction studies measure only the fast-conducting large-diameter fibres. Electromyography measures the electrical activity of muscle fibres. It is useful in diagnosing a number of muscle and myoneural junction diseases. The use of electromyography in the diagnosis of peripheral neuropathy is primarily in recognizing the loss of innervation of muscle fibres by large myelinated neurones. Loss of innervation leads to increased insertional activity, positive waves, fibrillation potentials, polyphasic motor unit potentials, and decreased recruitment patterns.

Generally, polyneuropathies are the result of lesions involving many peripheral nerves and result in autonomic neuropathies, sensory loss, or weakness. Mononeuropathies, as the name implies, involve a single nerve injury or entrapment. Carpal tunnel syndrome and Bell's palsy are common examples of mononeuropathies. Peripheral nerve disorders are also often classified as either hereditary or acquired. Charcot–Marie–Tooth syndrome is perhaps the most well-known hereditary form. Acquired nerve disorders are commonly associated with trauma or compression, diabetes, alcoholism, and other nutritional and metabolic problems. They may also be related to infectious causes such as Guillain–Barré syndrome, leprosy, Lyme disease, or HIV infection; or, they may be caused by toxic exposures to metals (e.g. lead, mercury) or industrial chemicals, or even by therapeutic drugs (e.g. antineoplastic agents) (Rowland and Merritt 1995).

Carpal tunnel syndrome

First characterized in 1880 by James J. Putnam, carpal tunnel syndrome is probably the most common neuropathy (Sternbach 1999). Carpal tunnel release surgery is also one of the most common hand surgeries performed in the United States (Rayan 1999). Franklin *et al.* (1991) reported that 'occupational' carpal tunnel syndrome resulting from repetitive, higher-impact actions may differ from carpal tunnel syndrome occurring in a non-occupational setting. Specifically, occupational carpal tunnel syndrome appeared to occur nearly equally among men and women and at a substantially lower mean age than had been reported for non-occupational carpal tunnel syndrome (37 versus 51 years). Based on workmen's compensation records over the period 1984 to 1988, an incidence of 1.74 per 1000 full-time equivalent jobs was observed (Franklin *et al.* 1991). Abbas *et al.* (1998) conducted a meta-analysis of work-related carpal tunnel syndrome. They showed that force and repetitive motion were important predictors of carpal tunnel syndrome after adjusting for study population and country of origin.

A general population estimate of carpal tunnel syndrome incidence was reported by Nordstrom *et al.* (1998). Medical records of all cases occurring in 2 years in a defined population were reviewed and classified as definite or probable carpal tunnel syndrome. In contrast to the occupational carpal tunnel syndrome incidence observed by Franklin *et al.* (1991), as well as other previous incidence estimates, Nordstrom *et al.* reported a carpal tunnel syndrome incidence of 3.46 per 1000 person-years. The apparent secular increase in incidence may reflect a true change in incidence or may be partially due to popular knowledge of the condition and diagnostic suspicion. Prevalence of symptoms in relation to true disease prevalence is also an important consideration (Atroshi *et al.* 1999). Reported carpal tunnel syndrome symptoms of tingling, pain, and numbness have shown a prevalence of about 14 per cent, whereas carpal tunnel syndrome was clinically and electrophysiologically confirmed in less than 3 per cent. Atroshi *et al.* (1999) conclude that symptoms of carpal tunnel syndrome are common but only about 1 in 5 of the persons complaining of symptoms is likely to actually have confirmed carpal tunnel syndrome.

Studying carpal tunnel syndrome patients recruited from physicians' offices, Katz *et al.* (1998) attempted to describe predictors of work absence. Approximately 70 per cent of the 315 patients had undergone surgery, the majority women. After 30 months of follow-up, those who began with worse functional status were more likely to have missed work. The other major predictor of work absence was reported to be having a 'contested Worker's Compensation claim'.

Non-occupational factors related to the occurrence and treatment of carpal tunnel syndrome were studied by Solomon *et al.* (1999) and Stallings *et al.* (1997). Solomon *et al.* found that carpal tunnel syndrome patients with inflammatory arthritis were about three times more likely to undergo carpal tunnel release surgery; patients with diabetes and hypothyroidism were also significantly more likely to receive surgery. Obesity has been reported as a risk factor for the occurrence of carpal tunnel syndrome, an association that was addressed in a case–control study by Stallings *et al.* (1997). Results indicated that obesity, as determined by body mass index, was significantly more common among cases than among control subjects.

Diabetes mellitus

Diabetes is a common, yet complex, cause of both mono- and polyneuropathies (Rowland and Merritt 1995). Peripheral neuropathy may affect more than 30 per cent of diabetes patients. More effective glucose control could reduce the risk to some extent (Boulton 1998*a*, *b*). Patients with diabetes have a higher hospital admission rate, length of stay, and mortality than non-diabetics (Currie *et al.* 1998), indicating the potential human and economic cost of the disease.

Dyck *et al.* (1997, 1999) developed a composite score for assessing the degree of diabetic polyneuropathy, then conducted a longitudinal study of 264 diabetics to determine how hyperglycaemia related to diabetic polyneuropathy. Microvessel disease, chronic hyperglycaemia, and type of diabetes were the most important predictors of polyneuropathy. Orchard *et al.* (1996) have also shown that among insulin-dependent diabetes mellitus patients diabetic autonomic neuropathy is strongly influenced by chronic hyperglycaemia and is associated with increased mortality. A study of diabetic peripheral neuropathy in 16 European countries identified several additional risk factors: elevated diastolic blood pressure, ketoacidosis, elevated fasting triglyceride level, and microabuminuria (Tesfaye *et al.* 1996).

Nutritional neuropathies

An epidemic of peripheral neuropathy was reported in Cuba during 1992 and 1993 (Roman 1994). That epidemic was said to affect over 50 000 Cubans and achieved a cumulative incidence rate of 461 per 100 000. An optic form and a peripheral form of the disease were observed. Extensive search for toxic exposures and a variety of other risk factors eventually lead to nutritional deficiency as the principal explanation for the outbreak. (Roman 1994; Hedges *et al.* 1997). Intervention and treatment with multivitamins, in particular B vitamins, acted to stop the outbreak.

HIV infection

Because of the prevalence of HIV in many countries, it is important to consider the prevalence of peripheral neuropathy among HIV-infected cases. This reached 44 per cent in one African study (Parry *et al.* 1997). Distal symmetrical polyneuropathy was predominant in persons with frank AIDS. One potential cause of that neuropathy is the AIDS therapy itself (Moyle and Sadler 1998). Specifically, nucleoside analogue reverse transcriptase inhibitors may act, in about 10 per cent of patients, to promote neuropathy. The severity of the neuropathy may then cause patients to discontinue the needed therapy.

Parkinsonism

Clinical overview

There are four cardinal features of parkinsonism: tremor, rigidity, bradykinesia, and postural gait changes. Though there are no established criteria, the diagnosis of parkinsonism usually requires two or more of these symptoms. The tremor of parkinsonism may take many forms. The most common form of tremor in parkinsonism has a frequency of 4 to 6 Hz. It is most prominent at rest, lessening with volitional movements. It has a somewhat rotary component with the 'pill rolling' tremor of the hands classically described. The hands are most prominently affected but the head, trunk, and legs may also be involved. Emotional stress may aggravate the tremor. The rigidity of parkinsonism is often described as 'lead pipe rigidity'. This rigidity is approximately equal in flexor and extensor muscles in contrast to the rigidity seen in spasticity, which is not equal. The rigidity is present throughout the full range of motion and is not dependent on speed of movement. The combination of rigidity with superimposed tremor constitutes 'cogwheeling', two of the four cardinal features of parkinsonism. Bradykinesia may take a number of forms, including the masked face with loss of blinking, wide-eyed staring, and loss of facial expression. Speech may be hypophonic, rapid, and without the usual modulations of pitch, enunciation, or emotion. Bodily movements become slowed with fewer spontaneous movements of the limbs. Rapid repetitive movements of the limbs are slowed. There may be a marked latency before planned movements are begun. Postural gait changes lead to a stooped posture with kyphosis, flexed arms, flexed legs, and loss of arm swing. The gait becomes unstable with patients being unable to reflexively recover from minor imbalances. The centre of balance may get progressively ahead of the patient as they walk leading to a 'festinating gait'. In severe cases, patients may be unable to move (freezing) when they encounter minor obstacles such as doorways or cracks (Rowland and Merritt 1995). While movement disorder specialists make the diagnosis of parkinsonism with some degree of confidence, Parkinson's disease usually requires histopathological confirmation. In an attempt to increase the accuracy and validity of clinical diagnosis, improvements in clinical diagnostic criteria have been proposed (Gelb *et al.* 1999; Jankovic *et al.* 2000).

Parkinsonism includes several major subclasses: idiopathic parkinsonism (Parkinson's disease), symptomatic parkinsonism (drug-induced, toxin-induced, and other specific causes), 'Parkinson-plus' syndromes (multiple system atrophy, progressive supranuclear palsy), and hereditary degenerative diseases (Hallervorden–Spatz disease, Huntington's disease). Parkinson's disease, or idiopathic parkinsonism comprises approximately 80 per cent of parkinsonism (Rowland and Merritt 1995).

Multiple system atrophy is sometimes misdiagnosed as Parkinson's disease; it is a relatively rare and very debilitating condition, usually involving progressive autonomic failure plus poor responsiveness to levodopa or cerebellar ataxia (Gilman *et al.* 1998; Kaufmann 1998; Lantos 1998; Austin *et al.* 1999; Oertel and Bandmann 1999; Siemers 1999; Swan and Dupont 1999). There is some speculation that multiple system atrophy may be a synucleinopathy (Goedert and Spillantini 1998; Wakabayashi *et al.* 1998; Dickson *et al.* 1999). The role of environmental toxins in the pathogenesis of multiple system atrophy has also been discussed but little evidence for such an association has been established to date (Hanna *et al.* 1999).

Incidence and prevalence of Parkinson's disease

Prevalence has been reported with dramatic inconsistency. Case ascertainment, age structure of the population, and study design may account for some part of the variability. Certainly door-to-door screening may find more disease than relying on medical records or death certificates. Decisions regarding the inclusion of institutionalized subjects in a screening effort may also impact obtained prevalence.

Consider that Parkinson's disease prevalence typically has been reported in the range of about 50 to 200 per 100 000 population, with a maximum of about 350 per 100 000. Examples in this range include 117.9 per 100 000 in Japan (Kusumi *et al.* 1996), 115 per 100 000 in Sweden (Fall *et al.* 1996), and 168 to 196 per 100 000 in Italy (Chio *et al.* 1998). Morgante *et al.* (1992) conducted a study in Sicily and found 63 Parkinson's disease cases among 24 496 persons in the population base, which results in a prevalence proportion of 257.2 per 100 000 (or 0.257 per cent). The Rotterdam Study (de Rijk *et al.* 1995) reported identifying a total of 97 Parkinson's disease cases from among 6969 enrolled subjects age 55 or older, for a crude prevalence of 1.39 per cent or 1392 per 100 000. Recently, the combined results of five European studies were published (de Rijk *et al.* 1997). These included 14 636 persons age 65 or older; after age-adjusting to the European 1991 standard population the prevalence of Parkinson's disease was reported as 1.6 per 100 population (presumably age 65 or older). This translates to about 1600 per 100 000. In addition, the age-specific prevalence of Parkinson's disease was reported to increase from 0.6 per cent in 65- to 69-year-olds to 3.5 per cent in 85- to 89-year-olds (or 600 to 3500 per 100 000) (de Rijk *et al.* 1997).

The example above is instructive. Not only must the reader attend to differences in case ascertainment when evaluating reported prevalence estimates, but also attention should be directed to the base from which the prevalence proportion is calculated. Limiting the base to only those subjects above a particular age can have dramatic effects on the reported proportion with disease. Furthermore, when restricted base figures are reported along with, perhaps, more conventional total population prevalence proportions, it may be easy for the reader to misinterpret findings.

Incidence rates for Parkinson's disease and parkinsonism carry many of the same caveats raised for prevalence. In addition, confusion is added by choosing to report incidence in terms of person-years, or per population per year, or perhaps as projected cumulative lifetime incidence. With some effort, or with some assumptions, conversions can be made, but this may not be obvious to the reader. For example, Kusumi *et al.* (1996) reported Parkinson's disease incidence in a Japanese city as 15.0 per 100 000 population per year (1989 to 1992); Fall *et al.* (1996) reported Parkinson's disease incidence in Sweden (age adjusted) as 7.9 per 100 000 person-years; and Hofman reported Parkinson's disease incidence in The Netherlands as 11 per 100 000 person-years. Bower *et al.* (1999) studied the incidence of parkinsonism and Parkinson's disease in Rochester, Minnesota, 1976 to 1990. The overall figures for Parkinson's disease showed an incidence rate of 10.8 per 100 000 person-years (i.e. based on the entire age distribution population). The age-specific incidence for ages 50 to 59 was 17.4 per 100 000 person-years, rising to 52.5 for ages 60 to 69, and peaking at 93.1 for ages 70 to 79 and 79.1 for ages 80 to 99. Parkinsonism showed an overall incidence rate of 25.6 per 100 000 person-years and rose from 26.5 at ages 50 to 59 to 304.8 per 100 000 person-years in those aged 80 to 99.

Age-specific incidence rates provide critical information not available from summary rates. The strong influence of age on the disease process is evident from the Rochester data: the incidence among those aged 0 to 29 is practically nil, while the incidence triples from 50 to 59 to 60 to 69, then nearly doubles again in the 70 to 79 age group (Bower *et al.* 1999). How ageing contributes to the degenerative process of Parkinson's disease or how aging increases susceptibility to genetic and environmental risk factors is important in describing the epidemiology of parkinsonism and Parkinson's disease.

Risk factors

A number of excellent reviews are available that discuss the epidemiology and risk factors for Parkinson's disease, for example Schoenberg (1987), Ben-Shlomo (1997), Langston (1998), Checkoway and Nelson (1999), and Tanner and Ben-Shlomo (1999).

The controversy over environmental and genetic causes of Parkinson's disease provides the current focus. Clear and consistent evidence of specific, strong, environmental risk factors has not been found. However, the possibility of environmental causes was increased by the observation that 1-methyl-4-phenyl-1,2,3,6-tetrahydropyridine, a 'designer' street drug, was observed to cause acute Parkinson's disease shortly after ingestion. Because the structure of this drug and its metabolism products are somewhat similar to some pesticides and herbicides, there was and is great interest in exploring the potential for those types of exposures as risk factors or causes of Parkinson's disease. Similarly, observations focusing on family history and familial cases, along with the rapid increase in information available on the human genome, has led to new interest in describing the genetics of Parkinson's disease.

Rural living, well-water consumption, and pesticide/herbicide exposure are reported relatively frequently as potential risk factors for Parkinson's disease, although neither critical time periods and duration for these exposures to influence onset, nor specific mechanisms have been identified. For example, a case–control study conducted by Gorell *et al.* (1998) found about a fourfold increase in risk of Parkinson's disease for exposure to herbicides and insecticides and nearly a threefold increase in risk of Parkinson's disease for those who had a farming occupation (but no increase for rural or farm residence, nor well-water use). Marder *et al.* (1998) found an association between farming, rural living, and well water in a multiethnic case–control study, but that association held only for African Americans and not for Hispanics. Kuopio *et al.* (1999) conducted a population-based case–control study in Finland and found no association between farming, drinking water, pesticide/herbicide use, and Parkinson's disease, but they did show that cases had a history of fewer domestic animals at home.

An association between exposure to metals and Parkinson's disease has been described by Gorell *et al.* (1999*a*, *b*). An association was noted with manganese exposure and with copper, also with combinations of lead and iron or copper. While interesting, it raises the question of whether the manganese association represented manganism rather than Parkinson's disease.

Smoking has been rather consistently associated with decreased risk of Parkinson's disease in reported reviews (Ben-Shlomo 1997; Langston 1998; Checkoway and Nelson 1999; Tanner and Ben-Shlomo 1999) and in individual studies (Tzourio *et al.* 1997; Rybicki *et al.* 1999; Taylor *et al.* 1999; Werneck and Alvarenga 1999). Reasons for the plausibility of such an association revolve around the potential action of nicotine on neurones. Although this is one of the more consistent findings it is not completely without alternative explanations. Most epidemiological studies of Parkinson's disease use 'prevalent' or existing cases in their studies. The low incidence of Parkinson's disease effectively precludes concentrating on only newly diagnosed cases in all but the largest of studies (or in very large cohort studies). When attempting to identify a cross-sectional sample of cases for enrolment into a case–control study, it can be shown that those patients who have had the disease the longest are the most likely to be included. The most severe, short duration, or rapidly declining cases tend to be missed. If Parkinson's disease cases who had a history of smoking were much more likely to die than non-smoking Parkinson's disease cases, and if, at the same time, the smoking–non-smoking mortality differential was somewhat less among the controls, the cross-sectional sampling of cases and controls could give the spurious impression of an excess of smoking among controls. The excess numbers of smokers among controls might then be misinterpreted as a causal protective effect.

Interest in pesticide exposure as a potential cause led to a new approach for evaluating the occurrence of susceptible persons. Specifically, some persons may be more, or less, able to metabolize environmental toxins because of polymorphic genes involved in metabolism. One of the family of cytochrome P-450 biotransformation genes, CYP2D6, is involved in metabolism of debrisoquine (structurally similar to pesticides); some polymorphic forms are 'poor' metabolizers and others are normal or rapid metabolizers of debrisoquine. Initial studies appeared to show that poor metabolizers were at increased risk of Parkinson's disease but later studies and meta-analyses fail to support this conclusion (Christensen *et al.* 1998; Joost *et al.* 1999; Sabbagh *et al.* 1999).

A similar approach has been taken to identify susceptibles focusing on polymorphic forms of glutathione transferases, which are involved in the metabolism of pesticides and other xenobiotics. Menegon *et al.* (1998) tested four different glutathione transferases classes and found the distribution of glutathione transferases (π) genotypes differed between cases and controls who had been exposed to pesticides. Another example of this ecogenetic approach was applied to the association between smoking and Parkinson's disease by testing the modifying effect of monoamine oxidase-B genotype (Costa *et al.* 1997; Checkoway *et al.* 1998*a*,*b*). Checkoway *et al.* (1998*b*) reported that smokers with one form of the monoamine oxidase-B gene appeared to have lowered risk of Parkinson's disease but that those with the other form did not. Recently, Mellick reported a different polymorphism of the monoamine oxidase-B gene as a relatively strong marker for Parkinson's disease in an Australian cohort. Monoamine oxidase-A genotype, on the other hand, has been shown to be *not* significantly associated with Parkinson's disease (Costa-Mallen *et al.* 2000). Continued efforts to identify gene–environment interaction in this way may eventually prove fruitful, but success is rather limited to date.

A relatively small subset of Parkinson's disease appears to be due to autosomal dominant (or recessive) gene or genes (Jones *et al.* 1998; Payami and Zareparsi 1998; Veldman *et al.* 1998; Wood 1998; Zareparsi *et al.* 1998). The α-synuclein gene on 4q and another autosomal dominant gene on 2q appear to be sufficient to cause a particular subtype of Parkinson's disease, but the familial form of the disease is quite rare (Vaughan *et al.* 1998). Similarly, 6q contains a recessive gene for 'juvenile parkinsonism'. Additional work is ongoing to describe the influence of mutations in the tau gene (17q) (Hardy *et al.* 1998; D'Souza *et al.* 1999; Hulette *et al.* 1999; Sperfeld *et al.* 1999). Genetic heterogeneity appears to be common in Parkinson's disease. With the increased progress in genetic research generally it is quite likely that additional genes will be found which may explain parts of parkinsonism and Parkinson's disease.

Public health impact

Parkinson's disease is progressive and debilitating. While initial treatments with levodopa and similar medications effectively quell most motor symptoms, their effectiveness begins to subside in about 50 per cent of patients after 3 to 5 years. With increasing motor problem comes increased health care cost and decreased quality of life (Chrischilles *et al.* 1998; Dodel *et al.* 1998; de Boer *et al.* 1999). For many patients, dementia also ensues as Parkinson's disease progresses (Marder and Mayeux 1991; Oertel 1995; Marder *et al.* 1999).

Multiple sclerosis

Clinical overview

Although multiple sclerosis is not as common as most of the neurological diseases previously discussed, it is an important cause of disability in young adults in developed countries, and is thus worthy of at least brief discussion here. The impact of this disease on society is disproportionately large because it strikes people 20 to 50 years of age. The impact of multiple sclerosis on wage earning is also notable, with only 21 per cent of multiple sclerosis patients having no work limitations and only 29 per cent remaining in the work force (Minden *et al.* 1993). In addition to the stresses the disease places on home life and employment, multiple sclerosis patients have substantial increases in medical costs compared to the general population (Minden *et al.* 1993). Because of lost earnings and increased health-care costs, multiple sclerosis is the third leading cause of significant disability in the 20 to 50 age range (Cobble *et al.* 1993).

Clinically, multiple sclerosis is characterized by demyelination of central nervous system white matter tracts including motor, sensory, cerebellar, visual, brainstem, autonomic, and spinal cord pathways. The symptoms may be episodic, with exacerbations and remissions, with symptoms remaining stable between exacerbations (relapsing/remitting disease). Alternatively, symptoms may slowly progress in the absence of exacerbations (primary progressive disease). Relapsing/remitting cases may change to include slow deterioration of the baseline in between attacks (secondary progressive disease). When the disease results in death, the immediate cause is usually infection, secondary to urinary tract involvement or pneumonia.

At present, corticosteroids are used to shorten the length of acute relapses. Interferon-β1a, interferon-β1b, glateramer acetate, and mitoxantrone have all been shown to slow the progression of the disease. In addition to disease-modifying therapy, symptomatic treatments are often required. New immunosuppressive treatments are being tested, and may prove to be efficacious in the future.

Definition

The criteria developed by Schumacher *et al.* (1965) and revised by Poser *et al.* (1991) are generally used for diagnosis. The criteria for clinically definite multiple sclerosis include two or more episodes of neurological deficit and evidence on neurological examination, MRI, or evoked potential of more than one site of involvement in the central nervous system.

Case ascertainment

Because of the necessity for neurological expertise and special studies to make reliable diagnoses, reported worldwide prevalences may not be completely comparable, especially where differences in the availability and quality of health care exist. The requirement for repeated attacks before a diagnosis is made leads to difficulties in determining exact incidence figures in a timely manner.

Prevalence

Disease prevalence—the number of cases present (alive) at a given time within a circumscribed population—is easier to determine than incidence. This is because all cases are included, regardless of disease duration, which can vary from as little as 1 year to more than 40 years, especially with treatment. The reported prevalence of multiple sclerosis varies widely with latitude, from 1 per 100 000 or less near the equator, to over 150 per 100 000 in some high-latitude areas. In the southern hemisphere less data are available, but studies in Australia and New Zealand support a similar gradient in prevalence (Skegg *et al.* 1987). Persons who migrate in childhood from high-risk to lower-risk areas seem to lower their risk of multiple sclerosis, while migrants over age 15 retain the risk associated with their areas of origin (Alter *et al.* 1966; Dean 1967; Detels *et al.* 1977).

Risk factors

Genetic susceptibility

There are several types of evidence for genetic influences on susceptibility. Asian, African, and aboriginal groups seem to have lower prevalence than Caucasians, regardless of latitude of residence. Because more research has been done on Caucasians, it has been shown in this group that some alleles of the HLA complex are associated with multiple sclerosis susceptibility (Multiple Sclerosis Genetics Group 1996). In addition, other groups of genes that influence the immune response or myelin structure have been investigated (Sadovnick *et al.* 1991). The extremely high rate of concordance in monozygotic twins also supports a genetic contribution to the disease (Xian-hao and McFarlin 1984). The higher rate of multiple sclerosis in females compared to males also supports involvement of the immune system.

Environmental factors

In the presence of inherent susceptibility, some external factors seem to be associated with multiple sclerosis. The lack of complete concordance in monozygotic twins supports an environmental factor. People with multiple sclerosis have a later age of exposure to common childhood exanthematous diseases, and lower birth orders (Allen and Brankin 1993). There have been reports of clusters of disease, thought to have been related to environmental exposures, but on investigation these supposed clusters have generally not been beyond expected variability. An apparent epidemic of multiple sclerosis following the British invasion of the Faeroe Islands has not yet been fully explained.

Overview

These genetic and environmental factors may result in an autoimmune destruction of myelin corresponding to the attacks that occur in multiple sclerosis. The positive effect of immunomodulating treatments supports this view of pathogenesis. However, much remains to be clarified about the mechanisms of the disease process.

Epilogue

Presenting current and useful research information on a number of neurological conditions is a difficult task. This chapter has addressed that challenge, for some selected neurological conditions. Conditions such as headache and back pain have substantial public health impact because of the age groups affected, their prevalence, and the lost productivity (or economic loss) related to them. Multiple sclerosis, a relatively uncommon neurological disease, can affect individuals in young adulthood, decrease their productivity, and ultimately make them dependent on others. Traumatic brain injury occurring in youth or young adulthood can cause years of extra medical care in addition to lost productivity among those who survive the immediate event. Epilepsy may have onset throughout life; it may result from trauma or may be caused by specific genes, among other causes. While there are intractable forms of epilepsy, great strides have been made in seizure control enabling patients to lead relatively full and normal lives. Neurodegenerative diseases, such as Parkinson's disease and Alzheimer's disease, rob older individuals of productivity, functional ability, and independence; they also force huge increases in health-care costs. Without question neurological diseases have substantial public health effects.

Determining the incidence and prevalence for most of the diseases and conditions in this chapter is quite an inexact science. The conditions are often difficult to define and detect in the population and for the most part they are not regarded as 'reportable' conditions. Therefore we gain insight as to disease occurrence primarily from limited but (hopefully) well-designed and conducted studies. As mentioned in the introduction to this chapter, the epidemiological study of neurological conditions is a complicated matter. Problems with diagnostic inaccuracy and insidious disease onset influence our ability to observe risk-factor associations; factors related to survival may be mistaken for risk/protective factors.

The recent identification of the code for the human genome foretells the increasing promise of genetic research. The contribution of genes that in and of themselves cause disease may be smaller than that of genes which act to metabolize or potentiate environmental exposures. The interaction between genes and environment will be increasingly well studied in the future. Descriptions of gene products and function may lead to specific drug therapies never before possible. The genetic information presented in this chapter, while relatively current, may become obsolete quickly. The fields of genetics and molecular biology are moving rapidly. It is also a challenge for epidemiologists to apply the knowledge gained by genetic researchers to the design and analysis of epidemiological studies. The diagnosis of neurological conditions may be made more accurately and earlier with genetic information. Science and the public health will benefit beyond even our current expectations, from the Human Genome Project.

Epidemiology must take advantage of these molecular advances. Many scholars have written on the advantages and disadvantages of reductionism in science. Much of epidemiology lies in its public health context, and the same is likely to be true for genetic influences on neurological diseases. Arrays of genes may identify susceptible individuals; however, those individuals may avoid disease unless met with specific environmental or behavioural exposures. The tasks of public health and epidemiology will still involve prevention, the non-random occurrence of disease, and its environmental context—in addition to heredity. The tools to address those tasks will continue to be refined.

References

Abbas, M.A., Afifi, A.A., Zhang, Z.W., and Kraus, J.F. (1998). Meta-analysis of published studies of work-related carpal tunnel syndrome. *International Journal of Occupational and Environmental Health*, **4**, 160–7.

Allen, I. and Brankin, B. (1993). Pathogenesis of multiple sclerosis: the immune diathesis and the role of viruses. *Journal of Neuropathology and Experimental Neurology*, **5**, 95–105.

Almkvist, O. and Winblad, B. (1999). Early diagnosis of Alzheimer dementia based on clinical and biological factors. *European Archives in Psychiatry and Clinical Neuroscience*, **249**, 3–9.

Almkvist, O., Basun, H., Backman, L., *et al.* (1998). Mild cognitive impairment—an early stage of Alzheimer's disease? *Journal of Neural Transmission*, **54** (Supplement), 21–9.

Alter, M., Leibowitz, U.S., and Peer, J. (1966). Risk of multiple sclerosis related to age of immigration to Israel. *Archives of Neurology*, **15**, 234–7.

Alvarez, V., Alvarez, R., Lahoz, C.H., *et al.* (1999). Association between an alpha(2) macroglobulin DNA polymorphism and late-onset alzheimer's disease. *Biochemical and Biophysical Research Communications*, **264**, 48–50.

American Psychiatric Association (1994). Task Force on DSM-IV. *Diagnostic and statistical manual of mental disorders* (4th edn). American Psychiatric Association, Washington, DC.

Anderson, G. (1981). Epidemiologic aspects on low-back pain in industry. *Spine*, **6**, 53–60.

Anderson, V.E., Hauser, W.A., and Rich, S.S. (1999). Genetic heterogeneity and epidemiology of the epilepsies. *Advances in Neurology*, **79**, 59–73.

Andersson, G. (1999). Epidemiological features of chronic low-back pain. *Lancet*, **354**, 581–5.

Annegers, J.F. (1994). Epidemiology and genetics of epilepsy. *Neurology Clinics*, **12**, 15–29.

Annegers, J.F. and Coan, S.P. (1999). SUDEP: overview of definitions and review of incidence data. *Seizure*, **8**, 347–52.

Annegers, J.F., Hauser, W.A., Coan, S.P., and Rocca, W.A. (1998). A population-based study of seizures after traumatic brain injuries. *New England Journal of Medicine*, **338**, 20–4.

Annegers, J.F., Beghi, E., and Begley, C.E. (1999). Cost of epilepsy: contrast of methodologies in United States and European studies. *Epilepsia*, **40**, 14–18.

Anonymous (1994). Clinical and neuropathological criteria for frontotemporal dementia. The Lund and Manchester Groups. *Journal of Neurology, Neurosurgery and Psychiatry*, **57**, 416–18.

Anonymous (1998). Rehabilitation of persons with traumatic brain injury. *NIH Consensus Statement 1998*, 26–28 October, **16**, 1–41.

Atroshi, I., Gummesson, C., Johnsson, R., Ornstein, E., Ranstam, J., and Rosen, I. (1999). Prevalence of carpal tunnel syndrome in a general population. *Journal of the American Medical Association*, **282**, 153–8.

Austin, M.T., Davis, T.L., Robertson, D., and Charles, P.D. (1999). Multiple system atrophy: clinical presentation and diagnosis. *Tennessee Medicine*, **92**, 55–7.

Baldereschi, M., Di Carlo, A., Lepore, V., *et al.* (1998). Estrogen-replacement therapy and Alzheimer's disease in the Italian Longitudinal Study on Aging. *Neurology*, **50**, 996–1002.

Beckett, L.A. and Evans, D.A. (1994). Estimating prevalence and incidence of chronic conditions in the elderly: design and sampling issues. *Alzheimer Disease and Associated Disorders*, **8**, S274–80.

Beghi, E., Brown, S., Capurro, D., *et al.* (2000). IBE Commission Report. Second Workshop on Epilepsy, Risks, and Insurance. *Epilepsia*, **41**, 110–12.

Begley, C.E., Annegers, J.F., Lairson, D.R., and Reynolds, T.F. (1999). Methodological issues in estimating the cost of epilepsy. *Epilepsy Research*, **33**, 39–55.

Begley, C.E., Famulari, M., Annegers, J.F., *et al.* (2000). The cost of epilepsy in the United States: an estimate from population-based clinical and survey data. *Epilepsia*, **41**, 342–51.

Behrens, V., Seligman, P., Cameron, L., *et al.* (1994). The prevalence of back pain, hand discomfort, and dermatitis in the United States working population. *American Journal of Public Health*, **84**, 1780–5.

Beilmann, A., Napa, A., Soot, A., Talvik, I., and Talvik, T. (1999). Prevalence of childhood epilepsy in Estonia. *Epilepsia*, **40**, 1011–19.

Ben-Shlomo, Y. (1997). The epidemiology of Parkinson's disease. *Baillière's Clinical Neurology*, **6**, 55–68.

Berg, A.T., Testa, F.M., Levy, S.R., and Shinnar, S. (1996). The epidemiology of epilepsy: past, present, and future. *Neurology Clinics*, **14**, 383–98.

Berkovic, S.F. (1997). Epilepsy genes and the genetics of epilepsy syndromes: the promise of new therapies based on genetic knowledge. *Epilepsia*, **38**, S32–6.

Bern, C., Garcia, H.H., Evans, C., *et al.* (1999). Magnitude of the disease burden from neurocysticercosis in a developing country. *Clinical Infectious Diseases*, **29**, 1203–9.

Berney, J., Froidevaux, A.C., and Favier, J. (1994). Paediatric head trauma: influence of age and sex. II. Biomechanical and anatomo-clinical correlations. *Childs Nervous System*, **10**, 517–23.

Bigos, S., Battie, M., Spengler, D., *et al.* (1991). A prospective study of work perceptions and psychological factors affecting the report of back injury. *Spine*, **16**, 1–6.

Birge, S.J. (1998). Hormones and the aging brain. *Geriatrics*, **53** (Supplement 1), S28–30.

Blacker, D., Wilcox, M.A., Laird, N.M., *et al.* (1998). Alpha-2 macroglobulin is genetically associated with Alzheimer disease. *Nature Genetics*, **19**, 357–60.

Boulton, A.J. (1998*a*). Guidelines for diagnosis and outpatient management of diabetic peripheral neuropathy. European Association for the Study of Diabetes, Neurodiab. *Diabete et Metabolisme*, **24** (Supplement 3), 55–65.

Boulton, A.J. (1998*b*). Lowering the risk of neuropathy, foot ulcers and amputations. *Diabetic Medicine*, **15**, S57–9.

Bower, J.H., Maraganore, D.M., McDonnell, S.K., and Rocca, W.A. (1999). Incidence and distribution of parkinsonism in Olmsted County, Minnesota (1976–1990). *Neurology*, **52**, 1214–20.

Braak, E., Griffing, K., Arai, K., Bohl, J., Bratzke, H., and Braak, H. (1999). Neuropathology of Alzheimer's disease: what is new since A. Alzheimer? *European Archives of Psychiatry and Clinical Neuroscience*, **249**, 14–22.

Brayne, C. (1991). The EURODEM collaborative re-analysis of case–control studies of Alzheimer's disease: implications for public health. *International Journal of Epidemiology*, **20**, S68–71.

Brayne, C., Gill, C., Huppert, F.A., *et al.* (1998). Vascular risks and incident dementia: results from a cohort study of the very old. *Dementia and Geriatric Cognitive Disorders*, **9**, 175–80.

Breitner, J.C. (1996). Inflammatory processes and antiinflammatory drugs in Alzheimer's disease: a current appraisal. *Neurobiology of Aging*, **17**, 789–94.

Brenner, D.E., Kukull, W.A., Stergachis, A., *et al.* (1994). Postmenopausal estrogen replacement therapy and the risk of Alzheimer's disease: a population-based case–control study. *American Journal of Epidemiology*, **140**, 262–7.

Breslau, N. and Davis, G.C. (1993). Migraine, physical health and psychiatric disorder: a prospective epidemiologic study in young adults. *Journal of Psychiatric Research*, **27**, 211–21.

Breslau, N., Davis, G.C., Schultz, L.R., and Peterson, E. L. (1994). Joint 1994 Wolff Award Presentation. Migraine and major depression: a longitudinal study. *Headache*, **34**, 387–93.

Breslau, N., Schultz, L.R., Stewart, W.F., Lipton, R.B., Lucia, V.C., and Welch, K.M. (2000). Headache and major depression: is the association specific to migraine? *Neurology*, **54**, 308–13.

Bressler, H., Keyes, W., Rochon, P., and Badley, E. (1999). The prevalence of low back pain in the elderly. *Spine*, **24**, 1813–19.

Breteler, M.M., Bots, M.L., Ott, A., and Hofman, A. (1998). Risk factors for vascular disease and dementia. *Haemostasis*, **28**, 167–73.

Brookmeyer, R., Gray, S., and Kawas, C. (1998). Projections of Alzheimer's disease in the United States and the public health impact of delaying disease onset. *American Journal of Public Health*, **88**, 1337–42.

Brown, J. (1975). Factors contributing to the development of low back pain in industrial workers. *Journal of the American Industrial Hygiene Association*, **36**, 26–31.

Bullido, M.J., Aldudo, J., Frank, A., Coria, F., Avila, J., and Valdivieso, F. (2000). A polymorphism in the tau gene associated with risk for Alzheimer's disease. *Neuroscience Letters*, **278**, 49–52.

Buring, J.E., Hebert, P., Romero, J., *et al.* (1995). Migraine and subsequent risk of stroke in the Physicians' Health Study. *Archives of Neurology*, **52**, 129–34.

Cady, R.K. (1999). Diagnosis and treatment of migraine. *Clinical Cornerstone*, **1**, 21–32.

Cady, L., Bischoff, D., O'Connell, E., *et al.* (1979). Strength and fitness and subsequent back injuries in fire fighters. *Journal of Occupational Medicine*, **21**, 269–72.

Caveness, W.F. (1979. Incidence of craniocerebral trauma in the United States in 1976 with trend from 1970 to 1975. *Advances in Neurology*, **22**, 1–3.

Celsis, P. (2000). Age-related cognitive decline, mild cognitive impairment or preclinical Alzheimer's disease? *Annals of Medicine*, **32**, 6–14.

Chang, C.L., Donaghy, M., and Poulter, N. (1999). Migraine and stroke in young women: case–control study. The World Health Organisation Collaborative Study of Cardiovascular Disease and Steroid Hormone Contraception. *British Medical Journal*, **318**, 13–18.

Checkoway, H. and Nelson, L.M. (1999). Epidemiologic approaches to the study of Parkinson's disease etiology. *Epidemiology*, **10**, 327–36.

Checkoway, H., Farin, F.M., Costa-Mallen, P., Kirchner, S.C., and Costa, L.G. (1998*a*). Genetic polymorphisms in Parkinson's disease. *Neurotoxicology*, **19**, 635–43.

Checkoway, H., Franklin, G.M., Costa-Mallen, P., *et al.* (1998*b*). A genetic polymorphism of MAO-B modifies the association of cigarette smoking and Parkinson's disease. *Neurology*, **50**, 1458–61.

Chio, A., Magnani, C., and Schiffer, D. (1998). Prevalence of Parkinson's disease in Northwestern Italy: comparison of tracer methodology and clinical ascertainment of cases. *Movement Disorders*, **13**, 400–5.

Chrischilles, E.A., Rubenstein, L.M., Voelker, M.D., Wallace, R.B., and Rodnitzky, R.L. (1998). The health burdens of Parkinson's disease. *Movement Disorders*, **13**, 406–13.

Christensen, P.M., Gotzsche, P.C., and Brosen, K. (1998). The sparteine/debrisoquine (CYP2D6) oxidation polymorphism and the risk of Parkinson's disease: a meta-analysis. *Pharmacogenetics*, **8**, 473–9.

Chui, H. and Gonthier, R. (1999). Natural history of vascular dementia. *Alzheimer Disease and Associated Disorders*, **13** (Supplement 3), S124–30.

Chui, H.C., Victoroff, J.I., Margolin, D., Jagust, W., Shankle, R., and Katzman, R. (1992). Criteria for the diagnosis of ischemic vascular dementia proposed by the State of California Alzheimer's Disease Diagnostic and Treatment Centers. *Neurology*, **42**, 473–80.

Chui, H.C., Mack, W., Jackson, J.E., *et al.* (2000). Clinical criteria for the diagnosis of vascular dementia: a multicenter study of comparability and interrater reliability. *Archives of Neurology*, **57**, 191–6.

Cobble N, Wangaard, C., Kraft, G., and Burks, J. (1993). Rehabilitation of the patients with multiple sclerosis. In *Rehabilitation medicine principles and practice* (ed. J. DeLisa and B. Gans), pp. 612–34. J.B. Lippincott, Philadelphia, PA.

Cockerell, O.C. (1996). The mortality of epilepsy. *Current Opinion in Neurology*, **9**, 93–6.

Colantonio, A., Dawson, D.R., and McLellan, B.A. (1998). Head injury in young adults: long-term outcome. *Archives of Physical Medicine and Rehabilitation*, **79**, 550–8.

Combs, C.K., Johnson, D.E., Karlo, J.C., Cannady, S.B., and Landreth, G.E. (2000). Inflammatory mechanisms in Alzheimer's disease: inhibition of beta-amyloid-stimulated proinflammatory responses and neurotoxicity by PPARgamma agonists. *Journal of Neuroscience*, **20**, 558–67.

Copeland, J.R., McCracken, C.F., Dewey, M.E. *et al.* (1999). Undifferentiated dementia, Alzheimer's disease and vascular dementia: age- and gender-related incidence in Liverpool. The MRC-ALPHA Study. *British Journal of Psychiatry*, **175**, 433–8.

Corder, E.H., Saunders, A.M., Strittmatter, W.J., *et al.* (1993). Gene dose of apolipoprotein E type 4 allele and the risk of Alzheimer's disease in late onset families. *Science*, **261**, 921–3.

Costa, P., Checkoway, H., Levy, D., *et al.* (1997). Association of a polymorphism in intron 13 of the monoamine oxidase B gene with Parkinson disease. *American Journal of Medical Genetics*, **74**, 154–6.

Costa, M.M., Reus, V.I., Wolkowitz, O.M., Manfredi, F., and Lieberman, M. (1999). Estrogen replacement therapy and cognitive decline in memory-impaired post-menopausal women. *Biological Psychiatry*, **46**, 182–8.

Costa-Mallen, P., Checkoway, H., Fishel, M., *et al.* (2000). The EcoRV genetic polymorphism of human monoamine oxidase type A is not associated with Parkinson's disease and does not modify the effect of smoking on Parkinson's disease. *Neuroscience Letters*, **278**, 33–6.

Croft, P., Papageorgiou, A., Thomas, E., Macfarlane, G., and Silman, A. (1999). Short-term physical risk factors for new episodes of low back pain. Prospective evidence from the South Manchester Back Pain Study. *Spine*, **24**, 1556–61.

Currie, C.J., Morgan, C.L., and Peters, J.R. (1998). The epidemiology and cost of inpatient care for peripheral vascular disease, infection, neuropathy, and ulceration in diabetes. *Diabetes Care*, **21**, 42–8.

Dean, G. (1967). Annual incidence, prevalence and mortality of MS in white South African-born and in white immigrants to South Africa. *British Medical Journal*, **2**, 724–30.

de Bittencourt, P.R., Adamolekum, B., Bharucha, N., *et al.* (1996). Epilepsy in the tropics: I. Epidemiology, socioeconomic risk factors, and etiology. *Epilepsia*, **37**, 1121–7.

de Boer, A.G., Sprangers, M.A., Speelman, H.D., and de Haes, H.C. (1999). Predictors of health care use in patients with Parkinson's disease: a longitudinal study. *Movement Disorders*, **14**, 772–9.

de Rijk, M.C., Breteler, M.M., Graveland, G.A., *et al.* (1995). Prevalence of Parkinson's disease in the elderly: the Rotterdam Study. *Neurology*, **45**, 2143–6.

de Rijk, M.C., Tzourio, C., Breteler, M.M., *et al.* (1997). Prevalence of parkinsonism and Parkinson's disease in Europe: the EUROPARKINSON Collaborative Study. European Community Concerted Action on the Epidemiology of Parkinson's disease. *Journal of Neurology, Neurosurgery and Psychiatry*, **62**, 10–15.

Delgado-Escueta, A.V., Medina, M.T., Serratosa, J.M., *et al.* (1999). Mapping and positional cloning of common idiopathic generalized epilepsies: juvenile myoclonus epilepsy and childhood absence epilepsy. *Advances in Neurology*,**79**, 351–74.

Demetriades, D., Murray, J., Sinz, B., *et al.* (1998). Epidemiology of major trauma and trauma deaths in Los Angeles County. *Journal of the American College of Surgeons*, **187**, 373–83.

Detels, R., Visscher, B.R., Malmgren, R.M., Coulson, A.H., Lucia, M.V., and Dudley J.P. (1977). Evidence for lower susceptibility to multiple sclerosis in Japanese Americans. *American Journal of Epidemiology*, **105**, 303–10.

Devereux, J., Buckle, P., and Vlachonikolis, I. (1999). Interactions between physical and psychosocial risk factors at work increase the risk of back disorders: an epidemiological approach. *Occupational and Environmental Medicine*, **56**, 343–53.

Deyo, R. and Bass, J. (1987). Lifestyles and low back pain: the influence of smoking, exercise, and obesity. *Clinical Research*, **35**, 577A.

Deyo, R. and Twui-Wu, Y. (1987). Descriptive epidemiology of low back pain and its related medical care in the United States. *Spine*, **12**, 264–8.

Dickson, D.W., Lin, W., Liu, W.K., and Yen, S.H. (1999). Multiple system atrophy: a sporadic synucleinopathy. *Brain Pathology*, **9**, 721–32.

Di Iorio, A., Zito, M., Lupinetti, M., and Abate, G. (1999). Are vascular factors involved in Alzheimer's disease? Facts and theories. *Aging (Milano)*, **11**, 345–52.

Dillane, J., Fry, J., and Katon, G. (1966). Acute back syndrome—a study from general practice. *British Medical Journal*, **2**, 82–4.

Dodel, R.C., Singer, M., Kohne-Volland, R., *et al.* (1998). The economic impact of Parkinson's disease. An estimation based on a 3-month prospective analysis. *Pharmacoeconomics*, **14**, 299–312.

Dodel, R.C., Du, Y., Bales, K.R., *et al.* (2000). Alpha2 macroglobulin and the risk of Alzheimer's disease. *Neurology*, **54**, 438–42.

Doll, R., Peto, R., Boreham, J., and Sutherland, I. (2000). Smoking and dementia in male British doctors: prospective study. *British Medical Journal*, **320**, 1097–102.

D'Souza, I., Poorkaj, P., Hong, M., *et al.* (1999). Missense and silent tau gene mutations cause frontotemporal dementia with parkinsonism-chromosome 17 type, by affecting multiple alternative RNA splicing regulatory elements. *Proceedings of the National Academy of Sciences of the United States of America*, **96**, 5598–603.

Duchowny, M. and Harvey, A.S. (1996). Pediatric epilepsy syndromes: an update and critical review. *Epilepsia*, **37**, S26–40.

Duggleby, T. and Kumar, S. (1997). Epidemiology of juvenile low back pain: a review. *Disability and Rehabilitation*, **19**, 505–12.

Durkin, M.S., Kuhn, L., Davidson, L.L., Laraque, D., and Barlow, B. (1996). Epidemiology and prevention of severe assault and gun injuries to children in an urban community. *Journal of Trauma*, **41**, 667–73.

Dyck, P.J., Davies, J.L., Litchy, W.J., and O'Brien, P.C. (1997). Longitudinal assessment of diabetic polyneuropathy using a composite score in the Rochester Diabetic Neuropathy Study cohort. *Neurology*, **49**, 229–39.

Dyck, P.J., Davies, J.L., Wilson, D.M., Service, F.J., Melton, III, L.J., and O'Brien, P.C. (1999). Risk factors for severity of diabetic polyneuropathy: intensive longitudinal assessment of the Rochester Diabetic Neuropathy Study cohort. *Diabetes Care*, **22**, 1479–86.

Elliott, A., Smith, B., Penny, K., Smith, W., and Chambers, W. (1999). The epidemiology of chronic pain in the comunity. *Lancet*, **354**, 1248–52.

Eriksen, W., Natvig, B., and Bruusgaard, D. (1999). Smoking, heavy physical work and low back pain: a four-year prospective study. *Occupational Medicine*, **49**, 155–60.

Evans, D.A., Funkenstein, H.H., Albert, M.S., *et al.* (1989). Prevalence of Alzheimer's disease in a community population of older persons. Higher than previously reported. *Journal of the American Medical Association*, **262**, 2551–6.

Fall, P.A., Axelson, O., Fredriksson, M., *et al.* (1996). Age-standardized incidence and prevalence of Parkinson's disease in a Swedish community. *Journal of Clinical Epidemiology*, **49**, 637–41.

Farrer, L.A., Cupples, L.A., Haines, J.L., *et al.* (1997). Effects of age, sex, and ethnicity on the association between apolipoprotein E genotype and Alzheimer disease. A meta-analysis. apolipoprotein E and Alzheimer Disease Meta Analysis Consortium. *Journal of the American Medical Association*, **278**, 1349–56.

Ferguson, R.J., Mittenberg, W., Barone, D.F., and Schneider, B. (1999). Postconcussion syndrome following sports-related head injury: expectation as etiology. *Neuropsychology*, **13**, 582–9.

Ficker, D.M., So, E.L., Shen, W.K., *et al.* (1998). Population-based study of the incidence of sudden unexplained death in epilepsy. *Neurology*, **51**, 1270–4.

Franceschi, M., Colombo, B., Rossi, P., and Canal, N. (1997). Headache in a population-based elderly cohort. An ancillary study to the Italian Longitudinal Study of Aging (ILSA). *Headache*, **37**, 79–82.

Franklin, G.M., Haug, J., Heyer, N., Checkoway, H., and Peck, N. (1991). Occupational carpal tunnel syndrome in Washington State, 1984–1988. *American Journal of Public Health*, **81**, 741–6.

Fratiglioni, L., De Ronchi, D., and Aguero-Torres, H. (1999). Worldwide prevalence and incidence of dementia. *Drugs Aging*, **15**, 365–75.

Frymoyer, J. (1988). Back pain and sciatica. *New England Journal of Medicine*, **318**, 291–300.

Frymoyer, J., Pope, M., Clements, J., Wilder, D., McPherson, B., and Ashikaga, T. (1983). Risk factors in low back pain. *Journal of Bone and Joint Surgery, American Volume*, **65A**, 213–18.

Gainotti, G., Marra, C., Villa, G., Parlato, V., and Chiarotti, F. (1998). Sensitivity and specificity of some neuropsychological markers of Alzheimer dementia. *Alzheimer Disease and Associated Disorders*, **12**, 152–62.

Geerlings, M.I., Deeg, D.J., Penninx, B.W., *et al.* (1999*a*). Cognitive reserve and mortality in dementia: the role of cognition, functional ability and depression. *Psychological Medicine*, **29**, 1219–26.

Geerlings, M.I., Schmand, B., Jonker, C., Lindeboom, J., and Bouter, L.M. (1999*b*). Education and incident Alzheimer's disease: a biased association due to selective attrition and use of a two-step diagnostic procedure? *International Journal of Epidemiology*, **28**, 492–7.

Gelb, D.J., Oliver, E., and Gilman, S. (1999). Diagnostic criteria for Parkinson disease. *Archives of Neurology*, **56**, 33–9.

Gervil, M., Ulrich, V., Kyvik, K.O., Olesen, J., and Russell, M.B. (1999). Migraine without aura: a population-based twin study. *Annals of Neurology*, **46**, 606–11.

Ghetti, B., Murrell, J., and Spillantini, M.G. (1999). Mutations in the Tau gene cause frontotemporal dementia. *Brain Research Bulletin*, **50**, 471–2.

Gibson, A.M., Singleton, A.B., Smith, G., *et al.* (2000). Lack of association of the alpha2-macroglobulin locus on chromosome 12 in AD. *Neurology*, **54**, 433–8.

Gilman, S., Low, P., Quinn, N., *et al.* (1998). Consensus statement on the diagnosis of multiple system atrophy. American Autonomic Society and American Academy of Neurology. *Clinical Autonomic Research*, **8**, 359–62.

Gilthorpe, M.S., Wilson, R.C., Moles, D.R., and Bedi, R. (1999). Variations in admissions to hospital for head injury and assault to the head. Part 1: Age and gender. *British Journal of Oral and Maxillofacial Surgery*, **37**, 294–300.

Gobel, H., Petersen-Braun, M., and Soyka, D. (1994). The epidemiology of headache in Germany: a nationwide survey of a representative sample on the basis of the headache classification of the International Headache Society. *Cephalalgia*, **14**, 97–106.

Goedert, M. and Spillantini, M.G. (1998). Lewy body diseases and multiple system atrophy as alpha- synucleinopathies (editorial; see comment). *Molecular Psychiatry*, **3**, 462–5.

Gordis, L. (1996). *Epidemiology*. W.B. Saunders, Philadelphia, PA.

Gordon, N. (1994). Review: juvenile myoclonic epilepsy. *Child Care Health Development*, **20**, 71–6.

Gorelick, P.B., Erkinjuntti, T., Hofman, A., Rocca, W.A., Skoog, I., and Winblad, B. (1999). Prevention of vascular dementia. *Alzheimer Disease and Associated Disorders*, **13** (Supplement 3), S131–9.

Gorell, J.M., Johnson, C.C., Rybicki, B.A., Peterson, E.L., and Richardson, R.J. (1998). The risk of Parkinson's disease with exposure to pesticides, farming, well water, and rural living. *Neurology*, **50**, 1346–50.

Gorell, J.M., Johnson, C.C., Rybicki, B.A., *et al.* (1999*a*). Occupational exposure to manganese, copper, lead, iron, mercury and zinc and the risk of Parkinson's disease. *Neurotoxicology*, **20**, 239–47.

Gorell, J.M., Rybicki, B.A., Cole Johnson, C., and Peterson, E.L. (1999*b*). Occupational metal exposures and the risk of Parkinson's disease. *Neuroepidemiology*, **18**, 303–8.

Goulding, J.M., Signorini, D.F., Chatterjee, S., *et al.* (1999). Inverse relation between Braak stage and cerebrovascular pathology in Alzheimer predominant dementia. *Journal of Neurology, Neurosurgery and Psychiatry*, **67**, 654–7.

Grunewald, R.A. and Panayiotopoulos, C.P. (1993). Juvenile myoclonic epilepsy. A review. *Archives of Neurology*, **50**, 594–8.

Guo, H., Tanaka, S., Halperin, W., and Cameron, L. (1999). Back pain prevalence in US industry and estimates of lost workdays. *American Journal of Public Health*, **89**, 1029–35.

Hachinski, V. (1983). Multi-infarct dementia. *Neurology Clinics*, **1**, 27–36.

Hachinski, V.C. (1990). The decline and resurgence of vascular dementia. *Canadian Medical Association Journal*, **142**, 107–11.

Hachinski, V.C. (1991). Multi-infarct dementia: a reappraisal. *Alzheimer Disease and Associated Disorders*, **5**, 64–8.

Hachinski, V. (1994). Vascular dementia: a radical redefinition. *Dementia*, **5**, 130–2.

Hall, K.S., Gao, S., Unverzagt, F.W., and Hendrie, H.C. (2000). Low education and childhood rural residence: risk for Alzheimer's disease in African Americans. *Neurology*, **54**, 95–9.

Hanna, P.A., Jankovic, J., and Kirkpatrick, J.B. (1999). Multiple system atrophy: the putative causative role of environmental toxins. *Archives of Neurology*, **56**, 90–4.

Hardy, J., Duff, K., Hardy, K.G., Perez-Tur, J., and Hutton, M. (1998). Genetic dissection of Alzheimer's disease and related dementias: amyloid and its relationship to tau. *Nature Neurosciences*, **1**, 355–8. (Erratum: *Nature Neurosciences*, **1**, 743, 1998.)

Haskell, S.G., Richardson, E.D., and Horwitz, R.I. (1997). The effect of estrogen replacement therapy on cognitive function in women: a critical review of the literature. *Journal of Clinical* Epidemiology, **50**, 1249–64.

Hauser, W.A. (1995). Epidemiology of epilepsy in children. *Neurosurgery Clinics of North America*, **6**, 419–29.

Hauser, W.A., Annegers, J.F., and Rocca, W.A. (1996). Descriptive epidemiology of epilepsy: contributions of population-based studies from Rochester, Minnesota. *Mayo Clinic Proceedings*, **71**, 576–86.

Hedges, III, T.R., Hirano, M., Tucker, K., and Caballero, B. (1997). Epidemic optic and peripheral neuropathy in Cuba: a unique geopolitical public health problem. *Surveys in Ophthalmology*, **41**, 341–53.

Henderson, V.W. (1997*a*). The epidemiology of estrogen replacement therapy and Alzheimer's disease. *Neurology*, **48**, S27–35.

Henderson, V.W. (1997*b*). Estrogen, cognition, and a woman's risk of Alzheimer's disease. *American Journal of Medicine*, **103**, 11S–18S.

Henderson, V.W., Paganini-Hill, A., Miller, B.L., *et al.* (2000). Estrogen for Alzheimer's disease in women: randomized, double-blind, placebo-controlled trial. *Neurology*, **54**, 295–301.

Hendrie, H.C. (1998). Epidemiology of dementia and Alzheimer's disease. *American Journal of Geriatric Psychiatry*, **6**, S3–18.

Hillier, S.L., Hiller, J.E., and Metzer, J. (1997). Epidemiology of traumatic brain injury in South Australia. *Brain Injury*, **11**, 649–59.

Hirano, M., Shtilbans, A., Mayeux, R., *et al.* (1997). Apparent mtDNA heteroplasmy in Alzheimer's disease patients and in normals due to PCR amplification of nucleus-embedded mtDNA pseudogenes. *Proceedings of the National Academy of Sciences of the United States of America*, **94**, 14894–9.

Hoogendoorn, W., van Poppel, M., Bongers, P., Koes, B., and Bouter, L. (1999). Physical load during work and leisure time as risk factors for back pain. *Scandinavian Journal of Work and Environmental Health*, **25**, 387–403.

Hu, X.H., Markson, L.E., Lipton, R.B., Stewart, W.F., and Berger, M.L. (1999). Burden of migraine in the United States: disability and economic costs. *Archives of Internal Medicine*, **159**, 813–18.

Hulette, C.M., Pericak-Vance, M.A., Roses, A.D., *et al.* (1999). Neuropathological features of frontotemporal dementia and parkinsonism linked to chromosome 17q21-22 (FTDP-17): Duke Family 1684. *Journal of Neuropathology and Experimental Neurology*, **58**, 859–66.

Hussain, I., Powell, D., Howlett, D.R., *et al.* (1999). Identification of a novel aspartic protease (Asp 2) as beta-secretase. *Molecular Cell Neuroscience*, **14**, 419–27.

Hutchin, T.P., Heath, P.R., Pearson, R.C., and Sinclair, A.J. (1997). Mitochondrial DNA mutations in Alzheimer's disease. *Biochemical and Biophysical Research Communications*, **241**, 221–5.

in 't Veld, B.A., Launer, L.J., Hoes, A.W., *et al.* (1998). NSAIDs and incident Alzheimer's disease. The Rotterdam Study. *Neurobiology of Aging*, **19**, 607–11.

Ingebrigtsen, T., Mortensen, K., and Romner, B. (1998). The epidemiology of hospital-referred head injury in northern Norway. *Neuroepidemiology*, **17**, 139–46.

International League Against Epilepsy (1997). The epidemiology of the epilepsies: future directions. International League Against Epilepsy Commission Report. *Epilepsia*, **38**, 614–18.

Jankovic, J., Rajput, A.H., McDermott, M.P., and Perl, D.P. (2000). The evolution of diagnosis in early Parkinson disease. Parkinson Study Group. *Archives of Neurology*, **57**, 369–72.

Jenny, C., Hymel, K.P., Ritzen, A., Reinert, S.E., and Hay, T.C. (1999). Analysis of missed cases of abusive head trauma. *Journal of the American Medical Association*, **281**, 621–6. (Erratum: *Journal of the American Medical Association*, **282**, 29, 1999.)

Jones, A.C., Yamamura, Y., Almasy, L., *et al.* (1998). Autosomal recessive juvenile parkinsonism maps to 6q25.2-q27 in four ethnic groups: detailed genetic mapping of the linked region. *American Journal of Human Genetics*, **63**, 80–7.

Joost, O., Taylor, C.A., Thomas, C.A., *et al.* (1999). Absence of effect of seven functional mutations in the CYP2D6 gene in Parkinson's disease. *Movement Disorders*, **14**, 590–5.

Jorm, A.F. and Jolley, D. (1998). The incidence of dementia: a meta-analysis. *Neurology*, **51**, 728–33.

Katz, J.N., Lew, R.A., Bessette, L., *et al.* (1998). Prevalence and predictors of long-term work disability due to carpal tunnel syndrome. *American Journal of Industrial Medicine*, **33**, 543–50.

Kaufmann, H. (1998). Multiple system atrophy. *Current Opinion in Neurology*, **11**, 351–5.

Kawas, C., Resnick, S., Morrison, A., *et al.* (1997). A prospective study of estrogen replacement therapy and the risk of developing Alzheimer's disease: the Baltimore Longitudinal Study of Aging. *Neurology*, **48**, 1517–21. (Erratum: *Neurology*, **51**, 654, 1998.)

Kelsey, J. (1975). An epidemiological study of acute herniated lumbar intervertebral disc. *Rheumatology and Rehabilitation*, **14**, 144–59.

Kelsey, J., White, A., Pastides, H., and Brobee, G. (1979). The impact of musculosketetal disorders on the population of the United States. *Journal of Bone and Joint Surgery*, **61**, 959–64.

Klein, B., Jenson, R., and Sandstrom, L. (1984). Assessment of workers' compensation claims for back strains/sprains. *Journal of Occupational Medicine*, **26**, 443–8.

Kramer, U. (1999). Epilepsy in the first year of life: a review. *Journal of Child Neurology*, **14**, 485–9.

Kramer, U., Nevo, Y., Neufeld, M.Y., Fatal, A., Leitner, Y., and Harel, S. (1998). Epidemiology of epilepsy in childhood: a cohort of 440 consecutive patients. *Pediatric Neurology*, **18**, 46–50.

Krause, N., Ragland, D., Fisher, J., and Syme, S. (1998). Psychosocial job factors, physical workload, and incidence of work-related spinal injury: a 5-year prospective study of urban transit operators. *Spine*, **23**, 2507–16.

Kuopio, A.M., Marttila, R.J., Helenius, H., and Rinne, U.K. (1999). Environmental risk factors in Parkinson's disease. *Movement Disorders*, **14**, 928–39.

Kurtzke, J. (1982). The current neurologic burden of illness and injury in the United States. *Neurology*, **32**, 1207–14.

Kusumi, M., Nakashima, K., Harada, H., Nakayama, H., and Takahashi, K. (1996). Epidemiology of Parkinson's disease in Yonago City, Japan: comparison with a study carried out 12 years ago. *Neuroepidemiology*, **15**, 201–7.

Lam, W.H. and MacKersie, A. (1999). Paediatric head injury: incidence, aetiology and management. *Paediatric Anaesthesia*, **9**, 377–85.

Langston, J.W. (1998). Epidemiology versus genetics in Parkinson's disease: progress in resolving an age-old debate. *Annals of Neurology*, **44**, S45–52.

Lantos, P.L. (1998). The definition of multiple system atrophy: a review of recent developments. *Journal of Neuropathology and Experimental Neurology*, **57**, 1099–111.

Larson, D.B., Lyons, J.S., Bareta, J.C., Burns, B.J., Blazer, D.G., and Goldstrom, I.D. (1989). The construct validity of the ischemic score of Hachinski for the detection of dementias. *Journal of Neuropsychiatry and Clinical Neurosciences*, **1**, 181–7.

Launer, L.J., Andersen, K., Dewey, M.E., *et al.* (1999). Rates and risk factors for dementia and Alzheimer's disease: results from EURODEM pooled analyses. EURODEM Incidence Research Group and Work Groups. European Studies of Dementia. *Neurology*, **52**, 78–84.

Lavados, P.M. and Tenhamm, E. (1997). Epidemiology of migraine headache in Santiago, Chile: a prevalence study. *Cephalalgia*, **17**, 770–7.

Leboeuf-Yde, C. (1999). A systematic literature review of 41 journal articles reporting 47 epidemiologic studies. *Spine*, **24**, 1463–70.

Lee, P.N. (1994). Smoking and Alzheimer's disease: a review of the epidemiological evidence. *Neuroepidemiology*, **13**, 131–44.

Leidy, N.K., Elixhauser, A., Vickrey, B., Means, E., and Willian, M.K. (1999). Seizure frequency and the health-related quality of life of adults with epilepsy. *Neurology*, **53**, 162–6.

Leppert, M.F. and Singh, N. (1999). Susceptibility genes in human epilepsy. (In Process Citation.) *Seminars in Neurology*, **19**, 397–405.

Levy Lahad, E., Tsuang, D., and Bird, T.D. (1998). Recent advances in the genetics of Alzheimer's disease. *Journal of Geriatric Psychiatry and Neurology*, **11**, 42–54.

Leys, D., Erkinjuntti, T., Desmond, D.W., *et al.* (1999). Vascular dementia: the role of cerebral infarcts. *Alzheimer Disease and Associated Disorders*, **13** (Supplement 3), S38–48.

Liao, A., Nitsch, R.M., Greenberg, S.M., *et al.* (1998). Genetic association of an alpha2-macroglobulin (Val1000lle) polymorphism and Alzheimer's disease. *Human Molecular Genetics*, **7**, 1953–6.

Lilius, L., Froelich Fabre, S., Basun, H., *et al.* (1999). Tau gene polymorphisms and apolipoprotein E epsilon4 may interact to increase risk for Alzheimer's disease. *Neuroscience Letters*, **277**, 29–32.

Linn, S., Smith, D., and Sheps, S. (1998). Epidemiology of bicycle injury, head injury, and helmet use among children in British Columbia: a five year descriptive study. Canadian Hospitals Injury, Reporting and Prevention Program (CHIRPP). *Injury Prevention*, **4**, 122–5.

Lipton, R.B. (1998). Comorbidity in migraine—causes and effects. *Cephalalgia*, **18** (Supplement 22), 8–11; discussion 11–14.

Loiseau, J., Picot, M.C., and Loiseau, P. (1999). Short-term mortality after a first epileptic seizure: a population-based study. *Epilepsia*, **40**, 1388–92.

Lopes-Cendes, I., Scheffer, I.E., Berkovic, S.F., Rousseau, M., Andermann, E., and Rouleau, G.A. (2000). A new locus for generalized epilepsy with febrile seizures plus maps to chromosome 2. (In Process Citation.) *American Journal of Human Genetics*, **66**, 698–701.

Lund and Manchester Groups (1994). Clinical and neuropathological criteria for frontotemporal dementia. *Journal of Neurology, Neurosurgery and Psychiatry*, **57**, 416–18.

Luukinen, H., Herala, M., Koski, K., Kivela, S.L., and Honkanen, R. (1999). Rapid increase of fall-related severe head injuries with age among older people: a population-based study. *Journal of the American Geriatric Society*, **47**, 1451–2.

McEwen, B.S. and Alves, S.E. (1999). Estrogen actions in the central nervous system. *Endocrine Reviews*, **20**, 279–307.

McGeer, P.L., Schulzer, M., and McGeer, E.G. (1996). Arthritis and anti-inflammatory agents as possible protective factors for Alzheimer's disease: a review of 17 epidemiologic studies. *Neurology*, **47**, 425–32.

McGugan, E.A. (1999). Sudden unexpected deaths in epileptics—a literature review. *Scottish Medical Journal*, **44**, 137–9.

McKeith, I.G., Perry, R.H., Fairbairn, A.F., Jabeen, S., and Perry, E.K. (1992). Operational criteria for senile dementia of Lewy body type (SDLT). *Psychological Medicine*, **22**, 911–22.

McKhann, G., Drachman, D., Folstein, M., Katzman, R., Price, D., and Stadlan, E.M. (1984). Clinical diagnosis of Alzheimer's disease: report of the NINCDS-ADRDA Work Group under the auspices of Department of Health and Human Services Task Force on Alzheimer's Disease. *Neurology*, **34**, 939–44.

MacMahon, B. and Trichopoulos, D. (1996). *Epidemiology: principles and methods* (2nd edn). Little, Brown, Boston, MA.

Marder, K. and Mayeux, R. (1991). The epidemiology of dementia in patients with Parkinson's disease. *Advances in Experimental Medical Biology*, **295**, 439–45.

Marder, K., Logroscino, G., Alfaro, B., *et al.* (1998). Environmental risk factors for Parkinson's disease in an urban multiethnic community. *Neurology*, **50**, 279–81.

Marder, K., Tang, M.X., Alfaro, B., *et al.* (1999). Risk of Alzheimer's disease in relatives of Parkinson's disease patients with and without dementia. *Neurology*, **52**, 719–24.

Mayeux, R., Saunders, A.M., Shea, S., *et al.* (1998). Utility of the apolipoprotein E genotype in the diagnosis of Alzheimer's disease. Alzheimer's Disease Centers Consortium on Apolipoprotein E and Alzheimer's Disease. *New England Journal of Medicine*, **338**, 506–11. (Erratum: *New England Journal of Medicine*, **338**, 1325, 1998.)

Mehta, K.M., Ott, A., Kalmijn, S., Slooter, A.J., van Duijn, C.M., Hofman, A., and Breteler, M.M. (1999). Head trauma and risk of dementia and Alzheimer's disease. The Rotterdam Study. *Neurology*, **53**, 1959–62.

Meier-Ruge, W.A. and Bertoni-Freddari, C. (1999). Mitochondrial genome lesions in the pathogenesis of sporadic Alzheimer's disease. *Gerontology*, **45**, 289–97.

Menegon, A., Board, P.G., Blackburn, A.C., Mellick, G.D., and Le Couteur, D.G. (1998). Parkinson's disease, pesticides, and glutathione transferase polymorphisms. *Lancet*, **352**, 1344–6.

Merchant, C., Tang, M.X., Albert, S., Manly, J., Stern, Y., and Mayeux, R. (1999). The influence of smoking on the risk of Alzheimer's disease. *Neurology*, **52**, 1408–12.

Merikangas, K.R., Whitaker, A.E., Isler, H., and Angst, J. (1994). The Zurich Study: XXIII. Epidemiology of headache syndromes in the Zurich cohort study of young adults. *European Archives in Psychiatry and Clinical Neuroscience*, **244**, 145–52.

Merikangas, K.R., Fenton, B.T., Cheng, S.H., Stolar, M.J., and Risch, N. (1997). Association between migraine and stroke in a large-scale epidemiological study of the United States. *Archives of Neurology*, **54**, 362–8.

Meyer, J.S., Rauch, G.M., Rauch, R.A., Haque, A., and Crawford, K. (2000). Cardiovascular and other risk factors for Alzheimer's disease and vascular dementia. (In Process Citation.) *Annals of the New York Academy of Sciences*, **903**, 411–23.

Minden, S., Marder, W., Harrold, L., and Dor, A. (1993). *Multiple sclerosis: a statistical portrait.* ABT Associates, Cambridge.

Mitchell, P., Wang, J.J., Currie, J., Cumming, R.G., and Smith, W. (1998). Prevalence and vascular associations with migraine in older Australians. *Australian and New Zealand Journal of Medicine*, **28**, 627–32.

Moceri, V.M., Kukull, W.A., Emanuel, I., van Belle, G., and Larson, E.B. (2000). Early-life risk factors and the development of Alzheimer's disease. *Neurology*, **54**, 415–20.

Moles, D.R., Gilthorpe, M.S., Wilson, R.C., and Bedi, R. (1999). Variations in admission to hospital for head injury and assault to the head. Part 2: Ethnic group. *British Journal of Oral and Maxillofacial Surgery*, **37**, 301–8.

Monahan, K. and O'Leary, K.D. (1999). Head injury and battered women: an initial inquiry. *Health and Social Work*, **24**, 269–78.

Morgante, L., Rocca, W.A., Di Rosa, A.E., *et al.* (1992). Prevalence of Parkinson's disease and other types of parkinsonism: a door-to-door survey in three Sicilian municipalities. The Sicilian Neuro-Epidemiologic Study (SNES) Group. *Neurology*, **42**, 1901–7.

Morris, M.C., Beckett, L.A., Scherr, P.A., *et al.* (1998). Vitamin E and vitamin C supplement use and risk of incident Alzheimer disease. *Alzheimer Disease and Associated Disorders*, **12**, 121–6.

Mortimer, J.A. (1998). New findings consistent with Alzheimer's-NSAIDs link. *Neurobiology of Aging*, **19**, 615–18.

Moyle, G.J. and Sadler, M. (1998). Peripheral neuropathy with nucleoside antiretrovirals: risk factors, incidence and management. *Drug Safety*, **19**, 481–94.

Muller-Spahn, F. and Hock, C. (1999). Risk factors and differential diagnosis of Alzheimer's disease. *European Archives in Psychiatry and Clinical Neuroscience*, **249**, 37–42.

Mulnard, R.A., Cotman, C.W., Kawas, C., *et al.* (2000). Estrogen replacement therapy for treatment of mild to moderate Alzheimer disease: a randomized controlled trial. Alzheimer's Disease Cooperative Study. *Journal of the American Medical Association*, **283**, 1007–15.

Multiple Sclerosis Genetics Group (1996). A complete genome screen for multiple sclerosis underscores a role for the major histocompatibility complex. *Nature Genetics*, **13**, 469–71.

Munoz, D.G., Ganapathy, G.R., Eliasziw, M., and Hachinski, V. (2000). Educational attainment and socioeconomic status of patients with autopsy-confirmed Alzheimer disease. *Archives of Neurology*, **57**, 85–9.

Murphy, Jr, R.X., Birmingham, K.L., Okunski, W.J., and Wasser, T. (2000). The influence of airbag and restraining devices on the patterns of facial trauma in motor vehicle collisions. (In Process Citation.) *Plastic Reconstructive Surgery*, **105**, 516–20.

National Institutes of Health (1998). Rehabilitation of persons with traumatic brain injury. *NIH Consensus Statement 1998 Oct 26–28*, **16**, 1–41.

Nee, L.E. and Lippa, C.F. (1999). Alzheimer's disease in 22 twin pairs—13-year follow-up: hormonal, infectious and traumatic factors. *Dementia and Geriatric Cognitive Disorders*, **10**, 148–51.

Nicoletti, A., Reggio, A., Bartoloni, A., *et al.* (1998). A neuroepidemiological survey in rural Bolivia: background and methods. *Neuroepidemiology*, **17**, 273–80.

Nicoletti, A., Reggio, A., Bartoloni, A., *et al.* (1999). Prevalence of epilepsy in rural Bolivia: a door-to-door survey. *Neurology*, **53**, 2064–9.

Nicoll, J.A., Mrak, R.E., Graham, D.I., *et al.* (2000). Association of interleukin-1 gene polymorphisms with Alzheimer's disease. *Annals of Neurology*, **47**, 365–8.

Nilsson, L., Tomson, T., Farahmand, B.Y., Diwan, V., and Persson, P.G. (1997). Cause-specific mortality in epilepsy: a cohort study of more than 9,000 patients once hospitalized for epilepsy. *Epilepsia*, **38**, 1062–8.

Nilsson, L., Farahmand, B.Y., Persson, P.G., Thiblin, I., and Tomson, T. (1999). Risk factors for sudden unexpected death in epilepsy: a case–control study. *Lancet*, **353**, 888–93.

Noebels, J.L. (1999). Single-gene models of epilepsy. *Advances in Neurology*, **79**, 227–38.

Nordstrom, D.L., DeStefano, F., Vierkant, R.A., and Layde, P.M. (1998). Incidence of diagnosed carpal tunnel syndrome in a general population. *Epidemiology*, **9**, 342–5.

Nourhashemi, F., Gillette-Guyonnet, S., Andrieu, S., *et al.* (2000). Alzheimer disease: protective factors. *American Journal of Clinical Nutrition*, **71**, 643S–649S.

Nyenhuis, D.L. and Gorelick, P.B. (1998). Vascular dementia: a contemporary review of epidemiology, diagnosis, prevention, and treatment. *Journal of the American Geriatric Society*, **46**, 1437–48.

Nyholt, D.R., Dawkins, J.L., Brimage, P.J., Goadsby, P.J., Nicholson, G.A., and Griffiths, L.R. (1998). Evidence for an X-linked genetic component in familial typical migraine. *Human Molecular Genetics*, **7**, 459–63.

O'Brien, B., Goeree, R., and Streiner, D. (1994). Prevalence of migraine headache in Canada: a population-based survey. *International Journal of Epidemiology*, **23**, 1020–6.

Octave, J.N., Essalmani, R., Tasiaux, B., Menager, J., Czech, C., and Mercken, L. (2000). The role of presenilin-1 in the gamma-secretase cleavage of the amyloid precursor protein of Alzheimer's disease. *Journal of Biological Chemistry*, **275**, 1525–8.

Oertel, W.H. (1995). Parkinson's disease: epidemiology, (differential) diagnosis, therapy, relation to dementia. *Arzneimittelforschung*, **45**, 386–9.

Oertel, W.H. and Bandmann, O. (1999). Multiple system atrophy. *Journal of Neural Transmission Supplement*, **56**, 155–64.

Olafsson, E. and Hauser, W.A. (1999). Prevalence of epilepsy in rural Iceland: a population-based study. *Epilepsia*, **40**, 1529–34.

Orchard, T.J., Ce, L.L., Maser, R.E., and Kuller, L.H. (1996). Why does diabetic autonomic neuropathy predict IDDM mortality? An analysis from the Pittsburgh Epidemiology of Diabetes Complications Study. *Diabetes Research and Clinical Practice*, **34** (Supplement), S165–71.

Osuntokun, B.O., Adeuja, A.O., Nottidge, V.A., *et al.* (1992). Prevalence of headache and migrainous headache in Nigerian Africans: a community-based study. *East Africa Medical Journal*, **69**, 196–9.

Ott, A., Breteler, M.M., van Harskamp, F., Stijnen, T., and Hofman, A. (1998). Incidence and risk of dementia. The Rotterdam Study. *American Journal of Epidemiology*, **147**, 574–80.

Ottman, R. (1997). Genetic epidemiology of epilepsy. *Epidemiology Reviews*, **19**, 120–8.

Ottman, R. and Susser, M. (1992). Data collection strategies in genetic epidemiology: The Epilepsy Family Study of Columbia University. *Journal of Clinical Epidemiology*, **45**, 721–7.

Ottman, R., Annegers, J.F., Risch, N., Hauser, W.A., and Susser, M. (1996). Relations of genetic and environmental factors in the etiology of epilepsy. *Annals of Neurology*, **39**, 442–9.

Palacio, L.G., Jimenez, I., Garcia, H.H., *et al.* (1998). Neurocysticercosis in persons with epilepsy in Medellin, Colombia. The Neuroepidemiological Research Group of Antioquia. *Epilepsia*, **39**, 1334–9.

Pantoni, L. and Inzitari, D. (1993). Hachinski's ischemic score and the diagnosis of vascular dementia: a review. *Italian Journal of Neurological Sciences*, **14**, 539–46.

Parry, O., Mielke, J., Latif, A.S., Ray, S., Levy, L.F., and Siziya, S. (1997). Peripheral neuropathy in individuals with HIV infection in Zimbabwe. *Acta Neurologica Scandinavica*, **96**, 218–22.

Payami, H. and Zareparsi, S. (1998). Genetic epidemiology of Parkinson's disease. *Journal of Geriatric Psychiatry and Neurology*, **11**, 98–106.

Pericak-Vance, M.A., Bass, M.P., Yamaoka, L.H., *et al.* (1997). Complete genomic screen in late-onset familial Alzheimer disease. Evidence for a new locus on chromosome 12. *Journal of the American Medical Association*, **278**, 1237–41.

Peroutka, S.J. (1998). Genetic basis of migraine. *Clinical Neurosciences*, **5**, 34–7.

Perry, I.J. (1999). Homocysteine and risk of stroke. *Journal of Cardiovascular Risk*, **6**, 235–40.

Petersen, R.C., Smith, G.E., Waring, S.C., Ivnik, R.J., Tangalos, E.G., and Kokmen, E. (1999). Mild cognitive impairment: clinical characterization and outcome. *Archives of Neurology*, **56**, 303–8. (Erratum: *Archives of Neurology*, **56**, 760, 1999.)

Phillips, H.A., Scheffer, I.E., Crossland, K.M., *et al.* (1998). Autosomal dominant nocturnal frontal-lobe epilepsy: genetic heterogeneity and evidence for a second locus at 15q24. *American Journal of Human Genetics*, **63**, 1108–16.

Phimister, B. (2000). Four companies announce discovery of beta-secretase gene. *Natural Biotechnology*, **18**, 16.

Picavet, H., Schouten, J., and Smit, H. (1999). Prevalence and consequences of low back problems in The Netherlands, working vs non-working population, the MORGEN-Study. Monitoring Project on Risk Factors for Chronic Disease. *Public Health*, **113**, 73–7.

Pine, D.S., Cohen, P., and Brook, J. (1996). The association between major depression and headache: results of a longitudinal epidemiologic study in youth. *Journal of Child and Adolescent Psychopharmacology*, **6**, 153–64.

Plaster, N.M., Uyama, E., Uchino, M., *et al.* (1999). Genetic localization of the familial adult myoclonic epilepsy (FAME) gene to chromosome 8q24. *Neurology*, **53**, 1180–3.

Poser, S., Scheidt, P., Kitz, B., *et al.* (1991). Impact of magnetic resonance imaging (MRI) on the epidemiology of MS. *Acta Neurologica Scandinavica*, **83**, 172–5.

Price, D.L., Tanzi, R.E., Borchelt, D.R., and Sisodia, S.S. (1998). Alzheimer's disease: genetic studies and transgenic models. *Annual Review of Genetics*, **32**, 461–93.

Puder, D.R., Visintainer, P., Spitzer, D., and Casal, D. (1999). A comparison of the effect of different bicycle helmet laws in 3 New York City suburbs. *American Journal of Public Health*, **89**, 1736–8.

Rayan, G.M. (1999). Carpal tunnel syndrome between two centuries. *Journal of the Oklahoma State Medical Association*, **92**, 493–503.

Reigo, T., Timpka, T., and Tropp, H. (1999). The epidemiology of back pain in vocational age groups. *Scandinavian Journal of Primary Health Care*, **17**, 17–21.

Riley, K.P., Snowdon, D.A., Saunders, A.M., Roses, A.D., Mortimer, J.A., and Nanayakkara, N. (2000). Cognitive function and apolipoprotein E in very old adults: findings from the Nun Study. (In Process Citation.) *Journal of Gerontology Series B, Psychological Sciences and Social Sciences*, **55**, S69–75.

Rivara, F.P., Thompson, D.C., and Thompson, R.S. (1997). Epidemiology of bicycle injuries and risk factors for serious injury. *Injury Prevention*, **3**, 110–14.

Rocca, W.A., Cha, R.H., Waring, S.C., and Kokmen, E. (1998). Incidence of dementia and Alzheimer's disease: a reanalysis of data from Rochester, Minnesota, 1975–1984. *American Journal of Epidemiology*, **148**, 51–62.

Rockwood, K., Bowler, J., Erkinjuntti, T., Hachinski, V., and Wallin, A. (1999). Subtypes of vascular dementia. *Alzheimer Disease and Associated Disorders*, **13** (Supplement 3), S59–65.

Rockwood, K., Wentzel, C., Hachinski, V., Hogan, D.B., MacKnight, C., and McDowell, I. (2000). Prevalence and outcomes of vascular cognitive impairment. Vascular Cognitive Impairment Investigators of the Canadian Study of Health and Aging. *Neurology*, **54**, 447–51.

Roks, G., Dermaut, B., Heutink, P., *et al.* (1999). Mutation screening of the tau gene in patients with early-onset alzheimer's disease. *Neuroscience Letters*, **277**, 137–9.

Roman, G.C. (1994). An epidemic in Cuba of optic neuropathy, sensorineural deafness, peripheral sensory neuropathy and dorsolateral myeloneuropathy. *Journal of the Neurological Science*, **127**, 11–28.

Roman, G.C. (1999*a*). A historical review of the concept of vascular dementia: lessons from the past for the future. *Alzheimer Disease and Associated Disorders*, **13** (Supplement 3), S4–8.

Roman, G.C. (1999*b*). Vascular dementia today. *Revue Neurologique (Paris)*, **155**, S64–72.

Roman, G.C., Tatemichi, T.K., Erkinjuntti, T., *et al.* (1993). Vascular dementia: diagnostic criteria for research studies. Report of the NINDS-AIREN International Workshop. *Neurology*, **43**, 250–60.

Roses, A.D. (1994). Apolipoprotein E is a relevant susceptibility gene that affects the rate of expression of Alzheimer's disease. *Neurobiology of Aging*, **15**, S165–7.

Roses, A.D. and Saunders, A.M. (1994). APOE is a major susceptibility gene for Alzheimer's disease. *Current Opinion in Biotechnology*, **5**, 663–7.

Rossignol, M., Suissa, S., and Abenhaim, L. (1988). Working disability due to occupational back pain: three-year follow-up of 2300 compensated workers in Quebec. *Journal of Occupational Medicine*, **30**, 502–5.

Rothman, K.J. and Greenland, S. (1998). *Modern epidemiology* (2nd edn). Lippincott-Raven, Philadelphia, PA.

Rowland, L.P. and Merritt, H.H. (1995). *Merritt's textbook of neurology* (9th edn). Williams and Wilkins, Baltimore, MD.

Rozenberg, S., Alcalay, M., Duplan, B., and Legrand, E. (1998). Risk factors for low back pain: an update. *Revue du Rhumatisme*, **65**, 275–8.

Rybicki, B.A., Johnson, C.C., Peterson, E.L., Kortsha, G.X., and Gorell, J.M. (1999). A family history of Parkinson's disease and its effect on other PD risk factors. *Neuroepidemiology*, **18**, 270–8.

Sabbagh, N., Brice, A., Marez, D., *et al.* (1999). CYP2D6 polymorphism and Parkinson's disease susceptibility. *Movement Disorders*, **14**, 230–6.

Sadovnick, A.D., Bulman, D.E., D'Hooghe, M.B., and Ebers, G.C. (1991). The influence of gender on the susceptibility to multiple sclerosis in sibships. *Advances in Neurology*, **48**, 586–8.

Sanchez, A.L., Lindback, J., Schantz, P.M., *et al.* (1999). A population-based, case–control study of Taenia solium taeniasis and cysticercosis. *Annals of Tropical Medicine and Parasitology*, **93**, 247–58.

Saunders, A.M., Schmader, K., Breitner, J.C., *et al.* (1993*a*). Apolipoprotein E epsilon 4 allele distributions in late-onset alzheimer's disease and in other amyloid-forming diseases. *Lancet*, **342**, 710–11.

Saunders, A.M., Strittmatter, W.J., Schmechel, D., *et al.* (1993*b*). Association of apolipoprotein E allele epsilon 4 with late-onset familial and sporadic Alzheimer's disease . *Neurology*, **43**, 1467–72.

Schoenberg, B.S. (1987). Descriptive epidemiology of Parkinson's disease: disease distribution and hypothesis formulation. *Advances in Neurology*, **45**, 277–83.

Schofield, P.W., Tang, M., Marder, K., *et al.* (1997). Alzheimer's disease after remote head injury: an incidence study. *Journal of Neurology, Neurosurgery and Psychiatry*, **62**, 119–24.

Schumacher, G.A., Beebe, G., Kibler R.F., *et al.* (1965). Problems of experimental trials of therapy in multiple sclerosis: report by the panel on the evaluation of experimental trials of therapy in multiple sclerosis. *Annals of the New York Academy of Sciences*, **122**, 552–68.

Schwartz, B.S., Stewart, W.F., and Lipton, R.B. (1997). Lost workdays and decreased work effectiveness associated with headache in the workplace. *Journal of Occupational and Environmental Medicine*, **39**, 320–7.

Senanayake, N. and Roman, G.C. (1993). Epidemiology of epilepsy in developing countries. *Bulletin of the World Health Organization*, **71**, 247–58.

Shackleton, D.P., Westendorp, R.G., Trenite, D.G., and Vandenbroucke, J.P. (1999). Mortality in patients with epilepsy: 40 years of follow up in a Dutch cohort study. *Journal of Neurology, Neurosurgery and Psychiatry*, **66**, 636–40.

Shafi, S., Gilbert, J.C., Loghmanee, F., *et al.* (1998). Impact of bicycle helmet safety legislation on children admitted to a regional pediatric trauma center. *Journal of Pediatric Surgery*, **33**, 317–21.

Shastry, B.S. and Giblin, F.J. (1999). Genes and susceptible loci of Alzheimer's disease. *Brain Research Bulletin*, **48**, 121–7.

Shelerud, R. (1998). Epidemiology of occupational low back pain. *Occupational Medicine*, **13**, 1–22.

Siemers, E. (1999). Multiple system atrophy. *Medical Clinics of North America*, **83**, 381–92.

Sinha, S., Anderson, J.P., Barbour, R., *et al.* (1999). Purification and cloning of amyloid precursor protein beta-secretase from human brain. *Nature*, **402**, 537–40.

Sisodia, S.S. (1999). Alzheimer's disease: perspectives for the new millennium. *Journal of Clinical Investigation*, **104**, 1169–70.

Skegg, D.C., Corwin, P.A., Craven R.S., Malloch, J.A., and Pollock, M. (1987). Occurrence of multiple sclerosis in the north and south of New Zealand. *Journal of Neurology, Neurosurgery and Psychiatry*, **50**, 134–9.

Slooter, A.J., Bronzova, J., Witteman, J.C., Van Broeckhoven, C., Hofman, A., and van Duijn, C.M. (1999). Estrogen use and early onset alzheimer's disease: a population-based study. *Journal of Neurology, Neurosurgery and Psychiatry*, **67**, 779–81.

Small, G.W., Scott, W.K., Komo, S., *et al.* (1999). No association between the HLA-A2 allele and Alzheimer disease. *Neurogenetics*, **2**, 177–82.

Solomon, D.H., Katz, J.N., Bohn, R., Mogun, H., and Avorn, J. (1999). Nonoccupational risk factors for carpal tunnel syndrome. *Journal of General Internal Medicine*, **14**, 310–14.

Sperfeld, A.D., Collatz, M.B., Baier, H., *et al.* (1999). FTDP-17: an early-onset phenotype with parkinsonism and epileptic seizures caused by a novel mutation. *Annals of Neurology*, **46**, 708–15.

Sperling, M.R., Feldman, H., Kinman, J., Liporace, J.D., and O'Connor, M.J. (1999). Seizure control and mortality in epilepsy. *Annals of Neurology*, **46**, 45–50.

St George-Hyslop, P.H. (2000). Molecular genetics of Alzheimer's disease. *Biological Psychiatry*, **47**, 183–99.

Stallings, S.P., Kasdan, M.L., Soergel, T.M., and Corwin, H.M. (1997). A case–control study of obesity as a risk factor for carpal tunnel syndrome in a population of 600 patients presenting for independent medical examination. *Journal of Hand Surgery*, **22A**, 211–15.

Steiner, H., Capell, A., Leimer, U., and Haass, C. (1999). Genes and mechanisms involved in beta-amyloid generation and Alzheimer's disease. *European Archives in Psychiatry and Clinical Neuroscience*, **249**, 266–70.

Steinlein, O.K. (1999). Gene defects in idiopathic epilepsy. *Revue Neurologique (Paris)*, **155**, 450–3.

Stern, Y., Albert, S., Tang, M.X., and Tsai, W.Y. (1999). Rate of memory decline in AD is related to education and occupation: cognitive reserve? *Neurology*, **53**, 1942–7.

Sternbach, G. (1999). The carpal tunnel syndrome. *Journal of Emergency Medicine*, **17**, 519–23.

Stewart, W.F., Lipton, R.B., Celentano, D.D., and Reed, M.L. (1992). Prevalence of migraine headache in the United States. Relation to age, income, race, and other sociodemographic factors. *Journal of the American Medical Association*, **267**, 64–9.

Stewart, W.F., Simon, D., Shechter, A., and Lipton, R.B. (1995). Population variation in migraine prevalence: a meta-analysis. *Journal of Clinical Epidemiology*, **48**, 269–80.

Stewart, W.F., Lipton, R.B., and Liberman, J. (1996*a*). Variation in migraine prevalence by race. *Neurology*, **47**, 52–9.

Stewart, W.F., Lipton, R.B., and Simon, D. (1996*b*). Work-related disability: results from the American migraine study. *Cephalalgia*, **16**, 231–8, 215.

Stewart, W.F., Kawas, C., Corrada, M., and Metter, E.J. (1997*a*). Risk of Alzheimer's disease and duration of NSAID use . *Neurology*, **48**, 626–32.

Stewart, W.F., Staffa, J., Lipton, R.B., and Ottman, R. (1997*b*). Familial risk of migraine: a population-based study. *Annals of Neurology*, **41**, 166–72.

Stratman, N.C., Carter, D.B., and Sethy, V.H. (1997). Ibuprofen: effect on inducible nitric oxide synthase. *Brain Research, Molecular Brain Research*, **50**, 107–12.

Strittmatter, W.J., Saunders, A.M., Schmechel, D., *et al.* (1993). Apolipoprotein E: high-avidity binding to beta-amyloid and increased frequency of type 4 allele in late-onset familial Alzheimer disease. *Proceedings of the National Academy of Sciences of the United States of America*, **90**, 1977–81.

Swan, L. and Dupont, J. (1999). Multiple system atrophy. *Physical Therapy*, **79**, 488–94.

Tang, M.X., Maestre, G., Tsai, W.Y., *et al.* (1996). Effect of age, ethnicity, and head injury on the association between APOE genotypes and Alzheimer's disease. *Annals of the New York Academy of Sciences*, **802**, 6–15.

Tanner, C.M. and Ben-Shlomo, Y. (1999). Epidemiology of Parkinson's disease. *Advances in Neurology*, **80**, 153–9.

Tanzi, R.E. (1999). A genetic dichotomy model for the inheritance of Alzheimer's disease and common age-related disorders. *Journal of Clinical Investigation*, **104**, 1175–9.

Tanzi, R.E., Kovacs, D.M., Kim, T.W., Moir, R.D., Guenette, S.Y., and Wasco, W. (1996). The gene defects responsible for familial Alzheimer's disease. *Neurobiological Disorders*, **3**, 159–68.

Taylor, C.A., Saint-Hilaire, M.H., Cupples, L.A., *et al.* (1999). Environmental, medical, and family history risk factors for Parkinson's disease: a New England-based case control study. *American Journal of Medical Genetics*, **88**, 742–9.

Tesfaye, S., Stevens, L.K., Stephenson, J.M., *et al.* (1996). Prevalence of diabetic peripheral neuropathy and its relation to glycaemic control and potential risk factors: the EURODIAB IDDM Complications Study. *Diabetologia*, **39**, 1377–84.

Thompson, D.C. and Patterson, M.Q. (1998). Cycle helmets and the prevention of injuries. Recommendations for competitive sport. *Sports Medicine*, **25**, 213–19.

Tietjen, G.E. (2000). The relationship of migraine and stroke. *Neuroepidemiology*, **19**, 13–19.

Tilley, L., Morgan, K., and Kalsheker, N. (1998). Genetic risk factors in Alzheimer's disease. *Molecular Pathology*, **51**, 293–304.

Tzourio, C., Tehindrazanarivelo, A., Iglesias, S., *et al.* (1995). Case–control study of migraine and risk of ischaemic stroke in young women. *British Medical Journal*, **310**, 830–3.

Tzourio, C., Rocca, W.A., Breteler, M.M., *et al.* (1997). Smoking and Parkinson's disease. An age-dependent risk effect? The EUROPARKINSON Study Group. *Neurology*, **49**, 1267–72.

Ulrich, V., Gervil, M., Kyvik, K.O., Olesen, J., and Russell, M.B. (1999). Evidence of a genetic factor in migraine with aura: a population-based Danish twin study. *Annals of Neurology*, **45**, 242–6.

Valkenburg, H. and Haanen, H. (1982. The epidemiology of low back pain. In *Symposium on idiopathic low back pain* (ed. A. White and S. Gordon), pp. 9–12. C.V. Mosby, St Louis, MO.

van Doorn, T. (1995). Low back disability among self-employed dentists, veterinarians, physicians and physical therapists in the Netherlands. *Acta Orthopaedica Scandinavica*, **66**, 1–64.

Vassar, R., Bennett, B.D., Babu-Khan, S., *et al.* (1999). Beta-secretase cleavage of Alzheimer's amyloid precursor protein by the transmembrane aspartic protease BACE. *Science*, **286**, 735–41.

Vaughan, J., Durr, A., Tassin, J., *et al.* (1998). The alpha-synuclein Ala53Thr mutation is not a common cause of familial Parkinson's disease: a study of 230 European cases. European Consortium on Genetic Susceptibility in Parkinson's Disease. *Annals of Neurology*, **44**, 270–3.

Veldman, B.A., Wijn, A.M., Knoers, N., Praamstra, P., and Horstink, M.W. (1998). Genetic and environmental risk factors in Parkinson's disease. *Clinical Neurology and Neurosurgery*, **100**, 15–26.

Wade, J. and Hachinski, V. (1986). Revised ischemic score for diagnosing multi-infarct dementia. *Journal of Clinical Psychiatry*, **47**, 437–8.

Wakabayashi, K., Hayashi, S., Kakita, A., *et al.* (1998). Accumulation of alpha-synuclein/NACP is a cytopathological feature common to Lewy body disease and multiple system atrophy. *Acta Neuropathologica (Berlin)*, **96**, 445–52.

Wallace, H., Shorvon, S., and Tallis, R. (1998). Age-specific incidence and prevalence rates of treated epilepsy in an unselected population of

2,052,922 and age-specific fertility rates of women with epilepsy. *Lancet*, **352**, 1970–3.

Wang, H. X., Fratiglioni, L., Frisoni, G. B., Viitanen, M., Winblad, B. (1999). Smoking and the occurrence of Alzheimer's disease: cross-sectional and longitudinal data in a population-based study. *American Journal of Epidemiology*, **149**, 640–4.

Waring, S.C., Rocca, W.A., Petersen, R.C., O'Brien, P.C., Tangalos, E.G., and Kokmen, E. (1999). Postmenopausal estrogen replacement therapy and risk of AD: a population-based study. *Neurology*, **52**, 965–70.

Weissbecker, K.A., Elston, R.C., Greenberg, D., and Delgado-Escueta, A.V. (1999). Genetic epidemiology and the search for epilepsy genes. *Advances in Neurology*, **79**, 323–40.

Werneck, A.L. and Alvarenga, H. (1999). Genetics, drugs and environmental factors in Parkinson's disease. A case–control study. *Arqivos de Neuropsiquiatriqua*, **57**, 347–55.

Wolf, H., Grunwald, M., Ecke, G.M., *et al.* (1998). The prognosis of mild cognitive impairment in the elderly. *Journal of Neural Transmission, Supplementum*, **54**, 31–50.

Wood, N.W. (1998). Genetic risk factors in Parkinson's disease. *Annals of Neurology*, **44**, S58–62.

Xian-hao, X. and McFarlin, D.E. (1984). Oligoclonal bands in CSF: twins with MS. *Neurology*, **34**, 769–74.

Xiong, L., Labuda, M., Li, D.S., *et al.* (1999). Mapping of a gene determining familial partial epilepsy with variable foci to chromosome 22q11-q12. *American Journal of Human Genetics*, **65**, 1698–710.

Yaffe, K., Sawaya, G., Lieberburg, I., and Grady, D. (1998). Estrogen therapy in postmenopausal women: effects on cognitive function and dementia. *Journal of the American Medical Association*, **279**, 688–95.

Yan, R., Bienkowski, M.J., Shuck, M.E., *et al.* (1999). Membrane-anchored aspartyl protease with Alzheimer's disease beta-secretase activity. *Nature*, **402**, 533–7.

Zareparsi, S., Taylor, T.D., Harris, E.L., and Payami, H. (1998). Segregation analysis of Parkinson disease. *American Journal of Medical Genetics*, **80**, 410–17.

Zarrelli, M.M., Beghi, E., Rocca, W.A., and Hauser, W.A. (1999). Incidence of epileptic syndromes in Rochester, Minnesota: 1980–1984. *Epilepsia*, **40**, 1708–14.

Ziegler, D.K., Hur, Y.M., Bouchard, Jr, T.J., Hassanein, R.S., and Barter, R. (1998). Migraine in twins raised together and apart. *Headache*, **38**, 417–22.

9.11 The transmissible spongiform encephalopathies

Stephen Palmer, Charles Hillier, and Roland Salmon

Introduction

The transmissible spongiform encephalopathies (**TSEs**) are a group of invariably fatal central nervous system neurodegenerative diseases affecting both animals and humans, and include scrapie, bovine spongiform encephalopathy, kuru, Creutzfeldt–Jakob disease (**CJD**), and the recently described variant Creutzfeldt–Jakob disease (**vCJD**) (Table 1). The term TSE derives from characteristic microscopic appearances of sponge-like vacuolation of neuropil of the brain and the fact that transmission occurs naturally within species and can be induced experimentally between species by parenteral injections of infected tissue and by oral challenge.

Although the oldest known form of TSE, scrapie in sheep, was described as early as 1732 (Pattison 1988), the nature of the agent causing the TSEs remains controversial. Certain characteristics unite the TSEs: they are caused by a highly resistant and unconventional agent, they have extremely long incubation periods, they are progressive and invariably fatal, and they cause degenerative changes in the brain without causing an inflammatory or immunological reaction.

It was traditionally believed that the TSEs were caused by 'unconventional transmissible agents', originally 'slow viruses', a term coined to emphasize their remarkable resistance to thermal and other physical factors (ultraviolet light, ionizing radiation (Alper *et al.* 1967), and the majority of chemical sterilization procedures (Dickinson and Taylor 1978)) that would be expected to inactivate conventional micro-organisms. This suggests that if the agents contain nucleic acid, it is either very small or extremely well protected. Treatment with nucleic acid denaturing enzymes does not alter the infectivity of the infective agent (Prusiner 1982), but infectivity is reduced by a number of procedures that modify or hydrolyse proteins.

Table 1 Animal and human spongiform encephalopathies

Disease	Species affected	Disease first described (year)	Transmission of disease first demonstrated (year)
Scrapie	Sheep, goat	1732	1936
Transmissible mink encephalopathy	Mink	1947	1965
Kuru	Humans	1957	1966
Sporadic CJD	Humans	1920	1968
Iatrogenic CJD	Humans	1974	1974
Chronic wasting disease	Mule deer	1978	1983
GSS	Humans	1936	1985
BSE	Cattle	1987	1988
Spongiform encephalopathy	Elk	1982	ND
	Nyala	1987	1992
	Greater kudu	1989	1992
	Gemsbok, oryx	1988	ND
Feline spongiform encephalopathy	Cat	1990	1992
Fatal familial insomnia	Humans	1986	1992
Variant CJD	Humans	1996	1996
Fatal sporadic insomnia	Humans	1999	1999

GSS, Gerstmann–Straussler–Schienker disease; ND, not demonstrated.

This evidence has been used to suggest that the agent does not contain nucleic acid and that the infectious agent consists solely of a protein. From the above discussion it can be appreciated that two fundamentally different categories of explanation describing the cause of these diseases have emerged. The 'prion' hypotheses (Prusiner 1982) (see below) propose that a particular membrane-bound host-coded protein, devoid of nucleic acid, causes disease. In contrast, the virus and the virino hypotheses predict that a yet-to-be-discovered replicating nucleic acid is the obligatory factor for transmission.

In 1982 biochemical purification of the scrapie agent from brain homogenate was achieved and produced evidence that this consisted solely of protein. The term 'prion' was introduced and defined as 'small proteinaceous infectious particles that resist inactivation by procedures which modify nucleic acids' (Prusiner 1982). Following this, the amino acid sequence of at least part of the protein was deciphered. Molecular techniques revealed that a single cellular gene was responsible for encoding prion protein (**PrP**), now routinely referred to as the prion protein gene (**PRNP**) and which is located on chromosome 20. This finding led to the recognition of two forms of the PrP, the normal cellular form, termed PrP^{C} (where C stands for cellular), and a pathological form present only in scrapie-infected organisms, termed **PrPSc** or **PrPRES** (where superscript Sc stands for scrapie and superscript RES for resistant form). The amino acid sequence of PrP encoded by the gene of a healthy animal does not appear to differ from that encoded by a scrapie-infected animal. This suggests that the different properties of PrP^{C} and PrP^{Sc} are due to post-translational change (Basler *et al.* 1986), that is, an alteration in the structure and behaviour of the protein after it has been synthesized.

Although the 'prion' hypothesis could account for the infectious agent, prions are as yet poorly defined, and 'for the most part this term is used as an operational term for the transmissible agent' (Chesebro 1998). Although it has been widely accepted throughout the scientific community, the 'prion hypothesis' still fails to explain the large number of different strains of disease seen in a species. Some feel the only explanation can be that the agent must contain an informational molecule (RNS/DNA). The major arguments for and against 'prion' versus 'virus' are eloquently argued by Chesebro (1998) and recommended to the reader.

Animal TSEs

Scrapie

Scrapie, affecting sheep and goats, was the first of the TSEs to be described and has been recorded in Europe for more than two centuries (Kimberlin 1981). Although its true prevalence is unknown in the United Kingdom, a rough estimate is 2 cases per 1000 sheep. Only Australia and New Zealand appear to be free of disease (Spongiform Encephalopathy Advisory Committee 1995). Most breeds and both sexes are affected and the age of peak incidence is about 3.5 years. The disease is characterized by rubbing of the poll and buttocks in response to pruritus, nervousness, or aggression, and hypersensitivity to sound or movement (Spongiform Encephalopathy Advisory Committee 1995).

In 1936, Cuille and Chelle formally transmitted scrapie to healthy sheep by intraocular injection of homogenized brain from clinically affected sheep. At about the same time an accidental natural experiment occurred in the United Kingdom through the use of contaminated louping-ill vaccine. The vaccine had been prepared from a suspension of brain, spinal cord, and spleen tissue from sheep and a large number of flocks were vaccinated in 1935. Two years later an epidemic of scrapie occurred in these flocks even though the louping-ill virus in the vaccine had been inactivated by the addition of formalin to the original suspension (Gordon 1946). Subsequent work by Gordon revealed resistance of scrapie agent to formalin and boiling, and showed that it would pass through 410-nm filters. In 1961 Chandler demonstrated that experimental transmission could occur between species when he successfully managed to produce a spongiform encephalopathy in mice by inoculating them with scrapie brain material, thus producing an inexpensive experimental model (Chandler 1961).

Transmissible mink encephalopathy

This disease, rare in ranch-raised mink, was first identified in Wisconsin in 1947 (Hartsough and Burger 1965), since when there have been 23 outbreaks worldwide (McKenzie *et al.* 1996). It was originally assumed that these sporadic outbreaks were attributable to the feeding of scrapie-infected sheep offal or carcass material, but the most recent outbreak in 1985 has raised the possibility that a previously unrecognized bovine agent might be involved (Marsh *et al.* 1991).

Chronic wasting disease

This disease of deer (family *Cervidae*) was first described in captive mule deer (Williams and Young 1980) in 1980 and then later in Rocky mountain elk (Williams and Young 1982). Cases have occurred primarily in captive animals but a few affected free-ranging animals have been identified in northeastern Colorado and southeastern Wyoming. A prevalence of 2.5 per cent has been estimated in wild deer in that area (Johnson and Gibbs 1998).

Bovine spongiform encephalopathy

Bovine spongiform encephalopathy (**BSE**) was first described in November 1986 in the United Kingdom (Wells *et al.* 1987), but it is believed that a few cases occurred as early as April 1985. A large-scale epidemic has since occurred in the United Kingdom, peaking in January 1993, and involving at least 186 000 cattle (Fig. 1). Since then the incidence has steadily fallen as predicted at the time of the feed ban (Spongiform Encephalopathy Advisory Committee 1995; Collee and Bradley 1997; Pattison 1998), although it is estimated that perhaps half a million infected animals entered the human food chain before control measures were introduced in November 1989, and a further 283 000 entered the food chain from December 1989 to December 1995. The disease has been reported in other countries, including Switzerland, France, Oman, the Falkland Islands, Denmark, Germany, Portugal, and Canada. In some of these cases affected cattle were exported from the United Kingdom (Oman, the Falkland Islands), but in other countries, notably Switzerland and France, no firm association with United Kingdom exports can be established (Bradley and Wilesmith 1993; Schreuder 1994).

BSE affects adult cattle of both sexes. The age of peak incidence and median incubation period is 4 to 5 years. Onset of disease is insidious

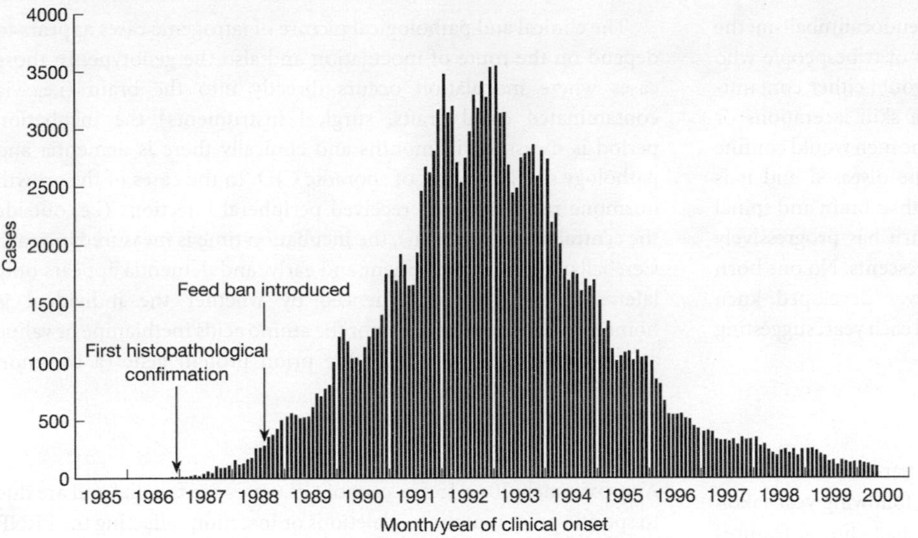

Fig. 1 Confirmed cases of BSE plotted by month and year of clinical onset.

and signs include changes in sensation with hyperaesthesia to touch or sound, excessive nose licking and teeth grinding, apprehension, frenzy, and nervousness of doorways. Abnormalities of posture with dropped head, arched back, splayed, stiff hind limbs, and ataxia of the hind limbs are all regularly described in affected animals. There are general signs such as loss of condition and weight and reduced milk yield in dairy cows. The duration of illness can be as short as 2 weeks but can last up to 1 year, with the average clinical course being several months.

Whether BSE originated as scrapie introduced into cattle, or whether BSE has always existed in cattle, has not definitely been established, but a series of case–control studies suggested that the epidemic spread of the disease occurred through the use of proprietary cattle dietary protein supplements containing contaminated meat and bonemeal prepared from abattoir waste (Wilesmith *et al.* 1988). It has been suggested, although not proved, that changes in the rendering industry in the late 1970s, which had led to decreased processing times, and a change from batch to continuous methods of processing, together with the abandonment of the use of organic solvents for fat extraction, allowed the introduction of the agent into feedstuff and its epidemic amplification by recycling infected bovine material (Pattison 1998). From computer simulation of the early incidence of the epidemic and analysis of the year of birth of cases, it was estimated that the date of the first exposures were in 1980 or 1981.

BSE has been transmitted experimentally to mouse, sheep, goat, and mink by the oral route and is probably responsible for spongiform encephalopathy in the exotic ungulates (see below), domestic cats, and humans (see below) (Bruce *et al.* 1997). To date only one BSE strain has been recognized after experimental transmission to sheep, and this was the strain identified in nyala, kudu, the domestic cat, and humans.

Spongiform encephalopathy in exotic ungulates

Since 1986, spongiform encephalopathy has been diagnosed in captive wild animals of six species (nyala, eland, greater kudu, Arabian oryx and scimitar horned oryx, cheetah, and puma) from eight zoological institutions in the United Kingdom. Temporal and geographical features coincided with the BSE epidemic, and animals were exposed to proprietary feeds containing ruminant-derived protein or consumption of cattle carcasses unfit for human consumption, and because brain homogenate induces BSE-like changes in mice, it is likely that BSE is responsible (Kirkwood and Cunningham 1994).

Feline spongiform encephalopathy

From 1990 to May 1998, 81 cases in domestic cats were reported over a wide geographical area in the United Kingdom (Pearson *et al.* 1993). It is estimated that the disease was probably under-reported before 1994, when feline spongiform encephalopathy was made a notifiable disease. Since that time the number of new cases has declined so that there were only four reported cases in the United Kingdom during 1998 and only one of these would have been born after the specified bovine offal ban in pet food in 1990. It is assumed that cats became infected through consumption of commercially produced cat feed that contained the BSE agent (Pattison 1998).

Human TSEs

Kuru

In 1957, Gajdusek and Zigas described kuru, an unusual progressive neurological disorder in the Fore tribe in the eastern highlands of Papua New Guinea (Gajdusek and Zigas 1957). 'Kuru' means shivering or trembling, and the disease was characterized clinically by cerebellar ataxia, tremor, dysathria, dysphagia, and finally dementia, progressing to death within one year of onset. Kuru is characterized pathologically by cerebellar atrophy, with spongiform change and neuronal cell loss evident throughout the central nervous system. Seventy per cent of brains affected contain characteristic plaques comprising a central eosinophilic core with a peripheral halo of radiating filaments, particularly in the cerebellum (Ironside 1996).

Early observation of the tribe revealed that the disease affected mainly the women, adolescent children of both sexes, and children, whilst the men seemed immune to the disease (Gajdusek 1977). It appears that the disease was spread by ritualistic endocannibalism; the women and children would prepare the bodies of tribespeople who had died, including removing the brain. They would either contaminate themselves by inoculation injury through skin lacerations or rubbing conjunctiva, or by eating brain tissue. The men would confine themselves to consuming skeletal muscle of the diseased and it is thought this tissue has a much lower infectivity than brain and spinal cord. Since the cessation of these practices, kuru has progressively disappeared, first among children and then adolescents. No one born in a village since cannibalism ceased has ever developed kuru (Prusiner 1993). However, cases are still reported each year, suggesting incubation periods of over 40 years.

Creutzfeldt–Jakob disease

In 1920, Creutzfeldt reported the case of a 23-year-old woman who had died of a neurodegenerative illness, and the following year Jakob reported five cases. At least two of the six cases had clinical features suggestive of the entity we now recognize as CJD. The following four forms of CJD are recognized: sporadic, familial, iatrogenic, and variant.

Sporadic

Sporadic CJD, which makes up about 85 per cent of all CJD cases, occurs worldwide with a reported incidence ranging from 0.06 to 1.6 per million of the population, with mean age of death of 65 years (Table 2). The annual reported incidence in the United Kingdom is 0.5 to 1 cases per million population. Most patients present with a rapidly progressive dementia with a mean clinical course of 4.5 months (Brown *et al.* 1994*a*), although up to 10 per cent may survive 2 years or more (Brown *et al.* 1994*a*). A wide range of neurological abnormalities has been described (de Silva 1996), but the commonest features include a subacute dementia with pyramidal and extrapyramidal signs. Myoclonus is present at some stage of the disease in up to 90 per cent. Electroencephalogram recordings show a characteristic periodic discharge in 60 to 80 per cent of cases.

Macroscopic examination of the brain in sporadic CJD may reveal no significant abnormality, particularly in cases with a short clinical history, but in most cases there is evidence of cortical atrophy. The most characteristic abnormality is spongiform change in the cerebral cortex, which consists of a fine vacuolation of the neuropil of the grey matter. The severity and distribution of this varies widely from case to case. Immunocytochemical staining for detection of disease-related protein may demonstrate plaques of abnormal protein similar in pattern to cases of kuru. Clinical (WHO 1998; Belay 1999) and pathological diagnostic criteria (Budka *et al.* 1995; Kretzschmar *et al.* 1996) for sporadic CJD have been established.

Iatrogenic

Iatrogenic CJD, making up less than 1 per cent of all cases, is spread from human to human via contamination of neurosurgical instruments, and by tissue grafts (such as the cornea) from infected donors; the latter have been reported since the mid-1970s (Duffy *et al.* 1974; Bernoulli *et al.* 1977). From the mid-1980s increasing numbers of cases associated with the use of infected cadaveric dura mater grafts were identified (Brown *et al.* 1992), but the most dramatic example of iatrogenic CJD is the continuing epidemic of cases in young adults treated for hypopituitarism with pooled growth-hormone extract.

The clinical and pathological picture of iatrogenic cases appears to depend on the route of inoculation and also the genotype. In those cases where inoculation occurs directly into the brain (i.e. via contaminated dural grafts, surgical instruments) the incubation period is measured in months and clinically there is dementia and pathology similar to that of sporadic CJD. In the cases of the growth hormone recipients who received peripheral injections (i.e. outside the central nervous system), the incubation time is measured in years. Cerebellar signs are prominent and early, and dementia appears only later. Susceptibility is influenced by whether the individual is homozygous or heterozygous for the amino acids methianine or valine at the codon position 129 of the prion protein gene (a common human PRNP polymorphism).

Familial

Approximately 10 to 15 per cent of CJD cases are familial and are due to specific point mutations, deletions or insertions affecting the PRNP located on chromosome 20. More than 20 different mutations in the PRNP have been discovered. Patients with sporadic CJD do not have a mutation deletion or insertion of this gene.

Familial CJD encompasses a wide range of clinical phenotypes, some with atypical features including dysautonomia and isolated spastic paraparesis. In general, familial CJD has an earlier age of onset and a longer duration than sporadic CJD.

Gerstmann–Straussler–Scheinker disease, first described by Gerstmann in 1936, contributes less than 2 per cent of all known human TSEs (Masters *et al.* 1981). Most cases are familial, exhibiting an autosomal dominant pattern of inheritance with almost complete penetrance. The clinical duration is from 2 to 10 years, much longer than for CJD.

Linkage studies suggested that substitution of leucine for proline at PrP codon 102 in the PRNP leads to the development of clinical disease in some families with Gerstmann–Straussler–Scheinker disease (Hsaio *et al.* 1989).

Fatal familial insomnia was first described in 1986 (Lugaresi *et al.* 1986), and is a dominantly inherited condition typified by a thalamic dementia with some pathological features of CJD in which insomnia, rather than dementia, is the dominant clinical feature. Over 21 affected families have been recognized worldwide (Brown *et al.* 1998; Budka *et al.* 1998; Gambetti and Lugaresi 1998; Julien *et al.* 1998; Kretzschmar *et al.* 1998; Pocchiari *et al.* 1998; Will *et al.* 1998*b*). The families have a PRNP mutation at codon 178 resulting in the substitution of the amino acid asparagine for aspartic acid, which when associated with the amino acid methionine at codon position 129 (a common human PRNP polymorphism) leads to this unique clinical phenotype (Medori *et al.* 1992).

Fatal sporadic insomnia was first described in 1999, in a total of six subjects (Parchi *et al.* 1998; Mastrianni *et al.* 1999). All subjects had a disease clinically similar and histopathologically virtually identical to fatal familial insomnia, but none had the PRNP mutation at codon 178. All were homozygous for the amino acid methionine at the codon 129 position of the PRNP.

Possible sources of sporadic CJD

The most commonly cited hypothesis for the cause of sporadic CJD is a spontaneous conformational change in PrP, in the absence of exogenous factors. However, there is evidence that exogenous

Table 2 National and regional CJD surveys

Country	Total no. of cases	Incidence per million total population	Period of survey
England and Wales			
Will *et al.* (1988)	46	0.09	1964–1973
Harries-Jones *et al.* (1988)	158	0.31	1970–1979
National CJD Surveillance Unit (1995)	120	0.49	1981–1989
Cousens *et al.* (1997*a*)	185	0.82	1990–1994
Austria			
Hainfeliner *et al.* (1996)	79	0.18	1986–1994
		0.67	1995
		1.38	1973–1977
Chile			
Galvez *et al.* (1980)	35	0.31	1973–1977
Araya *et al.* (1983)	46	0.69	1978–1993
France			
Brown *et al.* (1979)	178	0.81	1968–1977
Brown *et al.* (1988)	151	0.58	1978–1992
Will *et al.* (1998*a*)	146	0.84	1993–1995
Germany			
Harries-Jones *et al.* (1988)	NA	0.31	1979–1990
Will *et al.* (1998*b*)	122	0.55	1993–1995
Italy			
Masulio *et al.* (1988)	32	0.05	1958–1971
Will *et al.* (1998*a*)	79	0.09	1972–1986
	96	0.56	1993–1995
Israel			
Kahana *et al.* (1988)	NA	0.75	1963–1972
Neugat *et al.* (1979)		0.91	1963–1987
USA			
Masters *et al.* (1979)	265	0.26	1975–1979
Holman *et al.* (1995)	2614	0.90	1979–1990
Japan			
Tsuji and Kuroiwa (1983)	75	0.45	1975–1978
Akai *et al.*(1989)	9	0.99	1976–1986
Finland			
Kovanen and Haltia (1988)	30	0.57	1974–1984
Hungary			
Majtenyi (1988)	65	0.39	1979–1983
Australia			
Worthington 1995	29	0.66	1970–1980
New Zealand			
National CJD Surveillance Unit 1995	NA	0.88	1980–1989
Canada			
Anonymous (1996*a*)	334	1.60	1979–1993
Stratton *et al.*(1997)			
Slovakia			
Will *et al.* (1998*a*)	10	0.60	1993–1995
The Netherlands			
Will *et al.* (1998*a*)	37	0.81	1993–1995
Switzerland			
National CJD Surveillance Unit (1995)	NA	0.80	1980–1990
Sweden			
Lundberg (1998)	72	1.18	1985–1996

environmental factors may be important, an observation which is relevant to considering the aetiology of vCJD (Hillier *et al.* 2000). One observation difficult to reconcile to the prevailing hypothesis is the existence of clusters of cases of 'sporadic' CJD, even though some clustering may occur by chance, and that ascertainment of a first case may lead to better ascertainment of further cases (Raubertas *et al.* 1991). At least eight have been reported (Matthews 1975; Mayer *et al.* 1977; Will and Matthews 1982; Araya *et al.* 1983; Lechi *et al.* 1983). Matthews described three clusters in England. The first was of three cases in a small rural community in the Midlands over 7 years. The second involved five cases with onsets between 1969 and 1973 in four towns/villages in eastern England (separated by no more than 20 km), of whom at least three had lived locally since 1960. The third cluster involved two patients in 1965 and 1968 who lived within 250 m of each other and shared the same general practitioner. In 1980, a patient who lived mid-way between the two previous patients and within sight of both houses died of pathologically proven CJD. In Italy 11 cases of CJD, including five farmers, occurred in and around Parma, Italy, between 1975 and 1979. In Chile, four cases of histologically proven CJD in three farmers and one housewife occurred in 1982 and 1983. The four lived in small rural communities situated within a 20-km radius of the town. In addition to these clusters case-to-case transmission has been suggested in six reports.

Iatrogenic transmission

CJD can be transmitted from person to person by injecting or implanting CJD-infected instruments, tissue extracts, and organs (Brown 1988, 1995; Creange *et al.* 1995; Ricketts *et al.* 1997). Several points relevant to a wider understanding of the epidemiology arise. Firstly, the time from inoculation to disease onset is dependent on the route of entry. Two types of cases, those involving implantation of cerebral electrodes and corneal grafts, show the shortest incubation, of about 16 months. The longest incubation time is 30 years, following subcutaneous and intramuscular injection of growth-hormone extract and of gonadotrophins. Secondly, the route of transmission predicts the clinical appearance. Those infected directly into the central nervous system develop a global dementia, whereas those infected peripherally develop a progressive cerebellar syndrome. The genotype of the prion gene does not explain this difference. That the peripheral route of infection presents as a cerebellar syndrome would support the view that vCJD is acquired peripherally by diet, for example, as cerebellar signs are an early prominent feature of vCJD but not of sporadic CJD.

Blood transfusion

The infectivity of blood for TSEs in animals is well described (Brown 1995; Ricketts *et al.* 1997). Nevertheless, attempts to transmit CJD by infusing units of blood from patients with CJD to the chimpanzee have failed (Brown *et al.* 1994*a*). Although experimentally difficult, transmission of sporadic CJD and human growth-hormone related iatrogenic CJD to mouse, hamster, and guinea pig, by buffy coat and whole blood, has been demonstrated on four separate occasions (Brown 1995), but only after intracerebral injection. This suggests that transmission from human to human, via blood and blood products, is difficult but theoretically possible. A number of case reports have suggested that transmission by the transfusion of blood or a blood product has occurred in humans (Klein and Dumble 1993; Patry 1998).

One case–control study has examined blood transfusion in sporadic CJD. Esmonde (1993) identified 202 definite and probable United Kingdom cases of sporadic CJD between 1980–1984 and 1990–1992. Twenty-one patients had received blood and 29 had donated blood. This frequency of blood transfusion or donation did not differ from that in age- and sex-matched controls. The clinical features in patients with a history of blood transfusion were similar to those with a history of classical sporadic CJD, and clearly distinct from CJD in recipients of human growth hormone. However, since sporadic CJD is a rare disease and the number of potentially infected units of blood is small, any difference in the rate of receipt of transfusions between cases and controls will be small and a very large study would be needed to detect such a small difference.

Dietary factors

Several case reports and series have reported an apparent increase in the prevalence of CJD in populations of people who eat the brains of sheep or wild animals. There has been one case report of definite CJD in a Dutch man who ate occasional sheep brain and an annual feast of hog brain (Alter *et al.* 1975), and a case series of four patients from North America who all ate squirrel and other animal brains, including goat (Kamin and Patten 1984). A more recent case series obtained a history of eating squirrel brains in all five patients with probable or definite CJD seen over 3.5 years in a neurocognitive clinic in Western Kentucky (Berger *et al.* 1997). However, there are two reports of CJD in vegetarians. Matthews and Will (1981) described a case in a 62-year-old life-long vegetarian. Although she had never eaten meat, meat products, or offal, she had handled raw meat while preparing food for her husband. A study of seven patients from India (Singhal and Dastur 1983) revealed that two cases had been vegetarians but no further details are given.

Zoonotic transmission

CJD and scrapie exist together in many countries, but the incidence of CJD in countries where there is no scrapie, such as Australia, New Zealand, and Chile (Table 2), is no different from that in scrapie-endemic countries. In France, a detailed study looking at regional distribution of CJD and scrapie-infected flocks found there to be no relationship (Chatelain *et al.* 1981). The recent case of a 60-year-old Italian man and his cat (Zanusso *et al.* 1998) is of interest. The man developed CJD in November 1993 and died 3 months later. His cat developed a neurological disease at the same time and was killed at the time of her owner's death. Strain-typing suggested that the man was a case of sporadic CJD. The cat had the same strain, distinct from the feline spongiform encephalopathy strain, described in the United Kingdom in the early 1990s (Pearson *et al.* 1993). Zoonotic transmission would require that the cat had infected her owner whilst presymptomatic. A common source for both cat and man would seem more probable. The circumstances would be hard to explain without an exogenous source of disease. Matthews *et al.* (1979) described definite or probable CJD in four patients, all of whom kept ferrets for pets. One of the cases, who had also kept ferrets 30 years previously, had definitely been bitten by a ferret 2 years before disease onset. After his death the ferret was killed and examined histologically, but no spongiform change was found. In addition, the brain of the ferret was inoculated into four species of monkey and one cat, all of whom remained well. No such studies were performed with the other cases.

Occupational exposure

Case reports and series focus on two main occupational groups; health professionals and those who are exposed to farm animals, in particular sheep and cattle. There are at least 26 reports of sporadic CJD in health care workers worldwide (Maytenyi 1991; Berger and Noble 1993; Weber *et al.* 1993; Bobowick *et al.* 1973). These include seven physicians, including a neurologist, the head of an intensive-care unit, two neurosurgeons, an orthopaedic surgeon, and a pathologist, four dentists, nine nurses, three nursing assistants, and two histopathology technicians.

A wide range of other occupations have been reported among cases of sporadic CJD (Brown *et al.* 1979; Masters *et al.* 1979). Several case series quote an excess number of farmers and farmers' wives (Kovanen and Haltia 1988; Masullo *et al.* 1988). In an Italian study (Masullo *et al.* 1988), the incidence was three times the expected. An analysis of epidemiological surveillance data in the United Kingdom from 1970 to 1996 (Cousens *et al.* 1997*a*) revealed a statistically significant excess of cases among dairy-farm workers and their spouses, and among people with greater degrees of contact with live cattle infected with BSE. No such excess was found in abattoir workers, butchers, or meat cutters.

Case–control studies

To date there have been eight case–control studies of sporadic CJD in humans (Table 3). Such studies are particularly difficult to perform for two main reasons, the necessity of using proxy respondents for cases, and the long incubation period and therefore long recall period. The quality of these studies has been criticized particularly for control selection. Respondent-nominated controls, such as used in the first American study, may have lead to an overrepresentation of controls with similar occupations and social backgrounds (Masters *et al.* 1979). Selecting controls from relatives may obscure inherited risk factors for disease. Selecting from hospitals has the potential to mask associations with other medical and health care procedures, through overmatching, even though individuals with mental or neurological disease were generally excluded.

In one of the most important England and Wales studies in 1980 to 1984 (Harries-Jones *et al.* 1988), two control groups were selected, hospital patients with neurological disease (one group) and those with non-neurological disease (the other). Suitable controls were selected by questioning ward staff and accepting the first offered patient. The selection criteria used by staff were not described. In the 1993 to 1995 European study (van Duijn *et al.* 1998) the researchers simply state that control participants were recruited from the hospital where the patient who had sporadic CJD had been diagnosed and, apart from the exclusion of patients with dementia, no further information is given on selection. On stronger ground was the Australian study, where three community controls for every case were selected at random by using a random-dialling telephone survey, stratified by age, sex, and urban or rural residence.

Information bias is a major potential threat to the validity of these case–control studies since a spouse or close relative has to provide data for cases but, in many studies, the controls respond on their own behalf.

Despite these deficiencies, and given that the studies span Europe, Asia, Australia, and North America, it is of note that similar categories of risk factors do emerge: consumption of undercooked meat and offal products, contacts with various small biting animals, and working in, or receiving health care, notably surgical procedures (Table 4). It is surprising that the United Kingdom government's Spongiform Encephalopathy Advisory Committee (**SEAC**), when assessing the zoonotic potential of BSE, did not apparently pay much attention to these studies (Hillier and Salmon 2000). Significant associations with offal have consistently been dismissed as statistical artefacts.

As part of the National Surveillance Unit's work, a rolling case–control study has been ongoing since 1990 (National CJD Surveillance Unit 1995, 1997, 1998). Relatives of cases are interviewed by a clinician from the unit and a control is chosen who was a patient at the same hospital matched for sex and aged within 4 years of the case. An attempt is made to interview a relative of the control rather than the control him- or herself. However, use of hospital controls can lead to overmatching of exposures related to hospital admission. Selection of controls by ward staff could also introduce bias. Time available for interview is short and there is no attempt to validate histories of exposure by checking with other friends or relatives and by a systematic confirmation of exposure histories such as following up reported sources of foods eaten.

A total of 206 case–control pairs of sporadic CJD between 1990 and April 1997 were analysed (National CJD Surveillance Unit 1998). Significant associations were found with lifetime consumption of beef, venison, and veal. Also, dose–response relationships were found for beef, venison, and veal consumption. A significant association has been found for consumption of brain as well, with a strong dose–response, but not for other animal products.

Interpretation of these associations is particularly difficult since the study design means that data are particularly subject to bias arising from the fact that relatives of cases know both the diagnosis and publicity about the probable source of infection. To assess this bias researchers exploited the fact that relatives of cases were usually interviewed before the death of the case and therefore before pathological confirmation. Dietary histories for confirmed cases were compared with histories from patients who, though suspected initially to have CJD, were not subsequently confirmed. A comparison was made of 206 cases and 80 'non-cases'. The dose–response association for beef completely disappeared. For brain consumption, the odds ratios for eating it less than once a year, and for more than once a year, were raised (1.6 and 1.4) but the trend was not statistically significant ($p = 0.37$). These data suggest that the significant associations found in the case–control study are strongly influenced by information bias.

Variant Creutzfeldt–Jakob disease

In April 1996, the National CJD Surveillance Unit reported 10 cases of CJD in young people in the United Kingdom. It had a distinct clinical appearance characterized by an extended illness duration, a younger age at death, and predominantly psychiatric symptoms in the early stages including withdrawal, delusions, hallucinations, aggression, and depression (Zeidler *et al.* 1997*a*,*b*; National CJD Surveillance Unit 1998; Will *et al.* 1999, 2000). Neurological indications included cerebellar signs, dementia, involuntary movements, myoclonus, akinetic mutism, chorea, upgaze palsy, and dystonia. Electroencephalography changes characteristic of sporadic CJD with generalized bi/triphasic periodic complex (Brown *et al.* 1986) have not been reported in vCJD. The peak age of onset for sporadic CJD lies between 60 and 70 years of age, and in Britain only four cases of CJD had

Table 3 Case–control methods

Reference	No.	Case selection	Control selection and method of Information collection
1. Bobowick *et al.* (1973) USA	38	Biopsy or autopsy-proven cases diagnosed since 1966 were requested by writing to all members of American Association of Neuropathologists in USA and Canada plus all cases referred to NINDS	Nearest relative of the deceased asked to participate in structured interview and asked to select friend of the patient of the same age and sex to serve as control. All families visited in their home by same doctor and nurse
2. Kondo *et al.* (1982) Japan	60	902 neurological clinics asked to report cases between 1975 and 1977. Criteria of Masters used. Only definite and probable cases included. Study area, all Japan	Nearest relative of the deceased asked to participate in structured interview and asked to introduce a neighbour of the same age and sex as the patient. When necessary public health personnel allowed to serve as 'neighbour'
3. Kondo (1985) Japan	88	CJD cases retrieved from Annual or Pathological Autopsies in Japan, 1964–78	From the same register autopsies from craniocervical injuries, myocardial infarction, and pulmonary tuberculosis were selected as controls. Recorded information compared
4. Davanipour *et al.* (1985*a*,*b*, 1986) USA	26	Cases ascertained from records submitted to the Laboratory of Central Nervous System Studies between 1970 and 1981. Study restricted to Pennsylvania and surrounding mid-Atlantic states	Two control groups were selected. Hospital controls matched for age and sex were selected by writing to medical record departments. Ten case-notes of people admitted at the time of the patients' admission were selected. Random-number tables were used to select one of these cases. The other control group was family members. A questionnaire was administered by telephone
5. Harries- Jones *et al.* (1988) UK	92	Cases obtained from regional neurological centres in England and Wales by direct referral after repeated written requests for cases. In addition copies of all death certificates on which CJD or spongiform encephalopathy were mentioned were obtained from the Office of Population Censuses and Surveys	Two groups of hospital controls were selected by questioning ward staff and accepting the first proffered matched subject. One control had a 'neurological' diagnosis different from CJD and the other a non-neurological 'medical' diagnosis
6. van Duijn *et al.* (1998) Europe	405	Cases were obtained from the European national registers (19) which had been compiled by targeting professional groups, including neurologists, neurophysiologists, and neuropathologists, and asking for direct referrals	Control participants were recruited from the hospital where the patient who had CJD had been diagnosed. Data were collected by a structured interview. Control's next of kin was interviewed wherever possible
7. National CJD Surveillance Unit (1990) UK (ongoing)	473	Cases were obtained from direct referral by hospital physicians, neurologists, neuropathologists, and neurophysiologists	An age- and sex-matched hospital control was selected. Where possible the control's next of kin was interviewed.
8. Collins (1999) Australia	241	Cases were obtained from the Australian CJD registry, 1970–1993 retrospectively and 1993–1997 prospectively	For every case, three community controls were recruited and interviewed through a random-dialling telephone survey, with data collected using a questionnaire

NINDS, National Institute for Neurological Disorders and Stroke.

occurred in people under 35 between 1970 and the end of 1989. In contrast, six of the first ten cases of vCJD were younger than 30. Only fourteen cases of CJD under 30 years had ever previously been reported in the world (Will *et al.* 1996). Cases had no family history of prion disease and had no exposure to known transmitted CJD.

In addition to the United Kingdom cases of vCJD, one case occurred in a 26-year-old Frenchman who may have acquired infection from injecting the anabolic steroid bovine growth hormone somatotrophin, as an aid to body-building, prior to the July 1992 ban on its use.

The most striking and consistent neuropathological feature that helps separate vCJD from sporadic CJD is the presence of numerous large 'florid' amyloid plaques surrounded by spongiform change extensively distributed throughout the cerebral and cerebellar cortex, with smaller numbers in the basal ganglia, thalamus, and hypothalamus. Immunocytochemical staining for PrP shows strong staining of these plaque-like lesions. However, these lesions are not pathognomonic of this disorder (Ironside and Bell 1997) and have been occasionally reported in cases of iatrogenic CJD (Takashima *et al.* 1997).

Lymphoreticular tissues (68 tonsils, 64 spleens, and 40 lymph nodes) were obtained at autopsy from patients with 'prion' diseases, and from neurological and non-neurological controls, as well as tonsil samples from patients with suspected 'prion' disease. In

Table 4 Significant exposures from case–control studies

Exposure	Study	OR (CI)	p
Dietary—fish			
Raw seafood	1	4.02 (1.3–12.9)[a]	<0.05[a]
Raw oyster/clam	4	3.3	<0.10[b]
Dietary—meats			
Roast lamb	4	3.6	<0.10[b]
Roast/smoked pork	4	2.6	<0.10[b]
Scrapple	4	4.0	<0.10[b]
Pork chops (high versus never)	*4*	*6.6*	*<0.10*[b]
Ham (deli/canned)	*4*	*12.1*	*<0.01*[b]
Liver (ever versus never)	*4*	*5.9*	*<0.10*[b]
Meat (rare versus well done)	*4*	*8.0*	*<0.10*[b]
Raw meat	6	1.57 (1.1–2.2)	0.05[a]
Brain	6	1.63 (0.9–2.9)	0.1[a]
Beef (weekly)	7	2.37 (1.2–4.7)	0.01
Veal	7	1.69 (1.1–2.8)	0.005
Brain	7	3.1 (1.4–6.9)	0.005
Venison	*7*	*7.9 (1.8–34.9)*	*<0.005*
Zoonotic—hobbies and sports			
Involving fish	4	4.5 (1.6–)[c]	<0.005
Involving squirrel, skunk	4	4.4 (0.9–)[c]	<0.10
Deer (frequent versus none)	4	6.8 (1.1–)	<0.05[c]
Rabbit (frequent versus none)	4	6.0 (1.0)	<0.05[c]
Occupational			
Ever lived or worked on a farm or market garden, or been employed in an abattoir or butchery	8	2.6 (1.8–3.7)	≤0.001
Animal exposure (long versus none)	*4*	*8.6 (1.8–)*	*0.001*
Deer, monkey, squirrel	*4*	*9.0 (0.9–)*	*<0.005*[c]
Low (male exposure)	*4*	*5.7 (0.8–)*	*<0.10*[c]
Pet exposure			
Keeping cats	5	2.0 (1.2–3.6)	<0.01
Pets other than cats and dogs	5	4.4 (1.5–12.7)	<0.01
Ferret contact	5	2.1 (1.0–4.2)	0.05
Squirrel	*4*	*12.3 (1.1–)*	*<0.05*[c]
Mink contact	*5*	*8.6 (0.9–77.9)*	0.08
Animal product exposure	6	1.9 (1.1–3.3)	<0.05[a]
Frequent exposure to leather products	6	2.3 (1.3–3.9)	<0.005[a]
Exposure to fertilizer containing hoof and horn			
'Iatrogenic'			
Surgical operation	2/3	3.48 (1.3–9.4)	<0.01
Physical injury	2/3	2.53 (1.0–6.4)	<0.05
Organ resection	2/3	2.78 (1.0–6.5)[a]	Fisher's exact, <0.05
Head/face/neck trauma or operation	4	3.5 (1.0–13.5)[a]	<0.05
Other trauma	4	4.0 (1.2–14.6)[a]	<0.01
Suture	4	2.9 (0.9–9.9)[a]	<0.10
Zoster in adult life	5	2.6 (2.4–)	<0.005
Dementia in family	5	3.6 (1.8–7.1)	<0.0005
Surgical procedures (x 2)	8	1.7 (1.0–2.7)	<0.05
Surgical procedures (x 3)	8	2.1 (1.3–3.4)	<0.005
Tonometry (within 2 years of disease onset)	*4*	*9.2 (1.2–424)*	*Fishers exact, 0.02*[a]
Cataract/eye surgery	*8*	*6.1 (3.2–11.9)*	*<0.001*
Carpal tunnel surgery	*8*	*9.2 (2.5–34.1)*	*0.001*

OR, odds ratio; CI confidence interval. OR given is for 'case versus all controls' unless specified. Cases where OR > 5 are shown in italics.

[a] OR and *p* value calculated from original data using StatCalc (EpiInfo 6 version 6.04a).

[b] OR and *p* value provided in original data but without sufficient data to calculate CI.

[c] OR, *p* value, and lower limit of 95 per cent confidence interval are given in original paper, but insufficient data are provided to calculate upper limit.

lymphoreticular tissue, PrP^{Sc} was detected only in samples from individuals with confirmed vCJD. It was also detected from tonsil biopsy samples from all eight patients whose disease turned out to be vCJD. It was not detected in samples from patients with other forms of prion diseases, including iatrogenic and familial CJD (Hill *et al.* 1999). Tonsillar biopsy appears to be both an extremely specific and sensitive test for the antemortem diagnosis of vCJD and so far represents the only means of diagnosing vCJD before death without brain biopsy (Petersen 1999).

Prion strains can be typed using Western-blot protein analysis and strain typing links vCJD to BSE. Patterns of banding of protein fragments of PrP^{Sc} are determined by the degree of protein glycosylation. In humans four patterns have been recognized, designated Types 1–4. Most sporadic CJD is Type 2, most iatrogenic CJD is Type 3, but all vCJD is Type 4, the same pattern seen in BSE-infected cattle and in mice and macaques experimentally infected with BSE.

Unlike familial CJD, in which more than 20 different coding mutations have been found to be associated with the development of disease, no pathogenic mutations have been detected in the PRNP in cases of vCJD. However, in addition to the pathogenic mutations, there is a common polymorphism at codon 129 of the PRNP that results in the substitution of valine (**V**) for methionine (**M**) (Goldfarb *et al.* 1989). The codon 129 genotype is known to influence susceptibility to both sporadic CJD (Palmer *et al.* 1991) and iatrogenic CJD (Collinge *et al.* 1991; Brown *et al.* 1994*b*), and the disease phenotype of familial CJD can also be modulated by the codon 129 polymorphism (Goldfarb *et al.* 1992). All cases of vCJD so far studied have been homozygous for methionine (MM) at codon 129, which occurs in only around 37 per cent of normal controls and 79 per cent of sporadic cases of CJD. Interestingly, cattle are uniformly homozygous for methionine at codon 129 in the PRNP (Schätzl *et al.* 1997). If, as has been suggested, the ability to transmit disease from one species to another depends on the likeness of the infecting 'prion' to the hosts 'prion', then the MM genotype in humans might confer an increased susceptibility to bovine 'prions'. However, it would be premature to conclude that individuals who possess the codon 129 genotypes MV or VV cannot develop vCJD (Hill *et al.* 1997).

Up to October 2000 there have been 83 confirmed cases of vCJD in the United Kingdom (Table 5), one case from the Republic of Ireland, and two cases reported from France. Detailed demographic data have been made available on 52 of the vCJD cases that have occurred in the United Kingdom (National CJD Surveillance Unit 1999). Of the 52 cases, 28 were women. The median age at onset of disease was 28 years and the median age at death 29 years (compared with 65 years for the median age of death for sporadic CJD). The median duration of illness was 14 months (range 7 to 38) which is long when compared with 4.5 months in sporadic CJD. The median delay between onset of disease and confirmation of vCJD was 15 months (range 7 to 32 months). This has not decreased over time. Since the first case of vCJD, with onset in early 1994, there is now some evidence that the incidence of vCJD is increasing.

Table 5 Monthly Creutzfeldt–Jakob disease statistics

Year	Referrals	Sporadic	Iatrogenic	Familial	GSS	vCJD probable Still alive	vCJD probable Deaths awaiting PM results	nvCJD confirmed[a]	Total
1985	–	26	1	1	0	–			28
1986	–	26	0	0	0	–			26
1987	–	23	0	0	1	–			24
1988	–	22	1	1	0	–			24
1989	–	28	2	2	0	–			32
1990	53	28	5	0	0	–			33
1991	75	32	1	3	0	–			36
1992	96	43	2	5	1	–			51
1993	78	38	4	2	2	–			46
1994	116	51	1	4	3	–			59
1995	87	35	4	2	3	–		3	47
1996	134	40	4	2	4	–		10	60
1997	161	59	6	4	1	–		10	80
1998	154	63	3	4	1	–		18	89
1999	169	61	6	2	0	–	–	15	83
2000[a]	151	36	0	1	0	5	3	23	68

GSS, Gerstmann–Straussler–Schienker disease; PM., postmortem.

[a] To 1 December 2000: total number of definite and probable cases of vCJD is 87.

Source: Department of Health (2000).

Figure 2 shows the geographical distribution by place of residence at onset, of the 52 cases of vCJD with onset in the United Kingdom. Comparison of vCJD incidence rates in four northernmost regions (northwest, Yorkshire and Humberside, northern, Scotland) with those further south (southwest, southeast, Wales, West Midlands, East Midlands, East Anglia) according to place of residence in 1991 suggests that the incidence in the 'North' of the United Kingdom is twice that in the 'South'. There is no explanation as yet for this observation.

Initial concern over a cluster of four cases in east Kent led to speculation that there was a causal relationship between vCJD and a cattle-rendering plant in the vicinity (Chandrakumar 1998), but detailed investigation has suggested that the occurrence of four or more cases in a population of 1.5 million (approximately the population of east Kent) is not unexpected (Cousens *et al.* 1999). More recently, concern has been raised over a cluster of five cases in Leicestershire that are currently under investigation. Analysis of 48 vCJD cases by place of residence in 1991, as the likely time of peak exposure, provided no evidence of local clustering.

Cases of vCJD have not been the subject of intensive epidemiological field investigation, as might have been expected of a new disease cluster, but cases have been enrolled in the ongoing case–control study run by the CJD Surveillance Unit (National CJD Surveillance Unit 1996). Up until 1997, only hospital-based controls were recruited, but since then a decision has been made to change the study design to recruit four community controls per case, selected from general medical practices. The most recent data (National CJD Surveillance Unit 1999) present 51 cases but no community controls. Cases have been compared with 27 non-matched 'non-cases'. Cases were reported to have eaten beef more frequently than controls, but not significantly so. Interestingly, 51 per cent of the vCJD cases were reported to have eaten burgers, meat pies, and sausages likely to have contained mechanically recovered meat (**MRM**), compared to 41 per cent of controls. However, even if cases really have had a 10 per cent greater exposure to MRM, a case–control study would need to have 254 cases and 1016 controls to have an 80 per cent power to detect an increased odds ratio of 1.5 at the 95 per cent level of significance, a result reflecting the high exposure rate of the normal population to MRM.

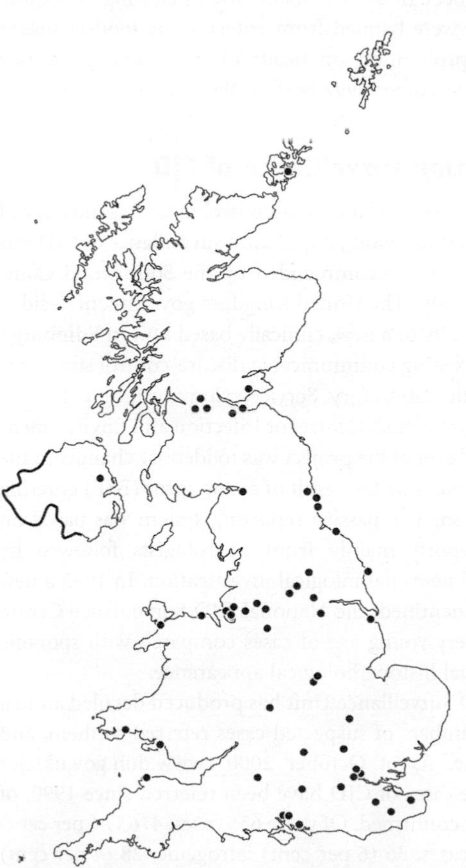

Fig. 2 The geographical distribution, by place of residence at onset, of the 52 cases of vCJD with onset in the United Kingdom.

Predicting the epidemic

Several attempts have been made to predict the size of the eventual vCJD epidemic. The first of these was by Cousens (1997*b*) based on the first 14 reported cases. In any calculation of this sort several fundamental assumptions have to be made. In the case of Cousens' predictions these were as follows.

- vCJD is due to exposure to the BSE agent.
- Until 1989 the number of people newly infected with the BSE agent each year was proportional to the number of cases of BSE in cattle with onset in that year.
- Individuals infected with the BSE agent develop vCJD after a long and variable incubation period (mean incubation periods of 10, 15, 20, and 25 years were used for these calculations).
- There were few (< 5) or no cases of vCJD before 1994.

Cousens used two sets of predictions for the number of BSE cases. The first set assumes that the degree of under-reporting of BSE changed little over time. The second set assumes that under-reporting was greatest early in the epidemic and reduced after BSE was made a notifiable disease.

Three models for predicting epidemic size were used, based on the distribution of incubation periods. These were lognormal, gamma, and Weibull. Assuming that there were fewer than five cases with onset before 1994, the Weibull model does not provide a good approximation to the incubation-period distribution.

Using the lognormal incubation-period distribution model the least number of cases expected would be 75 and the worst scenario would be 80 000 cases. Using the gamma incubation-period distribution model, the 'best' scenario would be 88 and the worst would be 13 000.

The actual number of confirmed cases with clinical disease onset in 1996, 1997, and 1998 were 10, 10, and 13 respectively (Ghani *et al.* 1998). These numbers would exclude Cousens' predicted worst-case scenarios and suggest that, based on the assumptions given above, the final size of the epidemic may well lie in the range of 75–450 cases.

Ghani *et al.* (1998) constructed a mathematical model to predict the magnitude of the vCJD epidemic based on data up to the end of 1997 (23 cases) and used the following assumptions to calculate a large number (5 million) of different scenarios. The following assumptions were made.

- vCJD is due to exposure (orally) to the BSE agent.

- Incubation-period distribution of vCJD is unimodal for the prion gene codon 129 methionine homozygous genotype (other genotypes were not considered in their calculations).
- There was no under-reporting of vCJD cases prior to 1995.
- There has been no human-to-human transmission.

The two epidemiological factors that had the greatest impact on the estimated epidemic size and duration were the average number of humans infected by one infectious bovine and the incubation-period distribution. From their calculations, the smallest epidemic would consist of just zero to 200 cases assuming that, on average, only 0.0001 humans are infected by one maximally infectious bovine. The worst-case scenario would be between 2 million and 10 million cases, assuming that over 100 persons are infected by one maximally infectious bovine. Ghani *et al.* (1998) address the issue of when it will be possible to narrow the range of possible outcomes. If the incidence of vCJD remains very low for the next 3 to 5 years, a small epidemic becomes more likely since it will become increasingly probable that the epidemic peak has been reached.

Based on the assumptions given above, and on the actual annual incidence of vCJD deaths in 1995 to 1999, Ghani *et al.* (2000) have reassessed their initial predictions using extensive scenario analyses. From the vCJD incidence in 1999 and the observed stable age structure of cases, they substantially reduce the upper limit of possible cases to 136 000.

A study by Cohen *et al.* (1999) attempted to predict the start date of the BSE epidemic and the consequent implications on any vCJD epidemic. Cousens has already made predications of the future vCJD epidemic based on the first human exposure to BSE taking place between 1983 and 1985 (Cousens 1997*b*). Cohen *et al.* applied an age-cohort model to BSE data between 1985 and 1996 to estimate the earliest possible date of the first unrecognized BSE cases. According to the models, BSE cases may have occurred as early as 1980, which implies a much smaller epidemic than that predicted by Cousens.

The public health response to BSE and variant CJD

Food safety

The epidemic of BSE in British cattle raised immediate concerns about its zoonotic potential and eventually in 1988 a working party was established under the chairmanship of Sir Richard Southwood (Table 6) (Southwood 1989).

The main task for this and subsequent committees was to decide whether the BSE agent would be transmitted to humans and what the possible pathways were. Thus the distribution of the agent in incubating and affected cattle needed to be known, as well as the ways in which products were processed and where they ended up. This proved to be immensely complex, since products of cattle such as gelatin may be used in cosmetic, pharmaceutical, and medical products. Southwood quickly recommended that BSE should be made a notifiable disease and that the practice of feeding ruminant protein to other ruminants should be banned. The order was made on 14 June 1988 but not implemented until 18 July 1988 in order to allow stocks of meat and bonemeal feed to be cleared. It is now clear that enforcement of this ban was inadequate (Patterson and Painter 1997). Cases continued to be seen in cattle born after the ruminant feed ban, and a case–control study suggested that this was due to ongoing feed contamination, possibly through cross-contamination of cattle feed by ruminant protein prepared in the same feed mills as for non-ruminants. (Only in March 1996 was the use of mammalian meat and bonemeal for any farm animal terminated.) Affected cattle were required to be slaughtered and carcasses incinerated or buried. However, until February 1990 compensation to farmers was set at only 50 per cent of the value of the cow, with the consequence that possibly infected animals would be sold for meat before a definite diagnosis was made.

In the United Kingdom in November 1989 certain bovine tissues (termed specified bovine offal (**SBO**)) believed to be potentially infectious, such as brain, spinal cord, intestines, tonsil, thymus, and spleen from cattle over 6 months of age, were banned from the human food chain. However, once again inadequate enforcement of the ban led to some of this material continuing to enter the food chain, particularly in the form of MRM (Patterson and Painter 1997). MRM from the vertebral column, which could contain fragments of spinal cord, was eventually banned only in December 1995. Therefore it seems probable that the British public was potentially exposed to the agent of BSE in presymptomatic cattle, via foods such as beefburgers and pies which use MRM, right up with the end of 1995.

The recognition of new variant CJD in 1996 led to further stringent control measures. In March 1996 the European Union banned the export of any British beef. In April 1996, in the United Kingdom, cattle over 30 months old were banned from entering the food chain. In September 1996 a prohibition on heads of sheep and goats was introduced, and in December 1997 beef on the bone was banned.

Human population surveillance of CJD

In parallel with the veterinary- and food-control measures introduced by MAFF in the United Kingdom, population surveillance of CJD was reinstated in May 1990 as recommended by the Southwood Committee (Southwood 1989). The United Kingdom government decided to give this responsibility to a new, clinically based unit in Edinburgh rather than use the existing communicable disease-control structures of the Public Health Laboratory Service, Communicable Disease Surveillance Centre or Scottish Centre for Infection and Environmental Health. The initial aim of the project was to identify changes in the pattern of CJD that might be the result of a new agent (BSE) entering the human population. The passive reporting system was based on receiving clinical reports mainly from neurologists followed by in-depth clinical and neuropathological investigation. In 1995 a new variant of CJD was identified; the National CJD Surveillance Centre was alerted by the very young age of cases compared with sporadic CJD and their unusual histopathological appearance.

The National CJD Surveillance Unit has produced detailed annual reports including numbers of suspected cases referred to them, and the clinical outcome. As of October 2000 (www.doh.gov.uk/cjd/stats/), 1261 possible cases of CJD have been referred since 1990, of which 639 have been confirmed. Of these 635 cases, 476 (74 per cent) have been sporadic cases, 36 (6 per cent) iatrogenic, 28 (4 per cent) familial, 15 (2 per cent) GSS, and 83 (13 per cent) vCJD. Trends in mortality since 1970 have been analysed, showing an increase in all age groups, a phenomenon seen in other European countries which is

Table 6 BSE: selected chronology of events, 1986–98

Date	Event
November 1986	BSE is identified by the Central Veterinary Laboratory
April 1987	Initial epidemiological studies start
5 June 1987	The Chief Veterinary Officer informs ministers about the new disease
15 December 1987	Epidemiological studies conclude that ruminant-derived meat and bone meal is the only viable hypothesis for the cause of BSE
21 April 1988	The setting up of the Southwood Working Party is announced
14 June 1988	The Bovine Spongiform Encephalopathy Order 1988 (SI 1988/1039) is made. Article 7, prohibiting the sale, supply, and use of certain feedingstuff for feeding to ruminants, comes into effect on 18 July
20 June 1988	The Southwood Working Party holds its first meeting
21 June 1988	The BSE Order 1988 makes BSE a notifiable disease
22 June 1988	Interim advice is received from Southwood to destroy affected cattle
7 July 1988	The decision to introduce a slaughter policy is announced
18 July 1988	The ruminant feed ban comes into force (included the BSE Order 1988)
8 August 1988	The Bovine Spongiform Encephalopathy (Amendment) Order 1988 (SI 1988/1345) and Bovine Spongiform Encephalopathy Compensation Order 1988 (SI 1988/1346) come into effect. These provide for a slaughter policy and compensation to be paid at 50 per cent value for confirmed cases, and 100 per cent for negative cases
October 1988	Transmission to mice following intracerebral inoculation is reported
15 November 1988	Advice from Southwood to extend the feed ban and destroy milk from infected cattle
22 December 1988	The Zoonosis Order 1988 designates BSE as a zoonosis, enabling powers under the Animal Health Act 1981 to be used to reduce the risk to human health from BSE
27 February 1989	The Southwood Report is published
27 February 1989	The Tyrrell Committee on research is established
10 June 1989	The government receives the Tyrrell Report
13 June 1989	The decision to introduce the offals ban is announced
28 July 1989	The European Union bans the export of cattle born before 18 July 1998 and of offspring or suspect animals
13 November 1989	The Bovine Offal (Prohibition) Regulations 1989 comes into force in England and Wales, banning the use of SBO for human consumption
9 January 1990	The Tyrrell Report is published
31 January 1990	Five antelopes succumb to a spongiform encephalopathy
3 February 1990	Transmission, cattle-to-cattle following intracerebral and intravenous inoculation of BSE brain tissue, and into mice via the oral route, reported in *The Veterinary Record*
14 February 1990	The Bovine Spongiform Encephalopathy Compensation Order (SI 1990/222). Full compensation for affected animals
1 March 1990	The European Union restricts exports of cattle to those which were slaughtered before 6 months of age
1 April 1990	The disease is made notifiable by the European Union
10 May 1990	Announcement about a cat with spongiform encephalopathy
25 September 1990	The Bovine Spongiform Encephalopathy (No 2) Amendment Order 1990 extends the ban on the use of SBO to any animal feed
27 March 1991	The first case of BSE in offspring born after the ruminant feed ban is announced
2 November 1994	The Bovine Offal (Prohibition) (Amendment) Regulations 1994 extends controls to include thymus and intestines of all bovine animals, except those under 2 months which have died
February 1995	SEAC publishes report *Transmissible Spongiform Encephalopathies—A Summary of Present Knowledge and Research*
15 August 1995	The Specified Bovine Offal Order 1995 takes effect. Main changes: dedicated lines for rendering plants processing SBO; a prohibition on the removal of brains and eyes; a prohibition on the removal of the spinal cord from the vertebral column apart from in slaughterhouses.
28 November 1995	The Specified Bovine Offal (Amendment) Order 1995 comes into effect, prohibiting the use of bovine vertebral column in the manufacture of all MRM, and also in the production of some other products for human consumption
15 December 1995	On advice from SEAC the government announces its decision to suspend use of bovine vertebral column in the manufacture of MRM
20 March 1996	SEAC announces that the CJD Surveillance Unit has identified a previously unrecognized and consistent disease pattern
27 March 1996	European Commission Decision 96/239—EU prohibits the export from the UK of live bovine animals, their semen and embryos; meat of bovine animals slaughtered in the UK; products obtained from bovine animals slaughtered in the UK which are liable to enter the animal-feed or human-food chain, and materials destined for use in medicinal products, cosmetics, or pharmaceutical products; and mammalian-derived meat and bone meal
28 March 1996	The government announces the calf slaughter scheme and financial aid for the rendering industry
31 May 1996	UK BSE Eradication Programme is sent to the European Commission
24 July 1996	Following SEAC advice, the government announces its intention to introduce controls to require the removal of sheeps' heads from the food chain, an interim measure pending EU-wide controls. This follows publication of evidence that BSE could be isolated from the spleen of sheep experimentally infected with BSE
1 August 1996	MAFF announces that SEAC has considered the interim results of MAFF research on maternal transmission (cohort study). SEAC concludes that very low levels of maternal transmission of BSE may have occurred
16 December 1996	The selective cull of cattle most at risk of BSE is announced.
3 December 1997	Following SEAC advice, the government announces its intention to consult on measures to require the deboning of all beef from cattle aged over 6 months before it is sold to the consumer.
16 December 1997	The Beef Bones Regulations 1997 (SI 1997/2959) comes into force, requiring the deboning of all beef derived from cattle both home-produced and imported aged over 6 months at slaughter before it is sold to customers.
22 December 1997	The government announces the Public Inquiry into BSE.
9 March 1998	Public hearings start in the Public Inquiry into BSE.
4 January 1999	BSE Offspring Slaughter Regulations (SI 1998/3070) comes into force, implementing a compulsory cull of offspring born on or after 1 August 1996 to BSE cases confirmed before 25 November 1998.
14 April 1999	The SEAC Subgroup publishes its report on research and surveillance for TSEs in sheep.

MAFF, Ministry of Agriculture, Fisheries, and Food
Source: www.maff.gov.uk

probably the result of improving surveillance and case ascertainment, and reporting.

In order to establish whether vCJD was really a new condition and not due to improved surveillance, a retrospective review of death certificates has been carried out (Majeed *et al.* 1998). A total of 1485 deaths from selected neurological disorders were identified in people aged 15 to 44 years in England from 1979 to 1996. Clinical records were traced for nearly half of the cases and reviewed. No new cases of sporadic or vCJD were identified, giving a strong measure of confidence in the completion of the surveillance system. A similar study in Wales also found no case of vCJD between 1985 and 1995, supporting the view that vCJD was a new disease entity rather than the result of better ascertainment.

Concern over the emergence of vCJD in the United Kingdom led the United States Centers for Disease Control and Prevention to set up an active CJD surveillance in April–May 1996 in the four established Emerging Infections Program sites and Atlanta (Schonberger 1998). The average annual death rate was stable from 1991 to 1995 at 1.2 per million population. No variant cases were identified and since then ongoing review of United States mortality data of CJD cases in younger adults has failed to identify variant cases.

Risk assessment, risk communication, and public confidence

Major issues of public policy have been highlighted by the BSE crisis (Maxwell 1999). The initial risk assessment of the threat to human health was based erroneously on the evidence that scrapie, though prevalent in the United Kingdom for centuries, had not seemingly been transmitted to humans, and that when experimentally transmitted to other animals the infectivity of scrapie via the oral route was low. The Southwood Report in 1989 concluded that 'it was most unlikely that BSE would have any implications for human health'. Patterson and Painter (1997) commented that:

> In their main report to Parliament in February 1989, the Southwood Committee acknowledged the paucity of evidence available to them. They advised that cattle were likely to prove a 'dead end host' for the disease agent and that it was 'most unlikely that BSE would have any implications for human health'. With the exceptions of baby foods and medicinal products no action was taken to reduce human exposure to high titre bovine tissues (such as brain and spinal cord) from preclinically infected cattle. This was despite prior health warnings about the consumption of BSE infected bovine brain, and concern that the inability to identify BSE infected cattle was a major threat to human disease control and to cattle exports from the UK.

Southwood did say that if his assumptions proved wrong 'the implications would be extremely serious'. However, Tyrrell, the first chairman of SEAC, set up in 1989, was even more convinced of the lack of risk and wrote that 'any risk as a result of eating beef or beef products is minute. Thus we believe that there is no scientific reason for not eating British beef and that it can be eaten by everyone' (Maxwell 1999).

Clearly, events have proved that judgement to be seriously in error and to lack the caution which the state of knowledge at the time required. Lack of evidence of a risk is to be distinguished from evidence of no risk. It is of great significance that up until 1997 the work of SEAC, like other government advisory committees, was not shared in any formal way with the public health profession or the public, contributing to the sense of distrust of MAFF and government advice (Anonymous 1996*b*). Further, its composition in the critical early years has been criticized for a lack of public-health experts who might have offered a more balanced approach to assessing population risk and the necessity to gain public confidence (Gore 1996). One editorial in the *Lancet* said:

> No sooner had a terse statement been made in the House of Commons ... than the lay and professional media swept into action, filling the information gap with variable accuracy. This reaction, condemned by some, was understandable since the scientific evidence that underpinned the announcement and subsequent advice had not been made publicly available ... The conclusions they reach and the recommendations they make are made public in short, bald statements that are distributed by the commissioning department. Only then might the data be offered for consideration for publication in a peer-reviewed journal; too late, perhaps, to contradict the baseless bluster that has already been given free space to shape opinion and policy. (Anonymous 1996*b*)

The identification of vCJD and the government statement that they were probably due to BSE led to a collapse of public confidence in both the United Kingdom and Europe, and a consequent collapse of the beef market (Palmer 1996). Just 14 weeks before the announcement of vCJD the official view of the Department of Health was that the risk to humans from eating beef was only theoretical. At the end of 1995 the report of two cases in young people was accompanied by a suggestion that this was ascertainment bias or a chance finding. The account on March 20 by SEAC with eight more young cases stated that 'on current data and in the absence of any credible alternative the most likely explanation at present is these cases are linked to exposure to BSE before the introduction of the SBO ban in 1989. This is cause for great concern.' But in the press release issued the same day by Stephen Dorrell, Secretary for Health, the statement is also made that 'There remains no scientific proof that BSE can be transmitted to man by beef.' 'No scientific proof' and 'cause for great concern' do not sit easily together and may have increased anxiety levels and decreased trust. Mr Dorrell's statement said in one paragraph that 'these new findings suggest that there may have been an association between eating bovine products' and CJD, and in the next paragraph states 'there remains, however, no scientific evidence that BSE can be transmitted by beef'. If the latter is true, then the expert scientific committee on whose advice government policy is based had no scientific evidence for its 'great concern'! There followed a robust appeal by at least one public-health advocate to 'have done with misleading the profession, the public, and the press with unqualified "no evidence of" statements. All evidence must be quantified' (Gore 1996).

The government, in an attempt to regain public confidence in its advice on food safety, announced its intention to set up a Food Standards Agency. Also, and in response to pressure from patients' families, an open enquiry into BSE was initiated under the chairmanship of Lord Phillips to 'establish and review the history of the emergence and identification of BSE and variant CJD and of the action taken in response to it up to 20 March 1996' and 'to reach conclusions on the adequacy of that response, taking into account the state of knowledge at the time.' This enquiry has broken new ground in the way in which access to information has been allowed. All proceedings have been conducted in public and all evidence has been made available as literal transcripts on the internet (www.bse.org.uk) within a few hours. Confidential government minutes of papers have been called as evidence and all these are available on the World Wide Web. Inquiry lawyers have sieved the huge volume of documentary evidence and have even compared draft documents and minutes with final versions to seek explanations for significant omissions. The key conclusions of the Phillips Inquiry are as follows.

- BSE has caused a harrowing fatal disease for humans.
- A vital industry has been dealt a body blow, inflicting misery on tens of thousands for whom livestock farming is their way of life. They have seen over 170 000 of their animals die or be destroyed, and the precautionary slaughter and destruction within the United Kingdom of very many more.
- BSE developed into an epidemic as a consequence of an intensive farming practice—the recycling of animal protein in ruminant feed. This practice, unchallenged over decades, proved a recipe for disaster.
- At the heart of the BSE story lie questions of how to handle hazard—a known hazard to cattle and an unknown hazard to humans. The government took measures to address both hazards. They were sensible measures, but they were not always timely nor adequately implemented and enforced.
- The rigour with which policy measures were implemented for the protection of human health was affected by the belief of many prior to early 1996 that BSE was not a potential threat to human life.
- The government was anxious to act in the best interests of human and animal health. To this end it sought and followed the advice of independent scientific experts, sometimes when decisions could have been reached more swiftly and satisfactorily within government.
- At times officials showed a lack of rigour in considering how policy should be turned into practice, to the detriment of the efficacy of the measures taken.
- At times bureaucratic processes resulted in unacceptable delays in giving effect to policy.
- The government introduced measures to guard against the risk that BSE might be a matter of life and death not merely for cattle but also for humans, but the possibility of a risk to humans was not communicated to the public or to those whose job it was to implement and enforce the precautionary measures.
- The government did not lie to the public about BSE. It believed that the risks posed by BSE to humans were remote. The government was preoccupied with preventing an alarmist over-reaction to BSE because it believed that the risk was remote. It is now clear that this campaign of reassurance was a mistake. When, on 20 March 1996, the government announced that BSE had probably been transmitted to humans, the public felt that they had been betrayed. Confidence in government pronouncements about risk was a further casualty of BSE.
- Cases of new variant CJD (vCJD) were identified by the National CJD Surveillance Unit, and the conclusion that they were probably linked to BSE was reached as early as was reasonably possible. The link between BSE and vCJD is now clearly established, though the manner of infection is not clear.

Of particular note for the public health management of the epidemic were the following conclusions of the Phillips Inquiry, released in November 2000.

1. The original risk assessment for human health was erroneously based on the view that BSE was introduced into cattle via feed derived from sheep infected with conventional scrapie. Since scrapie was not considered a human health hazard the potential threat to humans from BSE was underestimated.
2. There were significant communication problems within and between MAFF and the Department of Health, leading to significant delays in implementing control measures in relation to mechanically recovered meat, medicines, cosmetics, and occupational guidance. For example, 'By the end of 1987 MAFF officials had become concerned as to whether it was acceptable for cattle showing signs of BSE to be slaughtered for human consumption. However, the Department of Health was not asked to collaborate with MAFF in considering the implications that BSE had for human health. It should have been.'
3. Communication with the public 'failed to explain that the views expressed were subject to proper observance of the precautionary measures which had been introduced to protect human health against the possibility that BSE might be transmissible. These statements conveyed the message not merely that beef was safe but that BSE was not transmissible. The impression thus given to the public that BSE was not transmissible to humans was a significant factor leading to the public feeling of betrayal when it was announced on 20 March 1996 that BSE was likely to have been transmitted to humans.'
4. The Department of Health and MAFF were taken to task for overly relying on scientific committees.

   The Southwood Working Party considered that all reasonably practicable precautions should be taken to reduce the risks that would exist should BSE prove to be transmissible to humans. However, they did not make this plain in their Report and did not recommend that the possible risks from eating animals incubating BSE but not yet showing signs of the disease ("subclinical cases") called for any precautions, other than a recommendation that manufacturers should not include ruminant offal and thymus in baby food. This was a shortcoming in their Report.

   Because of a failure to subject the Southwood Report to an adequate review, MAFF and DoH failed to identify this shortcoming. Concern about the food risks posed by subclinical cases was, however, expressed by some scientists, by the media and by the public. With the agreement of DoH, MAFF reacted by announcing in June 1989 that those categories of offal of cattle most likely to be infectious (SBO) were to be banned from use in human food. The introduction of this vital precautionary measure was commendable. However, this ban was presented to the public in terms that underplayed its importance as a public health measure.

> Careful consideration was given by MAFF and DoH in 1989 to the terms of the human SBO ban, with one important exception. During the consultation process, concerns were raised about the practicality of ensuring the removal of all the spinal cord during abattoir processes, and about the practice of mechanical recovery of scraps left attached to the vertebral column for use in human food ('mechanically recovered meat' or MRM). However, MAFF officials discounted these concerns without subjecting them to rigorous consideration—in particular no advice was sought as to the minimum quantity of spinal cord that might transmit the disease in food.
>
> MAFF gave detailed consideration to spinal cord and MRM in 1990. A lengthy paper was submitted to SEAC, the Government's new expert advisory committee on TSEs. Unhappily, as a result of a breakdown in communications, MAFF officials understood that the members of SEAC were not concerned about the inclusion in human food of an occasional scrap of spinal cord, so that no action was called for. In fact the advice of some, at least, of the members of SEAC was premised on the false assumption that spinal cord could readily be removed from the carcass in its entirety, and would be so removed. This was one of a number of occasions that has given rise to lessons for the future about the proper use of expert committees by the Government.
>
> Not until 1995 was action taken in relation to MRM . . . Up to 1995, MRM was a potential pathway to the infection of humans with BSE, not merely because of the risk of inclusion of the occasional portion of spinal cord, but because the material recovered by the MRM process included dorsal root ganglia. These were peripheral nervous tissues which were not thought to be infectious at the time, but which have since been demonstrated to be infectious in the late stages of incubation.

Formal scientific risk assessment has continued. For example, the United Kingdom government's Advisory Committee on Dangerous Pathogens, together with SEAC, has reviewed the guidance for those who work with the agents of transmissible spongiform encephalopathies (Advisory Committee on Dangerous Pathogens 1996, 1998). A particular priority was to review advice to those in industrial workplaces such as slaughterhouses and carcass-dressing plants (Box 1). This was published in June 1996 (Advisory Committee on Dangerous Pathogens 1996), and in March 1998 revised guidance for those working in laboratories and hospitals, and handling animals, was published (Advisory Committee on Dangerous Pathogens 1998). However, a significant change in approach has been taken. Since 1997 a concentrated effort to conduct risk assessment more openly has led to the use of the World Wide Web to provide information on the agenda of SEAC, its advice, and government response.

The task for scientists estimating risks on usually limited evidence is considerable, especially so when the consequences of a wrong judgement may be grave, and particularly when conducted under the gaze of the media (www.doh.gov.uk/cjd/, 4 December 2000). At times the precautionary principle has been followed (such as the banning of beef on the bone) even when the estimated risk is minuscule. However, where the social and economic cost of such action is potentially huge, the precautionary principle is unrealistic. For example, of particular concern has been the discovery of PrP^{Sc} in lymphoid tissue and postmortem material from a patient with vCJD, and in appendix tissue removed 8 months before clinical onset, calling into question the safety of blood, blood products, and reusable surgical instruments (Collinge 1999). In September 1997 the United Kingdom Committee on Safety of Medicines recommended that blood products possibly obtained from confirmed CJD cases should be withdrawn. In November 1997 SEAC asked the Department of Health to commission an independent risk assessment on human-to-human transmission of vCJD via blood. Preliminary action has already been taken to remove white blood cells from all transfusion blood. An even more difficult issue is the potential for transmission via contaminated reused sterilized instruments, since prions are highly

Box 1 General basic protective measures for those working with BSE-infective animals

- Adhere to safe working practices and take extra care to avoid or minimize the use of tools and equipment likely to cause cuts, abrasions, or puncture wounds
- Where use of such equipment is unavoidable, wear suitable protective clothing (e.g. chain-mail gloves when using knives in the abattoir)
- Cover existing cuts, abrasions, and skin lesions on exposed skin with waterproof dressings
- If cuts or puncture wounds occur, encourage the wound to bleed, and then wash thoroughly with soap and water and cover with a waterproof dressing
- Use face protection (chiefly for eyes and mouth) if there is a risk of splashing, for example a visor or fixed screen
- If splashed in the eyes or face, wash with running water
- Take steps to avoid the generation of aerosols and dusts
- Wash hands and exposed skin before eating, drinking, smoking, taking any medication, using the telephone, or going to the toilet
- Wash down contaminated areas and equipment regularly with hot water and detergent
- Wash protective clothing thoroughly after use and store separately from other clothing; alternatively, use disposable clothing
- Use non-penetrative methods of stunning cattle if possible
- Discontinue pithing
- Avoid the use of reciprocating saws if the carcass has to be split through the spine
- Use low-pressure hoses to clean areas contaminated with specified bovine material
- Control exposure to dusts arising from greaves by use of engineering controls and/or standard personal protection measures
- For carcasses destined for disposal, we recommend acceleration of the development of alternative dressing techniques to avoid exposure of the spinal cord

Based on Advisory Committee on Dangerous Pathogens/SEAC (1998) resistant to conventional sterilization procedures. Use of new instruments for every patient will have huge cost implications.

The future

The BSE epidemic will continue to have major repercussions for the public's health. Firstly, the scale of the vCJD epidemic will become clear in the next few years, and there will be an increasing threat from person-to-person spread, both horizontally through surgical equipment, and vertically from mother to infant. Secondly, the question of whether there are exogenous risk factors for classical CJD remains open and new research may implicate other zoonotic exposures. Thirdly, the biology of prions will develop significantly. Will other prion-related diseases be identified? Fourthly, the procedures for public policy development, scientific risk assessment, and communication will be adapted to accommodate the recommendations of the Phillips report (www.bseinquiry.gov.uk).

References

Advisory Committee on Dangerous Pathogens (1996). *BSE (bovine spongiform encephalopathy): background and general occupational guidance.* HSE Books, London.

Advisory Committee on Dangerous Pathogens/SEAC (1998).*Transmissible spongiform encephalopathy agents: safe working and the prevention of infection.* HMSO, London.

Akai, J., Ishihara, O., and Higuchi, S. (1989). Creutzfeldt–Jakob disease in Japan: an epidemiological study done in a select prefecture between 1976 and 1986. *Neuroepidemiology*, **8**, 32–7.

Alper, T., Cramp, W.A., Haig, D.A., and Clarke, M.C. (1967). Does the agent of scrapie replicate without nucleic acid? *Nature*, **214**, 764–6.

Alter, M., Frank, Y., Doyne, H., and Webster, D.D. (1975). Creutzfeldt–Jakob disease after eating ovine brains? *New England Journal of Medicine*, **292**, 927.

Anonymous (1996*a*). Creutzfeldt–Jakob disease in Canada. *Canadian Communicable Disease Report*, **22-8**, 57–60.

Anonymous (1996*b*). Less beef, more brain. *Lancet*, **347**, 915.

Araya, G., Gálvez, S., Cartier, L., and Gajdusek, D.C. (1983). A spatiotemporal clustering of Creutzfeldt–Jakob disease in Chile. *Revista Chilena de Neuropsiquiatria*, **21**, 291–5.

Basler, K., Oesch, B., Scott, M., *et al.* (1986). Scrapie and cellular PrP isoforms are encoded by the same chromosomal gene. *Cell*, **46**, 417–28.

Belay E.D. (1999). Transmissible spongiform encephalopathies in humans. *Annual Review of Microbiology*, **53**, 283–314.

Berger, J.R. and Noble, J.D. (1993). Creutzfeldt–Jakob disease in a physician: a review of the disorder in health care workers. *Neurology*, **43**, 205–6.

Berger, J.R., Weisman, E., and Weisman, B. (1997). Creutzfeldt–Jakob disease and eating squirrel brains. *Lancet*, **350**, 642.

Bernoulli C., Siegfried, J., Baumgartner, G., *et al.* (1977). Danger of accidental person-to-person transmission of Creutsfeldt-Jakob disease by surgery. *Lancet*, **i**, 478–9.

Bobowick, A.R., Brody, J.A., Matthews, M.R., Roos, R., and Gajdusek, D.C. (1973). Creutzfeldt–Jakob disease: a case–control study. *American Journal of Epidemiology*, **98**, 381–94.

Bradley, R. and Wilesmith, J.W. (1993). Epidemiology and control of bovine spongiform encephalopathy (BSE). *British Medical Bulletin*, **49**, 932–59.

Brown, P. (1988). The clinical neurology and epidemiology of Creutzfeldt–Jakob disease, with special reference to iatrogenic cases. *Ciba Foundation Symposium*, **135**, 3–23.

Brown, P. (1995). Can Creutzfeldt–Jakob disease be transmitted by transfusion? *Current Opinion in Haematology*, **2**, 472–7.

Brown, P., Cathala, F., and Gajdusek, D.C. (1979). Creutzfeldt–Jakob disease in France: III. Epidemiological study of 170 patients dying during the decade 1968–1977. *Annals of Neurology*, **6**, 438–46.

Brown, P., Cathala, F., Castaigne, P., and Gajdusek, D.C. (1986). Creutzfeldt–Jakob disease: clinical analysis of a consecutive series of 230 neuropathologically verified cases. *Annals of Neurology*, **20**, 597–602.

Brown, P., Cathala, F., and Raubertas, R. (1988). Creutzfeldt–Jakob disease in France: epidemiologic data from 1968–1982. In *Unconventional virus diseases of the central nervous system* (ed. L.A. Court, D. Dormant, and P. Brown). Commissariat a l'Energie Atomique, Fontenay-aux-Roses.

Brown, P., Preece, M.A., and Will, R.G. (1992). 'Friendly fire' in medicine: hormones, homografts, and Creutzfeldt–Jakob disease. *Lancet*, **340**, 24–7.

Brown, P., Gibbs, Jr., C.J., Rodgers-Johnson, P., *et al.* (1994*a*). Human spongiform encephalopathy: the national institutes of health series of 300 cases of experimentally transmitted disease. *Annals of Neurology*, **35**, 513–29.

Brown, P., Cervenáková, L., Goldfarb, L.G., *et al.* (1994*b*). Iatrogenic Creutzfeldt–Jakob disease: an example of the interplay between ancient genes and modern medicine. *Neurology*, **44**, 291–3.

Brown, P., Cervenáková, L., and Powers, J.M. (1998). Fatal familial insomnia around the world: FFI cases from the United States, Australia, and Japan. *Brain Pathology*, **8**, 567–70.

Bruce, M.E., Will, R.G., Ironside, J.W., *et al.* (1997). Transmissions to mice indicate that 'new variant' CJD is caused by the BSE agent. *Nature*, **389**, 498–501.

Budka, H., Aguzzi, A., Brown, P., *et al.* (1995). Neuropathological diagnostic criteria for Creutzfeldt–Jakob disease (CJD) and other human spongiform encephalopathies (prion diseases). *Brain Pathology*, **5**, 459–66.

Budka, H., Almer, G., Hainfellner, J.A., and Jellinger, K. (1998). Fatal familial insomnia around the world: the Austrian FFI cases. *Brain Pathology*, **8**, 554.

Chandler, R.L. (1961). Encephalopathy in mice produced by inoculation with scrapie brain material. *Lancet*, 1378–9.

Chandrakumar, M. (1998). *An investigation of the local cases of Creutzfeldt–Jakob disease in East Kent.* Report, East Kent Health Authority.

Chatelain, J., Cathala, F., Brown, P., Raharison, S., Court, L., and Gajdusek, D.C. (1981). Epidemiologic comparisons between Creutzfeldt–Jakob disease and scrapie in France during the 12-year period 1968–1979. *Journal of the Neurological Sciences*, **51**, 329–37.

Chesebro, B. (1998). BSE and prions: uncertainties about the agent. *Science*, **279**, 42–3.

Cohen, C.H. and Valleron, A.-J. (1999). When did bovine spongiform encephalopathy (BSE) start? Implications of the prediction of a new variant Creutzfeldt–Jakob disease (nvCJD) epidemic. *International Journal of Epidemiology*, **28**, 526–31.

Collee, J.G. and Bradley, R. (1997). BSE: a decade on—Part 2. *Lancet*, **349**, 715–21.

Collinge, J. (1999). Variant Creutzfeldt–Jakob Disease. *Lancet*, **354**, 317–23.

Collinge, J., Palmer, M.S., and Dryden, A.J. (1991). Genetic predisposition to iatrogenic Creutzfeldt–Jakob disease. *Lancet*, **337**, 1441–2.

Collins, S., Law, M.G., Fletcher, A., Boyd, A., Kaldor, J., and Masters, C.L. (1999). Surgical treatment and risk of sporadic Creutzfeldt–Jakob disease: a case control study. *Lancet*, **353**, 693–7.

Cousens, S.N., Zeidler, M., Esmonde, T.F., *et al.* (1997*a*). Sporadic Creutzfeldt–Jakob disease in the United Kingdom: analysis of epidemiological surveillance data for 1970–1996. *British Medical Journal*, **315**, 389–96.

Cousens, S.N., Vynnycky, E., Zeidler, M., Will, R.G, and Smith, P.G. (1997*b*). Predicting the CJD epidemic in humans. *Nature*, **385**, 197–8.

Cousens, S.N., Linsell, L., Smith, P.G., and Will, R.G. (1999). Cluster of vCJD in Kent and its importance. *Lancet*, **353**, 18–21.

Creange, A., Gray, F., Cesaro, P., *et al.* (1995). Creutzfeldt–Jakob disease after liver transplantation. *Annals of Neurology*, **38**, 269–72.

Davanipour, Z., Alter, M., Sobel, E., Asher, D.M., and Gajdusek, D.C. (1985*a*). Creutzfeldt–Jakob disease: possible medical risk factors. *Neurology*, **35**, 1483–6.

Davanipour, Z., Alter, M., Sobel, E., Asher, D.M., and Gajdusek, D.C. (1985*b*). A case control study of Creutzfeldt–Jakob disease: dietary risk factors. *American Journal of Epidemiology*, **122**, 443–51.

Davanipour, Z., Alter, M., Sobel, E., Asher, D.M., and Gajdusek, D.C. (1986). Transmissible virus dementia: evaluation of a zoonotic hypothesis. *Neuroepidemiology*, **5**, 194–206.

de Silva, R. (1996). Human spongiform encephalopathy: clinical presentation and diagnostic tests. In *Prion diseases* (ed. H.F. Baker and R.M. Ridley), pp. 15–33. Humana Press, Totowa, NJ.

Dickinson, A.G. and Taylor, D.M. (1978). Resistance of scrapie agent to decontamination. *New England Journal of Medicine*, **229**, 1413–14.

Duffy, P., Wolf, J., Collins, G., DeVoe, A.G., Streeten, B., and Cowen, D. (1974). Possible person-to-person transmission of Creutzfeldt–Jakob disease. *New England Journal of Medicine*, **290**, 692–3.

Esmonde, T.G.F., Will, R.G., and Slattery, J.M. (1993). Creutzfeldt–Jakob disease and blood transfusion. *Lancet*, **341**, 205–7.

Gajdusek, D.C. (1977). Unconventional viruses and the origin and disappearance of kuru. *Science*, **197**, 943–60.

Gajdusek, D.C. and Zigas, V. (1957). Degenerative disease of the central nervous system in New Guinea: the endemic occurrence of 'kuru' in the native population. *New England Journal of Medicine*, **257**, 974–8.

Galvez, S., Masters, C., and Gajdusek, D.C. (1980). Descriptive epidemiology of Creutzfeldt–Jakob disease in Chile. *Archives of Neurology*, **37**, 11–14.

Galvez, S., Cartier, L., Monari, M., Araya, G. (1983). Familial Creutzfeldt–Jakob disease in Chile. *Journal of the Neurological Sciences*, **59**, 139–47.

Gambetti, P. and Lugaresi, E. (1998). Fatal familial insomnia around the world: conclusions of the symposium. *Brain Pathology*, **8**, 571–5.

Ghani, A.C., Ferguson, N.M., Donnelly, C.A., Hagenaars, T.J., and Anderson, R.M. (1998). Epidemiological determinants of the pattern and magnitude of vCJD epidemic in Great Britain. *Proceedings of the Royal Society of London*, **265**, 2443–52.

Ghani, A., Ferguson, N.M., Donnelly, C.A., and Anderson, R.M. (2000). Predicted vCJD mortality in Great Britain. *Nature*, **406**, 583–4.

Goldfarb, L.G., Brown, P., Goldgaber, D., *et al.* (1989). Patients with Creutzfeldt–Jakob disease and kuru lack the mutation in the PRIP gene found in Gerstmann-Straussler syndrome, but they show a different allele mutation in the same gene. *American Journal of Genetics*, **45**, A189.

Goldfarb, L.G., Petersen, R.B., Tabaton, M., *et al.* (1992). Fatal familial insomnia and familial Creutzfeldt–Jakob disease: disease phenotype determined by a DNA polymorphism. *Science*, **258**, 806–8.

Gordon, W.S. (1946). Advances in veterinary research: louping ill, tick-borne fever and scrapie. *Veterinary Record*, **58**, 516–21.

Gore, S.M. (1996). Bovine Creutzfeldt–Jakob disease? Failure of epidemiology must be remedied. *British Medical Journal*, **312**, 791–3.

Hainfellner, J.A., Jellinger, K., Diringer, H., *et al.* (1996). Creutzfeldt–Jakob disease in Austria. *Journal of Neurology, Neurosurgery, and Psychiatry*, **61**, 139–42.

Harries-Jones, R., Knight, R., Will, R.G., Cousens, S., Smith, P.G., Matthews, W.B. (1988). Creutzfeldt–Jakob disease in England and Wales, 1980–1984: a case control study of potential risk factors. *Journal of Neurology, Neurosurgery, and Psychiatry*, **51**, 1113–19.

Hartsough, G.R. and Burger, D. (1965). Encephalopathy of mink. 1. Epizootiologic and clinical observation. *Journal of infectious diseases*, **115**, 387–92.

Hill, A.F., Desbruslais, M., Joiner, S., *et al.* (1997). The same prion strain causes vCJD and BSE. *Nature*, **389**, 448–50.

Hill, A.F., Butterworth, R.J., Joiner, S., *et al.* (1999). Investigation of variant Creutzfeldt–Jakob disease and other human prion diseases with tonsil biopsy samples. *Lancet*, **353**, 183–9.

Hillier, C.E.M. and Salmon, R.L. (2000). Is there evidence for exogenous risk factors in the aetiology and spread of Creutzfeldt disease? *Quarterly Journal of Medicine*, **93**, 617–31.

Holman, R.C., Khan, A.S., Kent, J., Strine, T.W., and Schonberger, L.B. (1995). Epidemiology of Creutzfeldt–Jakob disease in the United States, 1979–1990: analysis of national mortality data. *Neuroepidemiology*, **14**, 174–81.

Hsiao, K., Baker, H.F., Crow, T.J., *et al.* (1989). Linkage of a prion protein missense variant to Gerstmann-Sträussler syndrome. *Nature*, **338**, 342–5.

Ironside, J.W. (1996). Human prion diseases. *J Neural Transm*, **47** (Supplement), 231–46.

Ironside, J.W. and Bell, J.E. (1997). Florid plaques and new variant Creutzfeldt–Jakob disease. *Lancet*, **350**, 1475.

Johnson, R.T. and Gibbs, Jr., C.J. (1998). Creutzfeldt–Jakob disease and related transmissible spongiform encephalopathies. *New England Journal of Medicine*, **339**, 1994–2004.

Julien, J., Vital, C., Delisle, M.B., and Géraud, G. (1998). Fatal familial insomnia around the world: the French FFI cases. *Brain Pathology*, **8**, 555–8.

Kahana, E., Alter, M., Braham, J., and Sofer, D. (1974). Creutzfeldt–Jakob disease: focus among Libyan Jews in Israel. *Science*, **183**, 90–1.

Kamin, M. and Patten, B.M. (1984). Creutzfeldt–Jakob disease: possible transmission to humans by consumption of wild animal brains. *American Journal of Medicine*, **76**, 142–5.

Kimberlin, R.H. (1981). Scrapie. *British Veterinary Journal*, **137**, 105–12.

Kirkwood, J.K. and Cunningham, A.A. (1994). Epidemiological observations on spongiform encephalopathies in captive wild animals in the British Isles. *Veterinary Record*, **135**, 296–303.

Klein, R. and Dumble, L.J. (1993). Transmission of Creutzfeldt–Jakob disease by blood transfusion. *Lancet*, **341**, 768.

Kondo, K. (1985). Epidemiology of Creutzfeldt–Jakob disease in Japan. In *Creutzfeldt–Jakob disease* (ed. T. Mizutanti and H. Khiraki), pp. 17–30. Wishmura/Wiigate/Elsevier, Amsterdam.

Kondo, K. and Kuroiwa, Y. (1982). A case control study of Creutzfeldt–Jakob disease: association with physical injuries. *Annals of Neurology*, **11**, 377–81.

Kovanen, J. and Haltia, M. (1988). Descriptive epidemiology of Creutzfeldt–Jakob disease in Finland. *Acta Neurologica Scandinavica*, **77**, 474–80.

Kretzschmar, H.A., Ironside, J.W., DeArmond, S.J., and Tateishi, J. (1996). Diagnostic criteria for sporadic Creutzfeldt–Jakob disease. *Archives of Neurology*, **53**, 913–20.

Kretzschmar, H.A., Giese, A., Zerr, I., *et al.* (1998). Fatal familial insomnia around the world: the German FFI cases. *Brain Pathology*, **8**, 559–61.

Lechi, A., Tedeschi, F., Mancia, D., *et al.* (1983). Creutzfeldt–Jakob disease: clinical, EEG and neuropathological findings in a cluster of eleven patients. *Italian Journal of Neurological Sciences*, **4**, 47–59.

Lugaresi, E., Medori, R., Montagna, P., *et al.* (1986). Fatal familial insomnia and dysautonomia with selective degeneration of thalamic nuclei. *New England Journal of Medicine*, **315**, 997–1003.

Lundberg, P.O. (1998). Creutzfeldt–Jakob disease in Sweden. *Journal of Neurology, Neurosurgery and Psychiatry*, **65**, 836–41.

McKenzie, D., Bartz, J.C., and Marsh, R.G. (1996). Transmissible mink encephalopathy. *Virology*, **7**, 201–6.

Majeed, A., Lehmann, P., Kirby, L., and Coleman, M.P. (1998). Mortality from dementias and neurodegenerative disorders in people aged 15–64 in England and Wales in 1975–1996. *British Medical Journal*, **317**, 320–1.

Majtenyi, C. (1988). Study on the cases of Creutzfeldt–Jakob disease in Hungary. In *Unconventional virus diseases of the central nervous system* (ed. L.A. Court, D. Dormant, and P. Brown). Commissariat a l'Energie Atomique, Fontenay-aux-Roses.

Marsh, R.F., Bessen, R.A., Lehmann, S., and Hartsough, G.R. (1991). Epidemiological and experimental studies on a new incident of transmissible mink encephalopathy. *Journal of General Virology*, **72**, 589–94.

Masters, C.L., Harris, J.O., Gajdusek, D.C., Gibbs, Jr., C.J., Bernoulli, C., Asher, D.M. (1979). Creutzfeldt–Jakob disease: patterns of worldwide occurrence and significance of familial and sporadic clustering. *Annals of Neurology*, **5**, 177–88.

Masters, C.L., Gajdusek, D.C., and Gibbs, Jr., C.J. (1981). Creutzfeldt–Jakob disease virus isolations from the Gerstmann–Straussler syndrome with an analysis of the various forms of amyloid plaque deposition in the virus-induced spongiform encephalopathies. *Brain*, **104**, 559–88.

Mastrianni, J.A., Nixon, R., Layzer, R., *et al.* (1999). Prion protein conformation in a patient with sporadic fatal insomnia. *New England Journal of Medicine*, **340**, 1630–8.

Masullo, C., Pocchiari, M., Neri, G., *et al.* (1988). A retrospective study of Creutzfeldt–Jakob disease in Italy (1972–1986). *European Journal of Epidemiology*, **4**, 482–7.

Matthews, W.B. (1975). Epidemiology of Creutzfeldt–Jakob disease in England and Wales. *Journal of Neurology, Neurosurgery and Psychiatry*, **38**, 210–13.

Matthews, W.B. and Will, R.G. (1981). Creutzfeldt–Jakob disease in a lifelong vegetarian. *Lancet*, **ii**, 937.

Matthews, W.B., Campbell, M., Hughes, J.T., and Tomlinson, A.H. (1979). Creutzfeldt–Jakob disease and ferrets. *Lancet*, **i**, 828.

Maxwell, R.J. (1999). The British Government's handling of risk: some reflections on the BSE/CJD crisis. In *Risk communication and public health* (ed. P. Bennett and K. Calman), pp. 95–107. Oxford University Press.

Mayer, V., Orolin, D., and Mitrová, E. (1977). Cluster of Creutzfeldt–Jakob disease and presenile dementia. *Lancet*, **ii**, 256.

Maytenyi, K. (1991). Creutzfeldt–Jakob disease in the last 5 years in Hungary. *European Journal of Epidemiology*, **7**, 457–9.

Medori, R., Tristschler, H.-J., LeBlanc, A., *et al.* (1992). Fatal familial insomnia, a prion disease with a mutation at codon 178 of the prion protein gene. *New England Journal of Medicine*, **326**, 444–9.

National CJD Surveillance Unit, and the Department of Epidemiology and Population Sciences London School of Hygiene and Tropical Medicine (1995). *Creutzfeldt–Jakob disease surveillance in the United Kingdom: fourth annual report*, pp. 1–53.

National CJD Surveillance Unit, and the Department of Epidemiology and Population Sciences London School of Hygiene and Tropical Medicine (1996). Creutzfeldt–Jakob disease surveillance in the United Kingdom: fifth annual report, pp.1–67.

National CJD Surveillance Unit, and the Department of Epidemiology and Population Sciences London School of Hygiene and Tropical Medicine (1997). *Creutzfeldt–Jakob disease surveillance in the United Kingdom: sixth annual report*, pp. 1–45.

National CJD Surveillance Unit, and the Department of Epidemiology and Population Sciences London School of Hygiene and Tropical Medicine (1998). *Creutzfeldt–Jakob disease surveillance in the United Kingdom: seventh annual report*, pp. 1–53.

National CJD Surveillance Unit, and the Department of Epidemiology and Population Sciences London School of Hygiene and Tropical Medicine. (1999). *Creutzfeldt–Jakob disease surveillance in the United Kingdom: eighth annual report*, pp. 1–51.

Neugat, R.H., Neugat, A.I., Kahana, E., Stein, Z., and Alter, M. (1979). Creutzfeldt–Jakob disease: familial clustering among Libyan-born Israelis. *Neurology*, **29**, 225–31.

Palmer, M.S., Dryden, A.J., Hughes, T., and Collinge, J. (1991). Homozygous prion protein genotype predisposes to sporadic Creutzfeldt–Jakob disease. *Nature*, **352**, 340–2.

Palmer, S.R. (1996). The BSE Crisis—an assessment. *Eurohealth*, **2**, 10–12.

Parchi, P., Capellari, S., Chin, S., *et al.* (1998). Creutzfeldt–Jakob disease (CJD) after blood product transfusion from a donor with CJD. *Neurology*, **50**, 1872–3.

Pattison, I.H. (1988). Fifty years with scrapie: a personal reminiscence. *Veterinary Record*, **123**, 661–6.

Pattison, J. (1998). The emergence of bovine spongiform encephalopathy and related diseases. *Emerging Infectious Diseases*, **4**, 390–4.

Patterson, W.J. and Painter, M.J. (1997). Bovine spongiform encephalopathy and new variant Creutzfeldt–Jakob disease: an overview. *Communicable Diseases and Public Health*, **2**, 5–13.

Pearson, G.R., Wyatt, J.M., Henderson, J.P., and Gruffydd-Jones, T.J. (1993). Feline spongiform encephalopathy: a review. *Veterinary Annual*, **33**, 1–10.

Petersen, R.B. (1999). Antemortem diagnosis of variant Creutzfeldt–Jakob disease. *Lancet*, **353**, 163–4.

Pocchiari, M., Ladogana, A., Petraroli, R., Cardone, F., and D'Alessandro, M. (1998). Fatal familial insomnia around the world. Recent Italian FFI cases. *Brain Pathology*, **8**, 564–6.

Prusiner, S.B. (1982). Novel proteinaceous infectious particles cause scrapie. *Science*, **216**, 136–44.

Prusiner, S.B. (1993). Genetic and infectious prion diseases. *Archives of Neurology*, **30**, 1129–53.

Raubertas, R., Brown, P., Cathala, F., and Brown, I. (1991). The question of clusters in Creutzfeldt–Jakob disease. *American Journal of Epidemiology*, **129**, 146–54.

Ricketts, M.N., Cashman, N.R., Stratton, E.E., and El Saadany, S. (1997). Is Creutzfeldt–Jakob disease transmitted in blood? *Emerging Infectious Diseases*, **3**, 155–63.

Schätzl, H.M., Wopfner, F., Gilch, S., von Brunn, A., and Jäger, G. (1997). Is codon 129 of prion protein polymorphic in human beings but not in animals? *Lancet*, **349**, 1603–4.

Schonberger, L.B. (1998). New variant Creutzfeldt–Jakob disease and bovine spongiform encephalopathy. *Emerging Infectious Diseases*, **12**, 111–21.

Schreuder, B.E.C. (1994). Animal spongiform encephalopathies—an update. Part II. Bovine spongiform encephalopathy (BSE). *Veterinary Quarterly*, **16**, 182–92.

Singhal, B.S. and Dastur, D.K. (1983). Creutzfeldt–Jakob disease in Western India. Observations in 7 patients. *Neuroepidemiology*, **2**, 93–100.

Southwood, R. (1989). *Report of the Working Party on Bovine Spongiform Encephalopathy*. HMSO, London.

Spongiform Encephalopathy Advisory Committee (1995). *Transmissible spongiform encephalopathies: a summary of present knowledge and research*. **1**, 1–95. HMSO, London.

Stratton, E.E., Ricketts, M.N., and Gully, P.R. (1997). The epidemiology of Creutzfeldt–Jakob disease in Canada: a review of mortality data. *Emerging Infectious Diseases*, **3**, 63–4.

Takashima, S., Tateishi, J., Taguchi, Y., and Inoue, H. (1997). Creutzfeldt–Jakob disease with florid plaques after cadaveric dural graft in a Japanese woman. *Lancet*, **350**, 865–6.

Tsuji, S. and Kuroiwa, Y. (1983). Creutzfeldt–Jakob disease in Japan. *Neurology*, **33**, 1503–6.

van Duijn, C.M., Delasnerie-Laupretre, N., Masullo, C., *et al.* (1998). Case–control study of risk factors of Creutzfeldt–Jakob disease in Europe during 1993–1995. *Lancet*, **351**, 1081–5.

Weber, T., Tumani, H., Holdorf, B., *et al.* (1993). Transmission of Creutzfeldt–Jakob disease by handling of dura mater. *Lancet*, **341**, 123–4.

Wells, G.A.H., Scott, A.C., Johnson, C.T., *et al.* (1987). A novel progressive spongiform encephalopathy in cattle. *Veterinary Record*, **121**, 419–20.

Wilesmith, J.W., Wells, G.A.H., Cranwell, M.P., and Ryan, J.B.M. (1988). Bovine spongiform encephalopathy: epidemiological studies. *Veterinary Record*, **123**, 638–44.

Will, R.G. and Matthews, W.B. (1982). Evidence for case-to-case transmission of Creutzfeldt–Jakob disease. *Journal of Neurology, Neurosurgery and Psychiatry*, **45**, 235–8.

Will, R.G., Matthews, W.B., Smith, P.G., and Hudson, C. A retrospective study of Creutzfeldt–Jakob disease in England and Wales 1970–1979. II: epidemiology. *Journal of Neurology, Neurosurgery, and Psychiatry* 1986, **49**, 749–55.

Will, R.G., Ironside, J.W., Zeidler, M., *et al.* (1996). A new variant of Creutzfeldt–Jakob disease in the United Kingdom. *Lancet*, **347**, 921–5.

Will, R.G., Alperovitch, A., Poser, S., *et al.* (1998*a*). Descriptive epidemiology of Creutzfeldt–Jakob disease in six European countries, 1993–1995. *Annals of Neurology*, **43**, 763–67.

Will, R.G., Campbell, M.J., Moss, T.H., Bell, J.E., and Ironside, J.W. (1998*b*). Fatal familial insomnia around the world: FFI cases from the United Kingdom. *Brain Pathology*, **8**, 562–3.

Will, R.G., Stewart, G., Zeidler, M., Macleod, M.A., and Knight, R.S.G. (1999). Psychiatric features of new variant Creutzfeldt–Jakob disease. *Psychiatric Bulletin*, **23**, 264–7.

Will, R.G., Zeidler, M., Stewart, G.E., *et al.* (2000). Diagnosis of new variant Creutzfeldt–Jakob disease. *Annals of Neurology*, **47**, 575–82.

Williams, E.S. and Young, S. (1980). Chronic wasting disease of captive mule deer: a spongiform encephalopathy. *Journal of Wildlife Disease*, **16**, 89–98.

Williams, E.S. and Young, S. (1982). Spongiform encephalopathy of Rocky Mountain elk. *Journal of Wildlife Disease*, **18**, 465–71.

WHO (World Health Organization) (1998). *Global surveillance, diagnosis and therapy of human transmissible spongiform encephalopathies: report of a WHO consultation*, pp. 1–30. WHO, Geneva.

Worthington, J.M. (1995). Epidemiology of Jakob-Creutzfeldt disease in Australia 1970–80. *Australian and New Zealand Journal of Medicine*, **25**, 243–4.

Zanusso, G., Nardelli, E., and Rosati, A. (1998). Simultaneous occurrence of spongiform encephalopathy in a man and his cat in Italy. *Lancet*, **352**, 1116–17.

Zeidler, M., Stewart, G.E., Barraclough, C.R., *et al.* (1997*a*). New variant Creutzfeldt–Jakob disease: neurological features and diagnostic tests. *Lancet*, **350**, 903–7.

Zeidler, M., Johnstone, E.C., Bamber, R.W.K., *et al.* (1997*b*). New variant Creutzfeldt–Jakob disease: psychiatric features. *Lancet*, **350**, 908–10.

9.12 Gastrointestinal disease: public health aspects

R.F.A. Logan, M.J.G. Farthing, and M.J.S. Langman

Introduction

This chapter considers the prospects for preventing infective and chronic digestive disease; cancer is discussed elsewhere.

Chronic gastrointestinal illness presents particular problems for applying public health measures to reduce the risk of contracting disease or ameliorating its impact. Our understanding of causes is rudimentary. The scarcity of reliable comparative data makes it difficult to decide if particular illnesses present special problems in one place or seldom cause significant disability elsewhere. Furthermore, the variety and precision of diagnostic measures are changing rapidly. Therefore it would be unwise to assume that illness, which in the past was primarily diagnosed by radiographic means but now is being increasingly assessed by fibre-optic methods, will necessarily represent the same range and proportions of severity in both periods.

If, despite these problems, the value of public health measures in prevention is to be examined, the strengths and frailties of individual indicators of disease presence and activity should be assessed. Thus for each disease where possible we have (i) reviewed the methods of measuring disease frequency before considering (ii) what is known of the environmental factors influencing occurrence and (iii) what prospects exist for prevention or improved control.

Intestinal infection

Infection is the most common affliction of the gastrointestinal tract worldwide. The major burden of intestinal infections is borne by individuals living in the developing world, where up to 4 million preschool children still die each year of acute dehydrating diarrhoeal disease of predominantly infectious aetiology (Farthing *et al.* 1993). Although prevalence is higher in the developing world, intestinal infection is now increasingly recognized in the majority of industrialized countries in which foodborne, and to a lesser extent waterborne infections are among the most common. Acute diarrhoea due to certain viruses is aetiologically important in infants and young children, although the mortality rate is extremely low. The vast majority of acute intestinal infections resolve without specific therapy providing there is adequate replacement of fluid and electrolyte losses (Farthing 1994). However, certain infections such as dysenteric shigellosis, invasive bacterial diarrhoea with systemic features, and some parasitic infections such as amoebiasis and giardiasis, do require specific antibiotic therapy (Farthing *et al.* 1992). Even chronic infections such as tuberculosis and schistosomiasis are amenable to drug therapy. Thus, although intestinal infections are numerically important in terms of disease morbidity worldwide and still produce an unacceptably high mortality in infants and preschool children, most are self-limiting and with appropriate public health interventions, the majority are preventable. Thus, intestinal infection continues to challenge clinicians and public health services; control and prevention of these diseases are achievable on the basis of current knowledge, providing appropriate infrastructures are put in place.

Methods of assessment

It is assumed that the local prevalence of intestinal infection is underestimated worldwide. There are marked geographic differences in the structures in place to collect such information, and even in those countries that attempt such an exercise, the quality of data collected is also variable. On a worldwide basis, the World Health Organization collects information on diarrhoeal diseases and publishes this on a yearly basis as a function of the Diarrhoeal Diseases Control Programme. In the United States, the Centers for Disease Control, Atlanta, produces regular reports on infectious diarrhoeal disease based on notifications and in-depth investigation of outbreaks. These processes are, of course, highly selective and only partially reflect the overall burden of infectious diarrhoeal disease. In the United Kingdom, the Communicable Disease Surveillance Centre, Colindale, functions in a similar way to the Centers for Disease Control and publishes the number of reported cases of specific infections on a yearly basis. Cholera, dysentery, food poisoning (with or without microbiological confirmation), typhoid fever, and tuberculosis are all statutorily notifiable infections in the United Kingdom. The Communicable Disease Surveillance Centre data for certain intestinal infections from 1980 to 1998 is shown in Fig. 1. The rise in *Salmonella* species and *Campylobacter* species infections, for example, is thought to be due to a true increase in the incidence of these diseases, rather than more vigorous reporting or efficient data collection. However, only a proportion of intestinal infections are notified to the Communicable Disease Surveillance Centre, and a substantial proportion are unlikely to even come to the notice of a general practitioner. A United Kingdom national study supported by the Department of Health has examined the background prevalence of a broad range of enteropathogens within the general practice setting in patients attending with and without diarrhoeal disease (Wheeler *et al.* 1999). The incidence of infectious intestinal disease was 19.4 per 100 person-years; however, only one in six people presented to a general practitioner. The ratio of cases in the community to cases reaching national surveillance was lower for bacterial pathogens than for viruses. Thus, the study indicates that there are about 9.4 million cases

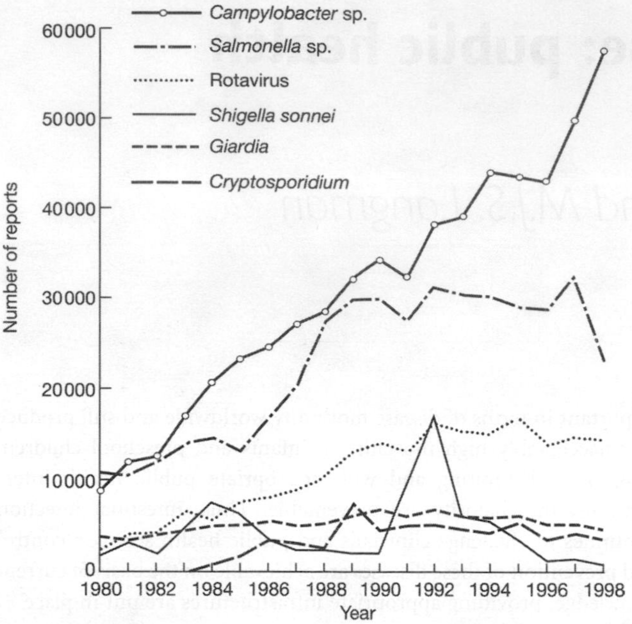

Fig. 1 Laboratory reports of selected gastrointestinal infections in England and Wales, 1980 to 1998.

of infective diarrhoea each year, although current surveillance methods markedly underestimate the size of the problem.

Disease patterns

Clinically, gastrointestinal infection can be classified on the basis of symptoms: (i) acute watery diarrhoea, (ii) diarrhoea with blood (dysentery), and (iii) chronic diarrhoea with or without evidence of steatorrhoea. The clinical presentation can often give an indication of the type of enteropathogen involved (Table 1) although this approach is by no means totally reliable. Acute watery diarrhoea is usually self-limiting and, provided that the illness begins to resolve within 5 to 7 days, no specific investigation or treatment is routinely required if fluid and electrolyte losses are replaced appropriately (Farthing 1994). However, it is wise to identify the enteropathogens responsible for dysentery and chronic diarrhoea as specific antimicrobial chemotherapy may be required. The prevalence of certain bacterial intestinal infections is increasing in the United Kingdom according to Communicable Disease Surveillance Centre data (Fig. 1). *Salmonella* species and *Campylobacter jejuni* dominate the bacterial causes of diarrhoea, a fact which has been attributed largely to the transmission of these organisms in food such as chickens and eggs (Telzak *et al.* 1990). Enterohaemorrhagic *Escherichia coli*, particularly serotype O157:H7 (also known as verocytotoxin-producing *E. coli*) has been responsible for a large number of community outbreaks of diarrhoea and dysentery associated with a significant mortality; major complications responsible for death include the haemolytic uraemic syndrome and thrombotic thrombocytopenic purpura.

Prevalence data on enteric viral infections is sparse because of the difficulties in making a firm diagnosis. However, clinical evidence would suggest that these infections (rotavirus and enteric adenovirus types 40 and 41) are extremely common in infants and young children, and worldwide are now the most common causes of acute diarrhoea in this age group. The small round structured viruses such as the

Table 1 Clinical patterns and aetiology of infective diarrhoea

Acute watery diarrhoea
Bacteria
Enterotoxigenic *E.coli*
Salmonella enteritidis
Shigella species (early phase of infection)
Vibrio cholerae
Vibrio parahaemolyticus
Viruses
Rotavirus
Enteric adenovirus (types 40 and 41)
Norwalk and related viruses
Protozoa
Cryptosporidium parvum
Microsporidium species
Bloody diarrhoea
Bacteria
Shigella species
Salmonella species
Enteroinvasive *E.coli*
Enterohaemorrhagic *E.coli*
Campylobacter jejuni
Yersinia enterocolitica
M. tuberculosis
Aeromonas species
Plesiomonas species
Protozoa
Entamoeba histolytica
Balantidium coli
Viruses
Cytomegalovirus (immunocompromised)
Helminths
Schistosoma species
Trichuris trichiura
Chronic diarrhoea
Bacteria
Enteropathogenic *E. coli*
Yersinia enterocolitica
M. tuberculosis
Protozoa
Entamoeba histolytica
Balantidium coli
Giardia lamblia
Cryptosporidium parvum
Microsporidium species
Cyclospora cayatenensis
Viruses
Cytomegalovirus (immunocompromised)
Helminths
Schistosoma species
Strongyloides stercoralis

Norwalk family of viruses are also common, but produce a milder illness often with vomiting as a major component. These infections affect adults and there is an extremely high secondary attack rate producing outbreaks in families and in other situations where humans live or work in close proximity.

Transmission

Intestinal infections are generally transmitted by the faecal–oral route. The organism itself or a protected, dormant form of the organism (cyst or oocyst) is excreted in faeces which can then be transmitted to other humans by (i) direct person-to-person contact or (ii) food and/or water. Thus, for many human intestinal infections, humans remain the major reservoirs. Certain infections such as amoebiasis and shigellosis are exclusively human pathogens, although under certain experimental circumstances, models of infection can be created in animals. However, some human enteropathogens, notably *Salmonella* species and *Campylobacter jejuni*, have large animal reservoirs, and thus these infections fulfil the criteria for a zoonosis. Similarly, certain parasitic infections such as cryptosporidiosis and possibly giardiasis are also carried by a variety of wild and domestic animals and can produce clinical disease. There is increasing concern that these animal reservoirs may be responsible for contamination of surface domestic water supplies and food products (Baird-Parker 1990). Molecular analysis has shown that there are at least two distinct strains of *Cryptosporidium parvum*: one which is only isolated from humans and does not colonize animals (type H), and another which is isolated from cattle but is also able to cause diarrhoea in humans (type C). Contamination of water supplies with cysts of *Cryptosporidium parvum* or *Giardia intestinalis* presents a major problem for domestic water suppliers since the cysts can survive for weeks or months in cool water and are unreliably inactivated or destroyed by the concentrations of chlorine that will render water acceptable with respect to coliform count (Porter *et al.* 1988; Sorvillo *et al.* 1992). There is some evidence to suggest that some enteric viruses such as small round structured viruses and possibly rotavirus are transmitted by aerosol created during vomiting (Reid *et al.* 1988). In this case, viral particles would be inhaled into the pharynx and then swallowed.

Seasonality

Enteropathogens vary in their prevalence in different seasons in the year. The majority of bacterial enteropathogens do not show marked variations in seasonality although in the developing world cholera outbreaks generally occur during times of heavy rainfall and flooding. Intestinal parasitic infections also tend to be more common in the cooler, wetter months of the year, situations which tend to favour the survival of cysts in the environment. Some enteric virus infections demonstrate seasonality with a dramatic increase in the cases of rotavirus infection during the winter months and a marked fall during the warm, dry summer months (Cukor and Blacklow 1984). However, enteric adenoviruses produce a similar number of cases throughout the year.

Geographic location

Intestinal infections are more common in developing countries than in the industrialized world where there has been more investment in sanitation and domestic water supplies. Other variables which increase the prevalence of intestinal infection include water shortages, which diminish the opportunity for maintenance of personal hygiene, crowded living conditions, the use of 'night soil' (human faeces) for fertilizing crops, and the proximity of humans to their domestic and farm animals. Certain infections such as cholera and those due to the intestinal helminths, hookworm, schistosomiasis, *Strongyloides stercoralis*, and others are limited almost exclusively to the tropics and subtropics and are usually only seen in the industrialized world as imported infections. The developing world thus carries the major burden of enteric infection, both with respect to case load and the spectrum of enteropathogens. Nevertheless, there is real concern that there has been true increase in the prevalence of intestinal infections in the industrialized world because of the increasing importance of foodborne disease and a variety of other risk factors outlined below.

Factors influencing disease frequency

Travel, immunodeficiency states, institutional residence or day-care attendance, reduced gastric-acid secretion, and extremes of age are the main factors known to increase susceptibility to intestinal infection. Travellers from the industrialized to the developing world are well recognized to be at risk of many of the infections shown in Table 1, although by far the most common is that due to enterotoxigenic *E. coli* (Farthing *et al.* 1992, 1993). Individuals with inherited or acquired immunodeficiency, particularly that relating to infection with HIV, are more commonly affected by the conventional bacterial enteropathogens and have a special susceptibility to the intracellular protozoa, *Cryptosporidium parvum* and *Microsporidium* species. These often produce chronic debilitating illnesses which are poorly responsive to medical therapy. Those at the extremes of age appear to be more susceptible to infection, presumably because of impaired immunological defences and the reduced ability to cope physiologically with the losses of fluid and electrolytes; morbidity from infection is increased in these individuals. People living in institutions or children attending day-centres appear to be more susceptible to enteric infections, largely because of the ease with which infection can be transmitted to large numbers of individuals living in close proximity to one another. This is particularly evident in shigellosis and giardiasis in which the infective dose may be as few as 10 organisms. The increased movement of individuals from the developing world to the industrialized countries has brought with it diseases that have previously not assumed great importance to those living in the developed world. Intestinal tuberculosis, for example, has increased dramatically in the United Kingdom, due almost exclusively to the increasing number of immigrants from the Indian subcontinent (Cook 1985). Similarly, some years ago a substantial number of cases of intestinal schistosomiasis was reported in New York City, again due exclusively to immigrants from the Caribbean. Finally, there is evidence that reduction in the concentration of gastric acid, either pharmacologically or following gastric surgery, results in an increased susceptibility to enteric bacterial infections. This has been demonstrated with *Salmonella* species where it appears that the elderly population are particularly at risk (Neal *et al.* 1994).

Other environmental and behavioural factors are also emerging as potential risk factors for the acquisition of intestinal infection. Seawater, freshwater lakes, and swimming pools have all been associated with the acquisition of intestinal infection, notably *Cryptosporidium parvum, Giardia intestinalis* and also enterohaemorrhagic *E. coli* (Walker 1992). Recent epidemiological analyses indicate that the relative risk of acquiring an infection is closely related to whether the swimmer swallows any of the water. Changes in eating habits in the West may also account for part of the increase in foodborne diarrhoeal disease. This includes the ingestion of raw fish, and of foods containing uncooked or partially cooked eggs such as mayonnaise, mousse, and certain Italian desserts.

Prevention

Primary prevention of gastrointestinal infection can be achieved by interruption of the faecal–oral transmission route. This involves the widespread availability of high quality potable water, adequate sanitation to ensure safe disposal of faeces, and clear guidelines on personal hygiene to minimize person-to-person transmission. The importance of these measures is emphasized by the frequent rapid development of epidemics of gastrointestinal infection in areas where the appropriate infrastructure is disrupted by natural disasters or by war. In addition, guidelines and, where necessary, legislation are required to ensure the highest standards in animal husbandry, food production, and subsequent food handling with regular surveillance procedures to ensure that these standards are maintained.

Chemoprophylaxis

There is compelling evidence that broad-spectrum antibiotics, taken at approximately half the therapeutic dose, can prevent certain bacterial infections of the intestine, notably the organisms that are responsible for travellers' diarrhoea and cholera (Farthing *et al.* 1992). Their use in travellers' diarrhoea remains highly controversial but, while not generally recommended, may be of value in certain situations, particularly in high-risk individuals. However, tetracycline is recommended for prophylaxis in family members during cholera outbreaks. Non-antibiotic approaches such as bismuth preparations have also been used to prevent travellers' diarrhoea, the most widely used being bismuth subsalicylate. This compound is less effective than broad-spectrum antibiotics but is free of the potential adverse effects of the latter, and does not increase the emergence of antibiotic resistant bacteria.

Probiotics

The concept that the gut can be colonized with harmless bacteria that will protect against the effects of bacterial and possibly viral enteropathogens has been considered for several decades. Lactobacilli, particularly those used to produce yoghurt, have been used empirically for this purpose, although the evidence of efficacy is extremely poor (Oksanen *et al.* 1990) or non-existent (Katelaris *et al.* 1995). However, a recent study using *Bifidobacterium bifidium* and *Streptococcus thermophilus* showed that these organisms do appear to protect infants from rotavirus infection (Saavedra *et al.* 1994). Further evidence is awaited to confirm the validity of this approach in the prevention of other intestinal infections.

Immunoprophylaxis

Although parenteral vaccines have been available for cholera and typhoid for many years, their efficacy is low. There have been major difficulties in developing effective oral vaccines but this approach is generally regarded as being the most effective for the production of protective immune responses in the gut, the site where they are most needed (Levine 1990). A whole cell-B subunit oral cholera vaccine has been subjected to extensive field trials and has been shown to produce moderately good but relatively short-lasting immunity to cholera (Peltola *et al.* 1991). More recently, a genetically engineered live oral cholera vaccine has been developed which appears to be as effective in a single dose, producing good protection without diarrhoea (Suharyono *et al.* 1992). There is some evidence to suggest that these cholera vaccines also protect against travellers' diarrhoea caused by other organisms and thus, their application may be wider than was initially envisaged (Peltola *et al.* 1991). Vaccines are also under development for *Salmonella* species, *Shigella* species, and enterotoxigenic *E. coli.* There have also been extensive efforts to develop a rotavirus vaccine that will be safe, effective, and affordable in the developing world. A 'tetravalent' rhesus assortment vaccine containing an RNA segment which encodes the major neutralization antigen of sertype 1, 2, or 4 human rotavirus has been subjected to field trials in the developing world and in the United States. Although there was initially great optimism, there is now evidence that this vaccine causes intussusception in well-nourished children in the United States, possibly as the result of an exaggerated immune response in Peyer's patches.

Peptic ulcer

Disability due to gastric or duodenal ulceration presents a major health problem in Western populations, where 10 per cent or more may be affected at some time in their lives. It is also a problem in many less-developed areas. Ulcer frequency varies greatly from time to time, and from place to place, reflecting the interplay of environmental and genetic influences, with environmental factors being of critical importance.

Methods of assessment

Mortality rates

Death usually occurs from ulcer complications or as a sequel to an operation. Few die as a result of a peptic ulcer, but mortality rates rise steeply with advancing age. In the United Kingdom the chance of dying from peptic ulcer is several hundred times greater in people over 65 years of age than in those under 35 (Table 2).

Those who die from ulcer are likely to do so because of the severity of complications, or because of innate inability to withstand the stresses of illness because of age or coincident disease.

Table 2 Ulcer of the stomach and duodenum 1991: death rates per million population for England and Wales

	Age (years)							
	15–	25–	35–	45–	55–	65–	75–	85+
Men	0	2	6	22	89	244	768	1812
Women	1	1	2	8	45	154	504	1480

Data from OPCS (1993).

Autopsy surveys

Careful scrutiny of the stomach and duodenum at autopsy can give reliable information about the current frequency of ulcer, and about past frequency as judged by stigmata of previous surgery. However, it may be difficult to decide if there is duodenal or gastric scarring due to previous ulceration, and individual judgement may vary. Matters are complicated in two more ways. First, the group of people in whom autopsy examination is performed do not necessarily form a reasonable sample of those dying. Second, the autopsy rate in many countries is falling steadily, and it would be dangerous to assume that the findings at a certain time when, say, two-thirds of all those dying in hospital were subjected to autopsy, can be simply related to findings at a time when a third or less are being so examined.

Hospital admission rates

Provided that hospital diagnostic indices are reliably compiled, admission rates can act as proxies for measures of disease occurrence. Data on peptic ulceration must be interpreted with particular caution. The introduction of highly effective pharmacological treatments has for all practical purposes eliminated the need for hospital admission for medical treatment, and elective surgery is now seldom needed.

Ulcer complication rates present attractions as measures. Perforation and severe haemorrhage are clinically obvious, and are mandatory reasons for hospital admission. However, in making comparisons it should be noted that the proportions of ulcers which bleed or perforate may vary from time to time, and from place to place.

Admission rates with ulcer complications are distinctly higher in the elderly than in the young in the United Kingdom and the United States, a pattern which may not necessarily be followed in non-European countries. Data obtained in the United Kingdom (Walt *et al.* 1986) and elsewhere suggest that ulcer-perforation rates have risen steeply in the elderly, particularly in women, and may have fallen greatly in the young (Table 3). A small proportion of the rise in the elderly may be attributable to the use of non-steroidal anti-inflammatory drugs, but most is not. One attractive hypothesis is that the elderly form a cohort exposed in youth to *Helicobacter pylori* who contracted infection and hence a lifelong susceptibility to ulcer. If this is true then it presupposes that those born more recently have for some reason failed to become infected. Interacting influences are also important because many more, amongst non-takers of non-steroidal anti-inflammatory drugs, become infected with *H. pylori* than develop peptic ulcers. Factors to be considered must plainly include smoking, although the elderly are not, in general, a group of heavy smokers. Outside predisposing factors remain poorly understood.

Diagnostic rates

Very few investigators have examined the overall frequency with which diagnoses are made over time, almost certainly because of doubts over the effects of changes in the type and intensity of application of diagnostic methods.

Sickness certification

Certified sickness rates are unsatisfactory proxies for true disease occurrence when symptoms are poor guides to the presence of specific disease, and when functional abdominal symptoms are very common.

Taking all these factors into account, the best comparator indices from time to time and place to place must be complication and death rates. Direct diagnostic figures are plainly the best measures in individual studies of, for instance, risk associated with infection or drug use, and can make valuable contributions within well-described stable study areas (Primatesta *et al.* 1994).

Factors influencing disease frequency or severity

The two influences which have emerged as being of particular importance in affecting ulcer occurrence or the development of complications have been infection with *H. pylori*, and use of non-steroidal anti-inflammatory drugs.

Table 3 Admission rates for gastric and duodenal ulcer perforation in England and Wales and the United States (per 100 000 population per year)

Ulcer type		Age (years)		
		15–44	45–64	65+
England and Wales 1978–1982[a]				
Gastric	Men	0.8 (–86)	4.4 (–72)	11.6 (–51)
	Women	0.6 (–25)	2.3 (–39)	10.1 (+20)
Duodenal	Men	6.9 (–62)	18.5 (–50)	39.1 (–13)
	Women	1.4 (–36)	6.6 (+38)	20.3 (+145)
United States 1979–1987[b]				
Gastric	Men	1.5	5.4	9.6
	Women	0.8	4.7	13.9
Duodenal	Men	3.7	12.7	27.8
	Women	1.3	4.0	18.0

[a] Data from Walt *et al.* (1986). The percentage change from 1958 to 1962 is given in parentheses.

[b] Data from Sonnenberg (1994).

Helicobacter pylori

Descriptions of gastric antral colonization by spiral-shaped organisms originally described as *Campylobacter*, and later recategorized as *H. pylori*, have been amply confirmed. The organism is an almost constant concomitant of duodenal ulceration in those who do not use non-steroidal anti-inflammatory drugs, it is detectable in a majority of those with gastric ulceration and a high proportion of those with antral gastric cancer, and it can also be found in many normal individuals who have, or tend to have, antral gastritis but not ulceration (Taylor and Blaser 1991; Labenz and Borsch 1994; Nomura *et al.* 1994). The evidence for a causal role in peptic, particularly duodenal, ulceration depends upon two main features. Firstly there is the almost constant association between ulcer occurrence and the presence of infection, and secondly eradication of infection by antibiotic therapy results in prolonged ulcer remission.

Unsolved questions include lack of understanding why infection in many people causes an acute or chronic gastritis, but no ulceration. This lack of ulceration does not seem wholly accounted for by the absence of other risk factors, notably smoking.

Although *Helicobacter* infection appears to be a substantial risk factor for gastric carcinoma, and distal carcinoma in particular, proximal disease and gastro-oesophageal reflux do not seem to be related, and attention has been drawn to opposing trends in the occurrence of peptic ulcer (falling) and of reflux disease (rising) in the United States (El Serag and Sonnenberg 1998).

Calculating the disease burden likely to be imposed by infection is hindered because the base upon which estimates should be founded is unclear. Serological studies using antibodies to *Helicobacter* as markers of infection, whether present or past, show clearly that in Western populations there is an increase with age in the proportions in whom raised titres can be detected, so that at age 60 half or more of all adults may have serological evidence of infection. Examination of age-stratified data indicates that positive serology is detectable in childhood in many individuals but that there is a cumulative increase with age. By contrast, in poorer and tropical populations seropositivity tends to be more frequent, and to be detectable at younger ages, the impression therefore being that infection is more easily acquired in infancy, in conditions where hygiene is poor; an analogy with infective diarrhoea is obvious (Klein *et al.* 1991; Mendall *et al.* 1992).

Analysis is complicated in at least two important ways. Firstly, since the frequency of ulcer is much lower than the frequency of infection, some explanation is needed of why most people who are infected do not develop ulcers. Secondly, comparison of results of serological studies conducted at different times indicates that the chances of becoming infected may have changed greatly, with a reduction in frequency in Western populations.

If such a reduction were generally occurring, and if there were a reasonably constant increment of risk of peptic ulceration imposed by infection, then one would predict that the peptic ulcer population would be tending to become progressively older as a cohort of the general population with a high rate of infection. There is evidence that this is what is happening. Thus in the United Kingdom the proportion of older individuals presenting with ulcer complications has risen (Walt *et al.* 1986).

The trend is clearly detectable in women; the difference from men is unexplained. It could perhaps be accounted for by a reduced rate in men as they smoke less with advancing age, but it does not seem to be accounted for by differential rates of non-steroidal anti-inflammatory drug use. Evidence that new infection, or reinfection, is uncommon in older people comes from two main sources. Firstly prolonged remission can be induced by antimicrobial therapy in ulcer patients and that remission is accompanied by evidence that active *Helicobacter* infection remains undetectable. Secondly, repeated serological examination at prolonged intervals has shown that few new infections were detectable serologically. Thus, in Busselton, Western Australia, comparison of serological evidence of infection in blood samples taken in 1968 and in 1990 showed that only 7 per cent of those aged 20 to 44 years in 1968 became positive in 1990 (Cullen *et al.* 1993).

If these findings are correct then they have important implications. Firstly, attempts to eradicate infection in those with established ulcer disease are clearly justified by the likely prolonged remission. Whether treating individuals who have evidence of infection but do not have peptic ulcer disease is worthwhile is harder to judge. In those who have abdominal symptoms but no detectable ulcer the results of antimicrobial therapy have been mixed, and often disappointing (Moayyedi *et al.* 2000; Laine *et al.* 2001). Thus in the United States no relationship could be found between the presence of infection, the activity of gastritis, and the occurrence of specific symptoms (Schubert *et al.* 1992).

A further factor to consider is whether eradication of infection, by reducing the risk of antral atrophic gastritis, would reduce the frequency of gastric cancer for which both atrophic gastritis and *Helicobactor pylori* infection appear to be risk factors, probably interdependently. Such treatment as a public health measure would imply a massive effort if up to half the adult population needed treatment, as seems likely. Furthermore, there are suggestions that eradication of *Helicobactor pylori* infection can enhance gastric acid secretion in patients with corpus gastritis, and so could make oesophageal reflux disease more likely. This, taken with evidence that reflux disease is an important predisposing factor to oesophageal adenocarcinoma (Lagergren *et al.* 1999), which is also increasing in frequency in Western countries (Pera *et al.* 1993; Devesa *et al.* 1998), makes the value of eradication in those without ulcer even more speculative.

Primary prevention of infection clearly must also be considered. Available evidence indicates that organisms can occasionally be found in dental plaque, but it is more likely that faecal–oral transmission takes place (Thomas *et al.* 1992). Risks of infection have been shown to be raised where sanitation has been poor during infancy (Mendall *et al.* 1992). The need for primary prevention measures may be less obvious in Western countries where the risk of infection appears to be falling rapidly (Parsonnet *et al.* 1992) than in those where clean water supplies and good sanitation may be lacking (Klein *et al.* 1991). Finally, consideration has to be given to intrinsic differences between varieties of *Helicobacter* (Covacci *et al.* 1993; Atherton *et al.* 1997).

Non-steroidal anti-inflammatory drugs

There is now ample evidence that takers of non steroidal anti-inflammatory drugs (**NSAIDs**) are at increased risk of peptic ulcer, hospitalization for the disease in general, or admission with ulcer complications. The development of ulcers during NSAID use has been clearly shown during the course of studies in which the value of drug prophylaxis against NSAID-associated ulcer has been examined. In addition, cohort and retrospective case–control studies have shown risks of varying size associated with NSAID treatment. Table 4 sets out odds ratios associated with the use of different agents. The size of the

Table 4 Risks of gastrointestinal hospital admission of ulcer complications associated with non-aspirin non-steroidal drug use

	Odds ratios			
	New Zealand[a]	UK[b]	Australia[c]	Spain[d]
Diclofenac	3.3	4.2	1.7	7.9
Ibuprofen	1.9	2.0	0.7	–
Indomethacin	13.9	11.3	2.5	4.9
Naproxen	5.1	9.1	2.8	6.5
Piroxicam	6.6	13.7	4.8	19.1

Selected data from case–control studies with data for at least four of the drugs examined, adjusted for non-prescribed drug use and social habits.

[a] Savage et *al.* (1993).

[b] Langman et *al.* (1994).

[c] Henry et *al.* (1993).

[d] Laporte et *al.* (1991).

apparent risk varies, sometimes markedly, from one to another, reflecting a varying mix of dose differences from one place to another, and of differing design features as well as simple chance effects as confidence intervals round point estimates are often wide. However, the consistency of data, associated with experimental verification and dose–response effects, indicate compellingly that the treatment is directly responsible.

The public health implications are complex. NSAIDs are used as analgesic and anti-inflammatory agents and in cardiovascular prophylaxis. Walt *et al.* calculated that about one-third of all peptic ulcer bleeding in the United Kingdom could be attributed to aspirin or non-aspirin NSAID use. Of this third about two-thirds were attributable to non-aspirin NSAID use, and a third to aspirin. NSAIDs are commonly used in managing patients with joint disease, apart from anti-ulcer-drug prophylaxis. Prevention depends on substituting safer selective selective NSAIDs (Langman *et al.* 1999). The disease burden imposed by NSAID treatment in these patients is nevertheless substantial. However, most treatment is given to patients with muscular and articular symptoms which may be ill-defined or associated with disease requiring simple analgesia, notably osteoarthritis. In such patients there is a strong case for using paracetamol, which is not ulcerogenic, or low doses of the least toxic NSAID, notably ibuprofen. Given current prescribing patterns for individual NSAIDs, such a policy should at least halve the number of ulcer complications attributed to NSAID use.

The position with aspirin cardioprophylaxis is more complex; most evidence showing its value relates to doses of 300 mg or more daily. However, there is clear evidence of substantially raised risks of upper gastrointestinal bleeding. The size of risk may be more than offset by the gain in terms of vascular disease prevented but it does emphasize the need to ensure that aspirin dosage is no greater than it need be. In this context risk appears to persist even when doses of 75 mg daily are in use (Weil *et al.* 1995).

Although it is plausible that *Helicobacter* infection might increases risks of ulcer associated with NSAID intake, evidence conflicts (Chan *et al.* 1997; Cullen *et al.* 1997).

Once *Helicobacter* infection and NSAID use have been taken into account, there remains major difficulty in deciding why ulceration develops. Thus, if over half of all those aged 60 and over in the general population have become infected by *Helicobacter*, and at least 30 per cent are takers of non-steroidal anti-inflammatory drugs or aspirin, then other reasons must explain why the prevalence of ulcer is of the order of 10 per cent. It is therefore reasonable to suggest that to develop an ulcer more than one factor must be operating, and that there are factors other than *Helicobacter* or drug use which are important.

Social factors

In the past, gastric ulcer was more common in the poor than in the rich, while the reverse was true of duodenal ulcer. However, the social class patterns for gastric and duodenal ulcer are now much the same. Table 5 compares mortality patterns according to social class in the United Kingdom. In general terms, ulcer death seems to be about twice as common in those of low social class (i.e. social classes IV and V).

The reasons for these patterns are not easily explained. Ulcer might be expected to cause death in those who are disadvantaged socially and hence less likely to obtain high-quality medical care. However, 50 years ago higher mortality rates for duodenal ulcer obtained in those of social class I than in those of low social class. A common trend of morbidity and mortality patterns suggests that they are describing real differences.

Examination of occupational data does not suggest any link with liability to ulcer. Smokers are in general more prone to peptic ulceration than non-smokers, and the social class distribution of ulcer might simply reflect heavier smoking in those of lower social class. However, when social class was judged by level of educational attainment, peptic ulceration was found to be more common in smokers than non-smokers at each educational level, and Massachusetts physicians who smoked were more liable to peptic ulceration than those who did not smoke (Monson and MacMahon 1969).

Stress

Despite many attempts to relate the development, complications, or exacerbations of ulcer to stress, no coherent body of evidence has emerged to support the concept. Polednak (1974) noted that certain somatic symptoms, notably palpitation and sleeplessness, were associated with later development of ulcer, but these were two amongst many, and Piper *et al.* (1978, 1981*a*), concluded that no association

Table 5 Ulcer mortality (SMR) in men aged 20–64 according to social class in UK

Mortality	Social class						
	I	II	IIIN	III	IIIM	IV	V
1959–1963							
Gastric	46	58		94		106	199
Duodenal	48	75		96		107	173
1979–1983							
Gastric	28	55	80		91	127	278
Duodenal	45	56	79		96	124	253

Data from Registrar General (1971) and OPCS (1986).

with stressful life events could be detected for either gastric or duodenal ulcer.

Smoking

There is clear evidence that smokers are more likely to die from peptic ulceration than non-smokers, that ulcer is likely to be found more often in smokers than non-smokers, and that duodenal ulcers are less likely to heal during histamine H_2 antagonist treatment if patients are smokers (Hammond and Horn 1958; Doll and Hill 1964; Friedman *et al.* 1974; Kratochvil *et al.* 1982). Examination of the smoking habits of Massachusetts physicians has suggested that those smokers who had an ulcer were likely to have smoked more heavily, and from an earlier age, than those who did not have ulcers (Monson 1970). The association of peptic ulcer with smoking is independent of other associations with consumption of coffee and cola-type soft drinks (Paffenbarger *et al.* 1974*a*).

By simple comparison of time trends in smoking habits and ulcer mortality in the United States, Kurata *et al.* (1986) estimated that most of the changes observed in mortality could be attributed to changed smoking patterns. This evidence has largely ignored the influence of infection by *H. pylori*. However, it is plausible that smoking is an important factor in converting the infected and non-ulcerated to the infected and ulcerated.

Diet

The role of nutritional factors is discussed more fully elsewhere. Despite the likelihood that dietary factors are of significance in affecting liability to upper gastrointestinal disease, there is little supportive evidence. Those who drink coffee and cola-type soft drinks may be relatively unprotected (Paffenbarger *et al.* 1974*b*). The buffering capacities of foods vary; proteins are better buffers but are more likely to stimulate gastric secretion, whilst carbohydrate foods are indifferent buffers but promote less acid output. No useful date are available to show whether specific dietary items or major changes in protein, carbohydrate, or fat intake materially alter liability to peptic ulceration. An increase in dietary fibre intake has been claimed to protect against the development of ulcer. This is based upon comparative analyses of ulcer frequency in places where dietary fibre intake is thought to differ markedly. A controlled clinical study suggested that relapse of duodenal ulcer is less likely to occur in those taking dietary fibre supplements (Rydning *et al.* 1982). Even if true, it is unclear whether it is the quantity or a specific quality of dietary fibre that is important.

A further possibility is that high polyunsaturated fat intake can, by modulating prostaglandin synthesis, reduce liability to peptic ulceration. Convincing evidence in favour of this suggestion is lacking.

Prospects for prevention

It already seems likely that reductions in the frequency of infection with *H. pylori*, with reductions in smoking, are having major influences on the frequency of gastric and duodenal ulceration. In addition, understanding that NSAID and aspirin actions on cyclooxygenase (**COX**) can be separated into two types, with receptor differentiation, one (COX-1) being constitutive and associated with mucosal protection and antiplatelet effects, and the other (COX-2) being inducible and associated with anti-inflammatory properties (Holtzman *et al.* 1992), has led to the design of novel NSAIDs devoid of COX-1 activity. These do not appear to induce peptic ulcer or its complications (Langman *et al.* 1999; Simon *et al.* 1999), and, if they can be targeted to susceptible patients, should substantially reduce the burden of non-*Helicobacter*-associated ulcer.

Inflammatory bowel disease

Materially the same problems exist for the examination of changes in the frequency of inflammatory bowel disease as for peptic ulceration. In addition, there are no absolute criteria by which Crohn's disease and ulcerative colitis can be separated with reliability. In the majority of cases the transmural inflammatory changes with the formation of giant cells and lymphoid aggregates, and the patchy distribution with, frequently, small intestine involvement of Crohn's disease can be distinguished from the uniform distal mucosal inflammation, particularly involving the rectum, of ulcerative colitis.

Methods of assessment

Mortality rates

Measurement of death rates concentrates upon severe and complicated disease, with postoperative deaths and deaths in the elderly forming particularly important groups. Despite difficulties of interpretation it is worth noting that, in the United Kingdom, death rates and hospital discharge rates for Crohn's disease have shown a similar upward trend (Miller *et al.* 1974; Langman 1979).

Hospital admission rates and other indices

It may no longer be true, given the range of medical treatments now available, that all patients with Crohn's disease are ultimately admitted to hospital. However, it is clear that only a minority of colitics are admitted because most have limited bowel disease. In consequence we are inevitably dependent in epidemiological studies upon data which are collected comprehensively from admission statistics, clinic attendances, and pathological records.

When all data sets are considered it is clear that Crohn's disease incidence rates rose markedly in the period between the 1960s and 1980s. This does not seem to represent diagnostic transfer, since ulcerative colitis incidence rates seem to have been stable. Crohn's disease incidence rates themselves may also have now stabilized (Logan 1998), and Table 6 shows representative recent datasets for both diseases.

Factors affecting disease patterns

We are largely ignorant of the causes of chronic inflammatory bowel disease. Both Crohn's disease and ulcerative colitis seem to be associated with Western cultural patterns, but it is difficult to be sure in countries where infective dysenteries are endemic that non-specific disease is not being misclassified as infective. The difficulty is compounded by the tendency for many tropical countries to have less sophisticated medical services than European and North American areas.

Within Western areas there appears to be a tendency, at least in some, for there to be pronounced urban-to-rural gradients for Crohn's disease, but probably not for colitis. However, there is no clear evidence of social class or occupational differences in disease frequency. Variations in sex ratio are of doubtful significance since data do not generally take into account smoking habits, which have been shown clearly to affect disease occurrence.

Diet

There is no conclusive evidence implicating dietary factors in the causation of ulcerative colitis or Crohn's disease. However, indications have appeared repeatedly that dietary sucrose, as judged by retrospective enquiries, was consistently greater in Crohn's disease patients than in matched controls (Martini and Brandes 1976; Thornton *et al.* 1979).

It seems likely, but is not certain, that dietary intakes antedate disease origin. However, a mechanism of action has not been identified, and modulation of dietary sucrose intake does not seem to influence disease behaviour.

Previous suggestions that milk intake could adversely affect disease behaviour were probably confounded by lack of understanding that those with intestinal hypolactasia would be prone to diarrhoea when consuming milk.

Other factors

There are unconfirmed suggestions that dietary sulphate could cause bowel damage—by conversion to sulphide (Gibson *et al.* 1991; Roediger *et al.* 1997). Butyrate enemata also seem to be beneficial in treating colitis but whether lack of short-chain fatty acids, a prime mucosal metabolic fuel in the bowel, precipitates disease is unclear.

Smoking

In 1982, Rhodes and his colleagues noticed that patients with ulcerative colitis were mainly non-smokers (Harries *et al.* 1982). Subsequent studies have confirmed and extended these observations. Although an increased proportion of disease occurring in non- or ex-smokers could reflect stopping smoking on medical advice after disease onset, that explanation seems untenable.

Ulcerative colitis has been clearly and repeatedly shown to occur not only in non-smokers but in ex-smokers, with disease onset coming after the cessation of smoking (Somerville *et al.* 1984). Plausibility is increased by evidence that the more patients smoke the greater the protection (Tobin *et al.* 1987) and that nicotine may be an effective treatment.

Table 6 Incidence of inflammatory bowel disease (data for selected studies) (rates per 100 000 per year)

	Crohn's disease		Ulcerative colitis	
	Study period	**Incidence**	**Study period**	**Incidence**
NW France[a]	1988–1990	4.9	1988–1990	3.2
NW Greece[b]	1988–1990	0.3	1988–1990	5.1
Leiden, The Netherlands[c,d]	1979–1983	3.9	1979–1983	6.8
Cardiff, UK[e,f]	1971–1975	4.8	1968–1977	7.2
Olmsted County, MN, USA[g,h]	1978–1982	4.3	1970–1979	14.3

[a]Data from Gower Rousseau *et al.* (1994).
[b]Data from Tsianos *et al.* (1994).
[c]Data from Shivananda *et al.* (1987*a*).
[d]Data from Shivananda *et al.* (1987*b*).
[e]Data from Mayberry and Rhodes (1986).
[f]Data from Morris and Rhodes (1984).
[g]Data from Stonnington *et al.* (1987).
[h]Data from Gollop *et al.* (1988).

In contrast, in Crohn's disease there is an increased proportion of smokers, and again retrospective enquiry suggests that the habit is established before disease onset (Table 7). The plausibility of a harmful effect of smoking is increased by evidence that progression of Crohn's disease is less obvious in those who do not smoke and in those persuaded to stop smoking (Cottone *et al.* 1994; Cosnes *et al.* 2001).

Perhaps the simplest explanation of this data is that smoking in some way directs the site of action of aetiological factors, or a factor, in inflammatory bowel disease in genetically susceptible individuals.

Drugs

Oral contraceptives

A relationship, albeit modest, has been suggested between oral contraceptive use and the occurrence of Crohn's disease (Vessey *et al.* 1986; Lesko *et al.* 1985; Logan and Kay 1989). The reasons are unclear, and the findings have been disputed (Lashner *et al.* 1989), although more recent evidence suggests that current smoking and oral contraceptive use are independent risk factors for relapse (Timmer *et al.* 1998). An association with smoking through a common relationship with a thrombotic tendency is possible. In this context it is noteworthy that patients with haemophilia and von Willebrand's disease appear to be protected from both colitis and Crohn's disease (Thompson *et al.* 1995).

Non-steroidal anti-inflammatory agents

Though once tested as possible treatments, there is clear evidence of these drugs causing intestinal ulceration, inflammation, perforation, and bleeding (Langman *et al.* 1985*b*; Bjarnason *et al.* 1993). Whether they cause exacerbation of chronic inflammatory bowel disease or precipitate it in the first place is uncertain.

Associated disease

A recent intriguing piece of evidence indicates the rarity with which colitic patients have had appendectomy performed (Rutgeerts *et al.* 1993). The association appears strong, but not as high as the initial odds ratio suggested (Duggan *et al.* 1998). The mechanism is unclear but the inverse association is only present when appendectomy is performed in childhood (Andersson *et al.* 2001).

Childhood factors and infection

Since both Crohn's disease and ulcerative colitis have maximal incidences in early adult life, it is natural to examine the relevance of childhood factors. Whilst some searches have been almost uniformly negative (Gilat *et al.* 1987), others have recently suggested that Crohn's disease, but not ulcerative colitis, is associated with poor domestic hygiene in childhood (Gent *et al.* 1994). The inevitable associated question would be whether the association reflects an infective cause. Searches for evidence of transmission of infection using mathematical techniques to look for space–time clusters have been uninformative (Miller *et al.* 1975, 1976). Suggestions that inflammatory bowel disease may be associated with autism as a consequence of measles, mumps, and rubella vaccination do not appear well-supported (Ter Meulen 1998; Committee on Safety of Medicines 1999).

Prospects for prevention

Given the lack of clear evidence about causal agents, advice on preventative methods is hard to construct. The single major exception is that advice to stop smoking should have valuable effects both in preventing Crohn's disease occurrence and in ameliorating its course. Calculating the actual value is impeded because the risks associated with smoking seem to vary from place to place.

Gallstones (cholelithiasis)

Cholelithiasis is extremely common in many countries, with a prevalence in the elderly of developed countries approaching a third or more (Table 8). As with colonic diverticular disease, the relationship between the presence of gallstones and the development of symptoms is poorly understood. If cholecystectomy rates are any guide, then symptomatic gallstone disease has been increasing in many countries (McPherson *et al.* 1985). Even so, recent surveys confirm that the numbers with asymptomatic disease exceed those with symptomatic disease, often by a factor of two to one or more (GREPCO 1984; Jorgensen 1987; Attili *et al.* 1995; Everhart 1999).

Gallstones contain varying proportions of cholesterol and bile pigments and by tradition have been classified as being cholesterol, pigment, or mixed stones. In Western countries the majority are mixed and by weight consist of 75 per cent or more of cholesterol. Few epidemiological studies distinguish types and the evidence available indicates that any recent increases have been in cholesterol-rich stones. Formation of cholesterol-rich stones is believed to be a four-stage process involving an individual with the genetic propensity or metabolic abnormality that encourages the production of bile saturated with cholesterol, the initiation of stone formation, and stone growth.

Table 7 Smoking and inflammatory bowel disease: relative risk for current smokers compared with never smokers at disease diagnosis or onset (data for selected studies)

	Ulcerative colitis	Crohn's disease
Milan, Italy[a]	0.61	2.9
Orebro, Sweden[b]	0.64	2.0
Nottingham, UK[c]	0.23	4.2
Baltimore, USA[d]	0.62	2.1

[a]Data from Franceschi *et al.* (1987).

[b]Data from Lindberg *et al.* (1988).

[c]Data from Logan *et al.* (1984); Somerville *et al.* (1984).

[d]Data from Calkins et *al.* (1984).

Table 8 Prevalence (in per cent) of gallstone disease in large ultrasound surveys

Population	Age group (years)							
	30–39		40–49		50–59		60–69	
	F	M	F	M	F	M	F	M
Bristol, UK 1988[a]	6	0	7	5	14	8	22	12
Copenhagen, Denmark 1983[b]	5	2	6	2	15	7	22	13
Bergen, Norway 1983[c]	15	13	25	18	29	25	41	37
Rome, Italy 1982[d]	6	2	11	7	18	15	25	14
Ten regions, Italy 1986[e]	10	3	17	7	21	12	30	17
Guadalajara, Spain 1992[f]	11	0	13	7	12	14	18	19
NHANES III, US 1999[g]	10	2	16	7	25	12	33	25
Kashmir, India 1988[h]	15	4	17	6	29	8	19	0
Okinawa, Japan 1984[i]	4	3	3	2	4	2	9	5

[a]Data from Heaton *et al.* (1991).
[b]Data from Jorgensen (1987).
[c]Data from Glamlek *et al.* (1987).
[d]Data from Attili *et al.* (1995).
[e]Data from GREPCO (1984).
[f]Data from De Pancorbo *et al.* (1997).
[g]Data from Everhart *et al.* (1999).
[h]Data from Khuroo *et al.* (1989).
[i]Data from Nomura *et al.* (1988).

Method of assessment

Surveys

Until the 1980s autopsy surveys were the main source of data on gallstone prevalence. Besides the obvious criticism that autopsied deaths may be unrepresentative, such surveys also depend on consistent examination and recording of the state of the gall bladder (Jorgensen *et al.* 1994). Abdominal ultrasound is now the method of choice for identifying gallstones and in the last 20 years there have been several large population surveys performed using ultrasound particularly in Europe (Table 8). In a few areas incidence has also been assessed by repeating the ultrasound survey some years after the first one. In one of these studies 5 per cent of those with gallstones identified in the first survey did not have them 5 years later, suggesting that asymptomatic passage or spontaneous dissolution may not be so uncommon (Jensen and Jorgensen 1991).

Hospital admission and operation rates

Measurement of disease using cholecystectomy rates seems logical, but the complex relationship between the presence of gallstones, development of symptoms, and eventual cholecystectomy creates problems. In approximately a third of cases, symptoms continue after cholecystectomy, indicating that gallstones were not the cause. Hospital admission data are further complicated by the fact that several admissions may occur before cholecystectomy is performed, which was normal practice until recently. Furthermore, the introduction of laparoscopic cholecystectomy has been followed by a rapid rise in cholecystectomy rates in several countries (Steiner *et al.* 1994; Lam *et al.* 1996). Nevertheless, McPherson *et al.* (1985) found a strong correlation between cholecystectomy rates and prevalence of cholelithiasis within Britain. In contrast, international comparisons of operation rates show a poor correlation with prevalence data.

Mortality rates

Death from cholelithiasis is now uncommon. In Dundee more patients died from postoperative complications of cholecystectomy than from the complications of untreated gallstones (Bateson and Bouchier 1975). Changes in mortality rates reflect a combination of improvements in medical care, declining case fatality, and the increasing frequency of cholecystectomy in the elderly, and therefore are of little value in assessing disease frequency.

Disease patterns

Geographic

The autopsy data suggested that there were great variations in gallstone prevalence, being high in Western countries, such as the United Kingdom, United States, and Scandinavia, and low in many African and Third World nations. This pattern has only partly been confirmed by ultrasound surveys (Table 8). While prevalence has been highest in elderly women in Western countries, prevalence has been almost as great in Kashmiri women. Figures for other developing countries are sparse, but in Uganda, Ghana, and Thailand autopsy series indicate that fewer than 5 per cent of elderly women have gallstones (Royal College of Physicians 1980). Gallstone disease was also a rare cause for hospital admission in Africa, India, and Arabia (Burkitt and Tunstall 1975), but cholecystectomy is now one of the most common operations performed in Saudi Arabia (Tamimi *et al.* 1990).

In the United Kingdom, a twofold variation (9 to 21 per cent) in standardized prevalence was found in a study of nine towns selected to represent various socio-economic conditions (Barker *et al.* 1979). Measures of affluence within high prevalence areas appeared not to be major determinants of gallstone prevalence.

Secular trends

What little data that exists on time trends suggests that the prevalence in many countries has shown considerable fluctuation over the past century (Bateson and Bouchier 1975; Telium 1990). In areas where gallstones are now common it is generally believed that prevalence has been increasing since 1900, with a more rapid increase since 1945, doubling in a decade in some areas (Holland and Heaton 1972; Fowkes 1980). This may partly reflect more aggressive investigation and surgery.

Age, sex, and race

As shown in Table 8, gallstones are more common in women; the difference is greatest in younger age groups, often being twice that of men. The almost linear increase in prevalence with age has led to suggestions that incidence is largely independent of age, at least between ages 30 and 70 (Opit and Greenhill 1974). Some ultrasound surveys support this hypothesis but one study found that the incidence rate in 30-year-olds was less than half the rate in those over 40 years old (Jensen and Jorgensen 1991). In most countries symptomatic gallstone disease is rare before age 20 years.

Gallstone prevalence is strongly influenced by racial factors, presumably reflecting genetic predisposition. This is well-illustrated by the findings of the large United States NHANES survey in which black men had a significantly lower prevalence of gallbladder disease (5.3 per cent) than white men (8.6 per cent) and Hispanic men (8.9 per cent), whereas in women Hispanics had the highest prevalence (27 per cent), compared with whites (17 per cent) and blacks (14 per cent) (Everhart *et al.* 1999).

Factors influencing disease frequency

Obesity

Obesity has long been recognized as a major risk factor for gallstone formation. Obesity is associated with excessive hepatic secretion of cholesterol, which results in obese individuals excreting bile that is more supersaturated with cholesterol than the non-obese. This abnormality reverses with weight reduction. Ultrasound surveys show obesity to be a more important risk factor for women than men (Jorgensen 1989; Everhart *et al.* 1999). In Copenhagen, for example, the prevalence of gallstone disease was four times greater in the heaviest women (> 30 kg/m^2) compared with the lightest (< 20 kg/m^2), while in men there was only a 1.6-fold difference. Similarly a sixfold increase in risk of developing symptomatic gallstones was found in the United States Nurses Health study when comparing women weighing greater than 32 kg/m^2 with those less than 20 kg/m^2 (Maclure *et al.* 1989). Paradoxically, persons losing weight also have an increased risk of developing gallstones and this is not entirely explained by the confounding effect of obesity. Ultrasound studies of people losing weight rapidly with very low-calorie diets have demonstrated the development of gallstones in up to 12 per cent within 4 months (Everhart 1993).

Diet

Although nutritional factors are obviously important in gallstone formation, it has been difficult to establish whether specific nutrients are involved. Total dietary fat and dietary cholesterol are not strongly associated but lack of dietary fibre has been implicated. In one survey of vegetarians, gallstone prevalence was half that of a matched control group of meat eaters (Pixley *et al.* 1985). Experimental studies have suggested that fibre can reduce the cholesterol saturation of supersaturated bile. Several studies have suggested that an excessive dietary energy intake occurs in patients with gallstones compared with controls (Sarles *et al.* 1970, 1978; Maclure *et al.* 1989). Others have disputed this finding, but this may reflect the frailties of dietary measurement.

A moderate alcohol intake has been associated with a modest reduction in frequency of clinical gallbladder disease (Friedman *et al.* 1966; Scragg *et al.* 1984; Maclure *et al.* 1989) and with fewer gallstones in population surveys (Jorgensen 1989; Everhart *et al.* 1999).

Parity

Although gallstone sufferers have been traditionally characterized as being 'fertile' as well as being fair, fat, and female, it is only recently that a clear effect of increasing parity has been disentangled from the confounding effects of obesity and age. During pregnancy bile becomes more saturated with cholesterol and the gallbladder tends to increase in volume and contract less.

Although some studies have shown an increasing risk of symptomatic gallbladder disease with parity (Friedman *et al.* 1966; Layde *et al.* 1982; Royal College of General Practitioners 1982; Scragg *et al.* 1984*b*), no significant relationship was found in the largest cohort (Maclure *et al.* 1989). However, ultrasound surveys have shown that after adjusting for the effects of age, obesity, and contraceptive use, a single pregnancy is associated with about a 25 per cent increase in overall prevalence of asymptomatic and symptomatic disease (GREPCO 1984; Jorgensen 1988).

Oestrogen therapy

Exogenous oestrogens increase the cholesterol saturation of bile, and oestrogens given as either oral contraceptives, or postmenopausal replacement, or when administered to men have been found to increase cholesterol saturation of bile (Bennion and Grundy 1978). Ultrasound surveys have found overall prevalence of gallbladder disease to be 36 per cent higher in ever compared with never users of oral contraceptives and cohort studies of oral contraceptive users have also found small (15 to 30 per cent) increases in incidence of symptomatic gallbladder disease (Thijs and Knipschild 1993; Murray *et al.* 1994). It seems likely that hormone replacement therapy will also increase gallstone formation but at present the size of this effect is unclear.

Exercise

It might be expected that physical activity would be associated with a reduced risk of gallstones because of its relationship to weight. Recent data from the United States have confirmed that physical activity in both men and women is associated with a reduction in symptomatic gallstones *independently* of obesity and of weight loss. Compared with the least active quintile the most active had a cholecystectomy rate about a third lower (Leitzmann *et al.* 1998, 1999).

Smoking

Most but not all studies have found smokers to have small increases in risk of less than twofold for gallbladder disease both asymptomatic and symptomatic. No mechanism is known and at present it is unclear whether this is a direct effect or a marker of some other risk factor (Logan and Skelly 2000).

Associated conditions

As with peptic ulcer, the increased surveillance of patients with gallstones probably accounts for early claims, now discounted, that gallstones are associated with disease such as peptic ulcer and hyperparathyroidism (Bennion and Grundy 1978). Clinical gallbladder disease is more common in diabetics (Maurer *et al.* 1990) and in population surveys diabetics have had a 50 to 100 per cent increase in prevalence of cholelithiasis (Jorgensen 1989; Everhart *et al.* 1999). In countries where gallstones are common, gallstones associated with cirrhosis of the liver, haemolytic disease, or resection of the ileum and biliary tract infection make only a small contribution to overall prevalence. In Japan biliary infection with roundworms appears to have been involved in pigment stone formation in the past, but this is no longer so.

Prospects for prevention

Cholesterol gallstone formation is strongly associated with Western lifestyles. Of the risk factors that can be modified, obesity is pre-eminent. Public health measures that reduce the prevalence of obesity might be expected to reduce gallstone formation. Although experimental studies suggest a beneficial effect from an increase in dietary fibre, at present there is insufficient evidence to support more specific dietary measures to reduce gallstone disease.

Appendicitis

Appendicectomy for acute appendicitis continues to be one of the commonest emergency operations performed in the United Kingdom and most other Western countries. For example, recent United States operation rates indicate that the lifetime risk of having an appendicectomy for appendicitis is about 9 per cent for 5-year-old boys and 7 per cent for girls (Addiss *et al.* 1990). Provided that allowance is made for removal of normal appendices and for elective appendicectomy, disease frequency can be monitored using operation rates. Several studies have found that a diagnosis of acute appendicitis can be confirmed in about three-quarters of acute appendicectomies (Donnan and Lambert 1976; Barker and Liggins 1981), the proportion being higher in men than women, who more often have their appendix removed for functional or gynaecological symptoms.

Mortality rates are not useful for disease monitoring, since case fatality rates are low, currently 0.5 per cent in younger age groups. In people aged over 65, case fatality rates rise to over 5 per cent and in 1985 accounted for two-thirds of the 501 deaths from appendicitis in the United States. In England and Wales mortality rates reached a peak in the 1930s and since have fallen steadily, at a time when operation rates were continuing to increase (Donnan and Lambert 1976). In the United States age-adjusted mortality from appendicitis has declined 10-fold from over 2 to less than 0.2 per 100 000 between 1950 and 1985 (Mendeloff and Everhart 1994).

Disease patterns

A striking feature of the epidemiology of the disease has been the rapid changes in incidence evident in Europe and North America during the twentieth century. In England and Wales, mortality rates between 1901 and 1915 rose from 40 to 70 per million at a time when better treatment was reducing case fatality rates, suggesting a severalfold rise in incidence.

The pattern of disease in countries where appendicitis is common is fairly uniform, the peak incidence being between the ages of 5 and 25 years, with incidence being slightly higher in men than women (Table 9). In Western countries appendicitis was initially more common in the more affluent socio-economic groups, but in the United Kingdom this gradient, as measured by mortality and operation rates, had disappeared by 1960 (Donnan and Lambert 1976; Barker and Liggins 1981).

In contrast, Burkitt (1971) has drawn attention to the rarity of acute appendicitis among natives of rural Africa and in other rural areas of the Third World. A survey of 17 000 16- to 18-year-olds in South Africa found the prevalence of appendicectomy to be 0.6 per cent in rural African, 0.7 per cent in urban African, 2.9 per cent in Indian, and 10.5 per cent in white populations (Walker *et al.* 1982). In countries such as Nigeria and Kenya, where the disease is now occurring in the native population, it is first being reported in the more affluent natives of urban areas (Burkitt 1971).

In many Western countries including the United Kingdom hospital discharges for appendicitis have been declining steadily since the 1950s (Barker 1985); in England discharge rates have almost halved since 1968 (Fig. 2). In the United States hospitalization data show appendicitis incidence to have fallen from 1 per 400 a year to 1 per 1000 over the past 30 years (Mendeloff and Everhart 1994*a*). Some of the early decline was the result of diagnostic transfer from appendicitis to abdominal pain, but there is no evidence that diagnostic transfer is continuing. By contrast, in Hong Kong discharge rates for appendicitis have doubled in 20 years (Donnan 1986).

Table 9 Hospital discharge rate per 100 000 for appendicitis (ICD-9, 540–543), England, 1985

	All ages	Age group (years)						
		0–4	5–14	15–44	45–64	65–74	75–84	85+
Men	111	16	234	143	40	40	36	44
Women	85	9	160	120	42	35	26	31

Data from OPCS (1985).

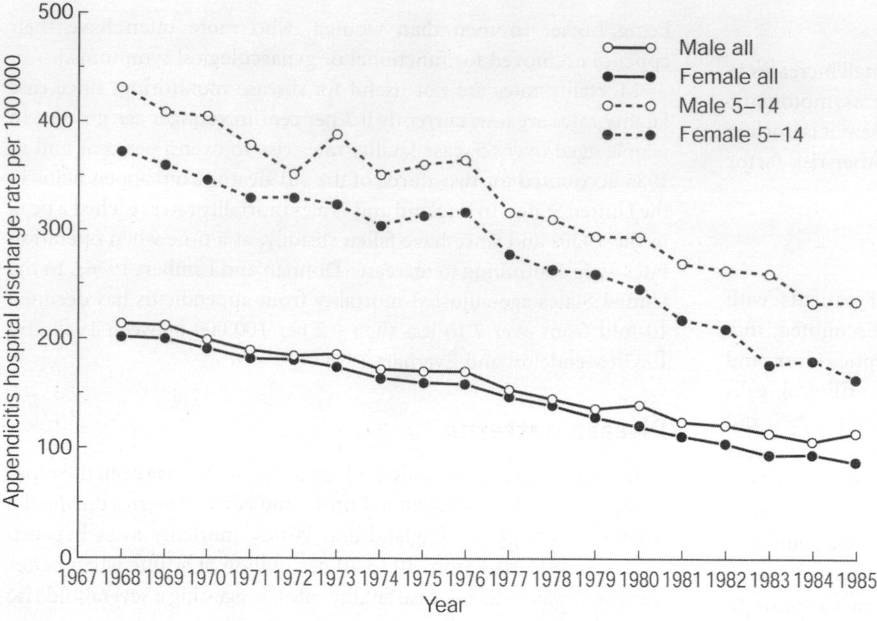

Fig. 2 Hospital discharge rate per 100 000 for appendicitis (ICD-8 and ICD-9 540–543), England and Wales, 1967–1985. (Data from OPCS 1985.)

Aetiological factors

Appendicitis is thought to result from obstruction of the appendix lumen with subsequent bacterial invasion of the ischaemic tissue. Obstruction is found in about one-third of all cases and may be due to faecoliths, which are possibly formed more readily on a low-fibre diet or to swelling of the lymphatic tissue surrounding the neck of the appendix in response to infection (Heaton 1987).

The low dietary fibre hypothesis remained largely untested until recently. Several case–control studies have now examined diet and although some have found slightly lower dietary fibre intakes in appendicitis cases compared with controls (Arnbjornsson 1983; Brender *et al.* 1985), others have found no significant differences (Nelson *et al.* 1984; Donnan 1986; Nelson *et al.* 1986). Furthermore, appendicitis rates in different parts of England and Wales have shown little correlation with cereal or total dietary fibre consumption but have been positively correlated with potato consumption and negatively with green vegetables and tomato consumption (Barker *et al.* 1986).

Barker (1985) has suggested that dietary changes correlate poorly with the time-trends for appendicitis in the United Kingdom and that the trends fit better with an infectious aetiology. On the basis of United Kingdom data correlating appendicitis rates with the provision of household amenities such as fixed baths, inside toilets, and running hot water, he attributes the rise and subsequent decline in appendicitis to improvements in domestic hygiene. With better hygiene early in life exposure to enteric infection is reduced, which in turn alters the response to later infection. This triggers appendicitis either by causing a greater lymphatic response around the appendix or by appendiceal mucosal damage allowing bacterial invasion. Further improvement in domestic hygiene results in even less enteric infection in childhood and adolescence and appendicitis rates then decline (Heaton 1987; Barker and Morris 1988; Barker *et al.* 1988).

Prospects for prevention

Although these rapid changes in appendicitis incidence underline the importance of environmental factors in its aetiology, primary prevention is clearly not possible on the basis of current knowledge. Indeed, if Barker's sanitation hypothesis holds true epidemics of appendicitis may be anticipated as a temporary consequence of improvements in domestic hygiene in some developing countries. While dietary factors are also likely to be involved no such factors have been consistently demonstrated.

Diverticular disease of the colon

In Western countries colonic diverticulosis is an increasingly common condition. In the United States almost 1 per cent of the population reported having diverticular disease in the National Health Interview Survey (Mendeloff and Everhart 1994*b*). Possibly only a tenth of cases will develop significant symptoms and for the remainder the condition is little more than an anatomical curiosity. It is not possible to predict if and when diverticulosis will produce symptoms.

Most estimates of prevalence have been obtained from either autopsy data or routine barium enema examinations. Both are usually performed on people with varying degrees of ill-health and are likely to overestimate prevalence (Mendeloff 1986). Accurate autopsy examination also requires cleaning and fixing of the colon before examination of the luminal surface with a hand lens. A radiographic technique suitable for population surveys, using oral barium and a single film at 48 h, has been described, but as yet has been used in only a few studies (Manousos *et al.* 1967, 1985; Foster *et al.* 1978).

Mortality data for diverticular disease are of limited value in assessing disease frequency since fatality rates are low, and changes in mortality are likely to reflect improvements in medical care and differences in diagnostic coding practices. Nevertheless, about 3000 deaths a year are attributed to diverticular disease in the United States, five times as many as for inflammatory bowel disease (Mendeloff and Everhart 1994*b*). Hospital discharge data are similarly difficult to interpret, particularly as the indications for admission to hospital and colectomy are ill-defined. In Scotland, depending on age, only 4 to 14 per cent of cases discharged from hospital with diverticular disease, even from surgical units, have had surgery performed (Chalmers *et al.* 1983).

Disease patterns

Like appendicitis, the striking feature of the epidemiology of diverticular disease is the great increase in prevalence that has taken place in Western countries in the twentieth century and the continuing low prevalence in less-developed countries. Between 1923 and 1963, the mortality from diverticular disease in England and Wales rose from 2 to 25 per million with a plateau during and immediately after the Second World War and food rationing (Painter and Burkitt 1971).

In countries where diverticular disease is common, the prevalence is similar in men and women, being rare before the age of 30 years and rising sharply at 60 years and over (Table 10). Although no relationship between presence of diverticular disease and socio-economic status has been established in the United States, self-reported disease is greater in those with higher incomes and twice as commonly reported by women despite hospitalization rates for United States women being only 20 per cent higher than men.

Although many of the estimates are anecdotal, diverticular disease is almost non-existent in rural Africans (Painter and Burkitt 1971). In these areas diverticulosis has been detected in less than one in 1000 autopsies or barium enemas. In urban-living Africans in South Africa and Kenya, diverticular disease is now being reported with increased frequency (Calder 1979; Segal and Walker 1982). Prevalence also appears low in the Oriental populations such as in Japan and Hong Kong, and when present tends to involve the right colon (Coode *et al.* 1985; Chia *et al.* 1991; Nakada *et al.* 1995).

Factors influencing disease frequency

To account for the geographical distribution, attention has focused mainly on dietary factors. Painter and Burkitt (1971) were the first to suggest that diverticular disease is the result of a fibre-deficient diet. In support of the importance of a low-fibre diet, a radiographic survey of English vegetarians with a high dietary fibre intake (41.5 g/day) found that the prevalence of asymptomatic diverticular disease was only 12 per cent, compared with 33 per cent in a matched control population (mean dietary fibre intake 21.4 g/day) (Gear *et al.* 1979). In case–control studies patients with symptomatic diverticular disease have been found to have lower dietary fibre intakes than controls and in the only prospective study United States male health professionals with a low fibre intake developed more symptomatic diverticular disease than those with a high intake (Brodribb and Humphreys 1976; Segal and Walker 1982; Manousos *et al.* 1985; Aldoori *et al.* 1994). Furthermore, in animal models rats have developed diverticulosis in inverse proportion to the amount of fibre in their feed (Fisher *et al.* 1985).

The role of other dietary components is not yet established; meat-eating has been implicated in diverticular disease in two studies (Manousos *et al.* 1985; Aldoori *et al.* 1994). Ingestion of non-steroidal anti-inflammatory drugs has also been implicated in the development of complications such as diverticulitis and diverticular bleeding in several British studies (Langman *et al.* 1985; Campbell and Steele 1991; Aldoori *et al.* 1998). In the United States health professionals study, physical activity, especially vigorous activity, appeared to protect from symptomatic disease (Aldoori *et al.* 1995). Other factors such as obesity, arteriosclerosis, and weakness of the colonic muscle, once considered responsible, are now regarded as secondary associations.

Table 10 Diverticular disease: prevalence by age in Oxford, England

Age (years)	Prevalence
45–49	12
50–54	20
55–59	30
60–64	33
65–69	48
70+	65

Data from Gear *et al.* (1979).

Prospects for intervention

The evidence for a central role for dietary fibre is stronger than for any other disease where it has been implicated. At least one randomized controlled trial has shown benefit in symptomatic diverticular disease (Brodribb and Humphreys 1976). On these grounds recommendations to increase dietary fibre intake can be supported.

Coeliac disease

Compared with other gastrointestinal diseases the aetiology of coeliac disease is well understood, as is indicated by its alternative name of gluten-sensitive enteropathy. Dietary gluten, the protein fraction of wheat, rye, and barley, is essential to the development of the disease. Oats also used to be proscribed but have now been shown not to be harmful. With avoidance of dietary gluten the characteristic intestinal villous atrophy recovers, often completely, and the disease remits. Gluten intolerance as demonstrated by the development of villous atrophy is believed to be lifelong, and in most coeliacs reintroduction of dietary gluten leads to recurrence of villous atrophy within 6 months.

A genetic predisposition to coeliac disease is well established. Family studies have consistently found that about 10 per cent of first-degree relatives have villous atrophy, which is often asymptomatic (Logan 1992). Strong associations with several genes within the HLA complex have been shown. Nevertheless, the difference in concordance rates between monozygotic twins and HLA identical siblings (70 per cent versus 30 per cent) implicates non-HLA genes as well.

Besides the appropriate genetic predisposition and dietary gluten, the importance of other unidentified environmental factors is underlined by the discordance of some monozygotic twin pairs (Polanco *et al.* 1981), and by the variable delay in recurrence of villous atrophy after gluten re-exposure (Bardella *et al.* 2000).

Methods of assessment

Mortality data are of no value in assessing disease frequency since the mortality rate of coeliacs is no more than twice that of the general population and death is rarely certified as being due to coeliac disease itself (Logan *et al.* 1989). Autopsy surveys are also not possible because of the effects of postmortem autolysis on the small intestinal mucosa. Investigation and diagnosis do not normally require hospital admission. Thus figures for incidence and prevalence were, until recently, derived from hospital-based case series and the steadily increasing prevalence reported for adults was generally assumed to reflect increased investigation rather than increased incidence (Logan 1992). Serological screening for coeliac disease is now possible using tests for the presence of antibodies to either gliadin, a cereal protein fraction, or to endomysium, a tissue antigen. Serological screening is now widely used in clinical practice and increasingly in population surveys (Catassi *et al.* 1994; Johnston *et al.* 1997; Meloni *et al.* 1999).

Patterns of disease

Depending on the measure used, the occurrence of clinical coeliac disease diagnosed in childhood shows a 10-fold variation across Europe (Fig. 3). Particularly striking is the recent doubling in incidence of childhood coeliac disease in Sweden where 3.5 of every 1000 births were being diagnosed as coeliac (Cavell *et al.* 1992). In contrast over a similar period the incidence in Denmark was constant at around 0.09 per 1,000 births (Weile and Krasilnikoff 1993). How much of this difference can be explained by differing proportions of subclinical undiagnosed disease is not known.

The increasing use of serological screening has shown that the prevalence of asymptomatic or subclinical (minor symptoms only) coeliac disease, first recognized in family studies, considerably exceeds previous estimates. In recent population surveys in children the prevalence has been as high as 1 per cent in Sardinia and 0.5 per cent in The Netherlands (Csizmadia *et al.* 1999; Meloni *et al.* 1999). In adults prevalence has been of a similar order at 0.8 per cent in Northern Ireland and 0.5 per cent in northern Sweden (Johnston *et al.* 1997; Ivarsson *et al.* 1999). What is clear is that the prevalence of undiagnosed coeliac disease in these areas is much greater than that already diagnosed, giving credence to the concept of a coeliac disease 'iceberg'. What is not known is the extent to which the hazards traditionally associated with untreated coeliac disease (osteoporosis and malignancy) apply to subclinical disease.

There are few figures on the occurrence of coeliac disease outside Europe. In North America the disease has been thought to be less common but preliminary serological surveys indicate that the prevalence as assessed by serology may be similar to Europe (Not *et al.* 1998).

Factors influencing disease frequency

In children the development of coeliac disease has been related to infant feeding practices. Case–control data implicate both bottle feeding and early introduction of dietary gluten (Greco *et al.* 1988). In the United Kingdom in the mid-1970s there was a sudden halving in incidence in children associated with a marked increase in mothers' breast feeding and delaying the introduction of dietary gluten (Littlewood *et al.* 1980; Dossetor *et al.* 1981; Logan 1992). The recent

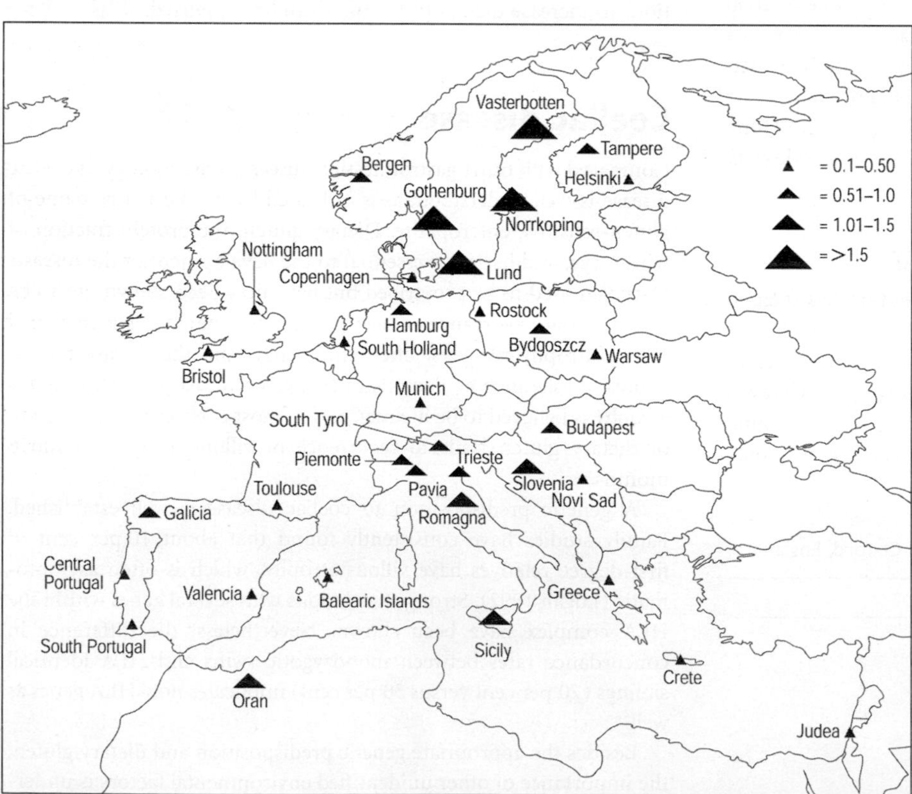

Fig. 3 Coeliac disease in children in Europe: cumulative incidence by age 15 (per 1000 live births). (Data from Greco *et al.* 1992.)

increase in Sweden, where there is already a high prevalence of breast feeding, occurred when there was an increase in the amount of gluten introduced at weaning, suggesting that relatively small changes in infant feeding either prevent disease developing or delay its development for many years (Juto *et al.* 1994; Ivarsson *et al.* 2000).

Prevention

If breast feeding and the amount and timing of gluten introduction are critical then measures to encourage the right pattern of infant feeding should reduce occurrence in childhood. Whether this will prevent the disease or merely postpone the onset of overt disease into adulthood remains to be determined.

Pancreatitis

The frequency of pancreatic disease is difficult to determine. Acute illness associated with grossly raised serum amylase levels is readily detected, but lesser varieties of acute disease may have no clear markers of occurrence, and the diagnosis of chronic disease in the absence of gross pancreatic calcification is dependent upon the use of sophisticated examination procedures of doubtful sensitivity and specificity. The few sets of data available give incidence rates for acute pancreatitis of between 5 and 25 per 100 000 per year with case-fatality rates of between 10 and 20 per cent. Thus, in the United States about 2700 deaths were certified annually to pancreatitis, mainly acute disease (Go and Everhart 1994). Data from non-European countries show that chronic disease may be common in tropical areas, such as South India, where gross calcific pancreatitis is regularly seen and is believed to be secondary to malnutrition.

Factors influencing disease frequency

Alcohol intake

In those areas where alcohol consumption is heavy, pancreatitis and liver cirrhosis tend to be common. But when clinical series from different areas are compared, the frequency with which disease is attributed to alcohol intake can vary from less than 5 per cent of acute disease in the United Kingdom to almost 90 per cent of chronic disease in France (Sarles *et al.* 1965). Chronic pancreatitis has also been associated with smoking independently of alcohol intake in several studies (Bourliere *et al.* 1991).

Gallstones

Gallstone migration along the common bile duct is an important cause of acute pancreatitis, accounting for one-third to one-half of all cases in Westernized countries depending on the prevalence of gallstones and alcohol abuse (Corfield *et al.* 1985). Biliary sludge or microlithiasis may also account for as many as one-half of otherwise idiopathic acute disease (Lee *et al.* 1992). There is no evidence that there are any special peculiarities about gallstone disease associated with pancreatitis.

Nutrition

No specific nutritional factors have been associated with liability to pancreatitis. Claims in Western countries of an association with protein or fat intake are inconsistent with the suggestion from tropical areas that malnutrition is of significance.

Drug-induced disease

Acute pancreatitis has been said to occur following treatment with, *inter alia*, corticosteroid drugs, analgesic agents, oral contraceptives, and diuretics. Almost all these claims rest upon anecdotal evidence, and taken overall it seems unlikely that drug-induced disease accounts for more than a very small proportion of the total. A single case–control study supports an association with diuretic use (Bourke *et al.* 1978).

Other factors

If there are other important environmental factors, and the general lack of aetiological information suggests that there must be, then they are unknown. It has been persistently suggested that viral infections can cause pancreatitis. Mumps virus could account for a very small proportion of cases of idiopathic non-gallstone non-alcoholic pancreatitis, but little is known about other possible causes.

Liver disease

Throughout the world morbidity and mortality from liver disease varies considerably. Comparative morbidity data are not available but in countries where liver disease is common, mortality can account for up to 5 per cent of all deaths, whereas in the United Kingdom, mortality from liver disease is less than 0.5 per cent of all deaths. Nevertheless, even in the United Kingdom liver disease ranks second only to peptic ulcer as a cause of digestive disease mortality, other than digestive cancers. In contrast in the United States around 1.5 per cent of all deaths are certified to chronic liver disease (32 000 in 1985) (Everhart 1994).

In the main, mortality results from infective liver disease including the acute viral hepatitides, hepatocellular cancer, and cirrhosis of the liver. In African countries such as Mozambique and Uganda, and also in developed countries like Greece and Japan, mortality is predominantly the result of hepatitis B virus infection and hepatocellular cancer. In Western countries hepatitis C infection has emerged as a major public health problem with 1.8 per cent of the United States population showing evidence of infection (Alter *et al.* 1999). Globally, prevalence of chronic infection is estimated to average 3 per cent and to account for 70 per cent of chronic hepatitis, 40 per cent of cirrhosis, and 60 per cent of hepatocellular cancer in Western Europe and North America (Proceedings of the European Association for the Study of the Liver 1999).

Of the other acute liver diseases, Reye's syndrome, first described in 1963, was estimated to account for almost a thousand cases per year in the United States in the 1970s (Sullivan-Bolyai and Corey 1981) (Fig. 4). The condition, which had a 50 per cent fatality rate, mainly affects children and produces an acute encephalopathy with cerebral oedema and liver failure due to hepatic steatosis. Case–control studies showing a strong association with aspirin ingestion led authorities in many countries to advise caution in the use of aspirin in children with viral illnesses. The incidence has subsequently shown a dramatic decline in both the United States and United Kingdom (Belay *et al.* 1999).

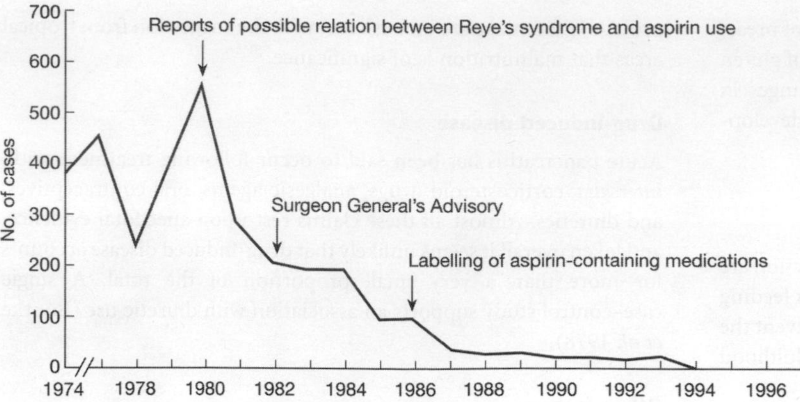

Fig. 4 Number of cases of Reye's syndrome reported in the United States.

Cirrhosis of the liver

The term 'cirrhosis' indicates an endstage histopathological state resulting from a wide range of causes. Death usually results from liver failure, often precipitated by gastrointestinal bleeding, or from development of an hepatocellular carcinoma once liver failure is established. Fewer than 15 per cent of cirrhotics survive 5 years, making mortality rates a reasonable measure of disease frequency. Nevertheless, liver failure is not an inevitable consequence of cirrhosis, as demonstrated in a British survey in which 11 per cent of cases were an incidental finding at autopsy (Saunders *et al.* 1981).

In Western countries alcohol abuse is the most common cause of cirrhosis and mortality from liver disease tends to correlate with levels of alcohol consumption (Fig. 5). The proportion of cirrhosis that is due to alcohol varies with the level of alcohol consumption in the population but even in populations where consumption has been low around a half of cases are alcohol-related.

In areas such as China, South East Asia and sub-Saharan Africa where hepatitis B infection is hyperendemic, hepatitis B infection is the major cause of cirrhosis. In these countries most adults have evidence of past infection and chronic carrier rates exceed 10 per cent (compared with < 0.2 per cent in blood donors in the United States and United Kingdom). Estimates as to what proportion of chronic carriers have a chronic hepatitis vary from 10 to 30 per cent, with higher rates for early ages of infection. Cirrhosis tends to develop only in those with more severe chronic infection (chronic active hepatitis) and in this group annual incidence has been found to be between 1.5 and 2.5 per cent. It has been estimated that worldwide there are around 300 million hepatitis B carriers (Dusheiko and Hoofnagle 1991). In comparison there are estimated to be around 150 million chronic hepatitis C carriers, of whom it is thought about 20 per cent will eventually develop cirrhosis 10 to 20 years after becoming infected (European Association for the Study of the Liver 1999).

Of the other causes of cirrhosis, a substantial number (half of non-alcoholic cirrhosis) are labelled cryptogenic and assumed to be the result of an autoimmune process such as chronic active hepatitis and primary biliary cirrhosis. Little is known of the aetiology of these autoimmune chronic liver diseases, which accounted for 70 per cent of non-alcoholic cirrhosis in Birmingham, United Kingdom (Saunders *et al.* 1981). Primary biliary cirrhosis is often asymptomatic but can be detected by testing for antimitochondrial antibodies and raised alkaline phosphatase levels in blood. In Europe, the prevalence of clinically diagnosed disease is 7 to 24 per 100 000, with incidence of around a tenth of prevalence (Lofgren *et al.* 1985; Metcalf *et al.* 1997).

Prospects for prevention

Despite the limited data available it is abundantly clear that alcohol abuse accounts for the majority of chronic liver disease in countries where drinking alcohol is popular. Measures that either reduce overall alcohol consumption or selectively reduce extreme consumption will reduce the incidence of chronic liver disease.

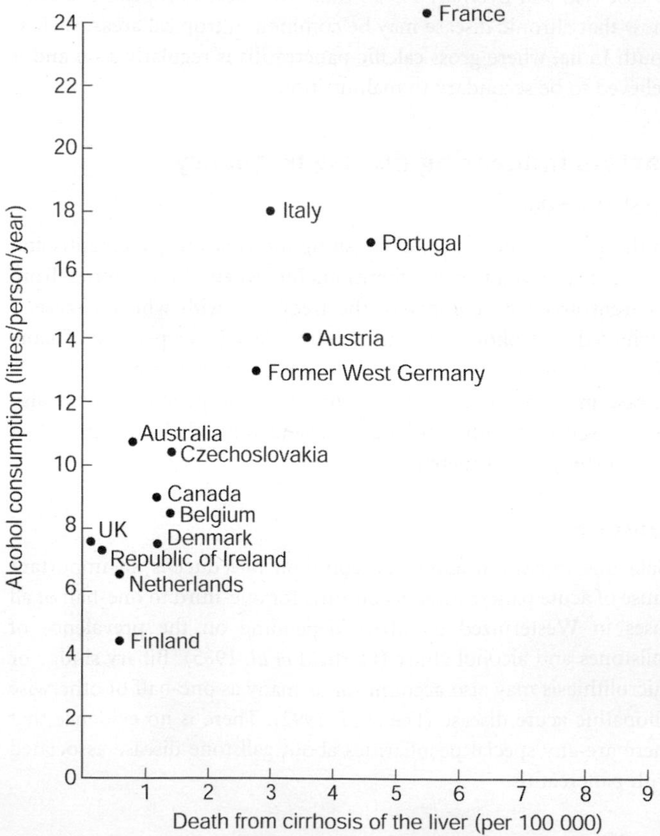

Fig. 5 Comparison of alcohol consumption and deaths from cirrhosis of the liver in 12 countries. (Data from Popham *et al.* 1975.)

Infection due to hepatitis B is a prime contributor to morbidity from cirrhosis and to mortality from hepatocellular cancer. The free availability of genetically engineered vaccines against the virus could make a crucial contribution to reducing the impacts of disease. The incidence of hepatitis C infection is already declining as transmission by blood products has virtually ceased. Increased awareness of the risks from intravenous drug use and needle exchange programs would reduce incidence further.

Prospects for the control of gastrointestinal disease in the new millennium

The rapid rise and fall in frequency of various digestive diseases worldwide is ample evidence of the importance of lifestyle and environmental factors in their causation. This suggests that the prevention of much gastrointestinal disease is a realistic objective.

For acute infective diseases which in many countries account for much of the burden of gastrointestinal disease, the prime requirement for control is the reliable provision of safe drinking water. In many developed countries modern methods of food production and preparation coupled with public complacency has lead to a resurgence of foodborne infections, emphasizing the need for continued surveillance and adequate legislation.

For chronic gastrointestinal disease the greatest rewards are likely to come from the control and prevention of *H. pylori* and hepatitis B and C virus infections. Recognition of the vital role of *H. pylori* in peptic ulceration and probably also in gastric carcinogenesis has thrown up the real possibility of producing substantial reductions in incidence of both conditions by the prevention of infection. However, public health action awaits a better understanding of the epidemiology of the infection, in particular the circumstances of its transmission. In contrast, the ability to prevent hepatitis B infection by screening and vaccination already exists and further public health action awaits the development of suitable strategies and resources.

Prospects for control of those diseases in which infection is not thought to be involved are less promising, mainly because understanding of their causation is rudimentary. Measures that reduce overall alcohol consumption will reduce the levels of liver and pancreatic disease, but reductions in tobacco consumption are likely to have little effect as smoking is only weakly related to most gastrointestinal diseases (the outstanding exception being oesophageal cancer). Measures that promote diets high in cereal or vegetable fibre and low in animal fat are likely to have a favourable impact on colonic disease as well as on vascular disease. On the debit side the rise in levels of inflammatory bowel disease may be a consequence of the lower rates of enteric infection that 'hygienic' Western lifestyles promote.

References

Addiss, D.G., Shaffer, N., Fowler, B.S., and Tauxe, R.V. (1990). The epidemiology of appendicitis and appendectomy in the United States. *American Journal of Epidemiology*, **132**, 910–25.

Aldoori, W.H., Giovannucci, E.L., Rimm, E.B., Wing, A.L., Trichopoulos, D.V., and Willett, W.C. (1994). A prospective study of diet and the risk of symptomatic diverticular disease in men. *American Journal of Clinical Nutrition*, **60**, 757–64.

Aldoori, W.H., Giovannucci, E.L., Rimm, E.B., *et al.* (1995). Prospective study of physical activity and the risk of symptomatic diverticular disease in men. *Gut*, **36**, 276.

Aldoori, W.H., Giovannucci, E.L., Rimm, E.B., Wing, AL., and Willett, W.C. (1998). Use of acetaminophen and nonsteroidal anti-inflammatory drugs: a prospective study and the risk of symptomatic diverticular disease in men. *Archives of Family Medicine*, **7**, 255–60.

Alter, M.J., Kruszon-Moran, D., Nainan, O.V., *et al.* (1999). The prevalence of hepatitis C virus infection in the United States, 1988 through 1994. *New England Journal of Medicine*, **341**, 556–62.

Andersson, R.E., Olaison, G., Tysk, C., and Ekbom, A. (2001). Appendectomy and protection against ulcerative colitis. *New England Journal of Medicine*, **344**, 808–14.

Arnbjornsson, E. (1983). Acute appendicitis and dietary fibre. *Archives of Surgery*, **118**, 868.

Atherton, J.C., Peck, Jr, R., Tham, K.T., Cover, T.L., and Blaser, M.J. (1997). Clinical and pathological importance of heterogeneity in vac A, the vacuolating cytotoxin gene of *Helicobacter pylori*. *Gastroenterology*, **112**, 92–9.

Attili, A.F., Carulli, N., Roda, E., *et al.* (1995). Epidemiology of gallstone disease in Italy: prevalence data of the Multicenter Italian Study on Cholelithiasis (MICOL). *American Journal of Epidemiology*, **141**, 158–65.

Baird-Parker, A.C. (1990). Foodborne salmonellosis. *Lancet*, **336**, 1231–5.

Bardella, M.T., Fredella, C., Prampolini, Marino, R., and Conte, O. (2000). Gluten sensitivity in monozygous twins: a long-term follow-up study. *American Journal of Gastroenterology*, **95**, 1503–5.

Barker, D.J.P. (1985). Acute appendicitis and dietary fibre: an alternative hypothesis. *British Medical Journal*, **290**, 1125.

Barker, D.J.P. and Liggins, A. (1981). Acute appendicitis in nine British towns. *British Medical Journal*, **283**, 1083.

Barker, D.J.P. and Morris, J. (1988). Acute appendicitis, bathrooms and diet in Britain and Ireland. *British Medical Journal*, **296**, 953.

Barker, D.J.P., Gardner, M.J., Power, C., and Hutt, M.S.R. (1979). Prevalence of gallstones at necropsy in British towns. *British Medical Journal*, **11**, 1389.

Barker, D.J.P., Morris, J., and Nelson, M. (1986). Vegetable consumption and acute appendicitis in 59 areas in England and Wales. *British Medical Journal*, **292**, 927.

Barker, D.J.P., Osmond, C., Golding, J., and Wadsworth, M.E.J. (1988). Acute appendicitis and bathrooms in three samples of British children. *British Medical Journal*, **296**, 956.

Bateson, M.C. and Bouchier, I.A.D. (1975). Prevalence of gallstones in Dundee: a necropsy study. *British Medical Journal*, **iv**, 425.

Belay, E.D., Bresee, J.S., Holman, R.C., Khan, A.S., Shahriari, A., and Schonberger, L.B. (1999). Reye's syndrome in the United States from 1981 through 1997. *New England Journal of Medicine*, **340**, 1377–82.

Bennion, L.J. and Grundy, S.M. (1978). Risk factors for the development of cholelithiasis in man. *New England Journal of Medicine*, **299**, 1221.

Bjarnason, I., Hayllar, J., MacPherson, A.J., and Russell, A.S. (1993). Side-effects of non steroidal drugs on the small and large intestine in humans. *Gastroenterology*, **104**, 1832.

Bourke, J.B., Mead, G.M., McIllmurray, M.B., and Langman, M.J.S. (1978). Drug-associated primary acute pancreatitis. *Lancet*, **i**, 706–8.

Bourliere, M., Barthet, M., Berthezene, P., Durbec, J.P., and Sarles, H. (1991). Is tobacco a risk factor for chronic pancreatitis and alcoholic cirrhosis? *Gut*, **32**, 1392–5.

Brender, J.D., Weiss, N.S., Koepsell, T.D., and Marcuse, E.K. (1985). Fiber intake and childhood appendicitis. *American Journal of Public Health*, **75**, 399.

Brodribb, A.J.M. and Humphreys, D.M. (1976). Diverticular disease: three studies. *British Medical Journal*, **i**, 424.

Burkitt, D.P. (1971). The aetiology of appendicitis. *British Journal of Surgery*, **58**, 695.

Burkitt, D.P. and Tunstall, M. (1975). Gallstones: geographical and chronological features. *Journal of Tropical Medicine and Hygiene*, **78**, 140.

Calder, J.F. (1979). Diverticular disease of the colon in Africans. *British Medical Journal*, **i**, 1465.

Calkins, B., Lilienfeld, A., Mendeloff, A., Garland, C.F., Monk, M., and Garland, F. (1984). Smoking factors in ulcerative colitis and Crohn's disease in Baltimore. *American Journal of Epidemiology*, **120**, 498.

Campbell, K. and Steele, R.J.C. (1991). Non-steroidal anti-inflammatory drugs and complicated diverticular disease: a case–control study. *British Journal of Surgery*, **78**, 190–1.

Catassi, C., Rätsch, I.-M., Fabiani, E., *et al.* (1994). Coeliac disease in the year 2000: exploring the iceberg. *Lancet*, **343**, 200.

Cavell, B., Stenhammar, L., Ascher, H., Danielsson, L., Dannaeus, A., Lindberg, T., and Lindquist, B. (1992). Increasing incidence of childhood coeliac disease in Sweden. Results of a national study. *Acta Paediatrica*, **81**, 589–92.

Chalmers, K., Wilson, J.M.G., Smith, A.N., and Eastwood, M.A. (1983). Diverticular disease of the colon in Scottish hospitals over a decade. *Health Bulletin*, **41**, 32–41.

Chan, F.K.L., Sung, J.J.Y., Chung S.C.S., *et al.* (1997). Randomised controlled trial of eradication of *Helicobacter pylori* before non-steroidal anti-inflammatory drug therapy to prevent peptic ulcers. *Lancet* , **350**, 975–9.

Chia, J.G., Chiantana, C.W., Ngoi, S.S., Goh, P.M., and Ong, C.L. (1991). Trends of diverticular disease of the large bowel in a newly developed country. *Diseases of the Colon and Rectum*, **34**, 498.

Committee on Safety of Medicines (1999). The safety of MMR vaccine. *Current problems in pharmacovigilance*, **25**, 9–10.

Coode, P.E., Chan, K.W., and Chan, Y.T. (1985). Polyps and diverticula of the large intestine: a necropsy survey in Hong Kong. *Gut*, **26**, 1045–8.

Cook, G.C. (1985). Tuberculosis—certainly not a disease of the past! *Quarterly Journal of Medicine*, **56**, 519–21.

Corfield, A.P., Cooper, M.J., and Williamson, R.C.N. (1985). Acute pancreatitis: a lethal disease of increasing incidence. *Gut*, **26**, 724–9.

Cosnes, J., Beaugerie, L., Carbonnel, F., and Gendre, J.P. (2001). Smoking cessation and the course of Crohn's disease—an intervention study. *Gastroenterology*, **120**, 1093–9.

Cottone, M., Rosselli, M., Orlando, A., *et al.* (1994). Smoking habits and recurrence in Crohn's disease. *Gastroenterology*, **106**, 643–8.

Covacci, A., Censini, S., Bugnoli, M., *et al.* (1993). Molecular characterization of the 120 kDa immunodominant antigen of *Helicobacter pylori* associated with cytotoxicity and duodenal ulcer. *Proceedings of the National Academy of Sciences of the United States of America*, **90**, 5791–5.

Csizmadia, C.G.D.S., Mearin, M.L., von Blomberg, B.M.E., Brand, R., and Verloove-Vanhorick, S.P. (1999). An iceberg of childhood coeliac disease in the Netherlands. *Lancet*, **353**, 813–14.

Cukor, G. and Blacklow, N.R. (1984). Human viral gastroenteritis. *Microbiology Reviews*, **48**, 157–79.

Cullen, D.J.E., Collins, B.J., Christiansen, K.J., Epis, J., Warren, J.R., Surveyor, I., and Cullen, K.J. (1993). When is *Helicobacter pylori* infection acquired? *Gut*, **34**, 1681.

Cullen, D.J.E., Hawkey, G.M., Greenwood, D.C., Humphreys, H., Shepherd, V., Logan, R.F.A., and Hawkey, C.J. (1997). Peptic ulcer bleeding in the elderly: relative roles of *Helicobacter pylori* and non-steroidal anti-inflammatory drugs. *Gut*, **41**, 459–62.

De Pancorbo, C.M., Carballo, F., Horcajo, P., *et al.* (1997). Prevalence and associated factors for gallstone disease: results of a population survey in Spain. *Journal of Clinical Epidemiology*, **50**, 1347–55.

Devesa, S.S., Blot, W.J., and Fraumeni, J.F. (1998). Changing patterns in the incidence of esophageal and gastric carcinoma in the United States. *Cancer*, **83**, 2049–53.

Doll, R. and Hill, A.B. (1964). Mortality in relation to smoking: 10 years observation of British doctors. *British Medical Journal*, **i**, 1399.

Donnan, S.P.B. (1986). *Appendicitis in Hong Kong in the aetiology of acute appendicitis*, pp. 16–19. Scientific Report 7, Southampton MRC Environmental Epidemiology.

Donnan, S.P.B. and Lambert, P.M. (1976). Appendicitis: incidence and mortality. *Population Trends*, **5**, 26.

Dossetor, J.F.B., Gibson, A.A.M., and McNeish, A.S. (1981). Childhood coeliac disease is disappearing. *Lancet*, **i**, 322–3.

Duggan, A.E., Usmani, I., Neal, K.R., and Logan, R.F.A. (1998). Appendicectomy, childhood hygiene, *Helicobacter pylori* status, and risk of inflammatory bowel disease: a case control study. *Gut*, **43**, 494–8.

Dusheiko, G. and Hoofnagle, J.H. (1991). Viral hepatitis. In *Oxford textbook of clinical hepatology* (ed. N. MacIntyre, J.P. Benhamou, J. Bircher, M. Rizzetto, and J. Rodes), Vol.1, pp. 571–92. Oxford University Press.

El Serag, H. and Sonnenberg, A. (1998). Opposing time trends of peptic ulcer and reflux disease. *Gut*, **43**, 327–33.

Everhart, J.E. (1993). Contributions of obesity and weight loss to gallstone disease. *Annals of Internal Medicine*, **119**, 1029–35.

Everhart, J.E. (1994). Overview. In *Digestive diseases in the United States: epidemiology and impact* (ed. J.E. Everhart), pp. 1–53. NIH Publication 94–1447, US Government Printing Office, Washington, DC.

Everhart, J.E., Khare, M., Hill, M., and Maurer, K.R. (1999). Prevalence and ethnic differences in gallbladder disease in the United States. *Gastroenterology*, **117**, 632–9.

Farthing, M.J.G. (1993). Pathophysiology of infective diarrhoea. *European Journal of Gastroenterology and Hepatology*, **5**, 796–809.

Farthing, M.J.G. (1994). Oral rehydration therapy. *Pharmacology and Therapeutics*, **64**, 477–92.

Farthing, M.J.G., Du Pont, H.L., Guandalini, S., Keusch, G.T., and Steffen, R. (1992). Treatment and prevention of travellers' diarrhoea. *Gastroenterology International*, **5**, 162–75.

Farthing, M.J.G., Katelaris, P.H., Dias, J., Munzer, D., and Popovic, O. (1993). Bacterial and parasitic intestinal infections in Europe. *Gastroenterology International*, **6**, 149–66.

Fisher, N., Berry, C.S., Fearn, T., Gregory, J.A., and Hardy, J. (1985). Cereal dietary fibre consumption and diverticular disease: a life-span study in rats. *American Journal of Clinical Nutrition*, **42**, 788.

Foster, K.J., Holdstock, G., Whorwell, P.J., Guyer, P., and Wright, R. (1978). Prevalence of diverticular disease of the colon in patients with ischaemic heart disease. *Gut*, **19**, 1054.

Fowkes, F.G.R. (1980). Cholecystectomy and surgical resources in Scotland. *Health Bulletin*, **38**, 126.

Franceschi, A., Panza, E., La Vecchia, S., Parazzini, F., Decarh, A., and Bianchi Porro, G. (1987). Non-specific inflammatory bowel disease and smoking. *American Journal of Epidemiology*, **125**, 445.

Friedman, G.D., Kannel, W.B., and Dawber, T.R. (1966). The epidemiology of gallbladder disease: observations on the Framingham study. *Journal of Chronic Diseases*, **19**, 273.

Friedman, G.D., Siegelaub, A.B., and Seltzer, C.C. (1974). Cigarettes, alcohol, coffee and peptic ulcer. *New England Journal of Medicine*, **290**, 469.

Gear, J.S.S., Ware, A., Fursdon, P., Mann, J.I., Nolan, D.J., Brodribb, A.J.M., and Vessey, M.P. (1979). Symptomless diverticular disease and intake of dietary fibre. *Lancet*, **i**, 511.

Gent, A.E., Hellier, M.D., Grace, R.H., Swarbrick, E.T., and Coggon, D. (1994). Inflammatory bowel disease and domestic hygene in infancy. *Lancet*, **343**, 766.

Gibson, G.R., Cummings, J.H., and Macfarlane G.T. (1991). Growth and activities of sulphate-reducing bacteria in gut contents of healthy subjects and patients with ulcerative colitis. *FEMS Microbiol Ecol*, **86,** 103–12.

Gilat, T., Hacohen, D., Lilos, P., and Langman, M.J.S. (1987). Childhood factors in ulcerative colitus and Crohn's disease: an international cooperative study. *Scandinavian Journal of Gastroenterology*, **22,** 1009.

Glambek, I., Kvaale, G., Arnesjö, B., Søreide, O. (1987). Prevalence of gallstones in a Norwegian population. *Scandinavian Journal of Gastroenterology*, **22,** 1089–94.

Go, V.L.W. and Everhart, J.E. (1994). Pancreatitis. In *Digestive diseases in the United States: epidemiology and impact* (ed. J.E. Everhart), pp. 691–712. NIH Publication 94–1447, US Government Printing Office, Washington, DC.

Gollop, J.H., Phillips, S.F., Melton III, L.J., and Zinsmeister, A.R. (1988). Epidemiological aspects of Crohn's disease; a population-based study in Olmsted County, Minnesota 1943–82. *Gut*, **29,** 49.

Gower-Rousseau, C., Salomez, J.L., Dupas, J.L., *et al.* (1994). Incidence of inflammatory bowel disease in Northern France (1988–1990). *Gut*, **35,** 1433.

Greco, L., Auricchio, S., Mayer, M., and Grimaldi, M. (1988). Case control study on nutritional risk factors in celiac disease. *Journal of Paediatric Gastroenterology and Nutrition*, **7,** 395–9.

Greco, L., Maki, M., Di Donato, F., and Visakorpi, J.K. (1992). Epidemiology of coeliac disease in Europe and the Mediterranean Area. In *Common food intolerances*. Vol. 1, *Epidemiology of coeliac disease* (ed. S. Auricchio and J.K. Visakorpi), pp. 25–44. Karger, Basel.

GREPCO (1984). Prevalence of gallstone disease in an Italian adult female population. *American Journal of Epidemiology*, **119,** 796–805.

GREPCO (1988). The epidemiology of gallstone disease in Rome, Italy. Part I. Prevalence data in men. *Hepatology*, **8,** 904–6.

Hammond, E.C. and Horn, D. (1958). Smoking and death rates-report on forty four months of follow up of 187,783 men. I. *Journal of the American Medical Association*, **166,** 1294.

Harries, A.D., Baird, A., and Rhodes, J. (1982). Non-smoking: a feature of ulcerative colitis. *British Medical Journal*, **284,** 706.

Heaton, K.W. (1987). Aetiology of acute appendicitis. *British Medical Journal*, **294,** 1632–3.

Heaton, K.W., Braddon, F.E.M., Mountford, R.A., Hughes, A.O., and Emmett, P.M. (1991). Symptomatic and silent gallstones in the community. *Gut*, **32,** 316–20.

Henry, D., Dobson, A., and Turner, C. (1993). Variability in the risk of major gastrointestinal complications from non-aspirin non-steroidal anti-inflammatory drugs. *Gastroenterology*, **105,** 1978.

Holland, C. and Heaton, K.W. (1972). Increasing frequency of gallbladder operations in the Bristol clinical area. *British Medical Journal*, **iii,** 627.

Holtzman, M.J., Turk, J., and Shornick, L.P. (1992). Identification of a pharmacologically distinct prostaglandin H synthase in cultured epithelial cells. *Journal of Biological Chemistry*, **267,** 21438–45.

Ivarsson, A., Persson, L.A., Juto, P., Peltonen, M., Suhr, O., and Hernell, O. (1999). High prevalence of undiagnosed coeliac disease in adults: a Swedish population-based study. *Journal of Internal Medicine*, **245,** 63–8.

Ivarsson, A., Persson, LA., Nyström, L., Ascher, H., Cavell, B., Danielsson, L., *et al.* (2000). Depidemic of coeliac disease in Swedish children. *Acta Paediatrica*, **89,** 165–71.

Jensen K.H. and Jorgensen, T. (1991). Incidence of gallstones in a Danish population. *Gastroenterology*, **100,** 790–4.

Johnston, S.D., Watson, R.G.P., McMillan, S.A., Sloan, J., and Love, A.H.G. (1997). Prevalence of coeliac disease in Northern Ireland. *Lancet*, **350,** 1370.

Jorgensen, T. (1987). Prevalence of gallstones in a Danish population. *American Journal of Epidemiology*, **126,** 912.

Jorgensen, T. (1988). Gallstones in a Danish population: fertility period, pregnancies and exogenous female sex hormones. *Gut*, **29,** 433–9.

Jorgensen, T. (1989). Gallstones in a Danish population: relation to weight, physical activity, smoking, coffee consumption, and diabetes mellitus. *Gut*, **30,** 528–34.

Jorgensen, T., Rossen, K., and Thorvaldsen, P. (1994). Are autopsy studies reliable in assessing gallstone prevalence in the community? *International Journal of Epidemiology*, **23,** 566–9.

Juto, P., Meeuwisse, G., and Mincheva-Nilsson, L. (1994). Why has coeliac disease increased in Swedish children? *Lancet*, **343,** 1372.

Katelaris, P.H., Salam, I., and Farthing M.J.G. (1995). *Lactobacilli* to prevent traveller's diarrhea. *New England Journal of Medicine*, **333,** 1360–1.

Khuroo, M.S., Mahajan, R., Zargar, S.A., Javid, G., and Sapru, S. (1989). Prevalence of biliary tract disease in India: a sonographic study in adult population in Kashmir. *Gut*, **30,** 201–5.

Klein, P.D., Graham, D.Y., and Gaillour, A. (1991). Watersource as a risk factor for *Helicobacter pylori* infection in Peruvian Children. *Lancet*, **337,** 1503.

Kratochvil, P., Gugler, R., and Rohner, H.G. (1982). Effect of smoking on duodenal ulcer healing with cimetidine and oxmetidine. *Gut*, **23,** 866.

Kurata, J.H., Elashoff, J.D., Nogawa, A.N., and Haile, D.M. (1986). Sex and smoking differences in duodenal ulcer mortality. *American Journal of Public Health*, **76,** 700.

Labenz, J. and Borsch, G. (1994). Evidence for the essential role of *Helicobacter pylori* in gastric ulcer disease. *Gut*, **35,** 19.

Lagergren, J., Bergstrom, R., and Lindgren, A. (1999). Symptomatic gastroesophageal reflux as a risk factor for esophageal adenocarcinoma. *New England Journal of Medicine*, **340,** 825–31.

Laine, L., Schoenfield, P., and Fennerty, B. (2001). Therapy for *helicobacter pylori* in patients with non-ulcer dyspepsia: a meta-analysis for randomised controlled trials. *Annals of Internal Medicine*, **134,** 361–9.

Lam, C.-M., Murray, F.E., and Cuschieri, A. (1996). Increased cholecystectomy rate after the introduction of laparoscopic cholecystectomy in Scotland. *Gut*, **38,** 282–4.

Langman, M.J.S. (1979). *The epidemiology of chronic digestive disease.* Edward Arnold, London.

Langman, M.J.S., McConnell, T.H., Spiegelhalter, D.J., and McConnell, R.B. (1985*a*). Changing patterns of coeliac disease frequency: an analysis of Coeliac Society membership records. *Gut*, **26,** 175–8.

Langman, M.J.S., Morgan, L., and Worrall, A. (1985*b*). Use of anti-inflammatory drugs by patients admitted with small or large bowel perforations or haemorrhage. *British Medical Journal*, **290,** 347–9.

Langman, M.J.S., Weil, J., Wainwright, P., *et al.* (1994). Risks of bleeding peptic ulcer associated with individual non steroidal anti-inflammatory drugs. *Lancet*, **343,** 1075.

Langman, M.J., Jensen, D.M., Watson, D.J., *et al.* (1999). Adverse upper gastrointestinal effects of rofecoxib compared with NSAIDs. *Journal of the American Medical Association*, **282,** 1929–33.

Laporte, J.R., Carne, X., Vidal, X., Morena, M., and Juan, J. (1991). Upper gastrointestinal bleeding in relation to previous use of analgesics and non-steroidal anti-inflammatory drugs. *Lancet*, **337,** 85.

Lashner, B.A., Kane, S.V., and Hanauer, S.B. (1989). Lack of association between oral contraceptive use and Crohn's disease: a community-based matched case–control study. *Gastroenterology*, **97,** 1442.

Layde, P.M., Vessey, M.P., and Yeates, D. (1982). Risk factors for gall-bladder disease: a cohort study of young women attending family planning clinics. *Journal of Epidemiology and Community Health*, **36,** 274.

Lee, S.P., Nicholls, J.F., and Park, H.Z. (1992). Biliary sludge as a cause of acute pancreatitis. *New England Journal of Medicine*, **326**, 589–93.

Leitzmann, M.F., Giovannucci, E., Rimm, E.B., Stampfer, M.J., Spiegelman, D., Wing, A.L., and Willett, W.C. (1998). The relation of physical activity to risk for symptomatic gallstone disease in men. *Annals of Internal Medicine*, **128**, 417–25.

Leitzmann, M.F., Rimm, E.B., Willett, W.C., *et al.* (1999). Recreational physical activity and the risk of cholecystectomy in women. *New England Journal of Medicine*, **341**, 777–84.

Lesko, S.M.N., Kaufman, D.W., Rosenberg, L., Helmrich, S.P., Miller, D.R., Stolley, P.O., and Shapiro, S. (1985). Evidence for an increased risk of Crohn's disease in oral contraceptive users. *Gastroenterology*, **89**, 1046–9.

Levine, M.M. (1990). Modern vaccines: enteric infections. *Lancet*, **335**, 958–61.

Lindberg, E., Tysk, C., Andersson, K., and Jarnerot, G. (1988). Smoking and inflammatory bowel disease: a case–control study. *Gut* **29**, 352.

Littlewood, J.M., Crollick, A.J., and Richards, I.D.G. (1980). Childhood coeliac disease is disappearing. *Lancet*, **ii**, 1359.

Lofgren, J., Jarnerot, G., Danielsson, D., and Hemdal, I. (1985). Incidence and prevalence of primary biliary cirrhosis in a defined population in Sweden. *Scandinavian Journal of Gastroenterology*, **20**, 647–50.

Logan, R.F.A. (1998). Inflammatory bowel disease incidence: up, down or unchanged? *Gut*, **42**, 309–11.

Logan, R.F.A. (1992). The epidemiology of coeliac disease. In *Coeliac disease* (ed. M.N. Marsh), pp. 192–214. Blackwell Scientific, Oxford.

Logan, R.F.A. and Kay, C.R. (1989). Oral contraception, smoking and inflammatory bowel disease—findings in the Royal College of General Practitioners Oral Contraception Study. *International Journal of Epidemiology*, **18**, 105.

Logan, R.F.A. and Skelly, M.M. (2000). Smoking and hepato-biliary disease. *European Journal of Gastroenterology and Hepatology*, **12**, 863–7.

Logan, R.F.A., Edmond, M., Somerville, K.W., and Langman, M.J.S. (1984). Smoking and ulcerative colitis. *British Medical Journal*, **288**, 751.

Logan, R.F.A., Rifkind, E.A., Turner, I.D., and Ferguson, A. (1989). Mortality in coeliac disease. *Gastroenterology*, **97**, 265–71.

Maclure, K.M., Hayes, K.C., Colditz, G.A., Stampfer, M.J., Speizer, F.E., and Willett, W.C. (1989). Weight, diet, and the risk of symptomatic gallstones in middle-aged women. *New England Journal of Medicine*, **321**, 563–9.

McPherson, K., Strong, P.M., Jones, L., and Britton, B.J. (1985). Do cholecystectomy rates correlate with geographic variations in the prevalence of gallstones? *Journal of Epidemiology and Community Health*, **39**, 179.

Manousos, O.N., Truelove, S.C., and Lumsden, K. (1967). Transit times of food inpatients with diverticulosis or irritable colon syndrome and normal subjects. *British Medical Journal*, **iii**, 760.

Manousos, O.N., Day, N.E., Tzonou, A., *et al.* (1985). Diet and other factors in the aetiology of diverticulosis: an epidemiologic study in Greece. *Gut*, **26**, 544.

Martini, G.A. and Brandes, J.W. (1976). Increased consumption of refined carbohydrates in patients with Crohn's disease. *Klinische Wochenschrift*, **54**, 367.

Maurer, K.R., Everhart, J.E., Knowler, W.C., Shawker, T.H., and Roth, H.P. (1990). Risk factors for gallstone disease in the Hispanic populations of the United States. *American Journal of Epidemiology*, **131**, 836–44.

Mayberry, J.F. and Rhodes, J. (1986). The changing incidence of Crohn's disease in Wales and the role of heredity in its aetiology. In *The genetics and epidemiology of inflammatory bowel disease* (ed. R.B. McConnell, P. Rozen, M. Langman, and T. Gilat), pp. 114–17. Karger, Basel.

Meloni, G., Dore, A., Fanciulli, G., Tanda, F., and Bottazzo, G.F. (1999). Subclinical coeliac disease in schoolchildren from northern Sardinia. *Lancet*, **353**, 37.

Mendall, M.A., Goggin, P.M., and Molineaux, N. (1992). Childhood living conditions and *Helicobacter* seropositivity in adult life. *Lancet*, **339**, 896.

Mendeloff, A.I. (1986). Thoughts on the epidemiology of diverticular disease. *Clinics in Gastroenterology*, **15**, 855.

Mendeloff, A.I. and Everhart, J.E. (1994). Acute appendicitis. In *Digestive diseases in the United States: epidemiology and impact* (ed. J.E. Everhart), pp. 457–67. NIH Publication 94–1447, US Government Printing Office, Washington, DC.

Mendeloff, A.I. and Everhart, J.E. (1994). Diverticular disease of the colon. In *Digestive diseases in the United States: epidemiology and impact* (ed. J.E. Everhart), pp. 551–65. NIH Publication 94–1447, US Government Printing Office, Washington, DC.

Metcalf, J.V., Bhopal, R.S., Gray, J., Howel, D., and James, O.F.W. (1997). Incidence and prevalence of primary biliary cirrhosis in the City of Newcastle upon Tyne, England. *International Journal of Epidemiology*, **26**, 830–6.

Miller, D.S., Keighley, A.C., and Langman, M.J.S. (1974). Changing patterns in epidemiology of Crohn's disease. *Lancet*, **ii**, 691.

Miller, D.S., Keighley, A., Smith, P.G., Hughes, A.O., and Langman, M.J.S. (1975). Crohn's disease in Nottingham: a search for time–space clustering. *Gut*, **16**, 454.

Miller, D.S., Keighley, A., Smith, P.G., Hughes, A.O., and Langman, M.J.S. (1976). A case control method for seeking evidence of contagion in Crohn's disease. *Gastroenterology*, **71**, 385.

Moayyedi, P., Feltbower, R., Brown, J., *et al.* (2000). Effect of population screening and treatment for *Helicobacter pylori* on dyspepsia and quality of life: a randomised controlled trial. *Lancet*, **355**, 1665–71.

Monson, R.R. (1970). Cigarette smoking and body form in peptic ulcer. *Gastroenterology*, **58**, 337.

Monson, R.R. and MacMahon, B. (1969). Peptic ulcer in Massachusetts physicians. *New England Journal of Medicine*, **281**, 11.

Morris, T. and Rhodes, J. (1984). Incidence of ulcerative colitis in the Cardiff region 1968–77. *Gut*, **25**, 846.

Murray, F.E., Logan, R.F.A., Hannaford, P.C., and Kay, C.R. (1994). Cigarette smoking and parity as risk factors for the development of symptomatic gall bladder disease in women: results of the Royal College of General Practitioners' oral contraception study. *Gut*, **35**, 107–11.

Nakada, I., Ubukata, H., Goto, Y., *et al.* (1995). Diverticular disease of the colon at a regional general hospital in Japan. *Diseases of the Colon and Rectum*, **38**, 755–9.

Neal, K.R., Brij, S.O., Slack, R.C.B., Hawkey, C.J., and Logan, R.F.A. (1994). Recent treatment with H_2 antagonists and antibiotics and gastric surgery as risk factors for *Salmonella* infection. *British Medical Journal*, **308**, 176.

Nelson, M., Barker, D.J.P., and Winter, P.D. (1984). Dietary fibre and acute appendicitis: a case–control study. *Human Nutrition: Applied Nutrition*, **38A**, 126.

Nelson, M., Morris, J., Barker, D.J.P., and Simmonds, S. (1986). A case–control study of acute appendicitis and diet in children. *Journal of Epidemiology and Community Health*, **41**, 316.

Nomura, A., Kashiwagi, S., Hayashi, J., *et al.* (1988). Prevalence of gallstone disease in a general population of Okinawa, Japan. *American Journal of Epidemiology*, **128**, 598–605.

Nomura, A., Stemmermann, G.N., Chyou, P., Perez-Perez, G.I., and Blaser, M.J. (1994). *Helicobacter pylori* infection and the risk for duodenal and gastric ulceration. *Annals of Internal Medicine*, **120**, 997.

Not, T., Horvath, K., Hill, I.D., Partanen, J., Hammed, A., Magazzu, G., and Fasano, A. (1998). Celiac disease risk in the USA: high prevalence of antiendomysium antibodies in healthy blood donors. *Scandinavian Journal of Gastroenterology*, **33**, 494–8.

Oksanen, P.J., Salminen, S., Saxelin, M., *et al.* (1990). Prevention of travellers' diarrhea by Lactobacillus. *Annals of Medicine,* **22,** 53–6.

OPCS (Office of Population Censuses and Surveys) (1985). *Hospital activity analysis.* OPCS, London.

OPCS (Office of Population Censuses and Surveys) (1986). *Decennial supplement occupational mortality 1979–80, 1982–3.* OPCS, London.

OPCS (Office of Population Censuses and Surveys) (1993). *Mortality statistics, cause 1991.* Series DH2, No. 18. HMSO, London.

Opit, L.J. and Greenhill, S. (1974). Prevalence of gallstones in relation to differing treatment rates for biliary disease. *British Journal of Preventive and Social Medicine,* **28,** 268.

Paffenbarger, R.S., Wing, AL., and Hyde, R.T. (1974*a*). Coffee, cigarettes and peptic ulcer. *New England Journal of Medicine,* **290,** 1091.

Paffenbarger, R.S., Wing, A.L., and Hyde, R.T. (1974*b*). Chronic disease in former college students. XIII. Early precursors of peptic ulcer. *American Journal of Epidemiology,* **100,** 307.

Painter, N.S. and Burkitt, D.P. (1971). Diverticular disease of the colon: a deficiency disease of Western civilisation. *British Medical Journal,* **ii,** 450.

Parsonnet, J., Blaser, M.J., Perez-Perez, G.I., Hargrett-bean, N., and Tauxe, R.V. (1992). Symptoms and risk factors of *Helicobacter pylori* infection in a cohort of epidemiologists. *Gastroenterology,* **102,** 41–6.

Peltola, H., Sitonen, A., Kyronseppa, H., *et al.* (1991). Prevention of travellers' diarrhoea by oral B-subunit/whole-cell cholera vaccine. *Lancet,* **338,** 1285–9.

Pera, M., Cameron, A.J., Trastek, V.F., Carpenter, H.A., and Zinsmeister, A.R. (1993). Increasing incidence of adenocarcinoma of the esophagus and esophagogastric junction. *Gastroenterology,* **104,** 510–13.

Piper, D.W., Greig, M., Shinners, J., Thomas, J., and Crawford, J. (1978). Chronic gastric ulcer and stress. *Digestion,* **18,** 303.

Piper, D.W., McIntosh, J.H., Ariotti, D.E., Calgiuri, J.V., Brown, R.W., and Shy, C.M. (1981). Life events and chronic duodenal ulcer: a case–control study. *Gut,* **22,** 1011.

Pixley, F. and Mann, J. (1988). Dietary factors in the aetiology of gallstones: a case control study. *Gut,* **29,** 1511.

Pixley, F., Wilson, D., McPherson, K., and Mann, J. (1985). Effect of vegetarianism on development of gallstones in women. *British Medical Journal,* **291,** 11.

Polednak, A.P. (1974). Some early characteristics of peptic ulcer descendants. *Gastroenterology,* **67,** 1094.

Popham, R.E., Schmidt, W., and de Lint, L. (1975). The prevention of alcoholism: epidemiological studies of the effect of government control measures. *British Journal of Addiction,* **70,** 125.

Porter, J.D., Ragazzoni, H.P., Buchanon, J.D., Waskin, H.A., Juranek, D.D., and Parkin, W.E. (1988). *Giardia* transmission in a swimming pool. *American Journal of Public Health,* **78,** 659–62.

Primatesta, P., Goldacre, M.J., and Seagroatt, V. (1994). Changing patterns in the epidemiology and hospital care of peptic ulcer. *International Journal of Epidemiology,* **23,** 1206.

European Association for the Study of the Liver (1999). Proceedings of the International Consensus Conference on Hepatitis C, Paris, France, 26–27 February 1999. *Journal of Hepatology,* **31** (Supplement 1), 1–268.

Registrar General (1971). Decennial supplement. *Occupational mortality tables for 1959–63.* HMSO, London.

Reid, J.A., Caul, E.O., White, D.G., and Palmer, S.R. (1988). Role of infected food handler in hotel outbreak of Norwalk-like viral gastroenteritis: implications for control. *Lancet,* **ii,** 321–3.

Roediger, W.E.W., Moore, J., and Babidge, W. (1997). Colonic sulfide in pathogenesis and treatment of ulcerative colitis. *Digestive Diseases and Sciences,* **42,** 1571–9.

Royal College of General Practitioners Oral Contraceptive Study (1982). Oral contraceptives and gallbladder disease. *Lancet,* **ii,** 957.

Royal College of Physicians (1980). *Medical aspects of dietary fibre.* Pitman, London.

Rutgeerts, P., D'Haens, G., Heile, M., Geboesk, and Vantrappen, G. (1994). Appendectomy protects against ulcerative colitis. *Gastroenterology,* **106,** 1251–3.

Rydning, A., Berstad, A., Aadland, E., and Odegaard, B. (1982). Prophylactic effect of dietary fibre in duodenal ulcer disease. *Lancet,* **ii,** 736.

Sarles, H., Sarles, J.C., Camatte, R., *et al.* (1965). Observations in 205 confirmed cases of acute pancreatitis, recurring pancreatitis and chronic pancreatitis. *Gut,* **6,** 545.

Sarles, H., Hawton, J., Planche, N.E., Lafont, H., and Gerolami, A. (1970). Diet, cholesterol gallstones and composition of bile. *American Journal of Digestive Diseases,* **15,** 251.

Sarles, H., Gerolami, A., and Bord, A. (1978). Diet and cholesterol gallstones. *Digestion,* **17,** 128.

Saunders, J.B., Walters, J.R.F., Davies, P., and Paton, A. (1981). A 20-year prospective study of cirrhosis. *British Medical Journal,* **282,** 263.

Savage, R.L., Moller, P.W., Ballantyne, C.L., and Wells, J.E. (1993). Variation in the risk of peptic ulcer complications with non-steroidal anti-inflammatory drug therapy. *Arthritis and Rheumatism,* **36,** 84.

Schubert, T.T., Schubert, M.A., and Ma, C.K. (1992). Symptoms, gastritis and *Helicobacter pylori* in patients referred for endoscopy. *Gastrointestinal Endoscopy,* **38,** 357.

Scragg, R.K.R., McMichael, A.J., and Baghurst, P.A. (1984*a*). Diet, alcohol, and relative weight in gallstone disease: a case–control study. *British Medical Journal,* **288,** 1113.

Scragg, R.K.R., McMichael, A.J., and Seamark, R.F. (1984*b*). Oral contraceptives, pregnancy and endogenous oestrogens in gall-stone disease: a case–control study. *British Medical Journal,* **288,** 1795.

Segal, I. and Walker, A.R.P. (1982). Diverticular disease in urban Africans in South Africa. *Digestion,* **24,** 42.

Shivananda, S., Pena, A.S., Mayberry, J.F., Ruiten, E.J., and Hoedemaeter, P.J. (1987*a*). Epidemiology of proctocolitis in the region of Leiden, the Netherlands. *Scandinavian Journal of Gastroenterology,* **22,** 993.

Shivananda, S., Pena, A.S., Mayberry, J.F., Ruiten, E.J., and Hoedemaeter, P.J. (1987*b*). Epidemiology of Crohn's disease in region Leiden, the Netherlands. *Gastroenterology,* **93,** 966.

Simon, L.S., Weaver, A.L., Graham, Dy., *et al.* (1999). Anti-inflammatory and upper gastrointestinal effects of celecoxib in rheumatoid arthritis: a randomised controlled trial. *Journal of the American Medical Association,* **282,** 1921–8.

Somerville, K.W., Logan, R.F.A., Edmond, M., and Langman, M.J.S. (1984). Smoking and Crohn's disease. *British Medical Journal,* **289,** 954.

Sonnenberg, A. (1994). Peptic ulcer. In *Digestive diseases in the United States: epidemiology and impact* (ed. J.E. Everhart), pp. 357–408. NIH Publication 94–1447, US Government Printing Office, Washington, DC.

Sorvillo, F.J., Fujoka, K., Nahlen, B., Tormey, M.P., Kebabjian, R., and Mascola, L. (1992). Swimming-associated cryptosporidiosis. *American Journal of Public Health,* **82,** 742–4.

Steiner, C., Bass, E.B., Talamini, M.A., Pitt, H.A., and Steinberg, E.P. (1994). Surgical rates and operative mortality for open and laparoscopic cholecystectomy in Maryland. *New England Journal of Medicine,* **330,** 403–8.

Stonnington, C.M., Phillips, S.F., Melton, III, L.J., and Zinsmeister, A.R. (1987). Chronic ulcerative colitis: incidence and prevalence in a community. *Gut,* **28,** 402.

Suharyono, S., Simanjuntak, C., Witham, N., *et al.* (1992). Safety and immunogenicity of single-dose live oral cholera vaccine CVD 103-HgR in 5–9 year old Indonesian children. *Lancet,* **340,** 689–94.

Sullivan-Bolyai, J.Z. and Corey, L. (1981). Epidemiology of Reyes' syndrome. *Epidemiologic Review,* **3,** 1.

Tamimi, T.M., Wosornu, L., Al-Khozaim, A., and Abdul-Ghani, A. (1990). Increased cholecystectomy rates in Saudi Arabia. *Lancet*, **336**, 1235–7.

Taylor, D.N. and Blaser, M.J. (1991). The epidemiology of *Helicobacter pylori* infection. *Epidemiologic Reviews*, **13**, 42.

Telium, D. (1990). Prevalence of gallstones at autopsy at the Institutes of Forensic Medicine in Aarhus and Copenhagen, Denmark, in 1944–1985. *Scandinavian Journal of Gastroenterology*, **25**, 401–4.

Telzak, E.E., Budnick, L.D., Greenberg, M.S.L., Blum, S., Shayegani, M., Benson, C.E., and Schultz, S. (1990). A nosocomial outbreak of *Salmonella* enteritidis infection due to the consumption of raw eggs. *New England Journal of Medicine*, **323**, 394–7.

Ter Meulen, V. (1998). Measles virus and Crohn's disease: view of a medical virologist. *Gut*, **43**, 733–4.

Thijs, C. and Knipschild, P. (1993). Oral contraceptives and the risk of gallbladder disease: a meta-analysis. *American Journal of Public Health*, **83**, 1113–20.

Thomas, J.G., Gibson, G.R., and Darboe, M.K. (1992). Isolation of *Helicobacter pylori* from human faeces. *Lancet*, **340**, 1194.

Thompson, N.P., Wakefield, A.J., and Pounder, R.E. (1995). Inherited disorders of coagulation appear to protect against inflammatory bowel disease. *Gastroenterology*, **108**, 1011–15.

Thornton, J.R., Emmett, P.M., and Heaton, K.W. (1979). Diet and Crohn's disease: characteristics of the pre-illness diet. *British Medical Journal*, **ii**, 762.

Timmer, A., Sutherland, L.R., Martin, F., and the Canadian Mesalamine for the Remission of Crohn's Disease Study Group (1998). Smoking, use of oral contraceptives, and medical induction of remission were risk factors for relapse in Crohn's disease. *Gastroenterology*, **114**, 1143–50.

Tobin, M.V., Logan, R.F.A., Langman, M.J.S., McConnell, U.R.B., and Gilmore, I.T. (1987). Cigarette smoking and inflammatory bowel disease. *Gastroenterology*, **93**, 316.

Tsianos, E.V., Masalas, C.N., Merkouropoulos, M., Kalekos, G.N., and Logan, R.F.A. (1994). Incidence of inflammatory bowel disease in north west Greece: rarity of Crohn's disease in an area where ulcerative colitis is common. *Gut*, **35**, 369.

Vessey, M., Jewel, D., Smith, A., Yeates, D., and McPherson, K. (1986). Chronic inflammatory bowel disease, cigarette smoking and use of oral contraceptives: findings in a large cohort study of women of childbearing age. *British Medical Journal*, **292**, 1101–3.

Walker, A. (1992). Swimming—the hazards of taking a dip. *British Medical Journal*, **304**, 242–5.

Walker, A.R.P., Walker, B.F, Duvenhage, A., Jones, J., Neongwane, J., and Segal, I. (1982). Appendicectomy prevalences in South African adolescents. *Digestion*, **23**, 274.

Walt, R., Katschinski, B., Logan, R., Ashley, J., and Langman, M.J.S. (1986). Rising frequency of ulcer perforation in elderly people in the United Kingdom. *Lancet*, **i**, 489.

Wheeler, J.G., Sethi, D., Cowden, J.M., *et al.* (1999). Study of infectious intestinal disease in England: rates in the community, presenting to general practice, and reported to national surveillance. *British Medical Journal*, **318**, 1046–50.

Weile, B. and Krasilnikoff, P.A. (1993). Extremely low incidence rates of celiac disease in the Danish population of children. *Journal of Clinical Epidemiology*, **46**, 661–4.

Weil, J., Colin Jones, D., Langman, M.J.S., *et al.* (1995). Prophylactic aspirin and risk of peptic ulcer bleeding. *British Medical Journal*, **310**, 827–30.

9.13 Sexually transmitted infections

Michael Adler and Frances Cowan

Introduction

Sexually transmitted infections (**STIs**) are those infections whose primary mode of transmission is through sexual contact. They present a major public health problem, and are among the most common causes of illness and even death in the world. STIs have far-reaching health, social, and economic consequences. The distribution of STIs within a community is dependent on the sexual behaviour of individuals within that community as well as the efficiency of transmission and the duration of infectiousness of the STI. The recognition that the presence of an STI, particularly those causing genital ulceration and/or inflammation within the genital tract, can enhance both the acquisition and transmission of the human immunodeficiency virus (**HIV**) has resulted increasingly in the development of integrated control programmes for HIV and STDs (Cohen *et al.* 1997; Fleming and Wasserheit 1999). Over and Piot (1991) reported that 70 per cent of HIV infection in Africa is found in patients with a sexually transmitted disease (**STD**) with lower, but increasing, levels of 15 to 30 per cent in Thailand amongst STD patients.

STIs (as well as HIV/AIDS) have a major demographic, economic, social, and political impact, particularly in sub-Saharan Africa and increasingly in Asia. The World Bank (in 1993) estimated that for those aged 15 to 44 years, STIs (excluding HIV) were the second most common cause of healthy life lost in women after maternal morbidity and mortality (Fig. 1).

What are the diseases/organisms?

The types of disease spread by sexual contact will vary in their incidence and clinical manifestations throughout the world. Traditionally, the venereal diseases comprised three bacterial infections, chancroid, syphilis, and gonorrhoea. However, over the last 30 years more and more micro-organisms have been recognized as spread by sexual intercourse or contact (Table 1).

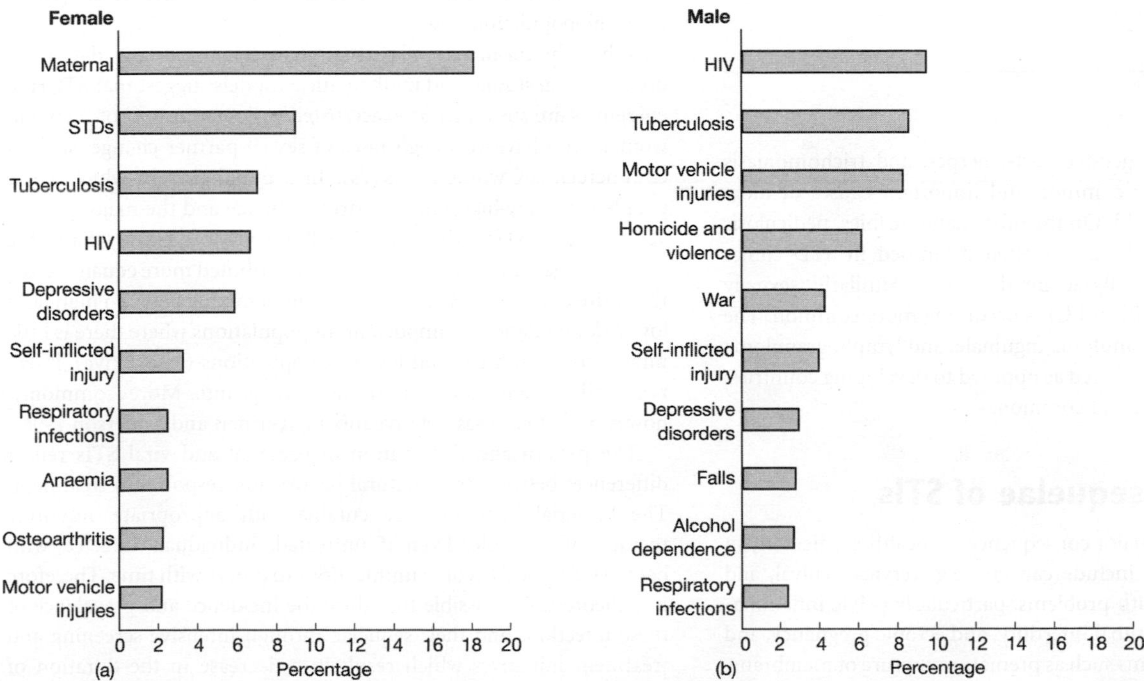

Fig. 1 Top ten causes of healthy life lost, ages 15 to 44 years: (a) females; (b) males.

Table 1 Micro-organisms that can be sexually transmitted

Bacteria
Chlamydia trachomatis
Neisseria gonorrhoeae
Gardnerella vaginalis
Treponema pallidum
Haemophilius ducreyi
Calymmatobacterium granulomatis
Shigella species
Mycoplasmas
Ureaplasma urealyticum
Mycoplasma hominis
Parasites
Sarcopetes scabiei
Phthirus pubis
Viruses
Herpes simplex virus types 1 and 2
Wart virus (papillomavirus)
Molluscum contagiosum virus (poxvirus)
Hepatitis A, B, and C virus
Cytomegalovirus
HIV-1 and HIV-2
Protozoa
Entamoeba histolytica
Giardia lamblia
Trichomonas vaginalis
Fungi
Candida albicans

Chlamydial infection, genital warts, herpes, and trichomoniasis have become increasingly common and important causes of morbidity throughout the world. On the other hand, scabies, pediculosis pubis, and vaginal candidiasis are often diagnosed in STD clinics although they are not usually acquired sexually. Similarly, sexually transmitted hepatitis (A, B, and C) is becoming more common. The incidence of chancroid, granuloma inguinale, and lymphogranuloma venereum is low in the developed as opposed to developing countries, where such conditions are still common.

Consequences/sequelae of STIs

Untreated STIs result in major consequences to health, particularly in women (Table 2). These include cancers (e.g. cervical, vulval, and penile), reproductive health problems, particularly pelvic inflammatory disease (salpingitis), tubal infertility, and ectopic pregnancy, and pregnancy-related problems such as premature rupture of membrane, preterm delivery, postpartum infection, and low birth weight. In addition, infection can be transmitted to the newborn either during pregnancy or at the time of delivery, resulting in conjunctivitis (*Chlamydia trachomatis*, *Neiserria gonorrhoeae*), pneumonia (*Chlamydia trachomatis*), neonatal herpes, and congenital abnormalities (syphilis).

The pattern and distribution of STIs around the world

The pattern and distribution of an STI within a population are dependent on the sexual behaviour of individuals within that community (including rate of partner change, extent of mixing between high- and low-risk populations, and barrier contraceptive usage), as well as the transmissibility and the duration of infectiousness of the micro-organism. The pattern and distribution can be expressed mathematically as set out below. The case reproduction rate R_0 represents the average number of new infections that result from an infected individual over the infectious period within a population:

$$R_0 = \beta c D$$

where β is the transmission probability, c is the average rate of acquiring partners (c is not the mean number, but is the mean m plus the variance-to-mean ratio σ^2/m of the relevant distribution of partner-change rates), and D is the duration of infectiousness.

It is possible to use this formula to predict or model the likely course of an STI epidemic, given various parameters, and to predict how altering these parameters might influence the epidemic. For example, in communities where the duration of infection is prolonged because of poor access to treatment facilities, an infection can be sustained, despite lower rates of partner change, than in a population where duration of infection is typically shorter. If the case reproduction rate R_0 is greater than unity, then the incidence of infection theoretically increases within the population while if it is consistently less than unity the incidence decreases and the infection disappears from the population.

While the mean rate of partner change is important, data from observational studies and mathematical models suggest that STI/HIV epidemics are sustained or exacerbated by ‘core groups’ of men and women who have very high rates of sexual partner change, such as commercial sex workers (**CSWs**). In a population in which a few people have very high rates of partner change and the majority have very low rates, STIs including HIV will spread more quickly than if the same average number of partners were distributed more equally across the entire population. Clearly, the extent of mixing between high- and low-risk populations is important. In populations where there is little mixing between high- and low-risk populations (assortative), infection will remain confined to the core group. More commonly, however, there is disassortative mixing (Garnett and Anderson 1996).

The pattern and distribution of bacterial and viral STIs reflect differences between their natural history and response to treatment. The bacterial infections are curable with appropriate antibiotic therapy, if available. Even if untreated, individuals infected with bacterial STIs will become uninfectious to others with time. Therefore it is theoretically possible to reduce the incidence and prevalence of these infections and their sequelae through intensive screening and treatment initiatives which result in a decrease in the duration of infectiousness. Indeed, in many developed countries, the rate of the bacterial STIs has dramatically reduced over the last 20 years.

Table 2 Major sequelae of STDs

Health consequence	Women	Men	Infants
Cancers	Cervical cancer Vulval cancer Vaginal cancer Anal cancer Liver cancer T-cell leukaemia Kaposi's sarcoma	Penile cancer Anal cancer Liver cancer T-cell leukaemia Kaposi's sarcoma	
Reproductive health problems	Pelvic inflammatory disease Infertility Ectopic pregnancy Spontaneous abortion	Epididymitis Prostatitis Infertility	
Pregnancy-related problems	Preterm delivery Premature rupture of membranes Puerperal sepsis Postpartum infection		Stillbirth Low birth weight Conjunctivitis Pneumonia Neonatal sepsis Acute hepatitis Congenital abnormalities
Neurological problems	Neurosyphilis	Neurosyphilis	Cytomegalovirus Herpes simplex virus Syphilis-associated neurological problems
Other common health consequences	Chronic liver disease Cirrhosis	Chronic liver disease Cirrhosis	Chronic liver disease Cirrhosis

However, in developing countries, with few resources for screening and treatment, infected individuals remain infectious for longer and rates of bacterial STIs and their sequelae remain high.

In contrast, the non-curable viral STIs are chronic and persist over years, in some cases for life, with those infected remaining potentially infectious to others over prolonged periods. In this circumstance, without effective primary prevention of infection either through behaviour modification or vaccination, the prevalence of viral STIs continues to rise in both developed and developing countries.

The recognition given and resources spent on control programmes and notification for STIs varies throughout the world. The World Health Organization (**WHO**) has been responsible for a series of estimates of the size of the problem represented by STIs, and they suggest an annual total of 333 million new infections per annum. The major focus for these is Southeast Asia, with an estimated 150 million new cases per year, and sub-Saharan Africa with 65 million. In Eastern Europe and Central Asia, the estimate is 18 million, and for Western Europe 16 million (Fig. 2). The estimated prevalence and incidence of STIs by region shows considerable variation. For example, the difference in prevalence and incidence rates between sub-Saharan Africa and Western Europe is fourfold and threefold respectively (Table 3).

Although notification of STIs is required in many European countries, the accuracy of this information is variable, and often suffers from the reluctance of private doctors or general practitioners,

Table 3 Estimated prevalence and incidence of STDs by region

Region	Prevalence (per 1000)	Incidence (per 1000)
Sub-Saharan Africa	208	254
South and Southeast Asia	128	160
Latin America and Caribbean	95	145
Eastern Europe and Central Asia	75	112
North America	52	91
Australasia	52	91
Western Europe	45	77
Northern Africa and Middle East	40	60
East Asia and the Pacific	19	28
Total	85	113

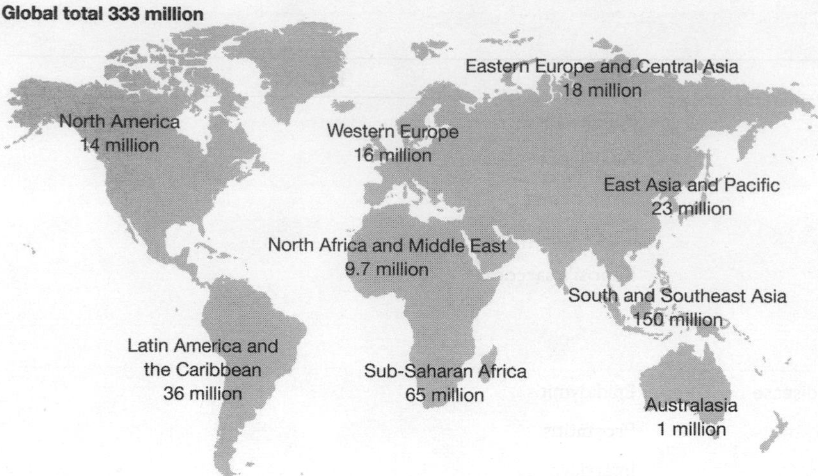

Fig. 2 Estimated new cases of curable STDs among adults (1995).

who in many European countries see the majority of patients, to notify these. For example, in Italy it is estimated that for each case of syphilis notified, 2.3 are not, and for each case of gonorrhoea notified, two are not. In The Netherlands under-reporting of gonorrhoea has been estimated in the past to run at 66 per cent. Because of these gross limitations it is difficult to obtain accurate data. Some countries have set up alternative systems for collecting this information which may not give total coverage. For example, STD clinics (United Kingdom, France, Italy), laboratory systems (Denmark, Sweden), and sentinel general practitioner systems (Belgium). However, these statistics do not cover patients who are treated in other facilities, for example family planning, gynaecology, and primary care. The majority of these surveillance systems are, however, only able to detect symptomatic STIs in individuals who present for clinical care. Many STIs are asymptomatic and are therefore unrecognized, particularly in women.

The lack of good data and notification systems has often been overcome by prevalence studies in particular countries. Such information is useful but is often of limited value as it is rarely based on a truly random sample of the community being studied. More often it is obtained from atypical, high-risk, and usually consulting groups of individuals and/or patients. Figure 3 indicates the prevalence of the common STDs in women in Africa in different settings. In CSWs, the prevalence of gonorrhoea can reach nearly 50 per cent and the prevalence of syphilis ranges from 2 to 30 per cent for acute or

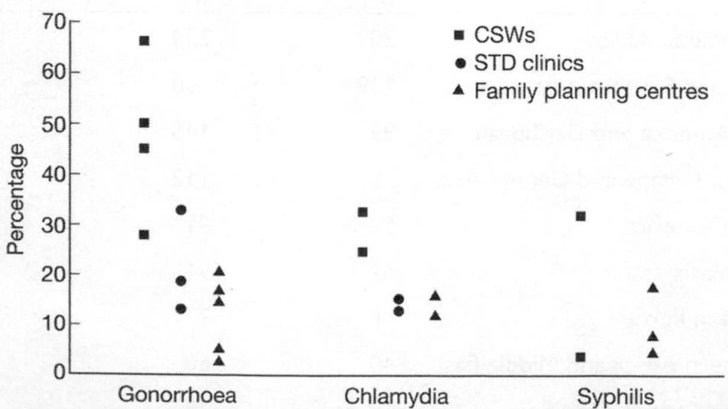

Fig. 3 STDs in women in Africa.

previous infection. Levels of *Chlamydia trachomatis* can be as high as 30 per cent. In the developing world, prostitution is a driving force for STDs and HIV. For example, in Kenyan urban STD clinics, 60 per cent of men with a gonococcal urethritis or chancroid reported commercial sex exposure as the probably source of infection. Other high-risk groups studied are men and women attending STD clinics, and, as expected, levels of infection are found to be high. Unfortunately, levels of infection can also be high in what can be termed as 'low-risk' groups, namely women attending antenatal clinics. One finds very high levels of gonococcal and chlamydial infection from various studies in other continents apart from Africa, for example Latin America and South and Southeast Asia. Studies of herpes simplex virus seroprevalence indicate very high levels of infection in many developing countries. For example, in Mwanza, Tanzania, over 40 per cent of teenage girls have evidence of infection with herpes simplex virus type 2 (**HSV-2**) (Obasi *et al.* 1999). Additionally, two random population studies from the United States indicate that the prevalence of HSV-2 antibody in non-institutionalized Americans has risen from 16.8 per cent in the period 1976–1978 to 21.2 per cent in 1988–1992 (Fleming *et al.* 1997). Studies from Europe suggest lower infection rates than those in the United States and developing countries.

Even though rates of STIs tend to be lower in Europe, there has been increasing concern over major epidemics of gonorrhoea and syphilis in Eastern Europe in the newly independent states of the former Soviet Union. Figure 4 indicates the high rates of gonorrhoea, the highest rates are seen in Estonia (166), Russia (139), and Belarus (125) per 100 000. Incidence rates for syphilis are now below 5 per 100 000 in nearly all Western European countries. However, Eastern Europe has not experienced this decline, and recently, as with gonorrhoea, there has been considerable concern about the epidemic of syphilis. In these countries, syphilis incidence in 1996 was between 140 and 254 per 100 000 (Fig. 5); increases are considerable in all age groups but particularly in older adolescents. Between 1986 and 1996, the incidence of syphilis in 18- to 19-year-old Russians increased from 6 to 607 per 100 000 in men and from 20 to 1321 per 100 000 in women. The increase between 1992 and 1996 was 20-fold in Russia, sixfold in Estonia, 12-fold in Latvia, and 14-fold in Lithuania (Fig. 6). It is unlikely that the epidemic is restricted to syphilis and gonorrhoea, and it is highly likely that there is also an epidemic of HIV infection.

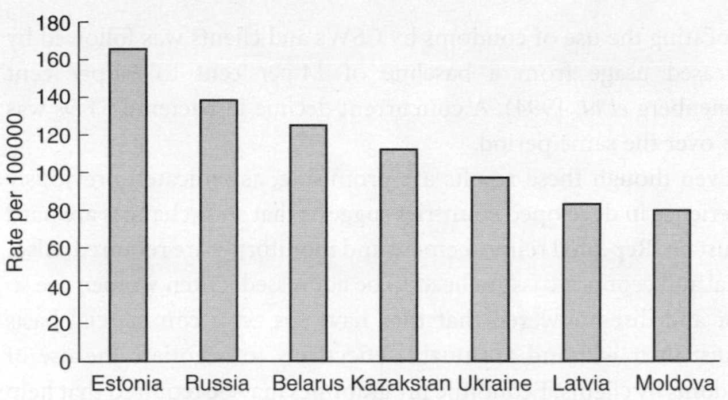

Fig. 4 Gonorrhoea rates per 100 000 Eastern and Central Europe (1996).

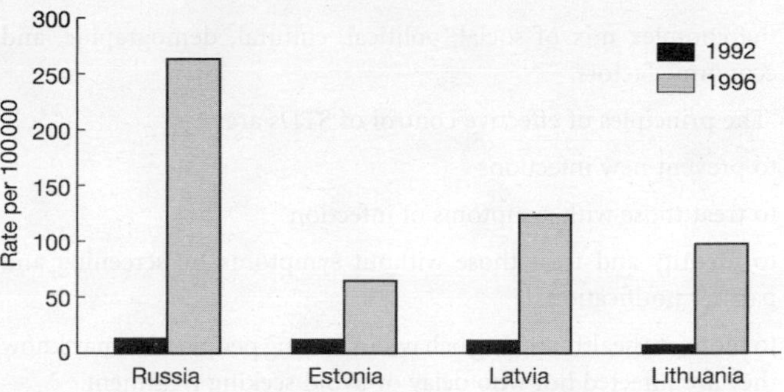

Fig. 6 New cases of syphilis in Russia and the Baltic States in the period 1992 to 1996 (rates per 100 000).

With recent outbreaks of HIV infection among intravenous drug users, particularly in Belarus, Russia, and Ukraine, and the very high incidence of syphilis and other STIs in the region, the stage is now set for a potentially rapid spread of HIV.

Interaction of STIs with HIV

There is strong evidence that STIs facilitate the transmission of HIV. Studies have shown that genital HIV viral shedding increases significantly in the presence of acute STIs, returning to preinfection levels following effective treatment (Cohen *et al.* 1997; Schacker *et al.* 1998*a*,*b*). In addition there is strong experimental evidence from the community-randomized trial in Mwanza, Tanzania, that it is possible to substantially reduce the incidence of HIV infection among adults by introducing effective STI control in the form of syndromic treatment for symptomatic bacterial STIs (Grosskurth *et al.* 1995). There is increasing evidence from cross-sectional studies and a few prospective studies of a strong association between HSV-2 infection and acquisition/transmission (Gwanzura *et al.* 1998; Fleming and Wasserheit 1999). In communities with high rates of STIs, it is likely that a considerable proportion of HIV infections are attributable to the effect of STIs on HIV transmission.

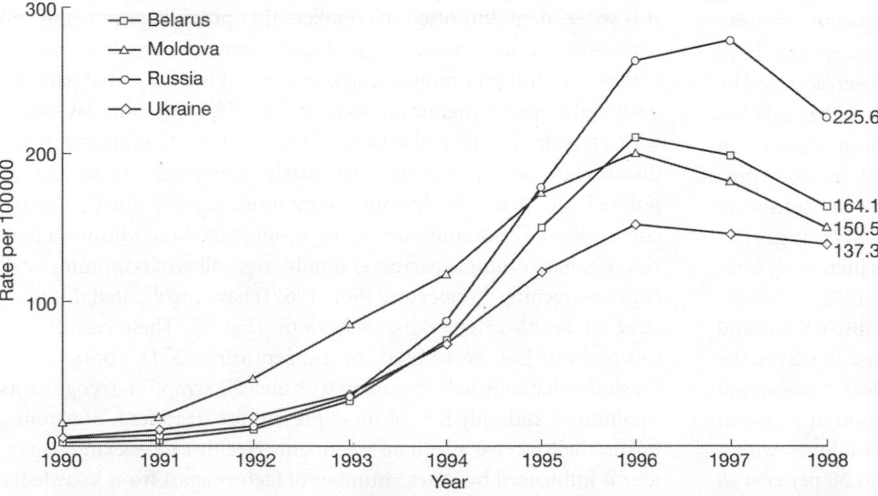

Fig. 5 Incidence of syphilis in Belarus, the Russian Federation, Moldova, and Ukraine during the period 1990 to 1998.

Control programmes

Control requires a broad-based approach which addresses prevention and low-cost/low-technology approaches to diagnosis, treatment, and care, which are often delivered by non-medical personnel in rural settings. The social, demographic, and economic causes and consequences of STDs need addressing since they have major consequences on productivity, social, and family structures. It follows from this that the medical model is too limited in controlling STDs. It is pointless to develop strategies for control if appropriate systems and public-sector financing are not in place for the delivery and adoption of services, health education, new technologies, etc. The institutional and infrastructural issues of public-sector financing, community development, and capacity building are pivotal to any control programme.

Particular issues for the control of STIs are as follows:

- high rates of infection among young adults, adolescents, and certain groups (CSWs and truck drivers)
- asymptomatic disease
- long-term morbidity, particularly in women
- increased acquisition of HIV in transmission
- women are disadvantaged/disempowered

- the complex mix of social, political, cultural, demographic, and economic factors.

The principles of effective control of STDs are:

- to prevent new infections
- to treat those with symptoms of infection
- to identify and treat those without symptoms by screening and partner notification
- to motivate health-seeking behaviour among people who may know they are infected but who delay or avoid seeking treatment.

These principles and aims can be achieved or attempted through two approaches.

- Primary prevention:
  health education
  provision of condoms
  social, cultural, and economic interventions.
- Secondary prevention:
  promotion of health-care-seeking behaviour
  case management
  early detection and treatment of symptomatic/symptomatic infections.

Primary prevention

Clearly it is best to avoid infection in the first place. The advent of AIDS has been a major influence in the increased awareness of the need for health education and the public acceptance of explicit messages and images. Programmes aimed at safer sexual practices and increased condom use have been widely advocated and implemented in both developed and developing countries. The success of such programmes is often difficult to assess and, sadly, initial modifications in behaviour are not always maintained over longer periods of time. This has been seen within both the United Kingdom and United States: initial and profound changes in sexual behaviour in homosexual men led to lower levels of STDs, but unfortunately this alteration in behaviour has not been universally sustained.

Programmes to market and encourage the use of condoms have been at the heart of many control programmes and are particularly useful since they reduce acquisition and transmission of both traditional STDs and HIV infection. In Africa there has been encouraging evidence that increased condom use has been accepted by high-risk groups such as CSWs and their clients, and that this has altered levels of infection. Examples of this have been reported in Africa and Southeast Asia. A 3-year programme of condom promotion and STD control in Zaire saw an increase in consistent condom use from 0 per cent to 68 per cent amongst CSWs (Laga *et al.* 1994). Social marketing of condoms in Zaire saw sales increasing from 20 000 to 18 million in a period of 3 years (Kyungu 1992). Multiple outlets were used, such as street traders, night clubs, CSWs, and pharmacists. In parallel with the increased condom use in CSWs, the incidence of gonorrhoea, trichomoniasis, genital ulcer disease, and HIV declined. In Zimbabwe a community intervention at a cost of $85 000 resulted in the distribution of 5.7 million condoms, with a suggested resulting decline in STDs ranging from 6 to 50 per cent in different areas. CSWs were found to have increased condom usage from 18 per cent prior to the programme to 72 per cent with their last client (World Bank 1993). In Thailand, an education programme advocating the use of condoms by CSWs and clients was followed by increased usage from a baseline of 14 per cent to 94 per cent (Hanenberg *et al.* 1994). A concurrent decline in bacterial STDs was seen over the same period.

Even though these results are promising, as indicated previously experience in developed countries suggests that such changes are hard to sustain. Repeated reinforcement and monitoring are required. Also, social and economic issues need to be addressed. Often women are so poor and disempowered that they have sex on a commercial basis against their will and are unable effectively to negotiate the use of condoms by clients. Economic programmes may be required that help reduce the necessity for women to earn or supplement their incomes by prostitution. At the same time women need to be taught skills that help them negotiate safer sex with clients and regular partners. This is particularly difficult with the latter since husbands and regular partners can see such negotiation as a reflection of themselves at the same time as suggesting that the woman has herself had multiple partners. The recognition of the substantial shift in cultural attitudes that are still necessary to establish wider condom use has led research workers to explore the use of vaginal virucides. Such an agent(s), if effective, would allow women more control. Raising the status of women in the developing world would be a crucial factor in the control of STDs and HIV, and can only be achieved through equality in the fields of education and employment.

Vaccination of susceptible individuals within a community is the other potential mechanism for primary prevention. To date the only effective vaccines for infections that are sexually transmitted are for the viral hepatitides. Concerted research efforts are underway to develop and test vaccines for other STIs, most notably for human papillomavirus infection and herpes simplex virus infection. For STIs, however, there is at least the theoretical possibility that an incompletely effective vaccine (which all vaccines are to some extent) could reassure vaccinees and result in increased sexual risk-taking, with all its adverse consequences.

Secondary prevention

Health-care-seeking behaviour

It is self-evident, but often overlooked, that providing screening and diagnostic services, however good and client friendly, is of no use within a control programme unless utilized. It is an essential part of a health education programme to point out the symptoms associated with a possible STD but also to reinforce an understanding that many diseases are asymptomatic, particularly in women. It should be pointed out that, ideally, once symptoms develop further sexual contact should cease and care be sought, and that those who are at high risk (e.g. have multiple partners) should, regardless of symptoms, seek regular screening. Waaler and Piot (1969)) have highlighted this basic issue of health-care-seeking behaviour (Fig. 7). Their cascade for tuberculosis has been used to conceptualize STD control, and illustrates that only half of women with an STD symptom recognize its significance and only half of these present for treatment, of whom a further half receive adequate treatment. Health-care-seeking behaviour is influenced by a large number of factors apart from knowledge and awareness. For example, economic structural adjustment programmes have been criticized, since the introduction of fees for medical care, which are forced upon governments to fulfil these

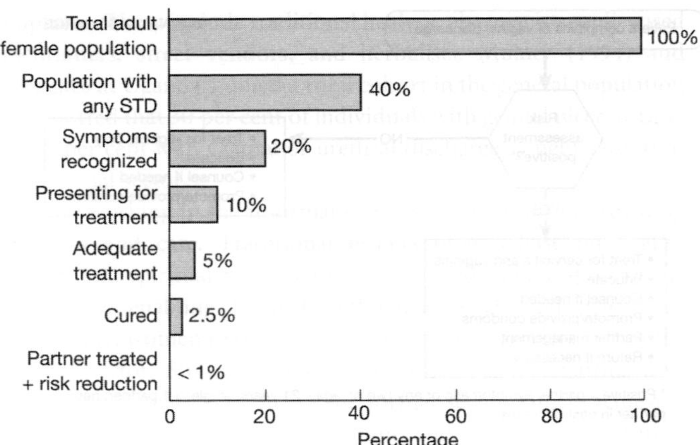

Fig. 7 Health-care-seeking behaviour in women with STDs.

programmes, affects uptake of services (Lurie *et al.* 1995). A documented example of this occurred in Nairobi's large STD clinic, where the introduction of fees was followed by a reduction in attendance of 60 per cent among men and 35 per cent among women (Moses *et al.* 1992).

Clinical services and case management

Once a client presents with an STI symptom, different methods of case management are available. Whichever method is used they should share the common objectives of providing diagnosis and treatment based on a clinical, laboratory, or syndromic approach, as well as promoting reduction of risk-taking behaviour and treatment of sexual partners. Whatever the chosen method of case management, it is essential to create a non-judgemental, sensitive, and user friendly environment which encourages clients to utilize services, whether they are provided in the formal or informal sector.

Vertical services for control

In resource-rich countries, the traditional approach to the diagnosis of a presumed STI is through aetiological diagnosis, established by microscopy and laboratory cultures and run by specialist doctors. This vertical approach has both advantages and disadvantages (Table 4). The main advantages are that the services provided by those who are specialists, well trained, and motivated to provide good services that are supported by accurate laboratory diagnoses to which appropriate treatment can be tailored. Such specialized facilities also offer the ability for good training, monitoring, surveillance, and research. However, this type of service has disadvantages, particularly in resource-poor settings, in that it is expensive, the use of laboratories for the definitive diagnoses inevitably means that there can be delays and therefore patients may not return for appropriate therapy, and that such services, usually based in urban settings, are of limited availability and do not give total coverage of the population. Since such services are usually specialist, they can create stigmatization. However, in countries such as the United Kingdom, this is no longer a major problem. A much more fundamental issue is that the expense of specialist vertical services mean that they are unsustainable in a resource-poor setting.

Integrated services

Thus it can be seen that the concepts for models of case management used in resource-rich countries are usually inappropriate for implementation in developing countries. In such situations care is provided in an integrated non-specialist manner through an array of services and individuals, including general hospital outpatient clinics, primary health centres, clinics, maternal and child health centres, family planning clinics, private practitioners, pharmacists, traditional healers, unqualified practitioners, and street vendors. Few of those providing STI care have specialist training or medical qualifications. As with vertical services, there are both advantages and disadvantages to the integrated approach (Table 5). The major advantages are immediate diagnosis by the non-specialists and an inexpensive service managed in a standardized way. The disadvantages relate to low sensitivity and specificity and the detection of asymptomatic infection, which is discussed under the section on syndromic case management.

Whilst all of these services and providers can work together in a complementary fashion, it is important that strategic decisions are taken about the most appropriate system to form the core and backbone of a control programme in any one country. It is likely that in the resource-poor countries, a different model from the vertical one described above will have to be used, and that is why the integrated approach using all types of potential providers is more sustainable and has led to the development of the syndromic approach.

WHO has placed increasing emphasis on integrated approaches, especially at the primary health centres level, using a syndromic approach for patient management (WHO 1991, 1994). This approach recognizes the limitation of resources for health-care and of specialist trained medical personnel. It is advocated for use particularly in high prevalence areas where there are inadequate laboratory facilities, lack

Table 4 Vertical services for STDs

Advantages	**Disadvantages**
Specialists	Expensive
Accurate laboratory diagnosis with appropriate treatment	Delays in diagnosis
	Limited availability
Reference laboratory	Limited coverage of population
Training	Stigmatization
Monitoring, surveillance, and research	Poor sustainability
Asymptomatic infection may be detected	

Table 5 Integrated services for STDs

Advantages	**Disadvantages**
Problem oriented	Low sensitivity/specificity for cervical gonococcal or chlamydial infection in women
Immediate presumptive diagnosis and treatment of possible aetiologies	
Non-specialist	Asymptomatic infection not detected but treatment possible by active partner notification and epidemiological treatment of partners
Inexpensive	
Standardization of management and monitoring of drug usage and antibiotic resistance	
	Not always acceptable to medical staff

Fleming, D.T. and Wasserheit, J. (1999). From epidemiological synergy to public health policy and practice: the contribution of other sexually transmitted diseases to sexual transmission of HIV infection. *Sexually Transmitted Infections*, **75**, 3–17.

Fleming, D.T., McQuillan, G.M., Johnson, R.E., *et al.* (1997). Herpes simplex virus type 2 in the United States 1976–1994. *New England Journal of Medicine*, **337**, 1105–11.

Garnett, G.P. and Anderson, R.M. (1996). Sexually transmitted diseases and sexual behavior: insights from mathematical models. *Journal of Infectious Diseases*, **174** (Supplement 2), S150–61.

Garcia, P., Gotuzzo, E., Hughes, J.P., and Holmes, K.K. (1998). Syndromic management of sexually transmitted diseases in pharmacies: evaluation and randomized intervention trial. *Sexually Transmitted Infections*, **74** (Supplement 1), S153–8.

Grosskurth, H., Mosha, F., Todd, J., *et al.* (1995). Impact of improved treatment of sexually transmitted diseases on HIV infection in rural Tanzania: randomised controlled trial. *Lancet*, **346**, 530–6.

Grosskurth, H., Mayaud, P., Mosha, F., *et al.* (1996). Asymptomatic gonorrhoea and chlamydial infection in rural Tanzanian men. *British Medical Journal,* **312**, 277–80.

Gwanzura, L., McFarland, W., Alexander, D., Burke, R.L., and Katzenstein, D. (1998). Association between human immunodeficiency virus and herpes simplex virus type 2 seropositivity among male factory workers in Zimbabwe. *Journal of Infectious Diseases*, **177**, 481–4.

Hanenberg, R.S., Rojanapithayakorn, W., Kunasol, P., and Sokal, D. (1994). Impact of Thailand's HIV control programme as indicated by the decline of sexually transmitted diseases. *Lancet,* **344**, 243–5.

Jackson, D.J., Rakwar, J.P., Bwayo, J.J., Kreiss, J.K., and Moses, S. (1997). *Trichomonas vaginalis* infection and HIV-1 transmission. *Lancet*, **350**, 1076.

Kahn, J.G. (1996). The cost effectiveness of HIV prevention targeting: how much more bang for the buck? *American Journal of Public Health*, **86**, 1709–12.

Kyungu, E. (1992). Condom and social marketing and mass media in Zaire. In *Proceedings of a Meeting on Effective Approaches to AIDS Prevention.* WHO, Geneva.

Laga, M., Alary, M., Nzila, N., *et al.* (1994). Condom promotion, sexually transmitted diseases, treatment and declining incidence of HIV infection in female Zairian sex workers. *Lancet*, **344**, 246–8.

Lurie, P., Hintzen, P., and Lowe, R.A. (1995). Socioeconomic obstacles to HIV prevention and treatment in developing countries: the roles of the International Monetary Fund and the World Bank. *AIDS*, **9**, 539–46.

Lutakome, M.D., *et al.* (1995). Traditional healers for HIV/AIDS prevention and care in Uganda. Abstract TUB109, 9th International Conference on AIDS and STDs in Africa, Kampala.

Mabey, D., *et al.* (1995). The role of a reference clinic in support of an integrated STD control programme in Tanzania. Abstract 080, 11th Meeting of the International Society for STD Research, New Orleans, LA.

McNagny, J.F., Parker, R.M., Zemlman, J.M., and Lewis, J.S. (1992). Urinary leukocyte esterase test: a screening method for detection of asymptomatic chlamydial and gonococcal infections in men. *Journal of Infectious Diseases*, **165**, 573–6.

Mayaud, P., Grosskurth, H., Changalucha, J., *et al.* (1995*a*). Risk assessment and other screening options for gonorrhoea and chlamydial infections in women attending rural Tanzanian antenatal clinics. *Bulletin of the World Health Organization*, **73**, 621–30.

Mayaud, *et al.* (1995*b*). Validation of a new clinical algorithm for the management of vaginal discharge using risk assessment in Mwanza, Tanzania. Abstract 213, 11th meeting of the International Society for STD Research, New Orleans, LA.

Moses, S., Plummer, F.A., Ngugi, E.N., Nagelkerke, N.J.D., Anzala, A.O., and Ndinya-Achola, J.O. (1991). Controlling HIV in Africa: effectiveness and cost effectiveness of an intervention in a high frequency STD transmitter core group. *AIDS*, **5**, 407–11.

Moses, S., Manji, F., Bradley, J.E., Nagelkerke, N.J., Malisa, M.A., and Plummer, F.A. (1992). Impact of user fees on attendance at a referral centre for sexually transmitted diseases in Kenya. *Lancet*, **340**, 463–6.

Mulder, D. (1994). Disease perception and health-seeking behaviour for sexually transmitted diseases. In *Prevention and management of sexually transmitted diseases in Eastern and Southern Africa: current approaches and future directions*, pp. 83–91. Network of AIDS Researchers of Eastern and Southern Africa, Nairobi.

Nzima, M., *et al.* (1995). Traditional healers' perception of sexually transmitted diseases in urban Zambia, Abstract TUB099, 9th International Conference on AIDS and STDs in Africa, Kampala.

Obasi, A., Mosha, F., Quigley, M., *et al.* (1999). Antibody to HSV-2 as a marker of sexual risk behaviour in rural Tanzania. *Journal of Infectious Diseases*, **179**, 16–24.

Over, M. and Piot, P. (1991). *HIV infection and sexually transmitted diseases.* Report HSPR 26, World Bank, Washington, DC.

Over, M. and Piot, P. (1993). HIV-infection and sexually transmitted diseases. In *Disease control priorities in developing countries*, (ed. D.T. Jamison, W.H. Mosley, A.R. Measham, and J.L. Bobadilla), pp. 455–528. Oxford University Press.

Oxman, A.D., Scott, E.A.F., Sellors, J.W., *et al.* (1994). Partner notification for sexually transmitted diseases: an overview of the evidence. *Canadian Journal of Public Health*, (Supplement 1), S41–S47.

Plummer, F.A., Nagelkerke, N.J.D., Moses, S., Ndinya-Achola, J.O., Bwayo, J., and Ngugi, E. (1991). The importance of core groups in the epidemiology and control of HIV-1 infection. *AIDS*, **5** (Supplement 1), S169–S176.

Rutayuga, J.B. (1995). Traditional medical practitioners coming together against the spread of HIV/AIDS in South Africa. Abstract TUB103, 11th International Conference on AIDS and STDs in Africa, Kampala.

Schacker, T., Ryncarz, A.J., Goddard, J., Diem, K., Shaughnessy, M., and Corey, L. (1998*a*). Frequent recovery of HIV-1 from genital herpes simplex virus lesions in HIV-1 infected men. *Journal of the American Medical Association*, **280**, 61–6.

Schacker, T., Zeh, J., Hu, H., Hill, E., and Corey, L. (1998*b*) Frequency of symptomatic and asymptomatic herpes simplex virus type 2 reactivations among HIV-infected men. *Journal of Infectious Diseases*, **178**, 1616–22.

Waaler, H.T. and Piot, M.A. (1969). The use of an epidemiological model for estimating the effectiveness of tuberculosis control measures: sensitivity of the effectiveness of tuberculosis control measures to the coverage of the population. *Bulletin of the World Health Organization*, **41**, 75–93.

Wawer, M.J., Sewankambo, N.K., Serwadda, D., *et al.* (1999). Control of sexually transmitted diseases for AIDS prevention in Uganda: a randomised community trial. *Lancet*, **353**, 525–35.

Woolhouse, M.E.J., Dye, C., Etard, J.F., *et al.* (1997). Heterogeneities in the transmission of infectious agents: implications for design of control programs. *Proceedings of the National Academy of Sciences of the United States of America*, **94**, 338–42.

WHO (1991). *Management of patients with sexually transmitted diseases: report of a WHO steering group.* WHO Technical Report Series 810, WHO, Geneva.

WHO (1994). *Management of sexually transmitted diseases.* Report WHO/GPA/TEM/94.1, WHO, Geneva.

World Bank (1993). *World development report 1993: investing in health.* Oxford University Press, New York.

World Bank (1997). *Confronting AIDS—public priorities in a global epidemic.* World Bank Policy Research Report. Oxford University Press.

9.14 Acquired immunodeficiency syndrome

Wiput Phoolcharoen and Roger Detels

History of the HIV/AIDS epidemic

Acquired immunodeficiency syndrome (**AIDS**) has been the most dramatic disease event of the second half of the twentieth century. It has been estimated that, by December 2000, 57.9 million individuals had been infected by the human immunodeficiency virus (**HIV**), including over 21.8 million who had died from AIDS (UNAIDS 2000). The majority of those infected have been in the most productive years of their life, causing a secondary economic impact beyond the cost of caring for them and creating a new cohort of orphans. The total number of deaths and expected deaths from HIV already exceeds the total killed in all the major wars of the twentieth century (Fig. 1). And the epidemic is still spreading! Its impact is particularly tragic because 95 per cent of HIV infections occur in developing countries that are least prepared to absorb the impact of the health and economic consequences.

AIDS was first recognized and reported in 1980 by an alert young physician, Michael Gottlieb, at the University of California Los Angeles School of Medicine, who realized that the unexplained immune deficiency that he observed in three young men represented a new disease (Gottlieb *et al.* 1981). Gottlieb reported his findings to the United States Centers for Disease Control and Prevention and published them in the *Morbidity and Mortality Weekly Report*, which resulted in the recognition by other physicians in San Francisco and New York that they were seeing the same unexplained immune deficiency. It soon became apparent that the disease occurred primarily in two groups—men who had sex with men and injecting drug users—but the infection soon spread to haemophiliacs.

The reasons for the sudden appearance of HIV infection and AIDS are not completely understood, but it is clear that both biological and sociological factors were involved (Gao *et al.* 1999). A report by Beatrice Hahn suggests that the biological parent of HIV-1 was present in chimpanzees. She gathered evidence that the virus spread to humans through exposure to chimps as pets and through butchering of infected animals for food. However, the virus has low infectivity and it is doubtful that it could have spread if there had not been a major change in sexual behavior towards greater acceptance of multiple sexual partners in the second half of the twentieth century. The change may have been due, in part, to the introduction of the contraceptive pill, which reduced the fear of pregnancy resulting from sexual intercourse, a major inhibitor of multiple partners and early sex in many parts of the world.

Although the disease was first recognized in the United States, that country has not been the primary focus of the epidemic. For the most part the early epidemic in the United States and the other developed countries was confined to men who have sex with men and the injecting drug-using population, who represent a relatively small proportion of the total population. In the developing world, however,

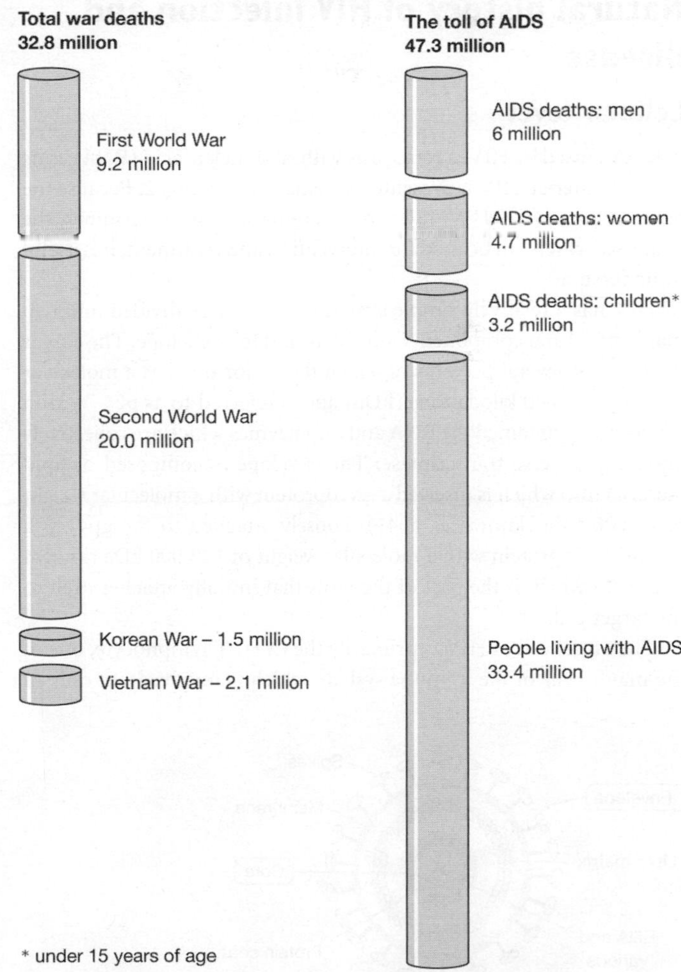

Fig. 1 The toll of AIDS (data from 1999). (Reproduced from Global Health Council 2000.)

it soon became apparent that the major mode of spread was through heterosexual intercourse. The countries of sub-Saharan Africa were the initial focus of the epidemic and this region continues to have the highest number of new infections. The epidemic soon spread to other countries as well, including Latin America, and in the late 1980s and early 1990s to South and Southeast Asia, currently the second most heavily involved region of the world. Although the prevalence of HIV is still low in both India and China, their large populations, representing 38 per cent of the world's population, and the increasing prevalence of sexual mixing and sexually transmitted diseases (**STDs**) suggest that it is only a matter of time before the epidemic establishes a firm stronghold in both these countries. The estimated number of HIV-infected individuals in India already exceeds the total estimated for all the rest of South and Southeast Asia. Clearly, dramatic steps must be initiated to prevent the further spread of HIV. However, the high proportion of silent infections and the stigma associated both with belonging to the most severely affected risk groups and being infected, combined with the reluctance of most societies to discuss sexual behaviours openly, make the implementation of effective intervention strategies very difficult, but not impossible; Thailand has successfully reduced the spread of HIV (Phoolcharoen *et al.* 1998).

Natural history of HIV infection and disease

Cellular level

AIDS is caused by HIV, a retrovirus with ribonucleic acid (**RNA**) as its genetic material. HIV is presented schematically in Fig. 2. Because the natural history of HIV infection is unusual and determines the strategies which can be used for intervention and treatment, it is useful to understand it.

HIV has a relatively simple structure that can be divided into two major structural components—the core and the envelope. The core is made up of several proteins of which the major one has a molecular weight of 24 000 kilodaltons (**kDa**) and is referred to as p24. Within the core are contained the RNA and the enzymes which are collectively known as reverse transcriptase. The envelope is composed of lipid material into which is inserted a glycoprotein with a molecular weight of 41 000 kDa (known as gp41). Loosely attached to the gp41 is a second glycoprotein with a molecular weight of 120 000 kDa (known as gp120) which is the part of the virus that initially attaches itself to the target cell.

The target cell of HIV is primarily the CD4$^+$ T lymphocyte, one of the major cells of the immune system, which is involved not only in

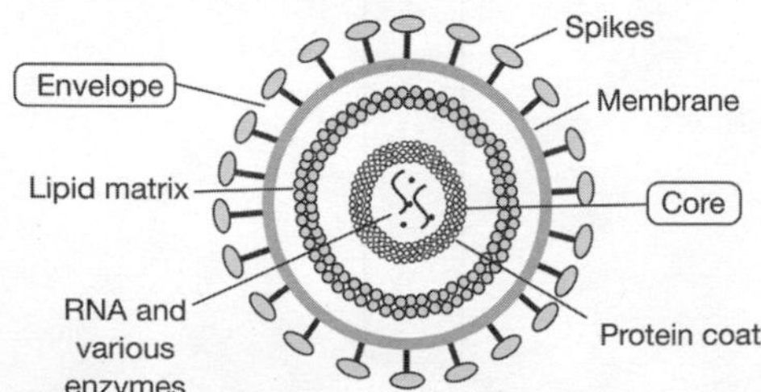

Fig. 2 HIV-1 virus.

the production of cellular immunity but also influences the production of antibodies. HIV can attach to any cell that has the CD4$^+$ receptor. Although these receptors are found primarily on the CD4$^+$ lymphocytes, they are also found on 40 per cent of mononuclear cells, including macrophages, 5 per cent of B cells, probably on mature CD8$^+$ cells, and the counterparts of these cells in the central nervous system.

The natural history of HIV infection of the CD4$^+$ cell is pictured in Fig. 3. The process of HIV replication begins with the attachment of the virus to the cell, which is accomplished primarily by attachment to two cell receptors: the CD4$^+$ receptor and either the CCR5 or the CRCX4 receptor. Early in the natural history of HIV infection, HIV will use the CCR5 receptor, but as the HIV undergoes changes within the infected individual from the so-called non-syncytium-inducing forms, found early in the course of disease, to the syncytium-inducing form in advanced disease, it also utilizes the CRCX4 receptor. There are other receptors that also influence the ability of HIV to attach to the cell, but the biology of these receptors is still under investigation.

Once HIV has successfully attached to the cell, the core of the virus is intruded into the cytoplasm of the cell and the viral RNA is transcribed into viral deoxyribonucleic acid (**DNA**) by the enzymes known collectively as reverse transcriptase. The transcription process, however, is imperfect and, on average, at least one mutation occurs per replication cycle. This is important because the human immune response to the virus is absolutely specific. Thus the immune system will not recognize the mutation and mounts a new immune response to the progeny virus, a process which may take several weeks, during which the HIV continues to infect other cells which produce more mutated virus. The 'errors' in this step are a major reason why HIV is able to escape the immune system and persist. Reverse transcription is blocked by the group of drugs known collectively as reverse transcriptase inhibitors.

Once transcription of the genetic material to viral DNA is completed, the viral DNA is integrated into the host cell DNA with the assistance of a viral enzyme known as integrase. After the viral DNA has been incorporated into the host DNA it is indistinguishable from the host DNA and is referred to as the 'provirus'. Each time the cell divides the viral DNA will also be passed on to the progeny cells. This is known as the 'latent' stage of the HIV replication cycle. The virus may remain in the latent stage for years.

The process of viral production begins with the production of two types of RNA: genomic RNA, which will be incorporated into the HIV that are produced by the cell, and messenger RNA, which directs the production of the viral proteins such as p24 and gp120. The viral proteins are produced in long chains that must be broken down into smaller components in order to be incorporated into the progeny HIV. This process is accomplished by the enzyme protease, which is also thought to be involved in the final maturation stage of the progeny HIV immediately after they are released from the cell. A second group of drugs, known collectively as the protease inhibitors, block this stage of the replication process. As the new HIV is extruded from the host cell, lipid from the cell wall is incorporated onto the virus and forms the envelope of the progeny virus. A single CD4$^+$ cell may produce hundreds of new HIV progeny.

It is important to realize that neither group of drugs, reverse transcriptase inhibitors nor protease inhibitors, actually result in the

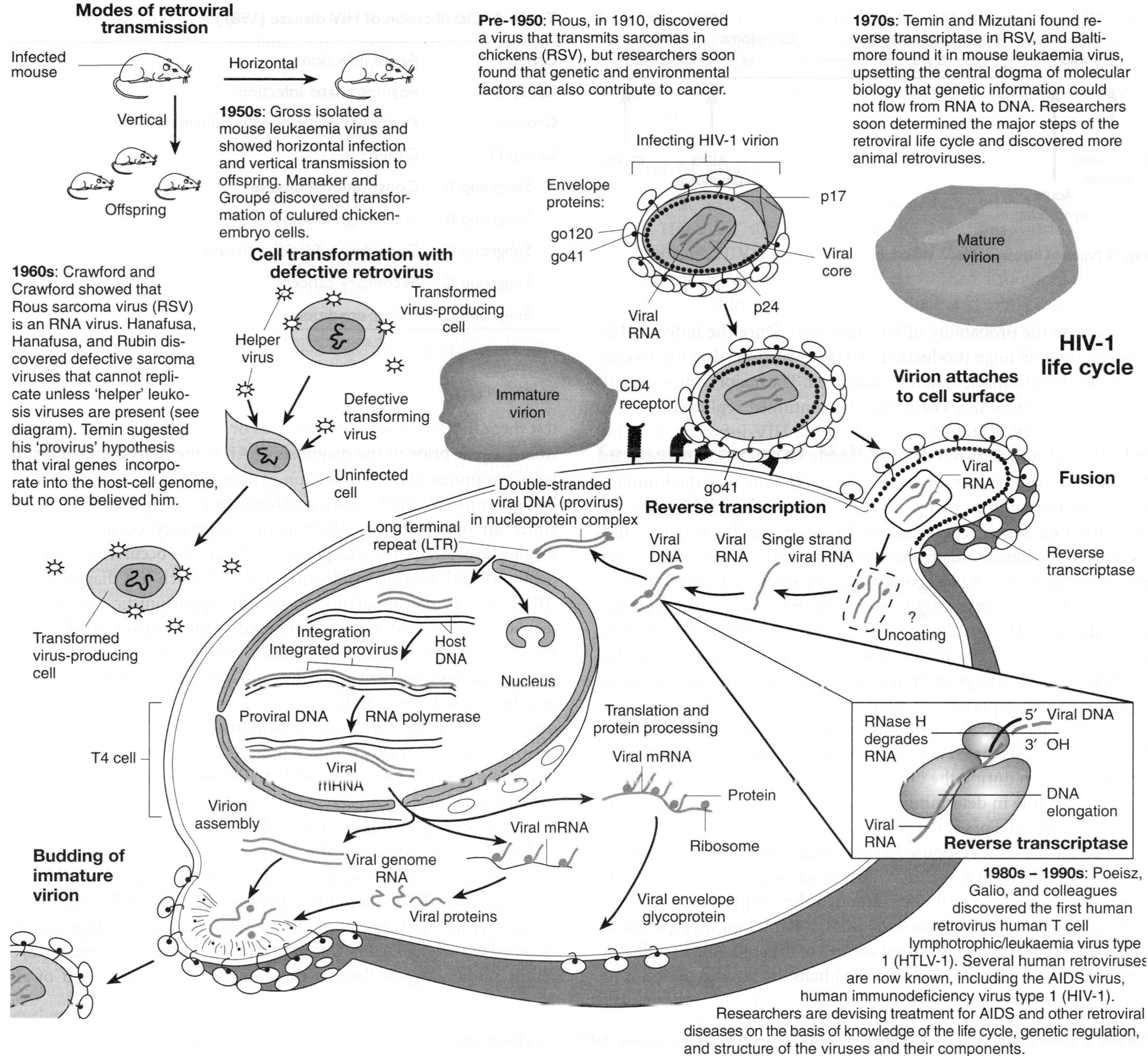

Modes of retroviral transmission
Infected mouse
Horizontal
Vertical
Offspring
1950s: Gross isolated a mouse leukaemia virus and showed horizontal infection and vertical transmission to offspring. Manaker and Groupé discovered transformation of culured chicken-embryo cells.
Pre-1950: Rous, in 1910, discovered a virus that transmits sarcomas in chickens (RSV), but researchers soon found that genetic and environmental factors can also contribute to cancer.
1970s: Temin and Mizutani found reverse transcriptase in RSV, and Baltimore found it in mouse leukaemia virus, upsetting the central dogma of molecular biology that genetic information could not flow from RNA to DNA. Researchers soon determined the major steps of the retroviral life cycle and discovered more animal retroviruses.
1960s: Crawford and Crawford showed that Rous sarcoma virus (RSV) is an RNA virus. Hanafusa, Hanafusa, and Rubin discovered defective sarcoma viruses that cannot replicate unless 'helper' leukosis viruses are present (see diagram). Temin sugested his 'provirus' hypothesis that viral genes incorporate into the host-cell genome, but no one believed him.
Cell transformation with defective retrovirus
Transformed virus-producing cell
Helper virus
Defective transforming virus
Uninfected cell
Transformed virus-producing cell
Infecting HIV-1 virion
Envelope proteins:
go120
go41
p17
Viral core
p24
Viral RNA
Mature virion
Immature virion
HIV-1 life cycle
Virion attaches to cell surface
CD4 receptor
go41
Fusion
Viral RNA
Reverse transcription
Double-stranded viral DNA (provirus) in nucleoprotein complex
Long terminal repeat (LTR)
Viral DNA
Viral RNA
Single strand viral RNA
Reverse transcriptase
Uncoating
Integration
Integrated provirus
Host DNA
Nucleus
Proviral DNA
RNA polymerase
T4 cell
Viral mRNA
Translation and protein processing
Viral mRNA
Protein
Ribosome
RNase H degrades RNA
5′ Viral DNA
3′ OH
DNA elongation
Viral RNA
Reverse transcriptase
Virion assembly
Viral mRNA
Budding of immature virion
Viral genome RNA
Viral proteins
Viral envelope glycoprotein
1980s – 1990s: Poeisz, Galio, and colleagues discovered the first human retrovirus human T cell lymphotrophic/leukaemia virus type 1 (HTLV-1). Several human retroviruses are now known, including the AIDS virus, human immunodeficiency virus type 1 (HIV-1). Researchers are devising treatment for AIDS and other retroviral diseases on the basis of knowledge of the life cycle, genetic regulation, and structure of the viruses and their components.

Fig. 3 Evolutions: retroviruses.

elimination of the virus. The viral DNA that has been incorporated into the host cell DNA will be unaffected and thus the infected individual is not 'cured'.

Studies by David Ho and George Shaw have suggested that the immune system, rather than being deficient in the initial stage of infection, actually produces as many as 2×10^9 $CD4^+$ cells per day in response to the virus (Ho *et al.* 1995; Wei *et al.* 1995). However, the production of more $CD4^+$ cells provides more opportunities for HIV to replicate and as many as 10^8 to 10^9 viruses may be produced per day. For a surprisingly long period the host immune system can maintain this huge production of $CD4^+$ cells, but eventually HIV production outpaces the productive power of the immune system. A number of factors, including infection with other viruses and sexually transmitted diseases, can alter this dynamic equilibrium allowing HIV to destroy the immune system.

Host level

The natural history of HIV infection in the host, as opposed to infection of the cells as described above, is pictured in Fig. 4. Successful infection of the host is actually a rare event, occurring, for example, in only approximately 1 per 1000 episodes of vaginal intercourse. The type of intercourse and the concurrent presence of other infections, especially sexually transmitted infections, however,

various combinations. The philosophy behind combination therapy was that doses of individual drugs given in combination could be lowered, reducing the probability of side-effects, while the probability of developing resistance to two different drugs was much lower than the probability of developing resistance to a single drug given alone.

The big treatment breakthrough came with the introduction of protease inhibitors in 1995 (Lewis *et al.* 1997). The recommended therapy became the use of three different drugs. This regimen was called highly active antiretroviral therapy (HAART) (Detels *et al.* 1998). The protease inhibitors block the assembly of the progeny HIV within the CD4$^+$ cell. The changing use of the different treatment regimens in homosexual men in the Multicenter AIDS Cohort Study (a large cohort study initiated in 1984 in the United States) is shown in Fig. 7. The addition of protease inhibitors to combination therapy resulted in a dramatic decline in the incidence of both AIDS and death as demonstrated in Table 6 (Detels *et al.* 1998, 2001). The efficacy of HAART has now been demonstrated in most groups, including women, injecting drug users, heterosexuals, and men who have sex with men. As a result of HAART the AIDS mortality rate among males 25 to 44 years in the United States has dropped from the leading cause of death in the late 1980s to number five in 1997. Nonetheless, HAART is not the final answer. Side-effects and intolerance to the drug combinations do occur and the efficacy of specific combinations of drugs does decline over time. Further, HAART requires taking 15 or more pills per day on different time schedules and with different restrictions. Thus compliance becomes a major issue. Skipping of drugs or irregular use of drugs increases the probability of drug resistance developing. Highly active antiretroviral therapy has been a major advance, but more drugs with fewer side-effects and improved ease of administration need to be developed. Thus the search for new drugs continues, especially drugs acting at different stages of the replication cycle. In the foreseeable future it is unlikely that a cure will be developed, but it is reasonable to hope that HIV/AIDS in the individual may be controlled much as high blood pressure and diabetes are controlled by effective medication.

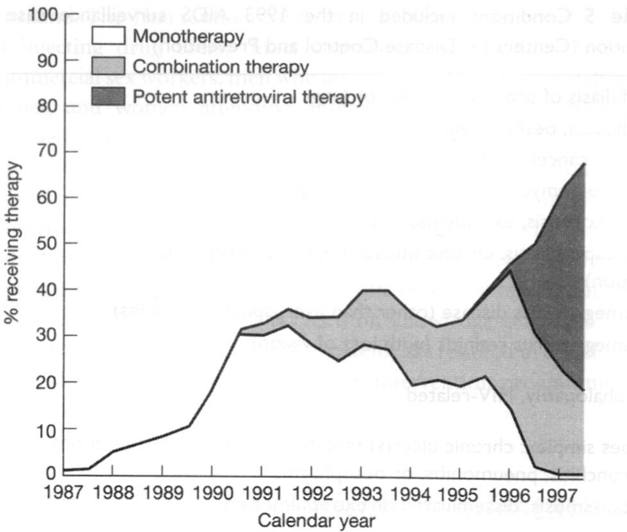

Fig. 7 Use of antiretroviral therapy by Multicentre AIDS Cohort Study seroconverters while free of AIDS. (Reproduced from Detels *et al.* 1998.)

Treatment in the developing countries

In the industrialized world, new treatment approaches can find their place with relative ease into the existing health-care systems, reaching most, although not all, potential beneficiaries. To make these therapies available to people living with HIV/AIDS in the developing world will require a major improvement in the number of qualified health-care providers and a willingness on the part of the drug manufacturers to use a different pricing strategy for developing countries or to allow developing countries to manufacture the drugs at cost. Most developing countries are only able to provide treatment or prophylaxis for the more common opportunistic infections and supportive care for symptomatic and dying patients. The clear need for improvement of HIV/AIDS care in developing nations, however, may create the opportunity and provide the impetus needed to reconsider resource

Table 6 Antiretroviral therapy and relative AIDS-free and survival times by calendar periods

Variable	Calendar period		
	1990–1993	**1993–July 1995**	**July 1995–July 1997**
Number seen while AIDS-free	414	370	288
Percentage of patients who received[b]			
No therapy	50	49	27
Monotherapy only	36	25	3
Combination therapy	14	26	21
HAART	0	0	49
Relative AIDS-free times (95% CI)[a, c]	1	0.97 (0.86–1.09)	1.63 (1.40–1.89)
Relative survival times (95% CI)[a, c]	1	1.01 (0.91–1.12)	1.21 (1.07–1.36)

CI, confidence interval.

[a]Estimates of relative times are adjusted by infection duration and age at seroconversion, and were obtained using log normal regression methods.

[b]Percentages of 347, 313, and 227 AIDS-free seroconverters for whom therapy could be assessed in the three calendar periods respectively.

[c]Relative time is the factor by which times are expanded or contracted.

Reproduced from Detels *et al.* (1998).

allocation and use in the economic and social development sectors as well as to redress the insufficiencies of existing health systems.

Historically, care for HIV-infected people has not been viewed as playing a preventive role in reducing HIV incidence. People with HIV must be seen as important partners in prevention; the virus can only be transmitted through them. However, if they feel abandoned by care services, they are less likely to understand the need for prevention and to be motivated to protect others (MacNeil and Anderson 1998).

Regardless of the effectiveness of prevention efforts being made today and new advances in treatments, the numbers of people becoming ill as a result of HIV infection will dramatically increase over the next few decades. In addition, increasing demand for, and access to, counselling and testing services will increase the number of HIV-infected persons who know their HIV status and will demand treatment. As the number of infections increases, demands for care will mount globally. As these demands mount, increasing consideration needs to be given to the mitigating effect care and social support can have on the epidemic, including its effect on prevention. While few health planners and providers would dispute the fact that both HIV prevention and care are necessary, the challenge confronting many developing countries is how to provide both in an environment with limited resources. Both developing and developed countries must be concerned with this issue.

HIV/AIDS intervention programmes need to recognize and understand the dynamics and existing strengths and weaknesses of household and community arrangements for care. In particular, home-based care programmes need to be made gender sensitive and designed so that they relieve the excessive caregiving burden on women. The emotional state of the women and their need to address their feelings of resentment and hatred should be recognized and given due importance in HIV/AIDS counselling. This is especially important when they are blamed for their partners' health condition and are culturally expected to provide care in sickness. At the community level, the social climate for those affected by HIV/AIDS needs to be improved. In the developing countries, the capacities of households and communities need to be strengthened to better manage care for their infected members.

Paediatric AIDS

One of the most tragic aspects of the HIV/AIDS pandemic has been the infection of infants. It is estimated that 30 to 50 per cent of HIV-infected pregnant women will give birth to an infected baby in the absence of treatment. The probability that the infant will be infected depends on the level of HIV, the stage of HIV infection, and the current phenotype of HIV (syncytium-inducing, non-syncytium-inducing) in the mother, her immune competence, premature birth, and chorio-amnionitis (Newell *et al.* 1997). Of infected infants, 30 to 50 per cent are infected during the birth process and another 15 to 20 per cent through breast feeding. Prior to the development of effective therapies, prevention depended on reducing the prevalence of HIV in women, reducing the exposure of the infant to blood during the birth process, not breast feeding the infant unless the mother was unable to obtain clean water and prepare safe formula, vaginal washing, topical and oral treatment of the infant, treatment with specific HIV-immune globulin, and delivery by Caesarean section (Bryson 1996). None of these efforts had a dramatic effect on reducing the risk of HIV infection to the infant. The most important determinant of maternal–fetal transmission is the level of HIV in the mother (Dickover *et al.* 1998).

Infants infected from their mothers follow one of two courses: rapid progression with early death within months of birth, or a slow course lasting years and in some cases into adolescence. Infants infected *in utero* tend to experience rapid progression whereas those infected during the birth process or infected through breast milk tend to experience a slower course, extending in many cases well beyond 2 years. The level of HIV in the infant during the first weeks to months is a better predictor of survival than $CD4^+$ level. There is also a very interesting subset of infants from whom HIV can be identified shortly after birth, but who apparently clear the virus and are no longer infected (Bryson 1995; Bryson *et al.* 1995). This last group is particularly interesting because identification of the mechanisms allowing the infant to clear the virus may provide clues to reversing infection in the majority of infants who cannot otherwise clear it.

In 1994 the results of a drug trial in which azidothymidine was given to infected women from the second trimester of pregnancy through delivery and to the infant for 1 month following birth demonstrated that the proportion of infants being infected could be reduced by three-quarters (Connor *et al.* 1994). Although this was good news to women in developed countries, the high cost of the long course of treatment was beyond the economic capacity of most developing countries. A 1998 study of azidothymidine given orally to mothers from 34 weeks of gestation through delivery and another study of nevirapine alone given orally at onset of labour both demonstrated a 50 per cent reduction in the prevalence of HIV among the infants (Guay *et al.* 1999; Shaffer *et al.* 1999; Wiktor *et al.* 1999). The cost of giving a single dose of nevirapine to the mother as well as the infant is US$4 to US$8. With the introduction of HAART given in the first trimester, the proportion of infants infected has been reduced to 5 per cent, and many investigators feel that the risk can be further reduced to 2 per cent (Bryson 1996).

The impact of HIV/AIDS

HIV/AIDS causes incalculable human suffering and social and cultural disruption, and has huge economic costs. The effects pervade the industrial, agricultural, and health-care sectors and permeate society, affecting individuals, families, and communities. The *World Health Report 1999* (WHO 1999) indicates that heart disease, strokes, and acute lower respiratory infections—typical causes of death in old age—are the only causes of death to surpass HIV/AIDS. HIV/AIDS is now the primary disease burden in developing countries, affecting primarily younger and middle aged people.

The impact on life expectancy and health

The most obvious impact of AIDS is on life expectancy. Measuring and predicting the impact on a society or nation, however, is difficult, not only because of the lack of quality data, but also because the magnitude of the impact depends on many factors, including the rate of spread and success in fighting other health problems. In the most severely affected countries, AIDS threatens to reverse a century of progress in the fight against infectious disease. Elsewhere, it is likely to account for an increased share of the infectious disease burden. But

AIDS is only one of many health problems confronting people in developing countries (World Bank Policy Research Report 1997).

Life expectancy is a basic measure of human welfare and of the impact of AIDS. From 1900 to 1990, dramatic successes in the fight against infectious disease raised life expectancy from 40 to 64 years in developing countries, narrowing the gap between these countries and the industrial countries from 25 to 13 years. AIDS has slowed, and in some countries reversed, this trend. Life expectancy in Burkina Faso, a mere 46 years, is 11 years shorter than it would have been in the absence of AIDS. In several other hard-hit countries, life expectancy also has been pushed back to levels of more than a decade ago. AIDS accounted for about 1 per cent of all deaths worldwide in 1990; this proportion is likely to rise to 2 per cent of all deaths in 2020 (Murray and Lopez 1996). However, the proportion of total deaths caused by a disease is an imperfect representation of its burden on society, because it ignores illness and does not distinguish among the deaths of people of different ages. The cost of diseases can be estimated in terms of disability-adjusted life years (**DALYs**). DALYs include the disability as well as the mortality effects of disease and use age weights to discount the importance of infant and elderly deaths. In 1990, poor health in developing countries resulted in the loss of 265 DALYs per thousand persons per year, almost twice the 124 DALYs per thousand per year lost in industrial countries. Because HIV/AIDS causes substantial disability before death and disproportionately strikes productive-age adults, it has a larger impact on health measured as DALYs than as a share of total deaths.

It was projected that HIV/AIDS would account for almost 3 per cent of all DALYs lost in developing countries in the year 2020, up from 0.8 per cent in 1990 (United States Bureau of the Census 1997). One reason that HIV/AIDS does not account for a larger percentage of lost DALYs is that other causes of death in developing countries also cause substantial disability and premature death. Further, some of the increased impact of HIV/AIDS is offset by the decreasing proportion of productive-age adults in the population associated with the demographic transition from high proportions of very young to greater proportions of elderly.

The economic impact

The economic impact of HIV/AIDS can be classified into macroeconomic and microeconomic effects. Macroeconomics describes economic systems and normally refers to a country's economy, while microeconomics examines individuals, groups, and firms.

Economic analysis during the first years of the HIV epidemic was speculative, and assumed that AIDS would adversely affect economies at all levels, from national to household. In 1988, the first international conference on the global impact of AIDS considered the impact on food production as well as on families and development (Fleming *et al.* 1988). It was recognized that AIDS would have a major impact since the infection is concentrated in the 20 to 40 age group, the age group which carries an enormous economic burden in societies in which nearly 50 per cent of the population is under 15 years of age.

In the early 1990s, studies began to demonstrate how AIDS might affect the economies of developing countries. The World Bank, using DALYs, demonstated enormous regional and global inequalities in health status (World Bank 1993). In sub-Saharan Africa in 1990, ill health and accidents led to the loss of 575 DALYs per 1000 population, of which HIV and sexually transmitted infections accounted for 8.8 per cent, whereas in industrialized countries only 117 DALYs were lost per 1000 population and HIV accounted for only 3.4 per cent of these. In extending the concept of DALYs to prevention and control, the study suggested that HIV in developing countries can be substantially reduced by interventions costing less than US$100 per DALY saved.

In sub-Saharan Africa, the macroeconomic impact of HIV/AIDS has been demonstrated in two ways (Over 1992). First, it has an impact on human capital, the skill base of an economy. Economic growth is closely correlated with increases in urban skilled populations. An adverse affect to these populations has a disproportionately negative impact on economic growth. Second, HIV/AIDS affects savings, which are essential for economic growth, as they allow new investment. Funds for AIDS treatment is taken from savings, so that investment and future growth suffer. Thus AIDS has the potential to slow economic growth significantly.

The effect of AIDS is felt first at the microeconomic, or household level. The next step occurs when economic activities, such as agriculture, transport, and mining are affected. Later, impacts on the national economy are detected.

The societal impact

In the period from 1981 to 1986, when the precise dimensions of the AIDS epidemic in the United States remained uncertain and the extent to which populations not initially infected might be exposed was unclear, analysts predicted that no geographical region and no aspect of social life would remain untouched. By 1985 the prospect of widespread heterosexual transmission of HIV in the United States caused anxiety. In the early 1990s, after more than a decade of living with AIDS, a very different, more subtle picture had emerged (Bayer 1996). The combination of a conservative national administration, and the fact that HIV occurred primarily in socially marginalized groups, shaped the impact of AIDS on the United States. The response to AIDS has been most successful where politics permitted gay men and their allies to press for changes, to elicit sympathetic responses, and to wrest, sometimes grudging, concessions.

The AIDS epidemic has had the unexpected impact of incorporating gay (homosexual) organizations into the pluralistic fabric of American political life (Altman 1988). Thus it was possible for gay groups to thwart widespread HIV testing without consent and to win the support of the Centers for Disease Control and Prevention for antidiscrimination and confidentiality (Bayer 1991) measures supporting both gay men and individuals with HIV/AIDS. Gay men have established a remarkable network of political, social, and service organizations to meet their needs and protect their interests.

In 1993, the National Research Council stated that the limited response to the AIDS epidemic could be explained because the absolute number of infected individuals, relative to the United States population, was not overbearing and because social institutions in the United States were strong, complex, and resilient. More important, the concentration of the epidemic was in socially marginalized groups and had only slowly spread to the mainstream heterosexual population. Thus those who continued to be affected were socially invisible, beyond the sight and attention of the majority population (National Research Council 1993).

HIV/AIDS has also impacted the cultures of Asia, but a different social impact was identified. Among the many factors influencing the ways in which households respond to HIV/AIDS in both India and Thailand are the economic situation of affected households and communities, prevailing gender relations and women's social status, local health beliefs, local health-care practices, and the stigma attached to HIV/AIDS (Bharat *et al.* 1998). While sociocultural contexts shape the ways in which households and communities respond to the epidemic, the epidemic itself is beginning to influence local practices and perceptions. This was evident from changes reported in funeral rituals and the ways in which illnesses are perceived as less or more threatening, depending on the severity of visible bodily symptoms. Gender biases were evident at the household level, where men received greater care and acceptance than women. This is not a surprising observation in the male-dominated, patriarchal culture of Asia where men's needs are considered more positively than those of women.

A major problem has been the apprehension of affected individuals and households of being stigmatized by their neighbours and relatives. Consequently, there is no openness about HIV status, resulting in an inability to tap the traditional sources of support and counselling such as village elders and extended family. Misconceptions about the epidemic have led to fear of discrimination and sometimes to suicide. The issue of stigmatization must be addressed if persons at risk of HIV are to be treated as individuals who need understanding, compassion, and access to treatment.

The global scope and extent of the AIDS-induced orphan situation is now better appreciated. Many of the countries in which the effects of HIV/AIDS have been most severe also have high adult mortality rates from other causes, including civil conflict and war. As a result, these countries already had many orphans even in the absence of HIV/AIDS. Since HIV/AIDS affects mainly young and middle-aged adults, AIDS causes a marked increase in the number of orphans, in some developing countries as much as 50 per cent (Ainsworth and Over 1992). The number of children who had been orphaned by HIV/AIDS by the year 2000 was estimated to be 13.2 million (UNAIDS 2000).

Three general observations about these orphans provide a basis for analysis and planning (Levine *et al.* 1996). First, most orphans are not infected with HIV. Second, the orphans create special stress on family and community resources, and third, they are highly vulnerable because families affected by HIV/AIDS usually have more than one ill or dying member. In African countries the HIV/AIDS pandemic has added a new group of orphans to the already serious problem of children who are parentless, but in industrialized countries the phenomenon of large numbers of children left parentless from a single disease is unprecedented. In Asia the rapid spread of HIV infection, especially among young women, presages a crisis around orphans.

Traditional family stuctures of people in developing countries, already stressed by poverty, poor health, and increased burdens of care, are in many instances reaching the breaking point. People with HIV/AIDS have received limited care by family members because of poverty, other responsibilities, and stigma. Some adult patients were cared for by children because there were no other adults in the home (Seeley *et al.* 1993). For those orphans, material assistance, such as food, bedding, medicine, and school fees, is needed to make up for lost income, but more than money is needed to overcome the burden of AIDS on families. Although the general 'safety net' for people with HIV/AIDS has gaps, the net for dependent orphaned children after the death of a parent is even looser. While many families have absorbed orphaned children out of love, custom, or moral obligation, they may not be able to do so indefinitely. An independent assessment is needed to determine the level of assistance required to promote family function. Assistance to orphans should not be viewed as a short-term project but rather as a long-term commitment to support local sustainable initiatives. The well being of children orphaned by the HIV epidemic, like children in distress from other causes, is the test of our future commitment to social stability, economic development, and human rights.

The role of stigmatization

One of the most difficult problems in controlling HIV/AIDS has been stigmatization of both groups at highest risk of HIV and of individuals who are infected. In the United States the home of a young haemophiliac infected with HIV was burned down in rural Florida because the youngster insisted on attending school. Sentinel surveillance, as mentioned above, plays an important role in providing information on which effective intervention programmes can be based. Stigmatization reduces the willingness of risk groups to be identified, making surveillance difficult, if not impossible. Thus the epidemic may rapidly increase in these groups and spread from them into the general population without the knowledge of public health professionals and policy-makers. The reluctance to diagnose AIDS on the part of physicians may also cause them to avoid reporting a diagnosis of AIDS in order to spare their patients embarrassment and stigmatization. But if the presence of AIDS in the community is hidden then public health officials are unable to take the necessary steps to prevent the further spread of HIV.

One of the most effective tools for altering risk behaviour is to provide individuals with the knowledge of their HIV infection status (Kalichman 1998). Thus HIV testing is an important intervention strategy. Unfortunately, many people are reluctant to be tested, fearing that they may test positive and have their HIV status revealed, subjecting them to discrimination, job loss, and loss of family. Further, many health officials and politicians feel that they must protect the HIV-infected person even at the expense of the uninfected. Even implementing such a simple strategy as premarital testing for HIV in countries with high levels of HIV infection in young persons has met with resistance from public health officials who seem to have forgotten that the most important task of public health is to protect the uninfected, albeit while doing the minimum amount of harm to the infected. Surely a young woman entering into marriage has a right to know that her husband will not kill her and their yet-to-be-born infants by infecting them with HIV (and vice versa). Rapid tests which can be interpreted by anyone are now available, but are blocked in many countries for political reasons. Making these 'risk-free' test kits available to individuals so that they can learn their HIV status without risk of disclosure should be a priority.

Because of the complication for control of HIV caused by stigmatization, a major effort should be directed towards reducing and eliminating stigmatization. This process, often called 'normalization of HIV', emphasizes the need to treat HIV/AIDS as an ordinary chronic disease such as diabetes or hypertension. This concept is appropriate for developed countries where HIV/AIDS patients can receive treatment and return to a relatively normal lifestyle, but is more difficult to apply in developing countries where treatment and return to a normal lifestyle are not usually a possibility due to economic constraints. Nonetheless, HIV/AIDS patients in developing countries need to be treated with understanding and compassion. Although a return to 'normalization' is not possible for HIV/AIDS patients in developing countries, they still need to obtain care and the social support which is an essential part of the compassionate treatment of chronic, fatal illnesses to which all human beings are entitled. To promote an understanding of this need in developing countries is a major challenge, but one that must be continually addressed.

Ethical and human rights issues

From the beginning of the epidemic in the early 1980s, ethical and human rights issues have been the subject of vigorous debate. One of the first issues was the question of whether to systematically identify and exclude homosexual men as blood donors in the United States in 1983 (Institute of Medicine 1995). The ethics of protecting the uninfected who might receive infected blood was in conflict with the rights of homosexual men to privacy. This basic conflict between the rights of the uninfected and the ethical public health obligation to protect the infected has persisted with the debate over whether to test pregnant women and/or infants for HIV infection and whether to require premarital testing in areas of high HIV endemicity.

Testing has been another area in which there has been considerable debate. Testing and counselling have been demonstrated to be an effective strategy for inducing behavioural change in people at risk for HIV infection (Fox *et al.* 1987; Kalichman 1998). Many public health professionals believe that individuals who test positive for HIV should be reported to the public health authorities by name to provide accurate information on which to determine the prevalence of infection in specific communities. Among those groups with a high prevalence of HIV, however, the concern has been that confidentiality cannot be maintained and naming could therefore result in disclosure to insurance companies and others who might take actions harmful to the individual. The issue of testing has now become even more complicated by the development of an effective treatment regimen that can delay onset of AIDS and extend life. For the treatment regimen to be most effective, however, treatment should begin before the onset of clinical AIDS. Thus the ethical rationale for promoting testing, especially to identify those who would benefit from treatment but do not suspect that they are infected, is even stronger than in the past.

The HIV/AIDS epidemic has also emphasized the ethical issues surrounding the rights of women to be able to protect themselves from HIV infection. The greatest HIV risk for many women, especially in developing countries, is their husband. The plight of the commercial sex worker not only raises the question of the forcing of women and men to become commercial sex workers in many societies (and in high-prevalence areas, assuring that they will become infected), but also the question of whether it is ethical to test commercial sex workers because the disclosure that they are infected causes an ethical dilemma for them. Should they stop working as a commercial sex workers and put themselves and their family back into poverty or continue to put their customers at risk?

The availability of an effective, but expensive treatment regimen raises the issue of the disparity between wealthy developed countries in which the prevalence of HIV/AIDS is low and the developing countries in which the vast majority of HIV/AIDS cases occur. HIV-infected individuals in the wealthy countries have access to effective treatment, whereas infected individuals in developing countries, which have 95 per cent of the infected persons, do not. What is the ethical responsibility of the drug companies and the wealthy nations to provide both the drugs and the health professionals capable of administering the drug regimen correctly?

Among many health professionals in the field of HIV/AIDS the philosophy has developed that the correct approach is to give the highest priority to protecting the rights of the infected. This policy has been called the policy of 'exceptionalism' to emphasize the idea that HIV/AIDS is different from other diseases and therefore should be treated as an exception and thus not be subject to the usual public health strategies for control of transmission. Given the magnitude of the epidemic and its continued rapid spread, particularly in countries least equipped to control the epidemic, it is time to recognize that although HIV/AIDS is an exceptionally severe disease associated with stigmatization, the public health principle of protecting the uninfected while doing the least possible harm to the infected should be observed. Only in this way will it be possible to control the HIV/AIDS epidemic.

Intervention and prevention strategies

HIV/AIDS prevention has progressed along two independent but related tracks (Mann and Kay 1991). One track is biomedical and uses research into the mechanisms of HIV and the human immune response to develop therapeutic and preventive technologies. The second track centres on individual and collective human behaviours to prevent HIV transmission. Efforts to prevent and control the pandemic of HIV/AIDS began worldwide as early as 1981. The dynamics of the epidemic, scientific progress, the experience of different population groups, and the variety of responses by a wide range of organizations in order to cope with the pandemic have provided considerable information about prevention strategies. A central theme emerges within each of these areas: HIV prevention requires efforts at the individual, community, and societal levels. Only a combination of all three will be sufficiently powerful to combat the pandemic.

An individual's capacity to change risky behaviour is strongly influenced by community and societal 'norms'. Therefore prevention activities should recognize the need to involve the community. Traditional public health approaches provide a framework to deal with the individual and the community, but should include promoting social awareness and concrete action.

Policy and structure for HIV/AIDS prevention

HIV/AIDS prevention has evolved through a number of stages since the beginning of the epidemic. The initial stage was characterized by programmes that focused on individual risk and responsibility through provision of information, awareness-raising campaigns, and sometimes delivery of fear-invoking messages. As the epidemic progressed, it was clear that effective messages needed to focus on sustaining safe behaviour. Greater understanding of the cultural and social dimensions of behaviour were crucial to developing more sophisticated responses aimed at facilitating community support for changed behaviour (Malcolm and Dowsett 1998). According to Jonathan Mann's conclusive study (Mann and Tarantola 1996), four policy approaches to HIV/AIDS prevention have evolved into preventive strategies, as outlined below.

Epidemiological information approaches

During the period of early response (1981–1984), individual risk reduction became codified as the central goal (WHO 1988). Epidemiological studies quickly identified the modes of HIV transmission even before the discovery of the virus, and identified the specific behaviours associated with increased risk of HIV spread (Tarantola 1995). In the early stages of the AIDS epidemic in the United States (Watney 1996), it was apparent to epidemiologists that gay and bisexual men were disproportionately affected. Accordingly, they were described as a risk group for AIDS together with other disproportionately affected people, including haemophiliacs and injecting drug users. The aim of defining such risk groups was to implement prevention activities, as well as to mobilize adequate and appropriate resources for those in greatest need.

Two factors initially led to the use of the term 'risk groups' in the early years of the epidemic. First, the mass media unfortunately used the phrase in such a way that named risk groups were seen to pose a risk to the rest of the population. This approach contributed to stigmatization and misunderstanding. Second, an exclusive focus on risk groups implied that HIV was not a risk for those who were not defined as members of risk groups. Public health professionals recognized that this promoted stigmatization and so they placed emphasis on risk behaviours facilitating the transmission of HIV. Thus the concept of risk behaviours became increasingly used in public health, and in HIV/AIDS education and prevention policies around the world. The shift from 'risk groups' to 'risk behaviours' suggested that everyone was at equal risk from HIV. However, the global epidemiology of HIV clearly demonstrates that HIV is not an 'equal opportunity' disease. Moreover, exclusive attention to risk behaviour increased the difficulty of prevention, since those at greatest risk could no longer be named, and therefore their entitlement to services and support was difficult to ascertain.

In the first period of response to HIV/AIDS, epidemiological information about risk formed the basis of informational campaigns, including some of the most aggressive and large-scale public information efforts ever undertaken in public health. Information campaigns based on risk activities were used worldwide as well as in developing countries.

The social intervention approach

A comprehensive programme to provide individuals with messages, education, and specific services that would help promote and support the process of individual behavioural change was initiated in the mid-1980s. Remarkable public health efforts, delivered through specific services and activities, were undertaken to support individual risk reduction. Overall this approach was guided by a three-part prevention programme model developed as part of the World Health Organization (**WHO**) Global AIDS Strategy (Mann and Tarantola 1996). Two of the three parts involved traditional public health ideas and one was innovative. Based on prior public health efforts to change various personal behaviours, HIV prevention programmes were designed to provide information and education, along with the health and social services needed to promote and support the recommended behavioural changes. These services included condom distribution, HIV testing and counselling, treatment for other STDs, needle exchange, treatment for injecting drug users, and the provision of safe blood and blood products.

A unique element in HIV prevention programmes was the recommendation that discrimination against persons with HIV/AIDS be prevented (WHO 1998). Field experience had demonstrated that the fear of profound personal and social consequences led those most likely to be infected to avoid participating in HIV prevention programmes, or even to be tested. Accordingly, stigmatization was identified as a tragic and counterproductive result of the epidemic that interfered with control efforts. Thus for the first time in public health's history prevention of discrimination against infected people became an integral part of a strategy to control an epidemic of an infectious disease.

Many of those who became infected had been labelled as socially undesirable before the beginning of the HIV epidemic. They included homosexual men and injecting drug users in developed countries (Watney 1996). In the developing world, they were commercial sex workers, injecting drug users, homosexual men, street children, prisoners, illegal migrants, and indigenous minority groups. It has become evident that the almost exclusive focus on individual risk reduction was too narrow to deal concretely with the social realities of the wide group of individuals at risk worldwide.

Another approach has considered the social influences on personal behaviour. This effort has taken many forms, from incorporating social context into sexual behaviour research, to proposals that pay greater attention to the influence of social norms and human development on individual behaviour. The WHO guidelines (1988) focused on the individual, but called for pragmatic societal support at the national level. Most official AIDS programmes are organized within institutions with a public health mandate, but even non-governmental efforts emphasize information and education to change individual behaviour. Thus WHO called for the establishment of national control programmes in all the countries to provide policies, education campaigns, and health and social services, as well as a central co-ordination and technical support to all involved partners.

The empowerment approach

Vulnerability is the converse of empowerment (Mann and Tarantola 1996). Vulnerability itself implies the extent to which individuals are incapable of making and implementing free and informed decisions about their life. A person who is genuinely able to make free and informed decisions is least vulnerable and most empowered; the person who is ill-informed, or unable to make informed decisions freely and carry them out is most vulnerable.

Personal vulnerability (Harvard School of Public Health 1993) to HIV/AIDS involves both cognitive and behavioural dimensions. Cognitive factors involve informational needs about HIV/AIDS, sexuality, and services for reducing vulnerability to infection. Behavioural factors can be considered in two overlapping categories: personal characteristics and personal skills. Personal characteristics include emotional development, perception of risk, attitudes towards risk-taking, personal attitudes towards sex and sexuality, and history of sexual and substance abuse. Personal skills are required to cope with risky situations such as the need to negotiate safe sexual practices, seek treatment for substance abuse, and practice safe sexual and drug-injecting behaviours.

Programmatic vulnerability has been defined broadly in terms of three major prevention elements:

- information and education
- health and social services
- non-discrimination towards people with HIV/AIDS.

Efforts to reduce pragmatic vulnerability have principally involved ensuring and strengthening the availability and success of key programme elements, the quality and content of each element, and the process through which the elements are designed, implemented, and evaluated.

Research and empirical observation (Catania *et al.* 1990) have demonstrated that societal factors profoundly influence and condition personal behaviour. To be effective it is necessary to influence the relevant societal factors (Frank 1995). For example, inferior economic and social status limits the ability of many women to refuse unwanted or unprotected sexual intercourse, regardless of how much they know about AIDS or wish to adopt recommended individual risk-reduction practices. Similarly, it has become evident that HIV/AIDS programmes are created within, and therefore are constrained by, the larger society. Thus in many countries, governmental refusal to inform the public about condom use for HIV prevention or allow harm-reduction strategies for injecting drug users severely handicaps their national AIDS programme.

The concept of societal vulnerability builds upon the insight that collective, societal factors strongly influence both personal vulnerability and pragmatic vulnerability. Societal vulnerability focuses directly on the contextual factors which define personal and pragmatic vulnerability, such as governmental structure, gender relationships, attitudes towards sexuality, religious beliefs, and poverty, all of which influence the capacity to reduce personal vulnerability to HIV, both directly and as mediated through programmes.

There have been several attempts to relate the causes of the HIV/AIDS epidemic to issues of income growth and distribution. The World Bank (1997) studied the influence of aggregate-level social conditions on the size of the epidemic in 72 developing countries. The analysis demonstrated that both low income and unequal distribution of income are strongly associated with high HIV infection rates. The authors concluded that the widespread poverty and unequal distribution of income that typify underdevelopment promote the spread of HIV. They therefore asserted that rapid and fair distribution of economic growth would slow the HIV epidemic. Gender-related factors, such as the ratio of males to females in urban centres and the gap between adult male and female literacy rates, also influence the epidemic. In addition, the accelerated labour migration, rapid urbanization, and cultural modernization that often accompany economic growth also facilitate the spread of HIV. For developing countries, the AIDS epidemic exacerbates the poverty and social inequality that promote the epidemic, thus creating a vicious cycle. Policy-makers who understand these links have the opportunity to break this cycle.

Empirical experience suggests that poverty is an important contextual issue in HIV/AIDS prevention; as poverty increases so does social vulnerability to HIV (O'Shaughnessy 1994). Poverty forces people, especially women, to engage in high-risk activities, creates a lack of disposable income for purchasing condoms, and limits access to health services and HIV prevention programmes. In addition, large gaps between the highest and lowest socio-economic strata (relative poverty) generate the conditions in which people adopt survival strategies which amplify their vulnerability to becoming HIV-infected (Panos Institute 1990). Such survival strategies involve providing unprotected sexual intercourse in return for money, lodging, food, or other necessities. The relationship of HIV/AIDS and poverty is a particularly strong example of the consistent global relationship between socio-economic status and health status (World Bank 1993). One of the most effective HIV prevention strategies would be reduction or elimination of poverty and the gap between the rich and the poor.

The ultimate aim of vulnerability reduction is to expand people's capacity to exert control over their own health. By identifying the larger social issues that constrain or promote this ability, contextual analysis stresses the need for positive and synergistic interaction between the individual services, programmes and other collective initiatives, and the social environment.

The human rights approach

Insight into the relationship of human rights to HIV vulnerability has been obtained through two lines of evidence (Mann 1995). First, a meta-analysis of the evolving HIV epidemics in countries around the world has revealed that people who are marginalized, stigmatized, and discriminated against have become, over time, those at the highest risk of HIV infection. Thus HIV is primarily a problem of people who live at the margins of society.

The second source of insight about human rights and HIV prevention is the detailed analysis of limits and failures in prevention programmes. For example, married and monogamous women who receive the normal benefits of HIV prevention programmes (information, education, access to testing and counselling, and condom availability) may nevertheless still be at risk of HIV infection. The recommendation to reduce the number of sexual partners as part of a risk-reduction approach fails in the real world for several reasons. First, women's risk is related to their male sexual partner's behaviour. Second, multiple sexual partnerships may be the only route of access to resources (for school, financial credit, or jobs). Third, women often lack control over their sexual relationships. In marriage, without legal recourse or legal rights to property, the pervasive threat of physical violence or divorce may totally disempower a woman, even if she knows about AIDS, that condoms are available, and that her husband is HIV-infected.

Therefore the central problem for HIV infection among women cannot be solved with risk-reduction approaches such as information campaigns or condom distribution systems. Since the central issue is the inferior role and subordinate status of women, the disadvantage created by society cannot be redressed through information and education or HIV-specific health and social services alone. To the extent that women's human rights and dignity are not respected, society creates and enhances their vulnerability to HIV and more generally to ill-health (Cook 1995). Many other groups also suffer vulnerability to HIV infection due to discrimination, including gay and lesbian people worldwide, commercial sex workers, and adolescents, whose competence and voice are rarely acknowledged in any meaningful way.

However, the concepts and language of modern human rights can be used to describe vulnerability and the societal meaning and impact of the epidemic's evolution (Mann *et al.* 1994). Guaranteeing human rights offers an extremely powerful approach to reduce marginalization, stigmatization, and discrimination. Indeed, the relationship of human rights to public health has been evolving rapidly in the context of HIV/AIDS. The HIV/AIDS epidemic has emphasized to public health professionals that human rights are an integral part of human well being.

International support

Prior to 1986, none of the industrialized nations funded AIDS prevention and care programmes in the developing world. Part of the responsibility for this delay lies with the United Nations system, which was slow to identify the AIDS pandemic as an important global problem (Finlay *et al.* 1992). However, the delay also reflected confusion within official development assistance agencies concerning the extent and seriousness of the AIDS pandemic, uncertainties about how to proceed in funding for AIDS prevention and care activities, and concern that AIDS would divert funding from existing health priorities and projects.

Global leadership and advocacy for HIV/AIDS prevention and control have been critical ingredients to progress. The WHO Global AIDS Strategy was established in 1986 to alert the world to HIV/AIDS. It was supported by official development assistance agencies, which transfer funds from the industrialized donor countries to international agencies and governmental and non-governmental organizations concerned with AIDS programmes in developing countries.

International funding for AIDS research, treatment, care, and programme management grew steadily from 1986 through the end of the decade. Total funding increased from US$200 000 in 1986, to about US$59 million in 1987, to over US$212 million in 1990 following the creation of the WHO Global Programme on AIDS. The total official development assistance funding assigned to AIDS increased rapidly through 1990. The annual rate of increase was 127 per cent between 1987 and 1988 but then declined to 4–11 per cent during 1990 to 1993 (Laws 1996).

The decline in international AIDS financing between 1991 and 1994 was explained by two main factors. First, the official development assistance agencies responded to increased competing demands for resources, which were compounded by economic recession. Second, donors' commitment to subsidizing HIV/AIDS programmes began to erode, which perhaps reflected scepticism about the efficiency and impact of past efforts to control the global HIV/AIDS pandemic.

In the early stages of the global mobilization, donors channelled most of their resources through WHO. However, donors have become dissatisfied with this funding strategy, which relies largely on multilateral channels. Consequently, there has been a major shift towards bilateral funding since 1990. Industrialized countries provided grants to specific recipient countries.

From 1986 to 1994, the World Bank awarded an increasing number of loans to developing countries for HIV/AIDS prevention and care, totalling approximately US$565 million. By mid-1995, 49 World-Bank-supported projects devoted partly or wholly to HIV/AIDS were in operation in 35 countries. The apparent shift from government grant money to government and private loans for HIV/AIDS programmes reflects two main factors. First, developing countries are turning to the World Bank as grant money is both becoming more difficult to obtain from other sources and is not increasing parallel to the growth of HIV/AIDS prevention and care needs in severely affected areas. Second, the World Bank has recognized the negative impact of HIV/AIDS on developing economies and is responding more favourably to loan requests for HIV/AIDS programmes than in the late 1980s.

Since 1989, the overall demand for development assistance has increased significantly. The combination of a shrinking pool of donor countries, rising demands for aid, and frustration by official development assistance agencies about the ability of developing countries to demonstrate progress towards the goals of development have led to a complex state of donor fatigue. Clear evidence of donor fatigue was revealed when the summit of heads of governments on AIDS, held in Paris in December 1994 with the aim of mobilizing significant international funds in support of the Global AIDS Strategy, did not succeed in generating the expected resources.

The Joint United Nations Programme on HIV/AIDS (**UNAIDS**) was established in 1995 to consolidate six organizations of the United Nations system (UNAIDS 1995). UNAIDS serves as the global AIDS programme for its six cosponsors (United Nations Children's Emergency Fund, United Nations Development Programme, United Nations Population Fund, United Nations Educational, Scientific, and Cultural Organization, the WHO, and the World Bank). At the country level, UNAIDS can be described as the joint action and collective resources of its cosponsoring organizations, co-ordinated by the UNAIDS central office in Geneva and UNAIDS country and regional staff.

The main focus of UNAIDS has been on strengthening national capacity for an expanded response. Thus UNAIDS works with government departments and ministries, people living with HIV, communities affected or threatened by the epidemic, non-governmental and community-based organizations, academic institutions, and the private sector, as well as bilateral and intergovernmental organizations. It has four mutually reinforcing roles: policy development and research, technical support, advocacy, and co-ordination.

However, while the HIV epidemic in most developing countries continues unabated, international funding for support of a global AIDS strategy is shrinking. Advocacy alone cannot overcome existing poor health and social infrastructures in ultra-low gross domestic product countries. Daunted by the lack of resources and other structural impediments to organized care for HIV, many in positions of power still shy away from the topic of care. The increase in the number of people in need of care globally, the limited capacity of health services, and the recognition that care needs go well beyond clinical therapies to psychosocial support and community-based care for the burgeoning populations with HIV/AIDS, especially in sub-Saharan Africa, can and does frighten some donors and governments.

Sexual behaviour change and condom use

The sexual behaviour of populations is still largely unknown in most of the countries in the world. The levels and forms of risk behaviour must be assessed in order to understand the potential for widespread HIV transmission, to monitor changes in behaviour, and to determine the magnitude of ongoing prevention needs. In only about 40 countries (UNAIDS/WHO 1998) have there been general population surveys which looked at sexual behaviour changes over time. Many factors contribute to the lack of behavioural data, including cost, reluctance to conduct such surveys for political or religious reasons, lack of personnel or technical resources, and concerns about the reliability and validity of data that might be gathered.

Without a complete picture of behavioural risk in a population it is difficult to prioritize prevention activities. Certain situations contribute disproportionately to HIV transmission, for example, commercial sex. Knowledge of important variations in sexual behaviours within populations is rare, so prevention efforts are not necessarily focused on those with the greatest risk behaviour. Populations, such as men having sex with men and sexually active youth, may be missed or under-represented, and other vulnerable groups such as factory workers, military personnel, fishermen, and truck drivers may not be included (Mills *et al.* 1998).

HIV risk reduction ranges from abstinence to the practice of safer sex. Both abstinence and safer-sex intervention reduce HIV sexual risk behaviours, but safer-sex interventions may be especially effective with sexually experienced adolescents and may have a longer-lasting impact (Jemmott *et al.* 1998). Abstinence intervention implies delaying sexual intercourse or reducing its frequency. Safer-sex intervention always stresses condom use. In the reproductive age population (Polacsek *et al.* 1999) the use of a condom with regular sex partners depends on their partners' reaction to condoms, perceived partner risk, length of relationship, sterility, cohabitation, perceived vulnerability to HIV infection, and perceived peer norms about condom use. When information, skills training, and services are made available to young people, they are often more likely to make use of them than their elders. Since sexual activity in youth is high, it is necessary to ensure that teenagers can exercise the right to protect themselves from risky sex.

Thailand has demonstrated a successful prevention programme, evolving from information through a public campaign (Phoolcharoen *et al.* 1998). A national survey of sexual behaviour conducted in 1990 found that a high proportion of men had sex outside marriage. The results of this survey were widely publicized, and government officials and the general public were made aware that their country was vulnerable to rapid spread of HIV. Although prostitution is illegal in Thailand, the state worked to set up partnerships with brothel owners to address the problem. With government support, brothel owners and sex workers enforced a policy of 100 per cent condom use in brothels to reduce transmission in what the evidence suggested was a focal point for infection in Thailand. In parallel, mass media campaigns encouraged respect for women and discouraged men from engaging in commercial sex, while young women were offered better educational and vocational opportunities to keep them out of the sex industry. These energetic campaigns have resulted in a reduction in risky sexual behaviours and decreased spread of the virus (Nelson *et al.* 1996).

In AIDS-endemic areas, it is complicated to promote safer sex by HIV-infected persons who have uninfected partners. The specific intervention (Norman *et al.* 1998) for these persons should emphasize communication skills and rehearsal of serostatus disclosure as well as risk-reduction discussions. Voluntary HIV testing with counselling in the community turned out to be a key strategy to support safer sex among those at risk, and has been made available in many countries.

Drug users

The importance of injecting drug use in many epidemics of HIV in many countries has been sporadically recognized. Although many discrete and interconnected epidemics of HIV infection among injecting drug users in various parts of the world have been well described, their role as epicentres for the wider epidemic, and their impact on whole communities, have undergone little formal investigation. Accordingly, public health responses to the specific issue of HIV among injecting drug users in developing countries have been slow to emerge. This issue is seen as secondary to the reduction of drug demand and the control of supply (Crofts *et al.* 1998).

For drug users in most parts of Asia, the move from smoking or inhaling to injecting of heroin, once established, is rarely seen to revert (Wu *et al.* 1996). The major factor for the transition to injecting is thought to be economic, but has not been deeply investigated. Among injecting populations, the sharing and reuse of injecting equipment is subject to many pressures, including scarcity and relative cost of equipment, social organization of drug use, and custom. A substantial proportion of injecting drug users have shared their needles and syringes with little effective cleaning beforehand. In many countries needles and syringes can be purchased from pharmacies, but carrying a needle can be seen as incriminating evidence of drug use and injecting drug users may therefore be reluctant to procure clean injecting equipment from a pharmacy.

The prevalences of HIV infection among injecting drug users in the countries of Southeast Asia are among the highest reported anywhere. Few signs exist of any major decrease in this epidemic. Various countries of this area have experienced the most rapid diffusion of HIV infection among injecting drug users found anywhere in the world. Within a period of approximately 12 months many areas reached a prevalence of HIV infection among injecting drug users of 40 per cent or greater (Sarkar *et al.* 1993).

The current consensus is that there is an urgent need to reduce the HIV risks associated with drug injecting to the users themselves, to their sex partners and children, and to society. One way to do this is through a comprehensive prevention programme based on the principle of 'harm reduction'. Just as in the case of sexual HIV transmission, the prevention of transmission through drug injecting calls for a package whose components operate simultaneously. A recent comparison of cities with high and low HIV prevalences in injecting drug users showed that those with success in averting a drug-user epidemic had three features in common. First, they used community outreach or peer education to reach and educate drug users, including those who would not otherwise receive HIV/AIDS information. Second, they ensured that drug users had cheap and easy access to sterile syringes through pharmacies or needle-exchange programmes. Third, they all started their prevention programmes early on, before HIV prevalence had risen past a critical point (UNAIDS/WHO 1998).

The best way for an individual to avoid HIV infection through drug injecting is to stop injecting. Many countries have responded to the HIV epidemic among injecting drug users by expanding drug treatment services. Evaluation of studies on the effectiveness of psychosocial interventions in reducing the risk of HIV infection in injecting drug users has showed that the existing programmes were not acceptably effective (Gibson *et al.* 1998).

Needle-exchange programmes, when part of a comprehensive harm-reduction approach, represent another way of combating the sharing of equipment. These programmes provide drug users with clean needles and syringes in exchange for used ones. HIV infection rates have been shown in various studies to be over three times lower in injecting drug users who participate in needle-exchange programmes than in those who do not (Des Jarlais 1993). The success of needle-exchange programmes is by no means limited to industrialized countries. There are currently programmes in the cities of Santos and Salvador in Brazil, the Nepalese capital of Kathmandu, and the Akha hill-tribe communities of northern Thailand, to name but a few. Most of these remain relatively small scale, however. Only a handful of countries, such as Australia and a few nations in Northern Europe, come close to meeting the demand.

Preventing vertical transmission

The overwhelming majority of children who die of AIDS acquired the infection from their mothers before or around the time of birth, or through breast milk. Most of these children with HIV live in the developing world. There are four major reasons for the difference between developed and developing countries. These are the higher proportion of HIV transmitted heterosexually, breast-feeding practices, limited access to drugs for reducing mother-to-child transmission, and the health infrastructure in each country.

Since it first became clear that HIV could be transmitted through breast milk, very few infected women in industrialized countries have chosen to breast feed their children, and so transmission of infection at the nipple is negligible. In developing countries, however, between one-third and one-half of all HIV infections in young children are acquired through breast milk. There are several reasons for this. First, more than nine out of ten HIV-positive women in developing countries do not know their HIV status. Secondly, a woman may choose to breast feed even if she knows about her infection, and knows she might pass it on through breast milk. Breast feeding protects the infant against a range of other infections, is convenient, is approved by most cultures, and is free. By choosing artificial feeding a woman may avoid passing on HIV, but where the water supply is unsafe she may expose her child to other deadly diseases. There are some governments, such as in Thailand, which distribute free or subsidized artificial milk to such women. But in many countries the critical first step remains to provide counselling, voluntary HIV testing, and information about safe infant feeding to all pregnant women.

In 1994, a study (Connor *et al.* 1994) demonstrated that giving an antiretroviral drug to women during pregnancy and delivery and to the infant after birth could reduce HIV transmission from mother to child by as much as two-thirds. This quickly became common practice in industrialized countries, but is not currently feasible in developing countries. The regimen is difficult to administer, involving regular drug taking over several months and an intravenous drip during delivery. The cost is around US$1000 per pregnancy.

A trial in Thailand (Shaffer *et al.* 1999) recently demonstrated that a short course of antiretroviral pills given to pregnant women during the last weeks prior to and during labour successfully reduced the rate of vertical transmission during pregnancy and delivery by half. The women were also given safe alternatives to breast milk and did not breast feed. A recent study that gave nevirapine at a cost of US$4 to US$8 at onset of labour and to the infants at birth also resulted in a 50 per cent reduction in HIV transmission to the infant (Guay *et al.* 1999).

The cost of treating HIV-positive women with a short course of antiretrovirals in late pregnancy and around the time of delivery compares well with that of many other health interventions. The cost-effectiveness varies according to the level of infection in a country. A study in Tanzania suggested that counselling, testing, and short-course antiretrovirals for pregnant women would cost under US$600 per HIV infection that is averted. This translates into around US$30 per healthy year of life gained. In high-prevalence areas of Thailand the cost per infection averted is around US$2800. With the use of nevirapine, the cost is reduced much further.

In Western countries it was shown that a positive attitude among health workers towards HIV testing contributes to lower anxiety among their pregnant patients (Boyd *et al.* 1999). However, in most developing countries the poorly developed health infrastructure has limited counselling for HIV-infected pregnant women. In some countries (Cartoux *et al.* 1999) this has been replaced by group pre- and post-test counselling. At the public health level, group pretest counselling can be easily integrated into existing sessions of antenatal care counselling routinely performed by the current clinic staff.

Control of sexually transmitted diseases

The presence of STD has repeatedly been shown to enhance the probability of HIV infection. Thus it seems reasonable that effective treatment of STDs would reduce the incidence of HIV, especially in very sexually active populations. Studies on the efficacy of STD treatment programmes on reducing the incidence of HIV have been conflicting. Grosskurth *et al.* (1995), working in Tanzania where the prevalence of HIV was still relatively low at the time of the study, found that improved treatment of STDs, including an adequate supply of drugs, lowered the incidence of HIV although not the prevalence of STDs. Presumably the period during which individuals were actively infected with an STD was shortened. On the other hand, a study in the Rakai district of Uganda, a district with a very high prevalence of HIV, found that periodic mass treatment of all residents for STDs every 10 months had no impact on the incidence of HIV (Wawer *et al.* 1999). Presumably the higher prevalence of HIV in the Rakai district, which increased the likelihood of exposure to HIV for sexually active people, lessened the impact of concurrent STDs on risk of HIV infection, although the difference in the therapeutic approaches may also have played a role. Nonetheless, at the individual level, diagnosis and treatment of STDs probably does reduce the risk of HIV infection.

Universal precautions and postexposure prophylaxis

Health workers are at risk for HIV transmission. Therefore intensive surveillance for health facilities began in some countries in 1985 (Weiss *et al.* 1985). According to studies of HIV exposure in health workers, the risk of HIV infection is 0.32 per cent per percutaneous exposure, 0.09 per cent per mucous membrane exposure, and zero per intact skin exposure (Bell 1997).

According to a collaborative study including the United States, France, Italy, and United Kingdom, the three main determinants for percutaneous infection are obvious exposure to infected blood, terminal illness in the source patient, and administration of antiretroviral postexposure prophylaxis.

The best prevention for health workers who may be exposed to HIV-infected specimens from clients is 'universal precautions'. This strategy imposes the burden of the increased cost of disposable and protective equipment that many developing countries cannot afford. However, even with universal precautions, there may be some accidental exposure to HIV-contaminated material. Thus postexposure antiretroviral prophylaxis is recommended for exposed health providers (Centers for Disease Control and Prevention 1995). In Western countries, a combination of three antiretroviral drugs has been recommended as prophylaxis for HIV-exposed health workers, but in most developing countries such a regimen is not affordable (Centers for Disease Control and Prevention 1996). Currently, postexposure antiretroviral prophylaxis has been accepted in coping with other causes of HIV exposure, such as after rape (Katz and Gerberding 1997). However, it is not recommended by any public health authority. HIV nosocomial transmission to patients may be a concern since there has been at least one report of transmission of HIV from health providers to their patients (Centers for Disease Control and Prevention 1991). The development of a DNA-sequencing capacity has facilitated the identification of the source of HIV transmission.

Vaccine

Vaccines have been demonstrated to be the most effective tool for controlling many infectious diseases. Unfortunately, development of a vaccine against HIV has not been accomplished as of the year 2002. The basic problem is that no natural immunity following infection has been demonstrated. There are thousands of variants of the virus and evoking an effective immune response appears to be specific to each variant. Inducing protection against the thousands of HIV variants is not feasible. Further, recovery with elimination of the virus and development of immunity, as occurs in most diseases for which a vaccine has been developed, has not been demonstrated in HIV except, possibly, in a few children. On the other hand, resistance to infection has been demonstrated in a few individuals and provides hope that resistance to infection can be induced, although not necessarily using the classic strategies for vaccine development (Imagawa and Detels 1991; Detels *et al.* 1994, 1996*a*,*b*).

In the late 1980s and early 1990s the scientific community was discouraged from working on vaccine development because of the formidable problems that had to be overcome. By the middle to late 1990s the urgent need for a vaccine overcame the previous discouragement and the National Institute of Allergy and Infectious Diseases, and private foundations such as the Rockefeller Foundation, provided funds to spur development of a vaccine. As a result many groups are now working on the development of a vaccine, but it will probably be well into the twenty-first century before an effective vaccine becomes available.

Summary and forecast

Twenty years after the identification of AIDS and 16 years after the discovery of HIV, more is known about the virus and the natural history of the disease than for the majority of other agents discovered many decades ago. And progress has been made towards control of HIV/AIDS. The incidence is declining in most developed countries, and several developing countries, including Thailand, Cambodia, and Uganda, have been successful in slowing the spread of HIV. Although science has not discovered a cure, the prognosis for HIV-infected and AIDS patients has improved and the prospects are good that the disease will become a chronic disease allowing an infected individual to lead a normal life, albeit requiring continuing medication. There has been considerable progress in the search for an effective vaccine although much more needs to be done before a vaccine is a reality.

But the epidemic continues. HIV continues to spread rapidly in both India and China, which contain 38 per cent of the world's population. In China there is evidence that HIV is now spreading to the heterosexual population. HIV continues to spread quickly in Africa and Asia, particularly in South and Southeast Asia, and has affected the longevity and productivity of the most severely affected countries in these regions. The challenge to control the epidemic is particularly great in the developing world where the epidemic is now concentrated, because of the lack of resources, health infrastructure, and trained manpower.

The epidemic can be controlled but to do so will require a better understanding of the sexual behaviour of populations at risk, improving the status of women (particularly in Asia and Latin America), increasing awareness of HIV/AIDS and prevention strategies, adoption of strategies to prevent transmission, including promotion of safer sex and condom use, decreasing the rate of sexual mixing, promoting 'risk-free' testing, and developing the political will to mandate more funds and a more effective health infrastructure to combat its spread. A key factor will be to reduce/eliminate stigmatization of groups at risk of HIV infection, HIV-infected individuals, and AIDS patients. The cycle of poverty promoting HIV transmission that in turn creates more poverty must be broken. Finally, the developed countries of the world need to recognize their responsibility to assist the developing countries to overcome this epidemic. If progress can be made in addressing these issues then the prospect for control of HIV/AIDS is good even in the absence of an effective vaccine.

References

Ainsworth, M. and Over, M. (1992). *The economic impact of AIDS: shocks, responses and outcomes*, Technical Working Paper 1, Report Number 11276, Population, Health and Nutrition Division, Africa Technical Department, World Bank, Washington DC.

Altman, D. (1988). Legitimacy through disaster. In *AIDS: the burdens of history* (ed. D. Fox and E. Fee). University of California Press, Berkeley, CA.

Anzala, A., Nagelkerke, N., Bwayo, J.J., *et al.* (1995). Rapid progression to disease in African sex workers with human immunodeficiency virus type I infection. *Journal of Infectious Diseases*, **171**, 686–9.

Bayer, R. (1991). Public health policy and the AIDS epidemic: an end to HIV exceptionalism? *New England Journal of Medicine*, **324**, 1500–4.

Bayer, R. (1996). Societal and political impact of HIV/AIDS. In *AIDS in the world II* (ed. J.Mann and D. Tarantola), pp. 117–28. Oxford University Press.

Bell, D. (1997). Occupational risk of human immunodeficiency virus infection in healthcare workers: an overview. *American Journal of Medicine*, **102** (Supplement 5B), 9–15.

Bennett, A. and Sharpe, A. (1996). AIDS fight is skewed by federal campaign exaggerating risks. *Wall Street Journal*, 1 May, pp. A1, A6.

Bharat, S., Singhanetra-Renard, A., and Angleton, P. (1998). Household and community response to HIV/AIDS in Asia: the case of Thailand and India. *AIDS*, **12** (Supplement B), S117–S122.

Boyd, F., Simpson, W., Johnstone, F., Goldberg, D., and Hart, G. (1999). Uptake and acceptability of antenatal HIV testing, *British Journal of Midwifery*, **7**, 151–6.

Bryson, Y.J. (1995). HIV clearance in infants—a continuing saga. *AIDS*, **9**, 1373–5.

Bryson, Y.J. (1996). Perinatal HIV-1 transmission: recent advances and therapeutic interventions. *AIDS*, **10** (Supplement 3), S33–S42.

Bryson, Y.J., Pang, S., Wei, L.S., Dickover, R., Diagne, A., and Chen, I.S. (1995). Clearance of HIV infection in a perinatally infected infant. *New England Journal of Medicine*, **332**, 833–8.

Bulterys, M., Nzabihimana, E., Chao, A., Bugingo, G., Musekera, J., Saah, A., and Van de Perre, P. (1993). Long-term survival among HIV-1 infected prostitutes. *AIDS*, **7**, 1269.

Cartoux, M., Sombie, I., Van de Perre, P., Meda, N., Tiendrebeogo, S., and Dabis, F. (1999). Evaluation of 2 techniques of HIV-pre-test counselling for pregnant women in West Africa. *International Journal of STD and AIDS*, **10**, 199–201.

Catania, J., Kegeles, S., and Coates, T. (1990). Toward an understanding of risk behavior: an AIDS risk reduction model. *Health Education Quarterly*, **17**, 53–72.

Centers for Disease Control and Prevention (1991). Transmission of HIV infection during an invasive dental procedure—Florida. *Morbidity and Mortality Weekly Report*, **40**, 377–81.

Centers for Disease Control and Prevention (1992). 1993 revised classification system for HIV infection and expanded surveillance case definition for AIDS among adolescents and adults. *Morbidity and Mortality Weekly Report*, **41**, 1–17.

Centers for Disease Control and Prevention (1995). Case–control study of HIV seroconversion in health-care workers after percutaneous exposure to HIV-infected blood—France, United Kingdom, and United States, January 1988–August 1994. *Morbidity and Mortality Weekly Report*, **44**, 929–33.

Centers for Disease Control and Prevention (1996). Provisional Public Health Service recommendations for chemoprophylaxis after occupational exposure to HIV. *Morbidity and Mortality Weekly Report*, **45**, 468–72.

Chamberland, M.E. (1998). Surveillance for transfusion-transmitted viral infections in the United States. *Biologicals*, **26**, 85–8.

Chesseman, S., Havlir, D., and McLaughlin, M. (1995). Phase I/II evaluation of nevirapine alone and in combination with zidovudine for infection with human immunodeficiency virus. *Journal of Acquired Immune Deficiency Syndromes and Human Retrovirology*, **8**, 141–51.

Connor, E.M., Sperling, R.S., Gelber, R., *et al.* (1994). Reduction of maternal-infant transmission of human immunodeficiency virus type 1 with zidovudine treatment. Pediatric AIDS Clinical Trials Group Protocol 076 Study Group. *New England Journal of Medicine*, **331**, 1173–80.

Cook, R. (1995). Gender, health and human rights. *Health and Human Rights*, **4**, 350–4.

Crofts, N., Reid, G., and Deany, P. (1988). Injecting drug use and HIV infection in Asia. *AIDS*, **12** (Supplement Bf), S69–S78.

Des Jarlais, D. (1993). Protective effects of syringe exchange against blood-borne virus infection among injecting drug users. *First National Conference on Human Retroviruses and Related Infections*, p. 178.

Detels, R., Liu, Z., Hennessey, K., *et al.* (1994). Resistance to HIV-1 infection. *Journal of Acquired Immune Deficiency Syndromes*, **7**, 1263–9.

Detels, R., Mann, D., Carrington, M., *et al.* (1996*a*). Persistently seronegative men from whom HIV-1 has been isolated are genetically and immunologically distinct. *Immunology Letters*, **51**, 29–33.

Detels, R., Mann, D., Carrington, M., *et al.* (1996*b*). Resistance to HIV infection may be genetically mediated. *AIDS*, **10**, 102–4.

Detels, R., Muñoz, A., Peng, Y., *et al.* (1997). Early versus deferred zidovudine monotherapy: impact on AIDS-free time and survival in the Multicenter AIDS Cohort Study. *Antiviral Therapy*, **2**, 21–9.

Detels, R., Muñoz, A., McFarlane, G., *et al.* (1998). Effectiveness of potent antiretroviral therapy on time to AIDS and death in men with known HIV infection duration. Multicenter AIDS Cohort Study Investigators. *Journal of the American Medical Association*, **280**, 1497–1503.

Detels, R., Tarwater, P., Phair, J.P., *et al.* (2001). Effectiveness of potent antiretroviral therapies on the incidence of opportunistic infections before and after AIDS diagnosis. *AIDS*, **15**, 347–55.

Dickover, R.E., Dillon, M., Leung, K.M., *et al.* (1998). Early prognostic indicators in primary perinatal human immunodeficiency virus type 1 infection: importance of viral RNA and the timing of transmission on long-term outcome. *Journal of Infectious Diseases*, **178**, 375–87.

Finlay, J., Mann, J., and Tarantola, D. (1992). Funding the Global AIDS Strategy. *In AIDS in the world* (ed. J. Mann, D.J.M. Tarantola, and T.W. Netter), pp. 511–35. Harvard University Press, Cambridge, MA.

Fleming, A., Carballo, M., Fitzsimmons, D., Bailey, M., and Mann, J. (1988). *Global impact of AIDS*. Alan R. Liss, New York.

Fox, R., Odaka, N.J., Brookmeyer, R., and Polk, B.F. (1987). Effect of HIV antibody disclosure on subsequent sexual activity in homosexual men. *AIDS*, **1**, 241–6.

Frank, J. (1995). The determinants of health: a new synthesis. *Current Issues in Public Health*, **1**, 42–65.

Gao, F., Bailes, E., Robertson, D.L., *et al.* (1999). Origin of HIV-1 in the chimpanzee *Pan troglodytes*. *Nature*, **397**, 436–41.

Gardner, L., Brudnage, J., McNeil, J., *et al.* (1992). Predictors of HIV-1 disease progression in early and late-stages patients: the US Army natural history cohort. *Journal of Acquired Immune Deficiency Syndromes*, **5**, 782–93.

Gibson, D., McCusker, J., and Chesney, M. (1998). Effectiveness of psychosocial interventions in preventing HIV risk behaviour in injecting drug users. *AIDS*, **12** (8), 919–29.

Global Health Council (2000). www.globalhealth.org/issues/hivaids.html

Goedert, J., Kessler, C., Aledort, L., *et al.* (1989). Prospective study of human immunodeficiency virus type 1 infection and the development of AIDS in subjects with haemophilia. *New England Journal of Medicine*, **321**, 1141–8.

Gottlieb, M.S., Schroff, R., Schanker, H.M., Weisman, J.D., Fan, P.T., Wolf, R.A., and Saxon, A. (1981). *Pneumocystis carinii* pneumonia and mucosal candidiasis in previously healthy homosexual men: evidence of a new acquired cellular immunodeficiency. *New England Journal of Medicine*, **305**, 1425–31.

Grosskurth, H., Mosha, F., Todd, J., *et al.* (1995). Impact of improved treatment of sexually transmitted diseases on HIV infection in rural Tanzania: randomised controlled trial. *Lancet*, **346**, 530–6.

Guay, L.A., Musoke, P., Fleming, T., *et al.* (1999). Intrapartum and neonatal single-dose nevirapine compared with zidovudine for prevention of mother-to-child transmission of HIV-1 in Kampala, Uganda: HIVNET 012 randomised trial. *Lancet*, **354**, 795–802.

Harvard School of Public Health (1993). *Towards a new health strategy for AIDS: a report of the global AIDS policy coalition*. Francois-Xavier Bagnoud Center for Health and Human Rights, Boston, MA.

Hira S.K, Ngandu, N., Wadhawan, D., *et al.* (1990). Clinical and epidemiological features of HIV infection at a referral clinic in Zambia. *Journal of Acquired Immune Deficiency Syndromes*, **3**, 87–91.

Ho, D.D., Neumann, A.U., Perelson, A.S., Chen, W., Leonard, J.M., and Markowitz, M. (1995). Rapid turnover of plasma virions and CD4 lymphocytes in HIV-1 infection. *Nature*, **373**, 123–6.

Ho, H.T. and Hitchcock, M.J. (1989). Cellular pharmacology of 2′, 3′-dideoxy-2′,3′-didehydrothymidine, a nucleoside analog active against human immunodeficiency virus. *Antimicrobial Agents and Chemotherapy*, **33**, 844–9.

Imagawa, D. and Detels, R. (1991). HIV-1 in seronegative homosexual men. *New England Journal of Medicine*, **325**, 1250–1.

Institute of Medicine (1995). *HIV and the blood supply: an analysis of crisis decisionmaking* (ed. L.B. Leveton, H.C. Sox, Jr, and M.A. Stoto). National Academy Press, Washington, DC.

Jaffe, H., Darrow, W., Echenberg, D., *et al.* (1985). Acquired immunodeficiency syndrome in a cohort of homosexual men: a six-year follow-up study. *Annals of Internal Medicine*, **103**, 210–14.

Jemmott, J., Jemmott, L., and Fong, G. (1998). Abstinence and safer sex HIV risk-reduction interventions for African American adolescents: a randomized controlled trial. *Journal of the American Medical Association*, **279**, 1529–36.

Kalichman, S.C. (1998). Influencing HIV transmission risk. *Focus*, **13**, 1–4.

Katz, M. and Gerberding, J. (1997). Postexposure treatment of people exposed to the human immunodeficiency virus through sexual contact or injection-drug use. *New England Journal of Medicine*, **336**, 1097–100.

Lanjewar, D.N., Anand, B.S., Genta, R., *et al.* (1996) Major differences in the spectrum of gastrointestinal infections associated with AIDS in India versus the West: an autopsy study. *Clinical Infectious Diseases*, **23**, 482–5.

Laws, M. (1996). International funding of the Global AIDS Strategy: official development assistance. In *AIDS in the world II* (ed. J. Mann and D. Tarantola), pp. 375–89. Oxford University Press.

Lee, C., Phillips, A., Efford, J., Miller, E., Bofill, M., Griffiths, P., and Kernoff, P. (1989). Natural history of human immunodeficiency virus infection in a haemophilic cohort. *British Journal of Haematology*, **73**, 228–34.

Lemp, G., Payne, S., Neal, D., Temelso, T., and Rutherford, G.W. (1990). Survival trends for patients with AIDS. *Journal of the American Medical Association*, **263**, 402–6.

Levine, C., Michaels, D., and Back, S. (1996). Orphans of the HIV/AIDS pandemic. In *AIDS in the World II* (ed. J. Mann and D. Tarantola), pp. 278–86. Oxford University Press.

Lewis, J.S., Terriff, C.M., Coulston, D.R., and Garrison, M.W. (1997). Protease inhibitors: a therapeutic breakthrough for the treatment of patients with human immunodeficiency virus. *Clinical Therapeutics*, **19**, 187–214.

Lifson, A., Buchbinder, S., Sheppard, J., Maule, A.C., and Miller, A.C. (1991). Long-term immunodeficiency virus infection in asymptomatic homosexual and bisexual men with normal $CD4^+$ lymphocytes counts: immunologic and virologic characteristics. *Journal of Infectious Diseases*, **163**, 959–65.

Lindan, C.P., Allen, S., Serufilira, A., *et al.* (1992). Predictors of mortality among HIV-infected women in Kigali, Rwanda. *Annals of Internal Medicine*, **116**, 320–8.

MacNeil, J. and Anderson, S. (1998). Beyond the dichotomy: linking HIV prevention with care. *AIDS*, **12** (Supplement 2), S19–26.

Malcolm, A. and Dowsett, G. (1998). *Prevention in practice: summation of guiding principles, partners in prevention: international cases studies of effective health promotion practice in HIV/AIDS*, pp. 58–66. UNAIDS, Geneva.

Mann, J. (1995). Public health and human rights. *Current Issues in Public Health*, **1**, 97–101.

Mann, J. and Kay, K. (1991). Confronting the pandemic: the World Health Organization's global programme on AIDS, 1986–1989. *AIDS*, **5** (Supplement 2), S221–9.

Mann, J. and Tarantola, D. (1996). From epidemiology to vulnerablity to human rights. In *AIDS in the world II* (ed. J.Mann and D. Tarantola), pp. 427–76. Oxford University Press.

Mann, J., Gostin, L., Gruskin, S. *et al.* (1994). Health and human rights. *Health and Human Rights*, **1**, 6–22.

Mellors, J.W., Muñoz, A., Giorgi, J.V., *et al.* (1997). Plasma viral load and $CD4^+$ lymphocytes as prognostic markers of HIV-1 infection. *Annals of Internal Medicine*, **126**, 946–54.

Mills, S., Ungchusak, K., Srinivasan, V., Utomo, B., and Bennett, A. (1998). Assessing trends in HIV risk behaviors in Asia. *AIDS*, **12** (Supplement B), S79–86.

Mulder, D., Nunn, A., Kamali, A., Nakiyingi, J., Wagner, H.U., and Kengeya-Kayondo, J.F. (1994*a*). HIV-1 incidence and HIV-1 associated mortality in a Ugandan rural population. *Lancet*, **343**, 989–90.

Mulder, D., Nunn, A., Wagner, H.U., Kamali, A., and Kengeya-Kayonda, J.F. (1994*b*). HIV-1 incidence and HIV-1 associated mortality in rural Ugandan population cohort. *AIDS*, **8**, 87–92.

Muñoz, A., Wang, M.C., Bass S. *et al.* (1989). Acquired immunodeficiency virus type 1 (HIV-1) seroconversion in homosexual men. *American Journal of Epidemiology*, **130**, 530–9.

Muñoz, A., Sabin, C.A., and Phillips, A.N. (1997). The incubation period of AIDS. *AIDS*, **11** (Supplement A), S69–76.

Murray, C. and Lopez, A. (1996). *The global burden of disease. Global burden of disease and injury series, WHO and Harvard School of Public Health*, Vol. 2. World Bank, Washington, DC.

Naglekerke, N., Plummer, F., Holton D., Anzala, A.O., Manjii, F., Ngugi, E.N., and Moses, S. (1990). Transition dynamics of HIV disease in a cohort of African prostitutes: a Markov model approach. *AIDS*, **4**, 743–7.

N'Galy, B., Ryder, R., Bila, K., *et al.* (1998). Human immunodeficiency virus infection among employees in an African hospital. *New England Journal of Medicine*, **319**, 1123–7.

National Research Council (1993). *Monitoring the social impact of AIDS in the United States.* National Academy Press, Washington, DC.

Nelson, K.E., Beyrer C., Eiumtrakol, S., Khamboonruang, C., and Celentano, D. (1996). Changes in sexual behavior and a decline in HIV infection amoung young men in Thailand. *New England Journal of Medicine*, **335**, 297–303.

Newell, M.L., Gray, G., and Bryson, Y.J. (1997). Prevention of mother-to-child transmission of HIV-1 infection. *AIDS*, **11** (Supplement A), S165–S172.

Norman, L., Kennedy, M., and Parish, K. (1998). Close relationships and safer sex among HIV-infected men with haemophilia. *AIDS Care*, **10**, 339–54.

Over, M. (1992). *Macroeconomic impact of AIDS in sub-Saharan Africa.* Technical Working Paper 3, Population, Health and Nutrition Division, Africa Technical Department, World Bank, Washington, DC.

O'Shaughnessy, T. (1994). *Beyond the fragments: HIV/AIDS and poverty, issues in global development 1.* World Vision, Australia Research and Policy Unit, Melbourne.

Panos Institute (1990). *Triple jeopardy: women and AIDS.* Panos Dossier, London.

Phoolcharoen, W., Ungchusak, K., Sittitrai, W., and Brown, T. (1998). Thailand: lessons from a strong national response to HIV/AIDS. *AIDS*, **12** (Supplement B), S123–35.

Polacsek, M., Celentano, D., O'Campo, P., and Santelli, J. (1999). Correlates of condom use stage of change: implications for intervention. *AIDS Education Preview*, **11**, 38–52.

Richman, D.D., Fischl, M.A., Grieco, M.H., *et al.* (1987). The toxicity of azidothymidine (AZT) in the treatment of patients with AIDS and AIDS-related complex. A double-blind, placebo controlled trial. *New England Journal of Medicine*, **317**, 192–7.

Sarkar, S., Das, N., Panda, S., *et al.* (1993). Rapid spread of HIV among injecting drug users in northeastern states of India. *Bulletin on Narcotics*, **16**, 17–23.

Sathapatayavong, B., Tansuphaswadikul, S., Kantiphong, P., Pornochaipoolthavee, S., and Chuchottaworn, C. (1997). In Prevalence of disseminated MAC in Thai AIDS patients. Abstract 5281, 20th International Congress of Chemotherapy, Sydney.

Seeley, J., Kajura, E., Bachengana, C., *et al.* (1993). Extended family and support for people with AIDS in a rural population in southwest Uganda: a safety net with holes? *AIDS Care*, **5**, 117–22.

Shaffer, N., Chuachoowong, R., Mock, P., *et al.* (1999). Short-course zidovudine for perinatal HIV-1 transmission in Bangkok, Thailand: a randomised controlled trial, *Lancet*, **353**, 773–80.

Simonsen, J., Plummer, F., Ngugi, E., *et al.* (1990). HIV infection among lower socioeconomic strata prostitutes in Nairobi. *AIDS,* **4**, 87–92.

Subhash, K.H., Gregory, D., and Sirisanthana, T. (1998). Clinical spectrum of HIV/AIDS in the Asia–Pacific region. *AIDS*, **12** (Supplement B), S145–54.

Tarantola, D. (1995). Structural and environmental influences on HIV risk behavior and vulnerability. Presented at USAID 3rd HIV/AIDS Prevention Conference, Washington, DC.

UNAIDS (1995). *Joint United Nations Programmes on HIV/AIDS: strategic plan 1996–2000.* Background document, Second Meeting of the Programme Coordinating Board. Document UNAIDS/PCB(2)/95.3, UNAIDS, Geneva.

UNAIDS (2000). *AIDS epidemic update.* www.unaids.org/hivaidsinfo/documents/html

UNAIDS/WHO (1998). *Global HIV/AIDS epidemic update.* www.unaids.org/hivaidsinfo/documents/html

United States Bureau of the Census (1997). *Recent HIV seroprevalence levels by county.* Research Note 23, Health Studies Branch, International Programs Center, Population Division, Washington DC.

Watanabe, M.E. (1999). China confronts AIDS: international help needed to stop the spread. *Scientist,* **13**, 1–6.

Watney, S. (1996). 'Risk groups' or 'risk behaviors'? In *AIDS in the world II* (ed. J. Mann and D. Tarantola), pp. 431–2. Oxford University Press.

Wawer, M.J., Sewankambo, N.K., Serwadda, D., *et al.* (1999). Control of sexually transmitted diseases for AIDS prevention in Uganda: a randomised community trial. Rakai Project Study Group. *Lancet*, **353**, 525–35.

Wei, X., Ghosh, S.K., Taylor, M.E., *et al.* (1995). Viral dynamics in human immunodeficiency virus type 1 infection. *Nature*, **373**, 117–21.

Weiss, S., Saxinger, W., Rechtman, D., *et al.* (1985). HTLV-III infection among health care workers: association with needle-stick injuries. *Journal of the American Medical Association,* **254**, 2089–93.

Weniger, B.G., Limpakarnjanarat, K., Ungchusak, K., *et al.* (1991). The epidemiology of HIV infection and AIDS in Thailand. *AIDS,* **5** (Supplement 2), S71–85.

Whitmore-Overton, S., Tillett, H., Evans, B., and Allardice, G. (1993). Improved survival from diagnosis of AIDS in adult cases in the United Kingdom and bias due to reporting delays. *AIDS*, **7**, 415–20.

Wiktor, S.Z., Ekpini, E., Karon, J.M., *et al.* (1999). Short-course oral zidovudine for prevention of mother-to-child transmission of HIV-1 in Abidjan, Cote d'Ivoire: a randomized trial. *Lancet*, **353**, 781–5.

World Bank (1993). *World development report. Investing in health.* World Bank, Washington, DC.

Ainsworth, M. and Over, M. (1997). AIDS: a challenge for government. World Bank policy research report. In *Confronting AIDS: public priorities in a global epidemic*, pp. 27–32. Oxford University Press, New York.

WHO (1988). *Guidelines for the development of national AIDS prevention and control programmes*, Technical Series Document 1, Global Programme on AIDS, WHO, Geneva.

WHO (1998). *Avoidance of discrimination against HIV-infected people and persons with AIDS. Resolution 41.24.* 41st World Health Assembly, WHO, Geneva.

WHO (1999). *World health report 1999. Making a difference.* WHO, Geneva. (www.who.int/whr/1999/en/pdf/whr99.pdf)

Wu, Z., Detels, R., Zhang, J., *et al.* (1996). Risk factors for intravenous drug use and sharing equipment among young male drug users in southwest China. *AIDS*, **10**, 1017–24.

Wu, Z., Rou, K., and Detels, R. (2001). Prevalence of HIV infection among former commercial plasma donors in rural eastern China. *Health Policy and Planning*, **16**, 41–6.

10

Prevention and control of public health hazards

10.1 Tobacco

Samara Asma, Gonghuan Yang, Jonathan Samet, Gary Giovino, Douglas W. Bettcher, A.D. Lopez, and Derek Yach

Introduction

Tobacco use is unique in terms of its current and projected future impacts on global mortality. If current trends continue, the number of people killed by tobacco use will more than triple to 10 million annually by the year 2020 (Murray and Lopez 1996). Despite this impending danger, there is also an opportunity—a lag between the precursors of the epidemic and its projection. While high smoking rates among men are nearly universal, the same is not true for women and children. Moreover, multiple disclosures of industry documents have had a significant impact in providing new information about the history and conduct of the tobacco industry. These documents have changed the way in which we perceive the tobacco debate (Bettcher and Yach 1998, 1999). Thus, in the face of the unprecedented toll caused by tobacco use and the worrying projections, there is also an opportunity to learn and apply vital lessons for the future of world health.

The purpose of this chapter is to explore that opportunity by (a) examining the history of tobacco use and dependence, and the current and projected pattern of the tobacco epidemic, (b) reviewing the structure, conduct, and strategies of the tobacco industry, and (c) proposing dynamic tobacco control strategies, already proven to be effective in some countries, which may have relevance throughout the world.

The tobacco epidemic

In this section we review the history of tobacco use and dependence, the epidemiological model, and the characteristics of the tobacco epidemic. The characteristics of the epidemic include production of tobacco, patterns of tobacco use, cessation, nicotine dependence, exposure to environmental tobacco smoke (**ETS**), and the burden of tobacco-related diseases.

History

The tobacco plant (*Nicotiana tabacum*) originates from South America, where tobacco habits were practised for ceremonial and shamanistic purposes long before Columbus arrived; however, it was not consumed regularly. By the arrival of Columbus in 1492, tobacco was being chewed, smoked, or snuffed in many areas of both North and South America. In the 1700s and the early 1800s, large quantities of tobacco were being snuffed by the aristocracy of Europe and chewed by the American settlers. By the middle of the 1800s the technology for making cigarettes and flue-curing tobacco had been developed, and the chewing of tobacco was beginning to be considered unhygienic. The converging development of several technologies between the late nineteenth and early twentieth centuries made the modern cigarette possible. New tobacco blends and curing processes were developed, which produced a tobacco product that, when burned, could be inhaled. Machinery for manufacturing cigarettes cheaply was perfected, the safety match was invented, and advertising and promotion techniques promoted the products of the tobacco industry. By the time of the First World War the mass production of cigarettes had begun and smoking among men in industrial countries began to rise dramatically. Cigarette smoking became increasingly accepted among women in industrial countries, starting about the time of the Second World War. At this time, smoking also began to rise in men in developing countries. Today, tobacco is cultivated commercially in more than 120 countries and is consumed in all countries of the world (Gold 1995).

Epidemiological model of tobacco use and dependence

The traditional epidemiological model of agent, host, vector, and environment facilitates the understanding of factors that influence patterns, determinants, and consequences of tobacco use (Orleans and Slade 1993).

An **agent** is traditionally defined as a factor whose presence is essential for the occurrence of disease (Last 1995). In this model, the myriad components of tobacco and tobacco smoke cause disease. Tobacco and tobacco smoke contain over 40 000 chemicals, including hundreds that are toxic or carcinogenic (USDHHS 1989; Hecht 1999). Tobacco also contains nicotine, an addictive compound that serves to maintain people's use of the agent even when they want to quit (USDHHS 1988; Giovino *et al.* 1995; FDA 1996). The bioavailability of nicotine can be influenced by the pH of the product (FDA 1996; Fant *et al.* 1999). In the United States, many tobacco products (e.g. so-called 'low tar' cigarettes) may appear to be less dangerous than others on the basis of 'tar' and 'nicotine' ratings derived from a smoking machine. However, such products are rated by a machine testing system that does not represent the way that smokers compensate for reduced nicotine yield, and their availability may undermine smokers' motivations to quit (USDHSS 1996; Kozlowski *et al.* 1998*a*,*b*).

The **host** in this model is the person who uses the product, i.e. one who smokes tobacco (through a cigarette, cigar, pipe, or other smoking device), chews or dips oral tobacco, or inhales snuff. Host factors found to be determinants of smoking include demographic characteristics, knowledge, attitudes, and behaviours, tobacco use by friends and family members, and susceptibility to addiction and disease (USDHHS 1989, 1994). One significant challenge to tobacco control lies in understanding why some people who experiment with smoking easily discontinue whereas others progress to become regular dependent users. Host factors can influence why some dependent smokers quit and others continue, and why some lifelong smokers develop smoking-attributable diseases while others do not.

Because **ETS** (the combination of sidestream smoke and exhaled mainstream smoke inhaled by non-smokers) causes disease in many exposed persons who do not consume tobacco products (USDHHS 1986; California Environmental Protection Agency 1997; SCOTH 1998; Samet and Wang 2000), the complete disease model also includes involuntary smokers as incidental hosts (DiFranza and Lew 1995). The **vector** serves to transport the agent to susceptible individuals (Last 1995). Just as we need to understand, for example, the role of the rat in the spread of the plague or the mosquito in the spread of malaria, we need to understand that tobacco has a vector—tobacco manufacturers. Thus, in the development of nicotine addiction and tobacco-attributable disease, tobacco manufacturers produce the agent and distribute it in ways that make the product appealing to both users and non-users. The industry uses packaging, advertising, and promotion to reach and influence as many people as possible. The price of the product (the lower the price, the more will be sold) and the ease with which it can be obtained (from vending machines, over-the-counter displays, and sales by street vendors) are also key distribution factors. In the case of tobacco, the vector also serves to undermine public health attempts to limit use by denying for decades the health consequences of use, and resisting many health-promoting programmes and policies (Hilts 1996; Kluger 1996; Jamieson 1998). This vector actively markets products that tacitly claim to be less hazardous, while simultaneously denying that any of their products cause disease and death (USDHHS 1996; Leavell 1999). Additionally, for decades the vector has manipulated the product in ways that have made it more addictive and potentially more harmful. For example, by the manipulation of pH, manufacturers have enhanced the bioavailability of nicotine to the smoker (FDA 1996; Hurt and Robertson 1998).

The **environment** includes diverse cultural, historical, economic, and political factors. In many countries, tobacco growing and tobacco product manufacturing have been, for decades, respected and lucrative businesses that wielded tremendous economic and political influence (World Bank 1999). When the health effects became known, and more recently when the industry's malfeasant activities became apparent, attitudes towards the industry changed precipitously. Nevertheless, the powerful effects of pro-tobacco forces have influenced many political decisions (Kluger 1996; Jamieson 1998). In addition, the industry often attempts to gain cultural and political favour by sponsoring cultural events and promoting smoking prevention campaigns (Tobacco Institute 1991; USDHHS 1998; *Charleston Gazette* 1999). Economic and cultural influences in regions where tobacco is grown and/or where tobacco products are produced often result in reduced support for tobacco control activities. Environmental factors also include efforts by the tobacco control community to counter pro-tobacco influences.

This model has proved useful for both research and intervention. Past and ongoing research addresses each of the components of this model, as well as the interactions among its elements. Most research has focused on host factors, although more recent attention has also turned to policy factors. With the widespread dissemination of industry documents, our understanding of the vector has increased.

Interventions address different levels in a continuum that extends from the individual smoker to the national and international levels. Some attempt to influence host factors, for example by educating people about the dangers of tobacco use, how to quit, and ways to resist pro-tobacco influences from the peers and the media. Recent activities attempt to influence the environment, for example by promoting policy changes and mass media interventions. The industry is changing the agent, for example by developing nicotine-delivery products that heat (as opposed to burn) tobacco. Regulatory efforts strive to control both the agent and the activities of the vector.

Characteristics of the tobacco epidemic

In this section we aim to provide an overview of the characteristics of the global tobacco epidemic, which will include tobacco production and its patterns of use. It will also describe tobacco use cessation and nicotine dependence, and discuss the exposure to ETS. Finally, it will conclude with a review of the literature of the patterns and burden of tobacco-related diseases.

Tobacco production

In this section we classify and describe the various tobacco products available, tobacco growing, and the world market in manufactured tobacco products.

Types of tobacco products

There are two main forms of tobacco in common use: smoking tobacco and smokeless tobacco. Smoking tobacco includes manufactured cigarettes (filter and unfiltered) and 'roll-your-own' cigarettes. *Kretek* (clove-flavoured cigarettes), from Indonesia, are sticks made from a local variety of sun-cured tobacco known as *brus* and wrapped in cigarette paper. *Bidis* (small hand-rolled cigarettes consisting of sun-dried tobacco wrapped in a *tendu* leaf) are smoked throughout Southeast Asia, particularly in India. Cigars are made of air-cured and fermented tobacco with a tobacco leaf wrapper, and come in many shapes and sizes, from cigarette-sized to 10-g double coronas. Pipes are used predominantly in Europe, the Americas, and Southeast Asia; for example, clay pipes known as *sulpa*, *chilum*, and *hookli* are common in Asia. Water pipes, also known as *hookah*, *gaza*, *narghile*, hubble-bubble, and *shisha*, are in common use in North Africa, eastern Mediterranean countries, and parts of Asia.

Smokeless tobacco products, consisting of tobacco leaf and a wide variety of flavouring and other ingredients, are used either orally or nasally. Smokeless tobacco includes chewing tobacco, used in Western Europe and North Africa, and snuff (dry and moist snuff). Chewing tobacco is produced by shredding tobacco leaf. The leaf can be consumed loosely, or by pressing into bricks (plugs), or by drying and forming twist. Snuff, which may be sniffed or placed in the mouth, has a much finer consistency than chewing tobacco and is made from powdered or finely cut tobacco leaves. Chewing tobacco is prevalent in the Eastern Mediterranean and South Asia. Moist snuff taken orally has been used for many years in Sweden and the United States. Smokeless tobacco is being actively marketed as a popular form of tobacco among children and adolescents in Canada, the United States (including Alaska), Scandinavia, and the United Kingdom (Peterson *et al.* 1990).

Tobacco growing

Tobacco is grown in more than 120 countries. In 1994, over 5 million metric tons of tobacco (dry weight) were produced worldwide (WHO 1997*a*), and by 1997 leaf production had increased to 8 million metric tons, up 25.9 per cent in 3 years (Table 1) (World Bank 1999). China is the world's leading producer of tobacco, with production increasing from 2.1 million metric tons in 1994 (36.3 per cent of total world output) to 2.4 million metric tons in 1997 (42.1 per cent of total world output). In 1997, the other seven leading producers were the United States, India, Brazil, Turkey, Zimbabwe, Indonesia, and Malawi.

Manufactured tobacco products

Although tobacco is mainly grown in developing countries, the world market is dominated by a handful of American, British, and Japanese companies, which have a controlling presence not only in all Western countries but throughout the developing world. China is an exception, with its tobacco products mainly used in the domestic market. About 5.5 trillion cigarettes were manufactured worldwide in 1994; four countries (China, the United States, Japan, and Germany) accounted for over half of global production (WHO 1997*a*).

During the late 1990s, two major trends emerged which were significant for the future of the tobacco industry. First, the multinationals merged into a few major conglomerates. Second, state monopolies were increasingly privatized and merged with multinationals. The international cigarette market has recently undergone a significant structural change: British American Tobacco (**BAT**) acquired Rothmans, Japan Tobacco purchased RJR Tobacco International (**RJRTI**), and France's Seita merged with Spain's Tabacalera to form Altadis. In 1998, Philip Morris's worldwide volume totalled 945 billion cigarettes (units), BAT–Rothmans volume stood at 922 billion units, and JT–RJRTI produced 451 billion units. These three companies controlled 65 per cent of the 3.8 trillion units that were sold outside of the People's Republic of China (Goldman 1999). Altadis has become the top producer of cigars, with a global market share of 24.7 per cent in 1998, while its cigarette wing showed a volume of 106 billion units (Seita 1999).

In some countries, state-owned tobacco companies continue to dominate within their own market; the most notable of these is the China National Tobacco Corporation, which is the largest tobacco company in the world in terms of number of cigarettes sold (WHO

Table 1 Output of tobacco leaf by world's 25 leading producers

Country	1994[a]		1997[b]		Difference between
	Output (1000 metric tons)	Share of world total (%)	Output (1000 metric tons)	Share of world total (%)	1994 and 1997 (%)
China	2088.0	36.3	3390	42.1	62.4
United States	641.2	11.2	746.4	9.3	16.4
India	475.2	8.3	623.7	7.8	31.3
Brazil	365.0	6.4	576.6	7.2	58.0
Turkey	176.4	3.1	296.6	3.9	68.1
Zimbabwe	152.9	2.7	192.1	2.4	25.6
Indonesia	137.0	2.4	184.3	2.3	34.5
Malawi	78.9	1.4	158.6	2.0	101.0
Greece	124.5	2.2	132.5	1.7	6.4
Italy	113.9	2.0	131.4	1.6	15.4
Argentina	61.7	1.1	123.2	1.5	99.7
Pakistan	95.7	1.7	86.3	1.1	–9.8
Bulgaria	30.0	0.5	78.2	1.0	160.7
Canada	64.3	1.1	71.1	0.9	10.6
Thailand	51.9	0.9	69.3	0.9	33.5
Japan	71.9	1.3	68.5	0.9	–4.7
Philippines	50.9	0.9	60.9	0.8	19.6
South Korea	88.7	1.5	54.4	0.7	–38.7
Mexico	60.4	1.1	44.3	0.6	–26.7
Bangladesh	52.8	0.9	44.0	0.6	–16.7
World	5747.4		8048.4		40.0

[a]Data from WHO (1997*a*).

[b]Data from World Bank (1999).

1999*a*). Increasingly, however, the multinationals are moving into countries formerly controlled by state monopolies and introducing aggressive marketing programmes. For example, in the 1980s the American tobacco companies relied upon the United States government—and the threat of trade sanctions—to open the cigarette markets in Japan, Taiwan, South Korea, and Thailand (Chaloupka and Corbett 1998). The shift in focus of the multinationals also comes at a time when they are under increasing attack in their home bases, particularly in the United States, as new disclosures become public detailing how the tobacco industry built and maintained its markets in the United States through decades of improper conduct. These disclosures, in addition to shedding important historical light on the tobacco industry, also provide sobering and relevant insights as the tobacco industry expands to conquer new markets.

Patterns of tobacco use

The continuum of tobacco use in a smoker's lifetime can be described in terms of five stages: pre-contemplation, contemplation, preparation, action, and maintenance (Prochaska *et al.* 1997). These dynamic processes are major contributors to a given population's patterns of tobacco use. (Differential mortality and immigration also contribute to a country's patterns of use, but to a lesser extent.)

Although the prevalence of smoking has decreased and quitting rates have increased in some developed countries in recent decades, the overall global pattern of tobacco consumption is of major public health concern. In 1995, nearly 1.1 billion people smoked cigarettes (including *bidis*), consuming a total of 5 trillion cigarettes. The current smoking rate for the world's population is 29 per cent: 47 per cent among males and 12 per cent among females. In developed countries, the prevalence of smoking for males and females is 39 per cent and 24 per cent respectively. In developing countries, the gender difference in smoking prevalence is larger, with 49 per cent of males and 7 per cent of females smoking (WHO 1997*a*).

The difference in smoking prevalence among regions is great, especially among women. The highest prevalence of smoking is 60 per cent in males in the Western Pacific Region; about 30 to 40 per cent of males smoke in other regions. The highest prevalence of smoking in females is in the Americas and Europe where over 20 per cent of women are regular smokers. In the Asian and Eastern Mediterranean regions the prevalence of smoking in females is lower, at about 4 per cent (WHO 1997*a*).

The prevalence of tobacco use by gender is shown for 87 countries in the report *Tobacco or Health: A Global Status Report* (WHO 1997*a*). Male smoking prevalence is 50 per cent or more in 22 countries and 60 per cent or more in eight countries: the Republic of Korea, China, Latvia, the Russian Federation, the Dominican Republic, Tonga, Turkey, and Bangladesh. The prevalence of smoking is lower (35 per cent or less) in Western and Northern European countries, North America, Australia, New Zealand, and Singapore. Female smoking prevalence is 25 per cent or more in 26 countries and 30 per cent or more in six countries: Denmark, Norway, the Czech Republic, Fiji, Israel, and the Russian Federation. Three countries—Fiji, Poland, and the Russian Federation—rank in the top 20 for both male and female smoking prevalence.

Trends in the consumption of tobacco

The global and regional trends in cigarette consumption per adult aged 15 years and over in 1970–1972 and 1990–1992 are given in Table 2.

Table 2 Annual consumption of cigarettes per adult (15 years and over) between 1970–1972 and 1990–1992, by region

WHO region	Cigarette consumption	
	1970–1972[a]	**1990–1992**[b]
Africa	460	590
The Americas	2580	1900
Eastern Mediterranean	700	930
Europe	2360	2340
Southeast Asia	850	1230
Western Pacific	1100	2010
More developed countries	2860	2590
Less developed countries	860	1410
World	1410	1660

[a]Data from WHO (1997*a*).

[b]Data from World Bank (1999).

Trends in consumption rates have varied worldwide. Overall, the world has seen an average annual increase of approximately 1 per cent in adult per capita consumption over the last two decades. The most rapid declines have been in countries such as Canada and the United Kingdom, where average annual decreases of 1.8 per cent and 1.6 per cent respectively have been recorded since the early 1970s. These have not been matched by equivalent declines in prevalence.

In contrast, over the same time period there have dramatic average annual increases in China (8 per cent), Indonesia (6.8 per cent), Syria (5.5 per cent), and Bangladesh (4.7 per cent). These high rates of increase are occurring from a low starting base, but China and Syria have already reached the per capita consumption levels of the United Kingdom and in both countries the rates of smoking among women remain low. There is growing concern about the efforts of the tobacco industry to increase smoking rates among women in developing countries (WHO 1997*a*).

In many countries, people begin smoking at young ages, with the median age of initiation usually being under 15 years. The prevalence of smoking in youth continues to increase in both developed and developing countries, even where the overall prevalence of tobacco use is declining (WHO 1997*b*).

In the United States, 1 226 000 persons aged under 18 years became daily smokers (smoking every day) in 1996 (CDC 1998). Data from the 1997 United States Youth Risk Behavior Survey indicate that the prevalence of current cigarette smoking among American high-school students increased from 27.5 per cent in 1991 to 36.4 per cent in 1997. In 1997, 42.7 per cent of high-school students had used cigarettes, smokeless tobacco, or cigars during the 30 days preceding the survey (CDC 1998).

In China, the regular smoking rate (proportion of people who smoked at least one cigarette daily among the whole population) in 1996 was 31 per cent—an increase of 3.4 per cent compared with 1984. Between the two surveys, the ages at which males and females reported starting to smoke dropped by about 3 years. For men, the average age of starting smoking in the 1996 data was about 19 years compared with about 22 years in 1984. For women, the age of starting to smoke dropped from 28 years of age to 25 years between the surveys (Yang 1997).

Many studies have shown that sociodemographic, environmental, behavioural, and personal factors are associated with the onset of tobacco use. Environmental factors include availability and advertising of cigarettes, the perception that tobacco use is the norm, peer and sibling attitudes, and lack of parental support during adolescence (Reid *et al.* 1995). Availability and ease of acquiring cigarettes are also environmental factors that can have an impact on smoking among adolescents. Parental attitudes toward smoking, and in particular towards their own children's smoking, has been shown to be related to adolescent smoking. Also important are school performance and psychosocial factors, including low academic achievement, rebelliousness, low self-esteem, alienation from school, and lack of skills to resist offers of cigarettes (Tyas and Pederson 1998). These findings are mainly from Western countries (Conrad *et al.* 1992; Tyas and Pederson 1998); a few studies from developing countries such as China have shown similar results (Zhu *et al.* 1996; S.Q. Wang *et al.* 1994).

Tobacco use by women

Tobacco use is one of the major causes of premature disease and death, and is an emerging global public health problem especially among girls and women. According to the World Health Organization (**WHO**), currently more than 200 million women smoke cigarettes worldwide and this figure excludes those using other forms of tobacco. It is estimated that between 80 000 and 100 000 young people start smoking everyday, and many of these are girls. An estimated 12 per cent of women smoke globally; about 24 per cent of women smoke in developed countries, while 7 per cent of women smoke in developing countries (WHO 1997*a*). Again, these statistics do not include forms of tobacco use other than cigarettes. For example, in India 75 per cent of men and only 10 per cent of women smoke. The prevalence of other forms of tobacco use, i.e. chewing tobacco, ranges from 15 to 67 per cent (Gupta 1996). Historically, smoking has been more common among men than among women in the majority of countries. In countries for which reliable data are available for assessing trends in smoking (primarily industrialized countries), peak prevalence among women occurred some years after it did so for men (Pierce *et al.* 1991). While there are minor gender differences in smoking rates in some industrialized countries (such as the United States, New Zealand, and Australia), disparities between male and female smoking rates in Asia are striking, specifically in Japan (61 per cent of men and 15 per cent of women), Korea (70 per cent of men and 5 per cent of women), and China (61 per cent of men 7 per cent of women).

Rates are also rising among young women in many countries in Asia and the Pacific regions, where smoking is a symbol of women's liberation and freedom from traditional gender roles. There is an even greater cause for alarm because statistics on cigarette consumption do not reflect the widespread use of smokeless tobacco among women in South Asia. For example, in Kerala, India, 22 per cent of rural women chew tobacco in a betel leaf. In the Bihar region and parts of Punjab and Harayana, women also smoke *bidis* and *hookahs*,. Rural Indian women in the state of Goa rub and plug burnt powdered tobacco inside their mouths (Aghi *et al.* 2001). It would be a major public health setback if women in all developing countries begin to smoke like women in developed countries and continued to use other forms of tobacco.

One of the contributing factors to this rising epidemic of tobacco use among women is the proliferation of seductive tobacco advertising worldwide which may lead women and girls to believe that smoking is socially desirable behaviour. Typically, women's brands in the developing countries feature slim glamorous Western models. Such models lend a sense of foreignness to the cigarette and can serve as symbols of prestige and modernity. To sell such images, tobacco companies in the United States spend in excess of US$5 billion annually on marketing and promotion. Japan will account for 56 per cent of spending in Asia and the Pacific region in 1999. In recent years, transnational tobacco companies have increasingly turned their focus to the developing world, with intensive marketing campaigns aimed at women and girls.

The Kobe Declaration adopted in 1999 by women and youth leaders, scientists and policy-makers 'demanded a global ban on direct and indirect advertising, promotion and sponsorship by the tobacco industry across all media and in all forms of entertainment; and demanded public funding for counter-advertising that disconnects women's liberation and tobacco use and that reaches women and girls in all cultural contexts' (WHO 1999*a*).

Tobacco use and indigenous people

Tobacco use is an important factor that impacts negatively on the health of indigenous peoples who have the highest rates of tobacco use in the world. It is not unusual for the rates of smoking of indigenous peoples to be twice that of the general population of the country in which they live. A survey among the Inuit of Greenland found that currently 82 per cent of Inuit men and 78 per cent of Inuit women are smokers. Further, in the area of Disko Bay, approximately 65 per cent of pregnant women were smokers (AMAP 1998). Therefore it is not surprising that the incidence and mortality of tobacco-related cancers are very high among the Inuit of Greenland (AMAP 1998). Similar patterns of smoking and smoking-related disease are evident among other groups of indigenous peoples, including the Maori of New Zealand, the First Nations and Inuit peoples of Canada, and the Aborigines and Torres Strait Islanders of Australia. By 1993, the rate of smoking among the Maori of New Zealand (46 per cent of Maori aged 15 years and over) was twice the rate of non-Maori New Zealanders. The rate for Maori women at this time was 58 per cent, with survey findings indicating that approximately 69 per cent smoke during pregnancy (Durie 1998). In 1997, 62 per cent of First Nations and Labrador Inuit adults (aged 15 years and over) were smokers. The ratio for indigenous and non-indigenous peoples of the Northwest Territories in 1996 was similar (S. Gauthier, unpublished report, 1999). The Aborigines and Torres Strait Islanders of Australia have twice the rate of smoking of the non-indigenous Australian population (54 per cent of indigenous men and 46 per cent of indigenous women, compared with 28 per cent and 22 per cent of non-indigenous men and women respectively (Australian Bureau of Statistics and the Australian Institute of Health and Welfare 1997).

Given the high level of tobacco use by many indigenous peoples around the world, it is essential that their distinctive needs are not lost in national and global public health efforts to control the tobacco epidemic. Tobacco control among indigenous peoples is not adequately addressed within the framework of minority groups or vulnerable populations. Specific approaches are needed to address their distinctive tobacco control needs.

Smoking cessation and nicotine dependence

Smoking cessation decreases health risks, even at older ages (USDHHS 1990). However, many smokers try to quit but fail. Nicotine dependence is the major reason for relapse after quitting. Nicotine, an alkaloid, is a constituent of all tobacco products and a drug that leads to addiction (USDHHS 1988). Nicotine administration can lead to tolerance and physiological dependence. Tolerance is indicated by the diminished response to repeated doses of nicotine. Nicotine-induced physiological dependence and withdrawal are specific to the administration or removal of nicotine itself. Cessation from tobacco following chronic use results in withdrawal symptoms, including a craving for nicotine, impaired ability to concentrate, disrupted cognitive performance, mood changes, and impaired brain function (Hatsukami *et al.* 1985).

Cessation of smoking is a dynamic process with a cyclical nature. Over the course of time, many people alternate between smoking and non-smoking. Smoking cessation is not a discrete process but rather a complex process involving several stages. The trans-theoretical model, which uses stages of changing to integrate processes and principles of change on people's behaviour, conceives behavioural change as a process involving progress through a series of five stages: pre-contemplation, contemplation, preparation, action, and maintenance (Prochaska *et al.* 1997). **Pre-contemplation** is defined as a stage in which current smokers have no intention to give up smoking within the next 6 months. During **contemplation** current smokers intend to give up smoking within the next 6 months. Current smokers in the **preparation** stage are seriously preparing to give up smoking within the next 30 days and take some steps in this direction, such as reading relevant materials. The **action** stage is defined as the first 6 months after smokers stop smoking. Lastly, **maintenance** continues from 6 months after stopping smoking until the person is a confirmed non-smoker without relapse.

There may be different stage profiles of smoking cessation in different countries and different population groups. Understanding the different stage profile might help public health officials to design messages and projects targeted more appropriately. For example, results from the 1990 California Tobacco Survey of 12 815 smokers and ex-smokers aged 18 years and older showed that 27.4 per cent of the respondents were in the pre-contemplation stage, 34.3 per cent in the contemplation stage, 11.8 per cent in the preparation stage, 5.9 per cent in the action stage, and 20.7 per cent in maintenance (Kaplan *et al.* 1993). The stage profile of cessation is different in developing countries. The 1996 National Survey on Smoking Patterns in China reported that 63.9 per cent of smokers never intended to give up smoking and only 15.7 per cent of smokers intend to quit (Yang 1997).

Environmental tobacco smoke exposure

Non-smokers inhale ETS, the combination of sidestream smoke that is released as the cigarette burns and the mainstream smoke exhaled by the active smokers (First 1985). Exposure to ETS is difficult to measure accurately as it is not a direct consequence of actions by the exposed subject. Indicators of exposure to the ETS range from surrogate indicators to direct measurements of exposure and of biomarkers.

In some countries, in which male smoking prevalence exceeds female smoking prevalence, one useful index is the husband's smoking status as an estimate of ETS exposure for wives. This is far from accurate because smoking by other family members may be important sources of ETS, the husband may smoke outside the home, and information about exposure before marriage is not captured (F.L. Wang *et al.* 1994). The indirect measures include self-reported exposure and description of the source of ETS in relevant microenvironments, most often the home and workplace, obtained by using questionnaires.

Nicotine and its metabolite cotinine have long been used as measures of tobacco smoke intake. The concentrations of serum and urinary cotinine in non-smokers increase significantly with the reported number of cigarettes smoked by their spouses; cotinine can be used to identify passive smokers and is sensitive to the extent of tobacco smoke exposure (Matsukura *et al.* 1984; Hackshaw 1998). However, cotinine provides a measurement for exposure within a few days and it cannot represent the long-term exposure to passive smoking.

The amount of ETS exposure of a non-smoker is influenced by the number of smokers in the indoor environment, the intensity of their smoking, the duration of exposure, the volume of the indoor environment, the ventilation characteristics, and the breathing pattern, as well as activity of the non-smoker (Samet *et al.* 1987). Homes, workplaces, and public places are all sources of ETS exposure, especially the home for women and children in many societies. The prevalence of ETS exposure can be very high, especially for women in countries where the prevalence of male smoking is very high. For example, in the survey of all current non-smokers in China in 1996, 54 per cent reported that they were exposed to ETS. The prevalence rate of ETS exposure in females (57 per cent) is higher than that in males (45 per cent). The highest exposure to ETS (up to 60 per cent) is in women of childbearing age, with higher exposure in the younger groups than in older age groups. The majority of passive smokers are exposed to ETS every day, with 71 per cent reporting exposure at home, 25.0 per cent reporting exposure in their work environments, and 33 per cent being exposed in public places.

Children's exposure to ETS is involuntary, arising from smoking, mainly by adults, in the places where they live, work, and play. WHO estimates that about 700 million, or almost half, of the world's children breathe air polluted by tobacco smoke, particularly at home (WHO 1999*b*). Data from a 1988 nation-wide survey of the United States show that about half of American children under the age of 5 years are exposed to tobacco smoke (Overpeck and Moss 1991). For more than a quarter of children, exposure begins before birth. Based on the survey data, 42 per cent of children in this age range were estimated to live in a household with a smoker. The proportion of ETS exposed children doubled from the highest income and maternal education groups to the lowest. In Shanghai, China, in the period 1986 to 1987, 58 per cent of newborn children were exposed to ETS, mainly from smoking by the father (Zhang and Ratcliffe 1993). For older children the proportion of ETS exposure ranges from 40 to 70 per cent (Overpeck and Moss 1991; Sherrill *et al.* 1992).

Patterns and burden of tobacco-related diseases

Toxicology of tobacco smoke

Tobacco smoke is generated by the burning of a complex organic material, tobacco, together with the various additives and paper, at a high temperature, reaching several thousand degrees Celsius. The resulting smoke, comprising numerous gases and also particles, includes many toxic components that can cause injury through inflammation and irritation, asphyxiation, carcinogenesis, and other mechanisms. Active smokers inhale mainstream smoke, i.e. the smoke that is drawn directly through the end of the cigarette. Passive smokers inhale smoke that is often referred to as ETS, comprising a mixture of mostly sidestream smoke, given off by the smouldering cigarette, and some exhaled mainstream smoke. Concentrations of ETS are far below the levels of mainstream smoke inhaled by the active smoker, but there are qualitative similarities between ETS and MS (USDHHS 1986).

Both active and passive smokers absorb tobacco smoke components through the lung's airways and alveoli, and many of these components, such as the gas carbon monoxide, enter into circulation and are distributed generally in the body. There is also uptake of some components, such as benzo[*a*]pyrene, directly into the cells that line the upper airways and the lung's airways. Some of the carcinogens undergo metabolic transformation into their active forms. The genitourinary system is exposed to toxins in tobacco smoke through the excretion of these compounds in the urine. The gastrointestinal tract is exposed through direct deposition of smoke in the upper airways and the clearance of smoke-containing mucus from the trachea through the glottis into the oesophagus. Not surprisingly, tobacco smoking has proved to be a cause of multisystem disease (USDHHS 1986).

There is a vast scientific literature on the mechanisms by which tobacco smoking causes disease (USDHHS 1989, 1994). This literature includes characterization of the many toxic components in smoke, which include well-known toxins such as hydrogen cyanide, carbon monoxide, and nitrogen oxides. The toxicity of smoke has been studied by exposing animals to tobacco smoke, in cellular and other laboratory toxicity assays, and by assessing smokers for evidence of injury by tobacco smoke using biomarkers such as tissue changes and levels of damaging enzymes and cytokines. The data from these studies amply document the powerful toxicity of tobacco smoke. For example, young smokers in their twenties already show evidence of permanent damage to the small airways of the lung (Niewoehner *et al.* 1974; PDAY Research Group 1990), and lavage of the lungs of smokers shows increased numbers of inflammatory cells and higher levels of markers of injury compared with non-smokers (USDHHS 1990). The new tools of molecular and cellular biologyhave provided evidence of tobacco-induced changes at the molecular level. For example, an activated tobacco-smoke carcinogen has been shown as binding to the same codon in the p53 gene where mutations are found in lung cancers in smokers (Denissenko *et al.* 1996) and a variety of genetic changes are found in epithelial cells in smokers' lungs (Wistuba *et al.* 1997).

Review of evidence on health risks of active smoking

The most useful epidemiological studies for assessing the health risks of tobacco were the cohort studies initiated in the 1950s, 1960s, and 1970s, together with the follow-up mortality analyses pertaining to this period (Lopez 1999). All are limited to the study of mortality, and all give quantitatively similar results for the relative risks of smoking for various diseases (and all causes of death), despite the fact that the cohorts were recruited from countries as diverse as the United States, Sweden, Japan, Canada, and the United Kingdom. These findings have complemented the results of numerous case–control studies, some including thousands of cases (USDHHS 1989).

In the United States, the United Kingdom, and Canada, where men had been smoking in large numbers for decades before these studies were carried out, smoking was typically associated with 70 to 80 per cent excess mortality from all causes (Peto *et al.* 1996). The relative risks varied substantially by disease, and were largest for cancers of the lung and upper aerodigestive tract (mouth, pharynx, larynx, and oesophagus), and lowest for vascular diseases that have complex multicausal aetiology. Typically, lung cancer death rates were 10 to 12 times higher in smokers than in non-smokers, with the notable exception of Japanese men and American women for whom the relative excess was three to four times that of non-smokers. Similarly, the all-cause mortality ratios (relative risks) were substantially lower in these two studies, reflecting the fact that tobacco use in the two populations had been much lower than for other cohorts. Relative risks from lung cancer for American women smokers versus lifelong non-smokers increased from 2.7 in 1959–1965 to 11.9 in 1982–1986, reflecting the dominant role of duration of exposure in determining lung cancer hazards (USDHHS 1989).

Two large cohort studies have produced more recent evidence on health hazards from smoking, which have emphasized the increasing hazards of smoking with longer duration of use. These two studies are the 40-year follow-up of the 1951 British doctors cohort (Doll *et al.* 1994) and the second American Cancer Society Cancer Prevention Study (CPS-II) cohort of over 1.2 million adults monitored since 1982, for which comparisons can be made with CPS-I, initiated 20 years earlier (Thun *et al.* 1997).

The alarming size of the hazards observable in populations that have been smoking for many decades is now apparent. In the first 20 years of follow-up of the British doctors cohort (1951–1971), smokers had, on average, about a 1.5- to twofold higher death rate at each age, similar to the excess reported in other studies around that time (Doll *et al.* 1994). With a longer duration of smoking, the death rates of smokers increase substantially, so that during the second period of follow-up (1971–1991) the death rate of middle-aged smokers was three times higher than that of non-smokers (Doll *et al.* 1994). A similar excess mortality ratio was found in the second American Cancer Society Cancer Prevention Study (CPS-II) cohort based on follow-up in the latter half of the 1980s. These relative risks suggest that, on average, a smoker who begins smoking in young adult life and continues to smoke has at least a 50 per cent chance of eventually being killed by tobacco in either middle or old age (Peto *et al.* 1994).

The evidence from these two studies of the disease-specific risks associated with smoking is similar (Lopez 1999). Current smokers have about a 20-fold higher death rate from lung cancer than never-smokers, among whom lung cancer death rates have remained low and constant. There is epidemiological evidence to suggest that this is also the case in other populations. For example, based on the two American Cancer Society studies with follow-up to 1959–1965 and 1982–1986 respectively, lung cancer death rates among lifelong non-smokers were remarkably constant at 15.4 and 14.7 per 100 000 (age-standardized) for men, and 9.6 and 12.0 for women; the rates for current smokers were 187.1 and 341.3 for men, and 26.1 and 154.6 for women (Thun *et al.* 1997). Smokers also incur a 10- to 20-fold excess mortality from chronic obstructive lung disease (primarily chronic bronchitis and emphysema), and a risk of death from major vascular diseases that is about twice that of non-smokers.

The excess mortality of smokers from vascular disease is particularly noteworthy. Vascular disease death rates are typically much higher than those for cancer or other causes associated with smoking. Therefore cardiovascular diseases (especially ischaemic heart disease and stroke) contribute more to smoking-attributable deaths at a population level than other causes, including lung cancer for which the relative risk is much higher, although this pattern will change as cardiovascular disease mortality declines. Finally, it is worth noting that the all-age excess mortality ratio of about 2 from cardiovascular diseases masks a very significant age gradient in relative risks. At younger ages (< 50 years), smokers have a five to six times higher death rate than non-smokers, with the relative excess declining with age. These data suggest that if a smoker dies from vascular disease before the age of about 50 years, there is a 70 to 80 per cent chance that death was caused by smoking, and that vascular disease is the chief mechanism through which smoking causes a threefold excess mortality rate in middle age (Parish *et al.* 1995).

Cigarette smoking is only one of several causative factors that produce disease. This is especially true for ischaemic heart disease where smoking interacts synergistically with other factors such as hypercholesterolaemia and hypertension to increase risk of heart disease substantially. Evidence suggests that the independent risk attributable to smoking is comparable with that of other major risk factors (USDHHS 1989). This interaction with dietary parameters probably explains the currently lower proportions of ischaemic heart disease attributable to smoking in populations such as China where low-fat diets have predominated (Liu *et al.* 1998).

Smoking by women also adversely affects reproduction. Smoking during pregnancy reduces birth weight by approximately 200 g on average (USDHHS 1990); the degree of reduction is dose-related. With successful cessation by the third trimester, much of the weight reduction can be avoided. Smoking also increases rates of spontaneous abortion, placenta previa, and perinatal mortality, and smoking during pregnancy is now considered to be a cause of sudden infant death syndrome. There is more limited evidence suggesting that smoking may increase childhood cancer incidence and congenital defects (Charlton 1996; SCOTH 1998).

Cigarettes have changed substantially over the last 50 years (USDHHS 1997). Filter cigarettes dominate the market, and tar and nicotine yields, as assessed by smoking machines, have declined substantially. Although tar and nicotine deliveries to smokers have little relationship to the machine levels (USDHHS 1997), epidemiological evidence comparing smokers of lower-delivery and higher-delivery products shows some reduction in risk for some cancers, particularly lung cancer, and for total mortality, but only a minor reduction for myocardial infarction (Peto *et al.* 1996; USDHHS 1997). Although rising relative risks of smoking have been documented across recent decades when the lower-delivery products came into widespread usage (Doll *et al.* 1994), this is due to a longer duration of exposure and not to a change in the hazard. For example, in the cohort study of British doctors, there was a substantial increase in mortality for smokers in the second 20 years of follow-up (Doll *et al.* 1994).

Health effects of passive smoking

Evidence on the health risks of passive smoking comes from epidemiological studies which have directly assessed the associations of ETS exposure with disease outcomes and also from knowledge of the components of ETS and their toxicities. Judgements as to the causality of association between ETS exposure and health outcomes are based not only on this epidemiological evidence, but also on the extensive evidence derived from epidemiological and toxicological investigation of active smoking. Additionally, studies using biomarkers of exposure and dose, including the nicotine metabolite cotinine and white cell adducts, document the absorption of ETS components by exposed non-smokers, adding to the plausibility of the observed associations of ETS with adverse effects.

ETS exposure of the infant and child has adverse effects on respiratory health, including increased risk for more severe lower respiratory infections, middle-ear disease, chronic respiratory symptoms, and asthma, and a reduction in the rate of lung function growth during childhood. There is more limited evidence suggesting that ETS exposure of the mother reduces birth weight and that child development and behaviour are adversely affected by parental smoking (Eskenazi and Castorina 1999; WHO 1999*b*). There is no strong evidence at present that ETS exposure increases childhood cancer risk.

In adults, ETS exposure has been causally associated with lung cancer and may also increase the risk of ischaemic heart disease. The association of ETS with lung cancer has now been evaluated in about 40 epidemiological studies. The most recent meta-analysis combined evidence from 37 published studies, and estimated the excess lung cancer risk for smokers married to non-smokers as 24 per cent (95 per cent CI, 13–36 per cent) (Hackshaw *et al.* 1997). Since 1986, other expert groups have also found ETS to be a cause of lung cancer in non-smokers (EPA 1992; California Environmental Protection Agency 1997; Australian National Health and Medical Research Council 1997; SCOTH 1998). Coronary heart disease has also been causally associated with ETS exposure on the basis of observational and experimental evidence (Glantz and Parmley 1995; California Environmental Protection Agency 1997; SCOTH 1998), although this is a more difficult relationship to assess. A meta-analysis by Law *et al.* (1997) estimated the excess risk from ETS exposure as 30 per cent (95 per cent CI, 22–38 per cent) at age 65 years. There is also evidence linking ETS to other adverse effects in adults, including stroke (Bonita *et al.* 1999), exacerbation of asthma, reduced lung function, and respiratory symptoms, but the associations have not yet been judged to be causal (California Environmental Protection Agency 1997; SCOTH 1998; Samet and Wang 2000).

Quantifying population-attributable mortality due to cigarette smoking

Estimates of the population-attributable risk for a given risk factor or exposure in a defined population are generally calculated using the classical attributable risk formula which relates the prevalence of exposure to the relative risk of death from a specific cause for those exposed compared with those not exposed (Levin 1953). While this may be theoretically correct, the practical application of this approach will always be difficult as observed population prevalence for any population is not an adequate representation of population exposure corresponding to an observed set of relative risks. For example, current smoking prevalence does not include other critical aspects of exposure to tobacco smoke such as duration, amount, degree of inhalation, etc., all of which affect relative risks for disease. From the point of view of relative risks, even if one has reliable estimates of smoking prevalence for a population, to what set of relative risks should this 'exposure' variable be applied?

Peto *et al.* (1994) have proposed an indirect method of estimating smoking-attributable mortality, which circumvents these theoretical difficulties with the attributable-risk approach. Their method is based on the assumption that the excess lung cancer rate(over and above non-smoker rates) observed in a population is the best indicator of cumulative population exposure to smoking hazards. A 'smoking-impact ratio' (**SIR**) is calculated as the relative excess of lung cancer in the observed population compared with the observed excess of smokers over non-smokers, calculated from the CPS-II follow-up for

Table 3 Estimated deaths caused by smoking in developed countries, 1950–2000

Mid-decade year	Men			Women		
	Deaths in mid-decade year	Percentage of all deaths	Percentage of deaths at ages 35–69	Deaths in mid-decade year	Percentage of all deaths	Percentage of deaths at ages 35–69
1955	447 000	10	20	26 000	<1	2
1965	793 000	17	28	70 000	2	4
1975	1 119 000	21	31	165 000	3	7
1985	1 369 000	24	35	317 000	6	11
1995	1 442 000	25	36	476 000	9	13
Total deaths caused by smoking (1950–2000)	52 million	20	30	10.5 million	4	7

Source: Peto *et al.* (1994).

1984 to 1988. SIR is then used to scale the relative risks from CPS-II in order to apply them to other populations. To allow for confounding, and in an attempt not to exaggerate the hazards of smoking, these 'scaled' relative risks are then halved and applied to the national cause-of-death data for those populations (all developed countries) where the assumptions of the method might be reasonably applicable.

The method is crude and somewhat arbitrary, but validation against national studies using the classical attributable-risk approach suggests that the results obtained are not implausible (Valkonen and van Poppel 1997). The advantage of the method is that it yields annual estimates of deaths from smoking by age, sex, and cause which have been calculated for all developed countries for the period 1955 to 1995 and published elsewhere (Peto *et al.* 1994).

A summary of the levels and trends of smoking-attributable mortality estimated from the application of the Peto–Lopez method to mortality data for developed countries is given in Tables 3 and 4.

Smoking is estimated to have been the cause of about 62 million deaths, mostly men (52 million) in the developed countries (Europe, including the former USSR, Australia, Japan, North America, and New Zealand) between 1950 and 2000. The annual mortality from smoking in the developed countries in 1995 was estimated to be about 1.9 million (1.44 million men and 0.48 million women), of which 1.2 million occurred in the established market economies and the remainder in the former socialist economies of Europe.

Estimates of current annual mortality from smoking in less developed regions are much more difficult to prepare, given the lack of representative and direct evidence from epidemiological studies on tobacco hazards. In view of the large background risks of lung cancer among non-smokers in many developing regions and the lack of reliable cause-of-death data, the Peto–Lopez method is not likely to be widely applicable in these countries without appropriate adjustment. The single exception is China where recent analyses of large

Table 4 Estimated percentage of deaths caused by smoking, sex, age, and major cause of death, all developed countries, 1995

Sex	Age (years)	All causes	All cancer	Lung cancer	Upper aerodigestive cancer[a]	Other cancer	COPD	Other respiratory disease	Vascular diseases	Other causes
Men	35–69	36	50	94	70	18	82	29	35	35
	70+	21	36	91	59	13	73	11	12	12
	All ages	25	43	92	66	15	75	14	21	18
Women	35–69	13	13	71	34	2	55	16	12	15
	70+	8	13	74	38	2	54	7	5	6
	All ages	9	13	72	36	2	53	7	6	7
Both sexes	35–69	28	35	89	65	10	73	25	28	27
	70+	13	25	86	52	7	65	9	8	8
	All ages	17	30	87	60	8	66	10	13	12

COPD, chronic obstructive pulmonary disease

[a]Cancers of the mouth, oesophagus, pharynx, and larynx.

Source: Peto *et al.* (1994).

retrospective and prospective evidence suggest that smoking is already killing about 800 000 people each year, mostly men (Liu *et al.* 1998). Data from a cohort study in Mumbai, India, found that all-cause mortality rates for smokers were higher than for non-smokers across all age groups in men and the difference was greater at younger ages. The relative risk was 1.39 for cigarette smokers and 1.78 for *bidi* smokers and there was a dose–response relationship. The relative risk among women in Mumbai, who were basically smokeless tobacco users, was 1.35. In this cohort, *bidi* smoking was as hazardous as cigarette smoking and smokeless tobacco also appeared to be related to excessive all-cause mortality (Gupta 1996).

Using a modification of the Peto–Lopez method, Murray and Lopez (1997*a*) have prepared estimates of smoking-attributable mortality for other developing regions. First, lung cancer mortality rates were estimated for each region, by age and sex, using methods reported elsewhere (Murray and Lopez 1997*a*). Next, the non-smoker lung cancer rates in each region were estimated on the basis of local epidemiological evidence, and the SIR in the Peto–Lopez method was adjusted (lowered) accordingly. These revised 'scalars' were then applied to estimated regional cause-of-death patterns in 1995 in the manner adopted by Peto *et al.* (1994).

To the extent that this method is reasonable for developing countries, smoking is estimated to cause about 1.6 million deaths each year in developing countries, half of them in China alone (Table 5). Most deaths in developing countries (1.4 million) occur among men, which is at least consistent with the sex differences in exposure described earlier. Annual mortality from smoking in developing countries is also much lower than in more developed regions, again a finding that is consistent with the observation that until recently cigarette consumption has been relatively low in much of the developing world. However, the pattern is changing rapidly. It is perhaps more relevant for public health to ask what the mortality will be in the future if current smoking trends persist than to estimate current smoking deaths (about 3.5 million) from past smoking levels. Based on projections of causes of death to 2020 and projections of lung cancer, Murray and Lopez (1997*b*) have estimated that smoking will cause about 8.4 million deaths annually by 2020, of which, on present trends, 6.0 million will occur in the developing world. Smoking is projected to be by far the leading cause of death in the world by the year 2020. A similar annual death toll has been forecast by Peto and Lopez (1990) using much cruder methods, with a prediction of 10 million deaths a year from smoking by about the late 2020s–early 2030s.

Summary

The tobacco epidemic undergoes four stages as it evolves within a country (Lopez *et al.* 1994). In the first stage, the prevalence of smoking among males is comparatively high, while among females it is low (about 15 per cent), which is largely because of sociocultural factors that discourage smoking among women. Death and disease due to smoking are not yet evident. In the second stage, the prevalence of smoking among men rises rapidly, reaching a peak of between 50 and 80 per cent. The proportion of ex-smokers is relatively low. Smoking prevalence among women typically lags behind that of males by 10 to 20 years, but increases rapidly. In the third stage, the prevalence of smoking among males begins to decline, falling to about 40 per cent by the end of this stage, which may last for several decades. The prevalence tends to be lower among middle-aged and older men, many of whom have become ex-smokers. Most importantly, the end of the third stage is characterized by an initial decline in smoking among females. There is also likely to be a marked age gradient in prevalence among women, with about 40 to 50 per cent of all young women being regular smokers but with relatively few smokers (about 10 per cent) among women above 55 to 60 years of age. Another characteristic of this period is the rapid increase in smoking-attributable mortality, which rises from about 10 per cent of all deaths in males to about 25 to 30 per cent within three decades. In middle age (35–69 years), the proportionate mortality of males due to tobacco is even higher (about one in three deaths). The tobacco-related death rate among women is still comparatively low (about 5 per cent of all deaths) but rising. In the fourth stage, smoking prevalence for both sexes continues to decline more or less in parallel, but only slowly, 20 to 40 years after reaching its peak.

History, structure, and conduct of the multinational tobacco industry

A distinguishing feature of the tobacco epidemic has been the role of major corporations—some of the largest in the world—in promoting smoking and, as a consequence, death and disease. This presents a

Table 5 Estimated number of deaths from tobacco by region, 1995

	Men	Women	Total
Developed countries	1 440 000	475 000	1 915 000
Established market economies	840 000	375 000	1 215 000
Former socialist economies of Europe	600 000	100 000	700 000
Developing countries	1 385 000	195 000	1 580 000
China	690 000	120 000	810 000
Other Asia and North Africa	500 000	40 000	540 000
Sub-Saharan Africa	90 000	5 000	95 000
Latin America and the Caribbean	105 000	30 000	135 000
World	2 825 000	670 000	3 495 000

Source: WHO (1997).

unique challenge for the public health community. The adversary is not only disease or natural forces. It also includes powerful corporations whose actions are antithetical to public health as discussed earlier in the chapter.

As the twenty-first century begins, these transnational tobacco corporations are increasing their global markets. While total consumption of cigarettes is falling in high-income countries, consumption in low and middle-income countries is increasing (Taylor *et al.* 2000).

Given the growing influence of the multinationals, an understanding of their history, conduct, and behaviour is essential to help guide strategies for tobacco control. In the mid- to late-1990s, the public health community gained an unprecedented view of the tobacco industry through the release of millions of pages of previously secret internal tobacco company documents. These documents were obtained primarily through pre-trial proceedings in lawsuits against the tobacco industry in the United States. Accordingly, the term 'industry' is used in this chapter to refer to the defendants in the United States lawsuits, i.e. the main United States cigarette companies and the BAT group of companies based in the United Kingdom.

The global corporate actors

While tobacco in diverse forms has been used since antiquity, the modern cigarette did not become a popular phenomenon until the twentieth century. Until the late 1800s, cigarette production remained a cottage industry. Then came the mechanical cigarette rolling machine—called the Bonsack machine, after its inventor—to replace the hand-rolling of cigarettes. With a dramatically increased production capacity, the first of the major tobacco corporations, the American Tobacco Company, took control of the United States market, and the modern tobacco industry began to come of age.

Indeed, since the beginning of the twentieth century, much of the world's cigarette market has been dominated by a handful of major corporations. In the early 1900s, the three major tobacco companies of the time agreed a pact to end their trade wars and to divide the world's cigarette trade. American Tobacco was to limit its trade to the United States, its dependencies, and Cuba. The Imperial Tobacco Company of Great Britain and Ireland agreed to limit its trade to the United Kingdom. British American Tobacco (**BAT**) agreed to take over the export business of the other two companies and operate in other countries around the world (*United States* v. *American Tobacco Co.* (1911), 221 US 106).

Decades of deceit

In the mid- to-late 1990s, millions of pages of previously secret internal documents from the files of the American tobacco companies (and BAT in the United Kingdom) were publicly released in the United States. Most of these documents—some 35 million pages—were produced by the tobacco companies in litigation in the State of Minnesota pursuant to multiple court orders. The documents paint a damning picture of an industry which, for decades, suppressed scientific research and information on the health hazards and addictiveness of smoking, manipulated the amount and/or form of nicotine to exploit the addictive potential of tobacco, and targeted marketing campaigns at youth. In 1995, the *Journal of the American Medical Association* (JAMA) devoted an issue (Volume 274, pp. 219–53) to some of the first disclosures of tobacco company documents (which came from a legal assistant who apparently stole several thousand documents while working for a law firm retained by the tobacco industry). It was concluded that the documents 'provide massive, detailed, and damning evidence of the tactics of the tobacco industry. They show us how this industry has managed to spread confusion by suppressing, manipulating, and distorting the scientific record' (JAMA 1995). It was also stated that 'analysis of these papers suggests that we would have seen a very different picture of tobacco use today if the group knowing the most about the dangers of tobacco use, the industry, had been honest with its customers ... We can only speculate how many lives would have been saved and how much suffering would have been averted' (JAMA 1995).

The tobacco company documents referred to in the following sections can be accessed at http://www.tobaccodocuments.org and http://www.tobaccoinstitute.com/documents.

The tobacco industry's public promises

In the United States, the tobacco industry was forced to confront the issue of the health hazards of smoking publicly in the early 1950s. The first solid scientific evidence on the health hazards of smoking to receive widespread public notice were epidemiological studies and mouse-back painting experiments (where the backs of mice were painted with tar condensate from cigarettes) in the early 1950s (Doll and Hill 1950; Wynder and Graham 1950; Wynder *et al.* 1953). These studies generated widespread public concern about the health hazards of cigarettes. Confronted with this evidence, and this threat to their business, the presidents of the leading United States tobacco companies met at an extraordinary gathering in the Plaza Hotel in New York City on 15 December 1953. This was the beginning of a concerted industry-wide effort to deny the health hazards of smoking and cover up the tobacco industry's own knowledge of the hazards. The tobacco company executives who met at the Plaza Hotel in 1953 viewed the problem as a public relations problem and 'as being extremely serious and worthy of drastic action' (*JH 000502*).

The industry leaders felt 'that the problem is one of promoting cigarettes and protecting them from these and other attacks that may be expected in the future', and that the industry 'should sponsor a public relations campaign which is positive in nature and is entirely"pro-cigarettes" ' (*JH 000502*).

On 4 January 1954, the tobacco industry took out full-page advertisements in every major newspaper in the United States. These advertisements were entitled 'A Frank Statement to Smokers' and stated (*CTRMN 11309817*):

- We accept an interest in people's health as a basic responsibility, paramount to every other consideration in our business.
- We believe the products we make are not injurious to health.
- We always have and always will cooperate closely with those whose task it is to safeguard the public health.

Over the years, the tobacco industry continued to renew the pledge set forth in the Frank Statement.

> We in the tobacco industry recognize a special responsibility to help science determine the fact. (*PM 1005136955*)
>
> In the interest of absolute objectivity, the tobacco industry has supported totally independent research efforts with completely non-restrictive funding...The findings are not secret. (*Tobacco Institute 0081352*)

> If our product is harmful, we'll stop making it. (*RJR 500324163D*)
>
> Since the first questions were raised about smoking as a possible health factor, the tobacco industry has believed that the American people deserve objective, scientific answers. The industry has committed itself to this task. (*B and W 670500618*)

The tobacco industry's public denials of the health hazards of smoking

Despite the pledges, year after year, decade after decade, the tobacco industry issued public statements creating doubt about the charges against cigarettes and denying that it has been proven that cigarettes cause any disease.

> There is no demonstrated causal relationship between smoking and any disease. (*B and W 670307882*)
>
> The deficiencies of the tobacco causation hypothesis and the need of much more research are becoming clearer to increasing numbers of research scientists. (*RJR 500015902*)
>
> The flat assertion that smoking causes lung cancer and heart disease and that the case is proved is not supported by many of the world's leading scientists. *RJR 500184776*)
>
> In our opinion, the issue of smoking and lung cancer is not a closed case. It's an open controversy. (*RJR 504638051*)

In fact, even as the twentieth century came to a close, some of the major players in the multinational tobacco industry refused to admit publicly that it had been proved that smoking causes any disease. In October 1999, Philip Morris publicly stated: 'there is an overwhelming medical and scientific consensus that cigarette smoking causes lung cancer, heart disease, emphysema and other serious diseases in smokers'. At the same time, the company stated: 'Cigarette smoking is addictive, as that term is most commonly used today'.

The tobacco industry's internal acknowledgement that smoking causes disease

In striking contrast to the tobacco industry's public statements, the newly disclosed internal tobacco company documents revealed that the tobacco industry had secretly acknowledged the health hazards of smoking. In fact, as early as 1958, most of the American industry apparently believed that smoking caused lung cancer. This was documented in a memorandum written in 1958 by three British scientists who visited the United States to meet top officials and scientists in the American tobacco industry. One object of their trip was to find out 'the extent in which it is accepted that cigarette smoke"causes" lung cancer'. Upon completion of their trip, these British scientists reported widespread acceptance of causation. In their trip report, they wrote:

> With one exception [an individual not affiliated with any tobacco company] the individuals with whom we met believed that smoking causes lung cancer if by 'causation' we mean any chain of events which leads finally to lung cancer and which involves smoking as an indispensable link. (*BAT 105408490*)

Some of the reasons for the tobacco industry's refusal to admit publicly that smoking causes disease were set out in a document written in 1980 by a tobacco industry lawyer. The document was written at a time when the BAT companies were considering changing their public stance on the issue of causation. The lawyer opposed such a change, and wrote:

> If we admit that smoking is harmful to 'heavy' smokers, do we not admit that BAT has killed a lot of people each year for a very long time? Moreover, if the evidence we have today is not significantly different from the evidence we had five years ago, might it not be argued that we have been wilfully killing our customers for this long period? Aside from the catastrophic civil damage and governmental regulation which would flow from such an admission, I foresee serious criminal liability problems. (*B and W 680051009*)

The tobacco industry's stance on addiction

The tobacco industry has also repeatedly denied that cigarettes are addictive and minimized the difficulties of quitting smoking. For example, in a 1988 press release, the tobacco industry stated:

> Claims that cigarettes are addictive contradict common sense... The claim that cigarette smoking causes physical dependence is simply an unproven attempt to find some way to differentiate smoking from other behaviors. (*Tobacco Institute 0019963*).

Once again, however, the internal documents show that the tobacco industry has long recognized that smoking is addictive. For example, a report of discussions with industry research directors in the 1950s, as the industry prepared to publish the Frank Statement, recorded among their conclusions: 'it's fortunate for us that cigarettes are a habit they can't break' (*JH 000493*). In 1961, a top industry scientist wrote: 'smokers are nicotine addicts' (*BAT 30108362*). In 1963, an industry lawyer wrote: 'Nicotine is addictive. We are, then in the business of selling nicotine, an addictive drug(' (*B and W 689033412*). In 1969, another industry scientist wrote:

> I would be more cautious in using the pharmic-medical model—do we really want to tout cigarette smoke as a drug? It is, of course, but there are dangerous F.D.A. [Food and Drug Administration] implications to having such conceptualizations go beyond these walls. (*PM 1003289921*).

In 1978, a tobacco executive wrote: 'very few consumers are aware of the effects of nicotine, i.e. its addictive nature and that nicotine is a poison' (*B and W 665043966*). In 1979, a tobacco executive considered the hypothesis that 'high profits...associated with the tobacco industry are directly related to the fact that the consumer is dependent upon the product' (*BAT 109872505*).

Again, one reason why the tobacco industry continued to deny publicly that smoking is addictive, despite these internal admissions, was to avoid legal accountability. As one internal document stated:

> Shook, Hardy [long-established tobacco industry law firm] reminds us, I'm told, that the entire matter of addiction is the

most potent weapon a prosecuting attorney can have in a lung cancer/cigarette case. (*Tobacco Institute TIMN 0107822*)

The tobacco industry's manipulation of nicotine

The internal documents also demonstrate that the tobacco industry intentionally designed cigarettes to exploit their addictive potential. While nicotine is a naturally occurring component of the tobacco plant, the modern cigarette is a highly engineered and sophisticated product in both manufacture and design. Decades ago, the tobacco industry began to control and manipulate nicotine in cigarettes in a variety of ways.

The tobacco industry has the capability of removing virtually all of the nicotine from the manufactured cigarette. However, it designs cigarettes to ensure that nicotine levels fall within parameters such that a sufficient dose is maintained for pharmacological and addictive purposes. As early as 1959, the tobacco industry noted the need to find the 'optimum offer' of nicotine to consumers, recognizing that lowering nicotine too much 'might end in destroying the nicotine habit in a large number of consumers and prevent it ever being acquired by new smokers' (*BAT 10009915*). By 1963, one tobacco company noted that 'Certainly, the nicotine level of Brown and Williamson cigarettes ... was not obtained by accident' and that 'even now ... we can regulate, fairly precisely, the nicotine and sugar levels to almost any desired level management might require' (*BAT 102630333*). Another tobacco company referred to the 'habituating level of nicotine' and asked 'how low can we go?' (*RJR 504210018*). At another tobacco company, scientists wrote 'we have shown that there are optimal cigarette nicotine deliveries for producing the most favorable physiological and behavioral responses' (*PM 2028813366*).

Another method developed by the tobacco industry to enhance nicotine delivery was to manipulate the form of nicotine by controlling the pH of cigarette smoke through the use of ammonia compounds. The introduction of ammonia or ammonia compounds in the manufacturing process can raise the pH. As the pH rises, the smoke becomes more 'basic' and results in an increased amount of 'free' nicotine, also referred to as 'free base' nicotine in the tobacco company documents. Free nicotine is more volatile and physiologically active than bound nicotine. As one tobacco company document explained:

> In essence, a cigarette is a system for delivery of nicotine to the smoker in an attractive, useful form. At 'normal' smoke pH, at or below about 6.0, essentially all of the smoke nicotine is chemically combined with acidic substances, hence is non-volatile and relatively slowly absorbed by the smoker. As the smoke pH increases above about 6.0, an increasing proportion of the total smoke nicotine occurs in 'free' form, which is volatile, rapidly absorbed by the smoker, and believed to be instantly perceived as the nicotine 'kick'. (*RJR 511223463*)

Tobacco industry scientists 'fully appreciated' that the addictive potential of a drug, such as nicotine, is enhanced if it is delivered to the brain more quickly (Hurt and Robertson 1998). For example, one tobacco company document states that 'free base nicotine is the most chemically and physiologically active form because it is most rapidly absorbed' (*BAT 500104402*). Eventually, almost the entire United States tobacco industry used some form of ammonia technology in some of their brands (Hurt and Robertson 1998).

The tobacco industry's targeting of youth

The tobacco industry is well aware of the fact that most smokers start smoking when they are young. In high-income countries, about eight of ten smokers begin smoking while in their teens. In low- and middle-income countries, most smokers start in their early twenties (World Bank 1999).

Publicly, the tobacco industry maintains that it does not want youth to smoke. However, the internal documents of the tobacco industry demonstrate that the tobacco industry has long recognized that the preservation of its market depends upon recruiting youth. As one document states:

> Younger adult smokers are the only source of replacement smokers... If younger adults turn away from smoking, the industry must decline, just as a population which does not give birth will eventually dwindle. (*RJR 501928462*)

Thus the tobacco industry documents are replete with discussions of marketing to youth.

> Evidence is now available to indicate that the 14 to 18 year old group is an increasing segment of the smoking population. RJR-T must soon establish a successful new brand in this market if our position in the industry is to be maintained over the long term. (*RJR 501630269*)
>
> To ensure increased and longer-term growth for CAMEL FILTER, the brand must increase its share penetration among the 14–24 age group which have a new set of more liberal values and which represent tomorrow's cigarette business. (*RJR 505775557*)
>
> Kool's stake in the 16–25 year old population is such that the value of this audience should be accurately weighted and reflected in current media programs. (*B and W 170052238*)
>
> The base of our business is the high school student. (*Lorillard 03537131*)
>
> Marlboro dominates in the 17 and younger age category, capturing over 50 per cent of this market. (*PM 2043828174*)
>
> It is suggested to develop a new RJR youth-appeal brand ... (*RJR 501166152*)

The tobacco industry's global strategies

The documents also shed light on the tobacco industry's global strategies and the industry's conduct around the world. Certainly, the tobacco industry views the world from a global perspective. As one internal document stated in a discussion of why a global strategy was needed for the industry to combat tobacco control measures: 'Experience tells us that no country is free from the influences of others in this area, and what is today's restriction in Norway could become tomorrow's in Malaysia' (*RJR 500629166*).

The American tobacco industry worked to achieve a common strategy throughout the world. One R.J. Reynolds document stated:

> It is recommended that RJR Tobacco International suggest to its overseas competitors that it would be beneficial for our Industry as a whole on a worldwide basis if a consensus could be developed on the Smoking and Health controversy... For historical reasons, the chief and earliest battleground for the Tobacco and

> Health controversy has been the United States. In the United States RJR Tobacco has more experience in this area than the other tobacco companies. We are therefore best equipped to take the initiative in trying to develop a common attitude among the various members of the worldwide cigarette manufacturing industries. (*RJR 500950279*)

The tobacco industry also set up a worldwide trade organization—known first as ICOSI and later as INFOTAB—to serve as an information clearing house and to ensure global co-ordination for the industry (*B and W 681510625*).

Another global strategy of the tobacco industry has been to attempt to thwart the tobacco control efforts of international agencies, such as the WHO. One document, in discussing the WHO, stated that:

> This organization has extraordinary influence on government and consumers and we must find a way to diffuse this and re-orient their activities to their prescribed mandate. (*PM 2021596422*)

Another document discussed the need to counter WHO activities aimed at combating youth smoking. The document stated:

> We need to identify the three countries in each region that the WHO will be targeting for special funding and muscle and, where it makes sense from a market standpoint, allocate the resources necessary to stop them in their tracks. We need ... a well-developed strategy for a number of issues to which the WHO has given priority status. Examples include ... juvenile smoking. (*PM 2500103969*)

Summary

As the multinational tobacco companies increasingly shift their attention to emerging markets, an understanding of the structure and behaviour of the tobacco industry becomes imperative as public health professionals attempt to fashion strategies to deal with a growing epidemic. These strategies cannot be formed and implemented in a vacuum. The tobacco industry is a major factor in the vector, and only by knowing its history and conduct—and taking measures to account for this—can public health strategies be effective. Thus a thorough understanding of the tobacco industry and its conduct will help tobacco-control efforts through regulation and legislation.

Tobacco control

The preventive potential for tobacco control to reverse the given forecast of a global tobacco epidemic is still high in many countries. We now have an improved understanding of the complexity of the tobacco epidemic, which will assist us to improve and activate interventions. The main focus of any strategy should be to prevent initiation of tobacco use, to promote quitting among the young and adults, and to eliminate non-smokers' exposure to tobacco smoke. Cost-effective strategies are available and have already been proved to make a positive impact in many countries. To build on those successes, a comprehensive tobacco control strategy can provide a road map for national and global action. In this section we explore the key components of a comprehensive tobacco control strategy that is applicable locally, regionally, and globally.

Components of a comprehensive strategy

A multifaceted strategy is needed to assure success of global tobacco control. The components of such a strategy will include (a) education and information, (b) legislative measures, (c) litigation, (d) economic measures, (e) cessation efforts, (f) crop substitution and diversification, (g) advocacy, and (h) administration and management. Also, it is essential that strong political support at a national level can be reinforced by supportive international agencies. Appropriate surveillance and evaluation mechanisms are essential to assess the effectiveness of specific interventions.

Education and information

Evidence about the addictive nature of nicotine, and other harmful effects of tobacco use, need to be widely disseminated. Consumers learn about the health effects of tobacco use in many ways. One is through published scientific and epidemiological research, which may be summarized in the media. They may also learn through educational initiatives, such as school and community programmes, through warning labels on the tobacco products, and through public information campaigns or counter-advertising. All of these have been shown to be effective to varying degrees.

School health education

Comprehensive school health programmes target multiple health risk factors, including tobacco, and combine education with public policy approaches. School-based tobacco use prevention programmes that teach skills to resist social influences to tobacco use can be successful if reinforced throughout the primary and secondary school years (USDHHS 1994). School antismoking programmes are widespread, particularly in high-income countries. However, not all programmes are effective. Success depends on adequate repetition and appropriate content. Results are optimal if they are accompanied by environmental measures such as mass media campaigns and appropriate legislative measures.

Warning labels

Warnings can have a positive impact on consumers, especially on starters and those contemplating quitting, if they are highly visible and provide specific information (USDHHS 1989). Some countries, for example Canada, have taken decisive action to set a new international standard for cigarette labelling. The Government of Canada proposed new regulations requiring tough messages and graphic full-colour images that cover 50 per cent of the front of cigarette packages. The warning labels provide detailed highly visible information about the magnitude of the health risks that smokers face and the practical steps that they could take to quit (Mahood 1999). Recent Polish evidence shows direct increases in awareness and reduction in consumption as a result of new warnings. In Poland, 3 per cent of male smokers and 4 per cent of female smokers reported quitting following the introduction of strong warnings (Zatonski *et al.* 1999). Similar evidence of the efficacy of warnings comes from South Africa (Aftab *et al.* 1999). Warnings may also be expected to have a greater impact in developing countries where there has been less education about tobacco risks.

Regulatory and legislative measures

Comprehensive regulation and legislation that prohibits advertising and promotion, smoking in public places, and underage tobacco

Cessation

Programmes that assist young and adult smokers t produce a quicker public health benefit. Smokers v age of 50 halve their risk of dying in the next 1 1990). In addition, the cost savings from reduced tc from the implementation of moderately priced an cessation interventions would more than pay for within 3 to 4 years (Wagner *et al.* 1995). Nicotine r increases the effectiveness of cessation efforts individual withdrawal costs. Yet, nicotine repla difficult to obtain in many countries, although evi it could increase demand for and effectiveness (Fiore *et al.* 1996). Under new proposals annou Kingdom government in December 1998, £60 mill available to set up a comprehensive service within Service to help people stop smoking. Proposals in week's supply of nicotine patches free to smoke (Anonymous 1998). Deregulation of nicotine re should permit governments to improve the success Such products are increasingly available in Wes they are much less available in developing countr

Crop substitution and diversification

Historically, tobacco is a highly attractive cr providing a higher net income yield per unit of l crops and substantially more than food crops. growing areas of Zimbabwe, tobacco is approxim profitable than the next best alternative crop. tobacco an attractive crop for more practical r global price of tobacco is relatively stable, th provides in-kind supports and loans to the farm perishable than many other crops, and the in delivery or collection (World Bank 1999).

There have been a number of experimental sc other crops for tobacco. However, there is no har Canada, that these schemes succeed. Crop subs place in broader diversification programmes, if tobacco farmers in their transition to other liveli 1999).

Advocacy

Advocacy for policy change is the cornerstone approach to tobacco control. The direction that t was set early. 'Tobacco is a killer. It should glamorized or subsidized,' said Dr Gro Harlem Br took over as Director General of the WHO in backed those words with immediate action. Initiative (**TFI**) was launched as a cabinet proje remit to negotiate the Framework Convention (**FCTC**)—the first set of legally binding rules d public health issue (WHO 2000*d*).

'Tobacco kills—don't be duped' is the leit 15-country media and non-governmental organi cacy programme, but it also emphasizes TFI's ba to expose tobacco industry tactics in subverting and public policy. Each of the 15 countries, w Brazil, Norway, Pakistan, Germany, India, and Ir insights to the FCTC process. The 'Don't Be D

access, coupled with limits on harmful substance, tar, and nicotine contents are discussed in the section below.

Advertising and promotion bans

Tobacco advertising and promotion activities stimulate adult consumption and increase the risk of youth initiation (USDHHS 1994). Children buy the most heavily advertised brands (USDHHS 1994) and are three times more susceptible to advertising than are adults (Pollay *et al.* 1996). In the light of these ubiquitous and sustained pro-tobacco use messages, counter-marketing efforts of comparable intensity are needed to alter the environmental context of tobacco use. Marlboro cigarettes are one of the most successful products in the world. Its advertising campaign is perhaps the most successful in history (Elliot 1995). Advertising associates smoking with independence, enjoyment, relaxation, health, vigour, and 'being cool'. The 'Marlboro man' is an outstanding and highly successful example.

Since 1972, most high-income countries have introduced stronger restrictions across more media and on various forms of sponsorship. A recent study of 22 high-income countries based on data from 1970 and 1992 concluded that comprehensive bans on cigarette advertising and promotion can reduce smoking, but more limited partial bans have little or no effect. The study concluded that if the most comprehensive restrictions were in place, tobacco consumption would fall by more than 6 per cent in high-income countries (World Bank 1999). Another study of 100 countries compared consumption trends over time in those with relatively complete bans on advertising and promotion and those with no such bans. In the countries with nearly complete bans, the downward trend in consumption was much steeper (World Bank 1999).

There are reasons to believe that young people are more receptive to advertising than are adults (Pierce *et al.* 1991; McCann 1992); hence an advertising ban may affect smoking incidence rates in the younger age groups more than it affects smoking cessation rates in adults. There is also growing evidence that the tobacco industry is directing increasing shares of its advertising and promotion activity toward markets where there is judged to be growth or potential for growth, including some youth markets and specific minority groups among whom tobacco use has been uncommon until recently.

Although Internet advertising is only a recent phenomenon, there are 50 million Internet access points at present around the world and growth to 500 million is expected by the end of 2000. Hong Kong has banned placing tobacco advertisements on the Internet. In Sweden, many use the Internet to purchase cigarettes by mail order from countries where prices are low. As companies advertise and sell tobacco products on the Internet, there is a need to ban this through a global process.

The European Union's ban on tobacco advertising and promotion in the 15-country European Union has been a successful milestone. In 1998, the European Commission adopted a directive stipulating that all direct and indirect advertising (including sponsorship) of tobacco products will be banned within the European Union, with full and final enforcement of all provisions by October 2006. The key points of the directive, which is now under implementation, are as follows.

- All member states of the European union must introduce national legislation by 30 July 2001.
- All advertisements in the print media must cease within one further year.
- Sponsorship (with the exception of events or activities organized at a global level) must cease with two further years.
- Tobacco sponsorship of world events, such as Formula One motor racing, may continue for a further 3 years, but must end by October 2006.
- Product information is allowed at points of sale.
- Tobacco trade publications may carry tobacco advertising.
- Third-country publications, not intended specifically for the European Union market, are not affected by the ban.

Clean indoor air laws

Clean indoor air laws in public places are important because they protect non-smokers from exposure to tobacco smoke, reduce smoker's consumption of cigarettes, and induce some smokers to quit (Brownson *et al.* 1997; Chapman *et al.* 1999). Many countries are implementing restrictions on smoking in public places such as public buildings, restaurants, schools, day-care centres, and transport facilities. Clean indoor air policies alter tobacco use behaviour in young adults. Chaloupka and Wechsler (1997) found that relatively strong restrictions on smoking in public places discourage college students from smoking. Evans *et al.* (1999) found that workplace smoking bans reduce smoking prevalence by 4 to 6 per cent and average daily consumption among smokers by 10 per cent. Furthermore, they found that workplace smoking bans have the largest impact on staff who work longer weeks and the smallest impact on part-time workers.

Youth access laws

Youth access laws limit the supply of tobacco products to youths who are too young to comprehend the risks of consuming tobacco products. Youth access laws are designed to limit the availability of tobacco to minors from commercial sources (stores, pharmacies, vending machines, samples from distributors). The rationale for governments enacting youth access restrictions rests primarily on the fact that minors should be protected from the inherent dangers of tobacco as they do not know how to access or accurately appreciate the risks of becoming addicted to nicotine (USDHHS 1994). Jurisdiction attempts to prohibit the sale of cigarettes to minors by establishing minimum age-at-sale laws, banning self-service displays, limiting vending machines to adult-only locations or banning them completely, banning the sale of loose cigarettes, and outlawing the distribution of free samples to minors. Additionally, some jurisdictions require retail vendors to be licensed to sell tobacco products, and some laws include revocation of the license if retailers repeatedly violate minimum age-at-sale laws. In general, youth restrictions are difficult to enforce, because youths often obtain cigarettes from their older peers and sometimes from their parents. There have been several unsuccessful attempts to impose restrictions on the sale of cigarettes to teenagers in many developed countries. In many developing countries where tobacco consumption is rising, the infrastructure and resources needed to implement and enforce such restrictions are not available.

The literature provides mixed evidence on the effectiveness of youth access laws in reducing youth smoking prevalence. Retailer compliance with laws prohibiting sales to minors can be increased through active enforcement (DiFranza and Brown 1992; Cummings *et al.* 1998; Forster and Wolfson 1998), educational interventions (Altman *et al.* 1991; Feighery *et al.* 1991; Gemson *et al.* 1998), and community involvement (Forster *et al.* 1998). Forster and Wolfson

al. 1996) had its origins in the long tradition of ethnography, community research, and outreach to drug users by researchers at the University of Chicago. In this particular project, ex-addicts, under the supervision of trained ethnographers, conducted outreach to IDUs not in treatment. Specific efforts were made to enrol influential persons (indigenous leaders) within drug-use networks into the project, and have them act to influence other IDUs to practice safer injection. This project thus utilized the naturally occurring social structure among IDUs to change HIV risk behaviours. A cohort research design was used, with subjects followed for 5 years. The subjects reported dramatic reductions in injection risk behaviour. At the start of the project, 95 per cent of subjects reported engaging in injection risk behaviour, and this declined to only 15 per cent of the subjects reporting injection risk behaviour in the fifth year of the study. (HIV incidence among subjects in this study is discussed below.)

One of the New York NADR projects involved 'self-organization' among IDUs (Friedman *et al.* 1992, 1993). The Dutch 'Junkie Bonds'—one of which had initiated the first syringe exchange programme in Holland—served as a model for how IDUs can act together to further their own health interests. In the New York project, outreach workers recruited IDUs and assisted them in developing self-help groups to address HIV transmission and other issues of importance to them. In particular, the subgroup of commercial sex workers among IDUs had a number of common interests. Regular group meetings were held to discuss how the participants could change peer norms about injection and sexual risk behaviours. Attending the meetings was strongly associated with both the subjects' own risk reduction and efforts to change the behaviour of other IDUs (Friedman *et al.* 1993).

Broadhead and colleagues (Broadhead *et al.* 1998) have developed a 'peer driven' outreach programme for IDUs. Individual IDUs are recruited into the study and provided with AIDS education. These initial subjects are then asked to recruit other IDUs into the study, and paid modest stipends for their recruiting efforts. The initial subjects are asked not only to recruit new subjects, but also to provide AIDS education to the new subjects. An AIDS information test is given to each of the peer-recruited subjects, and if the newly recruited subject passes the test, the original subject who did the recruiting and educating receives an increased stipend.

Latkin and colleagues have developed an AIDS risk reduction programme that utilizes naturally occurring peer networks of IDUs (Latkin *et al.* 1996). Existing peer networks are brought in for multiple sessions that not only provide information about HIV and AIDS, but also attempt to develop new social norms within the peer groups. These new norms emphasize practising safer injection and safer sex. These efforts have led to substantial reductions in risk behaviours.

Social change theories do not necessarily replace 'AIDS education' and psychological theories of health-related behaviour. Knowledge of HIV infection and AIDS and how to practise safer sex and safer injection are still important, as are perceptions of risk and a sense of efficacy in practising safer behaviours. Given the continuing developments in HIV/AIDS research (such as new therapies), AIDS education must also be done on a continuing basis.

Social change theories offer important additional power for reducing HIV risk behaviours, however. Influencing others to adopt new behaviours can also serve to strengthen the intentions of prevention programme participants to change their own risk behaviours. If social norms about injection and sexual behaviour can be changed, then it will be possible to change the behaviour of IDUs who do not directly participate in the prevention programme. Finally, the peer approval that comes with following the new norms can itself serve to reinforce safer injection and safer sex practices among IDUs.

Individual knowledge and motivation to reduce HIV risk and social support for reducing HIV risk may be critical to successful HIV prevention among IDUs. Having the means to reduce risk is also critical.

Providing the means for behaviour change

Reducing HIV risk behaviour often requires providing or facilitating access to means for behaviour change. Reducing sexual risk behaviours often requires access to condoms, reducing drug injection often requires access to drug abuse treatment, and reducing injection risk behaviour often requires access to sterile injection equipment, or to means for disinfecting HIV-contaminated injection equipment. In many developed countries, increasing legal access to sterile injection equipment was an important aspect of initial efforts to reduce HIV transmission among IDUs. For example, in 1985, the city of Amsterdam rapidly expanded existing syringe exchange services (previously implemented to reduce hepatitis B transmission) (Buning *et al.* 1988). In 1987 the United Kingdom implemented a nation-wide system of syringe exchange programmes (Stimson *et al.* 1988). In 1987, France repealed its laws requiring prescriptions for the sale of sterile injection equipment and set up a programme for encouraging pharmacists to sell injection equipment to IDUs (Espinoza *et al.* 1988; Ingold and Ingold 1989). Australia repealed its prescription requirement laws in 1984 and then established a system of syringe exchange programmes.

In many European countries, such as Italy, Germany, and Spain, there were no legal restrictions on the sale and possession of injection equipment prior to awareness of HIV infection among IDUs, and education programmes were implemented to educate and encourage IDUs to inject with sterile equipment. Many of these countries have since established syringe exchange programmes as a means for providing face-to-face outreach efforts to IDUs and to provide for safe disposal of the exchanged (potentially HIV-contaminated) injection equipment (Lurie *et al.* 1993). Providing legal access to sterile injection equipment, through expanded pharmacy sales, syringe exchange, or both, is now a standard aspect of HIV prevention in almost all industrialized countries.

In the United States, there was also some early consideration of providing legal access to sterile injection equipment as a method for reducing HIV transmission among IDUs (Des Jarlais and Hopkins 1985). Early exchanges were implemented by activists in the northeast and by community-based organizations in the northwest (see Lurie *et al.* (1993 and Normand *et al.* (1995) for histories of early syringe exchange efforts in the United States). There were many impediments to providing legal access to sterile injection equipment for IDUs in the United States (Des Jarlais and Friedman 1992; Lurie *et al.* 1993; Normand *et al.* 1995; Gostin 1998). The states with large numbers of IDUs (e.g. New York, California, and Illinois) had laws requiring prescriptions for the sale of injection equipment, and almost all states had laws criminalizing the possession of equipment for injecting illicit drugs.

Efforts to increase access by IDUs to sterile injection equipment, either through changing laws and/or by implementing 'underground' syringe exchanges in defiance of existing statutes, often generated intense controversy over whether this would increase illicit drug use and/or represent official 'condoning' of it (Lurie *et al.*1993; Normand *et al.* 1995). In some areas, racial/ethnic group antagonisms compounded the controversies (Anderson 1991). There is, however, no evidence that programmes to provide sterile injection equipment to IDUs has led to an increase in illicit drug use (Normand *et al.* 1995).

In 1989, federal legislation was enacted that prohibited the use of any federal funds to support syringe exchanges or other distribution of sterile injection equipment to persons who inject illicit drugs. This prohibition remains in effect.

Given the legal, political, and funding difficulties in providing legal access to sterile injection equipment, there was an obvious need to find some other means to assist IDUs in practising safer injection. Based on ethnographic interviews with IDUs, the Mid-City Consortium in San Francisco (Newmeyer *et al.* 1989) identified criteria for possible disinfection of HIV-contaminated drug injection: the disinfectant should be strong and readily available, the disinfection procedure should be very quick, should not harm the injection equipment, and should not harm the injector if small amounts of disinfectant were injected. Of the various possible disinfectants, household bleach appeared to be the closest to meeting these criteria. Outreach workers began distributing small bottles of bleach with instructions on how to use the bleach as a disinfectant (two rinses of the needle and syringe with bleach, followed by two rinses with clean water). The use of bleach was readily accepted by IDUs in San Francisco.

After the initial success in encouraging IDUs in San Francisco to use bleach as a disinfectant, many other outreach programmes adopted bleach distribution. The great majority of the NADR/ATOM programmes included bleach distribution.

Bleach distribution has also been adopted in developing countries such as India (Hanzo *et al.* 1997) where there is strong political opposition to having health workers provide IDUs with sterile injecting equipment.

While there is no doubt that bleach is a strong viricide, and that bleach has been readily accepted by IDUs as a method of disinfecting injection equipment, there is mixed evidence as to whether bleach distribution is effective as a method of reducing HIV transmission. There have been three studies of the effects of practising bleach disinfection that used HIV incidence as an outcome measure. In Baltimore (Vlahov *et al.* 1994) and New York (Titus *et al.* 1994), the self-reported use of bleach to disinfect injection equipment did not provide any protection against incident HIV infection, while a protective effect was found in Miami (McCoy *et al.* 1994). The reasons why bleach has not been more effective have not been fully determined. It is possible that the small spaces within a needle and syringe protect HIV from exposure to the bleach (perhaps through the formation of clots) or that there is not sufficient contact time between bleach and virus when bleach is used in field settings. At present, bleach is distributed in many projects throughout the world, but the use of bleach is considered only as a fallback method of HIV prevention. Using new needles and syringes is strongly preferred.

There have been a series of summary evaluations of syringe exchange programmes, including ones conducted by the United States National Commission on AIDS (1991), the United States General Accounting Office (1993), the University of California (Lurie *et al.* 1993), and the National Academy of Science (Normand *et al.* 1995). All of these evaluations have concluded that syringe exchange programmes do lead to reductions in injection risk behaviour and do not lead to increases in illicit drug use. There are now a moderately large number of studies that have used HIV incidence as an outcome measure for assessing syringe exchange programmes. Almost all studies, including studies from Tacoma, Washington (Hagan *et al.* 1995), Lund, Sweden (Ljungberg *et al.* 1991), Glasgow, Scotland (Frischer *et al.* 1993), the United Kingdom (Stimson *et al.* 1991; Stimson 1995), Portland, Oregon (Oliver *et al.* 1994), and New York (Des Jarlais *et al.* 1996), have shown low HIV incidence rates associated with syringe exchanges. In all these studies except for New Haven, the estimated HIV incidence among syringe exchange participants was less than 2/100 person-years at risk. The New York study may show the strongest protective effect of participating in a syringe exchange against new infections with HIV. The relative risk of becoming infected with HIV among consistent users of the syringe exchange programmes was 0.30 compared with IDUs who did not use the exchange.

The low incidence rates in areas with syringe exchange programmes may occur through both direct and indirect effects of syringe exchanges. Participants in the exchanges receive both supplies of sterile injection equipment and counselling and information about HIV. Since syringe exchanges tend to attract IDUs who would otherwise be at very high risk for HIV infection, reducing risk behaviour among the IDUs who come to syringe exchanges can have a partial 'herd immunity' effect that protects the local IDU population as a whole. Sterile injection equipment, information about HIV, and new social norms against sharing injection equipment may also diffuse outward from IDUs who directly participate in syringe exchange programmes to other IDUs in the community. Thus large-scale syringe exchange programmes should probably be considered as community-level interventions, whose protective effect extends beyond the IDUs who participate directly in the programmes.

The great majority of the studies of syringe exchange programmes have shown low HIV incidence associated with the programmes. There are also several studies of syringe exchange programmes that clearly did not provide sufficient protection against HIV infection for either their participants or for other IDUs in the community. In both Montreal (Bruneau *et al.* 1994) and Vancouver (Strathdee *et al.* 1997), HIV incidence exceeded 10/100 person-years at risk among syringe exchange participants. The reasons for these high incidence rates have not been determined, but likely factors include that the exchanges attracted very high-risk drug injectors and that the supplies of sterile injection equipment were not sufficient to protect against HIV transmission within contexts of very frequent cocaine injection.

NIH Consensus Development Conference

The National Institutes of Health held a Consensus Development Conference on methods to reduce HIV transmission (United States National Institutes of Health 1997). The conference included both sex- and drug injecting-related HIV transmission. With respect to methods of preventing injection-related transmission, the conference found three methods to be effective: community outreach, access to sterile injection equipment, including syringe exchange and pharmacy sales, and drug abuse treatment. This Consensus Development Conference can be viewed as an excellent summary of the first decade of research preventing HIV infection.

Second-generation research questions

The initial research questions in HIV prevention for IDUs have been answered: it is clear that drug users will change their risk behaviour to reduce their chances of developing AIDS, and it is clear that specific HIV prevention programmes can be effective in reducing HIV transmission. The data to date also show that programmes to increase 'safer injection' among drug users do not lead to any increases in illicit drug use (Normand *et al.* 1995).

A 'second generation' of research issues has now come to the fore (Des Jarlais 1997). First, how do we explain the wide variation in the apparent effectiveness of different HIV prevention programmes? As noted in the discussion of syringe exchange programmes, participants in the great majority of programmes have had low HIV incidence rates. There are also several notable exceptions, such as the Montreal and Vancouver programmes. There is also meaningful variation in HIV incidence rates among participants in different community outreach programmes (Friedman *et al.* 1995). At present, the most likely explanations are in terms of background HIV seroprevalence and a dose–response effect. From standard infectious disease control theory, as the number of potential disease transmitters increases within a local population, the incidence of new cases will increase. (With 'all other things being equal', and with many 'other things'). The implication of this principle is that more prevention efforts will be needed for higher HIV seroprevalence populations. Dose–response relationships for HIV prevention work can be expected in at least two areas. The more health care workers that encourage social reinforcement for risk reduction, the more likely that risk reduction will be maintained over time. The greater the numbers of sterile needles and syringes that are distributed within an IDU population, the less the need for sharing of needles and syringes within that population.

How should HIV prevention services be integrated with other health and social services for drug users? HIV prevention services were a major innovation in the drug abuse field in that many of the services were delivered in the community. Outreach and syringe exchange programmes have often uncovered large unmet needs among drug users, including needs for drug abuse treatment and primary medical care. Many of the outreach and syringe exchange programmes have set up mechanisms for referring drug users to other health and social services. Some programmes, particularly syringe exchange programmes operating from indoor sites, provide a rather wide variety of services, from screening for tuberculosis to women's support groups. The impression in the field is that providing onsite services greatly increases the likelihood that the drug users will actually receive the needed services. Providing onsite services for many different sites, however, can become quite expensive.

The hepatitis B and hepatitis C viruses are also spread through the sharing of drug injection equipment, and both are considerably easier to transmit than HIV. Whether syringe exchange programmes that are effective in controlling HIV will also be effective in controlling the hepatitis B and hepatitis C viruses remains to be determined. There is some evidence that syringe exchange programmes can reduce hepatitis B and hepatitis C virus transmission (Hagan *et al.* 1995), but there is also evidence for unacceptably high rates of hepatitis B and hepatitis C virus transmission among syringe exchange participants (Hagan *et al.* 1999). Given the variation in the effectiveness of syringe exchange programmes in controlling HIV, it is likely that there is even greater variation in the effectiveness of behavioural prevention programmes for controlling the hepatitis B and hepatitis C viruses among drug users. There is, of course, a highly effective vaccine for preventing hepatitis B virus infection. Very few countries, however, have been able to mount effective programmes to vaccinate IDUs or persons at high risk of becoming IDUs.

Finally, and perhaps most importantly, there is the question of how to increase implementation of HIV prevention programmes for drug users in many countries throughout the world. In some areas, simple lack of financial resources and local expertise are the determining factors. In other countries, there is 'denial' that either HIV/AIDS or illicit drug injection will ever be problems in their societies. Finally, the first policy response to illicit drug injection is often limited to law enforcement, without consideration of public health aspects of illicit drug use. Even in countries such as the United States, where a public health perspective is sometimes applied to psychoactive drug use, law enforcement predominates.

Implementing effective HIV prevention programmes for IDUs on a public health scale will probably require adopting a policy perspective on drug use that emphasizes public health concerns, without permitting full commercial exploitation of the profits to be made in selling psychoactive drugs. (The distribution of nicotine in cigarettes may be taken as the prototype for commercial exploitation of the profits to be made in marketing an addictive drug.) The 'Harm Reduction' movement (Berridge 1992; Des Jarlais *et al.* 1993*b*; Heather *et al.* 1993) is presently attempting to develop and elaborate a policy perspective that would emphasize public health concerns for policy decisions on psychoactive drug use.

Conclusions

Alcohol and drug use, abuse, and dependence are complex and require careful conceptual and empirical consideration. Their consequences are profound, including the substantial social costs in terms of lost productivity and the transmission of HIV, the causative agent for AIDS. The persistent and dynamic nature of alcohol and drug abuse in the United States illustrates the difficulties in identifying and implementing successful approaches to reduce abuse, dependence, and related consequences. As indicated by the discussion of the role of drug use in the worldwide AIDS epidemic, these difficulties are not limited by country or culture. Basic cross-cultural research on underlying causes and consequences of abuse and dependence is needed so that prevention and treatment efforts can be better informed. The selection and evaluation of the prevention and treatment approaches for a specific country or culture must consider how the social, economic, and political contexts may influence the utilization and effectiveness of the approach.

In the face of a worldwide AIDS epidemic, fuelled in large part by the sexual and injecting behaviours of drug abusers, increased support for collaborative cross-cultural research and development of effective intervention is needed. Such efforts should accelerate our ability to combat the AIDS epidemic while generating more effective approaches to reduce the persisting problem of alcohol and drug dependence.

References

Aaron, P. and Musto, D. (1981). Temperance and prohibition in America: a historical overview. In *Alcohol and public policy: beyond the shadow of prohibition* (ed. M.H. Moore and D.R. Gerstein). National Academy Press, Washington, DC.

American Psychiatric Association (1987). *Diagnostic and statistical manual of mental disorders* (3rd revised edn). American Psychiatric Association, Washington, DC.

Anderson, W. (1991). The New York needle trial: the politics of public health in the age of AIDS. *American Journal of Public Health*, **81**, 1506–17.

Aneshensel, C.S. and Huba, G.J. (1983). Depression, alcohol use, and smoking over one year: a four-wave longitudinal causal model. *Journal of Abnormal Psychology*, **92**, 134–50.

Annis, H.M. (1986). Is inpatient rehabilitation of the alcoholic cost effective, Con position. *Advances in Alcohol and Substance Abuse*, **5**, 175–90.

Armor, D.J., Polich, J.M., and Stambul, H.B. (1978). *Alcoholism and treatment*. Wiley, New York.

Babor, T.E. (ed.) (1986). *Alcohol and culture: comparative perspectives from Europe and America*. New York Academy of Sciences, New York.

Babor, T., Cooney, N., Hubbard, R., *et al.* (1988). The syndrome concept of alcohol and drug dependence: results of the secondary analysis project. In *Problems of drug dependence, 1987. Proceedings of the 49th Annual Scientific Meetin of the Committee on Problems of Drug Dependence* (ed. L.S. Harris). Research Monograph Series 81, National Institute on Drug Abuse, Rockville, MD.

Bachman, J.G., O'Malley, P.M., and Johnston, L.D. (1978). *Youth in transition*. Vol. VI, *Adolescence to adulthood—change and stability in the lives of young men*. Institute for Social Research, University of Michigan, Ann Arbor, MI.

Bale, R.N., Van Stone, W., Kuldau, J.M., Engelsing, T.M.J., Elashoff, R.M., and Zarcone, V.P. (1980). Therapeutic communities vs. methadone maintenance. *Archives of General Psychiatry*, **37**, 179–93.

Ball, A.L., Rana, S., Dehne, K.L., *et al.* (1998). HIV prevention among injecting drug users: responses in developing and transitional countries. *Public Health Reports*, **113** (Supplement 1), 170–81.

Bandura, A. (1977). *Social learning theory*. Prentice-Hall, Englewood Cliffs, NJ.

Becker, M.H. and Joseph, J.K. (1988). AIDS and behavioral change to reduce risk: a review. *American Journal of Public Health*, **78**, 394–410.

Berridge, V. (1992). Harm reduction: an historical perspective. Presented at 3rd International Conference on Reduction of Drug-Related Harm, Melbourne.

Botvin, G.J. (1983). Prevention of adolescent substance abuse through the development of personal and social competence. In *Preventing adolescent drug abuse: intervention strategies* (ed. T.J. Glynn, C.G. Leukefeld, and J.P. Ludford), pp. 115–40. Research Monograph 47, National Institute on Drug Abuse, Rockville, MD.

Brecher, E.M. and the Editors of Consumer Reports (1972). *Licit and illicit drugs: the Consumers Union report on narcotics, stimulants, depressants, inhalants, hallucinogens, and marijuana—including caffeine, nicotine, and alcohol*. Consumers Union, Mount Vernon, NY.

Broadhead, R.S., Heckathorn, D.D., Weakliem, D.L., *et al.* (1998). Harnessing peer networks as an instrument for AIDS prevention: results from a peer driven intervention. *Public Health Reports*, **113** (Supplement 1), 42–57.

Brown, B.S. and Beschner, G.M. (ed.) (1993). *Handbook on risk of AIDS: injection drug users and sexual partners*. Greenwood Press, Westport, CT.

Bruneau, J., Lamothe, E., Lachance, N., Soto, J., and Vincelette, J. (1994). HIV prevalence and incidence in a cohort of IDUs in Montreal, according to their needle exchange attendance, Abstract PD0496, 10th International Conference on AIDS, Yokohama.

Brunswick, A.F. and Boyle, J.M. (1979). Patterns of drug involvement: developmental and secular influences on age at initiation. *Youth and Society*, **2**, 139–62.

Bry, B.H. (1983). Empirical foundations of family-based approaches to adolescent substance abuse. In *Preventing adolescent drug abuse: intervention strategies* (ed. T.J. Glynn, C.G. Leukefeld, and J.P. Ludford), pp. 154–71. Research Monograph 47, National Institute on Drug Abuse, Rockville, MD.

Buning, E.C., van Brussel, G.H.A., van Santen, G., *et al.* (ed.) (1988). *Amsterdam's drug policy and its implications for controlling needle sharing. Needle sharing among intravenous drug abusers: national and international drug perspectives*. Research Monograph, National Institute on Drug Abuse, Rockville, MD.

Chaisson, R.E., Osmond, D., Moss, A.R., Feldman, H.W., and Biernacki, P. (1987). HIV, bleach and needle sharing. *Lancet*, **i**, 1430.

Clayton, R.R. (1985). Cocaine use in the United States: in a blizzard or just being snowed? In *Cocaine use in America: epidemiologic and clinical perspectives* (ed. N.J. Kozel and E.H. Adams), pp. 8–34. Research Monograph 61, National Institute on Drug Abuse, Rockville, MD.

Cloninger, R., Bohman, M., and Sigvardsson, S. (1981). Inheritance of alcohol abuse. *Archives of General Psychiatry*, **38**, 861–8.

Cook, C.C.H. (1988). The Minnesota Model in the management of drug and alcohol dependency: miracle, method, or myth? Part I: The philosophy and the programme. *British Journal of Addiction*, **83**, 625–34.

Day, N.A., Houston-Hamilton, A., Deslondes, J., and Nelson, M. (1988). Potential for HIV dissemination by a cohort of black intravenous drug users. *Journal of Psychoactive Drugs*, **20**, 179–226.

DeLeon, G. (1984). *The therapeutic community: study of effectiveness*. National Institute on Drug Abuse, Rockville, MD.

Des Jarlais, D.C. (1997). Fifteen years of research on HIV and injecting drug use. Presented at 4th Science Forum: Research Synthesis Symposium on the Prevention of HIV in Drug Abusers, Flagstaff, AZ.

Des Jarlais, D.C. and Friedman, S.R. (1988). HIV infection among persons who inject illicit drugs: problems and prospects. *Journal of the Acquired Immune Deficiency Syndromes*, **1**, 267–73.

Des Jarlais, D.C. and Friedman, S.R. (1992). The AIDS epidemic and legal access to sterile equipment for injecting illicit drugs. *Annals of the American Academy of Political and Social Science*, **521**, 42–65.

Des Jarlais, D.C. and Hopkins, W. (1985). 'Free' needles for intravenous drug users at risk for AIDS: current developments in New York City. *New England Journal of Medicine*, **313**, 1476.

Des Jarlais, D.C., Friedman, S.R., and Hopkins, W. (1985). Risk reduction for the acquired immunodeficiency syndrome among intravenous drug users. *Annals of Internal Medicine*, **103**, 755–9.

Des Jarlais, D.C., Friedman, S.R., and Strug, D. (1986). AIDS and needle sharing within the intravenous drug use subculture. In *The social dimensions of AIDS: methods and theory* (ed. D. Feldman and T. Johnson), pp. 111–25. Praeger, New York.

Des Jarlais, D.C., Friedman, S.R., Novick, D., *et al.* (1989). HIV-1 infection among intravenous drug users in Manhattan. *Journal of the American Medical Association*, **261**, 1008–12.

Des Jarlais, D.C., Friedman, S.R., Choopanya, K., Vanichseni, S. and Ward, T.P. (1992*a*). International epidemiology of HIV and AIDS among injecting drug users. *AIDS*, **6**, 1053–68.

Des Jarlais, D.C., Choopanya, K., *et al.* (1992*b*). Risk reduction and stabilization of HIV seroprevalence among drug injectors in New York City and Bangkok, Thailand. In *Science challenging AIDS* (ed. G.B. Rossi, E. Beth-Giraldo, L. Chieco-Bianchi, *et al.*), pp. 207–13. Karger, Basel.

Des Jarlais, D.C., Friedman, S.R., and Sotheran, J.L. (1992*c*). The first city: HIV among intravenous drug users in New York City. In *AIDS: the making of a chronic disease* (ed. E. Fee and D.M. Fox), pp. 279–95. University of California Press, Berkeley, CA.

Des Jarlais, D.C., Choopanya, K. Frischer, M., Lima, E., Friedmann, P, and Friedman, S.R. (1993*a*). Cross-cultural similarities in AIDS risk reduction among injecting drug users. Abstract WS-D09-3, 9th International Conference on AIDS, Berlin.

Des Jarlais, D.C., Friedman, S.R., and Ward, T.P. (1993*b*). Harm reduction: a public health response to the AIDS epidemic among injecting drug users. *Annual Review of Public Health*, **14**, 413–50.

Des Jarlais, D.C., Friedman, S.R., Sotheran, J.L., *et al.* (1994). Continuity and change within an HIV epidemic: injecting drug users in New York City, 1984 through 1992. *Journal of the American Medical Association*, **271**, 121–7.

Des Jarlais, D.C., Marmor, M., Paone, D., *et al.* (1996). HIV Incidence among injecting drug users in New York City syringe-exchange programmes. *Lancet*, **348**, 987–91.

Dole, V.P. and Joseph, H. (1978). Long-term outcome of patients treated with methadone maintenance. *Annals of the New York Academy of Sciences*, **311**, 181–9.

Edwards, G., Gross, M.M., Keller, M., and Moser, J. (1976). Alcohol-related problems in the disability perspective. *Journal of Studies in Alcohol*, **37**, 1360–82.

Elliott, D.S., Huizinga, D., and Ageton, S.S. (1985). *Explaining delinquency and drug use.* Sage, Beverly Hills, CA.

Espinoza, P., Bouchard, I., Ballian, P., and Polo DeVoto, J. (1988). Has the open sale of syringes modified the syringe exchanging habits of drug addicts? Abstract 8522, 4th International Conference on AIDS, 12–16 June, Stockholm.

Etheridge, R.M., Hubbard, R.L., Anderson, J., Craddock, S.G., and Flynn, P.M. (1997). Treatment structure and program services in the Drug Abuse Treatment Outcome Study (DATOS). *Psychology of Addictive Behaviors*, **11**, 244–60.

Etheridge, R.M., Craddock, S.G., Hubbard, R.L., and Rounds-Bryant, J.L. (1999). The relationship of counseling and self-help participation to patient outcomes in DATOS. *Drug and Alcohol Dependence*, **57**, 99–112.

Farrington, D.P. (1985). Predicting self-reported and official delinquency. In *Prediction in criminology* (ed. D.P. Farrington and R. Tarling), pp. 150–73. State University of New York Press, Albany, NY.

Fishbein, M. and Ajzen, I. (1975). *Belief, attitude, intention and behavior.* Addison-Wesley, Reading, MA.

Flay B.R. and Sobel, J.L. (1983). The role of mass media in preventing adolescent substance abuse. In *Preventing adolescent drug abuse: intervention strategies* (ed. T.J. Glynn, C.G. Leukefeld, and J.P. Ludford), pp. 535. Research Monograph 47 , National Institute on Drug Abuse, Rockville, MD.

Flynn, P.M., Kristiansen, P.L., Porto, J.V., and Hubbard, R.L. (1999). Costs and benefits of treatment for cocaine addiction in DATOS. *Drug and Alcohol Dependence*, **57**, 167–74.

Friedman, S.R., Des Jarlais, D.C., Sotheran J.L., Garbar, J., Cohen, G., and Smith, D. (1987). AIDS and self-organization among intravenous drug users. *International Journal of Addictions*, **22**, 201–9.

Friedman, S.R., Des Jarlais, D.C., Neaigus, A., *et al.* (1992). Organizing drug injectors against AIDS: preliminary data on behavioral outcomes. *Psychology of Addictive Behaviors*, **6**, 100–6.

Friedman, S.R., de Jong, W., and Wodak, A. (1993). Community development as a response to HIV among drug injectors. *AIDS*, S263–S269.

Friedman, S.R., Jose, B., Deren, S., *et al.* (1995). Risk factors for HIV seroconversion among out-of-treatment drug injectors in high- and low-seroprevalence cities. *American Journal of Epidemiology*, **142**, 864–74.

Frischer, M., Des Jarlais, D. C., Green, S., *et al.* (1993). Modeling AIDS awareness and behavior change among IDUs in Glasgow and New York. Presented at the 9th International Conference on AIDS, Berlin.

Fuller, R.K., Branchey, L., Brightwell, D.R., *et al.* (1986). Disulfiram treatment of alcoholism. *Journal of the American Medical Association*, **245**, 1449–55.

Goodstadt, M.S. (1980). Drug education—a turn on or a turn off? *Journal of Drug Education*, **10**, 89–93.

Goodstadt, M.S. (1981). Planning and evaluation of alcohol education programs. *Journal of Alcohol and Drug Education*, **26**, 1–10.

Goodwin, D.W. (1985). Alcoholism and genetics: the sins of the fathers. *Archives of General Psychiatry*, **6**, 171–4.

Gorsuch, R.L., Abbamonte, M., and Sells, S.B. (1976). Evaluation of treatments for drug users in the DARP: 1971–1972 admissions. In *The effectiveness of drug abuse treatment.* Vol. 4, *Evaluation of treatment outcomes for the 1971–1972 admission cohort* (ed. S.B. Sells and D.D. Simpson), pp. 210–51. Ballinger, Cambridge, MA.

Gostin, L. (1998). The legal environment impeding access to sterile syringes and needles: the conflict between law enforcement and public health. *Journal of Aquired Immune Deficiency Syndromes and Human Retrovirology* **18**, S60–70.

Grant, B.E, Harford, T.C., Chou, P., *et al.* (1991). Epidemiologic Bulletin 27. Prevalence of DSM-III-R alcohol abuse and dependence: United States, 1988. *Alcohol Health Research World*, **15**, 91–6.

Greenspan, S.I. (1985). Research strategies to identify developmental vulnerabilities for drug abuse. In *Etiology of drug abuse: implication for prevention* (ed. C.L. Jones and R.J. Battjes), pp. 136–54. Research Monograph 56, National Institute on Drug Abuse, Rockville, MD.

Hagan, H., Des Jarlais, D.C., Friedman, S.R., and Purchase, D., and Alter, M.J. (1995). Reduced risk of hepatitis B and hepatitis C among injecting drug users participating in the Tacoma syringe exchange program. *American Journal of Public Health*, **85**, 1531–7.

Hagan, H., McGough, J., Thiele, H., *et al.* (1999). Syringe exchange and risk of infection with hepatitis B and C viruses. *American Journal of Epidemiology*, **49**, 203–13.

Hanson, D. (1980). Drug education: does it work? In *Drugs and the youth culture* (ed. E. Scarpitti and S. Batesman). Sage, Beverly Hills, CA.

Hanzo, C., Chatterjee, A., Sarkar, S., *et al.* (1997). Reaching out beyond the hills: HIV prevention among injecting drug users in Manipur, India. *Addiction*, **92**, 813–20.

Harwood, H.J., Napolitano, D.M., Kristiansen, P.L., and Collins, J.J. (1984). *Economic costs to society of alcohol and drug abuse and mental illness: 1980.* Research Triangle Institute, Research Triangle Park, North Carolina.

Hawkins, J.D., Lishner, D.M., and Catalano, R.F. (1985). Childhood predictors and the prevention of adolescent substance abuse. In *Etiology of drug abuse: implications for prevention*, (ed. C.L. Jones and R.J. Battjes), pp. 75–126. Research Monograph 56, National Institute on Drug Abuse, Rockville, MD.

Hawkins, J.D., Lishner, D.M., Jenson, J.M., and Catalano, R.F. (1987). Delinquents and drugs: what the evidence suggests about prevention and treatment programming. In *Youth at risk for substance abuse* (ed. B.S. Brown and A.R. Mills), pp. 81–133. National Institute on Drug Abuse, Rockville, MD.

Heather, N., Wodak, A., Nadelmann, E., *et al.* (ed.) (1993). *Psychoactive drugs and harm reduction: from faith to science.* Whurr, London.

Hewitt, L.E. and Blane, H.T. (1984). Prevention through mass media communication. In *Prevention of alcohol abuse* (ed. P.M. Miller and T.D. Nirenberg), pp. 281–323. Plenum, New York.

Hilton, M.E. and Clark, W.B. (1987). Changes in American drinking patterns and problems, 1967–1984. *Journal of Studies in Alcohol*, **48**, 515–22.

Hoffman, N.G. and Harrison, P.A. (1987). *Chemical abuse treatment outcome registry, 1986 report: findings two years after treatment.* Comprehensive Assessment and Treatment Outcome Research (CATOR), St Paul, MN.

Holder, H.D. and Blose, J.O. (1986). Alcohol treatment and total health care utilization and costs. *Journal of the American Medical Association*, **256**, 1456–60.

Holland, S. (1982). *Residential drug-free programs for substance abusers: the effect of planned duration on treatment.* Gateway Houses, Chicago, IL.

Huba, G., Wingard, J., and Bentler, P. (1980). Applications of a theory of drug use to prevention programs. *Journal of Drug Education*, **10**, 25–38.

Hubbard, R.L., Bray, R.M., and Craddock, S.G. (1986). Issues in the assessment of multiple drug use among drug treatment clients. In *Strategies for research on drugs of abuse* (ed. M. Braude and H.M. Ginzburg), pp. 15–40. National Institute on Drug Abuse, Rockville, MD.

Hubbard, R.L., Brownlee, R.F., and Anderson, R. (1988). Initiation of alcohol and drug abuse in the middle school years. *Elementary School and Guidance Counselling*, **23**, 118–23.

Hubbard, R.L., Marsden, M.E., Rachal, J.V., Harwood, H.J., Cavanaugh, E.R., and Ginzburg, H.M. (1989). *Drug abuse treatment: a national study of effectiveness.* UNC Press, Chapel Hill, NC.

Hubbard, R.L., Craddock, S.G., Flynn, P.M., Anderson, J., and Etheridge, R.M. (1997). Overview of 1-year follow-up outcomes in the Drug Abuse Treatment Outcome Study (DATOS). *Psychology of Addictive Behaviors*, **11**, 261–78.

Ingold, E.R. and Ingold, S. (1989). The effects of the liberalization of syringe sales on the behavior of intravenous drug users in France. *Bulletin on Narcotics*, **41**, 67–81.

Institute of Medicine, Committee to Identify Research Effectiveness in the Prevention and Treatment of Alcohol Related Problems (1989). *Prevention and treatment of alcohol problems.* National Academy Press, Washington, DC.

Jackson, J. and Rotkiewicz, L. (1987). A coupon program: AIDS education and drug treatment. Presented at 3rd International Conference on AIDS, Washington, DC.

Jaffe, J.H. (1979). The swinging pendulum: the treatment of drug users in America. In *Handbook on drug abuse* (ed. R.L. DuPont, A. Goldstein, and J. O'Donnell), pp. 3–16. National Institute on Drug Abuse, Rockville, MD.

Jessor, R., Chase, J.A., and Donovan, J.E. (1980). Psychosocial correlates of marijuana use and problem drinking in a national sample of adolescents. *American Journal of Public Health*, **70**, 604–13.

Joe, G.W., Simpson, D.D., and Broome, K.M. (1999). Retention and patient engagement models for different treatment modalities in DATOS. *Drug and Alcohol Dependence*, **57**, 113–25.

Johnston, L.D., O'Malley, P.M., and Eveland, L. (1978). Drugs and delinquency: a search for causal connections. In *Longitudinal research on drug use: empirical findings and methodological issues* (ed. D. Kandel), pp. 137–56. Wiley, New York.

Johnston, L.D., O'Malley, P.M., and Bachman, J.G. (1984). *Highlights from drugs and American high school students 1975–1983.* National Institute on Drug Abuse, Rockville, MD.

Johnston, L.D., O'Malley, P.M., and Bachman, J.G. (1989). *Drug use, drinking, and smoking: national survey of results from high school, college, and young adult populations.* National Institute on Drug Abuse, Rockville, MD.

Johnston, L.D., O'Malley, P.M., and Bachman, J.G. (1994). *National survey results on drug abuse from the Monitoring the Future study, 1975–1993.* National Administration on Drug Abuse, Rockville, MD.

Johnston, L.D., O'Malley, P.M., and Bachman, J.G. (1999). *National survey results on drug use from the Monitoring the Future study, 1975–1998.* Vol. I, *Secondary school students.* NIH Publication 99–4660, National Administration on Drug Abuse, Rockville, MD.

Kandel, D.B. (1980). Drug and drinking behavior among youth. *Annual Review of Sociology*, **6**, 235–85.

Kandel, D.B. (1982). Epidemiological and psychosocial perspectives on adolescent drug use. *Journal of American Academy of Clinical Psychiatry*, **21**, 328–47.

Kandel, D.B. and Logan, J.A. (1984). Patterns of drug use from adolescence to young adulthood: I. Periods of risk for initiation, continued use, and discontinuation. *American Journal of Public Health*, **74**, 660–6.

Kandel, D.B. and Raveis, V.H. (1989). Cessation of illicit drug use in young adulthood. *Archives of General Psychiatry*, **46**, 109–16.

Kandel, D.B., Kessler, R., and Margulies, R. (1978). Antecedents of adolescents' initiation into stages of drug use: a developmental analysis. In *Longitudinal research in drug use: empirical findings and methodological issues* (ed. D.B. Kandel), pp. 73–99. Hemisphere-Wiley, Washington, DC.

Kandel, D.B., Simcha-Fagan, O., and Davies, M. (1986). Risk factors for delinquency and illicit drug use from adolescence to young adulthood. *Journal of Drug Issues*, **60**, 67–90.

Kaplan, H.B., Martin, S.S., and Robbins, C.A. (1982). Applications of a general theory of deviant behavior: self derogation and adolescent drug use. *Journal of Health and Science Behavior*, **23**, 274–94.

Kaplan, H.B., Martin, S.S., Johnson, R.J., and Robbins, C.A. (1986). Escalation of marijuana use: application of a general theory of deviant behavior. *Journal of Health and Social Behavior*, **27**, 44–61.

Kellam, S.G. and Brown, H. (1982). *Social adaptational and psychological antecedents of adolescent psychopathology ten years later.* Johns Hopkins University, Baltimore, MD.

Kinder, B., Pope, N., and Walfish, J. (1980). Drug and alcohol education programs: a review of outcome studies. *International Journal of Addiction*, **15**, 1035–54.

Latkin, C., Mandel, W., Vlahov, D., Oziemkowska, M., and Celentano, D. (1996). People and places: behavioral settings and personal network characteristics as correlates of needle sharing. *Journal of the Acquired Immune Deficiency Syndromes and Human Retrovirology*, **30**, 273–80.

Laundergan, J.C. (1982). *Easy does it: alcoholism treatment outcomes, Hazelden and the Minnesota Model.* Hazelden Foundation, Duluth, MN.

Ljungberg, B., Christensson, B., Tunving, K., *et al.* (1991). HIV prevention among injecting drug users: three years of experience from a syringe exchange program in Sweden. *Journal of the Acquired Immune Deficiency Syndromes*, **4**, 890–95.

Lurie, P., Reingold, A.L., and Bowser, B. (ed.) (1993). *The public health impact of needle-exchange programs in the United States and abroad*, Vol. I. Centers for Disease Control and Prevention, Atlanta, GA.

McAlister, A.L. (1983). Social-psychological approaches. In *Preventing adolescent drug abuse: intervention strategies* (ed. T.J. Glynn, C.G. Leukefeld, and J.P. Ludford), pp. 36–50. Research Monograph 47, National Institute on Drug Abuse, Rockville, MD.

McCoy, C.B., Rivers, J.E., McCoy, H.V., *et al.* (1994). Compliance to bleach disinfection protocols among injection drug users in Miami. *Journal of the Acquired Immune Deficiency Syndromes*, **7**, 773–6.

McGlothlin, W., Anglin, M., and Wilson, B. (1977). *An evaluation of the California Civil Addict Program.* DHEW Publication ADM 78–558, National Institute on Drug Abuse, Rockville, MD.

Meyer, R.E. (1989). Who can say no to illicit drug use? *Archives of General Psychiatry*, **46**, 189–90.

Miller, W.R. and Hester, R.K. (1986). Inpatient alcoholism treatment: who benefits? *American Psychologist*, **41**, 794–805.

Moskowitz, J.M. (1983). Preventing adolescent substance abuse through education. In *Preventing adolescent drug abuse: intervention strategies* (ed. T.J. Glynn, C.G. Leukefeld, and J.P. Ludford), pp. 233–49. Research Monograph 47, National Institute on Drug Abuse, Rockville, MD.

Myers, J.K., Weissman, M.M., Tischler, G.L., *et al.* (1984). Six-month prevalence of psychiatric disorders in three communities. *Archives of General Psychiatry*, **41**, 959–67.

Nash, G. (1976). An analysis of twelve studies of the impact of drug abuse treatment upon criminality. In *Drug use and crime: report of the Panel on Use and Criminal Behavior*, Appendix. Research Triangle Institute, Research Triangle Park, NC.

National Institute on Drug Abuse (1989). *Highlights from the National Household Survey on Drug Abuse: 1988.* National Institute on Drug Abuse, Rockville, MD..

Neaigus, A., Friedman, S.R., Curtis, R., *et al.* (1994). The relevance of drug injectors' social networks and risk networks for understanding and preventing HIV infection. *Social Sciences and Medicine*, **38**, 67–78.

Newmeyer, J.A., Feldman, H.W., Biernacki, P., *et al.* (1989). Preventing AIDS contagion among intravenous drug users. *Medical Anthropology*, **10**, 167–75.

Normand, J., Vlahov, D., Moses, L.E., *et al.* (ed.) (1995). *Preventing HIV transmission: the role of sterile needles and bleach.* National Academy Press/National Research Council/Institute of Medicine, Washington, DC.

Oliver, K., Maynard, H., Friedman, S.R., and Des Jarlais, DC. (1994). Behavioral and community impact of the Portland syringe exchange program. In *Proceedings of the Workshop on Needle Exchange and Bleach Distribution Programs*, pp. 35–9. National Academy Press, Washington, DC.

Pentz, M.A. (1983). Prevention of adolescent substance abuse through social skill development. In *Preventing adolescent drug abuse: intervention strategies* (ed. T.J. Glynn, C.G. Leukefeld, and J.P. Ludford), pp. 195–232. Research Monograph 47, National Institute on Drug Abuse, Rockville, MD.

Pentz, M.A., Cormack, C., Flay, B., Hansen, W.B., and Johnson, C.A. (1986). Balancing program and research integrity in community drug abuse prevention: Project STAR approach. *Journal of School Health*, **56**, 389–93.

Pentz, M.A., Dwyer, J.H., MacKinnon, D.P., *et al.* (1989). A multi-community trial for primary prevention of adolescent drug abuse. *Journal of the American Medical Association*, **261**, 3259–66.

Petrakis, P.L. (1985). *Alcoholism: an inherited disease*, DHHS Publication ADM 85–1426, National Institute on Alcohol Abuse and Alcoholism, Rockville, MD.

Polich, J.M., Armor, D.J., and Braiker, H.B. (1981). *The course of alcoholism.* Wiley, New York.

Project MATCH Research Group (1993). Project MATCH: rationale and methods for a multisite clinical trial matching patients to alcoholism treatment. *Alcoholism: Clinical and Experimental Research*, **17**, 1130.

Rachal, J.V., Guess, L.L., Hubbard, R.L., *et al.* (1982). Facts for planning no. 4: alcohol misuse by adolescents. *Alcohol Health and Research World*, **6**, 61–8.

Robert-Guroff, M., Weiss, S.H., Giron, J.A., *et al.* (1986). Prevalence of antibodies to HTLV-1, -2, and -3 in intravenous drug abusers from an AIDS endemic region. *Journal of the American Medical Association*, **255**, 3133–7.

Robins, L.N. (1980). The natural history of drug abuse. Evaluation of treatment of drug abusers. *Acta Psychiatrica Scandinavica*, **284** (Supplement 62), 7–20.

Robins, L.N. and Przybeck, T.R. (1985). Age of onset of drug use and other disorders. In *Aetiology of drug abuse: implications for prevention* (ed. C.L. Jones and R.J. Battjes), pp. 178–92. Research Monograph 56, National Institute on Drug Abuse, Rockville, MD.

Robins, L.N., Helzer, J.E., Weissman, M.M., *et al.* (1984). Lifetime prevalence of specific psychiatric disorders in three sites. *Archives of General Psychiatry*,**11**, 949–58.

Rounsaville, B.J., Spitzer, R.L., and Williams, J.B. (1986). Proposed changes in DSM-III substance use disorders: description and rationale. *American Journal of Psychiatry*, **143**, 463–8.

Saxe, L., Dougherty, D., Esty, K., and Fine, M. (1983). *The effectiveness and costs of alcoholism treatment.* Health Technology Case Study No. 22, US Congress Office of Technology Assessment, Washington, DC.

Schaps, E., DiBartolo, R., Moskowitz, J., Palley, C.S., and Churgin, S. (1981). A review of 127 drug abuse prevention program evaluations. *Journal of Drug Issues*, **11**, 17–43.

Schaps, E., Moskowitz, J., Malvin, J., and Schaeffer, G. (1984). *The Napa drug abuse prevention project: research findings.* DHHS Publication ADM 84–1339, National Institute on Drug Abuse, Rockville, MD.

Schuckit, M.A. (1980). Self-rating of alcohol intoxication by young men with and without family histories of alcoholism. *Journal of Studies in Alcohol*, **41**, 242–9.

Scitovsky, A. and Rice, D. (1987). Estimates of the direct and indirect costs of acquired immunodeficiency syndrome in the United States, 1985, 1986, 1990. *Public Health Reports*, **102**, 5–17.

Sells, S.B. (1979). Treatment effectiveness. In *Handbook on drug abuse* (ed. R.L. DuPont, A. Goldstein, and J. O'Donnell), pp. 105–18. National Institute on Drug Abuse, Rockville, MD.

Sells, S.B. and Simpson, D. (1976). *The effectiveness of drug abuse treatment*, Vols 1–5. Ballinger, Cambridge, MA.

Selwyn, P.A., Schoenbaum, E.E., Hartel, D., *et al.* (1987). Natural history of HIV infection in intravenous drug abusers (IVDAs). Presented at 3rd International Conference on AIDS, Washington, DC.

Skinner, H.A. and Horn, J.L. (1984). *Guidelines for using the Alcohol Dependence Scale (ADS)*. Addiction Research Foundation, Toronto.

Smart, R.G. (1976). Outcome studies of therapeutic community and halfway house treatment for addicts. *International Journal of Addiction*, **11**, 143–59.

Spencer B.D. (1989). On the accuracy of estimates of numbers of intravenous drug users. In *AIDS: sexual behavior and intravenous drug use* (ed. C.F. Turner, H.G. Miller, and L.E. Moses), pp. 429–46. National Academy Press, Washington, DC.

Stephens, R.C., Simpson, D.D., Coyle, S.L., McCoy C.B., and the National AIDS Research Consortium (1993). Comparative effectiveness of NADR interventions. In *Handbook on risk of AIDS* (ed. B.S. Brown and G.M. Beschner), pp. 519–56. Greenwood Press, Westport, CT.

Stimson, G.V. (1995). AIDS and injecting drug use in the United Kingdom, 1987–1993: the policy response and the prevention of the epidemic. *Social Science and Medicine*, **41**, 699–716.

Stimson, G.V., Alldritt, L.J., Dolan, K.A., Donoghoe, M.S., and Lart, R.A. (1988). *Injecting equipment exchange schemes: final report.* Monitoring Research Group, Goldsmith's College, London.

Stimson, G.V., Keene, J., Parry-Langdon, N., *et al.* (1991). *Evaluation of the syringe exchange programme, Wales, 1990–91. Final report to the Welsh Office.* Centre for Research on Drugs and Health Behavior, University of London.

Strathdee, S., Patrick, D., Currie, S.L., *et al.* (1997). Needle exchange is not enough: lessons from the Vancouver injection drug use study. *AIDS*, **11**, F59–F65.

Substance Abuse and Mental Health Services Administration (1999). Summary findings from the 1998 National Household Survey on Drug Abuse. Office of Applied Studies, Rockville, MD.

Tims, F.M. (1981). *Effectiveness of drug abuse treatment programs.* Treatment Research Report, DHHS Publication ADM 84–1143, National Institute on Drug Abuse, Rockville, MD.

Tims, E.M. and Ludford, J.P. (1984). *Drug abuse treatment evaluation: strategies, progress, and prospects.* Research Monograph 51, National Institute on Drug Abuse, Rockville, MD.

Titus, S., Marmor, M., Des Jarlais, D.C., Kim, M., Wolfe, H., and Beatrice, S. (1994). Bleach use and HIV seroconversion among New York City injection drug users. *Journal of the Acquired Immune Deficiency Syndromes*, **7**, 700–4.

Tobler, N.S. (1986). Meta-analysis of 143 adolescent drug prevention programs: quantitative outcome results of program participants compared to a control or comparison group. *Journal of Drug Issues*, **16**, 537–67.

Turner, C.E, Miller, H.G., and Moses, L.E. (ed.) (1989). *AIDS: sexual behavior and intravenous drug use.* National Academy Press, Washington, DC.

United States General Accounting Office (1993). *Needle exchange programs: research suggests promise as an AIDS prevention strategy.* Report to the Chairman, Select Committee on Narcotics Abuse and Control, US House of Representatives, Washington, DC.

United States National Commission on AIDS (1991). *Twin epidemics of AIDS and substance abuse.* US Government Printing Office, Washington, DC.

United States National Institutes of Health (1997). *Interventions to prevent HIV risk behaviors. NIH Consensus Statement.* National Institutes of Health, Washington, DC.

Vlahov, D., Astemborski, J., Solomon, L., and Nelson, K.E. (1994). Field effectiveness of needle disinfection among injecting drug users. *Journal of the Acquired Immune Deficiency Syndromes*, **7**, 760–6.

Watters, J.K., Estilo, M.J., Clark, G.L., and Lorvick, J. (1994). Syringe and needle exchange as HIV/AIDS prevention for injection drug users. *Journal of the American Medical Association*, **271**, 115–20.

Wiebel, W.W., Jimenez, A., Johnson, W., *et al.* (1996). Risk behavior and HIV seroincidence among out-of-treatment injection drug users: a four-year prospective study. *Journal of the Acquired Immune Deficiency Syndromes*, **3**, 282–9.

10.3 Alcohol*

Robin Room

Drinking and its effects

Alcoholic beverages have been consumed in most, but not all, human societies since the beginning of recorded history. Beverages containing ethanol (C_2H_5OH) can be fermented from most organic materials containing carbohydrates, and in one part or another of the world are prepared from fruits, berries, various grains, plants, honey, and milk. Under most circumstances, such fermented beverages can range up to about 13 per cent ethanol in content. The most widely commercialized fermented beverages are beers prepared from barley or other grains (usually 3–7 per cent ethanol), apple and other fruit ciders (usually 3–7 per cent), and grape wine (usually 8–13 per cent). Other fermented beverages are also prevalent in particular cultures, often both from home production and in commercial form; for example, sorghum or millet beers in eastern and southern Africa, palm wine toddy in west Africa and the Indian subcontinent, pulque (prepared from the maguey cactus) in Mexico, and rice wine (sake) in eastern Asia.

Distilled beverages, where ethanol is concentrated by evaporation and condensation from a fermented liquid, were a Chinese invention which came to Europe via Arabia in the Middle Ages. In Europe, their use was primarily medicinal at first, but by the 1600s popular use as a social beverage spread rapidly. Distilled beverages can be almost pure ethanol, but as sold for drinking most distilled beverages contain between 25 per cent and 50 per cent ethanol. Distilled alcohol is also added to wine, producing 'fortified wines' with about 20 per cent ethanol. Since distilled beverages and fortified wines do not readily spoil, they could be shipped long distances even before refrigeration and airtight packaging were available, and played a particularly important part in commerce and exploitation in the age of the European empires. Cultures vary in the strength at which they consume different alcoholic beverages, with water or a 'mixer' often being added to distilled beverages, and in some cultures also to wine and other fermented beverages.

Use-values for alcohol

Ethanol has many uses in human life. These include non-beverage uses as a fuel and as a solvent. Important use-values as a beverage include use as a medicine, as a religious sacrament, as a foodstuff, and as a thirst-quencher (Mäkelä 1983). But alcoholic beverages receive special attention as a public health hazard because of their psychoactive properties. These carry with them another set of use-values: in terms of psychopharmacology, ethanol is a depressant, and alcoholic beverages have long been used to affect mood and feeling. With enough consumption, alcohol becomes an anodyne, and indeed an anaesthetic; distilled spirits were used as an anaesthetic in surgical practice before the mid-nineteenth century. Many drinkers seek and appreciate levels of intoxication which lie between mild mood-alteration, at one end of the spectrum, and being comatose, at the other.

Decisions to drink and how much to drink are, however, often not made by the individual in isolation. Drinking is usually a social act, and the pace and level of drinking is often subject to collective influence. Drinking together is often an expression of solidarity and community. While drunkenness may be sought to relieve misery or loneliness, more commonly drunkenness is associated with sociable celebration.

Adverse effects

Alcohol consumption can have a variety of adverse effects. Some are acute effects associated with the particular drinking occasion. Drinking progressively impairs physical co-ordination, cognition and attention, resulting in an increased risk of accidents and injury. Above a threshold level, drinking also potentially affects intention and judgement, so that intoxication potentially plays a causal role in violent behaviour and crime (Graham *et al.* 1998). This relation appears to be culturally mediated, since there is substantial variation between cultures in the association of intoxication and violence and crime (MacAndrew and Edgerton 1969). Enough drinking may result in a potentially fatal overdose, by interrupting various autonomic bodily functions.

Other adverse effects of alcohol consumption are chronic effects of a repeated pattern of drinking. Alcohol consumption potentially adversely affects nearly every organ of the body, although some effects are not common. Chronic conditions in which alcohol is implicated as an important cause include liver cirrhosis, cancers of the upper digestive tract, liver and breast, cardiomyopathy, gastritis, and pancreatitis (English *et al.* 1995). Through a variety of mechanisms, alcohol is also implicated in the incidence of infectious diseases (NIAAA 1997).

Repeated heavy drinking can also adversely affect mental health. There are specific neurological disorders associated with sustained heavy drinking. More common concomitants include depression and affective disorders. Alcoholism—the experience of loss of control over drinking, along with other psychological and physical sequelae—has

* Portions of this chapter are adapted from Chapter 4.2.2.6, *New Oxford Textbook of Psychiatry* (ed. M.G. Gelder, J.J. López-Ibor Jr, and N. Andreasen), Oxford University Press, 2000.

also been considered a mental disorder in modern times. In current nosologies, alcoholism has been replaced by the terms alcohol dependence (in the *Fourth Revision of the Diagnostic and Statistical Manual of Mental Disorders* (DSM-IV)) or the alcohol dependence syndrome (in the *10th Revision of the International Classification of Diseases* (ICD-10)).

The impairment of co-ordination and of judgement produced by drinking potentially affects bystanders and the drinker's acquaintances, friends, and family, as well as the drinker him- or herself. The effects can be through impairment of co-ordination or judgement in the drinking event, resulting in injury or distress, or through impairment of performance in family, friendship, work, and other social roles, from recurring drinking episodes. It is the actual and potential adverse effects on others which have historically been the primary justification for alcohol controls and other societal responses to problematic drinking (Room 1996). Effects of drinking on the adult drinker's own health have been much less important in determining public policy on alcohol.

Positive effects

For the drinker, and sometimes also for those around the drinker, alcohol consumption also potentially has positive effects. We have already mentioned the different use-values of alcohol—effects which mean that drinkers are usually willing to pay more than the cost of production and distribution for the beverage. Apart from its valued effects on mental state, alcohol also potentially has some positive health effects. By far the most important of these, in terms of public health, is its potential effect in preventing cardiovascular disease. A fairly consistent finding in studies in several societies is that drinking at moderate levels is protective against cardiovascular disease (Klatsky 1999). Studies vary in findings of the upper limit of drinking for such protection; for that matter, not all studies find the protective effect (Leino *et al.* 1998). Taking the studies together, it appears that most of the protective effect can be gained with as little as one drink of an alcoholic beverage every second day (Maclure 1993). While about half of the effect seems to come from inhibiting the build-up of plaque in arteries, the other half seems to result from a relatively immediate effect in diminishing the likelihood of blood clots. To the extent this is true, an irregular or occasional drinking pattern is likely to have less of a protective effect.

While it has been argued that the protective effect comes primarily from red wine constituents, particularly resveratrol, rather than from the ethanol, the balance of evidence presently favours an ethanol effect (Klatsky 1999). But relatively little is known about how the ethanol effect interacts or overlaps with other risk and protective factors for coronary heart disease, such as regular exercise, diet, or taking aspirin or other pharmaceuticals (Criqui *et al.* 1998). The protective effect of alcohol appears to be higher for current cigarette smokers than for non-smokers (Kozlowski *et al.* 1994).

Drinking is not always good for the heart (Chadwick and Goode 1998; Poikolainen 1998). Some studies have found that a pattern of intermittent heavy drinking, such as getting drunk every weekend, is associated with an elevated rate of coronary death (Kauhanen *et al.* 1997), probably through such mechanisms as heart arrhythmias (Kupari and Koskinen 1998; McKee and Britton 1998). Recent data from countries of the former Soviet Union, where a pattern of intermittent intoxication is common, support a strong adverse effect of binge drinking on heart disease mortality. In a period of deliberate restriction of alcohol supplies in 1985 to 1988, the estimated per capita consumption in Russia, including the illicit alcohol market, fell from 14.2 litres in 1984 to 10.7 litres in 1987 (Shkolnikov and Nemtsov 1997), a fall of 25 per cent. The male rate of deaths from ischaemic heart disease in the same period fell by 10 per cent. The rate rose again when the restrictions lapsed, although in this period, unlike 1985 to 1988, other risk factors were also changing.

Net effects of drinking on the drinker's health

In most studies, the relationship of amount of drinking to overall mortality is a J-shaped curve, with abstainers (and often also very light drinkers) showing a higher mortality than those drinking a little more. In studies with these findings, a substantial part of the study population is older adults, and thus at risk of cardiovascular disease mortality. Studies limited to younger cohorts typically find a monotonic relation of amount of drinking with mortality (Andréasson *et al.* 1991; Rehm and Sempos 1995). Such a relation might be expected, too, in any population, such as in some developing societies, which have a low rate of cardiovascular disease.

The pattern of drinking is also potentially important in mortality. While this has long been obvious for casualty deaths, there is growing recognition of its potential importance also for other causes of death, as the Russian data just cited imply. But pattern of drinking has been little measured in the studies of alcohol and overall mortality. Variations between cultures in patterns of drinking may well partly explain why the J-curve relation of volume of drinking with mortality shows different low-points in different cultures.

The risks and potential benefits associated with a given drinking level thus vary with the age and sex of the drinker, and potentially with other sociocultural characteristics, as well as with the pattern and contexts of drinking. This has posed a considerable challenge when the political demand has arisen in a number of countries for guidance on 'low-risk drinking' or 'safe drinking' guidelines (Hawks 1994). While earlier guidelines tended to be stated in terms of volume of drinking, in line with the measurement methods of the medical epidemiology literature, more recent guidelines have also emphasized limits on the amount on an occasion or day (Bondy *et al.* 1999).

The current literature on the net effects of drinking on health relies substantially on summations of the prospective epidemiological literature such as that of English *et al.* (1995). Using meta-analyses of studies of the relation of volume of drinking to specific causes of death where alcohol was a risk or protective factor, English and coworkers derived attributable fractions for different levels of volume of drinking, and applied these to proportions of the population at different volumes of drinking to arrive at estimates of total lives and life-years lost and gained (Holman and English 1995). Reflecting the underlying literature that the study meta-analyses, the resulting estimates are based on a relatively narrow range of societies, and take no account of patterns of drinking. The method relies on an assumption which is thus problematic, that there is a single invariant mortality effect for a given range of volumes of drinking.

Drawing on the work of English and coworkers, but factoring in the estimated effects of intoxication as well as volume of drinking, Murray and Lopez (1996) have estimated the share attributable to alcohol of the global burden of disease. In these estimates, the projected protective effects of alcohol are subtracted from the negative burden. In addition to years of life lost, the study's most comprehensive indicator, disability-adjusted life-years (**DALYs**), includes a projection of the burden of disability attributable to alcohol.

According to the global burden of disease estimates, 3.5 per cent of the total burden of disease globally, as measured in DALYs, is attributable to alcohol (Murray and Lopez 1996). This compares with 2.6 per cent for tobacco and 0.6 per cent for illicit drugs. The alcohol share of the burden is highest in developed societies, and high also in Latin America and Eastern Europe. Although the alcohol share in all DALYs is lower in other developing regions, this fraction is calculated on the base of a higher total burden of disease and disability there. While the global burden of disease estimates must be regarded as a first rough-cut that will be refined in future, they do indicate that the global health burden attributable to alcohol is very substantial.

Net effects on the population level

Thus far we have been dealing with estimates of alcohol's effects based on individual-level data. The methodological difficulties in the studies underlying these estimates extend beyond those we have already discussed (Edwards *et al.* 1994). The estimates rely primarily on prospective epidemiological studies with alcohol consumption measured at one time-point; such a measurement is at best a poor surrogate for either of the main aspects of alcohol consumption as a risk factor—chronic effects of cumulated alcohol consumption or acute effects of intoxication in a specific event. In these studies, the effects of possible confounders are dealt with by statistically controlling for them in the analysis. But this can be problematic, if drinking and the potential confounder are causally intertwined, as for instance is true for hypertension or tobacco smoking. Consider, for instance, a person who only smokes when under the influence of alcohol; controlling for that person's smoking behaviour potentially controls out some of the alcohol effect.

From a public health perspective, it is the effects on the population level rather than the individual level which are the main concern. If drinking were entirely a matter of individual choice and behaviour, and if the effects of drinking happened only to the drinker, then effects at the population level would be a simple aggregation of effects at the individual level. But neither of these conditions is applicable. Drinking is in large part a social activity, and the drinking behaviour of one person is likely to influence and be influenced by those around the person. In a given population the amounts drunk by infrequent or light drinkers and by heavy drinkers tend to move up and down in concert. Thus, if there is some health gain when those at the bottom of the consumption spectrum increase their consumption, there will be health losses from an increase in consumption, too, at the top of the consumption spectrum. In view of this, it has been argued that the level of per-drinker consumption where the balance of health benefits and losses is optimized in a population is likely to be considerably lower than the optimum level of consumption for the individual drinker (Skog 1996). Skog argued, for instance, that the optimum level of alcohol consumption with respect to mortality was likely to be lower than the present-day per-capita consumption of any nation in Western Europe. His argument has recently been supported by the finding of a generally positive relationship with total mortality in time-series analysis of differenced data in 14 European countries (Norström 2001).

By their design, the prospective studies typically used for studies of alcohol's effects on mortality or morbidity do not measure the effects of drinking on others. Other types of individual-level studies, for instance of the effects of drinking–driving (Perrine *et al.* 1989) or studies of homicide and other crimes (Wolfgang 1958), document the importance of such effects in terms of death or injury. But the strongest evidence of the magnitude of such effects comes from aggregate-level studies of the covariation of changes over time in a given society or place. Differenced time-series analyses in European societies have suggested that a 1-litre change in per capita alcohol consumption produces about a 1 per cent change in the overall mortality rate (Norström 1996; Her and Rehm 1998). Here again, however, drinking patterns and social circumstances are likely to make a difference. The drop in Russian total mortality during the alcohol restrictions of 1985 to 1988, for instance, implies a decline of about 2.7 per cent in age-standardized mortality for each 1-litre drop in per capita consumption (recalculated from Shkolnikov and Nemtsov (1997) and Leon *et al.* (1998)). Even specifically for heart disease, any protective effects from changes in low-level drinking seem to be outbalanced in the population as a whole by negative effects from changes at high consumption levels, at levels of consumption typical in developed societies. Thus a time-series analysis of differenced data on coronary heart disease mortality in 14 European countries found positive and mostly significant relationships (Hemström 2001).

Alcohol as an issue in public health

Shifting societal responses to problematic drinking

Efforts to control problematic drinking date back to the beginning of recorded history. These efforts have been many-sided, including informal responses in the family and community, as well as governmental controls. Religious teachings and movements have often been directed against drinking or intoxication. Thus Muslims are forbidden by their faith to drink at all, and drinking is also discouraged or forbidden in at least some branches of all the major world religions.

In the last few centuries, European and Europe-derived societies have been hosts to conflicting trends in terms of alcohol issues. On the one hand, the production of alcoholic beverages became an important part of European economies, and of imperial domination and trade in the age of European colonization. Alcohol production and exports took on political importance not only in the wine cultures of southern Europe, but also in such countries as The Netherlands and Britain. In the British colonies in America in the late eighteenth century distilled spirits was the only profitable way to get grain to market (Rorabaugh 1979). In recent decades, alcohol beverage industries have become increasingly internationalized and concentrated (Jernigan 1997), and multinational companies, mostly based in Europe or North America, have pressed with considerable success to open up global markets for alcohol.

Starting in the early 1800s, there were substantial waves of popular and eventually governmental response to the problems which were resulting from the very heavy consumption of alcoholic beverages in English-speaking and northern European societies (Blocker 1989; Levine 1991). As a culmination of decades of popular temperance movements, in the early twentieth century alcohol prohibition was adopted in many of these countries, and stringent controls on the availability of alcohol in others. While alcohol's impact on public order and morals and on family life were more central to temperance movement thinking than public health issues, mainstream thought in medicine and public health acknowledged substantial adverse impacts of alcohol on health (Emerson 1932), and prohibition or an alternative, stringent control on the availability of alcohol (Catlin 1931), were often identified with the public health interest.

In the United States and other societies which had adopted alcohol prohibition, there was a strong reaction against it by the early 1930s, with middle-class youth in the lead (Room 1984*a,b*). In this cultural–political context, as the new generation moved into professional and research positions, adverse effects of alcohol were downplayed or denied (Herd 1992; Katcher 1993), and alcohol issues almost disappeared from view in public health textbooks and discourse. Any problems with drinking were seen as attributable to a relatively small cadre of alcoholics, unable to control their drinking because of a mysterious predisposing factor. As late as 1968, the main emphasis of the American Public Health Association in the alcohol field was on building treatment capacity for alcoholism (Cross 1968).

The 'new public health' approach

The last three decades of the twentieth century saw the rise of what has been termed in the alcohol literature the 'new public health' approach (Beauchamp 1976; Tigerstedt 1999) to alcohol issues. The approach brought together several strands of research and thinking. In contrast to a concept of the field in terms of 'alcoholism', the approach was premised on a disaggregated approach: there were a diversity of alcohol-related problems, fairly widely distributed among the population of drinkers (Knupfer 1967; WHO 1980). It was noted that for many problems, the heaviest drinkers accounted for only a minority of the instances of problems, since there were so many more drinking at somewhat lower levels (Moore and Gerstein 1981, pp. 30–2); picking up Rose's phrase (Rose 1981), Kreitman (1986) termed this the 'preventive paradox'. Attention was thus paid not just to the heaviest consumers, but to the whole range of drinking levels, and indeed to the distribution of consumption in the population (Ledermann 1956; de Lint and Schmidt 1968). What happens with moderate drinkers, it was argued, influences the social climate for heavy drinking, since drinking is largely a social activity, marked by mutual influences and norms of reciprocity (Bruun *et al.* 1975*a*, p. 39; Skog 1985). In a given population, it was found that rates of alcohol-related problems tend to rise and fall with changes in the level of alcohol consumption (Seeley 1960). Controls on the availability of alcohol, including taxes, affect the level of consumption, and thus also rates of alcohol-related problems (Seeley 1960; Terris 1967; Popham *et al.* 1976). The level of alcohol consumption in a population, and controls on alcohol availability, thus are seen as a public health concern, and part of a society's overall 'alcohol policy' (Bruun *et al.* 1975*a*).

In enumerating the elements of the 'new public health' approach, we have given references for early statements of each element. It will be seen that the strands of the approach were woven together gradually over a period of some years. A 1975 report by an international group of researchers (Bruun *et al.* 1975*a*) became a pivotal document for the approach. A few years later, the approach was given an authoritative endorsement in the United States by a committee of the National Academy of Sciences (Moore and Gerstein 1981). The most recent restatement of the approach by an international group of scholars appeared in 1994 (Edwards *et al.* 1994).

The approach has had considerable influence in WHO programmes in the alcohol field, particularly in the European Region (WHO 1980; Anonymous 1996). At national levels, there has been considerable variation in its influence on policy. In Sweden, where it is known as the 'total consumption' model, it attained hegemony as the basis of official policy (Sutton 1998). However, there is now considerable antipathy to the model in Swedish public discourse, and high-tax and other alcohol control policies based on it are being eroded as a consequence of Sweden's accession to the European Union (Holder *et al.* 1998). The approach also has had considerable currency in other Nordic countries.

In English-speaking countries, the approach has encountered substantial resistance in the cultural–political realm. Those allied with alcoholic beverage industry interests have strongly attacked the approach, both in analyses and polemics (Mott 1991; Grant and Litvak 1998) and through direct political action to remove official proponents (Room 1984*c*). An approach which contemplates government regulation and influence on private consumer choices is also unwelcome to those committed to consumer sovereignty and the primacy of individual choice (Peele 1987). Often, proponents of approaches seeking to 'domesticate' drinking—to reduce problems from drinking by integrating the drinking into everyday life—have portrayed the new public health approach as antithetical to this (Olsson 1990), although some researchers have noted that there is no necessary antithesis (Whitehead 1979).

In terms of the influence of the approach on policy, it has undoubtedly had some effect in strengthening the defence of existing control structures and regulations. But efforts to get the approach adopted as the practical base for policy have met resistance and failure in a number of countries (Baggott 1990; Hawks 1993). One response to this resistance has been some calls for an alternative approach (Stockwell *et al.* 1997), arguing that policy measures directed at heavy and problematic drinkers are more politically acceptable than measures directed at all drinkers.

The policy approach offered as an alternative is a focus on harm reduction, primarily by reducing instances of intoxication or insulating them from harm (Plant *et al.* 1997). An approach to prevention in terms of reducing total consumption is likened to 'draining the ocean to prevent shark attacks' (Rehm 1999). However, there is in fact usually no conflict between approaches aimed at total consumption and approaches aiming to reduce harm from heavy drinking. As Stockwell *et al.* (1997, p. 6) note, 'aggregate consumption levels are in fact likely to fall if effective [harm reduction] strategies are introduced'. Conversely, many measures which affect the whole drinking population—taxation is a good example—bear especially hard on heavier drinkers. Nor are targeted harm reduction measures necessarily more politically acceptable than measures which affect all drinkers. Old systems of rationing and individual buyer surveillance (Järvinen 1991), which were directed specifically at restraining heavy drinking, are now politically unacceptable in any developed society, though rationing, at least, was highly effective as a targeted prevention measure (Norström 1987).

Beyond its specific features, the controversy over the 'new public health' approach in the alcohol field replicates familiar patterns of controversy over public health approaches in general, particularly when those approaches impinge on familiar and valued patterns of behaviour, with substantial economic interests at stake. At the level of the knowledge base, the approach has had considerable success: the empirical evidence underlying the approach has considerably strengthened since the approach was first put forward. At a political level, however, the approach has had only limited success, and primarily in areas peripheral to its main focus—that is, in drinking–driving and minimum age limits for drinkers.

Strategies of prevention and control and their effectiveness

Simplifying somewhat, there are seven main strategies to minimize alcohol problems. One strategy is to educate or persuade people not to use, or about ways to use so as to limit harm. A second strategy, a kind of negative persuasion, is to deter drinking-related behaviour with the threat of penalties. A third strategy, operating in the positive direction, is to provide alternatives to drinking or to drink-connected activities. A fourth strategy is in one way or another to insulate the use from harm. A fifth strategy is to regulate availability of the drug or the conditions of its use. Prohibition of supply may be regarded as a special case of such regulation. A sixth strategy is to work with social or religious movements oriented to reducing alcohol problems. And a seventh strategy is to treat or otherwise help people who are in trouble with their drinking. We will consider these strategies, and the evidence on their effectiveness, in turn.

Education and persuasion

In principle, education can be offered to any segment of the population in a variety of venues, but it is usually education of youth in schools which first comes to mind in the prevention of alcohol problems. Community-based prevention programmes, which are often also directed at adults, also may include an educational component.

Education offers new information or ways of thinking about information, and leaves it to the listener to draw conclusions concerning beliefs and behaviour. However, most alcohol education programmes go beyond this. A commonplace of the North American evaluative literature on alcohol education is that 'knowledge-only' approaches do not result in changes in behaviour (Botvin 1995). School-based alcohol education has thus usually had a persuasional element, aiming to influence students in a particular direction.

Persuasion is directly concerned with changing beliefs or behaviours, and may or may not also offer information. Mass-media campaigns aimed at persuasion have been a very common component of prevention programmes for alcohol-related problems, but persuasion can be pursued also through other media and modalities.

In most societies, public health-oriented persuasion about alcohol must compete with a variety of other persuasional messages, including those intended to sell alcoholic beverages. The evidence that alcohol advertising influences teenagers and young adults towards increased drinking and problematic drinking is becoming stronger (Wyllie *et al.* 1998*a*,*b*). Even where alcohol advertising is not allowed on the mass media, these messages are often conveyed to consumers and potential consumers in a variety of other ways.

Evidence on effectiveness

The literature on effectiveness of educational approaches is dominated by studies from the United States on school-based education. This means that the alcohol education has usually been in the context of drug and tobacco education, and that the emphasis has been on abstention (Beck 1998), or at least on delaying the start of drinking, in cultural circumstances where the median age of actually starting drinking is about 13, while the minimum legal drinking age is 21. In general, despite the best efforts of a generation of researchers, this literature has had difficulty showing substantial and lasting effects (Paglia and Room 1999). There is a good argument from general principles for alcohol education in the context of consumer and health education, but there is little evidence from the formal evaluation literature at this point of its effectiveness beyond the short term.

Persuasional media campaigns have also been a favourite modality in many places in recent decades for the prevention of alcohol problems. In general, evaluations of such campaigns have been able to demonstrate impacts on knowledge and awareness about substance use problems, but can show only modest success in affecting attitudes and behaviours. As with school education approaches, there are hints in the literature that success may come more from influencing the community environment around the drinker—in terms of attitudes of significant others, or popular support for alcohol policy measures—than from directly persuading the drinker him- or herself. Thus, media messages can be effective as agenda-setting mechanisms in the community, increasing or sustaining public support for other preventive strategies (Casswell *et al.* 1989).

Deterrence

In its broadest sense, deterrence means simply the threat of negative sanctions or incentives for behaviour—a form of negative persuasion. Criminal laws deter in two ways: by general deterrence, which is the effect of the law in preventing a prohibited behaviour in the population as a whole, and specific deterrence, which is the effect of the law in discouraging those who have been caught from doing it again (Ross 1982). A law tends to have a greater preventive effect and to be cheaper to administer to the extent it has a strong general deterrence effect.

Prohibitions on driving after drinking more than a specified amount are now in effect in most nations (Hurst *et al.* 1997, pp. 555–6). In many societies, there have also been laws against public drunkenness (being in a public place while intoxicated), and against obnoxious behaviour while intoxicated. Other common prohibitions are concerned with producing or selling alcoholic beverages outside state-regulated channels, and with aspects of drinking under a specified minimum age.

Evidence on effectiveness

Drinking–driving legislation, such as *per se* laws outlawing driving while at or above a defined blood-alcohol level, has been shown to be effective in changing behaviour and reducing rates of alcohol-related problems (Ross 1982; Edwards *et al.* 1994, pp. 153–9; Hingson 1996). The effect is through both general and specific deterrence. The quickness and certainty of punishment, as well as its severity, are important in the deterrent value (too much severity tends to undercut the quickness and certainty). Drinking–driving is an ideal area for applying general deterrence, since the gains from breaking the law are limited, and automobile drivers typically have something to lose by being caught.

Many English-speaking and Scandinavian countries have had a tradition of criminalizing drinking in public places, or public drunkenness as such, but the trend has been to decriminalize public drunkenness. Though there are few specific studies, criminalizing public drunkenness may not be very effective in changing the behaviour of those who have little to lose.

Providing and encouraging alternative activities

Another strategy, in principle involving positive incentives, is to provide and seek to encourage activities which are an alternative to drinking or to activities closely associated with drinking. This includes such initiatives as making soft drinks available as an alternative to alcoholic beverages, providing locations for sociability as an alternative to taverns, and providing and encouraging recreational activities as an alternative to leisure activities involving drinking. Job-creation and skill-development programmes are other examples.

Evidence on effectiveness

'Boredom' and 'because there's nothing else to do' are certainly among the reasons that are given for drinking by some drinkers. And there are often good reasons of general social policy for providing and encouraging alternative activities. But as has been noted, the problem with alternatives to drinking is that drinking combines so well with so many of them. Soft drinks are indeed an alternative to alcoholic beverages for quenching thirst, but they may also serve as a mixer in an alcoholic drink. Involvement in sports may go along with drinking as well as replacing it. The few evaluation studies of providing alternative activities, again from a restricted range of societies, have generally not shown lasting effects on drinking behaviour (Moskowitz *et al.* 1983; Norman *et al.* 1997), though they undoubtedly often serve a general social purpose in broadening opportunities for the disadvantaged (Carmona and Stewart 1996).

Insulating use from harm

A major social strategy for reducing alcohol-related problems in many societies has been to separate the drinking, and particularly heavy drinking, from potential harm. This separation can be physical (in terms of distance or walls), it can be temporal, or it can be cultural (for example, defining the drinking occasion as 'time out' from normal responsibilities). These 'harm-reduction' strategies, as they are called in the context of illicit drugs, are often built into cultural arrangements around drinking, but can also be the object of purposive programmes and policies (Moore and Gerstein 1981, pp. 100–11), such as promotion of 'designated drivers', where one person in a social group is chosen to abstain and drive in the particular social situation (DeJong and Hingson 1998).

A variety of modifications of the driving environment affect casualties associated with drinking and driving, along with other casualties. These include mandatory use of seat belts, airbags, and improvements in the safety of road vehicles and roads. Many other practical measures to separate intoxication episodes from casualties and other adverse consequences have been put into practice, though usually without formal evaluation.

Evidence on effectiveness

Drinking–driving countermeasures are a prime example of an approach in terms of insulating drinking behaviour from harm, since they seek to reduce alcohol-related traffic casualties without necessarily stopping or reducing alcohol use (Evans 1991). There is substantial evidence of the success of a range of such countermeasures, including environmental change approaches as well as deterrence (Forsyth 1996; Zajac 1997; DeJong and Hingson 1998). Some environmental measures which reduce road casualties in general (e.g. requiring wearing of seatbelts in cars, or providing footpaths separated from the road) may prevent casualties associated with intoxication even more than other casualties.

Regulating the availability and conditions of use

In terms of the substantial harm to health and public order they can cause, alcoholic beverages are not ordinary commodities. Governments have thus often actively intervened in the markets for such beverages, far beyond usual levels of state intervention in markets for commodities.

Total prohibition can be viewed as an extreme form of regulation of the market. In this circumstance, where no one is licensed to sell alcohol, the state has no formal control over the conditions of the sales which nevertheless occur, and there are no legal sales interests, controlled through licensing, to co-operate with the state in the market's regulation.

With a general prohibition, typically the consumption of alcohol does fall in the population, and there are declines also in the rates of the direct consequences of drinking such as cirrhosis or alcohol-related mental disorders (Moore and Gerstein 1981; Teasley 1992). But prohibition also brings with it characteristic negative consequences, including the emergence and growth of an illicit market, and the crime associated with this. Partly for this reason, prohibition is not now a live option in any developed society, although it is in some other societies.

The features of alcohol control regimes which regulate the legal market in alcohol vary greatly. Special taxes on alcohol are very common, imposed often as much for revenue as for public health considerations. Many societies have minimum age limits forbidding sales to under age customers, and regulations forbidding sales to the already intoxicated. Often the regulations include limiting the number of sales outlets, restricting hours and days of sale, and limiting sales to special stores or drinking-places. Rationing of alcohol purchases—limiting the amount individuals can buy in a given time-period—has also been used as a means of regulating availability. Regulations restricting or forbidding advertising of alcoholic beverages attempt to limit or channel efforts by private interests to increase demand for particular alcoholic beverage products. Such regulations potentially complement education and persuasion efforts. State monopolization of sales of some or all alcoholic beverages at the retail and/or wholesale level has also been commonly used as a mechanism to minimize alcohol-related harm (Room 1993).

The effectiveness of specific types of regulation of availability

The last 25 years have seen the development of a burgeoning literature on the effects of alcohol control measures. Reference guides for communities, summarizing the research evidence and attuned to particular national or regional conditions, are becoming available

(Neves *et al.* 1998; Grover 1999). Specific types of regulation of the alcohol market, and the evidence on their effectiveness, are discussed below.

Minimum age limits

A minimum age limit is a partial prohibition, applied to one segment of the population. There is a strong evaluation literature showing the effectiveness of establishing and enforcing minimum age limits in reducing alcohol-related problems (Edwards *et al.* 1994, pp. 138–9). However, this literature is North America based, focuses mainly on youthful driving casualties, and mostly evaluates reduction from, and increases to, age 21 as the limit, a higher minimum age limit than in most societies. The applicability of the literature's findings in other societies and where youth cultures are less automobile-focused has been little tested.

Taxes and other price increases

Generally, consumers show some response to the price of alcoholic beverages, as of all other commodities. If the price goes up, the drinker will drink less; data from developed societies suggests this is at least as true of the heavy drinker as of the occasional drinker (Edwards *et al.* 1994, pp. 118–19). Studies have found that alcohol tax increases reduce the rates of traffic casualties, of cirrhosis mortality, and of incidents of violence (Cook 1981; Cook and Moore 1993).

Limiting sales outlets, and hours and conditions of sale

There is a substantial literature showing that levels and patterns of alcohol consumption, and rates of alcohol-related casualties and other problems, are influenced by such sales restrictions, which typically make the purchase of alcoholic beverages slightly inconvenient, or influence the setting of and after drinking (Edwards *et al.* 1994, pp. 125–42). Enforced rules influencing 'house policies' in drinking places on not serving intoxicated customers etc. have also been shown to have some effect (Saltz 1997).

Monopolizing production or sale

Studies of the effects of privatizing retail alcohol monopolies have often shown some increase in levels of alcohol consumption and problems, in part because the number of outlets and hours of sale typically increase with privatization (Her *et al.* 1999), and partly also because the new private interests typically exert political influence for further increases in availability. From a public health perspective, it is the retail level which is important, while monopolization of the production or wholesale level may facilitate revenue collection and effective control of the market.

Rationing sales

Rationing the amount of alcohol sold to an individual potentially directly impacts on heavy drinkers, and has been shown to reduce levels both of intoxication-related problems such as violence, and of drinking history-related problems such as cirrhosis mortality (Schechter 1986; Norström 1987). But while a form of rationing—the medical prescription system—is well accepted in most societies for psychoactive medications, it has proved politically unacceptable nowadays for alcoholic beverages in developed societies.

Advertising and promotion restrictions

Many societies have regulations on advertising and other promotion of sales of alcoholic beverages (Hurst *et al.* 1997, pp. 552–4). While it is well accepted that advertising can strongly affect consumer choices between products on the market, it has proved difficult to measure the effects of advertising on demand for alcoholic beverages as a whole, in part because the effects are likely to be cumulative and long term, making them difficult to measure. However, the evidence on the effects of advertising and promotion on overall demand has become stronger in the recent literature (Casswell 1995; Casswell and Zhang 1998; Saffer 1998).

Social and religious movements and community action

Substantial reductions in alcohol-related problems have often been the result of spontaneous social and religious movements which put a major emphasis on quitting intoxication or drinking. In recent decades, there have also been efforts to form partnerships between state organizations and non-governmental groups to work on alcohol problems, often at the level of the local community. There has been an active tradition of community action projects on alcohol problems, often using a range of prevention strategies (Giesbrecht *et al.* 1990; Greenfield and Zimmerman 1993; Holmila 1997; Holder 1998). School-based prevention efforts have also moved increasingly to try to involve the community, in line with general perceptions that such multifaceted strategies will be more effective (Paglia and Room 1999).

While some of the largest historical reductions in alcohol problem rates have resulted from spontaneous and autonomous social or religious movements, support or collaboration from a government can easily be perceived as official co-optation or manipulation (Room 1997). Thus there is considerable question about the extent to which such movements can or should become an instrument of government prevention policies.

Evidence on effectiveness

In the short term, movements of religious or cultural revival can be highly effective in reducing levels of drinking and of alcohol-related problems. Alcohol consumption in the United States fell by about one-half in the first flush of temperance enthusiasm during the period 1830 to 1845 (Moore and Gerstein 1981, p. 35). Rates of serious crime are reported to have fallen for a while to a fraction of their previous level in Ireland in the wake of Father Mathew's Temperance Crusade (Room 1983). The enthusiasm which sustains such movements tends to decay over time, though it often leaves behind new customs and institutions with much longer duration. For instance, though the days when the historic temperance movement in English-speaking societies was strong are long gone, the movement had the long-lasting effect of largely removing drinking from the workplace in these societies.

Treatment and other help

Providing effective treatment or other help for drinkers who find they cannot control their drinking can be regarded as an obligation of a just and humane society. The help can take several forms: a specific treatment system for alcohol problems, professional help in general health or welfare systems, or non-professional assistance in mutual-help movements. To the extent such help is effective, it is also a means of preventing or reducing future alcohol-related problems.

Treatments for alcohol problems need not be complex or expensive. The evaluation literature suggests that brief outpatient interventions aimed at changing cognitions and behaviour around drinking are as effective in most circumstances as longer and more intensive treatment (Finney and Monahan 1996; Long *et al.* 1998). Positive results from such interventions in primary health-care settings were shown in a WHO study that included a number of countries (Babor *et al.* 1994).

Evidence on effectiveness

In terms of the effects of treatment on those who come for it, there is good evidence for effectiveness of treatment for alcohol problems. Typically, the improvement rate from a single episode of treatment is about 20 per cent higher than the no-treatment condition. Further treatment episodes are often needed. Brief treatment interventions or mutual-help approaches usually result in net savings in social and health costs associated with the heavy drinker (at least where health-care is not self-paid), as well as improving the quality of life (Holder *et al.* 1992; Holder and Cunningham 1992).

The effectiveness of providing treatment as a strategy for reducing rates of alcohol problems in a society is more equivocal. In a North American context, it has been argued that the steep increase in alcohol problems treatment provision and mutual-help group membership in recent decades has contributed to reducing alcohol problems rates (Smart and Mann 1990). But the strength of the evidence for this contention is disputed (Holder 1997; Smart and Mann 1997). A treatment system for alcohol problems is an important part of an integrated national alcohol policy, but as an instrument of prevention—of reducing societal rates of alcohol problems—it is probably not cost-effective.

Building integrated alcohol policies

Alcohol policy at a community or societal level

Often the different strategies for preventing alcohol problems appear to be synergistic in their effects (DeJong and Hingson 1998). Controls of availability, for instance, are more likely to be adopted, continued, and respected when the public has been successfully persuaded of their effects and effectiveness. But strategies can also work at cross-purposes: a prohibition policy, for example, makes it difficult to pursue measures which insulate drinking from harm.

In a society where alcohol is a regular item of consumption, in view of the resulting rates of alcohol-related social and health problems, there is a strong justification for adopting a comprehensive policy concerning alcohol, taking into account production, marketing, and consumption, and the prevention and treatment of alcohol-related problems. In recent years, the idea that there should be an integrated alcohol policy at community or national levels, reaching across the many sectors of government and civil society which deal with alcohol issues, has become a common public health aim, although accomplishing this in practice has often proved difficult (Room 1999).

In terms of strategies we have reviewed for managing and reducing the rates of alcohol problems in society, there is a clear evidence for effectiveness and cost-effectiveness of measures regulating the availability and conditions of use, and measures which insulate use from harm. With respect to some aspects of alcohol problems, notably drinking–driving, deterrence measures also fall in the same category. Despite their perennial popularity, evidence of the effectiveness of education/persuasion and treatment strategies in reducing societal rates of problems is limited at best. Education and treatment are good things for a society and a government to be doing about alcohol problems, but they do not constitute in themselves a public health policy on alcohol. These strategies will be nevertheless be pursued in most societies, and they can be best pursued with attention to using cost-effective methods, and to integrating targets and messages with other aspects of alcohol policy.

Alcohol policy in a global perspective

Apart from agreements a century ago among the European colonial powers about control of the spirits trade in Africa (Bruun *et al.* 1975*b*), there is little tradition of collaboration on alcohol policy at the international level. It has been largely up to each nation to cope on its own with the serious social and health problems associated with drinking. Though alcohol smuggling has a long history, the nation-state could usually rely on distances and traditional trade barriers to keep alcohol issues largely a matter within its borders, in terms of the supply as well as of the problems.

The last 15 years of the twentieth century saw an accelerated rate of economic globalization that increasingly rendered obsolete the assumption that alcohol issues are local issues. This globalization affected alcohol issues in three main ways. The first of these was the influence of a global ideology of free markets. In its sweep, this ideology caught up and dismantled a variety of market arrangements which served to hold down and to structure alcohol consumption. State and provincial alcohol monopolies in North America were weakened or dismantled (Her *et al.* 1999). In Eastern Europe and the countries in transition, alcohol monopolies were swept away along with most other government intrusions in the market (Moskalewicz 1993). Many of the municipally run beerhalls in southern African countries were privatized (Jernigan 1997). In line with the general ideology, privatization of alcohol production and distribution was often suggested, abetted, or imposed on developing countries by international development agencies (White and Batia 1998).

Second, trade agreements, trade dispute mechanisms, and the growth of new sales media effectively reduced the ability of national and subnational governments to control their local alcohol markets. The influence of trade agreements and trade dispute decisions in breaking down alcohol controls, including control of price through taxation, has been most fully documented for North America (Ferris *et al.* 1993) and Europe (Tigerstedt 1990; Holder *et al.* 1998), but these mechanisms also operate in the developing world. For instance, the average tax on alcoholic beverages in South Korea is likely to be pushed down early in the 2000s as a result of complaints to the World Trade Organization by the European Union and the United States (Anonymous 1997, 1999). Sales of alcoholic beverages through the internet have become a fast-growing threat to national or local control of alcohol markets (Apple 1999).

Third, alcohol production, distribution, and marketing became increasingly globalized (Jernigan 1997). Transnational alcohol companies expanded rapidly into the developing world and the countries in transition in search of new markets, benefiting from weak policy environments and the sweeping tide of market liberalization. Though most alcoholic beverages are still produced in the country in which they are sold, industrially produced beverages were increasingly produced in plants owned, co-owned, or licensed by multinational firms. To promote increased sales, these firms have been able to transform and step-up the marketing techniques used in the national market, bringing to bear all the marketing resources and expertise they have developed in other markets.

In light of these converging trends, there is a growing need for mechanisms to express public health interests in alcohol issues at the international level, both in trade agreements and settlements of trade disputes, and in creating mutual obligations for one nation to back up rather than subvert the alcohol regulations and policies of another. If these needs are to be met, the public health interests may be expressed through the WHO or through new international bodies.

References

Andréasson, S., Romelsjö, A., and Allebeck, P. (1991). Alcohol, social factors and mortality among young men. *British Journal of Addiction*, **86**, 877–87.

Anonymous (1996). Europe unites in Paris. *Globe*, Issue 1/96, pp. 1–22.

Anonymous (1997). Pressure on liquor tax system mounts: US files complaint against Korea with WTO. *Korea Herald*, 27 May.

Anonymous (1999). Tax rate on soju still unresolved. *Korea Herald*, 31 October.

Apple, R.W. (1999). Zinfandel by mail? *New York Times*, 19 May.

Babor, T.F., Grant, M., Acuda, W., *et al.* (1994). Randomized clinical trial of brief interventions in primary health care: summary of a WHO project. *Addiction,* **89**, 657–78.

Baggott, R. (1990). *Alcohol, politics and social policy*. Gower, Aldershot, UK.

Beck, J. (1998). 100 years of 'just say no' versus 'just say know'. *Evaluation Review*, **22**, 15–45.

Beauchamp, D. (1976). Exploring new ethics for public health: developing a fair alcohol policy. *Journal of Health Politics, Policy and Law*, **1**, 338–54.

Blocker, J. (1989). *American temperance movements: cycles of reform.* Twayne, Boston, MA.

Bondy, S.J., Rehm, J., Ashley, M.J., Walsh, G., Single, E., and Room, R. (1999). Low-risk drinking guidelines: the scientific evidence. *Canadian Journal of Public Health*, **90**, 272–6.

Botvin, G.J. (1995). Principles of prevention. In *Handbook on drug abuse prevention: a comprehensive strategy to prevent the abuse of alcohol and other drugs* (ed. R.H. Coombs and D. Ziedonis), pp. 19–44. Allyn and Bacon, Boston, MA.

Bruun, K., Edwards, G., Lumio, M., *et al.* (1975*a*). *Alcohol control policies in public health perspective*. FFAS Vol. 25, Finnish Foundation for Alcohol Studies, Helsinki.

Bruun, K., Rexed, I., and Pan, L. (1975*b*). *The gentlemen's club*. University of Chicago Press.

Carmona, M. and Stewart, K. (1996). *Review of alternative activities and alternatives programs in youth-oriented prevention*. CSAP Technical Report 13, Center for Substance Abuse Prevention, Rockville, MD.

Casswell, S. (1995). Does alcohol advertising have an impact on public health? *Drug and Alcohol Review*, **14**, 395–404.

Casswell, S. and Zhang, J.F. (1998). Impact of liking for advertising and brand allegiance on drinking and alcohol-related aggression: a longitudinal study. *Addiction*, **93**, 1209–1217.

Casswell, S., Gilmore, L., Maguire, V., and Ransom, R. (1989). Changes in public support for alcohol policies following a community-based campaign, *British Journal of Addiction*, **84**, 515–22.

Catlin, G.E.G. (1931). *Liquor control*. Thornton Butterworth, London.

Chadwick, D.J. and Goode, J.A. (ed.) (1998). *Alcohol and cardiovascular diseases*. Wiley, Chichester.

Cook, P. (1981). Effect of liquor taxes on drinking, cirrhosis, and auto accidents. In *Alcohol and public policy: beyond the shadow of prohibition* (ed. M.H. Moore and D.R. Gerstein), pp. 255–85. National Academy Press, Washington, DC.

Cook, P.J. and Moore, M.H. (1993). Violence reduction through restrictions on alcohol availability. *Alcohol Health and Research World*, **17**, 151–6.

Criqui, M., *et al.* (1998) Discussion. In *Alcohol and cardiovascular diseases* (ed. D.J. Chadwick and J.A. Goode), pp. 122–4. Wiley, Chichester.

Cross, J.N. (1968). *Guide to the community control of alcoholism*. American Public Health Association, New York.

DeJong, W. and Hingson, R. (1998). Strategies to reduce driving under the influence of alcohol. *Annual Review of Public Health,* **19**, 359–78.

de Lint, J. and Schmidt, W. (1968). The distribution of alcohol consumption in Ontario. *Quarterly Journal of Studies on Alcohol*, **29**, 968–73.

Edwards, G., Anderson, P., Babor, T.F., *et al.* (1994). *Alcohol policy and the public good*. Oxford University Press.

Emerson, H. (ed.) (1932). *Alcohol and man: the effects of alcohol on man in health and disease*. Macmillan, New York.

English, D.R., Holman, C.D.J., Milne, E., *et al.* (1995). *The quantification of drug caused morbidity and mortality in Australia*. Australian Government Publishing Service, Canberra.

Evans, L. (1991). *Traffic safety and the driver*. Van Nostrand Reinhold, New York.

Ferris, J., Room, R., and Giesbrecht, N. (1993). Public health interests in trade agreements on alcoholic beverages in North America. *Alcohol Health and Research World*, **17**, 235–41.

Finney, J.W. and Monahan, S.C. (1998). Cost-effectiveness of treatment for alcoholism: a second approximation. *Journal of Studies on Alcohol*, **57**, 229–43.

Forsyth, I. (1996). Alcohol and drugs: the role of insurance in promoting effective countermeasures. In *Proceedings of the Conference on Road Safety in Europe and Strategic Highway Research Program (SHRP)*. VTI Conferens No. 4A, Part 3, pp. 45–63. Swedish National Road and Transport Safety Institute, Linköping.

Giesbrecht, N., Conley, P., Denniston, R., *et al.* (ed.) (1990). *Research, action and the community: experiences in the prevention of alcohol and other drug problems*. DHHS Publication (ADM) 89-1651, Office of Substance Abuse Prevention, Rockville, MD.

Graham, K., Leonard, K.E., Room, R., Wild, T.C., Pihl, R.O., Bois, C., and Single, E. (1998). Current directions in research on understanding and preventing intoxicated aggression. *Addiction*, **93**, 659–76.

Grant, M. and Litvak, J. (1998). Introduction: beyond per capita consumption. In *Drinking patterns and their consequences* (ed. M. Grant and J. Litvak), pp. 1–4. Taylor and Francis, Washington, DC.

Greenfield, T. and Zimmerman, R. (ed.) (1993). *Experiences with community action projects: new research in the prevention of alcohol and other drug problems*. DHHS Publication No. (ADM). 93-1976, Center for Substance Abuse Prevention, Rockville, MD.

Grover, P.T. (ed.) (1999). *Preventing problems related to alcohol availability: environmental approaches: reference guide*. DHHS Publication SMA 99-3298, Center for Substance Abuse Prevention, Washington, DC. (http://text.nlm.nih.gov/ftrs/dbaccess/csap)

Hawks, D. (1993). The formulation of Australia's National Health Policy on Alcohol. *Addiction*, **88** (Supplement), 19S–26S.

Hawks, D. (1994). A review of current guidelines on moderate drinking for individual consumers. *Contemporary Drug Problems*, **21**, 223–37.

Hemström, Ö. (2001). Per capita alcohol consumption and ischaemic heart disease mortality. *Addiction*, **96** (Supplement 1), S93–112.

Her, M. and Rehm, J. (1998). Alcohol and all-cause mortality in Europe 1982–1990: a pooled cross-section time-series analysis. *Addiction,* **93**, 1335–40.

Her, M., Giesbrecht, N., Room, R., and Rehm, J. (1999). Privatizing alcohol sales and alcohol consumption: evidence and implications, *Addiction*, **94**, 1125–39.

Herd, D. (1992). Ideology, history and changing models of liver cirrhosis epidemiology. *British Journal of Addiction*, **87**, 179–92.

Hingson, R. (1996). Prevention of drinking and driving. *Alcohol Health and Research World*, **20**, 219–26.

Holder, H. (1997). Can individually directed interventions reduce population-level alcohol-involved problems? *Addiction*, **92**, 5–7.

Holder, H.D. (1998). *Alcohol and the community: a systems approach to prevention.* Cambridge University Press.

Holder, H.D. and Cunningham, D.W. (1992). Alcoholism treatment for employees and family members: its effect on health care costs. *Alcohol Health and Research World*, **16**, 149–53.

Holder, H.D., Lennox, R.D.L., and Blose, J.O. (1992). Economic benefits of alcoholism treatment: a summary of twenty years of research. *Journal of Employee Assistance Research*, **1**, 63–82.

Holder, H.D., Kühlhorn, E., Nordlund, S., Österberg, E., Romelsjö, A., and Ugland, T. (1998). *European integration and Nordic alcohol policies.* Ashgate, Aldershot.

Holman, C.D.J. and English, D.R. (1995). Improved aetiologic fraction for alcohol-caused mortality. *Australian Journal of Public Health*, **19**, 138–41.

Holmila, M. (ed.) (1997). *Community prevention of alcohol problems.* Macmillan, Basingstoke.

Hurst, W., Gregory, E., and Gussman, T. (1997). *International survey: alcoholic beverage taxation and control policies.* Brewers Association of Canada, Ottawa.

Järvinen, M. (1991). The controlled controllers: women, men and alcohol. *Contemporary Drug Problems*, **18**, 389–406.

Jernigan, D.H. (1997). *Thirsting for markets: the global impact of corporate alcohol.* Marin Institute for the Prevention of Alcohol and Other Drug Problems, San Rafael, CA.

Katcher, B.S. (1993). The post-repeal eclipse in knowledge about the harmful effects of alcohol. *Addiction*, **88**, 729–44.

Kauhanen, J., Kaplan, G.A., Goldberg, D.E., and Salonen, J.T. (1997). Beer bingeing and mortality: results from the Kuopio ischaemic heart disease risk factor study, a prospective population-based study. *British Medical Journal*, **315**, 846–51.

Klatsky, A.L. (1999). Moderate drinking and reduced risk of heart disease. *Alcohol Research and Health*, **23**, 15–23.

Knupfer, G. (1967). The epidemiology of problem drinking. *American Journal of Public Health*, **57**, 973–86.

Kozlowski, L.T., Heller, D.A., Pillitteri, J.L., and Rovine, M. (1994). Tobaccco use, the health effects of moderate alcohol drinking, and the assessment of their interaction. *Contemporary Drug Problems*, **21**, 81–9.

Kreitman, N. (1986). Alcohol consumption and the preventive paradox. *British Journal of Addiction*, **81**, 353–63.

Kupari, M. and Koskinen, P. (1998). Alcohol, cardiac arrhythmias and sudden death. In *Alcohol and cardiovascular diseases* (ed. D.J. Chadwick and J.A. Goode), pp. 68–79. Wiley, Chichester.

Ledermann, S. (1956). *Alcool, alcoolisme, alcoolisation.* INED Cahier 29. Presses Universitaires de France, Paris.

Leino, E.V., Romelsjö, A., Shoemaker, C., *et al.* (1998). Alcohol consumption and mortality: II. Studies of male populations. *Addiction*, **93**, 205–18.

Leon, D.A., Chenet, L., Shkolnikov, V.M., *et al.* (1998). Huge variation in Russian mortality rates 1984–94: artefact, alcohol, or what? *Lancet*, **350**, 383–8.

Levine, H.G. (1991). Temperance cultures: concern about alcohol problems in Nordic and English-speaking cultures. In: *The nature of alcohol and drug related problems* (ed. M. Lader, G. Edwards, and D.C. Drummond), pp. 15–36. Oxford University Press.

Long, C.G., Williams, M., and Hollin, C.R. (1998). Treating alcohol problems: a study of program effectiveness and cost effectiveness according to length and delivery of treatment. *Addiction*, **93**, 561–71.

MacAndrew, C. and Edgerton, R.E. (1969). *Drunken comportment.* Aldine, Chicago, IL.

McKee, M. and Britton, A. (1998). The positive relationship between alcohol and heart disease in eastern Europe: potential physiological mechanisms. *Journal of the Royal Society of Medicine*, **91**, 402–7.

Maclure, M. (1993). Demonstration of deductive meta-analysis: ethanol intake and risk of myocardial infarction. *Epidemiologic Reviews*, **15**, 328–51.

Mäkelä, K. (1983). The uses of alcohol and their cultural regulation. *Acta Sociologica*, **26**, 21–31.

Moore, M.H. and Gerstein, D.R. (ed.) (1981). *Alcohol and public policy: beyond the shadow of Prohibition.* National Academy Press, Washington, DC.

Moskalewicz, J. (1993). Privatization of the alcohol arena in Poland. *Contemporary Drug Problems*, **20**, 63–275.

Moskowitz, J.M., Mailvin, J., Schaeffer, G.A., and Schaps, E. (1983). Evaluation of a junior high school primary prevention program. *Addictive Behaviors*, **8**, 393–401.

Mott, G. (1991). The anti-alcohol network, *Moderation Reader*, **5**, 6–20.

Murray, C.J.L. and Lopez, A.D. (1996). Quantifying the burden of disease and injury attributable to ten major risk factors. In: *The global burden of disease: a comprehensive assessment of mortality and disability from diseases, injuries and risk factors in 1990 and projected to 2020* (ed. C.J.L. Murray and A.D. Lopez), pp. 295–324. Harvard School of Public Health, Cambridge, MA.

NIAAA (1997). Alcohol and the immune system. In *Ninth special report to the US Congress on alcohol and health*, pp. 163–9. NIH Publication No. 97–4017, National Institute on Alcohol Abuse and Alcoholism, Rockville, MD.

Neves, P., de Pape, D., Giesbrecht, N., *et al.* (1998). *Communities take action! A practical guide for municipalities, enforcement agencies, community groups and others concerned about the impact of alcohol on public health and safety.* Addiction Research Foundation, Toronto.

Norman, E., Turner, S., Zunz, S.J., and Stillson, K. (1997). Prevention programs reviewed: what works? In *Drug-free youth: a compendium for prevention specialists* (ed. E. Norman), pp. 22–45. Garland, New York.

Norström, T. (1987). Abolition of the Swedish rationing system: effects on consumption distribution and cirrhosis mortality. *British Journal of Addiction*, **82**, 633–41.

Norström, T. (1996). Per capita consumption and total mortality: an analysis of historical data. *Addiction*, **91**, 339–44.

Norström, T. (2001). *Per capita alcohol consumption and all-cause mortality in 14 European countries. Addiction*, **96** (Supplement 1), S113–28.

Olsson, B. (1990). Alkoholpolitik och alkoholens fenomenologi: uppfattningar som artikulerats i pressen. (Alcohol policy and the phenomenology of alcohol: conceptions articulated in the press.) *Alkoholpolitik*, **7**, 184–95.

Paglia, A. and Room, R. (1999). Preventing substance use problems among youth: a literature review and recommendations. *Journal of Primary Prevention*, **20**, 3–50.

Peele, S. (1987). The limitations of control-of-supply models for explaining and preventing alcoholism and drug addiction. *Journal of Studies on Alcohol*, **48**, 61–77.

Perrine, M.W., Peck, R.C., and Fell, J.C. (1989). Epidemiologic perspectives on drunk driving. In *Surgeon General's Workshop on Drunk Driving: background papers*, pp. 35–76. US Department of Health and Human Services, Washington, DC.

Plant, M., Single, E., and Stockwell, T. (ed). (1997). *Alcohol: minimizing the harm—what works?* Free Association Books, New York.

Poikolainen, K. (1998). It can be bad for the heart, too—drinking patterns and coronary heart disease. *Addiction*, **93**, 1757–9.

Popham, R., Schmidt, W., and de Lint, J. (1976). The effects of legal restraint on drinking. In *The biology of alcoholism*, Vol. 4, *Social aspects of alcoholism* (ed. B. Kissin and H. Begleiter), pp. 579–625. Plenum Press, New York.

Rehm, J.T. (1999). Draining the ocean to prevent shark attacks? *Nordic Studies on Alcohol and Drugs*, **16** (English Supplement), 46–54.

Rehm, J. and Sempos, C.T. (1995). Alcohol consumption and all-cause mortality. *Addiction*, **90**, 471–80.

Room, R. (1983). Alcohol and crime: behavioral aspects. In *Encyclopedia of crime and justice*, Vol. 1 (ed. S. Kadish), pp. 35–44. Free Press, New York.

Room, R. (1984*a*). Alcohol control and public health. *Annual Review of Public Health*, **5**, 293–317.

Room, R. (1984*b*). A 'reverence for strong drink': the Lost Generation and the elevation of alcohol in American culture. *Journal of Studies on Alcohol*, **45**, 540–6.

Room, R. (1984*c*). Former NIAAA directors look back: policymakers on the role of research. *Drinking and Drug Practices Surveyor*, **19**, 38–42.

Room, R. (1993). The evolution of alcohol monopolies and their relevance for public health. *Contemporary Drug Problems*, **20**, 169–87.

Room, R. (1996). Alcohol consumption and social harm—conceptual issues and historical perspectives. *Contemporary Drug Problems*, **23**, 373–88.

Room, R. (1997). Voluntary organizations and the state in the prevention of alcohol problems. *Drugs and Society*, **11**, 11–23.

Room, R. (1999). The idea of alcohol policy. *Nordic Studies on Alcohol and Drugs*, **16** (English supplement), 7–20.

Rorabaugh, W.J. (1979). *The alcoholic republic.* Oxford University Press, New York.

Rose, G. (1981). Strategy of prevention: lessons from cardiovascular disease. *British Medical Journal*, **282**, 1847–51.

Seeley, J.R. (1960). Death by liver cirrhosis and the price of beverage alcohol. *Canadian Medical Association Journal*, **83**, 1361–6.

Ross, H.L. (1982). *Deterring the drinking driver: legal policy and social control.* Lexington Books, Lexington, MA.

Saffer, H. (1998). Economic issues in cigarette and alcohol advertising. *Journal of Drug Issues*, **28**, 781–93.

Saltz, R.F. (1997). Prevention where alcohol is sold and consumed: server intervention and responsible beverage service. In *Alcohol: minimizing the harm. What works?* (ed. M. Plant, E. Single, and T. Stockwell), pp. 72–84. Free Association Books, New York.

Schechter, E.J. (1986). Alcohol rationing and control systems in Greenland. *Contemporary Drug Problems*, **13**, 587–620.

Shkolnikov, V.M. and Nemtsov, A. (1997). The anti-alcohol campaign and variations in Russian mortality. In: *Premature death in the new independent states* (ed. J.L. Bobadilla, C.A. Costello, and F. Mitchell), pp. 239–61. National Academy Press, Washington, DC.

Skog, O.-J. (1985). The collectivity of drinking cultures: a theory of the distribution of alcohol consumption. *British Journal of Addiction*, **80**, 83–99.

Skog, O.-J. (1996). Public health consequences of the J-curve hypothesis of alcohol problems. *Addiction*, **91**, 325–37.

Smart, R.G. and Mann, R.E. (1990). Are increased levels of treatment and Alcoholics Anonymous large enough to create the recent reduction in liver cirrhosis? *British Journal of Addiction*, **85**, 1385–7.

Smart, R.G. and Mann, R.E. (1997). Interventions into alcohol problems: what works? *Addiction*, **92**, 9–13.

Stockwell, T., Single, E., Hawks, D., and Rehm, D. (1997). Sharpening the focus of alcohol policy from aggregate consumption to harm and risk reduction. *Addiction Research*, **5**, 1–9.

Sutton, C. (1998). Swedish alcohol discourse: constructions of a social problem. *Acta Universitatis Upsaliensis, Studia Sociologica Upsaliensia*, **45**.

Teasley, D.L. (1992). Drug legalization and the 'lessons' of Prohibition. *Contemporary Drug Problems*, **19**, 27–52.

Terris, M. (1967). Epidemiology of cirrhosis of the liver: national mortality data. *American Journal of Public Health*, **57**, 2076–88.

Tigerstedt, C. (1990). The European Community and the alcohol policy dimension. *Contemporary Drug Problems*, **17**, 461–79.

Tigerstedt, C. (1999). Alcohol policy, public health, and Kettil Bruun. *Contemporary Drug Problems*, **26**, 209–35.

White, O.C. and Batia, A. (1998). *Privatization in Africa.* World Bank, Washington, DC.

Whitehead, P.C. (1979). Prevention of alcoholism. In: *Alcohol problems* (ed. D. Robinson). Holmes and Meier, New York.

Wolfgang, M.E. (1958). *Patterns in criminal homicide.* University of Pennsylvania Press, Philadelphia, PA.

WHO Expert Committee on Problems Related to Alcohol Consumption (1980). *Problems related to alcohol consumption.* Technical Report Series 650, WHO, Geneva.

Wyllie, A., Zhang, J.F., and Casswell, S. (1998*a*). Positive responses to televised beer advertisements associated with drinking and problems reported by 18- to 29-year-olds. *Addiction*, **93**, 749–60.

Wyllie, A., Zhang, J.F. and Casswell, S. (1998*b*). Responses to televised advertisements associated with drinking behaviour of 10–17-year-olds. *Addiction*, **93**, 361–71.

Zajac, P.L. (1997). Can technology be used to intervene in behaviour in a human factors engineering approach to drunk driving deterrence? *Dissertation Abstracts International*, **57**, 4126A–7A.

10.4 Injury control: the public health approach

Corinne Peek-Asa, Bonnie Dean, and Jess F. Kraus

Introduction

In the last decades, decreases have been observed in almost all causes of injury death, although disparities among age, sex, and race/ethnic groups remain. In the last 75 years, the motor vehicle fatality rate per mile driven has decreased 90 per cent, yet despite this decrease motor vehicles remain the most common cause of injury death. After increasing 22 per cent from 1985 to 1993, the firearm-related mortality rate decreased 11 per cent from 1993 to 1995. These trends indicate that although great strides have been made in preventing injury deaths, changing risk patterns and disparity in exposures continue to challenge the field.

Observed decreases are due in large part to increasing activity in the systematic study of the causes of injury, and the broad application of this knowledge to prevention. This activity is known in sum as injury control, which is a multidisciplinary effort driven by public health to reduce the magnitude, severity, and consequences of injuries. Increased injury control activity was enabled by a slow change in how we think about risk and prevention. The very term 'accident', the most common reference to injurious events, evokes a feeling of chance and helplessness. However, injuries occur in predictable and usually preventable patterns, and our challenge is to identify and alter these patterns.

Injuries affect all human beings at some level. In fact, most of us sustain injuries from a very young age and continue to suffer from them throughout our lives. Perhaps this acceptance of injury as a part of everyday life delayed our efforts at prevention. However, the toll of injuries could not be ignored forever. Injuries take too many young lives suddenly and unexpectedly. Severe injuries can lead to lifelong disabilities and chronic pain which can restrict work, recreation, and leisure activities temporarily or permanently. Injuries can tear families, businesses, and communities apart, as was demonstrated in disastrous events such as Hurricane Mitch and the shooting at Columbine High School in Colorado. Individuals and societies can be left with enormous medical bills, extensive rehabilitation, major lifestyle adjustments, and post-traumatic stress and depression—losses that cannot easily, if ever, be recouped.

Although public awareness often focuses on events that cause many injuries at once, the toll of injuries climbs steadily every second of every day. The majority of injuries do not occur in mass events; for example, the annual number of deaths from motor vehicle crashes far exceeds that from airline crashes and natural disasters combined. Injuries disproportionately affect younger people more than the better-recognized threats to health such as cancer and circulatory disorders. The general public is unaware that injuries are a leading contributor to years of premature life lost, and missed days of work and school, and are one of the largest components of the medical care dollar spent per capita.

Despite successes in many areas of injury prevention, new risks and increasing population size constantly challenge the injury control community. Effective injury prevention strategies involve professionals from many fields working together. Modern injury control research combines ideas and skills from public health, biomechanics, engineering, behavioural sciences, law, law enforcement, medicine, and urban planning, among others.

This chapter will present a short public health history of injuries, examine the magnitude and distribution of injuries in the United States and the world, and outline approaches to injury control countermeasures. Injury control is a broad and complex field. This chapter will focus on injury prevention using public health models and how these models fit into the multidisciplinary field of injury control.

Public health history of injuries

Although injuries have been a leading cause of death throughout the history of humanity, they were not systematically studied until the twentieth century. The first formal safety organization, the National Safety Council, was chartered in 1913 with the primary goal of decreasing occupational fatality. The systematic study of injury incidence, risk factors, and successful prevention, however, was only beginning. One of the first epidemiological studies to document the effectiveness of an injury prevention strategy demonstrated that helmets decreased head injuries among motorcycle riders in the military (Cairns 1941; Cairns and Holbourn 1943). Cairns and his associates compared head injury incidence between helmeted and unhelmeted riders and were among the first to recognize the importance of studying defined populations using appropriate comparison groups.

John Gordon (1949) identified injury patterns by age, gender, and other demographic factors, noting that 'accidents' could be studied using epidemiological research methods similar to those in disease prevention. James Gibson (1961) defined energy and its many forms as the agent of injury. William Haddon Jr developed a framework for injury causation based on the infectious disease model (Haddon 1963;

Haddon *et al.* 1964). He recognized that injuries occur when energy delivered to a living host from a vehicle or vector exceeds human tolerance, and classified the agent–host interaction into two categories of human–energy interaction: (a) when energy is delivered in excess of human tolerance, such as mechanical energy in motor vehicle crashes or in falls; (b) when energy metabolism is interfered with and physiological functions are impeded, such as in drowning or poisoning. Haddon used these basic ideas as a framework to develop a comprehensive matrix of host–energy interactions, discussed later in this chapter.

The study of injury prevention was greatly advanced by combining expertise from engineering with epidemiology. In 1941, Hugh DeHaven survived a crash of his trainer aircraft and noticed that his abdominal injuries were related to the shape and riveting location of his safety belt. He then studied ways in which vehicle engineering could reduce the severity of injuries during crashes (DeHaven 1968). His work bred new studies on human tolerance to energy forces during many types of impacts.

The ability to identify the incidence and causes of injuries in populations has been an important development in injury research. Agencies such as the National Safety Council, the National Highway Traffic Safety Administration, and the National Center for Injury Prevention and Control have been instrumental in establishing national surveillance systems for certain injury mechanisms. As the high incidence and cost of injuries have become better recognized, hospitals and communities have established local injury surveillance systems. The first documented computerized trauma surveillance system was introduced in 1969 at Cook County Hospital in Chicago (Pollock and McClain 1989). In 1980, Massachusetts and Ohio were the first states to introduce emergency room surveillance, but most states have not been able to maintain such comprehensive databases because of prohibitive costs. Some areas, such as San Diego County in California, are combining information from hospitals, the Emergency Medical Service Authority, and police to form a comprehensive surveillance programme. The National Highway Traffic Safety Administration has since implemented statewide programmes to incorporate crash information with medical outcomes. International collaborations have been underway over the last several years and are now providing information to compare risks and prevention efforts in many different environments.

Legislation has been an important element of injury prevention in the United States. Among the first legislative actions to reduce injury risk was a 1927 bill prohibiting interstate mailing of firearms through the United States Postal Service (Institute of Medicine 1999). Some highly successful legislation includes the 1953 Flammable Fabrics Act, the 1970 Poison Prevention Packaging Act, and the 1973 Emergency Medical Services Systems Act. While some legislative efforts have been long-lasting, others have had more contested histories. Speed limits, motorcycle helmet use laws, and gun control measures are examples of legislation which continue to be highly debated, with compromises difficult to achieve.

The level of injury control activity has grown remarkably over the last two decades, with increases in prevention programmes, research, and funding at federal and local levels. This activity has led to decreases in injuries from many causes. Further growth of injury control activities will be an important factor in sustaining and further reducing injuries.

Causal model of injury control

The traditional epidemiological model for infectious diseases provided the framework for early epidemiological studies of injury (Fig. 1). At the centre of the causal pathway for injuries is the agent–host interaction. The agent, which in the case of injuries is energy, is absorbed by the host to cause injury. Energy can take many forms, such as mechanical, electrical, chemical, radiation, and thermal. An example of an agent–host relationship is a motor vehicle crash, in which the energy exerted on the individual is mechanical. The reservoir is the place in the environment where the agent is found. The potential for energy transfer exists everywhere, but its ability to cause injury is limited. For instance, the potential energy in a bullet causes injury only when the bullet is in motion and hits a human.

Vehicles and vectors are mechanisms which transport energy from the reservoir to the host. A vehicle is an inanimate object, such as a motor vehicle; a vector is animate, such as the dog that bites a child. For many injury causes, vehicles and vectors are both involved in energy transfer, such as when one individual (vector) stabs another with a knife (vehicle). The injury outcome is the trauma or injury sustained by the individual, and is influenced by host responses to the energy. Only energy transmitted beyond a host's tolerance causes an injury, and therefore not all exposures to energy result in noticeable injury. A human has some resistance to energy which can be increased through exercise or protective devices, or reduced through changes in intrinsic factors such as existing medical conditions or age, or through extrinsic factors such as fatigue and alcohol.

This model presents an easily understood framework for the causal pathway of injuries. However, it can appear deceptively simple. The interactions of vehicles, vectors, and hosts within the physical, social, economic, and cultural environment, as well as the factors which influence tolerance of the host and how severe the consequences of injuries to the host become, are extremely complex and ever-changing.

Data sources

Comprehensive and accurate data sources are the most important component in the cycle of surveillance, risk factor assessment, prevention, and evaluation. Data sources describing injuries are available on many levels, from broad national surveillance systems to local initiatives. In general, the detail in information provided decreases with the size of the surveillance system.

Increased efforts in injury surveillance are an exciting advancement in the field of injury control. A recent review by the Institute of

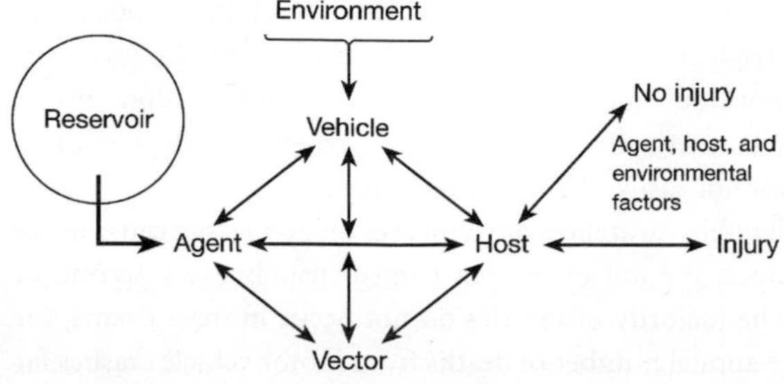

Fig. 1 The causal pathway for injuries.

Medicine (1999) identified 31 federally funded surveillance systems which address the incidence of injuries. The emergence of the Internet and improved computing power have made these databases easier to use and more accessible.

Specific data sources are described below.

Mortality

Incidence data of fatal injuries in the United States are available from 1900 through the present in the Vital Statistics Records collected by the National Center for Health Statistics. These data are collected from death certificates and classified by E-codes. The United States Vital Statistics Records are a good source for counts of fatal injuries by broadly defined causes as well as by age, race, and gender, but detailed information about the event and the types of injuries sustained is not available. Injury mortality rates can be obtained through CDC Wonder, an internet site maintained by the Centers for Disease Control and Prevention (http://wonder.cdc.gov). On-line queries of many databases can be conducted with instant results.

Most countries have some form of death certificate which is the source of official mortality counts. Deaths in developed countries have been accurately reported for many years. Mortality counts in less developed countries are less reliable and are often not available by cause. Although international comparisons of mortality statistics are routinely reported, the ability to compare international rates is limited by differing age distributions and exposures, as well as differences in reporting and coding criteria and data reliability.

In addition to overall injury mortality, several databases addressing specific causes of injury are maintained. A complete United States database on motor vehicle crash-related fatalities is found in the Fatal Accident Reporting System, developed in 1975 by the National Highway Traffic Safety Administration of the United States Department of Transportation. These standardized data on fatalities are collected from state and local police agency crash reports. Beginning in 1988, the General Estimates System was added to the Fatal Accident Reporting System database. The General Estimates System uses a nationally representative probability sample selected from all police-reported cases to estimate annual non-fatal crash injuries in the United States.

Work-related fatal injuries are collected by several sources. The National Traumatic Occupational Fatality System developed by the National Institute for Occupational Safety and Health was the first national system and uses United States death certificates for case identification. Work-related fatalities are determined by one item on the death certificate that indicates if the death occurred while the decedent was at work. The validity of this item to identify work-related fatalities varies by occupation, age, and gender. The specificity in correctly identifying all work-related fatalities may be low, leading to underestimates of work-related fatalities (Kraus *et al.* 1995). Since 1992, the Bureau of Labor Statistics has maintained the Census of Fatal Occupational Injuries. This census collects information from each state and may be the most accurate system currently in place because multiple data sources are used to identify and classify work-related injury. The National Safety Council also collects information on work-related fatalities. All three sources of work-related fatal injury data use different definitions of work, collect information from different populations of workers, and use different denominators for rate calculations.

National estimates of homicide deaths in the United States beginning in 1976 are maintained by the Federal Bureau of Investigations Uniform Crime Reporting System. Information on the victim, incident, and offender involved in the homicide are included. Data through 1996 are available to download from the Bureau of Justice Statistics web-page (http://www.ojp.usdoj.gov/bjs). Queries of databases describing perpetrators of crime are available on the same website through the Federal Justice Statistics Resource Center.

Morbidity

National estimates of injury morbidity are available from the National Health Interview Survey. Responses from sampled household interviews are weighted to estimate the incidence of all injuries in the United States, regardless of medical care received. Although this telephone interview provides valuable prevalence information, household telephone surveys often undersample severely injured individuals.

Information on hospital admissions, required for all accredited hospitals, is a source of national and community estimates of injury incidence. The National Hospital Discharge Survey conducted by the National Center for Health Statistics collects discharge data from each state to estimate national counts of injuries which require hospital admission. Discharge data are also usually available at the state and community level. These data represent only the most severe injuries. National estimates of emergency department visits and physician's office visits for injuries are available through surveys conducted by the National Center for Health Statistics.

Population-based surveys are conducted for information about risk-taking behaviours and injury events. One example is the National Health Interview Survey, which measures many aspects of health status including a few variables addressing injuries. The National Crime Victimization Survey is conducted annually to determine incidence and outcomes from crime victimization. The Behavioral Risk Factor Survey determines changes in perception of risk and the prevalence of behavioural risk factors such as wearing helmets and using seatbelts. The National Nursing Home Survey provides information about injuries sustained by older persons residing in nursing homes.

Many surveillance systems provide detailed information about specific types of injuries, exposures, and outcomes. The National Electronic Injury Surveillance System conducted by the United States Consumer Product Safety Commission gathers information about product-related injuries requiring hospital admission or emergency department treatment from a national sample of hospitals. National surveillance systems exist for burns, homicides and assaults, medicare claims, and child abuse and neglect. Periodic regional surveillance is commonly conducted for firearm injuries and traumatic brain injuries.

Most countries now have mortality statistics which identify injury deaths, and these have been used for new efforts in comparative analyses (see the discusion of international injury comparisons below). As these collaborative efforts progress, disparities in coding and reporting practices will be improved. Many countries which have an integrated hospital system have comprehensive injury surveillance programmes. For example, the New Zealand Health Information Service of the Ministry of Health has collected detailed information about all individuals admitted to a hospital in the country since 1979

(Langley 1995). Australia conducts the National Injury Surveillance Programme, which compiles injury hospitalizations for the entire country, and also conducts the National Health Survey, which is comparable with the United States National Health Interview Survey (McClure 1995). Canada has morbidity statistics available from 1979. Specific efforts in injury surveillance began in 1989 by co-ordinating emergency-room-based reporting from 10 Canadian paediatric hospitals. This programme has since grown to include all age groups and more hospitals (Sherman 1995). Sweden established a national discharge register in 1964, and began the National Injury Prevention Programme in 1986. This programme does not yet represent all counties of Sweden (Berg *et al.* 1995). Collaborative efforts among countries are leading to increased comparability and reliability among existing surveillance strategies, and helping establish surveillance systems in countries which do not yet have them.

Injury coding

Many features of injuries are necessary for a complete understanding of their causes, and the coding of injuries has been a complicated issue. The cause and nature of the injury as well as the acute and chronic physiological damage are each important issues. Injury causes are usually classified according to the International Classification of Diseases External Cause of Injury Codes (E-codes), and have traditionally been categorized as either unintentional or intentional. Unintentional injuries include motor and non-motor vehicle occupants, pedestrians, drowning, poisoning, falls, and suffocation, among others. Intentional injuries have included homicide and suicide. This system, however, combines cause with intent. For example, suicide, an intentional injury, can occur through drowning or poisoning. Recent improvements in injury classification schemes have separated intent and cause, and a matrix which separates E-codes by cause and intent is available (Fingerhut and Warner 1997). This classification approach is included in the 10th revision of the International Classification of Diseases. In this system, homicide and suicide are no longer causes of injury but are an intent. Firearms are now a cause of injury, for which the intent is divided into homicide, suicide, and unintentional. This system is much more informative and provides categories which are mutually exclusive.

There are two standard methods by which anatomical injuries are coded. The International Classification of Diseases system provides a complete taxonomy of injuries, categorized by anatomical location and type of damage. This system is used by most hospitals for their discharge data systems. However, the International Classification of Diseases system does not provide any information about the severity of injury. The Abbreviated Injury Scale (Association for the Advancement of Automotive Medicine 1990) categorizes injuries by the anatomical location and nature of damage, but also includes an index for injury severity. Scores for each individual injury can be combined through a defined algorithm to produce the Injury Severity Score, which is a single estimate of overall body damage from a given injury event. The Injury Severity Score was developed as a predictor of mortality in automotive crashes, but has become the main system for classifying overall injury severity.

Classifying long-term impairment and disability is very complex. Impairment refers to physical damage, such as loss of range of motion or inability to bear weight on a joint. Disability refers to the inability to perform tasks. The overall disability for an injured individual depends on many factors in addition to the physiological damage, such as occupation, activity level, and health status. For example, someone who lifts heavy objects at work will have a greater disability from a weight-bearing impairment than someone who does not need to perform lifting tasks. Impairments and disabilities occur on such a large spectrum that it is difficult to classify them in one scale. The Activities of Daily Living scale measures performance of the most basic tasks, such as feeding, transferring, and toileting and is often used to measure very severe disabilities. One of the most widely used measures of disability is the Functional Independence Measure, which includes at a minimum 13 motor and 5 cognitive measures rated on a seven-level scale (Granger 1998). The Functional Capacity Index was developed as a companion to the Abbreviated Injury Scale, and provides an estimate of the expected reduced functional capacity for each injury in the scale (MacKenzie *et al.* 1996). One advantage of the Functional Capacity Index is that independent assessments post-injury are not necessary.

Existing systems of injury classification have improved with increased knowledge about the causal pathway of injuries. The area of

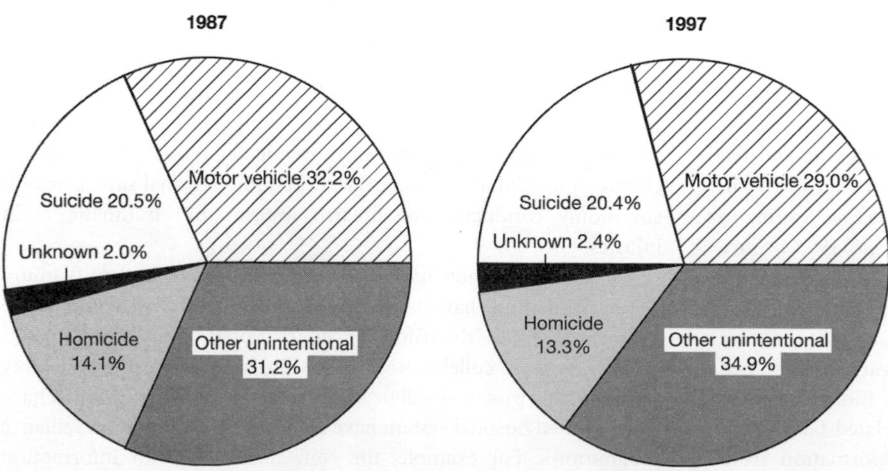

Fig. 2 Changes in the proportionate distribution of fatal injuries by type, United States, 1987 and 1997.

injury classification has made much progress, yet also holds many opportunities for further development.

Injury incidence and trends

Mortality

In 1997, unintentional injuries were the fifth leading cause of death in the United States, following heart disease, cancer, stroke, and pulmonary diseases. Suicide and homicide were the ninth and thirteenth leading causes respectively. However, unintentional injuries were the leading cause of death for those aged 1 to 44 years. Homicide was among the three leading causes of death for those aged 1 to 34 years, and suicide for the ages of 10 to 34 years. The three leading causes of death for those aged 15 to 24 years were unintentional injuries, homicide, and suicide (Hoyert *et al.* 1999).

Overall injury death rates have been decreasing since 1970, with the majority of the decline occurring among unintentional injuries. Figure 2 shows the change in the percentage of injury deaths by cause from 1987 to 1997. Although the rate of injury death has generally been decreasing, the proportionate causes of these deaths remained fairly stable. While unintentional injuries increased very slightly from 63.4 per cent to 63.9 per cent of all injury deaths, the proportion of motor-vehicle-related deaths decreased from 32.2 per cent to 29 per cent. This trend reflects a large decrease in the motor-vehicle-related fatality rate while other types of unintentional injuries, such as drowning and poisoning, have remained stable or increased slightly (Fingerhut and Warner 1997; Hoyert *et al.* 1999). The majority of the decrease in motor vehicle fatality rates has been for motor vehicle occupants, with less of an effect for other road users such as pedestrians. From 1987 to 1993, the motor vehicle crash rate decreased 19.4 per cent but remained relatively constant from 1993 to 1997. While motor vehicle deaths have decreased overall, these decreases have been less significant among children and the elderly (Brenner *et al.* 1999; Rivara 1999). Proper use and placement of child car seats and restraint of children who are too small for the shoulder harness and lap belt to fit properly are emerging focus areas. Further decreases in the motor vehicle death rates will require co-ordinated efforts at improving vehicle and road safety, public awareness campaigns, and new innovations in reducing alcohol and drug-involved crashes.

Homicides decreased from 14.1 per cent of injury deaths in 1987 to 13.3 per cent in 1997. Homicide deaths began decreasing in 1993, although the reasons for the decrease are not completely described. While increases in homicide rates since 1970 were attributed in part to increases in related crime, urban poverty, and inner city strife, as well as more accurate reporting of cause of death, recent decreases in homicide rates are attributed to the growing economy, community-based prevention programmes, increased and more effective law enforcement activities, and anticrime legislation (Sherman *et al.* 1997). The observed decreases are probably due in part to combinations of all of these as well as other undocumented factors. Suicide death rates remained at about 20.5 per cent of all injury deaths from 1987 to 1997. The most common and lethal method of suicide is the handgun. Increases in suicide death rates since 1950 are due almost exclusively to firearms, with the firearm death rate increasing 8.6 per cent from 1985 to 1995 (Fingerhut and Warner 1997). Increased access to firearms may lead to increases in suicide rates even if the number of attempts is stable, because attempts are more lethal. Non-complete suicide attempts are more commonly associated with poisoning and laceration (United States Department of Health and Human Services 1995).

Injury death rates have distinctive age patterns (Fig. 3). Non-motor-vehicle unintentional injuries are the leading cause of injury death from birth to age 5 and again after age 35, although the causes of these deaths differ. For those under 5 years the leading causes are suffocation, drowning, and fire/burns while the leading cause in the elderly is falls. Motor-vehicle-related deaths are the leading cause of injury death between the ages of 5 and 34 years and peak between the ages of 15 and 24 years. Those under 14 are more often killed as occupants in vehicles or as pedestrians, while the peak between the

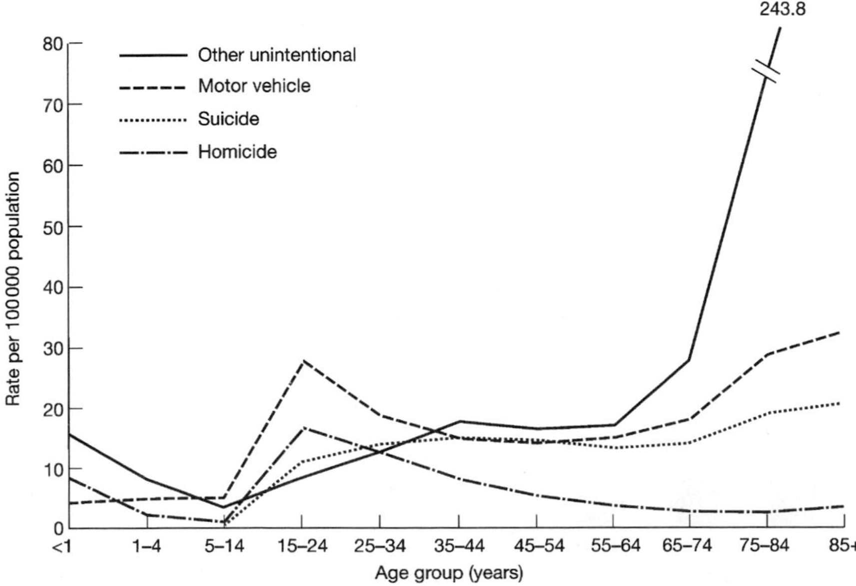

Fig. 3 Injury mortality rates by age, United States, 1997.

ages of 15 and 19 is largely due to the high fatal crash rate among younger drivers. Alcohol use is an important risk factor in motor vehicle crashes for all ages, but is a particular concern among drivers under 25. The elderly also have high pedestrian injury death rates.

Homicide is the second leading cause of injury death among infants and those aged 15 to 24 years. Although homicide has been decreasing in the last 5 years, these decreases have not occurred among those less than 18 years of age. Most homicides are committed with a firearm, occur during an argument, and are between acquaintances (United States Department of Health and Human Services 1995). Suicide rates are minimal until the age of 15 years, then increase steadily with increasing age. Trends indicate a reversal in the ranking of homicide and suicide deaths for persons over age 25, with suicide rates exceeding homicide rates.

Males have higher age-adjusted injury death rates than females for all causes of injury (Fig. 4). In 1997, the age-adjusted motor-vehicle-related death rate was approximately 53 per cent higher in males than females and showed similar gender variance in all age groups over age 5. The suicide rate was 76 per cent higher in males than in females, but diverged over age 65 when rates among males increased but for females remained constant. The homicide rate was 73 per cent higher for males than females. Homicide rates peak for males between the ages of 15 and 24 but for females peak between the ages of 25 and 34. While males are more likely to be killed by an acquaintance or stranger, females are overwhelmingly more likely to be killed by an intimate partner (Rennison 1999).

Death rates for injuries also vary by racial group. In 1995, Native Americans had the highest unintentional injury death rate and the highest suicide rate (Fingerhut and Warner 1997). African-Americans had the highest homicide rate, which was 123 per cent higher than the rate for Hispanics, who had the second-highest rate. Asian-Americans had the lowest death rates for both intentional and unintentional injury.

Recent improvements in the classification of injuries separate intent from mechanism. Figure 5 shows the leading causes of injury death rates in 1997 by mechanism. Motor vehicle deaths were predominantly unintentional with a small number of suicides. Over half of all firearm deaths were suicides and another 40 per cent homicides. Less than 5 per cent of firearm injuries were unintentional, but these occurred primarily among the young. Approximately 28 per cent of poisoning deaths were suicides, and this proportion increased with age. Among the young, poisoning deaths were mostly unintentional. Over 14 per cent of poisoning deaths had an unknown intent. Falls, drowning, and fire/burn deaths were predominantly unintentional. The intent for suffocation was most often suicide, but when examined by age, homicide is the main cause of suffocation for those

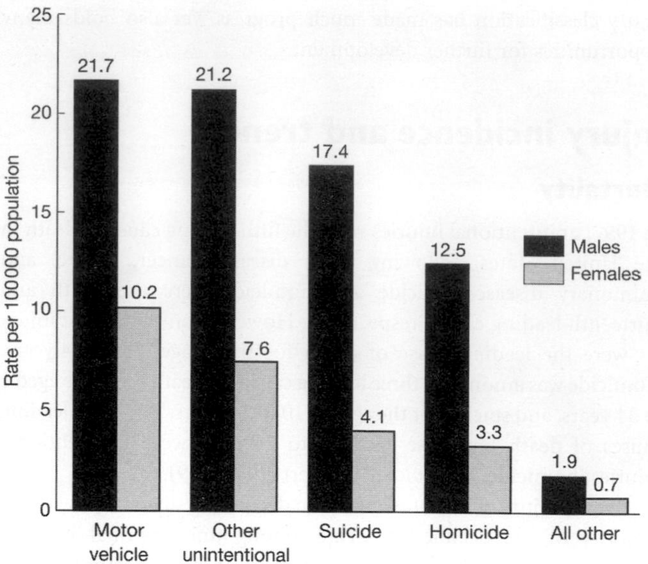

Fig. 4 Age-adjusted mortality rates for injuries by type and sex, United States, 1997.

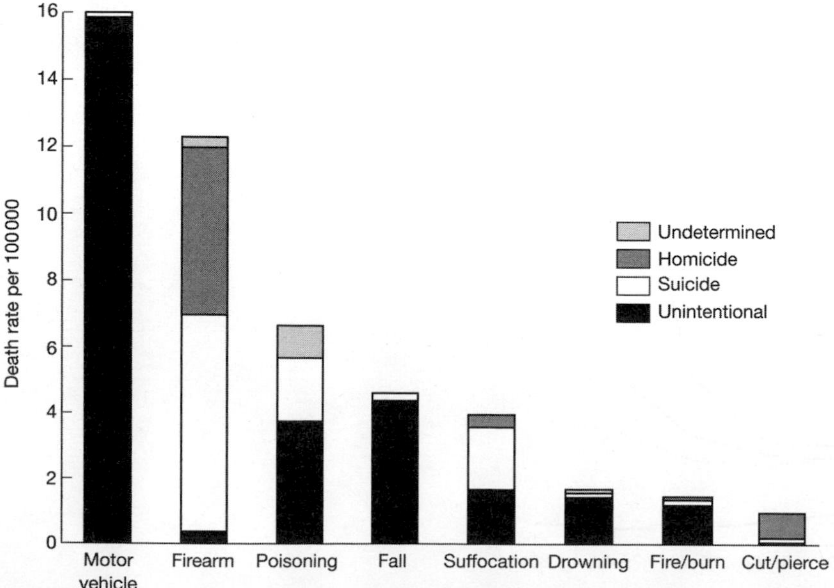

Fig. 5 Leading causes of injury mortality by intent, United States, 1997.

under the age of 1 year, unintentional suffocation was most frequent among those between 15 and 44, and suicidal suffocation increased with age. Cutting/piercing deaths were primarily homicides.

Hospital discharges

The injury pyramid is a common method for examining levels of injury severity including deaths, hospital admissions, emergency department visits, and office visits (Fig. 6) (McCaig and Stussman 1997; Woodwell 1997; Peters *et al.* 1998; Graves 1999). In 1996, the National Hospital Discharge Survey indicated that 2.55 million people were hospitalized in the United States for injuries (Graves 1999). This was a ratio of 17 hospital admissions for every death. For every death, 232 injured individuals (almost 35 million annually) were treated and released from hospital emergency departments and another 582 (almost 87.6 million annually) were treated in physicians' offices (McCaig and Stussman 1997; Woodwell 1997). The sum of all levels of the injury pyramid yielded over 125 million injuries requiring some level of medical care in 1996. In comparison to 1992, the ratio of hospital admissions and emergency department visits for every death has decreased, but the ratio of physician office visits increased. This pattern suggests either a reduction in the severity of injuries or changes in treatment practices. Reductions in injury severity could reflect effectiveness of secondary prevention measures aimed at reducing the severity of injuries once a potential injury-producing exposure has occurred. Increases in the use of outpatient care could also contribute to decreases in hospitalizations.

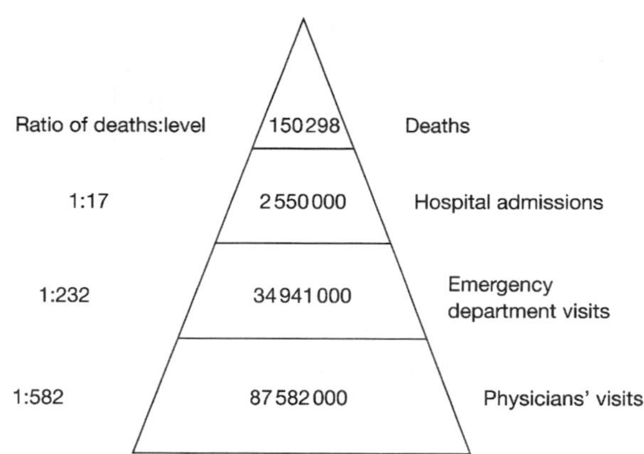

Fig. 6 Injury pyramid of treatment levels and mortality, United States, 1996.

Injuries were the fourth leading cause of hospitalization in 1996, following heart disease, respiratory disease, and digestive system diseases (Graves 1999). For about 8 per cent of all individuals hospitalized, or approximately 2.55 million persons, the primary reason for hospitalization was an injury.

Table 1 shows the first-listed primary injury diagnosis and length of stay among hospital admissions from the National Hospital Discharge Survey (Graves 1999). The first-listed diagnosis is principally used for billing purposes and is usually but not necessarily the most severe injury sustained, and approximates the total number of individuals injured. However, first-listed diagnoses do not reflect multiple injuries and therefore underestimate the total number of individuals sustaining particular types of injuries each year, in particular the less severe injuries.

The overall rate of hospital discharge for injuries in 1996 was 96.6 per 10 000 population with an average length of stay of 5.4 days. Fractures were the most common injury, with a rate of 38.9 per 10 000 population in 1993 to 1994, and required the longest average length of stay at 7.2 days. Poisoning, the second most frequent injury, occurred at a rate of 8.7 per 10 000 population and resulted in an average of 3.1 days in the hospital. Internal injuries, with a rate of 3.3, required the second longest hospital stay of 6.8 days. The rate of hospitalization for intracranial injuries was 5.9 and required an average of 6.5 days in the hospital.

Emergency department visits

Of the 94.9 million emergency department visits in the United States in 1997, 37 per cent were for injuries (Nourjah 1999). In addition to the fact that more injuries were presented to emergency departments than hospitals, the percentage of all emergency department visits attributable to injuries was far greater than the percentage of hospitalizations due to injuries. The rate of injury-related emergency room visits was 1311.9 per 10 000 persons per year.

Figure 7 shows the five leading injury-related complaints presented to emergency departments. About 6.4 million individuals were treated for falls, the leading cause of injury among emergency room visits. Over 4.8 million persons, or 13.7 per cent of all persons visiting the emergency department for injuries, were treated for injuries resulting from unintentionally being struck against or by objects or persons. More than 4.2 million people (12.2 per cent) were treated for motor vehicle crash injuries, almost 2.8 million (8.9 per cent) for unintentionally being cut by sharp or piercing objects, and an additional 2.16 million (6.1 per cent) for intentional-assault-related injuries.

Table 1 Rate per 10 000 population of first-listed injury diagnosis on hospital discharge data and average length of hospital stay, United States, 1993–1994

Diagnosis	Rate for first-listed diagnosis on discharge	Average length of hospital stay (days)
Internal injuries	3.3	6.8
Sprains and strains	5.1	2.8
Intracranial injuries	5.9	6.5
Open wounds and lacerations	6.3	3.6
Poisoning	8.7	3.1
Fractures	38.9	7.2
Superficial injuries	3.0	3.8

minority youth, were found to be far from goals stated for unintentional injuries. Child restraint and bicycle helmet usage, smoke detectors, and alcohol use were stated as priority areas. Currently, the United States Department of Health and Human Services (1998) is drafting health objectives for 2010. The number of injury-related goals has increased, and the new goals are focused on specific high-risk populations.

The Institute of Medicine has released several important reports addressing injuries and trauma care, the most recent of which was the report *Reducing the Burden of Injury*, produced in 1999. This report identified national priorities for surveillance, training and research, firearm prevention, trauma care systems, state infrastructure, and federal response. Recommendations from this report include expanding emergency department surveillance, the establishment of a national fatal intentional-injury surveillance system, expansion of training activities for both research and practice, and increased co-ordination and support for agencies leading the field of injury control.

Although these national priorities are vital to the growth and continued success of the field, the specific goals for prevention activities must occur locally. Each state, county, and community has different high-risk populations, injury risks, and attitudes towards prevention. These factors are a crucial element in the design of effective injury-prevention programmes. With increased recognition of the burden of injury as well as advances in our knowledge of the causes and consequences of injuries, the injury control field will continue to grow in an organized and informed manner.

References

Association for the Advancement of Automotive Medicine (1990). *Abbreviated Injury Scale: revision.* Association for the Advancement of Automotive Medicine, Des Plaines, IL.

Association for the Advancement of Automotive Medicine (1993). *Injury control in the 1990s: a national plan for action. Report to the Second World Conference on Injury Control.* Association for the Advancement of Automotive Medicine, Des Plaines, IL.

American College of Surgeons (1993). *Resources for optimal care of the injured patient.* American College of Surgeons, Chicago, IL.

Berg, L., Aberg, A., Schelp, L., and Svanstrom, L. (1995). Data needs for evaluation of injury prevention programs—experiences from Sweden. *Proceedings of the International Collaborative Effort on Injury Statistics*, Vol I, Chapter 19, pp. 1–9. Centers for Disease Control and Prevention, Department of Health and Human Services, Hyattsville, MD.

Blincoe, L.J. and Faigin, B.M. (1993). Economic impact of motor-vehicle crashes—United States, 1990. *Morbidity and Mortality Weekly Report*, **42**, 443–8.

Brenner, R.A., Overpeck, M.D., Trumble, A.C., DerSimonian, R., and Berendes, H. (1999). Deaths attributable to injuries in infants, United States, 1983–1991. *Pediatrics*, **103**, 968–74.

Burt, C.W. and Fingerhut, L.A. (1998). Injury visits to hospital emergency departments: United States, 1992–1995. *Vital and Health Statistics*, **13**, 1–76.

Cairns, H. (1941). Head injuries in motor-cyclists: the importance of the crash helmet. *British Medical Journal*, **ii**, 465–71.

Cairns, H. and Holbourn, H. (1943). Head injuries in motor-cyclists: with special reference to crash helmets. *British Medical Journal*, **i**, 591–8.

Chorba, T.L. (1991). Assessing technologies for preventing injuries in motor vehicle crashes. *International Journal of Technology Assessment in Health Care*, **7**, 296–314.

Cummings, P., Grossman, C.D., Rivara, F.P., and Koepsell, T.D. (1997). State gun safe storage laws and child mortality due to firearms. *Journal of the American Medical Association*, **278**, 1084–6.

DeHaven, H. (1968). Beginnings of crash injury research. In *Accident pathology* (ed. K. Brinkham), pp. 1–15. FH 11–6595, Department of Transportation, Washington, DC.

Dosenclos, J.C. and Hahn, R.C. (1992). Years of potential life lost before the age 65, by race, Hispanic origin, and sex—United States, 1986–1988. *Morbidity and Mortality Weekly Report*, **41**, 13–23.

Evans, L. (1985). *The effectiveness of safety belts in preventing fatalities.* General Motors Research, Warren, MI.

Fingerhut, L.A. and Warner, M. (1997). *Injury chartbook: health, United States, 1996–97.* National Center for Health Statistics, Hyattsville, MD.

Fingerhut, L.A., Cox, C.S., Warner, M., *et al.* (1998). International comparative analysis of injury mortality: findings from the International Collaborative Effort on Injury Statistics. *Advance Data*, **303**, 1–18.

Freed, L.H., Vernick, J.S., and Hargarten, S.W. (1998). Prevention of firearm-related injuries and deaths among youth: a product-oriented approach. *Pediatric Clinics of North America*, **45**, 427–38.

Gibson, J. (1961). The contribution of experimental psychology to the formulation of the problem of safety: a brief for basic science. In *Behavioral approaches to accident research* (ed. H.H. Jacobs), p. 77. Association for the Aid of Crippled Children, New York.

Gordon, F. (1949). The epidemiology of accidents. *American Journal of Public Health*, **39**, 504–15.

Graham, J.D. (1993). Injuries from traffic crashes: meeting the challenge. *Annual Review of Public Health*, **14**, 515–43.

Granger, C.W. (1998). The emerging science of functional assessment: our tool for outcome analysis. *Archives of Physical Medicine and Rehabilitation*, **79**, 235–40.

Graves, E. (1999). National Hospital Discharge Survey: annual summary, 1996. *Vital and Health Statistics*, **13**, 1–46.

Haddon, W., Jr (1963). A note concerning accident theory and research with special reference to motor-vehicle accidents. *Annals of the New York Academy of Sciences*, **107**, 635–46.

Haddon, W., Jr (1972). A logical framework for categorizing highway safety phenomena and activity. *Journal of Trauma*, **12**, 193–207.

Haddon, W., Jr, Schuman, E., and Klein, D. (1964). *Accident research: methods and approaches.* Harper and Row, New York.

Hedlund, J. (1985). Casualty reductions resulting from safety belt use laws. Presented at OECD Meeting, May, Washington, DC.

Hoyert, D.L., Kochanek, K.D., and Murphy, S.L. (1999). Deaths: final data for 1997. *National Vital Statistics Reports*, **47**, 1–104.

Institute of Medicine (1997). *Enabling America: assessing the role of rehabilitation science and engineering.* National Academy Press, Washington, DC.

Institute of Medicine (1999). *Reducing the burden of injury: advancing prevention and treatment.* National Academy Press, Washington, DC.

Kahane, C.J. (1986). *An evaluation of child passenger safety: the effectiveness and benefits of safety seats.* National Highway Traffic Safety Administration, Washington, DC.

Kraus, J.F. (1993). Epidemiology of head injury. In *Head injury* (3rd edn) (ed. P.R. Cooper), pp. 1–25. Williams and Wilkins, Baltimore, MD.

Kraus, J.F., Peek, C., McArthur, D., and Williams, A. (1994). The effects of the 1992 California Mandatory Motorcycle Helmet Use law on motorcycle crash fatalities and injuries. *Journal of the American Medical Association*, **272**, 1506–11.

Kraus, J.F., Peek, C., Silberman, T., and Anderson, C. (1995). The accuracy of death certificates in identifying work-related fatal injuries. *American Journal of Epidemiology*, **141**, 973–9.

Langley, J. (1995). Experiences using New Zealand's Hospital Based Surveillance System for injury prevention research. *Proceedings of the International Collaborative Effort on Injury Statistics*, Vol I, Chapter 9, pp. 1–8. Centers for Disease Control and Prevention, Department of Health and Human Services, Hyattsville, MD.

McCaig, L.F. and Stussman, B.J. (1997). National Hospital Ambulatory Medical Care Survey: 1996 emergency department summary. *Advance Data*, **293**, 1–20.

McClure, R. (1995). Injury and general practice in Australia. *Australian Family Physician*, **24**, 2059–63.

Mackay, M. (1985). Seat belt use under voluntary and mandatory conditions and its effect on casualties. In *Human behavior and traffic safety* (ed. L. Evan and R.C. Schwing), pp. 259–78. Plenum Press, New York.

MacKenzie, E.J., Damiano, A., Miller, T., and Luchter, S. (1996). The development of the functional capacity index. *Journal of Trauma*, **41**, 799–807.

Miller, T.R., Lestina, D.C., and Galbraith, M.S. (1994). Medical care spending—United States. *Morbidity and Mortality Weekly Report*, **43**, 581–6.

Murray, C.J.L. and Lopez, A.D. (1997*a*). Mortality by cause for eight regions of the world: Global Burden of Disease Study. *Lancet*, **349**, 1269–76.

Murray, C.J.L. and Lopez, A.D. (1997*b*). Global mortality, disability, and the contribution of risk factors: Global Burden of Disease Study. *Lancet*, **349**, 1436–41.

Murray, C.J.L. and Lopez, A.D. (1997*c*). Alternative projections of mortality and disability by cause 1990–2020: Global Burden of Disease Study. *Lancet*, **349**, 1498–1504.

National Center for Health Statistics (1991). Impairments due to injuries: United States, 1985–87. *Vital and Health Statistics*, **10**, 1–55.

National Committee for Injury Prevention and Control (1989). Injury prevention: meeting the challenge. *American Journal of Preventive Medicine*, **5** (Supplement).

National Highway Traffic Safety Administration (1984). *Final regulatory impact analysis: amendment to FMVSS 208 passenger car front seat occupant protection.* Department of Transportation, Washington, DC.

National Highway Traffic Safety Administration. (1992). *Economic costs of motor vehicle crashes 1990.* Department of Transportation, Washington, DC.

National Research Council (1985). *Injury in America.* National Academy Press, Washington, DC.

National Safety Council (1993). *Understanding and preventing violence* (ed. A.J. Reiss Jr and J.A. Roth). National Academy Press, Washington DC.

National Safety Council (1998). *Accident facts.* National Safety Council, Itasca, IL.

Nourjah, P. (1999). National Hospital Ambulatory Medical Care Survey: 1997 emergency department summary. *Advance Data*, **304**, 1–23.

O'Carroll, P.W., Rosenberg, M.L., and Mercy, J.A. (1991). Suicide. In *Violence in America: a public health approach* (ed. M.L. Rosenberg and M.A. Fenley), pp. 184–96. Oxford University Press, New York.

Partyka, S.C. and Womble, K.B. (1989). Projected lives saved from greater belt use. In *National Center for Statistics and Analysis Research Notes.* National Highway Traffic Safety Administration, Washington, DC.

Peters, K.D., Kochanek, K.D., and Murphy, S.L. (1998). Deaths: final data for 1996. *National Vital Statistics Reports*, **47**, 1–100.

Pollock, D.A. and McClain, P.W. (1989). Trauma registries: current status and future prospects, 1989. *Journal of the American Medical Association*, **262**, 2280–3.

Powell, E.C., Sheehan, K.M, and Christoffel, K.K. (1996). Firearm violence among youth: public health strategies for prevention. *Annals of Emergency Medicine*, **28**, 204–12.

Rennison, C.M. (1999). *Criminal victimization 1998: changes 1997–98 with trends 1993–98.* Bureau of Justice Statistics National Crime Victimization Survey NCJ 176 353, US Department of Justice, Washington, DC.

Rice, D., MacKenzie, E., *et al.* (1989). *Cost of injury in the United States: a report to Congress, 1989.* Institute for Health and Aging, University of California, San Francisco, and Injury Prevention Center, Johns Hopkins University, Baltimore, MD.

Rivara, F.P. (1999). Pediatric injury control in 1999: where do we go from here? *Pediatrics*, **103**, 883–8.

Sherman, G.J. (1995). Federal injury surveillance in Canada: filling the gaps. *Proceedings of the International Collaborative Effort on Injury Statistics*, Vol I, Chapter 10, pp. 1–5. Centers for Disease Control and Prevention, Department of Health and Human Services, Washington, DC.

Sherman, L.W., Gottfredson, D., MacKenzie, D., Eck, J., Reuter, P., and Bushway, S. (1997). *Preventing crime: what works, what doesn't, what's promising.* National Institute of Justice Report 165 366, US Department of Justice, Washington, DC.

Stambrook, M., Moore, A.D., Peters, L.C., Devianene, C., and Hawryluc, G.A. (1990). Effects of mild, moderate and severe closed head injury on long-term vocational status. *Brain Injury*, **4**, 183–90.

Tengs, T.O., Adams, M.E., Pliskin, J.S., *et al.* (1995). Five-hundred life-saving interventions and their cost-effectiveness. *Risk Analysis*, **15**, 369–90.

United States Department of Health and Human Services (1995). *Healthy People 2000, midcourse review and 1995 revisions.* US Department of Health and Human Services, Washington, DC.

United States Department of Health and Human Services (1998). *Healthy People 2010 objectives: draft for public comment.* US Department of Health and Human Services, Washington, DC.

Waller, J.A. (1985). *Injury control: a guide to the causes and prevention of trauma.* Lexington Books, Lexington, MA.

Woodwell, D.A. (1997). National Ambulatory Medical Care Survey: 1996 summary. *Advance Data*, **295**, 1–25.

Wright, M.A., Wintemute, G.J., and Rivara, F.P. (1999). Effectiveness of denial of handgun purchase to persons believed to be at high risk for firearm violence. *American Journal of Public Health*, **89**, 88–90.

Zador, P.L. and Ciccone, M.A. (1993). Automobile driver fatalities in frontal impacts: air bags compared with manual belts. *American Journal Public Health*, **83**, 661–6.

10.5 Interpersonal violence prevention: a recent public health mandate

Deborah Prothrow-Stith, Howard Spivak, and Robert D. Sege

Introduction

This chapter on public health approaches to interpersonal violence is a response to the epidemic of adolescent and young adult homicide in the United States, and the growing international attention and concerns about this problem. The chapter provides a short history of the efforts within public health to address violence, a definition and description of the problem, and a discussion of examples of public health approaches to violence prevention. While several types of violence are briefly discussed, the focus of the chapter is youth violence and the increase in youth homicide in the United States. The 1987 United States homicide rate for 15- to 24-year-old men of 22 per 100 000 was the highest among industrialized countries not at war in the period 1986 to 1987 (Fig. 1). By 1991, it had increased to 37 per 100 000. While high homicide rates also plagued South Africa at the same time, the political instability and violent freedom struggle made it an exception.

The public's demand for solutions to violence in the United States has generated increased multidisciplinary attention to the problem that goes beyond the traditional criminal justice responses of punishment and deterrence. In the past 25 years we have witnessed a dramatic effort led by public health professionals to confront violence in the United States. Leadership has emerged from the Centers for Disease Control (**CDC**), the Surgeon General's office, and many state and local health departments. Many international meetings, initially geared towards discussion of peace and ending war, now include interpersonal violence on their agendas.

In 1983 the CDC established the Violence Epidemiology Branch for the study of homicide and suicide. Initial *Morbidity and Mortality Weekly Reports* revealed that homicide is the leading cause of death for black men between the ages of 15 to 24 years and 25 to 44 years, and is the second leading cause of death for all adolescents (CDC 1982*a*,*b*, 1983*a*,*b*). Additional information concerning the characteristics of homicides was published for public health audiences, and indicated

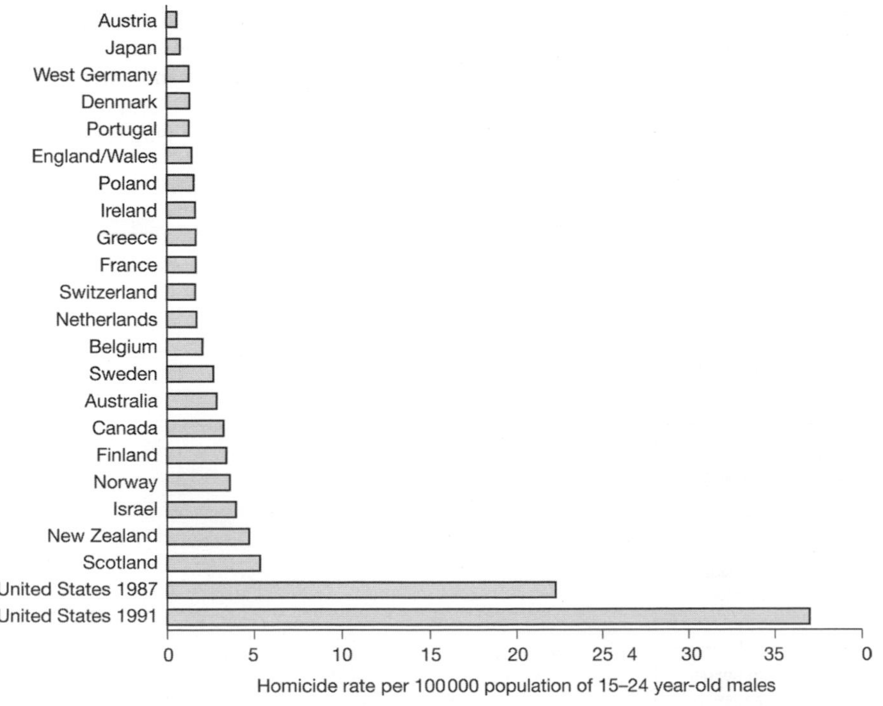

Fig. 1 International comparisons of homicide rate per 100 000 population (males, aged 15–24 years) in the period 1986 to 1987.

that 58 per cent of the victims knew their assailants, 47 per cent were precipitated by an argument, and only 15 per cent were a result of another felony (burglary, drug trafficking, etc.) (CDC 1983*a*,*b*). The application of basic epidemiology and reporting techniques became the impetus for public health professionals across the country to confront the issue.

In October 1985, C. Everett Koop convened an invitational meeting, the Surgeon General's Workshop on Violence and Public Health, in Leesburg, Virginia. The interdisciplinary meeting focused on assault and homicide, child abuse, rape and sexual assault, domestic violence, elder abuse, and suicide. The workshop and its published proceedings continue to fuel public health professionals' efforts to frame violence as a mainstream public health problem.

Today, public health endeavours to understand and prevent violence continue to grow with increasingly more programmes, publications, and presentations. In 1994, the CDC established the National Center for Injury Prevention and Control and every Surgeon General following Dr Koop has encouraged the public health community to use its strategies to better understand and prevent violence.

In the United States, a country-wide effort to prevent violence utilizing standard epidemiology, community outreach, screening, community-based programmes, health education, behaviour modification, public awareness, and education campaigns continues, involving every aspect of the United States Public Health Service. The movement to prevent violence in the United States is based upon similar multidisciplinary efforts to prevent lung cancer deaths, heart disease, and fatal car crashes.

Although embryonic and consisting of thousands of insulated programmes scattered across the country, this movement has the potential for the same level of success that public health professionals have had with reducing smoking and drink-driving in the United States. The analogy between violence prevention and other public health problems is not flawless, yet two decades of experience employing comparable techniques and strategies indicates enough similarity for success.

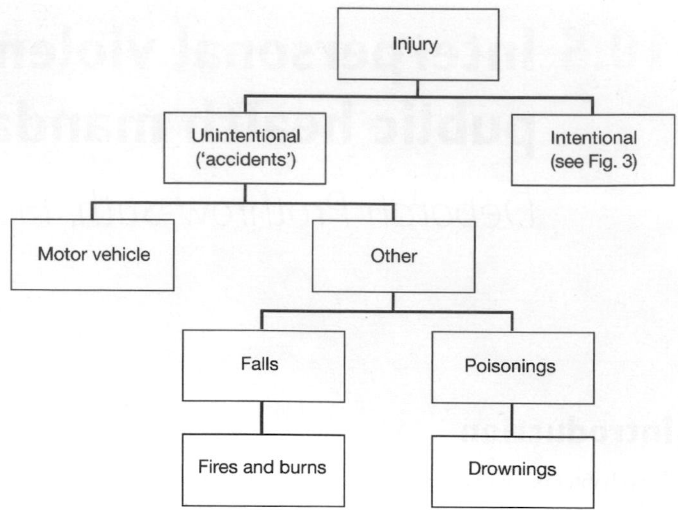

Fig. 2 Unintentional and intentional injury.

Definition and classification

The National Center for Injury Prevention and Control at the CDC classifies both unintentional injuries (accidents) and intentional injuries (violence) as public health problems, as illustrated in Fig. 2. Intentional injuries are divided into self-directed violence (suicides and suicide attempts) and interpersonal violence (assaults and homicides) (Fig. 3). Violence is defined by the CDC as 'the threatened or actual use of physical force or power against another person, against oneself, or against a group or community that either results or is likely to result in injury, death, or deprivation'.

Suicide, a more traditional problem for health and public health professionals, has several commonalities with interpersonal violence. Both often involve alcohol and other drugs, and the risk for both increases with the presence of a firearm. Media and entertainment values appear to have an impact on both. Adolescent suicide and homicide rates rose dramatically during the early 1980s. While suicide

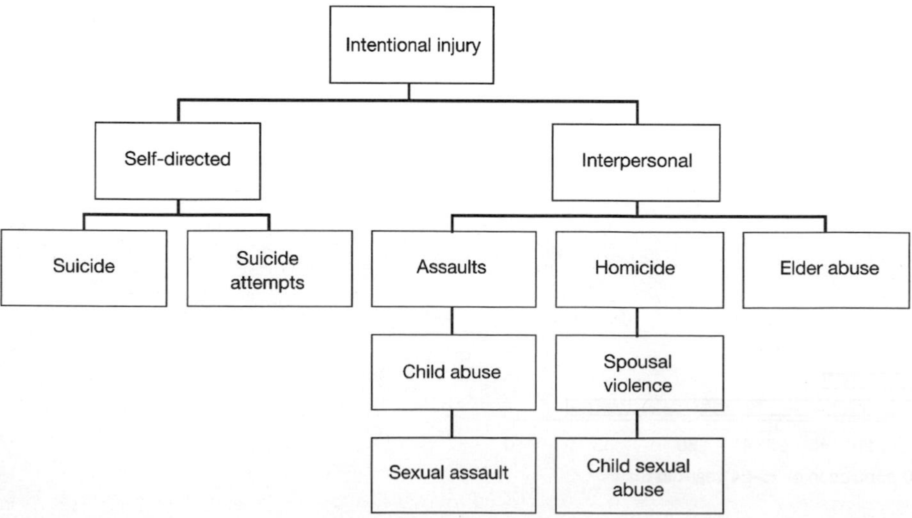

Fig. 3 Intentional injury—violence.

remains an important public health concern, recent efforts using public health strategies to address interpersonal violence have proliferated.

There are at least four reasons why interpersonal violence became an important concern for public health professionals in the United States: (a) the magnitude of the problem; (b) the characteristics of violence; (c) the contact that health professionals have with the victims and perpetrators of violence; (d) the application of public health strategies to both understanding and preventing violence.

Public health professionals have offered a unique approach to violence that has yielded significant contributions and offers further promise.

Data sources

There are several sources of data on violence in America which are accessible to the public or through community partnerships with academic institutions. The National Center for Education Statistics and the Bureau of Justice Statistics are the primary federal entities for collecting, analysing, and reporting data related to education and crime respectively in the United States and other nations. The Department of the Treasury, Bureau of Alcohol, Tobacco and Firearms publication *Commerce in Firearms in the United States* is an annual report of activities relating to the regulation of firearms. The Youth Crime Interdiction Initiative *Crime Gun Trace Analysis Reports: the Illegal Youth Firearms Market in 27 Communities* brings together federal, state, and local law enforcement officials to improve information about the illegal sources of guns recovered from juveniles and adult criminals.

The *Uniform Crime Reports*, published by the United States Federal Bureau of Investigation (FBI), is the most frequently cited source of national information on violent crime. These annual reports, which date back to 1930, use police data that are submitted to the FBI and which are aggregated into a national data source. Homicides are mandatorily reported in these datasets, but other crimes are reported voluntarily and therefore inconsistently. The reports give cursory information on homicides and assaults, including victim and perpetrator relationship, weapons used, location of the violent episode, and race of victim and perpetrator.

The magnitude of the problem

The FBI estimates that 1.8 million Americans are victims of violence each year. Adolescents are more likely than any other age group to be victims, mostly from their peers. A complete representation of the magnitude of violence is not available because there are no reliable and consistent measures of non-fatal episodes of violence. Homicides, the tip of the iceberg, are more accurately measured as they are mandatorily reported by the United States' local police departments to the FBI. Other countries have made their homicide rates available through the World Health Organization.

The magnitude of the problem of homicide in the United States is mind-boggling when compared with that of other industrialized nations not at war. Not only is the United States homicide rate 10 to 25 times higher than most industrialized nations, but the homicide rates rival those in some less developed countries facing war or considerable social, political, and economic turmoil (Wolfgang 1986).

The rate of youth violence in the United States is consistently higher than that of any other industrialized nation. In 1987, compared with 21 other developed countries, the United States had the highest homicide rate for males aged 15 to 24 years at 21.9 per 100 000 (Fingerhut and Kleinman 1990). Moreover, a study of 1985 homicide rates showed that the United States rate for both sexes, aged 1 to 19 years, was more than three times that of Canada which had the next highest rate (Williams and Kotch 1990).

Of the 16 914 murder victims in 1998, 94 per cent of the black victims were killed by black offenders and 87 per cent of the white victims were killed by white offenders. Firearms were used in six out of ten murders (FBI 1999). In 1997, the rate of homicide among males aged 15 to 19 years was 22.6 per 100 000—a decline of 12.4 per cent in one year. Homicide is the second leading cause of death for persons 15 to 24 years of age and is the leading cause of death for African Americans. Each month approximately 100 children die from gun violence (FBI 1997).

Non-fatal episodes of violence and assaults are not always reported to the police. Emergency departments captured a larger number of the assaults illustrated in the Northeast Ohio Trauma Study, where for every homicide there were 20 assaults reported to the police and 100 reported to the emergency rooms in one standard metropolitan statistical area in northeast Ohio. Many episodes of violence, particularly those occurring among friends and family, are not reported to the police or emergency departments.

The epidemic of youth violence in the United States is not limited to homicide. Police arrest data reveal an increase in non-fatal episodes of adolescent violence despite the limitations of the data set. The decade from 1980 to 1990 saw the juvenile violent-crime arrest rate for black adolescents increase by 19 per cent; for white adolescents it increased by 44 per cent, while the other-race category, despite a large increase in Asian youth, declined by 53 per cent (FBI 1992). Although minors make up less than 14 per cent of the United States population, they accounted for 37 per cent of homicide arrests, 28 per cent of rape arrests, and 51 per cent of robbery arrests in 1995. In 1982, 390 youths aged 13 to 15 years were arrested for homicide. By 1992, this figure had nearly doubled. Although these rates have been dropping since 1994, they are not dropping as quickly as adult violence rates (FBI 1997). The escalation of adolescent violent-crime rates in the last several decades cuts across race, class, and lifestyle, despite a common misconception that it is an urban black problem.

Adolescent violence

Violence involving youth has reached alarming levels in the United States. In 1991, the National Center for Health Statistics reported that homicide and legal intervention was the second leading cause of death for the group aged 15 to 24 years (22.4 deaths per 100 000, second only to motor vehicle accidents), at almost twice the rate for the overall United States population (11.7 deaths per 100 000) (CDC 1993*a*).

In 1997, 6146 people aged 15 to 24 years were victims of homicide. This amounts to an average of 17 youth homicide victims per day in the United States. Homicide is the second leading cause of death for persons aged 15 to 24 years, the leading cause of death for African Americans, and the second leading cause of death for Hispanic youths.

Furthermore, trends in adolescent mortality rates indicate that although overall death rates and death rates due to motor vehicle crashes both decreased for persons aged 10 to 24 years from 1979 to

1988, death rates for homicide increased by 6.7 per cent. The CDC estimates that by the year 2003 more Americans will die from firearms-related injuries than from motor vehicle accidents. This is already true in eight states (CDC 1994).

The 1990 National Crime Survey found that, even for non-fatal violent victimizations, age was one of the most important single predictors of an individual's risk, which peaks at age 16 to 19 for both men (95 per 1000) and women (54 per 1000) (Bureau of Justice Statistics 1992, 1993). Clearly, our nation's youth are at high risk for experiencing violence.

Dating violence is a form of adolescent and young-adult violence that is often overlooked, even within discussions of domestic violence. Very little research has been done and the general awareness of the problem of dating violence is relatively recent. A survey within a college population found that 21 per cent of the students admitted being in violent relationships, and 62 per cent knew personally of someone affected by a violent relationship (Makepeace 1981). Several studies indicate that between 12 and 19 per cent of high-school students are involved in dating violence, either as a victim or perpetrator. As with domestic violence, women are more often the victims.

School violence: more lethal

School suspension data offer another measure of the violence occurring, but there are several limitations. Suspension numbers may vary within a school depending upon the persons responsible for collecting the data. There are no standard criteria within or between school systems as to what behaviour will cause a student suspension.

Violence in schools is not new, but it is increasingly more severe and lethal. In the most recent Youth Risk Behaviour Survey conducted by the CDC, 18.3 per cent of students from the ninth to twelfth grades in the 50 states, including the District of Columbia and the Virgin Islands, reported carrying a weapon 30 days prior to the survey and 5.9 per cent reported that they had carried a gun. Seven per cent said they had been threatened or injured with a weapon while on school property in the 12 months before the survey. An estimated 74.2 separate incidents of weapon-carrying had occurred per 100 students 30 days prior to the survey. Among students nationwide, 36.6 per cent had been in a physical fight once or more during the 12 months preceding the survey.

The CDC survey also revealed that 4 per cent of the students said that they had missed at least one day of school in the previous month because they felt unsafe at school (no significant difference). In 1989, the United States Department of Justice found that 6 per cent of students report having to avoid certain places in school or on the way to or from school because they were afraid of being attacked. In a poll conducted by Metropolitan Life, 23 per cent of students said they never saw violent incidents at school. A Louis Harris Associates Poll of youth and guns conducted in 1993 of 2500 students in the sixth to twelfth grades showed that 15 per cent had carried a handgun to school in the past year, and 59 per cent said they could get a handgun if they wanted one. The addition of weapons to the typical school brawl has contributed significantly to the greater severity and mortality of school fights.

The CDC, the United States Department of Education, and the National School Safety Center are conducting a study of actual deaths in schools. Preliminary data show that 105 school-associated violent deaths (81 homicides, 19 suicides, and five unintentional firearm-related deaths) occurred in the school years 1992–1993 and 1993–1994. Sixty-six per cent of these occurred on school property and 75 per cent were committed with a firearm.

While the arrest rates for overall crime and violent crime are significantly lower for young women than for young men, recent increases in girls' arrests have narrowed the gap. From 1981 to 1995, there was a 129 per cent increase in the violent-crime arrest rate for young women compared with a 56 per cent increase over the same time period for young men. Now, girls account for 25 per cent of the juvenile arrests for violent crime—unheard of two decades ago. More girls are entering the juvenile justice system and are doing so at younger ages; there has been a 10 per cent increase in the numbers of 13- and 14-year-olds coming into juvenile court.

Some experts, including Meda Chesney-Lind at the University of Hawaii, believe that there has not really been a significant increase in the proportion of young women committing crimes. Rather, 'We're criminalizing a lot of schoolyard scuffles where, in the past, we'd call it a cat fight, we'd giggle and keep walking. Now we're calling the cops'.

Chesney-Lind and others also point to changes and biases within the juvenile justice system that they believe explain the increase in the number of girls being arrested. For example, girls are twice as likely as boys to be detained, with the detention period lasting five times longer for girls than for their male counterparts. Girls are more likely than boys to be charged with status offences, i.e. offences which, if committed by an adult, would not be considered a crime (e.g. running away from home, truancy, incorrigibility), and are more likely to be incarcerated for these offences than males.

Suicide

Historically, suicide in the United States was viewed as primarily a problem of older adult white men with clinical depression or other mental disorders; thus suicide prevention involved identifying and treating mental illness. A dramatic rise in the adolescent and young adult (15–24 years old) suicide rates, from 4.5 per 100 000 in 1950 to 20.5 per 100 000 in 1997, created the need for new prevention strategies. The rise was alarming particularly as research indicated that only one out of three of those who committed suicide fit the criteria for clinical depression or other mental illness (Shaffer *et al.* 1988).

Race and gender disparities in suicide rates are striking. The rates for adolescent girls and women have remained relatively stable over the last 30 years and the rates for white men have levelled since 1988. However, there has been a dramatic rise in the suicide rates for young black males (15–24 years old) since 1986 (Shaffer *et al.* 1994). While the suicide rates for white males remain higher than those for black males at each age cohort, the rates among black males increased at a faster rate than any other group.

The CDC convened a panel of experts and conducted a study of youth suicide prevention programmes. The study reviewed the existing programmes and delineated eight suicide prevention strategies.

1. School gatekeeper training: this type of programme is directed at school staff to help them identify and defer students at risk of suicide and to organize the response in case of a suicide.

2. Community gatekeeper training: this type of programme provides the same service to community staff, clergy, police, merchants, etc.

3. General suicide education: these programmes are school-based education on suicide, often incorporating self-esteem building or social competency exercises.
4. Screening programmes: screening involves administering an instrument to identify high-risk youth in order to provide services.
5. Peer support programmes: school- or community-based programmes to help adolescents develop competency in relationships and to help each other.
6. Crisis centres and hotlines: these programmes provide 24-hour emergency counselling.
7. Means restriction: strategies to restrict access to firearms, drugs, or other means of committing suicide.
8. Intervention after a suicide: commonly called postvention, these programmes are designed to help survivors and prevent suicide clusters.

Domestic violence

Domestic violence or partner violence is defined as violence between those involved in an intimate relationship. While it includes homosexual relationships and violence against men, it is usually the violence of a boyfriend, ex-boyfriend, husband, or ex-husband against a woman (Bureau of Justice Statistics 1994). It involves many kinds of attacks, physical, sexual, and verbal. Coercive control through degradation, malicious enforcement of petty rules, intermittent rewards, and isolations are examples of the methods employed to demonstrate and maintain power.

However, in family situations children under 12 years of age represent 62 per cent of all victims. Juveniles aged 12 to 17 comprise 30 per cent of the victims in overall offences and 23 per cent in family occurrences. Females are most frequently the victims of family and overall offences, comprising 74 per cent and 76 per cent of the victims of family and overall offences respectively (FBI 1998).

It is difficult to assess the amount of intimate violence that occurs, as most goes unreported. The Department of Justice regularly conducts the National Crime Victimization Survey showing that 2.5 million women annually report experiencing physical violence, two-thirds at the hands of an acquaintance or relation. The average annual victimization rates are 5 per 1000 by intimates, 1 per 1000 by other relatives, 8 per 1000 by acquaintances, and 5 per 1000 by strangers (Bureau of Justice Statistics 1994).

In 1985, the second large population-based study of domestic violence revealed that 3.4 per cent of adult women had been severely abused by an intimate partner, a prevalence of approximately 2 million. Minor acts of violence, pushing, shoving, or slapping, were reported by 11.6 per cent of the women.

In 1998, 27 per cent of those suffering family-related violence were reported to have been related to one or more of their offenders. A higher percentage of victims of family violence are over the age of 18 than are the victims of overall crimes of violence (80 per cent versus 76). Additionally, victims of family violence are overwhelmingly female (71 per cent for family violence and 58 per cent for overall violence) (FBI 1998).

Rape and sexual assault

In 1993, the FBI recorded 104 806 rapes for a national rate of 79 per 100 000 (FBI 1993). The National Crime Victimization Survey indicates that women report approximately 133 000 rapes each year, with half saying they reported them to the police and 55 per cent indicating that they knew the assailant.

Rape accounts for slightly less than 1 per cent of all violent offences. In particular, children under 12 comprise a larger portion of victims of family rape than all victims of rape (36 per cent versus 12) (FBI 1998).

Additional information is available from a national sample, the National Women's Study (Kilpatrick *et al.* 1992), suggesting a higher incidence and prevalence. According to this study, an estimated 683 000 women are raped each year, 60 per cent at ages younger than 18. The perpetrator was a stranger in only 22 per cent of the cases. This study estimates that 12.1 million American women are raped at some point in their lives. Only 16 per cent of them report the rape to the police.

Economic costs

Each year United States citizens pay about $53.5 billion for criminal justice interventions for violence, and an additional $158 billion for cost of lifetime care for victims of violence (medical treatment, rehabilitation, and lost productivity). These figures reflect only the monetary costs of violence, not the pain, suffering, and lost quality of life for victims. They do not reflect the cost for safety measures—the inability of children and adults to walk or play in their own neighbourhood, the cost of guard dogs and guns for 'protection', and an immeasurable sense of fear of crime victimization. In considering the impact of violence on society, it is also important to note the costs of violent crimes.

A framework model developed by Miller *et al.* (1993) was used to quantify costs of violent crime; it incorporated direct losses other than property losses (medical, mental health, and emergency services, insurance administration), productivity losses (wages, fringe benefits, housework), and non-monetary losses (pain, suffering, lost quality of life). Costs to victims of crimes resulting in injury were estimated to be $60 000 for rape survivors, $22 000 for assault survivors, and almost $2.4 million per murder (in 1989 dollars). Moreover, the lifetime costs of criminal victimizations for persons aged 12 and older were estimated to be $10 billion for rape, $96 billion for assault, and $48 billion for murder (Miller *et al.*1993).

Furthermore, these figures do not include property losses incurred during violent acts nor the mammoth costs incurred by collective society's reactive response to violence, including law enforcement, adjudication, victim services, and correctional expenditures.

In 1993, the costs of direct medical services, emergency services, and claims processed for the victims of gun violence nationwide totalled approximately $3 billion. Average hospital charges for treating one child wounded by gunfire were more than $14 000.

Taxpayers pay for gun violence. The average cost of medical treatments for the hospital stay of one gunshot-wound patient (all age groups) is more than $33 000. Approximately 80 per cent of patients who suffer from violence are uninsured and/or eligible for government medical care assistance.

The characteristics of violence

Contrary to the stereotype of violence as predominantly stranger-related, or occurring in the context of criminal behaviour such as racial harassment, robbery, or drug-dealing, much of the violence experienced in the United States is intimate and occurs in the context of personal relationships (Spivak *et al.* 1988). A typical homicide involves two people who know each other, who are under the influence of alcohol, and who get into an argument that escalates in the presence of a gun. Only 15 per cent of homicides occur in the course of committing a crime, as compared with over 50 per cent that stem from arguments among acquaintances (CDC 1982*a*,*b*). This 50 per cent takes place in family relationships (e.g. child abuse, elder abuse, spouse abuse) or friends (interpersonal peer violence). In the remaining 35 per cent, the relationship between victim and perpetrator is unknown.

The perpetrator and victim of violence share many traits. They are likely to be young, male, and of the same race. They are likely to be poor and to have been exposed to violence in the past—especially family violence. They may be depressed and use alcohol and or other drugs (Prothrow-Stith and Weissman 1991). This incongruity between public perception and actual circumstances has resulted in demands for resources and solutions that address only part—possibly the smaller part—of the problem. While certainly not discarding established anticrime and antiviolence strategies, we must recognize the diversity of violent circumstances that exist and must build a broader base of efforts that not only responds to violent events, but also focuses on preventive services as well.

A closer look at the demographic characteristics reveal certain noteworthy factors contributing to a complex picture of adolescent violence. Breaking down the 10- to 24-year age group further, 1997 homicide rates (deaths per 100 000) were considerably higher among 20- to 24-year-olds (19.0) and 15- to 19-year-olds (11.7) than among 10- to 14-year-olds (1.7); however, it is still important to note that the rates increased among all three groups from 1979 to 1988. In terms of gender, males greatly exceed females in the number of violent victimizations, with the exception of sexual assault, and are also more likely to be violent offenders and witnesses to violence.

Race and poverty

There appear to be extremely large racial differences in violence rates among young Americans. In 1991, homicide was the leading cause of death for black youth aged between 15 and 24; the homicide rate for black youth (both sexes) was nine times the rate for white youth aged between 15 and 24 (90.0 per 100 000 versus 10.8 per 100 000). National statistics concerning other ethnic minority groups, such as Latin Americans, Asian Americans, and Native Americans, are scant.

The racial data are not indicative of any biological or genetic factor because they are confounded by socio-economic status, urban living, gun availability, and racism. Using family income as the primary indicator of socio-economic status, the National Crime Survey found an inverse relationship between income and the risk of violent victimization (Bureau of Justice Statistics 1992). In 1988, the risk of victimization was found to be 2.5 times higher for people in low income families (under \$7500 per year), compared with high income families (\$50 000 per year).

It is important to note, however, that the relationship between violence and social factors is complex and still unclear. For example, multivariate studies have shown a complicated interaction between race and socio-economic status: at low socio-economic levels black individuals have a higher risk of homicide than white individuals, but at higher socio-economic levels the difference disappears. William Julius Wilson's work on neighbourhood poverty offers a possible explanation. Poor black people are much more likely than poor white people to live in neighbourhoods where the majority of the people are poor. Although it appears that race is a significant social predictor in certain studies, multivariate studies show a more complex situation.

Other studies have suggested that, in fact, socio-economic status is the major predictor and race is merely a marker. One study that used several markers for poverty, including number of people per square foot of housing, disaggregated the race and socio-economic variables. In this study overcrowded white people had the same high domestic homicide rates as did overcrowded black people. Less crowded members of both groups had the same lower rates (Centerwall 1984, 1993). In 1987, the homicide rate for young black men in the military was one-twelfth of their national rate, strongly indicating the influence of social, structural, cultural, and economic factors.

The contact that health professionals have with victims and perpetrators

The regular contact that physicians and nurses have with victims of violence, particularly in emergency departments, has caused many to begin to address this problem. The American College of Emergency Physicians has included violence prevention on the agenda of their annual meetings. *The Journal of the American Medical Association* has dedicated two special issues to the topic of violence, in parallel with the American Medical Association's publication of manuals for health providers on domestic violence, child abuse, and rape and sexual assault.

The Northeast Ohio Trauma Study illustrates the need for greater data from emergency departments, in showing that five times the number of assaults reported to the police were reported to hospital emergency departments. Not only are non-fatal violent episodes inadequately measured with police data, but the greater contact that health providers have with victims provides an opportunity to offer public health prevention and intervention strategies in the emergency department. Such programmes have been started at Boston City Hospital, Cook County Hospital in Chicago, Harborview Hospital in Seattle, and Washington and Grady Memorial Hospital in Atlanta, Georgia.

There is a substantial body of research which suggests that crime rates reflect 'community social disorganization'. Social disorganization theory was originally developed by the Chicago School researchers Clifford Shaw and Henry McKay in their classic work, *Juvenile Delinquency and Urban Areas*, published in 1942. Shaw and McKay demonstrated that the same socio-economically disadvantaged areas in 21 United States cities continued to exhibit high delinquency rates over a span of several decades despite changes in their racial and ethnic composition, indicating the persistent contextual effects of these communities on crime rates regardless of what populations experienced them. This observation led them to reject individualistic explanations of delinquency and to focus instead on community processes—such as disruption of local community organization and weak social controls—which led to the apparent transgenerational transmission of criminal behaviour. In general, social disorganization is defined as the 'inability of a community structure to realise the common values of its residents and maintain effective social controls'. The social organizational approach views local communities and neighbourhoods as complex systems of friendship, kinship, and acquaintanceship networks, as well as formal and informal associational ties rooted in family life and ongoing socialization processes. From the perspective of crime control, a major dimension of social disorganization is the ability of a community to supervise and control teenage peer groups, especially gangs. Thus Shaw and McKay argued that residents of cohesive communities were better able to control the youth behaviours that set the context for gang violence. Examples of such controls include the supervision of leisure-time youth activities, intervention in street-corner congregation, and challenging youth 'who seem to be up to no good'. Socially disorganized communities with extensive street-corner peer groups are also expected to have higher rates of adult violence, especially among younger adults who still have ties to youth gangs.

The application of public health strategies

Public health professionals have applied traditional public health strategies to violence prevention. They have brought a different perspective and orientation to bear on the problem. Applying public health techniques and strategies complements and strengthens the criminal justice approach.

Public health brings an analytic approach to problems that concentrates on identifying risk factors and important causes that could become the focus of preventive interventions. It also brings a record of accomplishment in controlling 'accidental' (unintentional) injuries through both environmental manipulations (e.g. seat belts and childproof caps on medicines), and behavioural change (e.g. laws and educational campaigns to reduce drink-driving).

Identification of risk factors

Major risk factors for youth violence have been identified. These factors can be broadly categorized as environmental or psychological. The major environmental risk factors include firearms, alcohol and other drugs, cultural factors, being a victim of child abuse, witnessing family violence, exposure to media violence, and exposure to high levels of peer and community violence. A consistent and strong environmental risk factor for homicide is the presence of poverty. The mechanism for this interaction is not completely understood, but may include the anger and frustration associated with not having money and essential commodities, the experience of classism, the probable absence of adult male role models, the scarcity of recreational, extracurricular, and after-school activities, and longer time spent watching television.

Corporal punishment is a controversial environmental factor that may be related to risk for violence. Certainly in its extreme form, abuse, there is evidence to suggest that it increases the risk of delinquency. Efforts to improve parenting and to reduce child abuse often focus on alternative disciplinary strategies. Other environmental risk factors for adolescents include peer pressure, the crack cocaine epidemic, and policing practices.

Child neglect and abuse

Child abuse and neglect are general terms used to encompass many harmful behaviours towards children. Verbal, emotional, and sexual abuse are included, as well as failure to meet a child's needs and outright physical violence. Child sexual abuse is most often considered separately, yet each state has its own definition and guidelines for protective custody.

Because child abuse has been a reportable crime for many years, better statistics are available. An annual 50-state survey estimated 2 million reports of child abuse and neglect in 1986. Over the decade of the eighties, the number of reports increased by 184 per cent (Daro and Mitchel 1987). The number of child sexual abuse reports increased dramatically as well, a 12-fold increase within the decade. It is obvious that researchers have the same problem in documenting both child abuse and child sexual abuse as they do in documenting other forms of violence: unreliable data sources, under-reporting by victims, inconsistent definitions, and failure to recognize an event as precipitated by violence.

With child abuse, reporting biases work in both directions to inflate or deflate the numbers. Episodes of child abuse occurring in families of middle class and professional parents are less likely to be reported, even with mandatory reporting laws, which will diminish the prevalence estimates. Yet greater awareness and sensitivity to child abuse, and the advent of mandatory reporting, no doubt increase the numbers. There is a struggle among child health and human service professionals to determine the way to maintain mandatory reporting and improve the effectiveness of the state protective services. An over-reliance on foster care without adequate attention to family preservation seems to have been the rule in the past.

The cycle of violence

The relationship between child abuse, neglect, and witnessing violence to adolescent and adult violence has been demonstrated in several studies. Existing studies suggest that there is a greater likelihood of abuse by parents if they were abused as children. Estimates of the percentage of abusive parents who were abused as children range from 7 per cent (Gil 1973) to 70 per cent (Egeland and Jacobvitz 1984). Among adults who were abused, up to one-third abuse their children (Straus and Gelles 1990).

A retrospective look at violent juvenile delinquents compared with non-violent juvenile delinquents showed a significantly higher rate of physical child abuse. Both interviews with the delinquents and medical chart reviews yielded evidence of greater victimization, skull fractures, emergency trauma visits, and other physical injuries.

A cohort study of abused or neglected children demonstrated a greater risk for delinquency, adult criminal behaviour, and violent criminal behaviour, even though the majority of such children do not demonstrate these behaviours. The abused children had a number of offences and began delinquent behaviour at earlier ages, regardless of race and gender (Widom 1989).

For black adolescents aged 11 to 19 years living in or around an urban housing project, the self-reported use of violence was associated with exposure to violence and personal victimization, hopelessness, depression, family conflict, and previous corporal punishments.

Those with a higher sense of purpose in life and less depression were better able to handle the exposure to violence in the home and community (Durant *et al.* 1994).

Children and exposure to media violence

The association between childhood exposure to media violence and subsequent aggressive behaviour has been firmly established over the past four decades. The American Psychological Association collected these data and decided unequivocally to pronounce the negative influence of the entertainment media violence (American Psychological Association Commission on Violence and Youth 1993). The Association expected the report to have an impact on parents and policy-makers. Other reviews of the literature have been done with similar conclusions (Dietz and Strasburger 1991; Sege and Dietz 1994).

Preschool children exposed to violent activity in a controlled setting were observed to imitate and repeat the violent behaviours (Bandura *et al.* 1963*a*,*b*). An actor appearing on screen attacked a Bobo-the-clown doll. Following this attack, in three separate video sequences the actor was either praised, ignored, or punished. Those preschool-aged viewers who saw the violent behaviour rewarded on screen were more likely than the other two groups to repeat the violent actions when shown a Bobo doll themselves. This experiment demonstrated that children can learn violent behaviours from television, and are especially likely to do so when these activities are depicted as socially acceptable.

Older children's behaviour is also heavily influenced by exposure to media violence. Meta-analysis of a series of experiences demonstrates conclusively that school-aged boys have more fights in the days following exposure to violent mainstream movies than they do in the days following exposure to less violent movies (Turner *et al.* 1986; Wood *et al.* 1991).

In a landmark cohort study involving children raised in Pennsylvania, Eron and Huesmann (1984) showed that preference for violent television programmes at age 8, as well as total hours of television viewing, predicted the severity of violent criminal convictions by age 30. However, this effect should be modified by parental interventions (Huesmann *et al.* 1983; Liebert 1988; Austin *et al.* 1990; Weaver and Barbour 1992; Sang *et al.* 1993).

Centerwall (1992) has shown that in three different countries (the United States, Canada, and South Africa), homicide rates doubled approximately 10 to 12 years after the introduction of English-language television. In the United States, homicide rates doubled first among those portions of the population exposed to television first (white urban dwellers), and only later among those segments of the population who received television later. He attributes approximately 10 000 deaths annually in the United States to the results of exposure to media violence.

Taken together, we believe that these studies satisfy most of the criteria for causality set forth in the Surgeon General's report on smoking and health (US Department of Health, Education, and Welfare 1964), and establish that exposure to media violence places children at risk for subsequent violence.

Public debate flourishes concerning the roles of video games and violence-oriented musical lyrics in encouraging violence. Currently, however, no definitive data are available on these issues.

Firearms

The United States has more firearms than any other industrialized nation not at war and the following facts extracted from the publication *Not Even One* (Carter Center 1994) are astounding.

- A gun in the home is 43 times more likely to kill a family member or friend than it is to be used in self-defence.
- In 1990, 4941 children in the United States under the age of 19 years died from gunshot wounds; 538 of these children were shot accidentally.
- From 1973 to 1991, the number of licensed firearms dealers increased by 95 000—the total had reached more than 225 000 by 1994. In 1992, nearly 92 000 Americans applied to get or renew a federal firearms licence. Only 52 were denied.
- In 1987, 1300 males under age 19 were murdered with guns in the United States. In the same year, fewer than 80 males under 19 were murdered with guns in Canada, Japan, France, West Germany, Australia, England, Wales, and Sweden combined.
- None of the federal revenues on guns are designated for the medical care of victims of gun violence. In fact, all of the revenues from the firearm excise tax are required to go to hunting-related activities.
- The firearm homicide rate for 15- to 19-year-olds increased 61 per cent from 1979 to 1989. The rate of homicide by all other methods remained stable or declined.
- In 1991, the Bureau of Alcohol, Tobacco, and Firearms performed compliance inspections on fewer than 4 per cent of all existing gun dealerships; 5967 violations were found but only 17 dealers' licences were revoked.
- Firearms are used in more than 80 per cent of teenage homicides and about 68 per cent of homicides by all ages.
- In 1990, 4.37 million guns were produced for the American market. That is 12 000 new guns every day. Although trigger lock loading indicators would save lives, few guns have them because no law requires them.
- Suicide is the third leading cause of death for adolescents and young adults in the United States, after car crashes and homicides. In 1990, 3165 youths aged 15 to 24 killed themselves with guns.
- Half of all Americans own guns. More than one-third of all male homicides are by firearms. Nearly half of all female homicides are by firearms.
- From 1953 to 1978, the suicide rate of young people tripled; this rise paralleled an increase in the firearm-caused suicide rate.
- From 1976 to 1987, more than twice as many American women were shot and killed by their husbands or boyfriends as by strangers using guns, knives, or any other means.
- Guns are used in 60 per cent of all teenage suicides. The youth firearm-suicide rate in an American city with minimal restrictions on gun ownership is more than three times higher than in a Canadian city with strict gun-control laws.

Teenage and young adult homicide is a uniquely American problem. The high rate of youth homicide in the United States has been attributed to the country's much higher rate of gun ownership. An international study of gun ownership and homicide found positive correlations between the rates of household gun ownership and the national rates and proportions of gun-related homicide (Lester 1988; Killias 1993).

Handgun availability appears to be playing an increasingly important role in youth homicides. As an example, the increasing trend seen in the total homicide rate among those aged 15 to 19 years between 1979 and 1989 is solely attributable to the increase in firearm homicides: the firearm-related homicide rate increased by 61 per cent (6.9 to 11.1 per 100 000), while at the same time the non-firearm-related homicide rates actually decreased by 29 per cent (3.4 to 2.4 per 100 000) (Fingerhut *et al.* 1992). From 1980 to 1989, over 65 per cent of the 11 000 homicides committed by high-school-aged youth were firearm related.

Handguns are widely accessible to adolescents in the United States. The national 1990 Youth Risk Behavior Survey found that about one in every 20 high-school students had carried a firearm at least once in the 30 days preceding the survey. The incidence was higher among males at 17 per cent. (CDC 1991). In another study of inner-city youths, as many as 35 per cent of males carried a gun outside of school (Sheley *et al.* 1992).

Firearms contribute to both the violent victimization of youth and the violent offences committed by youth. The presence of a weapon in the home is associated with a threefold increase in the likelihood of homicide compared with matched controls drawn from the neighbourhood surrounding the victim (Kellermann *et al.* 1993).

Comparisons of two cities (Seattle and Vancouver) which have similar demographic characteristics shows that Seattle's excess homicide rate is entirely attributable to firearm homicides (Sloan *et al.* 1988) (Fig. 4). Another study, designed to look at the effect of implementation of gun control legislation, showed a positive effect of the enactment of tougher gun control laws in the District of Columbia compared with both neighbouring states (Loftin 1991).

All these studies demonstrate that availability of firearms is strongly correlated with increased homicide rates. Logically, this result coincides with the earlier observation that most homicides result from conflicts among people who know each other well, including friends and acquaintances, as well as relatives and spouses. In a situation of passionate conflict, handgun availability appears to increase the likelihood of serious injury or death.

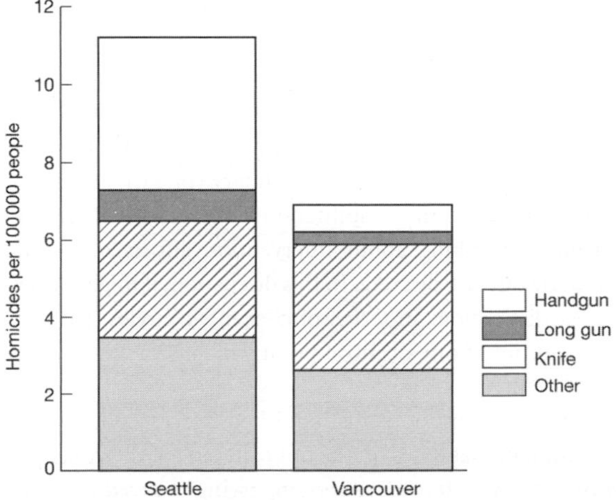

Fig. 4 Weapons and violence. (Source: Sloan *et al.* 1988.)

Psychological and behavioural factors

In pioneering studies conducted in the late 1980s, Slaby and Guerra (1988) demonstrated that adolescents involved in violence have habits of thought which lead them into violent confrontations. They examined the responses of three groups of teenaged boys to a specific scenario. One group of boys were in custody for the commission of violent crimes, a second group were identified by their teachers as being violence prone, and a third group were identified by their teachers as not being violence prone. Each boy was presented with the same scenario: he was going after school to work on his batting so that he could make the baseball team. As he arrived, another boy took the last bat. In understanding this scenario, the violence-prone boys were more likely to assign malicious intent to the boy who took the bat than were the less violent boys. The violence-prone boys were able to imagine fewer alternative means to resolve this situation.

Slaby and Guerra (1988) concluded from this study that the more violence-prone boys got into more fights because they were more likely to see harmful intent in a given situation, and, having seen such intent, were less likely to come up with a peaceful way to resolve the situation. These results have been confirmed with a large-scale study conducted in New York City schools (CDC 1993*b*). Boys who reported having been in serious fights were more likely than the general school population to suggest that carrying a weapon or threatening to use a weapon were good ways to stay out of fights; they were also far less likely than the overall population to say that one could avoid fighting by apologizing.

Witnessing violence

In addition to the young people directly injured by violence, increasing attention is being given to the scores more who are affected indirectly, as witnesses to violent acts or by exposure to chronic violent environments (Groves *et al.* 1993). Pynoos *et al.* (1987) examined the appearance of post-traumatic stress disorder symptoms in children who experienced a fatal sniper attack on their elementary school and reported a correlation between the type and number of post-traumatic stress disorder symptoms and proximity to the violent incident, as well as more severe symptoms in children who knew the deceased child.

In addition to acute incidents, other studies relate findings of correlations between exposure to chronic violence and distress symptoms (Fitzpatrick and Boldizar 1993; Freeman *et al.* 1993; Osofsky *et al.* 1993; Martinez and Richters 1993; Lorion and Saltzman 1993). In addition, Lorion and Saltzman (1993) described anecdotal reports from their research participants, including reports from teachers and administrators about children who lived in violent settings arriving at school in distress, who were unable to concentrate or maintain appropriate behaviour in class, and who hid in the classroom, afraid to return home or take the bus. Clearly, there is a need to address not only the physical threat of violence, but also the potential for psychopathological and/or emotional disturbances in both victims and bystanders (Emde 1993; Durant *et al.* 1994).

Approaches to violence prevention and control

Historically, society has relied almost exclusively on the criminal justice system both to respond to and to prevent violence. This tactic is rooted in the beliefs that violence is criminal, that those who commit violence should be punished, and that the threat of punishment is a potential deterrent to violent acts. A large, elaborate set of institutions has been developed to achieve these goals. That system includes police, prosecutors, public defenders, judges, probation officers, and prison guards. It is principally designed to respond to crimes after they have been committed by identifying, apprehending, prosecuting, punishing, and controlling the violent offender. It is guided not only by the practical goals of reducing crimes of all types (including violence), but also by the normative goal of assuring justice to victims and the accused.

The public health and criminal justice systems have been historically separate in their conceptualization of approaches to violence and the development of activities to reduce or prevent violence. The public health field has approached the issue through efforts to identify the risk factors related to violent behaviour. The field comes to this issue in reaction to the magnitude of intentional injuries that are present in health care settings. The criminal justice system has approached the issue through efforts to identify and assign blame for criminal behaviour, maintain public safety, and remove violent offenders from the community.

Viewed from the perspective of those interested in reducing violence, the criminal justice system's responses have had only limited success. Part of the reason is inherent limitations in the overall approach of the criminal justice system. First, it is more reactive than preventive in its basic orientation. True, deterrence may produce some preventive results. True too, the criminal justice system has sought to rehabilitate offenders through special programmes in prisons, and to prevent children from becoming violent offenders through the development of the juvenile justice system whose most fundamental goal is to prevent future criminal activity by children. Nonetheless, the criminal justice system comes into play only after a crime episode occurs.

Second, the criminal justice system—and particularly the police—is focused primarily on the predatory violence that occurs among strangers on the street. The violence that emerges from nagging frustrations and festering disputes, and takes place in intimate settings, is far more difficult for the criminal justice system to deal with than stranger-inflicted violence that arises from greed or desperate need and takes place in the open. Robbery and burglary, and the violence that attends these, are more traditional and central to the criminal justice system's business (and consciousness) than aggravated assaults that spring up among friends in bars, lovers in bedrooms, or teenagers at dances.

Public health and criminal justice: interdisciplinary challenges

Unfortunately, the collaboration of public health and criminal justice in the area of violence prevention has been fraught with tension. Some of this may stem from a basic failure in effectively reducing the problem of violence that has put both disciplines on the defensive—criminal justice for its failure to bring the problem under control and meet societal expectations, and public health for the slowness with which it has recognized and taken on the problem. However, much of this tension probably comes from the divergence of perspective of the two disciplines and the fact that there are inadequate resources directed to addressing violence, which has forced the disciplines to compete rather than collaborate.

Public health is primarily focused on identifying causality (or its approximation) and intervening to control or reduce the risk factors; it has little interest in assigning blame or meting out punishment, and does not discriminate between victim and offender. The public health community may agree that justice must be done, but is not professionally committed to the process. The criminal justice system, on the other hand, is deeply and morally rooted in 'justice', and the proper identification and punishment of criminal offenders. In this field there is less emphasis on the precursors or factors that may have led to the violent event. The criminal justice system is less likely to consider external factors that might have motivated the offender to engage in violence because it sees these issues as largely irrelevant to judgement of guilt and innocence. At worst, the claims that these other factors were causally important in the particular instance seems like a rationalization or an apology for what was a criminal deed. This rift is further exacerbated by the fact that the criminal justice profession continues to develop preventive agendas, such as first-offender programmes and community-policing initiatives, and probably feels that their 'thunder' and leadership are in jeopardy of being stolen by the entry of another professional player onto their turf.

This tension is clearly unproductive. It threatens effective collaboration and frustrates the opportunity to pool resources and expertise at a time when resources are seriously inadequate and the problem is increasing. Healing this rift requires a more collaborative spirit from both disciplines. The public health 'purists' must go beyond their science and recognize the invaluable contributions and practical experiences of the criminal justice professionals. The criminal justice 'moralists' must, in turn, recognize the limitations of a primary agenda of assigning blame and assuring justice is done.

If we are to get past these initial reactions and successfully exploit the complementary qualities of these two approaches to violence, it is essential to put aside professional jealousies. More important, we must better define the perspective, roles, and expertise both groups bring to the issue. This will not only lead to a more creative process but also to establishing productive working relationships.

Primary, secondary, and tertiary prevention

A conceptual framework that can alleviate interprofessional tension, facilitate definitions of roles in addressing the problem, and assist in developing a broader perspective on programmatic strategies, involves breaking the spectrum of violence into levels that reflect different points of intervention (Table 1). This framework, used frequently in public health circles, structures approaches to problems into three stages of prevention: primary, secondary (or early intervention), and tertiary (or treatment/rehabilitation). These distinctions have proved valuable in thinking about intervention efforts even though their boundaries are not discrete. In this discussion, it might be best to think of these distinctions in terms of concentric circles that widen out in space and time from a central point which is the occurrence of some violent event.

Tertiary prevention is distinguished from secondary and primary prevention in that it lies on the opposite side of the violent event from the other two. Its focus is on trying to reduce the negative consequences of a particular event after it has occurred, or on trying to find ways to use the event to reduce the likelihood of similar incidents

Table 1 Classification of preventive strategies

Primary prevention	Secondary prevention	Tertiary prevention
Reduced availability of guns (gun control)	Early identification and screening	Jail/prison
Reduced use of alcohol and drugs	Behaviour modification	Rehabilitation services
Reduced media violence	Early intervention in schools, emergency rooms, and juvenile justice system	Hospital services
Behavioural education; anger and conflict resolution	Counselling	
Promulgation of laws	Risk factor reduction	
Threat of punishment		
Parent education		
Street safety measures		
Social support services		
Community awareness		
Risk factor identification and reduction		

occurring in the future. Thus one might think of improved trauma care, on the one hand, and increased efforts to rehabilitate or incapacitate violent offenders, on the other, as tertiary prevention instruments in the control of or the response to violence.

Primary prevention, which by definition addresses the broadest level of the general public, might seek to reduce the level of violence that is shown on television or to promote gun control. This would be an effort directed towards dealing with the public values and attitudes that may promote or encourage the use of violence.

Secondary prevention is distinguished from primary prevention in that it identifies relatively narrowly defined subgroups or circumstances that are at high risk of being involved in or occasioning violence, and focuses its attention on them. Thus secondary prevention efforts might focus on urban poor young men who are at particularly high risk of engaging in or being victimized by violence, and educating them in non-violent methods of resolving disputes or displaying competence and power.

The relative risk level of groups or circumstances is a continuum—with some people and circumstances at very high risk (a person who has been victimized by violence in his or her own home, also surrounded by violence in school, entering a bar in which members of a rival gang are drinking), and others at relatively low risk (say, a happily married professor, who owns no weapon more lethal than a screwdriver, writing on her computer at home). Moreover, it is generally true that the higher-risk groups are smaller than the lower-risk groups.

Primary prevention instruments are those that can affect larger and larger populations, ideally at relatively low cost. Indeed, the need to reach very large populations requires primary prevention efforts to be low cost per individual reached. Thus primary prevention instruments tend to be those providing information and education on the problem of violence through the popular media, for example the recruitment of Bill Cosby to the cause of using the media to prevent adolescent violence, or Sarah Brady's efforts to advocate for gun control laws and educate the public about the risks of handguns, rather than providing non-violence training to the entire population. There are, of course, the ultimate long-term primary prevention goals that have to do with eliminating some of the root causes of violence such as social injustice and discrimination.

This public health model can be very useful when applied specifically to the issue of interpersonal violence. In the past, the criminal justice system has addressed each of the three points of intervention to varying degrees as represented, yet the bulk of the efforts have focused on the response to serious violent behaviour with moderate attention to early identification and intervention and limited efforts in the area of primary prevention.

The major activities of the criminal justice system have historically involved the roles of the police, the courts, and the prison system in responding to criminal or violent events. Most resources have been directed to investigating and punishing criminal behaviour. Tertiary prevention has generally involved incarceration. In the area of secondary prevention, the police have focused efforts on 'situated' crime prevention and the juvenile justice system has made attempts at early intervention with youthful offenders, although youths were frequently ignored by the courts and probation system until their criminal behaviour reached a relatively high level of concern. Primary prevention efforts have focused on elementary-school drug and violence prevention education by the police, as well as on controlling 'criminogenic' commodities such as drugs, guns, and alcohol.

With the more recent involvement of the public health system, attention has been broadened with enhanced efforts in the prevention arena. The public health agenda has focused primarily on prevention and early intervention, playing only a small role in the treatment of individuals with serious violence-related problems. The role and activities of the public health system are newer, less extensive, and therefore less evolved than that of the criminal justice system.

Traditionally, public health responded by treating the violence-related injury in the emergency setting. Today a new generation of committed health practitioners, community violence-prevention practitioners, social workers, and community activists have devised numerous intervention programmes to serve medium- to high-risk adolescents. At the primary prevention level, efforts have focused on gun control and safety, and enhanced public awareness of risk factors and the true characteristics of most violence to dispel myths and modify societal values around the use of violence. Additionally, some educational interventions (e.g. violence-prevention curricula) have been applied to broader, less high-risk settings. Again, much of this work is relatively recent and therefore has not yet established a long track record to assess fully its effects. Finally, public health has applied its analytical expertise to enhance greatly the understanding of risk factors, allowing for a broader vision in the planning and development of preventive approaches (Spivak *et al.* 1988; Prothrow-Stith and Weissman 1991).

In the area of secondary prevention, public health has been involved in the development of educational interventions specifically focused on behaviour modification of high-risk individuals, particularly children and youth. A number of curricula are currently in use addressing both the risks of violence in solving problems and conflict resolution techniques (Spivak *et al.* 1988; Prothrow-Stith and Weissman 1991).

It is important to note that the criminal justice system has increased its involvement with primary and secondary prevention efforts. For example, some criminal justice professionals have become increasingly involved in gun control initiatives. In 1974, the Juvenile Justice and Delinquency Prevention Act was passed and gave the Justice Department primary responsibility for delinquency prevention programmes. The Office of Juvenile Justice and Delinquency Prevention was designed in part to encourage development of model delinquency prevention programmes. One such programme is the Boys Clubs of America Targeting Programs for Delinquency Intervention. Other community groups refer at-risk boys to the programme, who are then recruited. Early evaluations of these programmes seem promising. Data indicate that 39 per cent of the boys did better at school and 93 per cent who completed the programme have not been reinvolved with the juvenile system (Boys Clubs of America 1986). These types of interventions reflect an important interface between the criminal justice and public health professions. With further attention, the dedication of resources of the public health system to this issue, and the broadening vision of criminal justice, a more reasonable balance between prevention and treatment can be achieved in the future. Efforts can be broadened to reflect more fully the range of efforts needed to both reduce the extent of violent behaviour and to respond to the violence that does occur. The emphasis of the public health system will be on prevention, with the criminal justice system prioritizing the response to violence, but with both disciplines working together across the spectrum.

Cigarette smoking reduction: a model for intervention

To illustrate the advantages of this approach, it is useful to review how it has worked successfully in other areas. One example, which on the surface appears to be a considerable stretch from violence, is the multidisciplinary approach that has been developed to deal with tobacco use. It is important to note that, while this example illustrates a collaboration between public health and the medical care system, it represents a useful analogy to the possible collaboration between public health and criminal justice.

Smoking is a major contributing factor to death and disability in this country. Significant inroads have been made in turning the tide on this major health threat. What was once a valued, sexy, and socially acceptable behaviour is now viewed as disgusting, unhealthy, and socially unacceptable. Heroes in the media used to smoke all the time; now they rarely do. Nationally, the number of people who smoke has declined dramatically, although smoking was and still is a learned behaviour—one that can be unpleasant or distasteful to start but is extremely difficult to stop.

The strategy to deal with smoking involved a three-pronged approach: primary prevention for those not yet smoking to teach the reasons for not starting and to support the decision not to start, secondary prevention to encourage stopping or reducing use for those who had already started smoking (often this involves helping individuals to identify alternative behaviours to replace the smoking), and treatment in the form of surgery, chemotherapy, and other medical interventions for those smokers who have developed cancer or other health consequences of their behaviour. Broad public initiatives to alter the societal values that encouraged smoking were also established to support the above efforts. This has been done through legislation (package labelling, advertising constraints, restrictions on sales to minors, establishment of smoke-free environments), public education, and pressure on media to change images and role models. Although, as stated earlier, this is an example of a public health–medical care interface, it represents an important success that has value when looking at the possibilities of a public health and criminal justice collaboration in addressing violence.

A similar approach could and should be taken with respect to violence. Primary prevention strategies and more targeted secondary prevention efforts need to be applied that proactively value and teach non-violent behaviours in response to anger and conflict. This is particularly important given the growing evidence that violence is a learned behaviour (Bandura *et al.* 1963*a*,*b*; Liebert *et al.* 1973; Slaby and Quarfoth 1980; Allen 1981; Eron and Huesmann 1984; Prothrow-Stith and Weissman 1991; Straus 1991; Vissing *et al.* 1991). Well-child health visits in neighbourhood health centres provide an ideal window of opportunity for early intervention. Peter Stringham, a paediatrician at the East Boston Neighborhood Health Center, incorporates a violence-prevention protocol for families, from the new-born visit to the teenage years. Social skills are as important to teach our children as the academic subjects we now emphasize in our society. This will in no way eliminate the underlying societal stresses that influence violent behaviour, but can affect and direct responses to these stresses towards a prosocial and productive outcome. Curricula that place emphasis on decision-making, non-violent conflict resolution, and self-esteem development currently exist but are extremely under-utilized and viewed as an 'add on' in academic settings rather than a basic component. A move to place more emphasis on the use of such curricula, with enhanced investment in social and support services for families and youth, will be an important step in countering the learned use of violence by our youth. Such a move would also require that the education, human service, and public health institutions play major roles in effecting these changes in our communities.

Indeed, the recognition that education designed to teach non-violent behaviours might be an important part of a combined public health–criminal justice response to the problem of violence helps to remind us that the modern view of how the law operates on behaviour in the society has become far more narrow that it once was. In our modern conceptions of the law, we imagine it operating on individual behaviour primarily through its incentive effects—the promise of punishment for misconduct made concrete and credible through individual prosecutions.

In the classic writings on laws, however, a great deal of attention was devoted not only to the passage of laws and to their application to individual cases, but also to their promulgation throughout the society (Friedman 1975). Extensive efforts to explain and educate citizens as to why the laws were necessary helped to ensure both their justice and their efficacy. Unless citizens knew about the law—its spirit as well as its letter—they could not reasonably be held accountable for failures to obey it. If the purpose of the law were not made clear, voluntary compliance—which was crucial to the law's effect—could not be counted upon.

The public health community's interest in non-violence education can be viewed as the modern rediscovery of the importance of explaining to and educating the public about violence, as well as simply having laws and applying them. It also incorporates an important modern discovery about the promulgation of obligations: it is often far easier to persuade people to comply with an important obligation when one can show individuals that it is in their best interests to do so, and when one can help them comply with the law. Persuasion and assistance are often more effective tools than accusation and blame. Still, it often helps in persuading and assisting if there is a broad social rule against violence that becomes part of the context for the education. Thus behavioural change may depend on a combination of education and laws that used to be called promulgation.

Gun control legislation efforts represent an important example of the interconnection between education and laws. Although there is growing support for increased handgun ownership restrictions as a primary prevention strategy, legislation alone is unlikely to create great change in violent injury rates in the foreseeable future. With over 60 million handguns in circulation in the United States (Bureau of Alcohol, Tobacco and Firearms 1991), an understanding and acceptance of the risks of handgun ownership and carrying is as important as legislative restrictions to reducing intentional handgun injuries.

Secondary level strategies require a more targeted effort. It requires early identification of individuals at high risk for, or already beginning to exhibit, violent behaviour and the development of treatment services for these individuals. This area represents an important interface between the human service and the criminal justice systems because the early identification of individuals at high risk for violence requires considerable collaboration. Points of early identification occur in schools, health facilities, police departments, courts, and a variety of other community institutions. Professional training in early identification and appropriate evaluation and treatment is necessary. This is not an easy process. Professional definitions and institutional boundaries have been established that encourage limited one-dimensional approaches.

Treatment interventions (tertiary prevention) for the most seriously affected individuals represent a key focal point for the criminal justice system. Violent behaviour cannot be condoned; punishment is an appropriate response to violent crimes or episodes and some individuals with serious pathology are not able to live in the general society. While it is essential that we understand how violent behaviour evolves, we must deal with it firmly to maintain safety within communities.

Although tertiary prevention falls most extensively into the criminal justice realm, with incarceration as the major strategy, public health needs to work along with the prison system in the area of rehabilitation. Without increased attention to rehabilitative efforts, including supportive services for those returning from prison to the community, most will continue to leave the prison system without the skills to avoid violence in the future. Public health must advocate for and support drug and alcohol treatment services, job training efforts, and conflict resolution and violence prevention skills, as well as the development of more extensive behaviour-change interventions. To date, successful rehabilitative efforts are limited, further reinforcing the need for more attention to be focused on this area as well.

Promising prevention programmes using public health strategies

Researchers Joy G. Dryfoos and Lisbeth Schorr both agree that the most effective programmes must be comprehensive, family and community oriented, and collaborative in nature. Some schools, communities, social agencies, and politicians around the country have incorporated this formula for success and have developed strategies to help children and their families prevent or cope with violence. These programmes offer the opportunity to learn from their successes and failures.

The Boston Violence Prevention Program

The Boston Violence Prevention Program, an intensive community-based outreach and education effort run by Boston's Department of Health and Hospitals, was launched in 1986 as part of its Health Promotion Program for Urban Youth. Much of its early work, supported by foundations, was focused on training teachers and youth services staff how to teach adolescents about the risks of violence, and discussing measures that can be employed to avoid fights using the Violence Prevention Curriculum for Adolescents. Regular training is offered for teachers, health workers, street outreach workers, and peer workers. The programme's peer leaders group is trained and actively participates in training sessions offered by the programme. A mass media campaign, Friends for Life Don't let Friends Fight, was developed to create a new community ethos in support of violence prevention. The programme has been part of the city budget for the last 5 years and has generated several spin-off activities.

Resolving Conflict Creatively Program—school-based conflict resolution programme in New York, California, and Alaska

The Resolving Conflict Creatively Program, a holistic school-based conflict resolution programme, works with the entire school structure to create safe schools. The K-12 curriculum, developed and refined since 1986, requires support from school administration although it does not mandate that every teacher be trained. Each of the 32 school districts in New York City that use the curriculum maintain a certain autonomy, leaving decision-making to the school community. After an intense 40-hour training on the curriculum, teachers incorporate the methods into their classrooms.

The progamme invites and encourages the participation of parents in training. Both teachers and administrators in these schools document fewer fights and a sense of peace. Students become peer mediators and receive special training to negotiate and mediate arguments that break out during school hours.

The programme provides a win–win situation. Not only do students develop leadership skills and a sense of responsibility for peace and respect, but teachers and administrators find practical use in their lives for conflict resolution skills. The programme also offers regular advanced training sessions in such topics as helping students deal with death and grief.

A walk through the hallways of the Satellite Academy High School in the Bronx gives the sense that, despite unsafe surroundings, the school offers an oasis of safety, a place of mutual respect—a place where learning takes place. Programme evaluations show that both teachers and students notice a positive change in the schools. A more comprehensive programme evaluation was recently funded through a grant from the CDC.

Save Our Sons and Daughters—a community-based programme working in Detroit public schools

Clementine Barfield Chism, Executive Director of the community-based programme Save Our Sons and Daughters (**SOSAD**), works daily to restore a sense of safety in a community that regularly experiences violence. She is one of the first in this country to recognize the feelings of children after a violent episode: 'They are scared. They see violence is a way of life so they act out. It is normal'. She cringes when she hears people talk about inner-city children experiencing post-traumatic stress disorder. To her, it is not a disorder, but a natural response to the chaotic violence around them.

After losing her son to violence, she founded SOSAD to provide grief counselling for her other sons. Over the past years, SOSAD activities have grown to include a K-12 curriculum—the Peace Program. The Peace Program was implemented in some Detroit schools in the communities most devastated by violence. The Peace Program teaches age- and culture-appropriate conflict resolution, and helps children and adolescents find a sense of empowerment in establishing and maintaining peace in their school by teaching them to become peacemakers. It also deals with the grief and pain that comes with losing someone to violence.

Peace Program schools proudly display a peace chain. Each child signs a peace pledge, and the chain links them all together. Early assessments indicate that teachers report improved school climates and that children are excited with their roles as peacemakers and peacekeepers.

The teachers of one particularly tough group of freshman girls, known for their physical fighting at one of Detroit's high schools, affirm the success of this programme. These girls have made a pledge not to fight. They are fully engaged in learning and practising the skills of peace.

School-based management—Comer method schools

More than 300 schools from around the country have adopted an educational model designed by Yale University's James P. Comer. A psychiatrist, Comer began his school-based work in one of New Haven's most troubled schools in 1968. He designed a multidisciplinary approach to school management. The programme stresses that a partnership between educators and parents is critical to a school's success. Its philosophy is based on the premise that each child is special and that schools should be places of learning.

Comer's model is also based on the premise that the initial relationship between schools and disadvantaged parents is too often wrought with mistrust and alienation. Comer schools require parental representation on all levels, including the school's management team. These parents also work to increase the involvement of other parents in the school's mission to educate all children.

Powerful Schools of Seattle, Washington

> I've been wanting to go to night school and learn how to use a computer, but when I get home after work, I just don't have the energy to drive half way across town, hunt for a parking place, and take a class at a community college . . . I really like the idea that the school buildings are being used full time. (A parent from Seattle's Powerful Schools programme)

Seattle's Powerful Schools used a collaborative community-based model to improve students' performance, 'to serve as a neighbourhood resource and empower parents, students, teachers and community'. This innovative coalition of four Rainier Valley elementary schools is a national leader in community-based school reform. These schools offer a wide variety of after-school programmes and classes for children and adults. Businesses and community groups help by planning field trips, providing support, and serving as a work-world contact for parents and students. The 30 to 40 classes offer reduced tuition fees and include topics such as gymnastics, blues harmonica, people's law school, and foreign languages.

A programme for students who exhibit emotional disturbances—Montgomery County, Maryland, public schools

A 20-member committee that included principals, teachers, and support services representatives in Montgomery County, Maryland, developed an interagency plan to serve students who exhibit violent behaviour. The co-operating agencies include public schools, department of social services, juvenile justice system, police, family resources services, recreation department, drug, alcohol, and mental health services, the State Attorney's Office, and the Office of Management and Budget.

The school district, mandated to serve students under the age of 16, has traditionally placed violent students in home instruction and provided 6 hours of instruction per week. The new plan includes creating centres that have school days longer than 8 hours and a half-day session. The longer school days coupled with the mandated Saturday sessions are meant to encourage students to return to public school.

The programme employs a case management approach. First, an assessment team evaluates the student to determine individual and family needs. The intense interagency programme is then implemented according to each student's identified needs. The school instructional day includes science and mathematics, life-skills building, physical education, group counselling, and English and social studies. The day also includes meetings with students, teachers, case managers, and counsellors. By co-ordinating existing resources and redirecting existing funds, the programme requires only moderate budget increase.

Overcoming Obstacles

Overcoming Obstacles, based in Los Angeles, is an education, jobs, and entrepreneurship programme that teaches young people the skills needed to succeed in education, find jobs, develop entrepreneurial skills, and involve themselves in the community. It is an example of business partnering with a community programme to give students a chance to succeed. This three-phased programme includes course work to:

- improve self-esteem
- develop a sense of personal responsibility
- instil a sense of pride in community
- set realistic goals
- develop communications and conflict resolution skills
- gain employment-seeking and retention skills.

An evaluation demonstrated positive behaviour change in successful students during the school year and after graduation.

After the first educational phase, high-school students move to a job placement phase. Through a network, part-time and summer employment is secured for students, while full-time employment is offered for programme graduates. One example is a special programme with ARCO Product Company/Prestige Stations Inc. Students working for this company receive a salary subject to increases and bonuses based on performance, and have the opportunity to attend college, paid for by ARCO.

Phase three encourages students to learn to become managers and owners of a business. Presently, funding has been provided for several businesses designed and managed by graduates of Overcoming Obstacles.

Co-ordinating coalitions

The Health Department of Contra Costa County, California, is widely known for its efforts to develop comprehensive programmes, harnessing existing resources, to alleviate poor health outcomes. Rather than designing and implementing their own stand-alone projects, the Contra Costa County Program co-ordinates and develops existing programmes to meet identified community needs. It serves as a lead agency for a number of health-related issues, including violence prevention. Some of its premises are that coalitions:

- offer more resources for less money
- can reach more people than a single organization
- provide greater credibility than single organizations
- offer more political clout
- serve a community networking function
- offer more diverse opinions and talents.

The Contra Costa County Program defines eight steps to building effective coalitions. An initial planning group should:

(1) analyse programme objectives and decide if a coalition is needed;

(2) recruit relevant and effective organizations/community representatives;

(3) develop preliminary objectives and activities;

(4) convene the group.

By using the input from the planning group, the coalitions should:

(5) develop a budget and structure;

(6) maintain coalition vitality (communications, public relations);

(7) evaluate programmes;

(8) based on evaluation, offer recommendations to improve programmes.

A guide further defining the eight-step process is available from the Contra Costa County Health Department.

A school-based planning model: Pittsburgh Safe Schools Project

The Safe Schools Project of the Pittsburgh Public Schools is a model for multidisciplinary violence prevention coalition. Members of the Pittsburgh Public Schools, the Jewish Healthier Foundation, the Western Psychiatric Institute and Clinic, the Center for Injury Research and Control at the University of Pittsburgh, and the Boys and Girls Club of Western Pennsylvania formed a working group that produced a Blueprint for Violence Reduction in Pittsburgh Public Schools. It is an action plan based on a sound theoretical framework, data collection and analysis, a commitment to understanding the causes of violence, and an analysis of state-of-the-art school violence prevention programmes.

The Blueprint contains a review of the project's components and discusses each step in a thorough manner, which lends itself to replication in other school districts. It also includes a set of valuable guiding principles for school-based program implementation:

- violence prevention must be a long-term priority for the school district
- adequate resources should be focused on very young children, particularly those at risk of developing aggressive lifestyles
- developmentally appropriate programmes should be integrated in a comprehensive approach for all grade levels
- students, teachers, and parents should participate in planning and assessing violence prevention activities
- activities should be culturally and racially appropriate
- prevention efforts should include home, school, and community co-ordination
- programme evaluation measures should be integrated into the programme design
- new programmes should be built upon successful existing programmes.

Conclusion

The contributions made by public health professionals towards efforts to prevent violence have been tremendous. The continued application of public health strategies to the understanding and prevention of violence assures success. The public health campaign to reduce smoking took 30 years after the first Surgeon General's report to have an effect. Violence reduction can be expected to take at least as long and require as many, if not more, diverse strategies.

References

Allen, N.H. (1981). Homicide prevention and intervention. *Suicide and Life Threatening Behavior,* **11**, 167–79.

American Psychological Association Commission on Violence and Youth (1993). *Violence and youth: psychology's response.* American Psychological Association, Washington, DC.

Austin, E.W., Roberts D.F., and Nass, C.I. (1990). Influences of family communication on children's television-interpretation processes. *Communication Research*, **4**, 545–65.

Bandura, A., Ross, D., and Ross, S.A. (1963*a*). Imitation of film-mediated aggressive models. *Journal of Abnormal Psychology,* **63**, 3–11.

Bandura, A., Ross, D., and Ross, S.A. (1963*b*). Vicarious reinforcement and imitative learning. *Journal of Abnormal Psychology,* **63**, 601–7.

Boys Clubs of America (1986). *Targeted Outreach Newsletter,* Vol. II-1.

Bureau of Alcohol, Tobacco and Firearms (1991). *Firearm census report.* US Treasury Department, Washington, DC.

Bureau of Justice Statistics (1992). *Criminal victimization in the United States, 1991.* US Department of Justice, Washington, DC.

Bureau of Justice Statistics (1993). *Highlights from 20 years of surveying crime victims: the national crime victimization survey, 1972–1992.* US Department of Justice, Washington, DC.

Bureau of Justice Statistics (1994). *Violence between inmates.* Report NCJ-149259, Office of Justice Programs, US Department of Justice, Washington, DC.

Carter Center (1994). *Not even one: a report on the crisis of children and firearms.* Carter Center, Atlanta, GA.

CDC (Centers for Disease Control) (1982*a*). Homicide. *Morbidity and Mortality Weekly Report,* **31**, 594.

CDC (Centers for Disease Control) (1982*b*). Homicide—United States. *Morbidity and Mortality Weekly Report,* **31**, 599–602.

CDC (Centers for Disease Control) (1983*a*). Violent deaths among persons 15–24 years of age—United States, 1970–78. *Morbidity and Mortality Weekly Report,* **32**, 453.

CDC (Centers for Disease Control) (1983*b*). *Homicide surveillance, high risk racial and ethnic groups—Blacks and Hispanics, 1970–83.* Public Health Service, US Department of Health and Human Services, Washington, DC.

CDC (Centers for Disease Control) (1990). Homicide among black males—United States, 1978–1987. *Morbidity and Mortality Weekly Report,* **39**, 869–72.

CDC (Centers for Disease Control) (1991). Weapon carrying among high school students—United States, 1990. *Morbidity and Mortality Weekly Report,* **40**, 681–4.

CDC (Centers for Disease Control) (1992). *Youth suicide prevention program: a resource guide.* National Center for Injury Prevention and Control, CDC, Atlanta, GA.

CDC (Centers for Disease Control) (1993*a*). Advance report of final mortality statistics, 1991. *Monthly Vital Statistics Report*, August. CDC, Atlanta, GA.

CDC (Centers for Disease Control) (1993*b*). Violence-related attitudes and behaviors of high school students—New York City, 1991. *Morbidity and Mortality Weekly Report,* **40**, 773–7.

CDC (Centers for Disease Control) (1994). Deaths resulting from firearm- and motor-vehicle-related injuries—United States, 1968–1991. *Morbidity and Mortality Weekly Report,* **3**, 37–42.

Centerwall, B.S. (1984). Race, socio-economic status, and domestic homicide, Atlanta, 1971–72. *American Journal of Public Health,* **8**, 813–15.

Centerwall, B.S. (1992). Television and violence: the scale of the problem and where to go from here. *Journal of the American Medical Association,* **267**, 3059–63.

Centerwall, B.S. (1993). Race, socio-economic status, and domestic homicide in New Orleans. Presented at the 2nd World Conference on Injury Control.

Daro, D. and Mitchel, L. (1987). *Deaths due to maltreatment soar: the results of the 1986 Annual Fifty State Survey.* National Center on Child Abuse Prevention Research, National Committee for Prevention of Child Abuse, Chicago, IL.

Dietz, W.H. and Strasburger, V.C. (1991). Children, adolescents and television. *Current Problems in Pediatrics,* **21**, 8–31.

Durant, R., Pendergast, R., and Cadenhead, C. (1994). Exposure to violence victimization and fighting behavior by urban black adolescents. *Journal of Adolescent Health,* **15**, 311–18.

Egeland, B. and Jacobvitz, D. (1984). Intergenerational continuity of parental abuse: cases and consequences. Presented at the Conference on the Bio Social Perspectives on Abuse and Neglect, York, ME.

Emde, R.N. (1993). The horror! The horror! Reflection on our culture of violence and its implication for early development and morality. *Psychiatry,* **56**, 119–23.

Eron, L. and Huesmann, L.R. (1984). Television violence and aggressive behavior. In *Advances in clinical child psychology* (ed. B. Lahey and A. Kardin). Plenum Press, New York.

FBI (Federal Bureau of Investigation) (1991). *Uniform crime report: crime in the United States.* US Department of Justice, Washington, DC.

FBI (Federal Bureau of Investigation) (1992). *Uniform crime report: crime in the United States.* US Department of Justice, Washington, DC.

FBI (Federal Bureau of Investigation) (1993). *Uniform crime report: crime in the United States.* US Department of Justice, Washington, DC.

FBI (Federal Bureau of Investigation) (1997). *Uniform crime report: crime in the United States.* US Department of Justice, Washington, DC.

FBI (Federal Bureau of Investigation) (1998). *Uniform crime report: crime in the United States.* US Department of Justice, Washington, DC.

FBI (Federal Bureau of Investigation) (1999). *Uniform crime report: crime in the United States.* US Department of Justice, Washington, DC.

Fingerhut, L.A. and Kleinman, J.C. (1990). International and interstate comparisons of homicide among young males. *Journal of the American Medical Association,* **24**, 3292–4.

Fingerhut, L.A., Ingram, D.D., and Feldman, J.J. (1992). Firearm and non-firearm homicide among persons 15 through 19 years of age. *Journal of the American Medical Association,* **22**, 3048–53.

Fitzpatrick, K.M. and Boldizar, J.P. (1993). The prevalence and consequences of exposure to violence among African American youth. *Journal of the American Academy of Child and Adolescent Psychiatry,* **32**, 424–30.

Freeman, L., Mokros, H., and Poznanski, E. (1993). Violent events reported by normal urban school-aged children: characteristics and depression correlates. *Journal of the American Academy of Child and Adolescent Psychiatry,* **32**, 419–23.

Friedman, L.M. (1975). *The legal system: a social science perspective,* pp. 56–66. Russell Sage Foundation, New York.

Gil, D. (1973). *Violence against children: physical child abuse in the United States.* Harvard University Press, Cambridge, MA.

Groves, B.M., Zuckerman, B., Marans, S., and Cohen, D.J. (1993). Silent victims: children who witness violence. *Journal of the American Medical Association,* **269**, 262–4.

Huesmann, L.R., Eron, L.D., Klein, R., Brice, P., and Fischer, P. (1983). Mitigating the imitation of aggressive behaviors by changing children's attitudes about media violence. *Journal of Personality and Social Psychology,* **44**, 899–910.

Kellermann, A.L., Rivara, F.P., Rushforth, N.B., *et al.* (1993). Gun ownership as a risk factor for homicide in the home. *New England Journal of Medicine,* **15**, 1084–91.

Killias, M. (1993). International correlations between gun ownership and rates of homicide and suicide. *Canadian Medical Association Journal,* **148**, 1721–5.

Kilpatrick, D.G., Edmunds, C.N., and Seymour, A.K. (1992). *Rape in America: a report to the nation.* National Victim Center, Arlington, VA.

Lester, D. (1988). Firearm availability and the incidence of suicide and homicide. *Acta Psychiatrica Belgica,* 387–93.

Liebert, R.M. (1988). *Early window: the effects of television on children and youth* (6th edn). Allyn and Bacon, Needham, MA.

Liebert, R., Neale, J., and Davidson, E. (1973). *Early window: the effects of television on children and youth.* Pergamon Press, New York.

Loftin, C., McDowall, D., Wiersema, B., and Cottey, T.J. (1991). Effects of restrictive licensing of handguns on homicide and suicide in the District of Columbia. *New England Journal of Medicine,* **325**, 1615–20.

Lorion, R.P. and Saltzman, W. (1993). Children's exposure to community violence: following a path from concern to research to action. *Psychiatry,* **56**, 55–65.

Makepeace, J.M. (1981). Courtship violence among college students. *Family Relations,* **30**, 97–102.

Martinez, P. and Richters, J. (1993). The NIMH community violence project. II: Children's distress symptoms associated with violence exposure. *Psychiatry,* **56**, 22–35.

Miller, T.R., Cohen, M.A., and Rossman, S.B. (1993). Datawatch: victim cost of violent crime resulting injuries. *Health Affairs (Millwood),* **12**, 186–97.

Osofsky, J., Wewers, S., Hann, D.M., and Fick, A.C.. (1993). Chronic community violence: what is happening to our children? *Psychiatry,* **56**, 36–45.

Prothrow-Stith, D. and Weissman, M. (1991). *Deadly consequences: how violence is destroying our teenage population and a plan to begin solving the problem,* pp. 1–203. Harper Collins, New York.

Pynoos, R.S., Frederick, C., Nader, K., *et al.* (1987). Life threat and post-traumatic stress in school-age children. *Archives of General Psychiatry,* **44**, 1057–63.

Sang, F., Schmitz, B., and Tasche, K. (1993). Developmental trends in television coviewing of parent–child dyads. *Journal of Youth and Adolescence,* **5**, 531–43.

Satcher, D. (1985). The public health approach to violence. presented at the National Education Association National Conference, Los Angeles, California.

Sege, R. and Dietz, W. (1994). Television viewing and violence in children: the pediatrician as agent for change. *Pediatrics,* **94**, 600–7.

Shaffer, D., Garland, A., Gould, M., Fisher, P., and Trautman, P. (1988). Preventing teenage suicide: a critical review. *Journal of the American Academy of Child and Adolescent Psychiatry,* **27**, 673–87.

Shaffer, D., Garland, M., and Hicks, R. (1994). Worsening suicide rate in black teenagers. *American Journal of Psychiatry,* **151**, 12.

Sheley, J., McGee, Z., and Wright, J. (1992). Gun-related violence in and around inner-city schools. *American Journal of Diseases of Childhood,* **146**, 677–82.

Slaby, R.G. and Guerra, N.G. (1988). Cognitive mediators of aggression in adolescent offenders: 1. Assessment. *Developmental Psychology,* **4**, 580–8.

Slaby, R. and Quarfoth, G. (1980). Effects of television on the developing child. *Advanced Behavioral Pediatrics,* **1**, 225–66.

Sloan, J.H., Kellerman, A.L., Reay, D.T., *et al.* (1988). Handgun regulations, crime, assaults, and homicide: a tale of two cities. *New England Journal of Medicine,* **319**, 1256–62.

Spivak, H., Prothrow-Stith, D., and Hausman, A. (1988). Dying is no accident: adolescents, violence, and intentional injury. *Pediatric Clinics of North America,* **35**, 1339–47.

Straus, M. (1991). Discipline and deviance: physical punishment of children and violence and other crime in adulthood. *Social Problems,* **38**, 137–54.

Straus, M. and Gelles, R. (1990). How violent are American families? Estimates from the National Family Violence Resurvey and other studies. In *Physical violence in American families: risk factors and adaptations to violence in American families: risk factors and adaptations to violence in 8145 families* (ed. M. Straus and R. Gelles). Transaction, New Brunswick, NJ.

Turner, C.W., Hesse, B.W., and Peterson-Lewis, S. (1986). Naturalistic studies of the long-term effects of television violence. *Journal of Social Issues,* 51–73.

United States Department of Health, Education, and Welfare (1964). *Smoking and health. Report of the Advisory Committee to the Surgeon General.* Public Health Service, Washington, DC.

Vissing, Y., Straus, M., Gelles, R., and Harrop, J. (1991). Verbal aggression by parents and psychological problems of children. *Child Abuse and Neglect,* **15**, 223–38.

Weaver, B. and Barbour, N. (1992). Mediation of children's televiewing: families in society. *Journal of Contemporary Human Services,* **4**, 236–43.

Widom, C.S. (1989). The cycle of violence. *Science,* **244**, 160–6.

Williams, B.C. and Kotch, B.J. (1990). Excess injury mortality among children in the United States: comparison of recent international statistics. *Pediatrics,* **86**, 1067–73.

Wolfgang, M. (1986). Homicide in other industrialized countries. *Bulletin of the New York Academy of Medicine,* **62**, 400–12.

Wood, W., Wong, F.Y., and Chachere, J.G. (1991). Effects of media violence on viewer's aggression in unconstrained social interaction. *Psychological Bulletin,* **109**, 371–83.

11

Intervention for special populations

11.1 Families

Michael J. Puma

Introduction

The family unit has been an integral part of our existence throughout recorded history. Even in prestate hunter–gatherer societies the family helped humans deal with the basic needs of our species. But what is a family? According to Mattessich and Hill (1987) it is a group of individuals related by kinship, residence, or close emotional attachments that display four common characteristics: (a) intimate interdependence and selective boundary maintenance; (b) the performance of certain key functions including physical maintenance, socialization and education, control of social and sexual behaviour, and sustaining family morale and motivation to perform roles inside and outside the family unit; (c) the acquisition of new members through procreation and the formation of sexual partnerships; (d) the launching of juvenile members from the family when they are mature. As the World Health Organization has noted (WHO 1985), the ability to perform these functions well '... is crucial for the attainment of health for all. As the basic social unit, the family has a determinant influence on the health and disease patterns of its members'.

An important context for understanding families today is the advent of the postindustrial 'information age' that is helping to drive profound social changes at the dawn of the twenty-first century, as did the transition to the industrial age in the late nineteenth century. For some, these changes spell disaster for the family institution. Pournelle, for example, warns that '... the family, at least as we know it, is under attack; and if trends continue the institution of the family will be greatly changed, greatly weakened, and may cease to exist' (Pournelle 1997, p. 491). For others, such as Fukuyama (1999), the trends that we are observing today are simply adjustments to a new postindustrial social order, in the same way that prior human transitions—from hunter–gatherer to agricultural to industrial—were associated with major social 'disruptions'. Only time will tell whether we are seeing the start of a decline in the family unit or a period of transition to a new evolving form.

In this chapter, we begin with an exploration of some of the major social and demographic changes affecting the family, and comment on the implications of these changes for health and well being. We then review some of the more important changes in government policies that are intended to alter or mediate the effect of these social transformations. The discussion is organized to begin with a focus on the United States, both because of the availability of a wealth of information and a rich base of research, and the current American position as a 'bellwether' of global social changes. This is then followed with a discussion of how similar trends have been seen in other industrial countries and, where possible, worldwide.

Social and demographic changes affecting families

Throughout most of the twentieth century, industrial nations had a shared idea of the ideal family. This symbol, what Goode (1993) has called the 'classical family of Western nostalgia', consisted of a married couple with a breadwinner father, a home-maker mother, and two or more children. By the end of the century, however, married couples in the United States with two or more own children only accounted for about 25 per cent of all households. Today, living arrangements, especially those involving children, have expanded to encompass a broad array of different situations reflecting significant transformations of the more traditional family structure. These changes are occurring in the United States and, to a greater or lesser degree, throughout the world, and have potentially important consequences for individual health and well being.

The trends shaping today's families include innovations in medical technology that have given women greater control over their own fertility, thereby diminishing the role of reproduction as seen in declining birth rates. As a consequence, the importance of kinship has also changed as seen by the decline in marriage, the increase in cohabitation, the increase in divorce, and the rise in non-marital childbearing. These changes have, in turn, led to an increase in female-headed households and a substantial decrease in the size of households, particularly the growth of single-person households. The nature of work has also changed as the information age increasingly rewards mental rather than physical labour propelling more women into the labour force and changing the traditional male–female roles of provider and home-maker. Taken together, these changes have substantially altered traditional family functions and roles.

Decline in birth and fertility rates

As noted above, one of the core functions of the family is reproduction. Yet, by the end of the twentieth century fertility rates had dropped substantially in nearly all industrialized countries, and these same trends have been seen worldwide. Several factors have led to this drop in fertility, especially in industrialized countries. First, increased demands for education have extended the time that young adults invest in their training prior to entering the work force. Today, few young adults can afford to marry and have children early in life—in an economy where a college education is necessary for many jobs, such family formation impedes the completion of one's education, especially for women. Second, there have been significant changes in equality for women. In most industrialized countries today, women are more highly educated, which improves their labour market opportunities and makes them more economically active and less financially dependent on their husbands. Finally, women are now more in control of their own fertility owing to the increasing awareness and use of birth control methods which, in many developing countries, has been supported by government policies encouraging smaller families (e.g. China's one child per family policy).

The United States

Birth and fertility rates

From 1936 to 1957 birth rates (i.e. the number of live births per 1000 women) rose by 67 per cent, largely as a result of the postwar baby boom, but rates then dropped by 55 per cent in the following two decades, reaching a low of 15.5 in 1983 (Janis 1997). Following a brief increase, United States birth rates have continued their downward slide, declining to a new low of 14.8 in 1996 (US Bureau of the Census 1998*a*). Overall, the birth rate has fallen by nearly 40 per cent since 1960. For women under the age of 25, those in the prime childbearing years, the number of births declined by 20 per cent just between 1980 and 1996 (US Bureau of the Census 1998*b*).

Another way to examine the decline in births is to look at changes in fertility rates which are defined as the number of live births per woman of childbearing age. At the end of the twentieth century, United States fertility rates have dropped to a point where they are now just over the level required to maintain the current level of population (i.e. the 'replacement level') at an average of 2.07 children per woman (US Department of Health and Human Services 1999). However, fertility rates for Hispanic Americans have remained high, and in combination with high rates of recent immigration have led to a rapid increase in the percentage of United States children who are non-white (US Department of Health and Human Services 1999). In 1980, 74 per cent of United States children were non-Hispanic white; by 1997 this percentage had declined to 66 per cent, and is projected to drop to 55 per cent by 2020 (US Department of Health and Human Services 1999). In fact, if it were not for immigration and the higher birth rates of foreign-born women, the United States birth rates would have fallen even more dramatically since 1960.

Sexual activity

Through the late 1980s, the pattern of falling birth and fertility rates in the United States was not accompanied by an associated decline in sexual activity. In 1970, 35 per cent of girls and 55 per cent of boys reported having had sex by age 18; by 1988, the percentages had increased to 56 per cent for girls and 73 per cent for boys (Popenoe 1998). More recent data, however, show a changing tide, with the proportion of females aged 15 to 19 who reported ever having sexual intercourse dropping to 50 per cent in 1995, although rates are higher for Hispanic and black teenagers (Federal Interagency Forum on Child and Family Statistics 1999).

At the same time, there have also been declines in the reported incidence of unprotected intercourse among teenagers and in the incidence of sexually transmitted diseases (**STDs**), in large part due to the adoption of more conservative attitudes by youth and the introduction of health education in schools (Ku *et al.* 1998). Many youth now report using condoms or other forms of contraceptive protection when they have sex, and over the past decade the substantial rise in condom use among teenagers has been one of the major public health success stories in the United States. Between 1979 and 1988, condom use reported by male teenagers in the United States more than doubled, and by 1995 the rate had increased again by one-fifth. Universal protection has not yet been achieved, however. In 1995, 27 per cent of male teenagers had had unprotected sex in the previous 12 months (Sonenstein *et al.* 1998).

Teenage pregnancy

The United States has historically had one of the highest rates of teenage pregnancy in the industrialized world. Each year, almost 1 million teenage girls in the United States become pregnant, and approximately 40 per cent of girls become pregnant at least once before reaching the age of 20 (Popenoe 1998). Such early childbearing in the United States is more common among girls from families of lower socio-economic status. For example, women in their twenties whose mothers did not finish high school were about five times more likely to have had a teenage birth than those whose mothers had a college education (US Department of Health and Human Services 1998).

However, in line with the reduction in teenage sexual activity, especially unprotected sexual intercourse, birth rates among United States teenagers have also fallen since 1991 after a substantial climb during the late 1980s. In 1997 the birth rate of 52.9 per 1000 among females aged 15 to 19 was at the same level last observed in 1988, and within three percentage points of the lowest rate observed in 1986. Birth rates have declined among both younger and older teenagers, among white, black, and Hispanic teenagers, and in all states except the District of Columbia (Ventura *et al.* 1998). Declines in the birth rate reflect real declines in pregnancy rates since rates of abortion have not increased at the same time.

These reductions in the incidence of early sexual activity are an important public health objective because sex at an early age is associated with more partners and more frequent sex, and the increased risks of STDs and HIV, and unintended pregnancy (National Center for Health Statistics 1999*a*). The extent to which early pregnancy has more far-reaching consequences for both mother and child has, however, been the subject of considerable debate, especially in the United States where research has shown that some young mothers end up doing rather well (Furstenberg *et al.* 1987; Duncan and Hoffman 1990). The problem has been trying to separate out the effects of early pregnancy from socio-economic conditions that existed prior to the pregnancy itself. That is, it is the case that, on average, teenage mothers are worse off on many dimensions than women who delay childbearing: teenage parenting is associated with lower educational attainment, lower earnings, and higher welfare dependency (Moore *et al.* 1995*a*, *b*), and teenage mothers are more likely to be poor at the end of their twenties, and more likely to raise their children alone (Furstenberg *et al.* 1987; Maynard 1997). But these conditions are not necessarily caused by the pregnancy itself. A recent review of the literature concludes that, although evidence on the socio-economic consequences of early pregnancy remains uncertain, it is clear that reducing early childbearing '... represents a potentially productive strategy for widening the pathways out of poverty or, at the very least, not compounding the handicaps imposed by social disadvantage' (Hoffman 1998, p. 8).

There is, however, a relationship between maternal age and birth outcomes, with babies born to very young teenage mothers (under age 15) being at higher risk than 25- to 29-year-olds for birth complications, prematurity, low birthweight, neonatal death, and developmental delays (Hayes 1987; Reichman and Pagnini 1997). Children born to teenage mothers are also at greater risk of physical abuse and accidental injury, do less well in school, and are more likely to be teenage parents themselves (Furstenberg *et al.* 1987; Manlove 1997; Maynard 1997).

Although the negative consequences of early childbearing for girls and their babies are now widely recognized, less attention has been paid to the consequences for their male partners who are required to make an 18-year commitment to support the child, now that the legal establishment of paternity is expected in the United States and can easily be accomplished using genetic tests.

Worldwide

Birth and fertility rates

Birth rates have dropped even more dramatically throughout most of Western Europe. At the end of the 1990s, the average birth rate across the 15 countries that comprise the European Union was 10.9 births per 1000 women compared with the new United States low of 14.8.

Birth rates have, in fact, declined so much in many European Union countries that fertility rates are now below replacement levels, leading to projections of declining populations and higher proportions of elderly persons. Across the European Union the average fertility rate has declined by 40 per cent, from an average of about 2.39 children per woman of childbearing age in 1970 to an average of 1.44 in 1998 (Eurostat 1999). Fertility rates are highest in Ireland at 1.87 (but down 52 per cent from 3.93 in 1970), and lowest in Spain and Italy at 1.18 and 1.17 respectively (Eurostat 1999). As a consequence, Italy, Spain, and Germany are estimated to lose up to 30 per cent of their population each generation, barring additions to the population through new immigration (Fukuyama 1999).

According to Rothenbacher (1996*b*), the factors driving these changes include the increased availability and use of birth control, rising female educational levels (and associated increases in workforce participation), increasing decisions by couples to have fewer children or to forego children altogether, and a rising age of first marriage (and of first birth). In particular, European women are increasingly delaying their first pregnancy—fertility rates for women aged 15 to 19 years fell by 50 per cent throughout the European Union between 1975 and 1998 (Eurostat 1999). Although there is some variation across countries in Western Europe, it is now increasingly rare for a woman to have a baby before the age of 20—the average age of having a first child has risen from 24 in 1970 to nearly 29 in 1995, and across the European Union countries only 1 per cent of women aged 15 to 19 have children (Eurostat 1999). Moreover, the younger the generation, the higher the proportion that is childless. For example, 15 per cent of German women born in 1950 are childless compared with 26 per cent of women born in 1959 (Eurostat 1998).

Declining birth and fertility rates have not, however, been confined to Western Europe; many East European countries have seen declines as well. For example, between 1975 and 1998 the birth rate dropped by a dramatic 54 per cent in the Czech Republic (from 19.6 to 8.96), 41 per cent in Hungary from (from 18.4 to 10.7), 41 per cent in Romania (from 15.8 to 9.3), and 48 per cent in Poland (from 18.9 to 9.8) United Nations 1997). In large part, these changes are due to the dramatic upheavals associated with the break up of the socialist states in 1989 and 1990 throughout central, eastern, and southeastern Europe (Rothenbacher 1996*a*). These regions have experienced a substantial loss of population due to both emigration (for employment) and very low birth rates (well below replacement levels). But there are exceptions, such as the agriculturally oriented countries of Albania and Macedonia where fertility rates are among the highest in Europe. For the most part, families in these countries remain close to the traditional household of the early to mid-twentieth century with nearly universal marriage rates, very low rates of non-marital childbearing, a high share of extended families, and a low incidence of people living alone.

Elsewhere in the industrialized world, birth rates have declined similarly to the trends seen in the United States and Europe. In Canada the age at which a woman has her first baby has risen from 23 in 1971 to 26 in 1989 (Vanier Institute of the Family 1994), and from 1975 to 1998 birth rates declined by 20 per cent in Australia (from 16.9 to 13.5), by nearly 30 per cent in Israel (from 28.2 to 20.0), by 40 per cent in Japan (from 17.2 to 10.3), by 19 per cent in New Zealand (from 18.4 to 14.9), and by 23 per cent in Singapore (from 17.8 to 13.8) (United Nations 1997).

Declining fertility is not restricted to the industrialized countries. Although fertility rates remain high in many developing nations, typically in excess of three children per woman, rates have dropped sharply since the early 1960s as a result of the wide availability of birth control, and improved educational and economic opportunities for women. Worldwide, between 1963 and 1993 there was a decline of 1.8 in the average number of children born to a woman of childbearing age (United Nations 1994). These declines, however, vary among the different regions of the world: sub-Saharan Africa, an average decline of 0.4 children (from 6.7 to 6.3); the Middle East and North Africa, 2.4 children (from 6.9 to 4.5); South Asia, 1.9 children (from 6.0 to 4.1); East Asia and the Pacific, 3.4 children (from 5.7 to 2.3); Latin America and the Caribbean, 2.8 children (from 5.9 to 3.1) (United Nations 1994). Countries that have cut their birth rate by 50 per cent or more since the early 1960s include Thailand (from 6.4 in 1963 to 2.1 in 1993), Columbia (from 6.7 to 2.7), Kuwait (from 7.3 to 3.1), Brazil (from 6.1 to 2.9), Mexico (from 6.7 to 3.2), Peru (from 6.8 to 3.4), and Venezuela (from 6.6 to 3.3) (United Nations 1994). China, in large part as a result of the government's one child limit, has seen a dramatic decline of an average of 3.6 births per woman between 1963 and 1993 (United Nations 1999). Even traditional Islamic countries have seen large declines, for example a decline in average births of 4.2 in Kuwait, 3.6 in Algeria, 3.2 in Egypt, and 2.5 in Jordan (United Nations 1999). For comparison, the average across all industrialized countries fell by 1.1 from 2.8 to 1.7 (United Nations 1994).

Teenage pregnancy

As noted above, teenage pregnancy is quite high in the United States at about 53 per 1000 women aged 15 to 19. Japan has the lowest rate among industrialized nations at about 4 per 1000, and rates are 10 or less per 1000 teenagers in Switzerland, The Netherlands, France, Italy, Belgium, and Denmark. But teenage pregnancy rates are also high in a number of East European countries: 59 per 1000 women aged 15 to 19 years in Bulgaria, between 40 and 50 per 1000 in the Czech Republic, Slovakia, Yugoslavia, the Ukraine, Macedonia, Romania, and Hungary, between 30 and 39 per 1000 in Moldova, Russia, Latvia,

Estonia, Bosnia, Lithuania, Croatia, and Slovenia, and 28 per 1000 in Belarus and Poland (United Nations 1994). The rate is 33 per 1000 in the United Kingdom, 35 per 1000 in New Zealand, 27 per 1000 in Canada, and 21 per 1000 in Australia (United Nations 1994).

Elsewhere in the world, the rates of teenage births are, in many instances, much higher than in most industrialized countries. For example, the average rate of births per 1000 females age aged 15 to 19 is 143 across sub-Saharan Africa, with rates in excess of 200 in Sierra Leone, Congo, Liberia, Niger, Somalia, Angola, and Guinea (United Nations 1997). The average in the Middle East and North Africa is 56, with the highest rates found in Yemen (101), Libya (102), Saudi Arabia (114), and Oman (122); average rates of 56 are also found in Asia and the Pacific (highest in Afghanistan at 152, India at 109, and Bangladesh at 115), and the average in the Americas is 68 (highest in Nicaragua at 133) (United Nations 1997). China, again as a consequence of strict government birth policies, has among the lowest teenage birth rates in the world at an average of 5 per 1000 females aged 15 to 19; similarly low rates are also found in Korea with an average of 4, and Singapore with an average of 8 (United Nations 1997).

Decline in the size of households

As Garrett (1997) points out, the trend towards lower birth rates, especially in industrialized nations, is not because procreation has become less desirable, but rather that there has been a significant shift in the desired number of children. Indeed, the average family size has fallen dramatically across most industrialized countries due, in many cases, to the rising cost of children as they move from being an 'economic asset', common through the nineteenth century and in many underdeveloped countries today (where child labour is common), to the 'emotional asset' of the postindustrial world.

The United States

Over 200 years ago, about two-thirds of all American households had five or more people. This proportion had dropped to 45 per cent by 1900, and to 14 per cent by 1997 (US Bureau of the Census 1998*a*). One reason for this decline in household size is that Americans have moved towards having fewer children. The percentage of women nationwide with one child has nearly doubled in the past 20 years to 19 per cent, and the rate is even higher for 'non-white' women at 22 per cent (O'Hanlon 1999). There are several reasons for this trend, including delayed marriage and first pregnancy, the high 'opportunity cost' of having a child (lost wages for women who stop or reduce work), changing lifestyles with a greater emphasis on adult fulfilment, and the high cost of child rearing. It is estimated, for example, that an average United States family with an annual income of $60 000 will spend $228 000 to raise a child, excluding the cost of college (O'Hanlon 1999).

There is also a growing percentage of United States families with no minor children of their own in their household. Between 1960 and 1997, the percentage of all families with no minor children rose from 43 to 51 per cent of all families, and only 34 per cent of all households now contain 'own' children (birth, adopted, or stepchildren) of the household head (US Department of Health and Human Services 1999). This trend is accompanied by an increase in the number of married couples under the age of 35 without own children under 18 from 23 per cent in 1970 to 29 per cent in 1997 (US Bureau of the Census 1998*b*). Families without own children under 18 at home are not necessarily 'childless', however. Some contain other related children (e.g. nieces/nephews, grandchildren, or foster children), while others contain adult children living at home or living away from home as part of their continuing education.

At the same time, the proportion of people living alone has risen dramatically from about 17 per cent of all households in 1970 to about 25 per cent in 1997 (US Bureau of the Census 1998*a*). In addition to the previously noted lengthening of young adulthood, these changes have been attributed to the rapidly increasing size of the elderly population driven by increasing longevity. For example, in the United States, children as a percentage of the total population have declined from a high of 36 per cent in 1960 to about 25 per cent; in contrast, the proportion of the population aged 65 and older has increased from 8 per cent in 1950 to 13 per cent in 1997, and is expected to grow to 16 per cent—nearly one out of six—by 2020 (US Department of Health and Human Services 1999).

Worldwide

As in the United States, other industrialized countries have also seen a decline in household sizes and a concomitant growth in single-person households. One cause, noted above, is delayed childbearing. Other causes include rising divorce rates (see below), increased time spent on education by young adults, and increased life expectancies, which have increased the number of elderly living alone, especially women. For example, single-person households now account for 28 per cent of all European Union households, up from 22 per cent in 1981 (Eurostat 1998). The averages are lower in the southern countries of Spain, Ireland, Portugal, and Italy, and higher in the northern countries of Denmark, Germany, Finland, and Sweden where they now account for more than one-third of the total household populations.

Although couples with children remain the most common family type, this pattern is being eroded throughout the European Union by the increasing number of single-parent families and childless couples, especially in the Scandinavian countries. In Denmark, for example, couples with children now account for 42 per cent of all households compared with more than 60 per cent in Spain, Ireland, and Portugal (Eurostat 1998). Single-parent families account for about 6 per cent of European Union households, with the highest rates in Ireland at 9 per cent; the majority of single parents are women, accounting for about 90 per cent of the total.

Similar changes are seen in Canada. In 1986, 52 per cent of families consisted of married couples with never-married children living at home, but in 1991, only 5 years later, this percentage had dropped to 48 per cent (Vanier Institute of the Family 1994). The proportion of families without children also increased during this same time period from 32 to 35 per cent, and single-parent families now account for 13 per cent of all Canadian families (Vanier Institute of the Family 1994).

Again, as in the United States, life expectancies have increased and this has given rise to more elderly persons in many European countries. In 1960, the elderly population (age 60 and older) accounted for an average of 17 per cent of the population across all European Union countries. By 1997, this proportion had risen to an average of 21 per cent, ranging from a low of about 15 per cent in Ireland to a high of about 23 per cent in Italy (Eurostat 1998). In fact, by the middle of the twenty-first century, current projections estimate that the proportion of elderly in Italy and Spain will reach about 37 per cent, fuelled by the previously discussed very low fertility rates in these countries.

Similar patterns are seen elsewhere in the world. For example, between 1960 and 1997 the proportion of the population over the age of 65 has increased from 8.5 to 12.1 per cent in Australia, from 10.2 to 13.5 per cent in the Czech Republic, from 5.7 to 15.7 per cent in Japan, and from 8.7 to 11.6 per cent in New Zealand (OECD 1999). In Canada, the proportion of the population aged 65 and over grew by about 80 per cent during the 1970s and 1980s (Vanier Institute of the Family 1994).

Marriage delayed

As noted by Goode, '... in our time people have been reducing their personal investment in the collectivity of the family ... a different structure of opportunities exists today, in which one's best interest is increasingly not to be found in the ... family ... better opportunities—for pleasure, self enhancement, advancement, even material goods—might be found elsewhere' (Goode 1993, p. 9). As a consequence, the last half of the twentieth century has seen a substantial transformation affecting the institution of marriage, and these changes are likely to continue into the new millennium.

The United States

Most Americans continue to prize marriage as a source of sexual faithfulness, emotional support, mutual trust, and lasting commitment, and most will marry at least once in their lifetime. Yet, overall fewer Americans today are choosing to marry than in the past. For example, the proportion of United States adults age 18 and older who are married dropped from 72 per cent in 1970 to 60 per cent in 1996 (US Bureau of the Census 1998*b*). These declines have been most dramatic for African-Americans; over this period, the proportion of married adults decreased from 73 to 63 per cent for white Americans, from 72 to 58 per cent for Hispanics, and from 64 to only 42 per cent for African-Americans (US Bureau of the Census 1998*b*). In contrast, the proportion of never-married adults has doubled in the United States since 1970, and now accounts for 23 per cent of all adults (US Bureau of the Census 1998*b*). The sharpest increases have been seen for adults in their late twenties and early thirties, with the proportion of 25- to 29-year-olds who had never married increasing by a factor of over 3 for women (from 11 to 38 per cent between 1970 and 1996), and more than doubling for men (from 19 to 52 per cent) (US Bureau of the Census 1998*b*).

In large part, these changes in marriage rates are due to decisions by young adults to delay marriage to much later in life. The median age of first marriage in the United States is now 25 for a woman and 27 for a man, compared with 20 and 23 respectively in 1960 (Popenoe and Whitehead 1999). In fact, the annual number of marriages per 1000 unmarried women declined by 43 per cent in the United States between 1960 and 1996 (Popenoe and Whitehead 1999). One consequence of this change is that marriage is no longer associated with first sexual intercourse—in the United States today just over half of young women have experienced intercourse by the age of 17, and teenage girls are sexually active for 7 or 8 years on average before marriage (Moore *et al.* 1998).

In addition, more adults in the United States are deciding to remain single for their entire lives. In 1960, 94 per cent of women had been married at least once by age 45, a percentage that had remained relatively stable since the nineteenth century. If current trends continue, fewer than 85 per cent of current young adults will marry (Popenoe and Whitehead 1999). In addition, the percentage of persons age 15 and older who were married dropped from 69 per cent for males and 66 per cent for females in 1960, to 58 per cent and 55 per cent respectively in 1998 (US Bureau of the Census 1998*b*). For African-American females the drop has been particularly precipitous, going from 60 to 39 per cent in the same time period.

As a consequence, marriage has increasingly become a means of satisfying adult sexual and emotional needs rather than its more traditional use as a way of increasing economic capacity and nurturing young children. This breaking of the tie between marriage and parenthood has also led to a growing recognition of same-sex partnerships, and parenthood is no longer viewed as an integral part of marriage. Parenting is increasingly being claimed as a right of same-sex couples through adoption and medically assisted fertility.

Worldwide

In Europe during the 1960s, nearly 90 per cent of adults of marriageable age were married (Golini and Silvestrini 1997). Like the United States, however, Europe saw a decline in marriage in the 1960s which began in Sweden and spread from north to south during the following decade, accompanied by an increasing trend towards cohabitation (see below). But the decline in Europe has been more severe, and average European Union marriage rates are now well below those of the United States. Overall, the marriage rate in European Union countries declined from about eight per year for every 1000 persons in 1970 to about five per year in 1997, compared with an average of 8.9 in the United States (Eurostat 1998). Sweden continues to have the lowest marriage rate at 3.8 per 1000 persons, but the greatest declines since 1970 were observed in France (down 72 per cent to 4.9), Finland (down 72 per cent to 4.6), Ireland (down 66 per cent to 4.3), and The Netherlands (down 64 per cent to 5.5) (Eurostat 1998). Canada, by comparison, was slightly above the European Union average in 1997 at 5.4 per 1000 persons, and Japan at 6.4 was much higher than the average for all European Union countries and on a par with Denmark (6.5) and Portugal (6.4) (Eurostat 1998).

Austria provides an interesting example of the kind of dramatic changes that have swept Western Europe. It is a predominantly Catholic country, and more than 90 per cent of women born between 1935 and 1945 married, and the two-child family was widely considered to be the ideal. Since the 1970s, however, trends have created dramatic changes in family structures: there has been a sharp drop in the birth rate from 2.82 per 1000 in the early 1960s to below replacement levels (1.37) in 1998, family sizes have declined (about one-third of all marriages are now childless), and there is a greater prevalence of never-married persons, divorced persons, single-parent families, and cohabiting couples (Schwenger 1999).

Declines in marriage rates have also been seen in Central and East European countries. Between 1990 and 1997, marriage rates (per 1000 population) fell 38 per cent in Bulgaria (from 6.7 to 4.1), 33 per cent in the Czech Republic (8.4 to 5.6), 22 per cent in Romania (8.3 to 6.5), nearly 30 per cent in Russia (8.9 to 6.3), and nearly 15 per cent in Yugoslavia (6.2 to 5.3) (United Nations 1997). Similar declines have been seen in other industrialized countries during the same period—a drop of 16 per cent in Australia (6.9 to 5.8), 20 per cent in Israel (7.0 to 5.6), and 24 per cent in New Zealand (7.0 to 5.3). In contrast, marriage rates in Japan have actually increased from 5.8 in 1990 to 6.3 in 1998 (United Nations 1997).

As in the United States, a major cause of these dropping marriage rates is the decision by young adults increasingly to delay their first marriage. As of 1996, two-thirds of European 20- to 24-year-olds, and one-third of 25- to 29-year-olds, have not left the parental home; rates are higher in the southern European countries, approaching 50 per cent of 25- to 29-year-olds in Spain, Italy, Greece, and Portugal, and are much lower in the northern countries at 17 per cent in the United Kingdom, 14 per cent in The Netherlands, and 8 per cent in Finland (Eurostat 1998). As a consequence, the average age of marriage in the European Union has dropped significantly from an average of 26 and 23 for men and women respectively in 1980, to 29 and 26 in 1995 (Eurostat 1998). Similarly, the age of marriage in Canada has also increased between 1970 and 1990 from 23 and 25 for women and men respectively, to 26 and 28 respectively (Vanier Institute of the Family 1994).

As in the United States, the European Union has seen an increasing trend towards same-sex partnerships, although there are substantial variations across Western European countries with the trends most stark in Denmark and The Netherlands where same-sex unions have become semi-institutionalized (Dumon 1997).

Increase in cohabitation

As Dumon (1997) points out, since the revolutionary period of the 1960s marriage has lost its role as a line of transition from parental home to the 'family of procreation'. Today, young adults are increasingly more likely to stay single (either living in their parental home or independently), or to enter into a cohabiting relationship (especially among more educated individuals with a higher socio-economic status). For example, cohabitation has become so prevalent in Scandinavian countries that the distinction between legitimate and illegitimate children has become meaningless, and with rates of non-marital childbearing in the range of 30 per cent in France and the United Kingdom, similar patterns may arise there as well (Dumon 1997).

The United States

In addition to the delay in first marriages, the decline in marriage in the United States is, at least in part, due to the growth in unmarried cohabitation which is increasingly replacing marriage as a significant early life experience for young adults. It is now estimated that about half of unmarried women aged 25 to 39 have lived at some time with an unmarried partner, and about half of the unmarried partners aged 25 to 34 living together have children in the household (Bumpass and Sweet 1989; Bumpass and Lu 1998; Manning and Lichter 1996). According to Waite (1999), many cohabiting adults behave more like room-mates, sharing a residence and expenses but maintaining separate social and economic pursuits. In fact, research has shown that individuals who cohabit prior to marriage have higher levels of divorce after marriage—women who cohabit with their spouses prior to marriage have divorce rates 80 per cent higher than women who do not (Bennett 1987).

Worldwide

As in the United States, cohabitation has increased throughout the European Union and now accounts for 8 per cent of all couples. As noted above, in Scandinavian countries cohabitation has become essentially a 'marriage substitute'. In most other European countries, where it exists, it is largely a temporary arrangement preceding marriage, especially for young adults (15 to 35 years) and divorced persons.

The highest rates of cohabitation are found in northern Europe, where rates range from highs of 25 per cent in Denmark, 14 per cent in France, 13 per cent in The Netherlands, and 11 per cent in the United Kingdom, to lows in the southern European countries of 2 per cent in Italy and Greece, and 3 per cent in Spain, Ireland, and Portugal. However, in all countries rates are highest for individuals under age 30. In Denmark, for example, 70 per cent of young couples are unmarried (Eurostat 1998). In Sweden cohabitation accounts for 75 per cent of all unions among people aged 20 to 24 years and 46 per cent of those aged 25 to 29 years, but drops to about 10 per cent among 45- to 49-year-olds (Golini and Silvestrini 1997).

In Canada, cohabitation has accounted for the greatest change in family structures: in the 5-year period from 1986 to 1991 the proportion increased from 7 to 10 per cent of all Canadian families (Vanier Institute of the Family 1994).

Increase in the divorce rate

Not only have marriages been delayed in the United States and most other industrialized countries, but also the rate of marriage dissolution has increased through divorce, a marked change from death as the previously more typical cause of the end of a marriage partnership. In part, this change has come about as a result of government policy changes that have increasingly allowed 'no fault' divorce.

One of the important consequences of rising marriage dissolution is the creation of newly organized families for which terms such as 'merged', 'blended', 'reconstituted', or 'serial' have been created, with adults and children from multiple marriages joining together to create new family units. Take, for example, the following pattern described by Golini and Silvestrini (1997): an individual is born into a family composed of a mother and a father (a 'traditional' nuclear family); following a divorce, the child lives with his or her mother alone (single-parent family) until she remarries to join a stepfamily, possibly consisting of stepbrothers and stepsisters (who may themselves be from prior marriages); when independent, he or she may live alone (a single-person household), then marry and have children (create own family), divorce and remarry (create own stepfamily), and end life as a widow or widower living alone (a single-person household). The variety of family formations—and the life experiences that are becoming more common—have created a changing system of family relationships that is likely to have profound effects as we move into the twenty-first century.

The United States

In 1920, there were 1.6 divorces per 1000 population in the United States, and this rose moderately to about 2.5 in the late 1960s. The rate of divorce then began to climb dramatically, along with changing divorce laws, peaking at 5.3 in the early 1980s, and since declining to 4.3 in 1997, but still at historically high levels (US Bureau of the Census 1998*b*). According to Popenoe and Whitehead (1999), these recent trends in the United States may be only temporary, owing to the aging of the American population, a decrease in the number of people of marriageable age, and some increase in marital stability.

As Garrett (1997) points out, although divorce rates have risen in the United States (and in many other industrialized countries), the rate of remarriage has gone up at almost the same rate, indicating a desire to get out of existing marriages but not to give up on the institution altogether. In particular, individuals who marry young and then divorce are more likely to remarry, thereby creating the newly emerging family forms noted above. Yet, there has still been an increase in the percentage of all United States adults who are currently divorced, from about 2 per cent and 3 per cent for males and females respectively in 1960, to about 8 per cent and 10 per cent respectively in 1998 (US Bureau of the Census 1998*b*). Overall, about 50 per cent of United States marriages are estimated to end in divorce (Popenoe and Whitehead 1999).

One of the important consequences of divorce in the United States (and elsewhere) is the increased poverty rate among women—American men who divorce experience an average 42 per cent *increase* in their standard of living, while separated women experience a 73 per cent *decline* after divorce (Garrett 1997). As a consequence, many previously married women are forced into the welfare system following divorce. In fact, a study by Antolin *et al.* (1999) in the United States, the United Kingdom, Canada, and Germany shows that divorce and separation are the main reasons for entry into poverty, and the length of stay in poverty, especially for female-headed households.

This fall into poverty following divorce has the greatest negative impact on the well being of any children created during the adult union. To begin with, conflict between mothers and fathers can affect the social and emotional well being of children, and this conflict often continues beyond the divorce separation (Peterson and Zill 1986). Children also experience strong reactions to the loss of contact with one parent through divorce (Wallerstein and Kelly 1980), and are affected by the change in parenting practices that also accompanies the family dissolution (Zill *et al.* 1993). Compared with children in two-parent families, children whose parents have divorced are more likely to drop out of school, to engage in premarital sex, and to become pregnant outside of marriage (Furstenberg and Teitler 1994). Moreover, there is evidence to suggest that remarriage does not necessarily lead to improved conditions for children (Zill and Rogers 1988; Whitehead 1993).

Worldwide

According to the United Nations Children's Fund (UNICEF 1997), '... 30–50 per cent of first marriages in developed countries, and 25 per cent of first marriages in developing countries are dissolved by the time women are 40–49 years old, many as a result of divorce or separation'. In general, divorce (and cohabitation) are more associated withthe middle- and upper-income classes than with the poor. But, as in the United States, in many countries the break-up of partnering relationships worsens the economic conditions of women and children as male financial support ends or dwindles away over time.

In Western Europe, the rate of divorce doubled from 1970 to 1997, but at an average of 1.8 divorces per 1000 population it is still well below the rates seen in the United States (Eurostat 1998). Average divorce rates are highest in the United Kingdom at 2.9 per 1000, Belgium at 2.6 (due to recently liberalized divorce laws), Finland (2.6), and Sweden (2.4). At present, more than half of all marriages in Belgium, and over 40 per cent of marriages in the United Kingdom and the three Scandinavian countries, end in divorce (Eurostat 1998). Alternatively, divorce rates are lowest in the southern European countries, especially Italy with the lowest rate in Western Europe at 0.6 per 1000 population, even though divorce was legalized in 1970 (Eurostat 1998). Divorce rates in Canada (2.6 per 1000), Japan (1.7), and the Czech Republic are comparable to those currently observed in Western Europe (Eurostat 1998). Finally, this trend is not confined to Western countries. Even China, with its long tradition of a strong family unit, has seen a dramatic increase in the divorce rate, coinciding with a rapidly growing economy and greater opportunities for women.

It should be noted, however, that making cross-national comparisons of divorce rates is very difficult. As Goode (1993) points out, there are the obvious data problems including a failure to collect data on divorces, and differences in the extent to which formal marriages are entered into. There are also strict religious rules that in many countries govern the ability to gain a divorce. For example, although many Catholic countries in Europe and Latin America have reduced prohibitions, prior laws did not necessarily prevent couples from seeking informal ways to dissolve their union. Finally, low rates of divorce do not necessarily indicate a more stable institution of marriage as '... we have no reason to believe that when rates are high, more people are unhappy with their family life. Nor do we believe that people in low-rate systems do not have divorce because they are content in marriage' (Goode 1993, p. 39).

Rise in non-marital childbearing

As noted above, marriage in many industrialized countries has declined as an early life experience for many young adults. As a consequence, marriage has lost its role as the primary entry point for sexual activity, and has increasingly been replaced by cohabitation between men and women as a vehicle for adult fulfilment. A recent Gallup International poll conducted in 16 countries (Saad 1997) explored opinions regarding whether non-marital childbearing is considered morally wrong. Overall, adults in Western Europe (particularly Germany, the United Kingdom, and Spain) are most liberal, whereas the most conservative opinions are found in Asia (Thailand, Taiwan, Singapore, and India), with the United States, France, and Canada in the middle. For example, the majority of adults in India (84 per cent), Singapore (69 per cent), and Taiwan (55 per cent) believe out-of-wedlock births are wrong. This contrasts with European adults: 20 to 25 per cent held a similar opinion in the United Kingdom and Spain, 16 per cent in Hungary and Lithuania, and less than 10 per cent in Germany, France, and Iceland. The United States is the most conflicted on this subject, with slightly less than half of all adults saying that births out of wedlock are morally wrong.

The United States

In 1940, only 3.5 per cent of all births in the United States were to unmarried women, and this statistic increased slightly to 5.3 per cent in 1960. Since then, the United States has seen a nearly sevenfold increase in the incidence of out-of-wedlock births to about 33 per cent in 1997 (US Department of Health and Human Services 1999). Although three-quarters of births to teenagers (aged 15 to 19) were to unmarried women, most of the non-marital births in the United States (about two-thirds) are to women over the age of 20 (US Department of Health and Human Services 1999).

Overall, nearly half of all pregnancies in the United States are estimated to be unintended (National Center for Health Statistics 1999*a*,*b*). Although this represents a decline of 12 per cent between

1988 and 1995, it is still much higher than in other developed countries. Canada's rate, for example, is 39 per cent, while it is only 6 per cent in The Netherlands (National Center for Health Statistics 1999*a*,*b*). Recent reports examining non-marital childbearing in the United States indicate that nearly 40 per cent of such pregnancies occur to cohabiting adults (Bumpass and Lu 1998). The evidence also suggests that some of the increase in non-marital births resulted from the higher probability that pregnancies would come to term rather than ending in abortion, i.e. less availability or lower social acceptance of abortion and higher social acceptance of illegitimacy (Moore *et al.* 1995*a*,*b*).

There are also important differences in non-marital childbearing by race and ethnicity in the United States, with the percentage of out-of-wedlock births at 16.3 per cent for Asian women, 25.3 per cent for white women, 40.8 per cent for Hispanics, 57.2 per cent for Native Americans, and a staggering 69.9 per cent for African-American women (US Department of Health and Human Services 1999). In fact, at least 80 per cent of all African-American children in the United States can expect to spend a significant part of their childhood apart from their fathers. In 1960, 78 per cent of African-American babies were born to married mothers, dropping to 58 per cent by 1970, and to 35 per cent by 1997; the rate for white women, by comparison, decreased from 90 per cent in 1960 to about 75 per cent in 1997 (Morehouse Research Institute 1999).

Children born to unmarried women are much more likely to grow up poor, to spend large portions of their lives without two parents, and to become single parents themselves (McLanahan and Sandefur 1994; Ventura 1995). Many have suggested that the rise in non-marital childbearing has led to a 'fatherlessness crisis' in America (Pearlstein 1997), with nearly 40 per cent of all American children residing in homes without their biological father (Blankenhorn 1995). Moreover, about 40 per cent of these fatherless children have not seen their father for at least a year, and only one in six see their father an average of once or more per week (Furstenberg and Nord 1985).

The consequences of living in the United States without the presence of a father are stark. American babies born out of wedlock are four to five times more likely to have received no prenatal care, almost half of unwed mothers go on public assistance within 1 year of the baby's birth, 70 per cent of incarcerated juveniles grew up in single- or no-parent families, three out of four teenage suicides occur in single-parent homes, and the infant mortality rate is higher for babies born out of wedlock (Horn 1995).

Worldwide

In line with increasing numbers of cohabiting adults in many European countries, there has been an associated increase in the proportion of out-of-wedlock births from an average of 10 per cent of all live births in 1980 to 22 per cent in 1998 (Eurostat 1999). However, the incidence of non-marital childbearing is quite variable among the different Western European countries, with the highest rates of illegitimacy, in excess of those in the United States, found in Scandinavian countries—54 per cent in Sweden, 46 per cent in Denmark, and 36.5 per cent in Finland—but rates are also high and comparable to the American experience in France (39 per cent) and the United Kingdom (36.7 per cent) (Eurostat 1998). Alternatively, the lowest rates of out-of-wedlock births are found in the southern European countries of Greece (3.3 per cent) and Italy (8.3 per cent) (Eurostat 1998).

Although the incidence of out-of-wedlock births varies among the European Union countries, the trend has moved in the same direction across Western Europe to the point that the population replacement level in many countries now depends on non-marital births (Dumon 1997). For example, the low fertility rate in Italy has been blamed on the low incidence of cohabitation and illegitimate births. Ireland provides another interesting example, as a strongly Catholic country in which abortion and divorce remain illegal. Not unexpectedly, Ireland has a relatively low level of unmarried couples but a surprisingly high proportion of births outside of wedlock (23 per cent) (Eurostat 1998). as a result of a high level of adult emigration to find employment and a relatively high fertility rate, Ireland now has 44 per cent of its population under the age of 25 (Quick 1995).

Elsewhere in the world, the rate of non-marital births in Canada (28 per cent) is comparable to that of many other industrial countries, but out-of-wedlock births are essentially non-existent in Japan, accounting for only about 1 per cent of all live births.

Growth in female-headed households

The combined trends of increased non-marital childbearing, divorce, and the dissolution of cohabiting relationships between parents (particularly common in Europe) have created a current situation in most developed countries in which ever smaller percentages of children will reach the age of 18 with both parents remaining in the household. According to Morris (1993), the bonds between unmarried women and their sexual partners are generally weak, and marriages resulting from unplanned pregnancies tend to be very unstable. Moreover, when teenagers have babies out of wedlock they do not receive the support or services they need during pregnancy, therefore negatively affecting their health and that of their baby. Father absence is also associated with higher rates of poor father–child relationships, increased teenage suicide, substance abuse, and early pregnancy.

The United States

In the past, single mothers were likely to be widowed or divorced, and the situation for those who bore children out of wedlock was often temporary. Today, single mothers are far more likely to have never married and are much more likely to remain single, making single motherhood a more permanent life situation.

In 1960 only about 9 per cent of all American children lived in single-parent families, a statistic that remained relatively stable for most of the twentieth century; by 1998, this had more than tripled to 28 per cent (US Bureau of the Census 1998*b*). Although the number of father-only families has grown, close to 90 per cent of these single-parent families are headed by women. At the start of the twenty-first century, nearly one out of four American children are living with their mother only (US Department of Health and Human Services 1999).

However, there are significant differences in the incidence of female-headed households in the United States by race and ethnicity. From 1970 to 1997 the percentage of white children living with both parents dropped from 90 to 75 per cent, for Hispanic children the decline was from 78 to 64 per cent, but for African-American children the percentage declined from 58 to 35 per cent (US Department of Health and Human Services 1999). Today, what some have called a crisis in American black families has led to a situation in which almost two-thirds of all African-American children are living in female-headed households.

We cannot say that a child in a two-parent family is necessarily doing better than a child in a single-parent family. In fact, the majority of United States children from single-parent families do well. But we do have considerable evidence that single-parent families are far more likely than two-parent families to be poor. United States children under the age of 18 living with only their mother are four times more likely to have a total family income of under $10 000 than children living with both parents, and about half of all children in female-headed households live below the United States defined poverty line (US Bureau of the Census 1998*a*). There is also accumulating evidence to indicate that children from single-parent families are less likely to experience healthy development than children from intact families—they are somewhat more likely to use alcohol and drugs, to become teenage parents themselves, to do poorly in school and/or fail to complete their education, and to have difficulty finding employment (McLanahan and Sandefur 1994; US Department of Health and Human Services 1999).

Divorce and non-marital childbearing can also affect a woman's earning capacity, and this is often exacerbated by the failure of many non-custodial parents to pay adequate child support. Fathers who live apart from their children also spend less time with their children (Wallerstein and Kelly 1980), and the added stress on mothers can negatively affect their parenting ability (McLeod and Shanahan 1993; McLoyd and Wilson 1993). Having another cohabiting adult enter the household can add further stress to children's lives. The lower incomes associated with single-parent families also keep them in poorer communities, with the concomitant risks of crime and violence, drug abuse, inadequate housing, and a deficiency of high-quality schools and other public services (Sandefur and Mosley 1997). They also experience high levels of mobility, which reduces community attachments and has been found to have a negative effect on a child's school performance (McLanahan and Sandefur 1994).

Worldwide

In general, the European Union countries have also seen a rise in single-parent families, due in part to increased rates of divorce and non-marital births, and lower rates of remarriage. Although the 'nuclear family' still predominates in the European Union, there is an increasing proportion of single-parent families and childless couples. In 1994, 9 per cent of children under the age of 16 were living in single-parent households, but rates were considerably higher in the United Kingdom (16 per cent), Sweden and Denmark (each at 14 per cent), and Ireland (12 per cent) (Eurostat 1998). This trend has been far less pronounced in the southern European countries of Italy, Spain, and Portugal, where marriage remains strongly institutionalized. Rates comparable to northern Europe are also found in Canada, where 14 per cent of children live with a single parent, most often the mother (Vanier Institute of the Family 1994).

Recent research examining poverty in the United States, the United Kingdom, Canada, and Germany clearly shows that single-parent, especially female-headed, households are consistently over-represented in poverty (Antolin *et al.* 1999). Whether the cause be non-marital childbearing, the dissolution of a cohabiting relationship in which children were present, or divorce, it is generally the case that women fare very poorly after a break-up and this has severe consequences for their health and well being and that of their children.

In other parts of the world, there have also been dramatic increases in the proportion of female-headed households. In the developing world in particular, war, disease, and political unrest have driven families apart, and a lack of economic opportunities have led many men to migrate away from their homes and in many instances to abandon their families. These conditions are especially severe in Latin America and Africa where women are increasingly forced to face higher economic burdens with limited economic opportunities.

More women in the labour force

Research by Micklewright and Stewart (1999) demonstrates that adult family member connectedness to the labour market determines in large part the overall well being of children. In addition, a lack of adult employment also causes tensions within the family, and may limit a child's aspirations and contacts.

The United States

Over the last 30 years, the proportion of women in the labour force has increased substantially, paralleling the increase in single-parent households. In particular, the employment rates for mothers with children under the age of 18 years rose from 53 per cent in 1980 to 66 per cent in 1996 (US Department of Health and Human Services 1999). As a result, there has been a substantial increase in the percentage of children who do not have a full-time parent at home; in 1997, 68 per cent of children had both parents, or their only resident parent, in the labour force, up from 59 per cent in 1985 (US Department of Health and Human Services 1999). The sharpest rise for women in the labour force has been for single-mother families with children under the age of 6 years, increasing from 49 per cent in 1980 to 65 per cent in 1997 (US Department of Health and Human Services 1999).

Americans have traditionally believed that at least one parent (usually the father) should work in a two-parent family because the added benefits almost always outweigh the benefits of having two parents at home. For low-income families in particular, a mother's income has provided an opportunity to raise a family's earnings out of poverty (Danziger and Gottschalk 1990; Bane and Ellwood 1994; McLanahan and Sandefur 1994). But American society has become increasingly ambivalent about whether the second parent—or the only resident parent—should work. However, as noted above, the reality is that most United States mothers are employed outside the home.

The research literature is inconclusive about the effect of parental employment on children's well being (Smith *et al.* 1997). When parents work their income almost always increases (the 'income effect'), but they also have less time to devote to their families, especially their children (the 'time effect' of work). In fact, Americans now surpass every other industrialized nation in terms of time spent on the job, and more and more children are expressing concerns about the quality of time that parents are able to devote to them (Grimsley and Salmon 1999).

Families in which mothers work have higher incomes, on average, than similar families in which mothers do not work outside the home. Higher incomes are important because poor children consistently fare worse on almost every outcome that social scientists have studied (Haveman *et al.* 1991; Brooks-Gunn and Duncan 1998). Gaining employment has also been found to be the main factor reducing the time spent in poverty in the United States and other industrialized countries, and households with multiple wage earners are better protected from poverty as they are better able to adjust their labour supply in response to job loss or reduction by one member (Antolin *et al.* 1999). Some have argued that the economic benefits of such work are often exaggerated, particularly when lost 'home production' is taken into account (P. Gottschalk and S.E. Mayer, unpublished work, University of Chicago, 1994). Furthermore, the added income may not benefit children as much as adults (Lazear and Michael 1988). However, others argue that employment makes parents better role models for their children.

The time effect of parental employment is difficult to measure as it depends on the quality of care provided by parents compared with that provided by others when parents are working. If the care is better, or if it provides new and different learning experiences, the child may benefit. This is why, in part, there has been greatly expanded demand for safe, affordable, and accessible child care arrangements in the United States. One in five part-time workers in the United States would, in fact, work more if reasonable child care were available to them, and one-third of poor women not working identified child care as a barrier to their workforce participation (Child Welfare League of America 1995).

However, increased workforce participation by parents has forced many children to negotiate the transition from home to school at a younger age, especially poor children. For most children, their initial exposure to schools used to occur when they entered kindergarten at age 5, or first grade a year later. Today the situation is quite different. In 1995, 60 per cent of children in the United States under the age of 6 years who were not in kindergarten received some form of care from adults other than their parents (Emig 1999). The incidence was nearly 90 per cent for women who worked full-time and 75 per cent for those employed part-time (Emig 1999).

Worldwide

There has been a similarly sharp worldwide increase in women's formal and informal employment as women are increasingly assuming jobs traditionally held by men, but often at lower wages. In the West the cost of children has increased substantially, placing greater demands on families and expanding the need for two wage earners. In developing countries, families have had to assume a greater share of their children's education in response to policy adjustments in poor debt-ridden countries. Working adults are also increasingly having to support elderly parents and extended family members as lifespans have increased due to improved health and sanitary conditions. Traditional family support networks have also become less stable as family sizes decline. The pandemic of AIDS, especially in sub-Saharan Africa, has led to situations where there are fewer adults able to provide care for children and the elderly.

Similar to the United States, women in European Union countries have moved in large numbers into the labour force, in parallel with declines in fertility rates, increases in educational opportunities for women, and changes in attitudes about the need for two wage earners. As of 1996, almost two-thirds of women between the ages of 25 and 59 in the European Union worked at least part-time (Eurostat 1998). Even though slightly lower, rates for women with children are also high. For example, for women aged 20 to 45 with one child, the rates of employment are near or over 80 per cent in France, Austria, Portugal, and Finland, and over 70 per cent in Denmark and the United Kingdom (Eurostat 1998). As in the United States, these changes have created the 'dual career family', which imposes a strong need for women to reconcile their work and family lives, including available and affordable child care, and 'family friendly' work arrangements. In contrast, The Netherlands has maintained the strength of the 'traditional family' model, despite high labour force participation by women, because nearly two-thirds of employed women are in part-time jobs (Rothenbacher 1998*b*).

Similar patterns of increasing employment by women, especially mothers, are also found elsewhere in the world. Between 1980 and 1995, female labour force participation for women age 15 to 64 has increased in Australia (from 52 to 65 per cent), Iceland (from 56 to 82 per cent), Japan (from 55 to 62 per cent), and New Zealand (from 45 to 66 per cent) (United States Bureau of the Census 1998*a*). Current rates are also high in the Czech Republic (65 per cent), Poland (61 per cent), South Korea (53 per cent), and Mexico (40 per cent) (United States Bureau of the Census 1998*a*). Even China, the fastest growing economy in the world over the last 20 years, has seen a dramatic rise in women's earnings from 20 per cent of average family incomes in 1950 to about 40 per cent today.

Changes in family functions

As noted at the start of this chapter, families at one time (and still in many parts of the world) performed a variety of functions that met most, if not all, of the needs of individual family members. Today, many of these same functions are met outside the family. For example, the workplace is now separate from one's place of residence, schools provide for the education of children, and economic assistance comes from banks or government rather than from other family members. Some have seen this transfer of functions as a decline in the viability and importance of the family; for others, this is really just allowing family members to focus more on what they can do best, such as nurturing and socializing the young, and supporting the development of adults (Garrett 1997).

As Dumon (1997) suggests, one of the important changes brought about by the entrance of women into the labour force is the changing functional roles of men and women, and the need to balance the often competing demands of work and family. Although women still bear the primary burden of domestic responsibilities, fathers and husbands are increasingly assuming housework chores and responsibility for child-rearing. In line with these changes, the 1994 United Nations International Conference on Population and Development in Cairo called for the promotion of gender equity, especially within the family where it can have an important effect on the well being of children.

As noted in a recent UNICEF publication, 'Traditional households with the father as provider and the mother as nurturer and caregiver are increasingly giving way to less conventional relationships and roles within the family. However, many families are not coping well with these changes, and the conditions of women and children have worsened' (UNICEF 1997). In many countries women have assumed a greater share of providing for the economic resources of the family without an associated decline in their domestic and child-bearing responsibilities. Evidence does indicate that when women are forced to balance these demands, child-caring tends to be the first obligation to be sacrificed.

Changing women's roles have also marginalized men and some have responded with higher levels of domestic violence. For example, the United States has seen increases in the number of children receiving child protective services. Between 1990 and 1996 the national rate of children who were subjects of reports of abuse or neglect increased from 41 to 44 children per 1000 (US Department of Health and Human Services 1998). Moreover, these numbers do not reflect reports of abuse and neglect screened out prior to investigation, a number that appears to be increasing (Petit and Curtis 1997). In 1996, child protective services agencies determined that almost 1 million children were identified as victims of substantiated or indicated abuse or neglect, an increase of approximately 18 per cent since 1990 (US Department of Health and Human Services 1998).

Similarly, the number of United States children entering foster care, and the total foster-care caseload, has continued to increase (American Public Welfare Association 1996). In 1998, 4 per cent of all United States children under the age of 18 lived in households in which there was no biological parent present, and the rate for African-American children is more than twice as high (US Bureau of the Census 1998). Many of these children live with relatives, with about two-thirds being cared for by grandparents, usually a grandmother. Compared with children being raised by their parents, children in such 'kinship care' are more disadvantaged on several measures: they are more likely to be cared for by a single woman, to have a caretaker who is over 50 years old, and to have a caretaker who is a high-school dropout. They are also substantially more likely to be poor and to be in families receiving government assistance.

Homelessness has also become an increasingly common aspect of life in many industrialized countries. It is estimated, for example, that 3 million people in the 15 countries that comprise the European Union lack a permanent home, while about three-quarters of a million are homeless in the United States (UNICEF 1999). Because women with children comprise the greater proportion of the poor in many industrialized countries, children are often most adversely affected by homelessness. For example, it is estimated that almost 250 000 young people between 16 and 24 became homeless in a single year in the United Kingdom (UNICEF 1999).

Health and social policy affecting families

The social and demographic trends described up to this point have been affected in various ways by government policies and programmes—in some cases, by the absence of government action. Government intervention in the family has a long history in human evolution, dating back to the first formal code of laws established by Hammurabi in the eighteenth century BC in Mesopotamia, which included rules governing the structure and maintenance of families and the institution of marriage. Today, government policies related to child support, cash assistance, and other efforts to help families can be the difference between poverty and self-sufficiency for many families (McLanahan and Garfinkel 1995).

The United States

Family support programmes in the United States date back to the creation of the Children's Bureau in 1912, but are most importantly tied to the post-Depression era with the passage of the landmark 1935 Social Security Act which, among other things, created the first national programme to provide Aid to Families with Dependent Children. Since then, a number of important legislative actions have been taken, particularly during the 1960s and 1970s, including the creation of Medicare (health care for the elderly), Medicaid (health care for the poor), Head Start (a preschool child-development programme for poor children), Food Stamps (nutrition assistance for low income families), and the creation of federal support for the education of disadvantaged children. However, as many have noted, there is no coherent 'family policy' in the United States as there is great division over the degree to which government should 'interfere' in personal family lives and decisions. For example, the United States is one of the very few industrialized nations that does not guarantee basic maternity and child health care for everyone.

Surprisingly, no comprehensive estimates of United States federal expenditures on children had been made until a recent effort by R.L. Clark and C.E. Steuerle (unpublished work, Urban Institute, 1999) which analysed trends in 66 separate federal programmes over a period of nearly 40 years. Their results show that United States federal expenditures on children increased by 251 per cent over this period, from $48.6 billion to $171 billion in 1997. However, this rate of increase lagged slightly behind the growth in the overall federal budget (which increased by 261 per cent), and closely matched the growth in the overall United States economy—as a percentage of gross domestic product, federal expenditures on children increased from 2 per cent in the late 1950s to 2.2 per cent in 1997. On a per capita basis, federal expenditures on children rose from $725 per individual aged 0 to 18 years to about $2300 in 1997. At the same time, the poverty rate for children increased from 17.6 per cent to almost 20 per cent.

Clark and Steuerle also examined federal expenditures by type of programme: tax credits and exemptions (the Earned Income Tax Credit, the dependent exemption, and exemptions for child care), income security (including the main welfare programme, Aid to Families with Dependent Children, Supplemental Security Income, and children's survivor benefits), education, nutrition assistance (including the Food Stamp Program, and the Special Supplemental Food Program for Women, Infants, and Children, and child nutrition programmes), health (including Medicaid), housing assistance programmes, social services (including Head Start, foster care assistance, and child care subsidies), and training programmes (including job training and summer youth employment). Their findings indicate that tax mechanisms, as a way of assisting children, declined in importance over the period studied, as did the relative share of federal expenditures for children through income security and education programmes. Alternatively, greater importance has been placed on nutrition and health assistance, and social services, primarily Head Start (a preschool education programme for low-income children), foster care, and child care subsidies.

In effect, two trends have characterized the United States federal role in assisting children since 1960: (a) a shift from efforts to help all children (especially children of parents with enough income to owe income taxes) to assistance targeted at poor children (and their families); (b) a shift from programmes that leave decisions about spending on children in the hands of parents (e.g. tax credits and exemptions, and cash assistance) to programmes that deliver 'in-kind' benefits (e.g. food stamps to purchase food, housing assistance, subsidized housing, and Medicaid health insurance). Choosing among these different approaches was the focus of much of the United States political debate during the last half of the twentieth century and is unlikely to go away in the near future. As Clark and Steuerle point out, broader efforts to help children, and those programmes that place discretion in the hands of parents, are favoured by proponents for their efficiency, but opponents point to the opportunity to purchase 'undesirable' goods and services that may not benefit children. On the other hand, more targeted programmes can place more money in the hands of poor families per dollar spent, but can have negative effects, particularly disincentives to work or marry because benefits are lost when income rises. With this as a backdrop, the following discussion examines current United States policies as they affect families, using the same trends as discussed above.

Childbearing

It has been estimated that over three-quarters of all unmarried teenage mothers begin receiving Aid to Families with Dependent Children within 5 years of the birth of their first child (Wertheimer and Moore 1998). As noted above, the United States has historically had one of the highest rates of teenage births among all industrialized countries, and the situation is especially serious for minority youth.

To deal with this problem, in 1996 the United States Congress, as part of the major overhaul of the American welfare programme, replaced the 60-year-old Aid to Families with Dependent Children programme with the new Personal Responsibility and Work Opportunity Reconciliation Act, which contained a number of provisions aimed at breaking the link between non-marital births and welfare, and reducing teenage childbearing. The legislation included restrictions on benefits to unwed teenage parents who do not live at home and do not attend school, bonuses to states with the highest decrease in out-of-wedlock childbearing (to be achieved without offsetting increases in abortion), an abstinence education programme that will invest $50 million in federal funds annually for 5 years, a requirement that states develop plans to reduce non-marital pregnancies with special emphasis on teenage pregnancies, establishment of national goals that 25 per cent of all United States communities have teenage pregnancy programmes in place, and a requirement that the Attorney General study the linkage between statutory rape and teenage pregnancy, and educate state and local criminal law enforcement officials on its prevention and prosecution.

Family formation

Many have called the Moynihan Report (Moynihan 1965) the most influential, and certainly most controversial, discussion of family breakdown in the United States. Its main conclusion was that the government's economic and social welfare policies were helping to destabilize families, especially African-American families. On the one hand, it has been argued that the loss of good entry-level jobs, particularly in the inner cities, has made many African-American men less marriageable, thereby helping to undermine the institution of marriage (Wilson 1987). On the other hand, it has been argued that Aid to Families with Dependent Children (the main welfare programme in the United States until the early 1990s) acted as an incentive for young women both to become pregnant and to remain apart from their child's father (Murray 1984; Gilder 1995).

The issue of social policy and the break-up of the American family surfaced in force in the early 1990s with a publication by Charles Murray (1993), which pointed to non-marital childbearing as the most devastating problem in America because, it was claimed, this was the root cause of most of the other social ills (e.g. crime, poverty, drug abuse, etc.). This argument coincided with Republican control of Congress and the rising power of political conservatives who subsequently pushed a social agenda based on 'family values' (Garrett 1997).

Although the research on the factors behind the rising incidence of non-marital childbearing is fairly sparse, changes in access to economic opportunity, the residential segregation of the poor in particular neighbourhoods, and shifts in values and norms are all implicated. One potential explanation that certainly drove the legislative intent of the 1996 welfare reform legislation that created the Personal Responsibility and Work Opportunity Reconciliation Act was that the availability of public assistance discourages marriage and encourages non-marital childbearing. However, a recent review of the literature by Moffitt (1998) concludes that '... the welfare system has some effect on marriage and childbearing, but the size of the effect is highly uncertain and unresolved.' Indeed Moffitt and others conclude that the size of the effect is probably small and that there is limited evidence that the long-term receipt of welfare in one generation increases non-marital childbearing in the next generation.

The Personal Responsibility and Work Opportunity Reconciliation Act contained numerous components aimed at decreasing non-marital childbearing and reducing the possible negative effect of welfare on family formation decisions. These include time-limited financial assistance (recipients can only receive benefits for a maximum of 5 years over their lifetime), allowing family caps (restricting welfare benefits for additional children), requiring that all able-bodied parents work or acquire training that will increase their employability, making it easier for states to serve married as well as unmarried parents, strengthening child support enforcement, and establishing $20 million bonuses for the five states showing the greatest decrease in births to unmarried women.

Working parents

As noted above, the movement of large numbers of women with children—especially very young children—into the labour force has significantly increased the demand for affordable, high-quality, and accessible child care (e.g. during the hours and days during which parents work, and close to either their home or place of employment). This has occurred even though overall birth rates have declined. Unlike many other industrial countries, however, the United States has failed to legislate comprehensive child care programmes, leaving a patchwork of federal, state, and local government and private-sector programmes (Bloom and Steen 1996).

The first forms of federal child care assistance in the United States date back to the Great Depression with the use of federal funds to establish child care centres and nursery schools (Bloom and Steen 1996). This effort expanded during the Second World War to accommodate the movement of large numbers of women into defence-related industries, but this programme was terminated in 1946 with the end of the war. Further assistance was provided in 1954 when Congress allowed parents to take a tax exemption on their annual income tax filings for certain types of child care expenses. This was replaced in 1976 with the Child and Dependent Care Tax Credit.

The first attempt to pass comprehensive legislation to assist working families with children (the Comprehensive Child Development Act in 1971) was subsequently vetoed by President Nixon. This action also stopped any further efforts until 1988, when growing concerns about the quality and availability of child care in the United States led to the introduction of more than 100 separate pieces of legislation dealing with child care (Bloom and Steen 1996). Although

Presidential resistance again led to the defeat of attempts at passing comprehensive legislation, in 1988 Congress passed the Family Support Act, which included an entitlement for child care assistance for families on welfare and families moving off welfare, and required states to match federal expenditures for this purpose. In 1990, federal involvement in child care assistance grew further with passage of the Child Care and Development Block Grant and At-Risk Grants to States which has several key provisions: expansion of the Earned Income Tax Credit (i.e. tax credits to the working poor), the provision of funds to states to improve the availability of child care (largely used to subsidize the cost of child care for poor families), funding to help states improve their licensing systems for child care provider, and increased funding for child care assistance including low-income families who do not qualify for the United States welfare system to help them avoid falling back into poverty.

Most recently, the primary focus of federal policy has been single mothers receiving public assistance as there has been increasing social acceptance of parental labour force participation. In particular, the 1996 Personal Responsibility and Work Opportunity Reconciliation Act, which represents the culmination of a decade-long trend altering 60 years of public assistance policy to low-income families, eliminated the Aid to Families with Dependent Children programme and replaced it with the Temporary Assistance to Needy Families block grant to the states. The most significant policy changes associated with this are the move towards a 'work first' approach to public assistance, and the removal of the entitlement status from federal cash aid (with limited exceptions, a family can receive federal cash assistance for a maximum of 60 months in a lifetime under Temporary Assistance to Needy Families). Recognizing that these changes would increase the demand for affordable child care among low-income parents, the Personal Responsibility and Work Opportunity Reconciliation Act also included increased funding for child care subsidies ($600 million in fiscal year 1997) and combined earlier subsidy programmes into a single block grant (the Child Care and Development Fund) to provide more flexibility to states in designing their child care assistance programmes.

In 1993, Congress provided further help to families with children with passage of the Family and Medical Leave Act, which requires most employers to provide up to 12 weeks of unpaid leave to employees at the birth of their child with the assurance that they will retain their job. This new law was a major step forward for the United States in creating a more family-friendly work environment, but still leaves it as one of only five countries that do not require paid maternity leave—the others are Australia, New Zealand, Lesotho, Swaziland, and Papua New Guinea (Emig 1999).

At the state level during the 1990s, support for child care also increased significantly due to a range of factors, including the federal matching requirements for funding, a growing interest in school readiness, and an increased understanding of child care as a necessary service to help low-income mothers into the labour force. As a result of this activity, this decade has closed with a child care subsidy system in every state, a broad range of funding and initiatives to improve the quality and supply of care, a significant expansion of state pre-kindergarten efforts, and an understanding of the importance of child care and early education by policy-makers and the public. As a result, there has been a significant increase in the use of more formal child care centres in the United States instead of the use of home care for children while their parents are at work. In 1991 nearly 25 per cent of mothers with children under the age of 5 years used a child care centre or a preschool as their primary care arrangement, compared with 13 per cent in 1977. In fact, a large majority of children in the United States now spend at least some portion of their childhood in the care of individuals other than their parents. Moreover, recent research has linked participation in formal child care and early education settings to school readiness, especially for children from families receiving welfare (Zaslow *et al.* 1998).

As a policy issue, the growing use of non-parental care has two important dimensions that will continue to frame political debate in the United States in the twenty-first century. First, child care is an essential support service for working parents, especially for single-parent and low-income families where the cost and availability of care can either support or undermine efforts to find or retain employment. The second dimension is the quality of the services that child care provides for children. Child care arrangements are the environments where many American preschool children now spend large portions of their day during critical developmental years, and the quality of this care plays a role in their social and cognitive development. This dimension of care is important regardless of work status since many parents in the United States now choose to have their child in some form of child care before they enter school even if one parent is at home. Among United States school-age children, there is also a growing interest in having before- and after-school programmes provide an environment where children can continue to learn (i.e. to expand the time spent in instruction), and where they are supervised at times of the day when the probability of their engaging in high-risk behaviours is highest.

Historically, federal and state efforts to address the two different dimensions of non-parental care have been characterized by separate policy processes. While this has been changing in recent years, policies dedicated to early childhood education (state pre-kindergarten and Head Start, for example) have often been developed with relatively little attention to child care policies and to the employment needs of the parents. Alternatively, child care policies have often been developed as an employment support service and focus much less on ensuring that children are provided with an environment which supports their social and cognitive development. These separate policy tracks present a number of challenges because they manifest the two different and sometimes competing policy priorities of child care. Furthermore, they create a distinction that does not exist when parents make decisions about child care, as parents look for child care programmes that allow them both to work and meet the needs of their children.

With regard to cost, child care is a major expense for most American families. In the autumn of 1993, for example, the average amount spent on child care for a preschool-age child was over $4000 (Casper 1995). While United States families above the poverty line spend an average of about 7 per cent of yearly earnings on child care, the financial burden is much greater for a low-income mother working at a minimum wage job who requires nearly 40 per cent of her income (Kisker and Ross 1997). While many low-income families find free sources of child care, significant numbers of low-income families do not have or do not want this option. The problem is particularly complicated for welfare mothers, because the skills of parents leaving welfare for work are low and their earnings are not expected to increase significantly over the long term (Burtless 1995, 1997). This problem has been recognized by federal and state governments in the United States, particularly since cost can create a major barrier to employment as well as a potential threat to the safety and well being of children when parents cannot afford decent quality care (Berger and Black 1992; US General Accounting Office 1994). As a consequence, there has been a significant expansion of public investment to reduce the child care cost faced by families, and in so doing to increase the range of child care settings parents can afford.

The quality of child care is another ongoing issue of concern, especially given evidence that it is inadequate in the United States (Adams 1990). A study of the quality of child care centres in four states, for example, found that only 14 per cent of the rooms provided good quality care (Helburn and Culkin 1995), and a study of the quality of family child care homes found similarly disturbing results (Galinsky *et al.* 1994). To address this concern, the federal government has started to require that states spend a portion of their funds on boosting quality. As a consequence, the last decade has seen a significant effort to improve the training and qualifications of child care providers, develop child care resource and referral networks, create salary-enhancement initiatives, provide targeted funds to improve quality and supply, and so forth. Moreover, policy-makers have continued to focus on the importance of such investment, as evidenced by the recent decision of Congress to earmark funds to improve the quality of care for infants and toddlers, as well as by the continued expansion of state efforts to improve quality (Blank and Adams 1997).

Head Start, started in 1965, serves the poorest American families by providing education, health, social services, and nutrition to over 800 000 children each year. Recent efforts have been made to significantly raise the quality of these programmes and these appear to be paying off. For example, a recent study of the health component of Head Start found that children who were enrolled in this preschool programme were more likely to have up-to-date immunizations, to have speech and language difficulties identified, and to have their dental problems identified and addressed (Keane *et al.* 1996).

The last area of policy concern, the supply of child care, has been a growing problem especially for certain types of child care, including care for some age groups (in particular, infant and toddler care, and school-age child care), children with disabilities, families who live in rural areas or high-density urban poverty areas, families who work non-traditional hours or have irregular schedules, and families with sick children (Siegel and Loman 1991; Clark and Long 1995; Fuller and Liang 1995; US General Accounting Office 1995). As a result, there has been growing interest in identifying effective ways to improve the supply of particular forms of child care. For example, federal government funding has allowed states to engage in a variety of supply-building initiatives, including targeted recruitment and training efforts, start-up grants or loans, other targeted loan programmes, efforts to finance construction and facility development, targeted grants or contracts, training initiatives to help welfare mothers become child care workers, public–private partnerships to increase the involvement of employers, and subsidy policies such as higher reimbursement rates for certain types of care.

Worldwide

The negative consequences of the family changes discussed in this chapter have been somewhat mitigated in most European countries because, unlike the United States, there has been a strong tradition of universal family-oriented policies and programmes rather than limited programmes targeted at low-income parents and/or children. Access to health care is nearly universal in most European Union countries, as is the provision of universal cash payments to families with children. Such family allowances date back to the nineteenth century in Europe, but generally grew after the Second World War thanks in large part to far less divisive attitudes about family assistance than those found in the United States. How different industrialized countries have dealt with families does, however, vary as we enter the twenty-first century.

The United Kingdom, Canada, Australia, and New Zealand have in recent years paralleled the United States as family policy today is more need based and less universal. This is not surprising, given their shared tradition of non-intervention in the personal life of individuals. Only the United Kingdom, like its European Union partners, continues to provide a universal child benefit, although the level of assistance is below that of the Scandinavian countries (Kamerman and Kahn 1998). All four nations provide family-related tax benefits, as does the United States (Kamerman and Kahn 1998).

Canada provides about 17 weeks of unpaid maternity leave, and 10 weeks of additional parental leave under the Unemployment Insurance Program (Kamerman and Kahn 1998). The United Kingdom's policies were relatively restrictive until forced to adopt the European Union standard of 14-week leave to all working women, with benefits at the level of sick pay (Kamerman and Kahn 1998). New Zealand provides 14 weeks of unpaid maternity leave and one year of unpaid parental leave (Kamerman and Kahn 1998). As noted above, in the United States a major political fight was required to adopt parental leave policies that are modest by European standards at 12 weeks of unpaid leave.

With regard to child care, the United Kingdom, like the United States, has emphasized the role of the marketplace in determining what types of services should be available, and has taken a view that government should not intrude in family decisions about the care of children (Fincher 1996). In the United Kingdom, for example, most children under the age of 3 years are cared for by a parent or a relative. Australia and Canada also lack a universal child care provision, with the political debate focusing on the potential negative effect of government regulation on the availability of child care choices (Fincher 1996). In Canada, for example, public nurseries were created during the Second World War, only to be terminated when the war ended. Later, a system was established which resembles that of the United States, with federal and state/provincial cost-sharing for the provision of subsidies to low-income families, and the regulation/licensing of providers delegated to the state/provincial governments (Fincher 1996).

Scandinavia presents a very different approach to government support to families. For example, Denmark, like all Scandinavian countries, provides health insurance for all workers, preventive health care services for children, and pre- and postnatal care for pregnant women. Maternity leave benefits are also well financed, providing for full salary coverage from 1 month prior to birth until 14 weeks afterwards (Soren 1990). All families with children under age 18 also receive a cash allowance, and this is extended to single parents and for out-of-wedlock children (Soren 1990). Child care is also subsidized.

Alternatively, Sweden's policies have been driven by a desire to encourage higher birth rates and women's participation in the labour force (Fincher 1996). By 1987, nearly half of all preschoolers were being cared for in the public child care system, though the cost and availability of care varied locally (Fincher 1996). Sweden has also developed a more comprehensive 'family' policy orientation that includes child care but which also provides for the most developed parental leave policy with a 90 per cent income-replacement rate, and policies to encourage equal parenting between men and women.

As was seen in the earlier discussion, the highest rates of illegitimacy are found in Sweden and Denmark, and it is argued by some that the very liberal approach to social benefits has encouraged this trend. These two countries cycle up to 50 per cent of their gross domestic product through the state. By comparison, Korea and Japan—with minimal welfare states—have two of the lowest rates of divorce and non-marital childbearing in the world.

Looking elsewhere in Western Europe, France has a national commitment to supporting families and allowances are provided to all families with at least two children under the age of 17 (or 20 if in school) without the limitation of a means test. There is also a young-child benefit paid for 5 months prior to birth through to 3 months after birth, and this is combined with a maternity benefit that provides 90 per cent of the mother's salary for 16 weeks (or 26 weeks for a third child or more) (Commaille 1990). Child care support is also provided and is among the highest in Europe, matching those found in Denmark and Sweden.

In part, this strong support of families is due to the unique position of France among European states. since its population actually declined during the post-War period when populations were growing throughout Europe. This led to a significant government focus on family-oriented policies during the last 40 years, leading to fertility rates that are now above the European Union average, and an above-average population growth rate (Rothenbacher 1998*a*). However, France also has a situation in which nearly 40 per cent of all births are conceived out of wedlock as part of non marital consensual partnerships.

In Spain, birth rates have been falling for the last 20 years and are now among the lowest in the world due, at least in part, to the dramatic changes in family law and policy that occurred in 1981—civil marriage became an option, responsibility for divorce shifted from the church to the state, abortion was legalized, and cohabiting and homosexual couples can now register their unions (Guerrero 1997). As a result, marriage has been increasingly delayed, there has been a dramatic drop in the birth rate, the divorce rate has risen, and female employment has increased (Guerrero 1997).

German family policy, like that of the United States, is primarily centred around the tax system with the leading government expenditures for families being the child tax allowances and other deductions (Bahle 1998). The next largest component of federal expenditures, accounting for 20 per cent of the total, is for family cash benefits, primarily the general child benefit (Bahle 1998). Direct services account for a relatively small share of all expenditures, especially child care subsidies which account for about 4 per cent of total expenditures (Bahle 1998).

Concluding remarks

The end of the twentieth century brought the globalization of markets and culture and, as shown in this chapter, surprisingly similar changes in the nature of the family unit. Although the magnitude of these trends differs across nations, largely in response to unique political and cultural factors, the common patterns may be signalling a fundamental social transformation. Birth rates are declining in response to changes in medical technology, the role of women in society, the costs (and benefits) of having children, and a variety of other social and lifestyle changes. Young adults are delaying marriage and pregnancy, often due to increased time spent on education and training, and once married the importance of having children has declined as has the desired family size. The dissolution of marriages has also become more common, as has cohabitation and non-marital childbearing, leading to an increasing variety of family forms and structures. Finally, women are increasingly playing important roles in the workforce and in society more generally, leading to significant changes in traditional gender roles and expectations. Such broad social changes are likely to have long-term social and economic consequences, especially for the more vulnerable members of society, particularly women and children.

Why have these changes occurred? Moralists point to negative changes in social norms and values, others to new economic competition associated with the postindustrial information age, and still others blame changes in public policies. In all likelihood there is no single cause. Moreover, it is not clear that these transformations are necessarily all bad, nor long term in their effect. Instead, it may be that we are seeing a 'temporary adjustment' to a new world order where information and knowledge, rather than physical prowess, determine economic well being. And the globalization of knowledge—spread at increasing speed and decreasing cost—may in fact improve the life chances for more people than may be harmed by these transitory adjustments.

As Skolnick (1997) points out, the great transformations that we are seeing are not that different from that which were observed during previous social upheavals. For example, during the change from a preindustrial agrarian society to the urban-centred industrial society in the late nineteenth century there was a breaking of the traditional tie between the place of work and family. With the advent of industrialization, fathers left home to go to work, thereby disrupting long-existing patterns of daily family life, as well as cultural and gender roles. In particular, the home was transformed from a place of work to a safe haven for mothers to raise children, and provide a place of domestic tranquillity for the working father. But the reality was that many individuals did not live in such ideal circumstances, especially the working class and ethnic minorities, in the United States and other Western nations. The 'traditional' notion of a breadwinner father and home-maker mother is actually an uncommon arrangement associated with the early stages of industrial development and primarily for middle-class families (Davis 1988). As industrialization grows, more and more women find employment in the service sector (offices, schools, hospitals, and stores) and this pattern is seen in different countries that are at different stages of industrialization (Davis 1988).

As a result, we are now seeing another evolution of marriage and family to what Skolnick (1997) calls the 'companionate style', where adult fulfilment is as important as childbearing. However, the importance of children may, in fact, be increasing as child mortality is now relatively uncommon in the industrialized world (compared with earlier periods). Parents today are far less inclined to have an 'extra' child as protection against the early loss of a child, and are more likely to use birth control as a way to plan families for the desirable (and affordable) number and spacing (e.g. not to have multiple costs of college at the same time) of children. Longer lifespans have also extended the potential length of marriages (and ironically increased the opportunity for divorce and separation), and the rising number of elderly has made the role of grandparents more prominent in the lives of children and young adults. At the time when marriage seems less desirable and more fragile, the importance of children and their involvement with 'family members' may actually be increasing.

These are profound changes and, as with the dawning of the information age, we do not know where these social transformations will lead. Nor is it clear whether these changes are, by themselves, good or bad. For example, lower birth rates and smaller families, and delayed marriage and childbearing, especially if tied to greater investments in human capital development, are not necessarily negative trends requiring some form of government policy intervention. Instead, the challenge for policy-makers is to find ways to harness these changes for good—for example, supporting the continuing growth in opportunity and equality for women—while at the same time providing sufficient protections for the well being of our most vulnerable populations: children, single mothers, working mothers, and the elderly. This may include a variety of programmes, including policies geared towards providing an economic 'safety net' as protection against poverty, supporting the provision of affordable and high-quality child care and health programmes, and supporting 'family friendly' work environments, especially for pregnant women and mothers with young children. Most important, governments need to be aware of the changes that are sweeping across society, and to be prepared to respond to the changing nature of the basic family unit. Families have endured throughout most of human history and, although they may look different in the future, are certain to maintain their role as the foundation of our daily lives.

References

Adams, G. C. (1990). *Who knows how safe? The status of state efforts to ensure quality child care.* Children's Defense Fund, Washington, DC.

American Public Welfare Association (1996). *Voluntary cooperative information system for child welfare.* American Public Welfare Association, Washington, DC.

Antolin, P., Dang, T., and Oxley, H. (1999). *Poverty dynamics in four OECD countries.* Organization for Economic Cooperation and Development, Paris.

Bahle, T. (1998). Family policy in Germany: towards a macro-sociological frame for analysis. *Eurodata Newsletter*, **7**, 21–8.

Bane, M.J. and Ellwood, D. (1994). *Welfare realities.* Harvard University Press, Cambridge, MA.

Bennett, N.G. (1987). Commitment and the modern union: assessing the link between non-marital cohabitation and subsequent marital stability. *National Bureau of Economic Research*, **26**, 3–20.

Berger, M.C. and Black, D.A. (1992). Child care subsidies, quality of care, and the labor supply of low-income, single mothers. *Review of Economics and Statistics*, **74**, 635–42.

Blank, H. and Adams, G. (1997). *State developments in child care and early education.* Children's Defense Fund, Washington, DC.

Blankenhorn, D. (1995). *Fatherless America: confronting our most urgent social problem.* Basic Books, New York.

Bloom, D.E. and Steen, T.P. (1996). Minding the baby in the United States. In *Who will mind the baby: geographies of child care and working mothers* (ed. K. England). Routledge, New York.

Brooks-Gunn, J. and Duncan, G.J. (1998). *Growing up poor: consequences for children and youth.* Russell Sage Foundation, New York.

Bumpass, L. and Lu, H.-H. (1998). *Trends in cohabitation and implications for children's family contexts.* University of Wisconsin, Madison, WI.

Bumpass, L. and Sweet, J. (1989) National estimates of cohabitation. *Demography*, **24**, 615–25.

Burtless, G. (1995). Employment prospects of welfare recipients.' In *The work alternative: welfare reform and the realities of the job market* (ed. D.S. Nightingale and R.H. Haveman), pp. 1–106. Urban Institute Press, Washington, DC.

Burtless, G. (1997). Welfare recipients' job skills and employment prospects. *Future of Children*, **7**, 39–51.

Casper, L. (1995). What does it cost to mind our pre-schoolers? *Current Population Reports*, P70–52. US Department of Commerce, Economics and Statistics Administration, Washington, DC.

Child Welfare League of America (1995). *Child day care fact sheet.* Child Welfare League of America, Washington, DC.

Clark, R. and Long, S. (1995). *Child care prices: a profile of six communities—final report.* Urban Institute, Washington, DC.

Commaille, J. (1990). Family policy and population policy. In *Family policy in EEC-countries. Luxembourg: Office for Official Publications of the European Communities* (ed. W. Dumon). Erlbaum, Mahwah, NJ.

Danziger, S. and Gottschalk, P. (1990). *How have families and children been faring?* University of Wisconsin, Madison, WI.

Davis, K. (1988). Wives and work: a theory of the sex role revolution and its consequences. In *Feminism, children, and the new families* (ed. S.M. Dornbusch and M.H. Strober). Guilford Press, New York.

Dumon, W. (1997). The situation of families in Western Europe: a sociological perspective. In *The family on the threshold of the 21st century: trends and implications* (ed. S. Dreman), pp. 181–99. Erlbaum, Mahwah, NJ.

Duncan, G. and Hoffman, S.D. (1990). Teenage welfare receipt and subsequent dependence among black adolescent mothers. *Family Planning Perspectives*, **22**, 16–20.

Emig, C. (1999). The changing American family. In *The forgotten half revisited: American youth and young families, 1988–2008* (ed. S. Halperin), pp. 41–57. American Youth Policy Forum, Washington, DC.

Eurostat (1998). *Social portrait of Europe.* Statistical Office of the European Commission, Luxembourg.

Eurostat (1999). *Social portrait of Europe.* Statistical Office of the European Commission, Luxembourg.

Federal Interagency Forum on Child and Family Statistics (1999). *America's children: key national indicators of well-being.* Federal Interagency Forum on Child and Family Statistics, Washington, DC.

Fincher, R. (1996). The state and child care: an international review from a geographical perspective. In *Who will mind the baby: geographies of child care and working mothers* (ed. K. England), pp. 143–68. Routledge, New York.

Fukuyama, F. (1999). *The great disruption: human nature and the reconstitution of social order.* Free Press, New York.

Fuller, B. and Liang, X. (1995). *Can poor families find child care? Persisting inequality nationwide and in Massachusetts.* Harvard University Press, Cambridge, MA.

Furstenberg, F.F. and Nord, C.W. (1985). Parenting apart patterns of child rearing after marital disruption. *Journal of Marriage and the Family*, **47**, 893–904.

Furstenberg, F.F. and Teitler, J.O. (1994). Reconsidering the effects of marital disruption: what happens to children of divorce in early adulthood? *Journal of Family Issues*, **15**, 173–90.

Furstenberg, F.F, Brooks-Gunn, J., and Morgan, S.P. (1987). *Adolescent mothers in later life.* Cambridge University Press.

Galinsky, E., Howes, C., Kunton, S., *et al.* (1994). *The study of children in family child care and relative care.* Families and Work Institute, New York.

Garrett, W.R. (1997). The 'decline-of-the-Western-family' thesis: a critique and appraisal. In *The family in global transition* (ed. G.L. Anderson). Professors for World Peace Academy, St. Paul, MN.

Gilder, G. (1995). End welfare reform as we know it. *American Spectator*, June, pp. 24–7.

Golini, A. and Silvestrini, A. (1997). Family change, fathers, and children in Western Europe: a demographic and psychosocial perspective. In *The family on the threshold of the 21st century: trends and implications* (ed. S. Dreman). Erlbaum, Mahwah, NJ.

Goode, W.J. (1993). *World changes in divorce patterns.* Yale University Press, New Haven, CT.

Grimsley, K.D. and Salmon, J.L. (1999). For working parents, mixed news at home. *Washington Post*, 27 September, pp. A1, A8.

Guerrero, T.J. (1997). Country profile: Spain. *Eurodata Newsletter*, **6**, 27–31.

Haveman, R., Wolfe, B., and Spaulding, J. (1991). Childhood events and circumstances influencing high school completion. *Demography*, **28**, 133–58.

Hayes, C.D. (ed.) (1987). *Risking the future: adolescent sexuality, pregnancy, and childbearing*, Vol. 1. National Academy Press, Washington, DC.

Helburn, S. and Culkin, M. (1995). *Cost, Quality, and Child Outcomes Study*. University of Colorado, Denver.

Hoffman, S.D. (1998). Teenage childbearing is not so bad after all ... or is it? A review of the literature. *Family Planning Perspectives*, **30**, 1–10.

Horn, W. (1995). *Father facts.* National Fatherhood Initiative, Lancaster, PA.

Janis, J. (1997). Families. In *Oxford textbook of public health* (3rd edn) (ed. R. Detels, W.W. Holland, J. McEwen, and G.S. Omenn), pp. 1339–53. Oxford University Press.

Kamerman, S.B. and Kahn A.J. (ed.) (1998). *Family change and family policies in Great Britain, Canada, New Zealand, and the United States.* Clarendon Press, Oxford.

Keane, M.J., O'Brien, R.W., Connell, D.C., and Close, N.C. (1996). *Descriptive study of the Head Start health component.* CDM Group, Washington, DC.

Kisker, E.E. and Ross, C.M. (1997). Arranging child care. *Future of Children*, **7**, 99–109.

Ku, L., Sonenstein, F., Lindberg, L., Bradner, C., Boggess, S., and Pleck, J. (1998). Understanding changes in sexual activity among young metropolitan men: 1979 to 1995. *Family Planning Perspectives*, **30**, 256–62.

Lazear, E. and Michael, R. (1988). *Allocation of income within the household.* University of Chicago Press.

McLanahan S.S. and Garfinkel, I. (1995). Single mother families and social policy lessons for the United States from Canada, France, and Sweden. In *Poverty, inequality, and the future of social policy* (ed. K.M. Lawson and W.J. Wilson). Russell Sage Foundation, New York.

McLanahan, S. and Sandefur, G. (1994). *Growing up with a single parent: what hurts, what helps.* Harvard University Press, Cambridge, MA.

McLeod, J.D. and Shanahan, M.J. (1993). Poverty, parenting, and children's mental health. *American Sociological Review*, **58**, 351–66.

McLoyd, V.C. and Wilson, L. (1993). The strain of living poor: parenting, social support, and child mental health. In *Children in poverty: child development and public policy* (ed. A.C. Huston). Cambridge University Press, New York.

Manlove, J. (1997). Early motherhood in an intergenerational perspective: the experiences of a British cohort. *Journal of Marriage and the Family*, **59**, 263–79.

Manning, W.D. and Lichter, D.T. (1996). Parental cohabitation and children's economic well-being. *Journal of Marriage and the Family*, **58**, 998–1010.

Mattessich, P. and Hill, R. (1987). Life cycle and family development. In *Handbook of marriage and the family* (ed. M.B. Sussman and S.K. Steinmetz), pp. 437–69. Plenum Press, New York.

Maynard, R.A. (ed.) (1997). *Kids having kids: economic costs and social consequences of teen pregnancy.* Urban Institute Press, Washington, DC.

Micklewright, J. and Stewart, K. (1999). *Is the well-being of children converging in the European Union?* UNICEF International Child Development Centre, Florence.

Moffitt, R.A. (ed.) (1998). *Welfare, the family, and reproductive behavior: research perspectives.* National Academy Press, Washington, DC.

Moore, K.A., Miller, B.C., Glei, D., and Morrison, D.R. (1995*a*). *Adolescent sex, contraception, and childbearing: a review of recent research.* Child Trends, Washington, DC.

Moore, K.A., Sugland, B., Blumenthal, C., Glei, D., and Snyder, N. (1995*b*). *Adolescent pregnancy prevention programs: interventions and evaluations.* Child Trends, Washington, DC.

Moore, K.A., Driscoll, A.K., and Lindberg, L.D. (1998). *A statistical profile of adolescent sex, contraception, and childbearing.* National Campaign to Prevent Teen Pregnancy, Washington, DC.

Morehouse Research Institute (1999). *Black fatherlessness: turning the corner on father absence in black America.* Morehouse Research Institute and the Institute for American Values, Atlanta, GA.

Morris, L. (1993). Determining male fertility through surveys: young adult reproductive health surveys in Latin America. Presented at the International Union for the Scientific Study of Population, Montreal.

Moynihan, D.P. (1965). A family policy for the nation. *America*, 18 September.

Murray, C. (1984). *Losing ground: American social policy, 1950–1980.* Basic Books, New York.

Murray, C. (1993). The coming white underclass. *Wall Street Journal*, 29 October.

National Center for Health Statistics (1999*a*). *Healthy People 2000 Review: 1998–99.* National Center for Health Statistics, Washington, DC.

National Center for Health Statistics (1999*b*). *Births: final data for 1997.* National Center for Health Statistics, Alan Guttmacher Institute, and National Campaign to Prevent Teen Pregnancy, Washington, DC.

OECD (Organization for Economic Cooperation and Development) (1999). *Labour force statistics: 1977–1997.* OECD, Paris.

O'Hanlon, A. (1999). When one child is just enough. *Washington Post*, 21 November, p. 1.

Pearlstein, M.B. (1997). Fatherlessness in the United States. In *The family in global transition* (ed. G.L. Anderson). Professors for World Peace Academy, St. Paul, MN.

Peterson, J.L. and Zill, N. (1986). Marital disruption and behavior problems in children. *Journal of Marriage and the Family*, **48**, 295–307.

Petit, M. and Curtis, P. (1997). *Child abuse and neglect: a look at the States.* Child Welfare League of America, Washington, DC.

Popenoe, D. (1998). Teen pregnancy: an American dilemma. Testimony before the US House of Representatives, Washington, DC, 16 July.

Popenoe, D. and Whitehead, B.D. (1999). *The state of our unions: the social health of marriage in America.* National Marriage Project, Rutgers University, New Brunswick, NJ.

Pournelle, J.E. (1997). The future of the family in an age of change. In *The family in global transition* (ed. G.L. Anderson). Professors for World Peace Academy, St. Paul, MN.

Quick, M. (1995). Country profile: Ireland. *Eurodata Newsletter*, **1**, 24–5.

Reichman, N.E. and Pagnini, D.L. (1997). Maternal age and birth outcomes: data from New Jersey. *Family Planning Perspectives*, **29**, 1–14.

Rothenbacher, F. (1996*a*). Social indicators for East European transition countries. *Eurodata Newsletter*, **4**, 19–21.

Rothenbacher, F. (1996*b*). European family indicators. *Eurodata Newsletter*, **3**, 19.

Rothenbacher, F. (1998*a*). Country profile: France. *Eurodata Newsletter*, **8**, 29–33.

Rothenbacher, F. (1998*b*). Country profile: Netherlands. *Eurodata Newsletter*, **8**, 23–5.

Saad, L. (1997). Family values differ sharply around the world. *Gallup Poll Monthly*, November, pp. 2–5.

Sandefur, G. D. and Mosley, J. (1997). Family structure, stability, and the well-being of children. In *Indicators of children's well-being* (ed. R.M. Hauser, B.V. Brown, and W.R. Prosser). Russell Sage Foundation, New York.

Schwenger, H. (1999). Country profile: Austria. *Eurodata Newsletter*, **9**, 17–23.

Siegel, G.L. and Loman, L.A. (1991). *Child care and AFDC recipients in Illinois.* Illinois Department of Public Aid, Chicago, IL.

Skolnick, A. (1997). The triple revolution: social sources of family change. In *The family on the threshold of the 21st century: trends and implications* (ed. S. Dreman). Erlbaum, Mahwah, NJ.

Smith, J.R., Brooks-Gunn, J., and Jackson, A. (1997). Parental employment and children. In *The family in global transition* (ed. G.L. Anderson). Professors for World Peace Academy, St. Paul, MN.

Sonenstein, F.L., Ku, L., Lindberg, L.D., Turner, C.F., and Peck, J.H. (1998). Changes in sexual behavior and condom use among teenaged males: 1988 to 1995. *American Journal of Public Health*, **88**, 956–9.

Soren, J. (1990). Danish family policy and the absence of a population policy. In *Family policy in EEC countries* (ed. W. Dumon), p. 33. Office for Official Publications of the European Commision, Luxembourg.

UNICEF (1997). *The role of men in the lives of their children.* UNICEF, New York.

UNICEF (1999). *The progress of nations: 1998.* UNICEF, New York.

United Nations (1994). *World population prospects.* United Nations, New York.

United Nations (1997). *Monthly bulletin of statistics, June 1997.* United Nations, New York.

US Bureau of the Census (1998*a*). *Statistical abstract of the United States: 1998.* US Bureau of the Census, Washington, DC.

US Bureau of the Census (1998*b*). *Current population reports, series P20–514; marital status and living arrangements: March 1998 (update).* US Bureau of the Census, Washington, DC.

US Department of Health and Human Services (1998). *Health, United States, 1998: socioeconomic status and health chart book.* US Department of Health and Human Services, Washington, DC.

US Department of Health and Human Services (1999). *Trends in the well-being of America's children and youth.* US Department of Health and Human Services, Washington, DC.

US General Accounting Office (1994). *Child care subsidies increase likelihood that low-income mothers will work.* US General Accounting Office, Washington, DC.

US General Accounting Office (1995). *Welfare to work: child care assistance limited: welfare reform may expand needs.* US General Accounting Office, Washington, DC.

Vanier Institute of the Family (1994). *Profiling Canada's families.* Vanier Institute of the Family, Ottawa.

Ventura, S.J. (1995). *Births to unmarried mothers: United States, 1980–1992.* US Department of Health and Human Services, Washington, DC.

Ventura, S.J., Martin, J.A., Curtin, S.C., and Mathews, T.J. (1998). Report of final natality statistics, 1996. *Monthly Vital Statistics Report*, **46** (115).

Waite, L.J. (1999). Cohabitation: a communitarian perspective. Presented to the Communitarian Task Force, Washington, DC.

Wallerstein, J.S. and Kelly, J.B. (1980). *Surviving the breakup: how children and parents cope with divorce.* Basic Books, New York.

Wertheimer, R. and Moore, K.A. (1998). *Childbearing by teens: links to welfare reform.* New Federalism: Issues and Options for States, Policy Brief Series A, No. A-24. Urban Institute, Washington, DC.

Whitehead, B.D. (1993). Dan Quayle was right. *Atlantic Monthly*, April, pp. 47–8.

Wilson, W.J. (1987). *The truly disadvantaged: the inner city, the underclass, and public policy.* University of Chicago Press.

WHO (World Health Organization) (1985). The health of the family: some key issues. *World Health Statistics Quarterly*, **38**, 254–5.

Zaslow, M.J., Oldham, E., Moore, K.A., and Magenheim, E. (1998). Welfare families' use of early childhood care and education programs, and implications for their children's development. *Early Childhood Research Quarterly*, **13**, 537–64.

Zill, N. and Rogers, C.C. (1988). Recent trends in the well-being of children in the United States and their implications for public policy. In *The changing American family and public policy* (ed. A.J. Cherlin). Urban Institute, Washington, DC.

Zill, N., Morrison, D.R., and Coiro, M.J. (1993). Long-term effects of parental divorce on parent–child relationships, adjustment, and achievement in young adulthood. *Journal of Family Psychology*, **7**, 91–103.

11.2 Women

Shaoxian Wang, Lin An, and Susan D. Cochran

Introduction

The field of women's health is broader than merely issues of fertility and reproductive health, or the biological differences between women and men, because there is growing recognition that social as well as biological factors strongly influence health outcomes in women (Goldman and Hatch 2000). This is because, despite the diversity of human experience globally, in all societies the ways in which men and women are treated differ (WHO 1998*a*). In most societies, human activities are divided into a 'public world of employment and politics', assigned principally to men, and a 'private arena of the family and household', which is the primary responsibility of women (WHO 1998*a*).

Traditionally, women undertake the burden of looking after children, husbands, and other members of the family. They are also responsible for nursing infants, preparing food for young children, cooking, sewing, and maintaining the household. In many countries, they must also assist in farming and other unpaid or underpaid physical labour and increasingly take part in the broader labour market at a financial disadvantage to men. Even in developed countries, where women participate in great numbers in paid employment, they still continue to bear the major burdens of family and household demands while receiving lower wages on average (United Nations 1995). Worldwide, women work longer hours than men, and girls enter the labour market at younger ages than boys (World Bank 1994).

The social inequalities engendered by this differential treatment directly or indirectly affect women's health and public health approaches to prevention and intervention (WHO 1995). For example, it is estimated that 70 per cent of those living in poverty worldwide are women (UNDP 1995), despite the fact that men slightly outnumber women in the world's population (United Nations 2000). This differential risk for poverty is seen in both developing and developed regions (UNDP 1995) and contributes to the well-documented health disparities that exist between women and men.

In addition, women's health and women's levels of health knowledge affect the health of their own children and families, owing to their primary caretaker role within the home. For example, in developing countries the death of a mother greatly increases mortality risk and risk for termination of formal education for young children, more so than the death of a father (World Bank 1994). Thus women's health plays a major role in the health and development of the family, the community, and ultimately the broader world. Nonetheless, in many parts of the world, men and children have priority over women for food and medical care. Women have less education and less chance to work for pay outside the family than men. When they fall ill, men and children have priority over women for the receipt of health care.

These gender biases exist not only within families but also in the broad health care sector where they influence the recommendations of health planners and providers. Thus some authors have asked: 'Where is the M in MCH (Maternal and Child Health)?' (Rosenfield and Main 1985). Recently, the World Health Organization (**WHO**) and other international agencies have called for increased attention to women's health, especially for research and medical resources directed to address the needs of women (FWCW 1995; WHO 1995).

Female mortality

Life expectancy at birth

Worldwide, women live longer than men, although the extent of this disparity varies between regions and especially between developed and developing countries (UN 1995) (Table 1). Generally, it is rare for men to outlive women, although there are exceptions (e.g. Bangladesh), and in southern Asia, men and women have similar life expectancies (WHO 1998*a*). The worldwide gender gap favouring women has not always existed (WHO 1998*a*). Historically, maternal morbidity and nutritional deficiencies resulted in lower female than male life expectancies. But over the last century, these causes of premature mortality among women have been reduced dramatically in many parts of the world through reductions in fertility rates, later age at first pregnancy, and improvements in prenatal health care and delivery (Goldman and Hatch 2000). For example, in the United States there was a 90 per cent reduction in maternal mortality between 1950 and 1989 alone (Bird and Rieker 1999). In contrast, improvements in male longevity have been mitigated by increasing prevalence of life-threatening behaviours that men are more likely to engage in than women, such as the widespread proliferation of tobacco use (Waldron 1995).

Reasons for the gender gap in life expectancy are not completely understood, although they are thought to be a mix of biological and social factors (UN 1995). Overall, mortality rates among infants, both male and female, are relatively higher than for other ages because infants are more vulnerable to environmental factors, especially infectious agents. As babies mature, the mortality rate decreases sharply through most of childhood. Above 55 years, the mortality rate increases more steeply. Furthermore, mortality rates in poor countries and regions are higher than in developed countries. But across strata,

Table 1 Gender differences in life expectancy for selected countries (1994–1997)

Country	Life expectancy at birth (years)		Life expectancy at 65 (years)	
	Male	Female	Male	Female
Ethiopia	48	52	–	–
Nigeria	51	54	–	–
Brazil	63	71	13	15
Philippines	67	70	12	14
Thailand	66	72	13	15
United States	73	80	15	19
United Kingdom	75	80	15	18
China	69	73	12	15
Japan	77	83	17	21

Source: Data at birth from UNFPA (1997) and State Statistical Bureau (1998); data at 65 years from United Nations (1997).

these effects are often more pronounced among males than females (Table 2).

Evidence indicating greater biological hardiness of females compared with males can be found in several quarters. Worldwide, there is a greater likelihood that female fetuses will be successfully carried to term than male fetuses (Waldron 1986). Also, in most geographical areas, particularly when male and female infants are treated equally, females are more likely than males to survive the first year of life (UN 1995) (Table 3). In developed countries, this advantage continues into childhood, although the same is not true in many developing countries. The underlying biological basis for these differences may be due to physiological differences linked to reproduction, including a stronger and more efficient immune system and an enhanced cardiovascular system protected by oestrogen premenopausally (Bird and Reiker 1999).

Social factors and the ways in which men's and women's lives differ also play a role. For example, men are more likely to be at risk of deaths from occupational or accidental causes than women (Waldron 1995). It has also been estimated than perhaps half of the gender-based difference in life expectancy in the United States and Sweden is a consequence of differential rates of smoking tobacco between women and men (Waldron 1986).

Major causes of mortality by sex

In most countries, there are few gender differences in the major causes of mortality (Table 4). Heart disease, cancer, cerebrovascular disease, and respiratory disease are the most common causes of death for both men and women.

Table 2 Mortality rates by age and sex in selected countries

Age (years)	Mauritius (1995)		Venezuela (1994)		Estonia (1995)		United States (1994)		Sweden (1995)		China (1995)	
	Male	Female	Male	Female	Male	Female	Male	Female	Male	Female	Male	Female
Total	775.3	566.8	536.3	388.7	1569.6	1264.1	915.0	837.6	1087.5	1034.8	719.2	594.2
<1	2208.4	1703.5	2765.2	2179.8	1649.7	1305.2	880.8	719.9	453.3	348.9	3127.8	3716.9
1–4	78.9	64.6	136.7	128.4	126.4	78.8	47.3	38.2	20.0	14.3	206.3	150.2
5–14	37.8	29.7	49.1	30.7	64.6	22.9	26.9	17.9	13.1	9.0	55.6	57.4
15–24	108.9	50.1	251.6	65.1	234.1	63.9	145.8	48.2	56.3	25.8	118.5	84.4
25–34	210.4	87.8	271.9	92.2	419.6	96.9	208.8	77.8	81.1	39.7	169.8	127.6
35–44	482.4	176.8	342.1	183.4	937.6	263.1	332.9	146.4	159.7	86.4	288.1	176.9
45–54	1078.7	494.0	606.8	373.5	1791.7	516.4	599.4	330.1	369.9	233.2	623.5	381.0
55–64	2424.2	1351.5	1515.1	937.6	3375.8	1120.5	1444.3	842.2	985.5	570.4	1668.1	1031.8
65–74	5198.0	2996.0	3306.3	2205.0	5564.3	2679.2	3332.3	1990.3	2834.9	1502.1	4196.1	2680.7
75+	12 541.7	8906.3	10 253.1	8724.8	13 292.8	10 920.1	9430.7	7449.2	10 075.4	7634.3	11 014.7	8605.1

Source: WHO (1998*d*) and State Statistical Bureau (1997).

Table 3 Infant and child mortality rates (1986–1993)

Region/country	Infant mortality	Child mortality
Developed regions (30 countries)	0.8	0.8
Northern Africa and Western Asia		
Egypt	0.9	1.4
Jordan, Morocco, Tunisia, Yemen	0.9	1.1
Sub-Saharan Africa (17 countries)	0.8	1.1
Latin American and Caribbean (10 countries)	0.8	1.0
Asia		
China	1.2	1.0
Pakistan	0.8	1.6
Indonesia, Philippines, Sri Lanka, Thailand	0.8	1.0

Source: UN (1995).

Maternal mortality

There are about 600 000 maternal deaths every year worldwide (WHO 1998*b*). Ninety-nine per cent of these occur in developing countries (Table 5). Estimates from the United Nations suggest that in developing countries one in every 48 women dies from maternal-related causes, with perhaps one in 16 women in Africa dying from these causes (Maine and McGinn 2000). In contrast, it is estimated that in northern Europe only one in 4000 women dies from maternal causes (Maine and McGinn 2000). Even within regions, women of lower socio-economic status are more at risk than women from higher socio-economic status, primarily because of limited access to health care.

Nevertheless, the causes of maternal mortality, such as haemorrhage, obstructed labour, sepsis, eclampsia, unsafe abortion, and severe anaemia, are similar in all countries and within regions, regardless of economic development (Rohde 1995). Worldwide, haemorrhage, obstructed labour, sepsis, and hypertensive disorders account for 60 per cent of maternal deaths (Maine and McGinn 2000). Unsafe abortions are blamed in approximately 13 per cent of deaths. Risk for maternal morbidity is greatest among women younger than 20 years or older than 35 years of age, but because parity is greatest among women in their twenties, this decade of life has the greatest absolute number of deaths.

Issues related to reproductive health

Health planners have typically defined women's reproductive health issues in terms of pregnancy and childbirth, focusing their interventions on medical considerations to solve issues arising out of these events. However, women's health has never been a simple biomedical issue. Both reproductive viability and patterns of reproduction are closely correlated with a woman's background. Many of the risks that women in developing countries face during pregnancy are a result of a lifetime of inadequate diet, illness, heavy work, poor education, and other social practices. For example, one major cause of obstructed labour is cephalopelvic disproportion. This obstetric complication is directly related to the body configuration of the puerperant. Underdeveloped configuration is the result of chronic nutritional deficiency, infectious disease, and cultural practices such as early marriage. Reproductive health risks for women cannot be underestimated. The period during which women are subject to these additional risks is very long, often 30 years or more, representing more than half the life expectancy of women in the poorest countries.

The International Conference on Population and Development (**ICPD**), held in Cairo in September 1994, and the Fourth World Conference on Women (**FWCW**), held in Beijing in September 1995, established the goals of reproductive health and women's reproductive rights. Both conferences noted that many women have no reproductive rights and often cannot access essential services. Many women worldwide suffer from poor physical and mental health. Hence the two conferences declared 'women's reproduction rights' to be the centre of the programme of action to promote good reproductive health worldwide. ICPD's programme of action defined reproductive health as follows (ICPD 1994):

> Reproductive health is a state of complete physical, mental and social well-being and not merely the absence of disease or infirmity, in all matters relating to the reproductive system and to its functions and processes.

This declaration implies that women should have both rights to safe pregnancies and healthy babies, and the freedom to decide when to have children and how often to do so. At the ICDP meeting, reproductive health was declared to include family planning, maternal and child health care, and prevention and treatment of infertility and sexually transmitted diseases, as well as improved education and social status for women. All these components were seen as essential for ensuring women's reproductive health.

Anaemia

Worldwide, more than a third of women and approximately half of pregnant women suffer from anaemia (UN 1995). This reduces physical productivity and also increases the risk of childbirth for women and newborns. Throughout the developing world, nutritionally related iron deficiency and the exacerbation of anaemia during pregnancy is a widespread problem. It is estimated, for example, that half of women in Africa are anaemic, increasing during pregnancy to perhaps two-thirds of women (Haslegrave 1995). Even higher rates have been estimated for women in south Asia where approximately 58 per cent women in general suffer from anaemia, rising to 75 per cent of women during pregnancy (UN 1995). In developed countries, rates are lower but, even so, approximately 12 per cent of women (18 per cent of pregnant women) experience anaemia.

Genital mutilation

Female circumcision or genital mutilation refers to several patterns of ritual cutting or altering of female genitalia (Izett and Toubia 2000). This cultural practice occurs primarily in the northeastern and northern sub-Saharan parts of Africa, in some Arab countries, including Yemen, and among immigrants from these regions. It is estimated that over 80 per cent of women in Sudan, Somalia, Djibouti,

Table 4 Ranking of top three causes of death and cause-specific death rates in selected countries

Country	Male		Female	
	Cause of death	**Death rate (per 100 000)**	**Cause of death**	**Death rate (per 100 000)**
Ghana (1994)				
1	CD	—	CD	—
2	IHD	—	IHD	—
3	RD	—	EMD	—
Paraguay (1994)				
1	CD	—	CD	—
2	MN	—	MN	—
3	IHD	—	IHD	—
Philippines (1994)				
1	RD	—	RD	—
2	IPD	—	IPD	—
3	MN	—	MN	—
China (1995)				
1	MN	156.35	CD	124.00
2	CD	133.66	MN	99.41
3	RD	94.85	RD	90.12
Estonia (1995)				
1	IHD	458.2	IHD	481.7
2	MN	265.6	CD	279.4
3	AC	208.1	MN	182.2
Sweden (1995)				
1	IHD	310.0	IHD	234.5
2	MN	246.2	MN	223.2
3	CD	97.0	IHD	128.2
UK (1995)				
1	IHD	289.7	MN	252.9
2	MN	286.5	IHD	233.3
3	RD	161.7	RD	184.7
USA (1994)				
1	MN	220.7	MN	190.5
2	IHD	193.1	IHD	177.2
3	RD	83.3	PD–CD–HD	87.0
Venezuela (1994)				
1	IHD	72.7	MN	61.6
2	AC	61.7	IHD	53.4
3	MN	59.5	CD	37.1

AC, accidental causes; CD, cerebrovascular disease; PD–CD–HD, pulmonary disease, circulatory disease, and other forms of heart disease; RD, respiratory disease; EMD, endocrine and metabolic diseases; IHD, ischaemic heart disease; IPD, infectious and parasitic diseases; MN, malignant neoplasms.

Source: WHO (1998).

Table 5 Maternal mortality rate in selected countries

Countries (year)	Maternal mortality rate (per 100 000 live births)
India (1990)	570.0
Australia (1995)	5.8
Afghanistan (1990)	1700.0
China (1995)	61.9
Hongkong, China (1996)	3.1
Japan (1995)	7.2
Philippines (1995)	179.7
Solomon Islands (1994)	549.0
Guinea (1990)	1600.0
Sierra Leone (1990)	1800.0
USA (1990)	12.0
UK (1990)	9.0
Sweden (1990)	7.0

Source: 1990 data from UNICEF (1998); other years from WHO (1998c).

Ethiopia, and Sierra Leone have undergone some form of female genital mutilation (WHO 1998*e*). Traditions surrounding the practice of genital mutilation vary, including the age at which it occurs, although typically girls are between 4 and 12 years of age. Female genital mutilation practices have been grouped into four major classifications (WHO 1998*e*): excision of the prepuce with or without partial or total excision of the clitoris, excision of the prepuce and clitoris with partial or total excision of the labia minora, excision of part or all of the external genitalia with infibulation, and other ritual practices including pricking, piercing, burning, and stretching of genitalia. It is estimated that 130 million girls and women worldwide have undergone one of these types of genital mutilation and that perhaps 2 million girls a year are at risk (UNICEF 1998).

Female genital mutilation poses a health risk for girls and women both physically and psychologically. Physically altering healthy genitalia results in impairment of normal functioning, the extent of which is dependent on the nature of the mutilation and the way in which it is performed. Most of these practices are conducted in unsanitary situations without anaesthetic. Among the immediate health consequences are pain, shock, haemorrhage, anaemia, infection, and death. Longer-term consequences include fistulae, faecal or urinary incontinence, dermoid cysts, keloidal scarring, neuromas, dyspareunia, ascending infections from the vulva, pelvic inflammatory disease, haematocolpus, and obstructed labour, depending on the pattern of genital alteration. One survey from Somalia, where most women undergo infibulation, found that 40 per cent experienced significant immediate complications and 40 per cent experienced long-term complications, excluding common difficulties with sexuality and delivery (UN 1995).

Psychological effects, too, reflect both the immediate and long-term consequences of female genital mutilation. Although less extensively documented than negative physical health outcomes, research suggests that the event is recalled as traumatic by girls and women who undergo it, with possible long-term disturbances in self-esteem and self-identity (Izett and Toubia 2000). Furthermore, chronic physical health difficulties arising from the procedure result in chronic or episodic psychological distress. Sexual responsiveness is impaired, depending upon the extent of the genital mutilation and the woman's prior experiences with sexual arousal (Izett and Toubia 2000).

Over the last two decades efforts to abolish the practice of female genital mutilation, particularly in Africa, have included intensive community-based campaigns (WHO 1998*e*) and widespread educational campaigns against this traditional cultural practice but they have had less success than was hoped for (PATH 1999). More recent efforts have focused on intervention strategies that enhance women's empowerment more generally in the hope of giving women the tools to decide if they wish to maintain or alter this cultural practice with the next generation (Izzett and Toubia 2000).

Fertility, contraception, and induced abortion

Fertility rates, or the rate of live births, has declined worldwide as a result of the development in the last 50 years of contraceptive strategies that allow people to regulate the timing and occurrence of pregnancies. For instance, in Bangladesh the total fertility rate (or the estimated number of live births that a girl will have from the age of 15 if she lives through her child-bearing years) declined from about 6.34 per woman in 1971 to 3.45 in 1995 (Jain *et al.* 1999). Similarly, the total fertility rate in China declined from 6.1 in 1949 to 1.5 in 1997 (State Family Planning Commission 1998). In the developed regions, where women have most ready access to contraception, total fertility rates range across countries between 1.2 and 2.2 (UN 1995). In contrast, rates range between 1.7 and 4.8 across countries in Latin America and the Caribbean, between 1.3 and 7.6 in Asia and the Pacific, and between 2.4 and 7.4 in Africa.

Despite these declines in total fertility rate, there are still millions of women with unmet contraceptive needs in developing countries (Table 6). There are more married women with an unmet contraceptive need about 31 million) in India than in any other country (Robey *et al.* 1996). Elsewhere, there are 5.7 million women married women with unmet contraceptive needs in Pakistan, 4.4 million in both Indonesia and Bangladesh, 3.9 million in Nigeria, 3.1 million in Mexico, 3.0 million in Brazil, and 2.5 million in the Philippines (Robey

Table 6 Total unmet contraceptive needs among married women of reproductive age in developing areas, 1996

Region	No. with unmet need (thousands)	Unmet need (% of MWRA)
Africa	22 200	26
Near East and North Africa	6200	16
Asia (except China)	62 100	19
Latin America	11 200	17
All developing areas (except China)	101 700	19

MWRA, married women of reproductive age.

Source: Robey *et al.* (1996).

et al. 1996). The proportion of all married women with unmet contraceptive needs in each country range from an estimated 11 per cent in Thailand and Turkey, to 36 per cent in Kenya and 37 per cent in Rwanda. On average 19 per cent of married women in developing countries, excluding China, have unmet contraceptive needs. Owing to the very strict birth control policy and widespread family planning services in China, contraceptives were available to 90 per cent of married women in 1997 (State Family Planning Commission 1998).

No contraceptive method is perfect. Hence, women facing an unwanted pregnancy may seek to induce an abortion. Of the 40 to 60 million induced abortions performed annually worldwide, approximately 20 million are estimated as being conducted under unsafe conditions, and 95 per cent of these occur in developing countries. According to WHO (1998*c*), at least 80 000 women die each year from induced abortions, and many others suffer lifelong physical or mental disorders as a consequence. Complications from unsafe abortions are among the leading causes of maternal mortality (WHO 1998*c*). The highest abortion rate is in Europe (48 per 1000 women aged 15–44 years) and the lowest is in North America and Oceania (21 and 22 per 1000 women aged 15–44 years) (Table 7). Africa, Asia, and Latin America had similar rates (Henshaw *et al.* 1999).

Almost all abortions are illegal in Latin America and Africa. For example, in Chile, 80 women were recently legally prosecuted and imprisoned for having abortions. Most of these women were adolescents or young adults and single mothers; eight of the 80 women had become pregnant after being raped. A great majority of them were reported to the police by the public hospital where they sought treatment for complications from an illegal abortion (Casas-Becerra 1997). Because the illegality of the procedure is the chief cause of unsafe abortions, both the ICPD (1994) and the FWCW (1995) expressed concerns that legal structures were jeopardizing women's health. The ICPD defined safe abortion as a component of essential reproductive health services (ICPD 1994), and asserted that, in circumstances where it is legal, abortion should be safe (ICPD 1994). The FWCW stressed the health risks of unsafe abortion and called for a review of laws that punish women who have undergone illegal abortions (FWCW 1995). Unfortunately, there are still many regions and countries where legal restrictions on abortion serve as barriers to women's access to safe abortions (Table 8). Even in countries where abortion is legal, restrictions on ready access to the procedure, including denial of public funding for abortion and requirements that minors obtain parental consent, can make it difficult for women to obtain abortions when needed (Fried 1997).

HIV/AIDS and other sexually transmitted diseases

In developing countries, sexually transmitted diseases are responsible for the second greatest number of disability-adjusted life years among women, second only to illnesses due to maternal causes (Padian 2000). By the end of 1999, less than two decades after AIDS was first recognized, 50 million people in the world had been infected with HIV and 14 million had died from AIDS. The number of individuals living with an HIV infection is about 34 million, with more than 95 per cent living in developing countries. UNAIDS/WHO also estimated that about 6 million people in the world were newly infected in 1998, a rate of almost 11 people per minute worldwide (UNAIDS 1999). Globally, 10 per cent of those infected were under the age of 15 years.

The number of HIV-positive women has also increased rapidly. In 1998, women accounted for 46 per cent of all infected people globally. The increasing risk for HIV is shared by women in developed and developing countries alike. For example, in France, the percentage of women among AIDS cases rose from 12 per cent in 1985 to 20 per cent by 1995. In Brazil, the figure rose from 1 per cent in 1984 to 25 per cent in 1994. Not surprisingly perhaps, the number of babies who acquire HIV from their infected mothers before or during birth or from breast feeding is also rising dramatically.

Why are women so vulnerable to HIV infection? Physiologically, compared with men, women have a larger and very thin surface area of mucosa exposed to their partner's sexual secretion during sexual intercourse. Moreover, semen infected with HIV typically contains a higher viral concentration than a woman's sexual secretion. Thus male-to-female transmission is more likely than female-to-male transmission. In addition, an untreated sexually transmitted disease in either of the partners enhances the risk of HIV transmission to the woman. Reproductive tract infections, most of which are sexually transmitted, are extremely common in developing countries. For example, a community-based survey in Egypt found that over half of women had one or more reproductive tract infections (World Bank 1994). Women are more likely than men to experience asymptomatic sexually transmitted diseases, and when symptoms are present women

Table 7 Estimated percentage of illegal abortions, abortion rate, and abortion ratio by region (1995)

Region	Illegal abortions (%)	Abortion rate[a]	Abortion ratio[b]
Total	44	35	26
Africa	99	33	15
Asia	37	33	25
Europe	12	48	48
Latin America	95	37	27
Northern America	—[c]	22	26
Oceania	22	21	20

[a]Abortions per 1000 women aged 15 to 44 years.

[b]Abortions per 100 known pregnancies.

[c]Less than 0.5 per cent

Source: Henshaw *et al.* (1999).

Table 8 Legal limitations on abortion by region and countries (1997)

The Americas and the Caribbean	**Central Asia, West Asia, and North Africa**	**East and South Asia and the Pacific**	**Europe**	**Sub-Saharan Africa**
To save the woman's life				
Brazil (R)	Afghanistan	Bangladesh	Ireland	Angola
Chile (ND)	Egypt (SA)	Indonesia		Benin
Colombia	Iran	Laos		Central African Republic
Dominican Republic	Lebanon	Myanmar		Chad
El Salvador (ND)	Libya (PA)	Nepal		Congo (Brazzaville)
Guatemala	Oman	Papua New Guinea		Cote d'Ivoire
Haiti	Syria (SA/PA)	Philippines		Democratic Republic of Congo (F)
Honduras	United Arab Emirates (SA/PA)	Sri Lanka		Democratic Republic of Gabon
Mexico (R)	Yemen			Guinea-Bissau (SA/PA)
Nicaragua (SA/PA)				Kenya
Panama (PA/R/F)				Lesotho
Paraguay				Madagascar
Venezuela				Mali
				Mauritania
				Mauritius
				Niger
				Nigeria
				Senegal
				Somalia
				Sudan (R)
				Tanzania
				Togo
				Uganda
Physical health grounds				
Argentina (R, limited)	Kuwait (SA/PA/F)	Pakistan	Poland (R/I/F)	Burkina Faso (R/I/F)
Bolivia (R/I)	Morocco (SA)	Republic of Korea (SA/R/I/F)		Burundi
Costa Rica	Saudi Arabia (SA/PA)	Thailand (R)		Cameroon (R)
Ecuador (R/I, limited)				Eritrea
Peru				Ethiopia
Uruguay (R)				Guinea
				Malawi (SA)
				Mozambique
				Rwanda
				Zimbabwe (R/I/F)
Mental health grounds				
Jamaica (PA)	Algeria	Australia	Northern Ireland	Botswana (F/R/I)
Trinidad and Tobago	Iraq (SA/F/R/I)	Malaysia	Portugal (PA/F/R)	Gambia
	Israel (F/R/I)	New Zealand (F/I)	Spain (F/R)	Ghana (F/R/I)
	Jordan		Switzerland	Liberia (F/R/I)
				Namibia (F/R/I)
				Sierra Leone
Socio-economic grounds				
		India (PA/R/F)	Finland (R/F)	Zambia
		Japan (SA)	United Kingdom (F)	
		Taiwan (SA/PA/I/F)		

Continued

Table 8 Legal limitations on abortion by region and countries (1997) (*Continued*)

The Americas and the Caribbean	Central Asia, West Asia, and North Africa	East and South Asia and the Pacific	Europe	Sub-Saharan Africa
Without restriction as to reason				
Canada (L)	Armenia[a]	Cambodia[b] (PA)	Albania[a]	South Africa[a]
Cuba[a] (PA)	Azerbaijan[a]	China (PA/L)	Austria[b]	
United States (PV)	Georgia[a]	Mongolia[a]	Belarus[a]	
Puerto Rico (PV)	Kazakhstan[a]	North Korea (L)	Belgium[b]	
	Kyrgyz Republic [a]	Singapore[c]	Bosnia-Herzegovina[a] (PA)	
	Tajikistan[a]	Vietnam (L)	Bulgaria[a]	
	Tunisia[a]		Croatia[a] (PA)	
	Turkey[a] (SA/PA)		Czech Republic [a] (PA)	
	Turkmenistan		Denmark[a] (PA)	
	Uzbekistan		Estonia[a]	
			France[a] (PA)	
			Germany[b]	
			Greece[a] (PA)	
			Hungary[a]	
			Italy[d] (PA)	
			Latvia[a]	
			Lithuania[a]	
			Macedonia[a] (PA)	
			Moldova[a]	
			Netherlands (PA)	
			Norway[a] (PA)	
			Romania[b]	
			Russian Federation[a]	
			Slovak Republic[a] (PA)	
			Slovenia[a] (PA)	
			Sweden[e]	
			Ukraine[a]	
			Yugoslavia[a] (PA)	

For gestational limits, duration of pregnancy is calculated from the last menstrual period, which is generally considered to occur 2 weeks prior to conception. Thus, statutory gestational limits calculated from the date of conception have been extended by 2 weeks.

F, abortion allowed in case of fetal impairment; I, abortion allowed in cases of incest; L, law does not indicate gestational limit; ND, existence of defence of necessity is highly doubtful; PA, parental authorization required; PV, law does not limit pre-viability abortions; R, abortion allowed in cases of rape; SA, spousal authorization required.

[a]Gestational limit of 12 weeks.

[b]Gestational limit of 14 weeks.

[c]Gestational limit of 24 weeks.

[d]Gestational limit of 90 days.

[e]Gestational limit of 18 weeks.

Source: Ranhman *et al.* (1998)

may have more difficulty attributing these to a sexually transmitted disease as opposed to common bodily changes (Padian 2000).

Another important factor is the greater social and economic vulnerability of women in comparison to men. Social inequalities between women and men serve to impair women's abilities to individually protect themselves from HIV infection. One effect of social inequality is lack of knowledge of how to prevent infection. Millions of young girls in developing countries have been raised with little understanding of their reproductive system or the mechanics of HIV/AIDS transmission and prevention. Although human sexuality courses are sometimes taught, this occurs in later grades when girls are already less likely than boys to have remained in school. A second effect is a lack of influential power in the sexual relationship. Condom use, when condoms are available, is primarily male-controlled and the opportunity to refuse sexual encounters that women might fear are high risk is obviated by social and economic pressures. Furthermore, in many societies, sex is the 'currency' for girls and women who must provide sexual services in order to survive. A third effect of social inequality is less access to resources that would make it less likely for HIV to be transmitted, such as treatment for other ulcerative sexually transmitted diseases. Often women dare not seek treatment for sexually transmitted diseases without male approval.

These problems have led UNAIDS (1997) to call for the empowerment of women in order to reduce rates of HIV infection. UNAIDS has suggested six ways of achieving this.

1. Combat ignorance: improve the access of girls to formal schooling and ensure they have information about their own bodies, education about AIDS and the other sexually transmitted diseases, and the skill to say no to unwanted or unsafe sex.
2. Provide HIV prevention services to women: ensure that girls and women have access to appropriate health care and HIV/AIDS prevention services at places and times that are convenient for them and expand voluntary HIV testing and counselling services.
3. Develop female-controlled HIV infection prevention methods: encourage the development of methods that are under the direct control of women that they can use in the absence of male approval or co-operation. Although the male condom currently is the only barrier method easily available for HIV prevention, UNAIDS is facilitating the development of and access to several such methods, including the female condom and vaginal microbicides—virus-killing creams or foams that women can insert vaginally before sexual intercourse.
4. Build safe norms: recognizing the power of social norms to protect individuals from pressure to engage in unwanted or unsafe behaviours, UNAIDS calls for support for women's groups and organizations to question traditional sexual norms and behaviours which have caused women to be infected with AIDS. This includes educating boys and men to respect girls and women, to be responsible in sexual behaviours, and to share responsibility for protecting themselves, their sexual partners, and their children from HIV and other sexually transmitted diseases.
5. Reinforce women's economic independence: economic independence allows women the option of risking disapproval in sexual negotiations. UNAIDS suggests building more opportunities for training and educational classes for women, setting up credit programmes and co-operatives, and include HIV/AIDS prevention activities in these programmes. For example, UNAIDS has supported Zambian women fish traders to form a co-operative which was given interest-free loans by UNAIDS. With such credit co-operatives, the fish-traders are able to resist the need to barter sexual favours with fish wholesalers or truck drivers who control their access to fish markets and to transportation.
6. Reduce women's vulnerability through changing social policies: current social policies from the community level up to the national level serve to maintain social inequalities. Social policies structured to protect women's rights and fundamental freedoms and to improve their economic independence and legal status will reduce women's vulnerability to HIV infection through altering behavioural risk patterns.

Reproductive health services

The 1994 ICPD in Cairo marked the historical turning point for women's reproductive health. Before the ICPD, many family planning programmes emphasized only demographic targets for family planning, neglecting the social and psychological components of the field of reproductive health services. In particular, women's concerns were overlooked. The programme of action from the ICPD declares:

> All countries should strive to make accessible through the primary health care system, reproductive health to all individuals of appropriate ages as soon as possible and no later than the year 2015. Reproductive health care in the context of primary health care should include: family-planning counseling, information, education, communication and services; education and services for prenatal care, safe delivery, and postnatal care, especially breast-feeding and infant and women's health care; prevention and appropriate treatment of infertility; abortion as specified in paragraph 8.25, including prevention of abortion and the management of the consequences of abortion; treatment of reproductive tract infections, sexually transmitted diseases and other reproductive health conditions; and information, education and counseling, as appropriate, on human sexuality, reproductive health and responsible parenthood. Referral for family-planning services and further diagnosis and treatment for complications of pregnancy, delivery and abortion, infertility, reproductive tract infections, breast cancer and cancers of the reproductive system, sexually transmitted disease, including HIV/AIDS should always be available, as required. Active discouragement of harmful practices such as female genital mutilation, should also be an integral component of primary health care, including reproductive health care programs.

This meeting reframed the goals of reproductive health services. Formerly, family planning programmes aimed solely at demographic targets, but now these programmes focus also on the needs and desires of individuals. In addition, ICPD's call for comprehensive reproductive health services specifically includes the involvement of women to serve women's needs and safeguard women's rights.

For example, Bangladesh was one of the first countries to adopt the Programme of Action drafted at the 1994 ICPD in Cairo (Hardee *et al.* 1999). Although Bangladesh is one of the poorest countries in the world, where both the literacy level and social status of women are very low, it increased contraceptive use by women from 3 per cent in the 1970s to 45 per cent in recent years. Its main intervention was to train 28 000 'on-the-spot' women workers who deliver oral contraceptives and contraceptive injections house by house (Schuler *et al.* 1995). Furthermore, the quality of reproductive health services in various departments was improved. For example, in one project in 1996, Bangladesh undertook a collaborative project with the Asia Foundation, the University of North Carolina, and USAID to train 20 county family planning officers in administration management. The objective was to enhance implementation of family planning programmes. Training included increasing levels of knowledge, skill, and competence among workers in the fields of family planning, statistics, epidemiology, demography, management, coalition building among persons and organizations, and professional standards and behaviour. Measured outcomes of this project found that the contraceptive prevalence rate increased in all the 19 counties served by an average of 5.47 per cent (Jain *et al.* 1999).

Other health issues

Maintaining health with limited resources

Overall life expectancy in most parts of the world is increasing, particularly in northern Africa, parts of Asia, and Central America (UN 1995). There are exceptions. For example, countries in Eastern Europe have experienced little gain in longevity and some in sub-Saharan Africa actually have suffered a decline in life expectancy due to increasing mortality from AIDS (UN 1995). One consequence of increasing longevity worldwide is that an increasing proportion of the world's population is older than in the past. Furthermore, because of the gender gap, with increasing age a greater and greater proportion of these individuals are women. For example, in the United States, 60 per cent of individuals over 65 years of age and 70 per cent over 85 years of age are women (Leveille and Furalnik 2000). For women, this represents more years at risk for experiencing age-related morbidity and decreasing likelihood of assistance from a spousal partner (UN 1995). Table 9 presents data from a survey in China demonstrating age-related increases in problems in one's ability to live independently. The table shows that, although ageing is not invariantly linked to disability, this becomes increasingly likely as one lives longer and women are more likely to experience this than men.

In both developed and developing countries, health status among older women is much worse than among older men. For example, in a 1993 household interview survey (Feng 1999) on the functional health status of rural elders aged 60 or over conducted in Henan Province, China, several indicators demonstrated that a greater proportion of women's later years are impaired by disabilities in comparison to men. As shown in Fig. 1, whether one measures activities of daily living, instrumental activities of daily living, or gross physical function, the number of years living with a disability are greater among women than men in all age groups above 60 years of age. The prevalence rate of disabilities in activities of daily living, instrumental activities of daily living, and gross physical function were 10.2 per cent, 30.3 per cent, and 33.5 per cent, respectively. Thus women in the older age groups experience greater rates of morbidity than men.

In most societies, women with physical disabilities face additional challenges in maintaining a healthy quality of life in the context of social inequalities resulting both from gender and physical disability. The Center for Research on Women with Disabilities (Nosek *et al.* 1997) in the United States conducted a nationwide survey concerning the impact of physical disabilities on women. They found that women with physical disabilities, in contrast with those without, have limited opportunities to establish relationships, lower likelihood of having children, and suffer more physical, social, and emotional abuse. This abuse can include withholding of necessary equipment (wheelchair, braces), medication, transportation, or essential assistance in daily living, such as dressing or getting out of bed. Another observation from the study was that women with disabilities seldom obtained information about sexuality and reproductive health tailored to their needs. A common misperception was that disabled women were not sexually active, even if they were. These women also are more likely to suffer from chronic diseases that have an earlier age of onset when compared with women who are not disabled (Table 10).

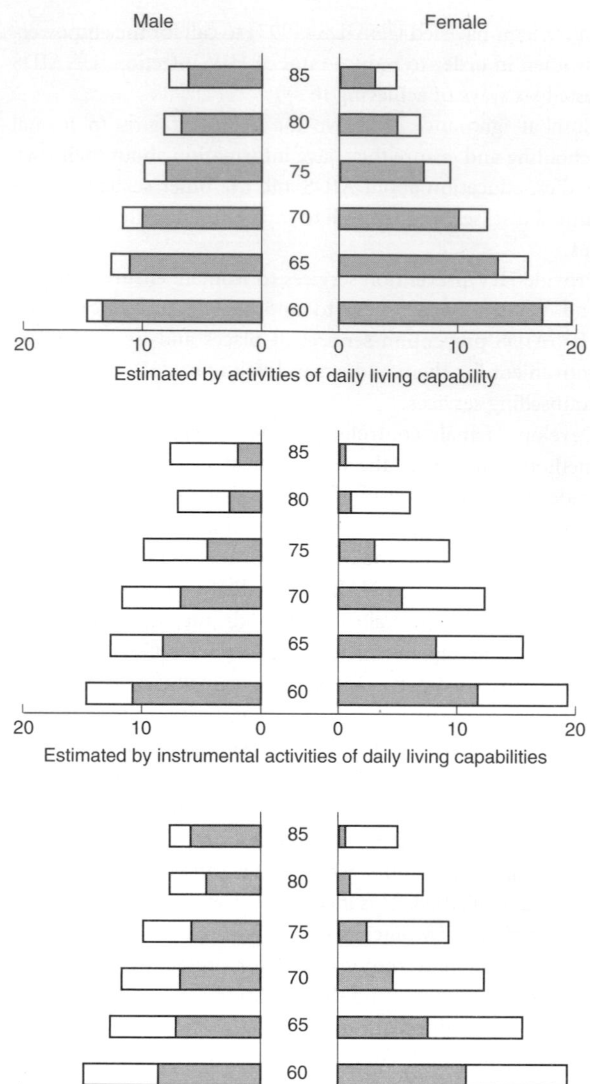

Fig. 1 Life expectancy, both years of disability and disability-free years, by age and sex estimated from a household survey in China in 1993.

Table 9 Results from a survey of people aged 60 years and older assessing ability to function independently (China, 1994)

Age	Total number	Number (percentage) unable to function independently	
60–64	25 612	653	(2.55)
65–69	19 535	867	(4.44)
70–74	13 999	1224	(8.74)
75–79	8100	1227	(15.15)
80–84	4231	1042	(24.63)
85–89	1453	490	(33.72)
90+	493	223	(45.23)

Source: State Statistical Bureau (1995).

Table 10 Survey estimating prevalence of chronic diseases in women with physical disabilities (United States)

Disease	Prevalence (%)
Chronic urinary tract infections	18
Major depression	17
Osteoporosis	12
Restrictive lung disease	6
Inflammatory bowel disease	6
Heart disease	5
Seizure disorder	5
Kidney disease	3

Source: Nosek *et al.* (1997).

Environmental and occupational health

Conceptualizing environmental and occupational health risks for women is complicated by both social and biological factors. The diversity of women's roles and their increasing participation in the broader labour market results in exposures that occur both in the household and the external workplace. The importance of workplace hazards for women is often overlooked despite the fact that toxins do exist in the home, women's occupations can and do bring them into contact with harmful chemicals and risk of physical injury, and many tools and machines are designed for larger and stronger average physiques (Silbergeld 2000*a*). For example, indoor cooking, an activity commonly undertaken by women in developing countries, represents a serious environmental hazard resulting in morbidity arising from acute and chronic exposure to smoke and toxic gases (World Bank 1994).

In addition, dietary, biological, and immunological differences between women and men may result in differential patterns of exposures and dissimilar responses to similar environmental exposures (Blair *et al.* 1999; Silbergeld 2000*b*). Men and women differ in their rates of contact with environmental toxins, the extent to which these substances are absorbed into or excreted from the body, and the rate at which they are metabolized. Levels of circulating hormones also influence the process. Within women, these rates are also altered by the biological changes associated with pregnancy, lactation, and menopause, leading to interactions between lifestage and the effects of toxins.

Despite these differences between women and men, very little research has focused on environmental and occupational health issues among women (Blair *et al.* 1999; Lindbohm 1999). The reasons for this are varied (Silbergeld 2000*b*). Many animal studies are limited to male animals. Most studies of environmental risks in humans have drawn respondents, primarily male, from occupational settings where there are intense and more easily measured exposures to toxins of interest. Furthermore, when surveys of women's health are conducted, such as the Women's Health Initiative in the United States, a large longitudinal cohort study of postmenopausal women, occupational experiences are not measured in sufficient detail. Nevertheless, the effects of toxins on some outcomes, such as gynaecological cancers, can only be studied in women and there are increasing concerns that results from studies using only male subjects do not generalize well to understanding health effects in women (Blair *et al.* 1999).

Violence against women

The effects of violence against women is another emerging area in women's health because of both directly attributable health consequences and the ways in which male violence against women expresses and reinforces the social inequalities that are known to impair women's health (WHO 1997). Worldwide, violence is often employed as a means by which control can be exerted over other human beings. Three current themes in today's worldwide patterns of violence are the greater importance of low-intensity conflicts in impoverished countries where civilian populations, including women, experience the brunt of the conflict, the high prevalence of deadly weapons, such as land mines, and the terrorization of the civilian population as a method of warfare (Desjarlais *et al.* 1995). Such violence impacts on both men and women, but women are also at risk for other forms of violence from intimate partners and members of their own family. Furthermore, social and community responses to the gender-based violence against women differs from violence where men are both perpetrators and victims (Miller and Downs 2000).

Gender-based violence against women is of many types including rape and sexual assault, physical battering, psychological abuse, forced abortions, female infanticide, and 'dowry death' (Desjarlais *et al.* 1995). Worldwide it is estimated that approximately 25 to 50 per cent of women, depending on the study, report being a victim of physical abuse from men (Heise *et al.* 1995) and 60 per cent of murders of women are linked to domestic violence (WHO 1997). Estimates of recent or lifetime prevalence of being sexually coerced by an intimate male sex partner vary worldwide from 6 per cent of women surveyed in London who reported forced sex in the past 12 months to more than half of women surveyed in a study from Turkey reporting on their lifetime experiences (WHO 2000). The World Bank estimates that a substantial portion of total morbidity among women is due to the effects of rape or domestic violence, accounting for 5 per cent of women's disease burden in developing countries and 19 per cent in developed countries (WHO 1998*a*).

Mental health

Among the 10 leading causes of disability worldwide in 1990, five were mental disorders (Murray and Lopez 1996). Between the ages of 15 and 54 years, there is little difference between women and men in rates of psychiatric disorders (Kessler *et al.* 1994; World Bank 1994), although the relative frequency of different disorders varies (Table 11). Women are more likely than men to experience depression and anxiety disorders, while men are more likely than women to evidence substance use disorders (Kessler *et al.* 1994; World Bank 1994; Desjarlais *et al.* 1995). The prevalence of major depression among women is 1.5 to 3 times higher than among men depending on the study and the time frame of reference (Kessler 2000). Although men are more likely than women to commit suicide, the female death rate from suicide is increasing, especially among women of child-bearing age. For example, suicides are the leading cause of death in women of child-bearing age in China (J. Yang, unpublished work, Beijing Medical University, 1999).

Surveys worldwide also document that women experience greater levels of depressive distress than men, sometimes reported as problems with 'nerves', 'heart distress', or intrusion of unwanted 'spirits' (Desjarlais *et al.* 1995). The reasons for this difference are generally attributed to the greater likelihood that women are impoverished in comparison with men, experience greater role strain and

Table 11 Gender differences in patterns of mental health disorders worldwide: relative contributions to disability-adjusted life years lost due to mental disorders

Disorder	Women (%)	Men (%)
Depression	25.6	10.4
Dementia	15.4	10.5
Self-inflicted injury	13.9	17.5
Epilepsy	8.7	9.9
Psychoses	7.2	6.5
Post-traumatic stress disorder	6.6	3.2
Alcohol dependence	3.4	19.2
Drug dependence	2.7	6.5
Other	16.5	16.3

Source: Desjarlais *et al.* (1995); adapted from World Bank (1993).

exhaustion, are more likely to experience abuse, particularly from intimate partners and family members, and have less of control over necessary resources (World Bank 1994; Desjarlais *et al.* 1995; Seaman and Wood 2000).

Promoting women's health

Two of the most important tenets of contemporary thinking about successful health development are that communities or constituencies must participate in decision-making, and that the non-health sector must work together with the health sector to achieve effective and sustained change. In promoting women's reproductive health and health in general, it is apparent that efforts to empower women are critical, because through empowerment women can participate in making the changes around them that are essential for their health. Without empowerment, they lack the tools and the freedom to create needed change. In developed countries, such as the United States and Australia, recognition of this need resulted in widespread social movements to alter the methods of health education and services delivery for women (Broom 1998; Seaman and Wood 2000). In developing countries, different models have been tried to create change. Two examples from China are described below.

Improving women's reproductive health

The Ford Foundation and Yunnan Province in China carried out a collaborative project on women's reproductive health and development beginning in 1991 (Wang and Li 1994). The major strategies adopted by the project are detailed below (Li and Wang 1998).

Empowerment of women

To motivate women to express their wishes and needs, the programme planners employed focus group discussions and photo novellas to encourage women to express their needs. The rural women identified two themes that were their most urgent needs. One stressed that their labour was too heavy and very hard. They said: 'Who *has* time to think about their health and suffering? We will be thankful if we will be given a little time to rest.' They wished to lighten the intensity of their labour. Another theme was that village women badly needed nurseries and kindergartens to provide care for their children. The village women had to do endless farm work and household duties. If there were no grandmothers to look after the young at home, mothers had to bring their babies to the field with them. When children reached the age of 2 or 3 years, they were frequently left at home unattended. Furthermore, these toddlers sometimes had to look after their younger brother or sister, and to perform other duties such as feeding the chickens.

Co-ordination of multiple sectors

Poverty and the overall low level of economic development made it unlikely that any intervention in the health sector alone will address the multiple causes of ill health among poor rural women. Women's health, and that of their families and communities, can be improved only if health interventions are integrated with efforts to improve women's educational and employment opportunities, to reduce gender bias in the distribution of nutritional, health, and other resources, to alleviate heavy workloads and the burdens of poverty, and to combat women's powerlessness so that they would have more effective control over their own lives. However, efforts to encourage co-ordination across domains of interest such as health care, education, and community resources, often devolve into conflicts surrounding competition for scarce resources. In this instance, the project worked specifically on evolving more synergistic relationships that could provide benefits for all.

Collaboration between multiple disciplines

The programme in Yunnan province involved collaboration between biomedical workers, sociologists, anthropologists, and others. Every one of the team members contributed their professional skill.

The programme developed over 40 projects ranging from midwifery training to the construction of water reservoirs to supply portable water to villages to promote pig raising and increase personal income. These experiences in Yunnan province demonstrated that empowerment for women to achieve better health outcomes requires co-ordination of various sectors and collaboration of diverse disciplines to promote women's reproductive health. Focusing only on reproductive issues would not have solved the health problems these women faced.

Decreasing maternal mortality rate

A second example of promoting women's health come from attempts to decrease the maternal mortality rate. Two methods of reducing the maternal mortality rate are to provide adequate antenatal care as well as performing clean and safe deliveries. Adequate antenatal care in the absence of safe childbirth is not sufficient because most obstetric complications occur abruptly and unexpectedly. If not treated in time, most women will die. Some authors assert that obstetric complications need to be treated at health organizations where blood transfusion, Caesarean section, placenta removal, and induced labour facilities are available (Rohde 1995). Some experts have called on the developed countries to assist developing countries in upgrading their emergency obstetric care facilities to ensure safe childbirth for women (Nowark 1995).

Although China is considered a developing country, in 1995 the maternal mortality rate was 61.9 per 100 000 live births, the lowest maternal mortality rate among the countries that have similar levels of economic development. The reason for this is that China started to organize primary health services in 1949. Gradually, a three-tier health system was established (Taylor *et al.* 1985). The three-tier health system covers even the remote areas in the country. As of 1998, every township had a health centre (a small hospital), and more than 90 per cent of the villages had a health post (Table 12). The three-tier health system is a guarantee of 'Health for All' (including reducing safe childbirth) at the functional level.

Because the rural areas enjoy governmental priority for improving health, the township health centres and village's health posts have been provided with essential equipment and personnel allowing in some instances blood transfusions and Caesarean sections, if needed. The existing gap in obstetric care between urban and rural areas is decreasing. By the end of 1997, about 93 per cent of deliveries in China were attended by trained health care workers (WHO 1998*c*).

In addition to addressing needs for safe childbirth, China also provides extensive family planning services. Indirectly, this also lowers the maternal mortality rate by allowing women to delay first pregnancy to older ages and to have fewer children. All contraceptives are provided free of charge and unmet contraceptive needs are rare. Countrywide, government agencies at all levels, from central to local, emphasize family planning. Nevertheless, the maternal mortality rate in rural areas is still higher than urban areas. Thus more needs to be done (Table 13).

Conclusion

One of the more interesting global facts about health is that women live longer than men, but experience greater morbidity (Goldman and Hatch 2000). This pattern of gender-associated differences in morbidity and mortality is a modern experience reflecting the gain in life expectancy for women from reducing the risks of childbirth and possibly the increasing mortality risks for men from tobacco use and other health risk related behaviours (Waldron 1995). Furthermore,

Table 12 The three-tier health system in China

Population	Organization[a]	Professional staff	Obstetric care capabilities
Level 1: Countywide			
70 000–1 million	Hospital (one or two hospitals) Maternal and child health centre Antiepidemic station Family planning service	University-trained specialists General practitioners	Blood transfusion Caesarean section High-risk deliveries
Level 2: Township			
20 000–70 000	Single health centre (small hospital including hospital services, maternal and child services, and antiepidemic services) Family planning services	General practitioners Nurse midwives Assistant doctors	Antenatal and postnatal care including clean safe delivery Administration of antibiotics and anticonvulsants Placenta removal Plasma expander Blood transfusion and Caesarean section are available in some health centres
Level 3: Local village			
1000–3000	Health post or clinic	Health workers Village doctors (6 months training) Personnel trained to provide clean safe delivery	Antenatal and postnatal care Clean safe delivery

[a]Health posts have been established in 90 per cent of the villages in the whole country, county hospitals and township health centres have been established in the whole country, and family planning service have been established in about 80 per cent of county hospitals and 60 per cent of township health centres.

Table 13 Maternal mortality rate in China (per 100 000 live births): national surveillance results

Year	Total	Urban	Rural
1989	94.7	49.9	114.9
1990	88.9	45.9	112.5
1991	80.0	46.3	100.0
1992	76.5	42.7	97.9
1993	67.3	38.5	85.1
1994	64.8	44.1	77.5
1995	61.9	39.2	76.0

public health interventions currently available and cost-effective in reducing human disability offer the potential for greater gains in reducing morbidity among women than men (World Bank 1994).

Over the last decade, it has become increasingly clear that further improvements in women's health, and collaterally in the health of their children and families, are dependent on successfully addressing the ill health effects generated by social inequality (ICPD 1994; World Bank 1994; FWCW 1995). Although women, unlike men, experience health risk associated with reproduction and child rearing, much of this additional risk is generated by women's lower social, educational, cultural, and economic status. Furthermore, women face additional threats to their health, such as relative lack of access to health care, greater risk of suffering, violence, and coercive, high-risk sexual encounters, that are not linked to reproduction but do stem directly from social inequalities.

Understanding women's health calls for an awareness of the biological differences between men and women, a focus on health matters specific to women's reproductive role, and an appreciation for the deleterious effects of social inequities. Improving the health of women will ultimately depend on the recognition of their rights to social, educational, cultural, and economic equality. A first step in achieving this goal is the empowerment of women in addressing their own health issues.

Evidence that this comprehensive view of women's health is taking hold can be seen in grassroots-level organization, national-level interventions, and international health efforts taking place worldwide (FWCW 1995; WHO 1995, 1998; Broom 1998*a*; UN 2000). Nevertheless these efforts, to date, have not remedied the problem. Tackling the complex issues raised by the field of women's health requires collaboration across many sectors in society, not just the health sector. The challenge for public health is to involve all parties in negotiation. This includes, in particular, the women themselves because interventions designed without the participation of women are likely to be ill informed, inefficient, or poorly accepted.

References

Bird, C.E. and Rieker, P.P. (1999). Gender matters: an integrated model for understanding men's and women's health. *Social Science and Medicine*, **48**, 745–55.

Blair, A., Zahm, S.H., and Silverman, D.T. (1999). Occupational cancer among women: research status and methodologic considerations. *American Journal of Industrial Medicine*, **36**, 6–17.

Broom, D.H. (1998). By women, for women: the continuing appeal of women's health centres. *Women and Health*, **28**, 5–22.

Casas-Becerra, L. (1997). Women prosecuted and imprisoned for abortion in Chile. *Reproductive Health Matters*, **9**, 29–36.

Desjarlais, R., Eisenberg, L. Good, B., and Kleinman, A. (1995). *World mental health.* Oxford University Press, New York.

Feng, Z. (1998). Study on active life expectancy of elderly aged of sixty years and over in rural area in Henan Province, China. *Journal of Information on Preventive Medicine*, **14**, 72–75.

Fried, M.G. (1997). Abortion in US: barriers to access. *Reproductive Health Matters*, **9**, 37–45.

FWCW (Fourth World Conference on Women) (1995). *Beijing Declaration and Platform for Action: FWCW.* United Nations General Assembly Document A/Conf. 177/20, United Nations, New York.

Goldman, M.B. and Hatch, M.C. (2000). An overview of women and health. In *Women and health* (ed. M.B. Goldman and M.C. Hatch), pp. 5–14. Academic Press, New York.

Hardee, K., *et al.* (1999). Reproductive health policies and programs in eight countries: progress since Cairo. *International Family Planning Perspectives*, **25** (Supplement), S2–S9.

Haslegrave, M. (1995). A global perspective on women's health. Presented at the 55th World Congress of Pharmacy and Phamaceutical Sciences, Stockholm, Sweden.

Heise, L., Moore, K., and Toubia, N. (1995). *Sexual coercion and reproductive health. A focus on research.* Population Council, New York.

Henshaw, S.K., *et al.* (1999). The incidence of abortion worldwide. *International Family Planning Perspectives*, **25** (Supplement), S30–8.

ICPD (International Conference on Population and Development) (1994). *Programme of action of the ICPD.*, United Nations General Assembly Document A/171/13, United Nations, New York.

Izett, S. and Toubia, N. (2000). Female circumcision/female genital mutilation. In *Women and health* (ed. M.B. Goldman and M.C. Hatch), pp. 404–19. Academic Press, New York.

Jain, S.C., *et al.* (1999). Improving family planning program performance through management training. *Journal of Health and Population in Developing Countries*, **2**, 1–25.

Kessler, R.C. (2000). Gender and mood disorders. In *Women and health* (ed. M.B. Goldman and M.C. Hatch), pp. 997–1009. Academic Press, New York.

Kessler, R.C., McGonagle, K.A., Zhao, S., *et al.* (1994). Lifetime and 12-month prevalence of DSM-III-R psychiatric disorders in the United States. *Archives of General Psychiatry*, **51**, 8–19.

Leveille, S.G. and Furalnik, J.M. (2000). Morbidity, disability, and mortality. In *Women and health* (ed. M.B. Goldman and M.C. Hatch), pp. 1147–54. Academic Press, New York.

Li, V.C. and Wang, S. (1998). *Collaboration and participation: women's reproductive health of Yunnan, China.* Beijing Medical University Press.

Lindbohm, M. (1999). Women's reproductive health. Some recent developments in occupational epidemiology. *American Journal of Industrial Medicine*, **36**, 18–24.

Maine, D. and McGinn, T. (2000). Maternal mortality and morbidity. In *Women and health* (ed. M.B. Goldman and M.C. Hatch), pp. 395–403. Academic Press, New York.

Miller, F.A. and Downs, W.R. (2000). Violence against women. In *Women and health* (ed. M.B. Goldman and M.C. Hatch), pp. 529–40. Academic Press, New York.

Murray, J.L. and Lopez, A.D. (ed.) (1996). *Global burden of disease.* Harvard University Press, Boston, MA.

Nosek, M.A., *et al.* (1997). *National study of women with physical disabilities.* Center for Research on Women with Disabilities, Department of Physical Medicine and Rehabilitation, Baylor College of Medicine, Waco, TX.

Nowark, R. (1995). New push to reduce maternal mortality in poor countries. *Science*, **269**, 780–2.

Padian, N.S. (2000) Sexually transmitted diseases. In *Women and health* (ed. M.B. Goldman and M.C. Hatch), pp. 269–71. Academic Press, New York.

PATH (Program for Appropriate Technology in Health) (1999). *Improving women's sexual and reproductive health. Review of female genital eradication programs in Africa.* World Health Organization, Geneva.

Rahman, A., *et al.* (1998). A global review of laws on induced abortion 1985–1997. *International Family Planning Perspectives*, **24**, 56–64.

Robey, B., *et al.* (1996). Meeting unmet need: new strategies. *Population Reports*, Series J, No. 43.

Rohde, J.E. (1995). Removing risk from safe motherhood. *International Journal of Gynecology and Obstetrics*, **50** (Supplement 2), S3–10.

Rosenfield, A. and Maine, D. (1985). Maternal mortality—a neglected tragedy. Where is the M in MCH? *Lancet*, **ii**, 83–5.

Schuler, S.R., *et al.* (1995). Bangladesh family planning success story: a gender perspective. *International Family Planning Perspectives*, **21**, 132–7.

Seaman, G. and Wood, S.F. (2000). Role of advocacy groups in research on women's health. *Women and health* (ed. M.B. Goldman and M.C. Hatch), pp. 27–36. Academic Press, New York.

Silbergeld, E.K. (2000*a*). Environmental exposures. In *Women and health* (ed. M.B. Goldman and M.C. Hatch), pp. 599–600. Academic Press, New York.

Silbergeld, E.K. (2000*b*). The environment and women's health: an overview. In *Women and health* (ed. M.B. Goldman and M.C. Hatch), pp. 601–6. Academic Press, New York.

State Family Planning Commission (1998). *China family planning yearbook.* State Family Planning Commission of the People's Republic of China, Beijing.

State Family Planning Commission (1995). *China population statistics yearbook.* State Family Planning Commission of the People's Republic of China , Beijing.

State Statistical Bureau (1997). *China population statistics yearbook.* State Statistical Bureau of the People's Republic of China, Beijing.

State Statistical Bureau (1998). *China population statistics yearbook.* State Statistical Bureau of the People's Republic of China, Beijing.

Taylor, C.E., *et al.* (1985). Public health policies and strategies in China. In *The Oxford textbook of public health* (2nd edn), pp. 261–9. Oxford University Press.

UN (United Nations) (1995). *The world's women 1995: trends and statistics.* Social Statistics and Indicators, Series K, No. 12. United Nations, New York.

UN (United Nations) (1997). *Demographic yearbook of United Nations.* United Nations, New York.

UN (United Nations) (2000). *Africa recovery briefing paper.* http://www.un.org/ecosocdev/geninfo/afrec/bpaper/maineng.htm.

UNAIDS (1997). *Women and AIDS: point of view.* UNAIDS, Geneva.

UNAIDS (1999). *AIDS 5 years since ICPD emerging issues and challenges for women, young people and infants.* UNAIDS Discussion Document, UNAIDS, Geneva.

UNFPA (1997). *World population situation in 1997.* UNFPA, New York.

UNDP (United Nations Development Programme) (1995). *Human development report 1995.* UNDP, New York

UNICEF (United Nations Children's Fund) (1998). *The state of the world's children.* Oxford University Press.

Waldron, I. (1986). What do we know about the causes of sex differences in mortality? *Population Bulletin on the United Nations*, **18**, 59.

Waldron, I. (1995). Contributions of changing gender differentials in behavior to change gender differences in mortality. In *Men's health and illness: gender, power and the body* (ed. D. Sabo and D. Gordon). Sage, London.

Wang, S. and Li, V.C. (1994). *Women's voice from rural Yunnan: needs assessment of reproductive health.* Beijing Medical University Press.

WHO (World Health Organization) (1995). *Women's health: improve our health, improve our world.* WHO Position Paper, Fourth World Conference on Women, WHO, Geneva.

WHO (World Health Organization) (1997). *Violence against women, information pack.* WHO/FRH/WHD/97.8, WHO, Geneva.

WHO (World Health Organization) (1998*a*). *Sex, gender and health.* Technical Paper. WHO, Geneva.

WHO (World Health Organization) (1998*b*). *Unsafe abortion: global and regional estimates of incidence of mortality due to unsafe abortion, with a listing of available country data.* WHO/RHT/MSM/97.16, WHO, Geneva.

WHO (World Health Organization) (1998*c*). *WHO for safe motherhood.* WHO in the Western Pacific Region, WHO, Geneva.

WHO (World Health Organization) (1998*d*). *World health statistics annual 1996.* WHO, Geneva.

WHO (World Health Organization) (1998*e*). *Female genital mutilation.* WHO, Geneva.

WHO (World Health Organization) (2000). *Prevalence of violence against women by an intimate male partner.* http://www.who.int/violence_injury_prevention/pages/table_physicalviole.htm

World Bank (1994). *A new agenda for women's health and nutrition.* http://www.worldbank.org/html/extdr/hnp/health/newagenda/whn.htm

Yang, J. (1999). Analysis of death of suicide in child-bearing women in China. Unpublished research paper, Beijing Medical University.

11.3 Child health

Carol Bellamy

The situation of children in the world

There have been major strides made in improving child health since the call for 'Health for All by the Year 2000' was first declared at the joint World Health Organization (**WHO**) and the United Nations Children's Fund (**UNICEF**) meeting at Alma Ata in 1978 (WHO 1978). The period following the Declaration of Alma-Ata witnessed revolutionary gains in life expectancy. Among today's high-income countries, life expectancy has increased by 30 to 40 years in the twentieth century. These health gains have transformed quality of life and created conditions favouring sustained fertility reductions and consequent demographic change. In many developing countries, for example, according to the WHO, the total fertility rate—the expected number of children a woman will bear over her lifetime—declined from over six in the late 1950s to about three at present. Life expectancy in developing countries today is greater that it was in any developed country at the start of this century (Murray and Lopez 1996).

The 1980s saw an acceleration of large-scale health projects in developing countries, focusing on immunization, control of diarrhoeal diseases, acute respiratory infections, and nutrition interventions. In the 1990s, clear and ambitious goals were established to reduce infant and child mortality rates and improve the overall well being and status of children in developing countries. Compared with 1990, a million more children now survive annually beyond their fifth birthday, polio is on the verge of elimination, and routine immunization coverage has reduced measles deaths by 85 per cent and deaths associated with neonatal tetanus by two-thirds. Mental retardation is no longer a risk for an estimated 12 million children every year as increasing numbers of people routinely consume iodized salt as part of their diet. In many parts of the world, children's overall resistance to infectious diseases and debilitating illnesses has been strengthened through increasing vitamin A intake, and blindness related to vitamin A deficiency has declined sharply. Improved breast-feeding practices in numerous countries have increased the chances of survival, growth, and development of millions of children.

Yet, despite this progress, 12 million children under the age 5 years still die annually from easily preventable causes and some 200 million children still suffer from malnutrition. Deaths from communicable diseases are expected to climb from 28.1 million a year in 1990 to 49.7 million in 2020, an increase in absolute numbers of 77 per cent. According to recent studies on the burden of disease among the global poor, communicable diseases caused 59 per cent of the deaths and disability among the world's poorest 20 per cent. Among the world's richest 20 per cent, non-communicable diseases caused 85 per cent of death and disability (Gwatkin *et al.* 1999). Seven million children continue to die every year in developing countries from just four conditions: pneumonia, diarrhoeal diseases, measles, and malaria. Some 1.2 million children under 14 years old are living with HIV/AIDS, approximately 90 per cent of whom have become infected through mother-to-child transmission during late pregnancy, labour, childbirth, or breast feeding. In southern and eastern Africa, HIV/AIDS is the leading cause of death for children. The impact of AIDS in eroding the gains made in infant and child mortality rates in the past 20 years is a serious threat. At the end of 1999, 33.6 million people were living with HIV/AIDS, more than 95 of them in developing countries. HIV/AIDS is the leading cause of death in Africa where more that 23 million people have died. A major obstacle to combating AIDS is that many nations have been slow to acknowledge the extent of the epidemic, which has left millions of children orphaned, with significantly reduced life expectancies, swamped health care services, and crippled economies.

The burden of infectious diseases falls most heavily on people living in poverty. Certain diseases are re-emerging as epidemics such as meningococcal meningitis, dengue fever, and cholera. Nearly one-quarter of the world's population, 1.3 billion people, continue to live in absolute poverty, earning less than US$41 per day. The 1993 World Development Report *Investing in Health* estimated loss of healthy life from over 100 of the most common diseases and injuries. Of the total global disease burden, 93 per cent is concentrated in low- and middle-income countries. The *State of the World's Children's Report 2000* (UNICEF 1999*b*) noted that, in 1960, the income gap between the richest one-fifth of the world's population and the poorest one-fifth was 30:1; in 1997, the gap was 74:1.

Children in many nations continue to be victims of war—losing their parents and their homes, losing their childhood and their opportunity for education, losing their limbs and their lives to the machinery of violence. Conflict-induced disruption in the public health system due to lack of adequate services and trained personnel willing to work in areas of conflict can severely affect the community. Interruption of immunization services is one of the most serious consequences of a fractured health system. This leaves children susceptible to rapid onset of diseases such as measles, but also the destruction of medical equipment and records, and lack of provision of services, can severely disrupt communities. To try to reduce the devastation as a result of the complete disruption of services and the impact on children who grow up in such chaos and violence, it is essential to ensure that some semblance of order is returned to their lives.

In the new millennium, more effort needs to be made to develop sustainable approaches to improve child health to reduce both mortality and morbidity if we are to ensure that children not only survive but also grow in a healthy environment with access to basic essential services. This calls for a more integrated approach to tackling child health and ensuring that communities and families are more actively involved in improving the health of their children and empowering them to be able to assist in this process. With the threat that is presently posed by HIV/AIDS and the likelihood that the disease will negate the gains made in child survival in large parts of the world, it is essential to develop a more integrated approach to address major health concerns. The challenge for the next 20 years is to ensure that mothers and children have access to the best health services that are available. This should include access to essential drugs and supplies, vaccines against all immunizable diseases, attendance by well-trained health professionals, access to the most recent and up-to-date health information, and a well-equipped health facility at a reasonable distance from their homes.

The most important and often neglected determinant of whether a child grows well or not is the quality of child care. Whether we are concerned with how well and how frequently a young child is fed, or about the degree of stimulation and interaction with parents, or about disease prevention and domestic hygiene, or use of health services and regular growth monitoring, the issue to which we are constantly returning is how well the child is cared for.

Although greater involvement by fathers in all countries and cultures is one of the most fundamental priorities for improving the care and upbringing of children, it is in practice the mothers who are the principal providers of care. However, regardless of how much a mother may care for her children, it is nearly impossible for her to provide high-quality child care if she herself is poor and oppressed, illiterate and uninformed, anaemic and unhealthy, has five or six other children, lives in a slum or shanty town, has neither clean water nor safe sanitation, and is without the necessary support from health services, from her society, or from the father of her children. We are therefore talking as much about care of the mother as care by the child. The care that is provided to a mother can determine the quality of child care and therefore the health and nutritional well being of children.

For the foreseeable future, hundreds of millions of children will continue to fall ill and will continue to be brought to clinics and health centres throughout the developing world. It is how those clinics, health workers, and families respond that will largely determine whether childhood illnesses will continue to seriously affect poor communities. At the moment, many health centres in developing countries are failing those children. Many die from preventable or treatable diseases even after they have been brought to clinics. And many parents leave without essential drugs and advice on how to prevent or treat the conditions that threaten the life and normal growth of their children. At all levels of primary care, health workers are too often badly trained, poorly supervised, underpaid, or absent from their posts. Parents with sick children may have to queue for hours, only to receive peremptory treatment or be told that no drugs are available. Also, there is often a weak system of referral for those cases where more qualified care is needed. It may be that this is due to cuts in government spending, perhaps as a result of economic adjustment programmes. Whatever the cause, the result is that many families in the developing world are abandoning public health services in favour of private practitioners who, in many cases, offer them the most expensive instead of the most appropriate treatment. Here, the opportunity for making available today's effective, inexpensive treatments and provision of vital information and advice is lost. Without an improved response from health workers and health clinics throughout the poor world, it will not be possible to finish the job and bring the ordinary diseases of childhood under control.

About 80 per cent of all children are suffering from just one or more of five common conditions—diarrhoea, measles, respiratory infections, malaria, or malnutrition—for which the treatment is relatively inexpensive and the advice needed by parents is relatively straightforward. In addition to the continuing effort to prevent disease and to enable families themselves to protect their children's health, the great challenge of the years immediately ahead is ensuring that any family taking a child to a clinic or health centre anywhere in the developing world will find a health provider who can examine and diagnose, make a decision on appropriate treatment, give basic drugs for the most common problems, refer the child to hospital if needed, and offer the right advice about how best to prevent and manage illness in the home.

Development of the child

Evidence suggests that early investments in development of the child can bring improvements in the life of a child and provide benefits to the entire society. Cumulative research indicates that most rapid mental growth occurs during infancy and early childhood and that, on the whole, the early years are critical in the formation and development of intelligence, personality, and social behaviour (Bundy 1996). Scientific research indicates that, given the decisive influence of children's early stimulation on physical, psychological, and social development, primary school and kindergarten programmes (for children 4 to 5 years old) may be too late to counteract some physical, neurological, psychological, and social factors closely associated with early deprivation and lack of adequate stimulation.

Early childhood, here defined as from birth to 8 years, is a particularly crucial period (Bundy 1996) when physical and nutritional elements have their most profound consequences. During the later years of life, even where remediation is possible, the rate of improvement is reduced because of the relative slowing of subsequent development.

The importance of attention to the mother and to the well being of the family, including measures to increase the mother's capacity to look after her children, building upon existing customs, is essential for early child survival and development. Survival, growth, and psychosocial and cognitive development are three intimately intertwined processes directed toward the overall well being of the child (UNICEF 1998). These processes occur simultaneously and mutually affect each other. The care that is provided to a child—by families, within communities, and/or through services and institutions—affects each of the child development outcomes. Survival is intimately connected with growth and development. The better the child's quality of life (involving good health, growth, development, and active social participation), the greater the chances of her/his survival. The bigger and stronger the child, the more likely the child is to survive, enjoy good health, and develop well. Conversely, a child who is physically healthy and who is developing well mentally, emotionally, and socially is more likely to grow well because his or her food intake will be better.

Psychosocial and cognitive development is the beginning of a lifelong process of human development in which people (and children) learn to handle increasingly complex levels of moving, thinking, feeling, and relating to others. Such development involves moving from simple to complex and from dependent to autonomous behaviour. The more advanced the development of a child, the greater the potential of that child to participate actively in life's events and to become empowered to affect others and the world around her. Attention to a child's development in all its dimensions can help to increase survival and growth, even as it enhances development and the quality of life.

At a conceptual level, recognition is needed that fostering a child's development affects survival and growth. There is general acceptance that health and nutrition must go together in order to affect survival, growth, and physical development, but we must now learn to include psychosocial (as well as physical) development in the equation (Eming Young 1994).

The challenge from experience gained

The World Summit for Children

The largest ever gathering of world leaders was held for the World Summit for Children (**WSC**), at the United Nations Headquarters in September 1990. Seventy-one heads of state or government, together with delegations from an additional 88 countries, met to consider the situation of children around the world and to issue a world declaration for children. The World Declaration and Plan of Action established a vision of a 'first call' for children by establishing seven major and 21 supporting health goals that were quantifiable and considered achievable by the year 2000 (Tables 1 and 2).

Convention on the Rights of the Child

The most widely ratified human rights treaty in history is the 1989 Convention on the Rights of the Child. The General Assembly of the United Nations adopted the text of the United Nations Convention, without modifications, on 20 November 1989. It entered into force as international law on 2 September 1990 after its ratification by the required 20 states. Today it is the most widely ratified human rights treaty in the world with all but two countries having ratified. The Convention is the most universally accepted human rights instrument in history—it has been ratified by every country in the world except two—and therefore it uniquely places children at the centre in the quest for the universal application of human rights. By ratifying this instrument, national governments have committed themselves to protecting and ensuring children's rights and they have agreed to hold themselves accountable for this commitment before the international community.

Built on varied legal systems and cultural traditions, the Convention on the Rights of the Child is a universally agreed set of non-negotiable standards and obligations. It spells out the basic human rights that children everywhere—without discrimination—have. These are the right to survival; to develop to the fullest; to protection from harmful influences, abuse, and exploitation; and to participate fully in family, cultural, and social life. The Convention protects children's rights by setting standards in health care, education, and legal, civil, and social services. These standards are benchmarks against which progress can be assessed. States that are party to the Convention are obliged to develop and undertake all actions and policies in the light of the best interests of the child.

The 54 articles of the Convention can be divided into four main parts. The key principles of the Convention are:

Table 1 Major goals for child survival and protection

Between 1990 and 2000, reduction of the infant and child mortality rate in all countries by one-third or to 50 and 70 per live births respectively, whichever is less
Between 1990 and the year 2000, reduction of the maternal mortality rate by one-half
Between 1990 and the year 2000, reduction of severe and moderate malnutrition among children under 5 years of age by one-half
Universal access to safe drinking water and to sanitary means of excreta disposal
By the year 2000, universal access to basic education and achievement of primary education by at least 80 per cent of primary schoolchildren
Reduction of the adult illiteracy rate (the appropriate age group to be determined in each country) to at least one-half of its 1990 level, with an emphasis on female literacy
Improved protection of children in especially difficult circumstances

Box 1 Convention on the Rights of the Child

The Convention incorporates the full spectrum of human rights—civil, political, social, cultural, and economic—and the ways that these should be made available to children:

- The definition of children as all persons less than 18 years of age, unless the legal age of majority in a country is lower.
- Civil rights and freedoms, including the rights to a name and nationality; to freedom of expression, thought, and association; to access to information; and the right not to be subjected to torture.
- Family environment and alternative care, including the right to live with parents, to be reunited with parents if separated from them, and to the provision of appropriate alternative care where necessary.
- Basic health and welfare, including the rights of disabled children, the right to health and health care, social security, child-care services and an adequate standard of living.
- The right to education, the aims of education, and the rights to play, leisure, and participation in cultural life and the arts.
- Special protection measures covering the rights of refugee children, those caught up in armed conflicts, children in the juvenile justice system, children deprived of their liberty and children in the juvenile justice system, children deprived of their liberty, and children suffering economic, sexual, or other exploitation.

Table 2 Major supporting goals for child survival and protection

Women's health and education
Special attention to the health and nutrition of the female child and to pregnant and lactating women
Access by all couples to information and services to prevent pregnancies that are too early, too closely spaced, too late, or too many
Access by all pregnant women to prenatal care, trained attendants during childbirth, and referral facilities for high-risk pregnancies and obstetric emergencies
Universal access to primary education with special emphasis for girls and accelerated literacy programmes for women
Nutrition
Reduction in severe, as well as moderate, malnutrition among children under 5 years to half of 1990 levels
Reduction of the rate of low birth weight (2.5 kg or less) to less than 10 per cent
Reduction of iron deficiency anaemia in women by one-third of 1990 levels
Virtual elimination of iodine deficiency disorders
Virtual elimination of vitamin A deficiency and its consequences, including blindness
Empowerment of all women to breast feed their children exclusively for 4 to 6 months and to continue breast feeding, with complementary food, well into the second year
Growth promotion and its regular monitoring to be institutionalized in all countries by the end of the 1990s
Dissemination of knowledge and supporting services to increase food production to ensure household food security
Child health
Global eradication of poliomyelitis by the year 2000
Elimination of neonatal tetanus by 1995
Reduction by 95 per cent in measles deaths and reduction by 90 per cent in measles cases compared with preimmunization levels by 1995, as a major step to the global eradication of measles in the longer run
Maintenance of a high level of immunization coverage (at least 90 per cent of children under 1 year of age by the year 2000) against diphtheria, pertussis, tetanus, measles, poliomyelitis, tuberculosis, and against tetanus for women of child-bearing age
Reduction by 50 per cent in the deaths due to diarrhoea in children under the age of 5 years and 25 per cent reduction in the diarrhoea incidence rate
Reduction by one-third in the deaths due to acute respiratory infections in children under 5 years
Water and sanitation
Universal access to safe drinking water
Universal access to sanitary means of excreta disposal
Elimination of guinea-worm disease (dracontiasis) by the year 2000
Basic education
Expansion of early childhood development activities, including appropriate low-cost family- and community-based interventions
Universal access to basic education, and achievement of primary education by at least 80 per cent of primary schoolage children through formal schooling or non-formal education of comparable learning standard, with emphasis on reducing the current disparities between boys and girls
Reduction of the adult illiteracy rate (the appropriate age group to be determined in each country) to at least half its 1990 level, with emphasis on female literacy
Increased acquisition by individuals and families of the knowledge, skills, and values required for better living, made available through all educational channels, including the mass media, other forms of modern and traditional communication and social action, with effectiveness measured in terms of behavioural change
Children in difficult circumstances
Provide improved protection of children in especially difficult circumstances and tackle the root causes leading to such situations

- the right to survival and development
- respect for the best interests of the child as a primary consideration
- the right of the child to express his or her views freely
- the right of all children to enjoy the rights of the Convention without any discrimination.

The Convention has been a major catalyst to the development of a children's rights movement across the world. It has provided a shared vision of the fulfilment of children's rights that has been accepted everywhere. However, deepening poverty, proliferating conflicts, the impact of HIV/AIDS, and rampant discrimination and disparities have stalled progress and further pose serious challenges to the improvement of the well being of children and the realization of their rights. Ten years after the World Summit, we should ensure that future actions for children are based on the commitments, unfinished business, and lessons of the past decade.

Mobilizing support for children in the future

Global health actions for children need to focus more on the reduction of child mortality, morbidity, and disability through the prevention and treatment of disease and illness in a more integrated way. The overarching aim of development co-operation for children should be to break the chains of disadvantage, impoverishment, and failed human development through actions that converge to promote capacities at critical times in the life of the mother and child.

- In pregnancy, since women's special reproductive health needs, especially in pregnancy, and child birth, have to be met if they are to fulfil their roles, especially with regard to family responsibilities, child care, and development—and if their children are to be born capable of achieving their full potential.
- In infancy and early childhood, since food, health, care, socialization, stimulation, and education in the earliest years of a child's life lay the foundation for subsequent human capabilities and development.
- In early adolescence, since children at this age are innovative, energetic, and are already contributing significantly to the care and well being of their families and the life of their communities. Yet these are the years of childhood when millions of children are abandoned by the formal education system, have no recognized role or status, and are exposed to forms of violence, exploitation and high-risk behaviours that threaten both their own lives and the lives of others. And these are the years that heavily influence when and how well they will assume their responsibilities as the next generation of adults and parents.

At the operational level, through programmes of co-operation, the world needs to continue to focus on protecting children from various forms of preventable death. In addition, it should place new emphasis on developing policies, institutional capacities, and social practices that will enable poor children to have access to further opportunities and to overcome barriers to their healthy growth, emotional well being, and intellectual development.

Reduction in child mortality and morbidity

The world's poorest populations live in the shadow of a group of old enemies—malnutrition, childhood infections, poor maternal and perinatal health, and high fertility. Approximately 65 per cent of all child deaths are from three causes (WHO 1999*c*).

- Acute respiratory tract infection now kills 3.6 million children each year.
- Diarrhoeal diseases are responsible for 3 million child deaths every year.
- Immunization-preventable diseases: measles, tuberculosis, tetanus, diphtheria, polio, and pertussis are responsible for some 2.1 million child deaths every year. Of these, almost 1 million are attributed to measles.

Two hundred million children under the age of 5 years still suffer from malnutrition. Every year 7.5 million children die during the perinatal period, primarily due to poor maternal health care, and 30 per cent of the world is still without safe water and sanitation. One in every 48 women dies from pregnancy-related causes in low- and middle-income countries (585 000 deaths per year) compared with 1 in 4000 in higher-income countries (UNICEF 2000).

Early childhood exposure to undernutrition, micronutrient malnutrition (iron, iodine, vitamin A), or infection (diarrhoea, malaria) often results in long-term or irreversible retardation of physical and cognitive development. These conditions are particularly devastating to the poor, whose children enter adulthood and the workforce handicapped by early life experiences.

Effective large-scale health interventions, such as immunization, the use of oral rehydration for treatment of diarrhoea, and early recognition and proper case management for pneumonia, have had a greater impact on mortality in the age group 1 to 4 years than in the first year of life. The number of deaths due to neonatal tetanus has been cut by a third since 1990, and measles as well as polio cases by over 80 per cent. The replacement and transport of cold-chain supplies and the purchase of vaccines are becoming more difficult due do the current economic crises in many countries. In countries with weak health systems, the Extended Programme for Immunization coverage is not very stable and is dependent on outreach, mobile teams, and conducting national immunization days. Measles epidemics still occur in most countries outside South America, despite high coverage rates. Routine reporting of measles cases is still weak in many countries, making accurate assessment of progress very difficult. Elimination of neonatal tetanus is constrained by low tetanus toxoid coverage in some countries such as China. Child mortality due to diarrhoeal dehydration has globally been reduced by about 25 per cent, but in many countries and also in marginal groups within low-income countries, diarrhoea, acute respiratory infections, and malaria still cause high numbers of deaths in children under 5 years old.

Protein-energy malnutrition affects 30 per cent of children globally, which amounts to more than 160 million children. The vast majority of these children are found in Asia. South Asia has the highest level (nearly 50 per cent) followed by East Asia and Africa each having levels of around 30 per cent in their children under 5 years of age. China displays large differences between geographical areas and population groups. In Asia the levels of malnutrition are generally decreasing, and severe malnutrition is becoming rare. However, the rate of improvement is slow and does not match the corresponding rates of global economic development. In Africa the reported rates are actually increasing.

Levels of maternal malnutrition (chronic energy deficiency) are also very high but show large variations. Incidence of low birth weight is equally significant suggesting a close relationship between maternal health and nutrition factors and infant and child malnutrition. The promotion and certification of 'baby friendly' hospitals advocating for improved breast-feeding practices has continued successfully in some countries. Despite very high rates for initiating breast feeding, exclusive breast-feeding rates remain low in many countries. Many countries have improved their high vitamin A supplementation coverage rates, especially of young children, often to over 90 per cent. Despite the capacity to iodize all edible salt in most countries, the key remaining challenge is to ensure that iodized salt is used by families in a sustainable way and to monitor the quality of iodization.

Immunization

Although vaccines are one of the most cost-effective ways in which to reduce child mortality, many children in the poor areas of the world do not have access to childhood vaccines. In some countries, only 30 per cent of children may be vaccinated (Fig. 1). Even fewer children

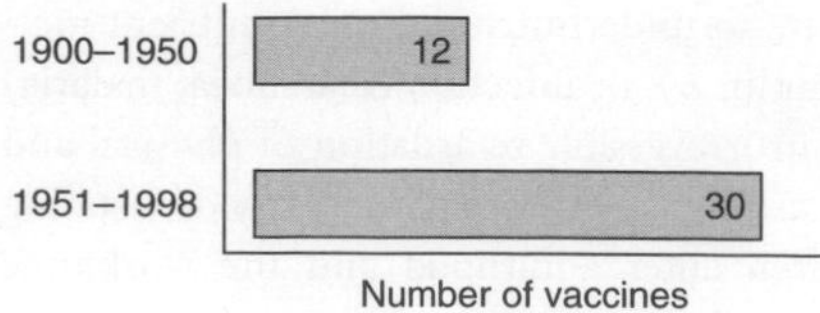

Fig. 1 Vaccines licensed since 1900.

have access to the recently licensed and expensive vaccines that are likely to have a major additional impact on decreasing child mortality such as vaccine for *Haemophilus influenzae* type B. This type has been shown to be a major cause of bacterial pneumonia in children and a significant cause of childhood meningitis. It is estimated to cause at least 3 million cases of serious disease and 400 000 to 700 000 deaths worldwide each year, in young children (WHO 1998).

Immunization has been one of the greatest public health success stories. Between 1980 and 1990, a massive effort raised coverage rates worldwide from 5 to 80 per cent. Deaths from six major childhood diseases (measles, tetanus, whooping cough, tuberculosis, polio, and diphtheria) have been slashed by 3 million a year. At least 750 000 fewer children are left blind, paralysed, or mentally disabled. Due to a successful global eradication campaign, polio is expected to follow smallpox into extinction by the year 2005, eliminating the need for vaccination and saving the governments of the world US$1.5 billion in vaccines, treatment, and rehabilitation costs every year. The campaign against polio has not only reduced the threat of the disease, but has also galvanized political commitment, brought in extra funding, and has increased awareness of the importance of routine immunization and other basic child health measures. For instance, countries are using National Immunization Days as an opportunity to distribute vitamin A supplements widely. Immunization and high-quality surveillance need to continue for a number of years after the last polio case has been detected before a region, and then eventually the world, is certified free of polio, and viruses are contained. The target date for certification of the world as polio free is 2005.

However, despite the low cost of the existing immunization package, many of the world's poorest children are not being reached, especially in sub-Saharan Africa. Many developing countries made spectacular progress throughout the 1980s but are finding it difficult to keep the momentum and to go the extra mile needed to reach the remaining children.

The Children's Vaccine Initiative, launched in 1990 (Fig. 2), aimed to improve the world's supply of existing vaccines. It was the idea of five sponsoring agencies: WHO, UNICEF, UNDP, the Rockefeller Foundation, and the World Bank. The initiative stimulated a global dialogue among governments, donors, and vaccine manufacturers, researchers, and immunization programme managers. The initiative encouraged governments to assume responsibility for their own vaccine needs. Many developing countries now procure more than half the vaccines used for national immunization programmes.

Newer vaccines, such as those for hepatitis B, *Haemophilus influenzae* type B, and yellow fever are now widely used in developed countries. While children in developing countries may have access to six or seven vaccines, children in industrialized countries can now expect to receive 11 or 12. Thus the gap between rich and poor children is widening.

In 1999, the Global Alliance for Vaccines and Immunization (**GAVI**) was formed. Members of GAVI include the WHO, UNICEF, the World Bank, representatives from bilateral agencies, the Rockefeller Foundation, the Bill and Melinda Gates Children's Vaccine Programme, and representatives from industry. The aim is to go beyond the goals of the Children's Vaccine Initiative to provide support to the poorest countries for the introduction of new vaccines and stimulate the necessary research and finance for the development of new vaccines. GAVI has established five strategic objectives: improve access to sustainable immunization services; expand the use

Box 2 World Summit for Children Goals for Immunization

The World Summit for Children set an end 1999 goal of achieving 90 per cent immunization coverage for children under 1 year of age against the six major child hood diseases as well as against tetanus for women of child-bearing age. The mid-decade goal of 80 per cent coverage has been reached and sustained. About 89 countries had achieved the end 1999 goal of 90 per cent by 1995. While overall coverage rates have been good, there is wide disparity between countries and several sub-Saharan countries have coverage rates below 50 per cent. Lessons learned include the following.

- Immunization efforts were sustained where there was planning and implementation at the local level with active support from national and subnational programme managers.
- The efforts made in the late 1980s to reach universal childhood immunization (UCI) goals led to coverage in the 1990s being at a much higher level than it would have been without such a global effort.
- Effective partnerships were developed between public and private sectors, between non-governmental organizations and governments as well as donors, and these were instrumental in raising the programme profile and committing everyone to a common outcome.
- The immunization programme strengthened primary health care programmes in many countries and became the vehicle for providing further child health interventions.

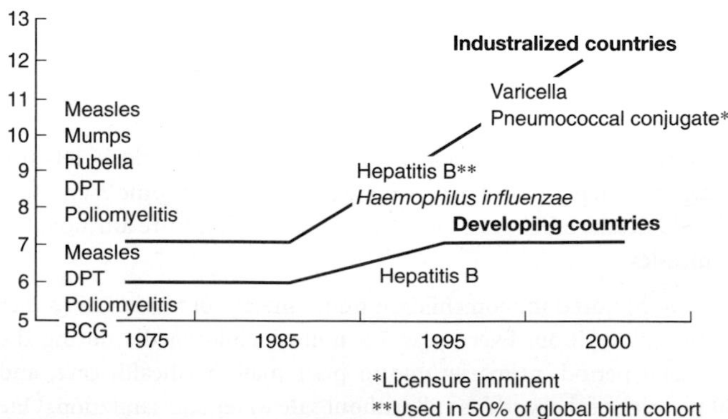

Fig. 2 The widening gap immunization gap: number of vaccines used in industrialized and developing countries (GAVI 2000).

Box 3 Global Alliance of Vaccines and Immunization (GAVI) milestones, 2000

During 2000, GAVI presented an analysis of current market and policy failures concerning levels of research, development, and commercialization of candidate vaccines for HIV/AIDS, malaria, and tuberculosis and made recommendations to overcome these problems

- By 2005, 80 per cent of developing countries will have routine immunization coverage of at least 80 per cent in all districts
- By 2002, 80 per cent of all countries with adequate delivery system will introduce hepatitis B vaccine and all countries by 2007
- By 2005, 50 per cent of the poorest countries with a high burden of disease and adequate delivery systems will have introduced *Haemophilus influenzae* type B vaccine

of all existing, safe, and cost-effective vaccines where they address a public health problem; accelerate the development and introduction of new vaccines and technologies; accelerate research and development efforts for vaccines needed primarily in developing countries; make immunization coverage a centrepiece in development efforts.

Strengthening of immunization services—as part of a comprehensive strategy to reduce child mortality and morbidity—will continue to play a major role in the promotion of early childhood care for child survival, growth, and development. However, governments need to ensure that strategies for immunization are informed by the lessons learned from the successes and shortcomings of programmes in the 1980s and 1990s, and are designed to contribute to strengthening health systems and overall health reform processes. It is also essential to ensure that immunization services are integrated with other important interventions such as improved breast-feeding practices, provision of micronutrients, and control of infectious diseases.

Prevention and treatment of communicable diseases

Until sufficient high-quality vaccines are available to protect against all major fatal diseases, countries must continue to exert efforts to prevent and treat communicable diseases seriously affecting children such as HIV/AIDS, malaria, diarrhoeal diseases, acute respiratory infections, and tuberculosis.

HIV/AIDS (see also Chapter 9.14)

HIV/AIDS is today the world's most rapidly spreading infectious disease for which science still has no cure. HIV/AIDS has reversed the survival, health, and wider human development gains of many countries and will continue to negatively affect all aspects of community life and children's well being in the regions most heavily affected for decades to come. Some 5.8 million people are newly infected each year. Nearly 12 million children have already been orphaned, mostly in Africa, and 50 per cent of all new infections are among young people aged 10 to 24 years. By the end of 1999, 33.6 million people worldwide were living with HIV, a 10 per cent increase over just a year before. According to UNAIDS/WHO estimates (UNAIDS/WHO 1999), 11 men, women, and children around the world were infected per minute during 1998, or 16 000 a day and close to 6 million people in all. Almost half of the new infections were in young people aged 15 to 24 years, and the epidemic is increasingly affecting women, young people, and children. Ninety-five per cent of HIV infections occur in developing countries.

In 1998, 43 per cent of all people over 15 years of age living with HIV/AIDS were women, up from 41 per cent the previous year. Mortality in infants and children under 5 years of age is expected to increase exponentially in the worst affected countries over the next years. Nearly 4.5 million children below the age of 15 years have been infected with HIV since the AIDS epidemic began, and more than 3 million of them have already died of AIDS. Today, on a global scale, children are becoming infected at about the rate of one child every minute of every day. In 1998, one in ten of all new infections was a child, and the vast majority of them acquired the virus from their infected mothers. Though Africa accounts for only 10 per cent of the world's population, it is home to 90 per cent of the world's HIV-infected children, largely as a consequence of high fertility rates combined with very high levels of HIV infection among women. However, the number of cases in India, China, and South-East Asia is rising rapidly.

The effects of the epidemic among young children are serious and far-reaching. AIDS threatens to reverse years of steady progress in child survival achieved through such measures as the promotion of breast feeding, immunization, and oral rehydration. UNAIDS believes that, by the year 2010, AIDS may have increased mortality of children under 5 years of age by more than 100 per cent in regions most affected by the virus. In Harare, Zimbabwe, for example, the death rate among infants in their first year of life increased from 30 to 60 per 1000 between 1990 and 1996. Deaths among 1 to 5 year olds, the age group in which the bulk of child AIDS-related deaths are concentrated, rose even more sharply—from eight to 20 per 1000—in the same period. In a growing number of countries, AIDS is now the greatest single cause of child death.

Mother-to-child transmission is by far the largest source of HIV infection in children below the age of 15 years (De Cock *et al.* 2000). In countries where blood for transfusion and blood products are regularly screened, and where clean syringes and needles are widely available in health centres and hospitals, mother-to-child transmission is virtually the only source of infection in young children. Therefore the extremely high rate of HIV infection among women of child-bearing age in some parts of the world—and the increasing risk of infection among women everywhere—is doubly concerning.

According to data from UNAIDS, there are very few places outside sub-Saharan Africa in which the prevalence of HIV infection among pregnant women has reached 10 per cent, let alone the extremely high figures seen in this region. However, this is partly because the epidemic in other badly affected countries is younger and less advanced than in sub-Saharan Africa.

The virus is spreading fastest among young people below the age of 24 years—at the peak of fertility. In places where the virus is spread predominantly through heterosexual intercourse—notably sub-Saharan Africa—young women outnumber young men among those becoming infected. Studies sponsored by UNAIDS show that in western Kenya nearly one girl in four between the ages of 15 and 19 years is living with HIV compared with one in 25 boys in the same age group. In Zambia in this age range, 16 times as many girls as boys are infected. Among 20- to 24-year-olds in rural Uganda, there are six young women who are HIV positive for every infected young man. It is these high rates of infection, coupled with high rates of pregnancy among women, that explain why Africa is also currently home to the vast majority of HIV-positive children.

The virus may be transmitted during pregnancy, childbirth, or breast feeding. Where no preventive measures are taken, the risk of a baby acquiring the virus from an infected mother ranges from 15 to 25 per cent in industrialized countries (most estimates are below 20 per cent), and from 25 to 45 per cent in developing countries (most estimates are between 30 and 35 per cent) (De Cock *et al.* 2000). Evidence suggests that the risk of transmission increases when the mother has a higher viral load (this is the case when a person is newly infected with HIV or is in an advanced stage of disease), or if the baby is highly exposed to the mother's infected body fluids during birth.

The difference in risk between developing and developed countries is due largely to feeding practices. Breast feeding is more common and usually practised for a longer period in developing countries than in the industrialized world. It is estimated that a child born uninfected to an HIV-positive mother has a 20 per cent chance of acquiring the virus from her milk if he or she is breast fed. In places where breast feeding is the norm, this route may account for more than one-third of mother-to-child transmissions of the virus.

Since there is a possibility of transmitting HIV through breast feeding, replacement feeding is an option for mothers. If an HIV-infected mother has access to an adequate supply of breast-milk substitutes, knows how to use them, has access to fuel and clean water, and the time to prepare breast-milk substitutes safely, refraining from breast feeding will reduce the risk of transmitting HIV through breast feeding. In countries where families live in poverty, have limited education, and poor access to the resources required to provide safe feeding alternatives to breast feeding, including counselling, the risk of death from diarrhoea, respiratory, and other infections associated with replacement feeding can be as great or greater than the risk of transmitting HIV through breast feeding.

Even if a mother has the means to feed her baby safely with a breast-milk substitute, she may face other dilemmas. In cultures where breast feeding is the norm, the very fact that she chooses not to breast feed may draw attention to her HIV status and invite discrimination or even violence and abandonment by her family and community.

In August 1997, the WHO, UNICEF, and UNAIDS issued a Joint Policy Statement on HIV and infant feeding. They subsequently prepared guidelines to help national authorities to implement the policy. These documents emphasize that it is the individual mother's right to decide how she will feed her child. The responsibility of health or social work professionals, who counsel HIV-positive women about infant feeding, is to give them the fullest available information on the risks associated with breast feeding. They should discuss breast feeding's feasibility and alternative feeding methods in the light of personal circumstances and give appropriate support to these women, for the course of action they choose. Women should have easy access to voluntary and confidential counselling and testing for HIV. Since the majority of pregnant and lactating women attending clinics are likely to be HIV negative, information on how to protect themselves from infection is also a vital component of routine care.

Breast feeding has been the cornerstone of child health and survival strategies for the past two decades and has played a pivotal role in reducing infant mortality in many countries. Even in the era of AIDS, breast feeding remains the best possible nutrition for the great majority of babies and it is important that the practice by women who are HIV negative or whose HIV status is unknown continues actively to be promoted, protected, and supported.

The recent study conducted in South Africa by Coutsoudis *et al.* (1999) suggested that children of HIV-infected mothers who are exclusively breast fed in their first 3 months of life are at no greater risk of contracting HIV than children fed solely on breast-milk substitutes. The Coutsoudis study looked at infant feeding in 549 women for 3 months after birth. At 3 months, there was no significant difference between the proportion of infants who became infected between the group which received any breast feeding (21.3 per cent) and those who were never breast fed (18.8 per cent). When the breast-fed group was divided according to whether the breast feeding was exclusive or partial, the infants who were exclusively breast fed from birth to 3 months had a significantly lower rate of infection (14.6 per cent) than those who received partial breast feeding along with other drinks or foods. Most of the experts that UNICEF has consulted regarding this study concede that it is very important, and that it certainly gives an indication that exclusive breast feeding may be protective. They caution, however, that because of limitations in the study design, notably the danger that the group of women who exclusively breast fed were not strictly comparable to the women who used formula, further studies are needed before the present policy adopted by the WHO, UNAIDS, and UNICEF is changed.

There are three complementary strategies for preventing mother-to-child transmission of HIV.

- The protection of children and women from HIV infection. This will minimize the risk that women of child-bearing age are carrying the virus in the first place. The strategy is sometimes referred to as 'primary prevention'. It involves promoting safe and responsible sexual behaviour in couples, providing them with knowledge about HIV/AIDS and how to prevent infection. It also means providing good-quality user-friendly prevention and treatment programmes for other sexually transmitted diseases, the presence of which increases the risk of HIV transmission up to 10-fold. Crucially, it means taking steps to deal with the cultural, legal, and economic factors that make girls and women especially vulnerable to HIV infection by limiting their autonomy and power to protect themselves.
- The provision of efficient and accessible family planning services to enable women to avoid unwanted pregnancies and births. The aim is to ensure informed reproductive choice.
- An integrated package of measures consisting of voluntary and confidential HIV counselling and testing, the provision of antiretroviral drugs for HIV-positive pregnant women (and sometimes their babies), counselling on infant feeding, and support for the feeding method(s) chosen by the mother. This package is often referred to as the antiretroviral drug strategy.

Until recently primary prevention measures and the provision of family planning were virtually the only options for limiting the number of HIV-infected children. However, in 1994, researchers in France and the United States reported the results of a major collaborative study (Connor *et al.* 1994) of mother-to-child transmission of HIV that offers a complementary strategy for HIV-positive women who want to give birth. The scientists found that when the antiretroviral drug zidovudine is given to HIV-positive women orally five times daily from the 14th week of pregnancy onwards, and intravenously during labour, and administered to their infants for 6 weeks after birth, the risk of transmitting HIV from mother to child is reduced by over two-thirds if breast feeding is avoided. However, the regimen is costly (approximately US$1000 per mother and child pair), and it is long and complicated to administer, which means that it is unsuitable for widespread use in developing countries.

Early in 1998, trials in Thailand sponsored by the country's Ministry of Public Health and the US Centres for Disease Control and Prevention (Shaffer *et al.* 1999) showed that a shorter and simpler course of zidovudine is able to cut the rate of mother-to-child transmission of HIV by at least half if the baby is not breast fed. The infection rate was just above 9 per cent compared with a rate of 19 per cent for babies of infected mothers who did not take antiretrovirals, but who also avoided breast feeding.

A study sponsored by the HIV Prevention Trials Network, supported through the American government, was conducted in Uganda to investigate the effectiveness of oral nevirapine and oral zidovudine administered to pregnant HIV-infected women during labour and to their infants during the first week of life (Guay *et al.* 1999). The study measured the number of new HIV infections in the infant. At 6 to 8 weeks of age, 11.9 per cent of infants in the nevirapine group were HIV infected compared with 21.3 per cent of infants in the zidovudine group. At 14 to 16 weeks of age, 13 per cent of infants in the nevirapine group were infected compared with 25 per cent in the zidovudine group. Ninety-five per cent of infants were breast fed to 14 weeks or longer.

The results of the study indicate that nevirapine is a low-cost drug that can achieve a superior reduction of transmission with only a single dose to the mother and a single dose to the baby within 3 days of birth. The nevirapine regimen costs around US$4 for each mother and child, and the drug can be easily stored in hot climates. Long-term follow-up of both the mothers and babies remain a high priority to assess any late drug toxicities as well as long-term survival (NIH 1999).

Box 4 Zambia needs more help to tackle HIV/AIDS

- Zambia, like its neighbours in sub-Saharan Africa, is grappling to cope with the devastating impact of the HIV/AIDS pandemic. It is estimated that one in five adults in Zambia is HIV positive and that by 1997, there were already 360 000 children under the age of 15 years who had lost their mother or both their parents to AIDS. The number of orphans is likely to increase, as more parents become ill and die
- A country already crippled by poverty and debt, Zambia is facing overwhelming challenges, as a generation of young people prepare to grow up without the love and support of their parents. Furthermore, many children experience the pain of watching their parents die one after the other. Although the majority of orphans are still being absorbed by the extended family, the number of children living or working on the streets is estimated at more than 90 000 and growing. UNICEF is working with the Zambian Government and non-governmental organizations to tackle the crisis. Efforts are underway to develop policies and strategies to increase the ability to cope with the disease. But preventing the further spread of HIV/AIDS and finding sustainable support for these children requires a dramatic increase in resources and political will from the international community

Programming needs to focus more on increasing youth participation in decision-making, promoting their rights and access to appropriate information and services, and creating supportive environments to reduce risk and vulnerability to HIV/AIDS. Voluntary and confidential counselling and testing are key elements in HIV prevention programmes targeting young people, and are services to which young people have a right to regular access. A number of priority actions are recommended for improving and accelerating the use of HIV counselling and testing with young people in the region, including improving understanding of the impact of HIV/AIDS on young people and expanding key services.

It is important to focus on identifying approaches that enable orphans with AIDS to remain within the community, especially approaches that strengthen families' capacity to cope and to find alternative models of care. Particular emphasis should be given to monitoring the impact of HIV/AIDS by identifying vulnerable children and improving orphan registration schemes, ensuring that children and families have access to essential health and social services, and co-ordinating the efforts of local organizations to provide practical support to children affected by AIDS.

Many countries, especially in Africa, are supporting the development of life skills and health education curricula, training of teachers and the production of materials for children with HIV/AIDS and children from families affected by HIV/AIDS, and to ensure that pregnant schoolgirls remain in school in a safe non-discriminatory environment. It becomes increasingly important to understand the socioculturally constructed gender roles of men and women in order to combat the causes and consequences of HIV/AIDS.

Communication is a critical tool for strengthening HIV/AIDS prevention and care, tackling stigma and discrimination, and addressing the social and cultural norms that influence sexual behaviour. Communication programming includes policy dialogue at global and national levels, to 'break the conspiracy of silence', emphasize the concerns of children, youth and women, and promote the rights of children and young people.

Malaria

This formidable tropical parasitic disease kills at least a million people annually, three-quarters of them children. Between 300 million and 500 million people suffer acute episodes of malaria in 100 developing countries each year. Of the more than a million people who die of malaria-related causes each year, 90 per cent are in Africa. This is a disease that is a major factor in Africa's high rate of infant and maternal mortality, the single largest cause of low birth weight among newborns, and the leading cause of school absenteeism, as well as low productivity in farming and other industries. The spread of chloroquine resistance in many countries, especially in Africa, has diminished the effectiveness of treatment with the most widely used drug leading to the risk of persistent parasitaemia and anaemia in young children (Shapira *et al.* 1993).

Malaria during pregnancy is a major public health problem in endemic areas, where pregnant women are the main adult risk group. *Plasmodium falciparium* infection during pregnancy has adverse health consequences for both the mother and her newborn. Non-immune pregnant women are at increased risk of severe malaria and death, spontaneous abortions, and stillbirths. In highly endemic areas where adults have a relatively high level of acquired antimalarial immunity, the risk of malaria is greatest during first and second pregnancies, with a gradual decrease in risk with subsequent pregnancies except in the presence of HIV infection. In these areas, malaria infection contributes to (severe) anaemia during pregnancy, putting the woman at risk of haemorrhage and death. Maternal anaemia and *P. falciparum* infection of the placenta increase the risk of low birth weight, the single greatest risk factor for neonatal mortality. Malaria in Africa is estimated to cause up to 15 per cent of maternal anaemia and 35 per cent of preventable low birth weight. HIV-infected pregnant women suffer from higher malaria parasite prevalence and densities at all parities, and infant mortality is increased. More detailed discussion of malaria in pregnancy can be found in Brabin (1991), Menendez (1995), Steketee *et al.* (1996), Nahlen (2000), USAID (2000), and WHO (2000*b*), and in *Annals of Tropical Medicine and Parasitology*, Vol. 93, Supplement 1, 1999.

For children, wherever malaria is common and access to diagnostic facilities scarce, it is important to treat any fever as if it were malaria. A full course of a recommended antimalarial drug should be given to the child immediately, even if the fever disappears rapidly. If treatment is not completed, malaria could recur and become more difficult to treat. Children with severe malaria symptoms such as fever or convulsions should be taken to a health facility as their case may be becoming complicated and they should be given extra liquids and food. Someone suffering from malaria should have prompt access to correct and affordable treatment within 8 hours of the onset of symptoms and should have access to a well-supplied and properly functioning health centre. Where this is not possible, governments will need to balance carefully the benefits against the risks of making good first-line malaria treatment readily available through shops or community organizations, which may be more accessible and less likely to run out of supplies.

Several field trials have evaluated the effectiveness of bed nets as a malaria prevention strategy. A meta-analysis of published reports of field trials that measured the incidence of infections was performed to provide a measure of the effectiveness of insecticide-treated bednets in preventing clinical malaria. Subset analyses were performed on 10 field trials to calculate pooled incidence rate ratios of infection among the study groups. The results showed that insecticide-impregnated bednets are effective in preventing malaria, decreasing the incidence rate ratio by approximately 50 per cent in field trails performed to date (Choi *et al.* 1995).

The WHO standard protocol was developed specifically for the testing of the therapeutic efficacy of antimalarial drugs against clinical infections with *P. falciparum* in infants and young children in areas of intense transmission (WHO 1996). It is based on the practical evaluation of a draft protocol, carried out in May 1996 by an international group of malaria workers in a district of Tanzania through a consensus of participants of meetings, intercountry workshops, and of several international malaria experts. It should be applied wherever a drug policy needs to be developed or revised with the intention of effective implementation and evaluation, and it implies the availability of appropriate antimalarial drugs at all levels of the health care system.

The impact of HIV/AIDS has compounded the crisis of malaria. Malaria affects most of the same desperately poor countries that are also reeling from the HIV/AIDS pandemic. Indeed, in many ways, Africa's future development is inextricably linked to the success of malaria and HIV/AIDS prevention and control. Malaria is a disease of poverty. It afflicts primarily the poor, who tend to live in malaria-prone areas, in dwellings that offer few, if any, barriers against mosquitoes. By sapping peoples' health, strength, and productivity, malaria generates still more poverty.

There is also a growing consensus on the need to expand malaria prevention and treatment programmes beyond the health infrastructure into communities and homes. The Roll Back Malaria Initiative, led by the WHO, the UNDP, the World Bank, and UNICEF, emphasizes the importance of forming strong partnerships—an objective to which UNICEF is committed. In recent years, there has been increasing involvement by a wider range of sector ministries and non-governmental and community organizations—and the pledging of more national and international financial resources.

Governments are helping by encouraging the commercial sector to make quality nets and insecticide more affordable and more available. They do this through a combination of incentives, such as exempting materials and manufacturing equipment from taxes and import duties, through tax credits for industries that wish to expand, and by creating demand for nets and insecticide through effective communication strategies.

Diarrhoea

Despite many advances, diarrhoeal diseases and the resulting dehydration continue to be responsible for 3 million child deaths every year. Approximately 50 per cent of these deaths are due to watery diarrhoea (WHO 1999*a*). This occurs either because of lack of access to oral rehydration solution and/or health facilities, or because of incorrect case management (home or health facility). Persistent diarrhoea (approximately 35 per cent) and dysentery (approximately 15 per cent) account for the remainder. While there are numerous diarrhoea-causing organisms, studies have shown that there are five organisms (WHO 1999*a*) primarily responsible: rotavirus was shown to be the only frequently isolated viral enteropathogen, *Escherichia coli*, *Shigella*, and *Campylobacter jejuni* were the most frequently isolated bacteria, and *Cryptosporidium* was the most frequent protozoan cause of diarrhoea.

It is most practical to base treatment of diarrhoea on the clinical type of the illness, which can easily be determined when a child is first examined. Laboratory studies are not needed. Four clinical types of diarrhoea can be recognized, each reflecting the basic underlying pathology and altered physiology (WHO 1999*a*).

- Acute watery diarrhoea (including cholera) which lasts for several hours or days: the main danger is dehydration; weight loss also occurs if feeding is not continued.
- Acute bloody diarrhoea, which is also called dysentery: the main dangers are intestinal damage, sepsis, and malnutrition; other complications, including dehydration, may also occur.
- Persistent diarrhoea which lasts 14 days or longer: the main danger is malnutrition and serious non-intestinal infection; dehydration may also occur.
- Diarrhoea with severe malnutrition (marasmus or kwashiorkor): the main dangers are severe systemic infection, dehydration, heart failure, and vitamin and mineral deficiency.

Diarrhoea is the passage of watery stools, usually more than three times in a 24-h period. However, it is the consistency of the stools rather than the number that is most important. Frequent passing of formed stools is not diarrhoea. Babies fed only breast milk often pass loose 'pasty' stools; this also is not diarrhoea. Mothers usually know when their children have diarrhoea and may provide useful working definitions in local situations. The management of each type of diarrhoea should prevent or treat the main danger(s) that each presents. Diarrhoea causes rapid depletion of water and sodium—both of which are necessary for life. If the water and salts are not replaced fast, the body starts to 'dry up' or become dehydrated. If more than 10 per cent of the body's fluid is lost, death occurs.

Diarrhoea can be prevented by pursuing multisectoral efforts: improving access to clean water and safe sanitation, promoting hygiene education, exclusive breast feeding, improved complementary feeding practices, immunizing all children especially against measles, using latrines, keeping food and water clean, washing hands with soap before touching food, and sanitary disposal of stools. The common thread that links these infectious diseases is the nutrition of the mother and child. Malnutrition predisposes children to disease, and diseases often result in worse nutritional status, and consequently a vicious circle of cause and effect is established.

Acute respiratory infections

Most children have about four to eight acute respiratory infections each year. Children with respiratory infections account for a large proportion of patients seen by health workers in health centres. These infections tend to be even more frequent in urban communities than in rural areas. Respiratory infections are infections in any area of the respiratory tract, including the nose, middle ear, throat (pharynx), voice box (larnyx, windpipe, trachea), air passages (bronchi or bronchioles), and lungs. Many areas of the respiratory tract can be involved, and there can be a wide variety of signs and symptoms of infection. These include cough, difficult breathing, sore throats, runny nose, and ear problems. Fever is also common in acute respiratory infections. Fortunately, most children with these respiratory symptoms have only a mild infection, such as a cold or bronchitis (WHO 1995).

A systematic and comprehensive study was carried out from 1991 to 1995 to identify interventions likely to be effective, feasible, and affordable for the prevention of childhood pneumonia. This study was also conducted in collaboration with the London School of Hygiene and Tropical Medicine, building on the methodological experience gained earlier (Kirkwood *et al.* 1995). Four interventions were found to be highly effective: reducing the prevalence of underweight and low birth weight, increasing measles immunization coverage, increasing breast feeding, and reducing indoor pollution. Improved breast-feeding practices are considered effective for prevention of childhood pneumonia. Breast feeding has long been believed to protect against acute respiratory illness in infants but studies have not consistently demonstrated that there is protection against infection. Victora *et al.* (1998) found that, in all regions except Latin America, interventions to prevent malnutrition and low birth weight appeared more promising than breast-feeding promotion. In Latin America, breast-feeding promotion appeared to have a similar effect to that of increasing birth weight. However, other more recent studies (Cushing *et al.* 1998) have indicated that breast feeding can reduce the severity of illness due to acute respiratory infection. One study (Cesar *et al.* 1999) found that breast feeding protects young children against pneumonia, especially in the first months of life. These results may be used for targeting intervention campaigns at the most vulnerable age groups.

Box 5 Outcome of review of interventions to prevent childhood deaths from pneumonia (1991–1995)

High effectiveness (potential impact more than 10 per cent)

- Pneumococcal vaccines
- Respiratory syncytial virus vaccines
- Reduction of indoor pollution
- Reduction of low birth weight
- Reduction of underweight

Medium effectiveness (potential impact 5–10 per cent)

- Increase in measles immunization
- *Haemophilus influenzae* type B vaccine
- Increase in breast feeding (Latin America only)

Some interventions showed no evidence of impact on pneumonia mortality or morbidity including:

- use of antibiotics for upper respiratory tract infections (although such use is widespread)
- prophylactic use of antibiotics in severely malnourished children
- vitamin A supplementation (except in relation to measles-associated pneumonia)
- treatment of helminth infections
- reduction of environmental tobacco smoke (although this is clearly implicated in other acute respiratory infections and childhood asthmas in developed countries).

Tuberculosis

Tuberculosis is a contagious disease. Like the common cold, it spreads through the air. Only people who are ill with pulmonary tuberculosis (tuberculosis of the lungs) are infectious. When infectious people cough, sneeze, talk, or spit, they propel tuberculosis germs known as bacilli into the air. A person needs only to inhale these to be infected. Left untreated, each person with active tuberculosis will infect on average between 10 and 15 people in each year. But people infected with tuberculosis will not necessarily become ill with the disease. The immune system 'walls off' the tuberculosis bacilli which, protected by a thick waxy coat, can lie dormant for many years. When someone's immune system is weakened, the chances of becoming ill are greater. Sputum smear microscopy is the most cost-effective method of screening pulmonary tuberculosis suspects referred to health services. It identifies sputum smear positive, highly infectious tuberculosis cases. Tuberculosis is diagnosed using patient history, clinical examination, and diagnostic tests. A sputum sample is submitted to the laboratory and the results of the microscopic examination are entered into the laboratory register. The goal is for all suspects to have a sputum smear microscopy examination and for all patients diagnosed with tuberculosis to be registered and treated (WHO 2000*a*).

- Someone in the world is newly infected with tuberculosis every second.
- Nearly 1 per cent of the world's population is infected with tuberculosis each year.
- Overall, one-third of the world's population is infected with the tuberculosis bacillus.
- Five to ten per cent of people who are infected with tuberculosis become ill or infectious at some time during their life.

Tuberculosis is the single largest killer of young women in the world, taking the lives of 750 000 each year as well as 250 000 children (UNICEF 2000). In addition to being a deadly killer, the stigma of tuberculosis often results in women being ostracized by their families and communities, which in turn has a devastating impact on the well being of their children. The result is that many thousands of upwardly mobile families are driven back into poverty, while those families that were already impoverished must struggle even harder just to survive. Children are especially vulnerable to the effects of tuberculosis, which is often difficult to diagnose in young children and therefore difficult to treat effectively. Children also suffer serious social consequences when someone in their family has tuberculosis. In India, for example, over 300 000 children are withdrawn from school each year either to go to work or to help their families bear the costs of tuberculosis care.

The method of directly observed treatment—short course (**DOTS**) has proved to be a successful, innovative approach to tuberculosis control in countries such as China, Bangladesh, Vietnam, Peru, and countries of West Africa (WHO 1999*b*). However, new challenges to the implementation of DOTS include health sector reforms, the worsening HIV epidemic, and the emergence of drug-resistant strains of tuberculosis. Short-course chemotherapy refers to a process treatment regimen lasting 6 to 8 months and uses a combination of powerful antituberculosis drugs. Standardized regimens are based on whether the patient is classified as a new case or a previously treated case. The most common antituberculosis drugs used are isoniazid, rifampicin, pyrazinamide, streptomycin, and ethambutol. Drug treatment of each patient needs to be observed for at least the first 2 months (WHO 1999*b*).

DOTS has been heralded as a breakthrough, and the achievements of such programmes in a wide range of settings are undoubtedly impressive. Globally, however, it is estimated that only 15 per cent of smear-positive tuberculosis cases are treated under a DOTS programme as recommended by the WHO. Coverage remains low because 'short-course' treatment is nonetheless protracted, and the burden of DOTS on patients and health services is quite substantial. Moreover, because marginalized groups such as women and migrant workers have difficulty in complying with DOTS, and incomplete treatment facilitates the spread of drug resistance. There is a danger that concerns about the spread of resistance and a desire to maintain high cure rates might lead to the exclusion of the poorest from tuberculosis programmes, which would exacerbate inequalities in health

Malnutrition

Malnutrition plays a very significant direct or indirect role in more than half of the nearly 12 million deaths each year of children under five in developing countries. It has multiple causes, including a lack of food, common and preventable infections, inadequate care, and unsafe water. In turn, malnutrition itself also exacerbates the symptoms of preventable illnesses. Strategies and interventions to improve the nutritional status of women and children aim to overcome many of the major health challenges posed by malnutrition.

About 20 per cent of babies born in developing countries weigh less than 2.5 kg (UNICEF 1997) which is an important factor contributing to the burden of malnutrition in developing countries. Few specific actions in developing countries have been supported to reduce the prevalence of low birth weight (Alnwick 1998). The lack of specific actions reflects the lack of any scientific consensus on the nature of effective interventions. The most effective interventions (Gulmezoglu *et al.* 1997) are considered to be smoking cessation, antimalarial chemoprophylaxis, and balanced protein-energy supplementation for the mother. Zinc, folate, iron, and magnesium supplementation in gestation and probably the reduction of teenage pregnancies merit further study.

Protecting, promoting, and supporting exclusive breast feeding for 4 to 6 months from birth and continued breast feeding with adequate complementary foods for 2 years or beyond is crucial in developing countries (Fig. 3). The cost of infant formula is often beyond the means of poor families, even when it is widely available. Besides, many families lack easy access to the knowledge, safe water, and fuel needed to prepare feeds safely, or simply have no time to prepare them. If used incorrectly—mixed with unsafe unboiled water, for example, or overdiluted—a breast-milk substitute can cause infections, malnutrition, and even death. Virtually all of the community-based programmes that have resulted in reductions in malnutrition have focused on improvements in infant feeding, especially the protection, promotion, and support of breast feeding. While community-based support for breast feeding is a major achievement, larger economic and institutional pressures can foil even the efforts of communities well aware of the central importance of breast feeding. Infant formula is an important product for the minority of children who for medical reasons cannot be breast fed. However, commercial pressures have often resulted in artificial feeding of children who would otherwise benefit from breast feeding.

Promotional activities, such as providing free or subsidized supplies of infant formula, bottles, and teats in maternity wards, have also undermined the best intentions and the confidence of new mothers to breast feed. In 1981, the World Health Assembly (**WHA**), which consists of the health ministers of almost all countries,

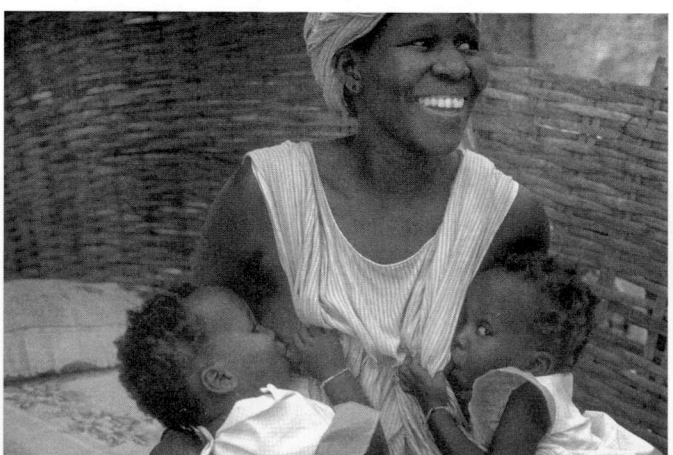

Fig. 3 Continued breast feeding.

responded vigorously to inappropriate promotional efforts of the infant-food industry by adopting the International Code of Marketing of Breastmilk Substitutes, drafted by the WHO, UNICEF, non-governmental organizations, and representatives of the infant-food industry. The Code and subsequent WHA resolutions establish minimum standards to regulate marketing practices by setting out the responsibilities of companies, health workers, governments, and others, and provides standards for the labelling of breast-milk substitutes. Among its provisions are that health facilities must never be involved in the promotion of breast-milk substitutes and that free samples should not be provided to pregnant women or new mothers.

Two global conferences which took place at the beginning of the last decade (World Summit for Children in 1990 and the International Conference on Nutrition in 1992) established for the first time specific global goals and targets for reducing micronutrient deficiencies and improving child nutrition. Only in the last decade has the world begun to realize the importance of micronutrients in saving and protecting children's lives. Foods and vitamin supplements in industrialized countries have been fortified with micronutrients like vitamin A and iodine for many years. However, it is only in recent years that their impact on child development in developing countries has been discovered. Some of the knowledge on the importance of micronutrients is now well established, like the effect of vitamin A on child survival, iodine's effect on learning ability, and iron's effect on productivity. Others, like the importance of vitamin A for reducing maternal mortality and of multiple micronutrient supplements for women and children's health, are beginning to emerge.

In areas where vitamin A deficiency exists, improving children's vitamin A status can increase their chances of survival by as much as 25 per cent. It is important to ensure that vitamin A capsules and fortified foods are available to women and children who need them. Ensuring that children consume enough vitamin A is a simple and effective child survival strategy. Adequate intake of vitamin A keeps children well; it is essential for the proper functioning of the body's immune system. In the past, vitamin A deficiency has been recognized as the leading cause of preventable childhood blindness. Recently, the international community has recognized that even so-called mild or moderate vitamin A deficiency, which does not result in eye damage or blindness, can impair children's ability to resist illness and can cause death.

Until recently, iodine deficiency was still the world's single greatest preventable cause of mental retardation. Even mild iodine deficiency can cause significant mental and physical retardation. In many parts of the world, people lack adequate amounts of iodine in their diet. The consequences of deficiency are most serious in pregnant women and young children. During pregnancy, iodine deficiency results in retarded fetal development, and severe iodine deficiency may result in fetal death or severe physical and mental growth retardation—a condition known as cretinism. In childhood, iodine deficiency can result in speech and hearing defects, delayed motor development, and impaired physical growth. In both adults and children, chronic iodine deficiency causes the disease known as goitre—a swelling of the thyroid gland. Grouped together, goitre, cretinism, and delayed physical and mental development due to iodine deficiency are known as iodine deficiency disorders.

Milder forms of goitre will disappear, and the mental and physical development of children mildly affected by iodine deficiency disorder will improve when iodine intake increases. But the severest forms of iodine deficiency disorder, such as cretinism, cannot be reversed; they must be prevented. The World Summit for Children set the goal of virtual elimination of iodine deficiency disorder by the year 2000. At the time of the Summit, 1.6 billion people—30 per cent of the global population—were still at risk of physical and mental retardation. Goitre affected 750 million people; 43 million have brain damage each year. Less than 20 per cent of those in affected countries had access to iodized salt. Currently about 70 per cent of the world's population has access to iodized salt, protecting millions of people from the negative impact of iodine deficiency.

Fifty per cent of all iron-deficiency anaemia occurs among pregnant women and preschool children. This condition greatly heightens women's risk of death during childbirth, and their newborns face a high risk of low birth weight, as well as poor growth and physical development. Pregnant women can receive a low-cost iron folate supplement that can reduce anaemia and contribute to improved maternal and infant health.

Iron-deficiency anaemia is perhaps one of the most prevalent global nutritional problems, affecting more than half of all women in developing countries and a large percentage of young children (Alnwick 1998). Worldwide, some 500 to 600 million people now suffer from iron-deficiency anaemia. Since it reduces work capacity and adversely affects productivity, iron-deficiency anaemia can have a profound impact on a family's ability to feed and care for its children. Children affected by iron-deficiency anaemia can also suffer from impaired cognitive abilities and reduced resistance to disease, impairing their right to achieve their fullest potential. The use of a simple, low-cost iron tablet could prevent these problems. Ensuring that pregnant women receive this dietary supplement can help prevent both maternal and infant deaths.

Measures to prevent iron deficiency should be part of an overall strategy to control anaemia and should be based on a combination of iron supplementation, dietary approaches including food fortification, and more general public health measures to address other causes of anaemia (WHO 2000*a*). It is encouraging to observe that more and more countries are embarking on iron fortification programmes.

Childhood disabilities

The rights of children with disabilities are clearly articulated in the Convention on the Rights of the Child. Article 2 calls on state parties 'to respect and ensure the rights set forth in the Convention to each child within their jurisdiction without discrimination of any kind, irrespective of the child's or his or her parent's race, colour, sex, language, religion, political or other opinion, national, ethnic or social origin, property, disability, birth or other status'. Article 23 goes on to state that all children should have access to rehabilitation services and the right to special care and assistance, appropriate to the child's condition.

It is estimated that between 300 to 500 million people live with a significant disabling condition. Of these, up to 120 million are children (WHO 2000*a*). According to the United Nations, 80 per cent of all individuals with a disability live in developing countries. More affluent countries may report higher rates of disability, both because of increased survival rates after a disability occurs and because census reports include individuals with mild or moderate disabling conditions. In many developing countries, some disabilities may not even be recorded due to poor data availability or, for example, poor recognition of milder disabilities such as dyslexia (UNICEF 1999*d*).

Developing countries often report higher disability rates for boys than girls. This may be due to work-related injuries. However, it is more likely to be due to the cultural preference for boys, and therefore the survival rate for disabled males will be higher than that for girls. For example in Nepal, the long-term survival rate for boys who suffered from polio was twice that for girls, although the chances of girls and boys being infected was equal.

Disability is more often considered a medical concern. However, it is increasingly being realized that most of the problems faced by the disabled are social, cultural, and economic rather than medical. Disabled people need to live in environments that are safe and supportive; they require education, health, and other basic services, and access to sports and recreation. They also need to develop skills that will allow them to earn a living.

Malnutrition and disability

The impact of malnutrition extends to the millions of survivors of malnutrition, who are left physically and psychologically crippled, chronically vulnerable to illness, and intellectually disabled. Child malnutrition is not only a problem of developing countries. In industrialized countries, widening income disparities, coupled with reductions in social protection, are resulting in increased vulnerability of children to malnutrition. In infancy and early childhood, iron-deficiency anaemia can delay psychomotor development and impair cognitive development.

Rehabilitative care

In industrialized countries, where long-term rehabilitative care is available, there is often a lack of comprehensive rehabilitative programmes that deal with both psychological and physical problems encountered. Hundred sof thousands of disabled children live in institutions. There, they are usually at greater risk of physical and emotional neglect and social isolation. They can also be at greater risk of abuse.

The most prominent unmet medical need identified for adolescents and youth with disabilities is the continuing lack of rehabilitation services. The United Nations estimates that, of those worldwide who need rehabilitation, only 5 per cent receive any sort of care. Moreover, rehabilitative services tend to be concentrated in urban areas and are often very expensive. Programmes that require long-term residency are also often unavailable to girls in societies where females are not allowed to travel unescorted or live on their own.

Prosthetic devices (artificial limbs, wheelchairs, hearing aids, spectacles, etc.) are often difficult and expensive to acquire, and a growing young person needs frequent replacements. A poorly fitting artificial limb has profound psychological and social implications for an already marginalized adolescent. A wheelchair that has become too small limits the ability of a young person to leave the house to attend school, do chores, or establish any measure of autonomy.

Children and land mines

Children face dangers form all sorts of weapons. However, the most dangerous is the threat of land mines. The 1997 international convention on banning land mines was a major step toward ridding the world of these terrible weapons. Children in 64 countries live amidst the contamination of 60 to 70 million land mines. Antipersonnel land mines kill or maim at least 2000 people each month with most of the victims being poor. In Cambodia, around 20 per cent of all children injured by mines die from their injuries. The rest have serious medical problems related to amputation. Around half of the world's mine-affected countries have had mine awareness programmes. It is important not only to tell the participants about the issues but also to try to involve them in the learning process. Programmes should address the specific needs of children, incorporating mine awareness into school curricula and providing teacher training.

UNICEF is the lead agency for mine awareness, and in co-operation with other partners has prepared international guidelines and developed a comprehensive package of mine awareness training materials and modules.

The damage caused by land mines stimulated an international campaign to ban their manufacture and use. In 1992, a global coalition of more than 1000 organizations in 60 countries formed the international campaign to ban land mines. The momentum triggered by this campaign led in 1997 to the Ottawa Convention related to the prohibition of the use, stockpiling, production, and transfer of antipersonnel mines and on their destruction. The Convention is now part of international law, and far fewer land mines are being produced and deployed. However, children continue to be killed and maimed by land mines each day, and resources for mine clearance and for the support and rehabilitation of victims are inadequate. Given sufficient determination and resources, countries should be able to eliminate all land mines in their territories within a decade, the timeframe set by the Ottawa Convention following ratification of the treaty.

Role of the mother

Every year, 1.4 million infants are stillborn and between 1.5 and 2.5 million infants die in the first week of life from complications related to their mothers' pregnancy or delivery—and those who survive their mother's death are at greater risk of malnutrition and death. These deaths constitute two-thirds of all the deaths of children under 1 year of age in developing countries (Fig. 4).

The toll of injury and disability from pregnancy-related causes is arguably the most neglected health problem in the world. For every woman who dies in childbirth, probably about 30 incur injuries and infections—many of which are often painful, disabling, embarrassing, and lifelong. Therefore it is likely that more than 15 million women a year fall victim to 'maternal morbidity', and that there are several hundred million women in the world today who have suffered or are suffering from the untreated and uncared-for consequences of injuries arising during pregnancy and childbirth. The percentage of women in developing countries who lose at least one child is still very high which has psychological and social consequences.

Each day worldwide some 1600 women die in pregnancy and childbirth—one death every minute—making complications of pregnancy and delivery the leading cause of death among reproductive-age women in developing countries. In addition to those who die, each year over 60 million women suffer acute complications from pregnancy. Most maternal deaths could be prevented if women had access to basic medical care during pregnancy, childbirth, and the

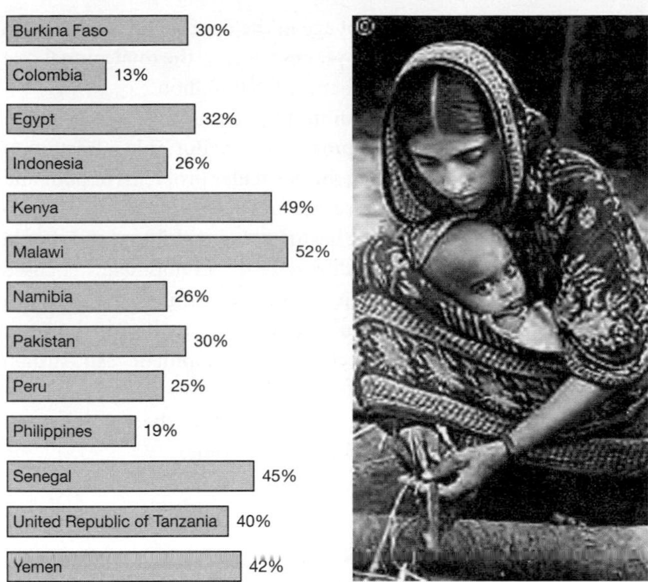

Fig. 4 The death of a child: percentage of women aged 15 to 49, married or previously married, who have had at least one child die.

postpartum period. This implies strengthening health systems and linking communities, health centres, and hospitals to provide care when and where women need it (UNICEF 1999*c*). Good-quality health care during the critical period of labour and delivery is the single most important intervention for preventing maternal and newborn mortality and morbidity. Lack of safe delivery care, late referral of complications, and low access to essential mother and child health services remain serious problems. Low accessibility and poor quality of emergency obstetric care, other reproductive health services, as well as treatment and prevention of general women's health problems (e.g. malaria, urinary tract infections, etc.), are some challenges that have to be addressed.

Distance and lack of transport is a great problem. In most rural areas, one in three women lives more than 5 km from the nearest health facility, and 80 per cent of rural women live more than 5 km from the nearest hospital. The scarcity of vehicles, especially in remote areas, and poor road conditions can make it extremely difficult for women to reach even relatively nearby facilities. Walking is the primary mode of transportation, even for women in labour.

Eighty per cent of maternal deaths all over the world are directly attributable to haemorrhage, sepsis, eclampsia, obstructed labour, and unsafe abortion. These direct factors are similar in all settings. However, multiple factors underlie women's capacity to survive pregnancy and childbirth. They include women's health and nutritional status, their access to and use of health services, household practices, and community behaviours with regard to women's health. The status of girls and women in society underlie all of the above.

Common barriers contributing to the low utilization of health services include the lack of compliance of services with defined standards, the shortage of supplies, infrastructure problems, deficiency in detection and management of complications or emergency cases, and poor client–provider interaction. Furthermore, services are also underutilized when they are perceived to be disrespectful of women's rights and needs, or are not adapted to the cultural contexts.

Women-friendly health services should provide accessible high-quality health care, be respectful of cultural and social norms, and empower users and motivate providers by involving them in decision-making, thereby enhancing all-around satisfaction. This approach builds upon existing concepts and recent experiences of countries, including all stakeholders involved in planning and implementing long-term country programmes. This is a rights-based approach to maternal and neonatal health care, which will enable governments and international agencies to monitor women's access to quality maternal and reproductive health services.

Vital to making maternal care accessible (prenatal, delivery, and postpartum care) is to ensure that no woman is denied care, even if she is unable to pay for it. The indicator for measuring affordability against the standard can be the proportion of women refused urgent essential obstetric care for financial reasons. Cultural barriers to health care relating to the lack of autonomy and decision-making power of women often constrain their access to health care. In some areas, for example, women are not allowed to leave home unaccompanied, while in others women are not permitted to be attended by male health care providers. Sometimes, the fear of not having her cultural values respected inhibits a woman from accessing the services she needs. To eliminate these barriers, health services should be organized in a way to respect women and their culture, religion, and beliefs.

Men often hold the financial as well as other assets. They are the decision-makers who determine what women can and cannot do, and consequently how they will be treated. Therefore, in order to improve women's health, men must be targeted with sufficient information on pregnancy and childbirth to make them more aware of their role and responsibilities.

Strengthening of child health services

The experience gained through dialogue on child survival programmes and the promotion and implementation of the Convention on the Rights of the Child has provided the necessary opportunities to review health policy issues with governments. The goal is to create health systems that can:

- improve health status
- reduce health inequalities
- enhance responsiveness to legitimate expectations
- increase efficiency
- protect individuals, families, and communities from financial loss
- enhance fairness in the financing and delivery of health care.

One of the keys to building more equitable and essential health services is the development of adequate financial mechanisms. Governments need to maintain an active dialogue with private health insurance companies and community-based insurance systems to ensure that they adhere to the principles of equity, non-discrimination, protection of women and children, and approaches to a better health status and lifestyle. In many countries where private health care providers are people's contact of choice, it is important to develop partnerships with these important actors. The role of the private sector is also crucial since they tend to focus more on purely curative care, and can sometimes neglect prevention, health education and promotion, and monitoring.

Box 6 Child health services

Strengthening of child health services should be considered at the following levels.

- **Policy level**: advocacy with governments and major donors for child-friendly movements, including national health systems management and financing strategies that ensure equitable access and quality of essential health care for marginal groups (including social safety nets/health insurance systems for the poor), especially in the context of privatization and decentralization, as well as review of policies on decentralization, cost-sharing, and co-management of health systems
- **District level**: improving access, quality, sustainability, and equity of health systems through child- and women-friendly movements can be instrumental to efforts being made in the regional context of privatization, decentralization, and economic crisis
- **Community level**: strengthening community links, which are essential to facilitate family care, referrals of obstetric complications and sick children, and increase health staff accountability for quality care and equity of access. This includes improving the capacity and motivation of primary health care staff (especially midwives), community health and social volunteers, teachers, and mass organizations to support family care. Improve capacities and motivation to identify limiting factors in family care practices and resources and develop appropriate communication and intersectoral support strategies to improve care and empower families
- **Family level**: improving family care practices, especially breast feeding, household-level integrated management of childhood illness, promotion of hygiene practices, use of bednets, and women's empowerment and psychosocial stimulation (which are not only essential for prevention of protein-energy malnutrition and sanitation but also for maternal mortality reduction and child mortality goals). This implies identifying limiting factors in family care practices and resources as well as developing appropriate communication and intersectional support strategies to improve care and to empower families

The rationale for health policy reform is based on the fact that, despite dramatic improvement in the health status of their population, life expectancy in the world's developing countries continues to be low and will continue to decrease in countries stricken with HIV/AIDS. Inadequate financial resources available for public health, combined with poor use of already scarce resources, have contributed to chronic drug shortages, inconsistent services, and a deterioration in health infrastructure.

The WHO and UNICEF have drawn up a list of the essential drugs required to deal with most of the common diseases of childhood. They include oral antibiotics for pneumonia, dysentery, and ear infections, an oral antimalarial drug, paracetamol for fever, oral rehydration salts for diarrhoeal dehydration, vitamin A for prevention of vitamin A deficiency and treatment of measles, mebendazole for intestinal parasites, tetracycline ointment for eye infections, and gentian violet for mouth ulcers and bacterial skin infections. The average cost for a full course of each treatment is approximately 15 cents. So even if every single child under 5 years of age in the developing world had to be given a course of drugs twice a year every year, the total annual cost would still be considerably less than US$200 million.

High-income countries now commit vast sums (over US$55 billion per year) to research and development efforts. But only a fraction of that amount is directed to solving the particular problems of poor and disadvantaged groups. Greater research and development can contribute significantly to improving the health status of children and should be an integral element of health system development. Focused investments by health systems on specific problems of the poor can generate major short- to medium-term gains in health; however increased investment in research and development can sustain medium- to long-term gains.

For strengthening of child health services, there are several remaining challenges which need to be overcome.

Box 7 Bamako Initiative

The Bamako Initiative, launched in 1987, has been recognized as the most cost-effective sustainable approach to revitalizing health systems in countries with poor primary health care structures. The strategy of the initiative was to revitalize public health systems by decentralizing decision-making from the national to the district level, reorganizing health care delivery, instituting community financing, and providing a minimum package of essential health services at the level of basic health units. By late 1994, the Initiative had been implemented in 33 countries, 28 in sub-Saharan Africa. Funds have been used mainly for the purchase of drugs to set up community revolving drug funds, for institution building at local levels and for the development of management capacity and logistic systems. The lessons learned from the actual experience confirm all the premises on which it was founded.

- **Service delivery**: experience demonstrates that utilization of health services increases once the quality of care improves. In Guinea, by mid-1994, 7 years after the launching of the Bamako Initiative, community co-financing and co-management had boosted the number of health centres to 295, covering approximately 80 per cent of the population and immunization coverage reached 74 per cent in the area
- **Resources for basic health services**: in areas where the Initiative has been implemented, it has contributed to making low-cost high-quality drugs accessible to the majority of the population. Community-managed health services have been able to generate sufficient resources to cover total essential drug costs and some small local expenses
- **Capacity building and empowerment**: the Bamako Initiative has contributed to developing managerial and organizational skills at all levels. Local decentralized management systems and district management capacity have been strengthened in many countries. At the national level, UNICEF has trained public health policy-makers and planners in Africa, Asia, and Latin America in health financing analysis and costing of services

Many countries in West and Central Africa are moving ahead to extend revitalization of health services nationally. This is largely due to the positive lessons of the Bamako Initiative

- Many health reform programmes continue to focus on user fees as an objective, with insufficient emphasis on conditions, management reform for efficiency, or co-management for accountability and empowerment. The best practices in community co-management need to be further documented and extended to other areas to improve the participation of health committee members and health centre users in monitoring and micro-planning. To make this possible, increasing emphasis should be placed on the training of communities and community health workers.
- The motivation of health professionals in public health centres is often poor due to low or unpaid salaries, insufficient supervision, and poor relationships with the communities where they are assigned. Rewards for good performance provide an impetus for hard work and good ethics.
- Although quality of care has improved in many health centres, there is still room for improvement. Improved drug policies and autonomous drug procurement units with associated distribution networks could vastly improve logistics and supply in most countries.

Since 1992 UNICEF and the WHO have been working on developing a strategy for reducing childhood mortality and morbidity associated with five major causes: acute respiratory tract infections, diarrhoeal diseases, measles, malaria, and malnutrition. This Initiative for the Integrated Management of Childhood Illness (**IMCI**) focuses on the prevention, early detection, and treatment of the leading childhood fatal diseases, recognizing that when children become ill they often have more than one illness. The initiative aims to improve the skills of health workers, the health system, including the availability of drugs, and family and community practices. Community-based actions to promote and protect child health and nutrition are complemented by improved management of childhood illness at health facilities.

The IMCI initiative incorporates many elements of diarrhoeal disease control and acute respiratory tract infection and some of the child-oriented aspects of malaria control and nutrition promotion. It also depends on the effective functioning of the Extended Programme for Immunization. In addition, it should also be noted that, as IMCI activities expand, single-disease programmes focusing on childhood diarrhoea and acute respiratory tract infection have been phased out.

Advocacy and communication for child health programmes

Communication strategies have provided a powerful means of accelerating action towards child health achievements and have proved effective in mobilizing social and individual change. Communication through news, entertainment, marketing and distribution of popular goods and services, community-level communication, interpersonal interactions, and awards programmes provide national scale channels that are compelling and influential. The development and implementation of skills-based health education in early childhood education and in primary and secondary schools should be supported. This includes strengthening the capacities of teachers to enable them to communicate better about health issues. In many

Box 8 Family and community practices

The following practices are promoted through the IMCI Initiative at the family and community level to improve child survival, growth and development.

Growth

- Breast feed infants exclusively for at least 6 months (taking into account WHO/UNICEF/UNAIDS policy and recommendations on HIV and infant feeding)
- Starting at about 6 months of age, feed children freshly prepared energy- and nutrient-rich complementary foods, while continuing to breast feed up to 2 years or longer
- Provide children with adequate amounts of micronutrients (vitamin A and iron, in particular) either in their diet or through supplementation
- Promote child's mental and social development by being responsive to the child's needs for care, and stimulating the child through talking, playing, and other appropriate physical and affective interactions

Disease prevention

- Dispose of faeces (including children's faeces) safely, and wash hands with soap after defecation, and before preparing meals and feeding children
- In malaria-endemic areas, ensure children sleep under recommended insecticide-treated mosquito nets
- Prevent child abuse/neglect and take appropriate action when it has occurred
- Adopt and sustain appropriate behaviour regarding prevention and care for people affected with HIV/AIDS, including orphans

Home care

- Continue to feed and offer more fluids to children when they are sick
- Give sick children appropriate home treatment for illness
- Take appropriate actions to prevent and manage child injuries and accidents

Care seeking

- Take children as scheduled to complete a full course of immunization (BCG, DPT, OPV, and measles)
- Recognize when sick children need treatment outside the home and take them to the appropriate providers for health care
- Ensure that every pregnant woman receives the recommended four antenatal visits, recommended doses of tetanus toxoid vaccination, and is supported by family and community in seeking appropriate care, especially at the time of delivery and during the postpartum/lactation period
- Ensure that men actively participate in provision of child care, and are involved in reproductive health initiatives

countries, assistance is provided for training adolescents to become peer educator trainers. A continuing priority is to strengthen the capacities of community- and workplace-based women's organizations for health promotion activities. This includes support for the incorporation of essential health information into organizations' activities and the creation of peer support mechanisms to motivate health action.

One of the prime examples of effective communication strategies has been the worldwide mobilization of all levels of society for child immunization. UNICEF was the driving force behind the social mobilization that led to the vast increase in vaccination coverage. The building blocks that led to the process of social mobilization were social marketing, advocacy, and forming strategic alliances. Social mobilization first came into prominence in connection with the Universal Child Immunization campaign, which was launched in 1984 with the objective of fully immunizing 80 per cent of the world's children by 1990. UNICEF was successful in generating political will for Universal Child Immunization in many countries, which was instrumental to the success of the programme. The success of Universal Child Immunization further led to the Global Polio Eradication Initiative with the goal of eradicating polio by the end of the twentieth century. The initiative has been largely successful with mass immunization campaigns such as National Immunization Days. The Days held in December 1998 and January 1999 in India constituted the largest public health campaign ever undertaken in a single country, immunizing about 134 million children. Such events require monumental co-ordination on the part of the government and public health authorities and the greatest challenge is to identify children who have not been reached by routine immunization.

Social mobilization and communication play an essential role in creating a demand for change. Through repeated messages such as speeches by political and religious leaders, messages from well-known personalities, media campaigns, slogans printed on caps and tee-shirts, radio and television spots, puppet shows, training sessions for village leaders, and conversations among neighbours, individuals and communities come to understand strategies that will improve their lives. Social mobilization and communication has been responsible for much of the dramatic success in efforts to improve child health in the past decade. Mobilizing people requires a thorough understanding of the local culture and the creativity to develop innovative strategies to respond to people's legitimate concerns.

Mobilizing resources for children

To achieve improved health outcomes for all children, development strategies and programmes need to focus far more on building the capacities of families and communities to provide for and protect the physical, emotional, and cognitive development of children. It is important to ensure universal access to good-quality basic social services for every child, and creating the national legal, policy, and budget framework to facilitate and promote the realization of children's rights to high-quality health services.

The challenges facing societies and the unfulfilled rights of children require broad participation and the commitment of many actors. Building an alliance of influential actors, governmental and non-governmental, who have the power to shape national laws, policies, budgets, institutions, and programmes, or who influence how societies behave towards children and adolescents, is essential.

UNICEF supports programmes to protect the rights and improve the health and welfare of children in over 160 countries. The leading international advocate for child survival and development, UNICEF works closely with other United Nations agencies such as the WHO, the World Food Programme, and the Joint United Nations Programme on HIV/AIDS. For more than 50 years, UNICEF has been helping governments, communities, and families make the world a better place for children. Part of the United Nations system, UNICEF has an enviable mandate and mission to advocate for children's rights and help meet their needs. UNICEF works in 161 countries, areas, and territories on solutions to the problems plaguing poor children and their families and on ways to realize their rights. Its activities are as varied as the challenges it faces, encouraging the care and stimulation that offer the best possible start in life, helping prevent childhood illness and death, making pregnancy and childbirth safe, combating discrimination, and co-operating with communities to ensure that girls as well as boys attend school.

Since the early 1980s UNICEF has been voicing its concern about the plight of children in the world's heavily indebted countries (UNICEF 2000), which are being driven by very high debt burdens to spend more on servicing their external debt than on basic health and other services. Unsustainable debt has implications for economic growth and equity as well as social sector financing. Debt, especially in the most heavily indebted countries, remains one of the greatest barriers to improving child health globally. UNICEF and Oxfam (UNICEF 2000) have developed a possible strategy for absorbing debt relief into the national poverty reduction strategy. The aim of this plan would be to provide a broad indication of expenditure plans, with special focus on longer-term development goals. It would be developed with bilateral donors, United Nations agencies, and the World Bank, and presented to national consultative groups.

The financial resources for child health are primarily within countries and therefore responsibility for success lies ultimately with governments. Only a fraction of resources for health in low- and middle-income countries originates in the international system—development banks, bilateral development assistance agencies, international non-governmental organizations, and foundations. According to the WHO, health spending in low- and middle-income countries in 1994 totalled about US$250 billion, of which only 2 or 3 billion dollars was from development assistance.

In recent years there has been growing pressure on donors to say how much of their aid goes to meet obvious basic needs—adequate nutrition, safe water and sanitation, basic health care, and primary education. At present, it is thought that only about 10 per cent of Official Development Assistance (**ODA**) is allocated to these basics. Five United Nations agencies—the UNDP, UNESCO, the UNFPA, UNICEF, and the WHO—have called for this to be increased to at least 20 per cent. An indicative target of 20 per cent of national budgets and 20 per cent of ODA was set to ensure universal access to basic social services. The purpose of the 20/20 Initiative is to provide adequate funding for universal access to basic social services for the achievement of the social goals that were set at the World Summit for Children, the International Conference for Population and Development and the World Summit for Social Development. The universal provision of basic social services is viewed as one of the most effective and cost-effective methods to address the worst manifestations of poverty. The initiative calls for greater collaboration among developing countries and their development partners in the financing of basic social services. This indicative allocation is not the only means to improve well being; the 20/20 Initiative also recognizes that better efficiency and more equity are required, which requires public action and entails adequate resources. Without universal coverage, the virtuous circle of social and economic development will remain elusive.

References

Alnwick, D. (1998). Combating micro-nutrient deficiencies: problems and perspectives. *Proceedings of the Nutrition Society*, **57**, 137–47.

Brabin, B.J. (1991). The risks and severity of malaria in pregnant women. In *Applied field research in malaria: report 1*, pp. 1–34. WHO, Geneva.

Bundy, D.A.P. (ed.) (1996). Health and early child development (abstract). *Investing in the Future: World Bank Conference on Early Child Development*. World Bank, Washington, DC.

Cesar, J.A., Victora, C.G., Barros, F.C., Santos, I.S., and Flores, A. (1999). Impact of breastfeeding on admission for pneumonia during postneonatal period in Brazil: nested case–control study. *British Medical Journal*, **318**, 1316–20.

Choi, H., Breman, J., Tuetsch, S., *et al.* (1995). The effectiveness of insecticide-impregnated bed nets in reducing cases of malaria infection: a meta-analysis of published results. *American Society of Tropical Medicine and Hygiene*, **52**, 377–82.

Connor, E.M., Sperling, R.S., Gelber, R., *et al.* (1994). Reduction of maternal–infant transmission of human deficiency virus type 1 with zidovudine treatment. *New England Journal of Medicine*, **331**, 1173–80.

Coutsoudis, A., Pillay, K., Spooner, E., Kuhn, L., and Coovadia, H.M. (1999). Influence of infant feeding patterns on early mother to child transmission of HIV in urban South Africa: a prospective cohort study. *Lancet*, **354**, 471–6.

Cushing, A.H., Samet, J.M., Lambert, W.E., *et al.* (1998). Breast-feeding reduces risk of respiratory illness in infants. *American Journal of Epidemiology*, **147**, 863–70.

De Cock, E., Fowler, M., Mercier, E., *et al.* (2000). Prevention of mother to child transmission in resource poor countries: translating research into policy and practice. *Journal of the American Medical Association*, **283**, 1175–82.

Eming Young, M. (1994). *Integrated early child development: challenges and opportunities*. World Bank, Washington, DC.

Guay, L.A., Musoke, P., Fleming, T., *et al.* (1999). Intrapartum and neonatal single-dose nevirapine compared with zidovudine for prevention of mother to child transmission of HIV-1 in Kampala, Uganda: HIVNET 012 randomised trial. *Lancet*, **354**, 795–802.

Gulmezoglou, M., Onis, M., and Villar, J. (1997). Effectiveness of interventions to prevent or treat impaired feotal growth. *Obstetrical and Gynaecological Survey*, **52**, 139–49.

Gwatkin, D.R. and Guillot, M. (1999). *The burden of disease among the world's poor: current situation, future trends, and implications for strategy*. World Bank and Global Forum for Health Research, Washington, DC.

Kirkwood, B.R., Gove, S., Rogers, S., Lob-Levyt, J., Arthur, P., and Campbell, H. (1995). Potential interventions for the prevention of childhood pneumonia in developing countries: a systematic review. *Bulletin of the World Health Organization*, **6**, 793–8.

Menendez, C. (1995). Malaria during pregnancy: a priority area of malaria research and control. *Parasitology Today*, **11**, 178–83.

Murray, C.J.L. and Lopez, A.D. (1997). Mortality by cause for eight regions of the world: Global Burden of Disease Study. *Lancet*, **349**, 1269–76.

Nahlen, B. (2000). Rolling back malaria in pregnancy. *New England Journal of Medicine*, **343**, 651–2.

NIH (National Institutes of Health) (1998). *HIV NET 012. Questions and answers*. News release, National Institute of Allergy and Infectious Diseases (NIH/NIAID), Washington, DC.

Shaffer, N., Chuachoowong, R., Mock, P.A., *et al.* (1999). Short-course zidovudine for perinatal HIV-1 transmission in Bangkok, Thailand: a randomised controlled trial. *Lancet*, **353**, 773–80.

Shapira, A., Beales, P.F., and Halloran, M.E. (1993). Malaria: living with drug resistance. *Parasitology Today*, **9**, 168–73.

Steketee, R.W., Wirima, J.J., Bloland, P.B., *et al.* (1996). Impairment of a woman's ability to limit *Plasmodium falciparum* by infection with human immunodeficiency virus type-1. *American Journal of Tropical Medicine and Hygiene*, **55** (Supplement 1), 42–9.

UN (United Nations) Joint Programme on HIV/AIDS (UNAIDS) (1998). *HIV and infant feeding: a policy statement developed collaboratively by UNAIDS, WHO and UNICEF*. WHO/FRH/NUT/CHD 98.1, WHO, Geneva.

UNAIDS/WHO Joint United Nations Programme on HIV/AIDS (1999). *AIDS epidemic update: December 1999*. WHO, Geneva.

UNICEF (United Nations Children's Fund) (1990). *World Declaration on the Survival, Protection and Development of Children and Plan of Action for Implementing the World Declaration on the Survival, Protection and Development of Children in the 1990s*. UNICEF, New York.

UNICEF (United Nations Children's Fund) (1993). *Towards a comprehensive strategy for the development of the young child*. Internal document, UNICEF, New York.

UNICEF (United Nations Children's Fund) (1995). *Health strategy: United Nations Children's Fund Executive Board*. E/ICEF/1995/11/Rev.1, UNICEF, New York.

UNICEF (United Nations Children's Fund) (1996). *The progress of nations*. UNICEF, New York.

UNICEF (United Nations Children's Fund) (1997). *The progress of nations*. UNICEF, New York.

UNICEF (United Nations Children's Fund) (1998). *Child development in UNICEF programming: a contribution to human development through early childhood care for survival, growth and development*. Programme Division, UNICEF, New York.

UNICEF (United Nations Children's Fund) (1999*a*). *The progress of nations*. UNICEF, New York.

UNICEF (United Nations Children's Fund) (1999*b*). *The state of the world's children report 2000*. UNICEF, New York.

UNICEF (United Nations Children's Fund) (1999*c*). *Programming for safe motherhood: guidelines for maternal and neonatal survival*. Health Section, Programme Division, UNICEF, New York.

UNICEF (United Nations Children's Fund) (1999*d*). *An overview of young people living with disabilities: their needs and their rights*. UNICEF, New York.

UNICEF (United Nations Children's Fund) (1999*e*). *The future global agenda for children—imperatives for the twenty-first century*. E/ICEF/1999/10, UNICEF, New York.

UNICEF (United Nations Children's Fund) (2000). *Children in jeopardy: the challenge of freeing poor nations from the shackles of debt*. Division of Evaluation, Policy and Planning, UNICEF, New York.

USAID Malaria and Pregnancy Network (2000). *Lives at risk: malaria and pregnancy* (Brochure).

Victora, C.G., Fuchs, S.C., Flores, J.A., Fonseca, W., and Kirkwood, B. (1994). Risk factors for pneumonia among children in a Brazilian metropolitan area. *Pediatrics*, **93**, 977–85.

WHO (World Health Organization) (1978). *Declaration of Alma-Ata*. WHO, Geneva.

WHO (World Health Organization) (1995). *CDD/ARI programme management: a training course.* WHO/CDR/95.12, WHO, Geneva.

WHO (World Health Organization) (1996). *Assessment of therapeutic efficacy of anti-malarial drugs for uncomplicated falciparum malaria in areas with intense transmission.* WHO/MAL/96.1077, WHO, Geneva.

WHO (World Health Organization) (1998). *Vaccines, immunisations and biologicals: 2000–2003 strategy.* Department of Vaccines and Biologicals, WHO, Geneva.

WHO (World Health Organization) (1999*a*). *The evolution of diarrhoea and acute respiratory disease control at WHO: Achievements 1980–1995 in research, development and implementation.* Department of Child and Adolescent Health, WHO, Geneva.

WHO (World Health Organization) (1999*b*). *Global tuberculosis control.* WHO/TB/99.259, WHO, Geneva.

WHO (World Health Organization) (1999*c*). *World health report.* WHO, Geneva.

WHO (World Health Organization) (2000*a*). *Global tuberculosis control.* WHO, Geneva.

WHO (World Health Organization) (2000*b*). WHO 20th Expert Committee on Malaria. *WHO Technical Report Series*, **892**, 1–74.

WHO/UNICEF/UNAIDS (1997). *Joint policy statement on HIV and infant feeding.* WHO, Geneva.

WHO/UNICEF/UNFPA (1999). *Women-friendly health services: experiences in maternal care. Joint Report of a WHO/UNICEF/UNFPA Workshop, Mexico City.* WHO, Geneva.

World Bank (1993). *World development report: investing in health.* World Bank, Washington.

11.4 Adolescence

*Joanne Barton and William Parry-Jones**

Introduction

Adolescence is popularly conceptualized as a period of good health. However, there are a small but significant number of young people for whom adolescence is associated with considerable morbidity and concerns about medical issues. There are also those who are in jeopardy because of their own risk-taking and health-compromising behaviours. Adolescence is also typically believed to be a period of emotional turmoil associated with conflict within families, irrational thought, and poorly controlled behaviour (Freud 1958; Blos 1962), and in some cases this would be an accurate representation of the period of transition from childhood to adulthood. For the majority of young people, however, adolescence is not a tumultuous developmental period fraught with conflict and rebellious antiauthoritarian behaviour. Most young people are well adjusted within their sociocultural environment and get on well with their families and peers (Offer and Schonert-Reichl 1992).

As noted in the first edition of this chapter there has been a lack of recognition of the special health care requirements of adolescents. Whilst there has been some improvement in this area, particularly in the developed world, there continues to be an inequality of health care provision for this age group compared with adults and children. *The Health of the Nation: A Strategy for Health in England* (DoH 1992) highlighted a number of targets for improving the health of children and young people. These included a reduction in smoking by one-third, halving the rate of pregnancy in girls under the age of 16 years, and reducing the number of accidents. Whilst some progress has been made in achieving these targets, there are areas in which little improvement has been made (Troop and Green 1997). Recent efforts to promote the health of young people have focused on schools with the Department of Health and the Department of Education working together to develop a policy for healthier schools (DoH 1998). The most recent governmental White Paper on health, *Saving Lives: Our Healthier Nation* (DoH 1999) dismisses the targets set out in *Health of the Nation* and instead claims to set tougher targets, addressing the 'main killers' of cancer, coronary heart disease and stroke, accidents, and mental illness. The specific health needs of young people are not addressed.

* This chapter represents a revision of the chapter on 'Adolescence' which appeared in the first edition of this book. I have been privileged to work on the original text written by my friend and mentor, William Parry-Jones, who died in July 1997 before work on the second edition was commissioned. It is a reflection of the rigorous and meticulous approach that William applied to all aspects of academic endeavour that I have had merely to update some sections of the text. His insights into the health needs of young people are as pertinent today as when the chapter was first published.

The provision of health care services for young people requires urgent attention; adolescents are important as they represent a significant proportion of the population. Considerable resources are invested in them in terms of their education and training. They have substantial commercial power and patterns of behaviour established during this period are likely to continue into adulthood. However, despite this, the special health requirements of adolescents have been, and continue to be, neglected relative to other age groups (Bennett 1982).

This chapter will provide an overview of the particular issues relating to adolescent health and behaviours that are important in the planning of comprehensive health care services for this age group. The specific aims are:

- to provide an overview of adolescent medical and surgical disorders, mental health problems, and risk-taking behaviours
- to review the range of adolescent health care services and health-promotion programmes and to consider the future development of service planning for this age group
- to reflect on teaching, training, and research in relation to adolescents.

The literature on adolescent health and related issues is extensive and it would not be possible to produce an exhaustive review in this context. This chapter is intended as a primer providing a basis for further study. The focus is the position in the United Kingdom, but drawing upon the extensive experience of our colleagues in the United States.

Definition and demography of adolescence

Hall's (1904) influential work at the turn of the last century identified adolescence as a distinct developmental stage although descriptions of adolescence have featured in earlier writings (Parry-Jones 1994). There was, however, comparatively little research into the adolescent age group until the last two decades when researchers became more interested in this developmental period. This interest has developed because of increasing recognition of the importance of this period and the impact of exposure to various stressors and influences on the risk of adverse outcomes.

However, a universally accepted definition of adolescence remains illusive. In many parts of the world adolescence is not clearly designated; children are introduced early to adult, social and economic responsibilities, with little transition between childhood and adulthood. From the physiological and psychological viewpoint, it is essential that the working definition used by clinicians takes into consideration the significance of two developmental transitions: that from childhood to adolescence, encompassing puberty, and that from an increasingly protracted adolescence and dependence, to adulthood. This coincides approximately with the age limits of 10 to 19 years used by the World Health Organization (WHO 1965), a period often subdivided into early, middle, and late adolescence. It is becoming evident that the transition to adulthood and the establishment of a fully mature relationship with parents, often in the mid or late twenties, can be more problematic than the intermediate adolescent years themselves. The increasing postponement of adolescent difficulties, associated particularly with the prolongation of formal education, and the delayed achievement of economic independence, heightens the obstacles to be overcome at the next developmental stage. Widening the age range of adolescence encourages the use of the alternative concept of youth, for young people aged 15 to 24 years (WHO 1989).

The world population currently stands at 5.9 billion persons and is growing at a rate of 1.33 per cent per year which represents an annual increase of 78 million people (UN 1998). The population of the United Kingdom is approximately 59 million of which 21 per cent are less than 16 years of age. Dramatic changes are taking place worldwide in the absolute and relative numbers of adolescents, especially in developing countries. Expected trends show increasing ageing of all populations, with wide variation in the proportions aged under 15 years. By the year 2025, for example, children and adolescents in more developed countries will form 19 per cent of the total population. In developing countries, the numbers will continue to rise, although the overall proportion will fall. The problems and health care priorities of adolescents, therefore, will continue to vary widely in terms of their geographical, social, economic, political, and cultural settings.

Mortality rates in the United Kingdom at ages less than 15 years have continued to fall. In developed countries the leading causes of death are accidents and suicide whilst in the United States, homicide is a major cause of death in the young (Frim Forman and Emans 1998). Cancer remains the next most common cause of death in young people in the West. In developing countries the picture is somewhat different with infection and pregnancy-related problems continuing to be a major cause of mortality.

Social value attached to adolescence and youth

The extent and adequacy of adolescent health care services and the scope for future development is inextricably linked with the relative significance attached by any society to adolescence as a distinct developmental period and to the health, welfare, education, and vocational training of teenagers. This includes the development of laws and policies covering health care and, while legislation focusing on adolescents has gathered momentum, this is still deficient in many countries (Paxman and Zuckerman 1987). In England and Wales, the Children Act of 1989 constituted a landmark in establishing the rights and interests of children up to the age of 18 years. It has considerable implications for health authorities, health professionals, and managers (DoH 1989).

Undoubtedly, the importance of the adolescent life period is becoming increasingly evident in all cultures of the world, especially as short, ritualized transitions from childhood to adulthood give way to more prolonged periods of adolescence in developing nations, consequent upon rapid industrialization, urbanization, and the erosion of traditional social structures. Although the demographic trend in Western society indicates falling numbers of young people, there is likely, nevertheless, to be a growing recognition of the social and economic importance of the health of teenagers. Furthermore, as child health interventions reduce mortality rates ensuring that most children reach adolescence, the quality of adolescent life assumes greater importance and the role of health care services, especially those concerned with mental health, increases correspondingly. Young people are being targeted increasingly by the music, fashion, and leisure industries, and this 'youth industry' shapes, to a considerable extent, the evolving patterns of youth culture. Despite such developments, however, adolescents are still likely to be perceived as a 'social problem' group, having negative correlations with disturbed behaviour, delinquency, drug taking, violence, and other manifestations of challenge to social order. This stereotyped image of the disturbed, and also disturbing, adolescent is more likely to result in public panic about the involvement of youth in sex, drugs, and crime and a call for tightening up 'law and order' in relation to this age group. It is less likely to generate pressures for enhanced health care programmes, or the modification of the environment in which adolescents are growing up.

Adolescent growth and development

Adolescence is characterized by rapid biological and psychological changes, intensive readjustment to the family, school, work, and social life, and an unrelenting process of preparation for adulthood. Emotional maturation carries with it growing understanding of the significance of affective experience and expression in oneself and others, the capacity to control impulses and to form meaningful emotional relationships. Cognitive changes include the acquisition of capability for abstract thought and hypothetical planning, and are associated with the often sudden development of spiritual, moral, and political thinking with the emergence of youthful idealism. Social maturation requires emancipation from the home; the establishment of an independent lifestyle, with a conscious sense of individual uniqueness; commitment to a sexual orientation and to a vocational direction; and the development of self-control. The achievement of these objectives requires experimentation with a variety of behaviour choices and role playing. If the process is to be successful, it calls for the confident acceptance of adult physiological, psychological and social experiences and roles, individual physical and personality characteristics, the ambiguity and frailty of human existence, and the responsibilities associated with personal autonomy. These processes take place gradually, involving a multiplicity of day-to-day decisions which carry identity-forming implications. Clinically, it is helpful to view adolescence as a sequence of stage-related developmental tasks, which have to be completed successfully if progress is to be made to the next stage. Although this approach is an oversimplification, it creates a frame of reference that health care professionals may find useful in structuring assessment and intervention. It requires a thorough familiarity with the phenomena and stages of normal adolescent development information about the lives of adolescents and their families in the context of their own communities and an appreciation of common internal and external stressors.

The profound maturational changes of this period can have far-reaching effects on the lives of young people and their families, with major implications for health and the planning of health care services. Although the theme of normal development appropriately pervades all aspects of adolescent medicine and psychiatry, it is not discussed at greater length in this chapter, since it receives comprehensive coverage in standard textbooks (Bancroft and Reinisch 1990; Coleman and Hendry 1990; Lewis and Volkmar 1990). Instead, emphasis is placed on the clinical aspects of adolescent development that have implications for causation, diagnosis, management of health problems, and also for the training of health care professionals.

Clinical significance of maturational stress

For most young people, the adolescent transition is one of natural orderly adjustment (Offer and Schonert-Reichl 1992) and not a time of storm, stress, identity crisis, and alienation. However, some degree of anxiety or stress is likely to be related to the need to cope psychologically with maturational changes and to rapidly develop a range of new capabilities, particularly since there are no clear-cut rules on how to progress to adulthood or to decide when this process is complete and the young person is fully grown up. Whilst unemployment rates appear to be falling in the United Kingdom, the labour market remains uncertain for many young people who therefore delay leaving the parental home, entering employment, and getting married, all of which are key symbols of adulthood. Furthermore, adolescents face a confusing range of legislation about the time at which the rights and obligations of full adult status are attained. Maturational stress is most likely to occur at times of transition, such as changing or leaving school, losing a close relationship, ending a period of being in institutional care, or the break-up of parental marriage. At such times, the anxiety of facing a new situation is added to other normative biological and psychological stresses. Therefore a range of adjustment difficulties, some of which may fulfil the criteria of mental disorder, can arise in response to adolescent development. For example, on entering puberty, children with pre-existing medical, psychiatric, developmental, or temperamental difficulties may experience particular problems. These may be related specifically to the timing of puberty, although all developmental changes have the capacity of being either stressful or supportive. Wide variation in age of onset and rate of growth spurt, for example, and the impact of both early and late physical development, may have positive or negative effects. In boys, delayed maturation can generate inferiority feelings and, in girls, early menarche may be experienced negatively or positively, because of the way it signifies maturity.

External stressors may operate within the family and, at all stages, adolescence is influenced by facilitating or obstructing family influences. In the assessment and management of adolescents therefore, this interactive process always needs consideration. Although a common occurrence, conflict between adolescents and parents is rarely long standing and generally parental influence remains significant throughout adolescence and young adulthood. Nevertheless, adolescent challenge to parental standards and attainments, which is an essential part of normal emancipation and detachment, may pose a major threat, because it can destabilize family homeostasis and lead to serious adjustment reactions, particularly in dysfunctional families. Therefore the parenting of adolescents can be demanding and stressful. Help-seeking is likely to be a more sensitive issue regarding adolescent problems than in relation to child-rearing difficulties, because it may expose a disabling sense of incompetence about parenting skills. Parents may seek help from a variety of sources, including family doctors, teachers, counsellors, books, and popular magazines. Parent-effectiveness training programmes have been developed and successful adolescent health promotion requires some intervention with parents.

Adolescent well being and the family

The role of the family in adolescent well being is increasingly recognized. The effect of family structure, family functioning, and parenting style on adolescent physical health, mental health, relational well being, and employment is the focus of increasing research attention (McFarlane *et al.* 1995; Spruijt and de Goede 1997). Many young people continue to live with their parents through their late teenage years and into early adulthood (Boyd and Noris 1999), thus, throughout adolescence, parents, especially mothers, continue to play an important role in the health of adolescents and in the identification of ill health The burden of adolescent ill health, particularly chronic illness, falls heavily on parents and siblings; families may be affected adversely and be at increased risks of psychiatric morbidity. Alternatively, family factors can precipitate, exacerbate, or maintain health-related problems in predisposed young people. In many situations, parents have to play a key part in supporting treatment, overcoming adolescent non-compliance, and as agents of change. Some degree of challenge and confrontation is appropriate to adolescent maturation. It is a considerable developmental challenge for parents to make the necessary adjustments to their perception of their child, who is becoming an adult, and to understand the challenges and conflicts, not as personal assaults, but as part of the process of maturation. A positive view of adolescence, as a creative force in the family, is beneficial, and parental morale and successful coping has to be fostered as part of adolescent health care and health-promotion programmes.

Problems in school

School is commonly the focus of adolescent disturbance, which may be characterized by disenchantment with conventional compulsory education, academic underachievement, disruptive behaviour, bullying, loneliness, association with delinquent peers, and truancy. It is not easy to assemble the profile of the disruptive teenager, because the causation is multifactorial (Parry-Jones and Gay 1984). From a clinical viewpoint, disruptiveness needs to be differentiated from both conduct disorder and maladjustment, in that it is usually a transient phenomenon, not necessarily reflecting individual psychopathology or forming part of identifiable antisocial behaviour. Although teachers commonly view disruptiveness as a consequence of the adolescent's abnormality and the dysfunctional home background, the ethos of the school and the management of disruptiveness by teachers themselves can play a significant part in the generation and perpetuation of problems.

Ethical and legal issues

In all aspects of adolescent health care, legal, and ethical issues need to be given thorough consideration. The maintenance of privacy and confidentiality, for example, are of vital importance in all professional interventions, with clarification of the extent to which any personal revelations made to health care professionals will remain private. Boundaries of personal and public thoughts and feelings in families need to be reflected explicitly in the stage-management of any individual and joint interviews. Nevertheless, reassurance about confidentiality has to be tempered by reality since, under certain circumstances, information may have to be disclosed to parents or others. When contacting schools or employers, written consent is always preferable.

The question of an adolescent's ability to seek, consent to, or refuse treatment without the knowledge or agreement of his or her parents is an important but highly controversial issue. There are wide cross-national differences in the legal rights of children and adolescents and health care practitioners have to develop familiarity with locally applicable legal and ethical principles and practices. In the United Kingdom, current practice has been influenced considerably by a number of high-profile cases such as the Gillick case in 1985 which concerned the prescription of contraceptive and pregnancy counselling services to under-16-year-olds. More recently controversy has surrounded issues such as heart transplantation and treatment for anorexia nervosa against the wishes of young people (Geist *et al.* 1996; Dyer 1999). Young people under the age of 16 years who are deemed capable of understanding the procedures involved can seek medical care and consent to treatment. Paradoxically this does not mean that treatment can be vetoed and courts have considerable over-riding powers.

The consent of 16- or 17-year-olds is sufficient in itself and separate permission from parent or guardian is unnecessary. Imposition of intervention without consent occurs only when emergency action is needed. It is conventional under such circumstances, with young people under 16 years, to accept the authority of a parent or guardian as an exercise of their parental responsibility. If such consent is absent and there is a psychiatric emergency with young people over 16 years, appropriate compulsory powers are provided by mental health legislation (Children's Legal Centre 1991).

Adolescent health concerns and knowledge

Adolescents hold diverse views about health and health problems depending on their developmental stage, gender, racial, social, economic, and educational status (Epstein *et al.* 1989), but generally their definitions of health and illness are similar to those of adults. During early and mid adolescence, normal heightened introspection can be associated with increased somatic concerns and many adolescents, especially females, are worried about their health. Their extensive interest in the subject is reflected in the proliferation of health-related articles in popular, teenage magazines. Younger adolescents are unlikely to acknowledge that they are having problems and usually find it difficult to seek help themselves. Self-referral is infrequent, but when help is sought the reasons are likely to reflect a pressing need for reassurance, guidance, explanation, protection, or relief. With progression through the teenage years, there is increasing acceptance of personal responsibility for health and recourse to health care services. Presenting complaints, however, may continue to mask underlying problems. Many studies have shown concerns about a wide range of general health issues, such as body shape and weight, acne, aches and pains, depression and other emotional problems, interpersonal relationships, adaptation to school, work and unemployment, dental problems, HIV/AIDS, and aspects of sexuality, particularly contraception (Porteus 1979; Millstein 1993). Concerns that are sensitive and more difficult to disclose are often undivulged and, therefore, tend to be ranked low. Adolescent girls report physical and psychological problems more frequently than boys, who tend to display disturbance by acting-out behaviour (Dubow *et al.* 1990; Offer and Schonert-Reichl 1992). The predominant 'personal' concerns are usually those bearing on immediate issues, such as appearance, peer relations, independence, and sexuality, rather than diagnosable clinical disorders with long-term health consequences, likely to be identified by health care professionals. This dichotomy has fundamental implications for the design and approach of health-promotion strategies. There may be mistrust of doctors and cynicism about the advice of 'experts', especially if the focus of health education is on the possibilities of harming health in the remote future. Therefore there are dangers of overselling health promotion and in mounting strategies that are counterproductive to long-term objectives (Challener 1990). Above all the attitudes and health concerns of adolescents need to be respected.

Risk-taking behaviours

High-risk behaviours such as violence, alcohol and substance use and abuse, sexual exploration, and associated risks of sexually transmitted disease and pregnancy, together with less typical behaviours such as financial risk-taking are characteristic of adolescence. Whilst they may be viewed as reactions to developmental and situational stress they are nevertheless anxiety provoking and can result in significant morbidity and mortality in this age group. Health care providers involved in the management of young people must therefore be aware of these behaviours and their associated risk factors.

It is a commonly held belief that adolescent risk-taking is mindless. However, in a study of 58 college-aged females Shapiro *et al.* (1998) found that risk-taking behaviour was largely goal oriented and that the behaviour was either a means to an end or reflected a preoccupation with a personal need. Males and females are equally likely to engage in risk behaviour but the reasons for engaging in such behaviour may reflect gender-specific issues (Sarigiani *et al.* 1999).

The number of homeless young people is increasing and they are more likely, out of necessity, to engage in health-compromising activities such as drug abuse and prostitution, thus exposing them to the risk of HIV infection. In general, this group tend not to seek help and to be underserved in terms of health and social welfare provision. Existing evidence suggests that the homeless population is characterized by higher levels of childhood adversity (particularly physical and sexual abuse) and psychiatric disorder (Craig and Hodson 1998).

Effective prevention of risk behaviours in young people requires comprehensive intervention. Of importance is the recognition that risk behaviours cluster: young people who smoke are likely to use alcohol and illicit drugs, to engage in unsafe sex, and to be violent. Therefore, targeting one risk behaviour is unlikely to promote healthy lifestyles overall. The role of individual, school, and community factors must be recognized; effective prevention and intervention programmes require collaborative endeavour by both social and behavioural scientists together with health-care professionals (Yach and Ferguson 1999).

Violence by and against young people

Young people perpetrate and are the victims of a great deal of violence. Between 1985 and 1994 arrests of people under the age of 18 years in the United States for murder increased by approximately 75 per cent. Similarly the rate of violent crime increased by 68 per cent in this age group between 1988 and 1992. Young people under the age of 18 years account for 19 per cent of violent crime, however, it is likely that this reflects an underestimate of youth criminal activity. Approximately half of all violent crimes are committed by young men (Cohall *et al.* 1998). Whilst the epidemic of youth homicide appears to be a predominantly American phenomenon, youth violence is a cause for concern internationally (Rae-Grant *et al.* 1999).

Risk factors for violence include experience of violence in the home and neighbourhood, drug and alcohol abuse, involvement in other criminal activities, and association with other delinquent adolescents. Youth violence is costly at a personal familial and societal level. It must also be remembered that delinquent youths present with high levels of psychopathology which must be treated.

A variety of prevention programmes have been described. In general evaluation of such intervention programmes is limited and there is a need for further rigorously executed investigation in this area. The most promising interventions to date would seem to be multisystemic therapy, a comprehensive intervention addressing the multiple determinants of delinquency and involving aggressive case management and family therapy (Borduin 1999).

There is limited information available regarding predictors of dangerousness in adolescents, most of the literature describes adult males. However, certain clinically determined factors are significantly associated with future risk of dangerousness in young people. Recent research has looked at the evaluation of short-term risk which is relevant to the day-to-day management of young people (Sheldrick 1999). Further research is required to improve our understanding of the causation of delinquent behaviour, including the biological basis, and to develop effective interventions.

Substance use and abuse

The use and abuse of substances such as tobacco, illicit and prescription drugs, inhalants, and alcohol is becoming more common. Substance use amongst eighth, tenth, and twelfth graders in the United States increased significantly for tobacco and illicit drugs, especially marijuana, and remained stable for alcohol between 1991 and 1997 (Windle and Windle 1999). Alcohol and cigarettes are the most commonly used and abused legal substances. The immediate risks of substance use include accidents, violence, risky sexual behaviour, and exposure to HIV. Clinicians working with youth must be aware of patterns of use, socio-environmental risk factors and comorbid behavioural disturbance (Bravender and Knight 1998).

Most young people who use drugs do not progress to substance use disorders. Methodological problems limit the studies which have examined the prevalence of substance use disorders but Cohen *et al.* (1993) found marijuana substance use disorder in 2.9 per cent of 17-year-olds surveyed. Comorbidity, particularly with conduct disorder and mood disorders is common.

The causation of substance use disorder is probably multifactorial but with increasing evidence for a neurobiological basis (Altman *et al.* 1996). Substance use, on the other hand, is more related to peer and social factors. Of increasing interest and importance is the identification of resilience or protective factors. Intelligence, problem-solving ability, a supportive family, and positive role models all seem to be important in this regard.

A variety of prevention programmes have been described (Blum 1997). School-based interventions utilizing an interactive rather than a didactic model and covering general lifeskills as well as resistance, combined with adequate follow-up periods of at least 2 years seem to be most effective (Tobler and Stratton 1997). Other forms of intervention have received less attention, particularly drug treatment. There is considerable evidence relating to the effectiveness of drugs such as methadone and naltrexone in the detoxification of adults but there is a paucity of clinical trials of these agents in the adolescent population.

Smoking

Cigarette smoking represents a significant threat to the health of young people. As many as 90 per cent of tobacco smokers begin their use before their eighteenth birthday, but if smoking does not start during adolescence, it is unlikely to occur. Even experimental smoking during adolescence increases the risk of adult smoking. Prevention of the onset of adolescent smoking is therefore of major importance. There are numerous studies describing the predictors of adolescent smoking (Williams and Covington 1997; Flay *et al.* 1998). The prevalence of smoking is increasing amongst children and young people with 33 per cent of girls and 25 per cent of boys becoming regular smokers by the age of 15 years. The likelihood of becoming a regular smoker increases between the ages of 11 and 15 years, but girls tend to smoke fewer cigarettes than boys (47 per week compared with 56 on average) (Office for National Statistics 1996).

Preventing smoking during childhood and adolescence is a vital component of an overall strategy to reduce mortality and morbidity from this dangerous habit. Various clinicians can play a role in smoking prevention by carrying out thorough assessments and counselling individuals (Sockrider 1997). Educational programmes have demonstrable short-term efficacy in reducing adolescent smoking, but their long-term effectiveness is less clear (Tyas and Pederson 1998). Certain components seem to be essential in order that sustained reduction in consumption can occur. These include policies to increase the price of tobacco, bans on advertising, limited availability, and readily available methods for supporting stopping smoking (Yach and Ferguson 1999).

Adolescent sexuality and sexual risk-taking

Adolescence is a critical period in the development of sexuality, attitudes to sex, and sexual behaviours. The sexual behaviour of young people may expose them to the risk of sexually transmitted diseases including HIV, unwanted pregnancy, date rape, and sexual violence. Despite increasing sexual liberation and more open discussion of sexual matters, coping with sexual development remains a silent solitary experience for many adolescents. They may feel anxious, frightened, and guilty about sexual thoughts and activities. The initial response to sexual development may take the form of denial of interest, withdrawal from all personal and social implications of genital sexuality, even to a self-abnegating lifestyle. Problems generated in this way, however, are much less likely to attract attention than difficulties in controlling sexual drives, in directing them into socially desirable channels, and in conforming to conventional sex roles.

Data regarding the occurrence of homosexuality during adolescence is limited, although a significant percentage of young people identify themselves as homosexual, or having had a sexual experience with a person of the same sex, or are confused about their sexual orientation. Specific sexual behaviours pose medical risks especially that of HIV/AIDS. In addition, stress related to isolation and stigma may predispose homosexual adolescents to social and emotional problems such as depression, school problems, running away, and illegal behaviour (Stronski Huwiler and Remafedi 1998).

Actual or anticipated promiscuity in girls, and fears about pregnancy or sexually transmitted diseases, may be an urgent reason for parents to seek help. In some respects, increased sexual permissiveness has complicated sexual adjustment, encouraging earlier sexual experimentation and coital experience. Such activities, entered into to test masculinity and femininity, may leave adolescents feeling guilty and disillusioned, but this needs to be differentiated from promiscuous behaviour which is typically symptomatic of emotional dysfunction and disturbed identity formation. From a medical viewpoint, problems associated with adolescent sexual activity are increasing, including sexually transmitted diseases and teenage pregnancy.

Pregnancy

Considerable progress has been made over the last two decades in the investigation of unprotected sex and pregnancy in the teenage years. As a result there is a better understanding of the epidemiology and demographics of teenage pregnancy, its complications, and the effects of improving adolescent knowledge of and access to contraception. What works in terms of intervention/prevention programmes is now better understood with programmes to reduce sexual risk-taking behaviour and teenage pregnancy. However, pregnancy amongst teenage girls continues to be a problem in most countries. The teenage birth rate is high in many developed and developing countries (United States, 5.3 per cent; United Kingdom, 3.2 per cent; The Netherlands, 0.6 per cent) although there is evidence that the rate has decreased over the last 6 years. The birth rate amongst unmarried teenagers has increased (Kirby 1999). The majority of teenage pregnancies are unwanted and may have medical, psychological, and social repercussions, including lack of appropriate prenatal care, disruption of the young person's life, disruption of family life and possible abandonment of the young person by their family, and abandonment of the baby.

As many as 50 per cent of teenage mothers in the United States will present with a repeat pregnancy within 2 years. Certain factors predict rapid repeat pregnancy including younger age, low socio-economic status, low education of the teenager's mother or head of household, marriage, and intended or wanted first pregnancy (Rigsby *et al.* 1998).

Sexually transmitted diseases

Adolescents are at risk of acquiring sexually transmitted diseases and high prevalence rates for the various sexually transmitted diseases make prevention programmes essential for this age group. In recurrent sexually transmitted diseases, HIV infection should always be considered. Information regarding trends in HIV incidence in young people are imprecise (Rosenberg and Biggar 1998) and it is likely that some adult patients with AIDS were exposed to the virus as teenagers. Many adolescents, particularly runaways, the homeless, and gay males, are exposed to HIV infection by risky sexual behaviour and drug abuse. Young male prostitutes are particularly vulnerable (Markos *et al.* 1994). This highlights the need to identify these youth and to develop effective behavioural change programmes. Adolescents are increasingly concerned about sexually transmitted diseases, particularly because HIV infection is becoming a reality among relatives, friends, and cult figures. Although most teenagers are likely to know that the disease is transmitted by sexual intercourse and reused needles, there may be continuing misconceptions and ignorance. The prevalence of unprotected or 'unsafe' sex is high (West *et al.* 1993) and knowledge about safer-sex practices is likely to be limited.

Extensive health education and preventive programmes are required to reduce sexually transmitted diseases, using the mass media-, school-, and community-based strategies, with sensitive consideration of the developmental needs of different age groups. These should aim at increasing awareness about the risks of HIV infection, discouraging promiscuity and promoting safer-sex practices through the use of condoms. Monitoring HIV/AIDS prevention programmes is methodologically difficult and probably the best measure is the occurrence of other sexually transmitted diseases (D'Souza and Shrier 1999).

Sexual offences

Although the physical and psychological consequences of sexual abuse in adolescents may be just as serious as those in children, they have attracted relatively less attention (Glaser 1993) and, by late adolescence, few young people remain on child protection registers. The prevalence of sexual abuse and assault of adolescents remains unclear because of under-reporting. Sexual offences by adolescents include rape and 'date rape', incest, paedophilia, sexual killing, and involvement in pornography and prostitution. The treatment of adolescent sex offenders and abusers presents major difficulties (Davis and Leitenberg 1987). Some obtrusive adolescent sexual problems, such as indecent exposure, generally reflect clumsy immature attempts to achieve sexual gratification and recognition. Cases of voyeurism and touching or fondling of strangers may be similarly explicable.

Adolescent and young adult women are more likely to be the victims of sexual assault than women of all other ages. Lifetime prevalence in adolescents varies from 20 to 68 per cent. Increased vulnerability is associated with younger age at first date, early sexual activity and earlier age at menarche, past history of sexual abuse or sexual victimization, and a greater acceptance of violence towards women. Other risk factors include alcohol and date behaviour, such as who initiated the date and who paid expenses. Further research is required to provide better understanding of sexual violence among adolescents and young adults (Rickert and Wiemann 1998).

Adolescent medical disorders

The range of physical disorders encountered in adolescence is covered in specialized textbooks of adolescent medicine (Friedman *et al.* 1992; Brook 1993) and is outside the scope of this chapter. Instead, the focus here will be on issues relating to medical disorders which occur in adolescence, or develop for the first time during this period including the impact of chronic illness on adolescent development.

Common medical problems encountered during this period include chronic disorders such as asthma, diabetes mellitus, and epilepsy either continuing from childhood or developing for the first time. Delayed or atypical pubertal maturation, functional menstrual disorders, sexually transmitted diseases, pregnancy, various musculoskeletal disorders, including overuse syndromes and sports injuries, obesity and eating disorders, and skin disorders, especially acne, are also seen.

In addition to providing appropriate medical and surgical intervention for the wide range of commonly presenting conditions, the management of adolescent patients requires special consideration of the potentially adverse psychological responses to, and treatment of, acute and chronic physical disorders. It is particularly necessary to consider the impact of chronic illness or disability, which affects 5 to 10 per cent of adolescents, since the numbers of subjects are growing as modern treatments modify previously fatal conditions, such as congenital heart disease and cancer. Improved long-term survival rates may be accompanied by psychosocial adjustment difficulties associated with uncertain life expectancy and ongoing treatment. Similarly conditions such as epilepsy, diabetes mellitus, asthma, chronic inflammatory bowel disease, and rheumatic disorders may be associated with psychological disturbance, such as lowering of self-esteem or the feeling of loss of control, and complex adjustment and compliance problems, although these are by no means inevitable. A range of both predisposing and protective factors may influence individual vulnerability (Mullins *et al.* 1997; Seiffge-Krenke 1998).

Response to chronic illness and hospital admission

Illness, especially when it is life-threatening or chronic, can provoke reactive psychopathology; it can also interfere less obviously with normal adolescent psychosocial maturation. Two aspects warrant special consideration.

1. **Prolongation of dependence on parents:** at home and in hospital, parents and staff are involved in doing things to, or for, the adolescent in ways that can foster increased dependence and encourage infantilization. In serious illness situations, parents tend to become more protective, more indulgent, and less strict. This can reach the stage when age-appropriate adolescent challenge and emancipation may be discouraged actively and ordinary, independent, teenage activities restricted unnecessarily. Such parental, and sometimes family, responses can generate behaviour problems that are very difficult to overcome at a later stage.
2. **Interference with peer group activities:** chronic illness and repeated hospital admission and treatment interfere in the teenager's involvement with other young people, particularly by prolonged school absences and restriction of ordinary socialization. Relationships may be complicated by fears of being thought of as weak, by embarrassment about appearance or the possibility of being regarded as physically unattractive, or even frightening, owing to treatment side-effects, such as hair loss or disfiguring operations like amputation.

The adolescent's coping capacity needs to be an important focus of clinical attention. The seriously or chronically ill adolescent who learns to live successfully with disability, develops for themself a number of effective coping responses to illness. Their acquisition is ill-understood but appears to be determined by personality, previous experiences, and family and social influences.

1. **Increased stress tolerance:** successful coping with mild stress strengthens the ability to cope subsequently and increases tolerance. This process probably explains why there may be less evidence of disruption when chronically ill adolescents have problems, than when healthy adolescents have to cope with relatively minor illnesses.
2. **Adaptive denial:** failure to 'take in' the threatening aspect of the reality of illness, or choosing not to do so, can contribute to a de-emphasis on illness and an apparent lack of concern about the diagnosis, even about death, that is often displayed by adolescents with life-threatening disorders. This process may be associated with overcompensation in other areas of life, such as school attainment or sporting activities. Younger adolescents are more likely than older patients to reject discussion and information about their illnesses, simply to avoid truths that might be distressing, especially in the acute phases. However, such denial needs to be viewed positively as a helpful part of effective adaptation, and should only become a matter of clinical concern if it is the adolescent's invariable response, or it interferes with treatment compliance.
3. **Intermittent regression:** all seriously ill young people may show childish, dependent, and manipulative behaviour at times of particular stress. Such regressive coping responses may be upsetting and annoying to parents and staff, but they may need to be recognized and permitted at particular times, such as immediately after diagnosis or during relapses.
4. **Intellectualization:** some teenagers may use intellectualization to help them overcome illness-related anxiety, by concentrating on the factual and rational aspects of a disorder in an apparently emotionally-detached fashion.

Surviving a potentially fatal illness presents significant challenges, not least of which may be the requirement that the young person copes with the sequelae of treatment including disfigurement, sterility, and the fear of recurrence. There may also be a protracted dependence on parents and a reluctance to form close relationships with others.

Scientific literature concerning terminal illness and death in adolescence is limited. During this period the adolescent and his or her family may continue to pursue aggressive therapies to prolong life and with ever-developing treatment protocols, this may be a possibility. This raises some ethical dilemmas in terms of the young person's ability to give informed consent to such interventions. The caring physician must assess and facilitate the adolescent's decision-making process and help families to accept the adolescent's point of view.

The primary concerns of the terminally ill adolescent focus commonly on worry about separation from friends, conflict about loss of control, concern about ordinary developmental needs and practical issues, such as how one actually dies, and funeral arrangements. Some adolescents may choose to talk about their impending death but many do not.

Adolescent surgery

The range of surgical procedures undertaken with adolescents varies little from those utilized with adults. Predictably, head injuries, especially resulting from motor vehicle accidents, are one of the main causes of morbidity and mortality in adolescents. Orthopaedic problems are common, especially in teenage athletes, and injury prevention and rehabilitation form major components of sports medicine (Nelson 1992). Plastic surgery may be sought in adolescence for the correction of birth defects, breast reconstruction, body contouring, or rhinoplasty. The preparation of teenagers for surgery needs to be pitched at an age-appropriate level and special attention given to the assessment, monitoring, and relief of postoperative pain since there may be a lack of familiarity with adolescent communication styles (Savedra *et al.* 1988). The hospital setting in the United Kingdom is likely to be either a paediatric or an adult ward, because there are very few separate surgical facilities for adolescents.

The increasing sophistication of transplant surgery (heart, lung, liver, renal, bone marrow, and so on) and the resultant prolongation of life expectancy of young people with previously terminal disorders poses a particular challenge to the clinician. The psychological functioning of young people before and after surgery and their subsequent adjustment must form part of the overall assessment and management of such young people (Tornqvist *et al.* 1999; Walker *et al.* 1999).

Adolescent mental disorder

There is a natural reluctance to diagnose mental disorder in adolescents from fears of the adverse effects of labelling, and of stigmatizing young people by identifying them as psychiatric patients. Nevertheless, a transition point has to be recognized at which what might be regarded as 'normal' mental health problems become mental 'disorders', despite the fact that this is difficult to operationalize. Applying the criteria for clinical significance in current psychiatric classification systems, the term mental disorder is used to refer to a clinically recognizable set of symptoms or behaviours associated with distress and interference with personal functions. This establishes a threshold for disorder and distinguishes those conditions and 'problems', which are not inherently pathological, and would not warrant labelling as disorder. This distinction is crucial in the planning of professional roles, approaches, and responsibilities within tiered multidisciplinary child and adolescent mental health services (NHS Health Advisory Service 1995).

Mood may fluctuate even in undisturbed adolescents, with periods of isolation and withdrawal alternating with bursts of energy and high spirits. Preoccupation with health, body shape, and complaints about cosmetic problems like acne are common. Feelings of sadness, apathy, emptiness, loneliness, boredom, and isolation from peer groups may appear in normally adjusted young people. Persistent low self-esteem, feelings of being different, of being unimportant in the lives of others, self-consciousness, and social sensitivity may all lead to periods of despondency. Furthermore, the prospect of leaving the security of home may result in regressive symptoms, such as sulking, temper tantrums, and obsessional activities. Therefore a fundamental task for the clinician confronted by alleged disturbance is disentangling essentially normal age-appropriate states of mind and behaviours from psychopathology.

The range of psychiatric disorders is encountered in adolescence, including those with onset specific to childhood and adolescence (emotional and behavioural, hyperkinetic, conduct, and pervasive developmental disorders) and those characterized under adult psychiatric disorders (anxiety, psychotic, eating, substance use, and adjustment disorders). During early adolescence, the main manifestations are of childhood disorder in conjunction with the emergence of disorders such as anorexia nervosa, substance use, and stress-related disorders accompanying biological and social change. By late adolescence disorders such as schizophrenia and manic–depressive disorder begin to emerge with their associated significant clinical continuities onwards from adolescence into adulthood (Robins and Rutter 1990).

No single theory provides a sound rationale for assessment, classification, and management in dealing with the diverse presentations encountered in adolescent psychiatry. Rather, the most satisfactory model is all-encompassing, involving interaction of biological, psychological, and social factors in the predisposition to, and the precipitation and maintenance of problems. There is growing evidence that early behavioural responses in childhood, such as aggressiveness and antisocial behaviour, are strong predictors of disorders occurring in adolescence and adulthood.

Prevalence rates for psychiatric disorders in the adolescent population range from 8 to 22 per cent. Estimation of the actual prevalence and incidence of adolescent mental health problems is difficult, especially in specific populations such as those with mental retardation or developmental disabilities. Variations in prevalence rates relate to differences in sampling methods, case definition criteria, and assessment procedures. Anxiety, conduct, hyperkinetic, and mood disorders are the most commonly encountered and comorbidity is frequent. Gender differences have been described, with depression and anxiety occurring more frequently in girls than boys whilst conduct disorder and hyperkinetic disorder are more common in boys.

Detailed descriptions of causation, presentation, and management of adolescent psychiatric disorders can be found in standard textbooks (Lewis 1991; Parry-Jones 1993; Rutter *et al.* 1994). Here, emphasis is placed on the distinctive features of adolescent presentations and on disorders prominent in this age group. Those disorders which attract attention, because the adolescent's behaviour becomes obtrusive, are described in the section on risk-taking behaviours.

Emotional problems and disorders

Anxiety and depression are common symptoms, especially in mid and late adolescence. Anxiety disorder may be amongst the most common psychiatric disorders in adolescence, affecting as many as 22 per cent of young people (Verhust *et al.* 1997). The features of anxiety disorder include excessive worrying, nervousness, irritability, sleep disturbance and fatigue, muscle tension, and other physical symptoms. Specific disorders include generalized anxiety disorder, post-traumatic stress disorder, obsessive–compulsive disorder, panic disorder, and phobias.

Major depressive disorder is identified in 3 to 9 per cent of adolescents (Lewinsohn and Hops 1993). Symptoms include sadness, irritability, reduced interest in activities, difficulties in concentrating, reduced or increased appetite, lack of energy, disturbed sleep (insomnia or hypersomnia), and low self-esteem. Depression in adolescents is also frequently associated with substance abuse and anxiety. Dysphoria is common amongst adolescents and therefore cannot be used *per se* as an indicator of mental health disturbance in this age group. Rather, the duration and pervasiveness of symptoms must be considered (Goodyer 1995). Serious mood disturbance may be associated with self-destructive ideation, self-mutilation, or attempted suicide.

Suicide and deliberate self-harm

The phenomena of suicide and deliberate self-harm or parasuicide have received considerable academic and political attention. The literature describing adolescent suicide and deliberate self-harm is extensive and the government in the United Kingdom have again identified a reduction in the rate of suicide as a priority (DoH 1999). However, suicide remains one of the leading causes of death in the adolescent age group (Rosewater and Burr 1998) and is therefore a cause for considerable concern (Barton 1995).

Thoughts of self-harm are common amongst adolescents; studies report that up to 40 per cent of adolescents will think about harming themselves at some point. Suicide before the age of 12 years is rare, but thereafter rates increase. Between 1980 and 1995, 1854 young people in England and Wales aged 11 to 19 years killed themselves (Roberts *et al.* 1998). The incidence of deliberate self-harm or parasuicide is difficult to determine in view of the fact that some parasuicidal activity will be concealed. In general, however, parasuicide attempts are between 10 to 20 times more common than actual suicides. Deliberate self-harm is more common in females whilst suicide is more common in males. Death by suicide is more common amongst young people who have tried to harm themselves in the past; 30 to 47 per cent of suicides occur in people who have tried to kill themselves before (Gunnell *et al.* 1995).

There are gender differences in the method of suicide. Males tend to use more violent methods such as jumping off buildings and hanging themselves; in the United States, where guns are more freely available, suicide by firearm is the most common method. Females are more likely to kill themselves by self-poisoning. Many suicides are completed under the influence of alcohol but very few young people who commit suicide have established psychiatric diagnoses or are in psychiatric treatment at the time of their deaths (J. Barton, unpublished data, 1995).

The range of motives described by young people who try to kill themselves includes relief from intolerable stress, retaliation, and manipulation in response to precipitating situations such as family rows, rejection by peers, break-up with a boy- or girlfriend, or some significant personal failure. There may have been feelings of being unwanted, unloved, persistently worthless, and socially alienated, and there may be evidence of uncharacteristically dangerous behaviour, risk-taking, or alcohol and drug abuse.

A variety of approaches to the management of adolescent suicidal behaviour have been described, including inpatient treatment programmes, school-based programmes, telephone hotlines, and pharmacological intervention (Greenhill and Waslick 1997). The most effective interventions are based on rigorous systematic screening which in turn has a high propensity for hospital admission (Shaffer and Craft 1999).

Reliable assessment of suicide risk in adolescents is difficult and, ideally, should be undertaken by psychiatrists or other experienced mental health professionals. All threats and warning signs of suicide need to be taken seriously, particularly when the adolescent displays an overwhelming sense of hopelessness, has attempted suicide before, and has difficulties in family and peer relationships. Admission to hospital for at least 24 hours should follow attempted suicide to permit full psychiatric and social assessment and family interviews. Assessment difficulties are compounded by the considerable geographical variation in the location of hospital departments and staff groups likely to be involved in catering for adolescents and young people. Parents have a key role in helping to prevent teenage suicides by encouraging adolescents to discuss what is bothering them, helping children to accept failure, reducing accessibility to the means for suicide, and trying to provide a role model for successful stress management.

Eating disorders

Concerns about weight and body shape are common amongst young people. Thirty to forty per cent of junior high school girls in the United States report worries about weight (Childress *et al.* 1993), and 40 to 60 per cent of high school girls have dieted to lose weight (Field *et al.* 1993). Problems concerned with eating and weight have increasingly become frequent reasons for the referral, or occasional self-referral, of young people (Steinhausen 1994). Anorexia nervosa is more common in girls especially during late adolescence and prevalence rates of 0.5 to 1.0 per cent have been recorded. Bulimia nervosa occurs chiefly in an older age range and has a prevalence of approximately 1 per cent in late adolescence.

The prevalence of obesity in young people is increasing, with 10.9 per cent of young people being above the 95th percentile for weight (Troiano *et al.* 1995; Hughes *et al.* 1997). Despite this, obesity remains an uncommon reason for referral to clinicians. Obesity is associated with significant short- and long-term health risks in addition to the effects on self-esteem and body image. The explanation for this trend requires careful consideration, but existing evidence suggests that a reduction in energy expenditure is the most important determinant of the increase in obesity in young people (Jebb 1997). The promotion of healthy lifestyles is an important challenge facing health care professionals with efforts to increase physical activity to address this problem.

Hyperactivity disorders

The term hyperactivity has become a familiar part of everyday language and thus its usefulness as a term to describe a symptom or syndrome has been greatly reduced. Attention-deficit hyperactivity disorder and hyperkinetic disorder are increasingly common reasons for referral to psychiatric clinics, and the assessment and management of these disorders in primary school-age children is well established. The literature describing their presentation and management in the adolescent age range is less extensive as it was thought that in many cases children outgrew hyperactivity disorders before they reached adolescence. However, it is increasingly recognized that these disorders can and do persist into adolescence, and may cause significant disability and dysfunction in terms of educational achievement and family and social functioning. Comorbidity is common especially with conduct disorder, and this combination has the worst prognosis (Hill 1998).

Anti-authority and antisocial behaviour

Antisocial behaviour in adolescents may arise initially in this age period or be a continuation from childhood. Its significance may be difficult to assess in that some degree of 'unreasonable' behaviour and poor impulse control is likely to occur during adolescence and complaints by adults may reflect their own low threshold of tolerance. Therefore common transient manifestations and occasional minor incidents of public disorder have to be distinguished from persistent and pervasive symptoms of antisocial behaviour that would justify the formal diagnosis of conduct disorder. Delinquency involves offences against the law and delinquent acts do not necessarily indicate the presence of conduct disorder. The clinical implications of antisocial behaviour become quite different if there is evidence of abnormally dangerous behaviour, such as fire-setting, long-standing aggression, or persistent delinquent activities, which warrant detailed psychiatric appraisal.

Conduct disorder is amongst the most common reasons for referral to psychiatry, representing up to 50 per cent of referrals in some clinics. It affects between 1.5 and 3.4 per cent of children and young people and is more common in males than females (sex ratio 5:1). Low socio-economic status and poverty are commonly associated with conduct disorder, although it is widely accepted that conduct disorder is a heterogeneous disorder where genetic liability may be triggered by environmental factors. Treatment of conduct disorder requires multimodal intervention, often over the long term. The best results seem to be achieved through the combination of intensive individual work and targeted family intervention (Steiner 1997).

Conduct disorder is amongst the most costly of psychiatric disorders in terms of cost to the affected individual, their family, and society. It is also one of the most difficult disorders to treat. The majority of young people affected by conduct disorder continue to experience dysfunction in some aspect of their lives and 40 per cent will go on to develop antisocial personality disorder.

Assessment and treatment

Assessment of mental health in young people includes the use of interviews, rating scales, and observational measures. Information should be obtained from as many perspectives as possible (the adolescent, their parent/guardian, and teachers).

A variety of treatment approaches have been applied to adolescent mental health problems (psychotherapy, family therapy, cognitive behaviour therapy, and pharmacotherapy). Evidence supports the fact that mental health treatment is better than no mental health treatment. However, there are insufficient rigorous evaluations to identify which treatments work best for which disorders presenting in which adolescents in which contexts (Weist *et al.* 1999).

Adolescent health care services

The general objectives of adolescent health care are the promotion of optimal physical and psychological development, the prevention of morbidity in adolescent or adult life, and the provision of services to achieve maximal physical and mental health. The attainment of these objectives necessitates a comprehensive multidisciplinary tiered approach to service provision and delivery, ranging from primary care and community-based health-promotion projects, to highly specialized hospital care. It requires continuity of care and good communication between health and other agencies. In this chapter, the status and effectiveness of these services are reviewed briefly.

Primary care services

Services delivered at primary level should be central to the health care of adolescents, offering the opportunity for prevention and early intervention. This is of particular importance since adolescent medicine is relatively undeveloped, yet family doctor consultation rates are low. Research, especially qualitative research examining the reasons why adolescents do not attend their primary care physician, is limited. Available evidence suggests that adolescents are concerned about issues such as being taken seriously, having their problems listened to, and being treated with respect (Rosenfeld *et al.* 1996). Many physicians feel ill equipped to deal with adolescent patients, acknowledging that their training in adolescent health care is inadequate (Veit *et al.* 1996). The nature of health service provision may be a further barrier to adolescents utilizing primary care. In private health care systems, adolescents are more likely to be uninsured or be part of a family insurance package such that they cannot gain access to health care without the knowledge of their family.

Adolescents may instead rely on the more anonymous accident and emergency department for their primary health care needs. This has implications for the training of accident and emergency staff who must be aware of the complex psychosocial needs of the adolescent as well as issues relating to consent (Melzer-Lange and Lyle 1996).

Guidelines produced recently in the United States have recommended the adoption of a staged approach to adolescent health care, describing three age groups: early (11–14 years), middle (15–17 years), and late (18–21 years). Analysis of primary care attendance by these age groups supports the targeting of services to these age groups (Ziv *et al.* 1999). During early adolescence the most common reasons for attendance are respiratory, dermatological, and musculoskeletal problems. Similar problems are responsible for attendance by middle and late adolescent males. Gynaecologial examination and diagnosis of pregnancy are the most common problems presented by middle and late adolescent females (Veit *et al.* 1996).

Various strategies have been employed to engage teenagers in the primary care system. School-based health centres have been reported to be highly successful in increasing adolescent utilization of medical, mental health and substance abuse counselling and intervention (Anglin *et al.* 1996; Kaplan *et al.* 1998).

Specialist medical services for adolescents and adolescent medicine

Children aged up to 13 or 14 years are customarily regarded as the responsibility of paediatric services. In some centres, older children may continue to be seen on an outpatient basis after the normal cut-off age, but the timing of transition to an adult clinic is likely to differ widely. Although the decline in childhood disorders is encouraging, paediatricians now need to divert more attention to adolescents. There is considerable variation in the extent to which adolescents are catered for on a separate basis, the majority being incorporated into general adult services. This means that in many medical specialties, the care of adolescents falls uneasily between paediatric and adult services.

The first steps in the organization of the special clinical care of adolescents began at the end of the nineteenth century and in the early decades of the twentieth century, following the emergence of the first scientific papers on adolescent growth and development. The establishment of the Medical Officers of Schools Associations in Great Britain in 1884 is often regarded as one of the first indicators of this process. However, subsequent progress took place largely in the United States (Heald 1992), where the Society for Adolescent Medicine was formed in 1968 and the clinical and professional boundaries of adolescent medicine began to be delineated (Blum 1987*a*). In 1980, the *Journal of Adolescent Health Care* began publication as the official voice of the Society. In the United Kingdom, despite explicit recommendations in numerous reports for specialized adolescent services (British Paediatric Association 1985), limited development has taken place. In general, professional interest and concern for adolescent health and welfare is reflected in growing scientific literature, textbooks and journals (Friedman *et al.* 1992; Brook 1993).

Teenagers require hospital admission for a wide variety of medical and surgical purposes (Henderson *et al.* 1993) and special consideration needs to be given to whether they should be nursed with younger children, with adults, or with other teenagers. The adult ward is generally inappropriate, especially for younger adolescents, because of possible juxtaposition with adults with degenerative and terminal disease, lack of a peer group, greater separation from parents through less flexible visiting arrangements, and staff unfamiliarity with age-appropriate responses and needs. Conversely, a paediatric setting can fail similarly to meet the psychological needs of teenagers in terms, for example, of independence, privacy, communication of feelings and information, consent to treatment, freedom from restrictive rules necessary for younger children, and even practical issues such as the size of the bed (Gillies and Parry-Jones 1992). Theoretically, services which assist in the transition from child to adult health care for young people with chronic disorders are identified as being of value. In practice they are limited in terms of their achievement of co-ordinated and integrated services (Scal *et al.* 1999).

Therefore there is a strong case for the use of separate purpose-designed adolescent wards, despite major implications for funding, human resources, and organizational and structural change. This view is supported by widespread experience in the United States and in the United Kingdom. In all outpatient or inpatient settings, there is a strong case for a multidisciplinary approach to the management of adolescents and their families, including input from child and adolescent psychiatrists, psychologists, psychiatric nurses, teachers, and social workers. Psychiatric liaison with adolescent services is much less frequent than with paediatrics and there are fewer examples of good practice (Black *et al.* 1990). The timing of transfer to adult services in adolescents who have built up strong attachment to their treatment teams, for example in cystic fibrosis or chronic renal failure, can generate problems. In general, the transfer date is best decided on an individual basis and needs to be backed by careful preparation. In many services problems are minimized by close liaison between paediatric or adolescent clinical teams and adult services.

Adolescent psychiatric services

Specialization in adolescent psychiatry has only a brief history (Parry-Jones 1994). During the second half of the nineteenth century, childhood mental disorders began to be described systematically, recognizing psychological and organic factors. Puberty became regarded increasingly as a physiological cause of mental disturbance, and pubescent or adolescent insanity began to be referred to frequently. Adolescents were admitted routinely to asylums and received no special age-related care until the late 1940s, when the first adolescent units opened. In the United Kingdom, exclusively adolescent inpatient services developed rapidly in the late 1960s in response to concern about the welfare of adolescents in adult mental hospital wards. Subsequently, there has been remarkable growth of adolescent outpatient, day patient, and inpatient services, and hospital treatment of serious adolescent psychiatric disorder is usually undertaken in age-appropriate surroundings. Nevertheless, significant deficiencies remain, reflecting the tendency for health services to be slower in providing for adolescents than for children or adults. Psychiatric services remain variable and incomplete, especially for acute disturbance, emergencies, rehabilitation and long-term care. Particular shortcomings include limited provision for older adolescents and young adults, the mentally retarded, aggressive conduct-disordered teenagers, and substance abusers, all of whom are difficult to place in other residential settings and who may need specialized secure facilities. Accessibility of services, especially inpatient units, is often unsatisfactory and overlap with adult services is inadequate and unplanned. Joint planning and co-ordination of services delivered by mental health, education and social services, and the voluntary organizations can be limited (Health Advisory Service 1986). The viability of inpatient units continues to challenge health care providers and many are threatened with closure (Parry-Jones 1995). Nevertheless, current guidelines for health service commissioning authorities in the United Kingdom (Health Advisory Service 1995) emphasize the fact that young people under the age of 16 years should only exceptionally be accommodated in adult wards and that commissioning or purchasing authorities should make provisions for the mental health problems of young people up to the age of 24 years.

Services for adolescents with disability

Good-quality services for adolescents with physical and learning disabilities requires a network of primary and specialist health care provisions, including rehabilitation facilities. It is particularly important to ensure the continuity of the health care of adolescents during the immediate postschool period as they transfer from child to adult services, and for there to be appropriate liaison with education authorities and social service departments (Fiorentino *et al.* 1998). The special health care requirements of adolescents with learning disability are complex and can only be provided on an individualized basis following assessment (Goh and Holland 1994).

Adolescent health-promotion and prevention programmes

Adolescence offers a unique opportunity for health promotion. The concept of adolescent health promotion, incorporating various prevention strategies, health education, and health protection programmes, is receiving increasing attention from health care policy-makers and providers, educators, and health and social scientists. In particular, significant morbidity and mortality amongst adolescents results from their participation in high-risk behaviours. Health-promotion activities have addressed these concerns in addition to the more conventional concern to prevent the development of disease in adulthood.

The subject is complex and compounded by inherent difficulties in the definition of health (especially mental health), uncertainty about the salience of health for adolescents, and controversy about the effectiveness of and justification for preventive intervention. It is not possible to establish a single set of universal objectives especially since health-promotion goals have to be seen in the perspective of the changing developmental stages of adolescence and the substantial influence of social, cultural, and economic factors. There is, for example, considerable evidence of the poor/non-poor differential in adolescent health status (Klerman 1993). The attitudes of teenagers to health advice and the response to information about what endangers health are extremely complex. Generally, it has proved difficult to gain access to the most vulnerable adolescent groups through health-promotion and health education programmes and, particularly, to demonstrate consistently the effectiveness of prevention and health-promotion programmes in reducing behavioural and lifestyle problems.

The interrelationship between health-promotion objectives and normal adolescent development is crucial and, in this context, Crockett and Petersen (1993) have suggested the following broad goals:

- to promote physical health and well being through proper nutrition and exercise, development of a positive body image and healthy sexuality, and adoption of a healthy lifestyle
- to promote cognitive maturity, including the capacity for abstract, formal reasoning, social-cognitive skills, and autonomous decision-making
- to promote self-esteem and a positive sense of personal identity, including positive future goals and a sense of self-efficacy and social responsibility
- to promote supportive relationships with family, peers, and other important adults
- to provide opportunities for educational and occupational success
- to avoid pitfalls that would interfere with the positive developmental outcomes.

Inevitably, such objectives are difficult to translate into large-scale prevention programmes.

There is a voluminous literature relating to prevention and health education. One prominent section is concerned principally with preventing or minimizing the adverse effects of risk-taking behaviours, such as dangerous driving, experimentation with smoking, drugs and alcohol, promiscuous sexual activity, and violence. The impact of intervention has often appeared to be disappointing, with particular difficulties in ensuring that the benefits of preventive programmes actually reach adolescents who come from impoverished, dysfunctional families or who are socially alienated. While the concept of the health-compromising lifestyle has been constructive, evidence of the effectiveness of intervention in such situations remains patchy. It may well be that since childhood behavioural responses predict psychopathological outcomes, the focus of intervention should be on a much earlier developmental stage. A second major section of the health-promotion literature is concerned specifically with the maintenance of sound general health, growth, and nutrition, and generally influencing attitudes to causes of future morbidity.

The application of health-promotion principles to adolescent mental health has been particularly challenging. Despite considerable advances in the understanding of the concept of mental health in this age group, there are formidable tasks facing mental health and other professionals in their efforts to promote optimal psychological development. These have to be based on an agreed definition of positive mental health, which Compas (1993) has described as 'a process characterized by development toward optimal current and future functioning in the capacity and motivation to cope with stress and to involve the self in personally meaningful instrumental activities and/or interpersonal relationships'. Optimal functioning is relative and depends on the goals and values of the interested parties, appropriate developmental norms, and one's sociocultural group. Intervention strategies based broadly on this model are usually concerned with lifeskills training and they have a particular role, for example in substance abuse prevention, by fostering skills for resisting social pressures to initiate abuse.

Many attempts have been made to identify factors and themes which contribute to successful programmes. In general terms, strategies should be acceptable to the individuals, cultural groups, and communities involved; adolescents should be involved actively in the process, and programmes should take into detailed consideration the needs of adolescents at different developmental stages (Hamburg *et al.* 1993). In an analysis of 100 prevention programmes for high-risk behaviours, Dryfoos (1990) identified a number of common strategies that appeared to contribute to success: one-to-one individual attention and support by trained staff, active involvement of parents, educational and non-educational interventions in schools, and finally, community-wide multiagency approaches. In general, the focus of intervention has to be on the antecedents of deviant behaviours, not the presenting problems. Health-promotion and education projects mounted simply at a local level are unlikely to be successful without the backing of substantial central government support for the enforcement of social policies. This may include laws against drunken driving and restrictions on cigarette advertising (Macfarlane 1993; Nutbeam *et al.* 1993).

Adolescent health promotion is a relatively new field for research. There is an urgent demand for better data, for example concerning the health status and the impact of health promotion on adolescents under conditions of poverty. There continues to be a need for exploration of the complex personal, interpersonal and sociocultural processes that encourage teenagers to persist with health endangering behaviours, despite having the relevant information about the risks involved. Evaluation studies remain an urgent priority.

Teaching and training of health care professionals

Many of the professionals involved in the health care of adolescents are unlikely to have day-to-day contact with members of this age group and have identified the need for more training at both undergraduate and postgraduate level in the management of adolescents. This compounds what appears to be a widespread neglect of teaching and training specifically about adolescent health issues, at either general professional or in-service training levels. There is an urgent need therefore to develop curricula for the training of physicians and other health care professionals that address the fact that adolescents present a spectrum of problems that extends beyond traditional medical practice (Blum 1987*b*). Training programmes need to cover a number of issues, including the following

- The changes associated with normal adolescent development and the way these affect and are affected by illness.
- Information about adolescents in the local community, causes of illness, disability, and death, specific health needs, and available resources.
- Preparation for the professional contact with adolescents and the all-important development of a therapeutic relationship. The face-to-face interview can be daunting for some adolescents and the clinician must be prepared to make imaginative use of anxiety-reducing moves, with particular attention given to establishing trust and confidence in adolescents who are withdrawn, uncommunicative, or fearful.
- The management of the full range of medical and surgical disorders, with particular emphasis on the psychological consequences of long-term illness.
- The management of the full range of psychosocial problems and mental disorders.
- Information about the most effective strategies for health promotion.

Conclusion

In this chapter, evidence is presented about the extent and the implications of physical, psychological, and social morbidity during adolescence and youth, and the slow, fragmented, and uneven response of health care providers. The magnitude of the psychological and social problems and health hazards facing adolescents and the existence of highly vulnerable groups of young people warrant urgent recognition by health care policy-makers, professionals, and managers. Worldwide, access for all adolescents to comprehensive age-appropriate health services must be a priority. In addition, programmes for reducing hazardous, high-risk behaviours and targeted interventions for the most vulnerable groups must be developed according to nationally determined priorities. Adolescent health care must be provided by specially trained professionals and designed to meet individual developmental, cultural, ethnic, and social needs. To meet this challenge, concerted action in relation to a set of central goals is imperative in order to improve the quality of adolescent health care throughout the world. These goals are set out below. Whilst they are universally applicable, priorities will be determined at national level.

- **Recognition of the social value attached to adolescence and youth:** the expansion and promotion of adolescent health care services is linked closely with the significance given by any society to adolescence as a distinct developmental period, and to the health, welfare, education, employment, and general status of teenagers.
- **Enhancement of the status of adolescent medicine:** the key to improving medical services for adolescents lies not only in enhancing the status of adolescent medicine as an independent specialty but also in addressing the needs of adolescents in the paediatric, general medical, and primary care setting.
- **Expansion of adolescent psychiatry:** when viewed in global perspective, adolescent psychiatry presents an extremely varied picture. Its establishment and expansion, in any country, depends on the funding for mental health services as a whole and on the legislative provisions for the care of mentally ill young people.
- **Accommodation of adolescent needs within service delivery:** adolescent needs should be recognized and met in all outpatient, inpatient, and community services. Some changes, such as the development of dedicated adolescent medical wards, will require substantial expansion of resources. Others, such as the improvement of facilities for adolescents, the establishment of outpatient services for young people suffering from the same medical disorder, joint hand-over clinics with adult specialists during a transitional period, and self-referral clinics, may require only modest additional funding and organizational change if existing services are reasonably well developed.
- **Inclusion of 'normal adolescence' and adolescent health issues in the teaching and training of health care professionals:** there is scope for at least an introduction to the special needs of normal adolescents in the teaching of all medical students, nurses, and other health care providers, as well as in postgraduate and in-service training. This provides an essential frame of reference for the identification, diagnosis, and management of adolescent health problems. In addition, all staff working directly with adolescents should receive specialized training.
- **Increased investment in prevention and health promotion:** the justification for early detection, preventive intervention, and health promotion in adolescence and young adulthood is powerful. However, adolescents are low users of health care; primary care

services frequently fail to meet their common health concerns and young people often prove difficult to engage. Therefore adolescents require imaginative, developmentally appropriate, and culturally sensitive school- and community-based programmes of health education and health promotion if their interest, trust, and commitment is to be gained.

- **Expansion of research:** there is extensive scope for research in adolescent medicine and adolescent health promotion, and for the assembly of reliable data on all aspects of adolescence and youth. Continuities and discontinuities with the health problems of childhood and adulthood, for example, need to be traced, with special emphasis on factors during childhood that influence adolescent and adult adaptation. Of fundamental importance is the continuing clarification of the developmental variation of medical and psychiatric disorders and the impact of normal development, maturational stress, and social and cultural factors on health care knowledge and attitudes, and response to illness. There needs to be verification of the nature and extent of the health problems and dysfunctional states experienced by adolescents in different cultures, the identification of the most vulnerable groups of young people and families, and the development of effective methods for the measurement of difficulty, distress, and quality of life. A major area of deficiency is the lack of information about what teenagers think about illness and the threat of disability or death. Hitherto, rigorous evaluation of preventive programmes has been lacking.
- **Collaboration between multiple agencies and services:** the problems and needs of adolescents impinge on many different agencies and services outside the health sector, involving schools, youth and social services, and a wide range of other community organizations. Consequently, in order to ensure comprehensive care, particularly as resources grow more scarce, there needs to be emphasis on the joint planning, co-ordination, and implementation of services.
- **Enhanced public policy considerations:** the need to raise the profile of adolescents and the improvement of adolescent health status on national political agendas calls for concerted representation and advocacy by all professional organizations concerned with their health and welfare. Innovative successful solutions for the improvement of adolescent health and the modification of high-risk behaviours are available and urgently await recognition, funding, and implementation. Many of the health-related problems of teenagers, especially those that make their behaviour obtrusive and disturbing within society, are associated with poverty, unemployment, homelessness, environmental deprivation, and racism. Therefore they are major public policy issues requiring intervention by governments followed by social change.

References

Altman, J., Everitt, B.J., Glautier S., *et al.* (1996). The biological, social and clinical bases of drug addiction: commentary and debate. *Psychopharmacology*, **125**, 285–345.

Anglin, T.M., Naylor, K.E., and Kaplan, D.W. (1996). Comprehensive school-based health care: high school students' use of medical, mental health, and substance abuse services. *Pediatrics*, **97**, 318–30.

Bancroft, J. and Reinisch, J.M. (1990). *Adolescence and puberty*. Oxford University Press.

Barton, J. (1995). A cause for public concern: suicide in children and young people. *Child Health*, **3**, 106–9.

Bennett, D.L. (1982). Worldwide problems in the delivery of adolescent health care. *Public Health*, **96**, 334–40.

Black, D., McFadyen, A., and Broster, G. (1990). Development of a psychiatric liaison service. *Archives of Disease in Childhood*, **65**, 1371–5.

Blos, P. (1962). *On adolescence*. Free Press, New York.

Blum, R. (1987*a*). Contemporary threats to adolescent health in the United States. *Journal of the American Medical Association*, **257**, 3390–5.

Blum, R. (1987*b*). Physician's assessment of deficiencies and desire for training in adolescent care, *Journal of Medical Education*, **62**, 401–7.

Blum, R. (1997). Adolescent substance use and abuse. *Archives of Pediatric and Adolescent Medicine*, **151**, 805–8.

Borduin, C.M. (1999). Multisystemic treatment of criminality and violence in adolescents. *Journal of the American Academy of Child and Adolescent Psychiatry*, **38**, 242–9.

Boyd, M. and Norris, D. (1999). The crowded nest: young adults at home. *Canadian Social Trends*, **52**, 2–5.

Bravender, T. and Knight, J.R. (1998). Recent patterns of use and associated risks of illicit drug use in adolescents. *Current Opinion in Pediatrics*, **10**, 344–9.

British Paediatric Association (1985). *Report of the working party on the needs and care of adolescents*. British Paediatric Association, London.

Brook, C.G.D. (ed.) (1993). *The practice of medicine in adolescence*. Edward Arnold, London.

Challener, J. (1990). Health education in secondary schools—is it working? A study of 1418 Cambridgeshire pupils. *Public Health*, **104**, 195–205.

Children's Legal Centre (1991). *Mental health handbook. Young people, mental health and the law—a handbook for parents and advisers*. Children's Legal Centre, London.

Childress, A., Brewerton, T., Hodges, E., and Jarrell, M. (1993). The kids eating disorder survery (KEDS): a study of middle school students. *Journal of American Academy of Child Adolescent Psychiatry*, **32**, 843–50.

Cohall, A., Cohall, R., and Bannister, H. (1998). Adolescents and violent crime. *Current Opinion in Pediatrics*, **10**, 356–62.

Cohen, P., Cohen, J., Kasen, S., *et al.* (1993). An epidemological study of disorders in late childhood and adolescence, I: age- and gender-specific prevalence. *Journal of Child Psychology and Psychiatry*, **34**, 851–67.

Coleman, J. and Hendry, L. (1990). *The nature of adolescence* (2nd edn). Routledge, London.

Compas, B.E. (1993). Promoting positive mental health during adolescence. In *Promoting the health of adolescents. New directions for the twenty-first century* (ed. S.G. Millstein, A.C. Petersen, and E.O. Nightingale), pp. 159–79. Oxford University Press, New York.

Craig, T.K. and Hodson, S. (1998). Homeless youth in London: I. Childhood antecendents and psychiatric disorder. *Psychological Medicine*, **28**, 1379–88.

Crockett, I.J. and Petersen, A.C. (1993). Adolescent development: health risks and opportunities for health promotion. In *Promoting the health of adolescents. New directions for the twenty-first century* (ed. S.G. Millstein, A.C. Petersen, and E.O. Nightingale), pp. 13–37. Oxford University Press, New York.

D'Souza, C.M. and Shrier, L.A. (1999). Prevention and intervention of sexually transmitted diseases in adolescents. *Current Opinion in Pediatrics*, **11**, 287–91.

Davis, G.E. and Leitenberg, H. (1987). Adolescent sex offenders. *Psychological Bulletin*, **101**, 417–27.

DoH (Department of Health) (1989). *The Children's Act (1989). An introductory guide for the NHS*. DoH, London.

DoH (Department of Health) (1992). *The health of the nation: a strategy for health in England*. DoH, London.

DoH (Department of Health) (1998). *On the state of the public health*. DoH, London.

DoH (Department of Health) (1999). *Saving lives: our healthier nation*. DoH, London.

Dryfoos, J. (1990). *Adolescents at risk. Prevalence and prevention.* Oxford University Press, New York.

Dubow, E.F., Lovko, R.R., and Kansch, D.F. (1990). Demographic differences in adolescents' health concerns and perceptions of helping agents. *Journal of Clinical Child Psychology*, **19**, 44–54.

Dyer, C. (1999). English teenager given heart transplant against her will. *British Medical Journal*, **319**, 209–19.

Epstein, R., Rice, P., and Wallace, P. (1989). Adolescent patients in an inner London general practice: their attitudes to illness and health care. *Journal of the Royal College of General Practitioners*, **39**, 247–9.

Field, A.F., Wolf, A.M., Herzog, D.B., *et al.* (1993). The relationship of caloric intake to the frequency of dieting among preadolescent and adolescent girls. *Journal of the American Academy of Child and Adolescent Psychiatry*, **32**, 1246–52.

Fiorentino, L., Datta, D., Gentle, S., *et al.* (1998). Transition from school to adult life for physically disabled young people. *Archives of Disease in Childhood*, **79**, 306–11.

Flay, B.R., Phil, D., Hu, F.B., and Richardson, J. (1998). Psychosocial predictors of different stages of smoking among high school students. *Preventive Medicine*, **27**, A9–18.

Freud, A. (1958). Adolescence. *Psychoanalytic Study of the Child*, **13**, 255–78.

Friedman, S.B., Fisher, M., and Schonberg, S.K.E. (1992). *Comprehensive adolescent health care.* Quality Medical Publishing, St Louis, MO.

Frim Forman, S. and Emans, S.J. (1998). Adolescent medicine. *Current Opinion in Pediatrics*, **10**, 337–7.

Geist, R., Katzman, D.K., and Colangelo, J.J. (1996). The Consent to Treatment Act and an adolescent with anorexia nervosa. *Health Law Canada*, **16**, 110–14.

Gillies, M.L. and Parry-Jones, W.L. (1992). Suitability of the paediatric setting for hospitalized adolescents. *Archives of Disease in Childhood*, **67**, 1506–9.

Glaser, D. (1993). Sexual abuse. In *The practice of medicine in adolescence* (ed. C.G.D. Brook), pp. 232–42. Edward Arnold, London.

Goh, S. and Holland, A.J. (1994). A framework for commissioning services for people with learning disabilities. *Journal of Public Health Medicine*, **16**, 279–85.

Goodyer, I.E. (1995). The depressed child and adolescent. In *Developmental and clinical perspectives.* Cambridge University Press.

Greenhill, L.L. and Waslick, B. (1997). Management of suicidal behavior in children and adolescents. *Psychiatric Clinics of North America*, **20**, 641–66.

Greve, J. and Currie, E. (1990). *Homeless in Britain.* Joseph Rowntree Memorial Trust, York.

Gunnell, D.J., Peters, T.J., Kammerling, R.M., and Brooks, J. (1995). Relation between parasuicide, suicide, psychiatric admissions and socioeconomic deprivation. *British Medical Journal*, **311**, 226–30.

Hall, G.S. (1904). *Adolescence: its psychology and its relations to phsiology, anthropology, sociology, sex, crime, religion and education.* Appleton, New York.

Hamburg, D.A., Millstein, S.G., Mortimer, A.M., Nightingale, E.O., and Petersen, A.C. (1993). Adolescent health promotion in the twenty-first century: current frontiers and future directions. In *Promoting the health of adolescents. New directions for the twenty-first century* (ed. S.G. Millstein, A.C. Petersen, and E.O. Nightingale), pp. 375–88. Oxford University Press, New York.

Heald, F.P. (1992). History adolescent medicine: a personal perspective. In *Comprehensive adolescent health care* (ed. S.B. Friedman and S.K. Schonberg), pp. xv–xviii. Quality Medical Publishing, St Louis, MO.

Henderson, J., Goldacre, M., and Yeates, D. (1993). Use of hospital inpatient care in adolescence. *Archives of Disease in Childhood*, **69**, 559–63.

Hill, P. (1998). Attention deficit hyperactivity disorder. *Archives of Disease in Childhood*, **79**, 381–5.

Hughes, J.M., Li, L., Chinn, S., and Rona, R.J. (1997). Trends in growth in England and Scotland. *Archives of Diseases in Children*, **76**, 182–9.

Jebb, S.A. (1997). Aetiology of obesity. *British Medical Bulletin*, **53**, 264–85.

Kaplan, D.W., Calonge, B.N., Guernsey, B.P., and Hanrahan, M.B. (1998). Management care and school-based health centers. Use of health services. *Archives of Pediatrics and Adolescent Medicine*, **152**, 25–33.

Kirby, D. (1999). Reflections on two decades of research on teen sexual behavior and pregnancy. *Journal of School Health*, **69**, 89–94.

Klerman, L.V. (1993). The influence of economic factors on health-related behaviors in adolescents. In *Promoting the health of adolescents. New directions for the twenty-first century* (ed. S.G. Millstein, A.C. Petersen, and E.O. Nightingale), pp. 38–57. Oxford University Press, New York.

Lewinsohn, P.M. and Hops, H. (1993). Adolescent psychopathology: I. Prevalence and incidence of depression and other DSM-III-R disorders in high school students. *Journal of Abnormal Psychology*, **102**, 133–13.

Lewis, M. (1991). *Child and adolescent psychiatry. A comprehensive textbook.* Williams and Wilkins, Baltimore, MD.

Lewis, M. and Volkmar, F.R. (1990). *Clinical aspects of child and adolescent development* (3rd edn). Lea and Febiger, Philadelphia, PA.

Macfarlane, A. (1993). Health promotion and children and teenagers. *British Medical Journal*, **306**, 81–89.

McFarlane, A.H., Bellissimo, A., and Norman, G.R. (1995). Family structure, family functioning and adolescent well-being: the transcendent influence of parental style. *Journal of Clinical Psychology and Psychiatry*, **36**, 847–64.

Markos, A.R., Wade, A.A.H., and Walzman, M. (1994). The adolescent male prostitute and sexual transmitted diseases. *Journal of Adolescence*, **17**, 123–30.

Melzer-Lange, M. and Lye, P.S. (1996). Adolescent health care in a pediatric emergency department. *Annals of Emergency Medicine*, **27**, 633–7.

Millstein, S.G. (1993). A view of health from the adolescent's perspective. In *Promoting the health of adolescents. New directions for the twenty first century* (ed. S.G. Millstein, A.C. Petersen, and E.O. Nightingale), pp. 97–118. Oxford University Press, New York.

Millstein, S.G., Igra, V., and Gans, J. (1996). Delivery of STD/HIV preventive services to adolescents by primary care physicians. *Journal of Adolescent Health*, 19, 249–57.

Mullins, L.L., Chaney, J.M., Pace, T.M., and Hartman, V.L. (1997). Illness uncertainty, attributional style, and psychological adjustment in older adolescents and young adults with asthma. *Journal of Paediatric Psychology*, **22**, 871–80.

Nelson, M.A. (1992). Sports medicine. In *Comprehensive adolescent health care* (ed. S.B. Friedman, M. Fisher, and S.K. Schonberg), pp. 1132–51. Quality Medical Publishing, St Louis, MO.

NHS Health Advisory Service (1986). *Bridges over troubled water.* HMSO, London.

NHS Health Advisory Service (1995). *Together we stand. The commissioning role and management of child and adolescent mental health services.* HMSO, London.

Nutbeam, D., Macaskill, P., Smith, C., Simpson, J., and Catford, J. (1993). Evaluation of two school smoking education programmes under normal classroom conditions. *British Medical Journal*, **306**, 102–7.

Offer, D. and Schonert-Reichl, K.A. (1992). Debunking the myths of adolescence: findings and recent research. *Journal of American Academy of Child and Adolescent Psychiatry*, **31**, 1003–14.

Office for National Statistics (1996). *Smoking among secondary school children survey.* HMSO, London.

Parry-Jones, W.L. (1993). Psychiatric disorders of adolescence. In *Companion to psychiatric studies* (ed. R.E. Kendell and A.K. Zeally) (5th edn), pp. 681–709. Churchill Livingstone, Edinburgh.

Parry-Jones, W.L. (1994). History of child and adolescent psychiatry. In *Child and adolescent psychiatry. Modern approaches* (3rd edn) (ed. M.

Rutter, E. Taylor, and L. Hersov), pp. 794–812. Blackwell Scientific, Oxford.

Parry-Jones, W.L. (1995). The future of adolescent psychiatry. *British Journal of Psychiatry*, **166**, 299–305.

Parry-Jones, W.L. and Gay, B.M. (1984). Disruptive incidents: causes and control in the secondary school classroom. In *Disruptive behaviour in schools* (ed. N. Frude and H. Gault), pp. 191–7. Wiley, London.

Paxman, J.M. and Zuckerman, R.J. (1987). *Laws and policies affecting adolescent health.* World Health Organization, Geneva.

Porteus, M.A. (1979). A survey of the problems of normal 15 year-olds. *Journal of Adolescence*, **2**, 307–23.

Rae-Grant, N. *et al.* (1999). Violent behaviour in children and youth: preventive intervention from a psychiatric perspective. *Journal of the American Academy of Child and Adolescent Psychiatry*, **38**, 235–41.

Rickert, V.I. and Wiemann, C.M. (1998). Date rape among adolescents and young adults. *Journal of Pediatric and Adolescent Gynecology*, **11**, 167–75.

Rigsby, D.C., Macones, G.A., and Driscoll, D.A. (1998). Risk factors for rapid repeat pregnancy among adolescent mothers: a review of the literature. *Journal of Pediatric and Adolescent Gynecology*, **11**, 115–26.

Roberts, I., Leah, L., and Barker, M. (1998). Trends in intentional injury deaths in children and teenagers (1980–1995). *Journal of Public Health Medicine*, **20**, 463–6.

Robins, L.N. and Rutter, M. (ed.) (1990). *Straight and devious pathways from childhood to adulthood.* Cambridge University Press.

Rosenberg, P.S. and Biggar, B.J. (1998). Trends in HIV incidence among young adults in the United States. *Journal of the American Medical Association*, **279**, 1894–9.

Rosenfeld, S.L., Fox, D.J., Keenan, P.M., Melchiono, M.W., Samples, C.L., and Woods, E.R. (1996). Primary care experiences and preferences of urban youth. *Journal of Pediatric Health Care*, **10**, 151–60.

Rosewater, K.M. and Burr, B.H. (1998). Epidemiology, risk factors, intervention, and prevention of adolescent suicide. *Current Opinion in Pediatrics*, **10**, 338–43.

Rutter, M., Taylor, E., and Hersov, L. (ed.) (1994). *Child and adolescent psychiatry. Modern approaches* (3rd edn). Blackwell Scientific, Oxford.

Sarigiani, P.A., Ryan, L., and Peterson, A.C. (1999). Prevention of high-risk behaviours in adolescent women. *Journal of Adolescent Health*, **25**, 109–19.

Savedra, M.C., Tesler, M.D., and Wegner, C. (1988). How adolescents describe pain. *Journal of American Academy of Child and Adolescent Psychiatry*, **9**, 315–20.

Scal, P., Evans, T., Blozis, S., Okinow, N., and Blum, R. (1999). Trends in transition from pediatric to adult health care services for young adults with chronic conditions. *Journal of Adolescent Health*, **24**, 259–64.

Seiffge-Krenke, I. (1998). Chronic disease and perceived developmental progression in adolescence. *Developmental Psychology*, **34**, 1073–84.

Shaffer, D. and Craft, L. (1999). Methods of adolescent suicide prevention. *Journal of Clinical Psychiatry*, **60**, 113–16.

Shapiro, R., Alexander, W., Siegel, L., Scovill, C., and Hay, J. (1998). Risk-taking patterns of female adolescents: what they do and why. *Journal of Adolescence*, **21**, 143–59.

Sheldrick, C. (1999). Practitioner review: the assessment and management of risk in adolescents. *Journal of Child Psychology and Psychiatry*, **40**, 507–18.

Sockrider, M.M. (1997). The role of the pediatrician in smoking prevention. *Current Opinion in Pediatrics*, **9**, 225–9.

Spruijt, E. and de Goede, M. (1997). Transitions in family structure and adolescent well-being. *Adolescence*, **32**, 897–911.

Steiner, H. (1997). Practice parameters of the assessment and treatment of children and adolescents with conduct disorder. *Journal of American Academy of Child and Adolescent Psychiatry*, **36**, 122S–39S.

Steinhausen, H.C. (1994). Anorexia and bulimia nervosa. In *Child and adolescent psychiatry* (ed. M. Rutter, E. Taylor, and L. Hersov), pp. 425–40. Blackwell Scientific, Oxford.

Stiller, C.A. (1994). Population based survival rates from childhood cancer in Britain. *British Medical Journal*, **309**, 1612–16.

Stronski Huwiler, S.M. and Remafedi, G. (1998). Adolescent homosexuality. *Advances in Pediatrics*, **45**, 107–44.

Tobler, N.S. and Statton, H.S. (1997). Effectiveness of school-based drug prevention programs: a meta-analysis of the research. *Journal of Primary Prevention*, **18**, 71–128.

Tornqvist, J., Van Broeck, N., Finkenauer, C., *et al.* (1999). Long-term psychosocial adjustment following pediatric liver transplantation. *Pediatric Transplant*, **3**, 115–25.

Troiano, R.P., Flegal, K.M., Kuczmarski, R.J., *et al.* (1995). Overweight prevalence and trends for children and adolescents: The national health and nutrition examination surveys, 1963 to 1991. *Archives of Pediatrics and Adolescent Medicine*, **149**, 1085–91.

Troop, P. and Green, S. (1997). The health of the nation 4 years on: what have we done, what must we do? *British Journal of Hospital Medicine*, **57**, 99–100.

Tyas, S.L. and Pederson, L.L. (1998). Psychological factors related to adolescent smoking: a critical review of the literature. *Tobacco Control*, **7**, 409–20.

UN (United Nations) (1998). *Revision of the world population estimates and projections.* Population Division, Department of Economic and Social Affairs, 1–2. United Nations, New York.

Veit, F.C., Sanci, L.A., Coffey, C.M., Young, D.Y., and Bowes, G. (1996). Barriers to effective primary health care for adolescents. *Medical Journal of Australia*, **165**, 131–3.

Verhust, F.C., van der Ende, J., Ferdinand, R.F., and Kasius, M.C. (1997). The prevalence of DSM-III-R diagnoses in national sample of Dutch adolescents. *Archives of General Psychiatry*, **54**, 329–9.

Walker, Z. and Townsend, J. (1998). Promoting adolescent mental health in primary care: a review of the literature. *Journal of Adolescence*, **21**, 621–34.

Walker, A.M., Harris, G., Baker, A., Kelly, D., and Houghton, J. (1999). Post-traumatic stress responses following liver transplantation in older children. *Journal of Child Psychology and Psychiatry*, **40**, 363–74.

Weist, M.D., Ginsburg, G., and Shafer, M. (1999). Progress in adolescent mental health. *Adolescent Medicine*, **10**, 165–75.

West, P., Wight, D., and Macintyre, S. (1993). Heterosexual behaviour of 18-year-olds in the Glasgow area. *Journal of Adolescence*, **16**, 367–96.

WHO (World Health Organization) (1965). *Health problems of adolescence: report of a WHO Expert Committee.* WHO, Geneva.

WHO (World Health Organization) (1989). *The health of youth.* WHO, Geneva.Williams, J.G. and Covington, C.J. (1997). Predictors of cigarette smoking among adolescents. *Psychological Reports*, **80**, 481–2.

Windle, M. and Windle, R.C. (1999). Adolescent tobacco, alcohol, and drug use: current findings. *Adolescent Medicine*, **10**, 153–63.

Yach, D. and Ferguson, B.J. (1999). Can we stop children and adolescents from smoking? *Social Science and Medicine*, 48, 757–8.

Ziv, A., Boulet, J.R., and Ap, G.B. (1999). Utilization of physician offices by adolescents in the United States. *Pediatrics*, **104**, 35–42.

11.5 Workers

Dean B. Baker and Philip J. Landrigan

Introduction

Workers constitute a large and important population. The World Health Organization (**WHO**) estimated in 1997 that the global labour force was about 2600 million with 75 per cent of these working people in developing countries (WHO 1997). The officially registered working population includes 60 to 70 per cent of the world's adult males and 30 to 60 per cent of the adult female population. In addition, the International Labour Organization (**ILO**) estimated that in 1996 there were 250 million children between the ages of 5 and 14 years who were engaged in economic activity—at least 120 million of them on a full-time basis (IPEC 1999). Most people between the ages of 22 and 65 spend approximately 40 per cent of their waking hours at work, so working is a central feature of most people's lives (Leigh *et al.* 1997).

Workers suffer a broad range of illness caused by hazards encountered in the workplace (Rom 1998; Stellman 1998). The illnesses include:

- lung cancer and mesothelioma in asbestos workers
- cancer of the bladder in dye workers
- leukaemia in workers exposed to benzene
- chronic bronchitis in workers exposed to dusts
- disorders of the nervous system in workers using solvents
- heart disease in workers exposed to carbon monoxide
- impairment of reproductive function in men and women using lead and certain pesticides
- chronic diseases of the musculoskeletal system in workers who suffer repetitive trauma.

National and international organizations, policies, and laws concerned with workplace safety and health have developed rapidly during the past three decades in response to concerns about workers' health. In the United States, the Occupational Safety and Health Act was passed by Congress in 1970. Its goal was 'to assure as far as possible every working man and woman in the nation safe and healthful working conditions'. In the United Kingdom, the first legislation pertaining to occupational health was the Act for Better Regulations of Chimney Sweeps and Their Apprentices, enacted in 1788. This Act was followed by passage of a series of protective laws through the nineteenth and early twentieth centuries. The Health and Safety at Work Act, enacted in 1974, provides a broad legislative framework for the protection of workers through specific regulations. The Control of Substances Hazardous to Health Regulations of 1988 oblige employers to control hazardous substances through comprehensive assessment and documentation of potential risks from using these substances in the workplace. The European Union adopted a policy in 1989 on the Fundamental Social Rights of Workers, emphasizing the need for safety and health protection in the workplace, improvements in living and working conditions, and provision of social protection for workers. The European Union has encouraged harmonization in occupational safety and health practices among member states through issuance of directives (Wright 1998). These directives provide guidance to nations worldwide on laws needed to protect workers. Laws governing workplace safety and health now exist in virtually all developed countries and in a growing number of developing countries.

Despite the passage of protective legislation, success in reducing work-related illness has remained elusive. For example, silicosis, a disease recognized since antiquity, is still the most widespread occupational lung disease (WHO 1999). Approximately 300 deaths are attributed to silicosis annually in the United States (OSHA 1996). It is found in as many as 25 per cent of Korean and Malaysian miners. Although used less frequently than in the past in many developed countries, global production of asbestos continues to increase, and it remains widely dispersed even in countries where new uses are banned. Sales of asbestos in the 1990s actually increased in a number of developing nations as a consequence of aggressive marketing campaigns which claimed misleadingly that some forms of asbestos are 'safe' (Landrigan *et al.* 1999). Occupational hazards are being relocated from countries with more protective laws to countries with less regulations or less enforcement (LaDou 1995). Finally, there is substantial uncertainty about possible risks to health of new technologies and changes in work organization associated with economic globalization.

Occupational diseases are highly preventable. They arise from man-made conditions and therefore can be prevented through alteration of those conditions. The fundamental public health techniques of surveillance, identifying groups at risk, and intervening to control the spread of disease may all be applied effectively in the control of work-related illness. Moreover, occupational disease is not necessarily restricted to the workplace. Toxic hazards may escape from the workplace or be released into the community environment to pollute the air, drinking water supply, or food chain. Also, occupational toxins have been transported home on the shoes and clothing of contaminated workers to cause such illnesses as lead poisoning, chloracne, and mesothelioma in children and other family members.

There is growing recognition of the close relationship between occupational and environmental health.

This chapter will review the impact of workplace hazards on workers' health, including changes associated with economic globalization and impacts on special populations of workers such as women and children. It will discuss approaches to more efficient identification and better surveillance of the illnesses caused by work. Finally, it will review and evaluate the hierarchy of techniques used for the prevention of occupational injuries and illnesses.

Extent of occupational injury and disease

In most nations there is no completely reliable source of information on the extent of work-related injuries and diseases. Even so, the ILO estimates that work-related injuries and illnesses kill 1.1 million people worldwide each year, including 300 000 worker fatalities from 250 million workplace accidents (WHO 1999). An estimated 160 million new cases of work-related diseases occur each year worldwide.

In the United States, employers reported 6.3 million work injuries and 515 000 cases of occupational illnesses in 1994 (NIOSH 1996). Because of limitations in using only employer reports to measure work-related injuries and illnesses, Leigh *et al.* (1997) used multiple data sources to develop more accurate estimates of the annual incidence and mortality associated with occupational injuries and illnesses in the United States. They aggregated national and regional datasets collected by the Bureau of Labor Statistics, the National Council on Compensation Insurance, the National Center for Health Statistics, the Health Care Financing Administration, and other government agencies. They applied an attributable risk proportion method to assess incidence of and mortality from occupational injuries and illnesses. For this method, they reviewed the scientific literature to derive conservative estimates for the proportion of specific injuries, diseases, or mortality that are work related. Examples of the proportions of mortality they attributed to occupational causes are cancer (6–10 per cent), cardiovascular and cerebrovascular disease (5–10 per cent among adults up to 65 years of age, or 0.6–1.2 per cent overall), chronic respiratory disease (10 per cent), pneumoconioses (100 per cent), nervous system disorders (1–3 per cent), and renal disorders (1–3 per cent). Based on this analysis, they estimated that there are approximately 6500 job-related deaths from injuries, 13.2 million non-fatal injuries, 60 300 deaths from occupational illness, and 862 200 new occupational illnesses annually in the United States workforce of 120 million persons (Leigh *et al.* 1997).

Estimates of cost and economic loss

Total economic losses due to occupational injuries and illnesses are large. The ILO estimated that overall economic losses from work-related injuries and illnesses in 1997 were approximately 4 per cent of the world's gross national product (WHO 1999). In 1992, the direct cost in compensation for work-related injuries and illnesses in European Union countries was 27 000 million ecus. The major categories of work-related injuries and diseases responsible for these costs were musculoskeletal (40 per cent), heart diseases (16 per cent), injuries (14 per cent), respiratory diseases (9 per cent), and central nervous system conditions (8 per cent).

To assess costs associated with work-related conditions in the United States, Leigh *et al.* (1997) used the human capital method that decomposes costs into direct categories such as medical and insurance administration expenses as well as indirect categories such as lost earnings, lost home production, and lost fringe benefits. They applied these costs to the estimated annual job-related deaths from injury and illnesses, non-fatal injuries, and illnesses cited above. The total annual cost for 1992 was estimated to be US$171 billion, comprising US$65 billion direct costs and US$106 billion indirect costs. Injuries cost US$145 billion and illnesses cost US$26 billion. These estimates are likely to be low because the numbers of occupational injuries and illness are probably undercounted in the national datasets and because they ignore costs associated with pain and suffering as well as within-home care provided by family members.

Causes of under-recognition of occupational disease

Although recording of workplace injuries is reasonably accurate in most developed countries, surveillance systems generally result in substantial underestimates of the actual cases of occupational illness. One explanation for under-recognition of occupational disease is the inherent difficulty in diagnosing occupational diseases and in establishing cause-and-effect relationships. The link between occupation and disease is often elusive, because most occupational diseases are not distinct clinically and pathologically from diseases associated with non-occupational aetiologies. For example, the skin cancer caused by polycyclic aromatic hydrocarbons is similar in appearance to that caused by sunlight. Similarly, solvent-induced encephalopathy may easily be attributed to old age and lead-induced nephropathy to high blood pressure or diabetes. Only in rare instances, such as the associations between asbestos and mesothelioma (Selikoff *et al.* 1964) and between vinyl chloride monomer and angiosarcoma of the liver (Creech and Johnson 1974), is the causal association between occupational exposure and disease readily established on clinical grounds alone.

A second cause of the under-recognition of occupational disease is that the majority of chemicals in commerce have never been evaluated with regard to their potential toxicity. Only about 12 000 of the estimated 70 000 chemicals commonly used in industry have been tested for toxicity in animals (LaDou 1997). Furthermore, the toxicity testing has concentrated primarily on high-dose, acute effects and on the long-term risk of cancer. Toxicity testing of reproductive, neurological, immunological, and other adverse effects remains quite limited.

The long latency which typically elapses between occupational exposure and onset of illness is a third factor which may obscure the occupational aetiology of chronic disease. For example, few occupational cancers appear within 10 or even 20 years of first exposure. Similarly, the chronic neurotoxic effects of solvents may become evident only after decades of exposure. A worker so affected may well have retired. In such a case, it is unlikely that the worker will be diagnosed as having a disease of occupational origin.

Lack of awareness among health practitioners about the hazards found at work is a fourth cause of underestimation of occupational disease, reflecting the fact that most physicians are not adequately trained to suspect work as a cause of disease (IOM 1988; Goldman *et al.* 1999). Very little time is devoted in most medical schools to teaching physicians to take a proper occupational history, to recognize the symptoms of common industrial toxins, or to recall the known associations between occupational exposures and disease.

Compounding this lack of medical awareness is the limited ability of many workers to provide an accurate report of their exposures. Workers may have had multiple toxic exposures in a variety of jobs over a working lifetime. In most countries, there are no requirements to inform workers of the nature or hazard of the materials with which they work. Even in the United States, employers' reporting requirements remain limited under the Hazard Communication Standard and under state right-to-know laws (National Research Council 1987). In many instances, an ill patient will simply not know about his or her past occupational exposures.

Finally, given the potential financial liability associated with the finding that a disease is of occupational origin, employers may be resistant to recognizing the work-relatedness of a disorder, especially in cases where personal habits or non-occupational pursuits are possible contributory factors. Since employers are often in the best position to recognize causal associations between workplace exposures and disease, this conflict of interest represents a major obstacle to obtaining accurate estimates of the burden of occupational illness.

Major types of occupational injury and disease

Occupational illness can affect virtually every organ system (Rom 1998; Stellman 1999). Occupational diseases of the lung and skin are common since these organs have substantial surface areas in direct contact with toxic substances. Noise induced hearing loss and musculoskeletal disorders are the most common disorders arising from physical factors in the workplace. Occupational cancer is a major concern because of the high mortality associated with many forms of cancer. Increasing attention has been paid in recent years to diseases affecting the neurological, reproductive, and immunological systems as sensitive measures have become available to demonstrate adverse effects of chronic low-level occupational exposures. The following examples illustrate major occupational injuries and diseases. Table 1 shows examples of occupational diseases associated with pertinent industries and toxic agents.

Occupational lung diseases

Occupational lung diseases are very important in the field of occupational medicine because the lung is an accessible target organ for airborne toxic substances. Major categories of lung disease include the 'dust diseases' of the lung or pneumoconioses, lung cancer, occupational asthma, industrial bronchitis and other effects of irritants, and infections. Silicosis is the most common pneumoconiosis worldwide. Exposure to silica occurs in a wide variety of occupations such as sandblaster, miner, miller, pottery worker, foundry worker, and workers using abrasives. The Occupational Safety and Health Administration (**OSHA**) estimates that there are over 2 million workers potentially exposed to silica dust in the United States, including 100 000 workers in high-risk jobs (OSHA 1996). The International Agency for Research on Cancer has classified crystalline silica as a known human carcinogen (IARC 1997).

Asbestos is also an important cause of pneumoconiosis and other lung diseases. Asbestos has been responsible for over 200 000 deaths in the United States and it will cause millions more deaths worldwide (Collegium Ramazzini 1999). All forms of asbestos cause asbestosis, a progressive fibrosis of the lungs. The preponderance of scientific evidence indicates that all forms of asbestos also cause lung cancer and malignant mesothelioma. Peto *et al.* (1999) estimate that deaths from malignant mesothelioma among men in Western Europe will increase from over 5000 in 1998 to about 9000 in 2018. They estimate that there will be more than half a million asbestos-related malignant mesothelioma cancer deaths in Western Europe over the next 35 years. Given the long latency, the future burden of mortality resulting from asbestos will be substantial even if all future exposures were to be eliminated completely.

Bronchial asthma affects about 5 to 10 per cent of the population in developed countries, and estimates in the United States suggest that occupational asthma accounts for up to 28 per cent of asthma in adults (NIOSH 1996). In some jurisdictions, occupational asthma has become the most prevalent occupational lung disease, exceeding silicosis and asbestosis. Even so, prevalence studies of occupational asthma usually underestimate the number of affected workers because these workers tend to quit jobs where they suffer such symptoms. Concern about occupational asthma has increased because studies have shown that many workers who develop occupational asthma do not recover completely even several years after removal from exposure (Venables and Chang-Yeung 1997; Perfetti *et al.* 1998; Ross and McDonald 1998).

Many gases, fumes, and aerosols are directly toxic to the respiratory tract by causing acute inflammation. Examples include soluble irritants such as hydrogen chloride, ammonia, and sulphur dioxide which produce effects in the eyes, nasopharynx, and large airways. Less soluble irritants such as nitrogen dioxide, ozone, or phosgene produce few upper respiratory symptoms, but in high exposure can cause a toxic pneumonitis. Long-term exposure can lead to lung fibrosis.

Occupational cancer

About 300 to 350 substances have been identified as occupational carcinogens (WHO 1997). They include chemical substances such as benzene and asbestos, physical hazards such as ionizing radiation, and biological hazards such as viruses. It is estimated that approximately 16 million workers in the European Union are exposed to carcinogens at work. The most common cancers due to these workplace exposures are cancers of the lung, bladder, skin, pleura (mesothelioma), liver, haematopoietic tissue, bone, and soft connective tissue.

Estimates of the fraction of cancers caused by occupational exposures vary from 4 to 40 per cent (Pearce *et al.* 1998). The large variability in the estimates arises from differences in the datasets used and the assumptions applied. The most commonly accepted estimate is 4 per cent with a plausible range, based on the best quality studies, being 2 to 8 per cent. However, if one considers not the whole population, but only the adult population in which exposure to occupational carcinogens almost exclusively occurs, the proportion of cancer attributed to occupation would increase to about 20 per cent among those exposed (Pearce *et al.* 1998).

Leigh *et al.* (1997) estimated that 6 to 10 per cent of the cancer mortality in the United States could be attributed to workplace exposures, accounting for 31 025 to 51 708 deaths annually. The

Table 1 Examples of occupational diseases and related hazards by occupation and agent

Condition	Industry/occupation	Agent
Pulmonary tuberculosis	Physicians, medical personnel	*Mycobacterium tuberculosis*
Plague, tularaemia, anthrax, rabies, and other infections	Farmers, ranchers, hunters, veterinarians, laboratory workers	Various infectious agents
Rubella	Medical personnel, intensive care personnel	Rubella virus
Hepatitis	Day-care centre staff, orphanage staff, medical personnel	Hepatitis A, B, and C virus
Ornithosis	Bird breeders, pet shop staff, poultry producers, veterinarians, zoo workers	*Chlamydia psittaci*
Malignant neoplasm of nasal cavities	Woodworkers, cabinet makers, furniture makers	Hardwood dust; formaldehyde
	Radium chemists and processors	Radium
	Nickel smelting and refining	Nickel
Malignant neoplasm of larynx	Asbestos industries and users	Asbestos
Malignant neoplasm of trachea, bronchus, and lung	Asbestos industries and users Topside coke oven workers Uranium and fluorspar miners Smelters, processors, users Ion exchange resin makers, chemists	Asbestos Coke oven emissions Radon daughters Chromates, nickel, arsenic *Bis*(chloromethyl)ether
Mesothelioma	Asbestos industries and users	Asbestos
Malignant neoplasm of bone	Radium chemists and processors	Radium
Malignant neoplasm of scrotum	Automatic lathe operators, metalworkers. Coke oven workers, petroleum refiners	Mineral/cutting oils Soots and tars
Malignant neoplasm of bladder	Rubber and dye workers	Benzidine, naphthylamine, auramine, 4-nitrophenyl
Leukaemia (lymphoid and myeloid)	Radiologists Rubber industry; chemical industry	Ionizing radiation Benzene
Erythroleukaemia	Rubber industry; chemical industry	Benzene
Non-autoimmune haemolytic anaemia	Whitewashing and leather industry Electrolytic processes, smelting Plastic	Copper sulphate Arsine Trimellitic anhydride
Aplastic anaemia	Chemical manufacture Radiologists, radium chemists	TNT, benzene Ionizing radiation
Agranulocytosis or neutropenia	Explosives and pesticide industries Pesticides, pigments, pharmaceuticals	Phosphorus Inorganic arsenic, benzene
Toxic encephalitis	Battery, smelter, and foundry workers	Lead
Parkinson's disease (secondary)	Manganese processing, welders	Manganese

Table 1 Examples of occupational diseases and related hazards by occupation and agent (*Continued*)

Inflammatory and toxic neuropathy	Pesticides, pigments, pharmaceuticals	Arsenic and arsenic compounds
	Furniture refinishers, degreasing operations	Hexane
	Plastics, rayon industries	Methyl butyl ketone, copper disulfide
	Battery, smelter and foundry workers	Lead
	Dentists, chloralkali plants, battery makers	Mercury
	Plastic industry, paper manufacturing	Acrylamide
	Radiologists	Ionizing radiation
	Blacksmiths, glass blowers, bakers	Infrared radiation
	Moth-repellent formulators, fumigators	Naphthalene
Hearing loss	Many industries	Excessive noise
Raynaud's phenomenon (secondary)	Lumberjacks, chain sawyers, grinders	Whole body vibration
	Vinyl chloride polymerization industry	Vinyl chloride monomer
Extrinsic asthma	Jewellery alloy, and catalyst makers	Platinum
	Polyurethane, adhesive, paint workers	Isocyanates
	Plastic, dye, insecticide makers	Phthalic anhydride
	Foam workers, latex makers, biologists	Formaldehyde
	Bakers	Flour
	Woodworkers, furniture makers	Wood dust
Pneumoconiosis of coal	Coal miners, power plant workers	Coal dust
Asbestosis	Asbestos industries, construction workers, demolition workers, building maintenance workers, fire fighters	Asbestos
Silicosis	Quarrymen, sandblasters, miners, silica processors, ceramic industries and foundries	Silica
Talcosis	Talc processors	Talc
Chronic beryllium disease of lung	Beryllium alloy workers, ceramic and cathode ray tube makers, nuclear reactor workers	Beryllium
Byssinosis	Cotton industry workers	Cotton, flax and hemp dust
Acute bronchitis, pneumonitis, and pulmonary oedema due to fumes and vapours	Alkali and bleach industries	Chlorine
	Silo fillers, arc welders	Nitrogen oxides
	Paper, refrigeration, oil industries	Sulphur dioxide
	Plastics industry	Trimellitic anhydride
Toxic hepatitis	Solvent users, dry cleaners, plastics industry	Carbon tetrachloride, chloroform
	Explosives and dye industries	Phosphorus, TNT
	Fumigators, fire extinguisher formulators	Ethylene dibromide
Acute or chronic renal failure	Battery makers, plumbers, solderers	Inorganic lead
	Electrolytic processes, smelting	Arsine
	Battery makers, jewellers, dentists	Inorganic mercury
	Fire extinguisher makers	Carbon tetrachloride
	Antifreeze manufacturers	Ethylene glycol
Male infertility	Pesticide formulators and applicators	Dibromochloropropane
Contact and allergic dermatitis	Leather tanning, poultry dressing plants, packing, adhesives and sealant industry, boat building and repair	Irritants and allergens (e.g. oils, solvents, acids, alkalis, allergens)

Adapted from Landrigan and Baker (1991).

work-related attributable proportion varies by cancer type. About 10 per cent of lung cancers, 21 to 25 per cent of bladder cancer, and nearly 100 per cent of mesotheliomas in the general population are related to occupational exposures (NIOSH 1996). For workers with exposure to specific carcinogens, the percentage of cancer attributed to the occupational exposure is even higher, approaching 50 per cent for asbestos in the development of lung cancer and 100 per cent for vinyl chloride in the development of angiosarcoma of the liver (NIOSH 1996).

Occupational skin disorders

Skin disorders are among the most commonly reported occupational diseases (Adams 1999). In 1997 the estimated rate of occupational skin disorders in the United States was 6.7 per 10 000 full-time workers, accounting for about 13 per cent of reported occupational diseases—second only to disorders associated with repeated trauma (BLS 1998). Contact dermatitis accounts for almost 90 per cent of these skin disorders, while about 5 per cent are due to skin infections. Although skin disorders are relatively easily diagnosed, occupational skin diseases are believed to be severely under-reported, so that the actual rate may be many times higher than officially reported (NIOSH 1996). Occupational skin disorders are unevenly distributed among industries. A worker in agriculture, forestry, fishing, or manufacturing has three times the risk of developing a work-related skin disease as a worker in other industries.

Occupational infectious diseases

Naturally much attention about infectious diseases has focused on health care settings, although infections can be transmitted in other workplaces such as research laboratories and animal processing facilities. Within health care settings, awareness has grown about the risk of infection by hepatitis (especially hepatitis B and hepatitis C virus), HIV, and tuberculosis (*Mycobacterium tuberculosis*). Before the widespread use of hepatitis B virus vaccine, approximately 8700 acute cases of hepatitis B virus infection were reported among health care workers each year in the United States (NIOSH 1996). The risk of hepatitis B virus infection following a needle-stick injury with a contaminated needle varies from 2 to 40 per cent, depending on the antigen status of the source patient. The risk of hepatitis C virus transmission ranges from 3.3 to 10 per cent. The potential for hepatitis B or hepatitis C virus transmission is greater than that for HIV, but the modes of transmission are similar. An increased risk of HIV infection has been shown to exist in settings in which workers may be exposed to blood or body fluids (NIOSH 1996).

Transmission of *M. tuberculosis* is a recognized risk in health care facilities. After years of declining incidence rates, multidrug-resistant tuberculosis re-emerged as a major occupational health problem during the 1990s in major cities in the United States which serve populations with high rates of multidrug-resistant tuberculosis (CDC 1999). The magnitude of risk for health care workers varies by the type of health care facility, the prevalence of tuberculosis in the community, the patient population served, and the effectiveness of the infection control programme. The rates of multidrug-resistant tuberculosis in health care facilities decreased by the end of the decade following implementation of the OSHA standard (OSHA 1991) designed to prevent exposure to infectious agents and strengthening of workplace tuberculosis control programmes (CDC 1999).

Infectious diseases can be especially prevalent in developing countries, resulting in higher risks for workers in these countries. Some of the infections result directly from the work, while others are indirectly related to work. Examples include vector-borne diseases like malaria, water- and food-borne diseases resulting from poor sanitation and inadequate potable water, and zoonoses among agricultural workers.

Occupational reproductive disorders

The overall contribution of occupational exposures to reproductive disorders is not known because there has been little research in this area until recently. More than 1000 workplace chemical have shown reproductive effects in animal studies, but most have not been studied in humans (NIOSH 1996). Furthermore, virtually no studies have been done on physical and biological agents that may affect fertility and pregnancy outcomes. Epidemiological research on occupational hazards to reproduction has expanded in recent years (Lindbohm 1999).

It has been well documented that lead and the pesticide dibromochloropropane cause testicular injury with resultant reduction in sperm count. Also lead can cross the placenta in a pregnant woman worker to cause neurological impairment in the fetus. Other substances associated with adverse reproductive outcomes for which human evidence is strong include methyl mercury, solvents such as carbon disulphide, oestrogens, anaesthetic gases, ethylene oxide, polychlorinated biphenyls, and physical agents such as ionizing radiation (Frazier and Hage 1998).

Occupational exposures can cause a wide range of reproductive disorders in both males and females. Effects of exposure in males include altered sperm number, shape, or function, altered sperm transfer, and altered hormones or sexual performance—all of which may lead to subfecundity or impaired capability to conceive a viable child (Lemaster 1998). Exposures in females may cause menstrual disorders, infertility, chromosomal aberrations, breast milk alteration, early onset of menopause, and suppressed libido.

Reproductive disorders also include adverse effects on the offspring of the exposed worker. Potential fetal effects from maternal exposure include preterm delivery, fetal loss, prenatal death, low birth weight, altered sex ratio, congenital malformations, childhood malignancies, infant or childhood illness, and developmental disabilities (Lemaster 1998). Less is known about male-mediated exposure effects on the offspring.

Musculoskeletal injuries

Musculoskeletal injuries include both acute and chronic injury to the musculoskeletal system, other than acute trauma. These conditions are one of the leading problems affecting workers. In the United States, back disorders account for 27 per cent of all non-fatal occupational injuries and illnesses involving days away from work (NIOSH 1996). More than half of the working population develop low back injury at some time in their working career. Musculoskeletal injuries are the principal cause of disability of people in their working years.

The incidence of musculoskeletal disorders associated with cumulative or repetitive work has increased dramatically in recent years to become the most commonly reported occupational disease. In 1997, 276 600 musculoskeletal disorders due to repeated trauma were reported in American workplaces (BLS 1998). This figure represents

64 per cent of all reported occupational illness cases in the United States. The most frequently reported upper extremity disorders affect the hand or wrist area, including the most widely recognized condition—carpal tunnel syndrome.

Severe occupational traumatic injuries

These injuries include such events as amputations, fractures, severe lacerations, eye losses, acute poisonings, and burns. The National Institute for Occupational Safety and Health (**NIOSH**) estimates that at least 10 million persons in the United States suffer traumatic injuries at work each year; the average annual occupational fatality rate for the United States workforce is 7 per 100 000 workers (CDC 1993). On average, 17 workers died each day during 1998 in the United States (BLS 1999). Major causes of deaths were highway motor vehicle crashes (24 per cent), homicides (12 per cent), falls (10 per cent), caught in or compressed by equipment or objects (6 per cent), electrocutions (7 per cent), and being struck by falling objects (5 per cent). The largest number of fatalities occurred among truck drivers, construction trades, farm occupations, and sales occupations. Occupations with the highest rates of fatal injuries were fishermen, timber cutters and loggers, aeroplane pilots and navigators, structural metal workers, taxicab drivers, and construction workers. Homicide and violence in the workplace have received increasing attention as major causes of occupational fatalities. Homicide is the leading cause of work-related death for females. Homicide is the leading cause of occupational fatalities in some of the largest and fastest growing industry sectors—retail trade, services, and finance/insurance/real estate.

Occupational exposure to noise

Noise is a widespread problem that has substantial impact on the prevalence of hearing loss among the working population. Estimates indicate that 30 million people in the United States work at sites where the level of noise, 85 dB or higher, presents an increased risk of noise-induced hearing loss (NIOSH 1996). One worker in four exposed occupationally to 90 dB of noise over a working lifetime will develop a hearing impairment caused by noise.

Economic globalization and workers' health

Rapid technological innovation and the proliferation of multinational organizations are driving the formation of a global economy that has a substantial impact on workers' safety and health. Technological change is creating fundamental transformations in the way corporations organize production, trade goods, invest capital, and develop new products (CAETS 1988). Technology allows virtually instantaneous communication among widely dispersed operations. Advanced manufacturing technologies have changed patterns of productivity and employment. Improved air and sea transportation has greatly accelerated the flow of people and goods. These technological developments have created greater interdependence among firms and nations. At the same time, the rapid rate of innovation means that competitive advantages are fleeting and companies must function with ever increasing efficiency to survive in the global economy.

The strategy is for corporations to be agile and rapidly responsive to market demands (Menzies 1998). This strategy has led to concepts such as re-engineering, computer-integrated manufacturing, just-in-time manufacturing, and lean production. Quality circles, total quality management, and other 'cultural training' programmes train workers to identify with the competitive goals of management. New technologies have been implemented to increase productivity and make flexible work schedules possible. However, these technologies can also mean loss of control for workers, increased work speed, and more repetitious work—each of which has been associated with increased job stress (Schnall *et al.* 2000). Employment is both more flexible and less secure as corporations use technology to ensure that individual workers are dispensable and that they conform to the competitive needs of the corporation. Consequently, there has been a dramatic growth in contracted work and non-standard forms of employment such as part-time and home-based work. Shift work and irregular work hours have increased significantly among those who are employed. The contingent workforce, which includes self-employed, temporary, and part-time workers, was estimated to include 34 to 42 million workers in 1996, or more than one in four workers in the United States (Department of Labor 1997). These workers typically have less training about hazards, less access to occupational health services, and less access to other social services such as medical and unemployment insurance or programmes. It is difficult under these circumstances for traditional forms of labour protection, such as government regulations and representation by unions, to function efficiently.

The global economy has also led to shifts in the distribution of occupational hazards among regions of the world. In the industrially developed nations, the principal shift has been from a manufacturing-based economy to an economy that is based on the provision of services and the transfer of information. In consequence, exposure to classic hazards such as silica, asbestos, and heavy chemicals are becoming less important in these nations, while exposure to new synthetic materials and solvents, as well as the ergonomic exposures associated with repetitive work before computer terminals, have become more important (Mustard 1997). In developing nations, by contrast, major hazards have resulted from the export of dangerous industries, materials, and occupations from the industrially developed to the developing nations. In some instances, this export can lead to devastating disasters such as the explosion in the chemical plant at Bhopal, India, that killed several thousand people. Another example is the international boom in the microelectronics industry, which now employs hundreds of thousands of workers worldwide under poorly controlled and highly exploitative conditions, producing products primarily for use in developed nations (LaDou 1995).

The global economy has led to the negotiation of trade agreements, such as the North American Free Trade Agreement, which define conditions of work in the context of trade facilitation and barriers. In some cases, agreements have led to standards that raise the level of protection to workers in countries where previously such protection was minimal; however, in many cases, agreements have encouraged de-unionization and movement away from work protections in order to 'harmonize' protections at a low, but common level among trading partners (Armstrong 1998). A major challenge for nations and international organizations is to implement policies that balance the demands of the global market economy with appropriate protections for workers' health and well being.

Special populations of workers

Recognition has increased that workplace hazards impact disproportionately on some worker populations—such as those in developing nations, as well as child labourers, women workers, and impaired workers (Frumkin and Pransky 1999; IPEC 1999). These populations are especially impacted because of the interaction between their work roles and broader roles in society, as well as by their particular exposures in the workplace. For example, workers in developing nations may be dually affected by hazards in the workplace and low sanitation in their communities. Children who work full time do not have access to education. Low literacy increases the potential that the children will be exposed to dangerous conditions in the workplace; at the same time, it is an obstacle to the children's future economic security as adults. Women workers in virtually all societies are expected to maintain dual roles as workers and primary caregivers in the home. The full impact of work on the health of these populations must be understood in the broader context of their roles in society and in the workplace.

Workers in developing nations

Approximately eight of 10 workers in the global workforce are from the developing world (Jeyrathnam 1998). Workers' health should be viewed in the context of national development. Occupational health policy-makers in many nations must consider a balance between adverse impacts on workers' health and the economic advantages of rapid development by allowing foreign investigators access to low-cost labour and conditions of weak labour protections.

The relationship between workers' health and development is complex for many reasons (Jeyrathnam 1998; Frumkin 1999). For example, workers in many developing countries may be affected by poor nutrition or endemic diseases, such as malaria, in which work may aggravate the condition, or which make the worker more susceptible to the effects of workplace exposures. Workers in these countries also generally have lower educational backgrounds and are often inadequately trained to handle the new technologies and potential hazards. There may be high turnover with little management investment in worker training. Consequently, workers may not be aware of health risks and safe practices.

Working conditions in developing countries may present special hazards because of tropical climates and poor, if any, building ventilation in production facilities. Much of the production equipment is imported from developed countries so that replacement parts and service may be unavailable. The machinery may be used or considered obsolete for use in the developed countries, while new and safer equipment may be unavailable or too expensive.

The social organization of work in developing countries also affects workers' health (Frumkin 1999). In addition to the large number of workplaces with a small number of workers, large proportions of the workforce work in the 'informal' sector, which consists of small, often home-based, businesses that have no government registration and oversight. For example, estimates of informal sector employment range from 49 to 99 per cent of the approximately 235 million total labour force in Africa.

Finally, countries of the developing world may have access to advanced technologies from the developed world without having developed legal or administrative infrastructure to control their adverse impacts on the workforce (Jeyarathnam 1998). Even if developing countries adopt standards and legislation from more developed nations, there is often a shortage of trained personnel to recognize and manage workplace hazards (Frumkin 1999).

Child labourers

Children are an important population of workers worldwide. The ILO estimated that, in 1996, 250 million children 5 to 14 years old were engaged in economic activities worldwide—at least 120 million of them on a full-time basis (IPEC 1999). Africa has the highest incidence of child labour, with 41 per cent compared with 22 per cent in Asia and 17 per cent in Latin America. Child labour also exists in many industrialized countries. Child labour has become an important issue because the children are often exploited in the workplace and denied basic human rights, such as access to education (IPEC 1999). In addition, many children work in dangerous jobs and they may be more susceptible to workplace hazards (CDC 1996; Warshaw 1998).

Poverty is the primary reason why children work. Poor households need the money, and children commonly contribute around 20 to 25 per cent of family income. Furthermore, families may have a tradition of children following in their parents' footsteps. If the family has a tradition of engaging in a hazardous occupation, it is likely that the children will continue in the trade.

The most common explanations about why employers hire children are the lower cost and specific skills afforded by children—the 'nimble fingers' argument. However, ILO research has concluded that the 'nimble fingers' argument is not valid (IPEC 1999). An actual reason is that employers believe that children are easier to manage because they are less aware of their rights, less troublesome, more compliant, more trustworthy, and less likely to be absent from work.

Many children work in hazardous occupations and are at greater risk of suffering ill effects than adult workers. These children may have greater exposure to hazards than adult workers in the same occupation because the children tend to be given the most menial jobs, which may involve higher exposures to toxic substances. Children are more susceptible to the same hazards faced by adult workers because they differ from adults in their anatomical, physiological, and psychological characteristics. Children using hand tools designed for adults run a higher risk of fatigue and injury. Personal protective equipment may also not fit and provide real protection. Furthermore, children may not be aware as adults of workplace dangers nor knowledgeable of the precautions to be taken at work (CDC 1996). Children are also more vulnerable to psychological and physical abuse than are adults, and suffer deeper psychological damage when they are denigrated or oppressed.

A resurgence of child labour is also occurring in developed nations. A Congressional Report documents a rise in the frequency of sweatshops employing children in the United States (General Accounting Office 1988). Each year in New York State, for example, more than 1000 children receive workers' compensation awards for injuries incurred on the job; over 40 per cent of these awards each year are for permanent disability (Belville *et al.* 1993). The most important reason for the re-emergence of child labour in the United States is the increase in poverty. The number of American children living in poverty has more than doubled in many areas of the nation since the early 1980s (Landrigan 1993). During the same time, there was a relaxation in federal government enforcement of labour laws, such as the ban on home piecework in the garment and electronic industries. Studies indicate that the risk of injuries is 10 times higher in illegal, exploitative work than in legally permissible employment.

The issue of child labour has received increasing attention (Warshaw 1998; IPEC 1999). This is reflected in the number of organizations involved in the cause of children and child workers. For example, the International Programme on the Elimination of Child labour (**IPEC**) was launched in 1992 and, as of 1999, developed into a 90-country alliance. The aim of IPEC is the elimination of child labour, giving priority to its worst forms. The 'worst forms' comprise all forms of slavery or practices similar to slavery; the use, procurement, or offering of a child for prostitution or production of pornography; the use, procurement, or offering of a child for illicit activities; and work which is inherently likely to harm the health, safety, or morals of children (IPEC 1999). Priorities to end child labour were defined through the Convention on the Worst Forms of Child Labour in 1999 (Convention No. 182). Withdrawing children from the worst forms of child labour requires improved legislation and enforcement, improved methodologies for identifying the children, rehabilitation of the children, provision of viable alternatives to the children, and awareness raising at all levels of society.

Women workers

Women are a special worker population because of the significant interplay between their roles in society, socio-economic condition, and occupation (Paltiel 1998). Women's roles in virtually all societies are defined in relation to their reproductive functions and responsibilities as family caregivers. Paid employment of women has increased in most countries, but this employment has increased the conflict between paid work and women's traditional family responsibilities. In many societies, early marriage, repeated child bearing, low education, and poverty all disproportionately impact on women workers (Loewenson 1999). The dual roles of women as workers and unpaid caregivers is especially challenging for sole-support mothers, who comprise 20 to 30 per cent of households worldwide.

Employment of women in most societies is characterized by occupational segregation, underemployment (doing seasonal and part-time work below their level of education), and barriers to advancement. Occupational segregation means that women tend to be clustered into a small number of occupations while being under-represented in most others (Stellman 1999). For example, professional women tend to be in teaching, nursing, and other health care specialties. In manufacturing, women tend to have jobs in assembly and small machine operations. Women in developing countries tend to be employed in sectors such as agriculture, textiles and clothing, food processing, and social services (Loewenson 1999). Compared with men, women work for smaller industries or organizations, are more often in informal work with little protection, have less opportunity for work control, and face the psychological demands of people-oriented or machine-paced work (Paltiel 1998). While some countries have enacted laws prohibiting gender discrimination, many countries have formal restrictions on women's employment.

Gender differences are observed in the rates of occupational injuries and illnesses, but these differences are primarily because of differences in the conditions of work or exposures rather than being due to genetic differences (Stellman 1999). As noted above, women tend to work in different occupations than men with a different distribution of hazards. Even when employed in the same industry, women generally do different jobs or different tasks than men so their exposures may be different. Even when doing the same task, women may have different levels of exposure because of variation in the effectiveness of engineering controls and personal protective equipment—which are generally designed for men.

The actual risks of occupational injuries and illnesses to women is not known because a large proportion of women work in the informal sector, and because there has been inadequate research on women workers. Women have higher rates of repetitive strain injuries, especially carpal tunnel syndrome, than men (Stellman 1999). This difference is because women's jobs typically involve more repetitive motion and more static effort. Women are also concentrated in health care occupations where there is greater risk of infections. In addition to toxic hazards, women also face sexual harassment and gender-based violence in the workplace.

There has been inadequate research on the effects of occupational hazards in women because much of past research has been done in industries for which women were largely excluded. It is possible to consider past research on male workers, but it may not be possible or justified to generalize the findings to women (Blair *et al.* 1999). For example, research on males cannot address the possibility of gynaecological disorders among women. It is also theoretically possible that there could be gender-specific responses, for example if the effects are hormonally mediated. Gender-specific effects have been seen for some carcinogens in animal studies (Blair *et al.* 1999). It is unclear whether gender-specific effects occur in humans, and so more attention must be given to studying occupational hazards in women.

Impaired workers

Many people can make constructive contributions in the workplace although they have some type of physical impairment. North American employers, generally in response to legal requirements for workplace human rights, are developing positive policies and strategies for management of a diverse workforce, including impaired workers. The United States has developed probably the most comprehensive legislation for disabled workers, including legislation regarding their entitlements in education, employment and all other spheres of living (Paltiel 1998). Reasonable accommodations are changes made to the work environment, job responsibilities, or conditions of work that provide opportunities for workers with special needs to perform essential job functions. Reasonable accommodation can cover the special needs of persons with impairments or those workers with chronic or recurrent disease, including persons with AIDS. Accommodation may include technical assistance devices, customization including personal protective equipment and clothing, and changes to processes, location, or timing for essential job functions.

In the United Kingdom, the Disability Discrimination Act 1995 prohibits employers from discriminating against applicants and employees with disabilities. Employers also should make reasonable accommodations for a known impairment.

Recognition of occupational disease

Recognition is the key initial step in preventing and managing occupational injuries and diseases in workers. Associations between occupational exposures and disease are typically recognized in three ways: clinical observation, epidemiological analysis, and toxicological evaluation of chemical substances.

Clinical recognition

The alert clinician is the key to clinical recognition of occupational disease. Historical examples of occupational illnesses which have been recognized by alert clinicians include angiosarcoma of the liver in workers exposed to vinyl chloride monomer (Creech and Johnson 1974), lung cancer in workers manufacturing *bis*(chloromethyl)ether (Figueroa *et al.* 1973), bladder cancer in aniline dye workers (Rehn 1895), and mesothelioma in asbestos workers (Selikoff *et al.* 1964).

Keys to the recognition of occupational illness are that the clinician is alert to the possibility that any patient may have an occupational disease and therefore obtains an adequate occupational exposure history on all patients, possesses basic knowledge about the pathogenesis and clinical presentation of the major types of occupational disease, and knows how to report suspected cases of occupational illness to public health authorities so that additional cases caused by the same exposures can be recognized or prevented. Table 1 can be used as a guide to medical conditions or potential occupational exposures for which the clinician should elicit a detailed occupational medical history for evaluation.

The occupational history

The occupational history is the principal clinical instrument for the diagnosis of occupational disease. It may not be possible to obtain a detailed occupational history on every patient. However, the clinician should routinely ask screening questions of every patient that provide an indication as to whether a complete occupational history is warranted. At a minimum, every patient should be asked about his or her current job, and about the longest held previous jobs, by industry and occupation. A general question should be asked about occupational exposures to chemicals, fumes, gases, dust, noise, radiation, and other physical hazards at work. If the patient reports exposure to any of these agents, it may be useful to ask if he or she thinks that there is a health hazard at work. In addition to these screening questions, the clinician should pay attention during the medical history and review of systems to any temporal relationships reported between work and the onset of symptoms.

If information from the routine interview suggests an occupational aetiology, the physician should obtain a more detailed history of exposures. Data on duration and intensity of exposures are particularly important. It is necessary to learn how the patient worked with the suspected toxin and to consider all jobs ever held, places of employment, products manufactured, and materials with which the patient worked.

If toxic exposures are identified or strongly suspected and an occupational cause seems likely, further follow-up enquiries may need to be made through the patient's labour union, companies where he or she has been employed, company physicians, or state or local health departments. Information on toxic substances used in a workplace may be legally available to patients under governmental 'right-to-know' laws.

Epidemiological analysis

All epidemiological study designs can be used to study occupational hazards, but some study designs are especially prominent in occupational epidemiology (Checkoway *et al.* 1989). Major strategies used by epidemiologists to recognize occupational diseases are the cross-sectional medical study, the proportional mortality study, the historical cohort mortality study, and secondary analysis of vital statistics and other population-based health data.

Cross-sectional studies

These studies, in which questionnaires are administered or physical examinations performed on a population of workers at a single point in time, are useful for the identification of acute short-latency conditions or stable conditions which do not result in workers leaving employment. A limitation inherent in cross-sectional studies is the difficulty of determining the temporal relationship between exposure and disease; review of exposure and medical records may be helpful in establishing the time sequence. Whenever possible, it is desirable to follow-up an initial cross-sectional evaluation and to continue clinical observations prospectively over time. Serial evaluations of a population of workers can provide extremely useful data about the development and causation of occupational disease.

Proportional mortality studies

These studies compare the pattern of causes of death among a group of workers with that in the general population or in another comparison population. They are relatively quick and inexpensive to perform, because they require information about only those employees who have died. This information is often available from pension or retirement plans. However, the proportional mortality study is susceptible to a variety of biases and should be considered a 'hypothesis-generating' approach preliminary to conducting more definitive cohort or case–control studies.

Historical cohort mortality studies

These studies are more common in occupational epidemiology than in other fields of epidemiology. This study design utilizes employment records to identify a cohort of workers at some time in the past. The subsequent mortality experience of the cohort is determined by reviewing death certificates and other sources of information. Cause-specific mortality rates are compared with those in the general population or with non-exposed members of the same cohort. The historical cohort mortality study is an important tool for establishing cause and effect associations between work exposures and fatal occupational disease and also for the quantitative assessment of occupational risks. These studies are particularly useful in worker populations, because these groups can generally be well defined through the use of employment records and seniority lists. Frequently, the limiting factor in historical cohort studies is the poor quality of the data on past exposures. However, nested case–control studies undertaken within a cohort can be used to examine past exposures in greater detail.

Epidemiological analysis of population-based health data

This approach can be useful for the surveillance of large populations of workers (such as all workers in a state) and for the recognition of new exposure–disease associations. An example is the use of population-based tumour registries to identify occupations with elevated risks of cancer, or of state-based vital record systems to assess occupation-specific factors, such as a high risk of death by electrocution in farmers. Data on occupational exposures in a registry may be limited simply to an occupation or industry code and investigators can group subjects with common exposures using the 'job-exposure matrix' technique (Hoar 1983). Case–control studies can then be performed on groups identified through the matrix to obtain detailed information from individuals about their past occupational exposures.

Toxicological evaluations

Toxicological analysis of chemical substances is an important means of assessing cause-and-effect relationships. The particular strength of toxicological analysis as a tool for disease prevention derives from the fact that it can precede occupational exposure. In contrast, medical and epidemiological studies can be undertaken only after exposure has already occurred. Thus chemicals found in laboratory tests to cause adverse health effects can be banned or strictly controlled to minimize the exposure of workers and community members.

Premarket testing is the most effective means of assessing the toxicity of new chemical compounds. However, until the passage of the Toxic Substances Control Act in 1976, there was no legal requirement in the United States for prospective evaluation of the toxicity of new industrial compounds. Many thousands of compounds whose introduction to commerce antedated passage of the Act remain untested. Also, testing procedures for new compounds have not been standardized; responsibility for deciding whether or not to test a new chemical and for the development of protocols for evaluating toxicity is left almost entirely to the discretion of manufacturers.

Research priorities

Research is an essential activity to further the recognition of occupational hazards. Governments are the single largest source of research funds, which are predominantly organized into national research programmes. In 1995, NIOSH initiated a nationwide planning process to guide occupational health research in the United States (NIOSH 1999). During the next few years, approximately 500 organizations and individuals provided input into the research agenda (Rosenstock *et al.* 1998). This process resulted in a framework for research and a list of priority research areas, which has been called the National Occupational Research Agenda. Priorities were identified by working groups with broad representation of employers, workers, safety and health professionals, public agencies, industry, and labour organizations. Criteria used to guide the evaluation of priorities included the following: seriousness of the hazard based on death, injury, disease, disability, and economic impact, number of workers exposed or magnitude of risk, potential for risk reduction, expected trend in importance of the research area, sufficiency of existing research, and probability that research will make a difference. The process identified 21 priority research areas which were divided into three categories: diseases and injuries, work environment and workforce, and research tools and approaches (Table 2). This framework has been used by NIOSH, other agencies, and private groups to prioritize funding for research. The planning process is now being used by a number of other countries to establish their research priorities (NIOSH 1999).

At the international level, there are, in addition to sections of the ILO and the WHO, research institutions such as the European Joint Safety Institute and the International Agency for Research into Cancer which carry out international programmes of research in occupational safety and health.

Surveillance of occupational disease

Surveillance is the collection, analysis and dissemination of results for the purpose of prevention (Halperin 1996). Hazard surveillance provides a means of assessing toxic occupational exposures to a population and thus of assessing risk (Wegman and Froines 1985; Markowitz 1998). A hazard surveillance system identifies chemicals in use, the industries and occupations where they are used, and the extent and magnitude of worker exposure. It also provides a means of identifying changes in patterns of exposure and of noting emerging toxic hazards. Disease surveillance provides a means of assessing the amount and types of occupational disease, time trends, and distribution according to geography, industry, and occupation. These two types of surveillance complement each other. Each is an integral component of a complete occupational health surveillance system.

Occupational hazard surveillance

Accurate assessment of the extent and resultant risk to populations of exposure to toxic occupational chemicals requires determination of the following parameters in a hazard surveillance system:

- identification of chemicals in use by industry
- description of each of the industrial processes in which these chemicals are used
- assessment of the number of workers exposed to particular substances by process
- assessment of current exposure levels in various processes
- identification of workplace settings in which there exists potential for increased risk owing to the synergistic effects of simultaneous exposures to several potential hazards
- assessment of the toxicity of specific agents (based on animal, human, or short-term test data)
- description and assessment of the effectiveness of controls to limit exposure.

Most countries do not have adequate systems for occupational hazard surveillance. The only systematic attempts in the United States to elicit most of the information described above were undertaken by NIOSH in national surveys conducted between 1972 and 1974 and between 1980 and 1983. The first of these surveys, the National Occupational Hazard Survey, was conducted in a sample of nearly 5000 industrial facilities across the United States. The second survey, the National Occupational Exposure Survey, was a geographically stratified probability sample of 4490 facilities covering nearly 2 million employees in over 500 different types of industries. The information provided by these two surveys has been valuable to estimate the number of workers exposed to specific agents in specific industries or occupations, but the information is now quite dated (Markowitz 1998). The fact that these surveys have not been repeated is evidence of the cost and effort involved in performing a large hazard surveillance survey.

Another approach to hazard surveillance in the United States has been use of the OSHA Integrated Management Information System (**IMIS**) (Markowitz 1998). The IMIS is a database of exposure measurements obtained in OSHA workplace inspections. The database has been used, for example, to identify the distribution and extent of exposure to lead (Froines *et al.* 1990) and wood dust (Teschke *et al.*

Table 2 United States National Occupational Research Agenda priority areas

Category	Priority research areas
Disease and injury	Allergic and irritant dermatitis
	Asthma and chronic obstructive pulmonary disease
	Fertility and pregnancy abnormalities
	Hearing loss
	Infectious diseases
	Low back disorders
	Musculoskeletal disorders of the upper extremities
	Traumatic injuries
Work environment and workforce	Emerging technologies
	Indoor environment
	Mixed exposures
	Organization of work
	Special populations at risk
Research tools and approaches	Cancer research methods
	Control technology and personal protective equipment
	Exposure assessment methods
	Health services research
	Intervention effectiveness research
	Risk assessment methods
	Social and economic consequences of workplace illness and injury
	Surveillance research methods

Source: NIOSH (1999).

1999) in American industries. The IMIS data are limited, however, because OSHA workplace investigations are not conducted on a representative sampling basis. Furthermore, OSHA concentrates its limited inspection resources on relatively few agents and industries so not many hazards can be evaluated using IMIS (Markowitz 1998). Clearly more systematic and ongoing programmes for occupational hazard surveillance are needed.

Occupational disease surveillance

Occupational disease surveillance has made significant gains in the United States during the past decade (Halperin 1996; Markowitz 1998). NIOSH has implemented several new programmes including the National Occupational Mortality Surveillance (**NOMS**), the Adult Blood Lead Epidemiology and Surveillance (**ABLES**), and the Sentinel Event Notification Systems for Occupational Risks (**SENSOR**) programmes. In addition, the Bureau of Labor Statistics, United States Department of Labor, compiles data on workers' compensation claims and has implemented the Census of Fatal Occupational Injuries based on legal reporting of work-related fatalities. These programmes show the various strategies and sources of data used for disease surveillance.

Under the NOMS programme, data from over 500 000 death certificates are collected annually from 23 states that record industry and occupation on the death certificate. These data are use to track occupation-specific conditions, such as pneumoconioses, and to identify occupation–disease associations using the proportional mortality study approach.

The ABLES programme obtains reports from over 25 states that have state-based registries of lead poisoning. These registries obtain most of the data from required reporting by medical laboratories of elevated blood lead levels.

The SENSOR programme is based on the concept of a sentinel health provider, which is a medical care provider or facility that is likely to provide medical care for workers. This subset of providers is then enrolled in an active occupational disease reporting system for a limited number of defined conditions—for example, silicosis (Maxfield *et al.* 1997), asthma (Jajosky *et al.* 1999), pesticides (Maizlish *et al.* 1995*b*), and carpal tunnel syndrome (Maizlish *et al.* 1995*a*). This approach is useful because specialist providers are more likely to recognize an occupational condition and it is not feasible to include all providers in an active reporting system.

Surveillance data reported by the Bureau of Labor Statistics are based on workers' compensation claims (BLS 1998). However, as discussed above, there are significant limitations in relying on official reporting of work-related diseases for occupational health surveillance. Because of these limitations, the annual Census of Fatal Occupational Injuries reported by the Bureau of Labor Statistics compiles data from multiple federal, state, and local sources, including death certificates, workers' compensation reports, reports to regulatory agencies, medical examiners reports, police reports, and even news reports (BLS 1999). Surveillance is more effective if the condition is discrete and clearly related to work, such as an on-the-job fatality, multiple sources of data are ascertained, and an active reporting system is implemented.

A limitation in these public health disease surveillance systems is that they rely on reporting mechanisms in which recognition of the problem occurs only after the fact. Primary and secondary prevention of occupational disease requires a more direct strategy in which disease surveillance is conducted in the workplace itself. Disease surveillance in the workplace uses the health history and the results of periodic physical and laboratory examinations of workers to estimate levels of exposure to toxins and to assess early effects of exposure. Direct surveillance in the workplace is valuable because many occupational standards are based on minimal amounts of human or animal data; thus, prior to the introduction of many chemicals to the workplace, it is unknown whether workers will be adequately protected. Also, health effects of workplace exposures may vary among workers depending on individual constitutional characteristics. Surveillance of individual workers in the workplace is therefore useful to identify unforeseen hazards and to protect workers who are at increased risk.

Prevention of occupational disease

Primary prevention of occupational disease requires the elimination or reduction of hazardous exposures. Such elimination of hazard is most efficiently accomplished prior to the release of a new chemical substance through premarket toxicological evaluation. Primary prevention with regard to chemicals requires either the elimination of toxic materials and their replacement by less hazardous substitutes or the use of tight processes and controls, such as complete enclosure or ventilation at the source of aerosol generation. Secondary prevention—the early detection of occupational disease in its presymptomatic stage where it can still be controlled or cured—is also feasible. It depends on the ability to identify work-related illness efficiently and effectively through screening workers at high risk for occupational disease using state-of-the-art biological markers. Tertiary prevention—the prevention of complication and disability of existing illness—depends on the development and wide application of appropriate diagnostic techniques for identification of persons with already established occupational illness. Prevention on all three levels requires solid information on the potential effects of specific occupational exposures, as well as data on the industries, occupations, and geographical areas in which hazardous substances are used. The hierarchy of strategies for preventing occupational diseases is shown in Table 3 (Schulte 1995).

The most important prevention strategy is the primary prevention of exposure to toxic chemical, physical, or biological agents. Reductions in exposure can be accomplished by using the techniques listed below, in descending order of preference.

Table 3 Hierarchy of strategies for the prevention of occupational disease

Reduce exposure (primary prevention)
1. Elimination or substitution
2. Engineering controls
3. Work practices
4. Administrative controls
5. Personal hygiene
6. Use of personal protective equipment
Reduce effects of exposure (secondary prevention)
1. Medical monitoring
(a) pre-exposure screening
(b) detection of evidence of excessive exposure
• biological tests of excessive exposure
• biological tests of early effect
2. Control of additive and synergistic exposures
Reduce effects of disease (tertiary prevention)
1. Medical treatment of disease (workers compensation)
2. Rehabilitation
3. Job re-entry

Modified from Schulte (1995).

Elimination or substitution

Elimination of a hazardous material or substitution with a thoroughly evaluated less hazardous material is the most efficacious method of controlling a workplace hazard. In some cases, this method may also be the least expensive. Several examples of effective materials substitution occurred in the late 1970s when outbreaks of neurological disease were documented from exposure to the neurotoxins, methyl-*n*-butyl ketone, dimethylaminopropionitrile and Lucel-7 (Horan *et al.* 1985). The aetiology of these episodes of chemicallyinduced neurological illness was recognized in clinical epidemiological studies, later buttressed by results of toxicological investigations. In each case, the manufacturer discontinued use of the product following identification of the neurotoxic agent. A less hazardous product was substituted.

Selection of a less hazardous process or equipment also represents a meaningful control strategy. For example, substitution of a continuous process for an intermittent process almost always results in a decrease of exposure. Where an entire process does not need to be changed to reduce hazards, equipment substitution may achieve the desired reduction in exposure. An example is use of a degreaser with a low-speed hoist rather than dipping parts by hand.

Engineering controls

The primary engineering controls used to reduce worker exposure to toxic substances are ventilation and process isolation or enclosure. Ventilation is one of the most effective and widely used control measures. Control of hazards by ventilation is usually further subdivided into two categories: local exhaust ventilation and general exhaust ventilation. The most effective approach for implementing ventilation controls is as follows: conduct an engineering study to evaluate sources of exposure; develop an engineering design; install a system based on the design; evaluate the completed system to ensure that the air contaminant has been effectively controlled.

Isolation is defined as the interposing of a barrier between a hazard and workers who might be injured or made ill by the hazard. Isolation may refer to storage of materials, such as flammable liquids, enclosure or removal of equipment to another area (such as noisy generators), or isolation of processes or of the workers themselves (e.g. by enclosing a sawmill worker in a sound-proof ventilated booth to protect him from noise and wood dust). For example, the petroleum industry uses automated remote processing in plants based on centralized computer control of process equipment. Thus workers are largely isolated from hazards except in maintenance operations and during process upsets.

Work practices

Alteration of work practices can help to reduce exposure to hazards. A common example is wet-sweeping rather than dry-sweeping dust. Another example is vacuuming cotton lint off spinning machines rather than blowing it off with compressed air, a practice which creates airborne dust particles.

Administrative controls

Administrative controls are methods of controlling total worker exposure by job rotation, work assignment, or time periods spent away from the hazard. With administrative controls, the level of exposure to the hazard is not diminished; instead, the duration of exposure is reduced and exposure is spread more widely among the workforce. For example, the current air standard for inorganic lead in the United States is 50 mg/m^3 based on an 8-h day. A worker could permissibly be exposed to 100 mg/m^3 for a total of 4 hours and then rotated to a job without lead exposure as an administrative control. The most common use in industry of administrative controls is to reduce overall noise exposure through rotation. Given the typical demands of production and the potential for misuse, administrative methods of controls are not an optimal mode of control.

Personal hygiene

Programmes for encouraging personal hygiene constitute another, although less efficient, approach to reducing exposure. In some instances, management may encourage or even require showers and a change to clean clothes at the end of the working day. Naturally, management should provide these showers, changing facilities, lockers, and work clothes if indicated; in fact, several American OSHA standards, such as the occupational lead standard, require management to provide such facilities.

A subtle but potentially important route of exposure is ingestion of toxic agents by eating, smoking, or applying cosmetics in the workplace. To prevent such exposure, management should provide separate eating facilities outside production areas. Workers should be encouraged to wash their hands before eating or smoking.

Use of personal protective equipment

Respirators, gloves, protective clothing, ear plugs, and muffs are all common forms of personal protective equipment in use throughout industry. They can play an important role, provided that carefully designed personal protective equipment programmes are in place and the equipment itself is frequently and regularly checked. It is important, however, to recognize that programmes of personal protection never constitute as efficient a means of protection as engineering or process controls. Personal protective equipment is intended to reduce exposures to toxic substances which have already been dispersed in the workplace as the result of inadequate ventilation or incomplete enclosure. The principal valid use of personal protective equipment as an approach to the prevention of occupational exposure is, therefore, during certain maintenance operations, in which static controls are not operating, or during process upsets. Unfortunately, programmes for personal protective equipment, such as respirator programmes, are often ill defined, given inadequate attention, and used instead of engineering controls, with poor maintenance of the necessary equipment.

Workers' compensation

Workers' compensation is a legal system designed to provide income support, medical payments, and rehabilitation payments to workers injured on the job, as well as to provide benefits to survivors of fatally injured workers (Ison 1998). Essentially all industrialized countries and many others have workers' compensation programmes (Barth 1995). However, the majority of countries in the developing world do not have such programmes. As of 1995, only 16 per cent of workers in Africa, 43 per cent in Latin America, and 23 per cent in Asia have protection from social security systems that include workers' compensation (Sekimipi *et al.* 1995). Each country has a different system with varying approaches to benefits, coverage of workers and medical conditions, eligibility criteria, financing, and administration. With the exceptions of the United States, Canada, Australia, and Germany, the programmes are administered or overseen nationally by the central government. In the United States, each of the 50 states, as well as three federal jurisdictions, has an autonomous workers' compensation system.

Internationally, workers' compensation programmes are structured along three lines (Barth 1995; Ison 1998). Perhaps the most common are those programmes that are embedded in a country's social security system. Since the country's social insurance programmes are integrated, permanent disability and survivor benefits and medical benefits are paid at levels that do not distinguish significantly between a work-related and non-work-related injury. The benefits are similar and therefore there is little need for controversy about the cause of an injury or illness. Thus these systems have little litigation related to workers' compensation. Another approach is one in which workers' compensation is funded and administered separately from that of the social security scheme, but the two programmes are closely related. An example of such links is where workers' compensation benefit is ended at the normal retirement age and old age benefits begin automatically. Germany has such an intermediate approach. At the other end of the continuum is the United States, where the social security programmes and the workers' compensation programmes have almost no links.

Although the many national systems are distinct, they have several characteristics in common (Barth 1995; Ison 1998, Plumb and Cowell 1998). Virtually all programmes provide some protection from income loss because of workplace injury or disease. The costs of health care are provided either through the workers' compensation programme or in conjunction with the country's social security and health care systems. An important general characteristic is that workers' compensation is a no-fault system. An injured worker does not need to prove that his or her injury was the result of employer negligence. For a worker to qualify for benefits, only three conditions usually must be met: (a) there must be an injury or illness; (b) the injury or illness must 'arise out of and in the course of employment'; (c) there must be medical costs, rehabilitation costs, lost wages, or disfigurement. If the claim is accepted, medical care and rehabilitation expenses are fully covered; lost wages are partially reimbursed. In most instances, specific benefit formulas are prescribed by law. Employers are legally responsible for paying most of these benefits to injured workers. Employers pay these costs through insurance premiums, social security payroll taxes, or self-insurance. The programmes in most countries operate through public insurance, but private insurers exist for some types of benefit programmes, especially in the United States.

Workers' compensation is structured theoretically as a no-fault system in order to minimize the amount of litigation that had developed under the common-law system used previously by workers seeking redress from employers for work-related injuries. Furthermore, workers' compensation has wider coverage than the common law system in that injuries and illnesses are compensated even if they are only partially work related. Generally, diseases are considered eligible for compensation if occupational exposure is the sole cause of the disease, is one of several causes of the disease, is aggravated by or aggravates a non-occupational exposure, or hastens the onset of disability. However, in exchange for this wider coverage and the introduction of a less litigious system, covered workers generally are not allowed to sue employers through common law. They also are given lower awards than those given through juries in negligence suits and cannot seek compensation for 'pain and suffering' beyond their physical injury.

Although intended to minimize litigation, workers' compensation systems do not actually eliminate the legal process. In some jurisdictions, such as most states in the United States, insurance carriers or employers have the right to contest a claim. The basis for contesting most claims is the question as to whether the injury is work related. Proof of work-relatedness is usually straightforward for acute injuries, and therefore relatively few claims for acute injury are contested. However, the great majority of claims for chronic occupational diseases are contested. The burden of proving that disease is occupational in origin lies with the worker. If a claim is contested, the worker must find a lawyer willing to represent him or her, and then identify physicians who can convince the referee who hears the case that the disease is work related. Although most of these cases are settled in favour of the injured worker, delay until settlement can be quite long. For example, the mean delay is 390 days for pneumoconiosis claims. Moreover, the injured worker may continue to work during this time, aggravating the injury. There is inherent difficulty in diagnosing an occupational disease and establishing a cause-and-effect relation, and therefore it may be difficult, if not impossible, to prove that a disease is work related. The legal process can be time-consuming and disheartening, discouraging the worker from filing a claim in the first place or encouraging an early settlement for substantially less than the defined benefit.

The amount of litigation associated with workers' compensation is much less in Europe than in the United States. Although the system is distinct in each country, there are generic characteristics that account for the contrast with the American experience. One factor is a heavier reliance on a schedule or list of covered diseases. While the definition of covered conditions varies among the countries, the use of a schedule within each system establishes a presumption of work-relatedness and reduces the proportion of controverted claims (Lesage 1998). Another distinction is that European workers' compensation systems do not utilize the adversarial system to resolve disputes, such as those involving questions of aetiology or extent of impairment. The common practice is to hold hearings to find the facts without using lawyers and often without the private insurer or employer challenging a claimant's position. Challenges to claims may arise, but they are handled by a governmental social insurance agency rather than by the private parties. A third distinction from the United States is that in European nations the determination of compensation in technically difficult claims is generally based on the position taken by professionals (such as physicians) who are employees or regular consultants to the compensation agency and not witnesses hired by the plaintiff or defendant. Thus the compensation administrator is not forced to reconcile different technical perspectives that may reflect the differing interests of the contending parties.

The most important difference between the workers' compensation experience in Europe and the United States is the availability in Europe of relatively generous alternatives to and supplements of workers' compensation benefits. In most of the world's industrialized countries, workers are entitled to publicly provided or required health care benefits regardless of the work-relatedness of the condition. Furthermore, income-maintenance programmes because of disability from illness or injury are common. The availability of universal medical care and strong social insurance programmes provides alternative sources of support that reduce the dependence of the injured worker on the workers' compensation system. Consequently, the determination as to whether an illness is work related is not critical to the worker's health and social security needs.

A concern expressed often about integrating workers' compensation programmes into broader social security programmes is that employers may have less incentive to provide a safe workplace. However, it is unclear whether workers' compensation costs, even in jurisdictions in which the employer is legally accountable, actually function as an effective incentive for employers to prevent the occurrence of occupational diseases. In developed countries, the costs on average to employers of workers' compensation are only about 2 to 3 per cent of payroll costs (Barth 1995). Consequently, a workers' compensation system at best can play a small role in discouraging unsafe or hazardous employer practices. The ideal system would provide both benefits for the injured worker and strong incentives for employers to prevent occupational injury and illness, but the first priority of a workers' compensation system should be to ensure prompt provision of full benefits to the injured worker.

Right to know

The 'right-to-know' concept refers to the mandatory sharing of information regarding workplace exposure to toxic substances between employers and workers, regulatory agencies, and in some cases communities near a workplace. The fundamental assumption in the right-to-know concept is that this transfer of information will prompt activity that will improve worker health (Ashford and Caldart 1985). In fact, there have been several instances of workers themselves playing a direct role in the discovery of occupational health problems.

Two examples are the discovery of lung cancer in workers exposed to *bis*(chloromethyl)ether (Figueroa *et al.* 1973) and sterility in workers exposed to dibromochloropropane (Whorton *et al.* 1977). Until recently, however, workers have remained largely ignorant of the potential hazards of the chemicals with which they work.

The right of workers to know about potential hazards necessarily implies a corresponding duty on employers to provide that information. Employers' duties can be considered in three categories. Firstly, the duty to generate or retain information means that an employer would be required to perform environmental or medical monitoring and to retain the records pertaining to that monitoring for a specified period of time. This duty is specified under some of the OSHA comprehensive standards, such as those for asbestos and lead. Secondly, the duty to disclose information on request means that an employer must provide copies of exposure or biological monitoring data to a worker or worker representative if that information is requested. For example, the OSHA Access to Employee Exposure and Medical Records Standard attempts to ensure that exposure, medical, and biological monitoring records are preserved and that workers or their representatives have access to them. Thirdly, the duty to inform refers to an employer's or manufacturer's obligation to disclose information about potential toxic substances in the workplace. Under the OSHA Hazard Communication Standard, employers have a duty to inform workers of the identity of the substances with which they work through labelling the product containers and disclosing the source of supply through the use of Material Safety Data Sheets. The standard also requires that workers must be trained in methods to detect the presence of hazardous chemicals, the hazards of the chemicals, and protective measures.

Workplace training programmes must be implemented effectively in order to assure workers of their 'right to know'. For example, Kahan *et al.* (1999) evaluated programmes established under workers' right-to-know regulations in Israel. They interviewed 552 workers and 33 safety officers employed at 50 industrial plants. They found that most of the worker's knowledge about work hazards was based on informal sources, and not on those stipulated by the regulations. Furthermore, 5 per cent of the workers were unable to read and another 22 per cent had educational levels below that necessary to understand technical material provided by the employer. In more than one-third of the cases, the workers and their safety officers disagreed about the existence of hazards in the workplace. This research demonstrates that employers must be more aware of the need to identify hazards and communicate effectively to their employees in understandable language and terms.

Workers have additional rights to information about toxic hazards through other federal statutes and regulations. For example, the Toxic Substances Control Act in the United States imposes requirements on chemical manufacturers and processors to develop health effects data. The Toxic Substances Control Act requires testing, premarket manufacturing notification, and reporting of information. Unfortunately, as noted above, the great majority of chemicals in commercial use were able to reach the market before requirements for premarket testing were promulgated. The Act does impose a duty to disclose to the Environmental Protection Agency any information which supports the conclusion that a substance or mixture presents a substantial risk of injury to health. Thus medical screening or biological monitoring data obtained by an employer indicating a substantial risk of injury must be reported to the Environmental Protection Agency. The National Labor Relations Act also provides a mechanism by which workers can gain access to information about hazardous working conditions. Since the National Labor Relations Act provides employees with a limited right to refuse hazardous work, it has been interpreted to mean that employees must be informed about those hazards. In addition, access is available to employees who are members of unions through the collective bargaining process. It has been held that unions have a right of access to exposure and medical records, so that they can bargain effectively with the employer regarding conditions of employment. Through legal avenues such as these, workers' access to information about potential hazardous exposures in the workplace has been expanded.

Conclusion

Workers suffer a broad range of injuries and illnesses caused by hazards encountered in the workplace. Despite the existence of protective legislation in many countries, the burden of injury and illness on workers remains significant. It is essential for medical practitioners and public health programmes to recognize, prevent, and manage work-related injuries and illnesses. There is a need for international co-ordination of occupational health protection for workers, given the increasing globalization of the world economy. Several approaches have been proposed to address this issue. For example, there should be harmonization of health, safety, and environmental standards in a way that does not unfairly impose a competitive disadvantage on the newly industrialized nations. Governments and multinational corporations should share the most advanced technologies and resources. Rather than allowing companies to manufacture products banned for use in their own country, governments in developed nations should provide financial incentives for their industries to develop and export safer products and technologies. At a minimum, international systems should be established to ensure complete notification of potential hazards, including labelling the contents of raw materials and products.

References

Adams, R.M. (ed.) (1999). *Occupational skin disease* (3rd edn). W.B. Saunders, Philadelphia, PA.

Armstrong, P. (1998). Transformation in markets and labour. In *Encyclopaedia of occupational health and safety* (ed. J. Stellman) (4th edn), pp. 24.15–17. International Labour Office, Geneva.

Ashford, N.A. and Caldart, C.C. (1985). The 'right-to-know'. Toxics information transfer in the workplace. *Annual Review of Public Health*, **6**, 383–401.

Barth, P.S. (1995). Compensating workers for occupational diseases: an international perspective. *International Journal of Occupational and Environmental Health*, **1**, 147–58.

Belville, R., Pollack, S.H, Godbold, J. H., and Landrigan, P.J. (1993). Occupational injuries among working adolescents in New York State. *Journal of the American Medical Association*, **269**, 2754–9.

Blair, A., Hoar Zahm, S., and Silverman, D.T. (1999) Occupational cancer among women: research status and methodologic considerations. *American Journal of Industrial Medicine*, **36**, 6–17.

BLS (Bureau of Labor Statistics) (1998). *Workplace injuries and illnesses in 1997.* Bureau of Labor Statistics, US Department of Labor, Washington, DC.

BLS (Bureau of Labor Statistics) (1999). *National census of fatal occupational injuries, 1998.* Bureau of Labor Statistics, US Department of Labor, Washington, DC.

CAETS (Council of Academies of Engineering and Technological Sciences) (1988). *Globalization of technology: international perspectives.* National Academy Press, Washington, DC.

CDC (Centers for Disease Control and Prevention) (1993). *Fatal injuries to workers in the United States, 1980–1989: a decade of surveillance.* CDC, NIOSH, Cincinnati, OH.

CDC (Centers for Disease Control and Prevention) (1996). Work-related injuries and illnesses associated with child labor—United States, 1993. *Morbidity and Mortality Weekly Report*, **45**, 464–8.

CDC (Centers for Disease Control and Prevention) (1999). Progress toward the elimination of tuberculosis—United States, 1998. *Morbidity and Mortality Weekly Report*, **48**, 732–6.

Checkoway, H., Pearce, N.E., and Crawford-Brown, D.J. (1989). *Research methods in occupational epidemiology.* Oxford University Press, New York.

Collegium Ramazzini (1999). Call for an international ban on asbestos. *American Journal of Industrial Medicine*, **36**, 227–9.

Creech, J.L., Jr and Johnson, M.N. (1974). Angiosarcoma of liver in the manufacture of polyvinyl chloride. *Journal of Occupational Medicine*, **16**, 150–1.

Department of Labor (1997). *Current population survey, 1996.* US Department of Labor, Washington, DC.

Figueroa, W.G., Raszkowski, R., and Weiss, W. (1973). Lung cancer of chloromethyl methyl ether workers. *New England Journal of Medicine*, **228**, 1096–7.

Frazier, L.M. and Hage, M.L. (ed.) (1998). *Reproductive hazards of the workplace.* Wiley, New York.

Froines, J.R., Baron, S., Wegman, D.H., and O'Rourke, S. (1990). Characterization of airborne concentrations of lead in US industry. *American Journal of Industrial Medicine*, **18**, 1–17.

Frumkin, H. (1999). Across the water and down the ladder: occupational health in the global economy. *Occupational Medicine*, **14**, 637–63.

Frumkin, H. and Pransky, G. (ed.) (1999). Special populations. *Occupational Medicine*, **14**.

General Accounting Office (1988). *Sweatshops in the US. Opinions on their extent and possible enforcement options.* Publication No.GAO/HRD-88-130BR, General Accounting Office, Washington, DC.

Goldman, R.H., Rosenwasser, S., and Armstrong, E. (1999). Incorporating an environmental/occupational medicine theme into the medical school curriculum. *Journal of Occupational and Environmental Medicine*, **41**, 47–52.

Halperin, W.E. (1996). The role of surveillance in the hierarchy of prevention. *American Journal of Industrial Medicine*, **29**, 321–3.

Hoar, S. (1983). Job exposure matrix methodology. *Journal of Toxicology. Clinical Toxicology*, **21**, 9–26.

Horan, J.M., Kurt, T.L., Landrigan, P.J., Melius, J.M., and Singal, M. (1985). Neurologic dysfunction from exposure to 2-*t*-butylazo-2-hydroxy-5-methylhexane (BHMH): a new occupational neuropathy. *American Journal of Public Health*, **75**, 513–17.

IARC (International Agency for Research on Cancer) (1997). *Working group on the evaluation of carcinogenic risks to humans: silica, some silicates, and coal dust and para-aramid fibrils.* IARC, Lyon, France.

IOM (Institute of Medicine) (1988). *Role of the primary care physician in occupational and environmental medicine.* National Academy Press, Washington DC.

IPEC (International Programme on the Elimination of Child Labour) (1999). *IPEC action against child labour – achievements, lessons learned and indications for the future (1998–1999).* ILO, Geneva.

Ison, T.G. (1998). Workers' compensation systems: overview. In *Encyclopaedia of occupational health and safety* (ed. J. Stellman) (4th edn), pp. 25.2–14. ILO, Geneva.

Jajosky, R.A., Harrison, R., Reinisch, F., *et al.* (1999). Surveillance of work-related asthma in selected U.S. states using surveillance guidelines for state health departments—California, Massachusetts, Michigan, and New Jersey, 1993–1995. *Morbidity and Mortality Weekly Report*, **48**, 1–20.

Jeyarathnam, J. (1998). Occupational health trends in development. In *Encyclopaedia of occupational health and safety* (ed. J. Stellman) (4th edn), pp. 20.2–4. ILO, Geneva.

Kahan, E., Lemesh, C., Pines, A., Mehoudar, O., Peretz, C., and Ribski, M. (1999). Workers' right-to-know legislation: does it work? *Occupational Medicine*, **49**, 11–15.

LaDou, J. (ed.) (1995). Special Issue: international issues in occupational health. *International Journal of Occupational and Environmental Health*, **1**, 76–222.

LaDou, J. (1997). The practice of occupational medicine. In *Occupational and environmental medicine* (ed. J. LaDou) (2nd edn), pp. 1–5. Appleton and Lange, Stamford, CT.

Landrigan, P.J. (1993). Child labor: a re-emergent threat. *American Journal of Industrial Medicine*, **24**, 267–8.

Landrigan, P.J. and Baker, D.B. (1991). The recognition and control of occupational disease. *Journal of the American Medical Association*, **266**, 676–80.

Landrigan, P.J., Nicholson, W.J., Suzuki, Y., and LaDou, J. (1999). The hazards of chrysotile asbestos. A critical review. *Industrial Health*, **37**, 271–80.

Leigh, J.P., Markowitz, S.B., Fahs, M., Shin, C., and Landrigan, P.J. (1997). Occupational injury and illness in the United States. Estimates of costs, mortality, and morbidity. *Archives of Internal Medicine*, **157**, 1557–68.

Lemaster, G.W. (1998). Occupational exposures and effects on male and female reproduction. In *Environmental and occupational medicine* (ed. W. Rom) (3rd edn), pp. 223–44. Lippincott–Raven, Philadelphia, PA.

Lesage, M. (1998). Work-related diseases and occupational diseases: the ILO international list. In *Encyclopaedia of occupational health and safety* (ed. J. Stellman) (4th edn), pp. 26.2–6. International Labour Office, Geneva.

Lindbohm, M.-L. (1999). Women's reproductive health: some recent developments in occupational epidemiology. *American Journal of Industrial Medicine*, **36**, 18–24.

Loewenson, R.H. (1999). Women's occupational health in globalization and development. *American Journal of Industrial Medicine*, **36**, 34–42.

Maizlish, N., Rudolph, L., Dervin, K., and Sankaranarayan, M. (1995*a*). Surveillance and prevention of work-related carpal tunnel syndrome: an application of the Sentinel Event Notification System for Occupational Risks. *American Journal of Industrial Medicine*, **27**, 715–29.

Maizlish, N., Rudolph, L., and Dervin, K. (1995*b*). The surveillance of work-related pesticide illness: an application of the Sentinel Event Notification System for Occupational Risks (SENSOR). *American Journal of Public Health*, **85**, 806–11.

Markowitz, S.B. (1998) The role of surveillance in occupational health. In *Environmental and occupational medicine* (ed. W. Rom) (3rd edn), pp. 19–29. Lippincott–Raven, Philadelphia, PA.

Maxfield, R., Alo, C., Reilly, M.J., *et al.* (1997). Surveillance for silicosis, 1993—Illinois, Michigan, New Jersey, North Carolina, Ohio, Texas, and Wisconsin. *Morbidity and Mortality Weekly Report*, **46**, 13–28.

Menzies, H. (1998). Globalizing technologies and the decimation/transformation of work. In *Encyclopaedia of occupational health and safety* (ed. J. Stellman) (4th edn), pp. 24.17–21. International Labour Office, Geneva.

Mustard, F. (1997). The economy and social equity in a period of major technoeconomic change. *Scandinavian Journal of Work, Environment and Health*, **23** (Supplement 4), 10–15.

National Research Council (1987). *Counting injuries and illnesses in the workplace. Proposals for a better system* (ed. E.S. Pollack and D.B. Keimig). National Academy Press, Washington DC.

NIOSH (National Institute for Occupational Safety and Health) (1996). *National occupational research agenda update.* DHHS (NIOSH) Publication No. 96-115, NIOSH, Cincinnati, OH.

NIOSH (National Institute for Occupational Safety and Health) (1999). *National occupational research agenda—May 1999.* DHHS (NIOSH) Publication No. 99-124, NIOSH, Cincinnati, OH.

OSHA (Occupational Safety and Health Administration) (1991). *Occupational exposure to bloodborne pathogens. Final rule: 29 CFR 1010.1030, 6 December 1991.* OSHA, Washington, DC.

OSHA (Occupational Safety and Health Administration) (1996). *OSHA fact sheet. Silica dust exposures can cause silicosis.* Fact Sheet OSHA 96–54, OSHA, Washington, DC.

Paltiel, F. (1998). Shifting paradigms and policies. In *Encyclopaedia of occupational health and safety* (ed. J. Stellman) (4th edn), pp. 24.2–5. International Labour Office, Geneva.

Pearce, N., Boffetta, P., and Kogevinas, M. (1998). Cancer—introduction. In *Encyclopaedia of occupational health and safety* (ed. J. Stellman) (4th edn), pp. 2.1–18. International Labour Office, Geneva.

Perfetti, L., Cartier, A., Ghezzo, H., Gautrin, D., and Malo, J.L. (1998). Follow-up of occupational asthma after removal from or diminution of exposure to the responsible agent: relevance of the length of the interval from cessation of exposure. *Chest*, **114**, 398–403.

Peto, J., Decarli, A., La Vecchia, C., Levi, F., and Negri, E. (1999). The European mesothelioma epidemic. *British Journal of Cancer*, **79**, 666–72.

Plumb, J.M. and Cowell, J.W.F. (1998) An overview of workers' compensation. *Occupational Medicine*, **13**, 241–72.

Rehn, L. (1895). Blasengeschwuelste bei Fuchsinarbeitern. *Archiv für Klinische Chirurgie*, **50**, 588.

Rom, W. (ed.) (1998). *Environmental and occupational medicine* (3rd edn). Lippincott–Raven, Philadelphia, PA.

Rosenstock, L., Olenec, C., and Wagner, G.R. (1998). The National Occupational Research Agenda: a model of broad stakeholder input into priority setting. *American Journal of Public Health*, **88**, 353–6.

Ross, D.J. and McDonald, J.C. (1998). Health and employment after a diagnosis of occupational asthma: a descriptive study. *Occupational Medicine*, **48**, 219–25.

Schnall, P.L., Belkic, K., Landsbergis, P., and Baker, D. (ed.) (2000). The workplace and cardiovascular disease. *Occupational Medicine*, **15**, 1–334.

Schulte, P.A. (1995). Introduction: the role of biomarkers in the prevention of occupational disease. In *Biomarkers and occupational health—problems and perspectives* (ed. M.L. Mendelsohn, J.P. Peeters, and M.J. Normandy), pp. 1–6. Joseph Henry Press, Washington, DC.

Sekimipi, D.K., Tambellini, A.T., and Trung, L.V. (1995). The global economy and occupational health. *International Journal of Occupational and Environmental Health*, **1**, 76–9.

Selikoff, I.J., Churg, J., and Hammond, E.C. (1964). Asbestos exposure and neoplasia. *Journal of the American Medical Association*, **188**, 22.

Stellman, J. (ed.) (1998). *Encyclopaedia of occupational health and safety* (4th edn). International Labour Office, Geneva.

Stellman, J.M. (1999). Women workers: the social construction of a special population. *Occupational Medicine*, **14**, 559–80.

Teschke, K., Marion, S.A., Vaughn, T.L., Morgan, M.S., and Camp, J. (1999). Exposures to wood dust in US industries and occupations, 1979 to 1997. *American Journal of Industrial Medicine*, **35**, 581–9.

Venables, K.M. and Chan-Yeung, M. (1997). Occupational asthma. *Lancet*, **349**, 1465–9.

Warshaw, L. (1998). Precarious employment and child labour. In *Encyclopaedia of occupational health and safety* (ed. J. Stellman) (4th edn), pp. 24.9–15. International Labour Office, Geneva.

Wegman, D.H. and Froines, J.R. (1985). Surveillance needs for occupational health. *American Journal of Public Health*, **75**, 1259–61.

Wright, F.B. (1998). Occupational health and safety: the European Union. In *Encyclopaedia of occupational health and safety* (ed. J. Stellman) (4th edn), pp. 23.31–34. International Labour Office, Geneva.

WHO (World Health Organization) (1997). Executive summary. *Health and environment in sustainable development: five years after the Earth Summit.* WHO, Geneva.

WHO (World Health Organization) (1999). *Occupational health: ethically correct, economically sound.* Fact sheet 84, WHO, Geneva.

Whorton, D., Krauss, R.M., Marshall, S., and Milby, T.H. (1977). Infertility in male pesticide workers. *Lancet*, **ii**, 1259–61.

11.6 Persons with physical disabilities: a rehabilitation approach

Anthony B. Ward

Introduction

With an increasingly ageing population, physical disability places greater demands on health care and society. According to a survey performed by the Office of Population Census and Surveys (**OPCS**) in 1988 and 1989 (Martin *et al.* 1988), people with disabilities account for 10 per cent of the United Kingdom population. Not only is the total proportion expected to rise, but the proportion of people with severe disabilities (OPCS grades 5 to 10) is also likely to increase. Great improvements have been made in reducing mortality, illness, and trauma, so that people can live longer even with the most severe disabilities. Their quality of life depends initially on health services, both in the acute phase and then in rehabilitation, but subsequently on social services, vocational services, and employment services to restore occupational activity and to make an accessible environment in which to live with as little difficulty as possible. Health professionals in rehabilitation, especially those involved in specialized rehabilitation, have an important role in the assessment of disability, treatment, and co-ordinating and involving professionals in other agencies to address the individual's needs.

Rehabilitation has developed considerably in recent years and it is important to describe the totality of rehabilitation rather than to confine it to just health-based activity. The establishment of a multiprofessional approach has concentrated expertise and led to a better understanding of what can be achieved. The use of new technology, particularly in the fields of electronics, computers, and informatics, is creating new possibilities for disabled people, their families and carers, and rehabilitation professionals. These developments are leading to greater participation for many disabled people and their carers.

The medical approach to physical disability has developed in a rather haphazard way. It is divided into services for children, adults, and elderly people. Paediatrics and geriatric medicine have taken on other activities, and only for adults is there a defined medical specialty called rehabilitation medicine. This is a relatively new specialty in the United Kingdom, created in 1984 and gaining Department of Health official designation in 1990. The specialty comes under a variety of names in different countries, ranging from physical medicine to rehabilitation medicine; the most commonly used term in Europe is physical and rehabilitation medicine. This chapter does not cover the history of the speciality, as this can be found elsewhere (Story 1992; Ward 1997).

Rehabilitation gained increasing importance after the First World War and established itself after the Second World War. Spinal cord injury units were founded at that time and the American Board of Physical Medicine and Rehabilitation was probably the first to start training and certifying doctors in the field from 1947 through the work of Krusen, Johnson, and others (Martin and Opitz 1997). The specialty has had a stable base in the United States through the American Academy of Physical Medicine and Rehabilitation and internationally two main medical organizations have represented national societies (the International Federation of and Rehabilitation Physical Medicine and Rehabilitation) and individual members (International Rehabilitation Medicine Association). They have now united to form the International Society of Physical Medicine and Rehabilitation, which aims to raise the international profile of medical rehabilitation.

Epidemiology

A major survey of disability in the United Kingdom during 1988 and 1989 showed an overall prevalence of 10 per cent of the population (Martin *et al.* 1988). This survey consisted of a number of reports, making a considerable contribution to the knowledge of disability and covering not only the numbers of disabled people, but also commenting on the situation of those living at home, children, services, transport, employment, and the financial circumstances of disabled adults living at home. It produced estimates of the prevalence of the 13 main domains of disability based on *International Classification of Impairments, Disabilities and Handicaps* (**ICIDH**) criteria and a new weighting scale of severity for each of these domains, ranging from 1 (least severe) to 10 (most severe). The survey found a prevalence of disability of 135 per 1000 population in adults aged 16 years and over, which increased to 142 per 1000 if people in institutional care were included. Table 1 shows the prevalence of the 13 domains of disability according to age. Over three-quarters (77 per cent) were found to have one or more of these physical disabilities, implying a prevalence rate of 104.1 per 1000 aged 16 years and over living in the community, and 109 per 1000 if those in institutions are included.

Difficulty with locomotion is the most common disability and has the highest prevalence for all age groups. Physical disability is likely to occur in combination with other types of disability, especially sensory disabilities. The combination of physical and mental disabilities appears to increase the severity of the disability more than physical disability alone and is the most likely to result in institutional care, as shown in Table 2.

In the United Kingdom most disability is due to musculoskeletal disorder (Table 3). Neurological conditions make up 13 per cent of

Table 1 Disability domains—estimates of prevalence of disability in the United Kingdom by type (ICIDH) and age per 1000 population

Type of disability	Age group			
	16–59	60–74	75+	All adults
Locomotion	31	198	496	99
Hearing	17	110	328	59
Personal care	18	99	313	57
Dexterity	13	78	199	40
Seeing	9	56	262	38
Intellectual function	20	40	109	34
Behaviour	19	40	152	31
Reaching and stretching	9	54	149	28
Communication	12	42	140	27
Continence	9	42	147	26
Disfigurement	5	18	27	9
Eating, drinking, and digesting	2	12	30	6
Consciousness	5	10	9	5

Source: Martin *et al.* (1988).

the total of disability in all ages, but have a higher impact in the more severe categories of the OPCS scale and in younger people, where they contribute to most of the severe disability seen. Therefore this should be reflected in services for specialized rehabilitation, which tends to concentrate on people severely disabled by neurological disease.

Severe disability is also associated with multiple pathologies and people over the age of 60 years are more likely to have two or more conditions. For instance, arthritis and hypertension coexisted in more than a quarter of people aged 60 or over. With each additional condition, there is an exponential rise in disability, typically found in older people. Rehabilitation is thus likely to be focused in this group at comorbid conditions—one of the main distinguishing features between rehabilitation for the elderly and younger adults, who are more likely to have a single condition.

There is also a geographical distribution of disease, and conditions seen commonly in some countries may be quite unusual even in near neighbours. The prevalence of multiple sclerosis rises as one travels further north in Europe, with high incidences and prevalences in Scotland and Scandinavia. The prevalence rises from 98 per 100 000 in Southampton, England, to 178 per 100 000 in the north of Scotland (BSRM 1993). The reasons for this are not known, but a combination of inherited and environmental factors are suggested. Services have to take this into account for the needs of the local population.

Table 3 provides further information on the types of disability caused by various disease groups. Most of the findings are to be expected, and confirm the great preponderance of musculoskeletal problems.

The data so far have been restricted to the impact of physical disability on society, but it is also important to look at the more common disease groups leading to physical disability. Rehabilitation medicine services for physically disabled people in the United Kingdom are primarily directed at neurological and musculoskeletal conditions, but also encompass an additional interest in people disabled by respiratory and cardiac diseases. Moreover they are also concerned with amputees, the provision of wheelchairs and special seating, and the development of assistive technology, particularly in the areas of communication aids and environmental controls.

Certain conditions, such as diabetes mellitus and hypertension, are common and do not always in themselves lead directly to much loss of personal functioning, but they have complications which have a significant impact on both acute and rehabilitation services. Therefore services for these groups of patients cannot be planned without taking into account the rehabilitation of complications such as stroke, myocardial infarction, peripheral vascular disease, visual impairment, tissue viability, etc. Wade and Langton-Hewer described four groups of neurological disease and disorders, for which a rehabilition response is required (Wade and Langton-Hewer 1987):

- those causing major physical disability affecting mobility, self-care, and everyday activities
- those causing disturbance of cognition and/or behaviour
- those causing pain
- those causing an episodic disturbance of consciousness and/or neurological function.

These groups are also applicable to other disorders and are therefore useful to service planners

All of these groups require health services, but rehabilitation is more focused on groups 1 to 3. Table 4 shows the incidence and prevalence of some of those in group 1, the most applicable to physical rehabilitation. They are mostly neurological, but some musculoskeletal conditions have been added.

Table 2 Types of disability by severity category expressed as a percentage within each severity group

Type of disability	Severity					
	1–2	3–4	5–6	7–8	9–10	Total
Other disability—not physical	38	26	17	5	0	23
Physical	39	35	31	25	18	33
Physical and sensory	21	31	30	36	28	28
Physical and mental ± sensory	2	8	24	34	56	18

Source: Martin *et al.* (1988).

Table 3 Frequency of disease groups causing physical disabilities and all disability for adults in private households (per 1000 population)

Disability (ICD group)	All groups	Locomotor	Disability type		
			Reaching and stretching	Dexterity	Disfigurement
Musculoskeletal	46	56	64	67	61
Ear	38	1	0	0	1
Eye	22	2	0	1	2
Circulatory	20	23	10	7	5
Mental	13	3	2	3	1
Nervous system	13	12	21	22	12
Respiratory	13	14	3	2	1
Digestive	6	2	2	1	5
Genitourinary	3	1	1	0	2
Neoplasms	2	1	3	2	4
Endocrine	2	2	1	1	1
Infections	1	1	1	1	3
Blood	1	0	0	0	0
Skin	1	1	0	0	4
Congenital	0	0	0	0	3
Other	6	2	3	4	1

Source: Martin *et al.* (1989).

Neurological conditions

Stroke

The annual incidence of first stroke is 200 per 100 000, of whom 80 will die in a year (one-third die within 3 weeks and half within 3 months); the most common cause of death is myocardial infarction. Sixteen per cent of those who survive for 3 months will die from a further stroke or cardiac disease, and this is age related. Thus the prevalence is around 550 per 100 000, of whom 300 will have a significant disability (Royal College of Physicians 1989). Around one-third of strokes are in people less than 60 years old.

In disability terms, 25 per cent improve rapidly during the first week, but an equal number deteriorate (Bamford *et al.* 1988; Wade 1992). More than half (50–70 per cent) are admitted to hospital; 25 per cent of those kept at home become severely disabled (Wade *et al.* 1985; Bamford *et al.* 1988). The resources required in the first 3 months are for effective management of motor, sensory, communication, and cognitive impairments, as well as for mood problems.

Multiple sclerosis

The prevalence is between 99 and 178 per 100 000 (BSRM 1993). The median survival of 35 years is now prolonged, but an increasing number of people require rehabilitation services for long periods of time, as rehabilitationists deal more effectively with disabling complications. The natural history is one of exacerbation and remission, with a gradual decline in recovery levels leading to impairment of mobility, dexterity, communication, cognition, continence, and nutrition, and the development of pressure sores, contractures, and emotional problems. Given the long and variable course of the disease, financial difficulties are common and carers require help (Martin and White 1988; Martin *et al.* 1989). Homes need adaptation and whole households are disrupted by the caring routines necessary. Marital breakdown is common, reducing the pool of potential carers. Intermittent hospital-based services are needed for the treatment of specific problems, but most people can be maintained at home with community nursing, maintenance rehabilitation therapy, and respite care.

Parkinson's disease

The annual incidence of 20 per 100 000 generally occurs in older people, but covers the age range of 55 years and above (Association of British Neurologists 1992). Of the 180 per 100 000 with the disease, about 40 per cent have severe disability, but they can be helped by new treatments which are becoming available. Their higher cost will increase the pressure on pharmacy budgets and there is an inequitable availability of them in the United Kingdom. The disease is still progressive and incurable, but patients can be helped with their mobility problems, communication, and bulbar and mental slowing. Patients can typically manage their impairments and disabilities quite well for many years, but more care is eventually required in a similar way to that for multiple sclerosis and other chronic diseases.

Motor neurone disease

The annual incidence of 2 per 100 000 and median survival of 1.5 years leads to a prevalence of 6 per 100 000 with severe disability

Table 4 Group 1 disorders

Disorder	Incidence[a]	Prevalence[a]	Prevalence of disability[a]
Stroke	550	1500	900
Parkinson's disease	45	400	342
Multiple sclerosis	10	300	225
Motor neurone disease	5	15	14
Traumatic brain injury	700	?	900
	20 severe		300 Severe
Spinal cord injury	3	150	150
Cerebral tumour	40	113	40
Guillain–Barré disease	3	60	12
Encephalitis—all forms	46.5	?	?
Cerebral palsy	2.7 per 1000 live births		2 per 1000 of school age
Spina bifida	0.38–3.5 per 1000 births		< 2 per 100 000 school leavers
Hydrocephalus	2.3–6 per 1000 births		
Friedreich's ataxia	5		5
Duchenne muscular dystrophy	1.3–3.3 per 10 000 live births	5–12	
Myasthenia gravis	1	10	10–25
Huntington's chorea		15	15
Rheumatoid arthritis	30	1000	130 severe
Osteoarthritis	300 knee	9500 knee	300 severe
	200 hip	3250 hip	
Back pain	5357 GP consultations	12 000	1000 severe

[a]Per 250 000 population unless stated otherwise

Source: Wade and Langton-Hewer (1987).

(Buckley *et al.* 1983). This disease is usually progressive and rapidly fatal, but some patients experience a milder attenuated course. Riluzole, an antiglutamate, is a new treatment which has been shown to slow the progression of disability and lengthen survival (Lacomblez *et al.* 1996). Despite this, motor neurone disease still rapidly advances to disability and death in the majority of cases. Management is aimed at preserving motor and functional skills through therapy and orthotics, and technology is most effective at maintaining quality of life until late in the disease (Cochrane 1989; Cox 1992). Carer support is particularly necessary because of the rapid progression of the disease and encompasses both practical help and emotional support. Because of the rapid nature of change, needs alter steadily and rehabilitation has to respond quickly. If a wheelchair or other specialist equipment takes 6 months to be provided, need soon outstrips provision, leading to a great potential for wasted resources and frustration in providing appropriate and effective rehabilitation. The direct input of a specialist rehabilitation team with a physician in rehabilitation medicine can ensure good forward planning for prospective disability and handicap.

Cerebral palsy, spina bifida, and the muscular dystrophies

While the incidences of cerebral palsy (2 per 1000) and muscular dystrophy (1.3 to 3.3 per 10 000 live births) have remained relatively constant, the prevalence (200 and 90 per 100 000 population, respectively) has increased with improved survival (Brett and Lake 1991; Lipkin 1991). There is renewed interest in the treatment of spasticity in young children with cerebral palsy. It is now possible to delay, and even in some circumstances avoid, the traditional treatment of surgery to the Achilles tendons through aggressive antispastic treatment, such as with botulinum toxin type A. Long-term longitudinal studies are underway to assess the abilities and participation of these young people as they leave school and progress into adulthood.

In contrast, the incidence of live births with spina bifida is decreasing, as it can now be diagnosed antenatally. The prevalence is declining and is probably less than 2 per 100 0000 school leavers (McBride and Ward 1991; Chamberlain *et al.* 1993; Ward 1994).

Trauma

Brain injury

The incidence of brain injury is also variable. Most authors describe an incidence of 250 minor brain injuries per 100 000 population (BSRM 1998), but many head- injured patients are 'lost' in other injuries. A study in 1989 in North Staffordshire (Barrett *et al.* 1995) indicated the true incidence to be 1330 per 100 000 population. The rate for severe and very severe injuries is 20 per 100 000 population (18 severe and 2 very severe) (BSRM 1998). More importantly in this context, the prevalence of persisting disability is 150 per 100 000 (Price and Ward 1997). Survivors have a normal lifespan in the absence of epilepsy, immobility (paticularly tetraplegia), and recurrent chest or urinary infections (Jennett *et al.* 1979; Ashwal *et al.* 1994). The most important aspects of the ensuing disability are cognitive and behavioural rather than physical. Most can be managed in the community, but a small number require inpatient treatment for severe behavioural disorders (Ward 1993). Access to neuropsychology, neuropsychiatry, and community psychiatric nursing is required. With better treatment and increased survivals, more people who would have previously died are now surviving in vegetative states. In very severe traumatic brain injury the prevalence is 1 to 14 per cent and survival is now reported at over 20 years (Andrews *et al.* 1996).

Spinal cord injury

In comparison with brain injury, this is relatively rare. However, numbers are boosted by middle-aged and elderly people developing spinal paralysis secondary to diseases such as metastases and central disc herniation. The annual incidence of traumatic spinal cord injury is 2 per 100 000 and life expectancy is virtually normal (Multi-Society Task Force on PVS 1994). Although initial and post-acute rehabilitation is carried out at designated specialist centres, follow-up and maintenance is often shared between the specialist unit and local provision. Long-term follow-up studies have shown the benefit of continued specialist input, particularly in the areas of bladder management, optimizing residual motor function, maternity and motherhood, and ageing (see below). Spinal cord injury units do call patients back, but this often involves long tiring journeys and the main requirements are disability equipment, particularly for activities of daily living and services to promote continence, tissue viability, and prevent complications, such as intercurrent illnesses, contractures, etc. Because these injuries tend to happen in younger populations, provision for family life and ageing is necessary. Non-traumatic spinal disease usually occurs in older patients, is due to tumour, infection, ischaemia, or vertebral problems, and can usually be managed locally.

Locomotor conditions

Arthritis

The prevalence of severe disability due to rheumatoid and osteoarthritis is 130 per 100 000 and 300 per 100 000 respectively (Kurtzke 1975). Rehabilitation is normally provided via the rheumatology or orthopaedic services, but close working with rehabilitation departments is necessary for wheelchair and orthotic provision. Community rheumatology and rehabilitation services bring specialist expertise of identification of patient needs closer to primary care teams as well as to disabled people and have shown benefits in close liaison with social services and community therapy services.

Amputation

The annual incidence of lower-limb amputation is 30 per 100 000, of whom 20 will require limb fitting (Bradley *et al.* 1984). In the same population there will be four or five upper-limb amputations. Many amputations are due to vascular insufficiency (64 per cent) or diabetes (21 per cent), and only a few (8.5 per cent) are traumatic (McColl 1986). Smoking is a major factor. Prospective amputees require access to expert advice and information on the rehabilitation programme, prosthetic options, and possible outcomes. In the immediate post-amputation phase, a fully comprehensive integrated rehabilitation package must be available with the aim of restoration of maximum self-care and independence. Prosthetic limbs are provided for appropriate patients and are maintained at subregional centres—approximately one per 1.5 million population. Satellite limb centres have been established where the population and local geography demand. The provision of some inpatient beds for appropriate patients requiring amputee rehabilitation is strongly recommended (Amputee Medical Rehabilitation Society 1992).

Cardiorespiratory conditions

This aspect of rehabilitation is outside the remit of this chapter and is mentioned for completeness. It forms an important area of rehabilitation activity and has been proven to be effective in improving abilities and participation. The principles behind cardiac and respiratory rehabilitation are similar to those for physical disability and reference is made elsewhere to this clinical activity (see Chapters 9.1 and 9.3).

Generic conditions

Rehabilitation differs from acute medicine by concentrating on the effect of the disease/injury on the functioning of individuals and their families rather than on the diagnosis. The family or 'significant others' invariably need rehabilitation as much as the patient and it is therefore additionally important to highlight some of the important impairments.

Pressure sores

The overall incidence is approximately 11 per cent (King's Fund Pressure Sore Study Group 1989) and around 25 per cent of those affected are aged 15 to 64 years (King's Fund Pressure Sore Study Group 1989). The prevalence is 5 per cent in general hospitals and a considerable number of younger disabled people contribute to this. The total cost of treating one significant pressure sore is now £38 000 at 1999 prices (Barbanel *et al.* 1977). Standardized scoring assessments of risk factors are now available but some need validation. All provider units should have prevention policies in operation (Thomas *et al.* 1980). The incidence in local provider units should be monitored as a routine and fundamental part of service quality assessment.

Incontinence

The prevalence of regular urinary incontinence is approximately 44 per 1000 population with a ratio of 2.9 females to each male (Stewart 1975). About four per 1000 will require active advice and treatment at any one time. Faecal incontinence is less common. While some sufferers require urodynamic assessment, the majority can be treated by community services.

Sexual problems

Many people with physical disabilities experience sexual dysfunction and/or associated emotional problems (King's Fund Consensus Statement 1988). Counselling services are required to deal with both the emotional aspects of partner attraction and body image, and the fears and physical difficulties of performing the sexual act, whether the disabilities are physical or psychological.

Speech, communication, and related disorders

Such disorders result from a wide range of diseases including stroke, multiple sclerosis, parkinsonism, traumatic brain injury, cerebral palsy, respiratory disorders, and laryngeal disease. Fifteen per cent of stroke survivors have a speech disorder (Lincoln *et al.* 1984). The beneficial effects of speech and language therapy have been demonstrated (Bax *et al.* 1988), and clear protocols should be available for patients requiring assessment by a speech therapist. Included here are assessment and treatment for related impairments such as swallowing disorders. Many patients have other disabilities, and multidisciplinary assessment is often required before treatment plans can be formulated. The most severely affected patients may require communication aids. Swallowing problems also come under the responsibility of speech and language therapists, as they often go together with communication dysfunction and severe disability.

Sensory—vision and hearing

The prevalence of impaired vision is 520 per 100 000 population and 200 people per 100 000 are severely deaf (Anonymous 1986). Thus sensory handicap may compound problems for people with other physical problems. Specialist service requirements for these deficits are outwith the scope of this chapter.

Disabled school leavers and young adults

Children with disabilities have traditionally been provided with their own distinct services, and moving into adult life at 16 years of age causes considerable difficulties. They are disadvantaged by a lack of health and social care and have decreased oppportunities for employment, education, and financial security. They make up about 1.7 to 2 per cent of the school population in England and Wales, and those in the more severe OPCS disability categories should have a transitional plan from the age of 13 years of age. Local authorities, in particular education and social services, have a statutory role to meet the conditions in Sections 5 and 6 of the Disabled Person Act 1986 (WHO 1980). The health service participates in some areas to ensure that there is a clear pathway in follow-up and disablity assessment and management as these young people move from paediatric to adult services. A report commissioned by the Department of Health outlines these responses clearly (Chamberlain *et al.* 1993). From a health perspective, the evidence shows that they have poorer vision and dentition than their abled-bodied peers, orthopaedic and foot problems, and poor knowledge of how to access services. Many cannot even get to a general practitioner and have never had a consultation without the presence of a parent; many have little idea about their own health and independent living with a disability. The dedicated services are patchy, but have reported improvements in many areas of life. A study will soon report on the outcomes of young people, who have been through two dedicated services in comparison with two areas where there have only been *ad hoc* arrangements (Ward and Houston 1993).

The rehabilitation process

Rehabilitation is a precise activity and the World Health Organization (**WHO**) definition of 1980 still applies today (WHO 1980). It is quite different from care and describes a goal-oriented activity. Similarly, it is quite different from 'therapy', which contributes to the rehabilitation process in individual recipients, but may not always be required for everyone. Therapy and rehabilitation are not synonymous.

Box 1 Rehabilitation—WHO definition (WHO 1980)

An active process, by which those disabled by injury/disease achieve a full recovery, or, if full recovery is not possible, realize their optimal physical, mental, and social potential and are integrated into their most appropriate environment

Health-based rehabilitation—working definition

A dedicated, designated, multiprofessional activity taking an active and holistic approach to care, which is centred on the individual needs of patients and carers, starts in earnest when the patient is medically stable, and continues through community reintegration and beyond, is goal orientated and is easily and appropriately accessible

Rehabilitation medicine (Ward and Houston 1993)

A consultant subacute specialty concerned with the secondary and tertiary management of the medical aspects of physical disability (especially in the fields of neurological and musculoskeletal disease, trauma, and amputation), which require specialist rehabilitation expertise

Rehabilitation therapy (Ward and Houston 1993)

Treatment provided by, or under the direction of, nurses, physiotherapists, occupational therapists, speech and language therapists, clinical psychologists, dietitians, chiropodists, and so on

Relationship between rehabilitation and disability

It is important to look further than the medical implications of physical disability, which may or may not confer a disadvantage and often have an impact on the social well being of the individual and carer. The terms mean different things to different groups and tend to be less specific for disability and handicap, and so this chapter will follow the philosophy behind the WHO definitions.

The original WHO report described four terms: pathology, impairment, disability, and handicap (WHO 1980). Medical practice is based on the concept of arriving at a diagnosis and providing a treatment, which aims to cure the patient. In the context of medical and social progress and the increasing importance of degenerative diseases. In medical practice, the relatively new concepts of improving quality of life and prevention of deterioration and complications have assumed greater priority. Disease and injury can cause the five scenarios described below. While rehabilitation is involved in all of them, the issue is to identify where it contributes to a better quality of life compared with that achieved if it had not taken place. The value of rehabilitation is discussed below, as is the risk to health if it does not take place.

Figure 1 shows the models or patterns of disease where rehabilitation has an impact. Rehabilitation is most effective in model 2 (post-stroke or brain injury with some recovery of function), model 3 (post-stroke or brain injury with no recovery of function), and model 4 (multiple sclerosis or rheumatoid arthritis with a relapsing course of

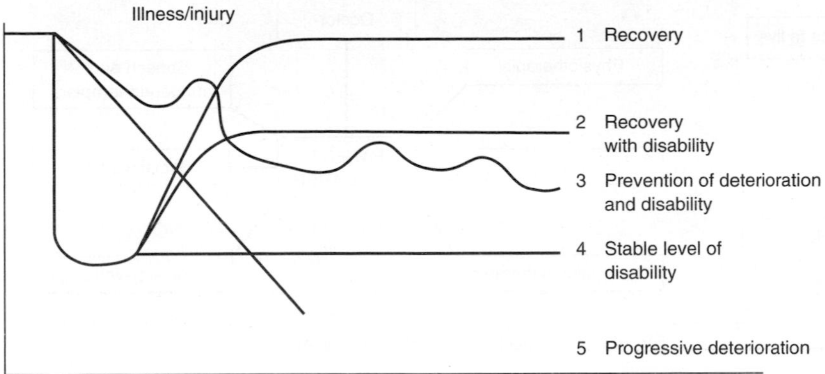

Fig. 1 Models of disease and disability.

improvement and deterioration), where its impact can preserve function, manage disability, and prevent complications of disability. It can also provide people with the means and education to live satisfying lives. In these people, rehabilitation can make an impact above that expected from natural recovery from a disease or injury, allowing people to gain more abilities because of the rehabilitative experience. Most people in group 1 (following limb fracture, where return of full function is expected) will improve despite rehabilitation, but may benefit from therapy, whereas people in group 5 (cancer, motor neurone disease) are going to deteriorate progressively despite the efforts of rehabilitation. However, there is much that can be done for both groups and for their carers in the areas of equipment provision, assistive technology, and education. Therefore rehabilitation units have to define their activity and their clientele if they are to be effective and successful.

The rehabilitation process uses different philosophies to assist people in achieving their aims. For instance, if the objective of rehabilitation is to allow someone to climb upstairs to gain access to the bathroom, there are several ways of achieving this:

- the underlying disease process could be treated to restore full function to the individual (pathology)
- the person could be trained to improve their strength through, for instance, fracture repair, pain relief, etc. (impairment)
- the person could be retrained to walk up and downstairs (disability)
- the person could be provided with a stairlift and two wheelchairs, one for upstairs and one for downstairs (handicap).

At this juncture, it is important to define and distinguish between the terms set out by the WHO in the ICIDH (WHO 1980).

- **Impairment:** any loss or abnormality of psychological, physiological or anatomical structure or function
- **Disability:** any restriction or lack (resulting from an impairment) of ability to perform an activity in the manner or within the range considered normal for a human being
- **Handicap:** a disadvantage for a given individual resulting from an impairment or disability, which limits or prevents the fulfilment of a role that is normal for age, sex, and social and cultural factors for that individual.

The WHO reported again in 1997 (ICIDH-2) because it was felt that the terms disability and handicap were somewhat negative and did not actually reflect the rehabilitative approach (WHO 1997). A more positive way to describe this was in the substitution of the terms 'disability' and 'handicap' for 'ability' and 'participation'. Figure 2 shows the role of impairment and ability in contributing to participation. Health service rehabilitation can thus be active in managing impairments and abilities, as well as in addressing societal issues.

Rehabilitation is much more than health based, and the relationships between health services in the United Kingdom and other agencies, such as employment and social services, have not developed together. A lack of both funding and volition has hampered the good work of the Prince of Wales Advisory Group on Disability and the King's Fund in the late 1980s, when a framework for action was published as part of the *Living Options in Practice* (Fiedler and Twitchin 1990). The essential elements of a comprehensive system of services for disabled people are listed below. Their definitions of disadvantage are different from those of health-based organizations and access to services is highlighted as the most significant blight to disabled people, no matter the cause of their disability (Fig. 3).

1. **A response point to users' needs:** a single point of entry to the service system, easily identifiable and easily accessible, offering information and advice on all aspects of disabled living, and help with the process of obtaining services through assessing, co-ordinating, and tracking requirements for, and delivery of, services.
2. **A place to live:** a range of housing options to suit individual lifestyles and life stages, including individually adapted dwellings, shared or clustered accommodation with support, and residential facilities offering 24-hour on-site support.

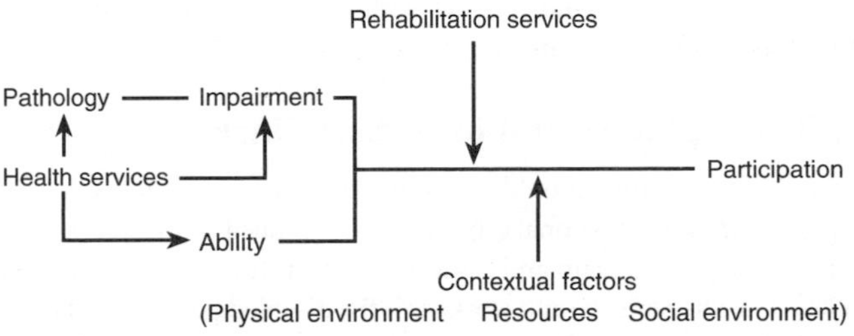

Fig. 2 The context of health and rehabilitation services on impairments, abilities, and participation.

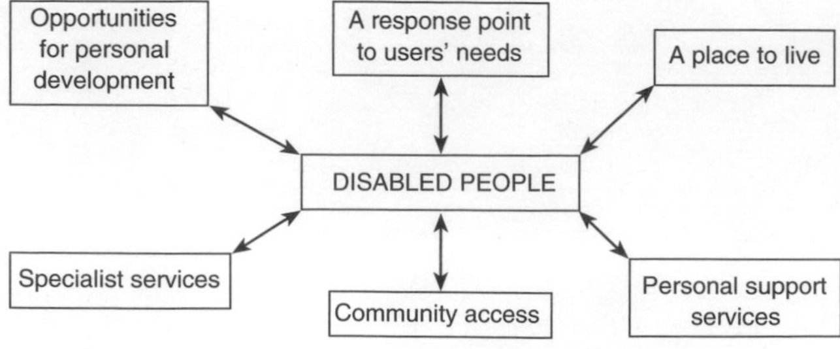

Fig. 3 Living options principles.

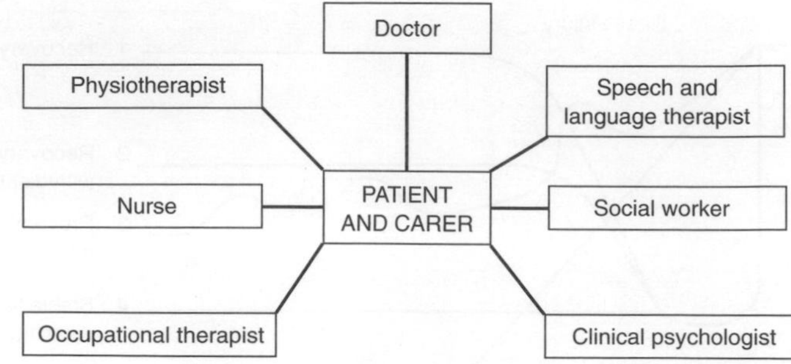

Fig. 4 A core specialist rehabilitation team.

3. **Personal support services:** appropriate, flexible, and sufficient assistance with personal care and daily living tasks, domestic/home-making duties and social/quality of life activities, enabling the individual to live as independently as he or she is able or wishes.
4. **Access to the community:** the opportunity to participate in all aspects of ordinary community life, including the availability of employment, education, leisure activities, transport, and health care.
5. **Specialist services:** a wide variety of services to minimize or overcome physical or sensory impairment—services that supplement and enable individuals to use ordinary community services.
6. **Opportunities for personal development:** training, counselling, and advocacy opportunities that enable individuals to aspire to and reach their full potential and take advantage of the opportunities available.

Rehabilitation teamwork

Rehabilitation is a multiprofessional activity that depends upon good communication between staff and the individual skills of the professionals involved. If it is to work, the team must have clear rehabilitation objectives for the patient, which should be created with the full co-operation of the patient and significant others. The value of teamwork in this setting is that the output of the team is greater than the summation of the individual professional inputs. Where teamwork scores is in the sharing of expertise and workload. There are fairly blurred margins between the roles of the team members, and successful teams thrive on everyone contributing despite professional boundaries.

Most rehabilitation teams for physical disability comprise a basic core of professionals who interact with each other. The professions most commmonly seen are shown in Fig. 4.

Multidisciplinary and interdisciplinary

Rehabilitation teams should be more than a simple collection of different health professionals. The individuals need to work as part of an interdisciplinary team and understand the roles and values of their colleagues. The team should work with the disabled person and family to set appropriate, realistic, and timely treatment goals within an overall co-ordinated rehabilitation programme. The goals of rehabilitation must be set with the active co-operation of the disabled person and family and need to be adjusted over time and according to progress. In other words, goals should be client centred and should not be set on a discipline-by-discipline basis. The team should not be asking 'What are the goals for the occupational therapist this week?' but 'What are the goals for the patient this week and how can the occupational therapist help to achieve them?' This is the difference between a multidisciplinary team and an interdisciplinary team. A multidisciplinary team is simply a collection of a number of disciplines working as separate individuals within their own discipline, albeit as part of a rehabilitation team. An interdisciplinary team is a collection of individuals who bring their own experience, professional skills, and expertise to the team and are prepared to work across professional boundaries. The case history below shows interdisciplinary teamwork in action and there are common actions for many professionals to work on. In addition, team members also have to get on with each other and good sociability is a key factor. In this way, rehabilitation is able to minimize and prevent disability and handicap by providing a co-ordinated source of information, advice, and treatment for the disabled person and the family, with the team acting as provider and catalyst.

Case history 1

BG is a 29-year-old married woman and mother of two small children: spontaneous pontine haemorrhage resulting in a locked-in syndrome; spontaneous improvement to spastic quadriplegia, worse on right than left. Problems include spastic quadriplegia, expressive dysphasia, spastic dysarthria, depressed and tearful, inappropriate emotional reactions, pain from spastic limbs and jaw, recurrent chest infections, and urinary incontinence.

Objectives and plans

1. Pain
   (a) Botulinum toxin to jaw muscles; analgesia and gabapentin for limb pain (doctor).
2. Mobility
   (a) Requires foot flat on ground; botulinum toxin to spastic calf muscles; stretch afterwards; cast lower leg (doctor/physiotherapist/occupational therapist). Antispastic medication (doctor/nurse).
   (b) Supply ankle–foot orthosis (doctor/orthotist).
   (c) Positioning in bed to hemiplegia (nurse).
   (d) Transfers—prevent inversion with ankle–foot orthosis (physiotherapist/occupational therapist).

(e) Powered indoor/outdoor wheelchair; seating required (Jay cushion); assess safety in chair (occupational therapist/nurse).

3. Transfers
   (a) Hoist initially; work on spastic limbs to effect transfers; reduce from three helpers to one within 3 months (physiotherapist/nurse).
   (b) Teach husband and parents safe transfers (physiotherapist/nurse).
   (c) Assess home (resettlement officer).

4. Tissue viability
   (a) Check pressure areas (nurse/occupational therapist).
   (b) Wheelchair service to measure seating pressures (occupational therapist).
   (c) Lie on bed for 2 hours between 1 and 3 p.m. to relieve pressure points (nurse).
   (d) Lose weight—1 kg per fortnight (nurse).

5. Communication
   (a) Assess comprehension; work on simple word production and needs on ward (speech and language therapist).
   (b) Letter board (speech and language therapist).
   (c) Litewriter communicator (speech and language therapist).
   (d) Claudius Converse telephone to contact children (speech and language therapist/occupational therapist).

6. Dysphagia
   (a) Percutaneous endoscopic gastrostomy feeding tube inserted; check feeds and weight (nurse).
   (b) Stimulate palatine and pharyngeal movements; check videofluoroscopy four times weekly (speech and language therapist).

7. Continence
   (a) Remove catheter; toilet training hourly (nurse).
   (b) Bowel management (nurse).

8. Mood/personality
   (a) Antidepressants given; reassess after 4 weeks (doctor).
   (b) Assess understanding; team support for consistent approach (clinical psychologist).

9. Environmental controls
   (a) Assess B when independently mobile in wheelchair and using communicator; ask at goal planning what she and husband want (occupational therapist).

10. Home
   (a) Meet husband (± parents) within 2 weeks (doctor).
   (b) Family education and information; assess home (nurse/resettlement officer/occupational therapist).
   (c) Assess family ability to cope with her at home (all).
   (d) Financial planning (social worker).
   (e) Family care, day care, B's role at home, etc. (social worker).

Organization of services

Rehabilitation must be a core service in each locality but there are some activities which are either very costly or require specific expertise, such that the logistics of providing them in each district would not be cost effective. Similarly, some conditions, such as motor neurone disease and spinal injuries, are too rare for each locality to develop the necessary skills to deal with them effectively. Therefore service delivery should be based on a pyramid with super-specialized services (low numbers/high activity and expertise) at the top and general rehabilitation (high numbers, e.g. after limb fracture) at the bottom (Fig. 5).

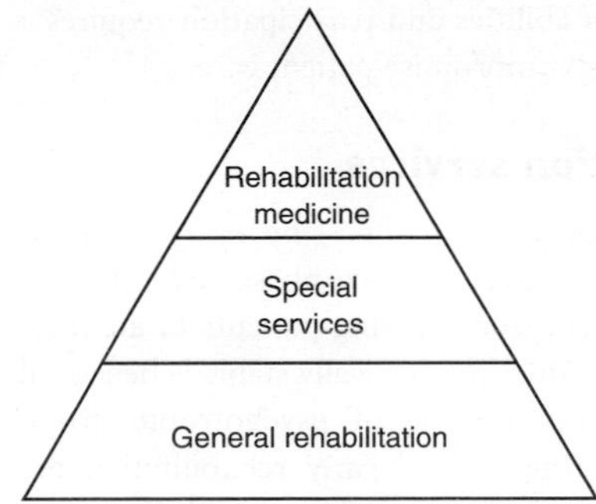

Fig. 5 Service organization

Description

Doctors should take the rehabilitative needs of their patients into account, but need themselves to dedicate time to take on specialized rehabilitation as an integral member of a multiprofessional team. Just as importantly, they need the expertise, aptitude, and experience of a formal training programme. Doctors with other responsibilities, such as acute medicine (e.g. geriatric medicine), or from other specialties (e.g. neurology or rheumatology) cannot properly dedicate themselves to medical rehabilitation. Their main specialty will always occupy most of their time. In addition, switching from dealing with

Box 2

- *General rehabilitation:* characterized by health professionals working within thier professional roles in relative isolation from others, that is in a polydisciplinary manner
- *Special services:* dedicated areas of working, where individual professionals have varying degrees of contact with others involved in the rehabilitation process. Typical examples are nurse advisors to continence and tissue viability services, dysphagia services, and so on. In some instances, this may involve multidisciplinary rehabilitation and the development of specialist multiple sclerosis nurses, Parkinson's disease nurses, back pain service co-ordinators are examples, where these individuals may have a general clinical role working within a team and an extra responsibility to these respective patients
- *Specialized rehabilitation:* dedicated multidisciplinary or interdisciplinary rehabilitation rehabilitation, where the team meets to define the rehabilitation objectives and activity and professionals work together to achieve the aims of the process. It is often inpatient based, but there are now a number of community teams working in this way

pathology and impairments to abilities and participation requires a shift of philosophy, which may compromise patient care.

Delivery of rehabilitation services

It should be stressed that, following acute illness or injury, rehabilitation should start in the immediate recuperative phase under the care of the admitting physician or surgeon. Moving patients to an acute rehabilitation facility as soon as they are medically stable is beneficial in the prevention of inappropriate use of psychotropic drugs, complications, and in promoting a good early rehabilitation experience (McLellan 1991). Stroke and brain injury units demonstrate this (Hall and Cope 1995) and the amount of therapy applied to these patients has a direct influence on their ability to lead an independent life (Shiel *et al.* 1999). Thereafter patients require an integrated approach to community living and the opportunity for life skills, work, education, and maintaining personal, emotional, and social contacts. In acute rehabilitation, they need to be under the care of the doctor and the rehabilitation team. There are good reasons for this, not least because the risk of deterioration and medical complications is still high, but rehabilitation activity also needs to be regarded as credible and valued by other specialties, and for this medical leadership is necessary.

However, people living at home or in an institution with a disability require an approach which will respond to their health and social needs. They require support in employment and, if that is not possible, in occupational activity. Their health and disability needs require regular review to ensure appropriate responses, and intermittent medical rehabilitation may be necessary to overcome intercurrent illness/deterioration or prevent complications. Above all, people need to live in a suitable place, have an income sufficient for their needs, understand the consequences of their condition on their lives, and learn how to maximize their opportunities in life.

Specialist centres

The standards proposed by the British Society of Rehabilitation Medicine for the numbers of beds required per district for rehabilitation medicine only account for younger adults (Turner-Stokes *et al.* 2000). The numbers required for older people and children is under debate at present and needs to be separated from acute beds for the elderly. In a climate of reduction of acute beds and redesign of community hospitals to meet the needs of the local primary care purchasing group or trust, it is imperative that sufficient attention is paid to the facilities for rehabilitation. This means not only beds, but also outpatient facilities; the criteria for inpatient rehabilitation are proposed below. There is a need to separate rehabilitation from care, and to develop an active goal-oriented programme to meet the patient's agreed objectives.

Criteria for inpatient rehabilitation

1. Patients who require 24-hour nursing and medical supervision for their rehabilitative needs.
2. Patients with neurological and locomotor disorders who have the capacity for, require, and will benefit from rehabilitation, i.e. patients in whom the evidence shows that active intervention improves function, life satisfaction, or prevents deterioration.
3. Severely disabled patients whose needs can only be met by a multiprofessional team practising interdisciplinary rehabilitation.
4. Patients with complex needs, i.e. requiring more than two professionals working in a team.
5. Some very severely disabled patients with little hope of improvement in personal functioning, but who require assessment and appropriate equipment and whose families require education for caring purposes.

People whose frailty or physical/mental health means that they are unlikely to cope with an active rehabilitation programme are probably unsuitable. However, they still often benefit from the educative process.

Rehabilitation services have traditionally been delivered in units reflecting recovery from illness and injury (Table 5). There are now a variety of models to choose from and, while each location may not have the need, finance, or expertise to develop a comprehensive provision of specialist services, a means of accessing them is necessary. However, a number of basic core services are required. For instance, the number of people disabled from arthritis, back pain, and brain injury would suggest that local services are necessary and it would be irresponsible to send residents from one area to another. The Royal College of Physicians of London first laid out some of the core local and regional services in its report *Physical Disability—1986 and Beyond* (Royal College of Physicians 1986), and in 1993 the British Society of Rehabilitation Medicine published a report entitled *Advice to Purchasers—Setting Contracts for Rehabilitation Medicine* (Ward

Table 5 Conditions requiring local rehabilitation services

Neurological	Trauma	Musculoskeletal	Cardiorespiratory
Stroke	Limb fractures	Back pain	Ischaemic heart disease
Multiple sclerosis	Brain injury	Other spinal pain	Chronic obstructive
Parkinson's disease		Fibromyalgia	pulmonary disease
Spinal paralysis		Inflammatory arthritis	
Motor neurone disease		Juvenile arthritis	
Cerebral palsy		Degenerative joint disease	
Spina bifida			
Other congenital conditions			

Table 6 Range of health services needed

Generic services	Specialized services
Local	
Rehabilitation therapy	Inpatient and outpatient rehabilitation
Wheelchair services	Community rehabilitation teams
Orthotics	Stroke services
Continence	Brain injury services
Tissue viability	Parkinson's disease, multiple sclerosis services, etc.
Dysphagia	
Information	Back pain services
Disability and sexual counselling	Complex wheelchair and special seating
Aids and equipment	Liaison with other specialties (e.g. neurology)
Communication aids	Liaison with other agencies (statutory and voluntary)
Rehabilitation engineering	
Supradistrict	
Disabled living centres	Spinal cord injury centres
Driving assessment centres	Neurobehavioural brain injury facilities
Rehabilitation research and development	Prosthetics centres
	Complex orthotics, seating, and wheelchair services
	Specialized communication aids centres
	Environmental control systems

and Houston 1993). The services described in these documents have been brought together in Table 6 and reflect what each district should be providing compared with those which are of a more specialized nature.

Models of delivery

With such a burden of physical disability in the population, adequate and equitable delivery of health care to the disabled population is clearly a major logistical problem. Services provided in most countries are patchy, fragmented, and inadequate. So what service delivery options are available?

Acute services

With increasing pressure on acute beds and the trend towards community-based services, one can argue that rehabilitation services should be outside acute facilities, but ready to assist in moving patients to definitive rehabilitation to meet their requirements. Some beds are required for specialized rehabilitation and certainly some will be required in the future for convalescence, as the acute facilities push patients out with increasing speed. Thus rehabilitation in the acute facility will be aimed at getting patients to the starting point where more definitive rehabilitation can take place and will by necessity be short-term and impairment driven rather than activity or participation focused. Therefore acute rehabilitation in community settings is possible and there will be a focus on more inpatient- and outpatient-based rehabilitation.

Medical clinics

The traditional model of managing people with disabilities through the hospital outpatient clinic is unsatisfactory for a number of reasons. There is often little continuity of care, with follow-up visits supervised by junior medical staff with little knowledge of the individual or of the disability. The numbers of people involved means that little time can be spent with any one person and the reappointment intervals tend to be long. This model provides little or no involvement by members of the rehabilitation team who were formally involved in the inpatient episode. It may have some relevance in certain conditions such as multiple sclerosis, Parkinson's disease, or chronic fatigue syndrome, but in general fails to meet the principles of service delivery outlined above and is widely known to be an unsatisfactory experience for both the doctor and disabled person.

Disease-specific clinics

Specific clinics and activities have recently been developed for managing certain long-term conditions, such as multiple sclerosis, epilepsy, Parkinson's disease, or inflammatory joint disease. In addition, back pain services have been set up and these clinics have the advantage of providing an expert multidisciplinary approach, which is familiar with the specific problems of that disorder. The team can supply information and counselling support and can act as a focus for self-help groups. Thus the clinic can provide a social as well as a medical function, and can also facilitate research. However, there are logistical problems of arranging a large number of such clinics to cover the whole range of disabilities and the possibility of ignoring rarer conditions. There is also the real danger of staff boredom and the problem of individuals seeing others with the same condition who are worse than themselves, with the consequent psychological stress both for them and their carers.

Community rehabilitation teams

Follow-up from the acute hospital-based rehabilitation team is essential for many people with significant disabilities to provide continuity of support and access to appropriate health resources after discharge. A community team can still work in a multi- or inter-disciplinary manner in the same way as the acute rehabilitation team, but tends to concentrate more on changing abilities and participation than on the relationship between impairments and abilities. A team is effective for a population of about 120 000 (Royal College of Physicians 1997). Teams may be peripatetic, based in health or community centres, or in community hospitals. Because regular review for large numbers of people would quickly place an unacceptable demand on the service, some teams operate an open-access service for self-referral which can counteract this problem. A self-referral review system can mean that preventable complications arise unrecognized by the disabled person and may only provide a health orientation to problems, potentially ignoring important social and vocational aspects of disability. There are examples of broader-based multidisciplinary teams with input from social services, employment, and other voluntary and statutory bodies. This requires a great deal of co-ordination and co-operation between different statutory and funding agencies which, at least within the present United Kingdom system, is difficult to achieve.

Primary care teams

A typical group general practice in the United Kingdom has a population of around 10 000. The numbers of disabled people are thus reduced within a primary care practice to a reasonable level. It is possible for the primary care team to keep a watching brief on the disabled people and make referrals to a local hospital-based team as appropriate. However, many disabilities are quite rare. For example, a general practitioner is likely to see only one new person with multiple sclerosis every 20 years. The level of expertise within the primary care team is thus limited and important points of management may be missed and questions left unanswered. It is likely that a system dependent on a primary care team will produce a rather unco-ordinated and fragmented service. In order to circumvent this problem the primary care team could be supported by visiting members of a specialist rehabilitation team. In one project a rehabilitation consultant and physiotherapist attended meetings of the primary care team to discuss management issues for people with Parkinson's disease. Such projects have potential but need further evaluation.

Case management

Disabled people, particularly those with severe and wide-ranging disabilities, will need a complex array of health and social services. The concept of case management has been developed as a way of assisting disabled people with the co-ordination of the necessary professional staff. Case management can include:

- simple co-ordination within a single agency
- co-ordination across agency boundaries
- service brokerage in which the case manager negotiates with the key agencies on the client's behalf
- budget-holding responsibility where services can be purchased on behalf of the client from statutory bodies or other voluntary or private agencies.

There have been very few controlled studies of the efficacy of case management, but it is widely practised within the United States and Canada, and probably provides a better and more coherent service, particularly for those who have a degree of cognitive impairment and are unable to find their own way through the maze of services (Beardshaw and Towell 1990; Shepherd 1990).

Links with other agencies

Health-based rehabilitation goes hand-in-hand with social and vocational rehabilitation and services need both formal and informal means to break down the artificial barriers between the participating agencies. Cross representation is neccessary at both the strategic and operational levels and disabled people need not only to be involved, but should also lead when and where it is appropriate. There is no single preferred model to suit every location and each will depend on the local facilities and assets of the participating individuals. However, all new services should take into account the living options principles (Fiedler and Twitchin 1990) (described in Table 7), and the views and advice of users' and disabled people's groups on disabled living should have a high priority (Fig. 6).

Joint commissioning of services for physical disability and rehabilitation works well and is the way forward. The distinction between the medical and social models of rehabilitation is probably not helpful and only serves to create barriers. Disabled people do not care who supplies or funds a service, just as long as it is provided, is timely and appropriate, and is in the right quantity. Service philosophies should be just as applicable in health-based or social rehabilitation settings, as long as the objectives of the rehabilitation intervention are clear. For instance if the aim is to achieve re-employment after injury, the individual will need to be fit to go to work, have the physical means to

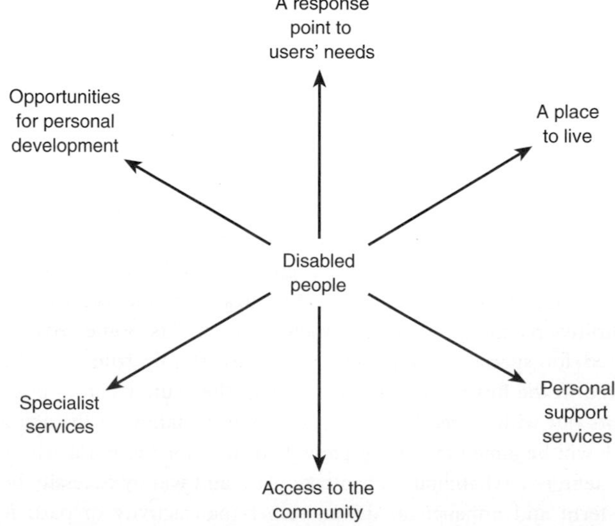

Fig. 6 The essential elements of a comprehensive service system for people with severe physical and sensory disabilities.

Table 7 Living Options Working Party key principles for disabled people

Choice	Of where to live and how to maintain independence without overprotection, or the risk of unnecessary hazards. This includes help in learning how to choose from the options available—a skill that needs to be acquired from an early age
Consultation	On services as they are planned and knowledge that such services will be based on the views of people with disability, their carers, families, and voluntary organizations with special expertise. Particular note should be taken of the views of those from differing cultural backgrounds
Information	Clearly presented and readily available to the most severely disabled consumers and their families, service providers, and those responsible for planning
Participation	In the life of local and national communities in respect of both responsibilities and benefits. Full integration can only exist when equal opportunities are available in the fields of access, housing employment, education, mobility, and leisure
Recognition	That long-term disability is not synonymous with illness and that the medical model of care is inappropriate in the majority of cases
Autonomy	Freedom to make decisions regarding the way of life best suited to an individual disabled person's circumstances

Source: Fiedler and Twitchin (1990).

get there, have the mental and physical capacity to do the job, and have the energy and good health to continue to attend on a regular basis thereafter. The discipline of travelling to and from work will need to be (re)learnt, as will the social skills to get on with colleagues, employers, and so on. This calls for a whole range of skills and a potential need for assistance and services. The best way to describe them is by means of the following case history.

Case history 2

JB is a 23-year-old man who was involved in a road traffic accident in 1995. He suffered a massive brain injury and was admitted to hospital with a Glasgow Coma Score of 5 (Teasdale and Jennett 1974). He was a right-handed man who suffered right frontoparietal lobe damage and a haematoma was evacuated. Following this, he developed intracranial hypertension and subsequently post-traumatic epilepsy. He had a left hemiplegia, left hemiaesthesia, a left homonynous hemianopia, visuospatial neglect, and a significant constructional dyspraxia and agnosia. He was resuscitated and transferred to rehabilitation.

He stayed in hospital for about 4 months and during that time made a remarkable physical recovery. He developed some increased tone on the left side, but had a good return of power, such that he could walk up- and downstairs unaided. He was quiet and withdrawn, but not clinically depressed, and had undergone a complete personality change. He had been an outgoing carefree man, who was married with a 2-year-old daughter. His dyspraxia and inertia were very evident and, despite a good physical recovery, he was unable to return to work. He would sit at home all day and while he admitted to being very frustrated, he did not have the means to express this.

He attended a post-head injury day therapy course and, although he enjoyed it, he did not really progress. His wife left him, as she found it difficult living with a man, who 'was not the man she married'. He went to live with his parents, and has been with them ever since. Shortly afterwards, he presented with grand mal epileptic fits and has become quite agoraphobic. He will not go out without his mother and develops regular panic attacks if he is in an open space. As a result, he has lost all contact with his friends and presents as a lonely man who is terrified of having a fit in public. He is on large doses of a single anticonvulsant, from which he has side-effects and occasionally is incontinent when he cannot find a toilet in time.

He is now reviewed jointly by the regional neurobehavioural unit and local rehabilitation centre, and his anticonvulsant medication has now been altered to two drugs in less toxic doses. He has undergone a period of inpatient rehabilitation in the neurobehavioural unit and a strategy for managing his agoraphobia has been started. During that time the staff from the physical rehabilitation unit have eliminated his incontinence and his fits are under better control. He still needs a lot of help and a claim for damages has been started. Unfortunately, there is a liability dispute, and this is producing a negative effect on his ability to move on. Financially, he is supported by his parents, but they are a little overprotective. He has thus rejected going out with social groups and has been only an intermittent attender at the local Headway House. If he gains independent financial support, it is planned to appoint a case manager who will employ some companions for him. With time and a consistent approach, it is hoped to get him out and to allow him to live eventually more independently of his parents. He will need continued help from the local rehabilitation unit, who will take advice from the regional neurobehavioural unit to access local services. He is unlikely to return to paid employment, but, in the first instance, the aim will be to get him to socialize more and just to get him out of his house. The local social services day centre has been offered by his social worker, who has co-operated closely with health professionals in trying to work with JB and his parents. The prognosis for independent living is not particularly favourable and it is possible that care services will be required when his parents are not in a position to look after him in the future.

Who is rehabilitation for?

As health services become better focused on effectiveness and care plans, they have looked more closely at where rehabilitation should be directed. The decision to accept people for inpatient and outpatient rehabilitation has been rather haphazard, without any objective assessment of therapeutic goals and without reference to explicit policies. Decisions about discharge also tend to be vague (Hass 1988). To make best use of resources, four questions need to be asked when assessing people for rehabilitation. They are more obvious when a patient is referred to a hospital rehabilitation programme, for example a stroke unit, but are equally applicable to outpatient or community settings.

- Is the rehabilitation resource (e.g. a hospital unit) designed for the person's needs?
- What is the effectiveness of rehabilitation?
- What is the benefit of rehabilitation?
- What will happen without rehabilitation?

Is the rehabilitation resource designed for the client's needs?

Clinical effectiveness and defined admission criteria to rehabilitation units have clarified the work of these facilities, but are more prevalent in hospital-based institutions than in community organizations (Royal College of Physicians 1997). Specific operational policies for hospital- and community-based rehabilitation programmes can be used when selecting patients for rehabilitation and again when deciding whether to continue the programme; for example, if the needs of a new referral have to be judged against those of someone else who is continuing to make gains during a prolonged inpatient rehabilitation episode. Difficulties most often arise when there are multiple disabilities involving combinations of physical, behavioural, and cognitive problems extending beyond the expertise of a specific rehabilitation team. The occurrence of this combination, for instance in head injury and schizophrenia, creates a strong argument for the existence of specialized units for such conditions. Units lacking the required expertise will be incapable of meeting all the client's needs and such people can only disrupt the efficiency and confidence of staff treating other people on the unit. Where a new area of need is defined, a unit must take a conscious decision to adapt its policies to accommodate it or, where necessary, to add its voice to demands for the development of new facilities.

One factor distinguishing the operational policies of different units is the pace or intensity of rehabilitation. Intensive programmes are not always required, even if they are available. Physical fitness and behavioural factors, such as attention span, influence an individual's ability to benefit from intensive therapy programmes. Elderly people and those with severe multiple disabilities sometimes benefit from a relatively slow pace of rehabilitation and the association with concomitant conditions distinguishes the rehabilitation pace for older and younger people above everything else. In establishing a unit's case mix, the needs of the rehabilitation staff must also be accommodated as they must feel confident and expert. Ongoing training of key staff is therefore essential in order for that expertise to be diffused downwards.

The geographical remoteness of regional units (spinal cord injury, brain injury) from where disabled people live show that the organization of services is critical for successful integration with other non-health services. However, the advantages of an intensive programme based in a regional centre to some people are outweighed by any remoteness from home. There are still major disadvantages in that there is limited access to the family, ignorance of the hospital's system of working, and difficulties in setting up appropriate post-discharge plans. People from outlying areas are sometimes impressed at first by the expertise of the large centre and then all the more disappointed by its inability to achieve outcomes which are relevant to the disabled person's own community. Nevertheless, it is impossible to mirror all the services in each district and regional organization along supra-district lines will always be necessary (Table 6).

As rehabilitation is heterogeneous, it is necessary for some units to specialize in certain areas. Therefore it may be difficult to compare one unit with another, and the British Society of Rehabilitation Medicine has recently published some clinical standards to cover what the basic standards the public can expect of inpatient rehabilitation (Turner-Stokes 1999). Thus peer review of rehabilitation units will be possible, albeit at a simple level at the moment. For instance, each unit should at least document on admission and discharge an outcome measure to reflect the patient's individual rehabilitation programme. This is a straightforward start and is achievable and easy enough to ensure full participation by all.

Effectiveness of rehabilitation

When a referral is appropriate, it is necessary to ask how and in what aspects the client will benefit from rehabilitation. There is now good data on clinical effectiveness in rehabilitation (Stroke Units Trialists Collaboration 1997). Stroke units save lives and reduce disability (Roth *et al.* 1998). There is an improvement in the abilities and participation of people undergoing stroke rehabilitation, even where there is not much change in the impairment (Wade *et al.* 1985). Much work has been done on the relationship between specific medical factors and outcome. A number of medical variables have been shown to predict poor outcomes—for example, in stroke (Bernspang *et al.* 1987). Such evidence from group studies is of limited value in predicting the rehabilitation potential of individuals. There are, however, neurological deficits which are intrinsically obstructive to the rehabilitation process. For example, a receptive aphasia limits the potential for verbally based education and there is evidence that high-order perceptual deficits following right hemisphere damage are associated with poorer outcomes (Stroke Units Trialists Collaboration 1997). Similarly, other physical deficits also disrupt the rehabilitation process and poor cardiac/respiratory reserve, loss of limb, obesity, and skin and joint problems are some examples. The ability to learn is crucial for rehabilitation potential (Tondat Carter *et al.* 1988), but it is often difficult to pick this up and the methods are not yet well developed. A number of studies, which show the benefit of rehabilitation and they are listed in Table 8.

In the light of this, it is possible to conclude that rehabilitation:

- reduces complications (e.g. the physical effects of neurological injury, immobility, etc.)
- optimizes the physical and social functioning of patients
- identifies cognitive and emotional complications of traumatic brain injury, even in the absence of physical sequelae
- improves the chances of living independently at home and returning to work
- concentrates therapy—more therapy input is associated with shorter hospital stays and improved outcomes (Shiel *et al.* 1999).

Benefits of dedicated rehabilitation

There is now considerable evidence that the process described above produces real benefits and improved outcomes. Reports of stroke

Table 8 Current evidence of effectiveness of rehabilitation in traumatic brain injury

Reference	Key findings
Benefits of rehabilitation	
Hall and Cope (1995)	Literature review of papers showing that designated rehabilitation facilities reduce preventable disability and complications with benefits to outcomes.
Roth *et al.* (1998)	Impairment and disability: their relationship during stroke rehabilitation. Applies to brain injury as well. The conclusion is that there is a greater change in disability measures than in impairment measures during rehabilitation programmes. Even in the absence of any change in impairment, there is still a benefit in patients' abilities following rehabilitation, indicating that the learning process and the therapeutic input has a direct effect on patient ability to carry out tasks and to gain in independence.
Early rehabilitation	
Cope and Hall (1982)	Compared two groups of patients, admitted early (< 35 days) and late (> 35 days). Similar levels of disability throughout rehabilitation episode. Late admission group required twice the length of stay of the early group. More problems with bowel, bladder. More psychological problems and bilateral damage.
Bishara *et al.* (1992)	Relationship of outcome to Glasgow Coma Scale score and post-traumatic amnesia duration. Latter more sensitive to outcome and rehabilitation intervention can thus be geared to this prognostic feature.
Tuel and Presty (1992)	Retrospective analysis of 49 cases of traumatic brain injury readmitted at least 1 year postinjury. With further therapy, the Barthel activities of daily living index increased in 53 per cent of cases and a third moved from dependence to assisted independence. Those in moderate range improved the most. The Barthel's ceiling effect prevented showing the improvement in the high range, but they improved also. Substantial savings in care provision suggested from this study.
Intensive therapy	
Blackerby (1990)	Intensity of rehabilitation and length of stay, which decreased by 31 per cent when the hours of therapy increased from 5 to 8 h/day every day.
Shiel *et al.* (1999)	Length of stay decreased and qualitative outcomes increased in proportion to the amount of therapy provided in acute rehabilitation
Dedication of facilities	
McLellan (1991)	The simple act of transferring patients from busy acute surgical wards to the calmer and quieter atmosphere of a rehabilitation unit decreased cognitive disturbance, the need for sedation, and improved overall outcomes in traumatic brain injury patients.
Prevention of complications	
Hall and Cope (1995)	Literature review of papers showing that designated rehabilitation facilities reduce preventable disability and complications.
Burbaud *et al.* (1996)	Use of botulinum toxin in treatment of spasticity in brain injury. Prevents the onset of deformities, contractures, and difficulties with providing nursing care, reduces pain, and improves self-esteem.
Spasticity Study Group (1997)	Systematic review of literature giving clinical guidance on management of spasticity, particularly in acquired brain injury. Identifies benefits to clinical care.
Booth *et al.* (1983)	Importance of casting in prevention of contractures in patients in traumatic brain injury. Beneficial outcomes in terms of mobility, posture, and pain levels.
Eames and Wood (1985)	Longitudinal study of 24 patients with challenging behaviour for 1 year postinjury made gains in quality of life and living arrangements.
Rapp *et al.* (1983)	Demonstrates loss of nutritional well being following brain injury and the effect of a sound rehabilitation programme to prevent and counteract this.
Temkin *et al.* (1991)	Outlines the evidence for management of post-traumatic epilepsy and the risk of management strategies on prevention.
Garland (1991)	Effects of severe brain injury on bone healing and on development of heterotopic ossification.
Kalisky *et al.* (1985)	Outlines the potential medical problems of severe traumatic brain injury. Ranges from the effect of the injury to the brain and subsequent endocrinological problems to the effects of immobility and concomitant injuries and disorders, for example psychiatric, cardiopulmonary (deep vein thrombosis/pulmonary embolism), musculoskeletal (heterotopic ossification), gastrointestinal, genitourinary, and immobilization (fluid and electrolytes) complications.
Post-acute rehabilitation	
Cope *et al.* (1991)	Follow-up of 145 patients 6–24 months postinjury. Residential status, productive activity, and hours of attendant care measured by independent assessors. Half were residential at time of readmission and this fell to 15 per cent by discharge. Those engaged in productive activity increased from 6 to 35 per cent and hours of care decreased from 10.2 to 3.8 h. A cost–benefit analysis using reduction in care alone suggests that the cost of rehabilitation is rapidly offset by the savings in provision of care, especially when the average life expectancy is 44 years or more.

Table 8 Current evidence of effectiveness of rehabilitation in traumatic brain injury (*Continued*)

Reference	Key findings
Malec and Basford (1996)	A post-acute brain injury programme established in Chicago showed a significant improvement in occupational activity, return to work, and overall outcomes in independence measures compared with previous practice in the same centre.
Johnston and Lewis (1991)	Report of patients discharged from nine different post-acute brain injury programmes. Outcomes assessed by telephone interview 1 year later using a 164-item questionnaire and a five-point hierarchical global rating of supervision of care. Highly significant change was reported. An institutional rate of 47 per cent fell to 7 per cent by discharge and the 72 per cent requiring constant supervision fell to 16 per cent. Adjustments for chronicity suggested that the findings were true even for those more than 1 year postinjury, so the effects were attributed to rehabilitation rather than to spontaneous recovery.
Wilson (1992)	Subjects using more memory aids than before the rehabilitation programme and more of these were back in some form of paid employment.
Therapy	
Faghri *et al.* (1994)	Functional electrical stimulation in hemiplegic arms prevents shoulder pain in a small randomized trial. Further evidence is about to be published on stimulating the common peroneal nerve in ambulant subjects.
Plus stroke evidence: cognitive retraining	
Oddy *et al.* (1985)	Of 43 patients admitted to Wolfson Rehabilitation Centre, only five had returned to their previous level of work at 2 years. Only one person not working at 2 years was working at 7 years. There is a willingness to accept any other job than that held before the injury.
Heiskanen and Sipponen (1970)	Age has a strong influence on the ability to return to work. Among patients who were unconscious for 24 h or more, 70 per cent of those $<$ 20 years of age were able to return to work. Over 50 years of age only 30 per cent were able to return. No one unconscious for 1 month was able to return to work. Over the age of 40, no one who had been unconscious for 1 week was able to return to work.
Ben Yishay *et al.* (1987)	94 patients on an outpatient cognitive retraining programme at an average of 3 years postinjury. 84 per cent of patients at the end of a 3-year follow-up were able to engage in productive employment, 63 per cent at a competitive level and 21 per cent in a subsidized capacity. Six patients who dropped out were not included and would have skewed the results downwards, but they are nonetheless impressive. Costs were high.
Evans *et al.* (1992)	536 patients followed for 1 year. 88 per cent returned to preinjury setting compared with only 33 per cent living at home on entry to study. Competitive employment increased from 5.6 to 50 per cent. Severity of disability not reported.
Prigatano *et al.* (1984)	Report on neuropsychological functioning, emotional distress, and productivity (employment and education) following a multidisciplinary programme. The treatment group showed increased productivity (50 per cent compared with 36 per cent) and decreased emotional stress. The study illustrates the variance one may see between outcome measured in terms of handicap with little or no change in impairment.
Cost-effectiveness	
Turner-Stokes *et al.* (1998)	Use of the Northwick Park Dependency Scale identifies nursing and care burden in acquired brain injury. This has been used to calculate costs of care for patients entered into an early rehabilitation programme at the Regional Rehabilitation Centre at Northwick Park Hospital compared with those admitted late. There were significant changes in the level of skilled nursing input and care required. Care provided by untrained staff was not signifiantly affected, but the patient population requires longer-term follow-up to identify further changes.
Livingston *et al.* (1985)	Significant dysfunction in families and partners of brain injured people. High carer burden and the most frequent predictor of relatives' psychiatric and social status was the level of patients' symptomatic complaints. This suggested the need for comprehensive rehabilitation of both patients and carers.
Cost of disability	
BSRM (1988)	Cost of disability huge. Cost of not providing rehabilitation not defined, but probably more expensive to country at large than providing services. Initial high costs to NHS diminishes ongoing costs with adequate rehabilitation.

rehabilitation trials (Indrevidavik *et al.* 1991) show that outcome is better for patients cared for in a specialist stroke unit than those cared for in a general medical ward. Those in stroke units were less likely to die and less likely to be living in institutions a year after the stroke. Stroke units also improved functional outcome following an intensive period of early rehabilitation (Strand *et al.* 1985; Indrevidavik *et al.* 1991). One large-scale overview of stroke rehabilitation in 3717 patients demonstrated that focused rehabilitation can improve functional performance (Ottenbacher and Jannell 1993). The best results were obtained with younger patients and those receiving rehabilitation early after their stroke.

Similar results, although with smaller patient numbers, have been demonstrated for rehabilitation after spinal cord and head injury (Yarkoney *et al.* 1987; Hall and Cope 1995). Most of these studies confirm the value of two different aspects of rehabilitation. Firstly, most studies documented improvements in functional outcome and speed of attaining such outcome. Secondly, disabled people going through rehabilitation units have less unnecessary complications. There are less unnecessary physical problems, such as those associated with spasticity, contractures, and pressure sores and less unnecessary psychological problems, such as untreated depression. There is clear evidence that an intensive period of rehabilitation after an acute event, such as head injury or spinal cord injury, produces clear, short-term functional gains (Cope and Hall 1982). However, there is also evidence that short-term gains are lost unless longer-term support is available (Garraway *et al.* 1980). Thus longer-term contact with the disabled person is important in order to provide rehabilitation until natural recovery is complete and to prevent the later development of unnecessary complications. Assessment of care costs should allow for continuing rehabilitation support.

There are clear benefits from early rehabilitation, but even if an individual has not received rehabilitation in the early stages after trauma, later rehabilitation should still not be considered a waste of time. Tuel and Presty (1992) demonstrated that just over half of 49 people with severe head injury seen by a rehabilitation team at least a year after the injury improved function regardless of age or injury severity. Benefit can be achieved in the alleviation of psychological, emotional, and behavioural problems. Eames and Wood (1985) showed a marked improvement in severe behavioural problems several years after severe head injury. Roth *et al.* (1998) showed that rehabilitation after stroke produced improvements in abilities and participation (independent living in this case), even when there was no sgnificant change in the severity of the impairment. It should also be considered that advantages can follow from access to rehabilitation for people with longer-term deteriorating conditons, such as multiple sclerosis. Rehabilitation has been shown not only to be efficacious (Larocca and Kalb 1992; Kidd *et al.* 1995) but also to be cost-effective (Feigenson and Scheinberg 1981). Once again, there is evidence that co-ordinated imput reduces physical and psychological problems and results in fewer unnecessary hospital admissions.

While the process of rehabilitation is clearly beneficial for the individual, it is also beneficial for the health service and society as a whole. Less unnecessary hospital admissions, shorter stays, and fewer physical and psychological complications all lead to cost reduction and a better service. More importantly, there is a reduction in hospital readmissions following rehabilitation for acute illness/trauma. Work in the United States has shown that a co-ordinated rehabilitation programme can lead to a better chance of returning to work (Ben-Yishay *et al.* 1987; Wehman *et al.* 1995) and such an outcome is clearly preferable to the individual and the family, and for the economy as a whole. Increased functional independence will lead to reduced care needs in the community. There can be significant long-term financial savings, which can more than offset the cost of a patient's initial rehabilitation, especially in traumatic brain injury where the expectation of life may be long lasting (Aronow 1987).

The process of interdisciplinary rehabilitation improves functional outcomes and reduces unnecessary complications. Research reveals that it is effective, but evaluation of its cost-effectiveness still needs further work. There are many indications of the latter, but we need to know which aspects of rehabilitation consistently produce the best outcome in relation to cost. The dilemma is that everyone knows that rehabilitation is vital, but new methodologies need to identify its true value. Randomized control trials are important, but may miss some of the most valuable and important observations of rehabilitation. Advantages can follow from access to rehabilitation for people with longer-term deteriorating conditions, such as multiple sclerosis.

What happens if rehabilitation does not take place?

A person's rehabilitation potential cannot be considered in isolation from what would have been the outcome without rehabilitation. Has the rehabilitation programme made the difference or has it all been left to chance? The natural history of the impairment and the consequent disabilities and disadvantages play a major role in the eventual outcome following rehabilitation. Some conditions recover spontaneously and early intervention may give the false impression that therapy has been efficacious (Dombovy *et al.* 1987; Legh Smith *et al.* 1987). Conversely, early intervention may be associated with an improved outcome where full recovery does not occur (Oakes *et al.* 1990).

The risk of recurrence or early death must be considered. In some cases, this is inevitable and, while the type of rehabilitation offered for the management of a cord lesion due to metastatic spinal disease is necessarily different from that of cord trauma, people with the former do nevertheless need rehabilitative programmes. Social and other premorbid factors (e.g. pre-existing personality, psychiatric, or medical disorders) may dominate the situation in such a way that the proposed rehabilitation input could only have a negligible effect on outcome. It is sometimes clear that the level of disadvantage (e.g. dependency) would be roughly the same with or without rehabilitation. For someone with a spouse/partner willing to act as carer, rehabilitation might make the difference between home life and institutional care, whereas a similar person with no family might be destined for a nursing home even after intensive rehabilitation. Giving priority to people with a wider range of possible outcomes may seem logical but is ethically hazardous since it leads to a 'what if' suggestion that some categories (e.g. 'old' single men without capital or income) are inherently less worthy of rehabilitation than others in more fortunate circumstances. To be effective, the rehabilitation plan must be tailored to individual needs, to enable people where possible to achieve or resume a lifestyle quality that meets their aspirations within the resources available.

The lives of people with persisting disabilities are also enhanced by rehabilitation but, more importantly, the consequence of them not having rehabilitation is to reduce their independent functioning and quality of life (Hall and Cope 1995). So what happens to people with complex physical disabilities in the absence of specialized planned rehabilitation? In the immediate period following injury, it is known that the simple act of transferring a brain injured patient from a busy surgical or neurosurgical ward to the calmer, quieter atmosphere of a rehabilitation ward has a therapeutic effect in itself and improvements in attention, irritability, and cognition are observed (McLellan 1985). In addition, patients on general wards are often inappropriately sedated during the irritable phase of their recovery and their behaviour is more difficult to manage in busy surgical wards, where the time and attention of the nursing staff must of necessity be devoted to other patients with urgent surgical problems. As a result, inappropriate referrals are made to psychiatric and other services. Acute general wards are not conducive to the practice of multiprofessional rehabilitation for patients with complex needs. Staff do not have the time, the expertise, or the resources to meet those needs properly and the net effect is to arrange discharge as quickly as possible. Many correctable problems, such as nutrition, swallowing, mobility, and equipment issues, are not addressed and the focus is on treating the impairment (e.g. wound healing) and freeing the bed for the next patient. In the absence of recognized rehabilitation, acute beds are blocked. Therefore patients are denied access to acute wards if their early discharge cannot be guaranteed. In the post-acute phase, all the problems of physical inactivity are seen in the absence of rehabilitation. While health services have a statutory duty to provide rehabilitation services to meet the health needs of patients, rehabilitation services and expertise is still very patchy (Anonymous 1990; Association of British Neurologists 1992). Therefore patients have very different experiences in the post-acute phase and in subsequent rehabilitation. Successful social integration depends not only on this but on many other factors, and some of the problems that arise in the absence of early rehabilitation are listed in Box 3.

Box 3

- Immobility including pressure sores, spasticity, contractures, and osteoporosis
- Pain
- Nutrition
- Swallowing problems
- Bladder and bowel problems:
  - constipation
  - incontinence
- Communication problems
- Mood and behavioural problems
- Systemic illness from a variety of causes, but in particular resulting from urinary tract and chest infections
- Complications of underlying condition

A lack of planned rehabilitation results in treatment activity being uncoordinated and inefficient, but this does not necessarily mean that the necessary services are not available. Treatments become ineffective either because the patient is not ready for them or because other things are not in place to ensure their success. Inappropriate disability equipment is provided and often may go unused, thereby cluttering up a household (Chamberlain 1988). Inappropriate use of equipment often leads to dissatisfaction and frustration aimed either at the person with the disability or the provider. In some cases, all that is required is a proper explanation of how to use a particular device or piece of equipment properly.

Without formal rehabilitation disabled people and their carers do not have the opportunity for gaining the necessary knowledge and information for independent living skills, which is vital for both. Later on, the full consequences of a lack of rehabilitation become apparent. As the disabled person moves into living in the community, the lack of follow-up leads to preventable health problems and social isolation. Carers become exhausted by the burden of care and many domestic situations break down. The first signs are an increase in the number of urgent calls to general practitioners or social workers, emergency admissions arranged to hospital, and eventually placements are made for residential or nursing home care (Edwards 1990). Review of those residents revealed in many cases conditions which could easily be managed in the community, given support (Martin and White 1988) and part of this package is the need to provide suitable daily care arrangements and opportunities for respite care. Skin breakdown is the most common, followed by urinary tract infections, pulmonary infections, and contractures (Shangraw *et al.* 1988). Inadequate personal assistance also leads to extended hospital stays, threats to safety, poor nutrition, and poor personal hygiene. The most significant feature of poor care is a total reliance on the family alone for assistance, the common adverse affects including burnout, family role changes, and economic strain (BSRM 1993).

Immobility

The consequences of immobility have a profound effect on physiology, health, and social well being. Even in the short term, loss of bone mineral content is observed (Krolner and Toft 1983). Sensory deprivation also occurs, and Leidermann *et al.* (1958) show that people confined to bed for prolonged periods suffer from disorientation, confusion, and delusions from decreased kinaesthetic, auditory, visual, and social stimulation. Sleep patterns change and loss of sleep impairs bladder control. In parkinsonian and other patients, memory and learning deteriorate (Parkes 1985) and this may occur to such an extent that irreversible dementia has been reported (Kelly and Feigenbaum 1982). Sleep is important not only for performance, but for healing of the impairment and conditions such as pressure sores as well.

Changes occur in muscle function and atrophy is seen by as much as 12 per cent in calf muscle bulk and 26 per cent in strength (Le Blanc *et al.* 1987), especially in antigravity muscles (Le Blanc *et al.* 1988). Neurological complications can occur in the form of compressive neuropathies of the lateral popliteal nerve at the head of the fibula and the ulnar nerve at the elbow as sites of particular risk. Also described is a devastating generalized sensory motor neuropathy seen in desperately ill people requiring intensive care treatment, characterized by generalized weakness, in which recovery may be poor (Warlow 1991). Changes also occur in the cardiovascular system with a greater likelihood of orthostatic hypotension (Greenleaf *et al.* 1985; Harper and Lyles 1988) which may take several months of ambulation to be corrected (Sandler *et al.* 1988). Deep vein thrombosis is a serious consequence of immobility and Warlow *et al.* (1976) identified an incidence of 50 per cent in a hemiparetic leg after stroke. The combination of stasis and vessel wall injury from abnormal posture and pressure—and the hypercoagulability that exists in conditions such as myocardial infarction, stroke, or surgery—is a powerful trigger for thrombogenesis (Thomas 1985). Prevention of formation and of embolization by adequate mobilization of the limb in a rehabilitation setting is necessary and early efficient mobilization is enhanced by an effective rehabilitation programme.

Pressure sores and contracture formation are two of the major consequences of a lack of rehabilitation. Rehabilitation experience drives general medical and nursing staff to develop pressure sore policies and quality standards are now a Department of Health recommendation (Department of Health 1993). While the creation of policies has raised standards, it has also opened up National Health

Service (**NHS**) Trusts to compensation claims in the event of patients developing sores. Contractures themselves are not only painful but lead to abnormal positioning and a greatly increased risk of pressure sore development. Yarkony and Sahgal (1987) found that contractures occurred in 84 per cent of patients requiring inpatient rehabilitation after traumatic brain injury and the number of contractures increased with coma duration. Most affected are the hips (81 per cent), shoulders (76 per cent), ankles (76 per cent), and elbows (44 per cent). These take time to develop and permanent limb deformity is often the consequence. Since this may take 2 to 3 years to develop (Blasier and Left 1989) there is time to organize their treatment.

Another major implication of immobility is the development of osteoporosis. The resultant loss of bone mass in immobility has been well studied in the context of paralysis, in weightlessness in space, and in people on bedrest (Albright *et al.* 1941; Krolner and Toft 1983; Stupakov *et al.* 1989). There is an increase in calcium excretion and breakdown products of bone collagen, which reach a peak between 3 and 6 months after injury. Even the resumption of exercise does not always counteract the loss of bone seen following bedrest as it is weight bearing that is important. Therefore people who may exercise hard need to spend time putting weight through their lower limbs and spine (Jessekutz *et al.* 1966; Schoutens *et al.* 1989). Hormone replacement and the advice on smoking and dietary intake of calcium appear to take second place in these people to the need to bear weight to prevent osteoporotic hip fractures (Law *et al.* 1991).

Nutrition

Most people become malnourished after major injury and some are frankly cachectic. The reasons for this are quite complex, but relate to poor feeding techniques on acute wards and a lack of awareness by staff of the metabolic needs of the recovering patient (Clifton *et al.* 1984; Gaddisseux *et al.* 1984). In addition, nurses do not give sufficient time to feed patients orally. Gisel and Patrick (1988) found that children with cerebral palsy took up to 12 times longer than normal children to chew pureed food and 15 times longer to chew solid food, and there is simply insufficient time on many acute wards for adequate feeding to occur. To confirm this, there is good evidence of increased nutritional requirements for people following brain injury, particularly those with very low Glasgow Coma Scale scores of 4 or 5 out of 15 (Robertson *et al.* 1984). Requirements increased during the initial 28 days and there was a correlation between proper nutritional support and recovery in severe traumatic brain injury (Young *et al.* 1992) with quicker earlier recovery in Glasgow Outcome Scale scores at 3 months.

The standard way of alternative feeding is now to switch as early as possible to fine-bore percutaneous endoscopy gastrostomy tube feeding. This method is beneficial (Wicks *et al.* 1992) and is generally more acceptable to patients and families (Llaneza *et al.* 1988). It is now the preferred method of feeding and many investigations support its superiority over other techniques (Himal and Schumacher 1987; Larson *et al.* 1987). Nutrients can either be given continually or intermittently by bolus feeding, and both have advantages. Certainly the latter can be easily incorporated into an active rehabilitation programme, and recovery of swallowing function can be easily assessed by videofluoroscopy (Splaingard *et al.* 1988). In addition, patients can still be treated for any communication disorders which would otherwise be inhibited by nasogastric tubing. This in itself highlights one of the benefits of rehabilitation to patients, which would not otherwise occur in its absence. Initially nasogastric tubes may be fitted on acute wards, but they are not now acceptable as longer-term solutions as they take a considerable time to achieve good nutrition and lead to the potential for increased irritability among confused patients, such as those following a traumatic brain injury. In addition, recovery of oral feeding may be inhibited by the presence of nasogastric tubes, and aspiration and oesophageal ulceration can occur. They are also cosmetically unpleasant for patients and their families, and many people find them very uncomfortable.

Swallowing

One of the main tasks in the rehabilitation of physically disabled people is the assessment and treatment of swallowing disorders. This is generally undertaken by speech and language therapists, in conjunction with the rest of the rehabilitation team, for it is important to rule out preventable and treatable causes such as those produced by the side-effects of medication. With modern techniques of imaging and early correction of the nutritional deficit by percutaneous endoscopy gastrostomy tube, there is reduced gastro-oesophageal regurgitation and thus less aspiration pneumonia. The latter is associated with a significant mortality and morbidity (Kiver *et al.* 1984), and in a rehabilitation setting the education of carers by staff leads to a better understanding of the importance of nutrition and its lack.

Bladder and bowel problems

Constipation

Another feature of rehabilitation is attention to constipation. Disabled people who do not receive formal specialist rehabilitation have a higher incidence of this condition and it is seen in those living in the community or in acute general wards. An audit of the North Staffordshire Rehabilitation Centre found severe colonic loading or faecal impaction in 35 per cent of patients admitted (Ward 1996). This is also found in spinal cord injured people (Andrews and Greenwood 1993). Chronic constipation is associated with, among other things, confusional states, pain, increased spasticity, and muscle spasm. It is a quality indicator in patient care and is thus indirectly associated with an increased incidence of problems such as pressure sores and contractures.

Incontinence

One of the considerations of a rehabilitation programme on constipation must also be to prevent the incidence of spurious diarrhoea. This still goes unrecognized in primary and secondary health care, and a lack of proper assessment causes antidiarrhoeal agents to be given when the patient requires bowel clearance instead. Similarly, urinary incontinence can be badly managed in the neurologically impaired person and there is often a lack of overall control and co-ordination in its prevention and management. The neurologenic bladder is not very well understood by many generalists and urological departments tend to concentrate, by sheer weight of numbers, on patients with mechanical bladder problems rather than those with neurological deficits. Real expertise has developed in this area in rehabilitation units.

Urinary and faecal incontinence are associated with skin problems and the development of pressure sores (Moolten 1972). If left untreated, both can be extremely handicapping, and they are two of the most common causes of disabled people remaining housebound. People describe planning their journeys around toilet facilities in order that they will not be 'caught short'. There is also inappropriate use of continence aids and equipment, and this is a crucial area for rehabilitation expertise.

Communication problems

Many people with communication disorders following neurological damage are isolated, misunderstood, and actively shunned. The rehabilitation process allows a better awareness of communication problems and helps patients, their families, and professionals to understand the importance of integrating sufferers back into society (Lincoln *et al.* 1984). The use of communication aids and other equipment, and the time given to understand communication disorders and individual patient's needs are important rehabilitation activities. Following a stroke, 35 per cent of patients have a communication problem and 15 per cent of these have a language difficulty. Following traumatic brain injury, half of all patients have communication difficulties which are, to a greater or lesser extent, involved with cognitive disturbance. It is very important to dissociate cognitive and communication problems, as their treatment may be quite different and assessment of one may be impossible without prior treatment of the other. Patients may present with good non-verbal communication skills yet have quite profound difficulties in understanding others and in expressing themselves. This leads to much confusion and can lead to profound mood and behavioural abnormalities.

Mood changes

Clinical depression is actively treated in the rehabilitation world and there is a great general awareness of its importance in producing well-adjusted patients. Similarly, the management of other mood disorders and of behavioural problems significantly affects outcome, even in conditions not affecting the brain. The successful management of pain, loss of limb, and chronic conditions, such as locomotor disorders, depends on the psychological well being of patients and their families. Assessment of life functioning is being developed in all these conditions, and outcome measures such as the General Health Questionnaire and the Life Satisfaction and Sickness Impact Profile are among those in common usage. Clinical psychologists are useful not only in the management of physically disabled people, but also in the prevention of these disorders which affect the rehabilitation process. The use of antidepressant medication has had a beneficial effect in rehabilitation units and, while the evidence of their benefit is variable, they are now quite safe drugs. The potential damage of missing a treatable depression appears to outweigh the risks of antidepressant medication in post-acute rehabilitation, particularly in people with traumatic and non-traumatic brain injury (Farm *et al.* 1995).

Pain

As with the management of depression, the management of chronic pain is crucial to the aim of producing a well-adjusted person, despite the limitations of his or her disability. Chronic pain is very common, occurring in people disabled by both neurological and locomotor disorders. For instance, shoulder pain occurs in up to 70 per cent of patients during the first year following a stroke and 25 per cent of patients develop the shoulder–hand syndrome, with or without a reflex sympathetic dystrophy (Van Ouwenaller *et al.* 1986). The management of pain is a multidisciplinary responsibility and combines a number of separate activities. There is a balance between analgesic medication, physical relief of pain (whether by therapeutic modalities or alteration of sensory nerve function), and by psychological means. It is important to achieve the right expectations and many patients with chronic pain have been mismanaged in the acute or early stages of their problem. The treatment of pain is an important facet of rehabilitation and should be instituted early. The use of transcutaneous electrical nerve stimulation, acupuncture, and complementary medicine may be beneficial to patients, but all concerned in the process should understand the rehabilitation goals. Pain is more frequent after non-dominant than dominant hemisphere stroke, and disorders of tone can also produce pain (Shahani *et al.* 1981; Poulin de Courval *et al.* 1990; Ko-Ko and Ward 1997). Although sensory neglect is found in non-dominant hemisphere stroke, it is itself not associated with pain.

Oral hygiene

The presence of caries resulting from poor oral hygiene or damage to teeth is directly associated with ill health and distant infection. Not only is it painful to eat, but certain foods cause further pain. Even when swallowing and chewing are normal, dental caries are more common in neurologically disabled people and those with a learning disability (Oreland *et al.* 1989). Injuries to the maxilla and to the brain cause malocclusion of teeth which can give rise to pain and headaches and lead to gum hyperplasia. The best known cause of this is the 1 per cent association with the anticonvulsant phenytoin (Grant *et al.* 1988). Oral hygiene, although time-consuming, should be strenuously managed. The presence of caries makes the fitting of foreign bodies, such as ventriculoperitoneal shunts, more risky, and there is a real association with endocarditis. Any potential infection will increase morbidity and may affect mortality, although the data for this are not robust. Certainly an important factor in rehabilitation is accessibility to a dentist.

Heterotopic ossification

One of the most restrictive complications of severe injury or surgery is the development of ectopic bone formation, which is most commonly recognized under the term heterotopic ossification. This is a condition in which mature laminar bone is formed in tissues that do not normally ossify, such as in muscles and ligaments around joints. It should not be confused with simple calcification of soft tissues (Damanski 1961). The cause of heterotopic ossification is mainly traumatic or neurogenic, or is due to a rare autosomal dominant congenital condition called myositis ossificans progressiva in which there is progressive ossification of muscles from early infancy, extending to all muscle groups. Traumatic heterotopic ossification is seen following musculoskeletal injury, such as after total hip arthroplasty, internal fixation of pelvic and femoral fractures, and following severe head injury, spinal cord injuries, and other disabling neurological insults. It affects the proximal limbs and joints with radiological evolution of heterotopic bone occurring over a 6-month period in the majority of patients (Garland 1991). Even in the absence of limb fractures, the brain injury itself can cause the development of heterotopic ossification and brain injured patients exhibit an abundant healing response to fractures leading to a significantly increased union (Spencer 1987).

Improvements in survival have led to better identification of its incidence. Spinal injured people tend only to develop this complication distal to the level of the cord injury; the incidence is 20 to 30 per cent of cases. However, limitation of joint movement is restricted to an incidence of 18 to 35 per cent (Stover *et al.* 1991) compared with an incidence following closed head injury of 10 to 20 per cent. Ten per cent of brain injured patients have a severe restriction of joint motion (Stover *et al.* 1991). Following total hip arthroplasty, heterotopic ossification is clinically significant in 2 to 7 per cent (Brooker *et al.* 1973; Kjaersgaard-Anderson and Ritter 1991) and as much as 15 per cent can be found following internal fixation of acetabular fractures (McLaren 1990). The male-to-female ratio is 2:1, and age over 60 years and previous formation of heterotopic ossification are established risk factors following total hip arthroplasty.

The most sensitive investigation of heterotopic ossification is the isotope bone scan, which becomes positive about 3 weeks after the injury. Serum alkaline phosphatase rises acutely and is still significantly raised up to 20 weeks after the initial injury (Wittenberg *et al.* 1992). The administration of anti-inflammatory drugs prior to and after hip replacement is probably protective. Intractable limb spasticity in neurologically impaired people has a direct effect on functional outcome and the possibility of recurrence of heterotopic ossification after excision treatment. Joint trauma or surgical repair of a fracture greatly increases its risk, as does a pressure sore around a proximal joint (Spencer 1987) . In spinal cord injuries, Frankel type A and B tetraplegics were more likely to have heterotopic ossification than paraplegics. Preventative measures with non-steroidal anti-inflammatory drugs and diphosphonate drugs are indicated in at-risk patients, but there is some controversy about the latter, as Thomas and Amstutz (1985) found the incidence of heterotopic ossification to be slightly higher in patients who had received diphosphonates following hip replacement. However, the general consensus is that they are useful and should be taken1 month before hip replacement and continued 3 months postoperatively. Similarly, they should be continued for 3 months after spinal or traumatic brain injury. Non-steroidal anti-inflammatory drugs are cheap and also effective, but cannot prevent the development of severe heterotopic ossification when started after the fifth day after surgery or injury.

Treatment of established heterotopic ossification should incorporate physiotherapy to mobilize the joints slowly and carefully, but overzealous treatment, particularly around the elbow joint, can itself lead to heterotopic ossification (Wilson 1974). Passive joint mobilization helps to maintain or increase joint mobility and can be more dynamic in neurologically impaired people. Surgery is of value to mature heterotopic bone formation, but can complicate the impairment if it is performed too early. Surgeons should wait until the ectopic bone has matured; serum alkaline phosphatase levels and plain radiographs are not particularly good indicators of this. The uptake from isotope bone scans decreases in proportion to the relative maturity of the new bone and it has been estimated that a 14-month period must elapse before the bone is sufficiently mature to allow surgical excision without significant recurrence of the problem. The difficulty is that people, particularly those with traumatic brain or spinal injuries, have often lost the opportunity for recovery of function in order to allow the bone to be dealt with. This has significant impact on outcome and can often delay good outcomes from a rehabilitation programme for up to 2 years. The importance of prophylaxis should be recognized and studies are now required to quantify the impact on activities of daily living after the development of heterotopic ossification.

Loss of limb

The United Kingdom has a long tradition in amputee rehabilitation, which first started with the artificial limb and appliance services. After the McColl Report, it was recognized that provision of limb-fitting and wheelchair services needed a wider approach to rehabilitation and the disablement services agency was an interim development to promote general rehabilitation for amputees and wheelchair users (McColl 1986). Services have been devolved to local trust level, although limb fitting itself has been organized on a regional basis. There is no doubt that there has been a distinct improvement in service and in artificial limb quality and that the total needs of amputees are being better met, one of which is the provision of an artificial limb.

Loss of limb is a devastating event in a young person or as a result of trauma, and compensation has traditionally appeared rather poor. Actuarial figures are available for such losses, and one can now be confident that loss of the lower leg need not necessarily be too great a handicap. The most common reason for amputation is peripheral vascular disease in elderly people and in diabetics, but road traffic accidents still represent the most frequent cause in young people. A previously fit person under the age of 40 can anticipate walking without a limb, skiing, and performing many sporting activities, and would only be impaired by a 25 per cent increase in energy consumption on normal walking speed. This rises to 55 per cent when extended to above knee amputations, but again for young relatively fit people, the impact on the quality of life is well understood in both rehabilitation and actuarial terms.

There is no doubt that the simple provision of a limb is not beneficial to every amputee. They have many needs, only one of which is a limb, and these need to be addressed via the rehabilitation process. McColl (1986) found in a review of the literature that there were many instances where a limb had been provided but was never used. It lay unused in the patient's home, and the patient was far better adapted to life in a wheelchair. One of the real values in the rehabilitation process has been the accurate assessment of the needs of the individual and his or her carers, and the quality of life of such individuals has been greatly improved by the enhancement of the rehabilitation service. In addition, new technologies, in particular computer-aided design and manufacture, have allowed the development of intelligent knees and ankles and sprung feet to improve energy absorption and the consequent gait pattem (BSRM 1994).

Disability equipment and new technologies

Inappropriate and untimely prescription of disability equipment is the result of poor or inaccessible rehabilitation and very often this results in expensive wastage of resources. Assessment of the need for equipment can be made by effective communication between staff, the patient, and the family. Equipment is designed to reduce handicap and is not necessary if the individual has the ability to carry out the function it was designed for. Rehabilitation also allows the experience of staff to help in the choice and appropriateness of equipment, since there is often a confusing array of items, some of which do not actually carry out the job they purport to do. Follow-up in rehabilitation is important and one of the benefits is regular assessment of needs as new equipment becomes available.

Disabled people benefit from exposure to and experimentation with new technologies. While a medical rehabilitation service is not always necessary for disabled people and their families to learn about new technologies, it does allow the education process by which the disabled person will understand his or her condition and the interaction with equipment to reduce handicap. Specific medical technologies are being developed all the time and they can significantly alter the quality of life for the affected individuals (Rushton 1997). Included in these are neurological endoprostheses. These have a multiplicity of functions and include bladder stimulators, intrathecal baclofen pumps, and muscle stimulator implants. More information on these appears constantly and there has been an excellent recent review of the whole subject of neuroprostheses, modulators, and stimulators (Rushton 1997).

Information

Accurate and up-to-date information is the key to empowerment for disabled people and their carers. The rehabilitation process allows contact with personnel and agencies who hold the key to the resource or to ways of accessing the necessary information process. Not only do professionals give advice, but they can also help disabled people and carers, making valued judgments about the quality of the advice and subsequent actions. Lack of contact with rehabilitation services means that disabled people have to find things out in an *ad hoc* rather than a structured manner, and much time and effort can be wasted.

Information should cover not only health matters, but benefits and allowances, community mobility, further education, training and employment, housing, leisure and recreation, and the formation of self-help groups, as well as a whole host of other activities which make up independent living. It is also important to have information about involving lawyers at an early stage of a potential claim for personal injury as they can become part of the rehabilitation team in these instances. However, information to disabled people and their carers must be coupled with practical advice in order to be really useful. A recent study of the activities of the North Staffordshire Rehabilitation Centre shows that the simple giving of information may increase the anxieties and stresses, as details of the potential difficulties in looking after a disabled person may overwhelm the family and carers unless practical solutions are given to methods of coping physically and emotionally with the needs of the disabled person (Ward and Wynn 1996).

Rehabilitation research

The evidence to show that rehabilitation works in populations is different from that in many other areas of health care, as it is tailored to the individual's needs and is not a standard item, like a drug. However, at a time when savings in health budgets have to be made, rehabilitation is an easy target. It has a low profile and little public appeal, as people are not seen to suffer directly through a lack of it. Rehabilitation services are thus currently under threat as hard evidence is required before they will be funded and there is a common belief that there is no good evidence to support rehabilitation. Obtaining research money is difficult both because of this low public appeal and because research in rehabilitation is thought to be difficult. As a result, finding a vehicle for publishing rehabilitation research can be difficult and publication tends to be in less widely read journals. This is not good for either rehabilitation or for patients. If rehabilitation is to develop, it is necessary to have a healthy research base to counteract these threats. Good, scientifically sound, and clinically convincing research should actually be no more difficult in rehabilitation than it is in other fields of health care. Furthermore, the confidence of the research world in rehabilitation should be boosted by the fact that many areas of medicine have less published evidence of their effectiveness than rehabilitation and examples include surgery, general medical care and many aspects of mental health.

Randomized and other controlled clinical trials give the best evidence (Sackett *et al.* 1991) and the Cochrane Collaboration has registered all randomized and controlled clinical trials relating to health care interventions, including rehabilitation. They have undertaken to identify and register all randomized clinical trials, as only a minority of all studies undertaken can be identified through searching Medline and other databases. This involves undertaking hand searches of journals to register all controlled trials on Medline. This has now been applied to articles published in *Clinical Rehabilitation* between 1987 and 1995 using the same criteria as those of the Cochrane Collaboration and by Medline for determining the nature of each study. A trial was considered to be a randomized controlled trial if the individuals (or other units such as limbs or treatment periods) were definitely or possibly assigned prospectively to one of two (or more) alternative forms of health care using random allocation, whereas a controlled clinical trial was classified if the same criteria apply but the allocation was more random (e.g. by date of birth, day of the week, etc.). Over the 9 years, 25 randomized controlled trials and 16 controlled clinical trials were published by all professions. This analysis shows that it is possible to judge good scientific research in rehabilitation (Wade 1995), but care should be taken that simple searching of Medline will give all the published data on a subject. Some studies by the very nature of the work and the samples available will be too small to give definitive answers and carrying out meta-analysis on studies in rehabilitation has led to some serious errors in conclusion (Anonymous 1992).

Randomized controlled trials have practical limitations in rehabilitation research (Andrews 1991), and trials examining packages of care are methodologically unsafe due to the heterogeneity of the needs of patients undergoing a rehabilitation programme (Tallis 1991). Thus single-case studies are helpful and allow for the examination of different aspects of rehabilitation intervention in smaller numbers of individual patients using baseline, treatment, and no-treatment phases over time (Ebrahim 1990). They should not be dismissed, but with the greater sophistication required and the need for rehabilitation to establish itself alongside the other main areas of health (and social) care, properly conducted controlled trials are required if rehabilitations are going to convince colleagues that theirs is a serious undertaking. Currently, careful evaluation of all studies is necessary in order to list the areas where controlled trials are most urgently required. This should span all areas of rehabilitation and involve all participating professionals, but should be carrried out where possible in a randomized controlled trials (Wade 1999*b*). The common weaknesses in design are listed in Box 4.

Box 4 Common weaknesses in the design of randomized controlled trials

- Inadequate trial size
- Lack (or poor choice) of controls
- Lack of definition of therapy
- Inappropriate outcome measurement
- Lack of blinding
- Poor generalizability
- Lack of cost information

In describing in greater detail the difficulties and some of the possible solutions in the context of stroke rehabilitation, the pitfalls are highlighted, particularly in defining the therapy inputs (Pollock *et al.* 1993), for it is unclear from many studies of stroke units whether it is the medical or therapeutic interventions that have led to change.

Rehabilitation outcome measures

In any clinical setting, outcome measurement is an important activity. Since rehabilitationists work in an environment of distinction between pathology, impairments, activities, and participation, it is also convenient to decribe relevant outcome measures along these lines. For instance, if the aim of a rehabilitation episode is to allow a disabled person to climb the stairs to access the bathroom, one can approach this problem in a number of ways. One could aim to alter the underlying pathological condition, in which case measures of this would be appropriate (e.g. erythrocyte sedimentation rate in inflammatory joint disease). If the pathology could not be changed, then diminishing impairments by restoring muscular strength to the individual and disability by practising stair climbing and walking would allow a return of function. Alternatively, it may be assumed that the patient will not achieve the goal by himself and the provision of two wheelchairs and a stair-lift in addition to finding a means of transfers will achieve the objective, but in a completely different manner. All are valid rehabilitation activities, but the range of skills and required outcome measures are quite different. Therefore a measure has to be chosen that will reflect not only the goal, but also the process by which that goal can be achieved.

There are a number of misconceptions in research for better outcome measures. The greatest is perhaps that better measures will lead automatically to better information and that a more satisfactory solution will result. One problem is also that outcomes are misunderstood. Patients present for rehabilitation with problems and rehabilitation is a problem-solving exercise. Outcomes here refer to the change in status of the person in need of intervention and for this one has to identify what the process is trying to achieve. The measure chosen should cover the whole of the area of concern and, as far as possible, should not include extraneous areas. The choice of outcome measures in the context of quality control needs to be discussed among the stakeholders. Service commissioners may well have different goals for rehabilitation (and therefore outcomes) than providers, and therefore measures should be put in the context of what the service is trying to achieve in the market place. Figure 7 shows the structure, process, and outcomes from rehabilitation episodes (Wade 1999*a*).

There are a number of appropriate measures, and *Measurement in Neurological Disability* (Wade 1992) is a useful *aide memoire*. It is not appropriate to list individual measures in detail, but there are a number of publications which highlight them. Measurement is a key area for setting standards in rehabilitation. No matter what the setting—be it a specialized rehabilitation centre or a community rehabilitation team—it is possible to identify a standard in multiprofessional working by some of the following standards.

1. Each rehabilitation team should work within written criteria for seeing and treating patients.
2. Each rehabilitation team should utilize appropriate outcome measures and should document at least one of these at admission and discharge for each patient.
3. Clear written goals should be identified for the patient's rehabilitation, which should actively involve the patient and family.

In conclusion, outcome measures are only tools and not solutions to better services and their value depends upon the validity of the process being examined. It is dangerous to draw conclusions from studies, be they research, audit, or daily clinical practice, until the context of the situation under examination is clear.

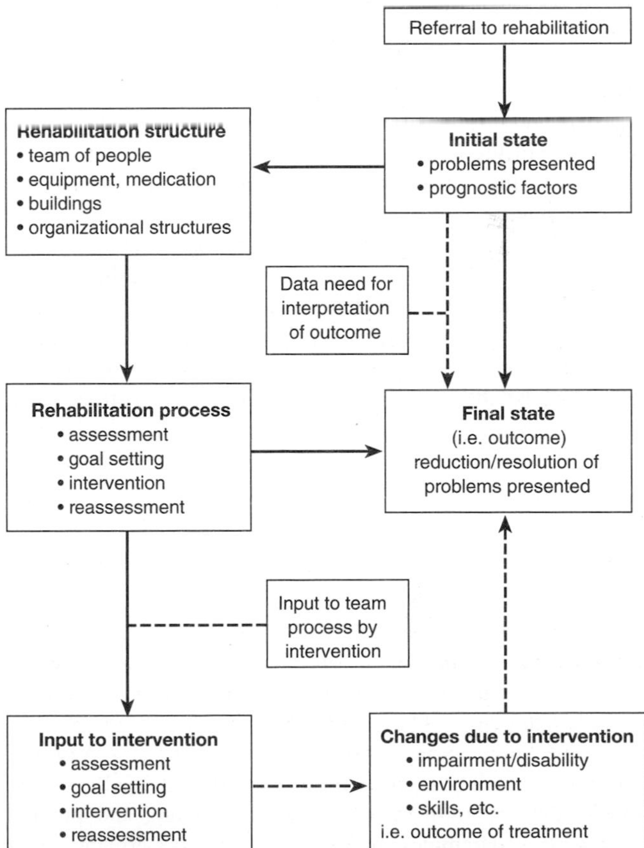

Fig. 7 Rehabilitation structure, process, and outcome. (Source: Pollock *et al.* 1993)

Conclusion

Rehabilitation has grown enormously over the last two decades, and is now becoming a part of the training of neurologists, rheumatologists, geriatricians, respiratory medicine physicians, and cardiologists. Formal training programmes are now established worldwide for specialists in physical and rehabilitation medicine and it now forms an important clinical and political activity in health care. However, where does it go from here? Not only does it have to embrace change, but there are also many challenges facing rehabilitation and physical disability four of which are highlighted here for their relevance to the field of public health.

New technologies

New technologies have changed the lives of disabled people, and *Rehabilitation Medicine* and the British Society of Rehabilitation Medicine has published several excellent reports on environmental controls, wheelchair equipment, neuroprostheses, and neuromodulators (Rushton 1997). The use of computers in rehabilitation will assume even greater importance in allowing patients to benefit from programmes to assist their own rehabilitation (Clegg and Turner-Stokes 1998). The use of the internet for shopping, banking, etc. will mean that disabled people will be able to manage many aspects of their lives from their sitting room; however, with this comes the spectre that many will not have to go outside at all which will have its own impacts.

Rehabilitation is all about opportunities for people within the context of their abilities and wishes. The squeeze on finances in health care will undoubtedly affect rehabilitation services to a greater extent than the more 'sexy' ones, as the cost of not providing them will be politically less damaging. Better organization of health and social care is necessary and it is hoped that joint commissioning of services will reduce some of the unnecessary costs. Achieving the right balance between reducing impairments, disabilities, and handicaps and promoting abilities and participation are important goals for service planners. While it is vital that people are encouraged to attain optimal physical functioning, there is a need to ensure that this is cost-effective. While it is obviously desirable for people to be given every opportunity for return of physical functioning, the selection of suitable candidates for rehabilitation will also be important. Not everyone will be able to or want to walk again after a stroke or an amputation; therefore investment in this activity may not be wise, especially if it is at the expense of providing disability equipment or home adaptations.

Vocational rehabilitation

Vocational rehabilitation has virtually ceased in the British health care system and there is little awareness of what is required, let alone how to ensure that people coming out of rehabilitation programmes have the opportunity to return to or take up employment. This has changed over the last 20 years and has resulted in the United Kingdom falling behind many countries in Europe, the United States, and Australia. Claims of about twice the rate of return to work after head injury are noted by the establishment of cognitive retraining and physical rehabilitation programmes in the United States, Germany, Switzerland, and Sweden, but there are differences in severity, social security benefits, etc. that make direct comparison difficult. The experience of Australia and the United States in dealing with the repetitive strain injury/disorder explosion of the 1970s and 1980s has meant that their guiding principles have moved away from a compensation culture to one of promoting rehabilitation to return people back to work. A comparative scale is required for success in disabled people returning to work after injury/illness and then staying in work. In order to achieve this, specialized centres of research and demonstration are required to look into the factors in bridging the gap between health, social, and employment rehabilitation. Government backing of such a project is required and discussions at departmental level are needed to work out a strategy for changing the face of rehabilitation in this area. The challenge is not only valuable, but is urgent and there are clear advantages to disabled people, rehabilitation professionals, and government itself in attempting to reduce expenditure on incapacity to work benefits.

Organization

As rehabilitation of elderly people becomes a greater priority, greater awareness is necessary of the different approaches required for general and specialized rehabilitation. Rehabilitation depends on clear therapeutic aims which are fundamental to health care responsibility. This applies equally to maintenance rehabilitation and to acute rehabilitation. Conversely, care is the means of maintaining safety and comfort. Rehabilitation professionals may be involved in periodic assessments of abilities and health status and an episode of rehabilitation may be triggered by the need to reverse functional deterioration of capitalize on any improvements. Clear outcomes must be identified in terms of therapeutic changes and shared between the participating health and social services professionals, the disabled person, and the family.

Academic base

Rehabilitation research is growing in activity and sophistication, but suffers from a lack of credibility in some circles because randomized controlled trials are difficult to perform in this field. Other methodologies may not provide as conclusive results, but are nonetheless of value and require support. While the effectiveness of treatments in many fields of medicine is not proved, much data about the effectiveness of rehabilitation is currently available. Data are now required on the value of rehabilitation through cost-effectiveness studies, some of which are underway (Turner-Stokes *et al.* 1999; P. Harding *et al.*, personal communication).

References

Albright, F., Burnett, C.H., Cope, O., and Parson, W. (1941). Acute atrophy of bone (osteoporosis) simulating hyperparathyroidism. *Journal of Clinical Endocrinology*, **1**, 711–16.

Amputee Medical Rehabilitation Society (1992). *Amputee rehabilitation, recommended standards and guidelines—report of a working party.* Amputee Medical Rehabilitation Society, London.

Andrews, K. (1991). The limitations of randomised controlled trials in rehabilitation research. *Clinical Rehabilitation*, **5**, 5–8.

Andrews, K. and Greenwood, R. (1993). Physical consequences of neurological disablement. In *Neurological rehabilitation* (ed. R. Greenwood, M.P. Barnes, T.M. McMillan, and C.D. Ward), pp. 199–218. Churchill Livingstone, Edinburgh.

Andrews, K., Murphy, R., and Littlewood, C. (1996). Misdiagnosis of the vegetative state: retrospective studies in a rehabilitation unit. *British Medical Journal*, **313**, 13–16.

Anonymous (1986). *Sections 5 and 6 of the Disabled Persons Act. Services, Consultation and Representation.* HMSO, London.

Anonymous (1990). *NHS and Community Care Act 1990.* HMSO, London.

Anonymous (1992). *Effective health care. Report 2: Rehabilitation after stroke.* University of Leeds.

Aronow, H.U. (1987). Rehabilitation effectiveness with severe brain injury: research into policy. *Journal of Head Trauma Rehabilitation*, **2**, 24–35.

Ashwal, S., Eyman, R.K., and Call, T.L. (1994). Life expectancy of children in persistent vegetative state. *Paediatric Neurology*, **10**, 27–33.

Association of British Neurologists, NeuroConcern Group of Medical Charities, British Society of Rehabilitation Medicine (1992). *Neurological rehabilitation in the United Kingdom—report of a working party.* British Society of Rehabilitation Medicine, London.

Badley, E.M., Wagstaff, S., and Wood, P.H.N. (1984). Measures of functional ability (disability) in arthritis in relation to impairment of range of joint movement. *Annals of Rheumatic Diseases*, **434**, 563–9.

Bamford, J., Sandercock, P., Warlow, C., and Gray, M. (1988). Why are patients with acute stroke admitted to hospital? *British Medical Journal*, **292**, 1369–72.

Barbanel, J.C., Jordan, N.M., Nicol, S.M., *et al.* (1977). Incidence of pressure sores in the Greater Glasgow Health Board Area. *Lancet*, **ii**, 548–50.

Barrett, K., Buxton, N., Redmond, A.D., Jones, J.M., Boughey, A.M., and Ward, A.B. (1995). A comparison of symptoms experienced following minor head injury and acute neck strain (whiplash injury). *Journal of Accident and Emergency Medicine*, **12**, 173–6.

Bax, M.C.O., Smyth, D.P.L., and Thomas, A.P. (1988). Health care of young physically handicapped adults. *British Medical Journal*, **296**, 1153–5.

Beardshaw, V. and Towell, D. (1990). *Assessment and case management: implications for the the implementation of 'Caring for People'.* King's Fund Institute, London.

Ben-Yishay, Y., Silver, S., Piasetsky, F., and Raft, J. (1987). Relationship between employability and vocational outcome after intensive holistic cognitive rehabilitation. *Journal of Head Trauma Rehabilitation*, **2**, 35–48.

Bernspang, B., Asplund, K., Erikson, S., and Fugl-Meyer, A.R. (1987). Motor and perceptual impairments in acute stroke patients: effect on self-care ability. *Stroke*, **18**, 1081–6.

Bishara, S.N., Partridge, F.M., Godfrey, H.P., and Knight, R.G. (1992). Post-traumatic amnesia and Glasgow Coma Scale related to outcome in survivors in a consecutive series of patients with severe closed-head injury. *Brain Injury*, **6**, 373–80.

Blackerby, W.F. (1990). Intensity of rehabilitation and length of stay. *Brain Injury*, **4**, 167–73.

Blasier, D. and Lefts, R.M. (1989). Pediatric update no. 7: the orthopaedic manifestations of head injury in children. *Orthopaedic Review*, **18**, 350–8.

Booth, B.J., Doyle, M., and Montgomery, J. (1983). Serial casting for the management of spasticity in the head-injured adult. *Physical Therapy*, **63**, 1960–6.

Brett, E.M. and Lake, B.D. (1991). Neuromuscular disorder: primary muscle disease and anterior horn cell disorders. In *Paediatric neurology* (ed. E.M. Brett) (2nd edn), pp. 121–45. Churchill Livingstone, Edinburgh.

Brooker, A.F., Bowerman, J.W., Robinson, R.A., and Riley, L.H. Jr (1973). Ectopic ossification following total hip replacement. Incidence and method of classification. *Journal of Bone and Joint Surgery, American Volume*, **55A**, 1629–32.

BSRM (British Society of Rehabilitation Medicine) (1988). *BRSM working party report.* British Society of Rehabilitation Medicine, London.

BSRM (British Society of Rehabilitation Medicine) (1993). *A working party report on multiple sclerosis.* British Society of Rehabilitation Medicine, London.

BSRM (British Society of Rehabilitation Medicine) (1994). *Prescription for independence.* Working party report of the BSRM Environmental Control Special Interest Group. British Society of Rehabilitation Medicine, London.

BSRM (British Society of Rehabilitation Medicine) (1998). *The management of traumatic brain injury.* A report of a working party. British Society of Rehabilitation Medicine, London.

Buckley, J., Warlow, C., Smith, P., Hilton Jones, D., Irvine, S., and Tew, J.R. (1983). Epidemiology of motor neurone disease. *Journal of Neurology, Neurosurgery and Psychiatry*, **46**, 197.

Burbaud, P., Wiart, L., Dubos, J.L., *et al.* (1996). A randomised, double blind, placebo controlled trial of botulinum toxin in the treatment of spastic foot in hemiparetic patients. *Journal of Neurology, Neurosurgery and Psychiatry*, **61**, 265–9.

Chamberlain, M.A. (1988). Disabled living centres: setting up and running a DLC. *International Disease Studies*, **10**, 89–91.

Chamberlain, M.A., Guthrie, S., Kettle, M., and Stowe, J. (1993). *An assessment of health and related needs of physically handicapped young adults.* Department of Health, London.

Clegg, F. and Turner-Stokes, L. (1998). Word processing assessment package for stroke. Abstract, British Society of Rehabilitation Medicine Meeting, Southampton.

Clifton, G.L., Robertson, C.S., Grossman, R.G., Hodge, S., Foltz, R., and Garza, C. (1984). The metabolic response to severe head injury. *Journal of Neurosurgery*, **60**, 687–95.

Cochrane, G.M. (1989). Motor neurone disease. *British Journal of Hospital Medicine*, **41**, 274–9.

Cope, D.N. and Hall, K. (1982). Head injury rehabilitation: benefit of early intervention. *Archives of Physical Medicine and Rehabilitation*, **63**, 433–7.

Cope, D.N., Cole, J.R., Hall, K.M., and Barkan, H. (1991). Brain injury: analysis of outcome in a post-acute rehabilitation system. Part 1: General analysis. *Brain Injury*, **5**, 111–25.

Cox, D.L. (1992). Perspectives of motor neurone disease. *Clinical Rehabilitation*, **6**, 333–9.

Damanski, M. (1961). Heterotopic ossification in paraplegia. *Journal of Bone and Joint Surgery, British Volume*, **43B**, 286–99.

Department of Health Working Group (1993). *Pressure sores—a key quality indication. A guide for NHS Purchasers and Providers.* Health Publications Unit, Heywood.

Dombovy, M.L., Basford, J.R., Whisnant, J.P., and Bergstrahl, E.J. (1987). Disability and use of rehabilitation services in Rochester, Minnesota, 1975–79. *Stroke*, **18**, 830–6.

Eames, T. and Wood, R. (1985). Rehabilitation after severe brain injury: a follow up study of a behaviour and modification approach. I. *Journal of Neurology, Neurosurgery and Psychiatry*, **48**, 613–19.

Ebrahim, S. (1990). *Clinical epidemiology of stroke.* Oxford University Press.

Edwards, F. (1990). *Health services for adults with physical disabilities—a survey of DHAs 1988–89.* Royal College of Physicians, London.

Evans *et al.* (1992). *Journal of Head Trauma Rehabilitation*, **7**, 24–36.

Faghri, P.D., Rodgers, M.M., Glaser, R.M., Bors, J.G., Ho, C., and Akuthota, P. (1994). *Archives of Physical Medicine and Rehabilitation*, **75**, 73–9.

Farm, J.R., Katon, W.J., Uomoto, J.M., and Esselman, P.C. (1995). Psychiatric disorder and functional disability in outpatients with traumatic brain injury. *American Journal of Psychiatry*, **152**, 1493–9.

Feigenson, J.S. and Scheinberg, L. (1981). The cost effectiveness of multiple sclerosis rehabilitation: a model. *Neurology*, **31**, 1316–21.

Fiedler, B. and Twitchin, D. (1990). *Living options in practice: a framework for action.* Project Paper 1, Prince of Wales Advisory Group on Disability and Community Living Development Team, King's Fund, London.

Gaddisseux, P., Ward, J.D., Young, A.F., and Becker, D. (1984). Nutrition and the neurosurgical patient. *Journal of Neurosurgery*, **60**, 219–32.

Garland, D.E. (1991). A clinical perspective on common forms of acquired heterotopic ossification. *Clinical Orthopaedics and Related Research* , **263**, 13–29.

Garraway, G.M., Akhtar, A.J., Prescott, R.J., and Hockey, L. (1980). Management of acute stroke in the elderly: follow-up of a controlled trial. *British Medical Journal*, **281**, 827–9.

Gisel, E.G. and Patrick, J. (1988). Identification of children with cerebral palsy unable to maintain a normal nutritional state. *Lancet*, **i**, 283–6.

Grant, R.H., Parsonage, M.J., and Barot, M.H. (1988). Phenytoin-induced gum hypertrophy in patients with epilepsy. *Current Medical Research and Opinion*, **10**, 652–5.

Greenleaf, J.E., Junos, L.T., and Young, H.L. (1985). Plasma lactic dehydrogenase activities in men during bed rest with exercise training. *Aviation, Space and Environmental Medicine*, **56**, 193–8.

Hall, K.M. and Cope, N. (1995). The benefits of rehabilitation in traumatic brain injury: a literature review. *Journal of Head Trauma*, **10**, 1–13.

Harper, C.I. and Lyles, Y.M. (1988). Physiology and complications of bed rest. *Journal of the American Geriatrics Society*, **36**, 1047–54.

Hass, J.F. (1988). Adnission to rehabilitation centers. Selection of patients. *Archives of Physical Medicine and Rehabilitation*, **69**, 329–32.

Heiskanen, O. and Sipponen, P. (1970). Prognosis of severe brain injury. *Acta Neurologica Scandinavica*, **46**, 343–8.

Himal, H.S. and Schumacher, S. (1987). Endoscopic vs surgical gastrostomy for enteral feeding. *Surgical Endoscopist*, **1**, 33–5.

Indrevidavik, B., Bakke, F., Solberg, R., Rosketh, R., Haaheim, L.L., and Holme, I. (1991). Benefit of a stroke unit: a randomised controlled trial. *Stroke*, **22**, 1026–31.

Jennett, B., Teasdale, G., and Braakman, R. (1979). Prognosis in a series of patients after severe brain injury. *Neurosurgery*, **4**, 283–9.

Jessekutz, B., Blizzard, J.J., Birkhead, N.C., and Rodahl, K. (1966). Effect of prolonged bed rest in urinary calcium output. *Journal of Applied Physiology*, **21**, 1013–20.

Johnston, M.V. and Lewis, F.D. (1991). Outcomes of community re-entry programmes for brain injury survivors. Part I: Independent living and productive activities. *Brain Injury*, **5**, 141–54.

Kalisky, Z., Morrison, D.P., Meyers, C.A., and von Laufen, A. (1985). Medical problems encountered during rehabilitation of patients with head injury. *Archives of Physical Medicine and Rehabilitation*, **66**, 25–9.

Kelly, J. and Feigenbaum, L.Z. (1982). Another cause of reversible dementia: sleep deprivation due to prostatism. *Journal of the American Geriatrics Society*, **30**, 645–6.

Kidd, D., Howard, R.S., Losseff, N.A., and Thompson, A.J. (1995). The benefit of inpatient neurorehabilitation in multiple sclerosis. *Clinics in Rehabilitation*, **9**, 198–203.

King's Fund Consensus Statement (1988). *The treatment of stroke.* King's Fund, London.

King's Fund Pressure Sore Study Group (1989). *The prevention and management of pressure sores. Report of a working party (Chairman, Professor B. Livesley).* Research for the Aged Trust, London.

Kiver, K.F., Hays, D.P., Fontin, D.F., and Maini, B.S. (1984). Pre- and post-pyloric enteral feeding: an analysis of safety and complications. *Journal of Parenteral and Enteral Nutrition*, **8**, 95.

Kjaersgaard-Andersen, P. and Ritter, M.A. (1991). Prevention of formation of heterotopic bone after total hip arthroplasty. *Journal of Bone and Joint Surgery, American Volume*, **73A**, 942–7.

Ko-Ko, C. and Ward, A.B. (1997). Management of spasticity. *British Journal of Hospital Medicine*, **58**, 400–8.

Krolner, B. and Toft, B. (1983). Vertebral bone loss: an unheeded side-effect of therapeutic bed rest. *Clinical Science*, **64**, 537–40.

Kurtzke, J.F. (1975). *Epidemiology of spinal cord injury. Experimental Neurology*, **48**, 197.

Lacomblez, L., Bensimon, G., Leigh, P.N., *et al.* (1996). Dose ranging study of riluzole in amyotrophic lateral sclerosis. *Lancet*, **ii**, 1425–31.

Larocca, N.C. and Kalb, R.C. (1992). Efficacy of rehabilitation in multiple sclerosis. *Journal of Neurological Rehabilitation*, **6**, 147–55.

Larson, D.E., Burton, D.D., Schroeder, K.W., and Di Magno, E.P. (1987). Percutaneous endoscopic gastrostomy: indications, success, complications and mortality in 314 consecutive patients. *Gastroenterology*, **93**, 48–52.

Law, M.R., Wald, N.J., and Meade, T.W. (1991). Strategies for prevention of osteoporosis and hip fracture. *British Journal of Medicine*, **303**, 453–9.

Le Blanc, A., Evans, H., *et al.* (1987). Changes in nuclear magnetic resonance (T_2) relaxation of limb tissue with bed rest. *Magnetic Resonance*, **4**, 487–92.

Le Blanc, A., Gogia, P., Schneider, V., Knebs, J., Schofield, F., and Evans, H. (1988). Calf muscle area and strength changes after five weeks of horizontal bed rest. *American Journal of Sports Medicine*, **16**, 624–9.

Legh Smith, J.A., Denis, R., and Enderby, P.M. (1987). Selection of aphasic stroke patients for intensive speech therapy. *Journal of Neurology, Neurosurgery and Psychiatry*, **50**, 1488–92.

Leiderman, H., Mendelson, J.H., Wexter, D., and Solomon, P. (1958). Sensory deprivation. *Archives of Internal Medicine*, **101**, 389–96.

Lincoln, N.B., McGuirk, E., Mulley, G.P., Leadrem, W., Jones, A.C., and Mitchell, J.R. (1984). Effectiveness of speech therapy for aphasic stroke patients: a randomised controlled trial. *Lancet*, **i**, 1197–200.

Lipkin, P. (1991). Epidemiology of developmental disabilities. In *Developmental disorders in infancy and childhood* (ed. A.J. Caputer and P.J. Accardo), pp. 5–21. Paul Brookes, Baltimore, MD.

Livingston, M.G., Brooks, D.N., and Bond, M.R. (1985). Patient outcome in the year following severe head injury and relatives' psychiatric and social functioning. *Journal of Neurology, Neurosurgery and Psychiatry*, **48**, 876–81.

Llaneza, P.P., Menendez, A.M., Roberts, R., and Dunn, G.D. (1988). Percutaneous endoscopic gastrostomy: clinical experience and follow-up. *Southern Medical Journal*, **81**, 321–4.

McBride, A. and Ward, A.B. (1991). *Developing services for physically disabled school leavers and young adults.* Hourds, Stafford.

McColl, I. (1986). *Review of artificial limb and appliance centre service. Report of an independent working party (Chairman, Professor I. McColl).* HMSO, London.

McLaren, A.C. (1990). Prophylaxis with indomethacin for heterotopic bone after open reduction of fractures of the acetabulum. *Journal of Bone and Joint Surgery, American Volume*, **72A**, 245–7.

McLellan, D.L. (1985). Targets for rehabilitation. *British Medical Journal*, **290**, 1514.

McLellan, D.L. (1991). Rehabilitation: achieving *Health of the Nation* targets. *British Medical Journal*, **303**, 355–7.

Malec, J.F. and Basford, J.S. (1996). Postacute brain injury rehabilitation. *Archives of Physical Medicine and Rehabilitation*, **77**, 198–207.

Martin, G.M. and Opitz, J.L. (ed.) (1997). *The American Board of Physical Medicine and Rehabilitation: the first 50 Years.* American Board of Physical Medicine and Rehabilitation. Rochester, MN.

Martin, J. and White, A. (1988). *The financial circumstances of disabled adults living in private households. Report 2: OPCS Surveys of Disability in Great Britain, 1988–89.* HMSO, London.

Martin, J., Meltzer, H., and Eliot, D. (1988). *The prevalence of disability among adults. Report 1: OPCS Surveys of Disability in Great Britain, 1988–89.* HMSO, London.

Martin, J., White, A., and Meltzer, H. (1989). *Disabled adults: services, transport and employment. Report 4: OPCS Surveys of Disability in Great Britain, 1988–89.* HMSO, London.

Moolten, S.F. (1972). Bed sores in chronically ill patients. *Archives of Physical Medicine and Rehabilitation*, **53**, 430–8.

Multi-Society Task Force on PVS (1994). Medical aspects of the persistent vegetative state: Parts 1 and 2. *New England Journal of Medicine*, **330**, 1499–1508, 1572–9.

Oakes, D.D., Wilmot, C.B., Hall, K.M., and Scherk, J.P. (1990). Benefit of early admission to a comprehensive trauma center for patients with a spinal cord injury. *Archives of Physical Medicine and Rehabilitation*, **71**, 637–43.

Oddy, M., Coughlan, T., Tyerman, A., and Jenkins, D. (1985). Social adjustment after closed head injury: a further follow-up seven years after injury. *Journal of Neurology, Neurosurgery and Psychiatry*, **48**, 564–8.

Oreland, A., Heijbel, J., Jagell, S., and Persson, M. (1989). Oral function in the physically handicapped with or without severe mental retardation. *Journal of Dentistry in Children*, **56**, 17–25.

Ottenbacher, K.J. and Jannell, S. (1993). Results of clinical trials in stroke rehabilitation research. *Archives of Neurology*, **50**, 37–44.

Parkes, J.D. (1985). *Sleep and its disorders.* W.B. Saunders, London.

Pollock, C., Freemantle, N., Sheldon, T., and Song, F. (1993). Methodological difficulties in rehabilitation research. *Clinical Rehabilitation*, **7**, 63–72.

Poulin de Courval, L., Bonanskas, A., *et al.* (1990). Painful shoulder in the hemiplegic and unilateral neglect. *Archives of Physical Medicine and Rehabilitation*, **71**, 673–6.

Price, D.J. and Ward, A.B. (1997) Traumatic brain injury. In *Medical aspects of personal injury litigation* (ed. M.P. Barnes, B. Braithwaite, and A.B. Ward), pp. 68–105. Blackwell Science, Oxford.

Prigatano, G.P., Fordyce, D.J., Zeiner, H.K., Roueche, J.R., Pepping, M., and Wood, B.C. (1984). Neuropsychological rehabilitation after closed head injury in young adults. *Journal of Neurology, Neurosurgery and Psychiatry*, **47**, 505–13.

Rapp, R.P., Young, B., Twyman, D., *et al.* (1983). The favorable effect of early parenteral feeding on survival in head-injured patients. *Journal of Neurosurgery*, **58**, 906–12.

Robertson, C.B., Clifton, G.L., and Grossman, R.G. (1984). Oxygen utilisation and cardiovascular function in head injured patients. *Neurosurgery*, **15**, 307–14.

Roth, E.J., Heinemann, A.W., Lovell, L.J., Harvey, R.L., McGuire, J.R., and Diaz, S. (1998). Impairment and disability: their relationship during stroke rehabilitation. *Archives of Physical Medicine and Rehabilitation*, **78**, 329–35.

Royal College of Physicians (1986). Physical disability in 1986 and beyond. *Journal of the Royal College of Physicians of London*, **20**, 160–94.

Royal College of Physicians (1989). *Stroke: towards better management.* Report, Royal College of Physicians, London.

Royal College of Physicians (1997). Report of a working group of the Royal College of Physicians Committee on Rehabilitation Medicine Model for the organisation of a community-based rehabilitation service. *Journal of the Royal College of Physicians of London*, **31**, 503–5.

Rushton, D. (1997). *Neuroprostheses, neuromodulators and stimulators.* Report, British Society of Rehabilitation Medicine, London.

Sackett, D.L., Haynes, R., Guyatt, G.H., and Tugwell, P. (1991). *Clinical epidemiology* (2nd edn). Little, Brown, Boston, MA.

Sandler, H., Popp, R.L., and Harrison, D.C. (1988). The haemodynamic effects of repeated bed rest exposure. *Aviation, Space and Environmental Medicine*, **59**, 1047–54.

Schoutens, A., Laurent, E., and Poortmans, J.R. (1989). Effects of inactivity and exercise on bone. *Sports Medicine*, **7**, 71–81.

Shahani, B.T., Kelly, E.B., and Glaser, S. (1981). Hemiplegic shoulder subluxation. *Archives of Physical Medicine and Rehabilitation*, **63**, 519.

Shangraw, R.E., Stuart, C.A., Prince, M.J., Peters, E.J., and Wolfe, R.R. (1988). Insulin responsiveness of protein metabolism *in vivo* following bed rest in humans. *American Journal of Physiology*, **255**, E548–58.

Shepherd, G. (1990). Case management. *Health Trends*, **22**, 59–61.

Shiel, A., Henry, D., Clark, J., McLellan, D.L., Wilson, B.A., and Burn, J. (1999). Effect of increased intervention on rate of functional recovery after brain injury: preliminary results of a controlled trial. *Clinical Rehabilitation*, **13**, 76.

Spasticity Study Group (1997). *Muscle and Nerve*, Supplement 6, S1–232.

Spencer, R.E. (1987). The effect of head injury on fracture healing. A quantitative assessment. *Journal of Bone and Joint Surgery, British Volume*, **69B**, 525–8.

Splaingard, M.L., Hutchins, B., Sulton, L.D., and Chaudhuri, G. (1988). Aspiration in rehabilitation patients: videofluoroscopy vs bedside clinical assessment. *Archives of Physical Medicine and Rehabilitation*, **69**, 637–40.

Stewart, W.F.R. (1975). *Sex and the physically handicapped.* Report, Committee on Sexual Problems of the Disabled, the National Fund for Research into Crippling Diseases, London.

Storey, G.O. (1992). *A history of physical medicine.* Royal Society of Medicine Services, London.

Stover, S.L., Niemann, K.M., and Tulloss, J.R. (1991). Experience with surgical excision of heterotopic bone in spinal cord injury patients. *Clinical Orthopaedics and Related Research*, **263**, 71–7.

Strand, T., Asplund, K., Eriksson, S., Hagg, E., Lithner, F., and Wester, P.O. (1985). A non-intensive stroke unit reduces functional disability and the need for long hospitalisation. *Stroke*, **16**, 29–34.

Stroke Units Trialists Collaboration (1997). Collaborative systematic review of the randomised trials of organised inpatient (stroke unit) care after stroke. *British Medical Journal*, **314**, 1151–9.

Stupakov, G.P., Kazeikin, V.S., and Mourkov, B.V. (1989). Micro gravity induced changes in human bone strength. *Physiologist*, **32** (Supplement 1), S41–4.

Tallis, R. (1991). Assessing outome in rehabilitation research. In *Horizons in medicine* (ed. C.A. Seymour and J.A. Summerfield), no. 3. Trans Medica, London.

Teasdale, G. and Jennett, B. (1974). Assessment of coma and impaired consciousness: a practical scale. *Lancet*, **ii**, 81–4.

Temkin, N.R., Dikmen, S.S., and Winn, H.R. (1991). Management of head injury. Posttraumatic seizures. *Neurosurgery Clinics of North America*, **2**, 425–35.

Thomas, B.J. and Amstutz, H.C. (1985). Results of the administration of diphosphonate for the prevention of heterotopic ossification after total hip arthroplasty. *Journal of Bone and Joint Surgery, American Volume*, **67A**, 400–3.

Thomas, D.P. (1985). Venous thrombogenesis. *Annual Review of Medicine*, **35**, 39–50.

Thomas, T.M., Flymat, K.R., Blannin, J., and Meade, W. (1980). The prevalence of urinary incontinence. *British Medical Journal*, **281**, 1243–5.

Tondat Carter, L., Oliveira, D.O., Duponte, J., and Lynch, S.V. (1988). The relationship of cognitive skills performance to activities of daily living in stroke patients. *American Journal of Occupational Therapy*, **42**, 449–54.

Tuel, S.M. and Presty, S.K. (1992). Functional improvement in severe head injury after re-admission for rehabilitation. *Brain Injury*, **6**, 363–72.

Turner-Stokes, L. (1999). The effectiveness of rehabilitation: a critical review of the evidence. Introduction. *Clinical Rehabilitation*, **13** (Supplement 1), 3–6.

Turner-Stokes, L., Tonge, P., Nyein, K., Hunter, M., Nielson, S., and Robinson, I. (1998). The Northwick Park Dependency Score (NPDS): a measure of nursing dependency in rehabilitation. *Clinical Rehabilitation*, **12**, 304–18.

Turner-Stokes, L., Nyein, K., and Halliwell, D. (1999). The Northwick Park care needs assessment (NPCNA): a directly costable outcome meaure in rehabilitation. *Clinical Rehabilitation*, **13**, 253–67.

Turner-Stokes, L., Williams, H., Abrahams, D., and Duckett, S. (2000). Clinical standards for inpatient rehabilitation services in the UK. *Clinical Rehabilitation*, **14**, 468–80.

Van Ouwenaller, C., Laplace, P.M., and Chantraine, A. (1986). Painful shoulder in hemiplegia. *Archives of Physical Medicine and Rehabilitation*, **67**, 23–6.

Wade, D.T. (1992). *Measurement in neurological disability.* Oxford University Press.

Wade, D.T. (1995). Editorial. Randomized and controlled clinical trials in clinical rehabilitation. *Clinical Rehabilitation*, **9**, 275–82.

Wade, D.T. (1999*a*). Outcome measurement and rehabilitation. *Clinical Rehabilitation*, **13**, 93–5.

Wade, D.T. (1999*b*). Randomised controlled trials—a gold standard? *Clinical Rehabilitation*, **13**, 454–5.

Wade, D.T. and Langton-Hewer, R. (1985). Hospital admission for acute stroke: who, for how long and to what effect? *Journal of Epidemiology and Community Health*, **39**, 347–52.

Wade, D.T. and Langton-Hewer, R. (1987). Epidemiology of some neurological diseases, with special reference to work load in the NHS. *International Rehabilitation Medicine*, **8**, 129–37.

Wade, D.T., Wood, V.A., and Langton Hewer, R. (1985). Recovery after stroke; the first three months. *Journal of Neurology, Neurosurgery and Psychiatry*, **48**, 7–13.

Ward, A.B. (1993). Rehabilitation after trauma. *Injury*, **24**, 363–4.

Ward, A.B. (1994). Disabilities—disabled school leavers. *Update*, **20**, 751–9.

Ward, A.B. (1997). Rehabilitation medicine in the United Kingdom. *Disability and Rehabilitation*, **19**, 355–8.

Ward, A.B. and Houston, A. (1993). *Advice to purchasers: setting NHS contracts for rehabilitation medicine.* British Society of Rehabilitation Medicine, London.

Ward, A.B. and Wynn, A.J. (1996). *A study of the activities of the North Staffordshire Rehabilitation Medicine Department.* Nuffield Provincial Hospitals Trust, London.

Warlow, C. (1991). *Handbook of neurology*. Blackwell Scientific, Oxford.

Warlow, C., Ogston, F., and Douglas, A.S. (1976). Deep vein thrombosis in the legs after stroke. *Lancet*, **i**, 1178–83.

Wehman, P.H., West, M.D., Kregal, J., Sherron, P., and Kreutzer, J.S. (1995). Return to work for persons with severe traumatic brain injury: a data-based approach to program development. *Journal of Head Trauma Rehabilitation*, **10**, 27–39.

WHO (World Health Organization) (1980). *International classification of impairments, disability, and handicap.* WHO, Geneva.

WHO (World Health Organization) (1997). *Revised international classification of impairments, disability and handicap.* WHO, Geneva.

Wicks, C., Gimson, A., *et al.* (1992). An assessment of the percutaneous endoscopic gastrostomy (PEG) feeding tube as part of an integrated approach to enteral feeding. *Gut*, **33**, 613–16.

Wilson, B. (1992). Recovery and compensatory strategies in head injured memory impaired people several years after insult. *Journal of Neurology, Neurosurgery and Psychiatry*, **55**, 177–80.

Wilson, D.H. (1974). Comparison of short wave diathermy and pulsed electromagnetic energy in the treatment of soft tissue injuries. *Physiotherapy*, **60**, 309–10.

Wittenberg, RH., Peschke, U., and Botel, U. (1992). Heterotopic ossification after spinal cord injury. Epidemiology and risk factors. *Journal of Bone and Joint Surgery, British Volume*, **74B**, 215–18.

Yarkoney, G.M. and Sahgal, V. (1987). Contractures: a major complication of craniocerebral trauma. *Clinical Orthopaedics and Related Research* , **219**, 93–6.

Yarkoney, G.M., Roth, E.J., Heinemann, A.W., Wu, Y., and Katz, R.T. (1987). The benefits of rehabilitation for traumatic spinal cord injury: a multi-varied analysis in 711 patients. *Archives of Neurology*, **44**, 93–6.

Young, B., Ott, L., *et al.* (1987). The effect of nutritional support on outcome from severe head injury. *Journal of Neurosurgery*, **67**, 668–76.

11.7 Mental retardation: public health approaches to intellectual impairment and its consequences

Tom Fryers

Introduction

The public health tradition arose from the need to protect the public from communicable disease. This required study of the epidemiology; a preventive approach to disease control which encompassed specific preventive measures, early diagnosis, and prompt, effective treatment; and a planned community overview of the provision of services.

Even for non-communicable disease, disorder, and disability, men and women living in the community are interdependent, and serious disadvantage in some members affects all of us in a broad commonality of health, disease, and disorder. A humane and compassionate society acknowledges this and our common responsibility, wherever possible, to improve health, to prevent, treat, and ameliorate disease and its consequences, to care for those most damaged and disadvantaged, and to share the burden which falls upon them. In the field of mental retardation, the burden to be shared falls not only upon the affected individuals, but also upon their immediate families to a disproportionate degree.

Therefore the three principle elements of public health concern are epidemiological elucidation of the nature and size of the problem, promotion of prevention, and provision of community-wide programmes of habilitation and care. Epidemiology will include searching for causes, studying the frequency of impairments, disabilities, and their consequences in different communities and at different times, and evaluating services. Preventive programmes offer many possibilities. Primary prevention can be implemented through mass screening, immunization, or control of the physical environment. Early assessment, and monitored programmes of habilitation help to facilitate development and minimize secondary disabilities. Social consequences can be reduced by organized support for the individual and the family, ameliorating adverse social conditions, and challenging stigmatizing attitudes and behaviours in the social environment. To plan community-wide habilitation and care requires an understanding of communities and cultures as well as the biology of intellectual impairment and its associated phenomena. A key problem will be co-ordination of many agencies and personnel.

Attitudes have changed a great deal in the past 30 years. Our inherited systems of care in industrialized countries were mostly based on large, remote, custodial, residential institutions, dominated by doctors, and capital intensive. These are alien to the basic philosophies of normalization, integration, human rights, and client choice which inform a modern public health approach to the disabled, the elderly, and the long-term sick. Programmes are necessarily multidisciplinary and labour intensive. The transformation of services has already proceeded a long way in many countries, not always adequately resourced or well managed, and not without problems, but changes on the scale required cannot be brought about overnight, or without commitment, conflict, and cost. They bring problems of a high order for the public health physician and his or her colleagues, which are amongst the most challenging on the current public health scene.

Concepts, classifications, terms, and labels

Mental retardation is neither a single entity nor a medical diagnosis, and the field is beset by serious problems of conceptualization, classification, and terminology. Promotion of normalization has led some to question the ethics of classifying people in terms of their disease, disorder, or disability because of the social consequences of 'labelling'. This concern is entirely proper, but planning requires categories, and scientific measurement requires clear definitions and a logical taxonomy. Moreover, however desirable the integration of disabled people into ordinary society, if they disappear from view they are likely to be ignored in the provision of the special help they need.

Disabled people do have special needs by definition. They cannot compete on equal terms with their fellows, and are unlikely, without help, to escape the low status and stigma which tends to be their lot. Normalization must not excuse invisibility and neglect, leaving the burden of care entirely on the disabled person and their immediate family. Epidemiology can clarify thinking about disabled people and their needs, and inform the planning of services and the allocation of resources.

For over a century, concepts and terms related to mental retardation have been debated and disputed. In earlier years, dominant concepts usually implied immutable pathologies, present at birth and largely inherited. More recently favoured concepts involve disrupted development caused by a variety of interacting physical and social determinants, with potential for further development. Underlying all of them is a common perception of people at the bottom of the scale of human competence who cannot survive independently.

But what are the criteria for survival in human society? Mental retardation engages the interests of paediatricians, geneticists, biochemists, psychologists, psychiatrists, educationalists, managers, social legislators, and others. Each group sees the client group, its needs, and problems differently, and each has promulgated its own definitions based on its own concepts. These are inherently difficult to reconcile: poor genetic potential, low measured intelligence, insufficiency in learned competencies, inadequate adaptation to society, social dependency, multiple physical and psychological disabilities, central nervous system damage or disorder, and specific pathological or aetiological entities.

Arising from this diversity of professional and scientific perspective, the literature of mental retardation provides a remarkable variety of terms, inconsistency of categories, and ambiguity of concepts. And for all these, measurement is problematic, especially in children, in whom we are implicitly trying to predict how they will function as adults. We must use age-related norms of function and behaviour which are not easily standardized across cultures or rendered precise in measurement. There are also difficulties of degree, since divisions are arbitrary, and milder expressions of developmental curtailment raise essentially different practical issues as they merge into 'normal'. In practice, most reported studies are small scale and pragmatic; they seldom discuss taxonomy or define the terms and categories used. Thus much of the literature is useless for comparison or application elsewhere.

Current classifications

The classification of mental retardation in the *International Classification of Diseases, 10th Revision* (**ICD-10**) (WHO 1992*a*) is simple but inadequate, depending upon intelligence quotient (**IQ**) criteria rarely available in practice. The classifications produced by the American Association on Mental Retardation (AAMR 1992) based upon their Adaptive Behaviour Scales (Grossman 1983) and in the *Diagnostic and Statistical Manual of Mental Disorders (Fourth Edition)* (**DSM-IV**) (APA 1980) are fairly closely related, using IQ data with qualifying criteria. The former is more precise, detailed, and standardized. Both tend to mingle concepts of impaired structure, disordered function, and social disadvantage, the discrimination of which is the great strength of the *International Classification of Impairments, Disabilities and Handicaps* (**ICIDH**) (WHO 1980). This conceptualization offers a useful framework for a general taxonomy for mental retardation, using the following definitions: 'impairment' is any loss or abnormality of psychological, physiological, or anatomical structure or function; 'disability' is any limitation of capacity to perform an activity in the manner or within the range considered normal for any human being; 'handicap' is any disadvantage which an individual experiences in the fulfilment of a social role that is considered normal for a person of his or her age and gender in that culture because of an impairment or disability.

The WHO classification has undergone revision (WHO 2001), changing both the concept boundaries and the terms used. 'Impairment' is retained but includes all loss of function below activities at the whole person level. The term 'disability' is used as an umbrella term for all imperfections and is replaced at the whole person level by 'limitation of activity'. 'Handicap' is replaced by 'restriction of participation' with a more overt emphasis on society's contribution to the experience of disadvantage. These changes were finally published in January 2001.

Other usages will continue and we cannot expect the new terms to be any less problematic than the old. Socially, an acceptable group 'label' may change to recognize changes in social perceptions, and to keep a step ahead of stigma. For example, in the United Kingdom, it has been 'mental deficiency', 'mental subnormality', and 'mental handicap' over the last 40 years, and is currently 'learning disabilities'. No doubt it will change again in the future. Other English-speaking countries use 'mental impairment', 'intellectual disability', 'developmental disability', 'learning handicap', and many others. The acceptability of terms to parents is as important as scientific study but does not necessarily follow the same logic, and scientific and social purposes differ. We have suffered very unscientific confusion, lack of compatibility, and waste of effort by professionals and researchers adopting whatever title is currently in use in their own community, assuming that definitions remain the same, and implying that there is no necessity for a standardized scientific taxonomy and terminology!

Lay and scientific use of terms should not be confused. Scientific categories are primarily for research into human groups. They can be applied to service planning, monitoring, and evaluation with care, but should be applied to individuals in service contexts only with great caution. To determine individual needs, individual assessment is required; it should not depend upon their allocation to a group or their acquisition of a group label. In this chapter, 'mental retardation' is used as the general title for the domain of scientific and professional activity, because it has long international usage and does not conflict with the ICIDH. Where applied (on behalf of all those other terms used in particular societies) to a group of people, it represents a category of social disadvantage. The terms used below, while based upon ICIDH concepts, are intended also to preclude conflict with ICIDH-2 in the future. To this end, 'handicap', the most contentious of the previous terms, has been avoided.

We should first distinguish between 'global' and 'partial' categories (Table 1). Global categories are those which purport to describe the client group as an entity entirely within the field of mental retardation, from one specified point of view or another. They imply a global or generalized impairment, disability, or social disadvantage (handicap) and to avoid ambiguity, 'generalized' is used in each case. Partial categories are those which are not exclusively related to or defined in terms of mental retardation, and thus encompass both individuals who are considered mentally retarded and those who are not. In principle there is no limit to the number of global or partial categories, but three of the former and five of the latter may be of most practical use (Fryers 1993).

Global categories

Generalized intellectual impairment

Intelligence—the capacity to learn, to apply learning, and to develop—can be operationalized broadly to include all aspects of learning, or narrowly to specify only one aspect. The organic basis of this capacity in the central nervous system, although not fully understood, may be conceived as a body system, called 'the intellect' analogous to biochemical systems to which the ICIDH applies the term 'impairment'.

Definitions are inextricably bound up with the means of measurement. Intelligence tests, the results of some of which can be summarized as an IQ, are far from consistent, do not entirely disentangle learned skills from underlying capacities, and can be misused, but nevertheless have validity and usefulness (Berger and Yule 1985). For individuals, they can provide a useful indication of current development if they are professionally administered and include subscores and commentary, but their predictive value is limited. Many children show increments of IQ as they mature,

Table 1 Taxonomies in mental retardation

Global (overall) categories	
Generalized intellectual impairment	
Criteria	Intellectual
Measures	Intelligence or developmental tests
Main categories	Severe
	IQ < 50 (sometimes divided into: profound, IQ < 20; severe, IQ 20 < 35; moderate, IQ 35–50)
	Mild
	IQ 50–69
Generalized learning disability (related to intellectual impairment)	
Criteria	Educational
Measures	Mostly of learning achievement as proxies for the learning process, such as memory recall, reading, number, problem solving, etc.
Main categories	In general, severe, moderate, and mild are used but in non-standard ways; often ill-defined
Generalized dependency (related to intellectual impairment) ('mental retardation' etc.)	
Criteria	Social—highly variable in different societies
Measures	Scales of dependency or maladaptation
Main categories	Severe
	Commonly limited to IQ < 50 and therefore coextensive with severe intellectual impairment
	Mild
	Used with very variable criteria of social selection
Partial categories	
Physical impairments, aetiological and pathological groups	
Criteria	Commonly pathological or aetiological diagnosis
Measures	Usually clinical and laboratory
Main categories	Mostly neurological impairments providing 'medical' diagnostic groups
Syndromes of impairments and/or disabilities	
Criteria	Grouping of signs and symptoms with epidemiological validation
Measures	Clinical, radiological, biochemical, etc.
Main categories	Epilepsies; cerebral palsies; autistic spectrum disorders; psychiatric disorders
Specific disabilities: losses of function	
Criteria	Defined deficits in normal functions
Measures	Standardized assessments where available
Main categories	Specific motor, sensory, intellectual, emotional, and behavioural dysfunctions
Social consequences: individual disadvantages	
Criteria	Social disadvantage
Measures	Measures: very few standard measures available
Main categories	Income, housing, employment, education, access, stigma, abuse, etc.
Carers concerns: parent and family disadvantages	
	Social disadvantages as for the disabled person

After Fryers (1991, 1993).

probably recovering from early lack of stimulation. Intelligence as measured is undoubtedly influenced by both nature and nurture, and determinants of impairment include general polygenic inheritance, specific genetic anomalies, organic damage, lack of education, emotional state, and social deprivation. Some of these are ameliorable.

IQs are entirely comparative, and a product of populations, showing essentially a statistically 'normal' distribution, but test means in particular populations change over time, subpopulations differ, and there is an excess at the lower end of the range due to brain damage and disorder. Any IQ band can be studied in its associations with any other characteristic of people in that population, their experience, or their environment. It is not unlike studying height, although IQs have no reference values outside human populations. People with very low IQs, like people with very low heights, are likely to have problems in society, and it is important to study their characteristics and needs.

Although particular IQ categories are arbitrary, the conventions of IQ < 50 for 'severe intellectual impairment' (IQ < 55 would have equal validity, but has been used much less in epidemiological research) and IQ 50–69 for 'mild intellectual impairment' carry considerable weight, especially the former. Subdivisions in the ICD and ICIDH of the IQ < 50 category into 'profound', 'severe', and 'moderate' have not proved very useful, as IQ measures below 35 are much less reliable (Fryers 1984, 1993). All people of IQ < 50, in all societies, will be considered learning disabled and mentally retarded, so IQ is the sole essential criterion. For IQ 50–69, additional criteria are always used to define the group in society. Mild mental retardation is never the same as mild intellectual impairment.

Generalized learning disability (related to intellectual impairment)

Where global impairment is of the intellect, global disability is of the function of learning, encompassing acquisition of knowledge, skills, and attitudes, mental development, and personality maturation. As commonly used in educational systems, specific categories of learning disability rarely match IQ categories. There are many reasons for children to be identified as having learning disabilities; current usage in the United Kingdom usually links these to a substantial degree of intellectual impairment, but American usage does not. If the criteria for selection and the measures used are stated, the relationship will be clear. All children of IQ < 50, i.e. those who are severely intellectually impaired, will always be identified as severely learning disabled, but children in the mildly intellectually impaired group may not be identified as learning disabled in some school contexts.

Determinants of generalized learning disability in populations may include, as well as intellectual impairment, motor and sense organ impairments, social and educational deprivation, childhood psychosis, highly selective school systems, inadequate teachers, administrative conventions, and legal requirements. Standard scientific categories are not available. Learning disability should be measured by tests of learning function, but tests usually provide proxy measures of the outcome of the learning process by testing performance of skills such as memorization and recall, reading, writing, and numeracy, and relating them to age and culture norms. It remains problematic to summate any collection of these as generalized learning disability.

For adults, measures of social maturity as in the Vineland Social Maturity Scale, and behavioural age, as derived from the American Association of Mental Deficiency Adaptive Behaviour Scales may also offer proxies for generalized learning disability. They have been much used and are standardized, although they should be applied to different populations with caution. Categories are independent of IQ, so offer a dimension which can be studied in relation to intellectual impairment. It is important to remember that there are groups of adults considered to have learning disabilities not closely related to intellectual impairment, especially prison inmates (BSU 1994).

Generalized dependency (related to intellectual impairment)

Social disadvantage associated with any impairment or disability is a very personal experience in a particular social context. Collectively, the principle general social disadvantage related to diminished intelligence shared by all those identified as mentally retarded (whatever the label) is lack of capacity for independence, or 'dependency'. This can be viewed as a summation of the 'major survival roles' in ICIDH. It offers six examples—orientation, physical independence, mobility, occupation, social integration, and economic self-sufficiency—but many more could be described.

Like learning disability, criteria for and measures of dependency need specifying. In the context of mental retardation, it is 'related to' intellectual impairment, but IQ has never been applied as the sole criterion. Prevalence differentials according to sex, social class, and race, and excess frequencies of sensory and motor deficits, psychiatric disturbance, challenging behaviour, and family disruption suggest that many social criteria are also applied.

It is these selection criteria—some overt, some covert—which determine who is perceived, categorized, registered, treated, or served as 'mentally retarded' in any one community. They will vary substantially from community to community, but are generally those which bring clients into contact with certain educational, medical and social services, or the law. Low intelligence—measured, guessed, or assumed—is usually, but not always, one overt factor, as are certain obvious medical diagnoses such as Down's syndrome. But many selection criteria are not overt, reflecting education, mental health, welfare and criminal law, and juridical practice; organizational characteristics of the services; professional conventions and perceptions; and government policies and public attitudes (Table 4). As Haywood (1970) wrote, 'Understanding the causes of handicap involves understanding the social system of which handicapped children are a marginal component.'

Selection, therefore, depends as much on the characteristics of services and society as of clients, but few studies have examined these to identify the selection processes adopted and the underlying social attitudes and societal context which created them. As human services emphasize normalization and integration of people with disabilities, such studies could be immensely useful.

A group of people with generalized dependency is identified and labelled, no doubt, in every society. If IQ < 50 is a criterion, severe intellectual impairment is being defined, but all such people will experience severe dependency too. This is not true for mild intellectual impairment; very few people of IQ 50–69 are selected as mentally retarded, and those who are usually exhibit challenging behaviour, mental illness, multiple physical disabilities, or contact with the criminal law. In some communities, people with similar problems but higher IQs may also be included.

Because mental retardation—generalized dependency related to intellectual impairment—is socially determined and very variable in population frequency (usually called 'administrative' prevalence), researchers have sometimes concluded that comparison is impossible but this is not so. Groups defined by IQ < 50 we can compare as severe intellectual impairment (Fryers 1984). Otherwise we must study the factors which determine selection and identification as 'mentally retarded' in different societies, the social processes involved, and the benefits and 'dis-benefits' for clients.

Partial categories

Persons with intellectual impairment may experience any disease or disorder, but some are commonly associated with intellectual impairment or commonly found in those selected as mentally retarded, and may be regarded as categories partially related to mental retardation. Serious investigation of causes and the potential for prevention requires studies of total human populations across all intelligence levels, not only of individuals identified as mentally retarded. Studies of the proportional composition of groups identified as mentally retarded, as regards aetiological diagnosis for example, are of limited value.

Any number of types of partial category could be described, but five types may be most useful as follows.

Physical impairments: aetiological and pathological groups

These mostly relate to neurological impairments. They are rarely limited to specific degrees of intellectual impairment or learning disability and many include people who would never be considered mentally retarded. Examples are phenylketonuria (including treated cases), Down's syndrome (including mosaics), and fragile X (including female carriers). Some common organ impairments are part of recognized syndromes also including diminished intelligence, such as rubella syndrome or fetal alcohol syndrome. Congenital cardiac defects and Alzheimer's dementia are found more commonly in Down's syndrome than the rest of the population. Congenital abnormalities tend to associate with each other in populations; trauma tends to produce multiple effects in individuals.

Syndromes of impairments and/or disabilities

These include the epilepsies, cerebral palsies, psychiatric disorders, and autistic spectrum disorders ('pervasive developmental disorders'); 'challenging behaviour' may be included here, although syndromes are less well defined. They are neither aetiological nor pathological entities, but are important in relation to mental retardation, showing higher frequencies than the general population, and posing serious problems for clinical and psychological assessment. The epidemiology of each of these groups of disorders is complex and difficult, and constantly interacts with that of intellectual impairment and mental retardation.

Specific disabilities: losses of function

Motor and sensory disabilities are common in people with severe intellectual impairment, and represent additional reasons for selection as mentally retarded in the presence of mild intellectual impairment. Similar losses arise in diverse ways, so disability categories do not correlate with IQ categories, organic impairments, or aetiological entities. Nor do similar disabilities always produce similar social consequences. Research demands a broad approach. Specific disabilities such as 'mobility' or 'inability to feed oneself' have been increasingly studied in recent years, and more guidance for habilitative practice is likely to emerge in the future. Some degree of standardization of measures is emerging (Fryers 1993). The 'academic skills disorders' of DSM-IV may be seen as specific learning disabilities related partially to intellectual impairment.

Social consequences: individual disadvantages

Specific disadvantages are poorly defined and little researched, although there is great potential in such studies for improving the lives of people identified as mentally retarded. Many social consequences of intellectual impairment are also experienced by other disabled people, the poor, and the disenfranchised. The social consequences depend upon the constellation of impairments and disabilities, abilities and aspirations, individual temperament and attitudes, and the demands, opportunities, and resources of the family and society in which he or she lives.

Some disadvantages, such as in housing, employment, and welfare benefits, have been much studied in general, but seldom including people with intellectual impairment. Few studies have examined marriage, friendship, social networks, employment, and leisure opportunities; a notable exception is the Aberdeen study following up all identified mentally retarded children in that Scottish city to observe a wide range of adult life patterns, opportunities and disadvantages (Koller *et al.* 1988; Richardson *et al.* 1988, 1993). More research is needed; it is social disadvantages which provoke the greatest frustrations and the greatest sense of alienation. The principle aim of services for people with intellectual impairment is the reduction of these disadvantages. Rarely can impairment be diminished; sometimes disability can be ameliorated; but most improvement in people's lives will come from addressing disadvantages directly through enhanced opportunities, extra assistance, positive discrimination, and political action.

Carers' concerns: parent and family disadvantages

The demands on parents caring for a severely intellectually impaired child has long been acknowledged, but many aspects are little researched (Twigg 1992; Beresford 1993; Keltner and Ramey 1993). As institutional care diminishes, more responsibility tends to fall on parents, siblings, and other family members, for adults who now frequently survive their parents. Community service agencies and professional staff are dependent upon such informal 'carers'. They should be considered partners in care programmes, but carers' own needs should not be ignored. Social scientists are only just beginning to address these issues.

Summary

Most classification systems have used a combination of IQ, educational failure, social adaptation, and medical diagnosis without precise relationships being specified. Imprecise and non-standard measures have increased the ambiguity. No single simple set of categories will suffice for all purposes within the field of mental retardation, but the basic concepts of the ICIDH offer multiple dimensions within a unified structure which resolves many of the difficulties.

Mental retardation probably remains the best general title for the field of study, with three sets of global categories—generalized intellectual impairment, generalized learning disability, and generalized dependency. These can be clearly defined by measurable criteria, and studied in relation to one another. Several sets of partial categories describe groups not exclusive to mental retardation and encompassing aetiological and pathological entities, clinical syndromes, specific disabilities, and social consequences for both individuals and carers. Causes of impairment, disability, and disadvantage, however defined, will be found in society as much as in individuals.

Research workers need to be wary and clear thinking; ambiguous definitions and imprecise measures waste time and resources. Service planners and managers need to understand the conceptual problems before applying simple criteria to their service situations. It is important that no classification system, however elegant to the epidemiologist or convenient to the manager, should be allowed to determine lifetime services for an individual! Lifetime institutionalization was the nightmare of labelling. Taxonomy is concerned with groups; individuals require thorough, multidisciplinary, professional assessment, constantly monitored and updated, and sensitively involving the client and his or her family where appropriate. This should help to avoid the problems of labelling, administrative determinism, institutional batch management and inflexible service structures, and ensure the best practical attention to constantly changing individual needs.

Descriptive epidemiology: frequencies in populations

Factors affecting frequencies

Incidence and prevalence of a heterogeneous category like mental retardation are highly dynamic. However defined, they are determined by the frequency of occurrence of very many disorders of widely varying genesis. Some disorders arise at conception and their causes must be looked for before conception; others arise in early fetal life, around birth, and in early postnatal life. New cases become progressively less frequent with age, and cumulative inception almost levels off by 4 or 5 years. But mortality of abnormal fetuses follows a similar dynamic, being concentrated in early fetal life, around birth and in early infancy, then almost levelling off. Prevalence at any age is determined by both inception rates and mortality rates before that age, although known prevalence also depends upon the identification rate (Fig. 1) Prevalence ratios are also susceptible to differential migration which changes the relationship between numerators and population denominators.

'Incidence' carries little meaning for the group as a whole, and 'true incidence' is difficult to establish even for individual syndromes. In Down's syndrome it must take account of the large proportion of naturally aborted fetuses, not easily estimated. In perinatal aetiologies it must encompass all similar adverse factors, whether or not the

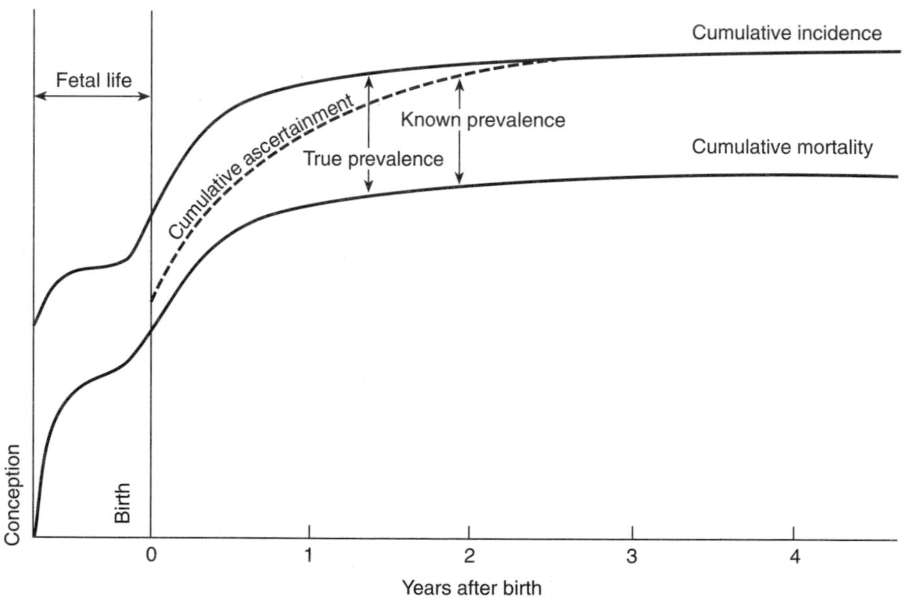

Fig. 1 Schematic diagram of the relationship between aetiology, mortality, and ascertainment in severe intellectual impairment. The two vertical lines represent conception and birth, respectively. The upper curve represents the cumulative incidence of disorders associated with severe intellectual impairment in a notional cohort of conceptuses. At conception, many individuals are already impaired; more arise early in fetal life, fewer later on. The perinatal period results in a relatively large increase in numbers, but incidence thereafter progressively diminishes. The lower curve represents the cumulative mortality of affected individuals within the cohort. Many impaired fetuses die early in fetal life, fewer later on. The perinatal period carries higher risks, but after birth mortality progressively diminishes. The vertical distance between the two curves represents the 'true prevalence' at any given age. Not all those impaired at birth are recognized at the time; ascertainment is progressively achieved, as represented by the dotted curve. The 'known prevalence' at any given age is represented by the vertical distance between the ascertainment curve and the mortality curve.

outcomes include intellectual impairment. The incidence of affected births varies with the current local population birth rate, so 'birth frequency' (or 'prevalence at birth': the proportion of cases in a continuous series of births in a given population) is used. Even this is difficult to know except for well-defined syndromes easily recognized at birth.

The dynamic processes of inception, mortality, and migration give rise to substantial variation in prevalence in different communities and at different times. There is substantial reliable research literature only with respect to groups defined by IQ < 50 (severe intellectual impairment, but usually called severe mental retardation, and so on). It reveals general characteristics summarized in Table 2 (Fryers 1984). The common assertion that prevalence ratios for severe mental retardation are 'stable' or consistent is not true, even for clearly defined severe intellectual impairment. It would, indeed, be very strange, given the social determinants of population frequency of the causes of neurological impairment, which vary so much between cultures and communities. These social factors (e.g. diet in neural tube defects; patterns of fertility in Down's syndrome; alcohol price and supply in fetal alcohol syndrome; consanguinity in recessive genetic disorders) are most likely to offer scope for prevention.

Severe intellectual impairment (IQ < 50)

This is coterminous with severe learning disability, mental retardation, or any other group which is defined as IQ < 50.

1. Point prevalence varies between similar birth cohorts (concurrent age groups) in different communities. Reliable studies found 1.62 per 1000 children born between 1951 and 1955 in Salford, United Kingdom, and 7.34 per 1000 children born in 1957 in Amsterdam, The Netherlands. Greater variation is expected in developing countries. Prevalence varies with genetic, cultural, economic, environmental, and service factors, largely by influencing the spectrum of biomedical causes and early mortality. Sometimes one cause dominates the scene, especially iodine deficiency disease, where more than 10 per cent of village populations can be affected by endemic congenital hypothyroidism ('cretinism'). In developed countries, Down's syndrome may be the most prevalent aetiological group in children, especially in communities with traditions of late marriage, large families, and taboos against contraception and/or abortion. But where early general mortality is high, few infants with Down's syndrome survive into later childhood. Congenital anomalies are relatively high in communities with traditions of consanguinous marriage, but few are associated with intellectual impairment. Mortality and survival are extremely variable often related to the 'development' status of the community.
2. Age-specific prevalence changes over time in the same community, because the spectrum of causes and the effects of early mortality change. In Salford, prevalence for children aged 5 to 9 years was 1.98 per 1000 in 1961, 5.54 per 1000 in 1971, and 3.86 per 1000 in 1980. The factors which explain differences between communities may explain changes over time in the same community.
3. A similar pattern of temporal change is seen throughout most of the developed world, with a low range of values for age-specific prevalence (1.8–4.0 per 1000) for children born in the early 1950s, a high range (3.3–5.5 per 1000) for those born in the mid-1960s, and falling prevalence ratios since then, at least well into the 1980s (Rumeau-Rouquette *et al.* 1997). There are exceptions: high recent frequencies in Northern Ireland, for example, are due to special cultural circumstances. In Fig. 2, reliable prevalence data for small age groups of children from many studies are plotted according to their period of birth to compare them as cohorts.

Table 2 Basic epidemiology of severe intellectual impairment: prevalence in developed communities

There is geographical variation within similar birth cohorts
Range at least 1.62–7.34 per 1000
There is temporal variation in successive birth cohorts in the same community
For example 1.98–5.54 per 1000 in Salford children aged 5–9 years (1961–1971)
There has been a similar pattern of temporal change in many developed countries
Low prevalence for children born in the early 1950s
High prevalence for children born in the early 1960s
Falling prevalence since then
There is variation by age due to variations in incidence and mortality of birth cohorts
Around 2002 the highest prevalence ratios will be in the age group 35–39 years
There is increased survival at all ages and into old age
There are more clients aged over 45 years than aged under 15 years
There is probably a social class gradient in both incidence and mortality
There are excesses in lower socio-economic groups
There are usually more males than females
However, there are no consistent patterns in the sex ratio

These features are typical of developed countries. They will be true to varying extent for communities in developing countries depending upon development and economic status, demographic characteristics, vital statistics, and many other social indicators

Increased prevalence can be related to a rapid decrease in early mortality associated with developments in neonatal care. This increased survival is well documented for Down's syndrome by life-table studies from birth (Table 3). Other aetiological groups are too rare or inconsistent in case definition to be studied in a similar way, but we can assume similar processes continue to increase survival.

The progressive decrease in prevalence in young children since the late 1960s reflects many different processes reducing inceptions. Large-scale oral contraception reduced both mean maternal age and, especially, conceptions in older women, which greatly reduced the incidence of Down's syndrome. In the 1980s, amniocentesis and abortion programmes began to reduce Down's syndrome even more, although the impact was diminished by the lack of conceptions in

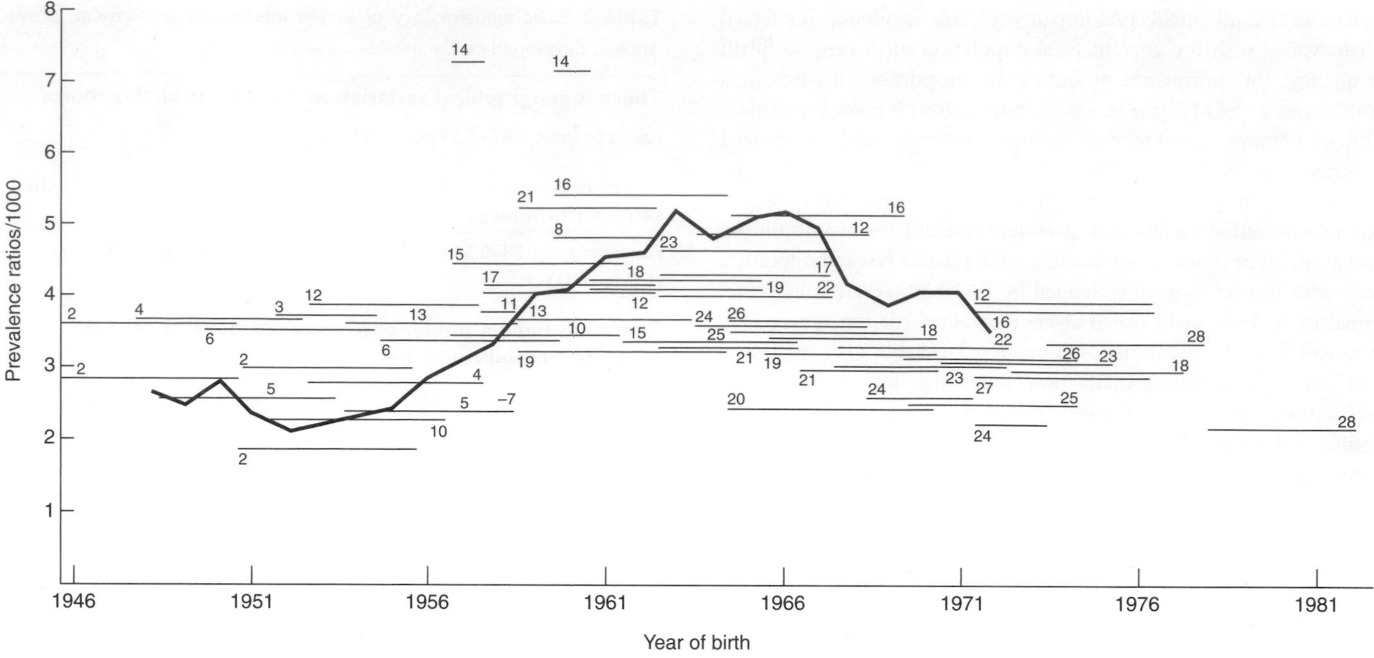

Fig. 2 Severe intellectual impairment (IQ < 50) from published studies in developed countries: age-specific prevalence ratios in school-age children related to years of birth. Each line represents the prevalence and years of birth for one age group of children in each study. The continuous line represents changing annual prevalence applied to years of birth, for 5–9- and 10–14-year-old children in Salford, United Kingdom, through 25 years (Fryers 1984, 1991).

older women. In the 1990s, the average age of conception has tended to increase again. This, together with new screening techniques applied at all maternal ages, increases the potential impact of abortion programmes.

Other contributions are very small because each aetiological group is small, but the cumulative effect may be significant. Postnatal screening programmes for inherited metabolic disorders and sporadic congenital hypothyroidism are very successful. Although conclusions are difficult to draw from the evidence, perinatal factors probably increased the number of babies with neurological impairments surviving in the 1970s but decreased them in the 1980s.

The reduction of encephalitis, encephalopathy, and rubella syndrome by effective immunization (and other measures for tuberculosis and bacterial meningitis) probably had a small effect in the 1970s and 1980s. However, a major impact can be anticipated in the 1990s in countries that achieve immunization rates sufficient to produce herd immunity for pertussis, measles, mumps, *Haemophilus influenzae* type B, and rubella.

The widespread adoption of early stimulation and training programmes for severely intellectually impaired infants, especially those with Down's syndrome may have removed a few individuals from the 'severe' group at later ages by improving their test performance, but the impact on prevalence rates would be extremely small and experienced only once in one community.

4. Prevalence varies by age. Age distributions change over time because of differences in birth cohorts and survival from early infancy. Although not 'in phase' everywhere, in many developed countries the highest age-specific prevalence is for those born in the early to mid-1960s. Thus, by 2000 the largest age group were approaching their mid-thirties. Younger age groups (i.e. later birth cohorts) have had progressively lower prevalence ratios. This has meant progressively fewer children throughout the last 20 years. The larger cohorts will, of course, move up the age range in future decades.

Prevalence also varies by age because reduced mortality has increased survival at all ages (McGrother *et al.* 2001). In most developed countries there are currently more adults over 45 than children under 15 years of age, and there are substantial numbers of elderly severely intellectually impaired people. Professionals and managers needs to recognize this.

5. From prevalence and mortality data, estimates can be made of age-specific prevalence ratios for severe intellectual impairment (IQ < 50) in developed countries. They assume a stable population over the last half century and no unusual factors affecting particular important aetiological groups. Figures for the youngest and oldest age groups are informed guesses. In Table 4, projections for a 'standard' United Kingdom District for 1.1.00 are more speculative than the original estimates for 1.1.90 because reliable recent data are few. The few recent studies are mostly consistent with them, and they should be useful guides for planning and resourcing community-based services, modifying the figures to take account of migration and other particular features of a real district.

6. There are usually more males than females at all ages, the ratio varying between 1 in 1 and 2 in 1, but with no clear pattern. It probably depends upon the particular spectrum of causes of central neurological damage and disorder in any population (some biomedical causes, such as fragile X, favour males), but

Table 3 Changes in survival in Down's syndrome: life tables, 1940–1980

Years of birth	*n*	Survival rates (%)						
		1 month	1 year	2 years	3 years	4 years	5 years	10 years
1942–52 Birmingham, UK	252	68.8	49.9	47.4	45.6	45.2	44.1	–
1944–55 London, UK	689	70.0	46.9	43.3	42.1	40.5	39.7	36.8
1948–57 Victoria, Australia	729	—	68.9	57.9	54.0	51.4	49.4	46.2
1953–58 Glasgow, UK	117	88.9	76.1	70.9	—	—	—	–
1950–66 Massachusetts, USA	2421	92.8	76.4	72.6	70.5	69.2	68.5	64.5
1952–71 British Columbia, Canada	927	—	89.4	87.3	85.8	85.2	84.9	82.1
1960–69 N Ireland, UK	101	—	64.4	—	—	—	—	–
1961–80 Salford, UK	59	89.8	81.4	81.0	79.2	77.3	77.2	70.7
1966–75 Japan	1052	—	93.6	90.4	89.0	88.1	87.1	86.0
1966–76 Western Australia	231	97.0	83.5	77.7	75.4	74.8	—	–

After Fryers (1984).

Table 4 Estimates of prevalence of severe intellectual impairment (IQ < 50) for a standard English district of stable population

Age (years)	Prevalence per 1000 at		
	1 January 1990	1 January 1995	1 January 2000
0–4	2.5?	2.50?	2.50?
5–9	3.0	2.25	2.25?
10–14	4.0	2.75	2.10
15–19	4.5	3.70	2.67
20–24	5.0	4.20	3.59
25–29	4.5	4.65	4.07
30–34	4.0	4.10	4.48
35–39	3.5	3.60	3.93
40–44	3.0	3.10	3.46
45–54	2.5	2.55	2.90
55–64	2.0	2.10	2.30
65–74	1.0	1.20	1.71
75+	Very few	Very few	0.80?

Estimates for 1990 and mortality expectations for 1990–1994 were derived from the available literature. Estimates for 2000 were derived by applying mortality data for 1995–1999 from the Leicestershire Learning Disabilities Information System (Case Register) (McGrother *et al.* 2001; McGrother and Thorpe, personal communication, 2001).

differential mortality may also play a part. Reduced mortality in recent years may have increased the male excess.

7. Severe intellectual impairment has often been found to be evenly distributed across socio-economic groups, a surprising finding given the social class differential of most measures of morbidity and mortality, and the social factors involved in the causes of severe intellectual impairment. Some more recent studies show the expected social class gradient and it is likely that a differential in inceptions, masked by a similar differential in early mortality, is revealed as mortality falls.

Mild intellectual impairment (IQ 50–69)

Using tests validated for specific populations, IQs approximate to a 'normal' statistical distribution. Test means and standard deviations, must be known from recent studies, because test means change over time with developments in education and other cultural changes. That is, the test mean for a particular population may not be 100, although tests were originally designed in this way. The prevalence of mild intellectual impairment (IQ 50–69) reflects almost entirely the statistical distribution. For a test of mean 100, standard deviation of 15, 2.27 per cent of the population will fall below IQ 70 (2 standard deviations below the mean), plus a small effect from specific pathologies influencing mostly the bottom of the range. The few populations providing data confirm this with figures of 25 to 30 per 1000 (Richardson and Koller 1985).

The proportion of children in this group (IQ 50–69) identified in schools as 'learning disabled' depends upon the particular features of a school system and its arrangements for 'special needs'. Children with higher IQs but a range of other problems may also be included, so the group as a whole may not relate closely to the IQ category. The relatively few adults with mild intellectual impairment identified as mentally retarded are those with the lowest IQs or those with serious additional motor, sensory, communication, or behavioural problems.

Although this group is never identified as a whole in services, it is important for research, especially studies of the effects on intelligence of exposure to hazards of birth, trauma, or environmental factors such as lead. Outcome must be assessed in relation to population norms in complete cohorts of births.

Mild learning disability and mild dependency related to intellectual impairment

Concepts of global disability and global handicap are commonly confused, and terminology is especially problematic. In the United States 'learning disability' is generally applied only to groups not exhibiting intellectual impairment, but in the United Kingdom it is the current general term for those identified as having some degree of intellectual impairment, i.e. what would be called 'mental retardation' in the United States. Other countries use yet other English terms for generalized learning disability and generalized dependency in the taxonomy described above. No doubt other languages experience similar problems.

In the context of the ICIDH, generalized learning disability is the appropriate term for the global disability experienced by people with intellectual impairment. Available statistics mostly record school or adult service groups characterized by certain levels of dependency, i.e. conceptually implying a generalized handicap definition. They do not commonly apply standardized measures and are therefore difficult to compare and interpret.

Such statistics expressed as population frequencies are usually called 'administrative prevalence' because they count those known to particular community service systems or derive from population registers related to service provision. They have been considered non-scientific, but if they are understood as frequencies of 'generalized dependency' (related to intellectual impairment), the characteristics and determinants of which in different societies can be examined and compared, they offer great potential for valuable research.

As noted above, terms purporting to describe severe learning disability and severe dependency (handicap) are frequently defined by measures of IQ. If a criterion of IQ < 50 is imposed upon either generalized learning disability or generalized dependency, the group defined is identical to, and should be identified as, severe intellectual impairment. This does not apply at lesser levels of intellectual impairment, although the same confusion prevails. The following discussion focuses, therefore, on the mild category, but the arguments apply also where mental retardation or an equivalent term is used without differentiation of degree. Because 'mild generalized dependency' has, as yet, no currency, the conventional term 'mild mental retardation' will be used, and readers must translate it into their own term of common use!

Mild mental retardation as identified in any community is never the same as mild intellectual impairment as defined above (all those with IQ 50–69 in the total population). Many individuals in that IQ range cope satisfactorily with society's demands and are never considered mentally retarded. Indeed, it might be said that the group exists mainly because of the demands of universal education; in communities without this, very few will be identified as 'different'. In other situations some people are considered mentally retarded in spite of an IQ above 69. Following up the British 1958 birth cohort, 10 per cent of all children were identified by teachers as needing special or remedial education, many with IQs above 69 (Fogelman and Wedge 1981).

The key to understanding this is to recognize that low intelligence, whether measured or merely clinically estimated, is only one of many criteria by which people are identified as different and dependent, and are therefore called mentally retarded (or equivalent term). Other social factors determine who is selected as mentally retarded to receive special services, and these often outweigh intelligence so that people with IQs over 69 may be included. It is important to recognize that mild mental retardation is always socially determined. The vast variation in reported prevalence for adults in the past 40 years (e.g. 2.97 per 1000 in Wessex, United Kingdom, and 77.91 per 1000 in Rose County, United States, both published in 1968), illustrates the variety of inclusion criteria. There is no standard definition, and there are no representative statistics for the prevalence of mild mental retardation.

Local 'registers' are valid measures if they fully record those for whom the label is perceived as appropriate in each community. We can only speak of 'underestimated' or 'hidden' mental retardation in respect of those who fulfil local criteria, but who have not been identified. In practice this is seldom known because many criteria are not overtly understood, are ambiguous, or are variable in application.

However, fruitful research is possible if the following crucial questions are recognized. Why are more people selected as mildly mentally retarded in one community than another? What are the different criteria, acknowledged and hidden, by which particular societies select people to be labelled mentally retarded? What are the consequences, good and bad, of selection or non-selection for individuals with mild intellectual impairment? Studies identifying the criteria for selection which operate in different communities and which determine prevalence, would help us to understand the social context of service provision, the variants and determinants of stigma and discrimination, the concomitants of labelling, and the advantages and disadvantages to vulnerable people of being excluded from the group. They would also guide community care planning.

Factors commonly influencing selection as mentally retarded are summarized in Table 5. Although perceived low intelligence and certain medical diagnoses may be overtly recognized, legislation, professional attitudes, and service structures and traditions may have much greater influence. For example, 'mild mental handicap' almost disappeared in the United Kingdom when social workers, who generally did not label people in that way, took the lead role from doctors who did. This can be justified in terms of normalization, but it may also mask unmet needs. It also renders epidemiological study very difficult.

People with mild intellectual impairment are more likely to be selected if they also have communication problems, multiple physical disabilities, mental illness, or challenging behaviour, and if they suffer unemployment, low socio-economic status, poor home environment, or inadequate parental care. In many countries, current services will have inherited some people, especially in or discharged from long-stay institutions, who have higher levels of intelligence and who would not now be labelled mentally retarded.

It is these selection criteria, recognized or unrecognized, which lead to the commonly observed characteristics of the mildly mentally retarded group. There are few cases with a precise aetiological diagnosis, but many with neurological impairments, major and minor, and many with motor and sensory disabilities. Epilepsy, cerebral palsy, autism, mental illness, and challenging behaviour, especially that which attracts the attention of the police and law courts, are more common than in the general population.

A very strong bias towards lower socio-economic groups has long been known, giving rise historically to terms such as 'sub-cultural retardation'. The interaction of low intelligence with poor stimulation and education, poor social environment, emotional deprivation or abuse, or lack of an effective, supportive family, will render a child or young adult very susceptible to identification as 'a problem', and to be labelled as mentally retarded. In a supportive family, a child of similar intelligence is likely to escape the attention of formal agencies outside school. Racial bias has also been demonstrated in some societies.

Sex distributions have always favoured males. X-linked disorders have some effect, and girls tend to be more mature than boys, age for age, but the excess is probably mostly the result of social selection of 'unacceptable' male-type behaviour in boys and young men of low intelligence. Dull girls tend towards more passive behaviour at school, and as young women tend to show less aggressive and criminal behaviour. They are often more protected at home, where they may be given satisfactory domestic occupation whereas men are perceived as unemployed. Many individuals have the basic capacity to be independent and to enjoy an essentially normal lifestyle. Successful rehabilitation, or simply maturing with increasing age, may move people out of the category as they get older.

Selection criteria change over time in all societies. In developed countries, changes in the philosophy of care, diversification of professional involvement, and diminishing reliance on legal control or formal classification have led to fewer people being labelled as mentally retarded. However, these factors and processes operate differently in different communities, and without understanding them we can offer no interpretation or explanation of differences in prevalence of mild mental retardation, nor can we plan appropriate services.

Table 5 Factors affecting selection as mentally retarded

Legislation: criminal, health, education, social welfare, and employment law
Service structures and traditions: in education, health, social welfare, etc.
Professional cultures: concepts, perceptions, expectations, labelling, etc.
Patterns of employment and unemployment: work and training opportunities
Social class and social attitudes: cultural expectations, deprivation, discrimination, etc.
Family support: structures and security of families
Historical service patterns: clients inherited from earlier situations; e.g. institutional care
Perceived very low intelligence: with or without valid measures
Perceived low intelligence with additional factors: e.g. antisocial behaviour, mental illness, motor, sensory or communication disabilities, multiple disabilities
Certain medical diagnoses: especially Down's syndrome

Central nervous system impairment: aetiological diagnosis and prevention of intellectual impairment

Known pathological processes and syndromes which contribute to intellectual impairment through damage or disorder of the central nervous system are very many and mostly rare. In mild intellectual impairment, few cases have a single clear biomedical cause; aetiology lies in the interaction of polygenic inheritance, neurological impairments, and social factors. In severe intellectual impairment, all cases have demonstrable pathology, although only 80 per cent or so will be diagnosed in life even with good paediatric assessment.

However, a diagnosis does not imply a fully understood cause, which is usually a complex of causal processes and causal factors related to particular outcomes. The rubella virus can be said to cause rubella syndrome, but what determines maternal infection, fetal infection, and fetal response to infection? In Down's syndrome we know much about the processes of causation, but little of the ultimate causal agents. The same processes and factors which may result in severe or mild intellectual impairment, may also diminish intelligence at higher levels, or result in a neurological impairment with no effect on intelligence. Aetiological studies must relate to particular causal factors and particular pathological outcomes; multiple exposure variables and multiple outcome variables almost always preclude clear conclusions, as illustrated by the many studies of perinatal factors.

Types and frequencies of organic syndromes

Table 6 orders organic syndromes by the period of development of the principle aetiological factors, with a brief description, estimates of frequency, relationship to intellectual impairment, and potential for prevention. A few syndromes are major contributors: iodine deficiency in some communities; fetal alcohol syndrome in some; Down's syndrome and fragile X in most. Other syndromes are rare, and small numbers make causal studies and evaluation of preventive programmes difficult, requiring enormous populations. Thus most frequency data are uncertain, approximate, and provisional. The three groups of organic causes are summarized below.

Pure primary disorders are present from conception, an autosome or sex chromosome aberration in one gamete producing an abnormal chromosome constitution. Trisomy 21 is the archetype, but trisomies 13, 17/18, and others also occur. Sex chromosome disorders are seldom associated with significant intellectual impairment. X-linked disorders gained prominence with the elucidation of fragile X syndrome.

Primary disorders with secondary neurological damage do not affect the general constitution, but a genetically determined specific defect affects development, with or without environmental provocation. Phenylketonuria is the most common (0.05 to 0.2 per 1000 births) of many inborn errors of metabolism, in which absence of an enzyme disrupts metabolism of proteins, carbohydrates, lipids, or mucopolysaccharides. Brain damage and severe intellectual impairment arise if the hazardous dietary component is not excluded from infancy. Sporadic congenital hypothyroidism leads to cretinism if not identified and treated with thyroxine (T_4) from infancy.

Pure secondary disorders arise from an environmental insult to a normal zygote any time after conception. Prenatal causes include neural tube defects, iodine deficiency disease, rhesus incompatibility, and the effects of communicable diseases and toxic agents such as alcohol, drugs, and radiation. Perinatal processes are complex; the main factors are hypoxia, hypoglycaemia, cerebral thrombosis and haemorrhage, and gross trauma. Factors increasing vulnerability in the baby include very large baby, very small baby, immaturity, and pre-existing abnormality. Other factors lie in the mother. Postnatal causes include encephalitis and encephalopathy from communicable disease, trauma, and metabolic disasters in infants.

Cause, frequency, and prevention

Causes in individuals must be considered differently from causes in populations. For an individual case, one asks what factors contributed to the damage or disorder observed; for a population, one asks what factors contribute to the prevalence in that population. This is particularly important when planning preventive interventions. However 'biological' a known cause of neurological impairment may be, there will be social and environmental factors which increase or decrease its frequency in populations. We may not be able directly to intervene in the causal process, but we may be able to influence factors which reduce prevalence. For example, we do not know the underlying cause of non-disjunction in Down's syndrome and cannot intervene, but the prevalence of Down's syndrome is influenced by age of marriage, family size, attitudes to contraception, economic circumstances, education, religion, and the law, which act variably on inception rates and mortality. Even if only maternal age is reduced, birth prevalence will decrease.

The prevalence of recessive genetic disorders is determined by consanguinity, religion, and isolation. Fetal alcohol syndrome depends upon cultural traditions, attitudes to alcohol consumption in pregnancy, and government tax policies. Perinatal damage reflects early nutrition of girls, traditions of child birth, and distribution of services.

Similarly accidents, infectious diseases, neural tube defects, iodine deficiency disorders, and others are determined by environments, traditions, attitudes, government policies, and other factors. For most people with intellectual impairment, a medical diagnosis offers little scope for treatment or any advantage for habilitation, but for communities, diagnosis may offer many practical options for reducing incidence and prevalence mainly by manipulating social factors.

Prevention of intellectual impairment may be one of many justifications for social action, for example to reduce road, industrial, and home accidents, all common in both developed and developing countries. General economic and social development is important, and especially the situation of women, their economic status and roles within the family. A co-ordinated efficient service infrastructure is probably more important than high technology, but an appreciation of scientific issues in policy-makers is helpful. Both the prevention of intellectual impairment and the development of rehabilitation services are dependent on social and political stability.

Specific aetiological groups: causal processes, treatment, and prevention of the most important syndromes

Down's syndrome

Down's syndrome is a universally common cause of intellectual impairment, with IQs falling mostly within the range 20 to 55. About 94 per cent are due to chromosome non-disjunction leading to trisomy 21, of which birth frequency increases with maternal age: about 0.5 per 1000 at age 20, 1 per 1000 at 30, 2.5 per 1000 at 35, 10 per 1000 at 40, 40 per 1000 at 45, and more than 150 per 1000 at 50, but with some racial variation (Huether *et al.* 1998). The most effective strategy for prevention is to reduce births to older women. This has happened in many countries by the widespread use of the contraceptive pill.

Fetal diagnosis by amniocentesis, followed by abortion, is available in most developed countries, usually targeted at older women. Prescreening with serum markers (four currently available) and ultrasound is increasingly common, but, if offered to all women, increases the total number of amniocentesis procedures with their attendant risks (Wald *et al.* 1998). Ethical issues are not easily resolved. Generally, no more than half of all Down's fetuses are detected, and women are offered only a calculated risk that they are carrying a Down's baby. Are they willing to undergo abortion if the tests reveal a high risk? Can they understand the basis on which the risk is calculated? At what level of risk should they be asked to decide on termination?

Until recently it was thought that 75 to 85 per cent of Down's syndrome was of maternal origin, but recent DNA polymorphic analysis suggests that it may be 90 to 95 per cent. Most non-disjunctions occur at the first meiotic division, during the mother's

Table 6 Aetiology of organic syndromes related to intellectual impairment (frequencies are approximate and sometimes insecure)

Primary disorders (chromosome aberrations which are present at conception)

Down's syndrome

Trisomy 21 (94% of all Down's syndrome): birth prevalence varies with maternal age

age 20: 0.5 per 1000	age 40: 10 per 1000
age 30: 1.0 per 1000	age 45: 40 per 1000
age 35: 2.5 per 1000	age 50: 150 per 1000

Trisomy mosaics (1%–3%): birth prevalence 0.03 per 1000

Translocation (3%–5%): birth prevalence 0.03 per 1000

(All except a few mosaics are intellectually impaired, generally in the IQ range 30–55)

Other autosomal anomalies: birth prevalence 2–4 per 1000

Includes Patau's, Edward's, and cri-du-chat syndromes

(Only occasionally severely or mildly intellectually impaired)

Sex chromosome disorders: birth prevalence 2–3 per 1000

(Only occasionally severely or mildly intellectually impaired)

Non-specific disorders associated with intellectual impairment

(a) Recessive: birth prevalence ?0.5 per 1000

(b) X-linked: birth prevalence 0.2–0.3 per 1000 (most boys but few girls are intellectually impaired; see text)

Doubtful aetiology

De Lange syndrome (always intellectually impaired)

Hypercalcaemia syndrome (usually intellectually impaired by later childhood)

Primary disorders with secondary neurological damage (specific impairments from conception but damage occurs later, with or without environmental provocation)

Defects of protein metabolism

Phenylketonuria: birth prevalence 0.05–0.2 per 1000

At least five others: aggregated birth prevalence 0.1 per 1000

(All severely intellectually impaired if untreated)

Defects of carbohydrate metabolism

Galactosaemia: birth prevalence 0.02 per 1000

(All severely intellectually impaired and die early if untreated)

Defects of lipid metabolism

Tay–Sachs disease: birth prevalence 0.04 per 1000 in Ashkenazi Jewish communities; rare elsewhere

Batten's disease: frequency uncertain

(All severely intellectually impaired and die early)

Defects of mucopolysccharide metabolism

Hurler's syndrome: birth prevalence 0.03 per 1000

(All severely intellectually impaired)

Defects of hormone system

Sporadic congenital hypothyroidism: birth prevalence 0.1–2.0 per 1000

(Intelligence variably but seriously affected unless treated from very early infancy)

Mechanism not clear

Epiloia (tuberous sclerosis): birth prevalence 0.01 per 1000

Neurofibromatosis (Von Recklinghausen): birth prevalence 0.33 per 1000

Some cases of microcephaly

(Effect on intelligence very variable)

Secondary disorders (a normal gamete is damaged after conception)

Antenatal factors

Iodine deficiency disorders: cretinism; frequency of severe intellectual impairment very variable; can be more than 10 per cent of whole populations

Neural tube defects: birth prevalence 1–8/1000, possibly 10 per cent intellectually impaired

Rhesus incompatibility: intellectual impairment varies

Communicable diseases: frequency of fetal infection, brain damage after infection, and intelligence after brain damage (Table 7 and text)

Alcohol: fetal alcohol syndrome; many cases severely intellectually impaired

Drugs; irradiation; heavy metals: no satisfactory data

Perinatal factors

Gross trauma, hypoxia, hypoglycaemia, and cerebral thrombosis

Often associated with cerebral palsy and epilepsy

(definitions are problematic and the frequency of damage is virtually unmeasurable)

Postnatal factors

Physical trauma; accidents

Communicable diseases; meningitis and encephalitis or encephalopathies

Chemical agents: lead may reduce intelligence a little

Nutritional/metabolic: high solute baby feeds combined with fever

(All very variable in frequency)

After Fryers (1984, 1991).

fetal life, remote from fertilization, and not susceptible to intervention. Increased incidence with maternal age may be related to ageing gametes within the ovary. There is some evidence that radiation could be a cause of non-disjunction at the second meiotic division. Those of paternal origin also arise just prior to fertilization; exposure to industrial toxins may be implicated, but intervention is not yet practicable. Of non-disjunctions 1 to 3 per cent show mosaicism, with a mixture of normal and abnormal cells and a variable picture of features, impairments, and disabilities. This probably explains the rare reports of a Down's person of normal intelligence and achievements. Three to five per cent of Down's syndrome is familial, due to gene translocation. Chromosome diagnosis is important to detect those for genetic counselling.

The typical features of Down's syndrome are recognizable in all races usually at birth, and include epicanthic folds over the eyes, a flattened upper nose, a narrowed cranium, and a small mouth, often with a protruding tongue. Hands and fingers are short, with only one prominent skin crease. Between 25 and 40 per cent have a serious heart defect, and many have increased vulnerability to infectious diseases, both major causes of early death. First-year mortality in developed countries has decreased from 50 to about 10 per cent, and many individuals now live at least into late middle age (Table 3) (McGrother and Marshall 1990; Hayes *et al.* 1997). In developing countries where early mortality is high, few Down's children survive. Hypothyroidism, leukaemia, and diabetes are relatively common in adults, and Alzheimer's dementia is common in those who reach middle age.

Fragile X syndrome

The prevalence at birth of this sex chromosome disorder is still subject to improving diagnostic techniques; recent studies suggest much lower figures than previously estimated, probably 0.2 to 0.3 per 1000 (Morton *et al.* 1997). A majority of affected boys have IQs below 70, but a minority of boys, and virtually no girls have IQs below 50. About 70 per cent of girls who carry and can transmit the genetic abnormality are otherwise unaffected; most of the others are mildly intellectually impaired. Clinical diagnosis is unreliable, but men with severe intellectual impairment show a variety of physical abnormalities including, commonly, large testes and long ears. They may show autistic behaviours. Screening of groups of mentally retarded men permits genetic counselling of family members about risks for future children. Population screening to detect carriers is barely feasible and not yet evaluated (Murray *et al.* 1997). Ethical and resourcing issues need addressing before the pressures of technical advance pre-empt them.

Inheritable metabolic disorders

Congenital hypothyroidism occurs sporadically in all communities (0.1–2.0 per 1000) unrelated to iodine deficiency, usually as a mutation.

Thyroid failure leads to cretinism, with severe intellectual impairment, if not detected and treated with T_4 before 3 months of age. In most cases early treatment will largely preserve intelligence, but irreversible damage may occur in some before birth. In the variety called thyroid agenesis, very low T_4 levels at diagnosis, and treatment as late as 3 weeks of age, may result in some loss of intelligence, although not enough to be identified as mentally retarded. Treatment is, therefore, extremely urgent. Comprehensive screening programmes are now widely adopted using a simple blood spot test and laboratory analysis immediately after birth.

Logistically, these have often been mounted on longer established blood screening programmes for phenylketonuria (0.05–0.2 per 1000 births) and several other very rare enzyme disorders. In these, a defective gene leads to an enzyme deficiency and accumulation of toxic byproducts from normal constituents of diet, resulting in progressive brain damage and severe intellectual impairment. A special diet can prevent serious damage and allow children to develop with their intelligence relatively unaffected. The diet is not easy to take and must be continued at least into late childhood. Loss of intelligence is related both to the age of starting the diet and the control of blood phenylalanine. It is therefore of great importance to identify children very soon after birth, to start the diet immediately, and to monitor and maintain it closely throughout childhood. Optimal screening and treatment leads to no measurable loss of intelligence. The diet must also be reinstated during pregnancy to protect the fetus (Friedman *et al.* 1996). Such programmes are demonstrably effective and cost beneficial in developed countries, and lessons can be learned from the longest established programmes, such as that of 25 years in the United Kingdom (Seymour *et al.* 1997; Streetly and Corbett 1998).

Recessive genetic abnormalities in general

Although each specific syndrome is very rare, collectively they are important. Physical anomalies often predominate and may be susceptible to surgical correction. There may be any degree of intellectual impairment or none. They are thought to be mostly mutations, but, in communities with a high degree of consanguinity, a substantial proportion may be familial. Consanguinity may be a cultural tradition, or a product of geographical isolation (e.g. remote mountain or island communities), social isolation (e.g. elite groups or those marginalized by poverty), or cultural isolation (e.g. immigrant groups). Prevention requires education, but without relief of isolation this may have little effect. Because of the frequency of mutations, the avoidance of mutagenic factors in the environment might be important, including protection of industrial workers and communities from chemical or radiation exposure.

Neural tube defects

Neural tube defects are sometimes associated with intellectual impairment, especially where there is hydrocephalus. Epidemiologically, they show a clear geographical variation in incidence in many countries, and dietary folate deficiency is established as an important cause, possibly reflecting a metabolic fault. Any supplement is required before conception, as the damage often occurs before pregnancy is recognized. Since the risk is greatly increased after one affected baby, folate supplements (4000 μg/day) should always be given to prevent second neural tube defects. Large-scale studies have shown that incidence can be reduced by changes in diet or specific folate supplementation (Locksmith and Duff 1998), and all women who are at risk of pregnancy should ensure adequate folate intake of 400 μg/day. Supplementation is cheap and tablets easy to take, but information and encouragement alone have proved inadequate (Rosano *et al.* 1999). Some countries are adding folate to common foods, such as cereals in the United States, but the adequacy of the amount is disputed (Daly *et al.* 1997). About a third of neural tube defects may be resistant to folates. Environmental lead may also be a causal factor (Watkins 1998).

Fetal alcohol syndrome

Frequencies are variable, with high incidence in some communities, for example native Americans on 'reserves' with seriously prejudiced cultures, lack of employment, and high consumption of alcohol. In some countries high risk will be limited to certain subgroups and deviant individuals; this may explain the apparently much higher rates in the United States than Europe (Abel 1995). It is not yet certain what dose of alcohol represents a calculable risk of the full syndrome including severe intellectual impairment. There is evidence that damage less than the full syndrome may also arise from alcohol consumption (Bradley *et al.* 1998). The best advice is still to avoid alcohol completely during pregnancy. Further prevention means tackling alcohol consumption in general (Forrest and Florey 1991; Alberman 1992).

Iodine deficiency disorders

Worldwide, iodine deficiency is the most common cause of mental retardation. Iodine is essential for the production of T_4, without which metabolism is slowed, and all growth and development inhibited. Adults obtain the 150 μg/day they need mostly from water, but in many upland areas it has been leached from the soil and is insufficient. Variation in individual response to environmental iodine is not understood; other minerals, goitrogenic toxins in food, and genetic factors may each play a part.

In 1985 the WHO estimated 6 million people with cretinism in the Southeast Asian region alone, not including China (WHO 1985). In China, more than 10 per cent of some rural populations can show frank 'cretinism' with many more exhibiting goitres and varying degrees of growth retardation, although preventive programmes are now changing this (Wang *et al.* 1997). The estimated populations at risk are over 1500 million worldwide, 29 per cent of the world population, with huge numbers in China, India, and other Himalayan, Asian, South American, and African countries. It is estimated that 50 to 100 million people are at risk in Europe. At least 110 countries have an iodine deficiency disease problem (WHO 1993, 1994).

Endemic congenital hypothyroidism (cretinism) combines intellectual impairment, stunting, deaf–mutism, and neuromuscular disorders in varying degrees. Treatment usually produces no clinical or intellectual improvement, although rehabilitation can improve quality of life. Whole communities suffer poor levels of economic performance, education, and social life, and need rehabilitation.

Prevention is technically simple, effective, and cheap. Unfortunately, it is not always logistically or culturally easy to introduce and maintain. To increase iodine (preferably iodates for stability) in the diet of a whole community, the most common vehicle is salt, used by everyone throughout the year. With a limited number of sources, costs in 1988 could be around US$20 to 40 per 1000 people per year. However, poor quality control, distribution delays, lack of acceptance, and use of alternative sources of salt threaten the effectiveness of many programmes (Dunn 1996).

Injections of iodized oil are logistically more demanding and expensive, but more certain, and especially suitable for remote communities and fertile or pregnant women in the first two trimesters. One injection can be effective for several years, there are few side-effects, and no cold chain is required. Experience is now being gained with oral iodized oil, which enters body fat stores from which iodine is slowly released, and appears successful. Supplementation of drinking water, irregation water, bread, and common sauces have also been used. In some communities oral potassium iodide tablets may be appropriate.

The prevention of iodine deficiency needs political and professional will for success. The world programme to eradicate it by 2000 has done well but is not complete; every country with iodine deficiency disease needs a strong campaign (van der Haar 1997). It will be a generation before cretinism disappears from a community, but tangible benefits will be perceived in only a few years, and in the long run, a successful programme will pay off abundantly (Hetzel 1989).

General nutrition

Although many have asserted that gross maternal or early infant undernutrition can damage the central nervous system and cause irreversible intellectual deterioration, this is not supported by the evidence. The known pattern of early brain development offers ready explanation of both fetal and infant protection. The second period of brain growth, from 20 months of fetal life to 2 years of postnatal life, permits repair of any spongioblast damage up to that age (Stein *et al.* 1975; Dobbing 1984; Fryers 1990).

However, generalized malnutrition contributes to increased fetal and infant vulnerability to micro-organisms and other hazards. It may also contribute to poor learning function and delayed development (Grantham-McGregor *et al.* 1991). Children who experience severe prolonged malnutrition and grossly deviant social rearing, may present as mentally retarded yet have the capacity to recover normal mental and social function, and it is very important to identify such children and treat them with food, stimulation, love, and care. This may not be easy; children may be assumed to be permanently intellectually impaired, especially if in institutions without informed professional supervision. Most permanently impaired children can also develop more than professionals generally expect, with appropriate help. The important lesson is that all retarded children should be fully assessed and given good physical, mental, emotional, and educational care from the earliest age possible, to maximize their potential and minimize their dependence. Signs of unexpected progress should prompt active reinvestigation.

Perinatal factors

During the perinatal period, a baby faces several hazards—anoxia, hypoglycaemia, thrombosis, and trauma. We rarely know its fitness for birth, although very low weight for age or gross prematurity are strong indicators, or the mother's preparedness for delivery, which varies with age, parity, health, and nutritional state. The result may be neurological impairment, such as cerebral palsy and epilepsy, as well as intellectual impairment. But many cases, particularly of cerebral palsy, are now thought to arise earlier in pregnancy, and similar syndromes may also arise in infancy from meningitis and encephalitis. In populations, the relationship between healthy survival, damaged survival, and death is dynamic. Where many babies are damaged, many also die. If conditions improve, fewer babies may be damaged but more damaged infants may survive; prevalence at subsequent ages will not necessarily be lower (Johnson *et al.* 1993).

The scientific evidence is difficult to evaluate (Fryers 1990; Escobar *et al.* 1991; Dammann and Leviton 1997), but perinatal factors, not least very low birth weight, are without doubt important causes of intellectual impairment, cerebral palsy, epilepsy, and mortality, and all may be reduced in frequency by effective antenatal and obstetric care. This may mean improving nutritional state of mothers and young girls, increasing access to early antenatal care, training traditional birth attendants, providing professional midwives, building up the primary health care system, and ensuring skilled hospital obstetrics where required.

Communicable disease

Damage to the fetal or infant brain may arise occasionally in many infections (Table 7), although establishing a causal relationship is often difficult.

Endemic and epidemic variation precludes even guideline incidence rates, but if a particular disease is very prevalent, especially in a poor community, it is reasonable to assume that there are risks, especially of meningitis and encephalitis. Some regions, particularly in Africa, have especially high rates of meningitis.

Cytomegalovirus is common and may cause more damage than generally realized, including intellectual impairment and deafness. We have as yet no specific means of prevention. Rubella syndrome can be prevented by immunization, and congenital syphilis by early diagnosis and treatment; intellectual impairment is rare. The vaccine for *Haemophilus influenzae* type B brings hope for further immunization against bacterial meningitis and encephalitis. Chemotherapy is still important. Encephalitis in infancy carries a high risk of intellectual impairment, cerebral palsy, epilepsy, and death, and careful clinical handling may both determine individual outcome and prevent secondary cases.

Toxoplasma gondii is a common protozoal infection spread from animal faeces or poorly cooked meat. Fetal infection does occur, but signs are variable and may be late. Any degree of intellectual impairment can result, but risks are difficult to compute (MDWG 1992). Incidence varies, and there is no consensus on screening policy; universally offered in France, it is still debated in the United Kingdom and United States. Otherwise, prevention relies on good hygiene, but antibiotics during pregnancy may help.

Malaria increases vulnerability to other infections, and may sometimes damage the fetal or infant brain directly. Measles can occasionally cause late-onset damage which may include intellectual impairment with subacute sclerosing panencephalitis. High levels of population immunization are effective in prevention (Miller *et al.* 1992; Aaby *et al.* 1993).

Prevention of intellectual impairment due to communicable disease largely depends upon general public health measures—provision of safe water, waste water treatment, control of vectors, general hygiene, case isolation, early diagnosis and effective treatment, and improved resistance through good nutrition. Specific prevention by immunization is important. It provides individual protection but, more importantly, herd immunity if immunization rates of at least 90 per cent and preferably 95 per cent can be achieved to restrict spread. The measles–mumps–rubella (**MMR**) vaccine is very successful; pertussis and tuberculosis are also important. Some vaccines, particularly pertussis and MMR have been alleged to cause brain damage as occasional side-effects. Evidence for this tends to be circumstantial, and extensive scientific reviews have failed to confirm these risks, but proof of no risk by epidemiological assessment is very difficult. The public health consensus is that if there are risks, they are extremely small and are far outweighed by the risks of damage from the wild virus in the absence of immunization.

New vaccines are constantly becoming available, but the effectiveness of immunization programmes is determined by the quality of primary health care and public health organization. For more detail, regularly updated handbooks of communicable disease (Benenson 1990) should be consulted.

Table 7 Principle infectious agents causing intellectual impairment

Intrauterine
Cytomegalovirus
Rubella
Varicella zoster
Herpes simplex
Listeriosis
Syphilis
Toxoplasmosis
Malaria
Trypanosomiasis
Cysticercosis
Cryptococcosis
Perinatal
Group B streptococci
Escherichia coli
Enteroviral infections
Herpes simplex
Other Gram-negative organisms
Postnatal
Bacterial meningitides
Pneumococcal
Meningococcal
Tuberculosis
Haemophilus influenzae
Bordetella pertussis
Viral encephalitides
Herpes simplex
Measles
Varicella
Mumps
Rubella
Arboviruses A and B
Echoviruses
Coxsackie A and B
Parasitic infections
Malaria
Trypanosomiasis
Cysticercosis
Cryptococcosis

Postnatal infection can trigger several different mechanisms to provoke brain damage, and some are better described as reactive encephalopathies rather than direct encephalitides.

After Dudgeon *et al.* (1985).

Commonly associated syndromes of impairments and/or disabilities

Certain complex syndromes, although separate entities, are frequently associated with significant degrees of intellectual impairment and are always prominent in groups of people defined as mentally retarded. Congenital abnormalities tend to occur together in populations and sometimes in individuals. Epilepsy and cerebral palsy commonly arise from the same aetiological process as intellectual impairment before, during, or after birth. Proportions vary with the way mentally retarded groups are defined, and with the spectrum of aetiologies in different communities, but epilepsy is reported in 20 to 50 per cent of people with severe intellectual impairment (IQ < 50) (Hannah and Brodie 1998). Many cases can be controlled with medication. It is a specific component of tuberose sclerosis. Cerebral palsy is reported in 15 to 40 per cent of those with severe intellectual impairment, depending on the thoroughness of neurological examination. There are few data from developing countries, but both cerebral palsy and epilepsy are likely to be common. Children with cerebral palsy and epilepsy need medical assessment, treatment, and supervision to minimize the physical disabilities so that optimal development of intellectual abilities, at whatever level, can be promoted.

Autistic spectrum disorders are often associated with intellectual impairment but, given the profound and complex communication problems characteristic of autism, this should not be assumed without specific evidence. Strictly defined, autism is probably only 2 to 4 per 10 000 of the child population in developed countries, 50 to 75 per cent of whom may be considered to be mentally retarded. Using broader case definitions, autistic spectrum disorders are more prevalent; some, like Asberger's syndrome, are less likely to be associated with intellectual impairment. Another syndrome has been described, the 'triad of social and language impairments' (Wing 1996). There is evidence of gender and race differences in patterns of disability and behaviour. Variable neurological response to similar environmental insults is possible.

Many studies have reported higher prevalence rates of psychiatric illness in those designated mentally retarded, but there are serious problems of interpretation when neither term is clearly or consistently defined. Non-psychotic disorder is probably common, related to brain disorder, experience of abnormal social and interpersonal environments, or other impairments and disabilities. People identified as mentally retarded tend to be subject to closer surveillance than the rest of the population, not least by psychiatrists, who thus have unusual opportunities to make diagnoses. However, psychiatric examination is often extremely difficult in people with severe intellectual impairment, and many psychiatric disorders described in the literature are minor or ambiguous, and overlap with categories of challenging behaviour (Smith *et al.* 1995).

Anxiety and depression are susceptible to treatment and are almost certainly recognized less frequently than they should be. Schizophrenia has often been said to be found in '3 per cent of the mentally retarded', but comparing lifetime prevalence has proved almost impossible since definitions of both groups are so variable, and the only good, full community study produced figures of 1 per cent like the rest of the population (Turner 1989).

Behaviour disorders are not necessarily comparable phenomena in people with and without serious central nervous system impairment. But there is no doubt about the importance of the relatively few intellectually impaired people who exhibit serious challenging behaviour, because of their impact on families, communities, and services. This is especially true for people with relatively high IQs who are also fully mobile (Mansell 1993).

Problems arise not only on account of ambiguous definitions, but also because the presence of several impairments and/or disabilities makes examination, diagnosis, and assessment extremely difficult. It should also be remembered that any concurrent disability, disease, or deviant behaviour may render an individual more likely to be identified as 'mentally retarded' by health workers, social workers, police, or the courts, so that such problems are inevitably over-represented.

Specific disabilities

Identification and assessment of mentally retarded people

As well as learning disabilities and the common disability syndromes, many people with intellectual impairment suffer motor and sensory disabilities which have a serious impact on their daily lives. Although many clinical assessments are available, scientific measurement and taxonomic development of disabilities have received relatively little attention. There are, indeed, formidable epidemiological problems in standardizing instruments and discriminating degrees of disability. Many instruments provide individual profiles of abilities and disabilities to inform individual programme planning, but do not permit comparative study. An exception, Wing's Handicaps, Behaviour and Skills Schedule has been used for comparative research in several countries (Wing 1980; Ort and Cooper 1984) and generated a short Disability Assessment Schedule suitable for studies in service settings (Holmes *et al.* 1982).

Those studies showed that mobility and degree of social interaction are better indicators of demanding behaviour and need for care, than IQ. Mobile children with poor social interaction are particularly difficult to manage in any setting, and those with higher IQs may be the most difficult of all. Prevalence rates in European-type populations are likely to be between 0.25 and 0.5 per 1000. About three-quarters of these are severely intellectually impaired; a few would have IQs above 70.

It has already been noted that epilepsy is found in 20 to 50 per cent, and cerebral palsy in 15 to 40 per cent of people with severe intellectual impairment. Many motor and sensory disabilities are commonly associated with intellectual impairment, increasing in frequency with lower IQ. Serious visual problems are found in 10 to 30 per cent of people with severe intellectual impairment (IQ < 50), hearing problems in up to 5 per cent, and serious problems with speech in 60 to 85 per cent. The communication problems which result from these often outweigh all other social consequences; they make assessment difficult to perform and services difficult to provide.

These features of the population must be taken fully into account when planning care, especially the provision of personnel, but these generalities do little to guide care for individuals. Thorough, individual assessment of all impairments, disabilities, and abilities is essential if individual children and adults are to be given help specific to their needs. Standard forms should be used wherever possible in order to promote clear thinking and encourage well-planned programmes of education, habilitation, treatment, and care, tailored to individual need and susceptible to rigorous monitoring. Clarifying variations in client behaviour and performance in different environments will also encourage evaluation of different interventions.

It should be noted that assessments of function in restrictive, institutional settings, or of people whose experience has been largely in such settings, may exaggerate problems and underestimate individual potential. It is a common experience in practice to find severely intellectually impaired people doing far better in community settings than expected, in terms of self-care, domestic skills, social competence, and degree of independence.

Consideration of the range of disabilities experienced by intellectually impaired people also implies that 'good medical care' means carefully planned, positive habilitation or rehabilitation, with clear objectives and professional techniques of intervention applied to all areas of disability. Professional contributions are required, where possible, from physiotherapy, speech therapy, occupational therapy, psychology, family doctor, paediatrician, and psychiatrist, as well as the skills of teachers, nurses, social workers, and carers. Medical and surgical treatment should not be neglected where specific functions can be improved. Behaviour modification and other psychology programmes should be professionally designed; they can crucially improve behaviour and permit learning and development otherwise inhibited. However, professional staff and family carers should also recognize the abilities and resources which intellectually impaired people bring to their own needs, and build upon them to extend the scope of their experience and enhance their lives.

In well-resourced services, many people are involved in the 'team', and there is a danger of unco-ordinated, poorly focused, and inefficient services. The family may be neglected as the principle source of care for many clients, but also in respect of their own needs. Even the client's needs and preferences may be lost sight of in the complexities of team work. The concept of the 'key worker' has proved invaluable in addressing these problems, especially in community-based, multidisciplinary, and multiagency services. But teams are necessary—sharing knowledge, skills, and experience is essential when disabilities are so wide ranging and so disadvantageous.

In developed countries, severely mentally retarded children will usually be identified in infancy through routine developmental examinations. In countries with few services for mentally retarded children, children may not be identified because there seems no advantage in doing so. However, mothers have usually observed developmental delay or other problems, and their anxieties need to be seriously addressed. Even where no schooling is available, parents can be supported and advised on early stimulation, play, and teaching that they can do at home. School systems frequently identify children with milder degrees of intellectual impairment, but in many developing countries obviously retarded children never start school.

In any culture, a sense of shame can drive parents to hide an obviously disabled child, sometimes with the collusion of officials and professionals. Conversely, special services for retarded children in many countries were started by parents themselves long before wider recognition of the need. This process continues in developing countries, but not all families are involved. Screening programmes or surveys to identify unknown cases should only be undertaken when services can be offered to those identified. When children are suspected of delayed development, parents need to be fully informed and involved throughout the processes of identification, diagnosis, and assessment. Once identified, parents need careful counselling to help them to come to terms with their new reality; this may be done by professionals, but carefully chosen parents who have been through a similar experience themselves can be very effective.

Assessment poses different problems in developed and developing countries. In the former, many professions claim specialist expertise. Each has a professional orthodoxy and each has a range of conventional assessment techniques and instruments. Co-ordination by a key worker is essential if children and families are not to get lost in the maze, and expensive resources are not to be wasted. In developing countries, the few specialists are usually confined to urban centres. For most children, assessment must come from primary health workers and local school teachers who need training in the recognition of mental retardation, in developmental and functional assessment, and in the potential for habilitation within the family and community.

Assessment should not be used to exclude people from services, but as a starting point for action. Assessments are always age related and compare performance with norms from a reference population (which is not always appropriate) in order to identify immediate needs, and to predict and monitor progress. It is important to assess abilities as well as disabilities, strengths as well as weaknesses, as these represent vital resources for the future. Where possible, assessment should include both formal testing and less structured observation in familiar environments. There are many scales, tests, and checklists; some are suitable for population screening, others for individual assessment. These are described in Mittler's (1992) wide-ranging summary and annotation, and Hogg and Raynes' (1987) critical review. Few tests are validated for developing country populations, and must therefore be used with caution.

Sensory assessment is important, as poor sight and especially deafness can prejudice the assessment of development and intelligence. Hearing tests need special equipment and training. Motor disabilities, epilepsy, cerebral palsy, and psychiatric illness should be fully assessed, for which standard protocols are increasingly used, as doctors are generally poorly trained in functional assessment.

Intelligence tests giving IQs have been in and out of fashion. Their potential and problems are usefully discussed in Graham and Lansdown (1992). They are not independent of education, experience, and culture, and should always be repeated, should include subscores, and be accompanied by an interview report. Shortened tests are available for use by less trained workers. Development tests use age-related 'milestones' for young children (e.g. Gesell, Griffiths, or Bayley tests). Few formal tests are standardized for developing country populations, and are thus of doubtful validity; behaviour checklists may be more useful to guide specific interventions, as in the Portage system.

Social adaptation is assessed to guide rehabilitation. The American Adaptive Behaviour Scale is relatively complex, examining personal independence and maladaptive behaviour in over 20 areas of social function such as self-direction, responsibility, and socialization. The Vineland Social Maturity Scale is simpler but more used for research. The Progress Assessment Chart (Gunzberg 1977) is used in developing countries successfully, providing a progressive visual record of mobility, self-care, practical skills, and communication. Others have been developed locally.

Social disadvantages can only be assessed in a specific cultural context; there are no standard methods. They often represent the greatest burdens and needs. Table 8 gives examples of key questions which should be addressed.

Table 8 Assessment of disadvantage—examples of questions to be asked

What social roles should a person of this age and sex be fulfilling in this society?
What social roles could this person be fulfilling even with his/her disabilities?
What would help to increase independence now and in the future?
What activities would he/she like to undertake in this particular social context?
What activities would the family like him/her to share in this community?
What barriers are there in the community to his/her participation in activities?
What barriers are there in him/her which inhibit participation?
What strategies can be adopted to improve the situation in each case?

Dependency: community needs and organization of services

History, organization, and philosophy of care

Since the latter part of the nineteenth century, intellectual impairment has gradually emerged as a distinct and significant problem in all communities. Severe mental retardation was discriminated from serious mental illness and the extension of primary education revealed those with serious learning disability. But the determinants of behaviour were ill-understood, and identified mental retardation was clearly associated with poverty and social deprivation. Eugenicists aroused fears of degradation of the population if such people were permitted to reproduce freely. In many countries, repressive legislation promoted special institutions, usually remote, custodial in character, and housing between 50 and 5000 or more people. They were generally poorly resourced and attracted poor quality and ill-trained staff, yet they constituted almost the only service available for people with mental retardation, hiding them from public view, and reinforcing stigma, prejudice, and pessimism.

Over the past 30 years or so, communities have been struggling to overcome this tragic inheritance and to build humane, individualized, and professional community-based services promoting self-esteem, dignity, independence, integration in ordinary society, and the enjoyment of normal lifestyles. Most of the dilemmas of current services reflect this radical change, which can be seen in almost all countries, although at different stages of development and with some cultural variation. The motivation for change came from increasing activity by parents and parents' associations, an increasing professional awareness of the human rights of people with intellectual impairment, and political responses to public exposure of scandalous practices and conditions in institutions.

Parents have frequently led the way towards modern services. Most parents never wanted their children removed into institutional care, but acceded to it in the absence of alternatives. They came together in local associations to provide mutual support, to demand better community services from the statutory authorities, and themselves to provide play groups, schools, day centres, workshops, respite care, leisure facilities, holidays, and other services. In many countries, these services were later adopted, funded in full or part, or partnered by government agencies, and many patterns of organization can be found. They particularly helped to stimulate the development of special education and adult day services, which made it so much easier for them to keep their sons and daughters at home.

It is common for intellectually impaired people to be the object of fear, ridicule, and discrimination, and for their families to experience shame and guilt. Segregated institutional services tend both to reflect and to reinforce negative images and attitudes in society, and such stigma permits devaluation and encourages maltreatment. The movement against institutions emphasized basic human rights and the necessity, not merely of improving standards of care in institutions, but of creating radically different services with objectives far beyond care: promoting satisfactory ordinary lifestyles for mentally retarded people, integrated in ordinary communities, participating in roles and activities valued in their own cultures, developing their abilities to the full, and in control of their own lives as far as possible.

These processes, and the philosophy which underpins them, are commonly called 'normalization', and operate according to the 'ordinary life' model. They require the overt presence of mentally retarded children and adults in communities: only when they are accepted as part of society's everyday experience will stigma be seriously challenged, and their and their families' rights to as fulfilling a life as lies within their capacity, begin to be realized.

To promote personal independence is an important principle for services, but is difficult for people with severe degrees of intellectual impairment or multiple disability. Parents must be fully involved, especially for children, but there can be conflict of interest for parents as principle caregivers, and as people with their own needs and aspirations. If such conflicts are to be sensitively resolved, professional support must be local and accessible, with no barriers of stigma, and mediated by personal workers well known to and accepted by the clients.

More recently, 'advocacy' has been promoted to guarantee legal and civil rights, to protect from abuse or degrading treatment, to demand information, and to assist very limited clients to make known their own desires and responses. 'Normalization' as a complete philosophy has its critics (Brown and Smith 1992) and it is probably best to see it as a set of valuable ideas and principles which must always be worked out pragmatically in particular situations and for particular people.

A revolution in care

Thus organizational development over the last 30 years has focused upon restricting new admissions to institutional care, relocating existing residents into 'the community', and building up a range of small-scale accommodation, education, work and leisure facilities, networks of social support, and access to generic services, which make 'the community' a practical reality.

The costs of this process are not negligible: high-quality community services may cost no more than high-quality institutional care, but most institutional care had been under-resourced and was not of high quality. Moreover, where most of the mental retardation budget was tied up in institutions, it could not be released for the development of alternatives until sections, and ultimately a whole institution could be closed. Thus extensive 'bridging' funds have been required. The process also required changes in location, training, and attitudes of staff, with important implications for professional recruitment, training, and organization. Nevertheless, many countries in Europe, North America, and Australasia have moved a long way towards total closure of the old institutions and their replacement with comprehensive community services, not least the United Kingdom where the national programme has been spread over 20 years. It must be emphasized, however, that closure must not precede the provision of alternatives, as has happened in some countries with dire consequences.

Professional rigidities and vested interests pose serious problems. It can be argued that medical, specifically psychiatric, domination, characteristic of institution-based services, has generally damaged the interests of intellectually impaired people and their families, despite much committed, compassionate, and imaginative work by some doctors. It is safer, healthier, and more creative for responsibility to be shared between the many professional groups who have a role in serving clients' needs.

Increasing professionalization has characterized both social workers and nurses, who find the relative independence of domiciliary work attractive, but other professionals are also involved in well-resourced services, each reflecting the emphases, limitations, and culture of their own profession's training and traditions, and the objectives and constraints of their own employing agencies. There is a danger of conflicting agendas, lack of co-ordination, and waste of resources. The need for multiprofessional and multiagency co-ordination, planning, and evaluation of an increasingly complex network of diverse services places mental retardation firmly in the domain of public health. The principles of human services are illustrated in Table 9.

Although there are many patterns of service organization, most have some form of local, multidisciplinary team to provide specialist advice, support, and counselling, to mediate access to services and welfare benefits, and to refer for medical and other specialist help. Some service systems do far more, controlling networks of residential and day care or managing a complex of services for a whole community. They frequently operate from a designated community centre, which may be a wide-ranging resource for mentally retarded people and their families. A key-worker system is favoured by many to combine personal access for clients with co-ordination of a team of several members.

Table 9 Principles of human services

Services should, as far as is possible, enable people to live ordinary lives by using means which are common, accepted and valued in their local community and culture
Services should enhance the status of disabled people by both what they do and how they do it
Services should acknowledge and respect disabled people as individual human beings with their own needs, preferences, abilities and social networks
Services should work with disabled people, who retain, as far as possible, the iniative, choice and direction of their own habilitation and lives
Disabled people should not be segregated from the rest of the community in housing, work, education or recreation
Special services should be available to meet needs inadequately served by ordinary means; these should be local and accessible to all relevant clients in the community served
Services should be professional in management and staffing, efficiently co-ordinated, and subject to effective quality control

Mentally retarded people's human needs are primarily the same as other people's: love and parental care, family life, a range of relationships, and opportunities for valued activities. Like others, they need access to professional help—teachers, doctors, and the like—but they may need more early stimulation, education, and training especially in self-care, practical literacy, social skills, and vocational skills. They usually need extra encouragement and support in establishing and maintaining themselves in any aspect of normal community life. A comprehensive community-based service complex will be coherent and co-ordinated within a definable community. It will encompass a home to live in, education, work and training for work, leisure, access to generic services, and provision of specialist services according to need. Each is discussed below.

Developing countries

Institutional models of care can be found in many developing countries, but almost everywhere, most retarded children and many adults, remain at home. Until recently, professionals and politicians largely ignored the needs of mentally retarded people and their families, and initiatives have come largely from parents and the organizations they have created. The International League of Societies for Mentally Handicapped Persons (now Inclusion International) helps member societies in many ways including 'partnerships' between those in developed and developing countries.

The International Year of the Disabled Person 1981 gave great encouragement; although situations vary greatly, the basic philosophy, principles, and elements of good practice are largely the same (Mittler and Serpell 1985). Developed countries may learn much from recent experience in developing countries, where limited funds have ensured appropriate local use of technology and the resources of families, social networks, and community volunteers, supported by specialists only when necessary.

The model has become known as community-based rehabilitation, and programmes often encompass all types of disability. Even where few specialist services exist, much can be achieved, and teaching and training materials are now available to guide those with little special experience. The model emphasizes appropriate technology and use of locally available people and resources, in the belief that effective local action which brings basic rehabilitation to many disabled people is better than waiting for sophisticated rehabilitation in urban centres serving few. Materials include the WHO manual *Training in the Community for People with Disabilities* (Helander *et al.* 1990), a collection of many simple and lucid 'training packages' which can be freely copied and distributed, the book *Disabled Village Children* (Werner 1987), and a regular newsletter *CBR News* from Healthlink Worldwide in London. These and many others also address rehabilitation for motor and sensory disabilities commonly associated with intellectual impairment.

An effective community-based rehabilitation programme would have community-level programmes for individual retarded people and their families run by local rehabilitation workers and supervisors. Special school facilities and day centres would offer a variety of training, sheltered work, and leisure opportunities. Specialist professionals from health centres, hospitals, colleges, and social welfare agencies, would support the programmes with guidance, staff training, and consultation, and provide access for some individuals to treatment or training in appropriate specialist centres. This model can be applied at many different levels of resourcing, but it always requires local community, professional, and political commitment.

Community-based rehabilitation projects have been set up in many countries by committed individuals, local non-governmental organizations, governments, and international agencies including the WHO and UNICEF. Evaluation is difficult, but experience is increasing understanding of the conditions for success. However, most programmes remain small scale and rural, and expanding to cover large populations has proved difficult, although there are now some examples, for example, in India. Some countries (e.g. Thailand) are grafting community-based rehabilitation onto a primary health care system. Even in cities, a community-based rehabilitation approach and overview may help to provide a rational structure for service development within which parents, professionals, and government services can co-operate.

Several training courses have been developed for community-based rehabilitation workers, but training should be as much as possible in the community where there is a community-based rehabilitation programme. It is important that disabled people and their families are involved in training their future professionals. Basic attitudes are important; selection is as important as training. Supervision and continuing training are essential, together with satisfactory career and pay structures, to ensure an appropriate status for them, their work, and their clients. Recommendations, with an outline curriculum, for training mid-level workers are available (WHO 1992*b*) which emphasize problem-solving approaches.

Components of community-based mental retardation services

Living in your own home

Intellectually impaired people have a right to enjoy a home of their own which promotes an 'ordinary lifestyle', minimizes stigma, and permits participation in the life of the community. Large residential institutions cannot provide this, and as they have diminished, we have rediscovered that almost all intellectually impaired adults can live in ordinary houses, within ordinary communities, as long as their special needs are met by support staff. Such staff may be only on call for those who are socially competent; they may visit regularly, attend during the day, or live-in, according to need. The best programmes limit the numbers living in one house to a 'family' size (usually a maximum of four to eight), but few large populations have yet achieved this comprehensively. Larger 'hostels', built in the first wave of anti-institutional enthusiasm, are now subject to similar criticisms and plans for closure.

Good programmes disperse their houses so that there is no aggregation in the community, and therefore no tendency to develop an enclave or ghetto which can mimic a large institution. People from institutions are generally relocated to their communities of origin, but some have ties elsewhere or nowhere. It may be more important to give them a home with friends. Homes may be provided by local authorities, charitable trusts, voluntary associations, or commercial agencies, but tenancies need careful working out, and management must be co-ordinated with the care and support services. Where there is an atmosphere of optimism, openness about intellectual impairment, and good support services, most parents will wish to care for their own sons and daughters at home at least into adulthood, but they do need a great deal of support. Their educational role with children is discussed below, but there are potential conflicts of interest later between their principle carer role and their own personal needs. This requires sensitive and skilled professional handling, and a range of services providing week-day activities outside the home, and a variety of respite care inside and outside the home.

Children and adults may be fostered or, in some countries, adopted; professional support is equally important in these situations. Some young adults will choose to leave the parental home early; others will continue to live with parents, but will eventually need a home of their own, and this should be anticipated and prepared well before the crisis of their parent's death or incapacity. Professional support for parents can be supplemented by volunteers and community networks, not least those created by the parents themselves through their local associations.

An alternative model favoured by some is the 'village community', where people with intellectual impairment may experience freedom of movement, self-care, maximal personal decision-making, and a wide range of relationships and activities including appropriate work, but in a protected and separated 'commune'. There is little integration or participation in other communities, and it shares some of the potential for ignorance and stigma with traditional institutions, but offers many elements of 'ordinary life' which may provide a satisfactory compromise for some adults.

Special needs for physical care can almost always be provided in ordinary home settings if staff are available, but some see a residual role for institutions in providing for those with serious behaviour disorders. These are few in any one community, and a linked network of small scattered units allows them to retain contact with their families and communities of origin. The most difficult are usually those with mild intellectual impairment, but there are no easy answers for seriously challenging behaviour, including those who commit serious offences.

Education and training

People with intellectual impairment have a right to education appropriate to their special needs. Early stimulation is of great benefit and can often be given in the home by parents. The Portage system and its many adaptations provide a model whereby parents are trained and assisted by a home visitor in teaching their own children, using developmental checklists, a special manual, and an inventory of parent teaching behaviours. Similar programmes are in use in many developed and developing countries and many translations are available. Other programmes use parent group workshops.

Special education for learning disabled children has made great strides in the last 25 years in most industrialized and many developing countries. Many school systems offer similar standards of provision as for other children, but separate schools are still common. The argument for integration into ordinary schools is not wholly won for those with severe learning disabilities, and many compromises exist.

For more able children, special schools and special classes in ordinary schools are gradually being replaced by full or partial integration of individual children into ordinary classes, with additional resources as required. Where the quality of ordinary schools is very poor, it will be better to create special education of higher quality even if separate.

Young Down's children may fit in relatively easily, although less so as they get older. Children with additional physical or behavioural problems pose serious difficulties for school staff, however well trained, resourced, and supported. Few school systems are willing to confront these problems on the scale of whole communities (as in Arrezzo, Italy). Children with autism, whether intellectually impaired or not, need special educational methods provided by specialist teachers.

Whatever schooling is created, it should be located within the culture of the community, and involve parents; the home remains a primary locus of learning. Wherever possible, parents should be partners with teachers and children in co-ordinated individual programmes. Such programmes need to extend beyond school leaving which is a stressful time for many. Further education and training in community colleges has become common in some countries, either as separate, specially designed courses or fully integrated. They include training in life-skills and leisure use, as well as vocational training, which may also be offered in schools.

Work and leisure

For many young mentally retarded people, vocational training is important to ease their way into ordinary work. But for those with severe intellectual impairment, an 'ordinary working life' in economic employment is not an option. However, they do need the dignity of work, a structure for each day, a satisfying occupation, and continuing education for their personal and social development. Occupational therapists are invaluable in directing the development of appropriate services. Sheltered, protected, or subsidized work situations are necessary; there are many examples of good practice, sometimes in ordinary workplaces.

Most, however, are day centres providing a variety of work, training, and leisure activities, and representing a daily focus for clients' social life and contact with professional services. Where work is the primary focus, they should reflect the appearance and location of other workshops in the community. Work activities should not be merely repetitive and boring, but provide interest and scope for development. The best examples achieve a reputation for high-quality products which not only improves the economics of the centre, but gives a positive message to the community. This is easier for more able clients, who may be capable of ordinary productive work, but who may be the least favoured employees when general unemployment is high. In some communities, co-operatives of disabled and non-disabled workers are successful.

Special centres for work activities and environments should be supplemented by job placement programmes. Personal contact with employers, negotiated individual placement, and assistance with on-the-job training and supervision, can achieve higher levels of employment. In some countries subsidies are offered to employers to accept less efficient disabled workers. Others have legal employment quotas for disabled workers in larger firms, although these are seldom effective, especially for people with intellectual impairment.

Severely intellectually impaired people may need to be taught how to gain satisfaction from leisure pursuits, participate in community activities, and gain access to leisure facilities. They need encouragement, advocacy, and sometimes active help to face the many barriers to community participation. But given the opportunities, many will enjoy swimming, horse riding, boating, and other active sports, as well as more passive outings and holidays, and the ambience of places where people generally meet in their particular community. Many will respond to careful introduction into the local public house or bar, leisure centre, arts centre, or church.

Access to generic and specialist health services

One of the benefits of community services is that people with intellectual impairment can have ordinary access to primary health care and the specialists in general hospitals. However, in practice, this may need the mediation of mental retardation professionals to make it happen. Family doctors and their nurse colleagues can be invaluable resources for clients, families, teams, schools, and centres, as there are many health problems encountered by intellectually impaired people. Dental treatment often poses problems, and particular dentists need to gain special experience, and establish relationships with clients.

However, many also have mental, emotional, and behavioural problems, physical deformities, speech and sensory defects, epilepsy, cerebral palsy, and others which need specialist medical attention as for other people in their community. Thus psychiatrists, orthopaedic surgeons, ear and eye specialists, and neurologists will be particularly needed, together with psychologists, physiotherapists, and speech therapists. Although rights to specialist health care, and problems of access will vary within the health-care system of different countries, access will often have to be negotiated because of stigma, stereotyping, ignorance, and prejudice amongst hospital staff. In many service systems, specialists have formal attachments so that clients and families can get to know them, and they can also advise staff of day centres and homes. In the United Kingdom, the establishment of general psychiatrists 'with a special interest' in mental retardation, has been very successful.

Monitoring and evaluation

Co-ordinating training and development activities in a variety of service settings can be difficult. Many services are operated without clear, stated goals or the means of monitoring progress. In recent years, individual programme plans, based on systematic assessments, agreed with the client, family, and care staff, which are written down and monitored, have been widely adopted (Table 10). The idea draws elements from the 'nursing process', management 'goal setting', behaviour therapy, and task-centred social work traditions, and assumes a developmental approach, asserting that all intellectually impaired people have potential for development.

Even where an individual programme plan system is very simple, it fosters discipline by using standard methods and records. It is especially needed where several staff members or centres concurrently serve one client; it should involve parents wherever possible. After assessment, precise short- and medium-term goals are agreed, trying to build on positive qualities and abilities, then the steps and tasks by which these objectives will be reached, and the people responsible for each one. Checklists may be used. The process is managed and supervised, and includes regular reviews, updating, and reassessment. It also allows ongoing evaluation of each client's programme.

Much more demanding as in-house evaluation is the Program Analysis of Service System (Wolfensberger and Thomas 1983), and its

Table 10 Individual programme planning

Features
Written assessments of an individual's developmental status, strengths, weaknesses, resources, and needs in a structured format, through a structured process:
in consultation with the disabled person and others significant in his or her life
specifying agreed short- and long-term goals
the means by which they will be tackled
who is responsible for action
how performance will be monitored
identifying service deficiencies which prevent or restrict achievement of goals
Strengths
Is an effective way of co-ordinating action by several people, facilities, or agencies
Promotes a view (and assessment) of the disabled person and his/her life as a whole
Encourages a positive approach by emphasizing strengths and realizable goals
Encourages an individual approach to care and rehabilitation—a 'needs led' service
Ensures a strong voice for the 'consumer'
Assigns clear accountability for action
Helps those involved to recognize and measure progress
Fosters an imaginative response to individual need
Provides aggregated information on service deficiencies

more recent modifications. This provides a means of measuring local services against a normalization ideal, and formal training is offered to staff to enable them to apply it in their own work setting.

Evaluation of services can be approached in many ways. Comparative descriptive studies, quantitative or qualitative, interpreted by involved professionals, are not very informative. More useful, normative evaluation sets long-term outcome goals for each element of the service against which performance is measured; checklists are available. Formative evaluation has long-term goals but also sets short-term goals which are monitored regularly, so that services may be adjusted to maintain the overall direction. It is desirable to measure both effectiveness (achieving desired outcomes) and efficiency (relating effectiveness to costs) of the means by which services are delivered, but process measures must often be used as proxies for outcomes. Evaluation protocols, with resources, should be built into any new services, as with the NIMROD Project in South Wales (Davies *et al.* 1990). Heron and Myers' thorough evaluation of services provided in the Sheffield Development Project is a rare example of a study of a complex service system (Heron and Myers 1983).

Accountability, including audit, is concerned with the proper use of resources and guaranteeing quality of care. Detailed costings are rarely available for specific elements of services where definitions may be very vague, and identifying discreet 'units' of care is not easy. Few cost–benefit studies have been done except for screening programmes. General agency audit tends towards oversimplification, but 'clinical audit' methods have greatly improved and have become generally accepted over the last few years. They should now be applied widely. It is difficult to take account of all cost elements, but potential benefits from the development of individual clients' performance and thus lower levels of dependency, should not be forgotten. High-quality services may be a good investment! More evaluation research is needed if we are to learn from present experience how better to serve people with intellectual impairment in the future.

Conclusion and summary

Generalized intellectual impairment, learning disability, and dependency represent distinct but overlapping concepts and classifications within the field of mental retardation. Rigour and clarity of thinking are required if progress is to be made in our understanding of these phenomena. Severe intellectual impairment is usually coextensive with categories called severe mental handicap or retardation because of a common IQ definition (< 50).

Prevalence is dynamic and changing, subject to many factors affecting incidence and mortality of the many contributing organic syndromes. It is equally subject to changes in population denominators. Prevalence at birth appears to be decreasing in most developed countries, but prevalence in adults is generally increasing due to increased survival. The largest cohort is currently in their mid-thirties. Mild mental retardation is socially determined, and to understand it, we must focus mainly upon the processes and factors determining selection as 'retarded' in particular communities.

Many organic aetiological factors are implicated, especially where intellectual impairment is severe. Some syndromes we can now prevent. The cost of public health programmes will usually be justified because of the devastating consequencies of these disorders, and the costs of lifetime dependency.

Needs are individual and varied, and thorough assessment of physical impairments and disabilities can be standardized and individual programmes monitored. Services should be guided by the general principles of 'normalization' and the 'ordinary life' model of care, which accord intellectually impaired people the same basic rights and privileges as others, to adopt roles and undertake activities valued in their community and culture, neither isolated nor alienated from their peers and neighbours. However, they should not be invisible to social policy-makers, service planners, or the providers of resources, for they necessarily need positive discrimination and affirmative action.

There is much to overcome from the past. Although intellectually impaired people have not offended, they have been placed in custodial care; although they pose no threat to the community, they have been removed to remote institutions; although they are not sick, their lives have been controlled by doctors and nurses. This is all changing. Increasingly the need for a home, education, work, leisure, and medical care is being judged on criteria similar to those for the rest of the population, and provided by the same agencies and the same personnel, in the same place and in the same manner. They and their families are people first, with a range of cultural expectations not easy to fulfil if you are intellectually impaired. Professional objectives are to help them to fulfil those aspirations as much as possible.

Care in the community, using the ordinary life model, is expensive, but probably no more expensive than high-quality institutional care. Community-based services are more demanding for personnel, but potentially more satisfying. However, it is difficult to maintain the necessary commitment, zest, imagination, and sensitivity without the full support of senior professionals and service managers, satisfactory conditions of pay and employment, and appropriate training. The public health challenge is to ensure a full range of social services to promote satisfactory lives for people of all ages with intellectual impairment, and for their personal carers, in a comprehensive, community-based service, with access to specialist care as individually required. Establishing new structures, making them work, and undertaking rigorous evaluation are all part of the challenge that currently makes the field of mental retardation in public health particularly exciting.

Useful addresses

Many important publications on services for people with intellectual impairment are available from these groups.

American Association for Mental Deficiency (AAMD), Washington, DC, USA

British Institute of Learning Disabilities (BILD), Kidderminster, UK

Campaign for People with Learning Disabilities (CPLD), London, UK

Disability Office, World Health Organization, Geneva

Healthlink Worldwide (formerly Appropriate Health Resources Technology Action Group (HRTAG)) London, UK

Inclusion International (formerly the International League of Societies for People with Mental Handicap (ILSMH)) Brussels, Belgium

International Association for the Scientific Study of Mental Deficiency (IASSMD)

Joseph Rowntree Foundation, York, UK

King's Fund Centre, London, UK

Lebenshilfe, Marburg, Germany

Mental Handicap in Wales Applied Research Unit, Cardiff, Wales, UK

National Institute for Mental Retardation (NIMR), Toronto, Canada

National Parents Associations

President's Committee on Mental Retardation (PCMR), Washington, DC, USA

Royal MENCAP, London, UK

Socialstyren, Stockholm, Sweden

Bibliography

General

Baine, D. (1988). *Handicapped children in developing countries.* Faculty of Education, University of Alberta, Edmonton.

Breuning, S.E., Matson, J.L., and Barrett, R.P. (ed.) (1985). *Advances in mental retardation and development disabilities.* JAI Press, Greenwich, CT.

Clarke, A.M., Clarke, A.D.B., and Berg, J.M. (ed.) (1985). *Mental deficiency: the changing outlook* (4th edn). Methuen, London.

Cooper, B. (ed.) (1981). *Assessing the handicaps and needs of mentally retarded children.* Academic Press, London.

Current Opinion in Psychiatry; Mental Retardation Current Science, London. (Reviews published literature from the previous year. *Mental Retardation* section published annually (October issue).)

Dobbing, J. (ed.) (1984). *Scientific Studies in Mental Retardation.* Royal Society of Medicine/Macmillan, London.

Emoe, R. and Harmon, R. (1985). *Continuities and discontinuities in development.* Plenum, New York.

Fryers, T. (1996). Mental retardation in the developing world. In *Psychiatry for the developing world* (ed. D. Tantam, L. Appleby, and A. Duncan). Gaskell Press, London.

International Review of Research in Mental Retardation. Academic Press, San Diego, CA. (An almost annual publication of commissioned reviews.)

Janicki, M.P. and Wisnievsky, H.M. (1985). *Aging and developmental disorders.* Brookes, Baltimore, MD.

Marfo, K., Walker, S., and Charles, B. (ed.) (1986). *Childhood disability in developing countries: issues in habilitation and special education.* Praeger, New York.

Russell, O. (1997). *Seminars in the psychiatry of learning disabilities.* Gaskell Press, London.

Snowden, L.R. (ed.) (1982). *Reaching the under-served: mental health needs of neglected populations.* Sage, Beverly Hills, CA.

Epidemiology

Belmont, L. (1984). *International epidemiological studies of childhood disability: final report.* Bishopp Becker Institute, Utrecht.

Durkin, M., Zaman, S., Thorburn, M., Hasan, M., and Davidson, L. (1991). Population-based studies of childhood disability in developing countries. *International Journal of Mental Health*, **20**, 47–60.

Farmer, R. (1992). *Dimensions of mental handicap.* Charing Cross and Westminster Medical School, London.

Fryers, T. (1997). Impairment, disability and handicap; categories and classifications. In *Seminars in the psychiatry of learning disabilities* (ed. O. Russell), pp. 16–30. Gaskell Press, London.

Fryers, T. and Russell, O. (1997). Applied epidemiology. In *Seminars in the psychiatry of learning disabilities* (ed. O. Russell), pp. 31–47. Gaskell Press, London.

Hogg, J. and Moss, S. (1993). Characteristics of older people with intellectual disabilities in England. In *International review of research in mental retardation* (ed. N.W. Bray), pp. 71–96. Academic Press, London.

Kiely, M. (1984). Descriptive epidemiology of cerebral palsy. *Public Health Review*, **12**, 79–87.

Kiely, M. (ed.) (1990). *Reproductive and perinatal epidemiology.* CRC Press, Boca Raton, FL.

Luckasson, R. (1992). *Mental retardation: definition, classification and systems of supports* (9th edn). AAMD, Washington, DC.

Richardson, S.A. (1987). The ecology of mental handicap. *Journal of the Royal Society of Medicine*, **80**, 203–11.

Richardson, S.A. (1989). Issues in the definition of mental retardation and the representativeness of studies. *Research in Developmental Disabilities*, **10**, 285–94.

Stanley, F. and Alberman, E. (1984). *The epidemiology of the cerebral palsies.* Spastics International and Blackwell Science, Oxford.

Specific syndromes, neurological impairments, and prevention

Aylward, G.P., Verhulst, S.J., and Bell, S. (1989). Correlation of asphyxia and other risk factors with outcome: a contemporary view. *Developmental Medicine and Child Neurology*, **31**, 329–40.

Aylward, G.P., Pfeiffer, S.I., Wright, A., and Verhulst, S.J. (1989). Outcome studies of low birth weight infants published in the last decade: a meta-analysis. *Journal of Pediatrics*, **115**, 515–20.

Baird, P.A. and Sadovnick, A.D. (1988). Maternal age-specific rates for Down syndrome: changes over time. *American Journal of Medical Genetics*, **29**, 917–28.

Berg, J.M. (1985). Biomedical amelioration and prevention. In *Mental deficiency: the changing outlook* (ed. A.M. Clarke, A.D.B. Clarke, and J.M. Berg) (4th edn), pp. 403–39. Methuen, London.

Boyages, S.C., Collins, J.K., Maberly, G.F., Jupp, J.J., Morris, J. and Eastman, C.J. (1993). Iodine deficiency impairs intellectual and neuromotor development in apparently normal persons. A study of rural inhabitants of north-central China. *Medical Journal of Australia*, **150**, 676–82.

Carter, C.H. (1979). *Handbook of mental retardation syndromes* (3rd edn). C.C. Thomas, Springfield, IL.

Carr, J. (1992). Longitudinal research in Down syndrome. In *International review of research in mental retardation* (ed. N.W. Bray), pp. 158–83. Academic Press, London.

Crocker, A.C. (1992). Data collection for the evaluation of mental retardation prevention activities; the fateful forty-three. *Mental Retardation*, **30**, 305–17.

Frith, U. (1991). *Autism and Asperger syndrome*. Cambridge University Press.

Gilbert, P. (1992). *The A–Z reference book of syndromes and inherited disorders*. Chapman & Hall, London.

Hosking, G. (1992). *Cerebral palsy; the child and the young person*. Chapman & Hall, London.

Lancet (1986). Prevention and control of iodine deficiency disorders. *Lancet*, **328**, 433–34.

Nadel, I. and Epstein, C.J. (ed.) (1992). *Down syndrome and Alzheimer disease: progress in clinical and biological research*. Wiley-Liss, New York.

Niswander, K.R. and Kiely, M. (1991). Intrapartum asphyxia and cerebral palsy. In *Reproductive and perinatal epidemiology* (ed. M. Kiely), pp. 357–70. CRC Press, Boca Raton, FL.

Palomaki, G.E. and Haddow, J.E. (1993). Is it time for population based prenatal screening for fragile X? *Lancet*, **341**, 373–4.

Smith, I., Beasley, M.G., and Ades, A.E. (1990). Intelligence and quality of dietary treatment in phenylketonuria. *Archives of Diseases in Children*, **65**, 472–8.

Turner, G., Robinson, H., Laing, S., *et al.* (1992). Population screening for fragile X. *Lancet*, **339**, 1210–13.

Disabilities and their consequences: identification and assessment

Bird, J. (1997). Epilepsy and learning disabilities. In *Seminars in the psychiatry of learning disabilities* (ed. O. Russell). Gaskell Press, London.

Bouras, N. (1994). *Mental health in mental retardation: recent advances and practices*. Cambridge University Press.

Emerson, E. (1995). *Challenging behaviour: analysis in people with learning disability*. Cambridge University Press.

Fraser, W.I. and Rao, J.M. (1991). Recent studies of mentally handicapped young people's behaviour. *Journal of Child Psychology and Psychiatry*, **32**, 79–108.

Fryers, T. (1986). Screening for developmental disabilities in developing countries: problems and perspectives. In *Childhood disability in developing countries: issues in habilitation and special education* (ed. K. Marfo, S. Walker, and B. Charles). Praeger, New York.

Nihira, K., Foster, R., Shellhaas, M., and Leland, H. (1974). *AAMD adaptive behaviour scale*. American Association on Mental Deficiency, Washington, DC.

Patel, P., Goldberg, D., and Moss, S. (1993). Psychiatric Morbidity in older people with moderate and severe learning disability; the prevalence study. *British Journal of Psychiatry*, **163**, 481–91.

Stein, Z., Durkin, M., Davidson, L., Hasan, M., Thorburn, M., and Zaman, S. (1992). Guidelines for identifying children with mental retardation in community settings. In *Assessment of people with mental retardation*. WHO, Geneva.

Zigman, W.B., Schupf, N., Zigman, A., and Silverman, W. (1993). Aging and Alzheimer disease in people with mental retardation. In *International review of research in mental retardation* (ed. N.W. Bray), pp. 41–70. Academic Press, London.

Overview of service provision: philosophy, law, planning, evaluation

Bewley, C. and Glendinning, C. (1994). *Involving disabled people in community care planning*. Joseph Rowntree Foundation, York.

Boswell, D.M. and Wingrove, J.M. (ed.) (1975). *The handicapped person in the community: a reader and sourcebook*. Open University Press, Milton Keynes.

Bradley, V.J. (1978). *De-institutionalisation of developmentally disabled persons: a conceptual analysis and guide*. University Park Press, Baltimore, MD.

Brechin, A. and Walmsley, J. (ed.) (1989). *Making connections: reflecting on the lives and experiences of people with learning difficulties*. Open University Press, Milton Keynes.

Disability Alliance (1995). *Disability rights handbook* (20th edn). Disability Alliance, ERA, London.

Flynn, R.J. and Nitsch, K.E. (ed.) (1981). *Normalisation, social integration and community services*. University Park Press, Baltimore, MD.

Fryers, T. (1983). *Standardisation of district mental handicap registers*. APMH, King's Fund Centre, London.

Fryers, T. (1989). *A curriculum for community rehabilitation workers*. Office of Rehabilitation, WHO, Geneva.

Glendinning, C. and McLaughlin, E. (1993). *Paying for care; lessons from Europe*. HMSO, London.

Independent Development Council (1982). *Elements of a comprehensive local service for people with mental handicap*. IDC, London.

Kavanagh, S. and Opit, L. (1998). *The cost of caring: the economics of providing for the intellectually disabled*. Politeia, London.

King's Fund (1988). *Ties and connections: an ordinary community life for people with learning difficulties*. King's Fund Centre, London.

Lindsey, M. (1998). *Signposts for success in commissioning and providing health services for people with learning disabilities*. National Health Service Executive, London.

McLaughlin, P.J. and Wehman, P. (1992). *Developmental disabilities: a handbook for best practice*. Butterworth Heineman, Oxford.

Malin, N. (ed.) (1994). *Implementing community care*. Open University Press, Milton Keynes.

Mansell, J. and Ericsson, K. (1995). *De-institutionalisation in Scandinavia, the USA and Britain: changing patterns of intellectual disability*. Chapman & Hall, London.

Matson, J.L. (1981). *Philosophy and care of the mentally retarded; a world wide status report*. Pergamon Press, Oxford.

Mittler, P. (1984). Evaluation of staff, services and training. In *Scientific studies in mental retardation* (ed. J. Dobbing), pp. 547–71. Macmillan, London.

Mittler, P. and McConachie, H. (1983). *Parents, professionals and mentally handicapped people; approaches to partnership*. Croom Helm, London.

National Health Service Management Executive (1992). *Health services for people with learning disabilities (mental handicap) health service guidelines*. HSG 92 42, Department of Health, London.

North Western Regional Health Authority (1982). *Services for people who are mentally handicapped; a model district service*. North Western Regional Health Authority, Manchester.

O'Brien, J. (1987). *A framework for accomplishment.* Responsive Systems Associates, Decatur, GA.

O'Brien, J. and Tyne, A. (1981). *The principle of normalisation; a foundation for effective services.* Campaign for Persons with Mental Handicap, London.

Oliver, M. (1990). *The politics of disablement.* Macmillan, London.

Raynes, N.V., Pratt, M.W., and Roses, S. (1979). *Organisational structure and the care of the mentally retarded.* Croom Helm, London.

Richardson, S.A. (1978). Careers of mentally retarded young persons; services, jobs, and inter-personal relations. *American Journal of Mental Deficiency*, **82**, 349–58.

Ryan, J. and Thomas, F. (1987). *The politics of mental handicap* (2nd edn). Free Association Books, London.

Shanley, E. and Starrs, T. (1993). *Learning disabilities: a handbook of care.* Churchill Livingstone, Edinburgh.

Shearer, A. (1986). *Building community with people with mental handicaps, their families and friends.* Campaign for Mentally Handicapped People, and King's Fund Centre, London.

Social Services Inspectorate (1995). *Planning for life: developing community services for people with multiple disabilities.* Social Services Inspectorate, Department of Health, London.

Swain, J., Finkelstein, V., French, S., and Oliver, M. (1993). *Disabling barriers, enabling environment.* Open University Press/Sage, Milton Keynes.

Towell, D. (1988). *An ordinary life in practice.* King's Fund, London.

Elements of care

Adams, F. (1990). *Special education in the 1990s.* Longman, London.

Beyers, S., Goodene, L., and Kilsby, M. (1997). *The costs and benefits of supported employment agencies.* HMSO, London.

Braddock, D. and Mitchell, D. (1992). *Residential services an developmental disabilities in the United States.* AAMR, Washington, DC.

Brewer, E.J., McPherson, M., Magreb, P.R., and Hutchins, V.I. (1989). Family centred, community based, co-ordinated care for children with special health care needs. *Pediatrics*, **83**, 1055–60.

Carr, J. (1995). *Helping your handicapped child: a step by step guide to everyday problems* (2nd edn). Penguin, London.

Centre for Educational Innovation and Research (1981). *Education of the handicapped adolescent: integration into school.* OECD, Paris.

Croxen, M. (1982). *Overview: disability and employment.* EEC, Brussels.

Gibson, D. and Harris, A. (1988). Aggregated early intervention effects for Down syndrome persons: patterning and longevity of benefits. *Journal of Mental Deficiency Research*, **32**, 1–18.

Golding, R. and Goldsmith, L. (1986). *The caring person's guide to handling the severely multiply handicapped.* Macmillan, London.

Gruenwald, K. (1984). *Day centres for mentally handicapped adults* (2nd edn). Socialstyren, Stockholm, and Inclusion International, Brussels.

Hatton, C. and Emerson, E. (1996). *Residential provision for people with learning disabilities: a research review.* Hester Adrian Research Centre, University of Manchester.

Howells, G.J.R. (1989). Down's syndrome and the general practitioner. *Journal of the Royal College of General Practice*, **39**, 470–5.

Kiernan, C. (1993). *Survey of Portage provision 1992/93.* National Portage Association, Yeovil.

King's Fund (1982). *An ordinary life: comprehensive, locally-based residential services for mentally handicapped people.* King's Fund Centre, London.

King's Fund (1984). *An ordinary working life: vocational services for people with mental handicap.* King's Fund Centre, London.

National Federation of Housing Associations (1987). *Housing: the foundation of community care.* NFHA and MIND, London.

Oswin, M. (1984). *They keep going away: a study of short term residential care.* King's Fund Centre, London.

Ovretveit, J. (1993). *Co-ordinating community care: organising multi-disciplinary teams and care management.* Open University Press, Milton Keynes.

Plank, M. (1982). *Teams for mentally handicapped people. A report of an enquiry into the development of multi-disciplinary teams.* Paper 10, Campaign for Mentally Handicapped People, London.

Porterfield, J. and Gathercole, C. (1985). *The employment of people with mental handicap. Progress towards an ordinary working life.* King's Fund Centre, London.

Raynes, N.V., Sumpton, R.C., and Flynn, M.C. (1987). *Homes for mentally handicapped people.* Tavistock, London.

Roos, P., McCann, B.M., and Addison, M.R. (ed.) (1980). *Shaping the future: community-based residential services and facilities for mentally retarded people.* University Park Press, Baltimore, MD.

Russell, O. and Ward, L. (1983). *Houses or homes? Evaluating ordinary housing schemes for people with mental handicap.* Centre on Environment for the Handicapped, London.

Werner, D. (1987). *Disabled village children.* Hesperian Foundation, Palo Alto, CA. (TALC edition, Institute of Child Health, London.)

White, M. and Cameron, S. (ed.) (1988). *Portage: progress, problems and possibilities.* NFER-Nelson, Windsor.

Wilcox, B.W. and Bellamy, G.T. (ed.) (1987). *The activities catalogue: an alternative curriculum for youth and adults with severe disabilities.* Brookes, Baltimore, MD.

References

Aaby, P., Andersen, M., and Knudsen, K. (1993). Excess mortality after early exposure to measles. *International Journal of Epidemiology*, **22**, 156–62.

AAMR (American Association on Mental Retardation) (1992). *Mental retardation: definition, classification and systems of supports.* AAMR, Washington, DC.

Abel, E.L. (1995). An update on incidence of FAS: FAS is not an equal opportunity birth defect. *Neurotoxicology and Teratology*, **17**, 437–43.

Alberman, E.D. (ed.) (1992). EUROMAC: maternal alcohol consumption and its relation to the outcome of pregnancy and child development at eighteen months. *International Journal of Epidemiology*, **21** (Supplement 1), 1–87.

APA (American Psychiatric Association) (1980). *Diagnostic and statistical manual of psychiatric disorder* (4th edn). APA, Washington, DC.

Benenson, A.S. (ed.) (1990). *Control of communicable disease in man* (15th edn). American Public Health Association, Washington.

Beresford, B. (1993). Resources and strategies: how parents cope with the care of a disabled child. *Journal of Child Psychology and Psychiatry*, **35**, 171–209.

Berger, M. and Yule, W. (1985). IQ tests and assessments. In *Mental deficiency: the changing outlook*, (ed. A.M. Clarke, A.D.B. Clarke, and J.M. Berg) (4th edn), pp. 53–96. Methuen, London.

Bradley, K.A., Badrinath, S., Bush, K., Boyd-Wickizer, J., and Anawat, B. (1998). Medical risks for women who drink alcohol. *Journal of General Internal Medicine*, **13**, 627–39.

Brown, H. and Smith, H. (ed.) (1992). *Normalisation: a reader for the nineties.* Routledge, London.

BSU (Basic Skills Unit) (1994). *Basic skills in prisons: assessing the need.* BSU, ALBSU, London.

Daly, S., Mills, J.L., Molloy, A.M., *et al.* (1997). Minimum effective dose of folic acid for food fortification to prevent neural-tube defects. *Lancet*, **350**, 1666–9.

Dammann, O. and Leviton, A. (1997). The role of peri-natal brain damage in developmental disabilities: an epidemiologic perspective. *Mental Retardation and Development Disorders Research Review*, **3**, 13–21.

Davies, L., Felce, D., Lowe, K., and de Pavia, S. (1990). *The evaluation of NIMROD, a community based service for people with mental handicap.* Mental Handicap in Wales Applied Research Unit, Cardiff.

Dobbing, J. (1984). Pathology and vulnerability of the developing brain. In *Scientific studies in mental retardation* (ed. J. Dobbing), pp. 89–106. Macmillan, London.

Dudgeon, J.A., Peckham, C.S., and Robinson, R.O. (1985). Infectious agents in the aetiology of mental retardation (and commentary). In *Scientific studies in mental retardation* (ed. J. Dobbing), pp. 203–32. Royal Society of Medicine/Macmillan, London.

Dunn, J.T. (1996). Seven deadly sins in confronting endemic iodine deficiency and how to avoid them. *Journal of Clinicial Endocrinology and Metabolism*, **81**, 1332–5.

Escobar, G.J., Littenberg, B., and Petitti, D.B. (1991) Outcome among surviving very low birth weight infants: a meta-analysis. *Archives of Diseases in Children*, **66**, 204–11.

Fogelman, K. and Wedge, P. (1981). The national child development study (1858 British cohort). In *Prospective longitudinal research* (ed. S.A. Mednick and A.E. Baert), pp. 30–42. Oxford University Press.

Forrest, F. and Florey, C. du V. (1991). The relation between maternal alcohol consumption and child development; the epidemiological evidence. *Journal of Public Health Medicine*, **13**, 247–55.

Friedman, E.G., Koch, R., Azer, C., *et al.* (1996). The international collaborative study on maternal phenyl- ketonuria: organisation, study design and description of the sample. *European Journal of Paediatrics*, **155** (Supplement 1), 158–61.

Fryers, T. (1990). Pre and peri-natal factors in the aetiology of mental retardation. In *Reproductive and peri-natal epidemiology* (ed. M. Kiely), pp. 171–204. CRC Press, Boca Raton, FL.

Fryers, T. (1984). *The epidemiology of severe intellectual impairment: the dynamics of prevalence.* Academic Press, London.

Fryers, T. (1991). Public health approaches to mental retardation: handicap due to intellectual impairment. In *Oxford textbook of public health* (ed. W.W. Holland, R. Detels, and E.G. Knox) (2nd edn). Oxford University Press.

Fryers, T. (1993). Epidemiological thinking in mental retardation: issues in taxonomy and population frequency. In *International review of research in mental retardation* (ed. N.W. Bray), pp. 97–133. Academic Press, London.

Graham, P. and Lansdown, R. (1992). The uses and abuses of psychological tests in childhood. In *Assessment of people with mental retardation.* WHO, Geneva.

Grantham-McGregor, S.M., Powell, C.A., Walker, S.P., and Himes, J.H. (1991). Nutritional supplementation, psychological stimulation and mental development of stunted children; the Jamaica study. *Lancet*, **338**, 1–5.

Grossman, H.J. (ed.) (1983). *Classification in mental retardation.* American Association on Mental Deficiency, Washington, DC.

Gunzberg, H.C. (1977). *Progress assessment charts.* MENCAP, London.

Hannah, J.A. and Brodie, M.S. (1998). Epilepsy and learning disabilities—a challenge for the next millenium. *Seizure*, **7**, 3–13.

Hayes, C., Johnson, Z., Thornton, L., *et al.* (1997). Ten year survival of Down's syndrome births. *International Journal of Epidemiology*, **26**, 822–9.

Haywood, H.C. (ed.) (1970). *Socio-cultural aspects of mental retardation.* Appleton-Century-Crofts, New York.

Helander, E., Nelson, G., Mendis, P., and Goertz, A. (1990). *Training in the community for people with disabilities.* WHO, Geneva.

Heron, A. and Myers, M. (1983). *Intellectual impairment: the battle against handicap.* Academic Press, London.

Hetzel, B.S. (1989). *The story of iodine deficiency.* Oxford University Press.

Hogg, J. and Raynes, N. (ed.) (1987). *Assessment in mental handicap; a guide to assessment practices, tests and checklists.* Croom Helm, London.

Holmes, N., Shah, A., and Wing, L. (1982). The Disability Assessment Schedule: a brief device for use with the mentally retarded. *Psychological Medicine*, **12**, 879–90.

Huether, C.A., Ivanovich, J., Goodwin, B.S., *et al.* (1998). Maternal age-specific risk rate estimates for Down's syndrome among live births in whites and other races from Ohio and Metropolitan Atlanta 1970–1989. *Journal of Medical Genetics*, **35**, 482–90.

Johnson, A., Townsend, P., Yudkin, P., Bull, D., and Wilkinson, A.R. (1993) Functional abilities at age four years of children born before 29 weeks of gestation. *British Medical Journal*, **306**, 1715–18.

Keltner, B. and Ramey, S.L. (1993). Family issues. *Current Opinion in Psychiatry*, **6**, 629–34.

Koller, H., Richardson, S.A., and Katz, M. (1988). Marriage in a young adult mentally retarded population. *Journal of Mental Deficiency Research*, **32**, 93–102.

Locksmith, G.J. and Duff, P. (1998). Preventing neural tube defects: the importance of periconceptional folic acid supplements. *Obstetrics and Gynecology*, **91**, 1027–34.

McGrother, C.W. and Marshall, B. (1990). Recent trends in incidence, morbidity and survival in Down's syndrome. *Journal of Mental Deficiency Research*, **34**, 49–57.

McGrother, C., Thorp, C., Taub, N., and Machado, O. (2001). *Prevalence, disability and need in adults with severe learning disability.* Tizard, London.

Mansell, J. (1993). *Services for people with learning disabilities and challenging behaviour or mental health needs.* HMSO, London.

MDWG (Multi-Disciplinary Working Group) (1992). *Pre-natal screening for toxoplasmosis in the UK.* Royal College of Obstetricians and Gynaecologists, London.

Miller, C., Farrington, C.P., and Harbert, K. (1992). The epidemiology of subacute sclerosing pan-encephalitis in England and Wales 1970–1989. *International Journal of Epidemiology*, **21**, 998–1006.

Mittler, P. (1992). Assessing people with mental retardation: an overview. In *Assessment of people with mental retardation.* World Health Organization, Geneva.

Mittler, P. and Serpell, R. (1985). Services: an international perspective. In *Mental deficiency: the changing outlook* (ed. A.M. Clarke, A.D.B. Clarke, and J.M. Berg) (4th edn), pp. 715–87. Methuen, London.

Morton, J.E., Bundey, S., Webb, T.P., Macdonald, F., Rindl, P.M., and Bullock, S. (1997). Fragile X is less common than previously estimated. *Journal of Medical Genetics*, **34**, 1–5.

Murray, J., Cuckle, H., Taylor, G., and Hewitson, J. (1997). Screening for fragile X syndrome. *Health Technology Assessment*, **1**, 4.

Ort, M. and Cooper, B. (1984). Relative contribution of medical and social factors to severity of handicap in mentally retarded children. In *Perspectives and progress in mental retardation* (ed. J.M. Berg), Volume 2, pp. 17–35. University Park Press, Baltimore, MD.

Richardson, S.A. and Koller, H. (1985) Epidemiology. In *Mental deficiency: the changing outlook* (ed. A.M. Clarke, A.D.B. Clarke, and J.M. Berg) (4th edn), pp 27–52. Methuen, London.

Richardson, S.A., Koller, H., and Katz, M. (1988). Job histories in open employment of a population of young adults with mental retardation I. *American Journal of Mental Retardation*, **92**, 483–91.

Richardson, S.A., Katz, M., and Koller, H. (1993). Patterns of leisure activities in young adults with mild mental retardation. *American Journal of Mental Retardation*, **97**, 431–42.

Rosano, A., Smithells, D., Cacciani, L., *et al.* (1999). Time trends in neural tube defects prevalence in relation to preventive strategies: an international study. *Journal of Epidemiology and Community Health*, **53**, 630–5.

Rumeau-Rouquette, C., Grandjean, H., Cans, C., du Mazaubrun, C., and Verrier, A. (1997) Prevalence and time-trends of disabilities in school-age children. *International Journal of Epidemiology*, **26**, 137–45.

Seymour, C.A., Thomason, M.J., Chalmers, R.A., *et al.* (1997). Newborn screening for inborn errors of metabolism: a systematic review. *Health Technology Assessment*, **1**, 11.

Smith, K., Shah, A., Wright, K., and Lewis, G. (1995). The prevalence and costs of psychiatric disorders and learning disabilities. *British Journal of Psychiatry*, **166**, 9–18.

Stein, Z.A., Susser, M.W., Saenger, G., and Marolla, F. (1975). *Famine and human development*. Oxford University Press.

Streetly, A. and Corbett, V. (1998). *The national newborn screening programme; An audit of phenyl-ketonuria and congenital hypothyroidism screening in England and Wales*. Department of Public Health Medicine, Guy's and St Thomas' Medical Schools, London.

Turner, T.H. (1989). Schizophrenia and mental handicap; an historical review with implications for further research. *Psychological Medicine*, **19**, 301–14.

Twigg, J. (ed.) (1992). *Carers: research and practice*. HMSO, London.

Van der Haar, J. (1997). The challenge of the global elimination of iodine deficiency disorders. *European Journal of Clinics in Nutrition*, **51** (Supplement 4), 3–8.

Wald, N.J., Kennard, A., Hackshaw, A., and McGuire, A. (1998). Ante-natal screening for Down's syndrome. *Health Technology Assessment*, **2**, 1.

Wang, J., Harris, M., Amos, B., Wang, X., Zhang, M., and Chen, J. (1997). A ten year review of the iodine deficiency disorder program of the People's Republic of China. *Journal of Public Health Policy*, **18**, 219–41.

Watkins, M.L. (1998). Efficacy of folic acid prophylaxis for the prevention of neural tube defects. *Mental Retardation and Developmental Disease Research Review*, **4**, 282–90.

Werner, D. (1987). *Disabled village children*. Hesperian Foundation, Palo Alto, CA. (TALC edition, Institute of Child Health, London.)

WHO (World Health Organization) (1980). *International classification of impairments, disabilities and handicaps*. WHO, Geneva.

WHO (World Health Organization) (1985). *Iodine-deficiency disorders in Southeast Asia*. SEARO Regional Health Papers 10, WHO, New Delhi.

WHO (World Health Organization) (1992*a*). *The ICD-10 classification of mental and behavioural disorders: clinical descriptions and guide-lines*. WHO, Geneva.

WHO (World Health Organization) (1992*b*). *The education of mid-level rehabilitation workers; recommendations from country experiences*. WHO, Geneva.

WHO (World Health Organization) (1993). *Global prevalence of iodine deficiency disorders*. Micro-nutrient Deficiency Information System, Working Paper 1. WHO, Geneva.

WHO (World Health Organization) (1994). *Indicators for assessing iodine deficiency disorders and their control through salt iodization*. WHO, Geneva.

WHO (World Health Organization) (1999). *International classification of functioning and disability (beta-2 draft; short version)*. WHO, Geneva.

Wing, L. (1980). MRC Handicaps, Behaviour and Skills (HBS) Schedule. *Acta Psychiatria Scandinavica, Supplementum*, **62**, 275–84.

Wing, L. (1996). *The autistic spectrum*. Constable, London.

Wolfensberger, W. and Thomas, S. (1983). PASSING (programme analysis of service systems). In *Implementation of normalisation goals. Normalisation criteria and ratings manual* (2nd edn), pp. 23–34. National Institute for Mental Retardation, Toronto.

11.8 Health of elderly people

Shah Ebrahim

In this chapter, population ageing and its determinants are described. The case for considering elderly people as a special needs group is discussed, together with the health problems they face. The available evidence of efficacy of preventive interventions, primary care and hospital services, long-term care and social support are reviewed.

Elderly people are a heterogeneous group comprising those who are still actively pursuing careers in industry or politics, enjoying a healthy retirement, caring for frail and dependent relatives or friends, and others who are themselves very frail and dependent. Such diverse people are frequently grouped together as 'the elderly' as if they had similar needs and would respond in the same way to interventions. It is essential to recognize this heterogeneity in defining need, assessing the effects and relevance of intervention, and planning for the future. It is common to define the 'young old' as aged 60 to 69 years, the 'old old' as aged 70 to 79 years, and the 'oldest old' as 80 years and over. In the past, United Nations and other international agencies used 60+ years as a criterion of 'the elderly', but more recently there is a growing consensus that 65+ years should be used.

Demographics and projections

The world population is around 6 billion (that is, 6×10^9) people of whom 385 million (6.5 per cent) were aged 65 years and over in 1997. The largest numbers of elderly people are found in the most populous countries of the world—China, India, the United States, Russia, and Japan—rather than in the more affluent postindustrialized countries.

Focusing on a single age threshold hides important trends in the numbers of the oldest old who tend to present major challenges for health and social services. Figures 1 and 2 show the numbers of people aged 65 years and over and 80 years and over, respectively, in the most aged countries in 1997 and projected to 2025. In developing countries the annual growth of people aged 65+ years is almost 3 per cent per year, whereas in industrialized countries it has fallen to below 2 per cent per year (Kinsella 1996). In industrialized countries the proportion of the oldest old is growing more rapidly than any other age group.

This growth in the numbers of elderly people is mirrored throughout most countries of the world but to different extents. The world can be divided into four main regional types. In type 1 countries of Europe, North America, Japan, Eastern Europe, and the former Soviet Union, the proportion of elderly people is high and will rise. Type 2 countries—China, Southeast Asia, Latin America, and the Caribbean—have a relatively small proportion of elderly people but rapid increases are predicted. Type 3 countries comprise India and the Middle East where the increase in the proportion of elderly people will be slower. The type 4 countries of sub-Saharan Africa are not expected to show any increase in the proportion of elderly people (Fig. 3).

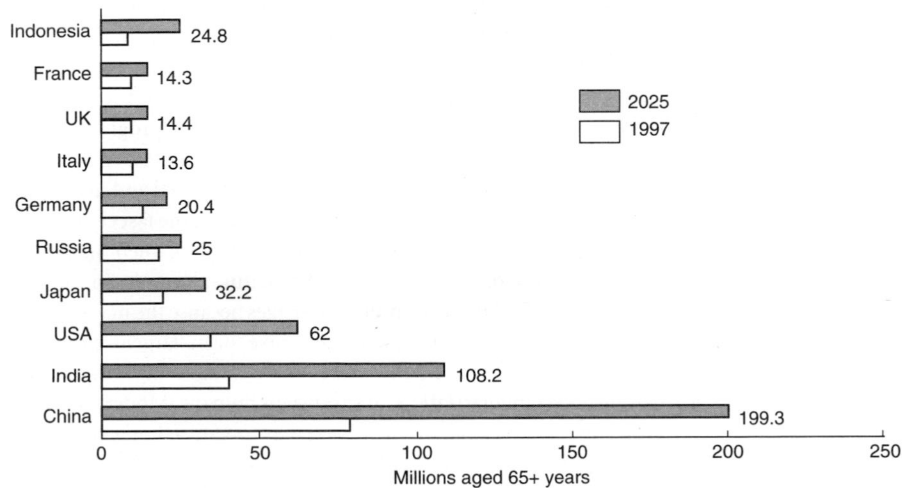

Fig. 1 Countries with the highest number of people aged 65+ years, 1997 and 2025. (Source: WHO 1998.)

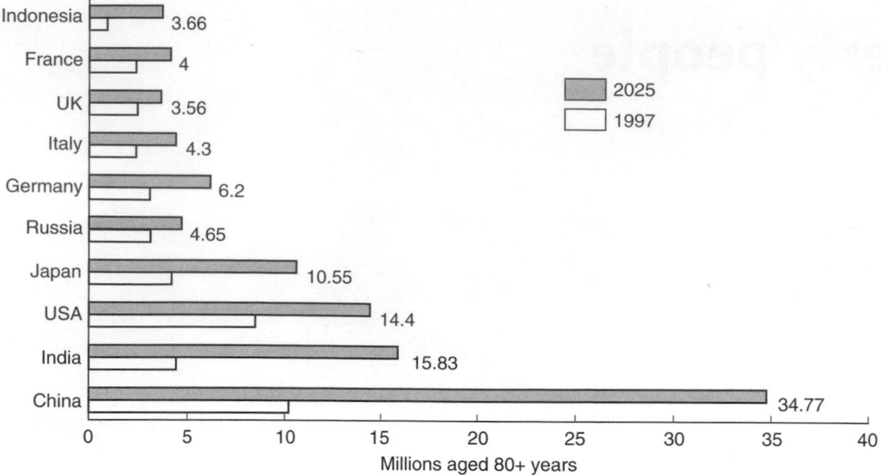

Fig. 2 Countries with the highest number of people aged 80+ years, 1997 and 2025. (Source: WHO 1998.)

Population ageing is an unprecedented phenomenon. It took over 100 years for Belgium to double the proportion of its 60+ population from 9 to 18 per cent. China will take 34 years and Singapore only 20 years to achieve the same population ageing. Projections suggest that the net world monthly gain in people aged 65 years and over by 2010 will be 1.1 million every month (Kinsella 1996), from a current level of about 800 000 every month (Fig. 4).

Projections of ageing of populations are important for planning services but are subject to error. Projections are particularly sensitive to assumptions about mortality rates at older ages and have always tended to underestimate the true numbers of older people. United Nations demographers give both high and low estimates for their projections.

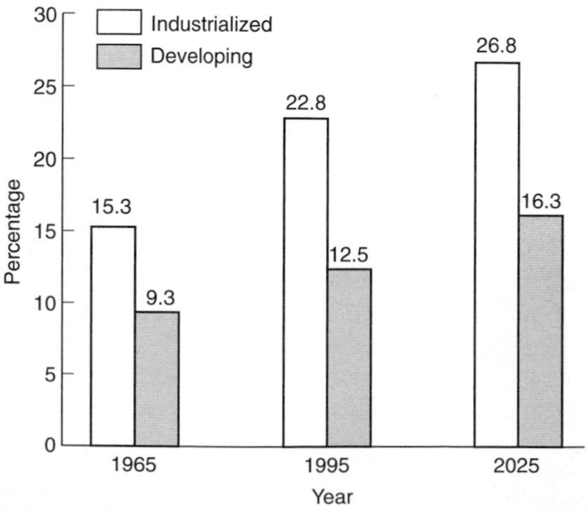

Fig. 3 Oldest old (80+ years) as a percentage of all people aged 65+ in industrialized and developing countries. (Source: Kinsella 1996.)

Determinants of population ageing

The major determinants of population ageing are declines in fertility and mortality. It is tempting to attribute the declines to improvements in medical care. In industrialized countries, such as the United Kingdom, falls in infant and childhood mortality began in the nineteenth century, predating the era of modern effective medical care by many decades. However, it was not until the 1950s that declines in mortality among those aged 75 years and over were achieved (Charlton and Murphy 1997). During the 1970s the rate of decline in mortality increased at all ages. The trends over the nineteenth and early twentieth centuries in the United Kingdom were probably due to general improvements in social and economic conditions resulting in better nutrition, the public health reforms of sanitation, clean water, and control of common communicable diseases. The more recent mortality declines may be attributable to medical care (Bunker 1994), although the evidence is not strong. However, even in the recent past, mortality declines have only been experienced by the better off in the United Kingdom, demonstrating the continuing influence of social and economic factors (Drever and Whitehead 1997). In developing countries the successful infant and child health programmes (growth chart monitoring, oral rehydration for diarrhoea, breast feeding, and immunization for common infections—the GOBI programme) are probably responsible for the very rapid rates of mortality decline at younger ages. Studies of survival of animals in the wild and in captivity show a striking similarity to the survival curves of the last century and the present. Animals in the wild seldom achieve their maximum lifespan because of predation and other natural hazards. In captivity they are capable of reaching much older ages because the major risks of predation, starvation, and accidents have been largely eliminated (Kirkwood 1999). Much the same phenomenon may explain the so-called 'rectangularization' of survival in humans. Modern society is protective to its weakest members, has organized means of distributing food, and is arguably safer than in the past (Fig. 5).

Declines in fertility are attributed to urbanization, industrialization, and social mobility which have all had an influence on family structures. In addition the emancipation of women, their greater

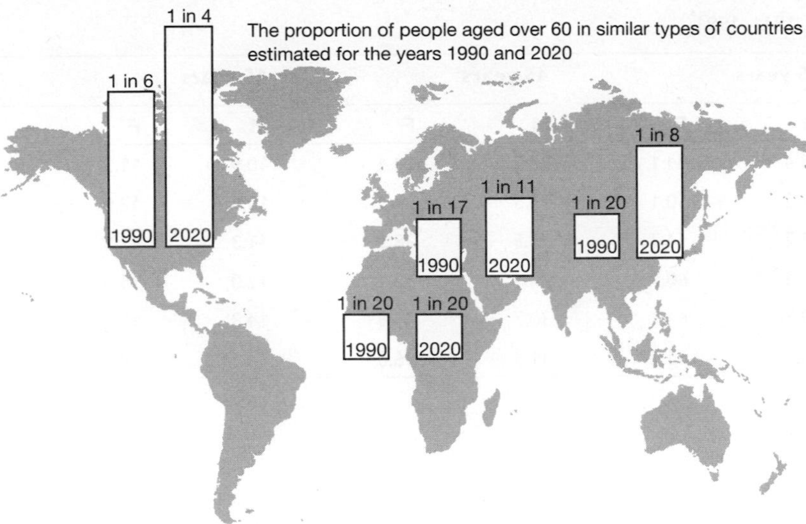

Fig. 4 The proportion of people aged over 60 years in similar types of countries estimated for the years 1990 and 2020. (Source: Dr M. Prince and Alzheimer's Disease International.)

chances for education, later age at marriage, and access to contraception have all played a part. In developing countries, it seems likely that education of women and access to contraception explain the very rapid rates of population ageing in countries such as China and those of Southeast Asia. Japan and the United Kingdom are among 61 countries that are not having enough babies to replace their populations (Anonymous 1999). Replacement fertility rates are 2.1 babies per women; the figures for the United Kingdom and Japan are 1.7 and 1.4 respectively, and Spanish women have the lowest fertility in the world at 1.15. Such trends in fertility are not confined to industrialized countries. Women in India are having fewer babies than American women had in the 1950s and China, Cuba, and Thailand are already below the replacement rate. These very sharp declines in fertility worldwide have resulted in reductions in forecasts for population growth. United Nations estimates suggested a total population of 9 billion people by 2050 but it might be as low as 7.5 billion.

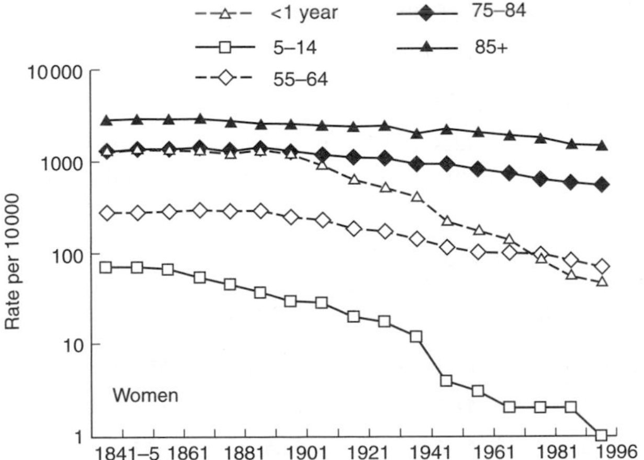

Fig. 5 Declines in mortality at different ages for women, United Kingdom, 1841–1994. (Source: Charlton and Murphy 1997; Office for National Statistics 1998.)

Demographic and epidemiological transitions

With a changing population structure came differing disease patterns, caused at least in part by the same factors that contributed to declines in mortality and fertility. In populations with high fertility, infections affecting those most susceptible, infants and children, were very common. As environmental conditions contributing to risk of infections improved, and as nutritional patterns changed from periods of starvation to a more plentiful food supply throughout the year, so were the seeds of chronic and degenerative diseases sown. These epidemiological transitions have been defined as the age of pestilence and famine, the age of receding pandemics, and the age of degenerative and man-made diseases. However, in the rapidly ageing developing countries the picture is not so clear-cut as in industrialized countries. Developing countries are experiencing the double burdens of both high levels of infectious diseases taking their toll on infants and children, and also emerging burdens of smoking- and diet-related diseases, in particular cardiovascular diseases, cancers, and diabetes mellitus.

Life expectancy

William Farr produced the first English life table using mortality data for 1841. At this time, life tables were valued by friendly societies who used then to calculate the survival prospects of people at different ages to determine how much they should pay (Charlton and Murphy 1997). The attraction of the life table, then as now, is that it provides a simple and easily understood summary of the mortality experience of a population. In 1841, life expectancy at birth was 42 years for women and 40 years for men, reflecting the prevailing high rates of infant mortality. William Farr calculated average life expectancies in 1841 for Liverpool, Surrey, and London which were 26, 45, and 37. By 1992, while the rank order by place of residence was much the same, life expectancy above the age of 85 years showed even greater variation in

Table 1 Life expectancy at different ages: England and Wales, 1841–1991

Year	Birth		15 years		45 years		65 years	
	M	F	M	F	M	F	M	F
1841	40.2	42.2	43.4	44.1	23.3	24.4	10.9	11.5
1901–10	48.5	52.4	47.3	50.1	23.3	25.5	10.8	12.0
1930–32	58.7	62.9	51.2	54.3	25.5	28.3	11.3	13.1
1960–62	68.1	74.0	55.3	60.9	27.1	32.1	12.0	15.3
1990–92	73.4	79.0	59.3	64.7	30.7	35.5	14.3	18.1
1994–96	73.4	79.6	60.1	65.2	31.5	36.0	14.8	18.4

Source: Charlton and Murphy (1997) and www.ons.gov.uk

1992 than it did in 1841! Gains in life expectancy have been most pronounced at younger ages, but even at older ages increases have occurred due to falling death rates. Table 1 shows life expectancy at different ages for men and women in England and Wales.

Information prior to the middle of the nineteenth century is difficult to find and interpret but supports a view that falls in infant and childhood mortality were the main driving forces in increased population growth during the period 1650 to 1850 (Gonner 1913), rather than increases in fertility (Wrigley and Schofield 1981). Comparisons between infant and child mortality among the British peerage and parishes (i.e. representative of the general population) in England show striking declines among both groups between 1650 and 1849; infant and childhood mortality showed a decline of about two-thirds among offspring of peers and about a third in parishes. Moreover, infant mortality among wealthy and poorer people showed little difference during the seventeenth and eighteenth centuries, suggesting that improvements in life expectancy were not driven by wealth but by reduced exposure to infectious diseases (Razzell 1998).

Life expectancy in England and Wales shows a marked social class gradient at birth and also at age 65 years. The difference in life expectancy at age 65 years between social classes I and II (professional and managerial) and IV and V (semi-skilled and unskilled manual) has increased from 1.4 years in 1972 to 2.6 years in 1987–1991 as shown in the Table 2. Similar, but less marked, gradients exist for women.

Life expectancy in the former USSR and Eastern European countries show stark declines among men since the political reforms (Leon *et al.* 1997; Chenet *et al.* 1998). The explanation for such trends is not clear, but sudden deaths due to binge alcohol drinking, increased risks of violent death, and suicide all play a part (Chenet *et al.* 1996). Reunification of the former East Germany with West Germany shows a somewhat different picture. In the decade since reunification, starting with the collapse of the Berlin Wall in 1989, mortality rates in the east have fallen towards those in the west among women but not in men (Haussler *et al.* 1995). Differences in life expectancy at birth between East and West Germany, which favoured East Germany at the start of division, have fallen since reunification (Table 3). These natural experiments in social and economic engineering provide examples of how public health is influenced by political change. It also reinforces the importance of social and economic factors as major forces in determining life expectancy.

Life expectancy can be calculated using either period death rates—that is, the age-sex specific death rates for a particular year—or cohort death rates. The latter provide better estimates of true life expectancy as they adjust for the fact that people in successive birth cohorts are becoming healthier and—age for age—have a lower risk of mortality than their predecessors. Period death rates make an unwarranted assumption that current death rates will prevail unchanged. In 1990, cohort life expectancy at birth was 77 years and 83 years for men and women respectively in the United Kingdom, about a 5 per cent increase on period life expectancy estimates (Charlton and Murphy 1997). At 75 years, the relative difference is far greater at 27 and 22 per cent increases for men and women, respectively, reflecting the major improvements in survival prospects for successive cohorts of older people.

Health expectancy

Life expectancy provides a crude monitoring tool for assessing the health status of a population. However, life expectancy does not tell

Table 2 Male life expectancy at birth and at age 65 years by social class, England and Wales, 1972–1991

	1972–6		1977–81		1982–86		1987–91	
	Birth	65 years	Birth	65 years	Birth	65 years	Birth	65 years
I and II	71.7	13.4	72.8	14.3	74.1	14.5	74.9	15.0
IIINM	69.5	12.6	70.8	13.3	72.2	13.6	73.5	14.1
IIIM	69.8	12.2	70.0	12.6	71.4	13.0	72.4	13.4
IV and V	67.8	12.0	68.3	12.0	69.8	12.3	69.7	12.4

Source: Drever and Whitehead (1997).

Table 3 Life expectancy in East and West Germany, 1949–1997

	Men			Women		
	West	East	Difference (East – West)	West	East	Difference (East – West)
1949–1953	64.6	65.1	+0.5	68.5	69.1	+0.6
1980	69.9	68.7	−1.2	76.8	74.6	−2.2
1990	72.7	69.2	−3.5	79.2	76.3	−2.9
1992–1994	73.4	70.3	−3.1	79.7	77.7	−2.0
1995–1997	74.1	71.8	−2.3	80.2	79.0	−1.2

Source: Anonymous (1999).

the whole story. A major goal of health and social policy in old age is the increase in life expectancy free of disease or disability—healthy active life expectancy (Evans 1993*a*). The generic term, health expectancy, is best used to describe the growing number of indicators: disease-free life expectancy, dementia-free life expectancy, impairment-free life expectancy, disability-free life expectancy, handicap-free life expectancy, and activity restriction-free life expectancy. The precise form of health expectancy used has a profound effect on the duration of life estimated as the rates of different conditions vary markedly. For example, dementia is comparatively rare compared with all types of disability. Table 4 shows some estimates of different types of health expectancy for China.

Compression of morbidity

Human lifespan, unlike average life expectancy, is fixed and is about 120 years. Accounts of people living very much longer than this have not been corroborated. Life expectancy is increasing dramatically and will eventually approximate to our fixed maximum achievable lifespan. If the age at onset of chronic disability is increasing then, with a fixed lifespan, the period of serious ill health and disability will be compressed into a smaller proportion of the lifespan—the compression of morbidity hypothesis (Fries 1980). Fries' original statement of the compression of morbidity hypothesis confused lifespan with life expectancy (the former is fixed and the latter is increasing) and he suggested that compression of morbidity would be apparent in populations where life expectancy was about 85 years (his 'ideal average lifespan'). Revisions of the compression of morbidity hypothesis have emphasized that decline in the incidence of morbidity and disability must increase at a faster rate than the decline in mortality rates if compression of morbidity is to be achieved (Fries 1989) (Fig. 6).

Fries *et al.* (1989) suggested that the compression of morbidity hypothesis was supported by evidence from randomized controlled trials of primary prevention that demonstrated no reduction in total mortality but reduction in the incidence of cardiovascular disease events. However, when all the evidence on the effects of primary prevention for cardiovascular disease is examined, no clear effects on morbidity or mortality are apparent (Ebrahim and Davey Smith 1997).

Alternative theories of expansion of morbidity and 'steady state' or equilibrium between morbidity and death have been put forward: the former on the assumption that increasing survival into old age will increase the numbers at risk of developing dementia syndromes (Olshansky *et al.* 1991). Manton's steady state hypothesis suggests that there will be an equilibration of the amount of morbidity through parallel declines in both disease incidence and total mortality (Manton 1982).

Evidence to support or refute these hypotheses is difficult to find and hard to interpret. Successive cross-sectional studies of the prevalence of disability over a period of time may be used to calculate health expectancy using Sullivan's method (Mathers and Robine

Table 4 Health expectancy at age 65 years, China 1987 and 1992: effect of criterion used

	Male		Female	
	1987	1992	1987	1992
Life expectancy	12.6	13.0	15.0	15.6
Disability-free life expectancy	9.0	—	10.2	—
Active life expectancy	9.6	11.9	11.5	13.7
Life expectancy in good perceived health	9.4	10.2	10.7	11.7
Disease-free life expectancy	—	4.2	—	4.4

Source: Robine and Romieu (1998).

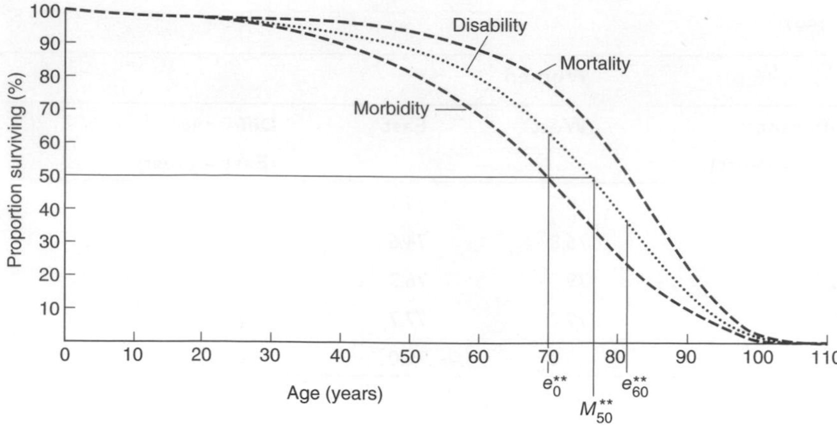

Fig. 6 The observed mortality and hypothetical morbidity and disability survival curves for females in the United States in 1980: e_0^{**} and e_{60}^{**} are the number of years of autonomous life expected at birth and at age 60 years respectively. M_{50}^{**} is the age to which 50 per cent of females could expect to survive without loss of autonomy. (Source: WHO 1984.)

1997). This makes the assumptions that disability is irreversible and that duration of disability remains constant over the time period examined. Trends in health expectancy may then be compared with life expectancy to determine which is increasing faster. Such data are rarely available as it is not common for regular surveys using similar sampling methods and criteria for disability to be performed. Trends are particularly sensitive to the indicator of disability used (Table 5).

Cross-sectional data from the United States and from England and Wales suggest that health expectancy may be increasing more rapidly than life expectancy (Manton and Stallard 1991; Bone *et al.* 1995) if more severe disability is used as the criterion to define 'health'. Figure 7(a) shows the trends in severe and milder levels of disability found in successive surveys in England and Wales, and Fig. 7(b) shows trends in limitation of activities among black and white people in the United States. In both England and Wales and the United States disability, however defined, is strongly age related. However, in England and Walse it appears that less severe disability—inability to get outdoors—shows no clear secular trend, whereas more severe disability—inability to manage basic self-care activities of daily living—show dramatic reductions in each age group over the same time period. In the United States, not only are disability rates higher among black than white people, but the trends between 1990 and 1996 show that white people have enjoyed a reduction in disability levels whereas black people have suffered an increase in levels (National Center for Health Statistics 1999). Unfortunately, such data are suspect owing to differences in the likelihood of selection bias in successive samples of older people and differences in how such questions on disability are interpreted by successive cohorts of older people. In the United States recent favourable trends in disability have been interpreted as demonstrating the effects of better health services (Manton *et al.* 1997). However, health services are unlikely to be the sole reason. Among university alumni followed up prospectively, those with high-risk health behaviours (i.e. smoking, high body mass index, lack of physical exercise) suffered twice the cumulative incidence of disability with the onset of disability postponed by an average of 5 years in those with low-risk health behaviours (Vita *et al.* 1998).

Trends in health expectancy are of major importance in monitoring health and social policy for older people. However, very few countries are capable of making reliable assessments over time, between geographic regions or socio-economic groups. Investment in research infrastructure is required to ensure that regular health and disability surveys using comparable methodology are established. The International Healthy Life Expectancy Network (REVES) has demonstrated the limitations of available data and have called for disability-

Table 5 Trends in disability-free life expectancy using different criteria of disability, England and Wales, 1976–1991

	Men				Women			
	DFLE – ADL		DFLE – IWO		DFLE – ADL		DFLE – IWO	
	65–69	80–84	65–69	80–84	65–69	80–84	65–69	80–84
1976	11.0	3.9	11.4	4.3	13.0	4.1	13.6	4.3
1980	11.8	4.4	11.8	4.7	15.0	5.7	13.5	4.2
1985	12.3	5.0	12.2	4.9	15.5	5.9	13.8	4.4
1991	13.6	5.6	13.2	5.0	16.9	7.3	15.2	5.6

ADL, activities of daily living (difficulty in bathing, dressing, and washing); DFLE, disability-free life expectancy; IWO, inability to walk outdoors

Source: Bone *et al.* (1995).

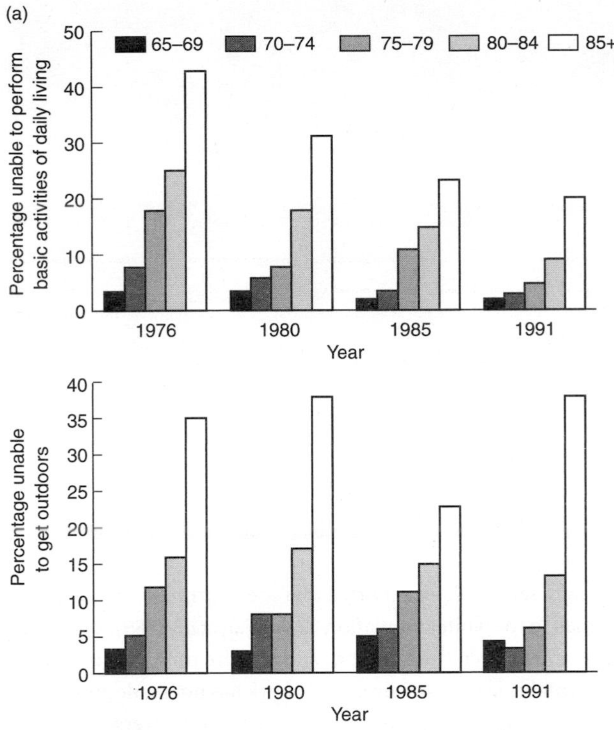

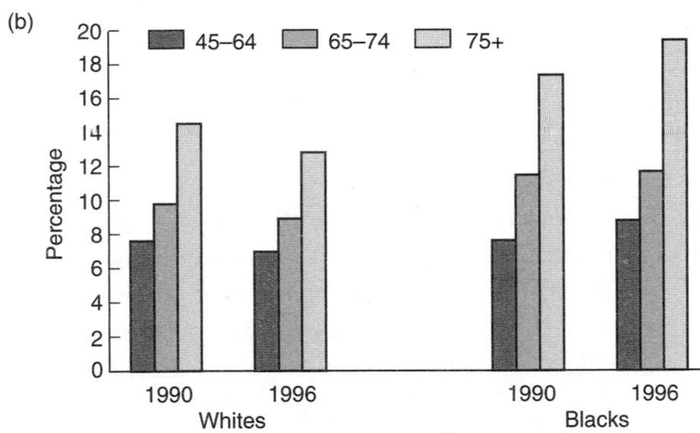

Fig. 7 (a) Trends in disability among older people in England and Wales, 1976–1991. (Source: Bone *et al.* 1995.) (b) Trends in disability among black and white people in the United States, 1990–1996 . (Source: national Centre for Health Statistics 1999.)

free life expectancy to be promoted internationally as a health indicator (Robine *et al.* 1992). Application of earlier and later disability prevalence rates will make a major difference to projections of disability and health burden over the next two decades (Khaw 1999).

Rural ageing

Population ageing is not uniform within most countries but tends to be geographically defined. For example, retirement communities have grown in areas of natural beauty and holiday resorts, and migration of younger people to cities has left older people behind in rural areas. The special circumstances of ageing in rural communities have not received much attention. However, the majority of the world's elderly people live in rural areas. Living in rural areas is generally associated with economic hardship, traditional culture and organization of society, and limited availability and range of services (transport, shops, health and social support). Migration of young adults away from rural areas diminishes opportunities for family support and is so extreme in northern Italian hill villages that many are unlikely to be viable within the next decade (Golini 1997). Of particular concern from a public health viewpoint are poverty and depopulation, particularly in developing countries, which make traditional rural development programmes focusing only on mothers and children inappropriate. Environmental factors, including lack of safe drinking water and poor sanitation, inadequate housing, and absence of electricity, and poor roads and transport make life increasingly difficult for elderly people. Distance from major urban centres of population further increases the ease of neglect by government and health services. Traditional values of self-reliance are unlikely to operate sufficiently to reduce disadvantage given depopulation. Lack of an agreed definition of 'rurality' has limited information on elderly people in rural areas and has hindered development of specific policies that might improve their access to services.

Ethnic minority elders

Immigration associated with trade, the colonial past, wars, and famine have produced complex multicultural societies in many countries. Different countries will have experienced immigration at different times and contexts which will affect how ethnic minorities are viewed, their place in society, and their absolute and relative numbers. In the United Kingdom, immigration of 'visible' Caribbean, Somali, south Asian, and Chinese people occurred at different times and for different reasons (Ebrahim 1996*a*,*b*). The 'push' factors of poverty, political instability, and oppression and 'pull' factors of economic gain explain most migration patterns. Ethnic minorities tend to settle in distinct towns and regions of towns reflecting relative safety in numbers and work opportunities. Ethnic minority populations that migrated to the United Kingdom and other European countries are now ageing rapidly and may be at 'triple jeopardy' owing to their age, cultural and racial discrimination, and lack of access to health, housing, and social services (Norman 1985) (Fig. 8).

Census information shows that older people from the major ethnic minority groups in the United Kingdom, with the exception of Chinese, appear to have more long-standing disability than the white majority. The explanations for excess morbidity may be found in poverty, poor housing and diet, and limited physical activity, all of which are likely to contribute to higher rates of cardiovascular disease, diabetes, and other chronic health problems. The aetiology of ethnic minority health problems may be classified as influences of the 'home' country, influences of the new adopted country, selection of who migrates, and the processes of adaptation and adjustment to migration (Marmot *et al.* 1984). However, once people from ethnic minorities reach old age the selective 'healthy migrant' factors tend to have worn off and they become prey to the common causes of chronic ill health in the wider population.

Interestingly, black people in the United States have better life expectancy than white populations beyond the age of 80 years, which may reflect survival of the fittest (Manton 1980). Disability levels among American black and white people also show complex patterns

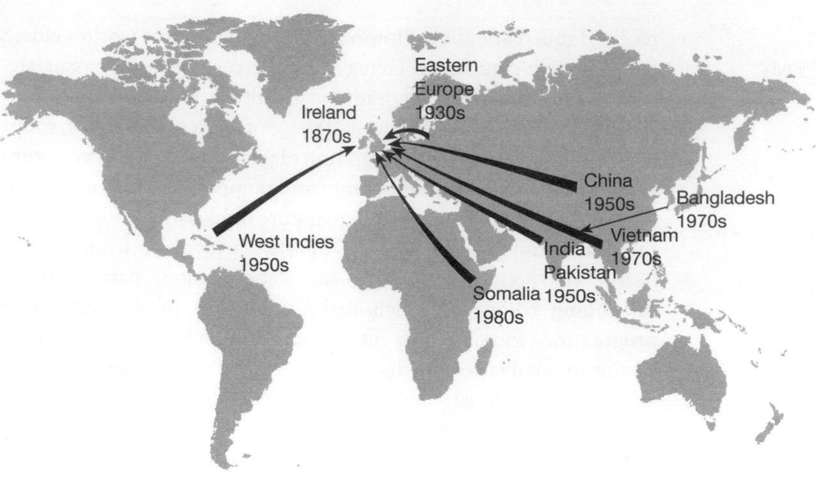

Fig. 8 Trends in world migration to the United Kingdom. (Source: Ebrahim 1996*a*.)

as shown by data from New Haven and North Carolina. Black people were more likely than white people to become disabled, particularly in New Haven. This increased risk was explained by social and economic factors in predominantly rural North Carolina but not urban New Haven. It is possible that unmeasured social and economic factors or residual confounding explain this latter finding. Alternatively, other factors (e.g. weak family or community support networks) associated with black ethnicity in New Haven, but not North Carolina, result in an increased risk of disability even after socio-economic adjustment (Mendes de Leon *et al.* 1997).

Examining need and use of health and social services for ethnic minority elders is beset with problems. Denominators are not accurately defined as classification of ethnicity tends to be based on country of birth that fails to capture aspects of culture, language, religion, diet, beliefs, and behaviour. For example, in the United Kingdom, the classification used in the census developed by the Office for National Statistics is dominated by skin colour, reflecting British views of ethnicity (Table 6).

Numerators for calculation of rates of morbidity are seldom complete owing to poor collection of information on ethnicity in routine health and social care settings. *Ad hoc* studies examining the use of health services have reported that use of primary care services is higher than in the white population (Balarajan *et al.* 1989), prompting concerns about 'over-consultation' and a desire to normalize rates to more acceptable levels. However, such work has not made appropriate allowance for higher levels of morbidity or more adverse social and economic factors which tend to have independent effects on primary care use. Inequality of access to primary health care may not occur but it is likely that more subtle barriers to referral, investigation, and treatment in secondary care exist (Ebrahim 1996*a*). For social services, it is far clearer that access is a major problem. Far fewer people from ethnic minorities receive social support services, yet from what is known of need, they should be represented in greater proportion. It is more likely that 'the family will cope' myth explains why fewer ethnic minority elders are deemed to need social services, together with culturally inappropriate and insensitive services (e.g. 'meat and two veg' meals on wheels, day care without appropriate religious observances). Much more work needs to be done to assess need in order to develop and evaluate more appropriate services for ethnic minority elders.

Table 6 Classification of ethnicity used in the United Kingdom Census 1991

White
Black—Caribbean
Black—African
Black—other
Indian
Pakistani
Bangladeshi
Chinese
Asian—other
Other

Source: Office of Population Census and Surveys (1991).

Older people as a special group

Like children, older people are often singled out for special status in public health plans and in prioritization exercises. While it is convenient for needs assessment to group older people by chronological age into young-old, old-old, and oldest-old, these groupings ignore very real differences in people and risk exacerbating the stereotyping of older people. People become more heterogeneous in their health status as they get older which would suggest that grouping elderly people together may be quite inappropriate. Indeed, much of the debate over geriatric versus general medical services for older people is due to the need to ensure that older people are treated decently and that they also obtain access to specialist services from which they are able to benefit. The physical and mental frailty of many older people, widespread ageism, and prejudicial views of their ability to benefit from health care increase the need for advocacy.

Icebergs of disease

Unrecognized health problems are more common among older than younger people and are caused by several distinct mechanisms: failure to report symptoms, denial of symptoms, underinvestigation, and poor diagnosis of disease by doctors. Under-recognition of health problems is particularly common in incontinence of urine, depression and dementia, visual and hearing impairment, and locomotor disability (Williamson *et al.* 1964). The implication of under-recognition is loss of potential health gain and attempts to improve under-recognition underpin much case-finding and screening for health problems in older people.

Multiple pathology

It is rare for any adult to have a single health problem. Typically most adults have a range of health problems, some of which are active, some inactive. In old age, it is more likely that such health problems will be active and will interact with each other, resulting in complicated patterns that tend to defy simple approaches to intervention. Multiple pathology is the rule rather than the exception and must be acknowledged in needs assessment and service delivery. At a population level, need is commonly assessed using mortality statistics. However, deaths are coded to a single underlying cause of death and routine mortality statistics do not use data from the second part of the death certificate on other diseases that may have contributed to the death. Indeed, such information is rarely complete, further limiting its value for assessing need. In developing countries it is common for a majority of deaths to be unattributed to International Classification of Disease groups. For example, in Thailand in 1996, 47 per cent of causes of death among people aged 60 years and over were recorded as 'senility' (R54), 6.7 per cent as 'ill-defined and unknown causes of mortality' (R95–R99), and 2.9 per cent were classed as 'symptoms, sign and abnormal clinical and laboratory findings, not elsewhere classified' (R00–R53; R55–R94).

From a therapeutic perspective, multiple pathology makes evaluation of interventions difficult as comorbidities may make treatment more hazardous or appear less effective. This may be a justification for excluding older people from randomized controlled trials but failure to include them perpetuates the current lack of evidence of benefits and harms of treatments for older patients.

Loss of adaptability

The physiological functional reserve capacity (e.g. in terms of muscle strength, cardiorespiratory fitness, skeletal integrity) of older people declines with increasing age (Young 1992). Older people have to cope with an increasing 'fitness gap' and it is this reduction in reserve capacity which places older people closer to thresholds that will limit their functional independence and will reduce their capacity to adapt to new challenges presented by disease and social and environmental factors (Gray *et al.* 1985; Evans 1990). Reduced adaptability makes elderly people vulnerable to increased risk of complications of disease and more likely to suffer a 'cascade of disasters' following an initial fairly trivial incident. Loss of adaptability also makes 'atypical' presentations of disease more common as thresholds for normal performance are so precarious that minor degrees of impairment,

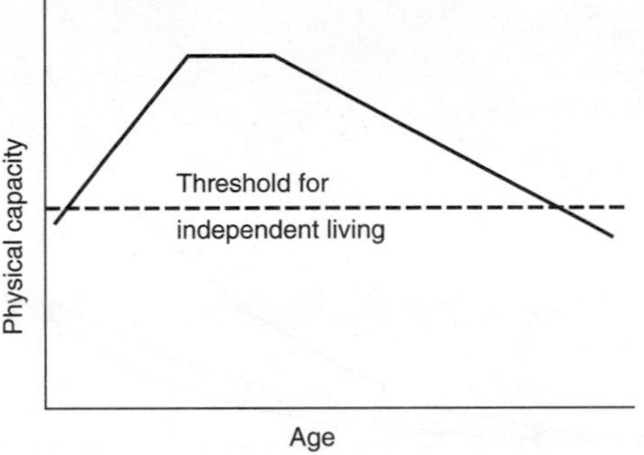

Fig. 9 Relationship between age and physical capacity showing the effects of a threshold for independent living.

regardless of the organ system involved, result in more general physical and mental disturbances (Fig. 9).

Loss of adaptability is of concern to public health in two main ways: firstly, maximizing functional reserve capacity through optimizing childhood and early adult life development will ensure that people cross thresholds that render them dependent at ever older ages. Secondly, public health should aim to identify and reduce social and environmental factors that present differential challenges to older people. For example, public transport in many countries is difficult to use without substantial reserves of lower-limb girdle muscle strength. Crossing a road within the time allowed on traffic light controlled crossings requires an average walking speed that is higher than that achievable by most 70-year-olds (Hoxie and Rubenstein 1994). Improving access to public transport and ensuring road crossings are safe for all should be part of wider public health concerns.

Costs of care

The potentially very high costs of care for older people make a compelling case for considering older people as a special group. However, the notion that health care costs increase inexorably with age is not supported by analyses examining the costs of care in relationship to proximity to death. Such analyses show that it is terminal illness that is expensive rather than age itself (Normand 1998). Very elderly people have lower costs than younger people with the same survival prospects (Himsworth and Goldacre 1999).

Nursing home costs in the United States have grown at a far faster rate since the 1960s than other sectors of health care spending (National Center for Health Statistics 1999), as shown in Fig. 10. British long-term care costs also dominate the overall projections over a period of decades, far outstripping primary care and hospital sector costs (Laing *et al.* 1991). Hotel 'board and lodging' costs make up a high proportion of long-term care costs and it is generally accepted that individual payment for these costs is acceptable (Royal Commission on Long Term Care 1999). Insurance schemes to meet long-term care costs have been introduced without much success. Commentators have noted that even with the most optimistic assumptions, long-term care insurance would meet only 10 per cent of total American government costs in this area (Weiner and Illson 1994).

Within the current health service system, both inequity of access to services and overuse of ineffective services occur. Older people who would benefit from specific interventions (e.g. coronary revascularization) do not receive them (Bowling 1999); simultaneously, acute

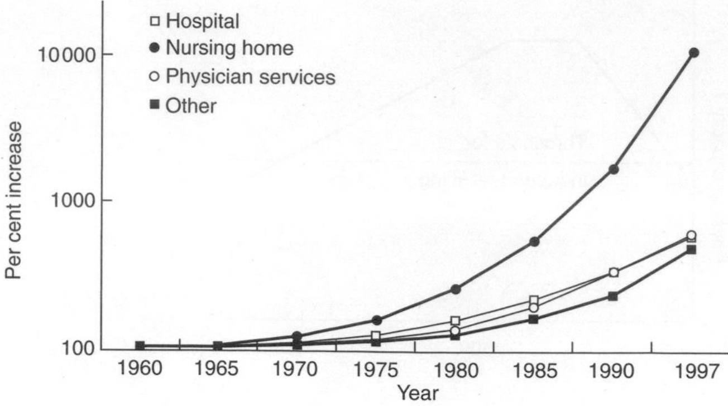

Fig. 10 Trends in different sectors of health care costs, United States, 1960–1997. (Source: National Centre for Health Statistics 1999.)

hospital beds are inefficiently used by older patients waiting for transfer to a different care sector, either their own homes or institutional accommodation. Increasing the barriers to gaining entry into secondary care for older people is an obvious, but misplaced response, as it exacerbates inequity for some. Ensuring that both health and social care costs are considered in economic appraisals, rather than just the costs of one or other system should ensure that the balance of care is of net benefit to society and not simply to one payer rather than another.

Health and social services for elderly people

The purpose of health and social services for elderly people are to prevent disease, save lives, reduce suffering and disability, avoid complications of disease, and to ensure that resources are used efficiently. 'Care in the community' is a broad strategic goal which cuts across these other goals as it is expected to be less expensive than care in the hospital and to make better use of a wider range of community services. It is important to recognize both the breadth of health and social services for elderly people and their interrelationships. It is useful to have a comprehensive approach to services and this is best achieved by grouping services according to area of activity: health promotion, primary care, community services, social services, residential and long-term care, and acute hospital services. Typically, acute hospital services occupy a disproportionate amount of time and resources compared with other areas. The very wide range of services that may be offered to elderly people may present considerable problems of planning and communication if 'seamless' care is to be achieved (Box 1).

Ideally, health and social services for elderly people would be jointly planned and funded from a single budget. In practice, the historical development of services has resulted in separate planning and funding with consequent gaps in provision, and geographical differences in custom and practice. A 'social bath', for example, would constitute a bathing service that health services will not pay for but social services might! Health care systems in which social care is entirely provided by families also require some form of joint planning. This is to ensure that gaps in provision do not occur and that family support is feasible within the constraints of other aspects of development such as the emancipation of women, urbanization, and economic change.

Major health sector reforms—increased user charges, cost containment through standard care pathways, separation of health and social components of care—implemented worldwide, will tend to reduce access to both primary and secondary care. Their effects will be felt disproportionately by the most vulnerable sections of society—children and elderly people.

Role of public health

Public health is concerned with improving the health of populations through assessing need, defining priorities with local stakeholders (including patients), identifying and implementing cost-effective interventions, and monitoring and evaluating their impact. Too often in the United Kingdom, public health has become a means of commissioning health services from the lowest-cost provider. The new public health movement in the United Kingdom emphasizes improving population health by working with agencies other than health services, the need to tackle inequalities in health and in access to health care, and should provide a new impetus for making progress. However, too often public health policies fail to consider older people, and if they do, exclude older people as unable to benefit from primary prevention, for example (Department of Health 1998). Public health medicine practitioners are not well trained in the issues caused by population ageing and are inexperienced in working with elderly people, particularly in developing countries where difficult resource use choices will have to be made. New training initiatives on public health for ageing populations are urgently needed (Ebrahim 1999).

Ageism and rationing

In a society that holds ambivalent but essentially negative values towards older people, manifest as ageism and paternalism, rationing through denial of services or 'knowing better' will occur. How much should be spent on care for elderly people can only be determined by reference to ethical principles. If no value is placed on life once economic productivity ceases, then logically resources should not be wasted on health services for elderly people. National values are shaped over time but may change rapidly in response to practices perceived to be unacceptable. For example, the transfer of frail, demented elderly people to private sector nursing homes to enable closure of old outdated British National Health Service (**NHS**) property was common and accepted as it was assumed that the care on offer would be better and cheaper than the NHS alternative. However, a 1992 television programme that examined the plight of 40 demented elderly patients with no immediate next-of-kin transferred from an East London hospital to a Yorkshire nursing home offering abysmal standards of care caused public and government outrage. In this case, public health values were out of step with national values that appeared to find lowest cost care unacceptable.

How much one generation should spend on supporting earlier generations remains to be tested. The 'fair innings' argument—after so many years, old people should not expect any more—is used by health economists to argue for transfers from old to young rather than vice versa (Williams and Evans 1997). An obvious flaw in such arguments is that we only get sick and in need of health and social care when we get old; the 'fair innings' does not relate to health status or to ability to benefit from health care, only to years lived. Considerable

Box 1 Health and social services for elderly people

Health promotion

- Primary care
- Primary prevention: immunization lowering blood pressure
- Case-finding and screening: generic cancers
- General practitioner services
- General dental services
- Opticians

Community care

- District nursing
- Community psychiatric nurse
- Bathing
- Chiropody
- Continence
- Health visiting
- Domiciliary rehabilitation
- Hospital-at-home schemes

Social services

- Day centre
- Meals-on-wheels
- Home help
- Respite care
- Good neighbour schemes
- Adult fostering
- Holidays
- Occupational therapy
- Home modification
- Residential care

Hospital

- Acute medical care
- Acute psychiatric care
- Early discharge schemes
- Specialist units: stroke, orthogeriatrics
- Day hospital: medical, psychogeriatric
- Rehabilitation
- Outpatient clinics
- Domiciliary visits
- Nursing home care
- Palliative care

Independent sector

- Family and informal carers
- Day care
- Lunch clubs
- Residential care
- Nursing home care
- Home care services

effort is being made by Age Concern in the United Kingdom to persuade government to remove age discrimination in society and within the NHS (Age Concern 1999; Rivlin 1999).

The ethics of state provision of any service is based on utilitarianism—the greatest good for the greatest number—and the British NHS was born out of the collectivist politics essential to surviving a world war. Health care policy should aim to target resources to where they will do most good rather than issue them in response to the distribution of disease. However, targeting requires relevant information on service inputs and health outcomes. In the face of inadequate information on costs and benefits—and the natural peacetime ethics of individualism (Evans 1997)—it seems inevitable that doing the best for the patient regardless of cost should gain hold over utilitarianism. With stronger evidence on the effects of pharmacological interventions, it is also inevitable that conflicts between groups holding different ethical precepts (and with different financial incentives) will emerge. Older people will stand to lose on two counts. Firstly, evidence is weakest and hardest to obtain for complex non-pharmacological interventions from which they may benefit. Secondly, the inherent ageism of society will ensure that elderly people will lose in an individual or collectivist fight for resources. In the United Kingdom, compared with European and North American countries, health care spending is now at such a low level that debates about age-based rationing are considered untenable until adequate resources for health services are found (Tonks 1999). However, without better and wider evidence of benefits of innovative patterns of care for elderly people, more resources will not necessarily mean better care.

Health outcomes

Deciding on appropriate health outcomes for the evaluation of services for elderly people is not a simple matter. As different services have different objectives, general outcomes, such as survival or quality-adjusted life years, do not have wide currency, nor do they help make choices between different areas of activity. Several factors determine what should be considered a benefit of health or social care: the ethical stance taken; the type of intervention; the type of patient; and the viewpoints of other 'stakeholders'—family, service providers, payers.

Interest in health-related quality-of-life indicators has increased as evaluation tools as their multidimensional approach and supposed focus on quality of life appear to tap into many of the objectives of health services for elderly people (Ebrahim 1995). Furthermore, health-related quality of life indicators are much more firmly rooted in patients' experience of disease and should increase the chances of more patient-centred care. The goal of many health-related quality of life indicators, including the Euro-QoL and the 36-Item Short Form (**SF-36**) health questionnaires (Brazier *et al.* 1993; Jenkinson *et al.* 1997; Ware and Gandek 1998), is to provide an index or profile of the value or utility of different health states.

Valuations of different health states may be obtained by time trade-off methods, standard reference gambles, or by simpler visual linear analogue scales. But should patient, professional, or general public valuations be used? For dimensions of pain and mobility, there appears to be little difference in valuations provided by older and younger people or disabled people (Ebrahim *et al.* 1991). In a patient-centred service, it would be logical to use not only patient valuations of health states but also to permit the individual to define the health states of interest and concern to them. Such patient-generated health outcome indicators have been developed (Ruta *et al.* 1994), but require further development work before they could be widely used in health service evaluations.

When pooled to provide utilities, health-related quality of life indicators fall into a potential trap of giving a number that may be less informative than responses to a profile of different dimensions. The items making up health-related quality of life indicators include a mixture of symptoms of pain and depression, difficulties carrying out everyday activities, and impact on social and work life. It is highly unlikely that a specific intervention would affect each area equally, consequently there is a risk of making false-negative inferences if health-related quality of life indicators are used as trial outcomes.

Impairment, disability, and handicap

An alternative model for examining the effects of interventions for older people is the impairment, disability, and handicap model (Harwood *et al.* 1994*b*). Impairment is defined as the loss or abnormality of psychological, physiological, or anatomical structure or function. Disability is any restriction or lack of ability to perform an activity in a normal manner. Handicap is the disadvantage experienced by the individual as a result of impairments and disabilities that limits performance of a normal role, taking account of age, sex, and cultural background (WHO 1980). Impairment, disability, and handicap provide clearly defined areas that might be improved by specific interventions. The classification also enables a distinction to be made between the intrinsic consequences of disease (i.e. impairment and disability) and the external factors that mitigate or accentuate the degree of disadvantage suffered by the individual (i.e. handicap). In evaluation of health services, these distinctions are essential. For example, an intervention comprising walking and kitchen aids together with practice in their use might be expected to improve performance in locomotor and kitchen abilities, and hence these areas would be logical to measure as outcomes. An intervention comprising social services support and benefits would aim to reduce disadvantage and consequently should be assessed by measurement of handicap. If either of these interventions were assessed using health-related quality of life indicators, it is quite possible that no benefits would be found as the indicator would be insensitive to the interventions under investigation.

Disability scales abound and the most commonly used in hospital practice are the Barthel Index of basic self-care activities (Mahoney and Barthel 1965) and the extended or instrumental activities of daily living scales (Nouri and Lincoln 1987) (both originally developed for use with stroke patients). Extended activities of daily living scales are more suitable for community evaluations where people may be less disabled. There is little to choose between various scales as they all share similar items and are scored in similar ways. A caution that should be noted is the practice of examining changes over time in terms of Barthel Index points per week (Shah *et al.* 1990, 1991). Such an approach makes the assumptions that an activities of daily living scale is a continuous variable with interval scaling properties and that a comparable initial baseline point for each patient can be obtained. Thus, patients seen very early in the course of their illness may score zero and be completely unable to perform any tasks but within a day, may be able to feed themselves. If the former baseline is used, changes over time will be exaggerated compared with using the latter baseline.

Handicap measures have not been widely developed owing to the difficulty in operationalizing a concept that is intrinsically individualistic. One way forward has been to produce a multidimensional handicap scale using dimensions suggested by the original World Health Organization (**WHO**) report (Harwood *et al.* 1994*a*). Semantics of disability and handicap have changed recently and the new WHO classification uses the terms impairment, ability (i.e. disability), and participation (WHO 1999). While these latter two terms are more positive, the term participation does not capture the same essential characteristic of disadvantage implicit in the term handicap. Operationalization of these new terms to produce outcome measures is underway but it will take time before the performance and value of these new concepts can be assessed.

Health service evaluations usually consider outcomes at fixed time points which fails to take account of the pattern of recovery or natural history of the diseases suffered.

Patients will experience very variable 'care careers' despite receiving treatment from the same services. For example, patients with heart failure may suffer episodes of profound disability alternating with periods of reasonable ability whereas patients with Parkinson's disease will tend to follow a progressive decline in ability. In these circumstances, it makes little sense to examine aggregated 'outcomes' of general services for elderly people. Heterogeneity between patients in their natural history and the goals of care make conventional evaluation methods much less robust and more likely to produce spurious data.

Information systems

Routine information in most health care systems has failed to keep pace with demographic and epidemiological transitions. Summary mortality statistics are still published with an upper age band of 75 years and over, although in the last decade the British Office of National Statistics uses an upper age band of 95 years and over but the American Bureau of the Census uses an upper band of 85 years and over. International agencies should agree which thresholds to use in varying circumstances so that comparisons may be made more easily.

While routine reporting of common infectious diseases has been maintained despite the falling mortality attributable to this cause, no efforts have been made to make common chronic diseases notifiable to national health statistics centres. Consequently, we have little idea of the incidence of coronary heart disease or stroke and sources of variation within and between countries. By contrast, routine cancer notification has been established in many countries and can make a useful contribution to monitoring trends. Such information is essential for health service planning for an ageing population.

Surveys of disability have been performed in many countries but few countries have invested resources in maintaining regular repeated national surveys of disability. In the United Kingdom, the first national disability survey (Martin *et al.* 1987) conducted in 1985 was repeated in 1996 (Devore 1998) but differences in sampling and methods make comparisons between the two surveys difficult. In particular the 1996 survey did not include institutionalized elders. Ideally, a series of nationally representative cohort studies should be established using internationally agreed methods of sampling and measurement. This information resource would enable national and regional differences in health and social policy to be examined in ecological analyses. Projections of future disability levels would be aided by information on transitions in and out of disabled states, leading to more accurate estimation of health expectancies and future health and social care needs.

Increasingly, useful sources of up-to-date information on population ageing and the effects of health care interventions can be found on the World Wide Web (Jenkins 1999) (Box 2).

Health promotion

Health promotion is concerned with three interrelated activities: primary prevention of disease, health education, and health protection (i.e. legislation or fiscal methods) (Downie *et al.* 1990). It can be argued that effective health promotion can only occur when all three areas are working optimally. Increasingly, there is a recognition and desire to include elderly people in health promotion programmes that were formerly targeted to younger people. Disease-specific programmes for cancer and heart disease prevention have typically involved middle-aged adults and little work has been carried out focusing specifically on elderly people. Such programmes of multiple risk factor intervention, typically including dietary and smoking cessation advice, exercise, and sometimes treatment of hypertension and raised blood cholesterol, do not appear to be effective in reducing the incidence of disease when tested in large-scale randomized controlled trials (Ebrahim and Davey Smith 1997). Alternative study designs using quasi-experimental methods have also failed to establish a clear role for current health promotion methods for cardiovascular disease prevention in middle-aged adults (Ebrahim and Davey Smith 1996). It seems unlikely that the same methods applied to older adults will deliver markedly better results.

By contrast similar multiple risk factor interventions applied to people who have already suffered a heart attack or angina are effective, reducing total mortality by about 20 per cent (Ebrahim and Davey Smith 1996). Secondary prevention is thus a major target for health promotion programmes and it is important that older people are allowed to take part in them. Reorientation of current primary prevention programmes is urgently required as resources are being wasted. It is also vitally important that these programmes are not sold to developing countries as the best means of coping with their increasing burdens of cardiovascular disease. Health protection appears to be more effective as shown by a recent account of the effects of a health promotion programme that achieved notable reductions in blood cholesterol only when the main source of cooking oil changed from palm oil to unsaturated oil (Dowse *et al.* 1995).

Smoking cessation advice amongst older people appears to be as effective as in younger adults (Vetter and Ford 1990; Vetter 1999), although in the United States brief interventions may not be as effective as in British primary care (Burton *et al.* 1995*a*). Contrary to popular belief, many older people do wish to stop smoking and do not view smoking as one of life's little pleasures but as a positive harm that may have ill effects on their grandchildren (Vetter *et al.* 1988). The British Doctors' Study highlights the years of life gained by avoiding smoking after the age of 35 years—over 7 extra years of life expectancy on average (Doll *et al.* 1994).

Exercise programmes are widely promoted among older people as a means of maintaining health. The supposed benefits of physical exercise are derived from observational epidemiological studies showing large differences in the rates of cardiovascular disease, depression, and osteoporosis in those taking moderate or greater levels of exercise (Fentem 1994; Wolman 1994; Tseng *et al.* 1995; NIH Consensus Development Panel on Physical Activity and Cardiovascular Health 1996; Buchner 1997; Rippe and Hess 1998; Fletcher 1999). However, attempts to test the effects of exercise in randomized controlled trials are less compelling (Hillsdon *et al.* 1995). Health benefits tend to be found in short-duration trials involving volunteers. Many older people do not wish to take part in exercise interventions, often because they feel too unwell or too busy to do so. Also, drop-out rates from trials are often large, emphasizing the difficulty of maintenance of increased levels of exercise, and have demonstrated that even brisk walking is not without adverse effects causing injury (Ebrahim *et al.* 1997). A systematic review has demonstrated that environmental interventions that encourage walking or cycling (e.g. safe cycle paths and walkways, local shops, and other amenities within walking distance) reach a greater proportion of the population than interventions aimed at increasing the use of exercise facilities (Hillsdon and Thorogood 1996).

Nutritional interventions for older people include the widespread 'healthy diet' approaches which have been modified over the years from low-fat low-cholesterol diets to fruit and vegetable diets.

Box 2 World Wide Web sources of information on ageing

Professional groups

http://www.americangeriatrics.org
http://www.bgs.org.uk/

Government statistics

http://pr.aoa.dhhs.gov/aoa/stats/statlink.html
http://pr.aoa.dhhs.gov/naic/
http://www.census.gov/
http://www.statistics.gov.uk/
http://www.nih.gov/nia/
http://www.who.int/m/healthtopics-a-z/en/index.html

Non-governmental sector

http://www.cpa.org.uk/
http://www.helpage.org/
http://www.ace.org.uk/
http://www.aarp.org/

Effectiveness of interventions

http://www.clinicalevidence.org

Evidence from randomized controlled trials of dietary advice provides limited support for the use of low-fat diets(Hooper *et al.* 2001) or antioxidant vitamins such as β-carotene (Egger *et al.* 1998). Among people with pre-existing heart disease, eating oily fish regularly has a significant and clinically important reduction in total and cardiovascular disease mortality (Hooper et *al.* 1999).

Age well programmes

More general health promotion programmes for elderly people have aimed to alleviate disengagement and loneliness and build on the perceived value of keeping active in old age. Examples abound and include programmes run by retirement associations and by voluntary sector charities such as Help Age International and Age Concern in the United Kingdom. Such programmes aim to provide opportunities for elderly people to participate in a range of activities that provide social engagement, role fulfilment, and physical and mental activity. In general, evaluation of these programmes has only been in terms of coverage and continued participation rates. Improvements in health status or in maintenance in the community have not been examined. Increasing the income of older people might be expected to increase health status from observational data showing social gradients in both disability and disease. Trials of increasing income have been conducted but appear not to have been targeted at older people (Connor *et al.* 1999). This is a major oversight and such trials are urgently required.

Cross-sectoral collaborative interventions aiming to improve environmental factors (e.g. transport, housing design) that contribute to disability have not been widely established or evaluated. Health improvement programmes are expected to involve local government departments and non-governmental agencies. These new alliances hold great promise for improving the health of older people. Evaluation of their costs and health benefits should be an integral component when establishing new programmes, but will be difficult (Judge 2000).

Primary care

Elderly people are high users of primary care services, reflecting their greater levels of disease and disability. In the United Kingdom, elderly people are more likely to see their general practitioner at home than at the surgery, probably reflecting the increased frailty of very elderly patients (Figs 11 and 12).

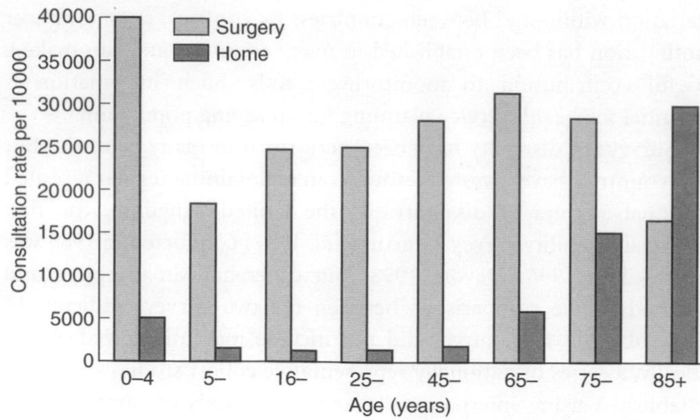

Fig. 11 Consultation rates in general practice by age and place of consultation. (McCormick *et al.* 1995, Table 2b.)

The major causes of consultations for elderly people do not show marked differences from those at younger ages. However, there is a tendency for ill-defined conditions to contribute relatively more at the oldest ages.

In many developing countries, the role of primary care is paramount as secondary level services are inaccessible, and often inappropriate, for a majority of elderly people. However, training in health care for elderly people is not a high priority in undergraduate medical or nursing curricula of developing country medical schools. Despite the undeniable importance of maintaining strong maternal and child health training programmes in developing countries, it is essential that recognition of the growing numbers of elderly people should be reflected in increased opportunities to learn about the health care of elderly people. European and North American models of geriatric medicine are heavily reliant on hospital services and do not have an appropriate balance of care for the needs of developing

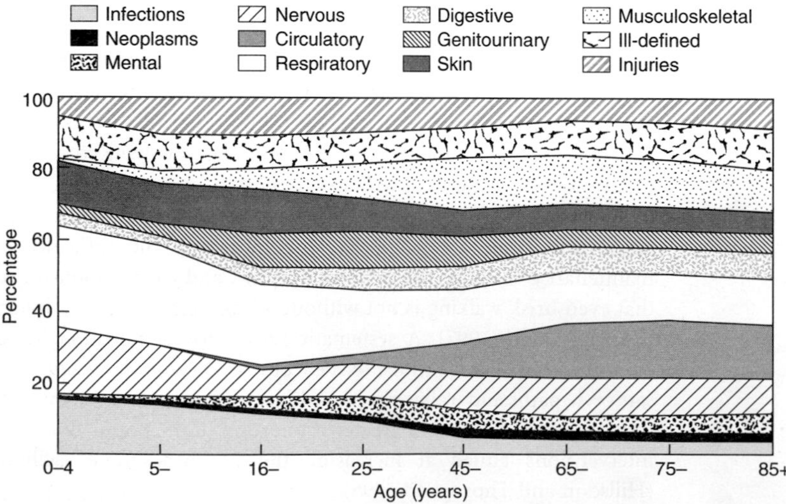

Fig. 12 Consultations in general practice by age and underlying diagnostic group. (McCormick *et al.* 1995, Table 19.)

countries. The first step is to examine the common health problems seen among older people in primary care and to match training to meeting these needs. Without appropriate training it is very likely that elderly people will simply receive a growing number of pills for each of their symptoms, running the risk of iatrogenesis, and their potentially diagnosable and treatable problems will be missed.

Primary prevention

Immunization

Immunization against influenza is strongly supported by evidence from cohort studies and randomized trials (Gross *et al.* 1995). It appears that elderly people who might benefit are frequently excluded or missed from immunization programmes (Centers for Disease Control and Prevention 1997; Watkins *et al.* 1999). In the United Kingdom, it has been suggested that immunization should be confined to high-risk and institutionalized elderly (Nicholson 1993). However, American cost-effectiveness studies demonstrated cost savings when universal, rather than selective policies of immunization were adopted (Mullooly *et al.* 1994; Nichol *et al.* 1994). It is likely that these findings would apply in most postindustrialized countries, and in 1999 British government medical advice was modified to bring it in line with many other countries, recommending the immunization of everyone aged 75 years and over (Watkins *et al.* 1999). It is probable that untargeted extension of immunization to those aged 65 years and over would also be cost-effective, given the problems associated with ensuring that high-risk people are identified. Additionally, there is trial evidence that health care workers in institutions for elderly people should be immunized against influenza, as this reduced the mortality risk among the residents (Potter *et al.* 1997).

Pneumococcal vaccination does not appear to give any protection against developing pneumonia or death when given to elderly people in the community (Fine *et al.* 1994). More recent trials confirm earlier findings (Koivula *et al.* 1997; Ortqvist *et al.* 1998) but suggest that those people at high risk of pneumonia (i.e. institutionalized, immobile, on immunosuppressive drugs, suffering with serious chronic diseases) would benefit. In cost-effectiveness analyses, a policy of widespread, untargeted vaccination of everyone aged 65 years and over was cost saving (Sisk *et al.* 1997). Further work is required to evaluate the cost-effectiveness of a combined strategy of universal vaccination of elderly people at different age thresholds with both influenza and pneumococcal vaccines compared with targeted vaccination to determine cost-effectiveness.

Case-finding and screening

Older people consult their general practitioner several times a year, which provides considerable opportunity for opportunistic case-finding. However, in areas such as high blood pressure, depression, and visual and hearing impairment, icebergs of unrecognized disease are common. Interestingly, non-consulters appear to be a fairly healthy group of elderly people and would not be a high priority for screening (Ebrahim *et al.* 1984). In the 1990 British general practitioner contract it was required that health checks be offered to people aged 75 years and over. These checks were expected to focus on mobility, mental state, hearing and vision, continence, general function, and medication review (Williams and Wallace 1993). While these areas are important and are the areas commonly causing problems to older people, the contractual obligation did not stretch as far as requiring any specific action to be taken in response to problems identified.

Health checks

The potential benefit of health checks amongst the over-75-year-olds has been assessed: more dementia, depression, incontinence, and immobility would be identified (Iliffe *et al.* 1991*a*), but the costs would be considerable, amounting to about 150 h of primary care time per year for a typical general practice of 2000 patients of whom 130 are over 75 years old (Iliffe *et al.* 1991*b*). The evidence to support the effectiveness of health checks or case-finding carried out in primary care is very limited, although a large British Medical Research Council trial comparing usual care with augmented health checks has been established but results have yet to be published.

Evaluations of case-finding in primary care have been systematically reviewed as part of a larger review of comprehensive geriatric assessment (Stuck *et al.* 1993). A total of seven randomized controlled trials (five performed in the United Kingdom and two in Scandinavian countries) were reviewed. The pooled results showed a statistically non-significant improvement in mortality (odds ratio 0.87, 95 per cent confidence intervals 0.71, 1.07), no difference in the chances of living at home at 12 months (odds ratio 1.07, 95 per cent confidence intervals 0.87, 1.31), and no difference in functional improvement at 12 months (odds ratio 0.96, 95 per cent confidence intervals 0.71, 1.29). Hospital readmissions were significantly reduced in those receiving health checks (odds ratio 0.84, 95 per cent confidence intervals 0.73, 0.96) but there was also significant heterogeneity between the trials suggesting that differences between the trials in the intervention studied contributed to this finding.

Since this review was published two further American trials, an Italian trial, and a Dutch trial have been reported. One American trial demonstrated that a home-based screening programme for people over 75 years was effective in reducing disability (Stuck *et al.* 1995). However, this analysis took no account of deaths and was based only on survivors. Reanalysis of the data using an intention to treat approach and combining deaths and disability produces a non-significant odds ratio of 0.73 (95 per cent confidence intervals 0.48, 1.12) which is consistent with the pooled data from the other seven trials. A Medicare preventive health care intervention offered to people aged 65 years and older found only 'modest health benefits'—a 25 per cent reduction in mortality (8.3 versus 11.1 per cent)—which was achieved at no increased cost to Medicare (Burton *et al.* 1995*b*; German *et al.* 1995). The Italian trial examined the effects of an integrated social and medical care and case management package among frail elderly people already in receipt of social support and found improvements in disability and reduced health service use over the period of a year (Bernabei *et al.* 1998). The Dutch trial failed to find any benefits associated with intervention, although a subgroup analysis showed some improvement in those people rating their health as poor (van Rossum *et al.* 1993). It is unlikely that findings on preventive health care can be generalized from systems of health care where financial barriers to consultation may exist to 'free at the point of use' services.

Screening for specific problems does not appear to be any more beneficial than attempting to deal with several problems together. For example, screening for visual problems is not associated with improvements in visual impairment (Smeeth and Iliffe 1998, 1999). Screening for mental health problems does not appear to improve quality of life or mood (Cole 1998). Screening for factors that might increase risk of falls, followed by targeting interventions at intrinsic and environmental factors may be of value but single interventions such as exercise or health education appear to have little value (Gillespie *et al.* 1999). An exercise intervention evaluated as part of a preplanned data pooling has demonstrated reductions in the risk of falls (Province *et al.* 1995). In each of these areas, trials are beset with methodological problems common to the evaluation of any complex intervention; of these problems, small sample sizes are the most common.

High blood pressure

Treatment of high blood pressure as a means of preventing stroke among relatively fit people up to the age of 80 years is supported by strong evidence from randomized controlled trials (Insua *et al.* 1994; Mulrow *et al.* 1994). Treatment of people over the age of 80 years has been examined in a subgroup analysis of the seven randomized controlled trials of drug treatments. Reductions in non-fatal cardiovascular events were found with no overall reduction in total mortality (Gueyffier *et al.* 1999). However, increased efforts to screen for high blood pressure, either by case-finding or screening, have not shown improvements in population coverage, in adherence to treatment, or better blood pressure control (Ebrahim 1998).

Cancer screening

Involving elderly women in routine breast and cervical cancer screening programmes is controversial. For women aged between 65 and 69 there is consistent evidence of benefit from breast cancer screening with a reduction in mortality of 30 per cent (95 per cent confidence intervals 50 per cent, 90 per cent) (Fletcher 1996). Among women over the age of 65 who have had a series of three negative cervical smears, further routine cervical screening is of no benefit (Fahs *et al.* 1992).

In summary, efforts to improve disability and to prevent disease through systematic case-finding are not supported by currently available evidence. It seems likely that failure to achieve benefits is due to inadequately specified actions to be taken in the light of problems detected by case-finding. Further work in this area needs to ensure that interventions are better planned and should evaluate how well the processes of care operate in addition to examining outcomes. Reliance on trials performed in different health care systems is unwise owing to the very different barriers to care, expectations of people, and differences in need. More data are required to guide policy on the application of trial evidence on treating hypertension and screening for cancers among elderly people.

Community and social care

The wide range of community and social services provided for elderly people (Box 1) are of potentially great importance in maintaining elderly people in their own homes and reducing inappropriate use of long-term institutional care or acute hospital care. Considerable resources are spent on social services for elderly people but there is no culture of evaluation comparable to that in health services. Community and home care services are characterized by problems of mismatch between needs and resources, inadequate assessment processes, lack of monitoring and review, and inflexibility of provision and lack of integration (Challis 1996).

In the United Kingdom, the use of care management was intended to bring greater coherence to planning by putting a single social worker in charge of building a 'package of care' for a patient. This package would be based on the patient's needs and would reduce the bias towards institutional care for frail elderly people. The research that underpinned this innovative approach had shown the importance of care manager training and experience and the need for discretionary budgets that would be controlled by care managers. Under these circumstances the need for institutional care was reduced, elderly people and their families were more satisfied, and the overall cost was no greater than usual patterns of care (Wolman 1994; Tseng *et al.* 1995). A before-and-after evaluation of the impact of community care reforms in Northern Ireland demonstrated that the use of institutional care was more targeted towards people with greater physical and mental disability after implementation of the reforms (Crawford *et al.* 1999).

Unfortunately, implementation of care management by social services departments in the United Kingdom has been difficult with many managers ill suited to the task and strapped for sufficient cash to make up viable packages of care. The principles of care management are sound but implementation requires greater commitment from senior managers.

Inevitably, the pattern of community and social services available in a locality will vary. Consequently, maintaining older people in their own homes may require available resources to be used in innovative and flexible ways. Public health medicine has a major role in ensuring better communication between service users, and the sectors paying for and providing services. In this way, local plans may be developed which would aim to cover the majority of needs. Research and development in community and social services is desperately needed to provide stronger evidence to support continued investment in services.

Hospital services

The variation in the organization of hospital services for physically ill elderly people, reflects differing beliefs and historical developments. In the United Kingdom, geriatric medicine grew out of the NHS and was initially a custodial service with responsibility for large long-stay care hospitals (Warren 1946). The first cohort of geriatricians managed to assess, rehabilitate, and discharge many of their long-stay patients, demonstrating the inadequacy of existing general medical services that had put patients in such places in the first place. These services grew into needs-based services which aimed to reduce the chances of elderly people being inappropriately treated by providing a rapid 'take-away' service for acute medical specialties. As the specialty of geriatric medicine grew, alternative models developed. Firstly, age-related services arose as a mechanism for obtaining better quality facilities in major, rather than peripheral, hospitals. These services agreed to manage all patients over a certain age and in return received a quota of acute beds. Next, integrated services arose as it became apparent that geriatric medicine was simply another subspecialty of medicine and should be organized no differently. In this model, all physicians take a share of all the acute medical admissions and only those elderly people with difficult problems are referred on to the physician with an interest in geriatric medicine (Evans 1983; Evans and Graham 1984).

As no good evidence exists to defend or support any of these three major models, considerable debate has occurred over which model best meets the needs of older people (Young 1989). As their needs are so variable, it is possible to make a compelling case for any model of care. And, with good communication and sensible referral of difficult cases, any model of care can be made to work to the benefit of patients and the hospital.

In developing countries where geriatric services seldom exist even in teaching hospitals, elderly patients are beginning to be experienced as 'problems' in acute wards and 'bed-blocking' has begun (Thamprechavai *et al.* 1992). The American hospital services have not had a history of geriatric medical services but have been in the forefront of performing randomized controlled trials to find out what is effective management for elderly patients (Stuck *et al.* 1993). This work, while not necessarily directly of general applicability to British or European services, does demonstrate the feasibility and importance of performing trials in circumstances of uncertainty.

Comprehensive geriatric services

A systematic review of comprehensive geriatric assessment examined the effects of hospital geriatric evaluation and management units and inpatient geriatric consultation services on mortality, place of discharge, and change in functional status (Stuck *et al.* 1993). In total, six trials of geriatric evaluation and management units and eight trials of inpatient geriatric consultation services were included in this review but one of the trials in each group was of patients with fractured neck of femur managed in orthopaedics or by geriatric services. As the focus was on comprehensive geriatric assessment applied to elderly patients admitted to hospital, it is debatable whether these two trials should be included when trials of specialist management of stroke patients were excluded. The review demonstrated short-term (6 months) improvements in mortality: odds ratios were 0.65 (95 per cent confidence intervals 0.46, 0.91) for geriatric evaluation and management units and 0.77 (95 per cent confidence intervals 0.62, 0.96) for inpatient geriatric consultation services, which had attenuated by 12 months. Interestingly, geriatric evaluation and management units were very successful at discharging people to their own homes and improving functional ability at 6 months (odds ratios of 1.80 and 1.63 respectively,) whereas inpatient consultation services did no better than usual care. This suggests that geriatric services that have direct responsibility for patient management do better than those that simply give advice.

A recent trial comparing inpatient assessment alone, assessment together with postdischarge home support, and usual care for elderly people admitted to hospital found that disability, readmissions to hospital, and institutionalization (but not mortality) were only improved by the combined assessment and home support service (Nikolaus *et al.* 1999).

Although the conclusions of this meta-analysis of trials of comprehensive geriatric assessment and the recent trial appear to support current working methods, there is always the possibility that publication bias has resulted in small negative trials remaining unpublished. This was examined in a study comparing the effect sizes derived from meta-analyses of small trials with definitive 'mega-trials' (Egger *et al.* 1997). The small trials appeared to overestimate the effect of geriatric care when compared with a large health maintenance organization trial of 2353 patients which found no improvements in survival or functional status (Reuben *et al.* 1995). The authors of the original meta-analysis suggest that one reason for the difference between their findings and those of the mega-trial was that patients in the usual care control arm of the mega-trial received greater geriatric medicine expertise than would typically be found outside of health maintenance organizations (Stuck *et al.* 1998). This explanation seems unlikely but does suggest that better characterization of the process of care in trials of complex interventions is essential for interpretation and implementation of findings (Beck and Stuck 1996).

Disease-specific services

Specialist services for patients suffering stroke have been evaluated in small randomized controlled trials and appear to be valuable, reducing mortality and institutionalization by about 20 per cent at 12 months (Stroke Unit Trialists' Collaboration 1999). However, these trials showed considerable statistical heterogeneity when meta-analysed which may be explained by differences in the precise nature of the stroke services or the types of patients included in the trials (Ebrahim and Harwood 1999). Although this evidence of benefit of organized stroke care is widely believed to be true, it is quite possible that the pooled evidence is misleading as it is derived from small, often poorly designed trials. In such circumstances it would be logical to perform a large, uniform protocol, multicentre trial to determine which patients benefit from organized stroke services and at what cost. Specialist services for fractured neck of femur patients (orthogeriatric services) have also been examined in systematic reviews of small randomized controlled trials; pooled effects show a non-significant trend towards improved survival and less dependence. However, the trials are very heterogeneous in terms of the interventions used and do not provide secure evidence for or against such services (Cameron *et al.* 1999).

Hospital-at-home and day hospitals

Various 'hospital-at-home' and early discharge schemes have been promoted in efforts to reduce demand on acute hospital services and several evaluations have been performed. Non-randomized evaluations were encouraging and several schemes were established in the United Kingdom, but systematic review of randomized controlled trial evaluations do not provide strong enough evidence to either support further development or discontinue existing schemes for elderly medical patients, patients who have had elective surgery, or those with a terminal illness (Shepperd and Iliffe 1999). A more recent trial has reported reductions in length of stay with associated cost-savings but no differences in health outcomes (Jones *et al.* 1999; Wilson *et al.* 1999).

Day hospitals that attempt to facilitate early discharge or to manage patients as an alternative to hospital admission show no survival or disability benefits when compared with comprehensive geriatric inpatient care and costs may be higher (Forster *et al.* 1999*a*,*b*).

Both comprehensive geriatric services and specialist hospital services are not well supported by available evidence and practice varies widely between countries. It is unlikely that evidence from trials of these complex interventions will be transferable from one health care system to another owing to the differing age distributions and comorbidities of patients and the selection effects introduced by different systems of social and health care. As the costs of investing in such services are high, evaluation of their cost-effectiveness should be a high priority.

Health services for mentally ill people

Unlike geriatric services, health services for elderly people suffering from functional mental illnesses (largely depressive illness) and organic brain syndromes (largely dementia) have followed the general trend of moving out of the psychiatric hospitals and into the community. In the United Kingdom, considerable energy and vision have been used to create a new specialty of psychogeriatrics as a direct response to the needs of an ageing population with an increased burden of dementia (Arie and Jolley 1998). Old age psychiatry services follow different models ranging from intergrated with geriatric medicine, separate old age services, or linked with adult psychiatry. Most services adopt common principles of attempting to be community orientated, comprehensive, available, and flexible (Lindesay 1996). Most have a common core of services including an acute assessment unit, a rehabilitation unit, a day hospital, and community liaison teams. As with hospital services for physically ill people, convincing evidence to support particular styles of practice in terms of costs and outcomes is not available. Current evaluations have focused on examining the processes of care and a disproportionate amount of research endeavour in the specialty is now devoted to drug trials rather than organization of service trials.

Community-based rehabilitation

Most rehabilitation received by elderly people is provided in the context of their acute admission to hospital and in day hospitals. The randomized controlled trials referred to above generally included some component of rehabilitation. This is often essential in the management of acute illness because of rapid deterioration in physical capacity. However, much less attention is given to rehabilitation outside hospital despite the importance to patients of rehabilitation in their own environments rather than those of the hospital (Young *et al.* 1999).

In developing countries that lack investment in hospital services for elderly people, community-based rehabilitation offers an alternative model that requires urgent evaluation. Establishing rehabilitation services outside hospitals is feasible and services are certainly more accessible and are probably cheaper for patients but probably not for health service providers (Jitapunkul *et al.* 1998). Services given in people's homes may be more effective in reducing handicap, optimal use of aids and appliances, and in ensuring that prevention of future problems is tackled. For stroke patients not admitted to hospital, community occupational therapy reduces disability and handicap (Walker *et al.* 1999). Specific issues that need study are the role of families in the process of rehabilitation, local low-cost production of disability aids and appliances, and education and training in rehabilitation for primary care teams. While there are good reasons for expecting community rehabilitation to have promise, only through systematic study of its costs and benefits will sound policy be developed.

Long-term care

Long-term care is often equated with institutional care rather than a more comprehensive definition of the care required by people to permit them to achieve their potential and maintain abilities in the face of chronic and often progressive disability (Kane and Kane 1991). In the United Kingdom, many long-term care institutions arose out of Poor Law workhouses that were originally set up to ensure that the destitute of every parish had somewhere to go (Townsend 1962). The level of provision had to be worse than that existing outside the workhouse to deter people from entering the workhouse. Standards of care in long-term care institutions are among the major concerns of elderly people and their carers (Counsel and Care 1991; Avebury 1996) (Table 7).

Costs of long-term care

The issue of who pays for long-term care is important as protection of health and social services budgets may not result in the optimal use of resources or good standards of care. Community care reforms have been introduced in many countries as a response to growing public concern over the costs of long-term care (Fig. 10). Projections suggest that long-term care costs will outstrip other health sector costs owing to the very large number of very elderly people who lack support (Laing *et al.* 1991). However, there is greater than fourfold variation between countries in the proportion of the elderly population aged 75+ receiving long-term institutional care which demonstrates that substitution of alternatives to institutions is feasible (Table 7). In all countries, the increasing trend of institutionalization with older age is apparent. In developing countries, there is a growth in institutions for elderly people and this is most marked in large towns and among more affluent sections of society. A move towards institutional care, rather than care at home, is likely to consume more resources and result in upward cost pressures and aspirations for more institutional care among less affluent people in the future. Unfortunately, much urban planning has ignored the needs of older people and is designed inappropriately (e.g. high-rise public housing), and is suited to small nuclear families rather than larger extended families.

The relationship between severity of dependency and cost of care is relatively flat for institutional care but increases approximately exponentially for care at home (Evans 1993*b*). Anyone can be looked after at home if sufficient resources are available; packages costing over £100 000 (US$165 000) a year have been set up for children and young adults with learning difficulties. Promoting care at home is a desirable policy but there comes a point where, within a cash limited budget, provision of home care for an individual becomes unethical if it is

Table 7 Age and prevalence of institutionalization in different countries

	65–69	70–74	75+
Austria	1.6	2.4	7.3
Belgium	2.0	3.1	9.0
Canada	2.7	4.6	17.5
Denmark	1.6	2.8	13.4
France	2.2	2.9	9.1
Italy	1.6	2.0	4.4
Japan	1.7	3.0	5.8
Luxembourg	2.7	4.4	11.6
Norway	0.9	2.1	11.0
Spain	1.2	1.8	3.7
Sweden	0.4	1.0	7.8
Switzerland	2.7	4.1	13.6
UK	1.2	1.9	7.8
USA	1.4	2.5	10.8

Source: Rubenstein and Nasr (1996).

accepted that the ethical perspective of purchasing is to achieve the greatest good for the greatest number.

Need for long-term care

The future need for long-term care will be determined by demographic trends, the strong relationship between age and disability, the extent to which community care permits people to stay at home, and the willingness of relatives to provide continued unpaid help. Most of these factors will tend to result in more rather than less need for long-term institutional care. In many countries, current levels of provision will be inadequate to meet future needs. Ignoring the problem is likely to have predictable consequences for waiting lists and admission of acutely ill elderly people as beds become clogged with people waiting for some alternative to an acute hospital bed.

Economic evaluations of private versus public sector residential homes suggest that the private sector is cheaper (Laing *et al.* 1991). Making these judgements is difficult and it is all too easy to make biased comparisons (Challis 1992). Variation in the costs of care depend on the following factors: levels of dependency, the number of residents and number of short-stay admissions, nursing qualified staff and supervisory staff, good physical standards, especially the proportion of single rooms, and local socio-economic status (Judge 1986). The cost advantages of private sector homes are probably attributable to the following points: small business enterprise, low rate of return on capital investment acceptable, lower wage rates, dependency may be managed more efficiently (i.e. with fewer staff), and a lower proportion of single rooms.

Evaluation of long-term care

Institutional care has had a chequered history, limiting its acceptability among many policy-makers. Goffman's early work was influential in raising public awareness of the inadequacies of institutions (Goffman 1961). He defined the total institution as working for itself rather than its inmates with characteristics of group rather than individual treatment, routines and depersonalization, and emotional distance between staff and residents. Consequently, most current philosophies of care have emphasized the need to avoid use of institutions, and if this is not possible, to defend the autonomy of individuals, promote choice, and the use of person-centred styles of care.

The majority of people who require and currently use long-term care are demented and need 24 h supervision. This has led to attempts to evaluate outcomes in a partial way, considering reduction of carer stress as a major outcome of long-term care, together with maintenance of dignity and provision of personal care as additional important aims of services (Melzer *et al.* 1992). While maintaining 'quality of life' is an obvious outcome of good long-term care, most of the indicators used in evaluations are insensitive to variation in the quantity and quality of care. Examining changes in these quality of life measures is complicated by deaths; the most severely ill die ensuring that improvements in survivors' abilities will be found. Satisfaction among relatives and staff may be far more important outcomes to consider.

Two randomized controlled trials have been conducted which aimed to compare care provided in purpose-built NHS nursing homes with more typical care in NHS long-stay wards. These trials illustrate the problems of applying 'objective' standardized measures of outcome. The first study randomized 464 residents and used the Crichton Royal Behavioural Rating Scale, a psychiatric assessment schedule, semistructured interviews of quality of care and self-rated health, life satisfaction index, and survival as outcomes (Bond *et al.* 1989*a*,*b*; Bond and Bond 1990). By 1 year, just under half the residents were dead and no differences were found in the outcomes measured. Non-participant observation demonstrated that there were differences in more subtle aspects of life in the two settings: calling staff by first names, later waking times, more positive feelings towards staff, residents' interaction, choice, and a more flexible day were hallmarks of NHS nursing home care. These findings were confirmed in the second, smaller trial (Clarke and Bowling 1990; Bowling *et al.* 1991).

Both trials demonstrated better processes of care and outcomes in terms of the residents' and staffs' everyday life in NHS nursing homes and that conventional outcomes (i.e. disability and behaviour scales) were not very useful in this context. Unfortunately, it is difficult to generalize from these trials to the wider world, and it would be wrong to conclude that any nursing home is better than a hospital ward. For health service commissioners, the message is clear—good quality care can be provided in state-run sectors and non-participant observation offers a powerful means of assessing standards of care.

The joint dangers of attempting to purchase sufficient low-quality long-term care places or of purchasing insufficient numbers of high-quality institutional places are self-evident. Neither option will do. The object of commissioning in this area is to ensure that both amount and standards are considered.

Donabedian (1989) has suggested that in evaluating health care for elderly people it is sensible to focus on processes of care rather than improvements in health (i.e. outcomes) because for elderly people, the cardinal principles of comprehensiveness, co-ordination, and continuity are more important than the outcomes themselves. Comprehensiveness means that care is not fragmented into social and health domains and implies an individual and holistic approach. Co-ordination is largely concerned with ensuring that everyone knows about and accepts responsibility for management and implies good communication. Continuity of care is achieved by maintaining the same staff and keeping the resident in the same place. Therefore, in the absence of efficacy studies (which are unlikely to be mounted because of cost and problems in defining sensible outcomes), it is appropriate to consider recommended standards in terms of their contributions to comprehensiveness, co-ordination, and continuity as goals in their own right.

Social support and informal carers

Observational epidemiological studies have demonstrated that social support is associated with improved survival, avoidance of institutionalization, reduced disability, and improved quality of life (Bowling and Browne 1991; Steinbach 1992; Mendes de Leon *et al.* 1999). The way in which social care resources are allocated shows considerable unexplainable variation. For example, in Sweden differences in allocation of resources such as home helps, sheltered housing, and institutional care places were found which could not be explained by differences in need for services (Lagergren and Johansson 1998). Evidence from controlled trials of the impact of social services schemes to provide social support are fairly rare and tend to be small scale. For example, a trial of outreach management of elderly people discharged from hospital failed to find any difference in quality of life or functional performance (Curtis *et al.* 1998). Similarly, social support interventions with stroke patients failed to demonstrate any effects (Friedland and McColl 1992). By contrast, an Italian trial of integrated social and medical care with case management did find reduced institutionalization and functional decline (Bernabei *et al.* 1998). Interpretation of small, often methodologically unsound, and underpowered negative trials is beset with problems. Much more work is required to develop both theoretically sound interventions and better methods of evaluation of these complex interventions.

Informal unpaid carers of frail elderly people provide a contribution to maintaining them at home that dwarfs state provision in any country (Travers 1996). It is estimated that there are at least 6 million carers in the United Kingdom (i.e. about one in ten of the population) (Smith 1994). Many caregivers are themselves elderly people. The causes of caregiver stress and breakdown have been well documented and include the type of care provided, living with the person cared for, coping with combined mental and physical problems, and ill health of the carer. Respite care (i.e. brief periods of admission to institutional care) does not appear to have any consistent effects or to moderate burdens (McNally *et al.* 1999). Other methods of carer support have been evaluated in specific contexts, particularly dementia, showing that an accurate diagnosis may help, as may family and individual counselling, and training (Schofield *et al.* 1998; Mittleman *et al.* 1996; Brodaty *et al.* 1997; Bamford *et al.* 1998).

The common belief—'families do not want to care for elderly relatives'—is not supported by European surveys which show that families do want to provide support to their parents and grandparents (McGlone and Cronin 1994). Willingness to give care is not related to employment status of women (Robison *et al.* 1995) but, perhaps inevitably, unmarried daughters tend to provide more direct care than married or divorced daughters (Brody *et al.* 1994) or sons. Informal carers, unlike formal sector services, are capable of providing very complex caring arrangements and are more flexible (Vetter *et al.* 1992). Therfore informal carers may substitute for inadequate formal sector provision or may act as a bridge, bringing elderly people into contact with services (Logan and Spitze 1994).

Health and social policy implications of population ageing

The WHO has highlighted the importance of 'active ageing'—the process of optimizing opportunities for physical, social, and mental well being throughout the life course in order to extend healthy life expectancy—as its major policy (Kalache 1999). Recognition of the contributions made by elderly people themselves to families, communities, and national wealth is an essential step in improving their situation and avoiding ageism. For frail sick elderly people, the major policies of care in the community, avoidance of long-term institutional care, and support for informal carers are essential elements. In developing countries, policy based on the assumptions that families will cope without support and that a tradition of respect for elders will be maintained seem doomed to failure. Greater efforts are needed to understand the best ways of maintaining health in old age, equipping primary care teams with appropriate skills in the management of health problems of elderly people and building support for families. Policy in the areas of education, employment, transport, social welfare, housing, and environment should be examined for its potential impact on elderly people so that the general goals of maintaining older people in their own homes and improving their health expectancy can be achieved.

References

Age Concern (1999). *Turning your backs on us.* Age Concern, London.

Anonymous (1999). *Statistical yearbook 1999 for the Federal Republic of Germany.* Statistisches Bundesamt, Wiesbaden.

Arie, T. and Jolley, D. (1998). Psychogeriatric services. In *Brocklehurst's textbook of geriatric medicine and gerontology* (ed. R. Tallis, H.M. Fillit, and J.C. Brocklehurst) (5th edn). Churchill Livingstone, Edinburgh.

Avebury, K. (1996). *A Better home life. A code of good practice for residential and nursing home care. Report of an Advisory Group.* Centre for Policy on Ageing, London.

Balarajan, R., Yuen, P., and Raleigh, V.S. (1989). Ethnic differences in general practitioner consultations. *British Medical Journal*, **299**, 958–60.

Bamford, C., Gregson, B.A., Farrow, G., Buck, D., Dowswell, T. and McNamee, P.B.J. (1998). Mental and physical frailty in older people: the costs and benefits of informal care. *Ageing and Society*, **18**, 317–54.

Beck, J.C. and Stuck, A. (1996). Preventing disability. Beyond the black box. *Journal of the American Medical Association*, **276**, 1756–7.

Bernabei, R., Landi, F., Gambassi, G., *et al.* (1998). Randomised trial of impact of model of integrated care and case management for older people living in the community. *British Medical Journal*, **316**, 1348–51.

Bond, S. and Bond, J. (1990). Outcomes of care within a multiple case study in the evaluation of the experimental NHS nursing homes. *Age and Ageing*, **19**, 11–18.

Bond, J., Gregson, B.A., Atkinson, A., and Newell, D.J. (1989*a*). The implementation of a randomised controlled trial in the evaluation of the experimental NHS nursing homes. *Age and Ageing*, **18**, 96–102.

Bond, J., Gregson, B.A., and Atkinson, A. (1989*b*). Measurement of outcomes within a multicentred randomised controlled trial in the evaluation of NHS nursing homes. *Age and Ageing*, **18**, 292–302.

Bone, M., Bebbington, A., Jagger, C., Morgan, K., and Nicolaas G. (1995). *Health expectancy and its uses.* HMSO, London.

Bowling, A. (1999). Ageism in cardiology. *British Medical Journal*, **319**, 1353–5.

Bowling, A. and Browne, P.D. (1991). Social networks, health, and emotional well-being among the oldest old in London. *Journal of Gerontology*, **46**, S20–S32.

Bowling, A., Formby, J., Grant, K., and Ebrahim, S. (1991). A randomized controlled trial of nursing home and long-stay geriatric ward care for elderly people. *Age and Ageing*, **20**, 316–24.

Brazier, J., Jones, N., and Kind, P. (1993). Testing the validity of the Euroqol and comparing it with the SF-36 health survey questionnaire. *Quality of Life Research*, **2**, 169–80.

Brodaty, H., Gresham, B., and Luscombe, G. (1997). The Prince Henry Hospital dementia caregivers' training programme. *International Journal of Geriatric Psychiatry*, **12**, 183–92.

Brody, E.M., Litvin, S.J., Albert, S.M., and Hoffman, C.J. (1994). Marital status of daughters and patterns of parent care. *Journal of Gerontology*, **49**, S95–103.

Buchner, D.M. (1997). Preserving mobility in older adults. *Western Journal of Medicine*, **167**, 258–64.

Bunker, J.P. (1994). Medicine's core values. Medical care does add to life expectancy. *British Medical Journal*, **309**, 1657.

Burton, L.C., Paglia, M.J., German, P.S., Shapiro, S., and Damiano, A.M. (1995*a*). The effect among older persons of a general preventive visit on three health behaviors: smoking, excessive alcohol drinking, and sedentary lifestyle. The Medicare Preventive Services Research Team. *Preventive Medicine*, **24**, 492–7.

Burton, L.C., Steinwachs, D.M., German, P.S., *et al.* (1995*b*). Preventive services for the elderly: would coverage affect utilization and costs under Medicare? *American Journal of Public Health*, **85**, 387–91.

Cameron, I., Finnegan, T., Madhok, R., Langhorne, P., and Handoll, H. (1999). Co-ordinated multidisciplinary approaches for inpatient rehabilitation of older patients with proximal femoral fractures

(Cochrane Review). In *The Cochrane Library*, Issue 4. Update Software, Oxford.

Centers for Disease Control and Prevention (1997). Missed opportunities for pneumococcal and influenza vaccination of Medicare pneumonia inpatients—12 western states 1995. *Journal of the American Medical Association*, **278**, 1307–8.

Challis, D. (1992). Providing alternatives to long-stay hospital care for frail elderly patients: is it cost-effective? *International Journal of Geriatric Psychiatry*, **7**, 773–81.

Challis, D. (1996). Community care. In *Epidemiology in old age* (ed. S. Ebrahim and A. Kalache). BMJ Publishing, London.

Charlton, J. and Murphy, M. (1997). *The health of adult Britain 1841–1994*. HMSO, London.

Chenet, L., McKee, M., Fulop, N., *et al.* (1996). Changing life expectancy in central Europe: is there a single reason? *Journal of Public Health Medicine*, **18**, 329–36.

Chenet, L., McKee, M., Leon, D., Shkolnikov, V., and Vassin, S. (1998). Alcohol and cardiovascular mortality in Moscow; new evidence of a causal association . *Journal of Epidemiology and Community Health*, **52**, 772–4.

Clarke, P. and Bowling, A. (1990). Quality of every day life in long-stay institutions for the elderly: an observational study of long stay hospital and nursing home care. *Social Science and Medicine*, **30**, 1201–10.

Cole, M.G. (1998). Impact of geriatric home screening services on mental state: a systematic review. *International Psychogeriatrics*, **10**, 97–102.

Connor, J., Rodgers, A., and Priest, P. (1999). Randomised studies of income supplementation: a lost opportunity to assess health outcomes. *Journal of Epidemiology and Community Health*, **53**, 725–30.

Counsel and Care (1991). *Not such private places*. Counsel and Care, London.

Crawford, V., Beringer, T.R., and Stout, R.W. (1999). Comparison of residential and nursing home care before and after the 1993 community care policy. *British Medical Journal*, **318**, 366.

Curtis, J.L., Millman, E.J., Struening, E.L., and D'Ercole, A. (1998). Does outreach case management improve patients' quality of life? *Psychiatric Services*, **49**, 351–4.

Department of Health (1998). *Our healthier nation: a contract for health*. HMSO, London.

Devore, D. (1998). *1996 disability survey. Follow up to the family resources survey*. Technical report, Office for National Statistics, London.

Doll, R., Peto, R., Wheatley, K., Gray, R., and Sutherland, I. (1994). Mortality in relation to smoking: 40 years' observations on male British doctors. *British Medical Journal*, **309**, 901–11.

Donabedian, A. (1989). Quality of care and the health care needs of the elderly patient. In *Care of the elderly patient. Policy issues and research opportunities* (ed. J.A. Barondess, D.E. Rogers, and K.N. Lohr), pp. 3–13. National Academy Press, Washington, DC.

Downie, R.S., Fyfe, C., and Tannahill, A. (1990). *Health promotion. Models and values*. Oxford University Press.

Dowse, G.K., Gareeboo, H., Alberti, K.G., *et al.* (1995). Changes in population cholesterol concentrations and other cardiovascular risk factor levels after five years of the non-communicable disease intervention programme in Mauritius. Mauritius Non-communicable Disease Study Group. *British Medical Journal*, **311**, 1255–9.

Drever, F. and Whitehead, M. (1997). *Health inequalities*. Decennial supplement DS No. 15, HMSO, Office for National Statistics, London.

Ebrahim, S. (1995). Clinical and public health perspectives and applications of health-related quality of life measurement. *Social Science and Medicine*, **41**, 1383–94.

Ebrahim, S. (1996*a*). Ethnic elders. *British Medical Journal*, **313**, 610–13.

Ebrahim, S. (1996*b*). Migration and ethnicity. In *Epidemiology in old age* (ed. S. Ebrahim and A. Kalache), pp. 201–9. BMJ Publications, London.

Ebrahim, S. (1998). Detection, adherence and control of hypertension for the prevention of stroke: a systematic review. *Health Technology Assessment*, **2**, 1–78.

Ebrahim, S. (1999). Demographic shifts and medical training. *British Medical Journal*, **319**, 1358–60.

Ebrahim, S. and Davey Smith, G. (1996). *Health promotion in older people for the prevention of coronary heart disease and stroke*. Health Education Authority, London.

Ebrahim, S. and Harwood, R.H. (1999). *Stroke: epidemiology, evidence and clinical practice*. Oxford University Press.

Ebrahim, S. and Davey Smith, G. (1997). Systematic review of randomised controlled trials of multiple risk factor interventions for preventing coronary heart disease. *British Medical Journal*, **314**, 1666–74.

Ebrahim, S., Hedley, R., and Sheldon, M. (1984). Low levels of ill health among elderly non-consulters in general practice. *British Medical Journal*, **289**, 1273–5.

Ebrahim, S., Brittis, S., and Wu, A. (1991). The valuation of states of illhealth: the impact of age and disability. *Age and Ageing*, **20**, 37–40.

Ebrahim, S., Thompson, P.W., Baskaran, V., and Evans, K. (1997). Randomized placebo-controlled trial of brisk walking in the prevention of postmenopausal osteoporosis. *Age and Ageing*, **26**, 253–60.

Egger, M., Davey Smith, G., Schneider, M., and Minder, C. (1997). Bias in meta-analysis detected by a simple, graphical test. *British Medical Journal*, **315**, 629–34.

Egger, M., Schneider, M., and Davey Smith, G. (1998). Spurious precision? Meta-analysis of observational studies. *British Medical Journal*, **316**, 140–4.

Evans, J.G. (1983). Integration of geriatric with general medical services in Newcastle. *Lancet*, **i**, 1430–3.

Evans, J.G. (1990). How are the elderly different? In *Improving the health of older people: a world view* (ed. R.L. Kane, J.G. Evans, and D. Macfadyen), pp. 50–68. Oxford University Press.

Evans, J.G. (1993*a*). Hypothesis: Healthy Active Life Expectancy (HALE) as an index of effectiveness of health and social services for elderly people. *Age and Ageing*, **22**, 297–301.

Evans, J.G. (1993*b*). Institutional care and elderly people. *British Medical Journal*, **306**, 806–7.

Evans, J.G. (1997). A correct compassion. The medical response to an ageing society. *Journal of the Royal College of Physicians of London*, **31**, 674–8.

Evans, J.G. and Graham, J.M. (1984). Medical care of the elderly: five years on. *Journal of the Royal College of Physicians of London*, **18**, 18–20.

Fahs, M.C., Mandelblatt, J., Schechter, C., and Muller, C. (1992). Cost effectiveness of cervical cancer screening for the elderly. *Annals of Internal Medicine*, **117**, 520–7.

Fentem, P.H. (1994). ABC of sports medicine. Benefits of exercise in health and disease. *British Medical Journal*, **308**, 1291–5.

Fine, M.J., Smith, M.A., and Carson, C.A. (1994). Efficacy of pneumococcal vaccination in adults: a meta analysis of randomized controlled clinical trials. *Archives of Internal Medicine*, **154**, 2666–77.

Fletcher, A. (1996). Breast cancer. In *Epidemiology in old age* (ed. S. Ebrahim and A. Kalache), pp. 317–23. BMJ Publishing, London.

Fletcher, G. (1999). Physical inactivity as a risk factor for cardiovascular disease. *American Journal of Medicine*, **107**, 10S–11S.

Forster, A., Young, J., Langhorne, P. and the Day Hospital Group (1999*a*). Medical day hospital care for the elderly versus alternative forms of care (Cochrane Review). In *The Cochrane Library*, Issue 4. Update Software, Oxford.

Forster, A., Young, J., Langhorne, P. and the Day Hospital Group (1999*b*). Systematic review of day hospital care for elderly people. *British Medical Journal*, **318**, 837–41.

Friedland, J.F. and McColl, M. (1992). Social support intervention after stroke: results of a randomized trial. *Archives of Physical Medical Rehabilitation*, **73**, 573–81.

Fries, J.F. (1980). Aging, natural death, and the compression of morbidity. *New England Journal of Medicine*, **303**, 130–5.

Fries, J.F. (1989). The compression of morbidity: near or far? *Milbank Quarterly*, **67**, 208–32.

Fries, J.F., Green, L.W., and Levine, S. (1989). Health promotion and the compression of morbidity. *Lancet*, **1**, 481–3.

German, P.S., Burton, L.C., Shapiro, S., *et al.* (1995). Extended coverage for preventive services for the elderly: response and results in a demonstration population. *American Journal of Public Health*, **85**, 379–86.

Gillespie, L., Gillespie, W., Cumming, R., Lamb, S., and Rowe, B.H. (1999). Interventions for preventing falls in the elderly (Cochrane Review). In *The Cochrane Library*, Issue 4. Update Software, Oxford.

Goffman, E. (1961). *Asylums*. Penguin, London.

Golini, A. (1997). Demographic trends and aging in Europe. *Genus*, **53**, 33–74.

Gonner, E.C.K. (1913). The population of England in the eighteenth century. *Journal of the Royal Statistical Society*, **58**, 261–96.

Gray, J.A.M., Bassey, E.J., and Young, A. (1985). The risks of inactivity. In *Prevention of disease in the elderly* (ed. J.A.M. Gray), pp. 78–94. Churchill Livingstone, Edinburgh.

Gross, P.A., Hermongenes, A.W., Sachs, H.S., Lau, J., and Levandowski, R.A. (1995). The efficacy of influenza vaccine in elderly persons: a meta-analysis and review of the literature. *Annals of Internal Medicine*, **123**, 518–27.

Gueyffier, F., Bulpitt, C.J., Boissel, J.P., *et al.* and for the INDIANA Group (1999). Antihypertensive drugs in very old people: a sub-group meta-analysis of randomised controlled trials. *Lancet*, **353**, 793–6.

Harwood, R., Rogers, A., Dickinson, E., and Ebrahim, S. (1994*a*). Measuring handicap: the London Handicap Scale, a new outcome measure for chronic disease. *Quality in Health Care*, **3**, 11–16.

Harwood, R., Jitapunkul, S., Dickinson, E., and Ebrahim, S. (1994*b*). Measuring handicap: motives, methods and a model. *Quality in Health Care*, **3**, 53–7.

Haussler, B., Hempel, E., and Reschke, P. (1995). Changes in life expectancy and mortality in East Germany after reunification (1989–1992). *Gesundheitswesen*, **57**, 365–72.

Hillsdon, M. and Thorogood, M. (1996). A systematic review of physical activity promotion strategies. *British Journal of Sports Medicine*, **30**, 84–9.

Hillsdon, M., Thorogood, M., Anstiss, T., and Morris, J. (1995). Randomised controlled trials of physical activity promotion in free living populations: a review. *Journal of Epidemiology and Community Health*, **49**, 448–53.

Himsworth, R.L. and Goldacre, M.J. (1999). Does time spent in hospital in the final 15 years of life increase with age at death? A population based study. *British Medical Journal*, **319**, 1338–9.

Hooper, L., Ness, A., Higgins, J.P.T., Moore, T., and Ebrahim, S. (1999). GISSI–Prevenzione trial. *Lancet*, **354**, 1557–9.

Hooper, L., Summerbell, C.D., Higgins, J.P.T., *et al.* (2001). Dietary fat intake and prevention of cardiovascular disease: systematic review. *British Medical Journal*, **322**, 757–63.

Hoxie, R.E. and Rubenstein, L.Z. (1994). Are older pedestrians allowed enough time to cross intersections safely? *Journal of the American Geriatrics Society*, **42**, 241–4.

Iliffe, S., Haines, A., Gallivan, S., Booroff, A., Goldenberg, E., and Morgan, P. (1991*a*). Assessment of elderly people in general practice. 1. Social circumstances and mental state. *British Journal of General Practice*, **41**, 9–12.

Iliffe, S., Haines, A., Gallivan, S., Booroff, A., Goldenberg, E., and Morgan, P. (1991*b*). Assessment of elderly people in general practice. 2. Functional abilities and medical problems. *British Journal of General Practice*, **41**, 13–15.

Insua, J.T., Sacks, H.S., Lau, T.S., *et al.* (1994). Drug treatment of hypertension in the elderly: a meta-analysis. *Annals of Internal Medicine*, **121**, 355–62.

Jenkins, R.D. (1999). Gerontology on the world wide web. *Reviews in Clinical Gerontology*, **9**, 289.

Jenkinson, C., Gray, A., Doll, H., Lawrence, K., Keoghane, S., and Layte, R. (1997). Evaluation of index and profile measures of health status in a randomized controlled trial. Comparison of the Medical Outcomes Study 36-Item Short Form Health Survey, EuroQol, and disease specific measures. *Medical Care*, **35**, 1109–18.

Jitapunkul, S., Bunnag, S., and Ebrahim, S. (1998). Effectiveness and cost analysis of community-based rehabilitation service in Bangkok. *Journal of the Medical Association of Thailand*, **81**, 572–8.

Jones, J., Wilson, A., Parker, H., *et al.* (1999). Economic evaluation of hospital at home versus hospital care: cost minimization analysis of data from randomised controlled trial. *British Medical Journal*, **319**, 1547–50.

Judge, K. (1986). Residential care for the elderly: purposes and resources. In *Residential homes for elderly people* (ed. K. Judge and I. Sinclair), pp. 5–20. HMSO, London.

Judge, K. (2000). Testing evaluation to the limits: the case of English Health Action Zones. *Journal of Health Services Research and Policy*, **5**, 3–5.

Kalache, A. (1999). Active ageing makes the difference. *Bulletin of the WHO*, **77**, 299–305.

Kane, R.L. and Kane, R.A. (1991). Special needs of dependent elderly persons. In *Oxford textbook of public health medicine* (ed. W.W. Holland, R. Detels, and G. Knox) (2nd edn), Vol. 3, pp. 509–21. Oxford University Press, New York.

Khaw, K.T. (1999). How many, how old, how soon? *British Medical Journal*, **319**, 1350–2.

Kinsella, K.G. (1996). Demographic aspects. In *Epidemiology in old age* (ed. S. Ebrahim and A. Kalache), pp. 32–40. BMJ Publishing, London.

Kirkwood, T. (1999). *The time of our lives: the science of human ageing.* Weidenfield and Nicolson, London.

Koivula, I., Sten, M., Leinonen, M., and Makela, P.H. (1997). Clinical efficacy of pneumococcal vaccine in the elderly: a randomized, single-blind population-based trial. *American Journal of Medicine*, **103**, 281–90.

Lagergren, M. and Johansson, P.-A. (1998). Are there differences in standard of care for the elderly? A comparative study of assistance decisions in Stockholm. *Scandinavian Journal of Social Welfare*, **7**, 340–9.

Laing, W., Hall, M., and Lumley, P. (1991). *Agenda for health. The challenges of ageing.* Association of the British Pharmaceutical Industry, London.

Leon, D.A., Chenet, L., Shkolnikov, *et al.* (1997). Huge variation in Russian mortality rates 1984–94: artefact, alcohol, or what? *Lancet*, **350**, 383–8.

Lindesay, J. (1996). Health service use in mental illness. In *Epidemiology in old age* (ed. S. Ebrahim and A. Kalache), pp. 96–105. BMJ Publishing, London.

Logan, J.R. and Spitze, G. (1994). Informal support and the use of formal services by older Americans. *Journal of Gerontology*, **49**, S25–S34

McCormick, A., Fleming, D., and Charlton, J. (1995). *Morbidity statistics from general practice. Fourth national study 1991–1992.* HMSO, London.

McGlone, F. and Cronin, N. (1994). *A crisis in care? The future of family and state care for older people in the European Union.* Family Policy Studies Centre, London.

McNally, S., Ben-Shlomo, Y., and Newman, S. (1999). The effects of respite care on informal carers' well-being: a systematic review. *Disability and Rehabilitation*, **21**, 1–14.

Mahoney, F.I. and Barthel, D.W. (1965). Functional evaluation: the Barthel Index. *Maryland State Medical Journal*, **14**, 61–5.

Manton, K.G. (1980). Sex and race specific mortality differentials in multiple cause of death data. *Gerontologist*, **20**, 480–93.

Manton, K.G. (1982). Changing concepts of morbidity and mortality in the elderly population. *Milbank Memorial Fund Quarterly—Health and Society*, **60**, 183–244.

Manton, K.G. and Stallard, E. (1991). Cross-sectional estimates of active life expectancy for the U.S. elderly and oldest-old populations. *Journal of Gerontology*, **46**, S170–S182.

Manton, K.G., Corder, L., and Stallard, E. (1997). Chronic disability trends in elderly United States populations: 1982–1994. *Proceedings of National Academy of Science of the United States of America*, **94**, 2593–8.

Marmot, M., Adelstein, A.M., and Bulusu, L. (1984). Lessons from the study of immigrant mortality. *Lancet*, **i**, 1455–7.

Martin, J., Meltzer, H., and Elliot, D. (1987). *The prevalence of disability among adults. OPCS surveys of disability in Great Britain*. HMSO, London.

Mathers, C.D. and Robine, J.M. (1997). How good is Sullivan's method for monitoring changes in population health expectancies? *Journal of Epidemiology and Community Health*, **51**, 80–6.

Melzer, D., Hopkins, S., Pencheon, D., Brayne, C., and Williams, R. (1992). *Epidemiologically based needs assessment: dementia*. NHS Management Executive, London.

Mendes de Leon, C.F., Beckett, L.A., Fillenbaum, G.G., Brock, D.B., Branch, L.G., Evans, D.A., and Berkman, L.F. (1997). Black–white differences in risk of becoming disabled and recovering from disability in old age: a longitudinal analysis of two EPESE populations. *American Journal of Epidemiology*, **145**, 488–97.

Mendes de Leon, C.F., Glass, T.A., Beckett, L.A., Seeman, T.E., Evans, D.A., and Berkman, L.F. (1999). Social networks and disability transitions across eight intervals of yearly data in the New Haven EPESE. *Journal of Gerontology. Series B, Psychological Sciences and Social Sciences*, **54**, S162–72.

Mittelman, M.S., Ferris, S.H., Shulman, E., Steinberg, G., and Levin, B. (1996). A family intervention to delay nursing home placement of patients with Alzheimer's Disease. *Journal of the American Medical Association*, **276**, 1725–31.

Mullooly, J.P., Bennett, M.D., Hornbrook, M.C., *et al.* (1994). Influenza vaccination programs for elderly persons: cost-effectiveness in a health maintenance organization. *Annals of Internal Medicine*, **121**, 947–52.

Mulrow, C.D., Cornell, J.A., Herrera, C.R., Kadri, A., Farnett, L., and Aguilar, C. (1994). Hypertension in the elderly. Implications and generalizability of randomized trials. *Journal of the American Medical Association*, **272**, 1932–8.

National Center for Health Statistics (1999). *Health, United States 1999*. National Center for Health Statistics, Hyattsville, MD.

Nichol, K.L., Margolis, K.L., Wuorenma, J., and Von Sternberg, T. (1994). The efficacy and cost effectiveness of vaccination against influenza among elderly persons living in the community. *New England Journal of Medicine*, **331**, 778–84.

Nicholson, K.G. (1993). Immunisation against influenza among people aged over 65 living at home in Leicestershire during winter 1991–2. *British Medical Journal*, **306**, 974–6.

NIH Consensus Development Panel on Physical Activity and Cardiovascular Health (1996). Physical activity and cardiovascular health. *Journal of the American Medical Association*, **276**, 241–6.

Nikolaus, T., Specht-Leible, N., Back, M., Oster, P., and Schlierf, G. (1999). A randomised trial of comprehensive geriatric assessment and home intervention in the care of hospitalised patients. *Age and Ageing*, **28**, 543–50.

Norman, A. (1985). *Triple jeopardy: growing old in a second homeland*. Centre for Policy on Ageing, London.

Normand, C. (1998). Ten popular health economic fallacies. *Journal of Public Health Medicine*, **20**, 129–32.

Nouri, F. and Lincoln, N.B. (1987). An extended activities of daily living scale for stroke patients. *Clinical Rehabilitation*, **1**, 301–5.

Office of Population Census and Surveys (1991). *Census for Great Britain 1991*. HMSO, London.

Olshansky, S.J., Rudberg, M.A., Carnes, B.A., Cassel, C.K., and Brody, J.A. (1991). Trading off longer life for worse health: the expansion of morbidity hypothesis. *Journal of Aging and Health*, **3**, 194–216.

Ortqvist, A., Hedlund, J., Burman, L.A., *et al.* (1998). Randomised trial of 23-valent pneumococcal capsular polysaccharide vaccine in prevention of pneumonia in middle-aged and elderly people. Swedish Pneumococcal Vaccination Study Group. *Lancet*, **351**, 399–403.

Potter, J., Stott, D.J., Roberts, M.A., *et al.* (1997). Influenza vaccination of health care workers in long-term-care hospitals reduces the mortality of elderly patients. *Journal of Infectious Diseases*, **175**, 1–6.

Province, M.A., Hadley, E.C., Hornbrook, M.C., *et al.* (1995). The effects of exercise on falls in elderly patients. A preplanned meta-analysis of the FICSIT Trials. Frailty and Injuries: Cooperative Studies of Intervention Techniques. *Journal of the American Medical Association*, **273**, 1341–7.

Razzell, P. (1998). The condundrum of eighteenth century English population growth. *Social History of Medicine*, **11**, 469–500.

Reuben, D.B., Borok, G.M., Wolde-Tsadik, G., *et al.* (1995). A randomized trial of comprehensive geriatric assessment in the care of hospitalized patients. *New England Journal of Medicine*, **332**, 1345–50.

Rippe, J.M. and Hess, S. (1998). The role of physical activity in the prevention and management of obesity. *Journal of the American Dietetic Association*, **98**, S31–S38.

Rivlin, M. (1999). Should age based rationing of health care be illegal? *British Medical Journal*, **319**, 1379.

Robine, J.M. and Romieu, I. (1998). *Healthy active ageing: health expectancies at age 65 in the different parts of the world*. REVES Paper 318, INSERM, France: Network on Health Expectancy and the Disability Process (REVES).

Robine, J.M., Blanchet M., and Dowd, J.E. (1992). *Health expectancy. First workshop of the International Healthy Life Expectancy Network (REVES)*. HMSO, London.

Robison, J., Moen, P., and Dempster-McClain, D. (1995). Women's caregiving: changing profiles and pathways. *Journal of Gerontology. Series B, Psychological Sciences and Social Sciences*, **50**, S362–S373.

Royal Commission on Long Term Care (1999). *With respect to old age: long term care—rights and responsibilities*, HMSO, London.

Rubenstein, L.Z. and Nasr, S.Z. (1996). Health service use in physical illness. In *Epidemiology in old age* (ed. S. Ebrahim and A. Kalache), pp. 106–25. BMJ Publishing, London.

Ruta, D.A., Garratt, A.M., Leng, M., Russell, I.T., and MacDonald, L.M. (1994). A new approach to the measurement of quality of life. The Patient-Generated Index. *Medical Care*, **32**, 1109–26.

Schofield, H., Murphy, B., Herrman, H.E., Bloch, S., and Singh, B.S. (1998). Carers of people aged over 50 years with physical impairment, memory loss and dementia: a comparative study. *Ageing and Society*, **18**, 355–69.

Shah, S., Vanclay, F., and Cooper, B. (1990). Efficiency, effectiveness and duration of stroke rehabilitation. *Stroke*, **21**, 241–6.

Shah, S., Vanclay, F., and Cooper, B. (1991). Stroke rehabilitation: Australian patient profile and functional outcome. *Journal of Clinical Epidemiology*, **44**, 21–8.

Shepperd, S. and Iliffe, S. (1999). Hospital-at-home versus in-patient hospital care (Cochrane Review). In *The Cochrane Library*, Issue 4. Update Software, Oxford.

Sisk, J.E., Moskowitz, A.J., Whang, W., *et al.* (1997). Cost-effectiveness of vaccination against pneumococcal bacteremia among elderly people. *Journal of the American Medical Association*, **278**, 1333–9.

Smeeth, L. and Iliffe, S. (1998). Effectiveness of screening older people for impaired vision in community setting: systematic review of evidence from randomised controlled trials. *British Medical Journal*, **316**, 660–3.

Smeeth, L. and Iliffe, S. (1999). Community screening for visual impairment in the elderly. In *Cochrane Review*. Cochrane Library, Issue 4. Update Software, Oxford.

Smith, J.P. (1994). Informal carers in Great Britain. *Journal of Advanced Nursing*, **20**, 787.

Steinbach, U. (1992). Social networks, institutionalization, and mortality among elderly people in the United States. *Journal of Gerontology*, **47**, S183–S190.

Stroke Unit Trialists' Collaboration (1999). Organised inpatient (stroke unit) care for stroke (Cochrane Review). In *The Cochrane Library*, Issue 4. Update Software, Oxford.

Stuck, A.E., Siu, A.L., Wieland, G.D., Adams, J., and Rubenstein, L.Z. (1993). Comprehensive geriatric assessment: a meta-analysis of controlled trials. *Lancet*, **342**, 1032–6.

Stuck, A.E., Aronow, H.U., Steiner, A., *et al.* (1995). A trial of annual in-home comprehensive geriatric assessments for elderly people living in the community . *New England Journal of Medicine*, **333**, 1184–9.

Stuck, A.E., Rubenstein, L.Z., and Wieland, D. (1998). Bias in meta-analysis detected by a simple, graphical test. Asymmetry detected in funnel plot was probably due to true heterogeneity. *British Medical Journal*, **316**, 469–1.

Thamprechavai, S., Somerville, K., Jitapunkul, S., Bunnag, S., and Ebrahim, S. (1992). Elderly bed-blockers in a Thai teaching hospital: is it a problem? *Journal of the Medical Association of Thailand*, **75**, 418–22.

Tonks, A. (1999). Medicine must change to serve an ageing society. *British Medical Journal*, **319**, 1450–1.

Townsend, P. (1962). *The last refuge*. Routledge and Kegan Paul, London.

Travers, A.F. (1996). Caring for older people. Carers. *British Medical Journal*, **313**, 482–6.

Tseng, B.S., Marsh, D.R., Hamilton, M.T., and Booth, F.W. (1995). Strength and aerobic training attenuate muscle wasting and improve resistance to the development of disability with aging. *Journal of Gerontology.Series A, Biological Sciences and Medical Sciences*, **50**, 113–19.

van Rossum, E., Frederiks, C.M., Philipsen, H., Portengen, K., Wiskerke, J., and Knipschild, P. (1993). Effects of preventive home visits to elderly people. *British Medical Journal*, **307**, 27–32.

Vetter, N.J. (1999). The impact of smoking in elderly people. *Reviews in Clinical Gerontology*, **9**, 273–80.

Vetter, N.J. and Ford, D. (1990). Smoking prevention among people aged 60 and over: a randomized controlled trial. *Age and Ageing*, **19**, 164–8.

Vetter, N.J., Charny, M., Farrow, S., and Lewis, P.A. (1988). The Cardiff Health Survey. The relationship between smoking habits and beliefs in the elderly. *Public Health*, **102**, 359–64.

Vetter, N.J., Lewis, P.A., and Llewellyn, L. (1992). Supporting elderly dependent people at home. *British Medical Journal*, **304**, 1290–2.

Vita, A.J., Terry, R.B., Hubert, H.B., and Fries, J.F. (1998). Aging, health risks, and cumulative disability. *New England Journal of Medicine*, **338**, 1035–41.

Walker, M.F., Gladman, J.R., Lincoln, N.B., Siemonsma, P., and Whiteley, T. (1999). Occupational therapy for stroke patients not admitted to hospital: a randomised controlled trial. *Lancet*, **354**, 278–80.

Ware, J.E.J. and Gandek, B. (1998). Overview of the SF-36 Health Survey and the International Quality of Life Assessment (IQOLA) Project. *Journal of Clinical Epidemiology*, **51**, 903–12.

Warren, M.W. (1946). Care of the chronic aged sick. *Lancet*, **ii**, 841–3.

Watkins, J., Rogers, C., and Evans, J. (1999). Implications of age-based policies for influenza immunisation. *Lancet*, **353**, 208–9.

Weiner, J. and Illson, L.H. (1994). Private insurance options for long term care financing. In *Community care: new agendas and challenges from the UK and overseas* (ed. D. Challis, B. Davies, and K. Traske), pp. 264–81. University of Kent Personal Social Services Research Unit, Canterbury.

Williams, A. and Evans, J.G. (1997). The rationing debate. Rationing health care by age. *British Medical Journal*, **314**, 820–5.

Williams, E.I. and Wallace, P. (1993). *Health checks for people aged 75 and over*, pp. 1–30. Occasional Paper, Royal College of General Practitioners, London.

Williamson, J., Stokoe, I.H., and Gray, S. (1964). Old people at home: their unreported needs. *Lancet*, **i**, 1117–20.

Wilson, A., Parker, H., Wynn, A., *et al.* (1999). Randomised controlled trial of effectiveness of Leicester hospital at home scheme compared with hospital care. *British Medical Journal*, **319**, 1542–6.

Wolman, R.L. (1994). ABC of sports medicine. Osteoporosis and exercise. *British Medical Journal*, **309**, 400–3.

WHO (World Health Organization) (1980). *International classification of impairments, disabilities and handicaps*. WHO, Geneva.

WHO (World Health Organization) (1984). *The uses of epidemiology in the study of the elderly. Technical Report Series 706*. WHO, Geneva.

WHO (World Health Organization) (1998). *World atlas of ageing*. WHO, Kobe, Japan.

WHO (World Health Organization) (1999). *International classification of impairments, activities and participation*. Beta version. WHO, Geneva.

Wrigley, E.A. and Schofield, R.S. (1981). *The population history of England, 1547–1871*. Cambridge University Press.

Young, A. (1989). There is no such thing as geriatric medicine, and its here to stay. *Lancet*, **ii**, 263–5.

Young, A. (1992). Strength and power. In *Oxford textbook of geriatric medicine* (ed. J.G. Evans and T.F. Williams), pp. 597–604. Oxford University Press.

Young, J., Brown, A., Forster, A., and Clare, J. (1999). An overview of rehabilitation for older people. *Reviews in Clinical Gerontology*, **9**, 183–96.

11.9 Refugees and other displaced populations

Mohamed Dualeh and Paul Shears

Introduction

Large-scale movements of refugees and other forced migrants have become a defining feature of the contemporary world. At few times in recent history have such large numbers of people in so many parts of the globe been obliged to leave their own countries and communities to seek safety elsewhere. The global refugee problem confronts the world with a range of practical and ethical dilemmas. Refugees and other displaced persons will continue to find refuge in remote regions (with limited infrastructures) where the provision of basic health care requires innovative approaches to the implementation of appropriate public health interventions.

The thrust of this chapter is to address the public health issues encountered by this population and how the international community can respond more effectively and expeditiously to large and sudden movements of displaced people. It provides a general framework of the priority health problems encountered by displaced people, and advocates the development of mutual awareness and shared understanding for a common approach.

Refugees are defined as people who have crossed international borders fleeing war or persecution for reason of race, religion, nationality, or membership of particular social and political groups. They are protected by several international conventions and protocols (UNHCR 1967). In contrast, persons who flee their homes for the same reason as refugees but who remain inside their own countries enjoy no such legal status. These 'internally displaced' persons are in a particularly precarious situation because they are often beyond the reach of international agencies, which rely on the co-operation of national governments to deliver relief aid. They are victims of civil strife or natural disaster within their own country (Fig. 1).

Other important categories of displaced populations include economic migrants, seasonal workers, illegal aliens, and migrants from rural areas to urban centres. These groups are displaced populations who have left their own area because of disaster, environmental deterioration, or economic hardship; all of which reasons fall outside the judicial definition of convention refugees. However, there are broad commonalties of the public health needs of all migrant populations, as they encounter similar conditions of displacement in their new environment.

Apart from the primary reasons which initiate migration (political, economic, social, etc.), other factors also influence population movement and mobility, and so further the risk of increased transmission of diseases. It is important to consider the influence of time in this process. Rapid migration will have less health impact than a journey of long duration. Internal migration is a common phenomenon in all continents, and particularly in developing countries. It is most marked in South and East Asia—China, India, Vietnam, and Myanmar. This is also true for Africa and Latin America. China now has internal migration on a large scale, with between 80 and 100 million persons travelling within the country (IOM 1998). Many of these so-called 'floating populations', or surplus rural labour, travel in search of work. Many live in shanty towns where there is no basic public health infrastructure—water, sanitation, garbage disposal, etc. The public health implications in these surroundings are enormous, as overcrowding, poor living conditions, and the lack of basic health services for these populations are common characteristics for migrant populations.

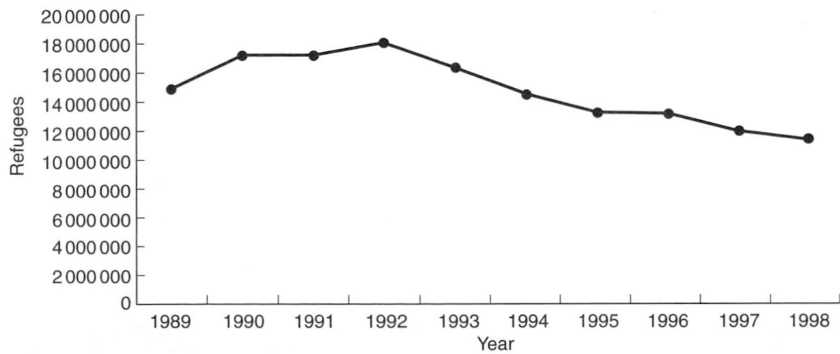

Fig. 1 Estimated numbers of convention refugees, 1989–1998.

Displaced people are victims of the political and social crises which affect our time; governments that refuse to respect human rights of their citizens; narrow-minded armed factions which use political goals as an impetus for personal or communal ambition, and social and religious groups which cannot tolerate alternative opinions and lifestyles. In addition, deep-rooted trends such as the growing inequality within and between nations; the rapid increase of the global population; and the depletion of the world's natural resources have a major impact on the movement of populations. Since the beginning of the 1990s, the world has witnessed a succession of internal armed conflicts that have led to major humanitarian emergencies and massive refugee movements; Iraq, Liberia, Rwanda, Somalia, Sri Lanka, and the former Yugoslavia are some of the most prominent examples. During the first quarter of 1998, the number of people of concern to UNHCR worldwide was 21.2 million. Most of these people were living in Africa, Asia, and Europe. Slightly more than half of them were refugees; the remainder were internally displaced persons, returnees, asylum seekers, and stateless persons. In addition, the international community has witnessed, during the twentieth century, an unprecedented development of mega-cities and big towns as a result of internal migration from rural areas to urban centres.

Analysis of trends in the global refugee population during the period 1989 to 1998 indicate that the estimated refugee population in 1998 was the lowest for the past 10 years. At the same time there has been a marked increase of the internally displaced in war-affected countries and population movements from least developing countries in the south to the more prosperous and highly industrialized countries in the north (Table 1).

Implications for public health

Displaced people are often suffering the devastating effects of exhaustion, bereavement, separation from loved ones, ill health or injury, separation from family and community, poor shelter, inadequate nutrition and food availability, poor water supplies, and impoverishment (Toole and Waldman 1993; Toole *et al.* 1993).

Over the past three decades the most common emergencies affecting the health of large populations in developing countries have been associated with famine and forced migration (CDC 1992). Public health, depending as it does on so many non-medical factors, is too large a subject to be left only to medical workers (UNHCR 1999). In an emergency, many refugees will be exposed to insecurity, poor shelter, overcrowding, and lack of sufficient safe water, inadequate or inappropriate food supplies and a possible lack of immunity to the diseases of the new environment. Furthermore, on arrival, displaced persons may be in a debilitated state from disease, malnutrition, hunger, fatigue, harassment, physical violence, and grief. Poverty, powerlessness, and social instability, conditions that often prevail for refugees and other displace populations, can also contribute to

Table 1 Refugees and others of concern to UNHCR , 31 December 1998[a]

Region	Refugees	Asylum seekers	Returnees	Others, including IDPs	Totals
Central Asia	42 000	5390	39 520	20	87 130
Central America and the Caribbean	59 060	90	7630	20 150	86 930
East Asia and the Pacific	573 800	7090	15 740	39 100	635 730
Eastern Europe	668 900	31 420	1850	2145 700	2847 870
East Africa and Horn of Africa	1121 340	6910	80 910	50 000	1259 160
Former Yugoslavia and Albania	595 000	6000	251 300	1374 100	2226 400
Great Lakes region	869 100	15 540	431 800	1156 700	2473 140
Middle East	208 610	14 330	22 500	166 500	411 940
North Africa	176 660	380	—	70	177 110
North America	636 800	546 200	—	—	1183 000
Southern Africa	195 100	22 960	75 640	—	293 700
South America	15 120	260	—	—	15 380
South Asia	333 930	100	40 310	717 700	1092 040
Southwest Asia	3133 800	170	193 000	343 700	3670 670
West and Central Africa	901 060	14 860	514 500	865 600	2296 020
Western and Central Europe	1934 760	211 080	—	268 700	2414 440
Total	11 465 240	882 780	1674 700	7148 040	21 170 760

IDP, internally displaced population.

[a]Statistics are provisional, subject to change.

increased sexual violence and spread of sexually transmitted diseases (**STDs**) including HIV.

In many conflict areas, the residual effect of land mines after the cessation of hostilities has resulted in a new and potentially devastating public health problem. As well as the physical components of public health, there is now an increasing awareness of the impact of displacement, insecurity, and refugee status on the mental health of affected communities. These various components of the wider concept of public health among refugee and displaced communities are described in this chapter.

Public health priorities

Displacement is a situation where needs are great, human and material resources are scarce, and action must be immediate. Health staff cannot deal with everything at once; they must assign priorities to problems. The emotional and physical stress of working in an emergency may cause intense anxiety and one of the survival mechanisms sometimes adopted unconsciously by inexperienced relief workers is to focus all of their energies upon conditions or activities with which they feel comfortable. Unfortunately, these often tend to be low-priority areas such as reconstructive surgery, tuberculosis control, or unreasonably detailed epidemiological studies often conducted by academics for research purposes only. Such misplaced emphasis is a gross error. The challenge is how to alleviate the suffering and prevent unnecessary loss of life with limited resources.

Health services for refugees and other displaced populations are based upon the well-known principles of primary health care, which normally underpin the pre-existing health structures of the national ministries of health. Another principle that must be woven through the fabric of the entire health programme is that of outreach. This principle means services must, as far as possible, be taken to the refugees and other migrant populations. Outreach is particularly important in non-camp situations where refugees or other displaced populations are scattered among local villages or in shanty towns located at the peripheries of major cities in the developing world. Cultural practices may preclude some portion of the population such as refugee women from attending clinics. This type of cultural obstacle is often exacerbated rather than relaxed in the context of a refugee or other displaced setting in which traditions are reinforced to counter rapid changes.

Whenever people are uprooted, for whatever reason, they are placed at an increased risk of disease and death. This holds true for persons suddenly fleeing their homes, but also, to a lesser extent, for refugees involved in voluntary repatriation. The sudden migration of people is associated with high mortality (Toole and Waldman 1997). The movement *per se* determines the risk. The public health consequences of mass population displacement have been extensively documented. The most severe consequences of population displacement have occurred during the acute emergency phase, when relief efforts are in the early stage. In some cases, deaths during this phase were 60 times the crude mortality rate among non-refugee populations in the country of origin (Toole and Waldman 1990). In the first few weeks, mortality rates were high in all Kurdish refugee camps with a rate 45 times higher than expected in the Iraqi citizen population (CDC 1991). The death rates in Zaire (34.1–54.5 deaths per 10 000 per day) were among the highest to be documented during recent population displacements (CDC 1994). Existing epidemiological data have effectively demonstrated those health problems that consistently cause deaths and severe morbidity. Even in normal migrations, recent studies showed also an increasing mortality among migrants to China: the crude death rate rose from 28.9 per 1000 in 1995, to 45.6 per 1000 in 1996, and to 56.0 per 1000 in 1997 (Robinson *et al.* 1999).

Health needs assessment

The initial assessment determines as accurately as possible the health and nutritional effects of a displacement, identifies the health needs, and establishes priority interventions for health programming. The refugees and other displaced populations, relief agencies, donors, and local authorities need to know that interventions are appropriate and effective. Analysis of the effects of the displacement and of the impact of the proposed health activities is therefore critical. If problems are not correctly identified and understood then it will be difficult, if not impossible, to implement the right response. Assessment of health needs of refugees and other displaced populations aim at:

- assessing the magnitude of the displacement
- determining major health and nutrition needs of the affected population
- initiating a health and nutrition surveillance system
- assessing the immediate needs and the local capacity
- identifying strengths and weaknesses of the existing co-ordination mechanisms
- ensuring the inclusion of local expertise (technical capacities) in the planning process
- defining existing constraints to expand and accelerate the response.

Assessments for emergency health projects aim to determine what the reality of the emergency situation is, which improvements are required, and the action needed to implement them. The initial assessment and subsequent health information analyses should demonstrate an awareness of underlying structural, political, economic, and environmental issues operating in the area. The current and pre-emergency living conditions of displaced and non-displaced people in the area and local resources must be considered. At every step the inclusion of local expertise and knowledge in data collection and analysis of resources, capabilities, vulnerabilities, and needs is important. The needs of groups that are at risk such as women, children, elderly people, and mentally disturbed persons must be considered (WHO 1996; IFRC 1998).

Communicable disease, nutrition, and public health

In emergencies that are characterized by large numbers of civilian casualties, including earthquakes, cyclones, and war, trauma-related injuries and deaths are the major causes of morbidity and mortality in the immediate aftermath of the disaster. However, in most situations of mass refugee exodus and population displacement, and in the weeks and months following acute disasters where infrastructure and health services are not immediately restored, communicable diseases and malnutrition represent the greatest risks to the affected communities. From the evidence of past refugee and displaced population crises, it is possible to categorize these risks into priorities for public health action.

The major contributing and causal factors of ill health are:

- overcrowded living conditions which facilitate increased transmission of infectious diseases
- poor nutritional status (and consequent lowered immunity) due to lack of adequate food before, during, and after displacement
- inadequate quantity and quality of water to sustain health and allow personal hygiene, and poor sanitation facilities.

It is self-evident that the trauma prior to and during their exodus is all-important in determining the health status of refugees on arrival in the country of asylum. Nevertheless, observers sometimes forget these rigours of flight. The possibly moribund condition of refugees and other displaced populations who may have just trekked for several weeks through war-torn and famished countryside can be falsely attributed to inadequate care on arrival. During flight, refugees and other migrant populations may have little or no food and no clean water; they may not be able to stop anywhere to cook or allow children or pregnant women to rest, and they may be exposed to rain or extremes of cold or heat for long periods. Harassment, physical violence, and grief will, in many cases, have added to the trauma of flight. All these elements combine to reduce the physical and emotional reserves of the affected population, and the natural resistance to disease is thus compromised.

Diarrhoeal diseases, measles, acute respiratory infections, malnutrition, and malaria constitute the top five recorded causes of morbidity and mortality (CDC 1992).

Diarrhoeal diseases

The crowded and insanitary conditions of refugees and displaced groups create an environment in which faecal–oral infections are rapidly transmitted. Studies in Somalia, Ethiopia, Mozambique, and Malawi have all demonstrated the high morbidity and mortality caused by diarrhoeal diseases in these communities (Shears 1991).

Epidemiology

In the early weeks of a refugee exodus, both water supplies and sanitation are likely to be inadequate. Natural water sources, such as rivers, wells, and ponds, rapidly become polluted as an increasing population uses them in an uncontrolled way. Excreta is invariably disposed of indiscriminately, with potential contamination of water supplies and the household environment, leading to contamination of both food and stored water.

The spread of enteric infections in such conditions has occurred in different refugee situations, ranging from mass exodus in tropical Africa to displacement in the former Soviet Union. The spectrum of diarrhoeal diseases ranges from increases in rates of infantile gastroenteritis to specific outbreaks of cholera, typhoid, and bacillary dysentery.

Gastroenteritis has been responsible for 30 to 40 per cent of all reported childhood illnesses in most refugee situations where surveillance data has been collected. Among malnourished children, mortality rates due to gastroenteritis have been as high as 30 per cent.

The massive outbreaks of cholera and dysentery that occurred among Rwandan refugees in 1994 in the former Zaire represent one of the greatest public health disasters reported among refugee communities. Over a period of 4 weeks, an estimated 80 000 cases, and 15 000 to 20 000 deaths, occurred from the use of polluted untreated water. The use of polluted untreated water, extreme difficulty of latrine construction in the rocky soil, and difficulties in organizing treatment centres all contributed to the high transmission and mortality rates (Goma Epidemiology Group 1995).

Control of diarrhoeal disease outbreaks among refugee and displaced populations requires both urgent public health interventions, and appropriate and timely case management. The public health priorities are the prevention of faecal contamination of water supplies, the provision of adequate quantities of water from protected natural sources, and the organization of simple but effective latrines (Medècins sans Frontières 1994).

In the majority of cases treatment of diarrhoea is based on early detection of cases and effective oral rehydration, preferably organized through community-level health workers, using standardized protocols according to the degree of dehydration.

Outbreaks of cholera may involve large numbers of patients initially requiring intravenous rehydration. Table 2 summarizes the rehydration strategies for diarrhoea and cholera cases. If appropriate intravenous therapy is implemented early in the course of cholera, mortality rates should be less than 3 per cent. However, where numbers overwhelm the medical staff and supplies are limited, as occurred in the early stages of the Goma epidemic, mortality rates in excess of 20 per cent may occur. Detailed analysis of the cholera management in Goma highlighted a number of reasons for the high mortality rates including delayed diagnosis, slow rates of rehydration, and inadequate experience of health work (Siddique *et al.* 1995).

Outbreaks of *Shigella dysenteriae* type 1 have been less extensive than cholera in refugee communities, but may be associated with significant morbidity and mortality. In Central Africa, outbreaks of *S. dysenteriae* type 1 among displaced communities have occurred in Burundi, Zaire, and Tanzania (Engels *et al.* 1995).

Shigella dysentery is highly contagious as only 10 to 100 organisms are required for transmission of disease. In crowded refugee camps with inadequate hygiene, attack rates may exceed 30 per cent.

In the absence of laboratory facilities, an appropriate clinical case definition should be agreed upon so that early detection of an increasing number of cases is possible. Where possible, stool specimens from representative cases should be collected to confirm the causative organism and determine antimicrobial resistance patterns. Multiple antimicrobial resistance in *S. dysentriae* is rapidly increasing globally. In outbreaks of shigellosis among refugees in Zaire and Burundi, strains resistant to all locally available antimicrobials, including nalidixic acid were responsible, requiring the use of fluoroquinolones such as ciprofloxacin.

Management of outbreaks of shigellosis requires early detection and treatment of cases, and improvements in hygiene both generally in the camp but particularly within refugee living areas as most transmission is within households rather than from a communal water or food source. Case management may involve using special treatment centres, with antimicrobial therapy for the most severe cases, and the young, elderly, and malnourished, and supportive therapy of hydration and nutrition for all cases. The use of antimicrobials must be decided according to the local conditions,

Table 2 Rehydration regimens for patients (more than 1 year old) with diarrhoea and cholera

Degree of dehydration	Clinical signs	Rehydration regimen
Mild	No obvious clinical signs,	Maintain hydration by replacing stool losses:
	but diarrhoea present	< 2 years 100 ml/loose stool
		2–9 years 200 ml/loose stool
		> 9 years (as required)
Moderate	Restless	Oral rehydration solution over 4 h:
	Sunken eyes	1–4 years 600–1200 ml
	Dry mouth	5–14 years 1200–2000 ml
	Thirsty, will drink	> 14 years 2000–4000 ml
	Reduced skin turgor	Maintain until adequate hydration
		Then maintain as in mild hydration
Severe	Lethargic	IV Ringer's lactate or normal saline 100 ml/kg in 3 h
	Sunken eyes/dry	Continue IV until hydration level moderate
	Dry mouth	Then give oral rehydration solution as indicated for
	Very reduced skin turgor	moderate dehydration
	Low urine output	
	Does not drink easily	

depending on the severity of illness, knowledge of antimicrobial sensitivity patterns of local strains, availability of antimicrobials, and likelihood of compliance with antimicrobial treatment. The World Health Organization (**WHO**) guidelines are to use a 5-day course of nalidixic acid as the mainstay of therapy. However, studies in recent epidemics have shown increasing resistance to nalidixic acid, requiring the use of ciprofloxacin. Control measures must involve improved hygiene within refugee living areas, particularly safe handling of food and water, the provision of soap, and attempts to improve safe disposal of faeces.

Epidemics of bloody diarrhoea caused by *Escherichia coli* 0157, initially thought to be shigellosis, have occurred in refugee communities in southern Africa. Laboratory investigations are necessary to distinguish the causative agent.

Measles

Measles has been consistently reported as one of the major causes of morbidity and mortality among children in refugee camps, particularly in Africa but also in other areas (Toole *et al.* 1989). Where there is a high prevalence of malnutrition, measles case-fatality rates may reach 30 per cent. Morbidity and mortality in measles are complicated by vitamin A deficiency, diarrhoeal disease, and lower respiratory tract infections (Shears *et al.* 1987).

Mass immunization against measles is an absolute priority in most refugee situations. In areas where displacement has occurred following several years of civil unrest, it is likely that recent immunization coverage rates will be low. Even where coverage rates are 60 to 80 per cent, there will be large numbers of non-immune children, with risk factors of malnutrition and crowding, resulting in high rates of measles transmission and morbidity.

Children with measles are at a high risk of worsening malnutrition, vitamin A deficiency, diarrhoea, and secondary respiratory infections, with each of these factors contributing to the high mortality rates that have occurred. The management of individual cases will require attention to the above medical complications, and demands a high degree of clinical staff input. It is for these reasons that effective measles immunization must be organized at a very early stage in the relief process.

There are now agreed strategies for implementing mass measles immunization campaigns among refugee and displaced communities (Toole *et al.* 1989) and 'immunization' kits, enabling the necessary cold chain to be maintained, and vaccine, needles, and syringes to be available in the most remote locations (Fig. 2).

Effective mass measles immunization in refugee communities should have as its target over 90 per cent coverage of all children aged between 6 months and 12 to 15 years. These recommendations differ from the standard Expanded Programme for Immunization recommendations, but are based on the epidemiological evidence of measles outbreaks in these communities, and the increased risk factors they face. Where numbers are overwhelming and resources are limited, an initial programme to achieve high coverage of children aged 6 months to 5 years may be justified, but it is essential that it is rapidly followed by a programme to cover the older age group.

As high coverage is essential for the measles immunization strategy to be effective, the immunization campaign must be based on an accurate census of the target population, full participation of the community, and accurate registration of the vaccines. There is no justification for an initial measles programme based on random clinic attendance, or unplanned house-to-house visiting.

It is recommended that vitamin A supplementation is linked to the measles immunization campaign, with a dose of 200 000 IU being

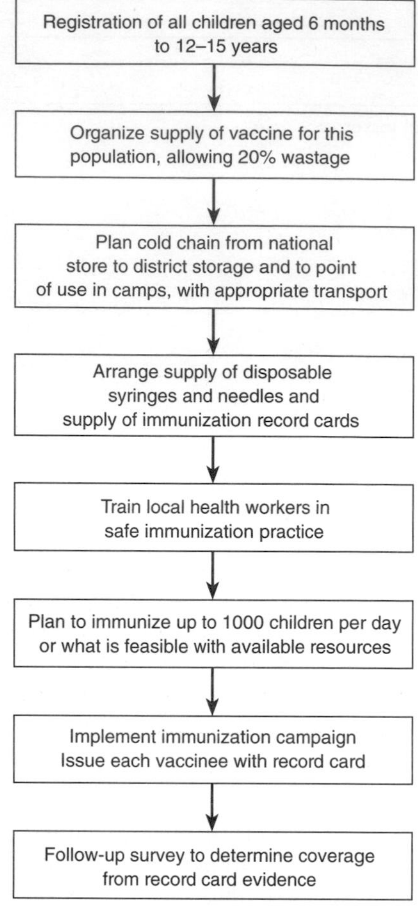
Registration of all children aged 6 months to 12–15 years
Organize supply of vaccine for this population, allowing 20% wastage
Plan cold chain from national store to district storage and to point of use in camps, with appropriate transport
Arrange supply of disposable syringes and needles and supply of immunization record cards
Train local health workers in safe immunization practice
Plan to immunize up to 1000 children per day or what is feasible with available resources
Implement immunization campaign Issue each vaccinee with record card
Follow-up survey to determine coverage from record card evidence

Fig. 2 Components of a mass measles immunization programme in refugee and displaced communities.

administered orally to each child at the time of immunization. Where the camps are receiving new arrivals, the immunization campaign must be extended to provide immunization on arrival.

The initial mass campaign must evolve into an ongoing campaign for the following groups:

- children missed by the initial campaign
- new arrivals
- children vaccinated in the age group 6 to 9 months who should receive a second dose after age 9 months
- new groups of children reaching the age of 6 months.

Follow-up of the immunization programme is essential to ensure that adequate coverage was achieved, and to locate children who may not have been included.

Acute respiratory infections

Acute respiratory infections are an important cause of morbidity and mortality among children in refugee camps in both tropical and temperate areas. Risk factors for increased morbidity include crowding, poor shelter, vitamin A deficiency, and malnutrition (Toole and Waldman 1990). Studies among displaced communities ranging from regions of Nepal and Iran to Africa and Central America have all shown acute respiratory infection to be responsible for 30 to 40 per cent of morbidity (Desenclos *et al.* 1990; Babille *et al.* 1994).

Strategies to reduce the morbidity of acute respiratory tract infections include both minimizing risk factors and providing appropriate accessible management.

In camps where crowding, malnutrition, measles, and pertussis are not controlled, acute respiratory infections will be responsible for excessive morbidity and mortality, even where treatment programmes are functioning, and emphasis must be given to preventing or minimizing these risk factors. Case management must be based on early recognition using an appropriate case definition, for example fever, cough, and respiratory rate greater than 50 breaths/min. While it will be difficult to differentiate virus and bacterial causes, standardized case management should include antimicrobial therapy, aimed at treating *Streptococcus pneumoniae* or *Haemophilus influenzae* infections.

For moderately ill children, the antimicrobial of choice is cotrimoxazole for ambulatory or home treatment. Supervision by community health workers to ensure antimicrobial compliance and adequate nutrition are essential. Severely ill children, particularly if malnourished, may initially require intravenous therapy, although the feasibility of this will depend on the staff and resources available.

Malnutrition

High rates of malnutrition among refugee and displaced communities are a major cause of increased morbidity and mortality. Malnutrition rates are likely to be highest among groups that have been displaced for extended periods in areas affected by crop failures resulting from drought or disease, and among war affected communities where agriculture and food distribution have been interrupted. Probably the single most important factor in predisposing refugees and other migrant populations to high mortality during the emergency phase is an inadequate food ration. Malnutrition has often been a major contributing factor to high death rates among refugees and internally displaced population. Conversely, as malnutrition takes weeks or months to develop, it does not occur in the early days following acute disasters such as earthquakes, floods, etc.

Malnutrition encompasses both protein-energy malnutrition, ranging from moderate malnutrition to severe cases of marasmus and kwashiorkor, and specific vitamin and mineral deficiencies.

Assessing nutrition status by cluster sample surveys is required to determine the prevalence of malnutrition and follow up nutrition monitoring of all children is required to plan feeding programmes.

Nutrition status may be assessed by a range of anthropometric techniques, the most practical of which are mid upper-arm circumference and weight/height. Standardized cut-offs are used, which may occasionally need to be modified for different ethnic groups. Table 3 shows cut-off values which are generally accepted for assessing nutrition status in refugee and displaced communities.

Malnutrition rates in excess of 30 per cent have been reported from refugees in the Horn of Africa and in earlier studies among Myanmar refugees in Bangladesh (Aall 1979). Several studies have demonstrated the increased mortality associated with malnutrition (Nieburg *et al.* 1992; Yip and Sharp 1993).

The management and prevention of malnutrition are based on the following strategies.

- An adequate general ration for the whole community.

Table 3 Cut-off values for assessment of protein-energy malnutrition for children aged 1 to 6 years

Method	Adequately nourished	Moderately malnourished	Severely malnourished
Mid upper-arm circumference[a]	> 13 cm	11–13 cm	< 11 cm or kwashiorkor
Weight/height (% of WHO/ NCHS standard)	> 80%	70%–80%	< 70% or kwashiorkor
Weight/height based on *Z* scores (number of SDs from median)	Within 2 SD	2–3 SD below	> 3 SD below

SD, standard deviation.

[a]Intended as a tool for community screening; it is not suitable for monitoring nutritional progress in individual children).

- Targeted (selective) feeding:
  - supplementary feeding for moderately malnourished children
  - therapeutic feeding to severely malnourished children
  - mass (blanket) supplementary feeding to all children if excessive malnutrition rates
  - inclusion of other groups (e.g. pregnant and lactating women) where appropriate
  - older persons and medically sick cases.

Random untargeted food distribution, often initiated by well-meaning groups with little effective refugee experience, should be avoided.

The general ration should aim to provide a minimum of 2100 kcal (UNHCR/WFP 1997), with vitamin and mineral fortification where necessary. Distribution should be based on a highly organized system, involving family registration and assuming availability of utensils, fuel, and dry storage facilities. These aspects are not the direct responsibility of the health workers, but should be monitored as part of the health surveillance programme.

Supplementary feeding to moderately malnourished children should aim to provide an additional 500 to 1000 kcal/day assuming that the children are also receiving appropriate general rations. Moderately malnourished children must be registered, and progress monitored by weekly or monthly weighing. They should continue to receive supplementary foods until they have achieved 85 to 90 per cent weight/height. Supplementary feeding may be provided in specific feeding centres providing on-site meals or, with adequate community participation, by home distribution of supplementary foods.

Therapeutic feeding of severely malnourished children is demanding in terms of staff, time, and clinical input. Many of the severely malnourished children will have associated infections, particularly acute respiratory infections or diarrhoeal diseases, and mortality rates may be high despite nutrition and medical interventions. Therapeutic feeding will require four to five feeds per day, often by nasogastric tubes. In both supplementary and intensive feeding programmes, the primary object must be a food mix containing sufficient calories. Most correctly balanced relief foods will contain appropriate amounts of protein and mineral nutrients. It is particularly important that this is understood for children with kwashiorkor. Specifically high-protein foods, which are often donated in relief supplies are not appropriate. The aetiology of kwashiorkor is more complex than simple protein deficiency, and provision of high-protein diets has been shown to worsen the metabolic derangement associated with kwashiorkor.

The problems associated with infant formulas, milk products, and feeding bottles are exacerbated in an emergency. Clean safe water is essential but rarely available in most situations, and careful dilution of the feeds is of critical importance but difficult to control. Infant formulas, if unavoidable, should be distributed in health facilities under strictly controlled conditions and proper supervision. It is mandatory not to distribute feeding bottles in emergency situations as the associated risk is very significant.

Malaria

High rates of malaria transmission have occurred in many refugee camps in endemic malaria areas. Malaria has been reported as a major cause of morbidity and mortality in Southeast Asia, central and southern Africa, Central America, and parts of Afghanistan and Central Asia (Suleman 1988; Toole and Waldman 1990).

Malaria morbidity and mortality may be particularly high where non-immune communities have been displaced into hyperendemic areas, as has occurred in migration from highland to lowland Ethiopia (Kloos 1990), and where crowding, poor environmental control, and the peak malaria transmission season coincide.

Surveillance is particularly important in providing a basis for the appropriate management and control of malaria. In the absence of laboratory diagnosis, case definitions for malaria are often non-specific and it is likely that other causes of fever will be included. Wherever possible, a basic laboratory for examination of blood films should be established at refugee camps where malaria is thought to be a major problem. In hyperendemic areas, a clinical case definition should be combined with laboratory findings.

Strategies for the prevention and control of malaria, which may include vector control and the use of impregnated bednets, must be planned effectively, with input from personnel experienced in malaria control.

Early detection and appropriate management of cases is essential. With the increasing prevalence of resistance to antimalarial drugs in many areas, local expertise should be utilized in planning treatment schedules, and attention given to WHO guidelines (WHO 1991).

Other health problems

While the above are the priority public health problems in many refugee and displaced communities, a wide range of other communicable disease and nutrition problems may occur and be responsible for significant morbidity and mortality. Some of these conditions only become apparent after camps have been in existence for some months, for example tuberculosis, micronutrient deficiencies, or vaccine-preventable diseases apart from measles. Other diseases may have specific geographical locations, including typhus/relapsing fever, viral haemorrhagic fevers, and leishmaniasis. The impact of these conditions on refugee and displaced communities, and strategies for prevention and control, are described in below.

Tuberculosis

The control and management of tuberculosis presents difficult problems in displaced and refugee communities who may remain in camps for only limited periods of time. Decisions on when to initiate a tuberculosis programme, case definitions for treatment, which treatment regimens to use, and the relevance of contact tracing and BCG prophylaxis are all more complex than in settled communities. While small numbers of cases may be present during the emergency phase of a refugee programme, it is often in the postemergency phase that tuberculosis may become a major public health problem, when crowding and high transmission rates produce clinical and infectious cases. Several studies have shown the importance of tuberculosis in refugee camps in the postemergency phase, and the difficulties in treatment and control.

In a study among refugees in Somalia in 1982, over 50 per cent of patients started on treatment were lost to follow-up and of the 50 per cent remaining over 25 per cent were intermittent defaulters. In camps with less mobile populations and greater health resources, improved follow-up and compliance are possible, but where such conditions are not met, poor compliance and treatment failures will continue.

The difficulties of effectively controlling and treating tuberculosis in such situations have led to the development of standardized guidelines for refugee and displaced communities (WHO 1997). The principal components of these guidelines are as follows.

- The emergency phase is over, and water, sanitation, nutrition, measles immunization, and essential clinical services are all adequately met.
- The stability of the camp is envisaged for at least 6 months, preferably longer, and the implementing organization, particularly if a foreign relief agency, is committed to maintaining the programme.
- The programme is based on passive case-finding and diagnosis by smear microscopy.
- Treatment by directly observed therapy (**DOT**) using short-course chemotherapy.
- Monitoring of tuberculosis patients by a standardized recording and reporting system.

It is important, where possible, that the decision to implement a tuberculosis control programme among refugee and displaced groups involves the national tuberculosis programme co-ordinators of the host country.

The recommended (adult) treatment regimen is that proposed within the WHO DOT guidelines:

- intensive phase (2 months): rifampicin, isoniazid, pyrazinamide, and ethambutol, under direct supervision, given daily or three times weekly
- maintenance phase (4 months) rifampicin and isoniazid given three times per week under direct supervision.

The priority in a tuberculosis control programme in refugee and displaced communities is to interrupt transmission by effectively treating sputum smear positive patients. Decisions to treat pulmonary smear negative and extrapulmonary cases must be made according to the local circumstances, but they should form only a small part of the tuberculosis programme.

Treatment of children with suspected tuberculosis, requires a careful assessment of each child, and often a trial period of supervised improved nutrition and management of other possible infections. The WHO guidelines provide a useful scoring system to assist the diagnosis and management of tuberculosis in children.

Meningococcal meningitis

Although limited to specific geographical areas, outbreaks of meningococcal meningitis (primarily *Neisseria meningitidis* serogroup A) have occurred among refugees in many locations ranging from the 'meningitis belt' of sub-Saharan Africa to camps in northern Thailand. The pattern of crowding, poor hygiene, and (often) delayed recognition of cases can result in extensive epidemics with significant mortality.

The greatest potential risk is among refugee and displaced communities in the African meningitis belt, particularly if the displacement is in a year and season when meningococcal transmission is likely to be high.

Prevention and control of meningococcal meningitis outbreaks is based on surveillance, case management, and, where appropriate, mass immunization.

Effective surveillance is essential if the first few cases, which may indicate the beginning of an epidemic, are to be detected. Case definitions must be appropriate to the resources that exist, but wherever possible should include laboratory confirmation by latex agglutination, Gram stain, or culture of the first reported cases (WHO 1995).

Several epidemiological studies have attempted to define epidemic 'threshold', based on the number of new cases per 100 000 in defined time periods, to predict the potential for an epidemic and the need to initiate mass immunization. In an extensive study in Burkina Faso, it was found a rate of 15 or more new cases per 100 000 per week, averaged over 2 consecutive weeks, had a high positive predictive value for detecting epidemic levels of disease. These data were determined from a large population base, not living in the crowded conditions of refugee camps, and modifications are required in displaced communities. In refugee camps with populations below 30 000 and where the occurrence of cases is not part of a wider epidemic, simple guidelines such as weekly doubling of cases over a 3-week period have been suggested (Moore *et al.* 1990).

Once a locally appropriate epidemic threshold has been reached, a mass immunization campaign must be implemented within 10 to 14 days if it is to have an impact on controlling the outbreak. Immunization should attempt to cover the age range from 6 months to 30 years. The decision to initiate a meningococcal immunization campaign must be weighed against other priorities within the camp health programme, particularly in the acute phase of an emergency, when measles, malnutrition, and inadequate water and sanitation may be much greater risk factors for morbidity and mortality.

Early detection and treatment of cases is essential to reduce morbidity and mortality. Cases may not be brought to health centres, and case-finding by community health workers will be necessary. Several studies have shown that a single intramuscular dose of long-acting chlorampherical is an effective treatment in the majority of cases, certainly in Africa meningococcal septicaemia and severe complications seem relatively uncommon.

Chemoprophylaxis of case contacts in refugee settings is not considered to be appropriate, as it is difficult in a crowded refugee camp to define 'close contacts', recolonization may occur rapidly in the crowded conditions, and with increasing prevalence of sulphonamide-resistant strains, widespread use of rifampicin would be required, which would be both expensive and undesirable in the context of restricting the availability of antimicrobials.

Relapsing fever and typhus

Relapsing fever (*Borrelia recurrentis* and *Borrelia duttoni*) and typhus fever (*Rickettsia* spp.) have limited geographical foci, but have occasionally caused outbreaks in refugee communities.

Both epidemic (louse-borne) relapsing fever and louse-borne typhus (*Rickettsia prowazeki*) are endemic in the highlands of Ethiopia, and have caused major epidemics among displaced communities in that area (Brown *et al.* 1988). In 1999, an epidemic of louse-borne relapsing fever was reported among displaced groups in war-affected areas of southern Sudan. Epidemic typhus has recently caused outbreaks among displaced communities in Burundi and Rwanda.

The prevention of both louse-borne relapsing fever and epidemic typhus is based on delousing the affected community and preventing further lice infestation by reducing crowding and improving hygiene. Delousing campaigns require major logistical input, and continued further surveillance to determine effectiveness (Thomson 1995).

Surveillance for possible cases is essential in detecting outbreaks, and ensuring appropriate case management. Because of the non-specific clinical picture, where possible initial relapsing fever cases should be confirmed by detection of *Borrelia* in blood films. Recommended antimicrobial treatment is a single oral dose of tetracycline or doxycycline. Because of the risk of a Herxheimer reaction, patients should be monitored during treatment. For epidemic typhus, treatment is a single dose of doxycycline or chloramphemicol.

Outbreaks of murine (flea-borne) and scrub (mite-borne) typhus have occurred in refugee camps on the Thai–Kampuchea border. Again, treatment is by a single dose of doxycycline, but where cases are sporadic and laboratory confirmation is not possible, rickettsial infections may be confused with other febrile infections.

Viral haemorrhagic fevers

Outbreaks of viral haemorrhagic fevers, including yellow fever, Rift Valley fever, and dengue, have been reported from several refugee and displaced communities. Because of the ecological and geographical occurrence of viral haemorrhagic fevers they are a potential risk only to refugee groups in selected areas. However, these risks may be increased where displaced groups move into new ecological zones, where environmental change leads to modified vector breeding habits, and where crowded conditions increase the rates of transmission.

Yellow fever outbreaks occurred on a large scale during population movements from Ethiopia into Sudan, and also during internal displacement of communities to new ecological zones in Ethiopia (Kloos 1990).

An extensive outbreak of Rift Valley fever occurred among Somali refugees in northern Kenya in 1995. The remoteness of the area, and uncertainties of diagnosis, resulted in an epidemic involving over 400 reported deaths (CDC 1998*a*). The epidemic had been preceded by increasing livestock mortality, and was associated with atypical heavy and prolonged rainfall, which may have increased vector-breeding sites. Dengue fever has affected refugee communities in endemic areas in Southeast Asia and has been reported, on the basis of serological evidence, among refugees in Somalia. Less common haemorrhagic fevers, including Congo–Crimean haemorrhagic fever in Iraq and haemorrhagic fever with renal syndrome in Kosovo have been reported among displaced communities.

Although outbreaks of Ebola haemorrhagic fever have not been reported from refugee or displaced communities, the presence of the infection in areas of central Africa, where population displacements are occurring, requires constant surveillance and contingency control planning.

For yellow fever outbreaks, mass immunization of the at-risk population, as has successfully been implemented in non-refugee populations in Africa, is the major control strategy to be implemented. If transmission is occurring in a camp setting, vector control, particularly in relation to breeding sites in water storage containers, should be implemented. Where refugees are displaced in small groups in forested areas, little can be done to control vector populations.

Dengue control should be primarily aimed at vector control within the refugee or displaced camps.

Hepatitis

Hepatitis in refugee communities presents two different issues. Enterically transmitted hepatitis (A and E) is a potential risk wherever water, sanitation, and hygiene are inadequate. In many tropical areas, a large proportion of the population will be immune at least to hepatitis A and few clinically apparent infections will occur. However, several outbreaks of hepatitis E virus have been reported, and more may be apparent as the epidemiology of this virus is understood in different areas.

Two extensive outbreaks of hepatitis E virus have occurred among Somali displaced groups: in north-western Somalia in 1985, and in northern Kenya in 1991. Transmission occurred both within households and from common water sources, reinforcing the importance of the need for adequate water and sanitation and improved hygiene in living areas.

The risks for hepatitis B and C are similar for refugee populations as for non-refugee communities in Africa and Asia, where 5 to 10 per cent of the population may be hepatitis B virus carriers. Risks of transmission may increase in the early days of refugee programmes through lack of clean medical equipment and transmission through injections. There is a definite risk to health care workers, particularly in disasters involving major trauma, and health care workers from non-endemic areas should be immunized.

Typhoid fever

Typhoid fever is endemic in most tropical areas, and in cooler areas where water and sanitation facilities are inadequate. Sporadic cases of typhoid fever may occur in any refugee setting. Relatively few outbreaks have been reported but in the absence of laboratory facilities, cases may be under-reported.

Outbreaks have been reported among Kurdish refugees in southern Iran and displaced persons in Bosnia-Herzegovina (Bradaric *et al.* 1996). In addition to these specific outbreaks, large increases in endemic cases have occurred in parts of the former Soviet Union. During 1996 and 1997, an epidemic of typhoid fever involving in excess of 20 000 cases were reported from Tajikistan, with over 8000 cases in the capital Dushanbe. The epidemic was characterized by multiple point sources of infection, overflow of sewage, contaminated water supplies, and person to person spread (CDC 1988*b*). The management of cases of typhoid fever is complicated by the increasing prevalence of multiple antimicrobial resistance in *S. typhi.* In Tajikistan, over 90 per cent of isolates of *S. typhi* were multidrug resistant (chloramphamicol, cotrimoxazole, ampicillin, and nalidixic acid) and, as the epidemic progressed, ciprofloxacin-resistant strains were isolated.

In refugee camps without access to laboratory investigations, management of individual cases should be in accordance with known treatment strategies in that locality. However, every effort should be made to confirm the diagnosis and monitor antimicrobial sensitivity patterns.

Prevention and control of typhoid is largely dependent on the provision of adequate water and sanitation facilities. For outbreaks in refugee camps, it may be necessary to undertake additional hygiene measures to attempt to interrupt transmission. Although oral typhoid vaccines have a high efficacy in individual cases, mass immunization is not currently recommended in most refugee and displaced communities, as compliance with the multidose vaccine may be poor and it may detract efforts from improving water, sanitation, and hygiene.

Leishmaniasis and trypanosomiasis

Among vector-bone parasitic diseases, in addition to malaria, major epidemics of visceral leishmaniasis and trypanosomiasis have been reported in displaced communities in southern Sudan and Uganda.

The leishmamiasis epidemic in the Western Upper Nile region of Sudan in 1988 to 1989 is estimated to have resulted in over 10 000 cases with high mortality. The epidemic was related to displacements among non-immune communities, high rates of malnutrition, and changes in local vector ecology (Seaman *et al.* 1996). Management of such large numbers of cases in a war-affected area with limited resources presented major difficulties. Field treatment centres in the villages treated over 3000 cases with a 30-day course of sodium stibogluconate.

Visceral leishmaniasis has a non-specific clinical presentation, and other disease of refugees including tuberculosis, typhoid fever, and chronic malaria must be considered. The outbreak in southern Sudan, despite the difficulty of access, was investigated and managed with a high degree of expertise, and is a model for how similar outbreaks should be managed.

Human African trypanosomiasis (sleeping sickness), although localized geographically, has been a major recent public health problem among displaced groups in the Democratic Republic of Congo and northern Uganda. The most documented outbreak, providing important information on the epidemiology of the disease in mobile and displaced communities, is an epidemic that occurred in northern Uganda between 1987 and 1992. The epidemic occurred in refugees returning to northern Uganda from a highly endemic area in southern Sudan. The return to the depopulated area, an increase in tsetse fly levels, and continuous in-migration of infected cases led to over 6000 cases being reported, with over 30 per cent of the community infected in some villages.

As with the outbreak of visceral leishmaniasis in southern Sudan, the control of trypansomiasis in displaced communities requires a high level of expertise in case-finding, management, and control.

HIV/AIDS and other sexually transmitted diseases

During the emergency phase of refugee camps, and among displaced communities, HIV/AIDS and STDs will reflect the pattern within the community prior to the refugee displacement period. In situations in which gross human rights violations have occurred, and where there may be large numbers of rape victims, HIV and/or other STDs present a major, acute, and complex medical and psychosocial problem, requiring very specific inputs (Toole and Waldman 1996).

In longer-term refugee camps, particularly where family and social structures may be disrupted, and when camps are part of a war-zone environment, STDs may become an important communicable disease problem. HIV spreads fastest in conditions of poverty, powerlessness, and social instability—conditions that are often at their most extreme during displacement (UNAIDS 1996). Mandatory testing is sometimes a reaction by authorities to the fear that a displaced population or refugee may infect a local population. However, mandatory testing in such situations does not stop the spread of infection from one population to another for the following reasons.

- HIV/AIDS is already present in all populations; testing itself does not stop the spread of the disease. Testing diverts resources from programmes for prevention, education, and information, management of STDs, and condom distribution, all of which are more effective in reducing the spread.
- Testing does not identify all those infected because of the false results and/or 'window period' during which a person may be infected and highly infectious but the antibodies to the disease have not yet developed and do not register on the test. Furthermore, a person who tests negative may become infected any time after the test.

Mandatory testing not only has no public health justification, but it also violates the rights of people, including the rights to privacy and security, as well as the ethical principles of autonomy, informed consent, and confidentiality. If HIV status is made known, HIV-positive people may be subject to discrimination, stigma, ostracism, harassment, and physical abuse (UNAIDS 1996). HIV/AIDS and STD prevention and treatment guidelines in refugee and displaced settings should follow standardized WHO recommendations. Because the risk of HIV transmission is greatly increased in the presence of other STDs, early establishment of STD-related services is a priority. STDs and their complications are a major cause of ill health and are usually grossly under-reported (UNAIDS 1996). The prevention of STDs involves the promotion of safer sex as well as early and effective case management and case-finding.

STD services should be user friendly and confidential. Appropriate and effective case management involves the following (UNAIDS 1996):

- guidelines for case management—case definition and management protocol
- training health care providers
- consistent availability of appropriate drugs
- consistent supply of condoms
- referral facilities
- monitoring.

All health care providers, including volunteer workers, should receive some training in prevention, be provided with information materials, and serve as channels for the distribution of condoms.

Micronutrient deficiencies

Nutrition programmes with refugee and displaced communities have generally been directed at monitoring and alleviating protein-energy malnutrition. However, deficiencies in micronutrients, particularly vitamin A deficiency, pellagra, scurvy, and beri beri, have been reported from a number of refugee and displaced communities dependent on food rations with little local supplementation (Toole 1994). Overall, vitamin A deficiency is potentially the most serious, as both insufficient vitamin A in the rations and coexisting malnutrition and measles can rapidly lead to severe vitamin A deficiency and xerophthalmia.

In any refugee and displaced communities where significant malnutrition exists, there should be a mass distribution of vitamin A to children aged 6 months to 15 years (200 000 IU), usually at the same time as measles immunization.

Outbreaks of scurvy (vitamin C deficiency) have been reported from refugee camps in Somalia and Ethiopia, generally becoming evident 3 to 4 months after the refugees arrived in the camps. In these programmes, the relief food was almost totally deficient in vitamin C and no fresh foods were available locally. Management of cases of scurvy requires vitamin C drug supplementation, but mass distribution as a preventive measure is unlikely to be successful as weekly distribution would be necessary and compliance may not be high. Food fortification is unlikely to be effective as vitamin C is destroyed by cooking. Food diversification, to introduce fresh foods into the diet, is the only effective long-term strategy.

Outbreaks of pellagra (niacin (vitamin B_3) deficiency) have occurred on a large scale among Mozambican refugees in Malawi, where the rations were based largely on maize, and groundnuts, which should have been in the rations, were unavailable. Beri beri (thiamine (vitamin B_1) deficiency) has occurred among Bhutanese refugees in Nepal (Upadhyay 1998) and among refugees in Thailand and West Africa, where the rations were based on polished rice with an inadequate amount of beans or groundnuts.

Prevention of pellagra and beri beri is primarily by ensuring that the distributed rations are sufficiently diversified to provide adequate amounts of B vitamins. Treatment of individual cases will require appropriate vitamin doses.

Vaccine-preventable diseases (excluding measles)

Among the vaccine-preventable diseases included in the Expanded Programme for Immunization (diphtheria, pertussis, tetanus, poliomyelitis, tuberculosis (BCG), and measles), only immunization against measles, described above, is a priority in the acute phase of health programmes with refugees and displaced communities.

Decisions on further immunizations in the Expanded Programme for Immunization in the postemergency phase are based on a number of different factors including:

- information on current immunization status
- short-term stability of the population
- resources available (a major logistic exercise only to be attempted if adequate coverage for the whole target population)
- relation to the host country national immunization programme
- difficulty of organization if refugees partially integrated into local community
- importance of registration and records.

While current strategies for poliomyelitis eradication are meeting with increasing success there have been small clusters of poliomyelitis cases in displaced communities in the past decade and in current war-affected communities, there may continue to be inadequately immunized cohorts of children. If there are a significant number of unimmunized children, crowding and poor sanitation will greatly increase the risk of transmission and subsequent cases. Any suspected cases must be assessed according to WHO guidelines as part of the global eradication programme. If cases occur, control involves oral poliomyelitis vaccine and improvements in water and sanitation.

Where there are significant numbers unimmunized children, pertussis is a risk in crowded, malnourished children. Outbreaks have not been specifically reported, but it is possible that pertussis has been underdiagnosed and under-reported. Management of individual cases is primarily supportive, through maintaining hydration and nutrition. If erythromycin if given before the paroxysmal stage, the severity of the disease may be reduced. Vaccination as an outbreak control measure will not be useful because of the time needed for immunity to develop.

Cases of neonatal tetanus may occur in displaced and refugee communities, particularly if conditions leading to the displacement had resulted in a breakdown of administration of tetanus toxoid in pregnancy. Apart from providing tetanus toxoid immunization as part of a wider immunization strategy in the postemergency phase, prevention will include assisting traditional birth attendants to ensure clean delivery techniques.

Although outbreaks of diphtheria have not recently been reported from refugee communities in tropical Africa or Asia, outbreaks that have occurred in states of the former Soviet Union are a reminder that such epidemics need to be considered, particularly in crowded communities where recent Expanded Programme for Immunization coverage has been reduced (Vitek and Wharton 1998).

BCG immunization should be included for newborns and for children below 5 years of age without an obvious BCG scar as part of the Expanded Programme for Immunization programme in the postemergency phase.

Unavoidable morbidity and mortality due to communicable diseases and malnutrition in refugee and displaced communities will only be achieved if interventions are based on the epidemiology of the particular crisis and on a systematic set of priorities. Figure 3 summarizes these as a strategic plan for public health intervention.

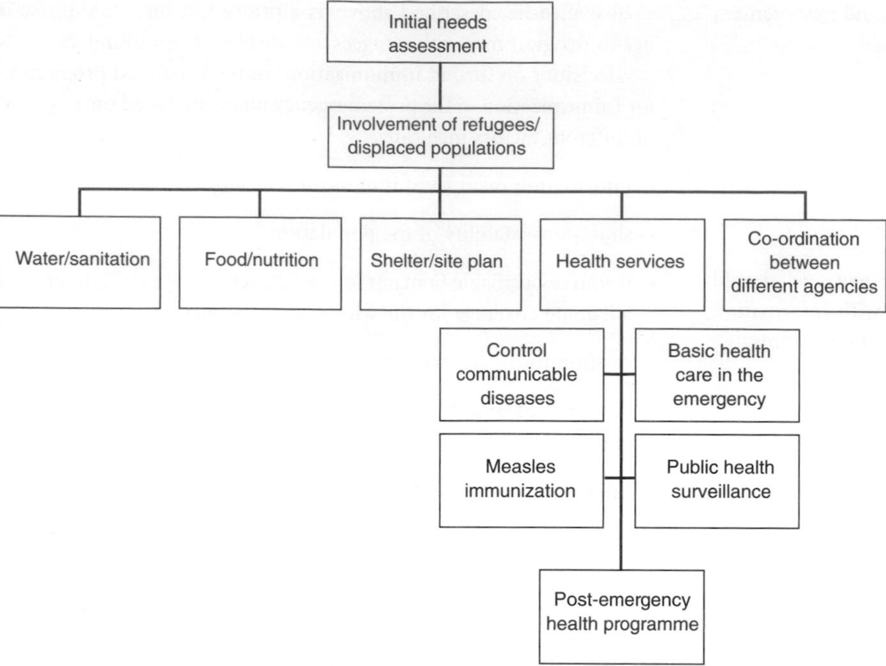

Fig. 3 Priorities for public health in refugee and displaced populations.

Reproductive health

Providing adequate food, clean water, shelter, sanitation, and primary health care are priority activities in an emergency. These interventions help to combat the major killers in displacement situation: malnutrition, diarrhoeal diseases, measles, acute respiratory infections, and malaria (where prevalent). However, reproductive health care is also crucial for the physical, mental, and social well being of any individual. As an integral part of primary health care, reproductive health care is important in overcoming such problems as:

- complications of pregnancy and delivery, which are the leading causes of death and disease among refugee women of child-bearing age
- malnutrition and epidemics which can further diminish the physiological reserves of pregnant or lactating women, thus endangering their health and that of their child
- an absence of law and order, commonly seen in refugee and other displaced settings, which, together with men's loss of power and status, leads to an increased risk of sexual violence; violence against refugee women, rape, sexual abuse, involuntary prostitution, domestic violence, and even physical assault during pregnancy have been found to be far more widespread than was previously acknowledged (UNHCR 1999).

Increasing numbers of refugees who have endured the terrible hardships of forced migration and long-term displacement desperately need reproductive health care. The needs and priorities of beneficiaries in situations of migration and displacement vary from region to region, and these must be fully studied and addressed. The majority of refugees are women, yet it is rarely women who determine what services are to be provided, and their very real public health problems often remain undetected.

Reproductive health care should be made available in all situations and be based on the needs and demands of the displaced population, particularly those of women (UNHCR 1999). The various religious beliefs, ethical values, and cultural backgrounds of the displaced population should be respected, in conformity with universally recognized international human rights. The major objectives of reproductive health care in a displacement situation are to:

- prevent and manage the consequences of sexual violence
- decrease HIV transmission by practising universal precautions and the availability of condoms
- prevent excess neonatal and maternal morbidity and mortality by providing clean home deliveries, ensuring clean and safe deliveries at health facilities, and managing complications by establishing a referral system
- plan for provision of comprehensive reproductive health services, integrated into primary health care, as soon as possible.

Men, women, and children can be victims of violence in conflict situations (including torture, rape, or solitary confinement) and suffer consequent trauma. Rape is a crime of violence, and is sometimes used as a systematic method of intimidation. Survivors of rape can be any age from the very young to the very old and can belong to any social group. It is documented that 25 per cent of women in a Burundian refugee camp in Tanzania had experienced sexual violence from the start of their flight to the time of the survey. Perpetrators of violence against women in refugee and displaced populations can be other refugees, including family members, or border guards, police, and soldiers. Types of violence include rape, and forced prostitution to obtain food and other basic amenities.

Another survey has shown that 22 per cent of women refugees between the ages of 12 and 49 years had experienced sexual violence since the start of the conflict in Burundi. UNHCR estimates that, because of the severe stigma attached to a woman who has been raped, the actual figures could be 10 times greater than the number of reported cases. There was a high rate of violence against Somali refugee women in Kenya when they left the camps to search for firewood. During a 1-month period there were 24 assaults on women ranging from 10 to 50 years old. Many of them were gang raped. They were also shot, knifed, severely beaten, and robbed. Sexual violence among refugees and other displaced populations is a major public health problem. It is of utmost importance to develop culturally appropriate public health measures to support and counsel women who have been raped. It is crucial that a safe environment is provided for women in camps.

Mental health and psychosocial needs

The shock of having to leave home and the circumstances of life as a displaced person, particularly in the early stages of displacement, create major emotional and social problems and exacerbate existing problems in the community. The trauma of flight and its aftermath may leave refugees confused, frightened, lonely, and insecure, facing an unknown future in a strange, sometimes hostile, environment. Separation from or loss of other family members as well as lack of community support are common in refugee emergencies, and causes emotional stress and problems for individuals and their community.

In every emergency, there will be refugee groups at risk with psychological or social problems that require particular attention. The most vulnerable are those with no family support who are dependent on external assistance for their daily survival. This dependence may be because of their age, physical condition, psychological condition, or socio-economic problems. The social disruption of emergencies causes these problems to be both aggravated and overlooked, while in stable non emergency situations the community itself meets many of the needs of groups at risk. The psychological impact of war in emergency situations is a new emerging public health problem that invites further research.

Post-trauma reactions to sexual violence include feelings of shame and guilt, anger, humiliation, nightmares, withdrawal, depression, and suicidal tendencies. Family, friends, and community support groups must be alerted to these possible reactions so that they can understand and assist the survivors of violence.

Social attitudes to rape are usually very judgemental. A woman who becomes pregnant by rape may need help in being accepted by her family and the community or in placing a child for adoption.

It is useful to consider the major psychosocial systems, both within the individual and across the community as a whole, that are disrupted or threatened by the refugee experience. A simplified framework suggests that five fundamental 'systems' can be identified (Silove 1999).

The attachment system

Traumatic losses and separation from close attachment figures affect many refugees. Disruptions to bonds are often of the most threatening nature, for example, being witness to the murder or kidnappings of close relatives. Such losses and bereavements are often unresolved, with the family member living in a state of uncertainty for prolonged periods of time, not knowing the fate or whereabouts of key relatives. The disruption of attachments poses major threats to particular groups such as unaccompanied minors and single women with children, since they do not have the capacity to 'repair' or 'substitute' for their losses. Unresolved grief, difficulties in forming and maintaining relations, separation anxiety, and other emotional difficulties are some of the psychosocial outcomes that may supervene if collective and individual coping mechanisms break down.

The security system

It is common for refugees to have witnessed or encountered successive threats to the physical safety and security of themselves and those close to them. Exposure to war, combat, bombardment, land mines, and torture all pose direct threats to life, involving the self and others. Post-traumatic stress disorder and its variants represent core psychic reactions to exposure to such experiences, but a range of other reactions may occur, for example severe anxiety (panic), depression, phobias, and reactive psychosis.

The identity/role system

The refugee experience poses a major threat to the sense of identity of the individual and the group as a whole. Loss of land, possessions, and professions divest individuals of a sense of purpose and status in society. Many have no defined role in the new camp environment, a problem that can be exacerbated by the idleness and inactivity that prevail in the refugee camps. Certain extreme reactions such as 'hysteria' and dissociation may have their roots in severe identity and role conflicts. The undermining of traditional cultures and the rapidity of cultural change also pose major threats to the integrity and identity of families and communities in general. Revisions of gender roles, responsibilities, and power relationships may be necessary to meet the demands of camp life. The loss of community leaders, elders, traditional healers, and group knowledge about traditions, customs, and rituals may further undermine the sense of group identity and empowerment.

The human rights system

Almost all refugees have been confronted with major challenges to their human rights. These include arbitrary and unjust treatment, persecution, brutality, and in some instances torture. Such experiences may provoke long-lasting feelings of dehumanization, outrage, anger, and resentment, especially if there are no mechanisms available to redress feelings of grievance. Thus violated groups may have limited trust in governing structures, being quick to react against perceived injustice or discrimination.

The existential-meaning system

The refugee experience poses a major threat to the sense of coherence and meaning that stable civilian life usually provides for most communities. Historical continuities linking past, present, and future have been radically disrupted by the upheavals associated with refugee experience, often leaving those affected in a state of bewilderment and uncertainty. Traditional meaning systems such as religion may no longer provide the sense of security and predictability that they once did in the home country. Alternatively, individuals may turn more fervently to religion and other sources of traditional meaning to re-establish a sense of coherence in their lives. The fantasy of resettlement may be elevated to an unrealistic status to the extent that life in the camp is seen as a state of paralysed waiting. Erosion of systems of values may loosen usual ethical and moral constraints in some individuals, making them more prone to antisocial behaviours.

By its nature, camp life risks eroding traditional value systems without offering a new sense of meaning or direction.

It is important to initiate mental health programmes during the emergency phase of a refugee crisis: local staff must be identified and trained, and time is required to understand the local cultural context and the need to become aware such help exists. Providing adequate response to the psychosocial and mental health needs of traumatized displaced population helps to restore the bond between the individual and the surrounding society. Simplified methods of assessing the mental health and psychosocial needs of refugees and other displaced people need to be refined and developed.

Land mines and public health

There is a growing concern about the problem of land mines as a leading cause of deaths and injuries in war-torn countries. Rates of 8.1 and 16.7 casualties per 1000 living people were found in Manica and Metuchuria (Mozambique) respectively. The prevalence of amputees was 3.2 per 1000 in Manica, and 2.3 in Metuchuria. The case-fatality rate was 48 per cent. Most of the victims were civilians (68 per cent) and were injured by antipersonnel mines. Sixteen per cent of victims were women, and 7 per cent were under 15 years of age (Ascherio *et al.* 1995). Similar situations have been documented in Cambodia, Afghanistan, Somalia, and many other countries in every continent.

Essential drugs management

Health information systems provide data which determine drugs and medical supplies needs. Procurement must be based on accurate assessment of needs.

When setting up an essential drugs programme in an emergency population it is important to integrate it into the essential drugs programme of the host country, if one exists. The provision of a different set of drugs from those in an established national programme is inappropriate. This integration minimizes disputes between health professionals from different backgrounds and facilitates the prompt implementation of health services. Among the points mentioned by Coninx (1988) as being crucial to the effective management of essential drugs, are co-ordination of expatriate input with the national system and use of a standard drug list and treatment protocols.

The new emergency health kit

The new emergency health kit, which was jointly developed by several United Nations agencies, includes written management principles based on an essential drugs list for emergency populations and treatment guidelines. Medical supplies for a population of 10 000 people for a period of 3 months are provided. The kit is made up of 10 basic kits of medical supplies and equipment and one supplementary kit of more specialized medical supplies and equipment, each for 1000 people for a period of 3 months. Use of the supplementary kit depends on the use of the basic kits within a primary health care management programme, based on the work of community health workers referring to secondary and tertiary levels of care.

This emergency health kit, which was developed and field-tested in the light of surveillance of common diseases and problems found in emergency populations, has continued to prove relevant to the major problems (Coninx 1988; Toole and Waldman *et al.* 1990, 1993). In the initial management phases of an emergency, the kits can be extremely useful. They are not meant to be used as a continuing source of supply. However, in the early stages, before information has been gathered, the contents of the kits can be used and drug use can be documented to form a basis for ongoing procurement of separate essential drugs.

Donation guidelines

Emergency situations requiring international help continue to occur. Problems caused by inappropriate donations are frequent. According to the *Guidelines for Drug Donations* (WHO 1999), existing national and WHO essential drugs lists should be respected by donors, and only donations of known good quality with a shelf-life 1 year beyond the estimated date of arrival should be offered. Generic names should be clearly included and packaging units of larger quantities are much preferred. For some donors a financial contribution may be more appropriate, as this can allow purchase of listed drugs and transport from procuring agencies closer to the scene at a fraction of the cost of the same products supplied from the donor countries.

Continuing experience with troublesome inappropriate donations in other refugee settings in Eastern Europe as well as in developing countries has led to more aggressive publication of the need for appropriate response to appeals (Forte 1994). Refugees do not need slimming aids and other inappropriate donations.

Monitoring and surveillance: the health information system

From the early stages of displacement, a health information system that is simple, reliable, and action oriented is a priority. It provides continuous information on the health status of displaced populations and comprises both on-going routine surveillance and intermittent community-based sample surveys. This health information system can be assessed periodically to determine its accuracy, completeness, simplicity, flexibility, and timeliness. Lack of reliable data impedes the efficient delivery of health care in displacement situations. To optimize care, the gathering and dissemination of epidemiological data, the development of laboratory facilities and treatment protocols, standardization of essential supplies, and the initiation of programmes for disease prevention deserve close attention and further research. The proper use of health information data by programme planners and key decision-makers is essential in order to:

- quantify the health and nutritional status of the displaced population
- follow trends in health status and monitor the impact and outcomes of the relief programme
- detect and respond to epidemics
- evaluate health programme effectiveness and service coverage
- ensure that resources are targeted to the greatest needs
- reorient the programme as necessary
- set programme priorities.

Instituting a sustainable health surveillances system to guide health planning for refugee and other displaced populations during the emergency phase of a relief programme is important (Marfin *et al.*

1994). The modern concept of surveillance was defined by Langmuir (1963) as 'the continued watchfulness over the distribution and trends of incidence (of disease) through the systematic collection, consolidation, and evaluation of morbidity and mortality reports and other data'. Even when data are incomplete, the systematic collection of information over time can detect changes in disease, assuming that methods of case ascertainment have remained constant.

Surveillance is a tool for continuous monitoring of changes in health status. The value of surveillance for rapidly assessing the health status of a large population of refugees was demonstrated in Thailand by Glass *et al.* (1982): the rapid collection of basic health data allowed for a co-ordinated health plan to be established, directed at eliminating preventable causes of death and severe illness. The use of a health surveillance system has also been shown to improve routine delivery of health services. On the basis of surveillance information, a highly targeted health delivery system was directed at those preventable causes of death identified by the system. The health information system should evolve as the need for information changes.

The planning and design of public health programmes need strong input from experienced technical specialists, academicians, and emergency management decisions need to be based on sound technical information (Toole and Waldman 1993). Timely public health and nutrition data need to be more widely disseminated.

Another form of input into the programming design is evaluation of lessons learnt from other emergencies. A key element of evaluation is balance and understanding of the conditions and constraints inherent to any particular emergency health programme. A high level of judgement and experience is required when evaluating on the basis of any set criteria and/or indicators. Indicators are measures of progress. They can be quantitative (numerical) or qualitative (non-numerical). Analysis of indicators can demonstrate changes in situation. They can be applied to show what performance has been achieved. When linked to desired results or objectives, they can be used to measure results.

Co-ordination of health services

Given the extraordinary human and material resources required to meet the public health needs of a mass influx or a major emergency operation, a concerted effort is required on the part of a number of agencies. A variety of agencies are involved in humanitarian aid for refugees and other displaced populations including United Nations organizations, bilateral agencies, non-governmental organizations, the military, the media, and the refugees themselves, to cite some examples. In order to respond in a cost-effective manner to the main health and nutrition needs of a refugee or displaced population, the activities of the various actors involved need to be well harmonized.

Effective co-ordination avoids gaps and unnecessary overlaps, and enables organizations from different backgrounds to adopt a complementary approach. The dual goals of emergency response are to ensure the protection of displaced populations and to reduce morbidity and mortality in the affected population. In theory, current technical knowledge is adequate to put in place effective programmes so as to reduce much of the disease burden related to complex emergencies. In reality, there are numerous constraints to the co-ordination of timely, efficient and effective relief programmes. Among the most important constraints are the following:

- political and conflicting interests
- lack of security and inaccessibility to the beneficiaries
- complex humanitarian emergencies
- lack of appropriate expertise among key players
- overlapping mandates
- increasing number and diversity of external agencies
- the commercialization of humanitarian aid
- competition for available resources
- Social constraints and cross-cultural barriers.

Effective co-ordination from the outset of any emergency will mean more effective and faster response on behalf of those who need it. It will also mean that precious health personnel and resources are not misdirected into areas which are already covered or which are non-essential in the first days of an emergency. Work in war-torn societies and in crisis and conflict situations in general is demanding and requires a special type and quality of staff, but current personnel and recruitment procedures and practices are not geared to this. Outside resources are complementary and supportive to the local initiatives, and they should not be devised as parallel systems to substitute and take over. Assistance should always be provided in such a way that it enhances rather than hinders the development of local capacity and the attainment of self-sufficiency by the people concerned. The role of outside help is primarily that of training, transfer of knowledge, and ensuring the application and implementation of best practices in public health interventions. This implies the involvement of experienced health workers in public health interventions at the onset of an emergency.

In theory, current technical knowledge and experience gained from previous refugee situations could enable us adequately to address much of the disease burden related to emergencies. However, it is difficult to achieve results as quickly as required without giving enough attention to the co-ordination elements of the health programme.

Co-ordination mechanisms in emergencies

An important and essential step is the establishment of a co-ordination meeting. There will be resistance from those professionals who see the need to act in life-threatening emergencies, rather than attend 'meetings, bloody meetings'. These meetings should include representatives of government structures, hospitals, etc., as well as key United Nations agencies and non-governmental organization personnel. If possible, health professionals from the refugee community should also participate. These meetings help to identify gaps, share information, and develop mutually agreed upon policies and priorities. They also reduce the risk of misunderstandings, agency jealousies, and overlap of work.

It is essential in an emergency to have a health co-ordinator. This co-ordinator is usually assigned to the UNHCR, which is the lead agency in refugee emergencies. Apart from involvement in the establishment and running of the meetings described above, this person has an important role in developing the policies for standardized treatment protocols and other medical response. He or she will also develop the strategy for health response and priorities. The co-ordinator will also have a responsibility to identify and attract additional international resources if needed, and act as an arbiter if there are agency disputes about modalities and assignment of tasks and geographical areas of responsibility.

There is a tendency to ignore or overlook local resources (government officials or resources within the refugee community) in an emergency when they can be perceived as having little relevant experience or capabilities. Co-ordination of these local and international inputs requires both a strong leadership and flexibility to work both for the displaced population and for the surrounding local population. The health co-ordinator will have an important role in encouraging their involvement and integration in the decision-making process. Steps taken early in the emergency will ensure a longer-term sustainability of health programmes.

It is also important to find a way to disseminate information on a regular basis. This can be achieved through co-ordination meetings, but also by other means that allow key players to keep informed about emerging problems, ongoing or new activities, etc. Co-ordination of the inputs of other sectors vital to the health and nutritional status of the populations should be ensured. These include water and sanitation, food security, shelter, and community services.

Conclusion

The effective management of refugee and other displaced population health activities rests on an understanding of the disease patterns which confront displaced populations, and focuses on the use of available health resources so that the greatest population coverage is achieved. The international community needs to address the issue of access to internally displaced and war-affected civilians in countries where the government either has ceased to function effectively or intentionally obstructs aid efforts (Toole and Waldman 1993).

Medical interventions must be based on the major causes of morbidity and mortality that have arisen from the crisis. Different disasters will cause different health and nutrition problems, and an initial assessment of needs is essential. Providing an adequate general ration, improving water and sanitation, and directing health resources to improving malnutrition and controlling communicable diseases should form the basis of the health intervention programme in the acute phase. Where refugee and displaced communities remain for extended periods of time in displaced or camp locations, a longer-term health programme based on the principles of primary health care must be planned and implemented.

There are several challenges to providing effective mental health services to refugees and other displaced persons. Some of the constraints are practical and logistical and relate to limitations in resources and skills. Others are attitudinal, for example the belief that mental health services are expensive, ineffective, and inappropriate, or require highly sophisticated skills. Yet, there is compelling evidence to support two key arguments from a public point of view: mental health problems associated with displacement may constitute some of the most important impediments to the long-term development of the community, and the advantages of providing a service far outweigh the costs—personal, familial, social, and in terms of human rights—of not doing so.

Ignoring the needs of the mentally ill, or conversely stigmatizing those with mental illness, are issues of central relevance to principles of equity and social justice. Whenever possible, efforts should be made to integrate indigenous methods of healing with 'Western' interventions. Traditional methods of healing appear to be used variably in different refugee settings and depend on levels of preserved knowledge and the availability of traditional healers and resources. Mental health services should be community based and be sensitive to gender and cultural issues and the needs of particular demographic groups (the young, the elderly, unaccompanied minors, widows, and single mothers) as well as high-risk groups such as the physically injured and disabled, the severely mentally disabled, and survivors of extreme trauma, torture, and sexual abuse.

Research focusing on practical issues is fundamental to establishing a knowledge base for future developments, but research endeavours should reflect a partnership model in which priorities in the refugee setting are given preferential attention. Objective methods of assessment of mental health needs in displacement situations and outcome evaluation are areas for further development.

References

Aall, C. (1979). Disastrous international relief failure: a report on Burmese refugees in Bangladesh from May to December 1979. *Disasters*, **3**, 429–34.

Ascherio, A., Biellik, R., Epstein, A., *et al.* (1995). Deaths and injuries caused by land mines in Mozambique. *Lancet*, **346**, 721–4.

Babille, M., De Colombani, P., Guerra, R., Zugaria, N., and Zanetti, C. (1994). Post-emergency epidemiological surveillance in Iraqi-Kurdish refugee camps in Iran. *Disasters*, **18**, 58–75.

Bradaric, N., Punda-Polic, V., Milas, I., Grgic, D., Radosovic, N., and Petric, I. (1996). Two outbreaks of typhoid fever related to the war in Bosnia and Herzegovina. *European Journal of Epidemiology*, **12**, 409–12.

Brown V., Larouze, B., Desve, G., *et al.* (1988). Clinical presentation of louse-borne relapsing fever among Ethiopian Refugees in northern Somalia. *Annals of Tropical Medicine and Parasitology*, **82**, 499–502.

CDC (Centers for Disease Control and Prevention) (1991). Public health consequences of acute displacement of Iraqi citizens, March–May 1991. *Morbidity and Mortality Weekly Report*, **40**, 443–6.

CDC (Centers for Disease Control and Prevention) (1992). Famine affected refugee and displaced populations: Recommendations for public health issues. *Morbidity and Mortality Weekly Report*, **41**, 1–76.

CDC (Centers for Disease Control and Prevention) (1994). Mortality and morbidity surveillance in Rwandan refugees—Burundi and Zaire 1994. *Morbidity and Mortality Weekly Report*, **45**, 104–7.

CDC (Centers for Disease Control and Prevention) (1998*a*). Rift Valley Fever, East Africa 1997–1998. *Morbidity and Mortality Weekly Report*, **47**, 261–4.

CDC (Centers for Disease Control and Prevention) (1998*b*). Epidemic typhoid in Dushanbe, Tajikistan. *Morbidity and Mortality Weekly Report*, **47**, 752–6.

Coninx, R. (1988). Essential drugs: a cornerstone to refugee health care. *Disasters*, **13**, 361–4.

Desenclos, J.C., Michel, D., Tholly, F., Magdi, I., Pecaul, B., and Desve, G. (1990). Mortality trends among refugees in Honduras 1984–1987. *International Journal of Epidemiology*, **19**, 367–73.

Engels, D., Madarcis, J., Nyandwi, S., and Murray J. (1995). Epidemic dysentery caused by *Shigella dysenteriae* type 1: a sentinel site surveillance of antimicrobial resistance patterns in Burundi. *Bulletin of the World Health Organization*, **73**, 787–91.

Forte, G. (1994). Private donations: an ounce of prevention is worth a pound of cure. *Essential Drugs Monitor*, **18**, 6–7.

Glass, R.L., Cates, W., Nieberg, P., *et al.* (1982). Rapid assessment of health status and preventive medicine needs of newly arrived Kampuchean refugees, SA Kaeo, Thailand. *Lancet*, **i**, 868–72.

Goma Epidemiology Group (1995). Public health impact of Rwandan refugee crisis: what happened in Goma, Zaire in July 1994? *Lancet*, **345**, 339–44.

IFRC (1998). *Sphere Project. Humanitarian charter and minimum standards in disaster response.* International Federation of Red Cross and Red Crescent Societies, Geneva.

IOM (International Organization for Migration) (1998). International migration. *Quarterly Review*, **36** (Special Issue).

Kloos, H. (1990). Health aspects of resettlement in Ethiopia. *Social Science in Medicine*, **30**, 643–56.

Langmuir, A.D. (1963). The surveillance of communicable diseases of national importance. *New England Journal of Medicine*, **268**, 182–92.

Marfin, A.A., Moore, J., Collins, C., *et al.* (1994). Infectious disease surveillance during emergency relief to Bhutanese refugees in Nepal. *Journal of the American Medical Association*, **272**, 377–81.

Medècins sans Frontières (1994). *Public health engineering in emergency situations.* Medècins sans Frontières, Paris.

Moore, P.S., Toole, M.J., Nieburg, P., Waldman, R.J., and Broom, C.V. (1990). Surveillance and control of meningococcal meningitis epidemics in refugee populations. *Bulletin of the World Health Organization*, **68**, 587–96.

Nieburg, P., Person-Karell, B., and Toole, M.J. (1992). Malnutrition—mortality relationships among refugees. *Journal of Refugee Studies*, **5**, 247–56.

Robinson, W.C., Ken Lee, M., Hill, K., and Burnham, G.M. (1999). Mortality in North Korean migrant households: a retrospective study. *Lancet*, **354**, 291–5.

Seaman, J., Mercer, A.J., and Sondorp, E. (1996). The epidemic of visceral leishmaniasis in southern Sudan. *Annals of Internal Medicine*, **124**, 664–72.

Shears, P. (1991). Epidemiology and infection in famine and disasters. *Epidemiology and Infection*, **107**, 241–51.

Shears, P., Berry, A.M., Murphy, R., and Nabil, M.A. (1987). Epidemiological assessment of the health and nutrition of Ethiopian refugees in emergency camps in Sudan 1985. *British Medical Journal*, **2295**, 314–18.

Siddique, A.K., Salaam, A., Islam, M.S., *et al.* (1995). Why treatment centres failed to prevent cholera deaths among Rwandan refugees in Goma, Zaire. *Lancet*, **345**, 359–61.

Silove, D. (1999). The psychosocial effects of torture, mass human rights violations, and refugee trauma: toward an integrated conceptual framework. *Journal of Nervous and Mental Disease*, **187**, 200–7.

Suleman, M. (1998). Malaria in Afghan refugees in Pakistan. *Transactions of the Royal Society of Tropical Medicine and Hygiene*, **82**, 44–7.

Thomson, M. (1995). *Disease prevention through vector control: guidelines for relief organisations.* Oxfam, Oxford.

Toole, M.J. (1994). Preventing micronutrient deficiency diseases. Presented at Workshop on the Improvement of the Nutrition of Refugees and Displaced People in Africa, Machakos, Kenya.

Toole, M.J. and Waldman, R.J. (1990). Prevention of excess mortality in refugee and displaced populations in developing countries. *Journal of the American Medical Association*, **263**, 3296–302.

Toole M.J. and Waldman, R.J. (1993). Refugees and displaced persons: war, hunger, and public health. *Journal of the American Medical Association*, **270**, 600–5.

Toole, M.J. and Waldman, R.J. (1997). The public health aspects of complex emergencies and refugee situations. *Annual Review of Public health*, **18**, 283–312.

Toole, M.J., Steketee, R.W., Waldman, R.J., and Nieburg, P. (1989). Measles prevention and control in emergency settings. *Bulletin of the World Health Organization*, **67**, 381–98.

Toole, M.J., Galson, S., and Brady, W. (1993). Are war and public health compatible? *Lancet*, **341**, 1193–431.

UNAIDS (1996). *Guidelines for HIV interventions in emergency settings.* UNAIDS, Geneva.

UNHCR (1999). *Reproductive health in refugee situations: an Inter-agency field manual.* UNHCR, Geneva.

UNHCR/UN (1967). *Protocol relating to the status of refugees.* UNHCR, Geneva.

UNHCR/WFP (1997). *WFP/UNHCR guidelines for estimating food and nutritional needs in emergencies.* UNAIDS, Geneva.

Upadhya, J. (1998). *Persistent micronutrient problems among refugees in Nepal.* Food and Statistical Unit, UNHCR, Geneva.

Vitek, C.R. and Wharton, M. (1998). Diphtheria in the former Soviet Union: re-emergence of a pandemic disease. *Emerging Infectious Diseases*, **4**, 539–50.

WHO (World Health Organization) (1991). *Management of severe and complicated malaria.* WHO, Geneva.

WHO (World Health Organization) (1995). *Control of epidemic meningococcal disease.* Fondation Marcel Merieux, Lyon.

WHO (World Health Organization) (1996). *Rapid health assessment in sudden population displacement.* WHO, Geneva.

WHO (World Health Organization) (1997). *Tuberculosis control in refugee situations: an inter-agency field manual.* WHO, Geneva.

WHO (World Health Organization) (1999). *Guidelines for drug donations* (2nd edn). WHO, Geneva.

Yip, R. and Sharp, T.W. (1993). Acute malnutrition and high childhood mortality related to diarrhoea. Lessons from the 1991 Kurdish refugee crisis. *Journal of the American Medical Association*, **270**, 587–90.

12

Public health functions

12.1 Public health—its critical requirements

Walter W. Holland

Introduction

An effective health service must identify and be responsive to major public health problems, and be effective in promoting strategies to combat them. If no well-attested solution is available, an effective service ensures that appropriate investigation is mounted in order to develop the body of knowledge and define the means of solving public health problems, and thus to identify appropriate methods of protecting the public's health. The intelligence system maintained by the service should provide appropriate mechanisms in order to undertake these public health tasks.

The preceding chapters in this book have attempted to outline the present status of public health in terms of both its functions and roles, and its potential. It is the purpose of this chapter to comment on some of the major current issues in the discipline of public health, and to consider how the discipline may require modification, expansion, and revision in order to be able to cope with the problems of the future.

Problem definition

A diagnostic surveillance system is essential to assess the situation and feed back to those involved in public health (particularly at the grassroots level) that a problem exists and requires solution.

The public health system ideally influences all sectors of society, not just those in immediate contact with the health care system. The preceding chapters of this textbook have identified numerous areas in which, given political will and professional freedom, the public's health can be influenced—for example, housing, the environment, the workplace, recreational facilities, social services support, and alcohol and tobacco policies. The public health service must strive toward this ideal.

Analysis of the problems identified and proposals for their solution

The service must have the ability to initiate action through mobilization of appropriate resources, or the ability to influence those responsible for executive action to undertake corrective or preventive activities. Public health permeates through all the social, environmental, and other activities of populations. It cannot be restricted to the actions of health practitioners. There are environmental and societal, as well as medical, solutions to public health problems. Thus, the activities of farmers in producing food or tobacco, to take two examples, may be as important as the activities of physicians that provide preventive or curative services, depending on the intervention deemed necessary.

Implementation of proposals and monitoring their effectiveness

There is a long-standing misunderstanding that curative medicine is the most important component of the maintenance of the health of the public. Since the middle of the last century, the objectives of the discipline of public health have been considered secondary to those of curative medicine, which is considered to have dramatic and immediate effects on health status. Lay people and politicians, in particular, have been led to believe that the major advances in medicine, and thus in health, are provided through hospital services. Meanwhile, the potential of public health to have long-term influence on health status goes largely unrecognized. Public health, as a discipline, has a responsibility to put pressure on those responsible for implementing health policy to resource adequately the most appropriate public health interventions they have identified. Generally, this will involve a change toward preventive and away from curative (resource-intensive) services. The ambitious primary care programme launched in 1979 by the World Health Organization (**WHO**) toward 'Health for All' is complementary to public health and should be integrated with public health (Mahler 1981).

When the major public health problems in the developed world were due to infectious and nutritional disease, the benefits of public health activity were obvious. In recent times, the need for effective action in public health has perhaps best been demonstrated by the emergence of the HIV infection and AIDS and its public health implications. Despite case-finding and quarantine, that is isolation of the affected, as methods of control, it is generally accepted that prevention has to be directed at effecting behavioural change, particularly among those engaging in high-risk activities.

The difficulties, however, lie in implementation and application. The problems of this infection are indicative of the problems of public health in general. The major emphasis has been placed on the investigation of the virus and the molecular basis of generation of the disease, its treatment, and the development of a vaccine to prevent the disease. Far fewer resources have been, or are being, devoted to the problems of understanding human behaviour, or the modification of human behaviour, and of thus influencing the rate and mode of transmission in Western, African, Asian, and other populations. Thus, once again, emphasis is being placed on the tail-end of the disease process—on treatment—rather than at the beginning, on prevention. Studies of the diffusion, incidence, and prevalence of the disease in various societies are hampered by the ignorance of both the public and governments, which inhibits the activity of those concerned with the implementation of public health (Quinn and Fauci 1998).

Public health, as a discipline, is failing to fulfil its role as outlined at the beginning of this chapter. Public health practitioners do not have the power to implement the policies they have identified. Thus they cannot, without political power, be held responsible for the health of the public. Nor can they, if their advice is ignored, be held to be accountable by politicians for the failure of public health policy.

This chapter sets out to elaborate on the three main issues outlined above, and, in the final part of the chapter, to describe in detail the potential impact of the discipline of public health on health status. Thus, the major issues facing public health in the future are:

- responsibility and accountability—how public health professionals can influence health care provision and become accountable for public health activities
- internal issues specific to the discipline of public health (human resources, training, research, centralization, etc.)
- the responsiveness of the discipline to a changing health environment
- a changing political, organizational, and financial environment.

Thus the major problems which public health needs to address are:

- outbreaks of disease caused by infectious toxic agents, for example, smallpox, typhoid, food poisoning, bovine spongiform encephalitis, radiation, etc.
- problems arising from social and environmental issues such as inadequate housing, unemployment, poverty, abortion, fluoridation of water, or even global environmental changes including climate change
- behavioural concerns such as smoking, excessive consumption of alcohol, drug misuse, and insufficient exercise, which have both individual and societal determinants
- health service issues including assessment of health care needs and outcomes, and the effectiveness and efficiency of particular services.

Issues of responsibility and accountability

Policy-making

Public health practitioners cannot act in isolation. They are always dependent on government, at central or local level, for the freedom to practice their discipline effectively. There is implicitly an underlying failure to recognize the nature of professional responsibilities for the public's health: in consequence, there is a failure to allow the public health professions a sufficient place or the power to determine and execute appropriate health policies. Often, public health knowledge and wisdom is counterintuitive to accepted practice. It is often difficult for the public health practitioner to convince health policy-makers of the most appropriate course of action. After all, Florence Nightingale advocated the miasmatic theory of contagion, whereas the public health practitioners of the day believed in the transmissibility of infection. However, Nightingale and her followers were influential in their views on hospital design, and, as a result, the advice of public health practitioners was neglected. More recently, many politicians believed that cervical cancer screening should be introduced for all women aged 16 to 64 years, thus (given limited resources) neglecting the fact that the major 'at-risk' group were those aged over 35 years, and that overdilution of effort would reduce the overall benefits of this service.

Often, financial or bureaucratic responsibilities are given too high a priority, and the public health suffers. Public health professionals are rarely given the necessary responsibility for the public's health—perhaps because their priorities would not necessarily reflect the priorities of government, and health services would no longer necessarily reflect government policy.

Determination of priorities

Thus, as a result of political interest, often perceived by professionals as interference, the public health practitioner is not free to determine his or her own priorities. In terms of the role of public health given at the beginning of this chapter, practitioners are not permitted to identify the problems freely, nor to devise and implement appropriate solutions. The media, and subsequently, public opinion, may affect the decision-making process, and newsworthy, but from a public health perspective trivial, problems may be given unwarranted attention. For example, recently, much attention focused on measures to reduce lead pollution from motor vehicle emissions in the United Kingdom, but none on the more serious impact of lead contamination of the water supply from lead pipes.

Health service organization

Public health medicine plays a vital role in the management and organization of health services. However, decisions about reorganizations are often beyond the realm of practitioners who, despite their specialized knowledge of health care provision, may later have to enforce inequitable methods of organization. Thus public health professionals are given responsibility for implementing operational decisions without being party to strategic planning. This lack of clearly allocated responsibilities and accountabilities is the paramount problem facing the public health services.

Public health practitioners are needed as part of an independent authority, not beholden to any specific interest group, but with an input into both strategic and operational decision-making in all forms of policy with an impact on health. Only if the public health practitioner is able and willing to provide uncomfortable, unwanted advice (even if later rejected) is it likely that the public health function can retain its integrity and can be adequately performed.

These conditions are now met, at least in theory, in the United Kingdom, by the division into purchaser–provider organizations, with the public health discipline represented in the purchaser domain.

The director of public health is an executive director, and thus a full responsible member of the body responsible for the health of a defined population. That authority is in the position to purchase services that promote health, including health services. Attempts are being made to develop methods to decide on the relative resources to be used for preventive, curative, and rehabilitative services for individual disease groups, for example coronary heart disease (O'Brien *et al.* 1997). The director of public health is also responsible for publishing an annual report on the health problems of the population for which he or she has responsibility, identifying both problems and solutions and, over time, recording what progress has been made. Although this report is intended to be independent, there are fears that it may be subject to some degree of censoring. However, the changes in structure, detailed in earlier chapters, enable an authority to take a much broader view and enables expenditure to be directed to, for example, road or housing improvements, rather than only accident and emergency facilities, to reduce the problem of accidents. A start in this direction is being made in some places (Holland 1995).

The public health professional must have an advisory as well as an executive capacity, and must be accountable for the advice he or she gives. The advice of a public health professional may conflict with that of a clinical medical practitioner, since priorities for the health of one individual may differ from priorities for populations. Co-ordination is thus necessary, and reconciliation of differing priorities is needed. The professional structure should allow the combination of executive and advisory functions, plus the necessary reconciliation with other professionals.

As long as public health remains totally enveloped within the current bureaucratic and administrative structure, the conflicts and difficulties are likely to be too great for it to be able to enforce appropriate methods of action and implementation of findings. However, there is danger that, were it removed from this structure, it would become even more remote. In many countries, such as the United Kingdom, public health is divided between two separate authorities: medical public health practitioners are enveloped within the medical hierarchy; non-medical public health practitioners are part of the local government. The conflict within each of these hierarchies, as well as the conflict between them, militates against an appropriate and effective public health function. In the United Kingdom attempts at developing a unified body are currently being made. In the past, public health has been separate from clinical medicine; but even then it aspired to have clinical functions in relation to individuals. Even at the start of public health activity, the subservience of public to bureaucratic domination existed. Thus, it is difficult to develop an entirely independent public health activity capable of influencing authorities at all levels. Only where public health was set to tackle major individual problems, as for example with tuberculosis, smallpox, and diphtheria, has it been able to act effectively. An example is the American Public Health Service (**USPHS**), which was accountable for overall achievements rather than specific activities.

Methodology

To fulfil the role identified at the beginning of this chapter, public health practitioners must develop an agreed methodology, based on evidence, for tackling public health problems. Methods of investigation and the risks of specific hazards have been set out in previous chapters in this book. Unless public health develops a more thorough, competent, professional methodology it is bound to have relatively small impact on the improvement of public health. The difficulties that practitioners face are numerous, and the development of professional expertise is the only hope so that they can fulfil their expected role and contribute constructively to the improvement of health policies.

No universal model of the detailed responsibilities of public health practitioners exists. Generally, public health practitioners are responsible for the maintenance of the health of populations and the evaluation and assessment of the needs for service of different population groups. This can take many forms. In some countries, for example the United States, The Netherlands, and France, the public health function is also concerned with the delivery of health services to individual population groups, for example indigent children. However, its major tasks should be:

- to assess the health status of the population
- from this, to evaluate the health care needs
- to determine the most appropriate way to satisfy the health care needs of individual population groups and to assess the effectiveness with which those needs are met
- the identification of specific health hazards, and their containment.

Thus the development of strategies for the promotion of health, the containment of ill health, and the deployment of human resources in order that the health hazards in the environment are appropriately investigated and contained are essential responsibilities of the public health service, as is the determination of priorities for health services. This discussion has illustrated some of the reasons why these functions are not presently achieved.

Dissemination of information

Dissemination of information and research findings is an essential function of the public health discipline, if progress is to be made using resources optimally. A number of means of dissemination are available to the public health practitioner, through the media or through the more traditional routes of journals, conferences, and seminars. In terms of the dissemination of information to the general public, there are often difficulties in the relationship between the media and practitioners because the media, despite their potential as a powerful tool in public health information and health-promotion campaigns, often neglect major public health issues.

The difficulties and deficiencies of providing information, both in the assessment of whether health services are performing adequately, determining how priorities can be determined, and how individuals and populations can improve their own health has been reviewed by Holland (1995).

Outbreaks of infectious disease, particularly of rare conditions such as *Legionella* infection or toxocariasis, are more dramatic than the containment of common diseases causing many more cases, for example influenza or acute respiratory infection. The concern that has been evoked through the AIDS epidemic is an example of the power of dissemination of information through the media. The lack of concern with, for example, road accidents or coronary heart disease mortality is an example of how the media may neglect non-sensational, although important, public health problems, but may report sensational stories which make 'good copy', although these may be less important from a public health perspective.

A major obstacle to dissemination is that the agendas of those responsible for public health may vary. The public health professional cannot always rely on governmental support for public health policy, since there are often vested interests at stake. For example, a restriction on smoking may affect employment, the economy, taxation revenue, and the cost of pensions provision—the priorities of a government will determine whether these are politically unacceptable prices to pay. There may also be conflict between clinical practitioners and public health practitioners since their priorities may differ—the former often placing an emphasis on curative activity, the latter on preventive.

Thus to fulfil their role effectively, public health practitioners have to perform certain functions.

- They have to be forthright in the advocacy of programmes that improve health and state clearly and openly the dangers and consequences of some actions, clinical, environmental, or political.
- They have to be able to influence the budget for public health activities and ensure that long-term public health issues are considered on a separate dimension from short-term clinical and practical issues which would otherwise always take precedence.
- They have to assume a clearly identifiable role in helping to influence and guide the policies, not only of health authorities but also of schools, environmental agencies, welfare agencies, housing departments, microbiological laboratories, and practising clinicians in hospital and general practice.

Internal specialty issues

Research

With the burden of death and disability from non-communicable disease increasing, research into the prevention of these conditions is receiving increased emphasis.

In many countries there is no coherent strategy for the maintenance of a stable research base. In the United Kingdom, for example, the National Health Service devotes far too small a part of its budget to seeking how to improve its own operations, and the pharmaceutical industry finances by far the largest part of funding for medical research. Inevitably, research priorities will be largely determined by the pharmaceutical market-place (House of Lords 1988; Secretaries of State for Health 1989*b*).

A second major problem stemming from this situation is the lack of human resources because of the absence of a stable career structure for those in research. Research standards can only be maintained by the development of a strong infrastructure for research in well-funded establishments, and through maintaining the supply of a well-trained and strongly motivated research community.

Public health research, by its very nature, can propose an alternative to traditional research priorities (for example, by concentrating on conditions such as influenza, which affect the population widely, as compared with more 'interesting' problems, such as rare metabolic disorders which, although serious, affect only small numbers of individuals). Thus it is in some ways in conflict with research supporting clinical activities. Since such research is allied to operational research, which is concerned with evaluating the effectiveness of new or existing treatments or technology, it may often arouse resentment among the medical professions, which may have a vested interest in those treatments or techniques. Public health research more often promotes prevention against cure.

For the development of appropriate public health research, a research strategy must be developed. This must include the gathering of intelligence on a broad front to determine main national priorities. These can be chosen by reference to alternative methodologies such as cost–benefit and cost-effectiveness analyses in the light of overall goals. Political and social values clearly enter into the determination of benefits and costs; but analytical tools must be used for more systematic and rational decisions to be made. Science is an aid to the art of policy-making, not an alternative.

An appropriate research structure is necessary in order that the tasks can be appropriately tackled. This implies a proper human resource development structure, with the involvement of educational institutions and government, and provision of adequate resources for such research.

Funding for health research is generally inadequate, and good research proposals are not always supported. Career prospects in research are often dismal, and the demands of patient care inhibit research activity. There is a lack of awareness of the importance of research and of the time and resources required to promote it. Findings of research are not always properly disseminated, and therefore duplication of research efforts cannot always be avoided.

Training and human resources

In order for public health to be generally accepted and developed as a valid influence on health status, appropriate training facilities are of vital importance. This implies specific skills in the application of public health, as well as an appreciation of the requirements for the subject. In the United Kingdom, the Faculty of Public Health Medicine has stressed the importance of a multidisciplinary approach to training in public health (Peach and Lakhani 1985; Faculty of Public Health Medicine 1992).

For an adequate education of medical graduates in public health, the subject must be given appropriate prominence in all parts of the undergraduate curriculum. Public health is a bridging subject which can integrate the various aspects of medical education. It is essential that future medical graduates have the ability to see common community problems, and they are able to appreciate the methods used by public health practitioners in the determination and evaluation of health care needs in order that they may see the relevance of individual components of the medical curriculum from a better perspective. They require a grounding in numerical and statistical concepts, as well as in social science theory and methods so they can understand both the need for and the applications of a variety of different techniques to the promotion of health. They should also have an understanding of the ways in which society changes in relation to the environment and other factors that are important in the determination of health and disease. Through a more realistic exposure to public health as a discipline, they should also be better able to understand the relative importance and place of diagnostic and therapeutic techniques in medicine, and the importance of preventing ill health rather than being concerned purely with its treatment.

Nurses, too, are a vital part of the public health team, and collaborate with the other professions in the provision of a service. Training in public health nursing covers basic nursing sciences and public health science. Nursing education has progressed in recent years, and nurses are increasingly achieving higher professional status. However, the nursing profession is still largely fighting for recognition of its potential for diagnoses and treatment, in addition to its traditional caring role, particularly in developed countries, where many aspects of health care have become highly medicalized.

For the non-medical graduate, public health as a discipline is particularly important to those students who are likely to become involved in environmental health, medical statistics, and the management of health and social services. Students of education and future teachers should also have some appreciation of the various ways in which their discipline can promote health and can contribute to improvement in health status.

It is vital that Schools of Public Health are multidisciplinary, since the nature of the public's health is determined by numerous factors which require input from a variety of disciplines. Only by the interaction of these is it possible that any improvement will occur in the future in the practice of public health (Omenn 1994).

There may also be a role for linking modern medical training to traditional practices in some developing countries. In this way modern and traditional methods can form a partnership, and thus increase the acceptability of newer practices.

Rapid changes in the public health sector warrant continuing training opportunities to confront the changing disease problems. Training opportunities are poor for non-medical staff in the public health sector in developed countries, and there may be skills shortages because of poor working conditions, poor pay, and poor professional status. These problems must be remedied to ensure the adequate skilled human resources to provide an adequate service.

In those countries that have a clear organizational structure in the health service and in local government, like the United Kingdom, it is important that the public health function is exercised by an appropriately trained workforce at each level, that is, at the centre (the government department or ministry of health), and in each district (the district health authority). An individual is unlikely to be effective alone, and there should be a team of individuals, having competence in the appropriate medical and non-medical disciplines, such as statistics, social science, and environmental science, in order for the public health professionals at all levels to fulfil their appropriate responsibilities.

In a less unified system, such as that existing in the United States, the public health service should be organized at each level or geographical area of government, for example at state and at county level. Although the public health service may not be involved in the provision of clinical services, it should be concerned with environmental control and the assessment of health care needs, so that it can advise national or local government on the provision of adequate services.

The workforce structure should be appropriately organized so that there are adequate training posts for both service and academics, in order that an appropriate cadre of well-trained individuals is available, both at present and in the future (IOM 1988).

The changing health environment

The population

The proportion of elderly people in the population is increasing, particularly those aged over 75 years. The elderly make greater and different demands on health services than the young. Demographic changes present new public health problems. In terms of the care of the elderly, the increasing dependence in society that accompanies care of the elderly, geographical variations in employment, skills shortages, unemployment, and poverty are all important determinants of health according to the WHO's Health for All indicators (WHO 1978).

Changes in medical and surgical techniques

The range of treatments available has increased significantly since the 1950s. Now there are effective drugs, such as antibiotics, which have revolutionized the treatment of infectious disease, and effective treatments are available for serious conditions, such as cardiac bypass operations for the treatment of coronary heart disease. However, many new treatments have not been properly evaluated. These treatments have increased patient expectations of the length and quality of life. Patients have become better informed, and expect a higher standard of care, which is often equated in the mind of the patient with highly medicalized care. Consequently, the public health practitioner finds himself evaluating technology which is already widely implemented. Difficulties exist in attempting to withdraw ineffectual technology once it has become accepted by physicians and patients.

Changes in social expectations and standards

There are still very major differences in access to health services within and between countries. There are sixfold or greater differences in case-fatality rates for conditions such as hernias, acute appendicitis, tuberculosis, and hip fractures in different parts of the United Kingdom alone (Holland 1997). This factor, together with changing demography, results in the emergence of a number of new public health problems (such as equity in health care provision, or the determination of national health priorities) which now have to be tackled.

The changing political environment

It is generally agreed that some level of public intervention is necessary to protect the health of the population. The chief factor which varies between countries of different political ideologies is the extent of this public intervention, often argued in terms of the extent of government intervention in public health.

Service organization and planning

There must be a public health presence at the centre in a planning role, as well as at the periphery. Public health practitioners are required at all levels of a health system, both in strategic planning and in an operational capacity to implement policies. All health systems are concerned with the promotion and maintenance of health, but many interpret this as a disease-treatment service, implying the provision of services only for the chronic sick. But the treatment of public health as a disease service implies its failure in its principal role—that of prevention and health promotion.

However, one of the main problems is the squeeze on the resources devoted to public health services. This has been clearly demonstrated in the United Kingdom, where in 1989 the government produced a White Paper which suggested major reorganization of the health service (Secretaries of State 1989*a*). The proposals outlined in this document affect all the essential aspects of a 'good' service which have already been described—the levels of responsibility of professionals, accountability, the ability of the service to respond to changing needs, degrees of political influence, and many issues internal to the specialty of public health. Resources available to promote public health must be allocated between all the disciplines necessary for the operation of the public health system. That is, in order for an appropriate public health function to be performed, support is required in terms of numerical, biological, bacteriological, and chemical services, which can be provided from appropriately staffed and equipped establishments. This has implications in terms of organization, for example of the provision of microbiological laboratories to investigate outbreaks of disease. The facilities required are different from those needed in a clinical laboratory dealing only with specimens from individual patients.

The future of public health

Public health is neither adequately funded nor suitably organized to confront the health problems facing the developed world in the twenty-first century. The public health system was designed to combat infectious disease and problems of undernutrition, hygiene, etc. The problems facing the developed world are now very different. We are faced with problems of plenty: inappropriate nutrition leading to heart disease; alcohol- and smoking-related illness reaching almost epidemic proportions; and a range of new occupational illnesses to replace the old. The problems are challenging in terms of preventive, therapeutic, and rehabilitative care.

Effective public health activities are essential to the general well being of the population, to ensure that the conditions in which people live and work are healthy. Public health activities can be undertaken by individuals, agencies, or governments; but governments, regardless of their political ideology, have a central role in ensuring that services are adequate (either by monitoring private services or by funding public services), and in collecting, analysing, and producing data. They have a responsibility to review regularly the status of the public health, to delineate clearly public health responsibilities, to ensure a unified service, and to bring public health services into line with the changing pattern of disease in the population. However, beyond this, it is the responsibility of the professionals to assist in the assessment of priorities and approaches to public health and solutions to its problems. Professionals must ensure that governments are aware of changing global disease patterns, and changing environmental problems.

It is often difficult to understand the resistance to public health and its practice. Part of this problem is that the activities of public health are difficult to comprehend in some instances, or in others appear so obvious that they are considered an extension of common sense. However, it must be recognized that public health permeates all human activity. The recent developments towards more appropriate nutrition and housing, and greater consciousness of environmental issues, have largely emerged as a response of communities to new environmental hazards and as a result of increased awareness of methods for preventing harm to individuals and communities.

It is easier to understand the functions of public health in areas of deprivation: the identification of major problems, the identification of methods for solving those problems, and then implementing those solutions. For example, where an outbreak of diphtheria occurs, it is essential to identify the source, to identify the means of containment, and then to set up the means of prevention. This is essentially what guided the activities of the WHO in eliminating smallpox. In developed countries this activity is more difficult to define. The sources of illness are more complex and multifactorial. Thus, public health has identified smoking as one of the major hazards for disease in the developed world. To implement appropriate antismoking activities involves all sectors of society, from those growing tobacco plants, to those selling the product, to those reaping the benefits from the sale of the product.

The role of public health in planning activities has often been confused. Public health practitioners perform a crucial role in this field in identifying major causes of illness and disease, and then devising appropriate methods of treatment or care, and thus identifying priorities.

The problem arises that many of their proposed solutions are difficult to implement, and often attack the current citadels of power. The results do not occur immediately, and are not as dramatic as those of curative medicine. It is only if the public health practitioner can deploy the resources of those in other sectors of society that truly effective activities can be developed. It is, however, important to appreciate that the risk of dying is but one concern of the practitioner. Thus, public health ought not only be concerned with the prevention of death, but must also be more concerned with the prevention of early death, and with the preservation of the quality of life of those who survive.

Thus public health is about the promotion of the health of the whole community. It is concerned with the prevention of disease, the prolongation of life, and the promotion of the quality of life of human populations, and aims to reduce the burden of ill health and disability.

This book has clearly shown the importance of various social, environmental, and industrial factors in the development of disease as well as in the promotion of health. That public health should straddle all of these aspects is essential, and its continued ability to influence all of them is the only way in which appropriate worldwide health policies can be maintained and developed.

Further reading

Beaglehole, R. and Bonita, R. (1997). *Public health at the crossroads.* Cambridge University Press.

Ciba Foundation (1973). *Medical research systems in Europe.* Wellcome Trust–Ciba Foundation Joint Symposium. Ciba Foundation Symposium 21. Associated Scientific Publishers, Amsterdam.

Council for Science and Society (1982). *Expensive medical techniques.* Council for Science and Society, London.

Holland, W.W. and Stewart, S. (1998) *Public health: the vision and the challenge.* Nuffield Trust, London.

Flook, E.E. and Sanazaro, P.J. (ed.) (1973). *Health services research and R & D in perspective.* Health Administration Press, Ann Arbor, MI.

IOM (Institute of Medicine) (1988). *The future of public health.* National Academy Press, Washington, DC.

Knox, E.G. (ed.) (1987). *Health-care information.* Report of a Joint Working Group of the Körner Committee on Health Services Information and the Faculty of Community Medicine. Nuffield Provincial Hospitals Trust Occasional Papers 8, Nuffield Provincial Hospitals Trust, London.

McGinnis, J.M. and Foege, W.H. (1993). Actual causes of death in the United States. *Journal of the American Medical Association*, **270**, 2207–12.

McLachlan, G. (ed.) (1971). *Portfolio for health. The role and programme of the DHSS in Health service research.* Nuffield Provincial Hospitals Trust/Oxford University Press.

McLachlan, G. (ed.) (1973). *Portfolio for health 2.* Nuffield Provincial Hospitals Trust/Oxford University Press.

McLachlan, G. (ed.) (1974). *Positions, movements and directions in health services research.* Nuffield Provincial Hospitals Trust/Oxford University Press.

McLachlan, G. (ed.) (1978). *Five years after. A review of health care research management after Rothschild.* Nuffield Provincial Hospitals Trust/Oxford University Press.

McLachlan, G. (ed.) (1985). *Data information and intelligence. A statement of needs and opportunities of relevance to the new NHS management procedures.* Report of a Nuffield Provincial Hospitals Trust Working Party. Nuffield Provincial Hospitals Trust Occasional Papers 4. Nuffield Provincial Hospital Trust, London.

Sheps, C.G. (Chairman) (1976). *Higher education for public health.* Prodist, New York.

US Department of Health and Human Services, Public Health Service (DHHS) (1994). *For a healthy nation. Returns on investment in public health.* Department of Health and Human Services, Washington, DC.

References

Faculty of Public Health Medicine of the Royal Colleges of Physicians of the United Kingdom (1992). *Handbook on training and the examination for membership.* Faculty of Public Health Medicine, London.

Holland, W.W. (1995). Achieving an ethical health service. What information do we need. *Journal of the Royal College of Physicians of London*, **29**, 325–34.

Holland, W.W. (ed.) (1997). *The European Community atlas of 'avoidable death'.* Commission of the European Communities Health Services Research Series No. 9, Oxford University Press.

House of Lords Select Committee on Science and Technology (1988). *Priorities in medical research.* Vol. 1: *Report.* HMSO, London.

IOM (Institute of Medicine) (1988). *The future of public health.* National Academy Press, Washington, DC.

Mahler, H. (1981). The meaning of 'health for all by year 2000'. *World Health Forum*, **2**, 5.

O'Brien, M., Halpin, J., Hicks, N., Pearson, S., Warren, V., and Holland, W.W. (1997), Health Care Commissioning Development Project. *Journal of Epidemiology*, **6** (Supplement), 589–92.

Omenn, G.S. (1994). *The context for a future school of public health committed to urban health needs.* Sun Valley Forum.

Peach, H. and Lakhani, A. (1985). Organization, training and staffing aspects of public health services in the United Kingdom. In *Oxford textbook of public health.* Vol. 2, *Processes for public health promotion* (ed. W.W. Holland, R. Detels, and E.G. Knox), p. 150. Oxford University Press.

Quinn, T.C. and Fauci, A.S. (1998). The AIDS epidemic and demographic aspects, population biology and virus evolution in emerging infections. In *Emerging infections* (ed. R.M. Krause), pp. 327–63. Academic Press, San Diego, CA.

Secretaries of State for Health, Scotland, Wales, and Northern Ireland (1989*a*). *White Paper. Working for patients'.* Cm. 555, HMSO, London,

Secretaries of State for Health, Education and Science, Scotland, Wales and Northern Ireland (1989*b*). *Priorities in medical research.* Cm. 902, HMSO, London.

Secretaries of State for Health, Social Security, Treasury, Home Office, Education and Employment, Trade and Industry, Agriculture, Fisheries and Food, Environment, Transport and the Regions, International Development (1999). *White Paper. Saving lives: our healthier nation.* Cm. 4386, HMSO, London.

WHO (World Health Organization) (1978). *Primary health care.* Report of the International Conference on Primary Health Care, Alma Ata, 6–12 September. WHO, Geneva.

12.2 Measuring health needs*

Gavin Mooney, Stephen Jan, and Virginia Wiseman

There is a beguiling simplicity about the proposition that health care services should be designed to meet the needs of the community. Faced with the obvious appetite for health care exhibited by virtually all communities exposed to it, it is traditional to distinguish between wants and needs: wants, by implication, being less rational, possibly even related to greed. Needs, by contrast, are seen as objective states, things that can be measured and agreed upon by rational people often on behalf of those who have them, as deserving attention.

The purpose of this chapter is first to explore the concept of need from several perspectives relevant to its interpretation within a public health framework. The purposes for which need might be measured—for action in the clinical and population settings and for planning—are then reviewed. Some currently available measures of need are then examined and some conclusions are drawn.

The concept of need within the context of public health

It is clear that need can be viewed in many different ways. A community experiencing high levels of infant mortality due to tetanus might be seen by a preventivist as one in need of the development of an effective maternal education programme focusing on hygiene at the time of the cutting of the umbilical cord and maternal immunization. Conversely, an intensive care physician may see the same phenomena and compute them in terms of needs for neonatal intensive care beds to effect rescue of the young victims. The individuals involved—the parents of the children affected—may have a third interpretation of what they need, which may have little to do with child survival.

These constructs of need—which is what they are, melding essentially the same 'facts' into different shapes—each have their legitimacy. Unless health is to be seen as something occupying a quiet biological space, independent of culture and society, then these different constructs need to be accepted. Each derives from the fact that any relevant concept of need is value laden. Definitions of need vary depending on whose perception, interpretation, and values are in play. There is also the question of whose values ought to come into play and in which circumstances. It is most unlikely that some universally valid construct of need can be adopted that will be apposite in all circumstances.

This becomes still more obvious when it is recognized that need cannot exist without addressing the question of 'need for what?' Need is thus best seen as being both value laden and requiring specification of the instrumentation for needs to be addressed or met. Health needs can be addressed and met through treatment services, rehabilitation services, caring services, prevention at an individual level, community health promotion activities, environmental protection, and in many other ways. Health needs are thus most commonly set in the context of a need for care, but in the wider context of public health, need may be more inclusive.

There is immediately a problem, seemingly at both an analytical level and a policy level, with respect to instrumentality (i.e. the instrument by which the need will be met). It is much easier—and relevant literature supports this view—to measure need when the instrument is health care than when the need is satisfied by an instrument using mechanisms not normally encountered within health services. It is with respect to non-health service, public health needs, that analysts and policy-makers seem to hit major problems of conceptualization (although given what has been said above this ought not to be the case) in particular with regard to assessment and quantification.

A fundamental point needs to be made at this juncture. Need is most frequently seen as being formed or perceived in the eyes of another, a third party. Thus, Liss (1990) wrote 'A need for health care exists when an assessor believes that health care ought to be provided'.

This statement neatly combines two important aspects of need. Firstly, it incorporates the notion of the instrumentality of need. The need is for health care but it is not health care that is the 'final goal or objective'. It is not, from the patient's point of view, health care *per se* that is wanted. The patient wants health and uses the 'instrument' of health care to try to obtain it. Secondly, Liss's statement embraced the notion of a third party doing the assessing. With this conceptualization of need it is not the patient who is doing the assessing but someone else, an agent (often a medical doctor), on behalf of the patient. (While it would be possible to deduce from the quote from Liss (1990) that need might be self-assessed, it is clear elsewhere in his and in much other literature in this area that is not what he intends.)

Such third-party assessment requires, for the assessment to have legitimacy, that wider concerns are at play. If a doctor, for example, assesses a patient's needs, this is only of interest if that assessment leads to rights for the patient or clarification or quantification of rights which then provide the patient with access to services which might be of assistance in addressing the problems indentified by the doctor. It is not the assessment by the doctor that provides the needs with their rights base, with their element of 'social legitimacy'. That can only come from the concept of a social contract. When it is claimed that

* We are grateful to Steve Leeder for allowing us to use materials included in the previous version of this chapter which he co-authored with GM.

individuals have a right to certain basic necessities, that is the language of a social contract. As Loewy (1990) stated 'Social contract consists of those things which"go without saying" and which we consider to be the legitimate expectations we have of others and of our community'.

Tension arises with respect to what sort of community it is in which we are trying to assess needs. As Loewy (1990) reminded us, according to the Aristotelian dictum, 'justice consists of giving everyone their due'. He continues, however:

> What is and what is not someone's due...is another matter. Minimalist communities which...accept freedom as an absolute condition of the moral life will see what is due quite differently than will more generously based communities. What is due in minimalist communities is doing each other no harm; what is due in broader based communities is a far more difficult matter and one which will ultimately be determined by an ongoing dialectic between communal values and individual interests.

It immediately follows that the separation of wants and needs, which for some seems so simple, in practice is far from simple. There is an astonishing lack of research into individuals or communities as to what they actually want from their health care services and so the pejorative view of wants as little more than expressions of greed by the ignorant is particularly unfortunate. Paternalistic professionalism has blocked progress in understanding how the community views health and health care and where they place them in the context of other things that they also want for their lives.

Distinctions between needs and wants are made still more difficult by the fact that different disciplines also use different definitions. A potentially useful set of constructs is provided by the discipline of economics. Wants are the preferences of individuals on behalf of themselves but do not have to be expressed through taking action to have the wants 'fulfilled'. 'Demands' are based on wants, that is on an individual's own preferences, by some action on the part of the individual in seeking to have the wants addressed. Thus, a want for better health can be expressed as a demand for health care if the individual visits a general practitioner. A need for health care would arise if the general practitioner were to agree that some relevant action could be taken by the health care services on behalf of the patient. It is clear that need could exist without want or demand, demand could exist without need but not without want, and want could exist without demand or need.

This distinction between need on the one side and wants and demands on the other emphasizes still further the value-laden nature of these phenomena. Such emphasis is merited. While wants and demands are normally readily recognized as being value laden, this is less commonly the case with the conceptualization of need.

Need is also likely to be dynamic over time. The need for care today, for example, is very different from the need for care 20 years ago. Partly, it is that the incidence and prevalence of diseases have changed. Also, expectations and values of both the population and the health professional have changed. Technological change and changing availability of services have also altered the extent and pattern of needs. Similarly, needs are likely to vary in moving from one culture or one society to another.

Policy and research in public health have not often adopted a multidisciplinary approach to the understanding of either wants or needs for health care. A great deal of ignorance thus lies undisturbed and the strengths and limits of the various public health sciences and discourses are thrown into relief when each comes to examine the nature of need. Epidemiology, with its reductionist roots, can provide a count of cases, deaths, and denominators, and can also provide insights into some of the causal pathways that manifest as these health states that we declare as needs. The social sciences can provide an interpretation of needs in terms of how society views departures from health—ranging from their perception as religious events through to secular phenomena that require government intervention that reinforces social values such as equity and efficiency. As indicated above, health economists can contribute to the understanding of health needs by setting them within the context of what demands individuals and society place upon the resources available to them, in terms of their individual and corporate happiness and satisfaction. For example, where do health needs fit in the total spectrum of needs, alongside the basic ones in the lower orders of the Maslow hierarchy (food, shelter, etc.) and in relation to the more sophisticated ones for education, justice, and freedom of speech?

Any simple interpretation of need must therefore be suspect. The reductionist quality of measures of need should be understood if we are to avoid making useless extrapolations from them. Nevertheless, reductionist measures of need share with much reductionist science a remarkable capacity to get the job done, things improved, wars won, and health status elevated. The major issue confronting those involved in public health, therefore, is not so much to search endlessly for an all-embracing definition of need, but to be willing to live with pared-down versions of need that may be useful within a particular context, whilst recognizing their limitations. The debate about measuring need therefore shares much with the debate about measuring the quality of life.

What is not to be applauded, however, are those interpretations of need which are driven by data availability rather than the purpose for which the need measure is required. There are too many examples in the literature of needs estimation based on inappropriate grasping at available numbers without due consideration as to whether in ordinal or cardinal terms the interpretation of the numbers does reflect the construct of need which is claimed implicitly or explicitly.

The purpose of measuring need

If we accept that the generic notion of need is complex and elusive we can proceed to identify different settings in which different measures of need, each with their limitations, may prove useful.

Need in the clinical setting

Within clinical practice, the measurement of need is an integral part of the daily routine. It is a necessary and accepted part of such practice.

The relevance of need and its usefulness in clinical decision-making are obvious and seemingly unchallenged and unchallengeable. Yet a challenge does arise from the extent to which there are substantial variations in such clinical practice for similar or even identical health conditions. At this level, seemingly similar problems—identified perhaps with respect to reduced health status—are interpreted quite differently by different clinicians in terms of what is needed to deal with them. Manifestations of such apparent variations in interpretation can be a function not only of diversity in respect of need but also of availability of resources to treat particular problems.

However, variations in the rates of performance of various surgical procedures exist to a very great extent even after allowing for or controlling for variations in the supply of resources and the qualities of the populations being served. There is little doubt that this is a function of differences in perception and/or interpretation of needs at a clinical level across different clinicians.

In the face of a value-laden concept of need, the 'medical model'—if A, then B—can appear somewhat mechanistic. Neither A (the diagnosis) nor B (the choice of therapy) are devoid of value judgements on the part of the clinician. Yet recently it was possible to read into the concept of need in clinical medicine something that appeared concrete, objective, and largely value free.

At the very heart of clinical medicine lies an increasing recognition of the extent to which medicine is about values, including the assessment and interpretation of needs.

At a clinical level there will be variations in interpretations of need across similar conditions but in different cultures. The fact that this occurs within cultures, and further, can very clearly be influenced by the nature and structure of incentive systems (and not just financial incentives), emphasizes still more the subjective nature of need. It is not possible to interpret the results of various studies on changes in remuneration systems in any other way. Need at a clinical level is a function, among other things, of how doctors are paid.

To point this out is not to criticize or to express regret about such a phenomenon. More importantly it is to recognize that there is potentially a useful tool for influencing clinical practice, in terms of not only the effectiveness of that practice but also its efficiency and its contribution to concerns for equity. Given the central place of need in clinical decision-making, the fact that need can be perceived differently within different remuneration systems (Krasnik *et al.* 1990) has to be an important consideration for policy-makers. Yet the potential for using the remuneration system for policy purposes has been underexploited to date.

Need at the level of the population

Although need may be considered in absolute terms, it is principally in relative terms that it finds its place in contemporary health service development and appraisal. Thus 'standardized mortality ratios', that is mortality rates standardized to some common population, are compared from one region or country to another and implications are drawn about need. A community that has a 10 per cent higher mortality rate from ischaemic heart disease than the national average is seen, in particular by the popular press, as being 'in need'—of more coronary care beds, or more preventive programmes, or more ambulances fitted with defibrillators, etc.

Need is defined in these settings as some correlate of mortality, in no small part because mortality statistics despite all their weaknesses are, like democracy, pretty good compared with anything else.

Where there is a problem at this level is with respect to answering the instrumentalist question: 'need for what?' Other things being equal, a higher level of mortality implies a higher level of need in some general rather unspecific sense—but greater need for what? It might be for health services but perhaps also for many other goods, services, or activities. We believe that in the continuing tension between, on the one hand, treatment services for meeting health needs and, on the other hand, public health services, one of the reasons why the latter may 'lose out' in resource allocation is the failure to specify needs adequately in terms of instrumentation. Instruments or interventions in treatment services tend to be of a much more specific and identifiable nature than is the case with public health measures. The former are also drawn from a defined set of health care services whereas public health interventions can be present in very many areas of the economy—transport, housing, the environment, food policy, etc.

Doctors working in the acute hospital sector always have seductively simple and clear instruments at hand. In the battle for meeting needs at that level as opposed to the public health level they have the imperative of current sickness to provide still more weight to their claims over a still greater share of society's scarce resources. The latter is difficult to push aside and there are arguments that in the context of rescue, there is no reason to push them aside. It is important, however, to decide the extent of influence since it cannot be the case that treating current sickness can be seen as an absolute or at least ought not to be.

Need from a planning perspective

There are two places where need impacts upon planning. The first is in relation to what economists refer to as 'allocative efficiency'. This involves first an acceptance that resources are scarce, and second that the over-riding goal is to maximize benefits with the available resources. In terms of needs this presumably translates as maximizing the needs met or the value of the needs met with the resources available.

The second place where need and planning converge is in the pursuit of equity. In relation to equity, issues of distribution are often set in terms of 'equal use for equal need' or 'equal access for equal need'.

For allocative efficiency the health service planner approaches need as but one ingredient in a complex equation which he or she is expected to solve. In this context, the planner may identify 'need' as being those margins of existing programmes for which additional resources might achieve more than similar sized investments in other programmes. A further implication of this is that there may be situations for which resources might be withdrawn and devoted elsewhere with greater well being than is currently derived from the system.

The following statement might be made: the returns to health of monies spent here, on this programme, in this location, on this group of patients, on this effort on prevention, are not high enough—the money would be better spent over there on that other programme, on that other group of patients over there. If it is possible to take $100 000 from the treatment of cancer patients and do still more good in treating the elderly for, perhaps, chronic arthritis, then it should be done. If the reverse is true then the direction of the resource shift should be reversed.

It is not enough to be able to say that resources which are scarce are being well spent; the issue is rather, could they be better spent? Are there more needs or more highly valued needs that resources could be used to address?

The idea of shifting resources to where they can meet the greatest need (or more correctly where they will do most good)—what economists call marginal analysis—is not difficult to grasp. If more good can be done than is being done, if more needs can be met with the same resources, then the argument is that that is what should be done.

It is here that the need for measurement of need becomes paramount as judgements have to be made about where resources will meet the greatest need. If, with the same amount of resources, pain, suffering, and death can be reduced still more, then let us do so. That is the simple notion of economic efficiency.

The concept of need incorporated into this planning framework is that of capacity to benefit (Culyer 1991). Here it is argued that if individuals have a capacity to benefit from a particular service then they have a 'need' for that service. This is a somewhat different type of need as compared with that which is used frequently at the population level and is interpreted in terms simply of the extent of illness and death in a population (as described above). Even if a health problem exists, if there is no capacity to benefit, under this definition there is no need.

This planning framework stands to benefit if we can obtain a picture of how resources are currently being spent and linked in an appropriate way to what the objectives and priorities are. This picture is what is known as a set of 'programme budgets'.

Most commonly in health care, expenditure data are available categorized by inputs, for example, expenditure on doctors, nurses, pharmaceuticals, and linen. In programme budgeting the interest is in categorization of sets of needs that we seek to alleviate or meet—the needs of the elderly, children, cancer patients, etc. The link is thus between expenditure and health objectives for relevant social or disease groupings.

Therefore, prior to proceeding with the marginal analysis or shifting resources, it is relevant to find out what is being spent on these groupings or 'programmes'. The two keys to designating programmes are first that the programmes together are comprehensive in that, first, all the health services—hospital, general practitioner, and community—are included, and second, the programmes are output or outcome orientated and not input orientated as is the case with most forms of budgeting.

This approach—programme budgeting plus marginal analysis—is what economists recommend for use in pursuing the meeting of needs at a planning level (Cohen 1994; *Health Policy* 1995). With respect to the marginal analysis part of the approach, trying to form a judgement about whether $1 million is better spent on maternity care rather than on care of the elderly is difficult. There are major measurement problems here and greater effort needs to be invested in developing appropriate measures to enable these comparisons to be made.

Quality-adjusted life year (**QALY**) league tables may be seen as a form of marginal analysis. Such tables allow comparisons to be made between conditions according to the impact they have on the quantity and quality of life of sufferers. As discussed in more detail below, the QALY, which discounts chronological survival according to the quality of life, has also been used as an output currency to compare what is attainable for investment in various health care procedures. Thus, for $10 000 spent on treatment for one condition one may purchase 300 QALYs, compared with 700 QALYs for the same price if one is treating a different condition. Yet QALY league tables have limited applicability in resource allocation contexts for several reasons (Gerard and Mooney 1993). For example, at the most practical level cost–utility studies, which form the basis of the QALY league tables, are relatively sparse.

The moves in, for example, the United States (through the Patient Outcome Research Team programme etc.), the United Kingdom (in particular Wales), New Zealand, and New South Wales in Australia, to plan health services with the focus on health outcomes or health gain, place emphasis on efficiency and equity in the context of needs. Such an emphasis demands that objectives be more precisely and explicitly stated and needs identified more carefully and quantified. It is to the quantification of needs that we will turn shortly.

Other possibilities exist at the planning level for meeting needs. For example, in the United Kingdom there is enthusiasm at present for 'needs assessment' by which the needs of the population are expressed in terms of the burden of illness attributable to several major diseases. Resources are then allocated in proportion to the size of the needs. However, this method appears to fail to consider the effectiveness of interventions to meet those needs. Nor does it directly confront the costs of interventions and so it is not clear how this method could achieve the most wise use of resources as discussed above. This thinking also underlies the World Health Organization (**WHO**) and World Bank initiatives on burden of disease. These issues are discussed more fully by Shiell *et al.* (1987), Mooney and Creese (1993), Murray and Lopez (1997), and Wiseman and Mooney (1998).

Attempts to reallocate limited Medicaid dollars to a wider pool of recipients in Oregon have attracted great attention, in no small part because need, effective therapy, and cost have been subject to public scrutiny in determining a pattern of resource expenditure for health care (Dixon and Welch 1991; Kitzhaber 1993). In 1991, after extensive consultation, a proposal was put forward that Medicaid coverage for the poor in Oregon should cease to cover everything possible for the poorest 200 000 recipients of aid and instead provide for 709 disease categories and paired treatments for an additional 100 000 recipients. The plan was approved by President Clinton on 19 March 1993.

Contrary to what many might have expected, the Oregon Health Plan still survives. Its resilience can be explained partly by its rather pragmatic adherence to the rationing criterion of restricting coverage to services above a cut-off point (Jacobs *et al.* 1999).

Teng (1996) argues that the compromises which led to the development of the list of services to be covered meant that the original objective of cost-effectiveness was largely undermined. Regardless of how the list was devised, however, it is doubtful whether cost-effectiveness is compatible, in general, with an approach to funding that partitions services above and below a fixed line. Its main limitation is that it takes no account of differences across individuals in terms of their capacity to benefit from the same treatment.

Despite this, the Oregon Health Plan has been successful in one of its major objectives: of increasing medical coverage across the state (Oregon Health Plan 1997; Jacobs *et al.* 1999; Leichter 1999). Conversely, it has been less successful in reducing overall health care expenditure and has relied to a large extent on funding from increases in tobacco taxes (Jacobs *et al.* 1999).

The second consideration that planners will be interested in concerns equity. One of the most problematical aspects of this is that there is so much confusion in health care policy circles as to what this word means. The chief contenders are 'equal health', 'equal use for equal need', and 'equal access for equal need'. Clearly the last two of these incorporate some view of need within them. Here our concern is restricted to the relationship between equity and need and, within that, the issue of resource allocation formulas.

The international industry of needs-based (or weighted capitation) resource allocation formulas began with the Resource Allocation Working Party (**RAWP**) in England whose report was published in 1976 (DHSS 1976). The approach has been used in several other places since (e.g. New South Wales in Australia and New Zealand) and has recently been reviewed in the United Kingdom (NSW Health Department 1996; DoH 1997, 1999).

What the original RAWP sought was a formula for allocating resources fairly to the 14 geographical regions of England based on the principle of equal access for equal need (although in practice it did not go beyond equal expenditure for equal need). The RAWP formula (and the various versions it has spawned) emphasized horizontal equity, i.e. equity that ensures that individuals with similar characteristics are treated equally. Vertical equity—the unequal treatment of unequals—is not included directly in the formulation except in so far as different needs are weighted by the cost of dealing with each.

A recent paper (Mooney 1998) argues that there may be a case for developing the notion of 'communitarian claims' to replace needs or at least to complement them. It is normally the case that need is conceptualized in terms of purely health and that in meeting need all nominally equal health gains (such as QALYs) be weighted equally. Communitarian claims, it is suggested, allow for other considerations (e.g. information or respect for patient dignity) to enter and for health gains to some recipients (e.g. those in particularly poor health) to be weighted more highly than others. A further claimed advantage is that it is the community who determine first what constitutes claim, and second the differential strengths of different claims. These would determine what health care resources were to be made available to different groups in society. These claims are communitarian not only in the sense that the responsibility to arbitrate over them lies with the community but also that it is beneficial to the community that they do so. For example, in Australia the overall community may feel better as a result of knowing that it has contributed to the betterment of the health of its indigenous peoples.

Measuring need—available instruments and their application

Needs-based formulas

In several countries measures of need have been constructed to guide the allocation of health care resources. The methods vary from allocating resources to geographical areas on the basis of prevailing patterns of mortality and social class, through to case-mix payment to hospitals on the basis of the need (in terms of diagnosis and severity) of patients admitted to their care.

The approach adopted in the RAWP (see above) aimed at measuring relative (and not absolute) need for health care in different regions. Such health care was divided into seven categories: non-psychiatric inpatient services, all day-patient and outpatient services, mental illness inpatient services, mental handicap inpatient services, community services, ambulance services, and administration of family practitioner (general practitioner) services, but not these services *per se*.

The relative need for each of these services in each region was calculated on the basis of a formula which weighted the population according to a number of factors. For example, the factors relevant to non-psychiatric inpatient services were size of population, age/sex composition, morbidity (although in practice this was actually the standardized mortality rate), cost, patient cross-boundary flows, medical education, and capital investment.

Relative need was calculated for each of the services listed and then weighted according to the national proportion of the total cost being spent on that service. These were then summed to give a regional overall weight. Thus, if a region with a population of, say, 5 million was above average in terms of need, for example to the extent of 10 per cent, then it would receive funding which assumed a weighted population of 5.5 million.

In 1993 in New Zealand, in the wake of the establishment of regional health authorities, the emphasis shifted from funding for individual services to funding for a region's needs. More attention was focused on providing resources for an equitable level of services across the country (New Zealand Ministry of Health 1998). This new way of funding health and disability services has continued even though the four regional health authorities have been merged to form the Health Funding Authority.

The total amount of funding for New Zealand's health and disability services is distributed between the four health funding authority regions using three population-based funding formulas—one for personal health, one for public health, and one for disability support services (New Zealand Ministry of Health 1998). The formulas are used to determine each region's population, broken down into age, sex, and ethnic groups, and to weight this population according to the cost of providing services to each of the age/sex/ethnic groups.

What these formulas assume is that the total relative need in a region and across regions is a meaningful entity and that is open to challenge. It further assumes that the relative total need can be measured sufficiently accurately by just a few factors. Thirdly, it assumes that using standardized mortality rates as a measure of relative morbidity is a valid measure (again a doubtful assumption as indicated previously).

We would not want to appear overcritical of this process. What we would emphasize is the desirability in many instances of trying to fund health services on an equitable basis and that using some concept of need is the way to follow. It remains the case, however, that the assumptions typically used in needs-based formulas and the problems of measurement are such that we are less than convinced that this is the best way to proceed. In particular we would submit that weighting different needs according simply to cost rather than social value remains problematical.

Measuring instruments

Measuring needs, as indicated above, is likely to be problematical for the various reasons already stated. Whatever process is adopted, it involves establishing a measure of some shortfall in health status which from some ideal, from some norm, from some achievable health status, or some measure of 'capacity to benefit'.

There are many ways of trying to measure needs which are severely deficient and reflect more the availability of data than any real attempt to grapple seriously with the conceptualization of needs as spelt out so far in this chapter. Various activity measures—numbers of hospital admissions, visits to general practitioners, vaccinations carried out, etc.—are sometimes used to measure need. Yet it is readily apparent that such indicators reflect not only need (although visits to general practitioners may perhaps be designated a measure of consumer demand, in particular first visits) but also supply side considerations such as availability and appropriateness of services.

Certainly there are a number of vehicles that can be adopted to allow measurement of need to take place. Most common here would be epidemiological and social surveys. The question then is how to measure needs within any such survey. Two possible measures here are the QALY and the Short Form 36 (**SF-36**).

The QALY, and its more recent 'stable mate' the healthy year equivalent, have been developed largely by economists (Williams 1985; Torrance 1986; Mehrez and Gafni 1989) to allow health status to be measured in various circumstances. Both are based on the concept of health-related utility which recognizes that health, as an output of health services and of other activities that promote health, is a function of both quantity of health and quality of health—or mortality and morbidity.

The QALY allows individuals, groups, or societies to 'trade-off' quantity of life against quality of life arguing, for example, that according to people's preferences 10 years living with a chronic condition which results in the individual being confined to his or her own home is equivalent to 8 years of full health. The implication is that the 'quality adjustment' for the chronic condition is 0.8. Furthermore, it is implied that intervening to cure the chronic condition would result in an improvement in quality of life of 0.2 per annum which over 10 years means 2 QALYs.

While there are various criticisms that can be made of QALYs (Loomes and McKenzie 1989), they do have considerable merit over the more conventional measures of health status and of need such as mortality rates or standardized mortality rates in that they do endeavour to combine both quantity of life and quality of health. The development of QALYs has helped to gain greater acceptance for the point that health status, and in turn need, have large subjective elements and are value laden. In practice, to date QALYs have been used to measure need, essentially marginal-met need, in the context of priority setting through QALY league tables, as discussed above.

The disability-adjusted life year (**DALY**) is a variant of the QALY. DALYs were first introduced by the World Bank in 1993 (World Bank 1993) as a means of calculating the burden of different diseases. The approach involves the measurement of health status (strictly lost health status) into a universal index of mortality and morbidity.

Specifically, the DALYs for a given condition or disease are the sum of years of life lost due to premature mortality and the number of years of life lived with disability, adjusted for the severity of the disability (Murray and Lopez 1997). In terms of the disability severity weights, these were originally based on the opinions of experts in international health and fell into six classes of severity ranging from 0 (for perfect health) to 1 (for death) but, more recently, social values have been incorporated in DALYs (Murray and Lopez 1997).

DALYs and their use as an aggregate measure of health status in the monitoring of population health, in the establishment of priorities between interventions, and as a guide to research priorities have been criticized by a number of authors. Prime among the criticisms made are that DALYs inadequately reflect social preferences for health, that all they reflect is health and not other possible outcomes or valued processes from the health care system, that the assumed or posited goals of health care systems are not validated, that such goals are constant across all societies, and that using DALYs, as is advocated, to measure the burden of disease to assist with priority setting is at best a misuse of analytical resources and at worst potentially misleading (Shiell *et al.* 1987; Mooney and Creese 1993; Mooney *et al.* 1997; Sayers and Fliedner 1997; Wiseman and Mooney 1998; Williams 1999).

The SF-36 was developed by the RAND Corporation in the United States for use in the Health Insurance Study Experiment/Medical Outcomes Study (Ware *et al.* 1993). It is a concise 36-item health-status questionnaire and has become one of the most widely used measures of subjective health status (Ware *et al.* 1993; Jenkinson *et al.* 1996; Jenkinson and Layte 1997).

The SF-36 contains 36 items which measure eight dimensions: physical functioning (ten items), role limitations due to physical problems (four items), role limitations due to emotional problems (three items), mental health (five items), energy/vitality (four items), social functioning (two items), pain (two items), and general health perception (five items). There is also a single item about perceptions of health changes over the past 12 months.

The validity and reliability of the SF-36 in patient populations has been confirmed in the United States (McHorney *et al.* 1992, 1993). For example, patients with chronic heart failure reporting oedema, orthopnoea, or dyspnoea on exertion were classified as having a serious medical condition. The SF-36 could detect differences in health status among these patient groups across all eight scales. Garratt *et al.* (1993) claim on the basis of their own empirical work in the United Kingdom that the SF-36 seems 'acceptable to patients, internally consistent, and a valid measure of the health status of a wide range of patients'.

However, not all studies have been favourable to the SF-36. For instance, it has been criticized for failing to detect low levels of morbidity in some patient groups (Bowling 1997). Kurtin *et al.* (1992) reported 'floor' effects in the role of functioning scales in severely ill patients, where 25 to 50 per cent of patients obtained the lowest score possible, the implication being that deterioration in condition will not be detected by the scale. Other studies have revealed that it has little discriminatory power among women receiving different treatments for stage II breast cancer (Levine *et al.* 1988; Guyatt *et al.* 1989). Detailed reviews of the instrument are given by Anderson *et al.* (1993) and Bowling (1997).

More recently, an abbreviated version of the SF-36, the SF-12, has been developed (Ware *et al.* 1995, 1996*a*,*b*). The SF-12 health survey generates the physical and mental component summary scores of the SF-36 'with considerable accuracy, while imposing less burden on the respondents' (Jenkinson and Layte 1997). However, there do appear to be trade-offs in terms of reliability. For example, Jenkinson and Layte (1997) warn that 'the questionnaire contains a number of areas of health tapped with only a single item...consequently the SF-36 will provide a more reliable profile of scores across the eight domains than could be gained using the SF-12'.

Moreover, the simple scoring algorithms used in most of the non-preference-based measures of health such as the SF-36 assume first that there are equal intervals between the response choices, and second that the items are of equal importance (Brazier *et al.* 1999). As Brazier *et al.* point out, the SF-36 physical functioning dimension assumes that being limited in walking has the same importance as being limited in climbing flights of stairs. There is no reason for this to be the case. The SF-36 has the advantage of taking only 5 to 10 minutes to apply; thus it is easier to use than QALY measures.

Which measure is to be preferred in measuring need is not only a function of why need is being assessed but also the context or environment in which it is being assessed. Many normative factors influence health perceptions including the health of others in the individual's community or group, the nature and severity of the illness, demographic characteristics, and social class (Festinger 1954; Berkowitz 1975; Twaddle and Hessler 1977; Wills 1981; Sen 1987; Crawford 1994). While many measurement efforts are mathematically sophisticated and some are reliable in the sense that they can reproduce the same results from one application to another, they tend to be of questionable validity in so far as they fail to recognize the importance of these normative factors. Currently, most health status indices do not take account of the variation in criteria that individuals or groups use to make health status judgements about their own health status.

The consistent underperception of ill health observed in many disadvantaged and marginalized groups has 'obvious implications for the design and implementation of public health programs particularly if these programs aim to bring treatment to those most in need of such help' (Wiseman 1999). Secondly, resource allocation decision-making which relies on subjective measures of health may provide a misleading picture of the resource requirements of some groups in society. This will have implications for estimating health care priorities and the funding and planning of health services. There is a need to learn more about the criteria of health which are relevant in judging the well being of these groups and to investigate alternative elicitation procedures which would allow for a more accurate reflection of the preferences of such groups.

Conclusion

The concept of need is elusive but useful. In confronting the notion of need, we acknowledge the value-laden quality of the community's expectation of health services, whether these be for the relief and treatment of illness or the preservation and maintenance of good health. Need derives its meaning from the instrumental pathways we can follow in meeting it and inevitably involves third parties in its definition.

Need is a critical concept in the pursuit of efficient health care and equally critical to the development of services which are equitable.

Once need is admitted into the health care decision-making environment, other things follow. In determining how to meet need in a setting of limited resources, the allocation of those resources must take account of the likely health gain and the cost of that achievement. Moving resources at the margins of our principal programmes of care and health development, according to estimates or measurement of the cost and outcome, offers ways in which we can move in the direction of the wisest use of those resources in meeting community need.

References

Anderson, R., Aaronson, N., and Wilkin, D. (1993). Critical review of the international assessments of health-related quality of life. *Quality of Life Research*, **2**, 369–95.

Berkowitz, L. (1975). *A survey of social psychology*. Dryden Press, Illinois.

Bowling, A. (1997). *Measuring health. A review of quality of life measurement scales* (2nd edn). Open University Press, Milton Keynes.

Brazier, J., Deverill, M., and Green, C. (1999). A review of the use of health status measures in economic evaluation. *Journal of Health Services Research and Policy*, **4**, 174–84.

Cohen, D. (1994). Marginal analysis in practice: an alternative to needs assessment for contracting health care. *British Medical Journal*, **309**, 781–4.

Crawford, R. (1994). The boundaries of the self and the unhealthy other: reflections on health, culture and AIDS. *Social Science and Medicine*, **38**, 1347–65.

Culyer, A.J. (1991). *Equity in health care policy*. Paper presented to the Ontario Premier's Council on Health, Well-Being and Social Justice. University of Toronto, Toronto.

DHSS (Department of Health and Social Security) (1976). *Report of the Resource Allocation Working Party (RAWP)*. HMSO, London.

Dixon, J. and Welch, H.G. (1991) Priority setting: lessons from Oregon. *Lancet*, **337**, 912–16.

DoH (Department of Health), NHS Executive (1997). *HCHS revenue resource allocation to health authorities weighted capitation formulas.* Department of Health, Resource Allocation and Funding Team, Leeds.

DoH (Department of Health), NHS Executive (1999). *Resource allocation weighted capitation formulas.* Department of Health, Leeds.

Festinger, L. (1954). A theory of social comparison processes. *Human Relations*, **7**, 117–40.

Garratt, A., Ruta, D., Abdalla, M., Buckingham, K., and Russell, I. (1993). The SF 36 Health Survey Questionnaire: an outcome measure suitable for routine use within the NHS? *British Medical Journal*, **306**, 1440–4.

Gerard, K. and Mooney, G. (1993). QALY league tables: handle with care. *Health Economics*, **2**, 59–64.

Guyatt, G., Nogradi, S., Halcrow, S., *et al.* (1989). Development and testing of a new measure of health status for clinical trials in heart failure. *Journal of General Internal Medicine*, **4**, 101–7.

Health Policy (1995). Special issue on programme budgeting and marginal analysis. *Health Policy*, **33**.

Jacobs, L., Marmor, T., and Oberlander, J. (1999). The Oregon Health Plan and the political paradox of rationing: what advocates and critics have claimed and what Oregon did. *Journal of Health Politics, Policy and Law*, **24**, 161–80.

Jenkinson, C. and Layte, R. (1997). Development and testing of the UK SF 12. *Journal of Health Services Research and Policy*, **2**, 14–18.

Jenkinson, C., Layte, R., Wright, L., and Coulter, A. (1996). *The UK SF-36: an analysis and interpretation manual.* Health Services Research Unit, Oxford.

Kitzhaber, J.A. (1993). Prioritizing health services in an era of limits: the Oregon experiment. *British Medical Journal*, **307**, 373–7.

Krasnik, A., Groenewegen, P., Pedersen, P.A., *et al.* (1990). Changing remuneration systems: effects on activity in general practice. *British Medical Journal*, **300**, 1698–1701.

Kurtin, P., Davies, A., Meyer, K., *et al.* (1992). Patient-based health status measurements in outpatient dialysis: early experiences in developing an outcomes assessment program. *Medical Care*, **30** (Supplement 5), MS136–49.

Leichter, H.M. (1999). Oregon's bold experiment: whatever happened to rationing? *Journal of Health Politics, Policy and Law*, **24**, 147–58.

Levine, M., Guyatt, G., Gent, M., *et al.* (1988). Quality of life in stage II breast cancer: an instrument for clinical trials. *Journal of Clinical Oncology*, **6**, 1798–1810.

Liss, P.E. (1990). *Health care need: meaning and measurement.* Linkoping University, Linkoping.

Loewy, E.H. (1990). Commodities, needs and health care: a communal perspective. In *Changing values in medical and health care decision making* (ed. U.J. Jensen and G. Mooney), pp. 17–31. Wiley, Chichester.

Loomes, G. and McKenzie, I. (1989). The scope and limitations of QALY measures. *Social Science and Medicine*, **28**, 299–308.

McHorney, C., Ware, J., Rogers, W., Raczek, A., and Lu, J. (1992). The validity an drelative precision of MOS short-and long-form health status scales and Dartmouth COOP charts: results from the medical outcomes study. *Medical Care*, **30** (Supplement), MS253–65.

McHorney, C., Ware, J., and Raczek, A. (1993). The MOS 36-item short form health survey. II: Psychometric and clinical tests of validity in measuring physical and mental health constructs. *Medical Care*, **31**, 247–63.

Mehrez, A. and Gafni, A. (1989). Quality adjusted life years, utility theory and healthy year equivalents. *Medical Decision Making*, **9**, 142–9.

Mooney, G. (1998). 'Communitarian claims' as an ethical basis for allocating health care resources. *Social Science and Medicine*, **47**, 1171–80.

Mooney, G. and Creese, A. (1993). Priority setting for health service efficiency: the role of measurement of burden of illness. In *Disease control priorities in developing countries* (ed. D. Jamison, W. Mosely, A. Measham, and J. Bobadilla). Oxford University Press, New York.

Murray, C. and Lopez, A. (1997). The utility of DALYs for public health policy and research: a reply. *Bulletin of the World Health Organization*, **75**, 377–81.

Mooney, G., Irwig, L., and Leeder, S. (1997). Priority setting in health care: unburdening from the burden of disease. *Australian and New Zealand Journal of Public Health*, **21**, 680–1.

New Zealand Ministry of Health (1998). *Population based funding formula—overview*. Ministry of Health, Wellington.

NSW Health Department (1996). *Implementation of the economic statement for health*. Structural and Funding Policy Branch, Policy Development Division, Sydney.

Oregon Health Plan (1997). *The uninsured in Oregon 1997*. Office for Oregon Health Plan Research, Salem.

Sayers, B.M. and Fliedner, T.M. (1997). The critique of DALYs: a counter-reply. *Bulletin of the World Health Organization*, **75**, 383–4.

Sen, A. (1987). *On ethics and economics*. Basil Blackwell, Oxford.

Shiell, A., Gerard, K., and Donaldson, C. (1987) Cost of illness studies: an aid to decision-making? *Health Policy*, **8**, 317–23.

Teng, T.O. (1996). An evaluation of Oregon's Medicaid rationing algorithms. *Health Economics*, **5**, 171–81.

Torrance, G.W. (1986). Measurement of health state utilities for economic appraisal. *Journal of Health Economics*, **5**, 1–30.

Twaddle, A. and Hessler, R. (1977). *A sociology of health*. C.V. Mosby, St Louis, MO.

Ware, J., Snow, K., Kosinski, M., and Gandek, B. (1993). *SF-36 health survey manual and interpretation guide*. Health Institute, New England Medical Center, Boston, MA.

Ware, J., Kosinski, M., and Keller, S. (1995). *How to score the SF-12 physical and mental health summary scales* (2nd edn). Health Institute, New England Medical Center, Boston, MA.

Ware, J., Kosinski, M., and Keller, S. (1996*a*). SF-12 An even shorter health survey. *Medical Outcomes Trust Bulletin*, **4**, 2.

Ware, J., Kosinski, M., and Keller, S. (1996*b*). A 12-item short-form health survey construction of scales and preliminary tests of reliability and validity. *Medical Care*, **34**, 220–33.

Williams, A. (1985). Economics of coronary artery bypass grafting. *British Medical Journal*, **49**, 825–31.

Williams, A. (1999). Calculating the global burden of disease: time for a strategic reappraisal? *Health Economics*, **8**, 1–8.

Wills, T. (1981). Downward comparison principles in social psychology. *Psychological Bulletin*, **90**, 245–71.

Wiseman, V. (1999). Culture, self-rated health and resource allocation decision-making. *Health Care Analysis*, **7**, 207–23.

Wiseman, V. and Mooney, G. (1998). Burden of illness estimates for priority setting: a debate revisited. *Health Policy*, **43**, 243–51.

World Bank (1993). *World development report 1993: investing in health*. Oxford University Press, New York.

12.3 Socio-economic inequalities in health in developed countries: the facts and the options

Johan P. Mackenbach

Introduction

The purpose of this chapter

Socio-economic inequalities in health, i.e. systematic differences in morbidity and mortality rates between those with a lower and a higher socio-economic status, have been studied extensively around the world in the past decades. Inequalities in health have been documented from the United States (Davey Smith *et al.* 1996) to the former Soviet Union (Dennis *et al.* 1993), from The Netherlands (Mackenbach 1992) to New Zealand (Pearce *et al.* 1991), and from Brazil (Duncan *et al.* 1995) to Bangladesh (Bairagi *et al.* 1993). The emphasis of research in this field has gradually shifted from description to explanation and, although the number of countries for which results of explanatory studies are available is still limited, a general understanding of the factors involved has emerged. Childhood circumstances, material factors, health-related behaviours, and psychosocial factors have all been shown to contribute significantly to the explanation of socio-economic inequalities in health (Carroll *et al.* 1993; Kaplan and Keil 1993; Davey Smith *et al.* 1994; Vågerö and Illsley 1995; Macintyre 1997).

More recently, a start has been made on the systematic development of strategies to reduce inequalities in health (Whitehead and Dahlgren 1991; Dahlgren and Whitehead 1992; Benzeval *et al.* 1995). It has become clear that waiting until all explanatory questions have been answered would imply that action will probably never occur, and so both researchers and health policy-makers have searched for sensible recommendations in the face of limited knowledge.

It is the purpose of this chapter to give a brief review of the available evidence on the description and explanation of socio-economic inequalities in health, and then to present the current (1999) state of the art with regard to the available options for reducing socio-economic inequalities in health.

Historical notes

Historical evidence suggests that socio-economic inequalities in health are not a recent phenomenon, but it is only relatively recently, during the nineteenth century and on the basis of mortality statistics, that socio-economic inequalities in health were 'discovered'. Before that time socio-economic inequalities in morbidity and mortality health went unrecognized, and there was even a general perception that all human beings were equal before death. This is illustrated by the Dances of Death or *Danses Macabres*, which were a favourite theme in western and central European literature and painting during the late Middle Ages (Mackenbach 1995*a*). These Dances of Death typically portray the living according to their social standing, and each of them is accompanied by a corpse or skeleton symbolizing death (Fig. 1). According to the historian Huizinga, the Dance of Death 'reminded the spectators of the frailty and the vanity of earthly things', but at the same time 'preached social equality as the Middle Ages understood it, Death levelling the various ranks and professions' (Huizinga 1976).

The awareness of socio-economic inequalities in health dates back to the nineteenth century, when great figures in public health such as Villermé in France, Chadwick in England, and Virchow in Germany devoted a large part of their scientific and practical work to this issue (Ackerknecht and Virchow 1953; Coleman 1982; Chave 1984). This was made possible by the availability of national population statistics, which permitted the calculation of, for example, mortality rates by occupation or by city district. The only reliable source of mortality data in the general population that existed before national population registers were implemented (i.e. generally before the nineteenth century) consists of parish registers of baptisms and burials. An analysis of socio-economic inequalities in mortality on the basis of data from seventeenth century Geneva shows that the life expectancy of children born in the lowest occupational class was only 18 years, and that of the highest occupational class was 36 years (Perrenoud 1975). Data for other European cities from the eighteenth century confirm this picture of huge differences in mortality rates between persons of higher and lower social rank (Schultz 1991).

It is not certain whether socio-economic inequalities in mortality also existed before the seventeenth or eighteenth centuries, but it is difficult to believe that they did not. The Middle Ages were a period characterized by frequent mortality crises, arising from three frequently interlinked causes, i.e. war, pestilence, and famine. Of the three causes, famine, or more generally undernutrition, provides the most obvious link with socio-economic conditions. The rich certainly had a lower risk of dying from undernutrition than the majority of the population, which was probably malnourished even in 'normal' years. In addition, anecdotal evidence suggests that mortality during epidemics, particularly the plague, was higher in the lower social classes. Reports of health commissions in plague-ridden towns frequently mention that there were large differences in mortality between rich and poor (Cipolla and Zanetti 1972). Therefore the notion, embedded in the Dances of Death, that all human beings were equal before death must primarily be interpreted in metaphysical terms.

Since the nineteenth century the magnitude of socio-economic inequalities in mortality has certainly declined in absolute terms;

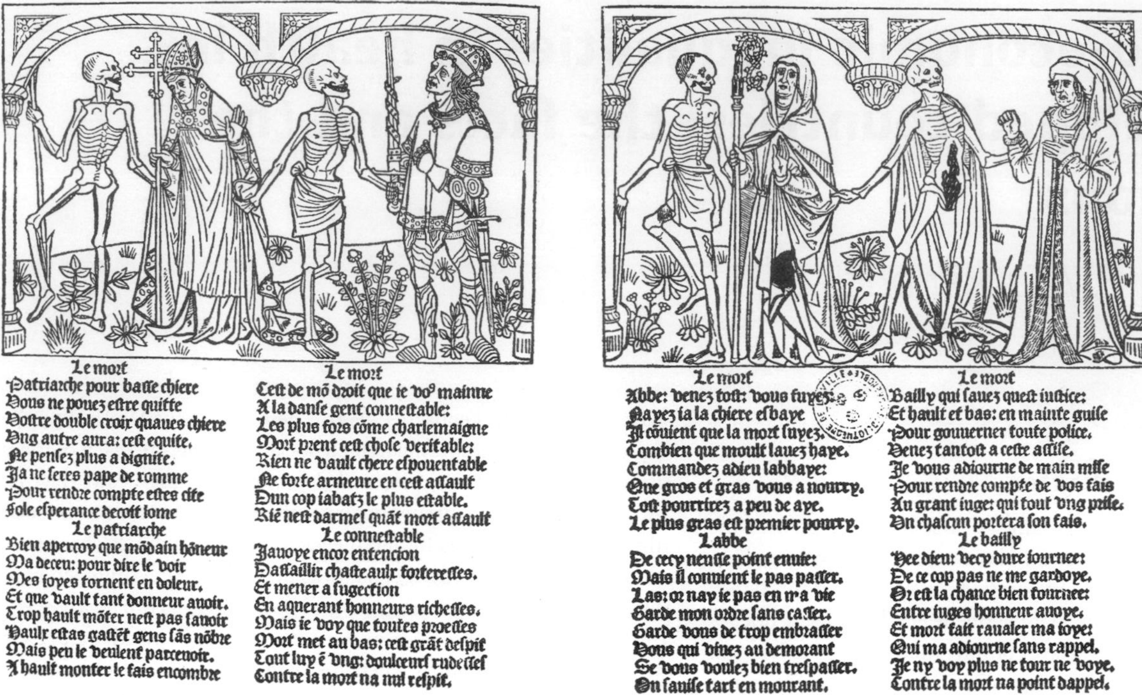

Fig. 1 The Dance of Death of Guillaume Marchant (fragment). (Source: Mackenbach 1995*a*.)

owing to the general decline of mortality, the absolute difference in mortality rates between those with a high and those with a low socio-economic position has become much smaller. It is less clear whether relative inequalities in mortality have also declined over time; relative risks of dying between those with a low and those with a high socio-economic position have remained remarkably stable. During recent decades there has even been a clear increase of relative inequalities in mortality in many developed countries (Valkonen 1993; Lang and Ducimetière 1995; Regidor *et al.* 1995; Vågerö and Lundberg 1995; van de Mheen *et al.* 1996; Drever and Bunting 1997). This is partly due to the social patterning of the ischaemic heart disease epidemic: this probably started in the higher socio-economic groups, then diffused into the lower socio-economic groups, and when the epidemic had reached its peak (about 1970) the decline also started in the higher socio-economic groups before diffusing into the lower socio-economic groups (Marmot *et al.* 1978; Stallones 1980; Marmot and McDowall 1986; Wing *et al.* 1986; Mackenbach *et al.* 1989).

As a result, at the start of the twenty-first century all developed countries are faced with substantial socio-economic inequalities in mortality (and many other indicators of health problems). These are perceived by many as unfair, and in any case as an enormous challenge to public health.

Outline of the chapter

The available evidence on the description and explanation of socio-economic inequalities will be reviewed briefly. Because of space limitations it will be impossible to give a complete survey of the international literature, for which the reader is referred to a number of recent review papers (Carroll *et al.* 1993; Kaplan and Keil 1993; Davey Smith *et al.* 1994; Vågerö and Illsley 1995; Macintyre 1997). Here, the emphasis will be on giving an internationally representative overview of socio-economic inequalities in morbidity and mortality in industrialized countries, and on presenting some explanatory frameworks that help to structure the available empirical evidence as well as the options for interventions and policies. The chapter then develops a systematic framework for a strategy to reduce socio-economic inequalities in health, highlighting the choices that have to be made in the areas of justification and objectives, choice of policies and interventions, and evaluation and monitoring. The final section illustrates some of these principles on the basis of recent examples from the United Kingdom and The Netherlands.

The facts: description

Morbidity

Many countries perform health interviews—level-of-living or multi-purpose surveys with questions on both socio-economic status (education, occupation, income) and self-reported morbidity (e.g. self-assessed health, chronic conditions, disability). Analysis of these data shows that inequalities in self-reported morbidity are substantial everywhere, and always in the same direction: persons with a lower socio-economic status have higher morbidity rates (Illsley and Svensson 1990; Mielck and do Rosario Giraldes 1993; Lahelma and Arber 1994; Kunst *et al.* 1995).

Within western Europe the risk of ill health is 1.5 to 2.5 times higher in the lower half of the socio-economic distribution than in the upper half. For example, in Sweden the risk of chronic conditions is 1.85 times higher among men with primary or lower secondary education than among men with higher secondary or tertiary education. When the extremes of the socio-economic distribution are compared (Fig. 2), the size of the inequalities becomes even more

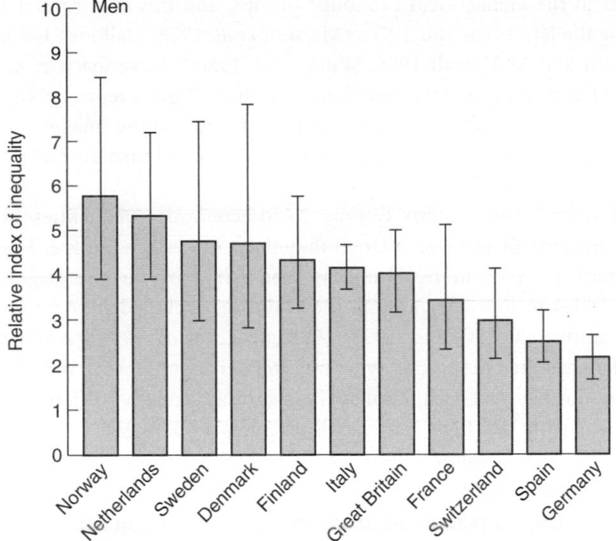

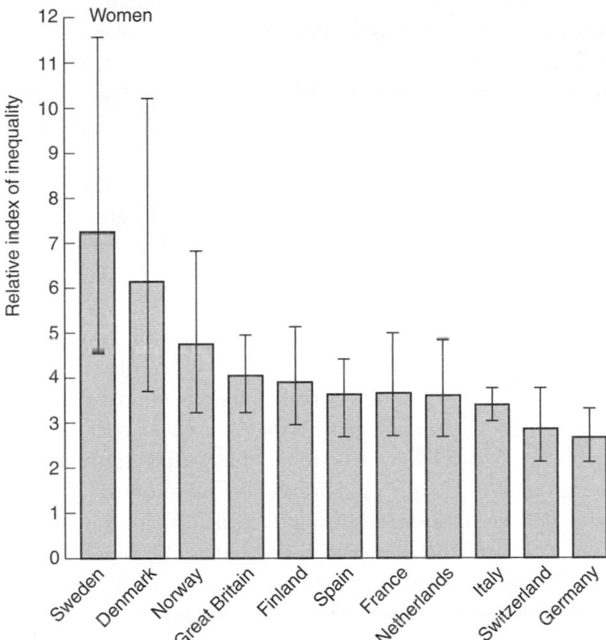

Fig. 2 Inequalities in less-than-good self-assessed health by level of education in 10 European countries, by sex (age range 25–69 years). The relative index of inequality represents the odds ratio of less-than-good self-assessed health for those at the bottom of the social hierarchy (here measured on the basis of educational achievement) compared with those at the top. (Source: Mackenbach *et al.* 1997.)

dramatic. Substantial inequalities in health are found in all countries included in this figure, from Spain to Finland and from Great Britain to Italy, emphasizing the tremendous importance of this public health problem. Surprisingly, substantial inequalities in self-reported morbidity are also found in the Nordic countries, with their long histories of egalitarian socio-economic and health care policies (Cavelaars *et al.* 1998*a*,*b*). Similar results are found in central and eastern Europe; for example, socio-economic inequalities in self-reported morbidity in the Czech Republic, Estonia, and Hungary are about the same as in most western European countries (Groenhof *et al.* 1996).

While these nationally representative data are based on self-reports, similar patterns are found in other studies using more objective assessments of morbidity, such as the incidence of ischaemic heart disease (Kaplan and Keil 1993; Lynch *et al.* 1996; Marmot *et al.* 1997) or cancer (Davey Smith *et al.* 1991; van Loon *et al.* 1995).

Mortality

Similar findings have been reported for mortality, the harder but rarer outcome measure,. Socio-economic inequalities in mortality of considerable magnitude are found in all countries with available data. For example, the excess risk of premature mortality among middle-aged men in manual occupations compared with those in non-manual occupations ranged from 33 to 71 per cent in a recent comparative study (Fig. 3(a)). On the basis of 'relative' differences there is no evidence for smaller inequalities in mortality in the Nordic countries,

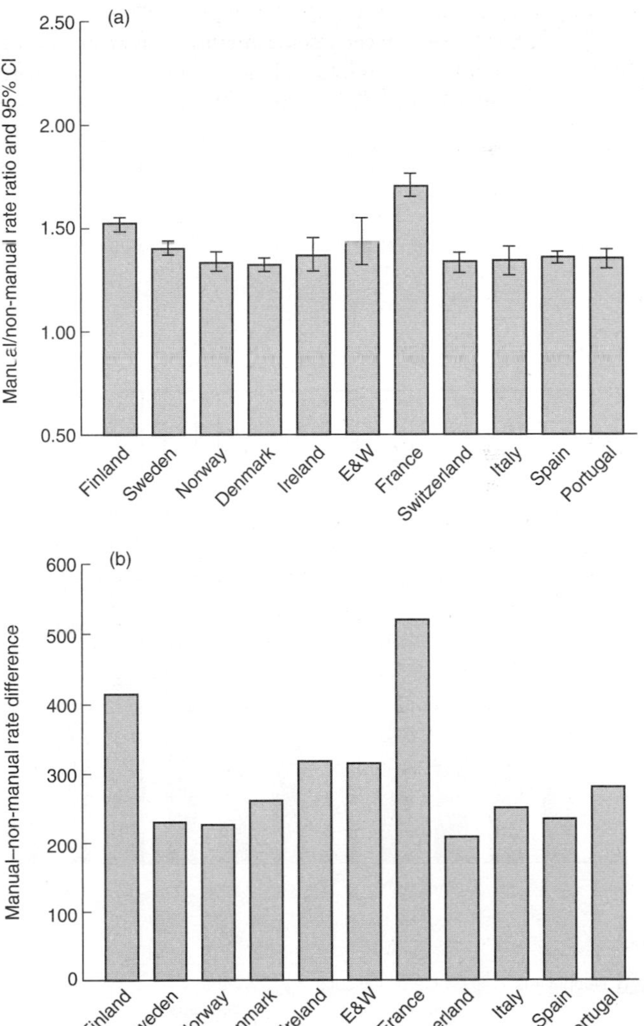

Fig. 3 Inequalities in total mortality by occupational class in 10 European countries, middle-aged men: (a) relative inequalities; (b) absolute inequalities. E&W, England and Wales. (Source: Kunst 1997.)

but Sweden does have rather low 'absolute' differences in mortality owing to its low average death rates (Fig. 3(b)) (Mackenbach *et al.* 1997).

Mortality data permit a breakdown by cause of death, which may help in exploring possible explanations of inequalities in mortality. An analysis by cause of death reveals a striking north–south pattern within western Europe (Fig. 4). In the Nordic countries, England and Wales, and Ireland, half or more of the socio-economic gap in total mortality is due to an excess risk of cardiovascular diseases in the lower socio-economic groups. In France, Switzerland, Italy, Spain, and Portugal cardiovascular diseases account for a small fraction of the higher risks of premature mortality in the lower socio-economic groups only, while cancers (but not lung cancer) and gastrointestinal diseases (such as liver cirrhosis) have a large share in the excess risks (Kunst *et al.* 1998, 1999). These data suggest that there are likely to be some differences in the explanations of socio-economic inequalities in mortality in the north and the south of Europe. Currently, cardiovascular risk factors such as smoking and intake of animal fat are likely to be important in northern Europe, with excessive alcohol consumption being important in the south (Cavelaars *et al.* 1997).

This international pattern can also be interpreted as an expression of different stages of epidemiological development. In northern Europe (and in the United States) mortality from cardiovascular diseases has not always been higher in the lower socio-economic groups. In the 1950s and 1960s ischaemic heart disease mortality was higher in the higher socio-economic groups, and this only reversed during the late 1960s and 1970s (Marmot *et al.* 1978; Stallones 1980; Marmot and McDowall 1986; Wing *et al.* 1986; Mackenbach *et al.* 1989). It is possible that the situation in southern Europe represents an earlier stage of epidemiological development, and that the smaller size of inequalities in cardiovascular disease mortality will turn out to be a temporary phenomenon.

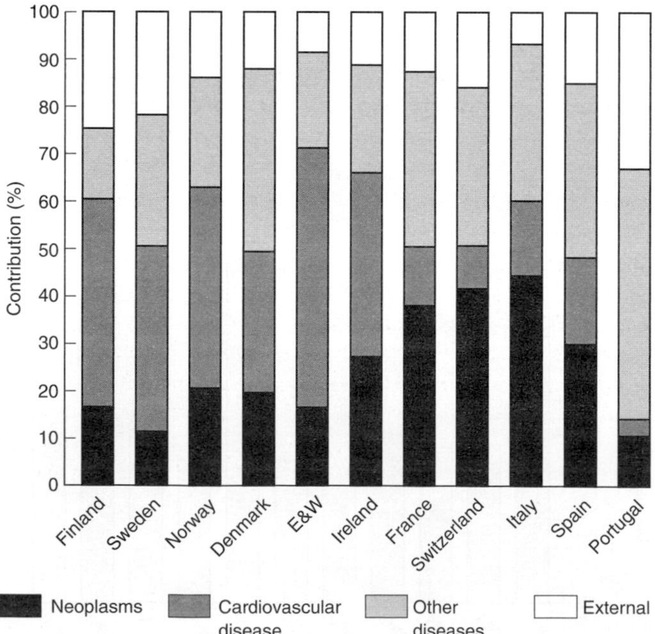

Fig. 4 Contribution of specific causes of death to inequalities in total mortality by occupational class in 10 European countries, middle-aged men. Contribution is measured as the proportion of the difference between manual and non-manual rates of total mortality which is due to a specific cause-of-death group. (Source: Kunst *et al.* 1998.)

In central and eastern Europe socio-economic inequalities in mortality are equally large or larger than those in western Europe. The real outlier seems to be Hungary, which had by far the largest inequalities in mortality among the countries included in a recent comparative study (Kunst 1997; Mackenbach *et al.* 1999). Among middle-aged men the risk of dying was 165 per cent higher in manual than in non-manual occupations. These very large relative differences combine with the high average death rates in Hungary to form extremely large absolute differences in mortality between the higher and lower socio-economic groups.

Substantial inequalities in mortality were also seen in the United States, but the size of these inequalities was not clearly different from those observed in western Europe. In view of the variations observed within Europe, it is tempting to speculate that the heterogeneity of the United States population, with its immigrants from all parts of Europe as well as from many other parts of the world, has averaged out the experience of subpopulations with larger and smaller inequalities in mortality (Kunst *et al.* 1999).

Many studies of socio-economic inequalities in mortality have been confined to men, partly because the most frequently used socio-economic classification, that based on occupation, can less easily be applied to women. From the studies that have included women, it has become clear that inequalities in mortality also exist among women but tend to be smaller than those among men (Moser *et al.* 1988; Dahl 1991; Koskinen and Martelin 1994; Martikainen 1995; Mackenbach *et al.* 1999). In studies that used occupational class as an indicator of socio-economic status this may be an artefact, but similar findings were reported from a few studies that used educational level or material living standards as socio-economic indicators. As Fig. 5 illustrates, women have smaller relative inequalities in mortality for most causes of death, including neoplasms, but not for cardiovascular diseases. The smaller inequalities in total mortality among women are the result of smaller inequalities for many causes of death, but also of differences between women and men in cause-of-death pattern. Neoplasms and cardiovascular diseases account for a large majority of all deaths among both men and women, but neoplasms, for which inequalities in mortality are relatively small among women and among men, have a larger share of total female mortality than of total male mortality (Koskinen and Martelin 1994; Mackenbach *et al.* 1999).

Nearly all causes of death have higher rates of mortality in the lower socio-economic groups. One of the very few exceptions is breast cancer, for which mortality rates tended to be higher among women in the higher socio-economic groups, perhaps because they adopted 'modern' fertility and breast-feeding practices that increase breast cancer risk before women in the lower socio-economic groups (van Loon *et al.* 1994). However, recent evidence suggests that this pattern is reversing, and that among younger generations of women risks are higher in the lower socio-economic groups (Heck and Pamuk 1997).

The international patterns highlighted in this section suggest not only that there are some differences between explanations of socio-economic inequalities in health in different countries, but also that

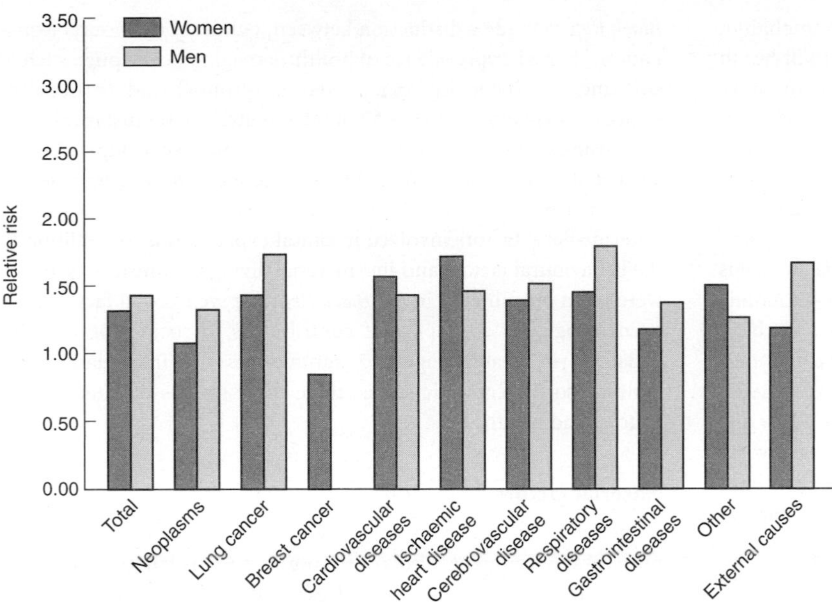

Fig. 5 Inequalities in cause-specific mortality by level of education among men and women in the United States: relative risk for up to lower secondary education versus upper secondary education and higher. (Source: Mackenbach *et al.* 1999.)

interventions and policies to reduce socio-economic inequalities in health may differ. Although the basic socio-economic structures are similar, the pathways through which low socio-economic status affects health are different, and therefore interventions targeting more proximal determinants of socio-economic inequalities in health should be adapted to the situation prevailing in the country.

Health expectancy

As was shown in the previous two paragraphs, both morbidity and mortality rates are higher in the lower socio-economic groups. These two health aspects combine in even larger inequalities in health expectancy, because people in lower socio-economic groups do not only live shorter lives but also spend a larger portion of their life in ill-health. While socio-economic inequalities in life expectancy usually amount to 3 to 7 years, differences in, for example, disability-free life expectancy amount to more than 10 years between the highest and lowest socio-economic groups (Valkonen *et al.* 1997; Sihvonen *et al.* 1998).

The facts: explanation

Selection versus causation

Research on explanations for socio-economic inequalities in health needs hypotheses, if not theories, and one important source of inspiration for such hypotheses has been the *Black Report*, published in 1980 in the United Kingdom by a committee chaired by Sir Douglas Black (Townsend *et al.* 1988*a*). In this report four types of explanation were proposed: artefact, social selection, cultural or behavioural, and materialist.

Artefact

Artefact explanations have largely been refuted by research carried out since the publication of the *Black Report*. Artefact explanations imply that the relationship between socio-economic status and health is produced by the process of measurement, and does not exist in reality. An example is inaccuracies in data on numerators and denominators used for the calculation of socio-economic inequalities in mortality, leading to an overestimation of mortality in the lower socio-economic groups. However, good-quality data, in which these and other problems have been avoided, show substantial socio-economic inequalities in health, and suggest that while bias may from time to time occur, the overall picture is not seriously distorted by measurement problems (Fox *et al.* 1985; Bloor *et al.* 1987).

Selection

The situation is slightly different with regard to social selection explanations. These imply that health determines socio-economic status, instead of socio-economic status determining health (Fig. 6). There is some evidence that during social mobility, i.e. changes in socio-economic position during an individual's life compared with either his or her parents (intergenerational mobility) or with him- or

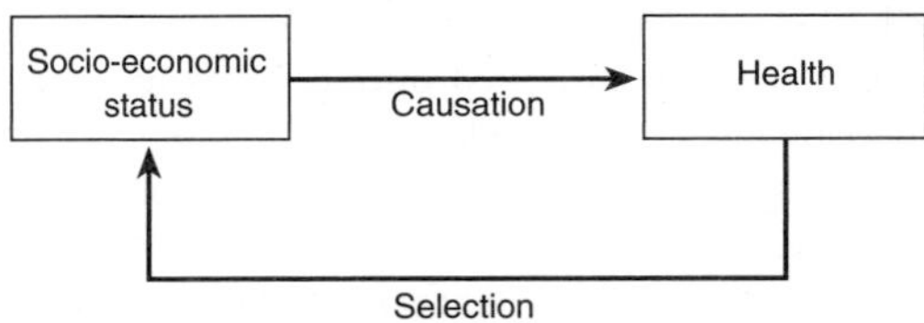

Fig. 6 'Selection' and 'causation' mechanisms in the explanation of socio-economic inequalities in health.

herself at an earlier point in time (intragenerational mobility), selection on (ill-)health may occur, with people who are in ill-health being less likely to move upward and/or more likely to move downward (Illsley 1955; Luft 1974; Stern 1983; Wadsworth 1986; van de Mheen *et al.* 1999). This is perhaps more likely with income as an indicator of socio-economic position than with occupational class or educational level; in the latter case, health problems in adult life cannot affect current level at all.

While the occurrence of health-related selection is undisputed, it is less clear what its contribution to the explanation of socio-economic inequalities in health is. It is only in a few studies that this has been investigated directly, and these have shown that the contribution to inequalities in health by occupational class is small (Fox *et al.* 1982; Wadsworth 1986; van de Mheen *et al.* 1999). This is at least partly due to the fact that while those who move downward do indeed have worse health than those who remain in their social class of origin, they have better health than those who are already in their class of destination (Goldman 1994).

More recently, a different form of selection has been proposed that may have a stronger impact on socio-economic inequalities in health—'indirect selection'. Indirect selection implies that social mobility is selective on determinants of health, not on health itself (West 1991). Intelligence could be an example; educational careers are partly dependent on intelligence, and intelligence is also likely to be a determinant of health, for example through sensible behaviour. Excessive alcohol consumption could be another example; employment and career prospects are negatively affected by alcohol abuse, which also may lead to health problems. There is very little empirical evidence yet on the occurrence and importance of indirect selection, and so it is difficult to assess its importance for the explanation of socio-economic inequalities in health. It is also important to take into account the fact that the health determinants on which indirect selection takes place, such as intelligence or excessive alcohol consumption, could themselves be related to living circumstances during the earlier stages of life. Indirect selection would then be part of a mechanism of accumulation of disadvantage over the life course (Davey Smith *et al.* 1994).

Implications for policy

The importance of selection mechanisms for socio-economic inequalities in health is not only a scientific issue, but is also relevant for public health and social policy. If ill-health leads to downward social mobility, and if this contributes to the higher rates of health problems in the lower socio-economic groups, then measures that limit the impact of ill-health on, for example, employment prospects or occupational careers will help in reducing inequalities in health.

Material, psychosocial, and behavioural factors

Longitudinal studies in which socio-economic status has been measured before health problems are present, and in which the incidence of health problems is measured during follow-up, show higher risks of developing health problems in the lower socio-economic groups, and suggest 'causation' instead of 'selection' as the main explanation for socio-economic inequalities in health (Rose and Marmot 1981; Fox *et al.* 1982, 1985; Marmot *et al.* 1991). This 'causal' effect of socio-economic status on health is likely to be mainly indirect, through a number of more specific health determinants that are differentially distributed across socio-economic groups. Here, the *Black Report* made a distinction between 'cultural/behavioural explanations' (a higher prevalence of health-damaging behaviours, such as smoking, in the lower socio-economic groups) and 'materialist/structural explanations' (less favourable material circumstances, such as housing conditions, in the lower socio-economic groups) (Townsend *et al.* 1988*a*). Since the publication of the *Black Report,* research has advanced considerably and produced a clearer view of the 'intermediary' factors involved in causal explanations. In addition to the behavioural factors and the 'material' living circumstances, which were given prominence in the *Black Report*, psychosocial factors have been recognized as important contributors to socio-economic inequalities in health. Figure 7 summarizes the interrelationships between socio-economic status, these three groups of intermediary factors, and health.

Material factors

'Material' factors, i.e. exposure to low income and to health risks in the physical environment, also contribute to the explanation of socio-economic inequalities in health. Despite the fact that low income is such a fundamental aspect of low socio-economic status, the evidence for its role in generating health inequalities is far from complete. Income-related indicators of socio-economic status, such as level of household income, house and car ownership, or area-based measures of deprivation, have been demonstrated to be relatively strong predictors of ill-health (Townsend *et al.* 1988*b*; Carstairs and Morris 1989; Goldblatt 1990; Davey Smith *et al.* 1994). How low income affects health, and the relative importance of pathways related to low income, is far from clear, however. It is obvious that income may affect exposure to a wide range of health determinants, either directly (through ability to purchase health-promoting goods, such as safe housing and a healthy diet) or indirectly (through the psychosocial effects of the experience of relative deprivation), but there has been surprisingly little empirical research into these mechanisms. Most of the recent research into the health effects of income inequality has focused on the aggregate relationship between the extent of income inequality in a population, and its average mortality level or life expectancy (Fig. 8) (Wilkinson 1992; Kaplan *et al.* 1996; Kennedy *et al.* 1996). This research has shown that after accounting for differences between populations in average income level, a wider disparity in income within a population is associated with a higher mortality level and a lower life expectancy. While this suggests that reducing income inequalities may not only reduce health inequalities but also improve the overall health level of a population, it is not yet clear how the

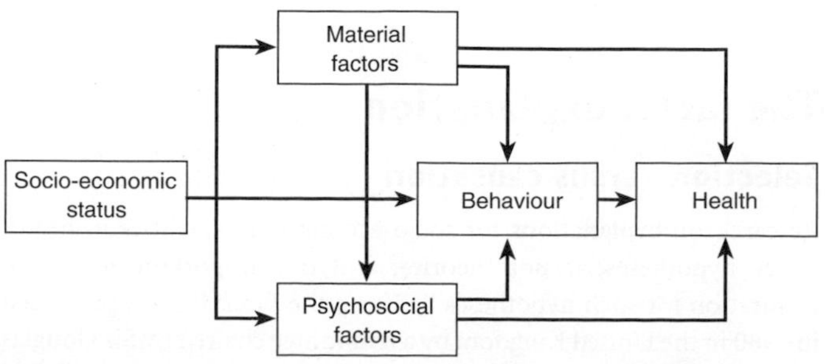

Fig. 7 The role of material, psychosocial, and behavioural factors in the explanation of socio-economic inequalities in health.

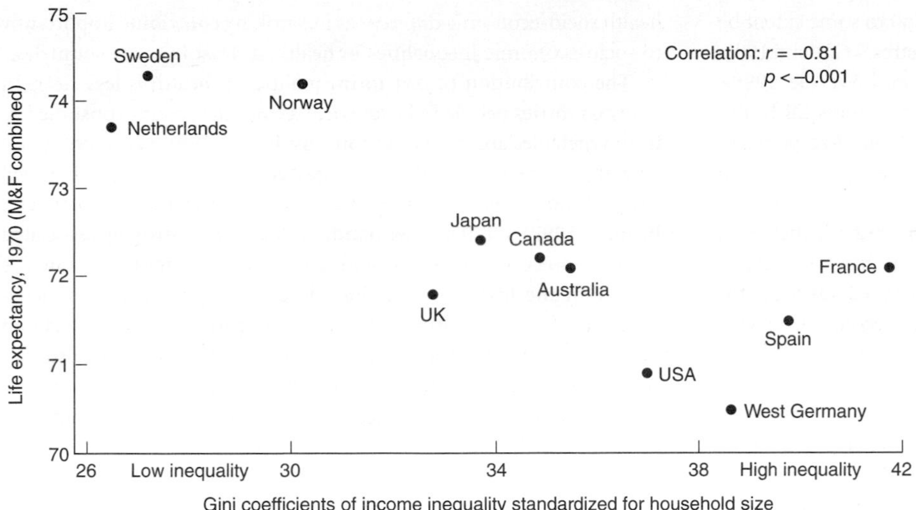

Fig. 8 The association between income inequality and life expectancy. (Source: Wilkinson 1996.)

association is to be explained. It may be due to psychosocial effects of income inequality (more relative deprivation, less social cohesion) or to the lack of investment in human resources, which is usually found in regions with more income inequality (when a more equal income distribution is the result of progressive taxation, there will be more public money for education, health care, etc.) (Wilkinson 1996; Lynch and Kaplan 1997).

Psychosocial factors

The recent interest in psychosocial pathways between low socio-economic status and ill-health has been stimulated by the observation that socio-economic inequalities in morbidity or mortality cannot be explained entirely by well-known behavioural or material risk factors for disease. This is particularly true for cardiovascular disease outcomes, where risk factors such as smoking, high serum cholesterol, and high blood pressure explain less than half of the socio-economic gradient in mortality (Rose and Marmot 1981; Davey Smith *et al.* 1990; Lynch *et al.* 1996). Together with the observation that inequalities in health have a generalized character, in the sense that the risks for diseases with widely different aetiologies are similarly socially patterned, this has given rise to the hypothesis that a lower socio-economic status may be associated with a higher 'generalized susceptibility' to disease (Marmot *et al.* 1984). This generalized susceptibility could be due to psychosocial factors; being in a low socio-economic position may be a psychosocial stressor, which, through biological or behavioural pathways, could lead to ill-health (Brunner and Marmot 1999).

One of the areas where there is clear evidence for psychosocial effects of being in a low socio-economic position is the work environment. Karasek's demand–control model predicts that a high level of psychological job demands combined with a low level of decision latitude (e.g. low level of decision authority) will lead to higher risks of stressful experience and subsequent physical illness, particularly ischaemic heart disease (Karasek *et al.* 1981). Jobs characterized by high demands and, particularly, low control are more prevalent in the lower socio-economic strata, and these psychosocial stressors in the work environment have indeed been shown to account for part of the social gradient in health (Fig. 9) (Marmot *et al.* 1997; Schrijvers *et al.* 1998).

In addition to the work environment, other spheres of life may also produce higher levels of stress in the lower socio-economic groups, as is evident from the higher prevalence of life events, chronic stressors, and daily hassles (Kessler and Cleary 1980; Stronks *et al.* 1998; Brunner and Marmot 1999). It is still unclear how psychosocial stress induces ill-health in the lower socio-economic groups. One possibility is that this is an indirect effect, through health-related behaviour; smoking,

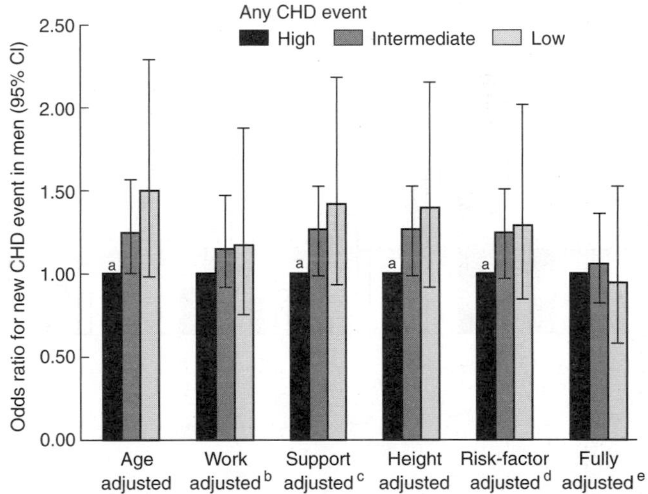

[a] p (trend test) < 0.05
[b] Job control and effort-reward imbalance
[c] Confiding/emotional support, practical support, negative characteristics, social network
[d] Smoking/serum cholesterol, body mass index, hypertension, and physical activity
[e] Early life, work, support, and risk factors

Fig. 9 The contribution of psychosocial job characteristics to the explanation of socio-economic inequalities in the incidence of coronary heart disease (CHD) in men. (Data from Marmot *et al.* 1997.)

excessive alcohol consumption, and obesity may all to some extent be a reaction to, or way of coping with, psychosocial stress (Graham 1995; Lynch *et al.* 1997; Stronks *et al.* 1997; Jarvis and Wardle 1999). Another possibility is that psychosocial stress induces ill-health directly, through biological mechanisms. The biological response to stress leads to release of adrenaline (through the sympatho-adrenal pathway) and cortisol (through the hypothalamic–pituitary–adrenal axis), and these have important effects on many organs, including blood pressure, blood clotting, and immunity. It has been hypothesized that such mechanisms underlie the elevated rates of, for example, cardiovascular disease in the lower socio-economic groups (Brunner and Marmot 1999).

Health-related behaviours

Health-related behaviours, such as smoking, diet, alcohol consumption, and physical exercise, are important 'proximal' determinants of socio-economic inequalities in health. As Fig. 10 shows, smoking is more prevalent in the lower socio-economic groups, at least in most European countries (van Reek and Adriaanse 1988; Pierce 1989; Cavelaars *et al.* 2000). However, there are some exceptions, particularly in southern Europe, where smoking seems to be more prevalent in the higher socio-economic groups, particularly among women. These patterns are likely to be related to differences between countries in the progression of the smoking epidemic. This started in northern Europe, among men and in the higher socio-economic groups, and then diffused into southern Europe, to women, and to the lower socio-economic groups. The cessation of smoking followed a similar pattern, and the 'reverse' patterns for women in southern Europe as seen in Fig. 10 are probably due to the fact that southern Europe is in an earlier stage of the smoking epidemic. Unfortunately, the situation in younger cohorts suggests that countries in southern Europe are catching up quickly. Because of the strong impact of smoking on health socio-economic differences in smoking contribute importantly to socio-economic inequalities in health, at least in some countries.

The contribution of diet to inequalities in health is less clear. In many countries people in lower socio-economic groups consume less fresh vegetables and fruits (Bolton-Smith *et al.* 1991; Osler 1993), but data on fat consumption do not suggest consistent differences between socio-economic groups (Hoeymans *et al.* 1996; Davey Smith and Brunner 1997). On the other hand, obesity is very strongly associated with socio-economic status, with much higher prevalence rates of obesity in the lower socio-economic groups, particularly in richer countries (Sobal and Stunkard 1989; Cavelaars *et al.* 1997). Data on socio-economic differences in alcohol consumption are also not always consistent, but frequently lower socio-economic groups have higher rates of both abstinence and excessive alcohol consumption (Cummins *et al.* 1981; Hupkens *et al.* 1993; Hoeymans *et al.* 1996; Cavelaars *et al.* 1997). Cause-of-death patterns suggest a substantial contribution of excessive alcohol consumption to inequalities in mortality in at least some countries, such as Finland (Mäkelä *et al.* 1997) and countries in southern Europe (Kunst *et al.* 1998). Finally, lack of leisure-time physical activity is more prevalent in the lower socio-economic groups (Holme *et al.* 1981; Tenconi *et al.* 1992; Lynch *et al.* 1997), but it is unclear to what extent this is compensated for by higher rates of work-related physical activity. It is unlikely that such compensation is substantial in the rich service economies of northern Europe, but it may still be in poorer countries.

Implications for policy

Following the publication of the *Black Report* there has been a sharp debate on the relative importance of material versus behavioural factors for the explanation of socio-economic inequalities in health. In some countries there has been a tendency among policy-makers to use evidence on the importance of health-related behaviour for arguing

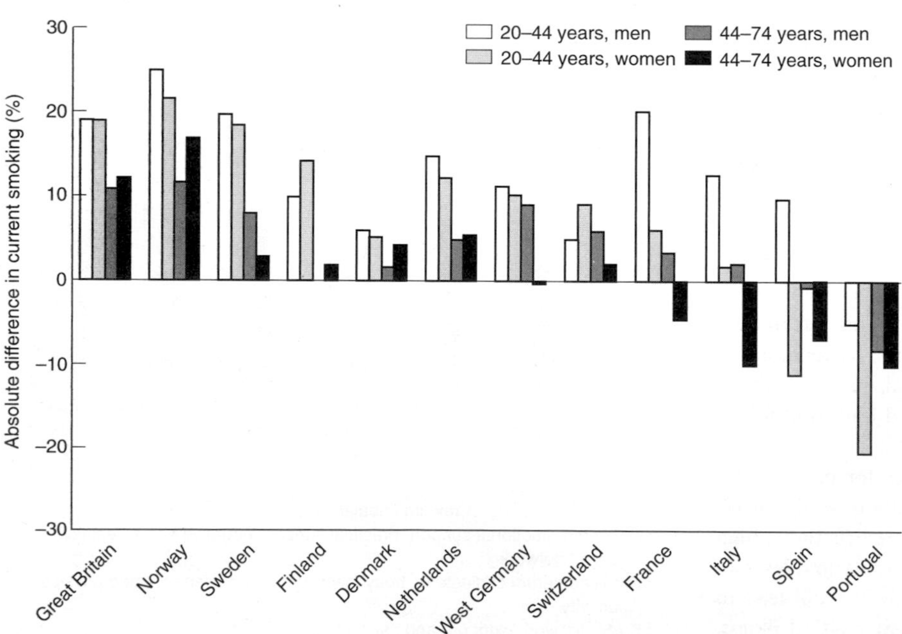

Fig. 10 Inequalities in smoking by level of education in 10 European countries, by sex and age group. Prevalence rate differences for up to lower secondary education versus upper secondary education and higher. Source: Cavelaars et al. 2000.)

that reducing inequalities in health is an individual instead of a public responsibility (Macintyre 1997). As a reaction, some researchers have tried to de-emphasize the importance of health-related behaviour. However, it can easily be shown that this is a false antithesis; the higher rates of smoking in the lower socio-economic groups may be a way of coping with unfavourable material circumstances (see Fig. 7) (Graham 1995; Stronks *et al.* 1997; Schrijvers *et al.* 1999). Health-related behaviour is a more 'proximal' risk factor, but may nevertheless be an important element of the causal chain linking low socio-economic status to ill-health.

This is clearly illustrated by the results of some of the international comparisons described above. Within Europe the Nordic countries are characterized by relatively large inequalities in cardiovascular disease mortality, and this is likely to be due to the strong social patterning of behavioural risk factors, which is seen in these countries (Kunst *et al.* 1998, 1999; Cavelaars *et al.* 2000). Egalitarian social and economic policies do not seem to protect a population against strong social gradients in health-related behaviour. There may even be a causal connection, in the sense that a reduction of inequalities in wealth and income reduces the opportunities for status acquisition on the basis of material advantage, which may lead to an increased tendency towards differentiation in cultural terms, for example in lifestyles (Bourdieu and Translated by Nice 1984). In any case, specific interventions and policies may be needed to reduce inequalities in health-related behaviour, even in the presence of maximum efforts to reduce inequalities in material factors.

Life-course perspective

Our discussion of the explanation of socio-economic inequalities in health has so far largely ignored the importance of time; disease usually occurs as a result of prolonged exposure to risk factors, and exposure to these risk factors may be the result of long individual life histories. Explanatory schemes such as those of Fig. 7, apply to a relatively small section of the life of an individual (e.g. middle age) and are based on explanatory studies, which also involve similarly short follow-up periods. Recently, the limitations of this approach for understanding socio-economic inequalities in health have been recognized, as a result of studies demonstrating an association between intrauterine and infant conditions and disease in middle age (Barker 1992) and of long-term follow-up studies of birth cohorts showing how health in adulthood reflects circumstances at earlier stages of life (Power *et al.* 1991).

Figure 11 illustrates how a life-course perspective could be applied to socio-economic inequalities in health. Socio-economic status in childhood (e.g. father's occupational class) determines socio-economic status in adulthood (despite social mobility many adults are in the same occupational class as their parents), and it has been shown that lifelong exposure to low socio-economic status carries higher risks of ill-health than exposure during one stage of life only (Davey Smith *et al.* 1997). Many health-related behaviours (e.g. smoking) are formed in adolescence, i.e. under the influence of socio-economic status in childhood, and it has been shown that socio-economic inequalities in health-related behaviour are partly the result of different exposures to low socio-economic status in childhood (van de Mheen *et al.* 1998*a*). The same is likely to apply to other intermediary factors, such as coping styles, locus of control, and other psychosocial factors (Bosma *et al.* 1999). Health may have a certain continuity

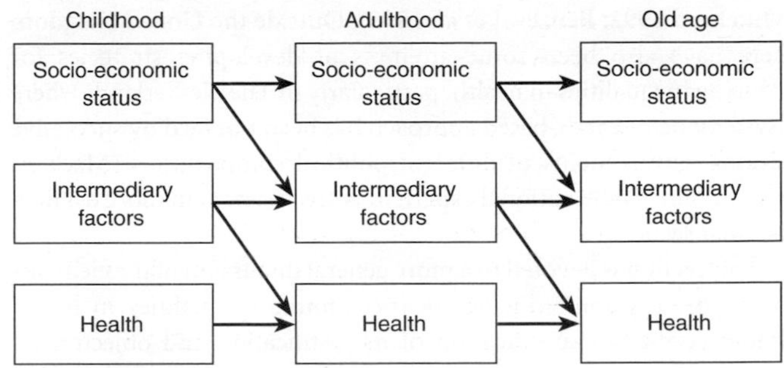

Fig. 11 A life-course perspective on the explanation of socio-economic inequalities in health.

across the life-course, with ill-health in adulthood tracking back to ill-health in childhood and therefore to determinants acting in earlier stages of life (Wadsworth 1997; van de Mheen *et al.* 1998*b*). Socio-economic inequalities in health may thus be due to the cumulative effect of disadvantage across the life-course.

Health during one stage of the life-course may also affect socio-economic status in a later stage, owing to processes of health-related selection (see the discussion of selection and causation above). The life-course perspective enables us to see more clearly the iterative nature of some of these processes and suggests a 'co-evolution' of social position and health, taking away the sharp contradiction between 'selection' and 'causation' explanations (Vågerö and Illsley 1995; van de Mheen *et al.* 1998*c*).

Implications for policy

At first sight, the life-course perspective suggests that interventions and policies targeting children and young adults should be prioritized. Many studies employing a life-course perspective have demonstrated that some of the roots of socio-economic inequalities in health can be found in the first decades of life. Interventions and policies aiming to reduce material or health disadvantage in childhood and adolescence, or breaking the chain between social and health development, are likely to contribute to smaller socio-economic inequalities in health over the entire life-course. On the other hand, the life-course perspective also suggests that all phases of the life-course are important. If it is true that the health disadvantage in the lower socio-economic groups is the result of cumulative health damage occurring over the entire life-course, then it is also important to reduce health damage occurring in later stages of life. There are critical periods, and while some of these are in early life (e.g. birth, move from primary to secondary school, entry into labour market), others are in later life (e.g. occupational change, onset of chronic illness, retirement). Social security systems have an important role to ensure that these critical periods do not result in cumulative disadvantage (Blane 1999).

The options: how to build a strategy to reduce inequalities in health?

Introduction

During the 1990s several attempts were made to develop strategies for reducing inequalities in health (Whitehead 1990; Dahlgren and

Whitehead 1992; Benzeval *et al.* 1995). Outside the United Kingdom there have also been some attempts at developing strategies for reducing inequalities in health, particularly in The Netherlands where a systematic research-based approach has been pursued by successive national governments of different political compositions (Mackenbach 1994*a*). These national experiences are reviewed in more detail in the final section.

This section is devoted to a more general discussion of the elements that a strategy for reducing socio-economic inequalities in health should contain: a specification of its justification and objectives, a package of policies and interventions, and facilities for evaluation and monitoring. Important choices have to be made for each of these elements.

Justification and objectives

What is a fair distribution of health?

It is important to note that it cannot be taken for granted that socio-economic inequalities in health are unfair. According to Whitehead's normative analysis, inequalities in health can only be labelled 'unjust' if they are perceived as both 'unacceptable' and potentially 'avoidable' (Table 1). Socio-economic inequalities in health which arise as a result of natural biological variation or of freely chosen health-damaging behaviour will not commonly be perceived as 'unacceptable'. However, inequalities in health resulting from health-damaging behaviour not chosen freely, or exposure to health hazards in the environment, or impaired access to health care services will be perceived as 'unacceptable' and are also potentially avoidable (Whitehead 1990).

This type of reasoning is generally accepted as a basis for policy-making on socio-economic inequalities in health. However, the 'perception' of acceptability of inequalities in health will very much be determined by one's theory of justice. Implicit in this type of reasoning is an egalitarian perspective, in which the fairness of a certain distribution of goods is judged on the basis of the equality of the outcome of the process of distribution. Regardless of how the process occurs (with only few exceptions, such as freely chosen health-damaging behaviour), more ill-health in the lower than in the higher socio-economic groups is seen to be unfair simply because some people have less of the highly valued good 'health' than others. In contrast, in a strictly libertarian perspective the justness of a certain distribution of goods is judged on the basis of characteristics of the process of distribution. The main criterion is whether the process of distribution is determined by 'freely negotiated transfers in the market-place'. Some people are more successful in using their opportunities than others; on the basis of their value in the employment market they obtain well-paid and safe jobs, and they can afford to live in comfortable houses in nice neighbourhoods. That others do not and as a result experience more ill-health can only be labelled unfair, in this view, if there has not been freedom of opportunity (de Jong and Rutten 1983).

It is important to analyse different political ideologies with regard to their implications for the judgement of socio-economic inequalities in health, and to choose one's normative justification carefully, if only because this may increase one's capacity for building broad coalitions. One interesting approach is to regard health as a 'resource', not as a 'good' or an end in itself (Sen 1985, 1990). Health then determines a person's capacity to operate in the various 'market-places' of society, and even a strict adherence to the libertarian theory of justice would probably agree that more ill-health in the lower socio-economic groups may be a danger to the free operation of markets. This is particularly the case when ill-health really determines a person's opportunities in life, as for children born to parents in lower social classes who because of ill-health may have less successful school careers. In the case of adults, one could argue that the higher frequency of ill-health in the lower social classes should be a reason for concern among libertarians, because ill-health is an important determinant of employment prospects.

What should the goal be?

There are also various options with regard to the (quantitative) specification of the objectives of policies and interventions to reduce socio-economic inequalities in health. The target agreed upon by the member states of the World Health Organization (**WHO**) European

Table 1 Whitehead's scheme for judging the (un)fairness of socio-economic inequalities in health

	Determinant of health differentials	Potentially avoidable	Commonly viewed as unacceptable
1.	Natural, biological variation	No	No
2.	Health-damaging behaviour if freely chosen	Yes	No
3.	Transient health advantage of groups who take up health-promoting behaviour first (if other groups can easily catch up)	Yes	No
4.	Health-damaging behaviour where choice of lifestyle is restricted by socio-economic factors	Yes	Yes
5.	Exposure to excessive health hazards in physical and social environment	Yes	Yes
6.	Restricted access to essential health care	Yes	Yes
7.	Health-related downward social mobility (sick people move down social scale)	Low income—yes	Low income—yes

Source: Whitehead (1990).

Region was that 'by the year 2000, the actual differences in health status ... should be reduced by at least 25 per cent, by improving the level of health of disadvantaged ... groups' (WHO 1985). Although this target has been immensely helpful in putting inequalities in health on the policy agenda, it has also been widely criticized because of its vagueness.

If one wants to be more precise, there is a large choice of possible measures for the size of socio-economic inequalities in health (Mackenbach and Kunst 1997). One of the most important distinctions is that between relative measures, such as rate ratios, and absolute measures, such as rate differences. This distinction is illustrated in Fig. 3 on the basis of an international comparison of inequalities in mortality among middle-aged men. Absolute inequalities are much smaller in Sweden than in Ireland, not because relative inequalities are smaller but because the average rate of mortality is smaller in Sweden. It can be argued that absolute inequalities are more relevant for public health policy than relative inequalities; it is the size of the absolute inequalities that directly influences a person's life chances, and therefore the primary aim should be to reduce absolute inequalities in health.

If one accepts this line of reasoning, and specifies objectives in terms of a reduction of absolute differences, the number of available policy options increases substantially. Any policy or intervention that reduces average rates of mortality or morbidity, without changing the size of the relative inequalities, will help in achieving this objective. Investing in overall improvements of population health, while taking care to achieve similar relative rates of improvement in higher and lower socio-economic groups, is a potentially powerful way of reducing inequalities in health and does not even require an explicit commitment to reducing inequalities in health.

What can realistically be achieved?

The WHO equity target was agreed upon in 1984 and has not been reached. Is this because national governments have not made serious efforts, or because the target was too ambitious? A recent review of policies and interventions to reduce socio-economic inequalities in health in Finland, The Netherlands, Spain, Sweden, and the United Kingdom has shown that, despite good intentions in some countries, the scale and intensity of the efforts have been very modest (Mackenbach and Droomers 1999).

One could also rightly argue that the target was far too ambitious. In many countries there is evidence of an, apparently spontaneous, widening of socio-economic inequalities in health. This widening has occurred not only in countries with increasing income inequalities, such as the United Kingdom, but also in countries with narrowing income inequalities, such as Finland (Valkonen *et al.* 1993). Although some of the widening of health inequalities may be an adverse effect of the introduction of libertarian economic policies, it is likely that the underlying 'spontaneous' trends would have counteracted any beneficial effect of serious efforts to implement the WHO equity target.

What can realistically be achieved is a function of, first, underlying 'spontaneous' trends and, second, the potential effect of interventions and policies that will be implemented. Making such estimates is a difficult exercise, and there is a great need for formal methods to estimate the potential effect of interventions and policies to reduce inequalities in health. Recently, the WHO renewed its equity target to be included in the new Health 21 Strategy (WHO 1999) (Box 1). While the target has become more specific, it is still very ambitious and is unlikely to be achieved unless spontaneous trends and systematic interventions and policies work together in the coming decades.

Box 1 Equity targets in the WHO Health 21 strategy (WHO 1999)

Target 2: equity in health

By the year 2020, the health gap between socio-economic groups within countries should be reduced by at least one-fourth in all member states, by substantially improving the level of health of disadvantaged groups.

In particular:

2.1 The gap in life expectancy between socio-economic groups should be reduced by at least 25%.

2.2 The values for major indicators of morbidity, disability and mortality in groups across the socio-economic gradient should be more equitably distributed.

2.3 Socio-economic conditions that produce adverse health effects, notably differences in income, educational achievement, and access to the labour market, should be substantially improved.

2.4 The proportion of the population living in poverty should be greatly reduced.

2.5 People having special needs as a result of their health, social, or economic circumstances should be protected from exclusion and given easy access to appropriate care.

Package of policies and interventions

Any attempt to reduce socio-economic inequalities in health should of course be based on an understanding of their causes. The explanatory models discussed earlier suggest the following options for intervention and policy:

- to reduce inequalities in education/occupation/income
- to reduce the effect of ill-health on education/occupation/income
- to reduce inequalities in specific determinants ('intermediary' material, psychosocial, and behavioural factors).

A fourth option could be added to this:

- to increase supply of health care in lower socio-economic groups (Mackenbach 1994*a*).

Choosing between these options, and between the specific interventions and policies within each option, may be a difficult task.

'Upstream' or 'downstream' solutions?

At first sight offering extra health care is not the most attractive option for reducing inequalities in health. It is expensive and can never totally eliminate the problem because people will have to fall ill before extra health care can repair the damage. Also, really effective health care interventions are scarce. It has all the disadvantages of a 'downstream' solution, with only one serious advantage—decisions about reallocation of resources within the health sector are at least partly under the control of health policy-makers.

In contrast, changing the basic socio-economic distributions is intuitively much more attractive. Where one knows the fundamental causes of health problems, it is appropriate to address these directly, and to try to reduce the prevalence of a low socio-economic status, by preventing children from leaving school with no or low qualifications, by increasing employment opportunities and abolishing low-status jobs, and/or by reducing poverty. It would seem that this is likely to have more leverage than addressing more immediate causes, let alone offering extra health care. Each fundamental cause is linked to a variety of more immediate causes, and through these to an even larger variety of health effects. Also, one avoids the possibility that after one of the more immediate causes has been eliminated, other immediate causes take its place because the same fundamental causes are still in operation. It has all the advantages of an 'upstream' solution, with only one serious disadvantage—decisions about basic socio-economic distributions are not taken by health policy-makers.

This intuitive comparison of 'downstream' and 'upstream' solutions may be theoretically valid, but it is important to note that there is no empirical evidence to support the claim that 'upstream' interventions are more effective for reducing health inequalities than 'downstream' interventions. Therefore choices will have to be made on other grounds as well, including well-documented effects on non-health-related outcomes of upstream policies or simply political feasibility.

Evidence-based policy-making?

Lack of evidence on effectiveness of interventions and policies is a general problem in this area. As the final section will show, policy-makers can choose from very large 'menus' of specific interventions and policies. These large menus certainly have positive aspects. They provide policy-makers with considerable decision latitude, which may increase their possibilities for political coalition building as well as for recruiting different organizations to achieve their objectives. On the other hand, these large menus also betray the uncertainty of their authors with regard to what would really help (Mackenbach 1995*b*). Recent reviews have shown that the evidence base for policy-making is rather unsatisfactory; evaluation studies reported in the international literature cover only a few of the options currently considered, suffer from methodological weaknesses, and do not always show positive effects of interventions (Arblaster *et al.* 1995; Gepkens and Gunning-Schepers 1996). An informal meta-analysis of studies fulfilling basic methodological criteria suggests that interventions that combine different approaches (e.g. health education combined with structural measures) are most effective in reducing inequalities in health (Table 2).

Evaluation and monitoring

How to evaluate?

As the earlier section on packages of policies and interventions has shown there is a great need here for 'evidence-based' policies and interventions. However, the complexity of evaluation should not be overlooked. This complexity follows from two specific characteristics of policies and interventions to reduce socio-economic inequalities in health.

The first is that the aim is not to reduce some average value of a health outcome, but to reduce a difference in health between groups. In the simpler case of interventions, which aim to reduce an average value, a minimum of four measurements is required: one 'before' and one 'after' measurement in an experimental and a control group. In this more complex situation, a minimum of eight measurements is required: one 'before' and one 'after' measurement in both higher and lower socio-economic groups in both the experimental and the control population (Mackenbach and Gunning-Schepers 1997). This design can only be simplified if some relatively strong assumptions are fulfilled. For example, if one can assume that the intervention does not influence the higher socio-economic groups, four measurements in the lower socio-economic group could be sufficient.

The second is that many policies and interventions will have to be 'collective' or population based in nature. This implies that assignment to the intervention or policy cannot be done on an individual basis, but only on a collective basis (e.g. schools, neighbourhoods, or even whole countries). Consequently, the randomized controlled trial will often not be the design of first choice. Sometimes the design of the community intervention trial can be used, when a select allocation of schools or neighbourhoods to either an experimental or control condition can be performed (Koepsell *et al.* 1992, 1995). With increasing levels of aggregation, however, experimentation becomes less and less feasible; in the extreme example of changes in national legislation a fully experimental evaluation of the policy is clearly impossible. This implies that experimental designs other than the classical type will frequently have to be employed. Quasi-experimental designs, in which the evaluator does not control the allocation of units to the experimental and control condition but chooses control units carefully to match the experimental units, are likely to be helpful alternatives (Campbell and Stanley 1963; Cook and Campbell 1979). The same applies to carefully designed observational studies, in which different types of evidence are creatively combined to support conclusions on effectiveness ('triangulation'). It is extremely import-

Table 2 Overview of evidence on effectiveness of interventions to reduce socio-economic inequalities in health

Types of intervention	Effective	Dubious	Ineffective	Total
Structural measures	11	4	1	16
Existing health care	5	3	3	11
Health education				
Providing information	6	6	4	16
Providing information + personal support	32	12	5	49
Health promotion + structural measures	2	1	—	3
Remainder	2	1	—	3
Total	58	27	13	98

Source: Gepkens and Gunning-Schepers (1996)

ant that the impossibility of employing classical experimental designs is not used as an excuse for not evaluating at all.

How to increase learning speed?

No single country has the capacity of contributing more than a fraction of the necessary knowledge to support strategies for reducing inequalities in health. This is not only a matter of restricted manpower or financial resources for research, but also of restricted opportunities for implementing policies and interventions. Some policies can be implemented in some countries, but not in others because they have already been implemented or are politically completely unfeasible. Different countries present different opportunities for evaluation, and therefore international exchange and perhaps co-ordination is necessary. There is an important role for international agencies, such as the European Union, to support this development.

How to remain visible?

Reducing inequalities in health requires systematic and prolonged action, and the likelihood of continuing commitment from policy-makers can be enhanced if socio-economic inequalities in health remain clearly visible to policy-makers as well as to the general public (including the media). Continuous monitoring of inequalities in health by bureaux of statistics and other agencies is likely to help in achieving this, as well as putting inequalities in health on the agendas of, for example, health research funding agencies (Gunning-Schepers 1989).

The options: experiences in the United Kingdom and The Netherlands

Introduction

In this section we will review the experiences of two countries, the United Kingdom and The Netherlands, in the field of interventions and policies to reduce socio-economic inequalities in health. These countries have been chosen because their experiences have been relatively well documented in the international literature, and also because they represent very different traditions. The United Kingdom is characterized by a long tradition of research in this area, dating back to the nineteenth century, which has resulted in a very rich knowledge base that has benefited researchers and policy-makers in many other countries as well. Another characteristic, perhaps not unrelated to this long tradition, is the strong political polarization of the debate on socio-economic inequalities in health in the United Kingdom. To their surprise, foreign observers will discover that different types of explanation have become linked to different political ideologies. In The Netherlands, on the other hand, there is a much shorter tradition of research on socio-economic inequalities in health, as in many other countries in continental Europe. Since the late 1980s a focused effort has been made to build a knowledge base for policy-making, and so far strong political polarization of the debate has not occurred. There is a broad consensus that inequalities in health are unfair, and that ways should be found to reduce inequalities in health. To their surprise, foreign observers will discover that the Dutch hope to find an engineering solution.

United Kingdom

The *Black Report* not only presented an influential explanatory framework, but also a set of recommendations, which has very much shaped the debate on reducing inequalities in health both inside and outside the United Kingdom (Macintyre 1997). Its recommendations focused on improving material living conditions and were very unwelcome to the Conservative government to which they were issued (Townsend *et al.* 1988*a*). For years there was little room for discussing policies to reduce inequalities in health, but in the early 1990s the political climate gradually changed. Whitehead's work for the WHO mentioned above (Whitehead 1990; Whitehead and Dahlgren 1991) was taken a step further in a King's Fund report (Benzeval *et al.* 1995), which discussed a wide range of policy options for one example in each of four different policy areas: physical environment (example: housing), social and economic influences (example: income maintenance), 'barriers to adopting a healthier personal lifestyle' (example: smoking), and 'access to appropriate and effective health and social services' (example: the role of the National Health Service).

When after many years of Conservative government a Labour government came to power in 1997, it made a clear commitment to reducing social inequalities, including socio-economic health inequalities. It asked a committee chaired by Sir Donald Acheson to perform an 'independent inquiry into inequalities in health' and to develop suggestions for policies aiming to reduce health inequalities. These were published in 1998 and subsequently partly incorporated in national (health) policies. The Acheson Report (Box 2) is the most comprehensive of all the reports cited so far. Interestingly, while it acknowledges the importance of health-related behaviour for the explanation of socio-economic inequalities in health, it does not include a chapter on lifestyle factors (these are treated as a component of other areas). Instead, and surprisingly, it has a chapter on mobility and transport, and discusses various target groups. It contains 123 recommendations in 11 areas for 'future policy development', and has been criticized for its resemblance to a shopping list (Davey Smith *et al.* 1998; Shaw *et al.* 1999).

To varying degrees, each of these reports published in the United Kingdom shows awareness of the need to provide evidence for its recommendations. Typically, this is observational evidence on the importance of the target factor for socio-economic inequalities in health, and not experimental evidence on the effectiveness of the proposed interventions and policies. The Acheson Report contains the most systematic attempt at reviewing the (quasi-)experimental evidence available to support its recommendations. Although such evidence is available for only a minority of the recommendations, the report clearly points the way to a more systematic evaluation of the interventions it recommends (Anonymous 1998).

Because the New Labour government that came into power in 1997 committed itself to the reduction of social inequality in general, the United Kingdom also offers interesting opportunities for evaluating social and economic policies with a potential impact on health. Table 3 gives a summary of a number of recent initiatives that may contribute to a reduction of socio-economic inequalities in health. Some of the measures, such as the introduction of a national minimum wage, have been taken in other countries long before 1997, but it would be interesting to all countries to know whether this has an

Box 2 A summary of the recommendations of the Acheson Report

Independent inquiry into inequalities in health
Chair: Sir Donald Acheson
Report: November 1998
Recommendations
I. General recommendations
II. Areas for future policy development
1. Poverty, income, tax, and benefits
2. Education
3. Employment
4. Housing and environment
5. Mobility, transport, and pollution
6. Nutrition and the Common Agricultural Policy
7. Mothers, children, and families
8. Young people and adults of working age
9. Older people
10. Ethnicity
11. Gender
III The National Health Service
Examples
We recommend:

- that all policies should be evaluated in terms of their impact on health inequalities...
- policies which will further reduce income inequalities...
- the further development of high quality pre-school education...
- good management practices which lead to increased control, variety and appropriate use of skills in the workforce...
- policies to improve insulation and heating systems
- measures to encourage walking and cycling
- policies which reduce the sodium content of processed foods
- increases in the real price of tobacco...
- development of services which are sensitive to the needs of ethnic minority groups...
- policies to reduce the fear of crime and violence...
- giving priority to a more equitable allocation of NHS resources

effect on inequalities in health. Other measures, such as the area-based programmes targeting different 'Action Zones', are innovations, which if successful may become a source of inspiration for many other countries (Graham *et al.* 1999).

The Netherlands

Socio-economic inequalities in health were a non-issue in The Netherlands until the early 1980s. In 1980, The Netherlands' Society for Social Medicine celebrated its fiftieth anniversary with a conference on socio-economic inequalities in health, which approximately coincided with the work on the *Black Report* in the United Kingdom. In the same year, the results of a study on inequalities in morbidity and mortality between neighbourhoods in Amsterdam were published, and to the surprise of many clearly demonstrated the existence of socio-economic inequalities in health in The Netherlands (Lau-Ijzerman *et al.* 1981). Although there was no direct follow-up to these initiatives, they laid the basis for the later adoption by The Netherlands' government of the Health for All policy targets of WHO, including the equity target. As a result, in 1986 the Ministry of Public Health included a paragraph on inequalities in health in a major policy document for the very first time.

From then on, initiatives were taken from inside the Ministry to put equity in health on the political as well as the research agenda (Gunning-Schepers 1989). In 1987 a conference was held under the aegis of the prestigious Scientific Council for Government Policy, and major press coverage was arranged for the publication of its proceedings (Wetenschappelijke Raad 1987). The report recommended, among other things, a national research programme which the Ministry launched in 1989. The main objective of this programme was to generate more knowledge on socio-economic inequalities in health in The Netherlands, both descriptive and explanatory. The programme was completed in 1994, and its results were reported widely in national and international journals, as well as in a book (Mackenbach 1994*b*) and a report to the Ministry (Programme Committee Socio-Economic Health Differences 1994). The latter contained a number of general policy recommendations covering all four areas mentioned above.

An evaluation of the research programme showed that it had a measurable impact on the scientific community, at least in the short run. Widespread involvement of research groups with socio-economic inequalities in health was generated. As a result the number of scientific publications on the topic had clearly increased, far more than could have been expected from studies directly funded from the programme. Also, the knowledge base had increased substantially. Not only the size and pattern of socio-economic inequalities in health in The Netherlands, but also the role of housing and working conditions, psychosocial factors, and lifestyle factors in the explanation of socio-economic inequalities in health, had been documented (Mackenbach 1994*a*).

The report on the programme also recommended launching a second programme focusing on the development and evaluation of interventions to reduce socio-economic inequalities in health. The new government, which came into power in 1994, adopted this

Table 3 Recent social and economic initiatives in the United Kingdom, which may help in reducing socio-economic inequalities in health

Employment-related initiatives
Welfare-to-work programme ('New Deal'): increasing the skills and employability of unemployed people
Working Family Tax Credit: more entitlements, more generous benefits
National minimum wage
Area-focused initiatives
Health Action Zones: 26 disadvantaged areas receive funding for innovative health policy
Initiatives to tackle social exclusion
National Strategy for Neighbourhood Renewal: 'New Deal for Communities'

Source: Graham *et al.* (1999).

Table 4 Overview of interventions evaluated in the second national research programme on socio-economic inequalities in health in The Netherlands

Projects in first round
Folic acid supplementation
Teeth brushing at school
Early intervention in social psychiatry
Brick-lifting machine for brick-layers
Education of Turkish diabetics
Projects in the second round
Community intervention in the city of Arnhem
Changes in work organization for elderly employees with physically demanding work
Practice nurse for general practices in deprived areas
Reduction of sickness absence among school pupils
School-based prevention of starting smoking among teenagers

recommendation, and sponsored a second national research programme, which ran from 1995 to 2000. Table 4 gives an overview of the interventions that were subjected to (quasi-)experimental evaluation. As is clear from this list, these are mostly small-scale interventions in specific settings. Although an attempt has been made to cover all the main policy areas, the focus is on interventions targeting specific determinants (intermediary factors). Results of evaluation studies will become available in 2000.

Conclusions

As this chapter has shown, socio-economic inequalities in health are a major challenge to public health. Inequalities in health are substantial and universal, and are unlikely to disappear spontaneously. Their explanation is only partly understood, and many of the factors are resistant to intervention. Nevertheless, the ambition has arisen to try to reduce inequalities in health. This requires systematic and prolonged efforts which in multiparty democracies will only be possible if broad coalitions can be built. Political will should be mobilized, not only to implement the recommendations for interventions and policies, but also to sponsor the research necessary to evaluate the effects. After documenting the existence of inequalities in health and studying their explanation, there is one further challenge to researchers in this area—assessing the effectiveness of interventions aimed at reducing these inequalities in health.

Attempts at reducing inequalities in health cannot but be illustrations of Rudolf Virchow's famous dictum 'Medicine is a social science, and politics is nothing than medicine at a grand scale' (Ackerknecht and Virchow 1953). Let us try to make this a rational form of medicine.

References

Ackerknecht, E.H. and Virchow, R. (1953). *Doctor, statesman, anthropologist.* University of Wisconsin Press, Madison, WI.

Anonymous (1998). *Independent inquiry into inequalities in health.* HMSO, London.

Arblaster, L., *et al.* (1995). *Review of the research on the effectiveness of health service interventions to reduce variations in health.* CRD Report No. 3, NHS Centre for Reviews and Dissemination, York.

Bairagi, R., Koenig, M.A., and Mazumder, K.A. (1993). Mortality-discriminating power of some nutritional, sociodemographic, and diarrheal disease indices. *American Journal of Epidemiology,* **138,** 310–17.

Barker, D.J.P. (1992). *Fetal and infant origins of adult disease.* BMJ Publishing, London.

Benzeval, M., Judge, K., and Whitehead, M. (1995). *Tackling inequalities in health; an agenda for action.* King's Fund, London.

Blane, D. (1999). The life course, the social gradient, and health. In *Social determinants of health* (ed. M. Marmot and R.G. Wilkinson). Oxford University Press.

Bloor, M., Samphier, M., and Prior, L. (1987). Artefact explanations of inequalities in health: an assessment of the evidence. *Sociology of Health and Illness,* **9,** 231–64.

Bolton-Smith, C., Smith, W.C., Woodward, M., and Tunstall-Pedoe, H. (1991). Nutrient intakes of different social-class groups: results from the Scottish Heart Health Study (SHHS). *British Journal of Nutrition,* **65,** 321–35.

Bosma, H., van de Mheen, H.D., and Mackenbach, J.P. (1999). Social class in childhood and general health in adulthood: questionnaire study of contribution of psychological attributes. *British Medical Journal,* **318,** 18–22.

Bourdieu, P. (1984). *Distinction. A social critique of the judgement of taste* (trans. R. Nice). Harvard University Press, Cambridge, MA.

Brunner, E. and Marmot, M. (1999). Social organization, stress, and health. In *Social determinants of health* (ed. M. Marmot and R.G. Wilkinson). Oxford University Press.

Campbell, D.T. and Stanley, J.C. (1963). *Experimental and quasi-experimental designs for research.* Rand McNally, Skokie, IL.

Carroll, D., Bennett, P., and Davey Smith, G. (1993). Socio-economic health inequalities: their origins and implications. *Psychology and Health,* **8,** 295–316.

Carstairs, V. and Morris, R. (1989). Deprivation and mortality: an alternative to social class? *Community Medicine,* 11, 210–19. (Erratum, *Community Medicine,* **11**(4).)

Cavelaars, A.E., Kunst, A.E., and Mackenbach, J.P. (1997). Socio-economic differences in risk factors for morbidity and mortality in the European Community: an international comparison. *Journal of Health Psychology,* **2,** 353–72.

Cavelaars, A.E., Kunst, A.E., Geurts, J.J., *et al.* (1998*a*). Differences in self reported morbidity by educational level: a comparison of 11 western European countries. *Journal of Epidemiology and Community Health,* **52,** 219–27.

Cavelaars, A.E., Kunst, A.E., Geurts, J.J., *et al.* (1998*b*). Morbidity differences by occupational class among men in seven European countries: an application of the Erikson–Goldthorpe social class scheme. *International Journal of Epidemiology,* **27,** 222–30.

Cavelaars, A.E., Kunst, A.E., Geurts, J.J., *et al.* (2000). Educational differences in smoking: an international comparison. *British Medical Journal,* **320,** 1102–7.

Chave, S.P.W. (1984). The origins and development of public health. In *Oxford textbook of public health* (ed. W.W. Holland, R. Detels, and G. Knox). Oxford University Press.

Cipolla, C.M. and Zanetti, D.E. (1972). Peste et mortalité differentielle. *Annales de Démographie Historique,* **3,** 197–202.

Coleman, W. (1982). *Death is a social disease; public health and political economy in early industrial France.* University of Wisconsin, Madison, WI.

Cook, T.D. and Campbell, D.T. (1979). *Quasi-experimentation: design and analysis issues for field settings.* Rand McNally, Skokie, IL.

Cummins, R.O., Shaper, A.G., Walker, M., and Wale, C.J. (1981). Smoking and drinking by middle-aged British men: effects of social class and town of residence. *British Medical Journal (Clinical Research Edition)*, **283**, 1497–502.

Dahl, E. (1991). Socioeconomic inequalities in mortality among women and among men: an international study. *Sociology of Health and Illness*, **13**, 492–505.

Dahlgren, G. and Whitehead, M. (1992). *Policies and strategies to promote equity in health.* World Health Organization, Copenhagen.

Davey Smith, G. and Brunner, E. (1997). Socio-economic differentials in health: the role of nutrition. *Proceedings of the Nutrition Society*, **56**, 75–90.

Davey Smith, G., Shipley, M.J., and Rose, G. (1990). Magnitude and causes of socioeconomic differentials in mortality: further evidence from the Whitehall Study. *Journal of Epidemiology and Community Health*, **44**, 265–70.

Davey Smith, G., Leon, D., Shipley, M.J., and Rose, G. (1991). Socioeconomic differentials in cancer among men. *International Journal of Epidemiology*, **20**, 339–45.

Davey Smith, G., Blane, D., and Bartley, M. (1994). Explanations for socio-economic differentials in mortality.Evidence from Britain and elsewhere. *European Journal of Public Health*, **4**, 131–44.

Davey Smith, G., Neaton, J.D., Wentworth, D., Stamler, R., and Stamler, J. (1996). Socioeconomic differentials in mortality risk among men screened in the Multiple Risk Factor Intervention Trial: I. White men. *American Journal of Public Health*, **86**, 486–96.

Davey Smith, G., Hart, C., Blane, D., Gillis, C., and Hawthorne, V. (1997). Lifetime socioeconomic position and mortality: prospective observational study. *British Medical Journal*, **314**, 547–52.

Davey Smith, G., Morris, J.N., and Shaw, M. (1998). The independent inquiry into inequalities in health is welcome, but its recommendations are too cautious and vague. *British Medical Journal*, **317**, 1465–6.

de Jong, G.A. and Rutten, F.F.H. (1983). Justice and health for all. *Social Science and Medicine*, **17**, 1085–95.

Dennis, B.H., Zhukovsky, G.S., Shestov, D.B., *et al.* (1993). The association of education with coronary heart disease mortality in the USSR lipid research clinics study. *International Journal of Epidemiology*, **22**, 420–7.

Drever, F. and Bunting, J. (1997). Patterns and trends in male mortality. In *Health inequalities* (ed. F. Drever and M. Whitehead). HMSO, London.

Duncan, B.B., Rumel, D., Zelmanowicz, A., Mengue, S.S., dos Santos, S., and Dalmaz, A. (1995). Social inequality in mortality in Sao Paulo State, Brazil. *International Journal of Epidemiology*, **24**, 359–65.

Fox, A.J., Goldblatt, P.O., and Adelstein, A.M. (1982). Selection and mortality differentials. *Journal of Epidemiology and Community Health*, **36**, 69–79.

Fox, A.J., Goldblatt, P.O., and Jones, D.R. (1985). Social class mortality differentials: artefact, selection or life circumstances? *Journal of Epidemiology and Community Health*, **39**, 1–8.

Gepkens, A. and Gunning-Schepers, L.J. (1996). Interventions to reduce socioeconomic health differences: a review of the international literature. *European Journal of Public Health*, **6**, 218–26.

Goldblatt, P. (1990). Mortality and alternative social classifications. In *Longitudinal study: mortality and social organisation* (ed. P. Goldblatt), pp. 163–192. HMSO, London.

Goldman, N. (1994). Social factors and health: the causation–selection issue revisited. *Proceedings of the National Academy of Sciences of the United States of America*, **91**, 1251–5.

Graham, H. (1995). Cigarette smoking: a light on gender and class inequality in Great Britain? *Journal of Social Policy*, **24**, 509–27.

Graham, H., Benzeval, M., and Whitehead, M. (1999). Social and economic policies in the UK with a potential impact on health inequalities. In *Interventions and policies to reduce socio-economic inequalities in health* (ed. J.P. Mackenbach and M. Droomers). Department of Public Health, Erasmus University Rotterdam.

Groenhof, F., *et al.* and the EU Working Group on Socioeconomic Inequalities in Health (1996). *Socio-economic inequalities in morbidity and mortality in Central and Eastern Europe: a comparison to some Western European countries.* Department of Public Health, Erasmus University Rotterdam.

Gunning-Schepers, L.J. (1989). How to put equity in health on the political agenda. *Health Promotion*, **4**, 149–50.

Heck, K.E. and Pamuk, E.R. (1997). Explaining the relation between education and postmenopausal breast cancer. *American Journal of Epidemiology*, **145**, 366–72.

Hoeymans, N., Smit, H.A., Verkleij, H., and Kromhout, D. (1996). Cardiovascular risk factors in relation to educational level in 36 000 men and women in The Netherlands. *European Heart Journal*, **17**, 518–25.

Holme, I., Helgeland, A., Hjermann, I., Leren, P., and Lund-Larsen, P.G. (1981). Physical activity at work and at leisure in relation to coronary risk factors and social class. A 4-year mortality follow-up. The Oslo study. *Acta Medica Scandinavica*, **209**, 277–83.

Huizinga, J. (1976). *The waning of the Middle Ages.* Penguin, Harmondsworth.

Hupkens, C.L., Knibbe, R.A., and Drop, M.J. (1993). Alcohol consumption in the European community: uniformity and diversity in drinking patterns. *Addiction*, **88**, 1391–404.

Illsley, R. (1955). Social class selection and class differences in relation to stillbirths and infant deaths. *British Medical Journal*, **ii**, 1520–4.

Illsley, R. and Svensson, P.G. (1990). Social inequalities in health. *Social Science and Medicine*, **31**, 223–40.

Jarvis, M.J. and Wardle, J. (1999). Social patterning of individual health behaviours: the case of cigarette smoking. In *Social determinants of health* (ed. M. Marmot and R.G. Wilkinson). Oxford University Press.

Kaplan, G.A. and Keil, J.E. (1993). Socioeconomic factors and cardiovascular disease: a review of the literature. *Circulation*, **88**, 1973–98.

Kaplan, G.A., Pamuk, E.R., Lynch, J.W., Cohen, R.D., and Balfour, J.L. (1996). Inequality in income and mortality in the United States: analysis of mortality and potential pathways. *British Medical Journal*, **312**, 999–1003. (Erratum. *British Medical Journal*, **312**, 1253.)

Karasek, R., Baker, D., Marxer, F., Ahlbom, A., and Theorell, T. (1981). Job decision latitude, job demands, and cardiovascular disease: a prospective study of Swedish men. *American Journal of Public Health*, **71**, 694–705.

Kennedy, B.P., Kawachi, I., and Prothrow-Stith, D. (1996). Income distribution and mortality: cross sectional ecological study of the Robin Hood index in the United States. *British Medical Journal*, **312**, 1004–7. (Erratum. *British Medical Journal*, **312**, 1194.)

Kessler, R.C. and Cleary, P.D. (1980). Social class and psychological distress. *American Sociological Review*, **45**, 463–78.

Koepsell, T.D., Wagner, E.H., Cheadle, A.C., *et al.* (1992). Selected methodological issues in evaluating community-based health promotion and disease prevention programs. *Annual Review of Public Health*, **13**, 31–57.

Koepsell, T.D., Diehr, P.H., Cheadle, A., and Kristal, A. (1995). Invited commentary: Symposium on Community Intervention Trials. *American Journal of Epidemiology*, **142**, 594–9.

Koskinen, S. and Martelin, T. (1994). Why are socioeconomic mortality differences smaller among women than among men? *Social Science and Medicine*, **38**, 1385–96.

Kunst, A.E. (1997). Cross-national comparisons of socio-economic differences in mortality. PhD Thesis, Erasmus University Rotterdam.

Kunst, A.E., Geurts, J.J., and van den Berg, J. (1995). International variation in socioeconomic inequalities in self reported health. *Journal of Epidemiology and Community Health*, **49**, 117–23.

Kunst, A.E., Groenhof, F., Mackenbach, J.P., *et al.* (1998). Occupational class and cause specific mortality in middle aged men in 11 European countries: comparison of population based studies. EU Working Group on Socioeconomic Inequalities in Health. *British Medical Journal*, **316**, 1636–42.

Kunst, A.E., Groenhof, F., Andersen, O., *et al.* (1999). Occupational class and ischemic heart disease mortality in the United States and 11 European countries. *American Journal of Public Health*, **89**, 47–53.

Lahelma, E. and Arber, S. (1994). Health inequalities among men and women in contrasting welfare states. Britain and three Nordic countries compared. *European Journal of Public Health*, **4**, 213–26.

Lang, T. and Ducimetière, P. (1995). Premature cardiovascular mortality in France: divergent evolution between social categories from 1970 to 1990. *International Journal of Epidemiology*, **24**, 331–9.

Lau-Ijzerman, A., Habbema, J.D.F., and van der Maas, P.J. (1981). *Vergelijkend buurtonderzoek Amsterdam*. GGD Amsterdam.

Luft, H.S. (1974). The impact of poor health on earnings. *Review of Economic Statistics*, **65**, 43–57.

Lynch, J.W. and Kaplan, G.A. (1997). Understanding how inequality in the distribution of income affects health. *Journal of Health Psychology*, **2**, 297–314.

Lynch, J.W., Kaplan, G.A., Cohen, R.D., Tuomilehto, J., and Salonen, J.T. (1996). Do cardiovascular risk factors explain the relation between socioeconomic status, risk of all-cause mortality, cardiovascular mortality, and acute myocardial infarction? *American Journal of Epidemiology*, **144**, 934–42.

Lynch, J.W., Kaplan, G.A., and Salonen, J.T. (1997). Why do poor people behave poorly? Variation in adult health behaviours and psychosocial characteristics by stages of the socioeconomic lifecourse. *Social Science and Medicine*, **44**, 809–19.

Macintyre, S. (1997). The Black Report and beyond: what are the issues? *Social Science and Medicine*, **44**, 723–45.

Mackenbach, J.P. (1992). Socio-economic health differences in The Netherlands: a review of recent empirical findings. *Social Science and Medicine*, **34**, 213–26.

Mackenbach, J.P. (1994*a*). Socioeconomic inequalities in health in The Netherlands: impact of a five year research programme. *British Medical Journal*, **309**, 1487–91.

Mackenbach, J.P. (1994*b*). *Ongezonde verschillen; over sociale stratificatie en gezondheid in Nederland*. Van Gorcum, Assen.

Mackenbach, J.P. (1995*a*). Social inequality and death as illustrated in late-medieval death dances. *American Journal of Public Health*, **85**, 1285–92.

Mackenbach, J.P. (1995*b*). Tackling inequalities in health. *British Medical Journal*, **310**, 1152–3.

Mackenbach, J.P. and Droomers, P.C.A. (1999). *Interventions and policies to reduce socioeconomic inequalities in health*. Erasmus University Rotterdam.

Mackenbach, J.P. and Gunning-Schepers, L.J. (1997). How should interventions to reduce inequalities in health be evaluated? *Journal of Epidemiology and Community Health*, **51**, 359–64.

Mackenbach, J.P. and Kunst, A.E. (1997). Measuring the magnitude of socio-economic inequalities in health: an overview of available measures illustrated with two examples from Europe. *Social Science and Medicine*, **44**, 757–71.

Mackenbach, J.P., Looman, C.W., and Kunst, A.E. (1989). Geographic variation in the onset of decline of male ischemic heart disease mortality in The Netherlands. *American Journal of Public Health*, **79**, 1621–7.

Mackenbach, J.P., Kunst, A.E., Cavelaars, A.E., Groenhof, F., and Geurts, J.J. (1997). Socioeconomic inequalities in morbidity and mortality in western Europe.The EU Working Group on Socioeconomic Inequalities in Health. *Lancet*, **349**, 1655–9.

Mackenbach, J.P., Kunst, A.E., Groenhof, F., *et al.* (1999). Socioeconomic inequalities in mortality among women and among men: an international study. *American Journal of Public Health*, **89**, 1800–6.

Mäkelä, P., Valkonen, T., and Martelin, T. (1997). Contribution of deaths related to alcohol use of socioeconomic variation in mortality: register based follow up study. *British Medical Journal*, **315**, 211–16.

Marmot, M.G. and McDowall, M.E. (1986). Mortality decline and widening social inequalities. *Lancet*, **ii**, 274–6. (Erratum. *Lancet*, **i**, 394 (1987).)

Marmot, M.G., Adelstein, A.M., Robinson, N., and Rose, G.A. (1978). Changing social-class distribution of heart disease. *British Medical Journal*, **2**, 1109–12.

Marmot, M.G., Shipley, M.J., and Rose, G. (1984). Inequalities in death—specific explanations of a general pattern? *Lancet*, **i**, 1003–6.

Marmot, M.G., Davey Smith, G., Stansfeld, S., *et al.* (1991). Health inequalities among British civil servants: the Whitehall II study. *Lancet*, **337**, 1387–93.

Marmot, M.G., Bosma, H., Hemingway, H., Brunner, E., and Stansfeld, S. (1997). Contribution of job control and other risk factors to social variations in coronary heart disease incidence. *Lancet*, **350**, 235–9.

Martikainen, P. (1995). Socioeconomic mortality differentials in men and women according to own and spouse's characteristics in Finland. *Sociology of Health and Illness*, **17**, 353–75.

Mielck, A. and do Rosario Giraldes, M. (1993). *Inequalities in health and health care. Review of selected publications from 18 western European countries*. Waxmann, Münster.

Moser, K.A., Pugh, H.S., and Goldblatt, P.O. (1988). Inequalities in women's health: looking at mortality differentials using an alternative approach. *British Medical Journal (Clinical Research Edition)*, **296**, 1221–4.

Osler, M. (1993). Social class and health behaviour in Danish adults: a longitudinal study. *Public Health*, **107**, 251–60.

Pearce, N., Marshall, S., and Borman, B. (1991). Undiminished social class mortality differences in New Zealand men. *New Zealand Medical Journal*, **104**, 153–6.

Perrenoud, A. (1975). L'inégalité sociale devant la mort a Genève au XVIIème siècle. *Population*, **39**, 211–43.

Pierce, J.P. (1989). International comparisons of trends in cigarette smoking prevalence. *American Journal of Public Health*, **79**, 152–7.

Power, C., Manor, O., and Fox, J. (1991). *Health and class: the early years*. Chapman & Hall, London.

Programme Committee Socio-Economic Health Differences (1994). *Research programme socio-economic health differences: final report and recommendations*. Ministry of Public Health, The Hague.

Regidor, E., Gutierrez-Fisac, J.L., and Rodriguez, C. (1995). Increased socioeconomic differences in mortality in eight Spanish provinces. *Social Science and Medicine*, **41**, 801–7.

Rose, G. and Marmot, M.G. (1981). Social class and coronary heart disease. *British Heart Journal*, **45**, 13–19.

Schrijvers, C.T., van de Mheen, H.D., Stronks, K., and Mackenbach, J.P. (1998). Socioeconomic inequalities in health in the working population: the contribution of working conditions. *International Journal of Epidemiology*, **27**, 1011–18.

Schrijvers, C.T., Stronks, K., van de Mheen, H.D., and Mackenbach, J.P. (1999). Explaining educational differences in mortality: the role of behavioral and material factors. *American Journal of Public Health*, **89**, 535–40.

Schultz, H. (1991). Social differences in mortality in the eighteenth century: an analysis of Berlin church registers. *International Review of Social History*, **36**, 232–48.

Sen, A. (1990). Justice: means versus freedoms. *Philosophy and Public Affairs*, **19**, 111–21.

Sen, J. (1985). Well-being, agency and freedom; the Dewey lectures 1984. *Journal of Philosophy*, **82**, 169–221.

Shaw, M., Dorling, D., Gordon, D., and Davey Smith, D.G. (1999). *The widening gap. Health inequalities and policy in Britain.* Policy Press, Bristol.

Sihvonen, A.P., Kunst, A.E., Lahelma, E., Valkonen, T., and Mackenbach, J.P. (1998). Socioeconomic inequalities in health expectancy in Finland and Norway in the late 1980s. *Social Science and Medicine*, **47**, 303–15.

Sobal, J. and Stunkard, A.J. (1989). Socioeconomic status and obesity: a review of the literature. *Psychological Bulletin*, **105**, 260–75.

Stallones, R.A. (1980). The rise and fall of ischemic heart disease. *Scientific American*, **243**, 53–9.

Stern, J. (1983). Social mobility and the interpretation of social class mortality differentials. *Journal of Social Policy*, **12**, 27–49.

Stronks, K., van de Mheen, H.D., Looman, C.W.N., and Mackenbach, J.P. (1997). Cultural, material, and psychosocial correlates of the socioeconomic gradient in smoking behavior among adults. *Preventive Medicine*, 26, 754–66.

Stronks, K., van de Mheen, H., Looman, C.W.N., and Mackenbach, J.P. (1998). The importance of psychosocial stressors for socio-economic inequalities in perceived health. *Social Science and Medicine*, **46**, 611–23.

Tenconi, M.T., Romanelli, C., Gigli, F., *et al.* (1992). The relationship between education and risk factors for coronary heart disease.Epidemiological analysis from the nine communities study.The Research Group ATS-OB43 of CNR. *European Journal of Epidemiology*, **8**, 763–9.

Townsend, P., Davidson, N., and Whitehead, M. (1988*a*). *Inequalities in health (the Black Report and the health divide)*. Penguin, Harmondsworth.

Townsend, P., Phillimore, P., and Beattie, A. (1988*b*). *Health and deprivation: inequality and the North.* Croom Helm, London.

Vågerö, D. and Illsley, R. (1995). Explaining health inequalities: beyond Black and Barker. *European Sociological Review*, **3**, 1–23.

Vågerö, D. and Lundberg, O. (1995). Socio-economic mortality differentials among adults in Sweden. In *Adult mortality in developed countries: from description to explanation* (ed. A.D. Lopez, G. Casselli, and T. Valkonen), pp. 223–42.Clarendon Press, Oxford.

Valkonen, T. (1993). Trends in regional and socio economic mortality differentials in Finland. *International Journal of Health Sciences*, **3**, 157–66.

Valkonen, T., Martelin, T., Rimpelä, A., Notkola, V., and Savel, S. (1993). *Socio-economic mortality differences in Finland 1981–1990.* Statistics Finland, Helsinki.

Valkonen, T., Sihvonen, A.P., and Lahelma, E. (1997). Health expectancy by level of education in Finland. *Social Science and Medicine*, **44**, 801–8.

van de Mheen, H., Reijneveld, S.A., and Mackenbach, J.P. (1996). Socio-economic inequalities in perinatal and infant mortality from 1854 till 1990 in Amsterdam, The Netherlands. *European Journal of Public Health*, **6**, 166–74.

van de Mheen, H., Stronks, K., Looman, C.W., and Mackenbach, J.P. (1998*a*). Does childhood socioeconomic status influence adult health through behavioural factors? *International Journal of Epidemiology*, **27**, 431–7.

van de Mheen, H., Stronks, K., Looman, C.W., and Mackenbach, J.P. (1998*b*). Role of childhood health in the explanation of socioeconomic inequalities in early adult health. *Journal of Epidemiology and Community Health*, **52**, 15–19.

van de Mheen, H., Stronks, K., and Mackenbach, J.P. (1998*c*). A lifecourse perspective on socio-economic inequalities in health: the influence of childhood socio-economic conditions and selection processes. *Sociology of Health and Illness*, **20**, 754–77.

van de Mheen, H., Stronks, K., Schrijvers, C.T., and Mackenbach, J.P. (1999). The influence of adult ill health on occupational class mobility and mobility out of and into employment in the The Netherlands. *Social Science and Medicine*, **49**, 509–18.

van Loon, A.J., Goldbohm, R.A., and van den Brandt, P.A. (1994). Socioeconomic status and breast cancer incidence: a prospective cohort study. *International Journal of Epidemiology*, **23**, 899–905.

van Loon, A.J., Brug, J., Goldbohm, R.A., van den Brandt, P.A., and Burg, J. (1995). Differences in cancer incidence and mortality among socio-economic groups. *Scandinavian Journal of Social Medicine*, **23**, 110–20. (Erratum. *Scandinavian Journal of Social Medicine*, **23**, 155.)

van Reek, J. and Adriaanse, H. (1988). Cigarette smoking cessation rates by level of education in five western countries. *International Journal of Epidemiology*, **17**, 474–5.

Wadsworth, M.E. (1986). Serious illness in childhood and its association with later-life achievement. In *Class and health, research and longitudinal data* (ed. R.G. Wilkinson). Tavistock Publications, London.

Wadsworth, M.E. (1997). Health inequalities in the life course perspective. *Social Science and Medicine*, **44**, 859–69.

West, P. (1991). Rethinking the health selection explanation for health inequalities. *Social Science and Medicine*, **32**, 373–84.

Wetenschappelijke Raad voor het Regeringsbeleid (Scientific Council for Government Policy) (1987). *De ongelijke verdeling van gezondheid.* Staatsuitgeverij, 's-Gravenhage.

Whitehead, M. (1990). *The concepts and principles of equity and health.* World Health Organization, Copenhagen.

Whitehead, M. and Dahlgren, G. (1991). What can be done about inequalities in health?. *Lancet*, **338**, 1059–63.

WHO (World Health Organization) (1985). *Targets for health for all.* WHO, Copenhagen.

WHO (World Health Organization) (1999). *Health 21—health for all in the 21st century.* WHO, Copenhagen.

Wilkinson, R.G. (1992). Income distribution and life expectancy. *British Medical Journal*, **304**, 165–8.

Wilkinson, R.G. (1996). *Unhealthy societies: the afflictions of inequality.* Routledge, London.

Wing, S., Hayes, C., Heiss, G., *et al.* (1986). Geographic variation in the onset of decline of ischemic heart disease mortality in the United States. *American Journal of Public Health*, **76**, 1404–8.

12.4 Reducing health inequalities in developing countries

Davidson R. Gwatkin

This is a review of current professional thinking about health inequalities in developing countries and how to reduce them. It is in four parts. The first provides a brief history of recent trends in concern about health inequalities and related issues. The second is a discussion of the concept of health inequalities, and of the similarities and differences between other distributional measures in current use. The third summarizes what is known about the dimensions and magnitude of health inequalities. The fourth presents a comparable summary of current thought about how best to reduce inequalities. The review closes with a brief conclusion.

Recent history

A concern about health inequalities and other distributional aspects of health status and service use has enjoyed varying degrees of attention over the years. During the 1970s and early 1980s, distributional concerns (i.e. a concern about the health status of different socio-economic groups within society as distinct from the overall societal average) were dominant in thought about international health. These concerns then receded for about a decade, from about the mid-1980s to the mid-1990s, as attention turned from equity to efficiency. Now, the pendulum has begun to swing back, and distributional concerns are on the rise.

Beginning in the early 1970s, in the field of general economic development, the traditional focus on overall per capita income growth was vigorously challenged by advocates of 'trickle-up' development with an emphasis on basic human needs. In the health field, a similar trend gave rise to what became known as the Health for All movement. Codified in the Alma Ata Declaration, named after the venue of a prominent conference organized by the World Health Organization (**WHO**) and UNICEF in 1978, the movement featured a strong emphasis on improving the health of the global poor, so that they might enjoy the health benefits already available to the better off. Given the epidemiological patterns then prevailing among the poor, inexpensive services provided by village-based paramedical personnel appeared particularly relevant for the achievement of this goal; these and other similar services came to play a central part in what became known as 'primary health care' (WHO 1978). Soon after, UNICEF added its strong advocacy of the 'child survival revolution' based on specific primary care measures (Grant 1982). In each case, the emphasis was on free services provided through government-supported health care services that were to be expanded to cover ever-increasing numbers of people.

By the mid-1980s, the situation had changed. To begin with, the overall development picture was clouded by the severe economic difficulties experienced by many poor countries, which made it clear that the cherished goal of free government health services for all was not going to be realized, at least not soon. In addition, the momentous changes in economic philosophy in the socialist countries of Eastern Europe and in China eroded the previous confidence in state-led approaches to development. These changes filtered into the health care field and began raising doubts about the appropriateness of a government's central role in health service provision. Also, reality began to replace the euphoria of the early days of Health for All, and a closer examination of the primary health care record, rightly or wrongly, led many to question its ability to produce the dramatic benefits initially expected of it.

Thus interest began to shift from Health for All and towards what became known as 'health sector reform'. The point can be overstated, as a concern for the distributional aspects of health status and service use continued to figure importantly in the prominent international health publications of the time, such as the World Bank's *1993 World Development Report* on health (World Bank 1993), WHO's first *World Health Report* (WHO 1995) and the *1995 Annual Report* of the Director of the Pan American Health Organization (Pan American Health Organization 1995). But increasingly, especially following the appearance of the World Bank's influential *Financing Health Services in Developing Countries* (World Bank 1987), the health of disadvantaged groups no longer monopolized the attention of those concerned with developing country health problems. Rather, the focus moved towards sustainability, as reflected in the intensive activity on health financing that took place, and towards efficiency, as seen in the push towards greater cost-effectiveness. In epidemiological terms, the attention moved from the disease burden of the poor to that of the world as a whole and settled on the demographic–epidemiological transition, which was producing new middle and upper classes in the poor countries and whose disease characteristics were more like those of the West than those of the global poor.

Then, beginning in the mid to late 1990s, came another shift, back towards a concern for the distributional dimensions of health status and service use. An early development was the emergence of over a dozen intercountry research projects on health, poverty, and equity, supported by a wide range of donors and covering over a hundred countries (Carr *et al.* 1999). Another indicator is the importance given to health of the poor in recent international agency statements and policy papers.

For example, in introducing the WHO's *1999 World Health Report*, Director-General Gro Brundtland opened her review of the challenges to be addressed in order to improve the world's health by indicating that 'first and foremost, there is a need to reduce greatly the burden of excess mortality and morbidity suffered by the poor' (WHO 1999*a*). In January 2000, she followed this up with a presentation to the WHO Executive Board outlining the strategy that WHO plans to follow in this regard (WHO 1999*b*) (see Chapter 12.11). More recently, a high-level WHO-appointed Commission on Macro-Economics and Health has been giving prominent attention to the needs of poor population groups in its work.

World Bank health policy statements have also been moving towards a greater emphasis on poor groups. A notable beginning was in 1997, when the Bank adopted its current strategy for work on health, nutrition, and population. According to this strategy, the Bank's first health, nutrition, and population priority is 'to work with countries to improve the health, nutrition and population outcomes of the world's poor' (World Bank 1997). This emphasis was subsequently reinforced by the World Bank's updated overall mission statement, which began by saying that the World Bank's principal objective is to 'fight poverty with passion and professionalism with lasting results' (www.worldbank.org/html/extdr/about/mission.htim).

Further movement in this direction came through the World Bank's 2000–2001 *World Development Report* (World Bank 2000), which included a notable shift in the definition of poverty that such reports have employed in the past. Earlier, the reports had followed the traditional World Bank practice of defining poverty almost exclusively in financial terms. But the 2000–2001 report broke with this tradition by viewing poverty in multidimensional terms, presenting a definition under which poor health (along with inadequate education, poor nutrition, and other social dimensions of development) is placed alongside inadequate income or financial assets as a core indicator of poverty. Under this formulation, poor health becomes an integral part of poverty, rather than simply a contributor to it.

The configuration of World Bank financial support for developing county health activities has begun to show signs of shifting to conform to the new orientation just described. The principal development so far has been provision of support for health initiatives through a program of debt relief for highly indebted poor countries, undertaken in co-operation with the International Monetary Fund (**IMF**). Under this program, the World Bank and the IMF invited 41 particularly poor and indebted countries to prepare poverty reduction strategy papers (**PRSPs**) designed to demonstrate, among other things, that any additional resources made available through debt forgiveness would be spent in a manner that would benefit the poor. As of March 2001, 35 of the country governments had prepared full or interim PRSPs, and the Bank and the IMF had agreed to some US$20 billion (in net present value terms) of debt relief for 22 of them. Approximately a quarter of these funds—some US$5 billion—had gone to health programmes. Plans are currently under development for extending the PRSP process to all 78 countries qualifying for subsidized lending through the World Bank's International Development Association (www.worldbank.org/hipc/hipc-review/hipc-review.html).

Other agencies have also been stressing the health of the poor. For example, in November 1997,the United Kingdom Department for International Development (**DfID**) issued a White Paper on international development committing itself to help achieve the internationally agreed target to halve the proportion of people living in extreme poverty by 2015, together with associated targets including basic health care provision and universal access to primary education by the same date (Secretary of State for International Development 1997). It followed this in November 2000 with a strategy paper outlining how it would reorient its health support in order to achieve this objective (Department for International Development 2000). Similarly, in 1999 the Rockefeller Foundation, whose Global Health Equity Initiative had already made a significant contribution, decided to make equity the principal theme for its future health work (Rockefeller Foundation 1999). In taking such steps, DfID and the Rockefeller Foundation joined organizations like the governments of The Netherlands and the Nordic countries and the many non-governmental agencies which had continued to give highest priority to reaching poor population groups throughout the earlier period when other agencies had turned more towards efficiency.

Thus, in brief, a concern for health inequalities and the health and the poor has once again come to occupy a central place in thinking about international health policies. The challenge now is for those concerned with distributional issues to take advantage of the opportunity that the current climate presents.

Concepts

While the principal focus of this paper is on health inequalities, it is important to recognize that such inequalities constitute only one of several indicators of interest to those dealing with the distributional aspects of health status and service use. Two others are health equity and the health of the poor.

These three indicators or concepts are similar in some ways, different in others. However, they all share a recognition that in health, as in many other fields, societal averages typically disguise as much as they reveal. Thus their interest is not in the health conditions that prevail in society as a whole, but in the condition of different socio-economic groups within society—especially the lowest or most disadvantaged groups.

But within this shared concern lie a number of distinctions. Those interested with the health of the poor are typically concerned primarily with improving the health of that group alone, rather than with reducing differences between poor and rich. For those oriented towards equality, the principal objective is the reduction of poor–rich health differences. Those concerned with health inequities are concerned with righting the injustice represented by inequalities or poor health conditions among the disadvantaged.

These similarities and differences can most easily be understood by considering each of the three indicators and concepts in turn, and then reviewing the practical implications of thinking in terms of one or the other.

The health of the poor

A concern for poor population groups has occupied a central role in established thinking about overall socio-economic development for over two decades. It emerged in the late 1960s and early 1970s in reaction to the then dominant emphasis on overall per capita income growth rates. At the time, a concern for distribution was thought likely to detract from the overall economic growth that was considered a necessary condition for the long-term alleviation of poverty. 'Concentrate first on overall growth', was the prevailing view. The result might be a rise in inequality over the short term, but eventually the benefits would trickle down to the poor and, in the long run, they would end up better off than under a development strategy oriented towards their immediate needs.

The 'trickle-up' and 'basic human needs' schools of thought, which emerged to counter the view just presented, advocated dealing directly with the poor as the best means of producing sustainable growth. The many discussions about how best to define the poor population groups of concern produced two approaches.

Absolute poverty

The first, based on what is often called 'absolute poverty', takes a universal perspective and defines poverty in terms of a given level of income or consumption, which is equally relevant for people wherever they may be. This is usually done by defining a 'poverty line' as the lowest amount of money sufficient to purchase the amount of food necessary for a minimally adequate diet (and still have enough left over to buy other essentials). A well-known practitioner of this approach is the World Bank, which has devoted a great deal of time and effort to defining a suitable international poverty line and estimating the number of people living below it. The current international poverty line stands at an average per capita consumption of just over US$1.00 per day (in 1993 dollars), adjusted for purchasing power differences between countries. The consumption level of about 1200 million of the world's population lies below this line. Almost all these people—who constitute just under a quarter of the world's total population—live in South Asia, sub-Saharan Africa, and China (World Bank 2000).

Relative poverty

The second approach, which is more country-specific, deals with what is frequently referred to as 'relative poverty'. The practice here is to define the poverty line in terms of relevance for a specific society. This is typically done in one of two ways. One way, analogous to the international approach just described, is to determine how much income one needs to live decently according to some locally established definition of decency. Poverty lines of this sort are used in the developed as well as the developing world. In the United States, for example, the Census Bureau estimates that a family of four requires US$16 000 annually to purchase a minimally adequate diet and meet other basic needs, and that 12.7 per cent of the population falls below this level (Uchitelle 1999). The second approach is simply to define the national poverty line as some proportion—often arbitrarily determined—of a society's average per capita income or expenditure. In the United Kingdom, a statistic frequently cited to document the prevalence of poverty refers to the proportion of the population (currently just under a quarter) with less than half the country's average per capita income (Anonymous 1999).

This distinction between absolute and relative poverty carries over into the field of health. For instance, a careful reading of the World Bank policy statement on health, nutrition, and population cited above reveals an absolute-poverty orientation through its reference to a concern for 'the world's poor', which is in line with the overall World Bank interest in people below the global poverty line as just described. However, others feel that relative poverty and deprivation are just as important, if not more so.

Inequality in health

While a concern for improving the health of the poor is widespread, it is by no means universally preferred. Many focus more on reducing inequalities, both in general and with respect to health in particular.

Such a focus has long occupied a particularly important place in thinking about international health issues. To say that the focus has been exclusively on inequality would be to overstate the case, for it is possible to cite expressions of concern for poverty in prominent international health documents from at least the time of the Alma-Ata Declaration (1978) onwards. However, it is rare for a prominent international health statement not to give at least equal, if not more, weight to inequality reduction. For example, at the same time as the Alma-Ata Declaration professed its concern for the unacceptable health conditions found among the hundreds of millions among the world's poor, it also advocated primary health care because of its potential 'to close the gap between the "haves" and the "have-nots" ', i.e. to lessen health inequalities (WHO 1978). The previously cited *World Health Report 1995* (WHO 1995), which had a great deal to say about the health of the poor, was subtitled *Bridging the Gaps*, referring to the inequalities between poor and rich. A recent major WHO publication in this area emphasizes the importance of being concerned with poor–rich health inequalities, rather than simply focusing on the health of the poor alone (WHO 1996).

Similarly, health inequalities have played a much more central part than the health of the poor alone in a long European tradition of concern. For instance, the well-known 1980 Black Report in the United Kingdom was entitled *Inequalities in Health* (Department of Health and Social Security 1980), as was the exercise that produced its successor, the 1998 Acheson Report (Department of Health 1998). In the same vein, the 1984 targets of the WHO Regional Office for Europe (EURO) were expressed in terms of reducing poor–rich disparities. 'By the year 2000', said the WHO document in which these targets were presented, 'the actual differences in health status between countries and between groups within countries should be reduced by at least 25 per cent, by improving the health of disadvantaged nations and groups' (Whitehead 1990).

However, just as there are different approaches to poverty alleviation, so too are there various views about the most appropriate strategies for the reduction of inequalities. Illustrative of the issues that arise in discussing the reduction of health inequalities are the following questions.

- **What dimensions of inequality matter most?** The most traditional approach has been to think of differences in health status according to an individual's income or economic standing. However, the economic dimension is by no means the only one that matters, and some would consider other dimensions even more important. Gender inequalities in health status have received a great deal of attention in recent years. Ethnic inequalities in health have been of particular concern in many areas, such as South Africa and the United States. Education and occupation have also been widely used as a basis for dividing populations in assessing intergroup health differentials, although often more as a proxy for economic status than as indicators of interest in their own right. Yet another approach might be called 'pure' health inequality, i.e. the ordering of people on the basis of their health status, from most to least healthy regardless of income or any other attribute, for the purpose of measuring health diversity in a society (Gakidou *et al.* 2000). In so doing, people applying this approach are drawing on a long tradition of studies with respect to income distribution.

- **How is inequality to be measured?** There are almost as many statistical definitions of inequality as there are statisticians, and the various definitions can produce very different interpretations of the same situation or trend. Until recently, one particular measure—the Gini coefficient—has been dominant, at least in economic thinking, supplemented by comparisons between the poorest and richest population quintiles (or between people above and below the poverty line) when the data available were insufficient for the calculation of the Gini coefficient. While the Gini coefficient probably remains the most frequently used indicator even now, its position is slipping. In health, as in economics, several other disparity indicators are under active consideration (Anand *et al.* 2001), with no clear consensus about a preferred alternative.
- **What aspects of inequality are most important?** There are many different views. Some would argue for looking at inequalities in health status as the outcome that counts; others favour focusing on health services as the determinant of health status that health professionals can most easily influence. Within each of these two streams of thought are further distinctions. Health status, for example, can be determined either through a physical examination or through self-assessment. (The two approaches can produce quite different results, in that people found to be relatively unhealthy through a physical examination do not always consider themselves to be less healthy than people whose health was determined by examination to be considerably better.) With respect to health services, there are distinctions between (a) use and financing, (b) among public, private non-profit, and private for-profit services, and (c) between preventive and curative services. Health services that come out ahead in one of these respects may lag from another perspective.
- **Should the focus be local or global?** A great deal of attention is currently being paid to inequalities within countries. However, there is also strong interest in some quarters in differences among countries and world regions.

Health equity

Poverty and inequality, as described above, are both primarily empirical concepts. Equity, by contrast, is a normative concept (a question of values) and closely associated with the concept of social justice. When applied to health, equity has traditionally been most often linked to the reduction of inequalities. Thus, one of the most widely cited definitions of health inequity is that it 'refers to differences in health which...are considered unfair and unjust'. In a similar vein, the WHO/EURO document on health equity cited above indicated that 'equity requires reducing unfair disparities...' and that 'pursuing equity in health and health care development means trying to reduce unfair and unnecessary social gaps in health and health care...' (Whitehead 1990).

However, equity need not be exclusively a matter of reducing inequalities. It can also be associated with poverty, as one could argue that it is unjust to allow people to continue living in poverty when adequate resources are available within the society at large to lift them out of it. Such a link figures prominently in general thinking about social justice, and it also appears in writings on health equity.

A particularly well-known example of poverty-oriented general thought about equity is the 'maximin' principle of distributive justice posited by John Rawls. That principle and others like it call for resources to be distributed in such a way that the worst-off people in society (i.e. those occupying the 'minimum' position) have the maximum possible amount of gain. What happens to the better-off through such a pattern of resource distribution is extraneous to the maximin principle (Rawls 1971). A variation on this theme, as applied to health, would consider any health gains among the rich in the course of implementing efforts to improve the health of the poor as welcome side-benefits, rather than regrettable because of the dilution in inequality reduction that they represent (Marchand *et al.* 1998).

While not many equality-oriented advocates of health equity seem prepared to go this far, almost all incorporate at least traces of such a poverty-oriented equity definition in their statements. The traces are to be seen most clearly in the tendency of equality-oriented discussions to disavow interest in one of the arguably more effective potential ways of reducing poor–rich health inequalities—assassination of the rich. Rather, the focus of all known inequality-oriented health equity proposals is on lessening poor–rich differences through special efforts to improve the health of the poor—a focus that makes the proposals sound suspiciously similar to what one might wish to do under a poverty-oriented health equity approach.

Thus, for instance, the previously cited inequality-oriented definition of health equity referring to the inequalities of health that are unjust and unfair was developed in conjunction with the WHO/EURO health equity objective, which called for a reduction in health disparities by improving the health of the disadvantaged (Whitehead 1990). The WHO's 1996 health equity document, while giving primacy to poor–rich health differences, also called for ensuring an adequate standard for the entire population, noting that, 'for some, "equity" means that all social groups should have a basic minimum level of well-being and services' (WHO 1996).

However, regardless of whether one considers health equity to be related more to equality or poverty, the introduction of normative or social justice considerations also raises questions.

- **When is an inequality unfair?** Not always, certainly. It is quite possible to imagine a situation marked by health inequalities that are not necessarily inequitable. One example is an inequality that is irremediable (Whitehead 1990). Another might be two population groups with similar incomes but marked differences in life expectancy attributable to different lifestyles. If the less healthy group adopts its lifestyle in full awareness of the risks involved, the resulting differences in life expectancy might be said to be simply a reflection of differences in the social preferences of the two groups rather than any fundamental inequity. Or, to illustrate the same point with a more general example, if two individuals are in fact unequal in capacity, equal treatment would be unfair to the more capable of the two. In such a case, equity might well call for unequal treatment. In other words, equity and equality are by no means synonymous and need to be carefully distinguished from one another.
- **On what basis can one decide when the resources in a society are adequate to alleviate poverty?** 'Adequacy' is not a binary concept, such that there is one level of resource availability above which availability is totally adequate, and below which it is completely inadequate. Rather, there is a spectrum running from a total lack to

infinite availability of resources, often with no obvious cut-off point along the way. Also, perceptions can differ—resources that seem adequate to one person may not be so to another.

The practical implications of the poverty–inequality–equity distinction

What has been said so far provides a basis for suspecting that, in general, there are only limited practical implications in adopting one or other of the three approaches covered here. As has been noted, even those who seem furthest apart (those giving highest priority to reductions in poor–rich health inequalities in the name of equity, and those concerned with improving the health of the poor) end up sounding rather similar, once one realizes that the approach preferred by advocates of inequality reduction looks primarily to improvements in the health of the disadvantaged.

A more careful look reinforces this view that the poverty–equality–equity distinction is often largely academic. The most obvious situation is in a low-income country where the most cost-effective measures available for the improvement of health in the society as a whole are also those that are especially beneficial to the poor. As pointed out in the *1993 World Development Report* (World Bank 1993), the contents of minimum service packages that feature such measures—management of the sick child, prenatal and delivery care, family planning, etc.—are especially relevant for low-income groups. Where this is the case, adoption of the approach that is most sensible for the poor is also more beneficial for the poor than for the rich, and can thus be expected to produce a reduction in poor–rich differences.

However, the record would not be complete without noting that there are at least some circumstances where an interest in improving the health of the poor can imply a different approach from that resulting from a concern for inequality reduction. Two examples can illustrate the point. One concerns inter-regional resource allocations by international agencies, and the other deals with disease priorities, whether at the global or the national level.

The inter-regional resource allocation example involves looking at the implications of different approaches as to where an international assistance agency might logically apply its health resources. Consider three alternatives.

- **An absolute-poverty approach** According to the World Bank figures cited earlier, some 90 per cent of the world's 1200 million people living below the poverty line live in Asia and Africa (World Bank 2000). This being the case, an international agency guided by an absolute-poverty objective would wish to put virtually all of its health resources into those regions. There would be much less justification for working in Latin America, and practically none at all for health activity in the Middle East or Eastern Europe, where hardly anyone is so poor as to lie below the international poverty line.
- **A relative-poverty approach** Relative poverty exists in every country. From this perspective, there could be as strong a justification for supporting pro-poor health activities in one region of the world as in any other.
- **An equality approach** Assuming that most of the existing health inequalities observed in the developing world are also inequitable and that inequality reduction interventions are equally effective, an equity approach would imply a particularly high priority for countries where health inequalities are greatest. Recent research points to the existence of large country-to-country differences in the degree of health inequality, which in turn suggests that some countries deserve much more attention than others from an equity perspective. According to one recent study (Wagstaff 2000), Brazil, Nicaragua, South Africa, and Nepal have large health-status inequalities and would thus be of high priority, while health-status inequalities are quite low in Ghana, Pakistan, and Vietnam which would accordingly merit a low priority.

With respect to the second set of examples, dealing with disease priorities, the available information is unfortunately inadequate to permit citation of 'real-world' experiences. However, the basic point can be demonstrated through two schematic illustrations, one from a global and one from a national perspective.

- **Global disease priorities** A global institution focusing on absolute poverty would logically devote primary attention and resources to communicable diseases, as they are the dominant causes of deaths and disability among the global poor (Gwatkin and Guillot 1999; Gwatkin *et al.* 1999). In an institution concerned with relative poverty, there would be a case for a much broader concern. Such an institution would be involved not only with the poor in Africa and Asia, but also with the disadvantaged populations in Eastern European countries, among whom non-communicable diseases may well be the dominant problem.
- **Disease priorities within advanced developing and transition countries** While communicable diseases are dominant among the global poor, chronic diseases in advanced developing and transition countries are, as just noted, likely to be responsible for the majority of deaths and disability among the poor—but, in all likelihood, for a smaller percentage of the poor than of the rich. The implications of such a situation can be illustrated by reference to a country where non-communicable diseases cause 60 per cent of deaths among the poor and 90 per cent of deaths among the rich. From a burden-of-disease perspective, such figures point to non-communicable diseases as a natural focus for a programme concerned with poverty alleviation, as such diseases cause the majority of deaths. But such a focus, if introduced on a society-wide basis, could well lead to an increase in inequality. This is because non-communicable diseases are even more important for the rich than for the poor, so that the benefit to the rich of any general evenly distributed decline in non-communicable diseases would be correspondingly greater. Thus, in a situation like this, burden-of-disease considerations would argue for the highest priority to be given to one type of disease (i.e. non-communicable diseases) from the perspective of improving the health of the poor, and to a different type of disease (i.e. communicable diseases) from an inequality-reduction perspective.

The second example is obviously oversimplified, ignoring cost-effectiveness and targeting considerations that may well be more important than disease burden factors in the establishment of health service priorities. However, while lessening the example's relevance for 'real-world' decision-making, the oversimplification is of value in facilitating understanding of the basic point that remains valid despite it: there is not an inevitable congruity between national-level policy prescriptions that are optimal for improving the health of the poor and those that are best for reducing health inequalities.

Inequalities

While the contents of the preceding section make it clear that a focus on inequalities is by no means the only one of relevance for approaching health differentials in developing countries, health inequalities remain of considerable interest and will be the topic of what follows. As space limitations prevent adequate coverage of the full range of health inequalities that might be considered, the discussion will focus on inequalities by socio-economic status. It will deal with the three following inequalities as illustrations of the different types that exist: (a) current intracountry inequalities in health status by economic class, (b) current intracountry inequalities in the use of government health care services, and (c) trends in intercountry health status inequalities.

Current intracountry inequalities in health status by economic class

Until recently, data limitations have prevented the direct examination of intracountry health inequalities by any of the three indicators typically employed by economists: income, consumption, or assets (wealth). Instead, as noted earlier, indicators such as father's occupation or mother's education have served as proxies for economic status, in addition to pointing to attributes of interest in themselves. This is changing, however, and a number of efforts are under way to provide more direct measures of economic status as a basis for assessing intracountry health differentials. Of particular relevance for the present discussion are findings from three multicountry comparative study programmes: country health and poverty reports, Living Standards Measurement Survey estimates, and WHO estimates.

Perhaps the most extensive of the programmes is the **country health and poverty report** project organized by the World Bank (Gwatkin *et al.* 2000). This project features preparation of tabulations, by asset or wealth quintile, for approximately 30 health, nutrition, population status, and service use indicators. The tabulations, designed primarily to provide basic distributional information for the use of policy-makers, are currently available for 44 countries in Africa, Asia, Latin America, and the Near East.

The information presented in the reports is drawn from household data collected through the Demographic and Health Survey programme sponsored by the United States Agency for International Development. This well-known programme of comparative country studies, typically covering 5000 to 10 000 households in each country investigated, is oriented especially to the collection of information about vital events and maternal/child health. It is considerably less strong with respect to information about economic status, as it contains no questions about income or consumption. However, its standard individual and household survey instruments include a number of questions about household assets—availability of electricity, possession of consumer goods (e.g. bicycle, radio), flooring material, source of drinking water, etc. Using principal components analysis, these can be combined into a single index of household assets or wealth which is of interest in its own right and approximates reasonably well the consumption measures that economists tend to prefer (Filmer and Pritchett 2001).

In preparing a report, a country's population is divided into quintiles on the basis of the asset index, and the value of each health, nutrition, or population indicator is tabulated for each population quintile. The status indicators include infant and under-5 mortality rates, total and adolescent fertility rates, and such commonly used indices of malnutrition as stunting and low weight-for-age. Typical of the service indicators are immunization rates, medical treatment for diarrhoea and acute respiratory infections among children, use of antenatal and professional delivery care, and contraceptive prevalence.

A summary of the available information about infant and under-5 mortality, to which the current discussion will be limited, appears in Table 1. The figures are expressed in terms of two indicators. The first is a poor–rich ratio, i.e. the ratio of infant or under-5 mortality in the poorest population quintile to that in the richest quintile. The second is a concentration index, which is a measure similar to the well-known Gini coefficient that is commonly used in measuring income

Table 1 Intracountry disparities in infant and under-5 mortality

Region	No. of countries	Poor–rich ratio		Concentration index	
		Mean	Range	Mean	Range
Infant mortality					
Sub-Saharan Africa	21	1.67	1.11 to 2.46	– 0.081	– 0.003 to – 0.141
Asia–Near East–North Africa	9	2.33	1.42 to 3.93	– 0.125	– 0.051 to – 0.195
Latin America–Caribbean	11	2.66	1.26 to 4.18	– 0.145	– 0.043 to – 0.251
Total	40	1.87	1.11 to 4.18	– 0.106	– 0.003 to – 0.251
Under-5 mortality					
Sub-Saharan Africa	21	1.79	1.27 to 2.60	– 0.095	– 0.040 to – 0.164
Asia–Near East–North Africa	9	2.69	1.69 to 4.60	– 0.147	– 0.084 to – 0.210
Latin America/Caribbean	11	2.99	1.55 to 4.67	– 0.167	– 0.071 to – 0.259
Total	40	2.06	1.27 to 4.67	– 0.124	– 0.040 to – 0.259

Source: Gwatkin *et al.* (2000).

inequalities. As in the case of the Gini coefficient, the value of the concentration index can range from –1.0 (if all infant or under-5 deaths occur in the poorest population quintile to +1.0 (if all deaths are in the richest quintile) (Wagstaff *et al.* 1991).

The unweighted poor–rich ratio for all countries together is about 1.9 for infant mortality and about 2.1 for under-5 mortality. This suggests that, on average, the newly born child in the poorest population quintile of a developing country is roughly twice as likely to die in infancy as is a child born into the richest quintile. The unweighted mean concentration indices are of the order of –0.11 or –0.12. This is modest compared with the range of about –0.2 to –0.5 typically found with respect to consumption as measured by the Gini coefficient. However, such modesty is not unexpected, given that mortality rates are much more tightly bounded variables than are consumption measures.

The data also point to considerable country-to-country variation. For instance, the low–high ratio for infant mortality ranges from 1.11 in Namibia to 4.17 in Bolivia. Differences in the concentration index are also large. The range is from –0.003 in Namibia to –0.251 in Brazil.

Regardless of which index is used, the data appear to support two generalizations about the variation that exists. First, intracountry inequalities seem larger for child (1–5) than for infant (0–1) mortality. This can be inferred from the modestly higher level of under-5 (i.e. 0–5) mortality relative to infant (0–1) mortality found for both inequality indices in each region (and also in 33 of the 40 individual countries covered). Infant mortality is nested within under-5 mortality and typically contains well over half the deaths on which under-5 mortality rates are based. Removal of less unequally distributed infant deaths in order to produce a child mortality rate would thus be likely to increase further the already larger poor–rich differences seen in the 0 to 5 rates. This would be consistent with current understanding about the pathogens to which poor children are exposed during the immediate post-weaning period. Second, intracountry socio-economic inequalities in infant and child mortality appear smaller in sub-Saharan Africa than in other parts of the world; in Latin America, they seem somewhat larger. This is readily visible from Table 1, where the average values for both the poor–rich ratio and the concentration index for sub-Saharan Africa (1.7 to 1.8; –0.08 to –0.10) are lower than the global mean (1.9 to 2.1; –0.11 to –0.12), and lower still than the Latin American average (2.7 to 3.0; –0.14 to –0.17). This can be explained rather easily for Latin America, given the high levels of inequality found in that region (Deininger and Squire 1996) and initial findings from other work that confirm the existence of a direct relationship between income and health inequality (Wagstaff 1999). The low degree of health inequality in sub-Saharan Africa is more difficult to understand, in the light of recent findings that income is almost as unequally distributed there as in Latin America (Deininger and Squire 1996).

However, these or any other conclusions that might be drawn from the infant or under-5 mortality data in the country health and poverty reports must be conditioned by at least two considerations. The first is the existence of rather large standard errors in many cases, which means that the concentration indices are statistically different from zero (as measured by a 5 per cent confidence interval) in only about half the countries covered. This occurred even though the tabulations were based on births during the 10 years prior to the survey, in order to increase the sample size. The second is the presence of regular or monotonic declines in mortality from the poorest to the richest quintiles in only approximately half the countries. The anomalies are usually quite small, often consisting of a high point in the next poorest quintile that is suggestive of under-reporting of mortality among the poorest population groups. However, in a few African countries there is a pronounced 'spike' in the middle quintiles that remains to be explained.

The results of the **Living Standards Measurement Survey estimates** are roughly in line with those discussed above. The study in question is by Adam Wagstaff of the World Bank and the University of Sussex (Wagstaff 2000). It is based on datasets for nine developing countries. Eight of the datasets are from the World Bank Living Standards Measurement Survey programme, which covers approximately 25 developing countries. The survey instruments are oriented towards the measurement of household consumption, so that Wagstaff was able to use consumption as his economic indicator, rather than the asset index featured in the work based on the Demographic and Health Survey described above. On the other hand, because of the less reliable mortality data available through the Living Standards Measurement Survey, Wagstaff was forced to employ estimation methods that were not necessary with the Demographic and Health Survey data.

Six of the nine countries that Wagstaff covered were among the 40 in the work based on the Demographic and Health Survey, making it possible to compare the concentration indices for these countries produced by the two studies. This comparison is presented in Table 2.

On average, the Wagstaff concentration indices are somewhat smaller than those resulting from the country health and poverty report exercise, although this is not the case for each country. Perhaps more significantly, there is an overlap between the 5 per cent confidence intervals for the two sets of estimates in 11 of the 12 cases presented (i.e. in all six countries for infant mortality, and in all countries except Vietnam for under-5 mortality). By this standard, the two sets of estimates can be considered mutually consistent, although, given the rather large size of the confidence intervals of the two studies, the standard can accommodate considerable variation among figures qualifying for mutual consistency status under it.

It remains to be seen whether such consistency exists between the country health and poverty reports and the Wagstaff estimates on the one hand, and the **WHO estimates** on the other. This third set of estimates, under preparation by the WHO, employs a very different method from those of the other two. Rather than relying on household data, as in the two previous studies, the WHO exercise is based on a cross-country dataset. The datasets used consist of two figures for each country included: the percentage of the population residing below the poverty line, and the country average for a particular health indicator of interest. The application of a statistical technique known as ecological inference makes it possible to derive from such data an estimate for the level of the health indicators among people above and below the poverty line in each country. For example, if one knows the percentage of the population above and below the poverty line and the average infant mortality for each country in a dataset, it is possible to estimate the infant mortality rate among people above and below the poverty line in each of the countries (Jamison 1997; WHO 1999*a*).

The first data from this exercise have been published, in an annex to the 1999 edition of the *World Health Report* (WHO 1999*a*); they provide estimates of the under-5 and 15–59 mortality for males and females and of tuberculosis prevalence for 49 developing and transition countries.

Table 2 Concentration indices for infant and under-5 mortality within six developing countries as measured by different studies

Country	Infant mortality		Under-5 mortality	
	Country health & poverty reports	Wagstaff	Country health & poverty reports	Wagstaff
Côte d'Ivoire	– 0.107	– 0.095	– 0.115	– 0.096
Ghana	– 0.093	+ 0.018	– 0.135	– 0.028
Nepal	– 0.060	– 0.109	– 0.096	– 0.132
Nicaragua	– 0.094	– 0.150	– 0.124	– 0.162
Pakistan	– 0.051	0.000	– 0.084	– 0.017
Vietnam	– 0.143	– 0.009	– 0.159	– 0.016
Unweighted mean	– 0.091	– 0.064	– 0.119	– 0.076

Sources: Wagstaff (2000), Gwatkin *et al.* (2000).

The figures most nearly comparable with those of the country health and poverty report and Wagstaff exercises discussed earlier are the under-5 mortality estimates. Here, the unweighted average poor–non-poor ratio for all 49 countries (male and female combined) is about 6.1:1. (Weighting by population size, in lieu of the number of births for which information is not provided, gives a ratio of 5.4:1.) About 30 per cent of the people in the 49 countries live below the absolute poverty line (whether calculated on a weighted or unweighted basis). Thus under-5 mortality among the poorest 30 per cent or so of the population is of the order of five to six times greater than that among the highest 70 per cent. This appears to be well above the poorest 30 per cent–richest 70 per cent ratio implied by the previously cited country health and poverty report finding that, on average, under-5 mortality among the poorest 20 per cent of a developing country's population is about twice as high as among the highest 20 per cent. This in turn suggests that the use of country-level household data, as in the country health and poverty report and Wagstaff exercises, is likely to produce intracountry differentials that are considerably smaller than indirect inferences based on country-level comparisons.

For the moment, however, this can be considered no more than a suggestion, to be confirmed or disproved on the basis of further more careful examination of the methodology and findings of all three study programmes. Also to be determined is the relevance for this particular issue of the common view that microlevel (household-level) data are more reliable—or, perhaps more accurately, less unreliable—than macrolevel (country-level) information for policy-oriented analyses.

Intracountry inequalities in use of government health care services by economic class

Concomitant with the rapid increase in research on intracountry socio-economic differentials in health status, as described in the preceding section, has come a growth in concern about differentials in access to health services. As access is difficult to define and measure, most work in this area has focused on the related issue of health service use. (Use is associated with access but differs from it in that one can have access to services but not use them for any of several reasons—for example, a lack of need for medical care because of continuing good health.)

Of particular interest has been the extent to which government health services have been able to reach disadvantaged population groups. This is being increasingly studied through the application of a technique called 'benefit–incidence analysis', borrowed from the field of public finance. Benefit–incidence analysis can be seen as an equity-oriented analogue of cost-effectiveness analysis used to study efficiency; while cost-effectiveness analysis is oriented towards determining how much output a health system produces per unit of input, benefit–incidence analysis seeks to assess how a health system's outputs are distributed across socio-economic classes.

Specifically, the benefit–incidence approach measures the financial subsidies accruing to different socio-economic groups through the use of government health services. It combines two types of information. The first consists of data from household surveys concerning the number and socio-economic status of people using different kinds of government services when ill. From these, it is possible to determine the number of per capita visits to a given type of government service, during a specified time period, for each socio-economic group of interest (such as income quintile of the population). The second is information from government financial reports about the total cost of the services in question (net of any income received from user fees), and from service statistics concerning the number of people using those services. These data permit an estimate of the unit cost of the different services, i.e. the average cost of providing the services in question to a single individual. The number of per capita visits to a given type of service is then multiplied by the unit cost of that service, and the results are aggregated to produce an estimate of the total financial benefit accruing to each socio-economic group through government expenditures on the range of services covered.

Information is currently available about benefit–incidence surveys on health that have been undertaken in 23 countries. This information is summarized in Table 3. The most reliable data come from sub-Saharan Africa, the site of a comparative study of seven countries organized by the World Bank (Castro-Leal *et al.* 2000). As each of the country exercises drew on household datasets collected through similar surveys undertaken by the Bank's Living Standards Measurement Survey programme, problems of intercountry comparability appear significantly lower than is the case with respect to the other studies for which findings are available.

Table 3 Percentage of financial subsidy from government health services accruing to poorest and richest quintiles of the population: regional averages

Region	Primary care		Hospital care						Total health care	
	Poorest quintile	Richest quintile	Outpatient		Inpatient		Total		Poorest quintile	Richest quintile
			Poorest quintile	Richest quintile	Poorest quintile	Richest quintile	Poorest quintile	Richest quintile		
Africa	15 (7)	23 (7)	12 (2)	36 (2)	16 (2)	34 (2)	10 (5)	33 (5)	12 (7)	30 (7)
Asia	21 (2)	16 (2)	7 (1)	41 (1)	5 (1)	41 (1)	13 (1)	22 (1)	19 (5)	21 (5)
Eastern Europe	16 (2)	22 (2)	—	—	—	—	12 (2)	29 (2)	13 (2)	27 (2)
Latin America	—	—	—	—	—	—	—	—	29 (8)	14 (8)

The number in parentheses indicates the number of countries included in the average.
Source: Gwatkin (2001*a*).

The findings from these studies make it clear that the rich benefit financially more than the poor from government health services in sub-Saharan Africa. This was the case in all seven of the countries covered by the principal systematic research effort thus far undertaken. The difference was particularly notable with respect to hospital services, but even primary care normally benefited the rich somewhat more than the poor. On average, the richest 20 per cent of the population received well over twice as much financial benefit as the poorest 20 per cent from overall government health service expenditures. In all but two of the seven countries, the richest 20 per cent also gained more than the poorest 20 per cent of the population from primary care expenditures.

In Asia, the situation appears mixed. On average, overall government health care expenditures in the five countries with available data appear to favour the rich slightly more than the poor. However, this is an average of very dissimilar situations: three (Indonesia, Mongolia, Vietnam) in which the rich gain far more than the poor, and two others (Malaysia, the Philippines) in which the poor receive larger financial benefits than the rich. It should be noted, however, that these findings may be less secure than that just cited for Africa. In part, this arises from the uncertain comparability of the studies cited, but more from the fact that the benefit–incidence tradition is less well established in Asia than in Africa or Latin America. Also, no fully published findings are available for the two largest countries, China and India.

To judge from the two countries in central Europe with available study data (Bulgaria and Romania), the situation appears similar to Africa. In each country, the rich gain more than the poor from primary as well as from hospital care. Overall, the financial benefit that government health services convey to the rich is nearly twice as large as that gained by the poor.

The situation in Latin America appears different. Information available for seven countries suggests that the poorest quintile gains more than the richest quintile in all but one (Brazil). On average, the poor in these countries receive twice as much benefit as the rich. However, these figures need to be viewed with caution, especially in comparison with those for Africa, cited above, for two reasons. One is that government-delivered health services represent a much smaller percentage of total government health expenditures than elsewhere. The health benefits that flow through social security systems, on which Latin American governments tend to spend almost as much as on health services they provide directly, are also important. (For example, according to one recent review about 17 per cent of government health expenditures were through social security systems, compared with 16 per cent for services provided directly by central governments and 9 per cent for local government services (R. Suarez-Berenguela, Pan American Health Organization, unpublished work, 1998).) As such programmes focus on formal sector employees, they tend to be oriented towards the middle and upper classes; when their benefit incidence is taken into account, the overall impact of government health care expenditures could well be regressive. A second consideration is technical. Many of the Latin American studies appear to be based on the benefits accruing to households rather than to individuals. As poorer families tend to be larger than rich ones, use of the household as the basis of analysis provides an impression of greater progressivity than do findings that refer to individuals.

In addition to the specific considerations indicated with respect to Asia and Latin America, the findings just described are affected by several general characteristics of the benefit–incidence approach that need to be taken into account. Five are particularly worthy of note.

1. In accordance with the tradition of the benefit–incidence literature, the findings are presented in terms of absolute rather than relative benefit (e.g. pesos per capita rather than percentage of per capita income). In relative terms, the poor are likely to benefit more than the rich because the incomes of the richest 20 per cent are normally many times greater than those of the poorest 20 per cent.

2. The conclusions are derived from estimates that cover only expenditures. These could differ quite significantly from conclusions that look at the revenue side as well, and measure only net benefits and incidence, i.e. the amount a given income group gains from government health expenditures relative to the amount of taxes that the group pays for those services. The potential difference results from the fact that, while the poor may gain less from government health services, they may pay substantially lower taxes as they live outside the organized economy.

3. The distribution of financial benefits covered by the figures is not necessarily the same as the distribution of therapeutic benefit, which is arguably more relevant. The two would not correspond when, for example, the services that the poor receive consist principally of primary interventions that, although inexpensive, are quite effective in treating illness, while the expensive tertiary care received by the rich is of limited therapeutic value.

4. The data provided cover only government curative health care services (hospitals, health posts, etc.). They do not include expenditures on government health education or preventative health programmes such as immunization campaigns. It remains unclear how much of a bias is introduced by the omission of such activities, as they typically represent a rather small portion of total government health expenditures and do not necessarily reach the poor all that more effectively than curative programmes. However, their omission at the very least significantly increases the possibility of inaccuracy in the benefit–incidence information available.
5. Figures for the financial benefit accruing to any specific economic group provide no guidance on how well that benefit corresponds to need. For example, to say that the financial benefit accruing to the poor is twice that accruing to the rich sounds progressive, but it may not be if the poor need, say, four times as large a financial benefit as required by the rich in order to compensate for the greater degree of illness that they experience.

Trends in intercountry health status inequalities

The data currently available can be used to assess trends in some types of country health inequalities, for example by gender or geographic area. However, they are not sufficient to support any assessment of trends in intracountry inequalities in health status or service use by socio-economic status, which is the focus of the current discussion.

However, it is possible to investigate trends with respect to inequalities by socio-economic status across countries. This can be done by looking at time series data for the average levels of infant mortality and life expectancy that are regularly published by such agencies as the United Nations Population Division, the World Bank, the WHO, and others.

What follows are two such investigations. One compares time trends in groups of countries. The second looks at changes over time in the distribution of infant mortality and life expectancy across individual countries.

Trends among country groups.

Table 4 presents the summary results of the first investigation, which is a simple exercise based on World Bank data for 1970, 1980, and 1990. The purpose is to provide an initial sense of changes over this period in the size of the infant mortality and life expectancy gaps between the rich and poor parts of the world. To this end, two types of comparison are presented: (a) between the rich industrialized countries and all others, and (b) between the same group of rich industrialized countries and the world's poorest countries (i.e. omitting the more advanced developing countries). In each case, the definitions of country groups are those of the World Bank. Intergroup boundaries are expressed in terms of per capita incomes, and countries were assigned to the appropriate group on the basis of the situation prevailing in 1990.

The results of the exercise vary according to the statistical measure and the indicator of health status used. In both types of comparison, infant mortality differences decline over time in absolute terms but rise in relative terms. For example, the comparison of the richest and poorest country groups shows that the absolute difference in infant mortality falls from about 125 in 1970 to about 95 in 1990. However, the infant mortality gap expressed in relative terms rises. While infant mortality in 1970 was about 6.5 times higher in the poorest countries than in the richest countries, it was over 11 times higher by 1990. The same is true for the comparison between the richest and all other countries. For life expectancy, both types of country group comparison show a decrease in inequality in both absolute and relative terms.

Trends among individual countries

Table 5 summarizes results of the second individual country exercise which is based on a World Bank dataset containing average infant mortality rates and life expectancies in all major countries of the world for 1970, 1980, and 1990. It features the measurement of changes in the degree of inequality among the countries in the dataset over the period from 1970 to 1990 through the application of a set of standard disparity indices: the standard deviation, the slope index of inequality, the relative index of inequality, the index of dissimilarity, and the concentration index. Two variants of the exercise were undertaken: the first covering all 130 countries, and the second dealing with only the developing and transition countries (approximately 100).

As with the earlier exercise, the results are mixed. This is particularly the case with respect to infant mortality, where in each variant the poor–rich country gap widens according to some

Table 4 Trends in health inequality between country groups, 1970–1990

Comparison	Percentage of global population[a]	Change in infant mortality rate disparity[b]		Change in life expectancy disparity[b]	
		Absolute	Relative	Absolute	Relative
High-income countries	Richest 16%				
vs.					
Low-, middle-, and upper- middle-income countries	Remaining 84 %	–	+	–	–
High-income countries	Richest 16%				
vs.					
Low-income countries	Poorest 56%	–	+	–	–

[a]Approximate 1990 figures.

[b] + Disparity increased between 1970 and 1990; – disparity decreased between 1970 and 1990.

Source: tabulations of World Bank data by N.R. Jones.

Table 5 Trends in health inequality among countries, 1970–1990

Comparison	Percentage of global population[a]	Indicator[b]				
		Standard deviation	Slope index of inequality	Relative index of inequality	Index of dissimilarity	Concentration index
Infant mortality						
All countries	100%	–	–	+	+	+
Developing countries only	Poorest 84%	–	–	+	+	+
Life expectancy						
All countries	100%	–	–	–	–	+
Developing countries only	Poorest 84%	–	+	–	–	+

[a]Approximate 1990 figures.

[b] + Disparity increased between 1970 and 1990; – disparity decreased between 1970 and 1990.

Source: tabulations of World Bank data by N.R. Jones.

indicators and narrows with respect to others. The trend in life expectancy is somewhat less ambiguous, narrowing in all but one of the 10 cases presented, although in some cases the figures show that the degree of narrowing was marginal.

Summary

All in all, the findings reported above are far from conclusive. The one possible exception is the moderately clear difference between infant mortality and life expectancy trends—the former are mixed, and the latter generally point to a narrowing gap. This hints at a narrowing in poor–rich country mortality differences at older ages that is faster than, and possibly in a direction different from, the trend at younger ages. But it is no more than a hint, as one cannot exclude the possibility that the difference is a statistical artefact, attributable to the subtleties of the relationship among mortality levels at different ages included in the life expectancy measure.

In brief, about all one can say with confidence is that any change in intercountry mortality inequalities between 1970 and 1990 period has not been dramatic enough to show up clearly through the application of standard disparity measurement approaches to the data available. Any more definitive statement will have to await more careful and sophisticated data analyses than have been possible within the limited scope of the current review.

Reducing inequalities

Thought about how to reduce the inequalities discussed in the preceding section has thus far lagged well behind the growing desire to reduce them that was described at the outset. The nature of this thought has also changed from that which prevailed in the late 1970s and early 1980s, when a concern for health inequalities and the health of the poor was last prominent in international health circles. As noted earlier, the emphasis at that time was on a single health-service-based approach—a set of relatively simple and inexpensive community-based interventions collectively known as primary health care. Current thought differs from this in two ways. First, at the conceptual or general strategic level, a much larger role is being accorded to general social and economic factors lying outside the health service sector. Second, at the operational level within the health sector, there exists a much more diverse set of ideas for helping the poor— many of them adapted from other sectors.

Enhanced place of general social and economic factors

The first of these changes—the more central place currently accorded general social and economic factors—can be seen in the documents of many agencies. Two of the more prominent documents, one each from the WHO and the World Bank, can serve as illustrations.

The WHO document is the four-part health and poverty strategy recently proposed by the Director-General (WHO 1999*b*). The first part is 'acting on the determinants of health by influencing development policy.' The second is 'reducing risks through a broader approach to public health', i.e. including not just basic public health services, safe and adequate food, clean water, and sanitation, but also the reduction of violence and environmental hazards, conflicts, and natural disasters. The more traditional health sector approaches come only later, in the third and fourth parts, which are 'focusing on the health problems of the poor,' and 'ensuring that health systems serve the poor more effectively'.

The World Bank document is the chapter on health, nutrition, and population in its *Poverty Reduction Strategy Sourcebook* (www.worldbank.org/poverty/strategies/sourctoc.htm), a massive document prepared in 1999–2000 as a reference work for developing country officials preparing the poverty reduction strategy papers described earlier. The chapter on health, nutrition, and population in this multifaceted volume is organized according to a framework that calls attention to three different sources of influence on health outcomes.

1. **Households and communities** At the household and community level, three sets of factors are described:
- household actions and risk factors, such as dietary, sanitary, and sexual practices
- household assets, human (such as education) as well as physical and financial
- community factors, such as the physical surrounding and degree to which the different members of the household feel responsible for one another's well being.

2. **Health system and related factors** Here, too, three sets of factors are laid out:
- health service provision, especially considerations like accessibility, quality, and price
- health financing, such as insurance or public subsidies for essential services
- supply in related sectors, covering issues such as the availability and quality of food, water, and energy.

3. **Government policies and actions** Two sets of factors are presented:
- health sector policies/actions, such as policies on essential drugs or towards private sector services
- policies/actions in other sectors, such as agriculture and education, which can have indirect but powerful side-effects on health.

In this World Bank framework, as in the WHO statement, the potential contribution of health services is duly noted, but such services constitute only one of the many factors that determine health status. For instance, they occupy only eight of the boxes that appear in the diagrammatic presentation of the framework, and only around 20 to 25 per cent of the text explaining the framework is devoted to them. Much more prominence is given to the other broader influences on health.

The extent to which such broader thinking in the headquarters of international agencies will affect what happens at the operational level remains unclear. At present, the impact appears limited. For example, to judge from reading the health chapters of country PRSPs, current plans do not look very different from the health strategies of two decades ago. There are occasional references to things like basic health insurance and private sector involvement that one would not have seen earlier, but typically the PRSP chapters feature measures like prenatal care, vaccinations, and essential drug provision that would have been at the centre of a strategy paper written at the height of the primary care movement of the early 1980s (Gwatkin 2001*b*). However, it is far too early to pass any final judgement, since the situation could well change over the years ahead if international thinking continues to be as influential in the formulation of developing country health policies as it has in the past.

Diverse sets of ideas within the health service sector

The second difference between earlier and current thought, concerning the diverse sets of ideas at the operational level within the health sector, can be illustrated with reference to four approaches that are currently in use or under active discussion. None of the four is exclusive to health. Rather, each represents the application to health of approaches being used in efforts to reduce inequalities in overall socio-economic status.

Two of the four—targeting and participatory approaches—are well established. The other two—protection against the financial risks of illness and the statement of health objectives in distributional terms—are much newer. Each appears sufficiently valuable or promising to merit careful consideration. However, none is a panacea and, on the basis on present knowledge, it is far from certain that even the four together would be strong enough to offset fully the current tendency of health programmes to reach the better-off more effectively than the disadvantaged, as described above in the section on inequalities in health service use.

Targeted health services

The expression 'targeting' refers to a set of techniques used to increase the percentage of benefits from a particular intervention that flows to the poor. Health is just one of the many sectors where these techniques are employed. Other common ones include the identification of individuals or groups qualified to receive subsidized food supplies, to obtain employment through government-supported public works programmes, or in some cases to qualify for subsidized loans through microcredit programmes.

Targeting has many supporters, but it also has detractors who are of two types. One type argues that, on the basis of findings like those cited below, targeting techniques do not work very well in distinguishing poor from rich and reaching the former. The second type is concerned with the 'top-down' nature of targeted measures, which deliver free or subsidized services or commodities. As such, they are thought to represent hand-outs that invite dependency rather than foster the initiative among beneficiaries seen as central for long-term poverty alleviation or health improvement (Sen 1994).

There are many different targeting techniques available, and many ways of categorizing them. One of the more common categorization approaches features a distinction between 'individual', 'direct', or 'narrow' targeting on the one hand, and 'indicator/characteristic', 'indirect', or 'broad' targeting on the other.

The former type refers to efforts to identify poor individuals and see that as much of the service concerned reaches as many of them as possible. The objective is to come as close as possible to the goal of 100 per cent coverage with zero leakage, i.e. seeing that all the poor are served and that all of those served are poor. The latter type of targeting deals with attributes rather than individuals. Rather than trying to identify individuals who are poor, for instance, it might feature the provision of services in slum areas in anticipation that the great majority of recipients will be poor. In doing so, it recognizes that it will not be able to reach all of the poor (some of whom live outside slums), and that at least some of those receiving services will not be poor (as not everyone living in a poor area is poor). However, it accepts these limitations as prices worth paying in order to attain two important advantages. One is administrative practicality or efficiency, through avoidance of the considerable effort typically required to distinguish between poor and non-poor individuals with even a modest degree of precision. The second is political—the belief that poverty-oriented service programmes are much more likely to gain the political support needed for survival if members of the middle and upper classes gain enough from them to have an incentive to defend their continuation.

These different targeting methods are not mutually exclusive and are often used in combination. There is no known instance of their achieving or even approaching perfection, but there is considerable evidence that, when employed with care and determination, they can increase the percentage of service benefits that accrue to the poor. The best-known instance of this comes from a set of studies covering nearly 50 government and private service programmes (including but not limited to health) in Latin America. These studies found that in the 18 carefully targeted programmes, some 70 to 75 per cent of benefits accrued to the poorest 40 per cent of households, compared with 55 to 60 per cent of the benefits from government primary health care and education projects and 30 to 35 per cent of the benefits from untargeted food distribution programmes. All three of the principal targeting methods used worked equally well, and the administrative costs of targeting were typically under 10 per cent of total programme expenses (Grosh 1994).

There are many specific targeting techniques available, each with unique features, strengths, and weaknesses. Three of them—individual targeting, geographic targeting, and disease targeting— can serve to illustrate the potential and limitations of the different options..

Individual targeting

Certain forms of individual targeting have long been practised in the health field. A common example is the use of simple diagnostic measures in screening programmes to identify individuals at high risk of serious illness and thus in need of priority attention. More recently, a great deal of attention has been given to the identification of poor individuals in order to exempt them from users' fees introduced in government health facilities of developing countries during health sector reforms.

The experience of efforts to identify individuals for this purpose has varied widely. There have been more reported failures than reported successes. But there have been successes as well, and rather clear differences in the design of the more and less successful efforts that can serve as guidelines for the design of future initiatives.

Towards the effective end of the effective–ineffective spectrum lie some of the Latin American projects noted above. Also instructive is the case of Thailand, which has been offering free medical care to low-income groups, through an initiative known as the Low Income Support Program, since 1975. The programme has been modified numerous times as the government has gained experience. In its present form, it is open to Thai families with monthly incomes of under 2000 baht, which constitutes about 25 per cent of the country's population. Local officials of the Ministry of Home Affairs determine who qualifies under the income criterion just noted and issue identity cards, valid for 3 years, to those families found eligible. The card-holders are exempted from fees at government health facilities. The cost is covered by a special allocation to the service-providing facilities from the Ministry of Public Health, which allocates about 8 per cent of its total budget to this end. The programme now covers some 11 million people, or about 20 per cent of the country's total population—equivalent to about 80 per cent of the eligible poor population. Independent surveys indicate that about 20 per cent of those covered are non-poor who are improperly included. Adjusting for this suggests that, in total, the programme covers about 65 per cent of Thailand's poor, with a leakage rate of 20 per cent (Khoman 1997).

At the other end of the spectrum are a series of casual efforts, especially in Africa. For example, according to a recent questionnaire study of 26 developing countries (most but not all in Africa), almost three-quarters of the countries responding reported at least some kind of official policy to exempt the poor from user fees. But, said the study organizers, 'there were numerous informational, administrative, economic, and political constraints to effective implementation of these exemptions' (Russell and Gilson 1997). For instance, in most countries policy guidelines on whom to exempt were quite vague, local exemption administrators found it very difficult to assess household incomes, and/or the potentially eligible were often unaware that exemptions were available. The findings of other reviews are similar: in general, found one such review, individual targeting efforts in sub-Saharan Africa 'have been compromised by a variety of difficulties, including excessive leakage, overly subjective exemption criteria, informal identification and verification procedures, and excessive costs' (H. Waters, unpublished work, 1995).

A plausible explanation of why some individual targeting programmes have been more successful than others emerges from a study of 29 such efforts in health. The study suggested two factors that differentiated between the nine efforts considered successful and the 20 that were not. One was the existence of clear, formal, and explicit criteria for eligibility. The second was the determination of eligibility by someone other than the health service provider, such as a village council (Willis 1993). A third factor might be hypothesized from the Thailand case cited above—the provision of a mechanism and of resources to reimburse health service providers for income foregone in providing free services.

Geographic targeting

The idea behind geographic targeting is straightforward—the poorer the area to which resources are allocated, the greater the likelihood that the individuals who benefit from those resources will be poor. Like individual targeting, geographic targeting is a generic approach, in the sense of being equally applicable to activities in almost any sector rather than being specific to health. Geographic targeting can be applied with widely varying degrees of precision. The amount of improved accuracy resulting from increases in precision will depend upon the spatial pattern of the distribution of poverty within the society concerned.

Perhaps the simplest and least precise form of geographic targeting is the emphasis often placed on rural areas, where the available information suggests that poverty is in general considerably more prevalent than it is in the cities. For example, World Bank data for the world's low-income countries indicated that in the mid-1990s the agricultural workers who constituted 66 per cent of the labour force produced only 27 per cent of the economic output. The same appeared to be the case in the middle-income countries, where 32 per cent of the workers were in the agricultural sector which accounted for 11 per cent of the national output (World Bank 1998).

Other more precise forms of targeting involve a focus on poor states or provinces, or subdivisions within these. Typically, these are identified on the basis of data for per capita income or output produced by government statistical offices. Several countries, particularly in Latin America, have sought to be even more precise by identifying villages or other small communities that are particularly poor. This has typically been done through the construction of a basic needs or similar index based on questions contained in national censuses such as literacy rates, education levels, and quality of housing.

Recently, there has been experimentation with techniques for identifying small areas on the basis of measures more obviously and directly related to consumption, traditionally the indicator preferred by economists concerned with poverty. The techniques concerned involve combining data from in-depth sample surveys, which ask many questions from a relatively small number of households, and from national censuses, which ask a few questions about all the households in a country. The basic idea is to identify those questions on the household survey instruments that are also included in the national census, and best predict the consumption levels of the households covered. Average values for the questions thus identified can then be calculated for individual villages covered by the census data in order to predict the average consumption levels prevailing in those villages, and the poorest villages can be selected on this basis. The use of such techniques is still in infancy, but initial experience with them has been promising in such widely varying settings as Burkina Faso, Ecuador, and South Africa (H. Alderman *et al.*, World Bank, unpublished work, 1999; Bigman *et al.* 2000; Hentschel *et al.* 2000).

Finding the areas with the greatest number of poor people is only part of the story, however. Equally important is the development of services that can reach the poor in those areas. This can be challenging, as poor areas frequently lack the capital and physical infrastructure necessary for effective programme initiation.

Targeting by disease

As with geographic targeting, two steps are involved in disease targeting. The first is to identify the diseases that are most important for the poor, and the second is to develop delivery mechanisms that reach the poor in order to lessen the impact of those diseases.

With respect to the first of these steps, a recent assessment has established that, at the global level, the diseases of greatest importance to the poor tend to be communicable. For example, among the 20 per cent of the global population living in the poorest countries, communicable and related conditions were responsible for about 59 per cent of all deaths in 1990, compared with 32 per cent caused by non-communicable diseases and about 9 per cent attributable to accidents and injuries. In that year, communicable and related diseases were responsible for over three-quarters of the global poor–rich mortality gap. Any acceleration in the rate of communicable disease decline, evenly distributed across all global social groups, would benefit the poorest 20 per cent some 10 times more than the richest 20 per cent. This stands in sharp contrast to the impact of a comparable acceleration in the fall of non-communicable diseases which would benefit the richest 20 per cent about three to four times as much as the poorest 20 per cent (Gwatkin and Guillot 1999).

Thus, at the global level, there is strong justification for emphasizing improved approaches for dealing with communicable diseases. However, the available evidence also indicates that there is a great deal of country-to-country variation relevant for the establishment of national policies. This is particularly the case in demographically advanced developing and transitional countries. In such settings, where overall mortality levels are generally low, it is quite possible for non-communicable conditions to be more important than communicable diseases even among the poor. At the same time, however, communicable diseases are still likely to be more important for the poor than for the rich, in the sense of being responsible for a larger minority of death and disability in the former group than in the latter.

The point can be illustrated by a study performed in Mexico in 1994 which provided estimates for rural and urban regions, using a combined mortality–disability measure called disability-adjusted life years (**DALYs**). Even in the rural population, presumably consisting primarily of poor people, more DALYs were lost as a result of non-communicable conditions than because of communicable diseases (44 per cent versus 37 per cent). However, communicable diseases, even though the minority cause of death and disability in rural areas, were still a considerably larger minority in the rural group than in the urban group (37 per cent versus 25 per cent of total DALYs lost) (Frenk *et al.* 1998).

In such a situation, which appears typical of that prevailing in much of Latin America and Eastern Europe, any country-wide emphasis on non-communicable diseases would be highly relevant for the poor. However, it would be more likely to increase than to decrease poor–rich disparities as non-communicable diseases are likely to be still more important for the rich. If the poor are to benefit more than the rich, it would be necessary to supplement disease targeting with some other targeting approach (such as individual or geographic targeting) to increase the proportion of total benefits reaching the needy. (One would also wish to incorporate cost-effectiveness considerations into any programme design in order to ensure the production of adequate health benefits overall.)

The situation is similar with respect to the second of the two issues posed above, concerning the effectiveness of intervention delivery systems in serving the poor. It is not safe to assume that a focus on diseases relevant for the poor will in itself lead to improvements in that group of a country's population, as those diseases also affect upper- and middle-income groups at least to some extent. It is quite possible to imagine a situation in which intervention programmes against diseases relevant for the poor fail to develop the outreach capacity required to reach the neediest, so that the programme benefits are limited primarily to better-off groups. The available information suggests that this is happening in many countries, although by no means all, and that, where this is happening, disease targeting will have to be supplemented by geographic, individual, or some other type of targeting if the poor are to be served.

The information containing such suggestions comes from data for the several intervention measures covered in the country health and poverty reports referred to above with respect to infant and under-5 mortality. Particularly relevant are the quintile-specific data for interventions directed against communicable diseases among children—diseases that, as suggested above, are especially important for the global poor. The interventions include immunizations against measles, diphtheria, whooping cough, and tetanus, and curative treatment of diarrhoea and acute respiratory diseases. Quintile-specific data are also available for antenatal care and deliveries attended by trained medical personnel, which deal with a condition which is not communicable, at least not in the traditional sense, but which turns out to be concentrated particularly among disadvantaged groups.

These data show that the situation varies greatly from country to country. For example, consider the data for the percentage of children immunized against all the diseases noted above, which are summarized in Table 6. Looking first at the percentage of children immunized among the poorest 20 per cent of the population, there is only a modest variation among the different regions—from 35 per cent in Africa to about 43 per cent in Asia, the Near East, and North Africa. However, the country-to-country variations within each region are dramatic, particularly in Sub-Saharan Africa where the range is from under 5 per cent (Niger) to over 70 per cent (Malawi, Zambia, Zimbabwe). A review of the poor–rich ratios and concentration indices, which permit a comparison of immunization rates among the poorest 20 per cent with those in higher socio-economic groups, reveals notably smaller disparities in Latin America than in other parts

Table 6 Levels and intracountry inequalities in immunization rates

Region	No. of countries	Immunization rate among poorest 20% of population (%)		Rich-to-poor ratio		Concentration index	
		Mean	Range	Mean	Range	Mean	Range
Sub-Saharan Africa	20	35.0	4.6–73.0	2.07	1.17–11.11	0.160	0.22–0.434
Asia–Near East–North Africa	9	42.8	17.1–69.3	1.71	1.05–3.80	0.117	0.012–0.262
Latin America–Caribbean	11	39.7	18.8–55.8	1.45	1.03–2.62	0.084	0.001–0.177
Total	39	37.1	4.6–73.0	1.84	1.03–11.11	0.128	0.001–0.434

Source: Gwatkin *et al.* (2000).

of the developing world. However, there are also very large country-to-country variations within each region. The reasons for the variations remain to be determined.

Participatory approaches to health service planning and delivery

As noted earlier, targeting is not universally popular among development professionals. To some, it is seen as an outgrowth of the tendency of many public health professionals to determine the most important health issues on the basis of the epidemiological considerations that are important to them; this is then done without pausing to determine whether the priorities thus established correspond with the priorities of the intended beneficiaries. An alternative approach, preferred by people holding this view, is to involve the prospective beneficiaries from the beginning. This means determining their priorities as the basis for project development and developing modes of service delivery that they are likely to find congenial. Such a 'consumer-oriented' or 'client-oriented' approach is often supported on pragmatic as well as conceptual grounds, through reference to the likelihood of increased utilization resulting from the provision of services that people want rather than those that outsiders think they need.

This approach has been present in development thought since at least the 1950s when it went by the name of development on the basis of prospective beneficiaries' 'felt needs.' Strong traces of it have also existed in international public health circles, among community medicine specialists who share many of the same concerns about technocratic epidemiology just expressed. The concern of such specialists can be seen in the strong emphasis on community-based approaches appearing in the Alma Ata Declaration of 1978.

At present, the approach is gaining strength. Work is going on in many venues, but recent trends are most clearly illustrated with reference to developments within the World Bank. While that institution remains better known for its technocratic orientation than for its participatory instincts, an incipient interest in participation can be seen through three streams of work. Two of these are analytical—identifying the poor through participatory poverty assessments, and determining what the poor want in the way of health services and what they think of the services they currently receive. The third is operational—increasing reliance on non-governmental or community organizations rather than government agencies to deliver health and other services.

Participatory poverty assessments

The basic premise underlying the participatory poverty assessment (**PPA**) approach is that villagers are much better able to define poverty and identify the poor among them than are outside government authorities. In a sense, PPAs can thus be seen from a technocratic perspective as a way of identifying people who deserve the highest priority under an individual targeting programme, although the information gathered goes well beyond this in helping determine how communities perceive poverty.

PPAs usually employ relatively non-quantitative methods based on guided discussions with village members. The discussions typically proceed in two stages. The first stage consists of reaching consensus about the appropriate indicators of wealth and poverty. The second consists of identifying individual families or people as rich or poor on the basis of the agreed-upon indicators.

By encouraging people first to establish criteria for poverty before identifying individuals who were poor, the PPA seeks to lessen the problem commonly attributed to village-based beneficiary approaches—the alleged proclivity of village leaders to identify their relatives, friends, and political supporters as those most deserving programme benefits. Just how well it succeeds in this regard remains unclear.

This approach has so far been applied in nearly 50 countries, especially in Africa, by the World Bank (Robb 1999), and no doubt in countless other locations by other agencies. Among the best-known is Tanzania, where discussions like those described above took place in 87 villages in different parts of the country and involved over 6000 village residents (Narayan 1997). In each village, the residents produced maps locating the dwellings of those they considered to belong to the poorest of five wealth categories. In the Dodoma region, for example, the poor were defined as (a) mostly old or disabled, (b) people who lived by begging, (c) childless women, and/or (d) people who were mentally unfit. In the Kilimanjaro region, participants defined the poor as people who were (a) landless, (b) did not plant crops, (c) depended upon relatives, and (d) lived in substandard housing. The percentage identified as poor by applying these criteria in the study villages closely approximated the percentage defined as living below the poverty line through more formal consumption-based methods, although there may have been differences in the particular individuals who qualified as poor.

Another multicountry PPA has been undertaken in connection with preparation of the World Bank's 2000–2001 *World Development*

Report, which is focusing on poverty. The exercise is known as Consultations with the Poor (Narayan *et al.* 2000*a*,*b*). It is in two parts: the first is a summary of some 80 earlier PPAs from around the world involving interviews with over 60 000 people; the second consists of 23 country studies, covering about 20 000 poor individuals. These new studies contain a great deal of information about how the poor perceive health and health services. They also cover a wide range of topics, including many which, strictly speaking, are more closely associated with the beneficiary assessments described in the following section than with PPAs.

Beneficiary assessments

While PPAs are oriented primarily (although not exclusively) towards determining just who is poor, beneficiary assessments focus more on what the poor want in the way of services and/or what they think of the services offered to them. Given this focus, they might be considered as a type of market research, designed to produce information of value to programme managers which can help them design programmes corresponding more closely to consumers' preferences.

Like PPAs, beneficiary assessments also tend to rely primarily on qualitative methods. Commonly used approaches include informal conversational interviews, participant observation, and focus group discussions. Upon occasion—as with the Voices of the Poor exercise described earlier—a particular qualitative study will include elements of both a beneficiary assessment and PPA, an indication of the fluidity of the distinction between them.

Beneficiary assessments appear to have been undertaken rather frequently in connection with health programmes, at least in connection with those receiving World Bank support. For example, a review of World Bank experience in 1995 listed some 20 beneficiary assessments made in the course of developing or evaluating health, population, and nutrition projects, more than twice the number prepared in any other sector of World Bank activity (Salmen 1995). An informal reading of subsequent World Bank project documents suggests that there have been many more since then. A systematic review of work done by individuals and agencies not associated with the World Bank would no doubt uncover many more. Also, in addition to studies considered as strictly defined beneficiary assessments, there exists a vast array of more general village-based anthropological and sociological literature about health which contains information about the health priorities of the poor that is of obvious relevance for programme development.

Virtually all of the beneficiary assessments known to have been performed to date have been undertaken for project preparation or evaluation rather than for formal publication. Such studies tend to disappear after having served their intended purpose, and this results in a problem of physical unavailability that makes it impossible to provide an overview of findings to see if there are common themes across countries. However, one can give a flavour of what the studies show through a few illustrations from recent studies that remain extant. For example, a focus group discussion in Bangladesh revealed that the major deterrent to the use of government facilities was the unpredictable volume of under-the-table payments requested by facility employees, thus making it difficult for the prospective clients to know in advance whether they could afford the services. A study conducted by participant observers in Lesotho found that the village health worker programme was having little impact because the workers were emphasizing preventive services which, while in line with professional thought, were of little interest to villagers. The villagers actually wanted curative services that the workers were not qualified to provide (Salmen 1995). In Ethiopia, policy-makers learned from a beneficiary assessment that the antenatal services they offered were being poorly used because of a cultural belief that pregnant women considered it improper to admit to any pain or discomfort during pregnancy (Salmen 1995). Anecdotal information based on such surveys in a number of countries suggests that the availability of drugs (and injections) is frequently a factor to which poor patients attract considerable importance.

Alternative delivery mechanisms

Frustration over the bureaucratic and political constraints that prevent government ministries from offering services that reach the poor effectively is giving rise to an interest in identifying alternative mechanisms. Typically, this means looking to agencies that have a larger degree of participation by, or at least are much closer to, the poor clients who are the intended beneficiaries. Most attention has thus far gone to two types of agency—non-government organizations and social funds.

With respect the former, there is a widespread belief that non-governmental organizations are much better than government health programmes at identifying and serving the poor. This is not inevitably the case: Tanzania and Zambia represent instances where the economic level of people served through the non-governmental health sector appears higher than that of patients in government facilities (F. Diop, unpublished work, WHO, 1997; Munishi 1997). However, where non-governmental organizations do reach the poor effectively, government grants to or contracts with non-governmental organizations for the delivery of services represent an alternative to efforts to target poor individuals through the government service system. This is not always easy for governments to do, given the resistance that can be expected from their employees who stand to lose if this practice becomes widespread. External agencies find it easier to move in this direction and appear increasingly interested in doing so. In Bangladesh, to cite perhaps the most prominent example, a massive volume of donor support has permitted the Bangladesh Rural Advancement Committee, which now employs some 25 000 to 30 000 people, to become one of the country's principal providers of health and other services in poor rural areas.

Another alternative to direct government health (and other) service delivery is a social fund, a relatively new form of quasi-governmental financial intermediary that channels funds directly to small-scale projects for poor and vulnerable groups operated by local governments, non-governmental organizations, or community groups. Social funds have been created in well over 30 countries, especially in Africa and Latin America, as a way around rigidities in traditional government ministries which prevent them from reaching the poor effectively. Thus far, the Inter-American Development Bank and the World Bank have made loans of over US$3.5 billion to more than 50 countries to support social funds (S. Jorgensen, World Bank, unpublished work, 1999). Roughly one-third of social fund support has traditionally gone to health, nutrition, and population (S. Carvalho, World Bank, unpublished work, 1995).

Data limitations prevent any clear assessment of just how well social funds have in fact reached the poor. But such information as exists suggests an overall picture quite similar to that presented above with respect to individual targeting in more traditional government programmes, i.e. social funds which adopt explicit carefully designed and implemented approaches to beneficiary identification work much better than those which do not (S. Carvalho, World Bank, unpublished work, 1995).

Protecting the poor from the financial consequences of illness

A third and more recent approach to dealing with health inequalities differs from the two just described in taking what might be called a financial orientation, i.e. the reason for being concerned with the health of the disadvantaged is not an interest in health *per se*, but rather the financial implications of poor health for the people concerned. Lessened health inequality through assistance to the disadvantage is seen less as an end in itself than as a means towards the end of reduced financial inequality. The rationale for such an approach lies in the belief, increasingly supported by empirical evidence, that the path out of poverty is not smooth. Families do not simply rise steadily out of poverty and, once out of it, follow a steadily upward trajectory. Rather, they often fall back, sometimes temporarily and sometimes permanently, as a result of external shocks over which they have little control.

Often, these external shocks are economic in nature, as in the case of the financial crisis that affected much of Asia in the mid-1990s. Sometimes, the shock is caused by civil strife, as in parts of Africa and the former Yugoslavia. But poor health also appears to play a significant role, partly because of the high costs of medical care, and partly because of the income lost in those cases where the sick person is a major breadwinner for the family.

The two most complete studies of this issue undertaken to date are from Bangladesh. One, carried out in an urban slum, found that over 40 per cent of people in the poorest quartile of the population had missed work during the preceding month, and that this had cost them an average of nearly 75 per cent of their family income in that period (Pryer 1989). The other, a survey of more than 60 villages, found that poor health was the principal cause of 15 to 20 per cent of the cases in which previously non-poor people had slipped into poverty. Many others avoided falling below the poverty line, measured in consumption terms, by drawing down their family assets (Sen 1997).

The three other known studies focused on medical costs, and dealt only indirectly with foregone income. Two cover poor rural areas in China. Each of these studies found that medical costs borne by poor families in the era following the collapse of rural medical co-operatives is extremely high. One study reported that medical costs represent over 15 per cent of the total expenditures among poor families. One-third of the families had to dip into assets in order to cover the costs; 70 to 90 per cent of the sick who did not seek care gave the high cost as the reason (W. Fu *et al.*, unpublished work, 1995). The other Chinese study found that the average cost of a one-time hospitalization equalled well over the annual income of a poor peasant, (b) costs of other care received by the poor cost them about 10 per cent of their incomes, and (c) 80 per cent of poor people needing hospitalization did not obtain it because of the expense. The study concluded that 'illness is a major reason why peasants become impoverished or (why) those who have made their way out of poverty revert to being poor' (Expert Committee for the Study of Policy and Administration 1996). The third study is from Mexico where over 4 per cent of the poorest 30 per cent of the population experienced medical expenses equal to over half of their incomes during the first 6 months of 1992—a percentage far higher than experienced at higher income levels (Frenk *et al.* 1998).

Beyond this are indications that, regardless of how important or unimportant the financial consequences of ill health might be when measured empirically, the poor worry a lot about them. In the interviews conducted with 20 000 poor people throughout the world in connection with the Consultations with the Poor study, the fear of ill health because of its potential financial implications arose again and again. In these interviews, ill health was the most frequently cited reason why families became impoverished (Narayan 2000).

Findings like these argue for a concern with protection against severe or catastrophic illness, whose costs, in the form of medical expenses and/or lost income, can easily drag families down into poverty or prevent their rising out of it. Several mechanisms for providing such protection are currently under consideration. They include the development of risk-pooling or insurance plans and subsidized or free secondary medical care for income-earning adults.

Establishing health objectives in distributional terms

A final and even more recent approach is oriented towards health planners and policy-makers at the national and international levels. Its focus is on the way that health objectives are established in macrolevel economic and health development plans. Typically, such health objectives are established in terms of society-wide averages—reduction of a country's overall infant mortality rate by x per cent, an increase in a society's average life expectancy by y years, etc. While averages like these are informative about conditions prevailing in a society as a whole, they say nothing about the inequalities that prevail in it. As a result, they are poorly suited for the development of strategies or the assessment of progress towards inequality reduction, or the improvement of conditions among the poor.

A recent exercise, based on a set of international development goals established in connection with the Global Social Summit conference held in Copenhagen in 1995, suggested that this is considerably more than an academic quibble. The health goals appearing in the set included a call for a two-thirds reduction in the average infant mortality rate in all countries by the year 2015. When examined from an intracountry inequality perspective, using the data on interquintile differences presented earlier, there proved to be several combinations of decline in different quintiles that could result in both a two-thirds reduction in overall infant mortality and a significant widening in interquintile differences. Under some circumstances, the two-thirds reduction in infant mortality could be attained without any significant decline in the rate prevailing in the poorest quintile (Gwatkin 2000).

This has led to an interest in finding an alternative way of stating health objectives in terms of, say, an x per cent reduction of the difference in infant mortality between the poorest and richest quintiles, or a y-year improvement in life expectancy among people below a society's poverty line. A statement of health objectives in such terms would be consistent with current thinking about economic development objectives, which are increasingly being expressed in poverty or distributional terms rather than with regard to societal averages. (The economic goals of the Social Summit, for instance, refer not to increasing average per capita incomes, as was the earlier convention, but rather to decreasing the numbers of people living in poverty.)

A restatement of goals would not in itself save lives, however. Restated goals would be of value only to the extent to which they succeed in directing the attention of policy-makers towards health inequalities and the health of the poor, thereby preparing the way for the development of effective interventions to deal with those issues. This implies a need not just for restated goals, but also for the use of these goals to shape policies and programmes.

Conclusions

This review began with the argument that a concern for health inequalities has recently begun to rise to prominence after a decade during which it attracted little attention. In closing, it is appropriate to ask what will be required to ensure that it remains at the centre of attention and leads to effective action.

Had this question been posed as recently asd 2 or 3 years ago, the temptation would have been strong to respond that effective action would require progress with respect to all three of the other topics covered in this review. That is, there appeared to be a clear need for closer agreement on what should be the governing concept for activities in this area—reducing health inequalities or improving the health of the poor, a better understanding of the magnitude and dimensions of health inequalities, and improved programme approaches for reaching the poor and improving their health, to supplement the approaches discussed in the section on reducing inequalities.

Now, however, the first and second of these three issues appear to constitute somewhat less formidable obstacles to progress than they did earlier. As noted in the section on concepts, the first issue, i.e. the distinction between reducing health inequalities and improving the health of the poor, is often (although admittedly not always) largely academic, with only limited policy implications. With respect to the second issue, the lack of understanding of health inequalities, the research findings reported in the section on inequalities have brought about a sharp increase in the amount of knowledge that exists.

This is not to argue that either of these issues has yet been by any means fully resolved, just that the amount of progress with respect to each of them has been considerably greater than that with respect to the third issue—the lack of proven policy and programmatic approaches. Thus, this third issue now stands out as the one most in need of attention.

Of course, overlying this issue is the much larger question of political commitment. If the importance currently being attached to poverty-oriented overall development is correct, major progress in reducing health inequalities will require not just a reorientation of the health sector, but also a broad social determination to alleviate poverty.

References

Anand, S., Diderichsen, F., Evans, T., Shkolnikov, V., and Wirth, M. (2001). Measuring disparities in health: methods and indicators. In *Challenging inequities in health: from ethics to action* (ed. T. Evans, M. Whitehead, F. Diderichsen, A. Bhuiya, and M. Wirth), pp. 49-67. Oxford University Press, New York.

Anonymous (1999). Labour's crusade. *Economist*, 25 September.

Bigman, D., Dercon, S., Giullaume, D., and Lambotte, M. (2000). Community targeting for poverty reduction in Burkina Faso. *World Bank Economic Review*, **14**, 167–93.

Carr, D., Gwatkin D., Fragueiro D., and Pande, R. (1999). *A guide to country-level information about equity, poverty, and health available from multi-country research programs.* World Bank, Washington, DC.

Castro-Leal, F., Dayton, J., Demery, L., and Mehra, K. (2000). Public spending on health care in Africa. Do the poor benefit? *Bulletin of the World Health Organization*, **78**, 66–74.

Deininger, K. and Squire, L. (1996). A new data set measuring income inequality. *World Bank Economic Review*, **10**, 565–91.

Department for International Development (2000). *Better health for poor people: strategies for achieving the international development targets.* Department for International Development, London.

Department of Health (1998). *Independent inquiry into inequalities in health (Acheson Report)*. HMSO, London.

Department of Health and Social Security (1980). *Inequalities in health.* Department of Health and Social Security, London.

Expert Committee for the Study of Policy and Administration (of the Chinese Ministry of Health) (1996). Policy proposals on enhancing health care development and reform in poor rural areas. *Health Work Bulletin*, 6 November.

Filmer, D. and Pritchett, L. (2001). Estimating wealth effects without expenditure data—or tears: an application of educational enrollments in states of India. *Demography*, **38**, 115–32.

Frenk, J., González Block, M., and Lozano, R. (1998). Seis tesis equivocadas sobre las politicas de salud en el combate a la pobreza. *Este Pais*, **84**, 28–36.

Gakidou, E., Murray, C., and Frenk, J. (2000). Defining and measuring health inequality: an approach based on the distribution of health expectancy. *Bulletin of the World Health Organization*, **78**, 42–54.

Grant J. (1982). *The state of the world's children, 1982–83.* Oxford University Press, New York.

Grosh, M. (1994). *Administering targeted social programs in Latin America: from platitudes to practice.* World Bank, Washington, DC.

Gwatkin, D. (2000). Health inequalities and the health of the poor: What do we know? What can we do? *Bulletin of the World Health Organization*, **78**, 3–18.

Gwatkin, D. (2001*a*). Poverty and inequalities in health in developing countries. In *Poverty, inequality, and health: an international perspective* (ed. D. Leon and G. Walt). Oxford University Press.

Gwatkin, D. (2001*b*). The need for equity-oriented health sector reforms. *International Journal of Epidemiology*, **30**, 720–3.

Gwatkin, D. and Guillot, M. (1999). *The burden of disease among the global poor:current situation, future trends, and implications for strategy.* World Bank and Global Forum for Health Research, Washington, DC.

Gwatkin, D., Guillot, M., and Heuveline, P. (1999). The burden of disease among the global poor. *Lancet*, **354**, 586–9.

Gwatkin, D.R., Rutstein, S., Johnson K., Pande, R., and Wagstaff, A. (2000). *Socio-economic differences in health, nutrition, and population in Bangladesh.* World Bank, Washington, DC. (See also comparable publications covering Benin, Bolivia, Brazil, Burkina Faso, Cameroun, Central African Republic, Colombia, Comores, Côte d'Ivoire, Dominican Republic, Ghana, Guatemala, Haiti, India, Indonesia, Kenya, Kyrgyz Republic, Madagascar, Malawi, Mali, Morocco, Mozambique, Namibia, Nepal, Nicaragua, Niger, Nigeria, Pakistan, Paraguay, Peru, Philippines, Senegal, Tanzania, Togo, Turkey, Uganda, Vietnam, Zambia, and Zimbabwe.)

Hentschel, J., Lanjuow, J., Lanjouw, P., and Poggi, J. (2000). Combining census and survey data to trace the spatial dimension of poverty: a case study of Ecuador. *World Bank Economic Review*, **14**, 147–65.

Jamison, D. (1997). The health of the poor: global and country-specific estimates for some indicators. Presented at World Bank Health, Nutrition, Population, and Poverty Seminar, 16 December.

Khoman, S. (1997). Rural health care financing in Thailand. In *Innovations in health care financing*, (ed. G. Schieber). World Bank, Washington, DC.

Marchand, S., Wikler, D., and Landesman, B. (1998). Class, health, and justice: health and society. *Milbank Memorial Fund Quarterly*, **76**, 449–67.

Munishi, G. (1997). *Private health care in Tanzania: private health sector growth following liberalization in Tanzania.* International Health Policy Program Working Paper, International Health Policy Program, Washington, DC.

Narayan, D. (1997). *Voices of the poor: poverty and social capital in Tanzania.* World Bank, Washington, DC.

Narayan, D. (2000). What do the poor have to say about health, nutrition, and population? Presented at World Bank Health, Nutrition, Population, and Poverty Seminar, 1 February.

Narayan, D., Patel, R., Schafft, K., Rademacher, A., and Koch-Schulte, S. (2000*a*). *Voices of the poor: can anyone hear us?* Oxford University Press, New York.

Narayan, D., Chambers, R., Shah, M., and Petesch, P. (2000*b*). Voices of the poor: crying out for change. Oxford University Press, New York.

Pan American Health Organization (1995). *The search for equity: annual report of the director.* Pan American Health Organization, Washington, DC.

Pryer, J. (1989). When breadwinners fall ill: preliminary findings from a case study in Bangladesh. *IDS Bulletin*, **20**, 49–57.

Rawls, J. (1971). *A theory of justice.* Harvard University Press, Cambridge, MA.

Robb, C. (1999). *Can the poor influence policy? Participatory poverty assessments in the developing world.* World Bank, Washington.

Rockefeller Foundation (1999). *A new course of action.* Rockefeller Foundation, New York.

Russell, S. and Gilson, L. (1997). User fee policy to promote health service access for the poor: a wolf in sheep's clothing? *International Journal of Health Services*, **27**, 359–79

Salmen, L. (1995). *Beneficiary assessment: an approach described.* World Bank Environment Department Paper 23, World Bank, Washington, DC.

Secretary of State for International Development (1997). *Eliminating world poverty: a challenge for the 21st century.* HMSO, London.

Sen, A. (1994). The political economy of targeting. In *Public spending and the poor: theory and evidence* (ed. D. van de Walle and K. Nead), pp. 11–24. World Bank/Johns Hopkins University Press, Baltimore, MD.

Sen, B. (1997). *Health and poverty in the context of development strategy: a case study on Bangladesh.* Macroeconomics, Health, and Development Series, No. 26, WHO, Geneva.

Uchitelle, L. (1999) More cash in hand, but poorer. *International Herald Tribune*, 19 October.

Wagstaff, A. (1999). Inequalities in infant and child mortality in the developing world: How large are they? How can they be reduced? Presented at World Bank Health, Nutrition, Population and Poverty Seminar, 30 March.

Wagstaff, A. (2000). Socioeconomic inequalities in child mortality: comparisons across nine developing countries. *Bulletin of the World Health Organization*, **78**, 19–29.

Wagstaff, A., Paci, P., and van Doorslaer, E. (1991). On the measurement of inequalities in health. *Social Science and Medicine*, **33**, 545–57.

Whitehead, M. (1990). *The concepts and principles of equity and health.* Document EUR/ICP/RPD/414, WHO Regional Office for Europe, Copenhagen.

WHO (World Health Organization) (1978). *Primary health care. Report of the International Conference on Primary Health Care, Alma-Ata, USSR, 6–12 September 1978.* WHO, Geneva.

WHO (World Health Organization) (1995). *World health report 1995: bridging the gap.* WHO, Geneva.

WHO (World Health Organization) (1996). *Equity in health and health care: a WHO/SIDA initiative.* Document WHO/ARB/96.1, WHO, Geneva.

WHO (World Health Organization) (1999*a*). *World health report 1999: making a difference.* WHO, Geneva.

WHO (World Health Organization) (1999*b*). *Poverty and health. Report by the Director General.* Document EB105/5 presented to the 105th session of the WHO Executive Board. WHO, Geneva.

Willis, C. (1993). *Means testing in cost recovery of health services in developing countries. Phase I: review of concepts and literature, and preliminary field work design.* Health Financing and Sustainability Major Applied Research Paper 7, Abt Associates, Bethesda, MD.

World Bank (1987). *Financing health services in developing countries: an agenda for reform.* World Bank, Washington, DC.

World Bank (1993). *World development report 1993: investing in health.* Oxford University Press, New York.

World Bank (1997). *Sector strategy: health, nutrition, and population.* World Bank, Washington, DC.

World Bank (1998). *1998 world development indicators.* World Bank, Washington, DC.

World Bank (2000). *World development report 2000–2001: attacking poverty.* Oxford University Press, New York.

12.5 Disease prevention and control of non-communicable diseases

Jørn Olsen

Introduction

In the year 2000 the Executive Board of the World Health Organization (**WHO**) recommended the 55th World Health Assembly:

(1) to formulate a global strategy for the prevention and control of non-communicable diseases.

(2) to recognize the enormous human suffering caused by cardiovascular diseases, cancer, diabetes, and chronic respiratory diseases, and the threats they pose to the economics of member states.

(3) to notice that these diseases are linked to common risk factors, namely, tobacco use, unhealthy diet, and physical inactivity, and being aware that these risk factors have economic, social, gender, political, behavioural, and environmental determinants.

Although, in principle the WHO knows how to prevent many of the most important non-communicable diseases in industrialized countries, in general it does not know how to implement this knowledge. Many of the proximal determinants of these diseases are known, and as the most important health determinants operate within the domain of lifestyle factors, behavioural changes will be needed (Roemer 1984; Koplan and Livengood 1994; Wynder and Andres 1994). Of course, these changes should be implemented without violating people's right to choose their own way of living. The ability to set up a preventive programme that is evidence based is limited, as the more distal determinants of lifestyle factors are not known, except that they are related to education, social conditions, peer pressure, role models, etc.

Lifestyle factors are closely related to our roles as consumers and we must realize that many actors are involved. An enormous amount of money is spent on influencing consumer behaviour on the market through advertising. Many people want to influence our lifestyle, yet there are few epidemiologists or public health workers and their financial resources are comparatively sparse. On the other hand, epidemiologists have a message that is of interest to the public and therefore to the media. Thus they have much more influence than their sparse financial resources would suggest. The problem in passing on the information is that when health consequences are addressed they are placed in a distant future—people are asked to give up habits that give them pleasure at present and no any guarantees are given that these changes will actually prevent the diseases in question. The concept of disease causation is used, which apparently is far away from a common-sense concept and therefore has low credibility (J. Olsen 1993).

Rose's paradox of prevention (Rose 1992) is well documented. Eliminating risk factors for those at highest risk who benefit the most from this intervention will only have limited impact at population levels as the majority of these diseases come from people with moderate risk who will personally benefit very little by avoiding the risk determinants in question. Furthermore, all individual-based health programmes are expected to have limited immediate effect and may increase social inequalities in health as the well educated are probably more likely to adapt to evidence-based disease prevention and health care than non-educated people.

Although many non-communicable diseases are preventable, a large proportion are not, even under optimal circumstances. Furthermore, many of the diseases we may prevent will not be prevented for ever. Prevention has to do with avoiding diseases at a premature stage, not necessarily preventing the diseases from occurring at any stage in life. In addition, the incidence of non-communicable diseases will increase with increasing life expectancy. Non-communicable diseases increase when clean drinking water is provided, poverty has been reduced, and malnutrition is gradually eliminated. Basic health care will lead to good-quality treatment of infections, and implementation of vaccination programmes will increase life expectancy; therefore the lifelong incidence of cancer, and probably of cardiovascular diseases, will increase. All of this is intended and desirable, but unfortunately this epidemiological transition is often followed by undesirable epidemics of chronic diseases. If elimination of environmental hazards is followed by physical inactivity, a high-fat diet, and increased smoking, the incidence of other diseases increases. The shift from communicable to non-communicable diseases in many developing countries is an achievement that cannot and should not be prevented as it is largely driven by forces that prevent premature death. The challenges lie in reducing the avoidable deaths and disabilities related to non-communicable diseases as much as possible with the available resources. What should be avoided is a community suffering acute diseases related to overcrowding and poverty, as well as chronic diseases related to overeating, alcohol abuse, and smoking.

Although wealthy countries spend 90 per cent of world health resources on 10 per cent of world health problems, history clearly shows that expenditure of health resources on treatment alone is not a very efficient way of reducing the number of non-communicable diseases (McKeown 1965; McKeown and Lowe 1974), simply because many of these diseases are not curable. There is no magic treatment that will make arteriosclerosis go away and it is unlikely that any cancer treatment will ever be able to eliminate the excess cancer mortality associated with smoking. Cancer treatment may in time be able to cure a growing number of cancer diseases, but many opportunities for prevention have been lost because we have waited in vain for this to happen.

Making changes in society that will make it easier to exchange unhealthy habits for more healthy ones will most likely have a large effect on life expectancy. Making it easy, safe, and pleasant to use the bicycle as a common means of transportation increases the number of people who take physical exercise every day, reduces air pollution, and saves fuel for more useful purposes. Accepting non-smokers' right to avoid passive smoke will reduce smoking habits as role models will have less influence when smoking is not performed in public places. Subsidizing healthy food or taxation on alcohol, tobacco, fat, and sugar may also facilitate a change towards a more prudent diet. One could envisage a taxation system where taxes are partly paid according to how much one's behaviour has negative consequences for the environment and to what extent one expects to need the health-care system to cure self-inflicted health problems.

Non-communicable diseases have only one common property—the diseases are non-transmittable directly from one person to another via a single external agent. However, transmission may occur via genetic factors from parents to offspring, or indirectly via role models, or by manipulating the determinants of the disease. This process does not necessarily operate from people with the disease to the non-diseased, and often the mechanism taks place via more distant determinants of the disease. Non-communicable diseases include arteriosclerosis, psychosocial diseases, low back pain, infertility, congenital malformations, poor visual acuity, hypertension, psoriasis, diabetes, etc. Some of these diseases may be caused by infection, but most are probably not.

It is not possible to cover all options for preventing these diseases in a single chapter. Therefore only certain aspects of prevention and health promotion will be discussed, and some of the most important risk factors will be presented.

Types of prevention

Prevention is often classified as primary, secondary, or tertiary. Primary prevention aims at lowering the occurrence rate of the event, i.e. the incidence rate of the disease. Secondary prevention aims at lowering the occurrence of the later and more severe stages of the disease, often by identifying diseases at a curable stage, as in screening, thus reducing the prevalence of the disease through treatment. Tertiary prevention aims at reducing the social consequences of the disease.

Although smoking cessation may be seen as a primary prevention of lung cancer, it could also be viewed as secondary prevention if lung cancer is seen as a disease that starts with a first-stage transformation in a multistage carcinogenic process. A screening programme would aim at diagnosing the disease at a stage where radical treatment is possible and thereby removing the patient from the pool of prevalent cases. Tertiary prevention would aim at securing work and income as long as possible and then to provide aid to reduce the losses following the disease, or to rehabilitate the patient to make it possible for him or her to work at a reduced physical or mental capacity.

In many cases, the distinction between primary, secondary, and tertiary prevention is not clear, because the disease has no clear onset in time but is a result of a process which may be lifelong (Kuh and Ben-Shlomo 1997). The distinction between disease and non-disease is not as clear as many believe, not even for many cancers, and certainly not for cardiovascular diseases or mental disorders. Without a clear demarcation it is difficult to base the taxonomy of prevention on the onset of certain stages of a disease, which may be unknown. For convenience, we often use the time when the clinician makes the diagnosis as a surrogate measure for the onset of disease.

For example, the periconceptual intake of folic acid to prevent neural tube defects is primary prevention (Berry *et al.* 1999). Prenatal screening for neural tube defects by ultrasound examination is secondary prevention if a finding leads to an induced abortion, which removes the child from the pool of prevalent cases at birth. High-quality surgical treatment followed by extensive physical and social training is tertiary prevention, aimed at reducing the social consequences for the affected child and the family.

Screening

Screening is usually considered to be secondary prevention as it aims at identifying those with diseases at a time when they will benefit from early treatment. Thus those with diseases are identified before reaching the critical point where only palliative treatment is available with the present technology. Screening consists of a programme, not just the application of a screening test, and it must be evaluated as a programme. Even in situations where a well-accepted screening test is available, a health benefit is expected, and the necessary health-care facilities are available, a screening programme must be carefully evaluated before it is implemented. The reason for this is not only that the screening programme takes up resources that could be spent in other areas, but also that a screening activity often has severe side-effects for some of the participants. When a screening test is applied to people without symptoms it aims at identifying the diseased before the critical point is reached. An illustration of the simplest possible outcome after using a screening test on a population without symptoms shows how participants fall into four groups (Table 1).

The true positives benefit from the screening if they are diagnosed before the critical point. Those who are diagnosed late may be harmed by the screening in some cases. The true negatives often benefit also as they do not have the disease and are reassured by the testing. The false negatives may have the normal diagnostic routines delayed as the test was negative, and the false positives may have to go through unpleasant and perhaps risky diagnostic routines due to the screening result. Therefore the validity of the screening test is a key parameter for the success of a screening programme. It is usually measured as sensitivity, i.e. the probability of being tested positive given that you have the disease, and as specificity, i.e. the probability of being tested negative given that you do not have the disease. Screening tests often have a sensitivity ranging from 30 to 95 per cent and a specificity ranging from 80 to 95 per cent. When such a test is applied to a population with a low prevalence of the disease to be screened, many

Table Illustration of the outcome of a screening test

Test result	Diseased	Not diseased
Positive	True positive	False positive
Negative	False negative	True negative

false-positive results are obtained, and not all with the disease are identified (Hugod and Fog 1992). Randomized control trials have shown a reduction in cause-specific mortality after screening for breast cancer and colorectal cancer (van Dam *et al.* 1995; Kronborg *et al.* 1996; Gyrd-Hansen 1999; Gotzsche and Olsen 2000; Jatoi 2000; De Koning 2000). It is also generally believed that screening for cervical cancer is useful in affluent societies. It is expected that more useful screening programmes will be available in cancer prevention in the future, but it would be dangerous to rely upon screening only in the fight against cancer.

Screening for hypertension and hypercholesterolaemia in preventing cardiovascular diseases seems to have a favourable cost–effect ratio, at least in high-risk groups (Schueler 1994; Littenberg 1995; Hughes 1997; Hedner 1998; Holloway *et al.* 1999).

Causation

The concept of prevention is as difficult as the concept of causation. Causation usually addresses proximal determinants of a disease because the cause must make a difference for at least some of the exposed (Lyon 1967). For example, we believe that tobacco smoking, asbestos, and some other exposures cause lung cancer, and by using counterfactual reasoning we believe that if we remove these causes we eliminate some of the expected cases from occurring. Very few of the proximal determinants are in themselves sufficient or necessary causes. Most of the necessary causes are made necessary by including the cause in the definition of the disease (J. Olsen 1993). However, the component causal model presents a framework for causal thinking that matches actual evidence (Mackie 1974; Rothman 1976).

Murray and Lopez (1999) have estimated that the five most important risk factors worldwide are malnutrition, tobacco, hypertension, poor water, and physical inactivity (in that order). These risk factors account individually for 11.7 per cent to 3.9 per cent of all deaths. Prevention should, if possible, aim at these proximal determinants directly, but in practice we may be more successful if we try to modify the determinants of, say, malnutrition or smoking (McMichael 1999). The first of these risk factors is to a large extent associated with poverty, and the second is to some extent associated with ignorance and powerful disease-provoking advertisement.

Although it is believed that specific subtypes of human papilloma virus are necessary causes of cervical cancer, dealing more distal risk factors, such as reducing the number of sexual partners or encouraging condom use, may be the only way of preventing cervical cancers while we wait for an efficient vaccine to be available for the public. Whether we should move upstream or downstream in the search for public health determinants remains an important topic for discussion (Olsen *et al.* 1999).

Health promotion

Health promotion includes activities that aim at improving health rather than preventing specific diseases. A prudent diet, physical exercise, better social networks, and a stimulating work environment will probably improve well being and lower the risk of several diseases.

In the past in developed countries, and now in many developing countries, communicable diseases were reduced by providing safe drinking water, avoiding crowding by reducing family size, and improving housing conditions and nutrition. Vaccination programmes have sustained this effect in developed as well as in developing countries (Holland 1995).

Preventing non-communicable diseases will, with our present technology, rest upon encouraging healthy habits such as non-smoking, more physical exercise, a better diet low in fat and rich in fruit and vegetables, and better stress control by improving social networks (WHO Europe 1999). However, poverty-related problems such as homelessness, drug and alcohol abuse, and physical violence, have not yet been eliminated, even in the most affluent societies. Basic needs concerning housing and food for all have not yet been secured, which makes health promotion meaningless for many people. We believe that a reduction in environmental exposures from pesticides, heavy metals, radon exposure, and other chemical and physical exposures are important, but at present these risk factors have a much smaller role than unhealthy lifestyle factors (Murray and Lopez 1999). As many of the non-communicable diseases develop over the entire lifespan prevention may be seen as a lifelong investment (Anonymous 1997). This enterprise should focus on a healthy diet (Glanz 1997), exercise (Gortmaker *et al.* 1997), and health promotion in general (Rijke 1997).

Changing lifestyle factors is more difficult and perhaps also more expensive than changing environmental factors. Not many people are willing to accept responsibility for their own health. Most would prefer to blame some external factor for their health problems—the environment in general, work conditions, or lack of social or personal support. Or they like to believe that medical treatment will solve all the problems that they may have in the future, perhaps not with the present technology but when they become patients in 10 to 20 years. The health care industry has in many ways promised more than it could deliver. How much influence these promises have on health promotion and disease prevention is not known, but the detrimental effect could be substantial.

It is not impossible to change lifestyle, and many private enterprises achieve this through repeatedadvertising. Usually large budgets are required as it is often necessary to create a perceived need and then to maintainit. Some health-related changes definitively benefit from being linked to profit-making enterprises, for example improving physical fitness is supported by an industry selling sport clothes and sport equipment. Commercial interest in selling smoking cessation tools may also be much more efficient in reducing smoking habits than traditional anti-smoking campaigns. Therefore public effort should concentrate on preventing young people from starting to smoke as no companies have any commercial interest in this aspect. Although it is important to make the best use of private health-promoting activities it is difficult or even impossible to co-ordinate these private activities and to set priorities.

Setting up a system that provided safe drinking water needed financial resources and political leadership in Europe in the nineteenth century (Holland and Stewart 1998). The same is true for organizing a well-functioning health-care system with a strong emphasis on health promotion, but we do not really know what kind of political leadership is necessary to improve health behaviour. Nor do we know who has the necessary instruments to provide leadership of this scale. Health insurance companies, public health activities, private and public health care, pharmaceutical companies, strong medical professions, etc. do not have the same interests or goals, and they are powerful players in the health field and difficult to co-ordinate.

Prevention and care

Usually only a small fraction of the budget for health care is spent on prevention and most of the money is spent on screening and regular health examinations (Cohen and Henderson 1988), although most experts agree that only changes in the most important lifestyle factors will succeed in substantially improving global health indicators in developed countries, and in improving social conditions, family size, and safe water supply in developing countries. Despite this, most political attention, in both developed and developing countries, is focused on improving treatment. Furthermore, it is difficult to see how this could change. Treatment deals with named patients in need. Prevention is about anonymous individuals who are at present healthy and who, in general, will not know whethet or not they have benefited from the preventive action.

Convincing circumstantial evidence indicates that changing the sleeping position in early childhood from a prone to a supine position has saved thousands of children from sudden infant death syndrome (Taylor and Emery 1990; Taylor 1991; Fleming 1994), but we do not know who were saved and thus we have no grateful parents who donate money to research or tell their member of parliament that prevention is an important activity to support. Prevention may be better then cure. Still, prevention will never be able to compete with cure on resources for many reasons, some of which are reasonable. A utilitarian approach to health care would allocate more resources to disease prevention, but a strictly utilitarian approach is not acceptable for ethical reasons and will be in conflict with the aim of equity in treatment (Jensen and Mooney 1990). In like manner it will not be acceptable to shift resources from necessary and efficient treatments to prevention. On the other hand, many treatments have little or no scientific justification and in these situations money is much better spent on evidence-based prevention. However, there is little or no attempt to make this change in health policy. Only in secondary prevention in the form of screening is there political pressure for spending money on prevention that matches the pressure to support better treatment.

A health-care system needs to be organized towards well-defined health goals to make any difference in the priority setting. This message was probably the most important result of the WHO Health for All policy. Still, day-to-day problem solving, where the media's treatment of case stories plays an important part, drives most health-care policy systems. In order to continue the discussion on setting priorities, the WHO (1999*a*) has decided to continue the Health for All strategy into the twenty-first century. A goal for chronic diseases has been set that aims at a 40 per cent reduction in mortality from cardiovascular diseases in people under 65, a 15 per cent reduction in cancer mortality under the age of 65, and a one-third reduction in diabetes-related amputations and pregnancy complications, and that 80 per cent of the children should be free of dental caries up to the age of 6. This goal is achievable even at our present level of knowledge.

While we do see political pressure to improve working conditions or the quality of drinking water, we cannot expect people to ask to be told what to do concerning their diet, smoking, and drinking habits. We may hope for support to make it easier to make healthy choices and for funding to provide information on the health consequences of the choices we make, but cannot demand much more than that.

Although prevention may be better than cure, few people act according to this precept. The health-care system is still organized to sweep up the water from an overflowing bathtub, and only a few people try to work out how to turn off the tap. It is unlikely that this will change substantially in the near future, which is why we should seize every opportunity to discuss and change unhealthy habits which do not provide personal satisfaction that justifies their negative health consequences. One such opportunity is illness. Stopping smoking after a myocardial infarction is late—too late in some cases, but not in all. Using secondary health-care institutions in prevention carries an important potential for lowering the disease burden. In most countries this potential resource has not been used to any large extent.

Reducing risk factors

Smoking is addictive. Addicts are strong advocates of their 'drug', whatever it may be, and smokers are no different from other addicts in this respect. Smokers may say that they smoke because they like smoking, but many like smoking because they dislike non-smoking. They have an urge for nicotine and fulfilling a need provides pleasure. Smokers often claim that they cannot think clearly without smoking; Sherlock Holmes described a difficult problem as a 'three-pipe problem'. Smoking may of course stimulate brain activity, but the mechanism might as well be that low levels of nicotine slow down brain activity among the addicted. Smokers need not like smoking but they clearly dislike not smoking. Whatever the reasons for pleasure, all agree that smoking causes more serious health problems than any other single avoidable exposure (Doll and Peto 1981; Murray and Lopez 1999). It is likely that even passive smoking causes cancer and perhaps also coronary heart disease (Lam and He 1997). Therefore reducing smoking habits is part of most preventive programmes. The most effective smoking cessation methods are expensive and man-power consuming since they are based on individual counselling. Labelling tobacco products with health warnings, health campaigns, increased taxation on tobacco, and trying to make teachers and health-care workers understand that they act as role models are all important methods but are not sufficient in most countries. The WHO (1999*b*) estimates that the worldwide mortality from tobacco will rise from 4 million deaths per year in 1998 to 10 million in 2030. Half of these deaths will occur in people aged between 35 and 69 years. Smoking removes people not only from nursing homes but also from golf courses.

Use of nicotine substitutes has proved effective for highly motivated smokers if they are under close surveillance (Rose 1996). As a 'stand-alone' treatment without close surveillance the effect is less convincing. Only one study has tried to estimate the effect of buying nicotine patches over the counter without being offered additional help or surveillance, and it showed only a moderate effect in the subgroup that received the largest dose of nicotine (Sønderskov *et al.* 1997). Use of incentives in public campaigns has shown a very modest long-term effect. However, it is inexpensive and, even if only 1 per cent quits smoking after these campaigns (Bains *et al.* 1998), may be highly cost-effective compared with other methods.

The WHO (1999*b*) advocates four principles of tobacco control that have been successful in many countries: public health information, advertising bans, taxes, and building tobacco control coalitions. The public has a right to know about the health consequences of smoking, and labelling or counter-advertising may be used together with evidence-based information. Despite public campaigns, few people know all the health consequences of smoking and many believe that smoking only shortens life among the oldest. Higher taxes seem to reduce consumption, as so do smoke-free workplaces. Nicotine replacement therapy may be useful for many, especially if accompanied by other support systems. Tobacco control coalitions may counterbalance the tobacco industry lobbying and try to help people who depend on their income from tobacco sales to find other sources of income.

It is also well accepted that substantial modification of diet may have important health benefits. Doll and Peto (1981) estimated that 35 per cent of all cancers are related to diet, and an inappropriate diet is believed to cause obesity, diabetes, and cardiovascular diseases for some. Most believe that the amount of fat, especially saturated fat, is of importance, although trials have not shown convincing benefit of lowering fat in order to reduce the incidence of coronary heart diseases, perhaps because the reduction of fat intake has been too small. Results have been more promising in secondary prevention by reducing cardiovascular case fatality (Oliver 1996). It is also generally accepted that people eating a diet rich in fruits and vegetables have a low risk of cardiovascular diseases. Whether this is due to antioxidant vitamins is not known, but at present the advice is to eat fruit and vegetables rather than taking vitamin tablets or other antioxidants (Oliver 1996). A moderate intake of alcohol appears to lower the risk of coronary heart diseases (Rimm *et al.* 1999), but advocating a moderate alcohol intake may increase alcohol abuse.

A high-energy diet is probably suitable for humans performing heavy physical work. Most people in the developed countries no longer perform such work, and lack of exercise is a major health problem. Physical exercise appears to have a beneficial effect on our psychological well being by reducing depression, anxiety, and stress (Scully *et al.* 1998). Exercise may also lower blood pressure, perhaps by reducing weight (Arroll *et al.* 1994), cardiovascular diseases, osteoporosis, muscular disorders, and breast cancer (Deuster 1996; Pina and Fitzpatrick 1996; Batty 1997).

Social determinants of health

It is expected that disease and death would be closely correlated to poverty. It is disappointing that social inequalities in health are strong even in welfare states that have eradicated poverty in a materialistic sense for almost everyone in their societies and provided access to health care for all. It is perhaps difficult to avoid the fact that chronic disease can lead to unemployment and loss of income, but it should be within our reach to limit the inequalities in health that follow differences in social status. This has been one of the key targets in the WHO plan for Health for All by the Year 2000. However, in many countries the trend has been the opposite (Cavelaars *et al.* 1998). Reasons for social inequalities could be genetic, due to differences in access to health care, or due to differences in exposures to health hazards in the working environment or in personal life. Poor social conditions may also lead to greater exposure to stress and more changes in social conditions and other life events. It is unlikely that genetic factors alone or differential access to health care can explain more than a small fraction of the social differences in health we see in most countries. Social inequality exists even in countries with free and equal access to care, and genetic factors do not explain some of the rapidly changing social inequalities that we see in some countries. In some of the East European states there has been a substantial decline in life expectancy in males over the past 10 to 15 years (Leon *et al.* 1997). From 1970 to 1990 the social gradient in suicides has increased dramatically in some countries (Drever *et al.* 1996), and it is unlikely that genetic factors are the only reasons for this change. Better treatment of depression for some is probably a more likely explanation (Mortensen *et al.* 2000).

Changes in the social classification system may explain some of the changes in social inequalities over time. If the population is classified into, say, quintiles according to a given social indicator, selection bias hardly explains changes in social inequalities. However, if the social classification system is based upon educational levels, or some other classification system that changes over time, those who remain in the lower social groups need not be comparable with those from the same level in the past. This type of selection bias is expected to be present in many societies where social grouping is based on, for example, educational levels (Cavelaars *et al.* 1998).

Gender roles have changed over the years in many countries, mainly as a consequence of better education for females. How we best describe social conditions for the family in relation to health is not well studied, but results do indicate (Olsen and Frische 1993) that the social status of both partners should be taken into consideration, not only the one with the highest social level. It is reasonable to assume that the educational level plays a part for health behaviour regardless of the social status of the family. It is also of interest to follow social inequalities in health for men and women. Some results indicate that women do not always obtain the health benefits that their higher social positions indicate (DIKE 1997).

Social indicators are usually developed within social research. Although there are many possible ways that social factors may impair health (Marmot and Wilkinson 1999), we still need to know how best to classify social conditions in relation to health. Income, housing and working conditions, health behaviour, and access to health care may be related to health through very different mechanisms that may change over time and be different in different societies. How all these factors should be included in a social classification system that addresses health issues is not well studied and therefore is not known.

It is likely that mandatory public health programmes, or programmes offered to all, such as vaccination programmes (Holland 1995), free school meals, or control of work exposures help to reduce social inequalities in health. Health campaigns and voluntary screening programmes may, on the other hand, be better accepted by the best educated. Health-care workers have an important task in providing information to be used in primary or secondary prevention in a way that is understood by all. This potential for health improvements in patients with lifestyle-related diseases has not been widely used in most countries.

The mapping of the human genome provides new tools and new challenges in epidemiology (Schulte and Perera 1993). For most of the non-communicable diseases, the genetic risk factors will probably be complex and their individual contributions will be small. We hope that stratifying the participants on genetic factors will make it easier to identify environmental and preventable causes of diseases, as has been shown for the Leiden V mutation and oral contraception (Appleby and Olds 1997). However, other gene–environment interactions may be much more difficult to detect. Important genetic determinants of breast cancer, colorectal cancer, and cardiovascular diseases have been identified, but the importance of these findings in primary prevention is still not clear (Lander and Schork 1994; Ruiz *et al.* 1994; Olschwang *et al.* 1997; Duval *et al.* 1999).

Epidemiology has had a strong link to public health. New research methods incorporating molecular biology have the potential to enhance the ability of epidemiologists to study disease processes; however, it is important for those epidemiologists using these new molecular tools to use them to help elucidate public health issues (Olsen *et al.* 1999). The development of diseases over time cannot be understood outside a social context. Diseases have causes and many of these causes are man-made and, therefore, often avoidable. Although these causes interact with genetic factors to produce their effect, it seems more appropriate to target or prevent these causes rather than change susceptibility, which may have unknown side-effects.

Environmental risk factors

Since Ramazzini published his book *De Morbis Artificium* about occupational diseases in the eighteenth century, many diseases have been accepted as occupational or environmental. Percival Pott was the first to identify an occupational cancer in 1775 when he recognized soot from chimney sweeping as the cause of scrotal cancer. Much later the culprit was identified as one of the polycyclic hydrocarbons. Now we know that 4-aminophenyl, arsenic, asbestos, benzene, benzidine, chromium, polyclorinated biphenyls, vinyl chloride, and other compounds cause cancer. The fraction of cancers attributable to specific occupations is probably small in most developing countries. Most countries have been successful in finding substitutes for some of the carcinogens or in reducing exposure levels to very low levels, but heavy metals and pesticides with very long biological half-lives are of concern, especially if they accumulate in human food chains. Asbestos exposure and exposure to radon daughter elements are still widespread and constitute important public health problems (Last 1998).

Environmental diseases have to be identified and their determinants described. Some diseases are so closely related to their causes that the task may be easy, such as cancer of the nose in furniture workers or liver cell angiosarcoma in people exposed to vinyl chloride. Most other diseases have environmental as well as non-environmental causes and thus are more difficult to detect despite the fact that they are much more frequent. Weak associations between exposure to high levels of electromagnetic fields and childhood leukaemia (UK Childhood Cancer Study Investigators 1999) have been difficult to interpret, as weak associations indicate that other causes of the disease are not included in the statistical model used. We can only hope that these alternative causes are equally distributed among the exposed and non-exposed.

Once the exposures of importance are identified, they may be replaced or they may be isolated or not transmitted to people by means of efficient ventilation or use of personal protection.

In countries with very poor occupational standards education may be the most cost-effective way of reducing exposures. Reducing environmental exposures need not be very expensive if the exposure levels are high. Exposure to, say, organic solvents may often be greatly reduced by minor rearrangements at the work site. Knowing what to do is often the first step to getting it done, but many newly industrialized countries lack the knowledge or the infrastructure to implement the knowledge.

Social support

Unemployment, divorce, widowhood, and rapid welfare changes are all characterized by the disruption of social support systems and may be associated with poor health (Dean and Holstein 1991). Therefore disease prevention should also aim at making strong social networks when existing ones break down. Unions, churches, social clubs, schools, and sport clubs all have had this role. The health-care system also has a part to play for people who, for reasons of age, diseases, racial discrimination, etc., fall outside these systems. Providing social support to the elderly in Denmark showed remarkably reduced mortality and morbidity in one Danish study (Dean and Holstein 1991), although these results could only partly be replicated in another Danish study (Gunnar-Svensson *et al.* 1984). We do not know how much social support is needed to prevent diseases and we expect the support required to depend upon the amount and level of external stressors.

The philosophy behind tertiary prevention of chronic diseases is that it is often possible to live with and die with these diseases, rather than dying from them (Lorig *et al.* 1996). Research in general has shown that it is possible to prolong the time period of optimal, physical functioning, and social activity by providing social support and self-management programmes (Katz 1983; Breslow and Somers 1988).

A boring job with few social contacts may increase plasma adrenaline at rest and thus blood pressure. Other cardiovascular changes are seen for unemployment (Arnetz *et al.* 1991). Prevention at the work site is thus more than making sure that the workplace is safe; it also involves establishing a stimulating work environment and making sure that the workplace creates social contacts which do not interrupt the family networks. A safe job is a job that you like which also makes it possible to develop socially and intellectually.

A life-course approach to disease prevention

It is well known that, for example, neurotoxic exposures in early life may permanently impair brain functioning as is the case in fetal alcohol syndrome (Abel 1998). Infections may also cause damage that is not detected clinically within a short follow-up period, but could cause chronic disease in adulthood. Cardiovascular diseases, type II diabetes, and cancer have been seen as diseases that were the result of high-fat intake, smoking, and lack of physical exercise in adult life for genetically susceptible people. It is quite a recent development to consider this susceptibility to be not only a function of genetic factors, but also a result of exposures that took place early in life (Forsdahl 1977; Bakketeig *et al.* 1991; Barker 1994, 1995; Kuh and Ben-Shlomo 1997). It is known from animal experiments that the functioning of some organs may be permanently altered if the diet is poor in nutritional components such as proteins, and this alteration is called 'programming' (Eriksson and Swenne 1993; Lucas *et al.* 1999; Nieuwenhuizen *et al.* 1999). However, the idea that programming may also play a part for humans is still based on circumstantial evidence, although the evidence is strong. The first evidence came from Forsdahl's (1977) studies in Norway showing that middle-aged males who were born in regions of high infant mortality at the time of their birth had a high mortality 50 years later, mainly due to cardiovascular diseases. Men born in regions with low infant mortality had a low risk of dying from cardiovascular diseases in middle-age. A similar ecological correlation was found to be present for serum cholesterol (Bakketeig *et al.* 1991). Barker (1995) followed up these ideas and established a link between birth weight and chronic diseases at the individual level in a series of important studies. In general, it was seen that low birth weight was associated with high blood pressure and high risk of other cardiovascular diseases in adult life, and the mechanism could operate via organ programming in fetal life (e.g. partly impaired liver functioning).

Low birth weight may be seen as a proxy measure of impaired fetal growth, although it is a very crude measure. Some neonates with low birth weight have grown to their full genetic potential, but others are growth retarded. If we are to look for fetal growth impairment at certain stages during pregnancy, it may be better to examine weight as a function of length (thinness), as it is done when estimating the Ponderal index (birth weight in kilograms divided by the cube of birth length in meters), which is, furthermore, a mathematical transformation that usually produces a symmetrical distribution of the index values. Birth weight and length are usually available in most birth records. On the other hand, in a search for growth retardation we should be looking for deviations from the birth weight that the fetus could have reached if it had access to use its full genetic growth potentials. Although this weight is unknown, we could calculate a predicted birth weight based on the gestational age and also on the parents' heights or even their birth weights. If the child has siblings, their birth weights can be included in the model used for prediction. There are results that suggest that a deviation between the observed birth weight and the expected birth weight is a much better predictor of perinatal health problems than birth weight itself (Bakketeig and Hoffman 1983). Whether it is also a better correlate of organ programming, should it exist, remains to be seen.

In any case, there is now overwhelming evidence that birth weight correlates with several adult diseases and functions. Organ programming may indeed explain some of these associations, but confounding by genetic or social factors cannot be excluded. Birth weight could be an epiphenomenon of something causing low birth weight and the disease in question, and the two outcomes need not be causally related. Most likely programming will be the explanation for some of these associations, but hardly for all. The next critical step will be to see what initiates the lack of growth of certain cells in organ development. Many candidates are available; not only nutritional components but also smoking, work-related exposures, drugs, stress, alcohol, etc. may impair fetal growth. Diseases during pregnancy may in like manner impair fetal growth directly or via interference with fetal nutrition such as we expect to see in hyperemesis or conditions such as Crohn's disease or ulcerative colitis (Fonager *et al.* 1998). Some of these growth-related factors may be preventable; others may not be. The major challenge in public health epidemiology is to identify those that are preventable and to use the information in the antenatal care system. Antenatal care will probably be an even more important part of disease prevention in the future than it is at present.

Although at present we do not know how important organ programming is for the most prevalent chronic diseases, most believe that it is of some importance. Unfortunately we do not know what activates the programming, but lack of nutrition has been part of most suggestions. In animal studies, specific nutrition components have been tested in most studies, especially a diet low in protein. In humans, lack of specific dietary components is also a possibility, although only components, such as n-3 fatty acids could explain the association seen for low birth weight and preterm delivery (S.F. Olsen 1993).

Diseases that could interfere with fetal growth or maternal nutrition, such as infections, hyperemesis, and placenta dysfunctions, could also play a part as well as external factors interfering with fetal growth, such as tobacco, alcohol, environmental exposures, or polluted drinking water or foods. We know that high levels of alcohol may permanently impair brain functioning, but probably not via programming (Vershuren 1993). We expect alcohol to be neurotoxic in high doses, and mercury may have a similar effect (Grandjean *et al.* 1999).

At present it is also believed that some cancers have a fetal aetiology, especially childhood cancers and cancer of the testis, but also breast cancers, ovarian cancers, and perhaps cancer of the prostate (Skakkebæk *et al.* 1987; Trichopoulos 1990; Ekbom *et al.* 1992, 1995; Adami *et al.* 1998; Ekbom 1998; Sabroe and Olsen 1998). The intrauterine hormonal level may be of importance for these cancers, especially oestrogen or the balance between oestrogen and progesterone, but again the evidence is circumstantial.

The number of Sertoli cells at birth determines sperm production, and male fecundity may similarly be affected by external or internal disrupters of the hormonal balance acting during the time period of organogenesis (Sharpe and Skakkebæk 1993). More than half of all pregnant women use medication during pregnancy. It is not known whether some types of medication have a programming effect or not.

However, whether or not these hypotheses are trueis not crucial to the life-course approach in preventing chronic diseases. We know that arteriosclerosis is a process that starts very early in life. We know that our dietary habits and our tendency to abuse alcohol, tobacco, or drugs depend upon social and psychological factors in our upbringing. We also know that obesity in childhood is strongly associated with obesity in adult life. Given these conditions, health promotion as well as disease management must focus on the longitudinal track of a given disease process on the health status of individuals as well as populations (Glassock 1997). Antenatal care is only the first process in a lifelong health promotion and disease prevention programme, and this programme needs to take into consideration not only diseases that surface to clinical detection shortly after the onset of the programme but also health in the long run. A health-care system strongly specialized within certain time periods of the lifespan or certain organ systems will not be well suited to meet the challenges raised by life-course research.

Non-communicable diseases in developing countries

Many developing countries are in a state of demographic balance with high fertility and a short life expectancy. The majority of the population are children or young adults. Improvements in social conditions usually decrease mortality and may increase fertility in the early stages (Taylor 1993), which leads to population growth before a new steady state is reached. This process is called the demographic transition, and it is usually followed by the epidemiological transition where the disease pattern changes from communicable to non-communicable diseases, although this pattern is not always seen. A deterioration of social conditions in industrialized countries in

Eastern Europe has been followed not only by increased incidence of infectious diseases but also by increased mortality due to violent death and non-communicable diseases, especially cardiovascular diseases. This has been followed by a substantial reduction in life expectancy, especially for males (Leon *et al.* 1997).

The Inuit in Greenland have undergone a substantial improvement in social conditions that has not been followed by the expected improvement in health, despite a comprehensive health-care system that focuses on treatment rather than prevention. Social stress as a function of cultural changes has been followed by an increased consumption of unhealthy foods and frequent use of alcohol and tobacco. As in other rapid developing countries, blood pressure begins to rise with age and hypertension becomes a problem, which was not the case in the past. This change has been related to obesity, lack of exercise, and an increased salt intake. More psychosocial stress related to the cultural changes is probably also important (Bjerregaard and Young 1998).

Type II diabetes is a rapidly growing problem in many developing countries, especially in Pacific populations and among native people in Australia and the United States. The 'thrifty genotype hypothesis' (Neel 1999) states that the genetic susceptibility to type II diabetes improves survival during time periods of famine. Hypersecretion of insulin, which facilitates transfer of glucose into the cell, is an advantage when food is short in supply, but when food is too plentiful hypersecretion of insulin leads to pancreatic β-cell failure and diabetes.

Shortage of nutrition to the fetus may also lead to β-cell failure, which may lead to diabetes in adult life in case of obesity. Fetal programming may be an alternative explanation of the epidemic of diabetes seen in many populations throughout the world. In both situations, control over obesity by reducing the fat content in the diet and increasing exercise will reduce the incidence of diabetes. If fetal programming plays a part, additional preventive measures during pregnancy may present new preventive options once we know what activates the programming.

The epidemic of diabetes does have external and avoidable causes acting on biological susceptibility that may be due to genes or programming or both.

The epidemiological transition also changes the cancer pattern. Cancers which have an infectious aetiology, such as liver cancer, oral cancer, nasopharyngeal cancer, cervix cancer, and gastric cancer, are caused mainly by food components that carry the agent. These cancers tend to occur less frequently when social conditions improve. The cancers that take over are usually lung cancer if the tobacco companies are free to move into the market, breast cancer, and colorectal cancers. It is expected that changes in fertility partly explain the changes in breast cancer risk, although this has not been well documented. Changes in dietary patterns may explain the rise in the incidence of colon cancer.

In developing countries a health plan with emphasis on treatment and screening is bound to fail. Restriction of tobacco smoking, limiting of a high-fat Western diet, and promotion of physical activities in the young will be the only way to reduce premature death due to smoking and overeating. Unfortunately, many developing countries do not only take over 'Western risk factors' but also the industrialized society's beliefs that better treatment in itself will solve all problems. However, the fight against AIDS has shown that prevention is possible, even in societies with a low level of background education. In many poor countries prevention is the only option available in fighting the disease burden of most importance.

Changes during the course of life

Critical changes occur in many countries which may permanently affect the health of a population. Individuals in all societies pass through critical stages during their life courses that may permanently determine future health. Social deprivation during childhood and lack of stimulation may not only lead to a low educational level and poverty, but may also have a direct biological affect on body development and disease susceptibility (Marmot and Wilkinson 1999).

Downward social mobility during a time period where the opposite is expected has been shown to be a stronger predictor for reproductive failures than low social status in itself (Basso *et al.* 1999). Social changes, like changes of schools, entry to the labour market, occupational changes, and retirement, may have positive or negative health effects depending on how well the individual copes with the psychological stress related to these events.

Unemployment is a risk factor for health in many situations, although research results have been ambiguous. Most studies have not been able to distinguish between health conditions leading to unemployment and health consequences of unemployment. Whether unemployment is a risk factor for health or not will depend on the social and psychological support provided to the unemployed as well as the working conditions present during employment. In some situations, unemployment will remove workers from high-risk exposures. We also expect the psychological stress to be less if many lose their job at the same time or if unemployment is common. Unemployment is probably worse for men if their roles in society are to be 'bread winners' in the family and if their social status depends upon their job. In any case, a policy that aims at reducing unemployment should also be supported for health reasons. Most research results indicate that unemployment may result in a deterioration in mental health, probably because a loss of job may be followed by a loss of a time structure to the day, a reduction in self-esteem, and lower social status.

Burden of chronic diseases

As indicated by the term 'chronic', these diseases do not show up in mortality statistics shortly after the onset and they need not lead to death. As only a few countries have reliable morbidity statistics, we do not know the global burden of chronic diseases in general, regardless of definition.

In order to get more information on chronic diseases that are not life threatening, several survey instruments have been developed. Most of these cover self-perceived physical and mental health problems leading to activity limitations (Hennessy *et al.* 1994; Lorig *et al.* 1996). In 1994 14 per cent of Danes reported health-related activity limitations. During a time period of 4 weeks 16 per cent reported reduced mental well being and 23 per cent said they had psychological problems leading to activity limitations. Poor health was reported more frequently in females than in males and poor health increased with age (Kjøller *et al.* 1999).

Murray and Lopez (1997*a*,*b*) have estimated the 30 leading causes of death worldwide and find that ischaemic heart diseases top the list, with cerebrovascular diseases in second place. Chronic obstructive pulmonary disease is sixth on the list, cirrhosis of the liver is thirteenth, and diabetes mellitus is sixteenth. In 1990 there were already 50 per cent more cancer deaths in less developed countries than in developed countries. Some diseases, such as diabetes, increase the risk of other diseases; compared with the estimated 580 000 deaths from diabetes in 1990, 2.8 million deaths were estimated to be attributable to diabetes. It is of interest that the probability of dying from a non-communicable disease was found to be higher in low-income regions such as Sub-Saharan Africa than in high-income regions (Murray and Lopez 1997*b*). If perinatal disease programming is a determinant of individual susceptibility, one can foresee a rapid growth in cardiovascular diseases in low-income regions following a higher life expectancy and better social conditions leading to sedentary work and a high-fat diet. This increase will exceed what is due to an increasing life expectancy and the age-adjusted predictions based upon current age- and sex-specific rates will underestimate the incidence.

While all accept that quality of life is at least as important as life expectancy in itself, it has been more difficult to agree upon an adjustment of the lost years of life for the quality aspect. Disability-adjusted life-years (**DALYs**) are now frequently used as a supplement to life expectancy measures (Murray and Lopez 1997*c*,*d*, 1999). DALYs are the sum of lost years of life due to death or disability adjusted for severity and as such are based upon value-loaded decisions. Murray and Lopez (1997*b*) estimated that in developed countries smoking is the leading cause of DALYs followed by alcohol, hypertension, and occupational risk factors. In developing countries malnutrition, poor water quality, unsafe sex, and alcohol were estimated to be the most important risk factors among the following: malnutrition, drinking water quality, unsafe sex, tobacco, alcohol, occupation, hypertension, physical inactivity, illicit drugs, and air pollution. However, they did not include overcrowding, unemployment, or social stress in their analyses. They did note that neuropsychiatric disorders were responsible for 10.5 per cent of the burden of diseases and injuries worldwide.

Health futures

'It is difficult to make predictions, especially for the future' was a statement made by the Danish writer Storm P with which most people will agree. On the other hand, all preventive activities try to change undesirable expected future events and therefore are, or should be, based on predictions for the future. Most preventive activities address elimination or reduction of known risk factors, but often without giving much consideration to other consequences of behavioural or environmental changes.

Most of the present predictions are based on what we know about the long-term consequences of present risk factors or long-term trends in, for example, life expectancy. Based on information of this type we expect most populations to age in developed as well as in many developing countries and we expect non-communicable disease morbidity to increase from 28 million deaths worldwide in 1990 to 50 million in 2020. During the same time period we expect tobacco-related mortality to increase from 3 million to more than 8 million deaths. In 2020 the five leading causes of DALYs worldwide are expected to be ischaemic heart diseases, unipolar major depression, road traffic accidents, cerebrovascular diseases, and chronic obstructive pulmonary diseases (Murray and Lopez 1997*b*). Although we know how some of these diseases may be prevented, we do not in general know how to implement this knowledge, nor do we know the related consequences if we manage to eliminate or reduce these risk factors. Predicting future trends rests upon many assumptions, guesses, and intuition that call for the use of many different sources of information coming from experts as well as non-experts. These methods include Delphi techniques, brainstorming, and simulation games, as well as quantitative approaches in time-series analyses, use of Markov chains, and many other related techniques (Garrett 1999; Kirchhoff *et al.* 1999).

Although futures research is a risky matter, as time will show if we are right or wrong, it is necessary because it emphasizes the need to imagine what will happen with or without the preventive activity we want to implement. We have to try to capture all consequences of our preventive activities by focusing upon the larger picture rather than just single outcomes. For example, it is a noble aim to reduce childhood accidents in day-care centres, but as accidents are an unavoidable part of the way in which children explore and learn about the environment, they should not be reduced at all costs. Eradication of disease is extremely important for diseases such as smallpox, even though this makes the smallpox virus a frightening biological weapon. Elimination of measles will also be valuable if the virus is not replaced with other more harmful infectious agents, or if the disease or vaccination against it have no beneficial effect on the immune system in general. If the disease or the vaccination have a non-specific beneficial effect on the immune system, the net outcome may be different or perhaps even negative.

As diseases have causes, and often several causes, and as some of these causes are man-made and therefore subject to manipulation, studies of health futures need to specify the conditions for a prediction in order for it to be testable. By specifying these conditions, priority setting in public health work provides an important input to setting up work priorities. When these conditions are established, it becomes easier to predict the most likely future together with other possible health scenarios, including more unlikely but still possible scenarios. This is done to set the boundaries between possible and impossible outcomes.

In fact, 'wild ideas' should be encouraged in order to cover as many scenarios as possible. The next step could be to identify the most likely scenarioss. Methods such as the Delphi method or other expert-based surveys may be used to predict the most likely future based on the insight and information these experts possess.

In most research, consensus is reached by a critical scrutiny of the evidence. When all other possible explanations of an association have been disregarded, what remains could be the truth, as stated by Sherlock Holmes (Olsen *et al.* 1991). In futures research criticism need not be part of the process in setting up likely or possible scenarios.

Use of futures health studies on prevention is especially necessary when preventive activities interfere with other risk factors, people's personal choice, or important social conditions. Use of hormonal replacement therapy not only prevents and causes a number of diseases, but also has an impact on sexual life and self-esteem. Taking such medicine regularly makes a healthy person a patient and has financial implications for women and perhaps also for society (Belchetz 1994).

Implementing a screening programme may bring more patients to treatment before their diseases reach a non-curable state, but may also delay treatment for those who are given a false-negative diagnosis. In adition, screening may induce anxiety among those who receive a false-positive result.

Screening programmes may replace primary prevention if it is believed that the health problem can be solved by early treatment. However, if a screening programme is followed by increased risk behaviour at work or in personal life, the net benefit may be less than expected and could even be negative.

Setting higher standards for automobile safety equipment leads to more expensive cars and may make it impossible for poor people to own a car, which could decrease job mobility and increase the risk of unemployment. Futures studies aim at bringing these problems into the open in order to minimize side-effects as much as possible by taking the appropriate actions in time.

The economy of prevention

Many countries declare that they want to give higher priorities to prevention in the future, but in general only little has been done in most countries. If priorities were set entirely upon how much health a unit of cost would produce, the health-care system would look very different from what we have at present. Few people would welcome such a radical approach as many other aspects have to be taken into consideration.

It is difficult to estimate how much money is actually spent on prevention as it will depend totally upon the definition of prevention. In the United Kingdom, attempts have been made to estimate the proportional distribution of the estimated 6 per cent spent on prevention in the National Health Service. Within the budget for prevention, it is found that 32.0 per cent is spent on the environment, 22.7 per cent on screening, 15.2 per cent on dental service, 7.7 per cent on maternal care, 7.6 per cent on occupational exposures, 5 per cent on family planning, 3.2 per cent on immunizations and vaccinations, and the remainder in other areas (Cohen and Henderson 1988).

Although it is likely that lasting improvements in health can secure considerable social and economic gains (WHO 1999*b*), priority setting should not be done on economic grounds only. Nor should prevention be implemented only if it saves resources elsewhere. We should accept that health in itself is a fair objective worth spending money on, and the decision process has to include intangibles and aim at equity.

Conclusions

Chronic diseases will increase in numbers when life expectancy is prolonged due to better social conditions, less crowding (Aaby and Samb 1994), better treatment of acute infections, and active immunization. However, chronic diseases may be delayed and the time period of active life prolonged. The length of good-quality life is what should concern us, not whether or not we contract the disease. This idea is accepted by most when we talk about death.

As prevention aims at improving true quality of life—to add life to years, rather than adding years to life—we should respect people's choices when selecting personal habits. We may be firmer when hazards that give no pleasure are to be removed from the environment, or when we try to make sure that everyone is able to live a socially acceptable life, to have a job, and to have access to education that is appropriate for his or her personal capacity and aspirations. Chronic disease must be prevented both within and outside the health-care sector. Most countries lack a high-ranking advocate for this activity—perhaps the time has come to have ministers for health promotion.

References

Aaby, P. and Samb, B. (1994). In *Health and diseases in developing countries* (ed. K.S. Lankinen, S. Bergström, P.H. Mäkelä, and M. Peltoman), pp. 166–76. Macmillan, London.

Abel, E.L. (1998). Prevention of alcohol abuse-related birth effects. II: Targeting and pricing. *Alcohol and Alcoholism*, **33**, 417–20.

Adami, H.O., Signorello, L.B., and Trichopoulos, D. (1998). Towards an understanding of breast cancer etiology. *Seminars in Cancer Biology*, **8**, 255–62.

Anonymous (1997). Guidelines for school health programs to promote lifelong healthy eating. *Journal of School Health*, **67**, 9–26.

Appleby, R.D. and Olds, R.J. (1997). The inherited basis of venous thrombosis. *Pathology*, **29**, 341–7.

Arnetz, B.B., Brenner, S.O., Levi, L., *et al.* (1991). Neuroendocrine and immunologic effects of unemployment and job insecurity. *Psychotherapy and Psychosomatics*, **55**, 76–80.

Arroll, B., Hill, D., White, G., Sharpe, N., and Beaglehole, R. (1994). The effect of exercise episode duration on blood pressure. *Journal of Hypertension*, **12**, 1413–15.

Bains, N., Pickett, W., and Hoey, J. (1998). The use and impact of incentives in population-based smoking cessation programs: a review. *American Journal of Health Promotion*, **12**, 307–20.

Bakketeig, L.S. and Hoffman, H.J. (1983). The tendency to repeat gestational age and birth weight in successive births, related to perinatal survival. *Acta Obstetricia et Gynecologica Scandinavica*, **62**, 385–92.

Bakketeig, L.S., Magnus, P., and Sundet, J.M. (1991). In *Problems and methods in longitudinal research*, (ed. D. Magnusson, L.R. Bergman, G. Rudinger, and B. Törestad). Cambridge University Press.

Barker, D.J.P. (1994). *Mothers, babies and disease in later life.* BMJ Publishing, London.

Barker, D.J. (1995). Fetal origins of coronary heart disease. *British Medical Journal*, **311**, 171–4.

Basso, O., Olsen, J., and Christensen, R. (1999). Study of environmental, social, and paternal factors in preterm delivery using sibs and half sibs. *Journal of Epidemiology and Community Health*, **53**, 20–3.

Batty, D. (1997). Review of interventions to prevent heart disease. *British Medical Journal*, **315**, 1468.

Belchetz, P.E. (1994). Hormonal replacement in postmenopausal women. *New England Journal of Medicine*, **330**, 1062–71.

Berry, R.J., Li, Z., Erickson, J.D., *et al.* (1999). Prevention of neural-tube defects with folic acid in China. *New England Journal of Medicine*, **341**, 1485–90.

Bjerregaard, P. and Young, T.K. (1998). *The circumpolar Inuit: health of a population in transition.* Munksgaard, Copenhagen.

Breslow, L. and Somers, A. (1988). The periodic health examination, and updates. *Canadian Medical Association Journal*, **4**, 617–26.

Brønnum-Hansen, H. (1999). How good is the Prevent model for estimating the health benefits of prevention? *Journal of Epidemiology and Community Health*, **53**, 300–5.

Cavelaars, A.E.J.M., Kunst, A.E., Geurts, J.J., *et al.* (1998). Differences in self reported morbidity by educational level: a comparison of 11 Western European countries. *Journal of Epidemiology and Community Health*, **52**, 219–27.

Cohen, D.R. and Henderson, J.B. (1988). *Health, prevention and economics.* Oxford University Press.

van Dam, J., Bond, J.H., and Sivak, M.V. Jr. (1995). Fecal occult blood screening for colorectal cancer. *Archives of Internal Medicine*, **155**, 2389–402.

Dean, K. and Holstein, B.E. (1991). In *Health promotion research* (ed. B. Bandura and I. Kickbusch). WHO European Series 37. WHO, Copenhagen.

De Koning, H.J. (2000). Breast cancer screening: cost-effective in practice? *European Journal of Radiology*, **33**, 32–7.

Deuster, P.A. (1996). Exercise in the prevention and treatment of chronic disorders. *Women's Health Issues*, **6**, 320–31.

DIKE (1997). *Danskernes sundhed mod år 2000. Sundhedsadfærd, sundhedstilstand, sygelighed, dødelighed, levekår.* DIKE, Copenhagen.

Doll, R. and Peto, R. (1981). *The causes of cancer. Quantitative estimates of avoidable risks of cancer in the United States today.* Oxford University Press.

Drever, F., Whitehead, M., and Roden, M. (1996). Current patterns and trends in male mortality by social class. *Population Trends*, **86**, 15–20.

Duval, A., Gayet, J., Zhou, X.P., Iacopetta, B., Thomas, G., and Hamelin, R. (1999). Frequent frameshift mutations of the TCF-4 gene in colorectal cancers with microsatellite instability. *Cancer Research*, **59**, 4213–15.

Ekbom, A. (1998). Growing evidence that several human cancers may originate in utero. *Seminars in Cancer Biology*, **8**, 237–44.

Ekbom, A., Trichopoulos, D., Adami, H.O., Hsieh, C-C., and Lan, S-J. (1992). Evidence of prenatal influences on breast cancer risk. *Lancet*, **340**, 1015–18.

Ekbom, A., Thurfjell, E., Hsieh, C.C., Trichopoulos, D., and Adami, H.O. (1995). Perinatal characteristics and adult mammographic patterns. *International Journal of Cancer*, **61**, 177–80.

Eriksson, U.J. and Swenne, I. (1993). Diabetes in pregnancy: fetal macrosomia, hyperinsulinism, and islet hyperplasia in the offspring of rats subjected to temporary protein-energy malnutrition early in life. *Pediatric Research*, **34**, 791–5.

Executive Board of the WHO (2000). *Prevention and control of noncommunicable diseases.* EB105.R12, 27 January 2000, WHO, Geneva.

Fleming, P.J. (1994). Understanding and preventing sudden infant death syndrome. *Current Opinion in Pediatrics*, **6**, 158–62.

Fonager, K., Sørensen, H.T., Olsen, J., Dahlerup, J.F., and Rasmussen, S.N. (1998). Pregnancy outcome for women with Crohn's disease: a follow-up study based on linkage between national registries. *American Journal of Gastroenterology*, **93**, 2426–30.

Forsdahl, A. (1977). Are poor living conditions in childhood and adolescence an important risk factor for arteriosclerotic heart disease? *British Journal of Preventive and Social Medicine*, **31**, 91–5.

Garrett, M.J. (1999). *Health futures.* WHO, Geneva.

Glanz, K. (1997). Dietary change. *Cancer Causes and Control*, **8**, S13–16.

Glassock, R.J. (1997). Optimizing disease management in the next 25 years. *Seminars in Nephrology*, **17**, 387–90.

Gortmaker, S.L., Mariani, A., Peterson, K., Cheung, L., and Wiecha, J. (1997). Exercise. *Cancer Causes and Control*, **8**, S17–19.

Gotzsche, P.C. and Olsen, O. (2000). Is screening for breast cancer with mammography justifiable? *Lancet*, **355**, 129–34.

Grandjean, P., Budtz-Jorgensen, E., White, R.F., *et al.* (1999). Methylmercury exposure biomarkers as indicators of neurotoxicity in children aged 7 years. *American Journal of Epidemiology*, **150**, 301–5.

Gunnar-Svensson, F., Ipsen, J., Olsen, J., and Waldstrøm, B. (1984). Prevention of relocation of the aged in nursing homes. *Scandinavian Journal of Primary Health Care*, **2**, 49–56.

Gyrd-Hansen, D. (1999). The relative economics of screening for colorectal cancer, breast cancer and cervical cancer. *Critical Reviews in Oncology/Hematology*, **32**, 133–44.

Hedner, T. (1998). Treating hypertension—effect of treatment and cost-effectiveness in respect to later cardiovascular diseases. *Scandinavian Cardiovascular Journal, Supplement*, **47**, 31–5.

Hennessy, C.H., Moriarty, D.G., Zack, M.M., Scherr, P.A., and Brackbill, R. (1994). Measuring health-related quality of life for public health surveillance. *Public Health Reports*, **109**, 665–72.

Holland, W.W. (1995). Advances in epidemiology and disease prevention. *Annals of the Academy of Medicine, Singapore*, **24**, 230–7.

Holland, W.W. and Stewart, S. (1998). *Public health. The vision and the challenge.* Nuffield Trust, London.

Holloway, R.G., Benesch, C.G., Rahilly, C.R., and Courtright, C.E. (1999). A systematic review of cost-effectiveness research of stroke evaluation and treatment. *Stroke*, **30**, 1340–9.

Hughes, K. (1997). Screening for and treatment of hypercholesterolaemia: a review. *Annals of the Academy of Medicine, Singapore*, **26**, 215–20.

Hugod, C. and Fog, J. (ed.) (1992). *Screening. Why, when and how?* National Board of Health, Denmark (English translation).

Jensen, U.J. and Mooney, G. (1990). *Changing values in medical and health care decision making.* Wiley, Chichester.

Jatoi, I. (1999). Breast cancer screening. *American Journal of Surgery*, **177**, 518–24.

Katz, S. (1983). Active life expectancy. *New England Journal of Medicine*, **11**, 1218–24.

Kirchhoff, M., Davidsen, M., Bronnun-Hansen, H., *et al.* (1999). Incidence of myocardial infarction in the Danish MONICA population 1982–1991. *International Journal of Epidemiology*, **28**, 211–18.

Kjøller, M., Rasmussen, N.K., and Keiding, L.M. (1999). Selvrapporteret sundhed og sygelighed blandt voksne danskere 1987–1994. *Ugeskrift for Laeger*, **16**, 2948–54.

Koplan, J.P. and Livengood, J.R. (1994). The influence of changing demographic patterns on our health promotion priorities. *American Journal of Preventive Medicine*, **10**, 42–4.

Kronborg, O., Fenger, C., Olsen, J., Jorgensen, O.D., and Søndergaard, O. (1996). Randomised study of screening for colorectal cancer with faecal-occult-blood test. *Lancet*, **348**, 1467–71.

Kuh, D. and Ben-Shlomo, B. (ed.) (1997). *A life course approach to chronic disease epidemiology. Tracing the origins of ill health from early to adult life.* Oxford University Press.

Lam, T.H. and He, Y. (1997). Passive smoking and coronary heart disease: a brief review. *Clinical and Experimental Pharmacology and Physiology*, **24**, 993–6.

Lander, E.S. and Schork, N.J. (1994). Genetic dissection of complex traits. *Science*, **265**, 2037–48.

Last, J.M. (1998). *Public health and human ecology.* Appleton and Lange, Stamford, CT.

Leon, D.A, Chenet, L., Shkolnikov, V.M., *et al.* (1997). Huge variation in Russian mortality rates 1984–94: artefact, alcohol, or what? *Lancet*, **350**, 383–8.

Littenberg, B. (1995). A practice guideline revisited: screening for hypertension. *Annals of Internal Medicine*, **122**, 937–9.

Lorig, K., Stewart, A., Ritter, P., González, V., Laurent, D., and Lynch, J. (1996). *Outcome measures for health education and other health care interventions.* Sage Publications, London.

Lucas, A., Fewtrell, M.S., and Cole, T.J. (1999). Fetal origins of adult disease—the hypothesis revisited. *British Medical Journal*, **319**, 245–9.

Lyon, A. (1967). Causality. *British Journal of the Philosophy of Science*, 1–20.

McKeown, T. (1965). *Medicine in modern society. Medical planning based on evaluation of medical achievement.* George Allen & Unwin, London.

McKeown, T. and Lowe, C.R. (1974). *An introduction to social medicine.* Blackwell Scientific, Oxford.

McMichael, A.J. (1999). Prisoners of the proximate: loosening the constraints on epidemiology in an age of change. *American Journal of Epidemiology*, **149**, 887–97.

Mackie, J.L. (1974). *The cement of the universe.* Oxford University Press.

Marmot, M. and Wilkinson, R.G. (1999). *Social determinants of health.* Oxford University Press.

Mortensen, P.B., Agerbo, E., Erikson, T., Qin, P., and Westergaard-Nielsen, N. (2000). Psychiatric illness and risk factors for suicide in Denmark. *Lancet*, **355**, 9–12.

Murray, C.J.L. and Lopez, A.D. (1997*a*). Alternative projections of mortality and disability by cause 1990–2020: Global Burden of Disease Study. *Lancet*, **349**, 1498–504.

Murray, C.J.L. and Lopez, A.D. (1997*b*). Global mortality, disability, and the contribution of risk factors: Global Burden of Disease Study. *Lancet*, **349**, 1436–42.

Murray, C.J.L. and Lopez, A.D. (1997*c*). Mortality by cause for eight regions of the world: Global Burden of Disease Study. *Lancet*, **349**, 1269–76.

Murray, C.J.L. and Lopez, A.D. (1997*d*). The utility of DALYs for public health policy and research: a reply. *Bulletin of the World Health Organization*, **75**, 577–81.

Murray, C.J.L. and Lopez, A.D. (1999). On the comparable quantification of health risks: lessons from the Global Burden of Disease Study. *Epidemiology*, **10**, 594–605.

Neel, J.V. (1999). Diabetes mellitus: a 'thrifty' genotype rendered detrimental by 'progress'. *Bulletin of the World Health Organization*, **77**, 694–703.

Nieuwenhuizen, A.G., Schuiling, G.A., Seijsener, A.F., Moes, H., and Koiter, T.R. (1999). Effects of food restriction on glucose tolerance, insulin secretion, and islet-cell proliferation in pregnant rats. *Physiology and Behavior*, **65**, 671–7.

Oliver, M.F. (1996). Which changes in diet prevent coronary heart disease? A review of clinical trials of dietary fats and antioxidants. *Acta Cardiologica*, **6**, 467–90.

Olsen, J. (1993). Some consequences of adopting a conditional deterministic causal model in epidemiology. *European Journal of Public Health*, **3**, 204–9.

Olsen, J. and Frische, G. (1993). Social differences in reproductive health. A study on birth weight, still births and congenital malformations in Denmark. *Scandinavian Journal of Social Medicine*, **2**, 90–7.

Olsen, J., Merletti, F., Snashall, D., and Vuylsteek, K. (1991). *Searching for causes of work-related diseases. An introduction to epidemiology at the work site.* Oxford University Press.

Olsen, J., Andersen, P.K., Sørensen, T.I.A., Melbye, M., and Aaby, P. (1999). The future of epidemiology. *International Journal of Epidemiology*, **28**, S996.

Olsen, S.F. (1993). Marine n-3 fatty acids ingested in pregnancy as a possible determinant of birth weight: a review of the current epidemiologic evidence. *Epidemiologic Reviews*, **15**, 399–413. (Erratum. *American Journal of Epidemiology*, **139**, 856 (1994).)

Olschwang, S., Hamelin, R., Laurent-Puig, P., *et al.* (1997). Alternative genetic pathways in colorectal carcinogenesis. *Proceedings of the National Academy of Sciences of the United States of America*, **94**, 12122–7.

Pina, I.L. and Fitzpatrick, J.T. (1996). Exercise and heart failure. *Chest*, **110**, 1317–27.

Rijke, R.P. (1997). Health promotion from an ecological viewpoint. *Oncologica*, **14**, 34–6 (in Dutch).

Rimm, E.B., Williams, P., Fosher, K., Criqui, M., and Stampfer, M.J. (1999). Moderate alcohol intake and lower risk of coronary heart disease: meta-analysis of effects on lipids and haemostatic factors. *British Medical Journal*, **319**, 1523–8.

Roemer, M.I. (1984). The value of medical care for health promotion. *American Journal of Public Health*, **74**, 243–8.

Rose, G. (1992). *The strategy of preventive medicine.* Oxford University Press.

Rose, J.E. (1996). Nicotine addiction and treatment. *Annual Review of Medicine*, **47**, 493–507.

Rothman, K.J. (1976). Causes. *American Journal of Epidemiology*, **104**, 587–92.

Ruiz, J., Blanche, H., Cohen, N., *et al.* (1994). Insertion/deletion polymorphism of the angiotensin-converting enzyme gene is strongly associated with coronary heart disease in non-insulin-dependent diabetes mellitus. *Proceedings of the National Academy of Sciences of the United States of America*, **91**, 3662–5.

Sabroe, S. and Olsen, J. (1998). Perinatal correlates of specific histological types of testicular cancer in patients below 35 years of age: a case-cohort study based on midwives' records in Denmark. *International Journal of Cancer*, **78**, 140–3.

Schueler, K. (1994). Cost-effectiveness issues in hypertension control. *Canadian Journal of Public Health*, **85**, S54–6.

Scully, D., Kremer, J., Meade, M.M., Graham, R., and Dudgeon, K. (1998). Physical exercise and psychological well being: a critical review. *British Journal of Sports Medicine*, **32**, 111–20.

Schulte, P.A. and Perera, F.P. (1993). *Molecular epidemiology: principles and practice.* Academic Press, San Diego, CA.

Sharpe, R.M. and Skakkebæk, N.E. (1993). Are oestrogens involved in falling sperm counts and disorders of the male reproductive tract. *Lancet*, **341**, 1392–5.

Skakkebæk, N.E., Berthelsen, J.G., Giwercman, A., and Müller, J. (1987). Carcinoma-*in-situ* of the testis: possible origin from gonocytes and precursor of all types of germ cell tumours except spermatocytoma. *International Journal of Andrology*, **10**, 19–28.

Sønderskov, J., Olsen, J., Sabroe, S., Meillier, L., and Overvad, K. (1997). Nicotine patches in smoking cessation: a randomized trial among over-the-counter customers in Denmark. *American Journal of Epidemiology*, **145**, 309–18.

Taylor, B.J. (1991). A review of epidemiological studies of sudden infant death syndrome in southern New Zealand. *Journal of Paediatrics and Child Health*, **27**, 344–8.

Taylor, E.M. and Emery, J.L. (1990). Categories of preventable unexpected infant deaths. *Archives of Disease in Childhood*, **65**, 535–9.

Taylor, R. (1993). Non-communicable diseases in the tropics. *Medical Journal of Australia*, **159**, 266–70.

Trichopoulos, D. (1990). Hypothesis: does breast cancer originate in utero? *Lancet*, **335**, 939–40.

UK Childhood Cancer Study Investigators (1999). Exposure to power-frequency magnetic fields and the risk of childhood cancer. *Lancet*, **354**, 1925–31.

Vershuren, P.M. (ed.) (1993). *Health issues related to alcohol consumption.* ILSI Europe, Brussels.

WHO (1999*a*). *Health 21. The health for all policy framework for the WHO European Region.* European Health for All Series 6, WHO, Copenhagen.

WHO (1999*b*). *The world health report 1999. Making a difference.* WHO, Geneva.

Wynder, E.L. and Andres, R. (1994). Workshop A: diet and nutrition research as it relates to aging and chronic diseases. *Preventive Medicine*, **23**, 549–51.

12.6 Screening

Anthony B. Miller and Vivek Goel

General principles of screening

Introduction

Ideally, the control of a disease should be achievable, either by preventing the disease from occurring or, if it does occur, by curing those who develop it with appropriate treatment. Completely successful prevention would make treatment obsolete. However, completely successful treatment would not make prevention obsolete, as there are costs and undesirable sequelae from the disease and treatment which patients and society would like to avoid if at all possible, especially from diseases such as cancer, diabetes, and hypertension. At present, neither prevention nor treatment is completely successful for most diseases. They will continue to complement each other while, for a number of conditions, another approach to control may prove to be appropriate and complementary to one or both of the other approaches. Such an approach is screening.

Because of the deep-rooted belief among physicians that 'early diagnosis' of disease is beneficial, many regard screening as bound to be effective. However, for a number of reasons this is not necessarily the case, as shown for example by the failure of screening for lung cancer using sputum cytology or chest radiographs to reduce mortality from the disease (Prorok *et al.* 1984). It is the purpose of this chapter to attempt to define some of the fundamental issues that are relevant to the consideration of screening in public health. In that context, we shall describe approaches to evaluating the efficacy of screening before it can be accepted as an established disease control measure and briefly consider the extent to which programmes proposed or underway for some diseases comply with these criteria.

It is often assumed that screening tests must involve some sort of technological procedure, such as a radiograph or laboratory test. However, screening can involve simple clinical examinations, such as assessment of blood pressure, or a history, such as the Michigan Alcohol Screening Test which is a set of questions (Selzer *et al.* 1979). However, it is the advent of expensive technologically based screening tests in the last few decades which has focused attention on the need for critical evaluation of screening and the importance of screening programmes. With the introduction of genetic susceptibility testing, as a result of the human genome programme, it becomes even more essential for public health practitioners to have a thorough understanding of the principles of screening.

Definition

Screening was defined by the United States Commission on Chronic Illness (1957) as 'the presumptive identification of unrecognized disease or defect by the application of tests, examinations or other procedures that can be applied rapidly.' A screening test is not intended to be diagnostic. Rather, a positive finding will have to be confirmed by special diagnostic procedures.

By definition, screening is offered to those who do not suspect that they may have a disease. This is subtly different from being asymptomatic. Symptoms may be revealed by careful questioning related to the organ of interest which may not be regarded by the screenee as being related to a possible disease. Furthermore, in a public health programme open to all comers, it may not be possible to determine that all subjects who enrol were truly asymptomatic. Indeed, many may enrol because they have a suspicion that they have the disease of interest, and they hope that their suspicion will not be confirmed. Thus although we, in common with others, will make the assumption subsequently that participants in screening programmes are asymptomatic, we do not imply that this is a necessary or an absolute prerequisite for participation in public-health-based screening programmes.

General principles governing the introduction of screening

The principles that should govern the introduction of screening programmes were first enunciated by Wilson and Junger (1968) and have since been refined by a number of authors (Miller 1978; Cuckle and Wald 1984; Miller 1996). These principles (in their refined form) are considered below.

The disease should be an important health problem. In practical terms this means that the disease prevalence should be high and the disease should be the cause of substantial mortality and/or morbidity. However, it is important to recognize that the life expectancy of a screened population may be changed little even if the programme is successful. For example, even if all cancer were to be eradicated in most technically advanced countries, the effect of other competing causes of death is such that life expectancy would be increased only by about 2.5 years. The benefits of cholesterol screening to prevent heart disease are measured, at the population level, in days of life expectancy gain per person screened (Kristiansen *et al.* 1991). It is not possible to provide a precise estimate for the level of burden necessary to mount a screening programme. The level of morbidity and mortality considered to be important will depend on a combination of factors such as the age distribution of the population affected, or the severity of the illness. There may be certain circumstances when the major benefit from screening may follow, not from reduction in mortality, but from reduction of morbidity consequent upon the diagnosis of the disease in a more treatable phase in its natural history. This could mean that the extent of treatment required and the possibility that treatment may be debilitating or mutilating would be much less. Such advantages may be difficult to quantify; however, as they may be considerable in psychological terms to individuals, and to communities in the lowering in the requirements for extensive rehabilitation services, they should not be overlooked.

The disease should have a detectable preclinical phase. It is important to recognize that this principle is not 'The natural history of the disease should include a phase with a detectable precursor'. For example for many cancers, including breast and prostate cancer, the detectable preclinical phase is largely asymptomatic invasive cancer rather than a precursor. Conversely, for cervix cancer the detectable preclinical phase probably includes the whole range from dysplasia through to occult invasive cancer. In screening for cardiovascular disease with cholesterol or hypertension, physiological markers of risk are being identified rather than detectable precursors. Nevertheless, such a point in time can be considered to be a preclinical phase. The key principle is that there should be a phase that screening detects prior to when clinical diagnosis of the disease is possible.

The natural history of the condition should be known. Ideally, such a requirement implies that it is known at what stage in the disease process progression, disability and/or death can no longer be prevented. If such information is available and the stage that the development of the disease had reached in individuals is determinable, it would be possible to decide precisely when a screening test should be applied in order to achieve maximum benefit and minimal overutilization of resources. Unfortunately it seems unlikely that knowledge will be accumulated to be able to determine the natural history of disease in individuals in such a precise fashion. It is recognized that the rate of progression of clinically detected disease from the point of diagnosis to cure or to death varies substantially in different individuals. The distribution of rates of progression of preclinically detectable disease that might be identified by screening is likely to be equally wide. Thus, although an objective for research on screening has to be to determine the extent of the distribution of the sojourn times of the detectable preclinical phase, in considering the introduction of screening programmes and the scheduling of tests within programmes, it is necessary to balance benefits with costs. This means that a schedule will have to be determined that will enable the detection of the maximal number of still curable cases compatible with the longest interval between tests.

It should also not be assumed that disease processes are inevitably progressive. For cancer of the cervix, for example, it has been determined that *in situ* carcinoma may undergo regression in a large proportion of cases (Boyes *et al.* 1982), as do most cases of mild and moderate dysplasia of the cervix (Holowaty *et al.* 1999). Such conclusions have substantial implications with regard to the optimum frequency of screening examinations. Designing a programme directed to those lesions that, in the absence of screening will progress and more rapidly escape curability, if they can be identified, will be the appropriate approach. Designing a programme which maximizes the detection of cases with good prognosis, but which in the absence of screening may be unlikely to progress, will waste resources.

The disease should be treatable, and there should be a recognized treatment for lesions identified following screening. This principle has been elaborated as follows:

> There should be evidence of the effectiveness of treatment of lesions discovered as a result of screening in reducing mortality and the level of improvement expected should be stated; [and secondly,] there should be reasonable expectation that recommendations for the appropriate management of the lesions discovered from a screening programme will be complied with both by the individual with the lesion and by the physician responsible for his (or her) health care. (Miller 1978)

Screening programmes should only be set up when there are adequate facilities for treating lesions discovered as a result of screening and functioning referral systems for securing such treatment. There is obviously no point in establishing a screening programme and identifying lesions that should be treated if the facilities are not available, or the infrastructure for referral, confirmation of diagnosis, and treatment is not in place. In general this is not a problem for technically advanced countries, but it can be for developing countries. Unfortunately problems allied to these have occurred. Thus on occasions it has not been certain whether or not lesions identified as a result of screening should be regarded as true disease precursors. When lesions are first identified in a screening programme, information may not be available as to their appropriate treatment, and special studies may be required. Otherwise, errors in terms of observation rather than treatment on the one hand, or too extensive treatment on the other, are possible. In prostate cancer screening, for example, if too radical treatment is applied in the elderly to the latent or good prognosis prostate cancers that may be identified in a screening programme, the morbidity in terms of incontinence and impotence, and even the mortality from treatment, could offset any benefit from the earlier detection of lesions with truly malignant potential (Chodak and Schoenberg 1989; Miller 1991; Krahn *et al.* 1994).

A different sort of difficulty could arise when, as a result of screening, lesions are diagnosed earlier in their natural history, but in spite of this, death is still inevitable. For example, if the available screening methods will not succeed in diagnosing disease before it is outside the range of current therapy, then screening to detect such disease is not worthwhile. The early studies of screening for lung cancer suggested that this was not a condition amenable to screening, probably for this reason (Prorok *et al.* 1984).

There is also a difficulty with the last two criteria when some different screening paradigms are considered. For example, with prenatal screening of the mother, as in maternal serum screening (or triple marker screening), a marker is being sought for risk of congenital anomaly in the fetus (Wald *et al.* 1997). A precursor to the disease is not sought, rather disease in the fetus is being identified. In the absence of truly effective fetal surgery for most of these conditions, treatment is not available. However, screening can lead to greater information for the family which can lead to better preparation for delivery or assist with decisions about termination of the pregnancy.

The screening test to be used should be acceptable and safe. In general, this implies a non-invasive test with high validity. Other criteria of a good screening test include ease of use and relatively low cost. These principles and various approaches to assessing validity will now be discussed.

The validity of a screening test

Two measures suffice to describe the validity of screening tests: sensitivity and specificity.

Sensitivity is defined as the ability of a test to detect all those with the disease in the screened population. This is expressed as the proportion of those with the disease in whom a screening test gives a positive result.

Specificity is defined as the ability of a test to identify correctly those free of the disease in the screened population. This is expressed as the proportion of people free of the disease in whom the screening test gives a negative result.

Table 1 illustrates how these measures can be derived. These two terms may be further expressed in terms of test results as follows: sensitivity is calculated as the true positives divided by the sum of the true positives and false negatives and expressed as a percentage; specificity is calculated as the true negatives divided by the sum of the true negatives and the false positives and expressed as a percentage.

In practice, difficulties with these measures arise over defining a positive result from the test as well as distinguishing the true positives from the false positives among those who test positive, and the true negatives from the false negatives among those who test negative. A relatively imperfect test of a quantitative continuously distributed measurement can be artificially given a very high sensitivity by setting the boundary between negative and positive to incorporate a high proportion of those who are eventually found to have the disease in the positive category, but at a substantial cost in terms of low specificity. Conversely, the same test can be made to appear highly specific, but will then become insensitive, if the boundary between positive and negative is shifted in the opposite direction.

If the test result is expressed in a quantitative form so that the boundaries between what is defined as positive and negative can be varied at will, it is possible to plot a receiver operating characteristic curve (Swets 1979). What is plotted is the sensitivity on the vertical axis and 1-specificity (proportion of false positives) on the horizontal axis. The point on the curve that is chosen as optimal is that furthest from the 45° diagonal. Receiver operating characteristics curves are most easily derived for blood tests, but have also been applied to mammography, by varying the extent to which different mammographic abnormalities were regarded as an indication of suspicion of malignancy (Goin and Haberman 1982). Such curves cannot be applied to a test with a dichotomous outcome. Furthermore, they imply a similar weight to sensitivity and specificity, which as discussed below may not be ideal.

Table 1 Derivation of the sensitivity and specificity of a screening test

	Disease present	Disease absent
Test positive	*a*	*b*
Test negative	*c*	*d*

Sensitivity (proportion with condition who test positive): $a/(a + c)$

Specificity (proportion without condition who test negative): $d/(b + d)$

Positive predictive value (proportion with positive test who have condition): $a/(a + b)$

Negative predictive value (proportion with negative test who do not have condition): $d/(c + d)$

The position of the boundaries that are set between what is regarded as disease and non-disease (or benign disease) can also considerably influence the numerical values placed on sensitivity and specificity. This arises because of uncertainty as to what truly constitutes an abnormality in the context of a screening programme. In order to come to such a decision it is essential that the conditions identified as a result of screening should have a known natural history. However, as discussed above, such knowledge may not be available at the initiation of a screening programme and may only be obtained as a result of careful study of findings from screening programmes.

Nevertheless, the definition as to what constitutes disease is crucial in order to determine sensitivity and specificity. Most people have a clear idea as to what they regard as disease in terms of that which surfaces in standard medical practice. By definition, screening is conducted on asymptomatic individuals, so that many conditions that are identified through screening are likely to be at an early stage and may not have the generally recognized clinical characteristics of relatively advanced disease. This difficulty should theoretically be overcome by having clearly defined definitions of disease. However, for cancer, diagnosis is usually made on histology, and histology only imperfectly characterizes behaviour, especially for lesions within the detectable preclinical phase. For cancer, one hope for the future is that some of the markers for prognosis currently being evaluated such as markers of oncogene expression or other markers of DNA change may serve to identify those precancerous or *in situ* components of the detectable preclinical phase that are likely to progress.

A common error in evaluating potential screening tests is to determine the sensitivity by utilizing the experience of the test in relation to people who have clinical disease. A test that may appear to be highly sensitive under these circumstances may later be found to be much less sensitive when its ability to detect the detectable preclinical phase is evaluated. A similar error is substituting an intermediate marker as the gold standard for calculating sensitivity and specificity. For example, the test characteristics for a thyroid assay may be compared with a putatively more accurate assay, rather than the presence of the condition in the individual tested. Therefore, in the screening context, sensitivity and specificity may vary according to whether they are estimated for early disease or preclinical lesions, and sensitivity for both should be determined in active screening programmes. To do so for specificity is very much easier than for sensitivity. This is because the diagnostic process put in train by a positive screening test generally fairly rapidly identifies those who have the disease and thus distinguishes the true from the false positives. As under most circumstances the proportion of those who have the disease in relation to the total population screened is low, a very good approximation to specificity is obtained by calculating the proportion of all those who tested negative of the sum of the test negatives and false positives. Including the unidentified false negatives in the numerator and denominator of this expression will in practice introduce little error.

However, sensitivity is a difficult measure to determine initially in a screening programme. The reason is that the false negatives are not immediately apparent, as there is no justification to retest all the test negatives just to identify a few false negatives. Only by following the total population who screened negative is it eventually possible to identify those who had the disease at the time the test was administered but were not so identified at the time of screening. This is facilitated if test materials are retained; for example, cervical smears or mammograms originally classed negative can be reassessed for those who are found to have disease at the next scheduled screen, or who develop disease during the interval between screens. Such reassessments should preferably be made blind to avoid bias. We have used such an approach in the assessment of the sensitivity of the 'reader error' for cervical cancer screening (Boyes *et al.* 1982) and in the assessment of the sensitivity of mammography in a trial of breast cancer screening (Baines *et al.* 1988).

When test materials cannot be retained, such as in the assessment of the sensitivity of physical examination as a screening test for breast cancer, and for what we have called the 'taker error and the biological component' of false negatives in cervical cytology, i.e. disease that was indeed present but was not incorporated in the smear or for some reason did not exfoliate (Boyes *et al.* 1982), a direct identification of false negatives will not be possible. The usual approach, which we used in estimating the sensitivity of physical examination (Baines *et al.* 1989), is to assume that disease occurring within a certain period are false negatives. However, a possibly more satisfactory approach is to assess the expected detection rate of disease on screening after repeated screens, assuming that most of the false negatives had by then been identified, and to regard the excess disease above this level at the second screen as a measure of the false negatives at the first screen. As a result of such an approach it was determined that the taker and biological component of false negatives was approximately equal to the directly measured reader error, so that the level of sensitivity for cervical cytology approximated to 78 per cent (Miller 1981).

In a workshop on screening for cancer (Miller 1978), two recommendations were made with regard to the validity of screening tests:

- the sensitivity and specificity of the screening test to be used should have been evaluated and their expected values stated
- there should be an acceptable programme of quality control to ensure that the stated levels of sensitivity and specificity are attained and maintained.

Quality control involves issues that concern not only the validity of the screening test but also its safety. For example, it is necessary to ensure that radiation exposure does not drift upwards in a mammography screening programme. Quality control encumbers the training of those who will actually administer and read screening tests, their supervision, and the introduction of procedures to check actively on the extent to which those positive or negative are misclassified.

Quality may suffer because of overwork and boredom. One of the reasons why a recommendation was made to change the frequency of examination for most women in cervical cytology screening programmes in Canada was to avoid repetitive rescreening of normal women, and the flooding of laboratories with unnecessary and unrewarding work (Task Force 1976). The Task Force described the mechanisms for ensuring appropriate quality control. It is relevant that these requirements had to be re-emphasized more than a decade later (Miller *et al.* 1991*a*).

That such issues are not simple was underlined by consideration of observer variation in mammography reading (Boyd *et al.* 1982). Relevant to all screening programmes is not only the accuracy with which abnormalities are identified, but also, if they are identified, the extent to which appropriate recommendations are made on their management. Our experience suggested that including a category of 'probably benign' in a screening mammography report increases the extent of observer variation. Readers differ substantially in the extent they use this category, the extent to which they recommend special observation of individuals placed in this category, and the extent to which they recommend biopsy. Dual reading helps to increase specificity without much, if any, loss of sensitivity. This permits the simplification of recommendations into two groups—'suspicious of malignancy' and 'satisfactory (normal)' examination—and results in far greater consistency. Furthermore, it is compatible with the appropriate separation of findings from screening tests into the probably abnormal (test positive) and probably normal (test negative) dichotomy. The probably abnormal group is subjected to diagnostic tests in the normal way. This approach to use of screening mammography was accepted with difficulty in North America, because of an initial tendency for most radiologists to regard mammography as a diagnostic rather than a screening test. This resulted in greater use of biopsy as a diagnostic test in North America than that reported from Europe (McLelland and Pisano 1992), where more use was made of diagnostic mammography subsequent to screening mammography (often called by European radiologists 'complete' mammography) with a consequent reduction in biopsies and a much lower benign to malignant ratio.

Most commentators in the past, when considering the relative weight to be placed on sensitivity and specificity, tended to encourage high sensitivity at the cost of relatively low specificity, as it was felt important to attempt to avoid missing individuals who truly had disease. One vigorous exponent of this view for breast cancer screening was Moskowitz, who coined the term 'aggressive screening', as he felt that 'minimal' breast cancers with an excellent prognosis would only be identified by such an approach (Moskowitz *et al.* 1976). However, there continues to be little evidence that such cancers are really responsible for the mortality reduction following breast cancer screening (Miller 2000*a*). Rather, there is much evidence that the early diagnosis of more advanced disease results in a benefit (Miller 1987, 1994). A disadvantage of aggressive screening was a high benign-to-malignant ratio and low specificity of the screen. Although the objective of screening is to identify disease in the detectable preclinical phase before it reaches the stage of escaping from curability, if a test is made so sensitive that it picks up lesions that would never have progressed in that individuals lifetime, there will be substantial additional costs for diagnosis and treatment (this is one consequence of the 'overdiagnosis' bias, which is more fully discussed in relation to survival of cases following screen detection below). There is no point in identifying through screening disease which would never have presented clinically, and little point (other than less radical therapy) in identifying early disease that would have been cured anyway if it had presented clinically. Similarly, identifying disease that results in death, even following screen identification and subsequent treatment, only results in greater observation time and no benefit to the screenee. It is only disease that results in death in the absence of screening, but which is cured following treatment after screen detection, from which the real benefit of a screening programme derives. Hence, if high 'sensitivity' is largely based on finding more good prognosis disease, but results in lowering specificity, the programme will incur much greater costs without corresponding benefit.

The process measure, as distinct from a measure of validity, that most clearly expresses this difficulty is the predictive value of a positive screen. This is defined as the proportion of those who test positive who truly have the disease. This measure is influenced not only by the sensitivity and specificity of the test, especially the latter, but by the prevalence of disease in the population, whereas sensitivity and specificity are invariant with regard to disease prevalence. If tests are administered under circumstances that incur a low predictive value positive, then not only may costs be high in terms of correctly identifying those who are falsely positive, but also the potential hazard may be high, as an individual classified as positive falsely derives no benefit and potentially a substantial risk from the associated diagnostic procedures. A test with a low predictive value positive rapidly enters into disrepute.

To complete discussion of process measures, the predictive value negative should be defined. This is the proportion of those who test negative who are truly free of the disease. This measure, like sensitivity, is dependent on identifying the false negatives, and therefore is rarely determined while being of little operational value. In practice, however, it is usually high.

As Day (1985) has pointed out, because of the difficulty in identifying false negatives, and because of the overdiagnosis bias, the usual approach to defining sensitivity is not ideal, nor particularly biologically meaningful. He suggested an alternative measure of sensitivity which can be derived if the expected incidence of disease in the absence of screening can be determined, ideally from the control group in a randomized trial, but sometimes in population based programmes from historical data or data from comparable unscreened populations. The method basically computes the extent a programme is successful in reducing the expected incidence of disease in the absence of screening. The lower the proportion of expected incidence occurring after screening the greater the sensitivity.

The acceptability of the test

One of the desirable attributes of a good screening test is that it should be acceptable to the population to which screening is offered and acceptable to those who will administer the test. In general, cervical cytology screening programmes have found acceptance with women and their physicians, except for women who tend to be at highest risk of the disease. This results in lower effectiveness of programmes than would be the case if all women were to be included. This lack of acceptance is largely related to lower socio-economic status, where presumably other health concerns take precedence over a long-term preventive manoeuvre such as screening.

Breast cancer screening has encountered different problems over acceptability, although this varies substantially in different countries, ranging from the 90 per cent acceptance with screening invitations in Sweden (Tabar *et al.* 1985) to the difficulties with both physician and women compliance in the United States (Howard 1987). In Europe, a median uptake of 74 per cent has been reported (European Society for Mastology 1993).

Screening for colorectal cancer also has its own difficulties, particularly in the inevitable distaste of individuals for a procedure that involves manipulation of faeces. In a number of pilot programmes, therefore, the return rates for haemoccult slides have been low, although they have been better in well-organized studies (Chamberlain and Miller 1988), and achieved approximately 75 per cent in the Minnesota Colon Cancer Screening Trial (Mandel *et al.* 1999).

Therefore a screening test has to be acceptable to the population in its widest sense. The test should be simple and as far as possible easily administered. It should involve procedures that are not unacceptable, and its use should not have unpleasant or potentially hazardous implications. There are also economic advantages in a test being administered or read by allied health professionals, such as use of technologists in initial screening of cervical cytology slides (Anderson 1985), or the use of nurses to perform breast examinations (Bassett 1985; Miller *et al.* 1991*b*).

The ethics of screening

In general medical practice the special nature of the relationship between patient and physician has dictated the need to build up a core of ethical principles that govern this relationship. Furthermore, it is generally accepted that additional issues arise when a patient becomes the subject of a research investigation that is superimposed upon his or her search for and receipt of appropriate medical care. However, it was not initially appreciated that screening opened up a completely new spectrum of issues, possibly requiring more restrictive boundaries of ethical behaviour than those applied in usual medical care. For example, when a patient goes to see a physician for relief of a symptom or treatment of an established condition, the physician is required to exercise his or her skills only to the extent that knowledge is currently available, while doing what is possible with available expertise and appropriate assistance to help the patient. Treatment may be offered without any implied guarantee that it is necessarily efficacious or will do more than just temporarily relieve the symptoms of which the patient complains. Thus the physician promises to do his or her best for the patient; there is no implied promise that the patient will be cured.

In screening, however, those who are approached to participate are not patients and most of them do not become patients. The screener believes that as a result of screening the health of the community will be improved. He or she does not necessarily intend to imply that the condition of every individual will be improved. However, screening is often promoted as if it implies a benefit to everyone who is screened. In fact, in some circumstances individuals included in a screening programme may be placed at a disadvantage, as discussed above. Furthermore, the harm from a screening test is not only related to the risk of being false positive or false negative. Those who are screened may also incur psychological consequences, sometimes merely from being labelled as being at risk of disease (Glanz and Gilboy 1995). Therefore, at the very least, those planning to introduce a screening programme should be in a position to guarantee overall benefit to the community and a minimum of risk that certain individuals may be disadvantaged by the programme. It was the inability to guarantee overall benefit and lack of disadvantage for those screened that led to the proscription of mammography in women under the age of 50 in the Breast Cancer Detection Demonstration Projects in the United States (Beahrs *et al.* 1979).

A second ethical issue, which is directed more to the obligations for appropriate care in the community than towards individuals, concerns how limited resources are equitably distributed across the whole community to obtain maximum benefit. Under certain circumstances the offer of screening could diminish the total level of health in a community. This may be a particular problem for developing countries by diverting resources intended for routine health care into screening. Thus resources diverted to a screening project, which might be regarded as prestigious, especially if involving high technology, could lower the resources available for other more pressing but also more mundane health problems. Although several screening programmes have been proposed for developing countries, there is a particular need for caution and care in order to ensure that they do not overbalance the health care system in the area in which they are introduced.

A final ethical dilemma for screening programmes is how to implement informed consent. Information about risks and benefits of tests and treatments are expected to be provided in usual clinical practice. For screening, providing information about the test alone is not sufficient. Information about the consequences of the test, the diagnostic assessment process and the diseases to be detected, and their treatments should also be presented, if a truly informed decision is to be made. Presenting such a large amount of information is obviously difficult, particularly in a primary care setting where several screening tests may be done at the same time. Furthermore, presenting such information becomes even more cumbersome when the evidence base for a screening test is controversial, such as the case with prostate screening.

Therefore screening programmes carry an ethical responsibility as least as great as that for medical practice in that approaches to participate are made to ostensibly healthy people. Indeed, the burden of proof for efficacy of the procedures and the necessity to avoid harm are greater than may be required for diagnostic or therapeutic procedures carried out when a patient presents with symptoms to a physician. In screening the physician or public health worker initiates the process and he or she bears the onus of responsibility to be certain that benefit will follow.

The population to be included in screening programmes

For a screening programme to be successful, the population to be included should be one in which it is known that the disease has a high prevalence. This will not only encourage a high predictive value for a positive test, but it will also tend to promote higher quality of performance and assessment of results of screening tests, and will result in lower costs per case detected. Thus in all screening programmes it is desirable to attempt to include only those who are at risk of the disease and to concentrate particularly on those who are at high risk of the disease. This approach was recognized by the Canadian Task Force on Cervical Cytology Screening Programs (Task Force 1976) which defined those whom it believed were at such low risk for the disease that they need not be included in cervical cytology screening programmes, thus defining the remaining 'at-risk' population on whom major efforts should be concentrated to bring them into screening. In the case of cardiovascular disease, family history and factors such as smoking have been used by some to define populations to be screened (Toronto Working Group 1990).

However, the known risk factors, apart from age, for other diseases may not suffice to distinguish adequately between those who should be considered for inclusion in screening programmes compared with those who should not. For breast screening, for example, although some discrimination using risk factors has been achieved (Schechter *et al.* 1986), this has not been sufficient to justify selection on this basis alone. However, age is an important predictor of risk, and for breast cancer in technically advanced countries, all women in the appropriate age group can be regarded as at high risk. Thus for breast cancer currently, it seems unlikely that any programme could justify routine screening of women under the age of 40, while screening women aged 40 to 49 with mammography is controversial.

One possible approach to concentrating on the relevant segment of the population for screening might be to administer a prescreening test, especially if for a marker for a factor necessary in the causation of the disease. Such a test can be envisaged for human papilloma virus infection as a prescreen for cancer of the cervix (Miller *et al.* 2000*b*), although a difficulty here is the high proportion of infections that are self-limiting without the development of high-grade cervical intraepithelial neoplasia. This means that the test is too non-specific if used among women under the age of 35. The development of genetic susceptibility testing opens up the possibility of prescreening for a range of diseases. For example, women found to carry genes showing susceptibility to breast cancer may undergo screening with MRI.

Hakama (1986) has pointed out that in programmes that attempt to select for screening on the basis of risk, there will usually be cases occurring in the unscreened group. Another consequence of such programmes, however, will be reduced numbers of false positives (in absolute terms) which with the increased prevalence of the disease will result in a higher predictive value positive of the screen. Hakama (1984) coined the terms 'programme sensitivity' and 'programme specificity' which help in understanding the effects of screening concentrating on high risk. The more a programme concentrates on 'high-risk' groups, the lower the programme sensitivity will be, as more and more cases will occur in unscreened people Conversely, however, the programme specificity will increase because of the increase in healthy people unscreened with a reduction in the costs of screening. The reduction in programme sensitivity will result in a reduction in the overall effectiveness of the programme because of the imprecision by which high-risk groups are identified, therefore the overall result of such an approach could be unacceptable.

One other approach to using risk factors is to help determine the optimal periodicity of rescreening. Once again, however, much of the necessary research is incomplete, and we do not know how appropriate such an approach may be. It will probably be necessary to calculate the marginal cost-effectiveness of extending screening from high- to low-risk groups (i.e. the additional cost for such an extension of screening related to the increase in effectiveness of the screening) in order to make the necessary policy decisions.

Diagnosis and treatment of the discovered lesions

As a screening test is not diagnostic, inevitably the success of the programme will ultimately depend upon the extent those identified as having an abnormal test result accept the procedures offered to them for further evaluation, and the effectiveness of the therapy offered.

A number of difficulties may arise. For example, in the initial phases of many breast cancer screening programmes, it was necessary to demonstrate to the general community of medical practitioners that the abnormalities identified were indeed of importance and that they required care and expertise to biopsy. Indeed, in the absence of skills in diagnosis and management, there can be unnecessary biopsy (potentially reducible by the use of diagnostic mammography and fine-needle aspiration biopsies) as well as failure to excise the lesion when biopsy is performed. This is part of the spectrum of problems that arise over the fact that lesions may be identified in screening programmes whose biological features, natural history, and other characteristics may be in doubt. The screening participants may require special education so that they understand the diagnostic process to reduce as far as possible one of the major adverse consequences of screening, the anxiety accompanying the identification of an abnormality, as well as ensuring that they comply with the recommendations for management. There may even be major disagreements over the histological interpretation of the excised lesions, with uncertainties over the borderline between benign and malignant. Thus the public and the professionals at all levels in a screening programme may require education and/or retraining dependent on their responsibilities. One mechanism of reducing difficulties in the professional area that should be encouraged is the provision of special diagnostic and treatment centres where the necessary expertise in diagnosis and management can be concentrated and where the necessary facilities are available (Miller and Tsechovski 1987). Such centres could be regionally based, serving a number of screening centres.

Evaluation of screening programmes

A number of issues have to be noted when evaluating screening programmes. Almost invariably individuals with disease identified as a result of screening will have a longer survival time than those diagnosed in the normal way. Four biases associated with screening explain this. The first is 'lead time', defined as the interval between the time of detection by screening and the time at which the disease would have been diagnosed in the absence of screening. In other words, it is the period by which screening advances the diagnosis of the disease. For example, if as a result of screening, the average point of diagnosis is advanced by 1 year, then inevitably cases diagnosed by screening will survive 1 year longer even if there is no long-term benefit. It is important to recognize that the lead time for different cases will vary, depending in part on the timing of the screening test in relation to the duration of the detectable preclinical phase in that case, as well as the rapidity of progression of the detectable preclinical phase in that individual. Thus there will be a distribution of lead times (Morrison 1985). The lead time for fatal cases will be fairly short, but in one study some fatal cases have been identified as having a lead time of a year or more following mammography screening (Miller *et al.* 1992).

The determination of lead time is complex, but models have been developed that do so providing there are control data that permit comparison of screen detection with that expected (Walter and Day 1983).

Differential lead time can be an important factor in comparing the outcome among cases detected by different screening modalities, making it almost impossible to make a comparison based on survival, unless it is possible to estimate and correct for differential lead time (Walter and Stitt 1987).

The second bias that accounts for improved survival of screen-detected cases is 'length-biased sampling'. This relates to the fact that individuals who have rapidly progressive disease will tend to develop symptoms that cause them to consult physicians directly. Thus only less rapidly progressive cases are likely to remain to be detected by screening. Yet the former have a poorer and the latter a better prognosis—hence the improved survival of screen-detected cases, over and above lead time. This bias is most obvious at the initiation of a screening programme, at the first or prevalent screen. However, length bias will also affect the type of cases detected at rescreening, with the more rapidly progressive cancers diagnosed in the intervals between screens. Hence in evaluating the total impact of programmes, the interval cases must be identified and taken into consideration as well as the screen-detected cases.

The third bias which can artefactually improve survival is selection bias. Those who enter screening programmes are volunteers, and almost invariably more health conscious than those who decline to enter. This means that, even in the absence of screening, they are likely to have a better outcome from their disease than the overall rates in the general population.

The fourth bias is overdiagnosis bias. This means that some lesions identified and counted as disease would not have presented clinically in those individuals during their lifetimes in the absence of screening. This is, in practice, an extreme example of length bias. It is difficult to obtain absolute confirmation of the existence of this bias, although it seems likely that it is at least in part an explanation for the substantial excess of cancers detected by prostate-specific antigen screening for prostate cancer.

The only design that effectively eliminates the effect of all these biases is the randomized controlled trial (Prorok *et al.* 1984), but only if mortality from the disease (i.e. deaths related to the person-years of observation) is used as the endpoint, rather than survival. Survival could be used in a randomized controlled screening trial only under special circumstances. These are that there is good evidence because of the equivalence in cumulative numbers of cases during the relevant period of observation that there is no overdiagnosis bias, and provided that the start of the period of observation of the cases is taken as the date of randomization, as that will eliminate differential lead time. This is the approach that will be used in a study of breast self-examination in Russia, where it will not be possible to follow all entrants to determine their alive and dead status at the end of the trial (Semiglazov *et al.* 1993). Length bias and selection bias are not issues, the latter having been equally distributed by the randomization, and the former by having started at the same point in time and by including all cases that occur during follow-up in the evaluation.

Outside a randomized trial, if the screening test detects a precursor, reduction in incidence of the clinically detected disease can be expected and evaluated. This effect has been well demonstrated in the Nordic countries in relation to screening for cancer of the cervix (Hakama 1982). If the screening test does not detect a precursor, or even if it does but the main yield is invasive cancer, then incidence can be expected to increase initially following the introduction of screening, and remain elevated while screening continues. Under such circumstances, when reduction in incidence cannot be anticipated, and improvement in survival cannot be relied upon because of the biases already discussed, the only valid outcome for assessment of results of a screening programme is mortality from the disease in the total population offered screening in comparison with the mortality that would be expected in the same population if screening had not been offered.

As already emphasized, the design of choice for evaluation of changes in mortality is the randomized controlled trial. This can be either an efficacy trial or an effectiveness trial. Efficacy trials are based on randomization of the screening test, which answers the biologically relevant question as to whether mortality is reduced in those screened. An effectiveness trial is based on the randomization of invitations to attend for screening, and more nearly replicates the circumstances that may eventually pertain in practice in a population. Both those who accept the invitation and those who refuse will have to be included in the assessment of outcome. Thus it tests the impact of introducing screening in a population. Some trials of this type involve randomization by cluster.

If for some reason randomization is believed inappropriate, a second-best method is the quasi-experimental study in which screening is offered in some areas, and unscreened areas as comparable as possible are used for comparison purposes. However, this design is not a cheap and easy way out but demands the same methodological accuracy as required for randomized trials. Furthermore, in view of the substantially larger populations that may have to be studied than in randomized trials, it may prove to be more expensive than the preferred design. In addition, difficulties in analysis may ensue if the baseline mortality in the comparison areas differ (United Kingdom Trial of Early Detection of Breast Cancer Group 1988).

Nevertheless, ethical issues may preclude the utilization of randomized trials, particularly for programmes that were introduced before the necessity of utilizing trials as far as possible for evaluation was appreciated. This has been the case for screening for cancer of the cervix for example. One approach under these circumstances is to compare the mortality in defined populations before and after the introduction of screening programmes, preferably with data available on the trends in acceptance of screening so that changes in mortality can be correlated with the mortality trends. Such a correlation study will be strengthened if other data that could be related to changes in the outcome variable are entered into a multivariate analysis (Miller *et al.* 1976).

A case–control study of screening is another approach that can be used to evaluate programmes that were introduced sufficiently long before the study that an effect can be expected to have occurred. Case–control studies depend on comparing the screen histories of the cases with the histories of comparable controls drawn from the population from which the cases arose. If sampled, individuals with early-stage disease would be eligible as controls, provided that the date of diagnosis was not earlier than that of the case, as diagnosis of disease truncates the screening history. However, a bias would arise if advanced disease is compared only with early-stage disease, as the latter is likely to be screen detected, although this is just a function of the screening process, not its efficacy (Weiss 1983). Cases have to reflect the endpoints used to evaluate screening, that is, those that would be expected to be reduced by screening. Thus cases are often deaths from the disease or advanced disease as a surrogate for deaths, or if a precursor of the disease is detected through screening, incident cases in the population. If incident cases are screen detected, the controls should be drawn from those screened in the same programme; if the cases are not screen detected, the controls should be population based (Sasco *et al.* 1986).

One difficulty with case–control studies of screening is that they may be affected by selection bias as the health conscious may select themselves for screening. This may be difficult to correct in the analysis, although such a correction should be attempted if the relevant data on risk factors for the disease (confounders) are available. However, such a bias may not be a problem if it can be demonstrated that the incidence of cancer in those who declined the invitation to the screening programme is similar to that expected in an unscreened population.

Even if data are available on risk factors for disease, control for them may not result in avoiding the effect of selection bias. For example, experience in studies of breast cancer in Sweden and the United Kingdom, where case–control studies were performed within trials, show that although those who refuse invitations for screening show a breast cancer incidence similar to that of controls, their breast cancer mortality experience is worse than that of controls. This means that the estimate of the effect of screening in such case–control studies will show a greater effect than could be expected in the total population (Miller *et al.* 1990; Moss 1991).

In addition to assessing effectiveness of screening, case–control studies may also be of use to assess other aspects of screening programmes. For example, a method has been proposed for estimation of the natural history of preclinical disease from screening data based on case–control methodology (Brookmeyer *et al.* 1986).

The cohort study design may also provide an estimate of the effect of screening. In this design the mortality from the cancer of interest in an individually identified and followed screened group (the cohort) is compared with the mortality experience in a control population, often derived from the general population. This approach has been used to evaluate the mortality experience in the United States Breast Cancer Detection Demonstration Project (Morrison *et al.* 1988) and in a cohort of women in Finland included in a breast self-examination program (Gastrin *et al.* 1994). In these studies it has to be recognized that those recruited into a screening programme are initially free of the disease of interest so that it is not appropriate to apply population mortality rates for the disease to the person-years experience of the study cohort. Rather, as is required in estimating the sample size required for a controlled trial of screening, it is first necessary to determine the expected incidence of the cases of interest, then apply to that expectation the expected case–fatality rate from the disease to derive the expectation for the deaths (Moss *et al.* 1987). In practice, a cohort study of screening suffers from the same problem of selection bias as for case–control studies, so the results have to be interpreted with caution.

Indirect indicators of effectiveness are often desired in evaluating screening programmes, especially one that would predict subsequent mortality. Compliance with screening, and rate of screen detection, as well as the ratio of prevalence and incidence can be indicators of potentially effective screens (Day *et al.* 1989). The cumulative prevalence (not the percentage distribution) of advanced disease is one such measure (Prorok *et al.* 1984). For example, reduction in advanced disease predicted subsequent breast cancer mortality reduction in a trial of mammography screening versus no screening in Sweden (Tabar *et al.* 1989). However, case detection frequency, numbers of small tumours, and stage shift in percentages of the total should not be used as indicators of effectiveness as they potentially reflect all four screening biases.

Organized screening programmes

There are a number of features of effective screening programmes that are largely related to good organization. Indeed, there is good evidence, at least for cancer of the cervix, that unorganized or opportunistic screening programmes, which depend on the willingness of individuals to volunteer for screening, and the extent to which their physicians offer screening, often to low-risk women, are far less successful (Hakama *et al.* 1985).

Hakama *et al.* (1985) defined certain essential elements of organized programmes:

- the target population has been identified
- the individual women are identifiable
- measures are available to guarantee high coverage and attendance such as a personal letter of invitation
- there are adequate field facilities for performing the screening tests
- there is an organized quality control programme on performing and reading the tests
- adequate facilities exist for diagnosis and for appropriate treatment of confirmed abnormalities
- there is a carefully designed and agreed referral system, an agreed link between the participant, the screening centre, and the clinical facility for diagnosis of an abnormal screening test, for management of any abnormalities found, and for providing information about normal screening tests
- evaluation and monitoring of the total programme is organized in terms of incidence and mortality rates among those attending and among those not attending, at the level of the total target population
- quality control of the epidemiological data should be established.

Although these elements are present in many European cancer screening programmes, especially in the Nordic countries, and contribute greatly to their success, several elements are missing from programmes elsewhere, especially those largely based on the private medical care system in North America. In Canada, there are opportunities for introducing some of them, such as the first three, and these were recommended by the two Canadian Task Forces on cervical cancer screening (Task Force 1976, 1982). Unfortunately, only three of the provincial health care authorities (Ontario, Manitoba, and British Columbia—the latter having accepted from the beginning the need for centralized laboratory services) have taken the initiative in establishing such programmes. However, all provinces that introduced breast-screening programmes accepted from the outset the necessity for them to be organized (Workshop Group 1989), thus attempting to replicate the organization of breast cancer screening that is proving successful in some of the Nordic countries, The Netherlands, and the United Kingdom.

Health-related quality of life and screening

An important evaluation measure for screening is the extent to which overall quality of life is improved or impaired by screening compared with usual care. Decision-making for health care policy is only possible if information is available on quality of life as well as health costs of screened and unscreened participants including mortality reduction from screening. For example, it requires an 'optimistic' estimate of screening effectiveness to derive an overall benefit from screening for prostate cancer (Krahn *et al.* 1994). Issues concerning health-related quality of life may well vary with different cultural value systems, and different health care systems.

Because of lead time, health-related quality of life events will tend to occur earlier in life than similar events associated with usual care. Given that the adverse quality of life associated with false-positive screening tests, and those associated with treatment will tend to occur relatively early, it could be easy to convince oneself (as it has convinced some commentators for prostate cancer screening already) that the health-related quality of life issues are overwhelming and that screening should not be conducted. It will require prolonged follow-up, probably more than 10 years, for the detriments associated with advanced disease late in life that may be prevented from occurring in the screened group, to appear in the non-screened group.

If the outcome of screening were to be a major benefit in terms of mortality reduction, the issues related to health-related quality of life would be overwhelmed. It is only if the outcome is a moderate to small mortality reduction that these issues become critical, and paradoxically then it would be necessary for them to have been measured with as much precision as was possible during screening, as, particularly for health-related quality of life, the decrements could not be measured retrospectively with precision. For this reason, in screening trials where adverse health-related quality of life can be anticipated, it is important for such events to be identified and quantified.

Health-related quality of life measurement is a new and developing field. There are many instruments available for assessing health-related quality of life. In the screening setting a range of instruments are often required. Disease-specific measures assess the impact of particular diseases, for example, prostate-specific symptoms can be assessed with the UCLA Prostate Cancer Index (Litwin *et al.* 1998). However, since many screening tests can have a range of effects, generic instruments are also often included in screening studies. The most widely used such instrument is the 36-item Short Form Health Survey (**SF-36**) (Ware and Sherbourne 1992). Such psychometric instruments are not easily applied in economic analysis, and so utility- or preference-based instruments are often used. The Patient Oriented Prostate Cancer Utility Scale (**PORPUS**) (Krahn *et al.* 1996) and Health Utility Index (Torrance *et al.* 1996) are examples of disease-specific and generic utility measures. The psychological impact of screening tests is often not assessed with these health measures and specific scales, such as the State-Trait Anxiety Inventory, have been used for such effects (Spielberger *et al.* 1970; Goel *et al.* 1998).

Economics of screening

Space does not permit a detailed evaluation of the various principles that have to be considered in assessing the economics of screening. In brief, it is necessary to determine the costs of the test and the subsequent diagnostic tests. The costs associated with any hazard of the test, as well as the costs of overtreatment, should also be included. These costs may be balanced by reduced costs of therapy of the primary condition, reduced costs associated with less expenditure on the treatment of advanced disease, and the economic value of the additional years of life gained. This can become quite complex when the value of treatment of disease in years of life gained, transfers such as pensions, and economic productivity are considered. The latter is often disputed, if not regarded with some distaste, so that often what is computed is the cost per year of life saved. The marginal costs of additional tests in relation to the benefit may be critical, especially when considerations of the frequency of rescreening arise.

Part of the difficulty in economic assessment is that costs are often incurred early, while benefits flow later, so that for proper comparisons of such costs they have to be discounted to the present day. Additional complexity ensues if attempts are made to assess quality of life in economic terms, while the calculations rarely attempt an economic assessment of the fact that if a death is prevented by screening, the relevant individual will inevitably die of some other condition, and that death could be more costly.

It is likely that economic assessments will increasingly guide policy decisions in the future, so that those interested in evaluation of screening must collect the necessary data. Although some economic assessments have suggested that cost-effective programmes are achievable (e.g. programmes of breast cancer screening using single-view mammography in Sweden (Jonsson *et al.* 1988)), others have suggested that programmes may not be cost-effective (e.g. breast cancer screening programmes for younger women in the United States (Eddy *et al.* 1988)). Economic analysis is particularly important for making decisions within screening programmes, for example around screening intervals or method of follow-up.

Screening programmes

Cancer

In this section, we shall summarize our conclusions on the appropriateness of screening for several cancer sites.

Screening for lung cancer

Both the UICC project (Prorok *et al.* 1984) and the American Cancer Society (1980) concluded that screening with sputum cytology and/or chest radiographs could not be recommended. The conclusive nature of the negative evidence from the three American controlled trials was such that the National Cancer Institute working guidelines (Early Detection Branch 1987) did not discuss screening for this site. However, there has been concern that screening using annual chest radiography has never been properly evaluated, and therefore this is being re-examined in a large study evaluating screening for a number of cancer sites (Gohagan *et al.* 1995). Furthermore, there is some indication that spiral CT scanning may diagnose lung cancers at a much earlier stage than conventional chest radiography (Henschke *et al.* 1999). Therefore it is possible that screening by this modality will be re-evaluated. The increasing proportion of lung cancers being diagnosed in ex-smokers in North America is adding a clinical imperative to the need for reconsideration of screening in those at high risk for lung cancer.

Screening for breast cancer

It has been recognized for some time that mass screening for breast cancer can reduce mortality from the disease (Day *et al.* 1986; Miller *et al.* 1990). Both single-view mammography alone and double-view mammography combined with physical examination are effective as screening modalities. Current data are insufficient to determine whether appreciable extra benefit in terms of mortality reduction derives from adding physical examination to mammography, or from double-view as distinct from single-view mammography. However, it now seems that mammography adds little extra benefit to screening by physical examination, a question raised by the working group to review the uncontrolled United States Breast Cancer Detection Demonstration Projects (Beahrs *et al.* 1979) and investigated in the Canadian National Breast Screening Study in women aged 50 to 59 on entry to the study (Miller *et al.* 1981, 1992).

The American Cancer Society guidelines for breast cancer detection are that every woman should be urged to practice breast self-examination every month from the age of 20, that women should have a breast physical examination every 3 years from the age of 20 and every year from the age of 40, and that mammography should be given every 1 to 2 years from 40 to 49 and every year from the age of 50 (Mettlin and Smart 1994) However, the United States Preventive Services Task Force (1996*c*) did not recommend mammography screening for women aged 40 to 49, and the National Cancer Institute, after accepting that the scientific evidence does not confirm efficacy of screening in women aged 40 to 49 (Kaluzny *et al.* 1994), reversed that position later despite the recommendations by a consensus conference (National Institutes of Health Consensus Development Panel 1997).

Organized breast screening programmes, all involving mammography and women aged 50 to 64 (or 69), have been set up in Canada and several European countries (e.g. Finland, The Netherlands, Sweden, the United Kingdom), but only some counties in Sweden actively invite women aged 40 to 49 for screening. The majority invite women to return every 2 years (every 3 years in the United Kingdom). It is still too early to judge the effectiveness of these programmes, but it is likely that mortality reductions attributable to screening will be seen within a few years in those programmes that have achieved the planned level of compliance (70 per cent or more), although these could be less than has been anticipated (Miller 2000).

The other screening test for which we currently have little evidence of effectiveness is breast self-examination. Only breast self-examination has the potential to improve the outlook for interval cancers, while its teaching probably goes some way to diminish false reassurance, and it has the potential to provide early diagnosis of breast cancer in many parts of the world (Miller *et al.* 1985). Two case–control studies have shown no overall benefit in the reduction of advanced disease (Muscat and Huncharek 1991; Newcomb *et al.* 1991), but one suggested benefit in breast self-examination compliers (Newcomb *et al.* 1991). A cohort study of breast self-examination compliers in Finland suggested a benefit in reducing breast cancer mortality (Gastrin *et al.* 1994), while a case–control study nested within the Canadian National Breast Screening Study also showed benefit from good breast self-examination practice in reducing breast cancer mortality and the cumulative prevalence of advanced (metastatic) breast cancer (Harvey *et al.* 1997).

Screening for cancer of the cervix

It is generally agreed that screening for cancer of the cervix is effective in reducing the incidence and mortality from the disease, but that for maximal effectiveness attention needed to be paid to the organizational aspects of screening (Hakama *et al.* 1985; Miller *et al.* 1990). The organized programmes that have shown the greatest effect, while using fewer resources than the unorganized programmes.

An IARC study, based on the records of a number of screening programmes in Europe and Canada (IARC Working Group on Cervical Cancer Screening 1986) indicated that starting at age 25 and stopping at age 64 with 3-year intervals gives 90 per cent of the maximal protection and only requires 13 tests a lifetime. Even screening starting at age 20 with annual screens gives only just over 90 per cent protection yet requires 45 tests per woman. The difficulty with annual screening, even in a wealthy country, is that it places emphasis on rescreening women already in programmes, while the emphasis needs to shift to bring women who are poorly screened, or not screened at all, into programmes if failures of screening policies are to be avoided (Task Force 1976; Chamberlain *et al.* 1986; Miller *et al.* 1991).

Another aspect of cervical cancer screening requires more attention. There are substantial costs associated with the management of the large numbers of cases of mild and moderate dysplasia found as a result of cervical cytology, the majority of which will regress spontaneously (Holowaty *et al.* 1999). A marker that may enable the identification of the lesions that would progress if left untreated is needed; tests for oncogenic types of human papilloma virus may provide this, but only in women over the age of 35 (Miller *et al.* 2000*b*). However, time is on the physician's side, and cytological surveillance is appropriate for mild if not moderate dysplasia (cervical intraepithelial neoplasia grade I or II) until it is clearer whether the lesion will regress spontaneously (Miller *et al.* 1991; Holowaty *et al.* 1999).

In developing countries there are often insufficient resources to support a cytology-based screening programme for cancer of the cervix. Therefore attention has shifted to attempts to detect early disease by visual inspection of the cervix with the naked eye using a speculum. Unaided visual inspection is too insensitive, and nonspecific, but visual inspection after acetic acid application to the cervix seems to have equivalent sensitivity to cervical cytology (Chirenje *et al.* 1999; Miller *et al.* 2000*b*). Although specificity is lower than for cytology, attempts are now being made to improve upon this.

Screening for gastric cancer

Screening programmes for gastric cancer were introduced in Japan over 20 years ago (Chamberlain *et al.* 1986). The screening test used has gradually been standardized and now comprises a photofluorographic barium meal technique with six standard views. Considerable observational evidence, including time trend analyses and case–control studies, has accumulated in Japan that the widespread application of screening has contributed to a fall in mortality, although its contribution is probably small in relation to that resulting from falling incidence (Chamberlain *et al.* 1986; Miller *et al.* 1990). In view of the uncertainty over its effectiveness, screening for gastric cancer in countries other than Japan cannot at present be recommended as public health policy.

Screening for colorectal cancer

In contradistinction to gastric cancer screening, a number of controlled trials of colorectal cancer screening have been conducted. The earliest evaluated rigid sigmoidoscopy as part of a multiphasic health screen. Although a reduction in mortality from colorectal cancer was seen in the study group, this is probably due to chance and not due to the effect of sigmoidoscopy (Selby *et al.* 1988).

Further evidence to support sigmoidoscopy as possibly appropriate for colorectal cancer screening has come from two case–control studies (Newcomb *et al.* 1992; Selby *et al.* 1992). The report of Selby *et al.* (1992) indicates an apparent benefit from sigmoidoscopy lasting for up to 10 years. However, as such studies cannot eliminate the effect of selection bias, benefit may have been overestimated. This is why there is a trial in the United States evaluating the effect of flexible sigmoidoscopy, initially conducted at 3-year intervals (Gohagan *et al.* 1995) and now every 5 years, and one in the United Kingdom evaluating one-time-only sigmoidoscopy (Aitkin *et al.* 1993).

All the other trials have evaluated the effect of the faecal occult blood test. Of these, two in the United States and two in Europe have reported mortality results. One of these, in New York, evaluated the effect of the addition of the faecal occult blood test to routine sigmoidoscopic screening (Flehinger *et al.* 1988; Winawer *et al.* 1993).

The other trial, in Minnesota, used the faecal occult blood test alone, annually in one group and biennially in another. The initial mortality result indicated that annual but not biennial faecal occult blood tests reduce mortality from colorectal cancer after about a 10-year period (Mandel *et al.* 1993). This was achieved at a substantial cost in terms of false-positive results. A more recent report, with follow-up to 18 years, confirmed the colorectal cancer mortality reduction from annual screening, but also showed mortality reduction at a lower level from biennial screening (Mandel *et al.* 1999). The trials in Europe also showed mortality reduction from biennial screening (Hardcastle *et al.* 1996; Kronborg *et al.* 1996).

It is clear, especially from the Minnesota trial, that a major difficulty with screening using the faecal occult blood test is lack of specificity, especially if the test is rehydrated. Furthermore, there seems to be a lack in sensitivity for adenomas.

Taken together, the faecal occult blood test trials suggest that, after an interval of about 10 years, there could be a reduction of up to 20 per cent in colorectal cancer mortality from biennial screening, and higher for annual screening. However, with the likelihood that the relatively high compliance achieved in the Minnesota trial could not be replicated in the population, the benefit that could be obtained would probably be much less.

Screening for prostate cancer

Screening for prostate cancer using the digital rectal examination is recommended by the American Cancer Society. However, it is not clear that this is a sensitive screening test for early disease. Other screening tests under consideration include the prostate-specific antigen and transrectal ultrasound, although the latter may be of more value as a diagnostic test (Miller *et al.* 1990). In the United States, the American Cancer Society recommends screening with prostate-specific antigen yearly from the age of 50 (Mettlin *et al.* 1993).

There are many obstacles in the way of an effective screening programme for a disease that is a relatively unimportant cause of premature mortality. Not only has an acceptable and valid screening test to be available, but an acceptable and effective treatment for the preclinical lesions found as a result of screening (Miller *et al.* 1990). This problem is particularly acute for prostate cancer because of the increasing frequency of latent prostate carcinoma with increasing age and the not inappreciable morbidity and mortality of the radical procedures usually used to treat prostate cancer. There is no question that it is necessary to establish the effectiveness of screening programmes for prostate cancer by well-designed randomized trials, before a recommendation on public health policy could be developed (IPSTEG 1999).

Other sites

Screening for bladder and mouth cancer (Prorok *et al.* 1984), endometrial and ovarian cancer (Hakama *et al.* 1985; Miller *et al.*

1990), oesophagus and liver cancer (Chamberlain *et al.* 1986), and melanoma, neuroblastoma, and nasopharyngeal carcinoma (Miller *et al.* 1990) cannot be recommended as public health policy. In the majority of instances this is because of the absence of a valid screening test, but the issue for oral cancer and melanoma is the lack of documented effectiveness of screening, especially, in the case of oral cancer, from developing countries where the disease is sufficiently common to propose programmes based on inspection of the mouth by allied health professionals. The Quebec Neuroblastoma Screening Project indicated no benefit from screening for this disease (Bernstein *et al.* 1996). Indeed, good evidence was derived that the results of earlier studies from Japan suggesting good survival from screen-detected cases were in fact due to overdiagnosis of neuroblastoma in 6-month-old children.

Cardiovascular disease

Unlike cancer, cardiovascular disease can be controlled by both primary and secondary means. Considerable controversy has existed as to whether or not a population-based approach using health education and promotion strategies or a high-risk approach, based on early detection and treatment, will result in the greatest reduction in cardiovascular diseases (Rose 1992). Two main approaches have been proposed for reducing the burden of cardiovascular disease—screening for hypertension and screening for hypercholesterolaemia.

Hypertension screening involves a simple test that can easily be incorporated as part of a routine clinical examination. There is clear evidence that detection of hypertension and its management can effectively reduce the subsequent risk of coronary heart disease, congestive heart failure, stroke, and renal failure (MacMahon *et al.* 1986; Collins *et al.* 1990). The test is acceptable to the population although compliance with treatments can be difficult, particularly when side-effects are encountered. However, there are problems with the test, particularly with respect to its reliability and intraobserver variability. There is also controversy over the exact level of blood pressure at which hypertension worthy of treatment should be diagnosed, and what treatments should be used. In particular, there is concern as to what the appropriate level for initiation of pharmacological interventions (United States Preventive Services Task Force 1996*b*). There is also controversy with respect to the age at which to initiate hypertension screening and the appropriate interval. Most guidelines recommend screening to commence in early adulthood (about the age of 30) with an interval of 3 to 5 years. However, blood pressure checks have become a routine part of every clinical examination, and are usually done far more frequently.

Cholesterol screening is similar in that there are also controversies regarding the appropriate level at which to consider a test to be positive and as to the need to initiate treatment with pharmacological agents for mild to moderate elevations (United States Preventive Services Task Force 1996*a*). Assessment of cardiovascular risk must be multifactorial, including behavioural factors such as exercise and smoking, clinical measures such as hypertension and family history. Preventive strategies need to be customized for the individual based on the risk profile, and not simply on a single test such as cholesterol. In the United States an aggressive approach to screening for cholesterol was taken ('know your number'), but other countries, such as the United Kingdom and Canada, have adopted more selective approaches.

Prenatal screening

Evaluation of screening prenatally requires applications of the general screening principles but does lead to some special considerations. As noted above, the disease condition is usually detected in the fetus, either directly, through a test such as ultrasound, or indirectly through a maternal marker such as maternal serum α-fetoprotein (Wald *et al.* 1997). Thus one difference from other screening tests is that the individual being tested is not necessarily the one affected with the disease. Secondly, treatment options are not usually available, although this is changing with the advent of fetal surgery. Thus ethical issues arise with the use of therapeutic abortion for the management of abnormalities detected.

Infectious disease

Screening for infectious disease is an important public health strategy. Unlike most of the screening tests for chronic disease, screening for infectious disease often affords the opportunity for benefit to the population as a whole, rather than just an individual through reduction in risk of disease transmission. Thus there may be situations when screening for infectious disease is warranted, even when not all the criteria for screening are met. For example, even if there is no treatment for a disease, screening may be warranted if effective infection control mechanisms are available. Such screening is being done in many tertiary care facilities for 'superbugs' such as methicillin-resistant *Streptococcus* type A (Cookson 1997).

However, screening for infectious disease often leads to considerable controversy, particularly when quarantine is the suggested control mechanism. Calls for population-wide screening for HIV have often included such proposals. The criteria for screening presented in this chapter can be very useful in assessing such proposals, in this instance quarantine becomes the treatment for the condition that is identified through screening.

Genetic susceptibility testing

The completion of mapping of the human genome holds great promise for disease control (Wadman 1999). At the same time, the availability of a range of markers for disease susceptibility will lead to increasing controversies about the use of screening tests (Goel 2001). While the general principles of screening outlined above will still apply, they will need to be modified and updated. Screening will identify individuals at risk of disease, rather than those with precursors or early-stage disease. Thus, rather than diagnostic assessment and treatment strategies, preventive strategies will be required. Ideally, primary prevention strategies will be available, but for many conditions the preventive strategies will be the application of other screening tests, further complicating the evaluation of these strategies.

Conclusion

There are a number of fundamental issues that have to be resolved when considering disease control by screening. The general principles that govern the introduction of screening programmes include the following:

- the disease should be an important health problem
- the disease should have a detectable preclinical phase
- the natural history of the lesions identified by screening should be known
- there should be an effective treatment for such lesions
- the screening test should be acceptable and safe.

The other issues range from ethics to economics. Critical issues include the population to be included in screening programmes and whether or not it is possible to introduce an organized screening programme. It cannot necessarily be assumed that a screening programme will benefit the population to which it is applied. Not only do ethics demand that only programmes with proven effectiveness be widely disseminated, it is also necessary to ensure that the programme is continually monitored to confirm that effectiveness is maintained. Furthermore, the benefits derived from the programme must be clearly shown to exceed the costs, both in terms of ill health induced by the test and accompanying procedures, and in economic terms.

Despite these caveats, screening carries the potential for a fairly rapid and important impact on mortality from disease, often exceeding what can currently be anticipated from other approaches to disease control. Hence there is continuing interest in, and expectation from, existing and potential programmes.

References

American Cancer Society (1980). Guidelines for the cancer-related check-up. Recommendations and rationale. *CA: A Cancer Journal for Clinicians*, **30**, 193–240.

Anderson, G.H. (1985). Cervical cytology. In *Screening for cancer* (ed. A.B. Miller), pp. 87–103. Academic Press, Orlando, FL.

Atkin, W.S., Cusick, J., Northover, J.M.A., and Whymes, D.K. (1993). Prevention of colorectal cancer by once-only sigmoidoscopy. *Lancet*, **341**, 736–40.

Baines, C.J., McFarlane, D.V., Miller, A.B., *et al.* (1988). Sensitivity and specificity for first screen mammography in 15 NBSS centres. *Journal of the Canadian Association of Radiologists*, **39**, 273–6.

Baines, C.J., Miller, A.B., Bassett, A.A., *et al.* (1989). Physical Examination; evaluation of its role as a single screening modality in the Canadian National Breast Screening Study. *Cancer*, **63**, 160–6.

Bassett, A.A. (1985). Physical examination of the breast and breast self-examination. In *Screening for cancer* (ed. A.B. Miller), pp. 271–91. Academic Press, Orlando, FL.

Beahrs, O.H., Shapiro, S., Smart, C., *et al.* (1979). Report of the working group to review the National Cancer Institute, American Cancer Society Breast Cancer Detection Demonstration Projects. *Journal of the National Cancer Institute*, **62**, 640–709.

Bernstein, M.L. and Woods, W.G. (1996). Screening for neuroblastoma. In *Advances in screening for cancer* (ed. A.B. Miller), pp. 149–63. Kluwer Academic, Boston, MA.

Boyd, N.F., Wolfson, C., Moskowitz, M., *et al.* (1982). Observer variation in the interpretation of Xeromammograms. *Journal of the National Cancer Institute*, **68**, 357–63.

Boyes, D.A., Morrison, B., Knox, E.G., *et al.* (1982). A cohort study of cervical cancer in British Columbia. *Clinical and Investigative Medicine*, **5**, 1–29.

Brookmeyer, R., Day, N.E., and Moss, S. (1986). Case–control studies for estimation of the natural history of preclinical disease from screening data. *Statistics and Medicine*, **5**, 127–138.

Chamberlain, J. (1986). Reasons that some screening programmes fail to control cervical cancer. In *Screening for cancer of the uterine cervix* (ed. M. Hakama, A.B. Miller, N.E. Day), pp. 161–8. IARC Scientific Publication 76. International Agency for Research on Cancer, Lyon.

Chamberlain, J. and Miller, A.B. (ed.) (1988). *Screening for gastrointestinal cancer.* Hans Huber, Toronto.

Chamberlain, J., Day, N.E., Hakama, M., *et al.* (1986). UICC workshop of the project on evaluation of screening programmes for gastrointestinal cancer. *International Journal of Cancer*, **37**, 329–34.

Chirenje, Z.M. *et al.* for the University of Zimbabwe/JHPIEGO Cervical Cancer Project (1999). Visual inspection with acetic acid for cervical-cancer screening, test qualities in a primary-care setting. *Lancet*, **353**, 869–73.

Chodak, G.W. and Schoenberg, H.W. (1989). Progress and problems in screening for carcinoma of the prostate. *World Journal of Surgery*, **13**, 60–4.

Collins, R., Peto, R., MacMahon, S., *et al.* (1990). Blood pressure, stroke, and coronary heart disease. Part 2, short-term reductions in blood pressure, overview of randomised drug trials in their epidemiological context. *Lancet*, **335**, 827–38.

Commission on Chronic Illness (1957). *Chronic illness in the United States: prevention of chronic illness.* Harvard University Press, Cambridge, MA.

Cookson, B. (1997). Is it time to stop searching for MRSA? Screening is still important. *British Medical Journal*, **314**, 664–5.

Cuckle, H.S. and Wald, N.J. (1984). Principles of screening. In *Antenatal and neonatal screening* (ed. N.J.Wald) Oxford University Press.

Day, N.E. (1985). Estimating the sensitivity of a screening test. *Journal of Epidemiology and Community Health*, **39**, 364–6.

Day, N.E., Baines, C.J., Chamberlain, J., *et al.* (1986). UICC project on screening for cancer, Report of the workshop on screening for breast cancer. *International Journal of Cancer*, **38**, 303–8.

Day, N.E., Williams, D.R.R., and Khaw, K.T. (1989). Breast cancer screening programmes: the development of a monitoring and evaluation system. *British Journal of Cancer*, **59**, 954–8.

Early Detection Branch (1987). *Working guidelines for early cancer detection.* Division of Cancer Prevention and Control, National Cancer Institute, Bethesda, MD.

Eddy, D.M., Hasselblad, V., McGivney, W., *et al.* (1988). The value of mammography screening in women under age 50 years. *Journal of the American Medical Association*, **259**, 1512–19.

European Society for Mastology (1993). Report of the European Society for Mastology Breast Cancer Screening Evaluation Committee. Presented at Consensus Conference on Breast Cancer Screening.

Flehinger, B.J., Herbert, E., Winawer, S.J., *et al.* (1988). Screening for colorectal cancer with fecal occult blood test and sigmoidoscopy, preliminary report of the colon project of Memorial Sloan-Kettering cancer center and PMI-Strang clinic. In *Screening for gastrointestinal cancer* (ed. J. Chamberlain and A.B. Miller), pp. 9–16. Hans Huber, Toronto.

Gastrin, G., Miller, A.B., To, T., *et al.* (1994). Incidence and mortality from breast cancer in the Mama program for breast screening in Finland, 1973–1986. *Cancer*, **73**, 2168–74.

Glanz, K. and Gilboy, M.B. (1995). Psychological impact of cholesterol screening and management. In *Psychosocial effects of screening for disease prevention and detection* (ed. R.T. Croyle), pp. 39–64. Oxford University Press, New York.

Goel, V., for Crossroads 99 Group (2001). Appraising organised screening programmes for testing for genetic susceptibility to cancer. *British Medical Journal*, **322**, 1174–8.

Goel, V., Glazier, R., Summers, A., and Holsapfels, S. (1998). Psychological outcomes following maternal serum screening, a cohort study. *Canadian Medical Association Journal*, **159**, 651–6.

Gohagan, J.K., Prorok, P.C., Kramer, B.S., *et al.* (1995). The Prostate, Lung, Colorectal, and Ovarian cancer screening trial of the National Cancer Institute. *Cancer*, **75**, 1869–73.

Goin, J.E. and Haberman, J.D. (1982). Comments on the logistic function in ROC analysis, Applications to breast cancer detection. *Methods of Information Medicine*, **21**, 26–30.

Hakama, M. (1982). Trends in the incidence of cervical cancer in the Nordic countries. In *Trends in cancer incidence* (ed. K. Magnus), pp. 279–92. Hemisphere, Washington, DC.

Hakama, M. (1984). Selective screening by risk groups. In *Screening for cancer* (ed. P.C. Prorok and A.B. Miller), pp. 71–9. UICC Technical Report Series, Vol. 78. International Union Against Cancer, Geneva.

Hakama, M. (1986). Cervical cancer, risk groups for screening. In *Screening for cancer of the uterine cervix* (ed. M. Hakama, A.B. Miller, and N.E. Day), pp. 213–16. IARC Scientific Publication 76. International Agency for Research on Cancer, Lyon.

Hakama, M., Chamberlain, J., Day, N.E., *et al.* (1985). Evaluation of screening programmes for gynaecological cancer. *British Journal of Cancer*, **52**, 669–73.

Hardcastle, J.D., Chamberlain, J.O., Robinson, M.H., *et al.* (1996). Randomised controlled trial of faecal-occult-blood screening for colorectal cancer. *Lancet*, **348**, 1472–7.

Harvey, B.J., Miller, A.B., Baines, C.J., and Corey, P.N. (1997). Effect of breast self-examination techniques on the risk of death from breast cancer. *Canadian Medical Association Journal*, **157**, 1205–12.

Henschke, C.I., McCaulay, D.I., Yankelevitz, D.F., *et al.* (1999). Early lung cancer action project, overall design and findings from baseline screening. *Lancet*, **354**, 99–105.

Holowaty, P., Miller, A.B., Rohan, T., and To, T. (1999). The natural history of dysplasia of the uterine cervix. *Journal of the National Cancer Institute*, **91**, 252–8.

Howard, J. (1987). Using mammography for cancer control, an unrealized potential. *CA: A Cancer Journal for Clinicians*, **37**, 33–48.

IARC Working Group on Cervical Cancer Screening (1986). Summary chapter. In *Screening for cancer of the uterine cervix* (ed. M. Hakama, A.B. Miller, and N.E. Day) pp. 133–42. IARC Scientific Publication 76. International Agency for Research on Cancer, Lyon.

IPSTEG (International Prostate Screening Trial Evaluation Group) (1999). Rationale for randomised trials of prostate cancer screening. *European Journal of Cancer*, **35**, 262–71.

Jonsson, E., Hakansson, S., and Tabar, L. (1988). Cost of mammography screening for breast cancer. Experiences from Sweden. In *Screening for breast cancer* (ed. N.E. Day and A.B. Miller), pp. 113–15. Hans Huber, Toronto.

Kaluzny, A.D., Rimer, B., and Harris, R. (1994). The National Cancer Institute and guideline development: lessons from the breast cancer screening controversy. *Journal of the National Cancer Institute*, **86**, 901–3.

Krahn, M.D., Mahoney, J.E., Eckman, M.H., *et al.* (1994). Screening for prostate cancer: a decision analytic view. *Journal of the American Medical Association*, **272**, 781–6.

Krahn, M.D., Naglie, G., Ritvo, P., Irvine, J., and Trachtenberg, J. (1996). Patient and expert quality of life ratings in the construction of an empirically derived domain-linked utility instrument for prostate cancer. *Medical Decision Making*, **16**, 470.

Kristiansen, I.S., Eggen, A.E., and Thelle, D.S. (1991). Cost effectiveness of incremental programmes for lowering serum cholesterol concentration, is individual intervention worth while? *British Medical Journal*, **302**, 1119–22.

Kronborg, O., Fenger, C., Olsen, J., *et al.* (1996). Randomized study of screening for colorectal cancer with faecal-occult-blood test. *Lancet*, **348**, 1467–71.

Litwin, M.S., Hays, R.D., Fink, A., Ganz, P.A., Leake, B., and Brook, R.H. (1998). The UCLA Prostate Cancer Index: development, reliability, and validity of a health-related quality of life measure. *Medical Care*, **36**, 1002–12.

MacMahon, S.W., Cutler, J.A., Furberg, C.D., *et al.* (1986). The effects of drug treatment for hypertension on morbidity and mortality from cardiovascular disease, a review of randomized, controlled trials. *Progress in Cardiovascular Disease*, **29S**, 99–118.

McLelland, R. and Pisano, E.D. (1992). The politics of mammography. *Radiology Clinics of North America*, **30**, 235–41.

Mandel, J.S., Bond, J.H., Church, T.R., *et al.* (1993). Reducing mortality from colorectal cancer by screening for fecal occult blood. *New England Journal of Medicine*, **328**, 1365–71.

Mandel, J.S., Church, T.R., Ederer, F., and Bond, J.H. (1999). Colorectal cancer mortality, Effectiveness of biennial screening for fecal occult blood. *Journal of the National Cancer Institute*, **91**, 434–7.

Mettlin, C. and Smart, C.R. (1994). Breast cancer detection guidelines for women aged 40–49 years: rationale for the American Cancer Society reaffirmation of recommendations. *CA: A Cancer Journal for Clinicians*, **44**, 248–55.

Mettlin, C., Jones, G., Averette, H., *et al.* (1993). Defining and updating the American Cancer Society guidelines for the cancer-related checkup, prostate and endometrial cancers. *CA: A Cancer Journal for Clinicians*, **43**, 42–6.

Miller, A.B. (ed.) (1978). *Screening in cancer.* A report of the UICC International Workshop in Toronto. UICC Technical Report Series, Vol. 40. International Union Against Cancer, Geneva.

Miller, A.B. (1981). An evaluation of population screening for cervical cancer. In *Advances in clinical cytology* (ed. L.G. Koss and D.V. Coleman), pp. 64–94. Butterworths, London.

Miller, A.B. (1987). Early detection of breast cancer. In *Breast diseases* (ed. J.R. Harris, I.C. Henderson, S. Hellman, *et al.*), pp. 122–34. J.B. Lippincott, Philadelphia, PA.

Miller, A.B. (1991). Issues in screening for prostate cancer. In *Cancer screening* (ed. A.B. Miller *et al.*), pp. 289–93. Cambridge University Press,

Miller, A.B. (1994). Screening for cancer, Is it time for a paradigm shift? *Annals of the Royal College of Physicians and Surgeons of Canada*, **27**, 353–5.

Miller, A.B. (1996). Fundamental issues in screening for cancer. In *Cancer epidemiology and prevention* (2nd edn) (ed. D. Schottenfeld and J.F. Fraumeni Jr), pp. 1433–52. Oxford University Press.

Miller, A.B. (2000). Effect of screening programme on mortality from breast cancer. Benefit of 30 per cent may be substantial overestimate. *British Medical Journal*, **321**, 1527.

Miller, A.B. and Tsechkovski, M. (1987). Imaging technologies in breast cancer control, Summary report of a World Health Organization meeting. *American Journal of Roentgenology*, **148**, 1093–4.

Miller, A.B., Howe, G.R., and Wall, C. (1981). The national study of breast cancer screening. *Clinical and Investigative Medicine*, **4**, 227–58.

Miller, A.B., Chamberlain, J., and Tsechovski, M. (1985). Self-examination in the early detection of breast cancer. A review of the evidence, with recommendations for further research. *Journal of Chronic Disease*, **38**, 527–40.

Miller, A.B., Chamberlain, J., Day, N.E., Hakama, M., and Prorok, P.C. (1990). Report on a workshop of the UICC project on evaluation of screening for cancer. *International Journal of Cancer*, **46**, 761–9.

Miller, A.B., Anderson, G., Brisson, J., *et al.* (1991*a*). Report of a National Workshop on Screening for Cancer of the Cervix. *Canadian Medical Association Journal*, **145**, 1301–25.

Miller, A.B., Baines, C.J., and Turnbull, C. (1991*b*) The role of the nurse-examiner in the National Breast Screening Study. *Canadian Journal of Public Health*, **82**, 162–7.

Miller, A.B., Baines, C.J., To, T., *et al.* (1992). Canadian national breast screening study. 2: Breast cancer detection and death rates among women age 50–59 years. *Canadian Medical Association Journal*, **147**, 1477–88.

Miller, A.B., Lindsay, J., and Hill, G.B. (1976). Mortality from cancer of the uterus in Canada and its relationship to screening for cancer of the cervix. *International Journal of Cancer*, **17**, 602–12.

Miller, A.B., To, T., Baines, C.J., and Wall, C. (2000*a*). Canadian National Breast Screening Study-2: 13-year results of a randomized trial in women aged 50–59 years. *Journal of the National Cancer Institute*, **92**, 1490–9.

Miller, A.B., Nazeer, S., Fonn, S., *et al.* (2000*b*). Report on consensus conference on cervical cancer screening and management. *International Journal of Cancer*, **86**, 440–7.

Morrison, A.S. (1985). *Screening in chronic disease*, pp. 48–63. Oxford University Press.

Morrison, A.S., Brisson, J., and Khalid, N. (1988). Breast cancer incidence and mortality in the breast cancer detection demonstration project. *Journal of the National Cancer Institute*, **80**, 1540–7.

Moskowitz, M., Pemmaraju, S., Fidler, J.A., *et al.* (1976). On the diagnosis of minimal breast cancer in a screenee population. *Cancer*, **37**, 2543–52.

Moss, S.M. (1991). Case–control studies of screening. *International Journal of Epidemiology*, **20**, 1–6.

Moss, S., Draper, G.J., Hardcastle, J.D., and Chamberlain, J. (1987). Calculation of sample size in trials of screening for early diagnosis of disease. *International Journal of Epidemiology*, **16**, 104–10.

Muscat, J.E. and Huncharek, M.S. (1991). Breast self-examination and extent of disease: a population-based study. *Cancer Detection and Prevention*, **15**, 155–9.

National Institutes of Health Consensus Development Panel (1997). Consensus statement. *Monographs of the National Cancer Institute*, **22**, vii–xviii.

Newcomb, P.A., Weiss, N.S., Storer, B.E., *et al.* (1991). Breast self-examination in relation to occurrence of advanced breast cancer. *Journal of the National Cancer Institute*, **83**, 260–5.

Newcomb, P.A., Norfleet, R.G., Storer, B.E., *et al.* (1992). Screening sigmoidoscopy and colorectal cancer mortality. *Journal of the National Cancer Institute*, **84**, 1572–5.

Prorok, P.C., Chamberlain, J., Day, N.E., *et al.* (1984). UICC workshop on the evaluation of screening programmes for cancer. *International Journal of Cancer*, **34**, 1–4.

Rose, G. (1992). *The strategy of preventive medicine.* Oxford University Press.

Sasco, A.J., Day, N.E., and Walter, S.D. (1986). Case–control studies for the evaluation of screening. *Journal of Chronic Disease*, **39**, 399–405.

Schechter, M.T., Miller, A.B., Baines, C.J., *et al.* (1986). Selection of women at high risk of breast cancer for initial screening. *Journal of Chronic Disease*, **39**, 253–60.

Selby, J.V., Friedman, G.D., and Collen, M.F. (1988). Sigmiodoscopy and mortality from colorectal cancer: the Kaiser Permanente multiphasic evaluation study. *Journal of Clinical Epidemiology*, **41**, 427–34.

Selby, J., Friedman, G.C.D., Quesenberry, C.P., Jr *et al.* (1992). A case–control study of screening sigmoidoscopy and mortality from colorectal cancer. *New England Journal of Medicine*, **326**, 653–7.

Selzer, M.L., Gomberg, E.S., and Nordhoff, J.A. (1979). Men and women's responses to the Michigan Alcoholism Screening Test. *Journal of Studies in Alcohol*, **40**, 502–4.

Semiglazov, V.F., Sagaidak, V.N., Moiseyenko, V.M., and Mikhailov, E.A. (1993). Study of the role of breast self-examination in the reduction of mortality from breast cancer. *European Journal of Cancer*, **29A**, 2039–46.

Spielberger, C.D., Gorsuch, R.L., and Kushene, R.E. (1970). *Manual for the State-Trait Anxiety Inventory*. Consulting Psychologists Press, Palo Alto, CA.

Swets, J.A. (1979). ROC analysis applied to the evaluation of medical imaging technologies. *Investigative Radiology*, **14**, 109–21.

Tabar, L., Fagerberg, C.J.G., Gad, A., *et al.* (1985). Reduction in mortality from breast cancer after mass screening with mammography: randomized trial from the breast cancer screening working group of the Swedish National Board of Health and Welfare. *Lancet*, **i**, 829–32.

Tabar, L., Fagerberg, G., Duffy, S.W., and Day, N.E. (1989). The Swedish two county trial of mammographic screening for breast cancer: recent results and calculation of benefit. *Journal of Epidemiology of Community Health*, **43**, 107–14.

Task Force (1976). Cervical cancer screening programs. The Walton Report. *Canadian Medical Association Journal*, **114**, 1003–33.

Task Force (1982). Cervical cancer screening programs. Summary of the 1982 Canadian task force report. *Canadian Medical Association Journal*, **127**, 581–9.

Toronto Working Group on Cholesterol Policy (1990). Asymptomatic hypercholesterolemia: a clinical policy review. *Journal of Clinical Epidemiology*, **43**, 1028–121.

Torrance, G.W., Feeny, D.H., Furlong, W.J., Barr, R.D., Zhang, Y., and Wang, Q. (1996). Multiattribute utility function for a comprehensive health status classification system. Health Utilities Index Mark 2. *Medical Care*, **34**, 702–22.

United Kingdom Trial of Early Detection of Breast Cancer Group (1988). First results on mortality reduction in the United Kingdom Trial of Early Detection of Breast Cancer. *Lancet*, **ii**, 411–16.

United States Preventive Services Task Force (1996*a*). Screening for high blood cholesterol and other lipid abnormalities. In *Guide to clinical preventive services 2*, pp. 15–38. Williams & Wilkins, Baltimore, MD.

United States Preventive Services Task Force (1996*b*). Screening for hypertension. In *Guide to clinical preventive services 2*, pp. 39–51. Williams & Wilkins, Baltimore, MD.

United States Preventive Services Task Force (1996*c*) Screening for breast cancer. In *Guide to clinical preventive services 2*, pp. 73–87. Williams & Wilkins, Baltimore, MD.

Wadman, M. (1999). Human Genome Project aims to finish 'working draft' next year. *Nature*, **398**, 177.

Wald, N.J., Kennard, A., Hackshaw, A., and McGuire, A. (1997). Antenatal screening for Down's syndrome. *Journal of Medical Screening*, **4**, 181–246.

Walter, S.D. and Day, N.E. (1983). Estimation of the duration of a pre-clinical disease state using screening data. *American Journal of Epidemiology*, **118**, 865–86.

Walter, S.D. and Stitt, L.W. (1987). Evaluating the survival of cancer cases detected by screening. *Statistics in Medicine*, **6**, 885–900.

Ware, J.E. and Sherbourne, C.D. (1992). The MOS 36-Item Short-Form Health Survey (SF-36). I: Conceptual framework and item selection. *Medical Care*, **30**, 473–83.

Weiss, N.S. (1983). Control definition in case–control studies of the efficacy of screening and diagnostic testing. *American Journal of Epidemiology*, **116**, 457–60.

Wilson, J.M.G. and Junger, G. (1968). *Principles and practice of screening for disease.* World Health Organization, Geneva.

Winawer, S.J., Flehinger, B.J., Schottenfeld, D., and Miller, D.G. (1993). Screening for colorectal cancer with fecal occult blood testing and sigmoidoscopy. *Journal of the National Cancer Institute*, **85**, 1311–18.

Workshop Group (1989). Reducing deaths from breast cancer in Canada. *Canadian Medical Association Journal*, **141**, 199–201.

12.7 Global strategies for control of communicable diseases*

Robert J. Kim-Farley

Ingenuity, knowledge, and organization alter but cannot cancel humanity's vulnerability to invasion by parasitic forms of life. Infectious disease which antedated the emergence of humankind will last as long as humanity itself, and will surely remain, as it has been hitherto, one of the fundamental parameters and determinants of human history. (William H. McNeill 1976)

Introduction and overview

Communicable, or infectious, diseases have been and continue to remain a leading cause of morbidity, disability, and mortality worldwide. Their control is a constant challenge that faces health workers and public health officials in both industrialized and developing countries. Only one infectious disease, smallpox, has been eradicated and stands as a landmark in the history of the control of infectious diseases. The international community is now well down the path towards eradication of poliomyelitis and dracontiasis (guinea-worm infection). Other infectious diseases, like malaria and tuberculosis, have foiled eradication attempts or control efforts and are re-emerging as increasing threats in many countries. Some infectious diseases, such as tetanus, will always be a threat if control measures are not maintained. Newer infectious diseases, like AIDS, demonstrate the truth of McNeill's statement that infectious disease will remain 'one of the fundamental parameters and determinants of human history'. The history of infectious diseases is an exciting story in itself and readers interested in the subject are referred to McNeill (1976) or to the comprehensive work on the history of human diseases (Kiple 1993).

In the organization of this chapter, a fundamental decision was taken to provide a global and comprehensive view of the control of infectious diseases through examination of the magnitude of disease burden, the chain of infection (agent, transmission, and host) of infectious diseases, the varied approaches to their prevention and control, and the factors conducive to their eradication as well as emergence and re-emergence. Although this chapter provides many examples of infectious diseases that illustrate modes of transmission and approaches to infectious disease control, this chapter does not attempt to be comprehensive in listing all infectious diseases. Detailed recommendations on control measures for any specific disease are outlined periodically in the updated reports of the American Public Health Association, *Control of Communicable Diseases Manual* (Chin 2000), the comprehensive two-volume work *Mandell, Douglas and Bennett's Principles and Practice of Infectious Diseases* (Mandell *et al.* 1995), and the textbook *Infectious Diseases* (Gorbach *et al.* 1998). For readers specifically interested in paediatric infectious diseases there is the comprehensive two-volume *Textbook of Pediatric Infectious Diseases* (Feigin and Cherry 1998), for infectious diseases in emergency medicine settings there is the textbook *Infectious Disease in Emergency Medicine* (Brillman and Quenzer 1998), and for tropical infectious diseases there is *Tropical Infectious Diseases: Principles, Pathogens, and Practice* (Guerrant *et al.* 1999). A comprehensive treatment of the worldwide distribution and diagnosis of infectious diseases is provided in *A World Guide to Infections: Diseases, Distribution, Diagnosis* (Wilson 1991). The Centers for Disease Control and Prevention (**CDC**) publishes up-to-date disease surveillance information for the United States and recommendations for control measures in the *Morbidity and Mortality Weekly Reports* and provides annual summaries of notifiable infectious diseases in the *Summary of Notifiable Diseases, United States* (CDC 1999). Many other countries have similar types of publications. The World Health Organization (**WHO**) publishes worldwide surveillance information and recommendations for control measures in the *Weekly Epidemiological Record*. A more detailed background on infectious agents as determinants of health and disease is provided in Chapter 2.6.

Definitions of infectious diseases and their control

Infection occurs when an infectious agent enters a body and develops or multiplies. Infectious agents are organisms capable of producing inapparent infection or clinically manifest disease and include bacteria, rickettsia, chlamydiae, fungi, parasites, viruses, and prions. An infectious, or communicable, disease is an infection that results in a clinically manifest disease. Infectious disease may also be due to the toxic product of an infectious agent, such as the toxin produced by *Clostridium botulinum* causing classical botulism. As this is a textbook of public health, the infectious diseases considered are those that manifest in human hosts and are a result of the interaction of people and their environment. Infectious diseases may be due to infectious agents exclusively found in human hosts such as rubella virus, in the environment such as *Legionella pneumophila*, or primarily in animals such as *Brucella abortus*.

Control of infectious diseases refers to the actions and programmes directed towards reducing disease incidence, reducing disease prevalence, or completely eradicating the disease. Control aimed at reducing the incidence of infectious disease can be considered as primary prevention of infectious disease. Primary prevention protects

* The author alone is responsible for the views expressed in this publication.

health through the effects of personal as well as community-wide measures, including such actions as maintaining good nutritional status, keeping physically fit, immunizing against infectious diseases, providing safe water, and ensuring the proper disposal of faeces.

Control aimed at reducing the prevalence by shortening the duration of infectious disease can be considered as secondary prevention of infectious disease. Secondary prevention corrects departures from good health through the effects of individual and community actions, including such actions as early detection of disease, prompt antibiotic treatment, and ensuring adequate nutrition. It should be noted that such control efforts in secondary prevention in a group of infected individuals may also result in primary prevention in uninfected persons, a good example being prompt specific drug therapy for tuberculosis patients to produce sputum conversion which renders them no longer a source of infection to others.

Control aimed at reducing or even eliminating long-term impairments of infectious disease can be considered as tertiary prevention of infectious disease. Tertiary prevention reduces or eliminates disabilities, minimizes suffering, and promotes adjustment to conditions that are not remediable through such actions as providing orthopaedic appliances, counselling and vocational training, and prevention of opportunistic infections. The prevention of opportunistic infections in HIV infection, for example, can be considered as tertiary prevention (Osterholm *et al.* 1995).

Global burden of infectious diseases

Infectious diseases remain a leading cause of morbidity, disability, and mortality worldwide. A WHO analysis of the global burden of disease estimated that 13.3 million deaths out of a total of 53.9 million deaths in 1998 were attributable to infectious diseases (WHO 1999*a*). Most of these deaths occurred in the economically developing group of countries. Infectious diseases contributed to approximately 25 per cent of all deaths globally, and one in two deaths in developing countries. This should not be construed to mean that infectious diseases are not significant in more developed countries. In the United States, for example, AIDS rose to become the leading cause of death in persons aged 25 to 44 years, and still ranks as an important cause of death in this age group.

The current magnitude of morbidity and mortality due to infectious diseases worldwide is highlighted by the WHO as follows (WHO 1999*a*).

- Acute respiratory infections, including pneumonia and influenza, result in 3.5 million deaths per year. These infections are the highest cause of infant and child mortality in developing countries with almost 2 million deaths in children under 5 years of age.
- Diarrhoeal diseases are also a major cause of morbidity and mortality in infants and children in developing countries. Each year there are 2.2 million deaths due to diarrhoeal disease, of which some 1.8 million are among children under 5 years of age.
- Malaria is estimated to cause 1.1 million deaths per year worldwide. Aprrroximately 800 000 deaths of children under the age of 5 years are attributable to malaria.
- Diseases preventable by vaccination, although in decline worldwide, still result in an estimated 1.6 million deaths each year. For example, there are still approximately 900 000 deaths due to measles each year in children under 5 years of age.
- *Mycobacterium tuberculosis*, the causative agent of tuberculosis, now infects about one-third of the world's population. It is estimated that there are approximately 1.5 million deaths due to tuberculosis each year.
- HIV has infected more than 58 million persons since the start of the HIV/AIDS pandemic and it is estimated that approximately 22 million persons with AIDS have died throughout the world.
- Sexually transmitted diseases other than AIDS are estimated to have a global annual incidence of some 333 million cases, occurring predominantly in developing countries.
- Hepatitis B virus infects some 2 billion people worldwide. There are approximately 350 million chronic carriers and the sequelae of their infections lead to over 1 million deaths per year, almost all avoidable by immunization.

Chain of infection: agent, transmission, and host

The chain of infection is the relationship between an infectious agent, its routes of transmission, and a susceptible host. The prevention and control of infectious diseases depend upon the interaction of these three factors that may result in the human host clinically manifesting disease.

Agent

The infectious agent is the first link in the chain of infection and is any micro-organism whose presence or excessive presence is essential for the occurrence of an infectious disease. Examples of infectious agents include the following.

- **Bacteria**: for example, spirochetes and curved bacteria such as *Borrelia burgdorferi* causing Lyme disease, Gram-negative rods such as *Yersinia pestis* causing plague, Gram-positive cocci such as *Streptococcus pyogenes* group A, causing erysipelas, and Gram-positive rods such as *Mycobacterium tuberculosis* causing tuberculosis.
- **Rickettsiae**: for example, *Rickettsia ricketsii* causing Rocky Mountain spotted fever, and *Rickettsia prowazekii* causing epidemic louse-borne typhus fever.
- **Chlamydiae**: for example, *Chlamydia psittaci* causing psittacosis, and *Chlamydia trachomatis* causing trachoma and genital infections.
- **Fungi**: for example, *Trichophyton schoenleinii* and *Microsporum canis* causing tinea capitis, and *Tinea rubrum*, *Tinea mentagrophytes*, and *Epidermophyton floccosum* causing tinea pedis.
- **Parasites**, for example, helminths such as *Trichinella spiralis* causing trichinosis, filaria such as *Brugia malayi* causing filariasis, nematodes such as *Enterobius vermicularis* causing enterobiasis (pinworm disease), trematodes such as *Clonorchis sinensis* causing clonorchiasis (oriental liver fluke disease), cestodes such as *Taenia solium* causing taeniasis (beef tapeworm disease), and protozoa such as *Trypanosoma cruzi* causing American trypanosomiasis (Chagas' disease).
- **Viruses**: for example, Paramyxoviridae such as measles virus which causes measles, Togaviridae such as the rubella virus which causes

rubella, and arthropod-borne viruses (arboviruses) such as dengue viruses which cause dengue fever.

- **Prions**, which are small proteinaceous infectious particles that cause diseases such as kuru, Creutzfeldt–Jakob disease (and its variant associated with exposure of humans to the bovine spongiform encephalopathy agent), and the Gerstmann–Straussler–Scheinker sydrome.

There is evidence that some infectious agents, often with cofactors, are associated with human tumours. Examples include *Shistosoma haematobium* with bladder cancer, *Shistosoma japonicum* with colorectal cancer, *Clonorchis sinensis* with cholangiocarcinoma, hepatitis B and C viruses with hepatocellular carcinoma, *Helicobacter pylori* with gastric cancer, and human papillomaviruses with cervical cancer.

Agents can be described by their ability to cause disease (pathogenicity) as well as their ability to cause serious disease (virulence). The pathogenicity of an infectious agent is the extent to which clinically manifest disease is produced in an infected population and is measured by the ratio of the number of persons developing clinical illness to the total number infected. Examples of highly pathogenic infectious agents are the measles virus and the human (α) herpesvirus 3 (varicella-zoster) causing measles and chickenpox, respectively, in which most infected susceptible persons will manifest disease.

The virulence of an infectious agent is the extent to which severe disease is produced in a population with clinically manifest disease. It is the ratio of the number of persons with severe and fatal disease to the total number of persons with disease. An example of a highly virulent infectious agent is HIV, whereby nearly all untreated persons with AIDS will die.

Characteristics of infectious agents that affect pathogenicity include their ability to invade tissues (invasiveness), produce toxins (intoxication), cause damaging hypersensitivity (allergic) reactions, undergo antigenic variation, and develop antibiotic resistance. An example of an infectious agent with high invasiveness is the *Shigella* organism that can invade the submucosal tissue of the intestine and cause clinically manifest shigellosis (bacillary dysentery). An example of an infectious agent that has a high degree of ability to produce toxins is the *Clostridium botulinum* organism that can elaborate toxins in inadequately prepared food and cause classical botulism. An example of an infectious agent that is highly allergenic is the *Mycobacterium tuberculosis* organism which can cause tuberculosis. An example of an infectious agent that has a high degree of antigenic variation is the type A influenza virus which frequently experiences minor antigenic changes—antigenic 'drift'. Influenza A viruses, on an irregular basis, may also undergo a major antigenic change creating an entirely new subtype—antigenic 'shift'. Antigenic shifts may result in an influenza pandemic when individuals immune to previous strains of influenza are exposed to the new strain. An example of an infectious agent that can develop antibiotic resistance that challenges control efforts is *Neisseria gonorrhoeae* that has both chromosomally mediated and resistance transfer plasmid mediated genetic factors for antibiotic resistance.

The infective dose of an infectious agent is the number of organisms needed to cause an infection. The infective dose may vary depending upon the route of transmission and host susceptibility.

Control measures for infectious diseases directed at inactivating the agent are designed according to the type of agent and its reservoirs and sources. An agent like *Vibrio cholerae*, for example, can be inactivated through adequate chlorination of the water supply. This is a chemical method for provision of safe water to control cholera. An agent like hepatitis B virus can be inactivated through adequate autoclaving of injection and surgical equipment. This is a sterilization method to control hepatitis B. Details of these and other methods of control directed at the agent are provided in the sections in this chapter on control measures applied to the agent and the environment.

Routes of transmission

Control efforts are often designed to break the routes of transmission, the mechanisms by which infectious agents are spread from reservoirs or sources to human hosts. A reservoir of an infectious agent is any person, other living organism, or inanimate material in which the infectious agent normally lives and grows. The source of infection for a host is the person, other living organism or inanimate material from which the infectious agent came. The routes of transmission have been summarized by Chin (2000) as follows.

Direct transmission

Direct and essentially immediate transfer of infectious agents to a receptive portal of entry through which human or animal infection may take place. This may be by direct contact as touching, biting, kissing or sexual intercourse, or by the direct projection (droplet spread) of droplet spray onto the conjunctiva or onto the mucous membranes of the eye, nose, or mouth during sneezing, coughing, spitting, singing, or talking (usually limited to a distance of about 1 m or less).

Indirect transmission

Vehicle-borne Contaminated inanimate materials or objects (fomites) such as (a) toys, handkerchiefs, soiled clothes, bedding, cooking or eating utensils, surgical instruments, or dressings, (b) water, food, milk, and biological products including blood, serum, plasma, tissues, or organs, or (c) any substance serving as an intermediate means by which an infectious agent is transported and introduced into a susceptible host through a suitable portal of entry. The agent may or may not have multiplied or developed in or on the vehicle before being transmitted.

Vector-borne

Mechanical Includes simple mechanical carriage by a crawling or flying insect through soiling of its feet or proboscis, or by passage of organisms through its gastrointestinal tract. This does not require multiplication or development of the organism.

Biological Propagation (multiplication), cyclic development, or a combination of these (cyclopropagative) is required before the arthropod can transmit the infective form of the agent to humans. An incubation period (extrinsic) is required following infection before the arthropod becomes infective. The infectious agent may be passed vertically to succeeding generations (transovarian transmission). Trans-stadial transmission indicates its passage from one stage of lifecycle to another, such as nymph to adult. Transmission may be by injection of salivary gland fluid during biting, or by regurgitation or deposition on the skin of faeces or other material capable of penetrating through the bite wound or through an area of trauma from scratching or rubbing. This transmission is by an infected non-vertebrate host and not simple mechanical carriage by a vector as a vehicle. However, an arthropod in either role is termed a vector.

Airborne transmission

The dissemination of microbial aerosols to a suitable portal of entry, usually the respiratory tract. Microbial aerosols are suspensions of particles in the air consisting partially or wholly of micro-organisms. They may remain suspended in the air for long periods of time, some retaining and others losing infectivity or virulence.

Droplet nuclei Usually the small residues that result from evaporation of fluid from droplets emitted by an infected host. They also may be created purposefully by a variety of atomizing devices, or accidentally as in microbiology laboratories or in abattoirs, rendering plants, or autopsy rooms. They usually remain suspended in the air for long periods of time.

Dust The small particles of widely varying size which may arise from soil (as, for example, fungus spores separated from dry soil by wind or mechanical agitation), clothes, bedding, or contaminated floors.

Control measures for infectious diseases directed at interrupting transmission are designed according to the type of transmission for the agent. Direct transmission of an agent like *Neisseria gonorrhoeae*, for example, can be reduced by using condoms as a barrier method of control of gonorrhoea. Vector-borne transmission of an agent like *Plasmodium falciparum* can be reduced by using a residual insecticide against *Anopheles* mosquitos as a chemical vector control method for malaria. Airborne transmission of an agent like *Mycobacterium tuberculosis* from sputum-positive pulmonary tuberculosis patients in hospital can be reduced by the use of special ventilation in the patient's room as an environmental method of control of tuberculosis. It should be recognized that some infectious agents may have more than one route of transmission. Poliovirus, for example, can be spread via direct transmission through the faecal–oral route and pharyngeal spread, or indirect transmission through contaminated food or other materials. Details of these and other methods of control directed at interrupting transmission are provided in the sections on control measures in this chapter.

Host

The host is the final link in the chain of infection. The infectious agent may enter the host through the following portals of entry.

- **Respiratory tract**: infectious agents can be inhaled into the respiratory tract and will be deposited at different levels of the pulmonary tree according to the size of the aerosol, droplet nuclei, or dust particles. Particles between 1 and 5 μm, for example, can reach to the alveoli of the lungs.
- **Intact skin**: some infectious agents, such as *Necator americanus* that may cause hookworm disease, can penetrate the intact skin.
- **Gastrointestinal tract**: an infectious agent such as *Vibrio cholerae* may enter via the gastrointestinal tract and result in cholera. Persons who have a compromised gastric function, such as gastric achlorhydria, may be at increased risk of disease.
- **Mucous membranes:** infectious agents, such as measles viruses, may be deposited on mucous membranes by droplet spread or by direct contact with infected persons or contaminated objects.
- **Urinary tract**: some infectious agents, such as *Escherichia coli*, can enter the urinary tract via an ascending route from the urethra colonized with the organism. Structural abnormalities of the urinary tract and procedures such as urinary catheterization may predispose the host to disease.
- **Placenta**: transplacental transmission is a direct route of transmission to the fetus for infectious agents such as rubella viruses.

Infectious agents also enter the host though mechanisms that get past the body's natural barriers, including wounds that break the integrity of the skin or mucous membranes; invasive procedures, parenteral injections, parenteral infusions, or organ transplants that may introduce an agent into the body; or insect vectors that may inject agents through the skin.

The most important host factors regarding developing clinically manifest disease and the severity of disease are immune status and age. Infants, young children, and the elderly are at generally higher risk from more severe disease due to immaturity or deterioration of immune systems, respectively.

Many host defence mechanisms help prevent infection or disease. Non-specific host defence mechanisms include the intact skin, nasal cilia, tears, saliva, mucus, and gastric acid. Specific host defence mechanisms include naturally acquired immunity from previous infection, tranplacentally acquired passive immunity in the newborn from the mother, artificially acquired active immunity from immunization, and artificially acquired passive immunity from immunoglobulins and antitoxins.

Host responses to infection that prevent or reduce the severity of infectious disease include (a) polymorphonuclear leukocytosis stimulated by some bacterial infections that increases the number of phagocytic cells, (b) fever that may slow the multiplication of some infectious agents, (c) antibody production that may neutralize some infectious agents or their toxins, and (d) interferon production that may block intracellular replication of viruses.

The manifestation of infection in the host may vary from inapparent (subclinical) infection to severe disease that may even result in death. The interaction between an infectious agent, routes of transmission and host factors determines the spectrum of signs and symptoms. Sometimes the host may become an asymptomatic carrier of the infectious agent and be a source of infection for others.

Control measures for infectious diseases directed at the host are designed according to the immune status of the host and the likelihood of host exposure to certain infectious agents. Measles disease, for example, can be prevented by active immunization with measles vaccine to develop host immunity. Pneumonic plague can be prevented in those in close contact with patients with plague pneumonia by using tetracycline or sulfonamide chemoprophylaxis. Details of these and other methods of control directed at the host are provided in the section on control measures applied to the host in this chapter.

Tools for control of infectious diseases

The primary concern of infectious disease control in public health, whether in developing or industrialized countries, is the reduction, elimination, or even eradication of infectious disease. This is accomplished by directing control measures to the host, the routes of transmission, or the agent. Such control measures include (a) identifying and reducing or eliminating infectious agents at their sources and reservoirs, (b) breaking or interfering with the routes of transmission of infectious agents, and (c) identifying susceptible populations and reducing or eliminating their susceptibility.

The tools for control of infectious diseases are related to the recognition and evaluation of the patterns of diseases and interventions to control them. The most important tool for the recognition and evaluation is surveillance of disease is defined as

> the continuing scrutiny of all aspects of occurrence and spread of a disease that are pertinent to effective control. Included are the systematic collection and evaluation of: (a) morbidity and mortality reports; (b) special reports of field investigations of epidemics and of individual cases; (c) isolation and identification of infectious agents by laboratories; (d) data concerning the availability, use, and untoward effects of vaccines and toxoids, immune globulins, insecticides, and other substances used in control; (e) information regarding immunity levels in segments of the population; and (f) other relevant epidemiological data. (Chin 2000)

Therefore surveillance is 'information for action'. More detailed information on surveillance and field investigations is given in Chapters 6.4 and 6.16.

There are many tools for control related to interventions:

- control measures applied to the host (e.g. active immunization, passive immunization, chemoprophylaxis, behavioural change, reverse isolation, barriers, and improving host resistance)
- control measures applied to vectors (e.g. chemical, environmental and biological control)
- control measures applied to infected humans (e.g. chemotherapy, isolation, quarantine, restriction of activities, and behavioural change)
- control measures applied to animals (e.g. active immunization, restriction or reduction, and chemoprophylaxis and chemotherapy)
- control measures applied to the environment (e.g. provision of safe water, proper disposal of faeces, food and milk sanitation, and design of facilities and equipment)
- control measures applied to infectious agents (cleaning, cooling, pasteurization, disinfection, and sterilization).

Achieving maximum impact on control of a specific infectious disease may involve more than one of these interventions. For example, the control of hepatitis A infection can be achieved through interventions that may include active immunization, passive immunization, food preparation and handwashing behaviours, provision of safe water, food sanitation, and proper disposal of faeces.

The tools for control can also be considered according to the level at which they are applied: individual, institutional, or community-based. At the individual level, control measures, usually initiated by a clinician, are directed towards the specific infectious disease threats to the particular individual. Examples include chemoprophylaxis to prevent wound infection, pre-exposure prophylactic immunization against rabies for a veterinarian, and use of diphtheria antitoxin in a patient with diphtheria. At the institutional level, control measures are directed to a group of people who are in close contact with each other, such as persons in day-care centres, schools, military barracks, hospital wards, nursing homes, and correctional facilities. Control activities in institutional settings are usually initiated by the officials of the institution. Examples includ administering amantadine hydrochloride or rimantadine for chemoprophylaxis or chemotherapy of influenza A in a high-risk institutional population, quarantining institutionalized young children during a measles outbreak, and hepatitis B immunization of staff and clients of institutions for the developmentally disabled. At the community level, control measures, usually initiated by local, state, or national public health agencies, are directed to the community at large. Examples include childhood immunization programmes, provision of safe water, and recall of contaminated food products. It should be noted that some control measures, such as immunization, may take place at all levels while others, such as the provision of safe water to the community, are more specifically applied at a particular level.

The tools for the control of infectious diseases and their relationship to the chain of infection are the main focus of the remainder of this chapter.

Control measures applied to the host

Control measures applied to the host range from relatively easily administered immunization to behavioural changes that may be extremely difficult for an individual to accept. This section details the types of control measures applied to susceptible hosts and gives examples of their application in the control of selected infectious diseases.

Active immunization

One of the most satisfactory control measures applied to a host is one that renders the host immune from infectious disease by an infectious agent. Active immunization is a cornerstone of public health measures for the control of many infectious diseases and is considered one of the most cost-effective methods of individual, institutional, and community protection for many infectious diseases. The most powerful example of the potential impact of active immunization against an infectious disease is that of smallpox vaccination. Mobilization of political will on a worldwide basis, coupled with full application of the strategies of active surveillance and containment immunization against smallpox, ultimately resulted in the complete global eradication of the disease and cessation of transmission of the infectious agent, variola virus.

Active immunization is usually considered synonymous with the term vaccination, and is the process of administration of an antigen that can induce a specific immune response that protects susceptible hosts from an infectious disease. Some draw a distinction between the two terms. Narrowly defined, vaccination is the process of administration of an antigen and immunization is the development of a specific immune response. Administering an antigen without evoking an immune response is possible, since no vaccine is 100 per cent effective. Conversely, someone can become immunized even if an antigen is administered to someone else (the live attenuated oral polio vaccine viruses, for example, can be transmitted from the recipient to other close contacts).

Active immunization can be accomplished through different types of antigens, including the following.

- **Inactivated toxins** Diphtheria toxoid is an example of a formaldehyde-inactivated preparation of diphtheria toxin that protects against clinically manifest disease, although the immunized person may still become infected with toxin-producing strains of *Corynebacterium diphtheria*. Tetanus toxoid and *Clostridium perfringens* toxoid (pig bel vaccine) are other examples of inactivated toxin preparations.
- **Inactivated complex antigens** Whole cell pertussis vaccine is an example of a heat or chemically treated preparation of killed whole pertussis bacteria that protects against clinically manifest disease even if the immunized person may still become infected with *Bordetella pertussis*. Other examples of inactivated vaccines include inactivated polio vaccine and influenza vaccine.
- **Purified antigens** Acellular pertussis vaccine is an example of a vaccine composed of isolated and purified immunogenic pertussis antigens. Other vaccines with purified components include polyvalent capsular polysaccharide pneumococcal, polysaccharide meningococcal, protein-polysaccharide conjugate *Haemophilus influenzae* type b, and plasma-derived hepatitis B vaccines.
- **Recombinant antigens** Hepatitis B recombinant vaccine is an example of a vaccine composed of hepatitis B surface antigen subunits made through recombinant DNA technology.
- **Live attenuated vaccines** Measles vaccine is an example of a vaccine containing live infectious agents that are of reduced virulence, but induce protective antibodies against measles viruses. Other live attenuated vaccines include oral polio, mumps, rubella, yellow fever, and bacille Calmette–Guérin (BCG) vaccines.

Protective antibody responses usually take 7 to 21 days to develop. Although most vaccines must be given before exposure to be effective, some vaccines may protect even if administered after exposure to an infectious agent. For example, measles vaccine may provide protection against measles disease if given within 72 hours of exposure.

Duration of protection varies from only months, such as with killed whole-cell cholera vaccine, to years, or even life with some live attenuated vaccines, such as measles vaccine. Some inactivated toxoids and vaccines, such as tetanus toxoid, may require a priming series of doses to be optimally effective and additional booster doses to maintain protective antibodies. Many new technologies are being explored that may increase the number and efficacy of vaccines available against infectious disease, including immune-stimulating complexes, live viral or bacterial vector vaccines, and timed-release vaccines.

It should be recognized that vaccines vary in their efficacy and no vaccine is 100 per cent effective. Vaccine efficacies vary with type of vaccine, storage and handling conditions, skill of administration, age of vaccination, and other host factors. Vaccines for routine use are safe. However, no vaccine is 100 per cent safe. Potential vaccinees, or their parents or guardians, should be screened for contraindications and be informed of potential side-effects.

Immunization schedules for the routine control of infectious diseases preventable by immunization vary between countries and are usually based on expert advice to governments and physicians. For example, in the United States recommended policies for immunization are provided by the Immunization Practices Advisory Committee and are published in the *Morbidity and Mortality Weekly Report* (ACIP 1994). In addition, the American Academy of Pediatrics periodically publishes comprehensive immunization recommendations in its *Report of the Committee on Infectious Diseases* (Committee on Infectious Diseases 2000). At the global level, the WHO publishes recommended immunization schedules (WHO 1995*b*) and recommendations on control of vaccine-preventable diseases are periodically updated by expert advisory groups and published in the WHO *Weekly Epidemiological Record*.

In outbreak settings, immunization schedules may be modified. For example, the age of immunization for measles may be lowered to 6 months during an outbreak. In such situations, persons receiving vaccine before the routinely recommended age of immunization should be immunized again at the recommended age since immunization at an earlier age may not have been optimally effective.

Immunization programmes include those for routine child, routine adult, travel, selected high-risk populations, and occupational settings. For example, tetanus toxoid is universally recommended, yellow fever vaccine is only recommended in geographical areas of epidemiological risk, typhoid fever vaccine is only recommended for individuals subject to unusual exposure to typhoid, including persons living in the same household as known carriers, and anthrax vaccine is only recommended for veterinarians and persons occupationally exposed to possibly contaminated industrial raw materials.

Besides protection of the individual, vaccination may also provide a degree of community protection. This phenomenon is known as herd immunity. Herd immunity is the relative protection of a population group achieved by reducing or breaking the chains of transmission of an infectious agent because most of the population is resistant to infection through immunization. Herd immunity is a complex phenomenon and varies according to the infectious agent, its routes of transmission, the degree to which immunization protects against infection versus only clinically manifest disease, and the distribution of immunity in the population. The mechanisms of herd immunity are several, including 'direct protection of vaccinees against disease or transmissible infection and indirect protection of non-recipients by virtue of surreptitious vaccination, passive antibody, or just reduced sources of transmission and, hence, risks of infection in the community' (Fine 1993).

A particularly difficult problem for vaccine-preventable infectious disease control programmes is complacency by the population that can result from the very success of the programmes. Low rates of vaccine-preventable infectious disease may mistakenly lead parents to consider that vaccination is no longer important for maintaining their children's health and may result in political leaders reducing funding for immunization programmes. Low disease rates may also focus undue attention on the relatively rare side-effects of vaccination in relation to current rates of disease. Such side-effects should only be compared in relation to rates of disease that would occur without immunization programmes.

A comprehensive discussion of active immunization is given by Plotkin and Orenstein (1999).

Passive immunization

Passive immunization is temporary immunity in a host due to the protection afforded by antibody produced in another host. Passive immunity may be acquired either naturally or artificially.

Naturally acquired passive immunity through transfer of maternal antibodies via the placenta is the way that newborn infants are provided with a temporary immunity against many infectious diseases for which the mother is immune. This immunity wanes over time and eventually leaves the infant susceptible to these diseases.

An important use of transplacental immunity as a control measure is in the prevention of tetanus neonatorum (neonatal tetanus) by immunization of women before or during pregnancy with tetanus toxoid. The disease typically occurs when the umbilical cord is cut with an unclean instrument contaminated with tetanus spores or when substances contaminated with tetanus spores are placed on the umbilical stump after delivery. Control by active immunization of the infant cannot be achieved in sufficient time since the average incubation period is only 6 days (with a range from 3 to 28 days). An adequately immunized mother, however, will usually effectively transfer maternal antibodies against tetanus to her newborn and prevent tetanus neonatorum.

Another example of naturally acquired passive immunity is the relative protection against measles disease in a young infant born to a mother who previously had the disease. Typically, such infants are immune for approximately 6 to 9 months or more after birth depending upon how much residual maternal antibodies are present at the time of pregnancy. Other diseases for which there is usually an effective transplacental immunity in infants, for variable amounts of time, include diphtheria, mumps, poliomyelitis, rubella, and varicella (chickenpox). It should be noted that if the mother is not immune, or if residual maternal antibodies have significantly waned, then the infant may be susceptible to disease.

Research is ongoing in other infectious diseases that may be preventable in the neonate or infant though immunization of the mother before or during pregnancy. Examples include *Haemophilus influenzae* type b, and group B streptococcal and meningococcal diseases (Insel *et al.* 1994). Many diseases, however, are not prevented by transplacental immunity.

Breast feeding is a form of naturally acquired passive antibody transfer to neonates and infants. Breast milk and colostrum contain secretory immunoglobin A antibodies that may play a protective role in the prevention of infections with such agents as respiratory syncytial virus, rotavirus, and *Haemophilus influenzae* type b.

Artificially acquired passive immunity through administration of an antibody-containing preparation, antiserum, or immune globulin, has a place in the control of certain infectious diseases. However, unlike active immunization that is appropriate for routine use in the general population, passive immunization is confined to special situations.

Examples of the use of artificially acquired passive immunity to control infectious disease include the following.

- **Rabies** Natural immunity to rabies in humans does not exist and therefore susceptible individuals bitten by an animal known or suspected to be rabid should receive rabies immune globulin to neutralize the rabies virus in the wound. It should be noted that, besides passive immunization with rabies immune globulin, such individuals should also receive active immunization with rabies vaccine.

- **Hepatitis A** In areas where sanitation is poor, hepatitis A infection commonly occurs at an early age and therefore most adults in developing countries are already immune. However, epidemics may occur in industrialized countries. Passive immunization with immune globulin may be given to all household and sexual contacts of patients with hepatitis A, other food handlers in an establishment where hepatitis A has occurred in a food handler, all individuals in an institution where a focal outbreak of hepatitis A has occurred, and persons from industrialized countries travelling to highly endemic areas. It should be noted that vaccines for active immunization for hepatitis A are now available.

- **Diphtheria** Treatment of this disease is an example of the use of an antibody-containing product (diphtheria antitoxin) produced in an animal (only diphtheria antitoxin from horses is available) administered as part of the treatment regimen for secondary prevention of disease. In suspected cases of diphtheria, the antitoxin must be given as soon as possible because it is only effective in neutralizing diphtheria toxins not yet bound to cells.

- **Other important infectious diseases, including hepatitis B, measles, tetanus, and varicella** Depending upon the circumstances of exposure, susceptibility of the host and status of the host's general immune system there are circumstances under which hepatitis B immune globulin, tetanus immune globulin, varicella-zoster immune globulin, or immune globulin may be warranted.

Chemoprophylaxis

Chemoprophylaxis is the prevention of infection or its progression to clinically manifest disease through the administration of chemical substances, including antibiotics. Chemoprophylaxis can also consist of the treatment of a disease to prevent complications of that disease (Solomon and Fraser 1998). Chemoprophylaxis may be specifically directed against a particular infectious agent or it may be non-specifically directed against many infectious agents. The use of antibiotics before surgical procedures is an example of non-specific chemoprophylaxis to prevent wound infections in the postoperative period. Examples of specific chemoprophylaxis are given below.

The use of chemoprophylaxis to prevent development of infection is illustrated by using chloroquine to prevent malarial parasitaemia caused by *Plasmodium vivax*, *Plasmodium ovale*, *Plasmodium malariae*, and chloroquine-sensitive strains of *Plasmodium falciparum*. For some chloroquine-resistant strains of *Plasmodium falciparum*, alternative regimes include the addition of pyrimethamine and sulfadoxine (Fansidar®), pyrimethamine and dapsone (Maloprim®), or mefloquine. To reduce the risk of a relapse from intrahepatic forms of *Plasmodium vivax* and *Plasmodium ovale* after chloroquine is stopped, primaquine may be given. Determination of a specific malaria chemoprophylactic regimen is complex. It must take into account the geographical area, the possibility of pregnancy, the weight of an individual (dose size for children is determined by body weight), and the risks of adverse reactions to the chemoprophylactic regimen.

Other examples of prevention of development of infection include the following:

- the use of silver nitrate, erythromycin or tetracycline instilled into the eyes of a newborn to prevent gonococcal ophthalmia by transmission of *Neisseria gonorrhoeae* from an infected mother during birth

- the use of tetracycline, sulfonamides (including sulfadiazine and trimethoprim-sulfamethoxazole), chloramphenicol, or streptomycin in close contacts of confirmed or suspected cases of plague pneumonia to prevent plague pneumonia by transmission of *Yersinia pestis*

- the use of benzathine penicillin in those in sexual contact with confirmed cases of early syphilis to prevent syphilis by transmission of *Treponema pallidum*.

An example of the use of chemoprophylaxis to prevent the progression of an infection to active manifest disease is the use of isoniazid to prevent the progression of latent infection with *Mycobacterium tuberculosis* to clinical tuberculosis. Persons less than 35 years of age who are tuberculin-test positive should receive isoniazid to prevent clinical tuberculosis. The decision to use isoniazid, especially in individuals more than 35 years of age, must be determined based on such information as length of infection, closeness of association with a current case, status of the immune system, presence of acute liver disease, possibility of pregnancy, and risk of adverse reactions.

Other examples of prevention of progression of an infection to active manifest disease include the following:

- use of co-trimoxazole or pentamidine to prevent subclinical latent infection with *Pneumocystis carinii* from progression to clinically manifest pneumocystis pneumonia in immunosuppressed persons such as HIV-infected individuals
- use of mebendazole, albendazole, or pyrantel pamoate to prevent infection with *Necator americanus*, *Ancylostoma duodenale*, and *Ancylostoma ceylanicum* progressing to the clinically manifest anaemia of hookworm disease
- use of pyrimethamine–sulfadiazine–folinic acid to prevent asymptomatic infants congenitally infected with *Toxoplasma gondii* from clinically manifest chorioretinitis and other sequelae of congenital toxoplasmosis.

In some situations, establishing screening programmes to detect and treat asymptomatic or unrecognized infections in defined populations is useful. An example is the screening for *Chlamydia trachomatis* in sexual partners of persons infected with *Chlamydia trachomatis*, women with mucopurulent cervicitis, sexually active women less than 20 years of age, and women 20 years of age or older who meet certain criteria. A more detailed background on screening as a public health function is given in Chapter 12.6.

An example of the use of chemoprophylaxis to treat an infectious disease to prevent complications of the disease is the use of penicillin (or erythromycin in penicillin-sensitive patients) to treat streptococcal sore throats caused by *Streptococcus pyogenes* group A to prevent acute rheumatic fever.

Other examples of prevention of complications of an infectious disease include the following:

- tetracycline for adults, or penicillin for children, for treatment of Lyme disease caused by *Borrelia burgdorferi* in the erythema chronicum migrans stage to prevent or reduce the severity of late cardiac, arthritic, or neurological complications
- benzathine penicillin for treatment of syphilis in its primary, secondary, or early latency period to prevent late manifestations of the disease such as cardiovascular syphilis
- ketoconazole for treatment of blastomycosis caused by *Blastomyces dermatitidis* in its early stages to prevent progression of chronic pulmonary or disseminated blastomycosis that may lead to death.

Potential problems with the use of chemoprophylaxis may include compromise of the host's own non-specific defence mechanisms, other replacement infectious agents causing disease by growing in the place of the infectious agent affected by the specific chemoprophylactic regimen, and emergence of resistant strains of the infectious agent. The development of antibiotic resistance can be reduced by using antibiotics only when needed, selecting the proper antibiotic (or, in some situations, the appropriate multidrug therapy) for the infectious agent, and ensuring compliance with the appropriate regimen for the duration of treatment.

Behavioural change

Perhaps the most challenging tool for the control of infectious diseases, and sometimes one of the most powerful and cost-effective, is behaviour change in the host that reduces or eliminates risk of exposure to an agent. Everyone has developed habits of living (lifestyles) that are not easily changed. Some of these behaviours are protective against infectious diseases. Others render the individual at higher risk of infection.

Examples of higher risk of exposure to infectious agents through behaviour, and behaviour changes that can have an impact on the chain of transmission, include the following.

Sexual behaviour

Many infectious agents are transmitted through the direct transmission route of sexual intercourse, including *Chlamydia trachomatis* causing chlamydial genital infections, *Neisseria gonorrhoeae* causing gonorrhoea, *Treponema pallidum* causing venereal syphilis, *Calymmatobacterium granulomatis* causing granuloma inguinale, *Haemophilus ducreyi* causing chancroid, herpes simplex virus causing herpes simplex, *Trichomonas vaginalis* causing trichomoniasis, human papillomaviruses causing condyloma acuminata, HIV causing AIDS.

Abstinence behaviour, i.e. refraining from sexual activity with other persons, eliminates the risk of transmission of these agents through sexual contact. The delaying of age of first sexual intercourse avoids the risk of transmission of these agents at an early age. Restricting sexual activity to having sex only between two uninfected persons who do not have sexual activity with any other persons virtually eliminates the risk of transmission of these agents through sexual intercourse. The exceptions are due to other routes of transmission of some of these agents (e.g. HIV acquired through intravenous drug use in one partner being transmitted through sexual intercourse to the other partner). Limiting the number of sexual partners, and limiting those sexual partners to persons who also have few sexual partners, reduces the risk of exposure. However, at the individual level, if one of these sexual partners has an infectious agent transmissible by sexual intercourse, the risk of transmission may still be high. Finally, condom use during sexual intercourse in high-risk situations will markedly reduce, but not eliminate, transmission. A more detailed background on sexually transmitted diseases is provided in Chapter 9.13.

Intravenous drug use behaviour

Injection of drugs using non-sterile needles and syringes previously used by other intravenous drug users may transmit infectious agents in blood through the vehicle-borne route of indirect transmission, including HIV causing AIDS, hepatitis B virus causing viral hepatitis B, and *Plasmodium vivax*, *Plasmodium malariae*, and *Plasmodium ovale* causing malaria.

Abstinence behaviour, i.e. refraining from intravenous drug use, eliminates the risk of transmission of such agents through contaminated needles and syringes. Using a sterile needle and sterile syringe for intravenous drug use will break the chain of transmission of these infectious agents through this route. Some community public health programmes, in addition to promoting drug abstinence and drug rehabilitation, conduct needle and syringe exchanges and education in methods of decontamination to help promote the use of sterile injection equipment among intravenous drug users.

Eating behaviour

Eating certain foods may result in exposure to infectious agents through the vehicle-borne route of indirect transmission. These behaviours include consuming raw molluscs by which an infectious agent like the hepatitis A virus can cause viral hepatitis A, eating raw eggs by which an infectious agent like a *Salmonella* serotype can cause salmonellosis, and consuming raw beef by which an infectious agent like *Taenia saginata* can cause beef tapeworm infection.

Although food and diet are strongly ingrained behaviours, modification of dietary patterns is possible. Cooking foods like beef, pork, and eggs can markedly reduce risk of transmission of infectious agents. In addition, reducing risks by elimination of infectious agents from the food may be possible (see the section on control methods applied to the environment). Handwashing before eating also reduces risk of transmission of many infectious agents, such as *Shigella dysenteriae*, *Shigella flexneri*, *Shigella boydii*, and *Shigella sonnei*, which are spread through direct or indirect routes of faecal–oral transmission.

Working behaviour

In certain occupations many behaviours may result in exposure to infectious agents and should be targets for control programmes in occupational health and safety. Specific examples include the following:

- dental workers improperly performing procedures with bare hands which may result in exposure to hepatitis B viruses from infected patients
- health workers improperly handling used needles which may result in needlestick injuries leading to exposure to HIV from infected patients
- hospital laboratory workers processing specimens containing infectious agents without proper glove or eyewear protection
- veterinarians who do not properly handle animals which may result in exposure to *Brucella abortus*, *Brucella melitensis*, *Brucella suis*, or *Brucella canis*.

Occupational hazards related to non-infectious materials may predispose an individual to increased risk of infectious diseases. For example, working conditions and behaviours in industrial plants and mines that lead to silicosis due to long-term inhalation of free crystalline silica dust will greatly increase the risk of developing tuberculosis.

Working behaviours appropriate for the particular occupational setting may include wearing protective clothing, eyewear, and gloves, handwashing and changing clothes after work, meticulous adherence to needle disposal and equipment sterilization procedures, and using hooded laboratory benches when handling certain specimens.

Other behaviours

Other behaviours may affect the transmission of infectious agents:

- scheduling outdoor activities at periods of low vector activity, applying insect repellents, and sleeping under bednets reduces the indirect transmission of vector-borne agents of infectious diseases like malaria
- searching oneself for attached ticks every 3 to 4 h when playing or working in tick-infested areas reduces the indirect transmission of vector-borne agents of infectious diseases like Rocky Mountain spotted fever
- avoiding sharing utensils, cups, toothbrushes, or towels reduces the indirect transmission of vehicle-borne agents of infectious diseases like mononucleosis
- wearing shoes reduces the direct transmission of infectious agents like those causing hookworm disease
- frequently bathing and regular washing of clothes in hot soapy water controls body lice
- breast feeding reduces diarrhoeal diseases in the infant, although it may transmit HIV from HIV-infected mothers
- large family sizes and crowding may facilitate airborne transmission of infectious agents in droplet nuclei for infectious diseases like tuberculosis.

Some of these other behaviours, like crowding, are conditioned by circumstances such as poverty that are not directly amenable to programmes promoting behavioural change.

A more detailed background on behaviour and behavioural modification is provided in Chapters 2.3 and 7.3 respectively.

Reverse isolation

Certain rare circumstances exist where a means of avoiding transmission of an infectious disease to a highly susceptible host is to provide reverse, or protective, isolation. Such isolation attempts to protect infection-prone patients from potentially harmful infectious agents. Reverse isolation procedures range from provision of a private room with the use of masks, gloves, and gowns by all persons entering the room, to elaborate facilities with laminar airflow rooms and sterilization of all food. Protective isolation is usually conducted for a limited time until the normal immune system recovers, a regimen of passive immunization is begun, or a bone marrow transplant has been successful. Examples of persons who may need periods of reverse isolation include those who have such diseases as X-linked agammaglobulinaemia, DiGeorge's syndrome, and severe combined immunodeficiency; or those who have received therapies, such as some forms of cancer chemotherapy, that have severely compromised the person's immune system in combating many infectious diseases.

Barriers

One tool of control that can be applied to the host is the use of barriers between the host and the infectious agent. The effectiveness of such barriers, however, may be dependent on the behaviour of the host to use them consistently. Examples of barriers include the following:

- screens, bednets (including bednets impregnated with benzyl benzoate), long-sleeved shirts and trousers (with the cuffs tucked into boots as a mechanical barrier), and repellents (such as diethyl-*m*-toluamide) to prevent transmission of malaria through the bite of infected female *Anopheles* mosquitoes

- condoms to prevent transmission of HIV and other sexually transmitted infectious agents through sexual intercourse
- masks to prevent transmission of tuberculosis through airborne droplet nuclei from patients with sputum-positive pulmonary tuberculosis.

General improvement in host resistance

Improving host resistance through general improvement of the immune system is a non-specific approach, but may be important in certain settings. Kwashiorkor, marasmus, and other forms of malnutrition debilitate the host's immune system and may make an individual more susceptible to some infectious diseases. Moreover, persons who are malnourished and succumb to an infectious disease are at higher risk of the disease being of greater severity and leading to other complications.

Malnutrition also encompasses micronutrient deficiencies. Vitamin A deficiency, for example, has been linked to higher rates of mortality associated with measles disease. Correcting vitamin A deficiency, through programmes of supplementation, fortification, and dietary modification in high-risk populations, can reduce mortality rates due to measles.

A complex interaction exists between infectious diseases, such as diarrhoeal diseases, and malnutrition. A downward spiral of infection may lead to malnutrition that, in turn, leads to more infections, and so on. If unchecked, especially in developing countries, this downward spiral can ultimately result in death.

International travel

The special situation of international travel combines many control measures applied to the host already mentioned. The increase in the numbers of travellers, the speed of travel, and the ability to reach areas previously infrequently visited have reduced the effectiveness of surveillance for infectious diseases at ports of arrival and increased infectious disease risks. Advice for prevention against infectious diseases must be both general and specific. General advice includes such issues as avoidance of eating and drinking potentially contaminated food or drink (including ice) and swimming or bathing in polluted water. Specific advice must be provided based on information about the area to be visited and may include such measures as active immunization against yellow fever, active or passive immunization against hepatitis A, chemoprophylaxis against malaria, repellents against potentially infected mosquitoes, and not walking barefoot in areas of risk for infection with hookworms *Strongyloides stercoralis* and *Strongyloides fuelleborni*. A more detailed background on international travel and health is provided in the annually updated WHO publication *International Travel and Health: Vaccination Requirements and Health Advice* (WHO 1999*b*).

Control measures applied to vectors

Vector-borne transmission is the only or main route of transmission for many infectious diseases. For example, there exist more than 100 arthropod-borne viruses that may produce clinically manifest diseases in humans. Control of vector-borne diseases include measures to change behaviour and create barriers to the susceptible host discussed above, to reduce or break the chain of transmission of the infectious agent from an infected host to the vector (which includes some of the same behaviour and barrier measures used to prevent infection in a susceptible host discussed above as well as some of the control measures applied to infected hosts discussed below), and to directly control the vector population itself. Chemical, environmental, and biological controls are the primary means of directly controlling the vector population.

Chemical control

Chemicals used in the control of vectors include minerals, natural plant products (botanicals), chlorinated hydrocarbons, organophosphates, carbamates, and fumigants. Chemical control measures include the following public health interventions.

- Spraying chemical insecticides such as organochlorine insecticides (for example, dichlorodiphenyltrichlorothane or **DDT**, and dieldrin), organophosphorus insecticides (for example, malathion and fenitrothion), and carbonate insecticides (for example, propoxur and carbaryl) to prevent malaria through control of mosquitoes.
- Spraying chemical biodegradable insecticides such as temephos (Abate®) to prevent onchocerciasis through control of *Simulium* fly vectors.
- Using traps impregnated with decamethrin to prevent African trypanosomiasis (sleeping sickness) through reduction of the population of infective species of *Glossina* (tsetse fly) vectors.
- Treating snail breeding places with chemical molluscicides to prevent schistosomiasis due to the free-swimming cercariae (larval forms) of *Schistosoma mansoni*, *Schistosoma haematobium*, and *Schistosoma japonicum* that develop in snails.
- Treating step-wells and ponds with chemical insecticides such as temephos (Abate®) to prevent dracontiasis due to infected cyclops (a crustacean copepod).
- Suppressing rat populations by poisoning, preceded or accompanied by measures to control fleas, as an additional measure to supplement environmental sanitation to control rodent populations to prevent human plague.

The use of spraying for control of mosquitoes has been complicated due to concerns of environmental contamination by chemicals such as DDT and dieldrin which have led to their being banned in many countries. In addition, the emergence of mosquito vectors resistant to the insecticides has diminished their effectiveness in many areas. New methods of application, such as ultra low-volume spraying of malathion, have reduced the amounts of insecticide used.

Environmental control

Environmental control of vectors includes the following public health interventions.

- Eliminating breeding sites of mosquito larvae by filling and draining areas where there is stagnant water and removing objects around houses that may collect water.

- Destroying the habitats of the tsetse fly vector.
- Properly implementing landfill procedures, placing lids on rubbish bins, covering food for human consumption, screening privies, cleaning up spilled food, and appropriately storing food.
- Placing cockroach and fly traps.
- Constructing rat-proof houses.
- Eliminating rodent habitats.

It is also important to note that certain development projects may have an impact on the environment that facilitates the growth of vector or intermediate host populations and results in increased infectious diseases. Construction of artificial waterways may serve as breeding sites for *Simulium* fly vectors that can transmit *Onchocerca volvulus* resulting in onchocerciasis. Irrigation schemes can foster the growth of snail intermediate hosts required for the transmission of *Schistosoma* species resulting in schistosomiasis. Carefully conducted environmental impact studies that include consideration of the impact of a construction project on the vector and intermediate host populations, and ways to modify the project to reduce such populations, are important environmental control measures.

Biological control

Biological control of vectors includes the following public health interventions.

- Introduction of predators and parasites: the introductions of *Gambusia affinis*, a small fish that feeds on mosquito larvae, and of *Coelomomyces*, a fungus, are examples of control measures that are effective against *Aëdes* mosquitoes.
- Insect growth regulators: the use of such regulators may result in death or sterility of vectors by interfering with normal insect development. An example is the use of methoprene (Altosid®) to control flood-water mosquitoes.

Control measures applied to infected humans

Control measures may be applied to infected persons in the community, institution, or hospital setting.

The hospital setting is a unique situation which requires special efforts to prevent and control nosocomial infections. Infection control programmes for hospitals should ideally include the following elements:

- an infection control committee responsible for overall co-ordination of infection control activities
- one or more infection control practitioners responsible for nosocomial disease surveillance, analysis of data, and consultation with and training of hospital staff
- a hospital epidemiologist to supervise the infection control practitioners, data collection and analysis, and carrying out of any necessary emergency infection control measures
- an engineer to direct engineering and preventive maintenance operations, especially ventilation equipment
- a sanitarian who helps to develop procedures for sanitation of water, ice, food, and proper disposal of liquid and solid wastes
- effective guidelines for patient care practices
- surveillance of patient care practices, patient infections, and environmental contamination by infectious agents
- co-ordination with other departments (microbiology laboratory, central services, housekeeping, food service, and laundry)
- vector control
- thorough investigation of problems.

Examples of specific control measures that may be applied to infected humans at the individual, institutional, and community levels are detailed below.

Chemotherapy

Treatment of persons with infectious diseases or subclinical infections may be a control tool for some infectious diseases. Such treatment may or may not have an impact on disease progression in the patient. It should be noted that rapid case detection and prompt application of appropriate chemotherapeutic agents are needed to limit infectivity.

Some important examples of control by chemotherapy include the following.

- Treatment of patients with sputum-positive pulmonary tuberculosis with appropriate multidrug therapy will usually result in sputum conversion rendering them non-infectious to others within a few weeks. Recommended treatment regimens include isoniazid combined with one or more of the following antibiotics: rifampin, streptomycin, ethambutol, and pyrazinamide. The WHO has recommended that adherence to a complete course of multidrug therapy be directly observed by another responsible person as part of the directly observed treatment, short-course (**DOTS**) global strategy for the control of tuberculosis.
- Patients with leprosy treated with appropriate multidrug therapy are considered no longer infectious within 3 months of regular and continued treatment. Recommended treatment regimens for multibacillary leprosy include the following antibiotics: rifampin, dapsone, and clofazimine.
- Treatment of patients with streptococcal sore throats with penicillin (or erythromycin for penicillin-sensitive patients) will usually no longer be infectious after 24 to 48 h.
- Patients with pertussis treated with antibiotics such as erythromycin or trimethoprim-sulfamethoxazole, although they may not affect the patient's symptoms, will usually result in the patient no longer being infectious after 5 to 7 days.

Of special note is the situation of treatment of persons who are carriers. A carrier is

> a person or animal that harbours a specific infectious agent without discernible clinical disease and serves as a potential source of infection. The carrier state may exist in an individual with an infection that is inapparent throughout its course (commonly known as healthy or asymptomatic carrier), or during the incubation period, convalescence, and postconvalescence of an individual with a clinically recognizable disease (commonly known as incubatory carrier or convalescent carrier). Under either circumstance the carrier state may be of short or long duration (temporary or transient carrier, or chronic carrier) (Chin 2000).

A chronic carrier of diphtheria, for example, may shed the infectious agent *Corynebacterium diphtheriae* for 6 months or more, but appropriate antibiotic therapy will usually promptly stop the carrier state. Another example is that of untreated patients with typhoid fever due to *Salmonella typhi.* Between 2 and 5 per cent of such patients will become permanent carriers. Treatment with appropriate antibiotics may be effective in ending the carrier state.

Antibiotic treatment may not always eliminate a carrier state for some infectious agents. For example, the treatment of persons with salmonellosis with an antibiotic may not terminate the period of communicability and can even result in emergence of antibiotic-resistant strains. However, antibiotic therapy may be still warranted under certain circumstances.

In some situations, establishing screening programmes in defined target populations for identification of asymptomatic or unrecognized infections that could be transmitted to others may be appropriate. Such screening should include the necessary follow-up with appropriate chemotherapy and counselling. An example would be screening close contacts of diphtheria patients with nose and throat cultures for the presence of *Corynebacterium diphtheriae.* Identified carriers with positive cultures should be treated with appropriate antibiotic therapy. See Chapter 12.6 on screening as a public health function.

Isolation

Isolation is the 'separation, for the period of communicability, of infected persons or animals from others in such places and under such conditions as to prevent or limit the direct or indirect transmission of the infectious agent from those infected to those who are susceptible to infection or who may spread the agent to others' (Chin 2000).

Category-specific isolation precautions in hospital settings have been summarized by Chin (2000) as quoted below. All categories have two common requirements: '(a) hands must be washed after contact with the patient or potentially contaminated articles and before taking care of another patient; and (b) articles contaminated with infectious material should be appropriately discarded or bagged and labelled before being sent for decontamination and reprocessing'. The specific categories are as follows.

- **Strict isolation** 'This category is designed to prevent transmission of highly contagious or virulent infections that may be spread by both air and contact. The specifications, in addition to those above, include a private room and the use of masks, gowns and gloves for all persons entering the room. Special ventilation requirements with the room at negative pressure to surrounding areas are desirable' (Chin 2000). Examples of infectious diseases for which patients are recommended to be placed under strict isolation precautions include the acute febrile period of Argentine haemorrhagic fever and Bolivian haemorrhagic fever caused by Junin virus and Machupo virus respectively, pharyngeal diphtheria caused by *Corynebacterium diphtheriae*, and pneumonic plague caused by *Yersinia pestis.*
- **Contact isolation** 'For less highly transmissible or serious infections, for diseases or conditions which are spread primarily by close or direct contact. In addition to the basic requirements, a private room is indicated, but patients infected with the same pathogen may share a room. Masks are indicated for those who come close to the patient, gowns are indicated if soiling is likely, and gloves are indicated for touching infectious material' (Chin 2000). Examples of infectious diseases for which patients are recommended to be placed under contact isolation precautions include cutaneous diphtheria caused by *Corynebacterium diphtheriae*, rubella, and disseminated herpes simplex caused by herpes simplex virus.
- **Respiratory isolation** 'To prevent transmission of infectious diseases over short distances through the air, a private room is indicated, but patients infected with the same organism may share a room. In addition to the basic requirements, masks are indicated for those who come in close contact with the patient; gowns and gloves are not indicated' (Chin 2000). Examples of infectious diseases for which patients are recommended to be placed under respiratory isolation precautions include pertussis caused by *Bordetella pertussis*, mumps caused by mumps virus, and patients in hospital with measles caused by measles virus through the fourth day of rash. Although isolation of patients with measles not in hospital is not practical in the general population, schoolchildren should remain out of school through at least the fourth day of rash.
- **Tuberculosis isolation** 'For patients with pulmonary tuberculosis who have a positive sputum smear or a chest X-ray that strongly suggests active tuberculosis. Specifications include use of a private room with special ventilation and closed door. In addition to the basic requirements, respirator-type masks are used by those entering the room. Gowns are used to prevent gross contamination of clothing. Gloves are not indicated' (Chin 2000).
- **Enteric precautions** 'For infections transmitted by direct or indirect contact with faeces. In addition to the basic requirements, specifications include use of a private room if patient hygiene is poor. Masks are not indicated; gowns should be used if soiling is likely and gloves are to be used for touching contaminated materials' (Chin 2000). Examples of infectious diseases for which patients are recommended to be placed under enteric precautions include acute diarrhoea caused by strains of *Escherichia coli* that are enterotoxigenic, enteroinvasive, or enteropathogenic, and patients in hospital with acute poliomyelitis caused by poliovirus. It should be noted that such enteric precautions for acute poliomyelitis patients in the home setting are of limited value since the highest risk of transmission would have already occurred during the prodromal phase of illness.
- **Drainage/secretion precautions** 'To prevent infections transmitted by direct or indirect contact with purulent material or drainage from an infected body site. A private room and masking are not indicated; in addition to the basic requirements, gowns should be used if soiling is likely and gloves should be used for touching contaminated materials' (Chin 2000). Examples of infectious diseases for which patients are recommended to be placed under drainage/secretion precautions include tularaemia with open lesions caused by *Francisella tularensis*, chlamydial genital infections caused by *Chlamydia trachomatis*, and brucellosis with draining lesions caused by *Brucella abortus*, *Brucella melitensis*, *Brucella suis*, or *Brucella canis.*

Chin (2000) also states that:

> [The] CDC has recommended that universal precautions be used consistently for all patients (in-hospital settings as well as outpatient settings) regardless of their bloodborne infection

status. This practice is based on the possibility that blood and certain body fluids (any body secretion that is obviously bloody, semen, vaginal secretions, tissue, cerebrospinal fluid, and synovial, pleural, peritoneal, pericardial, and amniotic fluids) of all patients who are considered infectious for HIV, HBV, and other bloodborne pathogens. Universal precautions are intended to prevent parenteral, mucous membrane, and non-intact skin exposures of healthcare workers to bloodborne pathogens. Protective barriers include gloves, gowns, masks and protective eyewear or face shields. A private room is indicated if patient hygiene is poor.

Quarantine of potentially infected persons

Quarantine is the 'restriction of the activities of well persons or animals who have been exposed to a case of communicable disease during its period of communicability (that is, contacts) to prevent disease transmission during the incubation period if infection should occur' (Chin 2000). Two categories of quarantine are as follows (Chin 2000).

- **Absolute or complete quarantine** The limitation of freedom of movement of those exposed to a communicable disease for a period of time not longer than the longest usual incubation period of that disease, in such manner as to prevent effective contact with those not so exposed.
- **Modified quarantine** A selective, partial limitation of freedom of movement of contacts, commonly on the basis of known or presumed differences in susceptibility and related to the danger of disease transmission. It may be designed to accommodate particular situations. Examples are exclusion of children from school, exemption of immune persons from provisions applicable to susceptible persons, or restriction of military populations to the post or to quarters. It includes: personal surveillance, the practice of close medical or other supervision of contacts to permit prompt recognition of infection or illness but without restricting their movements; and segregation, the separation of some part of a group of persons or domestic animals from the others for special consideration, control or observation; removal of susceptible children to homes of immune persons; or establishment of a sanitary boundary to protect uninfected from infected portions of a population.

Examples of diseases where quarantine may be considered include the following.

- Pneumonic plague: persons who have been in the same household or in face-to-face contact with patients with pneumonic plague and who do not accept chemoprophylaxis should be placed under absolute quarantine with strict isolation, including careful surveillance, for 7 days.
- Measles: although absolute quarantine is impractical, a modified quarantine is recommended in settings where young children are living in dormitories, wards, or institutions. When measles occurs in an institutional setting, strict segregation of infants is recommended.
- Lassa fever: close personal surveillance of all close contacts is recommended. Such persons include those who live or are in close contact with lassa fever patients as well as laboratory personnel testing specimens from such patients.

Restriction of activities

Controlling infectious disease transmission by restriction of the activities of a person in the community who is potentially infectious to others may be appropriate in certain circumstances. Examples of this include the following.

- Individuals with a diarrhoeal disease should be excluded from handling food and caring for patients in hospital, children, and elderly persons.
- Known carriers of *Salmonella typhi* should be excluded from foodhandling and care of patients.
- Persons with staphylococcal disease should avoid contact with debilitated persons and infants.
- Persons with rubella should be excluded from school or work for seven days after the onset of rash and from contact with pregnant women.

Behavioural change

Behaviour change in an infected person to protect others may be difficult to accomplish. However, this should be considered in preventing the transmission of infectious agents in the following situations.

Sexual behaviour

Examples of infectious agents transmitted through sexual intercourse are discussed in the section above on control measures applied to the host and in more detail in Chapter 9.13. Individuals who suspect that they may have a sexually transmitted disease should be encouraged to have health-seeking behaviours. Persons with a sexually transmissible infectious agent should be treated and co-operate with health officials to trace their sexual contacts. Patients with diseases such as lymphogranuloma venereum and syphilis, for example, should refrain from sexual contact until all lesions are healed. HIV-infected individuals should be counselled to treat genital ulcer disease promptly since such disease may increase transmissibility of HIV. Also, HIV-infected persons should avoid sexual intercourse with HIV-negative individuals or, if having sexual intercourse with HIV-negative individuals, use methods to reduce the risk of transmission, including condoms and a spermicide. For a more detailed overview of HIV and AIDS see Chapter 9.14.

Intravenous drug use behaviour

Besides counselling to abstain from intravenous drug use and establishing drug rehabilitation programmes to help individuals who wish to abstain, promoting behaviour change in the use of injection equipment is important. Discouraging the sharing of injection equipment and education on methods for the decontamination of needles and syringes for intravenous drug use reduces risks of transmission of infectious agents through contaminated injection equipment.

Food preparation behaviour

Individuals who should be restricted from handling food (e.g. carriers of *Salmonella typhi*) should be counselled regarding their condition and potential to infect others if they handle food. Foodhandlers who have an infectious disease that is potentially transmissible through the vehicle-borne means of food should be discouraged from handling food for others. The importance of handwashing, especially after defecation and before handling food, should be stressed.

Other behaviours that may reduce risk of transmission of infectious agents to other persons include the following:

- patients with infectious diseases directly transmitted by droplet spread or airborne transmitted by droplet nuclei (e.g. patients with sputum-positive tuberculosis) should cover their mouth and nose when coughing or sneezing
- persons suffering from dracontiasis should avoid entering a source of drinking water if they have an active ulcer or blister
- patients with the vector-borne disease of African trypanosomiasis (sleeping sickness) with trypanosomes in their blood should prevent tsetse flies from biting
- individuals who are infected with HIV or who have sexual and other behaviours that have placed them at increased risk for HIV infection should not donate blood, plasma, tissues, cells, semen for artificial insemination, or organs for transplantation.

Control measures applied to animals

'An infection or infectious disease transmissible under natural conditions from vertebrate animals to humans' is a zoonosis (Chin 2000). A detailed approach to zoonoses is given in the comprehensive *CRC Handbook of Zoonoses* (Beran and Steele 1994). Many approaches are used in the control of zoonoses, including the following.

Active immunization

An example of an infectious disease in animals in which some control can be achieved through immunization in selected animal populations is rabies. The reservoir of the rabies virus is varied and includes dogs, foxes, wolves, skunks, raccoons, and bats. Preventive measures include efforts to vaccinate all dogs.

Other examples of immunization of animals under certain conditions include immunization of young goats and sheep using a live attenuated strain of *Brucella melitensis* and calves using a strain of *B. abortus* in areas of high endemicity for brucellosis, and immunization of animals at risk for acquiring infection with *Bacillus anthracis* that could be transmitted to humans causing anthrax.

Restriction or reduction

The example of rabies can also be used to illustrate the use of restriction or reduction of an animal population to help control an infectious disease. Chin (2000) recommends a programme to:

> educate pet owners and the public that restrictions for dogs and cats are important (for example, that pets be leashed in congested areas when not confined on owner's premises; that strange-acting or sick animals of any species, domestic or wild, may be dangerous and should not be picked up or handled; that it is necessary to report such animals and animals that have bitten a person or another animal to the police and/or the local health department; that confinement and observation of such animals is a preventive measure against rabies); and that wild animals should not be kept as pets... Euthanize immediately non-immunized dogs or cats bitten by known rabid animals; if detention is elected, hold the animal in an approved secure pound or kennel for at least 6 months under veterinary supervision, and immunize against rabies 30 days before release. If previously immunized, reimmunize and detain (leashing and confinement) for at least 45 days... Cooperative programmes with wildlife conservation authorities to reduce fox, skunk, raccoon, and other terrestrial wildlife hosts of sylvatic rabies may be used in circumscribed enzootic areas near campsites and areas of human habitation. If such focal depopulation is undertaken, it must be maintained to prevent repopulation from the periphery.

In epizootic situations:

> in urban areas of the United States and other developed countries, strict enforcement of regulations requiring collection, detention and euthanasia of ownerless and stray dogs, and of non-immunized dogs found off owners' premises, and control of the dog population by castration, spaying or drugs have been effective in breaking transmission cycles. (Chin 2000)

Other examples of restricting or reducing animal populations include the following:

- rat-proofing dwellings and reduction of the rat population to prevent rat bites that may transmit the infectious agents *Streptobacillus moniliformis* and *Spirillum minus* causing the rat-bite fevers of streptobacillosis and spirillosis respectively
- rat suppression by poisoning (after achieving flea control) in rodent populations with a high potential for epizootic plague
- elimination of animals infected with *Brucella abortus*, *Brucella melitensis*, *Brucella suis*, and *Brucella canis* by segregation or slaughter to prevent brucellosis
- slaughtering dairy cattle that test positive for infection with *Mycobacterium bovis*, the infectious agent of bovine tuberculosis.

Chemoprophylaxis and chemotherapy

Psittacosis is an example of a zoonosis controlled by chemoprophylaxis or chemotherapy in selected animal populations. The infectious agent, *Chlamydia psittaci*, can be directly transmitted to humans from infected birds when the dried droppings, secretions, or dust from the feathers of such infected birds are inhaled. Imported psittacine species of birds should be placed under quarantine and receive an appropriate antibiotic chemotherapeutic regimen such as chlortetracycline administered in their feed for 30 days.

Another example is chemoprophylaxis in selected dogs at high risk of infection with *Echinococcus granulosus*. This infectious agent can be transmitted to humans through hand to mouth transmission of the tapeworm eggs from dog faeces causing echinococcosis due to *E. granulosus*, or cystic hydatid disease. Such high-risk dogs should periodically receive antihelminth treatment with a chemotherapeutic agent such as praziquantel (Biltricide®).

Control measures applied to the environment

Control measures applied to the environment are designed to interrupt the routes of transmission by which an infectious agent may be spread through the environment. Just as the routes of transmission are varied, so too are the control methods that can be applied. Control measures that affect transmission that can be applied to the host, agents, vectors, infected humans, and other animals are reviewed elsewhere in this chapter. Environmental factors may also have a direct impact on the host, agent, or vector. For example, low humidity may predispose to certain infections due to a greater permeability of mucus membranes in the host; cold, dry climates inhibit development of the infective larvae agent of hookworm disease; and higher altitudes and colder climates limit the mosquito vector.

The recognition of the relationship between disease and filth led to a sanitary revolution in industrialized countries that markedly reduced infectious diseases even before the arrival of the antibiotic era. Improved methods for storing and preserving food, better housing, and smaller families with a resultant decrease in the risk of infections in infancy all contributed to reductions in infant and child mortality rates.

This section focuses on general environmental control measures not mentioned elsewhere. Some of these methods, such as provision of safe water, have the potential to prevent several different infectious diseases and significantly reduce rates of disease in the community.

Provision of safe water

It has been estimated that about 1.3 billion people in the developing world lack access to clean and plentiful water (World Bank 1993). Contaminated drinking water, sometimes the result of poorly designed or maintained systems of sewerage, may lead to the water-borne indirect transmission of such infectious agents as *Giardia lamblia* causing giardiasis, pathogenic serotypes of *Salmonella* causing salmonellosis, and *Cryptosporidium* species causing cryptosporidosis.

Purification of water can occur though natural methods or human intervention. Examples of natural methods that contribute to water purification include the processes of evaporation and condensation, filtration through the earth, plant growth, aeration, and reduction and oxidation of organic material by bacteria. Purification of water for public consumption is conventionally done through such processes as coagulation of colloids by aluminium salts or with other techniques, filtration through such materials as coal, sand, or diatomaceous earth, and disinfection with such chemicals as chlorine derivatives. In special situations, boiling and distillation can be used for purification (Solomon and Fraser 1998).

Proper disposal of faeces

It has been estimated that nearly 2 billion people in the developing world do not have an adequate system for proper disposal of faeces (World Bank 1993). Infectious agents in faeces that may result in infectious diseases include poliovirus causing poliomyelitis, *Shigella dysenteriae*, *Shigella flexneri*, *Shigella boydii*, and *Shigella sonnei* causing shigellosis, and *Entamoeba histolytica* causing amoebiasis.

Infectious agents in faeces may be transmitted by the direct transmission route (including the faecal–oral mode), the vehicle-borne route (including water as noted in the previous section), and the vector-borne route (including the simple mechanism of flies carrying infected faeces on their feet). Public health environmental control measures to interrupt these routes of transmission by ensuring the proper disposal of faeces include appropriate on-site disposal through such means as properly constructed sanitary privies in rural areas with no sewerage systems, on-site disposal of domestic wastewater (such as use of septic tanks or cesspools), and sewerage systems with treatment of wastewater. Wastewater treatment may include preliminary treatment, sedimentation, chemical coagulation and flocculation, biological treatment (such as activated sludge units and trickling filters), stabilization ponds, sludge management, and disinfection (usually with chlorine) of effluents discharged into drinking, bathing, or shellfish-growing waters. The importance of personal health-promoting behaviours of using toilets, keeping toilets clean, and handwashing after defecation are a part of control efforts aimed at the proper disposal of faeces.

Food sanitation

Food-borne infectious diseases remain a problem in both industrialized and developing countries. In the United States alone, an estimated 76 million persons are affected each year resulting in some 5000 deaths annually. Significant food-borne outbreaks and sporadic cases continue to occur due to factors such as the following.

- Contamination of meat, poultry, and eggs with infectious agents, including pathogenic serotypes of *Salmonella*, *Yersinia pseudotuberculosis*, *Yersinia entercolitica*, and *Listeria monocytogenes*.
- Problems in food storage, handling, and preparation in commercial eating places and in homes.
- Larger and more centralized production and processing facilities, coupled with increasingly extensive distribution networks, which may result in transmission of infectious agents to many persons if a commercial product becomes contaminated.

Industrialized countries have significantly reduced the transmission of some infectious agents through major public health programmes in food sanitation, including inspection of eating and drinking establishments, meat and poultry inspection, shellfish sanitation, and promotion of adequate cooking, canning techniques, and refrigeration (Solomon and Fraser 1998).

Examples of vehicle-borne indirect transmission of infectious agents through food that can be controlled though a comprehensive public health food sanitation programme include the following.

- Pathogenic serotypes of *Salmonella* transmitted by ingesting food made from infected animals or contaminated by the infectious agent in faeces that may cause salmonellosis. Control is achieved through '(a) handwashing before, during, and after food preparation; (b) refrigerating prepared foods in small containers; (c) thoroughly cooking all foodstuffs derived from animal sources, particularly poultry, pork, egg products, and meat dishes; (d) avoiding recontamination within the kitchen after cooking is completed; and (e) maintaining a sanitary kitchen and protecting prepared foods against rodent and insect contanimation ... Inspect for sanitation and adequately supervise abattoirs, food-processing plants, feed-blending mills, egg-grading stations, and butcher shops' (Chin 2000).

- *Staphylococcus aureus* causing staphylococcal food intoxication by ingesting food containing the staphylococcal enterotoxin. Control is achieved through means to '(a) educate food handlers in strict food hygiene, sanitation and cleanliness of kitchens, proper temperature control, handwashing, cleaning of fingernails; and to the danger of working with exposed skin, nose, and eye infections and uncovered wounds; (b) reduce food handling time (initial preparation to service) to an absolute minimum, with no more than 4 hours at ambient temperature. Keep perishable foods hot (> 60°C) or cold (below 10°C; best is less than 4°C) in shallow containers and covered, if they are to be stored for more than 2 hours; and (c) temporarily exclude people with boils, abscesses, and other purulent lesions of hands, face, or nose from food handling' (Chin 2000).
- *Trichinella spiralis* transmitted by ingesting raw or improperly cooked meat or meat products, mainly pork, containing infectious encysted larvae that may cause trichinosis. Control is achieved through means to '(a) educate the public on the need to cook all fresh pork and pork products and meat from wild animals at a temperature and for a time sufficient to allow all parts to reach at least 71°C, or until meat changes from pink to gray, which allows a sufficient margin of safety. This should be done unless it has been established that these meat products have been processed either by heating, curing, freezing, or irradiation adequate to kill trichinae; (b) grind pork in a separate grinder or clean the grinder thoroughly before and after processing other meats; (c) adopt regulations to encourage commercial irradiation processing of pork products. Testing carcasses for infection with a digestion technique is useful. Immunodiagnosis of pigs with an approved ELISA test is also useful; (c) adopt and enforce regulations that allow only certified trichinae-free pork to be used in raw pork products that have a cooked appearance or in products that traditionally are not heated sufficiently to kill trichinea during final preparation; and (d) adopt laws and regulations to require and enforce the cooking of garbage and offal before feeding to swine' (Chin 2000).

Milk sanitation

Milk may be a vehicle for indirect transmission of such infectious agents as: *Mycobacterium bovis* causing tuberculosis, *Corynebacterium diphtheriae* causing diphtheria, *Listeria monocytogenes* causing listeriosis, and *Campylobacter jejuni* and *Campylobacter coli* causing *Campylobacter* enteritis.

Public health control measures to break the chain of transmission include the following:

- mechanization and sanitization of milking processes
- refrigeration of milk
- pasteurization of milk by high-temperature short-time, batch, ultra-pasteurization, or ultra-high-temperature methods
- monitoring milk quality by testing for bacteria using a standard bacterial plate count, by testing for density of coliform organisms, and by use of the phosphatase test to assay for pasteurization
- periodic testing of cows for tuberculosis and brucellosis.

The use of raw milk for human consumption and postpasteurization contamination may result in outbreaks of milk-borne diseases.

Design of facilities and equipment

The design and proper maintenance of buildings, rooms, and equipment can help break the chain of transmission of infectious agents. Laminar airflow hoods in laboratory workbenches, ventilation systems in hospitals, and disposable intravenous equipment are examples of systems designed to reduce risk of transmission. Routine maintenance needed to retain the original design standards for control of transmission of infectious agents include replacement of air filters, cleaning of cooling towers, monitoring of positive pressure rooms and airlocks, and replacement of indwelling peripheral venous catheters.

Examples of infectious agents whose transmission can be reduced through proper design and maintenance include the following.

- *Legionella* species, the infectious agents responsible for legionellosis, are usually transmitted through airborne transmission via aerosol production. Transmission of the agent from cooling towers can be reduced by periodically cleaning off any scale or sediment, routinely using biocides to kill slime-forming organisms, and draining such towers when not in use.
- *Staphylococcus aureus*, the infectious agent responsible for staphylococcal disease in medical and surgical wards, can be controlled by enforcing strict aseptic technique, including procedures to change intravenous infusion sites at least every 48 hours and replace indwelling peripheral venous catheters every 72 hours.
- *Bacillus anthracis*, the infectious agent responsible for anthrax, can be transmitted, among other ways, through inhalation of anthrax spores. Proper design of industrial plants that handle raw animal fibres include providing facilities for adequate ventilation and control of dust, washing and changing clothes after work, and eating away from the places of work.

Other methods

In addition to the environmental methods of control of transmission of infectious agents already mentioned, the following methods, some specific and some general, should also be noted.

- Improvement of housing conditions to reduce crowding (as measured by the number of persons per room and not total population density) is a general measure that can reduce the transmission of infectious agents, especially direct transmission from direct contact or direct projection (droplet spray).
- Improvement in working conditions can affect the risk of infectious disease. For example, control of particulate matter by proper ventilation in occupations such as textile mill workers, metal grinders, pottery factory workers, etc. can reduce inflammation of the lungs and thus decrease the risk of developing tuberculosis. Excessive physical exertion and the stress of exhausting work can also increase the risk of tuberculosis.
- Improved irrigation and agricultural practices and removing vegetation or draining and filling of snail-breeding sites can reduce or eliminate the freshwater snail hosts of such infectious agents as *Schistosoma mansoni*, *Schistosoma haematobium*, and *Schistosoma japonicum* that cause schistosomiasis in humans.

- Adequate screening of blood, serum, plasma, tissues, or organs can break the chain of vehicle-borne transmission from such biological products. Examples include screening for hepatitis B surface antigen and HIV antibodies in donated blood to prevent transmission of hepatitis B and HIV respectively.
- Installation of screened living and sleeping quarters and the use of bednets, including bednets impregnated with a synthetic pyrethroid such as permethrin, can reduce exposure to mosquitoes infected with the infectious agents of malaria.

Control measures applied to the agent

Control of some infectious diseases can be achieved through means that remove the infectious agents from the environment or inactivate the agents. Physical measures (such as heat, cold, ultraviolet light, and ionizing radiation) and chemical measures (such as liquid disinfectants and antiseptics, gases, and chlorination) can be used. Examples of control measures applied to infectious agents include the following.

- **Cleaning** is the removal of infectious agents from surfaces through such physical actions as vacuum cleaning or washing and scrubbing using soap or detergent and hot water. Cleaning also helps remove organic materials that might support the growth or survival of infectious agents.
- **Cooling** may inhibit bacterial multiplication, and some infectious agents, such as *Trichinella* cysts and *Taenia solium* larvae (cysticerci), can be killed by freezing temperatures.
- **Pasteurization** is the heating to a temperature of 75°C for 30 min to kill pathogenic vegetative bacteria. It does not inactivate bacterial spores. Pasteurization is a commonly used process to help ensure safety of milk and to prolong its storage quality.
- **Disinfection** is the reduction or killing of vegetative harmful bacterial infectious agents outside the body or on objects. Disinfection may not inactivate all bacterial spores and viruses. Disinfectants are used to eliminate pathogenic bacteria from the skin surface and from contaminated inanimate surfaces and include alcohols, halogens such as iodine and chlorine, surface-active compounds such as the quaternary ammonium compound benzalkonium chloride, phenolics, alkylating agents such as glutaraldehyde and formaldehyde. Antiseptics are a class of disinfectant that can be applied on body surfaces; they have a lower toxicity than environmental disinfectants and are usually less effective in killing micro-organisms.
- **Sterilization** is the complete removal or killing of all infectious agents in or on an object. Sterilization of equipment for surgery and wound dressings, during the parenteral administration of drugs, vaccines, or nutrients, during catheterization, and during dental work are all important means of controlling infectious diseases by killing infectious agents. Sterilization can be accomplished using fire, steam (such as in an autoclave), heated air, certain gases (such as ethylene oxide), ultraviolet light, ionizing radiation, liquid chemicals, and filtration. The method of sterilization chosen depends on the type of equipment to be sterilized.

The use of sterilized disposable equipment, such as disposable needles, syringes, and catheters, has the potential to reduce the risk of transmission of infectious agents. However, it must be ensured that such equipment is disposed of properly and is not reused. For example, disposable syringes cannot be properly resterilized because the plastic from which they are made cannot withstand the heat necessary for sterilization. Technologies such as the single-use disposable needle and syringe developed for immunization programmes help to ensure that such disposable equipment is not reused.

Control and prevention programmes

The preceding sections have considered the issues and given examples of control measures for infectious diseases at individual, institutional, and community levels and of the tools for control directed at the host, routes of transmission, and the agent. Control and prevention programmes using these tools must be developed according to a number of factors including the risk of disease, the magnitude of disease burden (as measured by mortality, degree of disability, morbidity, and economic costs), the feasibility of control strategies, the cost of control measures, the effectiveness of such measures (on current levels of disease and impact on future cases or outbreaks), the adverse effects or complications of the control measures, and the availability of resources. Public heath planning for the control of infectious diseases must consider these issues to design optimal rationally based control and prevention programmes.

The tools of disease surveillance for recognition and evaluation of the patterns of disease can provide the information on the risk and magnitude of disease burden to individuals, persons in institutions, subgroups of populations, and the community at large. Establishment and maintenance of the infrastructure for surveillance, including a system for the reporting of notifiable infectious diseases and unusual events, must be a high priority.

Feasibility of possible control and prevention strategies must be assessed through operational research, pilot projects, or from field experience. The fact that a particular measure can help control a disease does not mean it can be applied on a sufficient scale to have the desired impact. The cost of control activities (in both human and material resources) can be assessed through costing studies that can also provide the data needed to conduct more rigorous cost–benefit and cost-effectiveness analyses. A costly measure, even if it provides a high degree of control for an infectious disease, may not be affordable to the society or reasonable to apply in the light of other less expensive alternative strategies. Effectiveness of control measures may be assessed through epidemiological studies to find out their impact on reduction in the incidence or prevalence of disease.

The availability of resources for prevention and control programmes forces public health planners to set priorities by taking into account all these factors and then designing programmes that have maximum impact within available resources. Planners have a responsibility to mobilize additional necessary resources by raising public awareness and generating political will. Effective communication of disease burden and the results achievable through well-managed and effective control programmes can be a powerful tool for advocacy. Ideally, communities should actively participate in the planning, execution, and evaluation of public health programmes.

Prevention effectiveness is 'the measure of the impact on health (including effectiveness, safety, and cost) of prevention policies, programmes, and practices. The assessment of prevention effectiveness is the ongoing process of applying evaluation tools to prevention practices' (CDC 1995). Recognizing that systems for assessing the effectiveness of prevention strategies (including prevention strategies for infectious diseases) are weak or non-existent in both developing and industrialized countries alike, the CDC has suggested the following objectives for prevention effectiveness activities: 'evaluate the impact of prevention, use results of evaluation research to establish programme priorities, and establish or apply standardized methods to *compare* the benefits and effectiveness of alternative prevention strategies' (CDC 1995).

The current situation of international migration of many people worldwide presents an additional complexity to the design of programmes for the control of infectious diseases. Pertinent issues include refugee camps, legal status of migrants in recipient countries, and temporary return migration. Public health officials must consider the most effective mix of combined control measures applied to the host, agent, and routes of transmission when designing suitable control and prevention programmes (Gellert 1993).

International commerce and transportation are specific areas of concern for public health infectious disease control programmes, especially as the speed of travel has increased. The tools of control include measures such as spraying insecticides effective against mosquito vectors of malaria in aircraft before departure, in transit, or on arrival, and rat-proofing or periodic fumigation to control rats on ships, docks, and warehouses to prevent plague. Specific international control measures relating to aircraft, ships, and land transportation for infectious diseases have been specified in the *International Health Regulations* (WHO 1983).

The challenge facing infectious disease control programmes is to design an optimal set of interventions at local, institutional, and community levels supported and accepted by the political leadership and the persons to whom these measures are applied.

Eradication

A unique endpoint in the control of infectious diseases is that of eradication. Eradication is the cessation of all transmission of infection by extermination of the infectious agent. To date, only one infectious disease, smallpox, has been eradicated. The WHO World Health Assembly in May 1980 confirmed its global eradication some 3 years after the last naturally acquired case of smallpox in October 1977 (Fenner *et al.* 1988). The magnitude of this accomplishment is appreciated when one realizes that in the early 1950s it was estimated 50 million cases of smallpox still occurred each year in the world, some 150 years after Edward Jenner performed the first vaccination and wrote: 'it now becomes too manifest to admit of controversy, that the annihilation of the Small Pox, the most dreadful scourge of the human species, must be the final result of this practice' (Fenner *et al.* 1988).

The goal of global eradication has been set by the World Health Assembly for two other infectious diseases, poliomyelitis caused by wild poliovirus and dracontiasis, the latter caused by the infectious agent *Dracunculus medinensis*. A high level of sustained political will, aggressively applied disease surveillance, and effective control measures are the required elements to achieve eradication of the infectious agents for these diseases.

Impressive progress has been made towards the global eradication of poliomyelitis since the 1988 World Health Assembly set the goal for its eradication by the year 2000. The entire region of the Americas has succeeded in interrupting transmission of indigenous wild poliovirus since August 1991. The Western Pacific region has succeeded in interrupting transmission since 1997. In other regions of the world, countries endemic for poliomyelitis are carrying out the necessary strategies to eradicate the poliovirus. Poliomyelitis control measures that will lead to eradication include the following.

- Achieving and maintaining high levels of routine coverage of infants with at least three doses of oral polio vaccine.
- Mass application of oral polio vaccine in countries where poliomyelitis is endemic through national immunization days, usually by providing oral polio vaccine to every child less than 5 years of age twice each year, separated by 4 to 6 weeks, and conducted during the low season of poliovirus transmission.
- 'Mopping-up' operations after the use of national immunization days has reduced transmission of disease to defined focal geographical areas, usually by providing oral polio vaccine house-to-house to all children less than 5 years of age on two occasions separated by 4 to 6 weeks.
- Aggressive action-oriented surveillance for acute flaccid paralysis. Such surveillance includes case investigation, a laboratory network for isolation and characterization of polioviruses in suspect cases of poliomyelitis and people in close contact with them, and limited outbreak response immunization providing one house-to-house round of oral polio vaccine to children less than 5 years of age living in the same village or neighbourhood as the patient.

Significant strides in the eradication of dracontiasis have also been made. Over the last decade the total number of dracontiasis cases have declined by more than 95 per cent. The disease is now limited to only certain parts of some African countries in a band between the Sahara desert and the equator. India was certified as dracontiasis free in February 2000. Dracontiasis control measures that are leading to ultimate eradication include the following.

- Establishing a national programme office, conducting baseline surveys, and preparing and refining a national plan of action.
- Educating the population in endemic areas that the source of guinea-worm comes from their drinking water.
- Ensuring that persons with blisters or emerging worms do not enter sources of drinking water through behaviour changes and by converting step-wells into draw-wells.
- Promoting the boiling or filtering of water through a fine mesh cloth to remove copepods. Treating drinking water with chlorine or iodine will also kill the copepods and infective larvae.
- Providing non-infected water through construction of wells or rainwater catchments.
- In selected endemic villages, controlling copepod populations with temephos (Abate®) insecticide placed in reservoirs, tanks, ponds, and step-wells.
- Implementing an intensified surveillance and aggressive case-containment strategy as programmes get close to achieving eradication.

The eradication of a disease requires a unique set of conditions, including the following: the infectious agent must have a defined accessible reservoir; affordable and effective control measures that can interrupt the chain of infection directed at the host, agent, or route of transmission; a surveillance mechanism adequate to monitor and ultimately certify the disappearance of the infectious agent.

It is likely that measles may be targeted for global eradication in the future. Some countries and geographical regions have already targeted measles for elimination—a term sometimes used to describe the eradication of a disease from a large geographical area. Other diseases that may potentially be targeted for eradication in the future include mumps, rubella, hepatitis B, leprosy, and diphtheria.

Emerging infectious diseases

New, emerging, and re-emerging infectious diseases have become a focus for the attention of public health prevention and control programmes in both industrialized and developing countries. Such infectious diseases have thwarted any expectation that infectious diseases will soon be eliminated as public health problems and resulted in a widening spectrum of diseases, many of which were once thought to be almost conquered. Krause has reflected on this as follows:

> Microbes and vectors swim in the evolutionary stream, and they swim faster than we do. Bacteria reproduce every 30 minutes. For them, a millennium is compressed into a fortnight. They are fleet of foot, and the pace of our research must keep up with them, or they will overtake us. Microbes were here on earth 2 billion years before humans arrived, learning every trick for survival, and it is likely that they will be here 2 billion years after we depart. (Krause 1998)

Many factors contribute to the emergence of new diseases or the re-emergence of those previously known (Lederberg *et al.* 1992; CDC 1994; Murphy 1994), including the following.

- Human demographic change by which persons begin to live in previously uninhabited remote areas of the world and are exposed to new environmental sources of infectious agents, insects, and animals. A more detailed overview of population dynamics as a determinant of health and disease is provided in Chapter 7.2.
- Breakdowns of sanitary and other public health measures in overcrowded cities and in situations of civil unrest and war.
- Economic development and changes in the use of land, including deforestation, reforestation, and urbanization.
- Other human behaviours, such as increased use of child-care facilities, sexual and drug use behaviours, and patterns of outdoor recreation.
- International travel and commerce that quickly transport people and goods vast distances.
- Changes in food processing and handling, including foods prepared from many different individual animals and transported great distances.
- Evolution of pathogenic infectious agents by which they may infect new hosts, produce toxins, or adapt by responding to changes in the host immunity.
- Development of resistance of infectious agents such as *Mycobacterium tuberculosis* and *Neisseria gonorrhoeae* to chemoprophylactic or chemotherapeutic medicines.
- Resistance of the vectors of vector-borne infectious diseases to pesticides.
- Immunosuppression of persons due to medical treatments or new diseases that result in infectious diseases caused by agents not usually pathogenic in healthy hosts.
- Deterioration in surveillance systems for infectious diseases, including laboratory support, to detect new or emerging disease problems at an early stage.

Examples of emerging infectious disease threats include the following.

- Toxic shock syndrome, due to the infectious toxin-producing strains of *Staphylococcus aureus*, illustrates how a new technology yielding a new product, superabsorbent tampons, can create the circumstances favouring the emergence of a new infectious disease threat.
- Lyme disease, due to the infectious spirochete *Borrelia burgdorferi*, illustrates how changes in the ecology, including reforestation, increasing deer populations, and suburban migration of the population, can result in the emergence of a new microbial threat that has now become one of the most prevalent vector-borne diseases in the United States.
- Shigellosis, giardiasis, and hepatitis A are examples of emerging diseases that have become threats to staff and children in child-care centres as the use of such centres has increased due to changes in the work patterns of societies.
- Opportunistic infections, such as pneumocystis pneumonia caused by *Pneumocystis carinii*, chronic cryptosporidiosis caused by *Cryptosporidium* species, and disseminated cytomegalovirus infections, illustrate emerging disease threats to the increasing number of persons who are immunosuppressed because of cancer chemotherapy, organ transplantation, or HIV infection.
- Foodborne infections such as diarrhoea caused by the enterohaemorrhagic strain 0157:H7 of *Escherichia coli* and waterborne infections such as gastrointestinal disease due to *Cryptosporidium* species are examples of emerging disease threats that have arisen due to such factors as changes in diet, food processing, globalization of the food supply, and contamination of municipal water supplies.
- Hantavirus pulmonary syndrome, first detected in the United States in 1993 and caused by a previously unrecognized hantavirus, illustrates how exposure to certain kinds of infected rodents can result in an emerging infectious disease.
- Nipah virus disease, first detected in Malaysia in 1999 and caused by a previously unrecognized paramyxovirus, demonstrates how close contact with pigs can result in an emerging infectious disease.
- Emergence of the new toxigenic *Vibrio cholerae* 0139 strain of cholera in Asia is an example of a new strain of an infectious agent for which there is no protection from prior infection with other strains or with current vaccines.

Antimicrobial drug resistance as a major factor in the emergence and re-emergence of infectious diseases deserves special attention. Although significant reductions in infectious disease mortality have occurred since the introduction of antimicrobials for general use in the 1940s, antimicrobial drug resistance has emerged because of their widespread use in humans.

> Drugs that once seemed invincible are losing their effectiveness for a wide range of community-acquired infections, including tuberculosis, gonorrhoea, pneumococcal infections (a leading cause of otitis media, pneumonia, and meningitis), and for hospital-acquired enterococcal and staphylococcal infections. Resistance to antiviral (for example, amantadine-resistant influenza virus and acyclovir-resistant herpes simplex), antifungal (for example, azole-resistant *Candida* species), and antiprotozoal (for example, metronidazole-resistant *Trichomonas vaginalis*) drugs is also emerging. Drug-resistant malaria has spread to nearly all areas of the world where malaria occurs. Concern has also arisen over strains of HIV resistant to antiviral drugs. Increased microbial resistance has resulted in prolonged hospital admissions and higher death rates from infections; has required much more expensive, and often more toxic, drugs or drug combinations (even for common infections); and has resulted in higher health care costs. (CDC 1994).

Antimicrobial drug resistance has also emerged because of the use of antimicrobials in domesticated animals. For example, the use of fluoroquinolones in poultry has created a reservoir of quinolone-resistant *Campylobacter jejuni* that has now been isolated in humans.

An aggressive public health response to these new, emerging, and re-emerging infectious disease threats must be made to characterize them better and to mount an effective response for their control. For example, the outbreak of West Nile fever in New York City and surrounding areas in 1999 demonstrates how a viral encephalitis, initially classified as St Louis encephalitis and later confirmed to be due to West Nile-like virus, can reach far beyond its normal setting.

The WHO has outlined the following high-priority areas (WHO 1995*a*):

- strengthen global surveillance of infectious diseases
- establish national and international infrastructures to recognize, report, and respond to new disease threats
- further develop applied research on diagnosis, epidemiology, and control of emerging infectious diseases
- strengthen the international capacity for infectious disease prevention and control.

Another unfortunate source of a new or emerging disease threat is the spectre of biological warfare or bioterrorism, especially in an age where terrorist acts are frequent events (Christopher *et al.* 1997). Several countries are developing rapid-response capability to deal with such contingencies.

Only through worldwide concerted action will the effort to control infectious disease be effective. We have now entered an era where, as Nobel Laureate Dr Joshua Lederberg has stated, 'The microbe that felled one child in a distant continent yesterday can reach yours today and seed a global pandemic tomorrow' (quoted in CDC 1994). As Hans Zinsser stated over 60 years ago:

> Infectious disease is one of the few genuine adventures left in the world. The dragons are all dead and the lance grows rusty in the chimney corner ... About the only sporting proposition that remains unimpaired by the relentless domestication of a once free-living human species is the war against those ferocious little fellow creatures, which lurk in the dark corners and stalk us in the bodies of rats, mice and all kinds of domestic animals; which fly and crawl with the insects, and waylay us in our food and drink and even in our love. (Hans Zinsser 1934, quoted in Murphy 1994)

References

ACIP (Immunization Practices Advisory Committee) (1994). General recommendations on immunization. *Morbidity and Mortality Weekly Report*, **43**, RR1.

Beran, G.W. and Steele, J.H. (ed.) (1994). *CRC handbook of zoonoses* (2nd edn). CRC Press, Boca Raton, FL.

Brillman, J.C. and Quenzer, R.W. (ed.) (1998). *Infectious disease in emergency medicine* (2nd edn). Lippincott–Raven, Philadelphia, PA.

CDC (Centers for Disease Control and Prevention) (1994). *Addressing emerging infectious disease threats: a prevention strategy for the United States*. CDC, Atlanta, GA.

CDC (Centers for Disease Control and Prevention) (1995). *Prevention effectiveness: making prevention a practical reality*. CDC, Atlanta, GA.

CDC (Centers for Disease Control and Prevention) (1999). Summary of notifiable diseases, United States, 1998. *Morbidity and mortality weekly report*, **47** (53).

Chin, J. (ed.) (2000). *Control of communicable diseases manual* (17th edn). American Public Health Association, Washington, DC.

Committee on Infectious Diseases (2000). *American Academy of Pediatrics: report of the committee on infectious diseases* (25th edn). American Academy of Pediatrics, Elk Grove Village, IL.

Christopher, G.W., Cieslak, T.J., Pavlin, J.A., *et al.* (1997). Biological warfare: a historical perspective. *Journal of the American Medical Association*, **278**, 412–17.

Evans, A.S. and Kaslow, R.A. (ed.) (1989). *Viral infections of humans: Epidemiology and control* (4th edn). Plenum Press, New York.

Evans, A.S. and Brachman, P.S. (ed.) (1998). *Bacterial infections of humans: epidemiology and control* (3rd edn). Plenum Press, New York.

Feigin, R.D. and Cherry, J.D. (ed.) (1998). *Textbook of pediatric infectious diseases* (4th edn). W.B. Saunders, Philadelphia, PA.

Fenner, F., Henderson, D.A., Arita, I., Jecek, Z., and Ladnyi, I.D. (1988). *Smallpox and its eradication*. World Health Organization, Geneva.

Fine, P.E. (1993). Herd immunity: history, theory, practice. *Epidemiologic reviews*, **15**, 265–302.

Gellert, G.A. (1993). International migration and control of communicable diseases. *Social Science and Medicine*, **37**, 1489–99.

Gorbach, S.L., Bartlett, J.G., and Blacklow, N.R. (ed.) (1998). *Infectious diseases* (2nd edn). W.B. Saunders, Philadelphia, PA.

Guerrant, R.L., Walker, D.H., and Weller, P.F. (ed.) (1999). *Tropical infectious diseases: Principles, pathogens, and practice*. W.B. Saunders, Philadelphia, PA.

Insel, R.A., Amstey, M., Woodin, K., and Pichichero, M. (1994). Maternal immunization to prevent infectious diseases in the neonate or infant. *International Journal of Technology Assessment in Health Care*, **10**, 143–53.

Jamison, D.T., Mosley, W.H., and Bobadilla, J.L. (ed.) (1993). *Disease control priorities in developing countries*. Oxford University Press, New York.

Kiple, K.F. (ed.) (1993). *The Cambridge world history of human disease*. Cambridge University Press.

Krause, R.M. (ed.) (1998). *Emerging infections*. Biomedical Research Reports, Academic Press, New York.

Last, J.M. (ed.) (2001). *A dictionary of epidemiology* (4th edn). International Epidemiological Association. Oxford University Press, New York.

Lederberg, J., Shope, R.E., and Oaks, S.C., Jr (ed.) (1992). *Emerging infections: microbial threats to health in the United States*. National Academy Press, Washington, DC.

McNeill, W.H. (1976). *Plagues and peoples*. Anchor Press–Doubleday, Garden City, NY.

Mandell, G.L., Bennett J.E., and Dolin, R. (ed.) (1995). *Mandell, Douglas and Bennett's principles and practice of infectious diseases* (4th edn). Churchill Livingstone, New York.

Murphy, F.A. (1994). New, emerging, and reemerging infectious diseases. *Advances in Virus Research*, **43**, 1–52.

Osterholm, M.T., Hedberg C.W., and MacDonald, K.L. (1995). Epidemiology of infectious diseases. In *Mandell, Douglas and Bennett's principles and practice of infectious diseases* (4th edn) (ed. G.L. Mandell, J.E. Bennett, and R. Dolin), pp. 158–68. Churchill Livingstone, New York.

Plotkin, S.A. and Orenstein, W.A. (ed.) (1999). *Vaccines* (3rd edn). W.B. Saunders, Philadelphia, PA.

Ryan, K.J. (ed.) (1994). *Sherris's medical microbiology: an introduction to infectious diseases* (3rd edn), Elsevier Science, New York.

Solomon, S.L. and Fraser, D.W. (1998). Public health considerations. In *Textbook of pediatric infectious diseases* (ed. R.D. Feigin and J.D. Cherry) (4th edn), pp. 2803–25. W.B. Saunders, Philadelphia, PA.

WHO (World Health Organization) (1983). *International health regulations* (3rd edn). WHO, Geneva.

WHO (World Health Organization) (1995*a*). *Communicable disease prevention and control: new, emerging, and re-emerging infectious diseases*, No. A48/15. WHO, Geneva.

WHO (World Health Organization) Expanded Programme on Immunization (1995*b*). *Immunization policy*. WHO/EPI/GEN/95.3/ REV 2, WHO, Geneva.

WHO (World Health Organization) (1999*a*). *Report on infectious diseases: removing obstacles to healthy development*. WHO/CDS/99.1, WHO, Geneva.

WHO (World Health Organization) (1999*b*). *International travel and health: vaccination requirements and health advice*. WHO, Geneva.

Wilson, M.E. (1991). *A world guide to infections: diseases, distribution, diagnosis*. Oxford University Press, New York.

World Bank (1993). *World Bank development report: investing in health*. World Bank, Washington.

12.8 Environmental health practice

Lynn R. Goldman

Environmental health can be best understood within an overall context of health. In 1993, the World Health Organization (**WHO**) stated: 'environmental health comprises those aspects of human health, including quality of life, that are determined by physical, chemical, biological, social and psychosocial processes in the environment. It also refers to the theory and practice of assessing, correcting, controlling, and preventing those factors in the environment that can potentially affect adversely the health of present and future generations' (WHO 1993). Thus, as defined, environmental health encompasses a wide array of determinants that can impact on the health of the individual. A broad overview of environmental health and topics in environmental health science is given in the chapters in Part 8 of this textbook.

This chapter will focus on the practice of environmental health with respect to non-occupational environmental exposures. It will also focus on those aspects of the environment that are largely not under the control of individuals, such as contaminants in food, drinking water, and indoor and outdoor air. It will not cover voluntary exposures like smoking nor will it cover injury prevention and control of radiation hazards, which are covered in other chapters. It also will not cover occupational health; an overview is given in Chapter 8.6.

Many factors modify the relationship between environment and health. The practice of environmental health should take into account the variability in individual responses to the environment. Differences in age, gender, and individual genetic make-up influence both exposure and susceptibility to environmental agents. A challenge in environmental health is the consideration of all age groups, as well as the very ill and the very healthy, in evaluation of hazards. Behaviour is also important and can have a major impact on exposure. In addition, social differences can affect exposure. For example, diets vary greatly across different cultural groups. People who live in poverty may experience multiple environmental threats, dietary inadequacies, and other factors that contribute to increased risk from environmental exposures.

The practice of environmental health is inextricably involved with the prevention of chronic diseases such as cancers, asthma, and birth defects, as well as acute illnesses such as viral gastroenteritis. The general state of knowledge about causation of many chronic diseases is less advanced than for communicable diseases so that while outbreaks or statistical excesses (so-called 'clusters') of chronic disease are often attributed by the public to environmental exposures, in many cases the cause is unknown. Thus, practitioners of environmental health are often called upon to address not only known exposures and links to disease but also diseases of unknown aetiology and public concern about the potential for environmental links. How to investigate such issues is covered in Chapter 8.5. In the United States, the Centers for Disease Control (**CDC**), the National Center for Environmental Health, and the Agency for Toxic Substances and Disease Registries (**ATSDR**), as well as state and local public health agencies, are often called upon to address such community outbreaks.

From the outset it is important to emphasize that the practice of environmental health may differ greatly in industrialized nations versus countries in transition and developing countries. Certain environmental health problems are much more serious in developing countries; for example, drinking water contamination with micro-organisms and toxic substances is much more prevalent and consequent morbidity and mortality more serious. Indoor and outdoor air pollution are much more impacted by the burning of coal, wood, and other biomass fuel sources for cooking and heating homes. Air is much more polluted because many of the controls and technological changes that have been required in developed countries have not yet been applied. Chemical spills and plant accidents are more common and there are fewer means to protect nearby communities and passers by. Not covered in this chapter but very important worldwide is disaster prevention and management. Worldwide there are large numbers of unnecessary deaths and injuries due to earthquakes, storms, and floods, which are completely preventable with appropriate environmental measures like construction standards for homes and buildings. However, while the priority issues for environmental health management may differ in different countries, the general principles for environmental health practice do not.

In 1965, René Dubos noted that indices of environmental health are 'expressions of the success or failure experienced by the (human) organism in its efforts to respond adaptively to environmental challenges' (Dubos 1965). This effort to respond adaptively to environmental challenges becomes ever more complex as the environment is changed by humans at a very rapid pace. Despite the difficulty of adapting to an environment that has been changed dramatically within just a few generations, there is evidence of remarkable success in the twentieth century. The sanitation movement of the 1800s resulted in enormous reductions in mortality due to infectious diseases and marked increases in life expectancy. This has resulted in much of the increase in life expectancy in the United States, from 47 years in 1900 to almost 77 in 1997.

In the last 30 years, stronger environmental laws in the industrialized nations have resulted in cleaner air, safer drinking water, and recovery of some water bodies that in 1970 had unacceptable levels of pollution for fishing and recreation. In the United States, air lead levels are 98 per cent lower than 20 years ago, and from 1976 to 1993, the percentage of children 1 to 5 years old with elevated blood lead levels decreased from 88 per cent to 4 per cent. Reports to the nation's Toxic Release Inventory indicate that emissions of toxic wastes from American manufacturers decreased nearly 50 per cent between 1988 and 1996. Such successes are indicative of the important role of management of environmental health hazards.

At the same time, there are other trends in environmental health that are more disturbing and indicative of a failure to adapt to a changing environment (McMichael 1993). Globally, the trend for pollution of air and drinking water supplies is upward. In most of the world, population is exerting an enormous pressure on resources and contributing to pollution. Drinking water is under pressure both from pollution and from consumption, and in many parts of the world there are serious shortages of drinkable water. Even in the United States, there are shortages of potable drinking water in many parts of the country. In addition, overfishing and pollution of water bodies is posing an increasing threat to fish harvests. In most of the world there is little control of chemicals and pesticides in commerce and chemical waste disposal, even while development is moving forward at a very rapid pace. Even in developed nations, there are numerous challenges that remain. To a great extent the easiest problems have been addressed, leaving environmental threats that are much more difficult to control and require more participation from a broader range of society. Often the problems that must be faced involve multiple small sources of pollutants rather than a few large and visible ones. Many of these small sources are from sectors, like agriculture and small business, which are less familiar with environmental regulations and often resistant to change. Clearly, they will need to be involved, yet they do not have the resources of large industries to address environmental issues. As vehicle emissions become a larger component of air pollution, land use, transportation planning, and urban sprawl are becoming greater concerns. Furthermore, problems like non-point source pollution engage everyone in society from the farmer to the weekend car mechanic who needs to know how to properly dispose of used motor oil. All of this means that new tools for assessing and managing environmental hazards will be needed in order to continue to achieve gains in environmental health.

In 1988, the American Institute of Medicine published a report, *The Future of Public Health*, which defined three major functions for the practice of public health practice: assessment, policy development, and assurance (IOM 1988). This chapter will take this approach in describing the practice of environmental health.

Environmental health assessment

The weight-of-evidence approach employed in environmental health inevitably involves a multitude of disciplines. Toxicology is the study of how chemicals and pollutants can be hazardous to humans and other organisms. Environmental epidemiologists study and interpret the distributions and relationships among diseases and exposure in the environment. Exposure assessors and industrial hygienists have expertise in measuring and estimating human exposure to contaminants. Analytical chemical laboratories are important for measuring levels of pollutants whether in human blood and tissues or in environmental samples such as air, food, water, and soil. Statistics and modelling experts contribute an understanding of how to utilize the often immense quantity of data in order to inform decision-making. Many scientific disciplines, ranging from environmental and atmospheric chemistry to hydrogeology, which looks at the dynamics of flow of water in the environment, are needed to understand how pollutants move in the environment and the ultimate fate in terms of exposures to humans and ecosystems. Many fields of engineering are involved—chemical engineers who can design processes to minimize, eliminate, or treat wastes, sanitary engineers who can design treatment systems for wastewater, and so forth. Engineering may play a role not only in the management of environmental hazards but also in the development of standards, as described below.

Generally, the assessment of environmental health threats involves the identification of hazards that may lead to disease states, and measurement or monitoring of exposures or doses to the population. Hazard is a measure of the intrinsic ability of the stressor to cause harm. Dose is the amount of the stressor delivered to the person, organism, or ecosystem.

The principles are those used in the evaluation of epidemiology—the nine Bradford Hill principles—strength of association, consistency, specificity, temporality, biological gradient, biological plausibility, coherence of evidence, experimental evidence, and reasoning by analogy. A strong association between hazard and dose is one where the risk or odds of disease is relatively large. A consistent association is one that is demonstrated in different studies and perhaps using different methods. Specificity is the extent to which the effect is uniquely associated with a disease. For example, vinyl chloride is the only exposure known to cause a rare cancer, angiosarcoma of the liver. Temporality concerns the relationship between time of exposure and time of disease. Some diseases (e.g. cancer) may have long latency periods, as much as 10 or more years. Other diseases are caused by more immediate exposures; for example, pesticide poisoning from carbamates occurs within an hour of exposure. Biological gradient refers to the ability to demonstrate that there is a dose–response between the exposure and the disease. Biological plausibility is the extent to which the association is consistent with what is already known about the response to the exposure and/or the disease. Coherence of evidence concerns the fit between the studies and what else is known that is relevant to the association and experimental evidence is evidence from controlled experiments that is relevant. Reasoning by analogy is the extent to which the observed pattern is similar to known exposure–disease relationships. For example, knowledge about how benzene causes cancer has been helpful in interpreting data for similar compounds, with similar results from animal studies, but which lack the epidemiological information available for benzene.

Hazard identification

Hazard identification generally relies on two types of information: data from epidemiological studies, and data from animal testing and other scientific studies of animals. There are many sources of hazard information (Table 1). Environmental epidemiology is defined as 'the study of the effect on human health of physical, biologic, and chemical factors in the external environment, broadly conceived. By examining specific populations or communities exposed to different ambient environments, it seeks to clarify the relationship between physical, biologic or chemical factors and human health' (National Research Council 1991).

Environmental health surveillance is an important tool for community environmental health; it is defined as the ongoing systematic collection, analysis, and interpretation of data on specific health events

Table 1 Sources of hazard information

Data	Observational studies	Controlled studies
Human	Epidemiology	Dosing studies
	Case reports	Clinical trials
	Surveillance	
	Disease	
	Exposure	
	Case–control studies	
	Prospective studies	
Environmental/animal	Incident reports	*In vitro* studies
	Emissions inventories	General toxicity
	Field studies	Specialized toxicity
	Environmental	
	Monitoring	
	Ecological impacts	

affecting a population (Thacker and Stroup 1994). Surveillance of hazards and exposures, as well as diseases, is critical to the practice of environmental health (Wegman 1992). By tracking exposures and diseases we can identify and respond to different kinds of public health problems. Surveillance and monitoring are also essential to the assurance function, i.e. the follow-up to make sure that the treatment for the community is effective (Thacker *et al.* 1996). Examples of environmental health surveillance include air pollution monitoring, blood lead monitoring, poison centre surveillance for pesticide and chemical ingestions, pesticide illness reports, asthma surveillance, and birth defects registries. All of these are tools for monitoring trends, and identifying opportunities to prevent and control environmental disease and exposures. Another form of surveillance is post-market monitoring for adverse effects. In the United States, there are provisions under both the pesticide and chemicals laws for reporting adverse health (as well as environmental) effects of toxic chemicals to the Environmental Protection Agency (**EPA**). This can be an important safety mechanism for chemicals approved as a result of animal testing alone since such limited testing cannot detect effects that are expected to occur in a small percentage of the population, especially idiosyncratic effects that are not completely dose dependent.

It is important to recognize that environmental health monitoring is not the same as environmental quality monitoring. In the United States, a review of the available monitoring for environmental quality found that few of the data collected are useful for tracking status and trends in environmental health (Goldman *et al.* 1992). Although many of these data systems have other important uses for enforcement and administrative purposes as well as for assessment of ecological systems, it is clear that environmental health assessments need to be better informed by information about both exposure and disease rates in populations. There are examples of remarkable successes that have resulted in application of the public health model for surveillance in environmental health. The CDC surveillance of lead levels in children in the United States demonstrated the benefits of the EPA's phase-out of lead in petrol (gasoline) at a time when this was in doubt and there were efforts to overturn the decision. Despite this and other successes, the capacity for environmental surveillance at the federal, state, and local level is quite limited.

Environmental epidemiology suffers from some limitations. Firstly, it cannot detect risks of concern when there is little variation in exposure across the population. For example, dioxin exposures are difficult to evaluate in the general population because most people have dioxin body burdens within a narrow range. Secondly, epidemiology cannot be applied before approving the introduction into commerce of a chemical, product, or technology. Thirdly, studies of environmental exposures often rely on measurements for the ambient environment as a whole rather than measurements of individual exposures. Such studies are known as ecological studies and they are often the only feasible way to study exposures; air pollution is often studied this way. Generally, the larger the area over which exposures are averaged, the greater are the methodological limitations with these studies. The major limitation of ecologic studies is the ecological fallacy, which in some circumstances can result from making causal inferences based on ecological data (Morgenstern 1982).

Animal toxicity testing allows examination of a wide range of exposures, use of experimental controls to limit the possibility of confounding and premarket prediction of hazards. The principles of toxicology are described in Chapter 8.2. In the practice of environmental health, governments have established regulatory standards or guidelines to ensure that any testing required by the law meets strict standards for quality of the data generated. The international standard that is available, and employed by most industrialized nations, is the set of internationally harmonized guidelines developed by the Organization for Economic Co-operation and Development (**OECD**). Test guidelines attempt to assay toxic properties of chemicals in a manner that is valid, reproducible, standardized between different laboratories, and is as humane to laboratory animals as possible. In countries, specific requirements for testing vary with the type of substance and the statute under which the substance is covered. In the United States, the most highly tested substances are food-use pesticides, for which numerous health tests are required including tests of acute and chronic toxicity, neurotoxicity tests, cancer bioassays, and multiple generation studies to assess reproductive and developmental toxicity. In addition, there are new requirements for tests of immunotoxicity, developmental neurotoxicity, and endocrine toxicity that are being implemented by the EPA. The OECD is currently developing new and enhanced assays for endocrine disruption for oestrogen, androgen, and thyroid effects. Because most chemicals and pesticides are marketed in many countries, the OECD has also established an agreement for Mutual Acceptance of Data to avoid unnecessary duplication of tests.

Toxicity testing is done under good laboratory practices, standards established by governments to eliminate extraneous factors, such as poor nutrition of animals, sloppy laboratory practices, or unclean environments, which would tend to bias or distort the results of laboratory tests. These practices also include record-keeping requirements that allow intensive peer review of studies to ensure their quality. There is an internationally agreed upon set of good laboratory practice for chemicals adopted by the OECD.

Despite efforts to carry out accurate toxicity tests, these tests have limitations. To be cost-effective and humane, they are designed with as few animals as statistically possible, while dosing animals at high levels. Outcome measures have been refined over the years but may be cruder than the measurements that can be taken in humans; for example, a mouse cannot report a headache. There can be phenomena that occur in the high-dose groups that are not relevant to human risk assessment. Thus, expert judgement is needed to interpret such data and it is important that scientists review all of the evidence before making a judgement. Unfortunately, there is a perception that animal testing is irrelevant. When we have both epidemiological and animal testing data, there is a striking concordance between the two with respect to relevance to risk assessment. Furthermore, most chemicals that have been subjected to high dose testing do not cause cancer, refuting the often made assertion that 'everything causes cancer if you give a high enough dose'.

Despite the availability of accepted tests and practices to assess hazards, the truth is that we know very little about the chemicals used in commerce worldwide. In the United States a recent evaluation by the EPA found that even among the more than 2800 chemical produced at a total of at least 1 million pounds (about 500 000 kg) per year only one in five have a complete set of screening level hazard information and 40 per cent have none (US EPA 1998*a*).

Exposure assessment

Assessment of exposure involves numerous factors. Usually in risk assessment one does not have access to precise measurements of all these exposure attributes, and yet they are all important in being able to calculate an average daily lifetime exposure. It would be useful to know the rate and duration of exposure and the amount absorbed, as well as the body weight. In a laboratory experiment, a toxicologist has almost complete control over these factors.

Direct measurements of exposure to the human population are almost never available to decision-makers. It is recognized that such direct measurements, in combination with better information about environmental sources and levels, would be a vast improvement over the current methods for modeling and estimating exposure. In the United States the National Health Assessment and Nutrition Examination Survey (**NHANES**) has conducted some population monitoring of exposures, but, other than for lead, there are no national data available for trends.

As a practical matter, actual exposure measurements are often replaced by defaults. At the EPA, the policy is to assess a reasonable high-end exposure, i.e. an exposure at the upper 90th or 95th percentile. However, summation of numerous high-end exposures can greatly overestimate exposure. Exposure to pesticides in food is a good example of this. If one adds up the upper 90th percentile bound for all foods, a theoretical individual eats 5000 cal/day, not exactly a reasonable high-end estimate of exposure. If there are data on distributions of food consumption and on pesticide levels in the food, it is possible to use probabilistic modelling, which incorporates those distributions for all foods to compute the distribution of exposure to pesticide residues in the food. Most frequently, this is done using Monte Carlo modelling techniques, not only for pesticide residues on food but also for other aggregate exposure situations. Monte Carlo and other probabilistic modelling techniques simulate the distributions of individual combinations of multiple exposures, to produce a theoretical distribution of an aggregate exposure to the population.

Currently, there is no process under way for international harmonization of exposure assessment. This is probably because of the large differences (cultural, dietary, climatic, etc.) which can lead to differences in exposures for different countries. For example, there is more consumption of drinking water in a hot equatorial climate, and there is more consumption of marine mammals among traditional societies in the Arctic.

Risk assessment

A number of tools are used for integrating and summarizing information about environmental health hazards. Environmental health relies extensively on the use of risk assessment to evaluate environmental stressors. Use of risk assessment allows us to extrapolate either between human populations or from laboratory animals to humans. It involves weighing all the evidence in order to develop estimates of the risks to populations who may be exposed. The current practice of risk assessment in environmental health is largely based on a set of principles developed by the National Academy of Sciences in 1983. Risk is a function of hazard and dose. Four steps in risk assessment have been delineated: hazard identification, dose–response evaluation, exposure assessment, and risk characterization (National Research Council 1983). These are described in detail in Chapter 8.8. Some aspects of hazard and exposure assessment are addressed above. The section below discusses some aspects of dose–response evaluation and risk characterization that are important to the practice of environmental health.

As described in Chapter 8.8, the practice of dose–response assessment differs significantly between a carcinogen and a non-carcinogen. Cancer assessment is one of the most established areas of risk assessment. There are several authoritative bodies, all of which conduct cancer risk assessment in a similar fashion. On the international level, there is the International Agency for Research in Cancer (**IARC**), which publishes monographs on assessments of individual carcinogens. There are many bodies in the United States, but the most important is the National Toxicology Program, which reviews the evidence and lists substances likely to be carcinogenic in its *Biennial Report on Carcinogens.*

Hazard assessments for cancer are done in a roughly similar fashion worldwide. At the hazard assessment phase, all studies relevant to the assessment of cancer are reviewed. If there is definitive human evidence of cancer causation, all of these bodies rate the chemical as a human carcinogen. A substance can also be rated as a human carcinogen when the human evidence alone does not prove a causal relationship, but the weight of the evidence is convincing. (This is a change from the past, when only human data could be used to make this judgement.) When there is strong evidence, but not probative, of carcinogenicity to humans, the substance is considered to be a 'probable' human carcinogen. Most systems then have a category for 'possible' carcinogens, those with weaker evidence and non-carcinogens, chemicals that despite testing show no evidence for carcinogenicity.

At the dose–response assessment phase, the default assumption is that the dose–response curve is linear at low doses and starts at zero. This means that we assume that for every additional exposure there is additional cancer risk. In other words, we generally assume that if 20 out of 100 people exposed at 1 part per 1000 in air will get cancer, the risk for an exposure to a much lower level of 1 part per million would be 200 cancers for every 1 million people exposed. This relationship is assumed unless there is compelling evidence for a different dose–response relationship at low doses.

There are many mechanisms for carcinogenicity and it is believed that not all of these mechanisms have linear dose–response relationships at low doses. However, there are rigorous criteria for accepting arguments to depart from the low-dose linear model, and most carcinogens are still considered to have linearity at low doses. Whether from human or from animal data, the dose–response curve is modelled using statistical techniques that extrapolate from the higher doses in the occupational or laboratory setting to the lower doses that are often of concern in environmental settings. Because of the uncertainties in extrapolating from high to low doses, and to account for the variability in the general human population, the dose–response curve is plotted with 95 percentile confidence limits and the upper 95th percentile bound is generally used for risk assessment. This estimate is combined with the exposure assessment to give a probabilistic estimate of risk, for example 10^{-3}, 10^{-5}, or 10^{-6}.

There are alternatives to the risk assessment approach for regulation of carcinogens. One is the so-called Delaney Clause in the United States Federal Food, Drug and Cosmetics Act which applies, in part, to the regulation of cancer risks from pesticides in food. On the basis of a hazard identification alone (carcinogenicity in animals), it sets a standard of no allowable residues of that pesticide in processed food. Later scientific developments—in the form of increasingly sensitive methods in analytical chemistry, tools for quantitative risk assessment, and new understandings of cancer mechanisms—eventually led Congress to change its policy and remove pesticides from governance by the Delaney Clause. However, in the United States, the Delaney Clause still applies to food additives and colourants that are intentionally added to the food supply. Similarly, in the European Union pesticides that are both mutagens and carcinogens are not allowed in groundwater at levels above 1 ppm regardless of the level of risk.

Non-cancer risk assessment generally involves use of the reference dose or acceptable daily intake approach. The process of establishing such regulatory levels is described in Chapter 8.8. It is important for decision-makers to understand that a reference dose is a dose considered safe with a margin of uncertainty rather than a bright line for toxicity. A chronic reference dose is an estimate of a daily exposure to a population, which, over a 70-year lifespan, is likely to have no significant deleterious effects (Barnes and Dourson 1988). An acute reference dose considers a one-day exposure only. Generally, the reference dose for an acute exposure may be much higher than the reference dose for a chronic exposure but this is very much dependent on the nature of the chemical and effects under study.

Susceptible populations

Children and other susceptible populations pose a special challenge for assessment of environmental hazards. Children are not just small adults. They develop very rapidly in the first few years of life, their diets vary from those of adults, and they require more caloric intake, oxygen, and water for their body weights than adults. Children's metabolism changes over the first few years of life, affecting how their systems handle pharmaceuticals and toxic substances. Normal childhood behaviour includes intense exploration of the environment and hand-to-mouth activities that can lead to increased exposures to contaminants in soil and around the home. Children lack judgement and thus cannot avoid exposures unless adults ensure that their environments are safe (Rogan 1995).

These differences between children and adults influence toxicity and exposure assessments for children, as well as options for risk management. A National Research Council (**NRC**) committee in its 1993 report *Pesticides in the Diets of Infants and Children* concluded that the toxicity of, and exposures to, pesticides are frequently different for children and adults. It found that, despite a wealth of scientific information to warrant addressing risks to children, the EPA rarely did so in making regulatory decisions about pesticides. The committee advised the EPA to incorporate information about dietary exposures to children in risk assessments, and augment pesticide testing with new assessments of neurotoxicity, developmental toxicity, endocrine effects, immunotoxicity, and developmental neurotoxicity. It recommended that the EPA include cumulative risks from pesticides that act via a common mechanism of action and aggregate risks from non-food exposures when developing a tolerance for a pesticide. Since that time there has been a major undertaking by government to incorporate these recommendations into federal management of the use of pesticides (National Research Council 1993).

There are many other vulnerable populations as well, many of whom are not in the workplace. Those who live in poverty are very vulnerable because of the potential to multiple exposures, poorer diets, and lack of access to medical care (IOM 1999). For example, children who are relatively deficient in iron or calcium absorb more lead per gram of intake than children who have adequate nutrition. The elderly population may be particularly susceptible to some environmental exposures and may have slower elimination of many toxicants. Those who have chronic illnesses are often more susceptible as well. For example, people who have HIV or are immunosuppressed as a result of cancer therapy are much more at risk for serious infections from pathogens in drinking water or food. Pregnant women are at risk not only from the perspective of exposure of the developing child but also because of altered physiology and metabolism of many toxic agents. For women, menopause may be another time of vulnerability. For example, there is evidence that at the time of menopause BLLs increase because of liberation of stored lead from bones.

It is easy to conclude that the process of dose–response assessment has become ever more complex given considerations of the increasing sophistication in understanding of mechanisms of toxicity as well as increased appreciation that there are some in the population that are more vulnerable. This is creating challenges for practitioners in environmental health in developing a language that can be used and understood by stakeholders as well as decision-makers to achieve the public involvement and transparency that are so important in environmental health practice.

Risk characterization

Risk characterization is the final step of the risk assessment process. No additional scientific information is added during this phase, which involves estimating the magnitude of the public health or environmental problem. Much judgement is needed in appropriate selection of populations and exposure levels for analysis. In addition, it is important that relevant statistical and biological uncertainties are made clear at this stage. This part of the risk assessment process is the largest nexus between risk assessment and risk managers, and it is important that risk managers receive a complete set of information to guide decisions. This is where the very complex interactions between scientists, decision-makers, and the public occur, and yet where some of the most difficult communication issues occur as well.

The International Program for Chemical Safety, which is a collaborative effort between the WHO, the United Nations Environment Program (**UNEP**), the International Labor Organization (**ILO**), and the Food and Agriculture Organization (**FAO**), publishes Environmental Health Criteria documents which are intended to serve as international characterizations of risk for substances. In addition, there is information available in the ILO Chemical Safety Cards, in the WHO–FAO pesticide assessments and in summary form on UNEP's Global Information Network. Many nations make risk assessments widely available via the internet and other means but it is important to emphasize that the exposure assessment may differ between countries, as mentioned above.

Environmental health policy-making

Environmentally induced diseases and injuries are almost completely preventable, using pollution prevention, product design, engineering controls, personal protection, and education. So much of environmental health practice falls outside the realm of traditional medicine because the focus is generally on primary prevention, preventing exposures before the development of disease. At the same time, other interventions flow directly from a physician encounter that diagnoses the health problem and forms a connection between that problem and an environmental exposure (for example, childhood lead poisoning, pesticide poisoning, and asthma exacerbation by air pollution). As with occupational disease, single or small numbers of diagnosed cases can be sentinels for more widespread population exposures and disease. However, environmental health requires a broad range of disciplinary approaches and the application of engineering, sanitation, public health nursing, education and communication, epidemiology, toxicology, statistics, laboratory, administration, enforcement, and legal expertise as well as the expertise of public health generalists and physicians. Therefore this is a complex web of scientific expertise and information and much of the science of environmental policy-making involves the task of weaving together information from many disciplines to define problems and develop alternative approaches to solving them (Gordon 1997).

The 'players' in environmental health policy

Who makes environmental health policy? Nearly everyone at some level is involved with decisions related to the environment and health. At all levels, decisions about the planning of towns and cities, road building, and economic development all have an impact on environmental health. Much of the time, the policy-makers may not be aware of the environmental health implications of these decisions. Yet there is a need for more input of public health assessment data into such decision-making processes at all levels. For example, health experts are rarely engaged in discussions about transportation planning in the United States. Involvement of 'stakeholders', those with a stake in the outcome of decision-making, is important in environmental health policy-making. In a sense, since everyone wants to be able to breathe clean air, drink safe drinking water, and eat healthful food, all are stakeholders in environmental policy-making. Much of the art of environmental health practice is in not only informing but also involving stakeholders in all stages of the decision-making process, from problem definition through selection of alternative solutions to the problem (Omenn 1997). It also involves no small amount of political will to see solutions through, since by its very nature environmental health protection inevitably involves costs to taxpayers, or to industry, or to both. At the same time, environmental health practice usually creates winners as well as losers, and planning for transition from more to less polluting activities is at the heart of environmental health policy-making at its best.

Environmental health policy principles adopted by governments

In 1992, more than 100 nations signed the United Nations Commission on Environment and Development (**UNCED**) Treaty that formally adopted the goal of sustainable development and 27 principles of sustainable development (Table 2). Chief among these is Principle 1, which states: 'Human beings are at the center of concerns for sustainable development. They are entitled to a healthy and productive life in harmony with nature.' Principle 2 is also very fundamental: it describes a 'sovereign right' of states 'to exploit their own resources pursuant to their own environmental and developmental policies, and the responsibility to ensure that activities within their jurisdiction or control do not cause damage to the environment of other States or of areas beyond the limits of national jurisdiction' (UN 1992).

The precautionary principle is another UNCED principle for environmental policy-making. As governments agreed in 1992: 'In order to protect the environment, the precautionary approach shall be widely applied by States according to their capabilities. Where there are threats of serious or irreversible damage, lack of full scientific certainty shall not be used as a reason for postponing cost-effective measures to prevent environmental degradation' (UN 1992). For example, DDT was banned in the United States long before its precise mechanisms of action had been described by scientists.

Another important principle, adopted in many nations, is the principle of 'the polluter pays'. This means in essence that those who profit from pollution should pay the price for cleaning it up. More recently, this has evolved into the concept of economic instruments such as pollutant trading systems which employ market forces to shift the societal cost of pollution to the polluter, in order to bring down overall levels of pollution.

Environmental health policy tools

A number of tools are used in risk policy-making. Many environmental standards are based in whole or in part on best available technology, such as the air toxics Maximum Achievable Control Technology (**MACT**) standards under the American Clean Air Act and similar Best Available Technology standards in many European countries. Technology standards can be combined with risk-based standards. For example, for hazardous air pollutants the EPA was directed by Congress to regulate using MACT standards and then to assess the 'residual risks' and tighten the regulations if necessary.

Pollution prevention is another important principle of environmental policy; the rungs of the pollution prevention ladder go from the most preferable strategy, reduction of pollution at the source (source reduction), to waste minimization, reuse, recycling, emissions controls, and, least preferably, clean-up. It is generally less expensive

Table 2 UNCED principles of sustainable development most relevant to environmental health

Principle 1	Human beings are at the centre of concerns for sustainable development. They are entitled to a healthy and productive life in harmony with nature
Principle 2	In accordance with the Charter of the United Nations and the principles of international law, the sovereign right to exploit their own resources pursuant to their own environmental and developmental policies, and the responsibility to ensure that activities within their jurisdiction or control do not cause damage to the environment of other States or of areas beyond the limits of national jurisdiction
Principle 3	The right to development must be fulfilled so as to equitably meet developmental and environmental needs of present and future generations
Principle 4	In order to achieve sustainable development, environmental protection shall constitute an integral part of the development process and cannot be considered in isolation from it
Principle 5	All States and all people shall co-operate in the essential task of eradicating poverty as an indispensable requirement for sustainable development, in order to decrease the disparities in standards of living and better meet the needs of the majority of the people of the world
Principle 10	Environmental issues are best handled with the participation of all concerned citizens, at the relevant level. At the national level, each individual shall have appropriate access to information concerning the environment that is held by public authorities, including information on hazardous materials and activities in their communities, and the opportunity to participate in decision-making processes. States shall facilitate and encourage public awareness and participation by making information widely available. Effective access to judicial and administrative proceedings, including redress and remedy, shall be provided
Principle 11	States shall enact effective environmental legislation. Environmental standards, management objectives, and priorities should reflect the environmental and developmental context to which they apply. Standards applied by some countries may be inappropriate and of unwarranted economic and social cost to other countries, in particular developing countries
Principle 13	States shall develop national law regarding liability and compensation for the victims of pollution and other environmental damage. States shall also co-operate in an expeditious and more determined manner to develop further international law regarding liability and compensation for adverse effects of environmental damage caused by activities within their jurisdiction or control to areas beyond their jurisdiction
Principle 14	States should effectively co-operate to discourage or prevent the relocation and transfer to other States of any activities and substances that cause severe environmental degradation or are found to be harmful to human health
Principle 15	In order to protect the environment, the precautionary approach shall be widely applied by States according to their capabilities. Where there are threats of serious or irreversible damage, lack of full scientific certainty shall not be used as a reason for postponing cost-effective measures to prevent environmental degradation
Principle 18	States shall immediately notify other States of any natural disasters or other emergencies that are likely to produce sudden harmful effects on the environment of those States. Every effort shall be made by the international community to help States so afflicted
Principle 19	States shall provide prior and timely notification and relevant information to potentially affected States on activities that may have a significant adverse transboundary environmental effect and shall consult with those States at an early stage and in good faith
Principle 22	Indigenous people and their communities and other local communities have a vital role in environmental management and development because of their knowledge and traditional practices. States should recognize and duly support their identity, culture and interests and enable their effective participation in the achievement of sustainable development
Principle 24	Warfare is inherently destructive of sustainable development. States shall therefore respect international law providing protection for the environment in times of armed conflict and co-operate in its further development, as necessary
Principle 25	Peace, development, and environmental protection are interdependent and indivisible

to reduce pollution at the source and thus avoid costs of emissions controls and environmental cleanup.

In some cases an economic analysis of costs or feasibility in developing standards is an important driver in decision-making. Economic analyses can play a number of roles including assessing costs and benefits of an action (so-called cost–benefit analysis) weighing the relative cost-effectiveness of alternative solutions to a problem and identification of economic inequities in impact that can inform decision-making.

Pollution and its consequences are not distributed equally in society, and thus it is important to consider environmental justice issues in assessment of hazard (IOM 1999). Unfortunately, in the past there was a failure to do so, accounting for concentrations of polluting industries, sources of air pollution, and waste disposal operations in certain low-income and minority communities. In addition, there are higher rates of many diseases in poor and minority communities in the United States and elsewhere, lending support to the notion of differential exposure and risk.

Another important tool at a community level is an ecosystem-based approach or a community-based approach to environmental protection. In the United States, under the Clean Air Act, it has long been recognized that, for many communities, it would not be possible to meet standards unless management is undertaken for an entire air shed. This approach is now being adopted for the protection of large and complex watersheds both within countries and internationally. Increasingly it is recognized that non-point sources of pollution to air and water—i.e. sources that are diffuse rather than from large industrial incinerator stacks and water disposal outfalls—are important. Ecosystem-based approaches are more effective than individual permitting activities in controlling such sources. In the United States, of increasing concern is agricultural runoff from confined animal feeding operations, which can release harmful pathogens and nutrients to aquatic environments. The nutrients in turn have been associated with blooms of harmful organisms like *Pfiesteria*. Only watershed-based management schemes can address this kind of pollution.

Global environmental health policy issues

The threats of large-scale changes to the global environment, such as destruction of the tropospheric ozone layer and global climate change, are encouraging nations to co-operate on environmental policy issues. For example, air pollutants can persist and travel long distances, creating environmental damage. Hazardous wastes can be transported across borders and into nations with little or no capacity to handle them. Pollution to large water bodies like the Great Lakes or the Baltic Ocean can affect the quantity and quality of food available to neighbouring nations. Clearly when pollutants cross boundaries environmental decision-making must occur on an international basis. Agreements such as the United States–Canada joint agreement for the Great Lakes are beginning to govern how we manage resources that are shared by many nations (US EPA 1997).

Another international issue in environmental policy is the emergence of a global economy together with a global trading system that is more open than in the past. Although trading agreements have recognized past environmental agreements there is always the possibility of trade taking precedence over future environmental actions. Environmental policy-making must take into account not only national economic interests but international ones as well, while upholding the sovereign right of nations to establish their own health and environmental standards as agreed in UNCED.

Environmental health assurance

Environmental health assurance is a complex process that involves a multitude of players. In most nations, there are a number of governmental entities that carry out the process of providing environmental health protection. Generally there is a national environmental ministry that carries out most national environmental regulatory responsibilities. In the United States, this function is divided between the Department of the Interior and the EPA, but this is the exception rather than the rule. There are separate regulatory authorities for food safety that are either located in the health or agriculture ministry or, in the case of the United States, both. In addition, in many nations, the health or labour ministry also has some responsibility in the area of management of chemicals. There may be separate radiation safety and consumer products agencies as well. There may also be a justice agency (in the United States, this is the Department of Justice), with additional enforcement responsibilities.

In addition to agencies with direct responsibility for environmental health, there are many others who may become involved because of how regulations affect economic interests in society. Thus in the United States, the Departments of Energy, Commerce, Defense, Management and Budget, Small Business, and others all become involved where their interests may be affected by regulations. Therefore at a national level, assurance of environmental health involves a complex web and much of the practice of environmental health involves learning how to co-ordinate and work effectively within this kind of complex environment.

In most nations, environmental regulation is delegated to state and local government levels. For example, municipal waste disposal is primarily a state and local function in the United States. At a local level in the United States, environmental assurance primarily is in the hands of environmental health divisions within local health agencies. However, there are many other players, including those as diverse as environmental agencies, fire departments, and agriculture departments. Whereas activities at a national level may focus on assuring that there is a minimum standard for clean air, drinking water, and food, on a local level there are different responsibilities, such as inspection of food preparation establishments, rat control, sanitation services, spill clean-ups, lead poisoning prevention, and so on.

In the United States, in between the federal and local levels are state departments of environment and health who often administer yet another layer of standards established by state legislatures. Often states are delegated by the federal government to assure the compliance with federal standards as well (Gordon 1997). What is often missing at all levels is the function of monitoring the health of the public and the link between the practice of environmental health and real health improvements.

Command and control approaches to environmental health management

In most of the world, much environmental health assurance is via a command and control approach that involves the development and enforcement of laws, regulations, and standards. For example, there may be rules against leaking septic tanks or creating cross-connections between water and sewer lines in cities. In addition, for chemicals and pesticides there are licensing functions like new chemicals approvals and pesticide registrations. Environmental impact assessments allow the review of proposed projects to ensure compliance with environmental standards prior to the commitment of resources for new development and construction. Permitting of facilities for air emissions, water discharges, and waste disposal are essential to controlling point sources of pollution as is a strong environmental enforcement presence. Generally enforcement is targeted to specific goals—hopefully goals that are informed by priorities for protection of health and ecosystems. The first line of responsibility for enforcement is usually with local and state health and environmental agencies.

Environmental health management tools

There are a number of tools that are used in risk management. Environmental engineering has played a very important role in identifying alternative methods for pollution prevention and control.

Pollution prevention is an important tool for environmental management as well as for policy. Increasingly it is understood that trying to address environmental problems one medium at a time can result in just moving pollutants from water to air to land to water, without a net reduction in risk. So-called multimedia approaches look at all of the impacts of decisions. Pollution prevention can also be an important driver for decision-making. Changes that involve source reduction often occur over a longer production lifecycle than more incremental changes. In the United States pollution prevention is used in both regulatory and also voluntary approaches to environmental assurance. An example of the latter is the Design for Environment programme conducted in the United States by the EPA, which works with sectors in the economy to identify alternative means of production. For example, they established, with the American Chemical Society, a Presidential Award called the Green Chemistry Challenge, a contest in which companies and universities compete to be recognized for innovative new chemistries that reduce waste and are safer for health and the environment.

Environmental monitoring is also an important tool for evaluating the success of efforts and for targeting future regulatory and enforcement actions. Monitoring can involve reporting by regulated entities or actual sampling and analysis of pollutants in the air, water, food, and so on. Such monitoring can be enforcement driven or at random to reflect population exposure. While important for environmental health assurance, environmental monitoring that is directly relevant to human health can feed back into the assessment process and inform future environmental health practice.

The right to know and the power of information

Community right to know is a powerful driver for reducing pollution. It was first introduced at a national level in the United States with passage of the 1986 Emergency Preparedness and Community Right to Know Act and establishment of the Toxic Release Inventory (**TRI**), which initially required the manufacturing industry to report releases of some 300 chemicals to the public. In the rest of the world such reporting systems are called Pollutant Release and Transfer Registries. Like the material safety data sheets in workplaces, community right to know is designed to empower citizens to make informed decisions either as individuals or as a community. Community right to know is a powerful tool not only to inform citizens but also workers within plants as well as plant and corporate managers. In the United States, the TRI helped industry recognize that it often was more cost-effective to prevent the pollution by better managing the flows of materials into, in, and through facilities. In the United States the TRI was also the basis for a voluntary pollution reduction programme in which industry reduced TRI emissions of several toxic air contaminants by 33 per cent by 1992 and 50 per cent by 1995, giving rise to the name '30/50' for the programme, from the TRI baseline year of 1988. Overall industry met this target, and those enrolled in the 33/50 programme did so a year early. In 1996, the EPA reported an overall reduction of 45.6 per cent of all TRI releases for 'base' facilities and chemicals for a total of 2.4 billion pounds of chemicals released in the environment or transferred for disposal (US EPA 1998*b*).

Availability of information online is increasing the availability of information generally. A challenge for environmental health professionals will be keeping up with the available information, and helping communities and individuals sift through it to understand what is important and relevant for their communities and how to place it into perspective. Keeping up with and understanding these information sources is a critical part of environmental health practice. Industry has long been concerned that provision of information is damaging to competitiveness. There are other concerns that information can be easily taken out of context and misunderstood by communities. Clearly, while there is an appropriate balance between providing information and other concerns, right to know has proven to be a useful tool for environmental health protection. Since it is here to stay, an important role of environmental health practitioners is to promote the right to understand as well as the right to know, i.e. to provide the context for information so that communities can understand it as well as acquiring it.

Another powerful force in assuring environmental health is the private right of action. This varies with the legal system in place but in the United States the tort liability system sometimes has been a powerful driver towards the prevention of exposures to environmental pollutants. In some instances, American environmental statutes give the public the right to sue the EPA to enforce standards (called 'citizen suits' provisions). Completely unique in the United States is California's Proposition 65, which combined the right to know and the citizen suit approach. Briefly, companies must label products (a) if they may cause more than a one in 100 000 lifetime cancer risk, or (b) if they may cause reproductive toxicity and have exposures at levels greater than 1000 times the level where no effects are seen (the 'no observed effect level'). Citizens can sue the companies if they fail to provide such warning. Proposition 65 has prompted numerous product reformulations inspired by a desire to avoid having to use the label.

Environmental education also plays an important role in the management of environmental hazards. In the United States, hazards like radon gas in homes and environmental tobacco smoke have largely been managed, on a federal level, by providing education to the public. Environmental educators can also play an important role in helping to translate complex hazard and prevention information so that it is better understood by the public.

International agreements and the emergence of international standards

A number of international organizations are responsible for aspects of environmental health practice (Table 3). This is also a complex web of activity. Already mentioned are the roles of international organizations in the assessment and policy-making functions of environmental health practice. There are global and regional agreements to prevent climate change, control emission of ozone-depleting chemicals (Montreal Protocol), and decrease acid rain. There are chemical agreements on prior informed consent for import of certain toxic chemicals (UNEP 1998) and persistent pollutants (Long-Range Transport of Atmospheric Pollutants Persistent Organic Pollutants Protocol) (UN ECE 1998). In 2001, countries agreed to create a global agreement on persistent organic pollutants. Activity to agree upon a voluntary global system for classification and labelling of chemicals in commerce is also under way.

The Kyoto Climate Change Treaty was negotiated in 1998, and efforts are now under way for countries to begin to ratify and implement that agreement. In the United States, there continues to be debate about the urgency of addressing global climate change as a concern. There has been a gradual and subtle increase in the Earth's temperature over the last century, caused by the increased levels of

Table 3 International organizations involved in environmental protection

Acronym	Organization	Environmental health scope
UNEP	United Nations (UN) Environment Program	Environmental agreements, chemical information systems, technical assistance, right to know
WHO	World Health Organization	Toxicology and epidemiology, IARC, technical assistance
UNCED	UN Commission for Environment and Development	Implementation of Agenda 21 treaty signed in 1992
UNDP	UN Development Program	Sustainable development, growth, and population issues
FAO	Food and Agriculture Organization	Pesticides and other agricultural health issues. Food safety (Codex Alimentarius)
IMO	International Maritime Organization	Seafood safety and protection of the seas
OECD	Organization for Economic Co-operation and Development	Harmonization of chemicals testing and classification, good laboratory practices for chemicals, co-operation on waste disposal, climate and other issues
IPCC	International Program on Climate Change	Scientific assessment of climate change
IFCS	Intergovernmental Forum on Chemical Safety	Co-operation on global chemical safety issues
ILO	International Labor Organization	Workplace health and safety; chemicals labelling in the workplace
UNCTDG	UN Commission on Transport of Dangerous Goods	Harmonization of classification and labels for chemicals in transport

greenhouse gases, especially carbon dioxide, in the atmosphere. These gases act as an insulating blanket, reflecting back the heat of the sun in the same way that the glass of a greenhouse works. Warming of the Earth is predicted to have a number of adverse consequences. Firstly, many scientists believe that the climate is already more erratic than historically, increasing the likelihood of regional flooding, drought, and severe storm episodes. Secondly, as the polar ice caps melt, low-lying areas will be inundated. There is already some scientific evidence that this process is beginning to occur. The ultimate result would be flooding, with many coastal and low-lying areas becoming uninhabitable or requiring elaborate dikes and drainage systems. Thirdly, the ecosystem will not be able to adapt readily to a rapid shift in climate. This could result in the spread of vectors of infectious disease, poor health, death of forests and other ecosystems, disruption of agriculture in many areas, and concomitant effects on the health of other species and humans due to the spread of infectious disease and disruption of habitat and food supplies.

In some areas international standards are beginning to emerge. For the purpose of environmental health assurance the most important role these agencies play is in establishing either international treaties (UNEP) or agreements (some of a voluntary nature) that are beginning to form the foundation for global environmental health standards. However, it is important to emphasize that all environmental agreements in existence recognize the sovereign right and responsibility of nations to set their own standards and tend to get involved only with transboundary issues such as movement of pollutants, trade in hazardous goods, and trade in hazardous wastes. Another example is the voluntary system for harmonization of classification and labelling for industrial chemicals led by the ILO. In recognition of the widespread commerce in chemicals and the need for protection in transport, the workplace, and consumer products, nations have agreed to a voluntary system for hazard classification of chemicals and are working towards an agreement for standard labels. Implementation by nations will require several years but will be important for public health protection and right to know internationally.

References

Barnes, D. and Dourson, M. (1988). Reference Dose (RfD): description and use in health risk assessments. *Regulatory Toxicology and Pharmacology*, **8**, 471–86.

Dubos, R. (1965). *Man adapting*. Yale University Press, New Haven, CT.

Goldman, L.R., Gomez, M., Greenfield, S., *et al.* (1992). Use of exposure databases for status and trends analysis. *Archives of Environmental Health*, **47**, 430–8.

Gordon, L.J. (1997). Environmental health and protection. In *Principles of public health practice* (ed. F.D. Scutchfield and C.W. Keck), pp. 300–17. Delmar, Albany, NY.

IOM (Institute of Medicine) (1988). *The future of public health*. National Academy Press, Washington, DC.

IOM (Institute of Medicine) (1999). Committee on Environmental Justice: introduction and executive summary; health policy. In *Toward environmental justice: research, education and health policy issues*, pp. 1–10, 61–8. National Academy Press, Washington, DC.

McMichael, A.J. (1993). The health of populations. *Planetary overload: global environmental change and the health of the human species*, pp. 56–81. Cambridge University Press.

Morgenstern, H. (1982). Uses of ecologic analysis in epidemiologic research. *American Journal of Public Health*, **72**, 1336–44.

National Research Council (1983). *Risk assessment in the federal government: managing the process*. National Academy Press, Washington, DC.

National Research Council (1991). *Environmental epidemiology: public health and hazardous wastes.* National Academy Press, Washington, DC.

National Research Council (1993). *Pesticides in the diets of infants and children.* National Academy Press, Washington, DC.

Omenn, G.S. (Chair): Presidential/Congressional Commission on Risk Assessment and Risk Management (1997). *Framework for environmental health risk management.* US Government Printing Office, Washington, DC.

Rogan, W.J. (1995). Environmental poisoning of children—lessons from the past. *Environmental Health Perspective*, **103** (Supplement 6), 19–23.

Thacker, S.B. and Stroup, D.F. (1994). Future directions for comprehensive public health surveillance and health information systems in the United States. *American Journal of Epidemiology*, **140**, 383–97.

Thacker, S.B., Stroup, D.F., Parrish, R.G., and Anderson, H.A. (1996). Surveillance in environmental public health: issues, systems, and sources. *American Journal of Public Health*, **86**, 633–8 (Erratum. *American Journal of Public Health*, **86**, 1526.)

UN (United Nations) (1992). *The United Nations Conference on Environment and Development. Rio Declaration on Environment and Development*, Principle 15. UN, Rio de Janeiro.

UNECE (1998). *Protocol to the 1979 Convention on Long Range Transboundary Air Pollution on Persistent Organic Pollutants.* UNECE, Aarhus, Denmark.

UNEP (1998). *Convention on the Prior Informed Consent Procedure for Certain Hazardous Chemicals and Pesticides in International Trade.* UNEP, Rotterdam.

US EPA (United States Environmental Protection Agency) (1997). *Environment Canada. Canada–United States Strategy for the Virtual Elimination of Persistent Toxic Substances in the Great Lakes Basin.* Environmental Protection Agency, Washington, DC.

US EPA (United States Environmental Protection Agency) (1998*a*). *Chemical Hazard data availability study. What do we really know about the safety of high production volume chemicals?* Office of Pollution Prevention, Pesticides and Toxic Substances, Environmental Protection Agency, Washington, DC.

US EPA (United States Environmental Protection Agency) (1998*b*). *1996 Toxics release inventory: public data release—ten years of right-to-know.* US EPA, Office of Pollution Prevention Pesticides and Toxic Substances, Environmental Protection Agency, Washington, DC.

Wegman, D. (1992). Hazard surveillance. In *Public health surveillance* (ed. W. Halperin and E.J. Baker), pp. 62–75. Van Nostrand Reinhold, New York.

WHO (World Health Organization) (1993). *Consultation: Sofia, Bulgaria.* WHO, Geneva.

12.9 Structures and strategies for public health intervention

Don Nutbeam and Marilyn Wise

Introduction

The earlier chapters of this book confirm that the scientific base for public health is substantially developed. However, to be effective, the science of public health must be 'applied'. The twenty first century brings with it the need to improve the effectiveness of public health action further—to apply existing knowledge and strategies of public health intervention to all sectors in order to achieve improved health and well being for all.

To do this there needs to be health policy that links a nation's investment in its health sector with improved population health outcomes. Such policy should also provide a mandate for the use of the full range of public health strategies (as well as health care services) to achieve these outcomes. There must be an infrastructure for public health that provides public health leadership, and contributes directly to the policies, institutional development, and programmes that are necessary to deliver improvements in the health of populations, and to reduce the inequities in health, which have been identified and explored in other chapters.

This chapter describes key elements of health policy and strategy that have been found to be effective in guiding national public health action, and the components of an infrastructure that is necessary to enable countries and communities to design, deliver, and evaluate public health interventions.

Figure 1 provides an overview of the essential elements of the chapter. Based on analysis of experiences in several countries, Fig. 1 traces the steps which link identification of the determinants of health, through definition of priorities and development of policy, to the infrastructure and delivery system required by health sectors (and governments) to guide and implement effective public health action (National Health and Medical Research Council 1997*a*; International Union for Health Promotion and Education 1999).

Figure 1 illustrates the importance of establishing an infrastructure and delivery system for public health as the foundation that enables governments to apply public health science both to the analysis and investigation of public health problems, and to the design, delivery, and evaluation of public health interventions. The infrastructure includes the capacity to link evidence of the effectiveness of these public health actions to a process of regular review and redefinition of problems and priorities for public health and for related policy.

Following the structure in Fig. 1, the chapter explores the need for an initial analysis of the full range of determinants of public health problems—economic and social, alongside behavioural and environmental. This analysis can then be used to guide the selection of priority population health outcomes—expressed as goals and objectives. It goes on to explain the ways in which such measureable outcomes have been used as a benchmark against which investment in health (public and private) can be assessed. It also outlines ways in which goals and objectives have been helpful in guiding action with other sectors to develop public policy and to develop and implement tools such as health impact assessment.

The chapter concludes with an overview of the capacity needed by the health sector (and government) to direct and guide action to improve the health of populations. Examination of the history of public health in industrialized countries indicates the need for constant vigilance on the part of public health professionals and activists. This is to ensure that governments' investment in health continues to include a focus on action to protect and promote the health and well being of populations, and that governments maintain and develop their capacity to act effectively to achieve health for all.

Policies and interventions to address the determinants of health in populations

Earlier chapters describe a range of personal, social, and environmental factors that are related to increased risk of disease, and of adverse outcomes from disease. Analysis of the determinants of the health of populations is essential to clarify the relative importance of each, and to identify those that are modifiable through public health intervention. These determinants include individual characteristics and behaviours, such as smoking and diet, which have been the focus for the majority of public health interventions in developed countries to reduce the burden of non-communicable disease in the population.

Epidemiological analysis also reveals major differences in disease experience between different groups in the population with different social, economic, and environmental circumstances. Although some of these differences can be explained by differences in individuals' health-related behaviours (such as tobacco use and food choices), more of the difference is explained by the different social, economic, and environmental circumstances in which people live and work (Evans *et al.* 1994; Marmot and Wilkinson 1999).

In the case of coronary heart disease, Marmot's work in the United Kingdom has indicated that a high proportion of the variance in premature deaths between different social groups cannot be adequately explained by known behavioural and other personal risk factors (Marmot and Wilkinson 1999). Some other factors are at work,

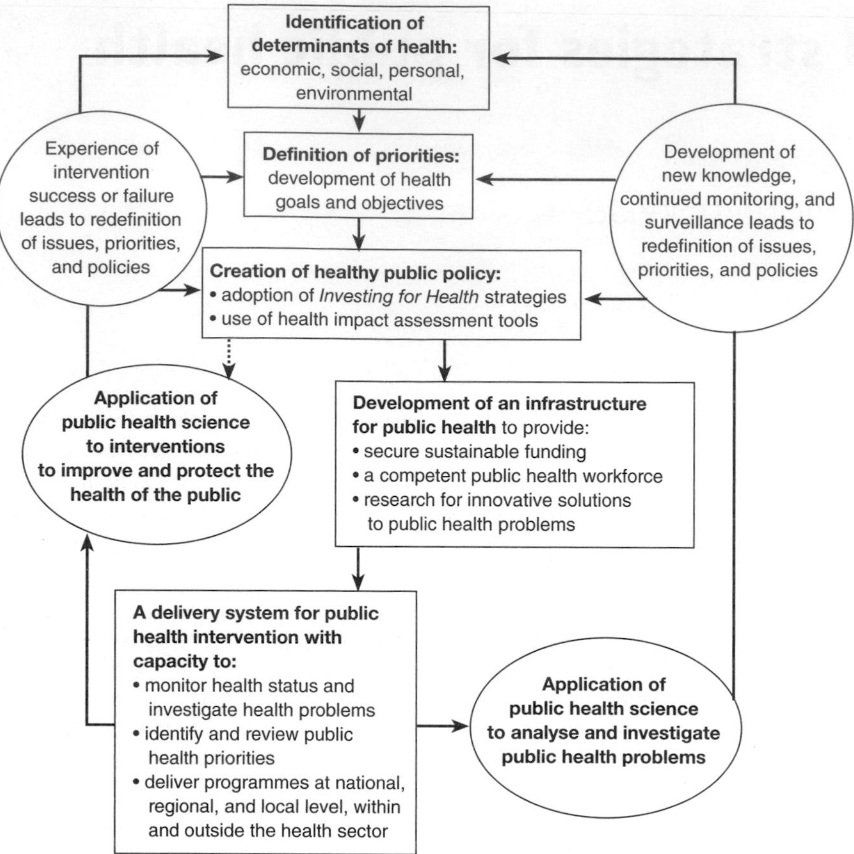

Fig. 1 Overview of an infrastructure for public health intervention.

and these appear to be related to differences in the social status and economic conditions of different populations.

Effective policies and interventions to modify these social, economic, and environmental conditions, have the potential to produce even greater gains in health status than those attributed to changes in lifestyles and improved health care in many developed countries in the past two decades.

In many ways this is not a new discovery. Creating supportive environments for health has been a major goal of public health policy and action for the past 150 years. Environmental interventions to provide clean water and waste disposal, safe food, and safe living and working conditions led to major improvements in public health in industrialized countries. The implementation of effective mass immunization programmes has been effective in reducing morbidity and mortality among children in many developing countries throughout the twentieth century.

However, during the twentieth century the very success of public health policy, research, and practice meant that it became 'invisible' in many countries. In industrialized countries, the policies, strategies, and structures that had been so effective in reducing mortality and morbidity across their populations were in decline by the middle of the twentieth century. The great proportion of health sector investment was (and remains) largely in biomedical intervention. Public health interventions have tended to become marginalized, and rather narrowly focused on the identification of biological and behavioural risk factors for non-communicable diseases—followed by interventions that aimed to change individuals' lifestyles.

By the late 1970s it was becoming increasingly obvious that national investment in health in most countries was, in reality, investment in services to diagnose and treat ill health. Progress towards improving the health of populations was limited, particularly in light of the fast-increasing expenditures on health care services. Limited public health interventions to address behavioural risks were having some impact on the lifestyles of those who were wealthier and better educated—those best placed to make change. In doing so, these interventions may also have had an unintended effect of exaggerating existing differences in health status between social groups.

In 1977, partly as a reaction to these developments in health systems, *Health for All* was developed as a concept, and adopted as the main social target of governments and the World Health Organization (WHO 1980). This resolution represented a commitment to explore new avenues to solve health problems and gave prominent attention to the need to reduce growing health inequalities between and within countries. *Health for All* has provided one focal point for a renaissance in public health, focused on addressing inequalities in health in many countries.

Finding ways of taking action that would effectively address these determinants of health represents a major challenge for governments and public health systems in all countries. This is especially the case in understanding how best to address the inequities in health between and within countries. For many, a significant turning point in the conversion of this renewed interest and understanding into public health action has come through the *Ottawa Charter for Health Promotion* (WHO 1986). The Charter advocated a 'new' approach to public health, where public health intervention has come to be understood as action which is directed towards improving people's control over all modifiable determinants of health. Thus public health interventions are not only directed at personal behaviours, but also the public policy, and living and working conditions which both influence behaviour indirectly, and have an independent influence on health.

This more sophisticated approach to public health action is based on accumulated evidence concerning the inadequacy of overly simplistic interventions of the past (National Health and Medical Research Council 1997*b*; International Union for Health Promotion and Education 1999). For example, efforts to communicate to people the benefits of not smoking, in the absence of a wider set of measures to reinforce and sustain this healthy lifestyle choice, are doomed to failure. A more comprehensive approach is required which explicitly acknowledges social and environmental influences on lifestyle choices, and addresses such influences alongside efforts to communicate with people. Thus, more comprehensive approaches to tobacco control are now adopted worldwide. Alongside efforts to communicate the risks to health of tobacco use, these also include strategies to reduce demand through restrictions on promotion and increases in price, to reduce supply by restrictions on access (especially to minors), and to reflect social unacceptability through environmental bans (US Department of Health and Human Services 1994*b*). This more comprehensive approach is not only addressing the individual behaviour, but also some of the underlying social and environmental determinants of that behaviour.

Developing the policies, strategies, and infrastructure needed to address these determinants of health has proved to be a challenge for governments and health systems worldwide. Although the links between social, economic, and environmental factors and different patterns of health and disease in populations are relatively easy to identify, the pathways through which to influence these are less well understood (Kawachi *et al.* 1999). In addition, social and economic conditions, and physical environments, are created by sectors other than health. The health sector's role in these is largely indirect. A total government approach is needed to develop sophisticated solutions to the complexities of this broader range of health determinants.

Encouragingly, there is evidence that the health policies and strategies of some nations (e.g. the United Kingdom and the United States (Department of Health 1999; US Department of Health and Human Services 1999*a*,*b*)) have been evolving in response to the growing understanding of the social, economic, and physical environmental determinants of health. There is also evidence of growing concern about inequalities in health on the part of governments and/or their health sectors. This can be seen in national and regional strategies for health in several countries, and most obviously in those countries that have adopted health goals and objectives to guide government policies to improve health (Nutbeam and Wise 1996). In Europe in particular, the WHO has promoted health targets as a mechanism for defining differences in health status between populations, and to target reductions in these differences—the central tenet of *Health for All* (WHO 1985, 1999).

Determining priority and direction: setting health goals and objectives

The identification of health objectives and targets is one of the more visible strategies that have been adopted by several regions, countries, and states since the late 1970s to direct the activities of their health sectors. Such a strategy provides a public statement of the direction and intent for health-related investment and activity by indicating the desired impact on the determinants of health, and intended outcomes in terms of disease incidence and prevalence, and population health and well being.

The United States was the first country to attempt this in a comprehensive format in 1980 (US Department of Health and Human Services 1980). In 1985, the WHO Regional Office for Europe published a set of targets for *Health for All* that were adopted by all member states (WHO 1985). These documents served as models for subsequent programmes in different countries and regions worldwide.

The use of goals and objectives to provide direction for public health intervention has evolved considerably in the past 20 years. The experience in several countries is well documented, and the examples from the United States, United Kingdom, and Australia presented here illustrate the evolution of different approaches that have been taken. Differences in approach can be seen to setting priorities, to the technical task of defining health targets, and the influence of political processes on the widely differing strategies adopted to achieve the targets.

The United States: *Healthy People*

During the period 1979 to 1980 the United States published *Healthy People: the Surgeon-General's Report on Health Promotion and Disease prevention* (US Department of Health and Human Services P1979) and *Promoting Health/Preventing Disease: Objectives for the Nation* (US Department of Health and Human Services 1980). Using a 'management-by-objectives' planning model, measurable national health goals and objectives were established for the first time. The United States adopted a 'life-stage' approach to analysing the health status of Americans, and 15 priority issues were identified. Measurable objectives were then set for each, using a standardized classification system.

Reviews of progress conducted in the following decades (US Office of Disease Prevention and Health Promotion 1986; US Department of Health and Human Services 1994*a*) indicated significant improvements in the health of the population in all major areas, but most notably in relation to infants and children. These reviews also highlighted new and outstanding challenges such as HIV/AIDS, and the relatively poor health of minorities. These new issues, in turn became important priorities for action in the future.

A revised set of objectives for the decade 1991 to 2000 was published in 1990 following a 3-year programme of consultation (US Department of Health and Human Services 1990). The 300 targets were organized into 22 priority areas with particular emphasis on achieving greater equity in health status. This report placed greater emphasis than the earlier document on strategies to achieve more substantial action in pursuit of the targets over the next decade. In particular, an implementation programme was based on the creation of a Healthy People Consortium of more than 350 organizations. In addition to the 54 state and territorial health departments, Consortium organizations represented older adults, racial and ethnic coalitions, educators, businesses, health care providers, and academic institutions. These organizations contributed to the development of the objectives in different ways and were encouraged to use the objectives to guide their own decision-making and action.

The most recently published objectives, *Healthy People 2010*, highlight the progress that has been achieved in relation to several key objectives (for all *Healthy People 2010* references visit the website http//www.health.gov/healthypeople/). This includes further progress in reducing infant mortality and increasing childhood immunization rates, as well as reductions in heart disease and stroke, and a levelling off in rates of smoking, alcohol, and illicit drug use. Outstanding challenges are also highlighted, including high rates of violence and abusive behaviour, high rates of obesity, and low levels of leisure time physical activity.

Healthy People 2010 also reflects further sophistication in understanding the determinants of health as well as the need for social action to address the determinants. It states:

> ...the underlying premise of *Healthy People 2010* is that the health of the individual is almost inseparable from the health of the larger community and that the health of every community in every State and Territory determines the overall health status of the Nation. That is why the vision for *Healthy People 2010* is 'Healthy People in Healthy Communities' (www.health.gov/healthypeople/Volume1/intro/, p.2)

This is reflected in the systematic approach to improving health summarized in Fig. 2, composed of four key elements: goals, objectives, determinants, and health status. *Healthy People 2010* has two overarching goals:

- to increase the quality and years of healthy life

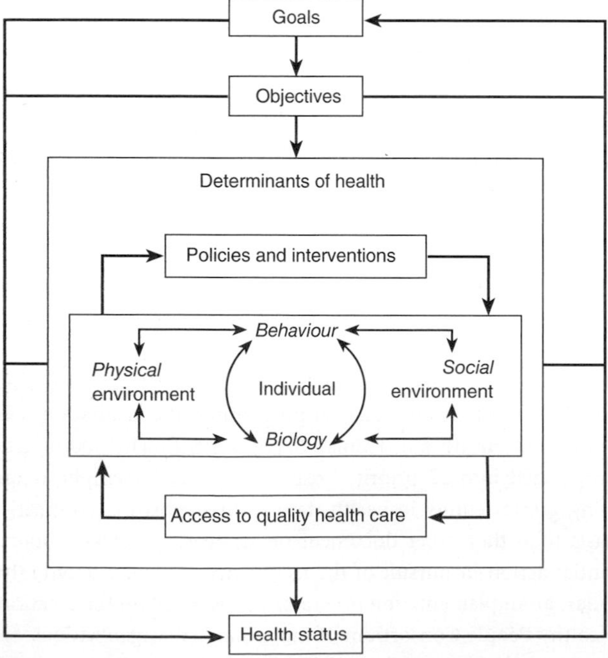

Fig. 2 Healthy people in healthy communities: a systematic approach to health improvement. (Source: US Department of Health and Human Services 1999*a*.)

- to eliminate health disparities.

Progress in achieving these goals will be monitored through 467 objectives in 28 focus areas. The majority of these objectives focus on reduction or elimination of illness, disability, or premature death among individuals or communities. Significantly, other objectives focus on broader issues such as improving access to high-quality health care, strengthening public health services, and improving the availability and dissemination of health-related information. The important influences of income and education on health is explicitly recognized in *Healthy People 2010* as key issues in achieving the goal of eliminating health disparities.

Healthy People 2010 is significantly different from the previous American health objectives in the extent to which it analyses the 'critical influences that determine the health of individuals and communities' (www.health.gov/healthypeople/Volume1/deter/,p.1). The document describes how individual biology and behaviours influence health through their interaction with each other and with individuals' social and physical environments. In addition policies and interventions can improve health by targeting factors related to individuals and their environments, including access to quality health care.

The outcomes expected of these processes are ultimately reflected in changes to health status, which are assessed by a range of measures including mortality and morbidity, life expectancy, and quality of life.

The implementation of policies and programmes to achieve the objectives remains substantially the responsibility of the states and the Consortium partners. This strategy contrasts with that adopted in other countries where governments have adopted a more direct role in action to address targets. Such differences in strategy undoubtedly reflect differences in social organization and in health systems between the United States and countries in Europe.

The process of developing the most recent health objectives was highly participatory and consultative in nature. This engagement has been essential to ensuring the continued commitment of the states and the Consortium partners to commit resources to actions directed towards achieving the objectives. Many of the Consortium partners have made use of the objectives to guide their priority setting and public health programmes. A new section in *Healthy People 2010* provides a 'toolkit' of:

> guidance, technical tools and resources to help States, Territories and tribes to develop and promote successful, state-specific Healthy People 2010 plans. (http://www.health.gov/healthypeople/state/toolkit/)

The toolkit provides ideas and guidance on how to obtain resources, engage community partners, set health priorities, and manage interventions intended to address local priorities. In addition, the objectives have been specified by the United States Congress as the measure for assessing the progress of the Indian Health Care Improvement Act, the Maternal and Child Health Block Grant, and the Preventive Health and Health Services Block Grant (http://www.health.gov/hpcomments/2010*f*ctsht.htm).

The evolution of health objectives in the United States illustrates well a progressively more sophisticated understanding of the determinants of health. The most recent objectives in *Healthy People 2010* reflect a much more comprehensive appraisal of the action required to address the major public health challenges in the United States, including the social and economic determinants of health alongside the behavioural and biological. It also goes further than ever before in advocating and mandating (where feasible) action to address the objectives.

Although the United States process is technically outstanding, a perceived weakness is the rather loose connection between the development of health objectives and the policies and resources that are required to address them. In contrast, approaches to health goal and objective setting in the United Kingdom and Australia have been more overtly linked to policy and public health programmes.

United Kingdom

Amidst the significant reforms of the National Health Service (**NHS**) in England and Wales during the 1980s, the government focused progressively on the need to redirect health policy and health services to the achievement of health. The *Health of the Nation* was published in 1992 (Department of Health 1992*b*). Five key areas were identified, goals and targets were set for each, and strategies for achieving the targets were included.

Unlike the American objectives, the targets in the *Health of the Nation* were overtly linked to the development of policy and programmes in tended to address the targets. A Ministerial Cabinet Committee was set up 'to oversee implementation, monitoring and development of the English strategy and to be responsible for ensuring proper co-ordination of United Kingdom-wide issues affecting health' (Department of Health 1992*b*). The role of the NHS was specified, making it clear that 'improving health should be the prime concern of every NHS authority and health professional and manager in the NHS' (Department of Health 1992*b*). A report outlining *First Steps for the NHS* was also published in 1992 (Department of Health 1992*a*).

The co-ordinated implementation programme included wide dissemination of the strategy throughout the community, oversight of its progress within government, action both within and outside the NHS, and action to ensure that monitoring, research, review, and reporting occur as required. Key Area Handbooks (Department of Health 1993) suggested actions that might be taken by the NHS, local authorities, employers, and schools.

A change in government in 1997 gave new impetus to these initiatives, culminating in publication of a strategy for public health, *Saving Lives: Our Healthier Nation*, in 1999 (Department of Health 1999). This strategy sets targets for improvements in health in four priority areas: coronary heart disease, cancer, injury, and mental health/suicide. It also seeks to address social inequalities in health by addressing the social, economic and environmental determinants of health. The report states that:

> While the roots of health inequality run deep, we refuse to accept such inequality as inevitable. Moreover, we fully accept the responsibility of Government to address such deep-seated problems. That is why we are committed to a wide-ranging programme of action, right across Government, to tackle them. (Department of Health 1999)

To emphasize this commitment, the report is signed by ministers from all relevant portfolios of government, rather than just the Minister for Health. The report specifies a range of programmes and policies to support action to achieve the targets. These include newly funded health system initiatives to improve individual access to health information and advice, stimulating local community action for health through health improvement programmes, and the creation of health action zones in geographical areas of greatest social need. These activities are combined with a strong emphasis on achieving high standards of practice, improved workforce training, and improved disease surveillance. In sectors other than the health sector, a commitment is made to health impact assessment of policies, although the tools for this remain somewhat underdeveloped (Scott-Samuel 1996; Department of Health 1999).

The British strategy overtly links targets for improving health to health system strategies, and to intersectoral action. It also reflects an understanding of the need to invest in the development of the infrastructure required to deliver effective programmatic responses. In these elements, the British approach represents a model of how to link target setting to policies and resources, which address both the underlying determinants of health, alongside behavioural and health system factors. The process of implementation and the effectiveness of these links will need to be carefully examined in the coming years.

Australia

The report *Health for All Australians* published in 1988 (Health Targets and Implementation Committee 1988) was Australia's 'first national attempt to compile goals and targets for improving health and reducing inequalities in health status among population groups'. Unlike other countries at the time, the Australian report contained a series of costed recommendations on strategies to address national health priorities.

Five priority areas were selected, including nutrition, cancer, and the health of older people. The Australian health ministers endorsed these and the *National Better Health Programme* was established with funding for 4 years to initiate strategies to achieve the targets in each of these areas. Although progress was made in building infrastructure for and improving resources for health promotion activity, the programme did not make the anticipated progress in achieving the targets. The reasons for this varied across the different elements of the programme. Progress was clearly limited by the nature of relations between the state and federal governments, which often delayed action, and by a failure to engage adequately the different sectors that needed to be involved in effective action to address these priorities (Commonwealth Department of Health, Housing and Community Services 1992).

In 1991 the Commonwealth Health Department commissioned a review of these targets. The review was intended to consider what progress had been made in relation to the 1988 targets and to examine options for extending the range of targets to reflect a 'social view of health'. This review process extended over 2 years, and included substantial technical consultations with academics and health professionals, and political discussions on the policy implications with individual state health ministers and their departments. The process led to proposals for major revisions in the report *Goals and Targets for Australia's Health in the Year 2000 and Beyond* published in 1993 (Nutbeam *et al.* 1993). This report included not only revisions to many of the originally proposed health targets concerning premature mortality and morbidity and behavioural risks, but also proposed two new categories of health targets concerned with personal health literacy and healthy environments.

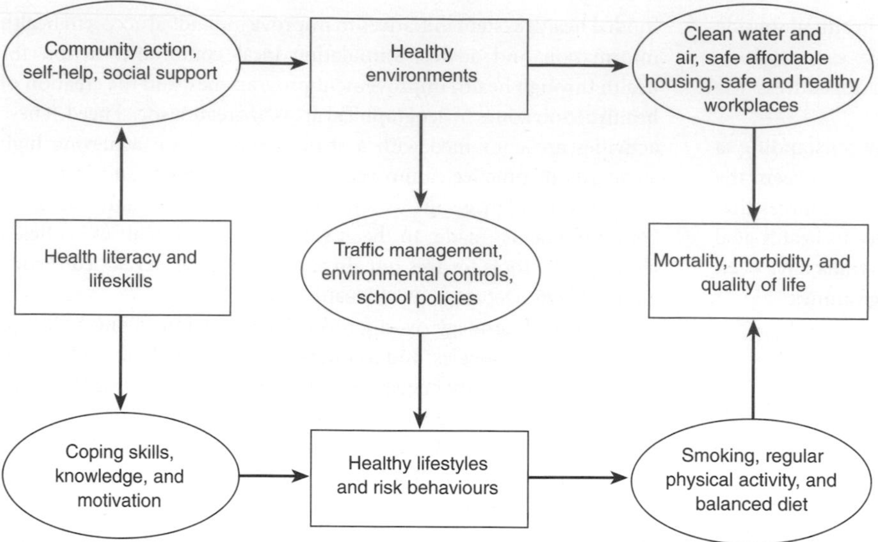

Fig. 3 Relationship between the four groups of health targets. Examples of targets are shown in oval boxes. (Source: Nutbeam *et al.* 1993.)

Figure 3 is derived from the report and provides an illustration of the framework for the targets and the relationship between the different types of targets that were proposed. It shows how each of three key determinants of health—health literacy, health behaviours, and healthy environments—is inextricably linked to the other two. The report made a strong case for co-ordinated public health action to address all of the determinants, particularly by adding to existing efforts to promote health literacy and healthy lifestyles with matching attention to the creation of healthy environments.

The section of the report on healthy environments reflected the greater attention and recognition being given to social, economic, and environmental determinants of health status. This part of the report was structured partly to reflect the way in which government was organized (e.g. housing, employment, environment), and partly to build upon existing working relations between the health sector and other sectors (e.g. health-promoting schools). Such an approach was seen as important both in defining the respective roles of the different sectors, in establishing a workable model for monitoring progress, and determining accountability for the achievement of targets (Nutbeam *et al.* 1993). At the time, this analysis and overt recognition of the links between socio-economic conditions and health was unique.

The subsequent history of this report and its proposals is somewhat mixed, although the initial responses were very positive (Pickering *et al.* 1994). The report served as a catalyst for the inclusion of a commitment to develop national health goals and targets as a part of the Medicare Agreement between the federal government, States, and Territories. Thus for the first time Australia had a statement concerning desired population health outcomes within the legislative agreement (Medicare Agreement) which governs the release of resources for the publicly funded health system. The Agreement committed the Commonwealth and States to a process leading to finalization of national health goals and targets in a limited number of priority areas within 1 year.

The product of this effort, *Better Health Outcomes for Australians* (Commonwealth Department of Human Services and Health 1994), was disappointing in many respects, particularly where it failed to encompass adequately the social, economic, and environmental determinants of health that were a prominent feature of the recommendations from the review which preceded it. No concrete plans were set down to link the targets to a strategy for their achievement. Rather, individual states and territories were left to interpret and act upon the priorities as seemed relevant to local circumstances. Changes in government at federal and state levels since the development of the report further blunted overt action to address these national priorities, but has resulted in greater attention being given to the development of an infrastructure for improving health through a national public health partnership (National Public Health Partnership 1998). This is referred to in greater detail below.

Stimulating action to address goals and objectives

As indicated above, health targets have been promoted by the WHO as a mechanism for defining differences in health status between populations, and to target reductions in these differences. In the three examples above, progressive improvements in routinely collected information and greater investment in research have provided both better data with which to define these differences and improved understanding of some of the determinants of health.

The strategic direction that can be defined by health goals and targets is ultimately dependent upon the quality of the data on which targets are set. This has restricted the priorities and directions that may be indicated by the development of objectives and targets. In Australia, for example, the first health targets in 1988 were restricted to those health indicators for which adequate national data existed—effectively ruling out specific targets to reduce key determinants of differences in health status among population groups. Similar restrictions have limited the targets and objectives adopted in the United States and United Kingdom. While more accurate data enable more precise goals and targets to be set, the limitations of existing national data can inhibit the setting of goals and targets, particularly those addressing social, economic, and environmental determinants.

There is now a better understanding of the need to achieve a balance between meeting the rigorous technical requirements of target setting, and the strategic purpose of providing policy direction. For example, in the United States the 2010 objectives have been expanded to include new areas where indicators do not currently exist in an agreed form, with the intention of stimulating action to develop appropriate indicators in areas such as 'health literacy' (US Department of Health and Human Services 1999*a*). This serves as a stimulus for action to address poor health literacy in the population even though widely accepted indicators and adequate surveillance are not yet in place.

Setting targets does not guarantee that any effective action to address them will follow. Indeed, the available evidence to link target setting to improved health is slim (Nutbeam and Wise 1996). Conceptually, health goals and targets are the proposed outcomes of a nation's entire investment in the health of its population. Therfore much of their potential benefit lies in the extent to which they are used to guide and measure the results of investments in health. To date this has rarely been the case.

Only the United States has had experience of using health targets to guide public policy over an extended period. In this case the process of development and review of the health objectives has offered some valuable technical and strategic lessons. Here, at the very least, the objectives have offered a benchmark against which changes in population health status could be observed over time, and act as a catalyst for response (US Department of Health and Human Services 1986, 1994*a*).

Direct government action to achieve targets and objectives can most easily be observed in the United Kingdom and Australia, where the development of targets has been directly managed by governments, and explicit commitments have been made to develop interventions to address the targets. Unfortunately, this link of health targets and objectives to political processes has not always been a stable base on which to build sustainable public health interventions. The examples from Australia confirm the political nature of public health intervention and the attendant risks.

A specific national programme was established to address the health goals and targets identified in 1988. Rather than being viewed as the responsibility of the whole of government, or even the health care system, the achievement of significant change in major non-communicable diseases and related behaviours was assigned to a modestly funded and poorly co-ordinated programme of activities (Commonwealth Department of Health, Housing and Community Services 1992).

Despite the comprehensive review that took place in the early 1990s—including extensive consultation across the country with politicians, public servants, public health practitioners, and communities—the political process that finally decided on priorities reverted to a narrow set of disease-specific goals and targets, ignoring the opportunity to take the riskier but ultimately necessary approach of identifying environmental and social mobilization goals and targets. By selecting the goals that were least threatening to established administrative and funding arrangements, the potentially more effective, but harder to achieve, health system reform and intersectoral action are ignored or given relatively limited emphasis.

This experience in Australia also indicates how a change in government, or even a change in minister, can lead to a reinterpretation of the nature and purposes of the targets, and substantial dislocation of any action to achieve the targets. Other examples of this experience can be observed in Canada, New Zealand, and The Netherlands (Beaglehole and Davis 1992; Nutbeam and Wise 1996).

Despite these chastening experiences, it is clear from the American experience that focusing on health outcomes and the determinants of health can act as a catalyst for public health interventions. However, comprehensive progress in relation to health objectives and targets will not be made until there are system-wide responses that are backed by resource incentives.

The American experience also suggests that national health objectives can survive changes in government provided that they are developed by a quasi-independent agency, are based on good technical support, and are supported by strong coalitions for action outside of government. Overall, in those countries that have adopted health objectives or targets, the objectives appear to have played an important role in focusing attention on the need for the following:

- a broad base for health policy across the different sectors of government
- changes in resource allocation to develop capacity for public health intervention
- the development of methods and structures which enable action to promote health and prevent disease.

In those countries that have adopted them, health objectives represent a public acknowledgement of the responsibility of governments to address the determinants of health. Health goals and objectives are not a substitute for health-oriented public policies and a viable public health infrastructure, but they can provide a powerful mechanism for public accountability and a substantial platform for the growth and development of public health programmes.

Developing public policy for health: the challenge to improve intersectoral action

Examination of the determinants of health provided in this and other chapters in this textbook has clearly demonstrated the important contribution that can be made by sectors other than the health sector to the achievement of improvements in health. These include the housing, education, transportation, and employment departments of government, as well as the activities of the departments of treasury and finance in relation to economic activity and income. In developing health targets, each of the countries referred to above has, to some extent, made the nature of this challenge explicit, and have provided a platform for concerted intersectoral action. In some cases this is through coalitions of government, non-government, and community organizations (such as in the United States), while in others it has led to the establishment of interdepartmental activity within government (as in the United Kingdom).

Experience in these examples has highlighted the dangers inherent in the health sector seeming to impose its priorities on other sectors. In general, the best strategy appears to be to focus on existing practical opportunities for collaboration by exploring the potential for integrating health goals to reduce risk and promote health into the work programmes of other sectors. This approach to building on existing common ground between sectors, combined with transparency in purpose, appears to offer a basis for developing the effective partnerships for health that are required to advance health and achieve greater equity in health by addressing its underlying determinants.

Experience in Australia, for example, has indicated that there are formidable obstacles, technical and political, to achieving a unified, national response to the complex problems of addressing the environmental, social, and economic determinants of health (Nutbeam and Harris 1994). Where progress has been achieved it has been through bilateral partnerships between the health services and other sectors. In the latter case such action is most achievable where there are clearly defined goals and targets of obvious mutual benefit, and where the roles and responsibilities of each sector and are clearly defined (Harris *et al.* 1996).

Investing for health as a model for intersectoral action

The patchy responses to the development of national health plans, goals, and objectives highlighted above are related to the frailty of the infrastructure for public health intervention in many countries. Encouragingly, the last two decades have seen a rejuvenation of interest and investment in public health in many countries. Although much of that investment has been *ad hoc*—in targeted programmes and services rather than in a well-defined public health system or infrastructure—it has represented a restatement by governments of the need to take an active role in protecting, promoting, and restoring the health of their populations. Even during this period of history in which neoliberal assumptions about the primacy of needs of the economy dominate governments' reform agendas (Mossialos and Permanand 2000), there has been acceptance that government is ultimately responsible for the health of the public (US Department of Health and Human Services 1999*a*).

The experiences of the last three decades have also confirmed that well-designed public health interventions, combined with significant community support and high levels of political commitment, can succeed in improving the health of populations (National Health and Medical Research Council 1997*b*). Analysis of these successes reveal that it is no longer possible or useful to develop interventions that attempt to persuade people to change their lifestyles and health behaviours in the absence of action to change the environments and institutions that shape people's choices. This is especially the case if improved health is to be experienced by all sections of society, not just those with greater wealth and education. Such an analysis also implies the need to link public health with economic and social policy (Mossialos and Permanand 2000), and for public health practitioners to become more fully engaged in the processes of public policy development and implementation.

Once again, this is hardly new. Any analysis of the determinants of health has shown that throughout history, the greatest improvements in people's health have mainly arisen from social and economic improvements that also promote health. The WHO have taken this argument much further by making the case that a healthier population can make a more productive contribution to overall development, requires less social support in the form of health care and welfare benefits, and is more able to support its community and avoid actions that, over the long term, damage its environment (WHO 2000). This logic dictates that investment aimed at securing positive health and well being also brings social and economic benefits for the whole community, and vice versa.

It is clearly established that priority social and economic policy areas—such as education, income maintenance, workplace regulation, housing, transport, agriculture, and communications—as well as private initiatives, have a profound influence on health. Governments have a great potential to improve or worsen people's health through their policy decisions in these areas. This increasingly applies to the private sector too. Great harm can be done to health by misguided public policies or private initiatives. For these reasons, actions to improve and protect the health of the public have to be grounded in a policy structure which:

- is sensitive to the impact on health of policy decisions across all government sectors
- maximizes opportunities for matching economic and social development goals with health development goals and objectives.

This logic is the basis for the WHO's *Investment for Health* strategy which offers a model for achieving a 'whole of government' approach to improving public health. Ziglio *et al.* (2000)describe this strategy as:

> a practical approach based on the rationale that resources are best applied in a way that not only addresses the main causes of ill-health in a credible, effective and ethical manner, but also furthers the achievement of goals for social and economic development

They state that:

> The ideas behind these principles are not new. We intuitively know them to be right. But very few (if any) countries or regions in the world systematically apply these principles to decisions about improving the health of their people.

Some of the key elements of the *Investment for Health* concept are described by Ziglio *et al.* as follows.

1. A focus on health—the objective is to achieve effective action to tackle the root causes of ill health and create opportunities for better health. Health improvement will not always be the primary policy goal, but there is a commitment to assess the population health impact (both positive and negative) of public policy decisions, development strategies and investment decisions, particularly those with social and economic implications. Economic development can be used as a means of improving both the social infrastructure and people's health. Tools for health impact assessment are essential to support this element of the strategy.
2. Genuine intersectoral working—in view of the importance for health of decisions and actions by sectors such as agriculture, education, finance, housing, social services, and employment, a sensible and effective strategy to improve health requires the active inclusion of all sectors to achieve the synergism required to improve population health. The adoption of mechanisms within government to enable intersectoral action for health is vital to support this strategy.

3. Equity focus—the WHO global strategy of achieving *Health for All* is fundamentally directed towards achieving greater equity in health between and within populations and between countries. Equity implies that all people will have equal opportunity to develop and maintain their health through a fair distribution of the resources and opportunities that support health. A mix of programmes to address fundamental differences in opportunity and access to resources, as well as targeted programmes for disadvantaged individuals and communities is required to support this element of the strategy.
4. Sustainability—in this context, this term has a dual significance, signalling firstly, the aim to create an *Investment for Health* process that is durable and resilient; and secondly, that investments are made and resources are managed in ways which do not compromise the health and well being of future generations. Mechanisms to embed the strategies within government, and to build and strengthen an infrastructure for public health are required to ensure the sustainability of the strategies and their effects.

Achieving such a substantial commitment to health is by no means an easy political task. The European Office of the WHO has carried out national *Investment for Health* appraisals in several countries including Slovenia, Hungary, Romania, and Malta (Ziglio *et al.* 2000). This has involved external appraisal, and reporting back to the Health Ministry and/or Parliament on:

- the strategy needed to improve the health status of the population
- the potential for investment for health in the country
- the infrastructure needed to build, support, and sustain *Investment for Health.*

Each part of the appraisal identifies the opportunities to promote health more effectively through key economic and social development policies. This strategy represents a sophisticated attempt to put into public health practice the logical consequences of contemporary analyses of what determines health in populations. Although the approach has not been widely adopted, or implemented over a prolonged period, it illustrates the important challenge facing public health advocates and practitioners. This challenge is to engage government and the private sector in a dialogue about the health impact of policies and practices, and to consider the scope for a synergystic relationship between health, economic, and social development strategies. Like health goals and targets, the *Investment for Health* strategy is not a substitute for investment in a public health infrastructure in countries. Rather, it is a mechanism that facilitates the dialogue needed to link investment for health with economic and social development, and support action across sectors to improve the health of the public. Underpinning such a strategy will be more formally organized systems and structures for public health interventions in different countries.

Developing infrastructure and delivery systems for public health interventions

To be effective, the science of public health must be 'applied'. The science, strategies, and tools used in public health are too often used only to describe and analyse public health problems, and to develop policy. To enjoy the fruits of this analysis, and of health-oriented public policy, it is essential that attention is also given to the development of the organizational capacity of the health sector, in particular, for effective public health intervention. These interventions include the health education and health promotion strategies described in previous chapters, as well as other forms of public health intervention required to assist people and communities to improve their control over the determinants of health.

Creating a sustainable infrastructure for public health has proved to be a complex undertaking for governments. The need for an effective public health service tends to be invisible both to governments and to the public except in times of crisis, and often oriented towards the control of infectious disease. There is relatively limited public demand for a strong public health service (compared with demand for health care services) in all but exceptional circumstances (Grossman and Scala 1993). However, the evolution of health policy to include recognition of the social determinants of health, and to commit governments to tackle non communicable disease, has stimulated action by a number of countries to review and strengthen their infrastructure for public health.

Although there remain significant unanswered questions about the most effective systems or structures through which to 'deliver' public health interventions, there are emerging models for defining priorities for action, for working across government to address determinants of health, and for establishing elements of an effective public health infrastructure. Such an infrastructure should have the capacity to effectively implement the policies and deliver the programmes indicated through the preceding sections of this chapter.

The range of activities and sectors in which practitioners need to act, and the broad range of disciplines that can be said to make up the field of public health have made it difficult to define the 'core business' of public health. Several recent initiatives have sought to identify these 'core functions of public health'. For example, the *Healthy People 2010* document includes a major new section on public health infrastructure (US Department of Health and Human Services 1999*a*). A 'Public Health Functions Project' has been established to address these issues. Among the priorities for the project is the intention to describe the essential services of public health, define public health workforce, training, and education, and improve public health data (US Department of Health and Human Services 1999*b*). Similarly, the National Public Health Partnership in Australia has defined core public health functions (National Public Health Partnership 2000).

Within these lists of core functions, essential services, and public health practices there is still a considerable lack of conceptual consistency. A mix of intended outcomes, interventions (or strategies), and principles for 'good practice' is represented in all the lists. To help untangle these conceptual inconsistencies the distinction is made in Fig. 1 between the essential infrastructure required to lead the development of policy and interventions to achieve priority health goals and targets, and the delivery system required to develop and execute public health interventions.

Key elements of infrastructure for public health

The components of public health infrastructure are similar to those needed by most organizations to conduct their core business—resources, a skilled workforce, and information from research, supported by a system through which to 'deliver' the service or product. In other words, infrastructure refers to the material and human resources that that are required to direct and support action to promote, protect, and maintain the health of the population.

Figure 1 highlights three essential components of an infrastructure for public health as follows.

Secure and sustainable funding

Aside from the *Investing for Health* strategy discussed above, secure, recurrent financial resources are required to support a public health infrastructure within the health sector. Without such investment in a dedicated infrastructure, experience has shown that the public health system can quickly lose capacity (National Health and Medical Research Council 1997*a*; US Department of Health and Human Services 1999*b*).

Public health will not work if left to market forces. Most countries have recognized the need to invest in a public health infrastructure as a 'public good'. In many cases these investments have provided capacity to analyse public health status, guide health decision-making, and respond to public health threats, especially infectious disease outbreaks. However, secure funding for the design, delivery, and evaluation of public health interventions directed to addressing non-communicable disease, and to tackling the social determinants of health has proved more elusive.

This 'programme funding' has proved to be much more difficult to sustain in many countries, particularly when interventions run counter to existing government policy or ideology, and especially when this contradicts economic policy (such as in relation to the sale of alcohol or tobacco, or nutritional programmes which conflict with agricultural practice). Providing a strong rationale for investing in public health interventions continues to be a major part of the role of public health professionals—requiring the use of both science (to demonstrate effectiveness) and political argument (to demonstrate professional and community concern).

The limited information available about the proportion of national recurrent health sector expenditure that is accounted for by public health infrastructure and programmes in different countries suggest that it is very small, relative to expenditure on acute and chronic health care services. Across several countries for example, it appears to be no more than 2 to 3 per cent of total health expenditure (Deeble 1999). While this does not include all the funding invested in public health it provide some indication of the minimal level of public investment through the health sector that might be expected to support public health infrastructure and intervention programmes.

In many countries it has proved necessary to find alternative sources of funding for public health interventions. The establishment of health promotion foundations has been one method used in some states in Australia, and now in some other countries. The funding for these organizations is generated by specific taxation levied by government on the sale of tobacco products. The legislation setting up the organizations originally required them to 'buy out' tobacco company sponsorship of sports, arts, and cultural events. After an initial phase during which funding was substantially applied for this purpose, most foundations have diversified their programmes and in some cases have been able to make a significant contribution to funding public health research and to actions to address social and environmental determinants of health.

The non-government and community sectors also play significant roles in funding research and interventions on issues such as cardiovascular disease prevention, tobacco control, or childhood injury prevention. Organizations such as heart foundations and cancer councils perform important roles in many countries, not only in raising money for research, but in direct community intervention to promote health and prevent disease. There are limitations imposed by their focus on single issues and by the level of funding that they are able to raise directly from their constituencies (in addition to government support). But their high levels of credibility among health professionals and community members mean that they can also be attractive as partners in developing and implementing public health interventions.

The private sector has also begun to take an increasing interest in contributing to public health and social development. In many cases the benefits of partnership are obvious and mutual. For example, in Australia the insurance industry has contributed significant levels of funding to specific programmes to reduce motor vehicle crashes, and the food industry has committed to a programme to improve consumers' recognition of low-fat foods.

It is important to recognize that private sector contributions, in particular, are linked to the needs of business for community support and to assist marketing of specific goods and products. These needs do not necessarily clash with public health goals, but the mutual benefit in partnerships with the private sector is not always as apparent as it could be. The WHO Jakarta Declaration provides some useful general guidance on this issue concerning the need for transparency in relationships and clearly defined mutual benefit (WHO 1998). In negotiating partnership agreements with the private sector it is important to ensure that there is no potential conflict between the outcomes required by the company and the intended public health outcomes.

Workforce and leadership within and outside the health sector

The delivery of essential public health services requires a skilled competent workforce, often working in partnership with other organizations and the community (Public Health Leadership Society 1998). In addition to a specifically trained public health workforce, professionals from many different sectors can be considered as part of the broad public health workforce. There is equal need to support education and professional development for both groups.

Most specialist public health training is provided at the post-graduate level through universities—usually through schools or departments of public health. In some countries medical qualifications have been a prerequisite for entry into public health training; in others a wide range of undergraduate qualifications is accepted. Many disciplines contribute to the body of knowledge that underpins the field, but there is growing agreement about the core competencies required of all members of the specialist public health workforce (Commonwealth Department of Health and Aged Care 2000; Ottoson *et al.* 2000; US Council on Linkages 2000). Within the field there are also several specialties that have developed advanced training programmes—epidemiology and biostatistics, health economics, and health promotion are three of the more common specialty groupings. Specific competencies are also being developed in these disciplines within public health (Howat *et al.* 2000; McCracken and Rance 2000).

In some countries, governments have recognized the need to invest in training programmes to ensure that there are adequate numbers of trained public health professionals. In Australia, for example, the

Public Health Education and Research Program (**PHERP**) was established by the Federal Department of Health and Aged Care in 1986 to fund universities to develop Master of Public Health programmes. Later, the PHERP was expanded to include funding to develop the quality and quantity of teaching and research in several specific areas of special need—environmental health, health promotion, mental health, health economics, and public health nutrition. This type of investment in the workforce has led to a rapid expansion in the quality and effectiveness of the public health workforce in Australia (Commonwealth Department of Health and Aged Care 1999).

Professional associations also make a significant contribution to workforce development. These include public health associations (linked through the World Federation of Public Health Associations), epidemiological associations (linked through the International Epidemiological Association), and health promotion and health education associations (linked through the International Union of Health Promotion and Education). The conferences and journals produced by these organizations are an essential component of workforce development infrastructure. Such associations are also important in the development of and advocacy for healthy public policy in many countries.

The opportunities that are offered by the Internet for collaboration among institutions have resulted in new possibilities to establish national and international programmes and standards of quality in public health workforce training. The Internet also offers students the opportunity to access a wider range of public health training, some of it across national borders (Davies *et al.* 2000).

Public health intervention requires special skills that are different to those required to analyse health problems in a population. Influencing health behaviour in populations, and influencing the structural and environmental determinants of health, requires public health specialists to have substantial knowledge and skills in the behavioural, social, and political sciences. This will require educational institutions to extend the range of current training in many cases.

This emphasis on intervention also highlights the need for a different style of leadership from senior public health practitioners. Earlier sections in this chapter have indicated some of the difficulties inherent in collaboration across sectors. Leadership for public health intervention requires practitioners to work more closely with other sectors, to advocate effectively for the development and adoption of healthy public policy, and to create, with communities, a shared vision for the public's health. There are few programmes that explicitly address the need for advanced training for public health leadership. One example is the Public Health Leadership Institute developed at the UCLA School of Public Health (Public Health Leadership Society 1998).

The training of other health professionals is gradually being adapted to provide them with basic knowledge of public health. Professionals in both the health sector (doctors, nurses, and allied health professionals) and other sectors (e.g. education, agriculture, or architecture) are increasingly being involved in developing policies and programmes that contribute to improvements in the health of the population. This is a major challenge and significant area for development in public health education in the next decade.

The education systems responsible for providing workforce development largely lie outside the ambit of the health sector. It is necessary that there are strong links between academic institutions and agencies responsible for public health. Examples of efforts to achieve this can be seen in the United States by the formation of the Council on Linkages between Academia and Public Health Practice, and in Australia by the National Public Health Partnership and the Public Health Education and Research Programme.

Supportive research, funding, and training

Public health research and development is central to continuous improvement in the relevance, quality, and impact of public health intervention. Research funding for public health can come from many sources. However, competition for health research funding is fierce, and public health research often competes poorly for funding which is dominated by biomedical and health services research. Within public health research, there is also a strong bias towards descriptive/investigative epidemiological research at the cost of adequate investment in intervention research. It is important to ensure that research addresses priority health/structural issues, population groups, and settings, and that it also addresses the need for methodological development specific to public health intervention.

One model used in Australia to enhance the quantity and quality of public health research was the establishment of a specific Public Health Research and Development Committee by the nation's principal health and medical research funding agency—the National Health and Medical Research Council. A designated level of funding was allocated to public health research—most of it investigator driven. Other funding agencies also experimented with such designated funding to encourage public health research.

Although these models have now been abandoned, there has been growing recognition of the need for research funding bodies to ensure a balance between biomedical and public health research funding. In Australia, the National Health and Medical Research Council has explicitly incorporated a funding stream that is intended to enhance and support a greater level of 'strategic' research that will, in turn, enhance public policy in relation to health (National Health and Medical Research Council 2000). There has also been some enhancement of capacity within research funding agencies to ensure that they include public health research among their funded projects and to provide high quality peer review for public health research. The focus on public health research also led to enhanced training opportunities for public health researchers.

Within the discipline of public health there has been tension between the twin intellectual approaches to public health practice, with many public health researchers focusing on the development of knowledge rather than on the actions required to solve public health problems (Hunter and Berman 1997). The most obvious manifestation of this can be seen in the overwhelming investments made in monitoring and surveillance, and in research focused on improving knowledge about public health problems and their causes, rather than on improving knowledge of effective action to resolve the problems. Policies of research funding agencies need to give greater weight to 'intervention' and evaluation research, and ensuring that the peer review process includes reviewers with appropriate knowledge and skills in such research.

Because effective public health interventions include a complex set of actions to bring about widespread social change there is a need for the development of research and evaluation methods that better 'fit' the demands of evaluating action to resolve these more complex problems (Nutbeam 1998; Chapman 1993). Several efforts are being made to identify frameworks and criteria to ensure that the quality of evidence to guide public health interventions meets the highest possible standards of scientific rigour within the context of the complex actions that are needed to bring about positive changes in the health status of the whole population (McQueen 2000).

An effective system for public health research is dependent upon national/organizational research policy that highlights the need for specific public health research—as distinct from biomedical research. It then depends upon there being funds available specifically for public health research, and upon a strong system of peer review by qualified public health researchers. Furthermore, the strength of the research system depends upon the availability of high-quality research training for young researchers, and upon a career development path for public health researchers.

The infrastructure for public health is not, on its own, sufficient to ensure that effective public health interventions are developed, delivered, and evaluated. The infrastructure must then work to develop organizational capacity within and beyond the health sector to create a delivery system for public health intervention referred to in Fig. 1. The components of the delivery system are as follows.

A system for population-wide health monitoring and surveillance

Understanding the complex and changing health status of the population is a cornerstone of public health. A national comprehensive system for population-wide health monitoring and surveillance is an essential component of public health infrastructure. (The Centers for Disease Control and Prevention is a widely recognized example of an organization providing such information.) Such a system should facilitate on-going systematic collection, analysis, and interpretation of national or state population data relevant to the national public health effort. Such data need to be collected at national or state levels repeatedly over time. This 'health intelligence' is needed to identify problems, to set priorities for action, and to monitor progress (National Health and Medical Research Council 1997*a*).

In many countries health information is largely restricted to data on mortality, morbidity, and health system use. This information is vitally important for epidemiological investigation, and to provide broad guidance on public health priorities and policy, but has limitations in its usefulness for planning and monitoring public health interventions (Nutbeam 1996). A much wider range of information, such as that outlined below, is needed for this purpose.

National health information (National Health and Medical Research Council 1997*a*) is either national in coverage or has relevance nationally and relates to:

- measures of health status in the population (including mortality and morbidity data)
- measures of the determinants of the population's health, including those in the external environment (physical, biological, social, cultural, and economic) and those internal to individuals (such as knowledge, behaviour, disease risk factors)
- health interventions or health services, including interventions provided directly to individuals and those provided to communities, covering information on the nature of interventions, management, resourcing, accessibility, use, and effectiveness
- the relationships among these elements.

Any type of health information system should enable analysis of the needs and progress of specific population subgroups with particular emphasis on disadvantaged groups. It must be capable of identifying inequalities in health status and their determinants.

The system for monitoring and surveillance should also be responsible for reporting on the 'state of the health of the population'—on progress towards achieving health goals and targets, and on emerging issues or gaps. There are some useful examples of such reports being used effectively to highlight progress and the need for specific investment in action to address the needs of social and economically marginalized populations (McGinnis *et al.* 1992; US Department of Health and Human Services 1994*a*; Department of Health 1999).

Examples of efforts to improve the relevance and range of health status indicators are beginning to emerge. To measure the influence of social, economic, and environmental factors on the health of populations an expanded range of information is needed in national systems of monitoring and surveillance. Examples of initiatives that are being explored include the Genuine Progress Indicator (Hamilton 1998), the Index of Social Health (Miringoff 1996), the Index of Leading Cultural Indicators (Bennett 1994), and some proposed sustainable development indicators (Interagency Working Group on Sustainable Development Indicators 1997). Although there is need for further research on the core concepts that contribute to social capital, there are some examples of large-scale efforts to measure group membership and levels of social trust across populations (Kawachi *et al.* 1997).

These approaches to health indicator development extend the fundamentally important datasets currently used for health surveillance in most countries, and offer a mechanism to align improvement (or regression) in health status with other indicators of social and economic development.

Identification of national, regional, and local priorities, regular review, and redefinition

The identification of priorities for investment in public health interventions remains one of the most contentious issues in contemporary public health. The use of different criteria for establishing priorities leads to very different priorities for action (Nutbeam 1996). Nationally determined priorities do not always resonate with local needs and perceptions of what actions are important to improve health.

Among the different approaches to priority development are those determined by epidemiological, economic, and community perspectives. Although not mutually exclusive, each of these perspectives places 'value' on different outcomes and processes.

To date, epidemiological analysis has dominated priority setting at national levels. The national health goals and targets identified by many nations and regions discussed above have given priority to leading causes of preventable deaths and morbidity. Analysis of the incidence, prevalence, costs to the health care system and to society associated with the disease/injury, and an assessment of the feasibility of acting to prevent or reduce the incidence or prevalence of the condition are criteria that have been used to identify these priorities. Actions that are linked through epidemiological analysis to a reduction in disease are valued in such an analysis.

Increasingly, economic principles of efficiency are being proposed as a means of identifying priorities for public health intervention (National Health and Medical Research Council 1997*a*). The term efficiency is used here to mean obtaining optimal gain from investment. However, to use the concept of 'efficiency' as a criterion for identifying public health priorities it is important to distinguish between two components of 'efficiency'. The first component concerns ensuring that the services to address a particular issue or problem (e.g. cardiovascular disease) are organized and resourced, which means placing investment across the range of interventions (preventive, curative, palliative, or all three) for a particular condition to maximize individual and community health gain. This is called 'technical efficiency'. It means giving the greatest proportion of investment to the 'part' of the service that produces the greatest health gains—sometimes this will be prevention, sometimes it will be treatment. The evidence is also continually changing, and needs to be applied to readjust the balance of investment. However, even if investment within a programme area (e.g. cardiovascular disease) is efficient, it is possible that investment across the range of health issues and population groups is not well balanced.

The second component of efficiency is 'allocative efficiency'. The analysis of the balance of investment based on assessment of allocative efficiency helps to identify priority issues or problems across the whole range of potential programme or service areas. At its most basic it is a tool for ensuring that a significant issue (such as mental illness) receives adequate resources compared with other, equally prevalent, severe issues. More sophisticated analyses will link investment in programme areas to predetermined population health outcomes, making decisions about the relative level of investment across different service/programme areas.

The third approach to priority setting reflects the growing evidence that the most effective and sustainable public health interventions have been characterized by high levels of community, organizational, and political support. This is particularly true at local level, which is also where national priorities are often seen to be remote from local concerns. Criteria for establishing priorities at local levels include extent of community concern about an issue, the capacity of the community to act to address the issue, and the capacity of local institutions, organizations, and people to contribute to action (Hancock and Minkler 1998). The process of participation in decision-making and perceived responsiveness to local priorities are valued through such an analysis.

These three perspectives on setting priorities are not mutually exclusive, and are best combined to achieve a sound basis for effective action which is nationally relevant, locally sensitive, and financially sound.

Furthermore, the development of priorities for public health intervention should not be considered a one-off event. The 'health intelligence' system established for defining priorities should also be capable of use in the review and redefinition of priorities. This is to ensure that there is capacity to redirect resources (as well as to increase the pool of resources) to address new priorities.

National, regional, and local programme delivery within and outside the health sector

As indicated above, epidemiological analysis of priorities for intervention has generally led public health intervention towards reducing risk factors and behaviours in individuals. This in turn has led frequently to highly differentiated vertical programmes within the health sector to tackle specific risks, such as tobacco use, or diseases such as coronary heart disease. Such programmes tend to have their own goals, resources, workforces, and research programmes (National Health and Medical Research Council 1997*a*). As a consequence, there has been limited scope for integrated programmes to address the social, economic, and physical environmental determinants of health. In contrast with disease/risk factor specific programmes, such integrated programmes are likely to focus more on policy and institutional change, in addition to the public information, education, and mobilization programmes.

In Europe and in Australia there are recent examples of processes being implemented that, amongst other things, are intended to encourage the redefinition of priorities to include greater emphasis on the underlying factors and environments that are 'shared' across different causes of disease and injury. In Australia, for example, instead of the public health funding from the Commonwealth to the states (providers) being distributed according to individual priority issues or population groups, a significant proportion of the 'vertical programme' funds is now pooled. States (providers) negotiate agreement with the Commonwealth (funder) on a specific range of public health outcomes that will be achieved within a specified period. In the United Kingdom the *Our Healthier Nation* strategy referred to above reflects an effort to shift the focus of public health programmes away from vertical programmes to address the underlying determinants of health (Department of Health 1999). Although vertical programmes remain the dominant organizational structure for public health intervention in both countries, these new initiatives are interesting attempts to link funding with the more contemporary analysis of determinants of health.

The comprehensive programmes that are needed to bring about the large-scale changes in the health of populations require public health infrastructure and action at national, regional, and local levels of jurisdiction. Experience has demonstrated the need for clear role delineation and mechanisms for co-ordinating activity, particularly where the focus of the activity is change in legislation (Bidmeade and Reynolds 1998), policy, or programmes in sectors other than health (National Public Health Partnership 1998). The exact nature of infrastructure needed at each level of jurisdiction has not been defined. However, there are examples of using the 'core functions' of public health as standards against which to assess local/regional and 'programme-specific' public health capacity (Turnock and Handler 1997).

In most countries the greater part of the systems for programme delivery are devolved to state, regional, or local levels. A significant factor in improving the infrastructure for programme delivery in some countries, including the United Kingdom and Australia, has been the establishment of subregional administrative structures within the health sector that are responsible for protecting, promoting, and maintaining the health of defined geographical populations. Within these structures, there have been initiatives to draw together the parts of the health care system that have the greatest 'affinity' with public health—divisions of population or public health. This has been an effective means of ensuring an ongoing public health service at local and regional levels. However, it has been less effective in refocusing public health action to address inequalities in health and the determinants of health, and it has not been an effective mechanism through which to increase the proportion of health sector spending on public health action.

In addition to its specialist public health services, the health sector has many other opportunities to make significant contributions to improving the health of the population—through its hospitals, general practitioners, nursing homes, and early childhood services, for example. The sector also has a more direct role in public health—as a major employer, as a consumer of non-renewable resources, and as a physical and social setting that can influence the health of patients, staff, visitors, and the community (Nutbeam *et al.* 1993). Mobilizing this significant untapped resource remains a major challenge for specialist public health practitioners.

As noted above, non-government, community, and professional organizations also play significant roles in the design and delivery of public health interventions. Many of these are linked to specific health issues, such as sudden infant death syndrome, HIV/AIDS, or schizophrenia. Others focus on the needs of specific population groups—older people, immigrants, or indigenous people. Such organizations have specific knowledge, experience, and access to individuals and communities that is often difficult for government agencies to obtain.

Local government also has a key role in public health. The Healthy Cities movement is largely based on this level of government. Municipal public health planning has been found to be an effective mechanism to bring together local government, communities, and key government agencies (including health) to define steps that each can take separately and together to improve the health of the population. In the United Kingdom a derivation of the Healthy Cities concept in the form of Health Action Zones represents a deliberate attempt to bring together the different agencies for public health at a local level. It is through this type of organizational structure that other sectors can be more successfully engaged in public health action. The health sector's role in such relationships varies, depending on the context and the issue being addressed (Harris *et al.* 1996). However, a nation's public health infrastructure must include people with the knowledge, skills, and resources (including power) to work effectively with other sectors. This is particularly important as the emphasis of public health action shifts from programmes developed and delivered by and within the health sector, to influencing public policy and organizations and programmes delivered by other sectors.

Systems for quality control, evaluation, and promotion of best practice

Public health interventions need to be evaluated. The frameworks for assessing the quality of evidence to guide public health interventions referred to above are a component of an effective public health infrastructure. However, such frameworks focus mainly on the quality of research design and methods, and less on the quality of the intervention (relevance, practicality of implementation, etc.) (Speller *et al.* 1997). There is a growing body of evidence that defines the characteristics of effective public health interventions (National Health and Medical Research Council 1997*b*; Malcolm and Dowsett 1998; Green and Kreuter 1999; International Union for Health Promotion and Education 1999). It is a base from which to develop standards of quality for the design and implementation of public health interventions in relation to specific issues or population groups. The Health Development Agency in the United Kingdom, the United States Task Force on Community Preventive Services (Task Force on Community Preventive Services 1999) in the United States, and the National Public Health Partnership in Australia are all working to develop further standards for application to national and regional intervention programmes. Use of such standards and guidelines in the development and implementation of public health interventions will be vitally important in improving the quality and impact of public health intervention in the future.

Conclusion

This chapter describes key elements of health policy and strategy that have been found to be effective in guiding national public health action, and the components of an infrastructure and delivery system required to design, deliver, and evaluate public health interventions. Public health intervention requires a complex mix of science, art (of practice), and politics. The emergence of non-communicable disease in most developed countries has required a radical reappraisal of what determines health, and what public health responses are most appropriate and effective. Four key challenges emerge from this chapter.

1. **Addressing all determinants of health**: it is increasingly apparent that, in many cases, public health practitioners need to expand the range of research methods used to identify public health problems and their causes. As well as using the traditional public health tools of epidemiology and demography, it is necessary to use the social, behavioural, and environmental sciences to obtain a more complete picture. More complex analysis of patterns of disease in populations, and of the determinants of disease will lead to better informed and potentially more effective interventions as a response. In addition, knowledge of current infrastructure and existing strengths in communities is a powerful platform from which to build effective public health interventions (Labonte 1999). Identifying this capacity within communities also requires the use of a wider range of research and consultation methods (McKnight and Kretzmann 1998). It also emphasizes the key role of communities in defining and prioritizing problems, and in developing solutions and is particularly important when working with communities that are disadvantaged or socially excluded.
2. **Gaining visibility for public health**: it is also clear from the analyses in this chapter that public health action often involves political processes. Public health practitioners need to use health data better to influence these political processes. Reporting on ever more sophisticated analyses of public health problems and their determinants will not, on its own, result in any action. However, this data is of great use in raising public and political awareness of health problems, and in highlighting the obligation of governments to develop policy that enables action to improve the health of the population. This includes engaging politicians in dialogue to identify priorities for efficient health sector investment, and when appropriate, advocating for action to support investment in public health interventions in the face of pressure for increased investment in health care services.
3. **Influencing policy and plans for improving public health**: the range of determinants of health means that public health practitioners will increasingly be required to provide technical advice on the impact on health of policies and practices in sectors other than the health sector. Health impact analysis is a relatively new and underdeveloped tool to assist this process. Such technical advice will inevitably lead to conflict in some cases that will require the public health practitioner to act as an advocate for health in the face of competing pressures. More positively, as evidence grows of the effectiveness of public health interventions it will be necessary for public health practitioners to operate across different sectors of government at national, regional, and local levels. Public health practitioners need skills in identifying the policy relevance of the evidence and in identifying the most

effective ways to ensure the use of evidence in the development and implementation of public policy.

4. **Working with people and organizations to improve health**: public health practitioners need to be able to engage people and organizations in practical action to address the determinants of health. Such action will often occur at a local level. The capacity to develop and deliver interventions within local communities and through different settings (such as schools and worksites) is an essential public health skill. Practical guidance on the type of skills and strategies required of public health practitioners to achieve change for public health at this level is provided in Chapter 7.3..

The development of effective organizational structures through which to bring together the components of an effective public health infrastructure within the health sector (in particular) to provide the capacity to 'orchestrate' public health action is a major challenge for the twenty-first century. However, it is important to reflect on the fact that having the technical capacity to develop and deliver effective interventions is not sufficient, on its own. Without political commitment, action to promote health is, at best, difficult—at worst, impossible. The national infrastructure for promoting health must include people and strategies aimed at building and maintaining political support both for public health in general as a key area of government activity, as well as for the specific actions that must be taken if we are to succeed in improving the health of the population.

References

Beaglehole, R. and Davis, P. (1992). Setting national health goals and targets in the context of a fiscal crisis: the politics of social choice in New Zealand. *International Journal of Health Services*, **22**, 417.

Bennett, W. (1994). *The index of leading cultural indicators: facts and figures on the state of American society.* Touchstone Books, New York.

Bidmeade, I. and Reynolds, C. (1997). *Public health law in Australia: its current state and future directions.* Australian Government Publishing Service, Canberra.

Chapman, S. (1993). Unravelling gossamer with boxing gloves: problems in explaining the decline in smoking. *British Medical Journal*, **307**, 429–32.

Commonwealth Department of Health and Aged Care (1999). *Independent review of the public health education and research program.* Department of Health and Aged Care, Canberra.

Commonwealth Department of Health and Aged Care (2000). *National public health education framework.* Public Health Education and Research Program, Commonwealth Department of Health and Aged Care, Canberra.

Commonwealth Department of Health, Housing and Community Services (1992). *Towards Health for All and health promotion: the evaluation of the National Better Health Program.* Australian Government Publishing Service, Canberra.

Commonwealth Department of Human Services and Health (1994). *Better health outcomes for Australians: national goals, targets and strategies for better health outcomes into the next century.* Australian Government Publishing Service, Canberra.

Davies, J., Colomer, C., Lindstrom, B., *et al.* (2000). The EUMAHP Project—the development of a European Masters programme in health promotion. *Promotion and Education*, **7,** 15–18.

Deeble, J. (1999). *Resource allocation in public health: an economic approach.* National Public Health Partnership, Melbourne.

Department of Health (1992*a*). *First steps for the NHS.* HMSO, London.

Department of Health (1992*b*). *The health of the nation.* HMSO, London.

Department of Health (1993). *The health of the nation: key area handbook. Coronary heart disease and stroke.* HMSO, London.

Department of Health (1999). *Saving lives: our healthier nation.* HMSO, London.

Evans, R., Barer, M., and Marmor, T. (ed.) (1994). *Why are some people healthy and others not? The determinants of health in populations.* Aldine de Gruyter, New York.

Green, L. and Kreuter, M. (1999). *Health promotion planning: an educational and ecological approach* (3rd edon). Mayfield, Mountain View, CA.

Grossman, R. and Scala, K. (1993). *Health promotion and organizational development: developing settings for health.* European Health Promotion Series 2, WHO Regional Office for Europe and IFF Health and Organizational Development, Vienna.

Hamilton, C. (1998). Measuring changes in economic welfare: the Genuine Progress Indicator for Australia. In *Measuring progress: is life getting better?* (ed. R. Eckersley), pp. 69–92. CSIRO, Melbourne.

Hancock, T. and Minkler, M. (1998). Community health assessment or healthy community assessment: whose community? Whose health? Whose assessment? In *Community organizing and community building for health* (ed. M. Minkler), pp. 139–56. Rutgers University Press, New Brunswick, NJ.

Harris, E., Wise, M., Hawe, P., Finlay, P., and Nutbeam, D. (1996). *Working together: intersectoral action for health.* National Centre for Health Promotion, Sydney, and Commonwealth Department of Human Services and Health, Canberra.

Health Targets and Implementation Committee (1998). *Health for All Australians.* Australian Government Publishing Service, Canberra.

Howat, P., Maycock, B., Jackson, L., Lower, T., Cross, D., Collins, J. and van Asselt, K. (2000). Development of competency-based university health promotion courses. *Promotion and Education*, **7,** 33 8.

Hunter, D. and Berman, P. (1997). Public health management. Time for a new start? *European Journal of Public Health*, **7**, 345–9.

Interagency Working Group on Sustainable Development Indicators (SDI Group) (1997). *Sustainable development indicators.* Council on Environmental Quality, Washington, DC.

International Union for Health Promotion and Education (1999). *The evidence of health promotion effectiveness. Shaping public health in a new Europe. A report for the European Commission* (2nd edn). European Commission, Brussels/Luxembourg.

Kawachi, I., Kennedy, B., Lochner, K., and Prothrow-Stith, D. (1997). Social capital, income inequality, and mortality. *American Journal of Public Health*, **87**, 1491–7.

Kawachi, I., Kennedy, B., and Wilkinson, R. (ed.) (1999). *Income inequality and health: a reader.* New Press, New York.

Labonte, R. (1999). Health promotion in the near future: remembrances of activism past. *Health Education Journal*, **58**, 365–77.

McCracken, H. and Rance, H. (2000). Developing competencies for health promotion training in Aoteoroa, New Zealand. *Promotion and Education*, **7**, 40–3.

McGinnis, M., Richmond, J., Brandt, E., Windom, R., and Mason, J. (1992). Health progress in the United States: results of the 1990 Objectives for the Nation. *Journal of the American Medical Association*, **268**, 2545.

McKnight, J. and Kretzmann, J. (1988). Mapping community capacity. In *Community organizing and community building for health* (ed. M. Minkler), pp. 157–74. Rutgers University Press, New Brunswick, NJ.

McQueen, D. (2000). Perspectives on health promotion: theory, evidence, practice and the emergence of complexity. *Health Promotion International*, **15**, 95–7.

Malcolm, A. and Dowsett, G. (ed.) (1998). *Partners in prevention: international case studies of effective health promotion practice in HIV/AIDS.* UNAIDS, Geneva.

Marmot, M. and Wilkinson R.(ed.) (1999). *Social determinants of health.* Oxford University Press.

Miringoff, M. (1996). *The 1996 Index of Social Health.* Fordham Institute for Innovation in Social Policy, New York.

Mossialos, E. and Permanand, G. (2000). *Public health in the European Union: making it relevant.* LSE Health, London School of Economics and Political Science, London.

National Health and Medical Research Council (1997*a*). *Promoting the health of Australians: a review of infrastructure support for national health advancement.* National Health and Medical Research Council, Canberra.

National Health and Medical Research Council (1997*b*). *Promoting the health of Australians. Case studies of achievements in improving the health of the population.* National Health and Medical Research Council, Canberra.

National Health and Medical Research Council (2000). *The inside guide to the National Health and Medical Research Council for the 2000–2003 triennium.* National Health and Medical Research Council, Canberra.

National Public Health Partnership (1998). *National strategies coordination.* National Public Health Partnership, Melbourne.

National Public Health Partnership (2000). *National Delphi Study on Public Health Functions in Australia.* National Public Health Partnership, Melbourne.

Nutbeam, D. (1996). Achieving 'best practice' in health promotion: improving the fit between research and practice. *Health Education Research*, **11**, 317–25.

Nutbeam, D. (1998). Evaluating health promotion—progress, problems and solutions. *Health Promotion International*, **13**, 27–44.

Nutbeam, D. and Harris, E. (1994) Creating supportive environments for health: A case study from Australia in developing national health goals and targets for healthy environments. *Health Promotion International*, **10**, 51–9.

Nutbeam, D. and Wise, M. (1996). Planning for *Health for All*: international experience in setting health goals and targets. *Health Promotion International*, **11**, 219–26.

Nutbeam, D., Wise, M., Bauman, A., Harris, E., and Leeder, S. (1993). *Goals and targets for Australia's health in the year 2000 and beyond.* Australian Government Publishing Service, Canberra.

Ottoson, J., Pommier, J., and Macdonald, G. (2000). The landscape in health education and health promotion training. *Promotion and Education*, **7**, 10–14.

Pickering, S., Bennett, J., and Ashpole, K. (1994). National health goals and targets—the Commonwealth Government's approach to achieving better health outcomes for all Australians. *Health Promotion Journal of Australia*, **4**, 5–8.

Public Health Leadership Society (1998). *Development of the Public Health Workforce: a preliminary compendium of national resources.* Public Health Leadership Society, Center for Health Leadership, McLean, VA (www.cfhl.org).

Scott-Samuel, A. (1996). Health impact assessment: an idea whose time has come. *British Medical Journal*, **313**, 183.

Speller, V., Learmonth, A., and Harrison D. (1997). The search for evidence of effective health promotion. *British Medical Journal*, **315**, 361–3.

Task Force on Community Preventive Services (2000). Introducing the Guide to Community Preventive Services: methods, first recommendations and expert commentary. *American Journal of Preventive Medicine*, **18** (Supplement), 1–142.

Turnock, B. and Handler, A. (1997). From measuring to improving public health practice. *Annual Review of Public Health*, **18**, 261–82.

US Council on Linkages (1999). *Competencies.* www.TrainingFinder.org/competencies

US Department of Health and Human Services (1979). *Healthy people: the Surgeon-General's Report on health promotion and disease prevention.* Department of Health and Human Services, Washington, DC.

US Department of Health and Human Services (1980). *Promoting health/preventing disease: objectives for the nation.* Department of Health and Human Services, Public Health Service, Washington, DC.

US Department of Health and Human Services (1986). *The 1990 objectives for the nation: a midcourse review.* Department of Health and Human Services, Washington, DC.

US Department of Health and Human Services (1990). *Healthy people 2000: national health promotion and disease prevention objectives.* Department of Health and Human Services, Public Health Service, Washington, D.C.

US Department of Health and Human Services (1994*a*). *Healthy people 2000 review 1993.* Department of Health and Human Services, Washington, DC.

US Department of Health and Human Services (1994*b*). *Preventing tobacco use among young people: a report of the Surgeon General.* US Department of Health and Human Services, Public Health Service, Centers for Disease Control and Prevention, National Center for Chronic Disease Prevention and Health Promotion, Office on Smoking and Health, Atlanta, GA.

US Department of Health and Human Services (1999*a*). *Healthy People 2010: objectives for the health of the nation.* http://www.health.gov/healthypeople/2010Draft/scripts

US Department of Health and Human Services (1999*b*). *The public health functions project.* http://www.health.gov/healthypeople/2010Draft

WHO (World Health Organization) (1980). *Global strategy for health for all.* WHO, Geneva.

WHO (World Health Organization) (1985). *Targets for health for all.* WHO Regional Office for Europe, Copenhagen.

WHO (World Health Organization), Health and Welfare Canada, Canadian Public Health Association (1986). *Ottawa Charter for Health Promotion.* WHO Regional Office for Europe, Copenhagen.

WHO (World Health Organization) (1998). *Jakarta Declaration on leading health promotion into the twenty-first century.* WHO, Geneva.

WHO (World Health Organization) (1999). *Health 21—health for all in the twenty-first century.* WHO, Cophenhagen.

WHO (World Health Organization) (2000). *Health is a precious asset. Accelerating follow-up to the World Summit for Social Development.* WHO, Geneva.

Ziglio, E., Hagard, S., McMahon, L., Harvey, S., and Levin L. (2000). Principles, methodology and practices of investment for health. *Promotion and Education*, **7**, 4–15.

12.10 Strategies for health services

Martin McKee and Josep Figueras

Introduction

At the outset it is necessary to ask why public health professionals should be interested in health services, and so set the agenda for this chapter. Those involved in the delivery of health services can have many different objectives. The growing numbers of for-profit chains of health maintenance organizations in the United States seek primarily to increase financial returns to their shareholders. In the European Union, the Amsterdam Treaty has recognized explicitly the contribution of health care to job creation. However, it is the view that health care offers a means of improving the health of a population that provides a justification for public health professionals to become involved in health services. As discussed below, this is leading to a growing recognition in many countries of the positive contribution that public health professionals can make to the organization and delivery of health care.

The content of this chapter follows from these arguments. Public health professionals, with their emphasis on improving population health, have a legitimate role in ensuring that the pursuit of health gain becomes a central objective of health care systems, whatever other objectives may be being pursued by others. To do so, they must promote the equitable use of interventions that are effective and appropriate for the population in question, reduce interventions that are ineffective or harmful, and thus maximize the health gains obtained with the available funding.

Health care systems in many countries are changing, for a variety of reasons (Saltman and Figueras 1997). This brings both opportunities and threats for public health professionals. On the one hand, change offers the possibility to challenge existing arrangements and maximize the contribution of health services to population health. On the other hand, it brings threats as those responsible for health policy seek other objectives, such as the narrow pursuit of profit.

Consequently, this chapter explores the changing nature of health services, the role that public health professionals can play in these processes, and the strategies that they can pursue to enhance health gain and promote equity. It does not seek to provide a description of the many different health services throughout the world or offer a blueprint for those wishing to design the perfect health system (if such a thing is possible). A critical review of texts covering these questions has been published elsewhere (McKee and Figueras 1997).

Before considering these matters, there is one question that must be addressed. This is whether health services actually make a meaningful contribution to population health. The view that they do is not universally accepted, and so before proceeding to examine what is known about how public health professionals can best contribute to the organization and delivery of health services, it is necessary to examine whether there is any evidence that such services actually do any good.

Do health services affect population health?

While most would agree that some interventions, most obviously immunization against diseases such as smallpox, poliomyelitis, and measles, but also some low-technology strategies such as integrated management of childhood illness (Lambrechts *et al.* 1999), have been remarkably successful in reducing mortality in many parts of the world, there is much less agreement about many other elements of health services.

At the risk of simplification, the debate has become somewhat polarized. If the major determinants of health lie outside the health care sector, is the involvement of public health professionals in the delivery of health care at best an irrelevance and, at worst, a diversion from the more important roles of advocacy and mobilizing inter-sectoral action (Whitty and Jones 1992)? Or have they a role in ensuring that health care is provided effectively and efficiently, on the basis that this will maximize population health?

A widely held view is that the weight of evidence supports the former position. This is associated most closely with McKeown (1979) who showed how three-quarters of the decline in mortality in England and Wales between 1841 and 1971 had been due to a reduction in deaths from infectious disease and that three-quarters of this reduction had preceded the widespread introduction of immunization or antibiotics. Thus, he argued, the main drivers of improvements in health had been nutrition, environment, and behaviour.

A different, but related, perspective is offered by those who argue that it is unrealistic to expect health care to contribute significantly to population health because so little of it has been adequately evaluated and found to be effective (Chappell 1993).

To others, however, it is not just that health care has little impact on health. Instead, it may actually damage it. This view receives some support from studies that have related health care inputs to outputs. If anything, these have suggested that there is an inverse association, with greater health care resources leading to worse overall health (Cochrane *et al.* 1978; Scheiber *et al.* 1993). One possible explanation is that scarce resources are being channelled into health care rather than sectors such as education where they would have a greater, albeit less immediately obvious, impact on health. Another is that health care has a direct and adverse effect on health, a view advanced by Illich (1976), who emphasized patients suffering from the side-effects of prescribed drugs, hospital-acquired infections, poorly performed surgery, and the consequences of following up spurious abnormalities found among increasing numbers of laboratory investigations.

These views have elicited a range of responses. Some physicians have simply dismissed them (Ingelfinger 1977), arguing that they are completely at odds with the everyday experience of clinicians who see the results of the care that they provide. In contrast, others, especially some health economists, have argued that the existing level of health care provision in some countries is excessive (Evans 1994; Lavis and Stoddart 1994) and that politicians should shift expenditure from health care to sectors such as education, housing, and employment (Smith 1994).

However, there is a compromise position which is that, while Illich and McKeown may have been correct in the 1960s and 1970s when they were developing their arguments, the intervening period has seen major changes, with many formerly fatal conditions now susceptible to treatment. Furthermore, many of the criticisms made by Illich concerning unnecessary and inappropriate investigations and treatment have now been addressed by the greater acceptance of evidence-based health care. In this scenario, health care, at least in industrialized countries, is seen, potentially, as one of the major determinants of health of a population and thus worthy of the attention of public health professionals.

Quantifying the contribution of health care to population health

Health care has changed remarkably in a relatively short time. Many new treatments have been introduced that have been shown, in high-quality evaluative research, to be able to prolong life. Examples include effective treatment for hypertension and heart failure, secondary prevention following myocardial infarction, and chemotherapy for many childhood cancers. There has also been, in many countries, a revolution in the approach to evidence in making treatment decisions.

These changes are part of a long-term trend. Beeson (1980) showed how many treatments advocated in a 1927 edition of a major textbook of medicine were, at the time he was writing, known to be either ineffective or harmful. The 1975 edition displayed a major shift to treatments that had been proven to be effective. However, the pace of change has accelerated during the 1980s and 1990s. There has been a much greater willingness to challenge professional judgement where it is not supported by evidence of effectiveness and to question whether clinical performance is optimal. This has led from early pioneers of the medical audit (Lembcke 1947; Neuhauser 1990) to the enormous expansion of evidence-based health care (see below). This encompasses a wide range of activities which together have helped to get rid of many interventions that do not work and have increased the uptake of those that are effective. Thus there is a case that if health care made little contribution to population health in the past, it may now be doing so. The following section asks whether this has actually happened.

Rutstein *et al.* (1976) addressed this question by asking an expert panel to identify a list of conditions from which death should not occur if appropriate medical care was provided. These deaths were deemed to be 'preventable' although subsequent writers have also used the terms 'avoidable' and 'amenable to medical care'. They argued that the decline in such deaths was a measure of the performance of the health care system. This concept has subsequently been adapted by other researchers and used to examine many different countries (Charlton and Velez 1986; Poikolainen and Eskola 1986; McKee and Bewley 1987; Malcolm and Salmond 1993) and in the production of regional atlases permitting cross-national comparisons (Holland 1991; Józan and Prokhorskas 1997).

These studies have consistently found that deaths due to causes amenable to medical care have fallen at a faster rate than other deaths, suggesting that medical care is now contributing to population health. This concept is not, however, without its critics. Carr-Hill *et al.* (1987) have argued that deaths amenable to medical care include only a small percentage of overall deaths. Furthermore, at a subnational level, there is no clear link with other measures of health care provision.

The first criticism arises largely because the original advocates of this concept adopted the somewhat arbitrary criterion that only deaths occurring under the age of 65 years could be considered amenable. This is inconsistent with life expectancies at birth in the high seventies or low eighties in many industrialized countries. Mackenbach and coworkers (Mackenbach *et al.* 1988; Mackenbach 1996) addressed this by increasing the age limit to 75 years. By also increasing the number of conditions classed as amenable, they considerably extended the concept of death amenable to medical care. They addressed the second criticism by relating changes in deaths from particular causes to the time that various interventions were introduced. By doing so, they were able to show that the impacts of specific treatments were observable as accelerating falls in mortality from the conditions they were intended to treat. They concluded that the health care interventions they examined added 2.9 years to life expectancy at birth for men in The Netherlands between 1950 and 1984 and 3.9 years for women.

The approach taken by Mackenbach had the advantage of bringing many more conditions under the umbrella of avoidability. However, the chain of events leading to death is complex and there is an advantage in separating those amenable to personal medical interventions from those amenable to wider government health policies. A study from Spain separated conditions amenable to personal medical care, such as tuberculosis, appendicitis, and asthma, that accounted for 11 per cent of all deaths, from conditions amenable to national policies, such as cirrhosis of the liver and motor vehicle accidents, that accounted for 19 per cent of total mortality (Albert *et al.* 1996). Deaths from causes amenable to personal medical care fell between 1975 and 1990 whereas those amenable to national health policies increased.

Support for this hypothesis also comes from studies of particular causes of death. Beaglehole (1986) estimated that 42 per cent of the decline in deaths from cardiovascular disease in New Zealand between 1974 and 1981 could be attributed to advances in medical care. The long-term decline in mortality from coronary heart disease in The Netherlands between 1969 and 1993 accelerated significantly after 1987 coinciding with the wider availability of interventions such as coronary care units and thrombolysis (Bonneaux *et al.* 1997). Deaths from testicular cancer in the German Democratic Republic fell following unification with the west and increased access to new treatments (Becker and Boyle 1997), and in childhood leukaemia in Russia where again modern treatments have recently become more widely available (Shkolnikov *et al.* 1999).

Notwithstanding these findings, it is pertinent to re-examine Illich's view that modern health care is generally harmful. Clearly some interventions are damaging to health. As the example of albumen, which has long been given to patients with burns and multiple trauma, shows, even treatments that seem intuitively likely to be beneficial may not withstand critical scrutiny (Cochrane Injuries Group Albumen Reviewers 1998). Increasingly, such interventions are being identified and withdrawn but this remains an unfinished agenda.

Health care and health equity

The health impact of health services raises the important issue of equity. When health care had little measurable impact on health, sociodemographic inequalities in access to care may have been of little importance. Indeed, it is arguable that the wealthy, exposed at considerable personal expense to such painful and ineffective treatments as leeches, cupping, and bleeding were actually disadvantaged compared with the poor. The present situation is quite different. If health care does contribute materially to population health, then lack of access to it will exacerbate health inequalities (Arblaster *et al.* 1996).

There is considerable evidence from many countries that such inequalities exist and that they have an impact on health. This is intuitive in health care systems where there is not universal access to care, such as the United States. For example, American research has found that people living in deprived areas with poor access to care have high rates of hospital admission with chronic medical conditions, such as asthma, heart failure, and diabetes that, if detected and treated early should not require admission to hospital (Bindman *et al.* 1995). But inequalities are also seen in countries offering universal coverage. In the United Kingdom, women (Petticrew *et al.* 1993), those from minority ethnic populations (Shaukat *et al.* 1993), and those living in deprived areas (Ben-Shlomo and Chaturvedi 1995) are all disadvantaged in access to surgical interventions for coronary artery disease. In New Zealand, social class gradients are substantially greater for causes amenable to medical care than other causes of death (Marshall *et al.* 1993). A study from Helsinki, Finland, found significantly higher death rates from causes amenable to medical care among those in the lowest social class or who were homeless (Poikolanen and Eskola 1995). Equitable access to effective health care becomes a matter of legitimate concern for public health professionals.

The findings discussed above suggest that, contrary to the situation before the 1960s, health services are now making an important contribution to overall improvements in life expectancies in industrialized countries. They may also be contributing to the differences in life expectancy between countries. Rates of treatment with interventions of known effectiveness vary considerably (Mulrow 1995). Even between otherwise similar countries, large differences may exist. Law and Wald (1999) have compared the uptake of secondary prevention among survivors following myocardial infarction in the United Kingdom and France (Table 1).

Table 1 Uptake of secondary prevention agents among survivors following myocardial infarction in the United Kingdom and France

Intervention	United Kingdom (%)	France (%)
Cholesterol-lowering agents	4	34
Aspirin	38	63
Anticoagulants	5	20
β-blockers	20	48

Data from Law and Wald (1999).

Boyle *et al.* (1996) argued that it would be possible to track trends in safer surgery and anaesthesia by means of a study of deaths from a common surgical condition, benign prostatic hypertrophy. They found that deaths had fallen in many countries between 1950 and 1990 the improvements were much greater in Northern Europe and North America than in Central and Eastern Europe and South America. Death rates from childhood cancers for which effective treatments are now available have decreased in most European countries although to a greater extent, and earlier, in Northern Europe than in Southern or Central Europe, arguably reflecting differences in the diffusion of new treatments (Levi *et al.* 1992).

The division of Europe prior to 1990 offers an opportunity to examine this issue further. The former communist countries of Central and Eastern Europe were relatively isolated from many modern health care developments. Noting that death rates from causes amenable to medical care were higher in these countries than in the west (Bojan *et al.* 1991; Boys *et al.* 1991). Velkova *et al.* (1997) sought to quantify their contribution to the East–West gap in life expectancy. Excluding early neonatal deaths, for which only incomplete data are available, they estimate that amenable causes accounted for 24 per cent of the gap in male life expectancy between birth and the age of 75 years in 1988. The corresponding figure for females was 39 per cent.

International comparisons in this field are intrinsically problematic because of differences in incidence of disease as well as definitional problems. However, these problems have, to a considerable extent, been overcome in a major comparative study of cancer survival in Europe, the Eurocare study. This has found large differences in cancer survival between countries, raising important questions about the organization and funding of cancer services in some countries (Coebergh *et al.* 1998) (Fig. 1). The implication, for public health professionals, is that international differences provide many natural experiments from which lessons can be drawn (McKee 1998). This process is increasingly being facilitated by initiatives such as the European Observatory on Health Care Systems (Figueras and Saltman 1998).

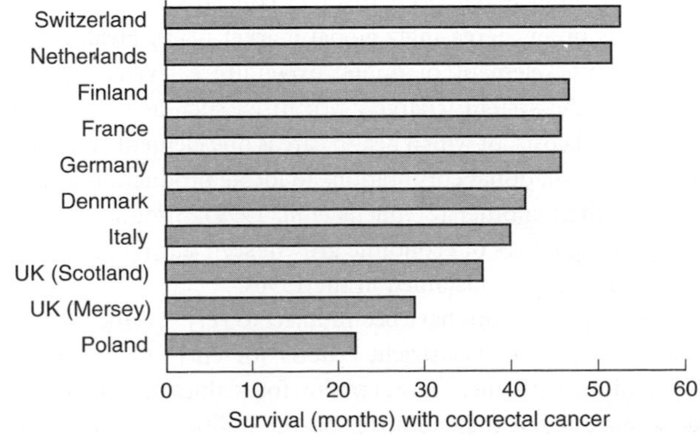

Fig. 1 Cancer survival in European countries. (Source: Sant *et al.* 1995).

Health care and health—a synthesis

The previous section showed that there is now considerable evidence that, unlike the situation prior to the 1970s, health care can make a substantial difference to population health. However, as the World Health Organization (**WHO**) noted in the Ottawa Charter (WHO 1986), health services are only one of the determinants of health, others being genetic predisposition, individual behaviour and lifestyle, and environmental circumstances. Public health professionals must look at the wider picture and take into account these other determinants. But it is important that, in taking a broad perspective, they do not loose sight of the contribution that health care can make to population health, ensuring that what care is provided is effective and is provided equitably. The remainder of this chapter explores the changing nature of health services, the impact that various policies have, and the role that public health professionals can play in maximizing the health gain that health services can provide.

Why are health systems changing?

Health care systems face a range of pressures, from both within and without (Saltman and Figueras 1997). External factors include the macroeconomic climate and the evolving framework of values of the society within which the system is located. Internal factors include the changing pattern of health in the population being served, upward pressures on expenditures arising from ageing populations and technological change, a search for improvements in the quality of health care that is delivered, and the expansion of information technology. These will be considered in turn.

Macroeconomic factors

The configuration of a health system is strongly influenced by its economic environment. While the costs of some inputs into health services reflect local market conditions, such as salaries for health care professionals, others, such as pharmaceuticals and technology, reflect world market prices. Indeed, co-ordinated purchasing policies mean that some products, such as insulin, may actually be substantially cheaper in industrialized than in developing countries. Consequently, the combination of labour, capital, and consumable elements in a health system can be expected to reflect each country's economic circumstances.

However, these circumstances are not static. During the 1990s, many health care policies had been driven by concerns about national competitiveness in an increasingly global market place. Health care represents a major element of public expenditure, even in those countries where the system is largely privatized such as the United States. High social costs, of which health care is one element, are cited as reasons for transnational corporations to locate production in one country rather than another (Stephens *et al.* 1999). Simultaneously, the historically high rates of economic growth seen during the 1960s and 1970s have not been sustained in the 1990s.

In addition, some regions have been subject to very specific factors. In Western Europe, the Maastricht criteria for entry to European Monetary Union, with their requirement for reductions in public sector debt, have had a major impact on the political environment within which decisions on public spending are made (Kanavos and McKee 1998). In the countries of Central and Eastern Europe, the collapse of established trading networks in the early 1990s led to deep economic recessions and wide-ranging reforms of the public sector. In the mid-1990s, the countries of Southeast Asia suffered a major economic crisis which has led to substantial changes in health care sector, a shift from private to public care, and the introduction of wide-ranging strategies aimed at cost containment (UNFPA 1998). Many developing countries have been faced by rising levels of debt and externally imposed structural adjustment policies with major implications for health services (Peabody 1996).

The importance of the macroeconomic environment for public health professionals, apart from the obvious need to be aware of the implications of macroeconomic change for population health, is primarily in the extent to which it influences the political decision-making process and, in particular, the allocation of resources to competing sectors. While, in most cases, public health professionals must work within the constraints that this creates, they also have a major role, as advocates for the public's health, in shaping the debate.

Norms and beliefs

A second set of factors driving change in health care systems relate to the underlying norms and beliefs of the society within which the system is embedded (Contandriopoulos *et al.* 1998). Health care systems act as mirrors that reflect deeply rooted social and cultural expectations of the population that they serve. Although these norms and beliefs are generated outside the formal structure of the health care system, they play a major role in defining the system's overall characteristics.

The impact of different norms and beliefs is apparent when comparing the United States, where health care is generally seen as a commodity to be bought and sold, and Europe, where health care is seen predominantly as a social or collective good, in which citizens benefit when an individual receives effective care. The latter model is associated the principle of solidarity, in which there are cross-subsidies between groups and population defined by age, wealth, health status, to enable access to health care to be available.

However, this dichotomy is oversimplified and, in reality, societies have dominant belief systems (Benson 1975). This does not imply that a single view is held by all members of that society; rather, the tension and negotiation that exists between various beliefs and values has some stability. A useful approach to understanding belief systems sees these tensions as grouped around four poles (Habermas 1987): values, understanding of phenomena, definition of jurisdictions and allocation of resources, and logic of regulation. Values include the tensions and trade-offs between equity, individual autonomy, and efficiency (Clark 1988). Understanding of phenomena relate to how concepts such as life, death, sickness, health, and pain are interpreted and thus viewed as relating to the objectives of a health care system (Gillett 1995). Definition of jurisdictions and allocation of resources comprise the perceptions of the role and functions of those working in the health care sector, as well as the allocation of resources between prevention and cure and between health care and broader determinants of health. The logic of regulation relates to how society chooses to regulate the delivery of health care (Contandriopoulos *et al.* 1998). This may be technocratic, with trained experts guiding the system on the basis of their knowledge and position within the hierarchy, professional self-regulatory, which has the physician, as the best agent of the patient, at the centre of the system, the market-based model, in which regulations reflect supply and demand in a competitive market, or the democratic model, in which the population, either directly or, more often, through elected or appointed representatives, is responsible for setting out the framework for delivery of health care.

Although dominant belief systems have some stability, they are in a state of constant tension as different classes and groups within a society struggle for ascendancy, a phenomenon most clearly seen in the fluctuating electoral success of political parties. In some societies, the process of change will be evolutionary and incremental. In others, as exemplified by the countries in Central and Eastern Europe after the collapse of communism, it will be abrupt.

An understanding of the dominant belief system in a society is important for public health professionals as it contributes to knowledge of why systems are as they are, how they have changed, and the objectives that individuals within the health care system are pursuing. It will also influence the choice of strategies that should be adopted to bring about change.

Changing burden of disease

Although it would be naive to think that the health needs of the population are the only factor driving the configuration of health services, they do play an important role. For example, the public health services in many industrialized countries are a direct result of the global epidemics of cholera in the mid-nineteenth centuries (Davies 1998). Recognition of the infectious nature of tuberculosis led, somewhat controversially, to the creation of sanitoria (Fairchild and Oppenheimer 1998). More recently, the discovery of the agent responsible for hepatitis B and, especially, the emergence of the HIV virus, have both had significant implications for the organization of systems designed to reduce cross-infection in health care facilities.

The burden of disease worldwide is dynamic (Murray and Lopez 1996). One factor is the changing age structure of the population. In many populations the number of old people, and especially the very old, is increasing. This is causing an increase in the frequency of patients with complex multiple pathology. Coupled with a growth in evidence of the effectiveness of organizational interventions, such as stroke units (Stroke Unit Trialists' Collaboration 1997) and integrated care teams, this will lead to a need for much closer working by different specialists and professional groups, and a consequent breaking down of many established hierarchies.

A second factor leading to changing patterns of disease is changing risk factors. Some of these, such as tobacco consumption, act over long periods, while others, such as alcohol or those leading to some infectious diseases, have consequences that appear almost at once.

In the space available it would be impossible to discuss the many different trends seen worldwide. They include, in industrialized countries, a long-standing decline in stomach cancer, most likely as a result of lower rates of infection with *Helicobacter pylori* in childhood (Pisani *et al.* 1997), more recent falls in ischaemic heart disease, mainly as a result of more healthy diets (Vartiainen *et al.* 1994), and a steady rise in smoking-related cancers among women (Peto *et al.* 1994). In developing countries falling death rates from some infectious diseases coincide with increases in the 'diseases of affluence', such as ischaemic heart disease (Bobadilla *et al.* 1993). In particular, many smoking-related disease will rise further (Barnum and Greenberg 1993). Many countries have also been severely affected by high levels of HIV infection and AIDS (Over and Piot 1993).

The key message is that the incidence and prevalence of many diseases are changing, creating a pressure for changes in health care systems. Public health professionals have a central role in tracking and predicting these emerging trends, in designing mechanisms that address them, and in supporting the changes in service delivery that are required.

Upward pressure on health care expenditure

Increased health spending constitutes the most important single factor leading to health systems change. At the core of many health care reforms is the need to contain costs. Figure 2 presents a snapshot of the growth of health care expenditure in a number of Western European countries. Several factors have combined in recent decades to exert upward pressure on health spending. These include the ageing of the population, the expansion of coverage and the development of more expensive health technologies combined with increased population expectations.

Ageing populations influence the demands on the health care system, especially as they often coincide with falling birth rates, leading to an increasing dependency ratio. Thus the demands on the system are increasing at a time when the number of people of working age, who are paying for it, is falling. These changes vary greatly between countries. Some, such as Germany and Japan, face substantial challenges while others, such as the United Kingdom, will be somewhat less affected, at least until the middle of the twenty-first century.

Although an ageing population is probably one of the most frequently cited causes of rising health care expenditure, it is necessary to enter a caveat. There is still considerable uncertainty about the extent to which health care costs actually do increase with age.

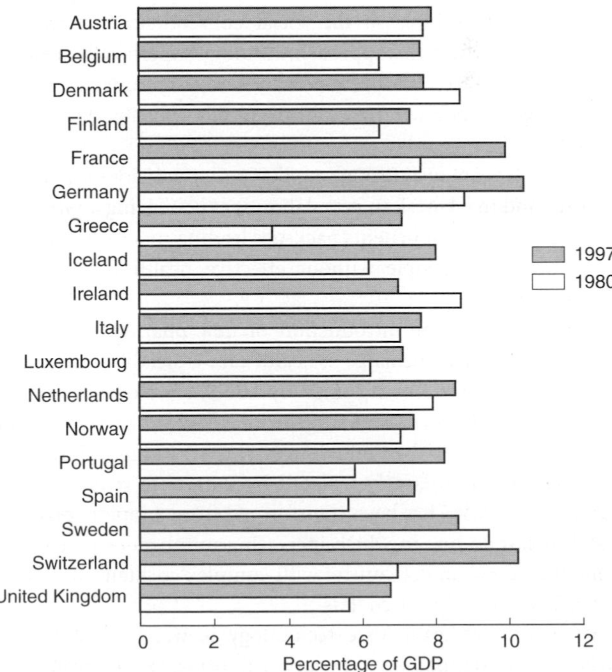

Fig. 2 Total expenditure on health as a percentage of gross domestic product, Western Europe, 1980 and 1997. (Source: OECD 1999).

Fuchs (1984) has argued that the elderly do not incur health care costs simply by being old. Rather it is that, with increasing age, more are in the last year of life, which is the true cause of high costs. This is supported by evidence from American Medicare data, which shows that payments associated with an additional year of death fall as age at death increases (Lubitz *et al.* 1995) and that the most costly patients are those who die young, possibly because, for a variety of reasons, they are more intensively treated (Scitovsky 1988). However, these studies did not include the cost of social or long-term care, unlike a study conducted in The Netherlands, which found that the total cost of health care rose exponentially with age from 50 to 95 years and over (Meerding *et al.* 1998).

Clearly, the relationship between ageing and health care costs is complex and depends partly on what is and is not included. In addition, it is at least plausible that the level of general health of the elderly in the future may be different from that of today, as they will have benefited from a lifetime of better nutrition and social conditions. For these reasons, simplistic extrapolations of cross-sectional data to a future population with a longer life expectancy is flawed.

A second factor exerting upward pressure on expenditure in some countries has been expansion of coverage, although the relationship with expenditure is complex, as illustrated by the case of the United States, which has the highest expenditure on health care but the lowest coverage of any industrialized country (Starr 1982; Rothman 1993).

In general, the twentieth century was characterized by an expansion of health care coverage. In 1960, only a few industrialized countries provided universal or near universal coverage through compulsory systems. By 1996, nearly all did. In Europe, for example, only Germany and The Netherlands do not, permitting or requiring the wealthiest segments of the population to opt for private coverage. Chile, under the Pinochet regime, permitted the wealthy to opt out of the Servicio Nacional de Salud (Reichard 1996). This had the effect of fragmenting the previous system and creating deep inequalities and offers a graphic example of the social consequences of reducing coverage. In particular, this approach, although superficially attractive because it appears to be reducing demands on the health care system, has adverse effects because the wealthy typically contribute more than they cost.

However, it is not just through explicit policy decisions that change takes place and the American population is experiencing an insidious process of reduction of benefits packages leading to a steady increase in the number of people without effective health care coverage (Kirkman-Liff 1997).

A third factor is the introduction of new pharmaceuticals and technology. The pace of change in health care is steadily accelerating. Hip replacements have been joined by knees, shoulders, and finger joint replacements. Transplant surgeons have added heart, liver, and pancreas transplants to their initial successes with kidneys. Surgery for peptic ulcer has been largely replaced by long-term treatment with H_2-antagonists. AIDS has been transformed from a rapidly progressive fatal disease to one in which increasing numbers of patients are keeping the disease under control with complex cocktails of antiviral therapy. The list is almost endless.

The growth of health care technology is widely held to have contributed substantially to the upward pressure on health care expenditure, for several reasons, although its precise contribution is controversial (Mossialos and Le Grand 1999). New technologies are often more expensive than the ones they replaced. Even where the actual technology is less expensive, it may lead to increased costs as other aspects of the service are reorganized to reflect changing patterns of treatment. The introduction of new treatments may lead to an expansion in the number of individuals with indications for treatment, either because a previously untreatable condition becomes treatable or, as side-effects or contraindications are reduced, the threshold for treatment falls. Finally, the diffusion of technology from tertiary centres, in some cases into primary care, can markedly reduce barriers to access and thus increase uptake.

In response to the increasing use of expensive new technologies, many countries have established health technology assessment facilities and related systems to control the introduction and diffusion of new technology although, in some, fragmentation of decision-making due to the introduction of market-based health sector reforms is making control more difficult.

Finally, consumers have increased their expectations about the services provided by the health care system. As noted above, the development of new and more expensive technologies coupled with the increased access to information by the general public, particularly with the appearance of new means of communication such as the Internet have led people to demand a wider range of services of high quality from health care providers. This factor is exerting a major pressure on health care costs. The role of information technology as a pressure for change in the health services and some of the reform strategies adopted to increase the role of the citizen in decision-making are dealt with below.

Each of these contributors to upward pressure on health care expenditure has implications for public health professionals and not only because of the importance of understanding the forces driving change in health services. The question of how health care costs change with ageing remains unresolved and more epidemiological and health economics research is urgently required. Public health professionals can also contribute to discussions on how health services can be reconfigured to meet the increasingly complex needs of an elderly population with multiple disease processes. Debates about health care coverage raise important questions for those seeking to address health inequalities. And discussions of new health technology require inputs from public health professionals, drawing on skill such as epidemiology and economics, to assess appropriateness and cost-effectiveness.

The quest for enhanced quality of care

Research undertaken in the 1970s and 1980s that drew attention to widespread geographical variations in the use of common procedures (McPherson 1989) gave way to a questioning of clinical judgements of appropriateness of health care interventions, with some authors suggesting that up to 30 per cent of clinical services may be ineffective (Chappell 1993). In conjunction with other work demonstrating large variations in the costs of apparently similar services and in the outcomes achieved, this has led to an emerging emphasis on the effectiveness and efficiency of health care. Increasing research on the effectiveness of interventions is casting doubt on the effectiveness of established treatments and is identifying gaps in knowledge. The International Cochrane Collaboration—an international grouping of researchers working in many countries worldwide, which undertakes systematic reviews of available evidence in the literature, agrees standardized methods, and disseminates information—has played a major part in this process (Chalmers and Altman 1995). Targeted programmes of research to fill these gaps are greatly increasing knowledge of what works and what does not, and in what circumstances. In parallel, work to increase research awareness among health policy-makers means that they are increasingly likely to ask for evidence that proposed innovations will actually achieve what they are intended to do.

While such research provides evidence of what health care interventions can achieve, there is also a growing recognition that this is not always achieved in practice. This has led many countries to introduce systems to assess and improve the quality of clinical care and, in some cases, to make the results of such assessments available to the public.

These developments reflect a change in dominant belief systems, challenging traditional models based on clinical autonomy. They are contributing to a range of changes in health care systems that include not only the elimination of ineffective treatments and adoption of effective ones but also new organizational structures to bring about change. Again, public health professionals have key roles to play because of their skills in health care evaluation and the management of change.

The information society

The 1980s and 1990s have seen an unparalleled revolution in the pace and volume of communication. The speed and storage capacity of computers has increased so that a machine which, a few decades ago, would have filled an entire room will now fit comfortably into a briefcase. Postal deliveries have given way to faxes, which have been supplanted by electronic mail. The Internet has vastly expanded the amount of information available to health professionals, patients, and the general public.

These developments are having profound impacts on the organization of health care, bringing benefits but also risks. E-mail offers scope to reduce delays between referral and treatment and between undergoing tests and receiving results. Telemedicine means that a primary care physician in the remotest corner of the world can have a radiograph or a skin lesion seen by the world expert in the condition in question (Wootton 1996). Patients can search for information on their conditions on the world wide web, drawing on the perspectives not only of physicians but also of other sufferers from their condition. However, those searching the web must be aware of its unregulated nature, publishing views of both Nobel laureates and quacks (Eysenbach *et al.* 1998; Sandvik 1999). Internet prescribing may offer price savings for some, but it may also circumvent regulatory safeguards designed to reduce risks to patients. Greater access to information on modalities of treatment in other countries, especially via the Internet, is increasing recognition of the wide variations between otherwise similar countries in the diffusion of technology and is fuelling public expectations, which may be difficult to meet.

The communications revolution is also changing the way in which health care is organized. Greater local access to information and to the capacity to analyse it is promoting more localized decision-making. Conversely, cascade fax systems and e-mail provide an opportunity for a more rapid flow of central directives and closer monitoring of subordinate units. The precise effects of the new technology in any particular system are difficult to predict but it is clear that they are changing the relationship between the centre and the periphery in many health care systems.

Emerging themes in health services

This section explores some of the themes that are emerging in the responses to these pressures for change in health services. Evolving norms and beliefs, coupled with the changing macroeconomic environment, have led to a reassessment of the relationship between the state and the market in health care in many countries. Changing beliefs, coupled with developments in information technology are challenging traditional hierarchies, stimulating new ways of organizing health systems, and focusing attention on empowerment of the public and patients' rights. These themes will be considered in turn.

The changing relationships between state and market in health care

During the 1980s and 1990s, many countries had begun to re-examine the role of the state in the funding and delivery of health care. In those countries in which the state has played a central role, new pluralistic solutions are being explored, with involvement of a range of actors at varying distances from the state. Where the state has played a less central role in the health sector, acting only as a source of regulation between competing private interests, a similar reassessment is taking place.

Before examining these trends in detail, it is important to recognize the limits to generalization. While governments do draw extensively on the experience of others, and many vested interests seek actively to export models of health care reform, it would be quite wrong to see these developments as a process of convergence to some ideal model of a health system. Instead, the situation in each country represents the complex interplay of interest groups and deep-seated cultural beliefs. Nonetheless, some observations are possible (Saltman and Figueras 1997). In some countries where the state traditionally has had a strong role, some functions are being devolved to local government or to statutory agencies at arm's length from government. Others are being transferred to private ownership. Conversely, in some countries in which the state has played a limited role, governments are now taking greater regulatory responsibility.

This debate is often characterized as a dichotomy between the state and the market but this is a gross oversimplification (Saltman and von Otter 1995). The terms 'state' and 'market' are often poorly defined and are used interchangeably to include very different mixes of public, quasi-public, statutory-regulated private, private non-profit, and private for-profit bodies. There is widespread agreement that a pure market in health care is unachievable (Roberts 1993), and so, in practice, the term 'market' is taken to mean the use of certain market mechanisms such as contracting. These can be applied at several levels (Frenk and Donabedian 1987; Saltman 1994): health care financing, the organizations delivering care, such as hospitals, individual health care professionals, the providers of health care infrastructure, or the provision of support services. Decisions may be taken on the basis of price, quality, or market share. In addition, the limitations of the market in health care have led some governments to introduce market mechanisms while retaining public ownership (Bartlett *et al.* 1998), sometimes termed quasi- or internal markets.

Although superficially attractive, the introduction of market mechanisms into the health sector creates a series of conceptual and practical difficulties. Conceptually, health care is considered in many societies as a social good, in which the provision of service to each individual is also valuable to the community as a whole, whether because of ideas of self-interest, as in the treatment of dangerous mental illness or contagious disease, or altruism. Such principles have led to the creation of systems to ensure universal coverage and solidarity. In contrast, market incentives are intrinsically based on the assumption that services provided are a commodity, with demand driven by individual preference.

The second difficulty is that the neoclassical concept of a market is based on the relationship between a buyer and a seller. However, health care systems typically comprise a more complex set of relationships involving the patient, various health professionals, a provider institution, and a payer, with health professionals acting as both suppliers of services and agents for the patient (Young and Saltman 1985). Finally, the assumption in neoclassical economic theory that cross-subsidies between different patients are inefficient is incompatible with the social function of the health care system based on solidarity in which there are substantial cross-subsidies between young and old, rich and poor, and healthy and sick.

While some may dismiss these conceptual difficulties as problems that can be resolved given sufficient imagination and determination, a more powerful critique is based on the experience of attempts to implement market mechanisms while at the same time seeking to maintain solidarity and contain costs. They include the failure to design effective systems to adjust for differences in risk of incurring future health care costs of those enrolling in competing health insurance systems, failure to achieve predicted savings after the introduction of competition between providers due to high transaction costs, and costly duplication of facilities to secure a competitive advantage (Saltman and von Otter 1995).

A related issue is the changing approach to state regulation. Traditional 'command and control' measures are giving way to market-derived incentive-based arrangements within the public sector. The appropriate balance between regulatory and competitive measures will depend on the objectives being pursued and the context in which they are implemented. Regulation is becoming more sophisticated, with greater recognition of the need to empower rather than constrain and of the scope, with poorly drafted regulations, for perverse incentives. It is most effective where the objectives can be clearly defined and operationalized, while maintaining sufficient flexibility to account for local circumstances. In general, it should focus on outcomes rather than inputs (Saltman and Figueras 1997).

Similarly, competitive measures also should be tailored to the specific objectives being pursued. These measures have been most successful where they have incorporated close monitoring and evaluation as well as a clear legal framework.

Regardless of the approach taken, public health professionals have an important role to play in ensuring that approaches based on either regulation or incentives are used to maximize health gain. Whichever model is employed, the increasing sophistication required from either regulation or use of incentives calls for an enhanced role for government (Kettl 1993).

Reorganizing the system: decentralization, recentralization, and privatization

Decentralization is a key element of health care policy in many countries (Mills *et al.* 1990). It is seen as a means of empowering those at local level to improve the delivery of services and of involving the population in decisions about priorities.

Decentralization has been defined as the transfer of authority from a high, or national, level to a lower, or subnational, level (Rondinelli 1981). It can take many different forms which, for convenience, can be considered under four headings (Rondinelli 1983) (Table 2).

Decentralization has become attractive because of disillusionment with the perceived failings of large centralized, bureaucratic institutions. These include inefficiency, lack of responsiveness, and failure to innovate. Decentralized institutions are seen to have several advantages. Those working in them are better equipped to identify changing circumstances and needs, and thus can respond more flexibly. They can be more innovative than centralized institutions and they can generate higher morale, more commitment, and greater productivity. Decentralization can also facilitate enhanced partnerships with the local population, thus increasing the democratic input into policy-making.

However, decentralization can have negative effects. These include fragmentation of services, loss of critical mass in central government functions, inequity, political manipulation to favour particular interests or stakeholders, and a weakening of the public sector (Collins and Green 1994).

Borgenhammer (1993) has identified certain social and cultural conditions that are necessary for successful decentralization. These include adequate local administrative and managerial capacity, ideological certainty in implementation of tasks, and readiness to accept several interpretations of a particular problem. Thus organizations undertaking decentralization must engage in a process of articulation of their mission, create internal cultures around core values, and establish mechanisms to monitor results (Osborne and Gaebler 1993).

Privatization requires separate consideration as it is fundamentally different, in several important aspects, from other types of decentral-

Table 2 Typology of decentralization

Type of decentralization	Definition
Deconcentralization	Decision-making is transferred to locally based elements of central government
Devolution	Decision-making is transferred to a subnational (regional or local) government authority
Delegation	Managerial responsibility for defined functions is transferred to organizations outside the formal government structure but under indirect government control
Privatization	Government functions are transferred to voluntary or private (for-profit or non-profit) organizations, with a varying degree of regulation

Source: Rondinelli (1983).

ization. Its advocates argue that it brings benefits from the introduction of economic incentives for greater efficiency and higher quality in the management of health care (Cabinet Office 1999). It is also attractive to some governments as a means of enticing private capital into the health sector, thus reducing demands on scarce public funds. Finally, the ability of governments to resist private sector involvement is being eroded by a series of international trade and development policies. The International Monetary Fund and World Bank have made private finance for public infrastructure a requirement for many structural adjustment loans (Gaffney *et al.* 1999*b*) and the World Trade Organization's Government Procurement Agreement requires public contracts in many countries to be opened to international competition (Thornton 1999).

However, these perceived benefits of privatization are being challenged by a growing body of evidence derived from experience of greater private sector involvement (Bennett 1992). Private competitive insurers have powerful financial incentives to engage in adverse selection on the basis of individual risk, thus undermining solidarity (Saltman and von Otter 1987). They can also go bankrupt, leaving governments as the insurer of last resort.

The suggested benefits of using private capital to build health care facilities have been examined in most detail in the United Kingdom, where the Private Finance Initiative enables consortia of private firms build and run hospitals. The National Health Service then pays an annual charge rather than having to find the initial cost of building. It is now clear that, as the consortia must secure financial returns consistent with those obtainable in other sections of the economy, the long-term cost is much greater than if the previous public sector procurement approach been adopted, despite highly creative accounting by those who have sought to justify the policy (Gaffney *et al.* 1999*a*). Other suggested benefits, such as transfer of risk to the private sector, have proved illusory because of creative wording of contracts.

A related issue, of greater relevance in those systems that are already highly pluralistic such as the United States, is the growth in for-profit health care chains at the expense of the non-profit sector. Health care is one of the most rapidly expanding sectors on the New York Stock Exchange. There is growing evidence that the increasing profits from this sector are accompanied by quality of care that is significantly lower than in the non-profit sector with, for example, lower rates of primary and secondary prevention activities (Himmelstein *et al.* 1999).

Three broad findings emerge from the debate on decentralization. The first is whether the advantages of decentralization outweigh the disadvantages, such as fragmented and duplicated services and high transaction costs, an issue that must be resolved on a case-by-case basis. Secondly, a policy of decentralization requires a series of measures to create an appropriate framework, including development of a shared vision and a means of monitoring outcomes. Thirdly, the suggestion that privatization is simply another form of decentralization and that, in practice, it is unimportant who provides the service, does not withstand scrutiny.

Enhancing citizens' rights, choice, and participation

A third theme emerging from the debate on health care systems is that of patient empowerment. This is fuelled by changing norms about the role of professional authority and expert judgement and, increasingly, greater access to information via media such as the Internet. Following in the path set by some well-educated vocal groups, patients in many countries are increasingly demanding a choice of who treats them, where, and how.

Enhanced patient participation can take many different forms and, in a given country, the debate will reflect the dominant belief system. One model involves taking the collective views of the public into account by means of increased participation in the policy-making process, thus making health care professionals and the health system more accountable. This view is commonly associated with the view that health care is a public good. A second model, which is more commonly associated with the view of health care as a commodity, focuses on enhanced individual patient participation. In some countries, a third model has emerged as part of the debate on rationing health care. Here, participation by the public involves being asked their views on priorities for health care. This is different from the first model in that the agenda is set by others and the role of the public is responsive rather than proactive. Finally, Saltman (1994) has proposed a democratic-political model in which patient choice is enhanced and used as a mechanism whereby individuals can exert more influence over what happens to them inside a publicly operating system.

These models can be placed on a continuum that moves from the least to the most empowered position for an individual patient. Beginning with moral persuasion, or the right to ask to be heard, it continues through legal remedies, patient selection of funder or provider, democratic control over finance and commission of services, to patient choice of treatment modality. In this typology, empowerment is signified by the degree of individual leverage by the patient over specific service delivery decisions.

While there is a general tendency in many countries to increase the participation of patients in health care systems, this is raising some complicated issues, bringing both challenges and opportunities for public health professionals (Saltman and Figueras 1997). One is whether choice is equally important in all health care decisions. In some circumstances, such as maternity care, many patients may be willing to invest the time and energy into collecting the information acquired to make an informed choice. This may not be so in other areas. The development of mechanisms for participation must take this into account. A related issue is that of the complexity of the information required to make judgement about quality of health care. Several countries have sought to inform the public by means of publication of rankings of outcomes by hospital or physician. However, these are subject to substantial methodological limitations and also provided scope for opportunistic behaviour, either to exclude patients and higher risk or to manipulate the data that are presented. Public health professionals, by virtue of their expertise in evaluating health care, have a role to play in addressing these problems. Finally, enhancing choice risks increasing health inequalities as those with the greatest command over resources will be most able to exercise choice. For these reasons, the concept of choice is a complicated one in the context of health care and it should not be assumed that policies that enhance it are inevitably desirable.

Strategies for health services

It is impossible in the space available to provide a comprehensive overview of every strategy that might be employed to enhance the performance of health services. Instead, a few areas have been selected on the basis of the contribution that public health professionals can make to them. Although there are many possible ways of categorizing strategies for health services, such as the objectives they seek to achieve (e.g. equity, effectiveness, or efficiency), what element of the health system they affect (e.g. funding, allocation of finance, or delivery of services), or which health sector actors they involve (e.g. the patient, third-party insurer, third-party purchaser, or service provider), this section draws on a taxonomy developed by Saltman and Figueras (1997) that combined these approaches. Evidence on the impact of different policy interventions is brought together into four broad categories. The first category includes strategies that address resource scarcity, which here includes the process of setting priorities for health care. The second category relates to health care funding, here focusing on the issue of equity and, specifically, the tension between competition and solidarity. The third category includes strategies designed to achieve a more effective allocation of resources, here including assessment of health care need and purchasing and contracting for health care. The final category includes strategies designed to achieve more cost-effective and higher-quality care, including achieving the optimal balance between the different levels of health care (primary, secondary, and tertiary), enhancing the quality of care, and reorienting the curative sector towards prevention.

Tackling scarcity of resources

Upward pressure on health care costs in the face of limited resources confronts governments with two options. One is to increase the resources for health care by shifting funds from other areas of public sector expenditure or by increasing taxation or social insurance contributions. The second is to seek to control health care expenditure by pursuing strategies that influence either the demand for or the supply of health care. Strategies that act on supply of health services include reducing the number of health care professionals or facilities, setting global budgets for providers (Schwartz *et al.* 1996), giving professionals incentives to reduce the amount of care provided, and reducing access to care (Abel-Smith *et al.* 1995).

Strategies acting on demand include priority setting to ration access to certain services, the use of cost-sharing, incentives to encourage greater private expenditure, such as tax concessions, and the right to opt out of the statutory system. Each of these measures seeks to reduce demand by shifting some portion of health care costs to the individual.

Each of these approaches has been discussed elsewhere (Abel-Smith *et al.* 1995; Mossialos and Le Grand 1999). Here only one approach, that of setting priorities, is considered as it is the one in which public health professionals have played the greatest role.

Setting priorities

Throughout the 1990s, many countries have addressed the issue of explicit rationing of publicly funded health care, in part as a result of the developments described above that have given the state a greater role in the health care system but also as a result of upward pressures on costs. The debate has been lengthy and complex (New 1997), with many different views. Perhaps the only issue where there is a degree of unanimity is that, in all health care systems, some form of rationing has always taken place although, in most cases, this was implicit, inextricably linked to clinical judgement. Beyond this, the consensus breaks down as illustrated by the situation in the United Kingdom where there has been a fundamental disagreement between politicians and others about even the choice of the terms 'rationing' or 'priority setting' as a means of describing the process (Klein 1998).

In this debate, some commentators have argued that rationing should not be necessary if either sufficient funding was made available, typically by redirecting it from other areas of public expenditure or raising taxes, or by ensuring that available resources are used more efficiently. However, others have argued that the continuing upward pressure on health care costs has made explicit rationing of effective care necessary. For these commentators, the key issue is transparency.

Concerns about the affordability of health care have led, in several countries, to initiatives that examine priority setting on a more systematic and explicit basis (Abel-Smith *et al.* 1995). These processes have brought together a wide range of individuals, including public health professionals, managers, politicians, economists, and philosophers.

Explicit setting of priorities involves making decisions at different levels within the health care system, ranging from the overall funding of health care to the treatments available to individual patients (Klein 1993). If explicit priority setting is to be undertaken, a co-ordinated, strategic approach is most effective to integrate decision-making at these different levels (Saltman and Figueras 1997). An example is provided by The Netherlands, where a national debate on a package of essential care has been combined with investment in technology assessment, the development of practice guidelines, and the establishment of criteria to control waiting lists.

Decisions may lead to blanket exclusions of interventions or of condition–intervention combinations, as in the approach taken in Oregon in the United States, or production of guidelines, as has been done in New Zealand (National Advisory Committee 1992) and by the National Institute of Clinical Excellence in the United Kingdom (Smith 1999).

The experience of Oregon has been especially interesting because of the technical and ethical issues it has raised (Oregon Health Services Commission 1991). It was designed to create a list of condition–intervention pairs, ranked on the basis of cost–benefit, with a cut-off point based on available resources below which combinations would not be funded. The idea was that this would maximize the return on resources invested in health care. However, the process was extremely problematic when it became clear that many of the data required were unavailable and some results were quite counterintuitive—for example, appendicectomy was rated lower than cosmetic dentistry. The process also raised important ethical questions as the exercise was confined to poor women and children in the Medicaid programme and services denied to them would remain available to others.

An alternative approach was used in The Netherlands. There the Dunning Committee (Dunning 1992) proposed four criteria that any intervention to be funded from social insurance should meet (Fig. 3). These were necessity, effectiveness, efficiency, and whether the condition is a matter of individual rather than community responsibility. As a result of this process, it was recommended that services such as dentistry for adults, homeopathic treatment, *in vitro* fertilization, and physiotherapy for sports injuries should be excluded.

From this debate has emerged a recognition that the priority-setting process must include government, providers, the public, and patients, as well as evidence on health needs and on the cost and effectiveness of available interventions (Fig. 4) (Ham 1993). Priority setting cannot be reduced to a technical exercise and should be

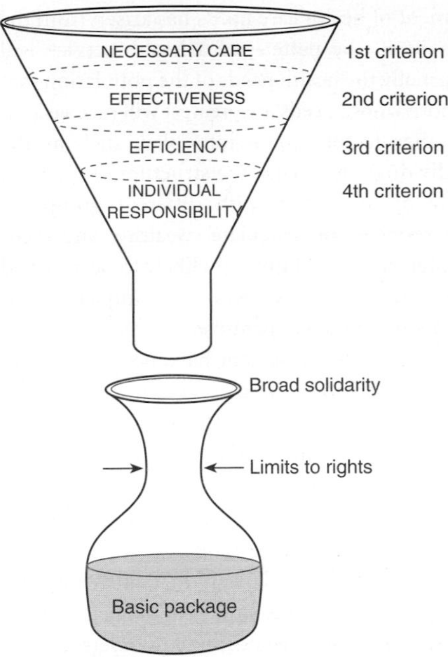

Fig. 3 Dutch criteria for inclusion within social insurance package. (Source: Dunning 1992).

combined with a thorough public debate about the choices to be made. This is seen in the approach taken in Sweden (McKee and Figueras 1996), which focused on the need to reach a shared view of the ethical basis on which priorities should be set. This rejected a narrow economic approach and gave priority to the treatment of life-threatening conditions. It also emphasized the importance of social solidarity.

Ultimately, while public health professionals have an important role in providing the evidence on which any debate on priority setting must be based and on examining the consequences of any decisions for equity, priority setting in a publicly funded system is the responsibility of politicians. Decision-making inevitably involves trade-offs between objectives as a balance is sought among universal coverage, comprehensiveness of services, equity, efficiency, cost containment, and broader social values.

Equitable funding of health systems

As Whitehead (1988) has shown, access to services is a key element of strategies designed to reduce health inequalities. Throughout the twentieth century the steady expansion of coverage in many countries has served to improve access to health care for those in greatest need. This has been associated with the growth of the principle of solidarity (Esping-Anderson 1990). As noted earlier, solidarity is based on 'risk pooling' in which those who remain healthy provide financial support for those who become sick and use health care services. In a system based on solidarity, individual financial contributions are related to ability to pay and are not dependent on the individual's health status.

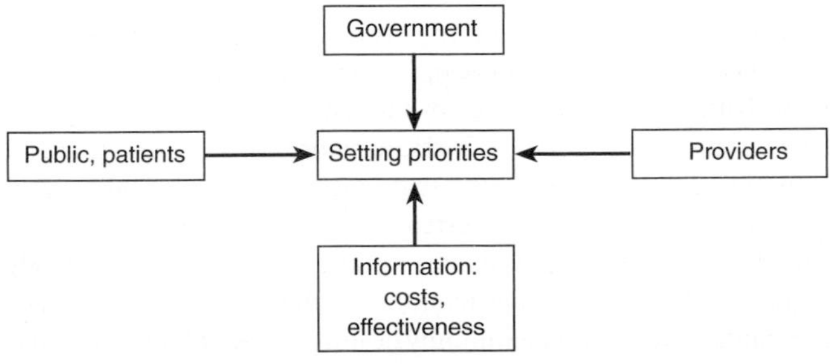

Fig. 4 Inputs into explicit priority setting. (After Ham 1993).

At present, however, certain developments threaten to undermine the principle of solidarity. One is the pressure from advocates of market-based policies to establish competition among health care insurers. A second is the development of information technology and, increasingly, the use of genetic profiling, enabling individual risks to be predicted more accurately and permitting exclusion or higher premiums for those at greatest risk, although this is raising enormous technical and ethical issues (Low *et al.* 1998). A third is the failure, by some governments, to collect sufficient taxes or social insurance contributions from the wealthy to fund the system. This has several causes. One is the prevailing global neoliberal agenda that argues that, for countries to attract inward investment and employment, they must reduce taxes. A second cause, which is especially problematic in, but not exclusive to, developing and middle income countries, is widespread tax avoidance by the wealthy. This is also an increasingly important issue in some industrialized countries as the Internet makes off-shore tax havens accessible to the middle classes.

Each of these issues has important implications for equity and thus for public health professionals. The third is beyond the scope of this chapter, but the first and second, which are linked in that competitive insurers have a strong incentive to identify the risks attached to those they accept, are relevant as public health professionals may have to work with such competitive systems. Furthermore, some of the issues that emerge have a wider relevance in, for example, systems in which there is competition between bodies that include both purchasing and provision of care, such as primary care groups in the United Kingdom (Goodwin *et al.* 1998).

Solidarity and competition

Competition between health insurers (whether private or public) tends to erode solidarity in health care financing, since health insurers seek to select good risks (Rothschild and Stiglitz 1976). In the absence of regulation, older people and those with pre-existing illness or even a strong family history of illness are either excluded from coverage or charged higher premiums. As noted above, advances in information technology and genetics are making this ever easier although this is raising enormous ethical issues (Danziger 1996). For example, should an insurer be permitted to know an individual's HIV status?

Two responses are open to policy-makers. One is mandatory open enrolment, so that insurers are unable to refuse coverage to an individual. This is typically linked to some regulation about the level of contributions, such as community ratings. The second is the use of risk-adjustment schemes that redistribute the health insurance system's revenue among competing health insurers on the basis of the risk profile of those enrolling with each insurer.

While these responses might work in theory, they are much more problematic in practice. Apparently open enrolment can be distorted in many subtle ways by targeting promotional activities or manipulating access so that insurers tend to 'cream skim' (de Roo 1995). Risk pooling requires development of valid formulas, which have proved elusive (van den Ven *et al.* 1994), with several systems relying purely on crude measures such as age.

If politicians choose to introduce competitive markets in health care financing, despite a widespread consensus from health economists and others that such initiatives are fraught with danger, public health professionals have an important role in monitoring and responding to any effects on equity. Maintaining solidarity in health care financing while introducing competition among insurers is an ambitious and difficult undertaking. The 'safety-net' for solidarity has to be designed very carefully, and such an undertaking requires experienced supervision of health care markets. Moreover, several crucial questions have not yet been answered. Whether competition among insurers really leads to more efficient and more effective health care has yet to be demonstrated (Chinitz *et al.* 1998), not least because of the need for expensive regulatory and risk adjustment systems, as has the question of whether mechanisms seeking to combine solidarity with competition can succeed.

Optimal allocation of resources

Upward pressure on costs and an increasing willingness of politicians, managers, and the public to challenge established patterns of care have placed an increased emphasis on the optimal allocation of scarce health care resources. Several strategies are available to health policy-makers. These include ensuring that the health services provided reflect the health needs of the population that they serve, enhance the efficiency with which services are delivered, and reduce the cost of key inputs such as pharmaceuticals and technology. Public health professionals can play an important role in both the assessment of health needs and, increasingly, in the process of intelligent purchasing of health care so as to maximize health gain for a given set of inputs.

Assessing need for health care

In this context, need is defined as the ability to benefit from health care. As such it is differentiated from demand, which arises when someone with a need for care expresses it. The relationship between need and demand is mediated by differing illness behaviours. Although it may seem obvious, it is also distinct from use of health care (Fig. 5). In reality, however, these two concepts are often confused, as when increased uptake of a widely advertised, but ineffective, intervention is described as need, or conversely where low uptake of an effective, but inaccessible, intervention is described as an absence of need (Stevens and Gabbay 1991).

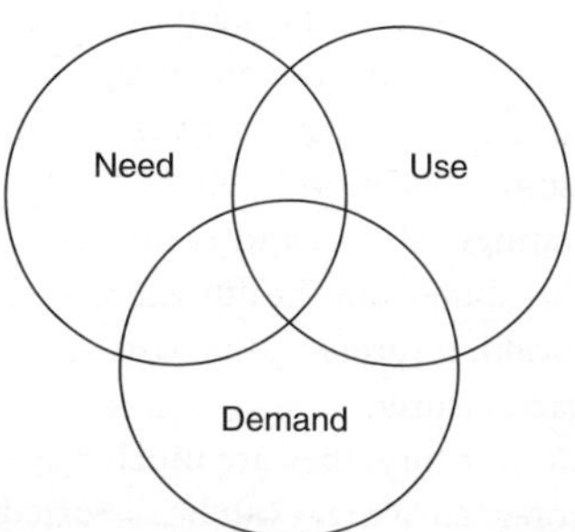

Fig. 5 Relationship between need, demand, and use. (Source: Stevens and Gabbay 1991).

Interest in the assessment of health care needs has arisen from the recognition that, left to itself, the pattern of a health service will frequently reflect only partially the health needs of the population that it is serving, and often those whose needs are greatest will receive least (Hart 1971). Instead, other factors come into play, such as the specialist interests of individual physicians, the structure of financial incentives, and the ease of interacting with different groups of patients. Consequently, services for articulate, wealthy, and well-educated patients with interesting conditions are likely to be supplied at the expense of those with low literacy who have unpleasant or uninteresting disease and who are uncooperative.

In practice, four types of needs assessment have been described: epidemiological, comparative, corporate, and pragmatic (Stevens and Raftery 1994). Epidemiologically assessed need involves selecting an intervention, such as a surgical procedure, defining indications for its use, operationalizing these into a survey instrument, and measuring the number of individuals in a population with those indications. Clearly, this is only possible for some conditions, typically surgical procedures where there is a straightforward means of identifying those with clinical indications. Examples include studies of the need for hip replacement (Wilcock 1979) and for prostatectomy (Sanderson *et al.* 1997).

Comparative need is defined as existing where the population of one area has a lower uptake of a particular intervention than that of another area, after adjustment for any differences in age or other population characteristics. While overcoming many of the technical difficulties involved in epidemiological assessment of need, it makes the assumption that the intervention rate in the area where it is higher is the correct one and fails to take account of either differences in disease prevalence rates or of previous treatment.

Corporate assessment of need is defined as a process whereby expert judgement is assembled to decide on either an appropriate level or configuration of services. Ideally, some system of formal consensus development would be used (Murphy *et al.* 1998) but clearly this approach risks legitimizing existing patterns of care that may have little rational basis.

The limitations of these approaches has led to the development of what has been described as the pragmatic approach to assessment of need (Stevens and Raftery 1994). This draws on data from a variety of sources. Information on the epidemiology of the condition in question is summarized, the range of possible interventions is defined, and evidence for the effectiveness of each one is summarized. Finally, an optimal model of care, taking into account the characteristics of the particular health care system and the dominant belief system, is generated. This approach accepts that there are gaps in the available evidence but takes the view that this should not preclude acting on what is available.

Each of these approaches requires a considerable amount of resources and, especially in developing and middle-income countries, they will often be inappropriate. An alternative model, rapid appraisal, offers certain advantages in such circumstances (Rikkin 1992). This is a multidisciplinary approach that incorporates flexibility and innovation and which draws extensively on the views of the local community. It is quick, as its name indicates, and it emphasizes timely insights and 'best bets' rather than final truths. It involves using key informants to build up a community health profile. This approach has also been used to enhance community involvement in developed countries (Ong *et al.* 1991).

Assessment of need for health care, using whichever of these models is most appropriate, is a prerequisite for optimal allocation of resources.

Intelligent purchasing

In an increasing number of countries intelligent purchasing is seen as an instrument to implement health policy objectives, including ensuring that health services closely reflect the health needs of the population that they serve (Øvretveit 1995). Purchasing acts as a co-ordinating mechanism that offers an alternative to a traditional command-and-control approach. Its essential characteristic is that it separates purchasers from providers but binds each party by means of contracts to explicit commitments, with creation of the economic motivation to fulfil these commitments.

The growth of purchasing health care is a result of the changing role of the state and the market described previously. Contracts have always been a feature of health care systems based on social insurance systems, with complex institutional structures developed to represent health insurers and physicians in negotiations over payment schedules. Governments have often played some role in these discussions, typically to ensure cost containment and preservation of solidarity. However, both insurers and governments are increasingly using contracts as a means of reorientating the focus of health services, to ensure that they reflect health needs and provide cost-effective care.

In contrast, in most tax-based systems, relationships between health authorities and providers have traditionally been based on hierarchies. This is also changing as policy-makers seek new ways of influencing provider behaviour, based on a clearer identification of the objectives of the health system, including explicit priority setting, while, at the same time, seeking ways of decentralizing decision-making (Ham 1997).

In systems based on private insurance, similar changes are taking place. Instead of simply reimbursing costs incurred retrospectively, insurers are introducing what is described as managed care, in which entitlements are defined in advance and treatment patterns are closely scrutinized (Corrigan *et al.* 1997).

From a public health perspective, interest in purchasing relates to whether or not it can achieve health gain and promote equity. Whether it does so will depend on both the objectives being pursued and on the quality of the contracting process. Contracts bring many potential benefits but also some risks.

For purchasing to promote health gain it must be based on an assessment of health needs coupled with a strong focus on the cost-effectiveness of clinical interventions and the organizational context within which they are delivered. Conversely, if, as seems increasingly to be the case in some American managed care systems, it is based primarily on cost-saving, it will reduce health gain.

Contracts can support equity if, through needs assessment, they take explicit account of vulnerable and disadvantaged groups as well as underserved communities. From this perspective, purchasers represent the interests of their populations, allocating resources and purchasing services in accordance with their needs. However, purchasing also carries the risk of undermining equity if providers are able to underemphasize or phase out services that are less profitable, rather than simply less efficient.

Purchasing also offers a means for enhancing participation by the population in the organization of health care, thus increasing the accountability of governments and the medical profession and making health policy more relevant to the needs and priorities of society.

In some countries, especially where public health professionals have played a central role in the contracting process, it has been possible to use contracts to develop intersectoral responses to health problems or to reorient health care providers so that they integrate prevention with curative care. The opportunities for doing so are discussed in more detail below.

Implementation of an intelligent purchasing system is a complex process requiring a high level of skills and well-developed information systems. At a minimum, information is required on patient flow, cost, and utilization information across specialties or diagnostic groups, and demographic and risk groups. It is important that expectations of what can be achieved are realistic (McKee and Clarke 1995). Medical care is extremely complex. Diagnostic labels are often imprecise and clouded by a degree of legitimate uncertainty. Decisions on clinical management incorporate values and beliefs relating to factors such as attitude to risk and the utility placed on different health states. Contracts must incorporate sufficient flexibility and reflect the views of all those concerned if they are to retain any credibility.

Purchasing also involves transaction costs to cover activities such as needs assessment, performance analysis, negotiating, and monitoring. A substantial increase in quality and efficiency is required to justify these additional costs. Increasingly, purchasers and providers are entering into long-term contractual relationships that reduce transaction costs (Rosen and McKee 1995).

If transaction costs can be minimized without compromising the pursuit of the objectives of equity and health gain, intelligent purchasing can provide a formidable instrument to promote population health.

Efficient service delivery

The increasing use of intelligent purchasing is focusing the attention of public health professionals on the delivery of health care. Evaluative research is highlighting the extent of use of treatments that are unsupported by evidence of effectiveness and the importance of appropriate organizational structures and cultures in the provision of high-quality care. This section examines three areas in which public health professionals can play an important role: the design of systems that ensure that patients are managed at the level of the health care system that is most appropriate, the creation of mechanisms that identify and promote high-quality clinical care, and the reorientation of curative services towards prevention.

Shifting interfaces

Health services are typically organized on different levels, reflecting the need to balance two competing objectives. On the one hand, dispersion permits easy access to those facilities in which most people receive care and where they can obtain an initial contact with the system. On the other hand, concentration of specialized resources required by relatively small numbers of patients optimizes scarce resources, with potential gains in effectiveness and efficiency, although the relationships are complex and often counterintuitive (Ferguson *et al.* 1997). Movement between the various levels (primary, secondary, tertiary, and community care) typically involves passage across an interface that is governed by rules of varying degrees of formality. Examples include referral to hospital by a primary care physician or discharge from an acute hospital to a long-stay facility.

The nature of these interfaces is steadily changing in the face of the new circumstances discussed above. Upward pressure on costs is causing policy-makers to ensure that patients are treated in the most cost-effective settings. Changing patterns of disease, coupled with evolving patient beliefs about the nature of health care, are challenging established ways of delivering care. New technologies in fields such as imaging, diagnosis, surgery, pharmaceuticals, and information are having a substantial impact on clinical practice. Health care professionals are developing new and different sets of skills (Coulter 1995).

These changes involve a process of substitution, by which there has been a continual regrouping of resources across care settings to exploit the best available solutions. This can take many forms. One typology differentiates three kinds of substitution: moving the location of care, introducing new technologies, and shifting the mix of staff and skills (Warner 1996). Examples include substituting hospital care with home care (e.g. hospital at home schemes and domiciliary renal dialysis) or with primary care (e.g. undertaking minor surgical procedures or the enhanced management of chronic diseases such as diabetes or asthma in primary care) (Fig. 6).

From a public health perspective, substitution brings the potential of both benefits and risks. Potential benefits include increased patient satisfaction, improved clinical outcomes, greater efficiency, and more appropriate management of certain diseases. Risks include fragmentation of services, loss of specialized skills, increased costs, and wasteful duplication of expensive technology. Each case must be assessed on its merits as initiatives that have seemed intuitively better than what they replaced have often, on detailed evaluation, failed to live up to the initial expectations (Hensher *et al.* 1996).

Effective substitution policies require co-ordination, with clear strategic objectives. A system-wide perspective is necessary to identify unintended consequences for other services (Checkland and Scholes 1990). Too often substitution involves simply changing the location, without an appropriate shift in skills and technology or without a reallocation of resources.

However, substitution offers a valuable tool to public health professionals to make services more accessible and appropriate to the population and to ensure that care is provided as cost-effectively as possible.

Improving outcomes

As noted above, former deference to medical judgement about how to deliver health care is giving way in the face of wide variations in how physicians actually provide care (McPherson 1989). The view expressed by the editor of *The Lancet* in 1951, that central guidance on clinical care should be rejected because of the harm that it would do to the sense of personal responsibility of the physician (Fox 1951), is no longer tenable.

Variations in clinical practice have many causes, the most important being clinical uncertainty about the most appropriate treatment in any given circumstance (Anderson and Mooney 1990). Studies of treatment pattern reveal both overtreatment, where patients receive treatments that are ineffective, and undertreatment, where those who would benefit are denied effective treatment. This has led to four related questions. Firstly, which treatments can be expected to produce improved health outcomes? Secondly, does a treatment that has been shown to be efficacious in evaluative research achieve the intended objective in routine clinical practice (Britton *et al.* 1999)? Thirdly, why are treatments of known effectiveness not used in circumstances where they would achieve health improvement? Finally, how does one change professional behaviour so as to ensure that the most effective, efficient, and humane treatments are provided (Freemantle 1996)? Together, these questions contribute to the quest for what is termed evidence-based health care.

Evidence-based health care includes a wide range of activities that have, as their common goal, the improvement of the outcome of health care. This 'outcomes movement' (Relman 1988) in its most developed form encompasses defining prioritized research questions, systematic reviews of available evidence on the corresponding topics, development of a research agenda to fill gaps in the knowledge, support to create a research infrastructure, and dissemination and implementation of the research findings in practice (Peckham 1991).

These activities draw on a multidisciplinary approach, with an emphasis on timeliness, relevance to the needs of the users, and the importance of changing policy and practice. Many countries have mechanisms to address some or all of these tasks. One example is the establishment of organizations for health technology assessment.

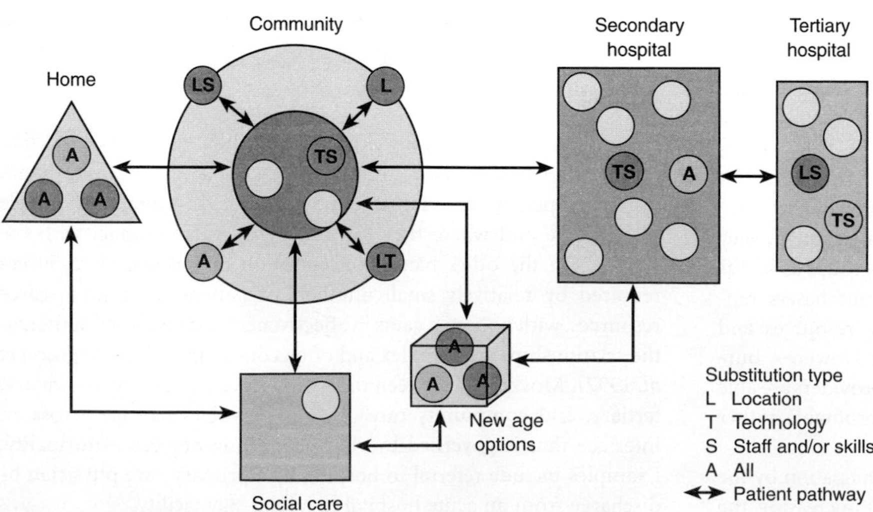

Fig. 6 Health and social care substitution. (Source: Warner 1996).

These typically undertake the early identification of emerging technologies, synthesis of available evidence, and commissioning of needed research. A detailed listing of organizations involved in these activities has been assembled elsewhere (University of York 1999).

The synthesis and dissemination of research-based evidence is at the core of these approaches to assuring the quality of clinical care. It is, however, also necessary to establish mechanisms to ensure that the available evidence is used by practitioners. These constitute what are usually described as quality assurance activities (Black 1992).

Three aspects of quality assurance are important. The first is that it is a continuous process, involving repeated cycles of setting standards, introducing change to meet those standards, and review of the results of change. The second is the existence of different types of quality measure (Donabedian 1966). Measures of structure relate to inputs such as facilities and the availability of trained staff. Measures of process include adherence to agreed good practice. Measures of outcome assess the extent to which the objectives of treatment are achieved. A third aspect involves the differentiation of internal and external approaches to quality assurance.

Quality assurance activities often deal with structures and processes of care rather than outcomes. Ideally, the focus would be on outcomes, but outcomes are typically more difficult to measure and may only become apparent long after the intervention took place. Some outcomes may also be rare and the sample size required to detect a deviation from what is expected may be very large. For example, Mant and Hicks (1995) have shown, on the basis of knowledge of effective treatment for myocardial infarction, that, in a comparison of two typical hospitals, it would take 73 years of data to detect a significant 3 per cent reduction in mortality whereas the corresponding difference in process measures, relating to uptake of treatments, would emerge after only 4 months. Where process or structure measures are used there should be evidence that they correlate with a good outcome. Measures based on structure can be of some value, based on the assumption that high-quality care cannot be provided in the absence of basic prerequisites, such as adequately trained staff, but this is a necessary rather than a sufficient measure and should normally be supplemented by measures of either process or outcome.

Internal and external forms of quality assurance have quite different characteristics. In the former, the activity is conducted by those undertaking the clinical activities concerned, such as the physicians in a hospital. They are responsible for setting standards and implementing change. This has the advantage of fostering a sense of ownership and is less open to opportunistic manipulation of results. However, it does require a culture in which it is accepted that clinical practice should be open to examination by one's peers. Professional bodies have often played a major role in promoting this approach.

External quality assurance involves a body outside the health care facility examining measures of quality. This typically focuses on structure, largely because this is so much easier to measure than process or outcome. A typical example is hospital accreditation (Scrivens 1997). Accreditation is especially important for countries seeking to establish a mix of private and public health services, as it offers a means of reassurance that all facilities meet an agreed minimum level of quality.

Perhaps the greatest challenge facing those seeking to improve the quality of health care is how to change clinical behaviour. An increasing volume of research on this topic is being brought together by the work of the Cochrane Collaboration on Effective Professional Practice. This has examined behavioural, financial, and organizational approaches to changing practice. It has shown how many traditional approaches, such as conferences and short educational events, are of little value (Thomson *et al.* 1997). Educational outreach visits have a small effect, and financial and organizational initiatives, such as the introduction of copayments, tend to reduce appropriate and inappropriate care to a similar extent. The most successful strategies involve combing a range of behavioural approaches, such as audit and feedback, production of guidelines, and, where appropriate, computer-generated reminders. However, the main conclusion of this research is that change is very difficult and requires carefully targeted sustained action.

Public health professionals have played a key role in the development of evidence-based health care, although its elements, from research through dissemination to implementation, are in place in only a few countries. Often the focus of health policy discussion remains focused on issues of financing and organization. The difficulties involved in integrating evidence-based health care with health sector reform should not be underestimated, although there is considerable scope for international co-operation, which is already well established through the Cochrane Collaboration.

Health services as a setting for promoting health

Public health professionals have a particularly important role in promoting the reorientation of health services to address the broader determinants of health. Health services are important settings in which it is possible actively to promote health through primary preventive strategies. Health professionals have an important role as opinion formers, both in individual patient encounters and, among the wider public, as respected advocates for healthy public policies (Chapman and Lupton 1994). Conversely, contradictory images, such as physicians and nurses smoking while they advise their patients to quit (Audet 1994), can do much to undermine public health messages.

Relatively simple approaches can often be very effective. One of every 37 patients given brief advice by a physician to stop smoking can be expected to quit, with those at most risk of smoking-related diseases most susceptible (Silagy and Ketteridge 1998). Women who receive brief advice on smoking during pregnancy are almost twice as likely to stop smoking than those who do not (Dolan-Mullen 1994), with a corresponding reduction in low-birth-weight babies. Brief interventions by a variety of health professionals have also been found to be effective in reducing problem drinking among men (Kahan *et al.* 1995). Such interventions are substantially more cost-effective than other strategies (Plans-Rubrio 1998; Meenan *et al.* 1998) (Table 3).

There is also some evidence to support a more proactive preventive role for health professionals in some areas. Assessment of elderly people by health professionals trained to identify risk factors is associated with a 20 per cent reduction in falls (Gillespie *et al.* 1998). However, this may simply require engagement in a process of patient empowerment. An enhanced process of self-management of asthma, involving self-monitoring and self-adjustment of medication, led to a fall of up to 50 per cent in hospital admission, unscheduled physician visits, and days off work or school (Gibson *et al.* 1998).

It is not sufficient to assume that such approaches are always going to be effective, and, as with treatment interventions, each must be assessed individually. For example, while advising patients to take more exercise or eat more nutritious food may seem intuitively beneficial, there is little evidence that it is effective (US Preventive

Table 3 Cost per life-year gained from interventions to reduce cardiovascular disease: Spain, 1998

Intervention	Cost (US$)	
	Men	Women
Smoking cessation	2608–3738	4482–5756
Treatment of moderate and severe hypertension	8564–38 678	9585–57 983
Treatment of mild hypertension	11 906–59 840	15 248–86 075
Dietary treatment	16 143–20 158	57 175–62 154
Drug treatment of hypercholesterolaemia	33 850–81 010	104 100–259 150

Source: Plans-Rubrio (1998).

Services Task Force 1996). There is no evidence that attempts to reduce the risk of coronary heart disease through multiple risk factor interventions have an impact on either total or coronary heart disease mortality (Ebrahim and Davey Smith 1997), and fiscal and legislative measures seem more appropriate.

However, it is important to recognize that interventions set in the health care sector may risk exacerbating health inequalities, especially where migrant workers and illegal immigrants are excluded from the formal health care system.

Many people come into contact with health care facilities, either as patients or staff. This provides an important opportunity to demonstrate support for health-promoting policies by means of an ethos based on healthy lifestyles. This includes bans on smoking, highlighting the importance of environmental tobacco smoke (Catford and Nutbeam 1983), and provision of cycle parks, gyms, and showers, so encouraging exercise, and ensuring that catering facilities provide healthy dietary choices (Clarkson and Nutbeam 1991). This approach forms one element of the WHO's Health-Promoting Hospitals project. This seeks to increase participation in health-promoting activities by patients, staff, and others outside the hospital, as well as improving communication and reorienting hospitals towards health promotion (WHO 1999). In contrast, failure to ban smoking or to promote healthy eating choices gives an implicit message that health promotion is not taken seriously. The obvious conflict between the culture of the organization and the advice given to patients will make behavioural change more difficult.

Finally, the contribution that health services can make to health by employing people should not be ignored. The adverse health effects of unemployment are well recognized (Bartley 1994), in particular the impact of job insecurity and anticipation of unemployment (Ferrie *et al.* 1995). Health services have always been labour intensive. Health care reforms in many countries have led to substantial reductions in staff numbers, either through redundancy or, in some countries, transfers to private sector agencies where levels of pay and conditions of service are substantially worse. While reducing the direct costs to the health service, such policies often increase overall government expenditure through increased social costs. However, some governments are recognizing the role of health services as a source of employment, as illustrated by the European Union's Amsterdam Special Action Programme, in which 10 billion Euros are being invested in job-creating projects, including health care (European Investment Bank 1999).

Health services as a threat to public health—the growth of antibiotic resistance

While, most commonly, public health professionals will focus on the issues raised in the preceding sections, one other issue requires specific attention. In some countries, the 1990s have seen a marked increase in the rate of resistance among hospital-acquired infections. Rates vary markedly between countries (Gruneberg and Felmingham 1996) and there is compelling evidence that they are related to the approach taken to the prescribing of antibiotics. Thus, hospitals and other health care facilities in which prescribing is uncontrolled and haphazard represent a threat to the wider population, and not only in the country concerned. Unfortunately, surveillance systems are often weak, even in many industrialized countries (Desenclos 1993).

The growth of iatrogenic antibiotic resistance creates a major challenge for public health professionals who must work in association with their clinical colleagues to change clinical behaviour (Frimodt-Møller 1998).

The contribution of public health to health services

This chapter began by showing how health care can no longer be regarded as peripheral to attempts to improve the health of populations. Notwithstanding the importance of tackling the wider determinants of health, modern clinical care offers new opportunities to reduce mortality and improve quality of life. Health care is also taking on a greater importance as evidence emerges of how differential access can increase health inequalities.

Health services are changing, bringing new opportunities for public health to increase its impact in this process by reorienting health services towards the maximization of health gain (McKee and Bojan 1998). However, if public health professionals are to take full advantage of these new opportunities they will need to have a thorough understanding of the contextual as well as the internal health sector pressures that are driving the health services change.

This chapter has highlighted the main health service themes that are emerging in response to these pressures for change. In particular, there is a changing relationship between the roles of the state and the market in health care with the introduction of a series of market incentives at different levels of the health system. However, the evidence does not lend support to a radical shift in the roles of state and market but to an incremental change leading to a more balanced model which retains key features of both approaches (Figueras *et al.* 1998). In fact the introduction of the market in health care has required not less government activity, but different activity including strategic planning, monitoring, and regulation. Two accompanying trends, partially reflecting the changing role of the state, have been decentralization of responsibility to lower levels within the public sector and an increasing role for the citizen and patient in various health service strategies including the development of patient rights legislation, increased patient choice of provider, and citizen participation in decision-making.

These three themes underlie many of the specific policies adopted at the different levels of health services and outlined above under a series of strategies to address cost containment, increase solidarity and sustainability of funding, achieve a more effective allocation of resources according to health need, and improve the efficiency in health service delivery. These various strategies can be summarized through a conceptual shorthand suggested by Saltman and Figueras (1998) which may help to better summarize the contributions of public health into the health services. This approach compresses the various categories into two traditional economic parameters: policy interventions instituted on the demand side as against those instituted on the supply side of the health care system.

The demand side incorporates all strategies that influence funding of the health care system and more specifically the relationships between the consumer and the third-party payers. A number of health system strategies have concentrated on the demand side by introducing measures shifting costs to the patient, such as cost-sharing arrangements or limiting the public package of care, and by introducing market competition incentives among third-party insurers. Many of these have led to equity problems. The role of public health here is twofold: first to ensure that solidarity of the health system is not harmed by these measures which tend to reduce access and coverage particularly for the most vulnerable groups in our society, and second to shift the policy-makers' agenda from these individual patient-based demand policies towards strategies dealing with aggregate population-based demand. Indeed, the latter is very much at the core of public health role.

The introduction of effective health promotion and primary prevention strategies should ultimately reduce the total demand for health care services and health care costs. However, the difficulties in measuring health promotion in terms of cost-effectiveness so that it can be compared with health services interventions, has meant that health promotion has not played a central role in health reform agenda. Public health professionals need to strive to develop more and better ways to evaluate health promotion that satisfy the needs of policy-makers, managers, and clinicians so the full potential of health promotion can be realized (McKee and Bojan 1998).

The supply side includes strategies forming a continuum that moves from the allocation of health resources to the delivery of health services. In the area of allocation these include efforts to change provider behaviour through the introduction of contracting within public operated health systems along the development of performance-based payment systems for providers. In the delivery area some of the key strategies include the introduction of quality-oriented strategies, the integration and substitution of services across the hospital and primary health care sectors, and the reorganization of health care providers in various types of public firms with more managerial independence and finance tied to production. In many instances, these reforms have met with considerable success (Saltman and Figueras 1998), but the extent of their success will depend on the availability of series of skills traditionally linked to the public health profession. These include assessing the health needs of the population, evaluating and monitoring interventions, assessing health outcomes, and reorienting health care delivery so that the focus is on prevention as well as cure (McKee and Bojan 1998).

Health services have an important contribution to play in improving the health status of populations. This chapter has identified mechanisms through which public health can have a major role in maximizing the health gain obtained from the health services, but much will depend on the ability of the public health profession to adapt and bring its portfolio of tools and skills to bear on rapidly changing health services.

References

Abel-Smith, B., Figueras, J., Holland, W., McKee, M., and Mossialos, E. (1995). *Choices in health policy: An agenda for the European Union.* Dartmouth Press/Office for Official Publications of the European Communities, Aldershot.

Albert, X., Bayo, A., Alfonso, J.L., Cortina, P., and Corella, D. (1996). The effectiveness of health systems in influencing avoidable mortality: a study in Valencia, Spain 1975–90. *Journal of Epidemiology and Community Health*, **50**, 320–5.

Anderson, T.F. and Mooney, G. (ed.). (1990). *The challenges of medical care variations.* Macmillan, Basingstoke.

Arblaster, L., Lambert, M., Entwistle, V., *et al.* (1996). A systematic review of the effectiveness of health service interventions aimed at reducing inequalities in health. *Journal of Health Services Research and Policy*, **1**, 93–103.

Audet, B. (1994). When it comes to smoking, Japanese MDs do not set a good example for their patients. *Canadian Medical Association Journal*, **150**, 1673–4.

Barnum, H. and Greenberg, E.R. (1993). Cancers. In *Disease control priorities in developing countries* (ed. D.T. Jameson, W.H. Mosley, A.R. Measham, and J.L. Bobadilla). Oxford University Press.

Bartlett, W., Roberts, J.A., and Le Grand, J. (1998). *A revolution in social policy: Quasi-market reforms in the 1990s.* Policy Press, Bristol.

Bartley, M. (1994). Unemployment and ill-health: understanding the relationship. *Journal of Epidemiology and Community Health*, **48**, 333–7.

Beaglehole, R. (1986). Medical management and the decline in mortality from coronary heart disease. *British Medical Journal*, **292**, 33.

Becker, N. and Boyle, P. (1997). Decline in mortality from testicular cancer in West Germany after reunification. *Lancet*, **350**, 744.

Beeson, P.B. (1980). Changes in medical therapy. *Medicine*, **59**, 79–84.

Bennett, S. (1992). Promoting the private sector: a review of developing country trends. *Health Policy and Planning*, **7**, 97–110.

Ben-Shlomo, Y. and Chaturvedi, N. (1995). Assessing equity in access to health care provision in the UK. Does where you live affect your chances of getting a coronary artery bypass graft? *Journal of Epidemiology and Community Health*, **49**, 200–4.

Benson, J.K. (1975). The interorganisational network as a political economy. *Administrative Science Quarterly*, **20**, 229–49.

Bindman, A.B., Grumbach, K., Osmond, D., *et al.* (1995). Preventable hospitalisations and access to health care. *Journal of the American Medical Association*, **274**, 305–11.

Black, N. (1992). The relationship between evaluative research and audit. *Journal of Public Health Medicine*, **14**, 361–6.

Bobadilla, J.L., Frenk, J., Lozano, R., Frejka, T., and Stern, C. (1993). The epidemiologic transition and health priorities. In *Disease control priorities in developing countries* (ed. D.T. Jamison, W.H. Mosley, A.R. Measham, and J.L. Bobadilla). Oxford University Press.

Bojan, F., Hajdu, P., and Belicza, E. (1991). Avoidable mortality. Is it and indicator of quality of medical care in Eastern European countries. *Quality Assurance of Health Care*, **3**, 191–203.

Bonneaux, L., Looman, C.W., Barendregt, J.J., and van der Maas, P.J. (1997). Regression analysis of recent changes in cardiovascular morbidity and mortality in The Netherlands. *British Medical Journal*, **314**, 789–92.

Borgenhammer, E. (1993). *At vårda liv: orgnisation, etik, kvalitet. (Looking after life: organisation, ethics, quality.)* SNS Förlag, Stockholm.

Boyle, P., Maisonneuve, P., and Steg, A. (1996). Decrease in mortality from benign prostatic hyperplasia: a major unheralded health triumph. *Journal of Urology*, **155**, 176–80.

Boys, R.J., Forster, D.P., and Jozan, P. (1991). Mortality from causes amenable and non-amenable to medical care: the experience of Eastern Europe. *British Medical Journal*, **303**, 879–83.

Britton, A., McKee, M., Black, N., McPherson, K., Sanderson, C., and Bain, C. (1999). Threats to applicability of randomised trials: exclusions and selective participation. *Journal of Health Services Research and Policy*, **4**, 112–21.

Cabinet Office (1999). *Modernising government.* HMSO, London.

Carr-Hill, R.A., Hardman, G.F., and Russell, I.T. (1987). Variations in avoidable mortality and variations in health care resources. *Lancet*, **i**, 789–92.

Catford, J.C. and Nutbeam, D. (1983). Smoking in hospitals. *Lancet*, **ii**, 94–6

Chalmers, I. and Altman, D.G. (1995). *Systematic reviews.* BMJ Publications, London.

Chapman, S. and Lupton, D. (1994). *The fight for public health.* BMJ Publications, London.

Chappell, N.L. (1993). The future of health care in Canada. *Journal of Social Policy*, **22**, 495.

Charlton, J.R.H. and Velez, R. (1986). Some international comparisons of mortality amenable to medical intervention. *British Medical Journal*, **292**, 295–301.

Checkland, P. and Scholes, J. (1990). *Soft systems methodology in action.* Wiley, Chichester.

Chinitz, D. Preker, A., and Wasem, J. (1998). *Balancing competition and solidarity in health care financing.* In *Critical challenges for health care reform* (ed. J. Figueras, R. Saltman, and C. Sakallarides). Open University Press, Buckingham.

Clark, D.G. (1988). Autonomy, personal empowerment and quality of life in long-term care. *Journal of Applied Gerontology*, **7**, 279–97.

Clarkson, J. and Nutbeam, D. (1991). Introducing healthy catering practice into hospitals: a case study from Wales. *Nutrition and Health*, **7**, 101–10.

Cochrane Injuries Group Albumen Reviewers (1998). Human albumin administration in critically ill patients: systematic review of randomised controlled trials. *British Medical Journal*, **317**, 235–40.

Cochrane, A.L., St Leger, A.S., and Moore, F. (1978). Health service 'input' and mortality 'output' in developed countries. *Journal of Epidemiology and Community Health*, **32**, 200–5.

Coebergh, J., Sant, M., Berrino, F., and Verdecchio, A. (1998). Survival of adult cancer patients in Europe diagnosed from 1978–1989: the Eurocare II Study. *European Journal of Cancer*, **34**, 2137–278.

Collins, C.D. and Green, A.T. (1994). Decentralisation and primary health care: some negative implications in developing countries. *International Journal of Health Services*, **24**, 459–75.

Contandriopoulos, A.P., Lauristin, M., and Leibovich, E. (1998). Values, norms, and the reform of health care systems. In *Critical challenges for health care reform* (ed. J. Figueras, R. Saltman, and C. Sakallarides). Open University Press, Buckingham.

Corrigan, J.M., Eden J.S., Gold, M.R., and Pickering, J.D. (1997). Trends toward a national health care marketplace. *Inquiry*, **34**, 11–28.

Coulter, A. (1995). Shifting the balance from secondary to primary care. *British Medical Journal*, **311**, 1447–8.

Danziger, R. (1996). An epidemic like any other? Rights and responsibilities in HIV prevention. *British Medical Journal*, **312**, 1083–4.

Davies, N. (1998). *Europe: a history.* Oxford University Press.

De Roo, A.A. (1995). Contracting and solidarity: market-orientated changes in Dutch health insurance schemes. In *Implementing planned markets in health care* (ed. R.B. Saltman and C. von Otter). Open University Press, Buckingham.

Desenclos, J.-C., Bijkerk, H., and Huisman, J. (1993). Variations in national infectious disease surveillance in Europe. *Lancet*, **341**, 1003–6.

Dolan-Mullen, P., Ramirez, G., and Groff, J.Y. (1994). A meta-analysis of randomized trials of prenatal smoking cessation interventions. *American Journal of Obstetrics and Gynecology*, **171**, 1328–34.

Donabedian, A. (1966). Evaluating the quality of medical care. *Milbank Memorial Fund Quarterly*, **44**, 169.

Dunning, A. (1992). *Choices in health care: a report by the Government Committee on Choices in Health Care.* Ministry of Welfare, Health and Culture, Rijkswijk, The Netherlands.

Ebrahim, S. and Davey Smith, G. (1997). Systematic review of randomised controlled trials of multiple risk factor interventions for preventing coronary heart disease. *British Medical Journal*, **314**, 1666–74.

Esping-Anderson, G. (1990). *The three worlds of welfare capitalism.* Princeton University Press.

European Investment Bank (1999). *EIB Initiative on Growth and Employment: Interim Review* (URL: http://www.eib.org/pub/news/asap_ir.htm).

Evans, R.G. (1994). Health care as a threat to health: defence, opulence, and the social environment. *Daedalus*, **123**, 21–42.

Eysenbach, G., Diepgen, T.L., Muir Gray, J.A., *et al.* (1998). Towards quality management of medical information on the Internet: evaluation, labelling, and filtering of information. *British Medical Journal*, **317**, 1496–502.

Fairchild, A.L. and Oppenheimer, G.M. (1998). Public health nihilism vs pragmatism: history, politics, and the control of tuberculosis. *American Journal of Public Health*, **88**, 1105–17.

Ferguson, B., Sheldon, T., and Posnett, J. (ed.) (1997). *Concentration and choice in health care.* Royal Society of Medicine Press, Glasgow.

Ferrie, J.E., Shipley, M.J., Marmot, M.G., Stansfield, S., and Davey Smith, G. (1995). Health effects of anticipation of job change and non-employment: longitudinal data from the Whitehall II study. *British Medical Journal*, **311**, 1264–9.

Figueras, J. and Saltman, R.B. (1998). Building upon comparative experience in health system reform. *European Journal of Public Health*, **8**, 99–101.

Fox, T.E. (1951). Professional freedom. *Lancet*, **ii**, 115–19.

Freemantle, N. (1996). Are health decisions taken by health care professionals rational? A non-systematic review of experimental and quasi experimental literature. *Health Policy*, **38**, 71–81.

Frenk, J. and Donabedian, A. (1987). State intervention in medical care: types, trends, and variables. *Health Policy and Planning*, **2**, 17–31.

Frimodt-Møller, N., Rosdahl, N., and Wegener, H.C. (1998). Microbiological resistance promoted by misuse of antibiotics: a public health concern. *European Journal of Public Health*, **8**, 193–4.

Fuchs, V.R. (1984). Though much is taken: reflections on aging, health, and medical care. *Milbank Memorial Fund Quarterly: Health and Society*, **62**, 143–66.

Gaffney, D., Pollock, A.M., Price, D., *et al.* (1999*a*). PFI in the NHS—is there an economic case? *British Medical Journal*, **319**, 116–19.

Gaffney, D., Pollock, A.M., Price, D., *et al.* (1999*b*). The politics of the private finance initiative and the new NHS. *British Medical Journal*, **319**, 249–53.

Gibson, P.G., Coughlan, J., Wilson, A.J., *et al.* (1998). The effects of limited (information only). patient education programs on the health outcomes of adults with asthma (Cochrane Review). *Cochrane Library, Issue 2.* Update Software, Oxford.

Gillespie, L.D., Gillespie, W.J., Cumming, R., Lamb, S.E., and Rowe, B.H. (1998). Interventions to reduce the incidence of falling in the elderly (Cochrane Review). *Cochrane Library, Issue 2.* Update Software, Oxford.

Gillett, G. (1995). Virtue and truth in clinical science. *Journal of Medical Philosophy*, **20**, 285–98.

Goodwin, N., Mays, N., McLeod, H., Malbon, G., and Raftery, J. (1998). Evaluation of total purchasing pilots in England and Scotland and implications for primary care groups in England: personal interviews and analysis of routine data. *British Medical Journal*, **317**, 256–9.

Gruneberg, R.N. and Felmingham, D. (1996). Results of the Alexander Project: a continuing, multicenter study of the antimicrobial susceptibility of community-acquired lower respiratory tract bacterial pathogens. *Diagnosis and Microbiology of Infectious Disease*, **25**, 169–81.

Habermas, J. (1987). *Théorie de l'agir communicationnel.* Fayard, Paris.

Ham, C. (1993). *Priority setting in the NHS: reports from six districts.* Rationing the action. BMJ Publications, London.

Ham, C. (1997). *Health care reform, learning from international experience.* Open University Press, Buckingham.

Hart, J.T. (1971). The inverse care law. *Lancet*, **i**, 405–12.

Hensher, M., Fulop, N., Hood, S., and Ujah, S. (1996). Does hospital at home make economic sense? Early discharge versus standard care for orthopaedic patients. *Journal of the Royal Society of Medicine*, **89**, 548–51.

Himmelstein, D.U., Woolhandler, S., Hellander, I., *et al.* (1999). Quality of care in investor-owned vs not for profit HMOs. *Journal of the American Medical Association*, **282**, 159–63.

Holland, W.W. (ed.) (1991). *European Community atlas of 'avoidable' death* (2nd edn). Oxford University Press.

Illich, I. (1976). *Limits to medicine.* Marion Boyars, London.

Ingelfinger, F.J. (1977). Health: a matter of statistics or feeling? *New England Journal of Medicine*, **296**, 448–9.

Józan, P.E. and Prokhorskas, R. (ed.) (1997). *Atlas of leading and 'avoidable' causes of death in countries of central and Eastern Europe.* Hungarian CSO, Budapest.

Kahan, M., Wilson, L., and Becker, L. (1995). Effectiveness of physician-based interventions with problem drinkers: a review. *Canadian Medical Association Journal*, **152**, 851–9.

Kanavos, P. and McKee, M. (1998). *Macroeconomic constraints and health challenges facing health systems in the European region.* In *Critical challenges for health care reform* (ed. J. Figueras, R. Saltman, and C. Sakallarides). Open University Press, Buckingham.

Kettl, D.F. (1993). *Sharing power: public governance and private markets.* Brookings Institution, Washington, DC.

Kirkman-Liff, B. (1997). The United States. In *Health care reform, learning from international experience* (ed. C. Ham). Open University Press, Buckingham.

Klein, R. (1993). Dimensions of rationing: who should do what? *British Medical Journal*, **307**, 309–11.

Klein, R. (1998). Puzzling out priorities. *British Medical Journal*, **317**, 959–60.

Lambrechts, T., Bryce, J., and Orinda V. (1999). Integrated management of childhood illness: a summary of experiences. *Bulletin of the World Health Organization*, **77**, 582–94.

Lavis, J.N. and Stoddart, G.L. (1994). Can we have too much health care? *Daedalus*, **123**, 43–60.

Law, M. and Wald, N. (1999). Why heart disease mortality is low in France: the time lag explanation. *British Medical Journal*, **318**, 1471–80.

Lembcke, P.A. (ed.) (1947). *Te Regional Hospital Plan—the second year's experience.* Council of Rochester Regional Hospital, Rochester, NY.

Levi, F., La Vecchia, C., Lucchini, F., Negri, E., and Boyle, P. (1992). Patterns of childhood cancer incidence and mortality in Europe. *European Journal of Cancer*, **28A**, 2028–49.

Low, L, King, S., and Wilkie, T. (1998). Genetic discrimination in life insurance: empirical evidence from a cross sectional survey of genetic support groups in the United Kingdom, *British Medical Journal*, **317**, 1632–5.

Lubitz, J., Beebe, J., and Baker, C. (1995). Longevity and medical care expenditures. *New England Journal of Medicine*, **332**, 999–1003.

McKee, M. (1998). An agenda for public health research in Europe. *European Journal of Public Health*, **8**, 3–7.

McKee, C.M. and Bewley, B.R. (1987). Preventable mortality in Northern Ireland. *Irish Medical Journal*, **80**, 229–31.

McKee, M. and Bojan, F. (1998). Reforming public health services. In *Critical challenges for health care reform* (ed. J. Figueras, R. Saltman, and C. Sakallarides). Open University Press, Buckingham.

McKee, M. and Clarke, A. (1995). Guidelines, enthusiasms, uncertainty and the limits to purchasing. *British Medical Journal*, **310**, 101–4.

McKee, M. and Figueras, J. (1996). Setting priorities—can Britain learn from Sweden? *British Medical Journal*, **312**, 691–4.

McKee, M. and Figueras, J. (1997). Comparing health systems: how do we know if we can learn from others? *Journal of Health Services Research and Policy*, **2**, 122–5.

McKeown, T. (1979). *The role of medicine: dream, mirage or nemesis?* Blackwell Scientific, Oxford.

McPherson, K. (1989). International comparisons in medical care practices. *Health Care Financing Review*, Annual Supplement, 9–20.

Mackenbach, J.P. (1996). The contribution of medical care to mortality decline: McKeown revisited. *Journal of Clinical Epidemiology*, **49**, 1207–13.

Mackenbach, J.P., Looman, C.W.N., Kunst, A.E., Habbema, D.F., and van der Maas, P.J. (1988). Post-1950 mortality trends and medical care: gains in life expectancy due to declines in mortality from conditions amenable to medical intervention in The Netherlands. *Social Science and Medicine*, **27**, 889–94.

Malcolm, M.S. and Salmond, C.E. (1993). Trends in amenable mortality in New Zealand 1968–1987. *International Journal of Epidemiology*, **22**, 469–74.

Mant, J. and Hicks, N. (1995). Detecting differences in quality of care: the sensitivity of measures of process and outcome in treating acute myocardial infarction. *British Medical Journal*, **311**, 793–6.

Marshall, S.W., Kawachi, I., Pearce, N., and Borman, B. (1993). Social class differences in mortality from diseases amenable to medical intervention in New Zealand. *International Journal of Epidemiology*, **22**, 255–61.

Meenan, R.T., Stevens, V.J., Hornbrook, M.C., *et al.* (1998). Cost-effectiveness of a hospital-based smoking cessation intervention. *Medical Care*, **36**, 670–8.

Meerding, W.J, Bonneaux, L., Polder, J.J., *et al.* (1998). Demographic and epidemiological determinants of health-care costs in Netherlands: cost of illness study. *British Medical Journal*, **317**, 111–15.

Mills, A., Vaughan, J.P., Smith, D.L., and Tabibzadeh, I. (1990). *Health system decentralization, Concepts, issues and country experience.* World Health Organization, Geneva.

Mossialos, E. and Le Grand, J. (1999). Cost containment in the EU: An overview. In *Health care and cost containment in the European Union* (ed. E. Mossialos and J. Le Grand). Ashgate, Aldershot.

Mulrow, C.D. (1995). Rationale for systematic reviews. In *Systematic reviews* (ed. I. Chalmers and D.G. Altman), pp. 1–8. BMJ Publications, London.

Murphy, M.K., Black, N.A., Lamping, D.L., *et al.* (1998). Consensus development methods and their use in clinical guideline development. *Health Technology Assessment*, **2**, 1–88.

Murray, C.J.L. and Lopez, A. (1996). *The global burden of disease.* Harvard University Press, Cambridge, MA.

National Advisory Committee (1992). *Core Services 1993/4.* National Advisory Committee, Wellington, New Zealand.

Neuhauser, D. (1990). Ernest Amory Codman, M.D., and end results of medical care. *International Journal of Technology Assessment of Health Care*, **6**, 307–25.

New, B. (ed.) (1997). *Rationing: talk and action in health care.* King's Fund/ BMJ Publications, London.

OECD (Organization for Economic Co-operation and Development) (1999). *OECD health data 1998.* OECD, Paris.

Ong, B., Humphris, S.G., Annett, H., and Rifkin, S. (1991). Rapid appraisal in an urban setting: an example from the developed world. *Social Science and Medicine*, **32**, 909–12.

Oregon Health Services Commission (1991). *Prioritization of health services.* Oregon Health Commission, Salem, OR.

Osborne, D. and Gaebler, T. (1993). *Reinventing government.* Addison-Wesley, Reading, MA.

Over, M. and Piot, P. (1993). *HIV infection and sexually transmitted diseases.* In *Disease control priorities in developing countries* (ed. D.T. Jameson, W.H. Mosley, A.R. Measham and J.L. Bobadilla). Oxford University Press.

Øvretveit J. (1995). *Purchasing for health.* Open University Press, Buckingham.

Peabody, J.W. (1996). Economic reform and health sector policy: lessons from structural adjustment programs. *Social Science and Medicine*, **43**, 823–35.

Peckham, M. (1991). Research and development for the National Health Service. *Lancet*, **338**, 367–71.

Peto, R., Lopez, A.D., Boreham, J., Thun, M., and Heath, C. (1994). *Mortality from smoking in developed countries 1950–2000.* Oxford University Press.

Petticrew, M., McKee, M., and Jones, J. (1993). Coronary artery surgery: are women discriminated against? *British Medical Journal*, **306**, 1164–6.

Pisani, P., Parkin, D.M., Muñoz, N., and Ferlay, J. (1997). Cancer and infection: estimates of the attributable fraction in 1995. *Cancer Epidemiology Biomarkers and Prevention*, **6**, 387–400.

Plans-Rubio, P. (1998). Cost-effectiveness of cardiovascular prevention programs in Spain. *International Journal of Technology Assessment in Health Care*, **14**, 320–30.

Poikolainen, K. and Eskola, J. (1986). The effect of health services on mortality: decline in death rates from amenable and non-amenable causes in Finland 1969–81. *Lancet*, **i**, 199–202.

Poikolainen, K. and Eskola, J. (1995). Regional and social class variation in the relative risk of death from amenable causes in the city of Helsinki 1980–1986. *International Journal of Epidemiology*, **24**, 114–18.

Reichard, S. (1996). Ideology drives health care reforms in Chile. *Journal of Public Health Policy*, **17**, 80–98.

Relman, A.S. (1988). Assessment and accountability: The third revolution in medical care. *New England Journal of Medicine*, **319**, 1220–2.

Rikkin, S. (1992). Rapid appraisal for health. *Rapid Appraisal Notes*, July, pp. 7–12.

Roberts, J. (1993). Managing markets. *Journal of Public Health Medicine*, **15**, 305–10.

Rondinelli, D. (1981). Government decentralisation in comparative theory and practice in developing countries. *International Review of Administrative Sciences*, **47**, 133–45.

Rondinelli, D. (1983). *Decentralisation in developing countries.* Staff Working Paper 581, World Bank, Washington, DC.

Rosen, R. and McKee, M. (1995). Short termism in the NHS. *British Medical Journal*, **311**, 703–4.

Rothman, D.J. (1993). A century of failure: health care reform in America. *Journal of Health Politics, Policy and Law*, **18**, 271–86.

Rothschild, M. and Stiglitz, J. (1976). Equilibrium in competitive insurance markets: an essay on the economics of imperfect information. *Quarterly Journal of Economics*, **90**, 629–49.

Rutstein, D.D., Berenberg, W., Chalmers, T.C., *et al.* (1976). Measuring the quality of medical care: a clinical method. *New England Journal of Medicine*, **294**, 582–8.

Saltman, R.B. (1994). Patient choice and patient empowerment in Northern European health systems: a conceptual framework. *International Journal of Health Services*, **24**, 201–29.

Saltman, R.B. and Figueras, J. (1997). *European health care reform: analysis of current strategies.* World Health Organization, Copenhagen.

Saltman, R.B. and Figueras, J. (1998). Analyzing the evidence on European health care reforms. *Health Affairs (Milwood)*, **17**, 85–108.

Saltman, R.B. and von Otter, C. (1987). Revitalising public health care systems: a proposal for public competition in Sweden. *Health Policy*, **7**, 21–40.

Saltman, R.B. and von Otter, C. (ed.) (1995). *Implementing planned markets in health care.* Open University Press, Buckingham.

Sanderson, C.F., Hunter, D.J., McKee, M., and Black, N. (1997). Limitations of epidemiologically based needs assessment: the case of prostatectomy. *Medical Care*, **35**, 669–85.

Sandvik, H. (1999). Health information and interaction on the Internet: a survey of female urinary incontinence. *British Medical Journal*, **319**, 29–32.

Sant, M., Capocaccia, R., Verdecchia, A., *et al.* (1995). Comparisons of colon-cancer survival among European countries: the Eurocare Study. *International Journal of Cancer*, **63**, 43–8.

Scheiber, G.J., Poulier, J.P., and Greenwald, L.M. (1993). Health spending, delivery, and outcomes in OECD countries. *Health Affairs (Milwood)*, **12**, 120–9.

Schwartz, F.W., Glennerster, H., and Saltman, R.B. (ed.) (1996). *Fixing health budgets—experience from Europe and North America.* Wiley, Chichester.

Scitovsky, A.A. (1988). Medical care in the last twelve months of life: the relation between age, functional status, and medical care expenditures. *Milbank Memorial Fund Quarterly: Health and Society*, **66**, 640–60.

Scrivens, E. (1997). Assessing the value of accreditation systems. *European Journal of Public Health*, **7**, 4–8.

Shaukat, N., De Bono, D.P., and Cruikshank, J.K. (1993). Clinical features, risk factors, and referral delay in British patients of Indian and European origin with angina matched for age and extent of coronary atheroma. *British Medical Journal*, **307**, 717–18.

Shkolnikov, V.M., McKee, M., Vallin, J., *et al.* (1999). Cancer mortality in Russia and Ukraine: validity, competing risks, and cohort effects. *International Journal of Epidemiology*, **28**, 19–29.

Silagy, C. and Ketteridge, S. (1998). Physician advice for smoking cessation (Cochrane Review). *Cochrane Library, Issue 2.* Update Software, Oxford.

Smith, R. (1994). Medicine's core values. *British Medical Journal*, **309**, 1247–8.

Smith, R. (1999). NICE: a panacea for the NHS? *British Medical Journal*, **318**, 823–4.

Starr, P. (1982). *The social transformation of American medicine.* Basic Books, New York.

Stephens, C., Leonardi, G., Lewin, S., and San Sebastian Chasco, M. (1999). The multilateral agreement on investment. Public health threat for the twenty-first century? *European Journal of Public Health*, **9**, 3–5.

Stevens, A. and Gabbay, J. (1991). Needs assessment, needs assessment. *Health Trends*, **23**, 20–2.

Stevens, A. and Raftery, J. (1994). *Health care needs assessment*, Vol. 1. Radcliffe Medical Press, Oxford.

Stroke Unit Trialists' Collaboration (1997). Collaborative systematic review of the randomised trials of organised inpatient (stroke unit). care after stroke. *British Medical Journal*, **314**, 1151–9

Thomson, M.A., Oxman, A.D., Davis, D.A., Haynes, R.B., Freemantle, N., and Harvey, E.L. (1997). Audit and feedback to improve health professional practice and health care outcomes. In *Collaboration on effective professional practice module of the Cochrane Database of Systematic Reviews* (ed. L. Bero, R. Grilli, J. Grimshaw, and A. Oxman) (updated 01 December 1997). Cochrane Collaboration, Issue 1. Update Software, Oxford.

Thornton, S. (1999). Accounting in an accrual world. *Public Finance*, 9 July, pp. 20–1.

UNFPA (1998). *Southeast Asian populations in crisis.* UNFPA, New York

University of York (1999). *Health technology assessment.* http://www.york.ac.uk/inst/crd/sites.htmhta

US Preventive Services Task Force (1996). *Guide to clinical preventive services.* Williams & Wilkins, Baltimore, MD.

Van den Ven, W.P.M.M., van Vleit, R.C.J.A., van Barnevald, E.M., and Lamers, L.L. (1994). Risk-adjusted capitation: recent experiences in The Netherlands. *Health Affairs*, **13**, 120–36.

Vartiainen, E., Puska, P., Pekkanen, J., Tuomilehto, J., and Jousilahti, P. (1994). Changes in risk factors explain changes in mortality from ischaemic heart disease in Finland. *British Medical Journal*, **309**, 23–7.

Velkova, A., Wolleswinkel-van den Bosch, J.H., and Mackenbach, J.P. (1997). The east-west life expectancy gap: Differences in mortality from conditions amenable to medical intervention. *International Journal of Epidemiology*, **26**, 75–84.

Warner, M. (1996). *Implementing health care reforms through substitution.* Welsh Institute for Health and Social Care, Cardiff.

Whitehead, M. (1988). *The health divide.* Penguin, Harmondsworth.

Whitty, P. and Jones, I. (1992). Public health heresy: a challenge to the purchasing orthodoxy. *British Medical Journal*, **304**, 1039–41.

WHO (World Health Organization) (1986). *Ottawa Charter for Health Promotion: an international conference on health promotion.* WHO Regional Office for Europe, Copenhagen.

WHO (World Health Organization) (1999). *Health promoting hospitals.* http://www.who.dk/tech/hs/recom.htm

Wilcock, C.K. (1979). The prevalence of osteoarthritis of the hip requiring total hip replacement in the elderly. *International Journal of Epidemiology*, **8**, 247–50.

Wootton, R. (1996). Telemedicine: a cautious welcome. *British Medical Journal*, **313**, 1375–7.

Young, D.W. and Saltman, R.B. (1985). *The hospital power equilibrium—physician behaviour and cost control.* Johns Hopkins University Press, Baltimore, MD.

12.11 Community health workers

Suwit Wibulpolprasert

Go to the people
Live among them, Learn from them
Plan with them, work with them
Start with what they know, build on what they have
Teach by showing, learn by doing
Not a showcase but a pattern
Not odds and ends but a system
Not piecemeal but integrated approach
Not to conform but to transform
Not relief but release

Y.C. James Yen

Introduction

Broad perspective of 'health' and the limitations of health professionals

The Executive Board of the World Health Organization (**WHO**) proposed redefining 'health' as 'A *dynamic* state of complete physical, mental, social and *spiritual* well-being, and not merely the absence of diseases and infirmity' (WHO 1998). The words in italics were added to the original definition as it appeared in the 1948 constitution of the WHO (WHO 1999*a*).

This new definition of 'health' further broadened the initial perspective to include the 'spiritual' dimension of health, and to stress its 'dynamicity'. Nevertheless, the new definition still affirms that health is 'a state of well-being'.

This broad perspective of health underscores its multifactorial nature. Health improvement depends much on the educational status (particularly of women), and other socio-economic development as on the development of the health-care systems (Roemer 1991; WHO 1999*b*) (Fig. 1).

As health is a state of well being, anyone who acts to improve well being can be broadly designated as a 'health worker'. Examples include

- mothers who try hard to nurse and protect their babies
- farmers who produce food for nutrition
- teachers who provide education to increase an individual's wisdom and to empower the community
- engineers who build roads and provide electricity to rural villages
- priests and monks who provide counselling to reduce mental stress, and encourage people to decrease their greed and selfishness, contribute significantly to improving the mental and spiritual dimension of health.

This holistic concept of health also emphasizes the intersectoral and participatory concept of 'All for Health' in addition to the human right concept of 'Health for All'. The holistic and broader perspective of health is usually neglected and seldom considered or taught among health professionals. They usually confine themselves within the narrow perspective of disease and medical technology oriented health-care systems.

With the advent of modern health-care systems, health professionals who possessed the modern medical knowledge rose to power at the expense of previously prevailing self-care practices and community healers. These modern health professionals, with their power of new wisdom and their financial and political power, sometimes played an important role in shaping the health-care systems of their country more towards professionalism than for public interest. Starr (1984) described clearly the role of the medical profession in structuring the American health-care system.

Training health professionals in sophisticated modern health technology is costly. Modern health professionals usually work in expensive technologically oriented urban health-care infrastructures. In addition, they usually come from better-off families and thus are reluctant to work in the remote rural areas or among the poor urban slum dwellers. Because of their narrow perspective, high cost, and inequitable distribution, most modern health professionals provide inadequate responses to community health demands, particularly in the remote areas and urban slums. Thus self-care practices and traditional community healers still exist both in remote rural areas and in urban communities. However, with misguided modern health legislation, these community healers often become illegal.

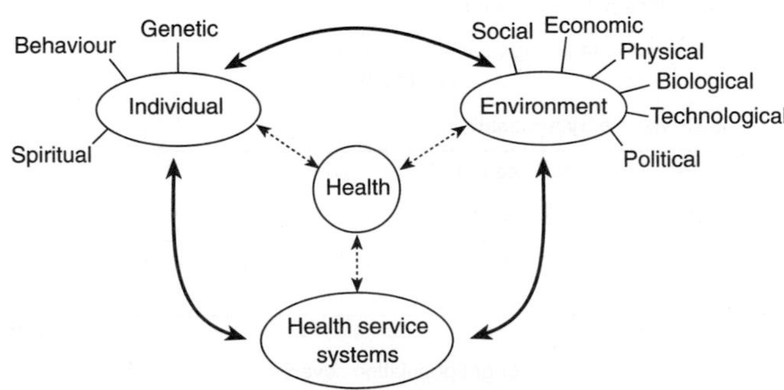

Fig. 1 Multifactorial relationship of health and its determinants.

The origin of community health workers

Accessibility to modern health-care services depends not only on its availability but also on its affordability, cultural acceptability, and its effectiveness (Fig. 2) (WHO 1984). Most developing countries cannot afford to build adequate modern health-care infrastructures to be accessed by every citizen. The existing public and private health facilities usually provide modern health services that are unaffordable for many, if not most. Those that provide free health services may provide substandard services which are unacceptable for the people. Finally many of these modern health services are not cost-effective because they are based on professional interests. Some even cause iatrogenic illnesses.

Countries usually respond to the problem of inadequate physical access to professional services first by providing a lower level of health personnel. For example, the posts of auxiliary midwives and junior sanitarians have been developed in Thailand since 1953. Apart from providing maternal and child care, and sanitation services, these auxiliary personnel also deliver basic medical care services. This inadequacy of professional services and the use of lower-level health personnel also occurs in more developed countries. In the United States and Canada, physician assistants and nurse practitioners have been developed since the mid-1960s (Jonas 1998). Nevertheless, even with the expanded services provided by these auxiliaries, basic health services are still not accessible by large number of rural villagers and poor people in urban slums. In many cases, rural health facilities have inadequate human resources or unqualified health personnel. Urban-trained health personnel, brought up in a different social and cultural background, also lack an understanding of the local community. Thus this problem is caused by multiplicity of complex socio-economic and cultural factors.

Inadequate access by a large part of the population to basic health services prompted many countries to start piloting the creation of systematically trained local community health workers. For example, in Thailand, the first pilot project to involve the community and appoint community health workers for sanitation activities, was started in 1960 (Vacharothai 1978). In the Democratic People's Republic of Korea, female sanitation monitors have been recruited and trained since 1955. However, a reliance on pilot or small-scale top-down projects not adapted to the local conditions, and a lack of community participation and consequently of local support and resources, have resulted in disappointments and failures. In the early 1970s, the health of the Chinese people improved spectacularly partly as a result of what we now call the nationwide primary health care approach. One of its guiding principles was the utilization of community health workers to:

- extend health services to the places where the people live and work
- support communities to identify their own health need
- help people to solve their own health problems.

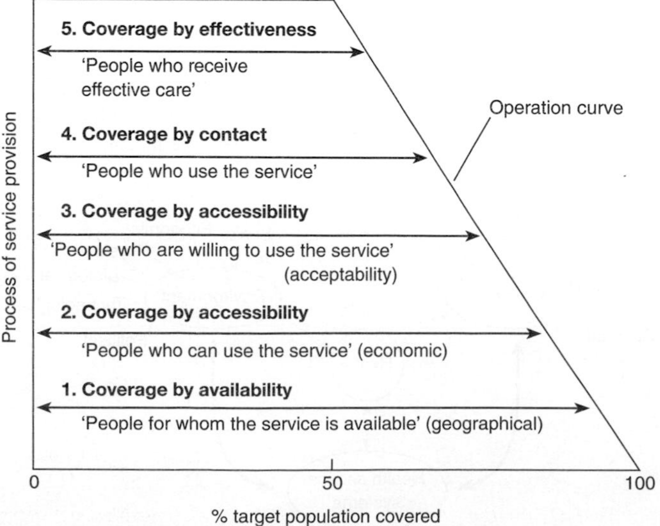

Fig. 2 Coverage of health services. (Adapted from WHO 1984.)

This new idea, that communities should assume substantial responsibility for their own health, brought a new dimension to the management of health-care services. It opened up an opportunity to redraft and expand basic health services.

The Alma-Ata International Conference on Primary Health Care in 1978, organized jointly by the WHO and the United Nations International Children's Emergency Fund (**UNICEF**), proposed the development of national community health worker programmes as an important strategy for improving access to primary health care (WHO 1978). Since then community health worker programmes have expanded to all developing countries. Table 1 provides the overall picture of community health workers in nine countries of the WHO's South-East Asia region.

After two decades of development, ample evidence has been published on the community health worker's role as a key agent in improving health. The World Bank (1994) described the importance of community health worker programmes to the success of health development in Africa. Walt (1990) concluded that community health workers not only provide basic health services but also promote the key principles of primary health care—equity, intersectoral collaboration, community involvement, and the use of appropriate technology. Community health workers have shown that they can reduce mortality and improve other indices of health status. In certain communities they can satisfy basic health-care needs which cannot realistically be met by other means (WHO 1989).

Definition and role of the community health worker

Community health workers are defined differently in different countries according to the needs of the country and the resources available for satisfying them. Their roles and responsibilities are also varied.

The WHO (1978) defined community health workers as people with limited education, trained in a short time to carry out either a wide range or restricted aspects of health-care services. They should come from the community in which they live and should be chosen by it. The WHO further defined community health workers as:

> Men and women chosen by the community, and trained to deal with the health problems of individuals and the community, and to work in close relationship with the health services. They should have had a level of primary education that enable them to

Table 1 Main categories of community health workers (CHW)/volunteers in nine countries of the WHO's South-East Asia region, by country

Country	Category	Date initiated	Ratio of CHW to population (pop) or households (hh)	Duration of training	Percentage of females	Numbers trained
Bangladesh	Village health volunteer	1988	1 to 30 hh	4 days	80	38 262
Bhutan	Village health volunteer/worker	1978–79	1 to 20–30 hh	12 days	10	1400
DPR Korea	Sanitation monitor	1955	1 to 20–30 hh	5 days	100	NA
India	Village health guides	1977	1 to 1000 pop	3 months	25	416 724 (1985)
	Anganwadi worker	1975	1 to 1000 pop	3 months	100	NA
Indonesia	Health cadre	1978	1 to 10 hh	3 days	100	1.8 million (1991)
Myanmar	Community health worker	1977	1 to 1000 pop	4 weeks	5	36 358
	Auxiliary midwife	1977	1 to 2266 pop	6 months	100	17 856 (1994)
	Ten-household health worker	1987	1 to 10 hh	7 days	90	41 643 (1994)
Nepal	Female village health volunteer	1988–89	1 to 400 hh (normal terrain) 1 to 250 hh (hill area) 1 to 150 hh (mountains)	12 days + 3 days refresher yearly	100	32 000
Sri Lanka	Volunteer health worker	1975–77	Cluster of hh	6 h (spread out)	66	40 000 (1996)
Thailand	Village health communicator	1979	1 to 10–15 hh	5 days	NA	598 908 (abolished in 1994)
	Village health volunteer	1979	1 to 80–150 hh	15 days	NA	642 532 (1998)
	Village sanitary craftsmen	1982	1 to 5–10 villages	15 days	NA	4132 (1990)
	Family health leaders	1996	1 to 1 hh	1 day	NA	1 177 464 (1998)

Many countries train traditional birth attendants as volunteer health workers (e.g. Thailand).

The numbers of community health volunteers enlisted are mainly those selected and trained in the government health-care system. Figures from non-governmental organizations are not included.

NA, not available.

Adapted and updated from WHO (1996).

read, write and do simple mathematical calculations. (WHO 1987)

Most community health workers are volunteers and receive short but systematic training. However, some receive longer-term training and even civil servant status, for example auxiliary midwives in Myanmar and community health aides in Jamaica.

To clarify further the definition of community health workers, a WHO study group (WHO 1989) proposed that community health workers should be:

- members of the communities where they work
- selected by the communities
- answerable to the communities for their activities
- supported by the health system but not necessarily a part of its organization
- have shorter training than professional workers.

Thus community health workers are generally part-time volunteers rather than full-time public employees.

Community health workers may have different job titles and have different responsibilities in different countries. They may be called community health workers, village health volunteers, village health communicators, health guides, sanitation monitors, barefoot doctors, Feldschers, and so on.

In India, the national community health worker programme, started in 1977, was changed to the Community Health Volunteer Scheme in 1979 to stress their 'volunteer' nature. In 1981, with the change in government, the programme was renamed the Health Guides Scheme (Bose 1983).

Table 2 shows the different categories of community health workers in response to the nine elements of primary health care in Thailand (Wibulpolprasert 1991).

Responsibilities of community health workers

Community health workers usually serve the role of educators, communicators, problem detectors, problem solvers, community organizers, and leaders for health. They serve as the link between the community and the health-care systems. They play an important role in galvanizing communities for action, and provide information that promotes individual and family self-care and responsibility as integral components of everyday life.

Some community health workers support delivery of general basic health services, for example village health volunteers in Bangladesh, Bhutan, and Thailand. Others play more specific roles, for example trained traditional birth attendants and village sanitary craftsmen in

Table 2 Categories of community health workers (CHWs) and community financing schemes for nine elements of primary health care, Thailand, 1988

Elements	CHWs[a]	Role	Financing schemes[b]
Health education	VHVs/VHCs	Village broadcasts/ education/motivation	—
Control of locally endemic diseases	Some VHVs/VHCs and malaria volunteers	Malaria surveillance Bleeding site control Provision of antimalarials	Mosquito Net Fund
Immunization (EPI)	VHVs/VHCs	Communication for immunization	Health Card Fund
Maternal and child health, family planning	VHVs/VHCs and trained traditional birth attendants	Advocate breast-feeding, supplementary diet, family planning and maternal and child health Distribute oral contraceptive pills and condoms	Health Card Fund
Nutrition	Model mother VHVs/VHCs	Nutritional surveillance Demonstration of supplementary diet	Nutrition Fund
Essential drugs and treatment of basic medical problems	VHVs/VHCs	Provision of essential drugs, first aid, and basic medical care	Village Drug Fund
Sanitation	Village sanitary craftsmen	Building latrines and water jars	Sanitation Fund
Dental health	VHVs/VHCs	Education and demonstration on regular and correct tooth brushing	Tooth-brush and Toothpaste Fund

VHCs, village health communicators; VHVs, village health volunteers.

[a]Only VHVs and malaria volunteers still existed in 1999.

[b]Most community financing schemes have faded away and been integrated into the multipurpose village development funds.

Adapted and updated from Wibulpolprasert (1991).

Thailand, and sanitation monitors in the Democratic People's Republic of Korea.

The specific role of community health workers has to be adapted to local situations and health demands. Nevertheless, their roles need to be specifically defined. Table 3 provides an example of the clearly defined specific responsibilities of village health communicators and volunteers in Thailand.

As community organizers and leaders for health, community health workers also play key roles in the establishment and management of community financing schemes for health development (Table 2). As a member (and leader) of the community, the community health worker can incorporate health into all community development activities, which is difficult for health professionals. In many countries community health workers combine service functions and developmental functions that are not just in the field of health. The relative importance of these two functions varies according to the socio-economic situation and the availability and accessibility of local health services. The service function is less important where there is ready access to health-care facilities. The developmental function is useful in all circumstances and is crucial in less developed communities.

Table 4 shows the duties of community health workers in 11 different countries (WHO 1987). Most community health workers have educational and motivational roles as well as delivering first-aid treatments and dispensing basic drugs. However, in some countries they provide more specific or sophisticated services. For example, community health workers in Columbia and Papua New Guinea also give injections, particularly for immunization. Community health workers in Botswana, Sudan, and Yemen provide regular school health activities. In Botswana, Jamaica, China, and Papua New Guinea they assist in health centre clinic activities.

Should community health workers provide medical services?

The preventive and health promotion roles of the community health workers are usually readily accepted by health professionals. However, their role in providing basic medical care is a controversial. Health professionals, particularly medical professionals, often allege that community health worker programmes, which train community health workers in basic medical care, promote quackery. Both scientific rationale and vested interests are involved in the professional movement against community health worker programmes.

Those who support community health worker training in basic medical care argue that the training not only provides more accessibility to villagers according to their need, but also creates social credit and acceptability for the community health workers so that providing other preventive and health promotion activities are much easier. In addition, knowledge and skills in basic medical care may help to prevent epidemics from breaking out through early case detection.

Training community health workers in basic medical care should thus be carried out cautiously with strong supervision to prevent them from overtreating patients, and particularly from providing care for

Table 3 Responsibilities of village health communicators and volunteers in Thailand

Responsibilities of village health communicators		
1.	To inform the villagers in their respective areas about information related to health	
2.	To collect information from the public regarding health and health-related matters such as births, deaths, migration, pregnancies, problems, and needs	
3.	To disseminate knowledge, advise and stimulate the public in the eight elements of primary health care as follows	
	3.1	Education concerning prevailing health problems and the methods of preventing and controlling them
	3.2	Promotion of food supply and proper nutrition
	3.3	Maternal and child health care, including family planning
	3.4	Adequacy of safe water supply and basic sanitation
	3.5	Immunization against major infectious diseases
	3.6	Prevention and control of locally endemic diseases
	3.7	Appropriate treatment of common diseases and injuries
	3.8	Provision of essential basic household drugs for the community
4.	To carry out and co-ordinate health development activities and join other intersectoral development activities	
Additional responsibilities of village health volunteers		
As well as assuming the tasks of a village health communicator, the village health volunteer has the following additional responsibilities		
1.	Weighing preschool children and distributing of supplementary foods for malnourished children	
2.	Providing simple symptomatic medical care by using home remedies or other medicines, which the Ministry of Public Health has given permission to use	
3.	Giving first aid treatment for fresh wounds, fractures, burns, etc.	
4.	Distributing birth control pills and condoms to the clients who have already been examined by the government health staff	

Adapted from Office of the Primary Health Care (1985).

Table 4 Duties of community health workers in different countries

Task summary	Benin	Botswana	Colombia	India	Jamaica	Liberia	Papua New Guinea	Philippines	Sudan	Thailand	Yemen
1. First aid, treat accidents, and simple illness	+	+	+	+	+	+	+	+	+	+	+
2. Dispense drugs	+	+	+ (including injections)	+	+	+	+ (including injections)	+	+	+	+
3. Pre- and post-natal advice, motivation	+	+	+	+	+	+	+	+	+	+	+
4. Deliver babies	+	×	+	×	×	×	×	×	×	× (trained TBA)	×
5. Child-care advice, motivation	+	+	+	+	+	+	+	+	+	+	+
6. Nutrition motivation, demonstration	+	+	+	+	+	+	+	+	+	+	+
7. Nutrition action	F	W	W	×	W, F	×	W	W, F	F	W, F	×
8. Immunization motivation, assistance during clinic	+	+	+	+	+	+	+	+	+	+	+
9. Immunization/ give injections	×	×	+	×	×	×	+	×	+	×	×
10. Family planning motivation	+	+	+	+	+	+	×	+	+	+	+
11. Family planning, distribute supplies	×	+	+	+	×	×	×	+	+	+	×
12. Environmental sanitation, personal hygiene, general health habits, motivation	+	+	+	+	+	+	+	+	+	+	+
13. Communicable disease screening, referral, prevention, motivation	+	+	+	+	×	+	+	+	+	+	+
14. Communicable disease follow-up, motivation of confirmed cases	+	+	+	+	×	Sometimes	+	+	+	+	Sometimes
15. Communicable disease action	×	D	D, M	M	×	×	D, M	TB sputum smear	D	D, M (malaria volunteers)	D
16. Assist health centre clinic activities (i.e. not in village)	Occasionally	+	Occasionally	×	+	×	+	×	Occasionally	Occasionally	×
17. Refer difficult cases to health centre or hospital	+	+	+	+	+	+	+	+	+	+	+
18. Perform school health activities regularly	×	/	×	×	×	×	×	×	+	×	+
19. Collect vital statistics	×	+	+	+	×	+	×	+	+	+	+
20. Maintain records, reports	+	+	+	+	+	+	+	+	+	+ (VHV only)	+
21. Visit homes on a regular basis	+	+	+	+	+	Sometimes	+	+	+	+	×
22. Perform tasks outside health sector (e.g. agriculture)	+	+	×	+	×	+	×	+	+	+	+
23. Participate in community meetings	+	+	+	+	+	+	+	+	+	+	+

+, Task performed by community health worker; ×, task not performed; D, provide drug resupply; F, distribute food supplements; M, take malaria slide; TB, tuberculosis; TBA, traditional birth attendant; W, weigh children, maintain chart.

Adapted from WHO (1987).

private benefits. It is clear that all community health worker programmes should include basic medical care as one of their core responsibilities (Table 4).

Community health workers: successes and failures

Over the past two decades many countries have experimented with the use of community health workers to provide primary health care. Although there is ample evidence of success, community health worker programmes have had some mixed results. Examples are discussed below of the successes and failures of the community health worker programmmes in both developing and developed countries.

Traditional birth attendants and maternal mortality

In the Gambia and Indonesia, studies have shown that traditional birth attendants who were not backed up by strong basic health services were unable to decrease the risk of maternal mortality (World Bank 1993). Conversely, in Bangladesh, a programme to train and support midwives to work with traditional birth attendants helped to lower maternal mortality by 60 per cent over a 10-year period (World Bank 1993). This is clear proof of the need for regular, systematic, and intensive supervision and support from existing basic health services. Strong support by the basic health services will ensure continuous motivation and continuity as well as a high quality of service. Community health worker programmes should thus be developed and strengthened along with the basic health services.

Organized community health workers in Jamaica

The Jamaican community health worker programme, launched in 1977, recruited many community health workers from different communities. A large group sought and obtained civil service benefits. In 1985 salaries for briefly trained community health workers were to be equivalent to two-thirds that of registered nurses with 3 years training. Shortages of higher-level staff prompted many health centres to substitute community health workers for nurses. Although they appear to be cost-effective, community health workers became increasingly linked to the health system, while their availability to the community diminished. For economic reasons, the programme has been greatly reduced. In 1989, in Hanover parish only one-third of the community health workers originally trained were still active. Fifty per cent had been laid off and the remainder had retired or emigrated in 1985 and 1986 (World Bank 1993; Kahssay *et al.* 1998).

Community health workers of non-governmental organizations

The Pastoral da Crianca, a community health worker programme instated in 1983 by the Catholic Church in Brazil, had 47 000 community health workers throughout the country in 1992, with 1.5 million children enrolled in the programme. It received strong support from Ministry of Health, UNICEF, and the Barnard Van Leer Foundation and other non-governmental organizations. Community health workers provided health education to low-income mothers, and monitored the growth of infants and young children. An evaluation carried out in 1990 found that health and nutritional indicators for young children enrolled in the programme were significantly better than indicators from similar communities in which the Pastoral da Crianca had no activities (World Bank 1993).

Sri Lanka Health Volunteer Corps

The building of a Health Volunteer Corps in Sri Lanka, begun in the early 1980s, had selected and trained 10 000 volunteers by the end of 1989. The continued training of volunteers boosted the volunteer force to 40 000 by 1996. They receive an initial 2-week training; review meetings and supervisory field visits by primary health care teams provide ongoing support. The success of this model is demonstrated by its adoption by non-governmental organizations and the plantation sector to improve the health of their workers and communities (WHO 1999*b*).

Community health workers in Thailand

Community participation was started in Thailand in 1960 in the nationwide sanitation programme (Vacharothai 1978). The Village Health Sanitation Project allowed, for the first time, many villagers to work alongside government officials. This success led to the project for training of traditional birth attendants and village health volunteers. In 1974, a comprehensive primary health care development project, the Lampang Health Development Project, was initiated, with support from the American Public Health Association, the University of Hawaii, and the USAID. It focused on the development of basic rural health infrastructures as well as community health workers. Its success and the Alma-Ata Declaration were the foundation for the development of the nationwide primary health care programme in 1979. Within 5 years, every village was provided with trained village health volunteers and communicators.

Extensive recruitment and training of the village health volunteers and communicators, together with the development of many community financing schemes and other specialized community health workers, successfully improved the coverage of many health service targets, such as family planning, maternal and child health, immunizations, sanitation, nutrition, and access to essential drugs. Nevertheless, problems in the selection, training, supervision, and incentives provided resulted in a high attrition rate. A 1988 evaluation found attrition rates of 62.4 per cent and 24.9 per cent for village health communicators and village health volunteers respectively (Hongwiwatana *et al.* 1988).

In the early 1990s, with rapid economic growth, massive urban migration of rural villagers, and even labour migration abroad, many community health workers had to be replaced and retrained. Most community health financing schemes faded away or were integrated into bigger multipurpose village development funds. In 1994, all village health communicators were upgraded to village health volunteers, and community run primary health care centres were set up in every village, supported by the health centre personnel. These primary health care centres were equipped with some basic equipment and drugs, for example, stethoscopes, sphygmomanometers, thermometers, urine test sticks, and basic essential drugs.

Village health volunteers are well recognized at a national level. They have special uniforms, receive free medical care (for their whole family), and receive daily allowances for their meetings. However, they are still volunteers. A National Health Volunteer Day on 20 March of each year was also established in 1995.

Kenyan experience in community-based health care in Saradidi

This project, which was started in 1981, recruited two community health workers from each village. They received intensive 2-week introductory training with further continuous training on analysis of priority health problems and some specific basic health skills. The community health workers contribute as much as 80 per cent of the project's voluntary time. Some of the very good community health workers become trainers of the newcomers. The project found that creating a new system of village health committees was inappropriate. It was best to strengthen and work within the existing leadership and community organization structures, such as clans, women, and other activity groups (Kaseje 1990).

Three-Generation Volunteer Corps (Komaki City, Japan)

The Three-Generation Volunteer Corps, a community volunteer organization, was formed in 1986 in Komaki City. It consisted of the Silver Volunteer Corps for the elderly, the Women's Volunteer Corps, and the Junior Volunteer Corps for junior high school children. Their activities focus mainly on the social dimensions of health, for example visits to bedridden elderly and elderly people living alone, litter gathering, road safety training, and fund raising. They try to nurture mutual understanding and exchange among volunteers in an effort to achieve communities where everyone can 'live without worry' in a friendly community atmosphere (Ministry of Health and Welfare 1994).

Attempts at community health worker development in the United States

Community health worker initiative in New York City

A conference called 'Learning from our Neighbours: Lessons for New York City from the Developing World' was convened in June 1997. The conference offered seven recommendations focused at supporting and strengthening community health worker activity in New York City. An advisory group has been established by the Department of Health to prioritize the conference recommendations and to develop a plan to move the community health worker agenda forward (Kahssay *et al.* 1998).

The National Community Health Advisor Study

The University of Arizona has completed a national study of the situation of community health worker programmes in the United States (the National Community Health Advisor Study). The study recommends the core role and competence of community health workers, career and field development for community health workers, community health worker evaluation strategies, community health worker's role in the changing health-care system, and the special needs of youth community health workers. The study proposed an evaluation framework including process and outcome measures on four levels: individual, programme–organization, community–agency, and external linkages (Kahssay 1998).

Community health workers: conditions for success

Early evaluations of community health worker programmes indicate four necessary (but difficult) conditions for success: community health workers must be well trained, well supervised, well provided with logistic support, and linked to well-functioning district health systems for referral when needed (World Bank 1993). These four conditions are relevant technical and managerial conditions which require clear policy and leadership support. Experience from many developing countries indicate the following conditions for the success of community health worker programmes.

Strong political support

Initiating a community health worker programme means accepting the Health for All policy based on primary health care. It means also that the limitations of health professionals and the potential of the community are well accepted. This inevitably means a decision to put more resources into primary health care, which include resources to support activities to establish and strengthen community health workers. It may also mean shifting resources from secondary and tertiary care in urban areas to support basic health services and primary health care in the rural settings. Shifting of resources is a painful process which requires strong political leadership. Strong political support is also needed for the community health worker programmes to overcome resistance and win acceptance from health professionals.

The Alma-Ata Declaration on the Health for All policy based on primary health care provided very strong political support for community health worker programmes in many developing countries. The Kenyan community-based health-care project initiated in 1979 is a good example of this (Kaseje 1990).

Political commitment for further and real decentralization of health services also allows more active participation by the community. At the local level, political leadership support from village leaders, religious leaders, teachers, and other informal leaders are crucial to the success of community health worker programmes.

In Thailand, political commitment towards rural development, including rural health development, during the early 1980s was so strong that significant resources were shifted from urban provincial hospitals to strengthen rural district hospitals, health centres, and community health worker programmes. In 1983, the budget of the district and subdistrict health programme, which used to be lower than those of the provinces, became higher (Fig. 3). At the same time the Ministry of Public Health announced a ministerial regulation allowing basic medical practices by rural health centre personnel including community health workers. Because of strong political support and social movement, there was very little resistance from the Medical Association.

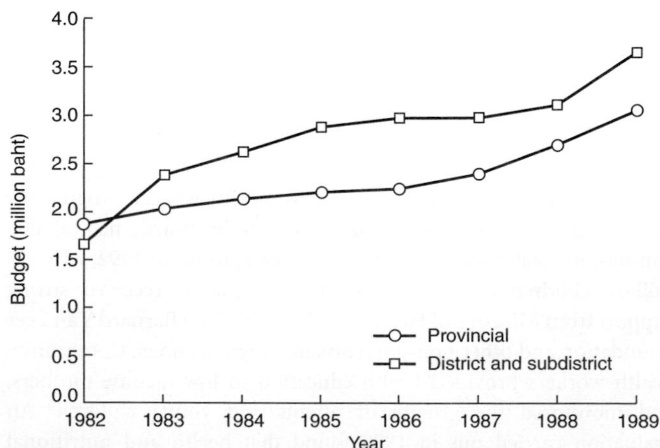

Fig. 3 Shift of budget allocation due to the strong political leadership in the rural development programme. (Adapted from Wibulpolprasert 1999.)

In India, the turbulent political scene between 1977 and 1980 placed severe constraints on the community health worker programme. The Health Minister, who initiated the programme in October 1977, was strongly attacked by the medical profession. Attacks on the minister were, in fact, attacks on the community health worker scheme itself. This was the worst possible political context for the new scheme, and its credibility suffered as a result. A drastic change in the funding arrangement from 100 per cent central funding in 1977 to 50 per cent in 1979 brought it to a grinding halt in several states. In December 1981, the government decided to make the scheme 100 per cent centrally financed in order to restore the programme (Bose 1983).

In Cuba, the national political leaders decided to focus on the equitable distribution of health professionals down to the grass root level. The community health worker programme was thus very weak and ineffective. However, with the success in building an equitable and widely accessible health-care system, in addition to other other socio-economic equities, the health of Cubans improved greatly (Werner 1983).

Intersectoral approach

The priorities of most rural communities are roads, water for agriculture, electricity, schools, and employment rather than health. In order to attract higher priority and more community involvement, community health worker programmes should be integrated into the overall community development programmes. This fulfils the holistic approach of the Health for All concept.

This intersectoral concept although not difficult to accept, is not easy to implement. In most developing countries, ministries usually have their own vested interests in maintaining a vertical bureaucracy. Vertical non-integrated activities are normal phenomena in different ministries or in different departments or divisions within one ministry. Thus it is not uncommon to see health, education, rural development, and agriculture ministries compete for the recruitment of volunteers in the villages.

During the height of primary health care development in Thailand in the mid-1980s, many vertical health activities existed in a single village. In many villages, the Village Drug Fund, Sanitation Fund, Nutrition Fund, Mosquito Net Fund, and Tooth-brush and Tooth Paste Fund, were implemented separately. They also created different categories of community health worker (Table 2). These fragmented community health activities created management confusion among villagers and community health workers. These vertical health activities were usually short lived and finally the many piecemeal community financing schemes were integrated into single multipurpose village health development funds (Wibulpolprasert 1991). All categories of community health workers were also integrated into the single category of village health volunteers.

In 1983, 5 years after the implementation of the primary health care programme in Thailand, a more integrated multisectoral development based on the basic minimum need approach and quality of life campaign was established (Fig. 4). This multisectoral approach started from the central level, under the National Rural Development Committee chaired by the Prime Minister, down to the village level under the Village Development Committee. Basic minimum need indicators became the basic tools to measure quality of life of the villagers, forming an information system shared by all ministries (Nittayarumphong 1990). Although the system changed over time and with changes in governments, the basic minimum need–quality-of-life concept and indicators remained. There has been an annual report on the basic minimum need indicators for each village since 1986. Those villages with the lowest basic minimum need indices are considered as having a lower quality of life and thus receive higher priority in public resources allocation (Ministry of Interior 1999).

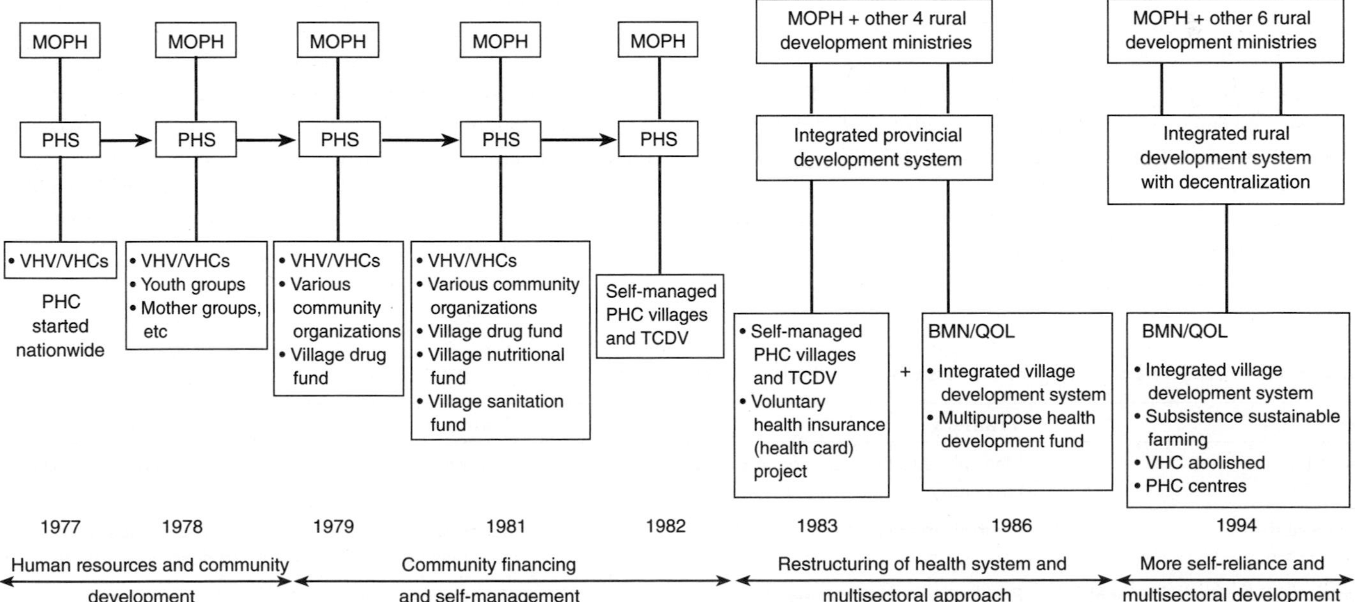

Fig. 4 The implementation of primary health care and integrated rural development in Thailand. BMN, basic minimum need; MOPH, Ministry of Public Health; PHS, provincial health service; QOL, quality of life; TCDV, technical co-operation among developing villages; VHVs/VHCs, village health volunteers and communicators. (Adapted and updated from Nittayaramphong (1990).)

Active community participation

Sustainability of community health worker programmes very much depends on acceptance by communities, its relevance to their demands, and their participation. Active community participation should be included in all activities of the community health worker programmes, from community preparation, selection of community health workers, decision on the types and strategies of health development activities, and management of the programmes.

Active community participation is not easy to achieve in the prevailing provider–client relationship between government officials and villagers of most rural communities. Reorientation of the health personnel perspective and the release of community potential are essential for its achievement. This requires not only community preparation but also active preparation of health personnel. Socio-economic and political reform of the country towards increasing decentralization and participatory democracy is also conducive to its success.

One approach to increasing active community participation is to make community health worker programmes more flexible. Most developing countries implement community health worker programmes on a single rigid top-down primary health care model. This approach usually leaves little room for the lower-level health personnel and the community to make adjustments to fit the local context. A rigid top-down primary health care model implemented on a nationwide scale may yield rapid impressive results, but is usually short lived.

One good example is the village drug funds in Thailand. This programme was started as a rigid top-down community financing scheme in 1981. Within 6 years, there were 27 135 village drug funds, covering 45 per cent of all rural villages. However, a census survey in 1998 found that only 15 per cent of the original village drug funds still existed. Those that survived were modified mainly by integrating into the multipurpose village grocery stores. These modifications were decided upon and implemented by active community leaders in consultation with the local health personnel.

Village leaders, either formal or informal, are important human resources who can actively participate in community health worker programmmes. Religious leaders, school teachers, youth leaders, and leaders of women's groups can also be active in community health worker programmes. Local health personnel should contact these leaders and seek their opinion and support for the success and sustainability of community health worker programmes.

Efficient management of community health worker programmes

Management makes the impossible possible. (Drucker 1977)

Although community health worker programmes may be rational and receive high political support, managing a community health worker programme is not an easy task. Several issues in the management of community health worker programmes need to be addressed.

Preparation of health personnel

This is one of the most crucial components of community health worker programmes. Health personnel, particularly at the district level, are the prime (and closest) trainers and supporters of community health workers. Their attitude and skills towards working in partnership with community health workers need to be developed and monitored. Two types of health personnel should be considered as follows.

Health personnel directly related to community health workers

These are mainly personnel at the district-level health infrastructures (e.g. district hospitals and health centres). They are in direct communication with community health workers and are responsible for community preparation and selection, and the training of community health workers, providing them with supervision and support. They need to be trained to become trainers themselves, primary health care supporters, and social advocators. Most important is the development of a positive attitude towards community health workers, and respect for the community's capabilities and community skills. They should be able to build up friendly working relations with community leaders, community health workers, and active members of the community. These skills will enable them to be efficient supporters of community health workers.

Their preparation can be achieved through short courses, on-the-job training in primary health care, community health worker programmes, and training methodology.

In the Thai primary health care programme, a three-tier training for trainers programme was started in 1977. The three tiers include central, provincial/district, and subdistrict trainers. It took 3 years to complete the training of all the subdistrict trainers in all 72 provinces. Table 5 summarizes the systematic three-tier training system.

Training materials and guidelines for health personnel should be locally prepared. They may be adapted from the one prepared by WHO (McMahon *et al.* 1980). Table 6 provides an example of the items for the training modules for Thailand.

Table 5 The three levels of training for trainers of primary health care programmes in Thailand

Level	Trainers	Trainees
Central	Medical education team from Chulalongkorn University	Staff members of departments and divisions concerned
Provincial/district	Central trainers	Health staff responsible for training and supervision from provincial health office and district health office
Tambon (subdistrict, commune)	Provincial/district trainers	Health personnel at *tambon* level
Village	*Tambon* trainers	VHCs/VHVs

VHCs, village health communicators; VHV, village health volunteers.

Adapted from Ministry of Public Health (1988).

Table 6 Items in the training for trainers of primary health care programmes in Thailand

Unit	Items
0	Motivation
1	Training and modules of training
2	Job analysis and performance discrepancy
3	Objectives of training and methods of evaluation during the period of training
4	Learning activities and planning of teaching/learning methods
5	Implementation of training
6	Training support and evaluation at the end of training programme

Adapted from Ministry of Public Health (1988).

Reorientation of basic education curricula to build up understanding, positive attitudes, and community skills for health professionals is also a very important undertaking.

In 1980, the Fourth National Medical Education Conference in Thailand concluded that all medical schools should produce doctors with four basic skills: clinicians, trainers, managers, and primary health care supporters. Since then the curricula of all medical schools have been reformed to incorporate community medicine in all courses as well as to establish a specific community medicine course for medical students. The curricula of other health professionals were also reformed towards more community orientation and a more primary health care approach. These reforms allowed students to have more exposure to real community health problems and contact with rural health personnel and community health workers. Almost all health professionals now have to spend at least 4 weeks in community hospitals and/or health centres. Many medical schools, nursing colleges, and public health colleges recruit their students from local provincial high school students. These students, after graduation, have more understanding of the community and work longer in their own locality.

In Mexico, the Autonomous Metropolitan University in Mexico City has adopted community-oriented medical education since the early 1980s. It consists of a series of 12-week problem-oriented multidisciplinary models. The medical students have opportunities to work with students from other disciplines, for example, nursing, social work, community planning, and agronomy. The students spend their fifth year of study in a rural setting. Students are assessed on both the adequacy of their clinical management skills and their community skills (Braveman and Mora 1987).

In India, the Christian Medical College and Hospital at Vellore has developed a programme to train 'basic doctors' who can function in any setting. The training has four phases. During the first phase in the preclinical years students are divided into groups of two or three and live for 2 weeks in a rural community. Each group is assigned 12 to 15 households to study in detail. They also work with community leaders and health workers in providing health services. The second phase lasts for 2 weeks in the first clinical year. The students, in groups of 10 to 12, undertake field investigations on morbidity and mortality in two to three villages. They also plan a programme for a defined health problem. The third phase lasts 2 to 3 weeks in the second clinical year. Students, in groups of five to six, evaluate the health status of a community and then plan, implement, and assess a programme. The last phase includes a 3-month community posting during the 1-year compulsory internship. They act as members of a health team and participate in all primary health care programme activities (Joseph 1985).

Other health personnel

Other specialized health professionals (e.g. medical specialists, laboratory and radiological technicians, hospital managers, and other supportive hospital personnel), although they do not relate directly with community health workers, also need an understanding and positive attitude towards them. They usually receive referred patients from health personnel and community health workers. They should also undergo short course training on primary health care and community health worker programmes. Activities, which allow them to participate in community health worker programmes (e.g. as trainers in basic medical care) will provide them with better understanding of the programme.

Selection of community health workers

The selection of the right community health worker is the beginning of a successful community health worker programme. Selecting wrong community health workers results in low productivity, a high drop-out rate, and many other problems as mentioned above in the case of Thailand.

Selection guidelines

Each country and community should establish its own selection guidelines for community health workers that best suit their needs and resources.

Some important qualities may be availability of time, community acceptability, social standing, long-term commitment to the community, and ability to influence community members particularly mothers. In situations where community health workers are to perform a wider range of services that require longer-term training, educational attainment may be an additional quality. All selection criteria should be clearly stated and agreed upon by the community. Table 7 gives an example of the selection criteria for community health workers in Thailand.

Selection method

Selection of community health workers may depend on a systematic sociometric approach or more preferably on a socioculturally accepted method determined by the community. In Thailand the early community health worker programme tried using a systematic sociometric method to identify village health communicators. Village health volunteers were further selected from among the communicators. Table 8 shows the questionnaire for the development of a 'sociogram' for identifying village health communicators in Thailand. Figure 5 shows an example of one such sociogram. Although it is a systematic approach, it is quite tedious and not easy to carry out. An assessment in 1986 found that sociograms were not always used. Village health communicators and volunteers were selected by simple village meetings or sometimes selected directly by the village leaders or health officers. The current selection method uses a more direct approach through community meetings or a meeting of the community committee.

Table 7 Selection criteria for village health communicators and volunteers, Thailand

Village health communicators

1. Be able to read and write
2. Live and work in the village
3. Be interested in health matters and be willing to help their fellow villagers without receiving any remuneration from the government
4. Availability of time

Village health volunteers

In addition to criteria for village health communicators, village health volunteers need to meet the following criteria

1. Have shown regular willingness in helping others and have enough free time for the public
2. Be trusted by the fellow villagers
3. Have their own occupation and be able to earn their own living
4. Live in a house easily accessible to the villagers
5. Not be a government official or the village headman

Adapted from Ministry of Public Health (1988).

Women as community health workers

Some countries (e.g. Indonesia, the Democratic People's Republic of Korea, and Nepal) select mostly female volunteers. The role of women in the family as health caregivers is known to be of great importance. A study of health-seeking behaviour in 16 developing countries found that women most often make decisions about health-care use, including self-care. At least 75 per cent of health-related decisions take place within the family. Involving women as volunteers enhances their confidence, skills, and status in the community, and thus contributes to the improvement of their own health as well as that of their families and the community (WHO 1999*b*).

Traditional healers as community health workers

In some instances, traditional healers accepted by most villagers, are good community health workers. Rural midwives or traditional birth attendants are useful community health workers. They are frequently one of the few workers to whom the community is willing to provide financial support. Community health workers who were traditional healers may function better than other community health workers.

A WHO evaluation of community health workers participating in a programme for the detection of malaria in northern Thailand found that traditional healer volunteers were more active in pursuing and identifying malaria cases than other volunteers and that they tended to remain in the programme longer because their service enhanced their standing in the community. Villagers indicated that they felt more confident about having someone they already knew as the village traditional healer draw their blood and administer treatment.

The WHO (1991) conducted a worldwide survey of 17 projects where traditional healers were trained and functioned as community health workers. These projects were located in all the regions of the WHO, except the European region. Eight of them had trained traditional birth attendants; others had trained traditional herbalists,

Table 8 Questionnaire for the development of a sociogram for selecting village health communicators (VHC), Thailand.

Village____________ *Tambon* (commune) ____________

District ____________ Province____________

Question: Who is the person in this cluster that you go to for advice most often and whom you respect?

House number	Name (best informed person)	Person (go for advice)	Name	House number/ owner of House	Hamlet number
		1.____________			
		2.____________			
		3. etc.____________			

Signature of the interviewer)____________ Date____________

This questionnaire is used for every household, the head of the household or the best informed person will be asked.

Adapted from Office of the Primary Health Care (1985).

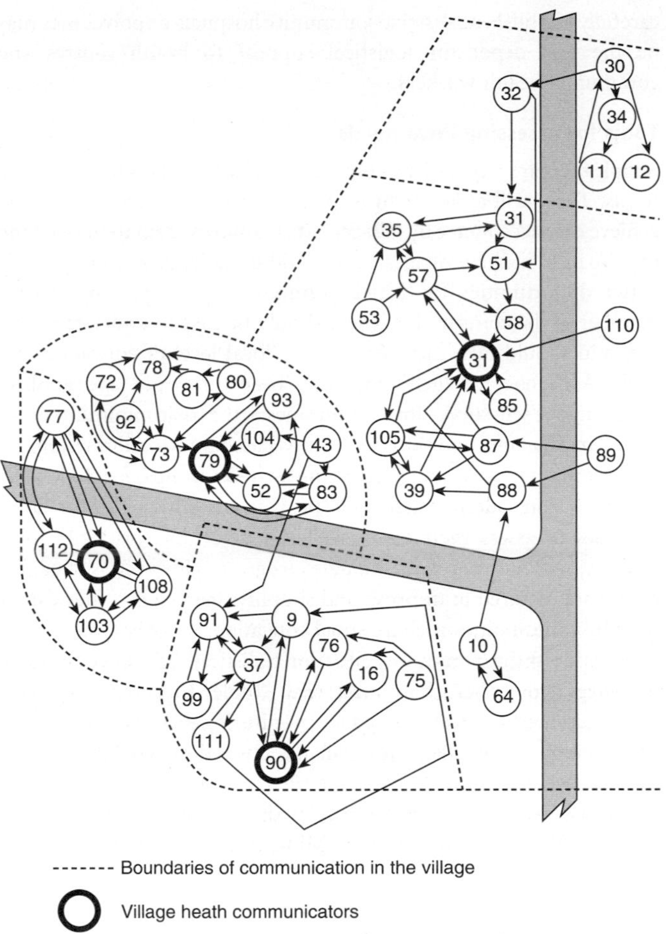

Fig. 5 Diagrammatic representation of the sociometric method of selecting village health communicators in Thailand: the broken lines indicate the boundaries of communication in the village; the circles indicate the village health communicators. (Source: Office of the Primary Health Care 1985.)

spiritual healers, and even bone-setters. Most were government sponsored.

This survey summarizes several advantages of using traditional healers as community health workers.

1. Traditional healers are willing to work in community health care and take on primary health care activities when they are given appropriate training. They can also establish good working relations with local health personnel. They are socioculturally accepted human resources with a good service attitude. Being community health workers usually boosts their acceptance by the community.

2. Traditional healers can be trained to perform a wide range of primary health care tasks. Appropriate knowledge and skills on the main elements of primary health care can be taught to traditional healers, from health education to providing basic medical care and essential drugs.

3. Traditional healers have produced several positive results. Projects that have attempted to evaluate the results of training have reported a number of positive outcomes. Most of the positive outcomes are changes in the attitude and practice of traditional healers, a high degree of acceptance by villagers, and an increase in coverage of basic health services. However, their success depends on strong support from basic health services.

Nevertheless, there are some obstacles and constraints of using traditional healers as community health workers.

1. Lack of policy directive: in many countries, traditional healers have been prohibited from practising. Dialogue with health personnel is usually missing and they sometimes become competitors. Without clear government policy, it may be difficult to overcome this problem.

2. Conflict with modern medical practices: harmful traditional practices are often a cause of conflict between traditional healers and modern medical practitioners. The contrast between the traditional holistic, spiritual healing orientation and the modern biomedical treatment-oriented approach is the second cause of conflict. Conflict of interest is also a component of the problem. However, these conflicts are not insurmountable if mutual respect and effective communication can be achieved. Clear role and communication systems, achievable through workshop meetings and group activities between health personnel and traditional healers, need to be formulated. This will reduce the opportunity for conflict and improve relationships. In Botswana, after a joint workshop with modern health workers, traditional healers agreed to promote the use of oral rehydration salt for the treatment of diarrhoea. They also agreed to refer patients with symptoms suggestive of tuberculosis or with bleeding during pregnancy.

3. Educational level of traditional healers: many traditional healers have a low level of literacy, which is a major obstacle to training. Special training methods, using pictorial learning materials and hands-on practical training are required, as demonstrated in community health worker programmes in Ghana and Swaziland. Conventional methods such as lectures and use of written materials were not appropriate.

Community preparation and involvement

It is very important that the community be adequately prepared before selection of community health workers. Health personnel at the peripheral health centres are usually assigned to perform this task. Preparation of the community should focus on creating an understanding regarding the functions and roles of community health workers, learning the expectations of the community, and formulating agreeable selection guidelines for community health workers. Formal selection guidelines should not override community choice and local circumstances. Community leaders and committees must participate actively in selecting community health workers.

Community preparation can be achieved through informal discussions with village leaders, discussions in village committees, and other more formal communication channels. Although this is a very important step, the local health personnel are usually not well trained enough to prepare the community adequately. Many of them use the traditional top-down approach, which usually results in selecting the wrong community health workers and leads to a high drop-out rate. Thus training local health personnel in community skills is one of the most important training modules.

Training and supervision of community health workers

Training

Community health workers usually received short-term training varying from a few days to a few weeks. Those that provide a wider range of services may receive a longer period of training. Training usually focuses on basic health issues covering elements of primary health care, such as basic medical care and essential drugs, nutrition, family planning, sanitation, immunization, maternal and child health, and control of local communicable diseases. Training material, particularly self-learning materials, are very helpful. The WHO (1977, 1987) has developed model learning and working materials that countries can adopt for the training and supervision of community health workers. Table 9 lists the self-learning modules for community health workers in Thailand. It is clear that apart from health issues, some health-related agricultural issues are also covered (modules 24–30). These self-learning modules are published and distributed to all community health workers.

Some community health workers with specific responsibilities may receive practical training on specific issues. For example, traditional birth attendants may be trained in maternal and child health and aseptic delivery, and village sanitary craftsmen in the building of latrines and water jars.

After initial training, continuous follow-up training is essential. In Thailand, after an initial training programme of 15 days, village health volunteers receive monthly/bimonthly visits, meeting, and training. Two- to three-day refresher courses are organized for all community health workers every year. Special monthly newsletters and journals for their continuing education plus other educational materials are regularly provided. Since 1979, the Folk Doctor Foundation, a non-governmental organization, has published the *Folk Doctor Magazine* monthly in support of community health workers as well as for the public. In some countries (e.g. Botswana, Jamaica, China, and Papua New Guinea), community health workers assist regularly in the health centres and receive continuous training.

Training, retraining, and activities to support continuous education are usually the main sources of expense in community health worker programmes.

Supervision and logistical support

Continuous supervision through regular visits, meeting, and training are important to maintain community health worker morale and skills. This requires strong basic health infrastructures at the district level. Thus basic health services need to be developed alongside primary health care and community health worker programme. Well-motivated and well-trained health personnel are the best supervisors and managers of community health worker programmes.

A regular schedule of supervision and meetings should be created which focuses on general as well as specific issues. Some forms of regular supervision are established in most community health worker programmes. The 'barefoot doctors' in China work in the local health centre every week and receive supervisory visits by health-centre staff.

Those community health workers who provide services which require logistical support, need to have their supplies replenished regularly (e.g. supplies of the contraceptive pill, condoms, and essential drugs). Good management systems to supply these materials regularly from the local health centres and hospitals have to be carefully established. District community hospitals or polyclinics may be the best depot for logistical support to health centres and community health workers.

Tools for assessing local needs

Simple tools are required for community health workers to assess local needs. These will allow them to play a more significant role and to achieve easy acceptance by villagers. It also allows them to understand the situation in their villages better. Additionally, these tools provide better opportunities for active community participation by each member of the community. These should be easy to understand and use, and should take into account the local level of education and skills. A number of such tools have been developed and applied, including the self-survey form in Indonesia, the basic minimum needs survey in Thailand, and the community-based information system for monitoring services and identifying at-risk groups for follow-up action in Bangladesh. Such tools provide methodologies for communities to assess their own problems, determine priorities, plan actions, and monitor and evaluate progress. However, substantial efforts are required to improve and simplify them so that they can be used by communities with minimal education.

To address the community situation holistically, these tools should be integrated rather than piecemeal. Table 10 shows the basic minimum needs indicators used for monitoring progress of quality of life development in villages in Thailand. It was developed in 1986 and has had several modifications. In the 1998 version, at least 20 out of the 39 indicators are directly health related; the rest are related to the overall well being of the villagers (Ministry of Interior 1999).

Incentives for community health workers

Community health workers are not government employees—they are volunteers. Adequate incentives in various forms increase their commitment and productivity. An evaluation of the community health worker programme in Thailand in 1988 found that the most important problem inhibiting community health workers' work is the inadequate financial reward. Community leaders and committees should play an active role in making decisions on the incentives for community health workers.

Social incentives

Social recognition and appreciation by health personnel are valuable incentives at little cost. The provision of certificates, badges, and uniforms enhances self-esteem and social status. Preferential reception for patients referred to the health service facilities by community health workers provides strong social recognition. In some countries (e.g. Thailand), the 'best performing' community health workers are given awards during the National Village Health Volunteer Day, and opportunities to travel within the country.

Financial incentives

Schemes based on financial incentives (e.g. the Jamaican community health worker programme) often collapse when the incentives are discontinued. Where financial incentives are necessary, the community should be consulted and decide on the suitable recompense. For sustainability and acceptance, financial incentives should come more from the community than from the government.

The WHO Study Group (WHO 1989) warned against a 'fee-for-service' arrangement, because of its tendency to concentrate on curative services, for which community health workers can charge

Table 9 Self-learning modules for village health communicators and volunteers, Thailand

VHCs		**Additional modules for VHVs**	
Code	**Module name**	**Code**	**Module name**
A	Public Health Problems to be Solved by the Community	33B	Oral Pills and Condoms
A1	Identification of Problems in the Village	34A	Maternal and Child Health
A2	Group Activities/Community Participation	34B	Postpartum Care
1	Utilization of Public Health Facilities	34C	Infant Care
2	Utilization of Household Drugs	36	Assisting Persons with Fever
3	Utilization of Traditional Herbal Medicines	37	Assisting Children with Fever and Rash and Red Spots
4	Dressing of Fresh Wounds	38	Assisting Persons with Cough
5	Assisting Persons with Fractures and Sprains	39	Assisting Persons with Headache
6	Assisting Fainting persons	40	Assisting Persons with Back Ache, Waist Ache and Ache all over the Body
7	Assisting Persons with Burns and Scars	41	Assisting Persons with Constipation
8	Assisting Persons with Convulsion	42	Assisting Persons with Stomach Ache
9	Assisting Drowning Persons	43	Assisting Persons with Diarrhoea
10	Assisting Persons Bitten by Snakes	44	Assisting Persons with Intestinal Worms
11	Assisting Persons Bitten by Dogs	45	Assisting Persons with Boils
12	Assisting Persons Taking Poisons	46	Assisting Persons with Skin Diseases
13	Provide Immunization Services	47	Assisting Persons with Dental Caries
14	Prevention of Tuberculosis	48	Assisting Persons with Conjunctivitis
15	Assisting Persons Suffering from Leprosy	49	Assisting Persons with Ear Ache
16	Potable Water and Water for Household Use	50	Assisting Persons with Beriberi
17	Construction of Sanitary Privies (latrines)	51	Assisting Persons with Anaemia
18	Garbage Disposal	52	Assisting Persons with Malaria
19	Sewage Disposal		
20	Mosquito, Fly and Cockroach Control		
21	House Mice and Rats Control		
22	Food Poisoning and Contaminated Foods		
23	Household Improvement		
24	Vegetable Preservation		
25	Fruit Preservation		
26	Kitchen Gardening		
27	Chicken Raising		
28	Duck Raising		
29	Fish Raising (Fishponds)		
30	Pig Raising		
31	Personal Hygiene		
32	Daily Diets		
33A	Family Planning Knowledge		
35A	Assisting Malnourished Children		
35B	Infant Food		
35 C	Infant Food Supplement		
35D	Food for Preschool Children		
1 (New)	Primary Health Care		
2 (New)	Village Health Planning		
3 (New)	Village Drug Fund		
4 (New)	Foods for Health Promotion and Energy		
5 (New)	Nutritional Surveillance		
6 (New)	Assisting Drug Addicts		

VHCs, village health communicators; VHVs, village health volunteers.

Source: Ministry of Public Health (1988).

Table 10 The basic minimum needs and indicators, Thailand, 1998

Indicators	Target for 2001 (%)	Result (1998)
Group 1: Healthiness		
(1) Pregnant women receive adequate antenatal care	80	97.8
(2) Appropriate delivery and postpartum service	95	98.6
(3) Birth weigh not less than 2500 g	93	97.5
(4) Breast-feeding for at least the first 4 months	30	81.3
(5) Comprehensive basic immunization for infants	95	99.3
(6) Good nutritional status of children under 5 years	80	96.1
(7) Good nutritional status of children 6–15 years	90	97.2
(8) Comprehensive immunization for children 6–12 years	100	98.9[a]
(9) Household with no consumption of raw meat/fish	90	88.1[a]
(10) Household with consumption of iodinated salt	60	93.7
(11) Household with consumption of FDA-approved food	85	96.7
(12) Household with rational use of drugs	60	92.4
Group 2: Appropriate shelter and environment		
(13) Houses are made of material of more than 5 years durability	95	97.4
(14) Household with sanitary latrine	95	98.0
(15) Household with adequate safe drinking water (5 litres/member/day)	95	90.0[a]
(16) Clean and orderly household	60	87.3
(17) Household without pollution	95	93.2[a]
Group 3: Educational coverage		
(18) Good child rearing (2–5 years of age)	90	93.5
(19) Coverage of compulsory education (6 years)	100	98.9[a]
(20) Percentage of children continuing to junior high school	98	91.0[a]
(21) Vocational training for those who do not continue their education	80	63.7[a]
(22) Literacy rate (14–50 years old)	99	97.7[a]
(23) Receive useful information at least three times per week	95	98.5
(24) Household with adequate knowledge on HIV/AIDS	80	98.2
Group 4: Happy family		
(25) Contraception prevalence	77	91.0
(26) Warm family	90	95.6
(27) Household with accident prevention	100	98.1[a]
(28) Household has security of life and possessions	100	99.4[a]
Group 5: Income		
(29) Family member income not less than 20 000 Baht/member/year	70	49.8[a]
Group 6: Participation in community development		
(30) Household becomes member of development group	90	87.9[a]
(31) Members of household use their right to vote in democratic activities	90	79.4[a]
(32) Household involved in maintaining public property	95	95.8
Group 7: Spiritual values		
(33) Practise religious activities at least once a week	90	94.8
(34) No addiction to alcohol	90	98.2
(35) No smoking of cigarettes	90	87.0[a]
(36) Participation in cultural events	90	98.5
(37) Elderly and disabled are well cared for	90	97.6
Group 8: Conservation of environment		
(38) Participation in activities to conserve natural resources	90	95.9
(39) Participation in activities to protect and control environment	90	96.0

[a]Indicators that have not yet achieved targets.

Adapted from Ministry of Interior (1998).

fees. However, fee-for-services for preventive and health promotion tasks may be allowed, for example, for the distribution of contraceptive pills and condoms.

Other additional incentives, such as free medical care for community health workers and their family members, and nominal profit from sales of essential drugs, may be given. Nevertheless, direct financial remuneration is usually counterproductive and is not recommended unless the time required to carry out the functions assigned requires a significant portion of the day.

Continuing education

Some community health workers with an adequate level of education may be good candidates to be recruited into health personnel training colleges. These students usually have a better attitude towards the community as well as better community skills. Nevertheless, this incentive may also have some detrimental effects and have to be carried out with great care and highly selectively. China's barefoot doctors provide a good example.

The barefoot doctors contributed greatly to the success of preventive health which had a proven effect on mortality and morbidity in China. In the late 1970s and 1980s, as a result of changes in economic policy and in the demand for medical care, they were offered the opportunity to become village doctors through training and qualifying examinations. They then provided more sophisticated services and, in many provinces, moved to a fee-for-service financing system. Thus a national community health worker programme evolved to become a private practice model free from any governmental guidance. The effect was a decline in preventive and promotion services (Rohde 1983; Zhu 1989; De Geyndt *et al.* 1992).

Resources support

Community health worker programes require quite high initial investment plus additional reinvestment in training, management, logistics, and supervision. Although the need for resources is quite high, it is nevertheless usually a small fraction of the total national health budget.

In Thailand, the budget for community health worker programmes increased from US$14 million to US$51 million and US$201 million for the fifth (1982–1986), sixth (1987–1991), and seventh (1992–1996) 5-year health development plans respectively, eqivalent to 0.79 per cent, 1.73 per cent, and 2.25 per cent of the total government health budget during the respective periods. During the economic crisis (1997 to 1999), there was a 17.3 per cent reduction in health budget. The budget for community health worker programmes, although protected, was reduced by 15 per cent in real terms (Ministry of Public Health 1999). This inevitably had a negative impact on community health worker programmes.

Clearly calculated and planned resource support is basic to the success of all community health worker programmes. Shifting of health resources requires strong political leadership. Apart from public resources, additional resources can be recruited from the community. Community financing schemes can be established to support various elements of primary health care, or to support integrated community health development activities. These additional resources may be used to provide incentives to community health workers. For example, in Thailand the multipurpose village development fund pays the village sanitary craftsmen to build latrines and water jars. The dividend from these community financing schemes, if substantial enough, may also encourage active community participation. However, these community financing schemes require good management under transparent and participatory community management structures. In many cases where the community structures are weak, there may be corruption and disruption of the activities.

Evaluation of community health worker programmes

Evaluating any health programme is a complex and difficult exercise, starting with the problem of methodology. Although there is general agreement on the measurements in terms of reductions in morbidity and mortality, the methodology for evaluating social impact is more complex. Qualitative phenomena such as community participation, behaviour, and perception are difficult to measure. Some subjectivity, and therefore criticism, are inevitable. No matter how complex and difficult, a built-in system of monitoring and evaluation of community health worker programmes is needed from formulation through to implementation. The evaluation is intended not only to measure the progress and the success but also to yield necessary proposals for further development. Necessary relevant, valid, and reliable indicators need to be developed to measure the inputs, processes, and outcomes of the programme. The WHO has developed handbooks on health programme evaluation, and the development of indicators for monitoring progress towards Health for All by the Year 2000 (WHO 1981*a*,*b*). Apart from the built-in system, some periodic external evaluations are needed to guide further development of the community health worker programme.

Information from the built-in monitoring and evaluation system of the Thai primary health care programme in 1986 revealed several constraints in the community health worker programme, such as high drop-out rates, low-levels of activity, and low morale. This led to a systematic external evaluation in 1988. This evaluation resulted in the abolishment of the village health communicators, an increase in social and financial incentives, and more involvement of village leaders and village committees, as well as the further strengthening of health service system support (Hongwiwatana 1988).

Community management structures

Community health workers should not be left alone in the community. Links to community infrastructure will not only result in higher levels of acceptability but also allow community health workers to access community resources conducive to health development. Community health workers should be included as members in the community development committee.

Some separate village health development committees have been set up. Top-down establishment of village health committees may be unsuccessful or even counterproductive. In the Saradidi project in Kenya, it was found that reorganizing the community or setting up a new leadership system of the village health committee was not appropriate. Village health committees proved to be a failure. It was best to strengthen and work within the existing leadership and community organization structures, such as clans, women's groups, and other community groups. It may be better to have task forces to undertake a specific activity for a very specific period of time. The task forces can report directly to the general meetings convened and chaired by a traditionally recognized and respected leader in the village.

Certain community financing schemes may provide a good basis for the activities of the community health workers in the community development committee. It can also increase their community management skills. The resources generated can be used for further development of community health workers and the community.

For example, including the Village Drug Revolving Fund as part of the Integrated Village Development Fund provides visible activity of community health workers and involvement of the community on the provision of essential drugs. Figure 6 shows the three important components for community health development—community health workers, committees, and community financing schemes (Wibulpolprasert 1991).

Community health workers during rapid socio-economic change

Rapid socio-economic change results in demographic and epidemiological transition, decentralization, health-care reform, and public sector reform. Economic development also causes changes in the demand for health care. More highly educated people require more professional services. These changes create incompatibility between the existing role and capacity of community health workers, the expectation of the community, and the real health problems.

Thus the role of community health workers in addressing new and emerging health challenges in a changing socio-economic and political environment is critical.

Demographic and epidemiological transition

There is a significant trend towards more elderly people and more chronic diseases, both communicable and non-communicable, in most countries. These chronic diseases (e.g. diabetes mellitus, hypertension, coronary heart diseases, cerebrovascular accidents, HIV/AIDS, malignancy, and mental health problems) require behavioural changes for prevention and long-term community care and support for treatment.

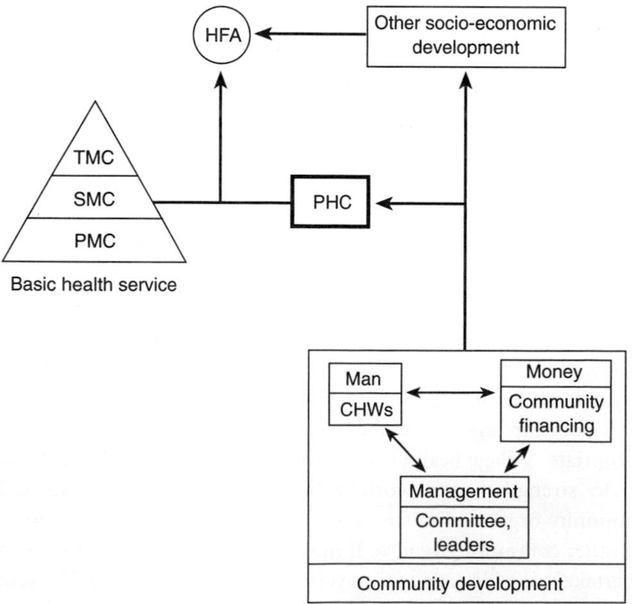

Fig. 6 Conceptual framework for community development in support of primary health care (PHC) and Health For All (HFA). CHWs, community health workers; PMC, primary medical care; SMC, secondary medical care; TMC, tertiary medical care.

Most community health workers were trained on the issues related to the eight main elements of primary health care. In many communities, these are now irrelevant to their actual health problems. In other communities, community health workers are facing the double burden of both types of disease at the same time.

The technologies and strategies used for the prevention and treatment of these chronic health problems require totally different knowledge and skills of community health workers. Thus retraining and retooling for community health workers is unavoidable. The retraining should be targeted not only at community health workers but most importantly also at the rural health personnel and health professionals who supervise them.

New forms of community setting and services may be a focus of campaigns, including advocacy for healthier lifestyles, consumer protection, and delivery of basic care for the chronically ill. Community health workers may be trained to monitor blood pressure, fasting blood sugar or urine sugar levels. Tuberculosis patients on a schedule of directly observed treatments may be monitored and supervised by community health workers. The primary health care centres in Thai villages are equipped with the necessary medical instruments and the community health workers (village health volunteers) are trained to do the job.

Changing demand of the community

Better-educated and better-off rural villagers demand better quality professional health services. Community health workers and health personnel need to be retrained and rearmed with more knowledge and skills relevant to the demand. This may require community health workers with a higher level of basic education. Nevertheless, it should be noted that higher educated and better-trained community health workers may focus more on curative services as in the case of China's barefoot doctors.

In the more developed communities, the health volunteer concept needs to be further extended to workplaces, schools, institutions, youth organizations, and among the elderly in order to develop the capacity of these various groups to assume responsibility for their own health and the health of their communities. Examples are the community health worker projects in Japan and the United States (Ministry of Health and Welfare 1994; Kahssay *et al.* 1998).

Decentralization of health services

Various degrees of decentralization, from deconcentration, delegation, devolution to privatization (Kolehmainen-Aiken and Newbrander 1997) greatly affect the role of community health workers. Those community health workers who are active members of local community committees or local government can influence the reform of the decentralized health services to be more responsive to local demand and more supportive of primary health care.

In the midst of the privatization movement, the focus of community health worker programmes on preventive and health promotion primary health care services, should be considered as 'public goods/services'. This means that they should not be forced to operate in an open and competitive market. Despite the possible changing role of the government from service provider to regulator, community health worker programmes should continue to be subsidized by the government and the community. The community health workers' spirit of volunteer work should be maintained.

New financing schemes

Governments, particularly those of the least developed countries pushed by the development banks, are placing too much hope on new resource schemes such as privatization, community financing, increasing or introducing user fees, and health insurance. If these changes are not carefully carried out, they may shift resources from preventive and health promotion activities towards high-technology curative services.

Community health workers may need to be trained to participate in the management of these new resource schemes, or even become the manager themselves. Retraining of community health workers and local health personnel in managing these new financing schemes are needed to maintain their efficiency and transparency.

Community health workers: not the end of Health for All–primary health care

Although community health workers may improve health under the Health for All–primary health care policy, they are the tools or means to arrive at Health for All. They are the 'change agents' for better health by promoting the capacity for self-care and community care.

The final goals or targets are the empowerment of the people to be able to take good care of their health and to be able to use and support health service systems efficiently and equitably. Thus we need to go beyond community health worker programmes to reach directly the families and the people. In Thailand, family health leaders have been recruited and trained since 1996. In 1998, there were 1 177 464 family health leaders.

Innovative strategies using mass media, public advocacy and campaigns, economic incentives, and legislation to empower individual self-care capacity are the new and challenging paradigm of primary health care.

References

Bose, A. (1983). The community health worker scheme: an Indian experiment. In *Practising Health for All* (ed. D. Morley, J. Rohde, and G. Williams), pp. 38–48. Oxford University Press.

Braveman, P.A. and Mora, F. (1987). Training physicians for community-oriented primary care in Latin America: model programmmes in Mexico, Nicaragua and Costa Rica. *American Journal of Public Health*, **4**, 485–90.

De Geyndt, W., Zhoa, X., and Liu, S. (1992). *From barefoot doctor to village doctor in rural China.* World Bank Technical Paper 187, World Bank, Washington, DC.

Drucker, P.F. (1977). *Management.* Harper's College Press, New York.

Hongwiwatana, T., Sri-ngernyuang, L., and Chuengsatiensap, K. (1988). *Alternatives to primary health care volunteers in Thailand.* Sangdad Publishing, Bangkok.

Jonas, S. (1998). *An introduction to the US health care system.* Springer, New York.

Joseph, A. (1985). Training doctors for primary health care: the Vellore model. *World Health Forum*, **6**, 118–21.

Kahssay, M.H., Taylor, M., and Berman, P. (1998). *Community health workers: the way forward.* WHO, Geneva.

Kaseje, D.C.O. (1990). Community-based health care: the Saradidi, Kenya experience. In *Why things work.* (ed. S. Halstead and J. Walsh), pp. 69–82. Adams, Boston, MA.

Kolehmainen-Aitken, R.-L. and Newbrander, W. (1997) *Decentralizing the management of health and family planning programs.* Management Sciences for Health, Boston, MA.

McMahon, R., Barton, E., and Piot, M. (1980). *On being in charge. A guide for middle-level management in primary health care.* WHO, Geneva.

Ministry of Health and Welfare (1994). *Annual report on health and welfare 1992–1993.* Japan International Corporation of Welfare Services, Tokyo.

Ministry of Interior (1999). *The 1998 quality of life of the Thai.* Perm Serm Kij Press, Bangkok.

Ministry of Public Health (1988). *The realization of primary health care in Thailand.* Amarin Printing Group, Bangkok.

Ministry of Public Health (1999). *Health in Thailand 1997–1998.* Veteran Press, Bangkok.

Nittayarumphong, S. (1990). Primary health care: the Thailand experience. In *Why things work* (ed. S. Halstead and J. Walsh), pp. 95–104. Adams, Boston, MA.

Office of the Primary Health Care, Ministry of Public Health (1985). *Primary health care in Thailand.* Veterans Press, Bangkok.

Roemer, M.I. (1991). *National health system of the world.* Vol. 1: *The countries.* Oxford University Press.

Rohde, J. (1983). Health for All in China: principles and relevance for other countries. In *Practising Health for All.* (ed. D. Morley, J. Rohde, and G. Williams), pp. 5–16. Oxford University Press.

Starr, P. (1984). *The social transformation of American medicine.* Basic Books, New York.

Vacharotai, S. (1978). *Lampang health development project: a Thai primary health care approach.* Amarin Press, Bangkok.

Walt, G. (1990). *Community health workers in national health programmes. Just another pair of hands?* Open University Press, Buckingham.

Werner, D. (1983). Health in Cuba: a model services or a means of social control-or both? In *Practising health for all* (ed. D. Morley, J. Rohde, and G. Williams), pp. 17–37. Oxford University Press.

Wibulpolprasert, S. (1991). Community financing: Thailand's experiences. *Health Policy and Planning*, **4**, 354–60.

Wibulpolprasert, S. (1999). Inequitable distribution of doctors: can it be solved? *Human Resources for Health Development Journal*, **1**, 1–22.

World Bank (1993). *World development report 1993. Investing in health.* Oxford University Press.

World Bank (1994). *Better health in Africa. Experiences and lessons learned.* World Bank, Washington, DC.

WHO (World Health Organization) (1977). *The primary health workers.* WHO, Geneva.

WHO (World Health Organization) (1978). *Primary health care.* WHO, Geneva.

WHO (World Health Organization) (1981*a*). *Development of indicators for monitoring progress towards health for all by the year 2000.* WHO, Geneva.

WHO (World Health Organization) (1981*b*). *Health program evaluation.* WHO, Geneva.

WHO (World Health Organization) (1984). *Evaluating primary health care in South-East Asia.* WHO/SEARO Technical Publication 4, WHO, South-East Asia Regional Office, New Delhi.

WHO (World Health Organization) (1987). *The community health worker.* WHO, Geneva.

WHO (World Health Organization) (1989). *Strengthening the performance of community health workers in primary health care. Report of a WHO study group.* WHO Technical Report Series 780, WHO, Geneva.

WHO (World Health Organization) (1991). *Traditional healers as community health workers*. Unpublished document WHO/SHS/DHS/91.6; available on request from Division of Analysis, Research, and Assessment, WHO, Geneva..

WHO (World Health Organization) (1996). *Role of health volunteers in strengthening action for health*. Unpublished document SEA/HSD/198; available on request from WHO Regional Office for South-East Asia, World Health House, Indraprastha Estate, Mahatma Gandhi Road, New Delhi 110002, India.

WHO (World Health Organization) (1998). *Executive Board Resolution EB101.R2 on the amendments to the constitution*. WHO, Geneva.

WHO (World Health Organization) (1999*a*). *Basic documents*. WHO, Geneva.

WHO (World Health Organization) (1999*b*). *Health Situation in the South-East Asia region*. WHO, South-East Asia Regional Office, New Delhi.

WHO (World Health Organization) (1999*c*). *The world health report 1999. Making a difference*. WHO, Geneva.

Zhu, N. (1989). Factors associated with the decline of the Cooperative Medial System and barefoot doctors in rural China. *Bulletin of the World Health Organization*, **4**, 431–41.

12.12 An international public health policy agenda for the twenty-first century*

Gro Harlem Brundtland

The world enters the twenty-first century with many advantages. Remarkable gains in health, rapid economic growth, and unprecedented scientific advance—all legacies of the twentieth century—stand as testament to enormous progress in human development. But darker legacies stand as stark reminders that the challenges ahead are just as great. Regional conflicts have replaced the global wars of the first half of the twentieth century as a source of continued misery. Half of the world's population lives on less than US$2 per day. The sustainability of a healthy environment is precarious. The Universal Declaration of Human Rights—now half a century old—is only a tantalizing promise for far too many people. The HIV/AIDS epidemic continues unchecked in much of the world, and it warns us against complacency about other, still unknown, microbial threats.

Human health—and its influence on every aspect of life—is central to the larger picture of human development. Improvements in health have made critical contributions to human and economic development in the past. Further progress in improving health would expand these benefits, especially to the world's poor. It would increase healthy life expectancy for all and reduce the burden of premature death and excessive disability for many of the world's poor. Wise investments in health may help to reduce poverty itself by increasing the productivity of the poor, ensuring the poor's access to health care, and preventing economic ruin as a result of high health expenditures.

This chapter explains the rationale and highlights the priorities for an international public health policy agenda in the twenty-first century. To do so, it first reviews the twentieth-century health revolution along with its demographic and economic consequences, and seeks explanations for their occurrence. We then turn to the epidemiological consequences of the health revolution that result from increasing longevity and ageing populations, while describing how the incompleteness of the health revolution has left perhaps a billion people suffering from completely preventable causes of illness and death. Addressing this 'double burden' is perhaps the central issue for health policy for the twenty-first century. The last section draws on the experiences of diverse countries in designing effective, efficient, and equitable health policies, in order to identify the fundamental principles and means by which health systems can meet the challenges of the twenty-first century.

* This chapter is drawn from material previously published in the WHO *World Health Report 1999*. It has been edited and updated for inclusion in this volume.

Health and development in the twentieth century

The twentieth century has seen a global transformation in human health unmatched in history. This section briefly describes this revolution and examines both its profound consequences for human demography and its contribution to the worldwide diffusion of rapid economic growth. It then explains why this revolution occurred.

Precipitous decline in mortality

The steady improvement in life expectancy that began in Europe in the late 1900s continued virtually without interruption throughout the twentieth century. Economic historians and demographers debate the genesis of these increases in life expectancy, but the increases appear at least partially linked to the economic changes resulting from the agricultural and industrial revolutions. One aspect of economic change—urbanization—actually affected health adversely by exposing an increasing proportion of the population to crowded conditions, thereby facilitating the spread of infection. Somewhat more than counterbalancing this effect, though, were increases in nutrient intake and improvements in sanitation resulting from higher income levels (McKeown 1976). Better health and nutritional status were both a result and a cause of income growth.

Although northern Europeans had began immunizing against smallpox by early in the nineteenth century, this was exceptional, and other specific knowledge and tools for improving health probably played only a limited role in the minor health improvements of the nineteenth century (Easterlin 1998). Mortality rates in European countries continued their decline in the twentieth century, and by the second half of the century, this mortality revolution had spread to the rest of the world.

The magnitude of this transformation can be illustrated by looking at the example of Chile. By the mid-1990s Chile had a per capita income of about US$4000 (adjusted for purchasing power currency), i.e. it had a high average standard of living, with an income level sufficient to provide its people with more than adequate food, shelter, and sanitation. Chilean women today have a life expectancy of 79 years—perhaps 25 years more than women in a country with a similar income level in 1900 and 46 years more than Chilean women had in the early 1900s. While Chile's progress in the twentieth century has been exceptional, most low- and middle-income countries have undergone (or are in the process of undergoing) a similar transformation of health and mortality levels. Recent exceptions to these favourable trends occur in AIDS-ravaged parts of Africa and, for a variety of reasons, among adult males in Central and Eastern Europe.

Mortality decline and the demographic transition

Although mortality declines have typically led to increases in population growth rates, these increases prove temporary. Fertility decline accompanies or soon follows mortality decline, bringing growth rates back to low levels of fertility. At mid-century, fertility rates were extremely high in most countries of the world (with the exception of the high-income countries). Total fertility rates—the expected number of children a woman would bear at the prevailing age-specific fertility rates—of 6 were not uncommon (a total fertility rate of 2 represents the population replacement level). Between 1950 and 1998, every region except Africa has experienced sharp declines in fertility. However, evidence is mounting that the decline in Africa has now commenced.

The world today is perhaps somewhat past the halfway point of a two-century period during which the demographic characteristics of the human population will have been totally transformed. This transformation (or demographic transition) entails a move from very high birth and death rates to low ones; a move from initially low population growth rates through a period of high rates and a vast increase in total population then back to low or zero growth rates; and a move from an age distribution with numerous young and few elderly to one with nearly equal numbers in most age groups. Enormous social, economic, and epidemiological changes follow the demographic transition, which is itself a consequence of the ongoing revolution in mortality.

Sources of mortality decline

Income improvements can lead to mortality reductions, and numerous studies have attempted to quantify this effect. The World Health Organization (**WHO**) analyses, for example, assessed the effects of national income on country-level health outcomes during the period 1952 to 1992. Figure 1 shows results from this analysis in curves relating the infant mortality rate to gross domestic product (**GDP**) per capita adjusted for purchasing power. Income increases do indeed correlate with mortality declines and there are good reasons to believe that the relation is causal in both directions.

How much of the remarkable decline in infant mortality rates has resulted from income growth during that period? The upper curve on Fig. 1 shows the income–mortality relation in 1952 and the lower one, for 1992, shows how much lower mortality rates had become by then for any given level of income. Figure 1 suggests that, however important income growth may be, the changing relation between mortality and other factors (e.g. access to health technology) is likely to be more important. Between 1952 and 1992, for example, per capita income increased by about two-thirds, on average, across the countries included in the analysis—from about US$1530 to US$2560. The upper curve in Fig. 1 shows that had the income–mortality relation remained as it was in 1952, the infant mortality rate would have declined from 144 to 116. In fact it declined further to only 55.

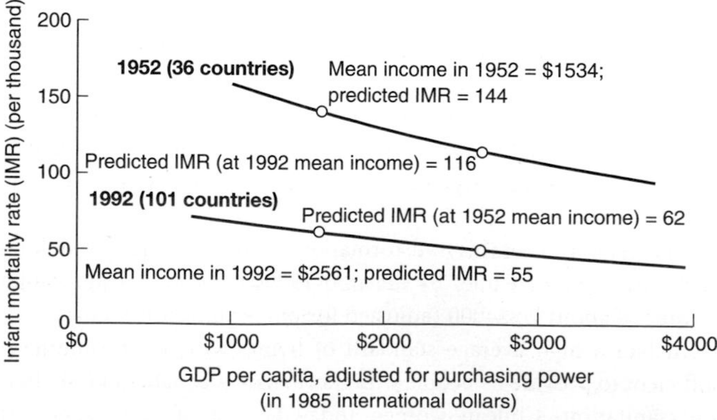

Fig. 1 The role of improvements in income in reducing infant mortality rates. Note: results are based on a cross-sectional time-series regression that relates, at 5-year intervals, the natural logarithm of infant mortality rate to the natural logarithm of income, the square of the natural logarithm of income, and indicator variables for time. Data sources are listed in Annex Table 6 of the *World Health Report 1999* (WHO 1999).

Table 1 reports the results of an attempt to quantify the relative importance of key determinants of mortality reduction. It draws on a statistical assessment of how the relation has changed over time between various health indicators and both income levels and average educational levels (of adult females). The table reflects a decomposition of the causes of improvement in health into three components: increases in average income levels, improvements in average educational levels among adult females, and a favourable shift in the underlying curve. This favourable shift is ascribed to the generation and application of new knowledge.

Other indicators of social welfare show a similarly modest relation to income growth along with favourable time trends at any given level of income (Easterly 1998). Much research remains to be done, however, in order to achieve a complete understanding of why the income–health relation has improved so much. Typically, half the gains in health between 1952 and 1992 result from access to better technology. The remaining gains result from movement along the curve (partially income improvements and, more importantly, better education). Figure 1 (which does not control for education changes) illustrates the magnitude of the effect of moving along the curve relative to shifts in the curve (Preston 1975, 1980). Higher levels of income and education affect health through a variety of mechanisms, often involving many sectors of the economy.

What conclusions can be drawn from this analysis? Firstly, it is clear that health system development is a key priority. The effects of economic growth on health, while real, are relatively weak and likely to be slow in coming. Rather than waiting for movement along the curve, countries should focus health system development on the task of joining the curve or going beyond it to the point of best practice.

Secondly, in the medium to long term, shifting the curve will underpin health improvements. The high-income countries now commit vast sums (over US$55 billion per year) to the research and development efforts that will shift the curve favourably. But only a fraction of that amount is directed to solving the particular problems of poor and disadvantaged people. Greater research and development commitments to such problems would be likely to pay off enormously in improving health. Ensuring an adequate commitment to research and development is an integral element of health system development, as discussed at the conclusion of this chapter.

There is every reason to expect, then, that focused investments by health systems on specific problems of the poor can generate major

Table 1 Sources of mortality reduction, 1960 to 1990[a]

Reduction	Percentage contribution of gains in		
	Income	Educational level of adult females	Generation and utilization of new knowledge
Under-5 mortality rate	17	38	45
Female adult mortality rate	20	41	39
Male adult mortality rate	25	27	49
Female life expectancy at birth	19	32	49
Male life expectancy at birth	20	30	50
Total fertility rate	12	58	29

[a]The results are based on analysis of data from 115 low- and middle-income countries.

Source: Wang *et al.* (1999).

short- to medium-term gains in health, and that investment in research and development can sustain medium- to long-term gains. Such gains are of immense intrinsic value. The association between income and health moreover suggests that health investments may have an economic pay-off as well. Supporting evidence for this assertion is presented below. Indeed, rather than continuing to indicate poverty as the root cause of ill health, decision-makers may come to focus on the two-way relationship between poverty and ill health, identifying the latter as one of the root causes of poverty—and one that is particularly amenable to public intervention.

Health and economic productivity

The global gains in health documented above arguably constitute humankind's most dramatic achievement. In our era it is possible for every individual to expect to live a long and substantially disease-free life. This accomplishment transcends the need for economic valuation. Health gains have intrinsic value. However, two particular reasons exist for assessing the economic consequences of better health.

1. Understanding health's economic role may help to understand the sources of one of humankind's other great accomplishments of the twentieth century—widespread rapid economic growth. To the extent that better health has contributed to increased growth rates, investing in health can become a tool of macroeconomic policy.

2. Conquering poverty constitutes the central task for development policy at the beginning of the twenty-first century. Despite rapid economic growth, over a billion humans still exist in absolute degrading poverty. Because ill health traps people in poverty, sustained investment in the health of the poor could provide a policy lever for alleviating persistent poverty.

Research has begun to provide clearer evidence of the economic benefits of improving health. But datasets underpinning the research—on characteristics of countries over time or on large numbers of households within a country at a given time—rarely permit conclusive determination of cause and effect. Therefore conclusions drawn from the literature remain suggestive rather than definitive. However, those conclusions do accord with common sense: healthier people are more productive. Health differences have played a significant role in determining why some countries have grown more rapidly than others, although technological advances and physical capital accumulation may have been even more important.

What is the evidence? This section summarizes the literature by firstly reviewing cross-country macroeconomic analyses, and then by turning to microeconomic comparisons across households. It closes with a brief discussion of the multiple pathways through which better health influences economic outcomes.

Macroeconomic evidence

Since the publication of Adam Smith's *The Wealth of Nations* over two centuries ago, economists have sought answers to the question of why some countries are wealthy and others poor. The main empirical tool now used to study economic growth is cross-country analysis of the relationship between economic growth (typically measured in terms of the growth rate of per capita GDP) and a range of variables believed to account for why growth rates differ (Barro 1997; Sachs and Werner 1997). Recent research has added several specific health indicators to these factors, and looked at the links between them and economic growth. There are direct links between economic performance and health indicators such as life expectancy. Some variables, such as geography and demography, indirectly link health with economic growth. Geography, particularly tropical location, is highly correlated with disease burden, which in turn affects economic performance (Gallup *et al.* 1998). Conversely, demography is determined in part by health status, and has a direct effect on economic growth through the age structure of the population, in particular the ratio of the working age to the total population.

Recent research shows that survival rates or life expectancy are powerful predictors of income levels or of subsequent economic growth. It finds a strong effect of health on economic levels or growth rates (Jamison *et al.* 1998). Health improvements also influence economic growth through their impact on demography. For example, in the 1940s, rapid improvements in health in East Asia provided a catalyst for demographic transition. An initial decline in infant and child mortality swelled the youth population, and somewhat later prompted a fall in fertility rates and a rise in the working-age population. This bulge in the age structure of the population created an opportunity for increased rates of economic growth. By introducing these demographic considerations into an empirical model of economic growth, analyses undertaken for the Asian Development Bank (**ADB**) were able to show that East Asia's changing demography can explain perhaps a third to half of the economic 'miracle' experienced between 1965 and 1990 (ADB 1997; Bloom and Williamson 1998).

The ADB study cautions that although a 'demographic gift' provides an opportunity for increasing prosperity, it by no means guarantees such results. East Asia's growth rates were achieved because government and the private sector were able to mobilize this burgeoning workforce by successfully managing other economic opportunities. The next phase for East Asia will involve less favourable dependency ratios consequent to population ageing. In contrast, both South Asia and Africa are now entering the period when demographic factors can enhance growth prospects.

Microeconomic analysis

Unlike macroeconomic studies, which compare the performance of countries over time, microeconomic analyses study the link between health and the income of households and individuals. Recent individual and household level studies have paid more attention to the impact of health (particularly nutritional aspects of health) on labour productivity (Strauss and Thomas 1998).

One example provides an indication of the results of this research. In Indonesia, men with anaemia were found to be 20 per cent less productive than men without it. In one of the few experimental studies in the literature, the anaemic men were randomly assigned to one of two groups in a clinical trial—they received either an iron supplement or a placebo. Those who were initially anaemic and received the iron treatment increased their productivity nearly to the levels of non-anaemic workers, and the productivity gains were large when weighed against the costs of treatment. Thus the effects of improved health were found to be greatest for the most vulnerable, i.e. the poorest and those with the least education.

At the household level, it is also possible to measure directly the economic burden created by particular diseases. For example, there are several ways in which tuberculosis affects economic outcomes. Tuberculosis-related morbidity directly increases household and public sector expenditures. It reduces labour inputs and can reduce human capital as a result of declines in school attendance. In a case study of costs of improving tuberculosis control in Thailand in 1995 (Easterly 1998), the cost of treatment was estimated to be US$343 per case. The researchers also estimated the total indirect cost of lost productivity in Thailand due to morbidity associated with treated and untreated cases of tuberculosis at US$57 million.

Pathways of influence

Delineating potential pathways of influence sheds light on health's role within the larger web of determinants of income levels and growth rates. There is evidence that adult health depends in part on child health and itself directly influences labour productivity. Per capita income is defined as the level of income generated by the productivity of the economically active population divided by total population. Clearly, the total population consists of economic dependants as well as the economically active. Improved adult health will improve the dependency ratio both by reducing mortality among the economically active and by reducing premature retirement that results from illness (Dwyer and Mitchell 1999). Better adult health directly affects productivity by increasing work output and reducing absenteeism. Less obviously, geographically specific diseases—onchocerciasis (river blindness) in West Africa is an example—deny communities access to valuable land or productive resources. And high levels of illness in a community may weaken links to the global economy (Radelet *et al.* 1997)—links that through the movement of ideas, goods, and capital help to create the conditions for more rapid growth.

Investments in both physical capital and education underpin labour productivity. A rapidly growing literature documents the effects of ill health on children's enrolment, learning, and attendance rates in school. Many of the conditions affecting school children (e.g. intestinal worm infections and micronutrient deficiencies) respond to inexpensive but effective interventions. Recent studies in the psychological literature point to steady, long-term gains during the twentieth century in the general intellectual ability of the populations of the high-income countries (where data were available to generate trends). One suggested determinant of this trend lies in improved health and nutritional status (Neisser 1998). The ADB's studies on Asia point strongly to the effect of better health on capital formation. Expectations of a longer life appear to stimulate savings.

This discussion fully recognizes the intrinsic value of health—and that today's health systems have the tools vastly to improve the welfare of the poor at modest cost. But simultaneously, the economic evidence underscores an important message—investing in health accelerates economic growth and is a viable approach to rolling back poverty.

The double burden: emerging epidemics and persistent problems

The twentieth century revolution in health—and the consequent demographic transition—led inexorably to major changes in the pattern of disease. This epidemiological transition has resulted in a major shift in causes of death and disability from infectious diseases to non-communicable diseases (Murray and Lopez 1996). As a result of the epidemiological transition, the distribution of causes of death at the end of the twentieth century differs markedly from the distribution of causes of death at the beginning of the century (Preston *et al.* 1972). Not only have the major causes of death changed, but also the average age of death has been steadily rising.

Despite the long list of successes in health achieved globally during the twentieth century, the balance sheet is indelibly stained by the avoidable burden of disease and malnutrition that the world's disadvantaged populations continue to bear. Some analysts have characterized a world of incomplete epidemiological transition, in which epidemiologically polarized subpopulations have been left behind (Frenk *et al.* 1989). Reducing the burden of that inequality is a priority in the international public health agenda.

Health policy-makers in the early decades of the twenty-first century will thus need to address a double burden of disease: firstly, the emerging epidemics of non-communicable diseases and injuries, which are becoming more prevalent in industrialized and developing countries alike; and secondly, some major infectious diseases which survived the twentieth century—part of the unfinished health agenda. This section describes this double burden of disease and describes cost-effective interventions that make it possible to complete substantially the unfinished agenda in the first decade of the twenty-first century.

Emerging epidemics of non-communicable diseases and injuries

The next two decades will see dramatic changes in the health needs of the world's populations. In the developing regions, non-communicable diseases such as depression and heart disease are fast replacing the traditional enemies, in particular infectious diseases and malnutrition, as the leading causes of disability and premature death. Injuries, both intentional and unintentional, are also growing in importance and by 2020 could rival infectious diseases worldwide as a source of ill health (Murray and Lopez 1996). The rapidity of change will pose serious challenges to health care systems and force difficult decisions about the allocation of scarce resources.

To provide a valid basis for such difficult health policy decisions, there is a great need for the development of reliable and consistent data on the health status of populations worldwide. As the WHO has argued (WHO 1996*b*, 1998), a new approach to measuring health status needs to be implemented—one that quantifies not merely the number of deaths but also the impact of premature death and disability on populations, and which combines them into a single unit of measurement. Several such measures have been developed in different countries, many of them being variants of the so-called quality-adjusted life year (**QALY**), which is principally used to measure gains from interventions. In contrast, the disability-adjusted life year (**DALY**) is a measure of the burden of disease.

DALYs express years of life lost to premature death and years lived with a disability, adjusted for the severity of the disability. One DALY is one lost year of healthy life. A 'premature' death is defined as one that occurs before the age to which the dying person could have expected to survive if he or she was a member of a standardized model population with a life expectancy at birth equal to that of the world's longest-surviving population, Japan. Disease burden is, in effect, the gap between a population's actual health status and some reference status.

Assessments of global disease burden using DALYs began in 1993 for the World Bank (1993) in collaboration with the WHO, with subsequent revisions for the year 1990 published more recently (Murray and Lopez 1996). The following data summarize new estimates of disease burden for the year 1998.

Non-communicable diseases

In 1998, an estimated 43 per cent of all DALYs globally were attributable to non-communicable diseases. In low- and middle-income countries the figure was 39 per cent, while in high-income countries it was 81 per cent. Among these diseases, the following took a particularly heavy toll:

- neuropsychiatric conditions, accounting for 10 per cent of the burden of disease measured in DALYs in low- and middle-income countries and 23 per cent of DALYs in high-income countries
- cardiovascular diseases, responsible for 10 per cent of DALYs in low- and middle-income countries and 18 per cent of DALYs in high-income countries
- malignant neoplasms (cancers), which caused 5 per cent of DALYs in low- and middle-income countries and 15 per cent in high-income countries.

One of the most surprising results of using a measure of disease burden which incorporates time lived with disability is the magnitude it ascribes to the burden of neuropsychiatric conditions. Because of the limited mortality consequences, this burden was previously underestimated. A large proportion of the burden of disease resulting from neuropsychiatric conditions is attributable to unipolar major depression, which was the leading cause of disability globally in 1990. The disease burden resulting from depression is estimated to be increasing both in developing and developed regions. Alcohol use is also quantified as a major cause of disease burden, particularly for adult men. It is the leading cause of disability for men in the developed regions and the fourth leading cause in developing regions.

These findings also highlight the 'hidden epidemic of cardiovascular disease'. Within cardiovascular diseases, which collectively are responsible for about one in eight DALYs lost globally, ischaemic heart disease and cerebrovascular disease (stroke) are the most significant conditions. It has been estimated that ischaemic heart disease will be the largest single cause of disease burden globally by the year 2020. Substantive evidence suggests that current programmes for cardiovascular disease risk factor prevention and low-cost case management offer feasible, cost-effective ways to reduce cardiovascular disease mortality and disability in populations both in developed and developing countries (Howson *et al.* 1998*a*). Implementation of such programmes should be a priority for health policy-makers as the burden of cardiovascular disease rises in all socio-economic groups and inflicts major human and economic costs on societies.

The third largest cause of disease burden within non-communicable conditions is cancer. Cancers are responsible for a large proportion of years of life lost and years lived with disability. Among cancers, the most significant cause of disease burden is lung cancer, which is projected to become ever more prevalent over the next few decades, if current smoking trends continue. Tobacco is a major risk factor for several other non-communicable diseases as well. Thus, tobacco control is one of the major public health priorities for the twenty-first century.

Non-communicable diseases are expected to account for an increasing share of disease burden, rising from 43 per cent in 1998 to 73 per cent by 2020, assuming a continuation of recent downward trends in overall mortality (which have yet to be realized in China and elsewhere) (WHO 1996*a*). The expected increase is likely to be particularly rapid in developing countries. In India, deaths from non-communicable causes are projected to almost double from about 4.5 million in 1998 to about 8 million a year in 2020.

The steep projected increase in the burden of non-communicable diseases worldwide—the epidemiological transition—is largely driven by population ageing, augmented by the rapidly increasing numbers of people who are at present exposed to tobacco and other risk factors, such as obesity, physical inactivity, and heavy alcohol consumption. This increase in non-communicable diseases induced by changes in age distribution poses significant problems. Health systems must adjust to deal effectively and efficiently with the globally changing nature of illness, and health policy-makers will be challenged to find the most cost-effective uses of their limited resources to control the rising epidemics of non-communicable diseases. In contrast with the limited number of conditions responsible for most of the excess disease burden among the poor, policy-makers will need to develop systems capable of responding to an enormous variety of conditions as the epidemiological transition matures.

Simultaneously, health policy-makers will need to respond to the unexpectedly persistent inequalities in health status within countries. This is a problem that affects disadvantaged populations in developed and developing countries alike. Traditionally, the focus of global health policy has been on the less developed nations. Recent studies have revealed surprisingly large inequalities within developed nations, and they highlight the need for policies that focus on disadvantaged populations throughout the world.

Injuries

Injuries, both intentional and unintentional, are a large and neglected health problem in all regions, accounting for 16 per cent of the global burden of disease in 1998. Road traffic accidents were the ninth leading cause of disease burden globally in 1998, and were fifth in the high-income countries and tenth in the low- and middle-income countries. For adult men aged 15 to 44 years, road traffic accidents are the greatest cause of ill health and premature death worldwide, and the second greatest in developing countries. The burden from road traffic accidents is projected to increase globally, and particularly in developing countries. In sub-Saharan Africa, partly because of the projected reduction of the burden from infectious diseases, injuries (primarily road traffic accidents, war, and violence) are expected to account for a large proportion of ill health.

Recent figures for homicides, suicides, and traffic accident deaths for countries in the Americas show that these rank as the main causes of death and disability. Every year, close to 120 000 people are killed, 55 000 commit suicide, and 126 000 die in traffic accidents in the Americas (PAHO 1998). At least 12 countries have homicide rates above 10 per 100 000 inhabitants.

Violence and self-inflicted injuries (including suicide) are a major public health concern because of their increasing significance within the global disease burden. Injuries primarily affect the younger age groups and often result in disabling conditions. In higher-income countries, road traffic accidents and self-inflicted injuries were among the 10 leading causes of disease burden in 1998 as measured in DALYs. In less developed countries, road traffic accidents were the most significant cause of injuries, ranking eleventh among the most important causes of lost years of healthy life. War, violence, and self-inflicted injuries were all among the leading 20 causes of such loss in those countries. Intentional injuries primarily affect young adults, with males in the age group of 15 to 34 years bearing a particularly large proportion of the burden.

Domestic violence, especially against women, is not always reflected in physical injury but may be apparent in psychological sequelae. Traditionally, violence has been classified as intentional injury. While it is clearly important to recognize violence as a cause of injury, particularly among women where the connection may not always be evident, the health consequences also need to be understood. So too does the different nature of the violence experienced by men, women, and children.

Globally, injuries are responsible for 1 in 6 years lived with disability. Nevertheless, injuries have often been a neglected area of public health policy. Therefore more attention needs to be focused on dealing with the growing problem of injuries—through more comprehensive prevention, improved emergency and treatment services, and better rehabilitation.

Persistent problems of infectious diseases and maternal and child disability and mortality

Despite the extraordinary advances of the twentieth century, a significant component of the burden of illness globally still remains attributable to infectious diseases, undernutrition, and complications of childbirth. These conditions are primarily concentrated in the poorest countries, and within those countries they disproportionately afflict populations that are living in poverty. The residual concentration of infectious diseases afflicting the poor is truly an avoidable burden, because inexpensive and effective tools exist to deal with much of it. In fact, it mostly results from relatively few conditions.

The disproportionate share of the burden of disease on the poor is demonstrated in Table 2, based on WHO analyses. Within countries, the disadvantaged fare much worse as measured by several health indicators than the better off. Those living in absolute poverty, compared with those who are not poor, are estimated to have a five times higher probability of death between birth and the age of 5 years, and a 2.5 times higher probability of death between the ages of 15 and 59 years. Overall, the poor fare worse than the better off in society on all health indicators studied while the converse is also true: the non-poor have a much higher overall health level than the poor.

These data illustrate another critical point. Some countries attain far better health conditions for their poor people than others. Poor children in China have less than a third of the risk of dying before their fifth birthday than comparably poor children in the United Republic of Tanzania. Poverty is not an insurmountable barrier to better health when policies are right. This further illustrates that much of the burden on the poor is unnecessary.

The unfinished agenda

The populations of developing countries, and particularly the disadvantaged groups within those countries, remain in the early stages of the epidemiological transition, where infectious diseases are still the major cause of death. Five major childhood conditions are responsible for 21 per cent of all deaths in low and middle-income countries: diarrhoea, acute respiratory infections, malaria, measles, and perinatal conditions. Almost all DALYs from these five conditions occur in developing countries. Less than 1 per cent are registered in high-income countries. Most of the DALYs among infants and young children are attributable to a limited number of conditions for which either preventive or curative interventions exist. Thus a priority for health systems is to achieve effective delivery of these interventions, delineated below.

Immunization programmes have yielded the most significant changes in child health in the last few decades. Although some vaccines represent the most cost-effective public health intervention of all, the world does not use them enough. At least 2 million children still die each year from diseases for which vaccines are available at low cost. Similarly, there exists a simple, inexpensive, and effective intervention for diarrhoeal disease—oral rehydration therapy. Diarrhoeal diseases and pneumonia together account for a high proportion of deaths of children in developing countries. Therefore in several developing countries diarrhoeal disease control programmes have been merged with a simplified approach to detecting acute respiratory infections (primarily pneumonia).

Table 2 Health status of the poor versus the non-poor in selected countries, around 1990

Country	Percentage of population in absolute poverty[a]	Probability of dying (females) per 1000				Prevalence of tuberculosis	
		Between birth and age 5		Between ages 15 and 59		Non-poor	Ratio of poor to non-poor
		Non-poor	Ratio of poor to non-poor	Non-poor	Ratio of poor to non-poor		
Aggregate[b]		38	4.8	92	4.3	23	2.6
Chile	15	7	8.3	34	12.3	2	2.6
China	22	28	6.6	35	11.0	13	8.0
Ecuador	8	45	4.9	107	4.4	25	3.8
India	53	40	4.3	84	3.7	28	1.8
Kenya	50	41	3.8	131	3.8	20	2.5
Malaysia	6	10	15.0	99	5.1	13	2.6

[a]Poverty is defined as income per capita of less than or equal to US$1 per day, expressed in dollars adjusted for purchasing power.

[b]The aggregate estimate refers to all countries listed in Annex Table 7 of the *World Health Report 1999* (WHO 1999).

See Explanatory Notes to the Statistical Annex for an explanation of the methods used to derive the estimates.

Source: Annex Table 7, *World Health Report 1999* (WHO 1999).

In adults, maternal conditions, HIV/AIDS, and tuberculosis are the three major causes of disease burden in developing regions. Together, they accounted for 7 per cent of all DALYs in 1998. Among maternal conditions, obstructed labour, sepsis, and unsafe abortion were among the 10 leading causes of death and disability among women aged 15 to 44 years in developing countries in 1998. The burden of maternal conditions has been difficult to quantify because of the lack of reliable data. But it is a major public health problem and represents a major and unnecessary burden for which policy-makers should increasingly be held accountable.

Persisting and evolving challenges

Despite the successful eradication of smallpox and the control of several infectious diseases in the twentieth century, there remain some significant threats that are particularly challenging because of the changing nature of the disease pattern and the ways it manifests itself in populations. A clear example is malaria. Public health efforts in the last four decades have been remarkably effective in reducing the burden of malaria in Southeast Asia and Latin America. Despite this achievement, malaria remains a major public health problem, particularly in Africa.

Malaria, along with HIV/AIDS and tuberculosis, can be classified among a group of diseases for which control efforts are being jeopardized by microbial evolution—the growing resistance of disease-causing organisms to antimicrobial drugs and other agents. A large proportion of the deaths occurring between the ages of 15 and 59 years in low- and middle-income countries can be attributed to HIV/AIDS and tuberculosis. Effective and cost-effective strategies for controlling tuberculosis exist, but standard treatment regimens require 6 or more months of chemotherapy and rely on well-organized services to achieve high rates of adherence. The interaction of HIV and tuberculosis is also an important public health matter, as individuals who are infected with both are more likely to die from tuberculosis than from other infections. During the period of active tuberculosis infection, they may transmit the infection to previously uninfected contacts. Because HIV infection is projected to increase over the next decade, the burden from tuberculosis may also increase unless there are energetic efforts to extend the reach of existing control measures with proven effectiveness and cost-effectiveness, as well as to invest in the development of new tools for tuberculosis control.

The challenge posed by these persisting and evolving conditions is that tools to control them have either not been developed or, if available, are not used effectively or, in some cases, are becoming increasingly ineffective (Harrison and Lederberg 1998). Antimicrobial resistance is a worrying phenomenon since it could have great adverse effects on the control and treatment of diseases such as pneumonia, tuberculosis, and malaria. These conditions emphasize the need, as discussed below, for health systems to invest in research and development strategies to develop cost-effective tools to control the remaining threats from infectious diseases.

Increases in international air travel, trade (particularly the food trade), and tourism mean that disease-producing organisms, the deadly as well as the commonplace, can be transported rapidly from one continent to another (WHO 1996*b*). This trend may threaten international public health security, although so far the consequences have remained quantitatively unimportant. To counter any such threat, the global surveillance of infectious diseases is being improved through an international information network. This should make it possible to recognize outbreaks faster.

The avoidable burden of disease

The most significant fact about this unnecessary burden is that it is concentrated on a few conditions, most of which are avoidable. There are many vaccines, drugs, and clinical algorithms that if employed globally would lead to a dramatic reduction in the burden of infectious diseases. That the infant mortality rate in low- and middle-income countries is higher in the most populous countries suggests the importance of focused international assistance. Health systems need to provide existing, cost-effective interventions to these populations so that the countries that are currently lagging behind can quickly catch up.

Immunization is the greatest public health success story in history (Henderson 1998). The basic vaccines are available to combat the six major diseases in children (measles, tetanus, pertussis, tuberculosis, poliomyelitis, and diphtheria). Immunization coverage falls far short of 100 per cent, and it is the world's poorest and most vulnerable children who remain unreached.

Poliomyelitis is an example of a disease for which eradication is possible. There have been remarkable reductions in the geographical spread of the disease since 1988. The last case caused by wild polio virus in the Western hemisphere occurred in Junin, Peru, on 23 August 1991. The last case in the Western Pacific Region was recorded in March 1997 near Phnom Penh in Cambodia. The only reason for the existence of remaining cases is insufficient coverage. The WHO initiated a 'final stretch' effort with the goal of stopping transmission globally by December 2000, of certifying this achievement by 2005, and of stopping immunization by 2010. The eradication effort illustrates two important points. Firstly, partnerships with non-governmental organizations can be very productive; Rotary International has made major commitments to polio eradication and its influence with local leaders plus financial contributions (about US$500 million) have been critical to success. Secondly, properly designed and highly goal-oriented programmes can contribute to health systems development.

The WHO has also promoted the provision of interventions against several other infectious diseases. The Integrated Management of Childhood Illness is a group of preventive and curative interventions. The strategy focuses on pneumonia, diarrhoea, measles, malaria, and malnutrition, as these account for 70 per cent of all childhood deaths globally, but it also addresses other serious infections (e.g. meningitis), other causes of febrile disease (e.g. dengue), and other associated problems (such as eye problems associated with measles or vitamin A deficiency, and ear infections). Preventive interventions including immunization, support for breast feeding, and other nutrition counselling are also emphasized.

Other similar initiatives are in different stages of development and implementation. For tuberculosis, the directly observed treatment, short course (**DOTS**) intervention has been shown to be highly cost-effective. Tuberculosis is highly concentrated in poor subgroups of populations, as indicated in Table 2. Prevalence of tuberculosis is estimated to be almost four times higher in populations living below the poverty line than in the better off. The Adult Lung Health initiative has grown out of the tuberculosis control activities of the WHO, recognizing that only a small proportion of adults presenting with a cough have tuberculosis and that adequate treatment or advice should be provided to individuals with other lung diseases. The initiative offers an integrated approach to detecting and treating tuberculosis, asthma, and chronic obstructive lung disease.

Maternal mortality risks, which are highly concentrated in developing countries, are also largely preventable and avoidable. The mother–baby package aims to reduce mortality and disability associated with maternal reproductive health, the risks of delivery for both mother and child, and the first weeks of life. The interventions needed to reduce the avoidable risks of childbirth are cost-effective. But expanding health system coverage is required; women must have access to skilled assistance during pregnancy and childbirth, and they must be able to reach a functioning health care facility when complications arise.

Syndromic treatment of sexually transmitted infections is another example of defining best practice in the face of resource constraints. By responding to the HIV/AIDS pandemic with urgency and commitment, successful interventions have been implemented to stop its transmission in Thailand and elsewhere in Southeast Asia.

Rationalization of drug use and the development of drug supply systems can similarly be aided by clearly defined standard guidelines where first- and second-line drugs for each level are specified. Revision of the regulations on who can use which drugs is often needed. For example, an injection of quinine for severe malaria or chloramphenicol for severe pneumonia, prior to referral to a higher level in the health system, may be life-saving. But health staff at first-level facilities may not be authorized to use injectable drugs or the drugs may be supplied regularly only to hospitals. Policies may need to be changed to accommodate broader use of certain drugs for defined purposes.

In addition to the disease-specific interventions and control programmes which are available, there is also a need to deal with a significant risk factor for disease, malnutrition, which is primarily concentrated in the world's poorest and most disadvantaged populations. Malnutrition is estimated to be the single most important risk factor for disease, being responsible for 16 per cent of the global burden in 1995, measured in DALYs (Murray and Lopez 1996). Malnutrition, either in the form of protein-energy malnutrition or micronutrient malnutrition, primarily of iron, vitamin A, and iodine, often contributes to premature death, poor health, blindness, growth stunting, mental retardation, learning disabilities, and low work capacity (WHO 1997). However, protein-energy malnutrition, as indicated by slow or incomplete physical growth is as much a consequence of disease as a cause. In many environments, infection may contribute more to malnutrition than dietary inadequacy. Hence disease control is important for reducing the malnutrition burden.

Interventions to reduce micronutrient malnutrition are likely to prove particularly cost-effective. Programmes can include four strategies—supplementation, fortification, food-based approaches leading to dietary diversification, and complementary public health control measures—to the degree appropriate and feasible (Howson *et al.* 1998*b*). The long-term goal of intervention should be to shift emphasis away from supplementation towards a combination of food fortification (e.g. universal salt iodization or iron-fortified flour) and dietary diversification.

In conclusion, the double burden of disease defines the complexity of the problems that health systems must address. The two elements of the double burden differ markedly in their implications for policy. The unfinished agenda deals with a limited number of conditions, highly concentrated on the poor and for most of which extremely cost-effective interventions are available. This burden on the poor is an unnecessary one that targeted programmes can alleviate. Conversely, epidemiological transition generates epidemiological diversity. This aspect of the double burden involves large numbers of conditions potentially affecting everyone, although again the poor suffer more. Interventions—whether preventive or curative—are less likely to be decisive, although there are important exceptions, such as tobacco. Health systems must be able to respond flexibly to this diversity.

Meeting the challenges: health systems development

In the early 1990s the world devoted about 9 per cent of its total product to the health sector (World Bank 1997*a*). This massive commitment of resources responds to the diversity of health challenges resulting from the demographic and epidemiological transition. Health systems now have the potential to reduce markedly the huge amount of excess disease that the poor and disadvantaged suffer. This burden is concentrated in a very limited number of conditions. Health systems could—and should—address those conditions for which effective tools already exist. In sharp contrast to the focus that health systems can bring to the particular problems of the poor they must also anticipate and respond to a bewildering variety of diseases and injuries. The tenth revision of the *International Classification of Diseases* (WHO 1992) runs to over 2000 pages. Although some of these conditions occur more frequently than others, health systems must have the financial means, organizational structures, and procedures to respond flexibly and efficiently to this diversity.

The development of science-based organized health systems is relatively recent, and very much in progress. Most countries have no single health system, but several distinct health financing and provision subsystems, embracing different types of traditional or alternative practice, as well as public, private, and not-for-profit hospitals and clinics, sometimes offering services for limited population subgroups such as civil servants.

Health systems in some countries perform well. Others perform poorly. An accumulation of applied research efforts and practical experience now suggests some reasons for these differences. Countries differ and lessons that are useful to one country may have little value to others. Furthermore, evidence about what has worked—and what has not—constitutes only one of several factors influencing the decisions that shape health systems. However, for many government officials, as for many clinicians, evidence does matter. But clearly, for national purposes, only national officials can judge the relevance and political feasibility of using evidence generated from other countries and other times. This last section summarizes accumulated evidence concerning a few key questions on health system finance and development.

Before turning to the evidence, it is worth listing the goals of health systems as the WHO sees them. Goals can be phrased in many ways, and each goal may have different relevance in different contexts. Yet the following core list of goals for health system development is likely to elicit broad agreement:

- improving health status
- reducing health inequalities
- enhancing responsiveness to legitimate expectations
- increasing efficiency
- protecting individuals, families, and communities from financial loss
- enhancing fairness in the financing and delivery of health care.

There are often trade-offs among these goals, given the limits to government involvement and government finance. One of the key policy questions becomes how best to achieve the right balance between systemic goals while recognizing budgetary and other limits. Furthermore, what incentives for providers of care will constrain cost escalation while motivating compassionate service of high quality? Independently of sources of finance, what are reasonable roles for private and public providers of care to play? How can research and development to underpin continued health improvement globally be sustained in a context where most health finance is national? Finally, and most important, what is the role of government in financing health services? Analytical and empirical work provides no specific answers to these questions but rather assembles the evidence on consequences resulting from the choices made in different countries at different times. The accumulated evidence may, in some cases, suggest that certain policies have worked well, while others have worked poorly.

Achieving greater efficiency

Efficiency concepts in health systems apply at several different levels. 'Macroeconomic efficiency' (Hurst 1992) refers to the total costs of health care in relation to aggregate measures of health status. Countries spend very different amounts of national resources on health, allocate those resources in very different ways, and achieve very different health outcomes in terms of health status, access, or satisfaction. Some of those outcome differences indicate differences in health system efficiency. China's performance (relative to national income) in reducing mortality in children under 5 years old fell sharply between the early 1980s and 1992, when incomes were rising but the rural medical system was deteriorating. Comparative work in Latin America suggests that a given level of health expenditure contributes positively to reductions in mortality in children under 5 years old if it is from public sources, but negatively if it is from private sources (Jamison *et al.* 1996).

Some governments have traditionally regarded health spending by the public sector as a pure consumption expenditure, and have wanted to minimize it. This is often the perspective of ministries of finance. Yet in many poor countries total health spending from all sources is very low—less than 2 per cent of GDP in Cameroon, Indonesia, Nigeria, Sri Lanka, and Sudan, for example—meaning that even the most inexpensive and effective health measures cannot be made available to the whole population. Even in Zambia, where over 3 per cent of GDP is allocated to health, the public per capita spending (government and external assistance) is only about half of the US$12 suggested by the World Bank as necessary to fund the cost of a basic package of preventive and curative interventions. The reality is that allocating an inadequate share of resources to health, from both public and private sources, perpetuates the cycle of poverty. Increased public financial support for cost-effective and equitable health services is overdue in many countries.

In middle- and upper-income countries, health financing policy is frequently driven by the need to increase co-ordination, reduce fragmentation, and exert better control over total health care costs. Countries in this group are often worried that their level of health spending will threaten economic growth and competitiveness by making their labour force, and therefore goods and services, more expensive. Argentina, France, Germany, Switzerland, and the United States, for example, are all spending in excess of 9 per cent of GDP on health, and in the United States the figure has risen to 14 per cent. While spending much more than 9 per cent of GDP may indicate macroeconomic inefficiency, countries spending less than 2 per cent are almost certainly investing too little in the health of their present and future population. Within this broad range there is no single economically efficient or 'correct' level of funding.

'Microeconomic efficiency' refers to the scope for achieving greater efficiency from existing patterns of resource use. Wastage and inefficiency occur in all health systems. Allocative inefficiency occurs when resources are devoted to the wrong activities. Spending large amounts of the health budget on hospital-based care for children with measles is clearly an allocative inefficiency: those children should have been immunized. Well-prioritized and universally accessible service packages, of the sort discussed above, can make major gains in the allocative efficiency of health systems of both rich and poor countries.

Technical inefficiency occurs when too many resources are used to achieve a given health intervention or outcome. An imbalance between the installed capacity of a health system (its buildings, equipment, and staff) and the recurrent resources needed for its proper functioning gives rise to a set of technical inefficiencies—with overstaffing and underemployment in relation to utilization levels becoming common, particularly at peripheral health facilities. Cost-effectiveness analysis is the key tool for guiding improvements in microeconomic efficiency.

Service quality falls when the required inputs (physical and human) are lacking, and when proper procedures are not used. Common symptoms in the public sector are a lack of essential drugs, inaccessible health facilities, absent staff, non-functioning vehicles and equipment, and dilapidated premises. Where these symptoms occur, health outcomes suffer. Perceptions of the fairness and responsiveness of government also suffer. Comparable difficulties abound in the private sector. In the large and inadequately regulated private sector of low- and middle-income countries, health workers are often unqualified, and diagnostic and prescribing practices are poor or even hazardous. Private sector treatment of tuberculosis, for example, often involves profitable but useless intervention while failing to achieve the high cure rates that have been attained in public facilities.

Setting priorities

Even the wealthiest countries may not be able to provide entire populations with every intervention that has medical value. Priorities have to be debated, agreed, and implemented, if universal access to affordable and effective health care is to be achieved. In most countries today, priorities are set in ways which exclude large numbers of people from access to organized care. Ability to pay appears increasingly to be the mechanism for rationing access to care (Ensor and San 1996). Governments can do better than this; indeed, an open and vigorous debate about how to set priorities in health has begun. Choosing public priorities, in terms of what governments will do and will not do, is how economic reality becomes an integral part of health system development and reform.

Explicit priority setting in health has taken several steps forward since the mid-1980s. National or regional guidelines have been debated, published, and—to differing degrees—implemented in The Netherlands, New Zealand, Norway, Sweden, and the State of Oregon (Ham 1997). Approaches differ. In Sweden, an explicit value base was proposed comprising three principles in descending order of importance: human dignity regardless of personal characteristics and social functions, need and solidarity, and cost-effectiveness. Several categories of political and clinical priority were defined. In Oregon and The Netherlands, the value bases for priority setting were also explicit. In all three countries they differed.

In developing countries, the debate on priorities has often been led by international agencies. From the early 1950s to the 1980s, global public health initiatives tended to focus on a single disease at a time, such as malaria or diarrhoeal disease control, and sometimes on a single intervention, such as DDT spraying or oral rehydration therapy. More recently, international advice has favoured grouped interventions, to achieve better outcomes and improve service quality. The Expanded Programme on Immunization groups vaccines aimed at preventing diphtheria, tetanus, pertussis, poliomyelitis, tuberculosis, and measles.

The *World Development Report 1993* (World Bank 1993) pushed forward debate on priority setting by introducing the notion of cost-effective intervention packages, tailored according to the public finance reality of each country. Numerous countries have designed such priority packages (Bobadilla and Cowley 1995). Bangladesh, Colombia, Mexico, and Zambia have begun implementation.

The clear definition of priorities facilitates planning, training, monitoring, and supervision of services in districts, provided the necessary investments are made in capacity building at this level. When packages of services for the most common conditions have been developed, health facilities can be reorganized to ensure shorter waiting times, more efficient patient flow, more standardized dispensing of drugs, and better communication with users of the services. In these ways, focused intervention priorities allow limited resources to have the greatest possible impact on service quality and health outcomes.

Focused approaches can reduce much of the excess disease burden of the poor. Cost-effectiveness measures are useful in that they summarize in a single measure the key scientific and technical evidence on health-improving actions. But without participatory processes to engage and sustain national and local debate on health priorities, the scientific information base will remain peripheral to actual implementation of resource allocation procedures in countries.

Rethinking incentives to providers

Two further influences on efficiency and service quality are the way in which service providers are paid, and the role of budget or fund-holding agencies with respect to service providers.

The likely incentive effects of many ways in which hospitals, clinics, or individual practitioners are paid have been well studied (Barnum *et al.* 1995; Newhouse 1996; Saltman and Figueras 1997). Prospective payment methods (e.g. budgets, capitation) transfer financial risk for delivering services from budget or fund-holding institutions (medical savings accounts, village or community prepayment schemes, commercial health insurance funds, health maintenance organizations, public budgets for health care) to providers. Retrospective payment methods (e.g. fee-for-service, case-based payment) reimburse providers for services rendered. It is clear from experiences in many countries at all income levels that pure fee-for-service methods (particularly those involving 'third-party' payment to providers) create incentives for overspending and inappropriate care. Without controls on utilization volume or quality of service, these systems are difficult to manage in the public interest and have created incentives for extravagant and wasteful care through oversupply of medication, overuse of diagnostic services, and excessive surgical intervention (Hsiao 1995; Medici *et al.* 1997; Yang 1997). Fee-for-service systems often create the wrong incentives for providers from a public policy perspective, and rapid but relatively unproductive growth in health expenditures (McGreevey 1988). Better choices exist, ranging from sophisticated prepayment methods to fee-for-service supplemented by relatively simple administrative controls to limit cost escalation (e.g. review of prescribing patterns to ensure compliance with an essential drug list). A major challenge for many countries is to ensure that poor quality and inefficient practice are not rewarded, whilst practice which is oriented to achieving health gain in populations is recognized in remuneration.

Prepayment means that fund-holding institutions are created: personal or family medical savings accounts, village or community schemes, private health insurance funds, health maintenance organizations, and public budgets for health. Many health funds have traditionally been passive financial intermediaries, failing to take full advantage of their financial power to promote changes in provider behaviour. However, currently there is a widespread tendency to explore contracting arrangements between public purchasers and different types of providers. In many countries, this extends to relations between different parts of the public sector, for example between central and local government health bodies. Competitive pressure has had a similar effect and has driven much of the 'managed care' reform in the United States; it is worth noting that the introduction of competition was in part due to state and local government attempts to contain cost growth in services purchased for their own employees, for the elderly, or for the poor.

In the health system reforms of New Zealand and the United Kingdom, and more recently in Kyrgyzstan and Zambia, the functional distinction between funding bodies and service providers has been formalized as a 'purchaser–provider split'. For public hospitals, autonomy over financial and managerial decisions is being introduced or increased in many countries, with benchmarks agreed for performance monitoring. Many health insurers are taking an active role in managing the provision of care to their beneficiaries. Budget allocations to district health managers in Ghana are now managed in much the same way as contracts, with prior agreement on performance indicators and the possibility of rewards or penalties in subsequent budget allocations. These experiences reflect the same trend—a more active use of the purchasing power of fund-holding agencies to control costs and improve the quality of services provided.

Payment incentives are not the only component of a more active purchasing role by insurers or public budget holding bodies. Other elements in active purchasing include primary care gatekeeping to improve the efficiency of the referral process, the maintenance of provider profiles so that the purchasing agent can more actively monitor individual provider behaviour, contracting with selected providers who meet defined quality and cost criteria, utilization review and quality assurance activities to reduce inappropriate care and improve quality, and the development of standard treatment protocols in drug prescribing or adherence to national essential drugs lists (Kane 1995).

Direct comparison between public and private providers of the same services, whether these are clinical or support services, opens the way for publicly managed competition between a wide array of possible providers. Competition for the delivery of health care to populations is an important means of empowering consumers *vis-à-vis* providers, as long as there is a well-informed and capable purchaser acting on behalf of consumers, using its financial power to induce changes in provider behaviour that improve the quality and efficiency of care for the population to which the purchaser is accountable.

Few ministries of health or public providers use mechanisms for assessing people's preferences or satisfaction with the way that health services are provided. Such unresponsiveness has been part of the environment in which private provision has flourished. Private providers have often ensured that their office locations and opening times are convenient for people. Greater accountability by the public sector requires much more concern with the way people are treated by health workers, both clinically and socially.

Clear policy guidance needs to be supported by an enabling set of institutions which offer the appropriate incentives. But there must be discretion in the interpretation of general policy guidelines to meet local circumstances, and an informed, consultative, and accountable chain of command from the peripheral clinic or health post to the minister's office. Achieving such a system often requires far-reaching change from the health system models in many countries, where the public sector is typically subject to centralized control while the private sector is virtually unsupervised.

Revitalizing progress towards universal coverage

A clear historical lesson emerges from health systems development in the twentieth century: spontaneous unmanaged growth in any country's health system cannot be relied upon to ensure that the greatest health needs are met (Arrow 1963; Barr 1993). Public intervention is necessary to achieve universal access. In any country, the greatest burden of ill health and the highest risk of avoidable morbidity or mortality is borne by the poor. While progress towards universal access to health care of an acceptable quality has been substantial in this century, as illustrated by global immunization coverage, the distribution of services in most countries of the world remains highly skewed in favour of the better off. The equity arguments for universal public finance are widely accepted; what is less well known is that this approach achieves greater efficiency as well.

Health care coverage

A historic WHO conference in Alma-Ata in 1978 established the goal of Health for All by the Year 2000. It defined this goal as 'the attainment by all peoples of the world by the year 2000 of a level of health that will permit them to lead a socially and economically productive life'. It encouraged the extension of basic primary health services to everyone as the major route for achieving the goal. In the decades following the Declaration of Alma-Ata, there have been enormous gains in life expectancy and many other key health status measures, indicating great progress towards better health for all. Inspiration and guidance from Alma-Ata contributed in no small measure to the health revolution, in addition to continued improvement in living standards, as well as the generation and application of new knowledge about diseases and their control. But problems and challenges remain.

The two decades since the Alma-Ata Declaration have not seen the realization of the wished-for rapid and sustained progress towards universally accessible basic health care. The global picture is very uneven, with many countries dismantling their social protection mechanisms in health rather than expanding them.

Major shifts in the 1990s in formerly socialist countries towards market economies have often been accompanied by a widespread movement of the health workforce into private practice, particularly in urban areas. In the decades up to the 1980s, many socialist countries had established universally accessible health care systems. Although these may have been inefficient, bureaucratic, and unresponsive to patient needs, basic care, and in many cases secondary and tertiary care as well, was effectively prepaid and available to almost the entire population for little or no payment at the time of need. Most people in these countries have found that they now have to pay more—officially or unofficially—for their health care, and access to care is increasingly reflecting the ability to pay. In just a decade, China dismantled its Rural Co-operative Medical System, built up from the 1950s to provide health insurance protection for the great majority, and in the 1980s made some four-fifths of the total population uninsured, in other words fully responsible for their own health care costs. In sub-Saharan Africa, user fees for health care have been instituted or increased in the great majority of countries (Nolan and Turbat 1995). Frequently, these policies missed opportunities to use fee revenues to improve the quality and availability of services. Attendance rates, particularly at public primary health facilities, are often already very low, indicating that most people now prefer to use traditional or private sector providers of primary care.

The industrialized countries have largely preserved their systems of near universally accessible and prepaid health care, sometimes (as in Canada, New Zealand, and the United Kingdom) implementing major organizational reform programmes. However, the fraction of the population under the age of 65 without private or public insurance protection in the United States has continued to grow, increasing from nearly 15 per cent in 1987 to nearly 18 per cent in 1996 (Hoffman 1998). And other countries have begun to shift payment responsibilities for long-term care directly onto patients and their families. Inequality in health outcomes between the poorest and best-off groups have widened in many industrialized countries. Yet some countries have made real progress towards universal coverage, such as the Republic of Korea which implemented universal health insurance in 1989, after a long period of rapid economic growth.

Policy choices

Some, but by no means all, health policy choices involve trade-offs among the six goals set out above. As the experience of China and Sri Lanka in the 1950s and 1960s has shown, in situations of great poverty it is possible to make dramatic improvements in equitable access to care and simultaneously to bring about major improvements in health outcomes, while still keeping total public spending on health at modest levels. Canada's shift to national health insurance simultaneously achieved both better health and economic gains. Ensuring that poor people benefit from the promotive, preventive, and curative interventions that are already available not only improves their access to health care, it substantially contributes to reducing the total burden of illness facing a region or a country. Opportunities now exist to make huge inroads into avoidable health problems, whilst cementing solidarity between different social strata.

To achieve this potential, the poorest and sickest people have to be reached by health promotion and prevention programmes, and they have to be able to get to clinics or health posts (private, public, or non-government) where the right kind of treatment is available for common local, treatable conditions. And there must be no significant price barrier at the time poor people need services. Universal coverage means that, irrespective of the source of funds, the health care system functions like a national health insurance system, prepaid either through tax revenues or through employment-based social insurance, to ensure the largest possible pool of risks. There has to be a shift in the mentality of the system from funding the 'needs' of the service delivery infrastructure to purchasing services according to the health care needs of the population. Instead of a series of independent and uncoordinated insurance and health financing schemes, each with its own beneficiaries, benefits, and sometimes with its own set of health facilities and professionals, a national health insurance system means a merging of risk protection responsibilities into the largest possible pool, or co-ordination of the benefit packages financed from different funding sources, with the ultimate aim of funding a comprehensive set of covered services from the resources of a single fund. A single fund for the pooling of risks allows for many options in the way incentives are set for individual providers of care, including the option of shifting risk to providers.

Figure 2 shows how risk pooling in health and the share of public spending in total increase as countries move away from out-of-pocket payment methods. Various institutional alternatives exist for achieving universal coverage. Recent comparative research, measuring equity in both the financing burden and the use of services by different income groups in countries, shows that the least organized and most inequitable way of paying for health care is on an out-of-pocket basis; people pay for their medical care when they need and use it. The financing burden falls disproportionately on the poorest (who face higher health care costs than the better off), and the financial barrier means that use of services is lower among the lower-income groups, although their need is typically higher (Doorslaer *et al.* 1993).

The market response to a user-fee-based system is through the development of private insurance. Insurers see a profitable opportunity. People prepay through insurance premiums, so that they do not have to live with unpredictable large health care bills. This method of financing entails some pooling of risks among the insured, but creates access inequities between the insured, who will have preferential access to better care, and the non-insured. Experience with commercial health insurance markets shows that they are both unstable and difficult to regulate, with each insurer constantly adjusting the risk profile of the beneficiary group in order to ensure that revenues are greater than expenditures.

In countries with a substantial percentage of the population employed in the formal sector of the economy, a larger pooling of risks

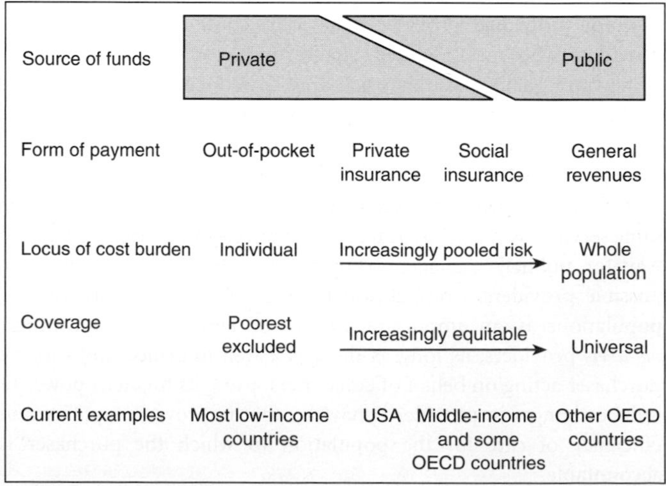

Fig. 2 Funding, risk pooling, and coverage patterns.

is possible through social insurance schemes, where mainly employed people and their immediate families are compulsorily enrolled in health insurance, and where premium payments are related to each member's income, rather than their actuarial risk of illness. In Costa Rica, Germany, and Japan, and in other countries where formal employment levels are high, this method of risk pooling forms the basis of the national health insurance system. In both its financing and in the access to health care that it allows, this type of system is more equitable than the two systems described above. But this conclusion does not necessarily hold true in countries where only a small percentage of the population works in the formal sector.

Most equitable of all in terms of the way the health financing burden is shared, and in allowing equal access to care for people with comparable need, are risk-pooling systems based on central government tax revenue financing, such as in Canada, Cuba, Denmark, New Zealand, Norway, Spain, Sweden, and the United Kingdom. The risk pool is the entire resident population, and the insurance function against the costs of health care is implemented by government, funded by taxes which, in a progressive system, take a larger share of income from the rich than from the poor.

There are, in essence, two policy routes open to countries in moving towards a higher level of prepayment for health. One can strive to increase private voluntary insurance schemes, in which government takes only a supportive financing role, as in Switzerland and the United States. Or, one can increase government responsibility for the development of a national prepaid system based on social insurance and public finance, as in France and Sweden.

What does each strategy entail for a developing country? The first is the market-oriented route, which may be preferred by better-off members of the population, but will exacerbate inequities in access. Its regulation, and overall expenditure control, will be problematic. And where formal employment levels are low as a percentage of total—as in most low- and middle-income countries—the level of coverage through prepayment will remain low. Only in upper-middle-income countries, or in situations of exceptionally high and sustained growth (over many decades in Germany and Japan, though dramatically shorter periods in the Republic of Korea, Taiwan, and China) when the employment structure shifts from rural self-employment to urban formal employment, have voluntary insurance schemes grown widely enough to become the basis for a national prepaid system.

The second strategy seeks to build prepayment systems through a combination of social insurance and public finance. Almost all countries already have elements of both, but these are seldom linked as part of an explicit health policy. Developing a national strategy for prepayment requires rethinking public finance for health into an integrated framework of finance for universal coverage. In this, employment-based, municipal, or community-based health insurance schemes would be linked with public subsidies, and guidelines given for the development of population-based coverage to ensure both equity and allocative efficiency.

Combining universal coverage with economic reality

Where do the values of the WHO lead when combined with the available evidence? The WHO remains firmly committed to the values and principles embodied in its Health for All policy. But the WHO believes that governments can no longer attempt to provide and finance everything for everybody. This 'classical' universalism, although seldom advanced in extreme form, shaped the formation of many European health systems. It achieved important successes. But classical universalism fails to recognize both resource limits and the limits of government in the current age.

At the same time, the WHO firmly refutes market-oriented approaches that ration health services according to the ability to pay. Not only do market-oriented approaches to finance lead to intolerable inequity with respect to a fundamental human right, but growing bodies of theory and evidence indicate them to be inefficient as well. Market mechanisms have enormous utility in many sectors and have underpinned rapid economic growth for over a century in Europe and elsewhere. But the very countries that have relied heavily on market mechanisms to achieve the high incomes that they enjoy today are the same countries that rely most heavily on governments to finance their health services. Therein lies a lesson. Health is an important component of national welfare. Achieving high health outcomes requires a combination of universal entitlement and tight control over expenditure.

Thus the WHO advocates a new and different type of universal coverage that recognizes government limits but retains government responsibility for the leadership and finance of health systems. Such systems would still be diverse, and some, subject to appropriate guidelines, would promote competition in the provision of services. At the same time, the WHO recognizes that if services are to be provided for all, then not all services can be provided. The most cost-effective services in a given setting should be provided first. Private providers would continue to be an important source of care in many countries, while private sector entities would supply service providers with drugs and equipment. Increased public and private investment is an essential ingredient in generating the new drugs, equipment, and vaccines that will underpin long-term improvements in health.

To maximize the efficiency and equity gains, and create 'win–win' situations in poorer countries with large burdens of illness, practical steps towards universal coverage need to be taken. There is no single blueprint available for replication by all countries. But a number of key design features for covering the most important health care services for everyone are now apparent.

Membership is defined to include the entire population, i.e. it is compulsory. Whether this is by citizenship or residence, the purpose is to ensure that the population covered is defined inclusively.

Universal coverage means coverage for all, not coverage of everything. The prepayment system, financed by government, corporations, and better-off individuals, will reflect a country's overall level of economic development. It will be a limited fund, not able to pay for all of those services that the population—and the health workforce—would like to see provided at no charge. Lower-priority services, which will vary between countries, will only be available for payment. A benefit package has to be clearly defined in the light of the resources available and the cost of top-priority health interventions, an assessment of the services and inputs for which individuals are able and willing to pay out of their own pockets, and the political feasibility of various choices.

Provider payment is not made by the patient at the time he or she uses the health service. Health care always has to be paid for. But the way it is paid for makes a major difference to who receives care and to overall levels of health. Out-of-pocket payments penalize the cash poor—those who work outside the cash economy, or who have only seasonal or occasional cash income, or who are unemployed. Heavy reliance on out-of-pocket payment sets the wrong incentives for both users and providers, and results in an inequitable financing burden and barriers to access for the poorest. Prepayment allows a wide range of incentive-setting methods for the efficient purchasing of services.

Services may be offered by providers of all types. Provided that health practices and health facilities meet certain quality standards and that they are subject to similar levels of managerial flexibility, their ownership status should not matter. A stronger purchaser setting standard rates of remuneration and enforcing a common set of quality and utilization regulations will enable the most efficient provider of services to flourish. Such arrangements will allow the very large numbers of private providers, who are essentially the first points of contact with the health system in many low-income countries, to be brought within a structured but pluralistic health care system, benefiting from its resources and subject to sanction and regulation by professional and public bodies.

Advice on health policy and financing from major global and regional development agencies is increasingly convergent and supportive of these same points (see, for example, recent reports from the World Bank (1997*a*), the Inter-American Development Bank (1996), and the ADB (1999)).

Providing for the future: the role of research and development

Most discussions of health systems and health finance focus on delivering services. This is in some respects appropriate since only about 3 per cent of health expenditures globally address the building of future capacity through research and development. Yet, the first part of this chapter indicated the generation and utilization of new knowledge as the dominant force underlying the twentieth-century revolution in health. Therefore health systems have a responsibility to provide for the generation of new knowledge.

Health research and development entails consequences for costs of health systems as well as for outcomes. A recent review (Pardes 1999) identified three established directions in research and development—a revolution in biotechnology enhanced efficiency in new pharmaceuticals development, and improved knowledge of how individuals can control their own health—which could stabilize expenditures on ageing populations. Even today's technologies, which are often expenditure enhancing, may result in less than anticipated cost increases as populations become more elderly. This results from a steady decline in disability rates among the aged and reduced health care costs in the final years of life among the very old relative to the old. In the United States, for example, health care expenditures in the final 2 years before a death at age 67 exceed those before a death at age 90 by a factor of 3. These trends combine with probable cost-saving (and health-enhancing) products in today's research and development pipeline to counter demographic pressures on health expenditures. Important among these products will be improved means for health promotion and delivery of preventive care (Fries *et al.* 1993).

A recent WHO report (1996*b*) indicates critical gaps in knowledge and needs for products, as well as to the growing productivity or capacity of the research and development enterprise itself. It presents an agenda for action that is partially at the national level and partially international. The report states the case for collaboration among national health systems as follows:

> Global challenges demand, in some sense, a global response. All nations share the fruits of research and development. Even though each country may invest a relatively modest sum towards collective goals, the aggregate effort potentially benefits all substantially. Collective action is the economically rational approach to public goods such as research and development; here, responsibility for catalysing collective action lies principally in the hands of the global community. Far from overshadowing action at the national level, global efforts help both to make national research and development efforts more productive and to lead to a global result that exceeds the sum of national ones. Thus, among the many competing demands on the funds allocated to international assistance for health, those contributing to generation of the new knowledge, products and interventions that can be shared by all have special merit.

One important step towards linking national health systems (and their research arms) into an international network has been the creation of the Global Forum for Health Research. The Forum's purposes included informed advocacy for reallocation of resources towards research and development, and improving the focus and efficiency of resources now being spent. The participation of national health systems in the generation of new knowledge provides dual benefits: it quickens the overall pace of advance, and it shortens the time it takes for results to be translated into practice. Hence the importance, in planning the financing and organization of health systems, of ensuring an adequate research and development base.

Conclusion

To enable the whole population of even the richest country to have access to effective care of good quality, many choices have to be made. These choices concern health interventions, as well as the way these interventions are delivered through health systems. In both cases, choices should take account of research into effectiveness in order to ensure the development of an optimal strategy. An open and informed debate about priorities in health is also a necessary part of this strategy. Informing this debate is a critical task for research. Unless these choices are made by responsible authorities, nationally and locally, and their implementation is monitored, service provision always tends to favour the better-off groups, both in terms of where services are available and what services are offered. The objectives enumerated earlier are more likely to be achieved when appropriate political and financial mechanisms complement performance data in making authorities accountable to the populations they are meant to serve. To select key interventions and to orient health services towards entire populations combines universal coverage with economic realism. Achieving this goal is necessary to ensure sustained and equitable improvements in health in the twenty-first century.

References

ADB (Asian Development Bank) (1997). *Emerging Asia*. ADB, Manila.

ADB (Asian Development Bank) (1999). *Policy for the health sector*. ADB, Manila.

Arrow, K.J. (1963). Uncertainty and the welfare economics of medical care. *American Economic Review*, **53**, 941–73.

Barnum, H., Kutzin, J., and Saxenian, H. (1995). Incentives and provider payment methods. *International Journal of Health Planning and Management*, **10**, 23–45.

Barr, N. (1993). *The economics of the welfare state* (2nd edn). Stanford University Press.

Barro, R.J. (1997). *Determinants of economic growth: A cross-country empirical study*. MIT Press, Cambridge, MA.

Bloom, D.E. and Williamson J.G. (1998). *Demographic transitions and economic miracles in emerging Asia*. Harvard Institute for International Development, Cambridge, MA.

Bobadilla, J. and Cowley, P. (1995). Designing and implementing packages of essential health services. *Journal of International Development*, **7**, 543–54.

Doorslaer, E., Wagstaff, A., and Rutten, F. (1993). *Equity in the finance and delivery of health care: An international perspective*. Oxford University Press.

Dwyer, D.S. and Mitchell, O.S. (1999). Health problems as determinants of retirement: are self-rated measures endogenous? *Journal of Health Economics*, **18**, 173–93.

Easterlin, R.A. (1998). *How beneficent is the market? A look at the modern history of mortality*. University of Southern California, Los Angeles, CA.

Easterly, W. (1998). *Life during growth*. World Bank, Washington, DC.

Ensor, T. and San, P.B. (1996). Access and payment for health care: the poor of northern Vietnam. *International Journal of Health Planning and Management*, **11**, 69–83.

Frenk, J., *et al.* (1989). Health transition in middle-income countries: new challenges for health care. *Health Policy and Planning*, **4**, 29–39.

Fries, J.F., Koop, C.E., Beadle, C.E., *et al.* (1993). Reducing health care costs by reducing the need and demand for medical services. *New England Journal of Medicine*, **329**, 321–5.

Gallup, J.L., Sachs, J.D., and Mellinger, A.D. (1998). *Geography and economic development*. Harvard Institute for International Development, Cambridge, MA.

Ham, C. (1997). Priority setting in health care: Learning from international experience. *Health Policy*, **42**, 49–66.

Harrison, P.F. and Lederberg, J. (ed.) (1998). *Antimicrobial resistance: issues and options*. Institute of Medicine. National Academy Press, Washington, DC.

Henderson, R.H. (1998). Immunization: going the extra mile. In *The progress of nations 1998*. UNICEF, New York.

Hoffman, C. (1998). *Uninsured in America: a chart book*. Kaiser Commission on Medicaid and the Uninsured, Washington, DC.

Howson, C.P., Reddy, K.S., Ryan, T.J., and Bale, J.R. (ed.) (1998*a*). *Control of cardiovascular diseases in developing countries. Research, development and institutional strengthening*. Institute of Medicine/National Academy Press, Washington, DC.

Howson, C.P., Kennedy, E.T., and Horwitz, A. (ed.) (1998*b*). *Prevention of micronutrient deficiencies: Tools for policymakers and public health workers*. Institute of Medicine/National Academy Press, Washington, DC.

Hsiao, W.C. (1995). The Chinese health care system: lessons for other nations. *Social science and medicine*, **41**, 1047–55.

Hurst, J. (1992). *The reform of health care: a comparative analysis of seven OECD countries*. OECD, Paris.

Inter-American Development Bank (1996). Making social services work. Special section in: *Economic and social progress in Latin America. Report of the IADB*. Johns Hopkins University Press, Baltimore, MD.

Jamison, D., *et al.* (1996). Income, mortality and fertility in Latin America: Country-level performance, 1960–1990 *Revista de Analisis Economico*, **11**, 219–61.

Jamison, D., Lau, L.J., and Wang, J. (1998). Health's contribution to economic growth, 1965–90. In *Health, health policy and economic outcomes*. Director-General's Transition Team, Health and Development Satellite, Final Report: 61–80. WHO, Geneva.

Kane, N. (1995). Costs, productivity and financial outcomes of managed care. In *Implementing planned markets in health care: balancing social and economic responsibility* (ed. R. Saltman and C. von Otter). Milton Keynes, Open University Press.

McGreevey, W.P. (1988). The high costs of health care in Brazil. *Bulletin of the Pan American Health Organization*, **22**, 145–66.

McKeown, T. (1976). *The role of medicine: dream, mirage or nemesis*. Nuffield Provincial Hospitals Trust, London.

Medici, A.C. *et al.* (1997). Managed care and managed competition in Latin America and the Caribbean. In *Innovations in health and financing* (ed. G. Schieber). Discussion Paper 365, World Bank, Washington, DC.

Murray, C.J.L. and Lopez, A.D. (ed.) (1996). *The global burden of disease: a comprehensive assessment of mortality and disability from diseases, injuries, and risk factors in 1990 and projected to 2020*. Harvard School of Public Health, Cambridge, MA, on behalf of the WHO and the World Bank.

Neisser, V. (ed.) (1998). *The rising curve: long-term gains in IQ and related measures*. American Psychological Association, Washington, DC.

Newhouse, J.P. (1996). Reimbursing health plans and health providers: Efficiency in production versus selection. *Journal of Economic Literature*, **34**, 1236–63.

Nolan, B. and Turbat, V. (1995). *Cost recovery in public health services in sub-Saharan Africa*. World Bank (EDI Technical Materials), Washington, DC.

PAHO (Pan American Health Organization) (1998). Health situation in the Americas: basic indicators 1998. PAHO/HDP/HDA/98.01, PAHO/WHO, Washington, DC.

Pardes, H., Manton, K.G., Lander, E.S., Tolley, H.D., Ullian, A.D., and Palmer, H. (1999). Effects of medical research on health care and the economy. *Science*, **283**, 36–7.

Preston, S.H. (1975). The changing relation between mortality and level of economic development. *Population Studies*, **29**, 213–48.

Preston, S.H. (1980). Causes and consequences of mortality declines in less developed countries in the 20th century. In *Population and economic change in developing countries* (ed. R.A. Easterlin), pp. 289–341. University of Chicago Press.

Preston, S.H., Keyfitz, N., and Schoen R. (1972). *Causes of death: life tables for national populations*. Seminar Press, New York.

Radelet, S., Sachs, J., and Lee, J.W. (1997). *Economic growth in Asia*. Development Discussion Paper 609, Harvard Institute for International Development, Cambridge, MA.

Sachs, J.D. and Werner, A.M. (1997). Fundamental sources of long-term growth. *American Economic Review*, **87**, 184–8.

Saltman, R.B. and Figueras, J. (ed.) (1997). *European health care reform: analysis of current strategy*. WHO Regional Publications, European Series No. 72, WHO Regional Office for Europe, Copenhagen.

Strauss, J. and Thomas, D. (1998). Health, nutrition and economic development. *Journal of Economic Literature*, **36**, 766–817.

Wang, J., *et al.* (1999). *Measuring country performance on health: selected indicators for 115 countries*. Human Development Network, Health, Nutrition and Population Series, World Bank, Washington, DC.

WHO (World Health Organization) (1992). *International statistical classification of diseases and related health problems (10th revision) (ICD-10)*. WHO, Geneva.

WHO (World Health Organization) (1996*a*). *Investing in health research and development*. WHO/TDR/Gen/96.1, WHO, Geneva.

WHO (World Health Organization) (1996*b*). *World health report 1996. Fighting disease, fostering development*. WHO, Geneva.

WHO (World Health Organization) (1997). *WHO global database on child growth and malnutrition*. WHO/NUT/97.4, WHO, Geneva.

WHO (World Health Organization) (1998). *World health report 1998. Life in the twenty-first century: a vision for all.* WHO, Geneva.

WHO (World Health Organization) (1999). *World health report 1999.* WHO, Geneva.

World Bank (1993). *World development report 1993. Investing in health.* Oxford University Press, New York.

World Bank (1997*a*). *Sector strategy: health, nutrition and population.* World Bank, Washington, DC.

World Bank (1997*b*). World development report 1997. The state in a changing world. World Bank, Washington, DC.

World Bank (1998). *World development report 1998–1999. Knowledge for development.* World Bank, Washington, DC.

Yang, B.M. (1997). The role of health insurance in the growth of the private health sector in Korea. In *Private health sector growth in Asia: issues and implications* (ed. W. Newbrander). Wiley, Chichester.

12.13 Bioterrorism

Frank Sorvillo, James R. Greenwood, and Roger Detels

Introduction

The terrorist attacks against targets in the United States, including the World Trade Center and the Pentagon, on 11 September 2001, coupled with the subsequent intentional dispersal of anthrax spores through mailed envelopes in New York, Florida, and Washington, DC (CDC 2001*a*) focused renewed attention on the potential for biological organisms to be used as agents of war and weapons of terror. Bioterrorism has important public health implications and, unlike other acts of terrorism, it will be public health professionals who will serve as frontline 'first responders' to a bioterrorist act (Bryan and Fields 2000). This chapter is not meant to be an exhaustive treatise on bioterrorism but rather an overview of the issue from the critical perspective of public health.

Bioterrorism basics

Bioterrorism is the intentional use of micro-organisms, or their products, to cause harm, and may be used to target humans, animals or crops. There are several characteristics of biological agents that may make them appealing to terrorists (Table 1) (Hughes 1999). Biological weapons are relatively inexpensive compared with conventional, chemical, and nuclear weapons. Many biological agents are readily available in nature, from laboratories, or through the numerous microbiological repositories throughout the world. Some organisms, particularly bacteria and parasites, are relatively easy to make or acquire in quantity. Bioweapons occupy little space and are easily concealed. They have delayed effects, requiring hours to weeks to manifest symptoms, which allows a perpetrator to escape undetected. Bioweapons, if prepared and disseminated effectively, can cause widespread and serious illness and exact a significant economic toll. Finally, biological agents have the capacity to cause widespread fear and panic.

Table 1 Characteristics of candidate biological agents for use by bioterrorists

Relatively inexpensive
Readily available
Easy to produce in quantity
Effective in causing injury
Easy to conceal and transport
Delayed effect
Secondary transmission possible
Significant economic impact
Ability to cause panic

History

While apprehension about bioterrorism has accelerated recently, the use of bioweapons is not a new phenomenon, and concern about bioterrorism had been heightened for several years preceding the terrorist attacks on the United States in the autumn of 2001 (Henderson 1999). Despite the often repeated refrain that 'It is not a question of *if* biological weapons will be used but *when* they will be used', bioweapons have been employed repeatedly by nations, groups, and individuals over the course of history (Table 2) (Phills *et al.* 1972; Harris 1994; Karlen 1995; Torok *et al.* 1997; *CBW Chronicle* 1999; Henderson *et al.* 1999). The catapulting of plague corpses over the walls of Kaffa in 1346 (Karlen 1995) and the transfer of blankets from smallpox victims to Native Americans by British troops in the United States (Henderson *et al.* 1999) are often cited as early examples of biowarfare. It is generally accepted that the Japanese military used bioweapons in occupied Manchuria in the 1930s and early 1940s (Harris 1994). These activities allegedly employed such agents as plague, anthrax, cholera, typhoid, and typhus against prisoners of war and the Chinese population. Testimony to the Truth and Reconciliation Commission in South Africa has indicated that biological agents, including those causing anthrax and cholera, were used against anti-apartheid forces (*CBW Chronicle* 1999). More recently, in the United States in 1984, the Rajneeshee cult, in an effort to influence local elections, contaminated salad bars in several restaurants in Wasco County, Oregon, with *Salmonella typhimurium* (Torok *et al.* 1997). This act resulted in 751 confirmed or presumptive cases. *Ascaris suum*, a roundworm of pigs, was used intentionally to infect four university students in Toronto, Canada, in 1971 who required hospitalization after consuming a meal that had been deliberately contaminated with a massive dose of eggs (Phills *et al.* 1972). Other acts of bioterrorism have been well documented (Tucker 1999). However, it is conceivable, and perhaps likely, that additional bioterrorist attacks, both successful and unsuccessful, have gone unrecognized and undetected.

Table 2 Examples of bioterrorist attacks[a]

Location	Perpetrator(s)	Agent	Number of cases/ deaths	Dissemination	Year
Eastern USA	Unknown	*Bacillus anthracis*	18/5[a]	Mailed envelopes	2001
Oregon	Rajneeshee cult	*Salmonella typhimurium*	751/0	Foodborne	1984
Texas	Individual	*Shigella dysenteriae*	12/0	Foodborne	1994
Toronto	Individual	*Ascaris suum*	4/0	Foodborne	1971
China	Japanese military	Several agents	Unknown	Various	1932–1944
South Africa	Governmental forces	Several agents	Unknown	Various	1980s

[a]As of November 2001

Potential for bioterrorism

Agents

Nearly every human microbial pathogen has the potential to be used as a bioweapon. However, the list of potential agents can be narrowed on such criteria as historical use, development by nations with extensive bioweapons programmes, availability of the agent, ease of preparation, dispersal requirements, and capacity for causing widespread and serious illness. The more sophisticated the terrorist or group, the greater the list of possible agents. The United States' Centers for Disease Control and Prevention (**CDC**) has classified potential bioterrorism agents into three priority categories, labelled A, B, and C (Table 3) (CDC 2000). Included in Category A are pathogens with the potential for high mortality, ready dissemination or transmission from person to person, and the capacity to cause public panic. Category B includes those agents or products that are moderately easy to disseminate and can cause moderate levels of morbidity but low mortality. Category C lists those emerging pathogens that could possibly be used as bioweapons because of availability, relative ease of production, and the potential for high morbidity and mortality. Detailed information on specific agents is available from a variety of sources.

Many potential bioterrorism agents (e.g. *Yersinia pestis, Bacillus anthracis, Salmonella* species) can be readily acquired in nature, through laboratories, or by ordering from microbiological repositories. Alternatively, it may be possible for a terrorist organization to obtain a bioweapon product from a state-sponsored biological weapons programme either directly or from someone who may have access to the agents. In general, viral agents (e.g. Ebola virus) are more difficult to acquire and may require special laboratory capabilities that are beyond the capacity of most terrorist organizations. All of the known successful historical users of bioweapons have employed bacterial or parasitic agents. In nation-sponsored biological weapons programmes, agent-screening procedures to evaluate such factors as virulence and environmental stability are pursued prior to large-scale production (Alibek 1999). Such screening efforts are probably outside the capability of most existing terrorist groups.

In addition to naturally occurring biological agents there is the potential, through genetic engineering, to create new microbes that may be resistant to antibiotics and current vaccines, possess increased virulence, and demonstrate improved environmental stability. Russian scientists reportedly engineered a strain of *Bacillus anthracis* resistant to the tetracycline and penicillin classes of antibiotics (Stepanov *et al.* 1996). Recent bioengineering of the mousepox virus resulted in the production of a highly virulent strain (Norazmi 2001).

Once an agent is acquired, it must then be produced in sufficient quantity, and maintained in a viable state, to be effectively disseminated. In general, bacterial agents are easier to culture than viral pathogens which require living cells, either tissue culture or live animals, in which to grow. Many bacterial organisms (e.g. *Bacillus anthracis*) can grow on a variety of readily available culture media (Inglesby *et al.* 1999). Transmissible stages of parasitic agents cannot be cultured and must be obtained from infected animals. Manufacturing pathogenic organisms presents a risk to those producing them, and sufficient expertise and appropriate laboratory equipment is necessary to avoid laboratory-acquired infection.

Dissemination

A biological weapon can be disseminated by several different methods, including aerosols (airborne), water, food, injection, infected vectors, and, as recent events have demonstrated, mailed envelopes. Release of an infectious micro-organism through the airborne route is the method of greatest concern since it has the potential to expose large numbers of people and has the capacity to induce more severe disease manifestations (Franz *et al.* 1999). A bioweapon aerosol is likely to be invisible and odorless, and therefore undetectable when released. However, aerosol transmission is difficult and necessitates overcoming a number of technical obstacles. Effective airborne dissemination requires that the preparation be of very small particle size. In order to remain suspended in air and to be respired deep into the respiratory tract, the product must be less than 5 μm in size. Moreover, even if a preparation can be created in the required size, it must then be effectively dispersed. Such dispersal requires a device capable of dispensing sufficient product into the air in a manner that will expose the targeted population. Aum Shinrikyo, the Japanese cult that perpetrated the sarin gas attack in the Tokyo subway system in 1995, attempted to release anthrax spores and botulinim toxin via aerosols on several occasions but failed each time (Olsen 1999). The fact that this terrorist group, despite significant financial resources and the successful recruitment of Ph.D. level scientists and engineers as members, could not disperse bioweapons through the airborne route demonstrates the difficulty of such dissemination. Nevertheless, some nations have developed sophisticated bioweapons programmes that have included effective aerosol delivery capability (Alibek 1999).

Table 3 US Centers for Disease Control and Prevention categorization of potential bioweapons

CDC Category A
Variola virus
Bacillus anthracis
Francisella tularensis
Yersina pestis
Ebola virus
Marburg virus
Lassa virus
Junin (and related) viruses
Clostridium botulinum toxin
CDC Category B
Coxiella burnetti
Brucella species
Burkholderia mallei
Salmonella species
Shigella dysenteriae
E. coli 0157:H7
Vibrio cholerae
Cryptosporidium parvum
Eastern encephalitis virus
Western encephalitis virus
Venezuelan encephalitis virus
Staphylococcus enterotoxin
Epsilon enterotoxin (*Clostridium perfringens*)
Ricin (castor bean)
CDC Category C
Nipah virus
Hantaviruses
Yellow fever
Tick-borne haemorrhagic fever viruses
Tick-borne encephalitis viruses
Mycobacterium tuberculosis (multidrug resistant)

Waterborne transmission is another possible mechanism of dispersal. However, most infectious agents would be inactivated or removed by the disinfection and filtration techniques employed by most municipal water systems (Khan *et al.* 2001). Consequently, such a method of dispersal would probably be limited to small water systems or sources.

Most of the successful bioterrorist events recognized to date have used food as a vehicle of dissemination, and, in all likelihood, foodborne transmission will remain the primary method of delivery. While it is possible for a contaminated food product to affect large numbers of people (Hennessy *et al.* 1996), most of the more virulent potential biological agents (e.g. smallpox virus, *Yersinia pestis*) cannot be effectively transmitted through foods. In addition, thorough heating will inactivate most agents or toxins and a contaminated food product is likely to be implicated rapidly in any large-scale epidemic.

The recent anthrax attacks on the east coast of the United States have demonstrated that mailed packages, such as envelopes, can be used as a method of dissemination. However, anthrax is the only significant agent with sufficient environmental stability to allow dispersal in such a fashion. Moreover, despite the occurrence of 18 cases and five deaths, the American anthrax cases had relatively limited casualties, and, coupled with existing data, this demonstates the relative inefficiency of such a method of dispersal.

Dissemination of a bioweapon via injection or through the use of vectors has limited utility.

Impact

The capacity of infectious agents to cause significant morbidity and mortality should not be underestimated. Infectious diseases remain the most important cause of mortality globally, accounting for an estimated 17 million deaths annually (Hinman 1998). Major infectious disease epidemics continue to occur even in industrialized countries. An outbreak of cryptosporidiosis in Milwaukee, Wisconsin, in 1993, linked to contaminated municipal water, affected an estimated 400 000 residents of the city (MacKenzie *et al.* 1994), and a multistate epidemic of salmonellosis caused by contaminated ice cream resulted in an estimated 250 000 cases in 1994 (Hennessy *et al.* 1996). Clearly, there exists the potential for a bioterrorist act to have considerable impact. However, while it is impossible to predict the nature and extent of future acts of bioterrorism, past events would suggest that such acts perpetrated by individuals or groups are likely to remain sporadic and result in limited outbreaks. Nevertheless, either a state-sponsored biological weapons attack or a bioweapon release by terrorist groups who have overcome the significant obstacles that currently exist, however implausible such an event may be, could inflict major casualties that might stretch or overload public health and medical capabilities. An estimate by a World Health Organization expert committee suggested that an aerosol release of 50 kg of anthrax spores upwind of a population of five million would infect 250 000 people with an estimated 100 000 deaths (WHO 1970; Alibek 1999). An attack of this extent is well beyond the scope of individuals or terrorist groups and could only be perpetrated by a nation with a sophisticated bioweapons programme. Such extreme scenarios, while improbable, nevertheless provide a sense of the potential magnitude of an intentional release of a bioweapon and its capacity to cause casualties. Depending on the agent employed, even a modest bioterrorist event would require rapid determination of persons at risk, effective distribution of appropriate prophylaxis, including antibiotics or vaccine when indicated, possible isolation and quarantine measures, co-ordination of medical support, and identification of sufficient hospital capacity.

While the biological impact of a bioterrorist event alone may be considerable, the use of infectious agents has the capacity to cause significant fear to the point of panic (DiGiovanni 1999; Holloway *et al.* 1999). The idea of being attacked by something invisible can induce considerable and, in some, uncontrollable anxiety. Such panic by the 'worried well' has the potential to overwhelm existing resources in demands for medical attention and therapeutic agents. Allaying public anxiety in the midst of a bioterrorist attack requires good communication, accurate information, co-ordination of all involved agencies, and a media that that will resist the impulse to sensationalize events.

A bioterrorist event, unlike a conventional, nuclear, or chemical attack, will unfold over time, probably over a period of days to weeks, and will be insidious in nature. Sporadic cases may occur over a wide geographic area and initially appear to be unrelated. The first to recognize and respond to such an occurrence will not be the traditional first responders but rather the medical and public health communities.

Elements of preparedness

Law enforcement and public health—forging new partnerships

Since the recent mail-related anthrax bioterrorism events in the United States, it has become increasingly clear that any response to bioterrorism, and consequently any preparedness effort, needs to be multifaceted and include organizations not traditionally related to public health disease control efforts. Public health and general law enforcement agencies now have a substantial area of overlap, particularly in the area of disease surveillance and the collection and analysis of evidence. Public health workers are not trained to treat infectious disease samples as evidence and have the potential to 'contaminate' these samples, from a law enforcement perspective, in the course of a routine investigation. Consequently, with the new possibility of bioterrorism, the larger issue becomes: When does a routine disease control investigation develop into a potential crime scene? Should public health and law enforcement collaborate every time there is an outbreak of a disease that starts with fever, malaise, and cough? It is now necessary to evaluate disease control efforts with this new world view in mind.

Partnerships of law enforcement and public health should be developed at all working levels, not just national and state agencies, but local jurisdictions as well. Inclusion of local public health is necessary because bioterrorist attacks involve biological material and control efforts usually must begin at the local level. Developing working relationships using standardized response protocols should ensure that future collaborative criminal and disease control investigations compliment rather than hinder the efforts of both groups.

Schools of public health also have a role in this new paradigm. Infectious disease epidemiology courses should be revised to include some aspects of law enforcement investigations as part of course offerings.

Enhancing public health surveillance and laboratory capabilities

The early recognition of a bioterrorist event is essential in ensuring effective containment and reduction of casualties (Kaufmann *et al.* 1997). Given the historically poor record of passive surveillance systems for most infectious diseases (Marier 1977), the rapid detection of a bioterrorist act will require enhanced disease surveillance activities using active surveillance methods. Active surveillance can include such measures as the use of sentinel primary care providers and emergency room physicians, assigning 'public health liaisons' to be stationed at selected health-care facilities, establishing collaborations with veterinarians for animal-based surveillance, employment of real-time Internet-based reporting, and conducting targeted surveillance activities during selected events such as political conventions or the Olympic Games. Other possible useful, albeit less timely, measures include accessing pharmaceutical databases and evaluation of medical examiner and mortality data for the occurrence of selected syndromes. Education of and close collaboration with local health-care providers and emergency medical system staff are essential to the success of any augmented surveillance system.

Early detection of bioterrorism also requires development of enhanced laboratory capabilities to ensure rapid diagnosis of bioterrorist agents. One example of this is the CDC multilevel laboratory response network in the United States which includes providing reagents, protocols, and training to local laboratory staff, typically public health laboratories (CDC 2000). Information is Internet-based and the system assigns a hierarchy of laboratories for the diagnosis of specific agents.

The World Health Organization (**WHO**) established a WHO Office in Lyon, France, in February 2001 to provide training and support of laboratory capabilities to enhance global security. The first group of international laboratory workers was trained in April 2001. The establishment of this office should improve the quality of public health laboratories which are essential for the establishment and continuing operation of effective surveillance programmes in all countries.

Once detected, effective response and mitigation of events requires epidemiological capability to conduct well-designed studies to implicate a source of infection quickly and to determine populations at risk. Such a capacity, which is lacking in many local jurisdictions, is essential to successfully direct implementation of control measures including provision of prophylactic antibiotics and vaccines as needed. Other control efforts may necessitate isolation and quarantine of patients and, to a lesser extent, disinfection and decontamination activities.

Enhancement of the existing public health infrastructure will require a commitment of funds and resources. However, any augmentation of public health systems for the purpose of responding to bioterrorism will have the added benefit of improving the quality of standard surveillance and response activities to naturally occurring infectious diseases.

Medical response

Training physicians to recognize and treat disease caused by bioterrorist agents

Before the recent bioterrorism attack in the United States, anthrax would not have been part of the differential diagnosis in a 46-year-old urban letter carrier presenting with fever, malaise, cough for 2 days, and the abrupt onset of severe dyspnoea. Now, however, the need for quick and accurate diagnosis of disease caused by bioterrorism agents has become part of the new reality facing physicians. Unfortunately, relatively few physicians have had experience with some of the agents listed earlier in this chapter (e.g. *Yersinia pestis, Clostridium botulinum, Coxiella burnetti*). Compounding this problem is the realization that many of the initial clinical manifestations of bioterrorism diseases overlap with common illnesses, and clustering of cases, which might raise the index of suspicion, might not occur because of delayed onset from exposure to a bioterrorism event and multiple sources of health care for exposed individuals.

Lack of case recognition is only one part of the problem. Treatment information for many bioterrorism agents is anecdotal at best and incorrect at worst. Many of the present medications and treatment modalities, while now considered standard treatment for many infectious diseases, have never been rigorously evaluated for the majority of bioterrorism agents. This also has obvious implications for the stockpiling of effective antimicrobial agents and vaccines, as will be outlined later in this chapter.

Key to an appropriate medical response is a trained cadre of emergency room physicians and primary care providers. These individuals would often be the first health-care providers to see individuals infected with bioterrorism agents. Consequently, they should be the primary recipients of medical education programmes to prepare them to recognize cases of infectious diseases most likely due to a bioterrorist attack. Although the list of potential agents is rather daunting, training should focus on those agents that most likely would be used and at a minimum should include the diagnosis and treatment of anthrax, smallpox, plague, botulism, tularemia, and the viral haemorrhagic fevers. Secondary training should include hospital infection control staff and ancillary staff. This training should be incorporated into medical center emergency response plans.

Upgrading hospital and quarantine capacities

Most experts in the field of bioterrorism feel that anthrax and/or smallpox would be the most likely agents used by terrorists. Of the two, smallpox has significant ramifications for hospital capacity. Because smallpox is highly contagious and most of the population has little or no immunity, even a small event could rapidly tax hospital capacity for handling infected patients. Infected patients must be confined to rooms with negative pressure and have exhaust air systems that are filtered to prevent the smallpox virus from exiting and then re-entering the air-handling system. Unfortunately, even in large metropolitan areas such as Washington, DC, there are probably less than 100 such isolation rooms available (Henderson 1999). Thus one of the first areas to receive serious review should be the capacity to isolate and treat smallpox-infected patients.

Concomitant with the review of isolation units should be an evaluation of the quarantine capacity in individual health jurisdictions. In addition to considering hospitals for primary quarantine areas, non-hospital sites, such as abandoned schools or old hotels should be considered as potential triage and quarantine locations. Public health quarantine laws and regulations need to be reviewed and updated as necessary so that little ambiguity will exist and restricting the mobility of exposed segments of the population can be implemented rapidly, if indicated. The concept of quarantine for containment of infectious diseases also needs to be reconsidered in the context of the feasibility of restricting movement in a highly mobile population, the nature of the disease threat, including the infectious characteristics of the agent (which may have been modified), the magnitude of the outbreak, and the nature of the outbreak. In conjunction with quarantine, the feasibility of post-exposure vaccination needs to be considered if an effective vaccine to the agent is available and the length of the incubation period is sufficient to permit artificial development of immunity post-exposure. For example, Meltzer *et al.* (2001) have suggested that a combination of quarantine and post-exposure vaccination is the most effective strategy to control a bioterrorist outbreak due to smallpox.

Another potentially useful tool for assessing capacity has been developed by the American Hospital Association (2001). This document presents a series of self-assessment questions that allow hospital managements to assess their own capacity for dealing with chemical and bioterrorism events. In addition to capacity, other major areas that are evaluated include communications and public affairs, access to care, business continuity plans, pharmaceuticals and equipment, medical treatment procedures, training and personnel, facility management/security, psychiatric services and crisis counselling, and diagnostic capabilities.

Stockpiling vaccines and antibiotics

One of the hallmarks of a good public health response to a man-made or natural disaster is preparedness. As an example, at the individual level, the public health message is for people who live in earthquake country to prepare for a disaster by storing food and water in case these supplies are not available for a few days after a major earthquake. At the community level, preparation might involve developing a disaster response plan and stockpiling supplies and tents to shelter, feed, and house people whose homes have been lost as a result of a disaster. Taken in this light, stockpiling of vaccines and appropriate antibiotics is good public health policy. However, in contrast to a natural disaster, the difficulty is knowing what and how much to stockpile. This is especially true if one is concerned about state-sponsored terrorism. For example, an announcement that ciprofloxacin is being stockpiled could lead a terrorist organization to develop ciprofloxacin-resistant strains, or at least to announce that they had done so in an attempt to further terrorize a population. Although it might be prudent not to publicise the details of what is being stockpiled, this is not feasible in an open society where the circle of those who need to know would be quite wide. Having sufficient antibiotics and vaccines on hand to control or limit outbreaks while calming the public is consistent with good public health policy.

Informing the public

The recent anthrax events in the United States have demonstrated how important it is for the public health community to provide accurate and timely information to the general public and news media about bioterrorism events. It was clear during the initial stages of the 2001 anthrax incidents in the United States that, in the absence of a strong, clear, and consistent message from the public health community, the news media and other less credible sources were eager to fill the information void. This resulted in inappropriate usage of antibiotics by large segments of the population who were not at risk of exposure to anthrax and the purchase of useless 'gas masks' to prevent anthrax inhalation.

The conflicting messages initially delivered by government health officials also undermined the confidence of the public and led to further feelings of insecurity. Therefore, to avoid confusion if there are more bioterrorism events, the public health community needs to develop 'consensus papers' on each of the potential agents that might be used. This information should be developed in a non-crisis mode and then distributed to state and local health departments and the media for use as specific situations develop. Part of this process should also be ongoing evaluation of treatment and prophylaxis for these agents. This information could then be sent to the local health-care community when necessary.

Safeguards

Mail system

The mail system has now been shown to provide a method for the delivery of anthrax spores. While it is not possible at this point to determine how efficient this mechanism is, there is no doubt that anthrax in letters has been responsible for widespread concern about the threat of anthrax and other forms of bioterrorism by the population of the United States. Based on the biology of most bioterrorism agents, it is extremely unlikely that the majority of them could be transmitted through contaminated letters. *Bacillus anthracis*, because it is a spore former, may be one of the few bioterrorism agents that has the potential to be transmitted through the mail.

The CDC has developed guidelines (CDC 2001*b*) to prevent the possible exposure of mail handlers to bioterrorism agents. Recommendations include the use of vinyl gloves when handling mail, particulate respirators (which would be difficult to implement), and other methods of avoiding contact with airborne particles. Longer-term disease control solutions have focused on the irradiation of mail to inactivate infectious materials that might be present within packages and letters.

Air intakes

There is no question that exposed air intakes make major buildings vulnerable to the deliberate introduction of biological and chemical agents. However, from a practical standpoint, most buildings do not have secured entries and the introduction of bioterrorism and chemical agents through the air-handling system is not the only way to contaminate a building that uses recirculated air. Consequently, the cost of any major alterations in air intakes, such as securing their location or raising ducts above ground level to avoid easy access to openings, needs to be balanced against potential threats to a building and its occupants versus other security provisions for limiting access. An alternative approach is to develop very efficient and affordable air-filtration systems capable of removing spores and biological agents.

One potentially promising approach for protecting higher-risk buildings or other essential facilities is the continuous air-sampling device. As envisaged, the quality of air entering or circulating within a building would be continuously tested for the presence of biological and chemical agents. If detected, the sensors would then be programmed to shut off intake air supplies or internal fan systems. To date these systems have had difficulty discriminating between dust particles and biological agents, but at some point technological advances should obviate this difficulty.

Water supplies

Water supplies to major cities and towns in the industrialized world are generally considered to be safe and secure from being used as a mechanism for the mass distribution of infectious agents. Because public health has had a historical role in developing drinking water that is free from infectious agents, treatment and monitoring systems are already in place to prevent such an occurrence. Most surface water supplies are presumed to be contaminated with infectious agents (e.g. *Cryptosporidium* or *giardia*) and are extensively filtered and chlorinated before water is distributed to individual users.

Preformed toxins, such as botulinum toxin, have been discussed as potential bioterrorism agents which could be distributed through a water system. However, because of the massive dilution of most metropolitan water supply systems, it is unlikely that sufficient quantities of toxin could be added to cause harm after dilution and treatment effects are taken into account. However, there is certainly a possibility that a determined terrorist could contaminate a small segment of a water-supply system by deliberately introducing infectious agents downstream from a water-treatment facility or by contaminating water to an individual building or group of buildings served by a single water main. In this case, if the attack were covert, it would be necessary for public health disease surveillance programmes to determine that an attack had taken place after non-deliberate modes of infection had been eliminated.

Food supplies

Food supplies are vulnerable to bioterrorism at multiple levels. The first of these is at the basic farm or production level where it is known that disease agents have been developed into weapons to infect growing crops and food animal production. Both the United States and the Soviet Union developed and experimented with smuts, rusts, and animal pathogens such as *Burkholderia mallei*, the causative agent of glanders in cattle (Alibek 1998; Carus 1998). It was the intention of these programmes to starve potential enemies and shift resources away from the production of military hardware to food. Delivery of such agents over a large area in the industrialized world, while possible, is still unlikely unless it is related to state-sponsored terrorism. Consequently, bioterrorism at the food-production level, if it is to take place at all, will more likely be limited to events designed to disrupt commerce and terrorize the population, rather than starving a military target.

Governmental surveillance systems and quarantine mechanisms are presently in place to monitor crop and animal health and to prevent the transportation of contaminated products. Many of these systems, especially as they relate to animal diseases, have recently been strengthened in many areas of the world in response to outbreaks of foot-and-mouth disease occurring in the late 1990s. However, it is obvious that these systems should now be re-evaluated to determine if they have the potential to detect and control the deliberate introduction of crop and animal diseases.

The next level of potential vulnerability in the food-supply system is related to modern commerce and the mass distribution of food. Multiple outbreaks (Tucker 1999) have demonstrated that foods contaminated with *Salmonella* or *E. coli* 0157, for example, can be widely distributed throughout a large geographical area by centralized food commissaries or other commercial food distribution networks. Thus it is entirely possible that food products at the commercial distribution level could be used deliberately to spread disease and cause terror among a population. Several obstacles prevent food at this level from becoming a major source of disease transmission. Multiple sources of similar foods are available to consumers and many of them are only distributed within local or regional areas. Thus it would be next to impossible to contaminate an entire regional milk supply. Also, many of the pathogens that could conceivably be used to contaminate foods are already considered to be part of the 'normal flora' of raw foods. Since these foods are cooked before they are consumed, the addition of more *Salmonella* to chicken or raw meat, for example, would be of little consequence. Nonetheless, many cases could be caused this way. Thus distribution procedures should be reviewed and strategies to protect against terrorist introductions of agents considered.

Detection of food-related bioterrorism events will require increased co-ordination between local, state, and federal regulatory and public health agencies. More active surveillance systems need to be developed and used to replace traditional passive reporting systems. Most importantly, public health will be required to adopt a new mindset in which the potential of terrorism will be one additional factor considered in any food-related disease outbreak.

Modelling potential threats

One of the major problems which the world must confront is the absence of knowledge. The pathogenicity and virulence of the naturally occurring potential organisms which would be used for bioterrorism are known, but these agents may be altered for use as a bioterrorist agent. For example, Russian scientists were able to develop anthrax strains that were resistant to penicillin and tetracycline and to increase the virulence of mousepox (Stepanov *et al.* 1996; Norazmi 2001). Further, their impact is dependent, in part, on the susceptibility of the population which depends on the prior exposure of the population to the organism, migration of susceptibles, and the proportion of individuals who have been immunized if, indeed, a vaccine exists for the particular organism. For example, some of the population who were alive prior to the eradication of smallpox in 1977 may have been vaccinated. But, in the absence of subsequent challenges to boost the level of artificial immunity, it is not know what proportion of even this population is immune. Those born since eradication will have no immunity to smallpox and the majority of the population will not have immunity to other potential bioterrorist agents.

A second problem is that several countries, and perhaps individuals, have conducted research to alter the basic properties of the agents to make them more pathogenic/virulent and to improve their potential for widespread transmission. An example of this is the attempt to reduce the size and electrostatic properties of the anthrax preparation to increase its ability to be aerosolized, thus enhancing its ability to infect a large number of individuals, especially in crowded congested situations such as a major subway station. Aerosolization of anthrax from letters has already been demonstrated in the bioterrorist episodes in Miami, Washington, DC, Connecticut, and New York in 2001, and involved transmission of spores at levels sufficient to cause infection of individuals who never came into direct contact with the originally infected letter, although relatively few cases occurred.

Given the variability of strains, the meteorological conditions existing when agents would be released (e.g. wind, temperature, and light conditions), the range of potential transporting media (e.g., water, air, food), the availability of treatment and vaccines, and the susceptibility of the population, how can responsible national and international agencies anticipate the magnitude of the threat and thus respond effectively? One approach is to model the potential episodes. Mathematical modelling has been used for a variety of infectious diseases, including estimates of the future of the HIV/AIDS epidemics in many countries and the impact of smallpox epidemics (see Chapter 6.14). Meltzer *et al.* (2001), from the CDC, developed a model to estimate the attack rate for smallpox following the deliberate release of the virus in a crowded situation. Not only were they able to estimate the number of secondary and subsequent cases that would occur, but they were also able to evaluate the relative contributions of a rapid vaccination response and quarantine on reducing the spread of the virus. The fact that the infectiousness of smallpox has already been established helped them in the development of their model. However, the relative infectiousness of many of the other potential bioterrorist agents, including those that have been altered, is not known. In this situation mathematical modelling can still be useful. Multiple models can be developed using different levels of infectiousness and different scenarios. The use of multiple models often reveals key determinants of rapid transmission.

Development of complex models is limited by the quality of the assumptions which may be incomplete or invalid. Moreover, it is difficult for any mathematical model to accommodate every possible contingency. Thus model predictions must be interpreted cautiously. Nonetheless, models can provide valuable information about the potential behaviour of agents in populations. The use of mathematical models can assist national and international agencies to prepare for potential bioterrorist episodes in the future. Although their accuracy will be difficult to evaluate in the absence of a real episode, the early stages of an episode will provide validation (or no validation) of each of the models which have been developed, providing an opportunity to select the most appropriate model.

Addressing the underlying causes of bioterrorism

When faced with a bioterrorist threat the tendency, even by governments, is to concentrate on the problem at hand and to ignore the underlying causes of bioterrorism. Yet, if we are to reduce the threat of bioterrorism effectively we must address its underlying causes. Terrorism may be the result of national policy, religious or political convictions, or a sense of unchangeable economic inequities, but may also be caused by a sense of alienation by a single individual. Perhaps a common thread among all these groups is the feeling of being disenfranchised by society. The terrorists feel that their only recourse when outnumbered and shunned by society is to engage in activities which can be implemented by only a few dedicated individuals but which will have a large impact. Examples include the Palestinians in Israel, the Catholics in Northern Ireland, and the al-Q'aida Muslims in Afghanistan. This perception on the part of nations, religious and political groups, and individuals may be due to psychological factors, political policies, economic disparities, and/or 'fanaticism'. However, fanaticism may also be the expression of or response to the feeling of being disenfranchised. Of course, there may well be other root causes of bioterrorism, as yet unknown, but which must be understood if we are to address the issue successfully.

The immediate response among individual victims, groups, and nations suffering the consequences of bioterrorism is usually to seek immediate revenge. But if bioterrorism is to be reduced it is also essential to step back from the immediacy of the problem to consider the underlying causes and how to address them. Addressing these root causes provides the best promise of a lasting strategy to reduce bioterrorism. Thus it is important, even in the midst of the terror and confusion caused by a bioterrorist incident, to study and identify the causes of the act by the nation, group, or individual perpetrating it. If we know the causes, we can attempt to address them and thereby reduce the likelihood of future incidents. It is important to realize that making the necessary changes may not be easy or popular, but it is the responsibility of national and international leaders to understand what needs to be done and to convince the public of the need.

International co-operation

The effort to prevent the threat of bioterrorism must be international. The threat of bioterrorism is not confined to one country. Bioterrorist attempts have been made in many countries, including the United States, Iran, and Japan. Although some bioterrorists act within their own country, others implement their activities in other countries. As observed by Horton (2001), terrorism is a consequence of wider political and social change and thrives in those countries undergoing state failure such as Afghanistan, Colombia, Northern Ireland, Sudan, and Iraq. But the activities are often directed at other countries. Thus international co-operation is essential to prevent these international bioterrorist activities. Further, a combined approach by many nations is more likely to be successful than uncoordinated attempts by individual countries. Joint antiterrorism efforts must include sharing of intelligence, co-ordinated diplomatic and financial pressures when indicated, close co-operation between national health authorities, including heightened surveillance for the rapid identification and communication of possible bioterrorist acts, and efforts to prevent terrorist groups acquiring biological agents from the numerous microbiological repositories and laboratories throughout the world.

The WHO publishes the *Weekly Epidemiologic Record* which reports disease outbreaks in member states. In order to upgrade the quality of the reports, the WHO has developed a manual for recommended surveillance standards in the field of communicable diseases. The *WHO Recommended Surveillance Standards* manual (WHO 1999) includes recommendations for diagnostic methods, case definitions, types of surveillance, minimum data elements, data analysis methods, principal uses of data for decision-making, and standardization of reporting and international data exchange based on the *International Classification of Disease (10th revision)* codes.

The *Weekly Epidemiologic Record* will be very helpful for identifying outbreaks of disease which may be caused by bioterrorism, but the utility of the system will depend on the quality of the surveillance in the various countries, the speed of reporting the outbreak, the honesty of the countries in both reporting the disease and providing an accurate estimate of the magnitude of the outbreak, and the ability of WHO to respond appropriately.

The member states of the United Nations recognized this need several decades ago by establishing a new instrument in 1972 to supplement the 1925 Geneva Protocol, the 'Convention on the Prohibition of the Development, Production and Stockpiling of Bacteriological (Biological) and Toxin Weapons and on their Destruction' (**BWC**) (United Nations 2001). Unfortunately, the absence of any formal verification protocol to monitor compliance severely limited its effectiveness. Recognizing this shortcoming, a group of governmental experts (VEREX) was established at the Third Review Conference of the BWC to identify and examine potential verification measures from a scientific and technical standpoint. Despite subsequent Review Conferences in 1996 and 2001, a system of verification that is acceptable to the signees has yet to be adopted by the signees (United Nations 2001).

The events of the latter half of 2001 have brought into sharper focus the need to adopt an international protocol which incorporates an effective verification strategy. At least equally important, however, is the need to address the underlying causes of bioterrorism. Thus an effort has to be made by the nations of the world to act together to reduce the feeling of alienation and disenfranchisement felt by some countries, especially smaller developing nations, and by groups both within individual countries and spanning many countries. It is clear that attempts of individual nations, even large powerful nations such as the United States, acting independently of other nations will fail. Thus the nations of the world must co-operate if the threat of bioterrorism is to be reduced and ultimately controlled. A united and co-ordinated antiterrorist strategy by the nations of the world may discourage rogue nations, groups, and individuals against using bioterrorism to achieve their goals.

References

Alibek, K. (1999). *Biohazard.* Random House, New York.

Alibek, K. (1998). Terrorist and intelligence operations: potential impact on the U.S. economy. Testimony provided before the Joint Economic Committee, 20 May 1998.

American Hospital Association (2001). *Chemical and bioterrorism preparedness checklist*, 3 October 1998. American Hospital Association, Washington, DC.

Bryan, J.L. and Fields, H.F. (2000). An ounce of prevention is worth a pound of cure – shoring up the public health infrastructure to respond to bioterrorist attacks. *Journal of the American Medical Association*, **283**, 242–9.

Carus, S. (1998). *Bioterrorism and biocrimes: the illicit use of biological agents in the 20th century.* Center for Counterproliferation Research, National Defense University, Washington, DC.

CBW Chronicle (1999). South Africa's apartheid-era germ warfare program investigated. January 1999.

CDC (Centers for Disease Control and Prevention) (2000*a*). Biological and chemical terrorism: strategic plan for preparedness and response. *Morbidity and Mortality Weekly Reports*, **49** (RR-4).

CDC (Centers for Disease Control and Prevention) (2000*b*). Notice to readers: Interim recommendations for protecting workers from exposure to *Bacillus anthracis* in work sites in which mail is handled or processed. *Morbidity and Mortality Weekly Reports*, **50**, 961.

CDC (Centers for Disease Control and Prevention) (2001). Recognition of illness associated with the intentional release of a biologic agent. *Morbidity and Mortality Weekly Reports*, **50**, 893–7.

DiGiovanni, C., Jr (1999). Domestic terrorism with chemical or biological agents: psychiatric aspects. *American Journal Psychiatry*, **156**, 1500–5.

Franz, D.R., Jahrling, P.B., Friedlander, D.J., *et al.* (1999). Clinical recognition and management of patients exposed to biological warfare agents. In *Biological warfare: limiting the threat*, pp. 37–79. MIT Press, Cambridge, MA.

Harris, S.H. (1994). *Factories of death: Japanese biological warfare, 1932–1944, and the American cover-up.* Routledge, New York.

Henderson, D.A. (1999). The looming threat of bioterrorism. *Science*, **283**, 1279–82.

Henderson, D.A., Inglesby, T.V., Bartlett, J.G., *et al.* (1999). Smallpox as a biological weapon: medical and public health management. *Journal of the American Medical Association*, **281**, 2127–37.

Hennessy, T.W., Hedberg, C.W., Slutsker, L., *et al.* (1996). A national outbreak of *Salmonella enteritidis* infections from ice cream. *New England Journal of Medicine*, **334**, 1281–6.

Hinman, A. (1998). Global progress in infectious disease control. *Lancet*, **16**, 1116–21.

Holloway, H.C., Norwood, A.E., Fullerton, C.S., Engel, C.C., Jr, and Ursano, R.J. (1999). The threat of biological weapons: prophylaxis and mitigation of psychological and social consequences. In *Biological warfare: limiting the threat* (ed. J. Lederberg), pp. 249–62. MIT Press, Cambridge, MA.

Horton, R. (2001). Public health: a neglected counterterrorist measure. *Lancet*, 358, 1112–13.

Hughes, J. (1999). The emerging threat of bioterrorism. *Emerging Infectious Diseases*, **5**, 494–5.

Inglesby, T.V., Henderson, D.A., and Bartlett, J.G., *et al.* (1999). Anthrax as a biological weapon: medical and public health management. *Journal of the American Medical Association*, **281**, 1735–45.

Karlen A. (1995). *Microbes and man.* Simon and Schuster, New York.

Kaufmann, A.F., Meltzer, M.I., and Schmid, G.P. (1997). *Emerging Infectious Diseases*, **3**, 83–94.

Khan, A.S., Swerdlow, D.L., and Juranek, D.D. (2001). Precautions against biological and chemical terrorism directed at food and water supplies. *Public Health Reports*, **116**, 3–14.

MacKenzie, W.R., Hoxie, N.J., Proctor, M.E., *et al.* (1994). A massive outbreak in Milwaukee of cryptosporidium infection transmitted through the public water supply. *New England Journal of Medicine*, **331**, 161–7.

Marier, R. (1977). The reporting of communicable diseases. *American Journal of Epidemiology*, **106**, 587–90.

Meltzer, M.I., Damon, I., LeDuc, J.W., and Millar, J.D. (2001). Modeling potential responses to smallpox as a bioterrorist weapon. *Emerging Infectious Diseases*, **7**, 959–69.

Norazmi, N.M. (2001). Possible mechanism for the enhanced lethality of an interleukin-4-expressing mousepox virus. *Journal of Medical Microbiology*, **50**, 936.

Olsen, K.B. (1999). Aum Shinrikyo: once and future threat? *Emerging Infectious Diseases*, **5**, 513.

Phills, J.A., Harrold, A.J., Whiteman, G.V., and Perelmutter, L. (1972). Pulmonary infiltrates, asthma and eosinophilia due to *Ascaris suum* infestation in man. *New England Journal of Medicine*, **286**, 965–70.

Stepanov, A.V., Mainin, L.I., Pomerantsev, A.P., and Staritsin, N.A. (1996). Development of novel vaccines against anthrax in man. *Journal of Biotechnology*, **44**, 155–60.

Torok, T.J., Tauxe, R.V., Wise, T.P., *et al.* (1997). A large community outbreak of salmonellosis caused by intentional contamination of restaurant salad bars. *Journal of the American Medical Association*, **278**, 389–95.

Tucker, J.B. (1999). Historical trends related to bioterrorism: an empirical analysis. *Emerging Infectious Diseases*, **5**, 498–504.

United Nations (2001). *The Biological Weapons Convention.* United Nations: Weapons of Mass Destruction Branch, Department for Disarmament Affairs. (www.un.org/depts/dda)

WHO (World Health Organization) (1970). *Health aspects of chemical and biological weapons*, pp. 98–9. WHO, Geneva.

WHO (World Health Organization) (1999). *WHO recommended surveillance standards* (2nd edn). WHO, Geneva.

Index

The page numbers in **bold** refer to major sections of the text.

Since the major subject of this title is public health, entries have been kept to a minimum under this key word and readers are advised to seek more specific references. Entries under specific countries have been limited to major topics. Additional statistics may be found within the text.

Indexing style
Alphabetical order. This index is in letter-by-letter order, whereby hyphens, en-rules and spaces within index headings are ignored in the alphabetization. Terms in brackets are excluded from initial alphabetization.

Abbreviations used in subentries (without explanation):
AIDS Acquired immunodeficiency syndrome
BSE Bovine spongiform encephalopathy
HIV Human immunodeficiency virus
STD Sexually transmitted diseases
WHO World Health Organization

F